DATE DUE

GAYLORD 353 CDD

BRENNER & RECTOR'S THE KIDNEY

Tenth Edition

VOLUME 1

Karl Skorecki, MD, FRCP(C), FASN
Annie Chutick Professor and Chair in Medicine (Nephrology)
Technion—Israel Institute of Technology
Director of Medical and Research Development
Rambam Health Care Campus
Haifa, Israel

Glenn M. Chertow, MD
Norman S. Coplon/Satellite Healthcare Professor of Medicine
Chief, Division of Nephrology
Stanford University School of Medicine
Palo Alto, California

Philip A. Marsden, MD
Professor of Medicine
Elisabeth Hofmann Chair in Translational Research
Oreopoulos-Baxter Division Director of Nephrology
Vice Chair Research, Department of Medicine
University of Toronto
Toronto, Ontario, Canada

Maarten W. Taal, MBChB, MMed, MD, FCP(SA), FRCP
Professor of Medicine
Division of Medical Sciences and Graduate Entry Medicine
University of Nottingham
Honorary Consultant Nephrologist
Department of Renal Medicine
Royal Derby Hospital
Derby, United Kingdom

Alan S.L. Yu, MD
Harry Statland and Solon Summerfield Professor of Medicine
Director, Division of Nephrology and Hypertension and The Kidney Institute
University of Kansas Medical Center
Kansas City, Kansas

SPECIAL ASSISTANT TO THE EDITORS
Walter G. Wasser, MD
Attending Physician, Division of Nephrology
Mayanei HaYeshua Medical Center
Bnei Brak, Israel;
Rambam Health Care Campus
Haifa, Israel

ELSEVIER

ELSEVIER

1600 John F. Kennedy Blvd.
Ste 1800
Philadelphia, PA 19103-2899

BRENNER AND RECTOR'S THE KIDNEY, TENTH EDITION ISBN: 978-1-4557-4836-5
Copyright © 2016 by Elsevier, Inc. All rights reserved. Volume 1 part number 9996096807
Volume 2 part number 9996096866

No part of this publication may be reproduced or transmitted in any form or by any means, electronic or mechanical, including photocopying, recording, or any information storage and retrieval system, without permission in writing from the publisher. Details on how to seek permission, further information about the Publisher's permissions policies and our arrangements with organizations such as the Copyright Clearance Center and the Copyright Licensing Agency, can be found at our website: www.elsevier.com/permissions.

This book and the individual contributions contained in it are protected under copyright by the Publisher (other than as may be noted herein).

Notices

Knowledge and best practice in this field are constantly changing. As new research and experience broaden our understanding, changes in research methods, professional practices, or medical treatment may become necessary.

Practitioners and researchers must always rely on their own experience and knowledge in evaluating and using any information, methods, compounds, or experiments described herein. In using such information or methods they should be mindful of their own safety and the safety of others, including parties for whom they have a professional responsibility.

With respect to any drug or pharmaceutical products identified, readers are advised to check the most current information provided (i) on procedures featured or (ii) by the manufacturer of each product to be administered, to verify the recommended dose or formula, the method and duration of administration, and contraindications. It is the responsibility of practitioners, relying on their own experience and knowledge of their patients, to make diagnoses, to determine dosages and the best treatment for each individual patient, and to take all appropriate safety precautions.

To the fullest extent of the law, neither the Publisher nor the authors, contributors, or editors, assume any liability for any injury and/or damage to persons or property as a matter of products liability, negligence or otherwise, or from any use or operation of any methods, products, instructions, or ideas contained in the material herein.

Previous editions copyrighted 2012, 2008, 2004, 2000, 1996, 1991, 1986, 1981, 1976.

Library of Congress Cataloging-in-Publication Data

Brenner & Rector's the kidney / [edited by] Karl Skorecki, Glenn M. Chertow, Philip A. Marsden, Maarten W. Taal, Alan S.L. Yu ; special assistant to the editors, Walter G. Wasser.—10th edition.
    p. ; cm.
  Brenner and Rector's the kidney
  Kidney
  Includes bibliographical references and index.
  ISBN 978-1-4557-4836-5 (hardcover : alk. paper)
    I. Skorecki, Karl, editor.   II. Chertow, Glenn M., editor.   III. Marsden, Philip A., editor.
IV. Taal, Maarten W., editor.   V. Yu, Alan S. L., editor.   VI. Title: Brenner and Rector's the kidney.   VII. Title: Kidney.
    [DNLM: 1. Kidney Diseases.   2. Kidney—physiology.   3. Kidney—physiopathology.   WJ 300]
    RC902
    616.6′1—dc23
                                                            2015033607

Content Strategist: Kellie Heap
Senior Content Development Specialist: Joan Ryan
Publishing Services Manager: Jeffrey Patterson
Senior Project Manager: Mary Pohlman
Senior Book Designer: Margaret Reid

Printed in United States of America.

Last digit is the print number: 9   8   7   6   5   4   3   2   1

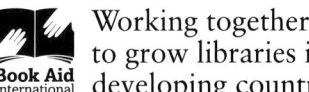

*Dedicated to our patients and to our students
—who provide us with the inspiration to learn,
teach, and discover.*

Contributors

Andrew Advani, BSc, MBChB(Hons), PhD, FRCP(UK)
Assistant Professor of Medicine
University of Toronto
St. Michael's Hospital
Toronto, Ontario, Canada
  Chapter 13, Vasoactive Molecules and the Kidney

Michael Allon, MD
Professor of Medicine
Division of Nephrology
University of Alabama at Birmingham
Birmingham, Alabama
  Chapter 70, Interventional Nephrology

Amanda Hyre Anderson, PhD, MPH
Assistant Professor of Epidemiology
Center for Clinical Epidemiology and Biostatistics
Perelman School of Medicine
University of Pennsylvania
Philadelphia, Pennsylvania
  Chapter 21, Demographics of Kidney Disease

Gerald B. Appel, MD
Professor of Medicine
Director of Clinical Nephrology
Division of Nephrology
Columbia University Medical Center
New York, New York
  Chapter 33, Secondary Glomerular Disease

Suheir Assady, MD, PhD
Director, Department of Nephrology and Hypertension
Rambam Health Care Campus
Haifa, Israel
  Chapter 79, Near and Middle East

Anthony Atala, MD
Director, Wake Forest Institute for Regenerative Medicine
William H. Boyce Professor and Chair
Department of Urology
Wake Forest School of Medicine
Winston-Salem, North Carolina
  Chapter 86, Tissue Engineering, Stem Cells, and Cell Therapy in Nephrology

Paul Ayoub, MD
Specialized Medicine
University of Montréal
Montréal, Quebec, Canada
  Chapter 69, Elimination Enhancement of Poisons

Kara N. Babaian, MD
Assistant Professor of Clinical Urology
Department of Urology
University of California, Irvine
Orange, California
  Chapter 41, Kidney Cancer

Colin Baigent, FFPH, FRCP
Professor of Epidemiology
Clinical Trial Service Unit
Nuffield Department of Population Health
Oxford, United Kingdom
  Chapter 56, Cardiovascular Aspects of Kidney Disease

Sevcan A. Bakkaloglu, MD
Professor of Pediatrics
Head, Division of Pediatric Nephrology and Rheumatology
Gazi University School of Medicine
Ankara, Turkey
  Chapter 74, Diseases of the Kidney and Urinary Tract in Children

George L. Bakris, MD
Professor of Medicine
Department of Medicine
University of Chicago Medicine
ASH Comprehensive Hypertension Center
Chicago, Illinois
  Chapter 47, Primary and Secondary Hypertension

Gavin J. Becker, MD, FRACP
Professor
Department of Nephrology
Royal Melbourne Hospital and University of Melbourne
Melbourne, Victoria, Australia
  Chapter 82, Oceania Region

Rachel Becker-Cohen, MD
Pediatric Nephrology
Shaare Zedek Medical Center
The Hebrew University School of Medicine
Jerusalem, Israel
  Chapter 76, Renal Replacement Therapy (Dialysis and Transplantation) in Pediatric End-Stage Kidney Disease

Theresa J. Berndt
Department of Medicine
Division of Nephrology and Hypertension
Mayo Clinic College of Medicine
Mayo Clinic
Rochester, Minnesota
  Chapter 7, The Regulation of Calcium, Magnesium, and Phosphate Excretion by the Kidney

Jeffrey S. Berns, MD
Professor of Medicine
Perelman School of Medicine
University of Pennsylvania
Philadelphia, Pennsylvania
   Chapter 21, Demographics of Kidney Disease

Prof John F. Bertram, BSc(Hons), PhD, FASN, DSc
Professor of Anatomy and Developmental Biology
Monash University
Clayton, Victoria, Australia
   Chapter 23, Nephron Endowment and Developmental Programming of Blood Pressure and Renal Function

Vivek Bhalla, MD
Assistant Professor of Medicine/Nephrology
Stanford University School of Medicine
Stanford, California
   Chapter 12, Aldosterone and Mineralocorticoid Receptors: Renal and Extrarenal Roles

Daniel G. Bichet, MD
Professor of Medicine and Physiology
University of Montréal
Nephrologist
Department of Medicine
Hôpital du Sacré-Coeur de Montréal
Montréal, Quebec, Canada
   Chapter 45, Inherited Disorders of the Renal Tubule

Alain Bonnardeaux, MD, PhD
Full Professor of Medicine
University of Montréal
Nephrologist
Hôpital Maisonneuve-Rosemont
Montréal, Quebec, Canada
   Chapter 45, Inherited Disorders of the Renal Tubule

William D. Boswell, Jr., MD, FACR
Professor and Chairman
Department of Radiology
City of Hope National Medical Center
Duarte, California
   Chapter 28, Diagnostic Kidney Imaging

Barry M. Brenner, MD, AM(Hon), DSc(Hon), DMSc(Hon), MD(Hon), Dipl(Hon), FRCP(London, Hon)
Samuel A. Levine Distinguished Professor of Medicine
Harvard Medical School
Director Emeritus, Renal Division, and Senior Physician
Department of Medicine
Brigham and Women's Hospital
Boston, Massachusetts
   Chapter 3, The Renal Circulations and Glomerular Ultrafiltration

Richard M. Breyer, PhD
Professor of Medicine
Professor of Biochemistry
Ruth King Scoville Chair in Medicine
Professor of Pharmacology
Vanderbilt University
Nashville, Tennessee
   Chapter 14, Arachidonic Acid Metabolites and the Kidney

Dennis Brown, PhD
Department of Medicine
Harvard Medical School
Center for Systems Biology
Program in Membrane Biology and Division of Nephrology
Massachusetts General Hospital
Boston, Massachussets
   Chapter 11, The Cell Biology of Vasopressin Action

Carlo Brugnara, MD
Professor of Pathology
Harvard Medical School
Director, Hematology Laboratory
Boston Children's Hospital
Boston, Massachusetts
   Chapter 57, Hematologic Aspects of Kidney Disease

Stéphan Busque, MD
Professor of Surgery (Abdominal Transplantation)
Director, Adult Kidney and Pancreas Transplant Program
Stanford University
Stanford, California
   Chapter 72, Clinical Management of the Adult Kidney Transplant Recipient

Juan Jesús Carrero, Pharm, PhD, MBA
Associate Professor
Karolinska Institutet
Stockholm, Sweden
   Chapter 58, Endocrine Aspects of Chronic Kidney Disease

Daniel Cattran, MD, FRCP(C), FACP
Professor of Medicine
University of Toronto
Senior Scientist
Toronto General Research Institute
Toronto General Hospital
Toronto, Ontario, Canada
   Chapter 34, Overview of Therapy for Glomerular Disease

James C. M. Chan, MD
Professor of Pediatrics
Tufts University School of Medicine
Director of Research
The Barbara Bush Children's Hospital
Maine Medical Center
Portland, Maine
   Chapter 75, Fluid, Electrolyte, and Acid-Base Disorders in Children

Anil Chandraker, MD
Associate Professor of Medicine
Harvard Medical School
Brigham and Women's Hospital
Schuster Family Transplantation Research Center
Boston, Massachusetts
Chapter 71, Transplantation Immunobiology

Katrina Chau, MBBS, FRACP
Department of Nephrology
University of British Columbia
Vancouver, British Columbia, Canada;
Department of Nephrology
Liverpool Hospital
Sydney, Australia
Chapter 26, Laboratory Assessment of Kidney Disease: Glomerular Filtration Rate, Urinalysis, and Proteinuria

Glenn M. Chertow, MD, MPH
Norman S. Coplon/Satellite Healthcare
Professor of Medicine
Department of Medicine, Division of Nephrology
Stanford University School of Medicine
Palo Alto, California
Chapter 84, Health Disparities in Nephrology

Devasmita Choudhury, MD
Associate Professor of Medicine
University of Virginia School of Medicine
Virginia Tech-Carilion School of Medicine
Chief of Nephrology
Director of Dialysis and Interventional Nephrology
Salem Veterans Affairs Medical Center
Salem, Virginia
Chapter 24, Aging and Kidney Disease

John F. Collins, MBChB, FRACP
Clinical Associate Professor of Renal Medicine
Auckland City Hospital
Auckland, New Zealand
Chapter 82, Oceania Region

H. Terence Cook, MB, BS, FRCPath
Professor, Department of Medicine
Centre for Complement and Inflammation Research
Imperial College London
Hammersmith Hospital
London, United Kingdom
Chapter 29, The Kidney Biopsy

Ricardo Correa-Rotter, MD
Head, Department of Nephrology and Mineral Metabolism
Instituto Nacional de Ciencias Médicas y Nutrición Salvador Zubirán
Mexico City, Mexico
Chapter 66, Peritoneal Dialysis

Shawn E. Cowper, MD
Associate Professor of Dermatology and Pathology
Yale University
New Haven, Connecticut
Chapter 60, Dermatologic Conditions in Kidney Disease

Paolo Cravedi, MD, PhD
IRCCS-Istituto di Ricerche Farmacologiche Mario Negri
Centro Anna Maria Astori, Science and Technology Park Kilometro Rosso
Bergamo, Italy
Chapter 35, Microvascular and Macrovascular Diseases of the Kidney

Vivette D'Agati, MD
Professor of Pathology
Columbia University College of Physicians and Surgeons
Director, Renal Pathology Laboratory
Columbia University Medical Center
New York, New York
Chapter 33, Secondary Glomerular Disease

Mogamat Razeen Davids, MD
Division of Nephrology
Stellenbosch University and Tygerberg Hospital
Cape Town, South Africa
Chapter 27, Interpretation of Electrolyte and Acid-Base Parameters in Blood and Urine

Scott E. Delacroix, Jr., MD
Assistant Professor of Urology
Director of Urologic Oncology
Department of Oncology
Louisiana State University School of Medicine
New Orleans, Louisiana
Chapter 41, Kidney Cancer

Bradley M. Denker, MD
Associate Professor of Medicine
Harvard Medical School
Clinical Chief, Renal Division
Beth Israel Deaconess Medical Center
Boston, Massachusetts
Chapter 68, Plasmapheresis

Thomas A. Depner, MD
Professor of Medicine
Department of Internal Medicine/Nephrology
University of California Davis Health System
Sacramento, California
Chapter 65, Hemodialysis

Thomas D. DuBose, Jr., MD
Professor Emeritus of Medicine
Department of Internal Medicine
Wake Forest School of Medicine
Winston-Salem, North Carolina
Chapter 17, Disorders of Acid-Base Balance

Vinay A. Duddalwar, MD, FRCR
Associate Professor of Clinical Radiology and Urology
Section Chief, Abdominal Imaging
Medical Director, Imaging
USC Norris Comprehensive Cancer Center and Hospital
University of Southern California
Keck School of Medicine
Los Angeles, California
   Chapter 28, *Diagnostic Kidney Imaging*

Kai-Uwe Eckardt, MD
Professor of Medicine
Chair of Nephrology and Hypertension
Friedrich-Alexander University Erlangen-Nürnberg
Erlangen, Germany
   Chapter 57, *Hematologic Aspects of Kidney Disease*

Meghan J. Elliott, MD
Nephrology Resident
Department of Medicine
University of Calgary
Calgary, Alberta, Canada
   Chapter 85, *Care of the Older Adult with Chronic Kidney Disease*

William J. Elliott, MD, PhD
Professor of Preventive Medicine
Internal Medicine and Pharmacology
Pacific Northwest University of Health Sciences
Yakima, Washington
   Chapter 47, *Primary and Secondary Hypertension*

David H. Ellison, MD
Professor of Internal Medicine
Oregon Health & Science University
Portland, Oregon
   Chapter 51, *Diuretics*

Michael Emmett, MD
Chief of Internal Medicine
Department of Internal Medicine
Baylor University Medical Center
Dallas, Texas;
Professor of Medicine
Internal Medicine
Texas A&M College of Medicine
Baylor University Medical Center
Denton, Texas;
Clinical Professor of Medicine
University of Texas Southwestern Medical School
Dallas, Texas
   Chapter 25, *Approach to the Patient with Kidney Disease*

Ronald J. Falk, MD
Chair, Department of Medicine
Director, UNC Kidney Center
The University of North Carolina
Chapel Hill, North Carolina
   Chapter 32, *Primary Glomerular Disease*

Harold I. Feldman, MD, MSCE
Professor of Epidemiology and Medicine
Perelman School of Medicine
University of Pennsylvania
Philadelphia, Pennyslvania
   Chapter 21, *Demographics of Kidney Disease*

Bo Feldt-Rasmussen, MD, DMSc
Professor and Head of Clinic
Department of Nephrology
Rigshospitalet University of Copenhagen
Copenhagen, Denmark
   Chapter 39, *Diabetic Nephropathy*

Robert A. Fenton, PhD
Professor of Molecular Cell Biology
Department of Biomedicine
Aarhus University
Aarhus, Denmark
   Chapter 2, *Anatomy of the Kidney*
   Chapter 10, *Urine Concentration and Dilution*
   Chapter 11, *The Cell Biology of Vasopressin Action*

Andrew Z. Fenves, MD, FACP, FASN
Inpatient Clinical Educator
Massachusetts General Hospital
Associate Professor of Medicine
Harvard Medical School
Boston, Massachusetts
   Chapter 25, *Approach to the Patient with Kidney Disease*

Kevin W. Finkel, MD, FACP, FASN, FCCM
Department of Internal Medicine
Director, Division of Renal Diseases and Hypertension
University of Texas Health Science Center at Houston
Department of Internal Medicine
Section of Nephrology
The University of Texas MD Anderson Cancer Center
Houston, Texas
   Chapter 42, *Onco-Nephrology: Kidney Disease in Patients with Cancer*

Paola Fioretto, MD
Associate Professor
Department of Medical and Surgical Sciences
University of Padova Medical School
Padova, Italy
   Chapter 39, *Diabetic Nephropathy*

Damian G. Fogarty, BSc, MD, FRCP
Consultant Nephrologist
Regional Nephrology and Transplant Unit
Belfast City Hospital at the Belfast Health and
   Social Care Trust
Belfast, Northern Ireland
   Chapter 62, *A Stepped Care Approach to the Management of Chronic Kidney Disease*

Denis Fouque, MD, PhD
Professor of Nephrology
Chief, Division of Nephrology
Université Claude Bernard and Centre Hospitalier Lyon Sud
Lyon, France
Chapter 61, Dietary Approaches to Kidney Diseases

Yaacov Frishberg, MD
Director, Pediatric Nephrology
Shaare Zedek Medical Center
The Hebrew University School of Medicine
Jerusalem, Israel
Chapter 76, Renal Replacement Therapy (Dialysis and Transplantation) in Pediatric End-Stage Kidney Disease

Jørgen Frøkiaer, MD, DMSci
Head of Department of Nuclear Medicine and Molecular Imaging
Department of Clinical Medicine
Aarhus University and Aarhus University Hospital
Aarhus, Denmark
Chapter 38, Urinary Tract Obstruction

John W. Funder, MD, PhD, FRCP, FRACP
Distinguished Scholar
Steroid Biology
Hudson Institute of Medical Research
Clayton, Victoria, Australia
Chapter 12, Aldosterone and Mineralocorticoid Receptors: Renal and Extrarenal Roles

Marc Ghannoum, MD
Associate Professor
Specialized Medicine
University of Montréal
Verdun Hospital
Montréal, Quebec, Canada
Chapter 69, Elimination Enhancement of Poisons

Richard E. Gilbert, MBBS, PhD, FRACP, FRCPC, FACP, FASN
Professor of Medicine
University of Toronto
St. Michael's Hospital
Toronto, Ontario, Canada
Chapter 13, Vasoactive Molecules and the Kidney

Paul Goodyer, MD
Professor of Pediatrics
McGill University
Montréal, Quebec, Canada
Chapter 23, Nephron Endowment and Developmental Programming of Blood Pressure and Renal Function

Yoshio N. Hall, MD, MS
Associate Professor of Medicine
Department of Medicine, Division of Nephrology
University of Washington
Seattle, Washington
Chapter 84, Health Disparities in Nephrology

Mitchell L. Halperin, MD
Division of Nephrology
St. Michael's Hospital
University of Toronto
Toronto, Canada
Chapter 27, Interpretation of Electrolyte and Acid-Base Parameters in Blood and Urine

Donna S. Hanes, MD, FACP
Clinical Associate Professor of Medicine
Clerkship Director, Internal Medicine
University of Maryland Medical Systems
Baltimore, Maryland
Chapter 50, Antihypertensive Therapy

Chuan-Ming Hao, MD
Professor
Medicine/Nephrology
Huashan Hospital Fudan University
Shanghai, China
Chapter 81, The Far East

David C. H. Harris, MD, BS, FRACP
Associate Dean and Head of School
Sydney Medical School—Westmead
The University of Sydney
Sydney, New South Wales, Australia
Chapter 82, Oceania Region

Peter C. Harris, PhD
Professor of Biochemistry/Molecular Biology
Professor of Medicine
Nephrology and Hypertension
Mayo Clinic
Rochester, Minnesota
Chapter 46, Cystic Diseases of the Kidney

Raymond C. Harris, MD
Ann and Roscoe Robinson Professor of Medicine
Chief, Division of Nephrology and Hypertension
Vanderbilt University School of Medicine
Nashville, Tennessee
Chapter 14, Arachidonic Acid Metabolites and the Kidney

Richard Haynes, DM, FRCP
Associate Professor
Clinical Trial Service Unit and Epidemiological Studies Unit
Nuffield Department of Population Health
Honorary Consultant in Nephrology
Oxford Kidney Unit
Churchill Hospital
Oxford, United Kingdom
Chapter 56, Cardiovascular Aspects of Kidney Disease

Brenda R. Hemmelgarn, MD, PhD
Professor of Medicine
University of Calgary
Calgary, Alberta, Canada
Chapter 85, Care of the Older Adult with Chronic Kidney Disease

Friedhelm Hildebrandt, MD
Warren E. Grupe Professor of Pediatrics
Harvard Medical School
Investigator, Howard Hughes Medical Institute
Chief, Division of Nephrology
Boston Children's Hospital
Boston, Massachusetts
Chapter 43, Genetic Basis of Kidney Disease

Michelle A. Hladunewich, MD, MSc
Associate Professor of Medicine
University of Toronto
Scientist, Sunnybrook Research Institute
Sunnybrook Health Sciences Centre
Toronto, Ontario, Canada
Chapter 34, Overview of Therapy for Glomerular Disease

Kevin Ho, MD
Associate Professor of Medicine & Clinical and
  Translational Science
Renal-Electrolyte Division
University of Pittsburgh
Pittsburgh, Pennsylvania
Chapter 87, Quality Improvement Initiatives in Kidney Disease

Ewout J. Hoorn, MD, PhD
Associate Professor
Department of Internal Medicine, Division of Nephrology
  and Transplantation
Erasmus Medical Center
Rotterdam, The Netherlands
Chapter 51, Diuretics

Thomas H. Hostetter, MD
Professor of Medicine
Case Western Reserve University School of Medicine
Vice Chairman, Research Services
University Hospitals Case Medical Center
Cleveland, Ohio
Chapter 54, The Pathophysiology of Uremia

Fan-Fan Hou, MD
Director of Guangdong Provincial Institute of Nephrology
Chief and Professor of Division of Nephrology
Nanfang Hospital
Professor of Medicine
Southern Medical University
Guangzhou, China
Chapter 81, The Far East

Chi-yuan Hsu, MD
Professor and Division Chief
Division of Nephrology
University of California, San Francisco
San Francisco, California
Chapter 20, Epidemiology of Kidney Disease

Raymond K. Hsu, MD
Assistant Professor of Medicine
Division of Nephrology
University of California, San Francisco
San Francisco, California
Chapter 20, Epidemiology of Kidney Disease

Holly Hutton, MBBS, FRACP
Department of Nephrology
University of British Columbia
Vancouver, British Columbia, Canada;
Department of Nephrology
Monash Health
Clayton, Victoria, Australia
*Chapter 26, Laboratory Assessment of Kidney Disease:
  Glomerular Filtration Rate, Urinalysis, and Proteinuria*

Hossein Jadvar, MD, PhD, MPH, MBA, FACNM
Associate Professor of Radiology
Associate Professor of Biomedical Engineering
University of Southern California
Keck School of Medicine
Los Angeles, California
Chapter 28, Diagnostic Kidney Imaging

J. Charles Jennette, MD
Kenneth M. Brinkhous Distinguished Professor and Chair
Department of Pathology and Laboratory Medicine
The University of North Carolina
Chapel Hill, North Carolina
Chapter 32, Primary Glomerular Disease

Eric Jonasch, MD
Associate Professor
Department of Genitourinary Medical Oncology
Division of Cancer Medicine
The University of Texas MD Anderson Cancer Center
Houston, Texas
Chapter 41, Kidney Cancer

Kamel S. Kamel, MD
Division of Nephrology
St. Michael's Hospital
University of Toronto
Toronto, Canada
*Chapter 27, Interpretation of Electrolyte and Acid-Base
  Parameters in Blood and Urine*

S. Ananth Karumanchi, MD
Professor
Department of Medicine, Obstetrics, and Gynecology
Harvard Medical School
Howard Hughes Medical Institute and Beth Israel
  Deaconess Medical Center
Boston, Massachusetts
Chapter 49, Hypertension and Kidney Disease in Pregnancy

Frieder Keller, MD
Professor of Nephrology
Department of Internal Medicine 1
Ulm University
Ulm, Germany
*Chapter 64, Drug Dosing Considerations in Patients with
  Acute Kidney Injury and Chronic Kidney Disease*

Carolyn J. Kelly, MD
Professor of Medicine
Associate Dean for Admissions and Student Affairs
University of California, San Diego School of Medicine
La Jolla, California
   Chapter 36, Tubulointerstitial Diseases

David K. Klassen, MD
Professor of Medicine
Division of Nephrology, Department of Medicine
University of Maryland School of Medicine
Baltimore, Maryland
   Chapter 50, Antihypertensive Therapy

Christine J. Ko, MD
Associate Professor of Dermatology and Pathology
Yale University
New Haven, Connecticut
   Chapter 60, Dermatologic Conditions in Kidney Disease

Harbir Singh Kohli, MD, DM
Professor, Nephrology
Post Graduate Institute of Medical Education and Research
Chandigarh, India
   Chapter 80, Indian Subcontinent

Curtis K. Kost, Jr., RPh, PhD
Associate Professor
Basic Biomedical Sciences
Sanford School of Medicine
University of South Dakota
Vermillion, South Dakota
   Chapter 3, The Renal Circulations and Glomerular Ultrafiltration

Jay L. Koyner, MD
Assistant Professor of Medicine
Division of Nephrology
University of Chicago Medicine
Chicago, Illinois
   Chapter 30, Biomarkers in Acute and Chronic Kidney Diseases

L. Spencer Krane, MD
Wake Forest Institute for Regenerative Medicine
Department of Urology
Wake Forest University School of Medicine
Winston-Salem, North Carolina
   Chapter 86, Tissue Engineering, Stem Cells, and Cell Therapy in Nephrology

Jordan Kreidberg, MD, PhD
Associate Professor of Pediatrics
Division of Nephrology
Boston Children's Hospital
Harvard Medical School
Boston, Massachusetts
   Chapter 1, Embryology of the Kidney

Rajiv Kumar, MBBS
Department of Medicine, Division of Nephrology and Hypertension
Department of Biochemistry and Molecular Biology
Mayo Clinic College of Medicine
Mayo Clinic
Rochester, Minnesota
   Chapter 7, The Regulation of Calcium, Magnesium, and Phosphate Excretion by the Kidney

Martin J. Landray, PhD, FRCP, FASN
Professor of Medicine and Epidemiology
Clinical Trial Service Unit and Big Data Institute
Nuffield Department of Population Health
Oxford, United Kingdom
   Chapter 56, Cardiovascular Aspects of Kidney Disease

Harold E. Layton, PhD
Professor, Department of Mathematics
Duke University
Durham, North Carolina
   Chapter 10, Urine Concentration and Dilution

Timmy Lee, MD, MSPH
Associate Professor of Medicine
Division of Nephrology
University of Alabama at Birmingham
Birmingham, Alabama
   Chapter 70, Interventional Nephrology

Colin R. Lenihan, MB BCh BAO, PhD
Clinical Assistant Professor of Medicine
Division of Nephrology
Stanford University
Stanford, California
   Chapter 72, Clinical Management of the Adult Kidney Transplant Recipient

Moshe Levi, MD
Professor of Medicine, Bioengineering, Physiology, and Biophysics
Division of Renal Diseases and Hypertension
University of Colorado AMC
Aurora, Colorado
   Chapter 24, Aging and Kidney Disease

Adeera Levin, BSc, MD, FRCPC
Professor of Medicine (Nephrology)
University of British Columbia
Vancouver, British Columbia, Canada;
Director
BC Provincial Renal Agency
British Columbia, Canada
   Chapter 26, Laboratory Assessment of Kidney Disease: Glomerular Filtration Rate, Urinalysis, and Proteinuria

Shih-Hua Lin, MD
Division of Nephrology
Department of Medicine
Tri-Service General Hospital
National Defense Medical Center
Taipei, Taiwan, R.O.C.
Chapter 27, Interpretation of Electrolyte and Acid-Base Parameters in Blood and Urine

Bengt Lindholm, MD, PhD
Adjunct Professor
Karolinska Institutet
Stockholm, Sweden
Chapter 58, Endocrine Aspects of Chronic Kidney Disease

Kathleen Liu, MD, PhD, MAS
Associate Professor
Departments of Medicine and Anesthesia
University of California, San Francisco
San Francisco, California
Chapter 67, Critical Care Nephrology

Valerie A. Luyckx, MBBCh, MSc
Associate Professor of Nephrology
University of Alberta
Edmonton, Alberta, Canada
Chapter 23, Nephron Endowment and Developmental Programming of Blood Pressure and Renal Function

David A. Maddox, PhD, FASN
Professor of Internal Medicine and Basic Biomedical Sciences
Sanford School of Medicine
University of South Dakota
Coordinator, Research and Development (retired)
VA Medical Center
Sioux Falls VA Health Care System
Sioux Falls, South Dakota
Chapter 3, The Renal Circulations and Glomerular Ultrafiltration

Yoshiro Maezawa, MD, PhD
Assistant Professor
Clinical Cell Biology and Medicine
Chiba University Graduate School of Medicine
Chiba, Japan
Chapter 1, Embryology of the Kidney

Karine Mardini, B.Pharm
Department of Pharmacy
University of Montréal
Montréal, Quebec, Canada
Chapter 69, Elimination Enhancement of Poisons

Peter W. Mathieson, MB, ChB(Hons), PhD, FRCP, FMedSci
President
President's Office
The University of Hong Kong
Hong Kong, China
Chapter 4, The Podocyte

Gary R. Matzke, PharmD
Professor and Founding Director, ACCP/ASHP/VCU Congressional Health Care Policy Fellow Program
Virginia Commonwealth University School of Pharmacy
Department of Pharmacotherapy and Outcomes Sciences
Richmond, Virginia
Chapter 64, Drug Dosing Considerations in Patients with Acute Kidney Injury and Chronic Kidney Disease

Ivan D. Maya, MD
Associate Professor of Medicine
Department of Medicine
University of Central Florida
Orlando, Florida
Chapter 70, Interventional Nephrology

Sharon E. Maynard, MD
Associate Professor
Department of Medicine
Lehigh Valley Health Network
University of South Florida
Morsani College of Medicine
Allentown, Pennsylvania
Chapter 49, Hypertension and Kidney Disease in Pregnancy

Alicia A. McDonough, PhD
Professor of Cell and Neurobiology
Keck School of Medicine
University of Southern California
Los Angeles, California
Chapter 5, Metabolic Basis of Solute Transport

Rajnish Mehrotra, MD
Section Head, Nephrology
Harborview Medical Center
Division of Nephrology
University of Washington
Seattle, Washington
Chapter 66, Peritoneal Dialysis

Timothy W. Meyer, MD
Professor of Medicine
Stanford University
Stanford, California;
Staff Physician
Department of Medicine
VA Palo Alto Health Care System
Palo Alto, California
Chapter 54, The Pathophysiology of Uremia

William E. Mitch, MD
Professor of Medicine and Nephrology
Baylor College of Medicine
Houston, Texas
Chapter 61, Dietary Approaches to Kidney Diseases

Orson W. Moe, MD
Professor of Internal Medicine, Division of Nephrology
University of Texas Southwestern Medical Center
Director
Charles and Jane Pak Center for Mineral Metabolism
 and Clinical Research
University of Texas Southwestern Medical Center
Dallas, Texas
  Chapter 8, Renal Handling of Organic Solutes
  Chapter 40, Urolithiasis

Sharon M. Moe, MD
Stuart A. Kleit Professor of Medicine
Professor of Anatomy and Cell Biology
Director, Division of Nephrology
Indiana University School of Medicine
Indianapolis, Indiana
  Chapter 55, Chronic Kidney Disease–Mineral Bone Disorder

Bruce A. Molitoris, MD
Professor of Medicine
Division of Nephrology, Department of Medicine
Director, Indiana Center for Biologic Microscopy
Indiana University School of Medicine
Indianapolis, Indiana
  Chapter 31, Acute Kidney Injury

Alvin H. Moss, MD
Professor of Medicine
Department of Medicine, Section of Nephrology
West Virginia University
Director
Center for Health Ethics and Law
West Virginia University
Medical Director
Supportive Care Service
West Virginia University Hospital
Morgantown, West Virginia
  Chapter 83, Ethical Dilemmas Facing Nephrology: Past, Present, and Future

David B. Mount, MD, FRCPC
Assistant Professor of Medicine
Harvard Medical School
Associate Division Chief, Renal Division
Brigham and Women's Hospital
Attending Physician, Renal Division
VA Boston Healthcare System
Boston, Massachusetts
  Chapter 6, Transport of Sodium, Chloride, and Potassium
  Chapter 18, Disorders of Potassium Balance

Karen A. Munger, PhD
Associate Professor of Internal Medicine
Sanford School of Medicine
University of South Dakota
Coordinator, Research and Development
VA Medical Center
Sioux Falls VA Health Care System
Sioux Falls, South Dakota
  Chapter 3, The Renal Circulations and Glomerular Ultrafiltration

Patrick H. Nachman, MD
Professor of Medicine
Division of Nephrology and Hypertension
Department of Medicine
UNC Kidney Center
The University of North Carolina
Chapel Hill, North Carolina
  Chapter 32, Primary Glomerular Disease

Saraladevi Naicker, MD, PhD
Professor
Department of Internal Medicine
University of the Witwatersrand
Johannesburg, South Africa
  Chapter 78, Africa

Sagren Naidoo, MD
Consultant Nephrologist
Department of Internal Medicine
Division of Nephrology
Charlotte Maxeke Johannesburg Academic Hospital
University of the Witwatersrand
Johannesburg, South Africa
  Chapter 78, Africa

Eric G. Neilson, MD
Vice President for Medical Affairs
Lewis Landsberg Dean
Professor of Medicine and Cell and Molecular Biology
Northwestern University Feinberg School of Medicine
Chicago, Illinois
  Chapter 36, Tubulointerstitial Diseases

Lindsay E. Nicolle, MD
Professor, Department of Internal Medicine and Medical
 Microbiology
University of Manitoba
Winnipeg, Manitoba, Canada
  Chapter 37, Urinary Tract Infection in Adults

Ann M. O'Hare, MD, MA
Associate Professor of Medicine
University of Washington
Staff Physician
Department of Medicine
Department of Veterans Affairs
Seattle, Washington
  Chapter 85, Care of the Older Adult with Chronic Kidney Disease

Daniel B. Ornt, MD
Clinical Professor
Department of Medicine
University of Rochester Medical Center
Vice President and Dean
College of Health Sciences and Technology
Rochester Institute of Technology
Rochester, New York
  Chapter 65, Hemodialysis

Manuel Palacín, PhD
Full Professor, Biochemistry and Molecular Biology
Universitat de Barcelona
Group Leader
CIBERER (The Spanish Network Center for Rare Diseases)
Group Leader
Molecular Medicine Program
Institute for Research in Biomedicine of Barcelona
Barcelona, Spain
Chapter 8, Renal Handling of Organic Solutes

Paul M. Palevsky, MD
Chief, Renal Section, VA Pittsburgh Healthcare System
Professor of Medicine and Clinical and Translational Science
Renal-Electrolyte Division, Department of Medicine
University of Pittsburgh School of Medicine
Pittsburgh, Pennsylvania
Chapter 31, Acute Kidney Injury

Suzanne L. Palmer, MD, FACP
Professor of Clinical Radiology and Medicine
Chief, Body Imaging Division
University of Southern California
Keck School of Medicine
Keck Hospital of USC
Los Angeles, California
Chapter 28, Diagnostic Kidney Imaging

Chirag R. Parikh, MD, PhD, FACP
Associate Professor of Medicine
Director, Program of Applied Translational Research
Yale University and Veterans Affairs Medical Center
New Haven, Connecticut
Chapter 30, Biomarkers in Acute and Chronic Kidney Diseases

Hans-Henrik Parving, MD, DMSc
Professor and Chief Physician
Department of Medical Endocrinology
Rigshospitalet Copenhagen
University of Copenhagen
Copenhagen, Denmark
Chapter 39, Diabetic Nephropathy

Jaakko Patrakka, MD, PhD
Assistant Professor
Department of Medical Biochemistry and Biophysics
Karolinska Institute, Nephrology Fellow
Division of Nephrology
Karolinska University Hospital
Stockholm, Sweden
Chapter 44, Inherited Disorders of the Glomerulus

David Pearce, MD
Professor of Medicine and Cellular and Molecular Pharmacology
University of California at San Francisco
Chief, Division of Nephrology
San Francisco General Hospital
San Francisco, California
Chapter 12, Aldosterone and Mineralocorticoid Receptors: Renal and Extrarenal Roles

Aldo J. Peixoto, MD
Professor of Medicine
Department of Medicine
Section of Nephrology
Yale University School of Medicine
New Haven, Connecticut
Chapter 47, Primary and Secondary Hypertension

William F. Pendergraft, III, MD, PhD
Assistant Professor of Medicine
Division of Nephrology and Hypertension
Department of Medicine
UNC Kidney Center
The University of North Carolina
Chapel Hill, North Carolina;
Visiting Postdoctoral Scholar, Hacohen Group
Broad Institute of Harvard and MIT
Cambridge, Massachusetts
Chapter 32, Primary Glomerular Disease

Norberto Perico, MD
IRCCS-Istituto di Ricerche Farmacologiche Mario Negri
Bergamo, Italy
Chapter 53, Mechanisms and Consequences of Proteinuria

Jeppe Praetorius, MD, PhD, DMSc
Professor of Medical Cell Biology
Department of Biomedicine
Aarhus University
Aarhus, Denmark
Chapter 2, Anatomy of the Kidney

Susan E. Quaggin, MD
Professor and Chief, Division of Nephrology and Hypertension
Department of Medicine
Director, Feinberg Cardiovascular Research Institute
Feinberg School of Medicine
Northwestern University
Chicago, Illinois
Chapter 1, Embryology of the Kidney

L. Darryl Quarles, MD
UTMG Endowed Professor of Nephrology
Director, Division of Nephrology
Associate Dean for Research, College of Medicine
University of Tennessee Health Science Center
Memphis, Tennessee
Chapter 63, Therapeutic Approach to Chronic Kidney Disease–Mineral Bone Disorder

Jai Radhakrishnan, MD, MS
Professor of Medicine
Columbia University Medical Center
Associate Division Chief for Clinical Affairs
Division of Nephrology
New York Presbyterian Hospital
New York, New York
 Chapter 33, Secondary Glomerular Disease

Rawi Ramadan, MD
Director, Medical Transplantation Unit
Department of Nephrology and Hypertension
Rambam Health Care Campus
Haifa, Israel
 Chapter 79, Near and Middle East

Heather N. Reich, MD CM, PhD, FRCP(C)
Associate Professor of Medicine
University of Toronto
Clinician Scientist and Staff Nephrologist
Medicine
University Health Network
Toronto, Ontario, Canada
 Chapter 34, Overview of Therapy for Glomerular Disease

Andrea Remuzzi, MD
University of Bergamo
IRCCS-Istituto di Ricerche Farmacologiche Mario Negri
Bergamo, Italy
 Chapter 53, Mechanisms and Consequences of Proteinuria

Giuseppe Remuzzi, MD, FRCP
IRCCS-Istituto di Ricerche Farmacologiche Mario Negri
Centro Anna Maria Astori, Science and Technology Park
 Kilometro Rosso
Unit of Nephrology and Dialysis
Azienda Ospedaliera Papa Giovanni XXIII
University of Milan
Bergamo, Italy
 *Chapter 35, Microvascular and Macrovascular Diseases
 of the Kidney*
 Chapter 53, Mechanisms and Consequences of Proteinuria

Leonardo V. Riella, MD, PhD, FASN
Assistant Professor of Medicine
Department of Medicine, Renal Division
Harvard Medical School
Brigham and Women's Hospital
Schuster Family Transplantation Research Center
Boston, Massachusetts
 Chapter 71, Transplantation Immunobiology
 Chapter 77, Latin America

Miquel C. Riella, MD, PhD
Professor of Medicine
Evangelic School of Medicine
Catholic University of Parana
Curitiba, Brazil
 Chapter 77, Latin America

Choni Rinat, MD
Pediatric Nephrology
Shaare Zedek Medical Center
The Hebrew University School of Medicine
Jerusalem, Israel
 *Chapter 76, Renal Replacement Therapy (Dialysis and
 Transplantation) in Pediatric End-Stage Kidney Disease*

Norman D. Rosenblum, MD, FRCPC
Staff Nephrologist and Senior Scientist
The Hospital for Sick Children, Toronto
Professor of Pediatrics, Physiology, and Laboratory
 Medicine and Pathobiology
Canada Research Chair in Developmental Nephrology
University of Toronto
Toronto, Ontario, Canada
 *Chapter 73, Malformation of the Kidney: Structural and
 Functional Consequences*

Peter Rossing, MD, DMSc
Professor and Chief Physician
Steno Diabetes Center
University of Copenhagen
Copenhagen, Denmark;
Aarhus University
Aarhus, Denmark
 Chapter 39, Diabetic Nephropathy

Dvora Rubinger, MD
Associate Professor of Medicine
Department of Nephrology
Hadassah Hebrew University Medical Center
Jerusalem, Israel
 Chapter 79, Near and Middle East

Piero Ruggenenti, MD
IRCCS-Istituto di Ricerche Farmacologiche Mario Negri
Centro Anna Maria Astori, Science and Technology Park
 Kilometro Rosso
Unit of Nephrology and Dialysis
Azienda Ospedaliera Papa Giovanni XXIII
Bergamo, Italy
 *Chapter 35, Microvascular and Macrovascular Diseases
 of the Kidney*

Ernesto Sabath, MD
Renal Department
Hospital General de Querétaro
Queretaro, Mexico
 Chapter 68, Plasamapheresis

Khashayar Sakhaee, MD
Department of Internal Medicine
Charles and Jane Pak Center for Mineral Metabolism
 and Clinical Research
University of Texas Southwestern Medical Center
Dallas, Texas
 Chapter 40, Urolithiasis

Vinay Sakhuja, MD, DM
Department of Nephrology
Post Graduate Institute of Medical Education and Research
Chandigarh, India
Chapter 80, Indian Subcontinent

Alan D. Salama, MBBS, PhD, FRCP
Professor of Nephrology
University College London Centre for Nephrology
Royal Free Hospital
London, United Kingdom
Chapter 29, The Kidney Biopsy

Jeff M. Sands, MD
Professor, Renal Division
Department of Medicine and Department of Physiology
Emory University School of Medicine
Atlanta, Georgia
Chapter 10, Urine Concentration and Dilution

Fernando Santos, MD
Professor of Pediatrics
Chair, Department of Medicine
University of Oviedo
Chairman of Pediatrics
Hospital Universitario Central de Asturias
Oviedo, Asturias, Spain
Chapter 75, Fluid, Electrolyte, and Acid-Base Disorders in Children

Anjali Saxena, MD
Clinical Assistant Professor of Medicine
Internal Medicine
Stanford University
Stanford, California;
Director of Peritoneal Dialysis
Internal Medicine
Santa Clara Valley Medical Center
San Jose, California
Chapter 66, Peritoneal Dialysis

Mohamed H. Sayegh, MD
Senior Lecturer, Harvard Medical School
Schuster Family Transplantation Research Center
Brigham and Women's Hospital
Boston, Massachusetts;
Dean and Vice President of Medical Affairs
Professor of Medicine and Immunology
Faculty of Medicine
American University of Beirut
Beirut, Lebanon
Chapter 71, Transplantation Immunobiology

Franz Schaefer, MD
Professor of Pediatrics
Head, Division of Pediatric Nephrology and KFH Children's Kidney Center
Heidelberg University Medical Center
Heidelberg, Germany
Chapter 74, Diseases of the Kidney and Urinary Tract in Children

John C. Schwartz, MD
Nephrology Division
Department of Internal Medicine
Baylor University Medical Center
Dallas, Texas
Chapter 25, Approach to the Patient with Kidney Disease

Rizaldy P. Scott, MS, PhD
Division of Nephrology and Hypertension
Department of Medicine
Feinberg School of Medicine
Northwestern University
Chicago, Illinois
Chapter 1, Embryology of the Kidney

Stuart J. Shankland, MD, MBA, FRCPC, FASN, FAHA, FACP
Professor of Medicine
Belding H. Scribner Endowed Chair in Medicine
Head, Division of Nephrology
University of Washington
Seattle, Washington
Chapter 4, The Podocyte

Asif A. Sharfuddin, MD
Associate Professor of Clinical Medicine
Division of Nephrology, Department of Medicine
Indiana University School of Medicine
Indianapolis, Indiana
Chapter 31, Acute Kidney Injury

Prabhleen Singh, MD
Assistant Professor of Medicine
Division of Nephrology and Hypertension
University of California, San Diego
VA San Diego Healthcare System
San Diego, California
Chapter 5, Metabolic Basis of Solute Transport

Karl L. Skorecki, MD, FRCP(C), FASN
Annie Chutick Professor and Chair in Medicine (Nephrology)
Technion—Israel Institute of Technology
Director of Medicine and Research Development
Rambam Health Care Campus
Haifa, Israel
Chapter 15, Disorders of Sodium Balance

Itzchak N. Slotki, MD
Associate Professor of Medicine
Hadassah Hebrew University of Jerusalem
Director, Division of Adult Nephrology
Shaare Zedek Medical Center
Jerusalem, Israel
Chapter 15, Disorders of Sodium Balance

Miroslaw J. Smogorzewski, MD, PhD
Associate Professor of Medicine
Division of Nephrology, Department of Medicine
University of Southern California, Keck School
 of Medicine
Los Angeles, California
> Chapter 19, *Disorders of Calcium, Magnesium, and Phosphate Balance*

Sandeep S. Soman, MD
Division of Nephrology and Hypertension
Henry Ford Hospital
Detroit, Michigan
> Chapter 87, *Quality Improvement Initiatives in Kidney Disease*

Stuart M. Sprague, DO
Chief, Division of Nephrology and Hypertension
Department of Medicine
NorthShore University HealthSystem
Evanston, Illinois;
Professor of Medicine
University of Chicago Pritzker School of Medicine
Chicago, Illinois
> Chapter 55, *Chronic Kidney Disease–Mineral Bone Disorder*

Peter Stenvinkel, MD, PhD, FENA
Professor of Renal Medicine
Karolinska Institutet
Stockholm, Sweden
> Chapter 58, *Endocrine Aspects of Chronic Kidney Disease*

Jason R. Stubbs, MD
Associate Professor of Medicine
Division of Nephrology and Hypertension
The Kidney Institute
University of Kansas Medical Center
Kansas City, Kansas
> Chapter 19, *Disorders of Calcium, Magnesium, and Phosphate Balance*

Maarten W. Taal, MBChB, MMed, MD, FCP(SA), FRCP
Professor of Medicine
Division of Medical Sciences and Graduate
 Entry Medicine
University of Nottingham
Honorary Consultant Nephrologist
Department of Renal Medicine
Royal Derby Hospital
Derby, United Kingdom
> Chapter 22, *Risk Factors and Chronic Kidney Disease*
> Chapter 52, *Adaptation to Nephron Loss and Mechanisms of Progression in Chronic Kidney Disease*
> Chapter 62, *A Stepped Care Approach to the Management of Chronic Kidney Disease*

Manjula Kurella Tamura, MD, MPH
Associate Professor of Medicine/Nephrology
Division of Nephrology, Stanford University School
 of Medicine
VA Palo Alto Health Care System Geriatrics Research
 Education and Clinical Center
Palo Alto, California
> Chapter 59, *Neurologic Aspects of Kidney Disease*

Jane C. Tan, MD, PhD
Associate Professor of Medicine
Division of Nephrology
Stanford University
Stanford, California
> Chapter 72, *Clinical Management of the Adult Kidney Transplant Recipient*

Stephen C. Textor, MD
Professor of Medicine
Division of Hypertension and Nephrology
Mayo Clinic College of Medicine
Mayo Clinic
Rochester, Minnesota
> Chapter 48, *Renovascular Hypertension and Ischemic Nephropathy*

Ravi Thadhani, MD, MPH
Professor of Medicine
Harvard Medical School
Chief, Nephrology Section
Massachusetts General Hospital
Boston, Massachusetts
> Chapter 49, *Hypertension and Kidney Disease in Pregnancy*

James R. Thompson, PhD
Department of Physiology, Biophysics, and Bioengineering
Department of Biochemistry and Molecular Biology
Mayo Clinic College of Medicine
Mayo Clinic
Rochester, Minnesota
> Chapter 7, *The Regulation of Calcium, Magnesium, and Phosphate Excretion by the Kidney*

Scott C. Thomson, MD
Professor of Medicine
University of California, San Diego
Chief of Nephrology Section
Department of Medicine
VA San Diego Healthcare System
San Diego, California
> Chapter 5, *Metabolic Basis of Solute Transport*

Vicente E. Torres, MD, PhD
Professor of Medicine
Nephrology and Hypertension
Mayo Clinic
Rochester, Minnesota
> Chapter 46, *Cystic Diseases of the Kidney*

Karl Tryggvason, MD, PhD
Professor of Medical Chemistry
Department of Medical Biochemistry and Biophysics
Karolinska Institutet
Stockholm, Sweden
Chapter 44, Inherited Disorders of the Glomerulus

Joseph G. Verbalis, MD
Professor of Medicine
Georgetown University
Chief, Endocrinology and Metabolism
Georgetown University Hospital
Washington, DC
Chapter 16, Disorders of Water Balance

Jill W. Verlander, DVM
Scientist
Director of College of Medicine Core Electron Microscopy Lab
Division of Nephrology, Hypertension, and Transplantation
University of Florida College of Medicine
Gainesville, Florida
Chapter 9, Renal Acidification Mechanisms

Ron Wald, MDCM, MPH
Associate Professor of Medicine
University of Toronto
Staff Nephrologist
Department of Medicine
St. Michael's Hospital
Toronto, Ontario, Canada
Chapter 67, Critical Care Nephrology

Walter G. Wasser, MD
Attending Physician, Division of Nephrology
Mayanei HaYeshua Medical Center
Bnei Brak, Israel;
Rambam Health Care Campus
Haifa, Israel
Chapter 50, Antihypertensive Therapy
Chapter 81, The Far East

I. David Weiner, MD
Professor of Medicine
Division of Nephrology, Hypertension, and Transplantation
University of Florida College of Medicine
Nephrology and Hypertension Section
North Florida/South Georgia Veterans Health System
Gainesville, Florida
Chapter 9, Renal Acidification Mechanisms

Matthew R. Weir, MD
Professor and Director
Division of Nephrology, Department of Medicine
University of Maryland School of Medicine
Baltimore, Maryland
Chapter 50, Antihypertensive Therapy

Steven D. Weisbord, MD, MSc
Staff Physician, Renal Section and Center for Health Equity Research and Promotion
VA Pittsburgh Healthcare System
Associate Professor of Medicine and Clinical and Translational Science
Renal-Electrolyte Division, Department of Medicine
University of Pittsburgh School of Medicine
Pittsburgh, Pennsylvania
Chapter 31, Acute Kidney Injury

David C. Wheeler, MD
Professor of Kidney Medicine
Centre for Nephrology
Division of Medicine
University College London
London, United Kingdom
Chapter 56, Cardiovascular Aspects of Kidney Disease

Christopher S. Wilcox, MD, PhD
Division Chief, Professor of Medicine
George E. Schreiner Chair of Nephrology
Director of the Hypertension, Kidney, and Vascular Research Center
Georgetown University
Washington, DC
Chapter 51, Diuretics

F. Perry Wilson, MD, MSCE
Assistant Professor of Medicine (Nephrology)
Yale School of Medicine
New Haven, Connecticut
Chapter 21, Demographics of Kidney Disease

Christopher G. Wood, MD
Professor and Deputy Chairman
Douglas E. Johnson, MD Endowed Professorship in Urology
Department of Urology
The University of Texas MD Anderson Cancer Center
Houston, Texas
Chapter 41, Kidney Cancer

Stephen H. Wright, PhD
Professor, Department of Physiology
University of Arizona
Tucson, Arizona
Chapter 8, Renal Handling of Organic Solutes

Jerry Yee, MD
Division Head
Division of Nephrology and Hypertension
Henry Ford Hospital
Detroit, Michigan
Chapter 87, Quality Improvement Initiatives in Kidney Disease

Jane Y. Yeun, MD
Clinical Professor of Medicine
Department of Internal Medicine, Division of Nephrology
University of California Davis Health System
Sacramento, California;
Staff Nephrologist
Medical Service
Sacramento Veterans Administration Medical Center
Mather, California
   Chapter 65, Hemodialysis

Alan S.L. Yu, MB, BChir
Harry Statland and Solon Summerfield Professor
   of Medicine
Director, Division of Nephrology and Hypertension
   and The Kidney Institute
University of Kansas Medical Center
Kansas City, Kansas
   *Chapter 19, Disorders of Calcium, Magnesium, and
   Phosphate Balance*

Ming-Zhi Zhang, MD
Assistant Professor of Medicine
Vanderbilt University
Nashville, Tennessee
   Chapter 14, Arachidonic Acid Metabolites and the Kidney

Foreword

Ten quadrennial editions and counting! This latest edition of Brenner and Rector's *The Kidney*, which comes 40 years after the first, is also the first in which I have had no formal role. The work of editing is now in the very capable hands of five exceptionally gifted and internationally dispersed former colleagues. It is perhaps fitting then to leave behind something of the history of how this textbook came into being. The year was 1972, the setting the Veterans Administration Medical Center at Fort Miley, perched on a high bluff overlooking the Golden Gate Bridge at the entrance to San Francisco Bay. I was then in my third year beyond renal physiology fellowship training, holding the position as Chief, Nephrology Section, overseeing a faculty of four and a single laboratory devoted to basic kidney research. Exploiting surface glomeruli in a unique strain of Wistar rats, using specially designed micropuncture techniques, our now classical studies of glomerular hemodynamics and permselectivity propelled me up the academic ladder such that a full professorship in the University of California system was soon earned. I was so self-confident and ambitious that new challenges and adventures were eagerly sought and considered.

But the one that presented itself on a Saturday morning in late 1972 could hardly have been imagined. After reviewing the week's laboratory data with my research team, I wandered, as I often did, into the nearby office of the Chair of Medicine, Marvin H. Sleisenger, whose warm and supportive words were always a treasured source of guidance and encouragement. On this particular morning's visit, I saw on his desk before him reams of long vertical galley proof of what was soon to become the first edition of a new textbook on gastroenterology, co-edited with John Fordtran. How wonderful it must feel, I remarked, to be in the position to oversee the organization and synthesis of a major field of internal medicine. He indeed expressed great pride and satisfaction in dealing with this challenge and, to my complete amazement, gazed up at me and suggested that this might be the appropriate time in my career to undertake a similar responsibility for a large-scale academic work in nephrology.

Flattered, of course, I left his office with little belief that I had the knowledge or capability to take on so formidable a challenge at this relatively early stage in my career. Not more than a week later, however, Albert Meier, Senior Editor at W.B. Saunders Publishing Company, was in my office urging me to set aside my reservations and undertake the responsibility for putting together a comprehensive compendium of nephrology, from basic science to clinical diagnosis and treatment of kidney disease. Weeks passed without decision into early 1973, when I learned that Floyd C. Rector, Jr., a world-renowned academic nephrologist, was moving to San Francisco to direct the Renal Division at the University of California, San Francisco. Imagine my excitement at the prospect of collaborating with this brilliant physician-scientist on a project of this magnitude and importance. Upon my sharing the notion with him, Dr. Rector was quick to agree that a two-volume textbook of nephrology based on fundamental physiologic principles was indeed needed, and we soon informed Saunders that a detailed outline of the scope and organization that reflected our combined personal insights and imagination would soon be forthcoming. All this was achieved in an informal 4-hour session in the living room of my Mill Valley home, where, over a lovely bottle of Napa Valley cabernet sauvignon and delicious, warm canapés prepared by my wife, Jane, we sketched out the five-section structure of a book that would remain unaltered over seven editions, namely, "Elements of Normal Renal Function," "Disturbances in Control of Body Fluid Volume and Composition," "Pathogenesis of Renal Disease," "Pathophysiology of Renal Disease," and "Management of the Patient with Renal Failure." Over the next few weeks, we added the filigree of specific chapter titles, prospective authors, timelines, and our shared editorial responsibilities and submitted the operational plan to Saunders for their executive consideration. Enthusiastic approval and contracts soon followed, and we were then busy with formal letters of invitation to authors (no e-mail in those days) for 49 chapters in nearly 2000 printed pages, with not a single turndown.

The first edition of *The Kidney* debuted at the ninth annual meeting of the American Society of Nephrology in November 1975, bearing the publication date of 1976. Acceptance was instantaneous and robust. Three subsequent editions with Dr. Rector appeared in 1980, 1984, and 1988, each extensively revised and expanded to reflect the remarkable progress in the field. I then served as sole editor for four editions, including an extensive structural redesign for the eighth edition, which consisted of 70 chapters in 12 sections. Among the newly crafted sections were the timely themes of "Epidemiology and Risk Factors in Kidney Disease," "Genetic Basis of Kidney Disease," and "Frontiers in Nephrology." The eighth edition also displayed cover art, tables, and figures redrawn in house in multicolor format and a fully functional electronic edition. In the preface to this eighth edition, which appeared in 2008, I wrote, "Just as blazing embers eventually grow dimmer, I recognize that now is the appropriate time to begin the orderly transition of responsibility for future editions…to a new generation of editors." An international team consisting of Glenn M. Chertow, Philip A. Marsden, Karl L. Skorecki, Maarten W. Taal, and Alan S. L. Yu joined me in crafting the ninth edition, to which two major new sections were added, "Pediatric Nephrology" and "Global Considerations in Kidney Disease." And for this tenth edition, which you are now reading, these five editors have operated fully independently in producing this extensively updated and further expanded latest edition, featuring several novel new chapters, by far the best ever!

In addition to the refinements mentioned, what has come to be known as the "Brenner and Rector" project has grown into a very well received library of nephrology, consisting of discrete companion volumes designed to delve more deeply into specific areas of readership interest, including *Therapy in Nephrology and Hypertension*; *Chronic Kidney Disease, Dialysis, and Transplantation*; *Hypertension*; *Acute Renal Failure*; *Acid-Base and Electrolyte Disorders*; *Diagnostic Atlas of Renal Pathology*; *Molecular and Genetic Basis of Renal Disease*; and *Pocket Companion to Brenner and Rector's The Kidney*.

Nephrology has evolved dramatically over these past 40 years and will surely continue at an ever-quickening pace in the future. This will necessitate a full thrust into multimedia electronic formats such that updating new developments will appear more and more as a continuum. This will surely require new tools and editorial flexibility not yet tested. But therein may lie the project's greatest challenge.

Looking back, I could hardly have imagined the enormous success and respect this textbook project has enjoyed. Of course, full credit rests entirely with the authors of the chapters in each edition, whose enormous commitments of time and effort provided the outstanding scholarship and synthesis their respective areas demanded, along with invaluable comprehensive bibliographies, all of which served our devoted readership so well. My gratitude to them, our editorial staff, and the readers for their generous feedback over the years is unbounded. Playing a part in documenting the ever-more complex and expanding disciplines of renal science and medicine is among my life's greatest pleasures and challenges. If only I could again be a young student and have this magnificent new edition introduce me to the kidney's many wonders and enigmas.

Barry M. Brenner, MD

Preface

The tenth edition of *The Kidney* represents a turning point in the more than 40-year history of what has rightfully become a classic in nephrology. Barry Morton Brenner, co–founding editor with his distinguished colleague, Floyd Rector, and sole editor for the fourth through eighth editions, has shepherded an orderly transition of editorial stewardship to five of his fortunate trainees. We served as co-editors with Dr. Brenner on the ninth edition, for which Maarten W. Taal was a lead editor, and have now been fully entrusted with this precious legacy, buoyed by the mentorship and training that we have each received from Dr. Brenner.

The same sense of honor, mixed with trepidation, responsibility, and pride, that accompanied each of us as we entered the vaunted nephrology clinical and research program in Dr. Brenner's division at Brigham and Women's Hospital now accompanies us as we accept into our hands this "labor of love." Although this is the first edition for which Dr. Brenner is not an editor, his presence is palpable throughout the book. A fascinating history of *The Kidney* is described in the foreword by Dr. Brenner, and the narrative very much follows the exciting history of scientific discovery and clinical advances in the rather young clinical specialty of nephrology and our emerging knowledge of kidney biology. Dr. Brenner's imprint is also evident in so many of his own scientific discoveries and insights that have transformed our understanding of all aspects of the kidney in health and disease, as described by the authors throughout all the sections of the book. *The Kidney* continues to combine authoritative coverage of the most important topics of relevance to readers worldwide with the excitement of "a work in progress" presenting novel and transformative insights based on basic and clinical research and clinical paradigms that inform and improve medical care to patients with kidney disease in every corner of the world.

The more than 200 authors with whom we have had the great privilege of working have succeeded in transmitting not only a wealth of information, but also a sense of passion for the topics at hand. We hope that the reader will readily identify for each author the specific attraction that draws the author closer to the subject. These are myriad and diverse, ranging from the sheer and exquisite beauty of the architecture, structure, and substructure of the renal system, to the intricacies of cellular and molecular function, alongside advances in our understanding of disease pathogenesis at the most fundamental level, coupled with the opportunity to offer lifesaving clinical management with a global health perspective. Indeed, the authors reflect an international fellowship of dedicated researchers, scientists, and health professionals who find their expression in narrative text, images, illustrations, Web links, review questions, and references that constitute this tenth edition of *The Kidney*.

Most of all, the book is imbued with the inspiration of Dr. Brenner. We feel that it is this ingredient that guarantees the continued success of *The Kidney* in an era when other textbooks in all specialties are supplanted by a morass of other information sources. We, the editors and publishers, together with our authors, believe in the cardinal importance of a coherent and updated source of empowering information for students and devotees of the kidney, whether in the professional, teaching, or research domain.

To this end, the ninth edition of *The Kidney*, with Maarten W. Taal as lead editor, introduced several major changes that have proven enormously successful. Therefore we have retained and extended these innovations in the tenth edition. As befitting a living textbook, all chapters have been extensively updated or entirely rewritten. All of the authors are authorities in their respective fields, and many have accompanied *The Kidney* for several editions. However, new authors have been invited to provide refreshing perspectives on existing topics or to introduce brand-new areas relevant to kidney biology and health. One of the many examples is thorough consideration of our completely transformed understanding of sodium balance, resulting from the discovery of sodium stores whose very existence had been unknown and whose fluxes are under complex hormonal and growth factor regulation. By combining the classical and authoritative with transformative discovery and perspectives, *The Kidney* has positioned itself as the "go-to" reference and also the leading learning resource for kidney health and disease throughout the world. For example, a section on pediatric kidney disease was included in the ninth edition, and the positive feedback we received resulted in greater emphasis in the tenth edition. The extension of *The Kidney* into pediatric kidney disease will allow individuals and institutions throughout the world, sometimes with limited resources, to access information from a learning resource that covers kidney health and disease from pre-conception, through fetal and infant health, childhood, adulthood, and into old age. Similarly, the section on global perspectives has been expanded, and the chapter on ethical challenges has been deepened.

A number of practical considerations were also taken into account in the production of the tenth edition. Positive feedback and reviews have reinforced the overall organization into 14 sections and 87 chapters that take the reader from normal structure and function through to current and future challenges in the concluding section.

The authors have been asked to choose 50 key references for their respective chapters, whose citations will appear in the print edition. The online edition will in turn offer access to the full repertoire of references for each chapter, allowing scholarly primary assessment of each subject. As a new resource, we have included a set of board review–style questions for those using *The Kidney* in preparation for certification and other examination purposes. As an educational resource, readers will be able to download figures for PowerPoint teaching purposes. We have also made an effort to adopt uniform terminology and nomenclature, in line with emerging consensus in the world kidney community. Thus, wherever possible, we have preferred terms such as *chronic kidney disease* and *acute kidney injury*, replacing the diverse and sometimes confusing terms that have peppered the literature in the past. Through Expert Consult, individuals who wish access to a physiology or disease topic at the most authoritative level will also be able to acquire separate chapters of interest, as might be the case for scientists and professionals outside of nephrology. Thus, through acquisition of *The Kidney*, individuals or institutions acquire a companion to accompany them on their journey in study, research, or patient care related to kidney health and disease.

Production of *The Kidney* is very much a team effort. The editors are indebted to the publication production team. Joan Ryan has served as our guide and lamppost beaconing the numerous contributors and providing expert input and support as Senior Content Development Specialist now for the ninth and tenth editions. Kate Dimock, Helene Caprari, and now Dolores Meloni have successfully assumed successive positions as Content Strategists, and Mary Pohlman as Senior Project Manager. These are but a few of the many members of the highly professional team at Elsevier, from whose wealth of experience the editors have benefited greatly.

None of this is possible without our authors, whose imprimatur, loyalty, and commitment to the highest standards continue to place *The Kidney* in its well-deserved position of international recognition. Through interactions with authors, we have also been able to strengthen long-standing bonds and to cultivate friendships. Most importantly, we owe a debt of gratitude to our readers, whose loyalty to and enthusiastic participation in each new edition energizes us as editors and reinforces our belief that the guiding spirit of Brenner and Rector for the subject matter and respect for the tradition initiated by the veritable "father" of *The Kidney*—Barry Morton Brenner—will continue to enliven this labor of love through many future editions.

On behalf of my co-editors, Maarten Taal, Glenn Chertow, Alan Yu, and Philip Marsden, I express tremendous gratification with the work that has become a major part of our lives and those of our families and friends and hope that the reader will also share this gratification upon partaking of *The Kidney*.

Karl Skorecki
Haifa, Israel

Contents

Volume 1

SECTION I NORMAL STRUCTURE AND FUNCTION, 1

1. Embryology of the Kidney, 2
   Rizaldy P. Scott | Yoshiro Maezawa | Jordan Kreidberg | Susan E. Quaggin

2. Anatomy of the Kidney, 42
   Robert A. Fenton | Jeppe Praetorius

3. The Renal Circulations and Glomerular Ultrafiltration, 83
   Karen A. Munger | David A. Maddox | Barry M. Brenner | Curtis K. Kost, Jr.

4. The Podocyte, 112
   Stuart J. Shankland | Peter W. Mathieson

5. Metabolic Basis of Solute Transport, 122
   Prabhleen Singh | Alicia A. McDonough | Scott C. Thomson

6. Transport of Sodium, Chloride, and Potassium, 144
   David B. Mount

7. The Regulation of Calcium, Magnesium, and Phosphate Excretion by the Kidney, 185
   Theresa J. Berndt | James R. Thompson | Rajiv Kumar

8. Renal Handling of Organic Solutes, 204
   Orson W. Moe | Stephen H. Wright | Manuel Palacín

9. Renal Acidification Mechanisms, 234
   I. David Weiner | Jill W. Verlander

10. Urine Concentration and Dilution, 258
    Jeff M. Sands | Harold E. Layton | Robert A. Fenton

11. The Cell Biology of Vasopressin Action, 281
    Dennis Brown | Robert A. Fenton

12. Aldosterone and Mineralocorticoid Receptors: Renal and Extrarenal Roles, 303
    David Pearce | Vivek Bhalla | John W. Funder

13. Vasoactive Molecules and the Kidney, 325
    Richard E. Gilbert | Andrew Advani

14. Arachidonic Acid Metabolites and the Kidney, 354
    Raymond C. Harris | Ming-Zhi Zhang | Richard M. Breyer

SECTION II DISORDERS OF BODY FLUID VOLUME AND COMPOSITION, 389

15. Disorders of Sodium Balance, 390
    Itzchak N. Slotki | Karl L. Skorecki

16. Disorders of Water Balance, 460
    Joseph G. Verbalis

17. Disorders of Acid-Base Balance, 511
    Thomas D. DuBose, Jr.

18. Disorders of Potassium Balance, 559
    David B. Mount

19. Disorders of Calcium, Magnesium, and Phosphate Balance, 601
    Miroslaw J. Smogorzewski | Jason R. Stubbs | Alan S.L. Yu

SECTION III EPIDEMIOLOGY AND RISK FACTORS IN KIDNEY DISEASE, 637

20. Epidemiology of Kidney Disease, 638
    Raymond K. Hsu | Chi-yuan Hsu

21. Demographics of Kidney Disease, 655
    Amanda Hyre Anderson | Jeffrey S. Berns | F. Perry Wilson | Harold I. Feldman

22. Risk Factors and Chronic Kidney Disease, 669
    Maarten W. Taal

23. Nephron Endowment and Developmental Programming of Blood Pressure and Renal Function, 693
    Valerie A. Luyckx | Paul Goodyer | John F. Bertram

24. Aging and Kidney Disease, 727
    Devasmita Choudhury | Moshe Levi

SECTION IV EVALUATION OF THE PATIENT WITH KIDNEY DISEASE, 753

25. Approach to the Patient with Kidney Disease, 754
    Michael Emmett | Andrew Z. Fenves | John C. Schwartz

26. Laboratory Assessment of Kidney Disease: Glomerular Filtration Rate, Urinalysis, and Proteinuria, 780
    Katrina Chau | Holly Hutton | Adeera Levin

27 Interpretation of Electrolyte and Acid-Base Parameters in Blood and Urine, 804
Kamel S. Kamel | Mogamet R. Davids | Shih-Hua Lin | Mitchell L. Halperin

28 Diagnostic Kidney Imaging, 846
Vinay A. Duddalwar | Hossein Jadvar | Suzanne L. Palmer | William D. Boswell, Jr.

29 The Kidney Biopsy, 915
Alan D. Salama | H. Terence Cook

30 Biomarkers in Acute and Chronic Kidney Diseases, 926
Chirag R. Parikh | Jay L. Koyner

SECTION V DISORDERS OF KIDNEY STRUCTURE AND FUNCTION, 957

31 Acute Kidney Injury, 958
Asif A. Sharfuddin | Steven D. Weisbord | Paul M. Palevsky | Bruce A. Molitoris

32 Primary Glomerular Disease, 1012
William F. Pendergraft, III | Patrick H. Nachman | J. Charles Jennette | Ronald J. Falk

33 Secondary Glomerular Disease, 1091
Gerald B. Appel | Jai Radhakrishnan | Vivette D'Agati

34 Overview of Therapy for Glomerular Disease, 1161
Daniel Cattran | Heather N. Reich | Michelle A. Hladunewich

35 Microvascular and Macrovascular Diseases of the Kidney, 1175
Piero Ruggenenti | Paolo Cravedi | Giuseppe Remuzzi

36 Tubulointerstitial Diseases, 1209
Carolyn J. Kelly | Eric G. Neilson

37 Urinary Tract Infection in Adults, 1231
Lindsay E. Nicolle

38 Urinary Tract Obstruction, 1257
Jørgen Frøkiaer

39 Diabetic Nephropathy, 1283
Peter Rossing | Paola Fioretto | Bo Feldt-Rasmussen | Hans-Henrik Parving

Volume 2

40 Urolithiasis, 1322
Khashayar Sakhaee | Orson W. Moe

41 Kidney Cancer, 1368
Kara N. Babaian | Scott E. Delacroix, Jr. | Christopher G. Wood | Eric Jonasch

42 Onco-Nephrology: Kidney Disease in Patients with Cancer, 1389
Kevin W. Finkel

SECTION VI GENETICS OF KIDNEY DISEASE, 1409

43 Genetic Basis of Kidney Disease, 1410
Friedhelm Hildebrandt

44 Inherited Disorders of the Glomerulus, 1421
Karl Tryggvason | Jaako Patrakka

45 Inherited Disorders of the Renal Tubule, 1434
Alain Bonnardeaux | Daniel G. Bichet

46 Cystic Diseases of the Kidney, 1475
Vicente E. Torres | Peter C. Harris

SECTION VII HYPERTENSION AND THE KIDNEY, 1521

47 Primary and Secondary Hypertension, 1522
William J. Elliott | Aldo J. Peixoto | George L. Bakris

48 Renovascular Hypertension and Ischemic Nephropathy, 1567
Stephen C. Textor

49 Hypertension and Kidney Disease in Pregnancy, 1610
Sharon E. Maynard | S. Ananth Karumanchi | Ravi Thadhani

50 Antihypertensive Therapy, 1640
Matthew R. Weir | Donna S. Hanes | David K. Klassen | Walter G. Wasser

51 Diuretics, 1702
Ewout J. Hoorn | Christopher S. Wilcox | David H. Ellison

SECTION VIII THE CONSEQUENCES OF ADVANCED KIDNEY DISEASE, 1735

52 Adaptation to Nephron Loss and Mechanisms of Progression in Chronic Kidney Disease, 1736
Maarten W. Taal

53 Mechanisms and Consequences of Proteinuria, 1780
Norberto Perico | Andrea Remuzzi | Giuseppe Remuzzi

54 The Pathophysiology of Uremia, 1807
Timothy W. Meyer | Thomas H. Hostetter

55 Chronic Kidney Disease–Mineral Bone Disorder, 1822
Sharon M. Moe | Stuart M. Sprague

56 Cardiovascular Aspects of Kidney Disease, 1854
Richard Haynes | David C. Wheeler | Martin J. Landray | Colin Baigent

57 Hematologic Aspects of Kidney Disease, 1875
Carlo Brugnara | Kai-Uwe Eckardt

58 Endocrine Aspects of Chronic Kidney Disease, 1912
Juan Jesús Carrero | Peter Stenvinkel | Bengt Lindholm

59 Neurologic Aspects of Kidney Disease, 1926
Manjula Kurella Tamura

60 Dermatologic Conditions in Kidney Disease, 1942
Christine J. Ko | Shawn E. Cowper

SECTION IX CONSERVATIVE MANAGEMENT OF KIDNEY DISEASE, 1955

61 Dietary Approaches to Kidney Diseases, 1956
Denis Fouque | William E. Mitch

62 A Stepped Care Approach to the Management of Chronic Kidney Disease, 1987
Damian G. Fogarty | Maarten W. Taal

63 Therapeutic Approach to Chronic Kidney Disease–Mineral Bone Disorder, 2019
L. Darryl Quarles

64 Drug Dosing Considerations in Patients with Acute Kidney Injury and Chronic Kidney Disease, 2034
Gary R. Matzke | Frieder Keller

SECTION X DIALYSIS AND EXTRACORPOREAL THERAPIES, 2057

65 Hemodialysis, 2058
Jane Y. Yeun | Daniel B. Ornt | Thomas A. Depner

66 Peritoneal Dialysis, 2111
Ricardo Correa-Rotter | Rajnish Mehrotra | Anjali Saxena

67 Critical Care Nephrology, 2137
Ron Wald | Kathleen Liu

68 Plasmapheresis, 2148
Ernesto Sabath | Bradley M. Denker

69 Elimination Enhancement of Poisons, 2166
Marc Ghannoum | Karine Mardini | Paul Ayoub

70 Interventional Nephrology, 2191
Timmy Lee | Ivan D. Maya | Michael Allon

SECTION XI KIDNEY TRANSPLANTATION, 2227

71 Transplantation Immunobiology, 2228
Mohamed H. Sayegh | Leonardo V. Riella | Anil Chandraker

72 Clinical Management of the Adult Kidney Transplant Recipient, 2251
Colin R. Lenihan | Stéphan Busque | Jane C. Tan

SECTION XII PEDIATRIC NEPHROLOGY, 2293

73 Malformation of the Kidney: Structural and Functional Consequences, 2294
Norman D. Rosenblum

74 Diseases of the Kidney and Urinary Tract in Children, 2308
Sevcan A. Bakkaloglu | Franz Schaefer

75 Fluid, Electrolyte, and Acid-Base Disorders in Children, 2365
James C.M. Chan | Fernando Santos

76 Renal Replacement Therapy (Dialysis and Transplantation) in Pediatric End-Stage Kidney Disease, 2402
Yaacov Frishberg | Choni Rinat | Rachel Becker-Cohen

SECTION XIII GLOBAL CONSIDERATIONS IN KIDNEY DISEASE, 2439

77 Latin America, 2440
Leonardo V. Riella | Miquel C. Riella

78 Africa, 2454
Saraladevi Naicker | Sagren Naidoo

79 Near and Middle East, 2468
Suheir Assady | Rawi Ramadan | Dvora Rubinger

80 Indian Subcontinent, 2494
Vinay Sakhuja | Harbir Singh Kohli

81 The Far East, 2510
Chuan-Ming Hao | Fan-Fan Hou | Walter G. Wasser

82 Oceania Region, 2538
Gavin J. Becker | John F. Collins | David C.H. Harris

SECTION XIV CHALLENGES IN NEPHROLOGY, 2557

83 Ethical Dilemmas Facing Nephrology: Past, Present, and Future, 2558
Alvin H. Moss

84 Health Disparities in Nephrology, 2574
Yoshio N. Hall | Glenn M. Chertow

85 Care of the Older Adult with Chronic Kidney Disease, 2586
Meghan J. Elliott | Ann M. O'Hare | Brenda R. Hemmelgarn

86 Tissue Engineering, Stem Cells, and Cell Therapy in Nephrology, 2602
L. Spencer Krane | Anthony Atala

87 Quality Improvement Initiatives in Kidney Disease, 2620
Sandeep S. Soman | Jerry Yee | Kevin Ho

NORMAL STRUCTURE AND FUNCTION

SECTION I

1 Embryology of the Kidney

Rizaldy P. Scott | Yoshiro Maezawa | Jordan Kreidberg | Susan E. Quaggin

CHAPTER OUTLINE

MAMMALIAN KIDNEY DEVELOPMENT: EMBRYOLOGY, 2
Development of the Urogenital System, 2
Development of the Metanephros, 3
Development of the Nephron, 4
The Nephrogenic Zone, 5
Branching Morphogenesis: Development of the Collecting System, 5
Renal Stroma and Interstitial Populations, 5
Development of the Vasculature, 6
MODEL SYSTEMS TO STUDY KIDNEY DEVELOPMENT, 6
Organ Culture, 6
Transgenic and Knockout Mouse Models, 9
Imaging and Lineage Tracing Studies, 19
Nonmammalian Model Systems for Kidney Development, 19

GENETIC ANALYSIS OF MAMMALIAN KIDNEY DEVELOPMENT, 21
Interaction of the Ureteric Bud and the Metanephric Mesenchyme, 21
Formation of the Collecting System, 25
Positioning of the Ureteric Bud, 27
Molecular Analysis of the Nephrogenic Zone, 28
Molecular Biology of Nephron Development: Tubulogenesis, 30
Molecular Genetics of the Stromal Cell Lineage, 31
Molecular Genetics of Vascular Formation, 32
The Juxtaglomerular Apparatus and the Renin Angiotensin Aldosterone System, 35
Nephron Development and Glomerulogenesis, 36
Maturation of Glomerular Endothelial Cells and Glomerular Basement Membrane, 39

Over the past several decades, the identification of genes and molecular pathways required for normal kidney development has provided insight into our understanding of obvious developmental diseases such as renal agenesis and renal dysplasia. However, many of the genes identified have also been shown to play roles in adult-onset and acquired kidney diseases such as focal segmental glomerulosclerosis. The number of nephrons present in the kidney at birth, which is determined during fetal life, predicts the risk of kidney disease and hypertension later in life; a lower number is associated with greater risk.[1-3] Discovery of novel therapeutic targets and strategies to slow and reverse kidney diseases requires an understanding of the molecular mechanisms that underlie kidney development.

MAMMALIAN KIDNEY DEVELOPMENT: EMBRYOLOGY

DEVELOPMENT OF THE UROGENITAL SYSTEM

The vertebrate kidney derives from the intermediate mesoderm of the urogenital ridge, a structure found along the posterior wall of the abdomen in the developing fetus.[4] It develops in three successive stages known as the *pronephros,* the *mesonephros,* and the *metanephros* (Figure 1.1), although only the metanephros gives rise to the definitive adult kidney. However, earlier stages are required for development of other organs, such as the adrenal gland and gonad, that also develop within the urogenital ridge. Furthermore, many of the signaling pathways and genes that play important roles in the metanephric kidney appear to play parallel roles during earlier stages of renal development, in the pronephros and mesonephros. The pronephros consists of pronephric tubules and the pronephric duct (also known as the precursor to the wolffian duct) and develops from the rostralmost region of the urogenital ridge at 22 days of gestation (humans) and 8 days post coitum (dpc; mouse). It functions in the larval stages of amphibians and fish, but not in mammals. The mesonephros develops caudal to the pronephric tubules in the midsection of the urogenital ridge. The mesonephros becomes the functional excretory apparatus in lower vertebrates and may perform a filtering function during embryonic life in mammals. However, it largely degenerates before birth. Prior to its degeneration, endothelial, peritubular myoid, and steroidogenic cells

CHAPTER 1 — EMBRYOLOGY OF THE KIDNEY

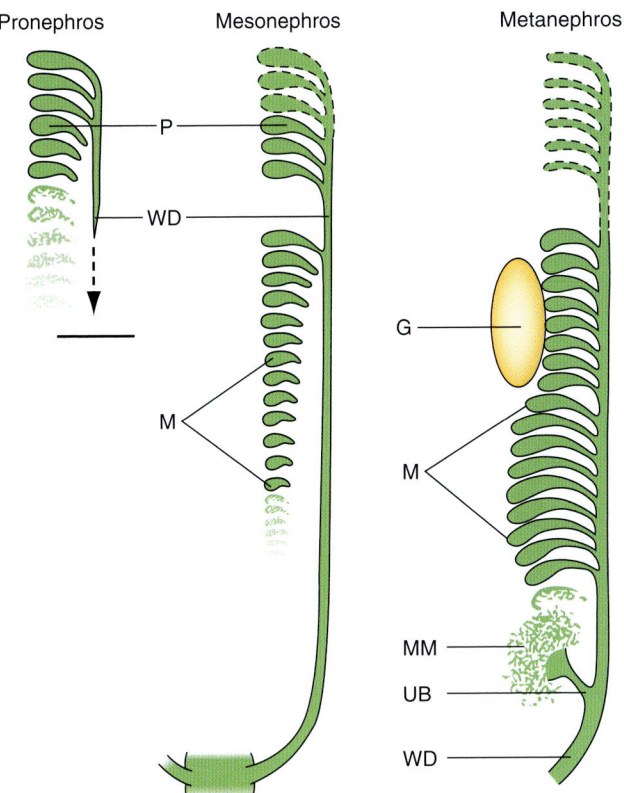

Figure 1.1 Three stages of mammalian kidney development. The pronephros (P) and mesonephros (M) develop in a rostral-to-caudal direction and the tubules are aligned adjacent to the wolffian or nephric duct (WD). The metanephros develops from an outgrowth of the distal end of the wolffian duct known as the ureteric bud epithelium (UB) and a cluster of cells known as the metanephric mesenchyme (MM). Cells migrate from the mesonephros (M) into the developing gonad (G), which develop in close association with each another. (Adapted from Saxen L: *Organogenesis of the kidney,* Cambridge, 1987, Cambridge University Press.)

from the mesonephros migrate into the adjacent adrenogonadal primordia, which ultimately form the adrenal gland and gonads.[5] Abnormal mesonephric migration leads to gonadal dysgenesis, a fact that underscores the intricate association between these organ systems during development and explains the common association of gonadal and renal defects in congenital syndromes.[6,7] In males, production of testosterone also induces the formation of seminal vesicles, tubules of the epididymis, and portions of the vas deferens from the wolffian duct.

DEVELOPMENT OF THE METANEPHROS

The metanephros, the third and final stage, gives rise to the definitive adult kidney of higher vertebrates; it results from a series of reciprocal inductive interactions that occur between the metanephric mesenchyme (MM) and the epithelial ureteric bud (UB) at the caudal end of the urogenital ridge. The UB is first visible as an outgrowth at the distal end of the wolffian duct at approximately 5 weeks of gestation in humans or 10.5 dpc in mice. The MM becomes histologically distinct from the surrounding mesenchyme and is found adjacent to the UB. Upon invasion of the MM by the UB, signals from the MM cause the UB to branch into a T-tubule (at around 11.5 dpc in mice) and then to undergo iterative dichotomous branching, giving rise to the urinary collecting duct system (Figure 1.2). Simultaneously, the UB sends reciprocal signals to the MM, which is induced to condense along the surface of the bud. Following condensation, a subset of MM cells aggregates adjacent and inferior to the tips of the branching UB. These collections of cells, known as *pretubular aggregates,* undergo mesenchymal-to-epithelial conversion to become the renal vesicle (Figure 1.3).

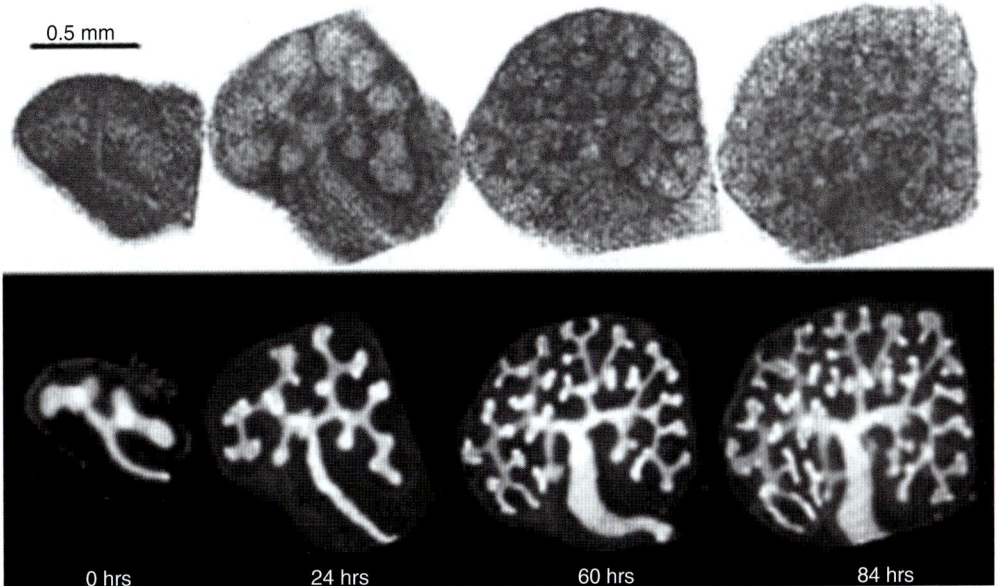

Figure 1.2 Organ culture of rat metanephroi dissected at T-tubule stage. Within 84 hours, dichotomous branching of the ureteric bud (UB) has occurred to provide the basic architecture of the kidney. *Bottom panel* is stained with *Dolichos biflorus* agglutinin—a lectin that binds specifically to UB cells. (Adapted from Saxen L: *Organogenesis of the kidney,* Cambridge, 1987, Cambridge University Press.)

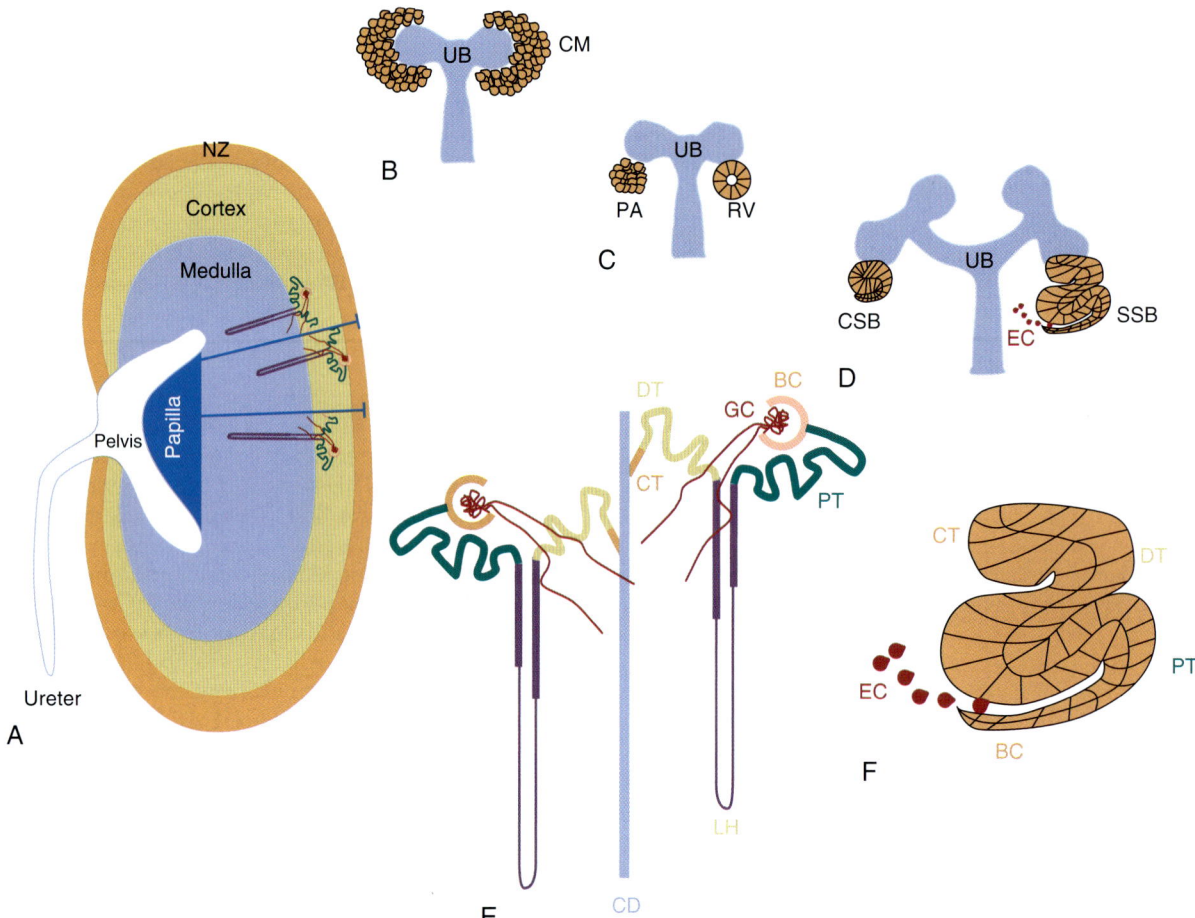

Figure 1.3 Overview of kidney development. A, Gross kidney histoarchitecture. NZ, nephrogenic zone. B through E, As described in the text, reciprocal interaction between the ureteric bud (UB) and metanephric mesenchyme results in a series of well-defined morphologic stages leading to formation of the nephron, including to the branching of the UB epithelium and the epithelialization of the metanephric mesenchyme into a highly patterned nephron. F, Distinctive segmentation of the S-shaped body defines the patterning of the nephron. BC, Bowman's capsule; CD, collecting duct; CM, cap mesenchyme; CSB, comma-shaped body; CT, connecting tubule; DT, distal tubule; EC, endothelial cells; LH, loop of Henle; PA, pretubular aggregate; PT, proximal tubule; SSB, S-shaped body.

DEVELOPMENT OF THE NEPHRON

The renal vesicle undergoes patterned segmentation and proceeds through a series of morphologic changes to form the glomerulus and components of the nephrogenic tubules from the proximal convoluted tubule, the loop of Henle, and the distal tubule. The renal vesicles undergo differentiation, passing through morphologically distinct stages starting from the comma-shaped body and proceeding to the S-shaped body, capillary loop, and mature stage, each step involving precise proximal-to-distal patterning and structural transformations (see Figure 1.3). Remarkably, this process is repeated 600,000 to 1 million times in each developing human kidney as new nephrons are sequentially born at the tips of the UB throughout fetal life.

The glomerulus develops from the most proximal end of the renal vesicle that is farthest from the UB tip.[8,9] Distinct cell types of the glomerulus can first be identified in the S-shaped body stage, in which presumptive podocytes appear as a columnar epithelial cell layer. A vascular cleft develops and separates the presumptive podocyte layer from more distal cells that will form the proximal tubule. Parietal epithelial cells differentiate and flatten to form Bowman's capsule, a structure that surrounds the urinary space and is continuous with the proximal tubular epithelium. Concurrently, endothelial cells migrate into the vascular cleft. Together with podocytes, the endothelial cells produce the glomerular basement membrane (GBM), a major component of the mature filtration barrier. Initially the podocytes are connected by intercellular tight junctions at their apical surfaces.[10] As glomerulogenesis proceeds, the podocytes revert to a mesenchymal-type phenotype, flatten, and spread out to cover the greater surface area of the growing glomerular capillary bed. They develop microtubule-based primary processes and actin-based secondary foot processes. During this time, the intercellular junctions become restricted to the basal aspect of each podocyte and eventually are replaced by a modified adherens junction–like structure known as the *slit diaphragm* (SD).[10] At the same time, foot processes from adjacent podocytes become highly interdigitated. The SDs are signaling hubs serving as the final layer of the glomerular filtration barrier.[11] Mesangial cell ingrowth follows the migration of endothelial cells and is required for development and patterning of the capillary loops that are found in normal glomeruli. The endothelial cells also flatten considerably, and capillary lumens are formed owing to apoptosis of a subset of endothelial cells.[12] At the capillary loop stage, glomerular endothelial cells develop fenestrae, which are semipermeable transcellular pores common in capillary beds exposed to high hemodynamic flux. Positioning of the foot processes on the GBM and spreading of podocyte cell bodies are still incompletely understood but share many features of synapse formation and neuronal migration.[13-15]

In the mature stage, glomerulus, the podocytes, fenestrated endothelial cells, and intervening GBM compose the filtration barrier that separates the urinary from the blood space. Together, these components provide a size- and charge-selective barrier that permits free passage of small solutes and water but prevents the loss of larger molecules such as proteins. The mesangial cells are found between the capillary loops (approximately three per loop); they are required to provide ongoing structural support to the capillaries and possess smooth muscle cell–like characteristics that give them the capacity to contract, which may account for the dynamic properties of the glomerulus. The tubular portion of the nephron becomes segmented in a proximal-to-distal order, into the proximal convoluted tubule, the descending and ascending loops of Henle, and the distal convoluted tubule. The distal tubule is contiguous with the collecting duct, a derivative of the UB. Imaging and fate mapping analysis reveal that this interconnection results from the invasion of the UB by cells from the distal segments of nascent nephrons (around the S-shaped body stage).[16]

Although all segments of the nephron are present at birth and filtration occurs prior to birth, maturation of the tubule continues in the postnatal period. Increased expression levels of transporters, switch in transporter isoforms, alterations in paracellular transport mechanisms, and the development of permeability and biophysical properties of tubular membranes have all been observed to occur postnatally.[17] Although additional studies are needed, these observations emphasize the importance of considering developmental stage of the nephron in interpretation of renal transport and may explain the age of onset of symptoms in inherited transport disorders; some of these issues may be recapitulated in acute kidney injury.

THE NEPHROGENIC ZONE

After the first few rounds of branching of the UB and the concomitant induction of nephrons from the MM, the kidney subdivides into an outer cortical region, where nephrons are being induced, and an inner medullary region, where the collecting system will form. As growth continues, successive groups of nephrons are induced at the peripheral regions of the kidney known as the *nephrogenic zone* (Figure 1.4). Thus, within the developing kidney, the most mature nephrons are found in the innermost layers of the cortex, and the most immature nephrons in the most peripheral regions. At the extreme peripheral lining, under the renal capsule, a process that seems to recapitulate the induction of the original nephrons can be observed, whereby numerous UB-like structures are inducing areas of condensed mesenchyme. Indeed, whether there are significant molecular differences between the induction of the original nephrons and these subsequent inductive events is not known. A subpopulation of self-renewing mesenchymal cells immediately

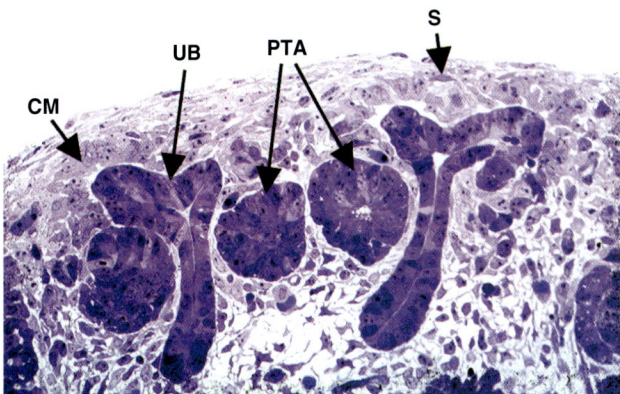

Figure 1.4 The nephrogenic zone. As described in the text, nephrons are continually produced in the nephrogenic zone throughout fetal life. CM, Condensing mesenchyme; PTA, pretubular aggregate; S, stromal cell lineage (spindle-shaped cells); UB, ureteric bud.

adjacent and inferior to the UB tips at the nephrogenic zone undergoes epithelial transformation, giving rise to new nephrons postnatally.[18,19]

BRANCHING MORPHOGENESIS: DEVELOPMENT OF THE COLLECTING SYSTEM

The collecting system is composed of hundreds of tubules through which the filtrate produced by the nephrons is conducted out of the kidney and to the ureter and then the bladder. Water and salt resorption and excretion, ammonia transport, and H^+ secretion required for acid-base homeostasis also occur in the collecting ducts, under different regulatory mechanisms and using different transporters and channels from those that are active along tubular portions of the nephron. The collecting ducts are all derived from the original UB (Figure 1.5). Whereas each nephron is an individual unit separately induced and originating from a distinct pretubular aggregate, the collecting ducts are the product of branching morphogenesis from the UB. Considerable remodeling is involved in forming collecting ducts from branches of UB, and how this occurs remains incompletely understood.[20] The branching is highly patterned; the first several rounds are somewhat symmetric, additional rounds of branching are asymmetric, in which a main trunk of the collecting duct continues to extend toward the nephrogenic zone but smaller buds branch as they induce new nephrons within the nephrogenic zone. Originally, the UB derivatives are branching within a surrounding mesenchyme. Ultimately, they form a funnel-shaped structure in which cone-shaped groupings of ducts or papillae sit within a funnel or calyx that drains into the ureter. The mouse kidney has a single papilla and calyx, but a human kidney has 8 to 10 papillae, each of which drains into a minor calyx, with several minor calyces draining into a smaller number of major calyces.

RENAL STROMA AND INTERSTITIAL POPULATIONS

For decades in classic embryologic studies of kidney development, emphasis was placed on the reciprocal inductive

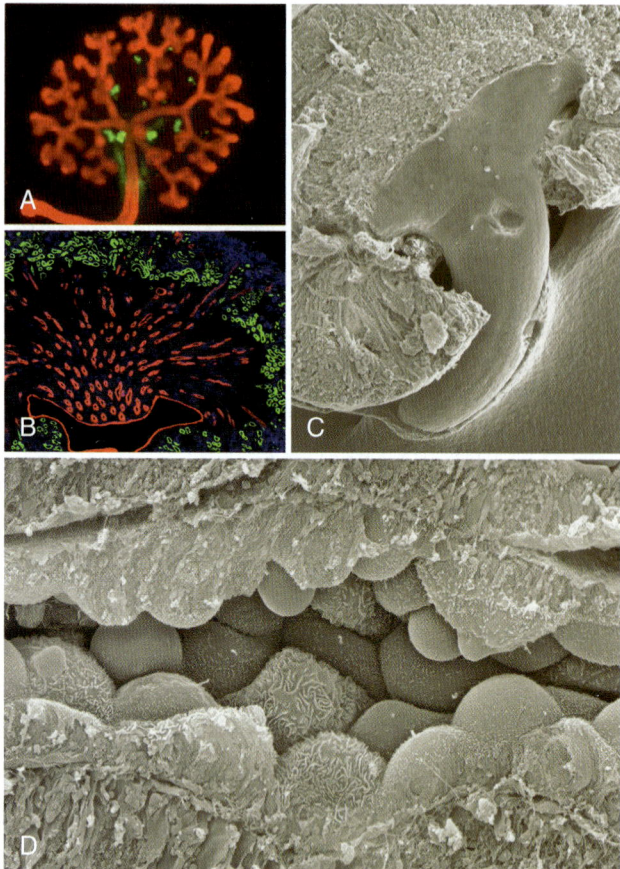

Figure 1.5 Collecting duct system. The branching ureteric epithelial lineage gives rise to the collecting duct system. **A,** E12.5 mouse embryonic kidney explant grown in vitro for 2 days and **B,** neonatal mouse kidney section, stained for the ureteric epithelium and collecting ducts (pan-cytokeratin, *red*) and the nascent proximal tubules (Lotus lectin, *green*). **C,** Scanning electron micrograph of a hemisected adult mouse kidney showing the funnel-shaped renal papillae. **D,** Scanning electron micrograph of a collecting duct showing smooth principal cells and reticulated intercalated cells.

signals between MM and UB. However, in later years, interest has arisen in the stromal cell as a key regulator of nephrogenesis.[9,21-23] Stromal cells also derive from the MM but are not induced to condense by the UB. Two distinct populations of stromal cells have been described: Cortical stromal cells exist as a thin layer beneath the renal capsule and medullary stromal cells populate the interstitial space between the collecting ducts and tubules (Figure 1.6). Cortical stromal cells also surround the condensates and provide signals required for UB branching and patterning of the developing kidney. Disruption or loss of these stromal cells leads to failure of UB branching, a reduction in nephron number, and disrupted patterning of nephric units with failure of cortical-medullary boundary formation. A reciprocal signaling loop from the UB exists to properly pattern stromal cell populations. Loss of these UB-derived signals leads to a buildup of stromal cells beneath the capsule that is several layers thick. As nephrogenesis proceeds, stromal cells differentiate into peritubular interstitial cells and pericytes that are required for vascular remodeling and for production of extracellular matrix responsible for proper nephric formation.[23] These cells migrate from their positions around the condensates to areas between the developing nephrons within the medulla. Although stromal cells are derived from the MM cells, it remains unclear whether stromal cells and nephric lineages arise from a common progenitor MM cell.

DEVELOPMENT OF THE VASCULATURE

The microcirculations of the kidney include the specialized glomerular capillary system responsible for production of the ultrafiltrate and the *vasa recta*, peritubular capillaries involved in the countercurrent mechanism. In the adult, each kidney receives 10% of the cardiac output. Vasculogenesis and angiogenesis have been described as two distinct processes in blood vessel formation. *Vasculogenesis* refers to de novo differentiation of previously nonvascular cells into structures that resemble capillary beds, whereas *angiogenesis* refers to sprouting from these early beds to form mature vessel structures including arteries, veins, and capillaries. Both processes are involved in development of the renal vasculature. At the time of UB invasion at 11 dpc (all timing given is for mice), the MM is avascular, but by 12 dpc a rich capillary network is present, and by 14 dpc vascularized glomeruli are present.

Transplantation experiments support a model whereby endothelial progenitors within the MM give rise to renal vessels in situ,[24] although the origin of large blood vessels is still debated. At 13 dpc capillaries form networks around the developing nephric tubules, and by 14 dpc the hilar artery and first-order interlobar renal artery branches can be identified. These branches will form the corticomedullary arcades and the interlobular arteries that branch from them. Further branching produces the glomerular afferent arterioles. From 13.5 dpc onward, endothelial cells migrate into the vascular cleft of developing glomeruli, where they undergo differentiation to form the glomerular capillary loops (Figure 1.7). The efferent arterioles carry blood away from the glomerulus to a system of fenestrated peritubular capillaries that are in close contact with the adjacent tubules and receive filtered water and solutes reabsorbed from the filtrate.[25] These capillaries have few pericytes. In comparison, the vasa recta, which surround the medullary tubules and are involved in urinary concentration, are also fenestrated but have more pericytes. They arise from the efferent arterioles of deep glomeruli.[26] The peritubular capillary system surrounding the proximal tubules is well developed in the late fetal period, whereas the vasa recta mature 1 to 3 weeks postnatally.

MODEL SYSTEMS TO STUDY KIDNEY DEVELOPMENT

ORGAN CULTURE

THE KIDNEY ORGAN CULTURE SYSTEM: CLASSIC STUDIES

Metanephric kidney organ culture (Figures 1.8 and 1.9) formed the basis for extensive classic studies of embryonic induction. Parameters of induction such as the temporal and physical constraints on exposure of the inductive tissue

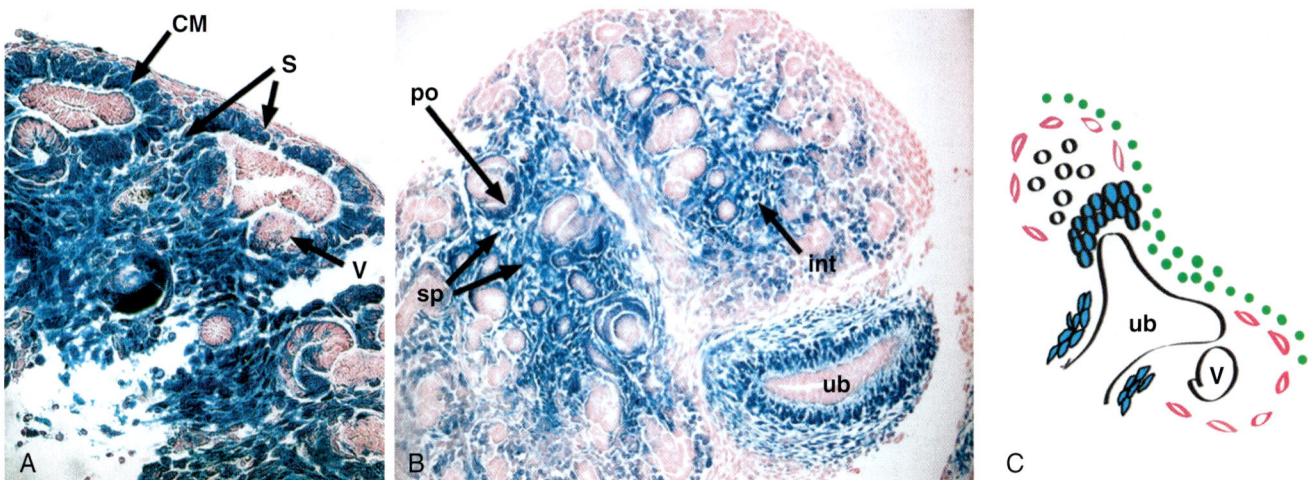

Figure 1.6 Populations of cells within the metanephric mesenchyme. As described in the text, these populations are defined by morphologic and molecular characteristics. Metanephroi from a 14.5 dpc Tcf21-LacZ mouse (**A**) and a 15.5 dpc Tcf21-LacZ mouse (**B**) are stained for β-galactosidase activity. Tcf21-expressing cells stain *blue*. Stromal cells (S; *pink* in **C**) are seen surrounding condensing mesenchyme (CM). Nephrogenic population (*green* in **C**) remains unstained. By 15.5 dpc a well-developed interstitial compartment is seen and consists of peritubular fibroblasts, medullary fibroblasts, and pericytes. Loose and condensed mesenchymal cells are also observed around the stalk of the ureteric bud in **B**. v, Renal vesicle; po, podocyte precursors; sp, stromal pericytes; int, interstitium. **C**, Schematic diagram of mesenchymal populations includes the nephrogenic precursors (in *green*), uninduced mesenchyme (*white*), condensing mesenchyme around the UB tips and stalk (*blue*), and stromal cell lineage (*pink*). (Reproduced with permission from *Developmental Dynamics*.)

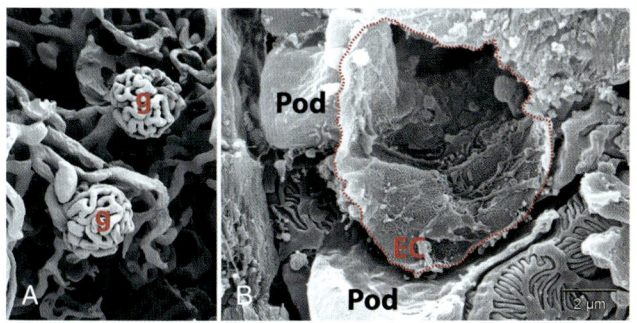

Figure 1.7 Renal vasculature. A, Corrosion resin cast of renal vasculature revealing the highly convoluted assembly of the glomerular capillaries (g). **B,** Scanning electron micrograph of a glomerulus with an exposed endothelial lumen (*dashed outlined*) showing fenestrations. EC, Endothelial cell; Pod, podocyte. (Corrosion cast electron micrograph courtesy of Fred Hossler, Department of Anatomy and Cell Biology, East Tennessee State University.)

to the mesenchyme were determined, as were the times during which various tubular elements of the nephron were first observed in culture.

MUTANT PHENOTYPIC ANALYSES

As originally shown by Grobstein, Saxen, and their colleagues in classic studies of embryonic induction, the two major components of the metanephric kidney, the MM and the UB, could be separated from each other, and the isolated mesenchyme could be induced to form nephron-like tubules by a selected set of other embryonic tissues, the best example of which is embryonic neural tube.[4,27] When neural tube is used to induce the separated mesenchyme, there is terminal differentiation of the mesenchyme into tubules, but not significant tissue expansion. In contrast, intact metanephric rudiments can grow more extensively, displaying both sustained UB branching and early induction of nephrons even when cultured for a week. The isolated mesenchyme experiment has proved useful in the analysis of renal agenesis phenotypes, in which there is no outgrowth of the UB. In these cases, the mesenchyme can be placed in contact with neural tube to determine whether it has the intrinsic ability to differentiate. Most often, when renal agenesis is due to the mutation of a transcription factor gene, tubular induction is not rescued by neural tube, as could be predicted for transcription factors which would be expected to act in a cell-autonomous fashion.[28] In the converse situation, in which renal agenesis is caused by loss of a gene function in the UB (e.g., *Emx2* in the mouse), it is usually possible for embryonic neural tube to induce tubule formation in isolated mesenchymes.[29] Therefore, the organ culture induction assay can be used to test hypotheses concerning whether a particular gene is required in the UB or the MM. As chemical inhibitors specific for various signal transduction pathways have been synthesized and become available, it has been possible to add them to organ cultures and observe effects that are informative about the roles of specific pathways in development of the kidney. Examples are the uses of drugs to block the Erk/MAP kinase, PI3K/Akt, and Notch signaling pathways in renal explant cultures.[30-32]

ANTISENSE OLIGONUCLEOTIDES AND siRNA IN ORGAN CULTURE

Several studies have described the use of antisense oligonucleotides and of siRNA (small interfering, or silencing, RNA) molecules to inhibit gene expression in kidney organ cultures. Among the earliest of these was the inhibition of the low-affinity nerve growth factor receptor, p75 or NGFR, by antisense oligonucleotides,[33] a treatment that decreased the growth of cultured embryonic kidneys. A subsequent study could not duplicate this phenotype,[34] although there were possible differences in experimental techniques.[35] An

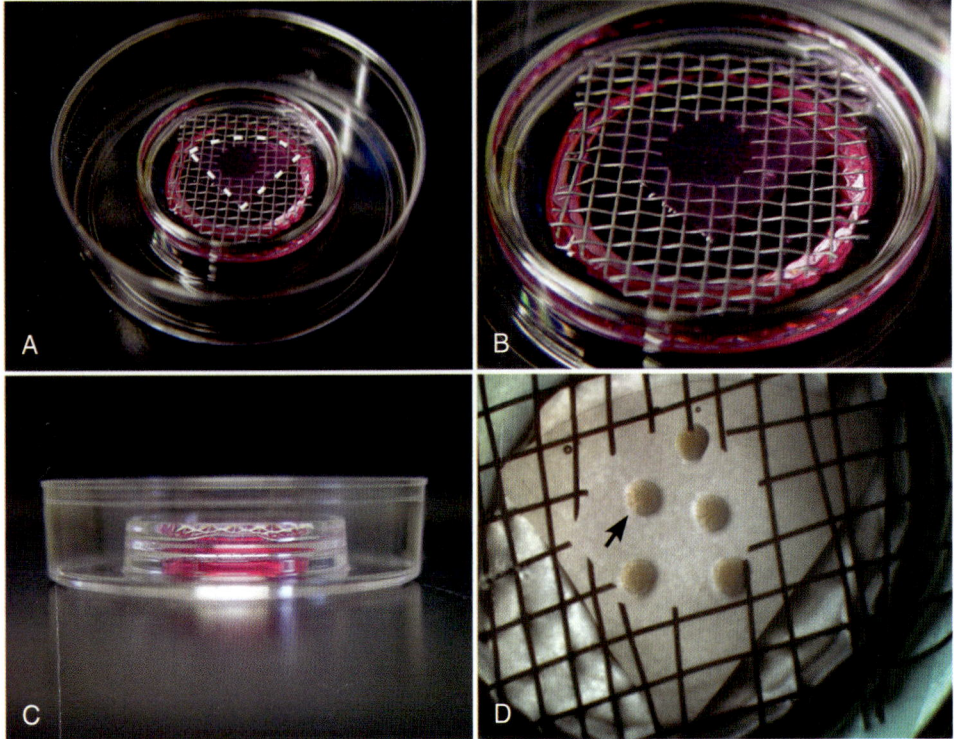

Figure 1.8 Metanephric organ explants Top **(A, B)** and lateral **(C)** views of a kidney organ culture in a center-well dish. Embryonic kidney explants are grown at the air-growth medium interface on top of a floating porous polycarbonate filter (*dashed lines* in **A**) supported on a metal mesh. **D,** Kidneys grown after 4 days of culture. (Reproduced with permission from Barak H, Boyle SC: Organ culture and immunostaining of mouse embryonic kidneys. *Cold Spring Harb Protoc* 2011[1]:pdb.prot5558, 2011.)

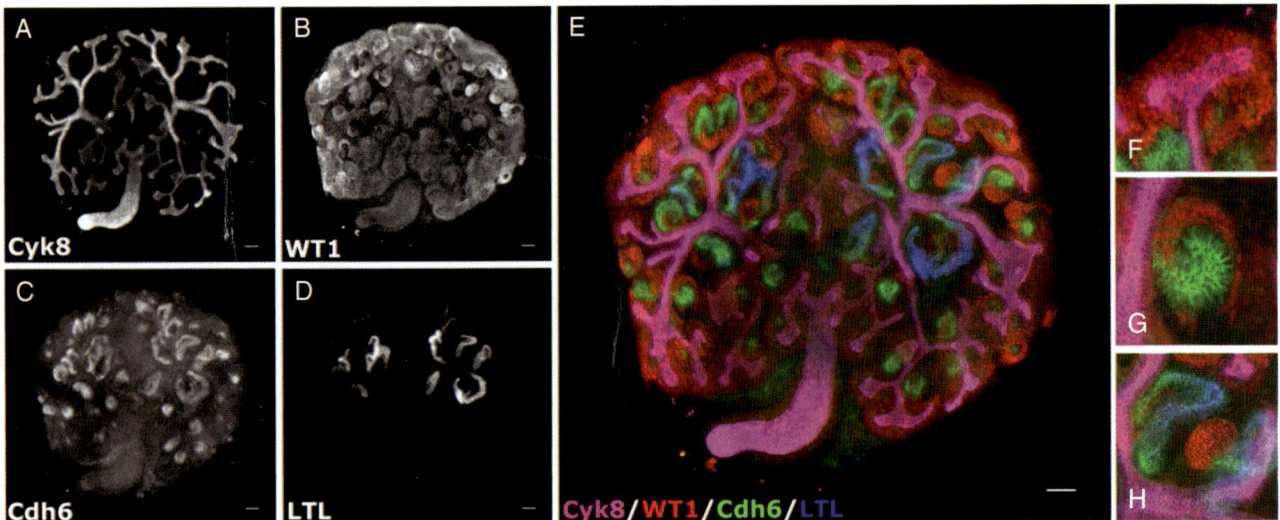

Figure 1.9 Recapitulation of branching and nephrogenesis in renal explant cultures. A, Ureteric tree stained for cytokeratin 8 (Cyk8). **B,** Condensed metanephric mesenchyme stained for WT1. **C,** Epithelial derivatives of the metanephric mesenchyme stained for E-cadherin (Cdh6). **D,** Proximal tubules stained with *Lotus tetraglobulus* lectin (LTL). **E,** Merged image of **A** through **D. F,** WT1-expressing cells represent the nephron progenitor cells that surround the ureteric bud. **G,** Cdh6-expression marks the mesenchyme-to-epithelial transformation of nephron progenitor cells. **H,** Early patterning of nascent nephrons along a proximodistal axis. **E-H,** Cyk8 (*magenta*), WT1 (*red*), Cdh6 (*green*) and LTL (*blue*). (Reproduced with permission from Barak H, Boyle SC: Organ culture and immunostaining of mouse embryonic kidneys. *Cold Spring Harb Protoc* 2011[1]:pdb.prot5558, 2011.)

additional study using antisense oligonucleotides to *Pax2* also showed this gene to be crucial in epithelialization of the MM.[36,37] Antisense morpholinos modified with an octaguanidine dendrimer moiety to facilitate cell uptake have been used to target Wilms' tumor-1 gene (*Wt1*) in kidney explant cultures. This morpholino-based knockdown strategy allowed the identification of WT1 transcriptional targets in nephron progenitors, which was technically impossible in conventional *Wt1* knockout mice because of renal agenesis.[38] Co-transported with synthetic delivery peptides, antisense morpholinos have also been used to investigate the negative regulation of ureteric branching morphogenesis by semaphorin3a (Sema3a).[39,40] Gene knockdown using siRNA has also been used to demonstrate the importance of *Wt1* and *Pax2* in nephrogenesis in whole organ and dissociated embryonic kidneys.[38,41,42] Similar siRNA-based knockdown strategies have been successfully used to demonstrate the importance of fibronectin, Dact2, and estrogen-related receptor γ (Esrrg) in ureteric branching in whole embryonic renal explant cultures.[43-45]

ORGAN CULTURE MICROINJECTION

Microinjection in kidney explant cultures can be used to selectively target gene expression using a variety of reagents (plasmid constructs, viruses, and siRNA) in either the MM or the branching ureteric epithelia, depending on the site of injection.[46,47] Retroviruses encoding mutants of polycystin-1 were used to demonstrate that polycystin-1 is required for normal ureteric branching patterns.[48] Microinjection followed by electroporation of DNA plasmid constructs has been used to overexpress *GDNF* (glial cell–derived neurotrophic factor), *Wt1*, *Pax2*, *Vegfa*, and *Robo2* in the MM and to assess the role of these genes in ureteric branching and early nephron induction.[47,49]

TRANSGENIC AND KNOCKOUT MOUSE MODELS

Over the past two decades, the generation and analysis of knockout and transgenic mice have provided tremendous insight into kidney development (Table 1.1).[50,51] Although homologous recombination to delete genes within the germline, also known as standard "knockout" technology, has provided information about the biologic functions of many genes in kidney development, it has several disadvantages. Disruption of gene function in embryonic stem (ES) cells may result in embryonic or perinatal death, precluding the functional analysis of the gene in the kidney that develops relatively late in fetal life. Additionally, many genes are expressed in multiple cell types, and the resulting knockout phenotypes can be complex and difficult or impossible to dissect. The ability to limit gene targeting to specific renal cell types overcomes some of these problems, and the temporal control of gene expression permits more precise characterization of a gene's function. A number of mouse lines may be used to target specific kidney cell lineages (Table 1.2; Figure 1.10). As with any experimental procedure, numerous caveats must be taken into account in the interpretation of data.[52,53] These include determining the completeness of excision at the locus of interest, the timing and extrarenal expression of the promoters, and general toxicity of expressed proteins to the cell of interest. In spite of these issues, tissue-specific conditional gene targeting strategies remain powerful tools to study gene functions. The next generation of targeting includes improved efficiency using bacterial artificial chromosome (BAC) targeting approaches, siRNA and microRNA (miRNA) approaches, and large genomewide targeting efforts already under way at many academic and pharmaceutical institutions.

In contrast to gene targeting experiments in which the gene is known at the beginning of the experiment (*reverse genetics*), random mutagenesis represents a complimentary phenotype-driven approach (*forward genetics*) to study the physiologic relevance of certain genes. Random mutations are introduced into the genome at high efficiency by chemical or gene trap mutagenesis. Consecutively, large numbers of animals are screened systematically for specific phenotypes of interest. As soon as a phenotype is identified, test breeding is used to confirm the genetic nature of the trait. Chromosomal mapping and positional cloning are then used to determine the identity of the culprit mutant gene. There are two major advantages of genomewide approaches over reverse genetics. First, most knockouts lead to major gene disruptions, which may not be relevant to the subtle gene alterations that underlie human renal disease. Second, many of the complex traits underlying congenital anomalies and acquired diseases of the kidney are unknown, making predictions about the nature of the genes that are involved in these diseases difficult.

One of the most powerful and well-characterized mutagens in the mouse is the chemical mutagen *N*-ethyl-*N*-nitrosourea (ENU). It acts through random alkylation of nucleic acids, inducing point mutations in spermatogonial stem cells of injected male mice.[54,55] ENU mutagenesis introduces multiple point mutations within the spermatogonia of the male, which is then bred to a female mouse of different genetic background. Resultant offspring are screened for renal phenotypes of interest (e.g., dysplastic, cystic) and

Text continued on p. 17

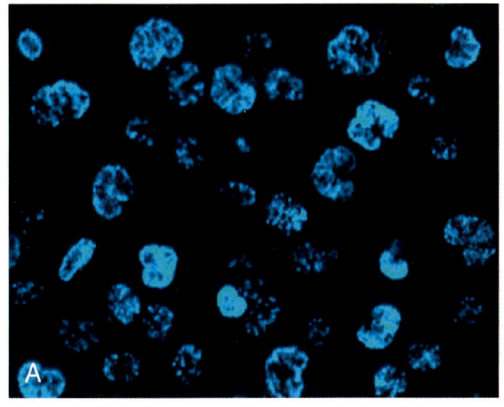

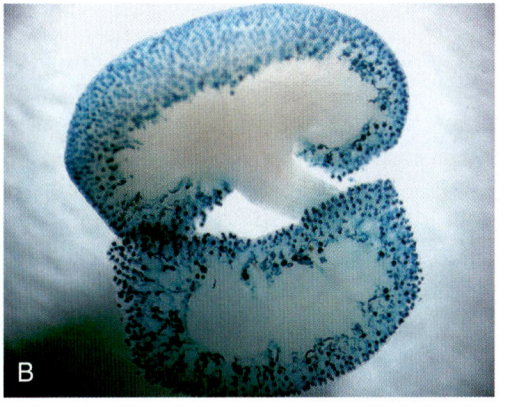

Figure 1.10 Glomeruli expressing **(A)** cyan fluorescent protein (CFP) or **(B)** β-galactosidase. Transgenic mice were generated using the nephrin promoter to direct expression of either CFP or β-galactosidase specifically in developing and mature podocytes.

Table 1.1 Summary of Knockout and Transgenic Models for Kidney Development

Gene Mutation or Knockout	Renal and Urogenital Tract Phenotypes, Other Tissues Affected	Associated Human Disease(s)	Reference(s)
Renal Aplasia (Variable)			
CTNNB1 (β-catenin)	Renal agenesis or severe renal hypoplasia, premature differentiation of UB epithelia (UB selective)	Colorectal cancer, hepatoblastoma, hepatocellular cancer	142
Emx2	Complete absence of urogenital system		29
Emx2, PAX2	Duplicated kidneys and ureter, ureteral obstruction	CAKUT, VUR	401
Etv4, Etv5	Renal agenesis or severe renal hypodysplasia		76, 166
EYA1 (Eyes absent-1)	Renal agenesis, lack of UB branching and mesenchymal condensation	Branchiootorenal syndrome (brachial fistulas, deafness)	96, 110
Fgf9, Fgf20	Renal agenesis		230
Fgf10, GDNF, Gfra1	Renal agenesis		172
Fgfr1, Fgfr2	Renal agenesis (MM selective)		240
FRAS1, FREM1, FREM2	UB failure, defect of GDNF expression	Fraser's syndrome (cryptophthalmos, syndactyly, CAKUT); Manitoba-oculotrichoanal (MOTA) syndrome	122, 123, 178-180
GATA3	Renal agenesis, gonad dysgenesis (null mutation); ectopic ureteric budding, kidney, hydroureter (UB selective)	Hypoparathyroidism, sensorineural deafness, and renal dysplasia (HDRS) syndrome; autoimmune disease (rheumatoid arthritis)	136, 137, 139, 140
Gdf11 (growth differentiation factor 11)	UB failure, skeletal defects		102, 402
GDNF, Gfra1, RET	Renal agenesis or rudimentary kidneys, aganglionic megacolon	Hirschsprung disease, multiple endocrine neoplasm type IIA/B (MEN2A/MEN2B), and familial medullary thyroid carcinoma (FMTC)	103-106, 118, 119, 403-406,
GLI3	Renal agenesis, severe renal agenesis, absence of renal medulla and papilla	Pallister-Hall (PH) syndrome (polydactyly, imperforate anus, abnormal kidneys, defects in the gastrointestinal tract, larynx, and epiglottis)	212, 213
Grem1 (Gremlin)	Renal agenesis; apoptosis of the MM		107
GRIP1	Renal agenesis	Fraser's syndrome	182-184
Hox-A11/D11	Distal limbs, vas deferens		407
Hs2st1 (heparan sulfate 2 O-sulfotransferase 1)	Lack of UB branching and mesenchymal condensation		408
Isl1 (islet1)	Renal agenesis, renal hypoplasia, hydroureter (MM selective)		409
ITGA8 (integrin α₈)	Renal agenesis, renal hypodysplasia	Fraser's syndrome	124
Itgb1 (integrin β₁)	Disrupted UB branching, bilateral renal agenesis, hypoplastic collecting duct system (collecting duct selective); podocyte dedifferentiation (podocyte selective)	Fraser's syndrome	134, 410, 411
Kif26b	Renal agenesis, failed UB attraction to the MM		125
Lamc1	UB failure, delayed nephrogenesis, water transport defects		185
LHX1/LIM1	Renal agenesis (null mutant); renal hypoplasia, UB branching defect, hydronephrosis, distal ureter obstruction (UB selective); arrested nephrogenesis, nephron patterning defects (MM selective)	Mayer-Rokitansky-Kuster-Hauser (MRKH) syndrome (müllerian duct agenesis)	97, 412, 413
LRP4	Delayed UB induction, failed MM induction, syndactyly, oligodactyly	Cenani-Lenz syndrome	414-417

Table 1.1 Summary of Knockout and Transgenic Models for Kidney Development (Continued)

Gene Mutation or Knockout	Renal and Urogenital Tract Phenotypes, Other Tissues Affected	Associated Human Disease(s)	Reference(s)
Npnt (nephronectin)	Delay of UB invasion into MM		126
Osr1/Odd1	Lack of MM, adrenal gland, gonads, defects in formation of pericardium and atrial septum		98, 109
PAX2	Renal hypoplasia, VUR	CAKUT, VUR, optic nerve colobomas	36, 37
PAX2, PAX8	Defect in intermediate mesoderm transition, failure of pronephric duct formation	CAKUT, VUR, optic nerve colobomas	418
PTF1A (pancreas transcription factor 1α subunit/Danforth short-tail)	Failure of UB induction; anal atresia, persistent cloaca, skeletal malformation	Pancreatic and cerebellar agenesis; diabetes mellitus	419-421
Retinoic acid receptors (Rara, Rarb2)	Renal hypoplasia, dysplasia, hydronephrosis, skeletal and multiple visceral abnormalities		7, 9, 68
SALL1	Renal agenesis, severe renal hypodysplasia	Townes-Brock syndrome (anal, renal, limb, ear anomalies)	99, 422
SHH (Sonic hedgehog)	Bilateral or unilateral renal agenesis, unilateral ectopic dysplastic kidney, defective ureteral stromal differentiation	Vertebral defects, anal atresia, cardiac defects, tracheoesophageal fistula, renal anomalies, and limb abnormalities (VACTERL) syndrome	209
SIX1	Lack of UB branching and mesenchymal condensation	Branchiootorenal syndrome	96, 110
SOX8, SOX9	Renal genesis, renal hypoplasia	Camptomelic dysplasia (limb and skeletal defects, abnormal gonad development)	423
WT1	Renal and gonadal agenesis, severe lung, heart, spleen, adrenal, and mesothelial abnormalities	Wilms' tumor, aniridia, genitourinary abnormalities, and retardation (WAGR) syndrome; Denys-Drash syndrome	28, 38, 337, 338
Hypoplasia/Dysplasia/Low Nephron Mass			
Adamts1	Hypoplasia of the renal medulla, hydronephrosis		250, 253
Adamts1, Adamts4	Hypoplasia of the renal medulla, hydronephrosis		254
Agtr2 (angiotensin II type-2 receptor)	Various collecting system defects	CAKUT	202, 321, 322
Ald1a2/Raldh2 (retinal dehydrogenase)	Renal hypoplasia, hydronephrosis, ectopic ureter		139
BMP1RA/Alk3	Hypoplasia of renal medulla, fewer UB branches (UB selective)	Juvenile polyposis syndrome	200
Bmp7	Reduced MM survival		225
Cdc42, Yap	Renal hypoplasia, oligonephronia, defects in mesenchyme to epithelial transition (CM selective)		424
Cfl1, Dstn (cofilin1, destrin)	Renal hypodysplasia, ureter duplication		425
CTNNB1 (β-catenin)	Severely hypoplastic kidney, lack of nephrogenic zone and S-shaped body (CM selective)	Colorectal cancer, hepatoblastoma	223
DICER1	Renal hypoplasia, dysplasia, cysts (UB selective); renal hypoplasia characterized by premature termination of nephrogenesis (MM selective)	Pleopulmonary blastoma	426
Dkk1 (Dickkopf 1)	Overgrown renal papilla (renal tubule and collecting duct restricted)		196
Dlg1, Cask	Renal hypoplasia and dysplasia, premature depletion of nephrogenic precursor cells		326, 427

Continued on following page

Table 1.1 Summary of Knockout and Transgenic Models for Kidney Development (Continued)

Gene Mutation or Knockout	Renal and Urogenital Tract Phenotypes, Other Tissues Affected	Associated Human Disease(s)	Reference(s)
Egfr (epidermal growth factor receptor)	Hypoplasia of the renal papilla, moderate polyuria, and urine concentration defects		194
Esrrg	Agenesis of renal papilla		43
Fat4	Failed nephrogenesis (mesenchyme-to-epithelial transition), expansion of nephrogenic precursor zone (stroma selective)		274
Fgf7	Small kidneys, reduction in nephron number		198
FGF8	Renal dysplasia, arrested nephrogenesis at pretubular aggregate stage (MM selective)	Kallmann's syndrome, hypogonadism	428, 429
Fgf10	Renal hypoplasia, multiorgan developmental defects including the lungs, limb, thyroid, pituitary, and salivary glands		199
Fgfr1, Fgfr2	Renal agenesis (MM selective)		240
Fgfr2	Renal hypoplasia, hydronephrosis (UB selective)		69
FOXC2	Renal hypoplasia	AD lymphedema-distichiasis syndrome	214, 430
Foxd1 (BF-2)	Accumulation of undifferentiated CM, attenuated UB branching, stromal patterning defects		22, 266, 268
Foxd1	Mild renal hypoplasia (UB selective)		431
Fzd4, Fzd8 (frizzled 4/8)	Impaired UB branching, renal hypoplasia		432
LGR4	Severe renal hypoplasia and oligonephronia; renal cysts	Aniridia–genitourinary anomalies–mental retardation syndrome	433, 434
LMX1B	Renal dysplasia, skeletal abnormalities	Nail-patella syndrome	334, 341
Mdm2 (murine double minute 2)	Renal hypoplasia and dysplasia, severely impaired UB branching and nephrogenesis (UB selective); depletion of nephrogenic precursors (MM selective)		435, 436
Mf2	Renal hypoplasia, oligonephronia		437
Pbx1	Reduced UB branching, delayed mesenchyme-to-epithelial transformation, dysgenesis of adrenal gland and gonads		438, 439
Plxnb2 (plexin B2)	Renal hypoplasia and ureter duplication		440
Pou3f3 (Brn1)	Impaired development of distal tubules, loop of Henle, and macula densa; distal nephron patterning defect		251
Prr (prorenin receptor)	Renal hypoplasia, renal dysplasia (UB selective)		441
Psen1, Psen2 (presenilins 1/2)	Severe renal hypoplasia, severe defects in nephrogenesis		247
Ptgs2 (prostaglandin endoperoxide synthase 2/cyclooxygenase-2)	Oligonephronia		442
Rbpj	Severe renal hypoplasia, oligonephronia, loss of proximal nephron segments, tubular cysts (MM selective)		248, 249
Shp2	Severe impairment of UB branching, renal hypoplasia		163

Table 1.1 Summary of Knockout and Transgenic Models for Kidney Development (Continued)

Gene Mutation or Knockout	Renal and Urogenital Tract Phenotypes, Other Tissues Affected	Associated Human Disease(s)	Reference(s)
Six1	Hydronephrosis, hydroureter, abnormal development of ureteral smooth muscle		309
Six2	Renal hypoplasia, premature depletion of nephrogenic precursors		235
Tbx18	Hydronephrosis, hydroureter, abnormal development of ureteral smooth muscle		307, 309
Tfap2b	MM failure, craniofacial and skeletal defects		443
TRPS1	Impaired UB branching, renal hypoplasia	Trichorhinophalangeal syndrome (skeletal defects)	444
Wnt4	Failure of MM induction		223
Wnt7b	Complete absence of medulla and renal papilla (UB selective)		190
Wnt9b	Vestigial kidney, failure of MM induction		191, 220
	Cystic kidney (collecting duct selective)		
Wnt11	Impaired ureteric branching, renal hypoplasia		165
Mislocalized or Ectopic UB/Increased UB Branching			
Bmp4, Bmp7	Ectopic UB, renal hypodysplasia, hydroureter, defective ureterovesical junction		218, 445
Cer1	Increased ureteric branching, altered spatial organization of ureteric branches		446
Foxc1	Duplex kidneys, ectopic ureters, hydronephrosis, hydroureter		214
HNF1B, PAX2	Renal hypoplasia, duplex kidneys, ectopic ureters, megaureter, hydronephrosis	CAKUT	447
Lzts2 (leucine-zipper putative tumor suppressor 2)	Duplex kidneys/ureters, hydronephrosis, hydroureter		448
Plxnb1 (plexin B1)	Increased ureteric branching		449
Plxnb2 (plexin B2)	Renal hypoplasia and ureter duplication		440
Sema3a	Increased ureteric branching (UB selective)		40
Slit2, ROBO2	Increased UB branching	CAKUT, VUR	215, 216
Spry1 (sprouty 1)	Supernumerary UBs, multiple ureters		70, 173
Cysts			
Aqp11 (aquaporin-11)	Abnormal vacuolization of proximal tubules; polycystic kidneys		450
Bcl2	Renal hypoplasia and cysts		451
Bicc1	Polycystic kidneys		452
Bpck/TMEM67	Polycystic kidneys, hydrocephalus	Meckel's syndrome (multicystic renal dysplasia, neural tube defects)	453
Erbb4	Renal cysts (overexpression in renal tubules)		454
	Dilated and mispolarized tubules, increased renal fibrosis (renal tubule deletion)		
FAT4	Renal cysts, disrupted hair cell organization in inner ear	Van Maldergem's syndrome (mental retardation, abnormal craniofacial features, deafness, skeletal and limb malformations, renal hypoplasia)	259, 455

Continued on following page

Table 1.1 Summary of Knockout and Transgenic Models for Kidney Development (Continued)

Gene Mutation or Knockout	Renal and Urogenital Tract Phenotypes, Other Tissues Affected	Associated Human Disease(s)	Reference(s)
GLIS3	Polycystic kidney, neonatal diabetes	Congenital hypothyroidism, diabetes mellitus, hepatic fibrosis, congenital glaucoma	456, 457
GPC3 (glypican-3)	Disorganized tubules and medullary cysts	Simpson-Golabi-Behmel syndrome	458-460
HNF1B	Polycystic kidney disease (tubular-selective)	Maturity-onset diabetes of the young type 5 (MODY5)	260, 261
Ift88/Orpk (intraflagellar transport 88/Oak Ridge Polycystic Kidney Disease)	Polycystic kidneys; defective left-right asymmetric patterning		461, 462
Invs (inversin)	Polycystic kidneys, inverted viscera		463, 464
Kif3A	Polycystic kidney disease (tubular-selective)		465
MAFB (Kreisler)	Decreased glomeruli, cysts, and tubular dysgenesis	Musculoaponeurotic fibrosarcoma	466, 467
MKS1	Renal hypoplasia and cysts	Meckel's syndrome (multicystic renal dysplasia, neural tube defect)	468
PKD1, PKD2	Renal cysts	ADPKD, ARPKD	469
PTEN	Abnormal ureteric bud branching, cysts (UB selective)	Cowden's disease, Bannayan-Riley-Ruvalcaba syndrome, various tumors	164
Taz/Wwtr1	Polycystic kidneys, emphysema		470, 471
VHL	Renal cysts (tubular-selective)	Von Hippel–Lindau syndrome	472
Xylt2 (xylosyltransferase 2)	Polycystic kidneys and liver		473
Later Phenotypes (Glomerular, Vascular, and Glomerular Basement Membrane)			
ACE (angiotensin-converting enzyme)	Atrophy of renal papillae, vascular thickening and hypertrophy, perivascular inflammation	Chronic systemic hypotension	203, 204
ACTN4 (α-actinin 4)	Glomerular developmental defects, FSGS	SRNS	349, 350
AGT (angiotensinogen)	Atrophy of renal papillae, vascular thickening and hypertrophy, perivascular inflammation	Essential hypertension, renal tubular dysgenesis	205, 326
AGTR1A (AT1A)	Hypertrophy of juxtaglomerular apparatus and expansion of renin cell progenitors, mesangial cell hypertrophy	Essential hypertension, renal tubular dysgenesis	474
AGTR1A, AGTR1B (AT1A, AT1B)	Atrophy of renal papillae, vascular thickening and hypertrophy, perivascular inflammation	Essential hypertension, renal tubular dysgenesis	206
AMPD (AMP [adenosine monophosphate] deaminase)	Podocyte foot process effacement, proteinuria	Minimal change nephrotic disease	475
Angpt1/ANG1 (angiopoietin 1)	Simplification and dilation of glomerular capillaries; detachment of glomerular endothelium from the GBM; loss of mesangial cells		286
Angpt2/ANG2 (angiopoietin 2)	Cortical peritubular capillary abnormalities (null allele) Apoptosis of glomerular capillaries, proteinuria (transgenic overexpression)		295, 296
ARHGDIA/RhoGDIα	FSGS	SRNS	351, 352
Bmp7	Hypoplastic kidney, impaired maturation of nephron, reduced proximal tubules (podocyte selective)		302
CD151	Podocyte foot process effacement, disorganized GBM, tubular cystic dilation	Nephropathy (FSGS) associated with pretibial epidermolysis bullosa and deafness	476, 477

Table 1.1 Summary of Knockout and Transgenic Models for Kidney Development (Continued)

Gene Mutation or Knockout	Renal and Urogenital Tract Phenotypes, Other Tissues Affected	Associated Human Disease(s)	Reference(s)
CD2AP	Podocyte foot process effacement, immunotactoid nephropathy	FSGS	387
Cdc42	Congenital nephrosis; impaired formation of podocyte foot processes (podocyte selective)		374
Cmas	Congenital nephrosis; impaired formation of podocyte foot processes, defective sialylation		478
COL4A1, COL4A3, COL4A4, COL4A5	Disorganized GBM, proteinuria	Alport's syndrome	479-482
Crk1/2, CrkL	Albuminuria, altered podocyte cytoarchitecture (podocyte selective)		483
Cxcl12/SDF1 (stroma-derived factor 1), CXCR4, Cxcr7	Petechial hemorrhage in the kidneys, glomerular aneurysm, fewer glomerular fenestrations, reduced mesangial cells, podocyte foot process effacement, mild renal hypoplasia	WHIM (warts, hypogammaglobulinemia, infections, and myelokathexis) syndrome	305, 306, 484
DICER1	Podocyte damage, albuminuria, end-stage kidney failure (podocyte selective); reduced renin production, renal vascular abnormalities, striped fibrosis (renin cell selective)	Pleuropulmonary blastoma	329, 396-398
Dnm1, Dnm2 (dynamin 1/2)	Podocyte foot process effacement and proteinuria (podocyte selective)		485
EphB4	Aberrant development of vascular shunts in glomerular arterioles (transgenic overexpression in renal tubules and parietal cells of Bowman's capsule)		300
Ephrin-B2	Dilation of glomerular capillaries		301
Fat1	Foot process fusion, failure of foot process formation		353
Flt1/VEGFR1	Nephrotic syndrome		395
Foxc2	Impaired podocyte differentiation, dilated glomerular capillary loop, poor mesangial migration		64
Foxi1	Distal renal tubule acidosis; absence of collecting duct intercalated cells		255
Fyn	Podocyte foot process effacement, abnormal slit diaphragms, proteinuria		382, 486
Gne/Mnk (glucosamine-2-epimerae/N-acetylmannosamine kinase)	Hyposialylation defect, foot process effacement, GBM splitting, proteinuria and hematuria		487
Ilk (integrin-like kinase)	Nephrotic syndrome (podocyte selective)		384
INSR (insulin receptor)	Podocyte effacement, GBM alteration, proteinuria (podocyte selective)	Diabetic nephropathy	488
Itga3 (integrin α_3)	Reduced UB branching, glomerular defects, poor foot process formation		195, 197
Itgb1 (integrin β_1)	Podocyte loss, capillary and mesangial degeneration, glomerulosclerosis (podocyte selective)		410, 411

Continued on following page

Table 1.1 Summary of Knockout and Transgenic Models for Kidney Development (Continued)

Gene Mutation or Knockout	Renal and Urogenital Tract Phenotypes, Other Tissues Affected	Associated Human Disease(s)	Reference(s)
Kirrel (Neph1)	Abnormal slit diaphragm function, FSGS		63
Lama5	Defective glomerulogenesis, abnormal GBM, poor podocyte adhesion, loss of mesangial cells		186
LAMB2	Proteinuria prior to the onset of foot process effacement	Pierson's syndrome	187, 489
LMX1B	Impaired differentiation of podocytes, cytoskeletal disruption in podocytes	Nail-patella syndrome	490-492
Mafb (Kreisler)	Abnormal podocyte differentiation		335
Mpv17 (mitochondrial inner membrane protein 17)	Nephrotic syndrome		493
Mtor/mTOR (mechanistic target of rapamycin)	Proteinuria, podocyte autophagy defects (podocyte selective)		494
MYO1E	Podocyte foot process effacement and proteinuria	SRNS	354, 495, 496
Nck1, Nck2	Failure of foot process formation (podocyte selective)		380
Nid1 (nidogen-1/entactin-1)	Abnormal GBM		497
NPHS1 (nephrin)	Absent slit diaphragms, congenital nephrotic syndrome	Congenital nephrosis of the Finnish type, childhood-onset steroid-resistant nephritic syndrome, childhood- and adult-onset FSGS	342
NPHS2 (podocin)	Congenital nephrosis, FSGS, vascular defects	SRNS, congenital nephritic syndrome	343, 498
NOTCH1, NOTCH2	Lack of glomerular endothelial and mesangial cells (standard knockout) Lack of podocytes and proximal tubular cells (MM selective); impaired nephrogenesis (cap mesenchyme selective)	Alagille's syndrome (cholestatic liver disease, cardiac disease, kidney dysplasia, renal cysts, renal tubular acidosis)	243, 244, 248, 499
Pdgfb/PDGFR-β	Lack of mesangial cells, ballooned glomerular capillary loop		332, 333
Pik3c3/Vps34	FSGS, defects in vesicular trafficking (podocyte selective)		500, 501
Prkci/aPKCλ/ι (atypical protein kinase C λ/ι)	Defect of podocyte foot processes, nephrotic syndrome (podocyte selective)		375, 376
PTPRO/GLEPP1 (glomerular epithelial protein phosphatase 1)	Broadened podocyte foot processes with altered interdigitation patterns	SRNS	487, 502
Rab3A	Albuminuria, disorganization of podocyte foot process structure		15
Rbpj	Decreased renal arterioles, absence of mesangial cells, and depletion of renin cells (stromal cell selective) Reduction in juxtaglomerular cells, impaired renin synthesis (renin cell selective)		310, 331
Rhpn1 (rhophilin-1)	FSGS, podocyte foot process effacement, GBM thickening		355
ROBO2	Abnormal pattern of podocyte foot process interdigitation, focal effacement of foot processes, proteinuria	CAKUT, VUR	503
SLC5A2/SGLT2 (sodium-glucose transporter 2)	Elevated urinary excretion of glucose, calcium, and magnesium	Glucosuria	504
Sh3gl1/2/3 (endophilin 1/2/3)	Podocyte foot process effacement and proteinuria, neuronal defects		485

Table 1.1 Summary of Knockout and Transgenic Models for Kidney Development (Continued)

Gene Mutation or Knockout	Renal and Urogenital Tract Phenotypes, Other Tissues Affected	Associated Human Disease(s)	Reference(s)
Sirpa/SIRPα	Irregular podocyte foot process interdigitation; mild proteinuria		505
Sox4	Oligonephronia, podocyte effacement, GBM defects (MM selective)		506
SOX17, SOX18	Vascular insufficiency in kidneys and liver; ischemic atrophy of renal and hepatic parenchyma; defective postnatal angiogenesis	HLT (hypotrichosis-lymphedema-telangiectasia) syndrome (hair, vascular and lymphatic disorder)	311, 314
Synj1 (synaptojanin 1)	Podocyte foot process effacement and proteinuria; neuronal defects		485
Tcf21 (Pod1/capsulin/epicardin)	Lung and cardiac defects, sex reversal and gonadal dysgenesis, vascular defects, disruption in UB branching, impaired podocyte differentiation, dilated glomerular capillary, poor mesangial migration		6, 264
Tie1	Tie1–null cells fail to contribute to the glomerular endothelium		297
TRPC6	Protected from angiotensin-mediated or proteinuria or complement-dependent glomerular injury (null mutation); podocyte foot process effacement and proteinuria (transgenic overexpression in the podocyte lineage)	SRNS, FSGS	356, 393, 394, 507-510
Vegfa	Endotheliosis, disruption of glomerular filtration barrier formation, nephrotic syndrome (podocyte selective)		279, 280, 511
VHL	Rapidly progressive glomerulonephritis (podocyte selective)	Von Hippel–Lindau syndrome	304

AD, Autosomal dominant; AR, autosomal recessive; CAKUT, congenital anomalies of the kidney and urinary tract; CM, cap mesenchyme; FSGS, focal segmental glomerulosclerosis; GBM, glomerular basement membrane; MM, metanephric mesenchyme; PKD, polycystic kidney disease; SRNS, steroid-resistant nephrotic syndrome; UB, ureteric bud; VUR, vesicoureteral reflux.

heritability. Mutations may be complete or partial loss of function, gain of function, or altered function and can have either dominant or recessive effect. The specific locus mutation frequency of ENU is 1 in 1000. Assuming a total number of 25,000 to 40,000 genes in the mouse genome, a single treated male mouse should have between 25 and 40 different heterozygous mutagenized genes. In the case of multigenic phenotypes, segregation of the mutations in the next generation allows the researcher to focus on monogenic traits. In each generation, 50% of the mutations are lost, and only the mutation underlying the selected phenotype is maintained in the colony. A breeding strategy that includes backcrossing to the female genetic strain enables rapid mapping of the ENU mutation that occurred on the male genetic background.

The screening in ENU mutagenesis experiments can focus on dominant or recessive renal mutations. Screening for dominant phenotypes is popular because breeding schemes are simple and a great number of mutants can be recovered through this approach. About 2% of all first-generation offspring mice display a heritable phenotypic abnormality.[56,57] One of the fruitful results obtained with this approach is the identification of a mutation in the aquaporin 11 gene *(Aqp11)* that causes severe proximal tubule injury and vacuolation of the renal cortex resulting in renal failure and perinatal death.[58] It is possible to design "sensitized screens" on a smaller scale, thereby improving the ability to identify genes in a pathway of interest. For example, in renal glomerular development, the phenotype of a genetic mouse strain with a tendency to development of congenital nephrosis (e.g., *CD2AP* haploinsufficiency) may be enhanced or suppressed by breeding a female of the strain to a mutagenized male.[59] The modifier gene may then be mapped using the approach outlined earlier. This approach has been successfully used to identify genes involved in neural development.[60,61]

Table 1.2 Conditional Mouse Lines for the Kidney

Promoter	Renal Expression	Extrarenal Expression	Reference(s)
11Hsd2 (11β-hydroxysteroid dehydrogenase-2)	Principal cells of collecting duct, connecting tubules	Amygdala, cerebellum, colon, ovary, uterus, epididymis, salivary glands	512
Aqp2 (aquaporin-2)	Principal cells of collecting duct	Testis, vas deferens	513
Atp6v1b1 (V-ATPase-B1)	Collecting ducts (intercalated cells), connecting tubule		514, 515
Bmp7	Cap mesenchyme		516
Cdh16/Ksp-cadherin	Renal tubules, collecting ducts, ureteric bud, wolffian duct, mesonephros	Müllerian duct	75, 517
Cited1	Cap mesenchyme		18
Emx1	Renal tubules (proximal and distal tubules)	Cerebral cortex, thymus	518
Foxd1/BF2	Stromal cells		519
Ggt1 (gamma-glutamyl transferase 1)	Cortical tubules		520
HoxB6	Metanephric mesenchyme	Lateral mesoderm, limb buds	409, 521
HoxB7	Ureteric bud, wolffian duct, collecting ducts, distal ureter	Spinal cord, dorsal root ganglia	209
Kap (kidney androgen regulated protein)	Proximal tubules	Brain	522
Klf3	Collecting ducts	Gonads	541
Nphs1 (nephrin)	Podocytes	Brain	523, 524
Nphs2 (podocin)	Podocytes		525
Osr2	Condensing metanephric mesenchyme; glomeruli	Palatal mesenchyme	526
Pax2	Pronephric duct, wolffian duct, ureteric bud, cap mesenchyme	Inner ear, midbrain, cerebellum, olfactory bulb	527
Pax3	Metanephric mesenchyme	Neural tube, neural crest	525, 528, 529
Pax8	Renal tubules (proximal and distal tubules) and collecting ducts (Tet-On inducible system)		530
Pdgfrb (PDGFR-β)	Mesangial cells, vascular smooth muscles	Pericytes, vascular smooth muscles	301, 531
Pepck	Proximal tubules	Liver	472
Rarb2	Metanephric mesenchyme		412
Ren1 (Renin)	Juxtaglomerular cells, afferent arterioles, mesangial cells	Adrenal gland, testis, sympathetic ganglia, etc.	319
Ret	Ureteric bud, collecting ducts	Dorsal root ganglion, neural crest	532
Sall1	Metanephric mesenchyme (tamoxifen-inducible system)	Limb buds, central nervous system, heart	533
Slc5a2/SGLT2 (sodium-glucose transporter 2)	Proximal tubules		534
Six2	Cap mesenchyme		19
Sox18	Cortical and medullary vasculature	Blood vessel and precursor of lymphatic endothelial cells	535-537
Spink3	Medullary tubules (distal or connecting tubules?)	Mesonephric tubules, pancreas, lung, liver, gastrointestinal tract	528, 529, 538
T (brachyury)	Whole kidney (both ureteric bud and metanephric mesenchyme)	Panmesodermal	428
Tcf21 (Pod1)	Metanephric mesenchyme, cap mesenchyme, podocytes, stromal cells	Epicardium, lung mesenchyme, gonad, spleen, adrenal gland	193
Umod (uromodulin/Tamm-Horsfall protein)	Thick ascending loops of Henle	Testis, brain	539
Wnt4	Renal vesicles, nascent nephrons (comma- and S-shaped bodies)		19, 540

Other genomewide approaches that have led to the discovery of novel genes in kidney development and disease are gene trap consortia[62,63] and genomewide transcriptome and proteome projects.[64-66] The interested reader is referred to the websites for the Centre for Modeling Human Disease (www.cmhd.ca), the International Gene Trap Consortium (www.genetrap.org), Knockout Resources to Conquer Human Disease (www.tigm.org), and the Human Kidney & Urine Proteome Project (www.hkupp.org).

IMAGING AND LINEAGE TRACING STUDIES

Detailed imaging of renal structures and morphogenetic processes has benefited significantly from the availability and development of multiple fluorescent proteins. The advent of genetically modified mice that express fluorescent proteins revolutionized cell lineage and mapping studies allowing high-resolution live visualization of morphogenetic events both in situ and in cultured organ explants. Targeted labeling of cells with fluorescent proteins can be achieved by driving expression of fluorescent proteins under direct control of a cell-specific promoter. Alternatively, a Cre driver mouse can be crossed with a fluorescent reporter animal, whereby Cre recombinase (an enzyme that triggers swapping, or recombination, of stretches of DNA in chromosomes) turns on the constitutive expression of a fluorescent protein. This Cre-driven strategy is particularly valuable in cell lineage tracking and fate mapping analysis because both the progenitor and its subsequent derivatives become fluorescently labeled. A third method involves spatiotemporal induction of fluorescent protein expression, allowing for the fluorescence to be turned on or off through administration of doxycycline or tamoxifen by either the tetracycline (Tet)- or estrogen receptor (ERT2)–dependent inducible system, respectively. This third method allows for the incomplete and pulse labeling of certain cell lineages, permitting the tracking of the fate and migratory behavior of individual cells in real time.

HoxB7-EGFP is the first fluorescent transgene developed to visualize renal development.[67] Enhanced green fluorescent protein (EGFP), placed under the control of the *HoxB7* promoter, specifically labels the wolffian duct and the ureteric epithelial lineage. *HoxB7-EGFP* has therefore proved to be invaluable in studying the rates and pattern of ureteric branching morphogenesis and ureteral development, including disruption of these events in the context of particular mutant backgrounds.[68-71] The *HoxB7–myr-Venus* transgene, designed to express a membrane-bound myristoylated variant of EGFP (myr-Venus), allows for the visualization of individual ureteric epithelial cells by confocal microscopy, thus facilitating observation of changes in cell shape and position.[72] Other fluorescent transgenes for imaging of ureteric epithelia are *Ret-EGFP* and *Ksp-cadherin* (*Cdh16-EGFP*). In *Ret-EGFP* mice, EGFP expression is most prominent in the ampullary tips of the UB.[73,74] In contrast, fluorophore expression is restricted in the UB trunk and stalk, and absent in the UB tips, in *Cdh16-EGFP* mice.[75] An ingenious strategy involving the creation of chimeric animals with wild-type epithelial cells expressing *HoxB7-EGFP* that are intermingled with cells derived from mutant ES cells engineered to express CFP (cyan fluorescent protein) under the control of *HoxB7-Cre* unraveled the distinctive dependence on genes such as *Ret*, *Etv4*, *Etv5*, and *Spry1* in the cellular sorting and rearrangement needed for ureteric branching (Figure 1.11).[76,77] Inducible transgene expression systems can be very useful in labeling a small subset of cells to enable the fate of the cells to be monitored temporally. A tamoxifen-inducible strategy to mark ureteric epithelial cells with myr-Venus has been cleverly used to observe the unique manner in which proliferating UB cells delaminate into the UB lumen and reposition themselves within the expanding UB ampullary tip.[78]

Lgr5-EGFP, *Cited1-EGFP*, and a variety of *Six2-EGFP* transgenes have been employed to characterize the self-renewing capacity and multipotency of nephron progenitor cells within the cap mesenchyme.[18,19,79] The mechanism by which nephrogenic and ureteric epithelia are physically conjoined via the invasion of the UB tip by distal nephron precursors has been imaged through the targeted expression of myr-Venus under the control of a *Six2-Cre* driver.[16] A wide variety of fluorescent protein transgenes and Cre transgenes are now available to characterize the development and organization of multiple compartments of the kidney (see Table 1.2).[80]

NONMAMMALIAN MODEL SYSTEMS FOR KIDNEY DEVELOPMENT

Organisms separated by millions of years of evolution from humans still provide useful models to study the genetic basis and function of mammalian kidney development. This continuing feature stems from the facts that all of these organisms possess excretory organs designed to remove metabolic wastes from the body and that genetic pathways involved in other aspects of invertebrate development may serve as templates to dissect pathways in mammalian kidney development. In support of the latter argument, elucidation of the genetic interactions and molecular mechanism of the Neph1 ortholog and nephrin-like molecules SYG-1 and SYG-2 in synapse formation in the soil nematode *Caenorhabditis elegans* is providing major clues to the function of their corresponding genes in glomerular and slit diaphragm formation and function in mammals.[81]

The excretory organs of invertebrates, which differ greatly in their structure and complexity, range in size from a few cells in *C. elegans* to several hundred cells in the malpighian tubules of the fly *Drosophila* to the more recognizable kidneys in amphibians, birds, and mammals. In *C. elegans*, the excretory system consists of a single large H-shaped excretory cell, a pore cell, a duct cell, and a gland cell.[82,83] *C. elegans* provides many benefits as a model system: the availability of powerful genetic tools including "mutants by mail," short life and reproductive cycle, publicly available genome sequence and resource database (www.wormbase.org), the ease of performing genetic enhancer-suppressor screens in worms, and the fact that they share many genetic pathways with mammals. Major contributions to our understanding of the function of polycystic and cilia-related genes have been made from studying *C. elegans*. The *PKD1* and *PKD2* homologs in *C. elegans*, *lov-1* and *lov-2*, are involved in cilia development and function of the mating organ required for mating behavior.[84,85] Strides in understanding the function of the slit diaphragm have also been made from studies of *C. elegans*, as described earlier.

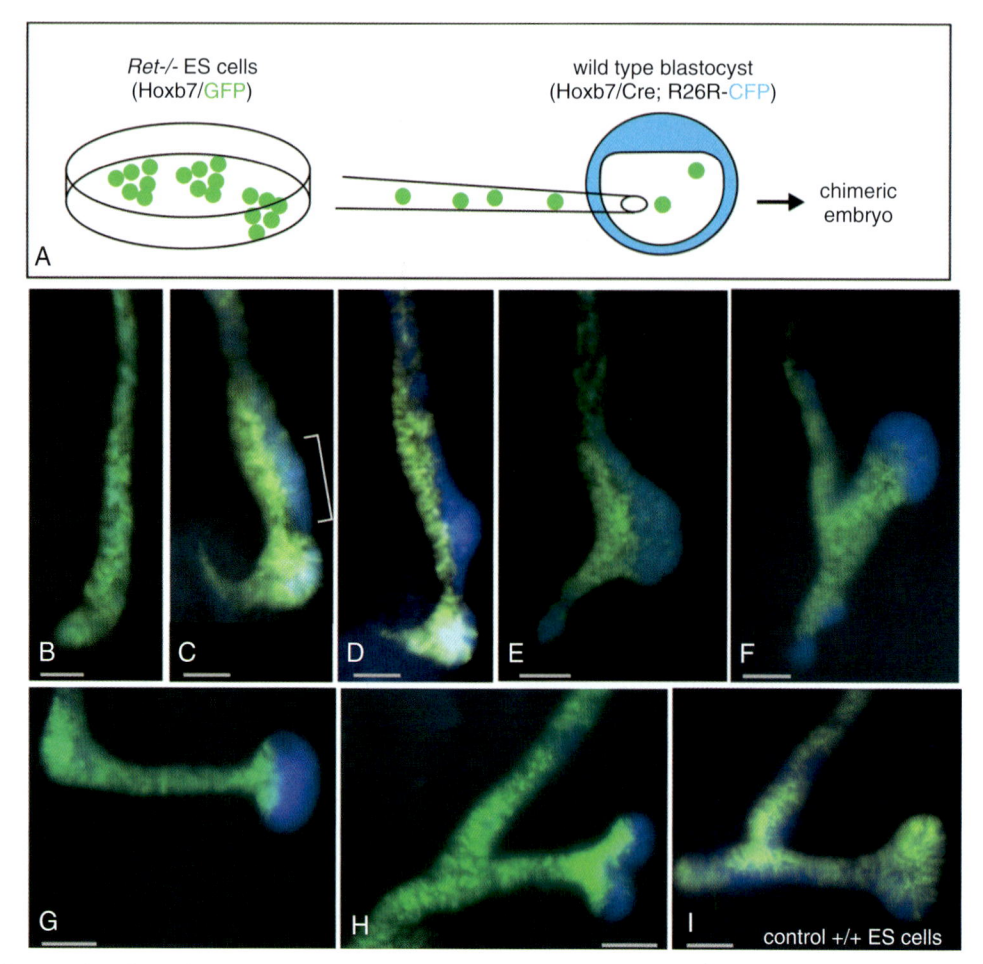

Figure 1.11 Cell fate tracing through genetic expression of fluorophores. Segregation of Ret-deficient cells in the outgrowth and branching of the ureteric bud (UB). **A,** Ret-null embryonic stem cells (ES) expressing HoxB7-GFP (green fluorescent protein) were mixed with a wild-type transgenic blastocyst (HoxB7-Cre: R26R-CFP [cyan fluorescent protein]). This process generates chimeric animals in which *Ret*-null cells exhibit GFP fluorescence and wild-type UB cells express CFP. **B,** At 9.5 dpc (days post coitum), *Ret*-null epithelial cells are intermingled with wild-type cells in the wolffian duct (WD). **C,** At 10 dpc, when the dorsal side of the WD begins to swell, the region where the UB will emerge becomes enriched with CFP-expressing but not *Ret*-null cells. **D** and **E,** At around 10.5 dpc, the UB is formed exclusively by wild-type cells. **F,** Upon elongation of the UB at 11 dpc, the bulbous distal tip of the UB is formed by wild-type cells but the *Ret*-null cells begin to contribute to the trailing trunk structure. **G** and **H,** During the initial branching of the UB at around 11.5 dpc, *Ret*-null cells are excluded from the distal ampullary UB tips. **I,** In contrast, control cells expressing Ret and GFP contribute to the whole branching UB structure. (Reproduced with permission from Chi X, Michos O, Shakya R, et al: Ret-dependent cell rearrangements in the Wolffian duct epithelium initiate ureteric bud morphogenesis. *Dev Cell* 17:199-209, 2009.)

In *Drosophila*, the "kidney" consists of malpighian tubules that develop from the hindgut and perform a combination of secretory, resorption, and filtering functions.[86] They express a number of mammalian gene homologs (e.g., *Cut*, members of the Wingless pathway) that have subsequently been shown to play major roles in mammalian kidney development. Furthermore, studies on myoblast fusion and neural development in *Drosophila*—two processes that may not appear to be related to kidney development at first glance—have provided major clues to the development and function of slit diaphragms.[87] Mutations in the fly *Neph* ortholog, irregular chiasm C-roughest (*irreC-rst*), are associated with neuronal defects and abnormal patterning of the eye.[88,89]

The pronephros, which is only the first of three stages of kidney development in mammals, is the final and only kidney of jawless fishes, whereas the mesonephros is the definitive kidney in amphibians. The pronephros found in larval stage zebrafish (*Danio rerio*) consists of two tubules connected to a fused, single, midline glomerulus. The zebrafish pronephric glomerulus expresses many of the same genes found in mammalian glomeruli (e.g., *Vegfa, Nphs1, Nphs2,* and *Wt1*) and contains podocytes and fenestrated endothelial cells.[90] Advantages of the zebrafish as a model system include its short reproductive cycle, transparency of the larvae with easy visualization of defects in pronephric development without sacrifice of the organism, availability of the genome sequence, the ability to rapidly knock down gene function with morpholino oligonucleotides, and the ability to perform functional studies of filtration using fluorescently tagged labels of varying sizes.[91] These features make zebrafish amenable to both forward and reverse genetic screens. Currently, multiple laboratories perform knockdown screens of mammalian homologs and genomewide mutagenesis screens in zebrafish in order to study renal function.

The pronephros of the clawed frog *Xenopus laevis* has also been used as a simple model to study early events in nephrogenesis. As in the fish, the pronephros consists of a single glomus, paired tubules, and a duct. The fact that *X. laevis* embryos develop rapidly outside the body (all major organ systems are formed by 6 days of age), the ease of injecting DNA, messenger RNA, and protein, and the ability to perform grafting and in vitro culture experiments establish the frog as a valuable model system for dissection of early inductive and patterning cues.[92] In addition, insights emerging from the use of the chick embryo as a model for mesonephros development have highlighted the role of the Vg1/Nodal signaling pathway in formation of the intermediate mesoderm as the embryonic source of all kidney tissue in vertebrates.[93]

GENETIC ANALYSIS OF MAMMALIAN KIDNEY DEVELOPMENT

Much has been learned about the molecular genetic basis of kidney development over the past 15 years. This understanding has been gained primarily through the phenotypic analysis of mice carrying targeted mutations that affect kidney development. Additional information has been gained by identification and study of genes expressed in the developing kidney, even though the targeted mutation, or knockout, either has not yet been performed or has not affected kidney development or function. This section categorizes the genetic defects on the basis of the major phenotype and stage of disrupted development. It must be emphasized that many genes are expressed at multiple points of renal development and may play pleiotropic roles that are not entirely clear.

INTERACTION OF THE URETERIC BUD AND THE METANEPHRIC MESENCHYME

The molecular analysis of the initiation of metanephric kidney development has included a series of classic experiments using organ culture systems that allow separation of the UB and the MM as well as a later analysis of many gene-targeted mice with phenotypes that included various degrees of renal agenesis. As previously mentioned, the organ culture system has been in use since the seminal experiments, beginning in the 1950s, of Grobstein, Saxen, and their colleagues.[27,94,95] These experiments showed that the induction of the mesenchymal-to-epithelial transformation within the MM required the presence of an inducing agent provided by the UB. The embryonic neural tube was found to be able to substitute for the epithelial bud, and experiments involving the placement of the inducing agent on the opposite side of a porous filter from the mesenchyme provided information about the degree of contact required between them. A large series of experiments using organ cultures provided information about the timing of appearance of different proteins normally observed during the induction of nephrons and about the intervals that were crucial in maintaining contact between the inducing agent and the mesenchyme to obtain induction of tubules.

The work with the organ culture system provided an extensive framework on which to base further studies of organ development, and the system remains in extensive use to this day. However, the modern era of studies on the early development of the kidney began with the observation of renal agenesis phenotypes in gene-targeted or knockout mice, the earliest among these being the knockout of several transcription factors, including the WT1, Pax2, Eya1, Osr1/Odd1, Six1, Sall1, Lhx1/Lim1, and Emx2.[28,29,37,96-101] The knockout of several secreted signaling molecules, such as GDNF, GDF11, gremlin (Grem1), and the receptors Ret and GFRα1 (GDNF family receptor alpha1), also resulted in renal agenesis, at least in the majority of embryos.[102-108]

EARLY LINEAGE DETERMINATION OF THE METANEPHRIC MESENCHYME

In most embryos exhibiting renal agenesis, an appropriately localized putative MM is often uninvaded by a UB outgrowth. Two exceptions are the *Osr1/Odd1* and *Eya1* mutant embryos, in which this distinct patch of MM is absent, suggesting that *Osr1* and *Eya1* represent the earliest determinants of the MM yet identified (Figure 1.12). Together, the phenotypes of these knockout mice have provided an initial molecular hierarchy of early kidney development.[96,109] *Osr1* is localized to mesenchymal cells within the mesonephric and metanephric kidney and is subsequently downregulated upon epithelial differentiation. Mice lacking *Osr1* do not form the MM and do not express several other factors required for metanephric kidney formation, including Eya1, Six2, Pax2, Sall1, and GDNF.[109] Other factors implicated in the earliest stages of MM cell fate determination are the Eya1/Six1 pathway. *Eya1* and *Six1* mutations are found in humans with branchiootorenal (BOR) syndrome.[110] It is now known through in vitro experiments that the proteins Eya1 and Six1 form a regulatory complex that appears to be involved in transcriptional regulation.[111,112] Interestingly, Eya1 was shown to have an intrinsic phosphatase activity that regulates the activation of the Eya1/Six1 complex.[112,113] Moreover, Eya and Six family genes are co-expressed in several tissues in mammals, *Xenopus,* and *Drosophila,* further supporting a functional interaction between these genes.[96,100,101,114,115] Direct transcriptional targets of this complex appear to include the pro-proliferative factor c-Myc.[112] In the *Eya1*-deficient urogenital ridge the putative MM is completely absent.[116] Consistent with this finding, Six1 is either absent or poorly expressed in the presumptive location of the MM of *Eya1*-null embryos.[112,114-116] These findings may identify *Eya1* as a gene involved in early commitment of this group of cells to the metanephric lineage. Although Six1 and Eya1 may act in a complex together, the Six1 phenotype is somewhat different, in that a histologically distinct mesenchyme is present at 11.5 dpc, without an invading UB, similar to the other renal agenesis phenotypes.[100,101] Eya1 is expressed in the *Six1*-null mesenchyme, suggesting that *Eya1* is upstream of *Six1*. Additionally, Sall1 and Pax2 are not expressed in the *Six1* mutant mesenchyme even though WT1 is expressed.[100,101,116] There are discrepancies in the literature about Pax2 expression in *Six1* mutant embryos, which may reflect the exact position along the anterior-posterior axis of the urogenital ridges of *Six1* mutant embryos from which sections are obtained.

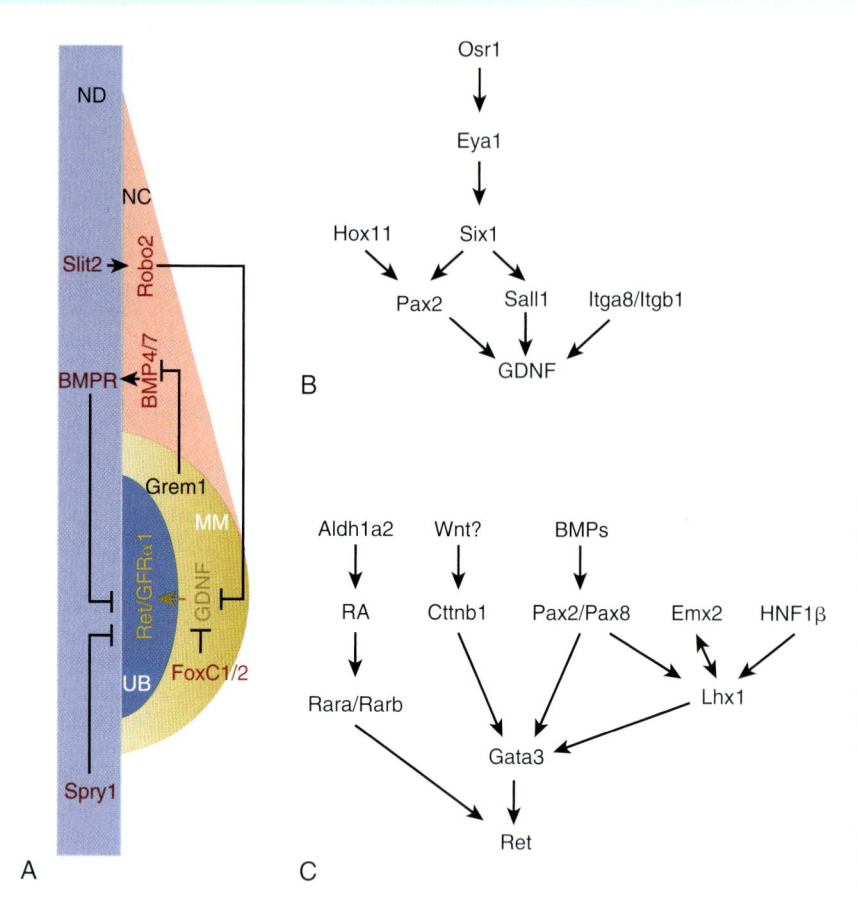

Figure 1.12 Genetic interactions during early metanephric kidney development. A, Regulatory interactions that control the strategically localized expression of GDNF (glial cell–derived neurotrophic factor) and Ret and the subsequent induction of the ureteric bud (UB). The anterior part of GDNF expression is restricted by Foxc1/2 and Slit/Robo2 signaling. Spry1 suppresses the post-receptor activity of Ret. BMP4/7-BMPR (bone morphogenetic protein 4/7–bone morphogenetic protein receptor) signaling inhibits the response to GDNF, an effect counteracted by gremlin 1 (Grem1). **B** and **C,** Genetic regulatory networks that control the expression of **(B)** GDNF and **(C)** Ret. MM, Metanephric mesenchyme; NC, nephrogenic cord; ND, nephric duct.

URETERIC BUD INDUCTION: TRANSCRIPTIONAL REGULATION OF GDNF

In many cases of renal agenesis, a failure of the GDNF-Ret signaling axis has been identified.[117] GDNF, a member of the tumor growth factor-β (TGF-β) superfamily and secreted by the MM, activates the Ret-GFRα1 receptor complex that is expressed by cells of the nephric duct and the UB. Activation of the Ret tyrosine kinase is of central importance to UB induction. Most mutant embryos lacking Gdnf, Ret, or Gfrα1 exhibit partial or complete renal agenesis owing to severe impairment of UB induction, whereas exogenous GDNF is suffice to induce sprouting of ectopic buds from the nephric duct.[103-106,118-121] Consistently, other genes linked to renal agenesis are known to regulate the normal expression of GDNF. These include genes encoding for transcription factors (e.g., Eya1, Pax2, Six1, Hox11 paralogs, and Sall1) and proteins required to stimulate or maintain GDNF expression (e.g., GDF11, Kif26b, nephronectin, $\alpha_8\beta_1$-integrin, and Fras1) (see Figure 1.12).[96,99,101,102,122-130]

As described earlier, *Eya1* mutants fail to form the MM. Pax2, a transcriptional regulator of the paired box *(Pax)* gene family, is expressed widely during the development of both UB and mesenchymal components of the urogenital system.[127] In *Pax2*-null embryos, Eya1, Six1, and Sall1 are expressed,[116] suggesting that the Eya1/Six1 is likely upstream of Pax2. Through a combination of molecular and in vivo studies, it has been demonstrated that Pax2 appears to act as a transcriptional activator of GDNF and regulates the expression of Ret.[128,131] Pax2 also appears to regulate kidney formation through epigenetic control because it is involved in the assembly of a histone H3, lysine 4 methyltansferase complex through the ubiquitously expressed nuclear factor PTIP (pax transcription activation domain interacting protein), which regulates histone methylation.[132] The *Hox* genes are conserved in all metazoans and specify positional information along the body axis. *Hox11* paralogs include *Hoxa11*, *Hoxc11*, and *Hoxd11*. Mice carrying mutations in any one of these genes do not have kidney abnormalities; however, triple-mutant mice for these genes demonstrate a complete absence of metanephric kidney induction.[129] Interestingly, in these mutants, the formation of condensing MM and the expressions of Eya1, Pax2, and WT1 remain unperturbed, suggesting that *Hox11* is not upstream of these factors. Although there seems to be some hierarchy, Eya1, Pax2, and Hox11 appear to form a complex to coordinately regulate the expression of GDNF.[133]

Sall1 indirectly controls the expression of GDNF. Sall1 is necessary for the expression of the kinesin Kif26b by the MM cells.[125] In the absence of either Sall1 or Kif26b, the nephronectin receptor $\alpha_8\beta_1$-integrin expressed by the MM mesenchyme is downregulated. The loss of Sall1, Kif26b, $\alpha_8\beta_1$-integrin, and nephronectin compromises the adhesion of the MM cells to the UB tips, ultimately causing loss of GDNF expression and failure of UB outgrowth.[124,126,134] Loss of the extracellular matrix protein Fras1—the gene which is linked to Fraser's syndrome and which is expressed selectively in the UB epithelium and nascent epithelialized nephrons but not the MM—causes loss of GDNF expression.[122] Fras1 likely regulates MM induction and GDNF expression via multiple signaling pathways. Fras1 deficiency results in downregulation of GDF11, Hox11, Six2, and α8-integrin, and an increase in bone morphogenetic protein 4 (BMP4), which cooperatively controls GDNF expression.[122]

NON-GDNF PATHWAYS IN THE METANEPHRIC MESENCHYME

Another pathway in early development of the MM involves WT1 and vascular endothelial growth factor A (VEGF-A).[49] Induction of the UB does not occur in *Wt1* mutants, although GDNF is expressed in the MM, indicating the existence of a GDNF-independent UB induction mechanism.[28] However, details of this pathway still remain to be clarified. A novel approach to the organ culture system involving microinjection and electroporation has also yielded insights as to a possible function of the *Wt1* gene in early kidney development. Overexpression of WT1 from an expression construct led to high-level expression of VEGF-A. The target of VEGF-A appeared to be Flk1 (VEGF receptor 2 [VEGFR2])–expressing angioblasts at the periphery of the mesenchyme. Blocking signaling through Flk1, if done when the metanephric rudiment was placed in culture, blocked expression of Pax2 and GDNF and, consequently, of the continued branching of the UB and induction of nephrons by the bud. Blockade of Flk1 after the organ had been in culture for 48 hours had no effect, indicating that the angioblast-derived signal was required to initiate kidney development but not to maintain continued development.[49] The signal provided by the angioblasts is not yet known, nor is it known whether WT1 is a direct transcriptional activator of VEGF-A. Flk1 signaling is also required to initiate hepatocyte differentiation during liver development. Numerous targets of WT1 in nephron progenitors have been identified though chromatin immunoprecipitation, providing a comprehensive catalog of genes particularly enriched for functions relating to transcription, multiorgan development, and cell cycle regulation. In addition, a number of these WT1 targets have special roles in remodeling of the actin cytoskeleton.[38]

GENES REQUIRED BY THE URETERIC BUD IN EARLY KIDNEY DEVELOPMENT

Several components of the genetic network supporting the development of the nephric duct and the UB have been identified (see Figure 1.12). *Pax2* and *Pax8* are required to maintain the expression of *Lhx1*.[135] *Pax2*, *Pax8*, and *Lhx1* altogether likely coordinate the expression of *Gata3*, which is necessary for elongation of the nephric duct.[136] *Gata3* and *Emx2*, which are required for the expression of Ret in the nephric duct, are both regulated by β-catenin, an effector of the canonical Wnt signaling pathway (for a discussion of Wnt, see section "Molecular Analysis of the Nephrogenic Zone").[29,137,138] Acting likely in parallel with *Gata3* to maintain Ret expression in the UB is *Aldh1a2 (Raldh2)*, a gene in the retinoic acid synthesis pathway.[139] Surprisingly, this genetic regulatory hierarchy cannot fully account for the distinctive phenotypes arising from the mutations of individual genes, suggesting that additional important components of the nephric duct genetic network have yet to be identified. Nephric duct specification fails in *Pax2/Pax8* mutants but not in the case of *Lhx1* deficiency, in which only the caudal portion of the nephric duct degenerates.[135] The absence of *Gata3* or *Raldh2* causes misguided elongation of the nephric duct, which terminates into either blind-ended ureters or abnormal connections between the bladder and urethra.[136] The curtailed caudal growth of the nephric duct when either *Lhx1* or *Gata3* is lost prevents the formation of the first UB and consequently causes renal agenesis.[136,140,141] The absence of *Aldh1a2* leads to the formation of ectopic ureters and hydronephrotic kidneys.[139] *Emx2* deficiency does not prevent caudal extension of the nephric duct toward the presumptive MM, but the evagination of the UB is aborted, thereby resulting in renal agenesis.[29] Without β-catenin, nephric duct cells undergo precocious differentiation into collecting duct epithelia.[142] Ret does not affect the nephric duct fate but has importance in later UB development and insertion of the nephric duct into the cloaca.[77,120,139] Identification of additional targets of Pax2, Pax8, Lhx1, Gata3, and β-catenin are necessary in order to fully understand these seemingly disparate mutant phenotypes.

UB induction and subsequent branching require a unique spatial organization of Ret signaling. The bulbous UB tip is a region enriched with proliferative ureteric epithelial cells, in contrast to the emerging stalk regions of the developing ureteric tree.[30,143] It is now well appreciated that receptor tyrosine kinase (RTK) signaling primarily through Ret is key to the proliferation of UB tip epithelia. Exogenous GDNF supplemented in explanted embryonic kidneys can cause expansion of the UB tip region toward the source of the ligand.[143-145] Erk kinase activation is prominent within the ampullary UB terminals, where Ret expression is elevated.[30] Consistently, chimera analysis in mice reveals that Ret-deficient cells do not contribute to the formation of the UB tips.[120] All together, these studies underscore the importance of strategic levels of Ret expression and activation of proliferative signaling pathways in the stereotypical sculpting of the nascent collecting duct network.

A ligand-receptor complex formed by GDNF, GFRα1, and Ret is necessary for autophosphorylation of Ret on its intracellular tyrosines (Figure 1.13). A number of downstream adaptor molecules and effectors have been identified to interact with active phosphorylated Ret, including the growth factor receptor–bound proteins Grb2, Grb7, and Grb10, ShcA, Frs2, phospholipase C$_{\gamma1}$ (PLC$_{\gamma1}$), Shp2, Src, and Dok adaptor family members (Dok4/5/6).[146-157] These downstream Ret effectors together are likely contributors to the activation of the Ras/SOS/Erk and PI3K/Akt pathways supporting the proliferation, survival, and migratory behavior of the UB epithelium.[30,32,158] Knock-in mutations of the interaction site for Shc/Frs2/Dok adaptors on the short isoform of Ret lead to the formation of rudimentary kidneys.[159-162] Specific mutation of the PLC$_{\gamma1}$ docking site on Ret leads to renal dysplasia and ureter duplications.[159] The loss of Shp2 in the UB lineage also causes severe renal hypoplasia, phenocopying that is observed in occasional Ret-deficient kidneys.[163] UB-specific inactivation of *Pten*, a target of the PI3K/Akt pathway, disrupts UB branching.[164] Taken together, these findings underscore the significance of Ret signaling in normal UB branching.

A number of transcriptional targets of Ret activation in microdissected UB stimulated with GDNF have been elucidated (see Figure 1.13).[76] Among these are Ret itself and Wnt11, which stimulates GDNF expression in the MM,[165] suggesting that a positive feedback loop exists for the GDNF-Ret signaling pathway. Ret activation also positively regulates

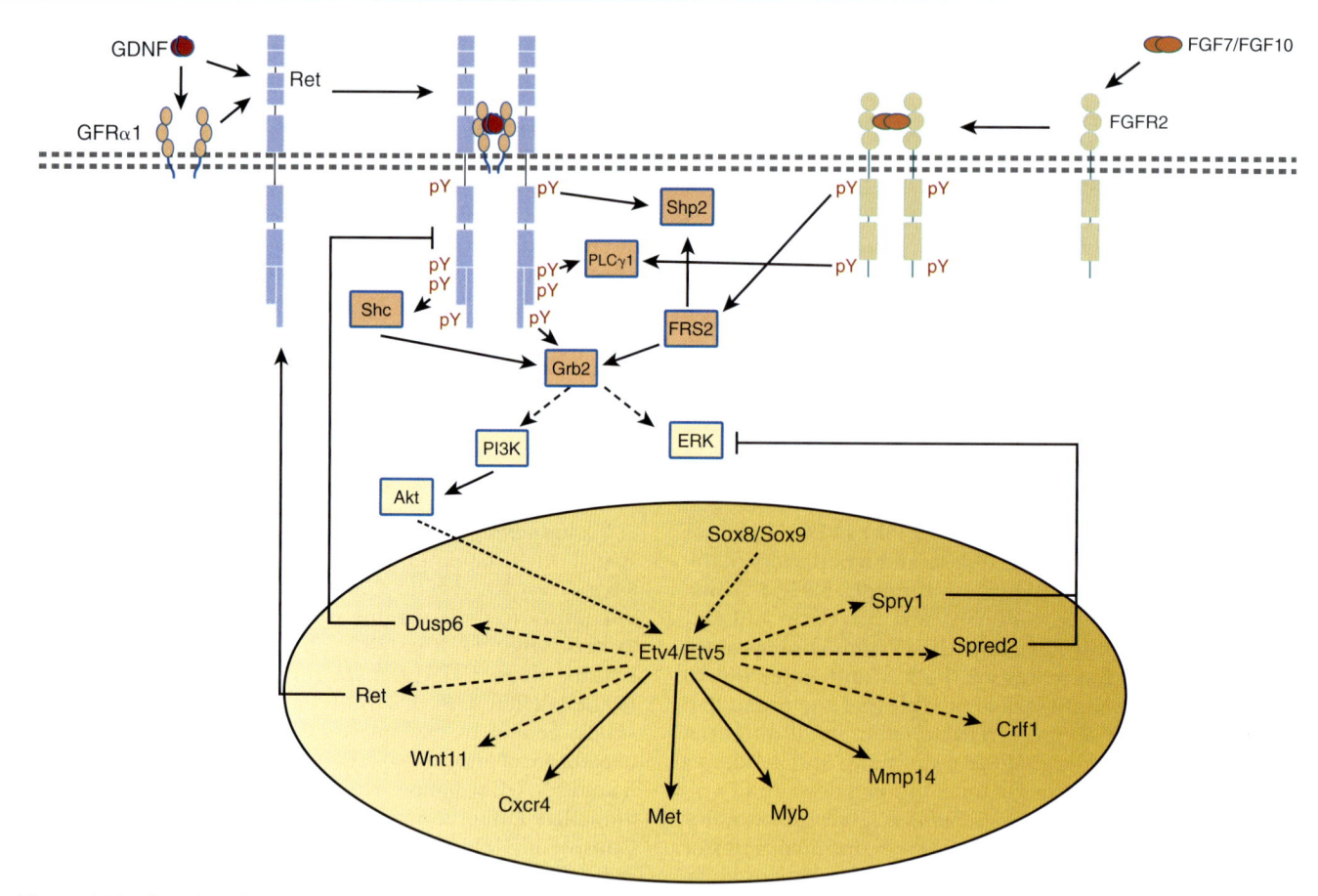

Figure 1.13 Ret signaling pathway. Ret is activated and becomes autophosphorylated on intracellular tyrosine residues (pY) upon association with GDNF GDNF (glial cell–derived neurotrophic factor) and its receptor GFRα1. Signaling molecules such as Grb2, Shc, FRS2, PLCγ1, and Shp2 bind directly to the phosphorylated tyrosine residues within the intracellular domain of Ret. Recruitment of Shc, FRS2, and Grb2 leads to activation of the ERK and PI3K/Akt pathways. GDNF-Ret signaling leads to the specific activation of a host of genes, some of which strongly depend on the upregulation of the transcription factors Etv4 and Etv5 *(solid arrows)*. Etv4/Etv5 activation requires activation of the PI3K/Akt but not the ERK pathway. Transcription factors Sox8 and Sox9 are believed to act in parallel to reinforce transcriptional responses to GDNF-Ret engagement. Some of these pathways are shared with the FGF7/10-FGFR2 receptor signaling system. The proteins Spry1 and Spred2 negatively regulate ERK signaling, whereas Dusp6 likely mitigates dephosphorylation of the Ret receptor, thus acting as part of a negative feedback regulatory loop. Other distinctive transcriptional targets of Ret activation include Crlf1, Cxcr4, Mmp14, Myb and Wnt11.

the ETS (E26 transformation-specific) transcription factors Etv4 and Etv5, which are also necessary for normal UB branching morphogenesis. *Etv4*-null homozygous mutants and compound heterozygous mutants for *Etv4* and *Etv5* manifest severe renal hypoplasia or renal agenesis, suggesting that these transcription factors are indispensable targets of Ret for proper UB development.[76] In chimeric animals Etv4/Etv5-deficient cells, just like Ret-deficient cells, fail to integrate within the UB tip domain.[120,166]

The gene *Sprouty* was identified as a general antagonist of RTKs and was discovered for inhibiting the fibroplastic growth factor (FGF) and epidermal growth factor (EGF) signaling pathways that pattern the *Drosophila* airways, wings, and ovarian follicles.[167-169] Of the four mammalian *Sprouty* homologs, *Spry1*, *Spry2*, and *Spry4* are expressed in developing kidneys.[170] *Spry1* is expressed strongly at the UB tips, whereas *Spry2* and *Spry4* are found in both the UB and the MM.[171] Sprouty molecules are thought to uncouple receptor tyrosine kinases with the activation of ERK pathway either through competitive binding with the Grb2/SOS complex or through the kinase Raf, effectively repressing ERK activation. Interestingly, *Spry1* expression is distinctively upregulated upon GDNF activation of Ret.[76] This finding suggests that Ret activates a negative feedback mechanism via Spry1 in order to control activated ERK levels and modulate cell proliferation in the UB. Studies on *Spry1*-knockout mice reveal some intriguing facets about Ret dependence of UB induction and branching.[70,72,172-175] *Spry1* deficiency leads to ectopic UB induction and can rescue renal development in the absence of either GDNF or Ret.[172,176] Germline inactivation of *Spry2* does not overtly affect renal development but can rescue renal hypoplasia in mice engineered to express *Ret* mutants impaired in activating the Ras/ERK pathway.[171] The transcriptional targets of Ret, such as Etv4, Etv5 and Wnt11, are retained in *Gdnf/Spry1* or *Ret/Spry1* compound null mutants.[172,176] These findings indicate that Ret signaling is not absolutely required for UB development. In fact, signaling via FGF10 and the receptor FGFR2 is sufficient for renal development despite the absence of GDNF or Ret, provided that *Spry1* is inactivated. Nevertheless, patterns of renal branching are distinctively altered in *Gdnf/Spry1* and *Gdnf/Ret* compound mutants, with UB tips often displaying more heterogeneous shapes and orientation. These findings indicate that there remain some distinctive roles of GDNF-Ret signaling that cannot be fully compensated by FGF10/FGFR2 during UB development.

ADHESION PROTEINS IN EARLY KIDNEY DEVELOPMENT

A current theme in cell biology is that growth factor signaling often occurs coordinately with signals from the extracellular matrix transduced by adhesion receptors, such as members of the integrin family. $\alpha_8\beta_1$-integrin is expressed by cells of the MM interacting with the novel ligand nephronectin expressed specifically by UB cells.[124,177] In most embryos with mutations causing absence of α_8-integrin, UB outgrowth is arrested upon contact with the MM.[124] In a small portion of embryos, this block is overcome, and a single, usually hypoplastic, kidney develops. Nephronectin gene (Npnt) knockout mice exhibit renal agenesis or severe hypoplasia.[126] Thus, the interaction of $\alpha_8\beta_1$-integrin with nephronectin must have an important role in the continued growth of the UB toward the MM. Phenotypes of both Itga8 and Npnt knockout mice appear to result from a reduction in GDNF expression.[126] The attraction of the UB to the mesenchyme is also governed by the maintenance of proper cell-cell adhesion within mesenchymal cells. Kif26b, a kinesin specifically expressed in the MM, is important for tight condensation of mesenchymal cells.[125] Genetic inactivation of Kif26b results in renal agenesis due to impaired UB induction. In Kif26b mutant mice, the compact aggregation of mesenchymal cells is compromised, resulting in distinctive loss of polarized expression of α_8-integrin and severe downregulation of GDNF expression. Hence, dysregulation of mesenchymal cell adhesion causes the failure to attract and induce the ureteric epithelia.

Genetic evidence further shows that nephronectin localization at the basement membrane of the UB is critical for GDNF expression by the MM. Genetic inactivation of basement membrane proteins associated with Fraser's syndrome (Fras1, Frem1/Qbrick, and Frem2) leads to renal agenesis characterized by severe downregulation of GDNF expression.[122,123,178-181] On the basis of interaction of nephronectin with Fras1, Frem1/Qbrick, and Frem2, it has been proposed that the Fras1/Frem1/Frem2 ternary complex anchors nephronectin to the UB basement membrane, thus stabilizing engagement with $\alpha_8\beta_1$-integrin expressed by the MM (Figure 1.14).[179] Grip1, a PDZ domain protein known to interact with Fras1, is required to localize the Fras1/Frem1/Frem2 complex on the basal aspect of the UB epithelium.[182] Grip1 mutations phenocopy Fraser's syndrome, including renal agenesis, thus further highlighting the importance of the strategic localization of nephronectin on the UB surface toward the opposing MM.[182-184]

The establishment of epithelial basement membranes during metanephric kidney development involves the stage-specific assembly of different laminin α and β subunits with a common laminin γ_1 subunit. The UB-specific inactivation of the gene Lamc1, which encodes for laminin γ_1, leads to impaired UB induction and branching, ultimately causing either renal agenesis or hypomorphic kidneys with water transport deficits.[185] Lamc1 deficiency prevents formation of basement membranes, causing downregulation of both growth factor (GDNF/Ret, Wnt11, and FGF2)–based and integrin-based signaling. This fact is another example of how signaling through the extracellular matrix intersects with growth factor signaling to influence morphogenesis. The importance of basement membrane assembly in the development of other renal structures is emphasized by genetic studies on the genes Lama5 and Lamb2, which encode for laminins α_5 and β_2, respectively. Loss of Lama5 causes either renal agenesis or disruption of glomerulogenesis, whereas deficiency of Lamb2 leads to a defective glomerular filtration barrier.[186,187]

The UB branching program is stereotypically organized so that the proliferative UB epithelial cells are largely confined to the bulbous UB tips but cell division is dampened within the elongated nonbranching UB stalks of the growing ureteric tree. TROP2/Tacstd2, an adhesion molecule related to epithelial cell adhesion molecule (EpCAM), is expressed prominently in the UB stalks, where it colocalizes with collagen-1.[188] TROP2, unlike EpCAM, which is expressed throughout the UB tree, is not expressed at the UB ampullary tips. Consistently, dissociated and sorted UB cells expressing high levels of TROP2 are nonproliferative and express low levels of Ret, GFRα1, and Wnt11, which are notable UB tip markers. Elevated expression of TROP2 is also associated with poor attachment of epithelial cells to collagen matrix and with suppression of cell spreading and motility, thus emphasizing the importance of this adhesion molecule in negative regulation of UB branching and the sculpting of the nascent collecting duct network. The formation of patent lumens within epithelial tubules of the kidney also depends on coordinated cell adhesion. β_1-integrin is tethered to the actin cytoskeleton via a ternary complex formed between integrin-like kinase (ILK) and parvin. ILK has been shown to be important in mediating cell cycle arrest and cell contact inhibition in the collecting duct epithelia.[189] The targeted ablation of Ilk expression in the UB does not cause remarkable defects in UB branching but does eventually lead to postnatal death due to obstruction of collecting ducts arising from dysregulated intraluminal cell proliferation. Thus, cell adhesion molecules may suppress cell division to regulate distinctive aspects of renal branching and tubulogenesis.

FORMATION OF THE COLLECTING SYSTEM

The overall shape, structure, and size of the kidneys are largely guided by the stereotypical branching of the UB and the subsequent patterning of the collecting duct system. During late gestation, past embryonic stage 15.5 dpc in the mouse, the trunks of the UB tree undergo extensive elongation to establish the array of collecting ducts found in the renal medulla and papilla. The radial arrangement of elongated collecting ducts together with the loops of Henle (derived from the nephrogenic mesenchyme) establishes the corticomedullary axis by which nephron distributions are patterned. Further elongation of the newly formed collecting duct network after birth is partly responsible for the postnatal growth of the kidney.

Elongation of the collecting ducts is regulated by oriented cell division, a process dependent on Wnt7b and Wnt9b.[190-192] Oriented cell division is characterized by the parallel alignment of the mitotic spindle of proliferating ductal epithelia with the longitudinal axis of the duct.

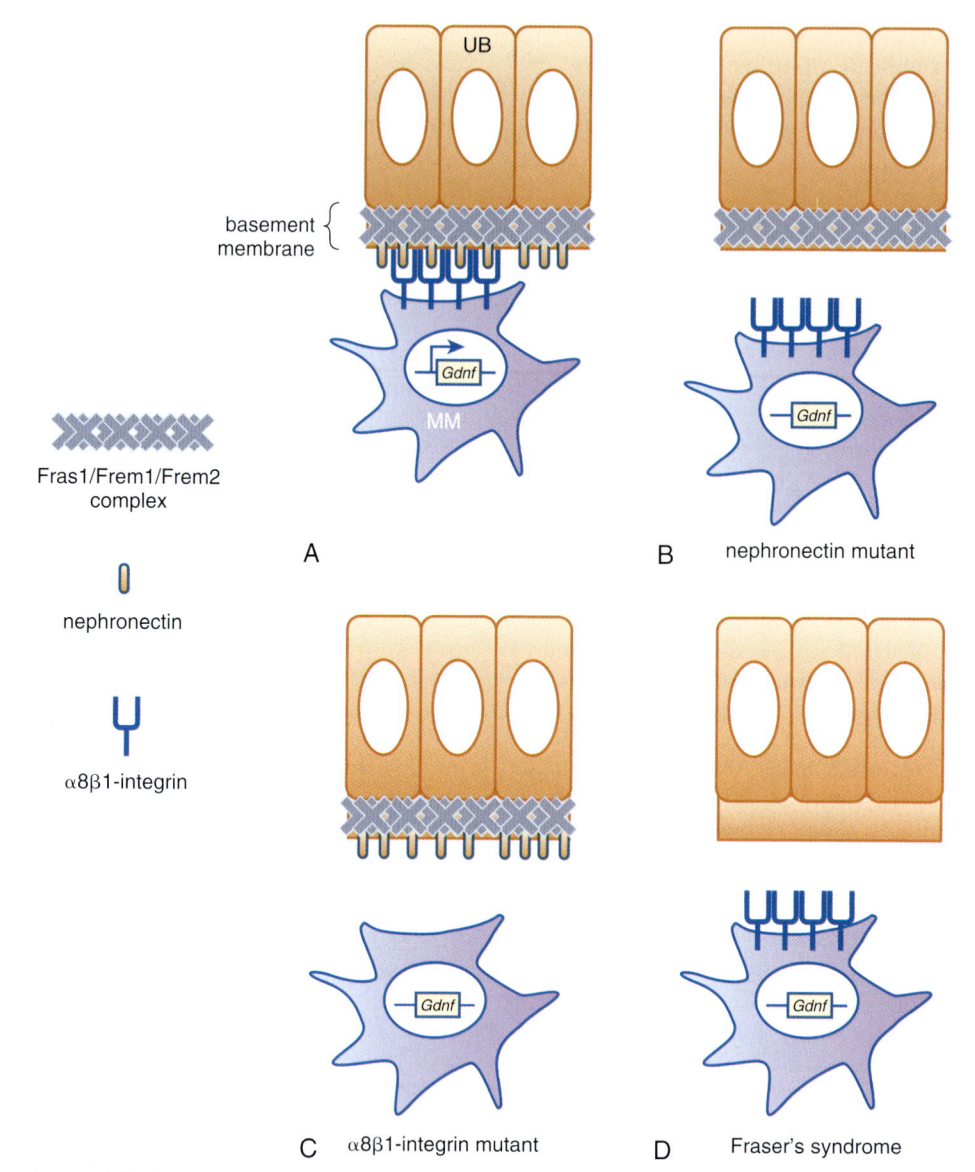

Figure 1.14 Molecular model of renal defect in Fraser's syndrome. A, Adhesion to the ureteric bud (UB) epithelium positively regulates the expression of glial cell–derived neurotrophic factor (GDNF) by the metanephric mesenchyme (MM). Adhesion and GDNF expression are impaired in the absence of **(B)** nephronectin (expressed by the UB), **(C)** α8β1 integrin (expressed by the MM), **(D)** or the Fras1/Frem1/Frem2 complex. Fras1, Frem1, and Frem2, which are implicated in Fraser's syndrome, are believed to coordinatedly anchor nephronectin to the UB basement membrane and stabilize the conjugation with α8β1 integrin. (Modified from Kiyosumi D, Takeichi M, Nakano I, et al: Basement membrane assembly of the integrin α8β1 ligand nephronectin requires Fraser syndrome-associated proteins. *J Cell Biol* 197:677-689, 2012.)

Oriented cytokinesis, therefore, guarantees that the daughter cells contribute to lengthening of the duct with minimal effect on tubular lumen diameter. The renal medulla and pelvis are nonexistent in mice lacking Wnt7b.[190] Notably, the collecting ducts and loops of Henle are stubbier, likely through disruption of oriented cell division. Wnt7b expression is restricted within the UB trunks and is absent in the ampullary UB tips. Oriented cell division of the collecting duct epithelia therefore requires reciprocal signaling with the surrounding interstitial stromal mesenchyme. Conditional inactivation of *Cttnb1 (β-catenin)* using a *Tcf21-Cre* transgene (which is expressed in the interstitial stroma) results in hypoplastic kidneys lacking medullary and papillary regions.[193] This is consistent with the possibility that the UB-stromal interaction via Wnt7b activates the canonical β-catenin–dependent Wnt signaling pathway. Wnt9b, another ligand expressed along the UB trunk region, has been identified as required for oriented cell division in collecting duct cells. In contrast, Wnt9b signals through a noncanonical Wnt pathway involving the activation of the small guanosine triphosphatase (GTPase) RhoA and the kinase Jnk.[191] Another mechanism that could contribute to elongation of the collecting ducts is convergent extension. Convergent extension involves the coordinated intercalation of elongated epithelial cells that thereby narrows and effectively lengthens the ducts. This mechanism was proposed on the basis of the reconfigured orientation of elongated cells in *Wnt9b* mutant collecting ducts.[191] How the interstitial stroma signals back to the UB to modulate oriented cell division and convergent-extension remains unknown.

The normal development of the collecting ducts also depends on cell survival cues provided by diverse ligands such as Wnt7b, EGF, and hepatocyte growth factor (HGF) and on interactions with the extracellular matrix.[190,194,195] Papillary collecting ducts display higher incidence of apoptosis in mice lacking Wnt7b or EGF receptor (EGFR).[190,194] Conversely, loss of Dkk1 (Dickkopf1), a secreted antagonist of Wnt7b, results in overgrowth of the renal papilla.[196] Conditional inactivation of *Dkk1* using the *Pax8-Cre* transgene (expressed in renal tubules and the collecting ducts) causes increased proliferation of papillary epithelial cells. The HGF receptor Met, $\alpha_3\beta_1$-integrin (*Itga3/Itgb1*), and laminin α_5 (*Lama5*) are all required to maintain the expression of Wnt7b and thus are likely to support the viability of collecting duct cells.[134,195,197]

Poor development of the renal medulla and papilla are also observed in mutant mice lacking FGF7, FGF10, FGFR2, BMPR1A (ALK3), the components of the renin angiotensin aldosterone system (RAAS), Shh (Sonic hedgehog), or the orphan nuclear steroid hormone receptor Esrrg. FGF7 and FGF10 are the cognate ligands of FGFR2. Renal hypoplasia observed when *Fgfr2* is conditionally removed from the ureteric lineage is more severe than in mutants lacking Fgf7 or Fgf10, suggesting that these related ligands may have some functional redundancy in the development of the UB and collecting ducts.[69,198,199] Kidneys lacking *Bmp1ra* show an attenuated phosphorylation of SMAD1, an effector of the BMP and TGFβ ligands, and a concomitant increase in expression of c-Myc and β-catenin.[200] Although the significance of these results are not clear, the elevation of β-catenin indicates a novel crosstalk between BMP and Wnt signaling pathways in collecting ducts. Signaling through angiotensin is relevant to both early UB branching and the morphogenesis of medullary collecting ducts.[201] Genetic inactivation of angiotensinogen, its processing enzyme angiotensin-converting enzyme (ACE), and its target angiotensin-II AT1R receptors (Agtr1a and Agtr1b) results in similar phenotypes characterized by hypoplastic kidneys with modestly sized renal papillae.[202-207] Furthermore, the postnatal growth and survival of renal papilla grown ex vivo depend on the presence of AT1R.[208] Interestingly, in cultures of renal papilla explants, angiotensin appears to regulate the Wnt7b, FGF7, and $\alpha_3\beta_1$-integrin signaling pathways such that the loss of endogenous angiotensin or pharmacologic inhibition of AT1R causes significant dampening of the expression of *Wnt7b*, *Fgf7*, *Cttnb1*, and *Itga3/Itgb1*.[208] *Shh* is expressed in the more distal derivatives of the UB, the medullary collecting ducts and the ureter.[209] The germline deletion of *Shh* results in either bilateral renal agenesis or a single ectopic dysplastic kidney.[210,211] It has been shown that *Shh* controls the expression of early inductive and patterning genes (*Pax2* and *Sall1*), cell cycle regulators (N-myc and cyclin D1), and signaling effectors of the Hedgehog pathway (*Gli1* and *Gli2*). Interestingly, genetic removal of *Gli3* on an *Shh*-null background restores the expression of *Pax2*, *Sall1*, cyclin D1, N-Myc, Gli1, and Gli2, providing physiologic proof for the role of *Gli3* as a repressor of the Shh pathway in renal development.[211] Frameshift mutations resulting in truncation of the expressed Gli3 protein is linked to Pallister-Hall syndrome and the presence of hydronephrosis and hydroureter in both humans and mice.[212,213] Esrrg has a strong and localized expression within collecting duct epithelia later in gestation, and its inactivation in mice causes complete aplasia of the renal medulla and papillae. However, the ligand of Esrrg remains to be identified, and little is known about its downstream targets.

POSITIONING OF THE URETERIC BUD

A crucial aspect of kidney development that is of great relevance to renal and urologic congenital defects in humans relates to the positioning of the UB (see Figure 1.12A). Incorrect positioning or duplication of the bud leads to abnormally shaped kidneys and incorrect insertion of the ureter into the bladder, with resultant ureteral reflux that can predispose to infection and scarring of the kidneys and urologic tract.

Foxc1 (Forkhead box C1) is a transcription factor of the Forkhead family, expressed in the intermediate mesoderm and the MM adjacent to the wolffian duct. In the absence of *Foxc1*, the expression of GDNF adjacent to the wolffian duct is less restricted than in wild-type embryos. *Foxc1* deficiency results in ectopic UBs, hypoplastic kidneys, and duplicated ureters.[214] Additional molecules that regulate the location of UB outgrowth are Slit2 and Robo2, signaling molecules best known for their role in axon guidance in the developing nervous system. Slit2 is a secreted factor, and Robo2 is its cognate receptor. Slit2 is mainly expressed in the Wolffian duct, whereas Robo2 is expressed in the mesenchyme.[215] In one study, UBs formed ectopically in embryos deficient in either Slit2 or Robo2 similar to those in the *Foxc1* mutant. However, in contrast to the *Foxc1* phenotype, ureters in the *Slit2/Robo2* mutants undergo remodeling allowing their insertion into the bladder.[215] Instead, the ureters remained connected to the nephric duct in *Slit2* or *Robo2* mutants. The domain of GDNF expression is expanded anteriorly in the absence of either *Slit2* or *Robo2*. Indeed, mutations in *Robo2* have been identified in patients with vesicoureteral junction defects and vesicoureteral reflux.[216] The expressions of *Pax2*, *Eya1*, and *Foxc1*, all thought to regulate GDNF expression, were not dramatically different in the absence of *Slit2* or *Robo2*, suggesting that Slit/Robo signaling is not upstream of these genes. It is possible that Slit/Robo signaling is regulating the point of UB initiation by regulating the GDNF expression domain downstream of *Pax2* or *Eya1*. An alternative explanation is that Slit2 and Robo2 act independently of GDNF and that the expanded GDNF domain is a response to rather than a cause of ectopic UBs.

Spry1, as described earlier, negatively regulates the Ras/Erk signaling pathway and is expressed strongly in the posterior wolffian duct and the UB tips.[217] Embryos lacking *Spry1* develop supernumerary UBs, but unlike mutants of *Foxc1*, *Slit2*, or *Robo2*, they do not display changes in GDNF expression.[173] The phenotype of *Spry1* mutants can be rescued by reducing the GDNF expression dosage.[173] *Spry1* deletion also rescues the renal agenesis defect in mice lacking either Ret or GDNF.[172] Consistently, renal agenesis and severe renal hypoplasia, in mice expressing Ret specifically mutated on a tyrosine phosphorylation site known to couple with the Ras/ERK pathway, can be reversed in the absence of *Spry1*.[176] Thus, *Spry1* appears to regulate UB induction site by dampening RTK-dependent proliferative signaling.

Another negative regulator of branching is BMP4, which is expressed in the mesenchyme surrounding the wolffian duct. *Bmp4* heterozygous mutants have duplicated ureters, and in organ culture, BMP4 blocks the induction of ectopic UBs by GDNF-soaked beads.[218] Furthermore, knockout of gremlin, a secreted BMP inhibitor, causes renal agenesis, supporting a role for BMP in the suppression of UB formation.[219]

MOLECULAR ANALYSIS OF THE NEPHROGENIC ZONE

The continued replenishment of the reservoir of nephron progenitors during kidney development is crucial to guarantee generation of a sufficient number of nephrons. Fate mapping studies in mice using Cre driven by *Cited1* and *Six2* promoters demonstrate that the condensed mesenchyme, which aggregates around the UB, represents a pool of multipotent progenitors that replenishes itself and differentiates to give rise to all epithelial components of the nephron from podocytes to distal tubules.[18,19] Signaling through Wnt, FGF, and the BMP family of ligands is critical to maintain the delicate balance between progenitor self-renewal and differentiation toward a nephrogenic fate.

Wnt11 and Wnt9b, two ligands belonging to the Wnt family of signaling molecules, are expressed by the UB. The Wnt family was originally discovered as the wingless mutation in *Drosophila* and, in mammals, as genes found at retroviral integration sites in mammary tumors in mice. Wnt11 is highly expressed at the UB tips and decreased branching occurs in its absence, although it has no known specific effect on the induction of the epithelial transformation of the MM.[165] Wnt11 is a downstream target of Ret and is necessary to sustain GDNF expression in the MM.[76,144,145,165] Hence, Wnt11 participates in an autoregulatory feedback loop that maintains GDNF-Ret signaling to promote UB branching.[165] In contrast, Wnt9b, which is expressed in the entire UB except the very tips, appears to be the vital molecule expressed by the UB that induces the MM.[220] Wnt9b is not essential for the early induction of the UB or for the initial condensation of the MM. Further UB branching fails beyond the initial branching step resulting in T-shaped tubule (T-stage), however, likely because of downregulation of GDNF in the MM. The MM condenses up to the T-stage but the expressions of *Pax2*, *Eya1*, *WT1*, *Bmp7*, and *Six2* are distinctively diminished by 12.5 dpc in *Wnt9b* mutant mouse embryos. This loss of MM markers leads to failed induction of renal vesicles and tubulogenesis. Thus, Wnt9b is the closest candidate identified to date, which is likely to be the crucial molecule produced by the bud that stimulates induction of the nephrons.

A third member of the Wnt family, Wnt4, is expressed in pretubular aggregates and is additionally required for the epithelial transformation of the MM.[220,221] In *Wnt4* mutant embryos, pretubular aggregates failed to epithelialize into the tubular precursor of the mature nephron.[221] *Wnt9b*-deficient MM could be sufficiently induced in vitro to undergo tubulogenesis when grown with Wnt4-expressing fibroblasts.[220] In contrast, another study using the same co-culture assay showed that Wnt9b could not compensate for the loss of Wnt4. These findings suggest that Wnt9b and Wnt4 likely bind distinctive receptor complexes, with Wnt4 acting downstream of Wnt9b. Thus, a model has been proposed whereby Wnt9b acts as a paracrine factor, priming the MM to develop into renal vesicles expressing Wnt4. Wnt4 in this model functions as an autocrine factor required for commitment to a tubulogenesis program (Figure 1.15).

Two major Wnt signaling branches exist downstream of the Frizzled receptor (Fz): a canonical β-catenin–dependent pathway and a noncanonical β-catenin–independent pathway.[222] In the canonical pathway, Wnt-mediated signaling suppresses a phosphorylation-triggered pathway of proteosomal degradation, enabling the stabilization of β-catenin, which results in the formation of a complex between β-catenin and TCF/LEF (T-cell factor/lymphoid-enhancing factor) DNA-binding proteins that directly regulates transcriptional targets. Numerous studies demonstrate the importance of the canonical Wnt pathway for renal development: Conditional deletion of β-catenin from the cap mesenchyme completely blocks renal vesicle formation as well as expression of markers of induction such as Wnt4,

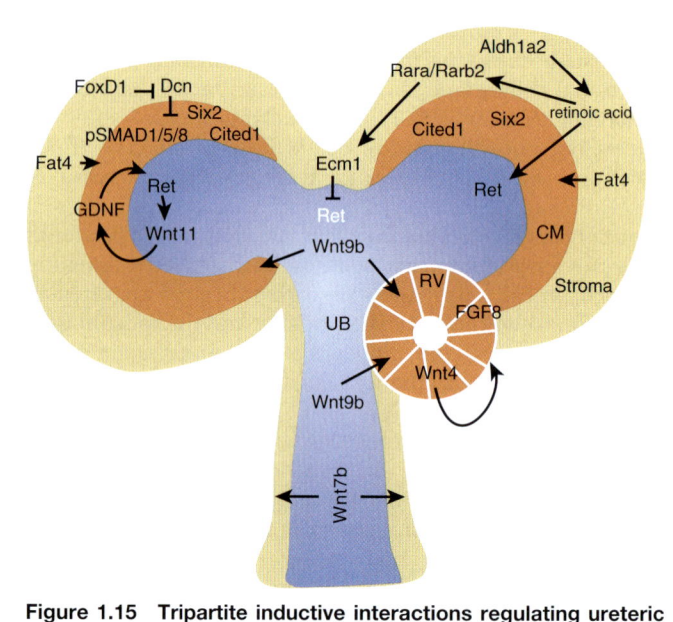

Figure 1.15 Tripartite inductive interactions regulating ureteric branching and nephrogenesis. Six2 and Cited1 are expressed in the self-renewing nephron progenitors within the cap mesenchyme (CM) surrounding the ureteric bud (UB). The UB tip domains express high levels of Ret, which is activated by glial cell–derived neurotrophic factor (GDNF) from the surrounding CM. Wnt11 is upregulated in response to Ret activation and stimulates GDNF synthesis in the CM. Wnt9b, expressed by the UB, and Fat4, expressed by the Foxd1-positive stroma, are required to initiate nephrogenesis from a subset of the CM. This results in the formation of a transient renal vesicle (RV) expressing FGF8 and Wnt4, factors that sustain epithelialization. The stroma expresses *Aldh1a2*, a gene required for retinoic acid synthesis, and genes for the retinoic acid receptors Rara and Rarb2. Retinoic acid signaling stimulates elevated expression of Ret in the UB tip domain while also suppressing Ret expression via Rara/Rarb2 and Ecm1 in the stroma to initiate bifurcation of the UB tip to generate new branches. Foxd1 in the cortical stroma also represses Dcn, thus relieving the Dcn-mediated suppression of BMP7-dependent signaling, which results in phosphorylation of SMAD1/5/8 (pSMAD1/5/8) and epithelialization of the cap mesenchyme. Wnt7b expressed in the UB stalk signals to the interstitial stroma and is an important factor that regulates cortico-medullary patterning of the kidney.

Fgf8, and Pax8.[223] By contrast, activation of stabilized β-catenin in the same cell population causes ectopic expression of mesenchymal induction markers in vitro and functionally rescues the defects observed in Wnt4- or Wnt9b-deficient mesenchymes. Inhibition of the kinase GSK3, a member of the β-catenin degradation complex, results in the ectopic differentiation of the MM.[224]

BMP7 is expressed in the UB and in the condensed MM.[225,226] Loss of BMP7 causes untimely depletion of the cap mesenchyme and nephrogenesis arrest.[225,226] BMP7 is thought to be a survival and proliferative factor for the cap mesenchyme, on the basis of organ culture experiments and the increased incidence of apoptosis observed within the presumptive nephrogenic zone of Bmp7-null kidneys.[226-229] The proliferative effect of BMP7 on nephron progenitors has been shown to depend on specific activation of the kinase Jnk leading to phosphorylation and activation of Jun and Atf2.[230] However, the cell-survival promoting functions of BMP7 are unlikely specific since BMP4 can functionally substitute for loss of BMP7 (based on phenotypic rescue in "knocked-in" mutants where Bmp4 cDNA was inserted next to the endogenous Bmp7 promoter).[231] The exact role of BMP4 in nephrogenesis is not known, although it has been described as important specifically within the UB lineage.[218] The transcription factor Trps1, an atypical member of the GATA family of transcription factors implicated in trichorhinophalangeal (TRP) syndrome, has been identified as a novel target of BMP7.[232] Trps1 expression is absent in Bmp7-null kidneys. Trps1-null mutant kidneys are hypoplastic and distinctively lacking glomeruli and renal tubules. Renal vesicle formation is distinctively compromised in the absence of Trps1, with a concomitant depletion of the cap mesenchyme. In cultured MM cells, the increased expression of E-cadherin following BMP7 stimulation is inhibited upon RNA interference–mediated knockdown of Trps1. Altogether these studies suggest that BMP7 acting through Trps1 is important for epithelialization of the cap mesenchyme.

The more primitive progenitors within the condensed mesenchyme express high levels of Cited1 and proliferate in a BMP7-dependent manner.[233] In response to BMP7, these Cited1-positive cells begin expressing Six2 and acquire responsiveness to Wnt9b. The exact role of Cited1 in the condensing mesenchyme remains poorly understood because Cited1- and compound Cited1/Cited2-knockout kidneys have apparently intact mesenchyme-to-epithelial transitions. It is not clear, however, whether the closely related Cited4 is upregulated and functionally compensates in the absence of Cited1 and Cited2.[234] Genetic inactivation of Six2 causes premature and ectopic nephrogenesis.[19,235] The precocious epithelialization combined with increased incidence of apoptosis in Six2-deficient cap mesenchyme rapidly depletes the pool of nephrogenic precursors. The defective maintenance of nephrogenic precursors impairs reciprocal inductive interactions between the cap mesenchyme and the UB, causing overall stunting of kidney growth. Overexpression of Six2, on the other hand, prevented epithelial differentiation of the cap mesenchyme. Six2, therefore, is required to maintain the undifferentiated, self-renewing progenitor states of nephron precursors. Nevertheless, epithelialization in Six2-null mutants remains dependent on Wnt9b induction.[19] In the absence of Wnt signaling, Six2 constitutively represses expression of renal vesicle markers within nephron progenitors.[223] In response to Wnt induction, Six2 forms a complex with β-catenin and Lef/Tcf factors that regulate the expression of multiple genes required to coordinate mesenchyme-to-epithelial transition, including the upregulation of Pax8, Fgf8, Wnt4, and Lhx1 and the attenuation of Six2 expression. A fine-tuned activity of Six2 is therefore required to balance the maintenance of a pool of self-renewing nephron progenitors and to prime these progenitors for commitment to an epithelial fate via a canonical Wnt-dependent pathway.

The multidomain scaffolding proteins Dlg1 and CASK, members of the MAGUK (membrane-associated guanylate kinase) family of proteins, have been shown to be important in maintenance of nephron progenitor cells.[236] Dlg1 and CASK prominently localize at the plasma membranes of polarized cells, where they coordinate cell junction formation and assembly of protein complexes that regulate cell polarity.[237] In neurons, they are known to be important for organization of synapses.[238] The global deletion of Dlg1 and Cask in mice led to severe renal hypoplasia and dysplasia with notable loss of the nephrogenic zone.[236] This renal phenotype was fully recapitulated when Dlg1 and Cask were removed conditionally using either Pax3-Cre or Six2-Cre, suggesting that the defects are inherent within the MM compartment, particularly the nephrogenic precursors. Although UB branching was also decreased in the global and MM double-knockout mice, this defect proved to be secondary to depletion of the nephrogenic zone, because targeted ablation of Dlg1 and Cask in the ureteric lineage using HoxB7-Cre did not cause renal hypoplasia or abnormal renal histology. Significantly diminished cell proliferation and increased apoptosis were observed in the nephrogenic zone in the absence of Dlg1 and Cask. Consistent with the loss of the nephrogenic zone is the decreased expression of BMP7, Cited1, Six2, and FGF8. GDNF expression is also notably decreased, a finding that could explain the secondary impairment in ureteric branching. The concomitant reduction in BMP7 and FGF8 levels correlates with the dampening of signaling events downstream of Ras, including Erk, Jnk, and p38 MAPK pathways, possibly accounting for the loss of cell proliferation in the nephrogenic zone of Dlg1/Cask double-knockout mice.

The extracellular cues regulating Dlg1 and CASK functions in the nephrogenic mesenchyme are not yet clear. One possibility invoked is the interaction between Dlg1 and CASK with the FGF pathway via syndecan-2.[237] FGF2 is known to mediate condensation of the MM, whereas FGF8 is important for transition to Wnt4-expressing pretubular aggregates and renal vesicles.[215,239] FGF9 and FGF20, on the other hand, are important to maintain the stemness of nephron progenitors.[230] The corresponding receptors, FGFR1 and FGFR2, are crucial for the survival of the MM without which renal agenesis ensues.[240] Dlg1 and CASK are also likely to mitigate the proper migration and condensation of the nephron precursors around the UB. In compound heterozygous/homozygous Dlg1/Cask knockout subjects, kidneys were only modestly hypoplastic but showed a distinctively loose aggregation of Six2-expressing condensing mesenchyme.[236] This result is consistent with those of other studies showing that Dlg1 is important for directed cell migration of Schwann cells.[241,242]

MOLECULAR BIOLOGY OF NEPHRON DEVELOPMENT: TUBULOGENESIS

Gene targeting and other analyses have identified many genes involved in the initial induction of the metanephric kidney and the formation of the pretubular aggregate, but much less is currently known about how the pretubular aggregate develops into a mature nephron, a process through which a simple tubule elongates, convolutes, and differentiates into multiple distinct segments with different functions. Discussions of how this segmentation occurs have considered whether similarities will be found to other aspects of development, such as the limb or neural tube, where there is segmentation along various axes.

The Notch group of signaling molecules has been implicated in directing segmentation of the nephron. Notch family members are transmembrane proteins, the cytoplasmic domains of which are cleaved by the γ-secretase enzyme upon the interaction of the extracellular domain with transmembrane ligand proteins of the Delta and Jagged families, found on adjacent cells.[243] Thus, Notch signaling occurs between adjacent cells, in contrast to signaling by secreted growth factors, which may occur at a distance from the growth factor–expressing cells. The cleaved portion of the Notch cytoplasmic domain translocates to the nucleus, where it has a role in directing gene expression. Mice homozygous for a hypomorphic allele of *Notch2* have abnormal glomeruli, with a failure to form a mature capillary tuft.[244,245] Because null mutants of Notch family members usually result in early embryonic death, further analysis of Notch family function in kidney development has made use of the organ culture model.

When metanephric rudiments were cultured in the presence of a γ-secretase inhibitor,[31,246] expression of podocyte and proximal tubule markers was diminished in comparison with expression of distal tubule markers and branching of the UB. When the γ-secretase inhibitor was removed, there seemed to be a better recovery of expression of proximal tubule markers than of podocyte differentiation markers. Similar results were observed in mice carrying targeted mutation of the *Psen1* and *Psen2* genes that encode a component of the γ-secretase complex.[247] Conditional deletion of *Notch2* in the MM resulted in hypoplastic kidneys that did not develop glomeruli and proximal tubules, despite the presence of distal tubules and collecting ducts. Interestingly, the condensed mesenchyme and pretubular aggregates initiated epithelialization expressing Pax2 and E-cadherin but did not proceed to form S-shaped bodies. By contrast, Notch1-deficient metanephroi are phenotypically wild type, suggesting that Notch1 is not critical for cell fate determination during early nephron formation. Taken together, these studies seem to indicate that local activation of Notch2 during tubule morphogenesis is critical to determining the proximal cell fate after the epithelialization of renal vesicle.[248] The transcription factor Rbpj, the homolog of the *Drosophila* gene Suppressor of Hairless, is a transducer of canonical Notch signaling. Genetic inactivation of *Rbpj* in the MM leads to pronounced renal hypoplasia characterized by significant paucity in nephrons and the development of tubular cysts.[248,249] Fate mapping analyses reveal that Rbpj-deficient nephrogenic precursors develop into podocytes and distal tubules but not proximal tubules.[249] These findings further reiterate the crucial importance of canonical Notch signaling via Rbpj in the specification of the proximal segment of nephrons and the likelihood that Notch signaling independent of Rbpj arbitrates the determination of podocyte fate. Consistently, overexpression of the constitutively active Notch1 intracellular domain (N1ICD) drives the acquisition of proximal tubule fate in nephron precursors but inhibits the development of podocytes.[248]

The specification of the distal nephron fate requires the POU domain–containing transcription factor Pou3f3 (Brn1) and the metalloprotease genes *Adamts1* and *Adamts4*.[250,251] The proneural basic helix-loop-helix (bHLH) factor Ascl1 (MASH1) binds cooperatively with Pou3f3 and the related Pou3f2 (Brn2) to the promoter of the Notch ligand Delta1 to synergistically activate the transcription of Delta1 and stimulate neurogenesis.[252] Whether Pou3f3 is involved in regulation of Notch signaling in renal development is not clear. Germline deletion of *Pou3f3* results in defective patterning of the distal nephron segments.[251] Pou3f3 expression is first detectable in renal vesicles and becomes localized to the distal aspects of the comma- and S-shaped bodies, regions destined to become the distal convoluted tubules, the macula densa, and the loop of Henle. Without Pou3f3, elongation of prospective loop of Henle and overall maturation of distal nephron segments are arrested. Although the development of glomeruli, proximal tubules, and collecting ducts is seemingly not affected by the absence of Pou3f3, the severity of the distal nephron abnormalities causes renal insufficiency and perinatal death. The products of *Adamts1* and *Adamts4* are secreted thrombospondin domain–containing metalloproteases known to cleave a class of proteoglycans called *lecticans*. Null mutation of *Adamts1* in mice leads to hydronephrosis and is characterized by the thinning of the renal medulla and a distinctive paucity in the loops of Henle.[250,253] Lack of *Adamts4* appears benign but can exacerbate the simplification of the renal medulla due to loss of *Adamts1*.[254] As a consequence, mice with a compound null mutation of *Adamts1* and *Adamts4* mostly perish perinatally. This finding suggests that *Adamts1* and *Adamts4* have overlapping importance in the development of the distal nephron segment by a mechanism yet to be identified.

There is one example so far of a transcription factor involved in the differentiation of a specific cell type in the kidney. The phenotype is actually found in the collecting ducts, rather than in the nephron itself, but is discussed in this section because it is demonstrative of the kinds of phenotypes expected to be found as additional mutant mice are examined. Two cell types are normally found in the collecting ducts—principal cells, which mediate water and salt reabsorption, and intercalated cells, which mediate acid-base transport. In the absence of the Foxi1 transcription factor, only one cell type is present in collecting ducts, and many acid-base transport proteins normally expressed by intercalated cells are absent.[255]

In addition to cell differentiation, spatial orientation of cells is essential for tubule elongation and morphogenesis. In epithelia, cells are uniformly organized along an apical-basal plane of polarity. However, in addition, cells in most tissues require positional information in the plane perpendicular to the apical-basal axis. This type of polarization, referred to as *planar cell polarity*, is critical for morphogenesis of metazoans.[256,257] A study using cell lineage analysis and close examination of the mitotic axis of dividing cells has shown that lengthening of renal tubules is associated with mitotic orientation of cells along the tubule axis, demonstrating intrinsic planar cell polarity.[192] Dysregulation of oriented cell division can give rise to cysts as a result of abnormal widening of tubule diameters.[258] To date, molecules implicated in planar cell polarity and tubule elongation include HNF1β-PKHD axis, Fat4, and Wnt9b.[191,192,259-263]

MOLECULAR GENETICS OF THE STROMAL CELL LINEAGE

The maintenance of reiterative ureteric branching and concomitant nephron induction largely accounts for the growth and enlargement of embryonic kidneys. Genetic studies reveal that interstitial stroma provides additional inductive cues that regulate UB branching and nephrogenesis (see Figure 1.15). These studies also underscore the pivotal role played by the stroma in establishing the stereotypical radial patterning of the kidney. In embryonic kidneys, the stroma is organized into two distinct zones, an outer stromal region within the nephrogenic zone expressing the winged helix transcription factor Foxd1/BF-2, and a deeper region expressing the basic helix-loop-helix transcription factor Tcf21 (Pod1/capsulin/epicardin).[22,23,264,265] Without either Foxd1 or Tcf21, UB branching and nephrogenesis are notably impaired, resulting in a distinctive perturbation of the corticomedullary renal histoarchitecture.[22,23,264]

The most prominent features of the genetic loss of Foxd1 include the thickening of the renal capsule and the formation of large metanephric mesenchymal condensates.[22,266] The morphologically altered renal capsule in *Foxd1* mutant kidneys has notably lost expression of *Aldh1a2/Raldh2* and *Sfrp1* (a regulator of Wnt signaling) and is abnormally interspersed with endothelial cells and Bmp4-positive cells.[266] The identity of these Bmp4-expressing cells populating the renal capsule in Foxd1-deficient kidneys is unknown, although on the basis of lineage tracing for Foxd1-promoter expression, the cells are clearly distinct from the presumptive medullary stroma. Bmp4 is a known chemotactic agent for endothelial cells,[267] so it is very likely that the ectopic Bmp4-positive cells account for the presence of endothelial cells within the broadened renal capsule of *Foxd1* mutant kidneys. The accumulation of the cap mesenchyme is also likely contributed in part by ectopic Bmp4 signaling in the absence of Foxd1, because Bmp4 has been shown to antagonize epithelialization of the cap mesenchyme.[267] Transcriptome analysis shows that the gene *Dcn*, which encodes for the collagen-binding proteoglycan decorin, is a specific target that is repressed by Foxd1 in the cortical interstitium.[268] *Dcn* expression is normally localized within the medullary stroma but is normally absent in the cortical stroma of wild-type kidneys. In the absence of Foxd1, decorin becomes abundantly expressed in the presumptive cortical stromal region. Functional cell-culture–based assays and epithelialization assays of mesenchymal aggregates demonstrate that decorin inhibits Bmp7 signaling and mesenchyme-to-epithelial transformation. The antagonistic effect of decorin on epithelial differentiation is further enhanced in vitro when the mesenchymal aggregates are grown in collagen IV, thus recapitulating the persistence of the cap mesenchyme as seen in Foxd1 mutant kidneys, in which both decorin and collagen IV are upregulated in the cortical interstitium. These findings are corroborated by the partial rescue of the *Foxd1*-null phenotype through genetic inactivation of *Dcn*.

Tcf21 (also called Pod1) is expressed in the medullary stroma as well as in the condensing MM.[264,265] Tcf21 is also expressed in a number of differentiated renal cell types that derive from these mesenchymal cells and include developing and mature podocytes of the renal glomerulus, cortical and medullary peritubular interstitial cells, pericytes surrounding small renal vessels, and adventitial cells surrounding larger blood vessels (see Figure 1.6).[193] The defect in nephrogenesis observed in *Tcf21*-null mice is similar to the defect seen in *Foxd1*-knockout mice, consisting of disruption of branching morphogenesis with associated arrest and delay in nephrogenesis. Analysis of chimeric mice derived from *Tcf21* mutant embryonic stem cells and EGFP-expressing embryos demonstrated both cell-autonomous and non–cell-autonomous roles for Tcf21 in nephrogenesis.[269] Most strikingly, the glomerulogenesis defect was rescued by the presence of wild-type stromal cells (i.e., mutant cells will epithelialize and form nephrons normally as long as they are surrounded by wild-type stromal cells). In addition, there is a cell-autonomous requirement for Tcf21 in stromal mesenchymal cells to allow differentiation into interstitial and pericyte cell lineages of the cortex and medulla, because Tcf21-null ES cells were unable to contribute to these populations.

Although many of the defects in the *Tcf21* mutant kidneys phenocopy those seen in the *Foxd1* mutant kidneys, there are important differences. Kidneys from *Tcf21*-null mice have vascular anomalies and defective pericyte differentiation that were not reported in *Foxd1* mutant mice. These differences might result from the broader domain of Tcf21 expression, which includes the condensing mesenchyme, podocytes, and medullary stromal cells in addition to the stromal cells that surround the condensates. In contrast to Foxd1, Tcf21 is not highly expressed in the thin rim of stromal cells found immediately beneath the capsule, suggesting that Foxd1 and Tcf21 might mark early and late stromal cell lineages, respectively, with overlap in the stroma that surrounds the condensates.[23] However, definitive co-labeling studies to address this issue have not been performed. Both Tcf21 and Foxd1 are transcription factors so it is interesting to speculate that they might interact or regulate the expression of a common stromal "inducing factor."

Retinoids secreted by the renal stroma are also recognized as important for the maintenance of a high level of Ret receptor expression in the UB tip, promoting the proliferation of UB epithelial cells and the growth of the ureteric tree.[9,270-272] One study concluded that the defective UB branching seen in *Foxd1*-null mutants is most likely a direct consequence of the loss of cortical expression of *Aldh1a2*, a gene involved in retinol (vitamin A) synthesis.[266] A later study has shown that renal stroma immediately around the UB tips is also important in regulating the bifurcation of the tips and the creation of new UB branches.[273] Autocrine retinoid signaling in the stromal cells juxtaposed to the UB tips stimulates the expression of extracellular matrix 1 (Ecm1). Ecm1 is specifically expressed at the UB cleft, where it suppresses and restricts Ret expression domains within the UB tips. In the absence of Ecm1, Ret expression in the UB tips

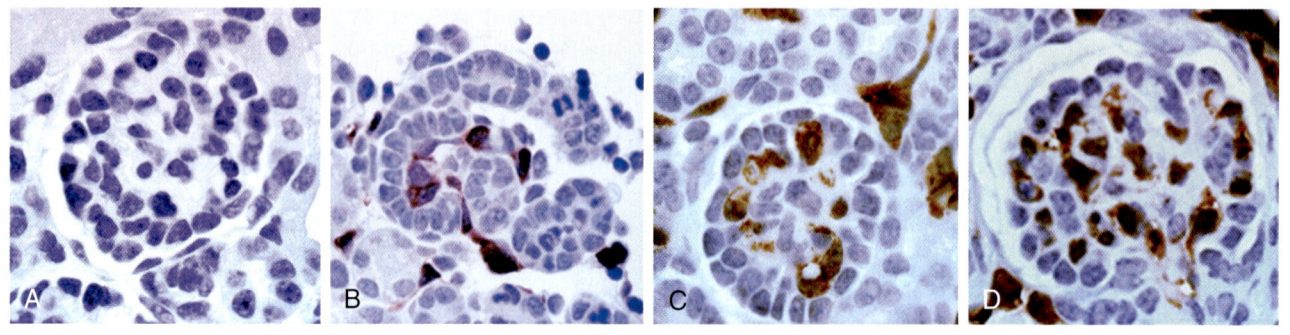

Figure 1.16 Developing glomeruli stained with an antibody to green fluorescent protein (GFP). Control glomerulus from a wild-type mouse. **A,** Comma-shaped body; **B,** S-shaped body; **C,** capillary loop stage; and **D,** mature glomeruli in the metanephros of an 18 dpc Flk1-GFP mouse strain. All endothelial cells express the GFP protein that is expressed under control of the endogenous Flk1/VEGFR2 promoter. (Reproduced with permission from the *Journal of American Society of Nephrology*.)

broadens, effectively attenuating UB branching through impaired formation of UB bifurcation clefts. Thus, stromal retinoids promote and confine Ret expression domains and, more likely, cell proliferation patterns within the UB tips.

A 2013 study has provided valuable insight into how stroma-based signaling intersects with UB-derived inductive cues to promote proper differentiation of the nephrogenic mesenchyme.[274] When the stromal lineage is selectively annihilated by Foxd1-Cre–driven expression of diphtheria toxin, the zone of condensing mesenchymal cells capping the UBs is abnormally broadened but the development of pretubular aggregates is strongly hindered. These findings reiterate those previously described in *Foxd1*-null mice, suggesting that regulation of nephrogenesis involves a crosstalk between stroma and UB-derived inductive signals. In particular, it was shown that Fat4-dependent Hippo signaling initiated by the stroma integrates with canonical Wnt signaling derived from the ureteric lineage in order to balance nephron precursor propagation and differentiation. The absence of Fat4 in the stromal compartment phenocopies the expansion of the nephrogenic precursor domain and failed epithelial differentiation of nephron progenitors seen in stroma-deficient kidneys. It was postulated that Fat4 acting through the Hippo pathway promotes the differentiation of the epithelial transition of nephrogenic precursors. This possibility was further reiterated by the rescue of the depletion of nephrogenic precursors by Fat4 deficiency in *Wnt9b*-knockout mice. Interestingly, the ablation of Vangl2, a signaling partner of Fat4 known to regulate renal tubular diameter,[259] fails to rescue the loss of nephron progenitors in *Wnt9b*-knockout animals, suggesting that Fat4-mediated signaling during early differentiation of nephrogenic precursors is independent of the planar cell polarity pathway.[274]

MOLECULAR GENETICS OF VASCULAR FORMATION

Vasculogenesis and angiogenesis both contribute to vascular development within the kidney. Endothelial cells may be identified through the expression of the tyrosine kinase receptor, VEGFR2 (Flk1/KDR).[275] Reporter mouse strains that carry β-galactosidase (lacZ) or GFP cDNA cassettes "knocked into" the *Vegfr2* locus permit precise snapshots of vessel development, because all the vascular progenitor and differentiated cells in these organs can be visualized either colorimetrically (with a β-galactosidase substrate) or by fluorescence (Figure 1.16). Use of other knock-in strains allows identification of endothelial cells lining arteriolar or venous vessels.[276]

Over the past decade, a number of growth factors and their receptors have been identified that are required for vasculogenesis and angiogenesis. Gene deletion studies in mice have shown that VEGF-A and its cognate receptor VEGFR2 are essential for vasculogenesis.[275,277] Mice that are null for the *Vegfa* gene die at 9.5 dpc from a failure of vasculogenesis, whereas mice lacking a single *Vegfa* allele (i.e., they are heterozygous for the *Vegfa* gene) die at 11.5 dpc, also from vascular defects.[277] These data demonstrate gene dosage sensitivity to VEGF-A during development. In the developing kidney, podocytes and renal tubular epithelial cells express VEGF-A and continue to express it constitutively in the adult kidney, whereas the cognate tyrosine kinase receptors for VEGF-A, VEGFR1 (Flt1), and VEGFR2 (Flk1/KDR) are predominantly expressed by all endothelial cells.[278] Which non-endothelial cells might also express the VEGF receptors in the kidney in vivo is still debated, although renal cell lines clearly do and MM cells express VEGFR2 in organ culture as outlined earlier.

Conditional gene targeting experiments and cell-selective deletion of *Vegfa* from podocytes demonstrated that VEGF-A signaling is required for formation and maintenance of the glomerular filtration barrier.[279,280] Glomerular endothelial cells express VEGFR2 as they migrate into the vascular cleft. Although a few endothelia migrated into the developing glomeruli of *Vegfa* podocyte conditional knockout mutants (likely because of a small amount of VEGF-A produced by presumptive podocytes at the S-shaped stage of glomerular development prior to Cre-mediated genetic deletion), the endothelia failed to develop fenestrations and rapidly disappeared, leaving capillary "ghosts" (Figure 1.17). Similar to the dosage sensitivity observed in the whole embryo, deletion of a single *Vegfa* allele from podocytes also led to glomerular endothelial defects known as endotheliosis that progressed to end-stage kidney failure at 3 months of age. As the dose of VEGF-A decreased, the associated endothelial phenotypes became more severe (Figure 1.18). Upregulation of the major angiogenic VEGF-A isoform (VEGFA[164]) in developing podocytes of transgenic mice led to massive proteinuria and collapse of the glomerular tuft by 5 days of age. Taken together, these results show a requirement for

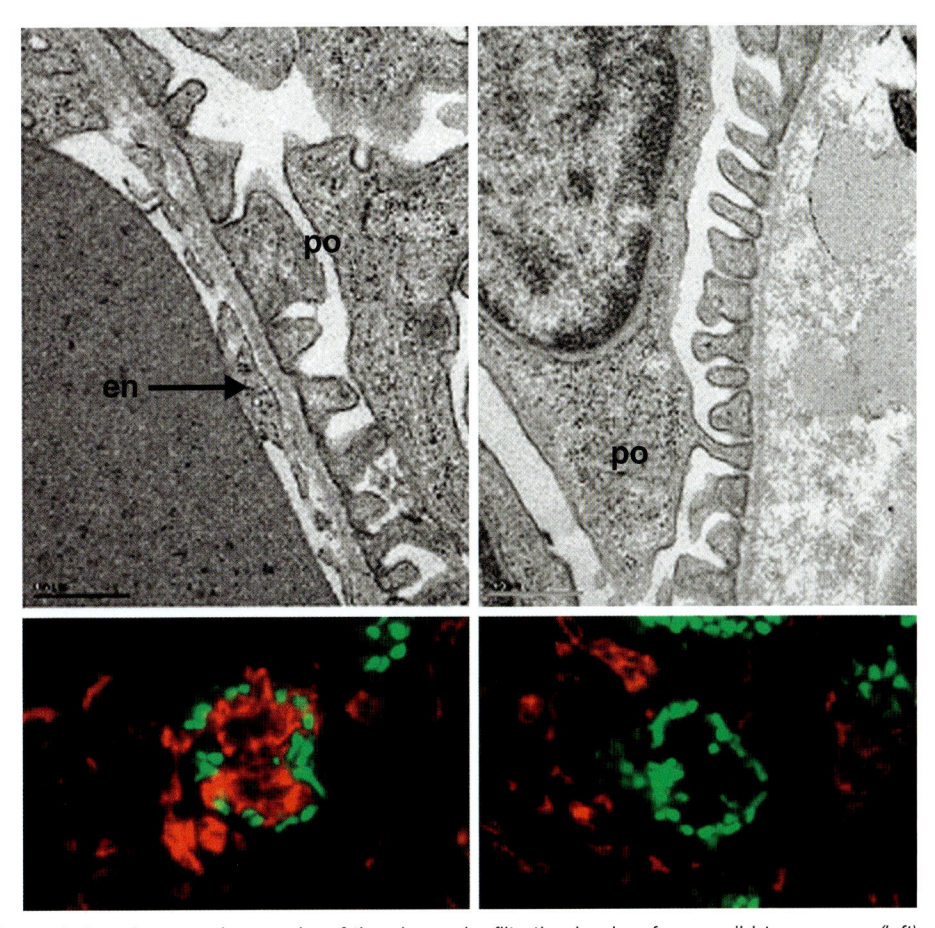

Figure 1.17 **Top,** Transmission electron micrographs of the glomerular filtration barriers from a wild-type mouse *(left)* and from a transgenic mouse with selective knockout of VEGF from the podocytes *(right)*. Podocytes (po) are seen in both but the endothelial layer (en) is entirely missing from the knockout mouse, leaving a "capillary ghost." **Bottom,** Immunostaining of the barriers for WT1 (podocytes/*green*) and PECAM (endothelial cells/*red*) confirms the absence of capillary wall in VEGF knockouts. (Adapted from Eremina V, Sood M, Haigh J, et al: Glomerular-specific alterations of VEGF-A expression lead to distinct congenital and acquired renal diseases. *J Clin Invest* 111:707-716, 2003.)

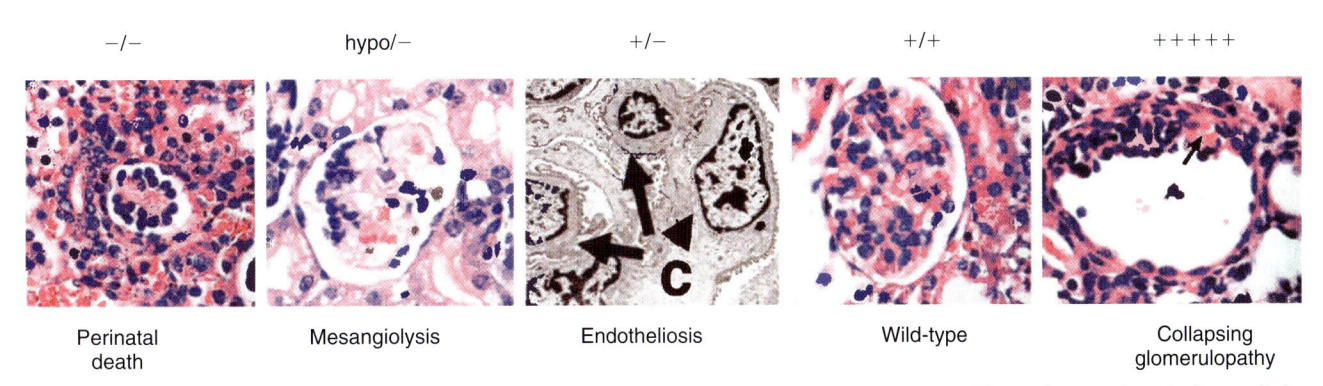

Figure 1.18 Effect of vascular endothelial growth factor dose on glomerular development. Photomicrographs of glomeruli from mice carrying different copy numbers of the VEGF gene within podocytes. A total knockout (loss of both alleles, –/–) results in failure of glomerular filtration barrier formation and perinatal death. A single hypomorphic allele (hypo/–) leads to massive mesangiolysis in the first weeks of life and death at 3 weeks of age. Loss of one copy (+/–) results in endotheliosis (swelling of the endothelium) and death at 12 weeks of age. Overexpression (20-fold increase in VEGF, +++++) results in collapsing glomerulopathy. (Adapted from Eremina V et al: Role of the VEGF-A signaling pathway in the glomerulus: evidence for crosstalk between components of the glomerular filtration barrier. *Nephron Physiol* 106:32-37, 2007.)

VEGF-A for development and maintenance of the specialized glomerular endothelia and demonstrate a major paracrine signaling function for VEGF-A in the glomerulus. Furthermore, tight regulation of the dose of VEGF-A is essential for proper formation of the glomerular capillary system. The molecular basis and mechanism of dosage sensitivity are unclear at present and are particularly intriguing, given the documented inducible regulation of VEGF-A by hypoxia-inducible factors (HIFs) at a transcriptional level. Nevertheless, it is clear that in vivo, a single *Vegfa* allele is unable to compensate for loss of the other. Immortalized podocyte cell lines express a variety of VEGF receptors, opening up the possibility that VEGF-A also plays an autocrine role in the developing glomerulus.[281-283] However, the functional relevance of these findings for the glomerulus in vivo is unclear at present.

A second major RTK signaling pathway required for maturation of developing blood vessels is the angiopoietin-Tie signaling system. Angiopoietin 1 (Angpt1) stabilizes newly formed blood vessels and is associated with loss of vessel plasticity and concurrent recruitment of pericytes or vascular support cells to the vascular wall.[284] The molecular switch or pathway leading to vessel maturation through activation of Tie2 (previously known as Tek), the major receptor for Angpt1, is not known and appears to be independent of the PDGF (platelet-derived growth factor) signaling system that is also required for pericyte recruitment. The importance of Angpt1 in promoting the development of the renal microvasculature was first suggested on the basis of observations that exogenous Angpt1 enhanced the growth of interstitial capillaries in mouse metanephric organ cultures.[285] Because *Angpt1*-null mice perish embryonically at around 12.5 dpc, the in vivo role of Angpt1 during renal development was gleaned through the use of an inducible knockout strategy.[286,287] Ablation of *Angpt1* at around 10.5 dpc resulted in general dilation of renal blood vessels, including the glomerular capillaries sometimes observed as simplified single enlarged loops.[286] A marked reduction of mesangial cells was also observed in *Angpt1*-deficient mutants. Without Angpt1, a few endothelial cells are seen to detach from the GBM, although the GBM itself appears otherwise normal directly beneath the podocytes, suggesting that the endothelium is primarily affected by loss of Angpt1.

In contrast, it is proposed that angiopoietin 2 (Angpt2) functions as a natural antagonist of the Tie2 receptor, because Angpt2 can bind to this receptor but fails to induce Tie2 phosphorylation in endothelial cultures.[288,289] Consistent with this hypothesis is the fact that overexpression of Angpt2 in transgenic mice resulted in a phenotype similar to the *Angpt1* or *Tie2* knockout mice. Angpt1, Angpt2, Tie2, and the orphan receptor Tie1 have all been shown to be expressed in the developing kidney.[290-294] Whereas Angpt1 is quite broadly expressed in condensing mesenchyme, podocytes, and tubular epithelial cells, Angpt2 is more restricted to pericytes and smooth muscle cells surrounding cortical and large vessels as well as in the mesangium. In one study, *Angpt2*-null mice were viable but exhibited defects in peritubular cortical capillary development; the mice died prior to differentiation of vasa recta, precluding analysis of the role of Angpt2 in these other capillary beds.[295] Podocyte-specific overexpression of Angpt2 has been found to cause proteinuria and increased apoptosis in glomerular capillaries.[296] Both angiopoietin ligands function in concert with VEGF, although the precise degree of crosstalk between these pathways is still under investigation. VEGF and Angpt2, for example, have been shown to cooperate in promoting endothelial sprouting. Chimeric studies showed that Tie1 is required for the development of the glomerular capillary system because *Tie1*-null cells failed to incorporate into the glomerular endothelium.[297]

The Ephrin-Eph family is a third tyrosine kinase–dependent growth factor signaling system that is expressed in the developing kidney; in the whole embryo, it is involved in neural sprouting and axon finding as well as in the specification of arterial and venous components of the vasculature.[298,299] Ephrins and their cognate receptors are expressed widely during renal development. Overexpression of EphB4 leads to defects in glomerular arteriolar formation, whereas conditional deletion of EphrinB2 from perivascular smooth muscle cells and mesangial cells results in glomerular vascular abnormalities.[300,301] How this latter effect occurs is not entirely clear because EphrinB2 has a dynamic pattern of expression in the developing glomerulus, beginning in podocyte precursors and rapidly switching to glomerular endothelial cells and mesangial cells.[276]

Dysregulation of BMP within the podocyte compartment also results in glomerular vascular defects. Overexpression of BMP4 leads to defects in endothelial and mesangial recruitment, and overexpression of noggin, a natural BMP2 antagonist, results in collapse of the glomerular tuft.[302,303] *Bmp4* haploinsufficiency, on the other hand, leads to dysplastic kidneys and glomerular cysts with collapsed capillary tufts.[303] Additional studies are required to fully understand the role of this family of growth factors in glomeruli.

An additional pathway that is likely to play a role in glomerular endothelial development and perhaps in development of the entire renal vasculature is the SDF1-CXCR4 axis. CXCR4, a G protein–coupled chemokine receptor, is expressed by bone marrow–derived cells but also by endothelial cells. SDF1 (CXCL12), the only known ligand for CXCR4, is expressed in a dynamic segmental pattern in podocytes and later in the mesangial cells of the glomerulus.[304] Embryonic deletion of either *Cxcl12* or *Cxcr4* does not preclude nephrogenesis but results in defective formation of blood vessels, notably an abnormal patterning of the renal vasculature and the development of a simplified and dilated glomerular capillary tuft.[305] Interestingly, genetic loss of CXCR7, which is thought to act as a decoy receptor for SDF1, phenocopies defective development seen in *Cxcl12* and *Cxcr4* mutant mice. Unlike CXCR4, CXCR7 is specifically expressed by podocytes and not endothelial cells.[306] It has been proposed that CXCR7, acting as a scavenger receptor, establishes an SDF1 morphogen gradient, preventing feedback inhibition of CXCR4 receptor expression in target cells such as the endothelium.[306] Consistent with this proposal, inactivation of *Cxcr7* distinctively causes downregulation of CXCR4 expression in the renal cap mesenchyme and the glomerular tuft. Thus, the spatial regulation of SDF1-CXCR4 signaling appears to be important for normal development of the glomerular vasculature.

The T-box transcription factor Tbx18 is strongly expressed during early urogenital tract development in the ureteral mesenchyme and in a subset of kidney stromal mesenchyme originating from Foxd1-positive precursor cells.[307,308] Later in renal development, Tbx18 expression is also found in the renal capsule, vascular smooth muscle cells, pericytes, mesangial cells, and the mesenchyme surrounding the renal papillae and calyces.[308] The most overt phenotype of Tbx18 inactivation is the onset of hydronephrosis and hydroureter due to impaired development of the ureteral smooth muscle cells.[307,309] This finding underscores the importance of Tbx18 in the normal differentiation of the ureteral mesenchyme. A detailed phenotypic characterization of *Tbx18*-null mutant kidneys reveals an additional significance of this transcription factor in the overall development of the renal vasculature.[308] The branching and overall density of the renal vasculature are notably reduced in the absence of Tbx18. Tbx18 is also specifically required in the normal development of the glomerular microvasculature. Loss of Tbx18 causes significant oligonephronia and dilation of glomerular capillaries. These vascular phenotypes likely result from the degeneration of the vascular mesenchyme and the failure to sustain the proliferation of mesangial precursors.

Mice carrying a hypomorphic allele of Notch2 that is missing two epidermal growth factor (EGF) motifs are born with a reduced number of glomeruli that also lack both endothelial and mesangial cells, as discussed in the section on nephron segmentation.[243,244] The transcription factor Rbpj, a common downstream target of Notch signaling pathways, has also been described as crucial to the proper development of the renal vasculature and the glomerular mesangium. Conditional inactivation of Rbpj in the Foxd1-expressing stromal lineage leads to profound renal maldevelopment and early postnatal death.[310] Rbpj deficiency in the renal stroma results in poor branching and simplification of the renal vascular network. Rbpj conditional mutant kidneys have a greater proportion of larger vessels and a concomitant reduction in microvascular density. Glomeruli are dilated and lack mesangial cells in Rbpj conditional knockout animal. Furthermore, loss of Rbpj results in loss of renin cells, abnormal thickening of blood vessels, and renal fibrosis. Altogether, these studies highlight the distinctive significance of Notch signaling in the establishment and organization of the renal vasculature.

Two transcription factors belonging to the large Sry-related HMG box (Sox) gene family, named *Sox17* and Sox18, have distinctive and overlapping expressions in vascular endothelial cells.[311] Complete loss of Sox17 is embryonically lethal in mice owing to endodermal dysmorphogenesis.[312] In mice, *Sox18* ablation results in a mild coat defect but does not cause cardiovascular abnormalities.[313] Nevertheless, a point mutation in *SOX18* in humans has been implicated in HLT (hypotrichosis-lymphedema-telangiectasia) syndrome, which affects hair, lymph, and blood vessel vasculature.[314] The more severe consequence of the human *SOX18* mutation, in comparison with the null mutation in mice, has been suggested to be due to a dominant-negative effect. *Sox17*, however, shows haploinsufficiency in a homozygous *Sox18* mutant background, affecting neovascularization in kidneys, liver, and the reproductive system and causing early postnatal death.[311] Kidneys from $Sox17^{-/+}$:$Sox18^{-/-}$ mice have hypoplastic and atrophying medullary regions. In these compound *Sox17*/*Sox18* mutants, the radiating outer medullary vascular bundles of the vasa recta are completely absent without apparent abnormalities in the inner medullary or cortical regions. These defects within the outer medullary region result in variable degrees of hydronephrosis. In livers from these mice, Angpt2 expression is elevated whereas Angpt1 expression is significantly attenuated, although Tie2 receptor expression in unchanged. Because Angpt1 and Angpt2 have distinctive roles in endothelial sprouting, vascular stabilization, and remodeling,[315] it can be argued that Sox17 and Sox18 play redundant or synergistic roles in coordinating normal postnatal angiogenesis.

There is evidence from other model systems that vascular development is required for patterning and terminal differentiation of adjacent tissues. For example, vascular signals and basement membrane produced by adjacent endothelial cells are required for differentiation of the islet cells of the pancreas.[316,317] In the kidney, it is possible that vascular signals are required for branching morphogenesis and patterning of the nephron and that this requirement may explain some of the defects observed in mice such as the *Tcf21* mutants. Understanding co-patterning between the vasculature and its immediate neighbors will be a challenging task, given the complex nature of various tissue-tissue communications involved, although progress in this effort will likely be facilitated by a growing arsenal of genetic tools.

THE JUXTAGLOMERULAR APPARATUS AND THE RENIN ANGIOTENSIN ALDOSTERONE SYSTEM

The juxtaglomerular apparatus consists of juxtaglomerular cells that line the afferent arteriole, the macula densa cells of the distal tubule, and the extraglomerular mesangial cells that are in contact with intraglomerular mesangium.[318] Renin-expressing cells may be seen in arterioles in early mesonephric kidneys in 5-week human fetuses and in metanephric kidneys by week 8, at a stage prior to hemodynamic flow changes within the kidney. Gomez and colleagues generated a *Ren1*–knock-in mouse that expresses Cre recombinase in the renin locus.[319] Offspring of matings between the Ren1-Cre and a reporter strain that expresses β-galactosidase or GFP showed that renin-expressing cells reside within the MM and give rise not only to juxtaglomerular cells but also to mesangial cells, epithelial cells, and extrarenal cells, including interstitial Leydig cells of the XY gonad and cells within the adrenal gland. Although most of these cells cease to express renin in the adult, they appear to reexpress renin in stress conditions and are recruited to the afferent arteriole.

The only known substrate for renin, angiotensinogen, is converted to angiotensin I and angiotensin II by ACE.[320] The renin angiotensin aldosterone axis is required for normal renal development. In humans, the use of ACE inhibitors during pregnancy has been associated with congenital defects including renal anomalies.[321,322] Two subtypes of angiotensin receptors exist: AT1 receptors are responsible for most of the classically recognized functions of the RAAS including pressor effects and aldosterone release mediated through angiotensin; functions of the AT2 receptors have been more difficult to characterize but generally seem to oppose the actions of the AT1 receptors.[323] Genetic deletion of angiotensinogen or ACE results in hypotension and defects in formation of the renal papilla and pelvis.[202-205] Humans have one *AT1* gene whereas mice have two, *Agtr1a* and *Agtr1b*. Mice carrying a knockout for either AT1 receptor alone exhibit no major defects,[324,325] but the combined deficiency phenocopies the angiotensinogen and ACE phenotypes.[206,207] Although AT2 receptor expression is markedly upregulated in the embryonic kidney, genetic deletion of the AT2 receptor does not cause major impairment of renal development.[326,327] However, an association between AT2 receptor deficiency and malformations of the collecting system, including vesicoureteral reflux and ureteropelvic junction obstruction, has been reported.[328]

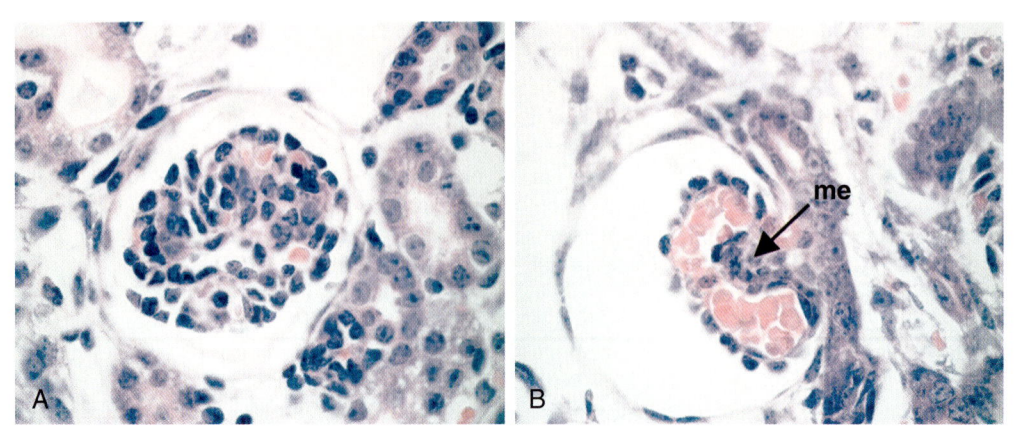

Figure 1.19 Glomeruli from a wild-type mouse **(A)** and a Tcf21 knockout mouse **(B)**. Note the dilated capillary loop and poor ingrowth of mesangial cells (me).

MiRNAs are regulatory RNAs that act as antisense post-transcriptional repressors by binding the 3′ untranslated region of target mRNAs. In eukaryotes, hundreds of miRNAs regulate the expression of thousands of mRNAs, thus implicating miRNAs in a myriad of events during development and disease including cell proliferation, differentiation, apoptosis, signaling and tumorigenicity. Dicer1 is an endoribonuclease that processes precursor miRNAs. Deletion of *Dicer1* from renin-expressing cells results in severe reduction in the number of juxtaglomerular cells, reduced renin production, and lower blood pressure. The kidney develops severe vascular abnormalities and striped fibrosis along the affected blood vessels, suggesting that miRNAs are required for normal morphogenesis and function of the kidney.[329]

Gene promoter analysis indicates that renin expression depends on the Notch signaling pathway. The intracellular domain of Notch (NIC) and the transcription factor Rbpj bind and cooperatively stimulate reporter gene expression from the renin promoter.[330] Genetic studies, however, indicate that Notch signaling has a broader role in the juxtaglomerular apparatus.[331] The conditional ablation of *Rbpj* in renin cells results in severe paucity of juxtaglomerular cells with consequential decrease in overall renin expression and the development of lower blood pressure. Lack of increase in apoptosis in *Rbpj* conditional mutant kidneys suggests that Rbpj may have altered the cell fate specification of renin cell precursors.

NEPHRON DEVELOPMENT AND GLOMERULOGENESIS

MESANGIAL CELL INGROWTH

Mesangial cells grow into the developing glomerulus and come to sit between the capillary loops. Gene deletion studies have demonstrated a critical role for PDGF-B/PDGFR-β signaling in this process. The absence of PDGF-B, which is expressed by glomerular endothelia, or of the receptor PDGFR-β, which is expressed by mesangial cells, results in glomeruli with single balloon-like capillary loops, instead of the intricately folded glomerular endothelial capillaries of wild-type kidneys. Furthermore, the glomeruli contain no mesangial cells.[332] Endothelial cell–specific deletion of *Pdgfb* results in the same glomerular phenotype and shows that production of PDGF-B by the endothelium is required for mesangial migration.[333] In turn, mesangial cells and the matrix they produce are required to pattern the glomerular capillary system. Loss of podocyte-derived factors such as VEGF-A also leads to failure of mesangial cell ingrowth, likely through primary loss of endothelial cells and failure of PDGF-B signaling.[280]

A number of other knockouts demonstrate defects in both vascular development and mesangial cell ingrowth. Loss of the transcription factors Tcf21 and Foxc2 causes defective migration of mesangial cells (Figure 1.19).[64,264] Mesangial abnormalities in *Tcf21-* and *Foxc2-*deficient mice are poorly understood in terms of the mesangium-specific transcriptional targets of Tcf21 and Foxc2. Nevertheless, these mutant phenotypes highlight the importance of cross-talk between cell compartments within the glomerulus.

GLOMERULAR EPITHELIAL DEVELOPMENT

Presumptive podocytes are located at the proximal end of the S-shaped body in apposition to the emerging vascular cleft (Figure 1.20). Immature podocytes are simple columnar epithelia expressing E-cadherin. Postmitotic mature podocytes, on the other hand, normally lose E-cadherin expression and atypically express vimentin, an intermediate filament protein more common among mesenchymal cells but absent in most epithelial cells. The most distinctive morphologic feature of a fully differentiated podocyte is its arborized and stellate appearance (Figure 1.21). Podocytes ensheathe the glomerular capillaries, with their foot processes effectively forming the final layer of the glomerular filtration barrier. Foot processes emanating from adjacent podocytes interdigitate in trans (i.e., a foot process from one podocyte is flanked by foot processes from its neighbouring podocyte) and form a unique and porous intercellular junction called the *slit diaphragm*, through which primary urinary filtrate passes.

The transcription factors WT1, Tcf21/Pod1, Mafb/Kreisler, Foxc2, and Lmx1b are highly expressed by developing podocytes and are important for the elaboration of podocyte foot processes and the establishment of slit diaphragms.[28,64,264,265,334,335] Complete loss of WT1 leads to renal agenesis.[28] However, specific loss of a WT1 splice isoform results in poor development of podocyte foot processes.[336] One study found that the *Wt1*-null phenotype in mice could also be rescued with use of a yeast artificial chromosome

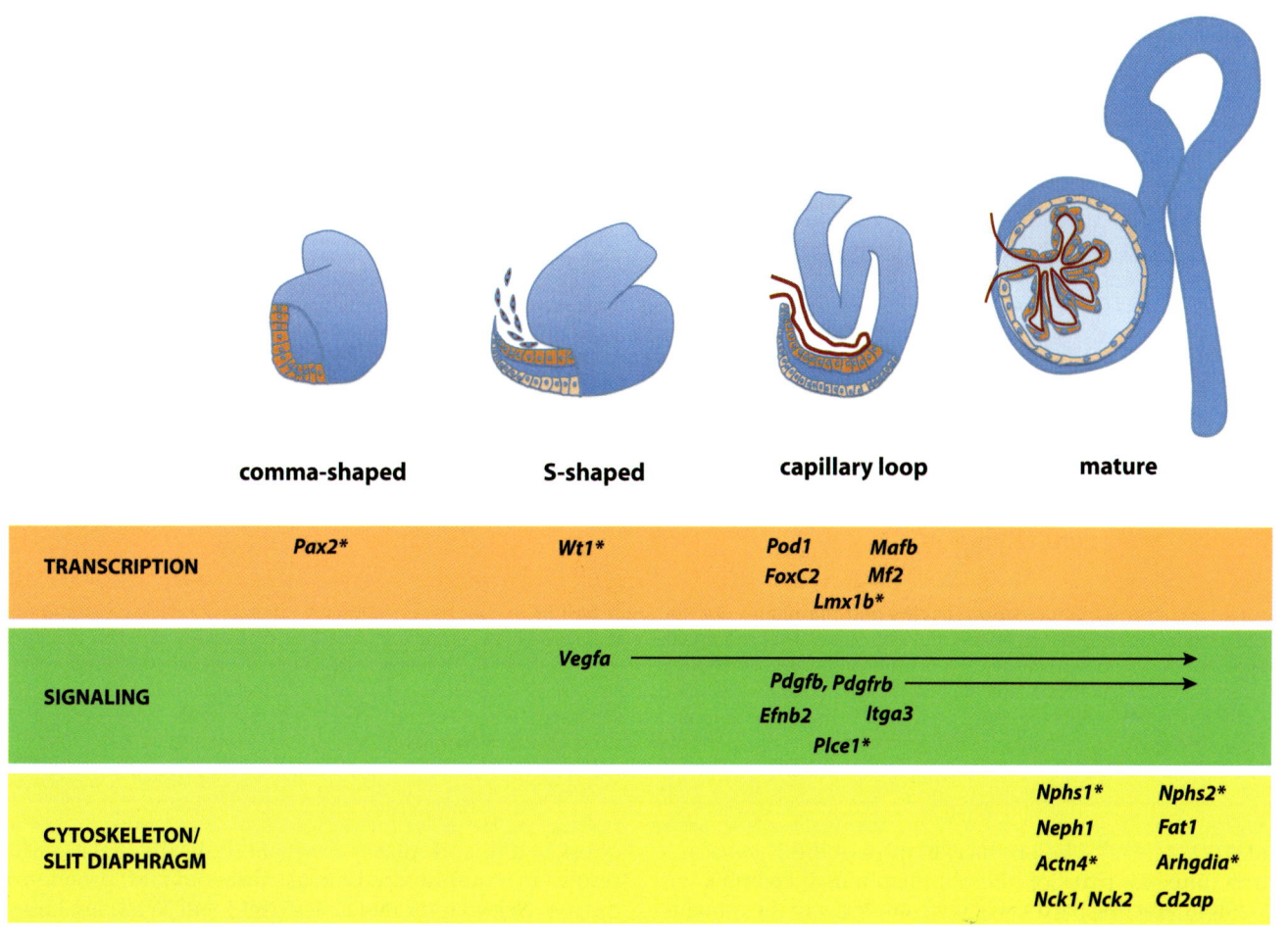

Figure 1.20 Molecular basis of glomerular development. Key factors are shown along with the time point where major effects were observed in knockout or transgenic mouse studies. Many factors play roles at more than one time point. Genes identified as mutated in patients with glomerular disease are marked by *asterisks*.

containing the human *Wt1* gene, and depending on the level of expression of *Wt1*, the mice developed a range of glomerular pathologies ranging from crescentic glomerulonephritis to mesangial sclerosis, clinical features observed in Denys-Drash syndrome arising from a mutant *WT1* allele in humans.[337] Transgenic mice expressing a Denys-Drash mutant *WT1* allele under the regulation of a podocyte-specific promoter also developed glomerular disease, with abnormalities observed in the adjacent endothelium.[338] Genetic inactivation of *Lmx1b*, *Tcf21*, *Mafb*, and *Foxc2* causes podocytes to remain as cuboidal epithelia and to fail to spread on the glomerular capillary bed.[64,264,335,339] Tcf21 likely acts upstream of Mafb, because the latter is downregulated in Tcf21-null mice.[335] Loss of Mafb and Lmx1b reduces the expression of Nphs1 (nephrin) and Nphs2 (podocin), whereas the absence of Foxc2 causes the specific downregulation of Nphs2 and α3α4α5 (IV) collagen.[64,335,340] *Lmx1b* mutations are linked to nail-patella syndrome in humans, with a subset of affected individuals manifesting nephrotic disease.[334,341] *WT1*, *Tcf21*, *Mafb*, *Foxc2*, and *Lmx1b* are expressed from the S-shaped stage onward and remain constitutively expressed in adult glomeruli. Proteinuria develops from loss of these genes, thus underscoring the importance of normal podocyte maturation in the establishment of the glomerular filtration barrier.

Genetic studies have also led to the identification of structural proteins crucial for normal podocyte function and the integrity of the glomerular filtration barrier. The seminal discoveries of the causal link between nephrotic diseases and mutations in podocyte-specific genes *NPHS1* and *NPHS2* set the stage for vigorous investigations that led to the appreciation of the key importance of podocytes in renal filtration.[342,343] Mutations in *NPHS1*, the gene that encodes for the protein nephrin, are associated with congenital nephropathy of the Finnish variety (CNF), a serious condition that requires early renal replacement therapy.[342] Glomeruli obtained from infants with CNF are devoid of slit diaphragms. Nephrin, a huge transmembrane adhesion molecule with multiple immunoglobulin-like motifs, has been shown to be a structural component of the slit diaphragm. *NPHS2*, whose product is the intracellular membrane–bound protein podocin, is the first gene identified as linked to steroid-resistant nephrotic syndrome (SRNS).[343] Podocin, which interacts with nephrin in cholesterol-rich membrane microdomains (also called *lipid rafts*), is also a vital and indispensable component of the slit diaphragm.[344-348] A number of other genes specifically expressed by podocytes have been associated with proteinuric diseases, including *CD2AP*, *Kirrel/Neph1*, *FAT1*, *ACTN4*, *TRPC6*, *MYO1E*, *ARHGAP24*, *ARHGDIA*, *Rhpn1*, *INF2*, *COQ2*, *COQ6*, *PLCE1*,

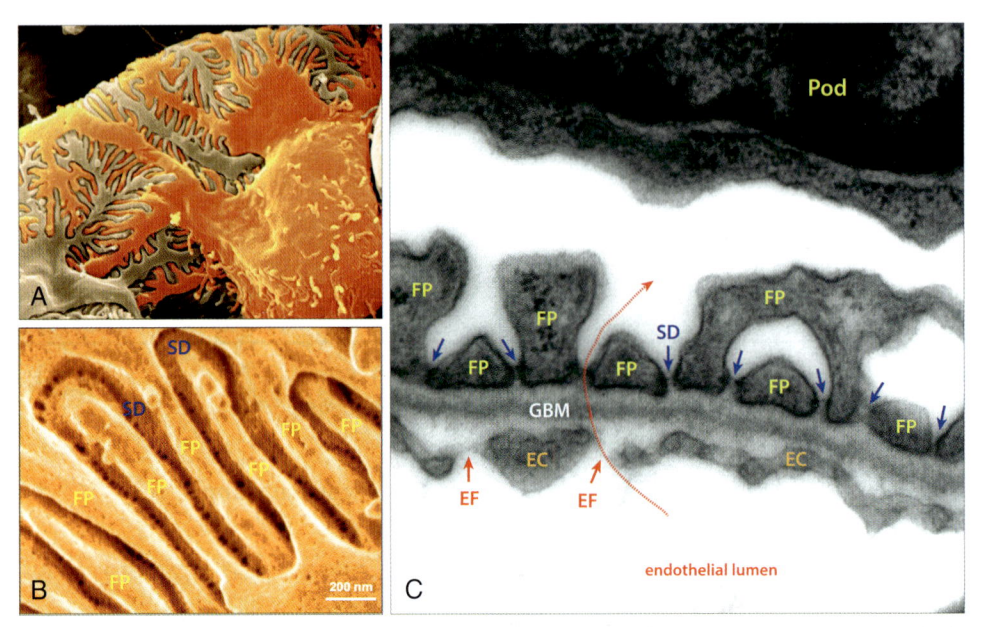

Figure 1.21 Ultrastructure of podocytes and the glomerular filtration barrier. A, Scanning electron micrograph of podocytes and their interdigitating foot processes (falsely colored to highlight the spatial relationships between neighboring foot processes). **B,** High-resolution image of podocyte foot processes (FP) and the porous slit diaphragms (SD) linking them. **C,** Transmission electron micrograph of the glomerular filter. Direction of filtration is indicated by the *dashed arrow*. EC, Endothelial cell; EF and *small red arrow*, endothelial fenestration; GBM, glomerular basement membrane; Pod, podocyte; SD and *blue arrows*, slit diaphragm. (Panel **B** is reproduced with permission from Gagliardini E, Conti S, Benigni A, et al: Imaging of the porous ultrastructure of the glomerular epithelial filtration slit. *J Am Soc Nephrol* 21:2081-2089, 2010.)

and *APOL1*.[63,349-366] The products of most of these genes are either integral parts of the slit diaphragm complex or directly interacting partners of the complex, and the remainder are important in regulating the development, viability, cytoskeleton, and distinctive morphology of podocytes.

The topologic organization of slit diaphragm components remains unknown but it is likely that the larger adhesion molecules nephrin and Fat1 bridge juxtaposed foot processes.[353,367-369] Smaller adhesion molecules within the slit diaphragms, such as Neph1, Neph3, and P-cadherin, may more likely associate in cis (within the same foot process surface).[370-372] Nephrin and the related protein Neph1 are known to interact with the polarity complex proteins Par3, Par6, and aPKCλ/ι, indicating a co-regulation between the polarized cell structure of podocytes and the compartmentalized assembly of the slit diaphragm complex along the foot processes.[373] Conditional inactivation in podocytes of aPKCλ/ι or the small GTPase Cdc42, which positively regulates the Par3/Par6/aPKCλ/ι complex, causes proteinuria characterized by abnormal, pseudo–slit diaphragms formed between effaced foot processes (Figure 1.22).[374-376] It has also been shown that inactivation of aPKCλλ/ι can specifically inhibit the localization of nephrin to the cell surface.[377]

Terminal foot processes of podocytes are longitudinally supported by parallel bundles of actin, setting them apart from the larger primary processes, which have a microtubule-based backbone.[378] The stereotypical response of podocytes to injury through either chemical insults or a detrimental gene mutation is effacement of foot processes. In effaced foot processes, the actin cytoskeleton has been remodeled into a meshlike network of randomly oriented filaments.[379] Genetic and biochemical studies provide evidence that the slit diaphragm is functionally coupled to the actin cytoskeleton and that perturbation of this relationship results in compromised renal filtration and proteinuric disease. Nck adaptor molecules (Nck1 and Nck2) are known to link tyrosine kinase receptors to signaling molecules that regulate the actin cytoskeleton. Podocytes lacking Nck1 and Nck2 are effaced and form abnormal slit diaphragms.[380] Cell culture studies demonstrate that clustered nephrin is phosphorylated at its cytoplasmic tail by the kinase Fyn, creating distinctive phosphotyrosine sites where Nck1 and Nck2 adaptors can bind directly. The association between nephrin and Nck adaptors consequently recruits N-WASP (neuronal Wiskott–Aldrich syndrome protein) and the Arp2/3 protein complex to mediate localized polymerization of actin.[380,381] Loss of Fyn causes congenital nephrosis, but podocyte-specific inactivation of N-WASP leads to proteinuric disease.[382,383] It is also very likely that Nck adaptors can mediate adhesion of podocytes to the GBM by virtue of their ability to interact with the PINCH-ILK-integrin complex.[384-386] Cdc42, in addition to its role in podocyte polarization, has been shown to be required for the coupling of actin polymerization to nephrin. CD2AP, a molecule known to stabilize actin microfilaments, is also indispensable in podocytes.[387-389] Mutations in *ACTN4*, *ARHGDIA*, *ARHGAP24*, *INF2*, and *MYO1E*, whose protein products are established regulators of the actin cytoskeleton, are also implicated in pathologic transformation of podocytes and proteinuric diseases.[349-352,354,358,360,363]

It has been proposed that the slit diaphragm likely functions in mechanotransduction in podocytes, allowing them to modulate renal filtration in response to hemodynamic changes within the glomerular microenvironment.[390,391] MEC-2, the *C. elegans* homolog of podocin, is a component of the touch receptor complex coupled to the ion channel

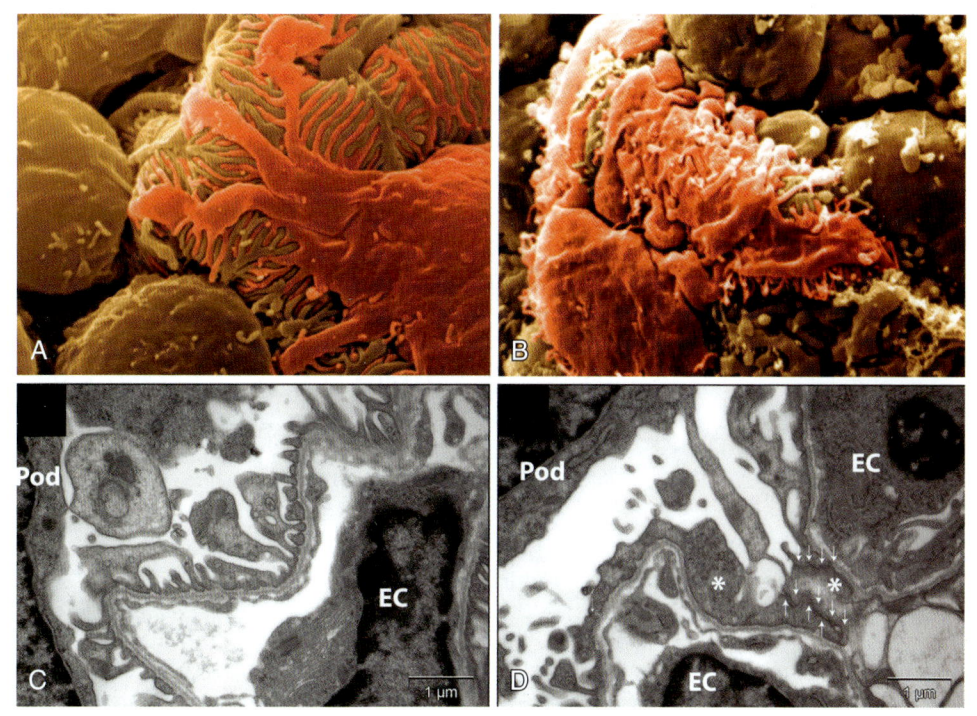

Figure 1.22 **Cdc42 inactivation in podocytes causes nephrosis. A** and **B,** Falsely colored scanning electron micrographs of glomeruli from neonatal kidneys: wild-type control podocytes showing normal interdigitated podocytes **(A)** and Cdc42-deficient mutant podocytes showing total effacement of foot processes **(B)**. **C** and **D,** Transmission electron micrographs of sectioned glomeruli: wild-type control, showing regularly interdigitating podocyte foot processes and basolateral slit diaphragms **(C)**, and podocyte-specific Cdc42-deficient mutant **(D),** showing mislocalized cell junctions (arrows) between effaced foot processes (asterisk). EC, Endothelial cell; Pod, podocyte. (Adapted from Scott RP, Hawley SP, Ruston J, et al: Podocyte-specific loss of Cdc42 leads to congenital nephropathy. J Am Soc Nephrol 23:1149-1154, 2012.)

MEC-4/MEC-10.[392] Loss of MEC-2 in worms leads to insensitivity to touch.[392] In podocytes, the ion channel Trpc6 forms an integral slit diaphragm component that directly interacts with podocin.[391] In diverse cell types such as myocytes, cochlear hair cells, and sensory neurons, Trpc6 channel opening is gated by mechanical stimuli. Mutations in *TRPC6* have been strongly linked to proteinuria.[356,393,394]

A novel lipid-dependent signaling pathway involving the VEGF receptor Flt1 (VEGFR1) has been described as crucial to the regulation of podocyte actin cytoskeleton and the maintenance of slit diaphragms. Genetic removal of *Flt1* from podocytes leads to foot process effacement and proteinuria.[395] Intriguingly, a kinase-inactive mutant of Flt1 is able to support normal podocyte development and function. In vivo, Flt1 is cleaved, releasing a soluble ectodomain (sFlt1). The secreted sFlt1 has been shown to act as an autocrine factor in podocytes, associating with glycosphingolipids and mediating podocyte cell adhesion, nephrin phosphorylation, and actin polymerization. It has been proposed that sFlt1 may function physiologically to stabilize the slit diaphragms and the attachment of podocytes to the GBM.

Three groups generated mice carrying a podocyte-specific deletion of Dicer1, thereby interfering with the production of functional miRNAs.[396-398] Podocyte-specific *Dicer1* knockout mice demonstrated albuminuria by 3 weeks of age and rapidly progressed to end-stage kidney failure by approximately 6 weeks. A number of potential miRNA targets were identified in these three studies, but their functional significance in the podocyte in vivo is yet unknown.

All of these studies indicate that intrinsic proteins and functions of podocytes play a key role in the development and maintenance of the permselective properties of the glomerular filtration barrier; however, as described earlier in the section on vascular development, podocytes also function as vasculature support cells, producing VEGF and other angiogenic growth factors. It is likely that endothelial cells also produce factors required for terminal differentiation of podocytes, although these factors are currently unknown.

MATURATION OF GLOMERULAR ENDOTHELIAL CELLS AND GLOMERULAR BASEMENT MEMBRANE

Following migration into the glomerular vascular cleft, endothelial cells are rounded and capillaries do not possess a lumen. Lumens form during glomerulogenesis through apoptosis of a subset of endothelial cells. Surviving endothelial cells flatten considerably and develop fenestrations and complex glycocalyces. Endothelial lumen formation depends on a TGFβ1-dependent signal, whereas fenestrations and the remodeling of the glycocalyx depend on VEGF-A and Angpt1, respectively.[12,279,399] Abnormal development of the glomerular endothelium, as in endotheliosis (see Figure 1.18), leads to disruption of the filtration barrier and protein loss, emphasizing that this layer of the filtration barrier plays a major role in perm-selectivity.

Although Chapters 2 and 44 in the book describes in detail the properties and development of the GBM, knockout models yielding information about this structure are listed in Table 1.1 for completeness. It is important to note that components are produced by both podocytes and glomerular endothelium and that a number of vital growth factors, such as VEGF-A, are stored and processed in the GBM.[400]

Complete reference list available at ExpertConsult.com.

KEY REFERENCES

19. Kobayashi A, Valerius MT, Mugford JW, et al: Six2 defines and regulates a multipotent self-renewing nephron progenitor population throughout mammalian kidney development. *Cell Stem Cell* 3:169–181, 2008.
29. Miyamoto N, Yoshida M, Kuratani S, et al: Defects of urogenital development in mice lacking Emx2. *Development* 124:1653–1664, 1997.
37. Torres M, Gomez-Pardo E, Dressler GR, et al: Pax-2 controls multiple steps of urogenital development. *Development* 121:4057–4065, 1995.
77. Chi X, Michos O, Shakya R, et al: Ret-dependent cell rearrangements in the Wolffian duct epithelium initiate ureteric bud morphogenesis. *Dev Cell* 17:199–209, 2009.
101. Xu PX, Zheng W, Huang L, et al: Six1 is required for the early organogenesis of mammalian kidney. *Development* 130:3085–3094, 2003.
120. Shakya R, Watanabe T, Costantini F: The role of GDNF/Ret signaling in ureteric bud cell fate and branching morphogenesis. *Dev Cell* 8:65–74, 2005.
124. Muller U, Wang D, Denda S, et al: Integrin alpha8beta1 is critically important for epithelial-mesenchymal interactions during kidney morphogenesis. *Cell* 88:603–613, 1997.
159. Jain S, Encinas M, Johnson EM, Jr, et al: Critical and distinct roles for key RET tyrosine docking sites in renal development. *Genes Dev* 20:321–333, 2006.
165. Majumdar A, Vainio S, Kispert A, et al: Wnt11 and Ret/Gdnf pathways cooperate in regulating ureteric branching during metanephric kidney development. *Development* 130:3175–3185, 2003.
172. Michos O, Cebrian C, Hyink D, et al: Kidney development in the absence of Gdnf and Spry1 requires Fgf10. *PLoS Genet* 6:e1000809, 2010.
173. Basson MA, Akbulut S, Watson-Johnson J, et al: Sprouty1 is a critical regulator of GDNF/RET-mediated kidney induction. *Dev Cell* 8:229–239, 2005.
177. Brandenberger R, Schmidt A, Linton J, et al: Identification and characterization of a novel extracellular matrix protein nephronectin that is associated with integrin alpha8beta1 in the embryonic kidney. *J Cell Biol* 154:447–458, 2001.
179. Kiyozumi D, Takeichi M, Nakano I, et al: Basement membrane assembly of the integrin alpha8beta1 ligand nephronectin requires Fraser syndrome-associated proteins. *J Cell Biol* 197:677–689, 2012.
180. Kiyozumi D, Sugimoto N, Sekiguchi K: Breakdown of the reciprocal stabilization of QBRICK/Frem1, Fras1, and Frem2 at the basement membrane provokes Fraser syndrome-like defects. *Proc Natl Acad Sci U S A* 103:11981–11986, 2006.
190. Yu J, Carroll TJ, Rajagopal J, et al: A Wnt7b-dependent pathway regulates the orientation of epithelial cell division and establishes the cortico-medullary axis of the mammalian kidney. *Development* 136:161–171, 2009.
191. Karner CM, Chirumamilla R, Aoki S, et al: Wnt9b signaling regulates planar cell polarity and kidney tubule morphogenesis. *Nat Genet* 41:793–799, 2009.
214. Kume T, Deng K, Hogan BL: Murine forkhead/winged helix genes Foxc1 (Mf1) and Foxc2 (Mfh1) are required for the early organogenesis of the kidney and urinary tract. *Development* 127:1387–1395, 2000.
215. Grieshammer U, Le M, Plump AS, et al: SLIT2-mediated ROBO2 signaling restricts kidney induction to a single site. *Dev Cell* 6:709–717, 2004.
218. Miyazaki Y, Oshima K, Fogo A, et al: Bone morphogenetic protein 4 regulates the budding site and elongation of the mouse ureter. *J Clin Invest* 105:863–873, 2000.
219. Michos O, Goncalves A, Lopez-Rios J, et al: Reduction of BMP4 activity by gremlin 1 enables ureteric bud outgrowth and GDNF/WNT11 feedback signalling during kidney branching morphogenesis. *Development* 134:2397–2405, 2007.
220. Carroll TJ, Park JS, Hayashi S, et al: Wnt9b plays a central role in the regulation of mesenchymal to epithelial transitions underlying organogenesis of the mammalian urogenital system. *Dev Cell* 9:283–292, 2005.
221. Stark K, Vainio S, Vassileva G, et al: Epithelial transformation of metanephric mesenchyme in the developing kidney regulated by Wnt-4. *Nature* 372:679–683, 1994.
223. Park JS, Valerius MT, McMahon AP: Wnt/beta-catenin signaling regulates nephron induction during mouse kidney development. *Development* 134:2533–2539, 2007.
228. Dudley AT, Godin RE, Robertson EJ: Interaction between FGF and BMP signaling pathways regulates development of metanephric mesenchyme. *Genes Dev* 13:1601–1613, 1999.
230. Barak H, Huh SH, Chen S, et al: FGF9 and FGF20 maintain the stemness of nephron progenitors in mice and man. *Dev Cell* 22:1191–1207, 2012.
233. Brown AC, Muthukrishnan SD, Guay JA, et al: Role for compartmentalization in nephron progenitor differentiation. *Proc Natl Acad Sci U S A* 110:4640–4645, 2013.
247. Wang P, Pereira FA, Beasley D, et al: Presenilins are required for the formation of comma- and S-shaped bodies during nephrogenesis. *Development* 130:5019–5029, 2003.
248. Cheng HT, Kim M, Valerius MT, et al: Notch2, but not Notch1, is required for proximal fate acquisition in the mammalian nephron. *Development* 134:801–811, 2007.
264. Quaggin SE, Schwartz L, Cui S, et al: The basic-helix-loop-helix protein pod1 is critically important for kidney and lung organogenesis. *Development* 126:5771–5783, 1999.
266. Levinson RS, Batourina E, Choi C, et al: Foxd1-dependent signals control cellularity in the renal capsule, a structure required for normal renal development. *Development* 132:529–539, 2005.
268. Fetting JL, Guay JA, Karolak MJ, et al: FOXD1 promotes nephron progenitor differentiation by repressing decorin in the embryonic kidney. *Development* 141:17–27, 2014.
269. Cui S, Schwartz L, Quaggin SE: Pod1 is required in stromal cells for glomerulogenesis. *Dev Dyn* 226:512–522, 2003.
270. Mendelsohn C, Batourina E, Fung S, et al: Stromal cells mediate retinoid-dependent functions essential for renal development. *Development* 126:1139–1148, 1999.
273. Paroly SS, Wang F, Spraggon L, et al: Stromal protein ecm1 regulates ureteric bud patterning and branching. *PLoS ONE* 8:e84155, 2013.
274. Das A, Tanigawa S, Karner CM, et al: Stromal-epithelial crosstalk regulates kidney progenitor cell differentiation. *Nat Cell Biol* 15:1035–1044, 2013.
279. Eremina V, Sood M, Haigh J, et al: Glomerular-specific alterations of VEGF-A expression lead to distinct congenital and acquired renal diseases. *J Clin Invest* 111:707–716, 2003.
319. Sequeira Lopez ML, Pentz ES, Nomasa T, et al: Renin cells are precursors for multiple cell types that switch to the renin phenotype when homeostasis is threatened. *Dev Cell* 6:719–728, 2004.
332. Lindahl P, Hellstrom M, Kalen M, et al: Paracrine PDGF-B/PDGF-Rbeta signaling controls mesangial cell development in kidney glomeruli. *Development* 125:3313–3322, 1998.
333. Bjarnegard M, Enge M, Norlin J, et al: Endothelium-specific ablation of PDGFB leads to pericyte loss and glomerular, cardiac and placental abnormalities. *Development* 131:1847–1857, 2004.
348. Schwarz K, Simons M, Reiser J, et al: Podocin, a raft-associated component of the glomerular slit diaphragm, interacts with CD2AP and nephrin. *J Clin Invest* 108:1621–1629, 2001.
380. Jones N, Blasutig IM, Eremina V, et al: Nck adaptor proteins link nephrin to the actin cytoskeleton of kidney podocytes. *Nature* 440:818–823, 2006.
381. Verma R, Kovari I, Soofi A, et al: Nephrin ectodomain engagement results in Src kinase activation, nephrin phosphorylation, Nck recruitment, and actin polymerization. *J Clin Invest* 116:1346–1359, 2006.
403. Srinivas S, Wu Z, Chen CM, et al: Dominant effects of RET receptor misexpression and ligand-independent RET signaling on ureteric bud development. *Development* 126:1375–1386, 1999.

405. Schuchardt A, D'Agati V, Pachnis V, et al: Renal agenesis and hypodysplasia in ret-k-mutant mice result from defects in ureteric bud development. *Development* 122:1919–1929, 1996.
412. Kobayashi A, Kwan KM, Carroll TJ, et al: Distinct and sequential tissue-specific activities of the LIM-class homeobox gene Lim1 for tubular morphogenesis during kidney development. *Development* 132:2809–2823, 2005.
428. Perantoni AO, Timofeeva O, Naillat F, et al: Inactivation of FGF8 in early mesoderm reveals an essential role in kidney development. *Development* 132:3859–3871, 2005.
429. Grieshammer U, Cebrian C, Ilagan R, et al: FGF8 is required for cell survival at distinct stages of nephrogenesis and for regulation of gene expression in nascent nephrons. *Development* 132:3847–3857, 2005.
491. Rohr C, Prestel J, Heidet L, et al: The LIM-homeodomain transcription factor Lmx1b plays a crucial role in podocytes. *J Clin Invest* 109:1073–1082, 2002.
492. Miner JH, Morello R, Andrews KL, et al: Transcriptional induction of slit diaphragm genes by Lmx1b is required in podocyte differentiation. *J Clin Invest* 109:1065–1072, 2002.

2 Anatomy of the Kidney

Robert A. Fenton | Jeppe Praetorius

CHAPTER OUTLINE

GROSS FEATURES, 42
THE NEPHRON, 44
Renal Corpuscle, 45
Endothelial Cells, 46
Glomerular Basement Membrane, 48
Visceral Epithelial Cells, 49
Mesangial Cells, 51
Parietal Epithelial Cells, 52
Peripolar Cells, 53
Juxtaglomerular Apparatus, 53
Juxtaglomerular Granular Cells, 53
Extraglomerular Mesangium, 53
Macula Densa, 54
Autonomic Innervation, 54
Tubuloglomerular Feedback, 55
Proximal Tubule, 55

Pars Convoluta, 55
Pars Recta, 60
Thin Limbs of the Loop of Henle, 61
Distal Tubule, 63
Thick Ascending Limb, 63
Distal Convoluted Tubule, 65
Connecting Tubule, 68
COLLECTING DUCT, 69
Cortical Collecting Duct, 70
Outer Medullary Collecting Duct, 73
Inner Medullary Collecting Duct, 74
INTERSTITIUM, 75
Cortical Interstitium, 77
Medullary Interstitium, 78
LYMPHATICS, 80
INNERVATION, 80

Knowledge of the complex structure of the mammalian kidney provides a basis for understanding the multitude of functional characteristics of this organ in both healthy and diseased states. In this chapter, an overview of the renal organization is presented through gross anatomical observations and ultrastructural information. Examples of the expression of selected molecules, such as channels, transporters, and regulatory proteins, are also provided, although this topic is covered in detail in later chapters.

GROSS FEATURES

The kidneys are paired retroperitoneal organs normally situated one on each side of the vertebral column. In the human, the upper pole of each kidney lies at a level corresponding to the twelfth thoracic vertebra, and the lower pole lies corresponding to the third lumbar vertebra. The right kidney is usually slightly more caudal in position than the left. The weight of a human kidney ranges from 125 to 170 g in the adult male and from 115 to 155 g in the adult female. The human kidney is approximately 11 to 12 cm in length, 5.0 to 7.5 cm in width, and 2.5 to 3.0 cm in thickness. When renal magnetic resonance imaging (MRI) is performed, the ranges of normal reference values (mean ± 2 SD) for male and female kidney lengths are 10.7 to 14.3 and 9.5 to 13.9 cm, respectively, and the ranges for male and female kidney volumes are 132 to 276 and 87 to 223 mL, respectively.[1] Located on the medial or concave surface of each kidney is a slit, called the hilum, through which the renal pelvis, the renal artery and vein, the lymphatics, and a nerve plexus pass into the sinus of the kidney. The organ is surrounded by a thin tough fibrous capsule, which is smooth and easily removable under normal conditions.

In the human, as in most mammals, each kidney is normally supplied by a single renal artery, although the presence of one or more accessory renal arteries is not uncommon. The renal artery enters the hilar region and usually divides to form an anterior and a posterior branch. Three segmental or lobar arteries arise from the anterior branch and supply the upper, middle, and lower thirds of the anterior surface of the kidney (Figure 2.1). The posterior branch supplies more than half of the posterior surface and occasionally gives rise to a small apical segmental branch. However, the apical segmental or lobar branch arises most commonly from the anterior division. No collateral circulation has been demonstrated between individual segmental or lobar arteries or their subdivisions. The kidneys often receive aberrant arteries from the superior mesenteric, suprarenal, testicular, or ovarian arteries. True accessory arteries that arise from the abdominal aorta usually supply the lower pole of the kidney. The arterial and venous circulations in the kidney are described in detail in Chapter 3 and are not discussed further in this chapter.

Two distinct regions can be identified on the cut surface of a bisected kidney: a pale outer region, the cortex, and a darker inner region, the medulla (Figure 2.2). In humans, the medulla is divided into 8 to 18 striated conical masses, the renal pyramids. The base of each pyramid is positioned at the corticomedullary boundary, and the apex extends toward the renal pelvis to form a papilla. On the tip of each papilla are 10 to 25 small openings that represent the distal ends of the collecting ducts (ducts of Bellini). These openings form the area cribrosa (Figure 2.3). A renal pyramid and the corresponding cortex are referred to as a renal lobe. In contrast to the human kidney, the kidney of the rat and of many other laboratory animals has a single renal pyramid with its overlying cortex and is therefore termed "unipapillate." Otherwise, these kidneys resemble the human kidney in their gross appearance. In humans, the renal cortex is about 1 cm in thickness, forms a cap over the base of each renal pyramid, and extends downward between the individual pyramids to form the renal columns of Bertin (see Figures 2.2 and 2.4). From the base of the renal pyramid, at the corticomedullary junction, longitudinal elements termed the "medullary rays of Ferrein" extend into the cortex. Despite their name, the medullary rays are actually considered a part of the cortex and are formed by the collecting ducts and the straight segments of the proximal and distal tubules.

In humans, the renal pelvis is lined by transitional epithelium and represents the expanded portion of the upper urinary tract. In rodents, the epithelium closely resembles that of the terminal part of the collecting duct. Two and sometimes three protrusions, the major calyces, extend outward from the upper dilated end of the renal pelvis. From each of the major calyces, several minor calyces extend toward the papillae of the pyramids and drain the urine formed by each pyramidal unit. In mammals possessing a unipapillate kidney, the papilla is directly surrounded by the renal pelvis. The ureters originate from the lower portion of the renal pelvis at the ureteropelvic junction, and in humans they descend a distance of approximately 28 to 34 cm to open into the fundus of the bladder. The mean size of ureters in adults is 1.8 mm, with a maximum width of 3 mm considered normal.[2] The papilla, the walls of the calyces, pelvis, and ureters contain smooth muscle that contracts rhythmically to propel the urine to the bladder.

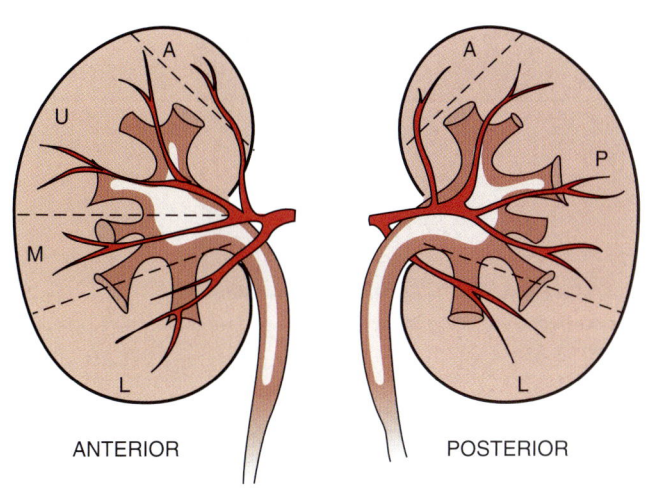

Figure 2.1 Diagram of the vascular supply of the human kidney. The **anterior half** of the kidney can be divided into upper (U), middle (M), and lower (L) segments, each supplied by a segmental branch of the anterior division of the renal artery. A small apical segment (A) is usually supplied by a division from the anterior segmental branch. The **posterior half** of the kidney is divided into apical (A), posterior (P), and lower (L) segments, each supplied by branches of the posterior division of the renal artery. (Modified from Graves FT: The anatomy of the intrarenal arteries and its application to segmental resection of the kidney. *Br J Surg* 42:132-139, 1954.)

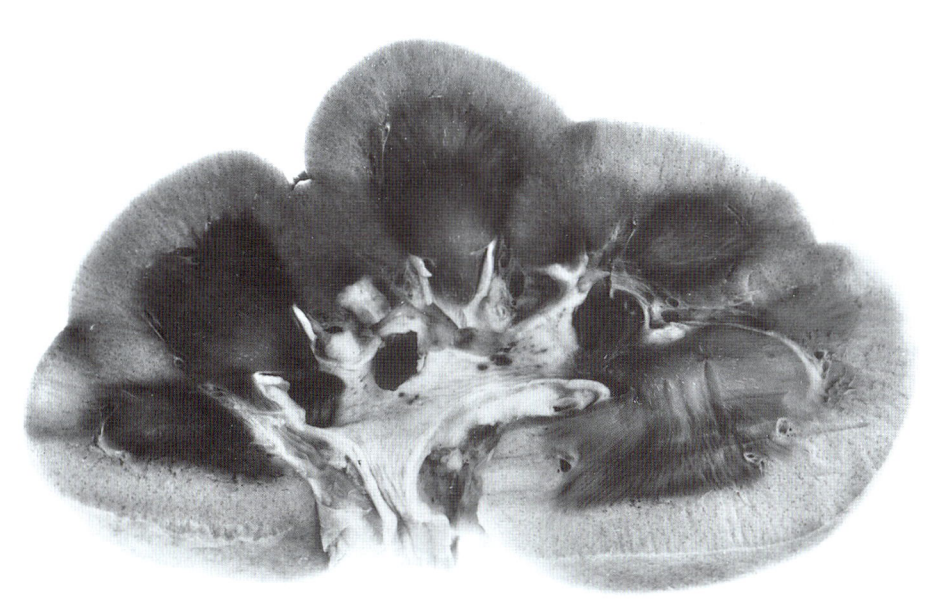

Figure 2.2 Bisected kidney from a 4-year-old child, demonstrating the difference in appearance between the light-staining cortex and the dark-staining outer medulla. The inner medulla and papillae are less dense than the outer medulla. The columns of Bertin can be seen extending downward to separate the papillae.

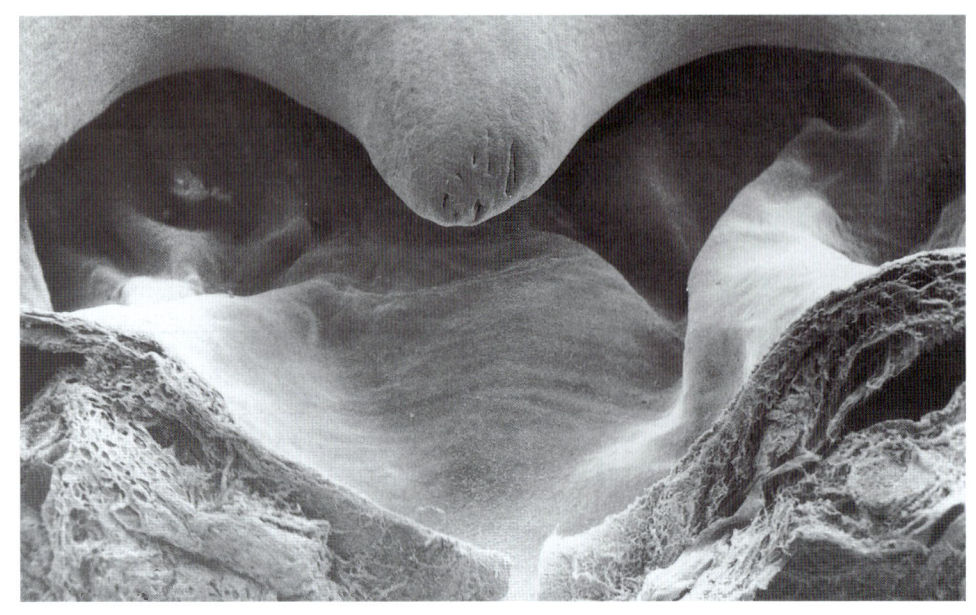

Figure 2.3 Scanning electron micrograph of papilla from a rat kidney **(upper center)**, illustrating the area cribrosa formed by slitlike openings where the ducts of Bellini terminate. The renal pelvis **(below)** surrounds the papilla. (×24.)

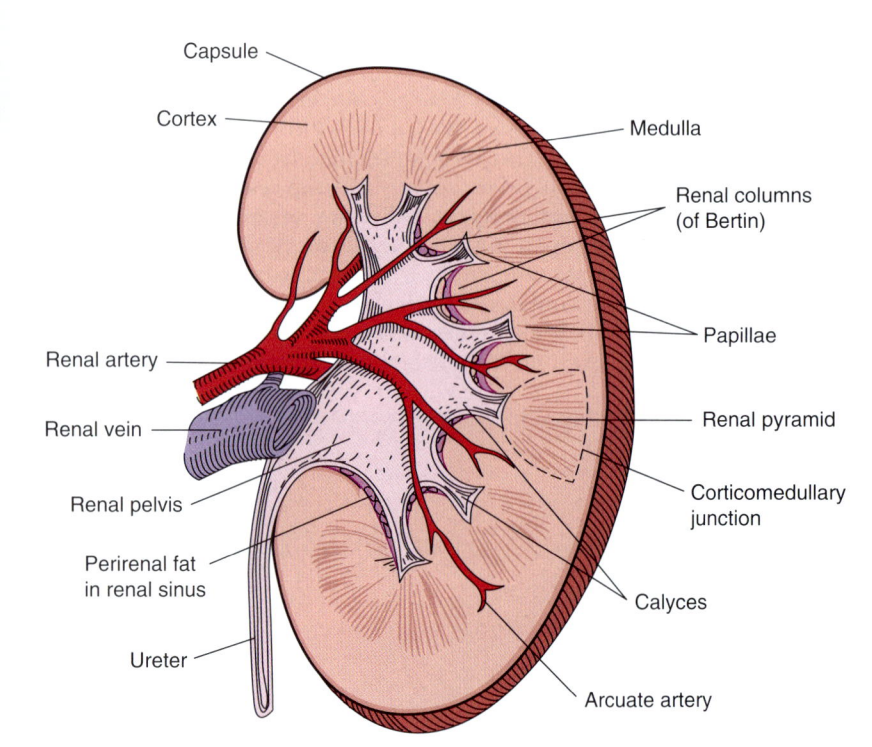

Figure 2.4 Diagram of the cut surface of a bisected kidney, depicting important anatomic structures.

THE NEPHRON

The nephron is often referred to as the functional unit of the kidney. Although the average nephron number in adult humans is approximately 900,000 to 1 million per kidney, numbers for individual kidneys range from approximately 200,000 to more than 2.5 million,[3-6] contrasting with the approximately 30,000 nephrons in each adult rat kidney.[7-9] The essential components of the nephron include the renal or malpighian corpuscle (comprising the glomerulus and Bowman's capsule), the proximal tubule, the thin limbs, the distal tubule, and the connecting tubule (Figure 2.5). The origin of the nephron is the metanephric blastema. Although there has not been universal agreement on the origin of the connecting tubule, it is now generally believed also to derive from the metanephric blastema.[10] The collecting duct system, which includes the initial collecting tubule/duct, the cortical collecting duct (CCD), the outer medullary collecting duct (OMCD), and the inner medullary collecting duct (IMCD), is not considered part of the nephron, because it arises embryologically from the ureteric bud. However, all of the components of the nephron and the collecting duct system are functionally interrelated. An

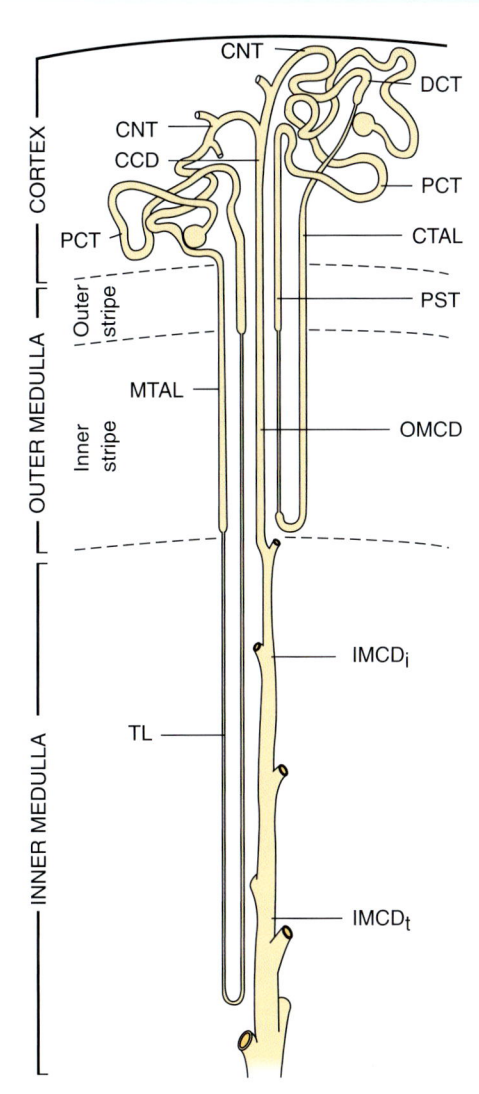

Figure 2.5 Diagram illustrating superficial and juxtamedullary nephron. CCD, cortical collecting duct; CNT, connecting tubule; CTAL, cortical thick ascending limb; DCT, distal convoluted tubule; IMCD$_i$, initial inner medullary collecting duct; IMCD$_t$, terminal inner medullary collecting duct; MTAL, medullary thick ascending limb; OMCD, outer medullary collecting duct; PCT, proximal convoluted tubule; PST, proximal straight tubule; TL, thin limb of loop of Henle. (Modified from Madsen KM, Tisher CC: Structural-functional relationship along the distal nephron. *Am J Physiol* 250:F1-F15, 1986.)

alternative structural/functional separation and a way to circumvent confusion in the literature are to use the terms (1) the renal corpuscle and (2) the renal tubular system.

Several populations of nephrons are recognizable in the kidney with varying length of the loop of Henle (see Figure 2.5). The loop of Henle is composed of the straight portion of the proximal tubule (pars recta), the thin limb segments, and the straight portion of the distal tubule (thick ascending limb [TAL], or pars recta). The length of the loop of Henle is generally related to the position of its parent renal corpuscle in the cortex. Most nephrons originating from superficial and midcortical locations have shorter loops of Henle that bend within the inner stripe of the outer medulla close to the inner medulla. A few species, including humans, also possess cortical nephrons with extremely short loops that never enter the medulla but turn back within the cortex.[11] Nephrons originating from the juxtamedullary region near the corticomedullary boundary have long loops of Henle with long descending and ascending thin limb segments that enter the inner medulla. Many variations exist, however, between the two basic types of nephrons, depending on their relative positions in the cortex. Three-dimensional (3D) reconstruction studies of the rat and mouse kidney have provided insight into the anatomical distribution of various nephrons.[12-16] These studies have highlighted that the ratio of long and short loop nephrons varies among species, with humans and rodents having a larger number of short looped than long looped nephrons. Owing to these anatomical differences, caution should be exercised in interpretation of micropuncture data for understanding the urinary concentrating mechanism, because the majority of this data arises from studies on short-looped nephrons.

On the basis of the segmentation of the renal tubules, the medulla can be divided into an inner zone and an outer zone, with the outer zone further subdivided into an inner stripe and an outer stripe (see Figure 2.5). The inner medulla contains both descending and ascending thin limbs and large collecting ducts, including the ducts of Bellini. In the inner stripe of the outer medulla, TALs are present in addition to descending thin limbs and collecting ducts. The outer stripe of the outer medulla of the human kidney contains the terminal segments of the pars recta of the proximal tubule, the TALs (pars recta of the distal tubule), and collecting ducts. By contrast, the renal cortex contains the renal corpuscles, segments of proximal tubules, and distal tubules as well as collecting ducts, but does not contain thin limbs of Henle's loop. The division of the kidney into cortical and medullary zones and the further subdivision of the medulla into inner and outer zones are of considerable importance in relating renal structure to the ability of an animal to form maximally concentrated urine.

RENAL CORPUSCLE

The initial part of the nephron is the renal corpuscle, which is composed of a capillary network lined by a thin layer of endothelial cells (glomerulus), a central region of mesangial cells with surrounding matrix material, the visceral epithelial layer of Bowman's capsule and the associated basement membrane, and the parietal layer of Bowman's capsule with its basement membrane (Figures 2.6 through 2.8). The *Bowman's space*, or the *urinary space*, is a narrow cavity between the two epithelial cell layers. Although *renal corpuscle* is anatomically correct when used to refer to the portion of the nephron composed of the glomerular tuft and Bowman's capsule, *glomerulus* is employed throughout this chapter because of its common use. At the vascular pole, the visceral epithelium is continuous with the parietal epithelium. This is where the afferent arteriole enters and the efferent arteriole exits the glomerulus. The parietal layer of Bowman's capsule continues into the epithelium of the proximal tubule at the so-called urinary pole. The average diameter of a glomerulus is approximately 200 μm in the human kidney and 120 μm in the rat kidney. However, the number of glomeruli and their size varies significantly with age, gender, birth weight, and renal health. The average glomerular volume is 3 to 7 million μm^3 in humans[3-5] and

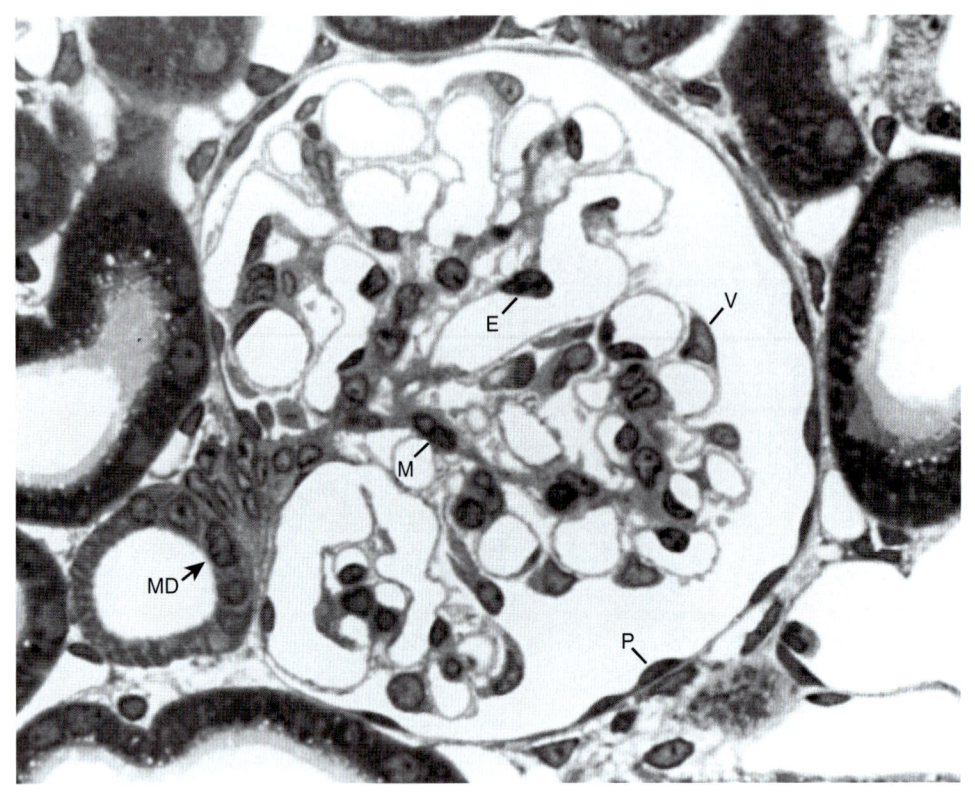

Figure 2.6 Light micrograph of a normal glomerulus from a rat, demonstrating the four major cellular components: endothelial cell (E), mesangial cell (M), parietal epithelial cell (P), and visceral epithelial cell (V). MD, macula densa. (×750.)

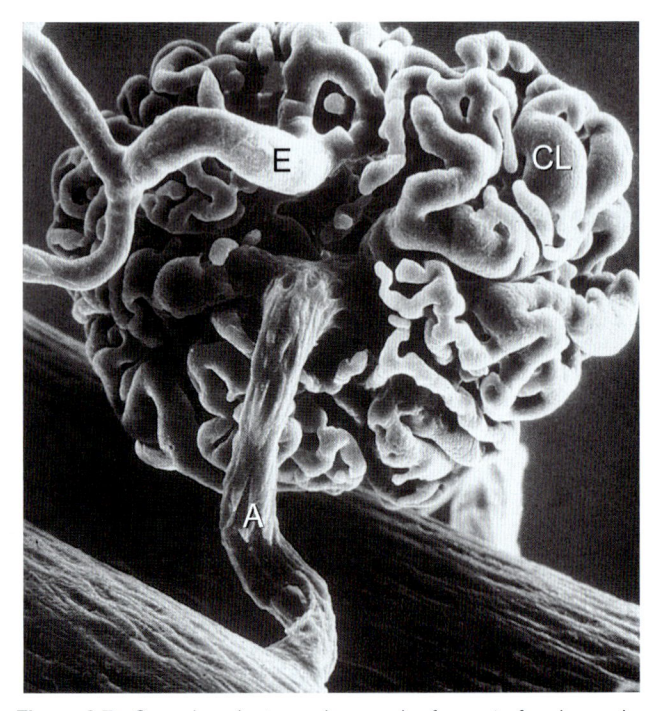

Figure 2.7 Scanning electron micrograph of a cast of a glomerulus with its many capillary loops (CL) and adjacent renal vessels. The afferent arteriole (A) takes its origin from an interlobular artery at **lower left**. The efferent arteriole (E) branches to form the peritubular capillary plexus **(upper left)**. (×300.) (Courtesy Waykin Nopanitaya, PhD.)

0.6 to 1 million μm^3 in rats.[7,8] Rat juxtamedullary glomeruli are larger than glomeruli in the superficial cortex; this is not the case in the human kidney.[17]

The main function of the glomerulus is production of an ultrafiltrate from plasma. The fenestrated endothelium, the peripheral glomerular basement membrane (GBM), and the slit pores between the foot processes of the visceral epithelial cells form the filtration barrier between the blood and the urinary space (Figure 2.9). In the human kidney, mean area of filtration surface per glomerulus is 0.203 mm^2,[18] and in the rat kidney, 0.184 mm^2.[19] Although the glomerular capillary wall functions as a "sieve" to allow passage of small molecules, it restricts the passage of larger molecules, such as albumin. The glomerular capillary wall possesses both size-selective and charge-selective properties.[20] To cross the capillary wall, a molecule must pass sequentially through the fenestrated endothelium, the GBM, and the epithelial slit diaphragm. The fenestrated endothelium, possessing a negatively charged glycocalyx, excludes formed elements of the blood and is important for determining access of proteins to the GBM.

ENDOTHELIAL CELLS

The glomerular capillaries are lined by a thin fenestrated endothelium (see Figures 2.9 and 2.10). These endothelial cells form the initial barrier to the passage of blood constituents from the capillary lumen to Bowman's space. Under normal conditions, the formed elements of the blood, including erythrocytes, leukocytes, and platelets, do not gain access to the subendothelial space.

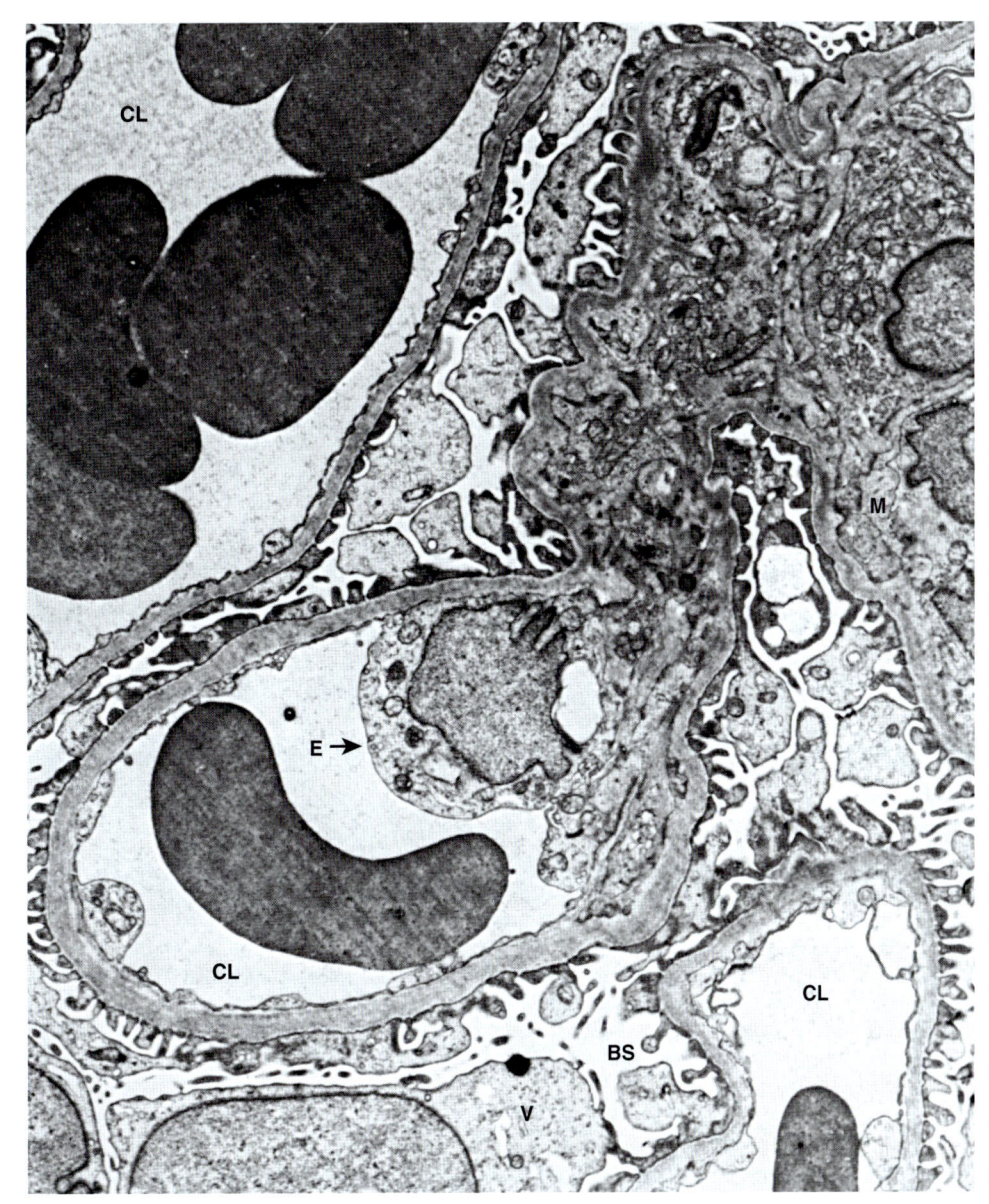

Figure 2.8 Electron micrograph of a portion of a glomerulus from a normal human kidney in which segments of three capillary loops (CL) are evident. The relationship between mesangial cells (M), endothelial cells (E), and visceral epithelial cells (V) is demonstrated. Several electron-dense erythrocytes lie in the capillary lumens. BS, Bowman's space. (×6700.)

The endothelial cell nucleus lies adjacent to the mesangium, with the remainder of the cell irregularly attenuated around the capillary lumen (see Figure 2.8). The endothelium contains pores or fenestrae that range from 70 to 100 nm in diameter in human (see Figure 2.10).[21] Thin protein diaphragms extend across these fenestrae, and filamentous sieve plugs have been observed in the fenestrae.[22] The function of these plugs remains to be fully established, and it is not known whether they represent a significant barrier to the passage of molecules. However, adult glomerular endothelial cells have been reported to lack these diaphragms, and instead diaphragmed fenestra are present predominantly in the embryo, where they may compensate for the functional immaturity of the embryonic glomerular filtration barrier.[23] Electron-dense filamentous material in the fenestrae and a thick filamentous surface layer on the endothelial cells have also been demonstrated.[24]

Nonfenestrated, ridgelike structures termed *cytofolds* are found near the cell borders.

An extensive network of intermediate filaments and microtubules is present in the endothelial cells and microfilaments surrounding the endothelial fenestrations.[25] The endothelial cells synthesize polyanionic glycosaminoglycans and glycoproteins, representing a glycocalyx, that coats the surfaces of the glomerular endothelial cells, providing a negative charge.[26] The endothelial cell glycocalyx contributes to the charge-selective properties of the glomerular capillary wall and constitutes an important part of the filtration barrier.[27]

The surfaces of glomerular endothelial cells express receptors for vascular endothelial growth factor (VEGF).[28] VEGF is synthesized by the glomerular visceral epithelial cells and is an important regulator of microvascular permeability.[28,29] VEGF increases endothelial cell permeability and

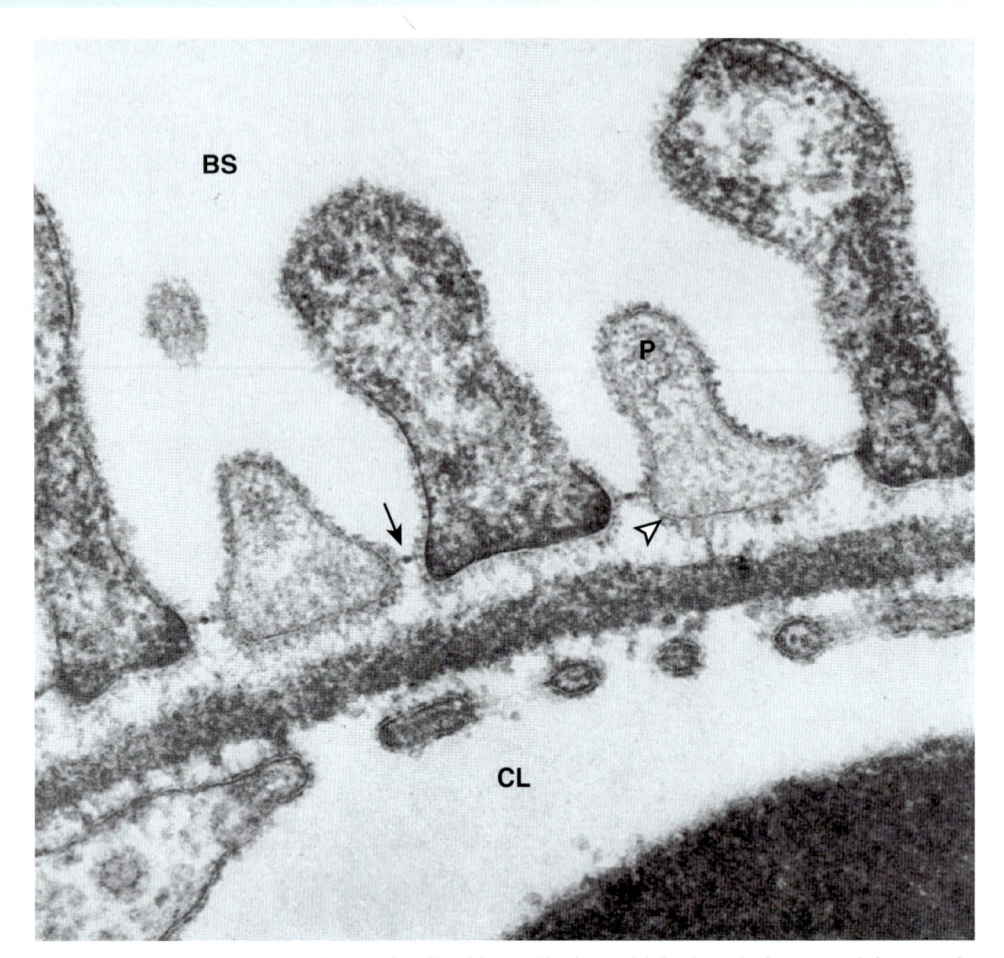

Figure 2.9 Electron micrograph of normal rat glomerulus fixed in a 1% glutaraldehyde solution containing tannic acid. Note the relationship among the three layers of the glomerular basement membrane and the presence of the pedicels (P) embedded in the lamina rara externa *(arrowhead)*. The filtration slit diaphragm with the central dense spot *(thin arrow)* is especially evident between the individual pedicels. The fenestrated endothelial lining of the capillary loop is shown below the basement membrane. A portion of an erythrocyte is located in the extreme **lower right** corner. BS, Bowman's space; CL, capillary lumen. (×120,000.)

induces the formation of endothelial fenestrations.[30,31] Gene deletion studies in mice have demonstrated that VEGF is required for normal differentiation of glomerular endothelial cells.[32,33] VEGF is also important for endothelial cell survival and repair in glomerular diseases characterized by endothelial cell damage.[34] Thus, VEGF produced by the visceral epithelial cells plays a critical role in the differentiation and maintenance of glomerular endothelial cells and is an important regulator of endothelial cell permeability.

GLOMERULAR BASEMENT MEMBRANE

The GBM is composed of a central dense layer, the lamina densa, and two thinner, more electron-lucent layers, the lamina rara externa and the lamina rara interna (see Figure 2.9). The latter two layers measure approximately 20 to 40 nm in thickness.[21] The layered configuration of the GBM results in part from the fusion of endothelial and epithelial basement membranes during development.[35] Although in the rat the width of the GBM has been found to be 132 nm,[36] the width of the human GBM has consistently been reported to be more than 300 nm[37,38] with a slightly thicker basement membrane in men (373 nm) than in women (326 nm).[39] Like other basement membranes in the body, the GBM is composed primarily of collagen IV, laminin, entactin/nidogen, and sulfated proteoglycans.[40-44] In addition, the GBM contains specific components, such as laminin 11, distinct collagen IV α chains, and the proteoglycans agrin and perlecan.[44-46] As reviewed by Kashtan,[47] six isomeric chains, designated α1 through α6 (IV), constitute the type IV collagen family of proteins.[48] Of these six chains, α1 through α5 have been identified in the normal GBM.[47] Mutations in the genes encoding α3, α4, and α5 (IV) chains are known to cause Alport's syndrome, a hereditary basement membrane disorder associated with progressive glomerulopathy.[47,49]

The exact contribution of the GBM to the glomerular filtration barrier remains somewhat controversial. Ultrastructural tracer studies provided evidence that the GBM constitutes both a size-selective and a charge-selective barrier.[50-52] Caulfield and Farquhar[53] demonstrated the existence of anionic sites in all three layers of the GBM. Additional studies revealed a lattice of anionic sites with a spacing of approximately 60 nm (Figure 2.11) throughout the lamina rara interna and lamina rara externa.[54] The anionic sites in the GBM consist of glycosaminoglycans rich in heparan sulfate.[55,56] Removal of the heparan sulfate side chains by enzymatic digestion resulted in an increase in the in vitro permeability of the GBM to ferritin[57] and to bovine

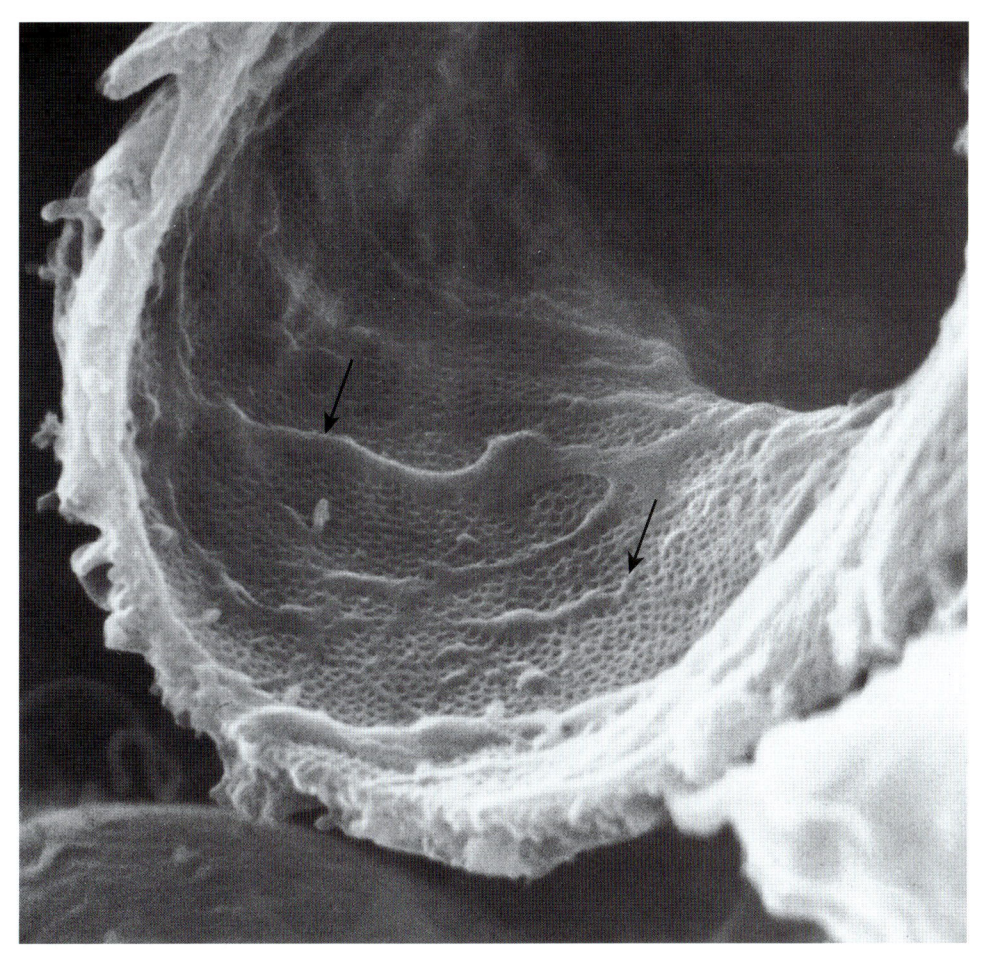

Figure 2.10 Scanning electron micrograph demonstrating the endothelial surface of a glomerular capillary from the kidney of a normal rat. Numerous endothelial pores, or fenestrae, are evident. The ridgelike structures *(arrows)* represent localized thickenings of the endothelial cells. (×21,400.)

serum albumin,[58] suggesting that glycosaminoglycans might play a role in establishing the permeability properties of the GBM to plasma proteins (see Figure 2.11). However, in vivo digestion of heparan sulfates with heparanase in rats did not result in proteinuria.[59] Furthermore, neither mice genetically engineered to lack agrin and perlecan heparin sulfate side chains,[60,61] nor collagen XVIII–deficient mice,[62] demonstrate significant proteinuria. Moreover, studies in the isolated GBM failed to demonstrate charge selectivity in vitro.[63] Nevertheless, a variety of genetic findings in humans and knockout studies in mice suggest that the GBM significantly contributes to the functional properties of the glomerular filtration barrier.[64] The strongest evidence for a specific role of the GBM in the filtration barrier is the finding that mice deficient in laminin β2, a major component of the GBM, have massive proteinuria,[65] as do patients with mutations in this gene.[66] Importantly, in the laminin β2 knockout mice, proteinuria is associated with increases in the permeability of the GBM that precede the onset of any abnormalities in the podocyte.[67]

VISCERAL EPITHELIAL CELLS

The visceral epithelial cells, also called podocytes, are terminally differentiated cells that do not replicate anymore. The podocytes are the largest cells in the glomerulus (see Figure 2.6) and are characterized by long cytoplasmic processes that extend from the main cell body. The primary processes divide into secondary and tertiary processes and finally into the individual foot processes, or pedicels, that come into direct contact with the lamina rara externa of the GBM (see Figures 2.8 and 2.9). By scanning electron microscopy, it is apparent that adjacent foot processes are derived from different podocytes (Figure 2.12). The podocytes contain well-developed Golgi complexes and are capable of endocytosis. Lysosomes are frequently observed, and their heterogeneous content most likely reflects the uptake of proteins and other components from the ultrafiltrate. Large numbers of microtubules, microfilaments, and intermediate filaments are present in the cytoplasm,[25] and actin filaments are especially abundant in the foot processes.[68] Despite a prominent motility in vitro, podocytes in the healthy glomerulus in vivo are rather stationary and maintain fixed positions of their cell bodies and microprojections as shown by intravital time-lapse microscopy of zebrafish larvae[69] and mouse kidneys.[70] However, podocyte motility drastically increases in the mice with glomerular damage induced by unilateral ureteral ligation and doxorubicin (Adriamycin) nephropathy.[70]

In a healthy glomerulus, the distance between adjacent foot processes near the GBM varies from 25 to 60 nm (see Figure 2.9). This gap, referred to as the filtration slit or slit

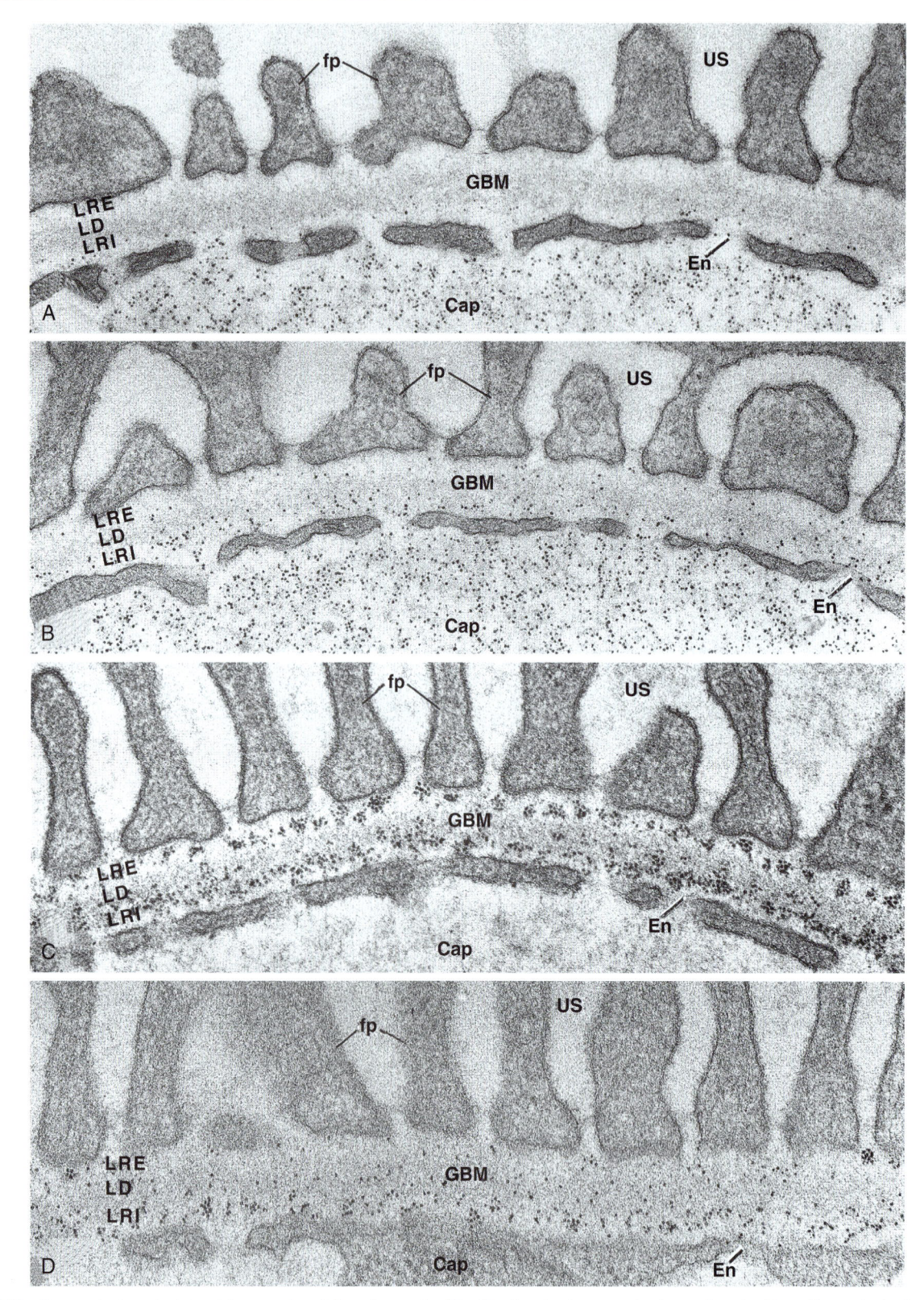

Figure 2.11 Transmission electron micrographs of the glomerular filtration barrier in normal rats perfused with native anionic ferritin (**A**) or cationic ferritin (**C**) and in rats treated with heparitinase before perfusion with anionic (**B**) or cationic ferritin (**D**). In normal animals, anionic ferritin is present in the capillary (Cap) but does not enter the glomerular basement membrane (GBM), as shown in **A**. In contrast, cationic ferritin binds to the negatively charged sites in the lamina rara interna (LRI) and lamina rara externa (LRE) of the GBM (see **C**). After treatment with heparitinase, both anionic (**B**) and cationic (**D**) ferritin penetrates into the GBM, but there is no labeling of negatively charged sites by cationic ferritin. En, endothelial fenestrae; fp, foot processes; LD, lamina densa; US, urinary space. (×80,000.) (From Kanwar YS: Biophysiology of glomerular filtration and proteinuria. *Lab Invest* 51:7-21, 1984.)

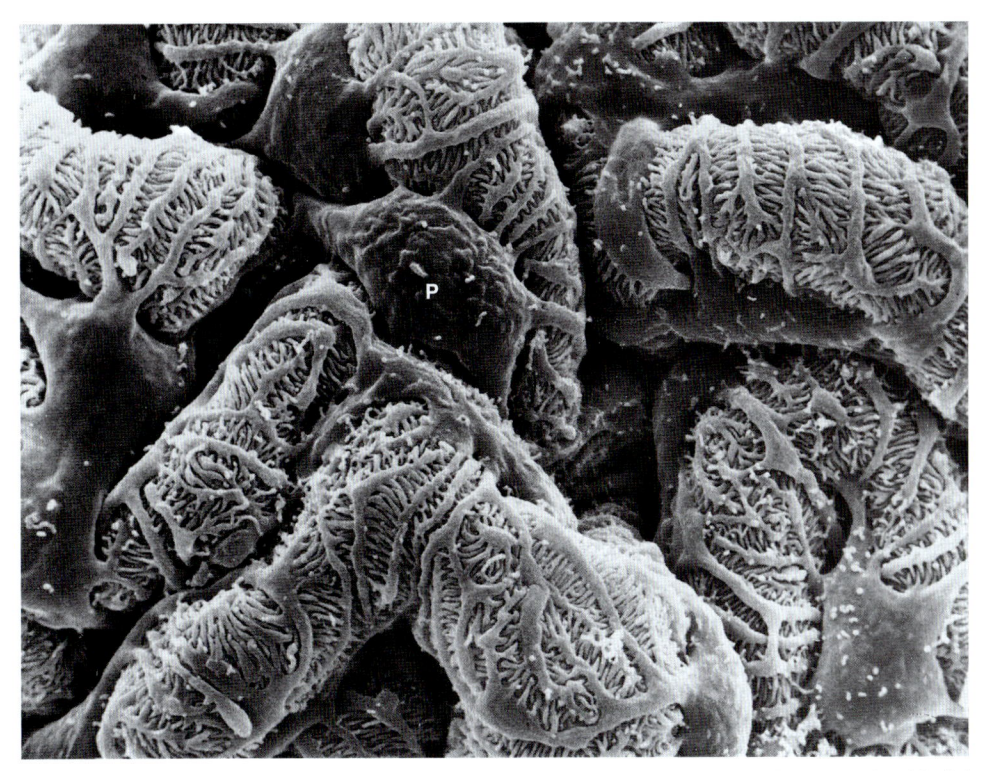

Figure 2.12 Scanning electron micrograph of a glomerulus from the kidney of a normal rat. The visceral epithelial cells, or podocytes (P), extend multiple processes outward from the main cell body to wrap around individual capillary loops. Immediately adjacent pedicels, or foot processes, arise from different podocytes. (×6000.)

pore, is bridged by a thin membrane called the *filtration slit membrane*[71,72] or *slit diaphragm*,[73] which is located approximately 60 nm from the GBM. A continuous central filament with a diameter of approximately 11 nm can be seen in the filtration slit diaphragm.[71] Detailed studies of the slit diaphragm in the rat, mouse, and human glomerulus have revealed that the 11 nm wide central filament is connected to the cell membrane of the adjacent foot processes by regularly spaced cross-bridges approximately 7 nm in diameter and 14 nm in length, giving the slit diaphragm a zipper-like configuration (Figure 2.13).[73,74] The slit diaphragm has the morphologic features of an adherens junction,[75] and the tight junction protein ZO-1 has been localized to the sites where the slit diaphragm is connected to the plasma membrane of the foot processes.[76]

The molecular components of the slit diaphragm and their role in determining the selective properties of the filtration barrier are now well established.[77-79] The slit diaphragm is formed by a complex of the transmembrane proteins nephrin, NEPH1-3, podocin, Fat1, VE-cadherin and P-cadherin. Mutations in nephrin and podocin cause inherited nephrotic syndrome,[80,81] and knockout of nephrin, NEPH1, and podocin causes proteinuria in mice.[82] In addition, mutations in linker proteins that connect the slit diaphragm to the actin cytoskeleton, such as CD2AP and Nck, also cause proteinuria.[83,84]

In many diseases associated with proteinuria, the interdigitating foot processes are replaced by rather broad adhesions of the cells to their GBM. This process is commonly referred to as *foot process fusion* or *effacement*. As reviewed by Kriz and associates,[85] foot process effacement is a rather complex structural response that involves profound cytoskeletal rearrangements that may finally prevent detachment of the podocyte from the GBM after injury.

MESANGIAL CELLS

The mesangial cells and their surrounding matrix constitute the mesangium, which is separated from the capillary lumen by the endothelium (see Figures 2.6 and 2.8). Light and electron microcopy studies have provided detailed descriptions of the mesangium.[21,86,87] The mesangial cell is irregular in shape, with a dense nucleus and elongated cytoplasmic processes that can extend around the capillary lumen and insinuate themselves between the GBM and the overlying endothelium (see Figure 2.8). In addition to the usual complement of organelles, mesangial cells possess an extensive array of microfilaments composed at least in part of actin, α-actinin, and myosin.[88] The contractile mesangial cell processes appear to bridge the gap in the GBM encircling the capillary, and bundles of microfilaments interconnect opposing parts of the GBM, an arrangement that is believed to prevent capillary wall distension secondary to elevation of the intracapillary hydraulic pressure.[88,89]

The mesangial cell is surrounded by a matrix that is similar to but not identical with the GBM; the mesangial matrix is more coarsely fibrillar and slightly less electron dense. Several cell surface receptors of the β-integrin family have been identified on the mesangial cells, including α1β1, α3β1, and the fibronectin receptor, α5β1.[90-92] These integrins mediate attachment of the mesangial cells to specific molecules in the extracellular mesangial matrix and link the matrix to the cytoskeleton. The attachment to the mesangial matrix is important for cell anchorage, contraction, and

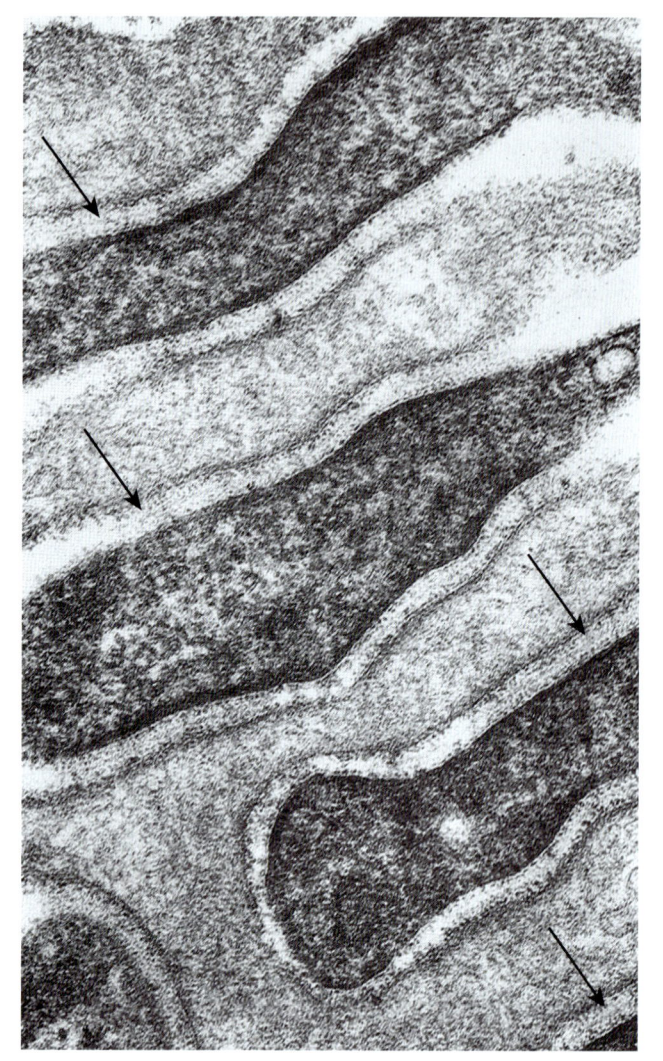

Figure 2.13 Electron micrograph showing the epithelial foot processes of normal rat glomerulus preserved in a 1% glutaraldehyde solution containing tannic acid. In several areas, the slit diaphragm has been sectioned parallel to the plane of the basement membrane, revealing a highly organized substructure. The thin central filament corresponding to the central dot observed on cross section (see Figure 2.9) is indicated by the *arrows*. (×52,000.)

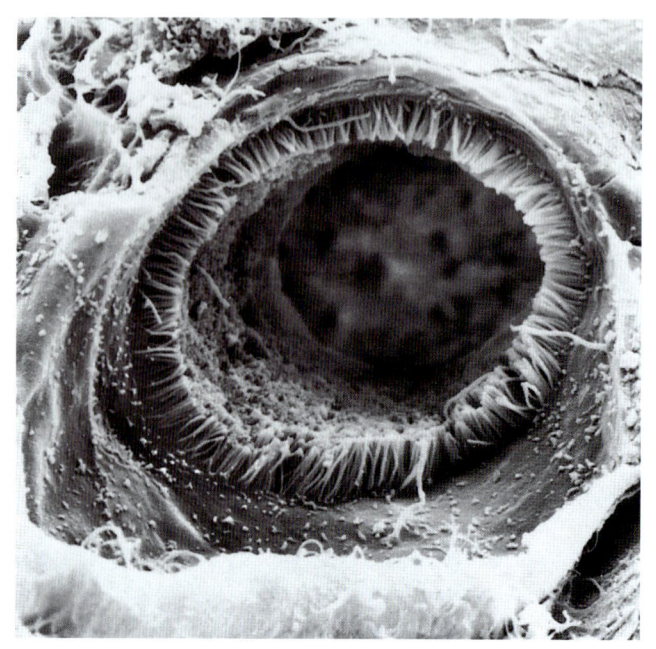

Figure 2.14 Scanning electron micrograph depicting the transition from the parietal epithelial cells of Bowman's capsule **(foreground)** to the proximal tubule cells, with their well-developed brush border, in the kidney of a rat. (×3200.)

Mesangial cells are also involved in the generation and metabolism of the extracellular mesangial matrix.[93,95] Because of both their distinct anatomic localization and their production of various vasoactive substances (e.g., nitric oxide [NO]), growth factors (e.g., VEGF, platelet-derived growth factor [PDGF], transforming growth factor [TGF]), and cytokines and chemokines (interleukins [ILs], chemokine [C-X-C motif] ligand 1 [CXCLs], chemokine [C-C motif] ligand [CCLs]), mesangial cells are also perfectly suited to mediate an extensive crosstalk to both endothelial cells and podocytes to control and maintain glomerular function.[99] As such, the mesangial cells also importantly contribute to a number of glomerular diseases, including immunoglobulin A (IgA) glomerulonephritis and diabetic nephropathy.

PARIETAL EPITHELIAL CELLS

The parietal epithelium, which forms the outer wall of Bowman's capsule, is continuous with the visceral epithelium at the vascular pole. The parietal epithelial cells are squamous in character, but at the urinary pole there is an abrupt transition to the taller cuboidal cells of the proximal tubule, which has a well-developed brush border (Figures 2.14 and 2.15). The parietal epithelium of the capsule was described in detail by Jørgensen.[21] The cells are 0.1 to 0.3 µm in height, except at the nucleus, where they increase to 2.0 to 3.5 µm. Each cell has a long cilium and occasional microvilli up to 600 nm in length. Cell organelles are generally sparse and include small mitochondria, numerous vesicles of 40 to 90 nm in diameter, and the Golgi apparatus. Large vacuoles and multivesicular bodies are rare. The thickness of the basement membrane of Bowman's capsule varies from 1200 to 1500 nm.[21] The basement membrane is composed of multiple layers, or lamellae, that increase in thickness with

migration; ligand-integrin binding also serves as a signal transduction mechanism that regulates the production of extracellular matrix as well as the synthesis of various vasoactive mediators, growth factors, and cytokines.[93,94]

As proposed by Schlondorff,[95] the mesangial cell may have some specialized features of pericytes and possesses many of the functional properties of smooth muscle cells. In addition to providing structural support for the glomerular capillary loops, the mesangial cell has contractile properties and is thought to play a role in the regulation of glomerular filtration.[95] The local generation of autacoids, such as prostaglandin E_2 (PGE_2), by the mesangial cell, may provide a counterregulatory mechanism to oppose the effect of vasoconstrictors.

Mesangial cells exhibit phagocytic properties and participate in the clearance of macro molecules from the mesangium,[95,96] as evidenced by the uptake of tracers such as ferritin,[86] colloidal carbon,[97] and aggregated proteins.[98]

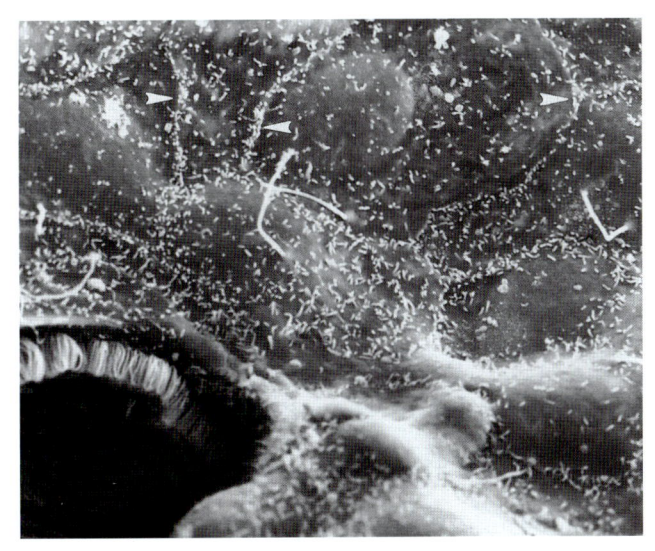

Figure 2.15 Scanning electron micrograph illustrating the appearance of the surface of the parietal epithelial cells adjacent to the early proximal tubule at the urinary pole **(lower left)**. Parietal epithelial cells possess single cilia, and their lateral cell margins are accentuated by short microvilli (*arrowheads*). (×12,500.) (Courtesy Jill W. Verlander, DVM.)

many disease processes. At both the vascular pole and the urinary pole, the thickness of Bowman's capsule decreases markedly.

The parietal epithelial cell functions as the final permeability barrier for the urinary filtrate. In experimental glomerulonephritis, this barrier is compromised, and macromolecules can leak into the space between the parietal cell and the basement membrane of Bowman's capsule and subsequently into the periglomerular space.[100] There is also evidence that the parietal epithelial cell can transdifferentiate into podocytes[101,102] and can even repopulate the glomerular tuft after extensive podocyte loss.[103] However, as reviewed by Shankland and associates, aberrant proliferation of parietal epithelial cells may also contribute to renal scarring or the formation of glomerular crescents in certain renal disease processes, such as rapidly progressive glomerulonephritis.[104]

PERIPOLAR CELLS

Ryan and colleagues have described a peripolar cell that is located at the origin of the glomerular tuft in Bowman's space and interposed between the visceral and parietal epithelial cells.[105] The peripolar cells are especially prominent in sheep, but they have also been identified in other species, including humans, and have been localized predominantly in glomeruli in the outer cortex.[106] The functional significance of these peripolar cells is unclear.

JUXTAGLOMERULAR APPARATUS

The juxtaglomerular apparatus is located at the vascular pole of the glomerulus, where a portion of the distal nephron comes into contact with its parent glomerulus. It represents a major structural component of the renin-angiotensin system and contributes to the regulation of glomerular arteriolar resistance and glomerular filtration.[107,108]

The juxtaglomerular apparatus has a vascular component and a tubular component. The vascular component is composed of the terminal portion of the afferent arteriole, the initial portion of the efferent arteriole, and the extraglomerular mesangial region. The tubular component is the macula densa, which is the terminal portion of the TAL and which is in contact with the vascular component.[109-111] The extraglomerular mesangial region, which has also been referred to as the *polar cushion (polkissen)* or the *lacis*, is bounded by the cells of the macula densa, the specialized regions of the afferent and efferent glomerular arterioles, and the mesangial cells of the glomerular tuft (the intraglomerular mesangial cells). Within the vascular component of the juxtaglomerular apparatus, two distinct cell types can be distinguished: the juxtaglomerular granular cells, also called *epithelioid or myoepithelial cells,* and the agranular extraglomerular mesangial cells, which are also referred to as *lacis cells*.

JUXTAGLOMERULAR GRANULAR CELLS

The granular cells are located primarily in the walls of the afferent and, to a lesser extent, the efferent arterioles.[109,111-113] They exhibit features of both smooth muscle cells and secretory epithelial cells and therefore have been called *myoepithelial cells*.[109] They contain myofilaments in the cytoplasm and, except for the presence of granules, are indistinguishable from the neighboring arteriolar smooth muscle cells. They also exhibit features suggestive of secretory activity, including a well-developed endoplasmic reticulum and a Golgi complex containing small granules with a crystalline substructure.[109,114]

The juxtaglomerular granular cells are characterized by the presence of numerous membrane-bound granules of variable size and shape (Figure 2.16),[113] which are thought to contain the aspartic protease renin.[115,116] In addition to these so-called specific granules, lipofuscin-like granules are commonly observed in the human kidney.[112,114]

The juxtaglomerular granular cells express both renin and angiotensin II, with activities being highest in the afferent arteriole.[117] Immunogold electron microscopy revealed that renin and angiotensin II colocalize in the same granules.[113] Enzyme histochemical and immunocytochemical studies also demonstrated the presence of lysosomal enzymes, including acid phosphatase and cathepsin B, in renin-containing granules, suggesting that these granules may represent modified lysosomes.[113] During renal development, a widespread expression of renin in the developing intrarenal arteries is seen. It later disappears from the larger arteries and arterioles and becomes restricted to the granular cells in the end portion of the afferent arteriole.[118] However, in response to extracellular volume depletion, renin expression may again extend into more proximal arterial portions,[119,120] suggesting that the renal arterial smooth muscle cells retain their ability to produce renin and can be recruited for renin secretion, depending on functional demand.

EXTRAGLOMERULAR MESANGIUM

Located between the afferent and efferent arterioles in close contact with the macula densa (see Figure 2.16), the

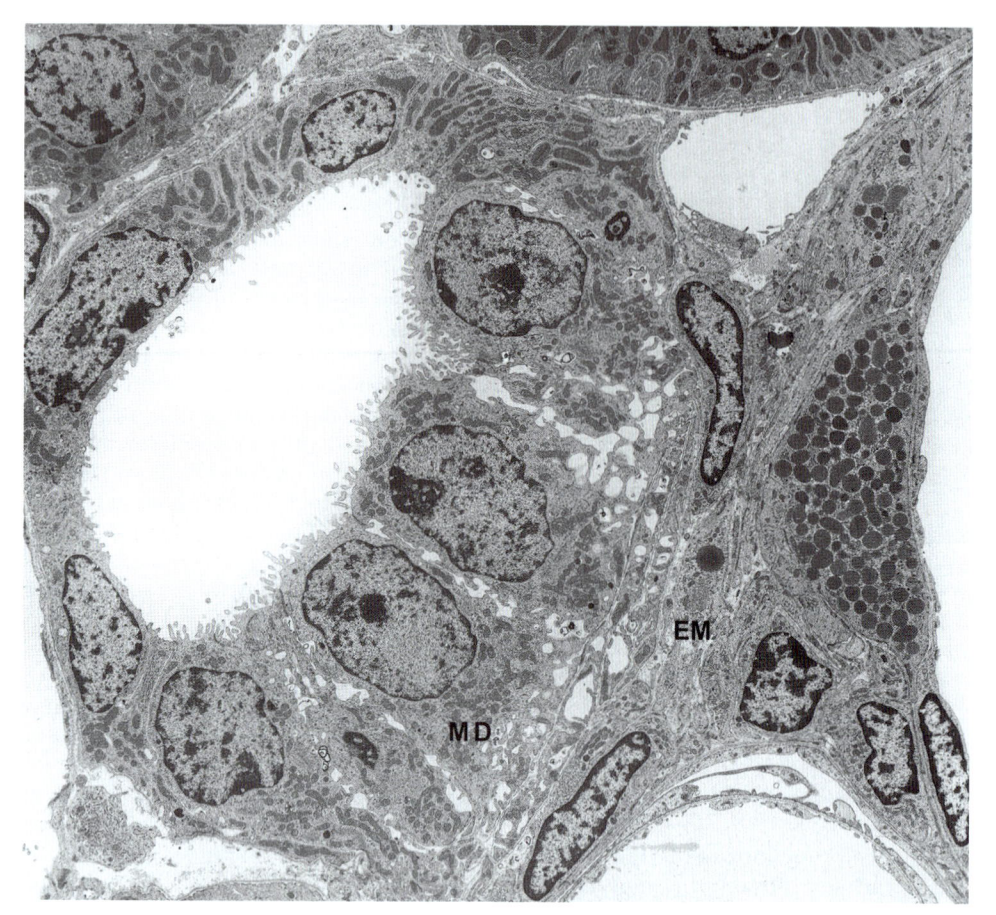

Figure 2.16 Transmission electron micrograph of juxtaglomerular apparatus from a rabbit kidney, illustrating macula densa (MD), extraglomerular mesangium (EM), and a portion of an arteriole (on the **right**), containing numerous electron-dense granules. (×3700.)

extraglomerular mesangium is continuous with the intraglomerular mesangium and is composed of cells that are similar in ultrastructure to the mesangial cells.[109,111] The extraglomerular mesangial cells possess long, thin cytoplasmic processes that are separated by basement membrane material. Under normal conditions, these cells do not contain granules; however, juxtaglomerular granular cells are occasionally observed in the extraglomerular mesangium. The extraglomerular mesangial cells are in contact with the arterioles and the macula densa, and gap junctions are commonly observed between the various cells of the vascular portion of the juxtaglomerular apparatus.[121,122] Gap junctions have also been described between extraglomerular and intraglomerular mesangial cells, suggesting that the extraglomerular mesangium may serve as a functional link between the macula densa and the glomerular arterioles.[122] Moreover, there is evidence that mesangial cell damage and selective disruption of gap junctions eliminate the tubuloglomerular feedback response.[123]

MACULA DENSA

The macula densa is a specialized region of the distal tubule adjacent to the hilum of the parent glomerulus (see Figure 2.16). Only those cells immediately adjacent to the hilum are morphologically distinctive from the surrounding cells of the TAL and are composed of columnar cells with apically placed nuclei. With electron microscopy, the cell base is seen to interdigitate with the adjacent extraglomerular mesangial cells.[109,110] Although mitochondria are numerous, their orientation is not perpendicular to the base of the cell, and they are rarely enclosed within foldings of the basolateral plasma membrane. The position of the Golgi apparatus is lateral to and beneath the cell nucleus. In addition, other cell organelles, including lysosomes, autophagic vacuoles, ribosomes, and profiles of smooth and granular endoplasmic reticulum, are located principally beneath the cell nucleus. The basement membrane of the macula densa is continuous with that surrounding the granular and agranular cells of the extraglomerular mesangial region, which in turn is continuous with the matrix material surrounding the mesangial cells within the glomerular tuft. Macula densa cells lack the lateral cell processes and interdigitations that are characteristic of the TAL. Ultrastructural studies have provided evidence that the width of the lateral intercellular spaces in the macula densa varies with the physiologic status of the animal.[124]

AUTONOMIC INNERVATION

The function of the juxtaglomerular apparatus is controlled by the autonomic nervous system. Electron microscopy demonstrated synapses between granular and agranular cells of the juxtaglomerular apparatus and autonomic nerve endings.[125] Nerve endings, principally adrenergic in type, were observed to be in contact with approximately one third of the cells of the efferent arteriole and with somewhat less than one third of the cells of the afferent arteriole, while the frequency of innervation of the tubule component of the juxtaglomerular apparatus was far less.[126] Consistent with the existence of neuroeffector junctions on renin-positive granular cells of the juxtaglomerular apparatus, renin secretion was shown to be modulated by renal sympathetic nerve activity.[127]

TUBULOGLOMERULAR FEEDBACK

The cells of the macula densa sense changes in the luminal concentrations of sodium and chloride, presumably via absorption of these ions across the luminal membrane by the Na^+-K^+-$2Cl^-$ cotransporter,[128,129] of which the NKCC2B and NKCC2A variants are expressed in the macula densa.[130,131] This sensing initiates the tubuloglomerular feedback response (see Chapter 3) by which signals generated by acute changes in sodium chloride concentration are transferred via the macula densa cells to the glomerular arterioles to control the glomerular filtration rate. Signals from the macula densa, generated in response to changes in luminal sodium and chloride, are also transmitted to the renin-secreting cells in the afferent arteriole.[108] Renin synthesis and secretion by the juxtaglomerular granular cells are also controlled by several other factors, including neurotransmitters of the sympathetic nervous system, glomerular perfusion pressure (presumably through arteriolar baroreceptors), and mediators in the macula densa.[108,132,133] There is increasing evidence that the macula densa control of renin secretion is mediated by NO, cyclo-oxygenase products such as PGE_2, and adenosine.[108,115,133-135] In addition to its inhibition of renin secretion, adenosine appears to serve as a mediator of the tubuloglomerular feedback response evoked by an increased NaCl concentration at the macula densa.[134]

PROXIMAL TUBULE

The proximal tubule consists of an initial convoluted portion, the pars convoluta, which is a direct continuation of the parietal epithelium of Bowman's capsule, and a straight portion, the pars recta, which is located in the medullary ray (see Figure 2.5). The length of the proximal tubule varies with species; for instance, it is 10 mm in rabbits,[136] 8 mm in rats, 4 to 5 mm in mice,[15] and 14 mm in humans.

In the rat[137] and the rhesus monkey,[138] three morphologically distinct segments—S1, S2, and S3—have been identified. The S1 segment is the initial portion of the proximal tubule; it begins at the glomerulus and constitutes approximately two thirds of the pars convoluta (see Figures 2.14 and 2.15). The S2 segment contains the final third of the pars convoluta and the initial portion of the pars recta. The S3 segment is the remainder of the proximal tubule, located in the deep inner cortex and the outer stripe of the outer medulla. These segments can be distinguished morphologically because of their structurally unique cells[137,139] (Figures 2.17 through 2.19). Cells in the S1 segment have a tall brush border and a well-developed vacuolar-lysosomal system. The basolateral plasma membrane forms extensive lateral invaginations, and lateral cell processes extending from the apical to the basal surface interdigitate with similar processes from adjacent cells. Elongated mitochondria are located in the lateral cell processes in proximity to the plasma membrane. The ultrastructure of cells in the S2 segment is similar to that in the S1 segment; however, the brush border is shorter, the basolateral invaginations are less prominent, and the mitochondria are smaller. Numerous small lateral processes are located close to the base of the cell. The endocytic compartment is less prominent than in the S1 segment, with the number and size of the lysosomes varying among species and between males and females.[136,137]

In cells from the S3 segment, the length of the brush border differs with species and can be rather short (in humans) or long (in rats). Lateral cell processes and invaginations are essentially absent, and mitochondria are small and randomly distributed within the cell. Species variation is also observed in the vacuolar-lysosomal compartment in the S3 segment. In rats[137] and humans,[140] endocytic vacuoles and lysosomes are small and sparse, whereas in rabbits, large endocytic vacuoles and numerous small lysosomes are present.[136] Peroxisomes are present throughout the proximal tubule, with progressively increased quantities toward the S3 segment. There are contrasts to the described morphology in different species. In rabbits, the S2 segment represents a transition between the S1 and S3 segments,[141,142] whereas in mice there is no structural segmentation along the proximal tubule.[15] In the nondiseased human kidney, only the pars convoluta and the pars recta have been positively identified and described.[140] To facilitate comparisons, the remainder of this chapter differentiates the proximal tubule into the convoluted and the straight portions, rather than the S1, S2, and S3 segments.

PARS CONVOLUTA

Cells of the pars convoluta are structurally complex (Figure 2.20).[143] Large primary ridges extend laterally from the apical to the basal surfaces of the cells. Large lateral processes, often containing mitochondria, extend outwards from the primary ridges and interdigitate with similar processes in adjacent cells (see Figure 2.20). At the luminal surfaces of the cells, smaller lateral processes extend outwards from the primary ridges to interdigitate with those of adjacent cells. Small basal villi that do not contain mitochondria are found along the basal cell surfaces (Figure 2.21). These extensive interdigitations result in a complex extracellular compartment, referred to as the *basolateral intercellular space* (see Figures 2.21 and 2.22), that is separated from the tubule lumen (apical cell surface) by the *zonula occludens* or *tight junctions*.[144] In parallel with a high-resistance pathway across the apical and basal plasma membranes of the proximal tubule cell, a low-resistance shunt pathway is also present.[145-147] Thus, the proximal tubule is often referred to as "a leaky epithelium" with low transepithelial resistance and high paracellular transport. Claudins, a diverse family of tight junction proteins with various ion permeability properties that are expressed throughout the renal tubule system, mediate the paracellular permeability properties of the tight junction (see Chapter 6).[148] Claudin-2 and claudin-10 are highly expressed in proximal tubule cells,[149] and claudin-2 forms high-conductance cation pores permitting large amounts of paracellular Na^+ transport.[150]

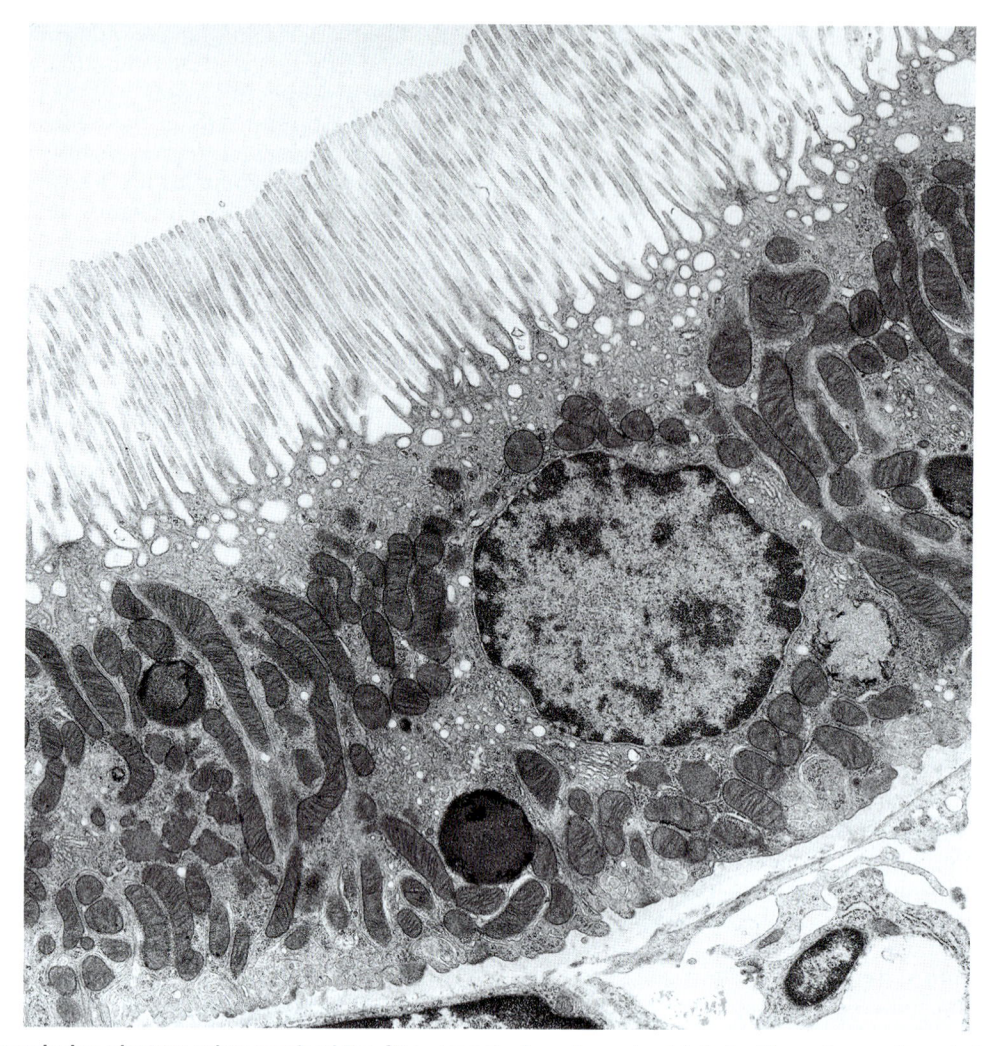

Figure 2.17 Transmission electron micrograph of the S1 segment of a rat proximal tubule. The cells are characterized by a tall brush border, a prominent endocytic-lysosomal apparatus, and extensive invaginations of the basolateral plasma membrane. (×10,600.)

Interestingly, claudin-2, which is frequently expressed in leaky epithelia, has been shown to be water permeable.[151] Below the tight junction lies the beltlike intermediate junction or *zonula adherens*,[144] which is followed by several desmosomes distributed randomly at variable distances beneath the intermediate junction. In mammalian and invertebrate renal proximal tubules, gap junctions are present in small numbers[19] and can provide a pathway for the movement of ions between cells and for cell-cell communication via a family of proteins known as *connexins*.[152] The lateral intercellular space of each pars convoluta cell is open toward the basement membrane, which separates the cell from the peritubular interstitium and capillaries. The thickness of the basement membrane gradually decreases along the proximal tubule, in the rhesus monkey, for example, from approximately 250 nm in the S1 segment to 145 nm in the S2 segment to 70 nm in the S3 segment.[138]

The lateral cell processes of pars convoluta cells combined with extensive invaginations of the plasma membrane increase both the intercellular space and surface area of the basolateral plasma membrane. Studies in rabbits have demonstrated that the area of the lateral surface equals that of the luminal surface and amounts to 2.9 mm^2 per mm of tubule.[153] Elongated mitochondria are located in the lateral cell processes in close proximity to the plasma membrane (see Figure 2.22), where the sodium-potassium adenosine triphosphatase (Na$^+$-K$^+$-ATPase) is located.[154,155] Mitochondria are often observed as rod-shaped and tortuous, but many mitochondria are branched and connected with one another.[156] A system of smooth membranes called the *paramembranous cisternal system*, thought to be in continuity with the smooth endoplasmic reticulum,[157] is often observed between the plasma membrane and mitochondria. The function of the paramembranous cisternal system is not known. Pars convoluta cells contain large quantities of smooth and rough endoplasmic reticulum, and free ribosomes are abundant in the cytoplasm. A well-developed Golgi apparatus, composed of smooth-surfaced sacs or cisternae, coated vesicles, uncoated vesicles, and larger vacuoles, is located above and lateral to the nucleus in the midregion of the cell (Figure 2.23). In addition, an extensive system of microtubules is located throughout the cytoplasm of proximal tubule cells.

Pars convoluta cells have well-developed brush borders at their luminal surfaces that are formed by numerous finger-like projections of the apical plasma membranes, the

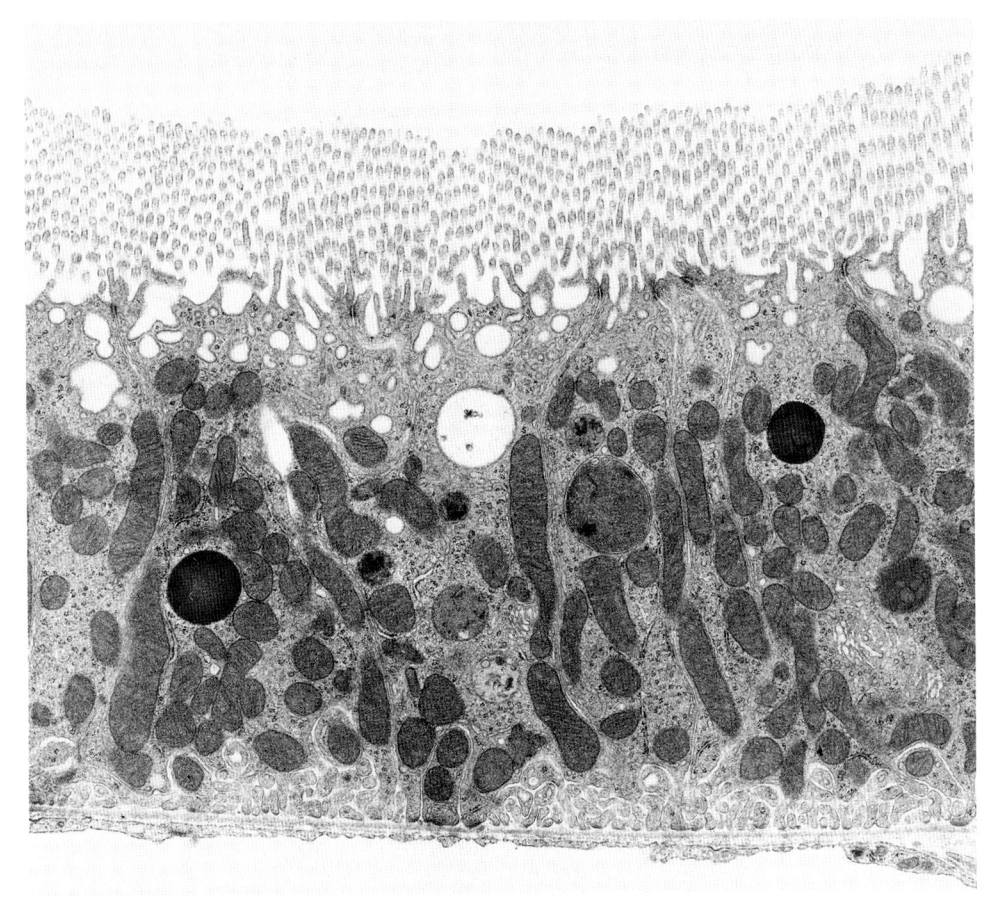

Figure 2.18 Transmission electron micrograph of the S2 segment of a rat proximal tubule. The brush border is less prominent than in the S1 segment. Note numerous small lateral processes at the base of the cell. (×10,600.)

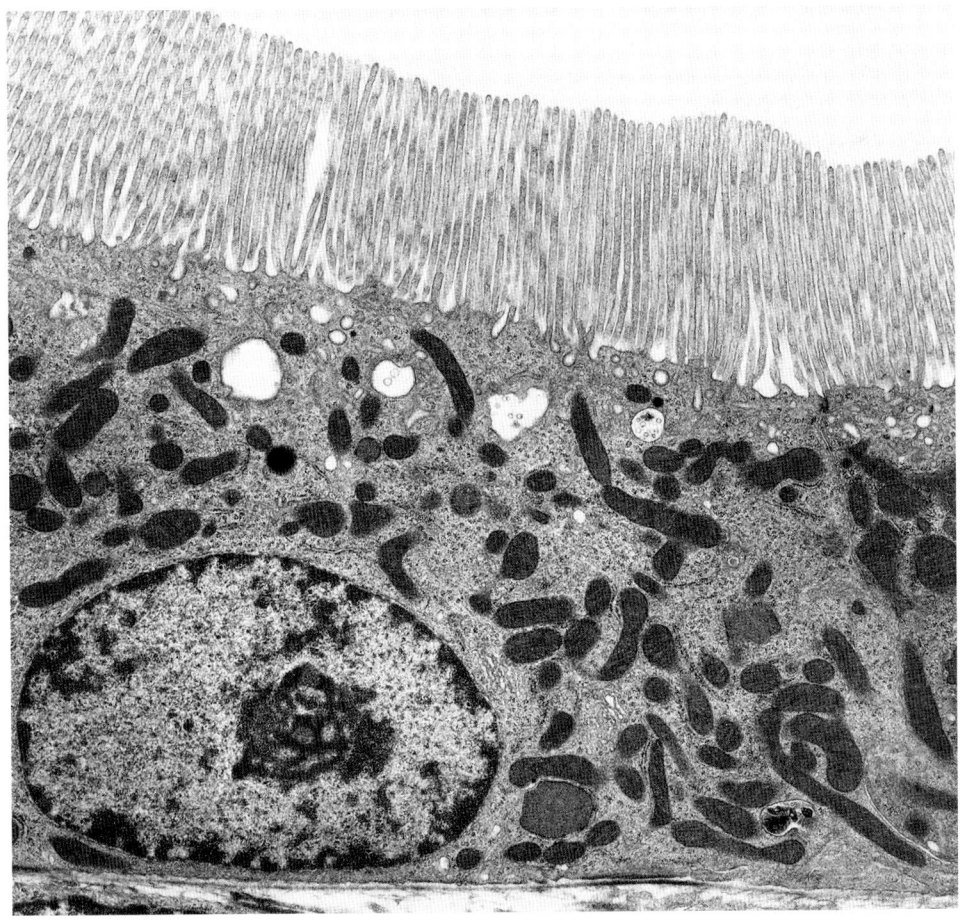

Figure 2.19 Transmission electron micrograph of the S3 segment of a rat proximal tubule. The brush border is tall, but the endocytic-lysosomal apparatus is less prominent than in the S1 and S2 segments. Basolateral invaginations are sparse, and mitochondria are scattered randomly throughout the cytoplasm. (×10,600.)

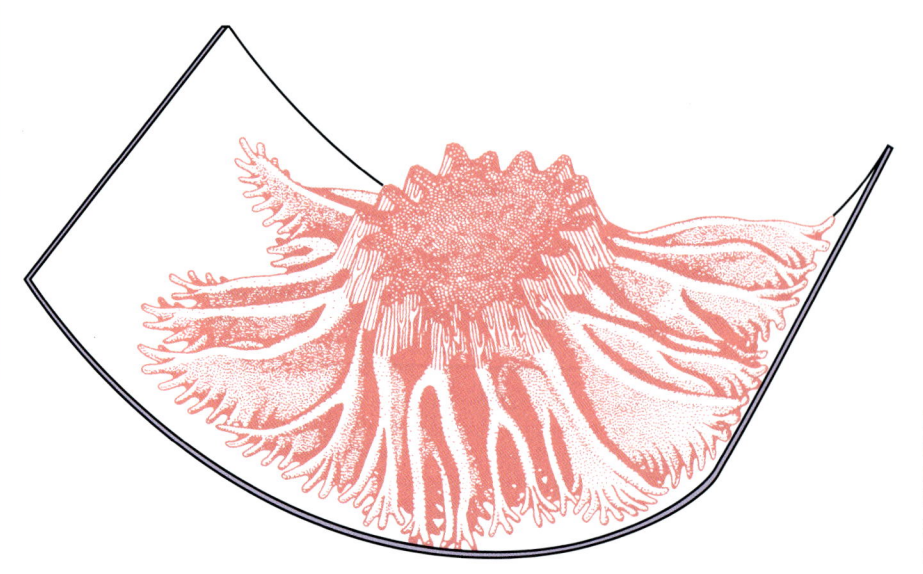

Figure 2.20 Schematic drawing illustrating the three-dimensional configuration of the proximal convoluted tubule cell. (From Welling LW, Welling DJ: Shape of epithelial cells and intercellular channels in the rabbit proximal nephron. *Kidney Int* 9:385-394, 1976.)

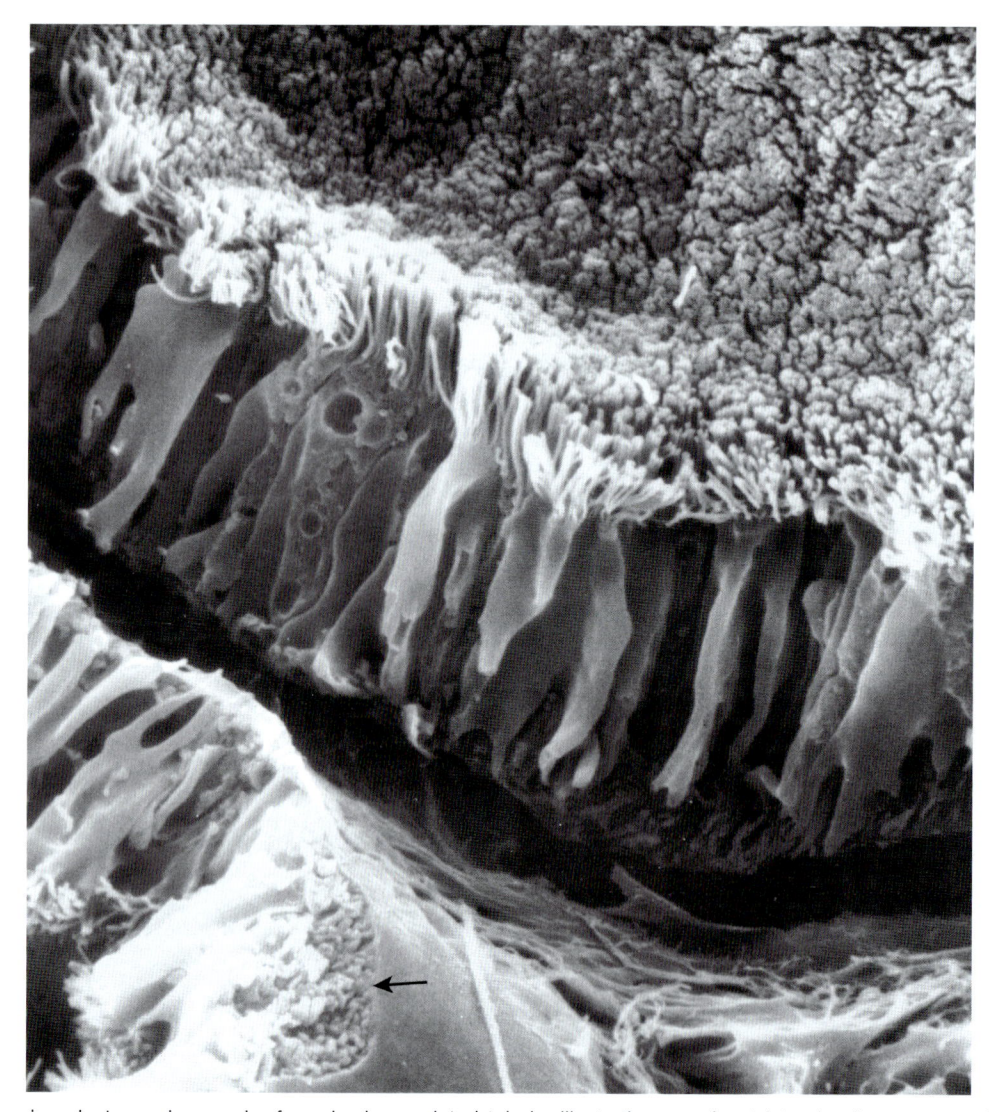

Figure 2.21 Scanning electron micrograph of proximal convoluted tubule, illustrating prominent lateral cell processes. *Arrow* on adjacent proximal convoluted tubule denotes small basal processes. (×8200.) (From Madsen KM, Brenner BM: Structure and function of the renal tubule and interstitium. In Tisher CC, Brenner BM, editors: *Renal pathology with clinical and functional correlations,* Philadelphia, 1989, JB Lippincott, p 606.)

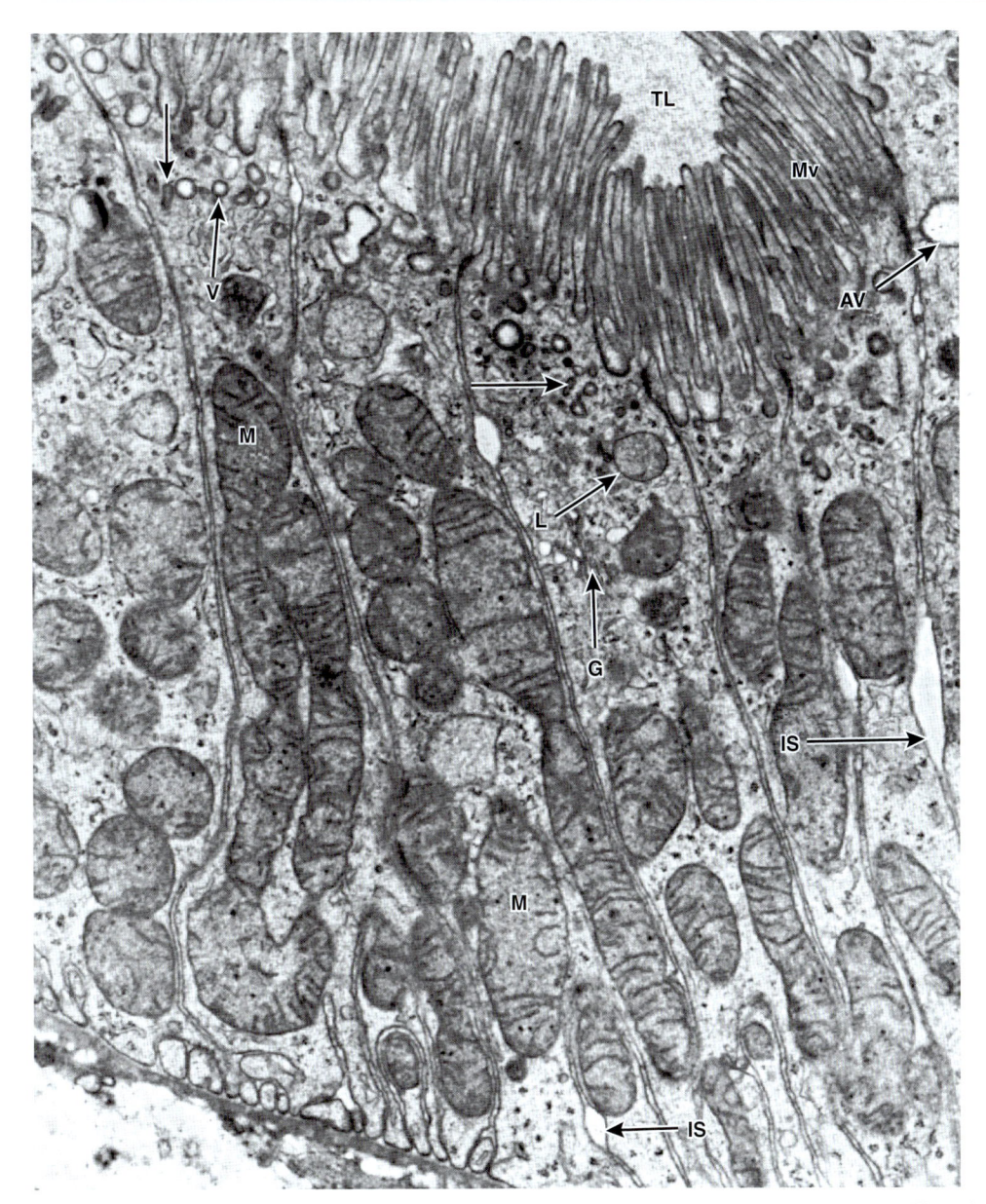

Figure 2.22 Electron micrograph of the pars convoluta of the proximal tubule from a normal human kidney. The mitochondria (M) are elongated and tortuous, occasionally doubling back on themselves. The endocytic apparatus, composed of apical vacuoles (AV), apical vesicles (V), and apical dense tubules *(arrows)*, is well developed. G, Golgi apparatus; IS, intercellular space; L, lysosome; Mv, microvilli forming the brush border; TL, tubule lumen. (×15,000.)

microvilli. The brush border serves to increase the apical cell surface, by 36-fold in rabbit kidneys.[153] Each microvilli contains 6 to 10 actin filaments of approximately 6 nm in diameter that extend downwards into the apical region of the cell for variable distances. A network of filaments containing myosin and spectrin,[158] called the *terminal web*, is located in the apical cytoplasm just beneath and perpendicular to the microvilli.[159] Each pars convoluta cell has a well-developed endocytic-lysosomal apparatus that is involved in the reabsorption and degradation of macromolecules from the ultrafiltrate.[160] The endocytic compartment consists of an extensive system of coated pits, small coated vesicles, apical dense tubules, and larger endocytic vacuoles without a cytoplasmic coat (Figure 2.24). The coated pits are invaginations of the apical plasma membrane at the base of the microvilli and contain clathrin[161] and megalin,[162,163] proteins that are involved in receptor-mediated endocytosis. The cytoplasmic coat of the small vesicles is similar in ultrastructure to the coat that is present on the cytoplasmic side of the coated pits.

A large number of lysosomes with variable size, shape, and ultrastructural appearance are present in cells of the pars convoluta (Figure 2.25).[160,164] Lysosomes are membrane-bound, heterogeneous organelles that contain a variety of acid hydrolases, including acid phosphatases, and various proteases, lipases, and glycosidases. Lysosomes are involved in the degradation of material absorbed by endocytosis (heterophagocytosis), and they often contain multiple electron-dense deposits that are believed to represent reabsorbed substances such as proteins (see Figure 2.25). Lysosomes

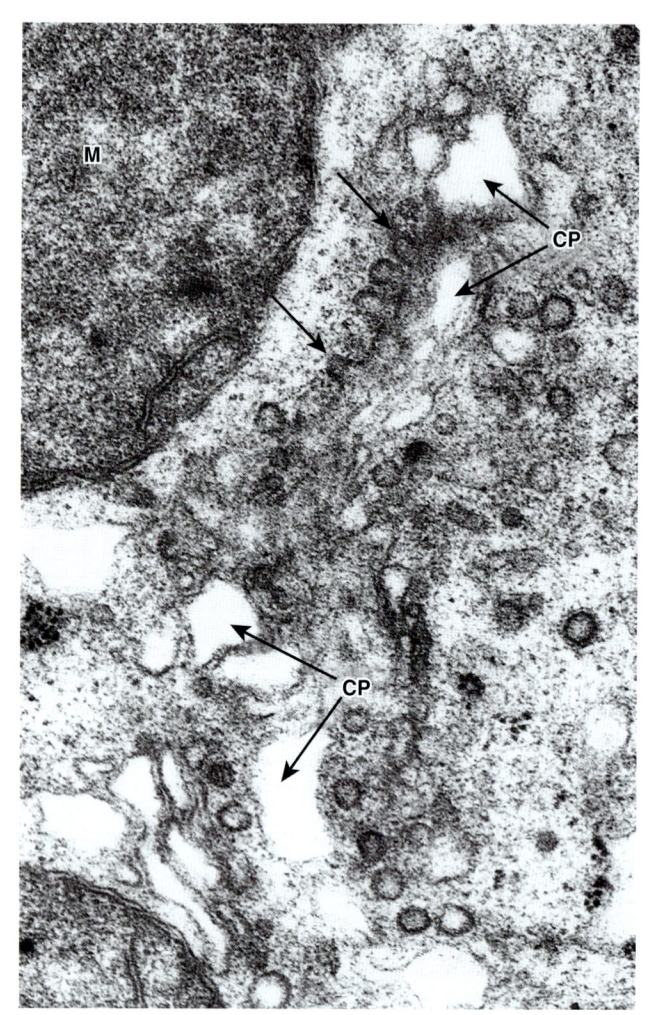

Figure 2.23 Electron micrograph of a Golgi apparatus from a normal human proximal tubule. Small vesicles *(arrows)* consistent with the appearance of primary lysosomes are seen budding from the larger cisternal profiles (CP). M, mitochondrion. (×32,900.) (From Tisher CC, Bulger RE, Trump BF: Human renal ultrastructure. I: Proximal tubule of healthy individuals. *Lab Invest* 15:1357-1394, 1966.)

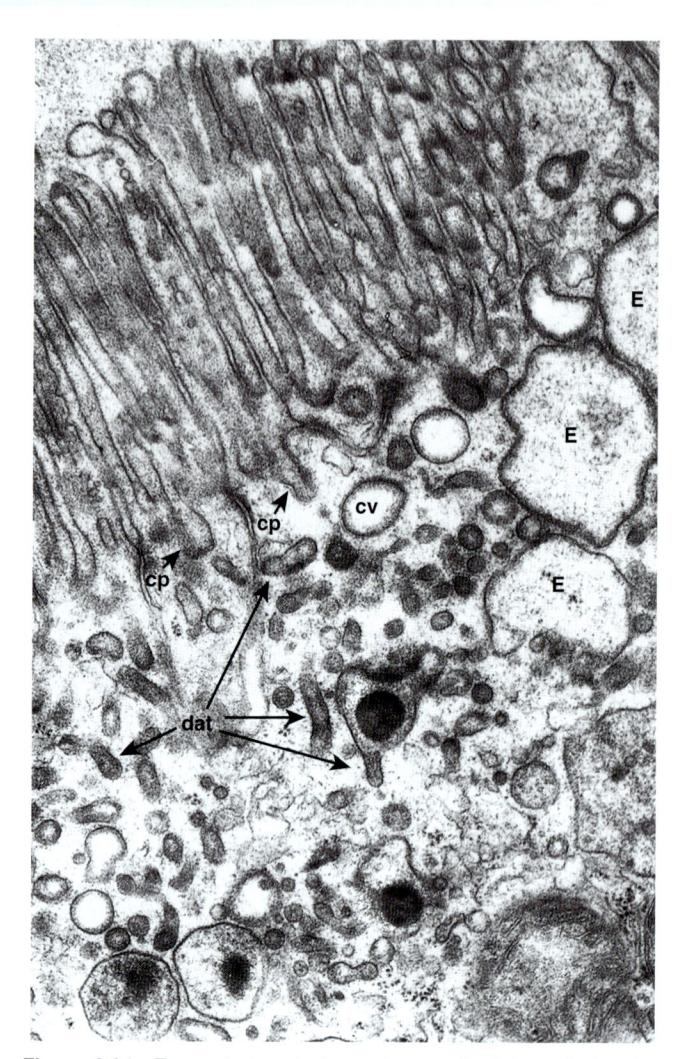

Figure 2.24 Transmission electron micrograph of the apical region of a human proximal tubule, illustrating the endocytic apparatus, including coated pits (cp), coated vesicles (cv), apical dense tubules (dat), and endosomes (E). (×18,500.)

also play a role in the normal turnover of intracellular constituents by autophagocytosis, and autophagic vacuoles containing fragments of cell organelles are often seen in pars convoluta cells.[164] Lysosomes containing nondigestible substances are called *residual bodies*, which can empty their contents into the tubule lumen by exocytosis. Multivesicular bodies (MVBs), which are part of the vacuolar-lysosomal system, are often observed in the cytoplasm of proximal convoluted tubule cells. MVBs were originally thought to be involved in membrane retrieval and/or membrane disposal, but later studies suggest that MVBs may provide an exit route for a variety of endocytically retrieved plasma membrane proteins (of both basolateral and apical membrane origin) and could also function as a signaling mechanism to downstream nephron segments.[165,166] The extensive vacuolar-lysosomal system of proximal tubule cells plays an important role in the reabsorption and degradation of albumin and low-molecular-weight plasma proteins from the glomerular filtrate.[160,167,168] Under normal conditions the vacuolar-lysosomal system is most prominent in the pars convoluta, but in proteinuric states large vacuoles and extensive lysosomes can be observed in the latter portions of the proximal tubule.[136,137]

PARS RECTA

The pars recta is the terminal portion of the S2 segment and the entire S3 segment. Pars recta morphology varies considerably between species, (e.g., in the rat, the microvilli of the brush border measure up to 4 μm in length, whereas in the rabbit and human kidney they are much shorter). The epithelium of the pars recta S3 segment is simpler than that of the S1 and S2 segments.[137,141] Invaginations of the basolateral plasma membrane are virtually absent, mitochondria are small and randomly scattered throughout the cytoplasm, and the intercellular spaces are smaller and less complex (see Figures 2.21 and 2.26). These morphologic characteristics are in agreement with studies demonstrating that Na^+-K^+-ATPase activity and fluid reabsorption are significantly less in the pars recta than in the pars convoluta.[169,170] In contrast to cells of the pars convoluta, the vacuolar-lysosomal system is less prominent in cells of the

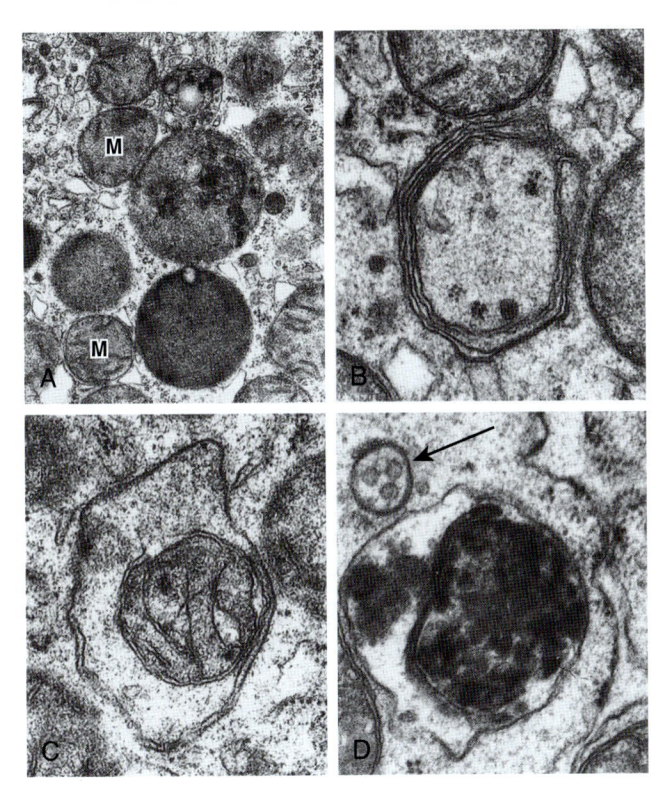

Figure 2.25 Electron micrographs illustrating the appearance of different types of lysosomes from human proximal tubules. **A,** Lysosomes. Several mitochondria (M) are also shown. (×15,500.) **B,** Early stage of formation of an autophagic vacuole. (×23,500.) **C,** Fully formed autolysosome containing a mitochondrion undergoing digestion. (×28,500.) **D,** Autolysosome, containing a microbody undergoing digestion. A multivesicular body *(arrow)* is also shown. (×29,250.) (From Tisher CC, Bulger RE, Trump BF: Human renal ultrastructure. I: Proximal tubule of healthy individuals. *Lab Invest* 15:1357-1394, 1966.)

S3 segment, although in both rabbits and humans, many small lysosomes with electron-dense membrane-like material can still be observed.[136,140] Peroxisomes are common in the pars recta. In contrast to lysosomes, peroxisomes are irregular in shape, are surrounded by a 6.5-nm-thick membrane, and do not contain acid hydrolases.[164] Peroxisomes within the pars recta vary considerably in appearance among species. In the rat, small, circular profiles can be observed just inside the limiting membrane, and rod-shaped structures often project outward from the organelle. In addition, a small nucleoid is often present in peroxisomes from the pars recta. The functional significance of peroxisomes in the kidney is not known with certainty; however, they are believed to be involved in lipid metabolism and fatty acid oxidation. They have a high content of catalase, which is involved in the degradation of hydrogen peroxide, and of various oxidative enzymes, including l-α-hydroxy-acid oxidase and D-amino acid oxidase.[171,172] Interestingly, mistargeting of the mutated peroxisomal enzyme EHHADH (enoyl-CoA hydratase–L-3-hydroxyacyl-CoA dehydrogenase) to proximal tubule mitochondria disrupts mitochondrial metabolism and leads to renal Fanconi's syndrome.[173]

The proximal tubule plays a major role in the reabsorption of Na^+, HCO_3^-, Cl^-, K^+, Ca^{2+}, PO_4^{3-}, water, and organic solutes such as vitamins, glucose, and amino acids. The aforementioned ultrastructural specializations of the proximal tubule cells aid in these transport processes. The transcellular transport of these substances occurs via specific transport proteins that have polarized expression in proximal tubule cells (see Chapters 6 through 9). Of note, the rate of fluid absorption from the proximal tubule to the peritubular capillaries is influenced by the hydraulic and oncotic pressures across the tubule and capillary wall. Changes in these parameters cause significant ultrastructural changes in the proximal tubule, especially in the configuration of the lateral intercellular spaces.[174,175]

THIN LIMBS OF THE LOOP OF HENLE

For an extensive review of the structure and function of the thin limbs of the loop of Henle, see the review by Pannabecker.[176] The thin limbs of the loop of Henle connect the proximal and distal tubules of the nephron. The transition from the proximal tubule to the descending thin limb of the loop of Henle is abrupt (Figures 2.27 and 2.28) and marks the boundary between the outer and inner stripes of the outer medulla. Short-looped nephrons originating from superficial and midcortical glomeruli have a short descending thin limb located in the inner stripe of the outer medulla. Close to the hairpin turn of the short loops of Henle, the thin limb continues into the TAL. Long-looped nephrons originating from juxtamedullary glomeruli have a long descending thin limb that extends into the inner medulla and a long ascending thin limb that continues into the TAL. The transition from the thin to the thick ascending limb forms the boundary between the outer and inner medulla (see Figure 2.5). Nephrons arising in the extreme outer cortex may possess short cortical loops that do not extend into the medulla. Variations on this basic organization have been highlighted in studies of different species.[13,16,177] The histotopographic organization of the renal medulla has been studied in several laboratory animals, including three-dimensional (3D) reconstruction studies of the nephron.[13,16] These studies have highlighted the complexity of organization of the medulla and are discussed in detail in Chapter 10.

Ultrastructural studies have shown that the cells of the initial part of the descending thin limb of Henle have extensive interdigitation with one another, whereas the cells of the ascending thin limb near the transition with the TAL, and thin limb cells in the inner medulla, are less complex in configuration. Four morphologically distinct segments of the thin limb of Henle, composed of four types of epithelia (types I through IV), have been described and classified on the basis of their ultrastructure and location within the medulla[141,178-182] (Figure 2.29). Type I epithelium is found exclusively in the descending thin limb of short-looped nephrons. Type II epithelium forms the descending thin limb of long-looped nephrons in the outer medulla and gives way to type III epithelium in the inner medulla. Type IV epithelium forms the bends of the long loops and the entire ascending thin limb to the transition into the TAL at the boundary between the inner and outer medulla. Type I epithelium is extremely thin and has few basal or luminal surface specializations, the latter in the form of microvilli (see Figure 2.29). There is a virtual absence of lateral interdigitations with adjacent cells, and cellular organelles are relatively sparse. Tight junctions between

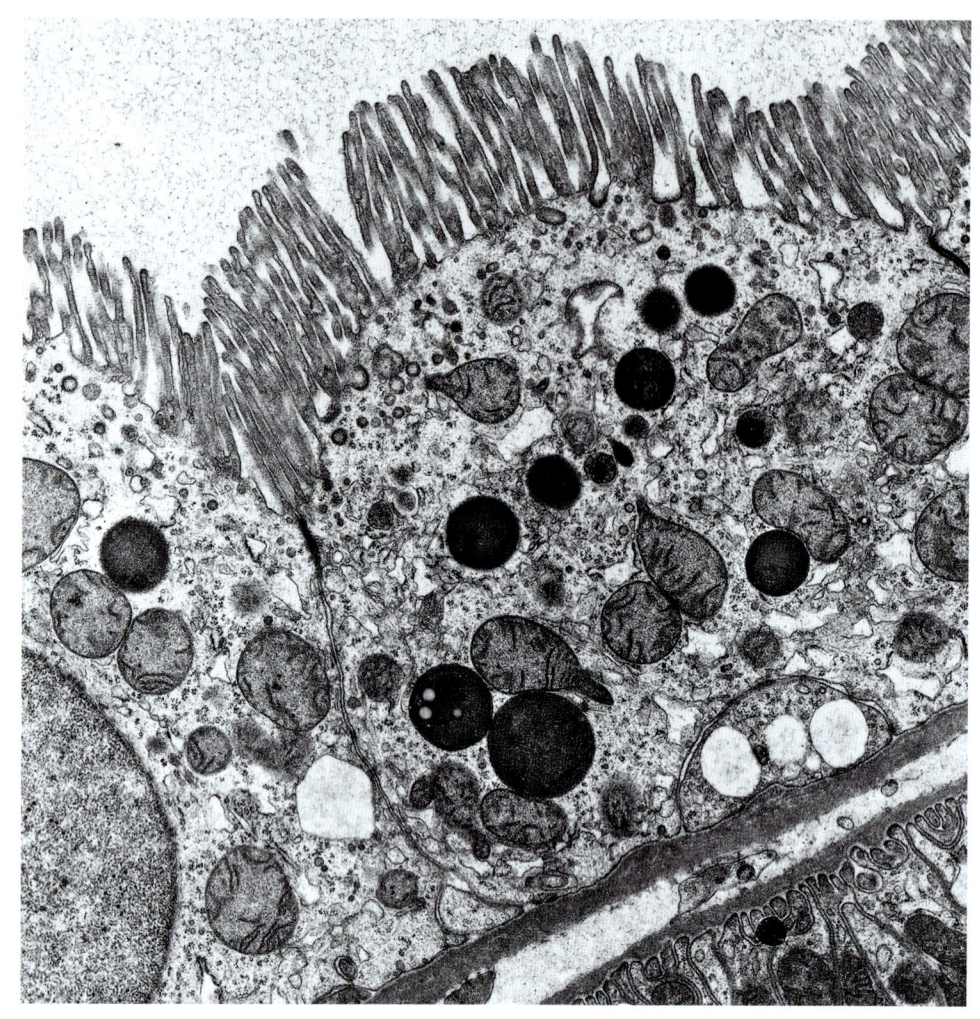

Figure 2.26 Low-magnification electron micrograph of a segment of the pars recta of a proximal tubule from a human kidney. The microvilli on the convex apical cell surface are not as long as those from the pars recta of the rat. The lysosomes are extremely electron dense. The clear, single membrane–limited structures at the base of the cell to the right represent lipid droplets. (×10,400.) (Courtesy R. E. Bulger, PhD.)

cells are intermediate in depth with several junctional strands, suggesting a tight epithelium.[183-185] Type II epithelium is taller and exhibits considerable species differences. In the rat,[186] mouse,[178] *Psammomys obesus*,[181] and hamster,[180] the type II epithelium is complex and characterized by extensive lateral and basal interdigitations and a well-developed paracellular pathway (Figure 2.30). The tight junctions are extremely shallow and contain a single junctional strand, characteristics of a "leaky epithelium." The luminal surface is covered by short blunt microvilli, and cell organelles, including mitochondria, are more prominent than in other segments of the thin limb. In the rabbit the type II epithelium is less complex[141]; lateral interdigitations and paracellular pathways are less prominent, and tight junctions are deeper.[184] In comparison with type II epithelium, type III epithelium is lower (thinner) and has a simpler structure. The cells do not interdigitate, the tight junctions are intermediate in depth, and fewer microvilli cover the luminal surface. Type IV epithelium (see Figure 2.29) is generally low and flattened and possesses relatively few organelles. It is characterized by an absence of surface microvilli but has an abundance of lateral cell processes and interdigitations. The tight junctions are shallow, characteristic of a leaky epithelium, and as such type IV epithelium has prominent paracellular pathways.

The basement membrane of the thin limb segments varies greatly in thickness from species to species and in many animals is multilayered. There is structural heterogeneity along the thin limb of the loop of Henle in the rat,[185] rabbit,[184] and *P. obesus*.[183] Segmental as well as species differences were found in the number of strands and the depth of the tight junctions. The most striking finding in these ultrastructural studies was the extremely high density of intramembrane particles in both the luminal and the basolateral membranes of type II epithelium. In the rat, type II epithelium has significant levels of Na^+-K^+-ATPase activity,[187,188] whereas little activity is detectable in other segments of the rat thin limb or in any segment of the rabbit thin limb.[189] Permeability studies of isolated perfused descending thin limbs from different species have demonstrated that type II epithelium has a higher permeability to Na^+ and K^+ in the rat and hamster than in the rabbit,[190] supporting the described differences in ultrastructure and biochemical properties of type II epithelium among species.

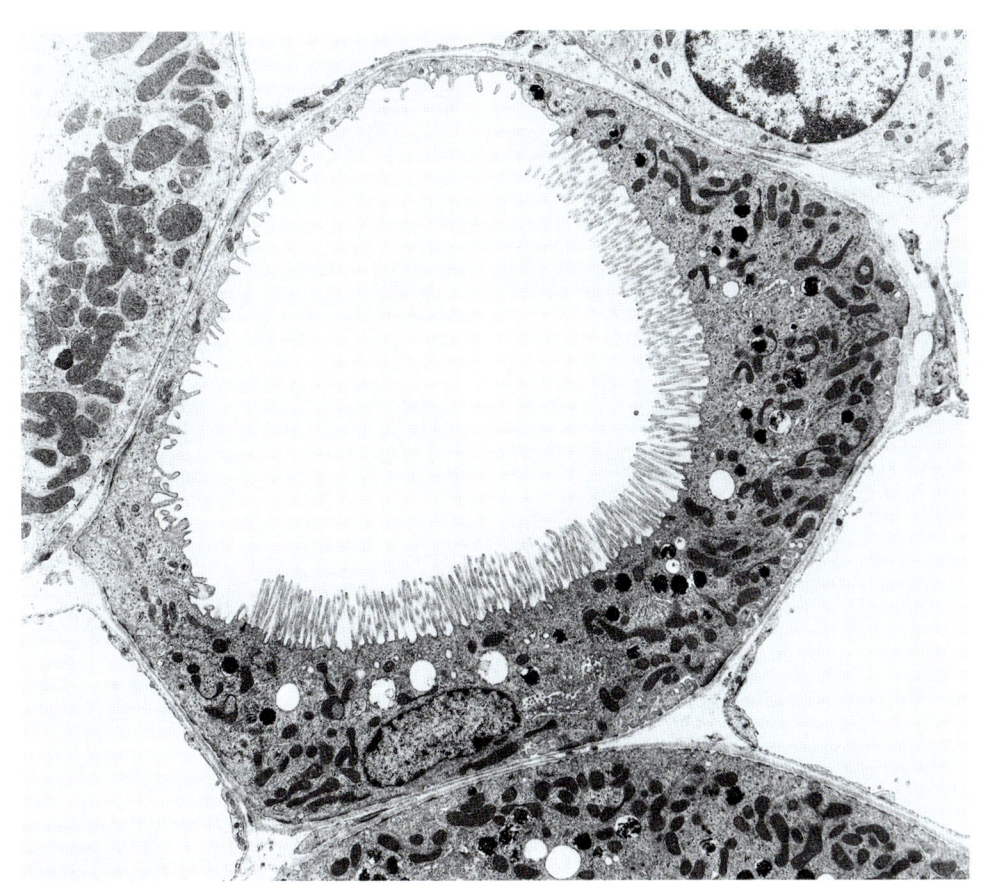

Figure 2.27 Transmission electron micrograph from rabbit kidney, illustrating the transition from the pars recta of the proximal tubule to the descending thin limb of the loop of Henle. (×4500.) (From Madsen KM, Park CH: Lysosome distribution and cathepsin B and L activity along the rabbit proximal tubule. *Am J Physiol* 253:F1290-F1301, 1987.)

It is generally accepted that the permeability properties of the thin limb epithelium are important for the maintenance of a hypertonic interstitium. The role of the thin limb in the maintenance of a hypertonic medullary interstitium and in the dilution and concentration of the urine via countercurrent multiplication is discussed in detail in Chapter 10.

DISTAL TUBULE

The distal tubule is composed of morphologically distinct segments: the TAL (pars recta), the macula densa, the distal convoluted tubule (DCT) (pars convoluta), and the connecting tubules. Some studies showed that the cortical TAL extends beyond the vicinity of the macula densa and forms an abrupt transition with the DCT at a slightly more distal position.[141,191] These data, combined with the observation that TAL proteins are observed by immunohistochemical methods even slightly distal to the macula densa, suggest that the macula densa is a specialized region within the TAL.

THICK ASCENDING LIMB

The TAL represents the initial portion of the distal tubule and can be divided into a medullary and a cortical segment (see Figure 2.5). In long-looped nephrons, there is an abrupt transition from the thin ascending limb to the TAL, which marks the boundary between the inner medulla and the inner stripe of the outer medulla. In short-looped nephrons, the transition to the TAL can occur shortly before the hairpin turn, but this is not the case in all species.[16] From its transition from the thin limb, the TAL extends upward through the outer medulla and the cortex to the glomerulus belonging to the nephron of origin, where the macula densa is formed. At the point of contact with the extraglomerular mesangial region, only the immediately contiguous portion of the wall of the tubule actually forms the macula densa. The transition from TAL to the DCT occurs shortly after the macula densa. The cells forming the medullary segment in the inner stripe of the outer medulla measure approximately 7 to 8 μm in height.[141,192] As the tubule ascends toward the cortex, cell height gradually decreases to approximately 5 μm in the cortical TAL of the rat[192] and to 2 μm in the terminal part of the cortical TAL of the rabbit. Welling and colleagues reported an average cell height of 4.5 μm in the cortical TAL of the rabbit kidney.[193]

The cells of the TAL are characterized by extensive invaginations of the basolateral plasma membrane and interdigitations between adjacent cells. The lateral invaginations often extend two thirds or more of the distance from the base to the luminal border of the cell. This arrangement is most prominent in the TAL of the inner stripe of the outer medulla (Figure 2.31). Numerous elongated mitochondria are located in lateral cell processes, and their orientation is perpendicular to the basement membrane. The mitochondria resemble those in the proximal tubule but contain very

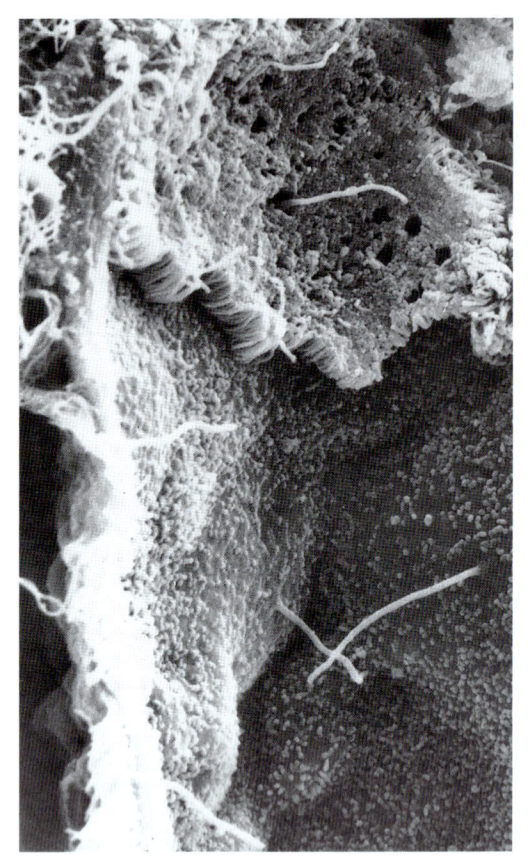

Figure 2.28 Scanning electron micrograph from a normal rat kidney, depicting the transition from the terminal S3 segment of the proximal tubule **(above)** to the early descending thin limb of Henle **(below)**. Note the elongated cilia projecting into the lumen from cells of the proximal tubule and the thin limb of Henle. (×4500.)

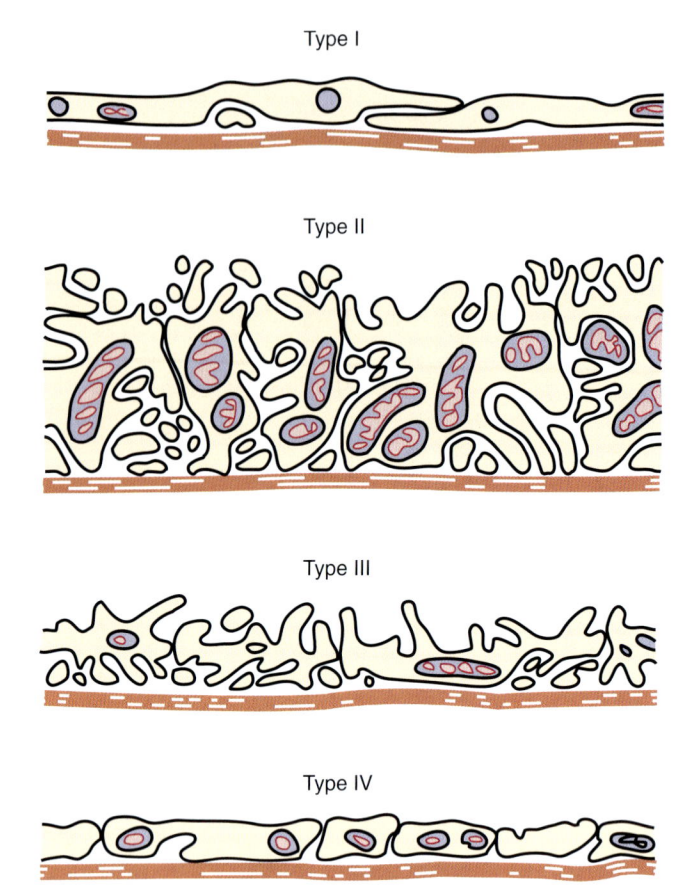

Figure 2.29 Diagram depicting the appearance of the four types of thin limb segments in a rat kidney. (See text for explanation.)

prominent granules in the matrix. Other subcellular organelles in this segment of the nephron include a well-developed Golgi complex, multivesicular bodies and lysosomes, and abundant quantities of smooth and rough endoplasmic reticulum. Numerous small vesicles are commonly observed in the apical portion of the cytoplasm. The cells are attached to one another via tight junctions that are 0.1 to 0.2 μm in depth in the rat.[144] Intermediate junctions are also present, but desmosomes appear to be lacking.

Scanning electron microscopy of the TAL of the rat kidney has revealed the existence of two distinct surface configurations of the luminal membrane.[191] Some cells have a rough surface because of the presence of numerous small microprojections, whereas others have a smooth surface that is largely devoid of microprojections except along the apical cell margins (Figure 2.32). Like all other cells from the parietal layer of Bowman's capsule to the terminal collecting duct (except intercalated cells), TAL cells possess a primary cilium. The rough-surfaced cells possess more extensive lateral processes radiating from the main cell body than do the smooth-surfaced cells. In contrast, small vesicles and tubulovesicular profiles are more numerous in the apical region of the smooth-surfaced cells. A predominance of cells with the smooth-surface pattern is observed in the medullary segment. As the thick limb ascends toward the cortex, the number of cells with a rough surface pattern increases, and luminal microprojections and apical lateral invaginations become more prominent. Consequently, the surface area of the luminal plasma membrane is significantly greater in the cortical TAL than in the medullary TAL.[192]

The TAL is involved in active transport of NaCl from the lumen to the surrounding interstitium. Because this epithelium is almost impermeable to water, the reabsorption of salt contributes to the formation of a hypertonic medullary interstitium and the delivery of a dilute tubule fluid to the DCT (see Chapter 6). In studies by Good and colleagues evidence is provided that in addition to NaCl reabsorption, the TAL is involved in HCO_3^- reabsorption in the rat.[194,195] Finally, the TAL is involved in the transport of divalent cations such as Ca^{2+} and Mg^{2+}.[196,197] The reabsorption of NaCl in both the medullary and the cortical segments of the TAL is mediated by a Na^+-K^+-$2Cl^-$ cotransport mechanism,[198-201] which is inhibited by loop diuretics such as furosemide and bumetanide.[201] The bumetanide-sensitive Na^+-K^+-$2Cl^-$ cotransporter (BSC-1 or NKCC2) is expressed in the cortical and medullary TAL,[130,202,203] where it localizes to the apical plasma membrane domains.[202,204,205]

The energy for reabsorptive processes in the TAL is provided by the Na^+-K^+-ATPase that is located in the basolateral plasma membrane. Biochemical[206] and histochemical[207] studies have demonstrated that Na^+-K^+-ATPase activity is greatest in the segment of the TAL from the inner stripe of the outer medulla, which also has a larger basolateral

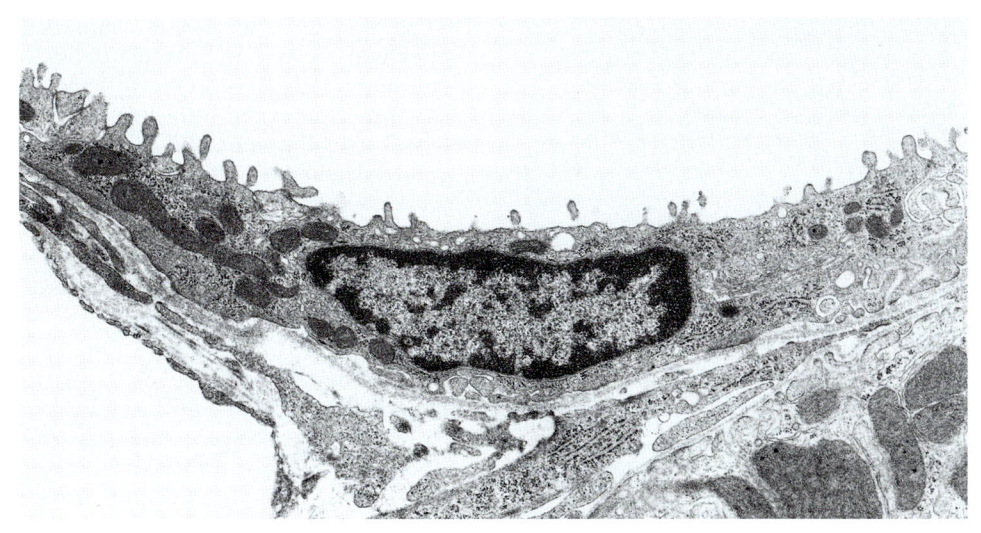

Figure 2.30 Transmission electron micrograph of type II epithelium of the thin limb of the loop of Henle in the inner stripe of the outer medulla of a rat kidney. (×11,800.)

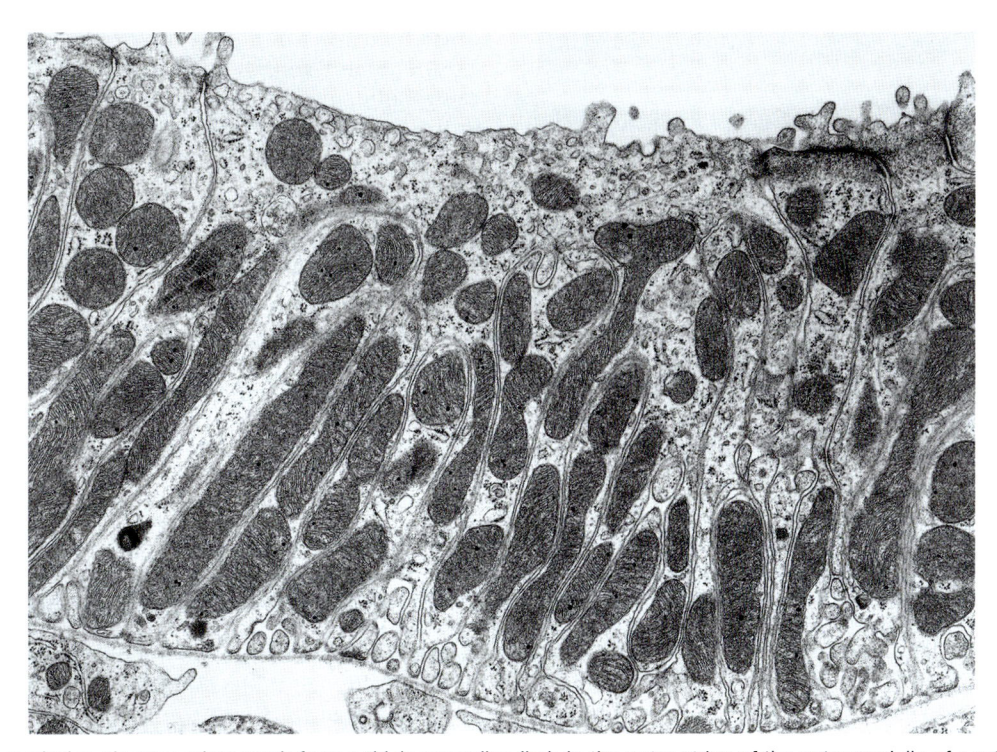

Figure 2.31 Transmission electron micrograph from a thick ascending limb in the outer stripe of the outer medulla of a rat kidney. Note the deep, complex invaginations of the basal plasma membrane, which enclose elongated mitochondrial profiles and extend into the apical region of the cell. (×13,000.)

membrane area and more mitochondria than does the remainder of the TAL.[192] In agreement with these observations, physiologic studies using the isolated perfused tubule technique have demonstrated that NaCl transport is greater in the medullary segment than in the cortical segment of the TAL.[208] However, the cortical segment can create a steeper concentration gradient and can therefore achieve a lower NaCl concentration and a lower osmolality in the tubule fluid.[209] Thus, an excellent correlation exists between the structural and functional properties of the TAL.

DISTAL CONVOLUTED TUBULE

The DCT measures approximately 1 mm in length[141,210] and extends to the connecting tubule, which connects the nephron with the collecting duct. The cells of the DCT resemble those of the TAL but are considerably taller (Figure 2.33). By light microscopy, the cells appear tall and cuboid, and they contain numerous mitochondria. The cell nuclei occupy an apical position just beneath the luminal plasma membrane. Scanning electron microscopy has

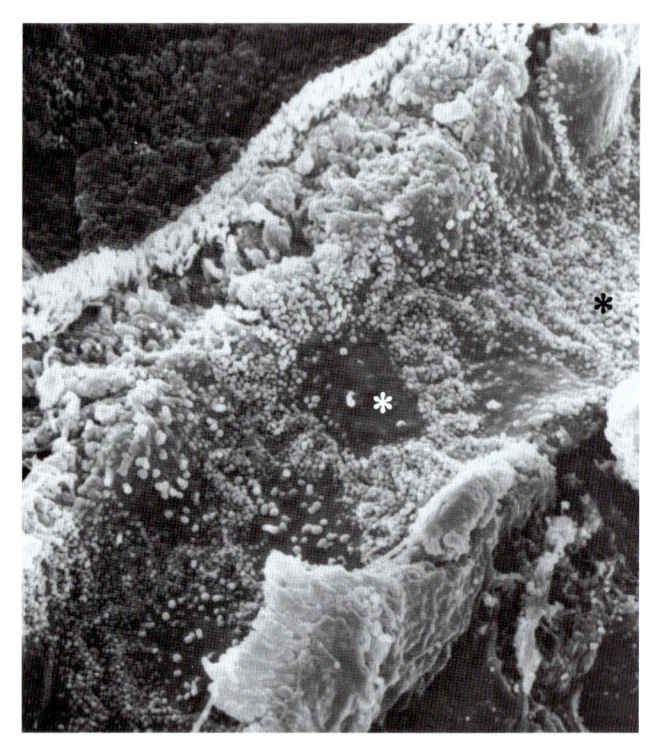

Figure 2.32 Scanning electron micrograph illustrating the luminal surface of a rat medullary thick ascending limb. The *white asterisk* denotes smooth-surfaced cells; the *black asterisk* identifies rough-surfaced cells. (×4300.) (From Madsen KM, Tisher CC: Structural-functional relationship along the distal nephron. *Am J Physiol* 250:F1-F15, 1986.)

demonstrated that the luminal surface of the DCT differs substantially from that of the TAL (Figure 2.34; compare with Figure 2.32). The DCT is covered with numerous small microprojections or microplicae. The individual cells each possess one centrally placed primary cilium on the apical surface. The epithelium of the DCT is characterized by extensive invaginations of the basolateral plasma membrane and by interdigitations between adjacent cells similar to the arrangement in the TAL. Transmission electron microscopy reveals numerous elongated mitochondria that are located in lateral cell processes and are closely aligned with the plasma membrane. They are oriented perpendicular to the basement membrane and often extend from the basal to the apical cell surface (Figure 2.35). The junctional complex in this segment of the nephron is composed of a tight junction, which is approximately 0.3 μm in depth and an intermediate junction.[144] Lysosomes and multivesicular bodies are observed but are certainly less common than in the proximal tubule. The Golgi complex is well developed, and its location is lateral to the cell nucleus. The cells contain numerous microtubules and abundant quantities of rough- and smooth-surfaced endoplasmic reticulum and free ribosomes. Numerous small vesicles are located in the apical region of the cells. Investigators working with micropuncture techniques arbitrarily defined the distal tubule as the region of the nephron that begins just after the macula densa and extends to the first junction with another renal tubule. With that definition, however, the distal tubule can be formed by as many as four different types of epithelia. In general, the "early" distal tubule corresponds largely to the DCT and, in some species, the short segment of the TAL that extends beyond the macula densa, whereas the "late" distal tubule actually represents the connecting tubule and the first portion of the collecting duct, which is sometimes referred to as the *initial collecting tubule* (Figure 2.36).[210,211] (A more detailed discussion of the anatomy of this region of the renal tubule can be found in the next section, which describes the connecting tubule.)

The DCT has the highest Na^+-K^+-ATPase activity of all nephron segments,[169,189] which provides the driving force for ion transport and explains the high mitochondrial density in this segment. Micropuncture and microperfusion studies in the rat demonstrated a net NaCl reabsorption in the distal tubule.[212,213] The apical transport pathway is the thiazide-sensitive Na^+-Cl^- cotransporter, NCC.[212] NCC is expressed exclusively in the DCT, where it localizes to the apical plasma membrane and subapical vesicles.[214-217] Kaissling and colleagues demonstrated that the ultrastructure and the functional capacity of the DCT and connecting tubule are highly dependent on the delivery and uptake of sodium.[218-221] Animals treated with a loop diuretic, furosemide, and given sodium chloride in their drinking water, which increases NaCl delivery to the tubule segments downstream of the TAL, exhibited a striking increase in epithelial cell volume, in the basolateral membrane area, and in cell proliferation in the DCT and connecting tubule. Consistent with these morphologic changes, NCC becomes upregulated[222] and the sodium transport capacity in these nephron segments rises.[223] Conversely, genetic deletion of NCC in mice[224] and pharmacologic inhibition of NCC by thiazides in rats[225] provoke marked DCT cell atrophy and apoptosis, respectively, supporting the idea that DCT cell structure largely depends on its ion transport activity.

The mineralocorticoid receptor as well as the enzyme that confers mineralocorticoid specificity, 11-β-hydroxysteroid dehydrogenase, are detected in the DCT, and NCC abundance is increased by mineralocorticoids.[226-228] However, in rat and mouse kidneys, the abundance of 11-β-hydroxysteroid dehydrogenase is rather low in the early DCT and prominent only in the late DCT,[227,229,230] suggesting that only a proportion of the DCT is sensitive to physiologic variations in circulating aldosterone levels. In fact, numerous morphologic studies (reviewed by Loffing and Kaissling[231]) have revealed a marked axial heterogeneity of the DCT in most species. Although rabbits show a clear morphologic demarcation between DCT and connecting tubule, the transition between these two segments is gradual in rats, mice, and humans, and the typical morphology of the DCT cells changes progressively to that of connecting tubule. Studies in the rat have distinguished between an early segment, DCT1, and a late segment, DCT2, on the basis of the observation that NCC is expressed throughout the DCT, whereas the Na^+-Ca^{2+} exchanger (NCX1) and a vitamin D-dependent calcium-binding protein, calbindin-D28K, are expressed at high levels only in DCT2 (as well as in the connecting tubule [CNT]) and not at all or only weakly in DCT1.[226,227] In mice[229,232] and humans[233] NCX and calbindin-D28K expression are seen along almost the entire DCT, making a sub-segmentation based on these markers difficult. Nevertheless, in all three species (i.e., rat, mouse, and human) the DCT can be subdivided into an early DCT that is only NCC-positive and a late DCT that expresses, in addition to the

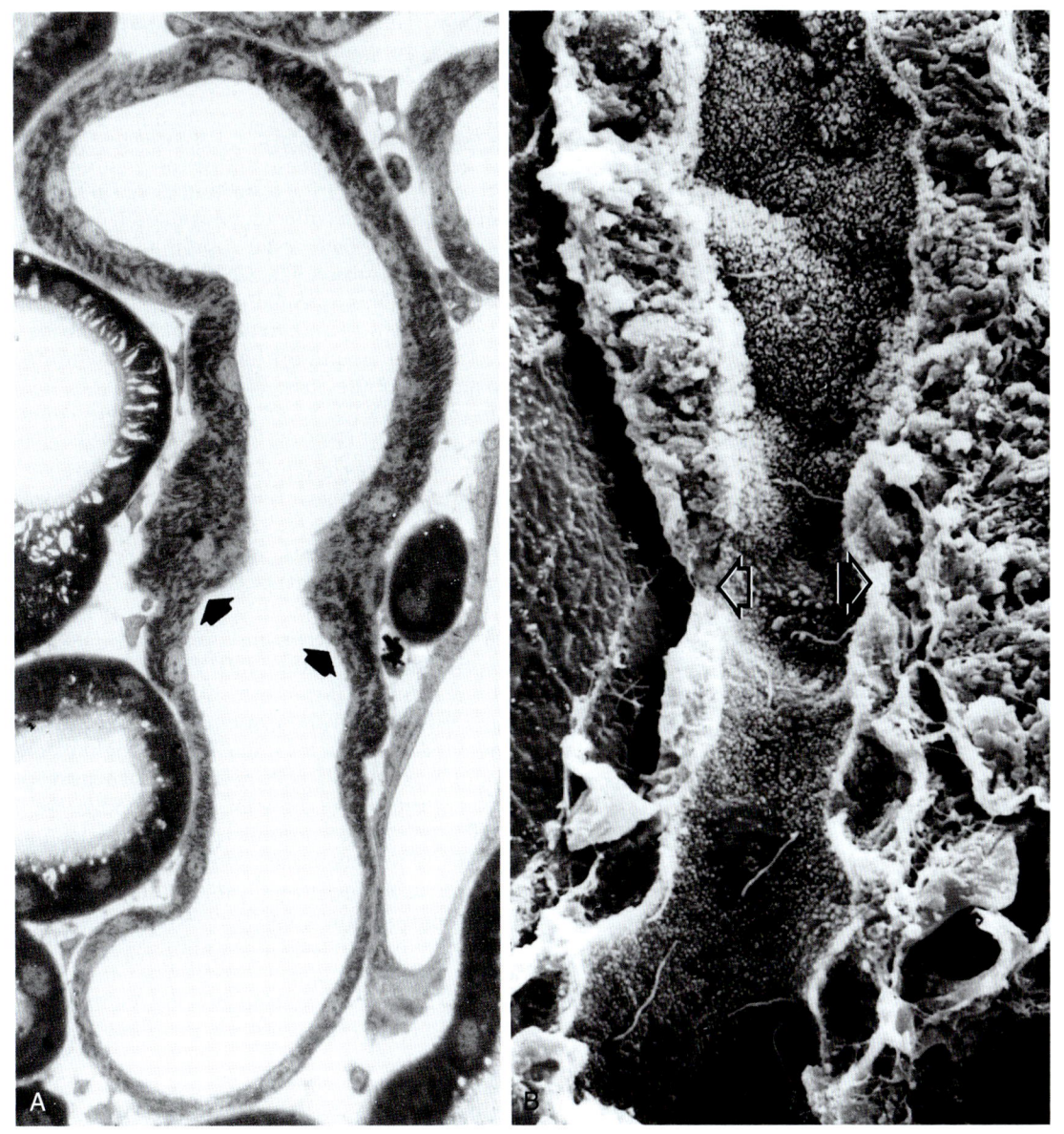

Figure 2.33 Micrographs depicting the abrupt transition (*arrows*) from the thick ascending limb of Henle **(below)** to the distal convoluted tubule **(above)**. **A,** Light micrograph of normal rat kidney. (×775.) **B,** Scanning electron micrograph of normal rabbit kidney. (×2700.) (**B** Courtesy Ann LeFurgey, PhD.)

thiazide-sensitive NCC, the amiloride-sensitive epithelial sodium channel (ENaC), which is the apical sodium entry pathway in the connecting tubule and the collecting duct.[231] Likewise, in mice and rats, the late DCT and the connecting tubule express the apical calcium channel TRPV5, which is absent from the early DCT,[234,235] and a Ca^{2+}-Mg^{2+}-ATPase in the basolateral plasma membrane.[236] Moreover, the DCT appears to specifically express the magnesium channel TRPM6 in its apical plasma membrane.[237] The high levels of expression of calcium- and magnesium-transporting proteins is consistent with suggestions from numerous functional studies that the DCT is involved in regulated reabsorption of Ca^{2+} and Mg^{2+} in the kidney (reviewed by Dimke and associates[238]). Immunohistochemical studies also demonstrated the co-localization of NCC with the secretory potassium channel ROMK in DCT cells of the rat,[239] although microperfusion studies did not detect significant K^+ secretion in early distal tubule portions (likely corresponding to the DCT).[213] Nevertheless, reports that a high dietary K^+ intake causes a rapid and persistent reduction of the phosphorylation and hence activity of NCC[240,241] indicate that the DCT does also participate in the control of K^+ homeostasis. Downregulation of NCC likely increases the delivery of Na^+ to the downstream collecting system, where the Na^+ can then be reabsorbed in exchange for secreted K^+.

The general consensus is that the DCT, like the TAL, is relatively impermeable to water. However, the DCT does express vasopressin receptors, and vasopressin positively regulates both Na^+ transport and NCC abundance/activity.[242-245] Furthermore, later studies have highlighted that adenylate cyclase 6 activity is essential for mediating the effects of vasopressin on NCC abundance/activity.[246] Several human diseases that result from abnormal distal tubule

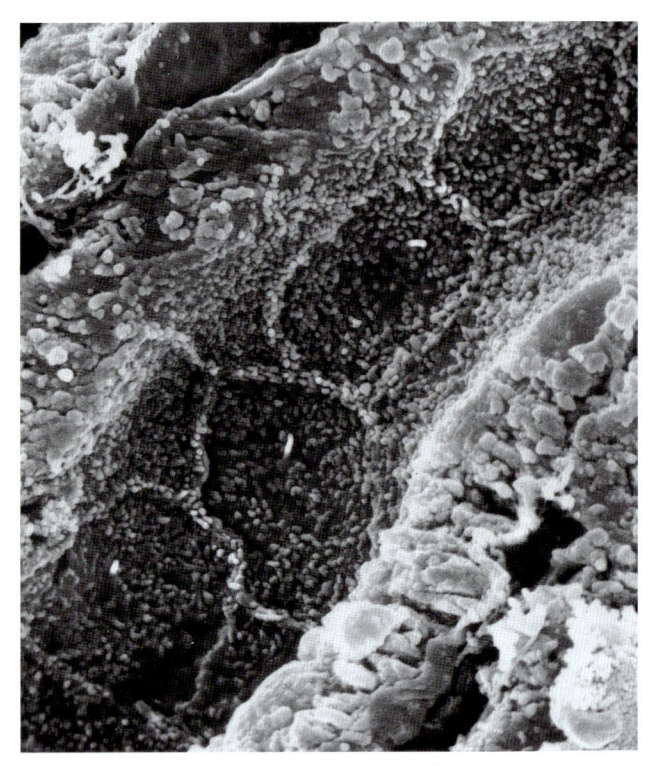

Figure 2.34 Scanning electron micrograph illustrating the appearance of the luminal surface of a distal convoluted tubule from a rat kidney. Microvilli are prominent, but there is a marked absence of lateral interdigitations in the apical region of the cells. The cell boundaries are accentuated by taller microvilli. (×3000.) (Modified from Madsen KM, Tisher CC: Structural-functional relationship along the distal nephron. *Am J Physiol* 250:F1-F15, 1986.)

function, such as Gitelman's syndrome, nephrolithiasis, and familial hyperkalemic hypertension (FFHt), emphasize the importance of this relatively short nephron segment.[212,247]

CONNECTING TUBULE

The CNT represents a transitional region between the distal nephron and the collecting duct, and it constitutes the main portion of the late distal tubule as defined in the micropuncture literature. The CNTs of superficial nephrons continue directly into initial collecting tubules, whereas CNTs from midcortical and juxtamedullary nephrons join to form arcades that ascend in the cortex and continue into initial collecting tubules (see Figures 2.36 and 2.37).[141,248] In the rabbit, the CNT is a well-defined segment composed of two cell types: the CNT cell and the intercalated cell.[141,249] In most other species, however, including rats,[210,211] mice,[249] and humans,[250] there is a gradual transition from the DCT to the CNT, and the CCD is not clearly demarcated from neighboring segments.

The CNT in the rat measures 150 to 200 μm in length.[211] It is composed of four different cell types: CNT cells, intercalated cells, DCT cells, and principal cells, which are similar to principal cells in the CCD. The CNT cell is characteristic of this segment. It is intermediate in ultrastructure between the DCT cell and the principal cell and exhibits a mixture of lateral invaginations and basal infoldings of the plasma membrane.[251] CNT cells are taller than principal cells and have apically located nuclei. Mitochondria are fewer in the CNT and more randomly distributed than in the distal tubule. In the rat, variations in the density of the cytoplasm of intercalated cells were reported in the CNT.[210] Two configurations of intercalated cells, type A and type B, were described in both the CNT and the CCD of the rat.[252] In the CNT, acid-secreting type A cells were more numerous than bicarbonate-secreting type B cells. A third type of intercalated cell was identified in the CNT of both rats and

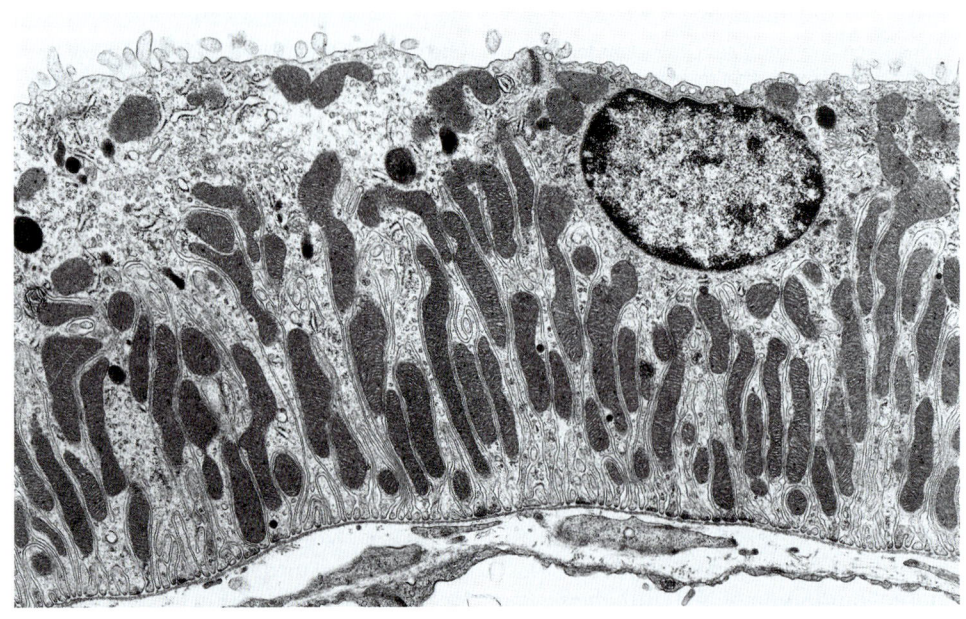

Figure 2.35 Transmission electron micrograph illustrating a typical portion of the pars convoluta segment of the distal tubule of a rat. The ultrastructural features closely resemble those of the pars recta of the distal tubule (see Figure 2.40). (×10,000.)

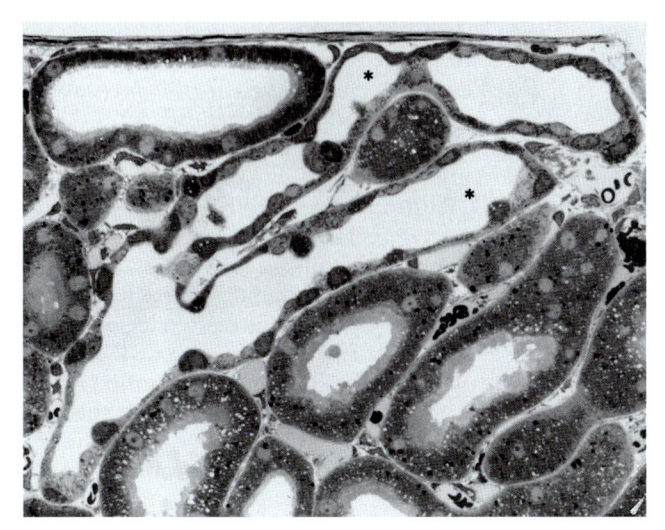

Figure 2.36 Light micrograph of initial collecting tubules (*asterisks*) of a cortical collecting duct in a rat kidney. One tubule is situated just beneath the surface of the capsule (**top** of picture) and hence is easily accessible to micropuncture. This segment of the cortical collecting duct corresponds to the so-called late distal tubule as defined with use of micropuncture studies. (×360.)

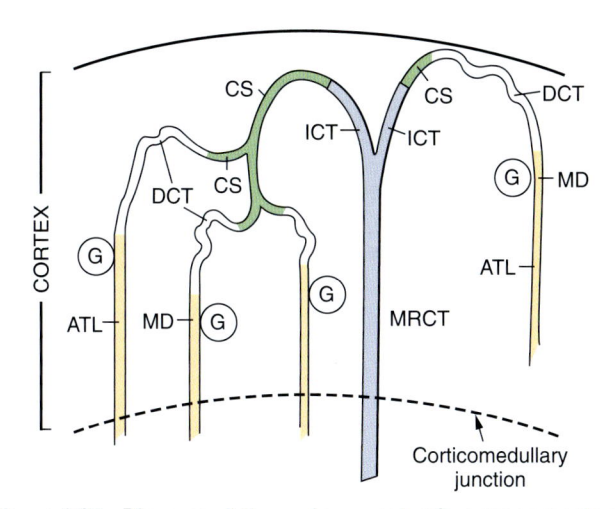

Figure 2.37 Diagram of the various anatomic arrangements of the distal tubule and cortical collecting duct in superficial and juxtamedullary nephrons. (See text for detailed explanation.) ATL, ascending thick limb (of Henle); CS, connecting segment; DCT, distal convoluted tubule; G, glomerulus; ICT, initial collecting tubule; MD, macula densa; MRCT, medullary ray collecting tubule.

mice.[253,254] This cell has been referred to as the nonA–nonB type of intercalated cell. In the mouse, this is the most prevalent form of intercalated cell in the CNT.[253] The functional properties and immunohistochemical features of the intercalated cells have been studied extensively and are described in Chapter 9.

Like the TAL and DCT, the CNT is an important site for regulation of Na^+ reabsorption, but unlike the TAL and DCT, it is also capable of transporting large amounts of water. Consistently, in rats, mice, and humans, not only the collecting duct but also the CNT expresses the vasopressin-sensitive water channel aquaporin-2 (AQP2). However, AQP2 is absent from the rabbit CNT.[231] The amiloride-sensitive sodium channel, ENaC, which is responsible for sodium absorption in the collecting duct, is also highly expressed in the CNT as well as in DCT2.[232] As described in the discussion of the DCT, the CNT is also an important site of calcium reabsorption. Immunohistochemical studies have demonstrated the presence of the Na^+-Ca^{2+} exchanger NCX1[215,255] as well as a Ca^{2+}-ATPase[236,256] in the basolateral plasma membrane of the CNT cells. Expression of a vitamin D–dependent calcium-binding protein, calbindin-D28K, and of the apical Ca^{2+} entry pathway, TRPV5, has also been demonstrated in the CNT cells.[256-259]

Immunohistochemical studies in rats showed that a subpopulation of cells in the late part of the DCT, at the transition to the CNT, expresses both the NaCl cotransporter NCC and the Na^+-Ca^{2+} exchanger, which are traditionally considered specific for DCT cells and CNT cells, respectively.[227,255] In the rabbit, the connecting tubule constitutes a distinct segment with respect to both structure and function, and there is no coexpression of NCC and the Na^+-Ca^{2+} exchanger in any cells in the DCT or CNT.[214] In all mammalian species investigated so far, the transition of the CNT to the CCD can arbitrarily be set to the region where the CNT exits the renal cortical labyrinth to fuse with the CCD running in the medullary ray. In rats, mice, and rabbits this transition coincides with a disappearance of the Na^+-Ca^{2+} exchanger, which is highly abundant in the basolateral plasma membrane of CNT cells but undetectable in the collecting duct principal cells.[231] Morphologic and physiologic studies have provided evidence that the CNT plays an important role in K^+ secretion, which is at least in part regulated by mineralocorticoids.[212] In a combined structural-functional study, Stanton and associates[260] demonstrated that chronic K^+ loading, which stimulates aldosterone secretion, causes an increase in K^+ secretion by the late distal tubule and a simultaneous increase in the surface area of the basolateral plasma membrane of CNT cells and principal cells of both the CNT and the initial collecting tubule, indicating that these cells are responsible for K^+ secretion. No changes were observed in the cells of the DCT. Studies in the rabbit showed a similar increase in the basolateral membrane area of the CNT cells after ingestion of a high-potassium, low-sodium diet.[249] Studies in adrenalectomized rats demonstrated a decrease in K^+ secretion in the superficial distal tubule[261] as well as a decrease in the surface area of the basolateral membrane of the principal cells in the initial CNT.[262] Both structural and functional changes could be prevented by aldosterone treatment, indicating that K^+ secretion in the CNT and initial collecting tubule is regulated by mineralocorticoids.

COLLECTING DUCT

The collecting duct extends from the connecting tubule in the cortex through the outer and inner medulla to the tip of the papilla. It can be divided into at least three regions, primarily on the basis of their location in the kidney: the CCD, the OMCD, and the IMCD. The inner medullary segments terminate as the ducts of Bellini, which open on the surface of the papilla to form the area cribrosa (see Figure 2.3). Traditionally, two types of cells have been described in the mammalian collecting duct: principal cells and intercalated cells. The principal cells are the major cell type; they were originally believed to be present in the entire collecting duct, whereas intercalated cells disappear at different points along the inner medulla collecting duct depending on the species. There is also both structural and functional evidence that the cells in the terminal portion of the inner medullary collecting duct constitute a distinct cell population, IMCD cells.[263] Furthermore, at least two, and in certain species, three configurations of intercalated cells have been described in the CCD,[252] highlighting the structural axial heterogeneity that exists along the collecting duct.

CORTICAL COLLECTING DUCT

The CCD can be further subdivided into two parts: the initial collecting tubule/duct (iCCD) and the medullary ray CD (rCCD) (see Figure 2.5). The cells of the initial collecting tubule are taller than those of the medullary ray segment, but otherwise no major morphologic differences exist between the two subsegments. The CCD is composed of principal cells and intercalated cells, the latter constituting approximately one third of the cells in this segment in the rat,[253,264] the mouse,[253,254] and the rabbit.[265] In electron micrographs, principal cells have a light-staining cytoplasm and relatively few cell organelles (Figure 2.38). They are characterized by numerous infoldings of the basal plasma membrane below the nucleus. The infoldings do not enclose mitochondria or other cell organelles, which causes the basal region to appear as a light rim by light microscopy. Lateral cell processes and interdigitations are virtually absent.[266] Mitochondria are small and scattered randomly in the cytoplasm. A few lysosomes, autophagic vacuoles, and multivesicular bodies are also present, as are rough and smooth endoplasmic reticulum and free ribosomes. Scanning electron microscopy of the luminal surface of the principal cells reveals relatively smooth membranes covered with short, stubby microvilli and single primary cilia (Figure 2.39).

Intercalated cells in the CCD have a dense-staining cytoplasm and therefore are sometimes referred to as *dark cells* (Figure 2.40). They are characterized by the presence of various tubulovesicular membrane structures in the cytoplasm and prominent microprojections on their luminal surfaces. In addition, numerous mitochondria and polyribosomes are located throughout the cells, which also contain well-developed Golgi apparatuses. Previous studies have described two distinct populations of intercalated cells, type A and type B, in the CCD duct of the rat,[252,267] each constituting approximately 50% of the intercalated cells in this segment (see Figure 2.40). Type A intercalated cells are similar in ultrastructure to intercalated cells in the OMCD. They have prominent tubulovesicular membrane compartments that include both spherical and invaginated vesicles and flat saccules or cisternae that appear as tubular profiles on section (Figure 2.41). The cytoplasmic faces of these membrane structures are coated with characteristic club-shaped particles or studs, similar to the coat that lines the cytoplasmic face of the apical plasma membrane.[268]

The ultrastructural appearance of the apical region of type A intercalated cells can vary considerably, depending on the physiologic state. Some cells have numerous tubulovesicular structures and few microprojections on their luminal surfaces, whereas other cells have extensive microprojections on their surfaces with only a few tubulovesicular structures in the apical cytoplasm. The type B intercalated cell has a denser cytoplasm and more mitochondria than the type A cell, giving it a darker appearance (see Figure 2.40). Numerous vesicles are present throughout the cytoplasm, but tubular profiles and studded membrane structures are rare in the cytoplasm of the type B cell. The apical membrane exhibits small, blunt microprojections, and often a band of dense cytoplasm without organelles is present just beneath the apical membrane. Morphometric analysis in the rat has demonstrated that type B intercalated cells have smaller apical membrane areas but a larger

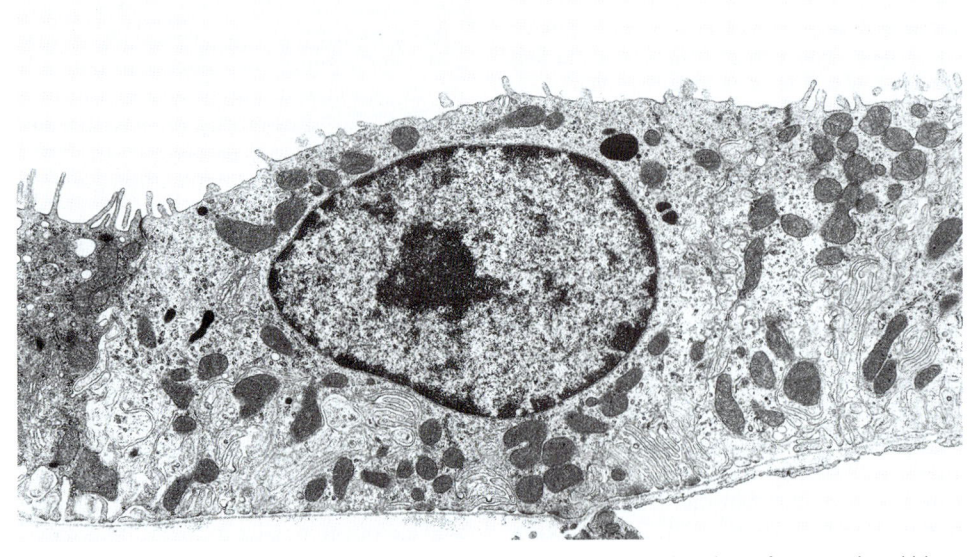

Figure 2.38 Transmission electron micrograph of a principal cell from the cortical collecting duct of a normal rat kidney. Note the extensive infoldings of the basal plasma membrane. (×11,000.) (From Madsen KM, Tisher CC: Structural-functional relationship along the distal nephron. *Am J Physiol* 250:F1-F15, 1986.)

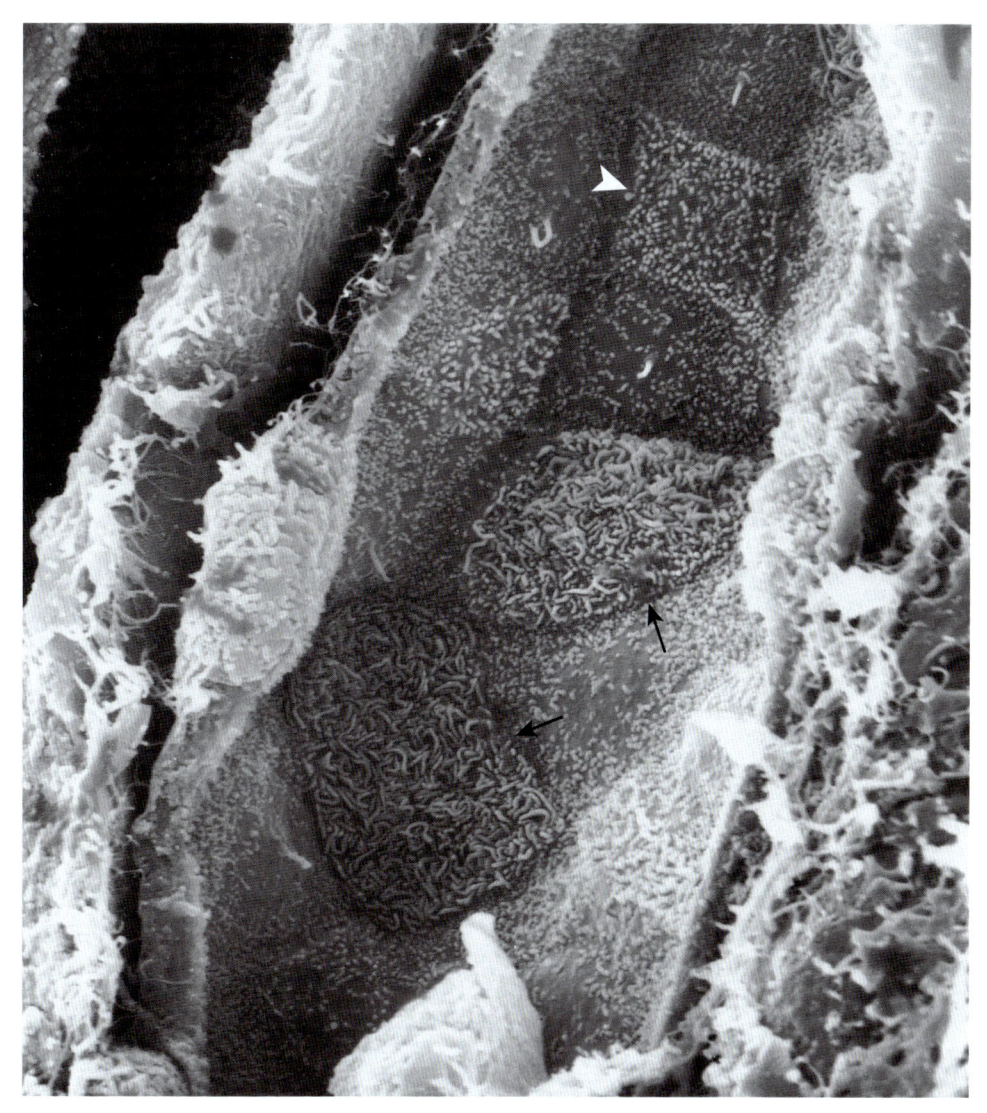

Figure 2.39 Scanning electron micrograph illustrating the luminal surface of a rat cortical collecting duct. The principal cells possess small, stubby microprojections and a single cilium. Two configurations of intercalated cells are present: type A *(arrows)*, with a large luminal surface covered mostly with microplicae, and type B *(arrowhead)*, with a more angular outline and a surface covered mostly with small microvilli. (×5900.) (From Madsen KM, Verlander JW, Tisher CC: Relationship between structure and function in distal tubule and collecting duct. *J Electron Microsc Tech* 9:187-208, 1988.)

basolateral membrane area than type A cells.[252] By scanning electron microscopy, two different surface configurations have been described in the rat.[252] The type A cell has a large luminal surface covered with microplicae or a mixture of microplicae and microvilli; the type B cell has a smaller, angular surface with a few microprojections, mostly in the form of small microvilli (see Figure 2.39).

Both type A and type B intercalated cells are present in the CCD of the mouse.[254] However, the type B cells are less common than in the rat. As previously mentioned, later studies have identified and characterized a third type of intercalated cell in both the rat[253] and the mouse.[253,254] This so-called nonA–nonB type of intercalated cell constitutes approximately 40% to 50% of the intercalated cells in the CNT and initial CCD of the mouse but is fairly rare in the rat.[253]

Kaissling and Kriz described both light and dark manifestations of intercalated cells in the collecting duct of the rabbit.[141] The light form was most commonly observed in the outer medulla, whereas the dark form was observed mainly in the cortex. Flat and invaginated vesicles were present in both cell configurations. The two manifestations of intercalated cells in the rabbit possibly correspond to type A and type B intercalated cells in the rat. Scanning electron microscopy has also revealed different surface configurations of intercalated cells in the collecting duct of the rabbit.[265] Cells with either microplicae or microvilli, or both, have been described, but their relationship to the two cell types has not been investigated. Cells with microvilli are prevalent in the cortex, however.

High levels of carbonic anhydrase are detectable in intercalated cells,[269-271] suggesting that these cells are involved in regulating tubule fluid acidity in the collecting duct. The CCD is capable of both reabsorption and secretion of HCO_3^-. Morphologic and immunocytochemical studies have provided evidence that the type A intercalated cells are

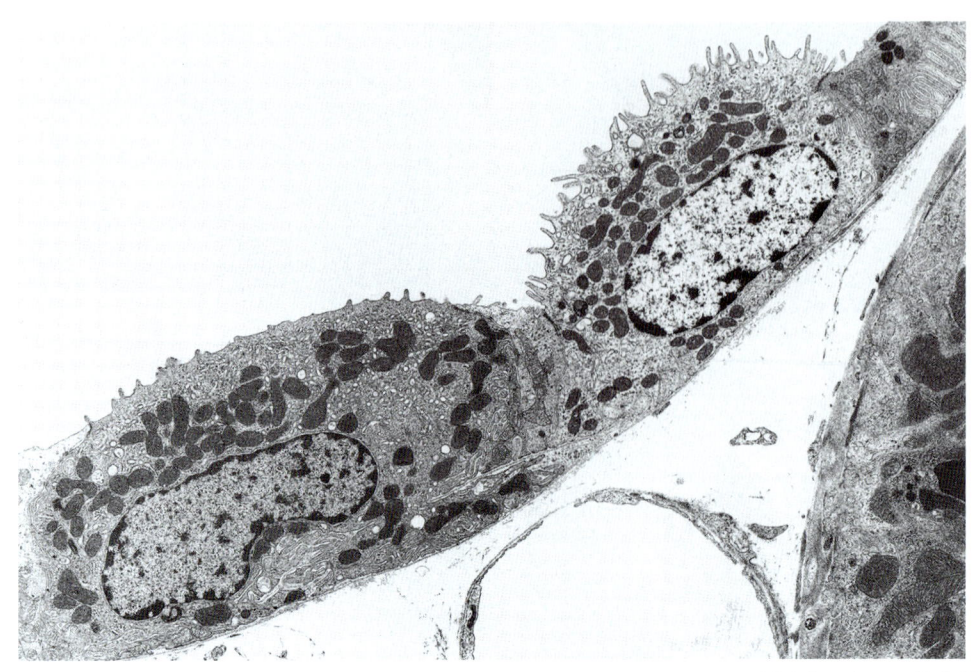

Figure 2.40 Transmission electron micrograph from rat cortical collecting duct illustrating type A **(right)** and type B **(left)** intercalated cells. Note differences in the density of organelles in the cytoplasm and the number of apical projections between the two cell types. (×5300.) (From Madsen KM, Verlander JW, Tisher CC: Relationship between structure and function in distal tubule and collecting duct. *J Electron Microsc Tech* 9:187-208, 1988.)

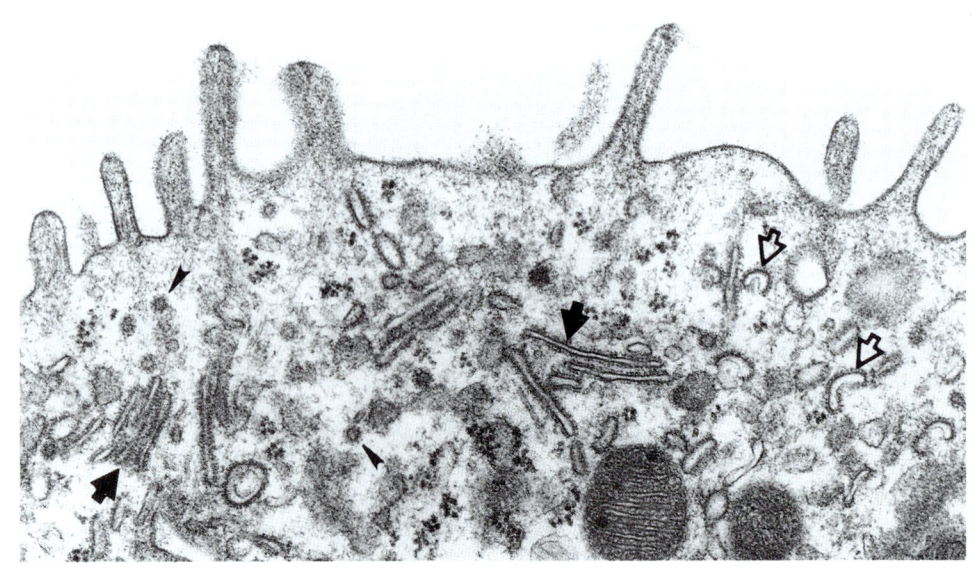

Figure 2.41 Higher-magnification transmission electron micrograph illustrating the apical region of an intercalated cell from a rat kidney. Note especially the large number of tubulocisternal profiles *(solid arrows)*, invaginated vesicles *(open arrows)*, and small coated vesicles with the appearance of clathrin vesicles *(arrowheads)*. (×38,000.)

involved in H^+ secretion in the CCD of the rat.[272] In a study of the effect of acute respiratory acidosis on the CCD of the rat, Verlander and colleagues demonstrated a significant increase in the surface area of the apical plasma membrane of type A intercalated cells.[252] No ultrastructural changes were observed in type B intercalated cells. Similar ultrastructural findings were reported in intercalated cells in the outer cortex of rats with acute metabolic acidosis; however, no distinction was made between type A and type B cells.[188] Immunocytochemical studies using antibodies to the vacuolar H^+-ATPase and the erythrocyte Cl^--HCO_3^- exchanger AE1 (band 3 protein) have confirmed the presence of two types of intercalated cells in the CCD in both mouse and rat. Type A intercalated cells have an apical H^+-ATPase (Figure 2.42)[253,254,273-277] and a basolateral AE1,[253,254,273,278,279] indicating that they are involved in H^+ secretion. In contrast, type B intercalated cells have the H^+-ATPase in the basolateral plasma membrane and in cytoplasmic vesicles throughout the cell, and they express pendrin rather than AE1 in the luminal membrane.[253,254,273,279-282]

In the CCD of the rabbit, AE1 immunoreactivity is located mainly in intracellular vesicles and multivesicular bodies in a subpopulation of intercalated cells, and there is little labeling of the basolateral plasma membrane.[283]

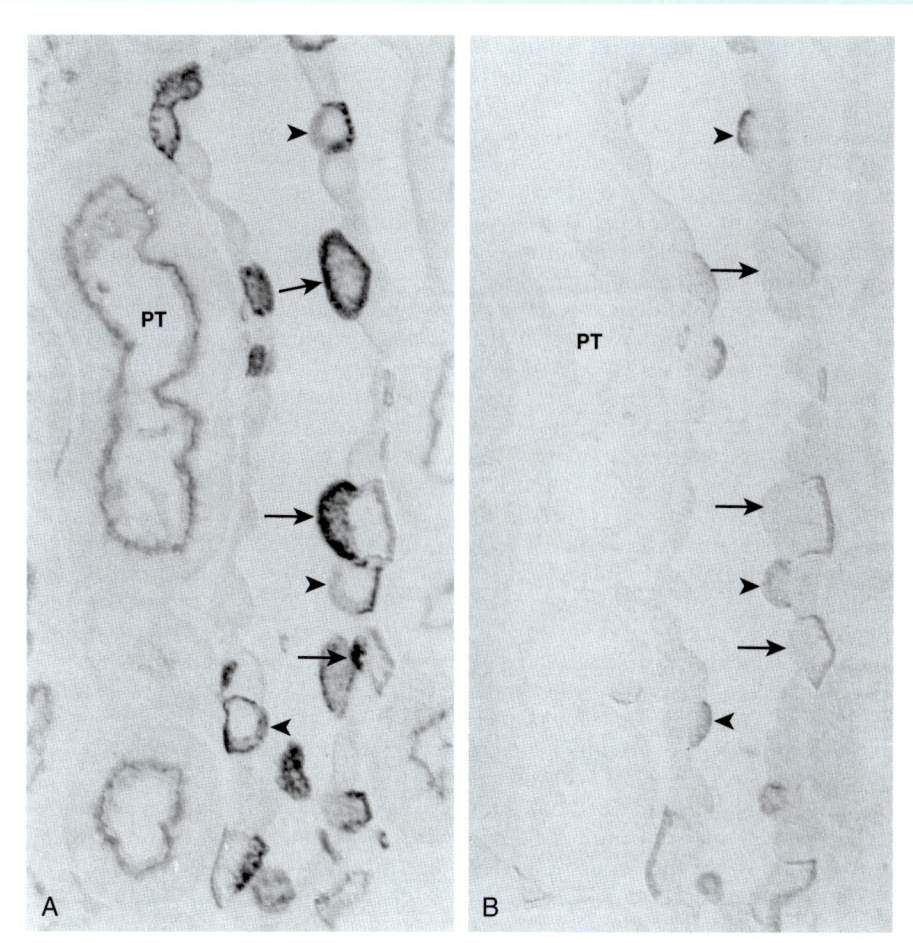

Figure 2.42 Light micrographs illustrating immunostaining for **(A)** the vacuolar H^+-ATPase and the anion exchanger, AE1, and **(B)** pendrin and AE1 in serial sections of the mouse cortical collecting duct with use of a horseradish peroxidase technique. In **A**, type A intercalated cells *(arrows)* have strong apical labeling for H^+-ATPase and basolateral labeling for AE1, whereas type B intercalated cells *(arrowheads)* have basolateral and diffuse labeling for H^+-ATPase and no AE1. In contrast, type B intercalated cells have apical labeling for pendrin **(B)**. PT, proximal tubule. (Differential interference microscopy; ×800.) (Courtesy Jin Kim, MD, Catholic University, Seoul, Korea.)

Immunocytochemical studies have demonstrated that the H^+-ATPase is located in intracellular vesicles in most intercalated cells in the rabbit CCD, and only a minority of intercalated cells in the apical plasma membrane have H^+-ATPase immunoreactivity characteristic of type A intercalated cells.[284] These observations suggest that, under normal conditions, most type A intercalated cells in the rabbit CCD are not functionally active.

In the CNT and collecting duct, sodium is absorbed through an amiloride-sensitive sodium channel, ENaC, which is located in the apical plasma membrane of CNT and principal cells.[285,286] The amiloride-sensitive sodium channel is composed of three homologous ENaC subunits, α, β, and γ, that together constitute the functional channel.[287] All three subunits are expressed in CNTs and principal cells in the collecting duct.[285,286] However, high-resolution immunohistochemistry and immunogold electron microscopy revealed that α-ENaC was expressed in both the apical plasma membrane and apical cytoplasmic vesicles, whereas β-ENaC and γ-ENaC appeared to be located in small vesicles throughout the cytoplasm.[286] The activity of ENaC in the collecting duct is regulated by aldosterone and vasopressin as well as other hormonal systems via mechanisms that involve complex signaling pathways and incorporate changes in expression and subcellular trafficking of ENaC subunits. The regulation of epithelial Na^+ transport by ENaC is complex, involving multiple mechanisms that control ENaC abundance at the apical cell surface. These mechanisms involve regulated exocytosis, endocytosis, and degradation and are reviewed in detail elsewhere.[288-291]

Another major function of the CCD is the secretion of K^+. This process is, at least in part, regulated by mineralocorticoids, which stimulate K^+ secretion and Na^+ reabsorption in the isolated perfused CCD of the rabbit.[292,293] Morphologic studies of the collecting ducts of rabbits given a low-sodium, high-potassium diet[249] and of rabbits treated with deoxycorticosterone[294] demonstrated a significant increase in the surface areas of the basolateral plasma membranes of the principal cells. The observed changes were similar to those reported in principal cells in the connecting segment and in the initial collecting duct of rats on a high-potassium diet,[260] indicating that these cells are responsible for K^+ secretion in the CNT and CCD.

OUTER MEDULLARY COLLECTING DUCT

The function and regulation of the medullary collecting ducts have been described in detail by Fenton and Praetorius.[295] In this section, the collecting duct segments in the outer and inner stripes of the outer medulla are abbreviated *OMCDo* and *OMCDi*, respectively. The homeostatic mechanisms of the OMCDs and the transport proteins responsible are discussed in detail in Chapters 5 to 11. The OMCDs are composed of principal cells and intercalated cells. In the rat and mouse, intercalated cells constitute approximately one third of the cells in both the OMCDo and the OMCDi.[254,264]

In the rabbit, although there is a similar ratio between principal cells and intercalated cells in the OMCDo, the number of intercalated cells varies in the OMCDi. This variation also applies to other species, and often intercalated cells are present only in the outer half of the OMCDi, where they constitute 10% to 15% of the total cell population.

Principal cells of the OMCD are similar in ultrastructure to those in the CCD. However, the cells become slightly taller and the number of organelles and basal infoldings decreases as the collecting duct descends through the outer medulla. Whether principal cells in the OMCDo are functionally similar to those in the CCD is a matter of debate. OMCDo cells express Na^+-K^+-ATPase in their basolateral plasma membranes[155] and ENaC in their apical plasma membranes,[285,286] and are believed to be involved in Na^+ reabsorption; however, there is no evidence that they secrete K^+ similarly to the CCD. In fact, in the rabbit, the OMCDi is a site of K^+ reabsorption.[296] Intercalated cells of the OMCD are similar in ultrastructure to type A intercalated cells of the CCD (Figure 2.43). In the OMCDi, the cells become taller and less electron-dense, and little difference in density of the cytoplasm exists between intercalated cells and principal cells. The main characteristics of the intercalated cells in the outer medulla include numerous tubulovesicular structures in the apical cytoplasm and prominent microprojections on the luminal surface. Intercalated cells are covered with microplicae and often bulge into the tubule lumen.

The OMCD plays an important role in urine acidification,[297] with H^+ secretion in the OMCDi occurring via an Na^+-independent electrogenic process.[298] After stimulation of H^+ secretion, ultrastructural changes occur in intercalated cells in the collecting duct; for example, in rats with acute respiratory acidosis[268] or chronic metabolic acidosis,[299] the surface areas of the apical plasma membranes of intercalated cells increased concomitant with a decrease in the number of tubulovesicular structures in the apical cytoplasm.

INNER MEDULLARY COLLECTING DUCT

The IMCD extends from the boundary between the outer and inner medullae to the tip of the papilla. As the IMCDs descend through the inner medulla, they undergo successive fusions, which result in fewer tubules that have larger diameters (Figure 2.44). The final ducts, the ducts of Bellini, open on the tip of the papilla to form the area cribrosa (see Figure 2.3). The epithelium of the ducts of Bellini is tall, columnar, and similar to that covering the tip of the papilla.[141,300] There are species differences in the length of the papilla, the number of fusions of the collecting ducts, and the height of the cells.[179,300] In the rabbit, the height of the cells gradually increases from approximately 10 μm in the initial portion to approximately 50 μm close to the papillary tip. In the rat, the epithelium is lower, and the increase in height occurs mainly in the inner half, from approximately 6 μm to 15 μm at the papillary tip.[263,300]

The IMCD has been subdivided arbitrarily into three portions: the outer third (IMCD1), middle third (IMCD2), and inner third (IMCD3).[263,301,302] IMCD1 is similar in ultrastructure to the OMCDi, but most of the IMCD2 and the IMCD3 appear to represent distinct segments.[302] Transport studies have provided evidence that the IMCD segments are functionally distinct: with an initial portion, the IMCDi, corresponding to the IMCD1, and a terminal portion, the IMCDt, including most of the IMCD2 and the IMCD3. In the following text, the terms IMCDi and IMCDt are used to distinguish these two functionally distinct segments of the inner medullary collecting duct.

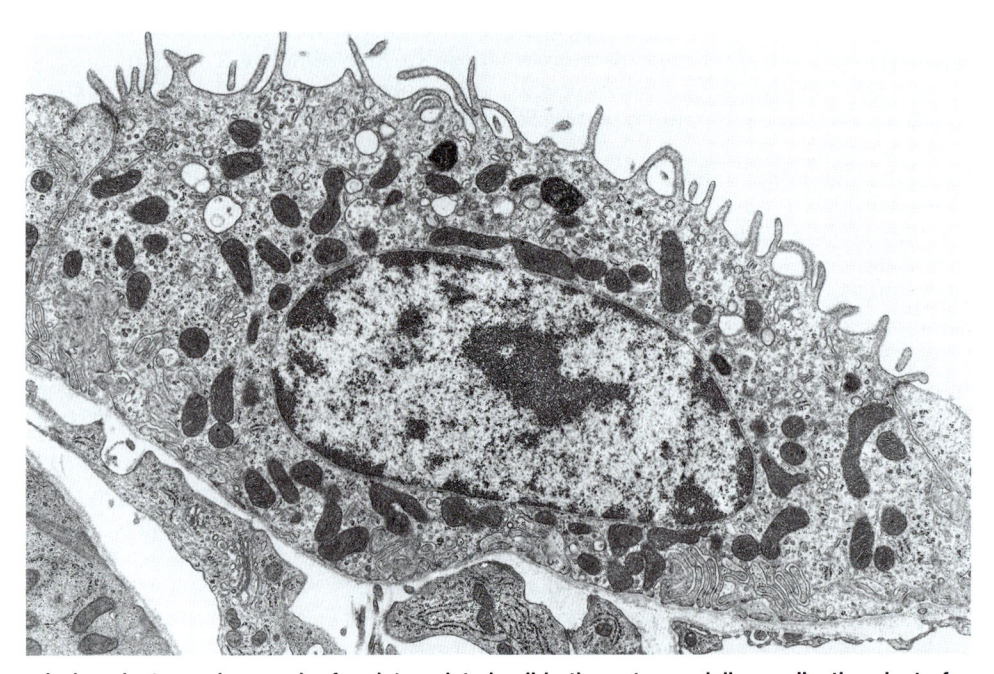

Figure 2.43 Transmission electron micrograph of an intercalated cell in the outer medullary collecting duct of a normal rat kidney. The cell has a prominent tubulovesicular membrane compartment and many microprojections on the apical surface. (×10,000.) (From Madsen KM, Tisher CC: Response of intercalated cells of rat outer medullary collecting duct to chronic metabolic acidosis. *Lab Invest* 51:268-276, 1984.)

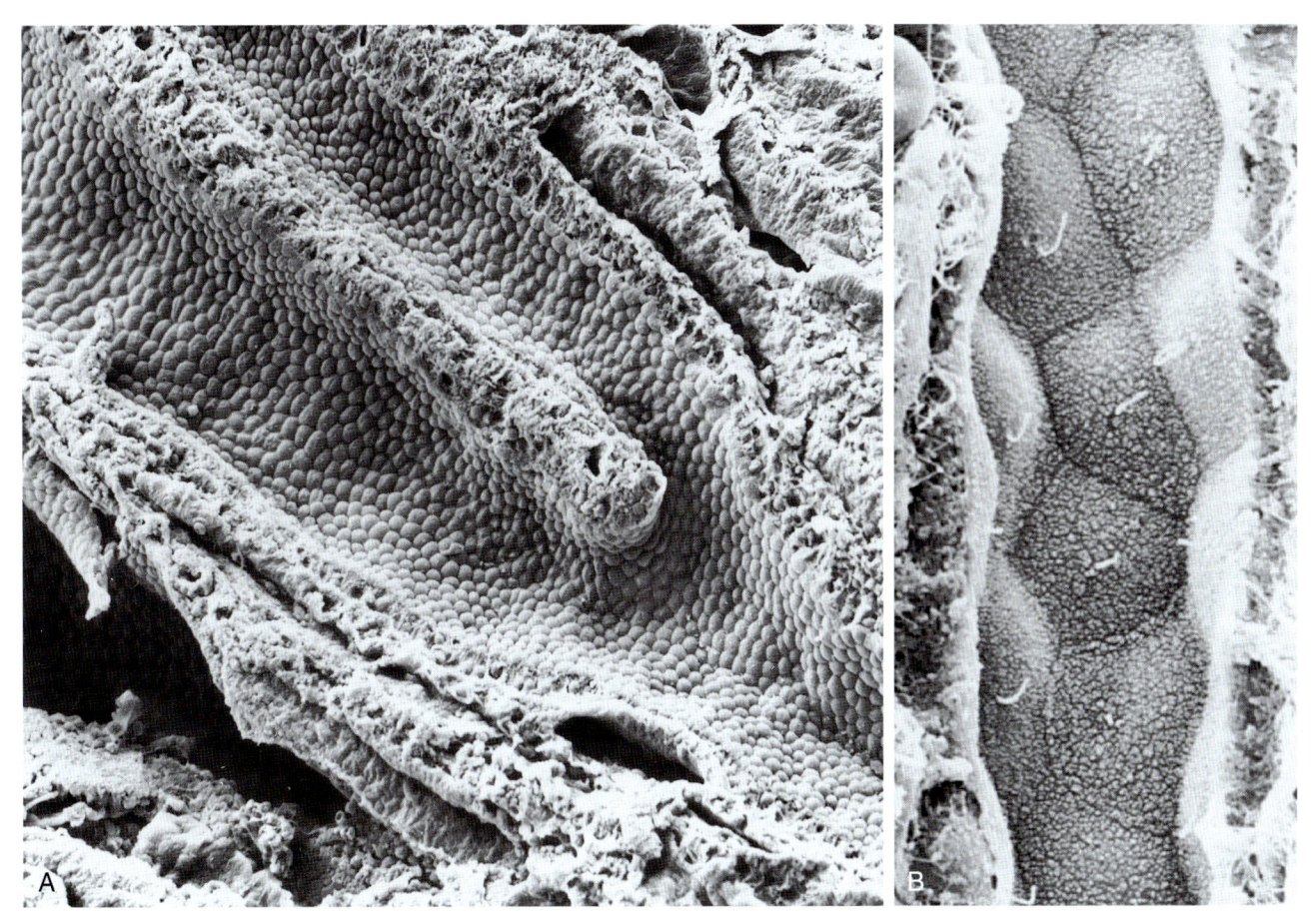

Figure 2.44 Scanning electron micrographs of the normal papillary collecting duct of a rabbit. **A,** The junction between two subdivisions at low magnification. (×600.) **B,** Higher-magnification view (×4250) illustrating the luminal surfaces of individual cells with prominent microvilli and single cilia. (**A** courtesy Ann LeFurgey, PhD; **B** from LeFurgey A, Tisher CC: Morphology of rabbit collecting duct. *Am J Anat* 155:111-124, 1979.)

In both rat[301] and mouse[254] species the IMCDi consists of principal cells (Figure 2.45) and intercalated cells, the latter constituting approximately 10% of the total cell population.[301] Both cell types are similar in ultrastructure to the cells in the OMCDi and are believed to have the same functional properties. In the rabbit, the IMCDi is often composed of only one cell type, similar in ultrastructure to the predominant cell type in the OMCDi.[141] However, in some rabbits, intercalated cells can be found in this segment.

In rats, the transition from the IMCDi to the IMCDt is gradual and occurs in the outer part of the IMCD2.[263,302] The IMCDt consists mainly of one cell type, the IMCD cell. It is cuboid to columnar with a light-staining cytoplasm and few cell organelles (Figure 2.46). It contains numerous ribosomes and many small coated vesicles resembling clathrin-coated vesicles. Small, electron-dense bodies representing lysosomes or lipid droplets are present in the cytoplasm, often located beneath the nucleus. The luminal membrane has short, microvilli that are more numerous than on principal cells, and they are covered with an extensive glycocalyx. Infoldings of the basal plasma membrane are sparse. By scanning electron microscopy, the luminal surfaces of IMCD cells are covered with numerous small microvilli (Figures 2.47 and 2.48), with only a proportion of cells possessing single central cilia.[302]

The functional properties of the IMCD have been studied by in vivo micropuncture of the exposed rat papilla by microcatheterization through a duct of Bellini[179,263] or the isolated perfused tubule technique. Use of these techniques has established that the IMCD is involved in the reabsorption of Na^+, Cl^-, K^+, urea, and water and the acidification of urine. The permeability properties of the epithelium and the various transport proteins responsible are discussed in detail in Chapters 6 and 10.

INTERSTITIUM

The renal interstitium is composed of interstitial cells and a loose, extracellular matrix consisting of sulfated and nonsulfated glucosaminoglycans.[303,304] The quantity of interstitial tissue in the cortex is limited, and the tubules and capillaries are often directly apposed to each other. The interstitium constitutes 7% to 9% of the cortical volume in the rat,[40,305] 3% of which is interstitial cells, and the remaining the extracellular space.[303] In the medulla, a gradual increase occurs in interstitial volume, from 10% to 20% in the outer medulla to approximately 30% to 40% at the papillary tip in both the rat and the rabbit.[300,306] The interstitial volume in the rat kidney constitutes

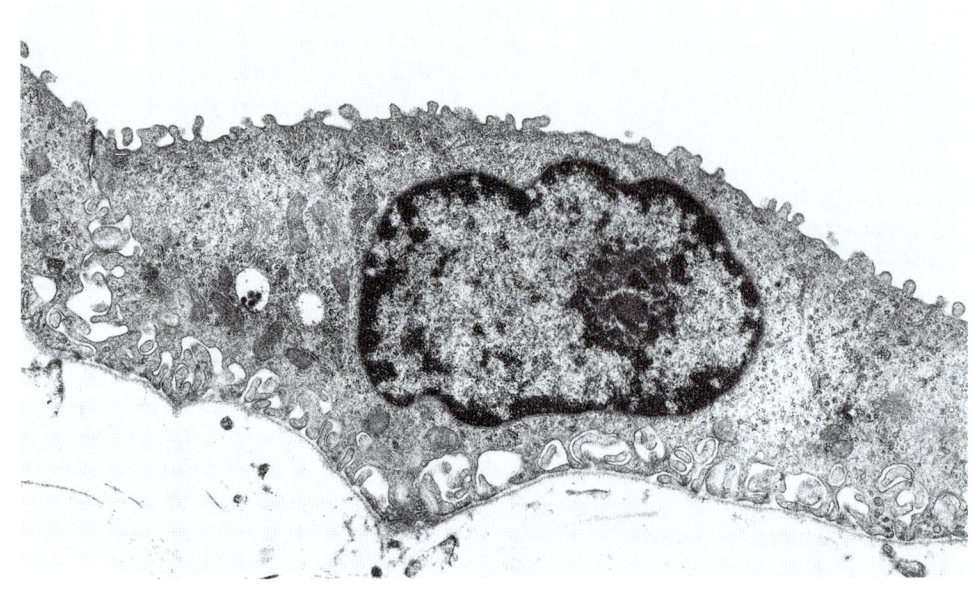

Figure 2.45 Transmission electron micrograph of a principal cell from the initial portion of the rat inner medullary collecting duct. Few organelles are present in the cytoplasm, and apical microprojections are sparse. (×11,750.) (From Madsen KM, Clapp WL, Verlander JW: Structure and function of the inner medullary collecting duct. *Kidney Int* 34:441-454, 1988.)

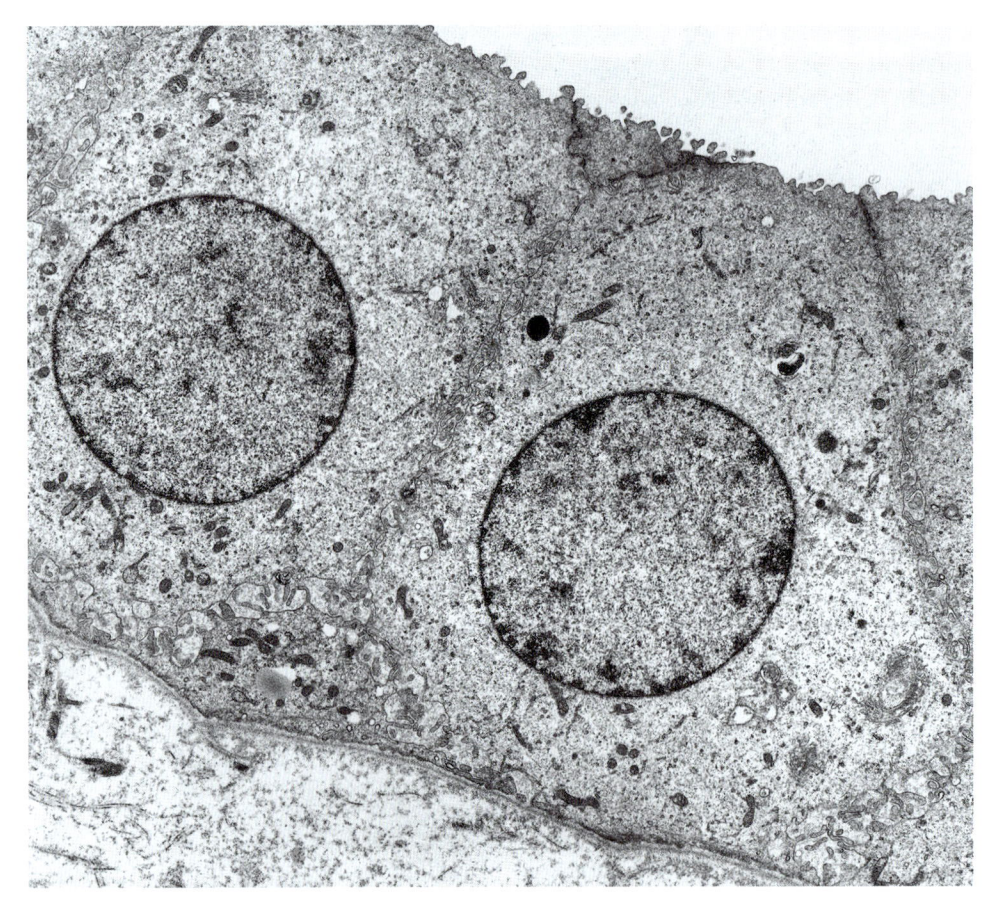

Figure 2.46 Transmission electron micrograph of cells from the terminal portion of the rabbit inner medullary collecting duct. The cells are tall, possess few organelles, and exhibit small microprojections on their apical surfaces. Ribosomes and small coated vesicles are scattered throughout the cytoplasm. (×7000.)

CHAPTER 2 — ANATOMY OF THE KIDNEY

approximately 13% of the total kidney volume; in the rabbit kidney, approximately 18%.[307]

CORTICAL INTERSTITIUM

The cortical interstitium can be divided into a wide interstitial space, located between two or more adjacent renal tubules, and a narrow or slitlike interstitial space, located between the basement membrane of a single tubule and the adjacent peritubular capillary.[308,309] Whether such a division has any functional significance is unknown; however, it is of interest that approximately two thirds of the total peritubular capillary wall faces the narrow compartment and that this portion of the vessel wall is fenestrated.[305] This relationship might facilitate the control of fluid reabsorption across the basolateral membrane of the proximal tubule via Starling forces.

There are two types of interstitial cells in the cortex: one that resembles a fibroblast (type 1 cortical interstitial cell) (Figure 2.49) and another, less common mononuclear or lymphocyte-like cell (type 2 cortical interstitial cell).[303,308] Type 1 cells are positioned between the basement membranes of adjacent tubules and peritubular capillaries. They have a stellate appearance and contain irregularly shaped nuclei and a well-developed rough- and smooth-surfaced endoplasmic reticula. Type 2 cells are usually round, with sparse cytoplasm and few cell organelles. Antigen-presenting dendritic cells are among the fibroblasts in the peritubular interstitium in both cortex and outer medulla of the normal rat kidney.[310] The interstitial space contains a loose, flocculent material of low density and small bundles of collagen fibrils. In humans, types I and III collagen and fibronectin are present in the interstitium of the cortex,[311] whereas type

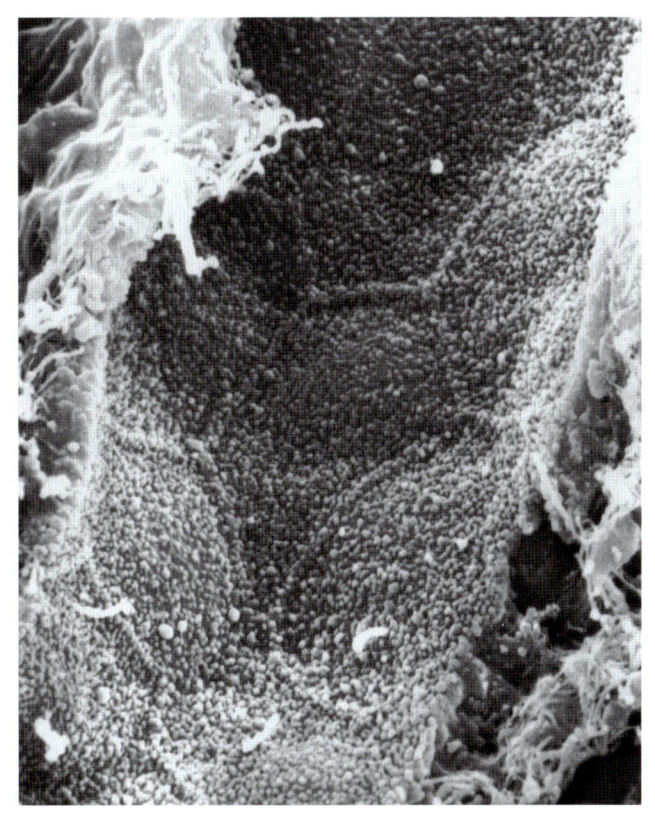

Figure 2.47 Scanning electron micrograph from the middle portion of the rat inner medullary collecting duct. The luminal surface is covered with small microvilli, and some cells possess single cilia. (×10,500.) (From Madsen KM, Clapp WL, Verlander JW: Structure and function of the inner medullary collecting duct. *Kidney Int* 34:441-454, 1988.)

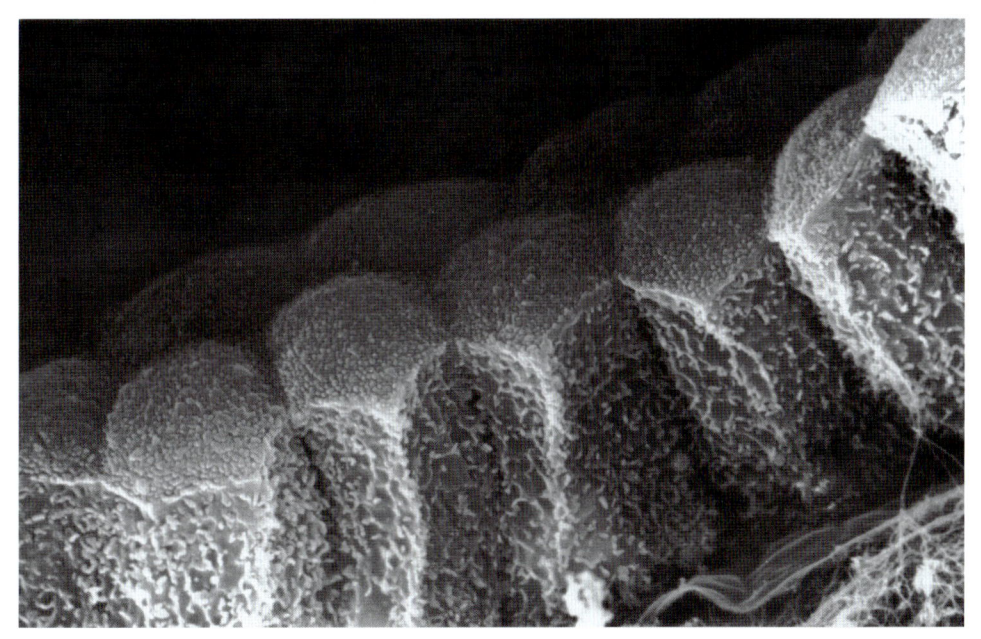

Figure 2.48 Scanning electron micrograph of the terminal portion of rabbit inner medullary collecting duct. The cells are tall and covered with small microvilli on their luminal surfaces. Small lateral cell processes project into the lateral intercellular spaces. (×6000.) (From Madsen KM, Clapp WL, Verlander JW: Structure and function of the inner medullary collecting duct. *Kidney Int* 34:441-454, 1988.)

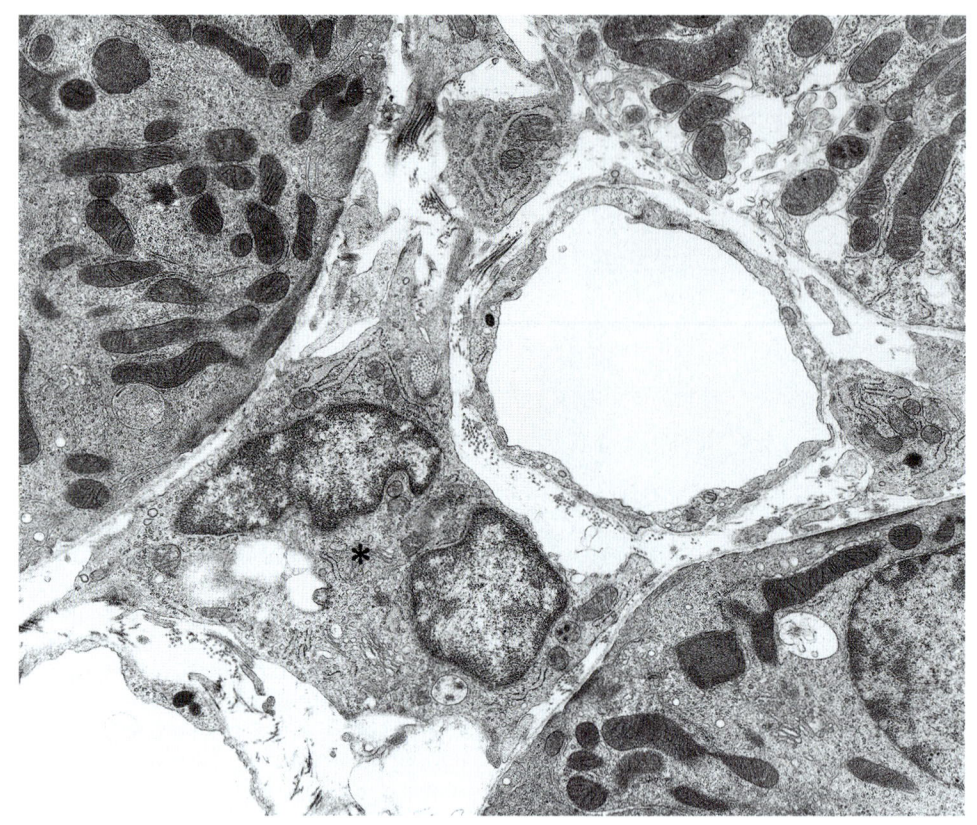

Figure 2.49 Transmission electron micrograph of type 1 cortical interstitial cell *(asterisk)* from a rat. A peritubular capillary is located at **right center**. (×9300.)

V collagen has been described in the cortical interstitium of the rat.[312] The peritubular, fibroblast-like interstitial cells express an ecto-5′-nucleotidase and are likely the site of erythropoietin production in the kidney.[313-315] The lymphocyte-like interstitial cells in the cortex are believed to represent bone marrow–derived cells. The morphology and functional aspects of the renal interstitium in the healthy and the fibrotic kidney have been reviewed elsewhere.[316,317]

MEDULLARY INTERSTITIUM

Three types of interstitial cells have been described in the renal medulla of the rat and the rabbit.[308,309] Type 1 cells are prominent, lipid-containing interstitial cells that resemble the type 1 cells in the cortex but do not express erythropoietin messenger RNA (mRNA) or contain ecto-5′-nucleotidase.[314,315] Type 1 cells are present throughout the inner medulla and are also found in the inner stripe of the outer medulla. The type 2 medullary interstitial cell is a lymphocyte-like cell present in the outer medulla and in the outer part of the inner medulla that is virtually identical to the mononuclear cell (type 2 interstitial cell) in the cortex. It is free of lipid droplets, but lysosome-like bodies are often observed. Type 2 cells are sometimes found together with type 1 cells. The type 3 cell is a pericyte that is located in the outer medulla and the outer portion of the inner medulla. It is closely related to the descending vasa recta, where it is found between two leaflets of the basement membrane.

Most interstitial cells in the inner medulla are the lipid-containing type 1 interstitial cells,[318] which are often referred to as the *renomedullary interstitial cells*. They have long cytoplasmic projections that give them an irregular, star-shaped appearance. The cells are often arranged in rows between the loops of Henle and vasa recta, with their long axes perpendicular to those of adjacent tubules and vessels, thus resembling the rungs of a ladder (Figure 2.50). The elongated cell processes are in close contact with the thin limbs of Henle and the vasa recta, but direct contact with collecting ducts is observed only rarely. Often, a single cell is in contact with several vessels and thin limbs.[309] The long cytoplasmic processes from different cells are often connected by specialized cell junctions that vary in both size and shape and contain elements of tight junctions, intermediate junctions, and gap junctions.[319,320]

The ultrastructure of the type 1 medullary interstitial cells has been described in rat,[309] rabbit,[308,318] and human kidneys. They contain numerous lipid inclusions or droplets in the cytoplasm that vary considerably in both size and number (Figure 2.51). An average diameter of 0.4 to 0.5 μm has been reported in the rat, but profiles of up to 1 μm in diameter were also observed.[321] The droplets have a homogeneous content and have no limiting membrane; however, they are often surrounded by smooth cytomembranes with a thickness of 6 to 7 nm. The cells contain large amounts of rough endoplasmic reticulum that often is continuous with elements of the smooth cytoplasmic membranes. Mitochondria are sparse and scattered randomly in the cytoplasm. A small number of lysosomes are present, but

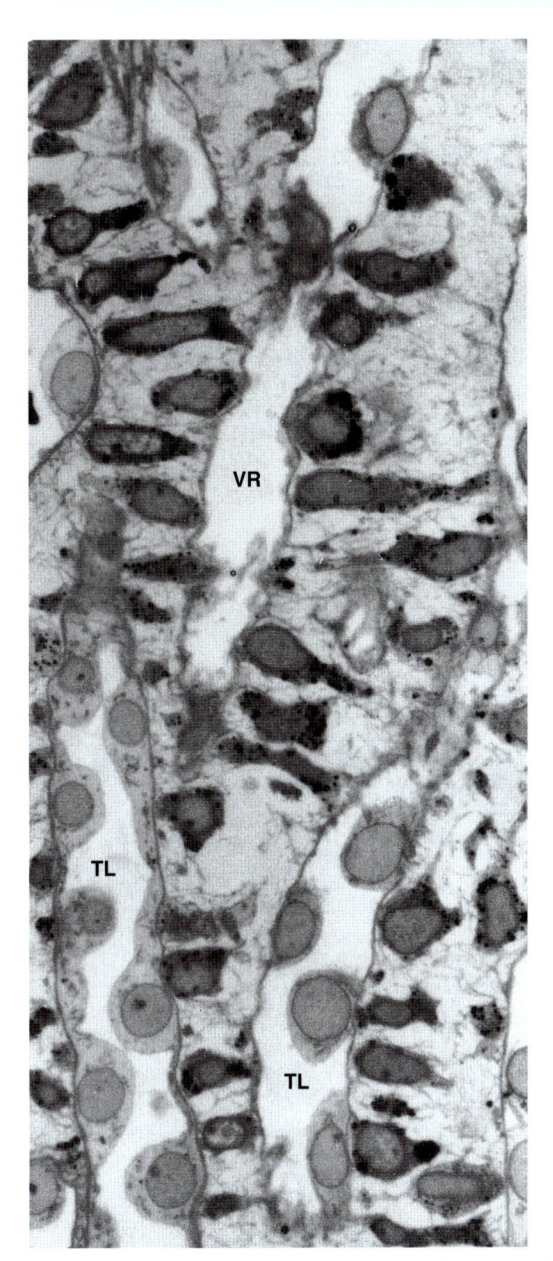

Figure 2.50 Light micrograph of the renal medullary interstitium from a normal rat. The lipid-laden type 1 interstitial cells bridge the interstitial space between adjacent thin limbs of Henle (TL) and vasa recta (VR). (×830.)

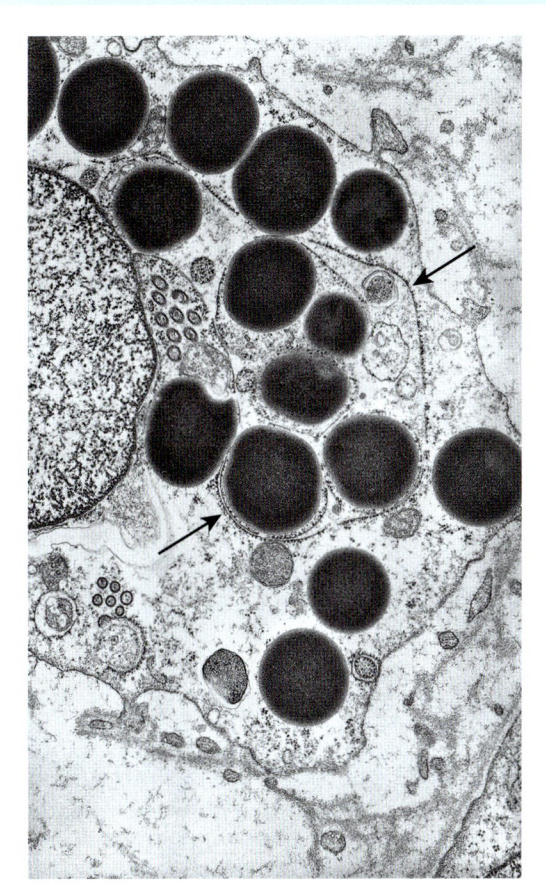

Figure 2.51 Higher-magnification electron micrograph illustrating the relationship between the electron-dense lipid droplets, which almost fill the type 1 medullary interstitial cells, and the granular endoplasmic reticulum *(arrows)*. Wisps of basement membrane–like material adjacent to the surfaces of the cells are contiguous with the basement membranes of the adjacent tubules **(lower right)**. (×12,000.)

endocytic vacuoles are sparse. An unusual type of cylindrical body, measuring 0.1 to 0.2 μm in diameter and up to 11 mm in length and believed to be derived from the endoplasmic reticulum, has been described in the type 1 interstitial cells.[303,322-324] These structures were observed originally in dehydrated rats and were believed to represent a response to severe dehydration,[322] but subsequent studies demonstrated their presence under normal conditions.[323] The walls of the cylinders consist of two triple-layered membranes, each measuring 6 nm in thickness, and connections between the walls and the membranes of the endoplasmic reticulum have been observed.[322] The functional significance of these cylindrical structures remains unknown. The number and size of the lipid inclusions in the type 1 medullary interstitial cells vary considerably, depending on the physiologic state of the animal[325,326] and on the species.[318] In the rat, lipid droplets constitute 2% to 4% of the interstitial cell volume, and the volume depends largely on the physiologic state of the animal.[321] The lipid droplets were originally reported to decrease in both size and number after 24 hours of dehydration,[326] but a later study could not confirm these findings.[321]

The functions of type 1 interstitial cells (renomedullary interstitial cells) are incompletely understood. The cells likely provide structural support in the medulla because of their special arrangement perpendicular to the tubules and vessels. The close relationship between type 1 interstitial cells and the thin limbs and capillaries also suggests a possible interaction with these structures. Owing to the well-developed endoplasmic reticulum and prominent lipid droplets, type 1 interstitial cells may also be secretory in nature.[327] The lipid droplets are not secretory granules in the usual sense, however, because they have no limiting membrane and there is no evidence that they are secreted by the cell. The droplets have been isolated from homogenates of the renal medulla of both the rat[328,329] and the rabbit.[330] They consist mainly of triglycerides and small amounts of cholesterol esters and phospholipids.[329] The triglycerides are rich in unsaturated fatty acids, including arachidonic acid.[328,330]

The renomedullary interstitial cells are a major site of prostaglandin synthesis, with the major product being PGE_2.[331] Prostaglandin synthesis in the renomedullary interstitial cells is mediated by cyclo-oxygenase-2 (COX-2),[332] which increases in expression in response to water deprivation or hypertonicity.[332-334] Binding sites for several vasoactive peptides, including angiotensin II, are also present in renomedullary interstitial cells,[335,336] and there is evidence that angiotensin may be involved in the regulation of prostaglandin production in the renal medulla.[337] Finally, the interstitial cells are responsible for the synthesis of the glycosaminoglycans, in particular hyaluronic acid, that are present in the matrix material of the interstitium.[338]

Little is known about the function of the type 2 and type 3 medullary interstitial cells. The type 2 cells are probably phagocytic,[303] but the function of type 3 cells remains unknown.

LYMPHATICS

Interstitial fluid can leave the kidney through two different lymphatic networks, a superficial capsular system and a deeper hilar system.[339,340] Our knowledge of the distribution of lymphatics is limited. Intrarenal lymphatics are embedded in the periarterial loose connective tissue around the renal arteries and are distributed primarily along the interlobular and arcuate arteries in the cortex.[339-341] Kriz and Dieterich[341] believed that the cortical lymphatics begin as lymphatic capillaries in the area of the interlobular arteries and that these capillaries drain into the arcuate lymphatic vessels at the region of the corticomedullary junction (Figure 2.52). The arcuate lymphatic vessels drain to hilar lymphatic vessels through interlobar lymphatics. Numerous valves have been described within the interlobar and hilar lymphatic channels.[340,341] In the horse, glomeruli are often completely surrounded by lymphatic channels, whereas in the dog, only a portion of the glomerulus is surrounded by lymphatics.[340]

In the dog, small lymphatic channels, in close apposition to both proximal and distal tubules, have been observed in addition to the interlobular arteries.[342] Furthermore, in the dog kidney the existence of cortical intralobular lymphatics closely associated with terminal arteries, arterioles, renal corpuscles, and tubule elements has been reported.[343] Morphometric analysis revealed that the cross-sectional area of interlobular lymphatics was almost twice that of intralobular lymphatics in the cortex, with the volume density of renal cortical lymphatics approximately 0.17%.[343] Similar morphometric studies in the rat, hamster, and rabbit revealed volume densities of cortical lymphatics of 0.11%, 0.37%, and 0.02%, respectively.[344]

A less extensive system of lymphatic vessels is present within and immediately beneath the renal capsule.[340,341] The lymphatic vessels of the renal capsule drain into subcapsular lymphatic channels that lie adjacent to interlobular arteries just beneath the renal capsule. These lymphatic vessels appear to provide continuity between the major intrarenal lymphatic vessels within the cortex (interlobular and arcuate lymphatic vessels) and the capsular lymphatic vessels; thus, in some animals, a continuous system of lymphatic drainage has been observed from the renal capsule, through the cortex, and into the hilar region (Figure 2.53). In the dog kidney, two types of tributaries have been described in association with the surface lymphatics.[345] So-called communicating lymphatic channels were found in small numbers, usually in association with an interlobular artery and vein; these lymphatics penetrated the capsule and appeared to represent a connection between the hilar and capsular systems. The second type of vessel, the so-called perforating lymphatic channel, penetrated the capsule alone or in association with a small vein; these channels appeared to represent a primary pathway for lymph drainage from the superficial cortex. From a study in the dog kidney, investigators concluded that medullary lymphatics do not exist in this species, and they suggested that interstitial fluid from the medulla may drain to the arcuate or interlobar lymphatics.[346] It has also been suggested that plasma proteins are cleared from the medullary interstitium through the ascending vasa recta.[347-349] Microscopic examination shows that the wall of the interlobular lymphatic vessel is formed by a single endothelial layer and does not have the support of a basement membrane.[341] The arcuate and interlobar lymphatic vessels are similar in appearance, although the latter possess valves.

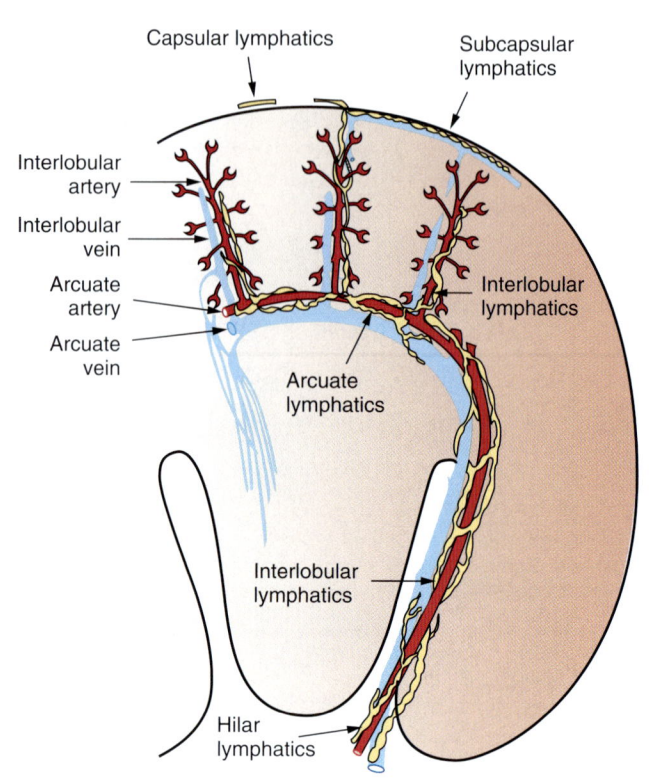

Figure 2.52 Diagram of the lymphatic circulation in the mammalian kidney. (Modified from Kriz W, Dieterich HJ: [The lymphatic system of the kidney in some mammals. Light and electron microscopic investigations]. *Z Anat Entwicklungsgesch* 131:111-147, 1970.)

INNERVATION

The efferent nerve supply to the kidney arises largely from the celiac plexus, with additional contributions originating from the greater splanchnic nerve, the intermesenteric plexus, and the superior hypogastric plexus.[350] The

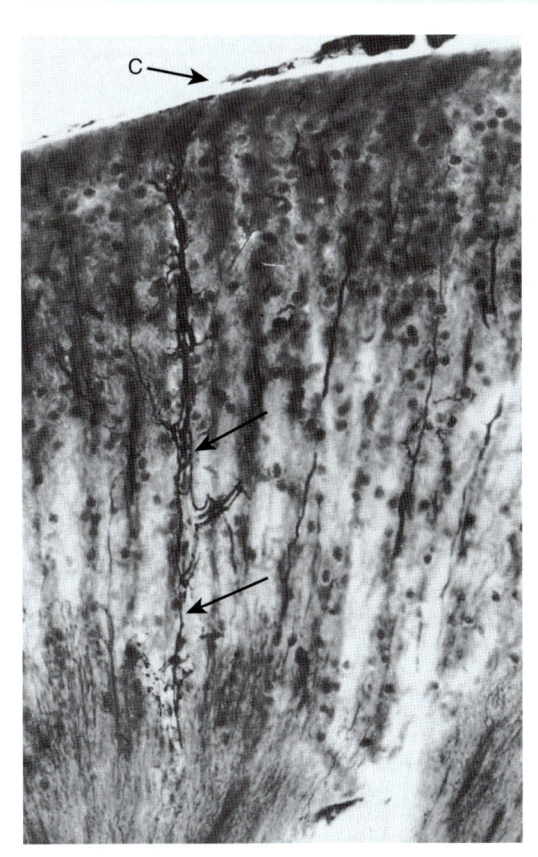

Figure 2.53 Light micrograph of a sagittal section through the cortex and outer medulla of a dog kidney. A capsular lymphatic (C) was injected with India ink. Intrarenal lymphatics *(arrows)* follow the distribution of the interlobular arteries in the cortex. (×10.) (From Bell RD, Keyl MJ, Shrader FR, et al: Renal lymphatics: the internal distribution. *Nephron* 5:454-463, 1968.)

postganglionic sympathetic nerve fiber distribution generally follows the arterial vessels throughout the cortex and outer stripe of the outer medulla.[351] Adrenergic fibers have been observed lying adjacent to smooth muscle cells of arcuate and interlobular arteries and afferent arterioles.[352-354] An extensive innervation of the efferent arteriolar vessels of the juxtamedullary glomeruli, which eventually divide to form the afferent vasa recta, has been described.[353,355] However, quantitation of monoaminergic innervation by autoradiography revealed a higher density of norepinephrine-containing nerves associated with the afferent than with the efferent arteriole.[354] The existence of large bundles of unmyelinated nerve fibers accompanying the efferent arterioles from the region of the juxtamedullary glomeruli to the level of the inner stripe of the outer medulla has also been reported.[355] Nerve fibers and nerve endings are not present at the convergence of smooth muscle layers of the efferent arterioles and arteriolae rectae, with pericytes surrounding the arterial vasa recta.[356]

Controversy has existed regarding the presence of direct tubule innervation in the renal cortex. Nerve bundles arising from perivascular nerves have been described in proximity to both proximal and distal tubules.[357] Structures termed *varicosities*, which are believed to represent nerve endings, have been described as being in close contact with proximal and distal tubules, often in the vicinity of the hilum of the glomerulus and the juxtaglomerular apparatus,[126,357,358] and in the connecting segment and the CCD.[359] Autoradiographic studies have also shown that injected tritiated norepinephrine is associated with both proximal and distal convoluted tubules, indicating monoaminergic innervation of these tubules.[19] The TAL receives the largest nerve supply.[19]

Myelinated and unmyelinated nerve fibers have been demonstrated in the corticomedullary region and in perivascular connective tissue.[360] Electron microscopic autoradiography revealed that tritiated norepinephrine is concentrated mainly on unmyelinated fibers, suggesting that these fibers are adrenergic in nature.[360] There is evidence that renal nerves possess fibers containing neuropeptide Y, a potent vasoconstrictor,[361,362] as well as immunoreactive somatostatin and neurotensin.[362] Vasoactive intestinal polypeptide immunoreactive nerve fibers are also well documented in the kidney.[362] Earlier studies describing cholinergic nerve fibers within the renal parenchyma have fallen into disrepute because the conclusions were based largely on the presence of acetylcholinesterase.[352]

The afferent renal nerves are found principally in the pelvic region, the major vessels, and the corticomedullary connective tissue.[358] Most, although not all, afferent renal nerves are unmyelinated.[363] Largely on the basis of immunocytochemical localization of calcitonin gene–related peptide, a marker of afferent nerve fibers, Barajas and associates[358] suggested that these immunoreactive nerve fibers may be involved in baroreceptor and afferent nerve responses to changes in arterial, venous, interstitial, or intrapelvic pressure.

ACKNOWLEDGMENTS

This chapter is a continuation of the chapters by Dr. C. Craig Tisher and Dr. Kirsten Madsen (8th edition) and Tae-Hwan Kwon, Jeppe Praetorius, Robert A. Fenton, and Søren Nielsen (9th edition).

The authors are grateful for the assistance of Takwa Shaiman Aroankins for help with reference formatting. Work from the laboratories of the authors was carried out with the support of the Danish Medical Research Council, the Novo Nordisk Foundation, the Lundbeck Foundation, the Carlsberg Foundation, and the Aarhus University Research Foundation. We thank our many excellent colleagues for their invaluable contributions to our research endeavors over the past several years.

Complete reference list available at ExpertConsult.com.

KEY REFERENCES

11. Christensen EI, Wagner CA, Kaissling B: Uriniferous tubule: structural and functional organization. *Compr Physiol* 2(2):805–861, 2012.
15. Zhai XY, Birn H, Jensen KB, et al: Digital three-dimensional reconstruction and ultrastructure of the mouse proximal tubule. *J Am Soc Nephrol* 14(3):611–619, 2003.
16. Zhai XY, Thomsen JS, Birn H, et al: Three-dimensional reconstruction of the mouse nephron. *J Am Soc Nephrol* 17(1):77–88, 2006.
23. Ichimura K, Stan RV, Kurihara H, et al: Glomerular endothelial cells form diaphragms during development and pathologic conditions. *J Am Soc Nephrol* 19(8):1463–1471, 2008.
30. Esser S, Wolburg K, Wolburg H, et al: Vascular endothelial growth factor induces endothelial fenestrations in vitro. *J Cell Biol* 140(4):947–959, 1998.

44. Miner JH: Renal basement membrane components. *Kidney Int* 56(6):2016–2024, 1999.
53. Caulfield JP, Farquhar MG: Distribution of annionic sites in glomerular basement membranes: their possible role in filtration and attachment. *Proc Natl Acad Sci U S A* 73(5):1646–1650, 1976.
64. Miner JH: The glomerular basement membrane. *Exp Cell Res* 318(9):973–978, 2012.
69. Endlich N, Simon O, Gopferich A, et al: Two-photon microscopy reveals stationary podocytes in living zebrafish larvae. *J Am Soc Nephrol* 25:681–686, 2014.
70. Hackl MJ, Burford JL, Villanueva K, et al: Tracking the fate of glomerular epithelial cells in vivo using serial multiphoton imaging in new mouse models with fluorescent lineage tags. *Nat Med* 19(12):1661–1666, 2013.
77. Grahammer F, Schell C, Huber TB: The podocyte slit diaphragm—from a thin grey line to a complex signalling hub. *Nat Rev Nephrol* 9(10):587–598, 2013.
79. Greka A, Mundel P: Cell biology and pathology of podocytes. *Annu Rev Physiol* 74:299–323, 2012.
85. Kriz W, Shirato I, Nagata M, et al: The podocyte's response to stress: the enigma of foot process effacement. *Am J Physiol Renal Physiol* 304(4):F333–F347, 2013.
94. Schlondorff D: The glomerular mesangial cell: an expanding role for a specialized pericyte. *FASEB J* 1(4):272–281, 1987.
99. Schlondorff D, Banas B: The mesangial cell revisited: no cell is an island. *J Am Soc Nephrol* 20(6):1179–1187, 2009.
100. Ohse T, Chang AM, Pippin JW, et al: A new function for parietal epithelial cells: a second glomerular barrier. *Am J Physiol Renal Physiol* 297(6):F1566–F1574, 2009.
103. Hakroush S, Cebulla A, Schaldecker T, et al: Extensive podocyte loss triggers a rapid parietal epithelial cell response. *J Am Soc Nephrol* 25(5):927–938, 2014.
105. Ryan GB, Coghlan JP, Scoggins BA: The granulated peripolar epithelial cell: a potential secretory component of the renal juxtaglomerular complex. *Nature* 277(5698):655–656, 1979.
115. Schnermann J, Briggs JP: Tubular control of renin synthesis and secretion. *Pflugers Arch* 465(1):39–51, 2013.
116. Kurtz A: Renin release: sites, mechanisms, and control. *Annu Rev Physiol* 73:377–399, 2011.
123. Ren Y, Carretero OA, Garvin JL: Role of mesangial cells and gap junctions in tubuloglomerular feedback. *Kidney Int* 62(2):525–531, 2002.
131. Castrop H, Schnermann J: Isoforms of renal Na-K-2Cl cotransporter NKCC2: expression and functional significance. *Am J Physiol Renal Physiol* 295(4):F859–F866, 2008.
135. Peti-Peterdi J, Harris RC: Macula Densa Sensing and Signaling Mechanisms of Renin Release. *J Am Soc Nephrol* 21:1093–1096, 2010.
140. Tisher CC, Bulger RE, Trump BF: Human renal ultrastructure. I. Proximal tubule of healthy individuals. *Lab Invest* 15(8):1357–1394, 1966.
141. Kaissling B, Kriz W: Structural analysis of the rabbit kidney. *Adv Anat Embryol Cell Biol* 56:1–123, 1979.
169. Katz AI, Doucet A, Morel F: Na-K-ATPase activity along the rabbit, rat, and mouse nephron. *Am J Physiol* 237(2):F114–F120, 1979.
176. Pannabecker TL: Structure and function of the thin limbs of the loop of Henle. *Compr Physiol* 2(3):2063–2086, 2012.
177. Zhai XY, Fenton RA, Andreasen A, et al: Aquaporin-1 is not expressed in descending thin limbs of short-loop nephrons. *J Am Soc Nephrol* 18(11):2937–2944, 2007.
192. Kone BC, Madsen KM, Tisher CC: Ultrastructure of the thick ascending limb of Henle in the rat kidney. *Am J Anat* 171(2):217–226, 1984.
205. Nielsen S, Maunsbach AB, Ecelbarger CA, et al: Ultrastructural localization of Na-K-2Cl cotransporter in thick ascending limb and macula densa of rat kidney. *Am J Physiol* 275(6 Pt 2):F885–F893, 1998.
208. Rocha AS, Kokko JP: Sodium chloride and water transport in the medullary thick ascending limb of Henle. Evidence for active chloride transport. *J Clin Invest* 52(3):612–623, 1973.
210. Crayen ML, Thoenes W: Architecture and cell structures in the distal nephron of the rat kidney. *Cytobiologie* 17(1):197–211, 1978.
212. Reilly RF, Ellison DH: Mammalian distal tubule: physiology, pathophysiology, and molecular anatomy. *Physiol Rev* 80(1):277–313, 2000.
218. Kaissling B, Bachmann S, Kriz W: Structural adaptation of the distal convoluted tubule to prolonged furosemide treatment. *Am J Physiol* 248(3 Pt 2):F374–F381, 1985.
227. Bostanjoglo M, Reeves WB, Reilly RF, et al: 11Beta-hydroxysteroid dehydrogenase, mineralocorticoid receptor, and thiazide-sensitive Na-Cl cotransporter expression by distal tubules. *J Am Soc Nephrol* 9(8):1347–1358, 1998.
228. Kim GH, Masilamani S, Turner R, et al: The thiazide-sensitive Na-Cl cotransporter is an aldosterone-induced protein. *Proc Natl Acad Sci U S A* 95(24):14552–14557, 1998.
231. Loffing J, Kaissling B: Sodium and calcium transport pathways along the mammalian distal nephron: from rabbit to human. *Am J Physiol Renal Physiol* 284(4):F628–F643, 2003.
232. Loffing J, Loffing-Cueni D, Valderrabano V, et al: Distribution of transcellular calcium and sodium transport pathways along mouse distal nephron. *Am J Physiol Renal Physiol* 281(6):F1021–F1027, 2001.
238. Dimke H, Hoenderop JG, Bindels RJ: Molecular basis of epithelial Ca2+ and Mg2+ transport: insights from the TRP channel family. *J Physiol* 589(Pt 7):1535–1542, 2011.
242. Fenton RA, Brond L, Nielsen S, et al: Cellular and subcellular distribution of the type-2 vasopressin receptor in the kidney. *Am J Physiol Renal Physiol* 293(3):F748–F760, 2007.
243. Pedersen NB, Hofmeister MV, Rosenbaek LL, et al: Vasopressin induces phosphorylation of the thiazide-sensitive sodium chloride cotransporter in the distal convoluted tubule. *Kidney Int* 78:160–169, 2010.
248. Morel F, Chabardes D, Imbert M: Functional segmentation of the rabbit distal tubule by microdetermination of hormone-dependent adenylate cyclase activity. *Kidney Int* 9:264–277, 1976.
250. Myers CE, Bulger RE, Tisher CC, et al: Human renal ultrastructure. IV. Collecting duct of healthy individuals. *Lab Invest* 16:655–668, 1966.
252. Verlander JW, Madsen KM, Tisher CC: Effect of acute respiratory acidosis on two populations of intercalated cells in rat cortical collecting duct. *Am J Physiol* 253(6 Pt 2):F1142–F1156, 1987.
253. Kim J, Kim YH, Cha JH, et al: Intercalated cell subtypes in connecting tubule and cortical collecting duct of rat and mouse. *J Am Soc Nephrol* 10(1):1–12, 1999.
259. Boros S, Bindels RJ, Hoenderop JG: Active Ca(2+) reabsorption in the connecting tubule. *Pflugers Arch* 458(1):99–109, 2009.
260. Stanton BA, Biemesderfer D, Wade JB, et al: Structural and functional study of the rat distal nephron: effects of potassium adaptation and depletion. *Kidney Int* 19(1):36–48, 1981.
295. Fenton RA, Praetorius J: Molecular physiology of the medullary collecting duct. *Compr Physiol* 1(2):1031–1056, 2011.
340. Bell RD, Keyl MJ, Shrader FR, et al: Renal lymphatics: the internal distribution. *Nephron* 5(6):454–463, 1968.
347. Michel CC: Renal medullary microcirculation: architecture and exchange. *Microcirculation* 2(2):125–139, 1995.

The Renal Circulations and Glomerular Ultrafiltration

Karen A. Munger | David A. Maddox |
Barry M. Brenner | Curtis K. Kost, Jr.

CHAPTER OUTLINE

MAJOR ARTERIES AND VEINS, 83
Hydraulic Pressure Profile of the Renal Circulation, 85
TOTAL RENAL BLOOD FLOW, 85
INTRARENAL BLOOD FLOW DISTRIBUTION, 87
Vascular-Tubule Relations, 87
Cortical Blood Flow, 87
Peritubular Capillary Dynamics, 89
Medullary Blood Flow, 90
Medullary Microcirculation, 90
Structure of the Glomerular Microcirculation, 92
DETERMINANTS OF GLOMERULAR ULTRAFILTRATION, 94
Hydraulic Pressures in the Glomerular Capillaries and Bowman's Space, 94
Glomerular Capillary Hydraulic and Colloid Osmotic Pressure Profiles, 94

Determination of the Ultrafiltration Coefficient, 96
Selective Alterations in the Primary Determinants of Glomerular Ultrafiltration, 97
REGULATION OF RENAL HEMODYNAMICS AND GLOMERULAR FILTRATION, 98
Vasomotor Properties of the Renal Microcirculations, 98
Role of the Renin-Angiotensin System in the Control of Renal Blood Flow and Glomerular Filtration Rate, 99
Endothelial Factors in the Control of Renal Hemodynamics and Glomerular Filtration, 101
Renal Autoregulation, 104
NEURAL REGULATION OF GLOMERULAR FILTRATION RATE, 110

Under resting conditions, blood flow to the kidneys represents approximately 20% of cardiac output in humans even though these organs constitute less than 1% of body mass. This rate of blood flow, approximately 400 mL per 100 g of tissue per minute, is significantly greater than that observed in other vascular beds considered to be well perfused, such as heart, liver, and brain.[1] From this enormous blood flow (1.0 to 1.2 L/minute), only a small quantity of urine is formed (1 mL/minute). Although the metabolic energy requirement of urine production is relatively high (approximately 10% of basal O_2 consumption), the renal arteriovenous O_2 difference reveals that blood flow far exceeds metabolic demands. In fact, the high rate of blood flow is essential to the process of urine formation as described later.

The kidney contains several distinct microvascular networks, including the glomerular microcirculation, the cortical peritubular microcirculation, and the unique microcirculations that nourish and drain the inner and outer medulla. In Chapter 2 the gross anatomy of the kidney and arrangement of tubular segments were described. In this chapter we consider the intrarenal organization of the discrete microcirculatory networks and regional renal blood flows as well as how this anatomy contributes to the physiologic factors that regulate renal blood flow (RBF) and glomerular filtration rate (GFR).

MAJOR ARTERIES AND VEINS

Blood supply for each kidney is provided by a renal artery that branches directly from the abdominal aorta. The human renal artery typically branches into multiple segmental vessels at a point just before entry into the renal parenchyma (Figure 3.1). Therefore, complete obstruction of an arterial segmental vessel results in ischemia and infarction of the tissue in its area of distribution. In fact, ligation of individual segmental arteries has frequently been performed in the rat to reduce renal mass and produce the remnant kidney model of chronic renal failure. Morphologic studies in this model reveal the presence of ischemic zones adjacent to the totally infarcted areas. These regions contain viable glomeruli that appear shrunken and crowded

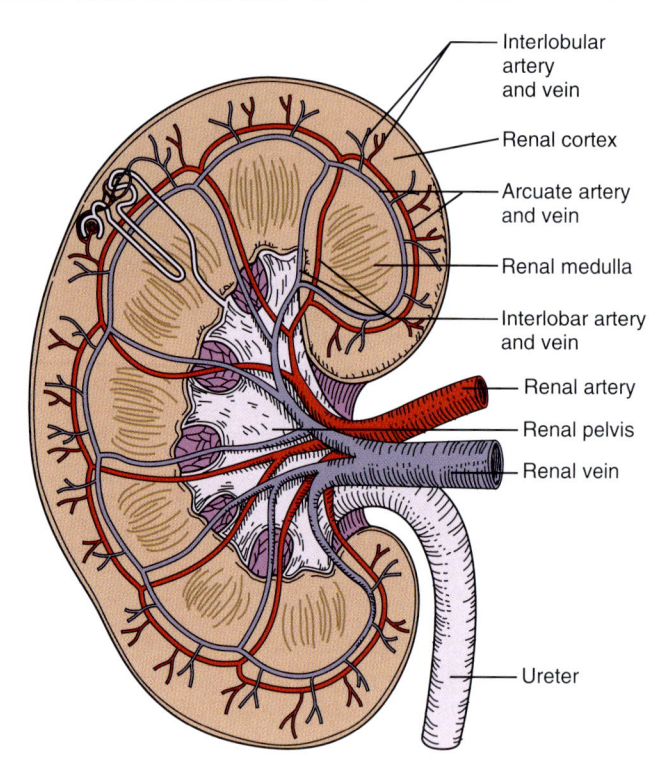

Figure 3.1 Simplified drawing of the human kidney in cross section, illustrating the organization of vasculature. A single nephron is also drawn to show the interlobular artery entering into the glomerular capillary network. (From Fox SI: *Human physiology*, ed 6, New York, 1999, McGraw-Hill, pg 529. Reproduced with permission of The McGraw-Hill Companies.)

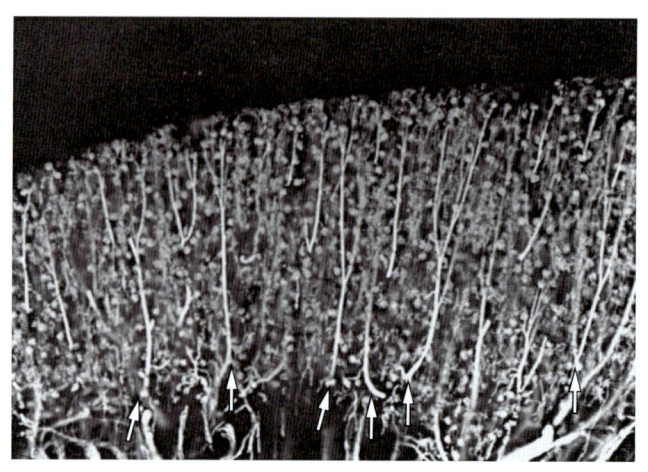

Figure 3.2 Low-power photomicrograph of silicone rubber-injected vascular structures in human renal cortex. The tissue has been made transparent by dehydration and clearing procedures after injection. Interlobular arteries (some indicated by *arrows*) arise from arcuate arteries *(not seen)* and extend toward the kidney surface. The glomeruli, visible as small round objects, arise from the interlobular vessels at all cortical levels. (×5.) (Courtesy of R Beeuwkes, PhD.)

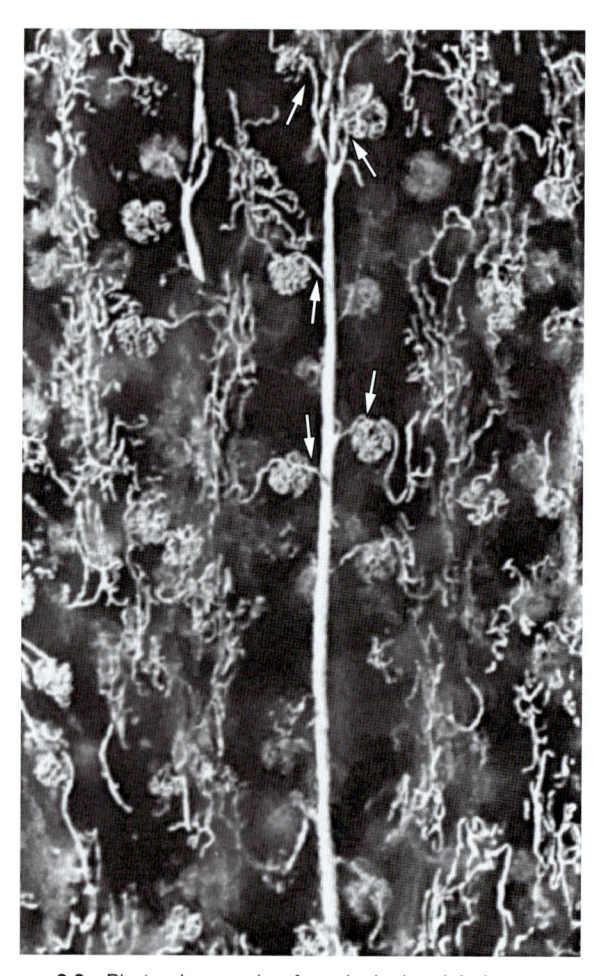

Figure 3.3 Photomicrograph of a single interlobular artery and glomeruli arising from it as seen in a cleared section of a silicone rubber–injected human kidney. Afferent arterioles *(arrows)* extend to glomeruli. Efferent vessels emerging from glomeruli branch to form the cortical postglomerular capillary network. The photomicrograph is oriented so that the outer cortex is at the **top** and the inner cortex is at the **bottom**. (×25.) (Courtesy R. Beeuwkes, PhD.)

together, demonstrating that some portions of the renal cortex may have partial dual perfusion.[2]

The anatomic distribution just described is most common; however, other patterns may occur.[3,4] Not infrequently, secondary renal arteries may result from division of the renal artery at the aorta. These vessels, which most often supply the lower pole,[5] may be the sole arterial supply of some part of the kidney.[6] Such additional arteries are found in 20% to 30% of normal individuals.

Within the renal sinus of the human kidney, division of the segmental arteries gives rise to the interlobar arteries. These vessels, in turn, give rise to the arcuate arteries, whose several divisions lie at the border between the cortex and medulla (see Figure 3.1). From the arcuate arteries, the interlobular arteries branch more or less sharply, most often as a common trunk that divides two to five times as it extends toward the kidney surface[7,8] (Figure 3.2). Afferent arterioles leading to glomeruli arise from the smaller branches of the interlobular arteries (Figure 3.3). Glomeruli are classified according to their position within the cortex as superficial (i.e., near the kidney surface), midcortical, or juxtamedullary (near the corticomedullary border). The capillary network of each glomerulus is connected to the postglomerular (peritubular) capillary circulation by way of the efferent arterioles. Both the nomenclatures and the patterns of the renal arterial system are similar in most of the mammals commonly used experimentally. For example, the main arterial branches that lie beside the medullary pyramid are called interlobar, even in animals such as rodents that have but a single lobe.

HYDRAULIC PRESSURE PROFILE OF THE RENAL CIRCULATION

The pressure drop between the systemic vasculature and the end of the interlobular artery in both the superficial and the juxtamedullary microvasculature can be as much as 25 mm Hg at normal perfusion pressures, with the majority of that pressure drop occurring along the interlobular arteries (Figure 3.4). However, on the basis of studies of the vasculature of a unique set of juxtamedullary nephrons, most of the preglomerular pressure drop between the arcuate artery and the glomerulus occurs along the afferent arteriole.[9,10] Approximately 70% of the postglomerular hydraulic pressure drop takes place along the efferent arterioles, with approximately 40% of the total postglomerular resistance accounted for by the early efferent arteriole (see Figure 3.4). Of note, studies of juxtamedullary nephrons perfused via the arcuate artery indicate that the very late portion of the afferent arteriole (last 50-150 µm) and the very early portion of the efferent arteriole (first 50-150 µm) provide a large portion of the total preganglionic and postglomerular resistance.[9,10] Indeed, elegant work by Peti-Peterdi and associates using multiphoton imaging indicate the presence of an intraglomerular precapillary sphincter[11,12] (Figure 3.5).

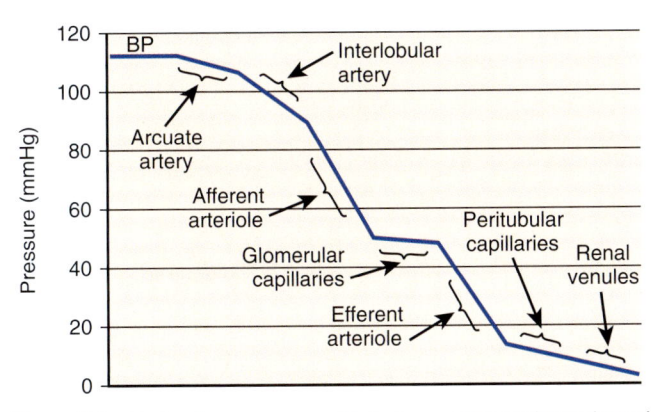

Figure 3.4 Hydraulic pressure profile in the renal vasculature based on a variety of micropuncture studies in superficial nephrons of the rat and squirrel monkey as well as values obtained by micropuncture of juxtamedullary nephrons in the rat. For these latter studies the arcuate artery was perfused with whole blood at normal arterial pressures, and hydraulic pressures were measured at downstream sites, including the interlobular artery, the proximal and distal portions of the afferent arteriole, the glomerular capillaries, the proximal and late segments of the efferent arteriole, the peritubular capillaries, and the renal vein. (See references 76 and 88 for sources of data used to generate the profile.)

TOTAL RENAL BLOOD FLOW

Total RBF in humans typically exceeds 20% of the cardiac output, or about 1 to 1.2 L/min for a man. The classic method of determining total RBF is first to determine renal plasma flow using the "clearance" of an indicator substance from blood passing through the kidney and its subsequent appearance in the urine. The simple formula for the clearance of any substance is as follows:

$$C_x = U_x V/P_x \quad (1)$$

where C_x is the clearance of a substance x, U_x is the urinary concentration of x, V is urine flow rate, and P_x is the plasma concentration of x.

If the substance is neither metabolized nor synthesized in the kidney then its rate of appearance in the urine equals its rate of extraction from the blood. The blood extraction rate is equal to the renal plasma flow rate multiplied by the difference between the arterial and renal venous plasma concentrations. This can be expressed mathematically as follows:

$$U_x V = (Art_x - Vein_x) \times RPF \quad (2)$$

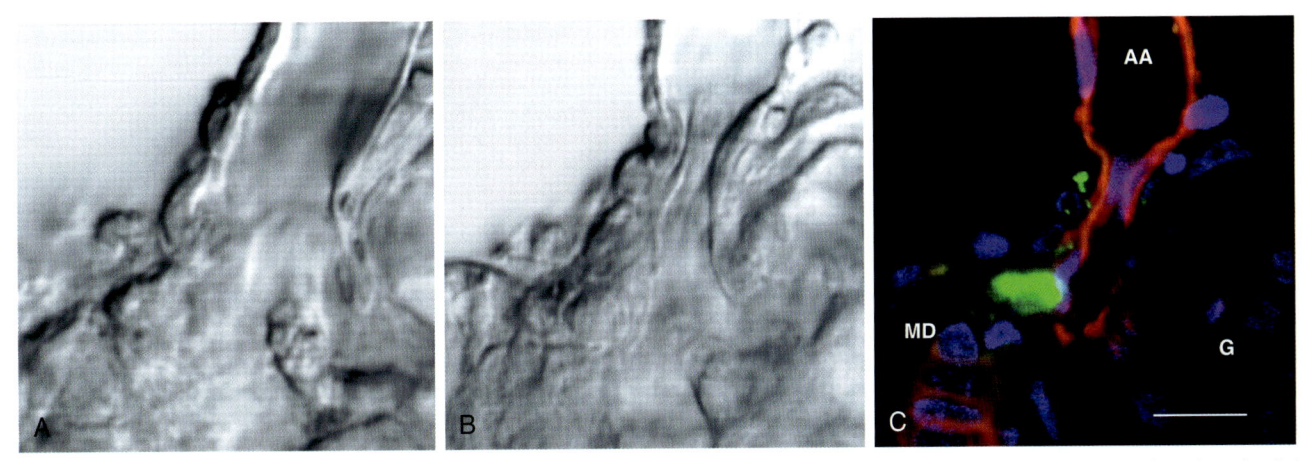

Figure 3.5 Constriction of the terminal afferent arteriole (AA), an intraglomerular precapillary sphincter, in response to elevations in distal tubular salt content. **A** and **B**, Transmitted light–differential interference contrast (DIC) images. **A**, Control, with NaCl concentration at the macula densa at 10 mM. **B**, NaCl concentration is increased to 60 mM, resulting in an almost complete closure of the AA. **C**, Fluorescence image of the same preparation as shown in **B**. Vascular endothelium and tubular epithelium are labeled with R18 *(red)*, renin granules with quinacrine *(green)*, cell nuclei with Hoechst 33342 *(blue)*. Note that renin-positive granular cells constitute the sphincter. MD, macula densa. Scale bar = 10 µm. (From Peti-Peterdi J: Multiphoton imaging of renal tissues in vitro. *Am J Physiol Renal Physiol* 288:F1079-F1083, 2005.)

where U_x is urine concentration of the indicator, V is urine flow rate, Art_x and $Vein_x$ are arterial and renal venous concentrations of the indicator, respectively, and RPF is renal plasma flow rate. Rearranging we get:

$$RPF = U_x V/(Art_x - Vein_x) \qquad (3)$$

RBF can then be calculated by dividing RPF by the plasma fraction of whole blood (from the hematocrit, Hct):

$$RBF = RPF/(1 - Hct) \qquad (4)$$

Historically, RBF has been estimated from determinations of renal plasma flow using *p*-aminohippuric acid (PAH) as the indicator. This substance is both filtered at the glomerulus and actively secreted by the tubules, resulting in the renal extraction of 70% to 90% of PAH from the blood. Not all the PAH is removed from the kidney circulation because of flow through regions of the kidney (e.g., medulla) that do not perfuse proximal tubule segments where secretion occurs, incomplete removal of PAH in (some) cortical regions, and the presence of periglomerular shunts (Figure 3.6). If the extraction is assumed to be equal to 100% (renal venous concentration equals zero) then the clearance of PAH, using equation 1 (($U_{PAH} \times V$)/Art_{PAH}), provides a simple, noninvasive approximation of RPF. This approximation is often termed "effective" renal plasma flow (ERPF) and provides an estimate of RPF without the need for a renal venous blood sample. However, this estimate of renal plasma flow is much less accurate in renal disease because extraction is further reduced by damage to proximal tubule segments involved in PAH secretion.[13] Figure 3.7 shows some typical values for ERPF and GFR in adult humans from a number of studies.

Micropuncture studies performed in vivo in experimental animals provide more accurate and detailed information about cortical blood flow but the medulla is less accessible to micropuncture, and thus the medullary blood flow has

Figure 3.6 **Anatomy of the medullary microcirculation.** In the cortex, interlobular arteries arise from the arcuate artery and ascend toward the cortical surface. Cortical and juxtamedullary glomeruli branch from the interlobular artery. The majority of blood flow reaches the medulla through juxtamedullary efferent arterioles; however, there is evidence that some may also be from periglomerular shunt pathways. In the outer medulla, juxtamedullary efferent arterioles in the outer stripe give rise to descending vasa recta (DVR) that coalesce to form vascular bundles in the inner stripe. DVR on the periphery of vascular bundles give rise to the interbundle capillary plexus that surrounds nephron segments (thick ascending limb, collecting duct, long-looped thin descending limbs *[not shown]*). DVR in the center continue across the inner-outer medullary junction to perfuse the inner medulla. Thin descending limbs of short-looped nephrons may also associate with the vascular bundles in a manner that is species dependent *(not shown)*. Inner medulla: Vascular bundles disappear in the inner medulla, and vasa recta become dispersed with nephron segments. Ascending vasa recta (AVR) that arise from the sparse capillary plexus of inner medulla return to the cortex by passing through outer medullary vascular bundles. DVR have a continuous endothelium *(inset)*. (From Pallone TL, Zhang Z, Rhinehart K: Physiology of the renal medullary microcirculation. *Am J Physiol* 284:F253-F266, 2003.)

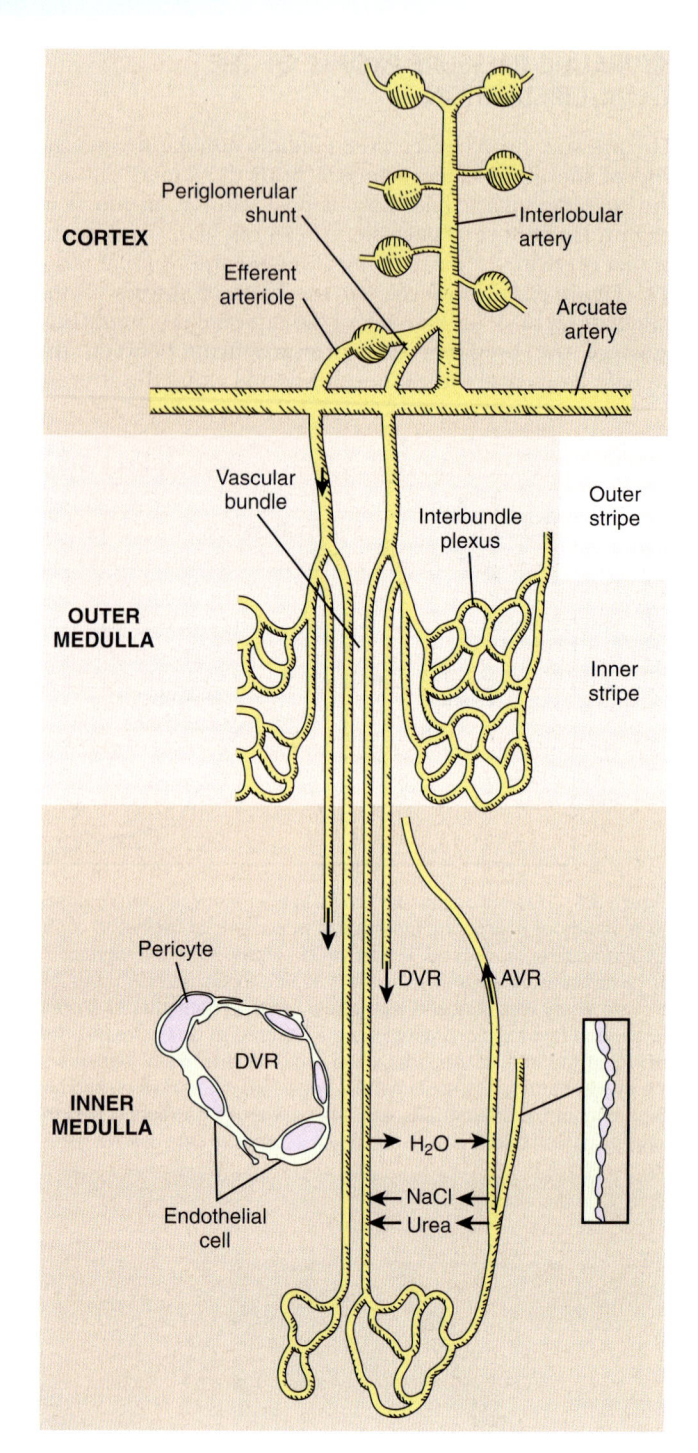

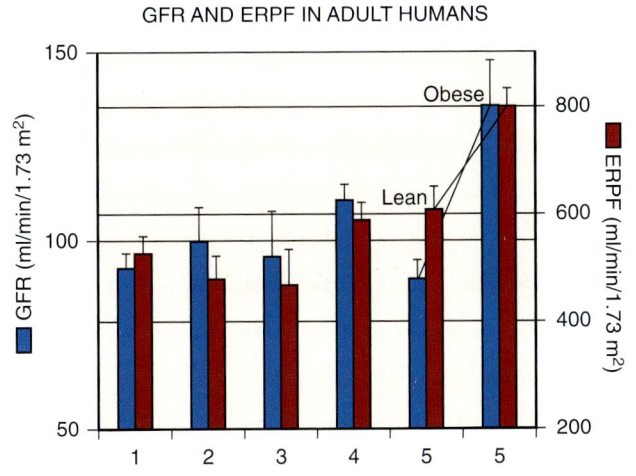

Figure 3.7 Typical values for glomerular filtration rate (GFR) and renal plasma flow (ERPF) from five studies in adult humans. Values from men and women were pooled. Numbers under each set of bars refer to the following studies: 1, Giordano and Defronzo[356]; 2, Winetz et al[357]; 3, Hostetter[358]; 4, Deen et al[359]; 5, Chagnac et al.[360] For studies 1 through 3 and 5, values were obtained after approximately 12 hours of fasting; subjects in study 4 were allowed food ad libitum. For study 5, values from lean subjects (average body mass index [BMI] = 22) were compared with those from obese nondiabetic individuals (BMI > 38) after a 10-hour fast, and those values were not corrected for body surface area.

been less studied. For detailed discussion of historical methods of RBF measurements, the reader is referred to Dworkin and Brenner.[13] Improved methods of RBF measurement have been introduced with laser Doppler flowmetry, video microscopy, and imaging techniques such as positron emission tomography (PET), high-speed computed tomography (CT), and magnetic resonance imaging (MRI).[13-17] These methods have been especially useful in determining regional blood flow as discussed later.

INTRARENAL BLOOD FLOW DISTRIBUTION

The cortex accounts for filtration and the majority of reabsorption, whereas the medulla's primary function is maintenance of a hypertonic gradient and urine concentration. Therefore, RBF to these regions is differentially regulated in response to the differing demands of these two kidney regions.[18] There are structural differences in vascular components of the cortex and the medulla that may account for differences in RBF, namely, the organization of the afferent and efferent arterioles of the cortical and juxtamedullary glomeruli. Studies conducted in rabbits demonstrated that cortical afferent arterioles have larger internal diameters than the efferent arterioles, whereas juxtamedullary afferent and efferent arterioles are significantly larger and the efferent arteriole is more muscular compared to the cortical arterioles.[18,19] In addition, the cortical peritubular capillaries, derived from efferent arterioles of cortical glomeruli, are about half the size of the medullary *vasa recta* derived from efferent arterioles of the juxtamedullary glomeruli

(Figure 3.8).[18] These features may partially explain the differential control of medullary and cortical blood flows. Additional factors include sympathetic nerve activity and hormonal influences.

VASCULAR-TUBULE RELATIONS

Cortical vascular-tubule relations have been described most completely in the canine kidney.[7,20,21] These studies show that, except for convoluted tubule segments in the outermost region of the cortex, the efferent peritubular capillary network and the nephron arising from each glomerulus are often dissociated. In addition, even though the blood supply of many superficial proximal and distal convoluted tubules is derived from peritubular capillaries arising from the parent glomerulus of the same nephron (Figure 3.9), the loops of Henle of such nephrons, descending in the medullary ray, are surrounded by blood vessels emerging from many midcortical glomeruli through efferent arterioles that extend directly into the ray. Nephrons originating from midcortical glomeruli have proximal and distal convoluted tubule segments lying close to the interlobular axis in the region above the glomerulus of origin. This region is perfused by capillary networks arising from the efferent arterioles of more superficial glomeruli. It is in the inner cortex, however, that this dissociation between individual tubules and the corresponding postglomerular capillary network is most apparent. The convoluted tubule segments of these nephrons lie above the glomeruli surrounded either by the dense network close to the interlobular vessels or by capillary networks arising from other inner cortical glomeruli.

Efferent vessel patterns and vascular-tubule relationships in the human kidney are similar to those in the dog kidney.[21,22] In general, a close association between the initial portions of peritubular capillaries and early and late proximal tubule segments of the same glomerulus has been shown.[23-25] However, this close association does not mean that each vessel adjacent to a given tubule necessarily arises from the same glomerulus. In fact, Briggs and Wright[26] found that although superficial nephron segments and vessels arising from the same glomerulus are closely associated, each vessel may serve segments of more than one nephron.

CORTICAL BLOOD FLOW

The majority of RBF perfuses the cortex. Vasoconstrictors such as angiotensin II, endothelin, and noradrenaline have much greater effects on cortical blood flow than on medullary blood flow, whereas vasodilators such as bradykinin and nitric oxide tend to selectively increase medullary blood flow.[18] There can be extensive redistribution of blood flow in the kidney under various conditions that may be important in physiologic and pathophysiologic conditions.[27] Studies by Trueta[28] of RBF distribution after hemorrhage were among the first performed. These studies indicated that during shock, RBF appeared to be shunted through the medulla. This phenomenon, observed more than 60 years ago in qualitative studies of the distribution of India ink and radiographic contrast media, was subsequently termed "cortical ischemia with maintained blood flow through the medulla."[29]

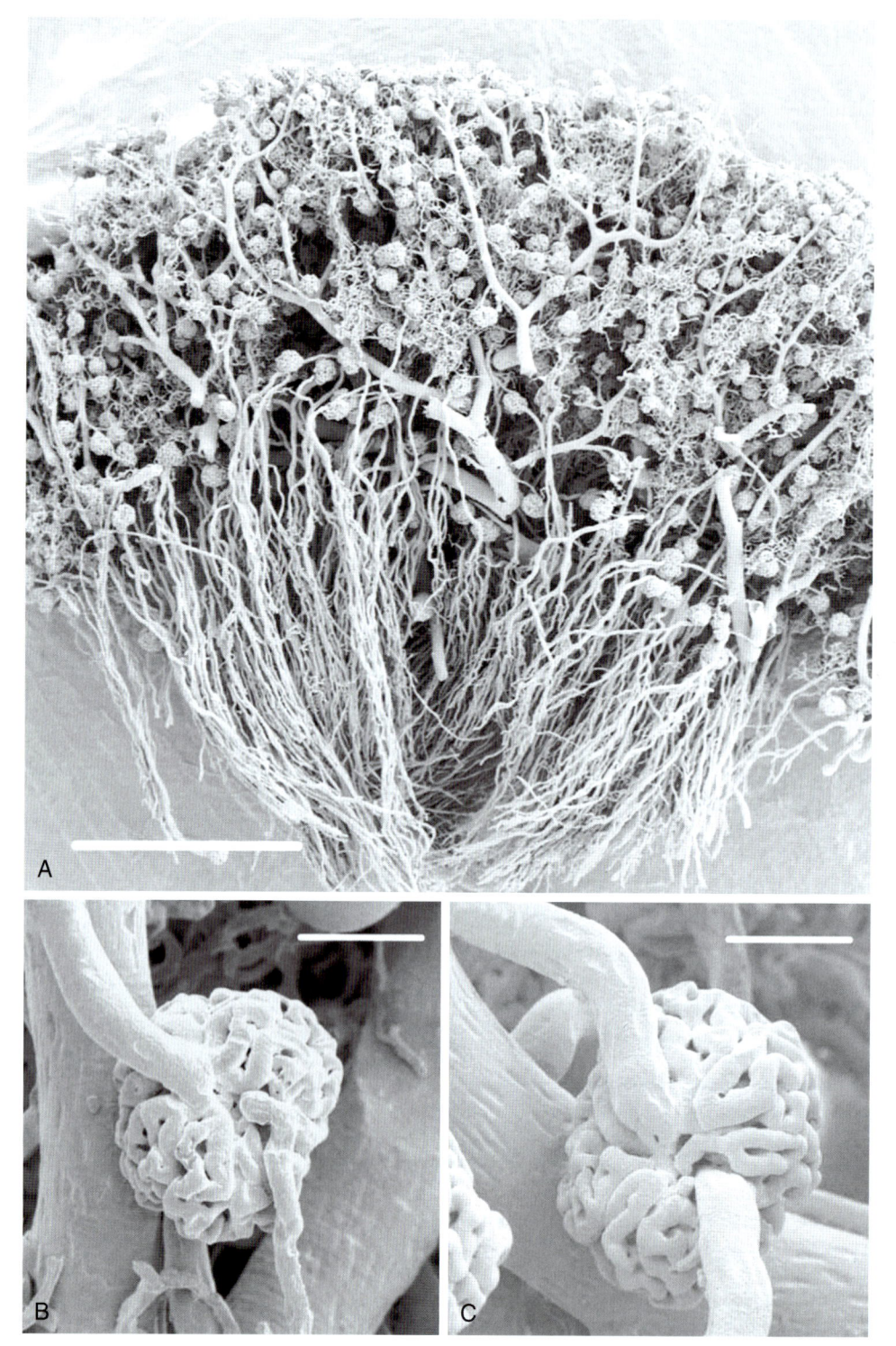

Figure 3.8 **A,** Resin cast of the renal vasculature of a rabbit, depicting both cortical and medullary vessels (scale bar = 1 mm). Note that the cortical peritubular capillaries are considerably smaller in diameter than the medullary vasa recta. **B,** Cortical glomeruli showing afferent *(upper vessel)* and efferent arterioles and the capillary tuft (scale bar = 60 μm). **C,** Juxtamedullary glomeruli showing afferent *(upper vessel)* and efferent arterioles and the capillary tuft (scale bar 60 = μm). Note that the juxtamedullary arterioles are larger in diameter than the cortical glomerular arterioles, particularly the efferent arterioles. (From Evans RG, Eppel GA, Anderson WP, Denton KM: Mechanisms underlying the differential control of blood flow in the renal medulla and cortex. *J Hypertens* 22:1439-1451, 2004.)

PERITUBULAR CAPILLARY DYNAMICS

The same Starling forces that control fluid movement across all capillary beds govern the rate of fluid movement across peritubular capillary walls. Owing to the relatively high resistance along the afferent and efferent arterioles, a large drop in hydraulic pressure occurs prior to the peritubular capillaries. In addition, as protein-free fluid is filtered out of the glomerular capillaries and into Bowman's space, the oncotic pressure of blood flowing into the peritubular capillaries increases because of "trapped" plasma proteins. The sum of these forces favors fluid movement into the peritubular capillaries. Alterations in the net driving force for reabsorption (i.e., the balance between the transcapillary oncotic and hydraulic pressure gradients) have significant effects on net proximal reabsorption.[30] The absolute amount of movement resulting from this driving force also depends on the peritubular capillary surface area available for fluid uptake and the hydraulic conductivity of the capillary wall. Values for the hydraulic conductivity of the peritubular capillaries are not as great as those for the glomerular capillaries, but this difference is offset by the much larger total surface area of the peritubular capillary network.

In the rat, it has been estimated that approximately 50% of the peritubular capillary surface is composed of fenestrated areas.[31] Unlike the glomerular capillaries, peritubular capillary fenestrations are bridged by a thin diaphragm[31] that is negatively charged.[32] Beneath the fenestrae of the endothelial cells lies a basement membrane that completely surrounds the capillary. For the most part, peritubular capillaries are closely apposed to cortical tubules (Figure 3.10), so that the extracellular space between the tubules and capillaries constitutes only about 5% of the cortical volume.[33] The tubular epithelial cells are surrounded by the tubular basement membrane, which is distinct from and wider than the capillary basement membrane (see Figure 3.10). Numerous microfibrils connect the tubular and capillary basement membranes, a feature that may help limit expansion of the interstitium and maintain close contact between tubular epithelial cells and the peritubular capillaries during periods of high fluid flux.[34] Thus, the pathway for fluid reabsorption from the tubular lumen to the peritubular capillary is composed, in series, of the epithelial cell, tubular basement membrane, a narrow interstitial region containing microfibrils, the capillary basement membrane, and the thin membrane bridging the endothelial fenestrae.[34]

Like the endothelial cells, the basement membrane of the peritubular capillaries possesses anionic sites.[32] The electronegative charge density of the peritubular capillary basement membrane is significantly greater than that observed in the unfenestrated capillaries of skeletal muscle and similar to that observed in the glomerular capillary bed. Although the function of the anionic sites in the peritubular capillaries is uncertain, it is likely, by analogy to the

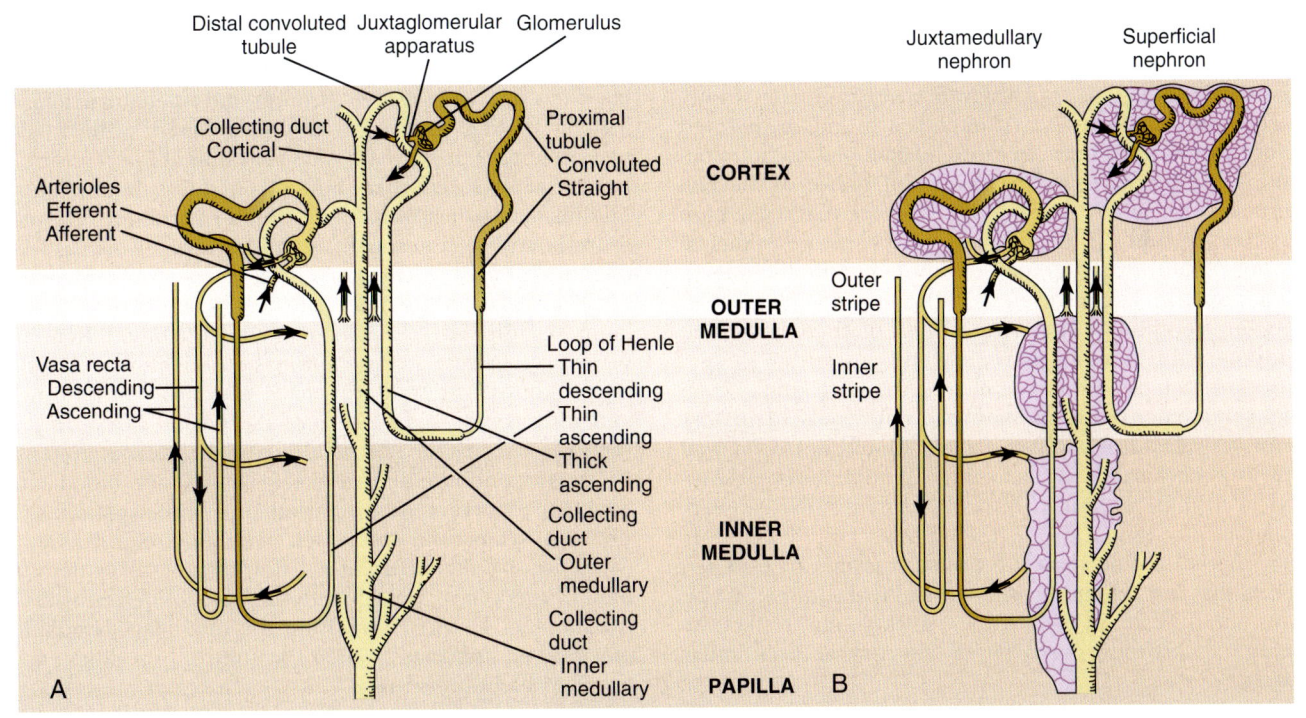

Figure 3.9 **A,** Superficial and juxtamedullary nephrons and their vasculature. The glomerulus plus the surrounding Bowman's capsule are known as the *renal corpuscle*. The beginning of the proximal tubule, called the *urinary pole*, lies opposite the vascular pole, where the afferent and efferent arterioles enter and leave the glomerulus. The early distal tubule is always apposed to the vascular pole belonging to the same nephron; the juxtaglomerular apparatus is located at the point of contact. **B,** Capillary networks have been superimposed on the nephrons illustrated in **A**. Both diagrams are highly schematic (for a more accurate portrayal, see Beewukes and Bonventre[21]), and they do not accurately reflect some relationships that probably have functional meaning. In the rat, for example, long thin descending limbs of Henle are located next to collecting ducts, and short thin descending limbs are closely associated with the vascular bundles made up of descending and ascending vasa recta in the outer medulla. (Drawings are based on Kriz and Bankir,[361] from Valtin H, Schafer JA: *Renal function*, ed 3, 1995, Philadelphia, Lippincott Williams & Wilkins).

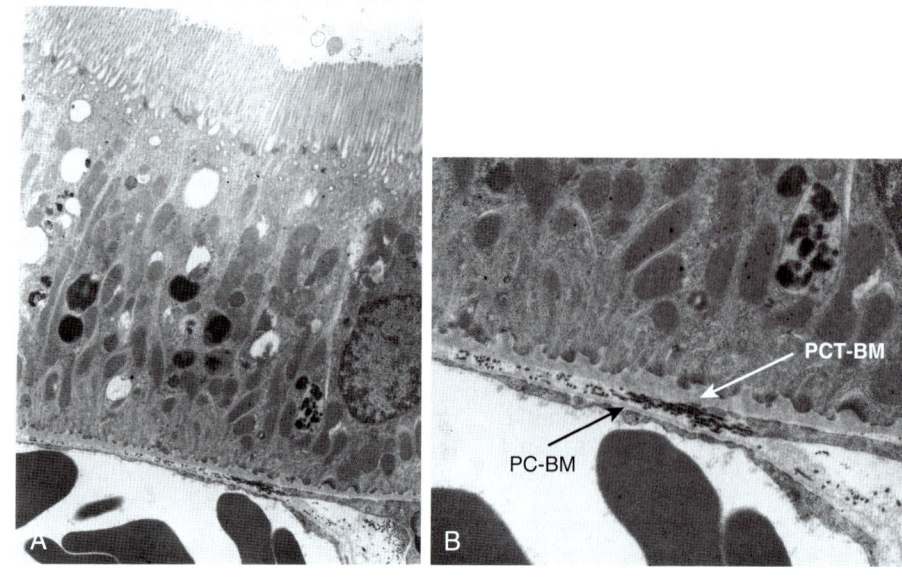

Figure 3.10 Electron micrographs (by DA Maddox) of a proximal tubule of a Munich Wistar rat. Tubule was perfusion-fixed with 1.25% glutaraldehyde thereby also fixing red cells in adjacent capillaries. **A,** The apposition of the basolateral surface of the tubular cells with the adjacent peritubular capillaries is close, leaving little interstitial space where the two come in contact. (≈ ×13,000.) **B,** The proximal tubule basement membrane (PC-BM) is relatively thick in comparison with the peritubular capillary endothelial basement membrane (PC-BM.) (≈×25,000.)

glomerulus, that they are an adaptation to compensate for the greater permeability of fenestrated capillaries, allowing free exchange of water and small molecules while restricting anionic plasma proteins to the circulation. In fact, some workers have reported that the renal peritubular capillaries are more permeable to both small and large molecules than are other beds.[35] This conclusion is based on tracer studies in which the renal artery was clamped or the kidney removed before fixation. However, because normal plasma flow conditions appear necessary for the maintenance of the glomerular permeability barrier,[36] it is possible that these high stop-flow peritubular permeabilities occur as an artifact of the unfavorable experimental conditions employed. Indeed, studies by Deen and associates[37] indicate that, at least under free-flow conditions, the permeability of these vessels to dextrans and albumin is extremely low.

Because the peritubular capillaries that surround a given nephron are derived from many efferent vessels, regulatory processes related to capillary factors should not be viewed only as a mechanism for balancing filtration and reabsorption in a single nephron. Instead, assuming that capillary dynamics throughout the cortex are the same, we may consider that all tubule segments are surrounded by capillary vessels that are operating in a similar reabsorptive mode. Thus, the function of the cortex as a whole may reflect the average reabsorptive capacity of all cortical peritubular vessels.

MEDULLARY BLOOD FLOW

Medullary blood flow constitutes about 10% to 15% of total RBF[13,38] and is derived from efferent arterioles of the juxtamedullary nephrons.[19,39] Although these medullary flows are less than one fourth as high as cortical flows, medullary flow is still substantial. Thus, per gram of tissue, outer medullary flow exceeds that of liver, and inner medullary flow is comparable to that of resting muscle or brain.[40] The fact that such large flows are compatible with the existence and maintenance of the inner medullary solute concentration gradient attests to the efficiency of countercurrent mechanisms in this region. The descending vasa recta have a continuous endothelium in which water moves across water channels and urea moves through endothelial carriers.[41,42] The ascending vasa recta are fenestrated, with a high hydraulic conductivity and water movement likely governed by transcapillary hydraulic and oncotic pressure gradients.[42] Medullary blood flow is highest under conditions of water diuresis and declines during antidiuresis.[38] This decrease depends, at least in part, on a direct vasoconstrictive action of vasopressin on the medullary microcirculation.[43] Vasodilatory factors act to preserve medullary blood flow and prevent ischemia. Acetylcholine,[44] vasodilator prostaglandins,[45] kinins,[46] adenosine,[47] atrial peptides,[48] bradykinin,[15] and nitric oxide[49] increase medullary RBF. In contrast to their vasoconstrictor effects in the renal cortex, angiotensin II[50-52] and endothelin [50] increase medullary blood flow, effects mediated in part by vasodilatory prostaglandins,[51,52] whereas vasopressin decreases medullary blood flow.[43,53] Alterations in medullary blood flow may be a key determinant of medullary tonicity and, thereby, solute transport in the loops of Henle. In addition the medullary circulation may play an important role in the control of sodium excretion and blood pressure.[54]

MEDULLARY MICROCIRCULATION

VASCULAR PATTERNS

The precise location of the boundary between the renal cortex and medulla is difficult to discern because the medullary rays of the cortex merge imperceptibly with the medulla. In general, the arcuate arteries or the sites at which the interlobular arteries branch into arcuate arteries mark this boundary. When considering the medullary circulation, most studies focus on its relation to the countercurrent mechanism as facilitated by the parallel array of descending and ascending vasa recta. However, although this configuration is characteristic of the inner medulla, the medulla also contains an outer zone, which consists of two morphologically distinct regions, the outer and inner stripes of the outer medulla (see Figure 3.9). The boundary between the outer medulla and inner medulla is defined by the beginning of the thick ascending limbs of Henle (see Figure 3.9). In addition to the thick ascending limbs, the outer medulla contains descending straight segments of proximal tubules (*pars recta*), descending thin limbs, and collecting ducts. The nephron segments of the inner stripe of the outer medulla include thick ascending limbs, thin descending limbs, and collecting ducts. Each of these morphologically distinct medullary regions is supplied and drained by an independent, specific vascular system.

The blood supply of the medulla is derived entirely from the efferent arterioles of the juxtamedullary glomeruli (see Figure 3.9).[21,55-57] Depending on the species and the method of evaluation, it has been estimated that from 7% to 18% of glomeruli give rise to efferents that ultimately supply the medulla.[57,58] Efferent arterioles of juxtamedullary nephrons are larger in diameter and possess thicker endothelium and more prominent smooth muscle layers than arterioles originating from superficial glomeruli.[18,59]

The vasculature of the outer medulla displays both vertical and lateral heterogeneity, but in general, both the outer and inner stripes contain two distinct circulatory regions: the vascular bundles, formed by the coalescence of the descending and ascending vasa recta, and the interbundle capillary plexus. Vascular bundles of descending and ascending vasa recta arise from the efferent arterioles of juxtamedullary glomeruli and descend through the outer stripe of the outer medulla to supply the inner stripe of the outer medulla and the inner medulla (Figure 3.11). Within the outer stripe, the descending vasa recta also give rise, via small side branches, to a complex capillary plexus. Early studies suggested that this capillary network was limited and, therefore, not the main blood supply to this region. Instead, it was thought that nutrient flow was provided by the ascending vasa recta rising from the inner stripe. This notion was further suggested by the large area of contact between ascending vasa recta and the descending proximal straight tubules within this zone.[31,58,60]

The outer medulla includes the metabolically active thick ascending limbs. Nutrients and O_2 to this energy-demanding tissue to the inner stripe are delivered by a dense capillary plexus arising from a few descending vasa recta at the periphery of the bundles. Approximately 10% to 15% of total RBF is directed to the medulla, and of this amount, probably the largest portion perfuses this inner stripe capillary plexus. The smooth muscle cells of the descending vasa recta are replaced by pericytes surrounding the endothelium with subsequent loss of the pericytes and transformation into medullary capillaries accompanied by endothelial fenestrations.[39,61]

The rich capillary network of the inner stripe drains into numerous veins, which for the most part do not join the vascular bundles but ascend directly to the outer stripe. These veins subsequently rise to the cortical-medullary

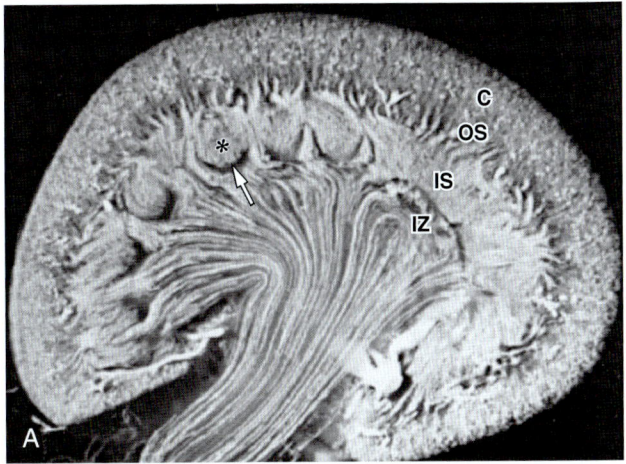

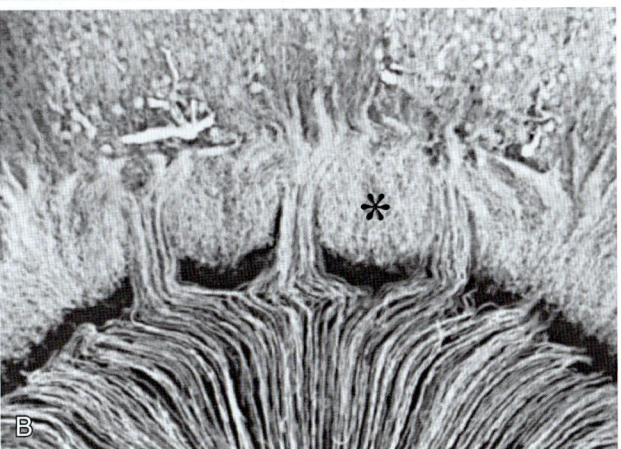

Figure 3.11 Longitudinal section of kidney of the sand rat *(Psammomys obesus)* after arterial injection of Microfil silicone rubber and clearing. **A,** The low-power magnification reveals distinct zonation of the kidney (C, cortex; OS and IS, outer and inner stripes of the outer medulla, respectively; IZ, inner medulla). The inner medulla is long and extends a short distance below the bottom of the picture. Giant vascular bundles, including a mixture of descending and ascending vasa recta, traverse the outer medulla to supply blood to the inner medulla. **B,** The outer medulla at a higher magnification. Between the vascular bundles (three are visible), a rich capillary plexus (*asterisk* in both views) supplies the tubule segments present in this zone. (From Bankir L, Kaissling B, de Rouffignac C, Kriz W: The vascular organization of the kidney of *Psammomys obesus*. *Anat Embryol* 155:149, 1979.)

junction, and the majority join with cortical veins at the level of the inner cortex.[61] A minority of the veins may extend within the medullary rays to regions near the kidney surface.[7,55,61] Thus, the capillary network of the inner stripe makes no contact with the vessels draining the inner medulla.

The inner medulla contains thin descending and thin ascending limbs of Henle, together with collecting ducts (see Figure 3.9). Within this region, the straight, unbranching vasa recta descend in bundles, with individual vessels leaving at every level to divide into a simple capillary network characterized by elongated links (see Figures 3.6 and 3.9).[39,58,61] These capillaries converge to form the venous vasa recta. Within the inner medulla, the descending and ascending vascular pathways remain in close apposition, although distinct vascular regions can no longer be clearly discerned. The venous vasa recta rise toward the outer medulla in parallel with the supply vessels to join the vascular bundles. Thus, the outer medullary vascular bundles include both supplying and draining vessels of the inner medulla. Within the outer stripe of the outer medulla, the vascular bundles spread out and traverse the outer stripe as wide, tortuous channels that lie in close apposition to the tubules, eventually emptying into arcuate or deep interlobular veins.[58] The venous pathways within the bundles are both larger and more numerous than the arterial vessels, suggesting lower flow velocities in the ascending (venous) than in the descending (arterial) direction.[62] The close apposition of the arterial and venous pathways within the vascular bundles is important for maintaining the hypertonicity of the inner medulla.

There are important differences in the structures of the ascending and descending vasa recta. The descending vasa recta possess a contractile layer composed of smooth muscle cells in the early segments that evolve into pericytes by the more distal portions of the vessels. Immunohistochemical studies demonstrate that these pericytes contain smooth muscle α-actin, suggesting that they may serve as contractile elements and participate in the regulation of medullary blood flow[63] as well as vascular-tubular crosstalk.[64] Each of these vessels also displays a continuous endothelium that persists until the hairpin turn is reached and the vessels divide to form the medullary capillaries. In contrast, ascending vasa recta, like true capillaries, lack a contractile layer and are characterized by a highly fenestrated endothelium.[65,66]

VASCULAR-TUBULE RELATIONS

The mechanism of urine concentration requires coordinated function of the vascular and tubule components of the medulla. In species capable of marked concentrating ability, medullary vascular-tubule relations show a high degree of organization favoring particular exchange processes by the juxtaposition of specific tubule segments and blood vessels.[61] In addition to anatomic proximity, the absolute magnitude of these exchanges is greatly influenced by the permeability characteristics of the structures involved, which may vary significantly among species.[67]

Most of our detailed knowledge of vascular-tubule relations within the medulla is based on histologic studies of rodent species.[56,60,61,63,68,69] As already discussed, the inner stripe of the outer medulla contains two distinct territories, the vascular bundles and the interbundle regions (see Figures 3.6 and 3.11). In most mammals, the vascular bundles contain only closely juxtaposed descending and ascending vasa recta running in parallel. The tubule structures of the inner stripe, including thin descending limbs, thick ascending limbs, and collecting ducts, are found in the interbundle regions and are supplied by the dense capillary bed described earlier.[61] Commonly, the interbundle territory is organized with the long loops of the juxtamedullary nephrons lying closest to the vascular bundles. The shorter loops arising from superficial glomeruli are more peripheral and therefore closer to the collecting ducts. The vascular bundles themselves contain no tubule structures.

MEDULLARY CAPILLARY DYNAMICS

The functional role of the medullary peritubular vasculature is basically the same as that of cortical peritubular vessels. These capillaries supply the metabolic needs of nearby tissues and are responsible for the uptake and removal of water extracted from collecting ducts during the process of urine concentration. However, because the urinary concentration process is based on the maintenance of a hypertonic interstitium, the countercurrent arrangement of medullary blood flow plays a vital role in maintaining the medullary solute gradient through passive countercurrent exchange.

STRUCTURE OF THE GLOMERULAR MICROCIRCULATION

The glomerulus and glomerular filtration are discussed in detail later in this chapter. Figure 3.12 shows a scanning electron micrograph of a resin-filled cast of a glomerulus with the afferent arteriole branching from the interlobular artery, the many loops of the glomerular capillaries, and the efferent arteriole emerging from the glomerular tuft. Elger and coworkers[70] published a detailed ultrastructural analysis of the vascular pole of the renal glomerulus. They described significant differences in the structure and branching patterns of the afferent and efferent arterioles as these vessels enter and exit the tuft. Afferent arterioles lose their internal elastic layer and smooth muscle cell layer prior to entering the glomerular tuft. Smooth muscle cells are replaced by renin-positive, myosin-negative granular cells that are in close contact with the extraglomerular mesangium.[71] As described by Eljer and coworkers,[70] upon entering Bowman's space, afferent arterioles branch immediately and are distributed along the surface of the glomerular tuft. These primary branches have wide lumens and immediately

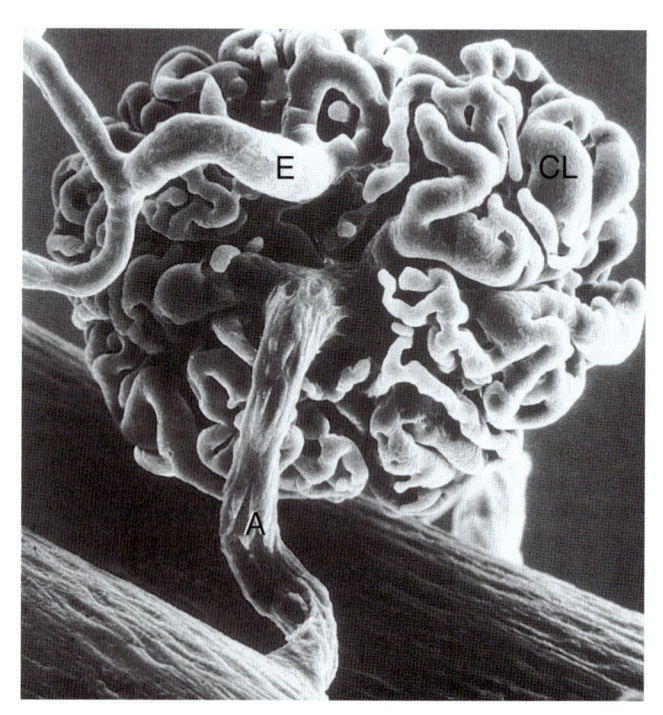

Figure 3.12 Scanning electron micrograph of a cast of a glomerulus showing the capillary loops (CL) and adjacent renal vessels. The afferent arteriole (A) is shown branching from an interlobular artery. The efferent arteriole (E) branches to form the peritubular capillary plexus *(upper left)*. (×300.) (Courtesy Waykin Nopanitaya, PhD.)

acquire features of glomerular capillaries, including a fenestrated endothelium, characteristic glomerular basement membrane, and epithelial foot processes. In contrast, the efferent arteriole arises deep within the tuft, from the convergence of capillaries arising from multiple lobules. Additional tributaries join the arteriole as it travels toward the vascular pole. The structure of the capillary wall begins to change even before the vessels coalesce to form the efferent arteriole, losing fenestrae progressively until a smooth epithelial lining is formed. At the arteriole's terminal portion within the tuft, endothelial cells may bulge into the lumen, reducing its internal diameter.

Typically, the diameter of the efferent arteriole within the tuft is significantly less than that of the afferent arteriole in the outer cortex. Efferent arterioles of the juxtamedullary nephrons, however, may be larger in diameter than the afferent arterioles and have thicker walls.[18] Moreover, both the efferent and afferent arterioles of the juxtamedullary nephrons appear to be larger in diameter than those of more superficial nephrons (see Figure 3.8).[18] Efferent arterioles acquire a smooth muscle cell layer, which is observed distal to the entry point of the final capillary. The efferent arteriole is also in close contact with the glomerular mesangium as it forms inside the tuft and with the extraglomerular mesangium as it exits the tuft. This precise and close anatomic relationship between the afferent and efferent arterioles and mesangium is consistent with the presence of the intraglomerular signaling system that participates in the regulation of blood flow and filtration rate.

The appearance of the vascular pathways within the glomerulus may change under different physiologic conditions. The glomerular mesangium has been shown to contain contractile elements (Figure 3.13)[70,72] and to exhibit contractile activity when exposed to angiotensin II.[73] Mesangial cells, which possess specific receptors for angiotensin II, undergo contraction when exposed to this peptide in vitro.[74] Three-dimensional reconstruction of the entire mesangium in the rat suggests that approximately 15% of capillary loops may be entirely enclosed within armlike extensions of mesangial cells that are anchored to the extracellular matrix.[75] Contraction of these cells might alter local blood flow and filtration rate as well as the intraglomerular distribution of blood flow and total filtration surface area. Many hormones and other vasoactive substances capable of altering glomerular filtration may bring about this adjustment, in part, by altering the state of contraction of mesangial cells.

In the outermost, or subcapsular, region of the cortex, the efferent arterioles give rise to a dense capillary network that surrounds the convoluted tubule segments arising from the superficial glomeruli (see Figure 3.9). There is evidence suggesting that this arrangement is of great importance for reabsorption of water and electrolytes in proximal tubule segments of superficial nephrons. In contrast, the efferent arterioles originating from the comparatively fewer juxtamedullary glomeruli extend into the medulla and give rise to the medullary microcirculatory patterns: an intricate capillary network in the outer medulla and long, unbranched capillary loops, the vasa recta, in the inner medulla. The arrangement of the medullary microcirculation plays an important role in the process of concentration of urine.

Venous drainage of the most superficial cortex is by way of superficial cortical veins.[7,57] In middle and inner cortex, venous drainage is achieved mainly by the interlobular veins. The dense peritubular capillary network surrounding the interlobular vessels drains directly into the interlobular veins through multiple connections, whereas the less dense,

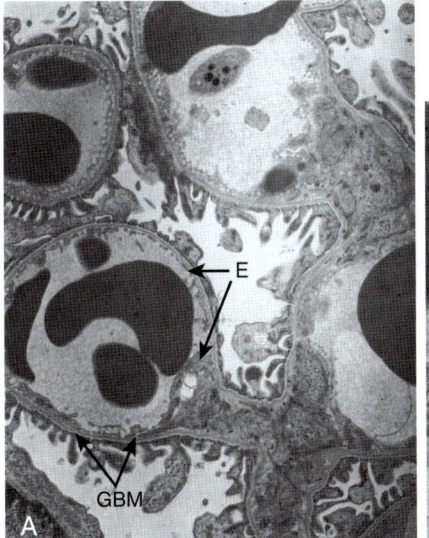

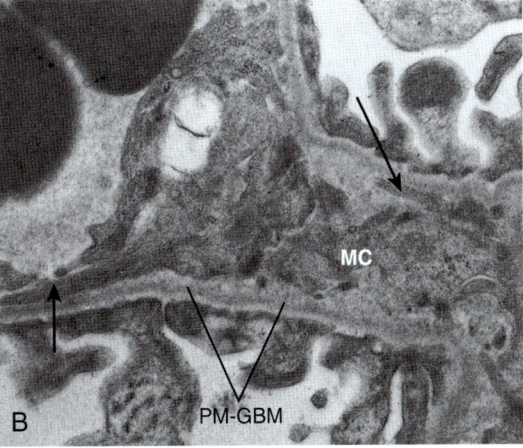

Figure 3.13 Electron micrographs of glomerular capillaries of a Munich-Wistar rat. **A,** An overview of several capillaries. (≈×14,500.) The majority of the glomerular capillary endothelium (E) is in contact with the glomerular basement membrane (GBM); only a small portion is in contact with the mesangium (M). At its outer aspect, the GBM is covered by podocyte foot processes. Note that there is no basement membrane separating the endothelium from the mesangium at their interface. **B,** The mesangial cell (MC) extends outward to meet the glomerular capillary. (≈×42,000.) Kriz and coworkers have suggested that within these cylinder-like stalks are contractile filament bundles *(short arrow)* that attach to the perimesangial glomerular basement membranes (PM-GBM) and extend to the GBM at the mesangial angles *(long arrow)*.[61,72] For this preparation the nephron was perfusion-fixed by micropuncture (DA Maddox) with 1.25% glutaraldehyde through Bowman's space, thereby yielding the fixation of glomerular structures as well as the red cells in the capillaries.

long-meshed network of the medullary rays appears to anastomose with the interlobular network and thus drain laterally. The medullary circulation also shows two different types of drainage: The outer medullary networks typically extend into the medullary rays before joining interlobular veins, whereas the long vascular bundles of the inner medulla (vasa recta) converge abruptly and join the arcuate veins. (See previous section on medullary circulation.)

DETERMINANTS OF GLOMERULAR ULTRAFILTRATION

Urine formation begins with filtration of a nearly protein-free fluid from the glomerular capillaries into Bowman's space. The barrier to filtration includes the fenestrated endothelial surface of the glomerular capillaries; the three layers of the glomerular basement membrane; the filtration slits between adjacent pedicels or foot processes of the visceral epithelial cells (podocytes) that surround the capillaries; and the filtration slit diaphragm that extends along the filtration slits and connects adjacent foot processes to form the ultimate barrier to filtration (see Chapter 2 and Figure 3.13). Water, electrolytes, amino acids, glucose, and other endogenous or exogenous compounds with molecular radii smaller than 20 Å are freely filtered from the blood into Bowman's space, whereas molecules larger than about 50 Å are virtually excluded from filtration.[30,76-80] At any given point of a glomerular capillary wall, the process of ultrafiltration of fluid is governed by the net balance among the transcapillary hydraulic pressure gradient (ΔP), the transcapillary colloid osmotic pressure gradient ($\Delta \pi$), and the hydraulic conductivity of the filtration barrier (k) on the basis of the Starling equation, as follows:

$$J_v = k(\Delta P - \Delta \pi)$$
$$= k[(P_{GC} - P_{BS}) - (\pi_{GC} - \pi_{BS})] \quad (5)$$

where J_v is the net movement between compartments, P_{GC} and P_{BS} are the hydraulic pressures in the glomerular capillaries and Bowman's space, respectively, and π_{GC} and π_{BS} are the corresponding colloid osmotic pressures. Because the protein concentration of the fluid in Bowman's space is essentially zero, π_{BS} is also zero. Total GFR of fluid for a single nephron (SNGFR) is equal to the product of the surface area for filtration (S), the hydraulic conductivity (k), and average values along the length of the glomerular capillaries of the right-side terms in equation 5, yielding the following expression:

$$SNGFR = kS(\Delta \bar{P} - \Delta \bar{\pi})$$
$$= K_f \bar{P}_{UF} \quad (6)$$

K_f, the glomerular ultrafiltration coefficient, is the product of S and k. $\bar{P}_{UF}$, the mean net ultrafiltration pressure, is the difference between the mean transcapillary hydraulic and colloid osmotic pressure gradients, $\Delta \bar{P}$ and $\Delta \bar{\pi}$, respectively.

On the basis of known ultrastructural detail and the hydrodynamic properties of the individual components of the filtration barrier, mathematical modeling suggests that only about 2% of the total hydraulic resistance is accounted for by the fenestrated capillary endothelium and the basement membrane accounts for nearly 50%.[81-83] The remaining hydraulic resistance resides in the diaphragm of the filtration slits.[82,83] A reduction in the frequency of intact filtration slits is an important factor in the deterioration of filtration in some disease states.[82,84]

HYDRAULIC PRESSURES IN THE GLOMERULAR CAPILLARIES AND BOWMAN'S SPACE

Direct measurements of glomerular capillary hydraulic pressure (P_{GC}) were first obtained in the Munich-Wistar rat more than 40 years ago by Brenner and associates,[85] who found that P_{GC} averaged 46 mm Hg. Subsequent studies confirmed the original observations, demonstrating that values for P_{GC} average 43 to 49 mm Hg (Figure 3.14), with similar values found in the squirrel monkey.[86] P_{GC} is nearly constant along the length of the capillary bed, resulting in a transcapillary hydraulic pressure gradient that averages 34 mm Hg in the hydropenic Munich-Wistar rat (see Figure 3.14). Coupling these hydraulic pressure measurements with determinations of systemic plasma protein concentration and efferent arteriolar protein concentrations of superficial nephrons permits determination of the hydraulic and oncotic pressures that govern glomerular ultrafiltration at the beginning and end of the capillary network.

The early direct measurements of $\bar{P}_{GC}$ were obtained in "hydropenic" rats, which exhibit a surgically induced reduction in plasma volume and GFR.[87] Subsequent studies in which plasma volume was restored to the "euvolemic" state, equal to that of the awake animal,[87] by infusion of isooncotic plasma, yielded SNGFRs substantially higher than those in hydropenic rats, primarily as a consequence of a marked increase in glomerular plasma flow (Q_A) associated with a fall in preglomerular (R_A) and efferent arteriolar (R_E) resistance values (see Figure 3.14). The use of the Munich-Wistar rat with superficial glomeruli allows direct determinations of hydraulic pressure drops and preglomerular and postglomerular blood flows and hence of R_A and R_E. Because surface glomeruli are not available in most experimental animals, the stop-flow technique has been used by a number of investigators to estimate P_{GC}. With this technique, fluid movement in the early proximal tubule is blocked, resulting in an increase in intratubular pressure until filtration at the glomerulus is stopped. At that point the sum of the hydrostatic pressure in the early proximal tubule plus the systemic colloid oncotic pressure is equal to the pressure in the glomerular capillaries (P_{GCSF}). Glomerular capillary pressures calculated using this stop-flow technique indicate that P_{GCSF} provides a reasonable estimate of $\bar{P}_{GC}$ with P_{GCSF} generally being about 2 mm Hg greater than that for $\bar{P}_{GC}$ measured directly.[88]

GLOMERULAR CAPILLARY HYDRAULIC AND COLLOID OSMOTIC PRESSURE PROFILES

Glomerular capillary hydraulic and oncotic pressure profiles for hydropenic and euvolemic Munich-Wistar rats are shown in Figure 3.15), which uses the mean values determined from the study data shown in Figure 3.14. By the time the blood reaches the efferent end of the glomerular

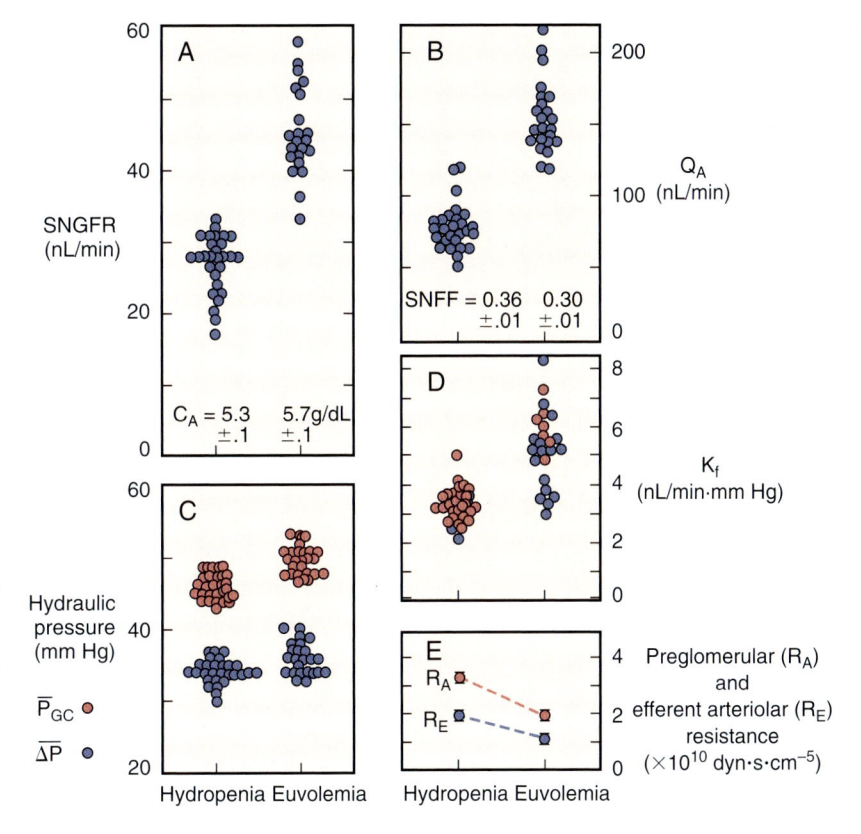

Figure 3.14 A to E, Glomerular ultrafiltration in the Munich Wistar rat. Each point represents the mean value reported for studies in hydropenic and euvolemic rats provided food and water ad libitum until the time of study. Only data from studies using male or a mix of male and female rats are shown. Values of the ultrafiltration coefficient, K_f (pink circles in D), denote minimum values because the animals were in filtration pressure equilibrium. Blue circles represent unique values of K_f calculated under conditions of filtration pressure disequilibrium ($\pi_E/\Delta\bar{P} \leq 0.95$). C_A, concentration in the afferent arteriole; $\Delta\bar{P}$, pressure gradient; $\bar{P}_{GC}$, pressure in the glomerular capillaries; Q_A, glomerular plasma flow rate; SNFF, single-nephron filtration fraction; SNGFR, single-nephron glomerular filtration rate. (Data from Maddox et al[76] and Deen et al[88].)

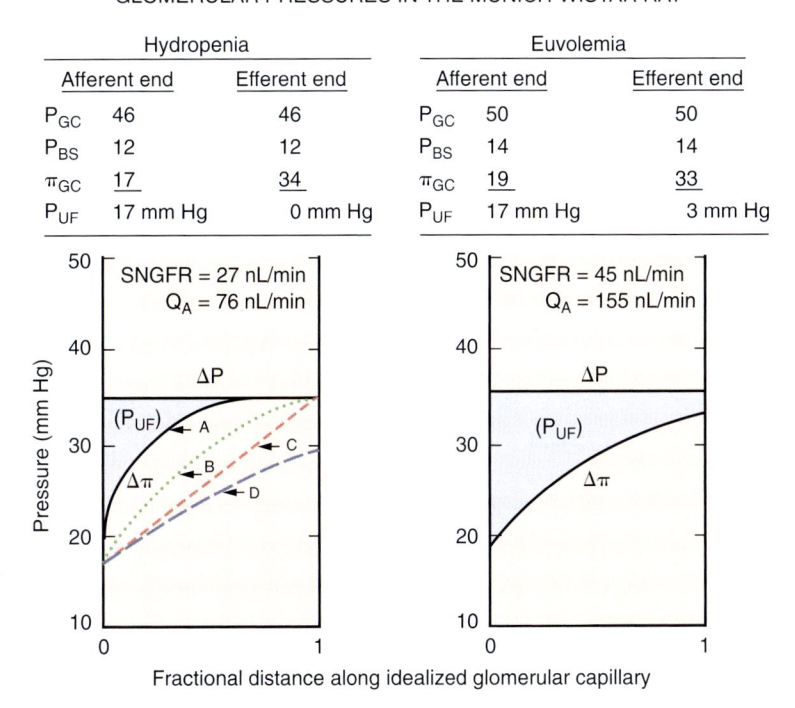

Figure 3.15 Hydraulic and colloid osmotic pressure profiles along idealized glomerular capillaries in hydropenic and euvolemic rats. Values shown are mean values derived from the studies shown in Figure 3.14. The transcapillary hydraulic pressure gradient, ΔP, is equal to $P_{GC} - P_T$, and the transcapillary colloid osmotic pressure gradient, $\Delta\pi$, is equal to $\pi_{GC} - \pi_T$, where P_{GC} and P_{BS} are the hydraulic pressures in the glomerular capillary and Bowman's space, respectively, and π_{GC} and π_T are the corresponding colloid osmotic pressures. Because the value of π_T is negligible, $\Delta\pi$ essentially equals π_{GC}. P_{UF} is the ultrafiltration pressure at any point. The area between the ΔP and $\Delta\pi$ curves represents the net ultrafiltration pressure, P_{UF}. **Left,** Lines A and B represent two of the many possible profiles under conditions of filtration pressure equilibrium. Line D represents disequilibrium. Line C represents the hypothetical linear $\Delta\pi$ profile. Q_A, glomerular plasma flow rate; SNGFR, single-nephron glomerular flow rate.

GLOMERULAR PRESSURES IN THE MUNICH-WISTAR RAT

	Hydropenia			Euvolemia	
	Afferent end	Efferent end		Afferent end	Efferent end
P_{GC}	46	46	P_{GC}	50	50
P_{BS}	12	12	P_{BS}	14	14
π_{GC}	17	34	π_{GC}	19	33
P_{UF}	17 mm Hg	0 mm Hg	P_{UF}	17 mm Hg	3 mm Hg

capillaries, plasma oncotic pressure (π_E) rises to a value that, on average, equals ΔP. As a consequence, the net local ultrafiltration pressure, P_{UF}, or $[P_{GC} - (P_T + \pi_{GC})]$, is reduced from approximately 17 mm Hg at the afferent end of the glomerular capillary network to essentially zero at the efferent end in hydropenic animals. The equality between π_E and ΔP is referred to as "filtration pressure equilibrium," As seen in Figure 3.15, filtration pressure equilibrium ($\pi_E/\Delta P \cong 1.00$) is almost always observed in the hydropenic Munich-Wistar rat but is present in only about 40% of the studies in the euvolemic rat, suggesting that the normal condition in the glomerulus is poised on the verge of disequilibrium.

The decline in P_{UF} between the afferent and efferent ends of the glomerular capillary network in the hydropenic animal is primarily due to the rise in π_{GC}, because ΔP remains nearly constant along the glomerular capillaries (see Figure 3.15). Curve A in Figure 3.15 shows that the decline in P_{UF} (the difference between the ΔP and $\Delta \pi$ curves) is nonlinear; the reasons are that (1) filtration is more rapid at the afferent end of the capillary where P_{UF} is greatest, and (2) the relationship between plasma protein concentration and colloid osmotic pressure is nonlinear (see Maddox and associates[76] and Maddox and Brenner[88]). Under conditions of filtration pressure equilibrium, the exact profile of $\Delta \pi$ along the capillary network cannot be determined, and curves A and B in Figure 3.15 are only two of many possibilities.

DETERMINATION OF THE ULTRAFILTRATION COEFFICIENT

As was shown in Equation 6, SNGFR equals the ultrafiltration coefficient (K_f) multiplied by the net driving force for ultrafiltration averaged over the length of the glomerular capillaries ($\overline{P}_{UF}$). Under conditions of filtration pressure equilibrium, a unique value of $\overline{P}_{UF}$ cannot be determined because an exact $\Delta \pi$ profile cannot be defined. If, however, a linear rise in $\Delta \pi$ between the afferent and efferent ends of the glomerular capillaries is assumed then a maximum value for $\overline{P}_{UF}$ can be determined (curve C, *dashed line* in Figure 3.15). With this maximum value for $\overline{P}_{UF}$ and measured values of SNGFR, a minimum estimate of K_f can be obtained. This minimum estimate of K_f in the hydropenic Munich-Wistar rat averages 3.5 ± 0.2 nL/(min • mm Hg) (see Figure 3.14*D*). In the euvolemic Munich-Wistar rat, K_f increases with age and little differences are noted between sexes when body mass is taken into account (see Figure 3.16).

Changes in Q_A (in the absence of changes in any other determinants of SNGFR) are predicted to result in proportional changes in SNGFR under conditions of filtration pressure equilibrium.[89] The reasoning is that an increase in Q_A slows the rate of increase of plasma protein concentration and therefore $\Delta \pi$ along the glomerular capillary network, shifting the point at which filtration equilibrium is achieved toward the efferent end of the glomerular capillary network. This process effectively increases the total capillary surface area exposed to a positive net ultrafiltration pressure and increases the magnitude of the local P_{UF} at any point along the glomerular capillary network. This situation is illustrated in Figure 3.15, which shows that even in the absence of changes in ΔP or plasma protein concentration, an increase in Q_A can result in a change in the profile from that seen with curve A to that of curve B while filtration pressure equilibrium is still achieved. For curve B, however, P_{UF} (the area under the curve) is significantly greater than with curve A, and hence SNGFR increases proportionately.

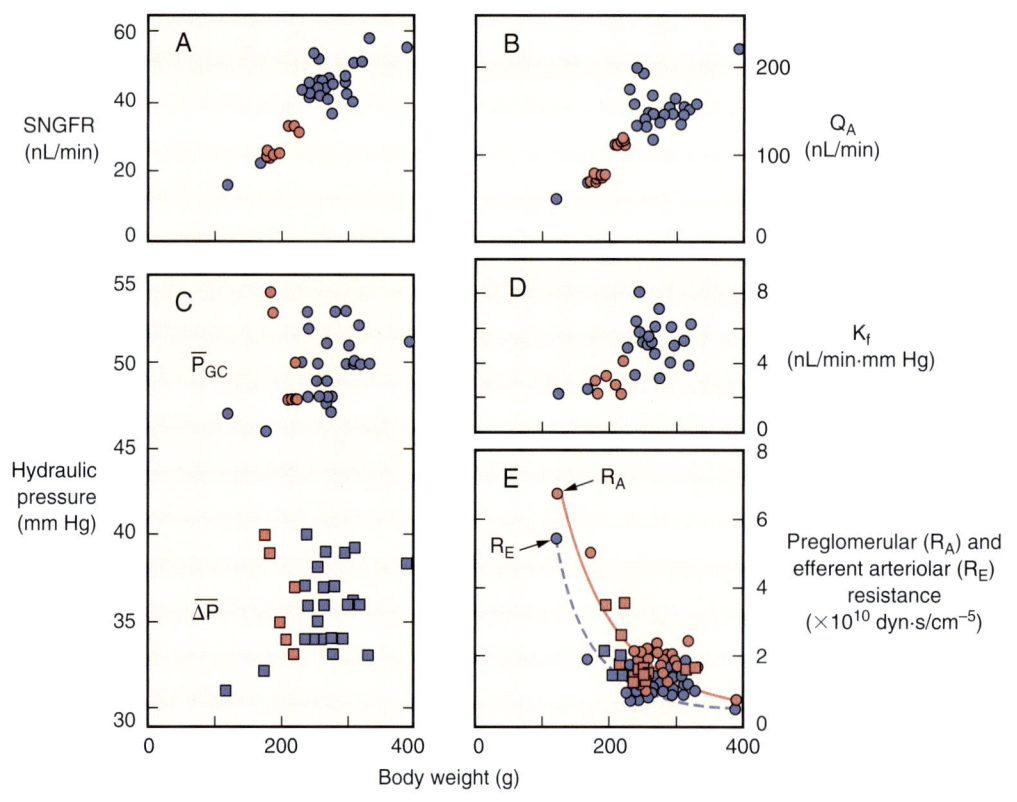

Figure 3.16 Maturational alterations in the determinants of glomerular ultrafiltration in the euvolemic Munich Wistar rat. In **A** through **D**, *pink symbols* denote values obtained from only female rats, and *blue symbols* denote values from studies of male or male plus female rats. In **E**, the *pink symbols* denote values of R_A, and *blue symbols* values of R_E.; *circles* are values from studies of male or male plus female rats, and *squares* values from studies of only female animals. Each point represents the mean value for a given study. K_f, ultrafiltration coefficient; $\Delta \overline{P}$, pressure gradient; $\overline{P}_{GC}$, pressure in the glomerular capillaries; Q_A, glomerular plasma flow rate; SNGFR, single-nephron glomerular filtration rate. (Data from Maddox et al[76] and Deen et al.[88])

Filtration pressure disequilibrium is obtained if Q_A increases enough so that $\Delta\pi$ no longer rises to the extent that efferent arteriolar oncotic pressure (π_E) equals ΔP.[89] A unique profile of $\Delta\pi$ can then be derived, $\overline{P}_{UF}$ can be accurately determined, and a unique value of K_f can be calculated.[89] Deen and colleagues used isooncotic plasma volume expansion to increase Q_A sufficiently to produce filtration pressure disequilibrium to obtain the first unique determinations of K_f in the Munich-Wistar rat.[89] Under these conditions the researchers observed that K_f exceeded the minimum estimate obtained in hydropenic rats by 37%, averaging 4.8 nL/(min • mm Hg). Because this value remained essentially unchanged over a twofold range of changes in Q_A, the data suggested that changes in Q_A per se did not affect K_f.[89]

The values of K_f for a large number of studies in euvolemic Munich-Wistar rats (shown in Figure 3.14) averaged 5.0 ± 0.3 nL/(min • mm Hg) and are similar to those obtained in plasma-expanded Munich-Wistar rats in which only unique values of K_f were obtained (4.8 ± 0.3 nL/(min • mm Hg)).[76,89] Although measured values of $\Delta\overline{P}$ are slightly higher in euvolemic rats than in hydropenic animals (see Figure 3.14), this difference is offset by higher plasma protein concentrations in the afferent arteriole (C_A and hence π_A), so that P_{UF} at the afferent end of the glomerular capillary network is nearly identical in euvolemia and hydropenia (see Figure 3.15). Thus, the higher SNGFRs observed in euvolemic rats are primarily the result of increases in Q_A (see Figure 3.14), yielding a greater value of P_{UF} (see Figure 3.15).

K_f is the product of the total surface area available for filtration (S) and the hydraulic conductivity of the filtration barrier (k). In the rat, total capillary basement membrane surface area per glomerulus (A_s) is approximately 0.003 cm² in superficial nephrons and 0.004 cm² in the deep nephrons.[90] Only the peripheral area of the capillaries surrounded by podocytes participates in filtration because a large portion faces the mesangium. This peripheral area available for filtration (A_p) is only about half that of A_s (≈0.0016-0.0018 and 0.0019-0.0022 cm² in the superficial and deep glomeruli, respectively).[90] With the use of a value of K_f of approximately 5 nL/(min • mm Hg), as determined by micropuncture techniques, these estimates of A_p yield a hydraulic conductivity (k) of 45 to 48 nL/(s • mm Hg • cm²). These estimates of k for the rat glomerulus are all one to two orders in magnitude higher than those reported for capillary networks in mesentery, skeletal muscle, omentum, and peritubular capillaries of the kidney.[76,88] As a consequence of this very high glomerular hydraulic permeability, filtration across glomerular capillaries occurs at very rapid rates despite mean net ultrafiltration pressures (P_{UF}) of only 5 to 6 mm Hg in hydropenia and 8 to 9 mm Hg in euvolemia.

SELECTIVE ALTERATIONS IN THE PRIMARY DETERMINANTS OF GLOMERULAR ULTRAFILTRATION

The four primary determinants of ultrafiltration are Q_A, ΔP, K_f, and π_A, and alterations in each of these affects GFR. The degree to which such alterations modify SNGFR has been examined by mathematical modeling[89] and compared with values obtained experimentally (see Maddox and Brenner[88]).

GLOMERULAR PLASMA FLOW RATE

Under normal conditions, protein is excluded from the glomerular ultrafiltrate, so the total amount of protein entering the glomerular capillary network from the afferent arteriole equals the total amount leaving at the efferent arteriole, as dictated by the conservation of mass:

$$Q_A C_A = Q_E C_E \quad (7)$$

where Q_A is afferent arteriolar plasma flow rate, Q_E is efferent arteriolar plasma flow rate, and C_A and C_E are the afferent and efferent arteriolar plasma concentrations of protein, respectively. This relationship can also be expressed as:

$$Q_A C_A = (Q_A - SNGFR) C_E \quad (8)$$

Rearranging Equation 8 yields

$$SNGFR = (1 - [C_A/C_E]) \times Q_A \quad (9)$$

with

$$SNFF = 1 - (C_A/C_E) \quad (10)$$

where SNFF is the single-nephron filtration fraction. Although the relationship between colloid osmotic pressure (π) and protein concentration deviates from linearity,[91] equation 9 can be approximated as follows:

$$SNGFR \cong (1 - [\pi_A/\pi_E]) \times Q_A \quad (11)$$

At filtration pressure equilibrium, $\pi_E = \Delta P$, so that:

$$SNGFR \cong (1 - [\pi_A/\Delta P]) \times Q_A \quad (12)$$

Under conditions of filtration pressure equilibrium, filtration fraction, approximately $1 - (\pi_A/\Delta P)$, is constant if π_A and ΔP are unchanged. SNGFR will then vary directly with changes in Q_A (Equation 12). If Q_A increases enough to produce disequilibrium (π_E less than ΔP), then C_E will fall, SNFF will decrease (Equation 9), and SNGFR will no longer vary linearly with Q_A. The first demonstration of the plasma flow dependence of GFR was provided by Brenner and colleagues.[91] As shown in Figure 3.17, increases in glomerular plasma flow are associated with increases in SNGFR in a number of studies of rats, dogs, nonhuman primates, and humans. Filtration pressure equilibrium was obtained in most studies at plasma flow rates less than 100 to 150 nL/min. Therefore, increases in Q_A result in proportional increases in SNGFR, and SNFF remains constant. Further increases in Q_A are associated with proportionately lower increases in SNGFR, resulting in decreased SNFF as filtration pressure disequilibrium is achieved.

TRANSCAPILLARY HYDRAULIC PRESSURE DIFFERENCE

Mathematical modeling also suggests that isolated changes in the glomerular transcapillary hydraulic pressure gradient affect SNGFR.[89] No filtration can take place until $\Delta\overline{P}$ exceeds the colloid osmotic pressure at the afferent end of the glomerular capillary. Once that point is reached, SNGFR increases as $\Delta\overline{P}$ increases. The rate of increase is nonlinear,

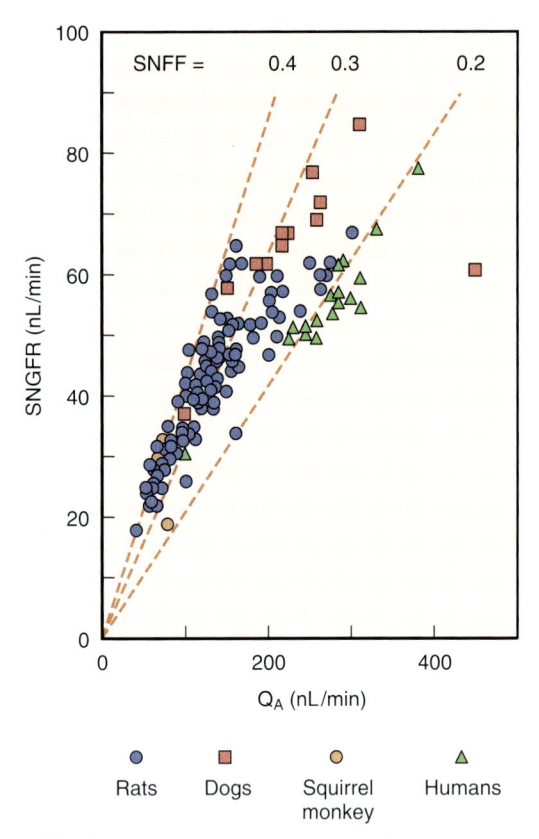

Figure 3.17 Relationship between single-nephron glomerular filtration rate (SNGFR) and glomerular plasma flow rate (Q_A) in three animal models and humans. The values for SNGFR and Q_A for humans were calculated by dividing whole kidney GFR and renal plasma flow by the estimated total number of nephrons/kidney (1 million). Each point represents the mean value for a given study. (Data from Maddox et al[76] and Deen et al.[88])

however, because the rise in SNGFR at any given fixed value of Q_A results in a concurrent (but smaller) increase in $\Delta\pi$. Because $\Delta\bar{P}$ is normally 30 to 40 mm Hg (see Figure 3.14), changes in $\Delta\bar{P}$ generally result in relatively minor variations in SNGFR.

THE GLOMERULAR CAPILLARY ULTRAFILTRATION COEFFICIENT

Glomerular damage from a variety of kidney diseases can result in a reduction in the glomerular ultrafiltration coefficient in part as a consequence of a reduction in surface area available for filtration. Studies of the hydraulic permeability of the glomerular basement membrane have demonstrated an inverse relationship to $\Delta\bar{P}$, indicating that K_f, the product of surface area and hydraulic conductivity, may be directly affected by $\Delta\bar{P}$.[92] The hydraulic conductivity of the glomerular basement membrane (GBM), and thus K_f, are also affected by the plasma protein concentration (see later). Filtration pressure equilibrium is generally observed at low values of Q_A, so reductions in K_f do not effect SNGFR until K_f is reduced enough to produce filtration pressure disequilibrium. At low Q_A values, increases in K_f above normal values move the point of equilibrium closer to the afferent end of the capillaries but have little affect on SNGFR.[88,89] At high Q_A values, filtration pressure disequilibrium occurs and there is a more direct relationship between K_f and SNGFR.[88,89]

COLLOID OSMOTIC PRESSURE

SNGFR and SNFF are each predicted to vary reciprocally as a function of π_A.[89] When Q_A, $\Delta\bar{P}$, and K_f are held constant, reductions in π_A will increase P_{UF}, leading to an increase in SNGFR. An increase in π_A should produce a decrease in SNGFR until π_A equals $\Delta\bar{P}$ (normally ~35 mm Hg), at which point filtration stops and SNFF is zero. In contrast to theoretical predictions, experimentally induced reductions in π_A do not lead to a rise in SNGFR. Studies in rats have shown a direct relationship between π_A and K_f when plasma protein concentrations were varied between 3.4 and 5.9 g/dL,[88] so that a reduction in π_A results in a reduction in K_f, thereby offsetting variations in P_{UF} that occur with changes in π_A.[88] Studies in isolated glomeruli, however, indicated that extremely low concentrations of albumin produce an increase in K_f while extremely high concentrations of albumin result in a decrease in K_f.[88] These divergent results of the effect of protein concentration on K_f can be partially explained by the results from studies of isolated glomerular basement membranes by Daniels and coworkers, who described a biphasic relationship between albumin concentration and hydraulic permeability.[92] They observed lower values of hydraulic permeability at albumin concentrations of 4 g/dL than at either 0 or 8 g/dL, but they did not study the effects of extremely high protein concentrations. Their studies suggest a primary effect of protein on hydraulic conductivity,[92] but the mechanism is unknown.

REGULATION OF RENAL HEMODYNAMICS AND GLOMERULAR FILTRATION

VASOMOTOR PROPERTIES OF THE RENAL MICROCIRCULATIONS

A variety of hormonal, neural, and vasoactive substances influence RBF and glomerular ultrafiltration.[76,88] The arcuate arteries, interlobular arteries, and both afferent and efferent arterioles are all influenced by such substances, thereby regulating the tone of preglomerular and postglomerular resistance vessels to control RBF, glomerular hydraulic pressure, and the transcapillary hydraulic pressure gradient. The glomerular mesangium is also the site of action and production of many such substances. Various growth factors can affect renal hemodynamics as well as promoting mesangial cell proliferation and expansion of the extracellular matrix, leading to obliteration of capillary loops and a reduction in the ultrafiltration coefficient. A number of vasoactive compounds may also affect K_f by changing the effective surface area for filtration through contraction of mesangial cells, causing shunting of blood to fewer capillary loops.[93,94] In addition, contraction of glomerular epithelial cells (podocytes), which contain filamentous actin molecules, may decrease the size of the filtration slit pores, thereby altering hydraulic conductivity of the filtration pathway and reducing K_f.[95]

Functional studies of reactivity of afferent and efferent arterioles to neural, hormonal, and vasoactive substances have, to a large part, come from micropuncture studies of glomerular hemodynamics. Other methods have included studies of renal tissue from neonatal hamsters grafted into the cheek pouches of adult hamsters, allowing access to afferent and efferent arterioles and the ability to examine the effects of local application of vasoactive agents.[96] Several other models have been developed to study functional responses of the preglomerular and postglomerular vasculature. Steinhausen and colleagues applied epi-illumination and transillumination microscopic techniques to the split, hydronephrotic rat kidney.[97] This preparation permits the arcuate artery, interlobular artery, afferent arteriole, and efferent arteriole to be visualized and studied in situ during perfusion with systemic blood, independent of tubular influences (e.g., tubuloglomerular feedback, as described later). Changes in diameter of these vessels have been measured in response to systemically or locally applied vasoactive substances.

Loutzenhiser and associates employed a modification of the hydronephrotic kidney technique in which the kidney is mounted and perfused in vitro to examine the response of the afferent arteriole to various stimuli.[98-100] In vitro perfusion of rat kidney has also been utilized to assess segmental vascular reactivity directly in the juxtamedullary nephrons that lie in apposition to the pelvic cavity.[101] Edwards developed an in vitro technique to study the reactivity of isolated segments of interlobular arteries and superficial afferent and efferent arterioles dissected from rabbit kidneys.[102] Ito and colleagues[103] further developed the in vitro approach to study changes in preglomerular resistance using the isolated perfused afferent arterioles with attached glomeruli. Thus a variety of techniques have been used to provide insight into the vasoactive properties of the preglomerular and postglomerular vasculature that control renal hemodynamics and GFR.

The renal vasculature and glomerular mesangium respond to a number of endogenous hormones and vasoactive peptides by vasoconstriction, reductions in RBF and GFR, and reductions in the glomerular capillary ultrafiltration coefficient. Among the vasoconstrictors are angiotensin II (Ang II), norepinephrine, leukotrienes C_4 and D_4, platelet activating factor (PAF), adenosine 5′-triphosphate (ATP), endothelin, vasopressin, serotonin, and epidermal growth factor. Similarly, vasodilatory substances such as endothelium-derived relaxing factor (nitric oxide [NO]), prostaglandins PGE_2 and PGI_2, histamine, bradykinin, acetylcholine, insulin, insulin-like growth factor, calcitonin gene–related peptide, cyclic adenosine monophosphate, and relaxin can increase RBF and GFR. However, in addition to having their own direct effects on blood flow and GFR, a number of these vasodilator substances stimulate Ang II production, masking their primary effects. In addition, vasoconstrictor substances such as Ang II can result in a feedback stimulation of renal vasodilator production, yielding a complex interaction for the control of renal hemodynamics. Cellular mechanisms of action of some of these compounds are covered in detail in other chapters.

ROLE OF THE RENIN-ANGIOTENSIN SYSTEM IN THE CONTROL OF RENAL BLOOD FLOW AND GLOMERULAR FILTRATION RATE

The renin-angiotensin system plays an important role in modulating RBF and filtration rate. Numerous studies indicate that preglomerular vessels, including the arcuate artery, interlobular artery, and afferent arteriole as well as the postglomerular efferent arterioles, constrict in response to exogenous and endogenous Ang II.[103-108] Figure 3.18 shows the effects of Ang II on diameters and estimated changes in resistance in these vessels. The efferent arteriole, however, has a 10- to 100-fold greater sensitivity to Ang II.[103,106-108] The vasoconstrictor effects of Ang II are blunted by the endogenous production of vasodilators, including the endothelium-derived relaxing factor nitric oxide as well as cyclo-oxygenase and cytochrome P450 epoxygenase metabolites, in the afferent but not the efferent arteriole.[99,103,108-113] Ang II–simulated release of NO in the afferent arteriole occurs through activation of the AT_1 receptors.[114,115] Ang II increases the production of prostaglandins in afferent arteriolar smooth muscle cells (both PGE_2 and PGI_2), and PGE_2, PGI_2, and cyclic adenosine monophosphate (cAMP) all blunt Ang II–induced entry of calcium into these cells,[110] potentially explaining, at least in part, the different effects of Ang II on vasoconstriction of the afferent and efferent arterioles.[109,110] PGE_2 has been found to have no effect on Ang II–induced vasoconstriction of the efferent arteriole.[99] The effects of PGE_2 on Ang II-induced vasoconstriction of the afferent arteriole are concentration-dependent, with low concentrations acting as a vasodilator via interaction with prostaglandin E_2 type 4 receptors (EP4), whereas high concentrations of PGE_2 act on type 3 receptors (EP3) to restore Ang II effects in that segment.[99] Ang II infusion alone has little effect on SNGFR, but when combined with cyclo-oxygenase inhibition, Ang II causes marked reductions in SNGFR as well as glomerular plasma flow rate (Q_A), suggesting an important role for endogenous vasodilatory prostaglandins in ameliorating the vasoconstrictor effects of Ang II.[116] Because Ang II increases renal production of vasodilatory prostaglandins, a feedback loop may exist to modulate the vasoconstrictor effects on Ang II under chronic conditions when the renin-angiotensin system is stimulated.[88]

In addition to causing renal vasoconstriction, reduced blood flow, and glomerular capillary hypertension, Ang II causes a decrease in K_f.[116] As noted earlier, glomerular Ang II receptors are found on the mesangial cells, glomerular capillary endothelial cells, and podocytes. Ang II causes contraction of mesangial cells,[117] so one possible cause for the changes in K_f is that contraction of the mesangial cells reduces effective filtration area by blocking flow through some glomerular capillaries; no direct evidence has been obtained, however, that would support this hypothesis. Alternatively the Ang II–induced decrease in K_f could be the result of a decrease in hydraulic conductivity rather than a reduction in the surface area available for filtration.[118] A role for glomerular epithelial cells in the effects of Ang II on K_f is suggested by the fact that the cells possess both AT_1 and AT_2 receptors and respond to Ang II by increasing cAMP production.[119] Alterations in neither epithelial structure nor the size of the filtration slits have been detected following infusion of Ang II at a dose sufficient to decrease GFR and K_f.[120]

The vasoconstrictive effect of Ang II on glomerular mesangial cells is markedly reduced by NO, which is often cited as "endothelium-derived relaxation factor" (EDRF) in older studies.[121] Mesangial cells co-incubated with endothelial cells have increased cyclic guanosine monophosphate

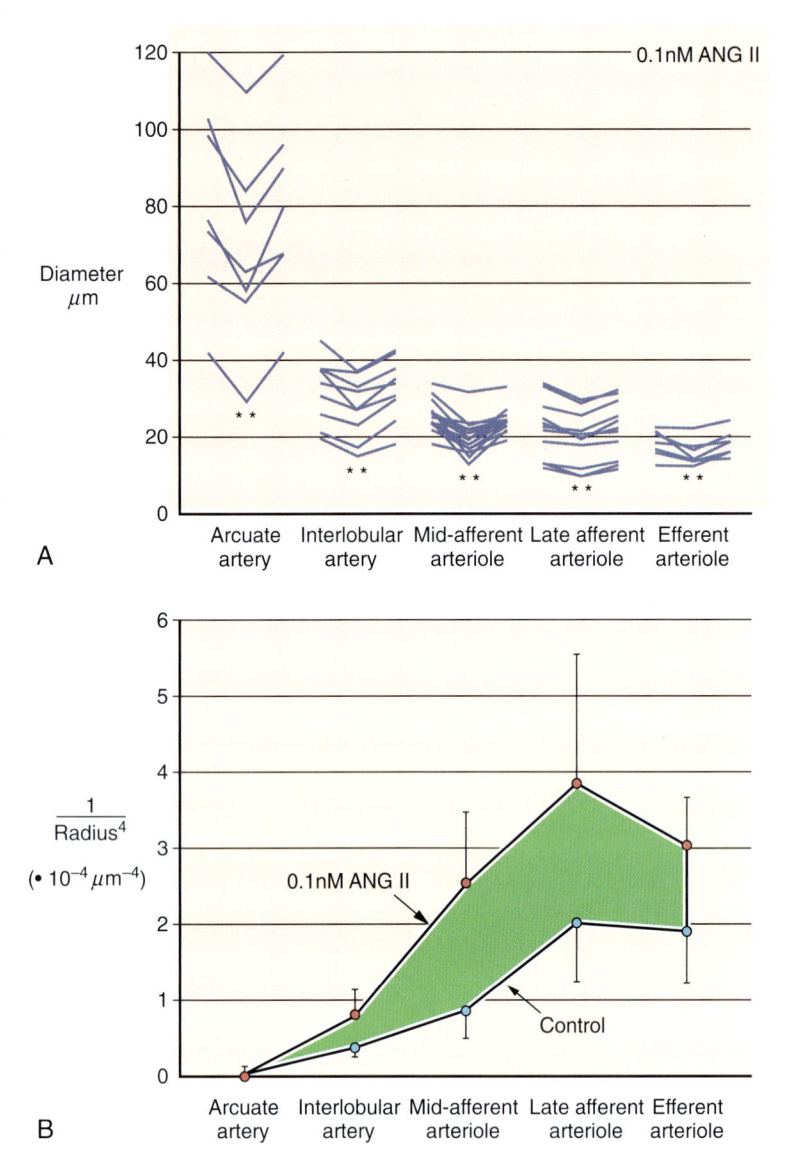

Figure 3.18 Effect of angiotensin II on the blood-perfused juxtamedullary nephron microvasculature. **A,** Vessel inside-diameter responses to angiotensin II (ANG II). Each line denotes observations of a single vessel segment during control, angiotensin II, and recovery periods. **B,** Estimation of angiotensin II–induced changes in segmental vascular resistance, calculated from data in upper panel. $P < 0.01$. (From Navar LG, Gilmore JP, Joyner WL, et al: Direct assessment of renal microcirculatory dynamics. *Fed Proc* 45:2851, 1986.)

(cGMP) production induced by NO release from the endothelial cells, decreasing the vasoconstrictive effects of Ang II, a finding that indicates that local NO production can modify the effects of agents such as Ang II.[121] Whether a similar effect would be observed for glomerular epithelial cells co-incubated with endothelial cells and whether either effect would translate into protection from Ang II–induced alterations of glomerular capillary surface area or hydraulic conductivity is not known, but inhibition of NO production in the normal rat does produce a marked decrease in K_f.[121-123] Arima and coworkers[124] examined Ang II AT_2 receptor–mediated effects on afferent arteriolar tone. When the AT_1 receptor was blocked, Ang II caused a dose-dependent dilation of the afferent arteriole that could be blocked by disruption of the endothelium or by simultaneous inhibition of the cytochrome P450 pathway. These data suggest that AT_2 receptor–mediated vasodilation in afferent arterioles is endothelium-dependent, possibly via the synthesis of epoxyeicosatrienoic acids via a cytochrome P450 pathway, counteracting the vasoconstrictor effects of Ang II at AT_1 receptors.[124,125]

In the past two decades, our understanding of the classical renin-angiotensin-aldosterone system (RAAS) has greatly evolved. For example, Ang II produces prohypertensive and renal vasoconstrictor effects via activation of AT_1 receptors, whereas activation of AT_2 receptors results in vasodilation as described previously.[124] Furthermore, fragments of the octapeptide Ang II that were once believed to be inactive have now been shown to have physiologic effects within the kidney, often opposing the actions of Ang II. Although findings from multiple laboratories and in various preparations have not always been consistent, the related peptide, angiotensin-(1-7) (Ang-[1-7]) has been shown to induce vasodilation of preconstricted renal arterioles.[126] These effects of Ang-(1-7) occur independent of binding to AT_1 or AT_2 receptors and appear to involve activation of the G protein–coupled Mas receptor,[127] which has been shown to be expressed in the afferent arteriole.[128] In addition, an isoform of angiotensin-converting enzyme (ACE) known as ACE2[129,130] appears to be involved in the formation of Ang-(1-7).[131] Ang-(1-7), ACE2, and the Mas receptor have all been detected within the kidney. The balance between opposing actions of the vasoconstrictor peptide, Ang II, and the vasodilator peptide, Ang-(1-7), may be influenced by the ratio of ACE to ACE2 and of AT_1 to Mas receptor contents within specific vascular regions (as well as tubular segments) of the kidney. In fact, cardiovascular and renal diseases may involve an imbalance of these peptides, enzymes, or receptors.[128]

There has been renewed interest in the hormone aldosterone. Once believed to be involved solely in salt and water balance manifested through tubular effects, aldosterone has been postulated to have direct renovascular effects, possibly via activation of rapid nongenomic mechanisms. Aldosterone has induced a rapid vasoconstriction that was not blocked by spironolactone in perfused arterioles isolated from rabbit kidneys.[132] These data are somewhat controversial, but other researchers have shown either no effect or a vasodilator effect of aldosterone in vasculature with intact endothelium, whereas a vasoconstrictor effect of aldosterone is consistently observed when endothelial function is impaired by inhibition of NO production (for review, see Arima[133] and Schmidt[134]). Finally, a novel peptide known as apelin was found to serve as an endogenous ligand for the orphan G protein–coupled receptor APJ, which shares significant homology with the AT_1 receptor.[135] Apelin immunoreactivity and APJ receptor messenger RNA have been detected in the kidney and are believed to play a counterregulatory role with respect to renovascular and tubular effects of the RAAS.[136,137]

ENDOTHELIAL FACTORS IN THE CONTROL OF RENAL HEMODYNAMICS AND GLOMERULAR FILTRATION

Endothelial cells were once considered "vascular cellophane," simple metabolically inactive cells that passively lined the vascular tree and provided a nonstick surface for blood cells. Thanks in large part to the pioneering work of Robert Furchgott, Louis Ignarro, Ferid Murad, and Masashi Yanigasawa, we now recognize that these cells produce a number of substances that can profoundly alter vascular tone, including vasodilators such as NO as well as vasoconstrictors such as the endothelins. These factors play an important role in the minute-to-minute regulation of renal vascular flow and resistance.

NITRIC OXIDE

In 1980, Furchgott and Zawadzki[138] demonstrated that the vasodilatory action of acetylcholine required the presence of an intact endothelium. The binding of acetylcholine and many other vasodilator substances to receptors on endothelial cells leads to the formation and release of an "endothelium-derived relaxing factor," which was subsequently determined to be NO.[139,140] NO is formed from L-arginine[141] by a family of enzymes that are encoded by separate genes called *nitric oxide synthases* that are present in many cells, including vascular endothelial cells, macrophages, neurons,[142] glomerular mesangial cells,[143] macula densa,[144] and renal tubular cells. Once released by the endothelium, NO diffuses into adjacent and downstream vascular smooth muscle cells,[145] where it activates soluble guanylate cyclase leading to cGMP accumulation.[121,146-150] Cyclic GMP modulates intracellular calcium concentration, in part, through a cGMP-dependent protein kinase (PKG)–mediated phosphorylation of targets believed to include IP_3 (inositol trisphosphate) receptors, calcium channels, and phospholipase A_2,[151] thereby reducing the amount of calcium available for contraction and hence promoting relaxation.[152] The breakdown of cyclic nucleotides such as cGMP as well as cAMP is catalyzed by a large superfamily of more than 50 phosphodiesterases (PDEs) that either are selective for cGMP or cAMP or are capable of metabolizing both.[153] Inhibitors of the PDEs are currently under investigation as potential therapeutic agents in kidney disease.

In addition to stimulation by acetylcholine, NO formation in the vascular endothelium increases in response to bradykinin,[121,154-157] thrombin,[158] platelet-activating factor,[159] endothelin,[160] and calcitonin gene–related peptide.[155,161-164] Increased flow through blood vessels with intact endothelium or across cultured endothelial cells, which results in increased shear stress, also increases NO release,[147,154,156,165-169] and elevated perfusion pressure/shear stress increases NO release from afferent arterioles.[170] Both pulse frequency and amplitude modulate flow-induced NO release.[165]

In the kidney, nitric oxide has numerous important functions, including the regulation of renal hemodynamics, maintenance of medullary perfusion, blunting of tubuloglomerular feedback, inhibition of tubular sodium reabsorption, modulation of renal sympathetic neural activity, and mediation of pressure natriuresis.[171] The net effect of NO in the kidney is to promote natriuresis and diuresis.[172] Indeed, pressure natriuresis in experimental models utilizing stepwise increases of both renal perfusion pressure and medullary blood flow involve increased medullary NO release,[173] which can exert direct tubular effects to promote sodium and water excretion. Although tubular epithelial cells are capable of releasing NO, the vasa recta may be a primary source of the NO produced during increased medullary flow, because Zhang and Pallone[174] observed flow-dependent increases in NO during microperfusion of isolated outer medullary vasa recta.

Experimental studies also support the presence of an important interaction among NO, Ang II, and renal nerves in the control of renal function.[175] Renal hemodynamics are continuously affected by endogenous NO production, as evidenced by the fact that nonselective NO synthase (NOS) inhibition results in marked decreases in RPF, an increase in mean arterial blood pressure (AP), and generally a reduction in GFR.[176-178] These effects are largely prevented by the simultaneous administration of excess L-arginine, the NOS substrate.[176] Selective inhibition of neuronal NOS (nNOS or type I NOS), which is found in the thick ascending limb of the loop of Henle, the macula densa, and efferent arterioles,[144,179] decreases GFR without affecting blood pressure or RBF.[180] Because eNOS (endothelial NOS or type II NOS) is found in the endothelium of renal blood vessels, including the afferent and efferent arterioles and glomerular capillary endothelial cells,[144] differences between the effects of inhibition of NO formation on RBF from generalized NOS inhibition and those from specific inhibition of nNOS appear to be related to the distinct distributions of eNOS and nNOS in the kidney.

Both short- and long-term inhibition of NO production results in systemic and glomerular capillary hypertension, an increase in preglomerular resistance and efferent arteriolar resistance, a decrease in K_f, and decreases in both Q_A and SNGFR.[122,123,181-183] As shown in Figure 3.19, acute administration of pressor doses of a blocker of NO production resulted in a decline in SNGFR, Q_A, and K_f and increases in both R_A and R_E. Administration of nonpressor doses of the inhibitor of NO formation through the renal artery yielded an increase in R_A and decreases in SNGFR and K_f but no effect on R_E (see Figure 3.19).[123] These studies suggested that the cortical afferent, but not efferent, arterioles were under tonic control by NO. However, other studies have found that the renal artery, the arcuate and interlobular arteries, and the afferent and efferent arterioles produce NO and constrict in response to inhibition of endogenous NO production.[103,108,145,184-187] In agreement with this finding, other investigators have reported that NO dilates both efferent and afferent arterioles in the perfused juxtamedullary nephron.[10,187]

Controversy exists regarding the role of the renin-angiotensin system in the genesis of the increase in vascular resistance that follows blockade of NOS. Studies of in vitro perfused nephrons[187] and of anesthetized rats in vivo[188] suggest that the increase in renal vascular resistance that follows NOS blockade is blunted when Ang II formation or binding is blocked. NO inhibits renin release, short-term Ang II infusion increases cortical NOS activity and protein expression and long-term Ang II infusion increases mRNA levels for both eNOS and nNOS.[188,189] Ang II increases NO production in isolated perfused afferent arterioles via activation of the AT_1 Ang II receptors.[114] On the other hand, Deng and colleagues reported that nonselective NOS inhibition increased renal oxygen consumption, an effect that was independent of Ang II.[190] Additionally, Baylis and associates reported that inhibition of NOS in conscious rats had similar effects on renal hemodynamics in both intact and angiotensin II–blocked states,[191] These findings show that the vasoconstrictor response of NOS blockade is not mediated by Ang II. In a later study, Baylis and associates showed that when the Ang II level was acutely raised by infusion of exogenous peptide, acute NO blockade amplified the renal vasoconstrictor actions of Ang II.[192] In agreement with this finding, Ito and coworkers[103] demonstrated that intrarenal inhibition of NO enhanced Ang II–induced constriction of afferent, but not efferent, arterioles in the rabbit. Similar results have also been obtained in dogs.[111] Although no clear consensus exists, these data suggest that NO modulates the vasoconstrictor effects of Ang II on glomerular arterioles in vivo, perhaps blunting Ang II's vasoconstrictor response in the afferent arteriole but not the efferent arteriole. As mentioned earlier, this difference may provide a mechanism for the proposed preferential vasoconstrictor response to Ang II in the efferent arteriole observed in settings where Ang II values are elevated.

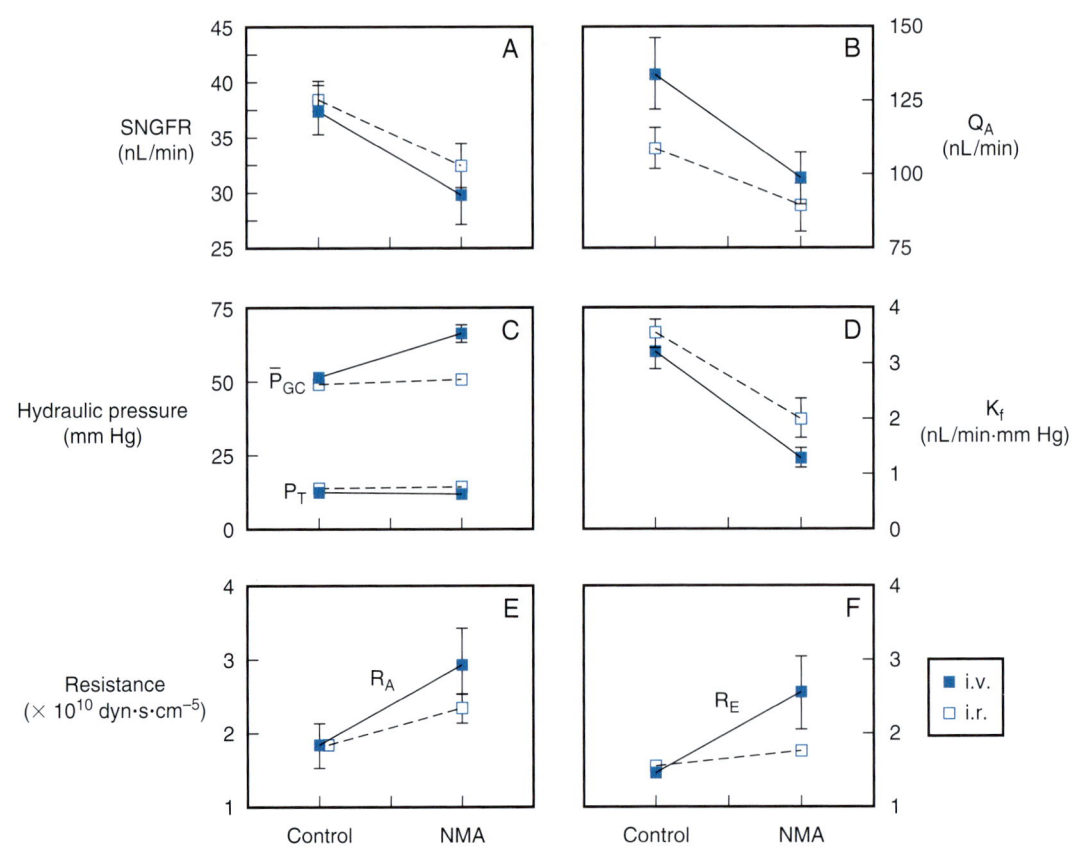

Figure 3.19 Role of endothelium-derived relaxing factor (EDRF = nitric oxide) in the control of glomerular ultrafiltration. Studies were performed in euvolemic Munich-Wistar rats either receiving intravenous pressor doses of the EDRF-blocker N-monomethyl-L-arginine (NMA) (i.v., *filled squares*) or nonpressor doses of NMA at the origin of the renal artery (i.r., *open squares*). K_f, ultrafiltration coefficient; $\bar{P}_{GC}$, pressure in the glomerular capillaries; P_T, pressure in the tubules; Q_A, glomerular plasma flow rate; R_A, preglomerular arteriolar resistance; R_E, efferent arteriolar resistance; SNGFR, single-nephron glomerular filtration rate. (Data [mean ± SE] obtained from Deng and Naylis.[123])

ENDOTHELIN

Endothelin, a potent vasoconstrictor derived primarily from vascular endothelial cells, was first described by Yanagasawa and colleagues.[193] There are three distinct genes for endothelin, each encoding distinct 21–amino acid isopeptides termed ET-1, ET-2, and ET-3.[193-195] Endothelin is produced after endothelin-converting enzyme cleaves the 38– to 40–amino acid proendothelin, which in turn is produced from proteolytic cleavage of pre-proendothelin (≈212 amino acids) by furin.[196,197] ET-1 is the primary endothelin produced in the kidney, including the arcuate arteries and veins, interlobular arteries, afferent and efferent arterioles, glomerular capillary endothelial cells, glomerular epithelial cells, and glomerular mesangial cells of both rats and humans,[198-209] and it acts in an autocrine or paracrine fashion or both[210] to alter a variety of biologic processes in these cells. Endothelins are extremely potent vasoconstrictors and the renal vasculature is highly sensitive to them.[211] Once released from endothelial cells, endothelins bind to specific receptors on vascular smooth muscle, the ET_A receptors that bind both ET-1 and ET-2.[210,212-215] ET_B receptors are expressed in the glomerulus on mesangial cells and podocytes with equal affinity for ET-1, ET-2, and ET-3.[214,215] There are two subtypes of ET_B receptors, the ET_{B1} linked to vasodilation and the ET_{B2} linked to vasoconstriction.[216] An endothelin-specific protease modulates endothelin levels in the kidney.[217]

Endothelin production is stimulated by physical factors, including increased shear stress and vascular stretch.[218,219] In addition a variety of hormones, growth factors, and vasoactive peptides increase endothelin production including transforming growth factor-β, platelet-derived growth factor, tumor necrosis factor-α, Ang II, arginine vasopressin, insulin, bradykinin, thromboxane A_2, and thrombin.[198,202,204,208,220-223] Endothelin production is inhibited by atrial and brain natriuretic peptides acting through a cGMP-dependent process[217,224] and by factors that increase intracellular cAMP and protein kinase A activation, such as β-adrenergic agonists.[204]

Typically, intravenous infusion of ET-1 induces a marked, prolonged pressor response[193,225] accompanied by increases in preglomerular and efferent arteriolar resistances and a decrease in RBF and GFR.[225] As shown in Figure 3.20, infusion of subpressor doses of ET-1 also decreases SNGFR, Q_A, and whole kidney RBF and GFR,[226-230] again accompanied by increases in both preglomerular and postglomerular resistances and filtration fraction.[226,228,231] Vasoconstriction of afferent and efferent arterioles by endothelin has been confirmed in the split, hydronephrotic rat kidney preparation[232,233] and in isolated perfused arterioles.[106,185,234] In both micropuncture[226] and isolated arteriole[106] studies, the sensitivity and response of the efferent arteriole exceeded those of the afferent vessel. Endothelin also causes mesangial cell contraction.[195,235] Finally, other studies have suggested that the vasoconstrictor effects of the endothelins can be modu-

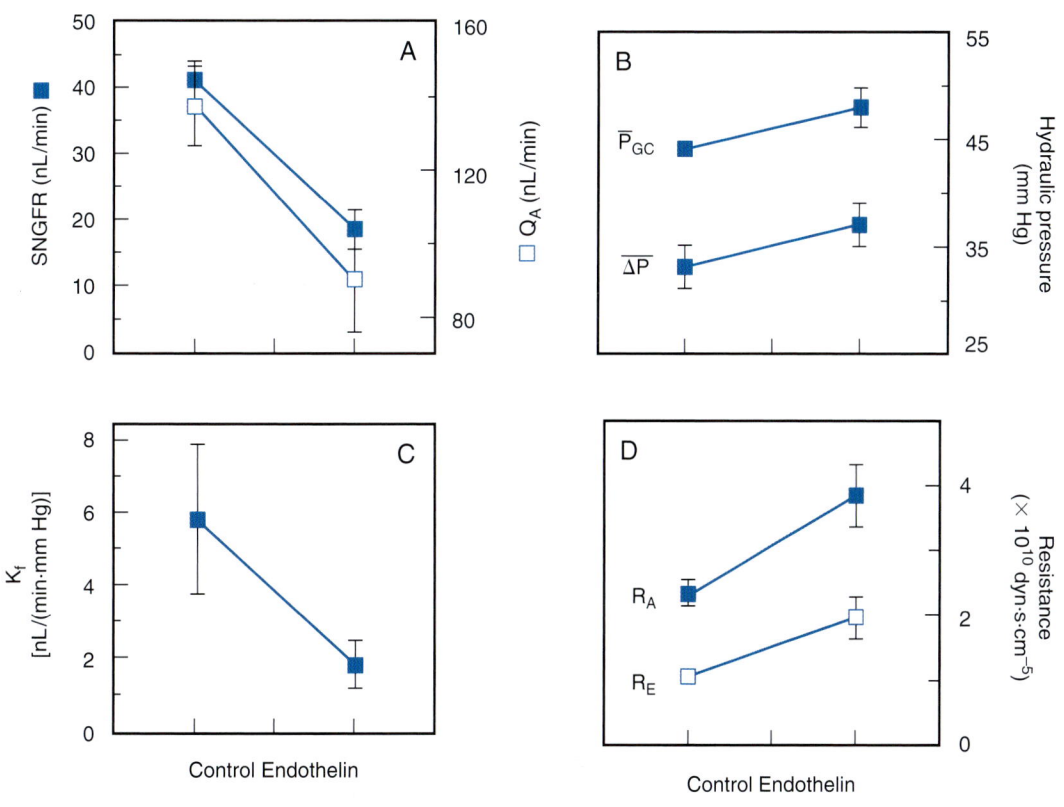

Figure 3.20 Effects of intravenous administration of endothelin (subpressor dose) on glomerular ultrafiltration. K_f, ultrafiltration coefficient; $\Delta \bar{P}$, pressure gradient; $\bar{P}_{GC}$, pressure in the glomerular capillaries; Q_A, glomerular plasma flow rate; R_A, afferent arteriolar resistance; R_E, efferent arteriolar resistance; SNGFR, single-nephron glomerular filtration rate. (Data [mean ± SE] obtained in euvolemic Munich-Wistar rats from Badr et al.[226])

lated by a number of factors,[213,236] including NO,[185,237] bradykinin,[238] PGE$_2$,[239] and prostacyclin.[239,240]

Although there are multiple endothelin receptors, most is known about the ET$_A$ and ET$_B$ receptors, which have been cloned and characterized.[215,241,242] According to the traditional view, ET$_A$ receptors, which are abundant on vascular smooth muscle, have a high affinity for ET-1 and play a prominent role in the pressor response to endothelin.[243] ET$_B$ receptors are present on endothelial cells, where they may mediate NO release and endothelium-dependent relaxation.[242] However, the distribution and function of ET$_A$ and ET$_B$ receptors vary greatly among species and, in the rat, even according to strain. In the normal rat, according to an immunofluorescence microscopy study by Wendel and associates, both ET$_A$ and ET$_B$ receptors are expressed in the media of interlobular arteries and afferent and efferent arterioles. In interlobar and arcuate arteries, only ET$_A$ receptors are present on vascular smooth muscle cells.[244] These workers found that ET$_B$ receptor immunoreactivity is sparse on endothelial cells of renal arteries, but strong labeling of peritubular and glomerular capillaries as well as vasa recta endothelium.[244] ET$_A$ receptors are evident on glomerular mesangial cells and pericytes of descending vasa recta bundles.[244] Another study in the rat suggested that endogenous endothelin may actually dilate the afferent arteriole and lower K$_f$ via ET$_B$ receptors.[245] However, ET$_B$ receptors on vascular smooth muscle also mediate vasoconstriction in the rat, an effect that is potentiated in hypertensive animals.[246]

Endothelin stimulates the production of vasodilatory prostaglandins,[229,237,240,247,248] yielding a feedback loop to modify the vasoconstrictor effects of endothelin. ET-1, ET-2, and ET-3 also stimulate NO production in the arteriole and glomerular mesangium via activation of the ET$_B$ receptor.[158,160,185,237,249] Resistances in the renal and systemic vasculature are markedly increased during inhibition of NO production, and these effects can be partially reversed by ET$_A$ blockade or inhibition of endothelin-converting enzyme, indicating the dynamic interrelationship between NO and endothelin effects.[250,251] The vasoconstrictive effects of Ang II may be mediated, in part, by a stimulation of ET-1 production that acts on ET$_A$ receptors to produce vasoconstriction.[220,223] Long-term administration of Ang II reduces RBF, and this effect is prevented by administration of a mixed ET$_A$/ET$_B$ receptor antagonist, suggesting that endothelin contributes importantly to the renal vasoconstrictive effects of Ang II.[220] Interestingly, antagonists of endothelin receptors may reduce proteinuria, demonstrating renoprotective effects in diabetic nephropathy. However, a clinical trial was halted early because of fluid retention and formation of peripheral edema in ET antagonist–treated patients with diabetic nephropathy. Currently, the endothelin antagonists have been approved by the U.S. Food and Drug Administration only for the treatment of pulmonary hypertension.[252]

RENAL AUTOREGULATION

Many organs are capable of maintaining relative constancy of blood flow in the face of major changes in perfusion pressure. Although the efficiency with which blood flow is maintained differs from organ to organ (being most efficient in brain and kidney), virtually all organs and tissues, including skeletal muscle and intestine, exhibit this property, termed "autoregulation." As shown in Figure 3.21, the kidney autoregulates RBF and GFR over a wide range of renal perfusion pressures.

Autoregulation of blood flow requires parallel changes in resistance and perfusion pressure. However, if efferent arteriolar resistance declined significantly when perfusion pressure was reduced, glomerular capillary pressure and GFR would also fall. Therefore, the finding that both RBF and GFR are autoregulated suggests that the principal resistance change is in the preglomerular vasculature. Studies using the Munich-Wistar rat, which has glomeruli on the renal cortical surface that are readily accessible to micropuncture, afforded an opportunity to observe the renal cortical microvascular adjustments that take place in response to variations in renal arterial perfusion pressure. Figure 3.22 summarizes the effects in the normal hydropenic rat of graded reductions in renal perfusion pressure on glomerular capillary blood flow rate, mean glomerular capillary hydraulic pressure ($\bar{P}_{GC}$), and preglomerular (R$_A$) and efferent arteriolar (R$_E$) resistance.[253] As shown in Figure 3.22, graded reduction in renal perfusion pressure from 120 to 80 mm Hg resulted in only a modest decline in glomerular capillary blood flow, whereas further reduction in perfusion pressure to 60 mm Hg led to a more pronounced decline. Despite the decline in perfusion pressure from 120 to 80 mm Hg, values of $\bar{P}_{GC}$ fell only modestly on average, from 45 to 40 mm Hg. Further reduction in perfusion pressure from 80 to 60 mm Hg resulted in a further fall in $\bar{P}_{GC}$ (from 40 to 35 mm Hg). Calculated values for R$_A$ and R$_E$ are shown in Figure 3.22. Autoregulation of glomerular capillary blood flow and $\bar{P}_{GC}$ as perfusion pressure decreased from 120 to 80 mm Hg was due to a pronounced decrease in R$_A$ with little change in R$_E$. Over the range of renal perfusion pressure from 120 to 60 mm Hg, R$_E$ tended to increase slightly. In that study, when plasma volume was expanded, R$_A$ declined while R$_E$ increased as renal perfusion pressure was

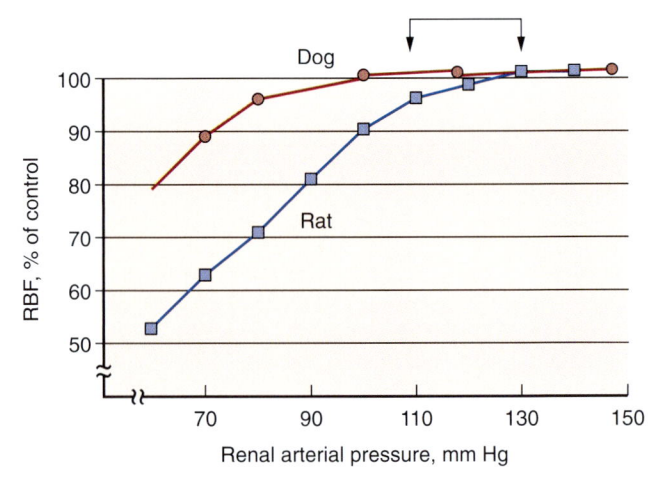

Figure 3.21 Autoregulatory response of total renal blood flow (RBF) to changes in renal perfusion pressure in the dog and rat. In general, the normal anesthetized dog exhibits greater autoregulatory capability to lower arterial pressure than the rat. (From Navar LG, Bell PD, Burke TJ: Role of a macula densa feedback mechanism as a mediator of renal autoregulation. *Kidney Int* 22:S157, 1982.)

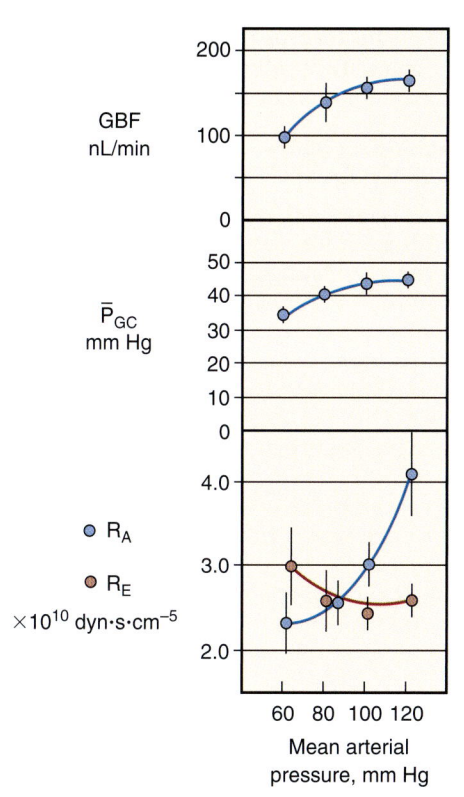

Figure 3.22 Glomerular dynamics in response to reduction of renal arterial perfusion pressure in the normal hydropenic rat. As can be seen, glomerular blood flow (GBF) and glomerular capillary hydraulic pressure ($\bar{P}_{GC}$) remained relatively constant as blood pressure was lowered from ≈120 mm Hg to ≈80 mm Hg, over the range of perfusion pressure examined, primarily as a result of a marked decrease in afferent arteriolar resistance (R_A). Efferent arteriolar resistance (R_E) was relatively constant. (Adapted from Robertson CR, Deen WM, Troy JL, Brenner BM: Dynamics of glomerular ultrafiltration in the rat. III: Hemodynamics and autoregulation. *Am J Physiol* 223:1191, 1972.)

large, preglomerular vessels in the autoregulatory response, Heyeraas and Aukland[258] reported that interlobular arterial pressure remained constant when renal perfusion pressure was reduced by 20 mm Hg, again suggesting that these vessels contribute importantly to the constancy of outer cortical blood flow in the upper autoregulatory range. A number of observations have provided evidence that the major preglomerular resistor is located close to the glomerulus, at the level of the afferent arteriole.[12,259-261] As in superficial nephrons, direct observations of perfused juxtamedullary nephrons revealed parallel reductions in the luminal diameters of arcuate, interlobular, and afferent arterioles in response to elevation in perfusion pressure. However, because quantitatively similar reductions in vessel diameter produce much greater elevations in resistance in small than in large vessels, the predominant effect of these changes is an increase in afferent arteriolar resistance.[259]

CELLULAR MECHANISMS INVOLVED IN RENAL AUTOREGULATION

Autoregulation of the afferent arteriole and interlobular artery is blocked by administration of L-type calcium channel blockers, inhibition of mechanosensitive cation channels, and a calcium-free perfusate.[262-265] The autoregulatory response thus involves gating of mechanosensitive channels, which produces membrane depolarization, and activation of voltage-dependent calcium channels, which leads to an increase in intracellular calcium concentration and vasoconstriction.[262,266,267] Calcium channel blockade almost completely blocks autoregulation of RBF.[268,269] The autoregulatory capacity of the afferent arteriole is attenuated by intrinsic metabolites of the cytochrome P450 epoxygenase pathway, and metabolites of the cytochrome P450 hydroxylase pathway enhance autoregulatory responsiveness.[270]

Autoregulation of both GFR and RBF has been found to occur in the presence of inhibition of NO, but values for RBF were reduced at any given renal perfusion pressure in comparison with control values.[177,271-273] In the isolated perfused juxtamedullary afferent arteriole, the initial vasodilatation observed when pressure was increased was of shorter duration when endogenous NO formation was blocked, but the autoregulatory response was unaffected.[267] Cortical and juxtamedullary preglomerular vessels in the split hydronephrotic kidney also perform autoregulation in the presence of NO inhibition.[184] The majority of evidence therefore suggests that NO is not essential, at least for the myogenic component of renal autoregulation, though it may play a role in tubuloglomerular feedback (see later).[274]

THE MYOGENIC MECHANISM FOR AUTOREGULATION

According to the myogenic theory, arterial smooth muscle contracts and relaxes in response to increases and decreases in vascular wall tension.[275] Thus, an increase in perfusion pressure, which initially distends the vascular wall, is followed by a contraction of resistance vessels, resulting in a recovery of blood flow from an initial elevation to a value comparable to the control level. Fray and coworkers presented a model of myogenic control of RBF based on the assumption that flow remains constant when the distending force and the constricting force, determined by the properties of the vessel wall, are equal.[276,277] The constricting force

lowered, so that $\bar{P}_{GC}$ and $\Delta \bar{P}$ were virtually unchanged over the entire range of renal perfusion pressures.[253] In plasma-expanded animals, the mean glomerular transcapillary hydraulic pressure difference ($\Delta \bar{P}$) exhibited nearly perfect autoregulation over the entire range of perfusion pressures because of concomitant increases in R_E as R_A fell.[253] These results indicate that autoregulation of GFR is the consequence of the autoregulation of both glomerular blood flow and glomerular capillary pressure.

The medullary circulation has also been shown to possess autoregulatory capacity.[254-256] The extent of autoregulation of the medullary circulation may be influenced by the volume status of the animal.[255] Preglomerular vessels, including the afferent arterioles and vessels as large as the arcuate and interlobular arteries, participate in the autoregulatory response. In the split, hydronephrotic rat kidney preparation, Steinhausen and coworkers observed dilation of all preglomerular vessels from the arcuate to interlobular arteries in response to reductions in perfusion pressure from 120 to 95 mm Hg.[257] The proximal afferent arteriole did not respond to pressure changes in this range but did dilate when perfusion pressure was reduced to 70 mm Hg. The diameter of the distal afferent arteriole did not change at any pressure. Also consistent with an important role of is envisioned to have both a passive and an active component, the latter sensitive to stretch in the vessel. Myogenic control of renal vascular resistance has been estimated to contribute up to 50% of the total autoregulatory response.[278]

Several lines of evidence indicate that such a myogenic mechanism is important in renal autoregulation. Autoregulation of RBF is observed even when tubuloglomerular feedback is inhibited by furosemide, suggesting an important role for a myogenic mechanism.[105] This myogenic mechanism of autoregulation occurs very rapidly, reaching a full response in 3 to 10 seconds.[105] Autoregulation occurs in all of the preglomerular resistance vessels of the in vitro blood-perfused juxtamedullary nephron preparation.[260,270,279-281] Of note, the afferent arteriole in this preparation has been shown to be able to constrict in response to rapid changes in perfusion pressure even when all flow to the macula densa was stopped by resection of the papilla, indicating an important role for a myogenic mechanism in autoregulation.[281] Isolated perfused rabbit afferent arterioles respond to step increases in intraluminal pressure with a decrease in luminal diameter.[102] In contrast, efferent arteriolar segments show vasodilation when submitted to the same procedure, probably reflecting simple passive physical properties. Autoregulation is also observed in the afferent arteriole and arcuate and interlobular arteries of the split hydronephrotic kidney,[184,262,264,265,282] but again the efferent arteriole did not show autoregulation in this model.[184] Further evidence that the renal vasculature is indeed intrinsically responsive to variations in the transmural hydraulic pressure difference was obtained by Gilmore and colleagues,[283] who provided direct evidence for myogenic autoregulation in renal vessels transplanted into a cheek pouch of the hamster. In this nonfiltering system, contraction of afferent but not efferent arterioles was observed in response to increased interstitial pressure in the pouch. However, it should be noted that, in vivo, efferent arteriolar resistance may increase in response to decreases in arterial pressure,[284,285] and this response may result from increased activity of the renin-angiotensin system. These data may also explain why autoregulation of GFR is more efficient than autoregulation of RBF.

The autoregulatory threshold can be reset in response to a variety of perturbations. Autoregulation in the afferent arteriole is greatly attenuated in the kidneys of subjects with diabetes and may contribute to the hyperfiltration seen early in this disease.[282] Autoregulation is partially restored by insulin treatment and/or by inhibition of endogenous prostaglandin production.[282] Autoregulation in the remnant kidney is markedly attenuated 24 hours after the reduction in renal mass and is again restored by cyclo-oxygenase inhibition, suggesting that release of vasodilatory prostaglandins may be involved in the initial response to increase SNGFR in the remaining nephrons after acute partial nephrectomy.[286] Much higher pressures than normal are required to evoke a vasoconstrictor response in the afferent arteriole during the development of spontaneous hypertension.[287] The intermediate portion of the interlobular artery of the spontaneously hypertensive rat exhibits an enhanced myogenic response, with a lower threshold pressure and a greater maximal response.[264] Both the afferent arterioles and the interlobular arteries of Dahl salt-sensitive hypertensive rats exhibit a reduced myogenic responsiveness to increases in perfusion pressure when the rats are fed a high-salt diet.[288] Thus, alterations in autoregulatory responses of the renal vasculature occur in a variety of disease states.

AUTOREGULATION MEDIATED BY TUBULOGLOMERULAR FEEDBACK

The nephron is uniquely organized so that the same tubule that descends from the cortex into the medulla eventually returns to the originating glomerulus to provide a regulatory mechanism known as *tubuloglomerular feedback* (TGF). There is a specialized nephron segment lying between the end of the thick ascending limb of the loop of Henle and the beginning of the distal convoluted tubule, known as the *macula densa*. The macula densa cells are adjacent to the cells of the extraglomerular mesangium, which fill the angle formed by the afferent and efferent arterioles of the glomerulus (Figure 3.23). This anatomic arrangement of macula densa cells, extraglomerular mesangial cells, arteriolar smooth muscle cells, and renin-secreting cells of the afferent arteriole is known as the *juxtaglomerular apparatus* (JGA). The JGA is ideally suited for a feedback system whereby a stimulus received at the macula densa may be transmitted to the arterioles of the same nephron to alter RBF and GFR. Changes in the delivery rate and composition of the fluid flowing past the macula densa have been shown to elicit rapid changes in glomerular filtration of the same nephron, with increases in delivery of fluid resulting in decreases in SNGFR and glomerular capillary hydraulic pressure (P_{GC}) of the same nephron.[289,290] This TGF system senses delivery of fluid to the macula densa and "feeds back" to control filtration rate, thus providing a powerful mechanism to regulate the pressures and flows that govern GFR in response to acute perturbations in delivery of fluid to the JGA.

The TGF mechanism has been suggested as an additional mechanism to the myogenic response to explain the autoregulation of RBF and GFR. Increased RBF or glomerular capillary pressure would lead to increased GFR, and therefore, delivery of solute to the distal tubule would rise. Increased distal delivery is sensed by the macula densa, which activates effector mechanisms that increase preglomerular resistance, reducing RBF, glomerular pressure, and GFR. A number of observations support this hypothesis. Perfusion of the renal distal tubule at increasing flows causes reduction in glomerular blood flow and GFR.[291] Furthermore, as reviewed by Navar and colleagues, a variety of experimental maneuvers that cause distal tubule fluid flow to decline or cease induce afferent arteriolar vasodilation and interfere with the normal autoregulatory response.[274,292] In addition, infusion of furosemide into the macula densa segment of juxtamedullary nephrons was found to significantly abrogate the normal constrictor response of afferent arterioles to increased perfusion pressure,[293] presumably by blocking the uptake of Na^+ and Cl^- from the tubule lumen.[294] A similar observation was made by Takenaka and coworkers.[260] These studies suggest that the autoregulatory response in juxtamedullary nephrons is mainly dependent on the TGF mechanism. Moreover, deletion of the A_1 adenosine receptor gene in mice to block TGF results in less efficient autoregulation, again indicating the role for TGF in the autoregulatory response.[295]

To examine the role of TGF in autoregulation, investigators have studied spontaneous oscillations in proximal

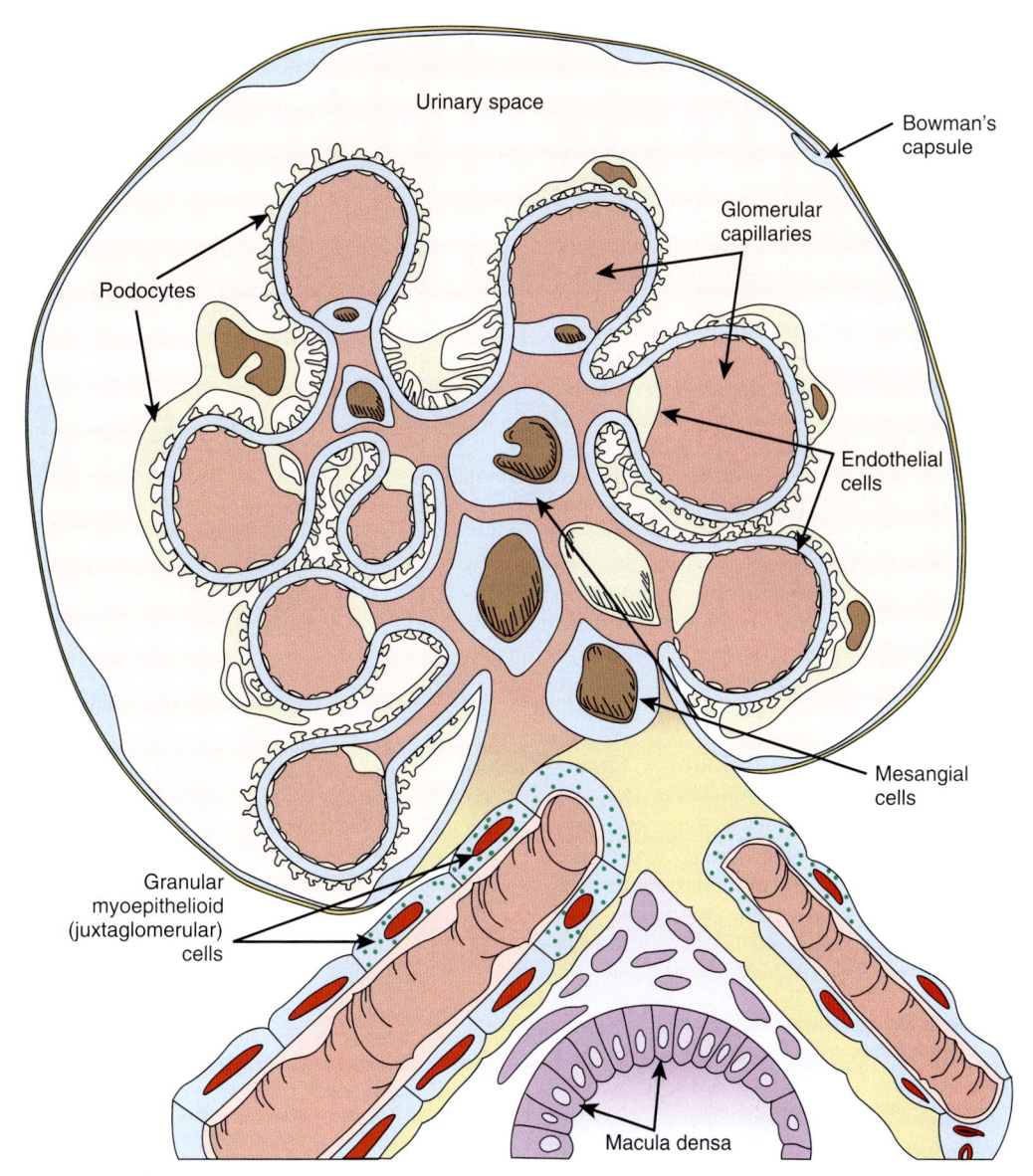

Figure 3.23 Schematic drawing of a cross section of a glomerulus, including the afferent and efferent arterioles, macula densa cells of the early distal tubule, glomerular capillaries, mesangial cells, and podocytes. (Drawing by DA Maddox.)

tubule pressure and RBF and the response of the renal circulation to high-frequency oscillations in tubule flow rates or renal perfusion pressure.[296] Oscillations in tubule pressure have been observed in anesthetized rats at a rate of about three cycles per minute that are sensitive to small changes in delivery of fluid to the macula densa.[297] These spontaneous oscillations are eliminated by loop diuretics,[298] findings consistent with the hypothesis that they are mediated by the TGF response. To examine this hypothesis, Holstein-Rathlou induced sinusoidal oscillations in distal tubule flow in rats at a frequency similar to that of the spontaneous fluctuations in tubule pressure.[296] Varying distal delivery at this rate caused parallel fluctuations in stop-flow pressure (an index of glomerular capillary pressure), probably mediated by alterations in afferent resistance, again consistent with dynamic regulation of glomerular blood flow by the TGF system. To investigate further, Holstein-Rathlou and colleagues examined the effects of sinusoidal variations in arterial pressure at varying frequencies on RBF in rats.[299] Two separate components of autoregulation were identified, one operating at about the same frequency as the spontaneous fluctuations in tubule pressure (the TGF component) and one operating at a much higher frequency consistent with spontaneous fluctuations in vascular smooth muscle tone (the myogenic component). Subsequently, Flemming and coworkers reported that renal vascular responses to alterations in renal perfusion pressure varied considerably according to the dynamics of the change and that rapid and slow changes in perfusion pressure could have opposite effects.[300] They suggested that slow pressure changes elicited a predominant TGF response, whereas rapid changes invoked the myogenic mechanism.

Despite these observations, the conclusion that the TGF system plays a central role in autoregulation is complicated by several factors. First, there is the process of glomerulotubular balance, by which proximal tubule reabsorption increases as GFR rises. This mechanism would tend to blunt the effects of alterations in GFR on distal delivery.

In addition, the persistence of autoregulatory behavior in nonfiltering kidneys[301] and in isolated blood vessels suggests that the delivery of filtrate to the distal tubule is not absolutely required for constancy of blood flow, at least in superficial nephrons. Consistent with this view, Just and associates demonstrated in the conscious dog that although TGF contributes to maximum autoregulatory capacity of RBF, autoregulation is observed even when tubuloglomerular feedback is inhibited by furosemide, suggesting an important role for a myogenic mechanism.[105,302] However, Wang and colleagues found that the myogenic responses of the afferent arteriole are affected by inhibition of the Na$^+$-K$^+$-2Cl$^-$ cotransporter with furosemide in the absence of tubuloglomerular feedback.[303] The myogenic and TGF mechanisms are not mutually exclusive, and Aukland and Oien have proposed a model of renal autoregulation that incorporates both systems.[304] Because the myogenic and TGF responses share the same effector site, the afferent arteriole, interactions between these two systems are unavoidable and each response is capable of modulating the other. The prevailing view is that these two mechanisms act in concert to accomplish the same end, a stabilization of renal function when blood pressure is altered.[278,305] Just suggested that the myogenic component of autoregulation requires less than 10 seconds for completion and normally follows first-order kinetics without rate-sensitive components.[278] Peti-Peterdi and colleagues reported that the response time for the tubuloglomerular feedback may be as short as 5 seconds,[261] although others have suggested it takes 30 to 60 seconds and shows spontaneous oscillations at 0.025 to 0.033 Hz.[278] The myogenic and tubuloglomerular feedback mechanisms account for the majority of the autoregulatory response.[278]

Mechanisms of Tubuloglomerular Feedback Control of Renal Blood Flow and Glomerular Filtration Rate

Several factors have been identified as tubular signals for TGF.[306] Changes in delivery of Na$^+$, Cl$^-$, and K$^+$ are thought to be sensed by the macula densa through the Na$^+$-K$^+$-2Cl$^-$ cotransporter (a.k.a. the NKCC2 or BSC1 cotransporter) on the luminal cell membrane of the macula densa cells.[307] Alterations in Na$^+$, K$^+$, and Cl$^-$ reabsorption result in inverse changes in SNGFR and renal vascular resistance, primarily in the preglomerular vessels. For instance, when the salt delivery increases to the distal tubule, the feedback mechanism decreases glomerular filtration. Agents such as furosemide that interfere with the Na$^+$-K$^+$-2Cl$^-$ cotransporter in the macula densa cells[294] inhibit the feedback response.[308] Adenosine, and possibly ATP, play a central role in mediating the relationship between transport of Na$^+$, K$^+$, and Cl$^-$, at the luminal cell membrane of the macula densa and the GFR of the same nephron, as illustrated in Figure 3.24.[290] According to this scheme, increased delivery of solute to the macula densa results in concentration-dependent increases in solute uptake by the Na$^+$-K$^+$-2Cl$^-$ cotransporter. These increases, in turn, stimulate Na$^+$-K$^+$-ATPase activity on the basolateral side of the cells, leading to the formation of adenosine diphosphate (ADP) and subsequent formation of AMP. Dephosphorylation of AMP by cytosolic 5′-nucleotidase or endo-5′-nucleotidase bound to the cell membrane yields the formation of adenosine.[290] Once adenosine leaves the macula densa cells or is formed in the adjacent interstitium, it interacts with adenosine A$_1$ receptors on the extraglomerular mesangial cells, resulting in an increase in $[Ca^{2+}]_i$.[309] The increase in $[Ca^{2+}]_i$ may occur, in part, via basolateral membrane depolarization through Cl$^-$ channels followed by Ca^{2+} entry into the cells via voltage-gated Ca^{2+} channels.[310] As indicated in Figure 3.24, gap junctions then transmit the calcium transient to the adjacent afferent arteriole, leading to vasoconstriction.[290] In addition, adenosine can directly constrict the afferent arteriole through calcium release from the sarcoplasmic reticulum; activation of calcium-dependent chloride channels; and influx of calcium through voltage-dependent calcium channels.[311] Macula densa cells respond to an increase in luminal [NaCl] by releasing ATP at the basolateral cell membrane through ATP-permeable large-conductance anion channels, possibly providing a communication link between macula densa cells and adjacent mesangial cells via purinoceptors receptors on the latter.[312]

Several lines of evidence support the role for adenosine in mediating TGF. Intraluminal administration of an

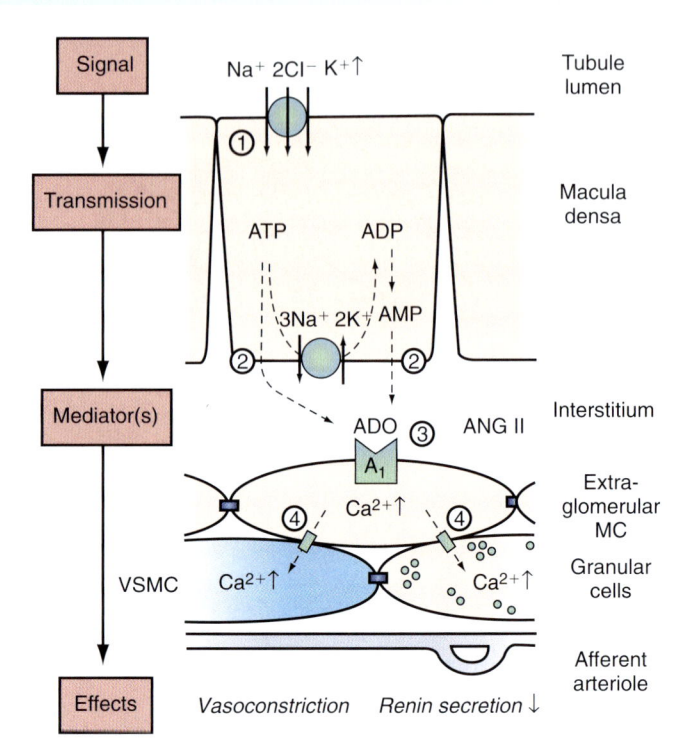

Figure 3.24 Proposed mechanism of tubuloglomerular feedback (TGF). The sequence of events (numbers in circles) are: (1) uptake of Na$^+$, Cl$^-$, and K$^+$ by the Na$^+$-K$^+$-2Cl$^-$ cotransporter on the luminal cell membrane of the macula densa cells; (2) intracellular or extracellular production of adenosine (ADO); (3) ADO activation of adenosine A$_1$ receptors, triggering an increase in cytosolic Ca^{2+} in extraglomerular mesangial cells (MCs); and (4) coupling between extraglomerular MCs and granular cells (containing renin) and smooth muscle cells of the afferent arteriole (VSMCs) by gap junctions, allowing propagation of the increased $[Ca^{2+}]_i$ (intracellular calcium concentration) and resulting in afferent arteriolar vasoconstriction and inhibition of renin release. Local angiotensin II and neuronal nitric oxide synthase (nNOS) activity modulate the response. ADP, adenosine diphosphate; AMP, adenosine monophosphate; ATP, adenosine triphosphate. (From Vallon V: Tubuloglomerular feedback and the control of glomerular filtration rate. News Physiol Sci 18:169-174, 2003.)

adenosine A_1 receptor agonist enhances the TGF response.[313] In addition, TGF is completely absent in adenosine A_1 receptor–deficient mice.[314,315] Blockage of adenosine A_1 receptors, or inhibition of adenosine synthesis via inhibition of 5′-nucleotidase, reduces TGF efficiency, and combining the two inhibitors nearly completely blocks TGF.[316] Addition of adenosine to the afferent arteriole causes vasoconstriction via activation of the adenosine A_1 receptor, and addition of an A_1 receptor antagonist blocks the effects of both adenosine and of high macula densa [NaCl].[317] Of note, these effects occur only when adenosine is added to the extravascular space and do not occur when adenosine is added to the lumen of the macula densa.[317] These results are consistent with the proposed scheme in Figure 3.24, which suggests that an increase in [NaCl] to the macula densa stimulates Na^+-K^+-ATPase activity, leading to increased adenosine synthesis followed by constriction of the afferent arterioles via A_1 receptor activation.[317]

Efferent arterioles preconstricted with norepinephrine vasodilate in response to an increase in NaCl concentration at the macula densa, an effect blocked by adenosine A_2 receptor antagonists but not by A_1 receptor antagonists.[318] The changes in efferent arteriolar resistance are in opposite direction to that of the afferent arterioles, which vasoconstrict in response to an increase in NaCl at the macula densa.[317,319] The net result is decreased glomerular blood flow, decreased glomerular hydraulic pressure, and a reduction in SNGFR.

Angiotensin appears to be another regulatory factor. TGF is blunted by Ang II antagonists and Ang II synthesis inhibitors and is absent in knockout mice lacking either the AT_{1A} Ang II receptor or angiotensin-converting enzyme (ACE). Furthermore, systemic infusion of Ang II in ACE knockout mice restores TGF.[320-325] Ang II enhances TGF via activation of AT_1 receptors on the luminal membrane of the macula densa.[326] Acute inhibition of the AT_1 receptor in normal mice blocks TGF and reduces autoregulatory efficiency.[321] There have also been studies showing the interaction of adenosine and angiotensin in feedback mechanisms. In these studies, adenosine A_1 receptor antagonist administration resulted in decreased afferent arteriolar resistance and increased transcapillary hydraulic pressure differences (ΔP), whereas pretreatment with an angiotensin AT_1 receptor antagonist prevented these changes.[327] Although it is known that Ang II is not the primary regulator of TGF, these results indicate that Ang II plays a prominent role in modulating TGF and that this response is mediated through the AT_1 receptor, which may also link to the adenosine regulation.

Neuronal nitric oxide synthase is present in the macula densa.[328] Nitric oxide derived from nNOS in the macula densa provides a vasodilatory influence on tubuloglomerular feedback, decreasing the amount of vasoconstriction of the afferent arteriole that otherwise would occur.[328,329] Increased distal NaCl delivery to the macula densa stimulates nNOS activity and also increases activity of the inducible form of cyclo-oxygenase (COX-2), which counteracts TGF-mediated constriction of the afferent arteriole.[328,329] Macula densa cell pH rises in response to increased luminal sodium concentration and may be related to the stimulation of nNOS.[330] Inhibition of macula densa guanylate cyclase increases the TGF response to high luminal [NaCl], further indicating the importance of NO in modulating TGF.[319] Ito and Ren, using an isolated perfused complete JGA preparation, found that microperfusion of the macula densa with an inhibitor of NO production led to constriction of the adjacent afferent arteriole.[186] When the macula densa was perfused with a low-sodium solution, however, the response was blocked, indicating that solute reabsorption is required.[186] Microperfusion of the macula densa with the precursor of NO, L-arginine, blunts TGF, especially in salt-depleted animals.[331-333] Therefore, it appears that the afferent arteriole vasodilates acutely in response to NO, thus blunting TGF. An increase in NO production may also inhibit renin release by increasing cGMP in the granular cells of the afferent arteriole,[334] thereby accentuating its vasodilatory effects. Of note, however, Schnermann and coworkers reported that when NO production is blocked long term in knockout mice lacking nNOS, TGF in response to acute perturbations in distal sodium delivery is normal.[322] These workers did observe, however, that the presence of intact nNOS in the JGA is required for sodium chloride–dependent renin secretion.[322] The TGF system, which elicits vasoconstriction and a reduction in SNGFR in response to acute increases in sodium delivery to the macula densa, appears to secondarily activate a vasodilatory response. Stimulation of NO production in response to increased distal salt delivery under conditions of volume expansion, by resetting tubuloglomerular feedback and limiting TGF-mediated vasoconstrictor responses, would be advantageous.

Tubuloglomerular feedback responses might be temporally divided into two opposing events. The initial, rapid (seconds) TGF response would yield vasoconstriction and a decrease in GFR and P_{GC} when sodium delivery out of the proximal tubule is acutely increased. The same increase in sodium delivery would be expected with time (minutes) to decrease renin secretion, which in the presence of a continued stimulus such as volume expansion would reduce Ang II production and allow filtration rate to increase, thereby helping raise urinary excretion rates. The rapid TGF system would prevent large changes in GFR under such conditions as spontaneous fluctuations in blood pressure that might otherwise occur, thereby maintaining tight control of distal sodium delivery in the short term.[322] Schnermann and coworkers hypothesized that the JG A functions to maintain tight control of distal sodium delivery only for the short term.[322] Over the long term, renin secretion is controlled by the JGA in accordance with the requirements for sodium balance, and the TGF system resets at a new sodium delivery rate.[322] The TGF system then continues to operate around this new set point. Over the long term, resetting of the TGF system may thus be the result of sustained increases in GFR and distal delivery.[322,335,336]

AUTOREGULATION MEDIATED BY METABOLIC MECHANISMS

The metabolic theory predicts that, given the relative constancy of tissue metabolism, a decrease in organ blood flow leads to local accumulation of a vasodilator metabolite, maintaining blood flow at or near its previous level, whether in tissues such as muscle or in kidney.[305,337,338] The TGF system is affected by compounds that are closely linked to cellular metabolism, ATP and its metabolites ADP and adenosine. These metabolites have important effects on renal vascular smooth muscle and thus may provide a metabolic link to autoregulation via the TGF mechanism.[272,339,340]

OTHER FACTORS INVOLVED IN AUTOREGULATION

Studies have shown that endothelium-dependent factors might play a role in the myogenic response of renal arteries and arterioles to changes in perfusion pressure. For example, in 1992 Hishikawa and coworkers reported that raised transmural pressure increased NO release by cultured endothelial cells.[341] In addition, Tojo and associates used histochemical techniques to demonstrate the presence of NOS in the macula densa, suggesting that NO also participates in the TGF response.[342] Other studies suggest that NO produced by the macula densa can dampen the TGF response.[331] In fact, studies have examined the role of this endothelial factor in the autoregulatory response. In dogs, inhibition of NO production leads to an increase in blood pressure and a decline in basal renal vascular resistance; however, autoregulatory ability is unimpaired.[177] On the other hand, Salom and colleagues reported that inhibition of NO production causes a greater decline in RBF in the kidneys of rats perfused at hypertensive than at normotensive pressure.[343] This finding suggests that increased NO production might modulate the vasoconstrictor response to an increase in perfusion pressure.

Elevations in transmural pressure also increase endothelin release by cultured endothelial cells, and this response was not altered by the presence of a calcium channel blocker, nifedipine, or a channel activator, gadolinium.[344] These findings suggest that endothelin, via a mechanism other than extracellular Ca^{2+} influx, may play a role in pressure-induced control of RBF. Of note, endothelin production is also stimulated by a rise in shear stress.[219] However, infusions of endothelin produce a prolonged constrictor response that is ill suited to an autoregulatory role,[345] and endothelin acting through ET_A receptors does not seem to play an important role in the autoregulation of RBF.[346]

NEURAL REGULATION OF GLOMERULAR FILTRATION RATE

The renal vasculature, including the afferent arteriole and the efferent arteriole, the macula densa cells of the distal tubule, and the glomerular mesangium, is richly innervated.[88,347] Innervation includes renal efferent sympathetic adrenergic nerves[347,348] and renal afferent sensory fibers containing peptides such as calcitonin gene–related peptide (CGRP) and substance P.[88,347] Acetylcholine is a potent vasodilator of the renal vasculature (discussed previously), suggesting a potential role for circulating acetylcholine in the control of the renal circulation. Sympathetic efferent nerves are found in all segments of the vascular tree from the main renal artery to the afferent arteriole (including the renin-containing juxtaglomerular cells) and the efferent arteriole[347,348] and play an important role in the regulation of renal hemodynamics, sodium transport, and renin secretion.[349] Afferent nerves containing CGRP and substance P are localized primarily in the main renal artery and interlobar arteries, with some innervation also observed in the arcuate artery, the interlobular artery, and the afferent arteriole, including the JGA.[347,348] Peptidergic nerve fibers immunoreactive for neuropeptide Y (NPY), neurotensin, vasoactive intestinal polypeptide, and somatostatin are also found in the kidney.[76] Neuronal nitric oxide synthase–immunoreactive neurons have now been identified in the kidney.[347] The NOS-containing neuronal somata are seen in the wall of the renal pelvis, at the renal hilus close to the renal artery, along the interlobar and arcuate arteries, and extending to the afferent arteriole, suggesting that they have a role in the control of RBF.[347] Such somata were also present in nerve bundles having vasomotor and sensory fibers, suggesting that they might modulate renal neural function.[347]

In micropuncture studies of the effects of renal nerve stimulation (RNS), RNS alone increased R_A and R_E, resulting in a fall in Q_A and SNGFR without any effect on K_f.[350] When prostaglandin production was inhibited by indomethacin, however, the same level of RNS produced even greater increases in R_A and R_E accompanied by very large declines in Q_A and SNGFR and decreases in K_f, P_{GC}, and ΔP.[350] When saralasin was administered as a competitive inhibitor of endogenous Ang II in conjunction with indomethacin, RNS had no effect on K_f, but both R_A and R_E were still increased and ΔP was slightly reduced.[350] The release of norepinephrine by RNS enhances Ang II production to yield arteriolar vasoconstriction and reduction in K_f. The increase in Ang II production may then increase vasodilator prostaglandin production,[350,351] partially ameliorating the constriction. Continued vasoconstriction by RNS during blockade of endogenous prostaglandins and Ang II suggests that norepinephrine has separate vasoconstrictive properties by itself. In agreement with this suggestion are the findings that norepinephrine causes constriction of preglomerular vessels.[109] Inhibition of NOS results in a decline in SNGFR in normal rats but not in rats with surgical renal denervation, suggesting that NO normally modulates the effects of renal adrenergic activity.[352] This modulation does not appear, however, to be related to sympathetic modulation of renin secretion.[353]

Renal denervation in animals undergoing acute water deprivation (48 hours duration) or with congestive heart failure produces increases in SNGFR, Q_A, and K_f.[354] This finding suggests that the natural activity of the renal nerves in these settings plays an important role in the constriction of the arterioles and reduction in K_f that were observed.[354] The vasoconstrictive effects of the renal nerves in both settings were mediated in part by a stimulatory effect on Ang II release, together with a direct vasoconstrictive effect on the preglomerular and postglomerular blood vessels.[354] These studies demonstrate the important role of the renal nerves in pathophysiologic settings. In fact, clinical trials have focused on whether catheter-based renal artery denervation reduces blood pressure in patients with resistant hypertension. The latest trial demonstrated a reduction in blood pressure of those patients who underwent renal denervation; however, the response did not differ from that of the sham-treated patients at 6 months after treatment.[355]

Complete reference list available at ExpertConsult.com.

KEY REFERENCES

14. Kost CK, Jr, Li P, Williams DS, et al: Renal vascular responses to angiotensin II in conscious spontaneously hypertensive and normotensive rats. *J Cardiovasc Pharmacol* 31:854–861, 1998.

19. Pallone TL, Robertson CR, Jamison RL: Renal medullary microcirculation. *Physiol Rev* 70:885–920, 1990.
22. Beeuwkes R, 3rd: The vascular organization of the kidney. *Annu Rev Physiol* 42:531–542, 1980.
33. Kriz W, Napiwotzky P: Structural and functional aspects of the renal interstitium. *Contrib Nephrol* 16:104–108, 1979.
38. Zimmerhackl B, Robertson CR, Jamison RL: The microcirculation of the renal medulla. *Circ Res* 57:657–667, 1985.
39. Pallone TL, Zhang Z, Rhinehart K: Physiology of the renal medullary microcirculation. *Am J Physiol Renal Physiol* 284:F253–F266, 2003.
61. Kriz W, Kaissling B: *Structural organization of the mammalian kidney*, Philadelphia, 2000, Lippincott, Williams & Wilkins, pp 587–654.
64. Peppiatt-Wildman CM: The evolving role of renal pericytes. *Curr Opin Nephrol Hypertens* 22:10–16, 2013.
71. Rosivall L, Peti-Peterdi J: Heterogeneity of the afferent arteriole–correlations between morphology and function. *Nephrol Dial Transplant* 21:2703–2707, 2006.
72. Kriz W, Elger M, Mundel P, et al: Structure-stabilizing forces in the glomerular tuft. *J Am Soc Nephrol* 5:1731–1739, 1995.
82. Deen WM, Lazzara MJ, Myers BD: Structural determinants of glomerular permeability. *Am J Physiol Renal Physiol* 281:F579–F596, 2001.
85. Brenner BM, Troy JL, Daugharty TM: The dynamics of glomerular ultrafiltration in the rat. *J Clin Invest* 50:1776–1780, 1971.
88. Maddox DA, Brenner BM: Glomerular ultrafiltration. In Brenner BM, editor: *Brenner & Rector's the kidney*, ed 7, Philadelphia, 2004, Saunders, pp 353–412.
89. Deen WM, Robertson CR, Brenner BM: A model of glomerular ultrafiltration in the rat. *Am J Physiol* 223:1178–1183, 1972.
91. Brenner BM, Troy JL, Daugharty TM, et al: Dynamics of glomerular ultrafiltration in the rat. II. Plasma-flow dependence of GFR. *Am J Physiol* 223:1184–1190, 1972.
101. Carmines PK, Morrison TK, Navar LG: Angiotensin II effects on microvascular diameters of in vitro blood-perfused juxtamedullary nephrons. *Am J Physiol* 251:F610–F618, 1986.
106. Lanese DM, Yuan BH, McMurtry IF, et al: Comparative sensitivities of isolated rat renal arterioles to endothelin. *Am J Physiol* 263:F894–F899, 1992.
108. Ito S, Arima S, Ren YL, et al: Endothelium-derived relaxing factor/nitric oxide modulates angiotensin II action in the isolated microperfused rabbit afferent but not efferent arteriole. *J Clin Invest* 91:2012–2019, 1993.
114. Patzak A, Lai EY, Mrowka R, et al: AT1 receptors mediate angiotensin II-induced release of nitric oxide in afferent arterioles. *Kidney Int* 66:1949–1958, 2004.
123. Deng A, Baylis C: Locally produced EDRF controls preglomerular resistance and ultrafiltration coefficient. *Am J Physiol* 264:F212–F215, 1993.
139. Ignarro LJ, Buga GM, Wood KS, et al: Endothelium-derived relaxing factor produced and released from artery and vein is nitric oxide. *Proc Natl Acad Sci U S A* 84:9265–9269, 1987.
140. Palmer RM, Ferrige AG, Moncada S: Nitric oxide release accounts for the biological activity of endothelium-derived relaxing factor. *Nature* 327:524–526, 1987.
171. Blantz RC, Deng A, Lortie M, et al: The complex role of nitric oxide in the regulation of glomerular ultrafiltration. *Kidney Int* 61:782–785, 2002.
182. Qiu C, Baylis C: Endothelin and angiotensin mediate most glomerular responses to nitric oxide inhibition. *Kidney Int* 55:2390–2396, 1999.
183. Zatz R, de Nucci G: Effects of acute nitric oxide inhibition on rat glomerular microcirculation. *Am J Physiol* 261:F360–F363, 1991.
187. Ohishi K, Carmines PK, Inscho EW, et al: EDRF-angiotensin II interactions in rat juxtamedullary afferent and efferent arterioles. *Am J Physiol* 263:F900–F906, 1992.
190. Deng A, Miracle CM, Suarez JM, et al: Oxygen consumption in the kidney: effects of nitric oxide synthase isoforms and angiotensin II. *Kidney Int* 68:723–730, 2005.
192. Baylis C, Harvey J, Engels K: Acute nitric oxide blockade amplifies the renal vasoconstrictor actions of angiotension II. *J Am Soc Nephrol* 5:211–214, 1994.
224. Munger KA, Sugiura M, Takahashi K, et al: A role for atrial natriuretic peptide in endothelin-induced natriuresis. *J Am Soc Nephrol* 1:1278–1283, 1991.
225. King AJ, Brenner BM, Anderson S: Endothelin: a potent renal and systemic vasoconstrictor peptide. *Am J Physiol* 256:F1051–F1058, 1989.
231. Kon V, Yoshioka T, Fogo A, et al: Glomerular actions of endothelin in vivo. *J Clin Invest* 83:1762–1767, 1989.
234. Edwards RM, Trizna W, Ohlstein EH: Renal microvascular effects of endothelin. *Am J Physiol* 259:F217–F221, 1990.
252. Speed JS, Pollock DM: Endothelin, kidney disease, and hypertension. *Hypertension* 61:1142–1145, 2013.
253. Robertson CR, Deen WM, Troy JL, et al: Dynamics of glomerular ultrafiltration in the rat. 3. Hemodynamics and autoregulation. *Am J Physiol* 223:1191–1200, 1972.
260. Takenaka T, Harrison-Bernard LM, Inscho EW, et al: Autoregulation of afferent arteriolar blood flow in juxtamedullary nephrons. *Am J Physiol* 267:F879–F887, 1994.
261. Peti-Peterdi J, Morishima S, Bell PD, et al: Two-photon excitation fluorescence imaging of the living juxtaglomerular apparatus. *Am J Physiol Renal Physiol* 283:F197–F201, 2002.
263. Davis MJ, Hill MA: Signaling mechanisms underlying the vascular myogenic response. *Physiol Rev* 79:387–423, 1999.
274. Navar LG: Integrating multiple paracrine regulators of renal microvascular dynamics. *Am J Physiol* 274:F433–F444, 1998.
289. Schnermann J, Wright FS, Davis JM, et al: Regulation of superficial nephron filtration rate by tubulo-glomerular feedback. *Pflugers Arch* 318:147–175, 1970.
290. Vallon V: Tubuloglomerular feedback and the control of glomerular filtration rate. *News Physiol Sci* 18:169–174, 2003.
292. Navar LG, Bell PD, Burke TJ: Role of a macula densa feedback mechanism as a mediator of renal autoregulation. *Kidney Int Suppl* 12:S157–S164, 1982.
293. Moore LC, Casellas D: Tubuloglomerular feedback dependence of autoregulation in rat juxtamedullary afferent arterioles. *Kidney Int* 37:1402–1408, 1990.
311. Hansen PB, Friis UG, Uhrenholt TR, et al: Intracellular signalling pathways in the vasoconstrictor response of mouse afferent arterioles to adenosine. *Acta Physiol (Oxf)* 191:89–97, 2007.
315. Sun D, Samuelson LC, Yang T, et al: Mediation of tubuloglomerular feedback by adenosine: evidence from mice lacking adenosine 1 receptors. *Proc Natl Acad Sci U S A* 98:9983–9988, 2001.
316. Thomson S, Bao D, Deng A, et al: Adenosine formed by 5′-nucleotidase mediates tubuloglomerular feedback. *J Clin Invest* 106:289–298, 2000.
327. Munger KA, Jackson EK: Effects of selective A1 receptor blockade on glomerular hemodynamics: involvement of renin-angiotensin system. *Am J Physiol* 267:F783–F790, 1994.
328. Wilcox CS, Welch WJ, Murad F, et al: Nitric oxide synthase in macula densa regulates glomerular capillary pressure. *Proc Natl Acad Sci U S A* 89:11993–11997, 1992.
331. Thorup C, Erik A, Persson G: Macula densa derived nitric oxide in regulation of glomerular capillary pressure. *Kidney Int* 49:430–436, 1996.
335. Thomson SC, Blantz RC, Vallon V: Increased tubular flow induces resetting of tubuloglomerular feedback in euvolemic rats. *Am J Physiol* 270:F461–F468, 1996.
355. Bhatt DL, Kandzari DE, O'Neill WW, et al: A controlled trial of renal denervation for resistant hypertension. *N Engl J Med* 370:1393–1401, 2014.

4 The Podocyte

Stuart J. Shankland | Peter W. Mathieson

CHAPTER OUTLINE

BIOLOGIC FUNCTIONS OF PODOCYTES, 112
ULTRASTRUCTURAL AND MOLECULAR ANATOMY OF PODOCYTES REQUIRED FOR NORMAL STRUCTURE AND FUNCTION, 113
Structure, 113
Slit Diaphragm Proteins, 113
Cytoskeleton, 113
GLOMERULAR DISEASES IN WHICH PODOCYTES ARE THE PRIMARY GLOMERULAR CELL TYPE INJURED, 113
MECHANISMS OF INJURY IN COMMON PODOCYTE DISEASES, 114
Minimal Change Nephropathy, 114
Focal Segmental Glomerulosclerosis, 116
Membranous Nephropathy, 116
Human Immunodeficiency Virus Nephropathy, 116
Diabetic Kidney Disease, 116
RESPONSES BY PODOCYTES TO DISEASE-INDUCED INJURY: LINKING STRUCTURE TO FUNCTION TO CLINICAL FINDINGS, 117
Effacement: A Histologic Change in Podocyte Shape Mediated by the Actin Cytoskeleton, 117
Proteinuria due to Reduced Size and/or Charge Properties, 118
Glomerulosclerosis and Reduced Kidney Function: A Correlation with Depletion in Podocyte Number, 118
EFFECTS OF EXISTING THERAPIES ON PODOCYTES, 119
Glucocorticosteroids, 119
Calcineurin Inhibitors, 119
Anti–B Cell Therapy, 119
Renin Angiotensin Aldosterone System Inhibitors, 119
IDENTIFICATION OF CANDIDATE THERAPEUTIC APPROACHES FOR THE FUTURE, 120
SUMMARY, 120

Normal human urine contains only tiny amounts of protein. The presence of increased amounts of urinary protein (proteinuria), especially albumin (albuminuria), is a cardinal feature of glomerular disease and an important prognostic marker in a wide variety of forms of kidney disease, including the most numerically and economically important form of kidney disease, diabetic nephropathy.[1] Perhaps not so widely appreciated is that albuminuria is also an important independent risk factor for cardiovascular mortality in both diabetic and nondiabetic populations.[2] Therefore the study of albuminuria, the factors that prevent it in the healthy state, the disease mechanisms that lead to its occurrence and its prognostic significance, and, perhaps most importantly, the therapeutic approaches to its modification, all have major clinical and health economic significance.

The healthy kidney limits the amount of albumin passing into the glomerular filtrate by virtue of the selective permeability of the glomerular capillary wall. In a 70-kg adult, approximately 180 L of water and small molecules such as salt, glucose, and amino acids pass relatively freely across the glomerular capillary wall into the primary urine in every 24-hour period. Yet, while allowing this massive permeability to water and small molecules, the glomerular capillary maintains relative impermeability to albumin. The structure of the glomerular capillary wall that serves this selective permeability comprises three interacting components: fenestrated glomerular endothelial cells on the inner (luminal) aspect, podocytes (also called glomerular visceral epithelial cells) on the outer (urinary) aspect of the capillary, and the highly negatively charged glomerular basement membrane (GBM) between these two cellular layers.[3] Each of these three components exerts an important influence on the selective permeability of the glomerular capillary wall to albumin and other proteins, and it is therefore unduly simplistic to think of any of the components in isolation. However, there are structural, scientific, clinical, and therapeutic reasons for focusing on the podocytes as the conductors of this orchestra, which is the purpose of this chapter.

BIOLOGIC FUNCTIONS OF PODOCYTES

The main biologic function of podocytes is to restrict the passage of albumin and other key proteins to the blood space within the glomerular capillaries and to prevent their passage into the extracapillary urinary space.[4] Additional functions include maintaining the shape of the underlying glomerular capillaries to which they adhere,[5] the production of extracellular matrix proteins for the development and likely subsequent maintenance of the GBM,[6] and the production and secretion of survival and angiopathic factors such as vascular endothelial growth factor (VEGF) and angiopoietin for the neighboring glomerular endothelial cells.[7,8] Alterations to one or more of these functions resulting from glomerular disease–induced injury lead to functional and structural changes that characterize podocyte injury, both clinically and pathologically. These will be discussed later.

ULTRASTRUCTURAL AND MOLECULAR ANATOMY OF PODOCYTES REQUIRED FOR NORMAL STRUCTURE AND FUNCTION

STRUCTURE

The complex podocyte ultrastructure comprises a cell body, from which extend long branching cellular processes. Major processes give rise to interdigitating secondary processes, which are arranged like the teeth of a zipper[9] (Figure 4.1). These minor processes end in foot processes, which attach podocytes to the underlying GBM. The gaps between these secondary processes form specialized and modified tight junctions called the slit diaphragms, through which glomerular filtration occurs (see Figure 4.1). This structure is analogous to a molecular sieve, which limits the passage of macromolecules based on size, in which the diameter of the sieve (40 nm) is smaller than that of albumin.[10] Foot processes are actively motile due to a well-organized and abundant actin cytoskeleton that is in direct communication with the slit diaphragm (see later). Multiple podocyte-specific proteins in the slit diaphragm enable this structure to serve several functions[11] (Figure 4.2). They include being a size, charge, and shape macromolecular filter to proteins (see later), anchoring the filter to the GBM, and communicating with the actin cytoskeleton in the foot processes to process cues appropriate for the regulation of podocyte shape and polarity.

SLIT DIAPHRAGM PROTEINS

Several classes of proteins make up the structure of the slit diaphragm, and each is required to accomplish specialized and diverse biologic functions in health (see Figure 4.2).[11] Perhaps the best known is the transmembrane protein nephrin, which spans the slit diaphragm across adjacent foot processes, giving rise to the characteristic zipper structure that participates in homotypic intercellular interactions.[10] Podocin helps anchor nephrin to the plasma membrane, whereas the family of Neph proteins ensures the *cis*-configuration of nephrin for proper function.[12] Nephrin, and likely additional slit diaphragm proteins, is further anchored to the actin cytoskeleton by the scaffold proteins CD2-associated protein (CD2AP),[13] zonula occludens 1 (ZO-1), and membrane-associated guanylate kinase, WW and PDZ domain–containing protein 2 (MAGI-2), and the actin-binding proteins α-actinin-4 and Ras activating-like protein IQGAP1 (IQGAP1). In addition, transient receptor potential cation channel, subfamily C, member 6 (TRPC6)[14] and TRPC5[15] are cationic sensing channels at the slit diaphragm. The protein structure of nephrin, and particularly its high number of intracytoplasmic tyrosine residues, strongly suggests a signaling function for this protein.[16] It has become apparent that slit diaphragm proteins play a key role in signaling to the podocyte actin cytoskeleton and in turn control the shape and structural integrity of the podocyte.[17] The slit diaphragm complex communicates actively with the rest of the podocyte to convey mechanical pressures and other signals to adapt to change. Phosphorylation of nephrin by Src family tyrosine kinases plays a role in signal transduction via phosphatidylinositol-3-kinase (PI3-K), Akt, and other pathways.[18]

CYTOSKELETON

The podocyte cytoskeleton ensures cell contractility, cell shape, and polarity. Foot processes contain long actin fiber bundles that run cortically and contiguously to link adjacent podocytes.[19] The cell body and major and secondary processes contain vimentin-rich intermediate filaments that assist in maintaining cell shape and rigidity, and large microtubules form organized structures along major and minor processes. Actin, α-actinin, and myosin form a contractile system in podocyte foot processes, and, along with the microtubule system, anchor podocytes to specific matrix proteins in the underlying GBM by way of integrins, vinculin, and talin.[20-22] Several Rho GTPases also regulate podocyte contractility[23]; actin is also regulated by podocyte-specific proteins, such as synaptopodin[24] and actinin-4, which are actin-binding proteins. Studies have shown that this well-orchestrated actin- and microtubule-cytoskeleton accounts for not only the shape of podocytes, but the ability to migrate.

GLOMERULAR DISEASES IN WHICH PODOCYTES ARE THE PRIMARY GLOMERULAR CELL TYPE INJURED

Certain types of proteinuric glomerular diseases are characterized by primary injury of podocytes.[25] The three leading primary glomerular diseases (defined as a kidney-specific disease) are focal segmental glomerulosclerosis (FSGS), membranous nephropathy (MN), and minimal change disease (MCD). "Nontraditional" podocyte diseases include diabetic kidney disease, amyloidosis, Fabry's disease, membranoproliferative glomerulonephritis and postinfectious glomerulonephritis. The inciting causes of each podocyte disease differ, and therefore each disease affects podocytes in different ways; in turn, the response to injury in each disease differs, leading to different histologic and clinical manifestations (Table 4.1). Yet, regardless of the inciting causes and their mediators of podocyte injury, several common clinical and pathologic responses occur, which will be highlighted later.

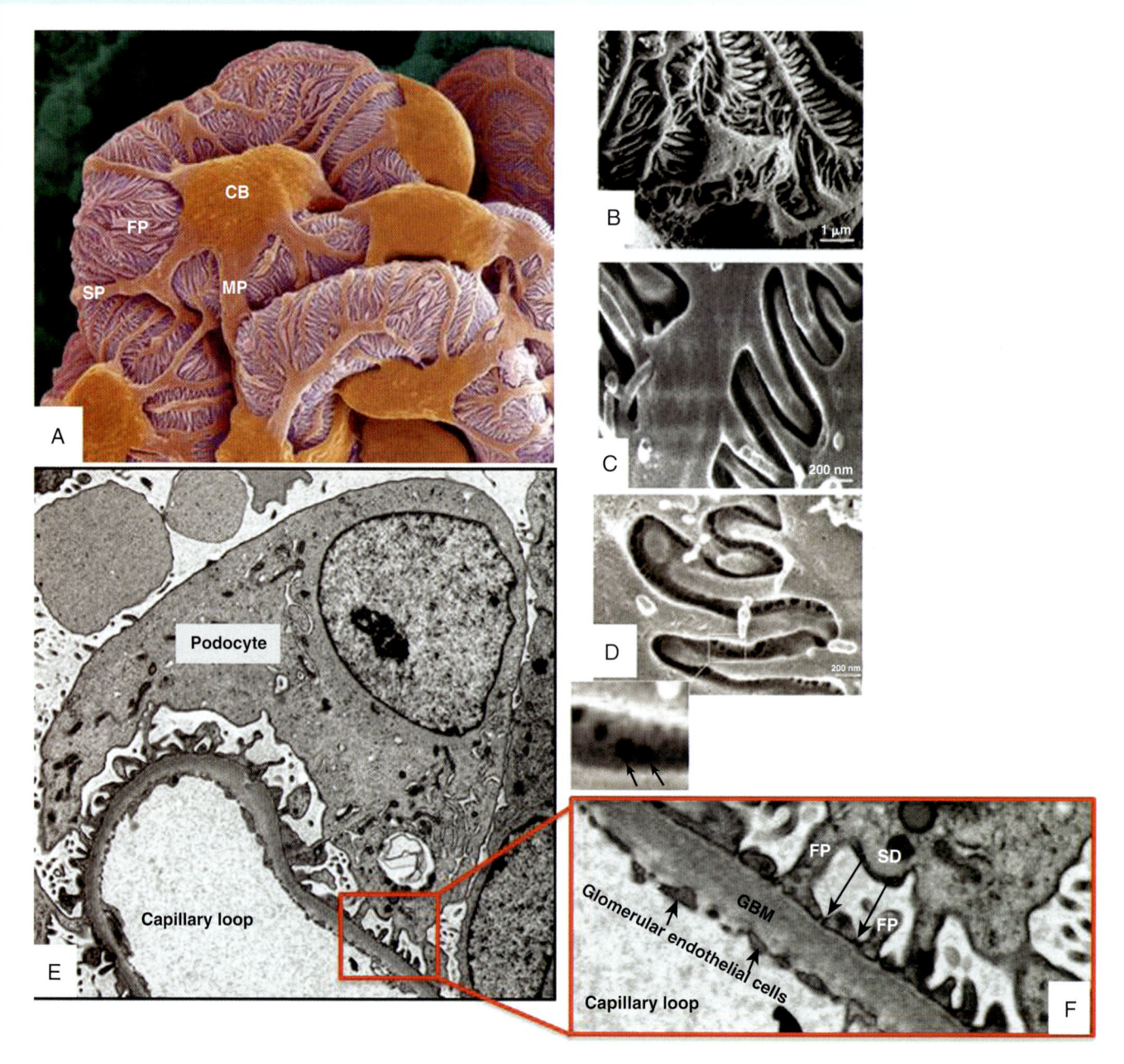

Figure 4.1 Podocyte ultrastructure. A, Scanning electron micrograph of podocytes (*orange*) covering the underlying capillary. From the cell body (CB), arise major processes (MP), from which arise secondary processes (SP), culminating in foot processes (FP). **B-D,** Visualization of interdigitating foot processes and epithelial filtration pores using an in-lens detector with scanning electron photomicrographs from a Wistar rat, taken at increasing magnifications (**B,** ×36,000; **C,** ×60,000; **D,** ×100,000). **E** and **F,** Scanning electron microscopy of a capillary loop covered by a podocyte. At higher power (**F**), the filtration barrier comprising the innermost glomerular endothelial cells, the middle glomerular basement membrane (GBM), and outermost podocyte foot processes (FP), between which are the slit diaphragms (SD). (**A** from Welsh GI, Saleem MA: The podocyte cytoskeleton—key to a functioning glomerulus in health and disease. *Nat Rev Nephrol* 8:14-21, 2011; **B-D** from Gagliardini E, Conti S, Benigni A, et al: Imaging of the porous ultrastructure of the glomerular epithelial filtration slit. *J Am Soc Nephrol* 21:2081-2089, 2010; **E** and **F** were provided by Dr. Behzad Najafian, University of Washington.)

MECHANISMS OF INJURY IN COMMON PODOCYTE DISEASES

The following is a brief overview of how each proteinuric glomerular disease leads to podocyte injury. Readers are referred to a more general discussion of these glomerular diseases in Chapter 32.

MINIMAL CHANGE NEPHROPATHY

The fact that the podocyte is the only glomerular cell that is structurally altered in MCD has led to the assumption that this disease is a "podocytopathy."[26] There are certainly changes in expression patterns of podocyte-specific genes, but it is difficult to be sure whether these are cause or effect. Unfortunately, there are no satisfactorily

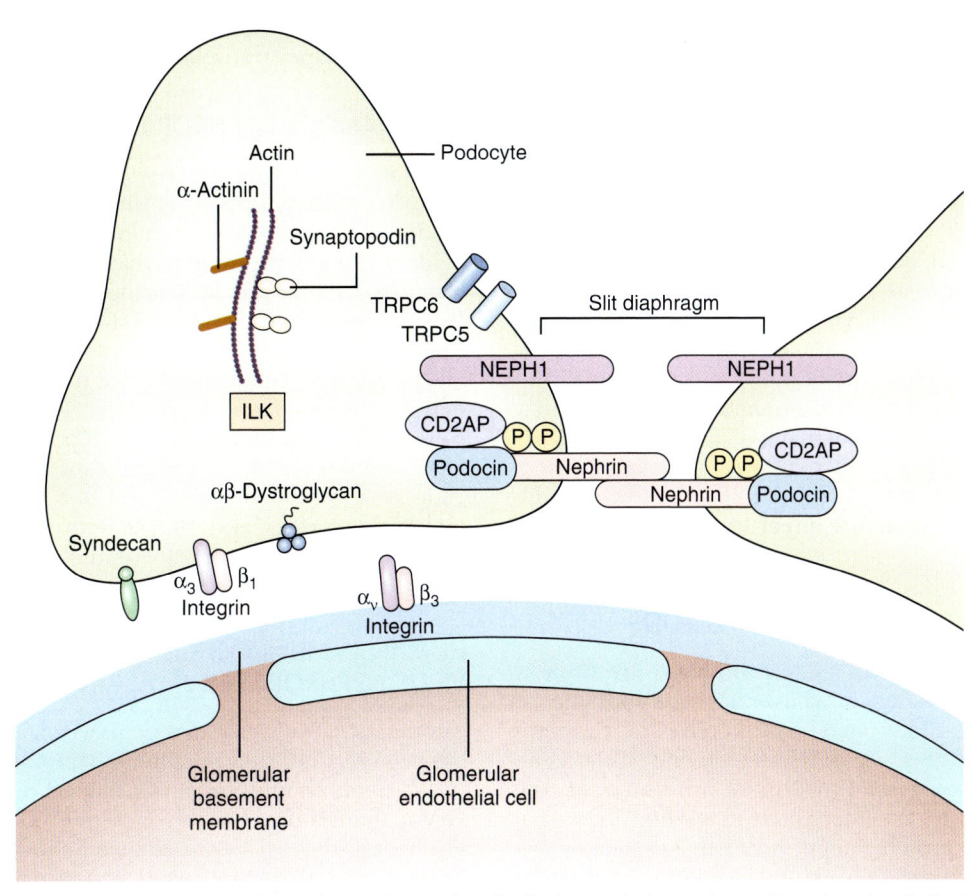

Figure 4.2 Podocyte molecular anatomy. The schema shows the slit diaphragm between two adjacent podocyte foot processes that are attached to the underlying glomerular basement membrane. Numerous constitutively expressed proteins are expressed within different geographic domains of the podocyte. CD2AP, CD2-associated protein; ILK, integrin-linked kinase; P, phosphate; TRPC5, transient receptor potential cation channel, subfamily C, member 5; TRPC6, transient receptor potential cation channel, subfamily C, member 6.

Table 4.1 Diseases of the Podocyte

Broad Classification of Podocyte Diseases	Disease	Mediators and Mechanisms of Inciting Injury to Podocytes
Traditional podocyte diseases—podocytes are considered the primary cell injured in disease	Focal segmental glomerulosclerosis	• Hereditary and congenital: due to mutations in structural podocyte proteins such as nephrin, podocin, CD2AP, TRPC6, and others • Circulating factors: candidates include suPAR • Drugs • Infections • Metabolic: obesity, hypertension
	Membranous nephropathy	• Primary: anti-PLA$_2$R antibodies • Secondary: antigen-antibody deposition, due to either preformed complexes or antibodies to existing antigens in podocytes
	Minimal change disease	• Cause unknown—circulating factors considered but not fully proven
Nontraditional podocyte diseases—podocytes considered injured as the primary or secondary cell by the disease process	Diabetic nephropathy	• Hyperglycemia • ROS • Systemic and local RAAS activation • Growth factors such as TGF-β, CTGF
	Mesangioproliferative glomerulonephritis Amyloidosis Fabry's disease Postinfectious glomerulonephritis	

CD2AP, CD2-associated protein; CTGF, connective tissue growth factor; PLA$_2$R, phospholipase A$_2$ receptor; RAAS, renin angiotensin aldosterone system; ROS, reactive oxygen species; suPAR, soluble urokinase-type plasminogen activator receptor; TGF-β, transforming growth factor-β; TRPC6, transient receptor potential cation channel, subfamily C, member 6.

specific animal models of MCD: administration of puromycin aminonucleoside causes similar morphologic changes, but puromycin aminonucleoside is a cellular toxin that is not specific for podocytes.[27] Administration of the antinephrin monoclonal antibody 5-1-6 in rats rapidly induces proteinuria with the glomerular structure initially remaining normal.[28] Perhaps the most exciting insights concern the production by podocytes of a hyposialylated version of a protein called angiopoietin-like 4, which seems to mediate proteinuria in rats overexpressing this protein selectively in their podocytes. The proteinuric animals had normal glomerular morphologic characteristics by light microscopy.[29] A later publication from the same group suggests that the normal form of angiopoietin-like 4 may actually be antiproteinuric but may explain the hypertriglyceridemia that is typically seen in nephrotic syndrome.[30] These observations strengthen the link between podocyte injury and MCD, but a direct causal link is not yet proven.

FOCAL SEGMENTAL GLOMERULOSCLEROSIS

The causes or mechanisms underlying FSGS are broadly considered as hereditary or congenital and sporadic or acquired in nature. Study of podocytes received new impetus in the late 1990s when the positional cloning of the gene responsible for congenital nephrotic syndrome of the Finnish type led to the identification of the archetypal podocyte-specific protein, nephrin.[31] This was rapidly followed by the identification of other proteinuric diseases linked to podocyte-specific single-gene disorders, including those affecting podocin,[14] Wilms' tumor 1,[32] CD2AP,[33] α-actinin-4,[34] TRPC6,[35] and phospholipase Cε_1 (PLCE1).[36] In each of these conditions it is generally accepted that proteinuria results directly from the disruption of these constitutively expressed genes in the podocyte, leading to FSGS. However, all these genetic disorders are rare, and a key question for practicing nephrologists is whether podocyte-specific gene mutations or polymorphisms play a role as predisposing factors for the much more common "sporadic" forms of proteinuric disease.

There is abundant evidence that podocyte injury and depletion lead to classical FSGS in experimental models (reviewed by D'Agati).[37] In human disease an opportunity to study the very earliest features of FSGS is afforded by studies of recurrence of this disease in transplanted kidneys: changes in podocytes can be seen in reperfusion biopsies and are predictive of full-blown FSGS recurrence.[38] An example of bringing the knowledge of podocyte biology to therapeutic application is afforded by the studies of the expression by podocytes of the protein B7-1 (also known as CD80, a protein originally thought to have its major role as a lymphocyte costimulatory protein). Upregulation of B7-1 on podocytes has been shown to be key to the development of nephrotic syndrome in various animal models,[39] and this led to the experiment in which abatacept, a fusion protein that targets B7-1, was used in the treatment of five patients with FSGS and led to marked reductions in proteinuria.[40] Another area of excitement in relation to FSGS concerns the possible role of a circulating mediator called soluble urokinase-type plasminogen activator receptor (suPAR),[41] which could also explain the recurrence of FSGS in a proportion of kidney transplants.

MEMBRANOUS NEPHROPATHY

The subepithelial (subpodocyte) location of the immune deposits in MN and analogies with the representative animal model of passive Heymann nephritis have led to attempts to identify podocyte antigens that are targets of the immune response.[42] Ronco and Debiec identified a podocyte antigen (neutral endopeptidase) that is the target of an alloimmune response in neonatal MN[43] but does not seem to explain idiopathic MN. The identification of autoantibodies to the M-type phospholipase A_2 receptor (PLA$_2$R) by Beck and colleagues in approximately 70% of patients with idiopathic MN[44] represents a very significant advance. PLA$_2$R is expressed by human podocytes, but its role in podocyte biologic processes and the causative link between anti-PLA$_2$R autoantibodies and the pathologic condition of MN require further study.

HUMAN IMMUNODEFICIENCY VIRUS NEPHROPATHY

Another acquired renal disease in which study of podocytes has been very informative is human immunodeficiency virus (HIV) nephropathy. Podocytes may be directly infected by HIV-1, though because they lack the cellular receptors for HIV that have been identified in lymphocytes, other mechanisms for uptake of HIV viral proteins may be involved.[45] Presence of HIV viral proteins leads to upregulation of the key mediator VEGF and its receptor.[46] Addition of exogenous VEGF to cultured podocytes leads to proliferation and dedifferentiation as seen in HIV nephropathy. HIV alters the shape of podocytes by disrupting the actin cytoskeleton. The kidney is known to act as a reservoir for HIV, and the podocyte may be a cell that is not easily accessible to antiviral defense mechanisms. Thus improved understanding of the relationship between HIV and the podocyte may be vitally important to the future success of anti-HIV therapeutic strategies.

DIABETIC KIDNEY DISEASE

Diabetic kidney disease, extensively covered in other parts of this edition, is the numerically and economically most important form of progressive kidney disease worldwide. The role of the podocyte therein has been the topic of much exciting literature. Podocyte number is a better predictor of prognosis in diabetic nephropathy than GBM thickness, mesangial proliferation or sclerosis, or any other feature of glomerular injury.[47-49] Podocyte abnormalities are detectable very early in the disease.[47,50] It seems that VEGF is key to understanding the importance of the podocyte in diabetic nephropathy[51] with chronic hyperglycemia leading to excessive production of VEGF by the podocyte and an abnormal crosstalk with the nitric oxide pathway. There may also be a link with insulin responsiveness of podocytes: insulin stimulates the production of VEGF by podocytes,[52] and the selective deletion of the insulin receptor from podocytes leads to progressive kidney disease with many features in common with diabetic nephropathy even though these animals are not diabetic.[53]

RESPONSES BY PODOCYTES TO DISEASE-INDUCED INJURY: LINKING STRUCTURE TO FUNCTION TO CLINICAL FINDINGS

The discussion of how podocytes may be injured in the common individual proteinuric glomerular diseases leads to the question "How does podocyte injury translate into the characteristic clinical findings in these diseases?" This requires that we focus on how the responses to podocyte injury lead to the characteristic histopathologic changes seen on renal biopsy, proteinuria (the clinical signature of podocyte injury), and glomerulosclerosis (which leads to reduced kidney function and progression of the disease).

EFFACEMENT: A HISTOLOGIC CHANGE IN PODOCYTE SHAPE MEDIATED BY THE ACTIN CYTOSKELETON

The podocyte depends for its normal functions on maintenance of the complex architecture of interdigitating secondary cell processes. Anything that disrupts this will lead to damage to the selective glomerular filter, with proteinuria being the demonstrable clinical consequence. Regardless of the underlying disease, a characteristic and almost predictable response to podocyte injury is a change in the shape of podocytes, called effacement (Figure 4.3).[54] On examination by electron microscopy, effaced podocytes appear flattened and even fused (although the latter does not happen functionally). Numerous studies have shown that effacement is an active process, due to changes in the actin cytoskeleton of the podocyte, which forms the "backbone" of these highly specialized cells.[17] Further evidence that effacement is an active process is that in some instances it can be reversed, such as in treatment-responsive patients with MCD. There has been debate whether effacement per se causes proteinuria, because proteinuria due to podocyte damage can occur independent of this change in shape. The relationship between podocyte foot process effacement and proteinuria has been questioned,[55] and it is clear that there is still much to learn about this long-recognized but still poorly understood ultrastructural phenomenon. Confusingly, effacement has also been reported (in the absence of proteinuria) in the protein-malnutrition state kwashiorkor,[56] suggesting that it may be a feature of hypoalbuminemia rather than of proteinuria per se. However, it is the view of the authors that effacement is a manifestation of serious podocyte injury, and that this histologic finding implies changes in either slit diaphragm proteins, actin binding and regulating proteins, podocyte attachment to the GBM, and/or other events. Therefore teasing out precisely the biologic role of effacement in the development and maintenance of proteinuria may not be important.

How does effacement occur? Several genetic studies in humans have been very instructive in understanding podocyte biology in general and the role of the actin cytoskeleton in particular (reviewed by Wang and von der Lehr).[57] For example, we now appreciate the importance of the gene encoding α-actinin-4, which plays an important role in actin polymerization. The mutant form of α-actinin-4 binds more avidly to actin and affects the mechanical properties of actin gels, providing an explanation for its effect on podocyte structure when mutated in autosomal dominant late-onset familial FSGS.[34] Experimental approaches have been employed to better understand the pathogenesis. To this end, the podocyte-specific transgenic expression of the mutant α-actinin-4 gene in mice leads to FSGS,[58] demonstrating that it is the effects of the gene in the podocyte rather than any other cell that is responsible for the disease. The final experimental proof of the causative role of the mutation came in experiments showing that when the mutant gene was "knocked in" in mice, the animals developed FSGS, showing that this gene defect alone is capable of causing the disease.[59] The mechanisms underlying the effects of the mutant protein were later demonstrated in detail,[60] and there is further evidence that the physicochemical characteristics of actin fibers formed with the mutant α-actinin-4 show altered flexibility that can explain the effects on the podocyte.[61] α-Actinin-4 protein mutants have been shown to mislocalize to the cell cytoplasm and lose their ability to associate with nuclear receptors and activate gene transcription.[62] Other groups have reported different gene mutations that affect the actin cytoskeleton and also cause FSGS. For instance, the gene encoding CD2AP encodes a protein that is important in linking to actin fibers.[33] Intriguingly, calcineurin antagonists and corticosteroids, discussed further in the section on therapeutic approaches, both have beneficial effects on the podocyte actin cytoskeleton, and this may be an important

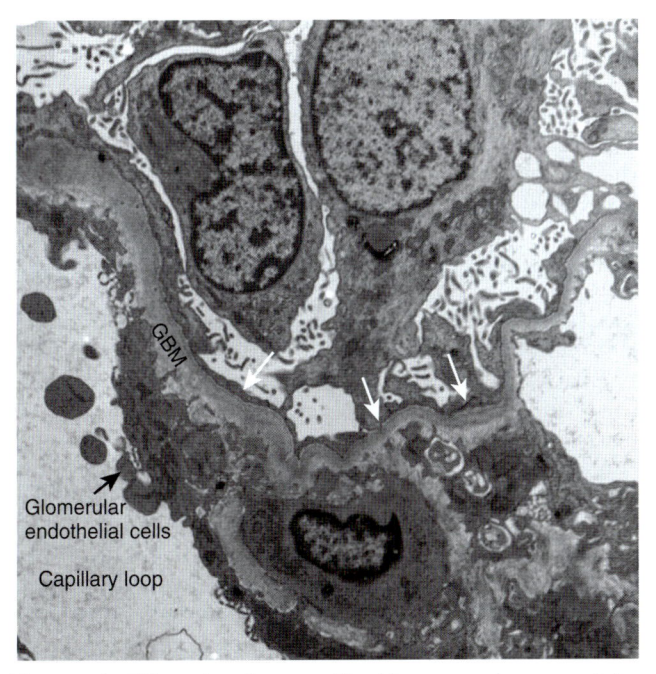

Figure 4.3 Effaced podocytes. The biopsy specimen was taken from a patient with focal segmental glomerulosclerosis. The electron micrograph shows that the foot processes appear flattened and give the impression that they are fused (*white arrows*). This ultrastructural change is called effacement. GBM, Glomerular basement membrane. (Figure was provided by Dr. Behzad Najafian, University of Washington.)

component of their mechanisms of action in proteinuric diseases.[63]

PROTEINURIA DUE TO REDUCED SIZE AND/OR CHARGE PROPERTIES

One of the most important biologic functions of podocytes is to limit the passage of plasma proteins into the urinary space. The podocyte slit diaphragm is a major size barrier to albumin and other proteins, and studies have suggested the possibility that this also serves as a charge barrier too. A hereditary or acquired defect of one or more structural proteins making up the slit diaphragm, such as nephrin, podocin, and TRPC6, leads to abnormal function, allowing increased passage of proteins across this barrier. In acquired diseases, either an absolute decrease in their levels or a change in their subcellular location is associated with proteinuria.[64] Moreover, given the complex interplay between proteins making up the slit diaphragm, a change in one slit diaphragm protein often leads to a cascading dysfunction of one or more of the other proteins.[65] The outer surface of podocytes is negatively charged due to the constitutive expression of proteins such as podocalyxin.[66] Although no known hereditary mutations have been described, reduced podocalyxin levels lead to proteinuria. Another mechanism for proteinuria is a decrease in podocyte number, which simply creates gaps in this layer, enabling proteins to escape through the cellular barrier.

A second mechanism underlying proteinuria from podocyte injury is its effect on the underlying GBM.[67] Recall that podocytes constitute the outermost layer of the glomerular filtration barrier, which includes the GBM to which it is anchored, and the innermost fenestrated and highly specialized glomerular endothelial cells. The GBM derives embryologically from both podocytes and glomerular endothelial cells. In adults, podocytes can alter GBM structure and function in disease as follows. In membranous and diabetic nephropathy, podocytes produce and secrete increased extracellular matrix proteins, which are laid down along the GBM, eventually leading to the characteristic thickening of the underlying GBM in these diseases.[68] The altered extracellular matrix composition leads to secondary changes (loss) in negative charge to the GBM, thereby enabling increased passage of proteins. In addition, increased production by and secretion from podocytes of reactive oxygen species and metalloproteinases leads to degradation of the GBM and proteinuria.

A third mechanism underlying proteinuria following podocyte injury is its effect on the glomerular endothelial cell. The survival of glomerular endothelial cells is dependent in part on VEGF produced and secreted from podocytes.[69] A decrease in production by podocytes, such as when podocyte number decreases, leads to secondary apoptosis of glomerular endothelial cells, which in turn is accompanied by a decrease in resistance of this layer of the glomerular filtration barrier.

In general, increased knowledge about genetic causes of nephrotic syndrome has so far had a disappointingly limited impact on understanding, prediction, or management of sporadic cases. In children with steroid-resistant nephrotic syndrome, with or without a positive family history, up to 20% may have mutations in *NPHS2*, the gene encoding podocin, particular mutations being strongly associated with early age of presentation.[70] In the other 80% of children, and in adult patients, the genetic contribution remains uncertain, although one study suggested that the most frequently reported variant of *NPHS2*, known as R229Q, increased the risk for sporadic FSGS in European-derived populations by 20% to 40%.[71] One small study of sporadic disease has reported that heterozygous mutations in one or more podocyte genes can predispose to FSGS[72]; this awaits confirmation in larger studies and in different populations. Analysis of podocyte genes as predisposing factors for diabetic nephropathy has so far produced negative results.[73] Studies of the increased susceptibility of African Americans to FSGS have implicated variants of another gene expressed in podocytes, apolipoprotein L1, although the causal mechanism remains obscure.[74-76]

Finding a genetic cause in a patient with apparently acquired nephrotic syndrome has implications for management. For example, a therapeutic response to steroids or immunosuppression is unlikely. Avoiding these drugs spares patients from unnecessary exposure to toxic therapies. Also, disease recurrence after transplantation is less likely. Regrettably, at present such information assists in the management of only a very small proportion of patients.

GLOMERULOSCLEROSIS AND REDUCED KIDNEY FUNCTION: A CORRELATION WITH DEPLETION IN PODOCYTE NUMBER

Many podocyte diseases such as FSGS, MN, and diabetic kidney disease are accompanied by a progressive decline in overall kidney function, measured clinically by a decrease in glomerular filtration rate. This is largely due to glomerulosclerosis, with or without tubulointerstitial fibrosis. Patterns of glomerulosclerosis histologically include a segmental form (a portion of an individual glomerulus is scarred) and the more extensive global form (the majority of an individual glomerulus scars). There are several mechanisms whereby injury to podocytes leads to glomerulosclerosis. First is the association of reduced podocyte number and scarring.[77] Several glomerular diseases are accompanied by podocyte apoptosis, necroptosis, necrosis, detachment, and dysregulated autophagy.[78] These lead to podocyte depletion. However, because podocytes are terminally differentiated epithelial cells, they are unable to adequately proliferate to replace those lost because of the events described earlier.[79] This is in part due to cell cycle arrest secondary to an increase in cyclin kinase inhibitors,[80] and/or mitotic catastrophe.[81] This imbalance (loss exceeding regeneration) ultimately leads to progressive podocyte depletion. The consequences of this have been well delineated experimentally as follows. When podocyte number is reduced by 20% of normal, mesangial cells begin to proliferate and undergo expansion.[82] When podocyte number is reduced by 40%, segmental glomerulosclerosis ensues, with global glomerulosclerosis when podocyte number is below 60% of normal.[82] A decrease in podocyte number is one of the best predictors for a poor outcome in clinical diabetic kidney disease. Studies have suggested that despite a lack of proliferation, podocyte number can be restored following certain therapies such as angiotensin-converting enzyme inhibition.[83] If podocyte regeneration does occur, then a possible source might be stem or progenitor cells derived from glomerular parietal epithelial cells[84] and/or cells of renin lineage,[85] although further studies are needed to fully validate these findings.

The cellular sources of the increase in extracellular matrix proteins in podocyte diseases derive from podocytes and also from their neighbors, the parietal epithelial cells. Studies have shown that podocytes produce increased matrix proteins in response to C5b-9, high glucose level, angiotensin II, and numerous other factors upregulated in disease.[68,86] This is mediated by cytokines such as transforming growth factor-β, connective tissue growth factor, and others. Later studies show that in diseases considered primarily podocyte in nature, the parietal epithelial cells become activated (defined as the de novo expression of CD44) and migrate from Bowman's capsule onto the glomerular tuft, where they produce and deposit extracellular matrix proteins. The composition of this extracellular matrix is related to that of Bowman's capsule.[87]

Finally, studies have shown that following podocyte depletion, the number of podocytes can be normalized under certain circumstances despite the absence of proliferation. Such findings would imply a regenerative pathway or pathways arising from another source. A study of kidneys transplanted from female donors into male recipients identified "male" (i.e., recipient)–derived podocytes in half the cases.[88] In humans, increasing evidence suggests that a subset of the neighboring glomerular parietal epithelial cells located at the tubular pole might serve as podocyte progenitors. Experimental data in mice do not support this at the time of writing this chapter. Experimental studies suggest that cells of renin lineage, normally residing in the juxtaglomerular compartment, might also serve as adult podocyte progenitors in states of podocyte depletion.[85]

EFFECTS OF EXISTING THERAPIES ON PODOCYTES

Regrettably no therapeutic approaches are currently available that specifically target podocytes in disease. However, several therapies have, in addition to their systemic effects, direct biologic actions on podocytes (i.e., pleiotropic actions), and these will be considered in the following sections.

GLUCOCORTICOSTEROIDS

Steroids are widely used in the treatment of proteinuric diseases, but their modes of action, especially in those forms of nephrotic syndrome, such as MCD, in which there is no inflammation remains completely unknown. Glucocorticoid receptor (GR) expression is ubiquitous. Therefore, in theory, any cell type could be affected by these drugs. The identification of the podocyte as the key cell type in proteinuric disease made it logical to examine whether effects of glucocorticoids on podocytes could explain their efficacy in nephrotic syndrome. Initial reports in murine[89] and human[90] podocytes showed that dexamethasone had potent biologic effects directly on podocyte structure and function. These include limiting podocyte apoptosis,[91] enhanced nephrin transport,[92] and effects on the actin cytoskeleton. It has been shown that GR-induced signaling pathways are functional in murine podocytes, having transcriptional and posttranscriptional effects on podocyte genes.[93] Dexamethasone increases phosphorylation of nephrin at a key intracellular tyrosine residue in cultured human podocytes, and this phosphorylation is blocked by a GR antagonist but not by a mineralocorticoid receptor antagonist.[94] It is assumed that phosphorylation of nephrin is important for its function, and the same group has shown[95] that nephrin phosphorylation is reduced in puromycin aminonucleoside nephrosis in rats and in human MCD. Thus an effect of corticosteroids to reverse these nephrin changes could provide a plausible mechanism of their action in MCD. Finally, studies have shown that administering corticosteroids to mice with FSGS following podocyte depletion does significantly increase podocyte number.[96] This is not due to proliferation and might be due to the augmentation of podocyte progenitors, although further studies are needed to better define this effect.[96]

CALCINEURIN INHIBITORS

The calcineurin inhibitors cyclosporine and tacrolimus are widely used in nephrotic syndrome, either alone or in combination with other therapies. An elegant study showed that the effects of cyclosporine on proteinuria are independent of its effects on the immune system and defined the calcineurin-dependent dephosphorylation of synaptopodin, which in turn leads to destabilization of the podocyte actin cytoskeleton, as the key reaction in podocytes that is inhibited by cyclosporine.[97] The net effect is that cyclosporine can stabilize the actin cytoskeleton in podocytes and thereby reduce proteinuria directly.[97]

ANTI–B CELL THERAPY

The specific anti–B cell monoclonal antibody rituximab, increasingly thought to be effective in proteinuric diseases even when they are not all obviously immune mediated, has been shown to have direct effects on podocytes, including stabilizing their actin cytoskeleton.[98] Although monoclonal antibodies are assumed to have very specific binding targets, they can also have "off-target" effects. In this case it seems that rituximab, as well as binding to the CD20 molecule that is its accepted molecular target, also binds to a podocyte protein called sphingomyelin phosphodiesterase acid-like 3b, (SMPDL-3b) and this protein stabilizes the actin cytoskeleton.

RENIN ANGIOTENSIN ALDOSTERONE SYSTEM INHIBITORS

The levels of tissue angiotensin II and the angiotensin subtype 1 receptor are increased in podocytes following injury in several glomerular diseases, including diabetic kidney disease.[99] The consequences include increased apoptosis, extracellular matrix protein accumulation, reactive oxygen species production and oxidative stress, alterations in several slit diaphragm proteins, increased calcium influx, cell cycle inhibition, detachment and inflammatory cytokine production, and other deleterious effects.[99,100] Angiotensin-converting enzyme inhibitors, AT_1R

antagonists, and mineralocorticoid receptor blockers are effective at reducing many of these deleterious effects on podocytes, independent of their blood pressure–lowering effects. For these reasons, inhibition of the renin angiotensin aldosterone system is currently the standard of care for lowering proteinuria.

IDENTIFICATION OF CANDIDATE THERAPEUTIC APPROACHES FOR THE FUTURE

In theory, any intervention that stabilizes the podocyte actin cytoskeleton or promotes podocyte recovery or repair should have therapeutic potential in proteinuric states; the challenge is to selectively target these effects to the podocyte. For example, hepatocyte growth factor appears to have reparative effects in podocytes injured by Adriamycin in vivo and in vitro[101] and in the glomerular injury induced by lipopolysaccharide.[102] Interferon-β reduces proteinuria in several experimental models of glomerulonephritis without apparently affecting inflammation and has marked effects on human podocytes and glomerular endothelial cells in vitro.[103] Inhibition of integrin-linked kinase protects podocytes in vivo and in vitro.[104] Inhibition of another kinase, focal adhesion kinase, prevents podocyte foot process effacement in vivo and reduces spreading and migration of podocytes in vitro.[105]

The great prize would be to develop podocyte protective therapies for diabetic nephropathy, this being the numerically most important cause of progressive kidney disease worldwide. In experimental diabetic nephropathy, blockade of the cannabinoid receptor 1 reduces albuminuria.[106] Targeting of the Notch pathway also looks likely to protect podocytes in diabetic nephropathy.[107] Targeting of insulin sensitizers to the podocyte could be a promising novel therapeutic approach: metformin[108] and rosiglitazone[109] have podocyte-protective effects. The critical role of VEGF in the balance of angiogenesis and anti-angiogenesis in diabetic nephropathy has already been discussed. Vasohibin-1, a negative regulator of angiogenesis, has been shown to have protective effects against the effects on podocytes of high glucose levels in vitro and in vivo, at least partly due to an interaction with VEGF.[110]

Specific targeting of therapeutic agents to any individual cell type is a familiar issue in all fields of medicine; the podocyte-specific gene expression profile that has been so informative in understanding podocytes in health and disease also holds out the possibility of targeted therapy.

SUMMARY

Much has been learned about podocytes in health and disease in the past 2 decades. The generation of "podocyte-specific" transgenic mice, as well as the development of several cell lines, has enabled investigators to better understand this dynamic and highly specialized, terminally differentiated epithelial cell. Podocytes constitutively express numerous cell-specific proteins required for normal function, and when these proteins are mutated genetically, or their levels and/or subcellular localization are altered in acquired diseases, the loss of normal function is manifest clinically. Moreover, these proteins are constantly communicating with one another through elaborate signaling pathways to ensure that they function properly to limit the passage of proteins from the blood compartment to the urinary space, while also maintaining a normal shape. Clearly podocytes do not function in isolation. Rather, they are critical for normal glomerular endothelial cell health, and likely GBM maintenance, and likely communicate with parietal epithelial cells by poorly understood pathways. Thus, when injured, they cause changes to other glomerular cells and structures to some extent, depending on the glomerular disease type. These changes can include mesangial proliferation, parietal epithelial cell activation, glomerular endothelial cell death, and/or GBM thickening. Our understanding of the causes of podocyte diseases, which except for diabetic kidney disease are rare, has improved substantially, as evidenced by the discovery of the anti-PLA$_2$R autoantibody in MN and the identification of genetic disorders underlying FSGS.

Several clinical and experimental challenges and opportunities lie ahead. Perhaps one of the biggest is podocyte regeneration, because these cells are simply unable to proliferate successfully or adequately to replace any depletion in their overall number. Designing and delivering therapeutic agents specific to podocytes is actively being pursued, both to enhance efficacy and to reduce systemic side effects. Noninvasive diagnostic testing is being keenly studied, such as measuring podocyte products in the urine, and markers in the serum and urine. Live video imaging is significantly advancing our understanding of the movement and behavior of podocytes under normal and stressed conditions beyond the traditional "fixed" pictures using conventional microscopy. Urinary and plasma biomarkers are being identified that it is hoped will translate into clinical practice. The past 2 decades have witnessed phenomenal advances in understanding podocyte biology in health and disease, and the future looks ever so bright too. There is definite hope for our patients.

Complete reference list available at ExpertConsult.com.

KEY REFERENCES

1. Jefferson JA, Shankland SJ, Pichler RH: Proteinuria in diabetic kidney disease: a mechanistic viewpoint. *Kidney Int* 74:22–36, 2008.
2. Gansevoort RT, Correa-Rotter R, Hemmelgarn BR, et al: Chronic kidney disease and cardiovascular risk: epidemiology, mechanisms, and prevention. *Lancet* 382:339–352, 2013.
3. Jefferson JA, Nelson PJ, Najafian B, et al: Podocyte disorders: core curriculum 2011. *Am J Kidney Dis* 58:666–677, 2011.
4. Brinkkoetter PT, Ising C, Benzing T: The role of the podocyte in albumin filtration. *Nat Rev Nephrol* 9:328–336, 2013.
5. Hohne M, Ising C, Hagmann H, et al: Light microscopic visualization of podocyte ultrastructure demonstrates oscillating glomerular contractions. *Am J Pathol* 182:332–338, 2013.
6. Byron A, Randles MJ, Humphries JD, et al: Glomerular cell crosstalk influences composition and assembly of extracellular matrix. *J Am Soc Nephrol* 25:953–966, 2014.
7. Jin J, Sison K, Li C, et al: Soluble FLT1 binds lipid microdomains in podocytes to control cell morphology and glomerular barrier function. *Cell* 151:384–399, 2012.
8. Jeansson M, Gawlik A, Anderson G, et al: Angiopoietin-1 is essential in mouse vasculature during development and in response to injury. *J Clin Invest* 121:2278–2289, 2011.

9. Gagliardini E, Conti S, Benigni A, et al: Imaging of the porous ultrastructure of the glomerular epithelial filtration slit. *J Am Soc Nephrol* 21:2081–2089, 2010.
10. Wartiovaara J, Ofverstedt LG, Khoshnoodi J, et al: Nephrin strands contribute to a porous slit diaphragm scaffold as revealed by electron tomography. *J Clin Invest* 114:1475–1483, 2004.
11. Grahammer F, Schell C, Huber TB: The podocyte slit diaphragm—from a thin grey line to a complex signalling hub. *Nat Rev Nephrol* 9:587–598, 2013.
12. Gerke P, Sellin L, Kretz O, et al: NEPH2 is located at the glomerular slit diaphragm, interacts with nephrin and is cleaved from podocytes by metalloproteinases. *J Am Soc Nephrol* 16:1693–1702, 2005.
13. Adair BD, Altintas MM, Moller CC, et al: Structure of the kidney slit diaphragm adapter protein CD2-associated protein as determined with electron microscopy. *J Am Soc Nephrol* 25:1465–1473, 2014.
14. Boute N, Gribouval O, Roselli S, et al: NPHS2, encoding the glomerular protein podocin, is mutated in autosomal recessive steroid-resistant nephrotic syndrome. *Nat Genet* 24:349–354, 2000.
15. Schaldecker T, Kim S, Tarabanis C, et al: Inhibition of the TRPC5 ion channel protects the kidney filter. *J Clin Invest* 123:5298–5309, 2013.
16. Mathieson PW: Nephrin sends us signals. *Kidney Int* 64:756–757, 2003.
17. George B, Holzman LB: Signaling from the podocyte intercellular junction to the actin cytoskeleton. *Semin Nephrol* 32:307–318, 2012.
18. New LA, Keyvani Chahi A, Jones N: Direct regulation of nephrin tyrosine phosphorylation by Nck adaptor proteins. *J Biol Chem* 288:1500–1510, 2013.
19. Welsh GI, Saleem MA: The podocyte cytoskeleton—key to a functioning glomerulus in health and disease. *Nat Rev Nephrol* 8:14–21, 2012.
20. Dandapani SV, Sugimoto H, Matthews BD, et al: Alpha-actinin-4 is required for normal podocyte adhesion. *J Biol Chem* 282:467–477, 2007.
21. Tian X, Kim JJ, Monkley SM, et al: Podocyte-associated talin1 is critical for glomerular filtration barrier maintenance. *J Clin Invest* 124:1098–1113, 2014.
22. Sachs N, Sonnenberg A: Cell-matrix adhesion of podocytes in physiology and disease. *Nat Rev Nephrol* 9:200–210, 2013.
23. Wang L, Ellis MJ, Gomez JA, et al: Mechanisms of the proteinuria induced by Rho GTPases. *Kidney Int* 81:1075–1085, 2012.
24. Asanuma K, Yanagida-Asanuma E, Faul C, et al: Synaptopodin orchestrates actin organization and cell motility via regulation of RhoA signalling. *Nat Cell Biol* 8:485–491, 2006.
25. Jefferson JA, Alpers CE, Shankland SJ: Podocyte biology for the bedside. *Am J Kidney Dis* 58:835–845, 2011.
26. Wiggins RC: The spectrum of podocytopathies: a unifying view of glomerular diseases. *Kidney Int* 71:1205–1214, 2007.
27. Pippin JW, Brinkkoetter PT, Cormack-Aboud FC, et al: Inducible rodent models of acquired podocyte diseases. *Am J Physiol Renal Physiol* 296:F213–F229, 2009.
28. Kawachi H, Koike H, Shimizu F: mAb 5-1-6 nephropathy and nephrin. *Microsc Res Tech* 57:236–240, 2002.
29. Clement LC, Avila-Casado C, Mace C, et al: Podocyte-secreted angiopoietin-like-4 mediates proteinuria in glucocorticoid-sensitive nephrotic syndrome. *Nat Med* 17:117–122, 2011.
30. Clement LC, Mace C, Avila-Casado C, et al: Circulating angiopoietin-like 4 links proteinuria with hypertriglyceridemia in nephrotic syndrome. *Nat Med* 20:37–46, 2014.
31. Kestila M, Lenkkeri U, Mannikko M, et al: Positionally cloned gene for a novel glomerular protein—nephrin—is mutated in congenital nephrotic syndrome. *Mol Cell* 1:575–582, 1998.
32. Jeanpierre C, Denamur E, Henry I, et al: Identification of constitutional WT1 mutations, in patients with isolated diffuse mesangial sclerosis, and analysis of genotype/phenotype correlations by use of a computerized mutation database. *Am J Hum Genet* 62:824–833, 1998.
33. Shih NY, Li J, Karpitskii V, et al: Congenital nephrotic syndrome in mice lacking CD2-associated protein. *Science* 286:312–315, 1999.
34. Kaplan JM, Kim SH, North KN, et al: Mutations in ACTN4, encoding alpha-actinin-4, cause familial focal segmental glomerulosclerosis. *Nat Genet* 24:251–256, 2000.
35. Winn MP, Conlon PJ, Lynn KL, et al: A mutation in the TRPC6 cation channel causes familial focal segmental glomerulosclerosis. *Science* 308:1801–1804, 2005.
36. Hinkes B, Wiggins RC, Gbadegesin R, et al: Positional cloning uncovers mutations in PLCE1 responsible for a nephrotic syndrome variant that may be reversible. *Nat Genet* 38:1397–1405, 2006.
37. D'Agati VD: Pathobiology of focal segmental glomerulosclerosis: new developments. *Curr Opin Nephrol Hypertens* 21:243–250, 2012.
38. Chang JW, Pardo V, Sageshima J, et al: Podocyte foot process effacement in postreperfusion allograft biopsies correlates with early recurrence of proteinuria in focal segmental glomerulosclerosis. *Transplantation* 93:1238–1244, 2012.
39. Reiser J, von Gersdorff G, Loos M, et al: Induction of B7-1 in podocytes is associated with nephrotic syndrome. *J Clin Invest* 113:1390–1397, 2004.
40. Yu CC, Fornoni A, Weins A, et al: Abatacept in B7-1-positive proteinuric kidney disease. *N Engl J Med* 369:2416–2423, 2013.
41. Smith HK, Nelson KL, Calaunan ES, et al: Effect of anaerobiosis on the antibiotic susceptibility of *H. influenzae*. *BMC Res Notes* 6:241, 2013.
42. Jefferson JA, Pippin JW, Shankland SJ: Experimental models of membranous nephropathy. *Drug Discov Today Dis Models* 7:27–33, 2010.
43. Ronco P, Debiec H: Target antigens and nephritogenic antibodies in membranous nephropathy: of rats and men. *Semin Immunopathol* 29:445–458, 2007.
44. Beck LH, Jr, Bonegio RG, Lambeau G, et al: M-type phospholipase A2 receptor as target antigen in idiopathic membranous nephropathy. *N Engl J Med* 361:11–21, 2009.
45. Bruggeman LA, Nelson PJ: Controversies in the pathogenesis of HIV-associated renal diseases. *Nat Rev Nephrol* 5:574–581, 2009.
46. Korgaonkar SN, Feng X, Ross MD, et al: HIV-1 upregulates VEGF in podocytes. *J Am Soc Nephrol* 19:877–883, 2008.
47. Meyer TW, Bennett PH, Nelson RG: Podocyte number predicts long-term urinary albumin excretion in Pima Indians with type II diabetes and microalbuminuria. *Diabetologia* 42:1341–1344, 1999.
48. Pagtalunan ME, Miller PL, Jumping-Eagle S, et al: Podocyte loss and progressive glomerular injury in type II diabetes. *J Clin Invest* 99:342–348, 1997.
49. Lemley KV: Diabetes and chronic kidney disease: lessons from the Pima Indians. *Pediatr Nephrol* 23:1933–1940, 2008.
50. Wolf G, Chen S, Ziyadeh FN: From the periphery of the glomerular capillary wall toward the center of disease: podocyte injury comes of age in diabetic nephropathy. *Diabetes* 54:1626–1634, 2005.
51. Tufro A, Veron D: VEGF and podocytes in diabetic nephropathy. *Semin Nephrol* 32:385–393, 2012.

5

Metabolic Basis of Solute Transport

Prabhleen Singh | Alicia A. McDonough | Scott C. Thomson

CHAPTER OUTLINE

THERMODYNAMIC APPROACH TO METABOLISM AND TRANSPORT, 123
Thermodynamic Analysis of Kidney Function, 123
Application of the Laws of Thermodynamics to Kidney Function, 123
ENERGY AND THE SODIUM PUMP, 124
Structure of the Sodium Pump, 124
Other Adenosine Triphosphatases, 124
Pump-Leak Process and the Sodium Potential, 124
Harnessing the Sodium Potential for Work, 125
CELL POLARITY AND VECTORIAL TRANSPORT, 126
METABOLIC SUBSTRATES FUELING ACTIVE TRANSPORT ALONG THE NEPHRON, 126
Metabolism Basics, 126
Whittam Model, 127
Energy Requirements and Substrate Use along the Nephron, 128
Renal Gluconeogenesis and Lactate Handling, 130

NEPHRON REGION–SPECIFIC METABOLIC CONSIDERATIONS, 132
Proximal Tubule, 132
Thick Ascending Limb, 132
Cortical Collecting Duct, 133
Medullary Collecting Duct, 133
CONTROL OF RENAL OXYGENATION, 133
Renal Blood Flow and Oxygen Consumption, 133
Tubuloglomerular Feedback, 135
Metabolic Cost of Sodium Reabsorption, 135
REGULATION OF METABOLIC EFFICIENCY OF TRANSPORT DURING NORMAL PERTURBATIONS AND DISEASE, 138
Physiologic Regulation: Filtration Fraction and Oxygen Consumption, 138
Hypoxia and Ischemia, 139
Adenosine Monophosphate–Activated Protein Kinase, 140
Mitochondrial Diseases, 142
SUMMARY, 142

The term *metabolism* refers to the entire set of interconnected chemical reactions within living organisms that form and maintain tissue and govern the storage and release of energy to sustain life. This chapter is dedicated to one aspect of kidney metabolism—namely the storage, release, and utilization of energy by the nephron as it transforms the glomerular filtrate into urine.

How much energy is required to make the urine? Of the major body organs, the kidney consumes the second highest amount of oxygen per gram of tissue (2.7 mmol/kg/min for the kidney vs. 4.3 mmol/kg/min for the heart).[1] Most of the potential energy provided by renal oxidative metabolism is committed to epithelial transport, which determines the volume and composition of the urine. It has been asserted that because the kidney reabsorbs 99% of the glomerular filtrate, it must use a lot of energy—but this logic is incorrect. The minimum net energy required for reabsorption does not depend on the amount of fluid that is reabsorbed. Forming a volume of urine with a solute composition equal to that of the body fluid from which it is formed is the thermodynamic equivalent of partitioning a bucket into two compartments by the use of a divider, which requires no net energy. On the other hand, energy is required to form a urine that differs in solute composition from that of the body fluids (e.g., plasma). To appreciate this, consider that the hypothetical remixing of urine with plasma would cause the formation of entropy, known as *mixing entropy*. Thus, energy is required to form urine from plasma and attain a state of reduced entropy. The minimum amount of energy required for this is equal to the temperature multiplied by the decrease in mixing entropy associated with the differential solute composition of urine versus plasma.

This chapter provides an overview of the interdependence of renal solute transport and renal metabolism, including the following: (1) role of the sodium pump,

Na⁺-K⁺-ATPase, in epithelial transport; (2) metabolic substrates fueling active transport along the nephron and regional metabolic considerations; (3) role of renal blood flow, glomerular filtration rate, and tubuloglomerular feedback in controlling fluid and electrolyte filtration and tissue oxygenation; (4) amount of oxygen consumed per sodium reabsorbed (Q_{O_2}/T_{Na}); and (5) metabolic efficiency of transport during normal perturbations and disease.

THERMODYNAMIC APPROACH TO METABOLISM AND TRANSPORT

THERMODYNAMIC ANALYSIS OF KIDNEY FUNCTION

Interest in kidney metabolism antedates most knowledge of the kidney's inner workings or of biochemistry. The theoretical minimum amount of energy required to make urine was determined from the laws of equilibrium thermodynamics nearly a century ago. For a human in balance on a typical diet, the cost of converting the glomerular filtrate into urine by an idealized process that is 100% efficient, infinitely slow, completely reversible, involves no backleak, and generates no entropy and heat is about 0.5 cal/min/1.73 m².[2] In reality, the kidney consumes more than 50-fold this amount of energy. On this basis alone, one might argue that the kidney is horribly inefficient, even after one subtracts the cost to the kidney of maintaining itself. On the other hand, added costs are imposed by the requirement to make urine in a finite amount of time, need for flexibility to alter the volume and composition of the urine rapidly, stoichiometric constraints of biochemistry, known limits on the thermodynamic efficiency of oxidative phosphorylation, and intrinsic permeabilities of tissues to electrolytes, gases, and urea.

The thermodynamic requirement may be a small fraction of the actual expenditure, but before one concludes that the body is unconcerned with thermodynamics, it may be noted that the thermodynamic energy required of the kidney to maintain salt and nitrogen balance with consumption of a typical diet is minimized with the usual water intake of 1 to 2 L/day. This is consistent with an evolutionary process geared to minimize the thermodynamic energy requirements of the kidney.

Moreover, the thermodynamic cost of excreting urea declines as blood urea nitrogen (BUN) concentration increases. Thus, as the BUN level rises in kidney disease, less energy is required to maintain the nitrogen balance. In kidney disease, the urine composition is also restricted to a narrower range. Using a classic thermodynamic approach, Newburgh suggested that the composition of the urine and body fluids in kidney disease are determined by the available free energy and noted that the declining flexibility of the diseased kidney to vary the urine composition could be predicted from the reduced free energy available for transport.[3]

APPLICATION OF THE LAWS OF THERMODYNAMICS TO KIDNEY FUNCTION

The macroscopic laws of equilibrium thermodynamics apply to kidney metabolism; any theory of metabolism is necessarily incorrect if it violates these laws. The laws of thermodynamics essentially describe transitions of a system from one state to another. The first law of thermodynamics states that total energy is conserved during any process that occurs in a closed system. When a system is open to its environment, the combined energy of the system plus environment remains constant. When the total internal energy, temperature, pressure, and volume of a system remain constant, any process that yields a change in free energy also yields a reciprocal change in entropy. Doing work on the system is equivalent to adding free energy to the system, which determines the upper limit of how much useful work the system can do against its environment.

The first law of thermodynamics stipulates that total energy is conserved throughout any process, but provides no other indication of whether a given process will occur spontaneously. The glomerular filtrate contains a mixture of salt and urea. The tubule partitions this into urine and reabsorbate. The urine has a different ratio of urea to salt than the reabsorbate, so the entropy has decreased. However, the total internal energy of the combined urine and reabsorbate is the same as the original filtrate. Hence, the first law would be satisfied if the urine were to form spontaneously from the filtrate. The fact that NaCl and urea never sort themselves spontaneously into regions of higher and lower concentration is a consequence of the second law of thermodynamics, which states that all spontaneous processes generate entropy. Conversely, all spontaneous processes dissipate free energy and will cease when the supply of free energy is exhausted. It is possible to reduce entropy or elevate free energy in a system, but only if the system imports energy from its surroundings, in which case there will be an increase in entropy of the surroundings that exceeds the decrease in entropy of the system. Some processes in the kidney, such as conversion of chemical to mechanical energy by Na⁺-K⁺-ATPase, are highly efficient and generate almost no entropy. Other processes, such as the countercurrent multiplier, are inefficient and generate a lot of entropy. As a rule, those processes that generate the least entropy work over short distances and short times.

The laws of equilibrium thermodynamics determine the direction of any spontaneous process, but they do not address the rate of change. Hence, the laws of equilibrium thermodynamics are not adequate for a full description of a living system that is displaced from equilibrium and characterized by flow of matter and energy within the system itself, as well as between the system and its environment. Thermodynamic principles are extended to incorporate time as a variable by the theory of nonequilibrium thermodynamics. Nonequilibrium thermodynamics entails certain assumptions and approximations that make it more of a tool and less of a foundation than classic equilibrium thermodynamics, but the theory performs well in many areas of physiology, including transport physiology. Basically, the theory asserts that the flow of any extensive property (e.g., mass, volume, charge) is the product of a driving force and a proportionality constant, which has units of conductance. It applies to macroprocesses and microprocesses involved in forming the urine. Examples include all mechanisms for secondary active transport and the conversion of chemical to translational free energy by adenosine triphosphatases (ATPases).

ENERGY AND THE SODIUM PUMP

Na^+-K^+-ATPase, also known as the *sodium pump*, is a ubiquitous plasma membrane protein that transports intracellular sodium out of the cell and extracellular potassium into the cell, thereby generating opposite concentration gradients for sodium and potassium ions across the cell membrane. This process of separating sodium from potassium across the cell membrane is fueled by the hydrolysis of adenosine triphosphate (ATP).[4,5] Each cycle of the pump consumes one ATP molecule while transporting three Na^+ and two K^+ ions across the cell membrane. The hydrolysis of ATP and the associated transport of ions are mutually dependent[4,5] and constitute an example of primary active transport. In this process, there is almost full conversion from chemical to mechanical energy, with minimal dissipation. The translational energy that develops after ATP hydrolysis results from electrostatic repulsion between the product ions, adenosine diphosphate (ADP) and inorganic phosphate (Pi), in accordance with Coulomb's law. Although this energy could be dissipated through subsequent collisions, such events are unlikely over very short time scales and short distances. For a relative kinetic energy of the phosphate of 0.6 electron volt (eV), for example, the phosphate ion moves about 0.1 nm in 0.3 picosecond. If no other collisions occur in that short time interval, the phosphate can then transfer its entire kinetic energy to the sodium pump in the form of a molecular strain. Given the intrinsic free energy of ATP hydrolysis, the pump can generate gradients that store up to approximately 0.6 eV of electrochemical potential per three Na^+ plus two K^+ ions. For a typical cell in a typical environment, about 0.4 eV is required to cycle the pump against the existing sodium and potassium gradients, which means that cells tend to operate with some reserve to reduce their sodium or increase their potassium concentrations further.

STRUCTURE OF THE SODIUM PUMP

The sodium pump is composed of an α-catalytic subunit, which hydrolyzes ATP and transports Na^+ and K^+ across the membrane, a β-subunit that is critical for functional maturation and delivery of Na^+-K^+-ATPase to the plasma membrane, and an FXYD protein that can modulate the kinetics of Na^+-K^+-ATPase in a tissue-specific manner[6] (Figure 5.1). There are multiple isoforms of each subunit. The $α_1β_1$ heterodimer is likely the exclusive Na^+-K^+-ATPase in renal epithelia,[7] whereas several FXYD protein subunits are expressed differentially along the nephron.[6-9] Biophysical models describing the turnover of the sodium pump through its functional cycle have been described in a review by Horisberger.[4]

OTHER ADENOSINE TRIPHOSPHATASES

In addition to Na^+-K^+-ATPase, additional ion-translocating ATPases are expressed in renal epithelia along the nephron,[10] including H^+-K^+-ATPase,[11,12] Ca^{2+}-ATPases,[13] and H^+-ATPases.[14,15] These transport ATPases play important roles in maintaining urinary acidification and calcium homeostasis, as discussed in Chapters 6, 7, and 9. These ATPases do not contribute significantly to the reabsorption of the bulk of the filtrate.

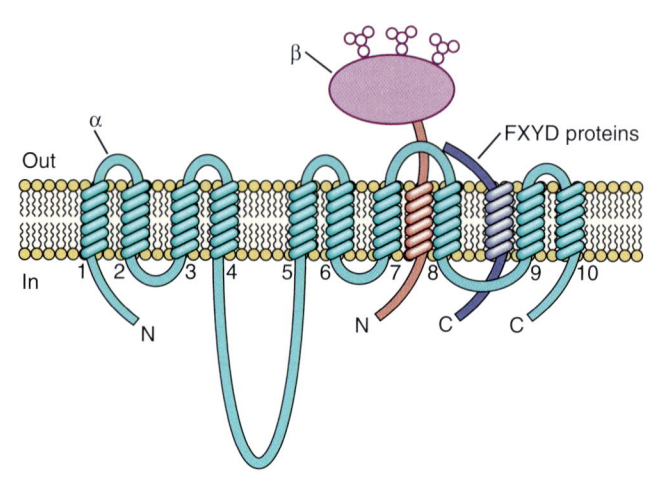

Figure 5.1 Na^+-K^+-ATPase is composed of a catalytic α-subunit (*teal*), an obligatory β-subunit (*pink*), and tissue-specific FXYD proteins (*blue*). The α-subunit has 10 transmembrane segments (1 to 10). It hydrolyzes ATP, is phosphorylated in the large cytoplasmic loop, and transports sodium and potassium. The β-subunit is a type II glycoprotein located close to M7/M10 that interacts with the extracellular loop between transmembrane segments M7 and M8 and with intracellular regions of the α-subunit. FXYD proteins are type I membrane proteins that interact with M9 with the β-subunit[4] and, in the case of FXYD1, with the intracellular lipid surface and cytoplasmic domain of the α-subunit. (From Geering K: Functional roles of Na,K-ATPase subunits. *Curr Opin Nephrol Hypertens* 17:526-532, 2008.)

PUMP-LEAK PROCESS AND THE SODIUM POTENTIAL

For a cell in steady state, the pumping of ions by the Na^+-K^+-ATPase must be offset by an equal and opposite diffusion of those ions back across the cell membrane. The backleak of ions is an example of electrodiffusion. This diffusion of ions generates an electric field to retard diffusion of the most mobile charged species, thereby transferring free energy from the chemical potential of the mobile species to an electrical potential acting on the less mobile species. If the electric field is constant within the cell membrane, then the electrical potential difference across the membrane is given by the Goldman voltage equation, which is shown here for a membrane that is permeable to Na, K, and Cl:

$$\psi = \frac{RT}{F} \ln\left(\frac{P_K [K]_o + P_{Na}[Na]_o - P_{Cl}[Cl]_o}{P_K [K]_i + P_{Na}[Na]_i - P_{Cl}[Cl]_i} \right)$$

where P_X is the permeability to X (X is Na, K, or Cl), $[X]_o$ is the concentration of X outside the cell, and $[X]_i$ is the concentration inside the cell. If the permeability to one ion dominates the others, then the membrane voltage approaches the Nernst potential for that ion, and the free energy is transferred to the electrochemical potential of the other ions. If chloride is not actively transported, then the second law of thermodynamics dictates that no free energy exists in the chloride gradient. Thus, for a membrane that actively transports Na and K and is primarily permeable to K, the membrane voltage approaches the Nernst potential for K, and the free energy provided by active transport is all transferred to the transmembrane Na difference.

To summarize, because cell membranes are generally more permeable to potassium than to sodium, potassium diffusion contributes more to the cell voltage than sodium diffusion, even though three sodium ions leak into the cell for every two potassium ions that leak out. Thus, diffusion of potassium out of the cell dominates the cell voltage, making it negative. The negative cell voltage, in turn, neutralizes the net driving force for further potassium egress and augments the net driving force for sodium entry. Because cell membranes are poor capacitors, an imperceptible charge imbalance suffices to form the entire membrane voltage. This allows the transmembrane concentration differences for sodium and potassium to remain almost equal and opposite in spite of the much greater permeability to potassium. The net outcome of this pump-leak process is that electrochemical potential, which originates with ATP hydrolysis, becomes concentrated in the transmembrane sodium gradient, whereas potassium resides close to electrochemical equilibrium.

HARNESSING THE SODIUM POTENTIAL FOR WORK

The difference in electrochemical potential for sodium across the cell membrane is available to drive the unfavorable passage of other solutes across the membrane by a variety of exchangers and cotransporters. Examples include the proximal tubule Na^+-H^+ exchanger, sodium-glucose–linked cotransporters (SGLTs), basolateral Na–α-ketoglutarate (α-KG) cotransporter, furosemide-sensitive Na^+-K^+-$2Cl^-$ cotransporter type 2 (NKCC2), and thiazide-sensitive Na^+-Cl^- cotransporter (NCC). Generically, transport that directly uses free energy from the sodium gradient to drive uphill flux of another solute is referred to as secondary active transport[16] (α-KG cotransport in Figure 5.2). Tertiary active transport refers to the net flux of a solute against its electrochemical potential gradient coupled indirectly to the Na^+ gradient (three transport processes working in parallel). An example of tertiary active transport is the uptake of various organic anions from the peritubular blood into the proximal tubular cell by the so-called organic anion transporters (OATs). Energy from the sodium gradient is converted into a gradient for α-KG to diffuse out of the cell by Na–α-KG cotransporter. OATs use this potential difference to exchange α-KG for another organic anion[17] (see Figure 5.2).

For tubular cells that actively reabsorb chloride, free energy is transferred from the Na potential to drive apical chloride entry and raise cell chloride above equilibrium. In the proximal tubule, the energy for apical chloride entry is derived circuitously via sodium-hydrogen exchange, which is coupled to oxalate, formate, or hydroxyl ion transport. In the thick ascending loop of Henle (TAL) and distal convoluted tubule (DCT), the energy transfer occurs by direct cotransport with Na via NKCC2 or NCC. In each case, raising cell chloride above equilibrium provides a driving force for chloride to diffuse out of the cell across the basolateral membrane, which is permeable to chloride. Raising cell chloride also makes the basolateral membrane voltage less negative, as is apparent from the Goldman equation. Because luminal voltage is the sum of voltage steps across the basolateral and apical membranes, raising cell chloride in a cell with basolateral chloride conductance will raise the lumen voltage (i.e., less negative), thus providing

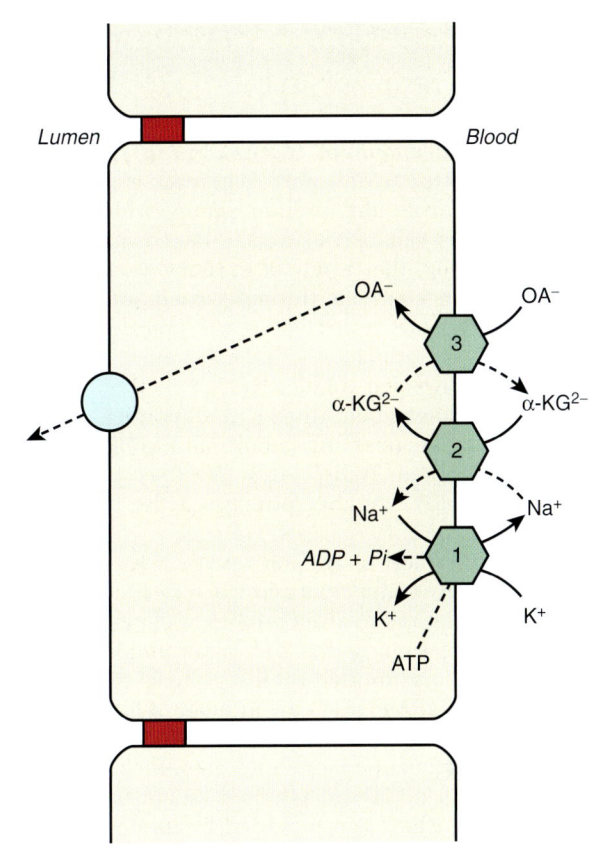

Figure 5.2 Different modes of active uphill transport as exemplified by organic acid (OA) secretion in proximal tubule epithelial cells. Transport across the basolateral membrane involves three steps functioning in parallel: **1**, primary active transport of Na^+ and K^+ by Na^+-K^+-ATPase coupled to the hydrolysis of ATP establishes the inwardly directed Na gradient; **2**, secondary active transport of α-ketoglutarate (α-KG) with Na^+ on an Na–α-KG cotransporter uses the inwardly directed Na gradient to drive α-KG into the cell; and **3**, tertiary active transport of OA with α-KG on an OA–α-KG antiporter uses the outward downhill transport of α-KG to drive the inward uphill transport of OA. The α-KG is recycled through the Na–α-KG cotransporter, which thus links the uphill transport of OA to the generation of the Na gradient by the Na^+-K^+-ATPase. Ultimately, OAs are secreted down the OA concentration gradient into the tubular lumen. (From Dantzler WH, Wright SH: The molecular and cellular physiology of basolateral organic anion transport in mammalian renal tubules. *Biochim Biophys Acta* 1618:185-193, 2003.)

free energy that can be dissipated by intercellular backleak of chloride, which would increase entropy, or be applied to do useful work of cation reabsorption, which would decrease entropy. The kidney uses the latter mechanism of energy transfer to augment Na reabsorption in the proximal tubule as well as calcium and magnesium reabsorption in the TAL.

For cells that express an amiloride-sensitive sodium channel (ENaC), opening these channels will depolarize the apical membrane, as can be seen from the Goldman equation. K^+ ions, which enter the cell via the basolateral Na pump, can leave the cell by K conductances in basolateral or apical membranes. Depolarizing the apical membrane will increase the fraction of K^+ ions leaving by way of the apical membrane conductance. This represents transfer of free energy from the Na^+-K^+-ATPase and apical Na potential to the useful work of K secretion.

CELL POLARITY AND VECTORIAL TRANSPORT

The polar arrangement of transporters in renal cells is essential for vectorial transport. Wherever it is expressed along the nephron, the sodium pump, which removes sodium from the cell, is restricted to the basolateral membrane. Meanwhile, the variety of exchangers, cotransporters, and sodium channels through which sodium enters the tubular cell are restricted to the apical membrane. These include the principal Na^+-H^+ exchanger (NHE3) and SGLTs in the proximal tubule, NKCC2 in the TAL, NCC in the distal convoluted tubule, and epithelial sodium channels in the connecting tubule and collecting duct. These apical sodium transporters effect secondary active transport coupled to the primary active transporter, Na^+-K^+-ATPase.

Close coordination of sodium uptake across the apical membrane with sodium extrusion across the basolateral membrane is required to avoid osmotic swelling and shrinking of the cell. Assuming that ATP is not limiting for basolateral exit, the magnitude of transepithelial transport is a function of the following: (1) the number of transporters in the plasma membrane, which can be varied by changes in synthesis or degradation rates and/or trafficking between intracellular and plasma membranes; and (2) the activity per transporter, which can be varied by covalent modification (e.g., phosphorylation, proteolysis) or protein-protein interaction (e.g., Na^+-K^+-ATPase kinetics are influenced by FXYD subunit association[6]). The rate of apical sodium entry is also subject to influence by the availability of substrates for cotransport. For example, the amount of sodium-glucose cotransport depends on the availability of glucose in proximal tubular fluid, and the sodium entry at a given point along the TAL is subject to variations in the local chloride concentration because NKCC2 has a relatively low affinity for chloride.

Many factors and hormones known to regulate renal sodium reabsorption (e.g., angiotensin II, aldosterone, dopamine, parathyroid hormone, blood pressure) act in parallel to affect the activity, distribution, or abundance of apical transporters and basolateral sodium pumps.[7,18] The molecular basis of this apical-basolateral crosstalk is not clearly understood, especially in the light of close cell volume control; however, there is evidence for a role of an elevated cellular calcium level in response to depressed sodium transport,[19] evidence for a salt-inducible kinase that responds to slight elevations in cell Na and Ca levels,[20] and evidence for the coupling of Na^+-K^+-ATPase to apical channel activity.[21]

METABOLIC SUBSTRATES FUELING ACTIVE TRANSPORT ALONG THE NEPHRON

It has been noted that[22]:

Biochemists generally accept the idea that metabolism is the cause of membrane transport. The underlying thesis of the hypothesis put forward here is that if the processes that we call metabolism and transport represent events in a sequence, not only can metabolism be the cause of transport, but also transport can be the cause of metabolism. Thus, we might be inclined to recognize that transport and metabolism, as usually understood by biochemists, may be conceived advantageously as different aspects of one and the same process of vectorial metabolism.

PETER MITCHELL

METABOLISM BASICS

Detailed accounts of cellular metabolism are provided in many excellent texts[23]; nonetheless, an abbreviated overview relevant to renal metabolism is warranted. Substrates enter the kidney via renal blood flow (RBF) and glomerular filtration rate (GFR) and enter renal epithelial cells by substrate transporters, often facilitated by the inward-directed Na^+ gradient created by the sodium pump (see Figure 5.2), as discussed thoroughly in Chapter 8. Oxygen is similarly delivered by RBF to the epithelial cells. Once in the cell, substrates face one of three fates: (1) transport across the epithelium back into the blood (reabsorption); (2) conversion into another substrate (e.g., lactate to pyruvate); or (3) oxidization to CO_2 in the process of cellular ATP production.[24] This section traces the road map that connects substrates to production of ATP in the mitochondrion and to ATP utilization by the sodium pump and the feedback connections between production and utilization.

Renal epithelia, except in the descending and thin ascending limbs of the loop of Henle, are packed with mitochondria (see Chapter 2). All the pathways of fuel oxidation take place in the mitochondrial matrix, except for glycolysis, which occurs in the cytosol. Substrates in the cytosol can freely cross the outer mitochondrial membrane through integral membrane porins. These substrates, as well as ADP and phosphate (the building blocks of ATP), cross the inner mitochondrial membrane into the mitochondrial matrix via specific substrate transporters driven by their respective concentration gradients or by the H^+ gradient created by the electron transport chain (Figure 5.3).

As illustrated in Figure 5.4, amino acids, fatty acids, and pyruvate are metabolized to acetyl coenzyme A and enter the citric acid cycle. With each turn of the cycle, three molecules of reduced nicotinamide adenine dinucleotide (NADH), one molecule of reduced flavin adenine dinucleotide ($FADH_2$), one molecule of guanosine triphosphate (GTP) or ATP, and two molecules of CO_2 are released in oxidative decarboxylation reactions. Electrons carried by NADH and $FADH_2$ are transferred into the mitochondrial electron transport chain, a series of integral membrane complexes located within the inner mitochondrial membrane, where the electrons are sequentially transferred, ultimately to oxygen, which is reduced to H_2O. NADH and $FADH_2$ oxidation provoke the transport of H^+ from the matrix to the inner mitochondrial space.

The release of the potential energy stored in the H^+ gradient across the inner mitochondrial membrane provides the driving force for ATP synthesis from ADP by the ATP synthase; H^+ is transported into the matrix coupled to the production of ATP from ADP and Pi; see Figure 5.3). These are the fundamental pieces of the chemiosmotic mechanism of oxidative phosphorylation proposed by Peter Mitchell in 1961.[22] The newly synthesized ATP is extruded from the matrix into the intermembrane space via the ADP-ATP countertransporter termed *adenine nucleotide translocase* and

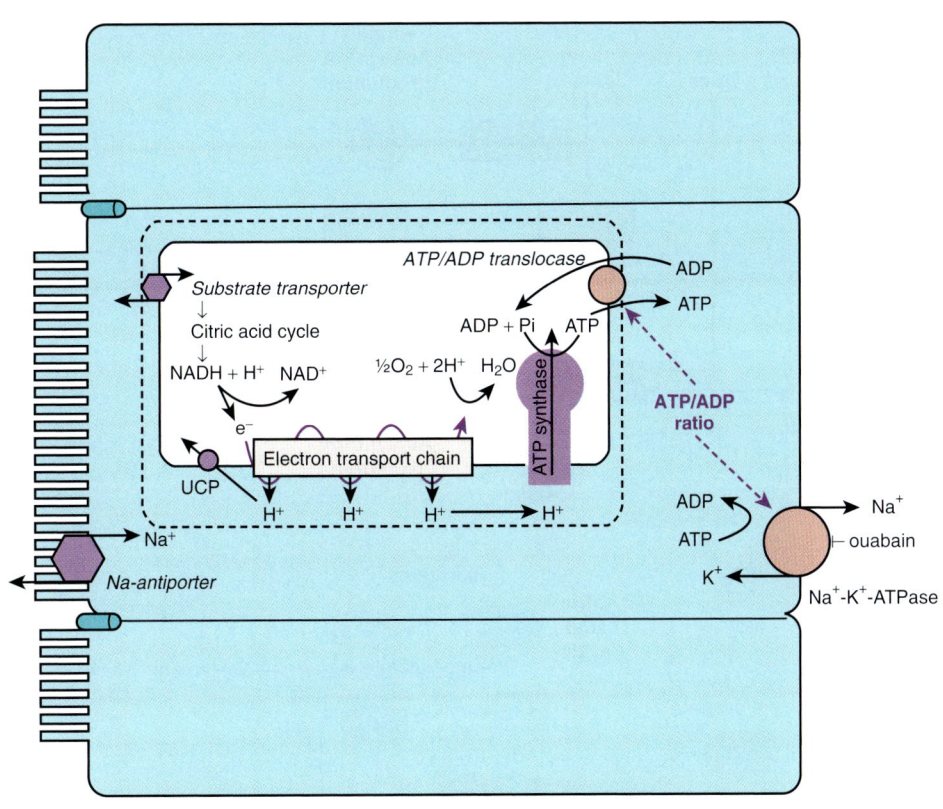

Figure 5.3 Whittam model showing the coupling of ATP utilization by Na^+-K^+-ATPase to ATP production by mitochondrial oxygen consumption (QO_2). Hydrolysis of ATP produces ADP plus inorganic phosphate (Pi), which lowers the ATP/ADP ratio, a signal to increase ADP uptake into the mitochondria and increase ATP synthesis. UCP, Uncoupling protein isoform.

then exits the mitochondria across the permeable outer membrane. In the cytosol, ATP is available to bind to ATPases such as plasma membrane Na^+-K^+-ATPase.

In summary, the flow of electrons through the electron transport chain generates a proton gradient across the inner mitochondrial membrane that provides the energy to drive ATP synthesis from ADP + Pi by ATP synthase and is also sufficient to extrude the ATP across the mitochondrial membrane.[23] Thus, the oxidation of substrates is coupled to ATP synthesis by an electrochemical proton gradient. This coupling can be influenced by uncoupling protein isoforms (UCPs) located in the mitochondrial inner membrane and expressed in a tissue-specific manner. Simply stated, UCPs create a proton leak that dissipates the proton gradient available to drive oxidative phosphorylation (see Figure 5.3). It has been reported that UCP-2 is expressed in the renal proximal tubule and TAL (not in the glomerulus or distal nephron) and that its expression is elevated in the kidneys of diabetic rats.[25] However, the physiologic consequences of the expression and regulation of UCP in kidneys have not been explored much experimentally.

WHITTAM MODEL

In the early 1960s, the coupling between active transport, respiration, and Na^+-K^+-ATPase activity was recognized by Whittam and Blond,[28,29] who tested the idea that inhibition of active ion transport at the plasma membrane would cause a fall in oxygen consumption (QO_2) in the mitochondria. Using brain or kidney samples studied in vitro, they demonstrated that inhibition of Na^+-K^+-ATPase activity by the removal of sodium or addition of the sodium pump–specific inhibitor ouabain (neither of which directly inhibits mitochondrial respiration) markedly reduced QO_2, which led the investigators to conclude that an extramitochondrial ATPase, sensitive to Na^+ and ouabain, as well as to K^+ and Ca^{2+}, is one of the pacemakers of respiration of the kidney cortex.[28,29]

A careful study by Balaban and colleagues 2 decades later[30] used a suspension of renal cortical tubules to reexamine this Whittam model (see Figure 5.3) in more detail by measuring the redox state of mitochondrial nicotinamide adenine dinucleotide (NAD), cellular ATP and ADP concentrations, ATP/ADP ratio, and QO_2 in the same samples. If transport and respiration are assumed to be coupled, inhibition of transport is predicted to provoke a mitochondrial transition to a resting state[31] accompanied by an increase in $NADH/NAD^+$ (reduced to oxidized NAD), increase in [ATP], decrease in [ADP] and [Pi], increase in ATP/ADP ratio, and decrease in QO_2. Stimulation of active transport would provoke the opposite pattern—decreased NADH, ATP, and ATP/ADP ratio, and increased QO_2. Predictably, incubating the renal cortical tubule suspension with the Na^+-K^+-ATPase inhibitor ouabain caused a 50% decline in QO_2, reduction of NAD to NADH, and 30% increase in the ATP/ADP ratio, all evidence for coupling of mitochondrial ATP production to ATP consumption via Na^+-K^+-ATPase. Similarly, in tubules deprived of K^+ (which is required for Na^+-K^+-ATPase turnover), adding 5 mmol/L of K^+ increased QO_2 by more than 50%, oxidized NADH to

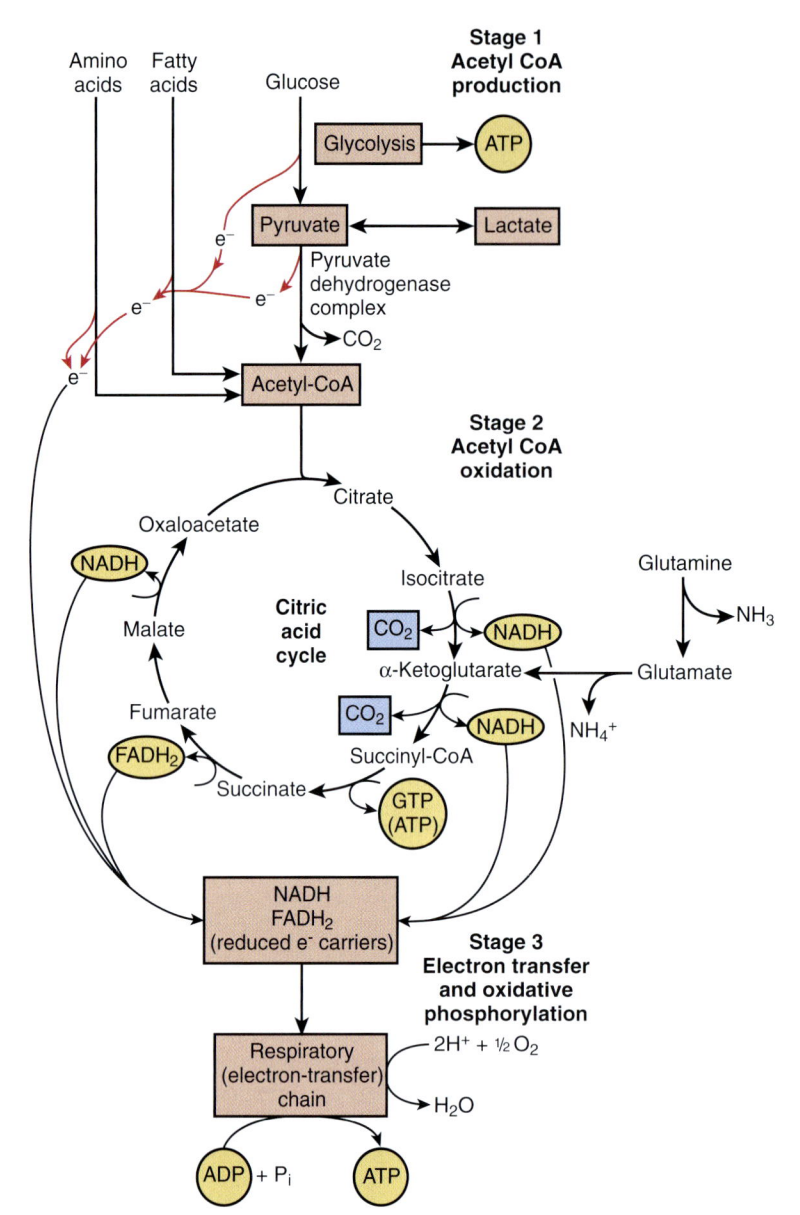

Figure 5.4 Catabolism of proteins, fats, and carbohydrates in three stages of cellular respiration. **Stage 1,** Oxidation of fatty acids, glucose, and some amino acids yields acetyl coenzyme A (CoA). **Stage 2,** Oxidation of acetyl groups in the citric acid cycle includes four steps in which electrons are abstracted. **Stage 3,** Electrons carried by reduced nicotinamide adenine dinucleotide (NADH) and reduced flavin adenine dinucleotide (FADH$_2$) are funneled into a chain of mitochondrial (or, in bacteria, plasma membrane–bound) electron carriers—the respiratory chain—that ultimately reduces O$_2$ to H$_2$O. This electron flow drives the production of ATP. Also shown are two proximal tubule pathways: (1) oxidation of lactate through pyruvate and acetyl CoA; and (2) glutamine conversion to glutamate and α-ketoglutarate in the mitochondria with the production of 2 mol NH$_3$, which is the main source of NH$_3$ secreted during acidosis. (Modified from Nelson DL, Cox MM: *Lehninger principles of biochemistry, ed 5,* New York, 2008, WH Freeman.)

NAD$^+$, and decreased the cellular ATP/ADP ratio by 50%. These results provide evidence for the coupling of both Na$^+$-K$^+$-ATPase and ATP production via ATP synthase to the cellular ATP/ADP ratio (see Figure 5.3).

ENERGY REQUIREMENTS AND SUBSTRATE USE ALONG THE NEPHRON

In all renal epithelial cells, from the proximal convoluted tubule to the inner medullary collecting duct (IMCD), the basolateral sodium pump uses the hydrolysis of ATP to drive primary active transport of Na$^+$ out of and K$^+$ into the cell, and the gradients created are used to drive coupled transport of ions and substrates across the apical and basolateral membranes.

In spite of consistent distribution and function, the relative abundance of Na$^+$-K$^+$-ATPase as a function of tubular location along the nephron is highly variable. Na$^+$-K$^+$-ATPase activity, ouabain binding, and Na$^+$-K$^+$-ATPase subunit abundance have been studied in dissected tubules and with imaging techniques. Na$^+$-K$^+$-ATPase expression patterns and ouabain binding patterns along the nephron are very similar.[10,32] The pronounced differences in activity can largely be accounted for by differences in sodium pump number, measured by ouabain binding or by immunoblot testing of subunits in dissected nephron segments (Figure 5.5).[33]

The patterns of Na^+-K^+-ATPase protein expression and activity as a function of tubule length are what is to be expected from what is understood of the physiology of the nephron segments—moderate levels are expressed in the proximal tubule, where two thirds of the sodium is reabsorbed across a leaky epithelium, and lower levels are expressed in the straight than in the convoluted segments, reflecting the amount of sodium transported in these two regions. Very low levels are detected in the thin limbs of the loop of Henle, whereas high levels are expressed in the medullary and cortical TALs (so-called diluting segments), which must reabsorb a significant fraction of NaCl without water against an increasingly steep transepithelial gradient. The Na^+-K^+-ATPase activity and expression in the DCT, which is responsible for reabsorbing another 5% to 7% of the filtered load against a very steep transepithelial gradient, is very high. In the collecting duct, which reabsorbs a smaller fraction of Na^+ via channels electrically coupled to the secretion of K^+ or H^+ and has variable H_2O permeability, the Na^+-K^+-ATPase is quite low, albeit sufficient to drive sodium reabsorption in this region. The distribution of the ATP-producing mitochondria along the nephron, reported as a percentage of cytoplasmic volume,[34] parallels the distribution of the ATP-consuming sodium pumps but is somewhat less variable, ranging from 10% or less of the cell volume in the thin loop of Henle and medullary collecting duct to 20% in the cortical collecting duct and proximal straight tubule to 30% to 40% of cell volume in the proximal tubule and TAL[34] (see Figure 5.5C).

Determining which substrates support ATP production and Na^+-K^+-ATPase activity along the nephron has been the subject of many studies and reviews.[24,35,36] To obtain nephron-specific information, investigators have dissected nephron segments and assayed for metabolic pathway enzyme distribution or examined how specific substrates affect ATP levels. Although these in vitro approaches lack the in vivo realities of blood flow, tubular flow, and autocrine-paracrine, hormonal, and nervous system inputs that are evident in the whole kidney, these studies do provide information about the metabolic potential of each segment under defined conditions.

Isolated nephron segments had been reported to have low levels of cellular ATP, so Uchida and Endou[37] reasoned that if the segments were incubated with fuels that could be used by the segment, their ATP levels should increase toward physiologic levels. They examined a range of substrates for their ability to maintain cellular ATP levels in microdissected glomeruli and nephron segments (excluding thin sections of loop of Henle and papillary duct). The substrates studied (all at 2 mmol/L) included L-glutamine, D-glucose, β-hydroxybutyrate (HBA), and DL-lactate. Because the preincubation did not fully deplete the TAL and distal nephron segments of ATP, the ionophore monensin was included in the incubation with the substrate to dissipate the Na^+ gradient and promote ATP consumption.

The change in ATP per millimeter of tubule (or glomerulus) as a function of substrate addition, shown in Figure 5.6,

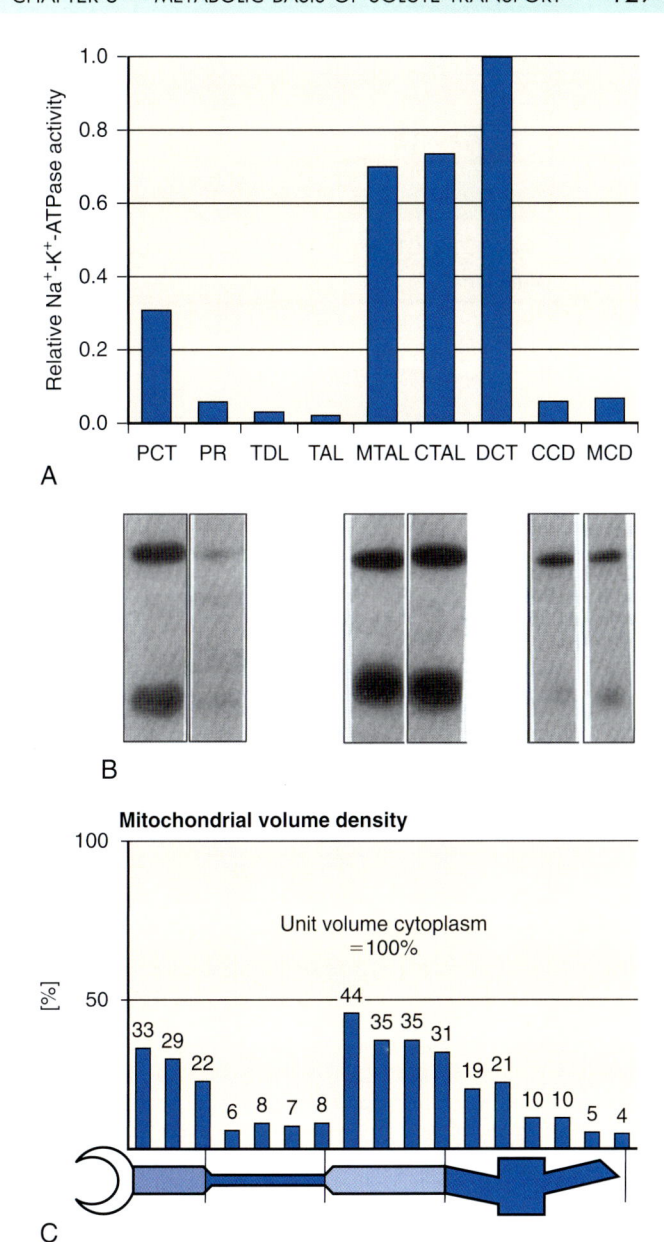

Figure 5.5 A, Relative levels of Na^+-K^+-ATPase activity measured in individual segments of the rat nephron. (Data are normalized to that of the distal convoluted tubule and expressed per unit length of the tubule segment.) **B,** Detection of Na^+-K^+-ATPase α_1- and β_1-subunits along the nephron. Tubule segments 40 mm long were resolved by sodium dodecyl sulfate–polyacrylamide gel electrophoresis (SDS-PAGE) and subjected to immunoblotting with subunit-specific antisera. Blots were placed below the corresponding tubule label indicated in **A. C,** Morphologic analysis of mitochondrial density relative to a unit of cytoplasm. CCD, Cortical collecting duct; CTAL, cortical thick ascending limb of the loop of Henle; DCT, distal convoluted tubule; MCD, outer medullary collecting duct; MTAL, medullary thick ascending limb of the loop of Henle; PCT, proximal convoluted tubule; PR, pars recta (proximal straight tubule); TAL, thin ascending limb of the loop of Henle; TDL, thin descending limb of the loop of Henle. (**A** redrawn from Katz AI, Doucet A, Morel F: Na^+-K^+-ATPase activity along the rabbit, rat, and mouse nephron, *Am J Physiol* 237:F114-F120, 1979; **B** based on data from McDonough AA, Magyar CE, Komatsu Y: Expression of Na[+]-K[+]-ATPase alpha- and beta-subunits along rat nephron: isoform specificity and response to hypokalemia. *Am J Physiol* 267:C901-C908, 1994; **C** based on data from Pfaller W, Rittinger M: Quantitative morphology of the rat kidney. *Int J Biochem* 12:17-22, 1980.)

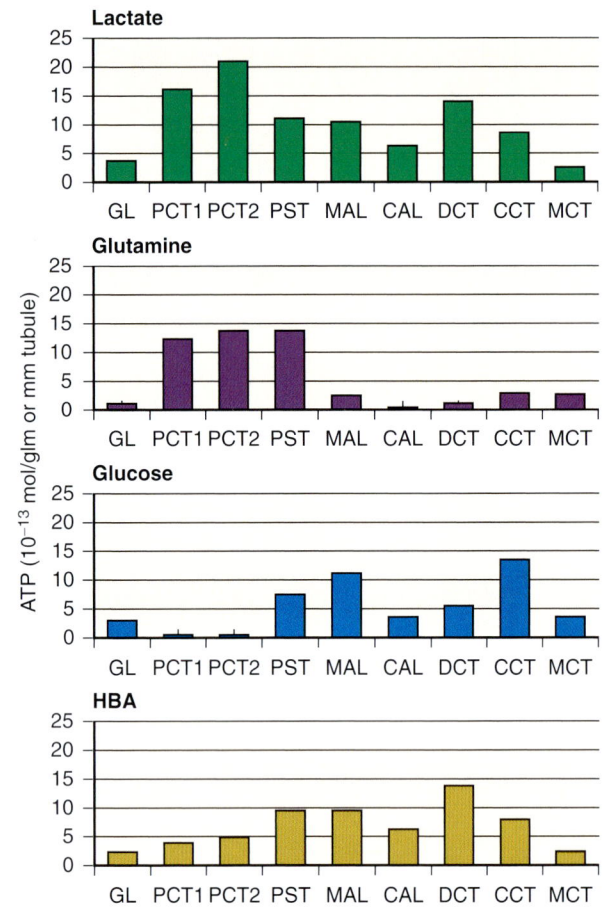

Figure 5.6 ATP production in glomeruli and dissected nephron segments as a function of substrates. In glomeruli and PCT1, PCT2, and PST segments, the values equal the differences in ATP content between samples incubated with and without each substrate for 30 minutes. In MAL, CAL, DCT, CCT, and MCT, the values equal the differences in ATP content between samples incubated with and without each substrate in the presence of monensin (10 pg/mL) for 15 minutes. CAL, Cortical ascending limb; CCT, cortical collecting tubule; DCT, distal convoluted tubule; GL, glomerulus; HBA, β-hydroxybutyrate; MAL, medullary thick ascending limb; MCT, medullary collecting tubule; PCT1, early proximal convoluted tubule; PCT2, late proximal convoluted tubule; PST, proximal straight tubule. (Data from Uchida S, Endou H: Substrate specificity to maintain cellular ATP along the mouse nephron. *Am J Physiol* 255[Pt 2]:F977-F983, 1988.)

illustrates that each segment has a distinct ability to use these substrates. Lactate was very effective at maintaining ATP levels in all nephron segments tested, notably in the proximal tubule. The S1, S2, and S3 segments of the proximal tubule all used glutamine effectively as a fuel, which is consistent with the role of the proximal tubule in ammoniagenesis. Glutamine is the main amino acid oxidized by the proximal tubule, where it is deaminated and converted to α-KG, yielding two NH_3 molecules that are secreted during acidosis, as illustrated in Figure 5.4 and discussed in Chapter 9. Glutamine is not a preferred fuel in the more distal nephron segments. Glucose is completely reabsorbed along the proximal tubule, but glucose is not an effective metabolic fuel for the S1 or S2 regions of the proximal tubule. In contrast, all the more distal segments tested readily used glucose to maintain cellular ATP. The ketone HBA was used effectively in all nephron segments tested; however, in the S1 and S2 segments of the proximal tubule, the capacity of HBA to support ATP production was far less than that provided by glutamine or lactate.

The distribution along the nephron of numerous enzymes involved in metabolic pathways, collated from many studies, has been summarized by Guder and Ross.[35] Their description of glycolytic (Figure 5.7A) and gluconeogenic (see Figure 5.7B) enzymes along the rat nephron[38-40] demonstrate very low glycolytic potential in the proximal tubule and high glycolytic potential from the medullary ascending limb to the medullary collecting tubule. In contrast, gluconeogenic enzymes are found almost exclusively in the proximal tubule.

In summary, the proximal tubule reabsorbs glucose and can synthesize glucose biosynthetically, but does not metabolize glucose. There are practical and theoretical explanations for the lack of glucose metabolism in this segment. The proximal tubule is specialized to reabsorb the filtered load of glucose from the tubular fluid back into the blood. Because of the enormous load of glucose moving through these cells, a proximal tubule hexokinase would need to have exceedingly low affinity for glucose, which would be difficult to regulate. In contrast, more distal regions of the nephron, such as the loop of Henle and distal nephron, normally have little or no glucose in their tubular fluid, have no sodium-glucose cotransporters in their apical membranes, and cannot synthesize glucose, but these regions use glucose delivered via RBF as a metabolic fuel (which could be provided by gluconeogenesis in the proximal tubule during fasting). A summary of substrate preferences along the nephron is provided in Figure 5.8.[36]

RENAL GLUCONEOGENESIS AND LACTATE HANDLING

In a review of renal gluconeogenesis, Gerich and colleagues[41] noted that the kidney can be considered two separate organs because the proximal tubule makes and releases glucose from noncarbohydrate precursors, whereas glucose utilization occurs primarily in the medulla. Because the kidney is a consumer and producer of glucose, net arteriovenous glucose differences across the kidney can be uninformative because glucose consumption in the medulla can mask glucose release by the cortex.

Gerich and colleagues[41] also made the case that the kidney is a significant gluconeogenic organ in normal humans based on the following:

1. In humans fasted overnight, proximal tubule gluconeogenesis can be as much as 40% of whole-body gluconeogenesis.[41]
2. During liver transplantation, endogenous glucose release falls to only 50% of control levels by 1 hour after liver removal.[42]
3. Pathologically, in type 2 diabetes, renal glucose release is increased by about the same fraction as hepatic glucose release.[43]

Zucker diabetic fatty rats also exhibit marked stimulation of gluconeogenesis compared with their lean littermate controls.[44]

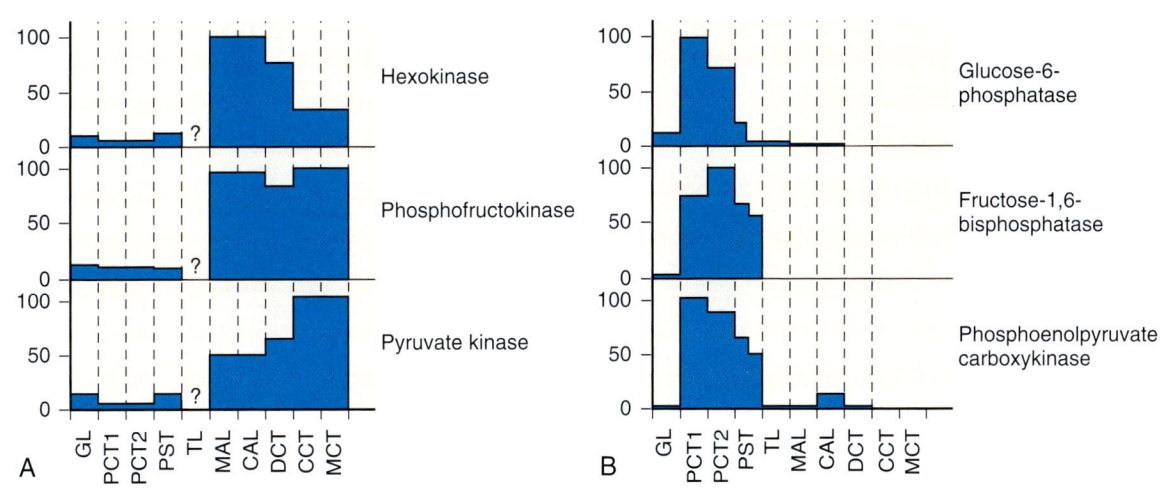

Figure 5.7 Distribution of glycolytic and gluconeogenic enzymes along the rat nephron. Nephron segments were dissected from fed (**A**) and starved (**B**) rats, respectively. The activity of hexokinase, phosphofructokinase, pyruvate kinase, glucose-6-phosphatase, fructose-1,6-bisphosphatase, and phosphoenolpyruvate carboxykinase were determined in individual segments. Enzyme activities are expressed as a percentage of the maximal value observed, based on the original activity per gram of dry weight. CAL, Cortical ascending limb; CCT, cortical collecting tubule; DCT, distal convoluted tubule; GL, glomerulus; MAL, medullary thick ascending limb; MCT, medullary collecting tubule; PCT1, early proximal convoluted tubule; PCT2, late proximal convoluted tubule; PST, proximal straight tubule; TL, loop of Henle, thin limbs. (Modified from Guder WG, Ross BD: Enzyme distribution along the nephron. *Kidney Int* 26:101-111, 1984.)

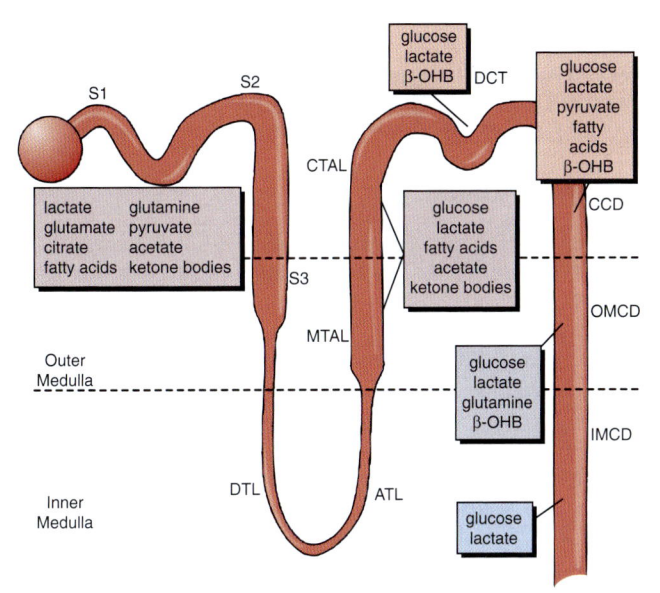

Figure 5.8 Substrate preferences along the nephron. Shown is a summary of preferred substrates to fuel active transport in nephron segments as gleaned primarily from studies using oxygen consumption (QO_2), ion fluxes, radioactive carbon (^{14}C)–labeled carbon dioxide generation from ^{14}C-labeled substrates, ATP contents, and reduced nicotinamide adenine dinucleotide (NADH) fluorescence. ATL, Ascending thin limb; β-OHB, β-hydroxybutyrate. CCD, cortical collecting tubule; CTAL, cortical thick ascending limb of the loop of Henle; DCT, distal convoluted tubule; DTL, descending thin limb; IMCD, inner medullary collecting duct; MTAL, medullary thick ascending limb of the loop of Henle; OMCD, outer medullary collecting duct. (From Kone BC: Metabolic basis of solute transport. In *Brenner and Rector's the kidney*, Philadelphia, 2008, Saunders.)

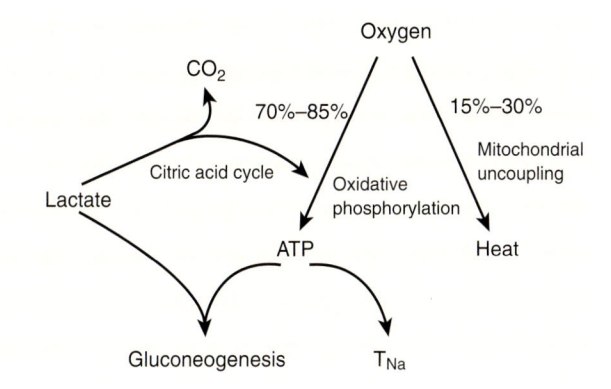

Figure 5.9 Fate of lactate and oxygen in renal metabolism. Oxygen can be used to generate ATP via oxidative phosphorylation or heat if mitochondrial uncoupling occurs. Lactate can act as a substrate for gluconeogenesis, which consumes energy, or enter into the citric acid cycle to generate energy. ATP is used for Na transport (T_{Na}) or consumed in the process of gluconeogenesis.

Lactate can reach the nephron by filtration or blood flow and can also be produced along the nephron. Within the kidney, lactate can either be oxidized to produce energy with generation of CO_2, a process that consumes oxygen but generates ATP, or be converted to glucose via gluconeogenesis in the proximal tubule, a process that consumes oxygen and ATP. This is shown in Figure 5.9. Studies by Cohen[45] in isolated whole kidney perfused only with lactate as a substrate demonstrated a change in ^{14}C-lactate utilization as a function of its concentration in the perfusate:

1. At low concentrations, all the lactate was oxidized (detected as CO_2) to fuel transport and basal metabolism.
2. When the lactate level in the perfusate was raised above 2 mmol/L, some of the lactate was used for synthesis of glucose (gluconeogenesis).
3. At a high lactate concentration in the perfusate, the metabolic and synthetic rates approached maximum, and some lactate was conserved (reabsorbed).

However, it is not the normal circumstance that lactate is the sole substrate, and it is now appreciated that the metabolism of lactate is affected by the presence of other substrates; for example, lactate uptake and oxidation are inhibited in the presence of fatty acids.[24,46]

The kidney's ability to convert lactate to glucose provides evidence that it can participate in cell-cell lactate shuttle, also known as the *Cori cycle*.[47] This cycle is important when oxidative phosphorylation is inhibited in vigorously exercising muscle, which becomes hypoxic. In the muscle, pyruvate is reduced to lactate to regenerate NAD^+ from NADH, which is necessary for ATP production by glycolysis to continue. Lactate is released into the blood and can be taken up by tissues capable of gluconeogenesis, such as liver and kidney. In the proximal tubule, the lactate that is not oxidized can be converted to glucose and, because this substrate is not used by the proximal tubule, glucose will be reabsorbed back into the blood, where it will be available for metabolism by the exercising muscle. Overall, this cycle is metabolically costly. Glycolysis produces two ATP molecules at a cost of six ATP molecules consumed in the gluconeogenesis. Thus, the Cori cycle is an energy-requiring process that shifts the metabolic burden away from the exercising muscle during hypoxia. This cell-cell lactate shuttle could also operate within the kidney between nephron segments that produce lactate anaerobically and the proximal tubule.

Renal medullary lactate concentration was explored in a 1965 study in rats by Scaglione and colleagues[48] to test the idea that the medulla uses glycolysis in the low-oxygen environment. Medullary lactate concentration is a function of delivery via blood flow, production in the medulla, and removal by blood flow, because there is no gluconeogenesis in this region to consume lactate. Because of the countercurrent arrangement of the vasa recta, lactate would be expected to be somewhat concentrated in the medulla. The study results indicate that lactate concentration is twice as high in the inner medulla as in the cortex and that during osmotic diuresis, the medullary lactate concentration doubled, whereas the cortical lactate level remained unchanged. The authors postulated that increased medullary lactate was evidence for increased glycolysis during osmotic diuresis because the diuresis and increased flow through the vasa recta would be expected to decrease the medullary lactate concentration if synthesis rates were unchanged. Sodium delivery to the distal nephron would also increase during osmotic diuresis, and the accompanying increased sodium reabsorption could drive the increased glycolysis.

Bagnasco and colleagues,[49] 20 years later, studied lactate production along the nephron in dissected rat nephron segments incubated in vitro with glucose, with or without antimycin A, an inhibitor of oxidative metabolism. The only pathway for lactate production in the kidney is from pyruvate via lactate dehydrogenase. Proximal tubules produced no lactate with or without antimycin A. The distal segments all produced lactate, and the production was significantly increased (approximately 10-fold in the TAL) during antimycin A incubation (Figure 5.10), which led the authors to conclude that significant amounts of lactate can be produced by anaerobic glycolysis during anoxia in the distal segments. The IMCD, a region with low oxygen tension

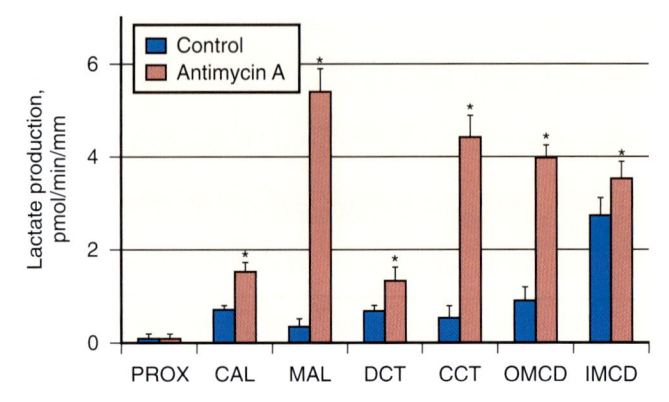

Figure 5.10 Lactate production by rat nephron segments under control conditions and in the presence of antimycin A. (From Bagnasco S, Good D, Balaban R, et al: Lactate production in isolated segments of the rat nephron. *Am J Physiol* 248:F522-F526, 1985.)

under control conditions, had high levels of lactate production, even without antimycin A, which indicates that it is primed for anaerobic glycolysis.

NEPHRON REGION–SPECIFIC METABOLIC CONSIDERATIONS

PROXIMAL TUBULE

Studies carried out in a number of laboratories have provided evidence that sodium transport and gluconeogenesis compete for ATP in the proximal convoluted tubule.[50-52] Friedrichs and Schoner[51] studied both processes in rat renal tubules and slices and found that ouabain inhibition of Na^+-K^+-ATPase increased renal gluconeogenesis by 10% to 40%, depending on the substrate, and that stimulating Na^+-K^+-ATPase activity with high extracellular K^+ inhibited gluconeogenesis. The authors concluded that inhibition of the sodium pump induces a higher energy state of the cell, which would favor energy-requiring synthetic processes.

Nagami and Lee[52] used an isolated perfused mouse proximal tubule preparation to address this issue. When tubules were perfused at higher rates, delivering more sodium to the proximal tubule, the glucose production rate was decreased by 50%, whereas when tubules were incubated with ouabain in the bath or perfused with amiloride (to inhibit apical transport), the glucose production rate increased above that seen in nonperfused tubules. The authors also verified that the reduction in glucose production seen at elevated perfusion rates does not result from increased glucose utilization and is not dependent on the presence of specific substrates.

THICK ASCENDING LIMB

The TAL has a very high rate of Na^+ transport against a steep concentration gradient, very high levels of Na^+-K^+-ATPase activity and expression and, perhaps not unexpectedly, 40% of its cytosolic volume occupied by mitochondria (see Figure

5.5). Although the TALs have a far greater capacity for anaerobic metabolism than the proximal tubules, this region still requires oxidative metabolism to maintain cellular ATP levels and active sodium reabsorption.[37,53]

CORTICAL COLLECTING DUCT

Cortical collecting duct (CCD) metabolism has been studied by Hering-Smith and Hamm.[54] This region is particularly interesting because it is made up of distinctly different cell types, such as principal cells that reabsorb sodium and intercalated cells that can secrete bicarbonate. Rabbit CCDs were microperfused, Na$^+$ reabsorption was measured by ^{22}Na$^+$ ion flux from lumen to bath, and bicarbonate transport was assayed by microcalorimetry in the presence of substrates, with and without inhibitors. Both Na$^+$ reabsorption and bicarbonate secretion were inhibited by antimycin A, which provides evidence for dependence on oxidative phosphorylation. However, neither was dependent on glycolysis or the hexose-monophosphate shunt pathways. A small component of sodium transport was supported by endogenous substrates. Na$^+$ reabsorption was supported best by a mixture of basolateral glucose and acetate, whereas HCO_3^- secretion was fully supported by glucose or acetate. HCO_3^- secretion (but not sodium transport) was supported to some extent by luminal glucose. In sum, this study indicates that principal cells and intercalated cells have distinct metabolic phenotypes.

MEDULLARY COLLECTING DUCT

Medullary collecting ducts contribute to final urinary acidification. Comparing the outer medullary collecting duct (OMCD) with the CCD, Hering-Smith and Hamm[54] found that bicarbonate secretion in the OMCD could be fully supported by endogenous substrates. This region has far less sodium transport and few mitochondria (see Figure 5.5). Stokes and colleagues[55] isolated IMCDs and examined their metabolic characteristics. In the absence of exogenous substrate, IMCD can maintain cellular ATP and respire normally, which is evidence for the presence of significant endogenous substrate. In the presence of rotenone, an inhibitor of oxidative phosphorylation, glycolysis increased 56%, which provides evidence for anaerobic metabolism, as supported by enzymatic profiles. Inhibition of sodium pump activity reduced QO_2 by 25% to 35%, which provides evidence for a requirement for a linkage between sodium pump activity and oxidative metabolism.

In studies that examined the metabolic determinants of K$^+$ transport in isolated IMCDs,[12] glucose increased oxygen consumption and cell potassium content by more than 10%, whereas an inhibitor of glycolysis promoted a release of cell potassium, and cell potassium content could not be maintained during the inhibition of mitochondrial oxidative phosphorylation. Thus, in the IMCD, glycolysis and oxidative phosphorylation are required to maintain optimal Na$^+$-K$^+$-ATPase activity to preserve cellular K$^+$ gradients. Given the low Po_2 and low density of mitochondria in this region, the collecting ducts have a higher reliance on anaerobic metabolism but still take advantage of oxidative metabolism to fully support transport.

CONTROL OF RENAL OXYGENATION

The kidneys are faced with the challenge of maintaining intrarenal oxygen levels to avoid both hypoxia, which leads to energy failure, and hyperoxia, which promotes oxidant damage.[56] Determinants of renal oxygenation and tissue oxygen tension (Po_2) include RBF and oxygen content of arterial blood, oxygen consumed by the cells, and arterial to venous (AV) oxygen shunting, which entails the diffusion of oxygen from preglomerular arteries to postglomerular veins without being available to the cell for consumption.

RENAL BLOOD FLOW AND OXYGEN CONSUMPTION

The kidney enjoys a high blood flow, almost 25% of the cardiac output, which is needed to sustain the GFR. Compared to other major body organs, renal oxygen consumption (product of RBF and renal oxygen extraction) per gram of tissue is high, second only to the heart (2.7 mmol/kg/min for the kidney vs. 4.3 mmol/kg/min for the heart).[1] Renal oxygen consumption is largely driven by the high RBF because renal oxygen extraction itself is low. It has been hypothesized that renal AV oxygen shunting is an adaptation to prevent hyperoxia in the setting of the high renal perfusion needed to sustain GFR. However, such shunting can be detrimental in conditions of oxygen demand and supply mismatch (Figure 5.11).[56]

The phenomenon of O_2 shunting from the descending to ascending vasa recta in the medulla has been accepted for decades. Evidence for AV O_2 shunting in the kidney cortex was provided when it was shown, by the use of oxygen-sensing microelectrodes, that the oxygen tension is substantially higher in the renal vein (50 mm Hg) than in efferent arterioles (45 mm Hg) or tubules (40 mm Hg).[57,58] The fraction of incident oxygen subject to AV O_2 shunting is estimated at 50%. This causes tissue oxygen pressure (Po_2) in the kidney cortex to be lower than otherwise expected and similar to that of other organs with a lower venous Po_2, in which perfusion is matched more closely to metabolic demand.

Noting the similarity of tissue Po_2 in the kidney and in other organs, some have argued that the renal AV O_2 shunt is an adaptive mechanism for preventing the exposure of cortical tubules to toxic levels of oxygen while permitting a high RBF, which is needed for clearance[59] (see Figure 5.11). As mentioned earlier, there is substantial shunting of oxygen from descending to ascending vasa recta in the renal medulla due to countercurrent flow in these vessels. Countercurrent flow in so-called hairpin loops formed by the vasa recta facilitates the recycling of solutes to the inner medulla, where a high osmolarity is essential to the formation of concentrated urine (see Chapter 10). As an inherent consequence of this countercurrent mechanism for maintaining a medullary osmotic gradient, there arises a negative oxygen gradient from the cortex to the inner medulla, where Po_2 falls to 10 mm Hg.[60] This results from the combination of slow blood flow through the vasa recta, O_2 consumption by active transport in the outer medullary TAL, and diffusion of O_2 from the descending to ascending vasa recta.[60] This leaves the medullary tissue at the brink of

Table 5.1 Mechanisms for Changing Amount of Oxygen Consumed per Work Performed

Dissociate glomerular filtration rate from renal blood flow.
Alter the amount of O_2 consumed per Na^+ reabsorbed.
Shift transport between tubular segments that make more or less use of passive reabsorption.
Alter backleak permeability of the tubule.
Change the coupling ratio of adenosine triphosphate generated to O_2 consumed by mitochondria.

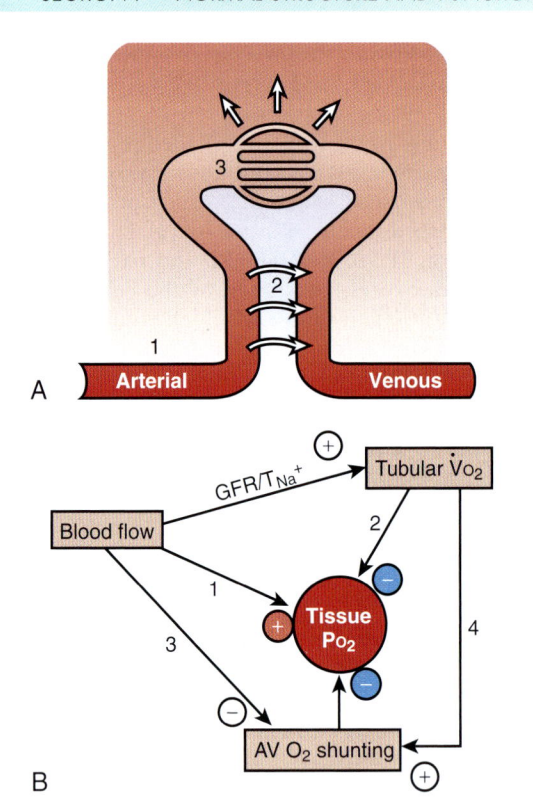

Figure 5.11 Control of intrarenal oxygenation. Renal arteriovenous (AV) oxygen shunting is a structural antioxidant mechanism that contributes to the dynamic regulation of intrarenal oxygenation. **A,** Because of AV oxygen shunting, much of the oxygen entering the kidney (1) never enters the renal microcirculation, instead diffusing from preglomerular intrarenal arteries to the closely associated veins (2). The O_2 content of downstream blood perfusing the peritubular capillaries (3) that supply the tissue with O_2 is low but sufficient to meet metabolic O_2 demands because of the high rate of renal perfusion. This mechanism helps maintain stable renal tissue oxygen tension. **B,** A model of the control of renal tissue oxygen tension (PO_2) is shown. Changes in renal blood flow (RBF) directly affect tissue PO_2 through changes in the supply of oxygen (1) but, at the same time, have an opposing effect on tissue PO_2 (2) by affecting the glomerular filtration rate (GFR), tubular sodium reabsorption (T_{Na^+}), and hence renal oxygen consumption ($\dot{V}O_2$). Each of these factors also affects the degree of AV O_2 shunting, which acts to limit delivery of oxygen to renal tissue. As RBF increases, circulatory transit time falls, which should limit the time available for AV diffusion and therefore the quantity of oxygen shunted (3). On the other hand, tubular ($\dot{V}O_2$) creates the driving force for AV oxygen shunting, the AV PO_2 gradient, so increased tubular ($\dot{V}O_2$) should increase shunting (4). (Modified from Evans RG, Gardiner BS, Smith DW, O'Connor PM: Intrarenal oxygenation: unique challenges and the biophysical basis of homeostasis. *Am J Physiol Renal Physiol* 295:F1259-F1270, 2008.)

distance from those vascular bundles. The model predicts steeply declining O_2 gradients from the vascular bundles to the corresponding TALs and a compromise between the TAL and inner medulla with respect to the provision of oxygen.[63]

In most organs, tissue oxygen can be stabilized by metabolic regulation of blood flow. In such an arrangement, vasoactive end products of metabolism due to increased metabolic activity and oxygen utilization produce a signal that results in more blood flow to that organ. A unique feature of renal oxygenation is that the kidney cannot rely on this simple mode of metabolic autoregulation because, unlike other organs that receive blood solely to supply the metabolic needs of the organ, the kidney also receives blood to perform the functions of glomerular filtration and tubule transport.

RBF creates its own demand, because it determines the GFR, which in turn determines the rate of tubular sodium reabsorption (T_{Na}), the main determinant of O_2 consumption ($\dot{Q}O_2$).[64,65] If the kidneys were to modulate RBF as a means of stabilizing renal O_2 content, this would create a vicious cycle of positive feedback in which increased O_2 delivery would increase O_2 consumption, which would call for more O_2 delivery. Positive feedback is inherently destabilizing, so this arrangement alone could not work to stabilize RBF or renal O_2 content. Hence, the kidney is compelled to invoke mechanisms that are more complex. There are two generic routes for the kidney to stabilize its O_2 content. One is to dissociate RBF from GFR. The other is to alter the metabolic efficiency of Na^+ transport (Table 5.1). Further details are discussed later.

Ultimately, the rate at which the kidney consumes oxygen must be linked to the GFR. This is true because the main use of oxygen is to reabsorb the filtered sodium, which is linked to GFR by glomerulotubular balance (GTB). GTB describes the direct effect of the filtered load on tubular reabsorption, and it operates in all nephron segments, although the mechanism differs among segments. In the proximal tubule, shear strain tied to increased tubular flow exerts torque on the apical microvilli, which leads to upregulation of apical sodium transporters.[66] In cases in which filtration fraction increases, the parallel increase in peritubular capillary oncotic pressure will increase the Starling force driving fluid reabsorption. In the TAL, flux through NKCC2 is limited by the chloride concentration, which declines more slowly along the TAL at high flow rates. However, although GTB applies to net reabsorption, an

hypoxia, especially the outer stripe of outer medulla, where the S3 segment of the proximal tubule and medullary TAL lie, making these segments most vulnerable to ischemic injury.

Consideration of O_2 transport was incorporated into a mathematical model of the rat outer medulla by Chen and colleagues.[61,62] This model takes into account fine details of the medullary anatomy, which includes positioning of the long descending vasa recta in the center of vascular bundles and the positioning of the TAL and collecting ducts at some increased flow rate in the tubule also shortens the time that a given sodium ion is exposed to the reabsorptive machinery. This leads to the prediction that GTB can do no better than maintain constant fractional reabsorption.[65]

TUBULOGLOMERULAR FEEDBACK

Significant fluctuations in RBF, GFR, and filtered Na$^+$ load would overwhelm the kidney's ability to match Na$^+$ and volume output accurately to input and compromise homeostasis of extracellular fluid volume. This does not normally occur because RBF and GFR are tightly controlled by the tubuloglomerular feedback mechanism (described in detail in Chapter 3). Thus, if RBF and/or GFR increases, and GTB maintains a constant fractional reabsorption along the proximal tubule, an increasing amount of salt will be delivered to the macula densa, which sets off the tubuloglomerular feedback response. Specifically, increases in apical NaCl delivery or flow to this region provoke the cells of the macula densa to release ATP into the interstitium surrounding the afferent arterioles. This response is dependent on the basolateral Na$^+$-K$^+$-ATPase to maintain the inward-directed Na$^+$ gradient.[67] ATP release is via maxi-anion channels.[68] Some fraction of the released ATP is converted to adenosine by local ecto-nucleoside triphosphate diphosphohydrolase 1 (ecto-NTPDase1) and ecto-5′-nucleotidase.[69] This adenosine activates A$_1$ adenosine receptors on the afferent arteriole, causing vasoconstriction. The arteriolar constriction reduces RBF and GFR in concert until Na$^+$ delivery to the macula densa is realigned. Thus, an inverse relationship is established between tubular NaCl load and the GFR of the same nephron.[64]

Because of the time it takes for information to pass through the tubuloglomerular feedback system, the system is prone to oscillate, with a period of around 30 seconds. Rhythmic oscillations of kidney Po$_2$ occur at the same frequency as tubuloglomerular feedback–mediated oscillations in tubular flow. This illustrates the simultaneous influence of tubuloglomerular feedback over minute to minute tubular flow rate and oxygen levels in the kidney.[70]

Adenosine mediates tubuloglomerular feedback as a vasoconstrictor. Adenosine-mediated vasoconstriction is unique to the afferent arteriole. In all other beds in which adenosine is vasoactive, it exerts a vasodilatory effect mediated by adenosine A$_2$ receptors. In addition to adenosine receptors, the afferent arteriole expresses P2X purinergic receptors, which also mediate a vasoconstrictor response, in this case to interstitial ATP. These P2X receptors are essential to pressure-mediated RBF autoregulation, but adenosine A$_1$ receptors are sufficient to explain the tubuloglomerular feedback response.[69]

Adenosine also plays an important role in stabilizing medullary energy balance through local adjustments in blood flow and transport, along with other autocrine and paracrine factors, including vasodilatory prostaglandins and nitric oxide, which increase medullary blood flow while inhibiting sodium transport in the TAL.[50,70,71] Adenosine, in particular, is a case study in local metabolic regulation by negative feedback in the medulla. When ATP levels decline, adenosine is released from TAL cells into the renal interstitium, where it binds to adenosine A$_1$ receptors and inhibits Na$^+$ reabsorption in the TAL and IMCD. This has the effect of increasing Po$_2$ by reducing Qo$_2$. The same pool of adenosine also activates vascular adenosine A$_2$ receptors in the deep cortex and medullary vasa recta to increase blood flow.[72,73]

By these mechanisms, the TAL looks after its own interests. However, because TAL sodium reabsorption normally exceeds the urinary sodium excretion by 40-fold, any significant decline in TAL reabsorption must be compensated for by increasing active transport somewhere else or by reducing the GFR through tubuloglomerular feedback. The activation of adenosine A$_1$ receptors in the glomerulus, proximal tubule, or TAL contributes to lessening the amount of work imposed on the hypoxic outer medulla, whereas activating adenosine A$_2$ receptors in the vasa recta supports O$_2$ delivery to the medulla (summarized in Figure 5.12).

METABOLIC COST OF SODIUM REABSORPTION

The cost of renal sodium transport can be estimated from the sodium pump stoichiometry and amount of oxygen required to produce ATP. Sodium pump stoichiometry dictates that hydrolysis of one ATP molecule is coupled to the transport of three Na$^+$ ions out of the cell and two K$^+$ ions into the cell,[4] and oxidative metabolism generates approximately six ATP molecules per O$_2$ molecule consumed (see Figure 5.4). In the 1960s, several investigators undertook to measure the metabolic cost of tubular reabsorption in various species of mammals. There is fair consensus among four oft-cited studies published between 1961 and 1966 that the relationship between Qo$_2$ and T$_{Na}$ is fairly linear, and that the kidney reabsorbs 25 to 29 Na$^+$ ions per molecule of O$_2$ consumed in the process.[74-77] A representative figure from one of these studies is shown in Figure 5.13.

If one assumes that kidney mitochondria make six molecules of ATP per molecule of O$_2$, the kidney must then reabsorb four or five Na$^+$ ions per ATP molecule. This exceeds the 3:1 stoichiometry of the Na$^+$-K$^+$-ATPase, which was known at the time.[78] Because there are thermodynamic difficulties with the idea of an undiscovered basolateral sodium pump capable of forcing five Na$^+$ ions from a tubular cell with energy from a single ATP molecule, it was surmised that a considerable fraction of overall sodium reabsorption must be passive and paracellular, as is now accepted.

It was later suggested by Cohen[45] and others that these calculated ratios of Qo$_2$/T$_{Na}$ actually underestimate the true efficiency of sodium reabsorption because a fraction of the oxygen consumed during sodium transport is also spent metabolizing organic substrates that enter the cell by sodium cotransport. The most important example of this is lactate, which is converted to glucose in the proximal tubule via the Cori cycle. The capacity for renal gluconeogenesis from lactate is large, and it has been estimated that the kidney can consume up to 25% as much energy converting lactate to glucose as it spends reabsorbing sodium.[45]

The metabolic cost of active sodium transport is expected to vary along the nephron. As reviewed earlier, the overall stoichiometry of Na$^+$ reabsorbed to O$_2$ consumed is estimated at 25 to 30 μEq Na$^+$/μmol O$_2$.[74,76] This ratio translates to five Na$^+$ ions reabsorbed for every ATP molecule consumed, which is much higher than the ratio of three Na$^+$ ions to every ATP molecule predicted by sodium pump stoichiometry. In fact, one might expect a ratio lower than

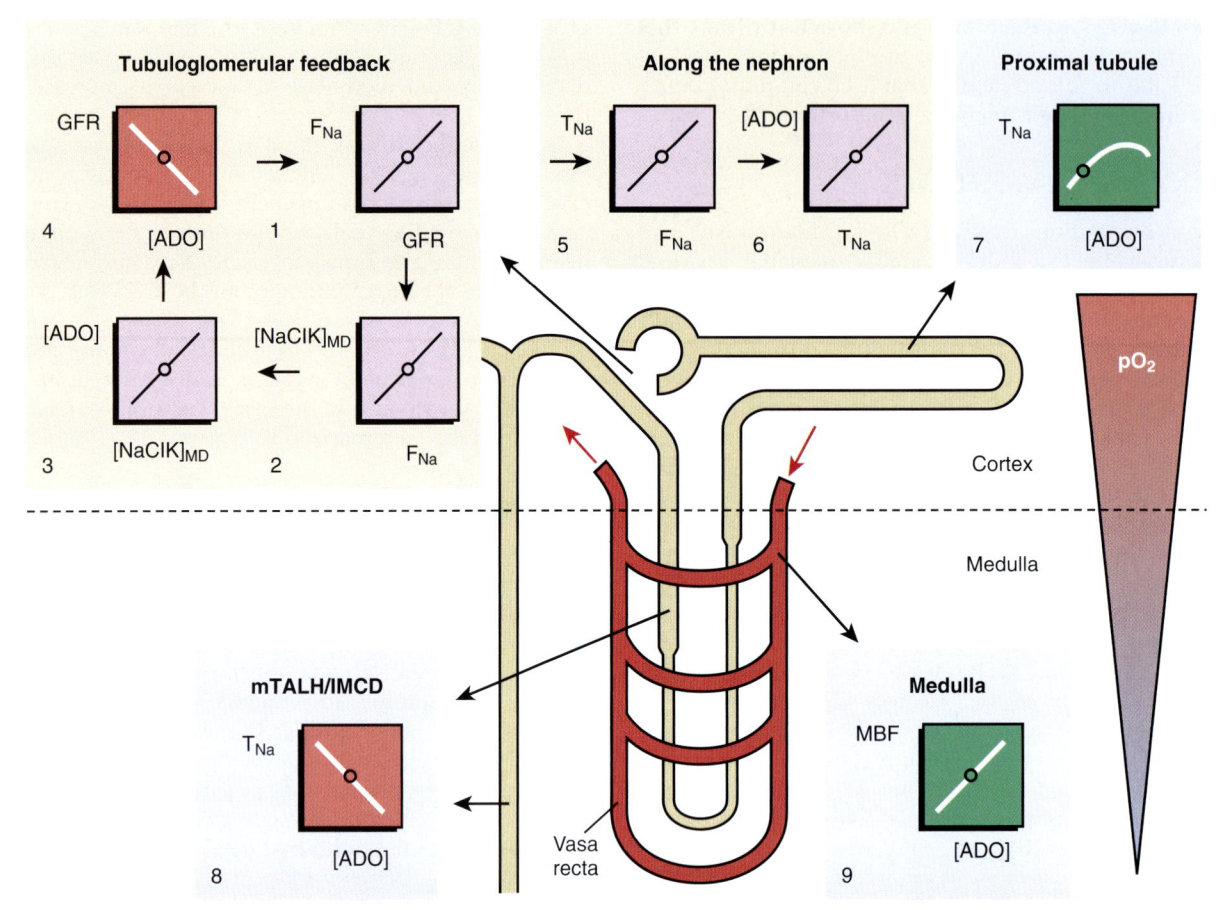

Figure 5.12 Role of extracellular adenosine (ADO) in protecting the renal medulla from hypoxia. The line plots illustrate the relationships between the given parameters. *Small circles* on these lines indicate ambient physiologic conditions. **1**, A rise in the glomerular filtration rate (GFR) increases the Na$^+$ load (F$_{Na}$) to the tubular system in cortex and medulla. **2**, This rise in F$_{Na}$ increases the salt concentration sensed by the macula densa ([NaClK]$_{MD}$). **3**, The increase in [NaClK]$_{MD}$, in turn, enhances local ADO. **4**, ADO lowers GFR and thus F$_{Na}$, which closes a negative feedback loop and thus provides a basis for an oscillating system. **5**, F$_{Na}$ determines Na$^+$ transport work (T$_{Na}$) and O$_2$ consumption in every nephron segment, so oscillations in F$_{Na}$ may help protect the medulla. **6**, A rise in T$_{Na}$ increases ADO along the nephron. **7**, In the cortical proximal tubule, ADO stimulates T$_{Na}$ and thus lowers the Na$^+$ load to segments residing in the medulla. **8**, In contrast, ADO inhibits transport work in the medulla, including the medullary thick ascending limb (mTALH) and inner medullary collecting duct (IMCD). **9**, In addition, ADO enhances medullary blood flow (MBF), which increases O$_2$ delivery and further limits O$_2$-consuming transport in the medulla. (Modified from Vallon V, Muhlbauer B, Osswald H: Adenosine and kidney function. *Physiol Rev* 86:901-940, 2006. © 2006 American Physiological Society.)

3:1 because of the basal metabolic functions of the kidney that are independent of sodium transport (i.e., insensitive to the Na$^+$-K$^+$-ATPase inhibitor ouabain; Figure 5.14) and because of tubular backleak.

One reason for this higher than expected efficiency of sodium reabsorption is that the kidney can leverage excess free energy in the gradients created by primary and secondary active transport to drive passive paracellular reabsorption of sodium chloride. Free energy for paracellular reabsorption is available in the midproximal tubule and early TAL.[78] In the proximal tubule, the driving force for the passive transport develops as a result of the preferential absorption of bicarbonate over chloride earlier in the tubule.[79,80]

The decline in tubular bicarbonate concentration is paralleled by a rise in chloride concentration as water follows Na$^+$, HCO$_3^-$, and organic osmoles across the leaky proximal tubule (see Chapter 6). This favorable lumen to blood Cl$^-$ gradient drives passive paracellular chloride reabsorption. The transepithelial voltage that arises from the electrodiffusion of chloride, in turn, drives passive sodium reabsorption. Because the NaCl reflection coefficient is less than that for NaHCO$_3$ in this region,[79] coupled sodium chloride reabsorption also occurs secondary to solvent drag.[81] Although estimates vary, this passive reabsorption may increase the number of Na$^+$ ions reabsorbed to O$_2$ molecules consumed in the proximal tubule from 18 to 48.[82]

Simultaneously blocking both cytosolic and membrane carbonic anhydrase with acetazolamide reduces bicarbonate reabsorption and Qo$_2$ in a 16:1 molar ratio, as expected for simple coupling to the sodium pump.[83] However, inhibiting bicarbonate reabsorption with a membrane-specific carbonic anhydrase inhibitor, which acidifies the tubular lumen, paradoxically increases Qo$_2$ both in vivo and in isolated proximal tubules, an effect that is prevented by also blocking the apical Na$^+$-H$^+$-exchanger isoform 3 (NHE3).[84] A simple explanation is lacking for why increasing the cell to lumen proton gradient should increase Qo$_2$ in the proximal tubule, but these results establish the phenomenon in vitro and in vivo.

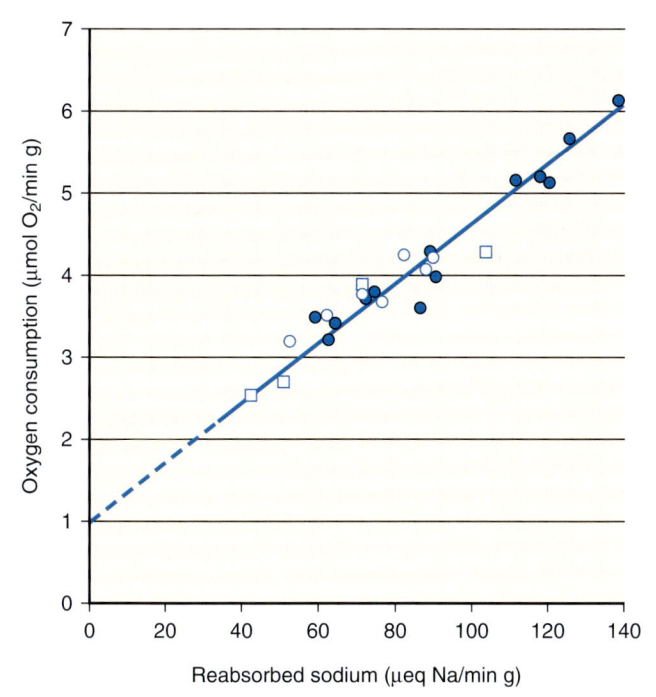

Figure 5.13 Oxygen consumption as a function of net sodium reabsorption in whole dog kidney. *Filled circles,* control; *open circles,* hypoxia; *squares,* hydrochlorothiazide. The slope of the line fitted to the data points represents Q_{O_2}/T_{Na} and is approximately 1/28. (Modified from Thurau K: Renal Na-reabsorption and O_2-uptake in dogs during hypoxia and hydrochlorothiazide infusion. *Proc Soc Exp Biol Med* 106:714-717, 1961; and Mandel LJ, Balaban RS: Stoichiometry and coupling of active transport to oxidative metabolism in epithelial tissues. *Am J Physiol* 240:F357-F371, 1981.)

Components of renal epithelial oxygen consumption

(Q_{O_2}) **Ouabain sensitive**
- Primary active transport
  - Na^+-K^+-ATPase
- Coupled transport
  - Secondary Na coupled transport
  - Tertiary coupled transport

Ouabain-insensitive (basal)
- Primary and secondary active transport *not* coupled to Na^+-K^+-ATPase
- Cell repair, growth
- Synthetic functions
  - Lipid synthesis
  - Gluconeogenesis
- Substrate interconversions

Figure 5.14 A large fraction of renal epithelial oxygen consumption (Q_{O_2}) in renal cells is sensitive to the Na^+-K^+-ATPase–specific inhibitor ouabain, and this Q_{O_2} drives primary active transport and transport coupled to sodium pump activity. The fraction of renal oxygen consumption that does not change in the presence of ouabain is, by definition, independent of Na^+-K^+-ATPase activity in the cell and is roughly equivalent to the basal Q_{O_2}, which fuels transport not coupled to sodium gradients, cell repair and growth, biosynthesis, and substrate interconversions.

The early portion of the TAL is also capable of paracellular sodium reabsorption. In this region, sodium can be transported transcellularly by the apical Na-K-2Cl cotransporter or apical Na^+-H^+ exchanger, secondary to a high density of Na^+-K^+-ATPase extruding sodium across the basolateral membranes. In addition, sodium can be reabsorbed paracellularly as long as there is a lumen-positive, transepithelial voltage sufficient to overcome the force for back diffusion associated with an unfavorable concentration difference. A lumen-positive voltage develops in the TAL because the apical membrane has a high concentration of sodium channels, whereas the basolateral membrane has both sodium and chloride channels. As predicted by the Goldman-Hodgkin-Katz voltage equation, the chloride conductance causes the basolateral membrane potential to be less negative than the apical membrane potential, which results in a positive transepithelial gradient.[85,86]

Further along the nephron in the distal tubule and collecting duct, the tubular fluid sodium concentration is too low to allow paracellular reabsorption of sodium. In those segments, a lower limit on the cost of sodium reabsorption is set by the 3:1 Na^+/ATP ratio of the sodium pump. Although active transport of sodium is a pacemaker for renal respiration, there are ways to reset the relationship of Q_{O_2} to sodium pump activity. Examples of this were provided by Silva and associates,[87] who measured O_2 consumption and Na^+-K^+-ATPase activity in rat kidney slices in which an increase in the latter had been induced by prior treatment of the animals with triiodothyronine (T_3), methylprednisolone, potassium loading, or subtotal nephrectomy. Although each of these maneuvers increased ex vivo sodium pump activity, only T_3 and methylprednisolone increased Q_{O_2}.

It has also been shown that the thermogenic effect of catecholamines, normally associated with brown fat and striated muscle, also occurs in the kidney, which responds to dopamine infusion with a near-doubling of overall metabolic rate, but minimal change in sodium reabsorption.[88] Dopamine inhibits sodium reabsorption in the proximal tubule,[89,90] thereby shifting the reabsorptive burden to less efficient downstream segments. However, heat accumulates in both the cortex and medulla during dopamine infusion, which suggests that the mechanism may be a direct effect of catecholamines on renal metabolism. In addition, an increase in RBF by dopamine could be responsible for the increased renal oxygen consumption, which is the product of RBF and renal oxygen extraction.

Weinstein and Szyjewicz[91,92] also examined Q_{O_2}/T_{Na} using 10% body weight short-term saline expansion as another way to inhibit proximal sodium reabsorption in rats. Using this maneuver, they were able to reduce fractional sodium reabsorption by 30% in the proximal tubule, leading to a GTB-mediated increase in net reabsorption downstream of the proximal tubule. However, overall Q_{O_2} did not increase but actually fell. It was conjectured that energy for this increase in downstream reabsorption was derived anaerobically, but the full details of this remain to be clarified. It appears that the energy cost of transport in the proximal versus distal nephron during inhibition of proximal tubule transport depends on the stimulus provoking the change in transport, as well as the metabolic environment.

REGULATION OF METABOLIC EFFICIENCY OF TRANSPORT DURING NORMAL PERTURBATIONS AND DISEASE

The kidneys have developed multiple mechanisms to minimize changes in oxygen delivery and to cope with a reduction in PO_2. Some of these are specific to the kidney, whereas others are generic to many tissues, as discussed next.

PHYSIOLOGIC REGULATION: FILTRATION FRACTION AND OXYGEN CONSUMPTION

As reviewed earlier, there are two generic routes for the kidney to achieve a stable content of O_2—dissociation of RBF from GFR and alteration of Qo_2/T_{Na} (see Table 5.1). Both routes are subject to regulation. Dissociating RBF from GFR equates to changing the glomerular filtration fraction. This can work to stabilize kidney O_2 because lowering the filtration fraction increases the ratio of supply to demand for O_2. For nephrons in filtration equilibrium, this requires independent control of the afferent and efferent arterioles, which can be achieved by modulating relative activities of purinergic, angiotensin, nitric oxide, and other signaling systems in the glomerulus. A full discussion of glomerular hemodynamics is available in Chapter 3, but a few features are noted here.

To begin, the filtration fraction can be lowered by constricting the afferent arteriole (which reduces net O_2 delivery) or dilating the efferent arteriole (which increases net O_2 delivery). Constricting the afferent arteriole confers initial energy savings by reducing the GFR faster than RBF, but there is a diminishing return as O_2 delivery declines toward the basal requirement. Dilating the efferent arteriole only reduces GFR when glomerular capillary pressure is low to begin with, such as during hypotension or with high afferent resistance.[93] When angiotensin II acts on the afferent and efferent arterioles to stabilize GFR in the presence of low blood pressure or high upstream resistance by preferentially constricting efferent arterioles, the kidney is accepting a decrease in the ratio of O_2 supply to O_2 demand. Conversely, adenosine signaling in the glomerulus decreases the filtration fraction and thus manages to stabilize nephron function without compromising the O_2 supply-demand balance. Adenosine in the nanomolar range constricts the afferent arteriole via high-affinity adenosine A_1 receptors. A higher adenosine concentration dilates the efferent arteriole via low-affinity adenosine A_2 receptors. The interstitial adenosine concentration rises as more NaCl is delivered into the nephron. The prototype for this is tubuloglomerular feedback signaling through the macula densa, although other sources are not precluded (see Figure 5.12). When the kidney is operating in the domain of modest distal delivery, increasing the tubuloglomerular feedback signal constricts the afferent arteriole. When the kidney is operating in the domain of high distal delivery, a further increase causes the efferent arteriole to dilate,[94] which can be viewed as a shift in priority toward maintaining the O_2 supply as the supply diminishes.

The second generic means for stabilizing kidney O_2 is to alter the Qo_2/T_{Na}. As mentioned earlier, studies in the 1960s established the linear relationship between Qo_2 and T_{Na}. Each adopted a similar standard, which was to express suprabasal renal Qo_2 as a function of T_{Na}. Suprabasal O_2 consumption was obtained by subtracting from total O_2 consumption the amount required for basal metabolism, which was determined by various methods. One method was to plot Qo_2 against T_{Na} and then extrapolate to the y-intercept to obtain basal Qo_2. Another approach was to reduce renal perfusion pressure to the point that glomerular filtration ceased, and then ascribe the residual measured Qo_2 to basal metabolism. These approaches for obtaining basal O_2 consumption have their unique limitations, and both require the dubious assumption that basal metabolism is static under most conditions and is unaffected by T_{Na} per se. Nonetheless, these studies attempted to measure and incorporate the contribution of basal Qo_2 to the total Qo_2. In recent studies,[95] the ratio of total Qo_2 to T_{Na} has been represented as an index of metabolic efficiency of transport, ignoring the contribution of basal Qo_2 to the total Qo_2. This can lead to inaccuracies, because estimates of basal metabolism have varied widely in the published literature, indicating its susceptibility to different experimental conditions. For example, the proximal tubule can devote considerable energy to gluconeogenesis, especially in the postabsorptive or fasting states, and in diabetes.[43,96,97] In light of the fact that oxygen can be diverted to do other work, an increase in Qo_2/T_{Na} is not necessarily due to "decreased transport efficiency."

The specific factors contributing to this Qo_2/T_{Na} stoichiometry, as well as to the basal metabolic rate in the kidney, have been the subject of numerous reviews.[98,99] It is theoretically possible to alter Qo_2/T_{Na} in a number of ways (see Table 5-1):

1. Transport could be shifted from the proximal tubule, where efficient use of energy from the Na^+-K^+-ATPase drives passive transport, to other segments, where all sodium reabsorbed passes through the Na^+-K^+-ATPase.
2. Tubular backleak permeability could change, which would affect the number of times that a given Na^+ ion must be reabsorbed to escape excretion into the urine.
3. The ratio of ATP produced per O_2 consumed could be altered by the regulated activity of UCPs (see Figure 5.3).[25]
4. ATP could be diverted to gluconeogenesis, such as during fasting.

The same neurohumoral factors that exert well-known effects on glomerular hemodynamics and O_2 supply, including nitric oxide, angiotensin II, adenosine, and catecholamines, also appear to participate in the regulation of kidney metabolism and Qo_2 by the tubule. It has been shown[100,101] that administration of nonselective nitric oxide synthase (NOS) inhibitors increases Qo_2/T_{Na}. Other experiments have suggested that NOS-1 is the specific isoform that regulates this action in vivo.[100] The changes in Qo_2 with NOS inhibition may occur because of the following: (1) a shift in the site of sodium reabsorption to a less efficient nephron segment; (2) decreased efficiency of transport in the proximal tubule (i.e., decrease in the passive component of reabsorption); or (3) less efficient use of O_2 by mitochondria. For example, nitric oxide given directly to a proximal tubular cell is a proximal diuretic[102] and competitive inhibitor of O_2 flux through the electron transport chain in mitochondria.[103]

Most effects of nitric oxide are mediated by cyclic guanosine monophosphate, but the mitochondrial effect is presumed to occur through the competitive inhibition of cytochrome c oxidase.[103-105] Studies in normal rats,[106] in rats with experimental diabetes,[107] and in rats with untreated hypertension[108,109] have found an antagonistic relationship between nitric oxide and angiotensin II in terms of glomerular hemodynamics and tubular reabsorption. Specifically, systemic NOS blockade causes renal vasoconstriction and activation of tubuloglomerular feedback, which can be prevented by angiotensin II blockers.

A similar antagonistic relationship also appears to exist in the control of kidney. Angiotensin II has been shown to be capable of increasing Q_{O_2}, in spite of lowering T_{Na}.[110] Rats and mice with angiotensin-induced hypertension exhibit stimulation of sodium transporters from the cortical TAL to the CD in regions with higher Q_{O_2}/T_{Na} and inhibition or no stimulation of sodium transporters in the proximal nephron, where Q_{O_2}/T_{Na} is lower.[111,112] Studies in spontaneous hypertensive rats have suggested opposing effects of angiotensin II and nitric oxide on the Q_{O_2}/T_{Na} ratio in the kidney.[113] Rats with angiotensin-induced hypertension demonstrated an increased Q_{O_2}/T_{Na} that was reversed by a mimetic of superoxide dismutase, which is consistent with the theory that many angiotensin II effects are mediated by upregulating the activity of reduced nicotinamide adenine dinucleotide phosphate (NADPH) oxidase.[110] In addition, there is evidence that angiotensin II contributes to mitochondrial dysfunction and oxygen consumption in aging rats.[114]

There is also evidence for a self-contained intrarenal renin angiotensin system that operates independently of the systemic renin angiotensin system (RAS).[115-118] It is possible to dissociate tubular and whole-kidney angiotensin II in the regulation of proximal reabsorption and salt homeostasis.[118] For example, a low-salt diet activates the systemic RAS and increases renal sodium reabsorption without any measurable increase in intrarenal synthesis of angiotensin II,[119] whereas a high-salt diet has a predictable inhibitory effect on plasma and whole-kidney angiotensin II; surprisingly, however, this leads to increased angiotensin II content of proximal tubular fluid. This finding explains why the tonic influence of endogenous angiotensin II over proximal reabsorption fails to decline with consumption of a high-salt diet. Thus, whereas the systemic RAS is oriented toward salt homeostasis, it appears that the tubular angiotensin II system is oriented toward a stable salt delivery beyond the proximal tubule.[118]

The role of angiotensin II in kidney metabolism is implicated in the ablation/infarction remnant kidney model of chronic kidney disease (CKD). Oxygen consumption factored for nephron number or T_{Na} has been shown to be elevated in this model[120-122] and lowered by various treatments, including angiotensin blockade.[120] A connection has also been established between local accumulation of the Krebs cycle intermediate succinate and activation of the RAS.[123] Succinate can accumulate extracellularly when oxygen supply does not match demand. In the extracellular fluid, it can bind to its G protein–coupled receptor, GPR91. P_{O_2} in the juxtaglomerular region is reduced in the hyperglycemia of diabetes, and succinate levels are very high in the urine and renal tissue of diabetic animals. Inhibition of the Krebs cycle's succinate dehydrogenase complex causes robust renin release. This effect is amplified in high-glucose conditions or with added succinate. In summary, GPR91-mediated signaling in the juxtaglomerular apparatus could modulate glomerular filtration rate and RAS activity in response to changes in metabolism (especially after a meal, when the glucose level is elevated). Pathologically, GPR91-mediated signaling could link metabolic diseases (e.g., diabetes) with RAS activation, systemic hypertension, and organ injury.

HYPOXIA AND ISCHEMIA

Intrarenal hypoxia has been proposed as a final common pathway to the progression of CKD.[124] In late stages of CKD, rarefaction of capillaries and other structural changes have been implicated in the decrease in oxygen supply leading to hypoxia. However, intrarenal hypoxia has been demonstrated in the early stages before any structural changes.[125] A high Q_{O_2}/T_{Na} has been postulated to be the cause of tubular hypoxia in the early stages of CKD.[120] In early experimental diabetes, decreased tissue oxygen tension (P_{O_2}) by blood oxygen level–dependent magnetic resonance imaging (BOLD MRI) has also been demonstrated prior to any structural changes associated with diabetic nephropathy.[126]

BOLD MRI has been used to measure blood flow, oxygen tension, and regional tissue oxygenation in the kidney cortex and medulla in humans with hypertension. The following were compared: kidneys with atherosclerotic renal artery stenosis, kidneys contralateral to the stenotic kidneys, and kidneys in individuals with essential hypertension, with no accompanying stenosis.[127,128] In the stenotic kidneys, as expected, tissue volume was decreased and blood flow was compromised; however, there was no significant decrease in P_{O_2} in the cortex or deep medulla compared with the contralateral kidney in the same person or compared with kidneys in individuals with essential hypertension. This led the authors to postulate that there was reduced oxygen consumption in the stenotic kidneys. Consistent with this interpretation, furosemide-suppressible Q_{O_2} in the medulla was significantly less in the stenotic kidney than in the contralateral kidney or in kidneys in those with essential hypertension.[128]

BOLD MRI has been found to be a useful technique for assessing whether renal artery stenosis is associated with tissue hypoxia and renal damage.[129] In diabetic and nondiabetic CKD patients, BOLD MRI has been used to demonstrate intrarenal hypoxia, with a good correlation with renal pathology.[130,131] It has also been used to assess alterations in renal oxygenation in acute transplant rejection.[132] It was also used recently to investigate the effect of sodium intake on renal tissue oxygenation.[133] In brief, 1 week of low sodium intake increased renal medullary oxygenation in normotensive and hypertensive subjects, whereas a high-sodium diet reduced medullary oxygenation. A recent study of humans with CKD and hypertension, as well as healthy controls, with BOLD MRI revealed tight regulation of renal oxygenation at rest, but an altered response to furosemide in the CKD and hypertension groups, suggesting early metabolic changes in hypertension.[134,135] In many of these studies, furosemide was administered to inhibit tubular reabsorption, which improved medullary oxygenation; this demonstrated the significant role of sodium reabsorption–driven Qo_2, even in established disease with structural alterations, which affect oxygen delivery.

Evans and colleagues[136] recently examined Po_2 during moderate renal ischemia, when changes in renal oxygen delivery and Qo_2 are mismatched. When renal artery pressure was reduced from 80 to 40 mm Hg, Qo_2 was reduced almost 40%, even though delivery was reduced by only 26%. Renal angiotensin II infusion reduced O_2 delivery by almost 40% and increased fractional oxygen extraction (renal venous Po_2 decreased). When renal arterial pressure was higher than 40 mm Hg, renal Po_2 remained remarkably stable. With these protocols, reductions in Qo_2 were proportionally less than reductions in T_{Na}. Thus, reducing renal Qo_2 can help prevent tissue hypoxia during mild ischemia; other mechanisms, not including increased efficiency of renal oxygen utilization for sodium reabsorption, apparently come into play to prevent a fall in renal Po_2 when renal Qo_2 is reduced less than O_2 delivery.

HYPOXIA-INDUCIBLE FACTOR

During hypoxia, the cellular interior becomes acidic, and the low cellular pH causes a small protein inhibitor called inhibitory factor 1 (IF_1) to dimerize. In the dimeric state, the IF_1 binds to two ATPase synthase molecules and inhibits their activity.[23] This is an important adaptation because, during low-energy states, ATPase synthase can actually operate in reverse (as an ATPase), which would cause further deterioration of the energy status of the cell. IF_1 inhibits the ATPase activity of ATP synthase, thereby preventing wasteful hydrolysis of ATP that could occur if there were insufficient oxygen to drive the electron transport chain. When oxygen delivery is normalized and cellular pH increases, the IF_1 dimer disassembles, and ATP synthase begins to operate in the ATP synthesis mode.[23]

In addition to the IF_1-mediated, rapid posttranscriptional adaptation to hypoxia, there is a transcriptional adaptive response to hypoxia mediated by hypoxia-inducible factor (HIF).[137] A great body of work by Semenza has described the role of HIF as a primary oxygen sensor and regulator of cellular oxygen homeostasis.[137-140] It accumulates in hypoxic cells, where it acts to regulate gene expression. HIF consists of a labile α-subunit (HIF-1α, HIF-2α, HIF-3α) and a constitutive β-subunit. These subunits heterodimerize to form a transcriptional complex that translocates to the nucleus and binds to hypoxia response elements of various hypoxia-responsive genes.[141,142] HIF-1α and HIF-2α have been well-studied, have similar structures, and have significant overlap in their actions on target genes; however, some target genes appear to be exclusively under the regulation of one or the other. Their renal tissue expression patterns also differ, with predominant expression of HIF-1α in the tubular epithelial cells and of HIF-2α in the interstitial fibroblasts and peritubular endothelial cells in the hypoxic kidney.[143,144] There is limited information regarding the function and actions of HIF-3α.

During adaptation to hypoxia, HIF-1α and HIF-2α regulate the expression of many genes that regulate oxygen delivery and consumption. Changes that culminate in a rise in erythropoiesis, vasodilation, and tissue vascularization all increase oxygen delivery.[145,146] Another set of responses conserves energy by decreasing substrate movement into the tricarboxylic acid cycle, increasing cellular glucose uptake and glycolytic enzymes to increase anaerobic ATP production and shifting the cell toward glycolytic metabolism.[140] HIF-1α also has significant effects on mitochondrial metabolism; specifically, it diminishes NADH supply to the electron transport chain (ETC), induces a subunit switch in complex IV of the ETC to optimize its efficiency in hypoxia, and represses mitochondrial biogenesis and respiration.[147,148] Finally, HIF-1α also induces mitochondrial autophagy as an adaptive metabolic response to prevent increased levels of reactive oxygen species (ROS) generation and cell death in hypoxia.[149]

HIF-1 α has also been recognized as a regulator of salt transport. High-salt intake increased HIF-1α expression in the renal medulla.[150] Inhibition of HIF-1α in the renal medulla decreased medullary blood flow and blunted urine flow and urinary Na excretion. In the presence of HIF-1α inhibitor, rats on a high-salt diet developed positive cumulative salt balance and higher blood pressure. Thus, medullary HIF-1α inhibition on high salt intake leads to the resetting of pressure natriuresis, sodium retention, and salt-sensitive hypertension.[151] HIF-1α expression has been reported in the medulla in a normal rat,[152] in which selective inhibition of medullary HIF-1 induced significant tubulointerstitial damage. Interestingly, HIF-1 expression appeared to correlate with salt transport; an increase was noted after an increase in medullary workload and a decrease in expression was noted after inhibiting sodium transport in the TAL by furosemide administration, which also increased medullary Po_2.[152]

HIF activity is regulated by proteasamal degradation during normoxia by a von Hippel-Lindau E3 ubiquitin ligase complex after being hydroxylated by prolyl-4-hydroxylase domains (PHDs). Of the three main identified PHDs (1, 2, and 3), PHD2 is the main enzyme that targets HIF for degradation under normoxia.[143] All three PHDs are expressed in the kidney and are found predominantly in the distal convoluted tubule, collecting duct, and podocytes, and levels are depressed during ischemia and reperfusion.[142,143] HIF activity is also regulated by factor-inhibiting HIF (FIH), which inhibits its transcriptional activity by hydroxylating an asparagine residue within the transactivation domain and preventing the binding of coactivators to the HIF transcriptional complex.[139] Although a tremendous amount of progress has been made in understanding how HIF helps maintain O_2 homeostasis, the study of this factor in the kidney under normal physiologic and pathophysiologic conditions is just in its infancy.

ADENOSINE MONOPHOSPHATE–ACTIVATED PROTEIN KINASE

The energy status of the cell can be detected by the ultrasensitive 5′-adenosine monophosphate (AMP)–activated protein kinase (AMPK), which is a ubiquitously expressed, highly conserved, key energy sensor and regulator of cellular metabolic activity.[153] AMPK is comprised of a heterotrimer of a catalytic subunit ($α_1$ or $α_2$), together with a beta ($β_1$ or $β_2$) and gamma ($γ_1, γ_2$, or $γ_3$) regulatory subunit.[153] Cellular energy stress, which can be due to a variety of conditions, such as nutrient or glucose deprivation, exercise, hypoxia, or ischemia, is detected as a rising concentration of AMP and an increase in the AMP/ATP ratio. AMPK is activated by phosphorylation of the α-catalytic subunit on threonine-172 (Thr172) by upstream kinases.[154] The binding of AMP to the γ-regulatory subunit of AMPK increases its activity in three ways: (1) conformational change in AMPK, which allows enhanced phosphorylation of the α-catalytic subunit on Thr172 by upstream kinases, thus activating AMPK; (2) inhibition of dephosphorylation of the catalytic subunit; and (3) direct allosteric activation. These three effects, working in concert, render the system exquisitely sensitive to changes in AMP, and all are antagonized by ATP—thus the importance of the AMP/ATP ratio. AMPK acts as a metabolic checkpoint to facilitate metabolic adaptation to cellular energetic stress by triggering ATP-producing pathways such as fatty acid oxidation, glucose uptake, and glycolysis while inhibiting ATP-consuming pathways such as fatty acid synthesis, protein synthesis, and potentially active transport[155] (Figure 5.15). AMPK also promotes cellular autophagy, an energy-conserving survival mechanism in low-energy states, by inhibiting the mammalian target of rapamycin (mTOR).[156,157]

There is abundant AMPK expression in the kidney, but the understanding of its impact on energy metabolism and transport in the kidney is just emerging. The role of AMPK in ion transport in the kidney has been recently reviewed.[158,159] Overall, AMPK becomes activated when ATP is limiting—that is, when the AMP/ATP ratio increases—and, once activated, it decreases ATP consumption and increases ATP synthesis. In the kidney, sodium transport is the major energy-consuming process, and there is increasing evidence regarding the role of AMPK in sodium transport in the kidney and other epithelial cells. AMPK has been shown to inhibit the activity of various transport proteins in lung, gut, and kidney, including the epithelial Na channel (ENaC) in the kidney collecting duct, NKCC2 in the TAL, and Na$^+$-K$^+$-ATPase in the alveolar epithelial cells, particularly during hypoxia.[159,160] Hallows and colleagues[158,159] have determined that AMPK activation depresses transport mediated by the cystic fibrosis transmembrane conductance regulator, epithelial sodium channel, vacuolar H$^+$-ATPase, and NKCC2 (see Figure 5.15). AMPK expression in the kidney is seen mainly in the cortical thick ascending limb and macula densa cells and in some DCTs and collecting ducts.[161] Recently, AMPK expression in the proximal tubule has also been reported.[162] Differing results in pAMPK expression in response to high salt intake has been observed with increased phosphorylated (activated) AMPK in one study[161] and reduced expression in another.[163] In vivo, pharmacologic activation of AMPK in rats fed a high-salt diet was shown to enhance the tubuloglomerular feedback (TGF) response and reduce sodium reabsorption in the proximal and distal tubules, but had no effects on these parameters in rats fed a normal-salt diet.[163] Whether these effects are driven by a change in cellular metabolism that results in an increase in AMP and ATP levels is not clear. Consumption of a high-salt diet decreases the fraction of the filtered load of sodium that is absorbed and, given the effect of AMPK activation in inhibiting transporters, the findings suggest that AMPK participates in salt and water homeostasis.

The AMPK pathway may provide another important layer of regulation between ATP production by mitochondria and ATP consumption by transporters. In the Whittam model illustrated in Figure 5.3, increased active transport provokes a decrease in the ATP/ADP ratio, which drives increased ATP production by the mitochondria. When ATP production by the mitochondria becomes limiting, however, AMPK is likely to be activated, which would drive a reduction in ATP consumption by active membrane transporters. Thus, AMPK may regulate the coupling of ion transport and energy metabolism in the kidney.

Acute renal ischemia provokes a rapid and powerful activation of AMPK, but its functional role in the response to ischemia remains unclear. There is conflicting evidence in the literature regarding the effects of AMPK activation in ischemia-reperfusion injury.[164-167] Similarly, although several studies have shown a beneficial effect of AMPK activation in myocardial ischemia-reperfusion, there are some conflicting studies demonstrating the deleterious effects of AMPK activation in ischemic injury in the heart and brain.[153] Hence, the effects of AMPK activation are likely to be time-, tissue-, and cell-dependent. Whether AMPK abundance or its phosphorylation is higher in the hypoxia-prone medulla than in the cortex has not yet been investigated, nor have studies been conducted examining the effect of AMPK activation on renal gluconeogenesis or glycolysis. A key question is whether renal AMPK activation suppresses

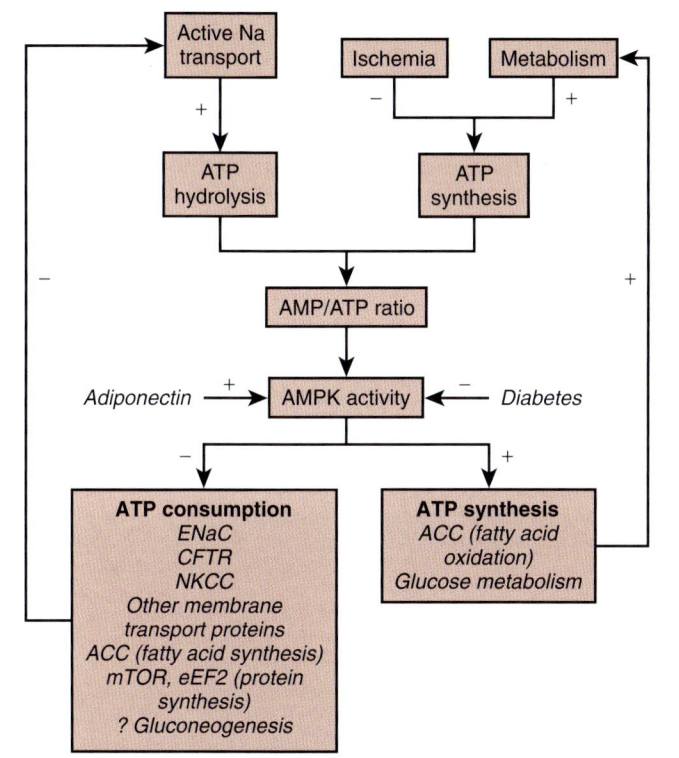

Figure 5.15 Proposed role of adenosine monophosphate–activated protein kinase (AMPK) in the kidney in coupling catabolic pathways requiring ATP hydrolysis (primarily sodium transport) with metabolic pathways leading to ATP synthesis (primarily fatty acid and glucose oxidation). +, Activating pathway; –, inhibitory pathway. ACC, Acetyl CoA carboxylase.; CFTR, cystic fibrosis transmembrane conductance regulator; eF2, elongation factor 2; ENaC, epithelial sodium channel; mTOR, mammalian target of rapamycin; NKCC, Na-K-chloride cotransporter. (From Hallows KR, Mount PF, Pastor-Soler NM, Power DA.: Role of the energy sensor AMP-activated kinase in renal physiology and disease. *Am J Physiol Renal Physiol* 298:F1067-F1077, 2010.)

Na$^+$-K$^+$-ATPase activity along the nephron. AMPK activation has been reported to inhibit lung cell Na$^+$-K$^+$-ATPase transport activity mediated by endocytosis,[168] but AMPK activation had no apparent effect on skeletal muscle Na$^+$-K$^+$-ATPase activity or distribution.[169] This leaves the question open for the kidney; one report has demonstrated that inhibition of AMPK induces the endocytosis of Na$^+$-K$^+$-ATPase in Madin-Darby canine kidney cells.[170]

MITOCHONDRIAL DISEASES

Given the central role of mitochondria in producing ATP via oxidative phosphorylation, it is not surprising that genetic mutations affecting mitochondrial function have renal manifestations. The mitochondrial genome is distinct from the nuclear genome, and it encodes 13 of the 88 protein subunits of ETC complexes I through V, as well as 22 mitochondrial-specific transfer RNAs (tRNAs) and two RNA components of the translational apparatus. The nuclear genome encodes the remaining respiratory chain subunits and most of the mitochondrial DNA replication and expression components.

Disorders affecting mitochondrial oxidative phosphorylation can arise from mutations in mitochondrial genes or nuclear genes encoding respiratory chain components, or ancillary factors involved in the maintenance of ETC function or the overall number of mitochondria.[171] The incidence of genetic mitochondrial disorders is estimated at about 1 in 5000 births, with the most common affecting the sequence of a mitochondrial tRNA for leucine. Such mutations affect mitochondrial function in all tissues. Symptoms are evident before 2 months of age, and the number of organ systems affected increases with age.

Impairment of mitochondrial oxidative phosphorylation results in increased levels of reducing equivalents (NADH, FADH$_2$), which, in the mitochondria, transform acetoacetate to 3-hydroxybutyrate and, in the cytosol, transform pyruvate to lactate. Thus, elevated levels of lactic acid, ketone bodies, and impaired redox status are suggestive of a mitochondrial defect disorder.[172] If the genetic cause of the impairment can be pinpointed, then an appropriate therapy, if available, can be implemented to treat these life-threatening disorders; for example, coenzyme Q$_{10}$ enzyme defects can be treated with coenzyme Q$_{10}$ supplementation.[171]

Myopathies and cardiomyopathies are the most common manifestations of mitochondrial disease, and central nervous system symptoms, including encephalopathies, are very common. Renal system impairment can be present, but is not seen without other system deficiencies and is usually reported in children. Although glomerular disease and tubulointerstitial nephropathy have both been reported, the most frequently observed is impairment of proximal tubule reabsorption, known as the de Toni-Debré-Fanconi syndrome, in which there are urinary losses of bicarbonate, amino acids, glucose, phosphate, uric acid, potassium, and water. All these symptoms can be explained by lack of ATP to fuel Na$^+$-K$^+$-ATPase sufficiently to drive transepithelial transport. The symptoms can range from mild to more severe and present in the neonatal period in most patients. Biopsy specimens show tubular dilations, casts, dedifferentiation, and cellular vacuolization. At the cellular level, there are enlarged mitochondria. Supplements of sodium bicarbonate, potassium, vitamin D, phosphorus, and water are called for if these symptoms are evident.[171,172]

SUMMARY

Most of the energy consumed by the kidney is traceable to the energy requirements for sodium reabsorption. Although all sodium reabsorption is linked to Na$^+$-K$^+$-ATPase, efficiency is achieved by leveraging Na$^+$-K$^+$-ATPase into transepithelial chloride or voltage gradients that allow some sodium to be reabsorbed without passing through the Na$^+$-K$^+$-ATPase itself. ATP production in the proximal tubule is solely by aerobic metabolism, whereas the medullary segments have additional capacity to produce energy by glycolysis. Transport activity regulates metabolism, metabolism may be rate-limiting for transport, and the efficiency of transport can be made to vary at multiple levels, from backleak permeability to the efficiency of mitochondrial respiration. With regard to metabolic autoregulation, the kidney faces a particular challenge because the usual mechanism for delivering more oxygen to the kidney also increases demand for that oxygen. Several intermediaries have been identified as parts of the complex network of interactions between transport and metabolism that allow the kidney to meet this challenge while balancing the risk of hypoxia against the risk of oxygen toxicity. These include adenosine, nitric oxide, prostaglandins, angiotensin II, dopamine, succinate, uncoupling proteins, HIF, and AMPK. A multiscale systems model that incorporates these elements, along with renal anatomy to recapitulate renal metabolism, is expected in the future.

Complete reference list available at ExpertConsult.com.

KEY REFERENCES

1. Cohen JJ, Kamm DE: Renal metabolism: relation to renal function. In Brenner BM, Rector BA, editor: *The kidney*, ed 2, Philadelphia, 1981, Saunders, p 147.
2. Rapoport S, Brodsky WA, West CD: Excretion of solutes and osmotic work of the resting kidney of hydropenic man. *Am J Physiol* 157:357–362, 1949.
16. Aronson PS: Identifying secondary active solute transport in epithelia. *Am J Physiol* 240:F1–F11, 1981.
18. McDonough AA: Mechanisms of proximal tubule sodium transport regulation that link extracellular fluid volume and blood pressure. *Am J Physiol Regul Integr Comp Physiol* 298:R851–R861, 2010.
22. Mitchell P: Coupling of phosphorylation to electron and hydrogen transfer by a chemi-osmotic type of mechanism. *Nature* 191:144–148, 1961.
24. Mandel LJ: Metabolic substrates, cellular energy production, and the regulation of proximal tubular transport. *Annu Rev Physiol* 47:85–101, 1985.
28. Blond DM, Whittam R: The regulation of kidney respiration by sodium and potassium ions. *Biochem J* 92:158–167, 1964.
33. McDonough AA, Magyar CE, Komatsu Y: Expression of Na(+)-K(+)-ATPase alpha- and beta-subunits along rat nephron: isoform specificity and response to hypokalemia. *Am J Physiol* 267:C901–C908, 1994.
35. Guder WG, Ross BD: Enzyme distribution along the nephron. *Kidney Int* 26:101–111, 1984.
37. Uchida S, Endou H: Substrate specificity to maintain cellular ATP along the mouse nephron. *Am J Physiol* 255:F977–F983, 1988.
41. Gerich JE, Meyer C, Woerle HJ, et al: Renal gluconeogenesis: its importance in human glucose homeostasis. *Diabetes Care* 24:382–391, 2001.

45. Cohen JJ: Relationship between energy requirements for Na+ reabsorption and other renal functions. *Kidney Int* 29:32–40, 1986.
46. Gullans SR, Brazy PC, Dennis VW, et al: Interactions between gluconeogenesis and sodium transport in rabbit proximal tubule. *Am J Physiol* 246:F859–F869, 1984.
49. Bagnasco S, Good D, Balaban R, et al: Lactate production in isolated segments of the rat nephron. *Am J Physiol* 248:F522–F526, 1985.
51. Friedrichs D, Schoner W: Stimulation of renal gluconeogenesis by inhibition of the sodium pump. *Biochim Biophys Acta* 304:142–160, 1973.
54. Hering-Smith KS, Hamm LL: Metabolic support of collecting duct transport. *Kidney Int* 53:408–415, 1998.
59. Evans RG, Gardiner BS, Smith DW, et al: Intrarenal oxygenation: unique challenges and the biophysical basis of homeostasis. *Am J Physiol Renal Physiol* 295:F1259–F1270, 2008.
60. Neuhofer W, Beck FX: Cell survival in the hostile environment of the renal medulla. *Annu Rev Physiol* 67:531–555, 2005.
64. Blantz RC, Deng A, Miracle CM, et al: Regulation of kidney function and metabolism: a question of supply and demand. *Trans Am Clin Climatol Assoc* 118:23–43, 2007.
65. Thomson SC, Blantz RC: Glomerulotubular balance, tubuloglomerular feedback, and salt homeostasis. *J Am Soc Nephrol* 19:2272–2275, 2008.
66. Du Z, Duan Y, Yan Q, et al: Mechanosensory function of microvilli of the kidney proximal tubule. *Proc Natl Acad Sci U S A* 101:13068–13073, 2004.
70. Schurek HJ, Johns O: Is tubuloglomerular feedback a tool to prevent nephron oxygen deficiency? *Kidney Int* 51:386–392, 1997.
73. Vallon V, Muhlbauer B, Osswald H: Adenosine and kidney function. *Physiol Rev* 86:901–940, 2006.
76. Thurau K: Renal Na-reabsorption and O2-uptake in dogs during hypoxia and hydrochlorothiazide infusion. *Proc Soc Exp Biol Med* 106:714–717, 1961.
78. Burg M, Good D: Sodium chloride–coupled transport in mammalian nephrons. *Annu Rev Physiol* 45:5335–5347, 1983.
81. Andreoli TE, Schafer JA, Troutman SL, et al: Solvent drag component of Cl- flux in superficial proximal straight tubules: evidence for a paracellular component of isotonic fluid absorption. *Am J Physiol* 237:F455–F462, 1979.
85. Hebert SC: Roles of Na-K-2Cl and Na-Cl cotransporters and ROMK potassium channels in urinary concentrating mechanism. *Am J Physiol* 275:F325–F327, 1998.
87. Silva P, Torretti J, Hayslett JP, et al: Relation between Na-K-ATPase activity and respiratory rate in the rat kidney. *Am J Physiol* 230:1432–1438, 1976.
95. Evans RG, Harrop GK, Ngo JP, et al: Basal renal O2 consumption and the efficiency of O2 utilization for Na+ reabsorption. *Am J Physiol Renal Physiol* 306:F551–F560, 2014.
98. Mandel LJ, Balaban RS: Stoichiometry and coupling of active transport to oxidative metabolism in epithelial tissues. *Am J Physiol* 240:F357–F371, 1981.
100. Deng A, Miracle CM, Suarez JM, et al: Oxygen consumption in the kidney: effects of nitric oxide synthase isoforms and angiotensin II. *Kidney Int* 68:723–730, 2005.
102. Yip KP: Flash photolysis of caged nitric oxide inhibits proximal tubular fluid reabsorption in free-flow nephron. *Am J Physiol Regul Integr Comp Physiol* 289:R620–R626, 2005.
106. De Nicola L, Blantz RC, Gabbai FB: Nitric oxide and angiotensin II. Glomerular and tubular interaction in the rat. *J Clin Invest* 89:1248–1256, 1992.
110. Welch WJ, Blau J, Xie H, et al: Angiotensin-induced defects in renal oxygenation: role of oxidative stress. *Am J Physiol Heart Circ Physiol* 288:H22–H28, 2005.
112. Nguyen MT, Lee DH, Delpire E, et al: Differential regulation of Na+ transporters along nephron during ANG II-dependent hypertension: distal stimulation counteracted by proximal inhibition. *Am J Physiol Renal Physiol* 305:F510–F519, 2013.
116. Navar LG, Harrison-Bernard LM, Imig JD, et al: Intrarenal angiotensin II generation and renal effects of AT1 receptor blockade. *J Am Soc Nephrol* 10(Suppl 12):S266–S272, 1999.
118. Thomson SC, Deng A, Wead L, et al: An unexpected role for angiotensin II in the link between dietary salt and proximal reabsorption. *J Clin Invest* 116:1110–1116, 2006.
120. Deng A, Tang T, Singh P, et al: Regulation of oxygen utilization by angiotensin II in chronic kidney disease. *Kidney Int* 75:197–204, 2009.
123. Toma I, Kang JJ, Sipos A, et al: Succinate receptor GPR91 provides a direct link between high glucose levels and renin release in murine and rabbit kidney. *J Clin Invest* 118:2526–2534, 2008.
128. Gloviczki ML, Glockner JF, Lerman LO, et al: Preserved oxygenation despite reduced blood flow in poststenotic kidneys in human atherosclerotic renal artery stenosis. *Hypertension* 55:961–966, 2010.
130. Inoue T, Kozawa E, Okada H, et al: Noninvasive evaluation of kidney hypoxia and fibrosis using magnetic resonance imaging. *J Am Soc Nephrol* 22:1429–1434, 2011.
134. Pruijm M, Hofmann L, Piskunowicz M: Determinants of renal tissue oxygenation as measured with BOLD-MRI in chronic kidney disease and hypertension in humans. *PLoS ONE* 9:e95895, 2014.
136. Evans RG, Eppel GA, Michaels S, et al: Multiple mechanisms act to maintain kidney oxygenation during renal ischemia in anesthetized rabbits. *Am J Physiol Renal Physiol* 298:F1235–F1243, 2010.
139. Semenza GL: Oxygen sensing, hypoxia-inducible factors, and disease pathophysiology. *Annu Rev Pathol* 9:47–71, 2014.
143. Haase VH: Mechanisms of hypoxia responses in renal tissue. *J Am Soc Nephrol* 24:537–541, 2013.
151. Wang Z, Zhu Q, Xia M, et al: Hypoxia-inducible factor prolyl-hydroxylase 2 senses high-salt intake to increase hypoxia inducible factor 1alpha levels in the renal medulla. *Hypertension* 55:1129–1136, 2010.
154. Hardie DG: AMP-activated protein kinase: maintaining energy homeostasis at the cellular and whole-body levels. *Annu Rev Nutr* 34:31–55, 2014.
160. Pastor-Soler NM, Hallows KR: AMP-activated protein kinase regulation of kidney tubular transport. *Curr Opin Nephrol Hypertens* 21:523–533, 2012.
163. Huang DY, Gao H, Boini KM, et al: In vivo stimulation of AMP-activated protein kinase enhanced tubuloglomerular feedback but reduced tubular sodium transport during high dietary NaCl intake. *Pflugers Arch* 460:187–196, 2010.

6 Transport of Sodium, Chloride, and Potassium

David B. Mount

CHAPTER OUTLINE

SODIUM AND CHLORIDE TRANSPORT, 144
Proximal Tubule, 144
Loop of Henle and Thick Ascending Limb, 156
Distal Convoluted Tubule, Connecting Tubule, and Collecting Duct, 165
POTASSIUM TRANSPORT, 174
Proximal Tubule, 175
Loop of Henle and Medullary K+ Recycling, 175

K+ Secretion by the Distal Convoluted Tubule, Connecting Tubule, and Cortical Collecting Duct, 176
K+ Reabsorption by the Collecting Duct, 178
Regulation of Distal K+ Transport, 179
Integrated Na+-Cl- and K+ Transport in the Distal Nephron, 182

SODIUM AND CHLORIDE TRANSPORT

Sodium (Na^+) is the principal osmole in extracellular fluid; as such, the total body content of Na^+ and chloride (Cl^-), its primary anion, determine the extracellular fluid volume. Renal excretion or retention of salt (Na^+-Cl^-) is thus the major determinant of the extracellular fluid volume, such that genetic loss- or gain-of-function in renal Na^+-Cl^- transport can be associated with relative hypotension or hypertension, respectively. On a quantitative level, at a glomerular filtration rate of 180 L/day and serum Na^+ of about 140 mmol/L, the kidney filters some 25,200 mmol/day of Na^+; this is equivalent to about 1.5 kg of salt, which would occupy roughly 10 times the extracellular space.[1] Minute changes in renal Na^+-Cl^- excretion can thus have massive effects on the extracellular fluid volume. In addition, 99.6% of filtered Na^+-Cl^- must be reabsorbed to excrete 100 mmol/L/day. Energetically, this renal absorption of Na^+ consumes 1 molecule of ATP per 5 molecules of Na^+.[1] This is gratifyingly economical, given that the absorption of Na^+-Cl^- is primarily, but not exclusively, driven by basolateral Na+-K+-ATPase, which has a stoichiometry of 3 molecules of transported Na^+ per molecule of adenosine triphosphate (ATP).[2] This estimate reflects a net expenditure, however, because the cost of transepithelial Na^+-Cl^- transport varies considerably along the nephron, from a predominance of passive transport by thin ascending limbs to the purely active transport mediated by the aldosterone-sensitive distal nephron (distal convoluted tubule, connecting tubule, and collecting duct). The bulk of filtered Na^+-Cl^- transport is reabsorbed by the proximal tubule and thick ascending limb (TAL; Figure 6.1), nephron segments that use their own peculiar combinations of paracellular and transcellular Na^+-Cl^- transport. Whereas the proximal tubule can theoretically absorb as much as 9 Na^+ molecules for each hydrolyzed ATP, paracellular Na^+ transport by the TAL doubles the efficiency of transepithelial Na^+-Cl^- transport (6 Na^+ per ATP).[1,3] Finally, the fine-tuning of renal Na^+-Cl^- absorption occurs at full cost (3 Na^+ per ATP) in the aldosterone-sensitive distal nephron while affording the generation of considerable transepithelial gradients.[1]

The nephron thus constitutes a serial arrangement of tubule segments with considerable heterogeneity in the physiologic consequences, mechanisms, and regulation of transepithelial Na^+-Cl^- transport. These issues will be reviewed in this section in anatomic order.

PROXIMAL TUBULE

A primary function of the renal proximal tubule is the near-isosmotic reabsorption of two thirds to three quarters of the glomerular ultrafiltrate. This encompasses the reabsorption of approximately 60% of filtered Na^+-Cl^- (see Figure 6.1), such that this nephron segment plays a critical role in the maintenance of extracellular fluid volume. Although all segments of the proximal tubule share the ability to transport a variety of inorganic and organic solutes, there are considerable differences in the transport characteristics and capacity of early, mid, and late segments of the proximal tubule. There is thus a gradual reduction in the volume of transported fluid and solutes as one proceeds along the proximal nephron. This corresponds to distinct ultrastructural characteristics in the tubular epithelium, moving from the S1

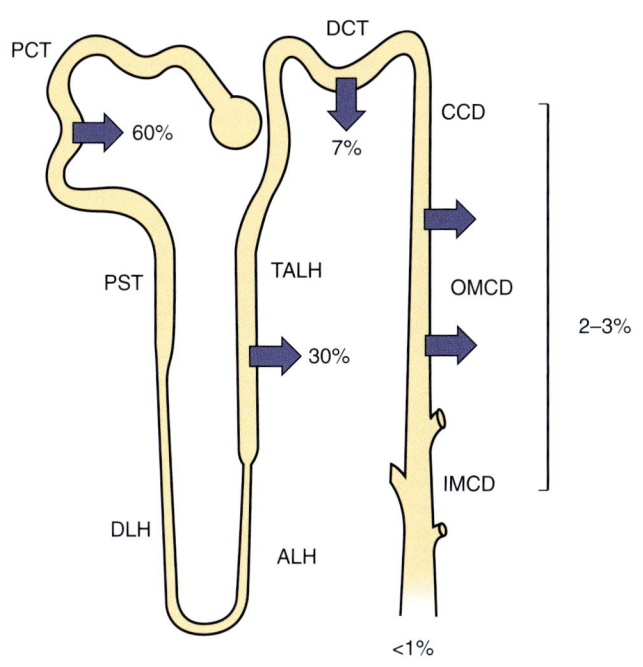

Figure 6.1 Percentage reabsorption of filtered Na⁺-Cl⁻ along the euvolemic nephron. ALH, Thin ascending limb of the loop of Henle; CCD, cortical collecting duct; DCT, distal convoluted tubule; DLH, descending thin limb of the loop of Henle; IMCD, inner medullary collecting duct; OMCD, outer medullary collecting duct; PCT, proximal convoluted tubule; PST, proximal straight tubule; TALH, thick ascending limb of the loop of Henle. (From Moe OW, Baum M, Berry CA, Rector FC, Jr: Renal transport of glucose, amino acids, sodium, chloride, and water. In Brenner BM, editor: *Brenner and Rector's the kidney*, Philadelphia, 2004, WB Saunders, pp 413-452.)

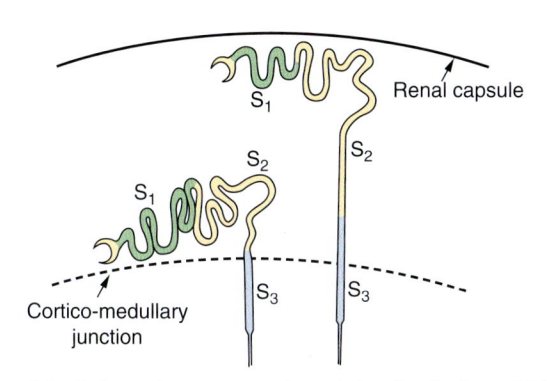

Figure 6.2 Schematic representation of the distribution of S1, S2, and S3 segments in the proximal tubules of superficial and juxtamedullary nephrons. (From Woodhall PB, Tisher CC, Simonton CA, Robinson RR: Relationship between para-aminohippurate secretion and cellular morphology in rabbit proximal tubules. *J Clin Invest* 61: 1320-1329, 1978).

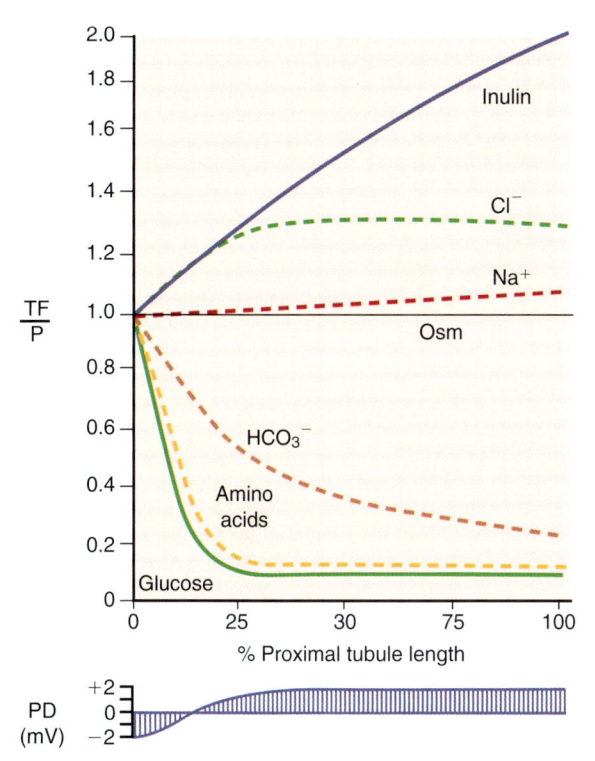

Figure 6.3 Reabsorption of solutes along the proximal tubule in relation to the transepithelial potential difference (PD). Osm, Osmolality; TF/P, ratio of tubule fluid to plasma concentration. (From Rector FC, Jr: Sodium, bicarbonate, and chloride absorption by the proximal tubule. *Am J Physiol* 244:F461-F471, 1983).

segment (early proximal convoluted tubule) to the S2 segment (late proximal convoluted tubule and beginning of the proximal straight tubule) and the S3 segment (remainder of the proximal straight tubule) (Figure 6.2). Cells of the S1 segment are thus characterized by a tall brush border, with extensive lateral invaginations of the basolateral membrane.[4] Numerous elongated mitochondria are located in lateral cell processes, with a proximity to the plasma membrane that is characteristic of epithelial cells involved in active transport. Ultrastructure of the S2 segment is similar, albeit with a shorter brush border, fewer lateral invaginations, and less prominent mitochondria. In epithelial cells of the S3 segment, lateral cell processes and invaginations are essentially absent, with small mitochondria that are randomly distributed within the cell.[4] The extensive brush border of proximal tubular cells serves to amplify the apical cell surface that is available for reabsorption; again, this amplification is axially distributed, increasing the apical area 36-fold in S1 and 15-fold in S3.[5] At the functional level, there is a rapid drop in the absorption of bicarbonate and Cl⁻ after the first millimeter of perfused proximal tubule, consistent with a much greater reabsorptive capacity in S1 segments.[6]

There is also considerable axial heterogeneity in the quantitative capacity of the proximal nephron for organic solutes such as glucose and amino acids, with predominant reabsorption of these substrates in S1 segments.[7] The Na⁺-dependent reabsorption of glucose, amino acids, and other solutes in S1 segments results in a transepithelial potential difference (PD) that is initially lumen-negative due to electrogenic removal of Na⁺ from the lumen (Figure 6.3).[8] This is classically considered the first phase of volume reabsorption by the proximal tubule.[9] The lumen-negative PD serves to drive both paracellular Cl⁻ absorption and a backleak of Na⁺ from the peritubular space to the lumen. Paracellular Cl⁻ absorption in this setting accomplishes the net transepithelial absorption of a solute such as glucose, along with equal amounts of Na⁺ and Cl⁻; in contrast, backleak of Na⁺

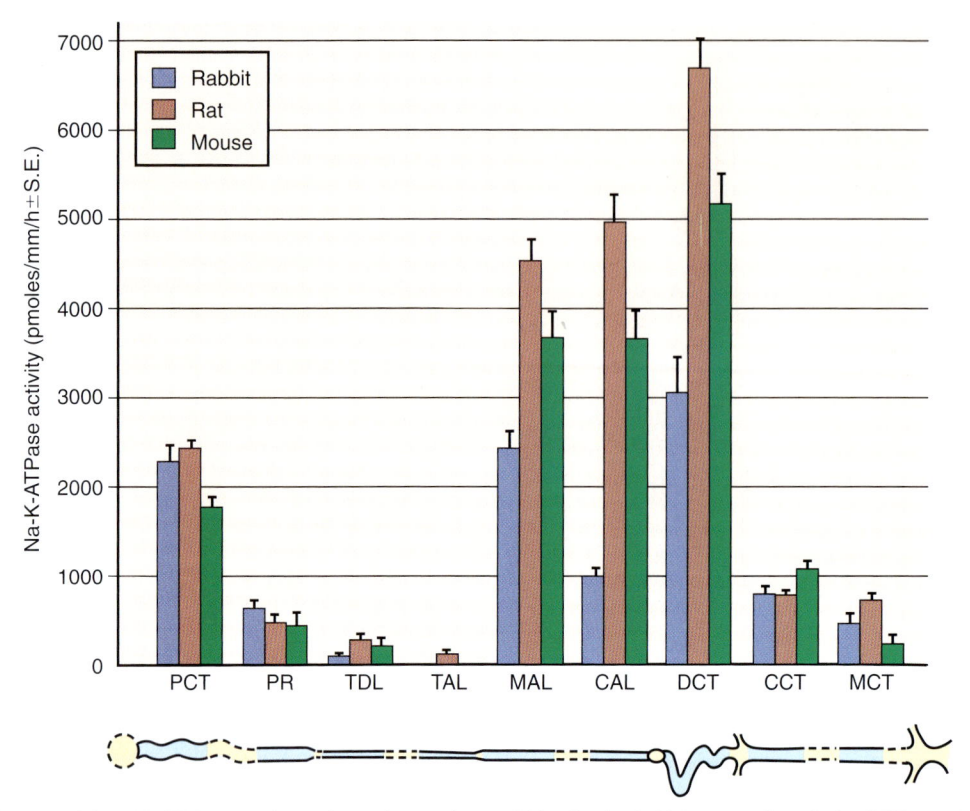

Figure 6.4 Distribution of Na^+-K^+-ATPase activity along the nephron. CAL, Cortical thick ascending limb; CCT, cortical collecting duct; DCT, distal convoluted tubule; MAL, medullary thick ascending limb; MCT, medullary collecting duct; PCT, proximal convoluted tubule; PR, pars recta; TAL, thin ascending limb of the loop of Henle; TDL, descending thin limb of the loop of Henle. (From Katz AI, Doucet A, Morel F: Na-K-ATPase activity along the rabbit, rat, and mouse nephron. *Am J Physiol* 237:F114-F120, 1979.)

leads only to reabsorption of the organic solute, with no net transepithelial transport of Na^+ or Cl^-. The amount of Cl^- reabsorption that is driven by this lumen-negative PD thus depends on the relative permeability of the paracellular pathway to Na^+ and Cl^-. There appears to be considerable heterogeneity in the relative paracellular permeability to Na^+ and Cl^-; for example, whereas superficial proximal convoluted tubules and proximal straight tubules in the rabbit are Cl^--selective, juxtamedullary proximal tubules in this species are reportedly Na^+-selective.[10,11] Regardless, the component of paracellular Cl^- transport that is driven by this lumen-negative PD is restricted to the very early proximal tubule.

The second phase of volume reabsorption by the proximal tubule is dominated by Na^+-Cl^- reabsorption via paracellular and transcellular pathways.[9] In addition to the Na^+-dependent reabsorption of organic solutes, the early proximal tubule has a much higher capacity for HCO_3^- absorption via the coupling of apical Na^+-H^+ exchange, carbonic anhydrase, and basolateral Na^+-HCO_3^- cotransport.[7] As the luminal concentrations of HCO_3^- and other solutes begin to drop, the concentration of Na^+-Cl^- rises to a value greater than that of the peritubular space.[12] This is accompanied by a reversal of the lumen-negative PD to a lumen-positive value generated by passive Cl^- diffusion (see Figure 6.3).[13] This lumen-positive PD serves to drive paracellular Na^+ transport, whereas the chemical gradient between the lumen and peritubular space provides the driving force for paracellular reabsorption of Cl^-. This passive paracellular pathway is thought to mediate about 40% of transepithelial Na^+-Cl^- reabsorption by the mid to late proximal tubule.[11] Of note, however, there may be heterogeneity in the relative importance of this paracellular pathway, with evidence that active (i.e., transcellular) reabsorption predominates in proximal convoluted tubules from juxtamedullary versus superficial nephrons.[14] Regardless, the combination of passive and active transport of Na^+-Cl^- explains how the proximal tubule is able to reabsorb about 60% of filtered Na^+-Cl^-, despite $Na+$-$K+$-ATPase activity that is considerably lower than that of distal segments of the nephron (Figure 6.4).[15]

The transcellular component of Na^+-Cl^- reabsorption initially emerged from studies of the effect of cyanide, ouabain, luminal anion transport inhibitors, cooling, and luminal-peritubular K^+ removal.[9] For example, the luminal addition of SITS (4-acetamido-4′-isothiocyanostilbene-2,2′-disulfonic acid), an inhibitor of anion transporters, reduces volume reabsorption of proximal convoluted tubules perfused with a high Cl^-, low HCO_3^- solution that mimics the luminal composition of the late proximal tubule; this occurs in the absence of an effect on carbonic anhydrase.[12] This transcellular component of Na^+-Cl^- reabsorption is clearly electroneutral. For example, in the absence of anion gradients across the perfused proximal tubule, there is no change in transepithelial PD after the inhibition of active transport by ouabain, despite a marked reduction in volume reabsorption.[16] Transcellular Na^+-Cl^- reabsorption is accomplished by the coupling of luminal Na^+-H^+ exchange or Na^+-SO_4^{2-}

cotransport with a heterogeneous population of anion exchangers, as reviewed below.

PARACELLULAR Na$^+$-Cl$^-$ TRANSPORT

A number of factors serve to optimize the conditions for paracellular Na$^+$-Cl$^-$ transport by the mid to late proximal tubule. First, the proximal tubule is a low-resistance, so-called leaky epithelium, with tight junctions that are highly permeable to both Na$^+$ and Cl$^-$.[10,11] Second, these tight junctions are preferentially permeable to Cl$^-$ over HCO$_3^-$, a feature that helps generate the lumen-positive PD in the mid to late proximal tubule.[12] Third, the increase in luminal Na$^+$-Cl$^-$ concentrations in the mid to late proximal tubule generates the electrical and chemical driving forces for paracellular transport. Diffusion of Cl$^-$ thus generates a lumen-positive PD, which drives paracellular Na$^+$ transport; the chemical gradient between the lumen and peritubular space provides the driving force for paracellular reabsorption of Cl$^-$.[13] This increase in luminal Na$^+$-Cl$^-$ is the direct result of the robust reabsorption of HCO$_3^-$ and other solutes by the early S1 segment, combined with the isosmotic reabsorption of filtered water.[7,17]

A highly permeable paracellular pathway is a consistent feature of epithelia that function in the near-isosmolar reabsorption of Na$^+$-Cl$^-$, including the small intestine, proximal tubule, and gallbladder. Morphologically, the apical tight junction of proximal tubular cells and other leaky epithelia is considerably less complex than that of tight epithelia. Freeze-fracture microscopy thus reveals that the tight junction of proximal tubular cells is comparatively shallow, with as few as one junctional strand (Figure 6.5); in contrast, high-resistance epithelia have deeper tight junctions, with a complex and extensive network of junctional strands.[18] At the functional level, tight junctions of epithelia function as charge- and size-selective paracellular tight junction channels, physiologic characteristics that are thought to be conferred by integral membrane proteins that cluster together at the tight junction. Changes in the expression of these proteins can have marked effects on permeability without affecting the number of junctional strands.[12,19,20] In particular, the charge and size selectivity of tight junctions appears to be conferred in large part by the claudins, a large (>20) gene family of tetraspan transmembrane proteins.[21-23] The repertoire of claudins expressed by proximal tubular epithelial cells may thus determine the high paracellular permeability of this nephron segment. At a minimum, proximal tubular cells coexpress claudin-2, -10, and -17.[12,24,25]

The robust expression of claudin-2 in the proximal tubule is of particular interest because this claudin can dramatically decrease the resistance of transfected epithelial cells.[20] Overexpression of claudin-2, but not claudin-10, also increases Na$^+$-dependent water flux in epithelial cell lines, suggesting that claudin-2 directly modulates paracellular water permeability.[26] Consistent with this cellular phenotype, targeted deletion of claudin-2 in knockout mice generates a tight epithelium in the proximal tubule, with a reduction in Na$^+$, Cl$^-$, and fluid absorption.[27] Loss of claudin-2 expression does not affect the ultrastructure of tight junctions, but leads to a reduction in paracellular cation permeability and secondary reduction in transepithelial Cl$^-$ transport.[27] Terminal differentiation of proximal tubular claudin-2 expression requires the integrin β$_1$-subunit, such that deletion of

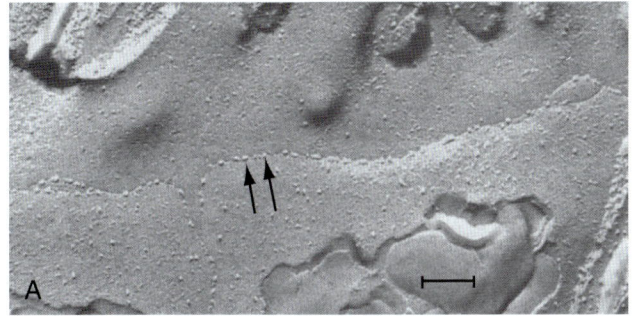

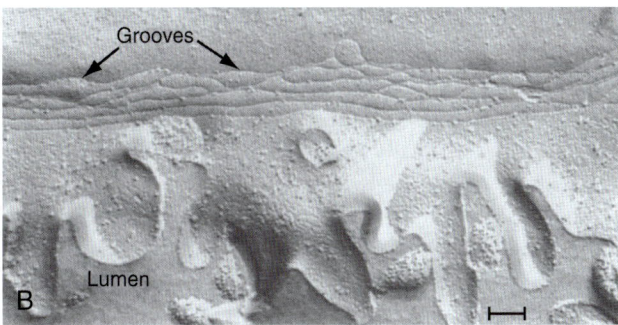

Figure 6.5 Freeze-fracture electron microscopy images of tight junctions in mouse proximal and distal nephron. **A,** Proximal convoluted tubule, a "leaky" epithelium; the tight junction contains only one junctional strand, seen as a groove in the fracture face (*arrows*). **B,** Distal convoluted tubule, a "tight" epithelium. The tight junction is deeper and contains several anastamosing strands, seen as grooves in the fracture face. (From Claude P, Goodenough, DA: Fracture faces of zonulae occludentes from "tight" and "leaky" epithelia. *J Cell Biol* 58:390-400, 1973).

this protein in mice converts the proximal tubule to a tight epithelium expressing low levels of claudin-2.[28]

The molecular identification of anion-selective claudins in the proximal tubule has remained a challenge. Recently, claudin-17 was found to generate a predominantly anion-selective paracellular conductance in Madin-Darby canine kidney (MDCK) C7 cells, whereas knockdown of the protein was able to reverse a predominantly cation-selective LLC-PK(1) epithelial cell line to an anion-selective cell line.[25] Claudin-17 appears to be expressed in proximal tubular cells, suggesting a significant role in paracellular chloride absorption by this nephron segment.

The reabsorption of HCO$_3^-$ and other solutes from the glomerular ultrafiltrate would be expected to generate an osmotic gradient across the epithelium, resulting in a hypotonic lumen. This appears to be the case, although the absolute difference in osmolality between the lumen and peritubular space has been a source of considerable controversy.[17] Another controversial issue has been the relative importance of paracellular versus transcellular water transport from this hypotonic lumen. These issues have been elegantly addressed through characterization of knockout mice with a targeted deletion of aquaporin-1, a water channel protein expressed at the apical and basolateral membranes of the proximal tubule. Mice deficient in aquaporin-1 have an 80% reduction in water permeability in perfused S2 segments, with a 50% reduction in transepithelial fluid transport.[29] Aquaporin-1 deficiency also results in a marked increase in luminal hypotonicity, providing definitive proof that near-isomotic reabsorption by the proximal tubule requires transepithelial water transport via aquaporin-1.[17] The residual water transport in the proximal tubules of aquaporin-1 knockout mice is mediated in part by aquaporin-7 and/or by claudin-2–dependent paracellular water transport.[27,30] Combined knockout of aquaporin-1 and claudin-2 in mice demonstrate sustained proximal tubule water reabsorption (25% of wild-type), suggestive of compensation from other pathways.[31] Alternative pathways for water reabsorption may include cotransport of H_2O via the multiple Na^+-dependent solute transporters in the early proximal tubule; this novel hypothesis is, however, a source of considerable controversy.[32,33] A related issue is the relative importance of diffusional versus convective (solvent drag) transport of Na^+-Cl^- across the paracellular tight junction; convective transport of Na^+-Cl^- with water would seem to play a lesser role than diffusion, given the evidence that the transcellular pathway is the dominant transepithelial pathway for water in the proximal tubule.[11,17,29,30]

TRANSCELLULAR Na^+-Cl^- TRANSPORT
Apical Mechanisms

Apical Na^+-H^+ exchange plays a critical role in the transcellular and paracellular reabsorption of Na^+-Cl^- by the proximal tubule. In addition to providing an entry site in the transcellular transport of Na^+, Na^+-H^+ exchange plays a dominant role in the robust absorption of HCO_3^- by the early proximal tubule; this absorption of HCO_3^- serves to increase the luminal concentration of Cl^-, which in turn increases the driving forces for the passive paracellular transport of Na^+ and Cl^-.[34] Increases in luminal Cl^- also help drive the apical uptake of Cl^- during transcellular transport. Not surprisingly, there is a considerable reduction in fluid transport of perfused proximal tubules exposed to concentrations of amiloride that are sufficient to inhibit proximal tubular Na^+-H^+ exchange.[12]

Na^+-H^+ exchange is predominantly mediated by the NHE proteins, encoded by the nine members of the SLC9 gene family; NHE3 in particular plays an important role in proximal tubular physiology.[35] The NHE3 protein is expressed at the apical membrane of S1, S2, and S3 segments.[36] The apical membrane of the proximal tubule also expresses alternative Na^+-dependent H^+ transporters, including NHE8.[35,37] NHE8 predominates over NHE3 in the neonatal proximal tubule, with subsequent induction of NHE3 and downregulation of NHE8 in mature, adult nephrons.[35] The primacy of NHE3 in mature proximal tubules is illustrated by the renal phenotype of *NHE3* null knockout mice, which have a 62% reduction in proximal fluid absorption and a 54% reduction in baseline chloride absorption.[38,39]

Much as amiloride and other inhibitors of Na^+-H^+ exchange have revealed an important role for this transporter in transepithelial salt transport by the proximal tubule, evidence for the involvement of an apical anion exchanger first came from the use of anion transport inhibitors; DIDS (4,4′-diisothiocyanostilbene-2,2′-disulfonic acid), furosemide, and SITS all reduce fluid absorption from the lumen of proximal (PT) segments perfused with solutions containing Na^+-Cl^-.[12] In the simplest arrangement for the coupling of Na^+-H^+ exchange to Cl^- exchange, Cl^- would be exchanged with the OH^- ion during Na^+-Cl^- transport (see Figure 6.6). Evidence for such a Cl^--OH^- exchanger was reported by a number of groups in the early 1980s that used membrane vesicles isolated from the proximal tubule.[40] These findings could not, however, be replicated in similar studies from other groups.[40,41] Moreover, experimental evidence was provided for the existence of a dominant Cl^--formate exchange activity in brush border vesicles in the absence of significant Cl^--OH^- exchange.[41] It was postulated that recycling of formate by the back diffusion of formic acid would sustain the net transport of Na^+-Cl^- across the apical membrane. Vesicle formate transport stimulated by a pH gradient (H^+-formate cotransport or formate-OH^- exchange) is saturable, consistent with a carrier-mediated process rather than diffusion of formic acid across the apical membrane of the proximal tubule.[42] Transport studies using brush border vesicles have also detected the presence of Cl^--oxalate exchange mechanisms in the apical membrane of the PT, in addition to SO_4^{2-}-oxalate exchange.[43,34] Based on differences in the affinities and inhibitor sensitivity of the Cl^--oxalate and Cl^--formate exchange activities, it was suggested that there are two separate apical exchangers in the proximal nephron, a Cl^--formate exchanger and a Cl^--formate-oxalate exchanger capable of transporting both formate and oxalate (see Figure 6.6).

The physiological relevance of apical Cl^--formate and Cl^--oxalate exchange has been addressed by perfusing individual proximal tubule segments with solutions containing Na^+-Cl^- and formate or oxalate. Both formate and oxalate significantly increased fluid transport under these conditions in rabbit, rat, and mouse proximal tubules.[39] This increase in fluid transport was inhibited by DIDS, suggesting involvement of the DIDS-sensitive anion exchanger(s) detected in brush border vesicle studies. A similar mechanism for Na^+-Cl^- transport in the distal convoluted tubule (DCT) has also been detected, independent of thiazide-sensitive Na^+-Cl^- cotransport.[45] Further experiments have indicated that the oxalate- and formate-dependent anion transporters in the PT are coupled to distinct Na^+ entry pathways, to Na^+-SO_4^{2-} cotransport and Na^+-H^+ exchange, respectively.[46] The coupling of Cl^--oxalate transport to Na^+-SO_4^{2-} cotransport requires the additional presence of SO_4^{2-}-oxalate exchange, which has been demonstrated in brush border membrane vesicle studies.[44] The obligatory role for NHE3 in formate-stimulated Cl^- transport was illustrated using *NHE3* null mice, in which the formate effect is abolished; as expected, oxalate stimulation of Cl^- transport is preserved in the *NHE3* null mice.[39] Finally, tubular perfusion data from superficial and juxtamedullary proximal convoluted tubules have suggested that there is heterogeneity in the dominant mode of anion exchange along the PT, such that Cl^--formate exchange is absent in juxtamedullary proximal convoluted tubule (PCTs), in which Cl^--OH^- exchange may instead be dominant.[12]

The molecular identity of the apical anion exchanger(s) involved in transepithelial Na^+-Cl^- by the proximal tubule has been the object of almost 3 decades of investigation. A key breakthrough was the observation that the SLC26A4 anion exchanger, also known as pendrin, is capable of Cl^--formate exchange when expressed in *Xenopus laevis* oocytes.[47] However, expression of SLC26A4 in the proximal tubule is minimal or absent in several species, and formate-stimulated Na^+-Cl^- transport in this nephron segment is unimpaired in

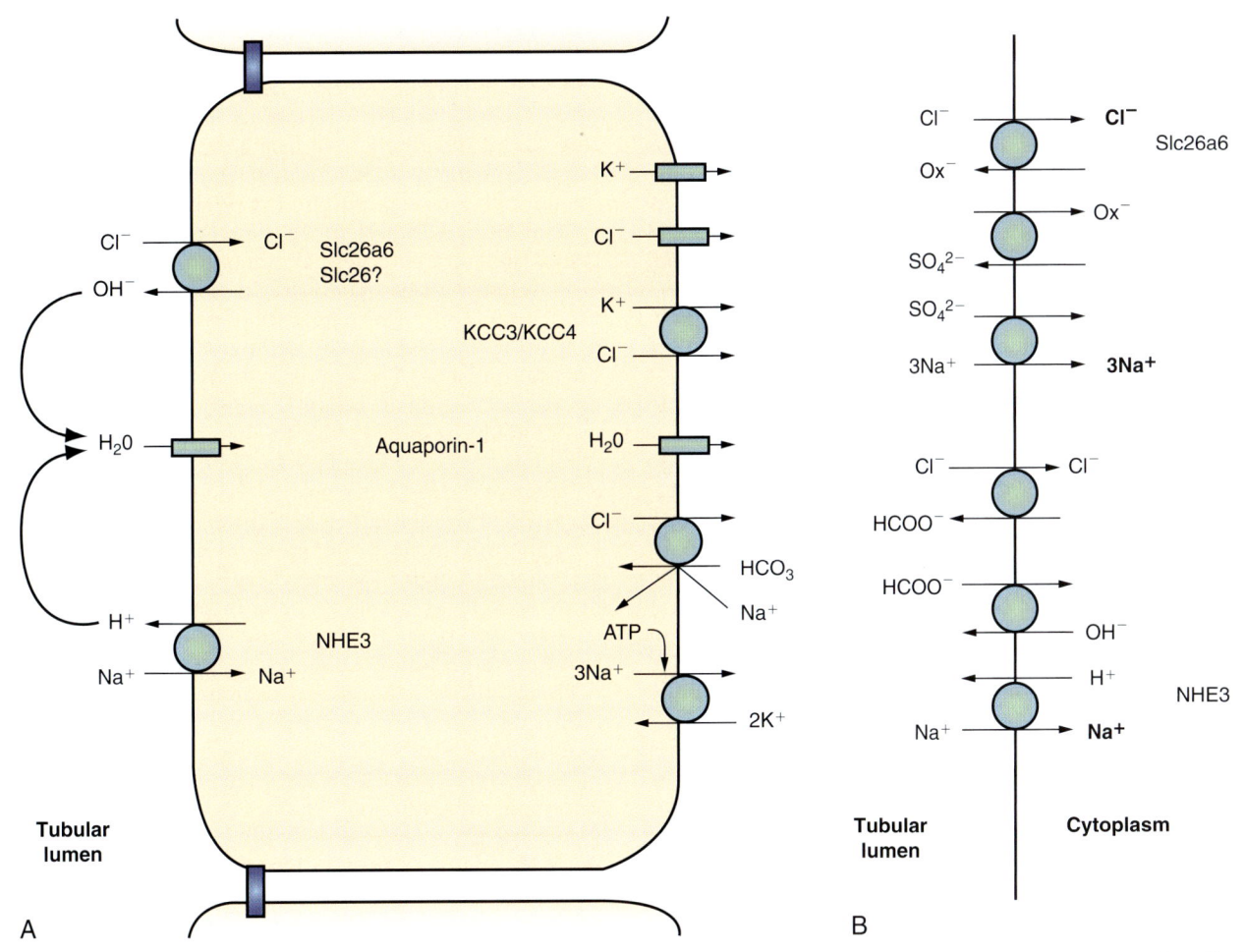

Figure 6.6 Transepithelial Na^+-Cl^- transport in the proximal tubule. **A,** In the simplest scheme, Cl^- enters the apical membrane via a Cl^--OH^- exchanger, coupled to Na^+ entry via NHE3. **B,** Alternative apical anion exchange activities that couple to Na^+-H^+ exchange and Na^+-SO_4^{2-} cotransport. See text for details.

SLC26A4 null mice.[12] There is, however, robust expression of SLC26A4 in distal type B intercalated cells; the role of this exchanger in Cl^- transport by the distal nephron is reviewed elsewhere in this chapter (see later, "Connecting Tubules and the Cortical Collecting Duct: Cl^- Transport").[48] Regardless, this data for SLC26A4 led to the identification and characterization of SLC26A6, a widely expressed member of the SLC26 family that is expressed at the apical membrane of proximal tubular cells. Murine Slc26a6, when expressed in *Xenopus* oocytes, mediates the multiple modes of anion exchange that have been implicated in transepithelial Na^+-Cl^- by the proximal tubule, including Cl^--formate, Cl^--OH^-, Cl^--SO_4^{2-}, and SO_4^{2-}-oxalate exchange.[49] However, tubule perfusion experiments in mice deficient in Slc26a6 did not reveal a reduction in baseline Cl^- or fluid transport, indicative of considerable heterogeneity in apical Cl^- transport by the proximal tubule.[50] Candidates for the residual Cl^- transport in Slc26a6-deficient mice include Slc26a7 and Slc26a9, which are expressed at the apical membrane of proximal tubules; however, these members of the SLC26 family appear to function as Cl^- channels rather than as exchangers.[51-53] SLC26A2 may also contribute to apical anion exchange in the proximal tubule.[54] It does, however, appear that Slc26a6 is the dominant Cl^--oxalate exchanger of the proximal brush border; the usual increase in tubular fluid transport induced by oxalate is abolished in Slc26a6 knockout mice, with an attendant loss of Cl^--oxalate exchange in brush border membrane vesicles.[50,55]

Somewhat surprisingly, Slc26a6 mediates electrogenic Cl^--OH^- and Cl^--HCO_3^- exchange, and most if not all the members of this family are electrogenic in at least one mode of anion transport.[12,49,53,56,57] This begs the question of how the electroneutrality of transcellular Na^+-Cl^- transport is preserved. Notably, however, the stoichiometry and electrophysiology of Cl^--base exchange differ for individual members of the family; for example, Slc26a6 exchanges one Cl^- for two HCO_3^- anions, whereas SLC26A3 exchanges two Cl^- anions for one HCO_3^- anion.[12,56] Coexpression of two or more electrogenic SLC26 exchangers in the same membrane may thus yield a net electroneutrality of apical Cl^- exchange. Alternatively, apical K^+ channels in the proximal tubule may function to stabilize membrane potential during Na^+-Cl^- absorption.[58]

Another puzzle is why Cl^--formate exchange preferentially couples to Na^+-H^+ exchange mediated by NHE3 (Figure 6.6), without evident coupling of Cl^--oxalate exchange to Na^+-H^+ exchange or Cl^--formate exchange to Na^+-SO_4^{2-} cotransport; it is evident that SLC26A6 is capable of mediating SO_4^{2-}-formate exchange, which would be necessary to support coupling between Na^+-SO_4^{2-} cotransport and formate.[39,49] Scaffolding proteins may serve to cluster these different transporters together in separate microdomains, leading to preferential coupling. Notably, whereas both Slc26a6 and NHE have been reported to bind to the scaffolding protein PDZK1, distribution of SLC26A6 is selectively impaired in PDZK1 knockout mice.[59] Petrovic and colleagues have also reported a novel activation of proximal Na^+-H^+ exchange by luminal formate, suggesting a direct effect of formate per se on NHE3; this may in part explain the preferential coupling of Cl^--formate exchange to NHE3.[60]

Basolateral Mechanisms

As in other absorptive epithelia, basolateral Na^+-K^+-ATPase activity establishes the Na^+ gradient for transcellular Na^+-Cl^- transport by the proximal tubule and provides a major exit pathway for Na^+. To preserve the electroneutrality of transcellular Na^+-Cl^- transport, this exit of Na^+ across the basolateral membrane must be balanced by an equal exit of Cl^-.[16] Several exit pathways for Cl^- have been identified in proximal tubular cells, including K^+-Cl^- cotransport, Cl^- channels, and various modalities of Cl^--HCO_3^- exchange (see Figure 6.6).

Several lines of evidence support the existence of a swelling-activated basolateral K^+-Cl^- cotransporter (KCC) in the proximal tubule.[61] The KCC proteins are encoded by four members of the cation-chloride cotransporter gene family; KCC1, KCC3, and KCC4 are all expressed in the kidney. In particular, there is very heavy coexpression of KCC3 and KCC4 at the basolateral membrane of the proximal tubule, from S1 to S3.[62] At the functional level, basolateral membrane vesicles from the renal cortex reportedly contain K^+-Cl^- cotransport activity.[61] The use of ion-sensitive microelectrodes, combined with luminal charge injection and manipulation of bath K^+ and Cl^-, suggest the presence of an electroneutral K^+-Cl^- cotransporter at the basolateral membrane of proximal straight tubules. Increases or decreases in basolateral K^+ increase or decrease intracellular Cl^- activity, respectively, with reciprocal effects of basolateral Cl^- on K^+ activity; these data are consistent with coupled K^+-Cl^- transport.[63,64] Notably, a 1-mmol/L concentration of furosemide, sufficient to inhibit all four of the KCCs, does not inhibit this K^+-Cl^- cotransport under baseline conditions.[63] However, only 10% of baseline K^+ efflux in the proximal tubule is mediated by furosemide-sensitive K^+-Cl^- cotransport, which is likely quiescent in the absence of cell swelling. Thus, the activation of apical Na^+-glucose transport in proximal tubular cells strongly activates a barium-resistant (Ba^{2+}) K^+ efflux pathway that is 75% inhibited by 1-mmol/L furosemide.[65] In addition, a volume regulatory decrease (VRD) in Ba^{2+}-blocked proximal tubules swollen by hypotonic conditions is blocked by 1-mmol/L furosemide.[61] Cell swelling in response to apical Na^+ absorption is postulated to activate a volume-sensitive basolateral K^+-Cl^- cotransporter, which participates in transepithelial absorption of Na^+-Cl^-.[12] Notably, targeted deletion of KCC3 and KCC4 in the respective knockout mice reduces VRD in the proximal tubule.[66] Furthermore, perfused proximal tubules from KCC3-deficient mice have a considerable reduction in transepithelial fluid transport, suggesting an important role for basolateral K^+-Cl^- cotransport in transcellular Na^+-Cl^- reabsorption.[67]

The basolateral chloride conductance of mammalian proximal tubular cells is relatively low, suggesting a lesser role for Cl^- channels in transepithelial Na^+-Cl^- transport. Basolateral anion substitutions have minimal effect on the membrane potential, despite considerable effects on intracellular Cl^- activity, nor for that matter do changes in basolateral membrane potential affect intracellular Cl^-.[63,64,68] However, as with basolateral K^+-Cl^- cotransport, basolateral Cl^- channels in the proximal tubule may be relatively inactive in the absence of cell swelling. Cell swelling thus activates both K^+ and Cl^- channels at the basolateral membranes of proximal tubular cells.[12,69,70] Seki and associates have reported the presence of a basolateral Cl^- channel in S3 segments of the rabbit nephron, wherein they did not see an effect of the KCC inhibitor H74 on intracellular Cl^- activity.[71] The molecular identity of these and other basolateral Cl^- channels in the proximal nephron is not known with certainty, although S3 segments have been shown to express mRNA exclusively for the swelling-activated CLC-2 Cl^- channel; the role of this channel in transcellular Na^+-Cl^- reabsorption is not as yet clear.[72]

Finally, there is functional evidence for Na^+-dependent and Na^+-independent Cl^--HCO_3^- exchange at the basolateral membrane of proximal tubular cells.[10,68,73] The impact of Na^+-independent Cl^--HCO_3^- exchange on basolateral exit is thought to be minimal.[68] First, this exchanger is expected to mediate Cl^- entry under physiologic conditions.[73] Second, there is only a modest difference between the rate of decrease in intracellular Cl^- activity and the combined removal of Na^+ and Cl^- versus Cl^- and HCO_3^- removal, suggesting that pure Cl^--HCO_3^- exchange does not contribute significantly to Cl^- exit. In contrast, there is a 75% reduction in the rate of decrease in intracellular Cl^- activity after the removal of basolateral Na^+.[68] The Na^+-dependent Cl^--HCO_3^- exchanger may thus play a considerable role in basolateral Cl^- exit, with recycled exit of Na^+ and HCO_3^- via the basolateral Na^+-HCO_3^- cotransporter NBC1 (see Figure 6.6). The molecular identity of this proximal tubular Na^+-dependent Cl^--HCO_3^- exchanger is not as yet known.

REGULATION OF PROXIMAL TUBULAR Na^+-Cl^- TRANSPORT

Glomerulotubular Balance

A fundamental property of the kidney is the phenomenon of glomerulotubular balance, wherein changes in the glomerular filtration rate (GFR) are balanced by equivalent changes in tubular reabsorption, thus maintaining a constant fractional reabsorption of fluid and Na^+-Cl^- (Figure 6.7). Although the distal nephron is capable of adjusting reabsorption in response to changes in tubular flow, the impact of GFR on Na^+-Cl^- reabsorption by the proximal tubule is particularly pronounced (Figure 6.8).[74] Glomerulotubular balance is independent of direct neurohumoral control and is thought to be mediated by the additive effects of luminal and peritubular factors.[75]

At the luminal side, changes in GFR increase the filtered load of HCO_3^-, glucose, and other solutes, increasing their reabsorption by the load-responsive proximal tubule and thus preserving a constant fractional reabsorption.[7] Changes

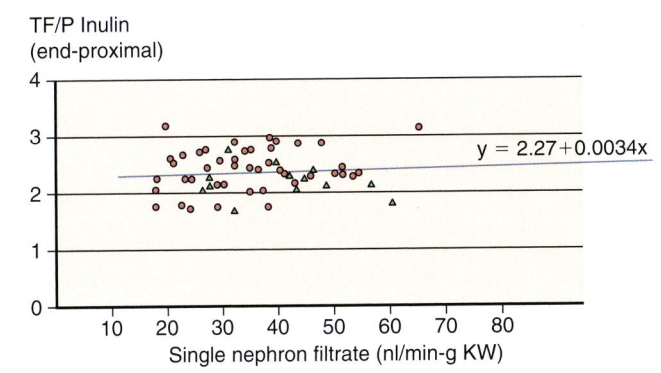

Figure 6.7 Glomerulotubular balance. The tubular fluid-to-plasma ratio of the nonreabsorbable marker, inulin (TF/P Inulin), at the end of the proximal tubule, which is used as a measure of fractional water absorption by the proximal tubule, does not change as a function of single nephron GFR. Measurements were done during antidiuresis (*triangles*) and water diuresis (*circles*). (From Schnermann J, Wahl M, Liebau G, Fischbach H: Balance between tubular flow rate and net fluid reabsorption in the proximal convolution of the rat kidney. I. Dependency of reabsorptive net fluid flux upon proximal tubular surface area at spontaneous variations of filtration rate. *Pflugers Arch* 304:90-103, 1968.)

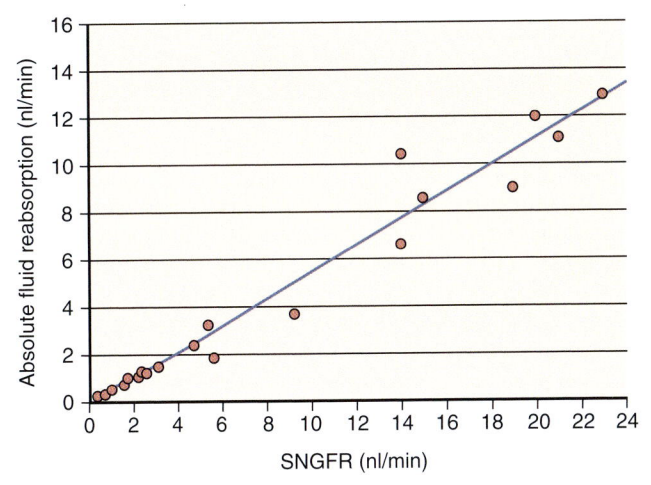

Figure 6.8 Glomerulotubular balance. Shown is the linear increase in absolute fluid reabsorption by the late proximal tubule as a function of single-nephron GFR (SNGFR). (From Spitzer A, Brandis M: Functional and morphologic maturation of the superficial nephrons. Relationship to total kidney function. *J Clin Invest* 53:279-287, 1974.)

in the tubular flow rate have additional stimulatory effects on luminal transport in both the proximal and distal nephrons.[74] In the proximal tubule, increases in tubular perfusion increase the rate of Na^+ and HCO_3^- absorption due to increases in the capacity of luminal Na^+-H^+ exchange, as measured in brush border membrane vesicles, with the opposite effect in volume contraction.[74]

Notably, influential experiments from almost 4 decades ago, performed in rabbit proximal tubules, failed to demonstrate a significant effect of tubular flow on fluid absorption.[76] This issue has been revisited by Du and coworkers, who reported a considerable flow dependence of fluid and HCO_3^- transport in perfused murine proximal tubules (Figure 6.9).[75,77] These data were analyzed using a mathematical model that estimated microvillus torque as a function of tubular flow; accounting for increases in tubular diameter, which reduce torque, there is a linear relationship between calculated torque and fluid and HCO_3^- absorption.[75,77] Consistent with an effect of torque rather than flow per se, increasing viscosity of the perfusate by the addition of dextran increases the effect on fluid transport; the extra viscosity increases the hydrodynamic effect of flow and thus increases torque. The mathematical analysis of Du and associates provides an excellent explanation of the discrepancy between their results and those of Burg and coworkers.[76] Whereas Burg and colleagues performed their experiments in rabbits, the more recent report used mice; other studies that had found an effect of flow used perfusion of rat proximal tubules, presumably more similar to mouse than rabbit.[74-77] Increased flow has a considerably greater effect on tubular diameter in the rabbit proximal tubule, thus reducing the increase in torque. Mathematical analysis of the rabbit data thus predicts a 43% increase in torque due to a 41% increase in tubule diameter at a threefold increase in flow; this corresponds to the statistically insignificant 36% increase in volume reabsorption reported by Burg and associates.[76]

Pharmacologic inhibition reveals that tubular flow activates proximal HCO_3^- reabsorption mediated by NHE3 and apical H^+-ATPase.[75] The flow-dependent increase in proximal fluid and HCO_3^- reabsorption is also attenuated in NHE3-deficient knockout mice.[75,77] Inhibition of the actin cytoskeleton with cytochalasin D reduces the effect of flow on fluid and HCO_3^- transport, suggesting that flow-dependent movement of microvilli serves to activate NHE3 and H^+-ATPase via their linkage to the cytoskeleton (see Figure 6.13 for NHE3). Fluid shear stress induces densely distributed peripheral actin bands and increases the formation of tight junctions and adherens junctions in cultured tubule cells; this junctional buttressing is hypothesized to maximize flow-activated transcellular salt and water absorption.[78] More recent studies have found that dopamine through the D_{1A} receptor and angiotensin II through the AT_{1A} receptor are able to inhibit the flow-dependent increase in sodium and bicarbonate transport, with no effects on the flow-dependent increase in H^+-ATPase activity.[79,80] Additionally, flow and torque were not found to have any effects on chloride absorption, suggesting no convective flow of chloride through the paracellular pathway.

Peritubular factors also play an important additive role in glomerulotubular balance. Specifically, increases in GFR result in an increase in filtration fraction and an attendant increase in postglomerular protein and peritubular oncotic pressure. It has long been appreciated that changes in peritubular protein concentration have important effects on proximal tubular Na^+-Cl^- reabsorption; these effects are also seen in combined capillary and tubular perfusion experiments.[75,81] Peritubular protein also has an effect in isolated perfused proximal tubule segments, where the effect of hydrostatic pressure is abolished.[75] Increases in peritubular protein concentration have an additive effect on the flow-dependent activation of proximal fluid and HCO_3^- absorption (see Figure 6.9). The effect of peritubular protein on HCO_3^- absorption, which is a predominantly transcellular phenomenon, suggests that changes in peritubular oncotic

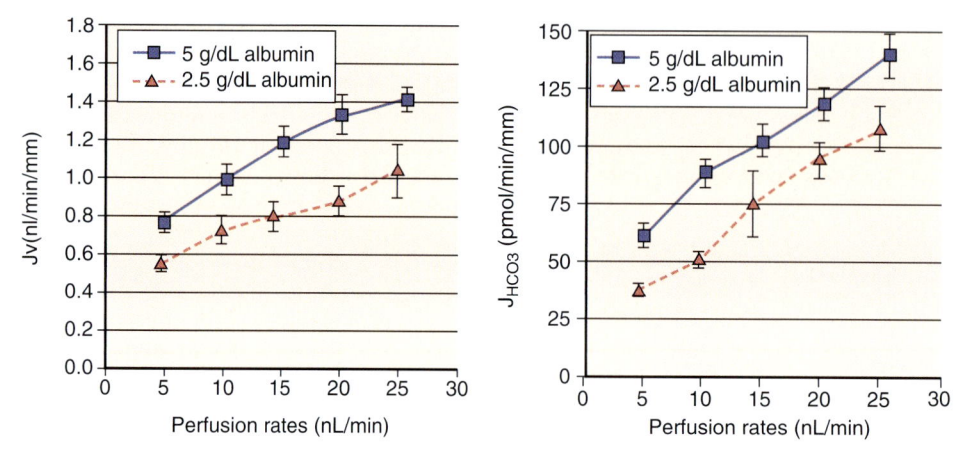

Figure 6.9 Glomerulotubular balance; flow-dependent increases in fluid (J_v) and HCO_3Cl^- (J_{HCO3}) absorption by perfused mouse proximal tubules. Absorption also increases when bath albumin concentration increases from 2.5 to 5 g/dL. (From Du Z, Yan Q, Duan Y, et al: Axial flow modulates proximal tubule NHE3 and H-ATPase activities by changing microvillus bending moments. *Am J Physiol Renal Physiol* 290:F289-F296, 2006).

pressure do not affect transport via the paracellular pathway.[12] However, the mechanism of the stimulatory effect of peritubular protein on transcellular transport is still not completely clear.[75]

Neurohumoral Influences

Fluid and Na^+-Cl^- reabsorption by the proximal tubule are affected by a number of hormones and neurotransmitters. The major hormonal influences on renal Na^+-Cl^- transport are shown in Figure 6.10. Renal sympathetic tone exerts a particularly important stimulatory influence, as does angiotensin II; dopamine is a major inhibitor of proximal tubular Na^+-Cl^- reabsorption.

Unilateral denervation of the rat kidney causes a marked natriuresis and a 40% reduction in proximal Na^+-Cl^- reabsorption, without effects on single-nephron GFR or on the contralateral innervated kidney.[82] In contrast, low-frequency electrical stimulation of renal sympathetic nerves increases proximal tubular fluid absorption, with a 32% drop in natriuresis and no change in GFR.[83] Basolateral epinephrine and/or norepinephrine stimulate proximal Na^+-Cl^- reabsorption via both α- and β-adrenergic receptors. Several lines of evidence suggest that $α_1$-adrenergic receptors exert a stimulatory effect on proximal Na^+-Cl^- transport via activation of basolateral Na^+-K^+-ATPase and apical Na^+-H^+ exchange; the role of $α_2$-adrenergic receptors is more controversial.[84] Ligand-dependent recruitment of the scaffolding protein NHERF-1 by $β_2$-adrenergic receptors results in direct activation of apical NHE3, bypassing the otherwise negative effect of downstream cyclic AMP (cAMP; see later).[85]

Angiotensin II (Ang II) has potent complex effects on proximal Na^+-Cl^- reabsorption. Several issues unique to Ang II deserve emphasis. First, it has been appreciated for 3 decades that this hormone has a biphasic effect on the proximal tubule in rats, rabbits, and mice; stimulation of Na^+-Cl^- reabsorption occurs at low doses (10^{-12} to 10^{-10} M), whereas concentrations greater than 10^{-7} M are inhibitory (Figure 6.11).[86] More recent data have found that this biphasic role of Ang II does not hold true for all species, and human proximal tubule samples obtained during nephrectomy surgeries concentrations up to 10^{-6} M Ang II stimulate Na^+-Cl^- reabsorption, primarily due to a stimulatory effect of the nitric oxide (NO)–cyclic guanosine monophosphate (cGMP) pathway on extracellular signal–regulated kinase (ERK) phosphorylation.[87] Further complexity arises from the presence of AT_1 receptors for Ang II at luminal and basolateral membranes in the proximal tubule.[88] Ang II application to the luminal or peritubular side of perfused tubules has a similar biphasic effect on fluid transport, albeit with more potent effects at the luminal side.[89] Traditionally, experiments using receptor antagonists and knockout mice have indicated that the stimulatory and inhibitory effects of Ang II are both mediated via AT_1 receptors due to signaling at the luminal and basolateral membranes.[90] However, recent work has identified that AT_2 receptors working through NO-cGMP pathway are able to downregulate NHE3 and Na^+-K^+-ATPase, leading to natriuresis and reduced blood pressure.[91] Finally, Ang II is also synthesized and secreted by the proximal tubule, exerting a potent autocrine effect on proximal tubular Na^+-Cl^- reabsorption.[92] Proximal tubular cells thus express mRNA for angiotensinogen, renin, and angiotensin-converting enzyme,[84] allowing for the autocrine generation of Ang II. Indeed, luminal concentrations of Ang II can be 100- to 1000-fold higher than circulating levels of the hormone.[84] Proximal tubular and systemic synthesis of Ang II may be subject to different control. Androgens increase proximal tubular Na^+-Cl^- reabsorption via marked induction of renal angiotensinogen, presumptively within the proximal tubule.[93] Thomson and colleagues have demonstrated that proximal tubular Ang II is increased considerably after a high-salt diet, with a preserved inhibitory effect of losartan on proximal fluid reabsorption.[94] They have argued that the increase in proximal tubular Ang II after a high-salt diet contributes to a more stable distal salt delivery.[94]

The proximal tubule is also a target for natriuretic hormones; in particular, dopamine synthesized in the proximal tubule has negative autocrine effects on proximal Na^+-Cl^- reabsorption.[84] Proximal tubular cells have the requisite enzymatic machinery for the synthesis of dopamine, using L-dopa reabsorbed from the glomerular ultrafiltrate.

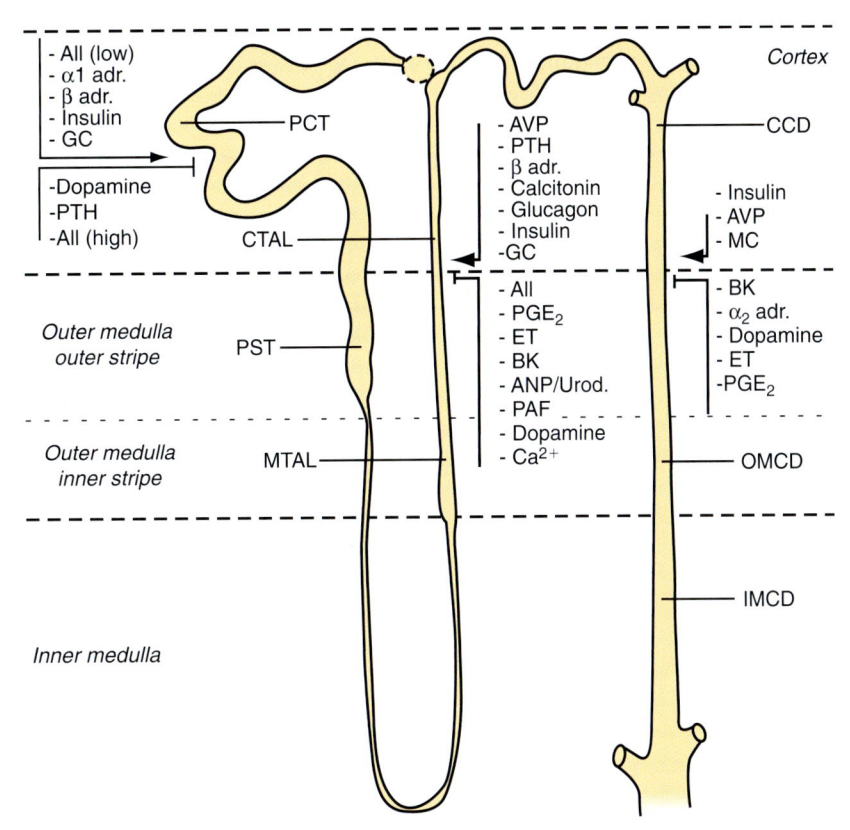

Figure 6.10 Neurohumoral influences on Na^+-Cl^- absorption by the proximal tubule, thick ascending limb, and collecting duct. Factors that stimulate (→) and inhibit (⊣) sodium reabsorption are as follows: α1 adr, $α_1$-Adrenergic agonist; ANG II, angiotensin II (low and high referring to picomolar and micromolar concentrations, respectively); ANP/Urod, atrial natriuretic peptide and urodilatin; AVP, arginine vasopressin; β adr, β-adrenergic agonist; BK, bradykinin; CCD, cortical collecting duct; CTAL, cortical thick ascending limb; ET, endothelin; GC, glucocorticoids; IMCD, inner medullary collecting duct; MC, mineralocorticoids; MTAL, medullary thick ascending limb of Henle's loop; OMCD, outer medullary collecting duct; PTH, parathyroid hormone; PAF, platelet-activating factor; PCT, proximal convoluted tubule; PGE_2, prostaglandin E_2; PST, proximal straight tubule. (From Feraille E, Doucet A: Sodium-potassium-adenosine triphosphatase-dependent sodium transport in the kidney: hormonal control. Physiol Rev 81:345-418, 2001.)

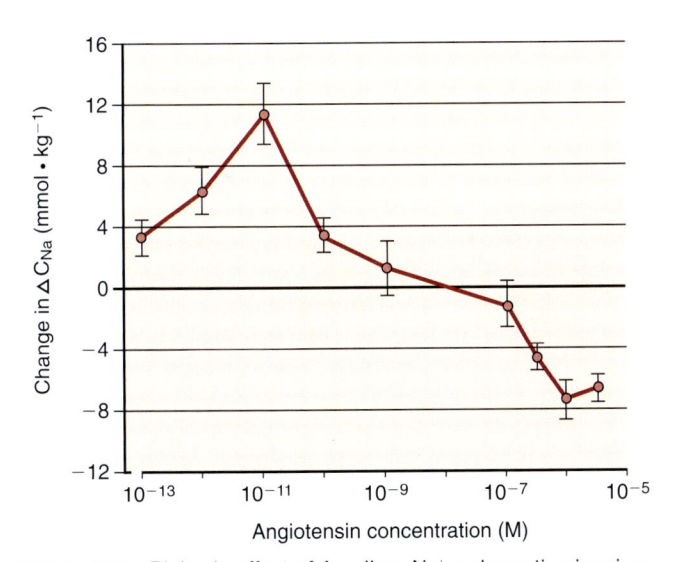

Figure 6.11 Biphasic effect of Ang II on Na^+ reabsorption in microperfused proximal tubules. The steady-state transepithelial Na^+ concentration gradient (peritubular-luminal), $ΔC_{Na}$, that developed in a stationary split droplet is used as an indication of the rate of active Na^+ reabsorption. This is plotted as a function of peritubular Ang II concentration; low concentrations activate Na^+ absorption by the proximal tubule, whereas higher concentrations inhibit it. (From Harris PJ, Navar LG: Tubular transport responses to angiotensin. Am J Physiol 248:F621-F630, 1985.)

Dopamine synthesis by proximal tubular cells and release into the tubular lumen is increased after volume expansion or a high-salt diet, resulting in a considerable natriuresis.[95,96] Luminal dopamine antagonizes the stimulatory effect of epinephrine on volume absorption in perfused proximal convoluted tubules, consistent with an autocrine effect of dopamine released into the tubular lumen.[95,97] Dopamine primarily exerts its natriuretic effect via D_1-like dopamine receptors (D_1 and D_5 in humans); as is the case for the AT_1 receptors for Ang II, D_1 receptors are expressed at the apical and luminal membranes of proximal tubules.[88,98] Targeted deletion of the D_{1A} and D_5 receptors in mice leads to hypertension by mechanisms that include reduced proximal tubular natriuresis.[99,100] The proximal tubular-specific deletion of aromatic amino acid decarboxylase (AADC), which produces dopamine, generates mice that are a vivid demonstration of the role of intrarenal dopamine. This intrarenal dopamine deficiency leads to upregulation of sodium transporters along the nephron, upregulation of the intrarenal renin angiotensin axis, decreased natriuresis in response to L-dopa, and reduced medullary cyclo-oxygenase-2 (COX-2) expression, with reduced urinary prostaglandin levels. These mice also exhibit salt-sensitive hypertension and ultimately a significantly shorter life span compared to wild-type mice.[101]

The natriuretic effect of dopamine in the proximal tubule is modulated by atrial natriuretic peptide (ANP), which inhibits apical Na$^+$-H$^+$ exchange via a dopamine-dependent mechanism.[12] ANP appears to induce recruitment of the D$_1$ dopamine receptor to the plasma membrane of proximal tubular cells, thus sensitizing the tubule to the effect of dopamine.[102] The inhibitory effect of ANP on basolateral Na+-K+-ATPase occurs via a D$_1$-dependent mechanism, with a synergistic inhibition of Na+-K+-ATPase by the two hormones.[102] Furthermore, dopamine and D$_1$ receptors appear to play critical permissive roles in the in vivo natriuretic effect of ANP.[12]

Finally, there is considerable crosstalk between the major antinatriuretic and natriuretic influences on the proximal tubule. For example, ANP inhibits Ang II–dependent stimulation of proximal tubular fluid absorption, presumably via the dopamine-dependent mechanisms discussed above.[12,103] Dopamine also decreases the expression of AT$_1$ receptors for Ang II in cultured proximal tubular cells.[104] Furthermore, the provision of L-dopa in the drinking water of rats decreases AT$_1$ receptor expression in the proximal tubule, suggesting that dopamine synthesis in the proximal tubule resets the sensitivity to Ang II.[104] Ang II signaling through AT$_1$ receptors decreases expression of the D$_5$ dopamine receptor, whereas renal cortical expression of AT$_1$ receptors is in turn increased in knockout mice deficient in the D$_5$ receptor.[105] Similar interactions have been found between proximal tubular AT$_1$ receptors and the D$_2$-like D$_3$ receptor.[106]

Regulation of Proximal Tubular Transporters

The apical Na$^+$-H$^+$ exchanger NHE3 and the basolateral Na+-K+-ATPase are primary targets for signaling pathways elicited by the various antinatriuretic and natriuretic stimuli discussed earlier; NHE3 mediates the rate-limiting step in transepithelial Na$^+$-Cl$^-$ absorption and, as such, is the dominant target for regulatory pathways.[77] NHE3 is regulated by the combined effects of direct phosphorylation and dynamic, C-terminal interaction with scaffolding proteins and signal transduction proteins, which primarily regulate transport via changes in trafficking of the exchanger protein to and from the brush border membrane (Figure 6.12).[35,107] Basal activity of the exchanger is also dependent on C-terminal binding of casein kinase 2 (CK2); phosphorylation of serine 719 by CK2 contributes significantly to the transport activity of NHE3 by modulating membrane trafficking of the transport protein.[108]

Increases in cAMP have a profound inhibitory effect on apical Na$^+$-H$^+$ exchange in the proximal tubule. Intracellular cAMP is increased in response to dopamine signaling via D$_1$-like receptors and/or parathyroid hormone (PTH)–dependent signaling via the PTH receptor, whereas Ang II–dependent activation of NHE3 is associated with a reduction in cAMP.[109] PTH is a potent inhibitor of NHE3, presumably so as to promote the distal delivery of Na$^+$-HCO$_3^-$ and an attendant stimulation of distal calcium reabsorption.[110] The activation of protein kinase A (PKA) by increased cAMP results in direct phosphorylation of NHE3; although several sites in NHE3 are phosphorylated by PKA, the phosphorylation of serine 552 (S552) and 605 (S605) have been specifically implicated in the inhibitory effect of cAMP on Na$^+$-H$^+$ exchange.[111] So-called phospho-specific antibodies, which specifically recognize the phosphorylated forms of S552 and S605, have demonstrated dopamine-dependent increases in the phosphorylation of both these serines.[112] Moreover, immunostaining of rat kidney has revealed that S552-phosphorylated NHE3 localizes at the coated pit region of the brush border membrane, where the oligomerized inactive form of NHE3 predominates.[112,113] The cAMP-stimulated phosphorylation of NHE3 by PKA thus results in a redistribution of the transporter from the microvillar membrane to an inactive submicrovillar population (see Figure 6.12).

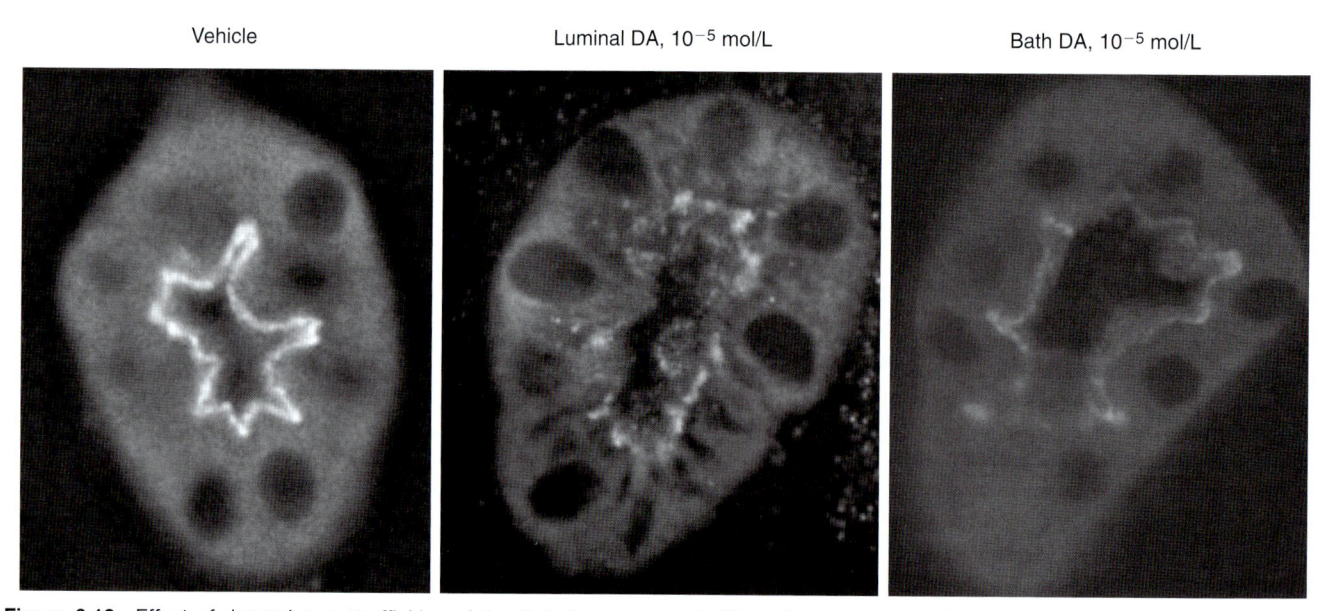

Figure 6.12 Effect of dopamine on trafficking of the Na$^+$-H$^+$ exchanger NHE3 in the proximal tubule. Microdissected proximal convoluted tubules were perfused for 30 minutes with 10^{-5} mol/L dopamine (DA), in the lumen or the bath, inducing a retraction of immunoreactive NHE3 protein from the apical membrane. (From Bacic D, Kaissling B, McLeroy P, et al: Dopamine acutely decreases apical membrane Na/H exchanger NHE3 protein in mouse renal proximal tubule. *Kidney Int* 64:2133-2141, 2003).

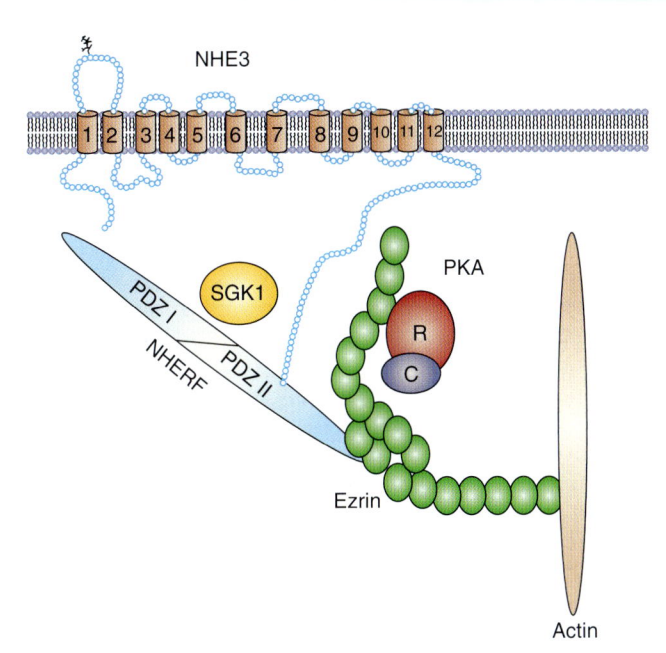

Figure 6.13 Scaffolding protein NHERF (Na⁺-H⁺ exchanger regulatory factor) links the Na⁺-H⁺ exchanger NHE3 to the cytoskeleton and signaling proteins. NHERF binds to ezrin, which in turn links to protein kinase A (PKA) and the actin cytoskeleton. NHERF also binds to SGK1 (serum- and glucocorticoid-regulated kinase 1), which activates NHE3. PDZ, Domain named for the PSD95, *Drosophila* disc large (*Drosophila*), and ZO-1 proteins; C, catalytic; R, regulatory.

Notably, however, phosphorylation of these residues appears to be necessary but not sufficient for regulation of NHE3.[35] A number of regulators of NHE3, including gastrin and uroguanylin, have been found to exert a functional effect through phosphorylation of S552 and/or S605.[114,115]

The regulation of NHE3 by cAMP also requires the participation of a family of homologous scaffolding proteins that contain protein-protein interaction motifs known as PDZ domains (named for the PSD95, *Drosophila* disc large, and ZO-1 proteins in which these domains were first discovered; Figure 6.13). The first of these proteins, NHE regulatory factor-1 (NHERF-1), was purified as a cellular factor required for the inhibition of NHE3 by PKA.[116] NHERF-2 was in turn cloned by yeast two-hybrid screens as a protein that interacts with the C-terminus of NHE3; NHERF-1 and NHERF-2 have very similar effects on the regulation of NHE3 in cultured cells. The related protein PDZK1 interacts with NHE3 and a number of other epithelial transporters and is required for expression of the anion exchanger Slc26a6 at brush border membranes of the proximal tubule.[59]

NHERF-1 and NHERF-2 are both expressed in human and mouse proximal tubule cells; NHERF-1 co-localizes with NHE3 in microvilli of the brush border, whereas NHERF-2 is predominantly expressed at the base of microvilli in the vesicle-rich domain.[116] The NHERFs assemble a multiprotein, dynamically regulated signaling complex that includes NHE3 and several other transport proteins. In addition to NHE3, they bind to the actin-associated protein, ezrin, thus linking NHE3 to the cytoskeleton; this linkage to the cytoskeleton may be particularly important for the mechanical activation of NHE3 by microvillar bending, as has been implicated in glomerulotubular balance (see above).[75,77,116] Ezrin also interacts directly with NHE3, binding to a separate binding site within the C-terminus of the transport protein.[107] Ezrin functions as an anchoring protein for PKA, bringing PKA into close proximity with NHE3 and facilitating its phosphorylation (see Figure 6.13).[116] Analysis of knockout mice for NHERF-1 has revealed that it is not required for baseline activity of NHE3; as expected, however, it is required for cAMP-dependent regulation of the exchanger by PTH.[116] One long-standing paradox has been that β-adrenergic receptors, which increase cAMP in the proximal tubule, cause an activation of apical Na⁺-H⁺ exchange.[84] This was resolved by the observation that the first PDZ domain of NHERF-1 interacts with the β₂-adrenergic receptor in an agonist-dependent fashion; this interaction serves to disrupt the interaction between the second PDZ domain and NHE3, resulting in a stimulation of the exchanger, despite the catecholamine-dependent increase in cAMP.[116]

As discussed above, at concentrations higher than 10^{-7} M (see Figure 6.11), Ang II has an inhibitory effect on proximal tubular Na⁺-Cl⁻ absorption.[86] This inhibition is dependent on the activation of brush border phospholipase A₂, which results in the liberation of arachidonic acid.[89] Metabolism of arachidonic acid by cytochrome P450 monooxygenases, in turn, generates 20-hydroxyeicosatetraenoic acid (20-HETE) and epoxyeicosatrioenoic acids (EETs), compounds that inhibit NHE3 and the basolateral Na+-K+-ATPase.[84,117] EETs and 20-HETE have also been implicated in the reduction in proximal Na⁺-Cl⁻ absorption that occurs during pressure natriuresis, inhibiting Na+-K+-ATPase and retracting NHE3 from the brush border membrane.[118]

Antinatriuretic stimuli such as Ang II acutely increase the expression of NHE3 at the apical membrane, at least in part by inhibiting the generation of cAMP.[109] Low-dose Ang II (10^{-10} M) also increases exocytic insertion of NHE3 into the plasma membrane via a mechanism that is dependent on phosphatidylinositol-3-kinase (PI3K).[119] Treatment of rats with captopril thus results in a retraction of NHE3 and associated proteins from the brush border of proximal tubule cells.[120] Glucocorticoids also increase NHE3 activity due to transcriptional induction of the NHE3 gene and an acute stimulation of exocytosis of the exchanger to the plasma membrane.[35] Glucorticoid-dependent exocytosis of NHE3 appears to require NHERF-2, which acts in this context as a scaffolding protein for the glucocorticoid-induced serine-threonine kinase SGK1 (see later, "Regulation of Na⁺-Cl⁻ Transport in the Connecting Tubule and Cortical Collecting Duct: Aldosterone").[121] The acute effect of dexamethasone has thus been shown to require direct phosphorylation of serine 663 in the NHE3 protein by SGK1.[122]

Finally, many of the natriuretic and antinatriuretic pathways that influence NHE3 have parallel effects on the basolateral Na+-K+-ATPase (see Feraille and Doucet[84] for a detailed review). The molecular mechanisms underlying inhibition of Na+-K+-ATPase by dopamine have been particularly well characterized. Inhibition by dopamine is associated with removal of active Na+-K+-ATPase units from the basolateral membrane, somewhat analogous to the effect on NHE3 expression at the apical membrane.[123] This inhibitory effect is primarily mediated by protein kinase C (PKC), which directly phosphorylates the α_1-subunit of Na+-K+-ATPase, the predominant α-subunit in the kidney.[84] The effect of dopamine requires phosphorylation of serine 18 of the α_1-subunit by PKC; this phosphorylation does not affect enzymatic activity of the Na+-K+-ATPase, but rather induces a conformational change that enhances the binding of PI3K to an adjacent, proline-rich domain. The PI3K recruited by this phosphorylated α_1-subunit then stimulates the dynamin-dependent endocytosis of the Na+-K+-ATPase complex via clathrin-coated pits.[123]

LOOP OF HENLE AND THICK ASCENDING LIMB

The loop of Henle encompasses the thin descending limb, thin ascending limb, and TAL. The descending and ascending thin limbs function in passive absorption of water and Na^+-Cl^-, respectively, whereas the TAL reabsorbs about 30% of filtered Na^+-Cl^- via active transport.[124,125] There is considerable cellular and functional heterogeneity along the entire length of the loop of Henle, with consequences for the transport of water, Na^+-Cl^-, and other solutes. The thin descending limb begins in the outer medulla after an abrupt transition from S3 segments of the proximal tubule, marking the boundary between the outer and inner stripes of the outer medulla. Thin descending limbs end at a hairpin turn at the end of Henle's loop. Short-looped nephrons that originate from superficial and midcortical nephrons have a short descending limb within the inner stripe of the outer medulla; these tubules merge abruptly into the TAL close to the hairpin turn of the loop (see also below). Long-looped nephrons originating from juxtamedullary glomeruli have a long ascending thin limb that then merges with the TAL. The TALs of long-looped nephrons begin at the boundary between the inner and outer medulla, whereas the TALs of short-looped nephrons may be entirely cortical. The ratio of medullary to cortical TAL for a given nephron is a function of the depth of its origin, such that superficial nephrons are primarily composed of cortical TALs, whereas juxtamedullary nephrons primarily possess medullary TALs.

TRANSPORT CHARACTERISTICS OF THE DESCENDING THIN LIMB

It has long been appreciated that the osmolality of tubular fluid increases progressively between the corticomedullary junction and papillary tip due to active secretion of solutes or passive absorption of water along the descending thin limb.[126] Subsequent reports have revealed a very high water permeability of perfused outer medullary thin descending limbs in the absence of significant permeability to Na^+-Cl^-.[127] Notably, however, the permeability properties of descending thin limbs vary as a function of depth in the inner medulla and inclusion in short- versus long-looped nephrons.[128,129] Descending thin limbs from short-looped nephrons contain type I cells, very flat, endothelial-like cells, with intermediate-depth tight junctions suggesting a relative tight epithelium.[128,129] The epithelium of descending limbs from long-looped nephrons is initially more complex, with taller type II cells possessing more elaborate apical microvilli and more prominent mitochondria. In the lower medullary portion of long-looped nephrons, these cells change into a type III morphology, endothelial-like cells similar to the type I cells from short-looped nephrons.[128] The permeability properties appear to change as a function of cell type, with a progressive axial drop in water permeability of long-looped descending limbs; the water permeability of descending thin limbs in the middle part of the inner medulla is thus about 42% that of outer medullary thin descending limbs.[130] Furthermore, the distal 20% of descending thin limbs have a very low water permeability.[130] These changes in water permeability along the descending thin limb are accompanied by a progressive increase in Na^+-Cl^- permeability, although the ionic permeability remains considerably less than that of the ascending thin limb.[129]

Consistent with a primary role in passive water and solute absorption, Na+-K+-ATPase activity in the descending thin limb is almost undetectable,[15] suggesting that these cells do not actively transport Na^+-Cl^-; those ion transport pathways that have been identified in descending thin limb cells are thought to contribute primarily to cellular volume regulation.[131] In contrast to the relative lack of Na^+-Cl^- transport, transcellular water reabsorption by the thin descending limb is a critical component of the renal countercurrent concentrating mechanism (see Chapter 10).[124,127]

Na^+-Cl^- TRANSPORT BY THE THIN ASCENDING LIMB

Fluid entering the thin ascending limb has a very high concentration of Na^+-Cl^- due to osmotic equilibration by the water-permeable descending limbs. The passive reabsorption of this delivered Na^+-Cl^- by the thin ascending limb is a critical component of the passive equilibration model of the renal countercurrent multiplication system. Consistent with this role, the permeability properties of the thin ascending limb are dramatically different from those of the descending thin limb, with a much higher permeability to Na^+-Cl^- and vanishingly low water permeability.[129,132] Passive Na^+-Cl^- reabsorption by thin ascending limbs occurs via a combination of paracellular Na^+ transport and transcellular Cl^- transport.[125,133-137] The inhibition of paracellular conductance by protamine thus selectively inhibits Na^+ transport across perfused thin ascending limbs, consistent with paracellular transport of Na^+.[133] As in the descending limb, thin ascending limbs have a modest Na+-K+-ATPase activity (see Figure 6.4); however, the active transport of Na^+ across thin ascending limbs accounts for only an estimated 2% of Na^+ reabsorption by this nephron segment.[138] Chloride channel blockers reduce Cl^- permeability of the thin ascending limb, consistent with passive transcellular Cl^- transport.[136] Direct measurement of the membrane potential of impaled hamster thin ascending limbs has also yielded evidence for apical and basolateral Cl^- channel activity.[137] This transepithelial transport of Cl^-, but not Na^+, is activated by vasopressin, with a pharmacologic profile that is consistent with direct activation of thin ascending limb Cl^- channels.[139]

Both apical and basolateral Cl^- transport in the thin ascending limb appear to be mediated by the CLC-K1 Cl^- channel in cooperation with the Barttin subunit (see also Na^+-Cl^- transport in the thick ascending limb; basolateral mechanisms). Immunofluorescence and in situ hybridization indicate a selective expression of CLC-K1 in thin ascending limbs, although single-tubule, reverse transcriptase polymerase chain reaction (RT-PCR) studies have suggested additional expression in the thick ascending limb, distal convoluted tubule, and cortical collecting duct.[140-142] Notably, immunofluorescence and immunogold labeling indicate that CLC-K1 is expressed exclusively at both the apical and basolateral membranes of thin ascending limbs, such that both the luminal and basolateral Cl⁻ channels of this nephron segment are encoded by the same gene.[137,140] Homozygous knockout mice with a targeted deletion of CLC-K1 have a vasopressin-resistant nephrogenic diabetes insipidus, reminiscent of the phenotype of aquaporin-1 knockout mice.[124,143] Given that CLC-K1 is potentially expressed in the TAL, dysfunction of this nephron segment might also contribute to the renal phenotype of CLC-K1 knockout mice; however, the closely homologous channel CLC-K2 (CLC-NKB) is clearly expressed in the TAL, where it can likely substitute for CLC-K1.[142] Furthermore, loss-of-function mutations in CLC-NKB are an important cause of Bartter's syndrome, indicating that CLC-K2, rather than CLC-K1, is critical for transport function of the TAL.[144]

Detailed characterization of CLC-K1 knockout mice has revealed a selective impairment in Cl⁻ transport by the thin ascending limb.[125] Whereas Cl⁻ absorption is profoundly reduced, Na⁺ absorption by thin ascending limbs is not significantly impaired (Figure 6.14). The diffusion voltage induced by a transepithelial Na⁺-Cl⁻ gradient is reversed by the absence of CLC-K1, from +15.5 mV in homozygous wild-type controls (+/+) to −7.6 mV in homozygous knockout mice (−/−). This change in diffusion voltage is due to the dominance of paracellular Na⁺ transport in the CLC-K1–deficient −/− mice, leading to a lumen-negative potential; this corresponds to a marked reduction in the relative permeability of Cl⁻ to that of Na⁺ (P_{Cl}/P_{Na}), from 4.02 to 0.63 (see Figure 6.14). Protamine, an inhibitor of paracellular Na⁺ transport, has a comparable effect on the diffusion voltage in −/− mice versus +/− and +/+ mice that have been treated with 5-nitro-2-(3-phenylpropylamino)-benzoate (NPPB) to inhibit CLC-K1; the respective diffusion voltages are 7.9 mV (−/− plus protamine), 8.6 mV (+/− plus protamine and NPPB), and 9.8 (+/+ plus protamine and NPPB). Therefore, the paracellular Na⁺ conductance is unimpaired and essentially the same in CLC-K1 mice when compared to littermate controls. This study thus provided elegant proof for the relative independence of paracellular and transcellular conductances for Na⁺ and Cl⁻, respectively, in thin ascending limbs.[125]

CLC-K1 associates with Barttin, a novel accessory subunit identified via positional cloning of the gene for Bartter's syndrome with sensorineural deafness (see later, "Na⁺-Cl⁻ Transport by the Thick Ascending Limb: Basolateral Mechanisms").[145] Barttin is expressed with CLC-K1 in thin ascending limbs, in addition to the TAL, distal convoluted tubule, and α-intercalated cells.[142,145] Rat CLC-K1 is unique among the CLC-K orthologs and paralogs (CLC-K1/2 in rodents, CLC-NKB/NKA in humans) in that it can generate Cl⁻ channel activity in the absence of coexpression with Barttin; however, its human ortholog CLC-NKA is nonfunctional in the absence of Barttin.[140,145,146] Regardless, Barttin co-immunoprecipitates with CLC-K1 and increases expression of the channel protein at the cell membrane.[142,146] This so-called chaperone function seems to involve the transmembrane core of Barttin, whereas domains within the cytoplasmic carboxy terminus modulate channel properties (open probability and unitary conductance).[146]

With respect to regulation in this nephron segment, vasopressin has stimulatory effects on Cl⁻ transport by the thin ascending limb, acting as in principal cells and TAL through V2 receptors and cAMP.[139] Water deprivation induces a four-fold increase in CLC-K1 mRNA, indicating transcriptional effects of vasopressin or medullary tonicity.[147] Basolateral

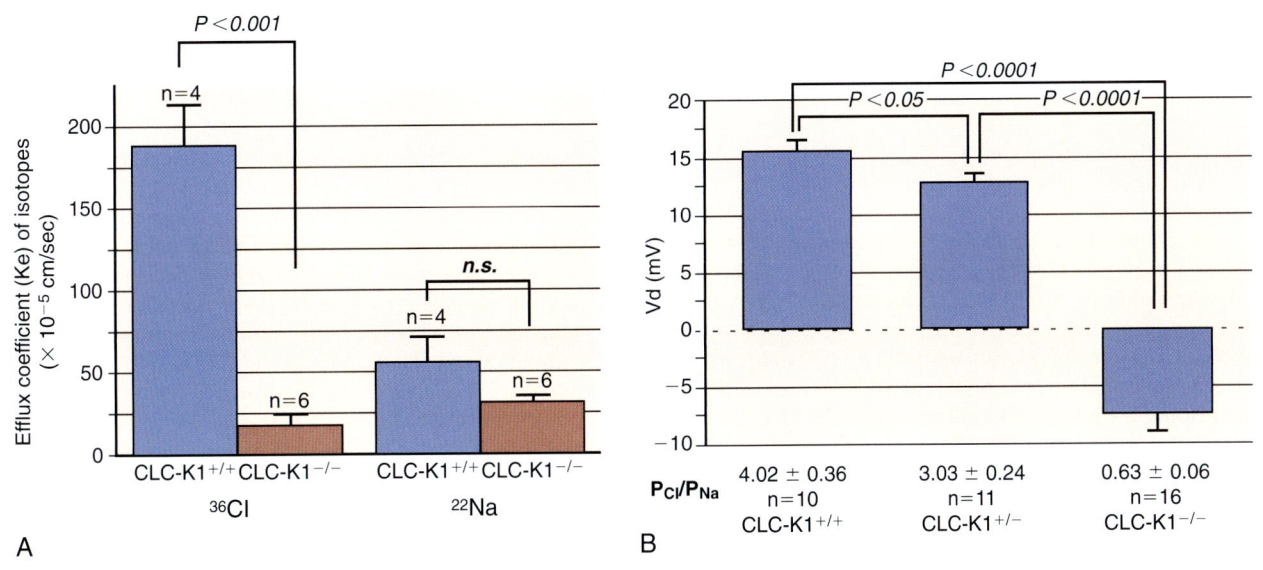

Figure 6.14 Role of the CLC-K1 chloride channel in Na⁺ and Cl⁻ transport by the thin ascending limbs. Homozygous knockout mice (CLC-K1⁻/⁻) are compared to their littermate controls (CLC-K1⁺/⁺). **A,** Efflux coefficients for ³⁶Cl⁻ and ²²Na⁺ in the thin ascending limbs. Cl⁻ absorption is essentially abolished in the knockout mice, whereas there is no significant effect of CLC-K1 deficiency on Na⁺ transport. **B,** The diffusion voltage (VD), induced by a transepithelial Na⁺-Cl⁻ gradient, is reversed by the absence of CLC-K1, from +15.5 mV in controls to −7.6 mV in homozygous knockout mice. This change in diffusion voltage is due to the dominance of paracellular Na⁺ transport in the CLC-K1–deficient −/− mice, leading to a lumen-negative potential; this corresponds to a marked reduction in the relative permeability of Cl⁻ to that of Na⁺ (P_{Cl}/P_{Na}), from 4.02 to 0.63. (From Liu W, Morimoto T, Kondo Y, et al: Analysis of NaCl transport in thin ascending limb of Henle's loop in CLC-K1 null mice. Am J Physiol Renal Physiol 282:F451-F457, 2002).

calcium in turn inhibits Cl⁻ and Na⁺ transport in the thin ascending limb via activation of the calcium-sensing receptor.[148]

Na⁺-Cl⁻ TRANSPORT BY THE THICK ASCENDING LIMB
Apical Na⁺-Cl⁻ Transport

The TAL reabsorbs about 30% of filtered Na⁺-Cl⁻ (see Figure 6.1). In addition to an important role in the defense of the extracellular fluid volume, Na⁺-Cl⁻ reabsorption by the water-impermeable TAL is a critical component of the renal countercurrent multiplication system. The separation of Na⁺-Cl⁻ and water in the TAL is thus responsible for the capability of the kidney to dilute or concentrate the urine. In collaboration with the countercurrent mechanism, Na⁺-Cl⁻ reabsorption by the thin and thick ascending limbs increases medullary tonicity, facilitating water absorption by the collecting duct.

The TAL begins abruptly after the thin ascending limb of long-looped nephrons and after the aquaporin-negative segment of short-limbed nephrons.[149] The TAL extends into the renal cortex, where it meets its parent glomerulus at the vascular pole; the plaque of cells at this junction form the macula densa, which function as the tubular sensor for tubuloglomerular feedback and tubular regulation of renin release by the juxtaglomerular apparatus. Cells in the medullary TAL are 7 to 8 μm in height, with extensive invaginations of the basolateral plasma membrane and interdigitations between adjacent cells.[4] As in the proximal tubule, these lateral cell processes contain numerous elongated mitochondria, perpendicular to the basement membrane. Cells in the cortical TAL are considerably shorter, 2 μm in height at the end of the cortical TAL in rabbits, with less mitochondria and a simpler basolateral membrane.[4] Macula densa cells also lack the lateral cell processes and interdigitations characteristic of medullar TAL cells.[4] However, scanning electron microscopy has revealed that the TAL of rat and hamster contains two morphologic subtypes, a rough-surfaced cell type (R cells) with prominent apical microvilli and a smooth-surfaced cell type (S cells) with an abundance of subapical vesicles.[4,150-152] In the hamster TAL, cells can also be separated into those with high apical and low basolateral K⁺ conductance and weak basolateral Cl⁻ conductance (LBC cells) versus a second population with low apical and high basolateral K⁺ conductance combined with high basolateral Cl⁻ conductance (HBC).[137,151] The relative frequency of the morphologic and functional subtypes in the cortical and medullary TAL suggests that HBC cells correspond to S cells and LBC cells to R cells.[151]

Morphologic heterogeneity notwithstanding, the cells of the medullary TAL, cortical TAL, and macula densa share the same basic transport mechanisms (Figure 6.15). Na⁺-Cl⁻ reabsorption by the TAL is thus a secondarily active process, driven by the favorable electrochemical gradient for Na⁺ established by the basolateral Na+-K+-ATPase.[12,153] Na⁺, K⁺, and Cl⁻ are cotransported across the apical membrane by an electroneutral Na⁺-K⁺-2Cl⁻ cotransporter; this transporter generally requires the simultaneous presence of all three ions, such that the transport of Na⁺ and Cl⁻ across the epithelium is mutually codependent, dependent on the luminal presence of K⁺.[12] Of note, under certain circumstances, apical Na⁺-Cl⁻ transport in the TAL appears to be K⁺-independent; this issue is reviewed below ("Regulation of Na⁺-Cl⁻ Transport by the Thick Ascending Limb"). Regardless, this transporter is universally sensitive to furosemide, which has been known for more than 3 decades to inhibit transepithelial Cl⁻ transport by the TAL.[154] Apical Na⁺-K⁺-2Cl⁻ cotransport is mediated by the cation-chloride cotransporter NKCC2, encoded by the SLC12A1 gene.[155] Functional expression of NKCC2 in Xenopus laevis oocytes yields Cl⁻- and Na⁺-dependent uptake of Rb⁺ (a radioactive substitute for K⁺) and Cl⁻- and K⁺-dependent uptake of ²²Na⁺.[86,155-157] As expected, NKCC2 is sensitive to micromolar concentrations of furosemide, bumetanide, and other loop diuretics.[155]

Immunofluorescence indicates expression of NKCC2 protein along the entire length of the TAL.[155] In particular, immunoelectron microscopy reveals expression in rough (R) and smooth (S) cells of the TAL (see above).[152] NKCC2 expression in subapical vesicles is particularly prominent in smooth cells, suggesting a role for vesicular trafficking in the regulation of NKCC2 (see later, "Regulation of Na⁺-Cl⁻ Transport by the Thick Ascending Limb").[152] NKCC2 is also expressed in macula densa cells, which have been shown to possess apical Na⁺-K⁺-2Cl⁻ cotransport activity.[152,158] This latter observation is of considerable significance, given the role of the macula densa in tubuloglomerular feedback (TGF) and renal renin secretion; luminal loop diuretics block tubuloglomerular feedback and the suppression of renin release by luminal Cl⁻.[12]

Alternative splicing of exon 4 of the SLC12A1 gene yields NKCC2 proteins that differ within transmembrane domain 2 and the adjacent intracellular loop. There are thus three different variants of exon 4, denoted "A," "B," and "F"; the variable inclusion of these cassette exons yields NKCC2-A, NKCC2-B, and NKCC2-F proteins.[155,157] Kinetic characterization reveals that these isoforms differ dramatically in ion

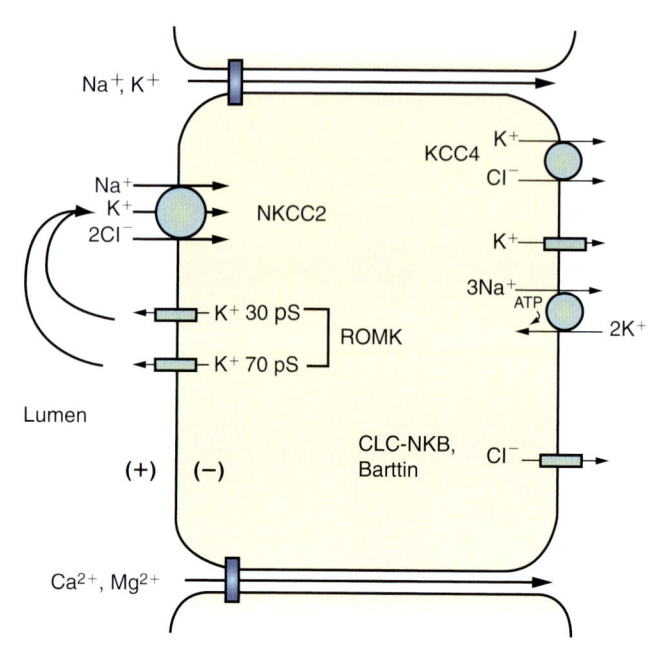

Figure 6.15 Transepithelial Na⁺-Cl⁻ transport pathways in the thick ascending limb (TAL). CLC-NKB, Human Cl⁻ channel, Barttin; KCC4, K⁺-Cl⁻ cotransporter-4; NKCC2, Na⁺-K⁺-2Cl⁻ cotransporter-2; ROMK, renal outer medullary K⁺ channel, Cl⁻ channel subunit.

affinities.[155,157] In particular, NKCC2-F has a very low affinity for Cl^- (K_m = 113 mmol/L) and NKCC2-B has a very high affinity (K_m = 8.9 mmol/L); NKCC2-A has an intermediate affinity for Cl^- (K_m = 44.7 mmol/L).[157] These isoforms differ in axial distribution along the tubule, with the F cassette expressed in the inner stripe of the outer medulla, the A cassette in the outer stripe, and the B cassette in cortical TAL.[12] There is thus an axial distribution of the anion affinity of NKCC2 along the TAL, from a low-affinity, high-capacity transporter (NKCC2-F) to a high-affinity, low-capacity transporter (NKCC2-B). Although technically compromised by the considerable homology between the 3′ end of these 96 base pair exons, in situ hybridization has suggested that rabbit macula densa exclusively expresses the NKCC2-B isoform.[12] Notably, however, selective knockout of the B cassette exon 4 does not eliminate NKCC2 expression in the murine macula densa, which also seems to express NKCC2-A by in situ hybridization.[159] The comparative phenotypes of NKCC2-A and NKCC2-B knockout mice are consistent with the relative Cl^- affinity of each isoform, with NKCC2-B functioning as a high-affinity, low-capacity isoform and NKCC2-A functioning as a low-affinity, high-capacity isoform. Thus, targeted deletion of NKCC2-A selectively reduces TGF responses at the higher range of tubular flow rates (a low-affinity, high-capacity situation), whereas NKCC2-B deletion reduces responses at low flow rates.[160] Loss of NKCC2-A almost abolishes the suppression of plasma renin activity by isotonic saline infusion, which is, if anything, more robust in NKCC2-B knockout mice than wild-type littermates.[160]

It should be mentioned in this context that the Na^+-H^+ exchanger NHE3 functions as an alternative mechanism for apical Na^+ absorption by the TAL. There is also evidence in mouse cortical TAL for Na^+-Cl^- transport via parallel Na^+-H^+ and $Cl^--HCO_3^-$ exchange, although the role of this mechanism in transepithelial Na^+-Cl^- transport seems less prominent than in the proximal tubule.[12] Indeed, apical Na^+-H^+ exchange mediated by NHE3 appears to function primarily in HCO_3^- absorption by the TAL.[161] There is thus a considerable upregulation of both apical Na^+-H^+ exchange and NHE3 protein in the TAL of acidotic animals, paired with an induction of AE2, a basolateral $Cl^--HCO_3^-$ exchanger.[162,163] NHE3 in the TAL is also upregulated by increased flow. However, this is not via shear stress, as demonstrated in the proximal tubule, but by the production of endogenous O_2^- and activation of PKC, a potential pathway for flow-stimulated bicarbonate reabsorption.[164]

Apical K^+ Channels

Microperfused TALs develop a lumen-positive PD during perfusion with Na^+-Cl^-.[165,166] This lumen-negative PD plays a critical role in the physiology of the TAL, driving the paracellular transport of Na^+, Ca^{2+}, and Mg^{2+} (see Figure 6.15). Originally attributed to electrogenic Cl^- transport, the lumen-positive transepithelial PD in the TAL is generated by the combination of apical K^+ channels and basolateral Cl^- channels.[12,153,166] The conductivity of the apical membrane of TAL cells is predominantly, if not exclusively, K^+-selective. Luminal recycling of K^+ via $Na^+-K^+-2Cl^-$ cotransport and apical K^+ channels, along with basolateral depolarization due to Cl^- exit through Cl^- channels, results in the lumen-positive transepithelial PD.[12,153]

Several lines of evidence have indicated that apical K^+ channels are required for transepithelial Na^+-Cl^- transport by the TAL[12,153]:

First, the removal of K^+ from luminal perfusate results in a marked decrease in Na^+-Cl^- reabsorption by the TAL, as measured by short circuit current; the residual Na^+-Cl^- transport in the absence of luminal K^+ is sustained by the exit of K^+ via apical K^+ channels, because the combination of K^+ removal and a luminal K^+ channel inhibitor (barium) almost abolishes the short circuit current.[12] Apical K^+ channels are thus required for continued functioning of NKCC2, the apical $Na^+-K^+-2Cl^-$ cotransporter; the low luminal concentration of K^+ in this nephron segment would otherwise become limiting for transepithelial Na^+-Cl^- transport.

Second, the net transport of K^+ across perfused TAL is less than 10% that of Na^+ and Cl^-; about 90% of the K^+ transported by NKCC2 is recycled across the apical membrane via K^+ channels, resulting in minimal net K^+ absorption by the TAL.[12,167]

Third, the intracellular K^+ activity of perfused TAL cells is about 15 to 20 mV above equilibrium due to furosemide-sensitive entry of K^+ via NKCC2.[168] Given an estimated apical K^+ conductivity of about 12 m/cm^2, this intracellular K^+ activity yields a calculated K^+ current of about 200 μA/cm^2, which corresponds quantitatively to the uptake of K^+ by the apical $Na^+-K^+-2Cl^-$ cotransporter.[153]

Fourth, the observation that Bartter's syndrome can be caused by mutations in renal outer medullary potassium (ROMK) provides genetic proof for the importance of K^+ channels in Na^+-Cl^- absorption by the TAL (see below).[169]

Finally, a novel ROMK inhibitor functions as a potent diuretic in vivo, primarily due to inhibition of TAL Na^+-Cl^- transport.[170]

Three types of apical K^+ channels have been identified in the TAL, a 30-pS (picosiemens) channel, a 70-pS channel, and a high-conductance, calcium-activated maxi-K^+ channel (see Figure 6.15).[171-173] The higher P_o and greater density of the 30-pS and 70-pS channels versus the maxi-K^+ channel suggest that these are the primary routes for K^+ recycling across the apical membrane; the 70-pS channel in turn appears to mediate about 80% of the apical K^+ conductance of TAL cells.[174] The low-conductance, 30-pS channel shares several electrophysiologic and regulatory characteristics with ROMK, the cardinal inward-rectifying K^+ channel that was initially cloned from renal outer medulla.[12] ROMK protein has been identified at the apical membrane of medullary TAL, cortical TAL, and macula densa.[175] Furthermore, the 30-pS channel is also absent from the apical membrane of mice with homozygous deletion of the gene encoding ROMK.[176] Notably, not all cells in the TAL are labeled with ROMK antibody, suggesting that ROMK might be absent in the co-called HBC cells with high basolateral Cl^- conductance and low apical, high basolateral K^+ conductance (also see above).[137,151] HBC cells are thought to correspond to the smooth-surfaced morphologic subtype of TAL cells (S cells)[151]; however, distribution of ROMK protein by immunoelectron microscopy has not as yet been reported.

ROMK clearly plays a critical role in Na^+-Cl^- absorption by the TAL, given that loss-of-function mutations in this gene are associated with Bartter's syndrome.[169] The role of ROMK in Bartter's syndrome was initially discordant with the data, suggesting that the 70-pS K⁺ channel is the dominant conductance at the apical membrane of TAL cells; heterologous expression of the ROMK protein in *Xenopus* oocytes had yielded a channel with a conductance of about 30 pS, suggesting that the 70-pS channel was distinct from ROMK.[12,174] This paradox has been resolved by the observation that the 70-pS channel is absent from the TAL of ROMK knockout mice, indicating that ROMK proteins form a subunit of the 70-pS channel.[177] ROMK activity in the TAL is clearly modulated by association with other proteins, such that co-association with other subunits to generate the 70-pS channel is perfectly compatible with the known physiology of this protein. ROMK thus associates with scaffolding proteins NHERF-1 and NHERF-2 (see earlier, "Proximal Tubule: Neurohumoral Influences") via the C-terminal PDZ-binding motif of ROMK; NHERF-2 is coexpressed with ROMK in the TAL.[178] The association of ROMK with NHERFs serves to bring ROMK into closer proximity to the cystic fibrosis transmembrane regulator protein (CFTR).[178] This ROMK-CFTR interaction is, in turn, required for the native ATP and glibenclamide sensitivity of apical K⁺ channels in the TAL.[179]

Paracellular Transport

Microperfused TALs perfused with Na⁺-Cl⁻ develop a lumen-positive, transepithelial PD generated by the combination of apical K⁺ secretion and basolateral Cl⁻ efflux.[12,153,165,166,168] This lumen-positive PD plays a critical role in the paracellular reabsorption of Na⁺, Ca²⁺, and Mg²⁺ by the TAL (see Figure 6.15). In the transepithelial transport of Na⁺, the stoichiometry of NKCC2 (1Na⁺:1K⁺:2Cl⁻) is such that other mechanisms are necessary to balance the exit of Cl⁻ at the basolateral membrane; consistent with this requirement, data from mouse TAL have indicated that about 50% of transepithelial Na⁺ transport occurs via the paracellular pathway.[3,180] For example, the ratio of net Cl⁻ transepithelial absorption to net Na⁺ absorption through the paracellular pathway is 2.4 ± 0.3 in microperfused mouse medullary TAL segments, the expected ratio of 50% of Na⁺ transport occurs via the paracellular pathway. In the absence of vasopressin, apical Na⁺-Cl⁻ cotransport is not K⁺-dependent (see "Regulation of Na⁺-Cl⁻ Transport by the Thick Ascending Limb"), reducing the lumen-positive PD; switching to K⁺-dependent Na⁺-K⁺-2Cl⁻ cotransport in the presence of vasopressin results in a doubling of Na⁺-Cl⁻ reabsorption, without an effect on oxygen consumption.[3,180] Therefore, the combination of a cation-permeable paracellular pathway and an "active transport," lumen-positive PD,[153] generated indirectly by the basolateral Na+-K+-ATPase, results in a doubling of active Na⁺-Cl⁻ transport for a given level of oxygen consumption.[3,181]

Unlike in the proximal tubule, the voltage-positive PD in the TAL is generated almost entirely by transcellular transport, rather than by diffusion across the lateral tight junction.[13] In vasopressin-stimulated mouse TAL segments, with a lumen-positive PD of 10 mV, the maximal increase in Na⁺-Cl⁻ in the lateral interspace is about 10 mmol/L.[180] Tight junctions in the TAL are cation-selective, with P_{Na}/P_{Cl} ratios of 2 to 5.[153,180] Notably, however, P_{Na}/P_{Cl} ratios can be highly variable in individual tubules, ranging from 2 to 5 in a single study of perfused mouse TAL.[180] Regardless, assuming a P_{Na}/P_{Cl} ratio of about 3, the maximal dilution potential in the mouse TAL is between 0.7 and 1.1 mV, consistent with a dominant effect of transcellular processes on the lumen-positive PD.[180]

The reported transepithelial resistance in the TAL is between 10 and 50 $\Omega \cdot cm^2$; although this resistance is higher than that of the proximal tubule, the TAL is not considered a tight epithelium.[12,153] Notably, however, water permeability of the TAL is extremely low, less than 1% that of the proximal tubule.[153] These hybrid characteristics—relatively low resistance and very low water permeability—allow the TAL to generate and sustain Na⁺-Cl⁻ gradients of up to 120 mmol/L.[12,153] Not unexpectedly, given its lack of water permeability, the TAL does not express aquaporin water channels; as in the proximal tubule, the particular repertoire of claudins expressed in the TAL determines the resistance and ion selectivity of this nephron segment. Mouse TAL segments coexpress claudin-3, -10, -14, -16, and -19.[12,182,183] Notably, the expression of claudin-19 in TAL cells is heterogeneous, analogous perhaps to the heterogeneity of ROMK expression (see above).[183]

Mutations in human claudin-16 (paracellin-1) and claudin-19 are associated with hereditary hypomagnesemia, suggesting that these claudins are particularly critical for the cation selectivity of TAL tight junctions.[12,182] Heterologous expression of claudin-16 (paracellin-1) in the anion-selective LLC-PK1 cell line markedly increases Na⁺ permeability without affecting Cl⁻ permeability; this generates a significant increase in the P_{Na}/P_{Cl} ratio (Figure 6.16).[184] LLC-PK1 cells expressing claudin-16 also have increased permeability to other monovalent cations. There is, however, only a modest increase in Mg²⁺ permeability, suggesting that claudin-16 does not form a Mg²⁺-specific pathway in the tight junction; rather, it may serve to increase the overall cation selectivity of the tight junction. Claudin-19 appears in turn to reduce P_{Cl} in LLC-PK1 cells, without having much effect on Mg²⁺ or Na⁺ permeability.[185] The claudin-16 and claudin-19 proteins interact in multiple systems, and coexpression of claudin-16 and claudin-19 synergistically increases the P_{Na}/P_{Cl} ratio in LLC-PK1 cells.[185,186] Knockdown of claudin-16 in transgenic mice increases Na⁺ absorption in the downstream collecting duct, with the development of hypovolemic hyponatremia after treatment with amiloride; claudin-19 knockdown mice exhibit an increase in fractional excretion of Na⁺ and a doubling in serum aldosterone levels.[186,187] In summary, therefore, claudin-16 and claudin-19 interact to confer the cation selectivity of tight junctions in the TAL, contributing significantly to the transepithelial absorption of Na⁺ in this nephron segment.

Other claudins expressed in the TAL modulate the function of claudin-16–claudin-19 heterodimers or have independent effects. Claudin-14 interacts with claudin-16, disrupting cation selectivity of the paracellular barrier in cells that also coexpress claudin-19.[188] Claudin-14 expression in the TAL is calcium-dependent via the calcium-sensing receptor, providing a novel axis for calcium-dependent regulation of paracellular calcium transport (see below).[188-190] Claudin-10 appears to modulate paracellular Na⁺ permeability specifically, with impaired paracellular Na⁺ transport in claudin-10 knockout mice.[191]

Basolateral Mechanisms

The basolateral Na+-K+-ATPase is the primary exit pathway for Na⁺ at the basolateral membrane of TAL cells. The Na⁺ gradient generated by Na+-K+-ATPase activity is also thought to drive the apical entry of Na⁺, K⁺, and Cl⁻ via NKCC2, the

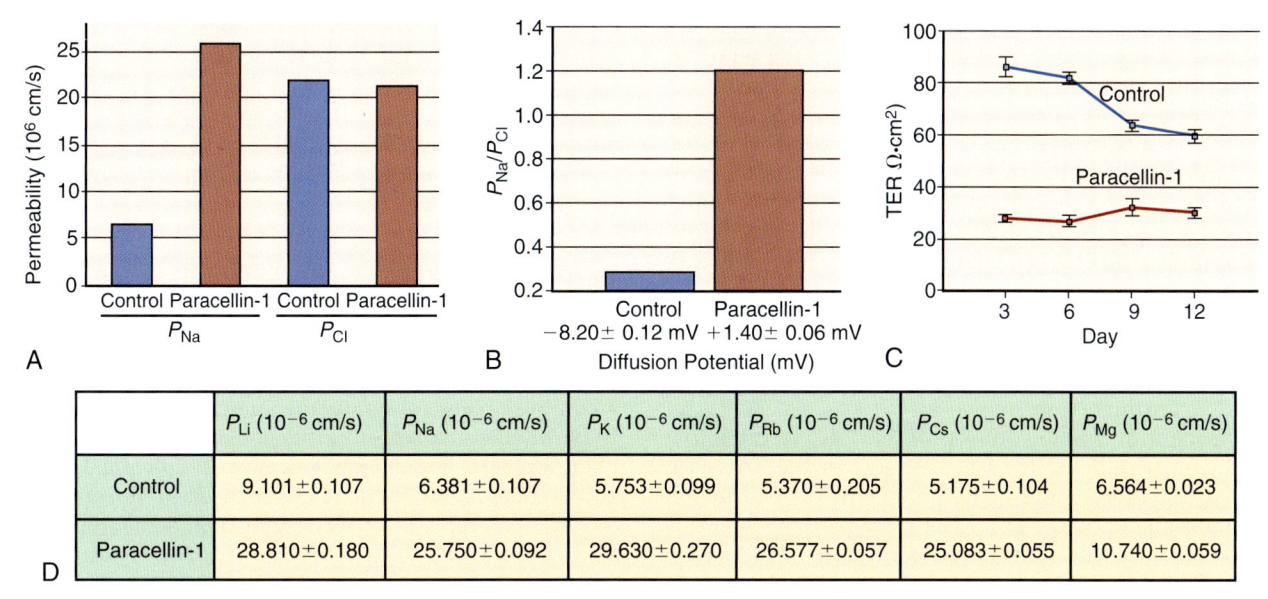

	P_{Li} (10⁻⁶ cm/s)	P_{Na} (10⁻⁶ cm/s)	P_K (10⁻⁶ cm/s)	P_{Rb} (10⁻⁶ cm/s)	P_{Cs} (10⁻⁶ cm/s)	P_{Mg} (10⁻⁶ cm/s)
Control	9.101±0.107	6.381±0.107	5.753±0.099	5.370±0.205	5.175±0.104	6.564±0.023
Paracellin-1	28.810±0.180	25.750±0.092	29.630±0.270	26.577±0.057	25.083±0.055	10.740±0.059

Figure 6.16 Effect of claudin-16 (paracellin-1) overexpression in LLC-PK1 cells. **A,** Effects of paracellin-1 on the permeability of Na⁺ and Cl⁻ in LLC-PK1 cells. **B,** Ratio of P_{Na} to P_{Cl} and diffusion potential (*bottom*) across an LLC-PK1 cell monolayer. **C,** Transepithelial resistance across an LLC-PK1 cell monolayer over a period of 12 days in cells expressing paracellin-1 and control cells. **D,** Summary of the effects of paracellin-1 on permeability of various cations in LLC-PK1 cells. (From Hou J, Paul DL, Goodenough DA: Paracellin-1 and the modulation of ion selectivity of tight junctions. *J Cell Sci* 118:5109-5118, 2005.)

furosemide-sensitive Na⁺-K⁺-2Cl⁻ cotransporter.[12] Inhibition of Na+-K+-ATPase with ouabain thus collapses the lumen-positive PD and abolishes transepithelial Na⁺-Cl⁻ transport in the TAL.[165,166,181] Basolateral exit of Cl⁻ from TAL cells is primarily but not exclusively electrogenic, mediated by Cl⁻ channel activity.[12,153,192] Reductions in basolateral Cl⁻ depolarize the basolateral membrane, whereas increases in intracellular Cl⁻ induced by luminal furosemide have a hyperpolarizing effect.[12] Intracellular Cl⁻ activity during transepithelial Na⁺-Cl⁻ transport is above its electrochemical equilibrium,[12] with an intracellular negative voltage of −40 to −70 mV that drives basolateral Cl⁻ exit.[12,153]

At least two CLC chloride channels, CLC-K1 and CLC-K2 (CLC-NKA and CLC-NKB in humans), are coexpressed in this nephron segment.[142,145] However, an increasing body of evidence has indicated that the dominant Cl⁻ channel in the TAL is encoded by CLC-K2. First, CLC-K1 is heavily expressed at the apical and basolateral membranes of the thin ascending limb, and the phenotype of the corresponding knockout mouse is consistent with primary dysfunction of thin ascending limbs, rather than the TAL (see Na⁺-Cl⁻ transport in the thin ascending limb).[3,125,140,143] Second, loss-of-function mutations in CLC-NKB are associated with Bartter's syndrome, genetic evidence for a dominant role of this channel in Na⁺-Cl⁻ transport in the TAL.[144] More recently, a very common T481S polymorphism in human CLC-NKB was shown to increase channel activity by a factor of 20; preliminary data have indicated an association with hypertension, suggesting that this gain-of-function in CLC-NKB increases Na⁺-Cl⁻ transport by the TAL and/or other segments of the distal nephron.[12,193] Finally, CLC-K2 protein is heavily expressed at the basolateral membrane of the mouse TAL, with additional expression in the DCT, connecting tubule (CNT), and α-intercalated cells.[194]

A key advance was the characterization of the Barttin subunit of CLC-K channels, which is coexpressed with CLC-K1 and CLC-K2 in several nephron segments, including TAL (see also "Na⁺-Cl⁻ Transport by the Thin Ascending Limb").[142,145] Unlike rat CLC-K1, the rat CLC-K2, human CLC-NKA, and human CLC-NKB paralogs are not functional in the absence of Barttin coexpression.[145,146] CLC-NKB coexpressed with Barttin is highly selective for Cl⁻, with a permeability series of Cl⁻ ≫ Br⁻ = NO_3^- > I⁻.[12,142,145] CLC-NKB/Barttin channels are activated by increases in extracellular Ca^{2+} and are pH-sensitive, with activation at an alkaline extracellular pH and marked inhibition at an acidic pH.[145] CLC-NKA/Barttin channels have similar pH and calcium sensitivities, but exhibit higher permeability to Br⁻.[145] Strikingly, despite the considerable homology between the CLC-NKA/NKB proteins, these channels also differ considerably in pharmacologic sensitivity to various Cl⁻ channel blockers, potential lead compounds for the development of paralog-specific inhibitors.[195]

Correlation between functional characteristics of CLC-K proteins with native Cl⁻ channels in TAL has been problematic. In particular, a wide variation in single-channel conductance has been reported for basolateral Cl⁻channels in this nephron segment.[196] This is perhaps due to the use of collagenase and other conditions for the preparation of tubule fragments and/or basolateral vesicles, manipulations that potentially affect channel characteristics.[196] There may also be considerable molecular heterogeneity of Cl⁻ channels in the TAL, although the genetic evidence would seem to suggest a functional dominance of CLC-NKB.[144] Notably, single-channel conductance has not been reported for CLC-NKB/Barttin channels because of the difficulty in expressing the channel in heterologous systems; this complicates the comparison of CLC-NKB/Barttin to native Cl⁻ channels. Single-channel conductance has, however, been reported for the V166E mutant of rat CLC-K1, which alters gating of the channel without expected effects on single-channel amplitude—coexpression with Barttin increases the single-channel conductance of V166E CLC-K1 from about 7 pS to 20 pS.[146] Therefore, part of the reported variability in native single-channel conductance may reflect heterogeneity in the interaction between CLC-NKB and/or CLC-NKA with Barttin. Regardless, a study using whole-cell recording techniques has suggested that CLC-K2 (CLC-NKB in humans) is the dominant Cl^- channel in TAL and other segments of the rat distal nephron.[196] Like CLC-NKB/Barttin, this native channel is highly Cl^--selective, with considerably weaker conductance for Br^- and I^-; CLC-NKA/Barttin channels exhibit higher permeability to Br^-.[12,142,145,196] This renal channel is also inhibited by acidic extracellular pH, but seems to lack the activation by alkaline pH seen in CLC-NKB/Barttin–expressing cells.[145,196]

Electroneutral K^+-Cl^- cotransport has also been implicated in transepithelial Na^+-Cl^- transport in the TAL (see Figure 6.15), functioning in K^+-dependent Cl^- exit at the basolateral membrane.[12] The K^+-Cl^- cotransporter KCC4 is thus expressed at the basolateral membrane of medullary and cortical TAL, in addition to the macula densa.[197,198] There is also functional evidence for K^+-Cl^- cotransport at the basolateral membrane of this section of the nephron. First, TAL cells contain a Cl^--dependent NH_4^+ transport mechanism that is sensitive to 1.5-mmol/L furosemide and 10-mmol/L barium (Ba^{2+}).[199] NH_4^+ ions have the same ionic radius as K^+ and are transported by KCC4 and other K^+-Cl^- cotransporters; KCC4 is also sensitive to Ba^{2+} and millimolar furosemide, consistent with the pharmacology of NH_4^+-Cl^- cotransport in the TAL.[199-201] Second, to account for the effects on the transmembrane potential difference of basolateral Ba^{2+} and/or increased K^+, it has been suggested that the basolateral membrane of TAL contains a Ba^{2+}-sensitive K^+-Cl^- transporter; this is also consistent with the known expression of Ba^{2+}-sensitive KCC4 at the basolateral membrane.[12,197,198,201] Third, increases in basolateral K^+ cause Cl^--dependent cell swelling in *Amphiuma* early distal tubule, an analogue of the mammalian TAL; in *Amphiuma* LBC cells with low basolateral conductance, analogous to mammalian LBC cells (see "Na^+-Cl^- Transport by the Thick Ascending Limb: Apical Na^+-Cl^- Transport"), this cell swelling was not accompanied by changes in basolateral membrane voltage or resistance, consistent with K^+-Cl^- transport.[137,151,202]

There is thus considerable evidence for basolateral K^+-Cl^- cotransport in the TAL, mediated by KCC4.[197,198] However, direct confirmation of a role for basolateral K^+-Cl^- cotransport in transepithelial Na^+-Cl^- transport is lacking. Indeed, KCC4-deficient mice do not have a prominent defect in function of the TAL, but exhibit instead a renal tubular acidosis.[198] The renal tubular acidosis in these mice has been attributed to defects in acid extrusion by H^+-ATPase in α-intercalated cells; however, this phenotype is conceivably the result of a reduction in medullary NH_4^+ reabsorption by the TAL due to the loss of basolateral NH_4^+ exit mediated by KCC4.[198,200,203]

Finally, there is also evidence for the existence of Ba^{2+}-sensitive K^+ channel activity at the basolateral membrane of the TAL, providing an alternative exit pathway for K^+ to that mediated by KCC4.[204-206] These channels may function in transepithelial transport of K^+, which is, however, only less than 10% that of Na^+ and Cl^- transport by the TAL.[167] Basolateral K^+ channels may also attenuate the increases in intracellular K^+ that are generated by the basolateral Na^+-K^+-ATPase, thus maintaining transepithelial Na^+-Cl^- transport.[204-206] In addition, basolateral K^+ channel activity may help stabilize the basolateral membrane potential above the equilibrium potential for Cl^-, thus maintaining a continuous driving force for Cl^- exit via CLC-NKB/Barttin Cl^- channels.[206]

REGULATION OF Na^+-Cl^- TRANSPORT BY THE THICK ASCENDING LIMB

Activating Influences

Transepithelial Na^+-Cl^- transport by the TAL is regulated by a complex blend of competing neurohumoral influences. In particular, increases in intracellular cAMP tonically stimulate ion transport in the TAL; the stimulatory hormones and mediators that increase cAMP in this nephron segment include vasopressin, PTH, glucagon, calcitonin, and β-adrenergic activation (see Figure 6.10). These overlapping cAMP-dependent stimuli are thought to result in maximal baseline stimulation of transepithelial Na^+-Cl^- transport.[84] For example, characterization of the in vivo effect of these hormones requires the prior simultaneous suppression or absence of circulating vasopressin, PTH, calcitonin, and glucagon.[84] This baseline activation is, in turn, modulated by a number of negative influences, most prominently prostaglandin E_2 (PGE_2) and extracellular Ca^{2+} (see Figure 6.10). Other hormones and autocoids working through cGMP-dependent signaling, including NO, have potent negative effects on Na^+-Cl^- transport within the TAL.[207] In contrast, Ang II has a stimulatory effect on Na^+-Cl^- transport within the TAL.[208]

Vasopressin is perhaps the most extensively studied positive modulator of transepithelial Na^+-Cl^- transport in the TAL. The TAL expresses type 2 vasopressin receptors (V_2Rs) at both the mRNA and protein levels, and microdissected TALs respond to the hormone with an increase in intracellular cAMP.[209] Vasopressin activates apical Na^+-K^+-$2Cl^-$ cotransport within minutes in perfused mouse TAL segments and also exerts a longer term influence on NKCC2 expression and function. The acute activation of apical Na^+-K^+-$2Cl^-$ cotransport is achieved at least in part by the stimulated exocytosis of NKCC2 proteins, from subapical vesicles to the plasma membrane.[210] This trafficking-dependent activation is abrogated by treatment of perfused tubules with tetanus toxin, which cleaves the vesicle-associated membrane proteins VAMP-2 and VAMP-3.[210] Activation of NKCC2 is also associated with the phosphorylation of a cluster of N-terminal threonines in the transporter protein; treatment of rats with the V_2 agonist desmopressin (DDAVP) induces phosphorylation of these residues in vivo, as measured with a potent phosphospecific antibody.[210] These threonine residues are substrates for SPAK (STE20/SPS1-related proline/alanine-rich kinase) and OSR1 (oxidative stress–responsive kinase 1), first identified by Gagnon and colleagues as key regulatory kinases for NKCC1 and other cation- chloride cotransporters.[211] SPAK and OSR1 are in turn activated by upstream WNK (*with no lysine* [*K*] kinases; see also "Regulation of Na^+-Cl^- Transport in the Connecting Tubule and Cortical Collecting Duct"), such that SPAK or OSR1 require coexpression with WNK4 to activate NKCC1 fully.[211] WNK kinases can, however, influence transport when coexpressed alone in *Xenopus* oocytes with cation-chloride cotransporters in the absence of exogenous SPAK/OSR1, reflective perhaps of the activation of endogenous *Xenopus laevis* orthologs of SPAK and/or OSR1. Regardless, coexpression with WNK3 in *Xenopus* oocytes results in activatory phosphorylation of the N-terminal threonines in NKCC2 that are phosphorylated in TAL cells after treatment with DDAVP.[210,212] The WNK3 protein is also expressed in TAL cells, although the link(s) between activation of the V$_2$ receptor and this particular kinase are as yet uncharacterized.[212]

The N-terminal phosphorylation of NKCC2 by SPAK and/or OSR1 kinases appears to be critical for activity of the transporter in the native TAL. The N-terminus of NKCC2 contains a predicted binding site for the SPAK kinase,[213] proximal to the sites of regulatory phosphorylation; the analogous binding site is required for activation of the NKCC1 cotransporter.[214] SPAK also requires the sorting receptor SORLA (sorting protein-related receptor with A-type repeats) for proper trafficking within TAL cells, such that targeted deletion of SORLA results in a marked reduction in N-terminal NKCC2 phosphorylation.[215] The role of the upstream WNK kinases is illustrated by the phenotype of a "knockin" mouse strain, in which the knocked-in mutant SPAK cannot be activated by upstream WNK kinases; these mice have a marked reduction in N-terminal phosphorylation of both NKCC2 and the thiazide-sensitive Na$^+$-Cl$^-$ cotransporter (NCC), with associated salt-sensitive hypotension.[216] The upstream WNK kinases appear to regulate SPAK and NKCC2 in a chloride-dependent fashion, phosphorylating and activating SPAK and the transporter in response to a reduction in intracellular chloride concentration.[217]

Of the two kinases, SPAK and OSR1, OSR1 is perhaps more critical for NKCC2 function in the TAL, given the loss of function of the TAL with reduced N-terminal NKCC2 phosphoprotein in mice with targeted, TAL-specific deletion of OSR1.[218] Some reports have also found an increase in NKCC2 N-terminal phosphorylation in SPAK knockout mice, suggesting overcompensation by OSR1.[219-221] However, in a more recent report, baseline Na$^+$ absorption by perfused TAL segments is profoundly impaired in SPAK-deficient mice, albeit with no evident effect on vasopressin-stimulated transport.[222] Truncated species of SPAK protein have also been detected in kidney due to generation of alternative mRNA species that lack the N-terminal kinase domain and to proteolytic degradation; both forms of SPAK function as dominant-negative inhibitors of the full-length kinase, abrogating the usual stimulatory effect on coexpressed NKCC2 or NKCC1.[221,223] Further complexity arises from the influence of the adaptor protein calcium-binding protein 39 (CAB39), which directly activates SPAK and OSR1 without the need for upstream phosphorylation by WNK kinases by promoting dimerization of the kinases.[224,225] WNK4 is also capable of direct interaction with CAB39, promoting activation of NKCC2 in the absence of SPAK or OSR1 expression.[226] Therefore, there appear to be three potential pathways for NKCC2 activation—a WNK4-dependent SPAK-OSR1 pathway, a WNK4-independent SPAK-OSR1 pathway, and a SPAK-independent WNK4 pathway.[226]

Vasopressin has also been shown to alter the stoichiometry of furosemide-sensitive apical Cl$^-$ transport in the TAL, from a K$^+$-independent Na$^+$-Cl$^-$ mode to the classic Na$^+$-K$^+$-2Cl$^-$ cotransport stoichiometry.[3] In the absence of vasopressin, ^{22}Na$^+$ uptake by mouse medullary TAL cells is not dependent on the presence of extracellular K$^+$, whereas the addition of the hormone induces a switch to K$^+$-dependent ^{22}Na$^+$ uptake. Underscoring the metabolic advantages of paracellular Na$^+$ transport, which is critically dependent on the apical entry of K$^+$ via Na$^+$-K$^+$-2Cl$^-$ cotransport (see above), vasopressin accomplishes a doubling of transepithelial Na$^+$-Cl$^-$ transport without affecting ^{22}Na$^+$ uptake (an indicator of transcellular Na$^+$-Cl$^-$ transport); this doubling in transepithelial absorption occurs without an increase in O$_2$ consumption, highlighting the energy efficiency of ion transport by the TAL.[3] The mechanism of this shift in the apparent stoichiometry of NKCC2 is not completely clear. However, splice variants of mouse NKCC2 with a novel, shorter C-terminus have been found to confer sensitivity to cAMP when coexpressed with full-length NKCC2.[227] Notably, these shorter splice variants appear to encode furosemide-sensitive, K$^+$-independent Na$^+$-Cl$^-$ cotransporters when expressed alone in *Xenopus* oocytes.[228] The in vivo relevance of these phenomena is not clear, however, nor is it known whether similar splice variants exist in species other than mouse.

In addition to its acute effects on NKCC2, the apical Na$^+$-K$^+$-2Cl$^-$ cotransporter, vasopressin increases transepithelial Na$^+$-Cl$^-$ transport by activating apical K$^+$ channels and basolateral Cl$^-$ channels in the TAL.[84,209] Details have yet to emerge of the regulation of the basolateral CLC-NKB/Barttin Cl$^-$ channel complex by vasopressin, cAMP, and related pathways. However, the apical K$^+$ channel ROMK is directly phosphorylated by protein kinase A on three serine residues (S25, S200, and S294 in the ROMK2 isoform). Phosphorylation of at least two of these three serines is required for detectable K$^+$ channel activity in *Xenopus* oocytes; mutation of all three serines to alanine abolishes phosphorylation and transport activity, and all three serines are required for full channel activity.[229] These three phospho acceptor sites have distinct effects on ROMK activity and expression.[230] Phosphorylation of the N-terminal S25 residue appears to regulate trafficking of the channel to the cell membrane, without effects on channel gating; this serine is also a substrate for the SGK1 kinase, which activates the channel via an increase in expression at the membrane.[230] In contrast, phosphorylation of the two C-terminal serines modulates open channel probability via effects on pH-dependent gating and on activation by the binding of phosphatidylinositol 4,5-bisphosphate (PIP2) to the C-terminal domain of the channel.[231,232]

Vasopressin also has considerable long-term effects on transepithelial Na$^+$-Cl$^-$ transport by the TAL. Sustained increases in circulating vasopressin result in marked hypertrophy of medullary TAL cells, accompanied by a doubling in baseline active Na$^+$-Cl$^-$ transport.[209] Water restriction or treatment with DDAVP also results in an increase in abundance of the NKCC2 protein in rat TAL cells. Consistent with a direct effect of vasopressin-dependent signaling, expression of NKCC2 is reduced in mice with a heterozygous deletion of the G$_s$ stimulatory G protein, through which the V$_2$R activates cAMP generation.[209] Increases in cAMP are thought to induce transcription of the *SLC12A1* gene that encodes NKCC2 directly, given the presence of a cAMP-response element in the 5′ promoter.[209,210] Abrogation of the tonic negative effect of PGE$_2$ on cAMP generation with indomethacin also results in a considerable increase in abundance of the NKCC2 protein.[209] Finally, in addition to these effects on NKCC2 expression, water restriction or DDAVP treatment increases abundance of the ROMK protein at the apical membrane of TAL cells.[233]

Inhibitory Influences

The stimulation of transepithelial Na$^+$-Cl$^-$ transport by cAMP-generating hormones (e.g., vasopressin, PTH) is modulated by a number of negative neurohumoral influences (see Figure 6.10).[84] In particular, extracellular Ca^{2+} and PGE$_2$ exert dramatic inhibitory effects on ion transport by this and other segments of the distal nephron through a plethora of synergistic mechanisms. Extracellular Ca^{2+} and PGE$_2$ both activate the G$_i$ inhibitory G protein in TAL cells, opposing the stimulatory, G$_s$-dependent effects of vasopressin on intracellular levels of cAMP.[234,235] Extracellular Ca^{2+} exerts its effect through the calcium-sensing receptor (CaSR), which is heavily expressed at the basolateral membrane of TAL cells; PGE$_2$ primarily signals through EP$_3$ prostaglandin receptors.[84,235,236] The increases in intracellular Ca^{2+} due to the activation of the CaSR and other receptors directly inhibits cAMP generation by a Ca^{2+}-inhibitable adenylate cyclase that is expressed in the TAL, accompanied by an increase in phosphodiesterase-dependent degradation of cAMP (Figure 6.17).[235,237] These negative stimuli likely inhibit baseline transport in the TAL; abrogation of the negative effect of PGE$_2$ with indomethacin results in a considerable increase in abundance of the NKCC2 protein, whereas targeted deletion of the CaSR in mouse TAL activates NKCC2 via increased N-terminal phosphorylation.[189,209]

Activation of the CaSR and other receptors in the TAL also results in the downstream generation of arachidonic acid metabolites, with potent negative effects on Na$^+$-Cl$^-$ transport (see Figure 6.17). Extracellular Ca^{2+} thus activates phospholipase A$_2$ (PLA$_2$) in TAL cells, leading to the liberation of arachidonic acid. This arachidonic acid is in turn metabolized by cytochrome P450 ω-hydroxylase to 20-HETE or by cyclo-oxygenase-2 (COX-2) to PGE$_2$; cytochrome P450 ω-hydroxylation generally predominates in response to activation of the CaSR in TAL.[235] 20-HETE has very potent negative effects on apical Na$^+$-K$^+$-2Cl$^-$ cotransport, apical K$^+$ channels, and the basolateral Na+-K+-ATPase.[84,235] PLA$_2$-dependent generation of 20-HETE also underlies in part the negative effect of bradykinin and Ang II on Na$^+$-Cl$^-$ transport.[84,235] Activation of the CaSR also induces tumor necrosis factor-α (TNF-α) expression in the TAL, which activates COX-2 and thus generation of PGE$_2$ (see Figure 6.17); this PGE$_2$ in turn results in additional inhibition of Na$^+$-Cl$^-$ transport.[235]

The relative importance of the CaSR in the regulation of Na$^+$-Cl$^-$ transport by the TAL is dramatically illustrated by the phenotype of a handful of patients with gain-of-function mutations in this receptor. In addition to suppressed PTH and hypocalcemia, the usual phenotype caused by gain-of-function mutations in the CaSR (autosomal dominant hypoparathyroidism), these patients manifest a hypokalemic alkalosis, polyuria, and increases in circulating renin and aldosterone.[238,239] Therefore, the persistent inhibition of

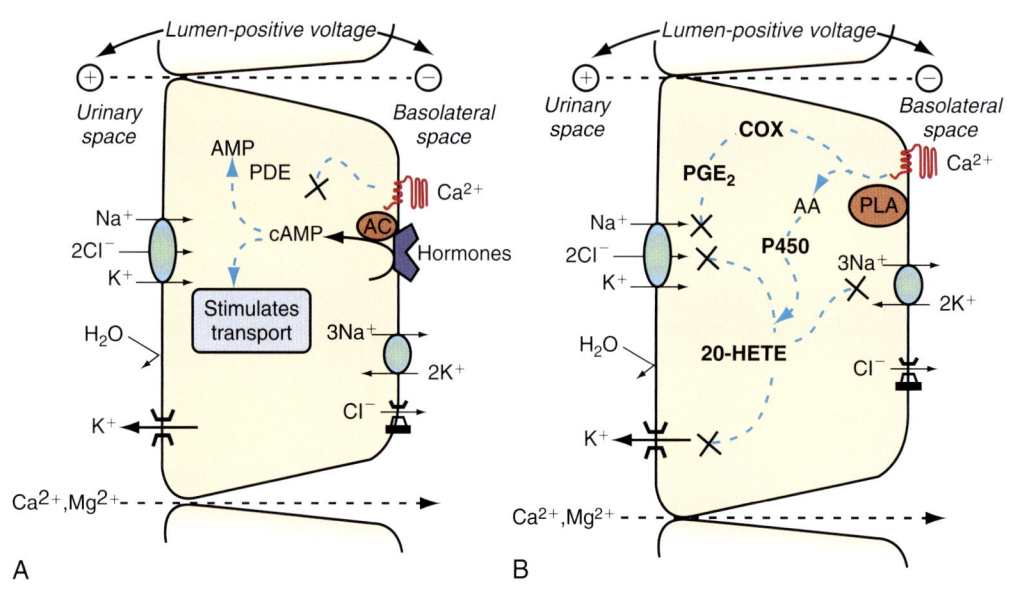

Figure 6.17 Inhibitory effects of the calcium-sensing receptor (CaSR) on transepithelial Na$^+$-Cl$^-$ transport in the TAL. **A,** Activation of the basolateral CaSR inhibits the generation of cAMP in response to vasopressin and other hormones (see text for details). **B,** Stimulation of phospholipase A$_2$ by the CaSR leads to liberation of arachidonic acid, which is in turn metabolized by cytochrome P450 ω-hydroxylase to 20-HETE (20-hydroxyeicosatetraenoic acid), or by cyclo-oxygenase-2 (COX-2) to prostaglandin E$_2$ (PGE$_2$). 20-HETE is a potent natriuretic factor, inhibiting apical Na$^+$-K$^+$-2Cl$^-$ cotransport, apical K$^+$ channels, and the basolateral Na$^+$-K$^+$-ATPase. Activation of the CaSR also induces tumor necrosis factor-α (TNF-α) expression in the TAL, which activates COX-2 and thus generation of PGE$_2$, leading to additional inhibition of Na$^+$-Cl$^-$ transport. (From Hebert SC: Calcium and salinity sensing by the thick ascending limb: a journey from mammals to fish and back again. *Kidney Int Suppl* 91:S28-S33, 2004).

Na$^+$-Cl$^-$ transport in the TAL by these overactive mutants of the CaSR causes a rare subtype of Bartter's syndrome, type V, in the genetic classification of this disease.[235]

Activation of the CaSR also affects claudin expression in TAL cells via downregulation of microRNAs, leading to PTH-independent hypercalciuria (see Chapter 7).[188-190,240]

Uromodulin

TAL cells are unique in expressing the membrane-bound, glycosylphosphatidylinositol (GPI)–anchored protein uromodulin (Tamm-Horsfall glycoprotein), which is not expressed by macula densa cells or the downstream DCT. Uromodulin is released by proteolytic cleavage at the apical membrane and is secreted as the most abundant protein in normal human urine (20 to 100 mg/day).[241] Uromodulin has a host of emerging roles in the physiology and biology of the TAL. A high-salt diet increases uromodulin expression, suggesting a role in ion transport.[241] In this regard, uromodulin facilitates membrane trafficking and function of the NKCC2 protein, with similar effects on apical ROMK protein.[242,243]

Autosomal dominant mutations in the *UMOD* gene encoding uromodulin are associated with medullary cystic disease type 2 and familial juvenile hyperuricemic nephropathy. Now referred to as uromodulin-associated kidney disease (UAKD), this syndrome includes progressive tubulointerstitial damage and chronic kidney disease (CKD), variably penetrant hyperuricemia and gout, and variably penetrant renal cysts that are typically confined to the corticomedullary junction.[241] The causative mutations tend to affect conserved cysteine residues within the N-terminal half of the protein, leading to protein misfolding and retention within the endoplasmic reticulum.[241,244] More common genetic variants in the *UMOD* promoter have recently been linked in genomewide association studies with a risk of CKD and hypertension.[241] These susceptibility variants have a high frequency (≈0.8) and confer an approximately 20% higher risk for CKD and a 15% risk for hypertension.[245] These polymorphisms are associated with more abundant renal uromodulin transcript and higher urinary uromodulin excretion due to activating effects on the *UMOD* promoter.[245,246] Overexpression of uromodulin in transgenic mice leads to distal tubular injury, with segmental dilation and an increased tubular cast area relative to wild-type mice; similar lesions are increased in frequency in older adults homozygous for susceptibility variants in *UMOD* when compared to those homozygous for protective variants.[245]

Uromodulin-transgenic mice also manifest salt-sensitive hypertension due to activation of the SPAK kinase and activating N-terminal phosphorylation of NKCC2. Human hypertensive subjects homozygous for susceptibility variants in *UMOD* appear to have an analogous phenotype, with exaggerated natriuresis in response to furosemide compared to those who are homozygous for protective variants.[245] These findings are compatible with the stimulatory effects of uromodulin on NKCC2 and ROMK—that is, a net gain of function in TAL transport.[242,243] Uromodulin excretion also appears to parallel transport activity of the TAL, with common polymorphisms in the *KCNJ1* gene encoding ROMK and two genes involved in regulating SPAK and OSR1 kinase activity (*SORL1* and *CAB39*).[246]

DISTAL CONVOLUTED TUBULE, CONNECTING TUBULE, AND COLLECTING DUCT

The distal nephron that extends beyond the TAL is the final arbiter of urinary Na$^+$-Cl$^-$ excretion and a critical target for natriuretic and antinatriuretic stimuli. The understanding of the cellular organization and molecular phenotype of the distal nephron continues to evolve and merits a brief review in this context. The DCT begins at a variable distance after the macula densa, with an abrupt transition between NKCC2-positive cortical TAL cells and DCT cells that express the thiazide-sensitive Na$^+$-Cl$^-$ cotransporter NCC. Considerable progress has been made in the phenotypic classification of cell types in the DCT and adjacent nephron segments, based on the expression of an expanding list of transport proteins and other markers.[247] This analysis has revealed considerable differences in the organization of the DCT, CNT, and cortical collecting duct (CCD) in rodent, rabbit, and human kidneys. In general, rabbit kidneys are unique in the axial demarcation of DCT, CNT, and CCD segments, at both a molecular and morphologic level; the organization of the DCT to CCD is considerably more complex in other species, with boundaries that are much less absolute.[247] Notably, however, the overall repertoire of transport proteins expressed does not vary among these species; what differs is the specific cellular and molecular organization of this segment of the nephron.

The early DCT (DCT1) of mouse kidney expresses NCC and a specific marker, parvalbumin, that also distinguishes the DCT1 from the adjacent cortical TAL (Figure 6.18).[248] Targeted deletion of parvalbumin in mice reveals that this intracellular Ca^{2+}-binding protein is required for full activity of NCC in the DCT.[249] Cells of the late DCT (DCT2) in mice coexpress NCC with proteins involved in transcellular Ca^{2+} transport, including the apical calcium channel, TRPV5 (previously ECaC1), the cytosolic calcium-binding protein calbindin D$_{28K}$, and the basolateral Na$^+$-Ca^{2+} exchanger NCX1.[248] NCC is coexpressed with ENaC in the late DCT2

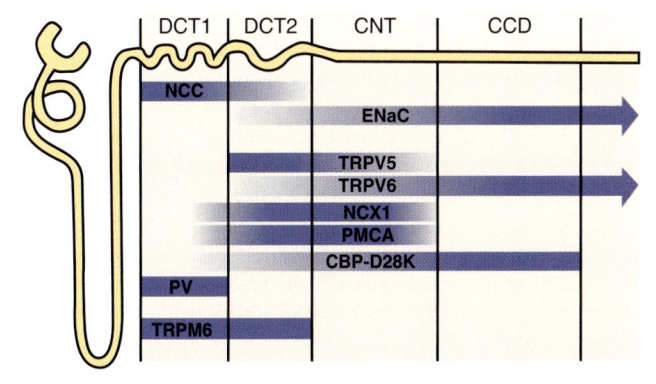

Figure 6.18 Schematic representation of the segmentation of the mouse distal nephron and distribution and abundance of Na$^+$-, Ca^{2+}-, and Mg^{2+}-transporting proteins. CB, Calbindin; CBP-D28K, calbindin-D28K; CCD, cortical collecting duct; CNT, connecting tubule; DCT1, DCT 2, distal convoluted tubules 1 and 2; ENaC, epithelial Na$^+$ channel; NCC, thiazide-sensitive Na$^+$-Cl$^-$ cotransporter; NCX1, Na$^+$-Ca^{2+} exchanger; PMCA, plasma membrane Ca^{2+}-ATPase; PV, parvalbumin; TRPM6, apical Mg^{2+} entry channel; TRPV5 and TRPV6, apical Ca^{2+} entry channels.[248,526,527]

of mouse, with robust expression of ENaC continuing in the downstream CNT and CCD.[248] In contrast, rabbit kidney does not have a DCT1 or DCT2 and exhibits abrupt transitions between NCC- and ENaC-positive DCT and CNT segments, respectively.[247] Human kidneys that have been studied thus far exhibit expression of calbindin D_{28K} all along the DCT and CNT, extending into the CCD; however, the intensity of expression varies at these sites. Approximately 30% of cells in the distal convolution of human kidney express NCC, with 70% expressing ENaC (CNT cells); ENaC and NCC overlap in expression at the end of the human DCT segment. Finally, cells of the early CNT of human kidneys express ENaC in the absence of aquaporin-2, the apical vasopressin-sensitive water channel.[247]

Although primarily contiguous with the DCT, CNT cells share several traits with principal cells of the CCD, including apical expression of ENaC and ROMK, K^+ secretory channel; the capacity for Na^+-Cl^- reabsorption and K^+ secretion in this nephron segment is as much as 10 times higher than that of the CCD (see also "Connecting Tubules and the Cortical Collecting Duct: Apical Na^+ Transport").[250] Intercalated cells are the minority cell type in the distal nephron, emerging within the DCT and CNT and extending into the early inner medullary collecting duct (IMCD).[251] Three subtypes of intercalated cells have been defined, based on differences in the subcellular distribution of the H^+-ATPase and the presence or absence of the basolateral AE1 Cl^--HCO_3^- exchanger. Type A intercalated cells extrude protons via an apical H^+-ATPase in series with basolateral AE1; type B intercalated cells secrete HCO_3^- and OH^- via an apical anion exchanger (SLC26A4 or pendrin) in series with basolateral H^+-ATPase.[251] In rodents, the most prevalent subtype of intercalated cells in the CNT is the non-A, non-B intercalated cell, which possesses an apical Cl^--HCO_3^- exchanger (SLC26A4 or pendrin) along with apical H^+-ATPase.[251] Although intercalated cells play a dominant role in acid-base homeostasis, Cl^- transport by type B intercalated cells performs an increasingly appreciated role in distal nephron Na^+-Cl^- transport (see "Connecting Tubules and the Cortical Collecting Duct: Cl^- Transport").

The outer medullary collecting duct (OMCD) encompasses two separate subsegments corresponding to the outer and inner stripes of the outer medulla, OMCDo and OMCDi, respectively. OMCDo and OMCDi contain principal cells with apical amiloride-sensitive Na^+ channels (ENaC); however, the primary role of this nephron segment is renal acidification, with a particular dominance of type A intercalated cells in OMCDi.[4,252] The OMCD also plays a critical role in K^+ reabsorption via the activity of apical H^+-K^+-ATPase pumps.[253-255]

Finally, the inner medullary collecting duct begins at the boundary between the outer and inner medulla and extends to the tip of the papilla. The IMCD is arbitrarily separated into three equal zones, denoted IMCD1, IMCD2, and IMCD3; at the functional level, an early IMCD (IMCDi) and a terminal portion (IMCDt) can be appreciated.[4] The IMCD plays a particularly prominent role in vasopressin-sensitive water and urea transport.[4] The early IMCD contains principal cells and intercalated cells; all three subsegments (IMCD1-3) express apical ENaC protein, albeit considerably weaker expression than in the CNT and CCD.[256] The roles of the IMCD and OMCD in Na^+-Cl^- homeostasis have been more elusive than that of the CNT and CCD; however, to the extent that ENaC is expressed in the IMCD and OMCD, homologous mechanisms are expected to function in Na^+-Cl^- reabsorption by the CNT, CCD, OMCD, and IMCD segments.

DISTAL CONVOLUTED TUBULE

Mechanisms of Na^+-Cl^- Transport in the Distal Convoluted Tubule

Earlier micropuncture studies that did not distinguish between early and late DCT indicated that this nephron segment reabsorbs about 10% of filtered Na^+-Cl^-.[257,258] The apical absorption of Na^+ and Cl^- by the DCT is mutually dependent; ion substitution does not affect transepithelial voltage, suggesting electroneutral transport.[259] The absorption of Na^+ by perfused DCT segments is also inhibited by chlorothiazide, localized proof that this nephron segment is the target for thiazide diuretics.[260] Similar thiazide-sensitive Na^+-Cl^- cotransport exists in the urinary bladder of winter flounder, the species in which the thiazide-sensitive Na^+-Cl^- cotransporter was first identified by expression cloning.[261] Functional characterization of rat NCC indicates very high affinities for both Na^+ and Cl^- (Michaelis-Menten constants of 7.6 ± 1.6 and 6.3 ± 1.1 mmol/L, respectively); equally high affinities had previously been obtained by Velazquez and associates in perfused rat DCT.[259,262] The measured Hill coefficients of rat NCC are about 1 for each ion, consistent with electroneutral cotransport.[262]

NCC expression is the defining characteristic of the DCT (Figure 6.19).[247] There is also evidence for expression of this transporter in osteoblasts, peripheral blood mononuclear cells, and intestinal epithelium; however, kidney is the primary expression site.[155,263] Loss-of-function mutations in the *SLC12A2* gene encoding human NCC cause Gitelman's syndrome, familial hypokalemic alkalosis with hypomagnesemia and hypocalciuria (see Chapter 45). Mice with homozygous deletion of the *Slc12a2* gene encoding NCC exhibit marked morphologic defects in the early DCT, with a reduction in the absolute number of DCT cells and changes in ultrastructural appearance.[264,265] Similarly, thiazide treatment promotes marked apoptosis of the DCT, suggesting that thiazide-sensitive Na^+-Cl^- cotransport plays an important role in modulating growth and regression of this nephron segment (see also "Regulation of Na^+-Cl^- Transport in the Distal Convoluted Tubule").[266]

Coexpression of NCC and ENaC occurs in the late DCT and CNT segments of many species, either in the same cells or in adjacent cells in the same tubule.[247] Notably, ENaC is the primary Na^+ transport pathway of CNT and CCD cells, rather than DCT. There is, however, evidence for other Na^+ and Cl^- entry pathways in DCT cells. In particular, the Na^+-H^+ exchanger NHE2 is coexpressed with NCC at the apical membrane of rat DCT cells.[267] As in the proximal tubule, perfusion of the DCT with formate and oxalate stimulates DIDS-sensitive Na^+-Cl^- transport that is distinct from the thiazide-sensitive transport mediated by NCC.[45] Therefore, a parallel arrangement of Na^+-H^+ exchange and Cl^- anion exchangers may play an important role in electroneutral Na^+-Cl^- absorption by the DCT (see Figure 6.19). Of note, the anion exchanger SLC26A6 is evidently expressed in the human distal nephron, including perhaps in DCT cells;

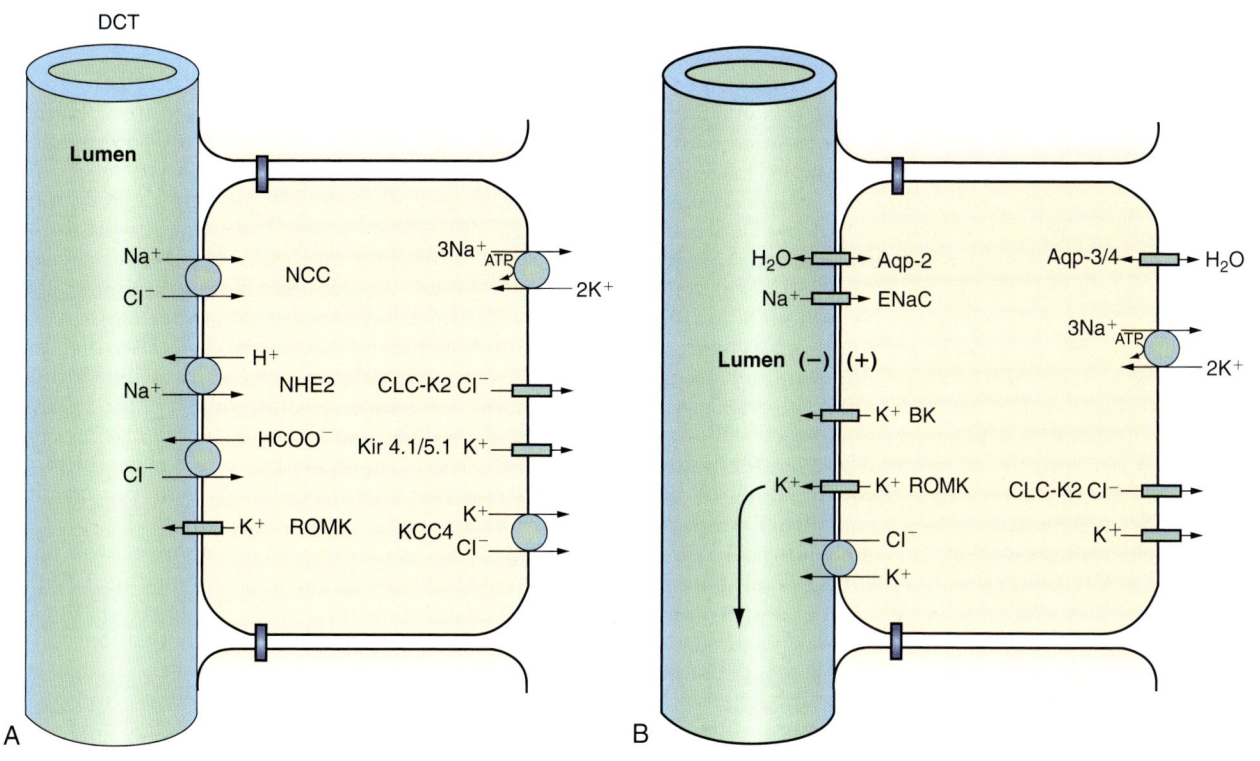

Figure 6.19 Transport pathways for Na$^+$-Cl$^-$and K$^+$ in DCT cells **(A)** and principal cells of the CNT and CCD **(B)**. Aqp-2, 3/4, Aquaporin-2, aquaporin-3/4. ENaC, Epithelial Na$^+$ channel; KCC4, K$^+$-Cl$^-$ cotransporter-4; NCC, thiazide-sensitive Na$^+$-Cl$^-$ cotransporter; NHE-2, Na$^+$-H$^+$ exchanger-2; ROMK, renal outer medullary K$^+$ channel.

NHE2 and SLC26A6 are thus candidate mechanisms for this alternative pathway of DCT Na$^+$-Cl$^-$ absorption.[267,268]

At the basolateral membrane, as in other nephron segments, Na$^+$ exits via Na$^+$-K$^+$-ATPase; bearing in mind the considerable caveats in morphologic identification of the DCT, this nephron segment appears to have the highest Na$^+$-K$^+$-ATPase activity of the entire nephron (see Figure 6.4).[15,247] Basolateral membranes of DCT cells in both rabbit and mouse express the K$^+$-Cl$^-$ cotransporter KCC4, a potential exit pathway for Cl$^-$.[197,269] However, several lines of evidence have indicated that Cl$^-$ primarily exits DCT cells via basolateral Cl$^-$ channels. First, the basolateral membrane of rabbit DCT contains Cl$^-$ channel activity, with functional characteristics similar to those of CLC-K2.[196,270] Second, CLC-K2 protein is expressed at the basolateral membrane of DCT and CNT cells; mRNA for CLC-K1 can also be detected by RT-PCR of microdissected DCT segments.[142,194] Third, loss-of-function mutations in CLC-NKB, the human ortholog of CLC-K2, typically cause Bartter's syndrome (dysfunction of the TAL); however, in some of these patients, mutations in CLC-NKB lead to more of a Gitelman's syndrome phenotype, consistent with loss of function of DCT segments.[144,271]

K$^+$ channels at the basolateral membrane of DCT cells play a critical role in the function of this nephron segment. Cell-attached patches in basolateral membranes of microdissected DCTs detect an inward rectifying K$^+$ channel, with characteristics similar to those of heteromeric KIR4.1/KIR5.1 and KIR4.2/KIR5.1 channels.[272] Basolateral membranes of the DCT express immunoreactive KIR4.1 and KIR5.1 protein, and DCT cells express KIR4.2 mRNA.[272-275]

Patients with loss-of-function mutations in the *KCNJ10* gene that encodes KIR4.1 develop a syndrome encompassing epilepsy, ataxia, sensorineural deafness, and tubulopathy (EAST or SeSAME syndrome).[274,276] The associated tubulopathy includes hypokalemia, metabolic alkalosis, hypocalciuria, and hypomagnesemia.[274,276] KIR4.1 knockout mice demonstrate a greater natriuresis than littermate controls, in addition to hypocalciuria; this can be attributed to reduced activation of NCC (see also below).[274,277] The KIR4.1/KIR5.1 and KIR4.2/KIR5.1 channels at the basolateral membrane of DCT cells are hypothesized to function in basolateral K$^+$ recycling, maintaining adequate Na$^+$-K$^+$-ATPase activity for Na$^+$-Cl$^-$ absorption and other aspects of DCT function. Notably, the calcium-sensing receptor co-associates with KIR4.1 and KIR4.2 proteins and inhibits their activity, providing a mechanism for the dynamic modulation of Na$^+$-Cl$^-$, calcium, and magnesium transport by the DCT.[273]

Regulation of Na$^+$-Cl$^-$ Transport in the Distal Convoluted Tubule

Considerable hypertrophy of the DCT occurs in response to chronic increases in delivery of Na$^+$-Cl$^-$ to the DCT, typically induced by furosemide treatment with dietary Na$^+$-Cl$^-$ supplementation.[247,257] These morphologic changes are reportedly independent of changes in aldosterone or glucocorticoid, suggesting that increased Na$^+$-Cl$^-$ entry via NCC promotes hypertrophy of the DCT; this is the inverse of the hypomorphic changes seen in NCC deficiency or thiazide treatment.[247,264,265] Notably, however, changes in aldosterone do have dramatic effects on the morphology of the DCT and expression of NCC.[247,278-280] The DCT is thus an aldosterone-sensitive epithelium, expressing both mineralocorticoid receptor and the 11β-hydroxysteroid dehydrogenase-2 (11β-HSD2) enzyme that confers specificity for aldosterone over glucocorticoids.[247] Mice with a targeted deletion of 11β-HSD2, with activation of the mineralocorticoid receptor by circulating glucocorticoid, exhibit massive hypertrophy of what appear to be DCT cells; this suggests an important role for mineralocorticoid activity in shaping this nephron segment.[278] Furthermore, NCC expression is dramatically increased by treatment of normal rats with fludrocortisone or aldosterone; adrenalectomized rats also show an increase in NCC expression after rescue with aldosterone, and treatment with spironolactone reduces expression of NCC in salt-restricted rats.[279,280]

Considerable insight into the role of NCC in the pathobiology of the DCT has emerged from the study of the WNK1 and WNK4 kinases.[281] WNK1 and WNK4 were initially identified as causative genes for familial hyperkalemic hypertension (FHHt; also known as pseudohypoaldosteronism type II or Gordon's syndrome). FHHt is in every respect the mirror image of Gitelman's syndrome, encompassing hypertension, hyperkalemia, hyperchloremic metabolic acidosis, suppressed PRA and aldosterone, and hypercalciuria.[282] Furthermore, FHHt behaves like a gain of function in NCC and/or the DCT in that treatment with thiazides typically results in resolution of the entire syndrome; however, simple transgenic overexpression of NCC in DCT cells does not replicate the phenotype in mice, indicating specific effects of the mutant WNK1 and WNK4 alleles.[282,283] Intronic mutations in WNK1 have been detected in patients with FHHt, leading to increased abundance of WNK1 mRNA in patient leukocytes; WNK4-associated FHHt is due to clustered point mutations in an acid-rich conserved region of the protein.[284] The WNK1 and WNK4 proteins are coexpressed within the distal nephron in DCT and CCD cells; whereas WNK1 localizes to the cytoplasm and basolateral membrane, WNK4 protein is found at the apical tight junctions.[284]

Consistent with the physiologic gain of function in NCC associated with FHHt,[282] WNK4 coexpression with NCC in *Xenopus* oocytes inhibits transport, and both kinase-dead and disease-associated mutations abolish the effect.[285,286] WNK1 was initially thought to have no effect on NCC, instead abrogating the inhibitory effect of WNK4.[287] However, more recent data using kidney-enriched splice forms of WNK1 have indicated that it activates NCC in a SPAK-dependent fashion in both a mouse model and heterologous expression systems.[288] WNK4 coexpression with NCC reduces transporter expression at the membrane of both *Xenopus* oocytes and mammalian cells, suggesting a prominent effect on membrane trafficking.[289,290] The WNK4 kinase activates lysosomal degradation of the transporter protein, rather than inducing dynamin- and clathrin-dependent endocytosis.[291,292] This occurs through effects of WNK4 on the interaction of NCC with the lysosomal targeting receptor sortilin and AP-3 adaptor complex.[291,292] Dynamin-dependent endocytosis of NCC is induced by ERK1/2 phosphorylation via activation of H-Ras, Raf, and MEK1/2, resulting in ubiquitination of NCC and endocytosis of the transporter; this plays a significant role in the downregulation of NCC by PTH.[293-295] Ubiquitination of NCC is catalyzed by the ubiquitin-ligase Nedd4-2, causing downregulation of NCC.[296]

To develop in vivo models relevant to FHHt and the physiologic role of WNK4 in the distal nephron, Lalioti and coworkers generated two strains of BAC-transgenic mice that overexpress wild-type WNK4 (TgWnk4^{WT}) or an FHHt mutant of WNK4 (TgWnk4^{PHAII}, bearing a Q562E mutation associated with the disease).[281] Consistent with the inhibitory effect of WNK4 on NCC, the blood pressure of TgWnk4^{WT} is lower than that of wild-type littermate controls; in contrast, TgWnk4^{PHAII} mice are hypertensive.[285,286] The biochemical phenotype of TgWnk4^{PHAII} is also similar to that of FHHt (i.e. hyperkalemia, acidosis, and hypercalciuria), with a suppressed expression of renal renin. TgWnk4^{PHAII} mice also exhibit marked hyperplasia of the DCT, compared to a relative hypoplasia in the TgWnk4^{WT} mice; the morphology and phenotype of the CCD were not particularly affected. Of particular significance, the DCT hyperplasia of TgWnk4^{PHAII} mice was completely suppressed on an NCC-deficient background, generated by mating TgWnk4^{PHAII} mice with NCC knockout mice.[264,265] Therefore, the DCT is the primary target for FHHt-associated mutations in WNK4. In addition, as suggested by prior studies, changes in Na$^+$-Cl$^-$ entry via NCC can evidently modulate hyperplasia or regression of the DCT.[247,264,265,281] Vidal-Petiot and colleagues have also generated mice that lack the orthologous intron of WNK1 involved in patients with FHHt, recapitulating the phenotype.[297] Treatment with the calcineurin inhibitor tacrolimus has a similar effect as in FHHt.[298]

Under certain conditions, a stimulatory effect of the WNK kinases appears to dominate. The WNK kinases appear to exert their effect on NCC and other cation-chloride cotransporters via the phosphorylation and activation of the SPAK and OSR1 serine-threonine kinases, which in turn phosphorylate the transporter proteins.[211,299,300] Specifically, in NCC, WNK-dependent phosphorylation and activation of SPAK or OSR1 leads to phosphorylation of a cluster of N-terminal threonines, resulting in the activation of Na$^+$-Cl$^-$ cotransport.[289,301]

A further level of complexity arises from the finding that most cases of FHHt are caused by mutations in cullin 3 (CUL3) or Kelch-like 3 (KLHL3), components of an E3 ubiquitin ligase complex that targets the WNKs for degradation.[302-304] Genetically, disease-associated mutations in KLHL3 abrogate binding to WNK4 and vice versa.[304] In turn, disease-associated mutations in CUL3 deplete levels of KLHL3, preventing WNK degradation.[305] Physiologically, phosphorylation of KLHL3 by protein kinase C, downstream of Ang II, also abrogates the interaction between KLHL3 and WNK4, leading to NCC activation.[306]

The various mechanistic models for the regulation of NCC by upstream WNK1, WNK4, and the SPAK-OSR1 kinases have recently been reviewed; interactions between WNK4 and both WNK3 and SGK1 also contribute to the complexity, as do CUL3 and KLH3.[289,302-304,306-309] Competing divergent mechanisms can be reconciled by the likelihood that the physiologic context determines whether WNK4 will have an activating or inhibitory effect on NCC. For example, the activation of NCC by the Ang II receptor type 1 (AT$_1$R) appears to require the downstream activation of SPAK by WNK4.[290,310] Changes in circulating and local levels of Ang II, aldosterone, vasopressin, and K$^+$ are thus expected to

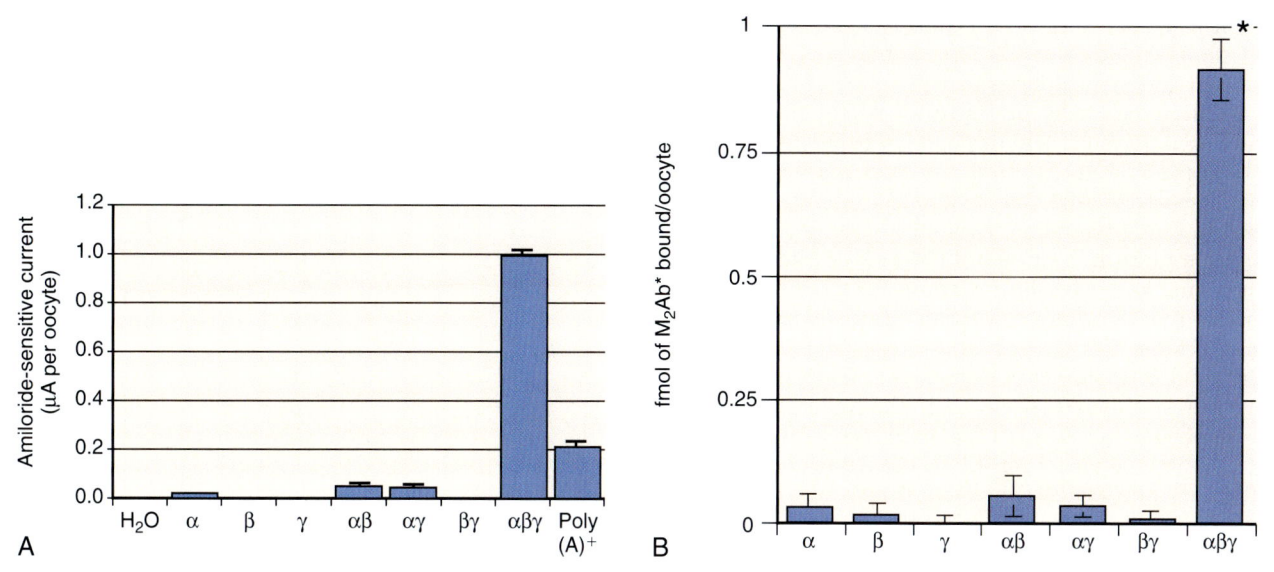

Figure 6.20 Maximal expression of the amiloride-sensitive epithelial Na$^+$ channel (ENaC) at the plasma membrane requires the coexpression of all three subunits (α-, β-, and γ-ENaC). **A,** Amiloride-sensitive current in *Xenopus* oocytes expressing the individual subunits and various combinations thereof. **B,** Surface expression is markedly enhanced in *Xenopus* oocytes that coexpress all three subunits. The individual cDNAs were engineered with an external epitope tag; expression of the channel proteins at the cell surface is measured by binding of a monoclonal antibody (M$_2$Ab*) to the tag. Poly A$^+$, Polyadenylated mRNA. (**A** from Canessa CM, Schild L, Buell G, et al: Amiloride-sensitive epithelial Na$^+$ channel is made of three homologous subunits. *Nature* 367:463-467, 1994; **B** from Firsov, D, Schild L, Gautschi I, et al: Cell surface expression of the epithelial Na channel and a mutant causing Liddle syndrome: a quantitative approach. *Proc Natl Acad Sci U S A* 93:15370-15375, 1996.)

have different and often opposing effects on the activity of NCC in the DCT (see also Figure 6.26 and "Integrated Na$^+$-Cl$^-$ and K$^+$ Transport in the Distal Nephron").[289,290,310-314]

Changes in intracellular chloride in particular play a key role in modulating the effect of the SPAK-OSR1 and WNK kinase pathway on NCC. A reduction in intracellular chloride thus activates the WNK isoforms.[315,316] For WNK1, chloride binds to the catalytic site of the kinase and inhibits autophosphorylation and activation of the kinase.[315] This chloride sensing has a major role in the potassium-sensing function of DCT cells. Reduction in potassium intake and/or hypokalemia lead to reduced basolateral K$^+$ concentration in the DCT; the subsequent hyperpolarization is dependent on basolateral KIR4.1-containing K$^+$ channels.[317] Hyperpolarization leads to chloride exit via basolateral CLC-NKB chloride channels and a reduction in intracellular chloride; the reduction in intracellular chloride activates the SPAK and OSR1-WNK cascade, resulting in phosphorylation of NCC and activation of the transporter.[317] These findings help explain the activating effect of potassium depletion on NCC and the inhibitory effect of potassium loading on NCC, and they go a long way to explain the critical role of the DCT and NCC in potassium homeostasis.[317]

CONNECTING TUBULES AND THE CORTICAL COLLECTING DUCT

Apical Na$^+$ Transport

The apical membrane of CNT cells and principal cells contain prominent Na$^+$ and K$^+$ conductances, without a measurable apical conductance for Cl$^-$.[196,250,318,319] The entry of Na$^+$ occurs via the highly selective epithelial Na$^+$ channel (ENaC), which is sensitive to micromolar concentrations of amiloride (see Figure 6.19).[320] This selective absorption of positive charge generates a lumen-negative PD, the magnitude of which varies considerably as a function of mineralocorticoid status and other factors (see also "Regulation of Na$^+$-Cl$^-$ Transport in the Connecting Tubule and Cortical Collecting Duct"). This lumen-negative PD serves to drive the following critical processes: (1) K$^+$ secretion via apical K$^+$ channels; (2) paracellular Cl$^-$ transport through the adjacent tight junctions; and/or (3) electrogenic H$^+$ secretion via adjacent type A intercalated cells.[321]

ENaC is a heteromeric channel complex formed by the assembly of separate, homologous subunits, denoted α-, β-, and γ-ENaC.[12] These channel subunits share a common structure, with intracellular N- and C-terminal domains, two transmembrane segments, and a large glycosylated extracellular loop.[12] *Xenopus* oocytes expressing α-ENaC alone have detectable Na$^+$ channel activity (Figure 6.20), which facilitated the initial identification of this subunit by expression cloning; functional complementation of this modest activity was then used to clone the other two subunits by expression cloning.[12] Full channel activity requires the coexpression of all three subunits, which causes a dramatic increase in expression of the channel complex at the plasma membrane (see Figure 6.20).[322] The subunit stoichiometry has been a source of considerable controversy, with some reports favoring a tetramer with ratios of two α-ENaC proteins to one each of β-, and γ-ENaC (2α:1β:1γ) and others favoring a higher order assembly with a stoichiometry of 3α:3β:3γ.[323] Regardless, the single-channel characteristics of heterologously expressed ENaC are essentially identical to those of the amiloride-sensitive channel detectable at the apical membrane of CCD cells.[12,320]

ENaC plays a critical role in renal Na$^+$-Cl$^-$ reabsorption and maintenance of the extracellular fluid volume (see also "Regulation of Na$^+$-Cl$^-$ Transport in the Connecting Tubule and Cortical Collecting Duct"). In particular, recessive loss-of-function mutations in the three subunits of ENaC are a cause of pseudohypoaldosteronism type I.[12,324] Patients with this syndrome typically present with severe neonatal salt wasting, hypotension, acidosis, and hyperkalemia; this dramatic phenotype underscores the critical roles of ENaC activity in renal Na^+-Cl^- reabsorption, K^+ secretion, and H^+ secretion. Gain-of-function mutations in the β- and γ-ENaC subunits are in turn a cause of Liddle's syndrome, an autosomal dominant hypertensive syndrome accompanied by suppressed aldosterone and variable hypokalemia.[325] With one exception, ENaC mutations associated with Liddle's syndrome disrupt interactions between a PPxY motif in the C-terminus of channel subunits with the Nedd4-2 ubiquitin-ligase leading to increased surface expression of the channel (see also "Regulation of Na^+-Cl^- Transport in the Connecting Tubule and Cortical Collecting Duct").[326]

The ENaC protein is detectable at the apical membrane of CNT cells and principal cells in the CCD, OMCD, and IMCD.[252,256] Notably, however, several lines of evidence have supported the hypothesis that the CNT makes the dominant contribution to amiloride-sensitive Na^+ reabsorption by the distal nephron:

1. Amiloride-sensitive Na^+ currents in the CNT are two- to fourfold higher than in the CCD; the maximal capacity of the CNT for Na^+ reabsorption is estimated to be about 10 times higher than that of the CCD.[250]
2. Targeted deletion of α-ENaC in the collecting duct abolishes amiloride-sensitive currents in CCD principal cells, but does not affect Na^+ or K^+ homeostasis; the residual ENaC expression in the late DCT and CNT of these knockout mice easily compensates for the loss of the channel in CCD cells.[327]
3. Na^+-K^+-ATPase activity in the CCD is considerably less than that of the DCT (see also Figure 6.4); this speaks to a greater capability for transepithelial Na^+-Cl^- absorption by the DCT and CNT.[15]
4. The apical recruitment of ENaC subunits in response to dietary Na^+ restriction begins in the CNT, with progressive recruitment of subunits in the downstream CCD at lower levels of dietary Na^+; although the CNT plays a dominant role in ENaC-mediated sodium transport, it does so primarily in an aldosterone-independent mechanism, with aldosterone-mediated sodium transport in the CCD involved in the finely tuned regulation of sodium transport.[328,329]

Cl^- Transport

There are two major pathways for Cl^- absorption in the CNT and CCD—paracellular transport across the tight junction and transcellular transport across type B intercalated cells (Figure 6.21).[251,330] The CNT and CCD are "tight" epithelia, with comparatively low paracellular permeability that is not selective for Cl^- over Na^+; however, voltage-driven, paracellular Cl^- transport in the CCD may play a considerable role in transepithelial Na^+-Cl^- absorption.[331] The CNT, DCT, and collecting duct coexpress claudin-3, -4, and -8; claudin-8 in particular may function as a paracellular cation barrier that prevents backleak of Na^+, K^+, and H^+ in this segment of the nephron.[12,332] Several lines of evidence have indicated that claudin-4 and claudin-8 interact to form a paracellular

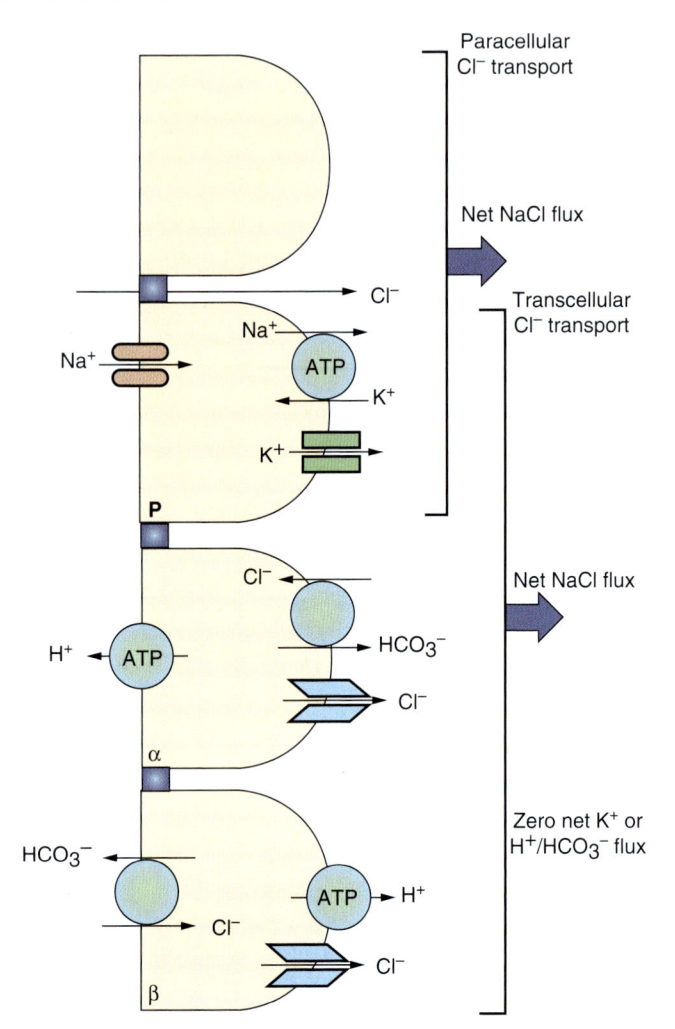

Figure 6.21 Transepithelial Cl^- transport by principal and intercalated cells. The lumen-negative PD generated by principal cells drives paracellular Cl^- absorption. Alternatively, transepithelial transport occurs in type B intercalated cells via apical Cl^--HCO_3^- exchange (SLC26A4/pendrin) and basolateral Cl^- exit via CLC-K2. (Modified from Moe OW, Baum M, Berry CA, Rector FC, Jr: Renal transport of glucose, amino acids, sodium, chloride, and water. In Brenner BM, editor: *Brenner and Rector's the kidney*, Philadelphia, 2004, WB Saunders, pp 413-452.)

pathway for Cl^- in the collecting duct, thus mediating transcellular Cl^- absorption via the paracellular pathway.[333] Moreover, CCD-specific knockout of claudin-4 in mice leads to NaCl wasting, hypotension, and hyperkalemia.[334] Regulated changes in paracellular permeability may also contribute to Cl^- absorption by the CNT and CCD. In particular, wild-type WNK4 appears to increase paracellular Cl^- permeability in transfected MDCK II cell lines; a WNK4 FHHt mutant has a much larger effect, with no effect seen in cells expressing kinase-dead WNK4 constructs.[335] Yamauchi and colleagues have also reported that FHHt-associated WNK4 increases paracellular permeability, due perhaps to an associated hyperphosphorylation of claudin proteins.[336] The claudin-4–mediated chloride conductance is also negatively regulated by cleavage in its second extracellular loop by channel-activating protease 1 (cap1).[334]

Transcellular Cl^- absorption across intercalated cells is thought to play a quantitatively greater role in the CNT and CCD than that of paracellular transport.[330] In the simplest scheme, this process requires the concerted function of type A and type B intercalated cells, achieving net electrogenic Cl^- absorption without affecting HCO_3^- or H^+ excretion[330] (see also Figure 6.21). Chloride thus enters type B intercalated cells via apical Cl^--HCO_3^- exchange, followed by exit from the cell via basolateral Cl^- channels. Recycling of Cl^- at the basolateral membrane of adjacent type A intercalated cells also results in HCO_3^- absorption and extrusion of H^+ at the apical membrane. The net effect of apical Cl^--HCO_3^- exchange in type B intercalated cells, leading to apical secretion of HCO_3^-, and recycling of Cl^- at the basolateral membrane type A intercalated cells, leading to apical secretion of H^+, is electrogenic Cl^- absorption across type B intercalated cells (see Figure 6.21).

At the basolateral membrane, intercalated cells have a very robust Cl^- conductance, with transport characteristics similar to those of CLC-K2/Barttin.[196] CLC-K2 protein is also detected at the basolateral membrane of type A intercalated cells, although expression in type B cells has not been clarified.[194] The basolateral Na^+-K^+-$2Cl^-$ cotransporter NKCC1 in adjacent type A intercalated cells also plays an evident role in transepithelial Cl^- absorption by the CCD.[337] At the apical membrane, the SLC26A4 exchanger (also known as pendrin) has been conclusively identified as the elusive Cl^--HCO_3^- exchanger of type B and non-A, non-B intercalated cells; this exchanger functions as the apical entry site during transepithelial Cl^- transport by the distal nephron.[251] Human SLC26A4 is mutated in Pendred's syndrome, which encompasses sensorineural hearing loss and goiter; these patients do not have an appreciable renal phenotype.[251] However, Slc26a4-deficient knockout mice are sensitive to restriction of dietary Na^+-Cl^-, developing hypotension during severe restriction.[338] Slc26a4 knockout mice are also resistant to mineralocorticoid-induced hypertension.[339] Pendrin has indirect effects on ENaC abundance and activity, apparently by modulating luminal ATP and HCO_3^- concentrations; pendrin and ENaC are also both coactivated by Ang II.[340-343] The overexpression of pendrin in intercalated cells thus causes hypertension in transgenic mice, with an increase in ENaC activity and activity of electroneutral Na^+-Cl^- absorption (see below).[344] Finally, dietary Cl^- restriction with provision of Na^+-HCO_3^- results in Cl^- wasting in Slc26a4 knockout mice and increased apical expression of Slc26a4 protein in the type B intercalated cells of normal littermate controls.[345] Several groups have reported that Slc26a4 expression is exquisitely responsive to changes in distal chloride delivery.[346] Therefore, Slc26a4 plays a critical role in distal nephron Cl^- absorption, underlining the particular importance of transcellular Cl^- transport in this process. Of broader relevance, these studies have served to underline the important role for Cl^- homeostasis in the maintenance of extracellular volume and pathogenesis of hypertension.[346]

Electroneutral Na^+-Cl^- Cotransport

Thiazide-sensitive Na^+-Cl^- cotransport is considered the exclusive provenance of the DCT, which expresses the canonical thiazide-sensitive transporter NCC (see earlier, "Mechanisms of Na^+-Cl^- Transport in the Distal Convoluted Tubule"). However, Tomita and coworkers demonstrated many years ago that approximately 50% of Na^+-Cl^- transport in rat CCD is electroneutral, amiloride-resistant, and thiazide-sensitive.[347,348] Thiazide-sensitive electroneutral Na^+-Cl^- transport has also been demonstrated in mouse CCD.[349] This transport activity is preserved in CCDs from mice with genetic disruption of NCC and ENaC, indicating independence from the dominant apical Na^+ transport pathways in the distal nephron. This thiazide-sensitive, electroneutral Na^+-Cl^- transport appears to be mediated by the parallel activity of the Na^+-driven SLC4A8 Cl^--HCO_3^- exchanger and SLC26A4 Cl^--HCO_3^- exchanger (pendrin; see above).[349] In particular, amiloride-resistant Na^+-Cl^- absorption is abolished in CCDs from Slc4a8 null knockout mice. Notably, however, heterologously expressed recombinant Slc4a8 and Slc26a4 are resistant and partially sensitive to thiazide, respectively, such that the in vivo pharmacology of this electroneutral Na^+-Cl^- absorption is not completely explained. Furthermore, immunolocalization of Slc4a8 within the CCD has been problematic; hence, it is unknown whether Slc4a8 and Slc26a4 are coexpressed in type B intercalated cells. Regardless, the combined activity of Slc4a8 and Slc26a4 appears to play a major role in Na^+-Cl^- transport within the CCD, with significant implications for Na^+-Cl^- and K^+ homeostasis (see also "Integrated Na^+-Cl^- and K^+ Transport in the Distal Nephron").

The apical entry of Na^+ via SLC4A8 requires a basolateral exit of Na^+ in type B intercalated cells, evidently mediated by the basolateral Na^+-HCO_3^- transporter SLC4A9.[2] Another puzzle was the energetics of transcellular Na^+-Cl^- transport in intercalated cells, which possess minimal, if any, detectable Na^+-K^+-ATPase activity. A series of elegant experiments has revealed that electroneutral Na^+-Cl^- transport in type B intercalated cells is energized by and thus dependent on the activity of the basolateral H^+-ATPase.[2] Type B intercalated cells are therefore unique among mammalian renal epithelial cells in that transcellular ion transport is driven by H^+-ATPase rather than Na^+-K^+-ATPase activity.

REGULATION OF Na^+-Cl^- TRANSPORT IN THE CONNECTING TUBULE AND CORTICAL COLLECTING DUCT

Aldosterone

The DCT, CNT, and collecting ducts collectively constitute the aldosterone-sensitive distal nephron, expressing the mineralocorticoid receptor and 11β-hydroxysteroid dehydrogenase-2 (11β-HSD2) enzyme that protects against illicit activation by glucocorticoids.[247] Aldosterone plays a dominant positive role in the regulation of distal nephron Na^+-Cl^- transport, with a plethora of mechanisms and transcriptional targets.[350] For example, aldosterone increases the expression of the $Na+$-$K+$-ATPase $α_1$- and $β_1$-subunits in the CCD, in addition to inducing Slc26a4, the apical Cl^--HCO_3^- exchanger of intercalated cells.[339,351] Aldosterone may also affect paracellular permeability of the distal nephron via posttranscriptional modification of claudins and other components of the tight junction.[352] However, particularly impressive progress has been made in the understanding of the downstream effects of aldosterone on synthesis, trafficking, and membrane-associated activity of ENaC subunits. A detailed discussion of aldosterone's actions may be found in Chapter 12; here we summarize the major findings of relevance to Na$^+$-Cl$^-$ transport.

Aldosterone increases abundance of α-ENaC via a glucocorticoid response element in the promoter of the *SCNN1A* gene that encodes this subunit.[353] Aldosterone also relieves a tonic inhibition of the *SCNN1A* gene by a complex that includes the Dot1a (disruptor of telomere silencing splicing variant *a*) and AF9 and AF17 transcription factors.[354] An aldosterone-dependent reduction in promoter methylation is also involved.[355] This transcriptional activation results in an increased abundance of α-ENaC protein in response to exogenous aldosterone or dietary Na$^+$-Cl$^-$ restriction (Figure 6.22); the response to Na$^+$-Cl$^-$ restriction is blunted by spironolactone, indicating involvement of the mineralocorticoid receptor.[280,356,357] At baseline, α-ENaC transcripts in the kidney are less abundant than those encoding β- and γ-ENaC[358] (see Figure 6.22). All three subunits are required for efficient processing of heteromeric channels in the endoplasmic reticulum and trafficking to the plasma membrane (see Figure 6.20), such that the induction of α-ENaC is thought to relieve a major bottleneck in the processing and trafficking of active ENaC complexes.[358]

Aldosterone also plays an indirect role in the regulated trafficking of ENaC subunits to the plasma membrane via the regulation of accessory proteins that interact with preexisting ENaC subunits. Aldosterone rapidly induces expression of a serine-threonine kinase denoted SGK-1 (serum and glucocorticoid-induced kinase-1); coexpression of SGK-1 with ENaC subunits in *Xenopus* oocytes results in a dramatic activation of the channel due to increased expression at the plasma membrane.[357,359,360] Notably, an analogous redistribution of ENaC subunits occurs in the CNT and early CCD, from a largely cytoplasmic location during dietary Na$^+$-Cl$^-$ excess to a purely apical distribution after aldosterone or Na$^+$-Cl$^-$ restriction (see Figure 6.22).[280,328,357] Furthermore, there is a temporal correlation between the appearance of induced SGK-1 protein in the CNT and the redistribution of ENaC protein to the plasma membrane.[357]

SGK-1 modulates membrane expression of ENaC by interfering with regulated endocytosis of its channel subunits. Specifically, the kinase interferes with interactions between ENaC subunits and the ubiquitin ligase Nedd4-2.[358] PPxY domains in the C-termini of all three ENaC subunits bind to WW domains of Nedd4-2[361]; these PPxY domains are deleted, truncated, or mutated in patients with Liddle's syndrome, leading to a gain of function in channel activity.[322,325] Coexpression of Nedd4-2 with the wild-type ENaC channel results in a marked inhibition of channel activity due to retrieval from the cell membrane, whereas channels bearing Liddle's syndrome mutations are resistant; Nedd4-2 is thought to ubiquitinate ENaC subunits, resulting in the removal of channel subunits from the cell membrane and degradation in lysosomes and the proteosome.[358] A PPxY domain in SGK-1 also binds to Nedd4-2, which is a phosphorylation substrate for the kinase; phosphorylation of

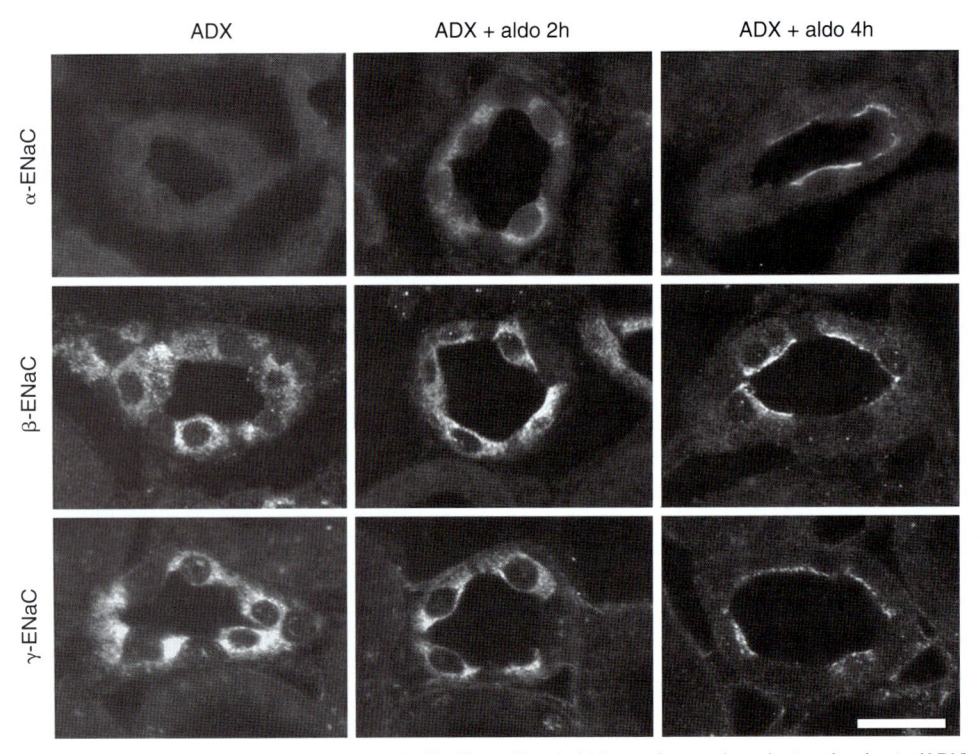

Figure 6.22 Immunofluorescence images of connecting tubule (CNT) profiles in kidneys from adrenalectomized rats (ADX) and from ADX rats 2 and 4 h after aldosterone (aldo) injection. Antibodies against the α-, β-, and γ-subunits of ENaC reveal absent expression of the former in ADX rats, with progressive induction by aldosterone. All three subunits traffic to the apical membrane in response to aldosterone. This coincides with rapid aldosterone induction of the SGK kinase in the same cells; SGK is known to increase the expression of ENaC at the plasma membrane (see text for details). Bar ≅ 15 μm. (From Loffing J, Zecevic M, Féraille E, et al: Aldosterone induces rapid apical translocation of ENaC in early portion of renal collecting system: possible role of SGK. *Am J Physiol Renal Physiol* 280:F675-F682, 2001.)

Nedd4-2 by SGK-1 abrogates its inhibitory effect on ENaC subunits.[362,363] Aldosterone also stimulates Nedd4-2 phosphorylation in vivo.[364] Nedd4-2 phosphorylation in turn results in ubiquitin-mediated degradation of SGK-1, suggesting that there is considerable feedback regulation in this system.[365] Aldosterone also reduces Nedd4-2 protein expression in cultured CCD cells, suggesting additional levels of in vivo regulation.[366]

The induction of SGK-1 by aldosterone thus appears to stimulate the redistribution of ENaC subunits from the cytoplasm to the apical membrane of CNT and CCD cells. This phenomenon involves SGK-1–dependent phosphorylation of the Nedd4-2 ubiquitin ligase, which is coexpressed with ENaC and SGK-1 in the distal nephron.[366] Of note, there is considerable axial heterogeneity in the recruitment and redistribution of ENaC to the plasma membrane, which begins in the CNT and only extends into the CCD and OMCD in Na^+-Cl^-–restricted or aldosterone-treated animals.[247,357] The underlying causes of this progressive axial recruitment are not as yet clear.[247] However, Nedd4-2 expression is inversely related to the apical distribution of ENaC, with low expression in the CNT and increased expression levels in the CCD. In all likelihood, the relative balance among SGK-1, ENaC, and Nedd4-2 figures prominently in the recruitment of the channel subunits to the apical membrane.[366]

Nedd4-2 and ENaC are part of a larger regulatory complex that includes the signaling protein Raf-1, stimulatory aldosterone-induced chaperone GILZ1 (glucocorticoid-induced leucine zipper-1), and scaffolding protein CNK3.[367,368] The mTORC2 (mammalian target of rapamycin complex 2) kinase complex is another component, catalyzing upstream activation of SGK1 and thus inducing activation of ENaC.[369,370]

Finally, aldosterone indirectly activates ENaC channels through the induction of channel-activating proteases, which increase open channel probability by cleavage of the extracellular domains of α- and γ-ENaC. Western blotting of renal tissue from rats subjected to Na^+-Cl^- restriction or treatment with aldosterone has revealed α- and γ-ENaC subunits of lower molecular mass than those detected in control animals, indicating that aldosterone induces proteolytic cleavage.[356,371] Proteases that have been implicated in the processing of ENaC include furin, elastase, and three membrane-associated proteases denoted CAP1-3 (channel activating proteases-1, -2, and -3).[372-374] Filtered proteases such as plasmin may also contribute to ENaC activation in nephrotic syndrome.[374] CAP1 was initially identified from *Xenopus* A6 cells as an ENaC-activating protease; the mammalian ortholog is an aldosterone-induced protein in principal cells.[375,376] Urinary excretion of CAP1, also known as prostasin, is increased in hyperaldosteronism, with a reduction after adrenalectomy.[376] CAP1 is tethered to the plasma membrane by a GPI linkage, whereas CAP2 and CAP3 are transmembrane proteases.[373,375] All three of these proteases activate ENaC by increasing the P_o of the channel, without increasing expression at the cell surface.[373] Proteolytic cleavage of ENaC appears to activate the channel by removing the self-inhibitory effect of external Na^+; in the case of furin-mediated proteolysis of α-ENaC, this appears to involve the removal of an inhibitory domain from within the extracellular loop.[372,377] Extracellular Na^+ appears to interact with a specific acidic cleft in the extracellular loop of α-ENaC, causing inhibition of the channel.[378] The structures of the extracellular domains of ENaC and related channels resemble an outstretched hand holding a ball, with defined subdomains termed the *wrist, finger, thumb, palm, β-ball,* and *knuckle*; functionally relevant proteolytic events target the finger domains of ENaC subunits.[374] Unprocessed channels at the plasma membrane are thought to function as a reserve pool, capable of rapid activation by membrane-associated luminal proteases.[372]

Vasopressin and Other Factors

Although not typically considered an antinatriuretic hormone, vasopressin has well-characterized stimulatory effects on Na^+-Cl^- transport by the CCD.[84,379] Vasopressin directly activates ENaC in murine CCD, increasing the open probability (P_o) of the channel.[380] In perfused rat CCD segments, vasopressin and aldosterone can have synergistic effects on Na^+ transport, with a combined effect that exceeds that of the individual hormones.[379] In addition, water and Na^+-restriction synergistically increase the P_o of ENaC in murine CCDs.[380] Prostaglandins inhibit this effect of vasopressin, particularly in the rabbit CCD; this inhibition occurs at least in part through reductions in vasopressin-generated cAMP.[84,379] There are, however, considerable species-dependent differences in the interactions between vasopressin and negative modulators of Na^+-Cl^- transport in the CCD, which include prostaglandins, bradykinin, endothelin, and α_2-adrenergic tone.[84,379] Regardless, cAMP causes a rapid increase in the Na^+ conductance of apical membranes in the CCD; this effect appears to be due to increases in the surface expression of ENaC subunits at the plasma membrane[381] in addition to effects on open channel probability.[380,382] Notably, cAMP inhibits retrieval of ENaC subunits from the plasma membrane via PKA-dependent phosphorylation of the phosphoacceptor sites in Nedd4-2 that are targeted by SGK-1; therefore, both aldosterone and vasopressin converge on Nedd4-2 in the regulation of ENaC activity in the distal nephron.[383] Analogous to the effect on trafficking of aquaporin-2 in principal cells, cAMP also seems to stimulate exocytosis of ENaC subunits to the plasma membrane.[382] Finally, similar to the long-term effects of vasopressin on aquaporin-2 expression and NKCC2 expression, chronic treatment with DDAVP results in an increase in abundance of the β- and γ-ENaC subunits.[209,384]

The activation of ENaC by vasopressin appears to have additional direct effects on water homeostasis. Hypernatremic mice treated with the ENaC inhibitor benzamil thus exhibit further increases in tonicity due to a reduction in urinary osmolality.[385] In adrenalectomized mice, which lack circulating aldosterone, vasopressin maintains ENaC activity in the distal nephron.[386] This vasopressin-dependent activation of ENaC may, by extension, play a role in generating hyponatremia in the setting of primary adrenal failure. Systemic generation of circulating Ang II induces aldosterone release by the adrenal gland, with downstream activation of ENaC. However, Ang II also directly activates amiloride-sensitive Na^+ transport in perfused CCDs; blockade by losartan or candesartan suggests that this activation is mediated by AT_1Rs.[387] Of particular significance, the effect of luminal Ang II (10^{-9}) was greater than that of bath Ang II, suggesting that intratubular Ang II may regulate ENaC in the distal nephron. Ang II also activates chloride absorption across intercalated cells via a pendrin (SLC26A4) and an H+-ATPase-dependent mechanism.[388] Stimulation of ENaC is seen when tubules are perfused with Ang I; this effect is blocked by angiotensin-converting enzyme (ACE) inhibition with captopril, suggesting that intraluminal conversion of Ang I to Ang II can occur in the CCD.[389] Notably, CNT cells express considerable amounts of immunoreactive renin versus the vanishingly low expression of renin mRNA in the proximal tubule.[390] Angiotensinogen secreted into the tubule by proximal tubule cells may thus be converted to Ang II in the CNT via locally generated renin and ACE and/or related proteases.[390]

Luminal perfusion with ATP or uridine triphosphate (UTP) inhibits amiloride-sensitive Na+ transport and reduces ENaC P_o in the CCD via activation of luminal P2Y$_2$ purinergic receptors.[391,392] Targeted deletion of the murine P2Y$_2$ receptor results in salt-resistant hypertension due in part to an upregulation of NKCC2 activity in the TAL; resting ENaC activity is also increased, but suppressed aldosterone and downregulation of the α-subunit of ENaC blunts the role of amiloride-sensitive transport.[392,393] Clamping mineralocorticoid activity at higher levels, via the administration of exogenous mineralocorticoid, reveals that P2Y$_2$ receptor activation may be a major mechanism for the modulation of ENaC P_o in response to changes in dietary Na+-Cl−.[394] Increased dietary Na+-Cl− thus leads to increased urinary ATP and UTP excretion in mice[392]; endogenous ATP from principal cells inhibits ENaC, and ENaC activity is not responsive to increased dietary Na+-Cl− in P2Y$_2$ receptor knockout mice.[392,394] In addition, the activation of apical ionotropic purinergic receptors, likely P2X$_4$ and/or P2X$_4$/P2X$_6$, can inhibit or activate ENaC, depending on luminal Na+ concentration; these receptors may also participate in fine-tuning ENaC activity in response to dietary Na+-Cl−.[395]

As in other segments of the nephron, Na+-Cl− transport by the CNT and CCD is modulated by metabolites of arachidonic acid generated by cytochrome P450 monooxygenases. In particular, arachidonic acid inhibits ENaC channel activity in the rat CCD via generation of the epoxygenase product 11,12-EET (epoxyeicosatrienoic acid) by the CYP2C23 enzyme expressed in principal cells.[396] Targeted deletion of the murine Cyp4a10 enzyme, another P450 monooxygenase, results in salt-sensitive hypertension; urinary excretion of 11,12-EET is reduced in these knockout mice, with a blunted effect of arachidonic acid on ENaC channel activity in the CCD.[397] These mice also became normotensive after treatment with amiloride, indicative of in vivo activation of ENaC. It appears that deletion of Cyp4a10 reduces activity of the murine ortholog of rat CYPC23 (Cyp2c44 in mouse) and/or related expoxygenases via reduced generation of a ligand for PPARα (peroxisome proliferator–activated receptor α) that induces epoxygenase activity.[397] The mechanism(s) whereby 11,12-EET inhibits ENaC are unknown as yet. However, renal 11,12-EET production is known to be salt-sensitive, suggesting that generation of this mediator may serve to reduce ENaC activity during high dietary Na+-Cl− intake.[396]

Finally, activation of PPARγ by thiazolidinediones results in amiloride-sensitive hypertension, suggesting in vivo activation of ENaC.[398,399] Thiazolidinediones (TZDs; e.g., rosiglitazone, pioglitazone, troglitazone) are insulin-sensitizing drugs used for the treatment of type II diabetes. Treatment with these agents is frequently associated with fluid retention, suggesting an effect on renal Na+-Cl− transport. Given robust expression of PPARγ in the collecting duct, activation of ENaC was an attractive hypothesis for this TZD-associated edema syndrome.[398,399] This appears to be the case, in that selective deletion of the murine PPARγ gene in principal cells abrogates the increase in amiloride-sensitive transport seen in response to TZDs.[398,399] TZDs appear to induce transcription of the *Sccn1g* gene encoding γ-ENaC in addition to inducing SGK-1; targeted deletion of SGK1 in knockout mice attenuates but does not abolish TZD-associated edema.[398,400,401] Notably, however, other studies have failed to detect an effect of TZDs on ENaC activity, which may instead activate a nonspecific cation channel within the IMCD.[402,403] Regardless, the beneficial effect of spironolactone in type II diabetics with TZD-associated volume expansion is consistent with in vivo activation of Na+-Cl− absorption in the aldosterone-responsive distal nephron.[404] In addition, the risk of peripheral edema is increased considerably in patients treated with both TZDs and insulin therapy. Notably, insulin appears to activate ENaC via SGK1-dependent mechanisms; PPARγ is required for the full activating effect of insulin on ENaC, such that this clinical observation may reflect synergistic activation of ENaC by insulin and TZDs.[402,405,406]

POTASSIUM TRANSPORT

Maintenance of K+ balance is important for a multitude of physiologic processes. Changes in intracellular K+ affect cell volume regulation, regulation of intracellular pH, enzymatic function, protein synthesis, DNA synthesis, and apoptosis.[12] Changes in the ratio of intracellular to extracellular K+ affect the resting membrane potential, leading to depolarization in hyperkalemia and hyperpolarization in hypokalemia. Thus, disorders of extracellular K+ have a dominant effect on excitable tissues, chiefly heart and muscle. In addition, a growing body of evidence has implicated hypokalemia and/or reduced dietary K+ in the pathobiology of hypertension, heart failure, and stroke; these and other clinical consequences of K+ disorders are reviewed in Chapter 18.

Potassium is predominantly an intracellular cation, with only 2% of total body K+ residing in the extracellular fluid. Extracellular K+ is maintained within a very narrow range by three primary mechanisms. First, the distribution of K+ between the intracellular and extracellular space is determined by the activity of a number of transport pathways—namely, Na+-K+-ATPase, the Na+-K+-2Cl− cotransporter NKCC1, the four K+-Cl− cotransporters, and a plethora of K+ channels. In particular, skeletal muscle contains as much as 75% of body potassium (see Figure 18.1) and exerts considerable influence on extracellular K+. Short-term and long-term regulation of muscle Na+-K+-ATPase play a dominant role in determining the distribution of K+ between the intracellular and extracellular spaces; the various hormones and physiologic conditions that affect the uptake of K+ by skeletal muscle are reviewed in Chapter 18 (see Table 18.1). Second, the colon has the ability to absorb and secrete K+, with considerable mechanistic and regulatory similarities to renal K⁺ secretion. K⁺ secretion in the distal colon is increased after dietary loading and in end-stage kidney disease (ESKD).[12,407,408] However, the colon has a relatively limited capacity for K⁺ excretion, such that changes in renal K⁺ excretion play the dominant role in responding to changes in K⁺ intake. In particular, regulated K⁺ secretion by the CNT and CCD play a critical role in the response to hyperkalemia and K⁺ loading; increases in the reabsorption of K⁺ by the CCD and OMCD function in the response to hypokalemia or K⁺ deprivation.

This section reviews the mechanisms and regulation of transepithelial K⁺ transport along the nephron. As in other sections of this chapter, the emphasis is on particularly recent developments in the molecular physiology of renal K⁺ transport. Of note, transport pathways for K⁺ play important roles in renal Na⁺-Cl⁻ transport, particularly within the TAL. Furthermore, Na⁺ absorption via ENaC in the aldosterone-sensitive distal nephron generates a lumen-negative potential difference that drives distal K⁺ excretion. These pathways are primarily discussed in the section on renal Na⁺-Cl⁻ transport; related issues relevant to K⁺ homeostasis per se will be specifically addressed in this section.

PROXIMAL TUBULE

The proximal tubule reabsorbs some 50% to 70% of filtered K⁺ (Figure 6.23). Proximal tubules generate minimal transepithelial K⁺ gradients, and fractional reabsorption of K⁺ is similar to that of Na⁺.[253] K⁺ absorption follows that of fluid, Na⁺, and other solutes, such that this nephron segment does not play a direct role in regulated renal excretion.[409,410] Notably, however, changes in Na⁺-Cl⁻ reabsorption by the proximal tubule have considerable effects on distal tubular flow and distal tubular Na⁺ delivery, with attendant effects on the excretory capacity for K⁺ (see later, "K⁺ Secretion by the Distal Convoluted Tubule, Connecting Tubule, and Cortical Collecting Duct").

The mechanisms involved in transepithelial K⁺ transport by the proximal tubule are not completely clear, although active transport does not appear to play a major role.[410,411] Luminal barium has modest effects on transepithelial K⁺ transport by the proximal tubule, suggesting a component of transcellular transport via barium-sensitive K⁺ channels.[412] However, the bulk of K⁺ transport is thought to occur via the paracellular pathway, driven by the lumen-positive potential difference in the mid to late proximal tubule (see Figure 6.3).[412,413] The total K⁺ permeability of the proximal tubule is thus rather high, apparently due to features of the paracellular pathway.[412,413] The combination of luminal K⁺ concentrations that are about 10% higher than that of plasma, a lumen-positive PD of about 2 mV (see Figure 6.3), and high paracellular permeability leads to considerable paracellular absorption in the proximal tubule. This absorption is thought to primarily proceed via convective transport—solvent drag due to frictional interactions between water and K⁺—rather than diffusional transport.[414] Notably, however, the primary pathway for water movement in the proximal tubule is conclusively transcellular via aquaporin-1 and aquaporin-7 water channels in the apical and basolateral membrane.[17,29,30] Therefore, the apparent convective transport of K⁺ would have to constitute so-called pseudosolvent drag, with hypothetical uncharacterized interactions between water traversing the transcellular route and diffusion of K⁺ along the paracellular pathway.[414]

LOOP OF HENLE AND MEDULLARY K⁺ RECYCLING

Transport by the loop of Henle plays a critical role in medullary K⁺ recycling (Figure 6.24). Several lines of evidence have indicated that a considerable fraction of K⁺ secreted by the CCD is reabsorbed by the medullary collecting ducts and then secreted into the late proximal tubule and/or descending thin limbs of long-looped nephrons.[415] In potassium-loaded rats, there is thus a doubling of luminal K⁺ in the terminal thin descending limbs, with a sharp drop after inhibition of CCD K⁺ secretion by amiloride.[416] Enhancement of CCD K⁺ secretion by treatment with DDAVP also results in an increase in luminal K⁺ in the descending thin limbs.[417] This recycling pathway (secretion in CCD, absorption in OMCD and IMCD, secretion in descending thin limb) is associated with a marked increase in medullary interstitial K⁺. Passive transepithelial K⁺ absorption by the thin ascending limb and active absorption by the TAL also contribute to this increase in interstitial K⁺ (see Figure 6.24).[167] Specifically, the absorption of K⁺ by the ascending thin limb, TAL, and OMCD exceeds the secretion by the descending thin limbs, thus trapping K⁺ in the interstitium.

The physiologic significance of medullary K⁺ recycling is not completely clear. However, an increase in interstitial K⁺ concentration from 5 to 25 mmol/L dramatically inhibits Cl⁻ transport by perfused thick ascending limbs.[167] By

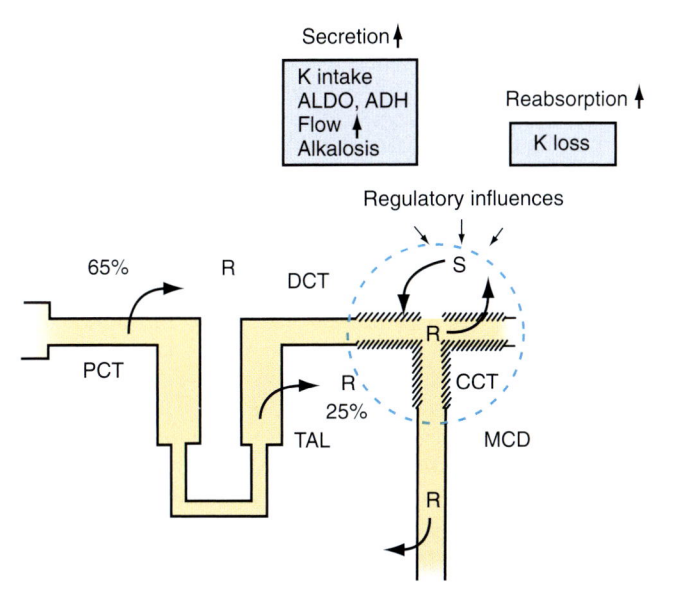

Figure 6.23 K⁺ transport along the nephron. Approximately 90% of filtered K⁺ is reabsorbed by the proximal tubule and the loop of Henle. K⁺ is secreted along the initial and cortical collecting tubule. Net reabsorption occurs in response to K⁺ depletion, primarily within the medullary collecting duct. ADH, Antidiuretic hormone; ALDO, aldosterone; CCT, cortical collecting tubule; DCT, distal convoluted tubule; ICT, initial connecting tubule; MCD, medullary collecting duct; PCT, proximal tubule; R, reabsorption; S, secretion; TAL, thick ascending limb.

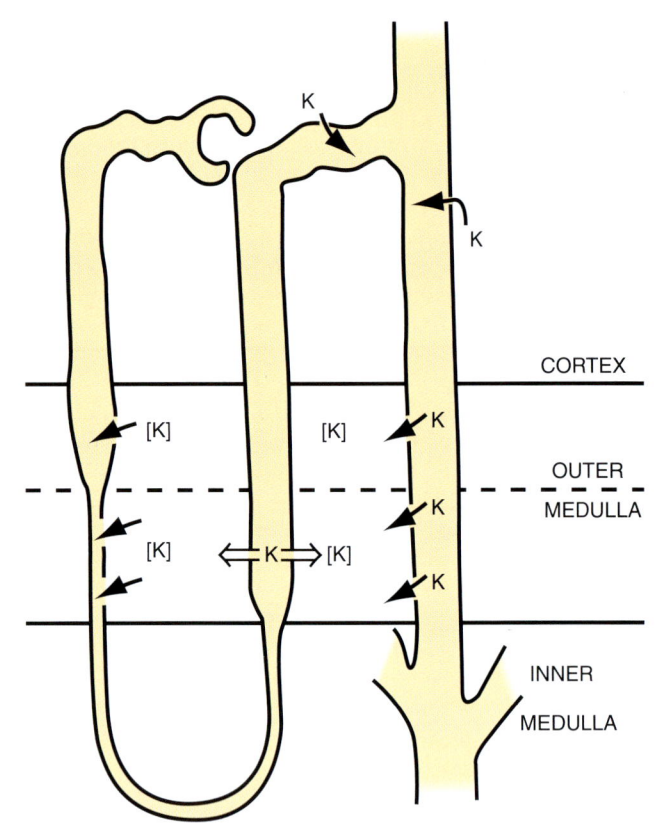

Figure 6.24 Schematic representation of medullary K+ recycling. Medullary interstitial K+ increases considerably after dietary K+ loading due to the combined effects of secretion in the CCD, absorption in the OMCD, TAL, and IMCD, and secretion in the descending thin limb. See text for details. (From Stokes JB: Consequences of potassium recycling in the renal medulla. Effects of ion transport by the medullary thick ascending limb of Henle's loop. *J Clin Invest* 70:219-229, 1982.)

K+ SECRETION BY THE DISTAL CONVOLUTED TUBULE, CONNECTING TUBULE, AND CORTICAL COLLECTING DUCT

Approximately 90% of filtered K+ is reabsorbed by the proximal tubule and loop of Henle (see Figure 6.23); the fine tuning of renal K+ excretion occurs in the remaining distal nephron. The bulk of regulated secretion occurs in principal cells within the CNT and CCD, whereas K+ reabsorption primarily occurs in the OMCD (see below). K+ secretion is initially detectable in the early DCT, in which NCC-positive cells express ROMK, the apical K+ secretory channel.[175,419] Generally, the CCD is considered the primary site for distal K+ secretion, partially due to the greater ease with which this segment is perfused and studied. However, as is the case for Na+-Cl− absorption (see "Connecting Tubules and the Cortical Collecting Duct: Apical Na+ Transport), the bulk of distal K+ secretion appears to occur prior to the CCD, within the CNT.[253,319]

In principal cells, apical Na+ entry via ENaC generates a lumen-negative PD, which drives passive K+ exit through apical K+ channels. Distal K+ secretion is therefore dependent on delivery of adequate luminal Na+ to the CNT and CCD, essentially ceasing when luminal Na+ drops below 8 mmol/L.[420-422] Dietary Na+ intake also influences K+ excretion, such that excretion is enhanced by excess Na+ intake and reduced by Na+ restriction.[420,421] Secreted K+ enters principal cells via the basolateral Na+-K+-ATPase, which also generates the gradient that drives apical Na+ entry via ENaC (see Figure 6.23).

Two major subtypes of apical K+ channels function in secretion by the CNT and CCD, with or without the DCT; a small-conductance (SK), 30-pS channel and a large-conductance, Ca^{2+}-activated, 150-pS (maxi-K or BK) channel.[176,319,423] The density and high P$_o$ of the SK channel indicates that this pathway alone is sufficient to mediate the bulk of K+ secretion in the CCD under baseline conditions—hence, its designation as the secretory K+ channel.[424] Notably, SK channel density is considerably higher in the CNT than in the CCD, consistent with the greater capacity for Na+ absorption and K+ secretion in the CNT.[31] The characteristics of the SK channel are similar to those of the ROMK K+ channel, and ROMK protein has been localized at the apical membrane of principal cells.[175,425] SK channel activity is absent from apical membranes of the CCD in homozygous knockout mice with a targeted deletion of the *Kcnj1* gene that encodes ROMK, definitive proof that ROMK is the SK channel.[176] The observation that these knockout mice are normokalemic, with an increased excretion of K+, illustrates the considerable redundancy in distal K+ secretory pathways; distal K+ secretion in these mice is mediated by apical BK channels (see below).[176,426] Of interest, loss-of-function mutations in human *KCNJ1* genes are associated with Bartter's syndrome; ROMK expression is critical for the 30- and 70-pS channels that generate the lumen-positive PD in the TAL (see Figure 6.15).[176,177] These patients typically have slightly higher serum K+ levels than those with other genetic forms of Bartter's syndrome, and affected patients with severe neonatal hyperkalemia have also been described; this neonatal hyperkalemia is presumably the result of a transient developmental deficit in apical BK channel activity.[12,169]

inhibiting Na+-Cl− absorption by the TAL, increases in interstitial K+ would increase Na+ delivery to the CNT and CCD, thus enhancing the lumen-negative PD in these tubules and increasing K+ secretion.[167] Alternatively, the marked increase in medullary interstitial K+ after dietary K+ loading serves to limit the difference between luminal and peritubular K+ in the CCD, thus minimizing passive K+ loss from the collecting duct.

K+ is secreted into the descending thin limbs by passive diffusion, driven by the high medullary interstitial K+ concentration. Descending thin limbs thus have a very high K+ permeability, without evidence for active transepithelial K+ transport.[418] Transepithelial K+ transport by ascending thin limbs has not to our knowledge been measured; however, as is the case for Na+-Cl− transport (see earlier, "Na+-Cl− Transport by the Thin Ascending Limb"), the absorption of K+ by the thin ascending limbs is presumably passive. Active transepithelial K+ transport across the TAL includes a transcellular component, via apical Na+-K+-2Cl− cotransport mediated by NKCC2, and a paracellular pathway (see Figure 6.15). Luminal K+ channels play a critical role in generating the lumen-positive PD in the TAL, as summarized earlier (see "Na+-Cl− Transport by the Thick Ascending Limb: Apical K+ Channels").

The apical Ca^{2+}-activated BK channel plays a critical role in flow-dependent K^+ secretion by the CNT and CCD.[423] BK channels have a heteromeric structure, with α-subunits that form the ion channel pore and modulatory β-subunits that affect the biophysical, regulatory, and pharmacologic characteristics of the channel complex.[423] BK α-subunit transcripts are expressed in multiple nephron segments, and channel protein is detectable at the apical membrane of principal and intercalated cells in the CCD and CNT.[423] The β-subunits are differentially expressed within the distal nephron. Thus, $β_1$-subunits are restricted to the CNT, with no expression in intercalated cells, whereas $β_4$-subunits are detectable at the apical membranes of the TAL, DCT, and intercalated cells.[423,427] Increased distal flow has a well-established stimulatory effect on K^+ secretion, due in part to enhanced delivery and absorption of Na^+ and to increased removal of secreted K^+.[420,421] The pharmacology of flow-dependent K^+ secretion in the CCD is consistent with dominant involvement of BK channels, and flow-dependent K^+ secretion is reduced in mice with targeted deletion of the $α_1$- and $β_1$-subunits.[423,428-430] Both mice strains develop hyperaldosteronism that is exacerbated by a high-K^+ diet, leading to hypertension in the $α_1$-subunit knockout.[430]

One enigma has been the greater density of BK channels in intercalated cells in both the CCD and CNT.[431,432] This has suggested a major role for intercalated cells in K^+ secretion; however, the much lower density of Na^+-K^+-ATPase activity in intercalated cells has been considered inadequate to support K^+ secretion across the apical membrane.[433] More recent evidence has revealed a major role for the basolateral Na^+-K^+-$2Cl^-$ cotransporter NKCC1 in K^+ secretion mediated by apical BK channels. NKCC1 is expressed almost exclusively at the basolateral membrane of intercalated cells, providing an alternative entry pathway for basolateral K^+ secreted at the apical membrane.[434,435] This still begs the question of how basolateral Na^+ recycles across the basolateral membrane in the absence of significant Na^+-K^+-ATPase activity; one possibility is an alternative basolateral Na^+ pump, the ouabain-insensitive furosemide-sensitive Na^+-ATPase, a transport activity that has been detected in cell culture models of intercalated cells.[434] At the apical membrane, BK-mediated K^+ secretion is only partially dependent on luminal Na^+; K^+ secretion would eventually hyperpolarize the membrane in the absence of apical Na^+ entry, which is mediated by ENaC in principal cells.[436] An intriguing possibility is that apical Cl^- channels allow for the parallel secretion of K^+ and Cl^- in intercalated cells.[437]

BK channels also play a critical role in cell volume regulation by intercalated cells, with indirect, flow-mediated influences on distal K^+ secretion. MDCK-C11 cells have an intercalated cell phenotype and express BK α- and $β_4$-subunits, as do intercalated cells; shear stress activates BK channels in these cells, leading to loss of K^+ and cell shrinkage.[427,438] Mice with a targeted deletion of the $β_4$-subunit exhibit normal K^+ excretion on a normal diet.[433] However, when fed a high-K^+ diet, which increases urinary and tubular flow rates and tubular shear stress, the $β_4$-knockout mice develop hyperkalemia with a blunted increase in K^+ excretion and urinary flow rates. Intercalated cells from $β_4$-knockouts fail to significantly decrease cell volume in response to high-K^+ diet. Intercalated cells thus function as so-called speed bumps that protrude into the lumen of distal tubules; flow-activated BK channels reduce the cell volume of intercalated cells after K^+ loading, reducing tubular resistance, increasing tubular flow rates, and increasing distal K^+ secretion.[433]

The physiologic rationale for the presence of two apical secretory K^+ channels, ROMK/SK and BK channels, is not completely clear. However, the high density and higher P_o of ROMK/SK channels is perhaps better suited for a role in basal K^+ secretion, with additional recruitment of the higher capacity, flow-activated BK channels when additional K^+ secretion is required.[423] Evolving evidence has also indicated that BK channels function in partially Na^+-independent K^+ secretion by intercalated cells, with ROMK functioning in ENaC- and Na^+-dependent K^+ excretion by DCT, CNT, and CCD cells. Regardless, at the whole-organ level, the two K^+ channels can substitute for one another, with BK-dependent K^+ secretion in ROMK knockout mice and an upregulation of ROMK in the distal nephron of $α_1$-subunit BK knockouts.[426,429]

Other K^+ channels reportedly expressed at the luminal membranes of the CNT and CCD include voltage-sensitive channels such as Kv1.3, the calcium-activated, small-conductance SK3 channel, and double-pore K^+ channels, such as TWIK-1 and KCNQ1.[439-441,443] KCNQ1 mediates K^+ secretion in the inner ear and is expressed at the apical membrane of principal cells in the CCD, whereas TWIK-1 is expressed at the apical membrane of intercalated cells.[442,443] The roles of these channels in renal K^+ secretion or absorption are not fully characterized. However, Kv1.3 may play a role in distal K^+ secretion in that luminal margatoxin, a specific blocker of this channel, reduces K^+ secretion in CCDs of rat kidneys from animals on a high-K^+ diet.[444] Other apical K^+ channels in the distal nephron may subserve other physiologic functions. For example, the apical Kv1.1 channel is critically involved in Mg^{2+} transport by the DCT, likely by hyperpolarizing the apical membrane and increasing the driving force for Mg^{2+} influx via TRPM6 (transient receptor potential cation channel 6); missense mutations in Kv1.1 are a cause of genetic hypomagnesemia.[445]

K^+ channels present at the basolateral membrane of principal cells appear to set the resting potential of the basolateral membrane and function in K^+ secretion and Na^+ absorption at the apical membrane, the latter via K^+ recycling at the basolateral membrane to maintain activity of the Na^+-K^+-ATPase. A variety of different K^+ channels have been described in the electrophysiologic characterization of the basolateral membrane of principal cells, which has a number of technical barriers to overcome.[446] However, a single predominant activity has been identified in principal cells from the rat CCD using whole-cell recording techniques under conditions in which ROMK is inhibited (low intracellular pH or presence of the ROMK inhibitor tertiapin-Q).[446] This basolateral current is tetraethylammonium (TEA)-insensitive, barium-sensitive, and acid-sensitive ($pK_a \cong 6.5$), with a conductance of about 17 pS and weak inward rectification. These properties do not correspond exactly to specific characterized K^+ channels or combinations thereof. However, candidate inward-rectifying K^+ channel subunits that have been localized at the basolateral membrane of the CCD include KIR4.1, KIR5.1, KIR7.1, and KIR2.3.[446] A more recent report suggested that KIR4.1 and KIR5.1 channels generate a predominant 40-pS basolateral K^+ channel in murine principal cells.[447] Notably, basolateral K^+ channel activity increases on a high-K^+ diet, suggesting a role in transepithelial K^+ secretion.[446]

In addition to apical K^+ channels, considerable evidence has implicated apical K^+-Cl^- cotransport (or functionally equivalent pathways) in distal K^+ secretion.[61,420,448,449] Thus, in rat distal tubules, a reduction in luminal Cl^- markedly increases K^+ secretion; the replacement of luminal Cl^- with SO_4^- or gluconate has an equivalent stimulatory effect on K^+ secretion.[450] This anion-dependent component of K^+ secretion is not influenced by luminal Ba^{2+}, suggesting that it does not involve apical K^+ channel activity.[450] Perfused surface distal tubules are a mixture of the DCT, connecting segment, and initial collecting duct; however, Cl^--coupled K^+ secretion is detectable in the DCT and in early CNT.[451] In addition, similar pathways are detectable in rabbit CCD, where a decrease in luminal Cl^- concentration from 112 to 5 mmol/L increases K^+ secretion by 48%.[452] A reduction in basolateral Cl^- also decreases K^+ secretion without an effect on transepithelial voltage or Na^+ transport, and the direction of K^+ flux can be reversed by a lumen to bath Cl^- gradient, resulting in K^+ absorption.[452] In perfused CCDs from rats treated with mineralocorticoid, vasopressin increases K^+ secretion; because this increase in K^+ secretion is resistant to luminal Ba^{2+} (2 mmol/L), vasopressin may stimulate Cl^--dependent K^+ secretion.[12,453] Pharmacologic study results of perfused tubules are consistent with K^+-Cl^- cotransport mediated by the KCCs; however, of the three renal KCCs, only KCC1 is apically expressed along the nephron.[61,449] Other functional possibilities for Cl^--dependent K^+ secretion include parallel operation of apical H^+-K^+-exchange and Cl^--HCO_3^- exchange in type B intercalated cells.[448]

A provocative study by Frindt and Palmer serves to underline the importance of ENaC-independent K^+ excretion, whether it is mediated by apical K^+-Cl^- cotransport and/or by other mechanisms (see also "Integrated Na^+-Cl^- and K^+ Transport in the Distal Nephron").[454] Rats were infused with amiloride via osmotic minipumps, generating urinary concentrations considered sufficient to inhibit more than 98% of ENaC activity. Whereas amiloride almost abolished K^+ excretion in rats on a normal K^+ intake, acute and long-term high-K^+ diets led to an increasing fraction of K^+ excretion that was independent of ENaC activity ($\approx$50% after 7 to 9 days on a high-K^+ diet).

K^+ REABSORPTION BY THE COLLECTING DUCT

In addition to K^+ secretion, the distal nephron is capable of considerable reabsorption, primarily during restriction of dietary K^+.[253-255] This reabsorption is accomplished largely by intercalated cells in the OMCD via the activity of apical H^+/K^+-ATPase pumps. Under K^+-replete conditions, apical H^+/K^+-ATPase activity recycles K^+ with an apical K^+ channel, without an effect on transepithelial K^+ absorption. Under K^+-restricted basolateral conditions, K^+ absorbed via apical H^+/K^+-ATPase appears to exit intercalated cells via a K^+ channel, thus achieving the transepithelial transport of K^+.[455]

H^+-K^+-ATPase holoenzymes are members of the P-type family of ion transport ATPases, which also includes subunits of the basolateral Na^+-K^+-ATPase.[456] $HK\alpha_1$ and $HK\alpha_2$ are also referred to as the gastric and colonic subunits, respectively; humans also have an $HK\alpha_4$-subunit.[456,457] A specific $HK\beta$-subunit interacts with the $HK\alpha$-subunits to ensure delivery to the cell surface and complete expression of H^+-K^+-ATPase activity; $HK\alpha_2$- and $HK\alpha_4$-subunits are also capable of interaction with Na^+-K^+-ATPase β-subunits.[12,458] The pharmacology of H^+-K^+-ATPase holoenzymes differs considerably, such that the gastric $HK\alpha_1$–subunit is typically sensitive to the H^+-K^+-ATPase inhibitors SCH-28080 and omeprazole and resistant to ouabain; the colonic $HK\alpha_2$-subunit is usually sensitive to ouabain and resistant to SCH-28080.[458] Within the kidney, the $HK\alpha_1$-subunit is expressed at the apical membrane of at least a subset of type A intercalated cells in the distal nephron.[457] $HK\alpha_2$-subunit distribution in the distal nephron is more diffuse, with robust expression at the apical membrane of types A and B intercalated cells and connecting segment cells and lesser expression in principal cells.[459-461] The human $HK\alpha_4$-subunit is reportedly expressed in intercalated cells.[457]

$HK\alpha_1$- and $HK\alpha_2$-subunits are both constitutively expressed in the distal nephron. However, tubule perfusion of K^+-replete animals suggests a functional dominance of omeprazole/SCH-28080–sensitive, ouabain-resistant H^+-K^+-ATPase activity, consistent with holoenzymes containing the $HK\alpha_1$-subunit.[462] K^+ deprivation increases the overall activity of H^+-K^+-ATPase in the collecting duct, with the emergence of ouabain-sensitive H^+-K^+-ATPase activity; this is consistent with a relative dominance of the $HK\alpha_2$-subunit during K^+-restricted conditions.[12] K^+ restriction also induces a dramatic upregulation of the $HK\alpha_2$-subunit transcript and protein in the outer and inner medulla during K^+ depletion; $HK\alpha_1$-subunit expression is unaffected.[12] Mice with a targeted deletion of the $HK\alpha_2$-subunit exhibit lower plasma and muscle K^+ than wild-type littermates when maintained on a K^+-deficient diet. However, this appears to be due to marked loss of K^+ in the colon rather than in the kidney, because renal K^+ excretion is appropriately reduced in the K^+-depleted knockout mice.[463] Presumably the lack of an obvious renal phenotype in $HK\alpha_1$- or $HK\alpha_2$-subunit knockout mice reflects the marked redundancy in the expression of $HK\alpha$-subunits in the distal nephron.[463,464] Indeed, collecting ducts from the $HK\alpha_1$-subunit knockout mice have significant residual ouabain-resistant and SCH-28080–sensitive H^+-K^+-ATPase activities, consistent with the expression of other $HK\alpha$-subunits that confer characteristics similar to the "gastric" H^+-K^+-ATPase.[465] However, data from $HK\alpha_1$- and $HK\alpha_2$-subunit knockout mice have suggested that compensatory mechanisms in these mice are not accounted for by ATPase-type mechanisms.[466]

The importance of K^+ reabsorption mediated by the collecting duct is dramatically illustrated by the phenotype of transgenic mice with generalized overexpression of a gain-of-function mutation in H^+-K^+-ATPase, effectively bypassing the redundancy and complexity of this reabsorptive pathway. This transgene expresses a mutant form of the $HK\beta$-subunit, in which a tyrosine-to-alanine mutation within the C-terminal tail abrogates regulated endocytosis from the plasma membrane; these mice have higher plasma K^+ than their wild-type littermates, with approximately half the fractional excretion of K^+.[467]

REGULATION OF DISTAL K+ TRANSPORT

MODULATION OF RENAL OUTER MEDULLARY POTASSIUM ACTIVITY

ROMK and other Kir channels are inward-rectifying—that is, K+ flows inward more readily than outward (Kir, inward rectifying renal K+ channel). Even though outward conductance is usually less than inward conductance, K+ efflux through the ROMK predominates in the CNT and CCD because the membrane potential is more positive than the equilibrium potential for K+. Intracellular magnesium (Mg^{2+}) and polyamines play key roles in inward rectification, binding and blocking the pore of the channel from the cytoplasmic side.[468-470] A single transmembrane residue, asparagine-171 in ROMK1, controls the affinity and blocking effect of Mg^{2+} and polyamines.[468,469] Intracellular Mg^{2+} in the TAL, DCT, CNT, and principal cells is thought to have a significant effect on ROMK activity because it inhibits outward ROMK-dependent currents in principal cells.[471] The blocking affinity of Mg^{2+} is enhanced at lower extracellular K+ concentrations, which should aid in reducing K+ secretion during hypokalemia and K+ deficiency.[471] A reduction of this intracellular Mg^{2+} block may also explain the hypokalemia associated with hypomagnesemia, wherein distal K+ secretion is enhanced.[470,471]

In addition to inward rectification, the endogenous ROMK channels in the TAL and principal cells exhibit a very high channel P_o. The high P_o of ROMK is maintained by the combined effects of binding of PIP2 to the channel protein, direct channel phosphorylation by PKA, ATP binding to the ROMK-CFTR complex, and cytoplasmic pH. PIP2 binding to ROMK is thus required to maintain the channel in an open state, whereas cytoplasmic acidification inhibits the channel.[472] PKA phosphorylates ROMK protein at one N-terminal serines and two C-terminal serines—S25, S200, and S294 in the ROMK2 isoform.[229] Phosphorylation of all three sites is required for full channel function. Phosphorylation of the N-terminal site overrides the effect of a carboxy-terminal endoplasmic reticulum retention signal, thus increasing expression of the channel protein at the cell membrane.[473] Phosphorylation of S200 and S294 maintains the channel in a high P_o state, in part by modulating the effects of PIP2, ATP, and pH.[179,231,232]

Because ROMK channels exhibit such a high P_o, physiologic regulation of the channel is primarily achieved by regulated changes in the number of active channels on the plasma membrane. The associated mechanisms are discussed in the context of the adaptation to K+ loading and hyperkalemia and K+ deprivation and hypokalemia.

ALDOSTERONE AND K+ LOADING

Aldosterone has a potent kaliuretic effect, with important interrelationships between circulating K+ and aldosterone.[474] Aldosterone release by the adrenal is thus induced by hyperkalemia and/or a high-K+ diet, suggesting an important feedback effect of aldosterone on K+ homeostasis.[475] Aldosterone also has clinically relevant effects on K+ homeostasis, with a clear relationship at all levels of serum K+ between circulating levels of the hormone and the ability to excrete K+.

Aldosterone has no effect on the density of apical SK channels in the CCD; it does, however, induce a marked increase in the density of apical Na+ channels in the CNT and CCD.[476] This hormone activates ENaC via interrelated effects on the synthesis, trafficking, and membrane-associated activity of the subunits encoding the channel (see "Regulation of Na+-Cl- Transport in the Connecting Tubule and Cortical Collecting Duct"). Aldosterone is thus induced by a high-K+ diet and strongly stimulates apical ENaC activity, which provides the lumen-negative PD that stimulates K+ secretion by principal cells.

The important relationships between K+ and aldosterone notwithstanding, it is increasingly clear that much of the adaptation to a high-K+ intake is aldosterone-independent. For example, a high-K+ diet in adrenalectomized animals increases apical Na+ reabsorption and K+ secretion in the CCD.[477] At the tubular level, when basolateral K+ is increased, there is significant activation of Na+-K+-ATPase, accompanied by a secondary activation of apical Na+ and K+ channels.[478] Increased dietary K+ also markedly increases the density of SK channels in the CCD, along with a modest increase in Na+ channel (ENaC) density; this is associated with changes in the subcellular distribution of the ROMK protein, with an increase in apical expression.[476,479] Notably, this increase in ENaC and SK density in the CCD occurs within hours of consuming a high-K+ diet, with a minimal associated increase in circulating aldosterone (Figure 6.25).[480] In contrast, a week of low Na+-Cl- intake, with almost a thousand-fold increase in aldosterone, has no effect on SK channel density, nor for that matter does 2 days of aldosterone infusion, despite the development of hypokalemia (see Table 6.1).[480] Of note, unlike the marked increase seen in the CCD, the density of SK channels in the CNT is not increased by high dietary K+.[319,476,480] This appears to be due to difficulties in estimating channel densities in small membrane patches, because measurement of whole cell currents using the ROMK inhibitor tertiapin-Q indicates an upregulation of ROMK activity in the CNT by a high-K+ diet.[481]

BK channels in the CNT and CCD play an important role in the flow-activated component of distal K+ excretion; these channels are also activated by dietary K+ loading.[423] Flow-stimulated K+ secretion by the CCD of mice and rats is thus enhanced on a high-K+ diet, with an absence of flow-dependent K+ secretion in rats on a low-K+ diet.[426,482] This is accompanied by the appropriate changes in transcript levels for α- and $β_{2-4}$-subunits of the BK channel proteins in microdissected CCDs ($β_1$-subunits are restricted to the CNT).[423] Trafficking of BK subunits is also affected by dietary K+, with a largely intracellular distribution of α-subunits in K+-restricted rats and prominent apical expression in K+-loaded rats.[482] Aldosterone does not contribute to the regulation of BK channel activity or expression in response to a high-K+ diet.[483]

The changes in trafficking and/or activity of the ROMK channel that are induced by dietary K+ appear in large part to involve tyrosine phosphorylation and dephosphorylation of the ROMK protein (see below). However, a series of reports have linked changes in expression of WNK1 kinase subunits in the response to a high K+ diet. WNK1 and WNK4 were initially identified as causative genes for familial hypertension with hyperkalemia (FHHt), also known as Gordon's syndrome or pseudohypoaldosteronism type II (see also "Regulation of Na+-Cl- Transport in the Distal Convoluted Tubule"). ROMK expression at the membrane of *Xenopus*

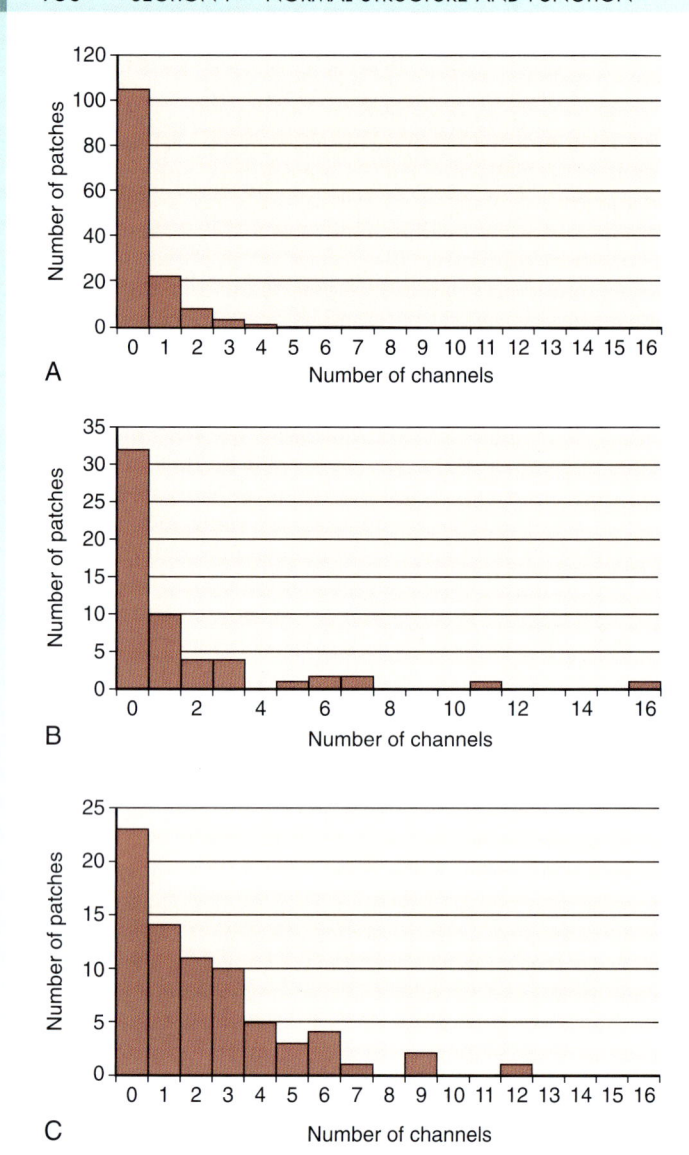

Figure 6.25 A high-K⁺ diet rapidly activates SK channels in the CCD, mediated by the ROMK (Kir 1.1) K⁺ channel. Histograms of channels/patch are shown for rats on a control diet **(A)**, a high-K diet for 6 hours **(B)**, and a high-K diet for 48 hours **(C)**. Each determination of N represents a single cell-attached patch. A high-K⁺ diet results in a progressive recruitment of SK channels at the apical membrane. (From Palmer LG, Frindt G: Regulation of apical K channels in rat cortical collecting tubule during changes in dietary K intake. *Am J Physiol* 277:F805-F812, 1999.)

oocytes is dramatically reduced by coexpression of WNK4; FHHt-associated mutations dramatically increase this effect, suggesting a direct inhibition of SK channels in FHHt.[484] The study of WNK1 is further complicated by the transcriptional complexity of its gene, which has at least three separate promoters and a number of alternative splice forms (Figure 6.26). In particular, the predominant intrarenal WNK1 isoform is generated by a distal nephron transcriptional site that bypasses the N-terminal exons that encode the kinase domain, yielding a kinase-deficient short form of the protein ("WNK1-S").[485] Full-length WNK1 (WNK1-L) inhibits ROMK activity by inducing endocytosis of the channel protein; kinase activity and/or the N-terminal kinase domain of WNK1 appear to be required for this effect, although Cope and colleagues have reported that a kinase-dead mutant of WNK1 is unimpaired.[486-488] WNK1 and WNK4 induce endocytosis of ROMK via interaction with intersectin, a multimodular endocytic scaffold protein.[489] Additional binding of ROMK to the clathrin adaptor protein termed *autosomal recessive hypercholesterolemia* (ARH) is required for basal and WNK1-stimulated endocytosis of the channel protein.[490] Ubiquitination of ROMK protein is also involved in clathrin-dependent endocytosis, requiring interaction between the channel and the U3 ubiquitin ligase POSH (*p*lenty *o*f *SH* domains).[491]

The shorter WNK1-S isoform, which lacks the kinase domain, appears to inhibit the effect of WNK1-L.[487,488] The ratio of WNK1-S to WNK1-L transcripts is reduced by K⁺ restriction (greater endocytosis of ROMK) and increased by K⁺ loading (reduced endocytosis of ROMK), suggesting that this ratio between WNK1-S and WNK1-L functions as a type of switch to regulate distal K⁺ secretion (see also Figure 6.26).[487,488,492] The inhibitory effect of WNK1-S tracks to the first 253 amino acids of the protein, encompassing the initial 30 amino acids unique to this isoform and an adjacent autoinhibitory domain.[493] Transgenic mice that overexpress this inhibitory domain of WNK1-S have lower serum K⁺ concentrations, higher fractional excretion of K⁺, and increased expression of ROMK protein at the apical membrane of CNT and CCD cells—all consistent with an important inhibitory effect of WNK1-S.[493]

The BK channel is also regulated by the WNK kinases. WNK4 thus inhibits BK channel activity and protein expression, whereas FHHt-associated mutations in WNK4 also enhance the inhibitory effect via ubiquitination.[494-496] WNK1 in turn activates the channel by reducing ERK1/2 signaling–mediated lysosomal degradation of the channel protein.[497]

K⁺ DEPRIVATION

A reduction in dietary K⁺ leads within 24 hours to a dramatic drop in urinary K⁺ excretion.[492,498] This drop in excretion is due to both an induction of reabsorption by intercalated cells in the OMCD and to a reduction in SK channel activity in principal cells.[12,254,255] The mechanisms involved in K⁺ reabsorption by intercalated cells are discussed above; notably, H⁺/K⁺-ATPase activity in the collecting duct does not appear to be regulated by aldosterone.[499]

Considerable progress has been made in defining the signaling pathways that regulate the activity of the SK channel (ROMK) in response to changes in dietary K⁺. Dietary K⁺ intake modulates trafficking of the ROMK channel protein to the plasma membrane of principal cells, with a marked increase in the relative proportion of intracellular channel protein in K⁺-depleted animals and clearly defined expression at the plasma membrane of CCD cells from animals on a high-K⁺ diet.[479,500] The membrane insertion and activity of ROMK is modulated by tyrosine phosphorylation of the channel protein, such that phosphorylation of tyrosine residue 337 stimulates endocytosis and dephosphorylation induces exocytosis; this tyrosine phosphorylation appears to play a key role in the regulation of ROMK by dietary K⁺.[501-503] Whereas the levels of protein tyrosine phosphatase-1D do not vary with K⁺ intake, intrarenal activity of the cytoplasmic tyrosine kinases c-src and c-yes are inversely related to dietary K⁺ intake, with a decrease under high K⁺ conditions and a marked increase after several days of K⁺ restriction.[12,504]

Table 6.1 Effect of High-K⁺ Diet, Aldosterone, and/or Na⁺-Cl⁻ Restriction on SK Channel Density in the Rat Cortical Collecting Duct

Parameter	K⁺ Channel Density (μm^2)	Plasma Aldosterone (ng/dL)	Plasma K (mmol/L)
Control	0.41	15	3.68
High-K⁺ diet, 6 hr	1.51	36	NM
High-K⁺ diet, 48 hr	2.13	98	4.37
Low-Na⁺ diet, 7 days	0.48	1260	NM
Aldosterone infusion, 48 hr	0.44	550	2.44
Aldosterone + high-K⁺ diet	0.32	521	3.80

NM, Not measured.
Modified from Palmer LG, Frindt G: Regulation of apical K channels in rat cortical collecting tubule during changes in dietary K intake. Am J Physiol 277:F805-F812, 1999.

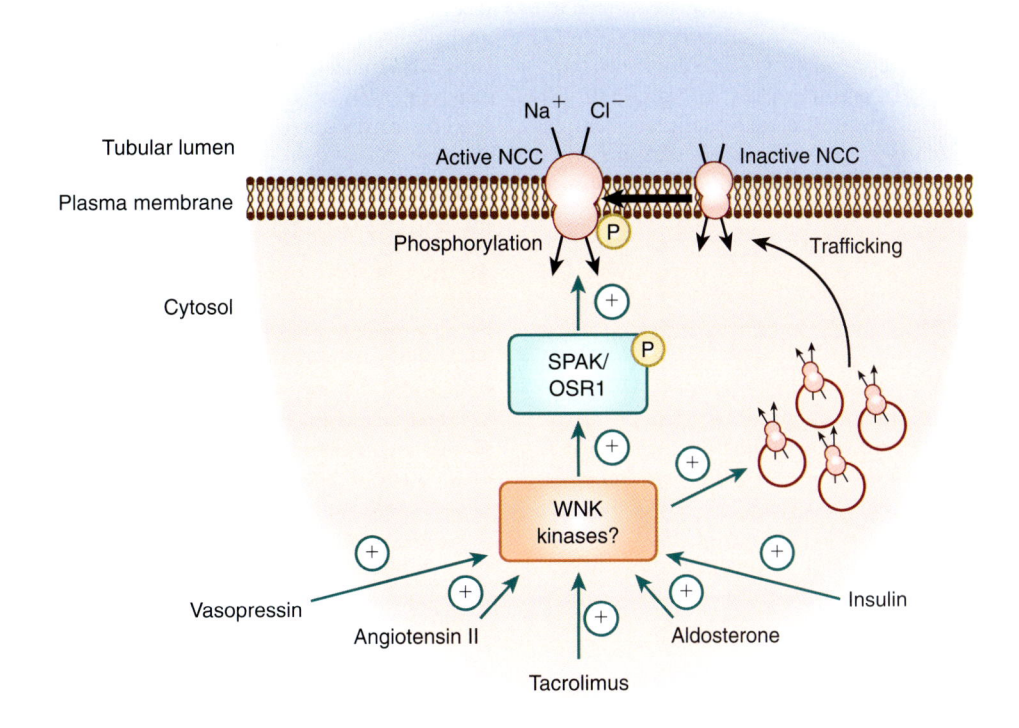

Figure 6.26 Model of NCC regulation by the WNK-SPAK/OSR1 signaling cascade. Several hormones are known to stimulate NCC phosphorylation at sites that are directly phosphorylated by SPAK and OSR1. The calcineurin inhibitor tacrolimus has similar effects, leading to thiazide-sensitive hypertension. The mechanisms likely involve activation of the upstream WNK kinases. In some cases, specifically aldosterone and angiotensin II, activation of the WNK-SPAK/OSR1 cascade is associated with increased trafficking of NCC to the apical membrane of DCT cells. NCC, Na⁺-Cl⁻ cotransporter. (From Subramanya AR, Ellison DH: Distal convoluted tubule. *Clin J Am Soc Nephrol* 9:2147-2163, 2014.)

Localization studies have indicated coexpression of c-src with ROMK in the TAL and principal cells of the CCD.[479] Moreover, inhibition of protein tyrosine phosphatase activity, leading to a dominance of tyrosine phosphorylation, dramatically increases the proportion of intracellular ROMK in the CCD of animals on a high-K⁺ diet.[479]

The neurohumoral factors that induce the K⁺-dependent trafficking and expression of apical ROMK and BK channels have only come into focus rather recently.[479,482,500] Several studies have implicated the intrarenal generation of superoxide anions in the activation of cytoplasmic tyrosine kinases and downstream phosphorylation of the ROMK channel protein by K⁺ depletion.[505-507] Potential candidates for the upstream kaliuretic factor include Ang II and growth factors such as insulin-like growth factor-1 (IGF-1).[505] Ang II inhibits ROMK activity in K⁺-restricted rats, but not rats on a normal K⁺ diet.[508] This inhibition involves downstream activation of superoxide production and c-src activity, such that the well-known induction of Ang II by a low-K⁺ diet appears to play a major role in reducing distal tubular K⁺ secretion.[509]

Reports of transient postprandial kaliuresis in sheep, independent of changes in plasma K⁺ or aldosterone, have suggested that an enteric or hepatoportal K⁺ sensor controls kaliuresis via a sympathetic reflex; tissue kallikrein has recently emerged as a candidate mediator for this postprandial kaliuresis (see below).[510] Regardless of the signaling involved, changes in dietary K^+ absorption have a direct anticipatory effect on K^+ homeostasis in the absence of changes in plasma K^+. Such a feed-forward control has the theoretical advantage of greater stability because it operates prior to changes in plasma K^+.[511] Notably, changes in ROMK phosphorylation status and insulin-sensitive muscle uptake can be seen in K^+-deficient animals in the absence of a change in plasma K^+, suggesting that upstream activation of the major mechanisms that serve to reduce K^+ excretion (reduced K^+ secretion in the CNT and CCD, decreased peripheral uptake, and increased K^+ reabsorption in the OMCD) does not require changes in plasma K^+.[512] Consistent with this hypothesis, moderate K^+ restriction, without an associated drop in plasma K^+, is sufficient to induce Ang II–dependent superoxide generation and c-src activation, leading to inhibition of ROMK channel activity.[509]

VASOPRESSIN

Vasopressin has a well-characterized stimulatory effect on K^+ secretion by the distal nephron.[417,513] Teleologically, this vasopressin-dependent activation serves to preserve K^+ secretion during dehydration and extracellular volume depletion, when circulating levels of vasopressin are high and tubular delivery of Na^+ and fluid is reduced. The stimulation of basolateral V_2Rs results in an activation of ENaC, which increases the driving force for K^+ secretion by principal cells; the relevant mechanisms have been discussed earlier in this chapter (see "Regulation of Na^+-Cl^- Transport in the Connecting Tubule and Cortical Collecting Duct: Vasopressin and Other Factors"). In addition, vasopressin activates SK channels directly in the CCD, as does cAMP.[424,514] The ROMK is directly phosphorylated by PKA on three serine residues (S25, S200, and S294 in the ROMK2 isoform), with phosphorylation of all three sites required for full activity in *Xenopus* oocytes (see "Regulation of Na^+-Cl^- Transport by the Thick Ascending Limb: Activating Influences"). Finally, the stimulation of luminal V_1 receptors also stimulates K^+ secretion in the CCD, apparently via activation of BK channels.[515]

TISSUE KALLIKREIN

The serine protease tissue kallikrein (TK) is involved in the generation of kinins, ultimately stimulating the formation of bradykinin.[516] Within the kidney, TK is synthesized in CNT cells and released into the tubular lumen and peritubular interstitium. Although TK-induced bradykinin has a number of effects on distal tubular physiology, more recent data have revealed a provocative role in postprandial kaliuresis.[516] Thus, oral K^+-Cl^- loading leads to a spike in urinary K^+ and TK excretion in rats, mice, and humans.[516] The increase in urinary TK after K^+ loading is not accompanied by changes in urinary aldosterone and can be detected in aldosterone synthase knockout mice.[517] Mice deficient in TK demonstrate postprandial hyperkalemia, indicating a role for the protease in postprandial kaliuresis. This transient hyperkalemia is accompanied by a marked increase in K^+ reabsorption by perfused CCDs due to an upregulation of H^+/K^+-ATPase activity and an increase in $HK\alpha_2$-subunit transcript. The addition of luminal but not basolateral TK inhibits the activated CCD H^+/K^+-ATPase activity in the TK knockout mice, consistent with direct proteolytic activation. There is also a marked increase in Na^+ reabsorption by perfused CCDs from TK knockout mice, without development of a lumen-negative PD; this is consistent with an increased activity of the electroneutral Na^+-Cl^- cotransport mediated by the Na^+-driven SLC4A8 Cl^--HCO_3^- exchanger and the SLC26A4 Cl^--HCO_3^- exchanger (see also below).[349] This electroneutral transport pathway had previously been shown to be inhibited by bradykinin; hence, the activation by TK deletion presumably reflected loss of tonic inhibition by TK-generated bradykinin.[347] Previous data had indicated that TK mediates proteolytic cleavage of the γ-subunit of ENaC, with reduced ENaC activity in TK-deficient mice; net Na^+ balance is thus neutral in these mice.[518]

In summary, TK secretion from CNT cells is induced by oral K^+-Cl^- loading, causing proteolytic activation of ENaC and thus an increase in ENaC-driven K^+ secretion, bradykinin-dependent inhibition of electroneutral Na^+-Cl^- cotransport in the CCD.[347,349,518] There is consequently a further augmentation of electrogenic Na^+ transport (favoring K^+ secretion), and direct luminal inhibition of H^+/K^+-ATPase activity and thus a decrease or tonic inhibition of K^+ reabsorption. TK may very well be the postprandial factor that functions in feed-forward control of plasma K^+.[510,511]

INTEGRATED Na^+-Cl^- AND K^+ TRANSPORT IN THE DISTAL NEPHRON

In the classic model of renal K^+ secretion, the lumen-negative potential difference generated by Na^+ entry via ENaC induces the exit of K^+ via apical K^+-selective channels. This general scheme explains much of the known physiology and pathophysiology of renal K^+ secretion, yet has several key consequences that bear emphasis. First, enhanced Na^+-Cl^- reabsorption upstream of the CNT and CCD will reduce the delivery of luminal Na^+ to the CNT and CCD, decrease the lumen-negative potential difference, and thus decrease K^+ secretion; K^+ secretion by the CCD essentially stops when luminal Na^+ drops below 8 mmol/L.[420-422] In this respect, the increasingly refined phenotypic understanding of FHHt, caused by kinase-induced gain of function of the DCT (see also "Regulation of Na^+-Cl^- Transport in the Distal Convoluted Tubule"), has served to underscore that variation in NCC-dependent Na^+-Cl^- absorption, just upstream of the CNT, has truly profound effects on the ability to excrete dietary K^+.[281] Second, aldosterone is a kaliuretic hormone, induced by hyperkalemia. However, under certain circumstances associated with marked induction of aldosterone, such as dietary sodium restriction, sodium balance is maintained without effects on K^+ homeostasis. This so-called aldosterone paradox—how does the kidney independently regulate Na^+-Cl^- and K^+ handling by the aldosterone-sensitive distal nephron?—is only recently beginning to yield to investigative efforts. The major factors in the integrated control of Na^+-Cl^- and K^+ transport appear to include electroneutral thiazide-sensitive Na^+-Cl^- transport within the CCD (see "Connecting Tubules and the Cortical Collecting Duct: Electroneutral Na^+-Cl^- Cotransport"), ENaC-independent K^+ excretion within the distal nephron, and the differential regulation of various signaling pathways by aldosterone, Ang II, and dietary K^+.[347-349,454,519,520]

Thiazide-sensitive electroneutral Na^+-Cl^- transport within the CCD is evidently mediated by the parallel activity of the Na^+-driven SLC4A8 Cl^--HCO_3^- exchanger and the SLC26A4

Cl⁻-HCO₃⁻ exchanger (see also "Connecting Tubules and the Cortical Collecting Duct: Electroneutral Na⁺-Cl⁻ Cotransport").[349] The molecular identity of this transport mechanism has only emerged rather recently, so regulatory influences are not fully characterized.[349] However, electroneutral Na⁺-Cl⁻ transport within the CCD is evidently induced by volume depletion and mineralocorticoid treatment.[347-349] This mechanism appears to mediate about 50% of Na⁺ reabsorption in the CCD under these conditions, all without affecting the luminal PD and thus without direct effect on K⁺ excretion. Therefore, electroneutral, thiazide-sensitive Na⁺-Cl⁻ transport affords the ability to increase the reabsorption of Na⁺ within the CCD without affecting K⁺ excretion. The converse occurs after several days accommodation to a high-K⁺ diet, which increases the fraction of ENaC-independent, amiloride-resistant K⁺ excretion to about 50%. Again, this presumptively electroneutral, aldosterone-independent pathway for K⁺ excretion serves to uncouple distal tubular Na⁺ and K⁺ excretion.[454]

In a landmark study in 2003, Kahle and coworkers established that the WNK4 kinase, encoded by a disease gene for FHHt, causes inhibition of ROMK activity in *Xenopus* oocytes; FHHt-associated mutations potentiated this effect.[484] This identified WNK-dependent signaling as a major pathway for integrating Na⁺-Cl⁻ and K⁺ transport within the distal nephron. Details of the relevant effects of WNK kinases on NCC and ROMK are discussed earlier (see Figure 6.26, "Regulation of Distal K⁺ Transport," and "Regulation of Na⁺-Cl⁻ Transport in the Connecting Tubule and Cortical Collecting Duct"). However, key findings include the differential influence of K⁺ intake on circulating Ang II, ROMK activity (i.e., K⁺ secretory capacity), ratio of WNK1 isoforms, and activity of NCC in the DCT. Thus, Ang II activates NCC via the WNK4-SPAK pathway, reducing delivery of Na⁺ to the CNT and limiting K⁺ secretion.[310,521,522] In contrast, Ang II inhibits ROMK activity via several mechanisms, including downstream activation of c-src tyrosine kinases.[507-509] Whereas K⁺ restriction induces renin and circulating Ang II, increases in dietary K⁺ are suppressive.[509,523] A decrease in circulating and local Ang II partially explains why NCC phosphorylation and activity is downregulated by a high-K⁺ diet; teleologically, this serves to increase delivery of Na⁺ to the CNT, thus increasing K⁺ secretion.[314] The DCT also clearly functions as a potassium sensor, directly responding to changes in circulating potassium. Reduction in potassium intake and/or hypokalemia thus lead to reduced basolateral [K⁺] in the DCT; the subsequent hyperpolarization is dependent on basolateral KIR4.1-containing K⁺ channels.[317] Hyperpolarization leads to chloride exit via basolateral CLC-NKB chloride channels and a reduction in intracellular chloride; the reduction in intracellular chloride activates the SPAK and OSR1/WNK cascade, resulting in phosphorylation of NCC and activation of the transporter.[317] Finally, within principal cells, increases in aldosterone induce the SGK1 kinase, which phosphorylates WNK4 and attenuates the effect of WNK4 on ROMK, while activating ENaC via Nedd4-2-dependent effects (see "Regulation of Na⁺-Cl⁻ Transport in the Connecting Tubule and Cortical Collecting Duct").[524] However, when dietary K⁺ intake is reduced, c-src tyrosine kinase activity increases under the influence of increased Ang II, causing direction inhibition of ROMK activity via tyrosine phosphorylation of the channel (see "Regulation of Distal K⁺ Transport").[501,503,525] The increase in c-src tyrosine kinase activity also abrogates the effect of SGK1 on WNK4.[520]

Complete reference list available at ExpertConsult.com.

KEY REFERENCES

2. Chambrey R, Kurth I, Peti-Peterdi J, et al: Renal intercalated cells are rather energized by a proton than a sodium pump. *Proc Natl Acad Sci U S A* 110:7928–7933, 2013.
3. Sun A, Grossman EB, Lombardi M, et al: Vasopressin alters the mechanism of apical Cl⁻ entry from Na+:Cl⁻ to Na+:K+:2Cl⁻ cotransport in mouse medullary thick ascending limb. *J Membr Biol* 120:83–94, 1991.
8. Kokko JP: Proximal tubule potential difference. Dependence on glucose, HCO₃, and amino acids. *J Clin Invest* 52:1362–1367, 1973.
9. Alpern RJ, Howlin KJ, Preisig PA: Active and passive components of chloride transport in the rat proximal convoluted tubule. *J Clin Invest* 76:1360–1366, 1985.
13. Barratt LJ, Rector FC, Jr, Kokko JP, et al: Factors governing the transepithelial potential difference across the proximal tubule of the rat kidney. *J Clin Invest* 53:454–464, 1974.
15. Katz AI, Doucet A, Morel F: Na-K-ATPase activity along the rabbit, rat, and mouse nephron. *Am J Physiol* 237:F114–F120, 1979.
27. Muto S, Hata M, Taniguchi J, et al: Claudin-2-deficient mice are defective in the leaky and cation-selective paracellular permeability properties of renal proximal tubules. *Proc Natl Acad Sci U S A* 107:8011–8016, 2010.
29. Schnermann J, Chou CL, Ma T, et al: Defective proximal tubular fluid reabsorption in transgenic aquaporin-1 null mice. *Proc Natl Acad Sci U S A* 95:9660–9664, 1998.
31. Schnermann J, Huang Y, Mizel D: Fluid reabsorption in proximal convoluted tubules of mice with gene deletions of claudin-2 and/or aquaporin1. *Am J Physiol Renal Physiol* 305:F1352–F1364, 2013.
36. Bacic D, Kaissling B, McLeroy P, et al: Dopamine acutely decreases apical membrane Na/H exchanger NHE3 protein in mouse renal proximal tubule. *Kidney Int* 64:2133–2141, 2003.
38. Schultheis PJ, Clarke LL, Meneton P, et al: Renal and intestinal absorptive defects in mice lacking the NHE3 Na+/H+ exchanger. *Nat Genet* 19:282–285, 1998.
45. Wang T, Agulian SK, Giebisch G, et al: Effects of formate and oxalate on chloride absorption in rat distal tubule. *Am J Physiol* 264:F730–F736, 1993.
74. Wang T: Flow-activated transport events along the nephron. *Curr Opin Nephrol Hypertens* 15:530–536, 2006.
94. Thomson SC, Deng A, Wead L, et al: An unexpected role for angiotensin II in the link between dietary salt and proximal reabsorption. *J Clin Invest* 116:1110–1116, 2006.
101. Zhang MZ, Yao B, Wang S, et al: Intrarenal dopamine deficiency leads to hypertension and decreased longevity in mice. *J Clin Invest* 121:2845–2854, 2011.
142. Waldegger S, Jeck N, Barth P, et al: Barttin increases surface expression and changes current properties of ClC-K channels. *Pflugers Arch* 444:411–418, 2002.
144. Simon DB, Bindra RS, Mansfield TA, et al: Mutations in the chloride channel gene, CLCNKB, cause Bartter's syndrome type III. *Nat Genet* 17:171–178, 1997.
145. Estevez R, Boettger T, Stein V, et al: Barttin is a Cl⁻ channel beta-subunit crucial for renal Cl⁻ reabsorption and inner ear K+ secretion. *Nature* 414:558–561, 2001.
166. Rocha AS, Kokko JP: Sodium chloride and water transport in the medullary thick ascending limb of Henle. Evidence for active chloride transport. *J Clin Invest* 52:612–623, 1973.
167. Stokes JB: Consequences of potassium recycling in the renal medulla. Effects of ion transport by the medullary thick ascending limb of Henle's loop. *J Clin Invest* 70:219–229, 1982.
175. Xu JZ, Hall AE, Peterson LN, et al: Localization of the ROMK protein on apical membranes of rat kidney nephron segments. *Am J Physiol* F739–F748, 1997.
177. Lu M, Wang T, Yan Q, et al: ROMK is required for expression of the 70-pS K channel in the thick ascending limb. *Am J Physiol Renal Physiol* 286:F490–F495, 2004.

211. Gagnon KB, England R, Delpire E: Volume sensitivity of cation-chloride cotransporters is modulated by the interaction of two kinases: SPAK and WNK4. *Am J Physiol Cell Physiol* 290:C134–C142, 2006.
236. Riccardi D, Hall AE, Chattopadhyay N, et al: Localization of the extracellular Ca2+/polyvalent cation-sensing protein in rat kidney. *Am J Physiol* 274:F611–F622, 1998.
245. Trudu M, Janas S, Lanzani C, et al; Swiss Kidney Project on Genes in Hypertension (SKIPOGH) team: Common noncoding UMOD gene variants induce salt-sensitive hypertension and kidney damage by increasing uromodulin expression. *Nat Med* 19:1655–1660, 2013.
247. Loffing J, Kaissling B: Sodium and calcium transport pathways along the mammalian distal nephron: from rabbit to human. *Am J Physiol Renal Physiol* 284:F628–F643, 2003.
277. Zhang C, Wang L, Zhang J, et al: KCNJ10 determines the expression of the apical Na-Cl cotransporter (NCC) in the early distal convoluted tubule (DCT1). *Proc Natl Acad Sci U S A* 111:11864–11869, 2014.
278. Kotelevtsev Y, Brown RW, Fleming S, et al: Hypertension in mice lacking 11beta-hydroxysteroid dehydrogenase type 2. *J Clin Invest* 103:683–689, 1999.
281. Lalioti MD, Zhang J, Volkman HM, et al: Wnk4 controls blood pressure and potassium homeostasis via regulation of mass and activity of the distal convoluted tubule. *Nat Genet* 38:1124–1132, 2006.
297. Vidal-Petiot E, Elvira-Matelot E, Mutig K, et al: WNK1-related familial hyperkalemic hypertension results from an increased expression of L-WNK1 specifically in the distal nephron. *Proc Natl Acad Sci U S A* 110:14366–14371, 2013.
299. Vitari AC, Deak M, Morrice NA, et al: The WNK1 and WNK4 protein kinases that are mutated in Gordon's hypertension syndrome phosphorylate and activate SPAK and OSR1 protein kinases. *Biochem J* 391:17–24, 2005.
302. Boyden LM, Choi M, Choate KA, et al: Mutations in Kelch-like 3 and cullin 3 cause hypertension and electrolyte abnormalities. *Nature* 482:98–102, 2012.
317. Terker AS, Zhang C, McCormick JA, et al: Potassium modulates electrolyte balance and blood pressure through effects on distal cell voltage and chloride. *Cell Metab* 21:39–50, 2015.
345. Verlander JW, Kim YH, Shin W, et al: Dietary Cl(−) restriction upregulates pendrin expression within the apical plasma membrane of type B intercalated cells. *Am J Physiol Renal Physiol* 291:F833–F839, 2006.
362. Snyder PM, Olson DR, Thomas BC: Serum and glucocorticoid-regulated kinase modulates Nedd4-2-mediated inhibition of the epithelial Na+ channel. *J Biol Chem* 277:5–8, 2002.
368. Soundararajan R, Ziera T, Koo E, et al: Scaffold protein connector enhancer of kinase suppressor of Ras isoform 3 (CNK3) coordinates assembly of a multiprotein epithelial sodium channel (ENaC)-regulatory complex. *J Biol Chem* 287:33014–33025, 2012.
374. Kleyman TR, Carattino MD, Hughey RP: ENaC at the cutting edge: regulation of epithelial sodium channels by proteases. *J Biol Chem* 284:20447–20451, 2009.
378. Kashlan OB, Blobner BM, Zuzek Z, et al: Na+ inhibits the epithelial Na+ channel by binding to a site in an extracellular acidic cleft. *J Biol Chem* 290:568–576, 2015.
380. Bugaj V, Pochynyuk O, Stockand JD: Activation of the epithelial Na+ channel in the collecting duct by vasopressin contributes to water reabsorption. *Am J Physiol Renal Physiol* 297:F1411–F1418, 2009.
385. Mironova E, Chen Y, Pao AC, et al: Activation of ENaC by AVP contributes to the urinary concentrating mechanism and dilution of plasma. *Am J Physiol Renal Physiol* 308:F237–F243, 2015.
397. Nakagawa K, Holla VR, Wei Y, et al: Salt-sensitive hypertension is associated with dysfunctional Cyp4a10 gene and kidney epithelial sodium channel. *J Clin Invest* 116:1696–1702, 2006.
398. Guan Y, Hao C, Cha DR, et al: Thiazolidinediones expand body fluid volume through PPARgamma stimulation of ENaC-mediated renal salt absorption. *Nat Med* 11:861–866, 2005.
432. Palmer LG, Frindt G: High-conductance K channels in intercalated cells of the rat distal nephron. *Am J Physiol Renal Physiol* 292:F966–F973, 2007.
433. Holtzclaw JD, Grimm PR, Sansom SC: Intercalated cell BK-alpha/beta4 channels modulate sodium and potassium handling during potassium adaptation. *J Am Soc Nephrol* 21:634–645, 2010.
449. Amorim JB, Bailey MA, Musa-Aziz R, et al: Role of luminal anion and pH in distal tubule potassium secretion. *Am J Physiol Renal Physiol* 284:F381–F388, 2003.
471. Yang L, Frindt G, Palmer LG: Magnesium modulates ROMK channel-mediated potassium secretion. *J Am Soc Nephrol* 21:2109–2116, 2010.
475. Palmer LG, Frindt G: Aldosterone and potassium secretion by the cortical collecting duct. *Kidney Int* 57:1324–1328, 2000.
476. Palmer LG, Antonian L, Frindt G: Regulation of apical K and Na channels and Na/K pumps in rat cortical collecting tubule by dietary K. *J Gen Physiol* 104:693–710, 1994.
480. Palmer LG, Frindt G: Regulation of apical K channels in rat cortical collecting tubule during changes in dietary K intake. *Am J Physiol* 277:F805–F812, 1999.
520. Yue P, Lin DH, Pan CY, et al: Src family protein tyrosine kinase (PTK) modulates the effect of SGK1 and WNK4 on ROMK channels. *Proc Natl Acad Sci U S A* 106:15061–15066, 2009.

The Regulation of Calcium, Magnesium, and Phosphate Excretion by the Kidney

Theresa J. Berndt | James R. Thompson | Rajiv Kumar

CHAPTER OUTLINE

CALCIUM TRANSPORT IN THE KIDNEY, 185
Role of Calcium in Cellular Processes, 185
Calcium Present in Serum in Bound and Free Forms, 186
Regulation of Calcium Homeostasis by the Parathyroid Hormone–Vitamin D Endocrine System, 187
Reabsorption of Calcium along the Tubule, 187
Regulation of Ca^{2+} Transport in the Kidney, 189
Regulation of Renal Calcium Transport by Novel Proteins, 191
Structures of Proteins Involved in the Transport of Calcium, 191
MAGNESIUM TRANSPORT IN THE KIDNEY, 193
Role of Magnesium in Cellular Processes, 193
Magnesium Present in Serum in Bound and Free Forms, 193
Regulation of Magnesium Homeostasis, 193
Reabsorption of Magnesium along the Tubule, 194
Regulation of Magnesium Transport in the Kidney, 195
Structures of Proteins Involved in the Transport of Magnesium, 195
PHOSPHORUS TRANSPORT IN THE KIDNEY, 196
Role of Phosphorus in Cellular Processes, 196
Phosphorus Present In Blood in Multiple Forms, 196
Regulation of Phosphate Homeostasis: An Integrated View, 197
Reabsorption of Phosphate along the Nephron, 198
Regulation of Phosphate Transport in the Kidney, 199
Structures of Proteins Involved in the Transport of Phosphorus, 202

In this chapter, we will discuss how the kidney regulates calcium, phosphorus, and magnesium balance and the manner in which various hormones and factors alter the efficiency with which these substances are reabsorbed by the kidney. The molecular processes responsible for the reabsorption of these substances by the kidney and the localization of the cognate molecular machinery along the nephron are unique for calcium, phosphorus, and magnesium. In the case of calcium and phosphorus, similar hormones regulate the efficiency of renal reabsorption, although specific factors for each substance also function to regulate reabsorption. With magnesium, the molecular mediators of reabsorption are poorly regulated, and the precise hormonal factors involved in the regulation of magnesium reabsorption by the nephron are less well defined.

CALCIUM TRANSPORT IN THE KIDNEY

ROLE OF CALCIUM IN CELLULAR PROCESSES

Calcium is an abundant cation in the body (Table 7.1). Several biochemical and physiologic processes, including nerve conduction and function, coagulation, enzyme activity, exocytosis, and bone mineralization, are critically dependent on normal calcium concentrations in extracellular fluid.[1-3] Not unexpectedly, intricate mechanisms exist to maintain extracellular fluid calcium concentrations within a narrow range and to maintain calcium balance. Significant decreases in serum calcium concentrations are associated with Chvostek's and Trousseau's signs, tetany and, when profound, generalized seizures.[4-6] A deficiency in calcium

Table 7.1 Composition of the Whole Body*

Body Weight (kg)	Water† (g)	Fat† (g)	Water (g)	N (g)	Na (mEq)	K (mEq)	Cl (mEq)	Mg (g)	Ca (g)	P (g)	Fe (mg)	Cu (mg)	Zn (mg)	B (mg)	Co (mg)
70	605	160	720	34	80	69	50	0.47	22.4	12.0	74	1.7	28	0.37	0.02

*As determined by chemical analysis (values per kilogram fat-free tissue, unless otherwise indicated).
†Per kilogram whole-body weight.

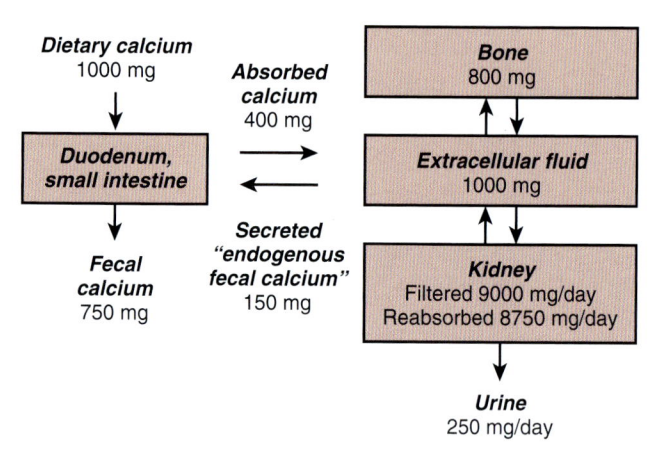

Figure 7.1 Calcium homeostasis in normal humans showing the amounts of calcium absorbed in the intestine and reabsorbed by the kidney.

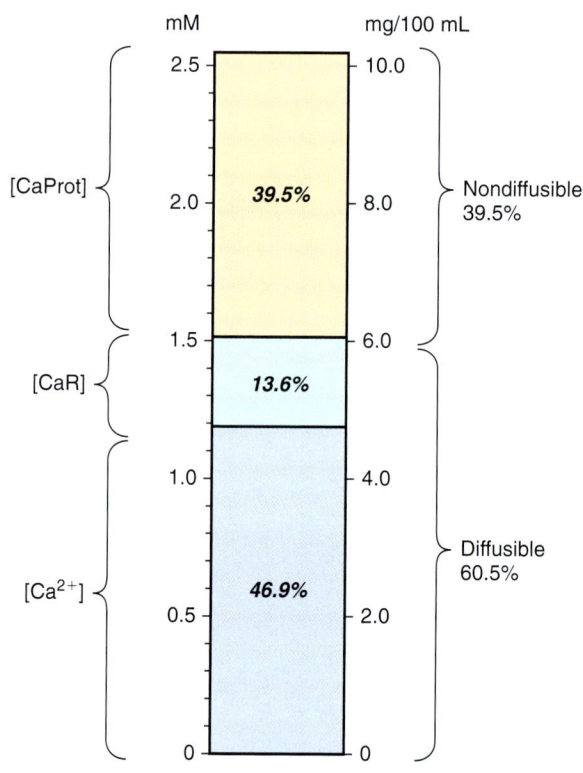

Figure 7.2 Components of serum total calcium assessed by ultrafiltration data in normal human subjects. CaProt, Protein-bound calcium; CaR, diffusible calcium complexes; Ca^{2+}, ionized calcium. (Redrawn from Moore EW: Ionized calcium in normal serum, ultrafiltrates, and whole blood determined by ion-exchange electrodes. *J Clin Invest* 1970;49:318-334, with permission of the publisher.)

absorption in the intestine, such as occurs in vitamin D deficiency, is associated with secondary hyperparathyroidism, hypophosphatemia, and rickets or osteomalacia.[5,6] Hypercalcemia, with attendant hypercalciuria, is associated with a reduced capacity to concentrate urine,[7-9] volume depletion, and nephrocalcinosis and renal stones.[10,11] As shown in Figure 7.1, the intestine and kidney are important in the absorption and reabsorption and excretion of calcium. Following absorption in the intestine, calcium in the extracellular fluid space is deposited in bone (the major repository of calcium in the body) and is filtered in the kidney. The concentration of calcium in serum varies with age and gender, with higher values being present in children and adolescent subjects than in adults.

CALCIUM PRESENT IN SERUM IN BOUND AND FREE FORMS

Calcium is present in plasma in filterable (60% of total calcium) and bound (40% of total calcium) forms. Filterable calcium is comprised of calcium complexed to anions such as citrate, sulfate, and phosphate (~10% of total calcium) and ionized calcium (~50% of total calcium; Figure 7.2).[12] The percentage of calcium bound to proteins (predominantly albumin and, to a lesser extent, globulins), and, the amount of filterable calcium, is dependent on plasma pH.[12] Alkalemia is associated with a reduction in free calcium, whereas acidemia is associated with an increase in free calcium. A 1-g/dL change in serum albumin is associated with a 0.8-mg/dL change in total serum calcium, and a 1-g/dL change in globulins is associated with a 0.16-mg/dL change in total serum calcium. An equation defining the amount of calcium (mmol/L) bound to albumin and globulins (g/L) as a function of pH is as follows[12]:

$$[CaProt] = 0.019[Alb] - [(0.42)([Alb]/47.3)(7.42 - pH)] + 0.004[Glob] - [(0.42)([Glob]/25.0)(7.42 - pH)]$$

If one assumes that all calcium is bound to albumin, the following equation applies:

$$[CaProt] = 0.0211[Alb] - [(0.42)([Alb]/47.3)(7.42 - pH)]$$

A nomogram describing this relationship is shown in Figure 7.3.

$$[CaProt] = [0.0211[Alb]] - [(0.42)\frac{[Alb]}{47.3}(7.42 - pH)]$$

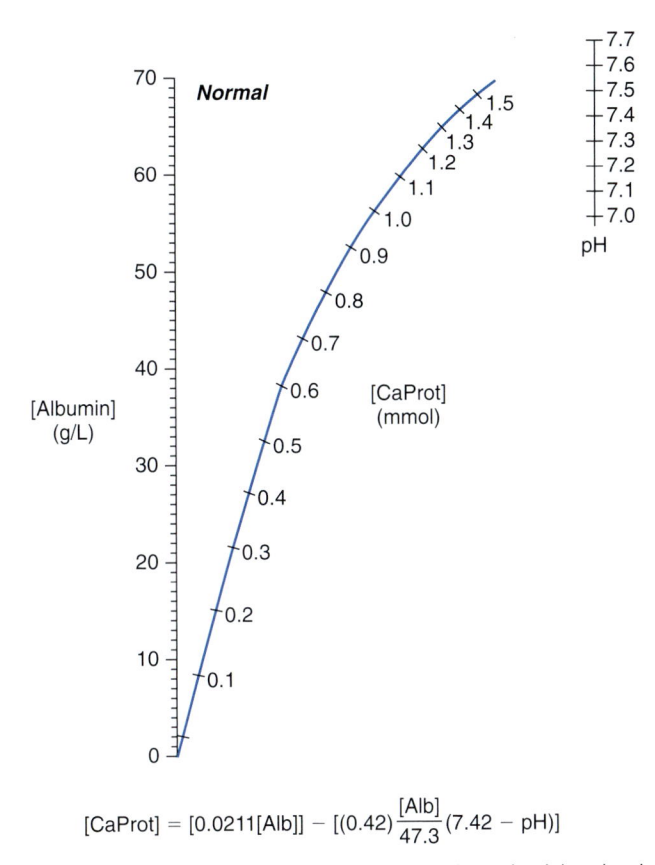

Figure 7.3 Nomogram for estimating protein-bound calcium levels [CaProt] in normal humans. [CaProt] is obtained by connecting observed albumin and pH values with a straight line and reading the point at which it intersects the curve. The equation describing the relationship among [CaProt], serum albumin concentrations, and pH is shown at the bottom of the graph. (Redrawn from Moore EW: Ionized calcium in normal serum, ultrafiltrates, and whole blood determined by ion-exchange electrodes. *J Clin Invest* 1970;49:318-334, with permission of the publisher.)

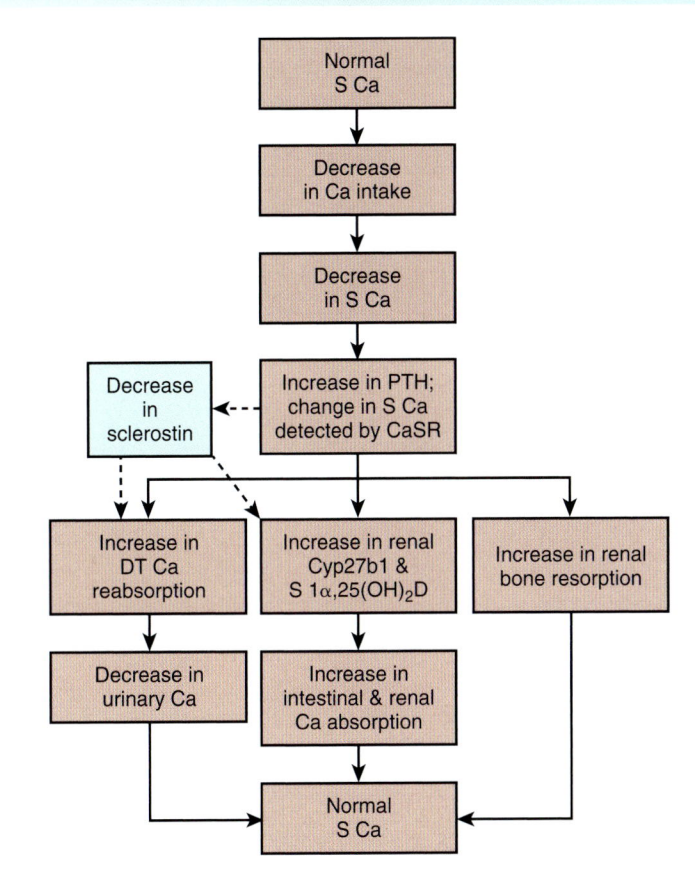

S = serum; Ca = calcium; CaSR = calcium-sensing receptor
Cyp27b1 = 25(OH)D_3–1-hydroxylase cytochrome P450;
DT = distal tubule

Figure 7.4 Changes in parathyroid hormone (PTH) and 1α,25-dihydroxyvitamin D 1α-25(OH)$_2$D and the subsequent physiologic changes in intestinal calcium absorption or renal calcium reabsorption following perturbations in serum calcium. The effects of PTH on sclerostin concentrations, and the effect of sclerostin *(green)* on tubular transport and 1α,25(OH)$_2$D synthesis, are also shown.

REGULATION OF CALCIUM HOMEOSTASIS BY THE PARATHYROID HORMONE–VITAMIN D ENDOCRINE SYSTEM

In states of neutral calcium balance, the amount of calcium absorbed by the intestine is equivalent to the amount excreted by the kidney.[13] The central role of the parathyroid hormone–vitamin D endocrine system in the regulation of calcium homeostasis is well recognized and is summarized in Figure 7.4.[14-16] In response to reductions in calcium intake and subsequent decreases in the serum calcium level, parathyroid hormone release from the parathyroid glands is increased. The change in serum calcium concentration is detected by the parathyroid gland calcium-sensing receptor, a G protein–coupled receptor, which alters parathyroid hormone release from the parathyroid cell.[17-20] Parathyroid hormone enhances the efficiency of calcium transport in the distal tubule of the kidney[21-23] and increases the activity of the renal 25-hydroxyvitamin D 1α-hydroxylase, which enhances the formation of 1α,25-dihydroxyvitamin D (1α,25(OH)$_2$D), the active metabolite of vitamin D.[24] The reader is referred to reviews by Kumar and colleagues[25] concerning details of the regulation of the synthesis of 1α,25(OH)$_2$D. 1α,25(OH)$_2$D increases the efficiency of calcium transport in the intestine[26-28] and in the kidney.[29-33] The effects of parathyroid hormone and 1α,25(OH)$_2$D restore calcium balance by increasing the amount of calcium accreted. At the same time, parathyroid hormone[34-36] and 1α,25(OH)$_2$D[37,38] increase bone calcium mobilization and help maintain serum calcium concentrations. The converse series of events occurs in hypercalcemic circumstances.

REABSORPTION OF CALCIUM ALONG THE TUBULE

The kidney reabsorbs filtered calcium in amounts that are subject to regulation by calciotropic hormones, parathyroid hormone (PTH), and 1α,25(OH)$_2$D.[15,25,39-44] The glomerulus filters 9000 to 10,000 mg of complexed and ionized calcium in a 24-hour period. The amount of calcium appearing in the urine is approximately 250 mg/day, and it is therefore evident that a large percentage of filtered calcium is reabsorbed. As a result of reabsorption processes that occur in both the proximal and distal tubules, only 1% to 2% of calcium filtered at the glomerulus appears in the urine.[41,43,44] Figure 7.5 shows the percentages of calcium reabsorbed along different segments of the nephron.

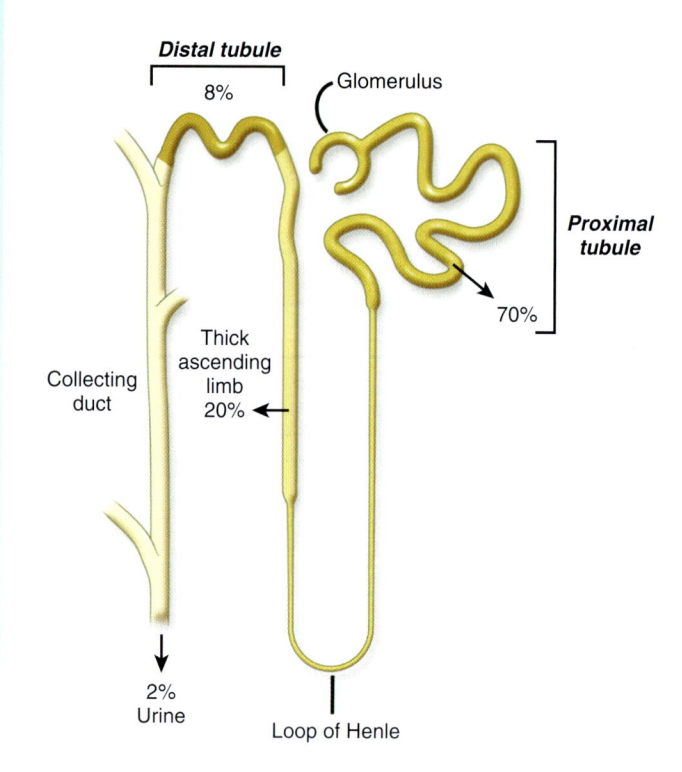

Figure 7.5 Percentages of filtered calcium reabsorbed along the tubule.

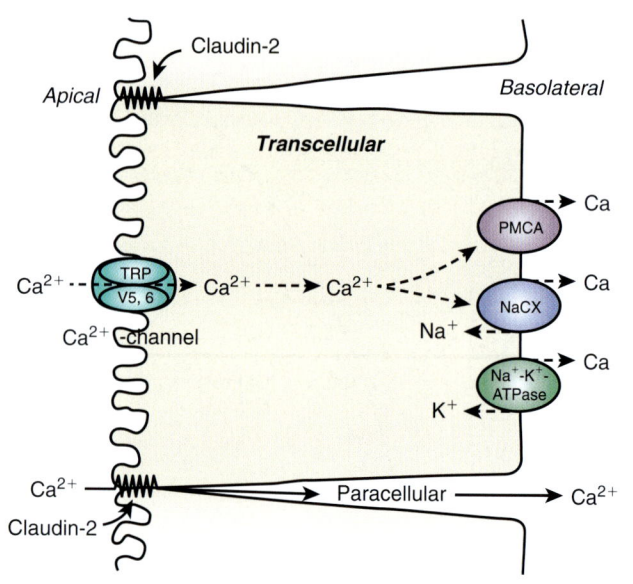

Figure 7.6 Mechanisms whereby calcium is transported in the proximal tubule. Most calcium is reabsorbed by paracellular mechanisms. A smaller percentage is reabsorbed by transcellular mechanisms.

Ca^{2+} REABSORPTION IN THE PROXIMAL TUBULE

This reabsorption is predominantly passive. As noted earlier, about 60% to 70% of total plasma calcium is free (not protein-bound) and is filtered at the glomerulus.[45,46] A large percentage (~70%) of filtered calcium (Ca^{2+}) is reabsorbed in the proximal tubule (PT), mainly by paracellular processes that are linked with Na^+ reabsorption.[45,47-50] In this nephron segment, the reabsorption of Na^+ and Ca^{2+} is proportional under a variety of conditions[49,51] and is not dissociated following the administration of several factors known to alter renal Ca^{2+} reabsorption, such as PTH, cyclic adenosine monophosphate (cAMP), chlorothiazide, furosemide, acetazolamide, or changes in the hydrogen ion content.[48,49,52,53] The precise cellular and molecular mechanisms responsible for the movement of Ca^{2+} from the lumen of the proximal tubule into the interstitial space are not clearly defined. Most Ca^{2+} is believed to move in between cells (paracellular movement), with a smaller, but significant, transcellular component (Figure 7.6). The components of the paracellular pathway include claudin-2. Ca^{2+} permeates through claudin-2[54] and simultaneously competitively inhibits Na^+ conductance.[55] A transcellular component of Ca^{2+} reabsorption may also be present in the proximal tubule. Undefined Ca^{2+} channels and intracellular Ca^{2+} binding proteins influence the movement of Ca^{2+} into and across the cell. The Na^+-K^+-ATPase has been implicated in transcellular Ca^{2+} transport in the proximal tubule,[56] and both the Na^+-Ca^{2+} exchanger[57] and isoforms 1 and 4 of the plasma membrane Ca^{2+} pump[58,59] are expressed in the proximal tubule and could be important in the movement of Ca^{2+} out of the proximal tubule cell. Although the proximal tubule reabsorbs large amounts of Ca^{2+}, primarily by paracellular processes, the rate of Ca^{2+} reabsorption is not influenced by factors or hormones that regulate calcium balance.[48,49,52] However, in conditions such as volume depletion, in which proximal tubule Na^+ reabsorption is increased, one also observes enhanced Ca^{2+} reabsorption, which can contribute to the hypercalcemia that is sometimes seen in such situations. The salutary effects of isotonic saline administration in patients with hypercalcemia are attributable to a reduction in Ca^{2+} reabsorption as a result of reduced Na^+ reabsorption.

Ca^{2+} REABSORPTION IN THE LOOP OF HENLE

The thin descending and thin ascending limbs of the loop of Henle do not transport significant amounts of Ca^{2+}.[60,61] Of filtered Ca^{2+}, 20% to 25% is reabsorbed in the thick ascending limb of Henle primarily by the paracellular route involving claudins 16 and 19.[45,60-71] Thick ascending limb cells express the furosemide-sensitive Na^+-K^+-$2Cl^-$ cotransporter, NKCC2,[72-75] which mediates the reabsorption of Na^+ and thereby contributes to the driving force for paracellular Ca^{2+} transport. A lumen-positive transepithelial potential is generated in the thick ascending limb of the loop of Henle through the activity of the NKCC2 (Na^+-K^+-$2Cl^-$ cotransporter)[76] by two mechanisms, secondary apical recycling of K^+ via the renal outer medullary potassium (ROMK) channel and a NaCl diffusion potential generated by reabsorbed NaCl establishing a concentration gradient across the Na-selective paracellular pathway. This transepithelial voltage provides the driving force for passive Ca^{2+} reabsorption through the paracellular pathway.

The specific role played by claudins in the tight junction of the thick ascending limb of Henle in Ca^{2+} reabsorption (and Mg^{2+} reabsorption, as discussed in the next section) is controversial. Together with claudin-19, claudin-16 forms a paracellular pore and a heteromeric claudin-16, and claudin-19 interaction is required to assemble and traffic to the tight junction and to generate cation-selective paracellular channels.[77,78] It has been postulated that these channels are themselves responsible for permeating divalent cations, Ca^{2+} and Mg^{2+}, via the paracellular route.[79,80] An alternative prevailing hypothesis is that claudins 16 and 19 form Na^+ channels and act primarily to establish the transepithelial NaCl diffusion potential, thus contributing to the driving force for divalent cation reabsorption.[77,78,81,82] Regardless of the mechanism, loss of function mutations in the genes encoding claudin-16 and claudin-19 result in familial hypomagnesemia with hypercalciuria and nephrocalcinosis, which is characterized by renal Ca^{2+} and Mg^{2+} wasting because of defective thick ascending limb divalent cation reabsorption. Similarly, mutations of NKCC2 are associated with the common form of Bartter's syndrome, which, like the other Bartter's forms, can be associated with hypercalciuria.[83]

There is considerable species heterogeneity with respect to responses to calcium-regulating hormones by the thick ascending limb; in the mouse, PTH and calcitonin (CT) stimulate Ca^{2+} transport in the cortical thick ascending limb,[64,66,84,85] whereas in the rabbit CT stimulates calcium reabsorption in the medullary thick ascending limb but not in the cortical thick ascending limb.[69] Extracellular fluid calcium also regulates calcium reabsorption in this segment through the Ca^{2+}-sensing receptor (see below).

Ca^{2+} REABSORPTION IN THE DISTAL TUBULE

This reabsorption is hormonally regulated, transcellular, and active and is mediated by specific channels, proteins, and pumps. In the distal convoluted tubule (primarily DCT2) and connecting tubule (together abbreviated as DT), 5% to 10% of filtered Ca^{2+} is reabsorbed[86-88] by active transport processes against electrical and concentration gradients. Ca^{2+} reabsorption in this segment of the nephron is regulated by PTH,[21-23] calcitonin,[84,85] and $1\alpha,25(OH)_2D_3$,[29-33] hormones that increase the efficiency of Ca^{2+} reabsorption in this nephron segment. Ca^{2+} reabsorption in the DT occurs via a transcellular pathway. Mediators of Ca^{2+} transport in the renal DT include apically situated, transient receptor potential cation channels, subfamily V, types 5 and 6 channels (TRPV5, TRPV6), which mediate the increase in Ca^{2+} uptake from the lumen into the cell[44,89-94]; micropuncture studies in knockout mice have indicated that TRPV5 is the gatekeeper of Ca^{2+} reabsorption in the accessible DT in mice (Figure 7.7A).[91] Intracellular Ca^{2+} binding proteins such as calbindin D9K and D28K facilitate the movement of Ca^{2+} across the cell,[40,95] and the basolateral plasma membrane calcium (PMCA) pump,[39,40,42] Na^+-Ca^{2+} exchanger (NaCX),[96-99] and Na^+-Ca^{2+}-K^+ exchanger (NaCKX)[100] increase the rate of extrusion of Ca^{2+} across the basolateral membrane (see Figure 7.7B and C). The Na^+ gradient for the activity of the NaCX and the NaCKX is provided by the Na^+-K^+-ATPase situated at the basolateral cell membrane (not shown).

REGULATION OF Ca^{2+} TRANSPORT IN THE KIDNEY

CALCIUM-REGULATING HORMONES

Calcium-regulating hormones alter the expression of calcium channels, calcium-binding proteins, calcium pumps, and exchangers in the kidney by varied mechanisms. PTH increases the activity of TRPV5 channels in the kidney by activating cAMP-PKA (protein kinase A) signaling and phosphorylating a threonine residue within the channel, resulting in an increase in the open probability of the channel.[100,101] PTH also activates the PKC pathway and increases the numbers of TRPV5 channels on the surface of tubular cells by inhibiting endocytosis of the caveolae in which the channels are located.[102] $1\alpha,25(OH)_2D_3$ enhances the expression of TRPV5 and TRPV6 channels present in the distal and connecting tubules and cortical collecting duct by increasing respective messenger RNA (mRNA) concentrations through increased binding of the vitamin D receptor to response elements in the gene promoters.[32,93] $1\alpha,25(OH)_2D_3$ increases the expression of calbindin D9K and D28K and the PMCA pump in the kidney and cultured renal cells.[32,59,103-112] The effect of PTH and $1\alpha,25(OH)_2D_3$ is to increase the expression of Ca^{2+} channels, binding proteins, pumps, and exchangers, thereby increasing the retention of calcium by the kidney.

EXTRACELLULAR CALCIUM

The level of extracellular calcium regulates renal Ca^{2+} reabsorption by signaling through the Ca-sensing receptor (CaSR). In the kidney, the CaSR is primarily expressed on the basolateral membrane of the thick ascending limb of the loop of Henle (TALH). Activation of the CaSR reduces renal tubular Ca^{2+} reabsorption and induces calciuresis in response to a Ca load.[113,114] One mechanism is by inhibition of NKCC2 expression[114] or activity. More recently, it has been suggested that CaSR acts primarily by regulating paracellular permeability. Loupy and colleagues have shown that a CaSR antagonist increases Ca^{2+} permeability in isolated perfused TALH, with no change in transepithelial voltage or Na flux.[115] This appears to be mediated by regulation of the expression of claudin-14. Activation of the CaSR causes robust upregulation of claudin-14,[116,117] which, through physical interaction, inhibits paracellular cation channels formed by claudin-16 and claudin-19.[116] The signaling mechanism seems to involve CaSR inhibiting calcineurin, a phosphatase that normally activates the nuclear factor of activated T cells (NFAT) to increase transcription of two micro-RNAs, miR-9 and miR-374, thereby downregulating claudin-14 expression.[116,118] The central role of claudin-14 is further supported by the finding that claudin-14 knockout mice are unable to increase their fractional excretion of calcium in response to a high-Ca^{2+} diet[116] and exhibit complete loss of regulation of urinary Ca^{2+} excretion in response to a CaSR agonist or antagonist.[118]

DIURETICS

Loop diuretics such as furosemide increase urinary calcium losses. The mechanism whereby furosemide causes hypercalciuria is linked to its ability to bind to and inhibit the furosemide-sensitive Na^+-K^+-$2Cl^-$ cotransporter type 2, NKCC2,[72-75] present in the TALH. NaCl absorption is diminished, as is potassium recycling, resulting in a reduction in lumen positivity that drives Ca^{2+} reabsorption. Subjects with the common form of Bartter's syndrome have inactivating mutations of the NKCC2, which are associated with calciuria.[83] Compensatory increases occur in the expression of distal tubule transport channels and proteins, such as the TRPV5 and TRPV6 channels and calbindin D28K following

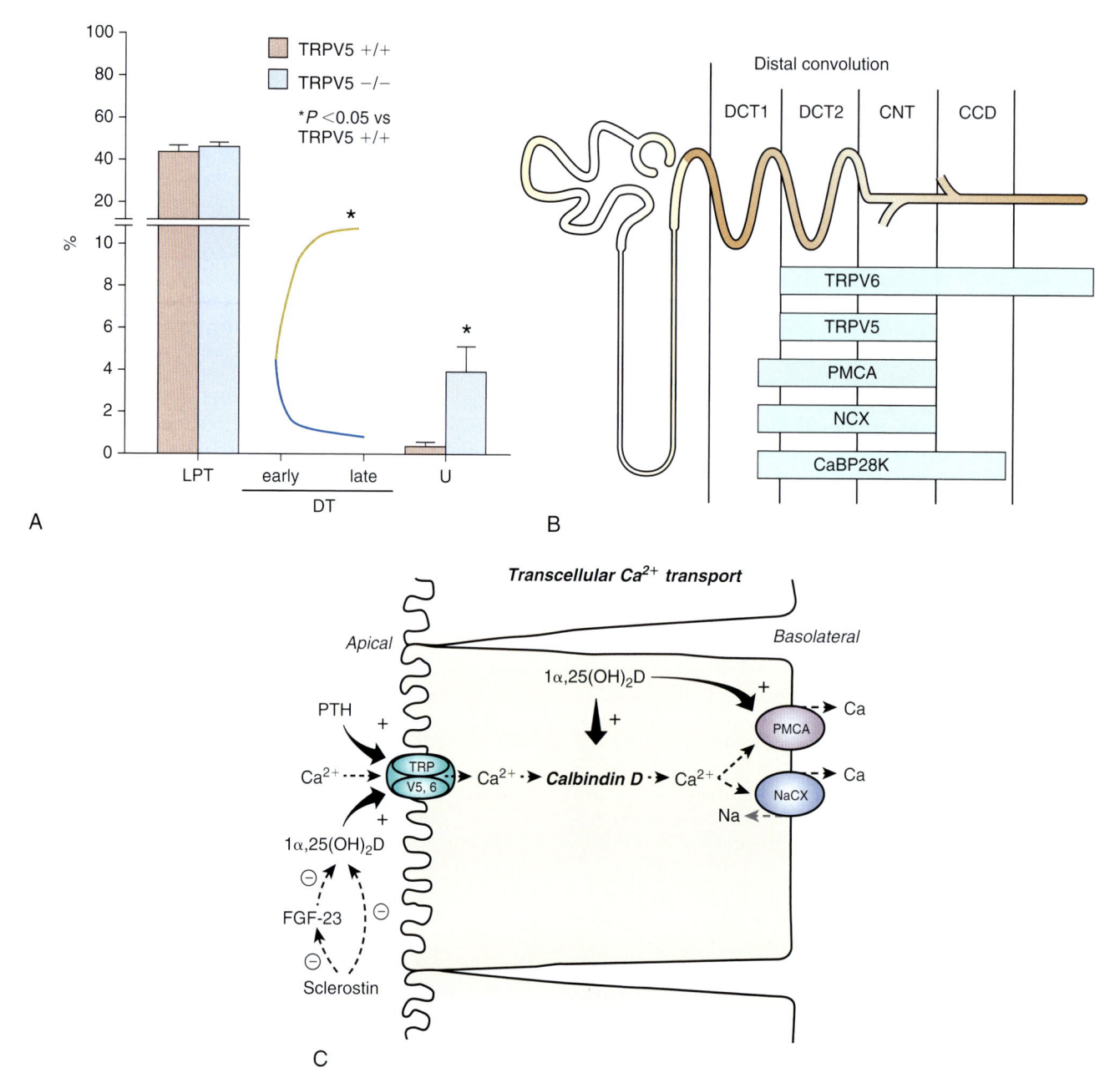

Figure 7.7 Mechanisms of calcium transport in the distal nephron. **A,** Role of TRPV5 investigated by micropuncture of kidneys from TRPV5 knockout mice. The figure shows fractional Ca^{2+} delivery to micropuncture sites in the late proximal tubule (LPT) to sites located along the distal convolution (DT) from early to late DT (as localized using tubular K$^+$ concentrations) and to the urine (U). Deletion of TRPV5 in mice prevents Ca^{2+} reabsorption along the DT, and there is even evidence for Ca^{2+} leaking back into the lumen, possibly by paracellular routes. TRPV6 may partially compensate in the collecting duct. **B,** Distribution of 1α,25(OH)$_2$D or parathyroid hormone (PTH)–sensitive channels and transporters along the distal convoluted tubules (DCT1 and DCT2), connecting tubule (CNT), and cortical and medullary collecting ducts (CCD and MCD). **C,** Ca transport in the DT occurs by transcellular mechanisms. Transcellular Ca transport is mediated by several channels, pumps, and exchangers located at the apical and basolateral portions of the cell. 1α,25(OH)$_2$D, 1α,25-dihydroxyvitamin D; FGF, fibroblast growth factor. (Modified from Kumar R, Vallon V: Reduced renal calcium excretion in the absence of sclerostin expression: evidence for a novel calcium-regulating bone kidney axis. *J Am Soc Nephrol* 25:2159-2168, 2014, with permission of the publisher.)

the administration of furosemide, but fail to compensate for the increase in excretion that occurs in the TALH.[119]

Thiazide diuretics, on the other hand, cause hypocalciuria,[93,120-122] and the effect appears to be independent of PTH in humans and rodents. Thiazides bind to and inhibit the Na-Cl cotransporter in the distal tubule.[72,123] Chronic thiazide use is associated with a reduction in extracellular fluid volume, which secondarily enhances Na$^+$ and Ca^{2+} reabsorption in the proximal tubule of the kidney.[53] Distal tubule Ca^{2+} transport is clearly unaffected by *chronic* thiazide use,[53] in contrast to older reports that thiazide *acutely* increases Ca^{2+} reabsorption in an isolated perfused DCT.[124] The development of hypocalciuria parallels a compensatory increase in Na$^+$ reabsorption secondary to an initial natriuresis following thiazide administration. These observations are supported by the upregulation of the Na$^+$-H$^+$ exchanger, responsible for most of the Na$^+$ and associated Ca^{2+} reabsorption in the proximal tubule, whereas the expression of proteins involved in active Ca^{2+} transport in the distal tubule was unaltered. Indeed, thiazide administration was associated with hypocalciuria in *Trpv5* knockout mice. Humans with Gitelman's syndrome and inactivating mutations of the thiazide-sensitive Na-Cl transporter have hypocalciuria, hypomagnesemia, and volume depletion,[88,125-127] findings that are recapitulated in Na-Cl cotransporter knockout mice.[128]

ESTROGENS

Estrogens influence calcium transport in the kidney because postmenopausal women have higher urinary Ca^{2+} excretion than premenopausal women.[129] In the early postmenopausal period, the administration of estrogen is associated with a decrease in urine Ca^{2+} excretion and an increase in serum PTH and 1α,25(OH)$_2$D levels.[130,131] Estradiol increases the expression of the TRPV5 channel in the kidney in a manner independent of 1α,25(OH)$_2$D$_3$.[132] These observations are supported by reduced duodenal TRPV5 channel expression in mice lacking the estrogen receptor alpha.[133]

METABOLIC ACIDOSIS AND ALKALOSIS

Metabolic acidosis is associated with hypercalciuria and, when prolonged, often results in bone loss and osteoporosis.[134] Metabolic acidosis and metabolic alkalosis decrease or increase the reabsorption of Ca^{2+} in the distal tubule,[52,135-138] expression of TRPV5 in the distal tubule,[139] and activity of TRPV5 channels.[140-142]

REGULATION OF RENAL CALCIUM TRANSPORT BY NOVEL PROTEINS

KLOTHO

Klotho is a co-receptor for the phosphaturic peptide, fibroblast growth factor 23 (FGF-23), with β-glucuronidase activity.[143-146] It is a kidney- and parathyroid gland–specific protein, which influences epithelial Ca^{2+} transport by deglycosylating TRPV5, thereby trapping the channel in the plasma membrane and sustaining the activity of the channel.[147] Further evaluation of serum Klotho concentrations and their association with changes in renal calcium excretion are required to establish a role for this factor in the regulation of renal calcium transport.

SCLEROSTIN

Sclerostin is an osteocyte-derived glycoprotein that influences bone mass.[148] Patients with sclerosteosis and its milder variant, van Buchem's disease,[149-151] have exceptionally dense bones and skeletal overgrowth that often constricts cranial nerve foramina and the foramen magnum, resulting in premature death. Sclerosteosis is caused by inactivating mutations of the sclerostin (*SOST*) gene, and the milder van Buchem's disease is caused by a 52-kb deletion of a downstream enhancer element of the sclerostin gene.[152] Mouse models of sclerosteosis have increases in skeletal mass similar to those found in patients with the disease[153-156] and, by using a *Sost* gene knockout model generated in our laboratory,[153] we have demonstrated that sclerostin, directly or indirectly, through an alteration in the synthesis of 1α,25(OH)$_2$D, influences renal calcium reabsorption in the kidney. Urinary calcium excretion and renal fractional excretion of calcium are decreased in *Sost*$^{-/-}$ mice.[153] Serum 1α,25(OH)$_2$D concentrations are increased without attendant hypercalcemia; renal 25(OH)D-1α hydroxylase (*Cyp27b1*) mRNA and protein expression are also increased in *Sost*$^{-/-}$ mice, strongly suggesting that the increase in serum 1α,25(OH)$_2$D concentrations was the result of increased 1α,25(OH)$_2$D synthesis. When recombinant sclerostin is added to cultures of proximal tubular cells, the expression of the messenger RNA for *Cyp27b1*, the 1α-hydroxylase cytochrome P450, is diminished. Serum 24,25(OH)$_2$D concentrations were diminished in *Sost*$^{-/-}$ mice, and PTH concentrations were similar in knockout and wild-type mice. The lack of change in PTH is consistent with previous studies in humans.[157] The data suggest that in addition to the hormones traditionally thought to alter calcium reabsorption in the kidney (PTH and 1α,25(OH)$_2$D), sclerostin plays a significant role in altering renal calcium excretion. Although PTH and 1α,25(OH)$_2$D decrease fractional excretion of calcium by increasing the efficiency of calcium reabsorption in the DT, sclerostin increases fractional excretion of calcium (the absence of sclerostin expression is associated with a reduced fractional excretion of calcium).[153] Thus, the adaptation to a reduction in calcium intake and resultant downstream alterations in hormones (see Figure 7.2 for current understanding) may need to be amended to include changes in sclerostin expression (see Figures 7.4 and 7.7C). In the modified scheme, reduced sclerostin expression, which can occur as a result of increases in PTH,[158-161] would enhance renal Ca^{2+} reabsorption directly or through changes in 1α,25(OH)$_2$D synthesis (see Figure 7.4). The change in 1α,25(OH)$_2$D synthesis might be direct or mediated through changes in FGF-23 concentrations. Clearly, further work needs to be performed to dissect the proximate drivers of increased sclerostin-mediated renal Ca$^+$ reabsorption.

STRUCTURES OF PROTEINS INVOLVED IN THE TRANSPORT OF CALCIUM

The structural analysis and molecular modeling of Ca^{2+} transporters and Ca^{2+}-binding proteins have revealed surprisingly diverse mechanisms whereby these proteins bind the metal ligand. Such information is important because it suggests how drugs might be designed to inhibit or enhance the activity of these Ca^{2+} transporters. As noted earlier, the TRPV5 channel, calbindin D28K, and plasma membrane calcium pump are important in the transport of Ca^{2+} across the cell. Figure 7.8A shows a homology model for the human TRPV5. The TRPV5 channel forms a tetramer. Each TRPV5 protomer, shown by a blue, green, red, and yellow trace of α carbon backbone atom positions, putatively contains six transmembrane helices that may traverse the phospholipid bilayer as drawn. Most of the tetramer, including the N- and C-termini, is intracellular. Residues of transmembrane helices 5 and 6 form a central pore *(black)*, where regulated calcium influx occurs. Residue D542 was reported as essential for Ca^{2+} selectivity[162] and likely creates the first of two calcium binding sites *(red spheres)* inside a funnel-like cavity within the pore's extracellular entry. Residue T539 may form another calcium binding site closer to the pore. N572 and I575 seemingly perform gatelike functions because the

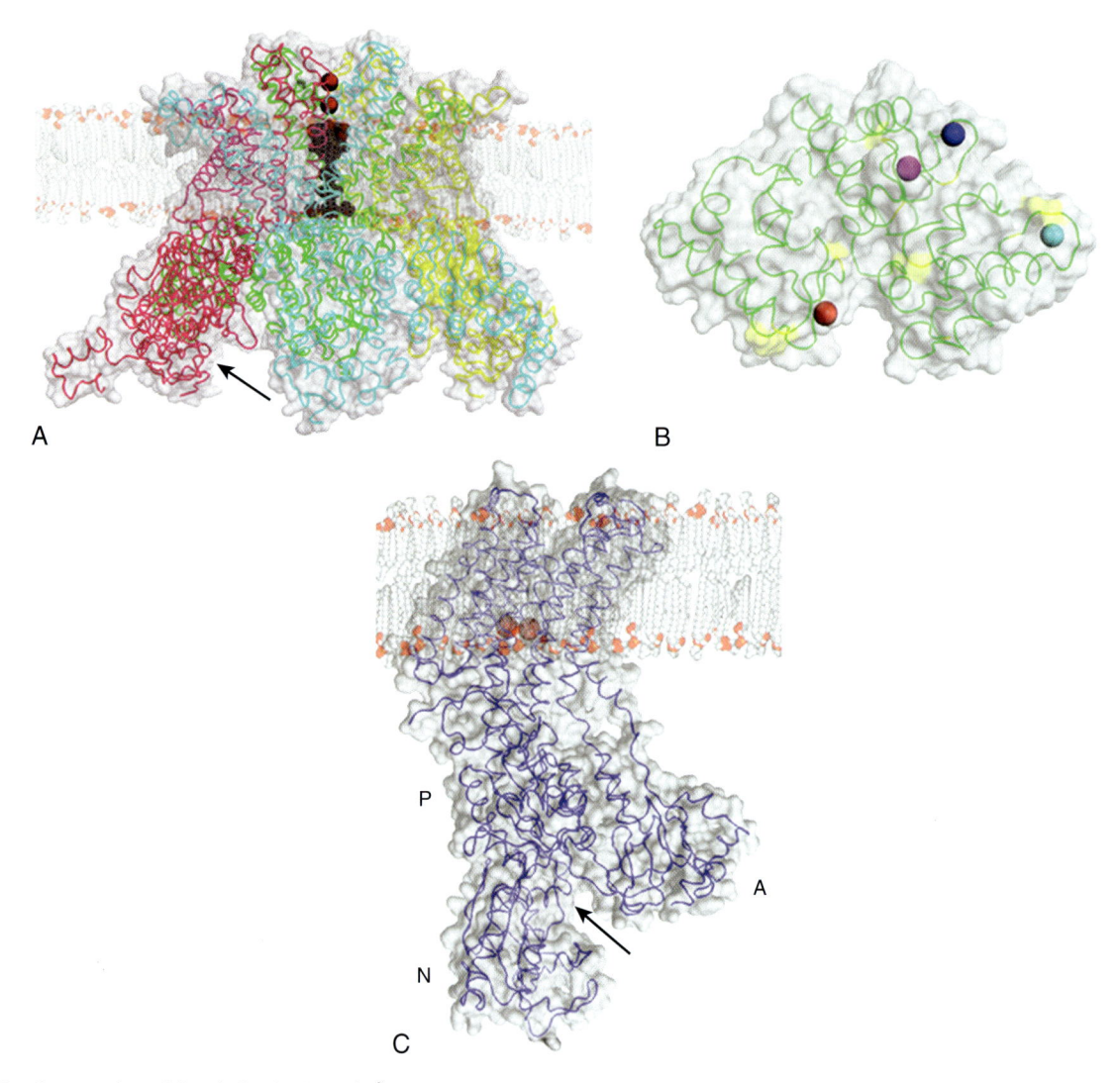

Figure 7.8 Structural models of distal tubule Ca^{2+} transport proteins. **A,** Human TRPV5 homology model made using Phyre 2 with atomic coordinates from PDB IDs 2B0O (chain F), 3J5P (chain B), and 2B5K (chain A). Each TRPV5 protomer, shown by a *blue, green, red,* and *yellow* trace of α carbon backbone atom positions, putatively contains six transmembrane helices that traverse the phospholipid bilayer as drawn. **B,** Surface and α carbon backbone atom trace of calbindin D28K (PDB ID 2G9B).[164] **C,** A homology model of human plasma membrane calcium pump A1 (PMCa1), created using Phyre 2 with atomic coordinates from PDB IDs 3IXZ (chain A), 3B9B (chain A), 2KNE (chain B), 3B8E (chain C), and 3B8C (chain B). (**B** from Kojetin DJ, Venters RA, Kordys DR, et al: Structure, binding interface and hydrophobic transitions of Ca^{2+}-loaded calbindin-D(28K). *Nat Struct Mol Biol* 2006;13:641-647.)

pore's diameter appears restricted by these residues. Ca^{2+} influx through TRPV5 is inhibited by a feedback mechanism when Ca^{2+}-bound calmodulin binds to amino acids 691 to 711 (*arrow*) between two TRPV5 protomers; the key contacts are the conserved R699, W701, L704, R705, and L709.[163] PTH-mediated PKA kinase activation leads to phosphorylation of T708 at this site, which stimulates TRPV5 by inhibiting calmodulin binding.

The structure of Ca-loaded calbindin D28K bound to Ca^{2+} has been solved (see Figure 7.8*B*).[164] Calbindin D28K contains six EF-hand motifs, which are canonical helix-loop-helix structures that coordinate Ca^{2+}. As shown, only four of the six EF hands in calbindin D28K bind Ca^{2+} ions with significant binding affinity—EF hand 1 (red Ca^{2+}), EF hand 3 (blue Ca^{2+}), EF hand 4 (purple Ca^{2+}), and EF hand 5 (cyan Ca^{2+}). The yellow surface patches indicate residues that display substantial chemical shifts when calbindin D28K is titrated with three peptides derived from other proteins known to interact. Unlike the conformation of many EF-hand proteins, such as calmodulin, Ca^{2+}-bound calbindin D28K forms one ordered domain. The apo calbindin D28K structure is also mostly ordered. However, EF hands 1 and 4, a segment prior to EF hand 1 and polypeptide between EF hands 4 and 5 and 5 and 6, are altered in conformation from the fully Ca^{2+}-bound form.[165,166] When only one, two, or three Ca^{2+} are bound, calbindin D28K is considerably more disordered.[165]

A model of the human plasma membrane calcium pump A1 (PMCA1) is shown in Figure 7.8*C*. The protein acts as a high-affinity, Ca^{2+}-H^+ P-type ATPase (cotransporter) that removes Ca^{2+} from cells at a slow rate against their electrochemical gradient.[2,167] The structural features of the PMCA1 are 10 transmembrane helices, with most of the polypeptide inside the cytoplasm (bottommost), organized into three domains, termed P, N, and A. The P, or phosphorylation domain, has the highly conserved catalytic core, with a canonical Rossmann fold common among ATPases. The N, or nucleotide-binding domain, is a region of β-sheet that oscillates among conformations to deliver bound ATP to the P domain's phosphorylation site. The A, or actuator domain, is also very mobile and actually consists of two subdomains, which may exist to protect the phosphoryl group from hydrolysis and sometimes block ion access or egress. The mechanism whereby the PMCA1 transports Ca^{2+} begins with Ca^{2+} binding to a site(s) in the transmembrane domain (key residues are N859, N891, and D895) made cytoplasmically accessible because helices 4 and 6 are structurally altered when the P domain is unphosphorylated. Two calciums, shown as red spheres, are modeled here based on a crystal structure of the homologous sarcoplasmic reticulum Ca^{2+}-ATPase.[168-170] ATP-Mg^{2+} binding to a site (arrow) that perturbs an important salt bridge between R646 and D248 brings the N domain into closer proximity with the P domain's residue D475. ATP hydrolysis leads to phosphorylation of D475 and large-scale conformational changes result, such as a 90-degree rotation of the A domain and rearrangement of transmembrane helices 4 and 6 to cause extracellular release of Ca^{2+}. There remains some debate about whether the ratio of calcium flux is one calcium per hydrolyzed ATP molecule. PMCA1 is autoinhibited by its C terminus; this regulation is relieved when calmodulin binds to a calmodulin-binding domain, also within the C terminus.[2,167] PMCA1 is also activated by acidic phospholipids, although a full understanding is lacking.[2,167]

MAGNESIUM TRANSPORT IN THE KIDNEY

ROLE OF MAGNESIUM IN CELLULAR PROCESSES

Magnesium is an abundant cation in the human body (Table 7.1).[171-176] It is required for a variety of biochemical functions.[177] The activities of magnesium-dependent enzymes are modulated by the metal as a result of binding to the substrate or of direct binding to the enzyme.[177-180] Enzymes of the glycolytic and citric acid pathways, exonuclease, topoisomerase, RNA and DNA polymerases, and adenylate cyclase are among the many enzymes regulated by magnesium.[177-181] Also, magnesium regulates channel activity.[177]

Given its role in such diverse biologic processes, it is not surprising that a deficiency or increase in serum magnesium concentration is associated with important clinical symptoms.[182] For example, a low serum magnesium concentration is associated with muscular weakness, fasciculations, Chvostek's and Trousseau's signs, and sometimes frank tetany.[182] The tetany of hypomagnesemia is independent of changes in the serum calcium level. On occasion, personality changes, anxiety, delirium, and psychoses may manifest. Hypocalcemia,[183-189] reduced PTH secretion,[190-195] and hypokalemia[196-199] are sometimes present in patients with hypomagnesemia. Cardiac arrhythmias and prolongation of the corrected QT interval[200,201] are sometimes observed. Conversely, hypermagnesemia seen in association with the administration of excessive amounts of magnesium in diseases such as eclampsia and in patients with renal failure is manifest as weakness of the voluntary muscles.

Table 7.2 Distribution and Concentrations of Magnesium in a Healthy Adult

Site	Whole-Body Mg (%)	Concentration and Content
Bone	53	0.5% of bone ash
Muscle	27	9 mmol/kg wet weight
Soft tissue	19	9 mmol/kg wet weight
Adipose tissue	0.012	0.8 mmol/kg wet weight
Erythrocytes	0.5	1.65-2.73 mmol/L
Serum	0.3	0.69-0.94 mmol/L

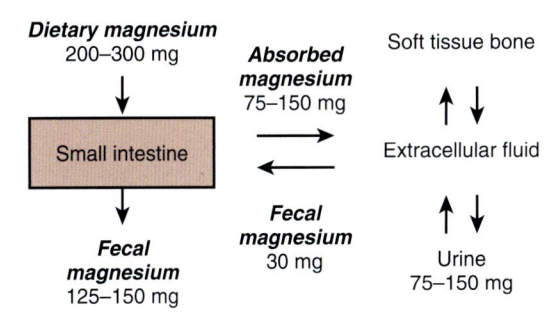

Figure 7.9 Magnesium homeostasis in normal humans showing the amounts of magnesium absorbed in the intestine and reabsorbed by the kidney.

MAGNESIUM PRESENT IN SERUM IN BOUND AND FREE FORMS

Most magnesium within the body is present in bone or within the cells (Table 7.2).[177] Approximately 60% of magnesium is stored in bone. The serum magnesium concentration varies slightly with age; in adults, it is 1.6-2.3 mg/dL (0.66 to 0.94 mmol/L). In plasma, about 70% of Mg is ultrafiltrable, 55% is free, and 14% of Mg is in the form of soluble complexes with citrate and phosphate.[202] Because Mg is present largely within cells and bone, there is some interest as to whether serum Mg concentration reflects tissue stores, especially when Mg is depleted or deficient. When rats[203-205] and humans[182,206] are placed on Mg-deficient diets, the serum Mg level decreases within 1 day in rats and in 5 to 6 days in humans. Bone Mg and blood mononuclear cell Mg concentrations correlate well with total body Mg and serum Mg levels.[206-209] The correlations between total body Mg stores and muscle or cardiac Mg, however, are not precise.[206]

REGULATION OF MAGNESIUM HOMEOSTASIS

The intestine and the kidney regulate magnesium balance (Figure 7.9).[177] A normal diet adequate in magnesium normally contains 200 to 300 mg of magnesium.[210] Of ingested dietary magnesium, 75 to 150 mg is absorbed in the jejunum and ileum, primarily by paracellular passive processes.[211-215] The Trpm6 protein (a mutant form of this protein is present in patients with familial hypomagnesemia) is localized to the apical membrane of intestinal epithelial cells and mediates transcellular magnesium absorption.[43,216] About 30 mg of magnesium is secreted into the intestine via pancreatic and intestinal secretions, giving a net magnesium absorption of approximately 130 mg/24 hr. Magnesium that is not absorbed in the intestine and is secreted into the intestinal lumen eventually appears in the feces (125 to 150 mg). Absorbed magnesium enters the extracellular fluid pool and moves in and out of bone and soft tissues. Approximately 130 mg of magnesium (equivalent to the net amount absorbed in the intestine) is excreted in the urine.

In experimental animals and humans, feeding a diet low in magnesium results in a rapid decrease in urinary and fecal magnesium and the development of a negative magnesium balance.[217-226] Conversely, the administration of magnesium is associated with an increase in the renal excretion of magnesium.[227-229] Unlike calcium and phosphorus, however, no hormones or molecules have been identified that alter magnesium transport in the intestine or alter the renal excretion of magnesium in response to changes in magnesium balance.[177,230,231]

REABSORPTION OF MAGNESIUM ALONG THE TUBULE

Approximately 10% of total body magnesium is filtered in glomeruli (≈3000 mg/24 hr). About 75% of total plasma magnesium is filterable. Because urinary magnesium excretion is about 150 mg/24 hr, a substantial fraction of filtered magnesium is reabsorbed along the tubule (≈95%). Fifteen percent to 20% of filtered magnesium is reabsorbed in the proximal tubule (Figure 7.10). The cellular and molecular mechanisms whereby magnesium is reabsorbed in the proximal nephron are unknown. However, it is speculated that reabsorption of magnesium in the proximal nephron occurs by paracellular mechanisms. The bulk of the filtered magnesium is reabsorbed in the TALH, again by a paracellular mechanism of which paracellin-1 or claudin-16 is a critical component.[77,81,232-239] As discussed earlier for Ca^{2+} transport, claudin-16 and claudin-19 form cation-selective paracellular channels[77,78] that directly mediate paracellular Mg^{2+} reabsorption or facilitate the generation of a NaCl diffusion potential that provides the driving force for paracellular Mg^{2+} reabsorption. Mutations of the *CLDN16* and *CLDN19* genes and the *SLC12A1*, *KCNJ1* and *CLCNKB* genes, which encode proteins required for normal thick ascending limb function, result in excessive magnesium losses in the urine and hypomagnesemia. Figure 7.11 shows the mechanism whereby magnesium is transported in the TALH.

Of filtered magnesium exiting from the thick ascending limb, 5% to 10% is reabsorbed in the distal convoluted tubule where proteins such as TRPM6 and HNF1 are localized.[43,88,92,216,240-242] Mutations of the *TRPM6*, *HNF1*, and *PCBD1* genes are associated with increased urinary magnesium losses and hypomagnesemia.[43,88,92,216,240-245] Figure 7.12 shows the cellular localization of these proteins in the DCT into the cell. It is unclear about the mode of exit of magnesium from the cell into the interstitial space. Precisely how these proteins interact with one another to regulate magnesium transport is currently under investigation. It has been suggested that PCBD1 binds HNF1B to costimulate the promoter of FXYD2, the activity of which is important in magnesium reabsorption in the DCT.[244]

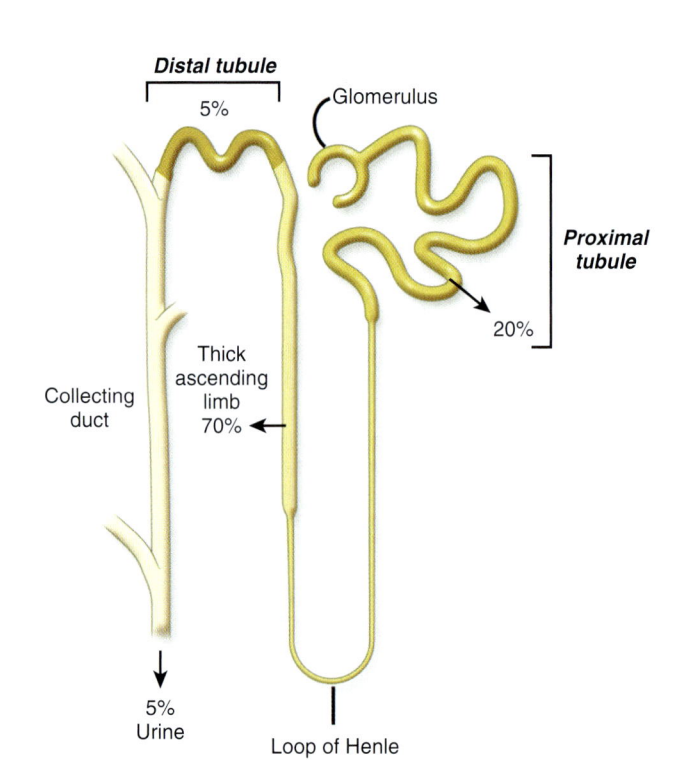

Figure 7.10 Percentages of filtered magnesium reabsorbed along the tubule.

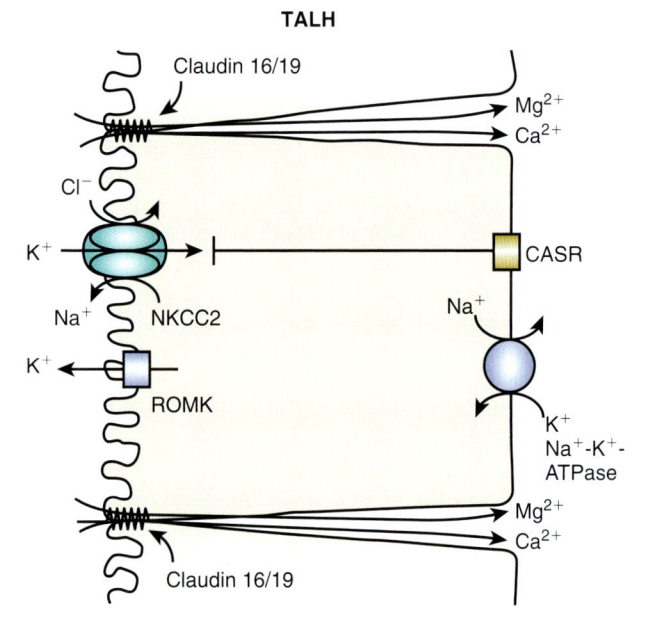

Figure 7.11 Mechanism whereby magnesium is transported in cells of the thick ascending limb of the loop of Henle (TALH). Most of the magnesium is reabsorbed by paracellular mechanisms. Claudin-16 and claudin-19 are depicted as directly transporting Ca^{2+} and Mg^{2+}, but it has also been hypothesized that their primary role is to allow backleak of reabsorbed Na^+ and thus establish a NaCl diffusion potential, thereby indirectly facilitating divalent cation reabsorption

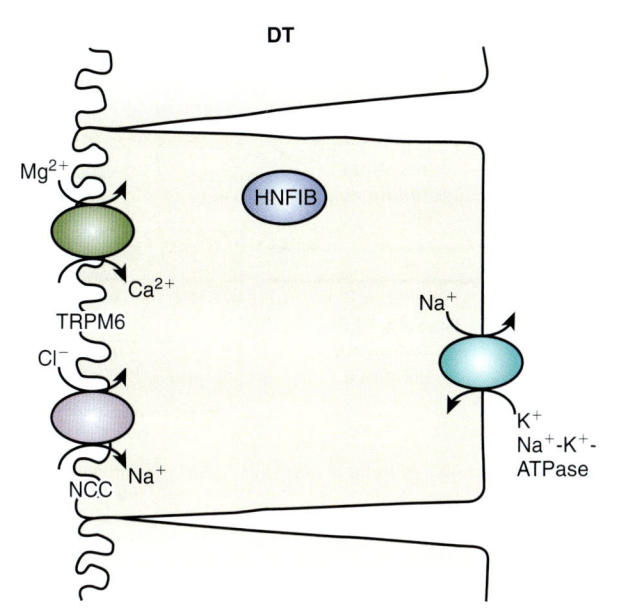

Figure 7.12 Mechanism whereby magnesium is transported in distal tubule (DT) cells. Most of the magnesium is reabsorbed by transcellular mechanisms mediated by the TRPM6 channel.

Table 7.3 Factors Altering the Uptake of Magnesium in the Kidney

Substance	Effect
Peptide hormones	
Parathyroid hormone[85,472-476]	Increase
Calcitonin[476-484]	Increase
Glucagon[485,486]	Increase
Arginine vasopressin[487]	Increase
Insulin[488]	Increase
β-Adrenergic agonists	
Isoproterenol[489]	Increase
Prostaglandins—PGE$_2$[490]	Decrease
Mineralocorticoids, aldosterone	Increase
1,25-Dihydroxyvitamin D$_3$[491]	Decrease
Magnesium	
Restriction[217-220,222]	Increase
Increase[227-229]	Decrease
Metabolic alkalosis[138,492,493]	Increase
Metabolic acidosis[138,492,493]	Decrease
Hypercalcemia[494]	Decrease
Phosphate depletion[495,496]	Decrease
Potassium depletion[497]	Unknown
Diuretics	
Furosemide	No effect
Amiloride[498,499]	Increase
Chlorothiazide[497,500]	Increase

Modified from Dai LJ, Ritchie G, Kerstan D, et al: Magnesium transport in the renal distal convoluted tubule. Physiol Rev 81:51-84, 2001.

REGULATION OF MAGNESIUM TRANSPORT IN THE KIDNEY

A variety of factors alter magnesium reabsorption in the kidney (Table 7.3). It should be emphasized that although effects on magnesium excretion in the urine are noted

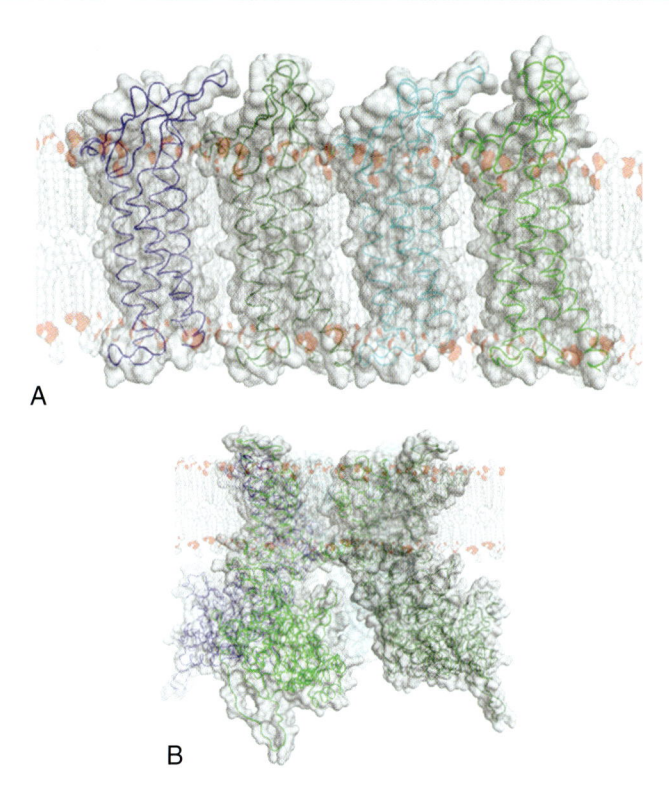

Figure 7.13 A, Claudin-16 and/or claudin-19 form permeable selective channels in the thick ascending limb of the loop of Henle. These proteins have four transmembrane helices with a short N-terminus and longer, more variable C-termini that associate with scaffold proteins intercellularly. When claudin-16 and claudin-19 are coexpressed, linear heteropolymeric fibrils develop within the plasma membrane, as shown (claudin-16, *dark-light green*; claudin-19, *blue-cyan*); this model is based on interactions observed in the mouse claudin-15 crystal lattice that are conserved in these human claudins. B, Model of the human transepithelial receptor potential melastatin 6 (TRPM6) channel kinase. The partial homology model for TRPM6 was initially created using Phyre 2, with atomic coordinates from PDB IDs 1YDA (chain A), 2Q4O (chain A), 3QUA (chain A), 2IZ6 (chain A), 3SBX (chain C), and 2Q4O (chain A). Modifications were then made based on another homology model created using a crystal structure of the kinase domain of TRPM7 (76% sequence identity) in complex with AMP-PNP (Adenylylimidodiphosphate) PDB ID 1IA9.

following the infusion of various substances or following blockade of their activity, it is not clear that such changes occur with physiologic changes in concentrations of these factors in vivo. Furthermore, it is clear that concentrations of the effector substances do not change in a physiologically appropriate manner following changes in serum concentrations of magnesium. Thus, hormonal homeostasis, in which concentrations of a hormone (e.g., PTH, glucagon, arginine vasopressin [AVP]) are altered following changes in the concentration of magnesium, and in turn alter the retention or concentrations of magnesium, are difficult to demonstrate.

STRUCTURES OF PROTEINS INVOLVED IN THE TRANSPORT OF MAGNESIUM

Claudin-16 and/or claudin-19 form permeable selective channels in the TALH (Figure 7.13*A*). These proteins have four transmembrane helices with a short N-terminus and longer, more variable C-termini that associate with scaffold proteins intercellularly. Where claudin-16 and claudin-19 are coexpressed, linear heteropolymeric fibrils may develop within the plasma membrane, as shown (claudin-16, dark-light green; claudin-19, blue-cyan), a model based on interactions observed in the mouse claudin-15 crystal lattice that are conserved in these human claudins.[246] This fibril model explains how human claudin-16 point mutants (L145P, L151F, G191R, A209T, and F232C) and claudin-19 mutants (L90P and G123R), which cause FHHNC, can disrupt fibril formation.[82] Tight junctions probably form when intramembrane fibrils of neighboring cells interact via the extracellular loops of claudin-16 and claudin-19.[82] A model for these interactions in the homologous claudin-15 has been published.[247] The first extracellular loop of claudin-16 contains negatively charged residues (D104S, D105S, E119T, D126S, and E140T) that appear to regulate cation permeability.[81] However, it is not now clear whether heteromeric claudin-16 and claudin-19 are selective for Na^+, and therefore influence Mg^{2+} and Ca^{2+} permeability indirectly, or whether they together have a degree of divalent cation selectivity. Interacting fibrils may also be later modified to achieve differentiation in the barrier function of these tight junctions.

A model of the human TRPM6 channel kinase is shown in Figure 7.13B. TRPM6 functions as a homotetramer. The transmembrane region is formed by six helices. The first four helices are likely to act as a sensor of transmembrane voltage. The last two, more highly conserved helices and their connecting loop constitute the pore. These helices most likely associate with the first four helices of a neighboring subunit in the homotetramer. The connecting loop for these last two helices probably contains a non–membrane-spanning α-helix that may have functional importance. The C-terminus of TRPM6 contains a kinase domain similar to other serine-threonine kinases. The mechanism of Mg^{2+} transport by the TRPM6 channel mechanism remains unclear, as does the role of its kinase domain. E1024 and E1029 are key residues that abolish Mg^{2+} and Ca^{2+} permeation and remove the pH sensitivity of TRPM6.[248] We are not able to model these residues.

PHOSPHORUS TRANSPORT IN THE KIDNEY

ROLE OF PHOSPHORUS IN CELLULAR PROCESSES

Phosphorus is a key component of hydroxyapatite, the major component of bone mineral, nucleic acids, bioactive signaling proteins, phosphorylated enzymes, and cellular membranes.[249-252] Prolonged deficiency of phosphorus and inorganic phosphate results in serious biologic problems, including impaired bone mineralization resulting in osteomalacia or rickets, abnormal erythrocyte, leukocyte, and platelet function, impaired cell membrane integrity that can result in rhabdomyolysis, and impaired cardiac function.[253-255] Phosphate balance is maintained through a series of complex hormonally and locally regulated metabolic adjustments. In states of neutral phosphate balance, net accretion equals net output. The major organs involved in the absorption, excretion, and reabsorption of phosphate are the intestine and kidney (Figure 7.14). A normal diet adequate in phosphorus normally contains approximately 1500 mg of phosphorus. Approximately 1100 mg of ingested dietary phosphate is absorbed in the proximal intestine predominantly in the jejunum. About 200 mg of phosphorus is secreted into the intestine via pancreatic and intestinal secretions, giving a net phosphorus absorption of approximately 900 mg/24 hr. Phosphorus that is not absorbed in the intestine or is secreted into the intestinal lumen eventually appears in the feces. Absorbed phosphorus enters the extracellular fluid pool and moves in and out of bone (and, to a smaller extent, in and out of soft tissues), as needed (~200 mg). Approximately 900 mg of phosphorus (equivalent to the amount absorbed in the intestine) is excreted in the urine.

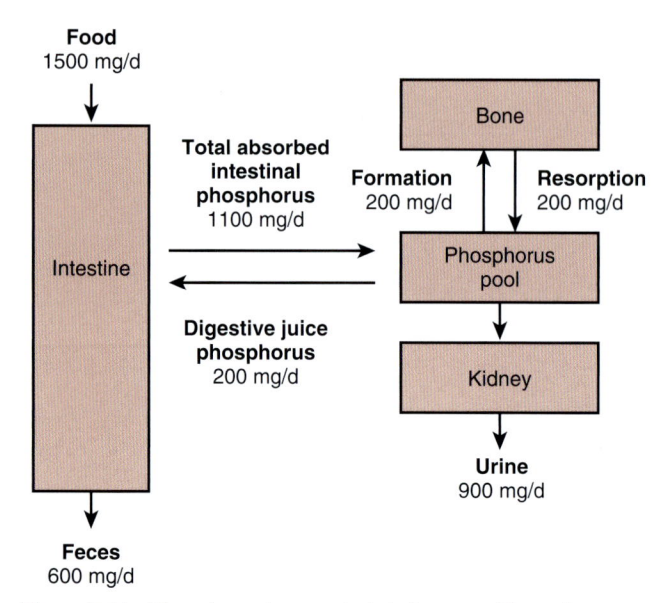

Figure 7.14 Phosphorus homeostasis in humans. The major organs involved in the absorption, excretion, and reabsorption of phosphate are the intestine and kidney.

PHOSPHORUS PRESENT IN BLOOD IN MULTIPLE FORMS

Phosphorus is present in almost every bodily fluid. In human plasma or serum, phosphorus exists in the form of inorganic phosphorus or phosphate (Pi), lipid phosphorus, and phosphoric ester phosphorus. Total serum phosphorus concentrations range from 8.9 to 14.9 mg/dL (2.87 to 4.81 mmol/L), inorganic phosphorus (phosphate, Pi) concentrations from 2.56 to 4.16 mg/dL (0.83 to 1.34 mmol/L) (this is what is usually measured clinically, referred to as the serum phosphorus, and the normal range changes with age),[256] phosphoric ester phosphorus concentrations from 2.5 to 4.5 mg/dL (0.81 to 1.45 mmol/L), and lipid phosphorus concentration from 6.9 to 9.7 mg/dL (2.23 to 3.13 mmol/L; Table 7.4).[257] Of phosphorus in the body, 85% is present in bones, 14% exists in cells from soft tissues, and 1% is present in extracellular fluids. In mammals, bone contains a substantial amount of phosphorus (≈10 g/100 g dry, fat-free tissue); in comparison, muscle contains 0.2 g/100 g fat-free tissue, and brain contains 0.33 g/100 g fresh tissue.[257]

REGULATION OF PHOSPHATE HOMEOSTASIS: AN INTEGRATED VIEW

Intestinal feed-forward and hormonal feedback systems (PTH–vitamin D endocrine system and the phosphatonins) are likely to be responsible for the control of phosphorus homeostasis (Figure 7.15). The short-term responses that occur within minutes to hours of feeding a high Pi meal are important in regulating phosphorus homeostasis via feed-forward mechanisms, whereas the longer term changes occur as a result of alterations in circulating concentrations of PTH, $1\alpha,25(OH)_2D_3$, and the phosphatonins, such as FGF-23.[258-262] Intestinal signals have been shown in rodents to alter renal Pi excretion rapidly in response to changes in duodenal Pi concentrations.[259]

PTH, $1\alpha,25(OH)_2D_3$ and the phosphatonin, FGF-23, control phosphorus homeostasis.[262,263] Concentrations of these hormones and factors are regulated by phosphorus in a manner that is conducive to the maintenance of normal phosphorus concentrations. Figure 7.16 shows the physiologic changes known to occur with low or high dietary intakes of phosphate. A decrease in serum phosphate concentration, as would occur with a reduced intake of phosphorus, results in increased ionized calcium concentration, decreased parathyroid hormone secretion, and a subsequent decrease in renal phosphate excretion. At the same time, by PTH-independent mechanisms, there is an increase in renal 25-hydroxyvitamin D 1α-hydroxylase activity, increased $1\alpha,25(OH)_2D_3$ synthesis, and increased phosphorus absorption in the intestine and reabsorption in the kidney.[264-273] Conversely, with elevated phosphate intake, there is decreased calcium concentration, increased parathyroid hormone release from the parathyroid gland, and increased renal phosphate excretion. An increased serum phosphate concentration inhibits renal 25-hydroxyvitamin D 1α-hydroxylase activity and decreases $1\alpha,25(OH)_2D_3$ synthesis. A reduced $1\alpha,25(OH)_2D_3$ concentration decreases intestinal phosphorus absorption and renal phosphate reabsorption. All these factors tend to bring serum phosphate concentrations back into the normal range. The vitamin D endocrine system, PTH, and the phosphatonins are responsible for the control of renal Pi reabsorption on a longer term basis (hours to days). PTH, by virtue of its phosphaturic effect in the kidney, decreases overall phosphate retention, whereas $1\alpha,25(OH)_2D_3$ increases phosphate retention by enhancing the efficiency of phosphorus absorption in the intestine and kidney.[30,274-285] PTH has two opposing effects; it increases urinary phosphate excretion but also increases the synthesis of $1\alpha,25(OH)_2D_3$ by stimulating the activity of the renal 25-hydroxyvitamin D 1α-hydroxylase. In turn, $1\alpha,25(OH)_2D_3$ increases the efficiency of phosphorus absorption in the intestine and kidney. The phosphatonins, FGF-23, and serum frizzled-related protein 4 (sFRP-4) modulate renal phosphate reabsorption.[286-295] They also decrease,[286,292,296-301] and insulin-like growth factor-1 (IGF-1)

Table 7.4 Distribution and Concentrations of Phosphorus (in mmol/L) in Adult Human Blood

Phosphorus Compounds	Erythrocytes	Plasma
Phosphate ester	12.3-19.0	0.86-1.45
Phospholipids	4.13-4.81	2.23-3.13
Inorganic phosphate	0.03-0.13	0.71-1.36

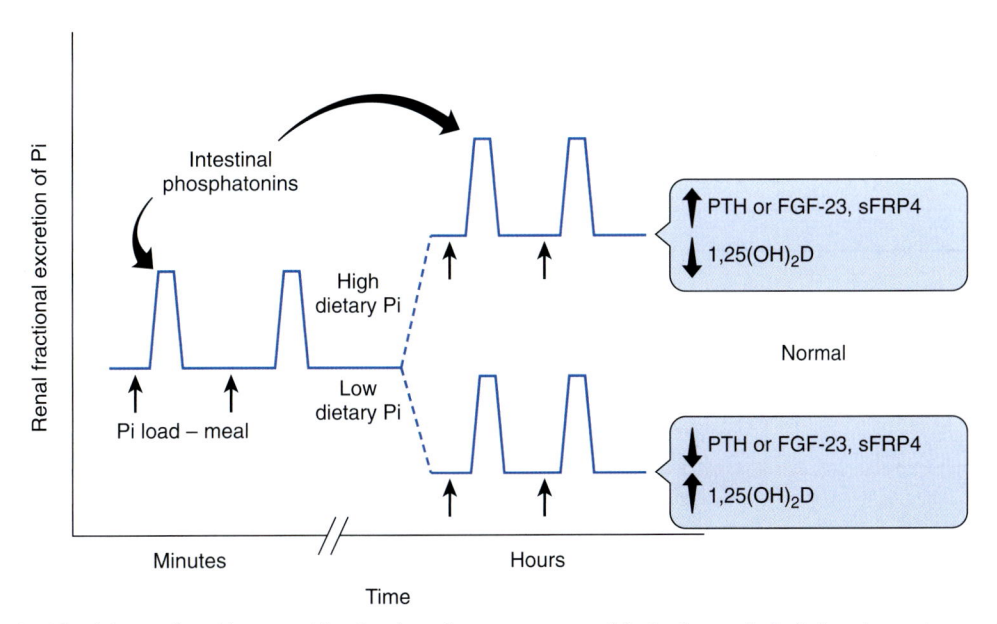

Figure 7.15 Intestinal feed-forward and hormonal feedback systems are responsible for the control of phosphorus homeostasis. Changes in intestinal luminal phosphate concentrations (Pi load meal) results in the elaboration of chemical signals (intestinal phosphatonins) that alter the fractional excretion of phosphate in the kidney over a time frame of minutes. Long-term changes in the amount of phosphate in the diet result in changes in the concentrations of parathyroid hormone (PTH), $1\alpha,25$-dihydroxyvitamin D, and phosphatonins, which influence the fractional excretion of phosphate in the kidney over a time frame of hours, as shown. Short-term changes mediated by feed-forward intestinal signals are proposed to be superimposed on this chronic baseline.

increases,[302] the activity of the 25-hydroxyvitamin D 1α-hydroxylase (growth factors in Figure 7.16). FGF-23 induces renal phosphate wasting in patients with tumor-induced osteomalacia (TIO),[289,303-305] autosomal dominant hypophosphatemic rickets (ADHR), X-linked hypophosphatemic rickets (XLH), and autosomal recessive hypophosphatemic rickets (ARHR).[287,292,294,306] From a physiologic perspective, it would be appropriate for FGF-23 and sFRP-4 concentrations to be regulated by the intake of dietary phosphorus and by the serum phosphate concentration. In humans, in the short term, the feeding of meals containing increased amounts of phosphate does not increase serum FGF-23 concentration, despite the induction of a robust and dose-dependent phosphaturia.[260,307] Other human studies conducted over a period of days or weeks, however, have shown changes in serum FGF-23 concentration following alterations in the content of phosphate in the diet.[308,309] In mice, Perwad and associates have shown that a high-phosphate diet increases and a low-phosphate diet decreases serum FGF-23 levels in these animals within 5 days of changing the dietary phosphate intake.[310] The changes in serum FGF-23 correlated with changes in serum phosphate concentration. Studies from our laboratory performed in rats fed a low-, normal-, or high-phosphate diet have demonstrated that serum FGF-23 levels significantly decrease in animals fed a low-phosphate diet and increase in animals fed a high-phosphate diet within 24 hours of altering dietary phosphate intake, but do not correlate with serum phosphate in the animals fed a high-phosphate diet.[295]

REABSORPTION OF PHOSPHATE ALONG THE NEPHRON

Almost all serum phosphate is filtered at the glomerulus.[311] Under conditions of normal dietary phosphate intake, and in the presence of intact parathyroid glands, approximately 20% of the filtered phosphate load is excreted. The other 80% of the filtered load of phosphate is reabsorbed by the renal tubules. The proximal tubules are the major sites of phosphate reabsorption along the nephron (Figure 7.17).[311] Little phosphate reabsorption occurs between the late proximal tubule and early distal tubule in animals with intact parathyroid glands.[312-320] In the absence of PTH, however, phosphate is avidly reabsorbed between the late proximal tubule and early distal tubule, reflecting phosphate reabsorption by the proximal straight tubule.[315] Phosphate transport rates are approximately three times higher in the proximal convoluted than in the proximal straight tubules.[321] Renal phosphate handling is characterized by intranephronal heterogeneity, reflecting segmental differences in phosphate handling within an individual nephron as well as internephronal heterogeneity.[312,316,321,322]

The uptake of phosphate is mediated by Na-phosphate cotransporters located at the apical border of proximal tubule cells (NaPi-IIa and NaPi-IIc).[323-346] The structure and physiology of these phosphate transport molecules have been extensively reviewed, and the reader is directed to other publications in this regard.[323-346] The Na-phosphate cotransporters are highly homologous and are predicted to

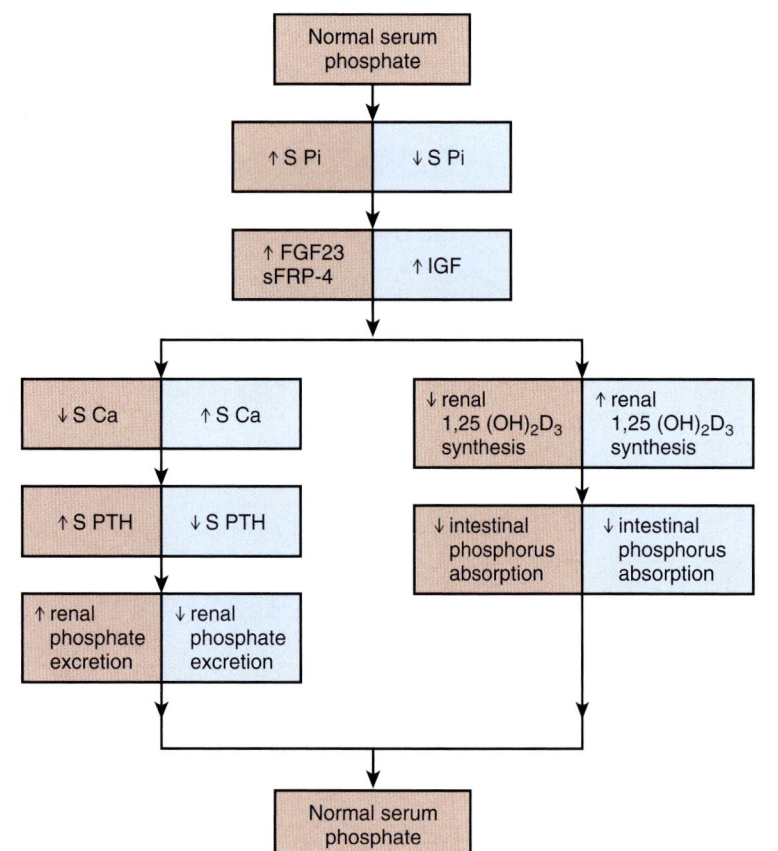

Figure 7.16 Shown are the changes in growth factors—fibroblast growth factor 23 (FGF-23), sFRP-4 (secreted frizzled related protein 4), insulin-like growth factor (IGF), parathyroid hormone (PTH), and 1α,25-dihydroxyvitamin D and the subsequent physiologic changes in intestinal or renal phosphate reabsorption following perturbations in serum phosphate levels.

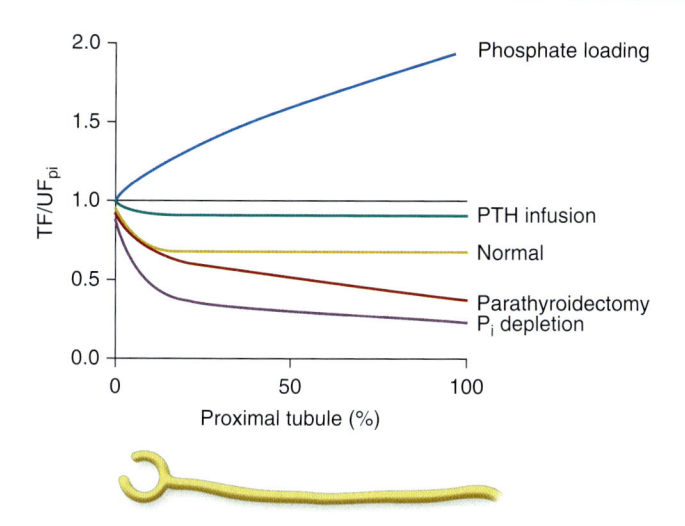

Figure 7.17 The proximal tubule is the major site of phosphate reabsorption along the nephron. The effects of dietary phosphate loading or deprivation, parathyroid hormone (PTH) infusion, or parathyroidectomy on phosphate absorption along the proximal tubule are shown. Proximal tubule %, distance along the proximal tubule as a percentage of total length; TF/UF$_{Pi}$, ratio of tubular fluid to ultrafiltrate phosphate concentration.

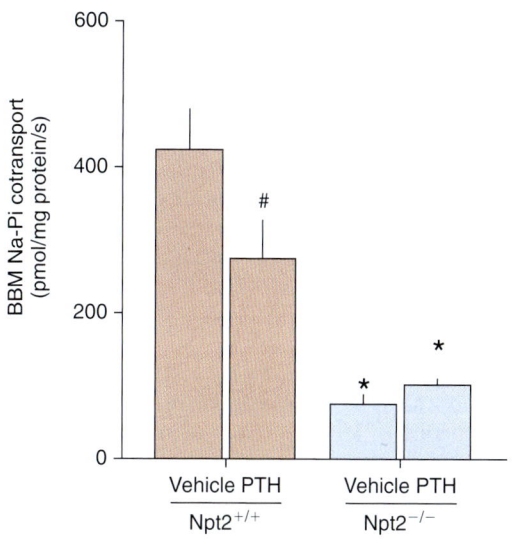

Figure 7.18 Mice with ablation of the NaPi-IIa gene exhibit renal phosphate wasting and fail to respond to parathyroid hormone (PTH). The effect of PTH or vehicle on brush border membrane (BBM) Na-Pi cotransport in Npt2$^{+/+}$ and Npt2$^{-/-}$ mice is shown. #, Effect of PTH in Npt2$^{+/+}$ mice, $P < 0.0015$. *, Effect of genotype in vehicle-treated mice, $P < 0.0001$; effect of genotype in PTH-treated mice, $P < 0.0041$. (Reprinted with permission from Zhao N, Tenenhouse HS: Npt2 gene disruption confers resistance to the inhibitory action of parathyroid hormone on renal sodium-phosphate cotransport. *Endocrinology* 141:2159-2165, 2000.)

have similar structures. Mice with ablation of the NaPi-IIa gene exhibit renal phosphate wasting, and it is estimated that the NaPi-IIa transporter is responsible for approximately 85% of proximal tubular phosphate transport, which contributes to the adaptive increase in tubular phosphate transport in animals fed a low-phosphate diet (Figure 7.18).[347,348]

REGULATION OF PHOSPHATE TRANSPORT IN THE KIDNEY

DIETARY PHOSPHATE

The influence of dietary phosphate intake on the urinary excretion of phosphate has been known for many years.[312,349-364] The reabsorption of phosphate is decreased in animals fed a high-phosphate diet, whereas animals with a low intake of phosphate reabsorb almost 100% of the filtered load of phosphate.[199,236-251] These changes in phosphate reabsorption are associated with parallel changes in the abundance of NaPi-IIa and NaPi-IIc.[365,366] In infants and children, phosphate reabsorption is high so as to maintain the positive phosphate balance required for growth.[367,368] Conversely, decreased phosphate reabsorption has been demonstrated in older adults.[369,370]

Although dietary phosphate deprivation results in marked changes in the plasma concentration of several hormones (see Figure 7.16) that contribute to the increases in phosphate reabsorption, the enhanced tubular reabsorption can also be demonstrated independently of changes in these hormones.[259,371-374] When a bolus of phosphate is instilled into the duodenum of intact rats, renal phosphate excretion increases within 10 minutes without a change in serum Pi concentration.[259] The change in Pi reabsorption in response to a high-Pi meal is independent of plasma Pi concentrations and filtered Pi load. Such changes are not elicited on the administration of NaCl into the duodenum. The increase in renal phosphate excretion is independent of PTH because thyroparathyroidectomy does not alter the process. Serum concentrations of PTH do not change, and serum concentrations of other phosphaturic peptides, such as FGF-23 and sFRP-4, are unchanged following the infusion of intraduodenal phosphate. Aqueous duodenal extracts contain a phosphaturic substance that is likely to be a protein. The processes or pathways whereby changes in luminal phosphate concentration within the bowel are detected have not been defined, although the presence of a so-called phosphate sensor has been postulated.[375] A recent study, however, suggests that such an intestinal phosphate-sensing mechanism may be absent in humans.[376]

Studies using cultured renal proximal tubular cells provide evidence of an intrinsic ability of these cultured cells to increase phosphate transport when exposed to a low phosphate concentration in the medium.[371-374] The mechanism of upregulation of Na-Pi cotransport in opossum kidney cells by low-Pi media involves two regulatory mechanisms, an immediate (early) increase (after 2 hours) in the expression of the Na-Pi cotransporter, independent of mRNA synthesis or stability, and a delayed (late) effect (after 4 to 6 hours), resulting in an increase in NaPi-4 mRNA abundance.[373,377] The enhanced Pi reabsorption of short-term Pi deprivation has been linked to decreased intrarenal synthesis of dopamine and/or stimulation of β-adrenoreceptors because infusion of dopamine or propranolol restores the phosphaturic response to PTH in short-term (<3 days) Pi deprivation.[378-380] Conversely, dopamine may also mediate the acute phosphaturic effect of a high-Pi diet.[381] The NaPi-IIa transporter is expressed in the brain and is regulated by dietary Pi, suggesting that dietary

Pi could regulate neural outputs to regulate renal Pi excretion.[382] Increasing cerebrospinal fluid Pi concentrations in the presence of low plasma Pi concentrations reversed the adaptations to feeding a low-Pi diet, suggesting that the Pi concentration in the brain regulates not only central but also renal expression of NaPi-IIa transporters. It should be remembered that alterations in serum Pi concentrations also alter $1\alpha,25(OH)_2D_3$ synthesis and serum concentrations.[264-273] Infusions of $1\alpha,25(OH)_2D_3$ increase the renal reabsorption of Pi, predominantly in the proximal nephron.[30,276,280,281,383-386]

PARATHYROID HORMONE

Parathyroidectomy decreases renal Pi excretion and, conversely, injection of PTH increases urinary Pi excretion[387-391] by altering Pi reabsorption along the proximal tubule (see Figure 7.17).[314-318,392] The proximal straight tubule is an important site of PTH action with respect to Pi transport and may be critical in the final regulation of Pi excretion.[313,319,322,393] Parathyroid hormone maintains Pi homeostasis by regulating NaPi cotransporters in the kidney. Renal NaPi cotransporters, which are internalized and degraded within the lysosomes,[333,338,394,395] are reduced in number along the apical borders of proximal tubular cells following the administration of PTH 1-34 but not by the administration of PTH 3-34.[343,344] Disruption of the *NaPi-IIa (Slc34a1)* gene in mice resulted in increased Pi excretion compared to wild-type mice and a resistance to the phosphaturic effect of PTH (Figure 7.18), although the cAMP response is normal.[396] Under conditions in which the phosphaturic effect of PTH is blunted or absent, such as following short-term Pi deprivation or acute respiratory alkalosis, the inhibitory effect of PTH on Pi reabsorption by the proximal convoluted tubule remains intact. However, the increased delivery of Pi is blunted by enhanced reabsorption by the proximal straight tubule.[319,322,393] These studies suggest that the regulation of Pi reabsorption by PTH in the proximal convoluted and proximal straight tubules may be mediated by different mechanisms. It should be noted that PTH has two opposing effects—PTH increases urinary Pi excretion but also increases the synthesis of $1\alpha,25(OH)_2D_3$ by stimulating the activity of the $25(OH)D_3$ 1α-hydroxylase enzyme in the kidney.[264-273]

VITAMIN D AND VITAMIN METABOLITES

Both PTH and $1,25(OH)_2D_3$ play important roles in calcium and Pi regulation (see earlier discussion regarding Ca homeostasis).[25] Decreases in plasma ionized calcium levels increase PTH levels, and PTH also stimulates the renal conversion of $25(OH)_2D_3$ to $1,25(OH)_2D_3$ by the $25(OH)D_3$ 1α-hydroxylase located in the proximal tubule of the kidney.[397-403] Dietary Pi deprivation or hypophosphatemia induces 25-hydroxyvitamin D_3 1α-hydroxylase.[264-273] Mice or rats, but not pigs, fed a low-Pi diet showed a decrease in the activity of the 25-hydroxyvitamin D_3 24-hydroxylase (a renal enzyme involved in the catabolism of $1,25(OH)_2D_3$) compared with rats fed a normal Pi diet within 24 hours of Pi restriction.[404-406] $1,25(OH)_2D_3$ decreases renal Pi excretion.[22,30,276,280,281,383]

Vitamin D receptor (VDR) mutant mice exhibit decreased serum Pi; however, Pi transport by renal cortical brush border membranes, Pi excretion, and/or NaPi-IIa or NaPi-IIc mRNA levels were not different between VDR null or wild-type mice, whereas NaPi-IIa protein expression and NaPi-IIa cotransporter immunoreactive signals were slightly but significantly decreased in the VDR mice compared with the wild-type mice.[366] When VDR knockout mice were fed a low-Pi diet, serum Pi concentrations were more markedly decreased in the VDR knockout mice than in the wild-type mice. Other studies performed in VDR and 25(OH)D 1α-hydroxylase null mutant mice have shown that both these knockout mice adapt to Pi deprivation with increased NaPi-IIa protein in a manner similar to that found in wild-type mice.[407] However, when these mice were fed a high-Pi diet, Pi excretion was less in the VDR and 25-hydroxyvitamin D 1α-hydroxylase null mutant mice compared to the wild-type mice. In vitamin D-deprived rats, NaPi-IIa transporter protein and mRNA levels were reported to be decreased in juxtamedullary but not superficial renal cortical tubules compared with normal rats.[408]

INSULIN, GROWTH HORMONE, AND INSULIN-LIKE GROWTH FACTOR

Insulin decreases plasma Pi and Pi excretion in human and animal models.[409-412] This enhanced renal Pi reabsorption can be demonstrated in the absence of changes in blood glucose, PTH, and Pi levels or urinary Na excretion. Micropuncture studies[410] have demonstrated enhanced Pi reabsorption in hyperinsulinemic dogs and somatostatin infusion, which decreases plasma insulin levels, increases Pi excretion.[413] Growth hormone decreases Pi excretion and has been postulated to contribute to the increased Pi reabsorption and positive Pi balance demonstrated in growing animals.[369,414] Administration of a growth hormone antagonist for 4 days to immature rats is associated with increased Pi excretion and a decreased transport capacity for Pi reabsorption.[415,416] In juvenile rats, suppression of growth hormone is associated with an increase in Pi excretion as a result of decreased NaPi-IIa expression.[417] Growth hormone administration increases Pi uptake by brush border membrane vesicles.[418] Because growth hormone increases renal IGF-1 synthesis,[419] the effects of growth hormone on Pi reabsorption may also be caused by IGF-1.[369,419-424]

RENAL NERVES, CATECHOLAMINES, DOPAMINE, AND SEROTONIN

Numerous studies have demonstrated that acute renal denervation or the administration of catecholamines alter Pi reabsorption independently of PTH.[378,425-437] The increase in urinary Pi excretion after acute renal denervation could be the result of both increased production of dopamine and decreased α- or β-adrenoreceptor activity because acute renal denervation was shown initially to increase renal dopamine excretion and almost completely abolish renal norepinephrine and epinephrine levels.[438,439] Epinephrine decreases plasma Pi, presumably by shifting Pi from the extracellular into the intracellular space. The hypophosphatemic response to isoproterenol infusion is blocked by propranolol, suggesting involvement of the β-adrenoreceptors. Infusion of isoproterenol markedly enhances renal Pi reabsorption in normal rats and hypophosphatemic mice.[436,440] The enhanced Pi reabsorption and attenuated phosphaturic response to PTH observed in acute respiratory alkalosis and Pi deprivation is blocked by infusion of propranolol, suggesting a possible role for stimulation of β-adrenoreceptors in these conditions. Stimulation of α-adrenoreceptors by the addition of epinephrine to opossum kidney (OK) cells blunts the PTH-induced increase in cAMP levels and the inhibition of Pi transport.[441]

Stimulation of α_2-adrenoreceptors in vivo has also been demonstrated to attenuate the phosphaturic response to PTH.[379] Dopamine infusion and the infusion of L-dopa, gludopa, or dopamine precursors increase Pi excretion in the absence of PTH.[442-444] Dopamine administration decreases Pi transport in OK cells and rabbit proximal straight tubules.[435,445-450] Increasing dietary Pi intake increases urinary dopamine excretion and Pi excretion.[451] Inhibition of endogenous dopamine synthesis by the administration of carbidopa to rats results in decreased dopamine and Pi excretion suggesting a role for endogenous dopamine in Pi regulation.[431,439] A paracrine role for dopamine in Pi regulation is strengthened by studies in OK cells showing that the addition of dopamine or L-dopa selectively decreases Pi uptake. Furthermore, Pi-replete OK cells produce more dopamine from L-dopa than Pi-deprived cells.[447] Dopamine inhibits Pi transport by multiple mechanisms, including activation of DA_1 and DA_2 receptors.[446,449,450] Dopamine induces the internalization of NaPi-IIa cotransporter molecules by activation of luminal DA_1 receptors.[445] Renal proximal tubules also synthesize serotonin from 5-hydroxytryptophan using the same enzyme that converts L-dopa to dopamine. Incubation of OK cells with serotonin or 5-hydroxytryptophan enhances Pi transport and raises the possibility that serotonin may also be involved in the physiologic regulation of renal Pi transport.[442,448,452,453]

PHOSPHATONINS (FGF-23, sFRP-4)

The term *phosphatonin* was introduced to describe a factor or factors responsible for the inhibition of renal phosphate reabsorption and altered 25(OH)D 1α-hydroxylase regulation observed in patients with tumor-induced osteomalacia.[304] Cai and coworkers[303] described a patient with tumor-induced osteomalacia (TIO) in whom the biochemical features of hypophosphatemia, renal phosphate wasting, and reduced serum $1\alpha,25(OH)_2D$ disappeared following removal of the tumor. Several factors have been identified that are associated with phosphate wasting, including FGF-23, sFRP-4, fibroblast growth factor 7 (FGF-7), and matrix extracellular phosphoglycoprotein (MEPE).

The most extensively studied phosphatonin is FGF-23, a 251–amino acid secreted protein.[256,287,293,454] Recombinant FGF-23 administered intraperitoneally to mice or rats induces phosphaturia and inhibits 25-hydroxyvitamin D 1α-hydroxylase activity.[256,287,293,454] The minimal sequence needed for phosphaturic activity resides between amino acids 176 and 210.[293] Transgenic animals overexpressing FGF-23 are hypophosphatemic and phosphaturic and show the presence of rickets and reduced serum $1\alpha,25(OH)_2D$ concentrations or 25-hydroxyvitamin D 1α-hydroxylase activity.[296,297,455] Conversely, mice in which the FGF-23 gene has been ablated demonstrate hyperphosphatemia, reduced phosphate excretion, markedly elevated serum $1\alpha,25(OH)_2D$ concentrations and renal 25-hydroxyvitamin D 1α-hydroxylase mRNA expression, vascular calcification, and early mortality.[297,456] The ablation of the VDR in FGF-23 null mice has been reported to rescue this phenotype, supporting an important role for vitamin D in the pathogenesis of the abnormal phenotype seen in FGF-23 null mice.[457] FGF-23 binds and signals through FGF receptors 1c, 3c, and FGFR4,[146] although this has not been established in mice in vivo.[458] A co-receptor, klotho, is necessary for FGF-23 to exhibit bioactivity.[146,459] The role of klotho in FGF-23 signaling is supported by the observation that klotho knockout mice have a phenotype identical to that of FGF-23 knockout mice.[460] FGF-23 synthesis is regulated by $1\alpha,25(OH)_2D$. Increasing doses of $1\alpha,25(OH)_2D$ increase FGF-23 concentrations in the serum within 24 hours, but statistically significant changes are observed 4 hours after $1\alpha,25(OH)_2D$ treatment.[461,462] In the physiologic sense, it is possible that FGF-23 is a negative feedback regulator of the 25-hydroxyvitamin D 1α-hydroxylase enzyme.

The Wnt antagonist, sFRP-4, is highly expressed in tumors associated with renal phosphate wasting and osteomalacia.[291] Recombinant sFRP-4 is phosphaturic in rats and prevents the upregulation of the 25-hydroxyvitamin D 1α-hydroxylase enzyme seen in the presence of hypophosphatemia.[286] sFRP-4 decreases Na^+Pi co-transporter abundance in the brush border membrane of the proximal tubule and reduces the surface expression of the Na^+Pi-IIa co-transporter in proximal tubules of the kidney, as well as on the surface of opossum kidney cells.[301] sFRP-4 expression is increased in bone samples and serum from X-linked hypophosphatemic mice and in mice with a global knockout of the *Phex* gene, but not in mice in which the *Phex* gene has been knocked out in bone alone.[463] sFRP-4 protein concentrations are increased in the kidneys of rats fed a high-phosphate diet for 2 weeks but not in animals fed a low-phosphate diet, suggesting a possible role for sFRP-4 during increases in phosphate intake.[464] This suggests that sFRP-4 concentrations are altered in the kidney of animals fed a high-phosphate diet and could play a role in the long-term adaptations to high phosphate intake.

MEPE is abundantly overexpressed found in tumors associated with renal phosphate wasting and osteomalacia.[465] Recombinant MEPE is phosphaturic and reduces serum phosphate concentrations when administered to mice in vivo.[466] The protein inhibits Na-dependent phosphate uptake in opossum kidney cells and has also been demonstrated to reduce intestinal Pi absorption directly.[467] MEPE also inhibits bone mineralization in vitro, and MEPE null mice have increased bone mineralization.[468] Thus, it is possible that MEPE is important in the pathogenesis of hypophosphatemia in renal phosphate wasting observed in patients with TIO. However, MEPE infusion does not recapitulate the defect in vitamin D metabolism seen in patients with TIO.[466] Infusion of MEPE reduces serum phosphate concentrations, and serum $1\alpha,25(OH)_2D$ concentrations increase following MEPE, as would be expected in the presence of hypophosphatemia. Thus, in patients with TIO, it is likely that MEPE contributes to the hypophosphatemia, but other products such as FGF-23 and sFRP-4 inhibit $1\alpha,25(OH)_2D$ concentrations by inhibiting the activity of the 25-hydroxyvitamin D 1α-hydroxylase. MEPE may play a role in the pathogenesis of X-linked hypophosphatemic rickets, in which there is phosphate wasting, and there is evidence for a mineralization defect that is independent of low phosphate concentrations in the extracellular fluid.[463] MEPE expression is increased in mice with the *Hyp*

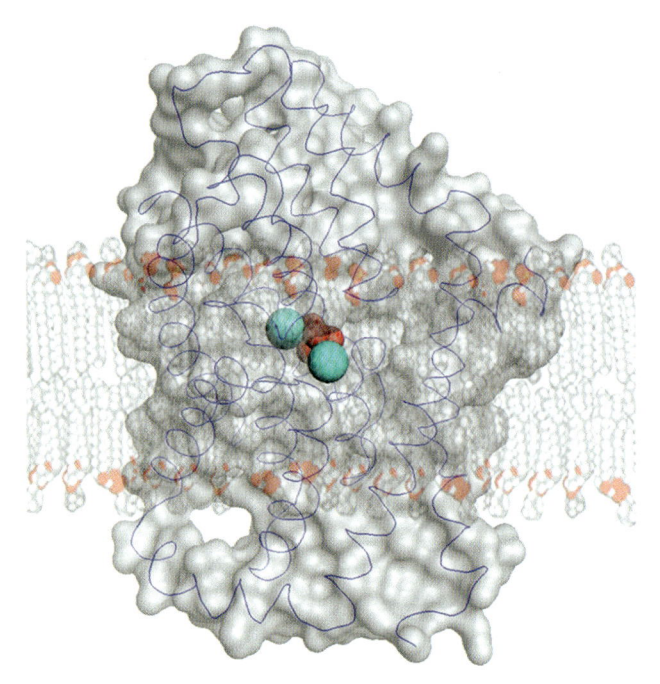

Figure 7.19 Model of the NaPi-IIa transporter. The extracellular region is shown topmost. The locations of two of three suspected Na$^+$ ion binding sites (*cyan* spheres) and for the Pi binding site (*red* spheres) are shown.

mutation and mice with a global knockout of the *Phex* gene but not in mice with a bone-specific knockout of the *Phex* gene. It is not known whether MEPE is regulated by phosphate concentrations, although Jain and colleagues have demonstrated that it is correlated with serum Pi concentration in normal humans.[469] Another growth factor, FGF-7, also known as keratinocyte growth factor, is overexpressed in tumors associated with phosphate wasting and osteomalacia.[470] FGF-7 inhibits Na-dependent phosphate transport in OK cells, and we have demonstrated that FGF-7 inhibits renal phosphate reabsorption in vivo. FGF-7 is present in normal plasma and is significantly increased in patients with renal failure (personal observations Kumar, R.). Whether or not FGF-7 is regulated by phosphate concentrations is unknown.

STRUCTURES OF PROTEINS INVOLVED IN THE TRANSPORT OF PHOSPHORUS

None of the structures of the mammalian renal phosphate transporters have so far been delineated. Shown in Figure 7.19 is a model of NaPi-IIa (Slc34a1) created using a sequence alignment described by Fenollar-Ferrer and colleagues[471] that uses part of the VcINDY crystal structure (PDB ID 4F35) as a template. The extracellular region is shown in Figure 7.19. Both the N- and C-termini are located within the cytosol. It was also demonstrated[471] that residues S164, T195, S196, S418, S419 and, to a lesser extent, R210 and Q417, are important for phosphate transport. The locations of two of three suspected Na$^+$ ion binding sites (cyan spheres) and for the Pi binding site (red spheres) in the NaPi-IIa transporter are shown.

Complete reference list available at ExpertConsult.com.

KEY REFERENCES

2. Brini M, Carafoli E: Calcium pumps in health and disease. *Physiol Rev* 89:1341–1378, 2009.
9. Marx SJ, Attie MF, Stock JL, et al: Maximal urine-concentrating ability: familial hypocalciuric hypercalcemia versus typical primary hyperparathyroidism. *J Clin Endocrinol Metab* 52:736–740, 1981.
12. Moore EW: Ionized calcium in normal serum, ultrafiltrates, and whole blood determined by ion-exchange electrodes. *J Clin Invest* 49:318–334, 1970.
14. DeLuca HF, Schnoes HK: Metabolism and mechanism of action of vitamin D. *Annu Rev Biochem* 45:631–666, 1976.
16. Wasserman RH, Smith CA, Brindak ME, et al: Vitamin D and mineral deficiencies increase the plasma membrane calcium pump of chicken intestine. *Gastroenterology* 102:886–894, 1992.
20. Brown EM, Pollak M, Hebert SC: The extracellular calcium-sensing receptor: its role in health and disease. *Annu Rev Med* 49:15–29, 1998.
39. Borke JL, Minami J, Verma A, et al: Monoclonal antibodies to human erythrocyte membrane Ca++-Mg++ adenosine triphosphatase pump recognize an epitope in the basolateral membrane of human kidney distal tubule cells. *J Clin Invest* 80:1225–1231, 1987.
43. Dimke H, Hoenderop JG, Bindels RJ: Molecular basis of epithelial Ca2+ and Mg2+ transport: insights from the TRP channel family. *J Physiol* 589:1535–1542, 2011.
45. Lassiter WE, Gottschalk CW, Mylle M: Micropuncture study of renal tubular reabsorption of calcium in normal rodents. *Am J Physiol* 204:771–775, 1963.
48. Agus ZS, Gardner LB, Beck LH, et al: Effects of parathyroid hormone on renal tubular reabsorption of calcium, sodium, and phosphate. *Am J Physiol* 224:1143–1148, 1973.
55. Yu AS, Cheng MH, Coalson RD: Calcium inhibits paracellular sodium conductance through claudin-2 by competitive binding. *J Biol Chem* 285:37060–37069, 2010.
72. Gamba G, Miyanoshita A, Lombardi M, et al: Molecular cloning, primary structure, and characterization of two members of the mammalian electroneutral sodium-(potassium)-chloride cotransporter family expressed in kidney. *J Biol Chem* 269:17713–17722, 1994.
77. Konrad M, Schaller A, Seelow D, et al: Mutations in the tight-junction gene claudin 19 (CLDN19) are associated with renal magnesium wasting, renal failure, and severe ocular involvement. *Am J Hum Genet* 79:949–957, 2006.
83. Hebert SC: Bartter syndrome. *Curr Opin Nephrol Hypertens* 12:527–532, 2003.
86. Costanzo LS, Windhager EE: Calcium and sodium transport by the distal convoluted tubule of the rat. *Am J Physiol* 235:F492–F506, 1978.
88. Dimke H, Hoenderop JG, Bindels RJ: Hereditary tubular transport disorders: implications for renal handling of Ca2+ and Mg2+. *Clin Sci (Lond)* 118:1–18, 2010.
90. Hoenderop JG, Nilius B, Bindels RJ: Calcium absorption across epithelia. *Physiol Rev* 85:373–422, 2005.
91. Hoenderop JG, van Leeuwen JP, van der Eerden BC, et al: Renal Ca2+ wasting, hyperabsorption, and reduced bone thickness in mice lacking TRPV5. *J Clin Invest* 112:1906–1914, 2003.
96. Magyar CE, White KE, Rojas R, et al: Plasma membrane Ca2+-ATPase and NCX1 Na+/Ca2+ exchanger expression in distal convoluted tubule cells. *Am J Physiol Renal Physiol* 283:F29–F40, 2002.
99. Yu AS, Hebert SC, Lee SL, et al: Identification and localization of renal Na(+)-Ca2+ exchanger by polymerase chain reaction. *Am J Physiol* 263:F680–F685, 1992.
123. Gamba G, Saltzberg SN, Lombardi M, et al: Primary structure and functional expression of a cDNA encoding the thiazide-sensitive, electroneutral sodium-chloride cotransporter. *Proc Natl Acad Sci U S A* 90:2749–2753, 1993.
147. Chang Q, Hoefs S, van der Kemp AW, et al: The beta-glucuronidase klotho hydrolyzes and activates the TRPV5 channel. *Science* 310:490–493, 2005.
153. Ryan ZC, Ketha H, McNulty MS, et al: Sclerostin alters serum vitamin D metabolite and fibroblast growth factor 23 concentrations and the urinary excretion of calcium. *Proc Natl Acad Sci U S A* 110:6199–6204, 2013.
164. Kojetin DJ, Venters RA, Kordys DR, et al: Structure, binding interface and hydrophobic transitions of Ca2+-loaded calbindin-D(28K). *Nat Struct Mol Biol* 13:641–647, 2006.

189. Wiegmann T, Kaye M: Hypomagnesemic hypocalcemia. Early serum calcium and late parathyroid hormone increase with magnesium therapy. *Arch Intern Med* 137:953–955, 1977.
191. Sherwood LM, Herrman I, Bassett CA: Parathyroid hormone secretion in vitro: regulation by calcium and magnesium ions. *Nature* 225:1056–1058, 1970.
192. Chase LR, Slatopolsky E: Secretion and metabolic efficacy of parathyroid hormone in patients with severe hypomagnesemia. *J Clin Endocrinol Metab* 38:363–371, 1974.
199. Whang R, Chrysant S, Dillard B, et al: Hypomagnesemia and hypokalemia in 1,000 treated ambulatory hypertensive patients. *J Am Coll Nutr* 1:317–322, 1982.
216. Voets T, Nilius B, Hoefs S, et al: TRPM6 forms the Mg2+ influx channel involved in intestinal and renal Mg2+ absorption. *J Biol Chem* 279:19–25, 2004.
237. Simon DB, Lu Y, Choate KA, et al: Paracellin-1, a renal tight junction protein required for paracellular Mg2+ resorption. *Science* 285:103–106, 1999.
241. Ferre S, Veenstra GJ, Bouwmeester R, et al: HNF-1B specifically regulates the transcription of the γa-subunit of the Na+/K+-ATPase. *Biochem Biophys Res Commun* 404:284–290, 2011.
243. Dimke H, Monnens L, Hoenderop JG, et al: Evaluation of hypomagnesemia: lessons from disorders of tubular transport. *Am J Kidney Dis* 62:377–383, 2013.
244. Ferre S, de Baaij JH, Ferreira P, et al: Mutations in PCBD1 cause hypomagnesemia and renal magnesium wasting. *J Am Soc Nephrol* 25:574–586, 2014.
254. Knochel JP: The pathophysiology and clinical characteristics of severe hypophosphatemia. *Arch Intern Med* 137:203–220, 1977.
256. Berndt T, Kumar R: Phosphatonins and the regulation of phosphate homeostasis. *Annu Rev Physiol* 69:341–359, 2007.
259. Berndt T, Thomas LF, Craig TA, et al: Evidence for a signaling axis by which intestinal phosphate rapidly modulates renal phosphate reabsorption. *Proc Natl Acad Sci U S A* 104:11085–11090, 2007.
289. Bowe AE, Finnegan R, Jan de Beur SM, et al: FGF-23 inhibits renal tubular phosphate transport and is a PHEX substrate. *Biochem Biophys Res Commun* 284:977–981, 2001.
290. De Beur SM, Finnegan RB, Vassiliadis J, et al: Tumors associated with oncogenic osteomalacia express genes important in bone and mineral metabolism. *J Bone Miner Res* 17:1102–1110, 2002.
292. Schiavi SC, Kumar R: The phosphatonin pathway: new insights in phosphate homeostasis. *Kidney Int* 65:1–14, 2004.
293. Berndt TJ, Craig TA, McCormick DJ, et al: Biological activity of FGF-23 fragments. *Pflugers Arch* 454:615–623, 2007.
303. Cai Q, Hodgson SF, Kao PC, et al: Brief report: inhibition of renal phosphate transport by a tumor product in a patient with oncogenic osteomalacia. *N Engl J Med* 330:1645–1649, 1994.
305. Shimada T, Mizutani S, Muto T, et al: Cloning and characterization of FGF23 as a causative factor of tumor-induced osteomalacia. *Proc Natl Acad Sci U S A* 98:6500–6505, 2001.
315. Greger R, Lang F, Marchand G, et al: Site of renal phosphate reabsorption. Micropuncture and microinfusion study. *Pflugers Arch* 369:111–118, 1977.
316. Haramati A, Haas JA, Knox FG: Nephron heterogeneity of phosphate reabsorption: effect of parathyroid hormone. *Am J Physiol* 246:F155–F158, 1984.
338. Murer H, Hernando N, Forster I, et al: Proximal tubular phosphate reabsorption: molecular mechanisms. *Physiol Rev* 80:1373–1409, 2000.
346. Werner A, Moore ML, Mantei N, et al: Cloning and expression of cDNA for a Na/Pi cotransport system of kidney cortex. *Proc Natl Acad Sci U S A* 88:9608–9612, 1991.
347. Beck L, Karaplis AC, Amizuka N, et al: Targeted inactivation of Npt2 in mice leads to severe renal phosphate wasting, hypercalciuria, and skeletal abnormalities. *Proc Natl Acad Sci U S A* 95:5372–5377, 1998.
454. Autosomal dominant hypophosphataemic rickets is associated with mutations in FGF23. *Nat Genet* 26:345–348, 2000.
463. Yuan B, Takaiwa M, Clemens TL, et al: Aberrant Phex function in osteoblasts and osteocytes alone underlies murine X-linked hypophosphatemia. *J Clin Invest* 118:722–734, 2008.
465. Rowe PS, de Zoysa PA, Dong R, et al: MEPE, a new gene expressed in bone marrow and tumors causing osteomalacia. *Genomics* 67:54–68, 2000.

8 Renal Handling of Organic Solutes

Orson W. Moe | Stephen H. Wright | Manuel Palacín

CHAPTER OUTLINE

GLUCOSE, 204
Physiology of Renal Glucose Transport, 204
Renal Glucose Handling, 205
Molecular Biology of Renal Glucose Transport Proteins, 205
Renal Glucose Transport in Disease States, 207
ORGANIC CATIONS, 210
Physiology of Renal Organic Cation Transport, 210
Molecular Biology of Renal Organic Cation Transport, 211
ORGANIC ANIONS, 215
Physiology of Organic Anion Transport, 215

Molecular Biology of Organic Anion Transport, 216
Clinical Relevance of Organic Anion Transporters, 219
Uric Acid, 220
AMINO ACIDS, 222
Physiology of Renal Amino Acid Transport, 222
Molecular Biology of Amino Acid Transport, 222
Structural Information of Amino Acid Transporters, 229

Most nephrons of lower organisms are largely secretory in nature. Kidneys in higher vertebrates transport solutes by combined filtration, reabsorption, and secretion. The handling of organic solutes involves all three of these; it spans a wide range from a clearance that exceeds the glomerular filtration rate (GFR) in the form of filtration-secretion (fractional excretion > 1) to filtration, followed by complete reabsorption (fractional excretion = 0), and everything in between.

The kidney adjusts the body fluid content as well as the concentration of specific solutes. To achieve these regulatory functions, there are sensing mechanisms for the pool size and concentration of the solute. Unlike inorganic solutes such as sodium or potassium, the total pool for organic solutes is difficult to define, because these solutes are constantly being absorbed, excreted, synthesized, and metabolized. For glucose, the maintenance of a discrete plasma concentration is clearly important. For amino acids and organic cations and anions, it is less clear whether plasma levels are that tightly regulated, so regulation of this latter group of organic solutes may be more concerned with external balance than maintaining concentration.

A filtration-reabsorption system is critical to maintain a high GFR, which is required for the metabolism and homeostasis of terrestrial mammals, because tubular reabsorption salvages all the valuable solutes that would otherwise be lost in the urine. Filtration-reabsorption commences by disposing everything and then selectively reclaiming and retaining substances that the organism needs to keep in the appropriate amount. This mechanism economizes on gene products required to identify and excrete the myriad of undesirable substances. In the secretion mode, the burden is on the kidney to recognize the substrates to be secreted and then secrete them. In contrast to glucose reabsorption, which is highly specific to certain hexose structures, organic anion and cation secretion can engage hundreds of structurally distinct substrates.

The reabsorption and secretion of organic solutes are primarily performed by the proximal tubule, with little or no contribution past the pars recta. This chapter summarizes the physiology, and cell and molecular biology of organic solute transport in the kidney. Although only renal mechanisms will be covered in this chapter, it is important to note that homeostasis of organic solutes involves the concerted action of multiple organs.

GLUCOSE

PHYSIOLOGY OF RENAL GLUCOSE TRANSPORT

Plasma glucose concentration is regulated at about 5 mmol/L, with balanced actions of glucose ingestion, glycogenolysis, and gluconeogenesis against glucose utilization

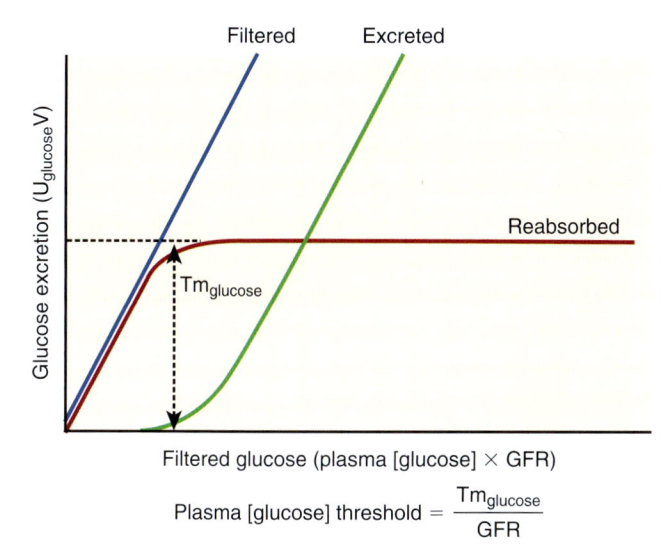

Figure 8.1 Urinary glucose excretion and tubular reabsorption as a function of filtered load. Tubular reabsorption increases linearly with filtered load as a part of glomerulotubular balance. When reabsorption reaches the tubular capacity ($Tm_{glucose}$), glucose starts appearing in the urine. Excretion is indicated by the *blue line*. The plasma glucose concentration for the given GFR is the glycosuric threshold.

$$\text{Plasma [glucose] threshold} = \frac{Tm_{glucose}}{GFR}$$

and, in some cases, renal glucose excretion. Although transient increments and decrements of plasma glucose are tolerated in postprandial and fasting states, neither hypoglycemia nor hyperglycemia is desirable for the organism. The metabolic rate of mammals mandates a high GFR, so the loss of glucose would be colossal if not reclaimed. The main physiologic task of the kidney is to retrieve as much glucose as possible so that normal urine is glucose-free, a phenomenon described by Cushny as early as 1917.[1] The proximal tubule is a major glyconeogenic organ,[2] so the glucose in the renal vein represents almost complete retrieval of glucose from the glomerular filtrate plus the glucose synthesized in the proximal tubule minus renal glucose utilization.

RENAL GLUCOSE HANDLING

Plasma glucose is neither protein-bound nor complexed, so it is filtered freely at the glomerulus. Glucose reabsorption by the proximal tubule increases as the filtered load increases (plasma [glucose] × GFR) until it reaches a threshold (tubular maximum, or $Tm_{glucose}$), which is the maximal reabsorptive capacity of the proximal tubule, beyond which glycosuria ensues (Figure 8.1). With a normal GFR, the value of plasma glucose for glycosuria to occur is about 9 to 11 mmol/L (162 to 200 mg/dL). One can predict that glycosuria will occur at a lower plasma glucose concentration in a physiologic state of hyperfiltration, such as pregnancy or a unilateral kidney (e.g., nephrectomy, transplant allograft). Conversely, in patients with a reduced GFR, it may take a higher plasma glucose concentration for glycosuria to occur if $Tm_{glucose}$ is relatively preserved. Some of the whole organism values for humans are as follows:

- Reabsorptive capacity ($Tm_{glucose}$), 1.7 to 2.0 mmol/min (2450 to 2880 mmol/day)
- Excretion rate—normally no more than 0 to 1 mmol/day

The maximal rate of glucose transport slows as one progresses from the early (S1) to late (S3) segments of the proximal tubule (Figure 8.2),[3] but the affinity for glucose rises, so the S1 segment reabsorbs glucose with a higher capacity but the S3 segment can decrease the luminal glucose concentration to a much lower level. Transport studies with brush border membrane vesicles and molecular cloning have established two transport systems with characteristics consistent with earlier microperfusion findings. Na^+ and glucose move as a net positive charge into the cell. Elimination of Na^+-glucose cotransport results in hyperpolarization of about 14 mV in the S1 and about 4 mV in the late S2 segment; Na^+-glucose transport accounts for approximately 15% of the apical membrane current and for 50% of the luminal negative potential difference (PD) in the early proximal convoluted tubule (PCT).[4] Crane first described the Na^+-coupled nature of glucose transport in the intestine,[5] and Aronson and Sacktor in renal brush border vesicles.[6,7] The two Na^+-glucose apical uptake systems have been defined by transport, biochemical, and molecular studies, with good internal agreement, and are summarized in Figure 8.3.

MOLECULAR BIOLOGY OF RENAL GLUCOSE TRANSPORT PROTEINS

CELL MODEL

Proximal tubule glucose reabsorption occurs in two steps: (1) carrier-mediated Na^+-glucose cotransport across the apical membrane; and (2) facilitated glucose transport and active Na^+ extrusion across the basolateral membrane (see Figure 8.3). Electroneutrality is maintained by paracellular Cl^- diffusion from the lumen or Na^+ back diffusion into the lumen, depending on the relative permeabilities of the intercellular tight junction to Na^+ and Cl^- (see Figure 8.3). Two Na^+-coupled carriers (sodium-glucose–linked cotransporters SGLT1 and SGLT2) are in the apical membrane (Table 8.1). The two SGLTs are part of a much larger SLC5 family, with 12 genes in humans expressed in a wide range of tissues with diverse functions encompassing plasma membrane Na^+-coupled cotransporters for glucose, galactose, mannose, fructose, myoinositol, choline, short-chain fatty acids, and other anions.[8]

Apical Entry

SGLT1. SGLT1 (SLC5A1) is an important brush border glucose transporter in the enterocytes for D-glucose and D-galactose,[8,9] as evidenced by studies of patients with glucose-galactose malabsorption and of mice with genetic ablations of SGLT1,[9,10] but its role in bulk glucose absorption in the kidney is likely smaller than that in SGLT2. Glucose transport is driven by the Na^+ electrochemical potential gradient using a model proposed by Wright and colleagues,[9] in which two extracellular Na^+ ions first bind to SGLT1, opening the external gate to permit sugar binding. After closure of the external gate, the internal gate opens to allow Na^+ and sugar to enter the cytoplasm site to permit the binding of external sugar. The sugar is then occluded from the aqueous phases by the closing of the external gate. The cycle is completed by the return of the protein conformation to the starting position. External phlorizin behaves

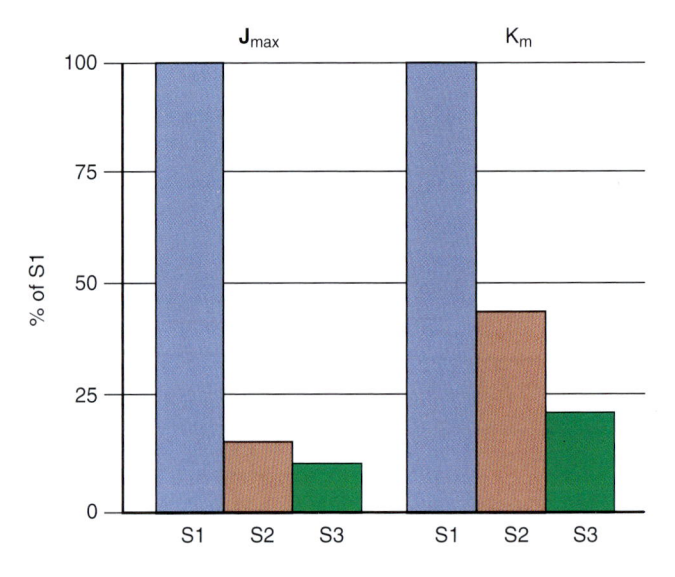

Segment		Capacity	Affinity	Glucose K_m	Na K_m	Stoichiometry Na:Glucose	Phlorizin inhibition
S1	PCT	High	Low	6 mmol/L	>200 mmol/L	1.1	1-2 mmol/L
S2							
S3	PST	Low	High	0.3 mmol/L	50 mmol/L	2.1	50 mmol/L

Figure 8.2 Relative magnitude of glucose transport characteristics in different segments of the proximal tubule. J_{max}, Maximal glucose transport rate; K_m, affinity constant for glucose. PCT, Proximal convoluted tubule; PST, proximal straight tubule. (Data from Barfuss DW, Schafer JA: Differences in active and passive glucose transport along the proximal nephron. *Am J Physiol* 241:F322-F332, 1981.)

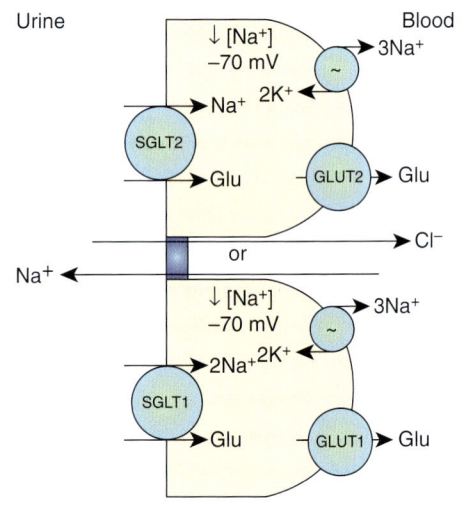

Figure 8.3 Model of proximal tubule glucose absorption. The Na$^+$-K$^+$-ATPase lowers cell [Na$^+$] and generates a negative interior voltage, driving uphill Na$^+$-coupled glucose entry from the apical membrane via the SGLT transporters 1 and 2. Glucose leaves the basolateral membrane via the facilitative glucose transporters GLUT1 and GLUT2 down its electrochemical gradient.

as a nontransported competitive inhibitor, with an inhibitor constant of 140 nM.[11]

In autosomal recessive glucose-galactose malabsorption (GGM), newborns present with life-threatening diarrhea (see later). Most mutations are missense mutations, but nonsense, frameshift, splice-site, and some promoter mutations have also been found. The functional effects include failure of the protein to reach the plasma membrane, which was also shown in patients by immunohistochemistry of jejunal biopsies. There are also allelic variants that are not associated with transport defects, such as Asn51Ser, His615Gln, and Ala411Thr.[9] The phenotype of GGM patients also may include a mild renal glucosuria that is reflective of the minor role that SGLT1 plays in glucose reabsorption in the kidney. Slc5a1$^{-/-}$ mice develop GGM but, surprisingly, this only occurs after weaning.[12]

SGLT2. SGLT2 (SLC5A2) is highly and specifically expressed in the early proximal tubule apical membrane in the S1 segment.[13] In subjects with familial renal glucosuria (Online Mendelian Inheritance in Man [OMIM] 233100), there is a correlation with mutations in the SGLT2 gene, and in knockout mice there is a massive glucosuria that is not observed in control mice.[13] This indicates that SGLT2 is the major protein responsible for the reabsorption of the filtered glucose. Transport properties of SGLT2 are distinct from those of SGLT1.[11] The Na$^+$ to glucose coupling is 1, not 2, rendering it with a lower power than SGLT1. In conjunction with the lower glucose affinity, it is not able to pick up all the glucose in the urine. Galactose is a poor substrate for SGLT2; this is understandable because the plasma concentration of galactose is only a few millimolar, and the filtered load of galactose is much smaller than that of glucose. Phlorizin is a more potent inhibitor of SGLT2 than SGLT1, with an inhibition constant, K_i of 11 versus 140 nM, respectively, and so is dapagliflozin. K_i is 100 to 1000 times lower for human SGLT2 than human SGLT1 (1 to 5 nM).[14,15] As

Table 8.1 Proximal Tubule Na⁺-Coupled Glucose Transporters*

Parameter	SGLT1	SGLT2
Gene (human chromosome)	*SLC5A1* (22p13.1)	*SLC5A2* (16p11.2)
Human genetic disease (OMIM)	Intestinal glucose-galactose malabsorption (182380)	Familial renal glycosuria (233100)
Mouse deletion	Glucose-galactose malabsorption	Massive glycosuria
Tissue distribution	Intestine, kidney liver, spleen	Kidney
Amino acids	664	672
Hexose selectivity	Glucose = galactose	Glucose ≫ galactose
Stoichiometry	2Na⁺ : glucose	Na⁺ : glucose
$K_{0.5}$ (mM)		
Glucose	0.4	2
Sodium	32	100
K_i phlorizin (nM)	140	11 nM

*Several other members of the SLC5 family (SGLT3, 4, and 5) are expressed in the kidney but there is little or no information on their role in renal glucose handling.

will be discussed later, SGLT2 inhibitors hold much promise for the treatment of type 2 diabetes.

Three other members of the SLC5 family with detectable transcripts in the kidney are glucose transporters based on in vitro substrate studies. SGLT3 (SLC5A, SAAT1) is likely a glucose-activated cation channel, and SGLT4 (SLC5A9) and SGLT5 (SLC5A10) are Na⁺-coupled glucose-mannose-fructose cotransporters.[8] Their protein localization and role in renal glucose transport are not yet defined.

A seminal achievement in this field was attained when Faham and associates solved the structure of the *Vibrio* Na⁺-galactose symporter (vSGLT1), which has a 32% identity and 60% similarity to SGLT1 in the presence of Na⁺ and galactose to approximately 3 Å resolution.[16] The predicted structure of the protein is shown in Figure 8.4. This structure was not predictable from the amino acid sequence of vSGLT but there is striking structural similarity to the leucine transporter, leuT, which shares almost no primary sequence similarity to vSGLT. The galactose binding site is interposed between hydrophobic residues that form intracellular and extracellular portals of entry. This 5 + 5 motif is discussed in more detail in the amino acid transport section later. An alternative access model was proposed to account for the translocation of the galactose and Na⁺ ions (see Figure 8.4). This should provide clues to the structure of the human SGLTs and guide further studies in transporter function and drug design.

Basolateral Exit

Proximal tubule basolateral membrane glucose transport is believed to be passive and is mediated by members of a large gene family termed *GLUT*. There are 18 known genes, of which 14 have known gene products (Table 8.2).[17] A thorough discussion is beyond the scope of this book; several excellent reviews are available.[17,18]

GLUT1 and GLUT2. The two isoforms believed to be important for renal transepithelial glucose transport are GLUT1 and GLUT2 (see Figure 8.3). GLUT1 was the first member of the GLUT family discovered in the red blood cell, with a 1- to 2-mM affinity for glucose ($K_{0.5}$), and is found at variable levels in almost all nephron segments.[19,20] It is probably also the principal mechanism for glucose exit in S3.[21] GLUT2 is a high-capacity, lower affinity basolateral transporter ($K_{0.5}$ = 15 to 20 mM) found in tissues with large glucose fluxes, such as intestine, liver, and pancreas and the S1 segment of the PCT.[20,21] GLUT4 is the insulin-responsive glucose transporter found in fat and muscle.[22,23] GLUT4 was found in glomeruli and renal microvessels but its role in tubular absorption is likely minimal.[24,25] The role of GLUT2 in renal glucose transport has been demonstrated by the presence of renal glycosuria in GLUT2⁻/⁻ mice[26] as well as in humans with GLUT2 mutations who present, interestingly, with the Fanconi syndrome, which is glycosuria accompanied by generalized proximal tubule dysfunction, possibly secondary to glycotoxicity.[27,28]

Transcripts of some of the other GLUT transporters have been detected in the kidney (see Table 8.2), but the location of their protein and their roles are unclear.

RENAL GLUCOSE TRANSPORT IN DISEASE STATES

MONOGENIC DEFECTS OF GLUCOSE TRANSPORT

Glucose-Galactose Malabsorption

The best-characterized monogenic disease in the SGLT family is glucose-galactose malabsorption due to an inactivating mutation of *SGLT1* (OMIM 182380).[25,29-32] This rare autosomal recessive disease presents in infancy with osmotic diarrhea, which resolves on cessation of dietary glucose, galactose, and lactose, substrates of SGLT1. The diarrhea returns when rechallenged with one or more of these substrates. The diagnosis of the disease can be readily confirmed by the administration of oral glucose or galactose followed by lactic acid determination in the breath. Patients with inactivating mutations of *SGLT1* exhibit some degree of renal glycosuria.[33] Because of redundancy in SGLT2, the glycosuria is mild, and reduction of $Tm_{glucose}$ is not always demonstrable. However, this is in keeping with the low-capacity, late proximal tubule SGLT1 transport system.

Renal Glycosuria

Because of the lack of intestinal defects and the renal-restricted distribution of SGLT2, the *SGLT2* gene is expected to be the perfect candidate for congenital renal glycosuria.

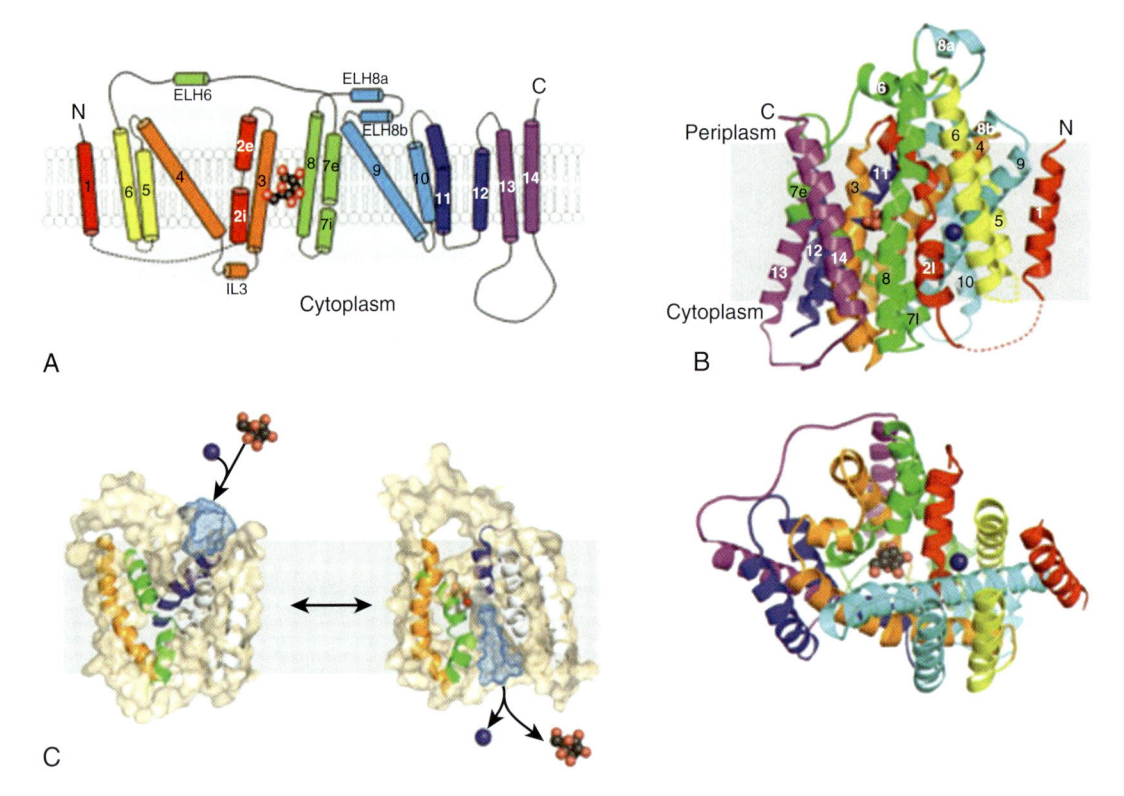

Figure 8.4 Structure of *Vibrio* sodium galactose transporter vSGLT. **A,** Topology. The protein has 14 transmembrane helices, with both termini in the extracellular space. A structural core is formed from inverted repeats of five transmembrane helices (TMII to VI and TMVII to XI). Galactose is at the central heart of the core seven helices (II, III, IV, VII, VIII, IX, XI). The two grey trapezoids represent the inverted topology of TMII-VI and TMVII-XI. Galactose traversing the central core is shown as *black* and *red spheres* (C and O atoms, respectively). **B, Top panel** shows the structure viewed in the membrane plane. The coloring scheme matches that of **A.** Bound galactose is shown as *black* and *red spheres*, as in **A.** Na$^+$ ion is shown as a *blue sphere*. **Bottom panel,** View from the intracellular side. **C,** Alternating accessibility. The protein on the **left** is a slice through the surface of the outward-facing model viewed from the membrane plane. An externally facing cavity is depicted by the *blue mesh*. The protein on the **right** shows a slice through the surface of the inward-facing structure of vSGLT in the membrane plane showing the internally facing cavity. Helices showing structural rearrangement during the transport cycle are colored *orange, green,* and *blue* for helices TMIII, TMVII, and TMXI. Helices with little movement during transport are *white*. The surface is shown in beige. Galactose is shown as *black* and *red spheres*. Na$^+$ ion is shown as *blue spheres*. (Adapted from Faham S, Watanabe A, Besserer GM, et al: The crystal structure of a sodium galactose transporter reveals mechanistic insights into Na$^+$/sugar symport. *Science* 321:810-814, 2008.)

Table 8.2 Facilitative Sugar Transporters

Protein	Gene	Class	Renal Expression	Extrarenal Expression
GLUT1	SLC2A1	I	All nephron segments; proximal tubule basolateral S2	Erythrocytes, brain
GLUT2	SLC2A2	I	Proximal tubule basolateral S1	Liver, islet cells, intestine
GLUT3	SLC2A3	I	Absent	Brain, testis
GLUT4	SLC2A4	I	mRNA in situ in thick ascending limb	Adipocyte, muscle
GLUT5	SLC2A5	II	mRNA in situ in proximal straight tubule	Testis, intestine, muscle
GLUT6	SLC2A6	III	Absent	Brain, spleen, leukocyte
GLUT7	SLC2A7	II	Unknown	Intestine, prostate, testis
GLUT8	SLC2A8	III	Absent	Testis, brain, adipocyte
GLUT9	SLC2A9	II	mRNA present	Liver
GLUT10	SLC2A10	III	mRNA present	Liver, pancreas
GLUT11	SLC2A11	II	Absent	Pancreas, placenta, muscle
GLUT12	SLC2A12	III	Unknown	Heart, prostate
GLUT 14	SLC2A14	I	Absent	Testis
HMIT	SLC2A13	III	Unknown	Brain
No gene product	SLC2A3P1	—		
No gene product	SLC2A3P2	—		
No gene product	SLC2A3P3	—		
No gene product	SLC2AXP1	—		

There is disagreement on the inheritance pattern (autosomal dominant vs. recessive), clinical classification of the reabsorptive defect (lowered glucose threshold vs. decreased maximal absorptive capacity, or both), and associated overlapping defects with aminoaciduria in this syndrome.[34,35]

To date, the strongest evidence that *SGLT2* is the major causative gene comes from the analysis of a patient with autosomal recessive renal glycosuria with a homozygous nonsense mutation in exon 1 of *SGLT2* and a heterozygous mutation in both parents and a younger brother.[36] In contrast, the linkage of the autosomal dominant form of renal glycosuria to the human leukocyre antigen (HLA) complex on chromosome 6 are not supportive of the SGLT transporters being causative.[37] Based on circumstantial evidence, an autoimmune mechanism has been proposed for this disease.[38] It is likely that this entity represents a heterogeneous group of disorders.

Diseases of Glucose Transporters

The first patient with Fanconi-Bickel syndrome[39] had hepatorenal glycogenosis and renal Fanconi's syndrome[40] who presented at age 6 months with failure to thrive, polydipsia, and constipation followed by osteopenia, short stature, hepatomegaly, and a proximal tubulopathy consisting of glycosuria, phosphaturia, aminoaciduria, proteinuria, and hyperuricemia. The liver was infiltrated with glycogen and fat. Disturbance of glucose homeostasis included fasting hypoglycemia, ketosis, and postprandial hyperglycemia. A mutation in *GLUT2* was demonstrated.[28] Most patients with the Fanconi-Bickel syndrome are homozygous for the disease-related mutations but some patients have been shown to be compound heterozygotes.[41]

The mechanism whereby *GLUT2* mutation causes the proximal tubulopathy is unclear. It is conceivable that impaired basolateral exit of glucose in the proximal convoluted tubule can lead to glucose accumulation and glycotoxicity.[42] *GLUT2* gene deletion in rodents leads to glucose-insensitive islet cells, but proximal tubulopathy was not described.[26] *GLUT1* mutations present with primarily a neurologic syndrome, with no documented renal involvement.[39,43,44]

Pharmacologic Manipulation of Sodium-Glucose–Linked Cotransporters

Antidiabetic therapy traditionally targets several broad levels—gut glucose absorption, insulin release, and insulin sensitivity. One additional strategy is to provide a glucose sink to alleviate hyperglycemia and the ravages of systemic glycotoxicity without actual direct manipulation of insulin secretion or sensitivity.[45] If one decreases the capacity of proximal absorption, the same filtered load will lead to higher glycosuria, resulting in a lower plasma glucose concentration (Figure 8.5).

In addition to providing a glucose sink, the proximal osmotic diuresis can potentially act via tubuloglomerular feedback and reduce the GFR, especially in the setting of diabetic hyperfiltration. One advantage of this approach is the self-limiting effect—increased filtered load from

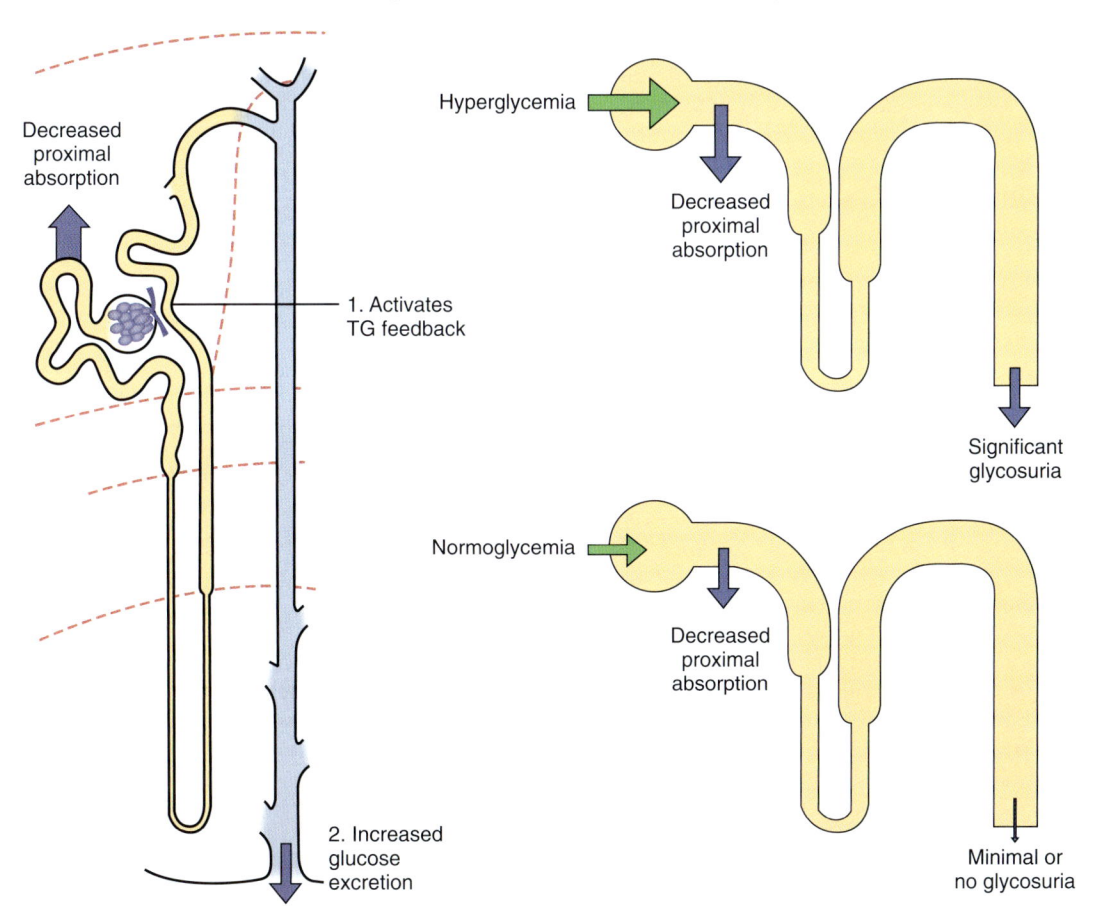

Figure 8.5 Effect of SGLT inhibition. **Left panel,** Inhibition of proximal absorption leads to increased glucose excretion. Proximal osmotic diuresis activates tubuloglomerular (TG) feedback and reduces hyperfiltration. **Right panel,** Self-adjusting features of the renal glucose sink. As the plasma glucose level falls, so does the filtered load, and glycosuria ceases, even though proximal absorption is still inhibited.

hyperglycemia in the presence of reduced proximal reabsorption increases glycosuria (see Figure 8.5). Once hyperglycemia is corrected and the filtered load is reduced, renal glucose leak ceases, even if the drug is still present (see Figure 8.5).[46-54] The long-term consequence of escalated glycosylation of epithelial proteins exposed to the urinary lumen has not been examined. Because hyperglycemia fluctuates, so does osmotic diuresis. The staccato natriuresis may present a challenge in control of the extracellular fluid volume. The increased renal glucose sink is also inducing higher glucagon and glucose production rates, which may or may not have undesired consequences.[55]

ORGANIC CATIONS

PHYSIOLOGY OF RENAL ORGANIC CATION TRANSPORT

The kidney clears the plasma of a vast array of organic solutes that share little in common other than a net positive charge at physiologic pH. These organic cations (OCs) include a structurally diverse array of primary, secondary, tertiary, or quaternary amines.[48,56] Studies using stop flow, micropuncture, and microperfusion have identified the renal proximal tubule as the principal site of renal OC secretion.[48] Although a number of endogenous OCs are actively secreted by the proximal tubule (e.g., N^1-methylnicotinamide [NMN], choline, epinephrine, dopamine[57]), an equal if not more important function is clearing the body of exogenous xenobiotic compounds.[48,56] These include a wide range of alkaloids and other positively charged heterocyclic dietary constituents, cationic therapeutic or recreational drugs, and cationic environmental toxins (e.g., nicotine). Importantly, the renal OC secretory pathway is also the site of clinically significant drug-drug interactions.[58]

RENAL ORGANIC CATION SECRETION

Renal OC secretion involves the concerted activities of a suite of distinct transport processes arranged in series in the basolateral and apical poles or in parallel within the same pole of renal proximal tubule cells. It is useful to consider the type I and II structural classifications of OCs originally developed to describe OC secretion in the liver.[47] In general, type I OCs are relatively small (generally, <400 Da) monovalent compounds such as tetraethylammonium and procainamide ethobromide. Most clinical cationic drugs are type I OCs, including antihistamines, skeletal muscle relaxants, antiarrhythmics, and β-adrenoceptor blocking agents. Type II OCs are usually bulkier (generally, >500 Da) and are frequently polyvalent, including D-tubocurarine, vecuronium, and hexafluorenium. Although the kidney plays a quantitatively significant role in the secretion of some type II OCs, the liver plays the most predominant role in excretion into the bile of these large hydrophobic cations. Renal excretion is the prime avenue for clearance of type I OCs,[59] and type I OCs will be focus of this discussion.

BASOLATERAL ORGANIC CATION ENTRY

Figure 8.6 shows a model for transcellular OC transport by the proximal tubule based on studies using intact proximal tubules and isolated membrane vesicles, subsequently

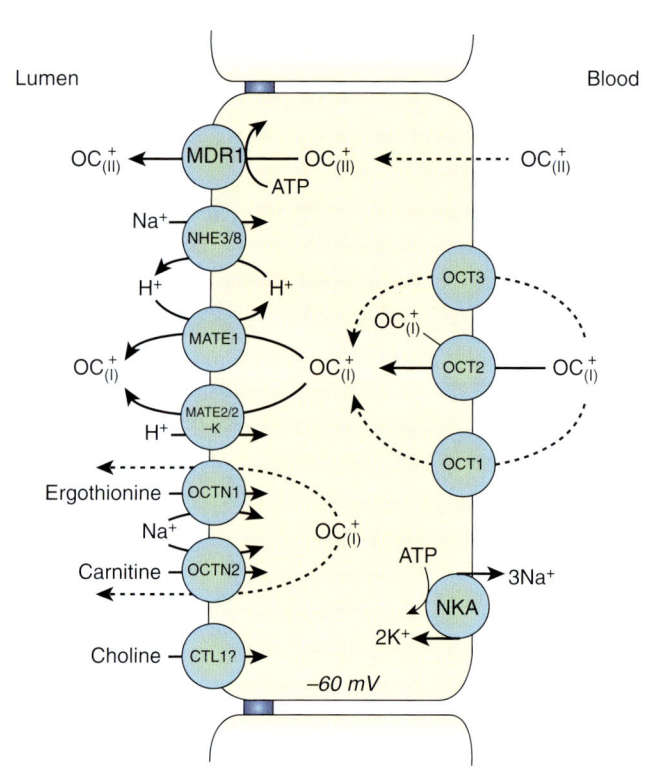

Figure 8.6 Schematic model of the transport processes associated with the secretion of organic cations (OCs) by renal proximal tubule cells. *Circles,* Carrier-mediated transport processes. *Arrows* indicate the direction of net substrate transport. *Solid lines* depict what are believed to be principal pathways of substrate transport; *dotted lines* indicate pathways believed to be of secondary importance; the *dashed line* indicates diffusive movement. Following is a brief description of each of the numbered processes currently believed to play a role, direct or indirect, in transepithelial OC secretion. Principal basolateral processes include the following: (1) Na^+-K^+-ATPase; maintains the K^+ gradient associated with the inside negative membrane potential and the inwardly directed Na^+ gradient, both of which represent driving forces associated with active OC secretion; (2) OCT1, OCT2, and OCT3—support electrogenic uniport (facilitated diffusion) of type I OCs from the blood (these processes are also believed to support electroneutral OC-OC exchange); (3) diffusive flux of type II OCs. The principal apical transport processes include the folllowing: (4) MDR1—supports the ATP-dependent, active luminal export of type II OCs; (5) NHE3 and NHE8—support the Na^+-H^+ exchange activity that sustains the inwardly directed hydrogen electrochemical gradient that, in turn, supports activity of MATE transporters; (6) MATE1 and MATE2-K—support the mediated electroneutral exchange of luminal H^+ for intracellular type I OCs; (7) OCTN1 and OCTN2—principally support electrogenic Na^+-dependent reabsorptive fluxes of ergothionine and carnitine, respectively; (8) physiologically characterized electrogenic choline reabsorption pathway (CTL1?).

supported by molecular data. For type I OCs, the basolateral entry step involves electrogenic uniport (facilitated diffusion) driven by the inside negative electrical potential[60] or electroneutral antiport (exchange) of OCs.[60] These two mechanisms can represent alternative modes of action of the same transporter(s).[61] The basolateral PD is approximately 60 mV (inside negative),[62] which is sufficient to account for an approximately 10-fold accumulation of OCs within proximal cells. A hallmark of peritubular OC uptake is its broad selectivity[63]; effective interaction of substrates and inhibitory ligands are largely defined by cationic charge and modest increases in solute hydrophobicity.[63] As will be discussed later, basolateral OC entry into human renal proximal tubules is likely dominated by the organic cation transporter OCT2.

The mechanisms for basolateral entry of type II OCs into the proximal tubule cells are less clear. The bulky ring structures render them substantially more hydrophobic than type I OCs. In the liver, type II OCs (e.g., rocuronium) tend to be substrates for the organic anion transporting polypeptide (OATP) superfamily of transporters (SLCO),[59] but these are poorly expressed in the proximal tubule.[64] Despite the presence of one or more cationic charges, the marked hydrophobicity of most type II OCs makes it likely that there is a substantial diffusive flux across the peritubular membrane that provides these compounds with a passive, electrically conductive avenue for entry into proximal cells.

APICAL ORGANIC CATION EXIT

Exit of type I OCs across the luminal membrane involves carrier-mediated antiport of OC for H^+ (see Figure 8.6), a process described in renal brush border membrane vesicles (BBMVs) in many species.[48] Importantly, net OC secretion does not require a transluminal H^+ gradient. Indeed, in the early proximal tubule, where the luminal pH is close to 7.4, tubular secretion exceeds that of later tubule segments,[65] in which an inwardly directed (lumen into cell) H^+ gradient is present.[66] The nonelectrogenic nature of the exchanger (obligatory 1:1 exchange of monovalent cations),[67] even in the absence of an H^+ gradient, will permit OCs to exit the cells and develop a luminal concentration as high as that in the cytoplasm. In the presence of an inwardly directed H^+ gradient, OCs can be moved uphill into the lumen. Net transepithelial secretion is a consequence of combining an electrically driven flux of OCs across the basolateral membrane and luminal OC-H^+ exchange. From an energy perspective, OC-H^+ antiport is the active step because it depends on the displacement of H^+ away from electrochemical equilibrium, primarily through the apical membrane Na^+-H^+ exchanger,[68] which derives electrochemical energy from the basolateral Na^+-K^+-ATPase. The inside negative membrane potential supports the concentrative uptake of OCs across the basolateral membrane and the inwardly directed Na^+ gradient that drives luminal Na^+-H^+ exchange. The primary contributor to apical OC-H^+ exchange activity includes MATE1 and MATE2-K, two novel members of the multidrug and toxin extrusion (MATE) family of drug resistance transporters.[69]

The SLC22 carriers are implicated in renal handling of selected cationic substrates. The so-called novel organic cation transporters, OCTN1 and OCTN2, are expressed in the luminal membrane of the proximal tubule[70] and were considered potential contributors to renal OC secretion.[71,72] However, these transporters were subsequently shown to support Na^+-dependent reabsorption of certain zwitterions, including ergothioneine (by OCTN1) and carnitine (by OCTN2),[73] and likely play little role in type I OC secretion. Although MDR1 (ABCB1) is linked to several aspects of renal function,[74] its quantitative influence on renal OC secretion is less clear. For example, whereas biliary excretion of the prototypic MDR1 substrate, doxorubicin, is markedly decreased in mdr1$^{-/-}$ mice, urinary clearance actually increases.[75] We will focus on OCTs and MATEs and renal OC transport.

ORGANIC CATION REABSORPTION

Whereas secretion dominates the net flux of OCs in the proximal tubule, net reabsorption has been reported for a few cationic substrates, most notably choline.[48] Also, although the secretory flux of metformin dominates in the proximal tubule, there is evidence for a modest reabsorption of metformin by the human renal proximal tubule that is associated with a modest expression of OCT1 in the luminal membrane of these cells.[76] The apical membrane of renal proximal tubule cells expresses an electrogenic uniporter that accepts choline and structurally similar compounds with relatively high affinity.[77,78] In contrast, the apical OC-H^+ exchanger has a low affinity (but high capacity) for choline.[78] Consequently, choline is effectively reabsorbed when plasma concentration is in the physiologic range (10 to 20 µmol/L) and is secreted when plasma concentrations exceed 100 µmol/L.[79] The molecular identity of the apical choline transporter is unknown, but expression patterns and the functional profile of a member of the SLC44 family of solute carriers, CTL1 (choline-like transporter 1), suggest that it may contribute to choline reabsorption.[80]

MOLECULAR BIOLOGY OF RENAL ORGANIC CATION TRANSPORT

The cloning of OCT1,[81] followed in close succession by the cloning of OCT2[82] and OCT3,[83] resulted in a rapid increase in understanding of the molecular and cellular bases of renal OC transport. Evidence supports the basolateral entry of type I OCs by species-specific combination of the activities of OCT1, OCT2, and OCT3. Although OCT1 and OCT2 both play major roles in basolateral OC transport in rabbits and rodents, the human kidney expresses very low levels of OCT1 and OCT3, and OCT2 appears to dominate basolateral OC transport.[84] Species differences are also found in the expression profile of apical OC transport. In humans, the apical exit of type I OCs uses a combination of MATE1 and MATE2/2-K, which are coexpressed along with OCT2[85] (Table 8.3). In contrast, rodent kidney only expresses MATE1.[86] The OCTs are members of the SLC22 family of solute carriers and share a common set of structural features that place them within the major facilitator superfamily (MFS) of transport proteins,[87] whereas the MATEs are part of the SLC47 family of solute carriers.[88]

BASOLATERAL ORGANIC CATION TRANSPORTERS: OCT1, OCT2, AND OCT3

Basolateral OC transport is dominated by the combined activity of three members of the SLC22A family—OCT1 (SLC22A1), OCT2 (SLC22A2), and OCT3 (SLC22A3).[89] The human genes for OCT1, OCT2, and OCT3 congregate within a cluster on chromosome 6q26-27, and each has 11 coding exons.[90] Several alternatively spliced variants of OCT1 have been described. Rat Oct1A lacks the putative transmembrane helix (TMH) types 1 and 2 and the large extracellular loop that separates these two TMHs, yet supports transport of TEA.[91] In humans, four alternatively spliced isoforms of OCT1 are present in glioma cells,[92] a long (full-length) form and three shorter forms. Only the long form (hOCT1G/L554) supports transport when expressed in HEK2 cells.[92,93]

Table 8.3 Renal Organic Cation Transporters

Name	Gene Name	Human Chromosome	Proximal Tubule Localization	Principal Transport Mode or Substrate
OCT Family				
OCT1	SLC22A1	6q26	Basolateral (low in human kidney)	Electrogenic uniport; type I OCs (e.g., TEA, MPP, clonidine)
OCT2	SLC22A2	6q26	Basolateral	Electrogenic uniport; type I OCs (e.g., TEA, MPP, metformin, cimetidine)
OCT3	SLC22A3	6q26-27	Basolateral (modest in human kidney)	Electrogenic uniport; type I OCs (e.g., MPP, catecholamines)
OCTN1	SLC22A4	5q31.1	Apical	Na-cotransport; ergothioneine
OCTN2	SLC22A5	5q31	Apical	Na-cotransport; carnitine
MATE Family				
MATE1	SLC47A1	17p11.2	Apical	H$^+$-driven exchange; type I OCs (e.g., TEA, MPP, metformin, cimetidine)
MATE2-K	SLC47A2	17p11.2	Apical	H$^+$-driven exchange; type I OCs (e.g., TEA, MPP, metformin, cimetidine)
MDR Family				
MDR1	ABCB1	7q21.1	Apical	ATP-dependent; type II OCs, neutral steroids, cardiac glycosides (e.g., doxorubicin, dexamethsone, digoxin)

MPP, 1-Methyl-4-phenylpyridium; TEA, tetraethylammonium.

The human kidney expresses at least one splice variant of OCT2, designated hOCT2A, that is characterized by a 1169-bp insertion from the intron between exons 7 and 8 of hOCT2,[93] resulting in a truncated protein missing the last three putative TMHs (10, 11, and 12). Despite the absence of the last three TMHs, hOCT2A retains the capacity to transport TEA and cimetidine, although guanidine transport is lost.

As MFS transporters, the OCTs share several structural characteristics, including 12 TMHs, cytoplasmic N- and C-termini, a long cytoplasmic loop between TMHs 6 and 7, and several conserved sequence motifs[94] (Figure 8.7). Several additional features are unique to the OCT members of SLC22A, including a long extracellular loop (~110 amino acid residues) between TMHs 1 and 2, as well as a distinguishing sequence motif just before TMH2.[95] The long extracellular loop between TMH1 and TMH2 contains three N-linked glycosylation sites in all three homologs. In OCT2, all three sites are glycosylated; their elimination is associated with decreased trafficking of protein to the membrane and changes in apparent affinity for substrate.[89]

The latter observation suggests that the configuration of the long extracellular loop influences the position of TMHs 1 and 2, which are elements of the hydrophilic binding cleft common to the OCTs and in which substrate is suspected to bind (discussed later).[96,97] The long extracellular loop also contains six conserved cysteine residues inaccessible to the aqueous medium supporting one or two disulfide bonds,[98,99] which influence the structure of the extracellular domain and stabilize the formation of functional homo-oligomers of OCTS (and OATS).[100-102]

Although the OCTs can support electroneutral OC-OC exchange (e.g., 1-methyl-4-phenylpyridium [MPP][103]), the predominant, physiologic mode of operation is electrogenic uniport.[61,104] Transport is independent of extracellular Na$^+$ and H$^+$, with membrane potential providing the driving force for concentrative uptake of cationic substrates.[104] Simultaneous measurement of rOCT2-mediated current versus radiolabeled OC flux has revealed charge-to-substrate ratios that vary between 1.5 and 4.0, depending on the substrate and membrane potential.[105] The excess charge-to-flux ratio appears to involve a nonselective cotransport (that does not involve energetic coupling) of OCs with cations, which could include molecules as diverse as Na$^+$ or lysine. Modeling of the outwardly directed surface of rOCT2 has revealed a binding region with more anionic residues than those accessible in the inward-facing mode of the transporter, thereby facilitating the parallel net influx of small charged cations with each transport cycle of conformational change.

OCT1, OCT2, and OCT3 display marked overlap in substrates but are nevertheless distinguishable by their selectivities for specific compounds. For example, the prototypic OC, tetraethylammonium, is transported with similar affinity by OCT1 and OCT2 but has very low affinity for OCT3, whereas epinephrine and norepinephrine are transported with similar affinities by OCT2 and OCT3 but interact poorly with OCT1.[106] In general, however, the three homologs all support transport of a structurally diverse array of type I OCs,[106] but can interact with a limited number of neutral and even anionic substrates.[107]

The molecular determinants of the interaction of substrates and inhibitors with OCTs have been assessed using computational methods. A screen of inhibition of OCT2 transport by 900 drugs was used to define three structural classes of inhibitory ligands.[108] Cluster I and cluster III

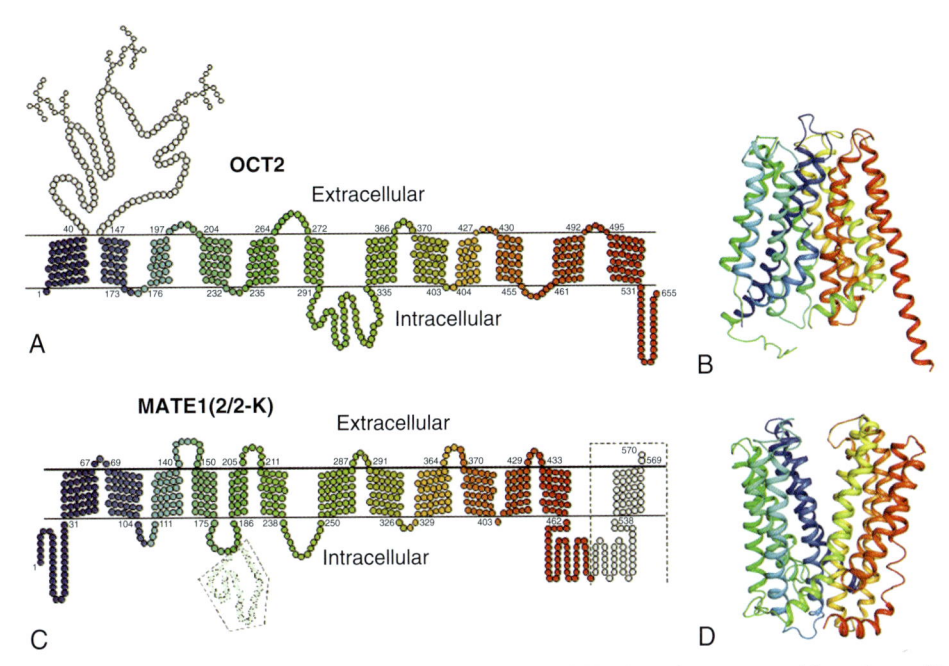

Figure 8.7 Model of the three-dimensional structure of the rabbit ortholog of OCT2 based on structural homology with the major facilitator superfamily (MFS) transporter, GlpT. **A,** Proposed secondary structure of OCT2, which is representative of all three OCT homologs. The human orthologs of OCT1, OCT2, and OCT3 contain 554, 555, and 556 amino acid residues, respectively, and several consensus sites for PKC-, PKA-, PKG-, CKII- and/or CaMII-mediated phosphorylation located within or near the long cytoplasmic loop between transmembrane helices (TMHs) 6 and 7, or in the cytoplasmic C-terminal sequence. **B,** Side view of OCT2, with the cytoplasmic face directed downward. The helices (TMHs 1 to 6) comprising the N-terminal half of the protein are shown in *blue*; the helices comprising the C-terminal half of the protein are shown in *cyan*. The lighter colored helices (1, 2, 4, 5, 7, 8, 10, and 11) border the hydrophilic cleft region formed by the juxtaposition of the N- and C-terminal halves of the protein. The amino acid residues that comprise the postulated substrate-binding region within the cleft are rendered as sticks with a *pink* van der Waals surface. D475 is rendered as a space-filling residue in *orange*. Note that residues from the long extracellular loop (between TMHs 1 and 2) and the cytoplasmic loop (between TMHs 6 and 7) were eliminated to facilitate homology modeling with the GlpT template.[97] **C,** Proposed secondary structure of MATE1 and MATE2/2-K. MATE1 is a 570-amino acid protein with 13 putative TMHs[139] and no N-linked glycosylation sites (in extracellular loops), and no splice variants have been described. MATE1 has three consensus PKG phosphorylation sites and no PKC, PKA, CKII, or CaMII sites, but current structural prediction suggests that the first three of these sites lie within TMH 8 or 9 and are probably inaccessible to modification. MATE2 is 602 amino acid residues in length, but MATE2-K is shorter (566 amino acid residues), the result of a deletion of 108 bp in exon 7 of hMATE2, probably due to alternative splicing.[130] MATE2/2-K has one PKC site, three PKG sites, and one MAPK site within putative cytoplasmic loops and these residues are within, or very close to, cytoplasmic loops in current homology MATE models, although no studies have examined the influence on MATE function of kinase activation to date. **D,** Side view of MATE1 with the cytoplasmic face directed downward. (Adapted from Zhang X, He X, Baker J, et al: Twelve transmembrane helices form the functional core of mammalian MATE1 [multidrug and toxin extruder 1] protein. *J Biol Chem* 287:27971-27982, 2012.)

consist primarily of nontransported inhibitors, which are large linear cations and globular neutral sterols. In contrast, cluster II contains most known OCT2 substrates, suggesting that they share the property of binding to the transport binding site. In addition, the kinetic mechanisms of inhibition of OCT2 activity, derived from representatives of the three clusters, are complex and include competitive, noncompetitive, and mixed-type interactions.[103] These observations are consistent with the view that ligand interaction of OCT2 (and, presumably the other OCTs), is not restricted to competition for a single binding site. It is therefore not surprising that the efficacy of the ligand inhibition of OCT transport is influenced by the identity of the substrate being transported. For example, trimethoprim is 12-fold more effective in inhibition of OCT2-mediated transport of the fluorescent organic cation, N,N,N-trimethyl-2-[methyl(7-nitrobenzo[c][1,2,5]oxadiazol-4-yl)amino]ethanaminium iodide (NBD-MTMA), than of MPP, and metformin is a threefold more effective inhibitor of OCT2-mediated transport of MPP than of NBD-MTMA.[109] Thus, efforts to model the structural basis of ligand interaction with OCTs and other multidrug transporters may require inclusion of the substrate identity as an additional factor.

Organic Cation Transporter Structure

The elucidation of the crystal structure of two MFS transporters, LacY and GlpT, and the fact that these two proteins share marked structural similarity of a common helical fold, despite low sequence homology (<15%), paved the way for homology modeling as a means to develop structural models for other MFS transporters.[110-112] LacY and GlpT served as templates for the modeling of OCT1[96] and OCT2,[97] respectively, and the models share a number of common structural features (partly because of shared structural features of the templates). These include a large hydrophilic cleft formed by the juxtaposition of the N- and C-terminal halves of the proteins comprised of the amino acid residues of the cleft-forming helices—TMH types 1, 2, 4, 5,7, 8, 10, and 11 (see Figure 8.7). Several residues in these helices predicted to face the cleft have been shown to influence substrate binding. In particular, an aspartate residue conserved in all OCT homologs (TMH 11 D475 in hOCT2) markedly influences substrate binding in rOCT1 and rOCT2 and is directed toward the hydrophilic cleft at a position within the protein that coincides closely to the binding site identified in GlpT111 and in LacY110 (see Figure 8.7).[113,114] Similarly, residues within TMHs 4 and 10 that influence substrate binding are also directed toward the cleft of OCT1[96] and OCT2,[97] including three residues in TMH10 that play a key role in defining the selectivity differences that distinguish OCT1 and OCT2.[96,97,115] The large extent of the pore or cleft region of OCTs ($20 Å \times 60 Å \times 80 Å$)[96] is consistent with the suggestion that the broad substrate selectivity of these proteins reflects binding interactions over a large surface that contains several distinct regions.[97,115] The external aspect of the binding cleft of all three OCTs also appears to include one or more inhibitory binding sites capable of interacting with specific OCs (e.g., nucleoside reverse transcriptase inhibitors), with dissociation constant, K_d values much less than 1 nM,[116] in addition to the lower affinity sites that appear to play predominant roles in substrate translocation (i.e., K_d values > 1 µmol/L). The influence of these very high-affinity sites on OCT transport activity is not clear, though the presence of high-affinity inhibitory ligands could influence the binding and translocation of other substrates.

At least 46 SNPs have been identified in the human *OCT2* gene. Of the 15 single-nucleotide polymorphisms (SNPs) in exons, nine are nonsynonymous and potentially influence OCT2 function. Primary focus has been directed toward the G808T (A270S) SNP, found in 7% to 16% of human populations (http://pharmacogenetics.ucsf.edu), in regard to the renal handling of metformin. The impact of this common SNP on metformin transport is controversial, with different groups showing significant or no changes in K_t and maximal glucose transport rate (J_{max}).[117] Similarly, clinical studies have reported decreased,[118] increased,[119] or no change[76] in renal clearance of metformin in subjects with the A270S variant. The failure to establish the A270S polymorphism consistently as a predictor of metformin pharmacokinetics may indicate that the influence of this variant is small in comparison to other factors, including age, gender, environmental influences, or genetic variations in other genes (e.g., other transporters involved in renal OC secretion).

It is interesting to consider the position of A270 within the current structural models of OCT proteins. A270 is within the small extracellular loop between TMHs 5 and 6[97] or in the middle of TMH 6.[117] Neither position is near the putative binding region within the hydrophilic cleft between the N- and C-terminal halves of OCT transporters. Thus, to the extent that the A270S polymorphism may influence ligand interaction with OCT2, this residue in fact resides far from the active sites of proteins but may be able to exert large effects on transporter activity.[117-120]

Regulation of OCT-Mediated Transport

OCT activity responds to short- and long- term regulation.[121] Human OCT2 is acutely downregulated following activation of protein kinase A (PKA), PKC, Ca^{2+}–calcium/calmodulin-dependent protein kinase (CaM), or phosphatidylinositol-3-kinase (PI3).[122] The kinase-mediated decrease in human OCT2 transport activity appears to reflect a decrease in the maximal rate of transport (i.e., K_t is not affected[123]). In rodents, Oct2 is regulated by sex steroids, with kidneys from male rats expressing higher levels of mRNA, protein, and transport function.[124] Moreover, treatment of male and female rats with testosterone significantly increases OCT2 expression in the kidney,[125] via androgen receptor–mediated transcription,[126] although similar profiles have not been seen in all species (e.g., rabbits[127]).

APICAL ORGANIC CATION TRANSPORTERS: MATE1 AND MATE2/2-K

The significance of MATEs in the apical secretion of OCs is evident from the Mate1$^{-/-}$ mouse, which displays 82% reduction of total renal clearance and 86% reduction in renal secretion of the cationic drug metformin.[128] In humans, the two MATE genes, each with 17 coding exons, are tandem-located on chromosome 17p11.2 and are designated as hMATE1 (*SLC47A1*) and hMATE2 (*SLC47A2*). MATE1 is expressed in the kidney and liver and is found in the apical and canalicular membranes, respectively, of renal proximal tubules and hepatocytes[69] (see Figure 8.6). Humans express at least three isoforms of MATE2. Expression of one of these is largely restricted to the kidney (hence, designated as MATE2-K), although by the reverse transcriptase polymerase chain reaction (RT-PCR), low levels of MATE2-K can be found in brain and testis.[129] The full-length isoform, MATE2, is also predominantly expressed in human kidney (MATE2 mRNA amounts to 39% of total mRNA for MATE2/2-K).[129] Antibodies that react with both MATE2 and MATE2-K have shown proximal tubule brush border expression.[90] MATE2 expression is more restricted to the kidney[69] and a splice variant (missing part of exon 7), resulting in the loss of 36 amino acids in the putative intracellular loop between TMHs 4 and 5 (see Figure 8.7). Both isoforms are functional, and their expression in human kidney is effectively comparable.[130] Figure 8.7C and D outline the structural characteristics of MATE1 and MATE2/2-K.

The principal mode of apical OC transport in intact renal tubules is OC-H^+ exchange, and it was the pH dependence of MATE-mediated OC transport that initially provided the evidence for MATEs serving as the OC-H^+ exchanger of renal (and hepatic) OC secretion.[69] MATE1 and MATE2/2-K uptake is *cis*-inhibited by extracellular H^+ and *trans*-stimulated by intracellular H^+, and MATE-mediated OC efflux is stimulated by inwardly directed H^+ gradients. The latter observation was confirmed in studies of transcellular OC transport across confluent MDCK cell monolayers stably expressing OCT in the basolateral membrane and MATE1 in the apical membrane. Acidification of the apical solution stimulates net transepithelial OC transport.[131] Proof that the pH sensitivity of MATE-mediated OC transport reflects a coupled exchange of H^+ for an OC was based on observations that membrane vesicles isolated from HEK2 cells expressing rat Mate1 or human MATE1 or MATE2-K support concentrative electroneutral accumulation of TEA driven by an outwardly directed H^+ gradient.[93,132,133] Together, the evidence strongly supports that mammalian MATEs can operate as secondary active OC-H^+ exchangers.

The ability to transport structurally diverse compounds is a defining characteristic of renal OC handling, and mammalian MATE transporters fulfill this description.[134] The multidrug acceptance of MATEs is evident in the observation that molecules as structurally dissimilar as cimetidine and MPP share a similar K_t and J_{max}. The diversity of effective ligand interaction with MATE transporters has been examined extensively. A study of the inhibitory efficacy of more than 900 prescription drugs has identified 84 (at concentration of 20 μmol/L) that reduced MATE1 transport activity by more than 50%. As seen with the OCTs, effective interaction of inhibitory ligands with MATE1 is positively correlated with increasing lipophilicity. However, compared to OCT2, MATE1 inhibitors tend to be larger (higher molecular weight, more bonds and rings, and longer circuits) and less electronegative molecules.[135] Predictive models of inhibitory ligand interaction with MATE1 also found correlations between half-maximal inhibitory concentration (IC_{50}) values and increasing lipophilicity, cationic charge, and number and placement of hydrogen donor and acceptor moieties.[136] However, the complex binding interaction of ligands (substrates and inhibitors) with the surface of a multidrug transporter (including MATEs and OCTs) makes it unlikely that a single molecular descriptor (e.g., log P or the number of hydrogen bond donors and acceptors) will provide an adequate means to predict drug-drug interactions.

It was also noteworthy that the structural characteristics of pharmacophores used to identify spatial correlations between the chemical features of an inhibitor and its inhibitory efficacy differed markedly, depending on the substrate used to assess MATE1 transport. The concept that profiles of ligand inhibition of transport activity display substrate dependence is not new. There has been growing recognition that ligand binding with multidrug-binding proteins involves interaction with spatially distinct sites within a larger binding surface. Similar observations have been reported for ligand interaction with the OCTs.[109] Also, the kinetics of ligand inhibition of Pgp-mediated transport shows a clear substrate-dependency,[137] as does the interaction of selected inhibitors with OATP-mediated transport.[138]

MATE Structure

Nonmammalian MATE proteins typically have 12 TMHs, but hydropathy analysis of the mammalian MATEs has suggested 13 TMHs (see Figure 8.7C), which has been confirmed by the mapping of heterologously expressed, epitope-tagged MATE1 (human, rabbit, mouse).[139]

Interestingly, elimination of the C-terminal (13th TMH) of MATE1 results in a protein that supports OC transport and has the same ligand inhibition profile as the full-length transporter.[139] Thus, the 13th TMH of the mammalian MATEs is not required for transport, and the functional core of the mammalian MATEs consists of the first 12 TMHs. Further evidence supporting the contention that the functional core of mammalian MATE is 12 TMHs was revealed in the Na$^+$-multidrug exchanger of *Vibrio*, NorM,[140] the prototypical prokaryotic MATE transporter. The structure of NorM, resolved to 3.65 Å, spans approximately 50 Å in the plane of the lipid bilayer and assumes an outward-facing conformation arranged as two bundles of 6 TMHs (1 to 6 and 7 to 12). The fold results in a large internal cavity with a volume of about 4300 Å^3 (almost two thirds that of the ABC exporter P gp), embedded within the lipid bilayer and open to the extracellular space. The N- and C-terminal halves of the protein display a pseudo–intramolecular twofold symmetry that is likely a result of gene duplication consistent with its protein sequence. The NorM (MATE) fold is unique among all known structures of transporters. This information was used to generate homology models of human MATE1 (see Figure 8.7) and MATE2-K. Several of the amino acid residues shown in site-directed studies to influence MATE1-mediated OC transport reside within the hydrophilic cleft between the N- and C-terminal halves of the protein (see Figure 8.7).

At least 57 SNPs have been identified in the human *MATE1* gene and 67 in the *MATE2* gene. Of these, 16 SNPs in MATE1 reside in exons and 12 are nonsynonymous changes altering the primary protein sequence. In MATE2/2-K, 15 SNPs reside in exons and six result in nonsynonymous changes. At least four of the MATE1 variants, and two of the MATE2/2-K variants, display reduced transport activity when expressed heterologously. The impact of these variants on renal clearance is unclear, but one intronic SNP (rs2289669 G>A) has been shown to be associated with changes in the glucose-lowering effect of metformin in humans, although the effect appeared to be correlated with MATE1-mediated export of metformin from hepatocytes.[141]

Regulation of MATE-Mediated Transport

Current efforts to understand the regulation of MATE expression has focused mainly on basal transcription. The constitutive expression of MATE1 appears to be under control of the general transcriptional factor SP1.[142] The promoter region of MATE1 also contains the sequence GTACTCA, which is similar to the consensus sequence recognized by activator protein 1 (AP-1) and the repressor AP-2rep.[143] AP-1 is a strong oncogene that mediates tumor invasion and is influenced by growth factors, cytokines, neurotransmitters, hormones, infections, and stress. The polymorphism g.-66T>C, present at a very high allele frequency in all major ethnic groups, is associated with reduction in the promoter activity of MATE1 and with lower expression levels of the transporter in the kidney, which are correlated with decreased binding of AP-1 and increased binding of AP-2rep.[143] The common variant of the basal promoter region of MATE2-K, G>A (rs12943590; >26% allele frequency) is associated in vitro with a significant increase in luciferase activity and reduces binding of the transcriptional repressor myeloid zinc finger 1 (MZF-1), which are correlated with a poor clinical response to metformin in patients homozygous for this variant.[144] In mice, the transcription factors aryl hydrocarbon receptor (AhR), constitutive androstane receptor (CAR), pregnane X receptor (PXR), peroxisome proliferator–activated receptor α (PPARα), and NF-E2–related factor 2 (Nrf2) do not appear to affect levels of Mate1 or Mate2.[86] It is not clear which, if any, of these regulatory pathways are involved in the decreased Mate1 expression in rat kidney associated with cisplatin-induced acute kidney injury[145] or to the decrease in cimetidine secretion associated with decreased expression of Mate1 in rats.[146]

ORGANIC ANIONS

PHYSIOLOGY OF ORGANIC ANION TRANSPORT

Organic anions (OAs) are another immensely broad group of solutes transported by the kidney. One can provide a general overview followed by a discussion of specific topics,

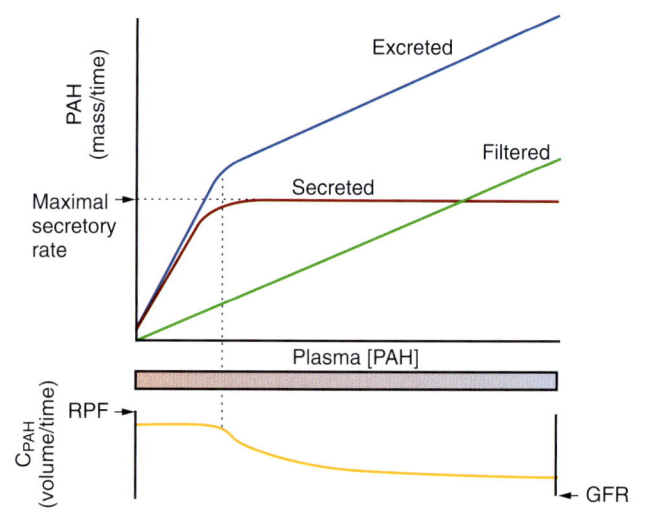

Figure 8.8 Illustration of filtration-secretion using *p*-aminohippurate (PAH) clearance. When plasma [PAH] is low, PAH clearance approximates that of renal plasma flow (RPF). When plasma [PAH] is high, it is less than RPF and higher than the glomerular filtration rate (GFR).

Table 8.4 Classes of Organic Anions Transported by the Proximal Tubule

Type of Agent	Examples
Endogenous	
Metabolic intermediates	α-Ketoglutarate, succinate, citrate
Eicosanoids	PGE_1, PGE_2, PGD_2, $PGF_{2α}$, PGI_2,
TXB_2 cyclic nucleotides	cAMP, cGMP
Others	Urate, folate, bile acids, oxalate, 5-HIA, HVA
Metabolic Conjugates	
Sulfate	Estrone sulfate, DHEAS
Glucuronide	Estradiol glucuronide, salicylglucuronide
Acetyl	Acetylated sulfonamide
Glycine	PAH, *o*-hydroxyhippurate
Cysteine	CTFC, DCVC, *N*-acetyl-*S*-farnesyl-cysteine
Drugs	
Antibiotics	β-Lactam, cepham, tetracycline, sulfonamide
Antiviral	Acyclovir, amantadine, adefovir
Antiinflammatory	Salicylates, indomethacin,
Diuretic	Loop diuretics, thiazides, acetazolamide
Antihypertensive	ACE inhibitors, ARBs
Chemotherapeutic	Methotrexate, azathioprine, cyclophosphamide, 5-FU
Antiepileptic	Valproate
Uricosuric	Probenicid
Environmental Toxins	
Fungal products	Ochratoxin A and B, aflatoxin G1, patulin
Herbicides	2,4-Dichlorophenoxyacetic acid

ACE inhibitor, Angiotensin-converting enzyme inhibitor; ARBs, angiotensin receptor blockers; CTFC, S-(2-chloro-1,1,2-trifluoroethyl)-L-cysteine; DCVC, S-(1,2-dichlorovinyl)-L-cysteine; DHEAS, dihydroxyepiandroesterone sulfate; 5-FU, 5-fluorouracil;. 5-HIA, 5-hydroxyindoleacetate; HVA, homovanillic acid; PAH, *p*-aminohippuric acid; PG, prostaglandin; TX, thromboxane.

without attempts to be exhaustive. An OA is any organic compound that bears a net negative charge at the pH of the fluid in which the compound resides. These can be endogenous substances or exogenously acquired toxins or drugs. The physiology can be poised for conservation, with an extremely low fractional excretion (FE); such is the case with metabolic intermediates such as monocarboxylates and dicarboxylates. The system can also be geared for elimination, with combined glomerular filtration and secretion. In addition to the large range of FEs, these transporters also have a broad array of substrates with completely disparate chemical structures. The field was opened by the seminal work of Marshall and coworkers who studied the elimination of dyes and concluded that mammalian renal tubules have a high-capacity secretory function.[147]

Smith has described the tubular secretion of *p*-aminohippurate (PAH) and provided a marker for estimating renal plasma flow (RPF) by PAH clearance.[148] Figure 8.8 illustrates the proximal tubule secretion using PAH as a surrogate. In low plasma concentrations, PAH has a FE of more than 1, and PAH clearance (C_{PAH}) approaches RPF because most of the PAH is removed from the plasma in a single pass. As plasma PAH increases, filtered and secreted PAH increase and C_{PAH} remains a good estimate of RPF. When the secretory maximum is reached and then exceeded, the increment in excretion is contributed solely by an increasing filtered load. At this stage, C_{PAH} starts to gradually drift below RPF toward the value of GFR (see Figure 8.8).

Classic studies using stop flow, micropuncture, and microperfusion[149-151] have demonstrated OA secretion in the proximal tubule. The secretory mode mandates energetic uphill transport and has broad substrate recognition. Table 8.4 is an illustrative but incomplete inventory of the spectra of OAs handled by the kidney; it is impossible to fathom any structural similarities among these compounds. In addition, the number of substrates far exceeds the number of proteins to excrete these substances. This is typical for these proteins, in which the ability to engage multiple compounds is intrinsic to their biologic function.[152,153] Fritzch and colleagues proposed a minimal requirement of a hydrophobic region in the anion to be a substrate.[154]

MOLECULAR BIOLOGY OF ORGANIC ANION TRANSPORT

The segregation into apical and basolateral classes of tandem transporters is not that distinct for OAs due to the assorted secretory and absorptive functions and the widespread use of anion exchange mechanisms; hence, the same family of transporters can be found on both membranes. Three families of solute transporters will be discussed here (Figure 8.9)—dicarboxylate-sulfate transporters (NaDC-NaS, SLC13 family, both apical and basolateral), OA transporters (OATs, SLC22 family, both apical and basolateral),

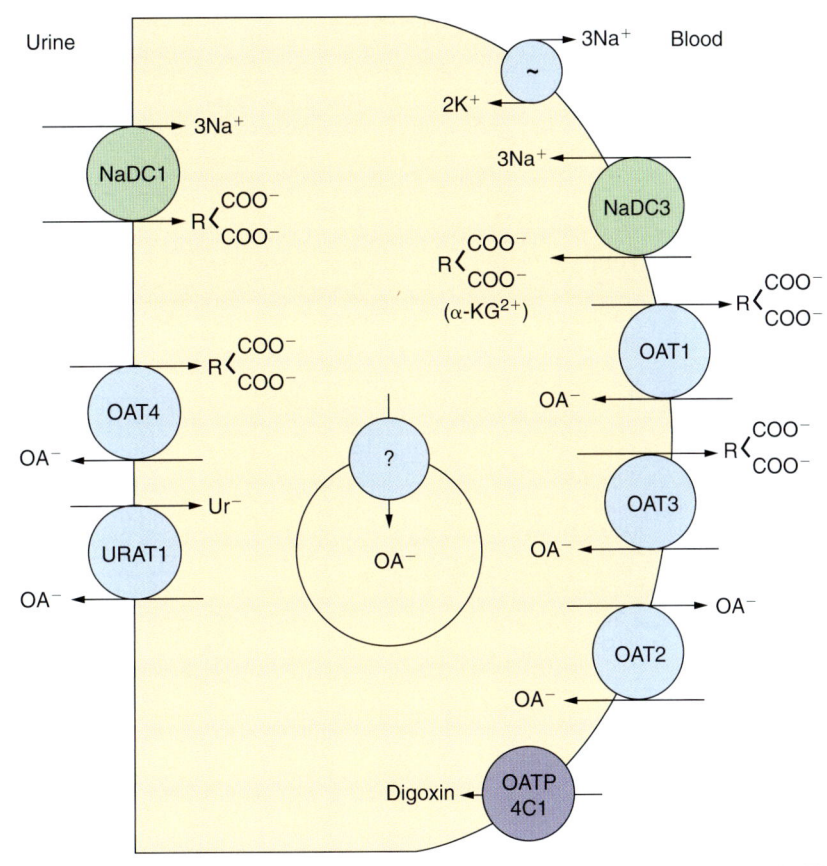

Figure 8.9 NaDC *(green)*, OAT *(blue)*, and OATP *(purple)* families of anionic transporters in the proximal tubule. The intracellular transport and sequestration of organic anions are not understood. OA, Organic anion; Ur, urate.

and OA-transporting polypeptides (OATP, SLC21 family, basolateral). Finally, we will consider uric acid separately.

NaDC FAMILY

Also designated as the SLC13A family, these proteins are functionally opposite to the secretory transporters because they mainly reclaim filtered solutes. The extended family is related by similarities in primary sequences but the members are quite distinct in their function (Table 8.5). NaS1 is a low-affinity sulfate transporter in the proximal tubule apical membrane (see Table 8.5) and is not an OA transporter; hence, it is not discussed here. NaS2 and NaCT are not expressed in the kidney (see Table 8.5). NaDC1 and NaDC3 are the main transporters of interest. An important aspect of citrate is that it is present in the urine in millimolar quantities; it is an important base equivalent in urine and also chelates calcium in a soluble form. Citrate is taken up into the proximal tubule cell from urine and plasma and extensively metabolized.

NaDC1

First cloned by Pajor and associates,[155] NaDC1 is on the apical membranes of the renal proximal tubule and small intestine, where it mediates absorption of tricarboxylic acid cycle intermediates from the glomerular filtrate and intestinal lumen. The preferred substrates are four-carbon dicarboxylates such as succinate, fumarate, and α-ketoglutarate. Citrate has six carbons and exists mostly as a tricarboxylate at plasma pH but, in the proximal tubule lumen, citrate^{3-} is titrated by H$^+$ (citrate^{3-}-citrate^{2-} pK = 5.7) and is taken up as citrate^{2-}. The Michaelis constant (K$_m$) for dicarboxylates ranges from 0.3 to 1 mmol/L, and one divalent anion is coupled to three Na$^+$ ions. Once across the apical membrane, cytosolic citrate is metabolized through adenosine triphosphate (ATP) citrate lyase, which cleaves citrate to oxaloacetate and provides a cytoplasmic source of acetyl coenzyme A or transported into the mitochondria, where it can be metabolized in the tricarboxylic acid cycle to neutral end products such as carbon dioxide (Figure 8.10).[156,157] When a divalent OA is converted to neutral products, two H$^+$ ions are consumed, which renders citrate^{2+} an important urinary base.[158] Gene deletion of NaDC1 in rodents leads to increased excretion of dicarboxylic acids in the urine, but the phenotype was not examined in regard to acid-base balance.[159]

NaDC3

NaDC3 has wider tissue distribution and broader substrate specificity than NaDC1. NaDC3 is on the basolateral membranes in renal proximal tubule cells[160] and in the liver, brain, and placenta. The basolateral localization signal of NaDC3 was mapped to a motif in its amino-terminal cytoplasmic domain.[161] The NaDC3 K$_m$ for succinate is lower than NaDC1 (10 to 100 mmol/L).[161] Similarly, NaDC3 displays a higher affinity for α-ketoglutarate than NaDC1.[162]

Like NaDC1, NaDC3 is Na$^+$-coupled and electrogenic, so it mediates citrate uptake from the peritubular space into the proximal tubule. It is also likely that NaDC3 serves a

Table 8.5 Organic Anion Transporters

Transporter Name	Gene Name	Human Chromosome	Renal Proximal Tubule Localization	Transport Mode or Substrate (Na$^+$-Dependent)
NaDC Family				
NaS1	SLC13A1	7q31-32	Apical	Sulfate, thiosulfate, selenate
NaDC1	SLC13A2	17p11.1-q11.1	Apical	Succinate, citrate, α-ketoglutarate
NaDC3	SLC13A3	20q12-13.1	Basolateral	Succinate, citrate, α-ketoglutarate
NaS2	SLC13A4	7q33	Absent	Sulfate
NaCT	SLC13A5	12q12-13	Absent	Citrate, succinate, pyruvate
OAT Family				
OAT1	SLC22A6	11q12.3	Basolateral	OA dicarboxylate exchange
OAT2	SLC22A7	6q21.1-2	Basolateral	OA dicarboxylate exchange
OAT3	SLC22A8	11q12.3	Basolateral	OA dicarboxylate exchange
OAT4	SLC22A11	11q13.1	Apical	OA dicarboxylate exchange
URAT1	SLC22A12	11q13.1	Apical	Urate OA exchange
OAT5	Slc22a19	(Murine)	—	—
OATP Family				
OATP4C1	SLCO4C1	5q21	PT—basolateral	Digoxin, ouabain, T$_3$
OATP1A2	SLCO1A2	12p12	CCD—basolateral	Bile salts, estrogen conjugates PGs, T$_3$, T$_4$, antibiotics, ouabain, ochratoxin A
OATP2A1	SLCO2A1	3q21	mRNA	PGs
OATP2B1	SLCO2B1	11q13	mRNA	Estrogen conjugates, antibiotics
OATP3A1	SLCO3A1	15q26	mRNA	Estrogen conjugates, antibiotics
OATP4A1	SLCO4A1	20q13.1	mRNA	Bile salts, estrogen conjugates, PGs, T$_3$, T$_4$, antibiotics

CCD, Cortical collecting duct; OA, organic anion (broad substrate specificity); PT, proximal tubule; PGs, prostaglandins; T$_3$, thyroid hormone; T$_4$, thyroxine.

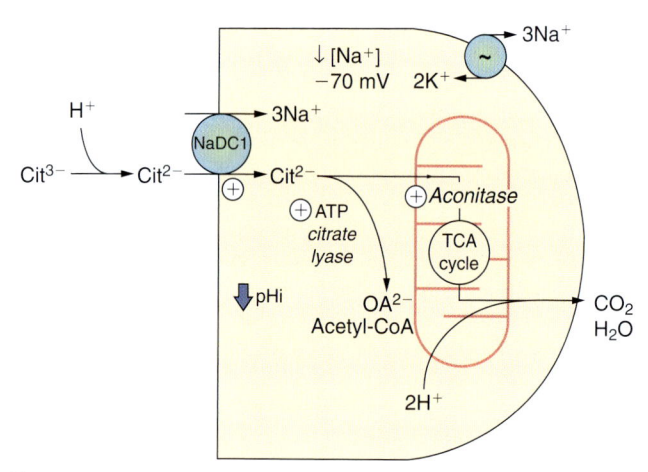

Figure 8.10 Proximal tubule citrate absorption and metabolism. The Na$^+$-K$^+$-ATPase generates the low cell [Na$^+$]. As a secondary active transporter, NaDC1 uses the electrochemical gradient to pick up filtered citrate, which is metabolized in the cytoplasm or the mitochondria. Ambient and cytoplasmic pH increase citrate uptake and metabolism. (1) Acidification of urinary lumen titrates citrate to the divalent transported species; (2) NaDC1 activity is directly activated by pH, and a chronic low pH increases the expression of NaDC1 (*circled plus symbol*); (3) intracellular acidification increases the expression of ATP citrate lyase and aconitase (*circled plus symbol*).

second function of supporting the outwardly directed α-ketoglutarate gradient required for OAT transporters to perform OA exchange (see later). NaDC3 supports approximately 50% of the OAT-mediated uptake of the organic anion across the basolateral membrane (see Figure 8.9) in isolated rabbit renal tubules,[163] with half of this effect reflecting the accumulation of exogenous α-ketoglutarate from the blood and the other half arising from recycling endogenous α-ketoglutarate that exited the cell in exchange for an OA substrate such as urate.

OAT FAMILY

Also known as *SLC22A*, these high-capacity transporters have tremendously diverse substrate selectivity (see Table 8.5), and are present on both membranes (see Figure 8.9). These proteins are important in rescuing the organism from succumbing to toxins. The uptake of substrates from the basolateral membrane of the proximal tubule is a thermodynamically uphill process using tertiary active transport. The Na$^+$ and voltage generated by the Na$^+$-K$^+$-ATPase drives the accumulation of α-ketoglutarate in the proximal tubule via NaDC3, which in a tertiary fashion (thrice removed from ATP hydrolysis) energizes the uptake of other OAs into the proximal tubule (see Figure 8.9). Endogenously produced α-ketoglutarate from deamination and deamidation of glutamine (ammoniagenesis) may also participate in the exchange. Some of the OAs transported may be endogenous or relatively innocuous exogenous compounds, but many of the substrates (see Table 8.4) are toxins. Although its function is to defend the body, the proximal tubule cells cannot afford a self-sacrificial approach because the end result can be destruction of the very mechanism that secretes these toxins. There is a detoxifying mechanism in the proximal tubule cell that protects the cell while the toxins are en route to the apical membrane to be disposed. The details of these mechanisms are still elusive, but current studies of isolated tubules and cell culture models have suggested that compartmentalization may serve to sequester the toxins from imparting their harmful effects.[164]

Basolateral OATs

More than a half-century after Homer Smith described PAH secretion into the urine,[148] the so-called PAH transporter was cloned by several laboratories almost contemporaneously.[165-168] OAT1 and OAT3 are present in the basolateral membrane of the proximal tubule (see Figure 8.9 and Table 8.5). OAT1-mediated uptake of PAH is stimulated by an outwardly directed gradient of dicarboxylates such as α-ketoglutarate, indicating that OAT1 is an OA exchanger.[169] The substrate selectivity of OAT1 is extremely broad with affinities comparable to those reported for the functional PAH transport system. OAT3 is localized in the basolateral membrane of the kidney and, like OAT1, has a broad extrarenal expression.[170] OAT3 also has a large substrate list comparable to that of OAT1. OAT2 was originally identified from the liver, and its expression in the kidney appears to be weaker than that of OAT1 and OAT3.[171] It transports PAH, dicarboxylates, prostaglandins, salicylate, acetylsalicylate, and tetracycline. Their role in uric acid transport is discussed later.

Apical OATs

There is no overlap of polarized expression of OATs in the proximal tubule. OAT4 was cloned from the kidney and is expressed in the apical membrane of the proximal tubule.[172] In oocytes, it transports PAH, conjugated sex hormones, prostaglandins, and mycotoxins in an OA-dicarboxylate exchange mode and is capable of bidirectional movement of OAs.[173] It is not known whether OAT4 represents an exceptional OAT-mediated luminal uptake. The role of OAT4 and OAT10 in facilitating luminal uric acid uptake as dicarboxylate and monocarboxylate exchangers is discussed later. The other apical transporter is URAT1, which is renal-specific in its expression.[174] Human URAT1 appears to be specific for urate transport[174] (see later).

OATP FAMILY

The OATPs are placed into their own family of transporters, designated SLCO (solute carrier OATP).[175] There are considerable interspecies differences that engender difficulties in extrapolating rodent data to humans. This family has 11 human members,[175] expressed widely in the brain, liver, heart, intestine, kidney, placenta, and testis and, like OATs, also has a wide spectrum of substrates.[176,177] The first member, Oatp1, was cloned from liver as a Na^+- independent bile acid transporter.[178] Substrates are diverse and include hormones and their conjugates, bile salts, and drugs such as the 3-hydroxy-3-methylglutaryl–coenzyme A (HMG-CoA) reductase inhibitors, cardiac glycosides, antimicrobials, and anticancer drugs. The presence of naturally occurring variations in human OATP genes renders this class of transporter a focus of pharmacogenomic research. Among human OATPs, only OATP4C1 is expressed in the kidney.

There is a myriad of rodent isoforms that have not been confirmed in humans.[175] One important substrate is the cardiac glycoside digoxin.[179] OATP4C1 is expressed in the basolateral membrane of proximal tubular cells and mediates the high-affinity transport of digoxin (K_m = 7.8 mmol/L) and ouabain (K_m = 0.38 mmol/L), as well as triiodothyronine (K_m = 5.9 mmol/L). The apical pathway for digoxin has been presumed, although not proven, to be an ATP-dependent efflux pump such as P-glycoprotein.

CLINICAL RELEVANCE OF ORGANIC ANION TRANSPORTERS

This field is obviously extremely broad and cannot be exhaustively covered. We will focus here on the transport of citrate, an anion with particular physiologic and clinical significance.

DISORDERS OF CITRATE TRANSPORT

The role of NaDC1 in physiology and pathophysiology has been well studied. Citrate exists in urine in millimolar quantities and has multiple functions in mammalian urine. The two most important are as a chelator for urinary calcium and as a physiologic urinary base.[158]

Calcium associates in a 1:1 stoichiometry. The highest affinity and solubility is a monovalent anionic (Ca^{2+}-citrate^{3-}) complex.[158] It is a tricarboxylic acid cycle intermediate, and most of the citrate reabsorbed by the proximal tubule is oxidized to electroneutral end products, so H^+ is consumed in the process, rendering citrate a major urinary base.

The final urinary excretion of citrate is determined by reabsorption in the proximal tubule, and the most important regulator of citrate reabsorption is the proximal tubule cell pH. Acidification of the cell increases citrate absorption by four mechanisms (see Figure 8.10):

1. Low luminal pH titrates citrate^{3-} to citrate^{2-}, which is the preferred transported species.[180]
2. NaDC1 is also gated by pH so that a low pH acutely stimulates its activity.[181]
3. Intracellular acidosis increases expression of the NaDC1 transporter[182] and insertion of NaDC1 into the apical membrane.
4. Intracellular acidosis stimulates enzymes that metabolize citrate in the cytoplasm and mitochondria.[183,184] This is a well-concerted response, and an appropriate response of the proximal tubule to cellular acidification is hypocitraturia.[185]

Although perfectly adaptive from an acid-base point of view, this response is detrimental to the prevention of calcium precipitation. All conditions that lead to proximal tubular cellular acidification (e.g., distal renal tubular acidosis, high-protein diet, potassium deficiency) are clinical risk factors for calcareous nephrolithiasis.[186] Hypocitraturia can cause kidney stones by itself or by acting with other risk factors such as hypercalciuria; therapy with potassium citrate reverses the biochemical defect and reduces stone recurrence.

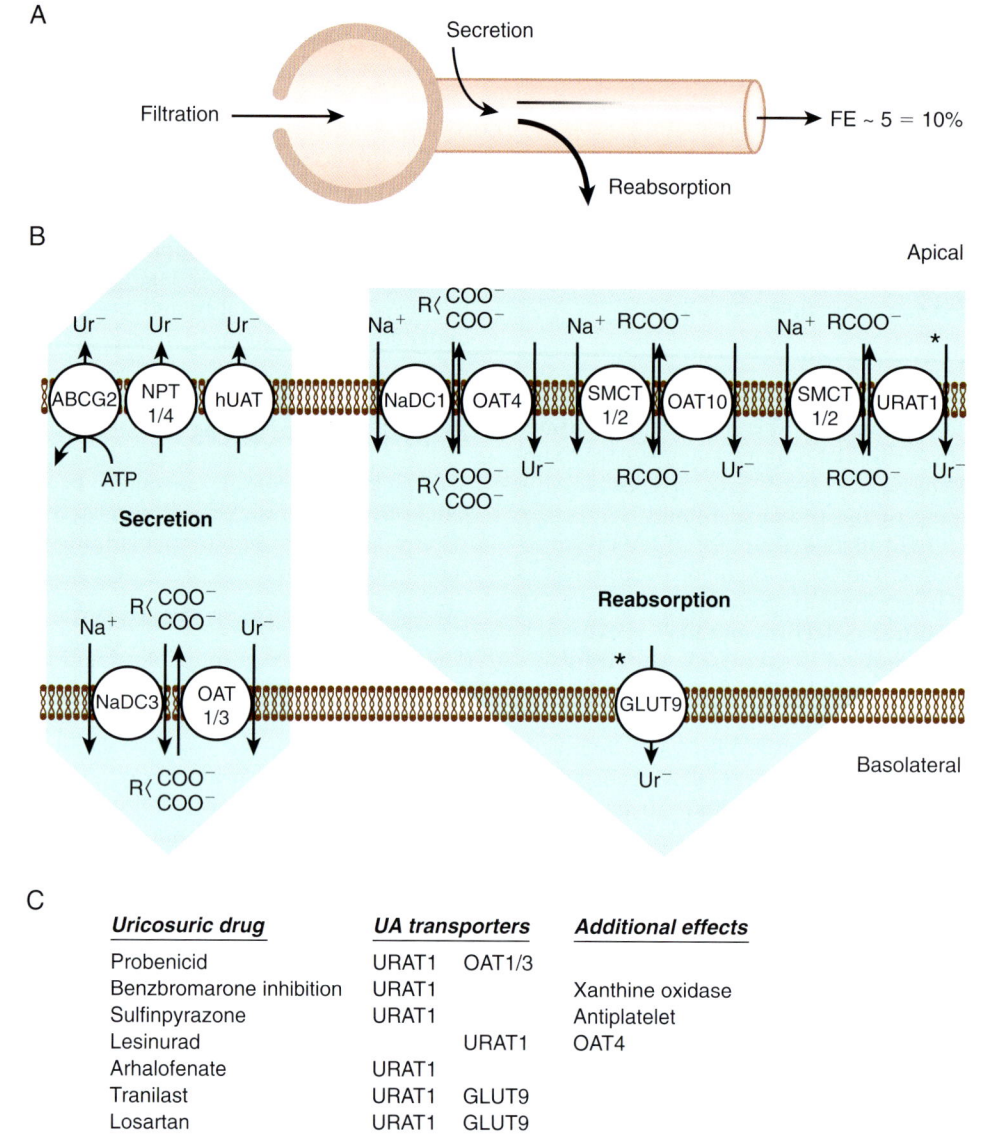

Figure 8.11 Uric acid transport. **A,** Filtration-reabsorption-secretion model of proximal tubule transport. **B,** UA transporters organized into whether they mediate secretion **(left)** or reabsorption **(right)**. **C,** Uricosuric drugs and their mechanism of action. All drugs target URAT1 and some have additional effects on other uric acid transporters and nontransport targets. *, denote the candidates with the strongest evidence; ABCG, ATP-binding cassette G; FE, fractional excretion; GLUT, glucose transporter; hUAT, human uric acid transporter; NaDC, Na-dicarboxylate cotransporter; NPT, Na-phosphate transporter; OAT, organic anion transporter; SMCT, Na monocarboxylate transporter; Ur, urate; URAT, uric acid transporter.

Uricosuric drug	UA transporters		Additional effects
Probenicid	URAT1	OAT1/3	
Benzbromarone inhibition	URAT1		Xanthine oxidase
Sulfinpyrazone	URAT1		Antiplatelet
Lesinurad		URAT1	OAT4
Arhalofenate	URAT1		
Tranilast	URAT1	GLUT9	
Losartan	URAT1	GLUT9	

URIC ACID

This is a highly complex field and will only be covered briefly here. More detailed recent reviews are available.[187,188] Several points will be highlighted. Genome-wide association studies (GWAS) have identified many loci linked to serum uric acid levels, and two surprising findings have emerged. The loci are remarkably reproducible across different geographic populations, and most of the loci are in fact uric acid transporters.[189,190] This highlights the important role that the kidney and uric acid transporters play in regulating serum uric acid levels.

The traditional four-phase model of renal uric acid handling is not supported by data and has been replaced by a simpler current model (Figure 8.11A).[187] This model has three components—glomerular filtration of uric acid, which occurs freely, and reabsorption and secretion, which are now believed to coexist along the entire length of the proximal tubule. Net tubular handling varies among mammalian species; in humans (like rodents), net reabsorption occurs so that the fractional excretion of uric acid averages 5% to 10%.

The reabsorptive and secretory transporters are depicted in Figure 8.11B. These candidates are based on multiple levels of data, but very few candidates satisfy all the criteria—immunolocalization in the proximal tubule, transport of urate when heterologously expressed, gene deletion in mice leading to the expected under- or overexcretion phenotype, GWAS loci linked to serum uric acid level or gout, Mendelian inheritance of functionally significant alleles, and

Table 8.6 Three Best Characterized Uric Acid Transporters[187,189,374]

Transporter	Uric Acid Transport in Expression Systems	Immunohistologic Localization to Proximal Tubule (PT)	Association with Uric Acid Level or Gout*	Evidence from Rodent Gene Deletion	Human Monogenic Disease or Direct Genotype-Phenotype Correlation
Absorptive					
URAT1 (SLC22A12)	Urate-lactate exchange; Xenopus oocytes inhibited by uricosuric drugs	Apical membrane	Yes		Renal hypouricemia 1 from loss-of-function mutation (OMIM 220150)
GLUT9 (SLC2A9)	Xenopus oocytes inhibited by some uricosuric drugs	GLUT9, long form (SLC2A9a), basolateral; GLUT9DN, short form (SLC2A9b), apical	Yes	Whole-body deletion—hyporuricemia, hyperuricosuria, urate nephropathy Liver-specific deletion—hyporuricemia, milder hyperuricosuria, no nephropathy	Renal hypouricemia 2 from loss-of-function mutation (OMIM 612076), urolithiasis, exercise-induced acute kidney injury
Secretory					
ABCG2 (ABCP)	Multisubstrate efflux transporter	Apical membrane in PT but also in intestine	Yes	Reduced gut and renal excretion, hyperuricemia	Hypofunctional single-nucleotide polymorphism Q141K—predisposes to gout

*In genome-wide association studies.

corresponding clinical phenotype. Of all the candidates shown in Figure 8.11B, GLUT9, URAT1, and ABCG2 currently fulfill all the criteria; a number of the features are shown in Table 8.6. Due to constraints in a number of references, a large number of original papers are not cited directly but are in the review articles mentioned in the table.

URIC ACID REABSORPTION

URAT1 is the dominant apical entry pathway for urate reabsorption.[174] It acts as an anion exchanger and reabsorbs urate in exchange for monovalent intracellular anions such as nicotinate, pyrazinamide, lactate, β-hydroxybutyrate, and acetoacetate, which enter the cell through Na-coupled monocarboxylate cotransporters, likely SMCT1 and SMCT2. Loss of function mutations in URAT1 cause renal hypouricemia.[172] Similarly, drugs such as probenecid and losartan inhibit URAT1, accounting for their uricosuric effect. However, probenecid does not entirely block urate reabsorption, suggesting the existence of other apical urate transporters. OAT4[191] and OAT10[192] have been postulated to fulfill these roles, but the evidence is incomplete. The dependence on filtered monocarboxylate anions potentially explains the development of hyperuricemia with diabetic, alcoholic, or starvation ketoacidosis and with nicotinic acid use.

The sole basolateral exit pathway for urate is believed to be GLUT9. Its properties are most consistent with its function as a urate uniporter or possibly as an electrogenic anion exchanger.[193,194] Loss-of-function mutations in GLUT9 cause renal hypouricemia with fractional urate excretion rates of about 150%, indicating complete loss of tubular urate reabsorption.[195] Interestingly, genetic variations within the SLC2A9 gene that encodes GLUT9 are the major determinant of serum uric acid levels in the general population.[193,196]

URIC ACID SECRETION

Urate entry from the basolateral side of the proximal tubule is likely mediated by members of the OAT family, particularly OAT1 and OAT3, in exchange for divalent anions such as α-ketoglutarate. Mice with double knockout of Oat1/3 have impaired renal urate secretion.[197] On the apical side, the major efflux pathway is through ABCG2, which functions as a high-capacity, ATP-dependent urate transporter.[198,199] Genetic variation in ABCG2 has been strongly associated with variation in serum uric acid levels.[200] Loss or reduced function in ABCG2 in mice and humans causes hyperuricemia although interestingly the mechanism seems to be primarily by reducing intestinal urate secretion.[201,202] Other transporters that have been postulated to play a role in apical uric acid efflux include NPT1, NPT4, and MRP, but the evidence for each of these is limited.

DRUGS THAT AFFECT RENAL URATE HANDLING

Antiuricosuric drugs raise serum and lower urine uric acid levels. These drugs include many diuretics, ethambutol, pyrazinoate, pyrazinamide, and aspirin. Uricosuric drugs do the exact opposite. The mechanisms whereby they are believed to inhibit uric acid reabsorbing transporters are depicted in Figure 8.11C.

AMINO ACIDS

PHYSIOLOGY OF RENAL AMINO ACID TRANSPORT

The amino acid cystine was discovered in the urine of a patient with urolithiasis by Wollaston in 1810.[203] Now we know that this was caused by failure of this patient's kidney to reabsorb cystine. Given a concentration of total free amino acids in the plasma of about 2.5 mmol/L,[204] the daily filtered load amounts to about 400 mmol. In 1917, Cushny recognized that reabsorptive mechanisms must be present in the tubular walls of the nephron to recover amino acids because almost none of the filtered load is lost in the urine.[204b]

The powerful techniques of stop flow, micropuncture, and microperfusion have identified the renal proximal tubule as the principal site of renal amino acid reabsorption.[204] Although net transepithelial reabsorption predominates, there is also a physiologically important influx of many amino acids from the blood into renal cells across the basolateral membrane. This is further complicated by tubular amino acid metabolism and synthesis. Renal glutamine breakdown, for example, plays a key role in acid-base balance by yielding NH_3, and renal conversion of citrulline to arginine is the most important source of this dibasic amino acid in the entire body.[205,206]

Contrary to the other transport processes highlighted in this chapter, which are restricted to the proximal tubule, all cells of the nephron express an array of distinct amino acid transporters that take up amino acids from the blood and support the metabolic needs of the cells. In addition, amino acid transporters in Henle's loop play critical roles in generating large medullary concentrations of certain amino acid, which protects the cells against the high ionic strength associated with concentrating mechanisms.[207-210] These features greatly complicate renal amino acid handling. The discussion of renal amino acid physiology at the tubular and organ levels from classic studies has been covered by Silbernagl.[204] We will focus on the molecular and cellular physiology of reabsorptive amino acid transport in the proximal tubule.

MOLECULAR BIOLOGY OF AMINO ACID TRANSPORT

OVERVIEW OF THE COMPLEXITY

Renal reabsorption of amino acids occurs mainly in the proximal convoluted tubule (S1 to S2 segments) and, to a lesser extent, in the proximal straight tubule (S3 segment),[204] somewhat akin to amino acid absorption in the small intestine.[211] Physiologic studies using substrate competition have defined distinct amino acid transport systems in renal and intestinal epithelial cells.[212] The molecular correlates of these functional transport systems were established in the early 1990s by cloning of mammalian amino acid transporters. Currently, we recognize that intestinal and renal epithelia have a remarkably similar set of plasma membrane amino acid transporters, but there are also divergent isoforms.[212,213] Amino acid transport in the kidney is more complex than in the gut because, for some amino acids, low-affinity and high-affinity systems are differentially distributed along the proximal convoluted and straight tubules, respectively.

Transepithelial flux of amino acids from the lumen to the interstitial space requires sequential transport through apical and basolateral plasma membranes (Figure 8.12). The easier experimental accessibility to apical membranes has allowed a more thorough knowledge of the transporters in the past, and this is still applicable in the age of genomes.

Apical transporters in the renal proximal tubule proven for reabsorption of neutral amino acids include B^0AT1, $IMINO^B$, B^0AT3, PAT2, and TauT; for dibasic amino acids, $rBAT/b^{0,+}AT$; and for dicarboxylic amino acids, EAAT3. Other transporters such as ASCT2 have been localized in the proximal apical membrane but their role in renal reabsorption is only suspected (see Figure 8.12).

Two basolateral transporters demonstrated to reabsorb dibasic and aromatic amino acids are $4F2hc/y^+LAT1$ and TAT1, respectively. Another basolateral transporter for neutral amino acids is $4F2hc/LAT2$. Other transporters in the basolateral plasma membrane (e.g., SNAT3 and EAAT2) might serve for the metabolic needs of the epithelial cells rather than reabsorption and are not addressed further here.[199] Different amino acid groups will be discussed separately.

NEUTRAL AMINO ACIDS

Apical Transporters

It is worthwhile to note that the cloning of these transporters, which really propelled the field forward, was achieved by multiple routes, including expression and homology cloning and bioinformatic screens. Differences among species complicate the study of amino acid transport in the kidney. For example, B^0AT2 is expressed in mouse kidney but, in humans, it is expressed in brain,[214,215] and B^0AT3 might not be a functional transporter at all in humans (see later).

B^0AT1 (SLC6A19). B^0AT1 corresponds to the major apical neutral amino acid transport system B^0 (or NBB, neutral brush border).[216-218] The main characteristics of B^0AT1 are as follows: (1) low-affinity amino acid symporter with Na^+, with 1:1 stoichiometry (K_m in the low millimolar range for L-leucine); (2) Cl-independent and therefore at odds with neurotransmitter transporters of the SLC6 family; (3) transports all neutral amino acids with preference for large aliphatic amino acids with higher apparent affinity and maximum velocity (V_{max}; e.g., proline is a slowly transported substrate, and glycine has low affinity); and (4) K_m values for amino acid and Na^+ are highly dependent on the concentration of the cotransported molecule. B^0AT1 is in the apical membranes of epithelial cells from the glomerulus to segments S1 and S2 (even some in S3) and in the small intestine.[216,219-221]

Hartnup's Disorder. Major support for the role of B^0AT1 in renal reabsorption has come from the fact that mutations in this transporter are associated with Hartnup's disorder (OMIM 234500; Table 8.7), an inherited aminoaciduria with hyperexcretion of all neutral amino acids except proline.[219-223] A total of more than 20 B^0AT1 mutations (missense, nonsense, frameshift, and splice-site) have been identified[224] in this autosomal recessive disease. The

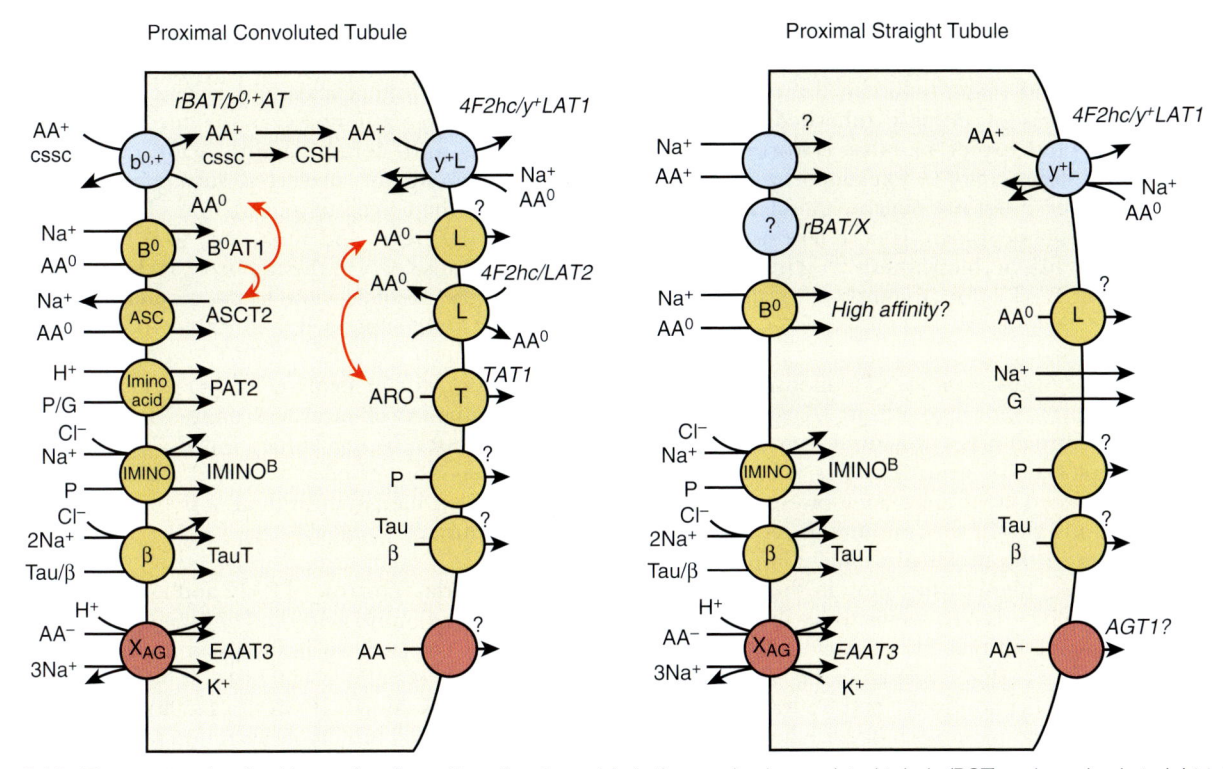

Figure 8.12 Transporters involved in renal reabsorption of amino acids in the proximal convoluted tubule (PCT) and proximal straight tubules (PST). *Red arrows* indicate possible functional cooperation between uniport and exchangers (between B⁰AT1 and rBAT/b⁰,⁺AT, B⁰AT1 and ASCT2, system L and 4F2hc/LAT2, and TAT1 and 4F2hc/LAT2 (see text for details). Efflux system L and efflux systems for proline, taurine, β-alanine, and anionic amino acids have been detected in the basolateral membrane but their molecular entity (indicated by ?) has not been identified. Basolateral Na⁺-dependent transporters with no clear function in renal reabsorption (e.g., EAAT2 for anionic amino acids in PCT and PST; SNAT3 for glutamine, histidine, and asparagine in PST and glycine transporter) are not depicted. Transporters are colored depending on the substrate—dibasic (*blue*), neutral (*gold*), and anionic (*red*). Letters inside the spheres refer to the amino acid transport systems and letters in italics refer to the molecular identity of the transporter. AA0, neutral amino acids; AA+, dibasic amino acids; AA–, anionic amino acids; ARO, aromatic amino acids; CSSC, cystine; CSH, cysteine; P, proline; G, glycine; Tau, taurine; β, β-alanine.

Table 8.7 Primary Inherited Aminoacidurias

Disorder	OMIM Code	Prevalence	Inheritance	Gene	Chromosome	Mutations	Transport System	Protein	Locale
Cystinuria*	220100	1:7000	AR/ADIP	SLC3A1	2p16.3	117	b⁰,⁺	rBAT	Apical
				SLC7A9	19q13.1	92	b⁰,⁺	b⁰,⁺AT	Apical
LPI	222700	~200 cases	AR	SLC7A7	14q11	49	y+L	y+LAT1	Basolateral
Hyperdibasic aminoaciduria type 1	222690	Very rare	AD	?	?	?	?	?	?
Hartnup's disorder	234500	1:26000	AR	SLC6A19	5p15	21	B⁰	B⁰AT1	Apical
Renal familial iminoglycinuria	242600	1:15000	Complex	SLC36A2	5q33	2	Imino acid	PAT2	Apical
				(SLC6A20)	3921	1	IMINO	IMINOB	Apical
				(SLC6A19)	5p15	1 Poly†	B⁰	B⁰AT1	Apical
Glycinuria	138500			(SLC6A18)	5p15	2 and 2 Poly†	?	XT2	Apical
Dicarboxylic aminoaciduria	222730	Very rare	AR?	SLC1A1	9p24	KO null‡	XAG -	EAAT3	Apical

*, Four phenotypes of cystinuria, depending on the obligate heterozygotes, are considered: type I (with AR inheritance), type non-I (ADIP inheritance), mixed type (combination of both), and isolated cystinuria. †, Poly, polymorphism. ‡, Slc1a1-null knockout mice present dicarboxylic aminoaciduria,[352] suggesting this gene as a candidate for the human disease. See text for details and references.

AR, Autosomal recessive; ADIP, autosomal dominant with incomplete penetrance; AD, autosomal dominant; AR? unclear but familial studies in the very few cases described for these diseases suggest an autosomal recessive mode of inheritance. Complex inheritance refers to autosomal recessive mode on inheritance of a major gene (SLC36A2) with other genes (SLC6A20, SLC6A19, SLC6A18) acting as modifiers indicated in parenthesis. LPI, Lysinuric protein intolerance.

B⁰AT1⁻/⁻ mouse has aminoaciduria resembling Hartnup's disorder.[225] Thus, B⁰AT1 is the predominant transporter for neutral amino acid reabsorption in the renal tubule. Clinical manifestations of primary inherited aminoacidurias are discussed in Chapter 45, but it is worth mentioning that most symptoms could be explained by tryptophan deficiency caused by intestinal malabsorption and defective renal reabsorption, which is a relevant precursor of serotonin and niacin biosynthesis.[226] This highlights the relevance of B⁰AT1 for tryptophan availability in humans.

B⁰AT3 (SLC6A18). Also known as XT2, mouse B⁰AT3 is a Na^+ and Cl^- symporter with high affinity (K_m in the micromolar range) for a broad range of neutral amino acids, with a stoichiometry of 1 amino acid (AA):$2Na^+$:$1Cl^-$.[221] Mouse B⁰AT3 is only expressed in the apical membrane of the renal proximal tubule and not in the intestine. B⁰AT3 shows an axial arrangement in the proximal tubule complementary to that of B⁰AT1 (i.e., higher expression in the more distal segments, S2 and S3).[227] B⁰AT3 seems to be the molecular correlate of the high-affinity B⁰-like activity in the proximal straight tubule (S3)[191] that reabsorbs the amino acids remaining after reabsorption by S1 and S2 transporters.[228] Indeed, the B⁰AT3⁻/⁻ mouse shows moderate defective renal reabsorption of several neutral amino acids, especially for glycine and glutamine.[229] Human B⁰AT3 may not be a relevant transporter for renal amino acid reabsorption because a considerable proportion of the human population carries a nonfunctional B⁰AT3 transporter (i.e., the stop codon variation Y318X has a frequency of 0.4 in French-Canadian, Australian, and Japanese populations), and functional expression of a human B⁰AT3 transporter in a heterologous expression system has not yet been reported.[230] Thus, the molecular correlate of the human high-affinity transporter for neutral amino acids is not known (see Figure 8.12).

Scriver and coworkers have revealed at least three transport systems for proline, hydroxyproline, and glycine in the proximal tubule brush border membrane[231]: (1) a system shared by these three amino acids (system imino acid); (2) specific systems for proline and hydroxyproline (system IMINO); and (3) glycine (system Gly). To our knowledge, the molecular correlate of the renal system Gly has not been unequivocally identified.

IMINO^B (SLC6A20). IMINO^B (SIT1, system imino transporter 1; XT3, STRP3, rB21A) is the molecular correlate of system IMINO.[232,233] Human IMINO^B transports proline, hydroxyproline, and N-methylated amino acids and analogues in a Na+- and Cl⁻-dependent manner, characteristic of the SLC6 family. The homologous genes with a syntenic location in the rat and mouse (*XT3s31* and *XT3*, respectively) have not been ascribed a transport function.[212] IMINO^B is expressed in brain and in the apical membrane of epithelial cells of the small intestine and kidney,[221] particularly in the S2 and S3 segments.[232] The role of IMINO^B in the renal reabsorption of proline is supported by the fact that mutations in this transporter combined with mutations in *PAT2* result in iminoglycinuria,[234] a primary inherited aminoaciduria characterized by hyperexcretion of proline, hydroxyproline, and glycine (see PAT2, later, and Table 8.7).

PAT2 (SLC36A2). PAT2 (proton amino acid transporter 2) is considered to be the molecular correlate of the common transporter for imino acids and glycine. It is an H^+ symporter with a high affinity (K_m in the micromolar range) for imino acids and neutral amino acids (1:1 stoichiometry).[235,236] Among the preferred substrates, glycine has a higher V_{max} than proline and alanine. PAT2 is expressed mainly in the heart and lung and, to a lesser extent, in kidney and muscle.[235] In the nephron, PAT2 localizes to the apical membrane of S1 close to the glomerulus.[234] Interestingly, PAT2 is not expressed in intestine. Another H^+–amino acid symporter of this family, PAT1, appears to be a lysosomal transporter in many cells, but is also found in the apical membrane of intestinal epithelial cells.[230] PAT1 is highly expressed in the kidney but its location along the nephron has not yet been reported. No *PAT1* mutations have been identified in individuals with iminoglycinuria and hyperglycinuria.[234]

Iminoglycinuria. The role of PAT2 and IMINO^B in the renal reabsorption of imino acids and glycine was elegantly demonstrated by the study of iminoglycinuria (OMIM 242600) and glycinuria (OMIM 138500; see Table 8.7 and Chapter 45).[234] Iminoglycinuria (OMIM 242600) is an autosomal disorder associated with hyperexcretion of proline, hydroxyproline, and glycine in the urine.[237] Large urine-screening studies have shown that iminoglycinuria is a benign condition[230] caused by several autosomal alleles, some of which are partially expressed in heterozygotes. In general, iminoglycinuria seems to be the recessive phenotype, whereas glycinuria is present in many, but not all, heterozygotes and thus can present as a dominant trait.[230] Individuals with iminoglycinuria have mutations in *SLC36A2*, *SLC6A20*, and *SLC6A19* that segregate with the phenotype.[234] The major gene involved in homozygous cases of iminoglycinuria is *SLC36A2* (renal transporter PAT2). Two types of mutations have been identified[230]: (1) a splice mutation (IVS1+1G→A) that inactivates the transporter by a premature stop codon and is not associated with intestinal malabsorption of imino acids and glycine; and (2) a nonsense mutation (G87V) that partially compromises transport and appears together with a mutated allele (missense mutation T199M) in *SLC6A20* (renal and intestinal transporter IMINO^B). T199M causes an almost complete inactivation of the transporter. In these cases, there are renal and intestinal phenotypes. The role of an *SLC6A19* polymorphism is not clear because it does not segregate completely with the phenotype (see Table 8.7).

TauT (SLC6A6). TauT is the molecular correlate of the amino acid transport system β, a Na^+- and Cl^--dependent, high-affinity transporter common for taurine, β-alanine, and γ-aminobutyric acid (GABA) in renal proximal tubule brush border membranes.[238-241] TauT mediates highly concentrative (three $\log_{10}$ orders of magnitude) taurine transport with K_m values of about 20 μmol/L and a stoichiometry of >$2Na^+$:$1Cl^-$:1 taurine.[242-245] TauT may have two functions in the kidney. Upregulation of TauT in Madin-Darby canine kidney (MDCK) cells on hypertonic stress suggests a role in osmotic regulation. TauT⁻/⁻ mice show an impaired ability to lower urine osmolality and increase urinary water excretion.[246] These animals excrete taurine to levels close to the filtered load, pointing to TauT as the major system for renal taurine reabsorption. A basolateral net efflux pathway for taurine has not been described in the renal proximal tubule (see Figure 8.12).

Other Transporters of Neutral Amino Acids: ASCT2 (SLC1A5). Two isoforms of the system ASC are ASCT1 (SLC1A4) and ASCT2 (SLC1A5, also called ATB^0). ASCT2 is the molecular correlate of intestinal ASC.[247,248] ASCT2 is a Na$^+$-dependent obligatory exchanger of neutral amino acids with variable stoichiometry for Na$^+$.[249] ASCT2 transports small neutral amino acids (e.g., alanine, serine, cysteine) with K$_m$ values of about 20 µmol/L and other neutral amino acids (e.g., glycine, leucine, methionine), with an order of magnitude lower affinity.[248] ASCT2 is expressed in the apical membrane of the proximal tubule.[250] In spite of its location, there is no evidence for a role of ASCT2 in renal reabsorption, and no knockout models have been reported. A functional cooperation between ASCT2 and B^{0}AT1 has been proposed but not demonstrated.[212] GlyT1 (SLC6A12) is a high-affinity Na$^+$ and Cl$^-$-dependent glycine symporter expressed in brain and kidney,[228] but the role of this transporter in kidney is unknown.

Ancillary Proteins for B^{0}AT1, B^{0}AT3, and IMINO^B. B^{0}AT1, B^{0}AT3, and IMINO transporters require collectrin (also called TMEM27 [transmembrane protein 27]) or ACE2 (angiotensin-converting enzyme 2) for cell surface expression in renal (B^{0}AT1, B^{0}AT3, and IMINO^B) and intestinal epithelial cells (B^{0}AT1 and IMINO^B).[220,251-254] Collectrin and ACE2 are type I membrane proteins, with an extracellular N-terminus and a single transmembrane domain. ACE2 inactivates angiotensin II,[241] but is also a carboxypeptidase that aids in the digestion of nutrient-derived peptides in the intestine.[220] ACE2 preferentially releases large neutral amino acids, which are the preferred substrates of the transporter B^{0}AT1. ACE2 does not modify the apparent substrates affinity (K$_m$) but complex formation with another general peptidase, aminopeptidase N (APN), decreases the K$_m$ of B^{0}AT1 for its substrates.[255] Thus, functional protein complexes between neutral amino acid transporters and peptidases could play a role in protein absorption by increasing local amino acid substrate concentration or affinity. In contrast, collectrin lacks the catalytic domain of ACE2 but shares sequence homology in the transmembrane and cytosolic regions.[241] Collectrin is thought to interact with the SNARE (soluble *N*-ethylmaleimide–sensitive fusion protein attachment protein receptor) exocytotic machinery.[256,257] Collectrin and ACE2 facilitate the fusion of vesicles containing transporters of the SLC6 family to the apical plasma membrane of the epithelial cells in the kidney (collectrin and ACE2) or small intestine (ACE2).

In accord with the differential tissue distribution of collectrin and ACE2, ablation of these proteins causes different phenotypes. Collectrin$^{-/-}$ mice show reduction of B^{0}AT1 expression and activity in renal brush border membranes but are otherwise normal.[252,253] These animals display tyrosine crystalluria and hyperexcretion of neutral amino acids, resembling Hartnup's disorder. In these mice, B^{0}AT1 expression was unaffected in the small intestine. ACE2$^{-/-}$ mice have a more complex phenotype, including cardiomyopathy and glomerulosclerosis, but have normal urinary amino acid levels.[251] These mice show no expression and transport function of B^{0}AT1 in brush border membranes from the small intestine, whereas expression of B^{0}AT1 in renal brush borders is not affected. Interestingly, there are some missense mutations that compromise interaction with ACE2, but not with collectrin, explaining patients with Hartnup's disorder affecting only the intestine.[251] In addition to B^{0}AT1 and B^{0}AT3, ablation of collectrin in mouse also depletes the renal brush border transporter IMINO^B.[252] Moreover, high-affinity, Na$^+$-dependent transport of L-proline, presumably via IMINO^B (*Slc6a20*), was absent in ACE2$^{-/-}$ mice.[254] Thus, both collectrin and ACE2 also seem to be trafficking proteins for transporter IMINO^B in the intestine and kidney.

Reabsorption requires a net basolateral efflux of neutral amino acids. These transporters were identified by homology (4F2hc/LAT2)[258-261] and expression cloning from rat small intestine (TAT1)[262] and MDCK cells in hypertonic medium (BGT1).[263] In addition to the TAT1 uniport specific for aromatic amino acids, no other neutral amino acids uniporters have been identified in the basolateral membrane of the small intestine and renal proximal tubule (see Figure 8.12). Orphan transporters from the monocarboxylate transporter family SLC16[264] and from the glycoprotein-independent, L-type transporter family SLC43[265,266] are candidates for such activities.

TAT1 (SLC16A10). TAT1 is the molecular correlate of system T (Na$^+$-independent uniport system for aromatic amino acids),[262] initially described in erythrocytes[267] Substrate affinity is low (K$_m$ in the micromolar range) and it also transports L-dopa and *N*-methylated aromatic amino acids.[262,268] TAT1 belongs to the H$^+$-monocarboxylate cotransporter family (SLC16).[269] TAT1, at variance with other SLC16 members,[270] neither cotransports H$^+$ nor needs ancillary proteins (e.g., basigin, embigin) to reach the plasma membrane and maintain the catalytic activity.

TAT1 is highly expressed in the basolateral membrane of the small intestine and renal proximal convoluted tubules (segments S1 and S2) in humans and mouse, but is curiously absent from rat kidney.[262,268] TAT1 likely has a direct role in the basolateral efflux of aromatic amino acids. Ablation of TAT1 in mouse results in aromatic aminoaciduria,[271] which is exacerbated and also involves other neutral amino acids when mice are fed with a high-protein diet. Intestinal absorption of phenylalanine is also reduced in the knockout mice.

4F2hc/LAT2 (SLC3A2/SLC7A9). A heavy (4F2hc) and light subunit (LAT2) linked by a disulfide bridge forming a heterodimer is a key feature of heteromeric amino acid transporters (HATs). No larger oligomeric state has been detected in kidney or cultured cells.[272] 4F2hc/LAT2 mediates a high-affinity (K$_m$ in the micromolar range) obligatory exchange of all neutral amino acids except proline with 1:1 stoichiometry.[258,259] This activity resembles the classic system L initially defined in nonepithelial cells,[273] but with broader substrate specificity, and fits with the Na$^+$-independent neutral amino acid transport defined in renal basolateral plasma membrane vesicles.[274] LAT2, in addition to several other tissues, is highly expressed in the kidney and small intestine.[258-260] LAT2 is expressed in the basolateral membrane in the small intestine and proximal convoluted tubule

b⁰,⁺AT: I120L, T123M, A126T, C137R
y⁺LAT1: L124P, A140P

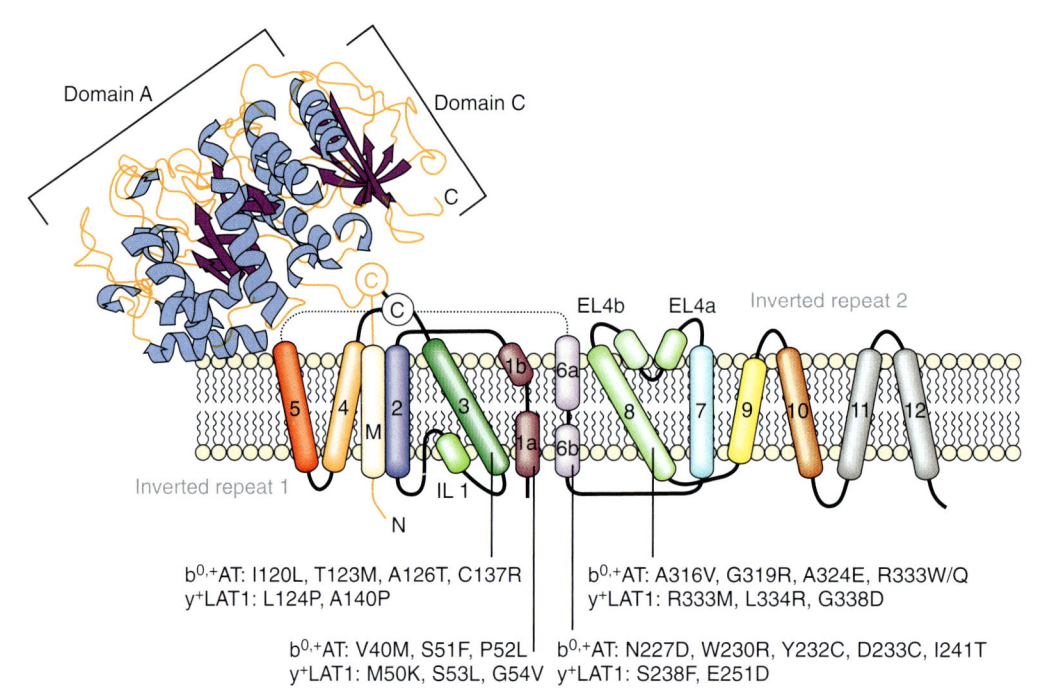

b⁰,⁺AT: A316V, G319R, A324E, R333W/Q
y⁺LAT1: R333M, L334R, G338D

b⁰,⁺AT: V40M, S51F, P52L
y⁺LAT1: M50K, S53L, G54V

b⁰,⁺AT: N227D, W230R, Y232C, D233C, I241T
y⁺LAT1: S238F, E251D

Figure 8.13 Schematic representation of heteromeric amino acid transporters (HATs) with indication of the membrane topology of the light subunits. HATs are composed of a heavy subunit and light subunit linked by a disulfide bridge between two conserved cysteine residues (C). The heavy subunit has a cytoplasmic N-terminus, a single transmembrane domain, TMD (M), and an ectodomain similar to that of bacterial glucosidases (for human 4F2hc, domain A, TIM barrel; domain C, all 8β; PDB code 2DH3). The light subunits share the LeuT fold and TMD1-5 and TMD6-10 correspond to the two inverted repeats. The C-terminal helices (TMD11 and TMD12) are not related symmetrically to the 5 + 5 inverted repeat. According to the atomic structure of the structural paradigm AdiC, TMD1 and TMD6 have unwound parts in the middle of the helices. The extracellular loop 4 (EL4) and intracellular loop 1 (IL1) are expected to occlude the substrate in the outward- and inward-facing conformations.[355] IL1 is accessible from the external medium in human xCT.[371] In the internal helices TMD1, TMD3, TMD6, and TMD8, most of the cystinuria (b⁰,⁺AT) and LPI (y⁺LAT1) missense mutations are located. The ectodomain of 4F2hc is located over the light subunit and not over the plasma membrane, according to the low-resolution structural model of human 4F2hc/LAT2.[369]

(segments S1 > S2 ≫ S3).[258] This distribution parallels the reabsorptive capacity for neutral amino acids along the nephron.[204] Knockdown of LAT2 in the proximal tubule-like OK cells resulted in increased intracellular cysteine content, lower transepithelial flux of cysteine, and decreased alanine, serine, and threonine content.[275] This suggests that 4F2hc/LAT2 likely plays a role in cysteine efflux, which is generated after the reduction of cystine by cytoplasmic glutathione.[276] Deletion of LAT2 in mice did not result in defective reabsorption of neutral amino acids,[277] possibly due to compensation by other transporters.

It has been speculated that the activity of 4F2hc/LAT2 (broad substrate specificity), in cooperation with the activity of a uniport with specificity for only a few neutral amino acids, could mediate the net basolateral efflux of any neutral amino acid by recycling the common substrates (Figure 8.13). TAT1 co-localizes with 4F2hc/LAT2 in the basolateral membrane of the human renal proximal convoluted tubule.[278,279] Coexpression of 4F2hc/LAT2 and TAT1 in *Xenopus* oocytes resulted in a net efflux of alanine, serine, glutamine, and asparagine, which are not normally TAT1 substrates.[279] Double-knockout models of TAT1 and LAT2 are needed to test this hypothesis.

Other Neutral Amino Acid Transporters

BGT1 (SLC6A12) is a Na⁺ and Cl⁻ cotransporter of GABA and betaine that is expressed in the liver, kidney, and brain.[263] In the kidney, BGT1 localizes to the basolateral membrane of the collecting ducts and thick ascending limbs of Henle's loop, precluding a role in reabsorption.[280] BGT1 expression responds to osmolarity changes, suggesting a protective role in osmotic stress. In contrast to this view, BGT1-deficient mice tolerate osmotic stress well, suggesting the existence of compensatory mechanisms.[280]

CATIONIC AMINO ACIDS

Apical Transporters

The molecular entity of one transporter for dibasic amino acids has been identified in the apical membranes of the renal proximal tubule, the heterodimer rBAT/b⁰,⁺AT. Expression cloning first identified rBAT (related to b⁰,⁺ amino acid transporter),[282,283] and 4F2hc-induced amino acid transport in oocytes.[282,283] 4F2hc needs accompanying proteins for transport activity in oocytes.[284] Coexpression cloning with 4F2hc[285] and coexpression of 4F2hc with orphan transporters[286] have identified LAT1 (system L exchanger) as the first light subunit of 4F2hc. Similarly, coexpression cloning identified xCT (system x_c^-).[287] The rest of the subunits associated with 4F2hc and rBAT were identified by homology, such as b⁰,⁺AT and y⁺LAT1.[288,289]

Transport studies have suggested Na⁺-dependent or Na⁺-modulated transport for cationic amino acids in the apical membrane. A defect in such a system may cause type I dibasic aminoaciduria (OMIM 222690), a disease affecting the kidney, but differs from cystinuria because of the absence of cystine hyperexcretion and from LPI because of the absence of hyperammonemia and protein intolerance.[290,291] The molecular identity of this transporter is unknown (see Table 8.7).

rBAT/$b^{0,+}$AT (SLC3A1/SLC7A9). This is the molecular correlate of the renal and intestinal cationic amino acid transport system $b^{0,+}$ named by Van Winkle initially in the mouse blastocyst[292] and that was detected in brush border membranes from the small intestine and kidney.[293,294] The heavy (rBAT) and light ($b^{0,+}$AT) subunits of the heterodimer are linked by a disulfide bridge, characteristic of HATs.[295] rBAT/$b^{0,+}$AT mediates the obligatory exchange of cationic amino acids, cystine (i.e., two cysteines bound by a disulfide bridge), and neutral amino acids (except imino acids) with 1:1 stoichiometry. The transport properties of the heterodimer has been studied mainly in oocytes injected with rBAT with the endogenous *Xenopus* $b^{0,+}$AT subunit with the following characteristics: (1) high affinity for cationic amino acids (lysine, arginine, and ornithine) and cystine (K_m values $\cong$ 100 µM) and slightly lower for other neutral amino acids; (2) apparent affinity that is three orders of magnitude higher in the extracellular than in the intracellular binding site; and (3) reversible electrogenic exchange of cationic and neutral amino acids.[296-299] The rBAT/$b^{0,+}$AT heterodimer is expressed in the apical membrane of the small intestine and S1 and S2 segments of the nephron,[300] where more than 90% of cystine reabsorption occurs.[191]

Under physiologic conditions, only cationic amino acids are absorbed via system $b^{0,+}$ in exchange with neutral amino acids, likely driven by the interior negative membrane potential. Similarly, system $b^{0,+}$ mediates the uptake of cystine from the lumen because, once in the epithelial cell, the amino acid is reduced to cysteine. Final proof came from the fact that mutations in system $b^{0,+}$ cause cystinuria,[288,301] characterized by defective renal reabsorption and intestinal malabsorption of cationic amino acids (lysine, arginine, and ornithine) and cystine, but not other neutral amino acids (see Table 8.7).[302] Cystine has low solubility and precipitates, forming cystine crystals and calculi. Moreover, mouse models with defective rBAT (D140G mutation)[303] or $b^{0,+}$AT (knockout)[304] and Newfoundland dogs with defective rBAT (natural nonsense mutation)[305] have cystinuria similar to that in humans.

Cystinuria. This is the most common primary inherited aminoaciduria (OMIM 220100), causing 1% to 2% of renal stones in adults and 6% to 8% in pediatric patients[306] (see also Chapter 45). Cystinuria is recessive in inheritance; homozygotes hyperexcrete large amounts of cationic amino acids (mainly lysine) and cystine.[307] A total of 133 mutations in rBAT (*SLC3A1*; cystinuria type A) and 95 mutations in $b^{0,+}$AT (*SLC7A9*; cystinuria type B) have been identified in humans, including missense, nonsense, splice-site, frameshift, and large rearrangements.[306] System $b^{0,+}$ mutations were identified in about 90% of the alleles studied and, in a small proportion of patients ($\approx$3%), no mutations have been identified. These cases may be due to mutations in promoter, regulatory, or intron regions. Alternatively, haplotypes with several $b^{0,+}$AT polymorphisms may contribute to cystinuria, as has been shown for the group of $b^{0,+}$AT heterozygotes who are cystine stone formers.[308] Brodehl and coworkers reported a family transmitting isolated cystinuria (hyperexcretion of cystine without cationic aminoaciduria).[309] A heterozygous $b^{0,+}$AT mutation (T123M) explains isolated cystinuria in this family and other individuals.[307,310] It is believed that all cases of classic and isolated cystinuria are caused by mutations in system $b^{0,+}$. Cystine clearance is close to the GFR in classic cystinuria (see Table 8.7).[289] Thus, system $b^{0,+}$ is the major transporter for cystine reabsorption in the proximal tubule apical membrane. In contrast, clearance of cationic amino acids is only partially affected (40 to 60 mL/min/1.73 m^2) in cystinuria,[311] suggesting that other apical transport systems participate in the renal reabsorption of these amino acids. Indeed, lysine transport has been reported in the human kidney, which was also present in patients with cystinuria.[312] The molecular identity of this transporter is currently unknown.

All $b^{0,+}$AT are covalently linked by a disulfide bridge to rBAT in kidney (segments S1 and S2) but not all renal rBAT heterodimerizes with $b^{0,+}$AT in mouse.[300] rBAT has the higher expression along the proximal tubule in the S3 segment,[313] where it forms disulfide-linked heterodimers (~140 kDa) with a yet unidentified light subunit.[300] This heterodimer (arbitrarily called rBAT-X) is clearly detected in renal brush border membranes from $b^{0,+}$AT knockout mice.[304] There is no experimental support for rBAT/X having a role in renal reabsorption. The mean and range (fifth to 95th percentile limits) of cystine, lysine, arginine, and ornithine in the urine of patients with mutations in rBAT and in $b^{0,+}$AT are almost identical.[307] This is expected because all $b^{0,+}$AT heterodimerizes with rBAT (system $b^{0,+}$) in renal brush border membranes and rules out the role of rBAT-X heterodimer in cystine and cationic amino acid reabsorption.

Oligomeric Structure and Biogenesis of rBAT/$b^{0,+}$AT. The native oligomeric state of system $b^{0,+}$ is a heterotetramer (dimer of heterodimers), in which each dimer independently catalyzes transport.[272] rBAT and $b^{0,+}$AT need to be coexpressed to reach the plasma membrane, but reconstitution of $b^{0,+}$AT alone conferred full transport activity, showing that it is the catalytic subunit.[299]

The mutations causing cystinuria that have been functionally studied agree with the proposed role of each subunit in the holotransporter $b^{0,+}$. Thus, mutations in rBAT cause trafficking defects,[314-316] whereas mutations in $b^{0,+}$AT cause trafficking defects and/or inactivation of the transporter.[299,317] The only exception to this rule is the rBAT mutation R365W, which affects both trafficking and transport.[316] The impact of cystinuria-specific rBAT mutations on system $b^{0,+}$ trafficking in transfected mammalian cells has been studied in more detail, allowing the proposal of a minimal working model for the biogenesis of the transporter.[314,318] Fast interactions of the transmembrane segment of rBAT with folded $b^{0,+}$AT determine formation of the heterodimer within the endoplasmic reticulum (ER). This interaction is drastically reduced by the cystinuria-specific mutation L89P, in the transmembrane domain of rBAT. Assembly with $b^{0,+}$AT is necessary for rBAT folding and blocks rBAT degradation via the ER-associated degradation (ERAD) pathway. These early steps do not require the calnexin chaperone system. After assembly, the rBAT extracellular domain folds within that chaperone system. Heterotetramerization proceeds immediately after completion of rBAT folding or is interspersed within the final folding steps. Only the heterotetramers exit the ER to the Golgi complex. Mutations of the extracellular domain of rBAT (T216M, R365W, M467T, M467K) disrupt or delay the postassembly folding, hindering stable oligomerization and leading to its degradation.

Cystinuria is classified clinically based on the urinary phenotype of the heterozygotes—type I are silent (without aminoaciduria) and those with moderate aminoaciduria (mainly lysine and cystine) are called type non-I.[307] rBAT heterozygotes are type I with the exception of some carrying the mutation dupE5-E9 (in-frame duplication of part of rBAT). Almost 90% of $b^{0,+}AT$ heterozygotes are type non-I. The remaining type I heterozygotes are associated with mild $b^{0,+}AT$ mutations. A low fraction of $b^{0,+}AT$ heterozygotes with the non-I phenotype present with cystine stones.[305] Like most patients, mice and dogs with defective rBAT transmit type I cystinuria,[303,305] whereas $b^{0,+}AT$ knockout mice transmit type non-I cystinuria.[304] Due to the role of $b^{0,+}AT$ in the biogenesis of system $b^{0,+}$, it is tempting to speculate that $b^{0,+}AT$ limits the amount of rBAT/$b^{0,+}AT$ heterotetramer leaving the ER, and half the genetic dose of $b^{0,+}AT$ is sufficient to result in moderate aminoaciduria.

Basolateral Transporters

4F2hc/y^+LAT1 is the only transporter for dibasic amino acids identified at the molecular level in the basolateral membranes of renal epithelial cells.[289,319]

4F2hc/y^+LAT1 (SLC3A2/SLC7A7). This is one of the two molecular correlates of system y^+L, initially described in erythrocytes and placenta,[320,321] and is the mediator of cationic amino acid efflux in epithelial cells.[295] The heavy subunit (4F2hc) and the light subunit (y^+LAT1) are linked by a disulfide bridge forming a heterodimer, characteristic of the HATs.[289,319]

4F2hc/y^+LAT1 mediates electroneutral, high-affinity (low micromolar range) exchange of cationic amino acids with neutral amino acids plus Na^+, with 1:1:1 stoichiometry.[289,319,322] The affinity of neutral but not cationic amino acids increases around two orders of magnitude in the presence of Na^+. 4F2hc/y^+LAT1 is highly expressed in the kidney, small intestine, placenta, spleen, and macrophages[323] (personal communication). In epithelial cells, the transporter has a basolateral location.[324] The other system y^+L isoform (4F2hc/y^+LAT2) is widely expressed, but less in the kidney and small intestine compared with 4F2hc/y^+LAT1.[323]

Under physiologic conditions, the high extracellular Na^+ concentration drives the efflux of cationic amino acids in exchange for neutral amino acids. In this mode, this electroneutral transporter mediates the efflux of cationic amino acids against the membrane potential (positive outside). Proof for this exchange mode is supported by the fact that mutations in y^+LAT1 cause lysinuric protein intolerance (LPI)[325,326] (see Table 8.7), characterized by urine hyperexcretion and intestinal malabsorption of cationic amino acids only.[327,328] Lysinuria is the most prominent aminoaciduria in patients with LPI, with renal clearance values of approximately 25 mL/min/1.73 m^2.

Lysinuric Protein Intolerance. LPI (OMIM 222700) is a rare recessive disease (~200 patients known), probably due partially to misdiagnosis. Impairment of intestinal and renal reabsorption of cationic amino acids in homozygotes causes a metabolic derangement characterized by a low cationic amino acid plasma concentration, which causes dysfunction of the urea cycle and leads to hyperammonemia and protein aversion (see Chapter 45). In contrast to disorders of apical amino acid transporters (Hartnup's disorder and cystinuria), the basolateral location of the LPI transporter cannot be bypassed by the apical intestinal absorption of peptides containing dibasic amino acids (PEPT1 (peptide transporter 1; *SLC15A1*).[329,330] Thus, patients fail to thrive normally. Similarly, y^+LAT1$^{-/-}$ mice that survive the neonatal lethality display identical metabolic derangements as LPI patients.[331] The pathophysiology of other symptoms of LPI, such as chronic kidney disease, lung alveolar proteinosis, and altered immune response are not understood.[332]

Fifty-four mutations (missense, nonsense, splice-site, frameshift deletions and insertions, and large rearrangements) have been described in y^+LAT1 in 149 patients from 115 independent families,[333,334] and some have been recently identified.[335-337] In addition to aminoaciduria, the other symptoms vary widely among patients, even when they harbor the same mutations, precluding genotype and phenotype correlations.[327] Only some LPI point mutations have been studied for functional defects.[326,338-340] Four mutations (E36del, G54V, F152L, L334R) showed defective system y^+L transport activity despite adequate plasma membrane expression in heterologous systems, indicating defective intrinsic transporter activity.[338,339]

As for other HATs, 4F2hc is needed to bring the heterodimer 4F2hc/y^+LAT1 to the plasma membrane,[338] and specifically to the basolateral membrane.[329] No mutations have been identified in 4F2hc in LPI, suggesting perhaps lethality and, indeed, 4F2hc knockout is lethal.[340] 4F2hc services six human amino acid transporter subunits (LAT1, LAT2, y^+LAT1, y^+LAT2, xCT, asc1)[295] and is necessary for proper β_1 integrin function.[341] Defective 4F2hc is likely incompatible with life.

ANIONIC AMINO ACIDS

Five transporters for anionic amino acids (EAAT1-5) are in the SLC1 family.[342] EAAT3 (EAAC1) was cloned from the kidney by functional expression.[343] The Na^+-dependent neutral amino acid transporters ASCT1 and ASCT2 are also part of the SLC1 family.[342] AGT1 is a light subunit (family SLC7) of HAT.[344]

EAAT3 (SLC1A1). EAAT3 is the molecular correlate of the neuronal and epithelial X-AG system, with transport activity fitting all properties of the high-affinity ($K_m < 20$ μmol/L), L-glutamate transporter described in the kidney and intestine.[342] EAAT3 cotransports $3Na^+$:glutamate:H^+, and the return of the transporters is facilitated by the binding of one K^+.[345,346]

The transporter shows preference for L-aspartate over L-glutamate and transports cystine with a K_m value of approximately 100 μmol/L. EAAT3 is expressed in the apical membrane of the S2 and S3 segments and weaker signals in the S1 segments, descending thin limbs of long-loop nephrons, medullary thick ascending limbs, and distal convoluted tubules.[347] This distribution agrees only partially with the reabsorption of glutamate along the nephron[348]; more than 90% occurs in segment S1, where EAAT3 expression is low, and remains significant until the distal convoluted tubules, which also express EAAT3.

Dicarboxylic Aminoaciduria. The role of EAAT3 in renal reabsorption is supported by the fact that mutations in *SLC1A1* cause human dicarboxylic aminoaciduria (OMIM 222730),[349] an extremely rare autosomal recessive disorder of glutamate and aspartate transport[350,351] (see Table 8.7). Two mutations (I395del and R445W) were identified in three patients from two families segregating with the phenotype and leading to the near absence of surface expression in a heterologous system.[349] The *Slc1a1*−/− knockout mouse also has dicarboxylic aminoaciduria.[352] In human and murine dicarboxylic aminoaciduria, hyperexcretion of cystine does not segregate with the genotype, suggesting that the role of EAAT3 in cystine reabsorption is minimal.

Basolateral AGT1. AGT1, also known as SLC7A13, is a light subunit of HAT in search of a heavy subunit. AGT1 has conserved cysteine residues responsible for disulfide bond formation. In contrast, none of the two heavy subunits identified (4F2hc, rBAT) resulted in function when coexpressed with AGT1 in *Xenopus* oocytes. In nonreducing conditions, AGT1 has a molecular weight compatible with that of a heterodimer, suggesting that a yet to be identified heavy subunit may heterodimerize with AGT. Fusion proteins of AGT1-4F2hc or AGT1-rBAT brought the transporter to the cell surface, and AGT1 showed Na$^+$-independent transport for acidic amino acids (K_m for L-aspartate and L-glutamate in the low micromolar range).[344] In contrast to the homologous Na$^+$-independent cystine-glutamate transporter xCT, AGT1 does not accept cystine, homocysteate, and l-α-aminoadipate. AGT1 is expressed in the basolateral membrane of the proximal straight tubules and distal convoluted tubules in mice; there are no data on human AGT1. In one report on AGT1 function, the mechanism of transport (uniport or exchanger) was not studied.[344] To date, there is no proof for AGT1 mediating renal amino acid reabsorption.

STRUCTURAL INFORMATION OF AMINO ACID TRANSPORTERS

Some information on protein structure was presented earlier on glucose and organic cation transporters, but there has been an eruption of new structural information in amino acid transporters. Since the beginning of the twenty-first century, the atomic resolution structures of prokaryotic models of several mammalian amino acid transporters have been reported and are summarized in Table 8.8. For reasons of brevity, we will focus only on transporters with the LeuT fold shared by SLC6 and SLC7 transporters, which are implicated in primary inherited aminoacidurias. PAT2 (SLC36 family) is considered to share the LeuT fold,[353] but structural homology models have not been reported to our knowledge.[234]

5 + 5 INVERTED REPEAT FOLD

The structure of the prokaryotic LeuT homologue from *Aquifex aeolicus* was solved by Gouaux's group.[354] The LeuT fold is characterized by a pseudosymmetry that relates two structurally similar repeats of five consecutive transmembrane domains (TMDs) by a pseudo–twofold axis of symmetry in the plane of the membrane—that is, five TMDs (first repeat) followed by five TMDs (second repeat) with an inverted topology in the membrane; this has been termed a *5 + 5 inverted repeat fold* (see Figure 8.13). The motif consists of two interior pairs of symmetry-related helices, surrounded by an arch of outer helices. The central part of the internal helices TMD1 and TMD6 are unwound (TMDs numbered according to LeuT, AdiC, or the light subunits of HAT). Thus, TMD1 and TMD6 each have two helices (e.g., TMD1a and TMD1b). To translocate substrate, LeuT fold transporters transit through different outward-facing and inward-facing conformations of apo, substrate-bound open and substrate-bound occluded states. When occluded, the substrate is blocked by a thin gate (side chain of a single residue) and thick gate (usually several TMDs; Figure 8.14), preventing the diffusion of the substrate to either side of the membrane.[355] Finally, release of the substrate to one or the other side of the membrane completes the alternate access mechanism of transport characteristic of secondary active transporters. Interestingly, the LeuT fold is shared by five transporter families, with no apparent primary amino acid homology between them (<10%).[356]

Six atomic structures of LeuT-fold transporters with a bound amino acid substrate have been reported: LeuT with L-leucine bound in the outward-facing state of the transporter,[354] AdiC with L-arginine bound in the outward-facing open state of the transporter,[357] AdiC with L-arginine bound in the outward-facing occluded state of the transporter,[358] and BetP, with betaine bound in a fully occluded state and inward-facing conformations.[359,360] Interestingly, a common feature in these structures is binding of the α-amino carboxyl moiety of the substrate to the unwound section of the first TMDs of each repeat and interaction of the side chain of the substrate to residues in the third TMD of each repeat (see Figure 8.14). In LeuT, the α-amino carboxyl moiety of L-leucine and the two Na$^+$ ions interact with (or next to) the unwound regions of TMD1 and TMD6. Specifically, one of the two Na$^+$ ions, Na1, connects the carboxyl group of L-leucine with TMD1 and TMD6 (see Figure 8.14). In AdiC, the α-amino carboxyl moiety of L-arginine interacts with the unwound regions of TMD1 and TMD6, and the main attractor of the guanidinium group is residue Trp293 in TMD8 (see Figure 8.13). A tilting movement of TMD6a in AdiC, and most probably in LeuT, positions residues Trp202 and Phe253 over L-arginine and L-leucine to occlude the substrates from the periplasm in the occluded, outward-facing conformations of AdiC and LeuT, respectively (see Figure 8.14).

SLC6 TRANSPORTERS

LeuT from *Aquifex aeolicus* presents an approximately 30% amino acid sequence identity to the mammalian SLC6 family, and good structural models have been made for human B^{0}AT1.[220,351] Based on the fact that the carboxyl group of leucine forms part of the Na1 site in LeuT, these models explain the mutual influence of substrate and Na$^+$ on each other's K_m, which has been observed in B^{0}AT1, B^{0}AT2, and IMINO^B.[212,361] Similarly, the Cl$^-$ binding site identified in GAT1 after the LeuT structure[362,363] is conserved in the SLC6 Cl$^-$-dependent transporters (e.g.,

Table 8.8 Prokaryotic Transporters as Structural Models of Mammalian Amino Acid Transporters

Transporter	Species	Description	Conformation*	PDB Code	Protein Family	Related Mammalian Transporter
GlpT[111]	Escherichia coli	Glycerol 3-phosphate exchanger	Apo, inward-facing, closed	1PW4	MFS	SLC16 members (e.g., TAT1)
GltPh[375]	Pyrococcus horikoshii	Sodium-dependent aspartate transporter	Substrate-bound, outward-facing	2NWL	DAACS	SLC1 members (e.g., EAAT3, ASCT2)
			Apo, inward-facing[376]	4P19		
LeuT[354]	Aquifex aeolicus	Sodium-dependent leucine transporter	Apo, outward-facing, open	3TT1	NSS	SLC6 members (e.g., B⁰AT1, B⁰AT2, IMINO, XT2, TauT) SLC36 members (e.g., PAT2)
			Substrate-bound, outward-facing, occluded[377]	2A65		
			Apo, inward-facing, open[378]	3TT3		
AdiC[379]	Salmonella sp.	Arginine-agmatine antiporter	Apo, outward-facing, open	3NCY	APC	SLC7 members (e.g., b⁰,⁺AT, y⁺LAT1)
	Escherichia coli[358]		Substrate-bound, outward-facing, open	3OB6		
	Escherichia coli[357]		Substrate-bound, outward-facing, occluded	3L1L		
ApcT[380]	Methanocaldococcus jannaschii	H⁺-coupled, broad specificity amino acid transporter	Apo, fully occluded	3GIA	APC	SLC7 members (e.g., b⁰,⁺AT, y⁺LAT1)
GadC[381]	Escherichia coli	Glutamate-GABA antiporter	Apo, inward-facing, open†	4DJK	APC	SLC7 members (e.g., b⁰,⁺AT, y⁺LAT1)

*APC transporters share the LeuT fold. Schematic representation of LeuT fold transporter conformations during the transport cycle is shown in Figure 8.14.
†This structure has the substrate binding site in a conformation that would be open to the cytosol were it not for blockade by the C-terminus of the transporter. Only structures with the highest resolution are indicated.
APC, Amino acid–polyamine–organocation family; Apo, without substrate-bound; DAACS, dicarboxylate amino acid cation symporter family; inward, the substrate binding site faces the cytosol; GABA, γ-aminobutyric acid; MFS, major facilitated superfamily; NSS, neurotransmitter sodium symporter family; open, occluded, refer to whether the substrate in the binding site is free to dissociate or is occluded; outward, the substrate binding site faces the extracellular medium; PDB code, protein database code of protein structures.

IMINO^B and TauT), but also in B⁰AT1 and B⁰AT2, which are not Cl⁻-dependent. This led to the suggestion that a static Cl⁻ ion stabilizes the structure of B⁰AT1 and B⁰AT2.[361]

LeuT-based B⁰AT1 structural models help in the understanding of the molecular bases of the defect in Hartnup's disorder. Functional analysis has shown that certain B⁰AT1 missense mutations that do not compromise protein expression (presumed functional defects) fall into three phenotypic categories.[220,251] In the first group (G93R and E501K), mutations abolish the intrinsic transport activity, irrespective of the presence of the auxiliary proteins collectrin and ACE2. Gly93 in TMD2 interacts with the intracellular part of TMD6b, and Glu501 in TMD10 interacts with one of two water molecules that hold the structure of the unwound residues between TMD6a and TMD6b, the domains that interact with the amino acid substrate and Na⁺ at the Na1 site. Thus, mutations E501K and G93R most probably affect the folding and position of this unwound region, compromising binding and eventually substrate translocation. In the second group of mutations (A69T and R240Q), neither collectrin nor ACE2 stimulated transport, in spite of physical interaction between the auxiliary proteins and the transporter. Interestingly, both residues are related to the extracellular loop TMD5-TMD6. Ala69 is located in the beginning of TMD2, interacting with loop TMD5-TMD6, and R240Q is located at the end of TMD5. This suggests that loop TMD5-TMD6 is involved in the functional interaction of B⁰AT1 with collectrin and ACE2. Finally, the third group of Hartnup mutants (the hypomorphic polymorphism D173N and mutation P265L) loses functional interaction with collectrin but not with ACE2. Interestingly, Pro[276] is located at the N-terminus of TMD6a in a similar location to the second group of mutants and is involved in defective interaction with collectrin and ACE2. Asp[174] is in the extracellular loop TMD3-TMD4, opposite to another extracellular loop, TMD5-TMD6, suggesting a complex functional interaction of B⁰AT1 with collectrin and ACE2 involving at least two extracellular loops.

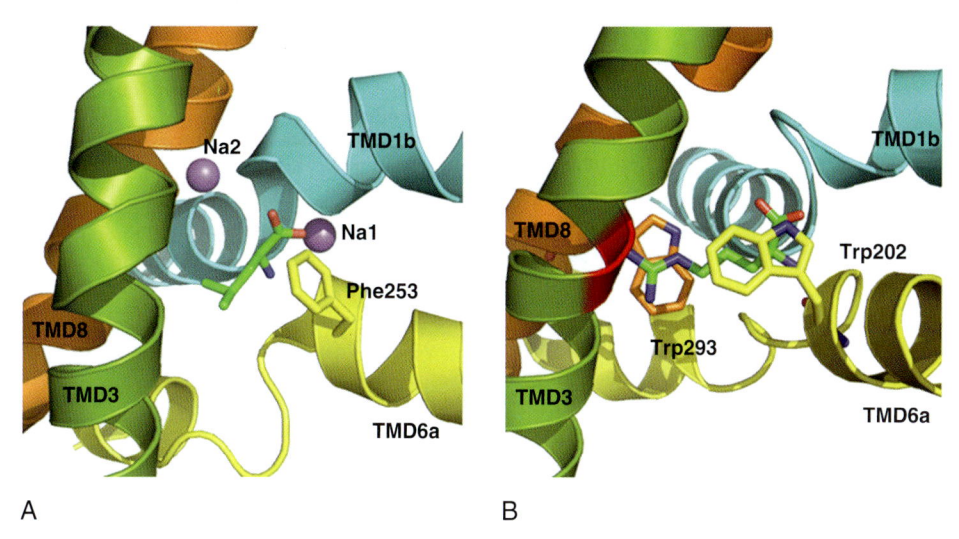

Figure 8.14 Binding pocket and substrate recognition in the bacterial L-leucine transporter LeuT **(A)** and in the L-arginine/agmatine antiporter AdiC **(B)**. View from the periplasmic side. Color codes for TMDs: TMD1, *cyan;* TMD3, *orange;* TMD6, *yellow;* TMD8, *green.* The α-amino carboxyl moiety of L-leucine (C atoms in *green* in **A**) and L-arginine (C atoms in *green* in **B**) interacts with the unwound regions of TMD1 and TMD6. Two Na+ ions (Na1 and Na2) are shown (*violet spheres*) in **A**. Na1 coordinates the carboxyl group of L-leucine with TMD1 and TMD6 residues of LeuT. Trp293 in TMD8 is the main attractor of the guanidinium group of L-arginine in AdiC in **B**. The region marked in *red* in TMD3 of AdiC corresponds to residue Gly100, homologous to residue Thr123 in b$^{0,+}$AT.[372] Residues Phe235 of LeuT and Trp202 of AdiC in TMD6a occludes the substrate from the periplasm (thin gate). The thick gate (occluding the substrate from the cytosol) is composed of several TMDs, including those depicted in the figure. For clarity, TMD4, TMD5, TMD7, TMD9, TMD10, TMD11, and TMD12 of LeuT and AdiC are not depicted. O and N atoms are depicted in *red* and *blue*, respectively. The atomic structures of LeuT and AdiC in the outward-facing substrate occluded conformation correspond to PDB codes 2A65 and 3L1L, respectively. (Adapted from Fotiadis D, Kanai Y, Palacin M: The SLC3 and SLC7 families of amino acid transporters. *Mol Aspects Med* 34:139-158, 2013.)

HETEROMERIC AMINO ACID TRANSPORTERS

HATs are composed of a heavy chain (rBAT or 4F2hc) linked by a disulfide bridge with a light subunit (in humans, b$^{0,+}$AT for rBAT; LAT1, LAT2, y$^+$LAT1, y$^+$LAT2, asc1, and xCT for 4F2hc; and AGT1 for an unidentified heavy subunit). HATs are, with the exception of 4F2hc/asc1, tightly coupled amino acid antiporters.[295]

rBAT and 4F2hc[364] share less than 30% of amino acid identity. The heavy subunits (molecular mass of ~90 and ~80 kDa for rBAT and 4F2hc, respectively) are N-glycoproteins with a single transmembrane segment, an intracellular N-terminus, and an extracellular C-terminal domain significantly homologous to insect and bacterial α-amylases (see Figure 8.13). X-ray diffraction of the extracellular domain of human 4F2hc has revealed an atomic structure similar to that of these enzymes—domain A, a triose phosphate isomerase (TIM) barrel [(αβ)8] and domain C, eight antiparallel β-strands at the C-terminal part (see Figure 8.13).[365] The conserved cysteine responsible for the intersubunit disulfide bridge is between the transmembrane segment and ectodomain.

In contrast to rBAT, 4F2hc has a dual role as a component of six amino acid transporters and as an enhancer of β$_1$ and β$_3$ outside-inside integrin signaling.[341] The structural information on the supramolecular organization of HAT is very scarce. Domain swapping and analysis of cystinuria point mutations have revealed that the rBAT transmembrane segment and cytoplasmic N-terminus are essential for amino acid transport function.[314,366] In contrast, the 4F2hc ectodomain might be necessary for interaction with the light subunits,[367] whereas the transmembrane segment and cytoplasmic N-terminus are essential for the stimulation of β$_1$ integrin signaling.[368] A low-resolution model (21 Å) of a human 4F2hc/LAT2 heterodimer positions the ectodomain of 4F2hc on top of LAT2, providing a structural basis for this ectodomain in recognition of the light subunit.[369]

Neither 4F2hc nor rBAT have α-amylase activity, and essential catalytic residues in α-amylases are missing in the 4F2hc ectodomain.[365] Therefore, the role of the large N-glycosylated ectodomains (~60 kDa) of rBAT and 4F2hc is unknown.

The light subunits are the catalytic components and confer specificity to the holotransporter, as revealed by reconstitution experiments of human b$^{0,+}$AT in the absence of rBAT[299] or functional expression of human LAT2 in *Pichia* yeast in the absence of 4F2hc.[369] Light subunits (~50 kDa) are highly hydrophobic and not glycosylated. Light subunits belong to the L-amino acid transporter (LAT) family within the large APC superfamily.[370] Cysteine scanning mutagenesis studies of xCT have supported a 12-transmembrane topology, with the N- and C- termini inside the cell and with the TMD2-TMD3 intracellular loop (IL1) accessible to the external medium (see Figure 8.13).[371] The 5 + 5 inverted repeat corresponds to the first 10 TMDs in the light subunits of HAT.[372] The conserved cysteine residue responsible for the intersubunit disulfide bridge is located in the TM3-TM4 extracellular loop.

In spite of the low amino acid sequence identity with LeuT (<10%) and AdiC (<20%), the design of the substrate-binding site seems to be conserved in LATs. Accordingly, residues in TMD8 seem to interact with the lateral chain of the substrate. Thus, thiol modification of Cys327 in TMD8 of the light subunit xCT suggests close proximity to the substrate binding site and permeation pathway.³⁷³ Furthermore, mutations of Lys295 in TMD8 (homologous to Trp293 in AdiC) broadened the substrate specificity of SteT, a bacterial LAT that exchanges L-serine and L-threonine.³⁷² Finally, the biochemical phenotype in some cystinuria and LPI mutations (e.g., T123M in b$^{0,+}$AT and G54V in y^{+}LAT1) also support a common substrate binding design. Mutation G54V completely abolishes the intrinsic transport activity of 4F2hc/y^{+}LAT1.³³⁸ According to homology models, residue Gly54 in y^{+}LAT1 is located in the unwound segment of TMD1, suggesting a substrate binding defect. Human carriers of mutation T123M in b$^{0,+}$AT present with isolated cystinuria, with hyperexcretion of cystine but not cationic amino acids in urine.³¹⁰ Homology modeling positions residue Thr123 in TMD3 close to the homologous substrate binding site in AdiC (see Figure 8.14). This location would be consistent with the observed altered substrate selectivity of T123M (defective binding for cystine but not for cationic amino acids) in isolated cystinuria. Finally, homology models of b$^{0,+}$AT and y^{+}LAT1 based on the AdiC structure show that almost half of the more than 60 missense mutations causing cystinuria and LPI are located in the two interior pairs of symmetry-related helices (TMD1 and TMD6 and TMD3 and TMD8), that are expected to participate in the substrate binding (see Figure 8.13). This highlights the relevance of the inner helices in the transport function of the light subunits of HAT as well.

Complete reference list available at ExpertConsult.com.

KEY REFERENCES

9. Wright EM, Loo DD, Hirayama BA: Biology of human sodium glucose transporters. *Physiol Rev* 91:733–794, 2011.
12. Gorboulev V, Schurmann A, Vallon V, et al: Na(+)-D-glucose cotransporter SGLT1 is pivotal for intestinal glucose absorption and glucose-dependent incretin secretion. *Diabetes* 61:187–196, 2012.
13. Vallon V, Platt KA, Cunard R, et al: SGLT2 mediates glucose reabsorption in the early proximal tubule. *J Am Soc Nephrol* 22:104–112, 2011.
14. Meng W, Ellsworth BA, Nirschl AA, et al: Discovery of dapagliflozin: a potent, selective renal sodium-dependent glucose cotransporter 2 (SGLT2) inhibitor for the treatment of type 2 diabetes. *J Med Chem* 51:1145–1149, 2008.
16. Faham S, Watanabe A, Besserer GM, et al: The crystal structure of a sodium galactose transporter reveals mechanistic insights into Na+/sugar symport. *Science* 321:810–814, 2008.
31. Martin MG, Turk E, Lostao MP, et al: Defects in Na+/glucose cotransporter (SGLT1) trafficking and function cause glucose-galactose malabsorption. *Nat Genet* 12:216–220, 1996.
36. van den Heuvel LP, Assink K, Willemsen M, et al: Autosomal recessive renal glucosuria attributable to a mutation in the sodium glucose cotransporter (SGLT2). *Hum Genet* 111:544–547, 2002.
56. Wright SH, Dantzler WH: Molecular and cellular physiology of renal organic cation and anion transport. *Physiol Rev* 84:987–1049, 2004.
69. Otsuka M, Matsumoto T, Morimoto R, et al: A human transporter protein that mediates the final excretion step for toxic organic cations. *Proc Natl Acad Sci U S A* 102:17923–17928, 2005.
70. Tamai I, Nakanishi T, Kobayashi D, et al: Involvement of OCTN1 (SLC22A4) in pH-dependent transport of organic cations. *Mol Pharm* 1:57–66, 2004.
76. Tzvetkov MV, Vormfelde SV, Balen D, et al: The effects of genetic polymorphisms in the organic cation transporters OCT1, OCT2, and OCT3 on the renal clearance of metformin. *Clin Pharmacol Ther* 86:299–306, 2009.
80. Traiffort E, O'Regan S, Ruat M: The choline transporter-like family SLC44: properties and roles in human diseases. *Mol Aspects Med* 34:646–654, 2013.
81. Grundemann D, Gorboulev V, Gambaryan S, et al: Drug excretion mediated by a new prototype of polyspecific transporter. *Nature* 372:549–552, 1994.
84. Motohashi H, Sakurai Y, Saito H, et al: Gene expression levels and immunolocalization of organic ion transporters in the human kidney. *J Am Soc Nephrol* 13:866–874, 2002.
85. Motohashi H, Inui K: Organic cation transporter OCTs (SLC22) and MATEs (SLC47) in the human kidney. *AAPS J* 15:581–588, 2013.
93. Urakami Y, Akazawa M, Saito H, et al: cDNA cloning, functional characterization, and tissue distribution of an alternatively spliced variant of organic cation transporter hOCT2 predominantly expressed in the human kidney. *J Am Soc Nephrol* 13:1703–1710, 2002.
96. Popp C, Gorboulev V, Muller TD, et al: Amino acids critical for substrate affinity of rat organic cation transporter 1 line the substrate binding region in a model derived from the tertiary structure of lactose permease. *Mol Pharmacol* 67:1600–1611, 2005.
103. Harper JN, Wright SH: Multiple mechanisms of ligand interaction with the human organic cation transporter, OCT2. *Am J Physiol Renal Physiol* 304:F56–F67, 2013.
106. Nies AT, Koepsell H, Damme K, et al: Organic cation transporters (OCTs, MATEs), in vitro and in vivo evidence for the importance in drug therapy. *Handb Exp Pharmacol* 201:105–167, 2011.
108. Kido Y, Matsson P, Giacomini KM: Profiling of a prescription drug library for potential renal drug-drug interactions mediated by the organic cation transporter 2. *J Med Chem* 54:4548–4558, 2011.
110. Abramson J, Smirnova I, Kasho V, et al: Structure and mechanism of the lactose permease of *Escherichia coli*. *Science* 301:610–615, 2003.
111. Huang Y, Lemieux MJ, Song J, et al: Structure and mechanism of the glycerol-3-phosphate transporter from *Escherichia coli*. *Science* 301:616–620, 2003.
118. Song IS, Shin HJ, Shim EJ, et al: Genetic variants of the organic cation transporter 2 influence the disposition of metformin. *Clin Pharmacol Ther* 84:559–562, 2008.
121. Ciarimboli G, Schlatter E: Regulation of organic cation transport. *Pflugers Arch* 449:423–441, 2005.
128. Tsuda M, Terada T, Mizuno T, et al: Targeted disruption of the multidrug and toxin extrusion 1 (mate1) gene in mice reduces renal secretion of metformin. *Mol Pharmacol* 75:1280–1286, 2009.
134. Tanihara Y, Masuda S, Sato T, et al: Substrate specificity of MATE1 and MATE2-K, human multidrug and toxin extrusions/H(+)-organic cation antiporters. *Biochem Pharmacol* 74:359–371, 2007.
135. Wittwer MB, Zur AA, Khuri N, et al: Discovery of potent, selective multidrug and toxin extrusion transporter 1 (MATE1, SLC47A1) inhibitors through prescription drug profiling and computational modeling. *J Med Chem* 56:781–795, 2013.
136. Astorga B, Ekins S, Morales M, et al: Molecular determinants of ligand selectivity for the human multidrug and toxin extruder proteins MATE1 and MATE2-K. *J Pharmacol Exp Ther* 341:743–755, 2012.
140. He X, Szewczyk P, Karyakin A, et al: Structure of a cation-bound multidrug and toxic compound extrusion transporter. *Nature* 467:911–914, 2010.
146. Nishihara K, Masuda S, Ji L, et al: Pharmacokinetic significance of luminal multidrug and toxin extrusion 1 in chronic renal failure rats. *Biochem Pharmacol* 73:1482–1490, 2007.
159. Ho HT, Ko BC, Cheung AK, et al: Generation and characterization of sodium-dicarboxylate cotransporter-deficient mice. *Kidney Int* 72:63–71, 2007.
165. Sekine T, Watanabe N, Hosoyamada M, et al: Expression cloning and characterization of a novel multispecific organic anion transporter. *J Biol Chem* 272:18526–18529, 1997.
166. Sweet DH, Wolff NA, Pritchard JB: Expression cloning and characterization of ROAT1. The basolateral organic anion transporter in rat kidney. *J Biol Chem* 272:30088–30095, 1997.
174. Enomoto A, Kimura H, Chairoungdua A, et al: Molecular identification of a renal urate anion exchanger that regulates blood urate levels. *Nature* 417:447–452, 2002.
175. Hagenbuch B, Meier PJ: Organic anion transporting polypeptides of the OATP/ SLC21 family: phylogenetic classification as OATP/

SLCO superfamily, new nomenclature and molecular/functional properties. *Pflugers Arch* 447:653–665, 2004.
190. George RL, Keenan RT: Genetics of hyperuricemia and gout: implications for the present and future. *Curr Rheumatol Rep* 15:309, 2013.
193. Vitart V, Rudan I, Hayward C, et al: SLC2A9 is a newly identified urate transporter influencing serum urate concentration, urate excretion and gout. *Nat Genet* 40:437–442, 2008.
194. Anzai N, Ichida K, Jutabha P, et al: Plasma urate level is directly regulated by a voltage-driven urate efflux transporter URATv1 (SLC2A9) in humans. *J Biol Chem* 283:26834–26838, 2008.
195. Matsuo H, Takada T, Ichida K, et al: Common defects of ABCG2, a high-capacity urate exporter, cause gout: a function-based genetic analysis in a Japanese population. *Sci Transl Med* 1:5ra11, 2009.
200. Dehghan A, Kottgen A, Yang Q, et al: Association of three genetic loci with uric acid concentration and risk of gout: a genome-wide association study. *Lancet* 372:1953–1961, 2008.
204. Silbernagl S: The renal handling of amino acids and oligopeptides. *Physiol Rev* 68:911–1007, 1988.
219. Kleta R, Romeo E, Ristic Z, et al: Mutations in SLC6A19, encoding B^{0}AT1, cause Hartnup disorder. *Nat Genet* 36:999–1002, 2004.
228. Singer D, Camargo SM: Collectrin and ACE2 in renal and intestinal amino acid transport. *Channels (Austin)* 5:410–423, 2011.
230. Broer S, Palacin M: The role of amino acid transporters in inherited and acquired diseases. *Biochem J* 436:193–211, 2011.
288. Feliubadalo L, Font M, Purroy J, et al: Non-type I cystinuria caused by mutations in SLC7A9, encoding a subunit (b$^{0,+}$AT) of rBAT. *Nat Genet* 23:52–57, 1999.
301. Calonge MJ, Gasparini P, Chillaron J, et al: Cystinuria caused by mutations in rBAT, a gene involved in the transport of cystine. *Nat Genet* 6:420–425, 1994.
303. Peters T, Thaete C, Wolf S, et al: A mouse model for cystinuria type I. *Hum Mol Genet* 12:2109–2120, 2003.
325. Borsani G, Bassi MT, Sperandeo MP, et al: SLC7A7, encoding a putative permease-related protein, is mutated in patients with lysinuric protein intolerance. *Nat Genet* 21:297–301, 1999.
357. Kowalczyk L, Ratera M, Paladino A, et al: Molecular basis of substrate-induced permeation by an amino acid antiporter. *Proc Natl Acad Sci U S A* 108:3935–3940, 2011.
380. Shaffer PL, Goehring A, Shankaranarayanan A, et al: Structure and mechanism of a Na+-independent amino acid transporter. *Science* 325:1010–1014, 2009.

9 Renal Acidification Mechanisms

I. David Weiner | Jill W. Verlander

CHAPTER OUTLINE

BICARBONATE REABSORPTION, 234
Proximal Tubule, 234
Loop of Henle, 238
Distal Convoluted Tubule, 238
Collecting Duct, 239
BICARBONATE GENERATION, 246
Titratable Acid Excretion, 246
Organic Anion Excretion, 247
Ammonia Metabolism, 248

Sulfatides, 255
ACID-BASE SENSORS, 256
Acid/Alkali–Sensing Receptors, 256
Kinases, 256
Bicarbonate-Stimulated Adenylyl Cyclase, 256
DIURNAL VARIATION IN ACID EXCRETION, 256

Acid-base homeostasis involves two separate but related processes, bicarbonate reabsorption and new bicarbonate generation. The first relates to the reabsorption of bicarbonate filtered by the glomerulus. The second relates to the need to generate "new bicarbonate" to replenish bicarbonate that is used to neutralize endogenous and exogenous fixed acid loads. Finally, a number of pathophysiologic conditions generate acid or alkali loads that the kidneys must respond to in order to maintain acid-base homeostasis.

BICARBONATE REABSORPTION

Bicarbonate reabsorption involves coordinated transport events in multiple nephron segments (Figure 9.1). The proximal tubule reabsorbs the majority of filtered bicarbonate. Little-to-no bicarbonate reabsorption occurs in the thin descending limb of the loop of Henle, moderate reabsorption occurs in the thick ascending limb of the loop (TAL), and the remaining filtered bicarbonate is reabsorbed in distal sites, including the distal convoluted tubule (DCT), connecting segment (CNT), initial collecting tubule (ICT), and collecting duct.

PROXIMAL TUBULE

GENERAL TRANSPORT MECHANISMS

Proximal tubule bicarbonate reabsorption involves several distinct, but interconnected, processes (Figure 9.2). First, protons (H^+) are secreted into the luminal fluid. Multiple proteins mediate H^+ secretion; the apical Na^+-H^+ exchanger, NHE3, and an apical H^+-ATPase (hydrogen ion adenosine triphosphatase) are the primary mechanisms of proton secretion in the adult kidney. In the neonatal kidney, the Na^+-H^+ exchanger, NHE8, appears to substitute for NHE3.[1] In the adult kidney, NHE3 is responsible for 60% to 70% of H^+ secretion, and H^+-ATPase accounts for the majority of the remainder.

Secreted H^+ combines with luminal HCO_3^- to form carbonic acid (H_2CO_3). Luminal carbonic acid dissociates to water (H_2O) and carbon dioxide (CO_2). Although this process can occur spontaneously, the spontaneous dehydration rate is inadequate to support normal rates of proximal tubule bicarbonate reabsorption. The dehydration reaction is catalyzed by carbonic anhydrase IV (CA IV), a membrane-bound carbonic anhydrase isoform present in the proximal tubule brush border.

Luminal CO_2 then moves across the apical plasma membrane into the cell. Although this process has traditionally been thought to occur through lipid-phase diffusion, the integral membrane protein, aquaporin 1 (AQP1), may mediate about 50% of CO_2 transport across the apical plasma membrane.[2] Cytosolic CO_2 is then hydrated, forming carbonic acid, through a process accelerated by the cytosolic carbonic anhydrase, carbonic anhydrase II (CA II). Cytosolic carbonic acid spontaneously dissociates to H^+ and HCO_3^-, "replenishing" the H^+ secreted across the apical plasma membrane by apical NHE3 and H^+-ATPase.

Cytosolic HCO_3^- is transported across the basolateral plasma membrane. In the S1 and S2 segments of the proximal tubule, the primary HCO_3^- transport mechanism is a sodium-coupled, electrogenic bicarbonate cotransporter, NBCe-1A.[3,4] Because NBCe-1A is electrogenic, generation and regulation of the transmembrane voltage between cytoplasm and interstitium are important and appear to be related to extracellular pH-dependent activation of the

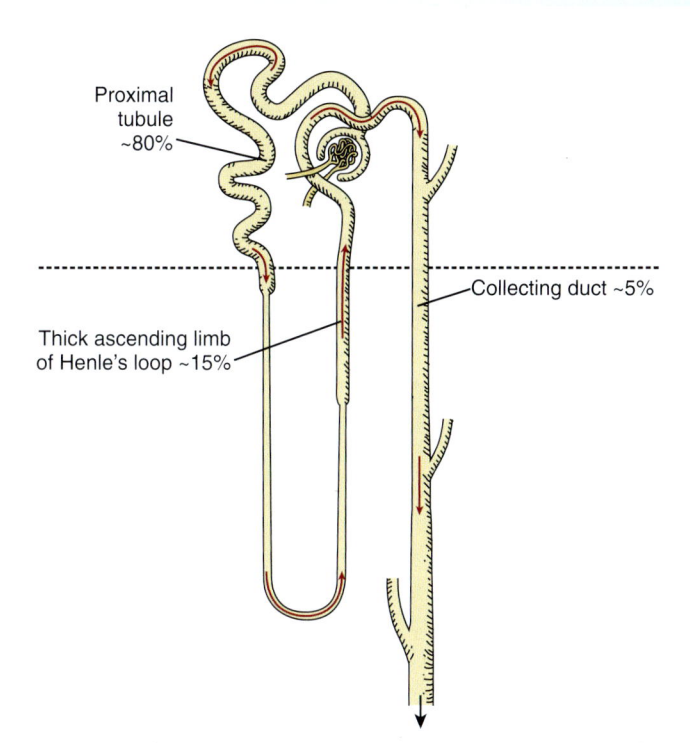

Figure 9.1 Summary of sites of bicarbonate reabsorption. The proximal tubule is the primary site quantitatively for filtered bicarbonate reabsorption. Minimal reabsorption occurs in the thin limb of the loop of Henle. The thick ascending limb of the loop of Henle reabsorbs the majority of the bicarbonate not reabsorbed in the proximal tubule. The collecting duct is the primary site for reabsorption of the remaining filtered bicarbonate.

(Proximal tubule ~80%; Thick ascending limb of Henle's loop ~15%; Collecting duct ~5%)

basolateral K^+ channel, TASK2.[5] In the S3 segment a Na^+-dependent, Cl^--HCO_3^- exchanger appears be the primary mechanism of basolateral HCO_3^- transport,[6] although NBCe-1A may also contribute.[7]

In addition to active or secondarily active H^+ secretion and bicarbonate reabsorption, the proximal tubule exhibits passive H^+ and bicarbonate transport. Because bicarbonate reabsorption decreases the luminal bicarbonate concentration and increases the luminal H^+ concentration relative to the peritubular space, this passive transport limits bicarbonate reabsorption and generation of an acidic luminal pH.[8] The molecular mechanisms of bicarbonate backleak are unclear, but several functional aspects are known. It is quantitatively less in newborn than in the adult kidney.[9] The backleak may be regulated; for example, the hormone angiotensin II (Ang II) decreases bicarbonate backleak.[10] Finally, it is known to be partially transcellular and involves specific membrane proteins, but it does not involve NHE3.[11,12]

TRANSPORTERS INVOLVED IN PROXIMAL TUBULE BICARBONATE REABSORPTION

Na^+-H^+ Exchangers

Na^+-H^+ exchangers (NHEs) are expressed widely in the kidney, where they function in intracellular pH regulation, transepithelial bicarbonate reabsorption, and vacuolar acidification. All utilize the extracellular-to-intracellular Na^+ gradient to enable secondary active, electroneutral H^+ secretion. Although the preferred ions are Na^+ and H^+, Li^+ can substitute for Na^+, and NH_4^+ can substitute for H^+.[13] The latter process, which enables Na^+-NH_4^+ exchange, is important in proximal tubule NH_4^+ secretion.[14]

NHE3, the primary apical Na^+-H^+ exchanger in the proximal tubule, mediates the majority of luminal bicarbonate reabsorption. Multiple mechanisms regulate NHE3. The best-studied hormonal mechanisms involve parathyroid hormone (PTH), dopamine, and Ang II. Both PTH and dopamine inhibit NHE3 activity, whereas Ang II has a biphasic effect, stimulatory at low concentrations and inhibitory at high concentrations. Both PTH and dopamine increase intracellular levels of cyclic adenosine monophosphate (cAMP), leading to decreased NHE3 activity,[15] and dopamine also has protein kinase C (PKC)–dependent effects.[16] Ang II decreases cAMP levels and activates PKC, tyrosine kinase, and phosphatidylinositol-3-kinase.[17]

NHE3 phosphorylation is an important regulatory mechanism. Serine 552 (in the rat sequence) is a consensus protein kinase A (PKA) phosphorylation site, and phosphorylation of this site causes localization to the coated pit region of the brush border membrane, where NHE3 cannot contribute to bicarbonate reabsorption.[18] Similarly, phosphorylation of rabbit serine 719 regulates insertion into the plasma membrane.[19] Dephosphorylation, mediated by the serine/threonine phosphatase 1 (PP1), but not PP2, at serines 552 and 605, and at other novel phosphorylation sites, stimulates NHE3 activity.[20]

Movement of NHE3 between different subcellular locations, including microvilli, intermicrovillar clefts, endosomes, and the cytoplasm, is an important regulatory mechanism. Only NHE3 in microvilli contributes to bicarbonate reabsorption. Redistribution within these domains is regulated by a variety of factors, including renal sympathetic nerve activity, glucocorticoids and insulin, Ang II, dopamine, and PTH.[15,21-24] This process involves a number of cellular proteins, including dynamin, NHE regulatory factor 1 (NHERF-1), clathrin-coated vesicles, calcineurin homologous protein-1, ezrin phosphorylation, G-protein alpha subunits and G-protein beta-gamma dimers.[25-27]

NHE8 is a second Na^+-H^+ exchanger found in the proximal tubule.[28] Under normal conditions, NHE8 is mostly intracellular in the adult kidney,[29] but in the absence of NHE3, NHE8 expression increases and the exchanger contributes to bicarbonate reabsorption.[1] In the neonatal kidney, NHE8 expression is increased and NHE3 expression is decreased, suggesting that NHE8 is the primary mechanism of apical Na^+-H^+ exchange activity in the neonatal kidney.[30]

H^+-ATPase

A second mechanism of proximal tubule apical H^+ secretion involves the vacuolar H^+-ATPase.[31] H^+-ATPase is expressed in the brush border microvilli, the base of the brush border, and apical invaginations between clathrin-coated domains.[32] In addition, H^+-ATPase acidifies proximal tubule endosomes and lysosomes, senses endosomal pH, and is involved in recruiting trafficking proteins to acidified vesicles, thereby assuring appropriate progression from early endosomes to lysosomes.[33] Proximal tubule H^+-ATPase activity is increased by Ang II, increased axial flow, and chronic metabolic acidosis.[34-36] H^+-ATPase has a direct binding interaction with aldolase, which may underlie the development of proximal

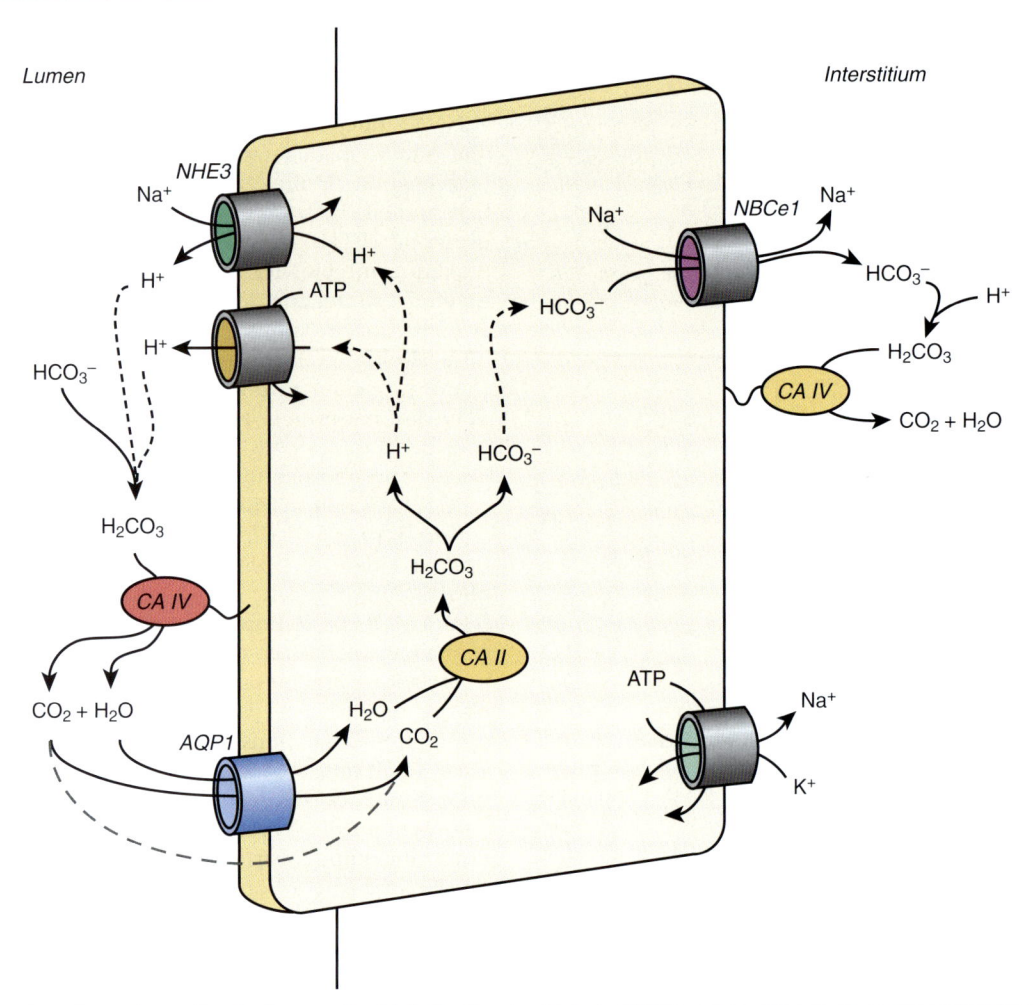

Figure 9.2 Bicarbonate reabsorption in the proximal tubule. Proximal tubule HCO_3^- reabsorption involves integrated function of multiple proteins. Protons are secreted by both the Na^+-H^+ exchanger, NHE3, and H^+-ATPase, and titrate luminal HCO_3^- to H_2CO_3. Luminal H_2CO_3 dehydration to H_2O and CO_2 is accelerated by luminal carbonic anhydrase activity mediated by carbonic anhydrase isoform CA IV. CO_2 enters the cell via aquaporin AQP1 and most likely also via passive lipid-phase diffusion, where its hydration to H_2CO_3 is accelerated by cytoplasmic CA II. H_2CO_3 rapidly dissociates to H^+ and HCO_3^-, thereby "replenishing" the secreted cytosolic H^+. Cytosolic HCO_3^- exits across the basolateral plasma membrane primarily by the electrogenic Na^+-HCO_3^- cotransporter, NBCe1.

renal tubular acidosis (RTA) in individuals with hereditary fructose intolerance.[37]

Electroneutral Sodium-Bicarbonate Cotransporter

Basolateral bicarbonate exit largely is mediated by the electroneutral sodium-bicarbonate cotransporter NBCe1-A. In humans, three splice variants of the *NBCe1* gene are known; only NBCe1-A, also known as kNBC1, is expressed in the kidney, where it is found exclusively in the basolateral plasma membrane in the proximal tubule.[4,38] In mice, two additional splice variants exist.[39] NBCe1-A has large cytoplasmic amino- and carboxy-termini tails, 14 transmembrane domains and two glycosylation sites.[40-43]

NBCe1-A in the proximal tubule mediates the coupled net movement of Na^+ and HCO_3^- in a 1:3 ratio of Na^+ and HCO_3^- equivalents. Under normal circumstances intracellular Na^+ and HCO_3^- concentrations are less than peritubular concentrations, meaning that reabsorption via NBCe1-A moves these solutes against their concentration gradients. Because the cytoplasm is negatively charged relative to the peritubular compartment, these electrical gradients provide the moving force. However, the coupling ratio of Na^+ and HCO_3^- is critically important: a 1:3 coupling mediates net HCO_3^- efflux, whereas with a 1:2 ratio the net electrochemical gradient favors HCO_3^- influx. Indeed, some cases of proximal RTA appear to result from NBCe1-A mutations that alter the coupling ratio.[44]

Metabolic acidosis increases proximal tubule HCO_3^- reabsorption and basolateral HCO_3^- transport activity but does not alter NBCe1-A expression.[45] Instead, phosphorylation regulates NBCe1-A activity in response to metabolic acidosis.[46] A number of signaling molecules regulate NBCe1-A. These include PKA, cAMP, PKC, Mg^{2+}, Ca^{2+}, adenosine triphosphate, carbonic anhydrases I through III, inositol 1,4,5-trisphosphate (IP_3) receptor (IP_3R)–binding protein released with IP_3 (IRBIT), and phosphatidylinositol 4,5-bisphosphate.[39]

Defects in NBCe1-A are the most common cause of autosomal recessive proximal RTA (pRTA).[39,44,47] In addition to causing severe pRTA, NBCe1 defects can cause growth and mental retardation, basal ganglia calcification, cataracts, corneal opacities (band keratopathy), glaucoma, elevations of serum amylase and lipase, and defects in the enamel suggestive of amelogenesis imperfecta.[39,47] In mice, homozygous NBCe1-A deletion causes a very severe phenotype, with severe metabolic acidosis, marked volume depletion, and death within a few weeks of birth. Heterozygous deletion gives rise to a milder phenotype but still causes development of pRTA.[48]

Carbonic Anhydrase

Carbonic anhydrases are a family of zinc metalloenzymes that catalyze the reversible hydration of CO_2 to form carbonic acid (H_2CO_3), reaction A in the following equation:

$$CO_2 + H_2O \overset{A}{\Leftrightarrow} H_2CO_3 \overset{B}{\Leftrightarrow} H^+ + HCO_3^- \qquad (1)$$

In the absence of carbonic anhydrase, the hydration/dehydration reaction (reaction A) is rate limiting.

Carbonic Anhydrase II. CA II, the predominant carbonic anhydrase in the kidney, is also the predominant carbonic anhydrase in the proximal tubule. It is expressed in the cytoplasm of the proximal tubule, in addition to multiple other sites in the kidney, including thin descending limb, TAL, and intercalated cells. In the mouse kidney, CA II is also expressed in collecting duct principal cells.

Carbonic Anhydrase IV. CA IV is found in the proximal tubule and in intercalated cells in the collecting duct.[49] CA IV is linked to the plasma membrane via a glycosylphosphatidylinositol lipid (GPI) anchor and extends into the extracellular compartment; the active site is thus extracellular, not intracellular.[50] In the proximal tubule, CA IV is expressed in both apical and basolateral plasma membranes where, by facilitating HCO_3^- interconversion with CO_2, it contributes to transepithelial bicarbonate reabsorption.[51]

REGULATION OF PROXIMAL TUBULE BICARBONATE REABSORPTION

Systemic Acid-Base

Changes in extracellular acid-base status profoundly alter proximal tubule bicarbonate reabsorption. Both metabolic acidosis and respiratory acidosis increase bicarbonate reabsorption, and alkalosis has the opposite effect. These changes occur with both acute and chronic pH changes, although the effect is substantially greater with chronic acidosis. It is important to note that these effects are mediated through changes in interstitial, that is, peritubular, HCO_3^- and pCO_2. Changes in luminal HCO_3^- have the opposite effect on proximal tubule bicarbonate transport, a manifestation of glomerular-tubular balance.

Studies have begun to elucidate the mechanisms through which extracellular bicarbonate and CO_2 regulate proximal tubule bicarbonate reabsorption. Changes in CO_2 and HCO_3^-, but not changes in pH when the other two components are constant, alter bicarbonate reabsorption.[52] These effects are specific to bicarbonate reabsorption, as fluid reabsorptive rates do not change. At least in part, this process involves members of the ErbB receptor tyrosine kinase family.[53] They also involve the intrarenal angiotensin system, because peritubular CO_2 stimulates intracellular production and luminal secretion of Ang II, which acts through an apical Ang II AT_1 receptor to stimulate bicarbonate reabsorption.[54,55]

Chronic metabolic acidosis increases proximal tubule bicarbonate reabsorption more than acute metabolic acidosis. This adaptive increase involves increased NHE3 expression and activity and increased H^+-ATPase activity,[34,56,57] but not detectable changes in NBCe1 expression.[45] Glucocorticoid levels rise with chronic metabolic acidosis,[58] and glucocorticoid receptor activation enhances acidosis-induced increases in NHE3 expression and apical trafficking.[59]

Luminal Flow Rate

Renal bicarbonate reabsorption changes in parallel with glomerular filtration rate and luminal flow.[60] Increased luminal flow enhances apical plasma membrane NHE3 activity.[61] In addition, increased flow minimizes changes in the luminal bicarbonate concentration, thereby maintaining a higher mean luminal bicarbonate concentration, which facilitates bicarbonate reabsorption.[62] Proximal tubule brush border microvilli may function as flow sensors, with drag force transmitted through the actin filament, altering cytoskeletal elements and regulating transport.[35]

Angiotensin II

Ang II is an important regulator of proximal tubule ion transport, including bicarbonate reabsorption. Low Ang II concentrations increase but high concentrations inhibit bicarbonate reabsorption.[63,64] Both luminal and peritubular low doses of Ang II stimulate bicarbonate reabsorption, mediated predominantly through apical and basolateral AT_1 receptors. An increase in AT_1 receptor expression due to acidosis may contribute to adaptive changes in bicarbonate reabsorption.[65]

Potassium

Chronic hypokalemia stimulates and chronic hyperkalemia inhibits proximal tubule bicarbonate reabsorption.[66] The inhibition is associated with parallel changes in apical Na^+-H^+ exchange and basolateral sodium-bicarbonate cotransport activity[67] and involves increased apical and basolateral plasma membrane AT_1 receptor expression.[68] Acute changes in extracellular potassium concentration, however, do not alter proximal tubule bicarbonate transport.[69]

Endothelin

Endothelin has important and direct effects on ion transport in a variety of renal epithelial cells, including the proximal tubule. Endothelin can be produced in the proximal tubule and exhibits an autocrine effect to stimulate NHE3.[70] In particular, metabolic acidosis–induced increases in NHE3 expression may require endothelin type B (ET-B) receptor activation.[71]

Parathyroid Hormone

PTH immediately inhibits proximal tubule bicarbonate reabsorption through activation of adenylyl cyclase and increased intracellular cAMP production.[72] Short-term systemic PTH administration leads to metabolic acidosis, but long-term administration to metabolic alkalosis.[73] The short-term effect is due primarily to increased urinary bicarbonate excretion, likely as a result of changes in proximal tubule bicarbonate reabsorption; the long-term effect is due to increased titratable acid excretion, which is likely a result of increased excretion of dihydrogen and hydrogen phosphate.[73]

Calcium-Sensing Receptor

The calcium-sensing receptor (CaSR) is present in the apical membrane in the proximal tubule. CaSR activation, through either increased luminal calcium or calcimimetic agents, increases bicarbonate reabsorption through a mechanism likely involving the activation of apical NHE3.[74] CaSR activation may modulate the effects of PTH in proximal tubule bicarbonate reabsorption; hypercalcemia resulting from excess PTH has the opposite effect of PTH alone on bicarbonate transport.

LOOP OF HENLE

The TAL reabsorbs approximately 15% of the filtered bicarbonate load. The overall schema in this loop is fundamentally similar to that in the proximal tubule. Apical Na^+-H^+ exchange and vacuolar H^+-ATPase secrete H^+. Quantitatively, apical Na^+-H^+ exchange activity is the major H^+ secretory mechanism; vacuolar H^+-ATPase activity is present but has at most a minor role in bicarbonate reabsorption.[75,76] Two Na^+-H^+ exchanger isoforms are present in the TAL, NHE2 and NHE3, but NHE3 appears to be predominant.[77,78] Secreted H^+ reacts with luminal HCO_3^-, forming H_2CO_3, which dissociates to CO_2 and H_2O. Whether luminal CA IV is present is unclear, as reports in the literature are conflicting.[51,79] Luminal CO_2 moves down its concentration gradient across the apical plasma membrane into the cell cytoplasm. Cytoplasmic CA II catalyzes CO_2 hydration to form H_2CO_3, which dissociates to H^+ and HCO_3^-, thereby recycling the H^+ secreted across the apical plasma membrane. Cytosolic HCO_3^- exits via basolateral Cl^-/HCO_3^- exchange—possibly anion exchanger 2 (AE2)—via an electroneutral sodium-bicarbonate cotransporter (NBCn1), and possibly via basolateral Cl^- channels.[80-82]

Several plasma membrane proteins either directly or indirectly alter bicarbonate reabsorption. Inhibiting the apical $Na^+-K^+-2Cl^-$ cotransporter, NKCC2, increases bicarbonate reabsorption.[75] This increase may occur because inhibiting NKCC2 decreases Na^+ entry, thereby decreasing intracellular Na^+ and increasing the Na^+ uptake gradient for apical Na^+-H^+ exchange. Inhibiting basolateral Na^+-H^+ exchange activity decreases bicarbonate reabsorption through cytoskeletal alterations that reduce apical NHE3 expression.[83,84]

REGULATION OF THICK ASCENDING LIMB BICARBONATE REABSORPTION

A variety of stimuli regulate TAL bicarbonate reabsorption. Metabolic acidosis increases TAL bicarbonate reabsorption,[85,86] but whether the effects are specific to metabolic acidosis or due to other mechanisms is not clear. Metabolic acidosis induced by NH_4Cl and chloride loading with NaCl have similar effects on bicarbonate transport, raising the possibility that chloride loads, not acid loads, regulate TAL bicarbonate transport.[86] Support for acidosis regulation of TAL bicarbonate transport comes from the finding that NH_4Cl-induced metabolic acidosis, but not equivalent chloride loading with NaCl, increases TAL NHE3 expression.[87] Further supporting a role of the TAL in acid-base regulation is the observation in experimental models that metabolic alkalosis decreases bicarbonate reabsorption.[88]

Several hormones regulate bicarbonate reabsorption. Ang II stimulates TAL bicarbonate reabsorption, likely through activation of AT_1 receptors.[89,90] Glucocorticoid receptors are present in the TAL, and glucocorticoids are necessary for normal bicarbonate reabsorption.[91] Mineralocorticoids, at high concentrations, stimulate bicarbonate reabsorption,[88] but their absence does not alter basal transport.[91] Arginine vasopressin (AVP) inhibits bicarbonate reabsorption through prostaglandin E_2–mediated inhibition of apical Na^+-H^+ exchange activity.[92,93] PTH inhibits bicarbonate reabsorption, but the effect is less than the effect of AVP.[93]

Cytokines regulate bicarbonate transport. Lipopolysaccharide (LPS) inhibits transport; this effect involves the cytokine receptor Toll-like receptor-4 (TLR4) as well as separate pathways activated by luminal and peritubular LPS. Luminal LPS involves the mTOR (mammalian target of rapamycin) pathway, whereas peritubular LPS functions through the MEK/ERK (mitogen-activated protein kinase/ extracellular signal–regulated kinase) pathway.[94,95]

Another important regulatory factor is the medullary osmotic gradient. Increased tonicity inhibits and decreased tonicity stimulates bicarbonate reabsorption; these effects occur through phosphatidylinositol 3-kinase–mediated changes in apical Na^+-H^+ exchange activity.[96,97] AVP, which contributes to the development of the medullary osmotic gradient, inhibits bicarbonate reabsorption.[93]

ACID-BASE TRANSPORTERS IN THE THICK ASCENDING LIMB

Many of the major H^+ and HCO_3^- transporters were discussed previously in relation to the proximal tubule and are not described again here.

Electroneutral Sodium-Bicarbonate Transporter 1

NBCn1 facilitates the electroneutral, coupled transport of Na^+ and HCO_3^- in a 1:1 ratio. In the kidney, NBCn1 is found in the basolateral plasma membrane in the TAL, the intercalated cells of the outer medullary collecting duct (OMCD), and the terminal inner MCD (IMCD).[45,98] Because the concentrations of Na^+ and HCO_3^- are generally lower in the cytoplasm than in the interstitium, basolateral NBCn1 likely mediates peritubular HCO_3^- uptake. Moreover, both metabolic acidosis and hypokalemia increase TAL NBCn1 expression.[45,99] Thus, NBCn1 is unlikely to mediate a critical role in bicarbonate reabsorption. Instead, it is likely to contribute to ammonia reabsorption, as discussed later.

DISTAL CONVOLUTED TUBULE

The DCT consists of two cell types, DCT cells and intercalated cells, which employ different mechanisms of bicarbonate reabsorption. DCT cells express apical NHE2,[100] and NHE2 inhibitors decrease bicarbonate reabsorption.[78] Basolateral HCO_3^- exit likely involves AE2.[80] A basolateral Cl^- channel that has limited HCO_3^- permeability may also contribute.[101] Cytosolic CA II is present, but not apical CA IV.[51] In the late DCT intercalated cells are present.[102] Quantitatively, intercalated cells constitute only a very small proportion of all cells in the DCT, about 4% and 7% in mouse and rat kidneys, respectively.[103] The majority of intercalated cells in the DCT are type A and non-A, non-B intercalated cells (see "Cell Composition").[103]

COLLECTING DUCT

The renal collecting duct, the final site of bicarbonate reabsorption, has the capacity to both reabsorb and secrete luminal bicarbonate. Specific proteins in specific epithelial cell types, which vary in type and frequency in different collecting duct segments, mediate these processes.

COLLECTING DUCT SEGMENTS

Technically, the collecting duct begins with the initial collecting tubule (ICT), immediately distal to the CNT, and extends through the IMCD. The CNT arises from a different embryonic origin from that of the ICT and the remainder of the collecting duct. However, the CNT is included in the discussion of the role of the collecting duct in acid-base regulation because it has cell types and acid-base transport mechanisms similar to those in the collecting duct. Different portions of the collecting duct are identified by where they reside: cortical collecting duct (CCD), outer medullary collecting duct in the outer stripe (OMCDo), outer medullary collecting duct in the inner stripe (OMCDi), and the IMCD.

CELL COMPOSITION

Collecting duct segments contain several distinct epithelial cell types, and the cellular composition differs in the various collecting duct segments. Two distinct cell types, intercalated cells and principal cells, are present. Principal cells account for about 60% to 65% of cells, and intercalated cells account for the remainder in the ICT, CCD, and OMCD. The proportion of intercalated cells is less in the IMCD and decreases progressively as one moves from the outer medullary–inner medullary junction to the papillary tip. In the terminal IMCD, the epithelium is composed of IMCD cells, a cell distinct from both intercalated cells and principal cells. The CNT contains both intercalated cells and a cell type specific to the CNT, termed the *connecting segment cell*; in some species, principal cells are also present.

At least three distinct intercalated cell subtypes exist; the type A intercalated cell, the type B intercalated cell, and the non-A, non-B intercalated cell (Figure 9.3). In the CNT, both type A and non-A, non-B intercalated cells are present, and type B intercalated cells are uncommon. In the CCD, both type A and type B intercalated cells are present, and the non-A, non-B cell is uncommon. In the OMCD and IMCD, only the type A intercalated cell is present under normal conditions.

Type A Intercalated Cell

The type A intercalated cell is involved in H^+ secretion, HCO_3^- reabsorption and ammonia secretion. The proteins involved in these processes are, in general, different from those in the proximal tubule and TAL (Figure 9.4).

Both vacuolar H^+-ATPase and P-type H^+-K^+-ATPases are involved in H^+ secretion. H^+-ATPase is abundant in the apical plasma membrane and in apical cytoplasmic tubulovesicles in type A intercalated cells. H^+-ATPase undergoes redistribution between the cytoplasmic compartment and the apical plasma membrane; this mechanism, rather than changes in total protein expression, appears to be the major adaptive response to acid-base disturbances.[104] In addition to having a major role in H^+ secretion, H^+-ATPase also has an essential role in cell volume regulation and maintenance of intracellular electronegativity, replacing the Na^+-K^+-ATPase which provides these functions in most other cell types.[105]

A second means of H^+ secretion is electroneutral, depends on luminal K^+, and is mediated by P-type H^+-K^+-ATPase proteins.[106] At least two H^+-K^+-ATPase α-isoforms are present. One, $HK\alpha_1$, is similar to the α-isoform involved in gastric acid secretion. The other, $HK\alpha_2$, is similar to the α-isoform in the colon. K^+ reabsorbed via apical H^+-K^+-ATPase can either recycle across the apical plasma membrane or exit the cell across the basolateral plasma membrane, and relative movement across the apical versus basolateral plasma membranes is regulated by dietary K^+ intake.[107]

A truncated isoform of the erythrocyte anion exchanger, the kidney anion exchanger (kAE1), is present in the basolateral plasma membrane and mediates basolateral

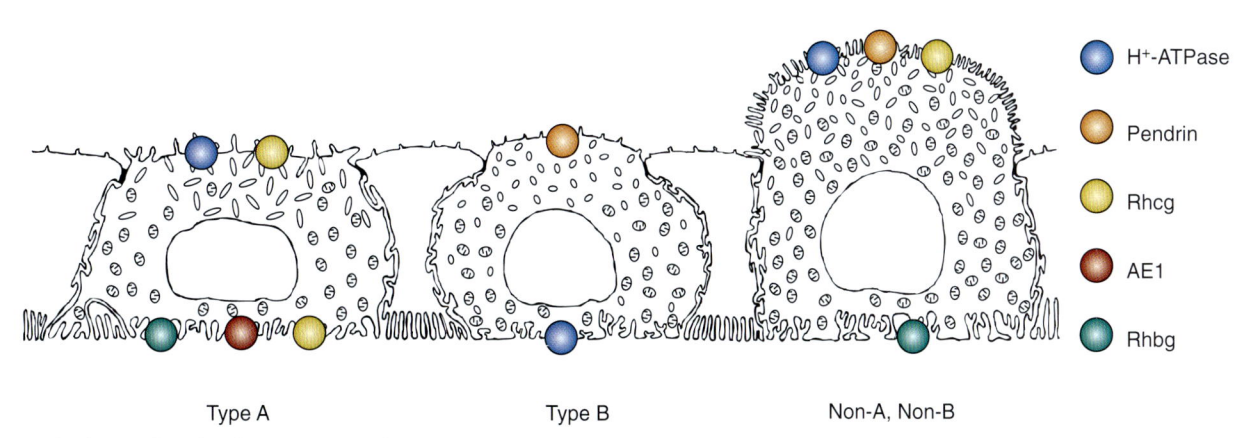

Figure 9.3 Intercalated cell subtypes in the distal nephron and collecting duct. The late distal convoluted tubule, connecting segment, initial collecting tubule, cortical collecting duct, outer and inner medullary collecting ducts have multiple distinct cell types. Three intercalated cell types can be distinguished on the basis of ultrastructural features and differential expression in plasma membrane domains of several proteins involved in renal acid-base transport, including H^+-ATPase, AE1, pendrin, Rhbg, and Rhcg. These specific intercalated cell subtypes occur at different frequencies specific to the various tubule segments. (Courtesy Ki-Hwan Han, MD, PhD, Ewha Womans University, Seoul, Korea.)

240 SECTION I — NORMAL STRUCTURE AND FUNCTION

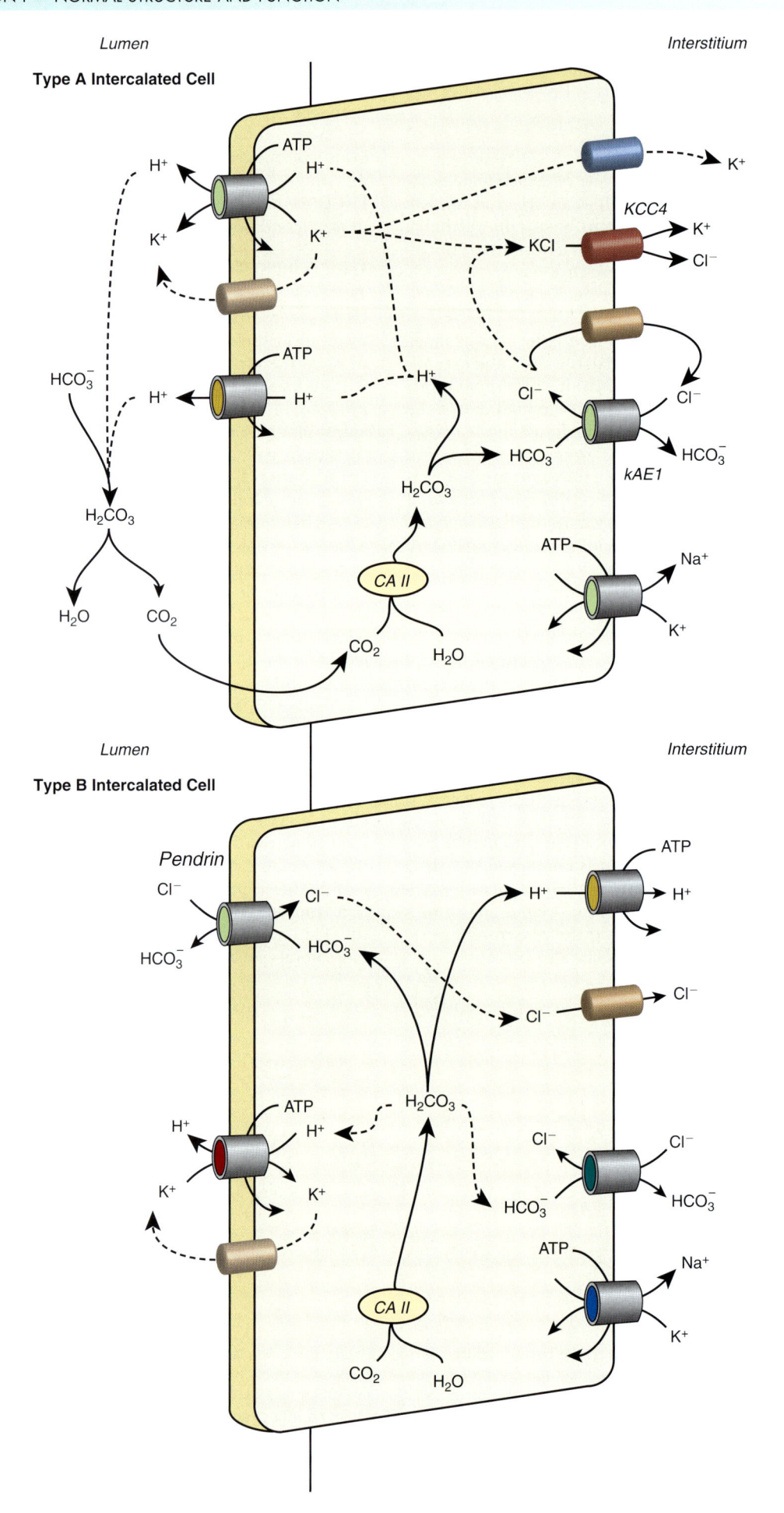

Type A Intercalated Cell

Lumen — *Interstitium*

Type B Intercalated Cell

Lumen — *Interstitium*

bicarbonate exit.[108] Cl⁻ that enters the cell via basolateral Cl⁻-HCO₃⁻ exchange exits via the KCl cotransporter, KCC4[109,110]; a basolateral Cl⁻ channel, presumably ClC-Kb in humans and ClC-K2 in rodents, also contributes to Cl⁻ recycling.[111]

Cytoplasmic CA II is abundant in type A intercalated cells and enables intracellular generation of H⁺, for apical secretion, and HCO₃⁻, for basolateral transport. In addition, membrane-associated carbonic anhydrases are present in the apical region (CA IV) and, at least in mouse and rabbit, in the basolateral region (CA XII) of intercalated cells.[112]

Type B Intercalated Cell

The type B intercalated cell mediates a major role in HCO₃⁻ secretion and luminal Cl⁻ reabsorption. It contains basolateral H⁺-ATPase and an apical Cl⁻-HCO₃⁻ exchanger, pendrin.[113] H⁺-ATPase is also present in vesicles throughout the cell, but it is not present in the apical plasma membrane. As in type A intercalated cells, H⁺-ATPase, rather than Na⁺-K⁺-ATPase, prevents cell swelling and maintains intracellular electronegativity in type B cells.[105] Type B intercalated cells also express H⁺-K⁺-ATPase.[114,115] In the rabbit and mouse an apical H⁺-K⁺-ATPase activity is present,[116,117] whereas in the rat a basolateral H⁺-K⁺-ATPase activity has been suggested.[118] The type B cell also has cytoplasmic CA II, which facilitates intracellular H⁺ and HCO₃⁻ production. Figure 9.4 summarizes the proteins involved in type B intercalated cell acid-base transport.

The type B intercalated cell also has the ability to secrete H⁺ and reabsorb luminal HCO₃⁻. As noted previously, most studies indicate that the type B intercalated cell has an apical H⁺-K⁺-ATPase activity, and functional studies have shown that all CCD intercalated cells with apical Cl⁻-HCO₃⁻ exchange activity, that is, all type B intercalated cells, also have basolateral Cl⁻-HCO₃⁻ exchange activity.[119]

The type B intercalated cell has several roles in acid-base and ion transport homeostasis. Genetic deletion of apical pendrin impairs HCO₃⁻ secretion, luminal Cl⁻ reabsorption, and, through a mechanism involving coordinated function with the principal cell, luminal Na⁺ reabsorption.[120-122] The type B intercalated cell may also contribute to H⁺ secretion and luminal HCO₃⁻ reabsorption. Ammonia, which is increased in metabolic acidosis and hypokalemia, increases apical H⁺-K⁺-ATPase and basolateral Cl⁻-HCO₃⁻ activity, a change that would result in increased net HCO₃⁻ reabsorption.[123]

Non-A, Non-B or Type C Intercalated Cell

A third intercalated cell subtype, generally termed the non-A, non-B cell (sometimes called the type C cell), is present in the CNT and ICT.[103,124] This cell has several features that distinguish it from both type A and type B intercalated cells. These differences include the expression of both pendrin and H⁺-ATPase in the apical plasma membrane and in apical cytoplasmic vesicles, the absence of basolateral plasma membrane H⁺-ATPase and basolateral AE1, the presence of apical but not basolateral Rhesus (Rh) glycoprotein Rhcg, and the absence of basolateral Rhbg (see Figure 9.3). Thus, this cell differs significantly from both type A and type B intercalated cells. Studies of the developing kidney show that non-A, non-B cells and type B intercalated cells arise simultaneously, but from different foci.[125,126] This cell type was termed "non-A, non-B cell" in early studies. However, its unique transporter expression, distribution, and developmental origin suggest it is a third distinct intercalated cell subtype.

Principal Cells

Principal cells have indirect and direct roles in acid secretion. Indirectly, principal cell–mediated Na⁺ reabsorption leads to luminal electronegativity, which facilitates H⁺ secretion by the electrogenic, and thus voltage-sensitive, H⁺-ATPase. In addition, principal cells have direct roles. Functional studies show that principal cells have apical H⁺ secretory and basolateral Cl⁻-HCO₃⁻ exchange activities,[127,128] and they express H⁺-ATPase[129,130] and both the HKα₁ and HKα₂ isoforms of H⁺-K⁺-ATPase.[106] In the mouse and rat kidney, principal cells in the OMCDi and IMCDi express both carbonic anhydrase activity and CA II protein.[131,132] Finally, the ammonia transporters Rhcg and Rhbg are both present in principal cells in the CCD and OMCD.[133]

IMCD Cell

The IMCD cell is a distinct cell type and is the predominant cell present in the terminal IMCD. It exhibits carbonic anhydrase activity,[132] both H⁺-ATPase and H⁺-K⁺-ATPase activity,[106,134] and basolateral Cl⁻-HCO₃⁻ exchange.[135] In vitro microperfusion studies have demonstrated directly that the IMCD secretes H⁺ and reabsorbs luminal HCO₃⁻.[136]

FUNCTIONAL ROLE OF DIFFERENT COLLECTING DUCT SEGMENTS

Connecting Tubule and Initial Collecting Tubule

Relatively little information is available on the functional role of the CNT and ICT in acid-base homeostasis. Morphologic and immunolocalization studies suggest that the CNT and ICT contain type A, type B, and non-A, non-B intercalated cells.[103,124,137] Under basal conditions, the CNT, at least in the rabbit, secretes bicarbonate through a Cl⁻-, carbonic

---

Figure 9.4 Bicarbonate transport by type A and type B intercalated cells. **Top panel** shows a model of acid-base transport by the type A intercalated cell. Two families of H⁺ transporters, H⁺-ATPase and H⁺-K⁺-ATPase, are present in the apical plasma membrane. Secreted H⁺ titrates luminal HCO₃⁻ to form H₂CO₃, which dehydrates to water (H₂O) and CO₂. Luminal carbonic anhydrase activity, most likely mediated by carbonic anhydrase isoform CA IV, is variably present in the collecting duct (see text for details). Cytosolic H⁺ and HCO₃⁻ are formed from CA II–accelerated hydration of CO₂ and rapid dissociation of H₂CO₃. Cytosolic HCO₃⁻ exits across the basolateral plasma membrane via the anion exchanger AE1. Cl⁻ that enters via the exchanger kAE1 recycles via a basolateral Cl⁻ channel. K⁺ that enters via apical H⁺-K⁺-ATPase can either recycle via an apical, Ba²⁺-sensitive K⁺ channel or be reabsorbed via a basolateral Ba²⁺-sensitive K⁺ channel. A basolateral Na⁺-H⁺ exchanger is present but does not contribute to bicarbonate reabsorption and is not shown. **Bottom panel** shows a model of acid-base transport by the type B intercalated cell. Apical pendrin is the primary mechanism of bicarbonate secretion. Chloride enters the cell via pendrin and exits across a basolateral chloride channel. Basolateral H⁺-ATPase extrudes protons into the peritubular compartment. Bicarbonate and protons are produced from CO₂ and water in a CA II–catalyzed reaction. In addition, an apical H⁺-K⁺-ATPase in series with a basolateral Cl⁻-HCO₃⁻ exchange activity is present and may contribute to bicarbonate reabsorption by the type B intercalated cell. ATP, adenosine triphosphate.

anhydrase–, and H$^+$-ATPase–dependent mechanism[138] that likely involves apical pendrin, cytosolic CA II, and basolateral H$^+$-ATPase.

Cortical Collecting Duct

Unlike the OMCD and IMCD, which can only secrete acid, the CCD both reabsorbs and secretes bicarbonate. The basal direction of bicarbonate transport varies among species, but both bicarbonate absorption and secretion can be induced in response to systemic acid or alkali loading.[139-141] The ability to secrete bicarbonate, which is not found in the OMCD or IMCD, correlates with the presence of type B intercalated cells in the CCD, but not in the OMCD or IMCD. Mineralocorticoids stimulate CCD bicarbonate secretion, likely in relation to generation of metabolic alkalosis and to stimulation of pendrin expression.[122,142]

Outer Medullary Collecting Duct

The OMCD is responsible for approximately 40% to 50% of the net acid secretion in the collecting duct. Both intercalated cells and principal cells contribute to acid secretion, although intercalated cells are believed to be the primary type responsible for OMCD acid secretion.[127,128]

Inner Medullary Collecting Duct

The IMCD secretes H$^+$ and reabsorbs luminal bicarbonate.[143] However, the number of type A intercalated cells is substantially less than in other collecting duct segments. In the rat they account for only 10% of cells in IMCD1,[144] and in all species examined the prevalence diminishes distally such that no intercalated cells exist in the distalmost portion of the IMCD (IMCD3). Nonetheless, bicarbonate reabsorption occurs in the terminal IMCD and basolateral Cl$^-$-HCO$_3^-$ exchange is present in cultured IMCD cells.[135] H$^+$ secretion is at least partly mediated by H$^+$-K$^+$-ATPase.[145] In rats fed a potassium-deficient diet, H$^+$-K$^+$-ATPase activities ware upregulated,[134] but H$^+$-K$^+$-ATPase accounts for only about 50% of bicarbonate reabsorption in the IMCD, indicating that other mechanisms of luminal acidification also contribute, likely including H$^+$-ATPase. The IMCD expresses carbonic anhydrase IV and luminal, cytoplasmic, and lateral membrane–associated carbonic anhydrase activity has been reported.[132,146]

PROTEINS INVOLVED IN COLLECTING DUCT H$^+$/BICARBONATE TRANSPORT

Collecting duct H$^+$ and HCO$_3^-$ transport involves the coordinated activity of multiple transporters in conjunction with specific carbonic anhydrase isoforms. This section reviews the specific proteins involved.

H$^+$-ATPase

Electrogenic apical H$^+$ secretion in acid-secreting intercalated cells and basolateral proton transport by bicarbonate-secreting intercalated cells are mediated by the vacuolar H$^+$-ATPase. Intercalated cells in the OMCD and initial IMCD and type A intercalated cells in the CCD contain H$^+$-ATPase in the apical plasma membrane and in an apical cytoplasmic vesicle pool, and redistribution between the cytoplasmic vesicle pool and the apical plasma membrane is a major mechanism regulating H$^+$ secretion. H$^+$-ATPase is also present in the apical region of principal cells and connecting segment cells, but its expression is much less than in intercalated cells. The role of apical H$^+$-ATPase in nonintercalated cells has not been clearly defined; it may be involved in endosomal trafficking and fusion,[147] and in the OMCDi it can also mediate apical H$^+$ secretion.[127]

Vacuolar H$^+$-ATPase is an assembly of multiple subunits that form two main domains; the V$_1$ domain is extramembranous and hydrolyzes ATP, and the V$_0$ domain is transmembranous and transports protons. The V$_0$ domain is composed of six subunits; the V$_1$ domain is composed of eight subunits and is linked to the V$_0$ domain via a stalk region comprising subunits from both V$_0$ and V$_1$. Distinct isoforms and splice variants have been identified for many of these H$^+$-ATPase subunits and their cell specific distribution may contribute to cell specific regulation of proton and bicarbonate transport.

Genetic defects in several H$^+$-ATPase subunit mutations can cause distal RTA (dRTA) in humans. Defects in the B1 subunit in the hydrolytic V$_1$ domain resulting from *ATP6V1B1* gene mutations can produce early-onset hearing loss with autosomal recessive, severe dRTA.[148-150] Mice with B1 subunit deletion have incomplete dRTA.[151] In these mice, the B2 subunit can substitute partially for the B1 subunit, enabling partial compensation.[152] Mutations in the a4 subunit (*ATP6V0A4*) in the H$^+$-translocating V$_0$ domain also produce recessive, severe early-onset dRTA, with variable onset of hearing loss.[150,153,154]

H$^+$-K$^+$-ATPase

The second mechanism of collecting duct H$^+$ secretion involves electroneutral H$^+$-K$^+$ exchange.[106] The active protein is a heterodimer composed of α- and β-subunits. The α-subunit is an integral membrane protein with multiple membrane-spanning domains and contains the catalytic portion of the enzyme. Two α-subunit isoforms have been identified. HKα$_1$, also termed the gastric isoform, was identified originally in the stomach. HKα$_1$ forms heterodimers with its specific β-subunit, HKβ. The β-subunit has only a single membrane-spanning region and is necessary for targeting of the α-subunit to the plasma membrane and for transport function.[106] HKα$_2$ was identified originally in the colon and is also referred to as the *colonic isoform*. Three splice variants of HKα$_2$ have been identified in the kidney. HKα$_2$ forms heterodimers with the β$_1$-subunit of Na$^+$-K$^+$-ATPase.

HKα$_1$, HKα$_2$, and HKβ are expressed throughout the collecting duct, with greater expression in intercalated cells than in principal cells.[155-157] Physiologic studies suggest that both HKα$_1$ and HKα$_2$ are present in type A as well as type B intercalated cells.[116,117,158] However, immunohistochemistry studies have yielded variable results with respect to the precise cellular distribution of the HKα$_1$ and HKα$_2$ isoforms. HKα$_1$ immunoreactivity was found in both AE1-positive (type A) and AE1-negative intercalated cells in both rat and rabbit kidneys,[115] but in human kidneys, diffuse HKα$_1$ immunoreactivity was present in both intercalated and principal cells.[159] HKα$_2$ immunoreactivity was consistently apical, but in different cell types in different studies. It was found exclusively in the connecting segment cell in rabbits in one study[160] and exclusively in the OMCD principal cell in rats in another.[161] A third study found the splice variant, HKα$_{2c}$, in intercalated cells, principal cells, and connecting segment cells from the CNT through the initial IMCD in rabbit kidneys.[114]

Multiple physiologic conditions alter H^+-K^+-ATPase expression and activity. Metabolic acidosis increases H^+-K^+-ATPase activity in the CCD and HKα_1 and HKα_2 mRNA expression in the OMCD, suggesting that H^+-K^+-ATPase contributes to H^+ secretion.[106] Specific studies have identified apical, but not basolateral, H^+-K^+-ATPase activity in both types A and type B intercalated cells in mouse and rabbit kidney.[117,158,162] Extracellular ammonia, which increases with both metabolic acidosis and hypokalemia, enhances apical H^+-K^+-ATPase–mediated H^+ secretion in both type A and type B intercalated cells in the CCD.[123,163]

Pendrin is an electroneutral Cl^--HCO_3^- exchanger present exclusively in type B and non-A, non-B intercalated cells. It is found in the apical plasma membrane and in apical cytoplasmic vesicles in type B and non-A, non-B intercalated cells in the CNT, ICT, and CCD. Under basal conditions, pendrin is predominantly expressed in the apical plasma membrane in non-A, non-B intercalated cells and in subapical cytoplasmic vesicles in type B intercalated cells, and redistribution between these two sites is an important regulatory mechanism.[164] Pendrin is regulated by Ang II, nitric oxide, and cAMP.[165,166] In addition to bicarbonate secretion, pendrin mediates an important role in extracellular fluid volume and blood pressure regulation. This role appears to involve participation in both transcellular Cl^- reabsorption and, through luminal alkalinization due to HCO_3^- secretion, activation of the principal cell epithelial Na^+ transporter, ENaC.[167,168]

Carbonic Anhydrase

Three carbonic anhydrase isoforms, CA II, CA IV, and CA XII, are present in the collecting duct. CA II is cytosolic in proximal tubular cells, discussed previously, in intercalated cells, and in principal cells in mouse collecting ducts.[169] CA II is present in all intercalated cell types, but expression is generally greater in the type A than in type B intercalated cells.

CA IV is an extracellular, membrane-associated carbonic anhydrase tethered to the membrane through a glycosylphosphatidylinositol (GPI) lipid anchoring protein. It is expressed apically in the majority of cells in the OMCD and IMCD and in type A intercalated cells in the CCD in rabbits.[170] In the OMCDi, luminal carbonic anhydrase inhibition decreases bicarbonate absorption, suggesting an important role for CA IV in acid-base homeostasis.[171]

CA XII is another extracellular, membrane-associated carbonic anhydrase found in the collecting duct.[112] In contrast to CA IV, CA XII is an integral membrane protein with a single membrane-spanning region.[112] Basolateral CA XII immunoreactivity has been reported in principal cells in human kidneys, and in the mouse, basolateral CA XII immunoreactivity is found in type A intercalated cells in the CCD and OMCD.[112,172]

Kidney Anion Exchanger 1

The major basolateral anion exchanger in type A intercalated cells is kAE1. In the human, rat, and mouse kidney kAE1 is expressed almost entirely in the basolateral plasma membrane. In the rabbit kidney under basal conditions, kAE1 is present in intracytoplasmic multivesicular bodies as well as in the basolateral plasma membrane; metabolic acidosis decreases intracellular kAE1 and increases basolateral kAE1, suggesting that regulated trafficking contributes to bicarbonate reabsorption.[173]

Several mutations in AE1 cause human autosomal dominant and autosomal recessive dRTA. Autosomal dominant dRTA can be caused by a trafficking defect leading either to mistargeting to the apical plasma membrane or to failure of plasma membrane insertion.[174,175] Autosomal recessive dRTA due to AE1 mutation is commonly due to mutations that lead to intracellular protein retention.[176]

KCl cotransporter KCC4 is a member of the SLC12 family of solute transporters and mediates electroneutral, coupled transport of K^+ and Cl^-. Basolateral KCC4 expression has been shown in the proximal convoluted tubule (PCT), TAL, DCT, CNT, and type A intercalated cells.[109,177] In the type A intercalated cell, KCC4 likely contributes to basolateral Cl^- recycling. Metabolic acidosis increases KCC4 expression in type A intercalated cells in the OMCD, suggesting a role in the response to metabolic acidosis,[110] and KCC4 deletion causes development of dRTA,[109] suggesting that KCC4 is necessary for both basal and acidosis-stimulated acid-base homeostasis.

Cl⁻ Channel

Cl^- entering via basolateral kAE1 recycles across the basolateral plasma membrane. In addition to KCC4, the Cl^- channel, ClC-K2, is present in the basolateral plasma membrane of type A intercalated cells and likely contributes to this recycling.[178]

Other Anion Exchangers

Several other anion transporters, including anion exchangers and sodium bicarbonate cotransporters, are present in the collecting duct, but their roles in acid-base homeostasis are less completely understood. AE2 is expressed in collecting ducts, particularly in the basolateral plasma membrane of IMCD cells.[179] Another Cl^--HCO_3^- exchanger, Slc26a7, is found in the basolateral plasma membrane of OMCD intercalated cells.[180] Slc26a7 messenger RNA (mRNA) and protein expression increases with acid loading, suggesting that it may contribute to regulated bicarbonate reabsorption.[181] Anion exchanger AE4 (Slc4a9) has been reported in the collecting duct, but both its location and function are in question. One study reported that AE4 immunoreactivity is exclusively apical in type B intercalated cells in rabbit kidneys,[182] whereas another found apical and lateral AE4 immunoreactivity in rabbit type A intercalated cells, and basolateral immunoreactivity in both type A and type B intercalated cells in the rat CCD.[183]

Sodium-Bicarbonate Cotransporters

Several sodium bicarbonate cotransporters (NBCs) are expressed in the collecting duct. NBC3 (Slc4a7) is found in the apical region of OMCD intercalated cells and type A intercalated cells in the CCD and in the basolateral region of type B intercalated cells.[184,185] It appears to contribute to intracellular pH regulation but not to transepithelial bicarbonate transport.[186] As previously mentioned, NBCn1, also an *SLC4A7* gene product, is an electroneutral sodium-bicarbonate cotransporter, and its basolateral expression is found in the terminal IMCD and in OMCD intercalated cells.[98] NBCe2 (Slc4a5), an electrogenic sodium-bicarbonate cotransporter, is apical in intercalated cells in the medullary collecting duct.[187]

REGULATION OF COLLECTING DUCT ACID-BASE TRANSPORT

The collecting duct is the final site controlling renal acid-base regulation. It responds quickly to physiologic conditions to increase acid or bicarbonate excretion as needed to maintain systemic acid-base homeostasis.

Acidosis

The collecting duct response to metabolic acidosis includes adaptations in all segments of the collecting duct and the connecting segment. Increased acid secretion in the collecting duct during acidosis is mediated primarily by H^+-ATPase. Both metabolic acidosis and respiratory acidosis increase apical plasma membrane H^+-ATPase expression and activity in acid-secreting collecting duct intercalated cells. Redistribution of H^+-ATPase from a subapical vesicle pool to the apical plasma membrane is the primary means of activation of proton secretion, and it involves vesicular trafficking that requires SNARE (soluble N-ethylmaleimide-sensitive factor attachment protein receptor) proteins and Rab GTPases (guanosine triphosphatases).[129,130] In most models of metabolic acidosis, total renal H^+-ATPase mRNA and protein expression do not change,[130,188] but examination of OMCD segments from acid-loaded mice found increased mRNA expression of several H^+-ATPase subunits, including the β1 and α4 subunits.[189]

During metabolic acidosis, AE1 mRNA and AE1 protein expression in the basolateral plasma membranes of OMCD and CCD type A intercalated cells is increased. In rats and mice, AE1 is present in the basolateral membrane under basal conditions, and the subcellular distribution does not change with metabolic acidosis.[190,191] In rabbits fed a normal diet, AE1 is in both intracellular multivesicular bodies and in the basolateral plasma membrane in type A intercalated cells. Metabolic acidosis increases the amount of AE1 immunoreactivity in the basolateral plasma membrane and reduces intracellular AE1.[173]

During metabolic acidosis, both net HCO_3^- secretion and type B intercalated cell–mediated unidirectional HCO_3^- secretion decrease. This decrease is associated with reductions of pendrin expression in type B and non-A, non-B cells as well as of apical Cl^--HCO_3^- exchange activity in type B intercalated cells in the CCD.[192-194] Reduced bicarbonate secretion by type B cells during acid loading thus contributes to increased net bicarbonate reabsorption.

Carbonic anhydrase activity and the expression of CA II and CA IV in the collecting duct are increased by metabolic acidosis.[112] CA IV expression is upregulated in the OMCD, whereas CA II expression is upregulated in the CNT, CCD, and OMCD.

The collecting duct response to respiratory acidosis appears to be similar to that to metabolic acidosis. Respiratory acidosis stimulates structural changes in OMCD and CCD type A intercalated cells that are consistent with translocation of H^+-ATPase–bearing membrane from the apical vesicle pool to the apical plasma membrane.[195] Respiratory acidosis also stimulates N-ethylmaleimide (NEM)–sensitive ATPase activity[130,196] and bicarbonate reabsorption in isolated CCDs,[197] a finding consistent with activation of H^+-ATPase–mediated proton secretion. In addition, chronic respiratory acidosis increases kAE1 mRNA.[198] Pendrin expression decreases during respiratory acidosis,[199] a decrease that likely mediates decreased bicarbonate secretion.

Alkalosis

Metabolic alkalosis induces coordinated changes in acid-base transport throughout the collecting duct. In the OMCD of bicarbonate-loaded animals, bicarbonate reabsorption is lower than in control animals[140] and in the IMCD, bicarbonate loading abolishes acid secretion.[200] In the CCD, bicarbonate loading in animals produces net bicarbonate secretion.[141] However, no studies have shown the development of HCO_3^- secretion by the OMCD or the IMCD in response to metabolic alkalosis, and absence of this development correlates with the lack of pendrin-expressing type B and non-A, non-B intercalated cells in these segments.

The cellular response to alkalosis in OMCD and CCD type A cells entails essentially the reverse of processes that occur to stimulate acid secretion. H^+-ATPase is redistributed from the apical plasma membrane into the apical vesicle pool, and basolateral AE1 immunoreactivity decreases.[191,201,202] Depending on the animal model, alkalosis increases pendrin expression and its apical distribution in type B and non-A, non-B intercalated cells as well as pendrin-mediated CCD bicarbonate secretion.[192,193] However, pendrin expression, subcellular location, and functional activity are regulated by other factors independent of acid-base status, particularly chloride balance and luminal chloride delivery.[203,204]

Hormonal Regulation of Collecting Duct Acid-Base Transport

In addition to extracellular pH, multiple other factors regulate collecting duct acid-base transport. Importantly, in vivo acid-base changes cause greater adaptations than equivalent in vitro changes, suggesting that in vivo regulatory mechanisms mediate a critical role in the response to acid-base disturbances.[205] Several hormones and receptors regulate bicarbonate transport in the collecting duct, particularly aldosterone and its analogs, and Ang II.

Aldosterone is an important regulator of collecting duct bicarbonate transport.[206] Both in vivo and in vitro mineralocorticoids increase OMCD bicarbonate reabsorption.[206] This increase involves, at least in vitro, increased H^+-ATPase activity and apical translocation in OMCD intercalated cells, stimulated through a nongenomic pathway not inhibited by mineralocorticoid receptor blockade.[207] Mineralocorticoids also increase CCD bicarbonate secretion; this increase depends on luminal chloride, is mediated by pendrin, and involves increased pendrin mRNA and protein expression and pendrin redistribution from cytoplasmic vesicles to the apical plasma membrane in type B intercalated cells.[121,122] Probably because of parallel stimulation of both acid and bicarbonate secretion, mineralocorticoid therapy usually has modest effects on systemic acid-base homeostasis.

Ang II exerts effects on the proximal tubule, TAL, DCT, and collecting ducts. The collecting duct expresses apical AT1 (AT_{1a}) receptors in both principal cells and intercalated cells.[208] In mouse OMCD and CCD, Ang II in vitro increases H^+-ATPase activity in acid-secreting intercalated cells by trafficking H+-ATPase to the apical plasma membrane.[208,209] In mouse OMCD, Ang II stimulates H+-ATPase activity through a G protein–coupled PKC pathway.[208] However, in other studies, Ang II in vivo and in vitro decreased bicarbonate reabsorption in rat OMCD but Ang II in vitro decreased H+-ATPase activity via AT1 receptors[210,211]; this apparent discrepancy has not been resolved.

Endothelin has important effects on collecting duct acid-base transport that are mediated partly by nitric oxide. Dietary protein intake stimulates urinary acidification through a process involving H+-ATPase activation, mediated by endothelin and nitric oxide.[212] Endothelin-1 (ET-1) is synthesized by the collecting duct,[213,214] and endothelin receptors ET-A and ET-B are present in the collecting duct.[215] ET-B activation regulates both type A and type B intercalated cell responses to metabolic acidosis.[216]

The calcium-sensing receptor (CaSR) is apical in inner medullary collecting duct cells and in type A intercalated cells[217] and mediates luminal Ca^{2+}-stimulation of H+-ATPase.[218] Luminal acidification stimulated by this pathway may inhibit calcium precipitation and minimize development of nephrolithiasis.[218]

Activation of the vasopressin type 1A (V1a) receptor is an additional regulatory mechanism. The V1a receptor is expressed in the medullary TAL (MTAL) and throughout the collecting duct,[219,220] with expression in both intercalated cells and principal cells in the CCD and only in intercalated cells in the OMCD.[219] Metabolic acidosis increases V1a receptor expression in the MTAL and the OMCD in the inner stripe.[219,221] Genetic deficiency of the V1a receptor causes development of type IV RTA and diminishes mineralocorticoid stimulation of H+-K+-ATPase and Rhcg.[222]

Several other hormones and drugs also alter collecting duct acid-base transport. Kallikrein inhibits bicarbonate secretion.[223] Calcitonin stimulates H+-ATPase–dependent bicarbonate reabsorption in the rabbit CCD.[224] Isoproterenol stimulates bicarbonate secretion by type B intercalated cells.[225]

Paracrine Regulation

Several compounds produced and/or transported in the proximal tubule and TAL have downstream effects that regulate collecting duct acid-base transport. Presumably, this arrangement enables these segments, which exist in an area with very high blood flow and thus rapid exposure to changes in systemic acid-base and potassium, to regulate transport in collecting duct segments in the outer medulla and inner medulla, sites of low blood flow and thus reduced exposure to changes in systemic acid-base and potassium homeostasis. The paracrine molecules most extensively studied are ammonia and α-ketoglutarate (α-KG).

Ammonia, discussed in detail later regarding its role in net acid excretion, is produced in the proximal tubule and undergoes regulated transport in both the proximal tubule and the TAL in response to both acid loading and hypokalemia. In addition to its roles in bicarbonate generation, ammonia stimulates CCD bicarbonate reabsorption in a concentration-dependent fashion.[163] Ammonia stimulates both type A intercalated cell acid secretion and inhibits type B intercalated cell bicarbonate secretion.[123,163] Its stimulation of proton secretion involves stimulation of H+-K+-ATPase, not H+-ATPase.[163,226]

The Krebs cycle intermediate, 2-oxoglutarate (α-KG), may have an important role in acid-base homeostasis. Changes in acid-base loading change the net direction of transport in the proximal tubule and the loop of Henle from reabsorption (acid-loaded) to net secretion (alkali loading).[227-229] In the CNT and CCD, luminal 2-oxoglutarate regulates net bicarbonate and sodium chloride reabsorption, acting through its receptor, Oxgr1, in type B and non-A, non-B intercalated cells.[229] Thus, 2-oxoglutarate can function as a paracrine mediator, enabling functional coordination of the proximal tubule and the TAL with the collecting duct.

CELLULAR ADAPTATIONS TO ACID-BASE PERTURBATIONS

In addition to changes in the abundance and subcellular distribution of membrane transporters, adaptive responses to some physiologic disturbances may involve changes in the numbers of intercalated cells. Several studies have shown that chronic metabolic acidosis and chronic hypokalemia increase intercalated cell numbers in medullary collecting ducts,[230-234] whereas others have found no change in intercalated cell number in these conditions.[137,190,235] Long-term administration of lithium or acetazolamide also increases intercalated cell numbers in the OMCD.[230,231,233]

Increases in intercalated cell numbers could result from intercalated cell proliferation or from principal cell proliferation followed by conversion into intercalated cells. Studies using proliferation markers show that metabolic acidosis, hypokalemia, and lithium administration are each associated with increased proliferation of collecting duct cells,[232,234,236] some showing increased proliferation in type A intercalated cells[234] and others showing the proliferating cells to be principal cells.[232,233,236] The latter studies suggest that principal cells and OMCD intercalated cells may interconvert on the basis of observations of rare cells with immunohistochemical and ultrastructural characteristics of both cell types.[232,233,236]

With respect to the CCD, some studies have suggested there may be interconversion of type A and type B intercalated cells. An early paper examining the rabbit isolated perfused CCD equated apical endocytosis with alpha (type A) intercalated cells and used apical peanut lectin binding as a marker of beta (type B) intercalated cells. Long-term NH_4Cl loading in vivo increased the number of intercalated cells exhibiting apical endocytosis in microperfused CCDs and decreased the number of cells that bound peanut lectin; the interpretation was that intercalated cell subtypes in the CCD could interconvert, with the type B intercalated cells reversing polarity to meet the physiologic demand for increased acid secretion.[237] Subsequently, some studies reported that acidosis, lithium administration, and carbonic anhydrase inhibition alter the relative numbers of intercalated cells identifiable as type A or type B, although none have shown cells in native tissue with either apical AE1, basolateral pendrin, or coexpression of these two transporters.[192,230,231,234,238] Other studies of acid-base disturbances find regulation of the abundance and distribution of transport proteins specific to the A and B intercalated cell types and changes in cell morphology, but no change in the relative or absolute numbers of specific intercalated cell subtypes.[104,137,191,195] The explanation for these different findings could include differences in the experimental models, species examined, sensitivity and specificity of intercalated cell identification, and cell quantitation methods.

In vitro studies have implicated the extracellular matrix protein hensin and the prolyl isomerase activity of cyclophilin in the process of intercalated cell remodeling.[239,240] In mice with intercalated cell–specific hensin deletion there is development of dRTA, lack of type A intercalated cells, and an increased number of type B intercalated cells.[241] Hensin's effects on type A intercalated cell development appears to require the activation of β_1 integrin.[241]

BICARBONATE GENERATION

Acid-base homeostasis requires not only reabsorption of filtered bicarbonate but also the generation of new bicarbonate to replace the bicarbonate used for buffering of endogenous and exogenous fixed acids. There are two major components of bicarbonate generation, titratable acid excretion and ammonia excretion. In addition, organic anion excretion is biologically important. Organic anions can be metabolized to form HCO_3^-; accordingly their excretion is physiologically equivalent to bicarbonate excretion.

TITRATABLE ACID EXCRETION

Titratable acids are urinary solutes that buffer secreted protons, enabling H^+ excretion without substantial changes in urine pH. Titratable acid excretion constitutes about 40% of net acid excretion under basal conditions. Metabolic acidosis increases titratable acid excretion by as much as 50% above baseline (Figure 9.5).[242,243]

Multiple buffers contribute to titratable acid excretion. An ideal urinary buffer has a pK_a lower than systemic pH, so that the majority of the filtered component is in the base form, and a pK_a higher than urine pH, so that the majority of the urinary component is in the acid form. Phosphate is the predominant titratable acid and typically accounts for more than 50% of total titratable acid.[242,244] Citrate and creatinine also contribute to titratable acid excretion, but to a lesser extent. Ammonia is frequently termed a urinary buffer, but because of its high pK_a it does not contribute substantially to titratable acid excretion. The role of ammonia in new bicarbonate generation is considered separately later. Figure 9.6 shows both the relative contributions of major urinary buffers to titratable acid excretion and the effect of changes in urine pH after the amount excreted under normal conditions and the pK_a of each buffer is taken into account.

PHOSPHATE AS A TITRATABLE ACID

Titratable acid excretion in the form of phosphate is the amount of HPO_4^{2-} that is filtered, not reabsorbed, and that buffers secreted H^+, forming $H_2PO_4^-$. Phosphate exists, under physiologically relevant conditions, in equilibrium between two forms, $H_2PO_4^-$ and HPO_4^{2-}. The relative amount of these two forms is given by the following formula:

$$10^{pH-6.8} = \frac{[HPO_4^{2-}]}{[H_2PO_4^-]} \quad (2)$$

The amount of $H_2PO_4^-$ in the urine ($H_2PO_4^-{}_{Urine}$) at any given pH can be calculated as follows:

$$H_2PO_4^-{}_{Urine} = \frac{U_{Phos}V}{10^{(pH_U - 6.8)} + 1} \quad (3)$$

where U_{Phos} is the urinary concentration of total phosphate. Filtered phosphate, at the typical serum pH of 7.4, is about 80% in the form of HPO_4^{2-} and 20% in the form of $H_2PO_4^-$.

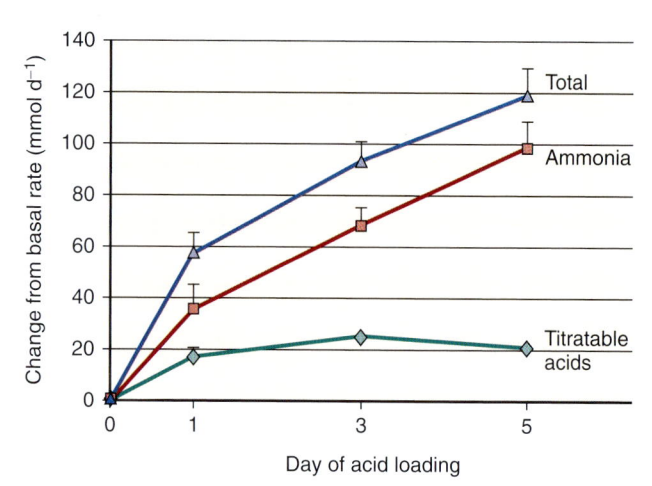

Figure 9.5 Relative contributions of titratable acid and ammonia excretion in the response to metabolic acidosis. Normal human volunteers were acid-loaded with approximately 2 mmol/kg/d of ammonium chloride, and changes in urinary ammonia and titratable acid excretion were quantified. (Data recalculated from Elkinton JR, Huth EJ, Webster GD, Jr, McCance RA: The renal excretion of hydrogen ion in renal tubular acidosis. *Am J Med* 36:554-575, 1960.)

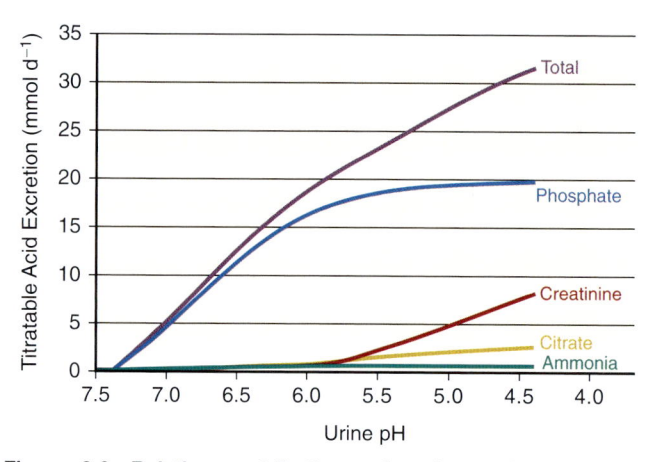

Figure 9.6 Relative contributions of various urinary buffers to titratable acid excretion. Ability of various urinary buffers to contribute to titratable acid excretion depends on the amounts excreted in the urine, their pK_a, and final urine pH. The figure shows titratable acid excretion accounted for by each of the four major urinary buffers—phosphate, creatinine, citrate, and ammonia—at differing urine pH. Rates were calculated with daily excretion rate and pK_a values, respectively, for phosphate, 25 mmol/d and 6.8; creatinine, 11 mmol/d and 4.9; citrate, 3 mmol/d and 5.6; and ammonia, 40 mmol/d and 9.15.

Thus, at any urine pH (pH_U), titratable acid excretion in the form of phosphate (TA_{Phos}) is given by the following formula:

$$TA_{Phos} = U_{Phos}V * \left(\frac{1}{10^{(pH_U - 6.8)} + 1} - 0.2\right) \quad (4)$$

These considerations indicate that titratable acid excretion as phosphoric acid is determined by phosphate excretion and by the ability to lower urine pH. Phosphate excretion is determined by the difference between the filtered load of phosphate and tubular phosphate reabsorption. Regulation of renal tubular phosphate transport is a complex process and is discussed in detail elsewhere in this text. Here, only the factors that regulate this process in response to acid-base disorders are reviewed.

The proximal tubule is the primary site of phosphate reabsorption and is where metabolic acidosis and other acid-base disorders regulate phosphate transport. Acid loading decreases proximal tubule phosphate reabsorption, leading to increased excretion. However, absolute changes in urinary phosphate excretion are usually rather modest, less than a twofold increase. The decrease involves decreased expression of sodium-dependent phosphate cotransporter NaPi-IIa protein and mRNA and changes in its subcellular distribution.[245,246] Interestingly, acid loading alters NaPi-IIa expression even if the acid load is completely compensated and there are no changes in systemic pH, suggesting that factors that precede changes in systemic pH regulate this response.[247] Metabolic acidosis also lowers luminal pH in the proximal tubule, thereby directly inhibiting phosphate uptake.[248,249] Finally, metabolic acidosis increases PTH release, also inhibiting phosphate reabsorption.

Other phosphate transporters besides NaPi-IIa, such as NaPi-IIc and Pit-2, are present in the proximal tubule apical plasma membrane. Whether NaPi-IIc changes with metabolic acidosis is unclear because some studies find decreased expression[247] and others do not.[250] Pit-2 expression, although regulated by dietary phosphate availability, is not altered in metabolic acidosis in phosphate-replete conditions but does increase in response to metabolic acidosis in conditions of phosphate depletion.[247]

Acidosis-induced changes in phosphate excretion depend on systemic phosphate availability. In the presence of dietary phosphate restriction, basal phosphate excretion is reduced, and the increase in urinary phosphate excretion in response to metabolic acidosis is blunted.[247] Similarly, changes in NaPi-IIa abundance are smaller.[245] In contrast to expression of NaPi-IIa, and to their response to metabolic acidosis in phosphate-replete animals, expression of NaPi-IIc and Pit-2 actually increases in phosphate-restricted animals exposed to metabolic acidosis.[247]

Increased renal phosphate excretion with metabolic acidosis is balanced by parallel increases in extrarenal phosphate transport. Metabolic acidosis increases small intestinal Na^+-dependent phosphate transport, and this increase is associated with greater expression of NaPi-IIb.[251] There is also increased phosphate release from bone in response to both acute and chronic metabolic acidosis.[252] These extrarenal effects minimize the changes in systemic phosphate levels that could otherwise develop from the higher phosphate excretion.

OTHER URINARY BUFFERS

Creatinine, typically used to assess glomerular filtration, has a pK_a of about 4.9 and is excreted in sufficient amounts—approximately 11 mmol • d^{-1}—that it can contribute to titratable acid excretion, particularly when urinary pH is 5.5 or less.[242] Uric acid, although it can function as a buffer, is typically excreted in such small amounts—approximately 4 mmol • d^{-1}—as to limit its role as a titratable acid. In ketoacidosis, β-hydroxybutyric acid and acetoacetic acid excretion increases, in turn increasing titratable acid excretion. However, because ketoacids can be metabolized to bicarbonate, their loss in the urine has no net effect on acid-base homeostasis.

ORGANIC ANION EXCRETION

Multiple organic anions in the urine can contribute to acid-base homeostasis. At least 95 different urinary organic anions have been identified, and many, including hippuric, erythronic, threonic, tartaric, and uric acids, are excreted in substantial quantities.[253] In general, their role in acid-base homeostasis is not as titratable acids. Instead, because their metabolism produces bicarbonate, their excretion enables alkali excretion without altering urine pH.

CITRATE EXCRETION

Citrate plays an important role in both acid-base homeostasis and urinary calcium excretion. The latter function, which relates to citrate's ability to complex calcium and enables excretion of high urinary calcium concentrations, is discussed elsewhere in this textbook. This chapter discusses citrate's role in acid-base homeostasis.

Citrate has two roles in acid-base homeostasis: (1) as a urinary buffer contributing to titratable acid excretion and, (2) as a substrate in the tricarboxylic acid cycle. Approximately 99% of plasma citrate is in the molecular form of citrate^{3-}, and at a urine pH of 5.6 about 50% of urinary citrate is in the form citrate^{2-}, thereby enabling citrate to function as titratable acid (see Figure 9.6). Citrate is also a key component of the tricarboxylic acid cycle, and its metabolism results in HCO_3^- generation. Thus, citrate excretion is functionally equivalent to HCO_3^- excretion through mechanisms independent of citrate's role as a titratable acid.

Multiple factors regulate renal citrate excretion. Metabolic acidosis decreases and alkalosis increases citrate excretion.[254] Decreased citrate excretion with metabolic acidosis reduces its availability as a titratable acid, but because citrate is also a metabolic alkali equivalent, decreased excretion results in decreased alkali equivalent excretion and is therefore beneficial for acid-base homeostasis. Hypokalemia reduces citrate excretion.[255,256] This effect is likely independent of systemic pH. The carbonic anhydrase inhibitor acetazolamide and high dietary intake of either NaCl or protein decrease citrate excretion.[257,258] Lithium chloride administered at equivalent therapeutic doses in animal models increases citrate excretion,[259] but this effect has not been found in studies in humans.[260]

Renal citrate handling determines renal citrate excretion. In humans, plasma citrate levels average about 0.1 mM, and changes in plasma levels are not an important regulatory mechanism. The proximal tubule reabsorbs 65% to 90% of filtered citrate, and reabsorption parallels the filtered load. Citrate transported into proximal tubule epithelial cells, whether across apical or basolateral plasma membranes, is metabolized, enabling citrate to serve as a significant component of renal oxidative metabolism.[257] There does not appear to be significant citrate transport in other renal sites.

Proximal tubule apical citrate uptake is a secondarily active process, involving electrogenic cotransport of 3 Na^+ with citrate^{2-}.[257] Apical citrate transport is believed mediated by the sodium-dicarboxylate cotransporter, NaDC-1, an integral membrane protein highly expressed in apical plasma membrane in the proximal tubule and in the small intestine.[261,262]

Multiple mechanisms regulate proximal tubule citrate transport. First, the transported citrate form is citrate^{2-}; luminal acidification, as present with metabolic acidosis, shifts the buffer reaction, citrate^{3-} + H^+ ↔ citrate^{2-}, towards citrate^{2-}, which facilitates citrate transport. Second, metabolic acidosis increases apical citrate transport capacity,[263] most likely by increasing NaDC-1 expression.[264] Both hypokalemia and starvation decrease citrate excretion, likely through stimulation of proximal tubule citrate transport.[265,266]

Basolateral citrate transport in the proximal tubule has different characteristics from those of apical transport. Uptake is pH-independent, Na^+-dependent, and electroneutral, appears to involve 3 Na^+ and 1 citrate^{3-},[257,267] and appears to be mediated by NaDC-3.[268] Approximately 20% of proximal tubule citrate uptake appears to be mediated by basolateral uptake. However, because the proximal tubule does not secrete citrate, basolateral citrate uptake does not regulate renal citrate excretion.

OTHER ORGANIC ANIONS

Humans excrete 26 to 52 mEq · d^{-1} of organic anions other than citrate. Because organic anions can be metabolized to bicarbonate, organic anion excretion is functionally equivalent to alkali excretion and thereby can contribute to acid-base regulation. The extent of change in these organic anions with acid-base disturbances is not clear. Some studies show that acid or alkali loading does not alter urinary organic anion excretion,[269] whereas other studies show that alkali loading increases and acid loading decreases organic anion excretion.[270]

Quantitatively, there are important species-dependent differences in the magnitude of organic anion excretion. In humans, basal organic anion excretion averages 0.3 to 0.7 mEq kg^{-1} · d^{-1},[269] whereas in the rat organic anion excretion is 2 to 8 mEq kg^{-1} · d^{-1}.[44,263,271,272] Studies in the dog report 1 to 2 mEq kg^{-1} · d^{-1},[273] and excretion in the rabbit averages 4 mEq kg^{-1} · d^{-1}.[272] This species-dependent variation may in part be due to differences in intestinal organic anion absorption.[372]

AMMONIA METABOLISM

Renal ammonia metabolism and transport constitute a predominant mechanism of the renal response to most acid-base disorders (see Figure 9.5). Ammonia metabolism involves integrated function of multiple portions of the kidney. Only a minimal amount of urinary ammonia derives from glomerular filtration, making urinary ammonia excretion unique among the major compounds present in the urine. Instead, the kidney produces ammonia, which is then selectively transported either into the urine or the renal vein, from where it is transported to the systemic circulation. Importantly, renal vein ammonia content exceeds arterial content, indicating that the kidney is a net producer of ammonia, even in the presence of significant urinary ammonia excretion. Selective ammonia transport involves integrated transport in the proximal tubule, the TAL, and the collecting duct (Figure 9.7).

AMMONIA CHEMISTRY

Ammonia exists in two molecular forms, NH_3 and NH_4^+. The relative amounts of each are governed by the following buffer reaction: $NH_3 + H^+ \leftrightarrow NH_4^+$. This reaction occurs essentially instantaneously and has a pK_a under biologically relevant conditions of about 9.15. Accordingly, the majority of ammonia is present as NH_4^+; at pH 7.4 only about 1.7% is present as NH_3. Because most biological fluids exist at a pH substantially below this pK_a, small changes in pH cause exponential changes in NH_3 concentration, but almost no change in NH_4^+ concentration (Figure 9.8).

NH_3, although uncharged, has an asymmetric arrangement of positively charged hydrogen nuclei around a central nitrogen, resulting in significant polarity (Figure 9.9). As a consequence, NH_3 has limited lipid permeability. Consequently, diffusion across plasma membranes is limited, and NH_3 transporters both accelerate NH_3 transport and provide important regulatory control.

NH_4^+ also has limited permeability across lipid bilayers in the absence of specific transport proteins. However, in aqueous solutions NH_4^+ and K^+ have nearly identical biophysical characteristics, enabling NH_4^+ to be transported at the K^+ transport site of many proteins.[274]

AMMONIA PRODUCTION

Almost all renal epithelial cells can produce ammonia, but the proximal tubule is the primary site for physiologically relevant ammoniagenesis.[275] Phosphate-dependent glutaminase (PDG) is involved in this process.[276] The proximal tubule accounts for 60% to 70% of total renal ammonia production under basal conditions and at least 70% to 80% in response to metabolic acidosis[275] (Figure 9.10).

Although multiple pathways for ammoniagenesis are present in the proximal tubule (Figure 9.11), the predominant pathway involves phosphate-dependent glutaminase (PDG).[277,278] PDG is an inner mitochondrial membrane–bound enzyme that metabolizes glutamine to glutamate, producing NH_4^+. Glutamate then undergoes further metabolism through multiple pathways. The major pathways involve glutamate dehydrogenase (GDH) with production of α-KG and release of NH_4^+. GDH-mediated metabolism is regulated in parallel with changes in total renal ammoniagenesis. Glutamate can be converted back to glutamine via the enzyme glutamine synthetase. This reaction utilizes NH_4^+ as a co-substrate, reducing net NH_4^+ formation. Glutamine synthetase is expressed in the proximal tubule and in intercalated cells, and its expression decreases in response to metabolic acidosis and, in the proximal tubule, with hypokalemia.[279]

α-KG can be metabolized through α-KG dehydrogenase and succinate dehydrogenase, forming oxaloacetic acid (OAA). OAA can serve as a substrate for phospho*enol*pyruvate carboxykinase (PEPCK) to form phospho*enol*pyruvate

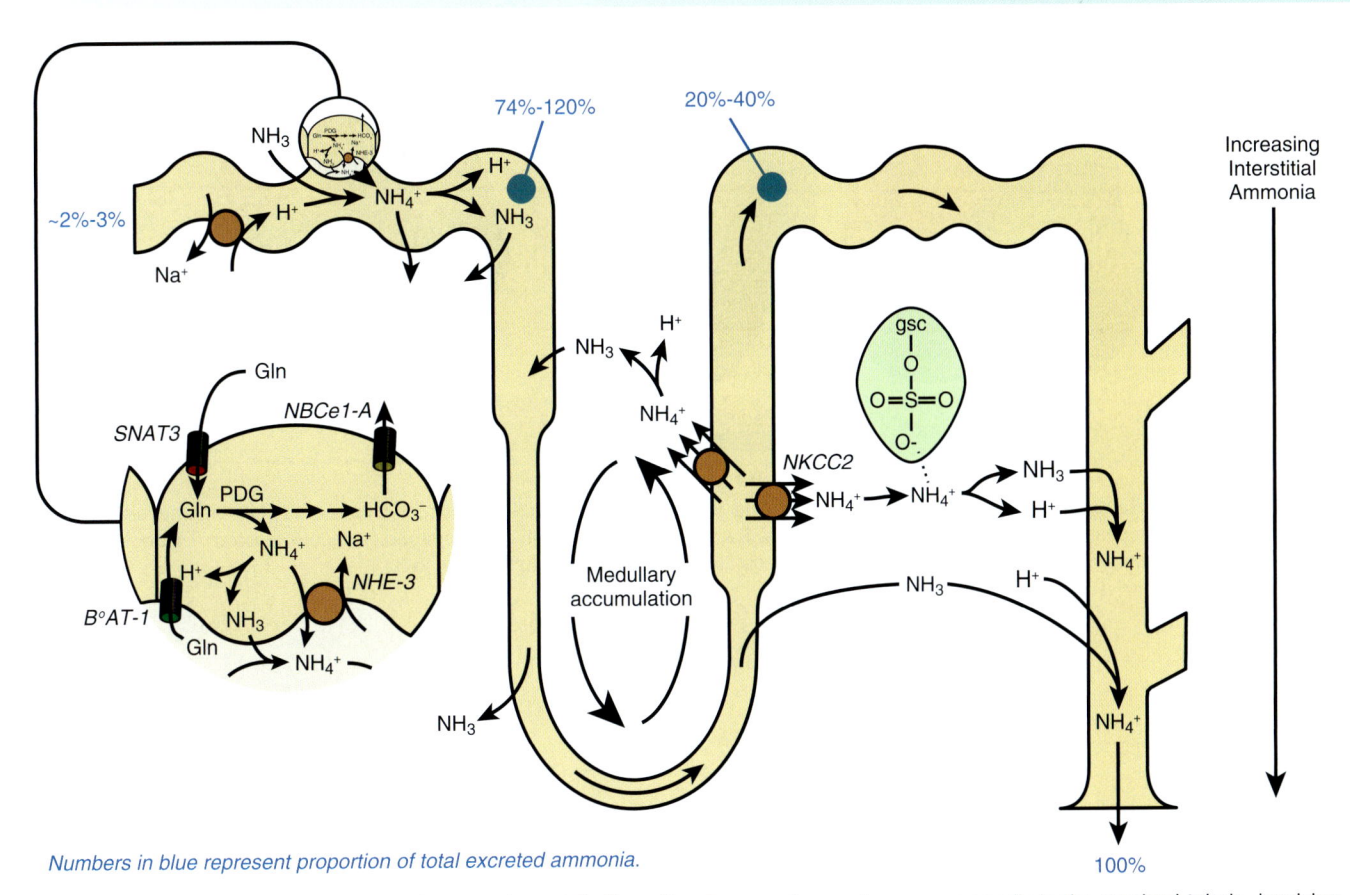

Figure 9.7 Integrated overview of renal ammonia metabolism. Renal ammoniagenesis occurs primarily in the proximal tubule, involving glutamine (Gln) uptake by transporters SNAT3 and B⁰AT-1, with glutamine metabolism forming ammonium and bicarbonate and apical NH_4^+ secretion involving the apical Na⁺/H⁺ exchanger NHE3 and parallel H⁺ and NH_3 transport. Ammonia reabsorption in the thick ascending limb, involving uptake mediated by apical Na⁺-K⁺-2Cl⁻ cotransporter NKCC2,, results in medullary ammonia accumulation. Medullary sulfatides (highlighted in *green*) reversibly bind NH_4^+, contributing to medullary accumulation. Ammonia is secreted in the collecting duct via parallel H⁺ and NH_3 secretion. Numbers in *blue* represent proportion of total excreted ammonia at each location. Gsc, Galactosylceramide backbone; NBCe1-A, electroneutral sodium-bicarbonate cotransporter; PDG, phosphate-dependent glutaminase.

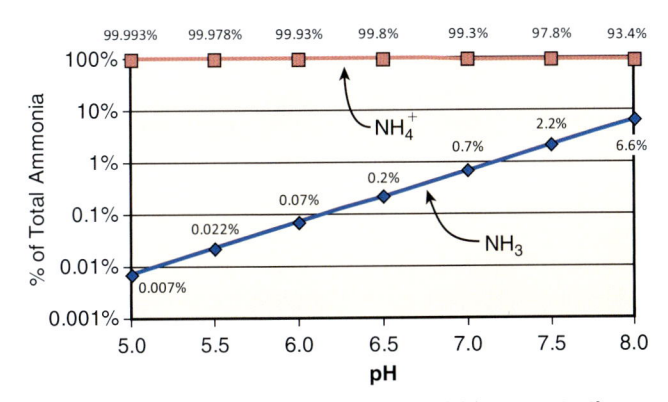

Figure 9.8 Relative changes in NH_3 and NH_4^+ concentration as pH changes. Contributions of NH_3 and NH_4^+ to total ammonia were determined from the buffer reaction, $NH_3 + H^+ \leftrightarrow NH_4^+$. A pK_a of 9.15 was used for calculations. Amounts shown are proportions of total ammonia present as NH_3 and NH_4^+. Note that the y-axis is log transformed. (From Weiner ID, Verlander JW: Renal ammonia metabolism and transport. *Compr Physiol* 3:201-220, 2013.)

(PEP), which is then utilized for gluconeogenesis. Conditions that increase ammonia increase flux through this pathway and stimulate renal gluconeogenesis. The net result is that complete glutamine metabolism results in production of 2 NH_4^+ and 2 HCO_3^- molecules per glutamine molecule in association with glucose production.

GLUTAMINE TRANSPORT IN AMMONIAGENESIS

Glutamine is the primary metabolic source for renal ammoniagenesis. Under normal acid-base balance conditions, the kidneys extract less than 3% of delivered glutamine. Acute metabolic acidosis induces a rapid, about twofold, rise in plasma glutamine levels; this rise results primarily from increased skeletal muscle and hepatic glutamine release.[280] In parallel, renal glutamine uptake increases to about 20% of delivered glutamine.[280,281] With chronic metabolic acidosis, renal extraction increases to as much as 50% of delivered glutamine.[281] Because glutamine uptake can exceed filtered glutamine, basolateral glutamine uptake is an important response element.

Filtered glutamine is almost completely reabsorbed in the PCT.[282] Multiple glutamine transporters are expressed in the apical membrane in the proximal tubule, including the Na⁺-dependent neutral amino acid transporters B⁰AT1

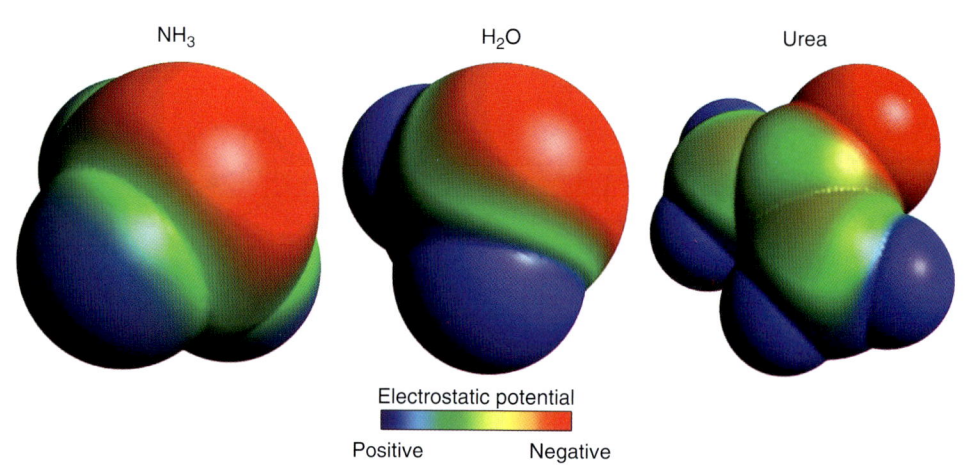

Figure 9.9 Electrostatic charge distribution in NH₃, H₂O, and urea molecules. Models of NH$_3$, H$_2$O and urea showing space-filling representation and surface pseudocolored to show surface charge. Each molecule, although an uncharged molecule, is polar. This polarity results in limited permeability across plasma membranes. (Models generated using Avogadro software, v1.0.3.)

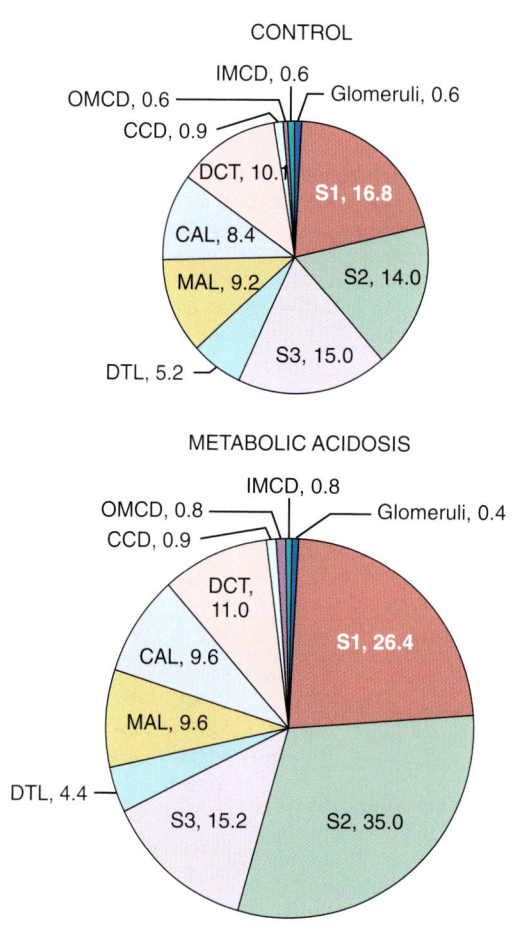

Figure 9.10 Ammonia production in various renal segments. Ammonia production rates in different renal components measured in microdissected components from rats eating control diets *(top)* and after induction of metabolic acidosis *(bottom)*. All segments tested produce net ammonia. Metabolic acidosis increases total renal ammoniagenesis, but only through increased production in proximal tubule segments (S1, S2, and S3). Rates (pmol/mm/min) calculated from measured ammonia production rates and mean length per segment as described in Verlander and associates.[122] Size of each pie graph is proportional to total renal ammoniagenesis rates. CCD, cortical collecting duct; CAL, cortical thick ascending limb of Henle's loop; DCT, distal convoluted tubule; DTL, descending thin limb of Henle's loop; IMCD, inner medullary collecting duct. MAL, medullary thick ascending limb of Henle's loop; OMCD, outer medullary collecting duct.

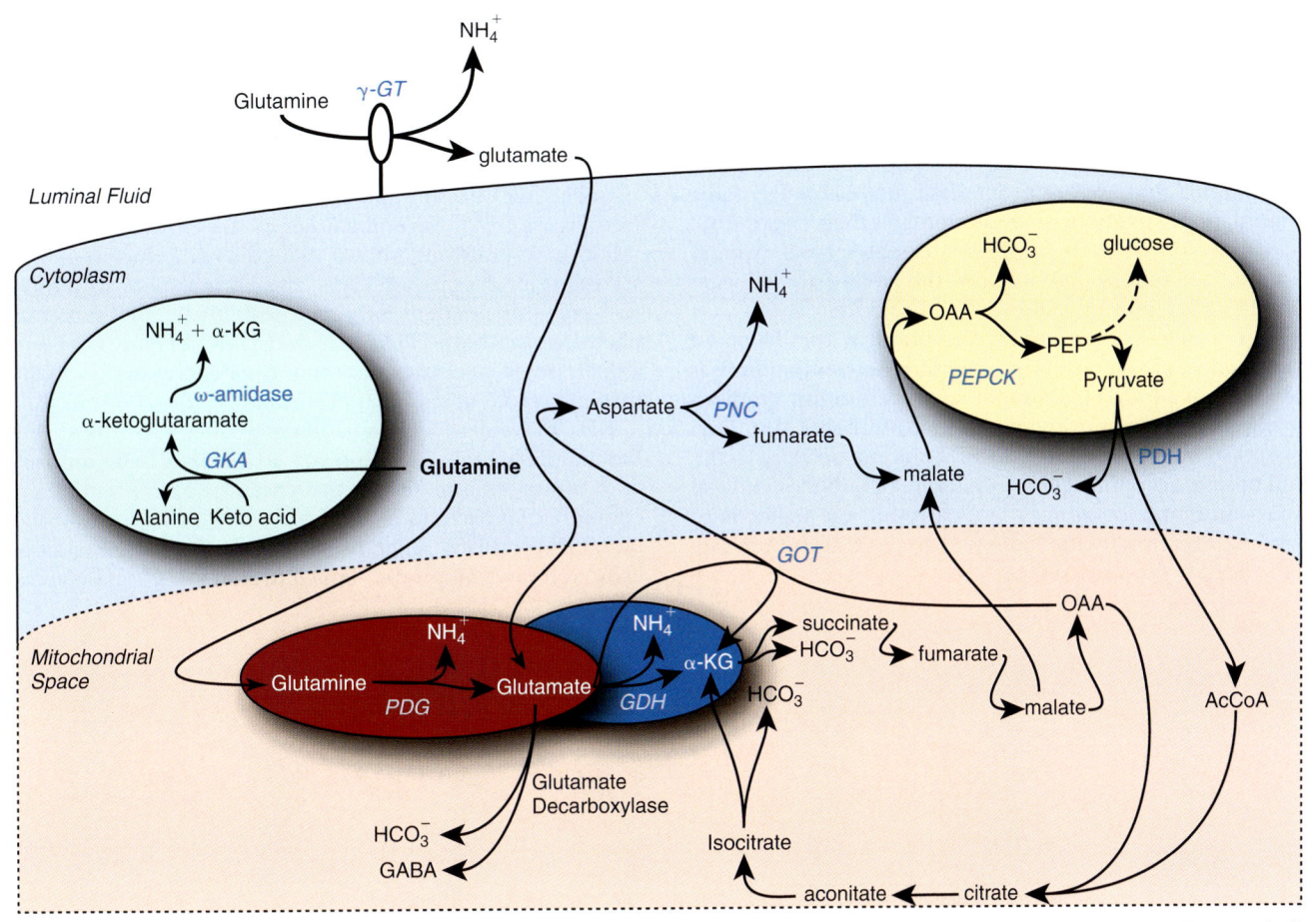

Figure 9.11 Mechanisms of ammoniagenesis. Multiple pathways for enzymatic ammonia production originating from glutamine metabolism are present in the proximal tubule. Glutamine metabolism through phosphate-dependent glutaminase (PDG) and glutamate dehydrogenase (GDH) and involving phospho*enol*pyruvate carboxykinase (PEPCK) is both the quantitatively most significant component of renal ammoniagenesis and the primary pathway stimulated in response to metabolic acidosis. AcCoA, Acetyl coenzyme A; GABA, gamma-aminobutyric acid; α-KG, α-ketoglutarate; OAA, oxaloacetic acid. (From Weiner ID, Verlander JW: Renal ammonia metabolism and transport. *Compr Physiol* 3:201-220, 2013.)

(SLC6A19) and B⁰AT3 (SLC6A18). Under basal conditions, relatively little glutamine reabsorbed in the proximal tubule is metabolized; instead it is transported across the basolateral membrane, resulting in glutamine reabsorption.

Chronic metabolic acidosis increases basolateral glutamine transport through a mechanism that likely involves glutamine transporter SNAT3.[283] Under basal conditions, basolateral SNAT3 is detectable only in the S3 proximal tubule segment, whereas conditions that increase ammoniagenesis, such as metabolic acidosis and hypokalemia, raise S3 segment expression and induce expression in the S2 proximal tubule segment.[284,285]

Because the initial enzyme involved in ammonia, PDG, is a mitochondrial enzyme, glutamine movement across the mitochondrial membrane is necessary. This process involves a specific transporter-mediated mechanism, is *trans*-stimulated and *cis*-inhibited by alanine, and is stimulated by metabolic acidosis.[286]

AMMONIA TRANSPORT

Ammonia produced in the proximal tubule is secreted preferentially into the tubule lumen. Preferential apical secretion is due to multiple factors, including NHE3-mediated Na^+-NH_4^+ exchange and luminal acidification, which facilitates "trapping" of secreted NH_3 as NH_4^+.[287,288] However, the role of NHE3 has been questioned by a study in which proximal tubule NHE3 deletion did not alter renal ammonia excretion.[289]

The proximal tubule also can reabsorb luminal ammonia; this reabsorption appears to occur primarily in the late proximal tubule.[290] This portion of the proximal tubule expresses glutamine synthetase, which catalyzes the reaction of NH_4^+ with glutamate to form glutamine.[291] Metabolic acidosis converts late proximal tubule ammonia transport from net reabsorption to net secretion[290]; the molecular mechanisms that underlie this conversion involve decreased glutamine synthetase–mediated NH_4^+ metabolism.[292,293]

The TAL reabsorbs luminal ammonia. The apical Na^+-K^+-$2Cl^-$ cotransporter NKCC2 mediates the majority of ammonium reabsorption.[294] Metabolic acidosis increases both TAL ammonia reabsorption and NKCC2 expression.[295] Intracellular NH_4^+ can dissociate into NH_3 and H^+, resulting in intracellular acidification. Ammonia exit across the basolateral plasma membrane appears to involve components of both diffusive NH_3 movement and basolateral NH_4^+ transport through NHE4 Na^+-NH_4^+ exchange activity.[278,296]

Some of the ammonia absorbed by the MTAL undergoes recycling into the thin descending limb of the loop of Henle. This results in countercurrent amplification of medullary interstitial ammonia concentration. Ammonia recycling predominantly involves NH_3 transport, with a smaller component of NH_4^+ transport.[297]

Interstitial ammonia appears to bind reversibly to medullary sulfatides. *Sulfatides* are highly charged, anionic glycosphingolipids that appear to increase medullary ammonia accumulation. Metabolic acidosis increases their expression, and disruption of their synthesis decreases basal urinary ammonia excretion and impairs the ability to increase ammonia excretion in response to an acid diet.[298]

The net effect of ammonia absorption by the TAL and passive ammonia secretion into the thin descending limb is development of an axial ammonia concentration gradient that parallels the hypertonicity gradient. Moreover, ammonia absorption by the MTAL results in ammonia delivery to the distal tubule, accounting for only about 20% to 40% of final urinary ammonia content.[242,299] As a result, the majority of ammonia excreted by the kidneys is secreted by tubule segments farther downstream.

There is likely to be a small component of ammonia secretion in the regions of the distal tubule prior to the CCD— that is, the DCT, CNT, and ICT. Studies in the rat show that ammonia secretion in the micropuncturable distal tubule could account for around 10% to 15% of ammonia excretion.[300,301]

Collecting duct ammonia secretion is a complex process (see Figure 9.12). Several studies of the CCD, OMCD, and IMCD have uniformly shown that collecting duct ammonia secretion involves parallel NH_3 and H^+ transport, with little-to-no pH-independent NH_4^+ permeability.[299,302] H^+ secretion likely involves both H^+-ATPase and H^+-K^+-ATPase. Carbonic anhydrase is necessary for ammonia secretion, probably through a role in supplying cytosolic H^+ for secretion.[303]

NH_3 movement across collecting duct cell apical and basolateral membranes appears to involve both diffusive and transporter-mediated movements. The nondiffusive component is Na^+ and K^+ independent, electroneutral, facilitated NH_3 transport, the predominant route at physiologically relevant ammonia concentrations.[304,305] Basolateral

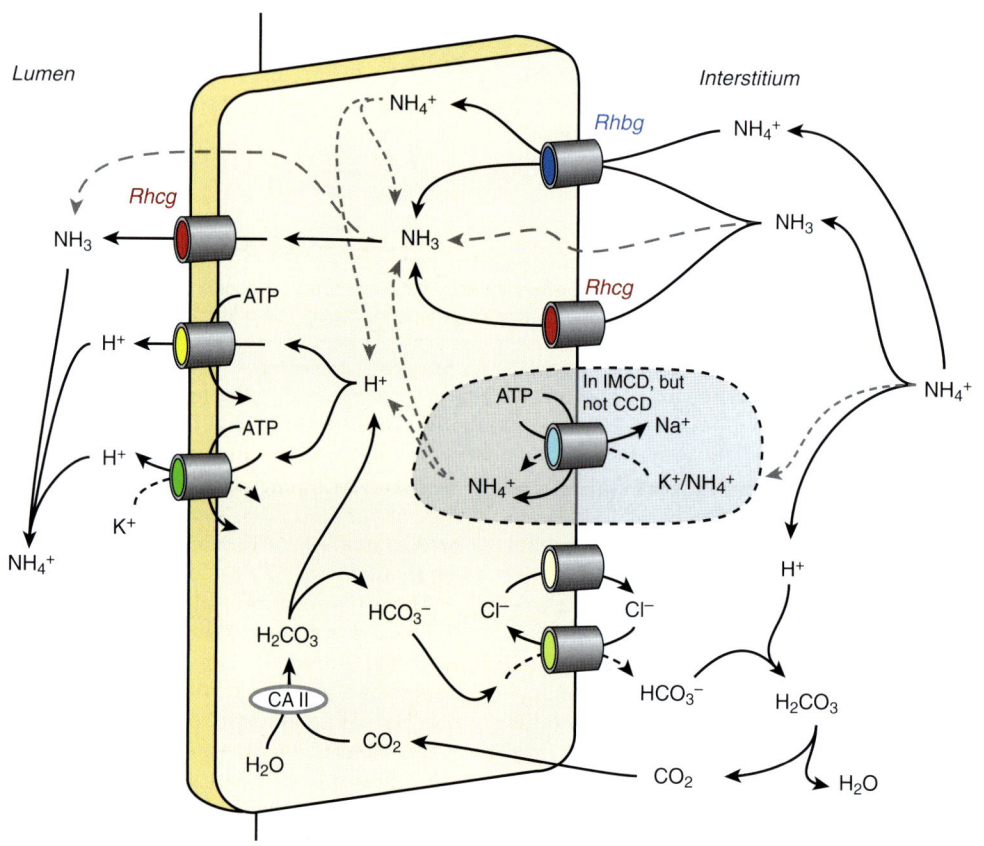

Figure 9.12 Mechanisms of collecting duct ammonia secretion. Rh glycoproteins Rhbg and Rhcg likely both contribute to basolateral ammonia uptake. As described in the text, whether Rhbg mediates transport of NH_4^+ or NH_3 remains controversial, but it is likely to mediate uptake of either ammonia molecular species across the basolateral membrane. Rhcg is generally believed to primarily mediate electroneutral NH_3 uptake across the basolateral plasma membrane. NH_3 is then secreted across the apical plasma membrane down its electrochemical gradient through processes involving both apical Rhcg transport and a separate, undefined mechanism. H^+ is secreted across the apical plasma membrane by both H^+-ATPase and H^+-K^+-ATPase. Cytoplasmic H^+ is supplied either by dissociation of NH_4^+ or via a carbonic anhydrase II (CA II)–dependent bicarbonate shuttle mechanism involving basolateral chloride-bicarbonate exchange and basolateral chloride channel–mediated bicarbonate shuttling. Also shown is NH_4^+ uptake by basolateral Na^+-K^+-ATPase, which contributes to ammonia secretion in the inner medullary collecting duct (IMCD),[346] where the majority of cells do not express Rh glycoproteins. Pharmacologic inhibitor studies indicate that Na^+-K^+-ATPase is unlikely to contribute to ammonia secretion by the cortical collecting duct (CCD).[173] *Not shown* is NH_4^+ uptake mediated by Na-K-Cl cotransporter NKCC1, because inhibitor studies suggest that this transport mechanism does not contribute substantially to collecting duct ammonia secretion.[348] *ATP*, Adenosine triphosphate.

NH$_3$ transport appears to involve Rhbg and Rhcg, and apical NH$_3$ transport involves Rhcg.

At least two basolateral NH$_4^+$ transport mechanisms are present. In the IMCD basolateral Na$^+$-K$^+$-ATPase contributes to basolateral NH$_4^+$ uptake.[306,307] However, in the CCD, basolateral Na$^+$-K$^+$-ATPase does not contribute to ammonia secretion.[308] Another possible NH$_4^+$ transport mechanism involves NKCC1. NKCC1 is present at the basolateral plasma membrane of medullary intercalated cells and IMCD cells and can transport NH$_4^+$ at the NKCC1 K$^+$ binding site.[309-312] However, inhibiting NKCC1 does not alter OMCD ammonia secretion, suggesting either that NKCC1 does not contribute to transepithelial ammonia secretion or that alternative transport mechanisms compensate in its absence.[303]

The absence or presence of luminal carbonic anhydrase activity impacts collecting duct ammonia secretion. In the absence of luminal carbonic anhydrase, H$^+$ secretion increases the luminal [H$^+$] above equilibrium because of relatively slow conversion of H$_2$CO$_3$ to CO$_2$ and H$_2$O. This is termed a luminal *disequilibrium pH*. The increased luminal acidification shifts the H$^+$ + NH$_3$ ↔ NH$_4^+$ reaction towards NH$_4^+$ and decreases luminal [NH$_3$]. The decreased luminal [NH$_3$] increases both the gradient for NH$_3$ secretion and net ammonia secretion. A luminal disequilibrium pH is found in the rat OMCD and terminal IMCD[146,313] and in the rabbit CCD and OMCDo,[308,314,315] but not in the rabbit OMCDi.[314]

SPECIFIC PROTEINS INVOLVED IN RENAL AMMONIA METABOLISM

Phosphate-Dependent Glutaminase

PDG is the initial enzymatic step in renal ammoniagenesis. It is located in mitochondria and catalyzes the reaction L-glutamine + H$_2$O → L-glutamate + NH$_4^+$. In the kidney, PDG activity is found primarily in the proximal tubule, although a lesser degree of activity is found in essentially all renal epithelial cells.[276,316,317] The physiologic role of this activity outside the proximal tubule is unclear. Some studies have found that metabolic acidosis increases PDG activity in the DTL, MTAL in the outer stripe, and DCT,[316] whereas others have found no change in activity in sites other than the proximal tubule.[317] Quantitative analyses suggest that the proximal tubule is the primary site of ammonia production, accounting for the majority of the increase in ammoniagenesis with metabolic acidosis.[277,278]

Multiple PDG isoforms exist. In humans, the gene for the kidney-type isoform gives rise to at least two transcripts, KGA and GAC.[318] A separate gene gives rise to an LGA isoform. The KGA protein is expressed ubiquitously in the kidney, including the renal proximal tubule, and is the source of the majority of renal PDG.

Metabolic acidosis increases proximal tubule PDG activity; these increases derive from multiple mechanisms. There is increased protein expression, which appears to be transcriptionally mediated.[319,320] The increase in PDG mRNA results from mRNA stabilization, not higher transcription rates.[321]

A second regulatory mechanism likely involves changes in intramitochondrial glutamate. Glutamate is a competitive inhibitor of PDG,[322] and decreases in intramitochondrial glutamate concentration, which occur during metabolic acidosis, likely in relation to increased GDH activity, increase PDG activity.[323]

Glutamate Dehydrogenase

GDH is a mitochondrial enzyme that catalyzes the reaction L-glutamate + H$_2$O + NAD$^+$ (or NADP$^+$) → α-KG^{2-} + NH$_4^+$ + NADH (or NADPH) + H$^+$. The two GDH isoforms are products of two different genes; GLUD1 is widely expressed, including in the kidney, whereas GLUD2 appears to be specific to neural and testicular tissues.[324,325]

Metabolic acidosis stimulates renal GDH activity,[326] both by altering its affinity for glutamate and by increasing protein and mRNA (GLUD1) expression.[323,327,328] Acidosis also decreases intramitochondrial α-KG concentration, a reduction which contributes to increased GDH activity.[322] Decreased α-KG accelerates GDH activity by relieving α-KG–mediated competitive inhibition of the enzymatic reaction and by inhibiting the reverse reaction.[329,330] Changes in mRNA expression occur through changes in mRNA stability, not transcription rate.[331]

Phospho*enol*pyruvate carboxykinase

Renal PEPCK is a cytosolic enzyme that is the product of the *PCK1* gene. In the kidney, as in extrarenal sites, including liver, adipose tissue, and small intestine, PEPCK is a key enzyme in gluconeogenesis through its role in conversion of oxaloacetate into PEP and CO$_2$. It also mediates an important role in the renal response to metabolic acidosis[332] coincident with increased renal gluconeogenesis. The adaptive increase in PEPCK activity and protein expression results from greater protein synthesis and mRNA expression.[327] In contrast to increases in PDG and GDH, the increase in PEPCK mRNA expression appears to result from increased gene transcription.[333]

γ-Glutamyl Transpeptidase

γ-Glutamyl transpeptidase (γ-GT) accounts for phosphate-independent glutaminase activity identified in many early enzymatic studies of renal ammoniagenesis. However, γ-GT is expressed primarily in the proximal straight tubule (PST),[276] and micropuncture studies suggest that glutamine is completely reabsorbed by the PCT, making PST ammoniagenesis via γ-GT unlikely to contribute significantly to renal ammoniagenesis.

Na$^+$-H$^+$ Exchanger 3

Multiple lines of evidence suggest that NHE3 secretes NH$_4^+$ through binding of NH$_4^+$ at the H$^+$ binding site. These data include evidence that proximal tubule brush border membrane vesicles exhibit NH$_4^+$-Na$^+$ exchange activity,[13] that combining a low luminal Na$^+$ concentration with Na$^+$-H$^+$ exchange inhibitor amiloride decreases ammonia secretion,[14] and that the Na$^+$-H$^+$ exchange inhibitor EIPA blunts ammonia secretion when alternative secretory pathways are blocked.[288] However, proximal tubule-specific NHE3 deletion does not alter either basal or acidosis-stimulated ammonia excretion.[289]

Apical NHE3 is also present in the TAL. However, because this transporter secretes NH$_4^+$, and the TAL reabsorbs NH$_4^+$, NHE3 is unlikely to mediate an important role in loop of Henle ammonia transport.

Changes in NHE3 expression and activity are important components of ammonia regulation. In response to chronic metabolic acidosis, changes in extracellular potassium and Ang II as well as in NHE3 expression and activity parallel changes in ammonia secretion.[56,334-336] In S2 and S3 segments, chronic metabolic acidosis increases AT_1 receptor–mediated stimulation of NHE3.[337-339] Increased ET-1 expression with subsequent activation of the ET-B receptor mediates an important role in raising both NHE3 expression and renal ammonia excretion in metabolic acidosis.[71]

Potassium Channels

At a molecular level, K^+ and NH_4^+ have nearly identical biophysical characteristics. In general, the relative conductance for NH_4^+ is 10% to 20% of that observed for K^+.[274] The primary evidence that K^+ channels contribute to proximal tubule ammonia transport comes from in vitro microperfusion studies showing that barium, a nonspecific K^+ channel inhibitor, inhibits proximal tubule ammonia transport.[288] Multiple K^+ channels are present in the apical membrane of the proximal tubule, including KCNA10, TWIK-1, and KCNQ1; which of these mediates ammonia transport is not known currently. In the TAL, K^+ channels can contribute to luminal NH_4^+ uptake when apical Na^+-K^+-$2Cl^-$ cotransport is inhibited.[294] However, NKCC2 inhibitors completely inhibit TAL ammonia transport, suggesting that apical K^+ channels are unlikely to mediate a quantitatively important role in TAL ammonia transport.[340]

Na$^+$-K$^+$-2Cl$^-$ Cotransport

NKCC1 is a widely expressed Na^+-K^+-$2Cl^-$ cotransporter family isoform that in the kidney is present in the basolateral membrane of intercalated cells in the OMCD and IMCD and in IMCD cells.[309,310,312] However, pharmacologic inhibitors do not alter either OMCD ammonia secretion or IMCD basolateral ammonia uptake.[303,306] Thus, NKCC1 appears unlikely to mediate a substantial role in renal ammonia secretion.

NKCC2 is a kidney-specific isoform expressed in the apical plasma membrane of the TAL and the major mechanism for ammonia reabsorption in the TAL.[340] Luminal NH_4^+ competes for binding with K^+ to the K^+-transport site, enabling alterations in luminal K^+ in hypokalemia and hyperkalemia to alter net NH_4^+ transport and lead to alterations in medullary interstitial ammonia concentration in conditions of altered potassium homeostasis. Metabolic acidosis increases NKCC2 expression, contributing to the higher ammonia reabsorption observed[86,295]; these changes appear related to a rise in systemic levels of glucocorticoid.[341]

Na$^+$-K$^+$-ATPase

Na^+-K^+-ATPase is present in the basolateral plasma membranes of essentially all renal epithelial cells. NH_4^+ binds to and is transported at the K^+-binding site, enabling Na^+-NH_4^+ exchange.[342,343] In the IMCD, Na^+-K^+-ATPase–mediated basolateral NH_4^+ uptake is critical for IMCD ammonia and acid secretion.[342,343] Reductions in interstitial K^+ levels during hypokalemia facilitate greater basolateral NH_4^+ uptake by Na^+-K^+-ATPase and contribute to increased NH_4^+ secretion rates.[344] In the CCD, in contrast, basolateral Na^+-K^+-ATPase does not appear to contribute to CCD ammonia secretion.[308]

H$^+$-K$^+$-ATPase

H^+-K^+-ATPase proteins, members of the P-type ATPase family, transport NH_4^+. The majority of evidence suggests NH_4^+ is transported at the K^+-binding site, such that these proteins mediate H^+-NH_4^+ exchange. Thus, H^+-K^+-ATPase is unlikely to contribute to collecting duct ammonia secretion. However, potassium deficiency increases expression of colonic H^+-K^+-ATPase, and it has been postulated that colonic H^+-K^+-ATPase mediates increased NH_4^+ secretion via transport at the H^+-binding site.[345]

Aquaporins

The aquaporin family is an extended family of proteins that facilitate water transport. Because H_2O and NH_3 have similar molecular sizes and charge distributions, several studies have examined the role of aquaporins in NH_3 transport. Importantly, many, but not all aquaporins transport ammonia.[346]

AQP1 was the first aquaporin shown to transport ammonia. Studies using AQP1 expression in *Xenopus* oocytes demonstrated that AQP1 expression increases NH_3 transport.[346,347] However, not all studies have confirmed NH_3 transport by AQP1.[348] AQP1 is present in the thin descending limb of the loop of Henle, suggesting it may contribute to ammonia permeability in this segment.

AQP3 is present in the basolateral membranes of collecting duct principal cells and, when expressed in the *Xenopus* oocytes, transports NH_3.[348] Whether AQP3 contributes to renal principal cell basolateral NH_3 transport has not been determined.

AQP8 is expressed in intracellular sites in the proximal tubule, CCD, and OMCD in the kidney, but not the plasma membrane.[349] AQP8's specific intracellular site in mammalian cells has not been determined, but it localizes to the inner mitochondrial membrane when expressed in yeast.[350] AQP8's role in renal ammonia metabolism is unclear. Genetic deletion alters hepatic ammonia accumulation, renal excretion of infused ammonia, and intrarenal ammonia concentrations but does not change serum chloride concentration, urine ammonia concentration, or urine pH either under basal conditions or in response to acid loading.[351,352]

Carbonic Anhydrase

Carbonic anhydrase, in addition to its role in bicarbonate reabsorption, contributes to ammonia secretion. Direct studies have shown that carbonic anhydrase inhibition, presumably through effects on CA II, block OMCD ammonia secretion.[303] Figure 9.12 shows the putative role of cytoplasmic CA II in facilitating transepithelial ammonia secretion.

CA IV, although functioning to increase bicarbonate reabsorption, likely reduces collecting duct ammonia secretion because it prevents a luminal disequilibrium pH. Apical CA IV expression has been demonstrated in the rabbit CCD type A intercalated cell, in the rabbit OMCD and IMCD,[170] in the human CCD and OMCD,[353] but not in the rat collecting duct.[51] This pattern is inconsistent with evidence of luminal disequilibrium pH in the rat CCD and OMCD[313,354] but consistent with the evidence of luminal disequilibrium pH in the rabbit CCD and OMCD outer stripe segments.[314,315]

Rh Glycoproteins

Rh glycoproteins are mammalian orthologs of Mep/AMT proteins, ammonia transporter family proteins present in yeast, plants, bacteria, and many other organisms. Three mammalian Rh glycoproteins are known, Rh A glycoprotein (Rhag), Rh B glycoprotein (Rhbg) and Rh C glycoprotein (Rhcg).

Rhag. Rhag is an essential component of the erythrocyte "Rh complex," which consists of Rhag in association with RhD and RhCE subunits in a 1:1:1 stoichiometric ratio.[355] Rhag transports ammonia in the form of NH_3, whereas RhD and RhCE do not transport ammonia.[356,357] In humans, RhAG deficiency leads to Rh_{null} disease, which is characterized by hemolytic anemia, spherocytosis, and lack of erythrocyte expression of RhAG, RhD, and RhCE.[358,359] Rhag protein is present in erythrocytes and in erythrocyte precursor cells present in the bone marrow and in rodent spleen, but it does not appear to be expressed in nonerythroid tissues. In particular, Rhag is not found in the kidney except in residual erythrocytes.[360,361]

Rhbg. Rhbg in the kidney is found exclusively in distal epithelial cell populations, with low-level basolateral expression in the DCT and higher-level basolateral expression in the CNT, CCD, OMCD, and IMCD.[169,362,363] The CNT and the collecting duct have heterogeneous epithelial cell populations; type A and non-A, non-B intercalated cells, principal cells, and connecting segment cells express Rhbg, but expression is greater in intercalated cells. Type B intercalated cells do not express detectable Rhbg immunolabeling.

Rhbg has important roles in the increase in ammonia excretion that occurs in response to both metabolic acidosis and hypokalemia. Both conditions increase Rhbg protein expression, and genetic deletion of Rhbg from intercalated cells impairs the change in ammonia excretion.[364,365] Another study using a different method of acid loading that resulted in lesser stimulation of ammonia excretion found no effect of Rhbg deletion.[366] This finding suggests that other mechanisms can compensate for the lack of Rhbg if only modest increases in ammonia excretion are needed but that greater degrees of adaptation require Rhbg expression.

A number of studies have addressed the issue as to whether Rhbg transports NH_3, NH_4^+, or both, with conflicting results.[367] Importantly, the electrochemical gradient across the basolateral plasma membrane is such that both electroneutral NH_3 transport and electrogenic NH_4^+ transport modes result in ammonia transport from the interstitium into the cell cytoplasm.[367]

Rhcg. Rhcg is expressed in the kidney exclusively in distal epithelial cells.[169,368-371] Rhcg is prominently expressed in the CNT, ICT, CCD, OMCD, and IMCD, weakly expressed in late DCT cells, and exhibits both apical and basolateral expression.[133,369-371] Rhcg expression differs among renal epithelial cell types. In general, type A intercalated cells express higher levels of Rhcg than principal cells. Rhcg is not detectable by immunohistochemistry in type B intercalated cells. In the CNT, apical Rhcg expression in non-A, non-B intercalated cells is similar to that in CNT cells, although non-A, non-B intercalated cells have very little or no basolateral Rhcg. IMCD cells do not express detectable Rhcg.

Rhcg has an important role in renal ammonia excretion in a wide variety of conditions, including basal acid-base homeostasis, metabolic acidosis, and hypokalemia. Gene deletion studies show that the absence of Rhcg impairs basal ammonia excretion.[372,373] Both metabolic acidosis and hypokalemia increase Rhcg expression, and Rhcg expression is necessary for the normal increase in ammonia excretion.[370,374] With reduced renal mass there is increased single-nephron ammonia excretion, and this increase involves greater polarization of Rhcg to the apical and basolateral plasma membranes.[375] Cyclosporine A can induce RTA, and this process involves altered Rhcg expression.[376] Aldosterone increases renal ammonia excretion, in association with increased Rhcg expression.[222]

Rhcg expression appears to be regulated through a variety of mechanisms. There are changes in total protein expression in several conditions; these are not associated with changes in steady-state mRNA expression, indicating a primary role for posttranscriptional regulation.[367] In addition, Rhcg is found in both apical and basolateral plasma membranes and in subapical sites, and changes in this subcellular distribution and expression are a prominent component of the response to metabolic acidosis, hypokalemia, and reduced renal mass.[364,371,375,377]

Multiple studies have addressed the molecular form of ammonia that Rhcg transports. Essentially all studies have found that Rhcg transports ammonia in the form of NH_3, although there is some controversy in this regard.[367]

CO_2 Transport by Rh Glycoproteins. Rh glycoproteins can transport molecules other than ammonia, specifically CO_2. Quantitative studies using human erythrocytes deficient in RhAG show that the absence of RhAG decreases CO_2 transport.[378,379] Studies using heterologous expression in *Xenopus* oocytes show that all Rh glycoproteins can transport CO_2.[346,380] However, the physiologic role of Rhbg- or Rhcg-mediated CO_2 transport in the kidney is not clear. Intercalated cells use cytoplasmic CO_2 to generate, through a CA II–catalyzed process, the intracellular H^+ used for urinary acidification. Several studies using Rhbg and/or Rhcg deletion show that Rhbg and Rhcg expression is not necessary for urine acidification.[365,366,372,373,381,382] However, these studies cannot exclude the possibility of either altered intrarenal CO_2 concentrations, which enable diffusive CO_2 movement in the absence of Rhbg and Rhcg, or adaptive changes in other CO_2 transport mechanisms.

SULFATIDES

Studies show that sulfatides, highly charged anionic glycosphingolipids, have an important role in renal ammonia metabolism. Sulfatides are highly charged anion glycosphingolipids that can reversibly bind NH_4^+. They are expressed throughout the kidney but at highest levels in the outer and inner medulla,[298] and they appear to have an important role in maintaining the high inner medullary ammonium accumulation and the increase in urinary acid elimination that develop during metabolic acidosis. Disruption of renal sulfatide synthesis, by a genetic approach along the entire renal tubule, led to lower urinary pH accompanied by lower ammonium excretion.[298] After acid loading, mice deficient in renal sulfatide synthesis showed impaired ammonia excretion, decreased ammonia accumulation in the papilla, and chronic hyperchloremic metabolic acidosis.[298] Thus, sulfatides, likely through their ability to reversibly bind interstitial NH_4^+, have an important role in renal ammonia handling, urinary acidification, and acid-base homeostasis.

ACID-BASE SENSORS

Several studies have begun to elucidate the molecular mechanisms through which the kidney recognizes alteration in systemic pH. Candidate molecular sensors have included acid/alkali–sensing receptors, tyrosine kinases, and bicarbonate-stimulated adenylyl cyclase.

ACID/ALKALI–SENSING RECEPTORS

G-PROTEIN–COUPLED RECEPTOR 4

Several G protein–coupled receptors (GPRs) are sensitive to extracellular pH, resulting in pH-dependent intracellular cAMP or IP_3 production.[383] Of these, GPR4 has been studied most extensively. It is expressed in the kidney, and GPR4 deletion results in mild metabolic acidosis, less acidic urine, and decreased ability to excrete an acid load.[384] Which renal cells express GPR4 has not been determined, but a preliminary report suggests that GPR4 is expressed in renal interstitial cells, not tubule epithelial cells.[385]

INSULIN RECEPTOR–RELATED RECEPTOR

Insulin receptor–related receptor (InsR-RR) is a member of the insulin receptor family and may have a role regulating collecting duct acid-base transport. It is found in the kidney in the basolateral plasma membranes of type B and non-A, non-B intercalated cells[386] and is activated by alkaline pH.[387] InsR-RR–deficient mice express lower levels of pendrin and have decreased ability to excrete an alkali load.[387]

KINASES

PYK2/ET-B RECEPTOR PATHWAY

The nonreceptor tyrosine kinase Pyk2 may function as a pH sensor in proximal tubular cells.[388] It is activated by extracellular acidosis, and through activation of proto-oncogene tyrosine-protein kinase c-Src, causes NHE3 activation.[388,389] A parallel pathway for proximal tubule NHE3 activation exists, involving activation of protein kinase ERK1/2 and proto-oncogene c-fos but not involving Pyk2.[390] These two pathways both increase expression of the endothelin gene, ET-1, which in turn activates the ET-B receptor and increases apical plasma membrane NHE3 expression.[391]

RECEPTOR TYROSINE KINASE

The proximal tubule responds to changes in peritubular HCO_3^- and CO_2 with altered rates of luminal HCO_3^- reabsorption. This activation involves a receptor tyrosine kinase, possibly a member of the erbB family,[53] and may involve heterodimerization of epidermal growth factor receptors ErbB1 and ErB2 and activation of receptor tyrosine phosphatase-γ.[390] Acute acidosis increases tyrosine phosphorylation of ErbB1 and ErbB2, consistent with a role in a signaling cascade that regulates HCO_3^- reabsorption.[392]

BICARBONATE-STIMULATED ADENYLYL CYCLASE

Another mechanism regulating renal acid-base homeostasis involves the soluble adenylyl cyclase (sAC). Its production of cAMP is directly stimulated by increases in cytoplasmic HCO_3^-,[393] and cAMP stimulates collecting duct H^+ secretion.[394] Soluble AC is widely expressed in the kidney, including the TAL, DCT, and collecting duct.[395,396] In collecting duct intercalated cells, sAC colocalizes with H^+-ATPase in both the type A and type B intercalated cells and it co-immunoprecipitates with H^+-ATPase, implicating sAC in regulation of H^+ secretion.[396] In clear cells of the epididymis, used as a model system of collecting duct intercalated cells, sAC regulates apical H^+-ATPase expression through changes in cAMP production.[395]

DIURNAL VARIATION IN ACID EXCRETION

There is a diurnal variation in renal acid excretion, which involves ammonia and titratable acid excretion and urine pH.[397] Circadian changes in NHE3 expression have been identified, particularly in the TAL in the outer medulla,[398] and are likely mediated by *Clock* and *BMAL1* genes.[399] There are also circadian changes in ENaC expression,[400] which by altering luminal electronegativity may alter voltage-sensitive H^+ secretion and urine acidification. Diurnal variation in net acid excretion is altered in uric acid stone formers and may contribute to the pathogenesis of nephrolithiasis in this condition.[401]

ACKNOWLEDGEMENTS

The authors thank the many talented investigators with whom we have been fortunate to work, the superb mentors who have supported, encouraged, and, in many cases, enabled our scientific endeavors, and our wonderful spouses and families who have supported all aspects of our lives. The preparation of this chapter was supported by funds from NIH R01-DK-045788 and the Department of Veterans Affairs (1I01BX000818-01).

Complete reference list available at ExpertConsult.com.

KEY REFERENCES

1. Baum M, Twombley K, Gattineni J, et al: Proximal tubule Na+/H+ exchanger activity in adult NHE8−/−, NHE3−/−, and NHE3−/−/NHE8−/− mice. *Am J Physiol Renal Physiol* 303:F1495–F1502, 2012.
14. Nagami GT: Luminal secretion of ammonia in the mouse proximal tubule perfused in vitro. *J Clin Invest* 81:159–164, 1988.
32. Brown D, Hirsch S, Gluck S: Localization of a proton-pumping ATPase in rat kidney. *J Clin Invest* 82:2114–2126, 1988.
33. Brown D, Paunescu TG, Breton S, et al: Regulation of the V-ATPase in kidney epithelial cells: dual role in acid-base homeostasis and vesicle trafficking. *J Exp Biol* 212:1762–1772, 2009.
34. Chambrey R, Paillard M, Podevin RA: Enzymatic and functional evidence for adaptation of the vacuolar H(+)-ATPase in proximal tubule apical membranes from rats with chronic metabolic acidosis. *J Biol Chem* 269:3243–3250, 1994.

42. Romero MF: Molecular pathophysiology of SLC4 bicarbonate transporters. *Curr Opin Nephrol Hypertens* 14:495–501, 2005.
47. Igarashi T, Inatomi J, Sekine T, et al: Mutations in SLC4A4 cause permanent isolated proximal renal tubular acidosis with ocular abnormalities. *Nat Genet* 23:264–266, 1999.
52. Zhou Y, Zhao J, Bouyer P, et al: Evidence from renal proximal tubules that HCO3– and solute reabsorption are acutely regulated not by pH but by basolateral HCO3– and CO2. *Proc Natl Acad Sci U S A* 102:3875–3880, 2005.
57. Preisig PA, Alpern RJ: Chronic metabolic acidosis causes an adaptation in the apical membrane Na/H antiporter and basolateral membrane Na(HCO3)3 symporter in the rat proximal convoluted tubule. *J Clin Invest* 82:1445–1453, 1988.
74. Capasso G, Geibel PJ, Damiano S, et al: The calcium sensing receptor modulates fluid reabsorption and acid secretion in the proximal tubule. *Kidney Int* 84:277–284, 2013.
83. Good DW, George T, Watts BA: III: Basolateral membrane Na+/H+ exchange enhances HCO3– absorption in rat medullary thick ascending limb: evidence for functional coupling between basolateral and apical membrane Na+/H+ exchangers. *Proc Natl Acad Sci U S A* 92:12525–12529, 1995.
89. Capasso G, Unwin R, Ciani F, et al: Bicarbonate transport along the loop of Henle. II. Effects of acid-base, dietary, and neurohumoral determinants. *J Clin Invest* 94:830–838, 1994.
104. Bastani B, Purcell H, Hemken P, et al: Expression and distribution of renal vacuolar proton-translocating adenosine triphosphatase in response to chronic acid and alkali loads in the rat. *J Clin Invest* 88:126–136, 1991.
105. Chambrey R, Kurth I, Peti-Peterdi J, et al: Renal intercalated cells are rather energized by a proton than a sodium pump. *Proc Natl Acad Sci U S A* 110:7928–7933, 2013.
106. Gumz ML, Lynch IJ, Greenlee MM, et al: The renal H+-K+-ATPases: physiology, regulation, and structure. *Am J Physiol Renal Physiol* 298:F12–F21, 2010.
108. Alper SL: Molecular physiology and genetics of Na+-independent SLC4 anion exchangers. *J Exp Biol* 212:1672–1683, 2009.
113. Alper SL, Natale J, Gluck S, et al: Subtypes of intercalated cells in rat kidney collecting duct defined by antibodies against erythroid band 3 and renal vacuolar H+-ATPase. *Proc Natl Acad Sci U S A* 86:5429–5433, 1989.
116. Lynch IJ, Rudin A, Xia SL, et al: Impaired acid secretion in cortical collecting duct intercalated cells from H,K-ATPase-deficient mice: role of HK isoforms. *Am J Physiol Renal Physiol* 294:F621–F627, 2008.
121. Royaux IE, Wall SM, Karniski LP, et al: Pendrin, encoded by the Pendred syndrome gene, resides in the apical region of renal intercalated cells and mediates bicarbonate secretion. *Proc Natl Acad Sci U S A* 98:4221–4226, 2001.
124. Teng-umnuay P, Verlander JW, Yuan W, et al: Identification of distinct subpopulations of intercalated cells in the mouse collecting duct. *J Am Soc Nephrol* 7:260–274, 1996.
140. Lombard WE, Kokko JP, Jacobson HR: Bicarbonate transport in cortical and outer medullary collecting tubules. *Am J Physiol* 244:F289–F296, 1983.
149. Karet FE, Finberg KE, Nelson RD, et al: Mutations in the gene encoding B1 subunit of H+-ATPase cause renal tubular acidosis with sensorineural deafness. *Nat Genet* 21:84–90, 1999.
151. Finberg KE, Wagner CA, Bailey MA, et al: The B1-subunit of the H+ ATPase is required for maximal urinary acidification. *Proc Natl Acad Sci U S A* 102:13616–13621, 2005.
168. Wall SM, Pech V: The interaction of pendrin and the epithelial sodium channel in blood pressure regulation. *Curr Opin Nephrol Hypertens* 17:18–24, 2008.
169. Verlander JW, Miller RT, Frank AE, et al: Localization of the ammonium transporter proteins, Rh B glycoprotein and Rh C glycoprotein, in the mouse kidney. *Am J Physiol Renal Physiol* 284:F323–F337, 2003.
173. Verlander JW, Madsen KM, Cannon JK, et al: Activation of acid-secreting intercalated cells in rabbit collecting duct with ammonium chloride loading. *Am J Physiol* 266:F633–F645, 1994.
175. Shayakul C, Alper SL: Defects in processing and trafficking of the AE1 Cl–/HCO3– exchanger associated with inherited distal renal tubular acidosis. *Clin Exp Nephrol* 8:1–11, 2004.
190. Huber S, Asan E, Jons T, et al: Expression of rat kidney anion exchanger 1 in type A intercalated cells in metabolic acidosis and alkalosis. *Am J Physiol* 277:F841–F849, 1999.
204. Verlander JW, Kim YH, Shin W, et al: Dietary Cl(−) restriction upregulates pendrin expression within the apical plasma membrane of type B intercalated cells. *Am J Physiol Renal Physiol* 291:F833–F839, 2006.
209. Pech V, Zheng W, Pham TD, et al: Angiotensin II activates H+-ATPase in type A intercalated cells. *J Am Soc Nephrol* 19:84–91, 2008.
245. Ambuhl PM, Zajicek HK, Wang H, et al: Regulation of renal phosphate transport by acute and chronic metabolic acidosis in the rat. *Kidney Int* 53:1288–1298, 1998.
250. Nowik M, Picard N, Stange G, et al: Renal phosphaturia during metabolic acidosis revisited: molecular mechanisms for decreased renal phosphate reabsorption. *Pflugers Arch* 457:539–549, 2008.
275. Good DW, Burg MB: Ammonia production by individual segments of the rat nephron. *J Clin Invest* 73:602–610, 1984.
277. Curthoys NP, Moe OW: Proximal tubule function and response to acidosis. *Clin J Am Soc Nephrol* 9:1627–1638, 2014.
284. Busque SM, Wagner CA: Potassium restriction, high protein intake, and metabolic acidosis increase expression of the glutamine transporter SNAT3 (Slc38a3) in mouse kidney. *Am J Physiol Renal Physiol* 297:F440–F450, 2009.
298. Stettner P, Bourgeois S, Marsching C, et al: Sulfatides are required for renal adaptation to chronic metabolic acidosis. *Proc Natl Acad Sci U S A* 110:9998–10003, 2013.
339. Nagami GT: Role of angiotensin II in the enhancement of ammonia production and secretion by the proximal tubule in metabolic acidosis. *Am J Physiol Renal Physiol* 294:F874–F880, 2008.
346. Musa-Aziz R, Chen LM, Pelletier MF, et al: Relative CO2/NH3 selectivities of AQP1, AQP4, AQP5, AmtB, and RhAG. *Proc Natl Acad Sci U S A* 106:5406–5411, 2009.
355. Gruswitz F, Chaudhary S, Ho JD, et al: Function of human Rh based on structure of RhCG at 2.1 Å. *Proc Natl Acad Sci U S A* 107:9638–9643, 2010.
356. Marini AM, Matassi G, Raynal V, et al: The human Rhesus-associated RhAG protein and a kidney homologue promote ammonium transport in yeast. *Nat Genet* 26:341–344, 2000.
365. Bishop JM, Verlander JW, Lee HW, et al: Role of the Rhesus glycoprotein, Rh B glycoprotein, in renal ammonia excretion. *Am J Physiol Renal Physiol* 299:F1065–F1077, 2010.
369. Han KH, Croker BP, Clapp WL, et al: Expression of the ammonia transporter, Rh C glycoprotein, in normal and neoplastic human kidney. *J Am Soc Nephrol* 17:2670–2679, 2006.
372. Biver S, Belge H, Bourgeois S, et al: A role for Rhesus factor Rhcg in renal ammonium excretion and male fertility. *Nature* 456:339–343, 2008.
380. Geyer RR, Parker MD, Toye AM, et al: Relative CO2/NH3 permeabilities of human RhAG, RhBG and RhCG. *J Membr Biol* 246:915–926, 2013.
390. Brown D, Wagner CA: Molecular mechanisms of acid-base sensing by the kidney. *J Am Soc Nephrol* 23:774–780, 2012.
391. Preisig PA: The acid-activated signaling pathway: starting with Pyk2 and ending with increased NHE3 activity. *Kidney Int* 72:1324–1329, 2007.
393. Chen Y, Cann MJ, Litvin TN, et al: Soluble adenylyl cyclase as an evolutionarily conserved bicarbonate sensor. *Science* 289:625–628, 2000.
394. Paunescu TG, Ljubojevic M, Russo LM, et al: cAMP stimulates apical V-ATPase accumulation, microvillar elongation, and proton extrusion in kidney collecting duct A-intercalated cells. *Am J Physiol Renal Physiol* 298:F643–F654, 2010.

10 Urine Concentration and Dilution

Jeff M. Sands | Harold E. Layton | Robert A. Fenton

CHAPTER OUTLINE

INDEPENDENT REGULATION OF WATER AND SALT EXCRETION, 258
CRITICAL ROLE OF PARALLEL ORGANIZATION OF STRUCTURES IN THE RENAL MEDULLA TO URINARY CONCENTRATING AND DILUTING PROCESS, 259
Renal Tubules, 259
Vasculature, 262
Medullary Interstitium, 262
Renal Pelvis, 264
URINE CONCENTRATION AND DILUTION PROCESSES ALONG THE MAMMALIAN NEPHRON, 264
Sites of Urine Concentration and Dilution, 264
Mechanism of Tubule Fluid Dilution, 265
Mechanism of Tubule Fluid Concentration, 265

MOLECULAR PHYSIOLOGY OF URINARY CONCENTRATING AND DILUTING PROCESSES, 273
Aquaporin-1 Knockout Mice, 273
Aquaporin-2 Knockout Mice, 276
Aquaporin-3 and Aquaporin-4 Knockout Mice, 276
UT-A1/3 Urea Transporter Knockout Mice, 276
Na^{++}-H^{++}-Exchanger Isoform 3 and Na-K-2Cl Cotransporter Type 2 Knockout Mice, 278
Epithelial Sodium Channel Knockout Mice, 278
Kidney-Specific Chloride Channel 1 Knockout Mice, 278
Renal Outer Medullary Potassium Channel Knockout Mice, 278
Type 2 Vasopressin Receptor Knockout Mice, 278

INDEPENDENT REGULATION OF WATER AND SALT EXCRETION

The kidney is responsible for numerous homeostatic functions. For example, body fluid tonicity is tightly controlled by regulation of renal water excretion; extracellular fluid volume is controlled by regulation of NaCl excretion; systemic acid-base balance is controlled by regulation of net acid excretion; systemic K^+ balance is controlled by regulation of K^+ excretion; and the body maintains nitrogen balance through regulation of urea excretion.

The independent regulation of water and solute excretion is essential for the homeostatic functions of the kidney to be performed simultaneously. This means that in the absence of changes in solute intake or metabolic production of waste solutes, the kidney is able to excrete different volumes of water upon changes in water intake. This ability to excrete the appropriate amount of water without marked perturbations in solute excretion (without disturbing the other homeostatic functions of the kidney) is dependent on renal concentrating and diluting mechanisms and forms the basis of this chapter (Figure 10.1).

Renal water excretion is tightly regulated by the peptide hormone arginine vasopressin (AVP; also named antidiuretic hormone). Under normal circumstances, the circulating vasopressin level is determined by osmoreceptors in the hypothalamus that trigger increases in vasopressin secretion (by the posterior pituitary gland) when the osmolality of the blood rises above a threshold value, approximately 292 mOsm/kg H_2O. This mechanism can be modulated when other inputs to the hypothalamus (e.g., arterial underfilling, severe fatigue, or physical stress) override the osmotic mechanism. Upon an increase in plasma osmolality, vasopressin is secreted from the posterior pituitary gland into the peripheral plasma. The kidney responds to the

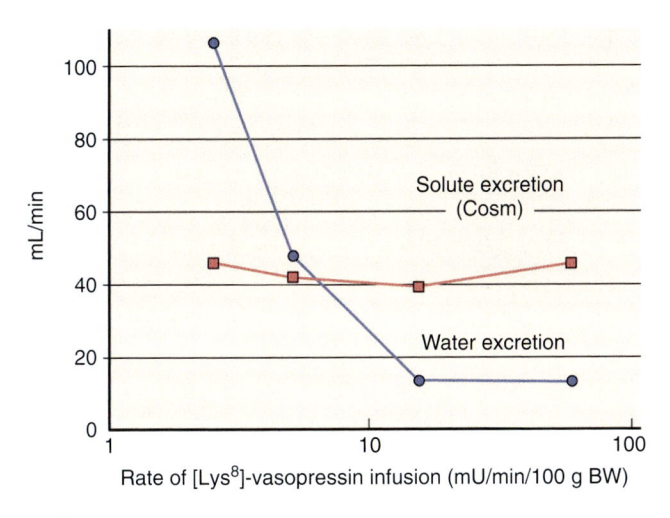

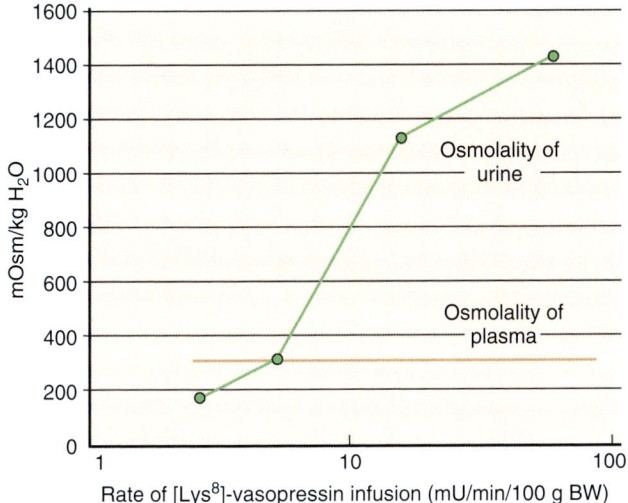

Figure 10.1 Steady-state renal response to varying rates of vasopressin infusion in conscious rats. A water load (4% of body weight [BW]) was maintained throughout the experiments to suppress endogenous vasopressin secretion. Although the urine flow rate was markedly reduced at higher vasopressin infusion rates, the osmolar clearance (solute excretion, Cosm) changed little. Concordantly, at higher vasopressin infusion rates, the osmolality of the urine increased significantly, whereas plasma osmolality remained constant. (Data from Atherton JC, Hai MA, Thomas S: The time course of changes in renal tissue composition during water diuresis in the rat. J Physiol 197:429-443, 1968.)

variable vasopressin levels by varying urine flow (i.e., water excretion). For example, during extreme antidiuresis (high vasopressin levels), water excretion is 100- or more-fold lower than during extensive water diuresis (low vasopressin levels). These major changes in water excretion are obtained without substantial changes in steady-state solute excretion. This phenomenon is dependent on the kidney's ability to concentrate and dilute the urine. During low circulating vasopressin levels, urine osmolality is less than that of plasma (290 mOsm/kg H_2O)—the diluting function of the kidney. In contrast, when the circulating vasopressin levels are high, urine osmolality is much higher than that of plasma—the concentrating function of the kidney.

CRITICAL ROLE OF PARALLEL ORGANIZATION OF STRUCTURES IN THE RENAL MEDULLA TO URINARY CONCENTRATING AND DILUTING PROCESS

The kidney's ability to vary water excretion over a wide physiologic range, without altering steady-state solute excretion, cannot be simply explained as a consequence of the sequential transport processes along the nephron.[1] The independent regulation of water and sodium excretion occurs in the renal medulla, where the nephron segments and vasculature (vasa recta) are arranged in complex but specific anatomic relationships, both in terms of which segments connect to which segments and their three-dimensional configuration. Thus it is necessary to consider the parallel interactions between nephron segments that occur as a result of its looped or hairpin structure. Figure 10.2 illustrates the regional architecture of the renal medulla and medullary rays.[2]

RENAL TUBULES

LOOPS OF HENLE

The kidney generally contains two populations of nephrons, long-looped and short-looped, which merge to form a common collecting duct system (see Figure 10.2). Both types of nephrons have loops of Henle that are arranged in a folded or hairpin configuration. Short-looped nephrons generally have glomeruli that are located more superficially in the cortex and have loops that bend in the outer medulla. Long-looped nephrons generally have glomeruli that are located more deeply within the cortex and have loops that bend at various levels of the inner medulla. Long-looped nephrons also contain a thin ascending limb, a segment that is not present in short-looped nephrons. Thin ascending limbs are found only in the inner medulla. The inner-outer medullary border is defined by the transition from thin to thick ascending limbs. Thus the outer medulla contains only thick ascending limbs, regardless of the type of loop. The long-looped nephrons bend at various levels of the inner medulla from the inner-outer medullary border to the papillary tip. Thus progressively fewer loops of Henle extend to deeper levels of the inner medulla. Some mammalian kidneys, such as human kidneys, also contain cortical nephrons, which are nephrons whose loops of Henle do not reach into the medulla.

The loops of Henle receive tubule fluid from the proximal convoluted tubules. Tubule fluid exits the thick ascending limbs of both long- and short-looped nephrons, and from cortical nephrons in species that have them, and flows into distal convoluted tubules (DCTs). Thus the descending and ascending limbs of the loops of Henle have a countercurrent flow configuration and are composed of several different nephron segments (see Figure 10.2). The descending portion of the loop of Henle consists of the S2 proximal straight tubule in the medullary ray, the S3 proximal straight tubule (or pars recta) in the outer stripe of the outer medulla, and the thin descending limb in the inner stripe of the outer medulla and the inner medulla. The descending thin limb of short-looped nephrons differs structurally

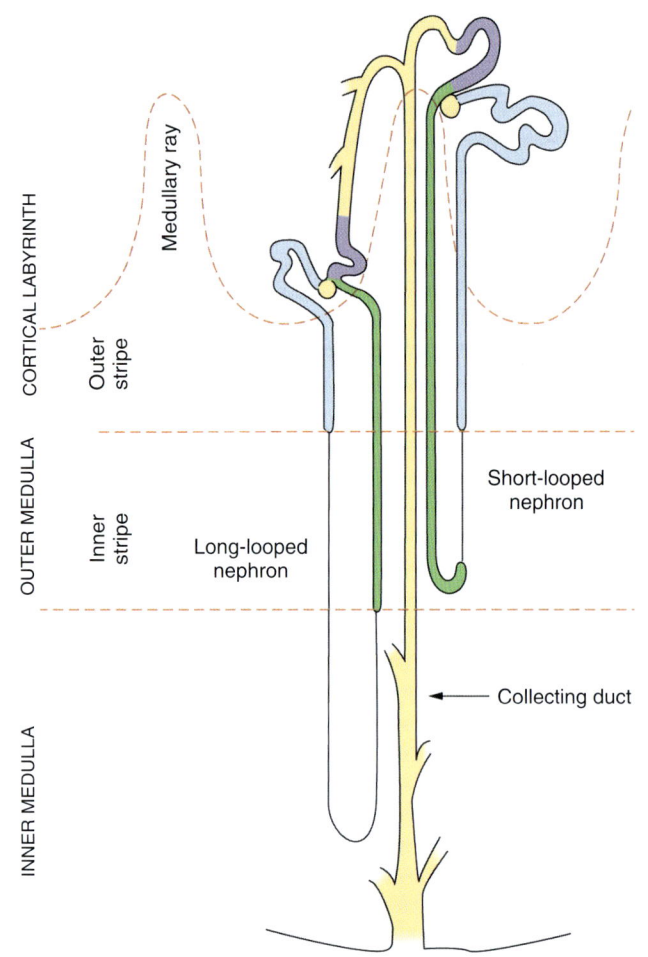

Figure 10.2 Mammalian renal structure. Major regions of the kidney are shown on the *left*. Configurations of a long-looped and a short-looped nephron are depicted. The major portions of the nephron are proximal tubules *(medium blue)*, thin limbs of loops of Henle *(single line)*, thick ascending limbs of loops of Henle *(green)*, distal convoluted tubules *(lavender)*, and the collecting duct system *(yellow)*. (Modified from Knepper MA, Stephenson JL: Urinary concentrating and diluting processes. In Andreoli TE, Hoffman JF, Fanestil DD, et al: *Physiology of membrane disorders*, ed 2, New York, 1986, Plenum, pp 713-726.)

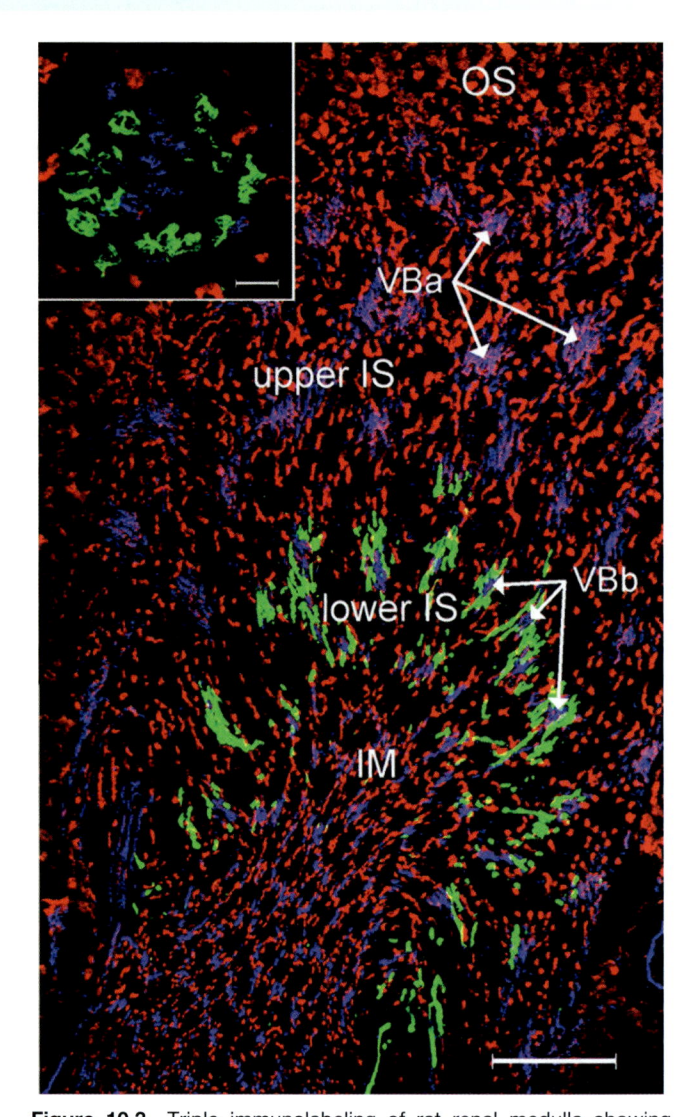

Figure 10.3 Triple immunolabeling of rat renal medulla showing localization of UT-A2 *(green)*, marking late thin descending limbs from short-looped nephrons, von Willebrand factor *(blue)* marking endothelial cells of vasa recta, and aquaporin-1 *(red)* marking thin descending limbs from outer medullary long-looped nephrons and early short-looped nephrons. *Inset* shows a cross section of a vascular bundle demonstrating that UT-A2–positive thin descending limbs from short-looped nephrons surround the vascular bundles in the deep part of the outer medulla. IM, Inner medulla; IS, inner stripe of outer medulla; OS, outer stripe of outer medulla; VBa, vascular bundles in outer part of inner stripe; VBb, vascular bundles in inner part of inner stripe. (From Wade JB, Lee AJ, Liu J, et al: UT-A2: a 55 kDa urea transporter protein in thin descending limb of Henle's loop whose abundance is regulated by vasopressin. *Am J Physiol Renal Physiol* 278:F52-F62, 2000.)

and functionally from the descending thin limb of long-looped nephrons.[3,4]

The location of the descending thin limb of short-looped nephrons within the outer medulla is illustrated in Figure 10.3 (labeled in green).[5] The descending thin limbs of short-looped nephrons surround the vascular bundles in the outer medulla and tend to be organized in a ringlike pattern (see Figure 10.3 *inset*). Thin descending limbs of long-looped nephrons in the outer medulla differ morphologically and functionally from thin descending limbs of long-looped nephrons in the inner medulla.[6-9] The histologic transition from the outer medullary to the inner medullary type of thin descending limbs of long-looped nephrons is gradual and often occurs at some distance into the inner medulla, rather than strictly at the inner-outer medullary border as is the case for the transition between thin and thick ascending limbs.

Pannabecker, Dantzler, and coworkers used immunohistochemical labeling and computer-assisted reconstruction to provide new detail about the functional architecture of the rat inner medulla.[10-13] Figure 10.4 shows a computerized reconstruction of the inner medullary portion of several long-looped nephrons from rats that are labeled using antibodies to the water channel aquaporin-1 (AQP1, shown in red) and the kidney-specific chloride channel 1 (ClC-K1; shown in green).[10-14] AQP1 is a marker of thin descending limbs of long-looped nephrons in the outer medulla, and AQP1 is detected in thin descending limbs of long-looped nephrons in the inner medulla for a variable distance.

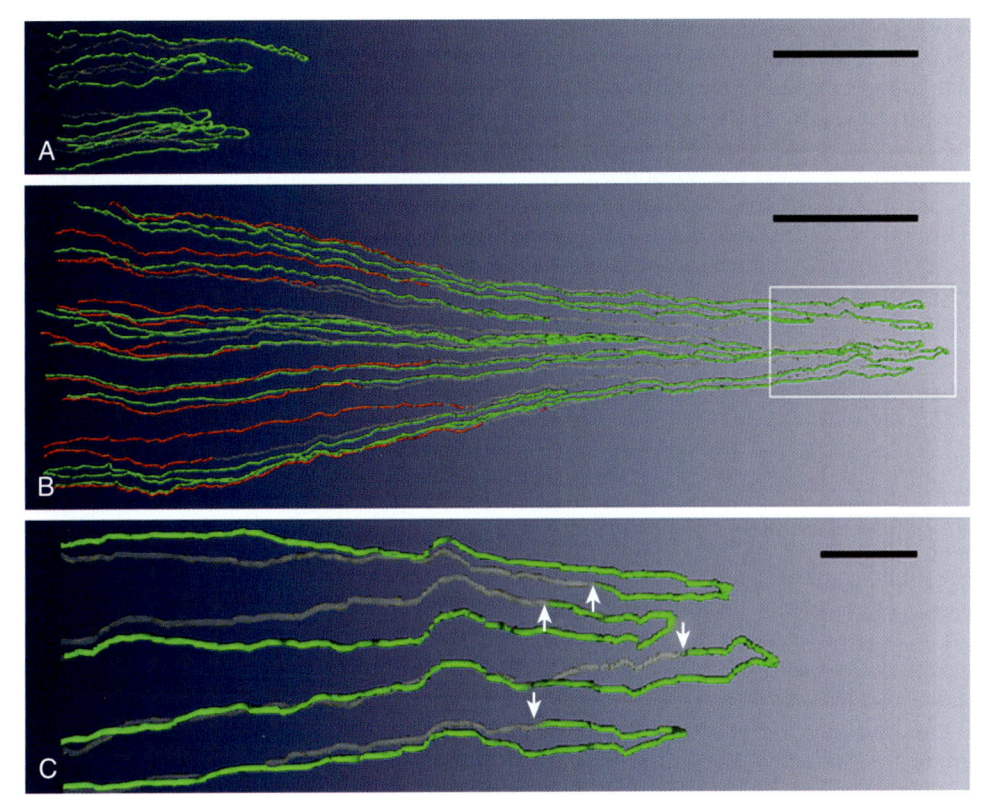

Figure 10.4 Computer-assisted reconstruction of loops of Henle from rat inner medulla showing expression of aquaporin-1 (AQP1; *red*) and kidney-specific chloride channel 1 (ClC-K1; *green*); *gray regions* (B-crystallin) express undetectable levels of AQP1 and ClC-K1. Loops are oriented along the corticopapillary axis, with the *left* edge of each image nearer the base of the inner medulla. **A,** Thin limbs that have their bends within the first millimeter beyond the outer-inner medullary boundary. Descending segments lack detectable AQP1. ClC-K1 is expressed continuously along the prebend segment and the thin ascending limb. **B,** Loops that have their bends beyond the first millimeter of the inner medulla. AQP1 is expressed along the initial 40% of each thin descending limb and is absent from the remainder of each loop. ClC-K1 is expressed continuously along the prebend segment and the thin ascending limb. **C,** Enlargement of near-bend regions of four thin limbs from *box* in **B**. ClC-K1 expression, corresponding to thin descending limb prebend segment, begins, on average, 165 μm before the loop bend *(arrows)*. Scale bars, 500 μm (**A** and **B**) and 100 μm (**C**). (From Pannabecker TL, Dantzler WH, Layton HE, et al: Role of three-dimensional architecture in the urine concentrating mechanism of the rat renal inner medulla. *Am J Physiol Renal Physiol* 295:F1271-F1285, 2008.)

However, AQP1 was not found in thin descending limbs of loops of Henle that turn within the upper first millimeter of the inner medulla. Correspondingly, Zhai and colleagues determined that AQP1 was not detectable along the entire length of thin descending limbs of short-looped rat nephrons.[15] In contrast, thin descending limbs of loops of Henle that turn below the first millimeter have three discernible functional subsegments: the upper 40% express AQP1, whereas the lower 60% do not. ClC-K1 is a marker of the thin ascending limb–type epithelium. It is first detected in the final approximately 165 μm of the thin descending limb. Thus, ClC-K1 is detected before the bend of the loops of Henle, consistent with several morphologic studies that demonstrate that the descending limb to ascending limb transition occurs before the loop bend. A substantial portion of the inner medullary thin descending limb of long-looped nephrons did not express either AQP1 or ClC-K1, as indicated in gray.

The deepest portions of descending thin limbs have low water permeability and reduced AQP1.[16] It has been proposed, but not demonstrated experimentally, that urine concentration would be improved by the presence of a urea-Na^+ or urea-Cl^- cotransporter in the AQP1-null portion of the thin descending limb.[17] These deep AQP1-null segments, prebend segments, and thin ascending limbs lie equally near the collecting ducts.[16] However, the distal 30% of thin ascending limbs of the longest loops of Henle lie distant from collecting ducts.[16] Based upon these findings, Pannabecker and colleagues hypothesize that descending and ascending thin limbs enter and exit collecting duct clusters in a manner that is important for the generation and maintenance of the osmolality gradient within the inner medulla.[19] These anatomic relationships result in isolated interstitial nodal spaces that may facilitate preferential mixing of solutes and fluid within the inner medulla.[18]

Pannabecker and colleagues have also found evidence for mixed descending- and ascending-type thin limbs of the loops of Henle in the inner medulla.[19] The ascending portions of the loops of Henle consist of the thin ascending limbs (which are present only in the long-looped nephrons of the inner medulla), the medullary thick ascending limbs in the inner and outer stripes of the outer medulla, and the cortical thick ascending limbs in the medullary rays.

DISTAL TUBULE SEGMENTS IN THE CORTICAL LABYRINTH

After tubule fluid exits the loop of Henle through the cortical thick ascending limb, it enters the DCT, which is located in the cortical labyrinth. In most mammalian species, several distal tubules merge to form a connecting tubule arcade.[20] The connecting tubular cells express both the vasopressin-regulated water channel, aquaporin-2 (AQP2), and the type 2 vasopressin receptor (V2R),[21] suggesting that the arcades are sites of vasopressin-regulated water reabsorption, similar to collecting ducts (see later). Tubule fluid exits the connecting tubules within the arcades and enters the initial collecting tubules, located in the superficial cortex, and then into the cortical collecting ducts. In most rodent species that have been studied, several nephrons merge to form a single cortical collecting duct.[3,22]

COLLECTING DUCT SYSTEM

The collecting duct system spans all regions of the kidney, starting in the cortex and running to the tip of the inner medulla (see Figure 10.2). The collecting ducts are arranged parallel to the loops of Henle in the medullary rays, outer medulla, and inner medulla. Like the loops of Henle, several morphologically and functionally discrete segments are contained within the collecting duct system. In general, the collecting ducts descend straight through the medullary rays and outer medulla without joining with other collecting ducts. However, several collecting ducts merge as they descend within the inner medulla, resulting in a progressive reduction in the number of inner medullary collecting ducts (IMCDs) from the inner-outer medullary border to the papillary tip.[22] The tapered structure of the renal papilla results from the reduction in collecting duct number, accompanied by a progressive reduction in the number of loops of Henle, reaching the deepest levels of the inner medulla.

Detailed studies of inner medullary structure, both by Kriz and coworkers and in later studies by Pannabecker and Dantzler, found that the IMCDs in the inner medullary base (initial IMCDs) form clusters that coalesce along the corticomedullary axis.[14,23-29] The thin descending limbs are predominantly present at the periphery of these clusters and appear to form an asymmetric ring around each collecting duct cluster, whereas the thin ascending limbs are distributed relatively uniformly among the collecting ducts and thin descending limbs.[28,30]

Pannabecker and Dantzler identified three population groups of loops of Henle in Munich-Wistar rats,[27] distinguished by the position of the thin ascending limb at the base of the inner medulla and by differing loop length (Figure 10.5). Group 1 loops have thin ascending limbs that are interposed between collecting ducts and reach a mean length of 700 μm into the inner medulla. Group 2 loops have thin ascending limbs that are adjacent to just one collecting duct and reach a mean length of 1500 μm. Group 3 loops have thin ascending limbs that lie more than 0.5 tubule diameters from a collecting duct and reach a mean length of 2200 μm. As the collecting ducts coalesce and the shorter loops of Henle disappear, the originating portions of the longer thin ascending limbs run alongside the collecting ducts for a substantial distance.[27]

VASCULATURE

For detailed descriptions of the renal vasculature, see Chapters 2 and 3. The major blood vessels that carry blood into and out of the renal medulla are named the *vasa recta*. Blood enters the descending vasa recta from the efferent arterioles of juxtamedullary nephrons and supplies it to the capillary plexuses at each level of the medulla. The outer medullary capillary plexus is denser and better perfused than the plexus in the inner medulla.[31] Blood from the inner medullary capillary plexus feeds into ascending vasa recta (ascending vasa recta are never formed directly from descending vasa recta in a looplike structure). Inner medullary ascending vasa recta traverse the inner stripe of the outer medulla in close physical association with the descending vasa recta in vascular bundles.[23] In many animal species, thin descending limbs of short-looped nephrons surround the vascular bundles, as shown in Figure 10.3. Here the thin descending limb segments are labeled with an antibody to the UT-A2 urea transporter,[5] suggesting a route for urea recycling from the vasa recta to the thin descending limbs of short-looped nephrons. The outer medullary capillary plexus is drained by vasa recta that ascend through the outer stripe of the outer medulla, separate from the descending vasa recta.[26] Computer-assisted digital tracing of mouse kidney combined with AQP1 immunohistochemistry has added to our knowledge of the arrangement of tubules and vessels in the vascular bundles being implicit in providing a lateral osmolality heterogeneity for urine concentration.[32]

The counterflow arrangement of the vasa recta in the medulla promotes countercurrent exchange of solutes and water, which is abetted by the presence of AQP1 and UT-B urea transporters in the endothelial cells of the descending portion of the vasa recta.[33-36] Countercurrent exchange provides a means of reducing the effective blood flow to the medulla while maintaining a high absolute perfusion rate.[37] The low effective blood flow that results from countercurrent exchange is thought to be important for the preservation of solute concentration gradients in the medullary tissue (see later).

In contrast to the medulla, the cortical labyrinth has a high effective blood flow. The rapid vascular perfusion to this region promotes the rapid return of solutes and water reabsorbed from the nephron to the general circulation. The rapid perfusion is thought to maintain the interstitial concentrations of most solutes at levels close to those in the peripheral plasma. The medullary rays of the cortex have a capillary plexus that is considerably sparser than that of the cortical labyrinth. Consequently, the effective blood flow to the medullary rays has been postulated to be lower than that of the cortical labyrinth.[1]

MEDULLARY INTERSTITIUM

The renal medullary interstitium connects the tubules and vasculature.[38] It is a complex space that includes the medullary interstitial cells, microfibrils, extracellular matrix, and fluid.[30,38,39] The interstitium is relatively small in volume in the outer medulla and the outer portion of the inner medulla, which may be important in limiting the diffusion of solutes upward along the medullary axis.[1,28,38] In contrast, the interstitial space is much larger in the inner half of the inner medulla.[1,28,38] Within this region, it consists of a gelatinous matrix containing large amounts of highly polymerized hyaluronic acid, consisting of alternating N-acetyl-D-glucosamine and D-glucuronate moieties.[40] Theories have been proposed in which the hyaluronic acid interstitial

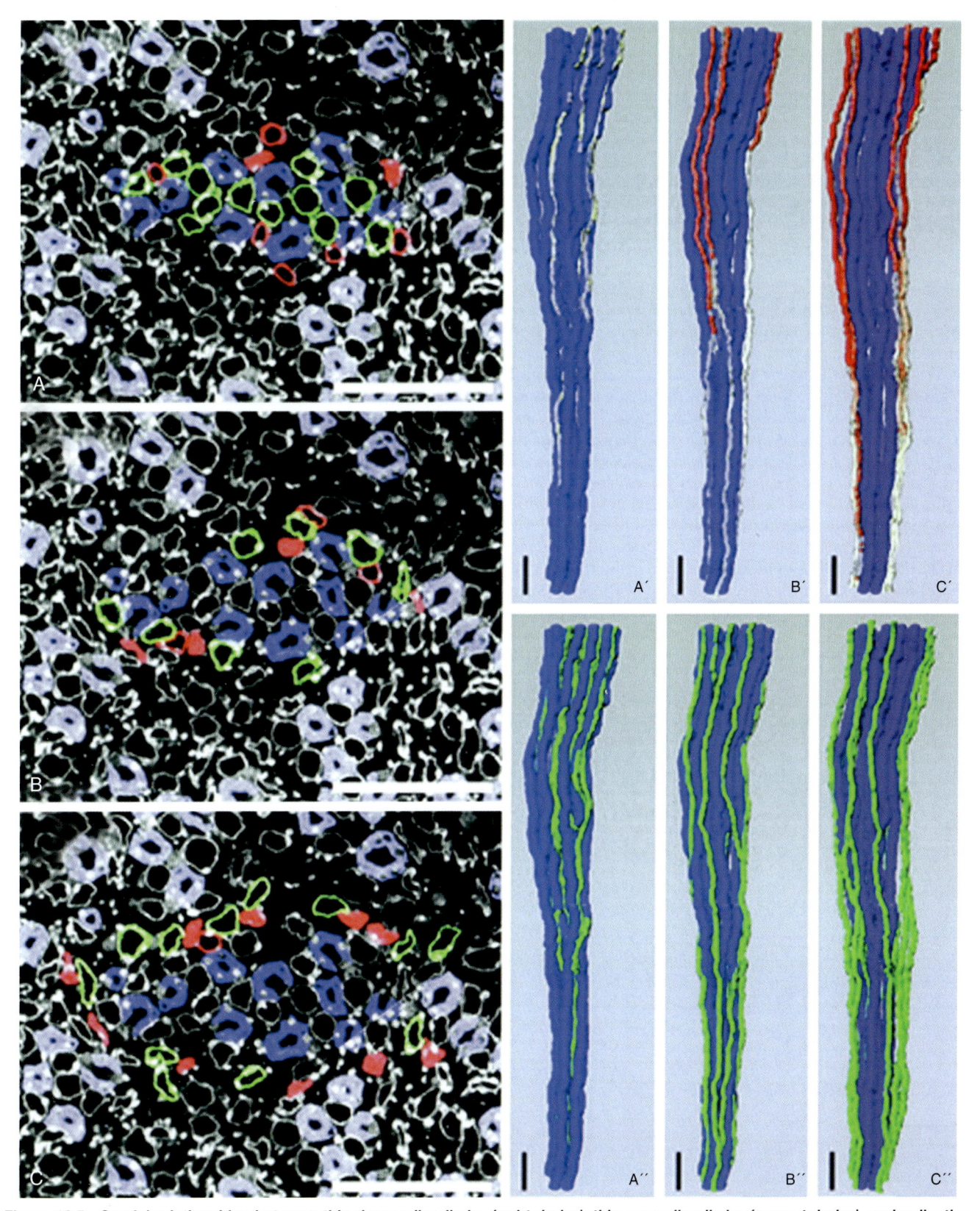

Figure 10.5 Spatial relationships between thin descending limbs *(red tubules)*, thin ascending limbs *(green tubules)*, and collecting ducts *(dark blue tubules)*. Thin ascending limbs were categorized into three groups related to their lateral proximity to collecting ducts. Members of each group are shown in a transverse section located at the base of the inner medulla. **A,** Group 1. **B,** Group 2. **C,** Group 3. **A-C,** *Open red figures* represent aquaporin-1 (AQP1)–null thin descending limbs, *solid red figures* represent AQP1-expressing thin descending limbs, *white outlined figures* represent thin ascending limbs not associated with the collecting duct cluster, and *light blue figures* represent collecting ducts not associated with the collecting duct cluster. Two prebend segments from group 1 are included in **A**. One thin ascending limb from each of groups 2 and 3 (**B** and **C**) extends below the region of reconstruction, and their thin descending limbs were therefore not reconstructed. **A′**, **B′**, and **C′** show thin descending limbs and collecting ducts. *Gray tubules* represent AQP1-null thin descending limbs. **A″**, **B″**, and **C″** show thin ascending limbs and collecting ducts. Scale bars, 100 μm. (From Pannabecker TL, Dantzler WH: Three-dimensional lateral and vertical relationships of inner medullary loops of Henle and collecting ducts. *Am J Physiol Renal Physiol* 287:F767-F774, 2004.)

matrix plays a direct role in the generation of an inner medullary osmotic gradient through its ability to store and transduce energy from the smooth muscle contractions of the renal pelvis (see later).[40]

RENAL PELVIS

Urine exits the collecting duct system through the ducts of Bellini at the papillary tip and enters the renal pelvis (Figure 10.6). The renal pelvis (or calyx in multipapillate kidneys) is a complex intrarenal urinary space that surrounds the papilla. The renal pelvis (or calyx) has portions that extend into the outer medulla, which are called fornices and secondary pouches. Although a transitional epithelium lines most of the pelvic space, the renal parenchyma is separated from the pelvic space by a simple cuboidal epithelium.[41] It has been proposed that water and solute transport could occur across this epithelium, thereby modifying the composition of the renal medullary interstitial fluid.[42] There are two smooth muscle layers within the renal pelvic (calyceal) wall.[43] Contractions of these smooth muscle layers generate powerful peristaltic waves that appear to displace the renal papilla downward with a "milking" action.[44] These peristaltic waves may intermittently propel urine along the collecting ducts. The contractions compress all structures within the renal inner medulla, including the interstitium, loops of Henle, vasa recta, and collecting ducts.[45] Theories have been proposed whereby these contractions furnish part of the energy for concentrating solutes, and hence concentrating urine, within the inner medulla,[40] as discussed later.

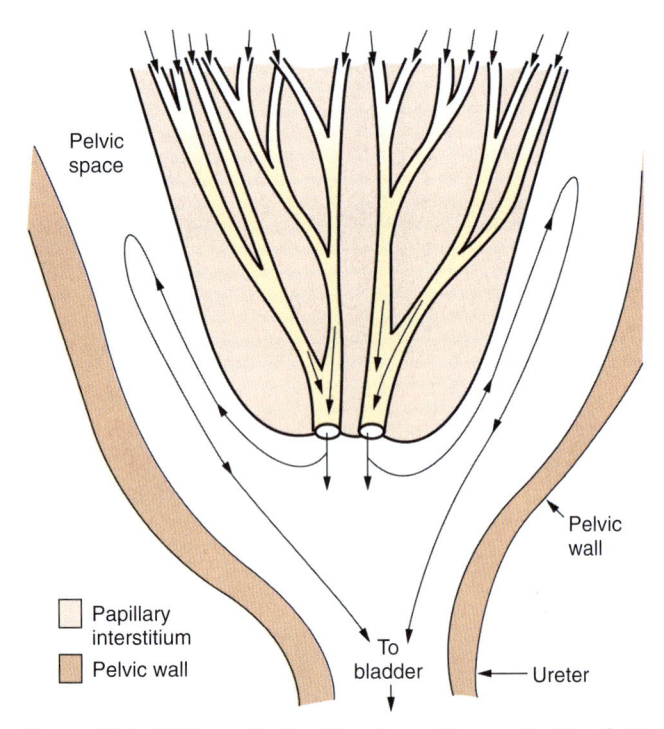

Figure 10.6 Pattern of urine flow in papillary collecting ducts and renal pelvis. Urine exits the papillary collecting ducts (ducts of Bellini) at the tip of the renal papilla and is carried to the urinary bladder by the ureter. Under some circumstances, a fraction of the urine may reflux backward in the pelvic space and contact the outer surface of the renal papilla. Solute and water exchange across the papillary surface epithelium has been postulated (see text).

URINE CONCENTRATION AND DILUTION PROCESSES ALONG THE MAMMALIAN NEPHRON

SITES OF URINE CONCENTRATION AND DILUTION

Micropuncture studies of the mammalian nephron have determined the major sites of tubule fluid concentration and dilution (Figure 10.7). Proximal tubule fluid is always isosmotic with plasma, regardless of whether the kidney is diluting or concentrating the urine.[46] In contrast, the fluid in the early DCT is always hypotonic, regardless of the final osmolality of the urine. Indeed, during both antidiuresis and water diuresis, the earliest nephron segment where

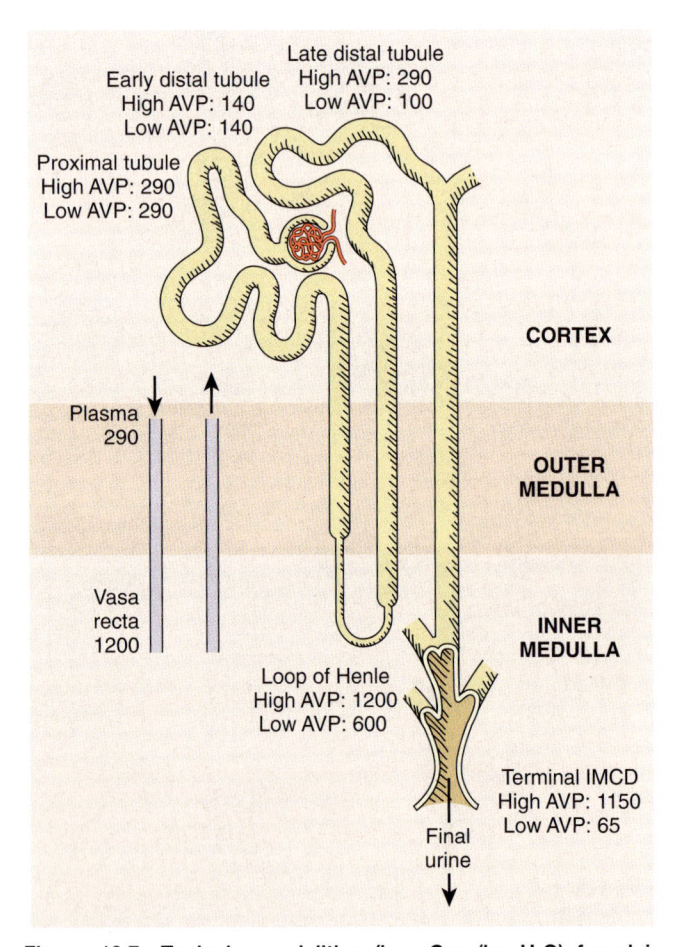

Figure 10.7 Typical osmolalities (in mOsm/kg H$_2$O) found in various vascular (*left*) and renal tubule (*right*) sites in rat kidneys. Fluid in the proximal tubule is always isosmotic with plasma (290 mOsm/kg H$_2$O). Fluid emerging from the loop of Henle (entering the early distal tubule) is always hypotonic. Osmolality in the late distal tubule increases to plasma level only during antidiuresis. Final urine is hypertonic when the circulating vasopressin (AVP) level is high, and hypotonic when the AVP level is low. A high osmolality is always maintained in the loop of Henle and vasa recta. During antidiuresis, osmolalities in all inner medullary structures are nearly equal. Osmolalities are somewhat attenuated in the loop and vasa recta during water diuresis (not shown). (Based on micropuncture studies; see text.) IMCD, Inner medullary collecting duct.

significant differences in tubule fluid osmolality can be detected is the late distal tubule. During water diuresis, the fluid in the distal tubule remains hypotonic. During antidiuresis, the fluid in the distal tubule becomes isosmotic with plasma, and the osmolality between the end of the late distal tubule and the IMCD rises to a level greater than that of plasma. Thus the conclusion from micropuncture studies is that the loop of Henle is the major site of dilution of tubule fluid, and that dilution processes in the loop occur regardless of whether the final urine is dilute or concentrated. Further dilution of the tubule fluid can occur in the collecting ducts during water diuresis.[47] In contrast, the chief site of urine concentration is beyond the distal tubule (i.e., in the collecting duct system). The mechanisms of urinary dilution and of urinary concentration are discussed in the following sections.

MECHANISM OF TUBULE FLUID DILUTION

Micropuncture studies in rats have shown that the fluid in the early distal tubule is hypotonic, due mainly to a reduction in luminal NaCl concentration relative to that in the proximal tubule.[48] The low luminal NaCl concentration could result either from active NaCl reabsorption from the loop of Henle or from water secretion into the loop of Henle. Micropuncture measurements in rats, performed using inulin as a volume marker, demonstrated net water reabsorption from the superficial loops of Henle during antidiuresis, thereby ruling out water secretion as a potential mechanism of tubule fluid dilution.[49] Thus one can conclude that luminal dilution occurs because of NaCl reabsorption from the loops of Henle, in excess of water reabsorption. Classic studies of isolated perfused rabbit thick ascending limbs established the mechanism of tubule fluid dilution.[50,51] NaCl is rapidly reabsorbed by active transport, which lowers the luminal osmolality and NaCl concentration to levels below those in the peritubular fluid. The osmotic water permeability of the thick ascending limb is very low, which prevents dissipation of the transepithelial osmolality gradient by water flux.

The tubule fluid remains hypotonic throughout the distal tubule and collecting duct system during water diuresis, aided by the low osmotic water permeability of the collecting ducts when circulating levels of vasopressin are low. Even though the tubule fluid remains hypotonic in the collecting duct system, the solute composition of the tubule fluid is modified within the collecting duct, mainly by Na^+ absorption and K^+ secretion. Active NaCl reabsorption from the collecting duct results in a further dilution of the collecting duct fluid, beyond that achieved in the thick ascending limbs.[47]

MECHANISM OF TUBULE FLUID CONCENTRATION

When circulating vasopressin levels are high, net water absorption occurs between the late distal tubule and the collecting ducts.[49] The reader is referred to Chapter 11 for a detailed discussion of the cell biology of vasopressin action. Because water is absorbed in excess of solutes, with a resulting rise in osmolality along the collecting ducts toward the papillary tip,[52] it can be concluded that collecting duct fluid is concentrated chiefly by water absorption, rather than by solute addition.

An axial osmolality gradient in the renal medullary tissue, with the highest degree of hypertonicity at the papillary tip, provides the osmotic driving force for water absorption along the collecting ducts. This osmolality gradient was initially reported by Wirz and colleagues.[53] In a classic study they demonstrated, in antidiuretic rats, the existence of a continuously increasing osmolality gradient along the outer and inner medulla, with the highest osmolality in the deepest part of the inner medulla, the papillary tip. In addition, within the medulla the osmolality of the collecting ducts was as high as in the loops of Henle, and the osmolality of vasa recta blood, sampled from near the papillary tip, was virtually equal to that of the final urine.[53] Taken together these results demonstrated that the high tissue osmolality was not simply a manifestation of a high osmolality in a single structure, namely, the collecting duct. Micropuncture studies by Gottschalk and Mylle based on the superficial and thus accessible tubules and vessels confirmed that the osmolality of the fluid in the loops of Henle, the vasa recta, and the collecting ducts is approximately the same (see Figure 10.7),[46] supporting the hypothesis that the collecting duct fluid is concentrated by osmotic equilibration with a hypertonic medullary interstitium. Furthermore, in vitro studies demonstrated that collecting ducts have a high water permeability in the presence of vasopressin,[54,55] as is required for osmotic equilibration. The mechanism by which the corticomedullary osmolality gradient is generated is considered in the next section.

Although the final axial osmolality gradient within the renal medulla is due to the combined gradients of several individual solutes, as initially demonstrated using tissue slice analysis by Jarausch and Ullrich,[56] the principal solutes responsible for the osmolality gradient are NaCl and urea (Figure 10.8). The increase in the NaCl concentration gradient along the corticomedullary axis occurs predominantly in the outer medulla, with only a small increase in the inner medulla. In contrast, the increase in urea concentration occurs predominantly in the inner medulla, with little or no increase in the initial outer medulla. The mechanisms for generating the NaCl gradient in the outer medulla and urea accumulation in the inner medulla are discussed in the next section.

GENERATION OF THE AXIAL SODIUM CHLORIDE GRADIENT IN THE RENAL OUTER MEDULLA

A sustained osmolality gradient is maintained along the corticomedullary axis of the outer medulla (see Figure 10.8); that gradient, which is present in both diuresis and antidiuresis,[57] arises mostly from an accumulation of NaCl. The gradient is generated by the concentrating mechanism of the outer medulla. General considerations circumscribe the nature of that mechanism. Because the axial osmolality gradient is present in both diuresis and antidiuresis (in which the outer medullary collecting duct is water permeable to varying degrees), the accumulation of NaCl in the outer medulla cannot depend on a sustained osmolality difference across the collecting duct epithelium. Thus the concentrating mechanism must depend on the loops of Henle, on the vasculature, and on their interactions within the outer medulla. Moreover, mass balance of water and NaCl

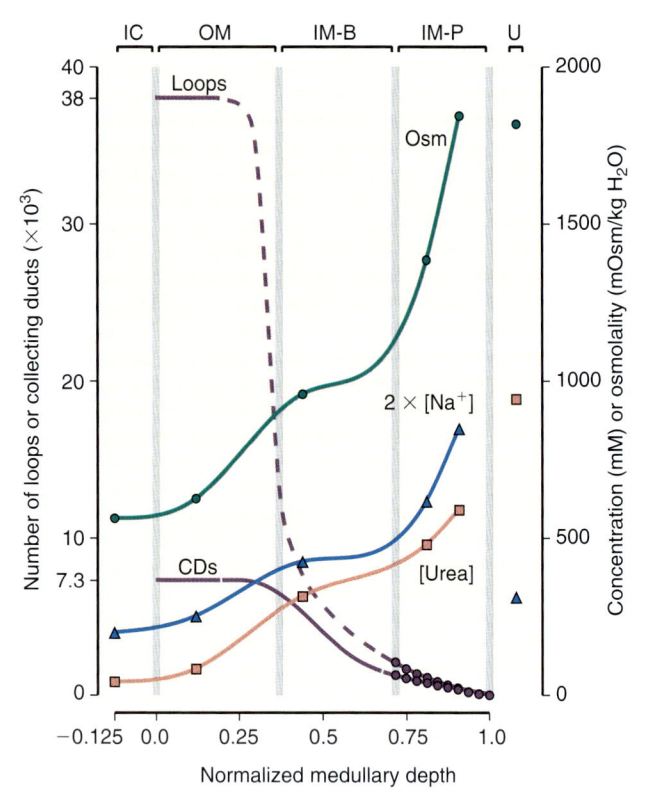

Figure 10.8 Data from rat kidney in an antidiuretic state. Osmolality, urea concentration, and sodium concentration plus its anion are shown (scale at **right**); also, loop of Henle and collecting duct (CD) populations (scale at **left**). Loop of Henle and CD populations decrease in inner medulla because CDs merge and loops turn back. The osmolality gradient is larger in the outer medulla (OM) and papilla than in the outer part of the inner medulla. The gradient is largest in the papilla, where the osmolality and concentration profiles appear to increase exponentially. The shape of the sodium profile has been corroborated by electron microprobe measurements.[200] IC, Inner cortex; IM, outer part (base [B]) of inner medulla; P, papilla or inner part (tip) of inner medulla; U, urine. Figure based on published data. *Curves* connecting data points are natural cubic splines, computed by standard algorithms.[201] *Dashed curve segments* are interpolations without supporting measurements. Tubule populations in papilla are from Han and colleagues[202]; tubule populations in outer medulla are based on estimates in Knepper and associates.[22] Concentrations and osmolalities are from tissue slices and urine samples collected 4.5 hours after onset of vasopressin infusion at 15µ /min per 100 g body weight. Data are from Figure 5 in Atherton and coworkers and Figures 1, 3, and 9 in Hai and Thomas[57,203]; slice locations were given in Chou and Knepper.[8] The osmolality reported in the inner cortex seems high relative to the reported plasma concentration of 314 mOsm/kg H$_2$O. The osmolality and concentration profiles, as drawn in Hai and Thomas, apparently do not take into account relative distances between tissue sample sites.[57] (From Sands JM, Layton HE: The urine-concentrating mechanism and urea transporters. In Alpern RJ, Caplan MJ, Moe OW, editors: *The kidney: physiology and pathophysiology,* ed 5, San Diego, 2013, Academic Press, pp 1463-1510.)

It has long been believed that the osmolality gradient of the outer medulla is generated by means of countercurrent multiplication of a single effect ("Vervielfältigung des Einzeleffektes"). In this paradigm, proposed by Kuhn and Ryffel in 1942,[58] osmotic pressure is raised along parallel but opposing flows in nearby tubes that are made contiguous by a hairpin turn (Figure 10.9): a transfer of solute from one tubule to another (i.e., a single effect) would augment (multiply), or reinforce, the osmotic pressure in the parallel flows. Thus, by means of the countercurrent configuration, a small transverse osmotic difference would be multiplied into a relatively large difference along the axes of flow. In support of this paradigm, Kuhn and Ryffel provided both a mathematical model and an apparatus that exemplified countercurrent multiplication.

As anatomic and physiologic understanding of the renal medulla increased, the countercurrent multiplication paradigm was reinterpreted and modified. In 1951 Hargitay and Kuhn put the paradigm in the context of specific renal tubules.[59] The loop of Henle was identified with the parallel tubes joined by a hairpin turn as proposed by Kuhn and Ryffel. Thus the loops of Henle were proposed as the source of the outer medullary gradient, and that gradient was hypothesized to draw water out of water-permeable collecting ducts. In 1959 Kuhn and Ramel used a mathematical model to show that active transport of NaCl from thick ascending limbs could serve as the single effect.[60] Subsequent physiologic experiments confirmed the active NaCl transport and the osmotic absorption of water from collecting ducts.[49-52] Experiments indicating high water permeability in hamster descending limbs of short loops and in descending limbs of long loops suggested that the accumulation of NaCl from thick limbs concentrated descending limb tubule fluid by osmotic water withdrawal, rather than by NaCl addition (see Figure 10.9).[6,7,9,61]

Doubts have arisen about whether the paradigm of countercurrent multiplication provides an accurate representation of the means by which the gradient is generated in the mammalian outer medulla. Several weaknesses have been noted:

1. The descending limbs of short loops are anatomically separated from ascending limbs, with inner stripe portions of short loops near (or within) the vascular bundles and thick limbs near the collecting ducts.[23,62] This configuration is not consistent with direct interactions between counterflowing limbs.
2. In short-looped rat nephrons, Wade and associates found that AQP1 is not expressed in portions of descending limb segments in the distal inner stripe.[5] Zhai and colleagues found that AQP1 is not expressed in descending limbs of short loops in the inner stripes of mice, rats, and humans.[15] The absence of AQP1 suggests that the assumption of high water permeability in descending limbs of short loops merits further experimental study. (Dantzler and coworkers have found that the AQP1-null segments of descending limbs in the inner medulla are essentially impermeable to water.[63])
3. Using transport rates based on measured sodium-potassium adenosine triphosphatase (Na$^+$-K$^+$-ATPase) activities, mathematical models predict substantial transepithelial NaCl gradients along the medullary portions

must be maintained; thus, for example, concentrated fluid that flows into the inner medulla must be balanced by dilute fluid that, in the presence of vasopressin, is absorbed from the cortical collecting duct, dilutes the cortical interstitial fluid, enters the cortical vasculature, and thus participates in maintaining an appropriate systemic level of blood plasma osmolality.

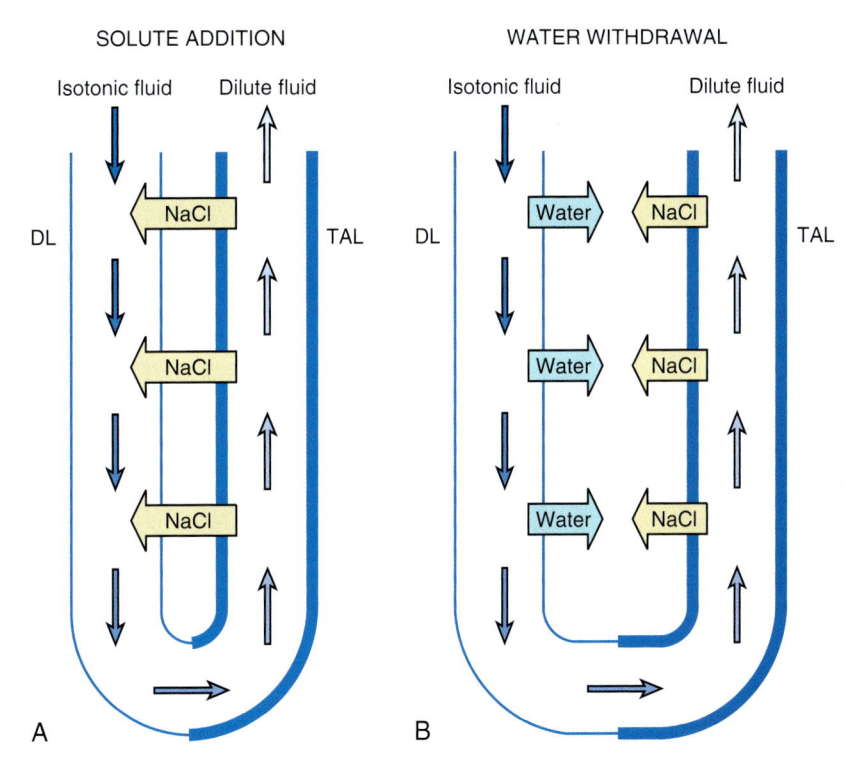

Figure 10.9 A, Countercurrent multiplication by means of NaCl transfer from an ascending flow to a descending flow. **B,** Countercurrent multiplication by means of water withdrawal from a descending flow. NaCl transport from the ascending flow into the interstitium raises interstitial osmolality; this results in passive water transport from the descending flow, which has lower osmolality than the interstitium. In both panels, tubule fluid flow direction is indicated by *blue arrows*; increasing osmolality is indicated by *darkening shades of blue*. Ascending flow may be considered to be in the thick ascending limb of Henle (TAL) and descending flow in the descending limb of Henle (DL). *Thick blue lines* indicate that a tubule is impermeable to water; *thin lines* indicate high permeability to water.

of thick limbs[64]; this seems contrary to the notion of a small single effect.
4. It may well be that the concentrating mechanism of the outer medulla is placed under increased load, not less, if it has to concentrate water flowing in, and absorbed from, the descending limbs of short loops.[65]
5. The absorption of water from the outer medullary portions of long loops has sometimes been considered to participate in a generalized form of countercurrent multiplication, and this may be the case for long loops that extend for sufficiently short distances into the inner medulla. However, in sufficiently long loops, tubule fluid is likely to be much altered by urea secretion and passive NaCl absorption within the inner medulla.

From these considerations, it seems reasonable therefore to hypothesize that the outer medullary osmolality gradient arises principally from vigorous active transport of NaCl, without accompanying water, from the thick ascending limbs of short- and long-looped nephrons. The tubule fluid of the thick limbs that enters the cortex is diluted well below plasma osmolality, and thus, the requirement of mass balance is met. In rats and mice, the thick limbs are localized near the collecting ducts[66]; mathematical models suggest that at a given level of the outer medulla, the interstitial osmolality will be higher near the collecting ducts than near the vascular bundles.[64,65] This higher osmolality will facilitate water withdrawal from the descending limbs of long loops and from collecting ducts. Descending vasa recta are thought to be found only in the vascular bundles. Thus the ascending vasa recta will act as the collectors of any NaCl that is absorbed from loops of Henle and water that is absorbed from the descending limbs of long loops and from collecting ducts.

The countercurrent configuration of the ascending vasa recta, relative to the descending limbs and collecting ducts, is likely to participate in sustaining the axial gradient: as ascending vasa recta fluid ascends toward the cortex, its osmolality will exceed that in the descending limbs of long loops and in the collecting ducts. Thus ascending vasa recta fluid will be progressively diluted as that fluid contributes to the concentrating of fluid in descending limbs of long loops and in collecting ducts, by giving up NaCl to, and absorbing water from, the interstitium (Figure 10.10).

The previous summary appears to account for the elevation of osmolality in the outer medulla without invoking a role for countercurrent multiplication. However, a question remains: why does the osmolality gradient increase along the outer medulla as a function of increasing medullary depth? The answer likely lies in the local balance of NaCl absorption from thick limbs and water absorption from descending limbs of long loops and from collecting ducts. At deeper medullary levels, the rate of NaCl absorption from thick limbs may be higher than at shallow levels, owing to a higher Na^+-K^+-ATPase activity at deeper levels and to a saturation of transport proteins by the higher NaCl concentration in thick limb tubule fluid before dilution.[67] Moreover, because of the water already absorbed in the upper outer medulla, the load of water presented to the thick limbs deep in the outer medulla by descending limbs of long loops and by the collecting ducts is much reduced.

A caveat is in order. Our understanding of the outer medulla is mostly based on information obtained from heavily studied laboratory animals, especially rats and mice. Outer medullary function and structure are likely to vary substantially in other species. For example, the human kidney has limited concentrating capability (relative to many other mammals), and only approximately one seventh of the loops of Henle are long[68]; the mountain beaver *(Aplodontia rufa)* has mostly cortical loops of Henle and essentially

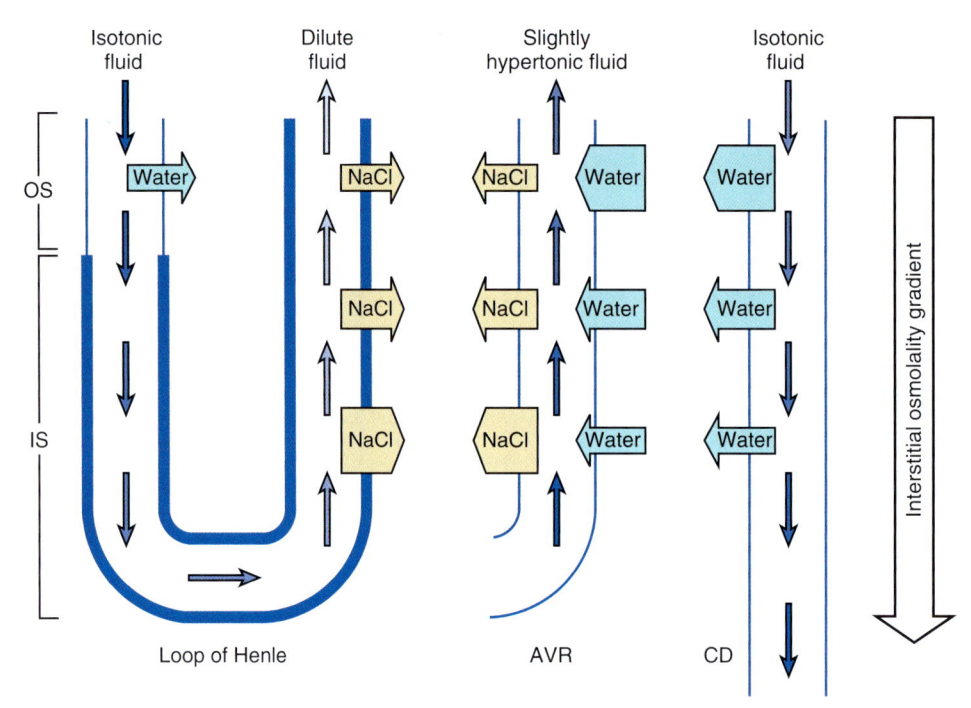

Figure 10.10 **Outer medullary concentrating mechanism based on NaCl addition to the interstitium but without water absorption from descending limbs of short loops.** *Arrows* indicate water *(cyan)* and NaCl *(yellow)* transepithelial transport; *arrow widths* suggest relative transport magnitudes. Isotonic fluid is considered to have the same osmolality as blood plasma. Flow entering the ascending vas rectum (AVR) is assumed to arise from a descending vas rectum that is in, or near, a vascular bundle. Outflow from collecting duct (CD) enters the inner medullary CD. Tubule fluid flow direction is indicated by *blue arrows*; increasing osmolality is indicated by *darkening shades of blue*. *Thick blue lines* indicate that a tubule is impermeable to water; *thin lines* indicate high permeability to water. IS, inner stripe; OS, Outer stripe.

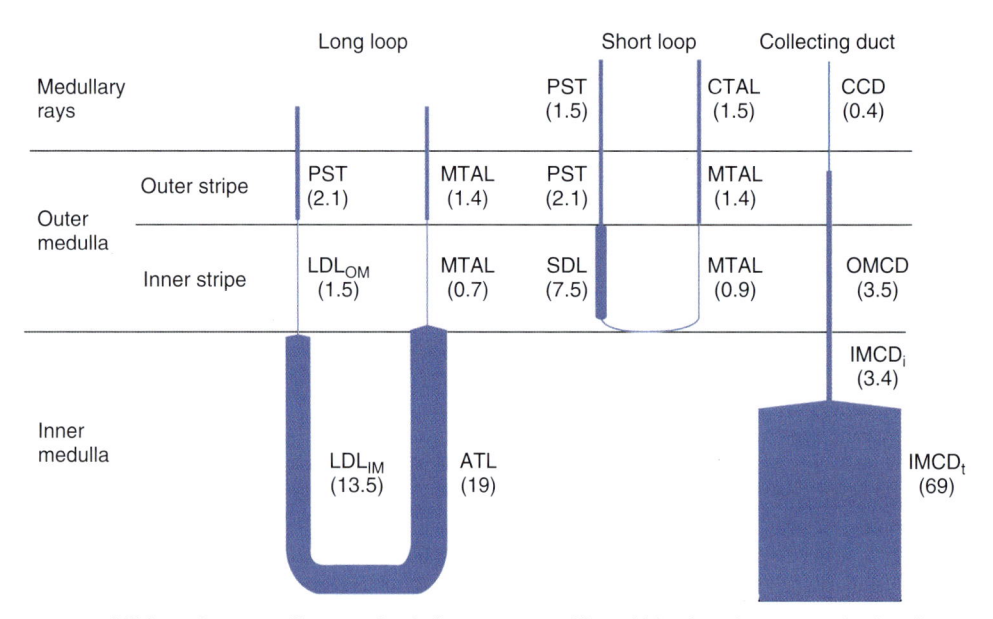

Figure 10.11 **Urea permeabilities of mammalian renal tubule segments.** The width of each segment in the diagram is distorted to be proportional to the urea permeability of that segment. Numbers in parentheses are measured values for the permeability coefficient ($\times 10^{-5}$ cm/sec). Values are from isolated perfused tubule studies. ATL, Ascending thin limb; CCD, cortical collecting duct; CTAL, cortical thick ascending limb; IMCDi, initial inner medullary collecting duct; IMCDt, terminal inner medullary collecting duct; LDL, long-loop thin descending limb; MTAL, medullary thick ascending limb; OMCD, outer medullary collecting duct; PST, proximal straight tubule; SDL, short descending limb.

no inner medulla.[69] It seems likely that the outer medullary structure in these species differs substantially from that in rats and mice. Finally, it should be acknowledged that the paradigm formulated earlier is similar to that proposed by Berliner and coworkers in 1958.[37]

ACCUMULATION OF UREA IN THE RENAL INNER MEDULLA

Urea accumulation within the inner medulla is partly dependent on variable urea permeabilities along the collecting duct system (Figure 10.11). Within the collecting duct system, only the terminal portion of the IMCD possesses high urea permeability,[70] which can be further increased by vasopressin.[55,71,72] The effects of vasopressin are mediated (at least in part) by the secondary messenger cyclic adenosine monophosphate (cAMP).[73] Urea-specific transporters are localized to the apical and basolateral plasma membranes of the IMCD cells and are responsible for the high urea permeability of the terminal portion of the IMCD.

The mechanisms of urea accumulation in the renal medulla are depicted in Figure 10.12. Accumulation of urea is predominantly a result of passive urea reabsorption from the IMCD. Tubule fluid entering the collecting duct system in the renal cortex has a relatively low urea concentration. However, during antidiuresis, water is osmotically reabsorbed from the urea-impermeable parts of the collecting duct system in the cortex and outer medulla, causing a progressive increase in the luminal urea concentration along the connecting tubules, cortical collecting ducts, and outer medullary collecting ducts. Thus, when the tubule fluid reaches the highly urea-permeable terminal IMCD (due to the presence of urea transporters), urea rapidly exits from the lumen to the inner medullary interstitium, where it is "trapped" by countercurrent urea exchange between descending and ascending flows in both vasa recta and loops of Henle. Under steady-state conditions, and in the continued presence of vasopressin, urea nearly equilibrates across the IMCD epithelium and thus osmotically balances the urea in the collecting duct lumen, preventing possible instances of osmotic diuresis (Figure 10.13).

The descending and ascending vasa recta are in close association with each other in the inner medulla, facilitating countercurrent exchange of urea between the two structures.[37] In the ascending vasa recta, aided by the extremely high ($>40 \times 10^{-5}$ cm/sec) permeability to urea, the concentration of urea exiting the inner medulla is similar to the concentration of urea in the descending vasa recta.[35,55] This minimizes the washout of urea from the inner medulla. However, countercurrent exchange cannot completely eliminate loss of urea from the inner medullary interstitium, because the volume flow rate of blood in the ascending vasa recta exceeds that in the descending vasa recta.[74] During antidiuresis, water is added to the vasa recta from both IMCDs and descending limbs, resulting in a higher volume flow rate and an increased mass flow rate of urea. This ensures that the inner medullary vasculature continually

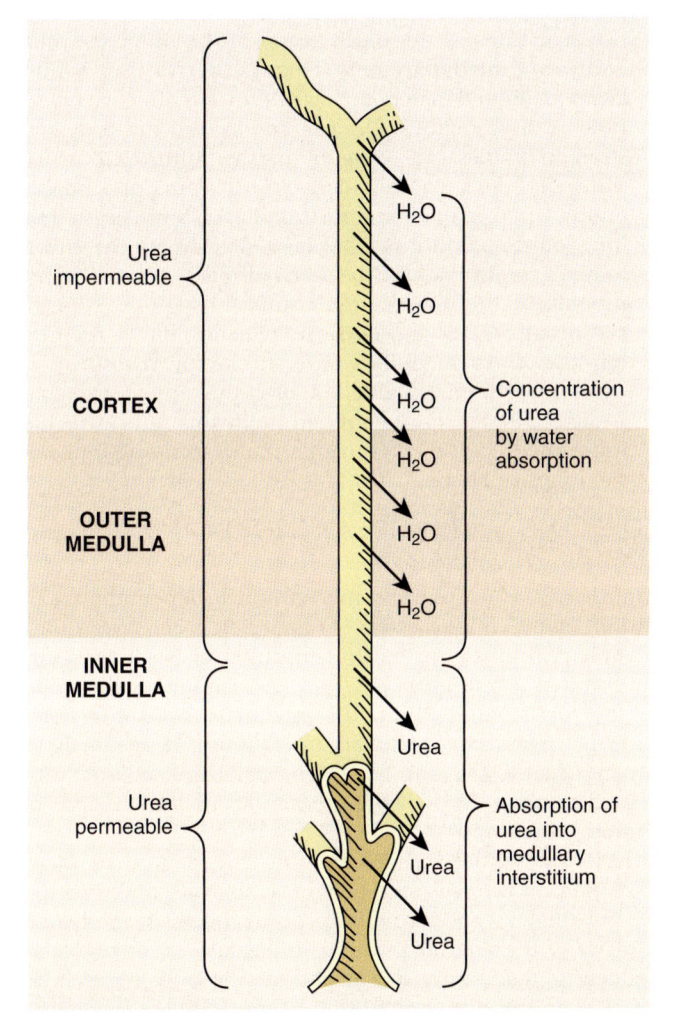

Figure 10.12 **Schematic representation of the mammalian collecting duct system showing principal sites of water absorption and urea absorption.** Water is absorbed in the early part of the collecting duct system, driven by an osmotic gradient. Because urea permeabilities of the cortical collecting duct, outer medullary collecting duct, and initial inner medullary collecting duct (IMCD) are very low, the water absorption concentrates urea in the lumen of these segments. When the tubule fluid reaches the terminal IMCD, which is highly permeable to urea, urea rapidly exits from the lumen. This urea is trapped in the inner medulla as a result of countercurrent exchange.

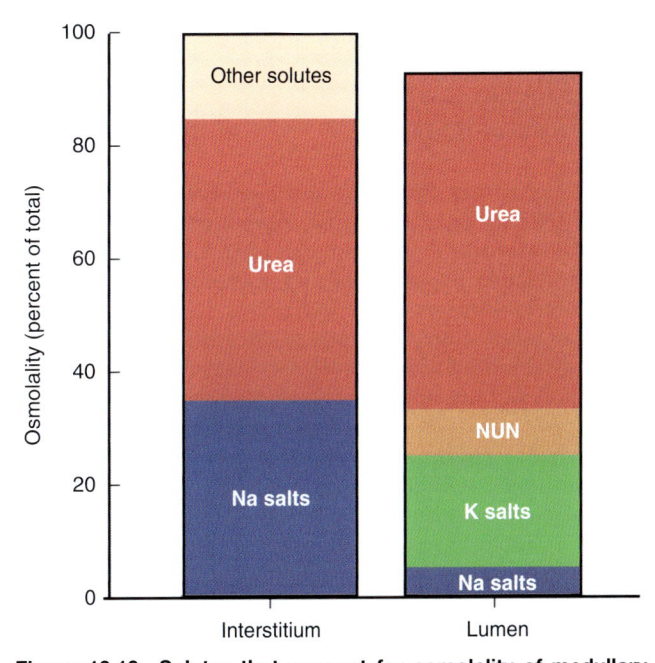

Figure 10.13 **Solutes that account for osmolality of medullary interstitium and tubule fluid in the inner medullary collecting duct (IMCD) during antidiuresis in rats.** Urea nearly equilibrates across the IMCD epithelium as a result of rapid facilitated urea transport. Although the osmolalities of the fluid in the two spaces are nearly equal, the nonurea solutes can differ considerably between the two compartments. Typical values in untreated rats are presented. Values can differ considerably in other species and in the same species with different diets. NUN, Nonurea nitrogen.

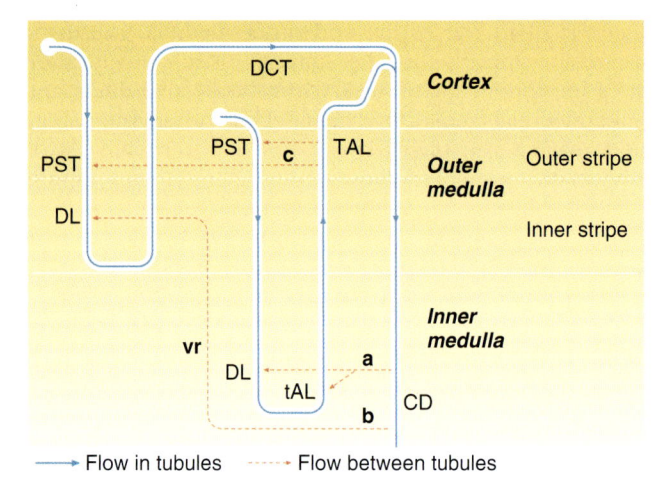

Figure 10.14 Pathways of urea recycling in renal medulla. *Solid blue lines* represent a short-looped nephron **(left)** and a long-looped nephron **(right)**. Transfer of urea between nephron segments is indicated by *dashed red arrows* labeled *a*, *b*, and *c*, corresponding to recycling pathways described in the text. CD, Collecting duct; DCT, distal convoluted tubule; DL, descending limb; PST, proximal straight tubule; TAL, thick ascending limb; tAL, thin ascending limb; vr, vasa recta. (From Knepper MA, Roch-Ramel F: Pathways of urea transport in the mammalian kidney. *Kidney Int* 31:629-633, 1987.)

removes urea from the inner medulla. Quantitatively, the most important loss of urea from the inner medullary interstitium is thought to occur via the vasa recta,[75] but urea recycling pathways play a major role in limiting the loss of urea from the inner medulla. These pathways have been further elucidated via the use of knockout mouse models (see later).[76-78] Three major urea recycling pathways are described in the following list, and an overview of these is shown in Figure 10.14.

1. *Recycling of urea through the ascending limbs, distal tubules, and collecting ducts.* Urea that escapes the inner medulla in the ascending limbs of the long loops of Henle is carried back through the thick ascending limbs, DCTs, and early portions of the collecting duct system by the flow of tubule fluid.[49] When it reaches the urea-permeable part of the IMCDs, it passively exits into the inner medullary interstitium and starts the cycle again.
2. *Recycling of urea through the vasa recta, short loops of Henle, and collecting ducts.* The delivery of urea to the superficial distal tubule exceeds the delivery out of the superficial proximal tubule.[49,79,80] This implies that net urea addition occurs somewhere along the short loops of Henle. One possible mechanism is that the urea leaving the inner medulla in the vasa recta is transferred to the descending limbs of the short loops of Henle and is subsequently carried through the superficial distal tubules back to the urea-permeable part of the IMCDs,[79] where it passively exits, completing the recycling pathway. The close physical association between the vasa recta and the descending limbs of the short loops in the vascular bundles of the inner stripe of the outer medulla would facilitate this transfer of urea from the vasa recta to the short loops of Henle.[26,81] Furthermore, the existence of a facilitative urea transporter, UT-A2, in the thin descending limb of the short loops of Henle provides further support for this mechanism.[5,82] However, later studies on UT-A2 knockout mice and UT-A2/UT-B knockout mice have raised doubts about the importance of this pathway.[83,84]
3. *Urea recycling between ascending and descending limbs of the loops of Henle.* The urea permeability of thick ascending limbs from the inner stripe of the outer medulla is low.[85,86] However, the urea permeability of thick ascending limbs from the outer stripe of the outer medulla and the medullary rays is relatively high.[85,87] Based on this, a urea recycling pathway has been proposed in which urea is reabsorbed from thick ascending limbs and is secreted into neighboring proximal straight tubules, forming a recycling pathway between the ascending limbs and the descending limbs of the loop of Henle.[1,75] Urea recycling from the thick ascending limbs and the proximal straight tubules is facilitated by the parallel relationship of these two structures in the outer stripe of the outer medulla and in the medullary rays. This transfer of urea is also likely to depend on a relatively attenuated effective blood flow in these regions. Urea secretion into the proximal straight tubules can occur by passive diffusion,[87] active transport,[88] or a combination of both. Urea presumably enters the proximal straight tubules of both short- and long-looped nephrons. The urea that enters the short-looped nephrons will be carried back to the inner medulla by the flow of tubule fluid through the superficial distal tubules and cortical collecting ducts, reentering the inner medullary interstitium by reabsorption from the terminal IMCD. The urea that enters proximal straight tubules of long-looped nephrons returns to the inner medulla directly through the descending limbs of the loops of Henle.[75]

COLLECTING DUCT WATER ABSORPTION AND OSMOTIC EQUILIBRATION

The urinary concentrating mechanism is dependent upon two independent processes: (1) generation of a hypertonic medullary interstitium by concentration of NaCl and urea via countercurrent processes, and (2) osmotic equilibration of the tubule fluid within the medullary collecting ducts with the hypertonic medullary interstitium. In reality these two processes are not truly separable, particularly with regard to urea. The following describes the mechanism of osmotic equilibration.

AVP is essential for determining the degree of water excretion for two reasons: (1) it increases NaCl reabsorption via the thick ascending limb and thus increases the hypertonicity of the medullary interstitium; and (2) it regulates collecting duct water permeability, allowing removal of water from the tubule fluid via diffusion. When circulating vasopressin levels are low, for example during water diuresis, the water permeability of the collecting ducts is also extremely low and relatively little water is reabsorbed from the tubule fluid. The dilute tubule fluid that exits from the loops of Henle remains dilute as it passes through the collecting duct system, yielding a large volume of hypotonic urine. In contrast, high circulating levels of vasopressin increase the water permeability of the collecting ducts to very high levels. At the same time, vasopressin increases the permeability of the apical membrane of the thick ascending limb to NaCl, leading to an increase in the osmolality of the peritubular interstitium (due to countercurrent multiplication). These effects combined result in water being rapidly reabsorbed from the cortical and outer medullary portions of the collecting duct system via aquaporin water channels (discussed later), resulting in the production of a small volume of hypertonic urine, with osmolality approaching that of the inner medullary interstitium.

Micropuncture studies indicate that the late distal tubule (the late DCT, the connecting tubule, and the initial collecting tubule) is the earliest site along the renal tubule where water absorption increases during antidiuresis (see Figure 10.7).[89] Although the DCT does not express any water channels, it does express V_2R, and vasopressin regulates NaCl transport in this segment via increasing the activity of the NaCl transport protein, Na-Cl cotransporter (NCC).[90,91] In contrast, the connecting tubule and the cortical collecting duct express the V_2R and the vasopressin-regulated water channel AQP2.[92] Thus it is likely that the connecting tubule and the cortical collecting duct segments are the earliest sites of distal tubular osmotic equilibration.

The volume of water absorption in the connecting segment and initial collecting tubule required to raise tubule fluid to isotonicity is considerably greater than the additional amount required to concentrate the urine above the osmolality of plasma in the medullary portion of the collecting duct system.[1] Consequently, during antidiuresis most of the water reabsorbed from the collecting duct system enters the cortical labyrinth, where the effective blood flow is high enough to return the reabsorbed water to the general circulation without diluting the interstitium. In contrast, if such a large volume of water were reabsorbed along the medullary collecting ducts, it would have a significant dilution effect on the medullary interstitium and thus impair concentrating ability.[93,94]

During water diuresis a modest corticomedullary osmolality gradient persists,[95,96] and the water permeability of the collecting ducts is low but not zero.[72,97] Consequently, some water is reabsorbed by the collecting ducts during water diuresis, driven by the small transepithelial osmolality gradient. The majority of this water reabsorption occurs in the terminal IMCDs, where the transepithelial osmolality gradient is highest. In fact, more water is absorbed from the terminal IMCDs during water diuresis than during antidiuresis owing to a much greater transepithelial osmolality gradient.[93] Water reabsorption from the IMCDs is thought to contribute to the reduction of the medullary interstitial osmolality during water diuresis due to its dilutional effect.[94,98]

DETERMINANTS OF CONCENTRATING ABILITY

The overall concentrating ability of the kidney arises from interactions among several differing components. In addition to the active transport of NaCl from the thick ascending limbs and the water permeability of the collecting ducts, two other factors play a significant role in determining the osmolality of the final urine. One important determinant is the delivery rate of NaCl and water to the loop of Henle, which sets an upper limit on the amount of NaCl actively reabsorbed by the thick ascending limb to drive the outer medullary concentrating mechanism. Another important determinant is the volume of tubule fluid delivered to the medullary collecting duct, which has an underappreciated effect on the concentrating process. Too much fluid delivery saturates water reabsorption processes along the medullary collecting ducts, leading to interstitial dilution due to rapid osmotic water transport. In contrast, too little fluid delivery to the medullary collecting ducts, even in the absence of vasopressin, results in sustained osmotic equilibration across the collecting duct epithelium owing to the nonzero osmotic water permeability of the IMCD.[72,93,97]

AN UNRESOLVED QUESTION: CONCENTRATION OF SODIUM CHLORIDE IN THE RENAL INNER MEDULLA

Tissue slice studies have demonstrated that the corticomedullary osmolality gradient is made up largely of a NaCl gradient in the outer medulla and a urea gradient in the inner medulla (see Figure 10.8). Accordingly, in the previous sections we have emphasized the processes that concentrate NaCl in the outer medulla and the processes responsible for urea accumulation in the inner medulla (passive urea absorption from the IMCD plus countercurrent exchange of urea via diffusion). The concentrating mechanism described earlier functions only in the renal outer medulla and medullary rays of the cortex. The ascending limbs of the loops of Henle that reach into the inner medulla are thin walled and do not actively transport NaCl[55,99,100]; nonetheless, in antidiuresis a substantial axial osmolality gradient is generated in the inner medulla of many mammals. For nearly 50 years, controversy has persisted regarding the nature of the mechanism that generates the inner medullary osmolality gradient. Moreover, the energy source for the concentrating of nonurea solutes in the inner medullary interstitium is not known. General analysis of inner medullary concentrating processes indicates that, to satisfy mass balance requirements, either an ascending stream (thin ascending limbs or ascending vasa recta) must be diluted relative to the inner medullary interstitium, or a descending stream (descending thin limbs, descending vasa recta, or collecting ducts) must be concentrated locally relative to the inner medulla.[40,101]

Three major hypotheses have been proposed for the concentrating mechanism of the inner medulla:

1. The "passive" countercurrent mechanism of Kokko and Rector and of Stephenson,[102,103] in which the absorption of urea and accompanying water from the IMCDs results in a transepithelial NaCl gradient that promotes NaCl absorption from the water-impermeable ascending thin limbs without a significant compensatory secretion of urea into those limbs
2. The external solute hypothesis, proposed by Jen and Stephenson and extended by Thomas and colleagues,[104-107] in which a net generation of osmotically active particles in the inner medulla raises the osmolality of the inner medulla
3. The mechano-osmotic induction hypothesis,[40,108] in which energy from the peristaltic contractions of the renal pelvic wall is used to concentrate solutes in the descending limbs and collecting ducts by water withdrawal, or, alternatively, the peristaltic contractions reduce sodium activity in the hyaluronan matrix of the interstitium resulting in the reabsorption of hypotonic fluid from that matrix into ascending vasa recta

These hypotheses are described in more detail in the following sections.

The "Passive Mechanism"

Kokko and Rector and Stephenson simultaneously and independently proposed a model by which the osmolality in the thin ascending limb could be lowered below that of the interstitium entirely by passive transport processes in the inner medulla.[102,103] This mechanism is generally referred to as the "passive model" or the "passive countercurrent multiplier mechanism." The passive mechanism depends on the separation of urea and NaCl that is accomplished by NaCl absorption from the thick ascending limbs; indeed, this absorption is the hypothesized energy source for the passive mechanism. In this model, rapid urea reabsorption from the IMCD generates and maintains a high urea concentration in the inner medullary interstitium, causing the osmotic withdrawal of water from the thin descending limb. This concentrates NaCl in the *descending* limb lumen and results in a transepithelial gradient favoring the passive reabsorption of NaCl from the thin *ascending* limb of Henle's loop. In addition, if the ascending limbs have extremely low urea permeability, then any NaCl that has been reabsorbed from the ascending thin limb will not be replaced by urea. Thus the ascending limb fluid will be dilute relative to the fluid in other nephron segments generating a "single effect" analogous to active NaCl absorption from thick ascending limbs. This single effect can then be multiplied by the counterflow between the ascending and descending limbs of the loops of Henle. This model requires that the thin descending limbs be highly permeable to water but not NaCl or urea, whereas the thin ascending limb would have to be permeable to NaCl but not water or urea. Several objections to the passive mechanism have been made, both because of the high urea permeabilities that have been measured in the thin descending limb and thin ascending limb (summarized in Gamba and Knepper),[109] and studies in urea transporter knockout mice in which urea accumulation in the inner medulla was largely eliminated, but inner medullary NaCl accumulation was not affected (discussed in the "UT-A1/3 Urea Transporter Knockout Mice" section).[92,110,111]

Layton and colleagues reevaluated the passive mechanism in the context of the emerging information coming from the studies by Pannabecker and Dantzler.[112] This study showed that water absorption from descending limbs was not a requirement for the passive mechanism to generate an osmolality gradient. That study also identified a second concentrating passive mode in which the loops of Henle are highly urea permeable and serve as a highly effective countercurrent urea exchanger. However, neither mode was able to fully account for the high urine osmolalities attained by some animals.

Nawata and colleagues, by means of isolated perfused tubule studies conducted using with tubules taken from Munich-Wistar rats,[113] found that lower portions of long-loop thin descending limbs in the inner medulla (approximately 2.5 mm in length) have little or no osmotic water permeability but exhibit high urea permeability (e.g., ≈200 × 10^{-5} cm/sec). Conversely, upper thin descending limb segments (those extending approximately 0.5 to 2.5 mm below the outer medulla) exhibited high osmotic water permeability (e.g., ≈3200 μm/sec) and low urea permeability (e.g., 40 × 10^{-5} cm/sec). Long-loop thin ascending limbs, which have previously been shown to exhibit no water permeability,[114] were found to have high urea permeability (e.g., ≈204 × 10^{-5} cm/sec) in the upper thin ascending limbs and somewhat higher urea permeability (e.g., 265 × 10^{-5} cm/sec) in the lower thin ascending limbs. The significance of these findings is that they are inconsistent with the passive mechanism for concentrating the inner medulla proposed by Kokko and Rector and by Stephenson,[102,103] because the passive mechanism requires that thin descending limbs in the inner medulla have high water permeability whereas thin ascending limbs are required to have low urea permeability (much less than the NaCl permeability in thin ascending limbs).

Concentrating Mechanism Driven by External Solute

Jen and Stephenson proposed that the concentrating mechanism of the inner medulla depends on a solute other than NaCl and urea.[104] By means of a mathematical model, they demonstrated, in principle, that the continuous addition of small amounts of an unspecified, but osmotically active, solute to the inner medullary interstitium could produce a substantial axial osmolality gradient. Such a solute would have to be generated in the inner medulla by a chemical reaction that produces more osmotically active particles than it consumes. The mechanism of concentration is similar to that driven by urea in the "passive" models proposed by Kokko and Rector and by Stephenson: the thin descending limbs of inner medulla are assumed impermeable to the solute (thus it is an "external" solute), and as a result, water is withdrawn from the descending limbs and the concentration of NaCl is raised in descending limb tubule fluid.[102,103] Beginning at the loop bend, elevated NaCl concentration within the loop will result in a substantial NaCl efflux that will dilute the ascending flow and that is sufficient to generate the axial gradient.

The feasibility of this mechanism was subsequently confirmed by Thomas and Wexler in the context of a more detailed mathematical model.[107] In further modeling studies, Thomas and Hervy proposed that lactate, generated by anaerobic glycolysis (the predominant means of adenosine triphosphate [ATP] generation in the inner medulla), could serve as the solute.[105,106] Two lactate ions are generated per glucose consumed:

$$\text{glucose} \rightarrow 2 \text{ lactate-} + 2\, H^+$$

However, as pointed out by Knepper and colleagues,[40] the net generation of osmotically active particles depends on which buffering anions are titrated by the protons. If the protons titrate bicarbonate, there may be a net removal of osmotically active particles; if instead the protons titrate other buffers (e.g., phosphate or NH_3), there will be a net generation of osmotically active particles.

A mathematical model developed by Zhang and Edwards predicted that vascular countercurrent exchange would tend to restrict significant glucose availability into the outer medulla and the upper inner medulla,[116] thus limiting the rate of lactate generation in the deep inner medulla where the highest osmolalities are found. Findings by Dantzler and associates present an additional challenge to the external solute hypothesis: in a perfused tubule study, they found that the deepest 60% of inner medullary thin descending limbs (those limb portions that lack measurable AQP1) have essentially no osmotic water permeability.[63]

Hyaluronan as a Mechano-osmotic Transducer

Hyaluronan (or hyaluronic acid) is a glycosaminoglycan (GAG). GAGs consist of unbranched polysaccharide chains composed of repeating disaccharide units. In contrast to other GAGs, which are produced in the Golgi apparatus, hyaluronan is synthesized at the plasma membrane by an integral membrane protein, hyaluronan synthase (HAS).[117,118] Three mammalian HAS genes have been identified: *HAS1*, *HAS2*, and *HAS3*. All three HAS proteins produce hyaluronan on the cytoplasmic side of the plasma membrane and transport it across the plasma membrane to the extracellular space. Because of the importance of GAGs in the structure of connective tissues (e.g., cartilage, tendon, bone, synovial fluid, intervertebral disks, and skin), the physiochemical properties of GCGs have been extensively investigated.[119]

Hyaluronan is abundant in the interstitium of the renal inner medulla.[120,121] Other GAGs are also present, but in much lower amounts. The hyaluronan in the inner medulla is produced by a specialized interstitial cell (the type 1 interstitial cell), which forms characteristic "bridges" between the thin limbs of Henle and the vasa recta.[122] These bridges may delimit, above and below, the nodal compartments identified by Pannabecker and Dantzler.[29] Thus the inner medullary interstitium may be considered to be composed of a compressible, viscoelastic, hyaluronan matrix.

Several hypotheses have been advanced that depend on the peristalsis of the papilla as an integral component of the concentrating mechanism of the inner medulla.[78,123] Knepper and colleagues proposed that the periodic compression of the papilla, and the effects of that compression on the hyaluronan matrix, could explain the osmolality gradient along the inner medulla.[40]

Two hypotheses were proposed. In the first hypothesis, which was suggested in part by Schmidt-Nielsen,[124] compression of the hyaluronan matrix stores some of the mechanical energy from the smooth muscle contraction that gives rise to the peristaltic wave. In the postwave decompression, the matrix exerts an elastic force that promotes water absorption from thin descending limbs and collecting ducts and thereby increases tubule fluid osmolality. Water absorption from the descending limbs would raise tubule fluid NaCl concentration and thus promote a vigorous NaCl absorption from the loop bends and early ascending limbs. However, if, as is apparently the case in the rat, the lower 60% of inner medullary descending limbs are water impermeable,[63,113] water is unlikely to be absorbed from descending limbs in the deep portion of the inner medulla where the highest osmolalities are achieved.

The second hypothesis involves special properties of hyaluronan.[125] Hyaluronan is a large polyanion (1000 to 10,000 kDa). Its charge is due to the carboxylate (COO) groups of the glucuronic subunits. Hyaluronan is hydrophilic and assumes a highly expanded, random-coil confirmation that occupies a large volume of space relative to its mass. This extended state arises partly from electrostatic repulsion between carboxylate groups (which maximize the distances between neighboring negative charges) and partly from the extended conformations of the glycosidic bonds.

When hyaluronan is compressed, the repulsive forces of neighboring carboxylate groups are overcome in part by a condensation of cations (mainly Na^+), and a localized crystalloid structure is formed. Thus compression of the hyaluronan gel results in a decrease of the local sodium ion activity in the gel.[40] In aqueous solutions that are in equilibrium with the gel, the NaCl concentration will decrease as a consequence of the compression-induced reduction in Na^+ activity within the gel. Therefore, the free fluid that is expressed from the hyaluronan matrix during the contraction phase will have a lower total solute concentration than that of the gel as a whole. The slightly hypotonic fluid expressed from the matrix is likely to escape the inner medulla via the ascending vasa recta, the only structure that remains open during the compressive phase of the contraction cycle.[124] As a consequence, the ascending fluid within ascending vasa recta would have a lower osmolality than the local interstitium, and therefore, fluid in collecting ducts and descending vasa recta would be concentrated.

This mechanism is consistent with the nodal compartments found by Pannabecker and Dantzler: these compartments, which are likely rich in hyaluronan, are in contact with collecting ducts, thin ascending limbs, and ascending vasa recta.[29] Thus they are well configured to be sites of transduction, that is, sites where the mechanical energy of peristalsis is harnessed to generate an ascending flow that is dilute relative to average local osmolality. However, no quantitative analyses or mathematical models have examined the mass balance consistency or the thermodynamic adequacy of hypotheses that depend on the peristaltic contractions.

MOLECULAR PHYSIOLOGY OF URINARY CONCENTRATING AND DILUTING PROCESSES

Figure 10.15 shows a schematic representation of the mammalian nephron with the localization of major water channels (aquaporins), urea transporters, and ion transporters important to the urinary concentrating process. Figure 10.16 shows which of these transporters and channels are molecular targets for regulated vasopressin action, either in abundance or activity, and thus likely to play a role in urine concentration. The function and regulation of several of these transporters are explained in detail elsewhere in this book, with Chapter 11 providing a detailed discussion of the cell biology of vasopressin action.

The functions of several of the transporters and channels shown in Figure 10.15 have been evaluated in mice using gene deletion techniques (see Fenton and Knepper for a comprehensive review of these mouse models and other knockout models with urinary concentrating defects).[84] The phenotypes of these mice have been informative with regard to the role of these proteins in the urinary concentrating and diluting mechanisms. A brief overview of the studies in these mice with respect to the urinary concentrating mechanism is provided here.

AQUAPORIN-1 KNOCKOUT MICE

AQP1 is abundantly expressed in and responsible for water reabsorption along the proximal tubule and the descending

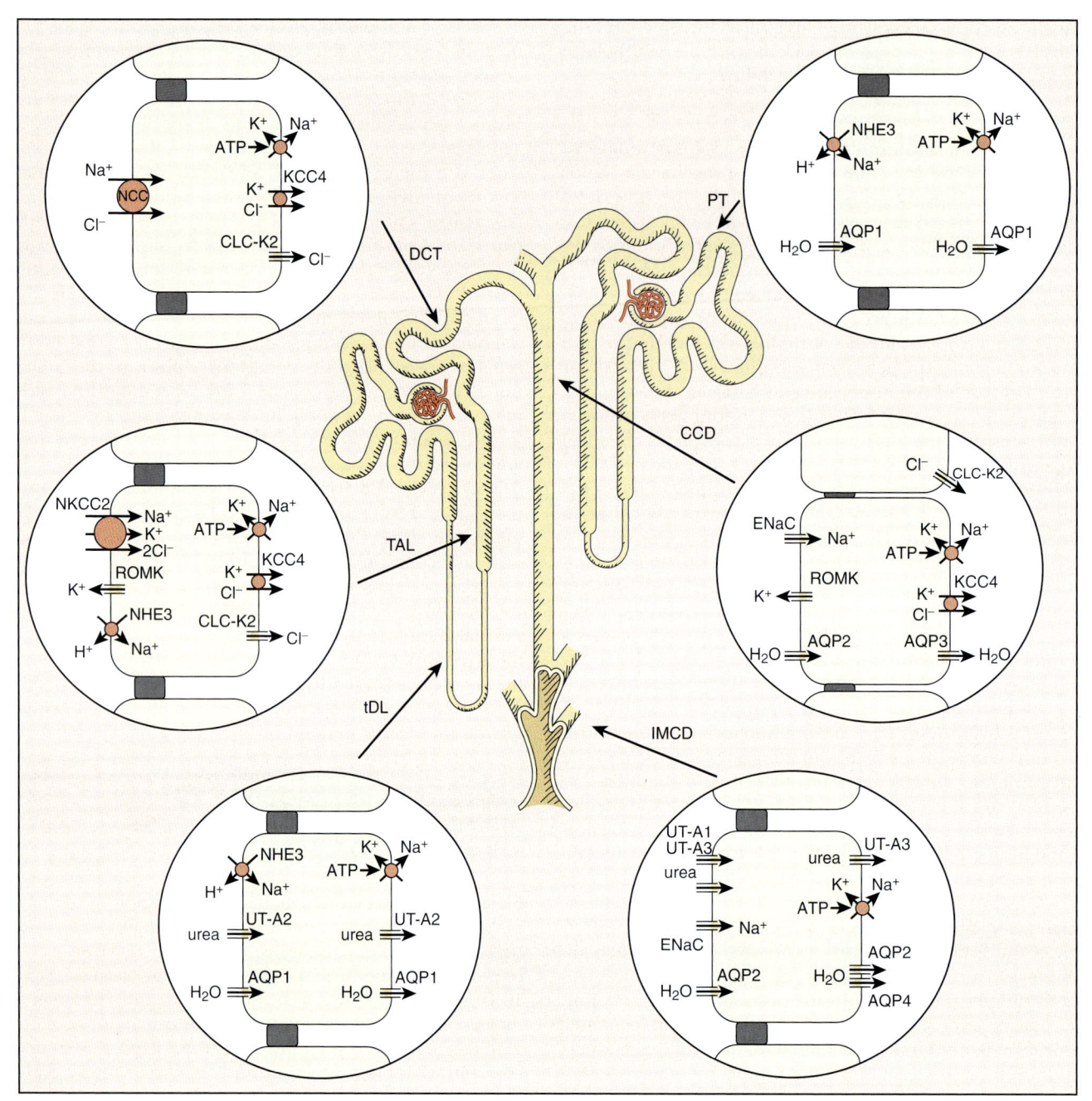

Figure 10.15 Major aquaporins, urea transporters, and ion transporters/channels that are important to the urinary concentrating and diluting process. Schematic overview of a mammalian kidney tubule, showing the solute and water transport pathways in the proximal tubule (PT), thin descending limb of the loop of Henle (tDL), thick ascending limb (TAL), distal convoluted tubule (DCT), cortical collecting duct (CCD), and inner medullary collecting duct (IMCD). Tubule lumen side is always on the left-hand side of the cell, whereas the interstitium is on the right-hand side. *Arrows* represent direction of movement. (See text for details.) AQP1, Aquaporin-1; ATP, adenosine triphosphate; ClC-K2, kidney-specific chloride channel 2; ENaC, epithelial sodium channel; KCC4, K+-Cl− cotransporter 4; NHE3, Na+-H+-exchanger isoform 3; NKCC2, Na-K-2Cl cotransporter type 2; ROMK, renal outer medullary potassium. (Adapted from Fenton RA, Knepper MA: Mouse models and the urinary concentrating mechanism in the new millennium. *Physiol Rev* 87:1083-1112, 2007.)

limbs of long-looped nephrons.[7,126,127] However, AQP1 is absent along the entire length of thin descending limbs of 90% of short-looped nephrons,[15] suggesting that the mechanisms of water transport in the thin descending limbs of short-looped nephrons and the roles of AQP1 in the countercurrent multiplier and water conservation may need to be readdressed. AQP1 knockout mice have increased urine volume and reduced urinary osmolality that does not increase in response to water deprivation.[128] The concentrating defect is so severe that their average body weight decreases by 35% and serum osmolality increases to greater than 500 mOsm/kg H$_2$O after 36 hours of water deprivation. Proximal tubule fluid absorption is markedly impaired in AQP1 knockout mice, but distal delivery of water and NaCl is not impaired due to a reduction in glomerular filtration rate (GFR) via the tubular-glomerular feedback mechanism.[129] The osmotic

CHAPTER 10 — URINE CONCENTRATION AND DILUTION

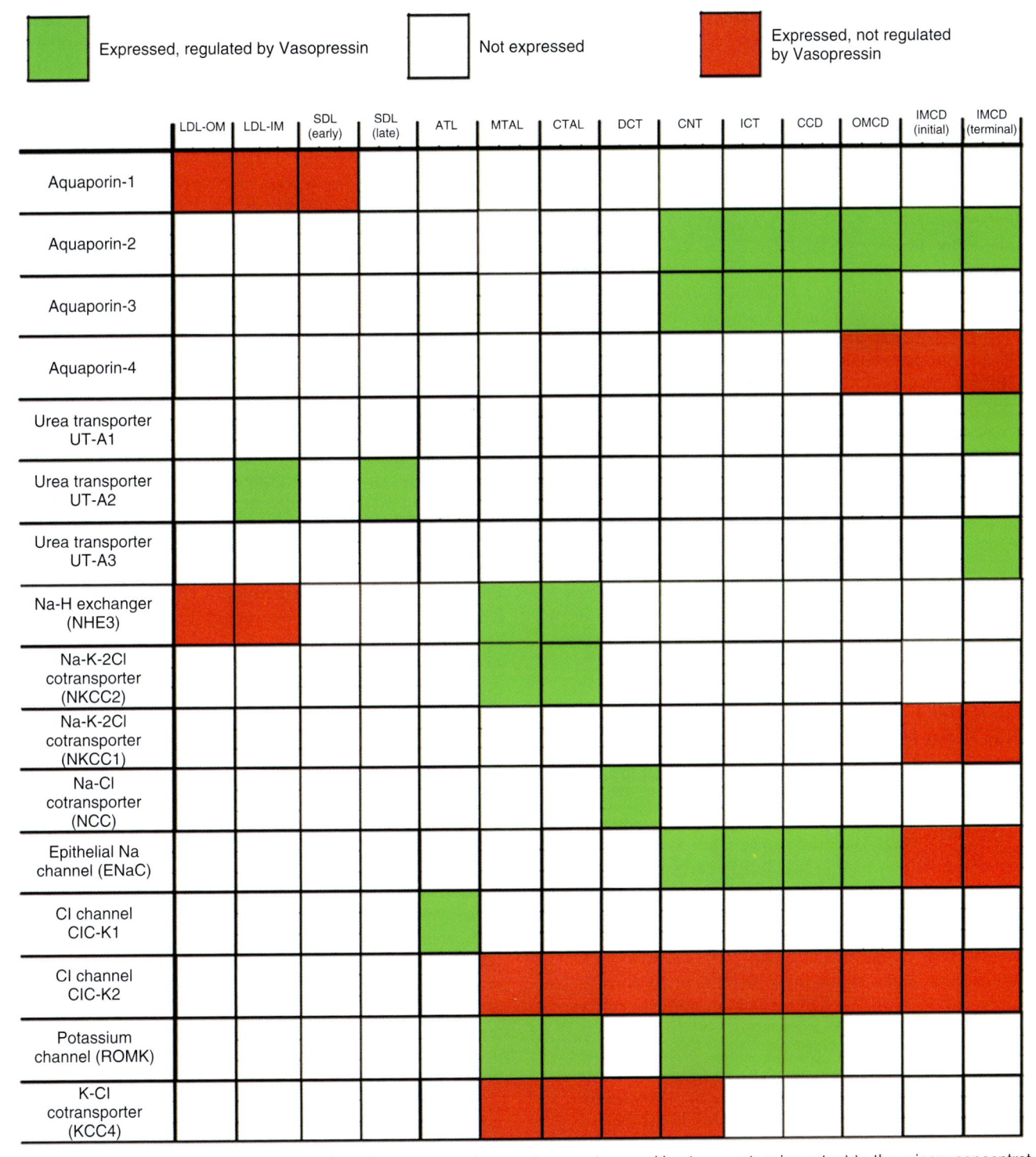

Legend: 🟩 Expressed, regulated by Vasopressin ⬜ Not expressed 🟥 Expressed, not regulated by Vasopressin

	LDL-OM	LDL-IM	SDL (early)	SDL (late)	ATL	MTAL	CTAL	DCT	CNT	ICT	CCD	OMCD	IMCD (initial)	IMCD (terminal)
Aquaporin-1	🟥	🟥	🟥											
Aquaporin-2									🟩	🟩	🟩	🟩	🟩	🟩
Aquaporin-3									🟩	🟩	🟩	🟩		
Aquaporin-4												🟥	🟥	🟥
Urea transporter UT-A1														🟩
Urea transporter UT-A2		🟩		🟩										
Urea transporter UT-A3														🟩
Na-H exchanger (NHE3)	🟥	🟥				🟩	🟩							
Na-K-2Cl cotransporter (NKCC2)						🟩	🟩							
Na-K-2Cl cotransporter (NKCC1)													🟥	🟥
Na-Cl cotransporter (NCC)								🟩						
Epithelial Na channel (ENaC)									🟩	🟩	🟩	🟩		
Cl channel ClC-K1					🟩									
Cl channel ClC-K2						🟥	🟥	🟥	🟥	🟥	🟥	🟥	🟥	🟥
Potassium channel (ROMK)						🟩	🟩		🟩	🟩	🟩			
K-Cl cotransporter (KCC4)						🟥	🟥	🟥						

Figure 10.16 Grid showing sites of expression of water channels, urea transporters, and ion transporters important to the urinary concentrating process. (See text for details.) ATL, Ascending thin limb; CCD, cortical collecting duct; CNT, connecting tubule; CTAL, cortical thick ascending limb; DCT, distal convoluted tubule; ICT, initial collecting tubule; IMCD, inner medullary collecting duct; LDL-IM, inner medullary long-loop thin descending limb; LDL-OM, outer medullary long-loop thin descending limb; MTAL, medullary thick ascending limb; OMCD, outer medullary collecting duct; SDL, short descending limb.

water permeability of isolated perfused thin descending limbs from AQP1 knockout mice was markedly reduced compared to control animals.[130] Because rapid water absorption from the long-loop thin descending limbs is essential for countercurrent multiplication processes in the outer medulla, the reduced water reabsorption from the long-loop thin descending limbs is one factor responsible for the concentrating defect in AQP1 knockout mice. Descending vasa recta, a second renal medullary site of AQP1 expression, also displayed a marked reduction in osmotic water permeability in AQP1 knockout mice,[33,34] and thus, countercurrent exchange processes are also likely to be impaired in AQP1 knockout mice. The results from studies in these mice show that AQP1 in the renal medulla is essential for the urine concentrating mechanism.

AQUAPORIN-2 KNOCKOUT MICE

AQP2 is a major target for vasopressin action in the connecting tubule and throughout the collecting duct system, where its function is regulated acutely, via regulated AQP2 trafficking, or long-term, via alterations in AQP2 protein abundance. The biology of AQP2 is reviewed extensively in Chapter 11 and various review articles.[131-133] A number of different genetic models have been generated to assess the role of AQP2 in the urinary concentrating mechanism, including inducible and nephron-specific models of AQP2 deletion, models where essential phosphorylation sites in AQP2 are modified, and models of autosomal dominant nephrogenic diabetes insipidus (NDI).[134-143] The major phenotype in these models is severe polyuria; however, with free access to water, plasma concentrations of electrolytes, urea, and creatinine are not different in knockout mice compared to controls. In contrast, a mouse model with connecting tubule–specific AQP2 deletion has indicated a role of the connecting tubule in regulating body water balance under basal conditions,[144] but not for maximal concentration of the urine during antidiuresis. Taken together, these mouse models confirm that AQP2 is responsible for the majority of transcellular water reabsorption in the connecting tubule and collecting duct system.

AQUAPORIN-3 AND AQUAPORIN-4 KNOCKOUT MICE

The basolateral component of water transport across connecting tubular cells and collecting duct principal cells is mediated by aquaporin-3 (AQP3) and aquaporin-4 (AQP4).[145,146] AQP3 is the dominant basolateral water channel in the connecting tubule and early parts of the collecting duct system, whereas AQP4 predominates in the outer medullary and inner medullary collecting ducts. The abundances of AQP3 and AQP4 can be increased by the long-term action of vasopressin.[145-147] The osmotic water permeability of the basolateral membrane of cortical collecting duct cells from AQP3 knockout mice is reduced by greater than threefold compared to wild-type control mice.[148] Consequently, AQP3 knockout mice are markedly polyuric (10-fold greater daily urine volume than controls), with an average urine osmolality of less than 300 mOsm/kg H_2O. In contrast to AQP1 or AQP2 knockout mice, AQP3 knockout mice can slightly increase their urine osmolality after either water deprivation or vasopressin treatment, indicating that other basolateral AQPs may partially compensate for loss of AQP3. The relatively severe polyuria in AQP3 knockout mice is consistent with data from micropuncture studies indicating that the majority of post–macula densa fluid reabsorption is from the cortical portion of the collecting duct system, where AQP3 is normally the predominant basolateral water channel.[1]

AQP4 knockout mice have a fourfold decrease in IMCD osmotic water permeability, indicating that AQP4 is responsible for the majority of water movement across the basolateral membrane in this segment.[149,150] Despite this reduced IMCD water permeability, AQP4 knockout mice have relatively normal serum electrolyte concentrations and, compared to wild-type controls, have no difference in urine osmolality. However, after 36 hours of water deprivation, AQP4 knockout mice have a significantly reduced maximal urine osmolality that cannot be further increased by vasopressin administration. This modest decrease in urinary concentrating ability in AQP4 knockout mice, compared to the profound concentrating defect in AQP3 knockout mice, is likely due to the normal distribution of water transport along the collecting duct,[1] with much greater osmotic reabsorption of water in the cortical portion of the collecting duct system (where AQP3 is predominant) than in the medullary collecting ducts (where AQP4 is the predominant basolateral water channel).

UT-A1/3 UREA TRANSPORTER KNOCKOUT MICE

Urea plays a central role in the urinary concentrating mechanism. Urea's importance has been appreciated since 1934, when Gamble and colleagues initially described "an economy of water in renal function referable to urea,"[151] findings that were confirmed and advanced in UT-A1/A3 knockout mice (discussed later).[152] Many studies show that maximal urine concentrating ability is decreased in protein-deprived or malnourished humans (and other mammals), and that urea infusion restores urine concentrating ability (reviewed in Sands and Layton).[78] Urine concentrating defects have been demonstrated in UT-A1/3, UT-A2, UT-B, and UT-A2/UT-B knockout mice.[83,110,153-156] Thus an effect due to urea or urea transporters must be part of the mechanism by which the inner medulla concentrates urine.

UT-A1 and UT-A3 are major targets for vasopressin action in the IMCD (Figure 10.17), where its function is regulated acutely via phosphorylation and changes in plasma membrane accumulation. Hyperosmolality also increases the phosphorylation and the plasma membrane accumulation of both UT-A1 and UT-A3, similar to the effects of vasopressin. The biology of UT-A1 and UT-A3 is reviewed extensively in various review articles.[76-78,157]

A mouse model in which the two IMCD urea transporters UT-A1 and UT-A3 were deleted ($UT\text{-}A1/3^{-/-}$ mice) was generated in 2004.[77,158,159] These mice have a complete absence of phloretin-sensitive and vasopressin-regulated urea transport in the IMCD.[110] $UT\text{-}A1/3^{-/-}$ mice fed a normal or high-protein diet have a significantly greater fluid intake and urine flow, resulting in a decreased urine osmolality, compared to wild-type mice.[110,111] Under these dietary conditions, after an 18-hour water restriction, $UT\text{-}A1/3^{-/-}$ mice are unable to reduce their urine flow to levels below those observed under basal conditions, resulting in volume depletion and loss of body weight. In contrast, on a low-protein diet (4%), $UT\text{-}A1/3^{-/-}$ mice did not show a substantial degree of polyuria and can reduce their urine volume to a similar level as control mice after water restriction. On a low-protein diet, hepatic urea production is low and urea delivery to the IMCD is predicted to be low, thus rendering collecting duct urea transport largely immaterial to water balance. Thus, the concentrating defect in $UT\text{-}A1/3^{-/-}$ mice is due to a urea-dependent osmotic diuresis, results that are compatible with a model of urea handling proposed in the 1950s by Berliner and colleagues.[37]

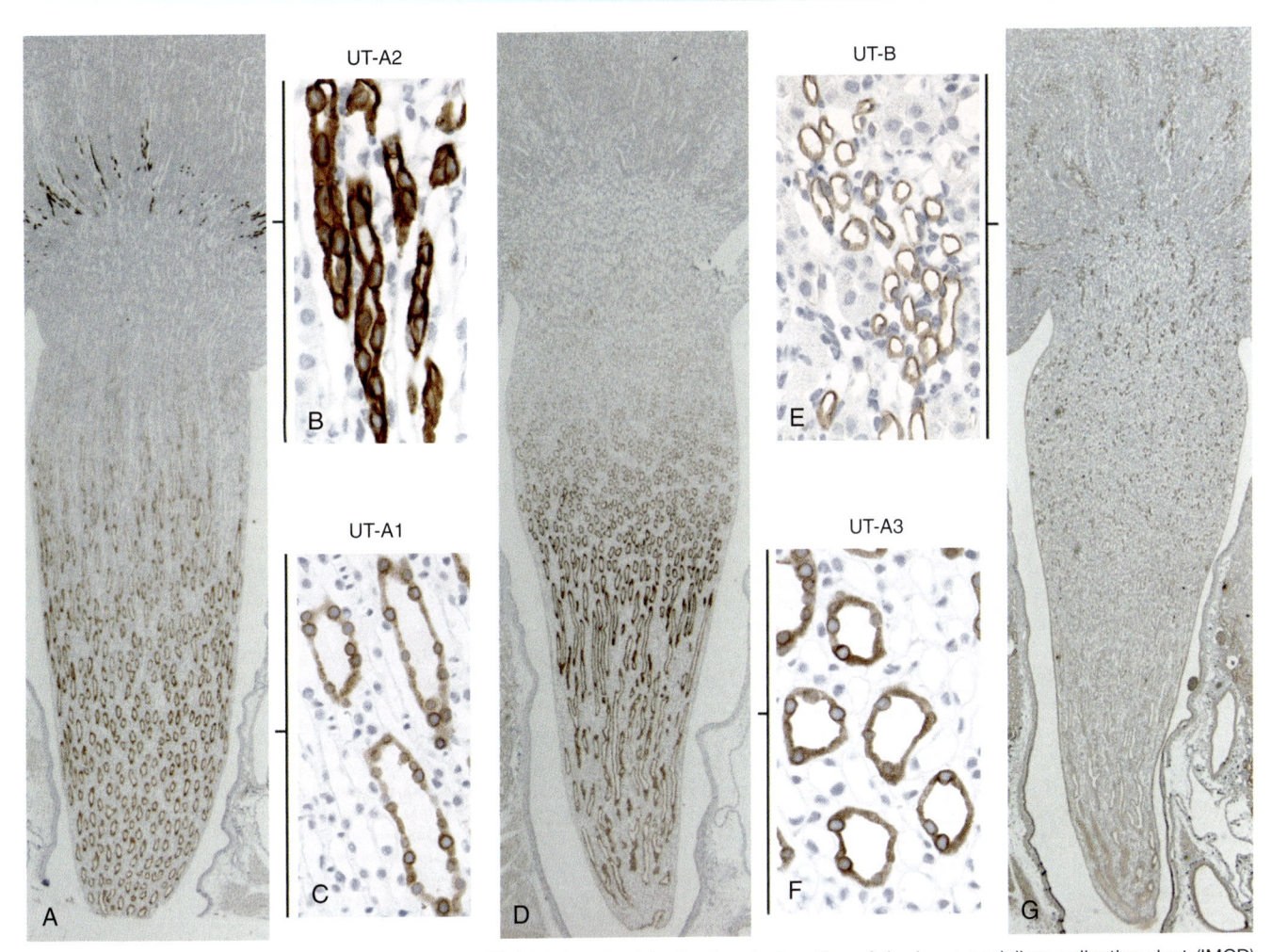

Figure 10.17 Localization of urea transporters. UT-A1 is localized to the terminal portion of the inner medullary collecting duct (IMCD), whereas UT-A2 is localized to the thin descending limbs of the loop of Henle in the inner stripe of outer medulla (**A**). Higher magnification shows that both UT-A2 (**B**) and UT-A1 (**C**) are predominantly intracellular. UT-A3 is localized to the terminal portion of the IMCD (**D**) and is both intracellular and in the basolateral membrane domains (**F**). UT-B is expressed in the descending vasa recta (**G**), where it is localized to the basolateral and apical regions (**E**). (Adapted from Fenton RA, Knepper MA: Urea and renal function in the 21st century: insights from knockout mice. *J Am Soc Nephrol* 18:679-688, 2007.)

$UT\text{-}A1/3^{-/-}$ mice have also been exploited to study the models proposed in 1972 by Stephenson and by Kokko and Rector for concentration of Na$^+$ and Cl$^-$ in the inner medulla in the absence of active transport (see earlier discussion).[102,103] In these models, generally referred to as the "passive model" or the "passive countercurrent multiplier mechanism," the passive electrochemical gradient that drives Na$^+$ and Cl$^-$ exit from the thin ascending limb is indirectly dependent on rapid reabsorption of urea from the IMCD (see earlier for a full description). However, despite a profound decrease in inner medulla urea accumulation in $UT\text{-}A1/3^{-/-}$ mice, three independent studies failed to demonstrate the predicted decline in Na$^+$ and Cl$^-$ concentrations in the inner medulla.[77,110,151,159] Based on these results alone, the passive concentrating model in the form originally proposed does not appear to be the only mechanism by which NaCl is concentrated in the inner medulla. However, mathematical modeling analysis of these same data concluded that the results found in the $UT\text{-}A1/3^{-/-}$ mice are consistent with what one would predict for the passive mechanism.[10] Thus the issue remains unresolved at present.

Another hypothesis regarding urea and the urinary concentrating mechanism was described nearly 75 years ago as "an economy of water in renal function referable to urea" and affectionately known as the Gamble phenomenon.[151] Gamble described that (1) the water requirement for excretion of urea is less than for excretion of an osmotically equivalent amount of NaCl, and (2) less water is required for the excretion of urea and NaCl together than the water needed to excrete an osmotically equivalent amount of either urea or NaCl alone. In $UT\text{-}A1/3^{-/-}$ mice both elements of the Gamble phenomenon were absent, indicating that IMCD urea transporters play an essential role.[152] When wild-type mice were given progressively increasing amounts of urea or NaCl in the diet, both substances induced osmotic diuresis, but at different excretion levels (6000 μosmol/day for urea; 3500 μosmol/day for NaCl). Mice were unable to increase urinary NaCl concentrations above 420 mM. Thus, the second component of the Gamble phenomenon derives from the fact that both urea and NaCl excretion are saturable, presumably resulting from an ability to exceed the respective reabsorptive capacity for urea and NaCl, rather than a specific interaction of urea transport and NaCl transport at an epithelial level.

Na$^+$-H$^+$-EXCHANGER ISOFORM 3 AND Na-K-2Cl COTRANSPORTER TYPE 2 KNOCKOUT MICE

Knockout of Na$^+$-H$^+$-exchanger isoform 3 (NHE3) or Na-K-2Cl cotransporter type 2 (NKCC2), the major apical transporters mediating Na$^+$ entry in the thick ascending limb,[160-163] results in drastically different effects on the urinary concentrating mechanism.[164,165] NHE3 knockout mice have a marked reduction in proximal tubule fluid absorption, with a compensatory decrease in GFR owing to an intact tubuloglomerular feedback (TGF) mechanism.[166] On ad libitum water intake, NHE3 knockouts manifest a moderate increase in water intake associated with lower urinary osmolalities.[167] In contrast, NKCC2 knockout mice die before weaning due to renal fluid wasting and dehydration—highlighting the essential role of NKCC2 in the urinary concentrating mechanism.[165] Why does deletion of NKCC2 result in such a severe phenotype, when deletion of NHE3, a transporter responsible for reabsorption of far more Na$^+$, results in a viable mouse capable of maintaining extracellular fluid volume? The answer appears to be in the special role that NKCC2 plays in the macula densa in the mediation of TGF. TGF allows NHE3 knockout mice to maintain a relatively normal distal delivery through a decrease in GFR, whereas NKCC2 mice cannot compensate in this manner because the transporter is necessary for the feedback to occur. Indeed, mice with isoform-specific deletion of NKCC2 have been generated that may be useful for examining the tubular versus TGF role of NKCC2 in the urinary concentrating mechanism.[168,169]

EPITHELIAL SODIUM CHANNEL KNOCKOUT MICE

Epithelial sodium channel (ENaC) is localized to the late DCT, connecting tubule, initial collecting tubule, and throughout the collecting duct.[170,171] Vasopressin treatment results in increased protein abundance of NCC and the β- and γ-subunits of ENaC.[172-174] Acute vasopressin exposure also increases Na$^+$ reabsorption in the cortical collecting duct by increasing apical Na$^+$ entry via ENaC,[175-177] due to adenylyl cyclase 6–dependent stimulation of ENaC open probability and apical membrane channel number.[178] Deletion of any of the ENaC subunits results in a severe phenotype with neonatal death.[179-182] In ENaC knockout mice, early death appears to be due to failure to adequately clear fluid from the pulmonary alveoli after birth, whereas the β- and γ-ENaC knockout mice appear to die of hyperkalemia and sodium chloride wasting.[179,180,182] α-ENaC deletion from the collecting ducts alone, leaving intact ENaC expression in the connecting tubule and nonrenal tissues, resulted in viable mice that had little or no difficulty in maintaining salt and fluid homeostasis.[183] In contrast, α-ENaC deletion from the connecting tubule and collecting duct together results in a mouse model with increased urine volume and decreased urine osmolality,[184] indicating that α-ENaC expression within the connecting tubule and collecting duct is crucial for sodium and water homeostasis.

KIDNEY-SPECIFIC CHLORIDE CHANNEL 1 KNOCKOUT MICE

ClC-K1 is localized to both the apical and basolateral plasma membranes of thin ascending limbs.[185] In addition, CLC-K1 messenger RNA has been detected in both the thick ascending limb and DCT.[186] In isolated perfused tubules, chloride conductance of the thin ascending limb is increased by vasopressin exposure, a result of either increased unit conductance or altered cellular localization of ClC-K1 chloride channels.[187] Microperfusion studies of ClC-K1 null mice (*Clcnk1*$^{-/-}$) determined that there was drastically reduced transepithelial chloride transport in the thin ascending limb of knockout mice.[188] *Clcnk1*$^{-/-}$ mice had significantly greater urine volume and lower urine osmolality compared to controls, and even after water deprivation, or vasopressin administration, knockout mice were unable to concentrate their urine. This observed polyuria was due to water diuresis and not osmotic diuresis. Inner medulla concentrations of Na$^+$ and Cl$^-$ from *Clcnk1*$^{-/-}$ mice were approximately half those of controls, resulting in a significantly reduced osmolality of the papilla. These studies demonstrate that the ClC-K1 chloride channel is necessary for maintenance of a maximal osmolality in the inner medullary tissue. The findings in the *Clcnk1*$^{-/-}$ mice emphasize the importance of rapid chloride exit (and presumably sodium exit) from the thin ascending limb in the inner medullary concentrating process and provide support for the passive mechanism (see earlier).

RENAL OUTER MEDULLARY POTASSIUM CHANNEL KNOCKOUT MICE

The renal outer medullary potassium (ROMK) channel (Kir 1.1), an ATP-sensitive inwardly rectifier potassium channel, localizes to the thick ascending limb, DCT, connecting tubule, and collecting duct system, where it is predominantly associated with the apical plasma membrane (see Figure 10.15).[189-193] Chronic vasopressin treatment increases ROMK abundance in the thick ascending limb, thus contributing to the long-term effect of vasopressin to increase NaCl transport in this segment.[194,195] The majority of ROMK knockout mice die before weaning due to hydronephrosis and severe dehydration.[196] Although 5% of these mice survive the perinatal period, adults manifest polydipsia, polyuria, impaired urinary concentrating ability, hypernatremia, and reduced blood pressure, consistent with the known role of ROMK in active NaCl absorption in the thick ascending limb. From these animals, a line of mice has been derived that has a greater survival rate and no hydronephrosis in adult animals; yet the concentrating defect still persists.

TYPE 2 VASOPRESSIN RECEPTOR KNOCKOUT MICE

A mouse model of X-linked NDI (XNDI) has provided insight into the role of the V$_2$R in the urinary concentrating mechanism.[197] Male V$_2$R mutant mice (*V$_2$R$^-$/y*) die within 7 days after birth, with 3-day mice displaying severe hypernatremia, drastically increased serum Na$^+$ and Cl$^-$ levels, and significantly lower urine osmolality. The V$_2$R agonist desmopressin (DDAVP) had no effect in V_2R^-/y mice. Adult, female $V_2R^{+/-}$ mice have an approximately 50% decrease in total vasopressin binding capacity and a 50% decrease in DDAVP-induced intracellular cAMP levels, resulting in polyuria, polydipsia, and a reduced urinary concentrating ability. The expression of multiple other gene products, including those of the renin-angiotensin-aldosterone system, are altered in V_2R-deficient mice.[198]

Mice have been generated in which the V_2R gene can be conditionally deleted during adulthood by administration of 4-OH-tamoxifen.[199] Upon V_2R deletion, adult mice displayed all characteristic symptoms of XNDI, including polyuria, polydipsia, and resistance to the antidiuretic actions of vasopressin. These models are consistent with the general view that the antidiuretic effects of vasopressin result from an initial interaction between vasopressin and the V_2R, resulting in increased intracellular cAMP and eventually promoting water reabsorption in the kidney collecting duct via aquaporins. Furthermore, they demonstrate that there is no other significant compensatory event that can generate cAMP and increase water permeability in the renal collecting duct.

ACKNOWLEDGMENTS

This work was supported by National Institutes of Health grants R01-DK41707, R01-DK89828, and R21-DK91147 to JMS. RAF is supported by the Danish Medical Research Council, the Novo Nordisk Foundation, the Carlsberg Foundation (Carlsbergfondet), and the Lundbeck Foundation.

Complete reference list available at ExpertConsult.com.

KEY REFERENCES

10. Pannabecker TL, Dantzler WH, Layton HE, et al: Role of three-dimensional architecture in the urine concentrating mechanism of the rat renal inner medulla. *Am J Physiol Renal Physiol* 295(5):F1271–F1285, 2008.
12. Pannabecker TL: Comparative physiology and architecture associated with the mammalian urine concentrating mechanism: role of inner medullary water and urea transport pathways in the rodent medulla. *Am J Physiol Regul Integr Comp Physiol* 304(7):R488–R503, 2013.
17. Layton AT, Dantzler WH, Pannabecker TL: Urine concentrating mechanism: impact of vascular and tubular architecture and a proposed descending limb urea-Na+ cotransporter. *Am J Physiol Renal Physiol* 302(5):F591–F605, 2012.
18. Layton AT, Gilbert RL, Pannabecker TL: Isolated interstitial nodal spaces may facilitate preferential solute and fluid mixing in the rat renal inner medulla. *Am J Physiol Renal Physiol* 302(7):F830–F839, 2012.
37. Berliner RW, Levinsky NG, Davidson DG, et al: Dilution and concentration of the urine and the action of antidiuretic hormone. *Am J Med* 24:730–744, 1958.
46. Gottschalk CW, Mylle M: Micropuncture study of the mammalian urinary concentrating mechanism: evidence for the countercurrent hypothesis. *Am J Physiol* 196:927–936, 1959.
49. Lassiter WE, Gottschalk CW, Mylle M: Micropuncture study of net transtubular movement of water and urea in nondiuretic mammalian kidney. *Am J Physiol* 200:1139–1146, 1961.
54. Grantham JJ, Burg MB: Effect of vasopressin and cyclic AMP on permeability of isolated collecting tubules. *Am J Physiol* 211:255–259, 1966.
55. Morgan T, Berliner RW: Permeability of the loop of Henle, vasa recta, and collecting duct to water, urea, and sodium. *Am J Physiol* 215:108–115, 1968.
64. Layton AT, Layton HE: A region-based mathematical model of the urine concentrating mechanism in the rat outer medulla. I. Formulation and base-case results. *Am J Physiol Renal Physiol* 289(6):F1346–F1366, 2005.
65. Layton AT, Layton HE: A region-based mathematical model of the urine concentrating mechanism in the rat outer medulla. II. Parameter sensitivity and tubular inhomogeneity. *Am J Physiol Renal Physiol* 289(6):F1367–F1381, 2005.
70. Sands JM, Knepper MA: Urea permeability of mammalian inner medullary collecting duct system and papillary surface epithelium. *J Clin Invest* 79:138–147, 1987.
71. Rocha AS, Kudo LH: Water, urea, sodium, chloride, and potassium transport in the in vitro perfused papillary collecting duct. *Kidney Int* 22:485–491, 1982.
72. Sands JM, Nonoguchi H, Knepper MA: Vasopressin effects on urea and H_2O transport in inner medullary collecting duct subsegments. *Am J Physiol* 253:F823–F832, 1987.
76. Klein JD, Blount MA, Sands JM: Urea transport in the kidney. *Compr Physiol* 1(2):699–729, 2011.
78. Sands JM, Layton HE: The urine concentrating mechanism and urea transporters. In Alpern RJ, Caplan MJ, Moe OW, editors: *Seldin and Giebisch's The kidney: physiology and pathophysiology*, ed 5, San Diego, 2013, Academic Press, pp 1463–1510.
84. Fenton RA, Knepper MA: Mouse models and the urinary concentrating mechanism in the new millennium. *Physiol Rev* 87:1083–1112, 2007.
85. Knepper MA: Urea transport in isolated thick ascending limbs and collecting ducts from rats. *Am J Physiol* 245:F634–F639, 1983.
86. Rocha AS, Kokko JP: Permeability of medullary nephron segments to urea and water: effect of vasopressin. *Kidney Int* 6:379–387, 1974.
90. Elalouf JM, Roinel N, de Rouffignac C: Effects of antidiuretic hormone on electrolyte reabsorption and secretion in distal tubules of rat kidney. *Pflugers Arch* 401(2):167–173, 1984.
91. Pedersen NB, Hofmeister MV, Rosenbaek LL, et al: Vasopressin induces phosphorylation of the thiazide-sensitive sodium chloride cotransporter in the distal convoluted tubule. *Kidney Int* 78(2):160–169, 2010.
102. Kokko JP, Rector FC: Countercurrent multiplication system without active transport in inner medulla. *Kidney Int* 2:214–223, 1972.
103. Stephenson JL: Concentration of urine in a central core model of the renal counterflow system. *Kidney Int* 2:85–94, 1972.
110. Fenton RA, Chou C-L, Stewart GS, et al: Urinary concentrating defect in mice with selective deletion of phloretin-sensitive urea transporters in the renal collecting duct. *Proc Natl Acad Sci U S A* 101(19):7469–7474, 2004.
111. Fenton RA, Flynn A, Shodeinde A, et al: Renal phenotype of UT-A urea transporter knockout mice. *J Am Soc Nephrol* 16(6):1583–1592, 2005.
112. Layton AT, Pannabecker TL, Dantzler WH, et al: Two modes for concentrating urine in rat inner medulla. *Am J Physiol Renal Physiol* 287(4):F816–F839, 2004.
113. Nawata CM, Evans KK, Dantzler WH, et al: Transepithelial water and urea permeabilities of isolated perfused Munich-Wistar rat inner medullary thin limbs of Henle's loop. *Am J Physiol Renal Physiol* 306(1):F123–F129, 2014.
128. Ma TH, Yang BX, Gillespie A, et al: Severely impaired urinary concentrating ability in transgenic mice lacking aquaporin-1 water channels. *J Biol Chem* 273(8):4296–4299, 1998.
132. Fenton RA, Pedersen CN, Moeller HB: New insights into regulated aquaporin-2 function. *Curr Opin Nephrol Hypertens* 22(5):551–558, 2013.
140. Moeller HB, Olesen ET, Fenton RA: Regulation of the water channel aquaporin-2 by posttranslational modification. *Am J Physiol Renal Physiol* 300(5):F1062–F1073, 2011.
144. Kortenoeven ML, Pedersen NB, Miller RL, et al: Genetic ablation of aquaporin-2 in the mouse connecting tubules results in defective renal water handling. *J Physiol* 591(Pt 8):2205–2219, 2013.
150. Chou C-L, Ma TH, Yang BX, et al: Fourfold reduction of water permeability in inner medullary collecting duct of aquaporin-4 knockout mice. *Am J Physiol Cell Physiol* 274(2):C549–C554, 1998.
151. Gamble JL, McKhann CF, Butler AM, et al: An economy of water in renal function referable to urea. *Am J Physiol Renal Physiol* 109:139–154, 1934.

152. Fenton RA, Chou CL, Sowersby H, et al: Gamble's "economy of water" revisited: studies in urea transporter knockout mice. *Am J Physiol Renal Physiol* 291(1):F148–F154, 2006.
158. Fenton RA: Urea transporters and renal function: lessons from knockout mice. *Curr Opin Nephrol Hypertens* 17:513–518, 2008.
164. Schultheis PJ, Clarke LL, Meneton P, et al: Renal and intestinal absorptive defects in mice lacking the NHE3 Na^+/H^+ exchanger. *Nat Genet* 19:282–285, 1998.
180. Hummler E, Barker P, Gatzy J, et al: Early death due to defective neonatal lung liquid clearance in alpha-ENaC-deficient mice. *Nat Genet* 12:325–328, 1996.
181. Hummler E, Barker P, Talbot C, et al: A mouse model for the renal salt-wasting syndrome pseudohypoaldosteronism. *Proc Natl Acad Sci U S A* 94:11710–11715, 1997.
188. Matsumura Y, Uchida S, Kondo Y, et al: Overt nephrogenic diabetes insipidus in mice lacking the CLC-K1 chloride channel. *Nat Genet* 21:95–98, 1999.
196. Lorenz JN, Baird NR, Judd LM, et al: Impaired renal NaCl absorption in mice lacking the ROMK potassium channel, a model for type II Bartter's syndrome. *J Biol Chem* 277:37871–37880, 2002.
197. Yun J, Schöneberg T, Liu J, et al: Generation and phenotype of mice harboring a nonsense mutation in the *V2 vasopressin receptor* gene. *J Clin Invest* 106(11):1361–1371, 2000.
203. Atherton JC, Hai MA, Thomas S: Acute effects of lysine vasopressin injection (single and continuous) on urinary composition in the conscious water diuretic rat. *Pflugers Arch* 310:281–296, 1969.

The Cell Biology of Vasopressin Action

11

Dennis Brown | Robert A. Fenton

CHAPTER OUTLINE

VASOPRESSIN—THE ANTIDIURETIC HORMONE, 282
THE TYPE 2 VASOPRESSIN RECEPTOR—A G PROTEIN–COUPLED RECEPTOR, 282
Interaction of Type 2 Vasopressin Receptor with Heterotrimeric G Proteins and β-Arrestin, 282
Fate of the Type 2 Vasopressin Receptor after Internalization—Delivery to Lysosomes, 284
Diabetes Insipidus (Central and Nephrogenic), 285
THE AQUAPORINS—A FAMILY OF WATER CHANNEL PROTEINS, 286
Other Permeability Properties of Aquaporins, 286
Aquaporin-2: The Vasopressin-Sensitive Collecting Duct Water Channel, 286
An Overview of Vasopressin-Regulated Aquaporin-2 Trafficking in Collecting Duct Principal Cells, 287
Use of In Vitro Systems to Examine Aquaporin-2 Trafficking and Function, 288
Expression of Multiple Basolateral Aquaporins (Aquaporin-2, Aquaporin-3, and/or Aquaporin-4) in Principal Cells, 289
A Role of Basolateral Aquaporin-2 in Cell Migration and Tubule Morphogenesis, 290
INTRACELLULAR PATHWAYS OF AQUAPORIN-2 TRAFFICKING, 291
Role of Clathrin-Coated Pits in Aquaporin-2 Recycling, 291
Aquaporin-2 Localization in Intracellular Compartments during Recycling, 291
Aquaporin-2 Is a Constitutively Recycling Membrane Protein, 291

REGULATION OF AQUAPORIN-2 TRAFFICKING, 291
Role of Kinases and A-Kinase Anchoring Proteins in Aquaporin-2 Trafficking, 292
Importance of the S256 Residue for Aquaporin-2 Membrane Accumulation, 293
Other Phosphorylation Sites (S261, S264, S269) Are Modified by Vasopressin, 293
Role of Phosphorylation in Exocytosis and Endocytosis of Aquaporin-2, 293
Phosphorylation of S256 Modulates Aquaporin-2 Interaction with Endocytotic Proteins, 293
Role of the Actin Cytoskeleton in Aquaporin-2 Trafficking, 294
Identification of Actin-Associated Proteins Potentially Involved in Aquaporin-2 Trafficking, 294
Microtubules and Aquaporin-2 Trafficking, 295
SNARE Proteins and Aquaporin-2 Trafficking, 295
LONG-TERM REGULATION OF WATER BALANCE, 296
Acquired Water Balance Disorders, 297
Lithium Treatment, 297
Electrolyte Abnormalities: *Hypokalemia and Hypercalcemia*, 299
Obstruction of the Urinary Tract, 299
Acute and Chronic Renal Injury, 299
Liver Cirrhosis and Congestive Heart Failure, 299
Novel Approaches for X-Linked Nephrogenic Diabetes Insipidus Therapy, 300
Vasopressin Receptor–Independent Membrane Insertion of Aquaporin-2—Potential Strategies for Treating Nephrogenic Diabetes Insipidus, 300

The small peptide hormone vasopressin (AVP) and its type 2 receptor (V_2R) play a central role in the urinary concentrating mechanism. V_2R activation results in the accumulation of a water channel, aquaporin-2 (AQP2), on the plasma membrane of collecting duct (CD) principal cells, thus increasing their permeability to water. This event permits the collecting duct luminal fluid to equilibrate osmotically with the surrounding interstitium in the kidney, resulting in water reabsorption and urine concentration. In humans the glomerulus filters approximately 180 L/day of fluid from plasma, of which 90% is returned to the circulation by reabsorption in the proximal tubule and descending limb of Henle's loop. Most of the remaining 18 L is delivered to the CD system and is reabsorbed under the regulation of AVP. Dysfunction of this reabsorptive mechanism in the CD results in the production of large amounts of dilute urine, up to 18 L per day—a disease known as diabetes insipidus (DI). The antidiuretic hormone, AVP, plays a multifaceted role in the urinary concentrating process in mammals. In addition to activating the V_2R and increasing plasma membrane AQP2 levels, AVP stimulates NaCl reabsorption by thick ascending limbs of Henle. AVP also stimulates urea transport in terminal portions of the CD, which allows high levels of urea to be excreted without reducing urinary concentrating ability. The urinary concentration mechanism therefore requires the tight coordination of cellular and molecular events within the context of renal architecture and fluid dynamics in the vasculature. This chapter will focus on the AVP-activated renal concentrating mechanism and will address how the V_2R and the AQP2 water channel interact via intracellular signaling pathways to regulate CD water reabsorption and urine concentration.

VASOPRESSIN—THE ANTIDIURETIC HORMONE

The antidiuretic hormone of most mammals is a nine–amino acid peptide, AVP. Secretion of AVP from the posterior pituitary is stimulated by an increase in plasma osmolality, but also by a reduction in plasma volume (see Chapter 16). A change in osmolality as small as 1% can cause a significant rise in plasma AVP levels. AVP then activates regulatory systems necessary to retain water and restore osmolality to normal. In contrast, a 5% to 10% decrease in volume is required to stimulate AVP secretion, but AVP nevertheless has important clinical applications in the control of vasodilatory shock.[1] The effects of AVP occur through the stimulation of receptors that are located on different cell types. The V_1 receptor activates a Ca^{++} pathway and is involved in the pressor effect of AVP, whereas the V_2R activates a cyclic adenosine monophosphate (cAMP) pathway that regulates transepithelial water transport in the kidney.[2,3] In situations when it becomes critical to distinguish V_1 from V_2 receptor effects, a modified form of AVP, known as 1-desamino-8-D-arginine vasopressin (DDAVP) is used, which is specific for the V_2R and has little or no V_1-related pressor effect. The remainder of this discussion will focus on the V_2R in renal epithelial cells.

THE TYPE 2 VASOPRESSIN RECEPTOR—A G PROTEIN–COUPLED RECEPTOR

The V_2R is a member of the family of seven membrane-spanning domain receptors that couple to heterotrimeric G proteins (GPCRs).[4,5] In the kidney it is expressed in segments from the thick ascending limb of the loop of Henle through to the CD principal cells.[6-10] Most studies on V_2R recycling, downregulation, and desensitization have been performed in cell culture using epitope-tagged V_2R constructs. When AVP binds to the V_2R, adenylyl cyclase (AC) activity is stimulated and cytosolic cAMP levels increase.[11] This activates protein kinases, leading to the phosphorylation of several proteins, including AQP2. This water channel then accumulates in the apical plasma membrane of CD principal cells, thus increasing transepithelial water permeability and facilitating osmotically driven water reabsorption (Figure 11.1). AQP2 contains several C-terminal residues whose phosphorylation status changes upon AVP treatment of V_2R-expressing cells. Intracellular calcium is also increased by AVP via a mechanism involving calmodulin[12]; this is also involved in the regulated trafficking of AQP2.[13,14]

INTERACTION OF TYPE 2 VASOPRESSIN RECEPTOR WITH HETEROTRIMERIC G PROTEINS AND β-ARRESTIN

The V_2R has been cloned from several mammalian species, and the sequences are more than 90% identical. Upon ligand binding, the V_2R assumes an active configuration and the bound heterotrimeric G protein, Gs, dissociates into Gsα and Gsβγ subunits.[11] This G protein is localized on the basolateral plasma membrane of the thick ascending limb of Henle, distal convoluted tubule, and CD principal cells.[15,16] AC is stimulated by activated Gsα, and cAMP levels are increased. The predominant AC isoform in the adult rat kidney is AC-6, but several other AC isoforms are expressed at lower levels, including AC-4, AC-5, and AC-9 and calmodulin-sensitive AC-3.[17] Knockout mice lacking the AC-6 isoform have significant nephrogenic DI (NDI),[18,19] confirming its key role in the V_2R-mediated signal transduction pathway. Liganded V_2R interacts with Gs via its cytosolic domain, and a peptide corresponding to the third intracellular loop of the V_2R inhibits signaling through Gs.[20]

The AVP/V_2R association increases cellular cAMP, which initiates a cascade of events that increases CD water permeability by changing the phosphorylation pattern of AQP2 and causing its accumulation at the cell surface. Termination of this response depends on the internalization of the V_2R after AVP binding and its delivery to and degradation in lysosomes (Figure 11.2A and D). Many accessory proteins are involved in V_2R downregulation, including inhibitory G_i proteins,[11,21,22] proteins involved in clathrin-mediated endocytosis,[23,24] and proteins of the so-called retromer complex.[25] In addition to less receptor at the cell surface, the level of V_2R messenger RNA (mRNA) also decreases rapidly after elevation of plasma AVP.[26] Additional mechanisms that downregulate the AVP response include destruction of cAMP by cytosolic phosphodiesterases[27] and inhibition by prostaglandins,[28] dopamine,[29,30] adenosine

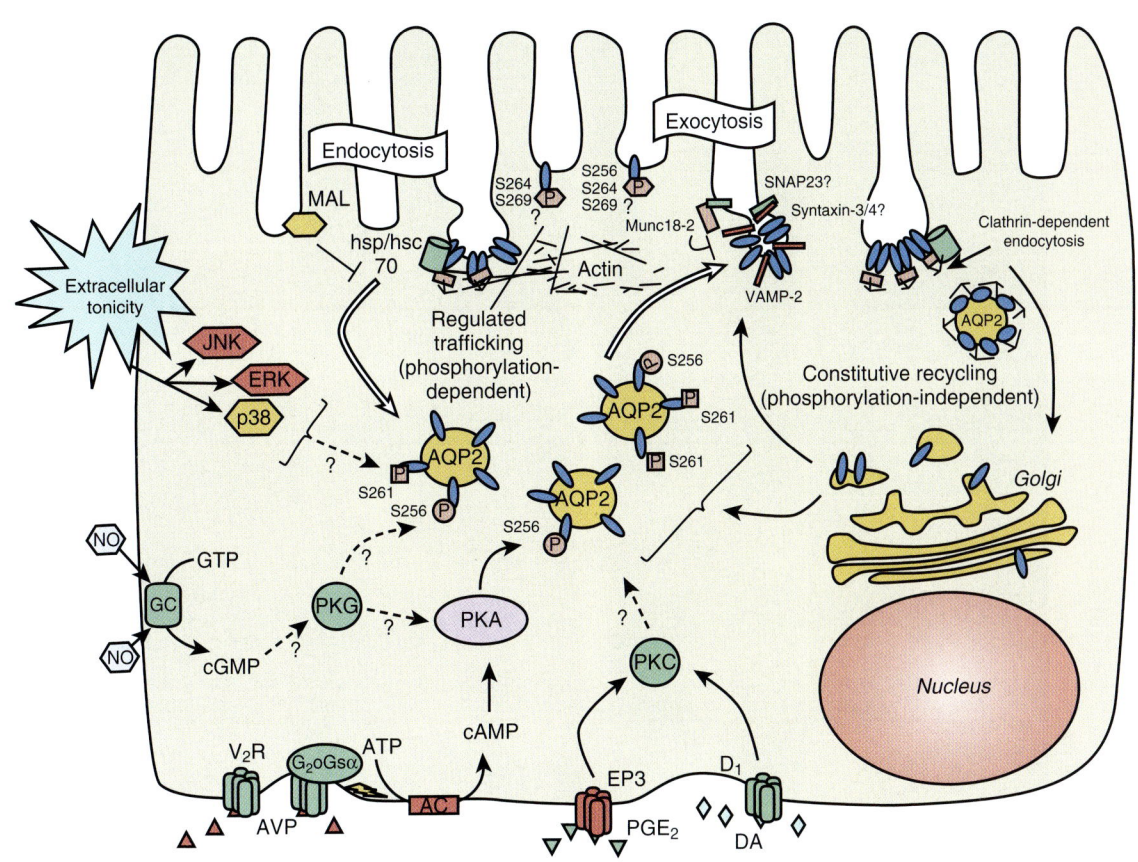

Figure 11.1 Key events that contribute to the regulation of aquaporin-2 (AQP2) trafficking. The canonical pathway involves interaction of vasopressin (AVP) with the type 2 receptor (V_2R) on the basolateral surface of the principal cell. This increases cyclic adenosine monophosphate (cAMP) formation after $G_{\alpha s}$ stimulation of adenylyl cyclase (AC). Phosphorylation of AQP2 occurs initially on residue S256, via protein kinase A (PKA) activation. After AVP stimulation, residue S261 on AQP2 is dephosphorylated, and residues S264 and S269 phosphorylation is increased. During exocytosis AQP2 interacts with soluble N-ethylmaleimide–sensitive factor attachment protein receptor (SNARE) proteins and their regulatory proteins such as Munc18-2, and these interactions may be regulated by phosphorylation. At the cell surface, phosphorylated AQP2 is present in endocytosis-resistant domains, and its interaction with heat shock protein/heat shock cognate 70 (hsp/hsc70) which is required for clathrin-mediated endocytosis, is inhibited. The myeloid and lymphocyte protein (MAL) also is involved in AQP2 endocytosis by an as-yet-unknown mechanism. Endocytosis of AQP2 is also facilitated by protein kinase C (PKC) activation (but possibly not by direct phosphorylation of AQP2), as well as by activation of dopamine (DA, D_1), prostaglandin E_2 (PGE_2), and PGE_2 receptor type 3 (EP3). However, constitutive exocytosis of AQP2 occurs without AVP stimulation and does not require AQP2 phosphorylation on residue S256. Accumulation of AQP2 at the plasma membrane is increased by inhibiting clathrin-mediated endocytosis. AQP2 phosphorylation can also be increased by stimulating the cyclic guanosine monophosphate/protein kinase G (cGMP/PKG) pathways using, for example, nitric oxide (NO). Extracellular hypertonicity activates the mitogen-activated protein (MAP) kinase pathway, and c-Jun N-terminal kinase (JNK), extracellular signal–regulated kinase (ERK), and p38 MAP kinase activities are all required for AQP2 surface accumulation after acute hypertonic shock. Finally, AQP2 trafficking involves the actin cytoskeleton, and actin depolymerization results in cell surface accumulation of AQP2 without the need for AVP stimulation. ATP, Adenosine triphosphate; GC, guanylyl cyclase; GTP, guanosine triphosphate; SNAP23, synaptosomal-associated protein 23; VAMP-2, vesicle-associated membrane protein 2.

receptor stimulation,[31] adrenergic agonists,[32] endothelin-1,[33] bradykinin,[34] and epidermal growth factor.[35] However, data have shown that cAMP levels in AVP target cells remain elevated for a considerable time after stimulation, and that the V_2R continues to signal from endosomes after internalization.[25]

Changes in receptor conformation after AVP binding are followed by receptor phosphorylation, desensitization, internalization, and sequestration. One critical step in this process is the binding of β-arrestin to the V_2R,[36] which is triggered by phosphorylation of the V_2R by kinases, including G protein–coupled receptor kinases (GRKs). Interestingly, different cellular responses to receptor phosphorylation can be dissected depending on the kinase that is involved in the phosphorylation process. Thus phosphorylation of V_2R with GRK2 and GRK3 results in AVP-dependent desensitization and recruitment of β-arrestins. In contrast, GRK5 and GRK6 phosphorylation is involved in extracellular signal–regulated kinase activation.[37]

Arrestin-receptor complexes recruit the clathrin adaptor protein AP-2, an important component of the endocytotic mechanism,[22] and the complex is then internalized via clathrin-mediated endocytosis.[23,38,39] Arrestins also uncouple GPCRs from heterotrimeric G proteins, producing a desensitized receptor.[40] After downregulation, restoration of prestimulation levels of V_2R at the cell surface requires several hours.[41-43] In contrast, prestimulation levels of the β2-adrenergic receptor (β2AR) are restored on the cell surface

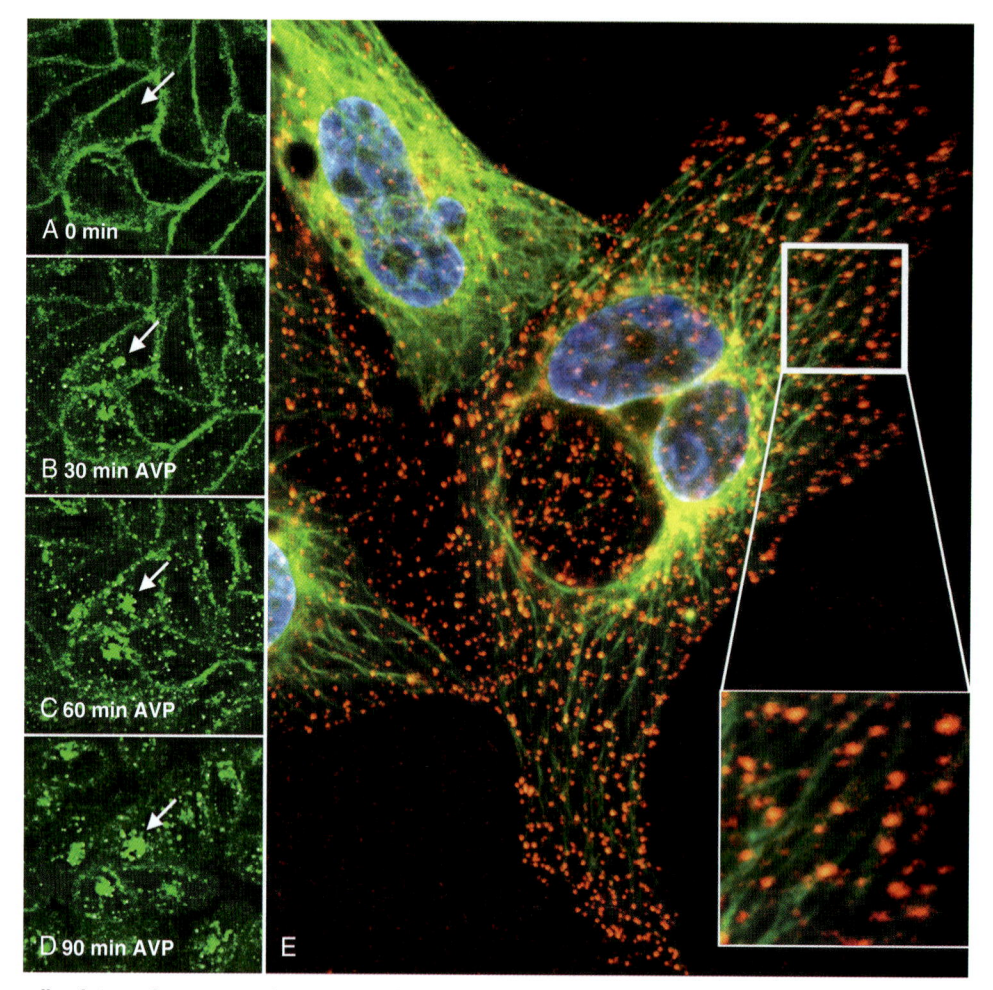

Figure 11.2 Internalized type 2 vasopressin receptor (V_2R) is trafficked along microtubules to lysosomes for degradation. **A** to **D**, Spinning disk confocal microscopy (live imaging of the same cells over time) of LLC-PK$_1$ cells stably expressing type 2 vasopressin receptor (V_2R)–green flourescent protein (GFP) seen at various times (0 to 90 minutes) after addition of vasopressin (AVP). Initially most of the V_2R-GFP is located on the plasma membrane (**A**). After AVP treatment, the V_2R-GFP is downregulated from the cell surface and is progressively internalized (**B, C,** and **D**) into a perinuclear compartment that is seen as a bright fluorescent patch (indicated with an *arrow* in each panel). **E,** LLC-PK$_1$ cells expressing GFP-tubulin after incubation with a fluorescent derivative of AVP, AVP-tetramethylrhodamine (AVP-TAMRA). Endocytotic vesicles containing the internalized ligand align along GFP-labeled microtubules *(inset)* and are eventually delivered to the perinuclear region for degradation in lysosomes. (Adapted from Brown D: Imaging protein trafficking. *Nephron Exp Nephrol* 103:e55-e61, 2006; Bouley R, Lin HY, Raychowdhury MK, et al: Downregulation of the vasopressin type 2 receptor after vasopressin-induced internalization: involvement of a lysosomal degradation pathway. *Am J Physiol Cell Physiol* 288:C1390-C1401, 2005; and Chen S, Webber MJ, Vilardaga JP, et al: Visualizing microtubule-dependent vasopressin type 2 receptor trafficking using a new high-affinity fluorescent vasopressin ligand. *Endocrinology* 152:3893-3904, 2011.)

within an hour of internalization.[42] This difference has been correlated with the association characteristics of the receptor/β-arrestin complex. The V_2R forms a more stable interaction with β-arrestin than the β$_2$AR. This interaction is responsible for the intracellular retention of the V_2R[38,42] and its continued signaling from intracellular vesicles,[25] but it does not dictate the final cellular destination of the receptor.[44]

FATE OF THE TYPE 2 VASOPRESSIN RECEPTOR AFTER INTERNALIZATION—DELIVERY TO LYSOSOMES

After AVP stimulation, there is a rapid β-arrestin–dependent ubiquitination of the V_2R, followed by internalization and increased degradation.[45] Much of the V_2R that is internalized with the AVP ligand enters a lysosomal degradation compartment.[46-48] Real-time microscopy of transfected LLC-PK$_1$ cells shows that after ligand binding, V_2R–green fluorescent protein (GFP) moves along microtubules (Figure 11.2*E*) to perinuclear late endosomes and lysosomes for degradation.[46,49,50] Restoration of prestimulation levels of the V_2R at the cell surface is greatly inhibited by cycloheximide, indicating that new protein synthesis is involved in the resensitization process.[46] However, the V_2R can continue to signal even after internalization, because of the presence of the requisite array of signal transduction proteins on endosomes.[25] This can extend the duration of cAMP elevation in cells, in contrast to oxytocin, which stimulates a cAMP pulse of much shorter duration. This prolonged cAMP signaling via the V_2R may be an adaptation to the unusually harsh (high osmolality, low pH) conditions in the renal medulla, which, combined with low circulating levels of AVP that allow only low receptor occupancy, might otherwise lead to only a small cAMP response.

In summary, the V_2R—classified as a "slow-recycling" GPCR—continues to signal after internalization and is then largely degraded in lysosomes. This pathway may allow the V_2R to function in the harsh environment of the renal medulla, which can be acidic and of high osmolality.[51,52] Receptor-ligand pairs often separate in the acidic environment of endosomes, but AVP must actually associate with the V_2R in the acidic renal medulla, indicating that it is at least partially resistant to pH-induced dissociation. Delivery of both the ligand and receptor to lysosomes may be required to terminate the physiologic response to AVP.[52]

DIABETES INSIPIDUS (CENTRAL AND NEPHROGENIC)

DI is characterized by excessive urinary water loss (up to 18 L of dilute urine/day) via the kidneys.[53,54] Central DI (CDI), results from loss of AVP, whereas in NDI the kidneys no longer respond to circulating AVP. Both types can be either acquired or inherited. Failure of water reabsorption in the CD is associated with most cases of DI. If not detected and corrected early in life, DI can result in severe dehydration and damage to the central nervous system, hypernatremia, and bladder enlargement. The most common cause of NDI is in bipolar patients treated with lithium, which results in NDI in approximately 20% of treated patients.[55] Other acquired causes of NDI include hypokalemia, hypercalcemia, and ureteral obstruction. Both acquired and congenital forms of NDI have been linked to defects in AVP signaling and AQP2 trafficking. Although the inherited forms of DI are much rarer, their molecular basis has been largely elucidated following identification and characterization of the key proteins involved: the V_2R,[4,5] the AVP-sensitive CD water channel, AQP2,[56] and the gene coding for the AVP/neurophysin/glycopeptide precursor protein from which active AVP is generated.[57,58] Chapters 16 and 45 provide more extensive details on the pathophysiology of this disease, and several review articles have covered this topic in depth.[59-61]

CENTRAL (NEUROHYPOPHYSEAL) DIABETES INSIPIDUS

CDI results from a defect in the production and release of functional AVP.[62,63] Acquired CDI is often idiopathic but can also result from damage to the AVP-producing and AVP-secreting cells in the hypothalamus/pituitary, for example from trauma or infection. Hereditary forms of familial diabetes insipidus have been linked to over 66 different mutations of the gene encoding the AVP-neurophysin II precursor.[61] Absence of functional AVP can be generally treated by administration of AVP or DDAVP, usually via nasal aerosol.[64] However, AVP is also involved in stimulating AQP2 transcription; AQP2 levels are significantly lower than normal in Brattleboro rats—a valuable, but now difficult to obtain, animal model of CDI that does not produce functional AVP because of a single amino acid mutation in the neurophysin domain of the AVP gene.[57,65] It is likely, therefore, that the beneficial effect of AVP in CDI results from increased sodium reabsorption in the thick ascending limb of Henle, increased AQP2 trafficking (see later), and increased AQP2 protein levels following transcriptional activation of the AQP2 gene.

NEPHROGENIC DIABETES INSIPIDUS

The loss of an appropriate renal response to AVP in NDI usually reflects a functional defect in either the V_2R or AQP2 protein. Administration of AVP is not, therefore, usually sufficient to rectify the concentrating defect. However, the mutated V_2R may have a reduced affinity for AVP in some patients, and they may respond if circulating AVP levels are increased sufficiently.

NDI can be of a rare congenital/hereditary nature or, more commonly, an acquired disease.[61] A variety of gene mutations that result in defective targeting and/or function of the V_2R or the AQP2 water channel result in several distinct forms of NDI. The predominant form (type 1) affecting the V_2R is an X-linked recessive trait resulting from mutations in the AVP receptor type 2 gene (AVPR2).[66,67] Mutations in AVPR2 represent approximately 90% of hereditary NDI cases. Over 225 mutations that result in NDI have been identified in the V_2R protein,[61] and these are discussed in more detail in Chapter 45. These mutations can be divided into five classes.[68] Class I mutations lead to improperly processed/unstable mRNA, frameshifts, or nonsense mutations resulting in truncation of the receptor.[68] Class II mutations result in misfolding of the receptor and retention in the endoplasmic reticulum (ER). Class III mutations cause misfolding of the V_2R, reduced interaction of the V_2R with G proteins, and impaired cAMP production. Class IV mutations also lead to misfolding, with the V_2R able to reach the plasma membrane yet unable to interact properly with AVP. Class V mutations are missorted to an incorrect cellular compartment. Novel approaches for X-linked NDI therapy are discussed later in this chapter.

Type II NDI is a much less common autosomal recessive disease caused by mutations in the AQP2 gene,[54,68] representing approximately 10% of NDI cases. Currently 49 mutations in the AQP2 gene, resulting in two different molecular outcomes, have been described. First, mutations in AQP2 can affect the routing of functional AQP2 to the membrane. Second, some AQP2 mutations result in a defect in the formation of the pore-forming structure of AQP2, resulting in a lack of water channel function. In addition to these recessive forms, 10% of autosomal NDI cases are inherited in a dominant manner. The defect in these cases is due to mutations in the C-terminal tail of AQP2, which is essential for correct intracellular routing of the channel. In this case, heterotetramers of AQP2 monomers may be formed between the wild-type and the mutated form, causing misrouting of AQP2,[69] retention in the Golgi apparatus, or sorting of AQP2 to late endosomes, lysosomes, or the basolateral plasma membrane.[70] Thus the mutations act by a dominant negative mechanism. Because the condition is only partial, some wild-type AQP2 forms functional homotetramers,[71-74] and fluid restriction or desmopressin (DDAVP) administration increases urine osmolality except in severe cases.[75]

Although specific treatments for non–X-linked NDI are not available, various novel approaches have been proposed (see later). In addition, therapeutic guidelines include the use of a low-salt diet, combined with hydrochlorothiazide and amiloride treatment. In addition, inhibitors of cyclo-oxygenases, such as indomethacin, are often prescribed, despite their involvement in gastrointestinal disturbances.[61]

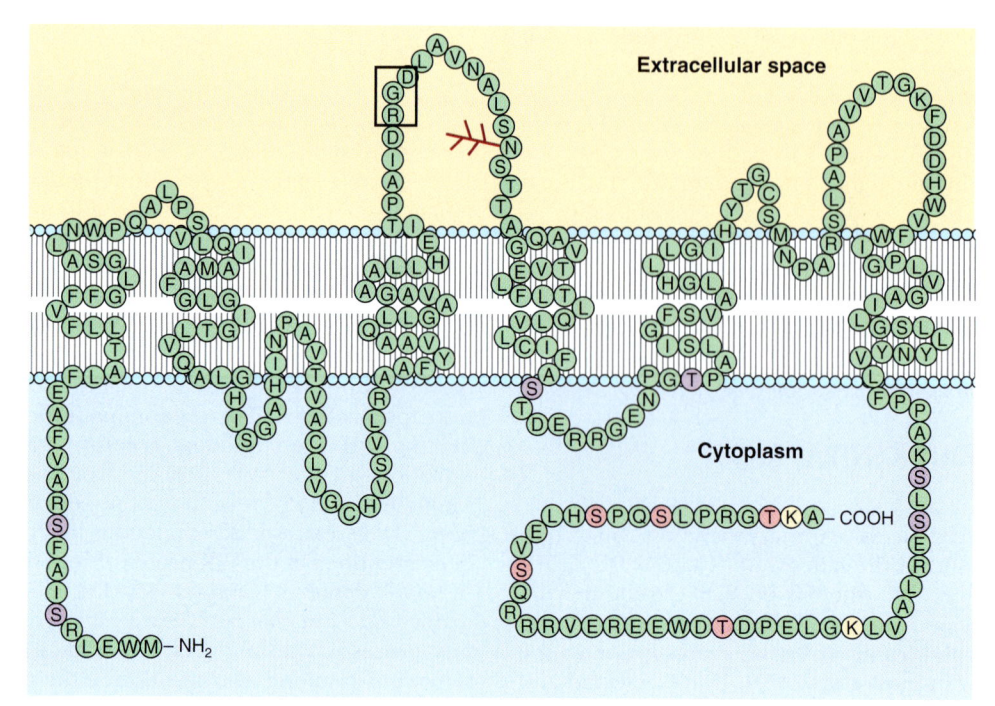

Figure 11.3 **Membrane topology of the aquaporin-2 (AQP2) water channel.** This 271–amino acid protein spans the lipid bilayer six times. Both N and C termini are in the cytoplasm. Five confirmed phosphorylation sites in the C-terminal region are shown in *red*, T244, S256, S261, S264, and S269. The S256 site is a target for protein kinase A (PKA), protein kinase G (PKG), and potentially other kinases and was originally shown to be required for AQP2 membrane accumulation after vasopressin stimulation. It is now believed to be a "master regulator" for the other adjacent phosphorylation sites in the C terminus. Other potential AQP2 phosphorylation sites, based on motif analysis by bioinformatics, are shown in *purple*, but they have not yet been confirmed experimentally. Two AQP2 ubiquitinylation sites are shown in *yellow*, of which only the penultimate residue in the C terminus, K270, has been shown to be functionally important at the time of writing. The single N-glycosylation site in the second extracellular loop is indicated by a *red branched symbol*. Finally, the arginine-glycine-aspartic acid (RGD) integrin–binding site, also in the second extracellular loop, is enclosed in a *black rectangle*.

THE AQUAPORINS—A FAMILY OF WATER CHANNEL PROTEINS

A total of 12 mammalian aquaporin homologs are known, and dozens more have been identified in virtually all organisms, including invertebrates, plants, and microbes. The first water channel (AQP1) was identified in 1991 by Peter Agre and his associates[76-79] and the CD AVP-sensitive water channel, AQP2, was cloned in 1993.[56] AQP1 is expressed in many cells and tissues with high constitutive water permeability, including proximal tubules and thin descending limbs of Henle's loop in the kidney.[80,81] AQP2 is the principal cell water channel that is involved in AVP-regulated urinary concentration in the kidney.[82-87] The membrane topography and some key features (e.g., phosphorylation sites) of AQP2 are illustrated in Figure 11.3.

OTHER PERMEABILITY PROPERTIES OF AQUAPORINS

The single channel water permeability of different aquaporins varies greatly,[88] and some aquaporins, including AQP3, AQP8, and AQP9—referred to as aquaglyceroporins—even allow the passage of molecules, including urea, glycerol, ammonia, and other small solutes. However, all aquaporins are impermeable to protons, a property that was first demonstrated using isolated apical endosomes from rat kidney papilla.[89,90] Crystallographic evidence has shown that the central region of the aqueous channel with charged residues lining a constricted region renders the passage of protons energetically unfavorable.[91-94] Physiologically the impermeability of aquaporins, including AQP2, to protons is important because the CD luminal fluid is acidic due to proton secretion and can reach a pH close to 4.5. It would be problematic if the cytosol of the principal cells equilibrated with the low pH of the tubule lumen simultaneously with an increase in apical membrane water permeability.

AQUAPORIN-2: THE VASOPRESSIN-SENSITIVE COLLECTING DUCT WATER CHANNEL

AQP2 is the AVP-regulated water channel in kidney CD principal cells.[56] AVP stimulation of the kidney CD results in the accumulation of AQP2 on the plasma membrane of principal cells (Figure 11.4). This involves the recycling of AQP2 between intracellular vesicles and the cell surface.[82-84,87,95-98] However, both AQP3 and AQP4, which are found in the basolateral membrane of principal cells,[99,100] are also regulated at the expression and possibly functional level by AVP and/or dehydration.[100-103]

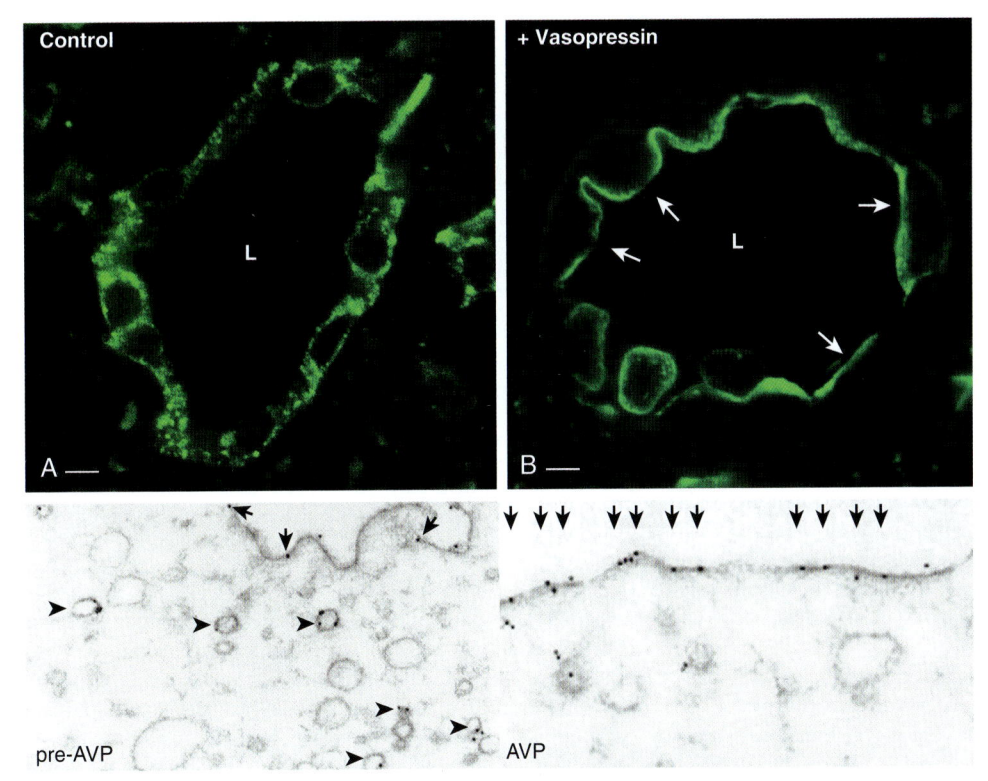

Figure 11.4 Increased plasma membrane expression of AQP2 in principal cells of VP-deficient Brattleboro rat kidney inner medullary collecting duct injected with AVP for 15 minutes. Kidneys were then fixed, sectioned and immunostained using anti-AQP2 antibodies. Under control conditions **(A)**, AQP2 has a cytosolic distribution in principal cells. After perfusion with VP **(B)**, AQP2 shows an increased apical localization in principal cells (arrows). A weaker basolateral localization of AQP2 in principal cells is also visible in this section. The **lower two panels** show the effect of VP on AQP2 distribution by immunogold electron microscopy. Tubules were perfused with 4nM DDAVP for 60 minutes The **left panel** (pre-VP) shows the apical region of a principal cell, with gold particles (detecting AQP2) distributed on cytoplasmic vesicles, as well as a few on the apical plasma membrane (arrows). After VP treatment, the number of gold particles on the apical plasma membrane is greatly increased (arrows), and the number of labeled cytoplasmic vesicles (arrowheads) is decreased. L, Tubule lumen. Bar equals 5 μm. (Lower panels adapted from Nielsen S, Chou CL, Marples D, et al: Vasopressin increases water permeability of kidney collecting duct by inducing translocation of aquaporin-CD water channels to plasma membrane. *Proc Natl Acad Sci U S A* 92:1013-1017, 1995.)

The AVP-induced change from a low-to-high permeability state of CD principal cells, and vice versa, involves the reversible redistribution of AQP2 from cytoplasmic vesicles to the apical plasma membrane. Because the basolateral membrane of these cells always has high water permeability due to the presence of AQP3 and/or AQP4, the luminal fluid then equilibrates osmotically with the surrounding interstitium. The osmolality in the renal inner medulla reaches approximately 1200 mOsm/kg in humans, and the urine can reach the same concentration in the presence of AVP. However, this mechanism also functions in the cortical CDs, in which a lumen (approximately 100 mOsm/kg) to interstitial (approximately 300 mOsm/kg) osmotic gradient results from NaCl extraction (luminal dilution) in the thick ascending limbs of Henle. Approximately 60% of the distally delivered water load is reabsorbed in the cortical CD system, or approximately 12 L/day.

AN OVERVIEW OF VASOPRESSIN-REGULATED AQUAPORIN-2 TRAFFICKING IN COLLECTING DUCT PRINCIPAL CELLS

Early freeze-fracture electron microscopy studies using amphibian urinary bladder and skin suggested that clusters of water channels are located on intracellular vesicles that fuse with the apical plasma membrane upon AVP stimulation. The water channels are internalized back into the cell by endocytosis after AVP washout.[104-108] Following the identification of aquaporins, specific antibodies allowed direct testing of the mechanism by which membrane water permeability is increased in AVP target cells, both in the kidney and in cell culture models. AQP2 is located in the apical plasma membrane of CD principal cells, as well as in intracellular vesicles.[56,109,110] In vitro and in vivo studies correlated the AVP-stimulated increase in CD water permeability and urinary concentration with relocalization of AQP2 from intracellular vesicles to the plasma membrane of principal cells (see Figure 11.4).[110-113] This relocation was reversible upon AVP washout and in animals either infused with a V_2R antagonist or subjected to water loading to reduce circulating AVP levels.[114-116] These and other data indicated that AVP acutely regulates the osmotic water permeability of CD principal cells by inducing a reversible shift in the steady state distribution of AQP2. One unexpected observation from initial studies was that significant amounts of AQP2 were present on principal cell basolateral membranes in some kidney regions, and that this staining tended to increase after AVP treatment. This issue will be addressed in more detail later in this chapter.

The internalized AQP2 that accumulates in endosomes after AVP withdrawal follows a complex intracellular pathway before reinsertion into the plasma membrane.[97,117-119] Recycling of the existing cohort of AQP2 can occur even when protein synthesis is inhibited, indicating that de novo protein synthesis is not required for sequential responses to AVP stimulation.[120] However, not all AQP2 is recycled. A significant amount of AQP2 also accumulates in multivesicular bodies (MVBs) after treatment of rats with an AVP antagonist.[114] This pool of AQP2 can then be directed to lysosomes for degradation, be transferred to a recycling compartment, or be directly transported to the cell surface via transport vesicles that derive from the MVBs. The fate of internalized AQP2 seems to be at least in part regulated by ubiquitinylation, and this pathway will be discussed later.

At least some of the MVBs can fuse with the apical membrane of principal cells and release small vesicles known as exosomes into the tubule lumen. These exosomes contain AQP2 on their limiting membranes,[121,122] as well as AQP2 mRNA and many other mRNAs and microRNAs within their lumen.[123,124] AQP2 protein can be detected in urine, and the amount increases in conditions of antidiuresis, when more AQP2 is present in the apical membrane of principal cells. The physiologic relevance, if any, of this urinary excretion of AQP2 and other membrane proteins in exosomes remains unknown, but the amount of exosomal AQP2 can be increased by AVP and urinary alkalinization.[125] It has also been shown that exosomes from DDAVP treated rats can induce increased AQP2 expression and water permeability in mCCD11 cells in culture,[124] implying a role in cell-cell communication. Interestingly, urinary AQP2 correlates with the severity of nocturnal enuresis in children, and lowering urinary calcium levels (by a low-calcium diet) has a beneficial effect in reducing the severity of the enuresis and reducing AQP2 secretion in hypercalcemic children treated with DDAVP.[126]

USE OF IN VITRO SYSTEMS TO EXAMINE AQUAPORIN-2 TRAFFICKING AND FUNCTION

EXPRESSION OF AQUAPORINS IN *XENOPUS* OOCYTES

Xenopus oocytes were the first model protein expression system that allowed the identification of AQP1 as a functional water channel using an oocyte swelling assay.[79,127] This system has also been valuable in assessing the function and regulation of mutated aquaporins[128] and addressing the role of oligomerization and phosphorylation of both wild-type and mutated AQP2 on its function.[129] In this way, many of the mutant AQP2 proteins resulting in NDI were shown to have folding defects that cause retention and ultimate degradation in the rough endoplasmic reticulum and/or retention in the Golgi.[73,130]

EXPRESSION OF AQUAPORINS IN NONEPITHELIAL CELLS

Chinese hamster ovary (CHO) and other nonpolarized cells, although not being appropriate models for studying the polarized expression of aquaporins in epithelia, can be used to measure functional and physical properties of aquaporins. For example, freeze-fracture studies on CHO cells revealed that AQP1 assembles in the lipid bilayer as a tetramer,[131,132] in agreement with biochemical cross-linking data[133] and cryomicroscopy and atomic force microscopy.[134-136] Important information was gathered concerning the abnormal intracellular location and the defective functional activity of AQP2 mutations.[130] CHO cells were also used to demonstrate that chemical chaperones could increase the delivery of misfolded AQP2 protein to the cell surface.[137]

TRANSFECTED POLARIZED CELLS EXPRESSING EXOGENOUS AQUAPORIN-2

Several laboratories developed stably transfected cells to dissect AQP2 trafficking and V_2R signaling. These include LLC-PK$_1$ cells (Figure 11.5),[120] rabbit CD epithelial cells,[138]

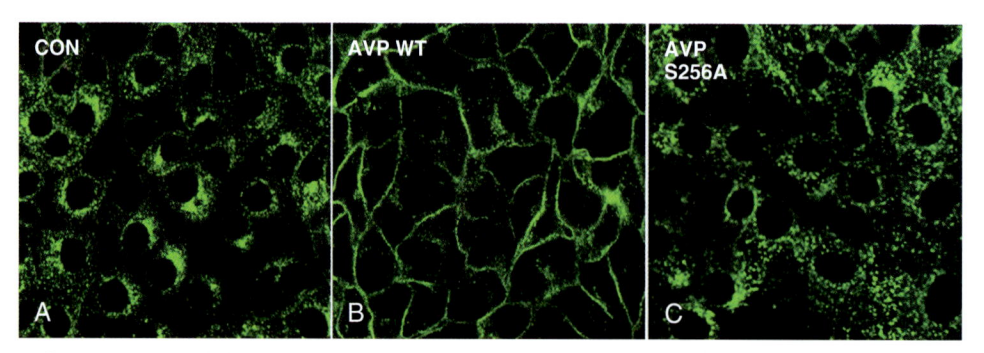

Figure 11.5 Immunofluorescence staining showing aquaporin-2 (AQP2) expressed in LLC-PK$_1$ cells. Under control (CON) conditions (**A**), AQP2 is located on perinuclear and more diffusely distributed intracellular vesicles, with very little plasma membrane staining. After vasopressin (AVP) treatment for 10 minutes, AQP2 accumulates on the plasma membrane of cells expressing wild-type (WT) AQP2 (**B**) but remains mainly on intracellular vesicles after AVP treatment of cells expressing AQP2-S256A, a mutation that prevents protein kinase A–mediated phosphorylation of this critical amino acid (**C**). Bar equals 5 μm.

Madin-Darby canine kidney (MDCK) cells,[139] and primary cultures of inner medullary CD (IMCD) cells.[140] Transfected LLC-PK₁ and MDCK cells showed constitutive plasma membrane expression of AQP1, similar to its pattern of expression in vivo, whereas AQP2 accumulation at the cell surface was increased by AVP or forskolin.[120,141] Similar data were obtained using transformed rabbit CD epithelial cells.[138] Since their initial development, AQP2-expressing cultured cell lines have proven to be reliable cell models that in most cases predict the in vivo behavior of the AVP-stimulated AQP2 trafficking pathway.

CELLS EXPRESSING ENDOGENOUS AQUAPORIN-2

Some cell lines, including mpkCCD(cl4) cells, express endogenous AQP2[142] and can be used to examine factors regulating AQP2 transcription. These include studies on the tonicity-responsive enhancer–binding protein (TonEBP) and the nuclear factor-kappaB pathway regulating AQP2 expression in response to hypertonicity and lipopolysaccharide,[143] showing that the effect of lithium on AQP2 downregulation was unrelated to AC activity,[144] demonstrating the role of exchange protein activated by cAMP (Epac) in long-term regulation of AQP2 transcription,[145] and showing that angiotensin II increases AQP2 protein expression.[146] Other studies using mpkCCD cells to address issues of AQP2 expression and trafficking have also used this cell line.[147-149]

USE OF KIDNEY TISSUE SLICES AND ISOLATED COLLECTING DUCT TO EXAMINE AQUAPORIN-2 TRAFFICKING

Kidney slices and isolated tubules have been extremely valuable tools to study AQP trafficking.[112,147,150-153] Although there may be potential issues of oxygen, nutrient, and drug diffusion into 150- to 200-μm–thick slices, dozens of samples can be prepared from the same kidney and treated simultaneously in paired studies. Isolated perfused tubules provide invaluable data, but the procedure is technically demanding and is accessible to only a few laboratories. Finally, isolated, microdissected CDs in suspension have been exploited as a system to study AQP2 recycling,[154] as well as to provide a pure IMCD cell population for detailed proteomic analysis of IMCD cells before and after exposure to AVP.[155]

EXPRESSION OF MULTIPLE BASOLATERAL AQUAPORINS (AQUAPORIN-2, AQUAPORIN-3, AND/OR AQUAPORIN-4) IN PRINCIPAL CELLS

The presence of AQP3 and/or AQP4 renders the basolateral plasma membranes of CD principal cells constitutively permeable to water. AQP3 expression is predominant in the cortex and decreases toward the inner medulla, with the reverse pattern for AQP4, which is most abundant in the inner medulla.[100,156] Interestingly, AQP2 is also localized in the basolateral plasma membrane of these cells in some regions of the CD.[109] The bipolar expression of AQP2 is most evident in the cortical connecting segment (Figure 11.6A) and the inner medulla (Figure 11.6B)[111,157-159] but is also detectable in other regions, including the outer medullary CD. An example of AQP2 and AQP4 staining in the same principal cells from an outer medullary CD is shown in Figure 11.7. In the inner medulla, basolateral expression of AQP2 is greatly increased by AVP (see Figure 11.6B) and oxytocin,[160,161] with hypertonicity in the medulla playing a modulating role.[161] Basolateral AQP2 expression is increased by long-term (6 days) aldosterone or AVP treatment of rats in the cortical CD.[158,162,163] Importantly, basolateral membrane water permeability in this region is increased in a mercurial-sensitive manner by AVP treatment, ruling out the contribution of the mercurial-insensitive AQP4 to this process.[164]

A frameshift mutation in AQP2 that results in NDI in humans also results in basolateral targeting when the mutated protein is expressed in polarized MDCK cells.[69] This shows that an increased basolateral expression of AQP2 is not sufficient to increase transepithelial water permeability in the CD. Based on new data (see later), it now appears that the basolateral AQP2 represents a transient step in an indirect apical targeting pathway for the AQP2 protein.[165]

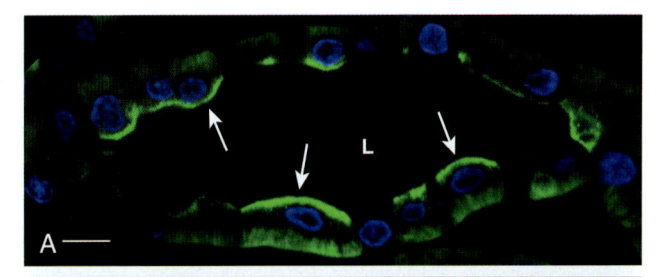

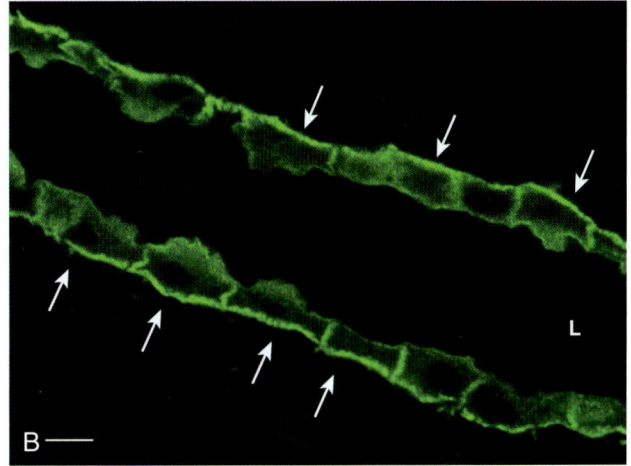

Figure 11.6 Immunofluorescence localization of aquaporin-2 (AQP2) in apical and basolateral plasma membranes of epithelial cells in the cortical connecting segment (CNS) (**A**) and the inner medullary collecting duct (IMCD) (**B**) of rat kidney. In the CNS, cells positive for AQP2 show a sharp apical band of staining *(arrows)*. The basolateral staining appears broader, due to the relatively deep basolateral infoldings present in these CNS cells. The IMCD segment shown here is from the central portion of the papilla and is from a tubule that was exposed to AVP for approximately 15 minutes before fixation and staining. In this region AVP induces a marked basolateral accumulation of AQP2 *(arrows)*. This basolateral AQP2 may be important in cell migration and tubulogenesis in the kidney. Nuclei are stained *blue* with 4′,6-diamidino-2-phenylindole (DAPI) in **A**. L, Tubule lumen. Bar equals 5 μm.

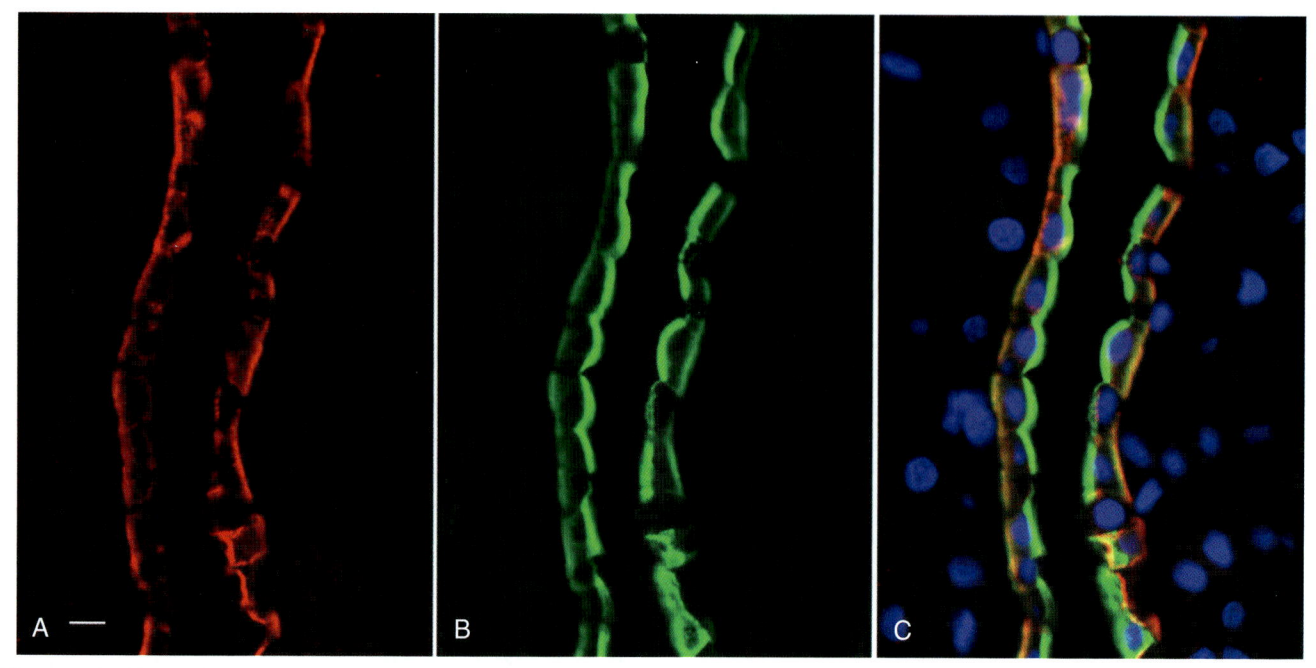

Figure 11.7 Example of a collecting duct from the outer medulla (outer stripe) of a rat kidney, immunostained for aquaporin-2 (AQP2) *(green)* and aquaporin-4 (AQP4) *(red)*. The merged image in **C** shows that AQP2 is largely apical in this region, but both AQP2 and AQP4 are present on basolateral membranes. This is best seen in the individual images in **B** (AQP2) and **A** (AQP4). All principal cells have some basolateral AQP2 staining at about the same intensity, whereas the basolateral staining for AQP4 varies somewhat among different, even adjacent, principal cells in this segment. Intercalated cells are not stained with either antibody and appear as darker gaps among the other cells. In **A**, nuclei are stained with 4′,6-diamidino-2-phenylindole (DAPI). Bar equals 10 μm.

A ROLE OF BASOLATERAL AQUAPORIN-2 IN CELL MIGRATION AND TUBULE MORPHOGENESIS

Because other water channels are basolaterally localized, the additional role of basolateral AQP2 in principal cell water transport remains unclear. However, studies have suggested that basolateral AQP2 may have a role in cell migration and tubulogenesis.[166] The extracellular domain of AQP2 contains an arginine-glycine-aspartic acid (RGD) domain that is involved in interaction with some integrins.[166,167] Many transgenic or knockout mice that lack AQP2 expression have a defect in kidney structure, most evident in the medulla, which can lead to premature death (Figure 11.8). These phenotypes are similar to those seen in a β1 integrin knockout mouse.[168] The structural alterations in AQP2 knockout mice were previously attributed to increased urine flow due to an AQP2-related concentrating defect. However, based on analysis of the phenotypes of various mice with NDI, the kidney structural defects may instead be due to the absence of normal AQP2/integrin/extracellular matrix interactions during renal development and perhaps adulthood.[166] This morphogenic effect seems to be independent of the water-transporting activity of AQP2. In contrast, the effects of AQP1 expression on cell migration were attributed to its role in increasing membrane water permeability.[169,170]

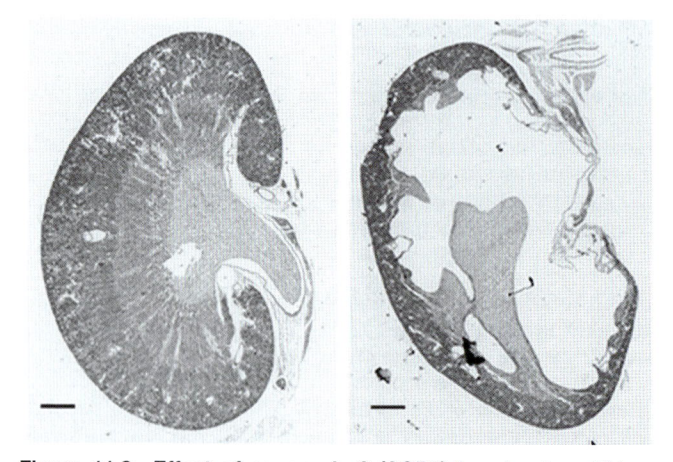

Figure 11.8 Effect of aquaporin-2 (AQP2) knockout on kidney morphology. Compared to the wild-type mouse kidney section *(left)*, the kidney from an AQP2 knockout mouse *(right)* has severe morphologic abnormalities 5 weeks after birth. Bar equals 1 mm. (From Chen Y, Rice W, Gu Z, et al: Aquaporin 2 promotes cell migration and epithelial morphogenesis. *J Am Soc Nephrol* 23:1506-1517, 2012.)

INTRACELLULAR PATHWAYS OF AQUAPORIN-2 TRAFFICKING

AQP2 is continually (constitutively) recycling between intracellular vesicles and the cell surface even in the absence of AVP stimulation. Membrane accumulation of AQP2 can then be achieved by a combination of stimulation of exocytosis and inhibition of endocytosis.[171,172] This pattern of trafficking has been described for some other membrane transporters, including the insulin-regulated glucose transporter 4 (GLUT4)[173] and cystic fibrosis transmembrane conductance regulator (CFTR).[174]

ROLE OF CLATHRIN-COATED PITS IN AQUAPORIN-2 RECYCLING

Clathrin-coated pits concentrate and internalize many plasma membrane proteins, including receptors,[22] transporters, and channels.[171] Clathrin-coated pits are critical for the internalization of both AQP2 and the V_2R.[23,38,175] When clathrin-mediated endocytosis is inhibited by the expression of a mutated dominant negative form of the protein dynamin in LLC-PK$_1$ cells, AQP2 accumulates on the plasma membrane and is depleted from cytoplasmic vesicles.[175] Dynamin is a GTPase that is involved in the formation and pinching off of clathrin-coated pits to form clathrin-coated vesicles.[176] The cholesterol-depleting drug methyl-β-cyclodextrin (MBCD) also blocks clathrin-mediated endocytosis. Exposure of both AQP2-expressing cell cultures and intact kidneys (using an isolated perfused kidney preparation) to MBCD results in AQP2 accumulation on the plasma membrane within 15 minutes (Figure 11.9).[177,178] Taken together, these data demonstrate the central role of clathrin-coated pits in AQP2 endocytosis. A later study proposed a role for caveolae as an alternative endocytotic pathway for AQP2 in cultured cells,[179] but under normal conditions, caveolae and caveolin are not present on the apical pole of principal cells in vivo.[180] Therefore, if caveolae are indeed involved in apical endocytosis in vitro, this is probably an artifact of cell culture. It has already been shown that several endocytotic events attributed to caveolae in proximal tubular cell cultures are not relevant to the in vivo situation. Proximal tubules do not express caveolin under normal conditions, but expression is induced in proximal tubular cell cultures.[181]

AQUAPORIN-2 LOCALIZATION IN INTRACELLULAR COMPARTMENTS DURING RECYCLING

Recycling of AQP2 was directly demonstrated in cycloheximide-treated, AQP2-transfected LLC-PK$_1$ cells, in which several rounds of exocytosis and endocytosis of AQP2 occurred despite the inhibition of de novo AQP2 synthesis.[120] After internalization via clathrin-coated pits, AQP2 enters an early endosomal antigen 1 (EEA1)–positive compartment.[182] This subapical recycling compartment is distinct from organelles such as the Golgi, the trans-Golgi network (TGN) and lysosomes,[182] does not contain transferrin receptor, and is distinct from vesicles that contain GLUT4 (another recycling protein) in adipocytes that coexpress AQP2 and GLUT4.[183] Whether vesicles containing recycling AQP2 represent a novel "organelle" or whether AQP2 usurps an already existing pathway in cultured cells and modifies it based on intrinsic signals within the AQP2 sequence remains unclear. It is probable that as newly synthesized AQP2 is loaded into transporting vesicles as it exits the TGN, the fate of the vesicles is indeed determined by signals on the AQP2 protein itself.

However, when recycling of AQP2 is interrupted by lowering the incubation temperature of the cells to 20°C, or by incubating cells with bafilomycin (an inhibitor of the vacuolar hydrogen ion adenosine triphosphatase [H^+-ATPase]), AQP2 can be concentrated in a clathrin-positive, Golgi-associated compartment.[118] This accumulation occurs even in the presence of cycloheximide, indicating that recycling AQP2 is also accumulating in this juxtanuclear compartment. The 20°C block prevents exit of proteins from the TGN,[184] and clathrin-coated vesicles are enriched in this cellular compartment.[185] However, some portions of the so-called recycling endosome, which is located in a similar juxtanuclear region of some cells, also have clathrin-coated domains.[186] Therefore, the AQP2 could be recycling either via the TGN, through a specialized clathrin-coated recycling endosome, or both. Indeed recycling AQP2 is partially co-localized with rab11, a marker of the recycling endosomal compartment, in subapical vesicles.[187,188]

AQUAPORIN-2 IS A CONSTITUTIVELY RECYCLING MEMBRANE PROTEIN

As discussed earlier, AQP2 recycles continually between intracellular vesicles and the cell surface, both in cultured cells and in principal cells in situ.[83,117] This provides the opportunity to modulate the plasma membrane content of AQP2 by increasing the rate of exocytosis, decreasing endocytosis, or both. Such a dual action of AVP was predicted by Knepper and Nielsen by comparing mathematical models of AVP-induced permeability changes to experimental data from perfused CDs.[172] Constitutive recycling was subsequently shown experimentally by blocking the AQP2 recycling pathway either in an intracellular perinuclear compartment identified as the TGN as discussed earlier,[118] or at the cell surface.[175,177] When clathrin-mediated endocytosis is arrested using dominant negative dynamin or MBCD, AQP2 accumulates at the plasma membrane in an AVP-independent manner (see Figure 11.9).[175,177,189,190] Importantly, MBCD also causes a rapid and significant accumulation of AQP2 in the apical membrane of CD principal cells in situ (see Figure 11.9E and F).[178] This observation raises the possibility that inhibition of endocytosis is a potential pathway by which AQP2 can be accumulated at the cell surface of CD principal cells in patients with X-linked NDI.

REGULATION OF AQUAPORIN-2 TRAFFICKING

Our understanding of AQP2 recycling continues to evolve in parallel with new discoveries related to the targeting and trafficking of membrane proteins in general. These include the discovery of alternative signaling pathways for AQP2 trafficking in addition to the "conventional" cAMP pathway,

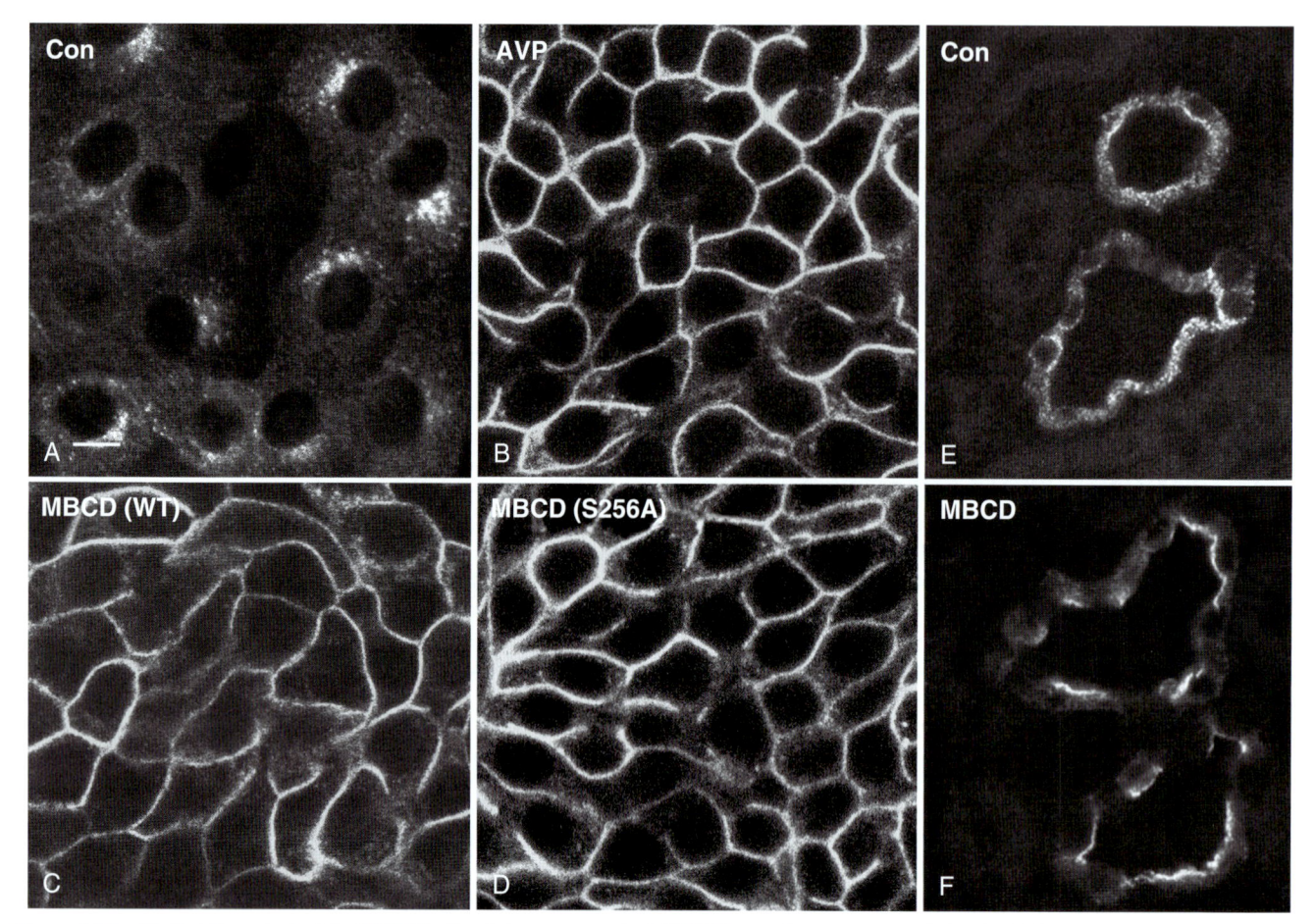

Figure 11.9 Methyl-β-cyclodextrin (MBCD) stimulates aquaporin-2 (AQP2) membrane accumulation in LLC-PK₁ cells (A to D) and collecting duct principal cells in situ (E and F). Immunofluorescence staining for AQP2 in LLC-PK₁ cells expressing wild-type AQP2 (A to C) or a mutant in which the S256 residue has been replaced by alanine (S256A) (D). Under baseline conditions, wild-type AQP2 is located mainly on intracellular vesicles, often concentrated in the perinuclear region of the cell (A). After vasopressin (AVP) treatment, wild-type AQP2 relocates to the plasma membrane (B). When endocytosis is inhibited by application of the cholesterol-depleting drug MBCD, both wild-type and S256A AQP2 accumulate at the cell surface in the absence of AVP (C and D). This result shows that both wild-type AQP2 and S256A AQP2 are constitutively recycling between intracellular vesicles and the plasma membrane, and that inhibiting endocytosis with MBCD is sufficient to cause membrane accumulation, even in the absence of S256 phosphorylation of AQP2. In collecting duct principal cells (inner stripe of outer medulla) in situ, AQP2 is located on vesicles scattered throughout the cytoplasm after perfusion of intact kidneys in vitro (E). However, after perfusion of kidneys for 60 minutes with 5 mmol/L MBCD, increased apical plasma membrane expression of AQP2 is seen (F). This finding indicates that AQP2 is constitutively recycling through the apical plasma membrane in principal cells in situ, and that membrane accumulation can be induced by blocking endocytosis (with MBCD) even in the absence of AVP. Con, Control.

the role of phosphorylation by various kinases, the involvement of the actin cytoskeleton, and the gradual discovery of accessory interacting proteins, including phosphorylation-dependent AQP2-binding proteins.

ROLE OF KINASES AND A-KINASE ANCHORING PROTEINS IN AQUAPORIN-2 TRAFFICKING

Phosphorylation of the C-terminal tail of AQP2 plays a complex regulatory role in trafficking and compartmentalization of the protein. AQP2 contains several putative phosphorylation sites for kinases (see Figure 11.3), including protein kinase A (PKA), protein kinase G (PKG), protein kinase C (PKC), Golgi casein kinase, and casein kinase II. The majority of work has focused on the role of PKA-induced phosphorylation of S256 in the AVP-induced signaling cascade, because this site is critical for the AVP-induced membrane accumulation of AQP2.[191,192] However, S256 is part of a polyphosphorylated region at the C terminus of AQP2, which contains three further AVP-regulated phosphorylation sites: S261, S264, and S269 (threonine in humans),[193,194] as well as a threonine at position T244.[195] The rise in intracellular cAMP following activation of AC by AVP/ V₂R results in recruitment of PKA to AQP2-containing vesicles by A-kinase-anchoring proteins (AKAPs).[196] The co-localization of vesicular AQP2 with AKAP 18δ makes this the most likely isoform to mediate this event.[197,198] Inhibition of the cAMP-specific phosphodiesterase 4D (PDE$_{4D}$) with rolipram increases AKAP-tethered PKA activity in AQP2-bearing vesicles and enhances AQP2 trafficking,[187] indicating that a novel, compartmentalized cAMP-dependent signal transduction pathway consisting of anchored PDE$_{4D}$, AKAP18δ, and PKA plays an essential role in AQP2 translocation. Furthermore, AKAP Ht31 directly interacts with the actin-modifying GTPase RhoA, which plays a crucial role in modulating AQP2 trafficking (see later).

IMPORTANCE OF THE S256 RESIDUE FOR AQUAPORIN-2 MEMBRANE ACCUMULATION

Phosphorylation is certainly involved in the regulated accumulation of AQP2 in the plasma membrane; phosphorylation of S256 and S269 prevent or reduce AQP2 endocytosis (see later). Whether the actual water permeability of AQP2 is also modulated by phosphorylation—by analogy with some of the plant aquaporins[199,200] and AQP4[201,202]—is controversial.[203,204] In addition, PKA-dependent phosphorylation of AQP2 in purified endosomes had no effect on single channel water permeability.[205] In contrast, regulation of membrane permeability by AQP2 trafficking has been established in a variety of experimental systems. Following PKA activation, phosphorylation of AQP2 on S256 is critical for AVP-induced cell-surface *accumulation* of AQP2 (see Figure 11.5).[191,192] In oocytes, S256 phosphorylation is required for AQP2 trafficking to the plasma membrane.[206] A mouse strain with an amino acid substitution at S256 (S256L), which prevents phosphorylation of this residue and inhibits AQP2 accumulation on the plasma membrane, has polyuria and congenital progressive hydronephrosis.[207] The importance of S256 phosphorylation was shown in humans by the identification of a mutation in AQP2 (S254L), which destroys the PKA phosphorylation site at S256 and results in NDI.[71]

OTHER PHOSPHORYLATION SITES (S261, S264, S269) ARE MODIFIED BY VASOPRESSIN

The role of three other phosphorylation sites in the AQP2 C terminus, S261, S264, and S269, remains uncertain, although the pS269 form of AQP2 is exclusively detected in the apical plasma membrane, suggesting a regulatory role of this phosphorylation site directly in the plasma membrane, perhaps by inhibiting endocytosis.[208,209] S256 seems to be the "master" phosphorylation site, because downstream phosphorylation of S264 and S269 requires prior PKA-mediated phosphorylation of S256,[193] whereas S261 phosphorylation is independent of any of the other sites.[204] Acute AVP exposure normally decreases the abundance of pS261 but increases that of both pS264 and pS269. All three phosphorylated forms are localized to some degree in the plasma membrane in vivo,[103,208,210,211] but cell-culture studies have demonstrated that S261 phosphorylation is not required for either AVP-stimulated AQP2 trafficking or constitutive recycling.[212,213] Preventing dephosphorylation of AQP2 with the phosphatase inhibitor okadaic acid increases cell surface accumulation of AQP2 in cultured cells, although this effect was also unexpectedly found in the presence of the kinase inhibitor H89, suggesting an effect that is not dependent on AQP2 phosphorylation by PKA.[214] However, there is a complex interaction between S261 phosphorylation and AQP2 ubiquitinylation that plays a role in modulating AQP2 trafficking.[215] As for other proteins with multiple kinase target sites, dissecting their individual contributions to AQP2 trafficking is likely to be a complex and difficult process, made even more complicated by the superimposition of AQP2 ubiquitinylation events that contribute to the regulation of AQP2 trafficking.

ROLE OF PHOSPHORYLATION IN EXOCYTOSIS AND ENDOCYTOSIS OF AQUAPORIN-2

Although phosphorylation has clearly been shown to inhibit endocytosis of AQP2, its role in exocytosis is much less clear. An S256A mutant, from which the PKA phosphorylation site is absent, readily accumulates on the plasma membrane upon inhibition of endocytosis with either K44A dynamin or MBCD (see Figure 11.9),[177] suggesting that the exocytotic pathway is intact under these conditions. Using a fluorescence-based exocytosis assay, Nunes and associates showed that AVP increases exocytosis of vesicles in AQP2-expressing cells whether or not AQP2 is phosphorylated at S256.[216] Thus, although AVP-induced *accumulation* of AQP2 at the cell surface requires S256 phosphorylation, exocytotic *insertion* of AQP2 into the plasma membrane is probably independent of this phosphorylation event.

Although phosphorylation of AQP2 is usually required for AVP-induced cell surface expression of AQP2, the internalization of AQP2 may not be dependent on its phosphorylation state at S256. Prostaglandin E_2 (PGE_2) stimulates removal of AQP2 from the surface of principal cells when added after AVP treatment[217] but does not appear to alter the S256 phosphorylated state of AQP2. This conclusion was based on whole-cell examination, however, and it remains possible that the cohort of AQP2 that is internalized does in fact undergo dephosphorylation. Resolving this issue will require immunolabeling of individual endocytotic events/vesicles, either by electron microscopy or superresolution fluorescence imaging. However, the S256D-AQP2 mutant—which mimics a phosphorylated S256 residue—is constitutively expressed predominantly at the cell surface,[218] and internalization can be induced by either PGE_2 or dopamine, but only after preexposing cells to forskolin. This suggests that PGE_2 and dopamine induce internalization of AQP2 independently of AQP2 S256 dephosphorylation,[219] but that preceding activation of cAMP production is necessary for PGE_2 and dopamine to cause AQP2 internalization. These data imply that phosphorylation of another intracellular target(s) (presumably by forskolin-stimulated elevation of cAMP) is necessary for AQP2 endocytosis to occur (see later). However, other data suggest that the effect of PGE_2 on AQP2 recycling depends on which PGE_2 receptor (EP receptor) it acts upon, because EP2 and EP4 receptor stimulation is able to increase intracellular cAMP levels and presumably AQP2 membrane insertion.[153,220] In a similar manner, the fact that AVP-induced exocytosis of AQP2 also seems to be independent of S256 phosphorylation[216] also suggests that AVP acts on other targets within the cell to stimulate vesicle exocytosis. One such target is the actin cytoskeleton (see later).

PHOSPHORYLATION OF S256 MODULATES AQUAPORIN-2 INTERACTION WITH ENDOCYTOTIC PROTEINS

The mechanism by which phosphorylation of AQP2 affects the steady-state redistribution of AQP2 is slowly being unraveled. One report has suggested that a Golgi casein kinase–mediated phosphorylation of S256 is necessary for the passage of AQP2 through the Golgi apparatus in its biosynthetic pathway.[221] However, this conclusion is not supported by studies showing that S256A AQP2 can recycle and accumulate at the cell surface when endocytosis is inhibited.[177] Nonetheless, accumulating evidence suggests that phosphorylation of AQP2 mediates its interaction with other proteins. For example, phosphorylation modifies AQP2 interaction with key proteins of the endocytotic machinery, including heat shock cognate/heat shock protein 70 (hsc/hsp70).[222] AQP2 is present in "endocytosis-resistant" membrane domains after AVP treatment,[49] probably because the interaction of AQP2 with hsc/hsp70 and other key proteins, such as dynamin and clathrin itself, that are required for clathrin-mediated endocytosis is greatly reduced by phosphorylation of AQP2 at S256.[213,222] AQP2 membrane accumulation was increased in cells expressing a dominant negative mutation of hsc70, which blocks clathrin-mediated endocytosis.[222] A comparative proteomic approach determined that several proteins, including hsp70 isoforms 1, 2, and 5 (hsp70-1, hsp70-2, hsp70-5), and annexin 2, differentially interact with AQP2 depending on its phosphorylation status.[103] The myelin and lymphocyte protein (MAL) is an AQP2-interacting protein that enhances AQP2 cell surface accumulation by reducing AQP2 internalization. MAL associates less with AQP256A than with wild-type AQP2.[223]

ROLE OF THE ACTIN CYTOSKELETON IN AQUAPORIN-2 TRAFFICKING

It has been appreciated for many years that the actin cytoskeleton is important for AQP2 trafficking. G-actin associates directly with non–S256-phosphorylated AQP2,[224-226] and both β- and γ-actin are associated with AQP2-containing vesicles.[227] Early studies conducted in rat inner medulla and toad urinary bladder demonstrated that AVP induces a reduction in F-actin in apical regions of cells[228,229] in parallel with the accumulation of water channels on apical membranes.[230] Later studies in mpkCCD14 cells have confirmed these findings and demonstrated that in response to AVP, F-actin disappears from near the center of the apical plasma membrane while consolidating laterally near the tight junction in a calcium-dependent manner.[231] Furthermore, AVP-induced apical AQP2 trafficking and forskolin-induced water permeability increases were blocked by F-actin disruption.

The potential role of actin in AQP2 trafficking was directly examined in transfected cells in culture. Exposure of cells to *Clostridium* toxin B, which inhibits Rho GTPases that are involved in regulating the actin cytoskeleton,[232] resulted in actin depolymerization and accumulation of AQP2 in the plasma membrane.[230] AQP2 translocation was also seen in cells treated with the downstream Rho kinase inhibitor, Y-27632.[230] Conversely, expression of constitutively active RhoA in these cells induced stress fiber formation, indicating actin polymerization, and inhibited the AQP2 translocation in response to forskolin. The actin cytoskeleton has varied and complex effects on several aspects of vesicle trafficking, including an involvement in endocytosis in some systems.[233,234] This mechanism is probably responsible for the effects of actin depolymerization on AQP2 membrane accumulation.

Noda and colleagues showed that AQP2 phosphorylation results in release of AQP2 from G-actin and an increased affinity of AQP2 for tropomyosin 5b (TM5b).[225] This causes a reduction of TM5b bound to F-actin, inducing F-actin destabilization and subsequent AQP2 trafficking to the plasma membrane. These findings also suggest a novel mechanism of protein trafficking in which the channel protein itself critically regulates local actin reorganization to initiate its movement. This idea is supported by data showing that AVP induces a burst of exocytosis only in cells expressing AQP2, and not in cells that are AQP2 null.[216] In addition, AVP induces significant actin depolymerization in LLC-PK$_1$ cells and MDCK only when they express AQP2.[235] Thus the presence of AQP2 influences the cellular effect of AVP on target cells, despite the fact that cAMP levels are similarly increased under all conditions. Further evidence for the involvement of actin in AQP2 trafficking comes from work using statins. After acute application to cells, statins cause the inhibition of RhoA, actin depolymerization, and AQP2 membrane accumulation due to inhibition of endocytosis.[236,237]

In contrast to the data showing membrane accumulation of AQP2 after actin depolymerization, a study using transfected MDCK cells reported that AQP2 was concentrated in an EEA1-positive early endosomal compartment upon actin filament disruption by either cytochalasin D or latrunculin.[188] These contrasting effects may reflect the use of different model systems. The physiologic role played by actin on AQP2 trafficking in renal principal cells in situ is still not clear, but apical fluid shear stress has been reported also to depolymerize the apical actin cytoskeleton and cause AQP2 membrane accumulation in IMCD cells,[238] suggesting that luminal flow might also be implicated in this response in vivo.

IDENTIFICATION OF ACTIN-ASSOCIATED PROTEINS POTENTIALLY INVOLVED IN AQUAPORIN-2 TRAFFICKING

Many studies have implicated actin and associated proteins such as the myosins, as well as microtubules (see later), in sequential transport steps of vesicle trafficking.[239,240] Myosin I, an actin-associated motor protein, was localized on AQP2-containing vesicles by electron microscopy,[241] and various other myosin isoforms, including nonmuscle myosins IIA and IIB, myosin VI, and myosin IXB, were identified by mass spectrometry using these vesicles.[227] Coupling of motor proteins to vesicles requires multiple Rab proteins, and myosin VB has been suggested to play a role in the AQP2 shuttle by Rab11-family interacting protein 2–dependent recycling through a perinuclear Rab11 compartment.[187] Quantitative proteomics has revealed a network of 14 actin regulatory proteins whose abundance is changed in cortical CD cells after AVP stimulation.[231] Myosin light-chain kinase, the myosin regulatory light chain, and nonmuscle myosin IIA and IIB isoforms have also been detected in rat IMCD cells and implicated in a calcium/calmodulin-regulated pathway leading to AQP2 membrane accumulation.[242] These results support previous data that Ca^{2+} release from ryanodine-sensitive stores plays an essential role in AVP-mediated AQP2 trafficking via a calmodulin-dependent mechanism.[13] A role of Epac, which is expressed in the CD,[243] in AVP-induced calcium mobilization, and AQP2 exocytosis in perfused CDs, has also been shown.[244] Epac has also been implicated in extending the AQP2 transcriptional response to AVP when cAMP levels are no longer elevated.[145] However, the role of calcium in the AVP response was questioned by another group who provided capacitance data in support of a cAMP-dependent but calcium-independent exocytotic process after AVP stimulation.[245]

Immunoaffinity isolation of AQP2 followed by protein mass spectrometry has been used to identify a "multiprotein complex" containing ionized calcium–binding adapter molecule 2, myosin regulatory light-chain smooth muscle isoforms 2A and 2B, α-tropomyosin 5b, annexin A2 and A6, scinderin, gelsolin, α-actinin-4, αII-spectrin, and myosin heavy-chain nonmuscle type A.[246] Interestingly, the gelsolin-like protein adseverin is much more highly expressed in CD principal cells than gelsolin (which is abundant in intercalated cells), indicating that it might be a physiologically important player in calcium-activated actin remodeling.[247] In addition to myosins, members of the ERM (ezrin-radixin-moesin) family of scaffolding proteins, have also been implicated in the apical trafficking process.[248] Ezrin expression is significantly upregulated in the CDs of lithium-treated rats,[249] indicating that actin remodeling might occur. The GTPase Rap1 and the signal-induced proliferation–associated gene 1 (SPA-1) may also have a role in regulating AQP2 trafficking.[250] Activation of Rap1 was found to inhibit AQP2 plasma membrane targeting, possibly by increasing actin polymerization mediated by SPA-1.

Based on these studies, it is clear that actin and its complex array of regulatory proteins play critical roles in the membrane accumulation and recycling of AQP2. However, with few exceptions, the precise steps in the pathway, and how these processes are regulated by AVP (e.g., via protein phosphorylation) have not been established in any detail.

MICROTUBULES AND AQUAPORIN-2 TRAFFICKING

Intracellular vesicles can move along microtubules, driven by microtubule "mechanoenzymes" or motors.[251-253] It is therefore not surprising that microtubule-depolymerizing agents such as colchicine and nocodazole partially inhibit the AVP-induced water permeability increase in target epithelia.[254-256] Colchicine and combretastatin treatment disrupt the apical localization of AQP2 in rat kidney principal cells, resulting in AQP2 scattering in vesicles throughout the cytoplasm.[110,257-258] Furthermore, cold treatment, which depolymerizes microtubules, also inhibits the AVP response, indicating that caution must be exercised in the interpretation of data from cell or tissue preparations that involve a cold incubation step as part of the experimental procedure.[152]

Two large protein families are critically involved in microtubule-based vesicle movement. These are ATPases known as motor proteins, the dyneins[259] and the kinesins.[260] Minus end–directed motors (dyneins) transport vesicles toward the microtubule-organizing center, whereas plus end–directed motors (kinesins) transport vesicles in the opposite direction.[261,262] Dynein and dynactin, a protein complex thought to link dynein to microtubules and vesicles, are associated with AQP2-bearing vesicles.[263] The effect of AVP on transepithelial water flow in toad bladder and CDs was only partially inhibited by microtubule disruption (approximately 65% in CDs).[255] These data support the idea that microtubules are involved in the long-range trafficking of vesicles toward the plasma membrane, but that the final steps of approach and fusion are microtubule independent. Upon AVP exposure the microtubule network is reversibly reorganized with increased formation of microtubules in the cell periphery.[258] In the same study, depolymerization of microtubules prevented the perinuclear positioning of AQP2 in resting cells, but, after internalization of AQP2 following AVP washout, forskolin stimulation still caused a redistribution of AQP2 to the plasma membrane,[258] in agreement with previous data. These results suggest that the microtubule-dependent translocation of AQP2 is predominantly responsible for trafficking and localization of AQP2 inside the cell after internalization, but not for its exocytic translocation. Microtubules are also critical for the trafficking of the V_2R to lysosomes after ligand-induced internalization, as described earlier (see Figure 11.2).[50]

Later studies demonstrated a role of microtubules in the basolateral to apical transcytosis of AQP2.[165] Data from MDCK cells suggest that AQP2 trafficking to the apical recycling endosome and ultimately the apical plasma membrane can occur via an indirect pathway through the basolateral membrane of epithelial cells (Figure 11.10). It is possible that this pathway is in some way disrupted or absent in LLC-PK$_1$ cells, in which AQP2 is inserted into the basolateral membrane both constitutively and after stimulation by AVP or forskolin.[177,264]

SNARE PROTEINS AND AQUAPORIN-2 TRAFFICKING

The membrane docking and fusion steps of AQP2 vesicle exocytosis are mediated by vesicle-targeting proteins similar to those described in many other cell types. Vesicle tethering, docking, and fusion involve a complex series of protein-protein interactions that are combined under the name "the SNARE hypothesis."[265-268] This requires a complex interaction between integral membrane proteins, the SNAREs (soluble N-ethylmaleimide–sensitive factor attachment protein receptors), present in the vesicle (v-SNAREs) and the target membrane (t-SNAREs). In the CD principal cell, several proteins of the SNARE complex are associated with AQP2-containing vesicles and/or the apical plasma membrane of principal cells. The SNARE protein VAMP-2 (vesicle-associated membrane protein 2, also known as synaptobrevin-2) is associated with AQP2 vesicles,[269,270] and disruption of VAMP-2 with tetanus toxin diminishes cAMP-dependent AQP2 trafficking.[271] Further SNARES that co-localize with AQP2 include VAMP-3 (cellubrevin), SNAP23 (synaptosomal-associated protein 23), and the ATPase Hrs-2, which may regulate exocytosis via interaction with SNAP25.[271,273,274] The t-SNARE syntaxin 4 is present in the apical plasma membrane of CD principal cells,[275] and SNAP23 is associated with syntaxin 4 and VAMP-2.[276] The interaction of AQP2 and the t-SNARE complex may be mediated by the protein snapin[277] and/or by the angiotensin-converting enzyme 2 homolog collectrin, which has been implicated in salt-sensitive hypertension.[278] Furthermore, other proteins that are involved in exocytotic processes in other cell types, such as members of the Rab GTPase family Rab3 and Rab5a,[279] have been identified in AQP2-containing vesicles and may also play a role in vesicle docking and

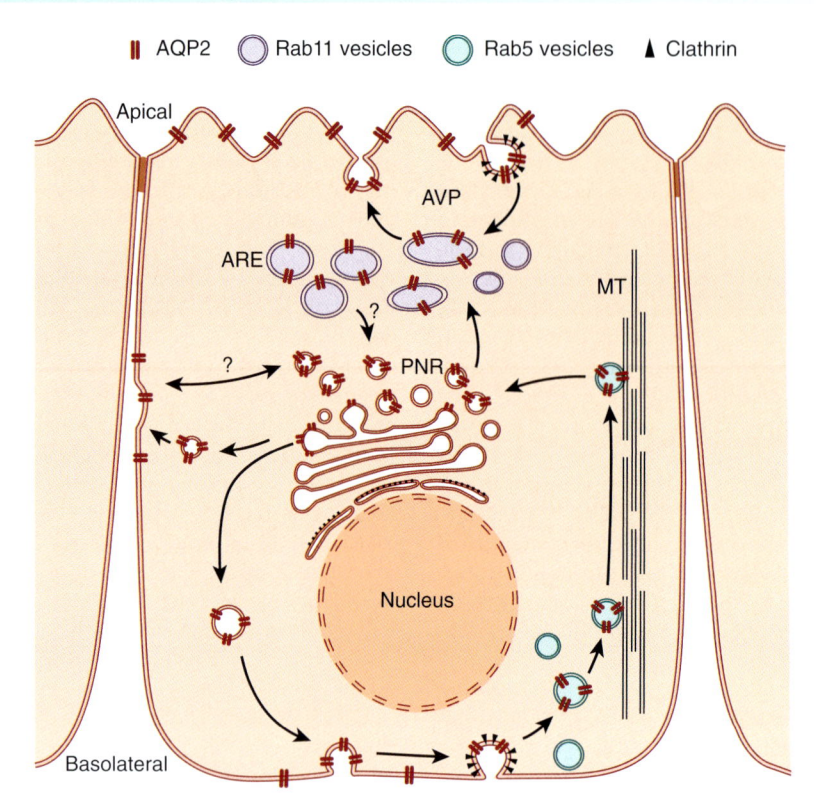

Figure 11.10 Aquaporin-2 (AQP2) follows a transcytotic pathway before apical membrane delivery. From vesicles in the perinuclear region (PNR), probably originating from the trans-Golgi network, AQP2 can be delivered to the basolateral plasma membrane before reaching the apical surface of epithelial cells. From there, it is retrieved by clathrin-mediated endocytosis into Rab5-positive endosomes *(green)*, which move in a microtubule (MT)-dependent manner to the PNR and ultimately to Rab11-positive apical recycling endosomes (AREs, *purple*). These Rab11-positive vesicles are involved in recycling AQP2 constitutively to and from the apical plasma membrane. The endocytotic branch of this recycling pathway is inhibited by the methyl-β-cyclodextrin treatment shown in Figure 11.9, resulting in cell surface accumulation of AQP2. The physiologic stimulus, vasopressin (AVP), increases apical AQP2 expression in two ways. It increases exocytosis from the Rab11 compartment and also inhibits clathrin-mediated endocytosis of AQP2 from the apical plasma membrane. The delivery of AQP2 to the basolateral membrane of collecting duct principal cells may be important for collecting duct tubulogenesis,[166] whereas apical AQP2 is necessary for urine concentration. (From Yui N, Lu HA, Chen Y, et al: Basolateral targeting and microtubule-dependent transcytosis of the aquaporin-2 water channel. *Am J Physiol Cell Physiol* 304:C38-C48, 2013.)

fusion. Several additional SNARE proteins, including syntaxin 7, syntaxin 12, and syntaxin 13, were identified in a proteomic screen using vesicles immunoisolated using anti-AQP2 antibodies.[227] However, such isolated vesicles represent a mixed population that contain AQP2 but are not all in the exocytotic pathway. A study using small interfering RNA has shown that VAMP-2, VAMP-3, syntaxin 3, and SNAP23 are a complementary set of SNAREs responsible for AQP2-vesicle fusion into the apical plasma membrane, and Munc18b is a negative regulator of the SNARE complex.[280] Finally, VAMP-8–null mice have hydronephrosis, and AQP2 exocytosis is impaired in VAMP-8–null CD cells.[281] This study also showed that VAMP-8 interacts with both syntaxin 3 and syntaxin 4.

LONG-TERM REGULATION OF WATER BALANCE

The actions of AVP on the kidney CD are mediated by two different but convergent mechanisms. As described earlier, AVP-mediated short-term regulation of CD water permeability is highly dependent on AQP2 trafficking events. Of equal importance are the effects of long-term AVP exposure. Prolonged dehydration increases urinary concentrating ability to a similar extent as acute AVP treatment,[282] whereas chronic water loading reduces urinary concentrating capacity. The consequences of long-term dehydration are complex and probably result from numerous adaptational changes. For example, in addition to changes in circulating AVP levels, dehydration alters circulating levels of glucocorticoids and prostaglandins, in addition to causing adaptational changes in the kidney, such as reducing glomerular filtration rate. However, one aspect of long-term regulation can be ascribed to changes in CD water permeability. Lankford and colleagues demonstrated that isolated perfused CDs isolated from water-restricted rats displayed a much higher AVP-stimulated osmotic water permeability than tubules from water-loaded rats,[283] suggesting an adaptation in CD principal cells. One such adaptation is that AQP2 expression markedly increases in response to water restriction with a greater abundance of AQP2 in the apical plasma membrane,[109] and long-term AVP exposure results in increased abundance of several forms of phosphorylated AQP2.[103,210,284] It was shown that the cAMP responsive element pathway is involved in the initial rise in AQP2 levels after DDAVP stimulation, but not in the long-term effect of DDAVP.[145] Instead, long-term regulation of AQP2 may involve the activation of Epac. In addition, both AVP-dependent and AVP-independent pathways probably play a role in these changes,[111,285-288] with evidence suggesting that both secretin[289] and oxytocin[290,291] are important for AVP-independent AQP2 translocation and expression. Also, the long-term effects of AVP on medullary hyperosmolality should not be underestimated, because extracellular tonicity, through activation of the tonicity-responsive enhancer–binding protein, increases AVP-induced AQP2 transcription and subsequent whole-cell AQP2 abundance.[292]

ACQUIRED WATER BALANCE DISORDERS

In addition to the rare hereditary forms of NDI, resulting in the inability of the kidney to respond to AVP and produce a concentrated urine, acquired forms of NDI occur much more frequently and arise as a consequence of drug treatments, electrolyte disturbances, and urinary tract obstruction (Table 11.1). These conditions are discussed extensively in other chapters, and only an overview is provided here.

In most manifestations of acquired NDI, dysregulation of AQP2, either in terms of protein abundance or in AQP2 membrane targeting, plays a fundamental role in the development of polyuria.[70,293] Quantitative data on AQP2 levels in various experimental conditions resulting in acquired NDI are summarized in Figure 11.11. Downregulation of AQP2 observed in acquired NDI is most likely the primary cause of the NDI, rather than being a secondary event (e.g., as a consequence of the increased urine production or reduction in interstitial osmolality). For example, in models of hypokalemic and lithium-induced NDI, the changes in AQP2 expression in the kidney cortex are identical to those seen in the inner medulla,[294-296] which indicates that interstitial tonicity is not a major factor. Moreover, washout of the medullary osmotic gradient for 1 or 5 days using the loop diuretic furosemide has no effect on AQP2 expression,[288,296] which indicates that high urine flow in itself is not responsible for the reduced AQP2 expression in experimental NDI. Here, we summarize a number of causes of acquired NDI, focusing on new developments in the field and potential new strategies for NDI treatment that have arisen from experimental research. Readers are directed toward other chapters of this book or extensive review articles[98] for further information.

LITHIUM TREATMENT

Approximately 0.5% of the Western population is currently receiving lithium therapy for treatment of bipolar affective disorders.[297] Unfortunately, up to 40% of treated individuals develop NDI as a side effect.[298] Lithium treatment can result in a reduced capacity to concentrate urine as early as 8 weeks after onset of treatment, with prolonged use (over 10 years) being linked to chronic kidney disease in some patients.

Lithium is filtered and reabsorbed by the kidney similarly to sodium and can enter the CD principal cells. AQP2 expression in principal cells is greatly decreased by lithium treatment (Figure 11.12). Several sets of data indicate that lithium exerts its effects by entering principal cells through

Table 11.1 Physiologic or Pathophysiologic Conditions Associated with Altered Abundance and/or Targeting of Aquaporin-2

Reduced Abundance of AQP2	Increased Abundance of AQP2
With Polyuria	**With Expansion of Extracellular Fluid Volume**
Genetic defects	Vasopressin infusion (SIADH)
Brattleboro rats (central DI)	Congestive heart failure
DI $^{+/+}$ Severe mice (low cAMP)	Hepatic cirrhosis (CCl4-induced noncompensated)?
AQP2 mutants (human)	Pregnancy
Vasopressin type 2 receptor variants (human)*	**With Polyuria**
Acquired NDI (rat models)	Osmotic diuresis (DM model in rat)
Lithium treatment	
Hypokalemia	
Hypercalcemia	
Postobstructive NDI	
Bilateral	
Unilateral	
Low-protein diet (urinary concentrating defect without polyuria)	
Water loading (compulsive water drinking)	
Chronic renal failure (5/6 nephrectomy model)	
Ischemia-induced acute renal failure (polyuric phase in rat model)	
Cisplatin-induced acute renal failure	
Calcium channel blocker (nifedipine) treatment (rat model)	
Age-induced NDI	
With Altered Urinary Concentration without Polyuria	
Nephrotic syndrome models (rat models)	
PAN-induced	
Adriamycin-induced	
Hepatic cirrhosis (CBL, compensated)	
Ischemia-induced acute renal failure (oliguric phase in rat model)	

*Reduced vasopressin type 2 receptor density has a profound effect on AQP2 targeting and expression.
AQP2, Aquaporin-2; cAMP, cyclic adenosine monophosphate; CBL, common bile duct ligation; CCl4, carbon tetrachloride; DI, diabetes insipidus; DM, diabetes mellitus; NDI, nephrogenic diabetes insipidus; PAN, puromycin aminonucleoside; SIADH, syndrome of inappropriate antidiuretic hormone secretion.

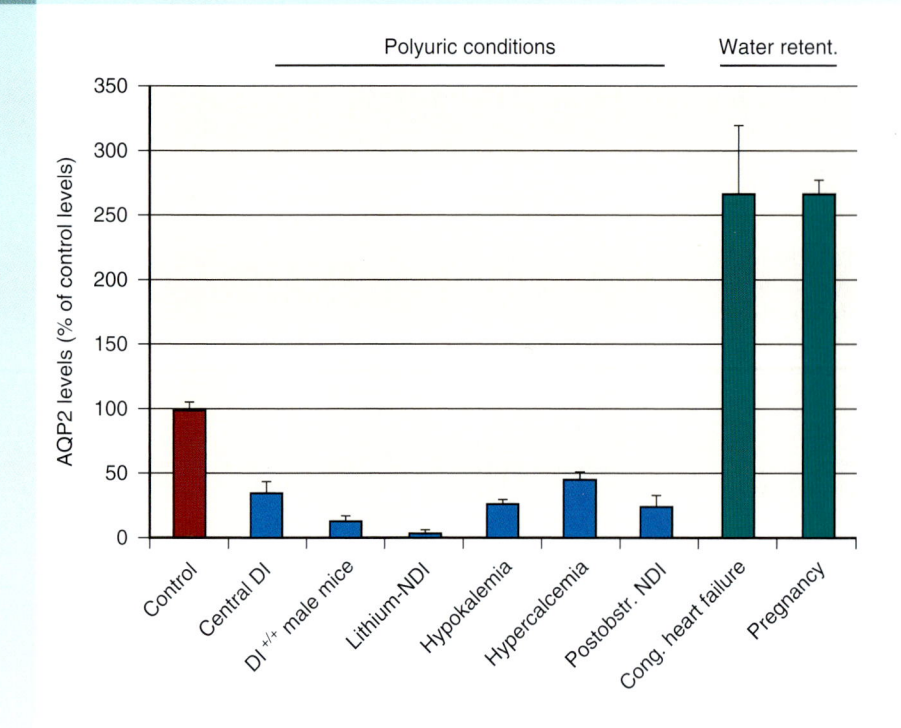

Figure 11.11 Quantitation of aquaporin-2 (AQP2) levels in various conditions of fluid and electrolyte imbalance, including acquired nephrogenic diabetes insipidus (NDI). DI, Diabetes insipidus.

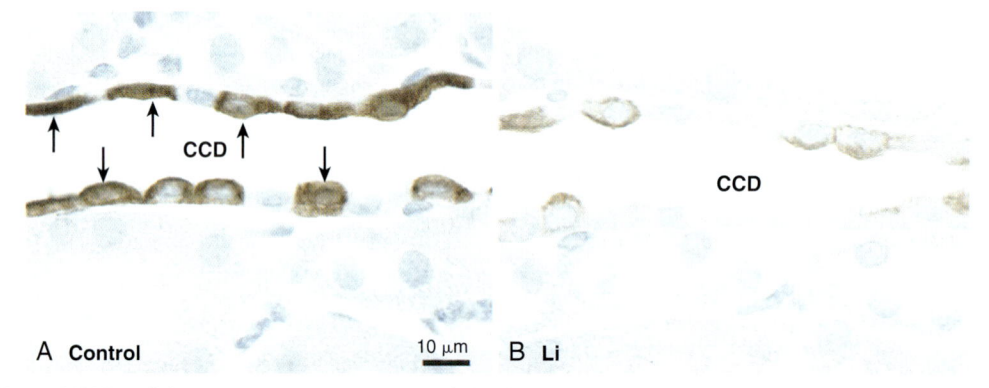

Figure 11.12 Effect of lithium (Li) treatment on aquaporin-2 (AQP2) expression and cellular composition of rat medullary collecting ducts. AQP2 levels in control rat kidneys (**A**, *arrows*) are considerably greater than after treatment with lithium for 4 weeks (**B**), when levels of AQP2 fall dramatically, and some principal cells (PCs) show little or no immunoperoxidase staining. In parallel, the number of PCs is reduced in collecting ducts of lithium-treated rats, whereas the number of intercalated cells is increased (not shown).[383] CCD, Cortical collecting duct. (Figure courtesy Soren Nielsen, Aarhus University, Aarhus, Denmark.)

the epithelial sodium channel (ENaC). ENaC has a higher permeability for lithium than for sodium,[299] the ENaC blocker triamterene increases lithium excretion,[300] and it has been shown in rats[301] and in a limited number of lithium-NDI patients that blocking ENaC with amiloride significantly reduces urine volume and increases urine osmolality.[302] In addition, in the mouse CD cell lines mCCD$_{c11}$ and mpkCCD, co-incubation of lithium with the ENaC blockers amiloride or benzamil prevented the lithium-induced AQP2 downregulation and decreased the intracellular lithium concentration,[303] showing that ENaC is the major cellular entry pathway for lithium. Confirming the ENaC-mediated lithium entry pathway in CD principal cells, CD-specific α-ENaC knockout mice do not demonstrate polyuria or a reduction in urine osmolality when treated with lithium.[304]

In contrast to these effects in the CD, the use of connecting tubule–specific AQP2 knockout mice has demonstrated that the connecting tubule is not involved in the pathogenesis of lithium treatment.[305]

The mechanisms behind the *onset* of lithium-induced NDI and the molecular mechanisms behind lithium-induced effects on AQP2 have been long sought, but these mechanisms are likely to be multifactorial.[293] One hypothesis derived from early cell studies suggests that lithium causes decreased AQP2 transcription.[144,306] Lithium-based interruption of normal AVP signaling and impaired cAMP production would result in drastically reduced AQP2 expression levels and/or targeting.[307-310] However, studies in mpkCCD cells contradicted this hypothesis and demonstrated that lithium decreases AQP2 transcription without changes in cAMP levels.[144] Other factors involved in the effects of lithium on water balance could be altered PGE_2 production or secretion, cyclo-oxygenase-2 (COX-2)–mediated signaling, AVP-independent mechanisms, β-catenin–mediated gene transcription or glycogen synthase kinase type 3β–mediated cell signaling.[293,298,311,312] Thus, it is likely that the diuretic effect of lithium is not simply a direct effect on AQP2, but a complex cascade of events that results from alterations in various signaling pathways, cell death, cell proliferation, altered principal cell morphology, and cellular organization of the tubular system.[310,313-316]

Treatment strategies for lithium-induced NDI include treatment with thiazide and amiloride[317,318] or modulation of the renin-angiotensin-aldosterone system via captopril (angiotensin-converting enzyme inhibitor), spironolactone (mineralocorticoid receptor blocker), or candesartan (angiotensin II receptor antagonist).[293]

ELECTROLYTE ABNORMALITIES: HYPOKALEMIA AND HYPERCALCEMIA

Hypokalemia and hypercalcemia are both associated with significant AVP-resistant polyuria.[296,319] In rat models of hypokalemia the condition is associated with decreased AQP2 mRNA and protein expression.[296,320] Besides AQP2, hypokalemia also decreases the expression of renal urea and sodium transporters in the distal nephron, which may contribute to the urinary concentrating defect by reducing interstitial tonicity.[321,322] Hypercalcemia decreases AQP2 protein levels independently of AQP2 mRNA, suggesting that the effects are independent of AQP2 transcription and may result from increased AQP2 degradation or decreased AQP2 translation.

Hypercalcemia also affects AQP2 membrane targeting,[323] the expression levels of AQP1 and AQP3, and the AVP-regulated Na-K-2Cl cotransporter type 2 (NKCC2) and renal outer medullary potassium[324]; probably all of these effects contribute to the decreased urine concentrating ability. The effects of hypercalcemia on AQP2 have been ascribed to activation of the apical calcium-sensing receptor (CaSR), which might be a defense mechanism to reduce the risk for calcium renal stone formation in states of high luminal calcium. Activation of the CaSR by high extracellular calcium antagonizes AQP2 translocation to the plasma membrane and AQP2 expression in cultured cells, which suggests that hypercalcemia-induced activation of the CaSR in vivo may have a similar effect, resulting in subsequent urine concentration defects.[126,325-327]

OBSTRUCTION OF THE URINARY TRACT

Chronic urinary outflow obstruction with impaired ability of the kidney to concentrate the urine is a common condition among elderly men. Moreover, acute obstruction in all age groups results in a similar concentrating defect. Several experimental animal models have been developed to study the physiology of this disorder. Experimental bilateral ureteral obstruction (BUO) for 24 hours results in dramatically reduced expression of AQP1 to AQP4, key sodium transporters/channels, and urea transporters.[328-330] BUO is associated with COX-2 induction and cellular infiltration of the renal medulla.[331,332] Indeed, treatment with a specific COX-2 inhibitor prevents downregulation of AQP2 and reduces postobstructive polyuria.[332] The renin-angiotensin system is also involved in the pathophysiologic changes of BUO,[333] and angiotensin II type 1 receptor blockade prevents downregulation of NaPi2, NKCC2, and AQP2 following BUO release.[334] In contrast to BUO, unilateral ureteral obstruction does not result in changes in the absolute excretion of water and solute, because the nonobstructed kidney is able to compensate.[328,330] However, there is still a pronounced reduction in AQP1 to AQP4 in the obstructed kidney, suggesting that local factors, such as prostaglandins, may play a role.[332,334] Inflammatory cytokines have also been implicated in ureteral obstruction,[335] and α-melanocyte–stimulating hormone treatment of rats with ureteral obstruction or release of obstruction markedly prevents the downregulation of several aquaporins and sodium transporters.[336]

ACUTE AND CHRONIC RENAL INJURY

As discussed in detail in Chapter 16, polyuria and impaired urinary concentration are seen in patients with acute and chronic renal injury. In both conditions, various abnormalities contribute to the renal dysfunction. A widely used experimental animal model for acute kidney injury (AKI) is ischemia and reperfusion,[337,338] which are a major cause of AKI in humans.[338] AKI is complicated by defects of both water and solute reabsorption in the proximal tubule and CD,[339-341] where AQP1 expression and AQP2 and AQP3 expression are decreased in AKI, respectively.[342] Hemorrhagic shock–induced AKI is also associated with decreased expression of AQP2 and AQP3.[343] In patients with chronic kidney disease (CKD), administration of AVP has no effect on the dilute urine, suggesting a defect in the receptor response.[344] Rat models of CKD have reduced AVPR2 mRNA[345] and downregulated AQP2 and AQP3 expression,[346] providing a molecular mechanism for the impaired concentrating function.

LIVER CIRRHOSIS AND CONGESTIVE HEART FAILURE

Hepatic cirrhosis and congestive heart failure (CHF) are just two conditions resulting in extracellular fluid expansion and hyponatremia due to sodium and water retention. In experimentally induced CHF, a marked increase in AQP2 expression and apical targeting was observed.[347,348] Administration of the V_2R antagonist OPC 31260 (Mozavaptan) in this model significantly increases diuresis, decreases urine osmolality, and reduces the observed increase in AQP2 levels, supporting the view that dysregulation of AQP2 plays a significant role in the development of water retention and hyponatremia in CHF. Interestingly, restoration of prestimulation levels of the V_2R on the surface of principal cells occurs within 30 minutes in CDs from CHF rats, compared to several hours in control rats.[349] This implies that the V_2R acquires the capacity to recycle rapidly (like the β2AR [see earlier]) in this experimental model, explaining the high sensitivity to AVP and the increased AQP2 expression levels in this condition. It should be emphasized that other mechanisms, including changes in NaCl transporter expression, are also likely to play a major role in the development of sodium and water retention in CHF.[350] Treatment of CHF rats with Losartan normalizes the levels of NKCC2 and AQP2, resulting in normalization of daily sodium excretion and partially improved renal function.

In experimental models of severe hepatic cirrhosis, AQP2 protein abundance is greatly increased,[351,352] whereas in models of compensated biliary hepatic cirrhosis AQP2 expression is reduced.[353] Thus it appears that, unlike in CHF, the changes in AQP2 levels vary considerably between different experimental models of hepatic cirrhosis. Concordantly, some studies of cirrhosis patients have demonstrated greater AQP2 levels in the urine compared to control subjects,[354,355] whereas other studies have demonstrated no increase, or even a decrease, in urinary AQP2 in cirrhosis patients.[355,356] Although an explanation for these differences remains to be determined, it is well known that the dysregulation of body water balance depends on the severity of cirrhosis.[293] Thus the downregulation of AQP2 observed in milder forms of cirrhosis may represent a compensatory mechanism to prevent development of water retention. In contrast, the increased levels of AVP seen in severe noncompensated cirrhosis with ascites may induce an inappropriate upregulation of AQP2 that would in turn participate in the development of water retention.

NOVEL APPROACHES FOR X-LINKED NEPHROGENIC DIABETES INSIPIDUS THERAPY

Our increased understanding of V_2R cell biology and signaling pathways have led to the consideration and development of several potential therapeutic strategies for X-linked NDI. For example, the aminoglycoside antibiotic G418 (Geneticin) promotes a cAMP response from a V_2R mutant resulting from a premature stop codon.[357] In the case of the most prevalent *AVPR2* mutations (class II) that result in misfolding of the receptor and ER/Golgi retention, a variety of approaches to induce the cell surface delivery of mutated receptors (which may be functional) have been attempted. These include the use of chemical chaperones, such as glycerol and dimethylsulfoxide, or drugs that modify cellular calcium levels, such as thapsigargin/curcumin or ionomycin. However, these approaches have had limited success with surface expression of only one V_2R mutant (V206D) increased using these reagents.[358] In contrast, the use of V_2R antagonists to increase cell surface expression and functionality of mutant V_2R protein seems more promising,[359-361] with small, cell-permeable nonpeptide antagonists (e.g., satavaptan, lixivaptan, mozavaptan, and tolvaptan) able to rescue the cell surface appearance of eight mutant receptors.[360] Importantly, the antagonist SR49059, which was shown to be effective in three patients harboring the R137H V_2R mutation, acts by improving the maturation and cell surface targeting of the mutant receptor.[362] Furthermore, the pharmacologic V_2R antagonist SR121463B resulted in greater maturation and surface expression of the V_2R mutations V206D and S167T than chemical chaperones.[358] However, when clinically relevant drug concentrations are considered, high-affinity nonpeptide antagonists such as OPC 31260 and OPC 41061 are the best potential candidates to treat NDI.[363] The alternative membrane-permeable peptides, penetratin and its synthetic analogue KLAL, could increase surface expression of the Y205C mutant that has a post-ER defect, whereas plasma membrane delivery of the L62P mutant is not influenced by either peptide.[364] The use of small nonpeptide compounds that also act as agonists have also been proposed.[365] However, despite their promise, there are several considerations that need to be addressed for the potential use of pharmacologic chaperones: (1) effects of chaperones are often significantly dependent on the nature of the mutation,[366,367] (2) if the compound is not a completely selective V_2R agonist, side effects via other receptors may arise, (3) the need for sufficient receptor binding combined with easy release from the receptor may constitute a weak point in this treatment strategy, (4) stimulation of V_2R by AVP promotes termination of the response by inducing receptor internalization and its delivery to and degradation in lysosomes. In the presence of high levels of AVP, this could counteract the effect of the rescued receptor.

Another exciting approach for X-linked NDI (XNDI) treatment is the use of cell-permeable nonpeptide agonists, which do not necessarily have to elicit translocation of the V_2R to the plasma membrane. For example, VA999088, VA999089, and OPC 51803 can enter the cell, reach the mutant V_2R, and initiate a cAMP response and AQP2 translocation,[366,368] because the V_2R can signal even when on intracellular vesicles.[25] However, some agonists (e.g., MCF14, MCF18, and MCF57) can also rescue membrane expression of the V_2R and thus provide additional beneficial effects (e.g., antagonistic effects on β-arrestin recruitment that would downregulate V_2R signaling).[365]

VASOPRESSIN RECEPTOR–INDEPENDENT MEMBRANE INSERTION OF AQUAPORIN-2 — POTENTIAL STRATEGIES FOR TREATING NEPHROGENIC DIABETES INSIPIDUS

Important progress has been made in the last few years in our understanding of intracellular signaling or alternative trafficking pathways that bypass the V_2R-cAMP-PKA cascade, allowing membrane accumulation of AQP2 even in the absence of a functional V_2R. This is especially important for the generation of novel strategies to alleviate the symptoms of X-linked NDI, in which a mutated V_2R is defective for a number of reasons (see earlier). Renal principal cells in these patients may still produce AQP2, but the defective V_2R signaling mechanism means that it does not accumulate at the cell surface to increase urine concentration upon an increase in circulating AVP levels. Later developments in understanding the cell biology of AQP2 trafficking have provided some hope that AQP2 can in fact accumulate at the cell surface independently of AVP signaling in CDs of these patients. Various treatment strategies have been extensively reviewed,[61,117] and an overview is provided here.

PHOSPHODIESTERASE INHIBITORS

Increasing either cyclic guanosine monophosphate (cGMP) or cAMP levels in principle will lead to increased AQP2 phosphorylation and trafficking. Intracellular cGMP levels can be increased by sodium nitroprusside, L-arginine, and atrial natriuretic peptide. All these substances can increase AQP2 abundance in the apical plasma membrane.[117,150,369] The selective cGMP phosphodiesterase (PDE_5) inhibitor sildenafil citrate (Viagra) prevents degradation of cGMP,

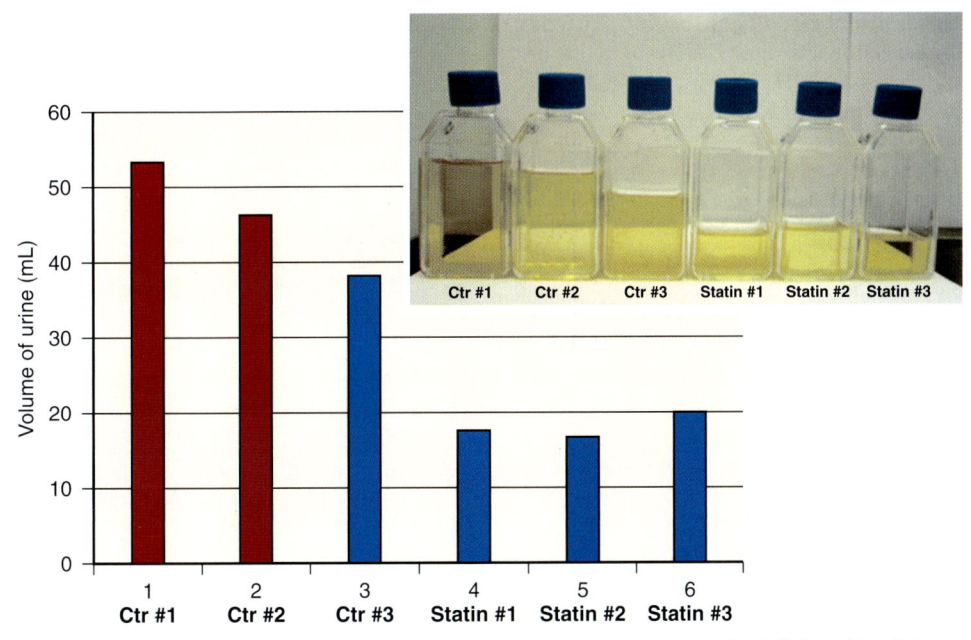

Figure 11.13 **Statins increase urine concentration and reduce urine volume in vasopressin-deficient Brattleboro rats.** Six-hour urine volumes produced by untreated, vasopressin-deficient rats (Ctr #1 to #3), compared to rats treated with simvastatin for 6 hours. *Inset*, The actual urine specimens from these animals. (Adapted from Li W, Zhang Y, Bouley R, et al: Simvastatin enhances aquaporin-2 surface expression and urinary concentration in vasopressin-deficient Brattleboro rats through modulation of Rho GTPase. *Am J Physiol Renal Physiol* 301:F309-F318, 2011.)

resulting in increased membrane expression of AQP2 in vitro and in vivo.[151] Sildenafil citrate also reduces polyuria in rats with lithium-induced NDI.[370] In comparison, rolipram, a PDE_4 inhibitor, increased cAMP and AQP2 trafficking in cell culture and urine osmolality in a mouse model of autosomal dominant NDI, whereas PDE_3 and PDE_5 inhibitors had no significant effects.[371] However, rolipram treatment of two male patients suffering from NDI due to V_2R mutations did not result in any relief of symptoms.[372]

CALCITONIN AND SECRETIN

Calcitonin is a 32–amino acid linear polypeptide hormone that is produced in humans primarily by the parafollicular cells of the thyroid. Calcitonin acts via a seven transmembrane spanning (7TM) GPCR, which is coupled to $G_{\alpha s}$ and can increase intracellular cAMP levels. Calcitonin induces AQP2 membrane accumulation in vitro and in vivo via a cAMP-mediated mechanism.[373,374] Secretin is another hormone that acts via a GPCR to increase cAMP and induce AQP2 membrane expression in principal cells.[289] A study has combined secretin with fluvastatin (see also later) to ameliorate the symptoms of NDI in mice with X-linked NDI.[375] Secretin may also influence AVP release from the hypothalamus, and defects in this regulation could be involved in some cases of syndrome of inappropriate secretion of antidiuretic hormone secretion.[376]

STATINS

Statins inhibit the activity of 3-hydroxy-3-methylglutaryl–coenzyme A reductase, which results in decreased biosynthesis of cholesterol, and they are most commonly associated with treatment of hypercholesterolemia. Statins have also been proposed for treatment of NDI. Acute exposure to simvastatin, fluvastatin, or lovastatin increased apical membrane AQP2 in cultured cells.[236,237,377] In addition, simvastatin increased AQP2 trafficking in principal cells of Brattleboro rats in parallel with increased urine concentration (Figure 11.13),[236] and fluvastatin increased AQP2 expression and water reabsorption in mouse kidney in an AVP-independent manner.[377] The molecular mechanism behind these effects is not fully understood but has been attributed to changes in prenylation of Rho family proteins that are involved in AQP2 trafficking and regulation of the cell cytoskeleton.[236,377] Importantly, a later study demonstrated that atorvastatin administration significantly improved urinary concentration in BUO-induced NDI by reversing the downregulation of AQP2.[378] Whether the effect of statins is specific for AQP2 or whether all other classes of membrane channels/transporters are influenced by statin treatment remains to be resolved.

PROSTAGLANDINS

Although PGE_2 antagonizes AVP-induced water permeability, PGE_2 increases CD water permeability in the absence of AVP stimulation, probably via activation of its receptors EP2 and/or EP4.[379-381] Agonists specific for EP2 (butaprost) and EP4 (CAY10580) increase AQP2 trafficking in MDCK cells.[153] The EP4 agonist ONO-AE1-329 increased urine osmolality, decreased urine volume, and increased AQP2 expression in a mouse model for XNDI, whereas the EP2 agonist butaprost reduced urine volume and increased urine osmolality in rats treated with a V_2R antagonist.[153,220] Furthermore, long term, the ONO compound increased AQP2 protein abundance in XNDI.[220] Together these data suggest that specific EP2 or EP4 agonist administration could be a promising treatment strategy for NDI.

HEAT SHOCK PROTEIN 90

Heat shock protein 90 (hsp90) is considered an ER-resident/cytoplasmic "molecular chaperone" that aids proper folding of proteins.[363] An hsp90 inhibitor (17-allylamino-17-demethoxygeldanamycin) partially corrected NDI in a mouse model of autosomal recessive NDI in which the mutant, AQP2-T126M, was retained in the ER.[382]

ACKNOWLEDGMENTS

Work from the laboratories of the authors was carried out with the support of National Institutes of Health grants PO1 DK38452 and RO1 DK096586 (DB) and a grant from the Danish Medical Research Council (RAF), Novo Nordisk Fond (RAF), and the Lundbeck Foundation (RAF). We thank our many excellent colleagues for their invaluable contributions to our research endeavours over the past several years.

Complete reference list available at ExpertConsult.com.

KEY REFERENCES

1. Landry DW, Oliver JA: The pathogenesis of vasodilatory shock. *N Engl J Med* 345:588–595, 2001.
3. Sugimoto T, Saito M, Mochizuki S, et al: Molecular cloning and functional expression of a cDNA encoding the human V1b vasopressin receptor. *J Biol Chem* 269:27088–27092, 1994.
4. Birnbaumer M, Seibold A, Gilbert S: Molecular cloning of the receptor for human antidiuretic hormone. *Nature* 357:333–335, 1992.
5. Lolait SJ, O'Carroll AM, Konig M, et al: Cloning and characterization of a vasopressin V2 receptor and possible link to nephrogenic diabetes insipidus. *Nature* 357:336–339, 1992.
18. Rieg T, Tang T, Murray F, et al: Adenylate cyclase 6 determines cAMP formation and aquaporin-2 phosphorylation and trafficking in inner medulla. *J Am Soc Nephrol* 21:2059–2068, 2010.
25. Feinstein TN, Yui N, Webber MJ, et al: Noncanonical control of vasopressin receptor type 2 signaling by retromer and arrestin. *J Biol Chem* 288:27849–27860, 2013.
36. DeWire SM, Ahn S, Lefkowitz RJ, et al: Beta-arrestins and cell signaling. *Annu Rev Physiol* 69:483–510, 2007.
38. Oakley RH, Laporte SA, Holt JA, et al: Association of beta-arrestin with G protein-coupled receptors during clathrin-mediated endocytosis dictates the profile of receptor resensitization. *J Biol Chem* 274:32248–32257, 1999.
45. Martin NP, Lefkowitz RJ, Shenoy SK: Regulation of V2 vasopressin receptor degradation by agonist-promoted ubiquitination. *J Biol Chem* 278:45954–45959, 2003.
49. Bouley R, Hawthorn G, Russo LM, et al: Aquaporin 2 (AQP2) and vasopressin type 2 receptor (V2R) endocytosis in kidney epithelial cells: AQP2 is located in "endocytosis-resistant" membrane domains after vasopressin treatment. *Biol Cell* 98:215–232, 2006.
56. Fushimi K, Uchida S, Hara Y, et al: Cloning and expression of apical membrane water channel of rat kidney collecting tubule. *Nature* 361:549–552, 1993.
61. Moeller HB, Rittig S, Fenton RA: Nephrogenic diabetes insipidus: essential insights into the molecular background and potential therapies for treatment. *Endocr Rev* 34:278–301, 2013.
67. Rosenthal WA, Seibold A, Antaramian A, et al: Molecular identification of the gene responsible for congenital nephrogenic diabetes insipidus. *Nature* 359:233–235, 1992.
76. Denker BM, Smith BL, Kuhajda FP, et al: Identification, purification and partial characterization of a novel Mr 28,000 integral membrane protein from erythrocytes and renal tubules. *J Biol Chem* 263:15634–15642, 1988.
79. Preston GM, Carroll TP, Guggino WB, et al: Appearance of water channels in Xenopus oocytes expressing red cell CHIP28 protein. *Science* 256:385–387, 1992.
105. Brown D, Orci L: Vasopressin stimulates formation of coated pits in rat kidney collecting ducts. *Nature* 302:253–255, 1983.
112. Nielsen S, Chou CL, Marples D, et al: Vasopressin increases water permeability of kidney collecting duct by inducing translocation of aquaporin-CD water channels to plasma membrane. *Proc Natl Acad Sci U S A* 92:1013–1017, 1995.
121. Pisitkun T, Shen RF, Knepper MA: Identification and proteomic profiling of exosomes in human urine. *Proc Natl Acad Sci U S A* 101:13368–13373, 2004.
128. Deen PM, Verdijk MA, Knoers NV, et al: Requirement of human renal water channel aquaporin-2 for vasopressin-dependent concentration of urine. *Science* 264:92–95, 1994.
153. Olesen ET, Rutzler MR, Moeller HB, et al: Vasopressin-independent targeting of aquaporin-2 by selective E-prostanoid receptor agonists alleviates nephrogenic diabetes insipidus. *Proc Natl Acad Sci U S A* 108:12949–12954, 2011.
157. Christensen BM, Marples D, Wang W, et al: Decreased fraction of principal cells in parallel with increased fraction of intercalated cells in rats with lithium-induced NDI. *J Am Soc Nephrol* 13:270A, 2002.
166. Chen Y, Rice W, Gu Z, et al: Aquaporin 2 promotes cell migration and epithelial morphogenesis. *J Am Soc Nephrol* 23:1506–1517, 2012.
172. Knepper MA, Nielsen S: Kinetic model of water and urea permeability regulation by vasopressin in collecting duct. *Am J Physiol* 265:F214–F224, 1993.
175. Sun TX, Van Hoek A, Huang Y, et al: Aquaporin-2 localization in clathrin-coated pits: inhibition of endocytosis by dominant-negative dynamin. *Am J Physiol Renal Physiol* 282:F998–F1011, 2002.
177. Lu H, Sun TX, Bouley R, et al: Inhibition of endocytosis causes phosphorylation (S256)-independent plasma membrane accumulation of AQP2. *Am J Physiol Renal Physiol* 286:F233–F243, 2004.
182. Tajika Y, Matsuzaki T, Suzuki T, et al: Aquaporin-2 is retrieved to the apical storage compartment via early endosomes and phosphatidylinositol 3-kinase-dependent pathway. *Endocrinology* 145:4375–4383, 2004.
191. Fushimi K, Sasaki S, Marumo F: Phosphorylation of serine 256 is required for cAMP-dependent regulatory exocytosis of the aquaporin-2 water channel. *J Biol Chem* 272:14800–14804, 1997.
192. Katsura T, Gustafson CE, Ausiello DA, et al: Protein kinase A phosphorylation is involved in regulated exocytosis of aquaporin-2 in transfected LLC-PK1 cells. *Am J Physiol* 272:F817–F822, 1997.

12

Aldosterone and Mineralocorticoid Receptors: Renal and Extrarenal Roles

David Pearce | Vivek Bhalla | John W. Funder

CHAPTER OUTLINE

GENERAL INTRODUCTION TO ALDOSTERONE AND MINERALOCORTICOID RECEPTORS, 304
ALDOSTERONE SYNTHESIS, 305
MECHANISMS OF MINERALOCORTICOID RECEPTOR FUNCTION AND GENE REGULATION, 306
Mineralocorticoid Receptor Function as a Hormone-Regulated Transcription Factor: General Features and Subcellular Localization, 306
Domain Structure of Mineralocorticoid Receptors, 307
Mineralocorticoid Receptor Regulation of Transcription Initiation: Coactivators and Corepressors, 310
REGULATION OF SODIUM ABSORPTION AND POTASSIUM SECRETION, 310
General Model of Aldosterone Action, 310
Aldosterone and Epithelial Sodium Channel Trafficking, 311
Basolateral Membrane Effects of Aldosterone, 312
Activation of the Epithelial Sodium Channel by Proteolytic Cleavage, 312
Potassium Secretion and Aldosterone, 312
Separation of Sodium Absorption and Potassium Secretion by the Aldosterone-Sensitive Distal Nephron, 313
Aldosterone-Independent ENaC-Mediated Sodium Reabsorption in the Distal Nephron, 314
Sites of Mineralocorticoid Receptor Expression and Locus of Action Along the Nephron, 315

NONRENAL ALDOSTERONE-RESPONSIVE TIGHT EPITHELIA, 315
Colon, 316
Lung, 317
Exocrine Glands and Sensors, 317
ROLE OF SERUM- AND GLUCOCORTICOID-REGULATED KINASE IN MEDIATING ALDOSTERONE EFFECTS, 317
Induction of SGK1 by Aldosterone, 317
Molecular Mechanisms of SGK1 Action in the Aldosterone-Sensitive Distal Nephron, 318
11β-HYDROXYSTEROID DEHYDROGENASE TYPE 2, 320
11β-HSD2: An Essential Determinant of Mineralocorticoid Specificity, 320
Sites of 11β-HSD2 Expression, 320
Impact of 11β-HSD2 on Mineralocorticoid Receptor Activity, 320
Apparent Mineralocorticoid Excess: A Disease of Defective 11β-HSD2, 320
Role of 11β-HSD2 in Blood Vessels, 320
Summary of 11β-HSD2 Roles, 321
NONGENOMIC EFFECTS OF ALDOSTERONE, 321
DISEASE STATES, 321
Primary Aldosteronism, 321
Congestive Heart Failure, 322
Chronic Kidney Disease, 322
NONEPITHELIAL ACTIONS OF ALDOSTERONE, 322

In mammals, the control of extracellular fluid volume and blood pressure is intimately intertwined with the regulation of epithelial ion transport. Aldosterone, which is essential for survival, is the central hormone regulating the relevant epithelial transport processes, particularly of ions such as Na^+, K^+, and Cl^-. All circulating aldosterone is generated in the adrenal glomerulosa, where its synthesis and secretion are under the control of angiotensin II and potassium, and its major epithelial actions occur in the distal nephron and colon. The former extends from the late distal convoluted tubule (DCT) through the connecting segment and the entire cortical and medullary collecting ducts. These segments, rich in mineralocorticoid receptor (MR), are often referred to as the *aldosterone-sensitive distal nephron* (ASDN).[1] Most if not all effects of aldosterone are mediated by MR, a hormone-regulated transcription factor related closely to the glucocorticoid receptor and more distantly to other members of the nuclear receptor superfamily. The physiologic effects of aldosterone on epithelia entail direct gene regulatory actions of MR. Thus, a sound foundation for understanding aldosterone's physiologic effects on the extracellular fluid, blood pressure, and electrolyte concentrations can be had through familiarity with MR-dependent effects on the transcription of various genes, which, in turn, alter epithelial ion transport. Aldosterone actions in certain disease states involve both genomic and nongenomic effects in both epithelial and nonepithelial tissues. This chapter addresses the cellular and molecular mechanisms underlying aldosterone action, focusing primarily on its effects on ion transport in epithelia but also highlighting key aspects of nonepithelial actions, which are of particular importance to its pathophysiologic effects.

GENERAL INTRODUCTION TO ALDOSTERONE AND MINERALOCORTICOID RECEPTORS

Steroid hormones are derived from cholesterol and produced in systemically relevant amounts in a relatively narrow range of tissues (adrenal glands, gonads, placenta, and skin). In mammalian physiology, six classes of steroid hormones are commonly recognized: mineralocorticoid, glucocorticoid, androgen, estrogen, progestin, and the secosteroid vitamin D_3. This classification was based on observed effects of these hormones and has proven robust despite current appreciation of a much more diverse physiology of steroid hormones over and above their classical roles. In further support of this original classification is the characterization of six intracellular receptors (mineralocorticoid, MR; glucocorticoid, GR; androgen, AR; estrogen, ER; progestin, PR; vitamin D_3, VDR). As further addressed later, it is now appreciated that a one-to-one relationship between receptor and hormone does not hold, and this is particularly the case for MR. Aldosterone was isolated and characterized in 1953. Crucial for its isolation was the application of radioisotopic techniques to measure $[Na^+]$ and $[K^+]$ flux across epithelia in the laboratory of Sylvia Simpson, a biologist, and Jim Tait, a physicist.[2,3] Because of this, the active principle was initially called *electrocortin;* the name was soon changed to *aldosterone* when its unique aldehyde (rather than methyl) group at carbon 18 was discovered in collaborative studies between investigators in London and Basel.[4] Aldosterone is commonly depicted so as to highlight this aldehyde group (Figure 12.1, *right*). In vivo, the very reactive aldehyde group cyclizes with the β-hydroxyl group at carbon 11 to form the 11,18 hemiacetal and, in addition, may exist in an 11,18 hemiketal form. This cyclization of the 11β-hydroxyl group protects aldosterone from dehydrogenation by the enzyme 11β-hydroxysteroid dehydrogenase in epithelial tissue, which enables it to activate epithelial MR and thus regulate ion transport at very low (subnanomolar) circulating levels.[5,6] There is broad evidence that aldosterone is not the only cognate ligand for MR, its essential effects via MR on epithelial ion transport notwithstanding. MR is found in high abundance in the hippocampus and cardiomyocytes, and in such nonepithelial tissues—which lack 11β-hydroxysteroid dehydrogenase type 2 (11β-HSD2; see "11β-Hydroxysteroid Dehydrogenase Type 2" section)—are essentially constitutively occupied by glucocorticoids (cortisol in humans, corticosterone in rodents). This is due to the comparable affinity and markedly higher plasma free levels (≥100-fold) of glucocorticoids compared with those of aldosterone. In terms of evolution, MR appeared well before aldosterone synthase (e.g., in fish).[7] It was commonly assumed that MR and GR share a common immediate evolutionary precursor,[8] although this has recently been challenged on sequence grounds,[9] which implicate MR as the

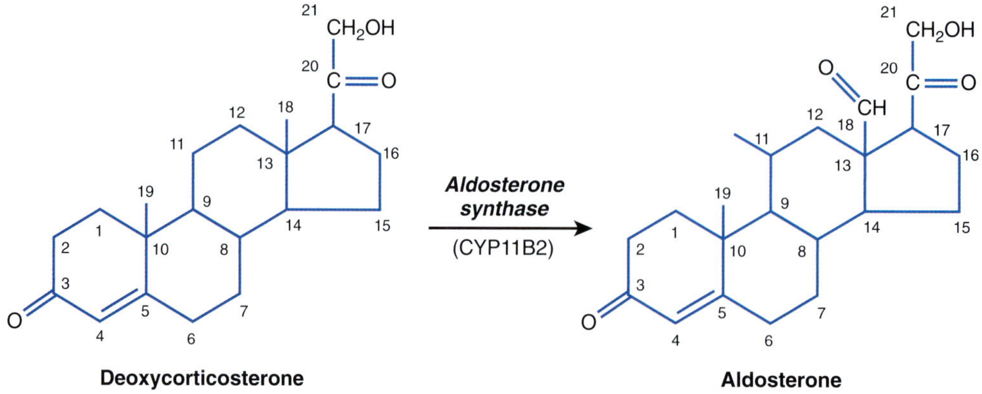

Figure 12.1 Final step in aldosterone synthesis. Note that the aldehyde form of aldosterone is shown. Most aldosterone (>99%) exists as the hemiacetal form, which is cyclized and does not allow access of 11β-hydroxysteroid dehydrogenase type 2 (11β-HSD2) to the 11-hydroxyl. See text for details.

first of the MR/GR/AR/PR subfamily to branch off an ancestral receptor. A final reason not to equate MR and aldosterone action derives from a comparison of the MR knockout and aldosterone synthase knockout (AS$^{-/-}$) phenotypes. MR knockout mice (which lack all functional MR) cannot survive sodium restriction; AS$^{-/-}$ mice (which have no detectable aldosterone) survive even stringent sodium restriction but die when their fluid intake is restricted to that of wild-type animals.[10] The survival of AS$^{-/-}$ mice on a low Na$^+$ intake may reflect, in part, Na$^+$ retention via renal tubular intercalated cells, in which MRs (not 11β-HSD2 protected) are activated by glucocorticoids in the context of high ambient angiotensin concentrations.[10a,10b] Their inability to survive fluid restriction suggests an as yet poorly defined dependence on aldosterone for vasopressin action.[11]

ALDOSTERONE SYNTHESIS

Aldosterone is synthesized in the adrenal cortex, which has three functional zones. The outermost layer of cells represents the zona glomerulosa, which is the unique site of aldosterone biosynthesis. Cortisol is synthesized in the middle zone, the zona fasciculata, and the innermost zona reticularis secretes adrenal androgens in many species, including humans, but not in rats or mice. Normally the glomerulosa secretes aldosterone at the rate of 50 to 200 μg/day, to give plasma levels of 4 to 21 μg/dL; in contrast, secretion of cortisol is at levels 200- to 500-fold higher. Underlying the separate synthesis of cortisol and aldosterone is expression of the enzyme 17α-hydroxylase uniquely in the zona fasciculata and that of aldosterone synthase uniquely in the glomerulosa.

In most species, aldosterone synthase, or cytochrome P450 (CYP) enzyme 11B2, is responsible for the conversion of deoxycorticosterone to aldosterone in a three-step process of sequential 11β-hydroxylation, 18-hydroxylation, and 18-methyl oxidation, to produce the characteristic C18-aldehyde from which aldosterone derives its name (Figure 12.2, *left*). Although CYP11B2 is distinct from CYP11B1 (11β-hydroxylase) in most species,[12,13] in some species (e.g., bovine), only a single CYP11B is expressed. How this enzyme is responsible for the three-step process of aldosterone synthesis in the glomerulosa but not the fasciculata is yet to be determined.

Figure 12.2 also shows key steps in biosynthesis of cortisol to illustrate the overlap and similarities with that of aldosterone. The genes encoding CYP11B1 and CYP11B2 lie close to one another on human chromosome band 8q24.3, so that an unequal crossing over at meiosis has been shown to be responsible for the syndrome of glucocorticoid-remediable aldosteronism (now known as familial hyperaldosteronism type I), in which the 3′ end of the CYP11B1 is fused to the 5′ end of CYP11B2. The chimeric gene product[14] is expressed in the fasciculata and responds to adrenocorticotrophic hormone (ACTH) with aldosterone synthesis, producing a syndrome of juvenile-onset hyperaldosteronism and hypertension.

Normal glomerulosa secretion of aldosterone is primarily regulated by angiotensin II in response to posture and acute lowering of circulating volume, to plasma [K$^+$] in response to elevated potassium, particularly in settings of Na$^+$ deficiency,[15] and to ACTH to the extent of entrainment of the circadian fluctuation in plasma aldosterone levels with those of cortisol. Aldosterone secretion is lowered by high levels of atrial natriuretic peptide and by the administration of

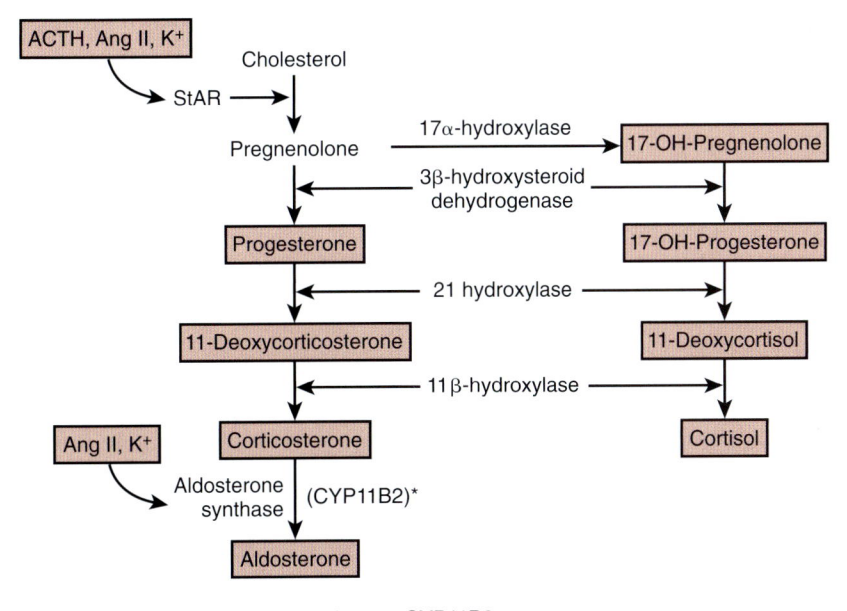

Figure 12.2 Overview of aldosterone synthetic pathway showing key regulatory nodes. Note that adrenocorticotropic hormone (ACTH), angiotensin II (Ang II), and K$^+$ regulate steroidogenic acute regulatory protein (StAR), which stimulates cholesterol uptake by mitochondria and thus substrate availability for synthesis of all of the steroid hormones. Aldosterone synthase (AS; gene name *CYP11B2*), which is selectively expressed in the adrenal glomerulosa, mediates the final step in aldosterone synthesis. It is also regulated by Ang II and K$^+$. Aldosterone synthesis is shown on the *left*. Cortisol synthesis is also shown (*right*) to emphasize the interconnections and similarities between these pathways.

heparin, somatostatin, and dopamine. As yet, incompletely characterized molecules of adipocyte origin have been shown to stimulate aldosterone secretion in vitro, and roles in the metabolic syndrome have been proposed on this basis.[16]

Angiotensin and plasma [K+] stimulate aldosterone secretion primarily by increasing the expression and activity of key steroidogenic enzymes as well as the steroidogenic acute regulatory protein (StAR).[17] StAR is required for cholesterol transport into mitochondria and hence is available for steroid synthesis.[18] Regulated steroidogenic enzymes include side-chain cleavage enzyme, 3β-hydroxysteroid dehydrogenase, and, most notably, aldosterone synthase, which mediates the final step in aldosterone synthesis. Common to the mechanism of stimulation by angiotensin II and [K+] is elevation of intracellular [Ca^{2+}]. Angiotensin activates angiotensin type I receptors in the glomerulosa cell membrane, which in turn activate phospholipase C. Elevated [K+] increases intracellular [Ca^{2+}] by depolarizing the cell membrane and activating voltage-sensitive Ca^{2+} channels.[19,20] Subsequently, the pathways diverge, with the [K+] effect but not the angiotensin effect dependent on Ca^{2+}/calmodulin kinase. Patients taking angiotensin-converting enzyme inhibitors or angiotensin receptor blockers usually show a degree of suppression of aldosterone secretion, reflected in a modest (0.2 to 0.3 mEq/L) elevation in plasma [K+]. This is often sufficient to establish a new steady state, with plasma aldosterone levels rising into the normal range, a process best termed *breakthrough* rather than *escape*, given the time-honored usage of the latter for escape from progression of the salt and water effect of mineralocorticoid excess in the medium and long term.[21]

Recent data have shed new light on the regulation of aldosterone production by the adrenal glomerulosa in health and disease. Choi and associates found recurrent somatic mutations in the K+ channel Kir3.4 (encoded by the gene *KCNJ5*), which were present in more than a third of human aldosterone-producing adenomas studied.[22] These mutations increased Na+ conductance through Kir3.4 and resulted in increased Ca^{2+} entry and enhanced aldosterone production and glomerulosa cell proliferation. Interestingly, an inherited mutation in *KCNJ5* is associated with hypertension associated with marked bilateral adrenal hyperplasia (now known as familial hyperaldosteronism type III [FH-III]).[23] These findings suggest that *KCNJ5* may provide tonic inhibition of aldosterone production and glomerulosa cell proliferation. In glomerulosa cells harboring the mutant channel, both proliferation rate and aldosterone synthesis are increased. These initial studies have been continued and extended by a much wider survey by Boulkroun and colleagues[24]; more recently, less common but similarly somatic mutations in the adrenal cortex (*ATP1A1, ATP2A3, CACNA1D*) have been associated with hyperaldosteronism caused by adrenal adenomas.[25,26]

MECHANISMS OF MINERALOCORTICOID RECEPTOR FUNCTION AND GENE REGULATION

Mammals cannot survive without MR, except with substantial NaCl supplementation. This member of the nuclear

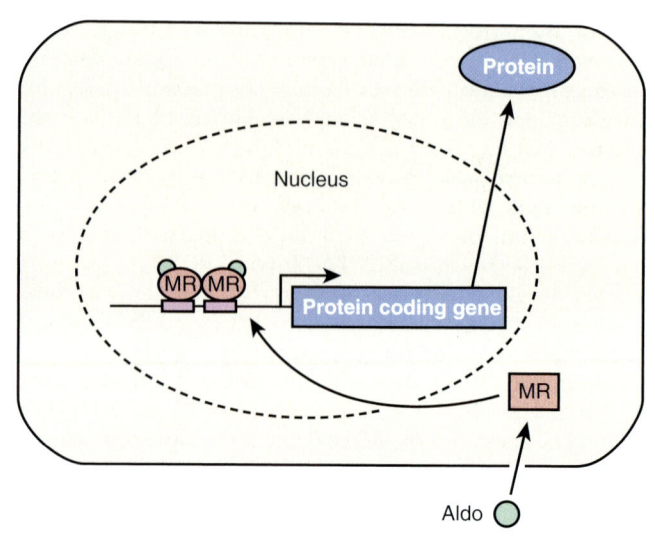

Figure 12.3 General mechanism of aldosterone action through the mineralocorticoid receptor (MR). This simple schematic shows the general features of MR regulation of a "simple" hormone response element (HRE), common to a large subset (but not all) of aldosterone-stimulated genes. Note that in the absence of hormone, MR is found in both nucleus and cytoplasm (see Figure 12.4). Aldosterone triggers nuclear translocation of cytoplasmic MR, binding as a dimer to HREs, and stimulation of transcription initiation complex formation (*arrow* upstream of "protein coding gene" defines the site of transcription initiation). See text for further details.

receptor superfamily appears to have both genomic and nongenomic actions; however, the latter do not appear to play a significant role in the control of epithelial ion transport. This section thus focuses exclusively on the function of MR as a hormone-regulated transcription factor.

MINERALOCORTICOID RECEPTOR FUNCTION AS A HORMONE-REGULATED TRANSCRIPTION FACTOR: GENERAL FEATURES AND SUBCELLULAR LOCALIZATION

In the presence of agonists, MR binds to specific genomic sites and alters the transcription rate of a subset of genes. Figure 12.3 shows the fundamental paradigm of MR function. All nuclear receptors shuttle in and out of the nucleus; however, in the absence of hormone, some, such as the estrogen and the vitamin D receptors, are predominantly nuclear, whereas others, like GR, are almost exclusively cytoplasmic. In the absence of hormone, MR is distributed relatively evenly between nuclear and cytoplasmic compartments, but in the presence of hormone, it is highly concentrated in the nucleus (Figure 12.4).[27,28] It is also notable that in addition to this marked change in MR cellular distribution, its subnuclear organization and protein-protein interactions are also changed.[28] Like its close cousin the GR, the unliganded MR (in the absence of hormone) is complexed with a set of chaperone proteins, which include the heat shock proteins hsp90, hsp70, and hsp56, and immunophilins.[29,30] This chaperone complex is essential for several aspects of MR function, notably high-affinity hormone binding and trafficking to the nucleus.[30] It was thought for many years that after binding hormone, the hsp90-containing chaperone complex is jettisoned. However, it has become clear that this complex

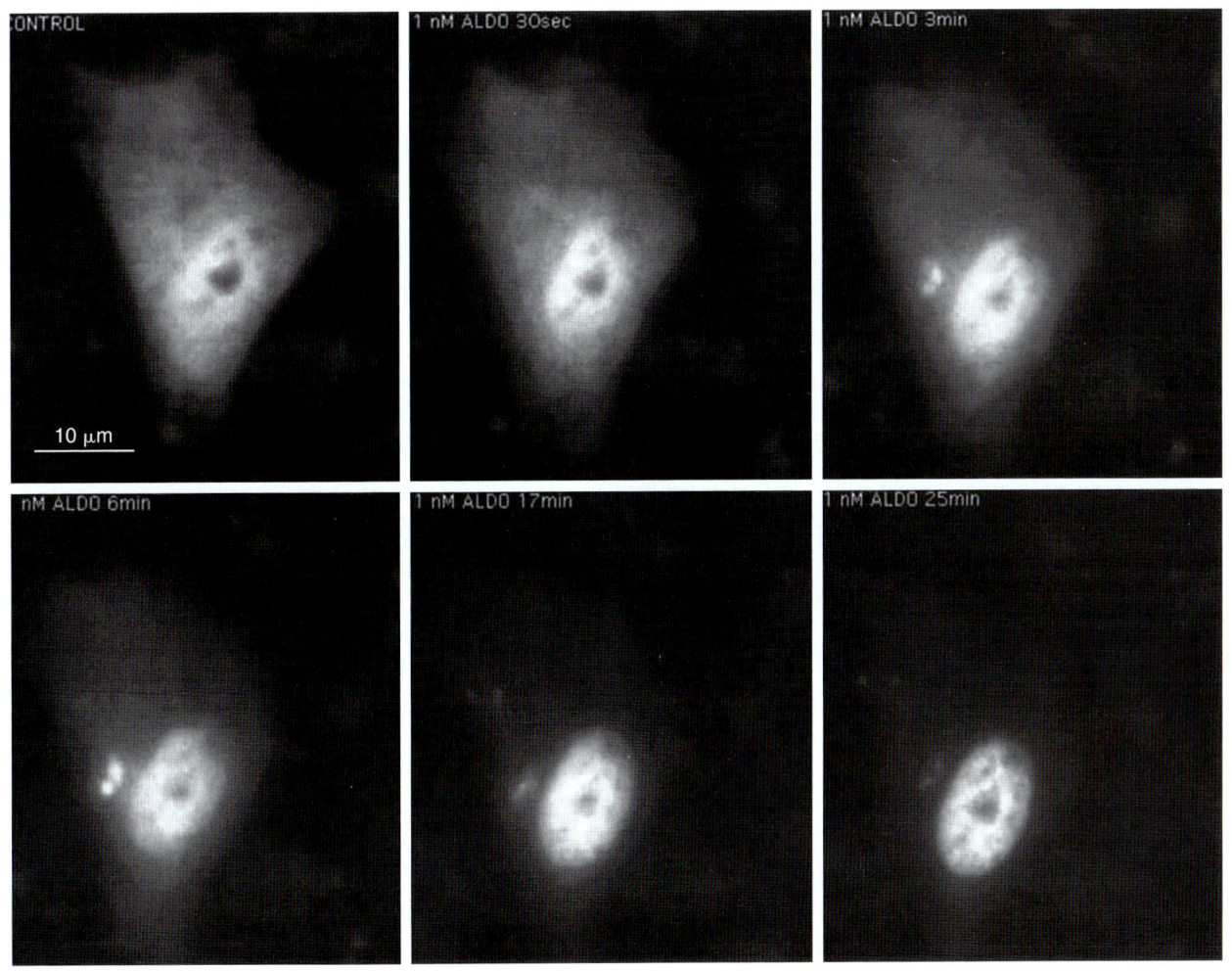

Figure 12.4 Time-dependent nuclear translocation of the mineralocorticoid receptor (MR) in the presence of aldosterone. Cultured cells expressing green fluorescent protein–MR fusion protein (GFP-MR) were grown in a steroid-free medium and treated with 1 nmol/L aldosterone. Translocation of GFP-MR was followed in real time, and images were captured at indicated times. It is notable that nuclear accumulation of GFP-MR started within 30 sec, was half-maximal at 7.5 min, and was complete by 10 min. Control: MR distribution prior to addition of aldosterone. (From Fejes-Toth G, Pearce D, Naray-Fejes-Toth A: Subcellular localization of mineralocorticoid receptors in living cells: effects of receptor agonists and antagonists, *Proc Natl Acad Sci U S A* 95[6]:2973-2978, 1998, Figure 3.)

remains associated with the receptor and plays an important role in nuclear trafficking.[29] Several members of the immunophilin family, including FKBP52, FKBP51, and CyP40, are present in the chaperone complex and provide a bridge between hsp90 and the cytoplasmic motor protein dynein, which moves the receptor-hsp90 complex retrogradely along microtubules to the nuclear envelope.[30] Here, the receptor is handed off to the nuclear pore protein, importin-α, and translocated into the nucleus, where it functions as a transcription factor, stimulating transcription of certain genes and repressing the transcriptional activity of others. In the regulation of ion transport, stimulation of key target genes is paramount. Transcriptional repression may be essential for effects in nonepithelial cells, including neurons, cardiomyocytes, smooth muscle cells, and macrophages.[31]

DOMAIN STRUCTURE OF MINERALOCORTICOID RECEPTORS

The MRs of all vertebrates are highly conserved. There are only minor differences between MRs in rodents and MRs in humans.[31] In general, the steroid and nuclear receptors have been divided into three major domains (Figure 12.5): (1) an N-terminal transcriptional regulatory domain, (2) a central DNA-binding domain (DBD), and (3) a C-terminal ligand/hormone-binding domain (LBD). Each of these broadly defined domains has more than one function, and not all of the functions can be neatly assigned to separate distinct domains; however, much of what MRs do can be understood from this point of view. In the following sections, the domains are described roughly in the historical order in which they were characterized, which also parallels the clarity of functional and structural knowledge about them.

DNA-BINDING DOMAIN

The sine qua non of MR function as a transcription factor is its ability to bind specifically to DNA. This protein-DNA interaction is mediated by the receptor's compact modular DBD (amino acids 603 to 688 of human MR; Figure 12.5 shows a strip diagram and two-dimensional structure), which forms a variety of contacts with a specific 15-nucleotide

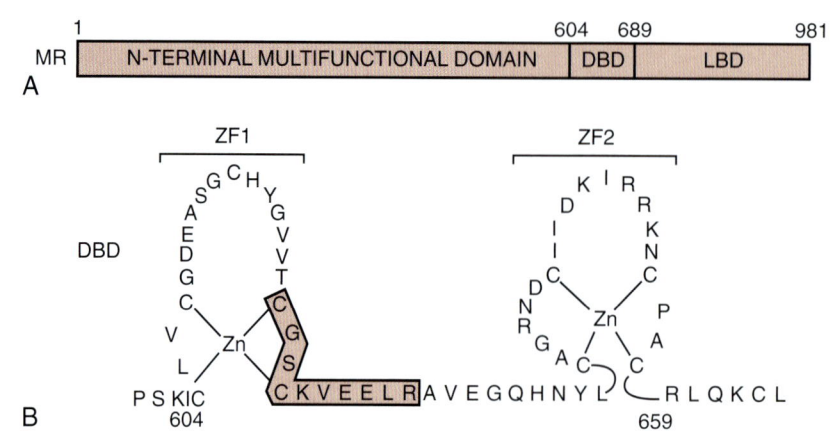

Figure 12.5 Domain structure of the mineralocorticoid receptor (MR). Three major domains have been defined, which are common to all steroid/nuclear receptors. Further refinements have led some to use a six-letter system, which is shown; however, this adds little to the understanding of receptor structure or function, and the authors prefer the three global domain system. These large receptor sections should not be confused with the many small functional domains that have been identified, as discussed in the text. The size and amino acid designations used here are for rat MR (981 amino acids total); they apply with minor variations to human MR (984 amino acids total). **A,** Strip diagram of MR. N terminus is to the *left,* C terminus to the *right.* **B,** Schematic of MR DNA-binding domain (DBD), showing the two zinc fingers, and the positions of the coordinating Zn ions. *Boxed region* is the α-helix, which intercalates into the major groove of the DNA and provides the major protein-DNA interaction contacts. The dimerization interface comprises amino acids within the second zinc finger, which form van der Waals and salt bridge interactions. *LBD,* Ligand/hormone-binding domain.

DNA sequence termed a *hormone response element* (HRE). Receptor binding to the HRE in the vicinity of regulated genes promotes the recruitment of coactivators and components of the general transcription machinery, such as the TATA-binding protein, which binds to the thymidine- and adenosine-rich DNA sequence found upstream of many genes and is required for correct transcription initiation. These types of HREs have been identified near or in many of the key MR-regulated genes, such as serum- and glucocorticoid-regulated kinase 1 *(SGK1),* glucocorticoid-induced leucine zipper *(GILZ),* and amiloride-sensitive sodium channel subunit α *(α ENaC).* Although in many cases, differential binding to HREs is a key determinant of the specificity of many transcription factors, it should be noted that some steroid receptors (notably MR and GR) have only minor (<10%) differences within this domain and have identical DNA-binding properties.[32] Specificity in these cases is determined through other mechanisms.[31,33]

The canonical MR HRE is a 15-nucleotide sequence that forms a partial palindrome (inverted repeat), which binds a receptor homodimer. A dimer interface embedded within the DBD is essential for MR to form these requisite homodimers, as well as to form heterodimers with GR.[34,35] Mutations that disrupt this interface have complex effects on receptor activity in animals[36] and cultured cells,[37] and similar mutations in other receptors (AR in particular) result in disease states.[38] Also, in at least one kindred of the autosomal dominant form of pseudohypoaldosteronism type I, an MR DBD mutation appears to be causative, although the mechanistic basis has not been elucidated.[39]

In addition to supporting DNA binding and dimerization, the DBD also harbors a nuclear localization signal,[40,41] as well as surfaces that contact distant parts of the receptor and that mediate interactions with other proteins, as has been shown for GR and, in some cases, MR.[42-44]

LIGAND/HORMONE-BINDING DOMAIN

The MR LBD comprises amino acids 689 to 981 (see Figure 12.5A). Like the DBD, the LBD has multiple functions: in addition to binding with high affinity to various MR agonists and antagonists, it also harbors interaction surfaces for coactivators, dimerization, and N-C interactions.[45-47] MR is distinct from GR in that it binds with equal, high affinity to cortisol, corticosterone (the physiologic glucocorticoid in rats and mice), and aldosterone. Indeed, as discussed later, MR appears to function as a high-affinity glucocorticoid receptor in some tissues, including the brain and the heart.

High-resolution representations of the crystal structures of wild-type and mutant MR have identified the structural features of the LBD and specific amino acid contacts involved in binding to the mineralocorticoid desoxycorticosterone (Figure 12.6).[48,49] Key features include the following: (1) The LBD of MR, like that of other nuclear receptors, is arranged into 11 α-helices and four small β-strands. (2) The C-terminal α-helix, H12, contains the activation function AF2. (3) Ligand is deeply embedded into a pocket comprising α-helices H3, H4, H5, H7, and H10, and two β-strands; numerous contacts are made between amino acids of the pocket and the hormone. This accounts for the slow off rate and high affinity of aldosterone, corticosterone, and cortisol for MR.[48] The crystal structure of the mutant (S810L) MR, in which progesterone acts as an agonist rather than an antagonist,[50] reveals that H12 is stabilized with AF2 in the active conformation.[49] The crystal structure of wild-type MR LBD also provides insight into the mechanisms underlying some forms of pseudohypoaldosteronism type I. Notably, MR/S810L has an LBD mutation in helix 5, which is predicted to disrupt interaction with the steroid ring structure,[51] whereas Q776R and L979P have

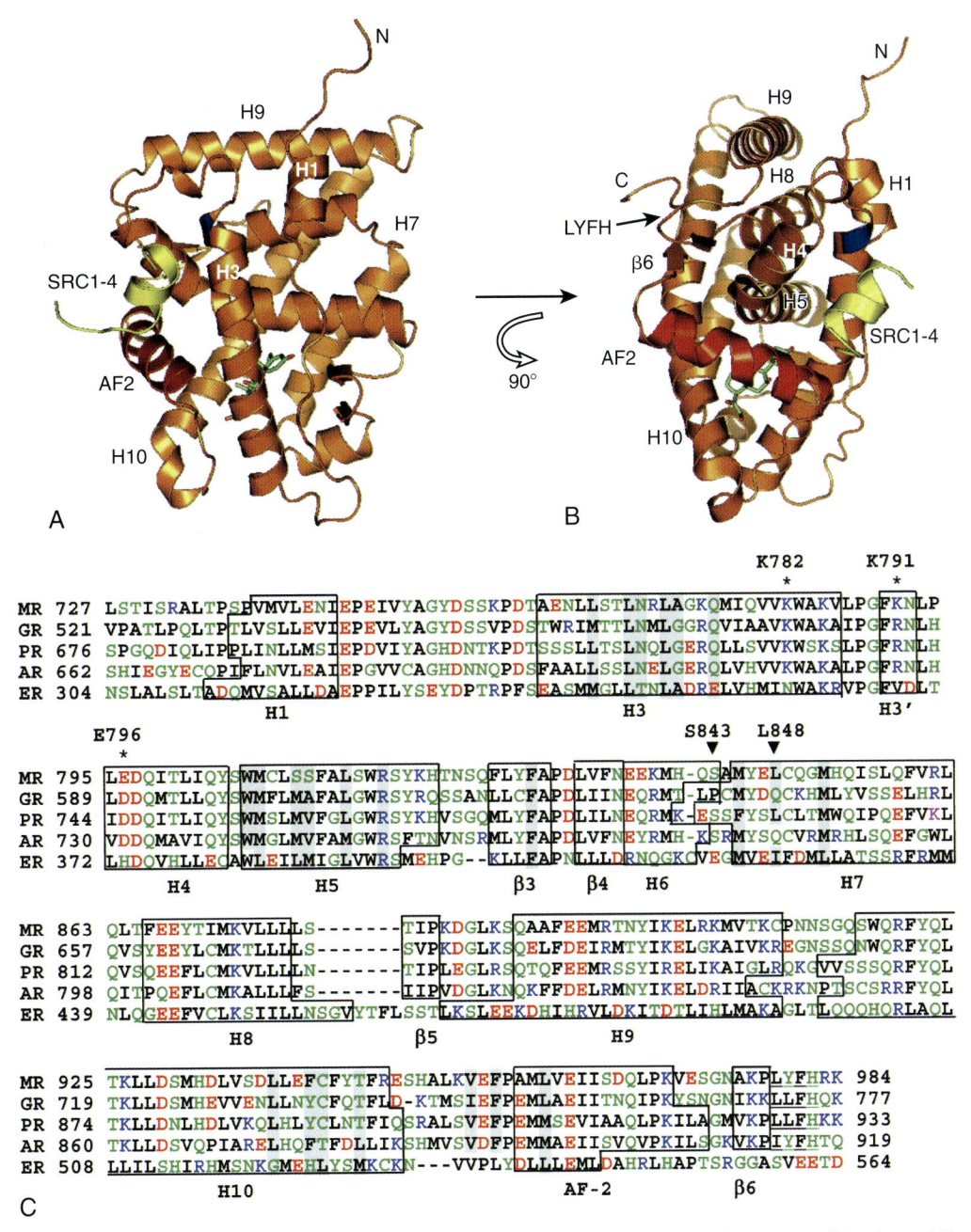

Figure 12.6 **Mineralocorticoid receptor (MR) ligand/hormone-binding domain (LBD) crystal structure.** Structure of the MR LBD bound to corticosterone and coactivator peptides (SRC1-4). **A** and **B**, Two views of the complex (rotated by 90 degrees about the vertical axis) are shown in ribbon representation. MR is colored in *gold* and SRC1-4 peptide in *yellow*. Corticosterone, which binds MR with an affinity comparable to that of aldosterone, is shown in *ball and stick* representation. Note that hormone is located in a deep pocket formed by helices 3, 5, and 7 (H3, H5, and H7), which explains the slow off rate and high affinity. **C,** Sequence alignment of the human MR LBD with other steroid hormone receptors (GR, glucocorticoid; AR, androgen; PR, progesterone; and ER, estrogen). Residues that form the steroid-binding pockets are shaded in *gray*. Key structural features for the binding of SRC peptides are noted with *stars,* and the residues that determine MR/GR hormone specificity are labeled by *arrowheads*. See Li and others[381] for further details. (From Li Y, Suino K, Daugherty J, et al: Structural and biochemical mechanisms for the specificity of hormone binding and coactivator assembly by mineralocorticoid receptor. *Mol Cell* 19:367-380, 2005.)

been demonstrated to have markedly reduced aldosterone binding.[39] Structural analysis reveals that Q776 is located in helix H3 at the extremity of the hydrophobic ligand-binding pocket and anchors the steroid C3-ketone group.

MR binds cortisol and corticosterone with an affinity similar to that of aldosterone. 11β-HSD2 is an essential determinant of aldosterone specificity, through its effect in metabolizing glucocorticoids to their receptor-inactive keto-congeners in collecting duct principal cells, as discussed later. In tissues that do not coexpress 11β-HSD2, the physiologic ligand for MR is cortisol (corticosterone in rats and mice).[52-54] The extent to which such "unprotected" MR can be pathophysiologically activated in aldosterone excess states is discussed in the "Primary Aldosteronism" section under "Disease States" and in the "Nonepithelial Actions of Aldosterone" section.

N-TERMINAL DOMAIN

As its noncommittal name implies, the N-terminal region of MR has diverse functions, which appear to revolve primarily around protein-protein interactions and recruitment of coactivators and corepressors. It has two potent transcriptional regulatory motifs, usually termed *AF1a* and *AF1b*.[45,55] This domain bears some functional and sequence similarity to the homologous region of GR and is capable of stimulating gene transcription when fused to an unrelated DBD.[45] Overall, however, MR and GR differ markedly in the N-terminal domain, and this region of the receptor is a central determinant of specificity.[56] Recent evidence supports the idea that this domain has functional sequences that limit receptor activity through recruitment of corepressors, in addition to transcriptional activation functions.[44,57] Its role in coactivator and corepressor recruitment is addressed further in the following section.

MINERALOCORTICOID RECEPTOR REGULATION OF TRANSCRIPTION INITIATION: COACTIVATORS AND COREPRESSORS

The major mechanism of MR action is its effects on transcription initiation; however, there may also be effects on transcript elongation.[58,59] Much has been learned about the generation of an initiation complex and the particular roles that steroid receptors play in this process. Several review articles and book chapters provide in-depth examinations of the biochemistry of the general transcription machinery, transcription initiation, promoter escape, and processive elongation.[60-62] Most of the coactivators identified so far interact with the C-terminal AF2 domain and include the prototypical GRIP1/TIF2 and SRC,[63,64] which sequentially recruit a series of different components of the transcriptional machinery and result in the formation of a preinitiation complex (PIC). This PIC includes all of the key components of the transcription machinery, including RNA polymerase II. A detailed picture of MR-dependent PIC formation has not been obtained. However, the general features are likely similar to those for ER[65] and involve the sequential recruitment by the receptor of (1) chromatin-remodeling SWI/SNF and CARM1/PRTM1 proteins, which promote chromatin remodeling and initiation of complex formation; (2) histone acetylase CBP/P300 (cyclic adenosine monophosphate [cAMP]–responsive element–binding protein), which promotes an active chromatin conformation[61]; and (3) direct or indirect recruitment of the TATA-binding protein and other components of the general transcription machinery.[65]

The aforementioned mechanisms are generic and are used by many transcription factors, including all steroid receptors, through interactions with the C-terminal AF2 domain. The N-terminal region of MR, which harbors the AF1 domain, diverges from the other steroid receptors, and recent evidence has identified coregulators that interact selectively with this receptor domain. ELL (eleven-nineteen lysine-rich leukemia factor) is a coactivator for MR that specifically interacts with AF1b and assists in PIC formation.[58] It was originally identified as an elongation factor, and it may also affect transcript elongation. Other specific coregulators include the synergy inhibitory protein PIAS1,[57] Ubc9,[66] and p68 RNA helicase.[67]

REGULATION OF SODIUM ABSORPTION AND POTASSIUM SECRETION

GENERAL MODEL OF ALDOSTERONE ACTION

Aldosterone enters the cell passively, binds to MR, triggers changes in gene transcription (as addressed in the "Mechanisms of MR Function and Gene Regulation" section), and potentially has nongenomic effects. Aldosterone effects in the ASDN have been divided into three major phases: latent, early, and late.[1] This designation goes back to the early observations by Ganong and Mulrow that after aldosterone infusion into experimental animals, no effect was observed for at least 15 to 20 minutes.[68] A similar delay was observed in isolated epithelia.[69] The early phase, which is now known to involve primarily MR-dependent regulation of signaling mediators such as SGK1, culminates in increased apical localization—and possibly increased probability of the open state—of ENaC. In the late phase, aldosterone stimulates transcription of a variety of effector genes, including those that encode components of the ion transport machinery, notably the ENaC and Na^+-K^+–adenosine triphosphatase (Na^+-K^+-ATPase) subunits. The major direct effect is to increase Na^+ reabsorption, which is accompanied variably by Cl^- reabsorption and/or K^+ secretion, and ultimately water reabsorption. Aldosterone's actions in the principal cells of the connecting segment and collecting duct (Figure 12.7) are of primary significance; however, it also has been shown to influence fluid and electrolyte transport in other tubule segments, as well as in other organs. These actions of aldosterone can be surmised from the clinical features of individuals with aldosterone-secreting tumors; they have volume expansion with high blood pressure and are commonly ($\approx 50\%$) hypokalemic.[70,71] In general, the effects of aldosterone on Na^+ absorption and K^+ secretion work together. However, there are ways that these actions can be separated, as discussed later.

The two basic cell processes that aldosterone regulates—Na^+ absorption and K^+ secretion—are depicted in Figure 12.7. Most aspects of this mechanism are relevant to the various aldosterone target tissues.

Na^+-K^+-ATPase, located on the basolateral membrane (blood side), establishes the essential electrochemical gradients that drive ion transport (see Chapters 5 and 6). The most important, rate-limiting step is that of Na^+ entry into the cell via the epithelial Na^+ channel, ENaC. The discovery of the molecular composition of ENaC in 1993[72,73] opened the door to understanding how aldosterone functions to regulate this critically important ion channel. Most Na^+ transporters are encoded by a single gene product. In contrast, ENaC is composed of three similar but distinct subunits, each encoded by a unique gene. All three subunits come together (the stoichiometry is controversial) to form an ion channel with unique biophysical characteristics, the most striking of which is the relatively long time it stays open or closed.[74] The complete loss of any one of these subunits in mice is incompatible with life.[75-77]

The entry of Na^+ into the cell via ENaC in the apical membrane is the rate-limiting step in both Na^+ absorption and K^+ secretion.[78] Na^+ enters the cell down a steep electrochemical gradient; intracellular [Na^+] is approximately

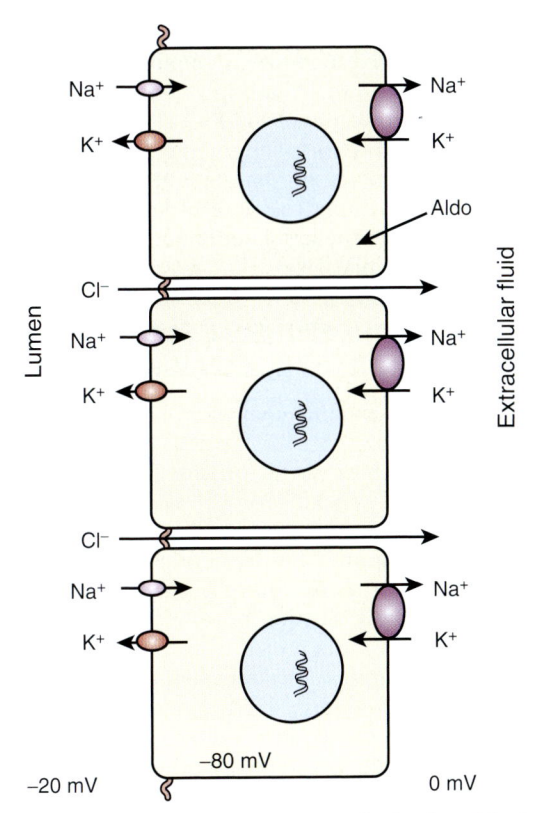

Figure 12.7 Schematic of principal cells in the aldosterone-sensitive distal nephron (ASDN). The ASDN includes the distal third of the distal convoluted tubule (DCT), the connecting tubule (CNT), and the collecting duct. The Na$^+$-K$^+$–adenosine triphosphatase (Na$^+$-K$^+$-ATPase) establishes the gradients for passive apical entry of sodium through the epithelial sodium channel (ENaC). Transport of sodium through the ENaC creates a negative lumen potential that drives potassium secretion into the lumen. Potassium is also recycled at the basolateral surface, which facilitates potassium exchange across the Na$^+$-K$^+$-ATPase. Chloride (Cl$^-$) moves via paracellular and transcellular pathways. There is evidence to support aldosterone actions in other segments, particularly the sodium-chloride cotransporter (NCC)—expressing portions of the DCT (DCT1 and DCT2).

10 mmol/L, and the membrane voltage is strongly negative inside the cell. The Na$^+$ inside the cell is pumped out across the basolateral membrane by Na$^+$-K$^+$-ATPase, as addressed in detail in Chapter 6. Most epithelial cells have a greater density of K$^+$ channels on the basolateral membrane and thus recycle K$^+$ back into the blood. The distal nephron is unique in that it has an unusually high density of K channels on the apical membrane (primarily Kir 1.1 [renal outer medullary potassium (ROMK)] and BK channels).[79,80] This distribution of K$^+$ channels permits a large amount of K$^+$ that enters the cell via Na$^+$-K$^+$-ATPase to exit the cell into the lumen and be excreted into the urine. The vast majority of K$^+$ that appears in the urine is secreted by the distal nephron.

Much attention has been focused on the early phase of aldosterone action because it appears to be more tractable to dissection and the majority of change in Na$^+$ current occurs during this phase. This separation is probably somewhat artificial, however, and there is considerable overlap in events that define the early and late phases. Moreover, many efforts to manipulate mediators of the early phase (through overexpression and knockdown experiments) have been evaluated after prolonged alteration. Nevertheless, there is some heuristic value in considering early and late phases of aldosterone action separately.

In cultured collecting duct cells deprived of corticosteroids and then exposed to high concentrations of aldosterone, an increase in ENaC-mediated Na$^+$ transport can be observed in well under an hour, which is consistent with animal studies.[68,81] Na$^+$ transport continues to increase for 2 to 3 hours, then plateaus for a few hours, and then gradually increases over the next several hours. After 12 hours of exposure to saturating aldosterone concentrations, the increase in ENaC activity is near maximal. The molecular basis for this increase in ENaC activity has been intensively investigated, and several key events are now apparent.

For aldosterone to increase ENaC activity, a change in gene transcription must occur. One of the earliest response genes is *SGK1*.[82-84] This discovery has had a major impact on the direction of research on aldosterone action, and this gene is addressed separately—together with its major target, Nedd4-2—later in this chapter. *SGK1* is particularly important for the early actions of aldosterone.[85,86] An important consideration in evaluating our understanding of this molecular pathway is that the genetic disease Liddle's syndrome provided the first clues that the C-terminal portions of the ENaC subunits were essential in regulating ENaC surface expression[87,88] (see Chapter 45).

ALDOSTERONE AND EPITHELIAL SODIUM CHANNEL TRAFFICKING

The major action of aldosterone is to increase the number of functional ENaC units on the apical membrane. This process can involve an increase in the number of channel complexes on the surface, or activation of existing complexes, or both. There is evidence to support both, although the bulk of evidence favors the idea that change in the number of ENaC complexes predominates.[89-91] The redistribution of ENaC to the apical membrane can be detected in less than 2 hours after aldosterone exposure.[81]

It is less well established whether the number of ENaC complexes is increased through increased insertion, decreased removal, or both. Aldosterone probably contributes to both processes. Rapid insertion of ENaC complexes is best understood with regard to the actions of cAMP.[92] The extent to which the molecules involved in cAMP-mediated insertion are also involved in aldosterone action is uncertain, but some common mechanisms probably are used. Trafficking to the apical membrane appears to involve hsp70,[93] SNARE (soluble NEM-sensitive factor attachment protein receptor) proteins,[94] and the aldosterone-induced protein melanophilin.[95] The mitogen-activated protein kinase pathway may also be involved, because interruption of ERK phosphorylation by GILZ[96] increases ENaC surface expression.

Considerably more is known about how ENaC complexes are retrieved from the apical membrane. This understanding is the direct result of dissecting the molecular consequences of Liddle's syndrome, in which mutations in the C terminus of ENaC lead to increased residence time in the apical membrane.[87,88] The missing or mutated domains in the β- or γ-subunit of ENaC in this syndrome normally bind to Nedd4-2, a ubiquitin ligase, which ultimately is responsible for initiating endocytosis and degradation.[97,98] The interaction of Sgk1 and Nedd4-2 in the actions of aldosterone is discussed later. ENaC is internalized via clathrin-coated vesicles and processed into early endosomes, then further processed into recycling endosomes and late endosomes.[99,100] Degradation is via lysosomes or proteasomes.[101,102] The processing of ENaC by vesicular trafficking and its regulation by aldosterone has been reviewed.[103]

Phosphatidylinositol-3-kinase (PI3K)–dependent signaling is essential for epithelial Na^+ transport. It controls SGK1 activity (addressed later) and also appears to have independent effects on ENaC open probability through direct actions of 3-phosphorylated phosphoinositides, particularly phosphatidylinositol (3,4,5) trisphosphate.[104,105] Ras-dependent signaling may also regulate ENaC and the pump in complex ways that depend on downstream signaling through Raf, MEK and ERK, as well as through PI3K.[106-111]

The late phase of ENaC activation by aldosterone is less well understood than the early phase. A simple evaluation of the late phase is that aldosterone increases the transcription and protein abundance of the ENaC subunits. This idea comes from the fact that aldosterone increases the mRNA and protein abundance of α-ENaC in the kidney[90,112] after a lag of several hours.[113] However, whereas aldosterone produces an increase in α-subunit expression in the kidney, it produces an increase of β- and γ-subunits in the colon.[113,114] Dietary Na^+ restriction, a physiologically relevant maneuver that increases aldosterone secretion, clearly increases ENaC surface expression in the renal distal nephron.[91] However, there appear to be some important differences between chronic aldosterone administration to an Na^+-replete animal and chronic dietary Na^+ restriction.[112,115] The role of increased expression of α-ENaC in the long-term actions of aldosterone has been questioned, because overexpression of this subunit does not increase ENaC activity in models of collecting duct and lung epithelia.[116] It appears that increased expression of α-ENaC may be important for the consolidation of the increase, but it is not sufficient to reproduce the steroid-mediated increase in ENaC activity.

BASOLATERAL MEMBRANE EFFECTS OF ALDOSTERONE

Over the years, research on aldosterone action has focused with varying degrees of intensity on apical effects,[117,118] basolateral effects,[119-121] and effects on metabolism.[69] There is general agreement now that the early effects of aldosterone are on apical events, primarily on ENaC, and that basolateral and metabolic effects come later. In addition, although it is somewhat less settled whether the basolateral effects are direct or result indirectly from the enhanced entry of Na^+ into cells, the bulk of evidence favors the latter view. Notably, increased Na^+ entry has been found to control more than 80% of increased Na^+-K^+-ATPase activity and basolateral membrane density in the rat[122,123] and rabbit[123] cortical collecting tubule. Furthermore, striking increases in basolateral membrane folding and surface area occur in aldosterone-treated animals,[124] an effect that is markedly attenuated in animals fed a low-Na^+ diet. This result strongly suggests that apical Na^+ entry is required for basolateral changes to occur. However, good evidence exists for direct transcriptional stimulation of Na^+-K^+-ATPase subunit expression,[125,126] as well as reports supporting some direct effects of aldosterone in increasing basolateral pump activity[119,127] or at least in constituting the pool of latent pumps, which are then recruited to the basolateral membrane in response to a rise in intracellular $[Na^+]$.[128]

ACTIVATION OF THE EPITHELIAL SODIUM CHANNEL BY PROTEOLYTIC CLEAVAGE

There is now clear evidence that when ENaC is delivered to the apical membrane, it can be activated by proteolytic cleavage. The first hint of this process was the demonstration that rats fed a low-Na diet or given aldosterone over the long term showed the appearance of a proteolytic fragment of the γ-ENaC subunit.[90] Subsequently, investigators have shown that both the α- and the γ- but not the β-ENaC subunits can be cleaved. Furthermore, cleavage at each site apparently initiates a degree of activation of the channel complex. ENaC complexes are activated by cleavage because specific regions of the large extracellular domain (26 residues in the α-ENaC and 46 residues in the γ-ENaC) are excised. These regions contain inhibitory sequences that, when introduced exogenously, can inhibit ENaC function. Removing these regions by proteolytic cleavage releases this inhibition.[129]

Several proteases can cleave either the α- or γ-ENaC subunits. Among them are furin, prostasin, CAP2, kallikrein, elastase, matriptase, plasmin, and trypsin. It is not clear whether activation of ENaC by proteolytic cleavage can be regulated by aldosterone, but the idea certainly has attractive features. Were aldosterone able to regulate expression of one or more rate-limiting proteases, it would be able to regulate both the number of complexes in the apical membrane and the ability of the channel complex to be active. It appears that aldosterone may regulate the expression of prostasin.[130] Aldosterone may also regulate the expression of the protease, nexin-1 (an inhibitor of prostasin), and other proteases.[131]

The discovery of ENaC activation by cleavage helps to explain how aldosterone might increase ENaC activity by increasing both surface expression and the activity of a single ENaC complex. By phosphorylating Nedd4-2 via SGK1 and reducing its ability to bind to the PY domains of the ENaC subunits, aldosterone increases ENaC residence time on the apical membrane. This additional time permits proteolytic activation by one or more endogenous proteases.[132]

POTASSIUM SECRETION AND ALDOSTERONE

One of the major effects of aldosterone is to increase K^+ secretion (and thus excretion). This phenomenon has been demonstrated in countless patients with aldosterone-secreting tumors and in hundreds of studies in animals given excess amounts of aldosterone. The general mechanism whereby aldosterone increases K^+ secretion is depicted in Figure 12.7. The key feature of this process involves the increased absorption of Na^+ via ENaC. The dependence of

K+ secretion on Na+ absorption is the basis of the action of the "K-sparing" diuretics, amiloride and triamterene, both of which inhibit ENaC. These drugs have no direct effect on the apical K+ channels.

Increasing ENaC activity produces two major secondary effects that, in turn, enhance K+ secretion. First, the enhanced Na+ conductance of the apical membrane produces depolarization of that membrane and hence a more favorable electrical driving force for K+ efflux into the lumen. The second effect relates to the activity of the Na+-K+ pump on the basolateral membrane. The more Na+ that enters across the apical membrane, the more that must be extruded by the pump. Since the stoichiometry of the pump is constant (3Na+ and 2K+), more K+ enters the cell. In isolated, perfused cortical collecting ducts, the amount of secreted K+ is highly related to the amount of absorbed Na+ when the stimulus for Na+ absorption is mineralocorticoid hormone.[133]

Two kinds of K+ channels are found in the apical membrane of the ASDN: small conductance (SK, 30 to 40 picosiemens) channels encoded by the *ROMK* gene, and large conductance (BK, 100 to 200 picosiemens) channels found in many kinds of cells, including the apical membrane of the colon. The majority of the K+ channels on the apical membrane of the principal cells appear to be SK, at least as far as can be assessed by patch clamp analysis. The activity of either channel is not increased by aldosterone.[134,135]

A feature of K+ secretion is that although apical K+ channels are abundant in the proximal portion of the ASDN (connecting tubule and cortical collecting duct), they are strikingly less abundant in the medullary collecting duct.[136-138] Because apical K channels are not regulated by aldosterone, their absence in the medullary collecting duct might uncouple aldosterone-regulated Na+ reabsorption from K+ secretion in this segment.

Recent advances in understanding genetic forms of hypertension have uncovered an important role for a family of kinases that lack an otherwise conserved lysine residue in the catalytic domain. These kinases, called *WNK* (*w*ith *n*o lysine; *K* is the one-letter code for lysine), have potent effects on pathways regulating Na+ and K+ transport in the distal nephron. An important feature of one member of this family, WNK4, is its ability to modulate the activity of ROMK.[139,140] The activity of ROMK can be regulated via WNK4 by signaling events activated by aldosterone but modulated by serum [K+], Na balance via angiotensin II, and SGK1 activity. The importance of this synthesis is that it provides a molecular mechanism for the collecting duct separately to regulate Na+ absorption via ENaC and K+ secretion via ROMK.

SEPARATION OF SODIUM ABSORPTION AND POTASSIUM SECRETION BY THE ALDOSTERONE-SENSITIVE DISTAL NEPHRON

The preceding sections establish a picture that parsimoniously accounts for the effect of aldosterone to stimulate, pari passu, Na+ reabsorption and K+ secretion. The simple stimulation of electrogenic Na+ reabsorption (via ENaC) is sufficient to stimulate K+ secretion, which fits well for organisms faced with a combined low-Na+, high-K+ diet, which was maintained most of the time through millions of years of vertebrate evolution. However, organisms do not ingest a fixed amount of Na+ and K+, so inexorable linkage between Na+ absorption and K+ secretion by the ASDN cannot possibly occur all the time. Investigators have proposed several possibilities to explain how these processes can be separated.

ROLE OF DISTAL TUBULE FLUID DELIVERY

A traditional view for differential Na+ and K+ handling stems from the differing role that aldosterone plays in potassium secretion depending on the tubular flow (and thus "sodium flow") rate. Studies from adrenalectomized dogs have demonstrated that the primary regulators of potassium excretion are serum potassium concentration and tubular flow rate. A higher serum potassium concentration yields a higher filtered load of potassium. Hyperkalemia also stimulates natriuresis from upstream segments of the nephron.[141,142] This latter effect can increase tubular flow rate, which, in turn, diminishes potassium concentration in the lumen and activates flow-stimulated BK channel–mediated potassium secretion in the collecting duct. In the setting of sufficient distal delivery of sodium, potassium loading will not yield a higher steady-state concentration of aldosterone, as the two mechanisms previously mentioned are sufficient to normalize serum potassium.[143] However, under conditions of sodium depletion, proximal Na+ reabsorption is increased, which further diminishes distal delivery of sodium and hence tubular flow rate.[144] This diminishes flow-mediated potassium secretion, so that aldosterone secretion is necessary to normalize potassium balance.

INDEPENDENT REGULATION OF SODIUM AND POTASSIUM TRANSPORTERS

Other possible mechanisms have been suggested, which involve separate regulation of sodium and potassium transport (e.g., ENaC and ROMK) by specific stimuli depending on the state of Na+ and K+ intake. With a constant Na+ intake, one could envision that a high-potassium diet could enhance the activity of ROMK, while a low-potassium diet would reduce its activity. Such an effect would cause more or less of the K+ entering the cell via the Na+-K+ pump to be recycled across the basolateral membrane. This mechanism, although probably very complex in its execution, is appealing in its simplicity. The actions of WNK4 may be central to the regulation of ROMK.[140]

ELECTRONEUTRAL VERSUS ELECTROGENIC SODIUM REABSORPTION

Other appealing possibilities invoke the differing nature of Na+ and K+ transport along the distal nephron. For example, DCT absorbs Na+ and Cl− via the electroneutral Na-Cl cotransporter (NCC), and enhanced activity in this segment would not stimulate K+ secretion. Such a situation occurs in pseudohypoaldosteronism type II or familial hyperkalemic hypertension (also referred to as Gordon's syndrome).[145] Indeed, potassium, independent of aldosterone, is known to regulate the NCC. A high-potassium diet inhibits this transporter[141,142] and would thus promote aldosterone-mediated sodium reabsorption only through ENaC (rather than both NCC and ENaC), while favoring potassium secretion via ROMK and also potassium and flow-induced K+ secretion via BK channels.[146]

SHIFT TO MEDULLARY COLLECTING DUCT

Another possibility involves modulation of Na^+ absorption by the medullary collecting duct, a segment that has little capacity to secrete K^+. The environment of the renal medulla is very different from that of the cortex, and endogenous paracrine factors such as prostaglandins E_2 and transforming growth factor–β, both of which have potent inhibitory effects on Na^+ transport, are increased in response to a high-NaCl diet.[147,148]

REGULATION OF CHLORIDE TRANSPORT

A fifth possibility involves the independent regulation of Cl^- transport by the collecting duct. Cl^- can be absorbed by the paracellular pathway (i.e., between cells) driven by the lumen-negative voltage across the epithelium. This pathway can be influenced by aldosterone.[149] Cl^- can also be absorbed through the cells by specific transporters. One example of a Cl^- transporter in the collecting duct is pendrin, an anion exchanger present on the apical membrane of intercalated cells. Mice that lack this transporter do not tolerate NaCl restriction as well as normal mice.[150] This transporter seems not to be upregulated by aldosterone, but is dependent on Cl^- delivery to the distal nephron and is upregulated by angiotensin II.[151,152]

DIFFERENTIAL REGULATION OF INTERCALATED CELL MINERALOCORTICOID RECEPTOR

A recent study has highlighted a sixth possible mechanism allowing distinct responses to volume depletion versus hyperkalemia.[153,154] The central feature of this proposed regulation is differential phosphorylation of the MR LBD in intercalated cells, as shown schematically in Figure 12.8. When phosphorylated at S843 in the LBD, MRs cannot bind aldosterone or cortisol and thus cannot be activated. This phosphorylation, which is stimulated by hyperkalemia, occurs selectively in intercalated cells but not principal cells. Angiotensin II, on the other hand, induces S843 dephosphorylation in intercalated cells, markedly increasing ligand binding and, therefore, activation. Intercalated cells are known predominantly to mediate H^+ transport; however, recent studies have implicated them in electroneutral NaCl transport via the combined actions of Na^+-dependent Cl^--HCO_3^- exchanger (NDCBE) [155] and the apical Cl^--HCO_3^- exchanger, pendrin.[156,157] Thus, when MR is active in these cells (S843 dephosphorylated), electroneutral NaCl transport occurs, without enhancing the driving force for K^+ secretion. Since intercalated cells lack 11β-HSD2, under these conditions, it is cortisol that binds to and activates MR. When intercalated cell MR is inactive (S843 phosphorylated), aldosterone acts in principal cells to stimulate ENaC-dependent electrogenic Na^+ transport, which enhances K^+ secretion.

ALDOSTERONE-INDEPENDENT ENaC-MEDIATED SODIUM REABSORPTION IN THE DISTAL NEPHRON

The term *aldosterone-sensitive distal nephron* emphasizes the primacy of this key steroid in the control of ion transport in this region of the nephron. However, ENaC activity and aldosterone sensitivity exhibit axial heterogeneity from the

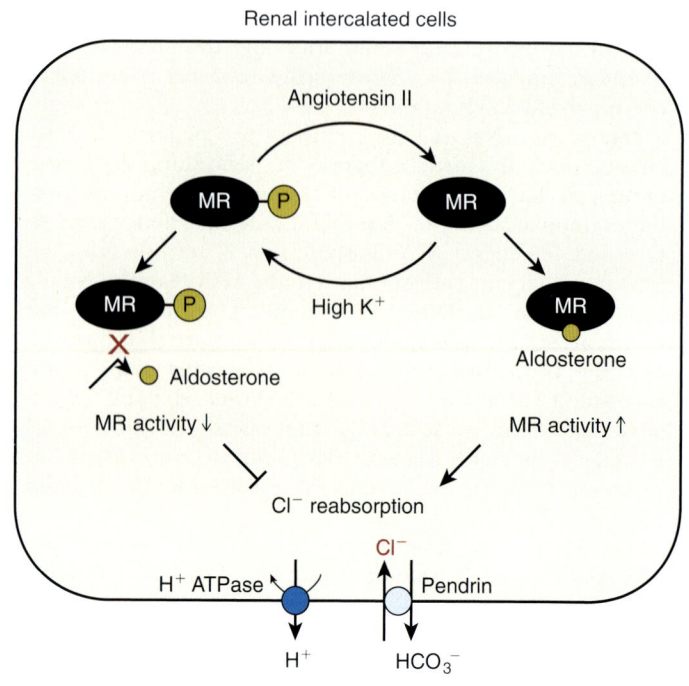

Figure 12.8 The role of mineralocorticoid receptor (MR) ligand/hormone-binding domain (LBD) phosphorylation in controlling chloride reabsorption by intercalated cells. When phosphorylated at Ser-843 in the LBD, MR cannot bind ligand and hence cannot be activated. This phosphorylated state of MR is found only in intercalated cells, not in neighboring principal cells. In states of volume depletion, elevated angiotensin II decreases MR phosphorylation at Ser-843, allowing activation. In intercalated cells, MR mediates stimulation of both the proton pump and Cl^--HCO_3^- exchangers, thereby increasing Cl^- reabsorption and promoting increased plasma volume while inhibiting K^+ secretion. In contrast, in states of hyperkalemia, phosphorylation of Ser-843 is increased, and hence Cl^- reabsorption by intercalated cells is decreased, and principal cell-dependent K^+ secretion is increased. (Reprinted with permission from Shibata S, Rinehart J, Zhang J, et al: Regulated mineralocorticoid receptor phosphorylation controls ligand binding and renal response to volume depletion and hyperkalemia. *Cell Metab* 18[November 5]:660-671, 2013.)

late distal convoluted tubule (DCT2) through the connecting tubule to the cortical collecting duct and, finally, to the medullary collecting duct. In mice on a standard salt diet, total ENaC expression increases with progression from the DCT2 to the connecting tubule,[158] although ENaC apical localization and activity are higher in the DCT2. Only under conditions of low-sodium diet or aldosterone administration does the primacy of the connecting tubule in particular, and to a lesser extent the cortical collecting duct, emerge. The total luminal surface area in the DCT2 and connecting tubule is several-fold higher than in the cortical collecting duct,[159] and together these two segments appear to be sufficient to maintain sodium balance, even in the absence of detectable ENaC along the collecting duct. Mice lacking ENaC selectively in the collecting duct come into balance, even on a low-sodium diet.[160] Congruent with these findings, deletion of α-ENaC from the DCT2, connecting tubule and collecting duct results in severe sodium wasting.[161] Notably, it is the connecting tubule that appears to be most important in the response to aldosterone, while DCT2 has the highest baseline transport in the absence of MR activation.[162] The cortical collecting duct is not as critical as was originally thought for either baseline or aldosterone-stimulated sodium reabsorption, probably due to its smaller surface area compared with the DCT2 and connecting tubule.

As we continue to traverse the nephron, further sodium reabsorption is minimal in the medullary collecting duct, under standard sodium diet conditions, and not significantly stimulated by aldosterone.[133]

SITES OF MINERALOCORTICOID RECEPTOR EXPRESSION AND LOCUS OF ACTION ALONG THE NEPHRON

ALDOSTERONE-SENSITIVE DISTAL NEPHRON

In the kidney, MR is expressed at the highest levels in distal nephron cells extending from the last third of the DCT through the medullary collecting duct,[163] which is frequently referred to as the *aldosterone-sensitive distal nephron* (ASDN) (Figure 12.9).[1] This pattern of expression was first demonstrated using labeled hormone–binding studies performed before the cloning of MR[164] and has been confirmed since by several methods, including polymerase chain reaction,[165] in situ hybridization,[166] and immunohistochemical analysis.[167] Effects of aldosterone on electrogenic Na^+ and K^+ transport in principal cells have been found consistently in these nephron segments,[163] which also express ENaC, and 11β-HSD2, as addressed in detail earlier. Collecting duct intercalated cells also express MR and respond specifically to aldosterone and alter proton secretion. Aldosterone directly increases the activity of the H^+-ATPase in the collecting duct, and its absence results in decreased proton secretion.[168-170] Interestingly, nongenomic stimulation of H^+-ATPase activity in type A intercalated cells has been demonstrated in isolated murine collecting ducts.[171] Consistent with these effects, aldosterone deficiency results in distal renal tubular acidosis type 4, and excess aldosterone results in metabolic alkalosis.[172] It should be noted that aldosterone also stimulates H^+ secretion due to effects on principal cell Na^+ transport, which alter the electrical gradient. These older studies must also now be interpreted in the context of more recent data,[153] which, as noted earlier, demonstrate that the effect of aldosterone on intercalated cells depends on the genesis of the signal.

OTHER SITES OF EXPRESSION

MR has been identified at some level in all parts of the nephron examined, including the glomerulus.[165,173-178] Its effects, at least at some of these sites, are likely to be physiologically relevant in states of volume depletion and acid-base disturbances; however, the data are not as robust and consistent as those for the ASDN.

Glomerulus

MR (but not 11β-HSD2) is expressed in glomerular mesangial cells, where it is thought to affect proliferation and production of reactive oxygen species[179,180] and to have profibrotic effects through SGK1.[181] These effects have been suggested to be important in the progression of renal damage, particularly in diabetic nephropathy,[182] where glucocorticoids mimic the activity of aldosteronism in the context of tissue damage. However, the physiologic role of mesangial cell MR is uncertain.

Proximal Convoluted Tubule

Hierholzer and Stolte showed, through elegant microperfusion studies, that the sodium reabsorptive capacity of the proximal convolution was decreased in adrenalectomized animals and restored by administration of aldosterone.[183] Chronic volume depletion increases sodium reabsorption in the proximal convoluted tubule, which is in part mediated by MR. The mechanisms of action in this nephron segment are controversial. Recent studies indicate an MR-dependent increase in the activity of Na^+-H^+-exchanger isoform 3, possibly through an increase in trafficking of the transporter to the membrane.[184-187] This transporter contributes to sodium and bicarbonate reabsorption. MR activation, in turn, may activate the Na^+-K^+-ATPase in the basolateral membrane of the proximal convoluted tubule to maintain a gradient for sodium reabsorption.[188-191]

Medullary Thick Ascending Limb

In the medullary thick ascending limb, mineralocorticoids but not glucocorticoids increase sodium and chloride reabsorption. In rodents, adrenalectomy impairs reabsorption of NaCl in the medullary thick ascending limb, and aldosterone restores this process.[192,193] This reabsorptive defect may contribute to the urinary concentrating and diluting abnormality measured in patients with Addison's disease and in mice lacking aldosterone synthase.[169,183,194] The medullary thick ascending limb also participates in the regulation of acid-base balance by reabsorbing most of the filtered HCO_3 that is not reabsorbed by the proximal tubule. In this context, aldosterone has been shown to stimulate the Na^+-H^+ exchanger in amphibian thick ascending limb, possibly through a rapid nongenomic effect.[195] Recent evidence has also implicated regulation of the Na-K-2Cl cotransporter type 2 in the thick ascending limb—as well as the NCC in the DCT (see later)—by oxidative stress response kinase 1 (OSR1) and STE20/SPS1-related proline/alanine–rich kinase (SPAK) (OSR1/SPAK).[196,197]

Distal Convoluted Tubule

The DCT is also capable of mineralocorticoid specificity.[198,199] Hormone studies in rodents demonstrate that aldosterone increases expression of the NCC and its apical membrane abundance[200-202] without changes in mRNA expression.[202,203] The recently described family of WNK kinases may play a pivotal role in mediating this effect. Aldosterone acts through MR to increase NCC phosphorylation, which appears to be important for the changes in its expression and apical targeting.[204,205] Recent evidence supports the idea that aldosterone-induced NCC phosphorylation occurs through a signaling cascade in which SGK1 phosphorylates WNK4,[206,207] which, in turn, phosphorylates OSR1 and SPAK.[204,208,197] OSR1/SPAK then directly phosphorylates NCC at three serine/threonine sites,[209] which results in increased activity. It is interesting to note that SGK1 may also be a target of WNK1.[210]

NONRENAL ALDOSTERONE-RESPONSIVE TIGHT EPITHELIA

The mineralocorticoid effects of aldosterone have predominantly been studied in the distal nephron, but do influence

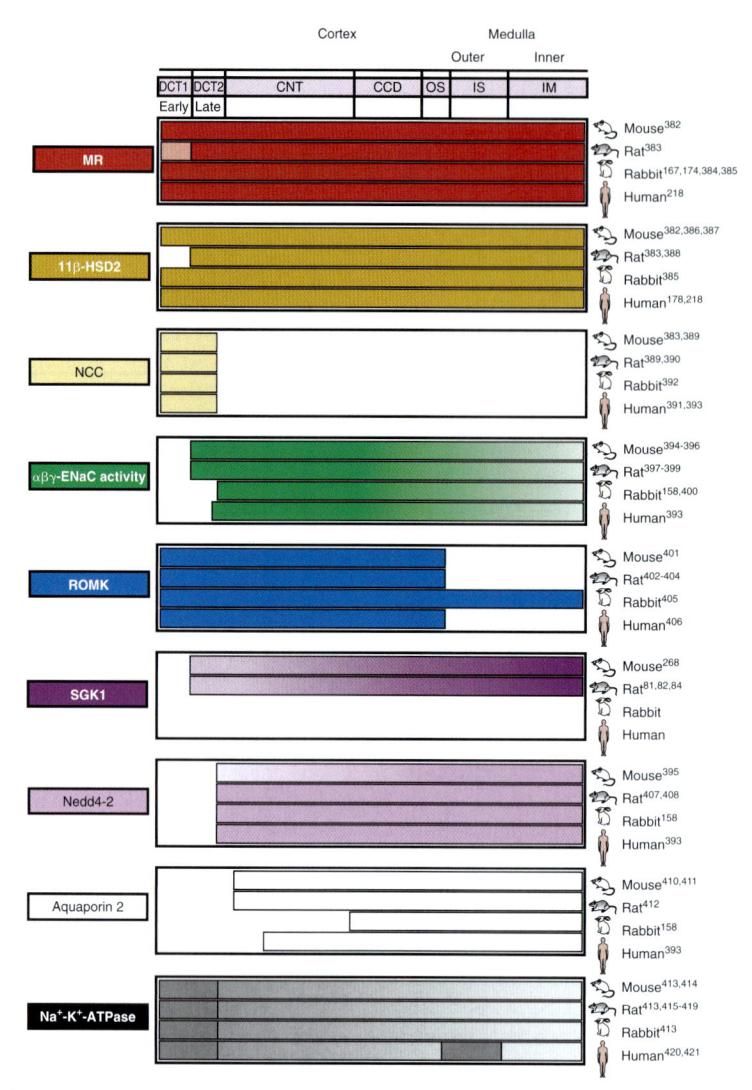

Figure 12.9 Expression and/or activity of the mineralocorticoid-dependent transport machinery in principal cells along the mature aldosterone-sensitive distal nephron (ASDN). Mineralocorticoid specificity is conferred by the presence of the mineralocorticoid receptor (MR) and 11β-hydroxysteroid dehydrogenase type 2 (11β-HSD2) beginning primarily from the latter part of the distal convoluted tubule (DCT). The thiazide-sensitive sodium-chloride cotransporter (NCC) is expressed exclusively in the DCT, but after the transition from the DCT to the connecting tubule (CNT), sodium reabsorption is distinctly determined by amiloride-sensitive sodium channel (ENaC) activity. ENaC activity is strongest in the CNT and decreases down to the inner medulla collecting duct. Variation in gene expression or activity along the nephron is indicated by the intensity of shading. Note that there is some variation in gene expression from mouse to human. However, the machinery for sodium reabsorption in the ASDN is predominantly conserved across species. Each nephron segment is drawn to scale, but expression of channels/transporters in intercalated cells is omitted. Expression and/or activity is based on messenger RNA, protein, and biochemical studies. G, Glomerulus; PCT, proximal convoluted tubule; ROMK channel, renal outer medullary potassium; SGK1, serum- and glucocorticoid-regulated kinase 1. (Adapted from Loffing J, Korbmacher C: Regulated sodium transport in the renal connecting tubule [CNT] via the epithelial sodium channel [ENaC]. *Pflugers Archiv* 458[1]:111-135, 2009.)

other—mostly ENaC-expressing—tight epithelia. ENaC is present in visceral epithelial cells of the distal colon, distal lung, salivary glands, sweat glands, and taste buds.

COLON

Under physiologic conditions, approximately 1.3 to 1.8 L of electrolyte-rich fluid is reabsorbed per day from the colonic epithelium, which accounts for about 90% of the salt and water that enter the proximal colon from the terminal ileum. In nonmammalian vertebrates, sodium conservation by the colon plays an even more significant role.[211] This transport is regulated by several transporters and channels, including ENaC. Like the nephron, the proximal colon reabsorbs sodium via an electroneutral, ENaC-independent process. In the distal colon, electrogenic Na+ absorption via ENaC channels is the predominant mode of sodium transport.[212-215] In disease states such as inflammatory bowel disease, ENaC-mediated sodium reabsorption can be reduced,[216] although in diarrheal states, elevated aldosterone levels may attenuate sodium and water loss from the colon.[217] It should be noted that in the colon, as in the distal nephron, MR signaling is aldosterone selective, reflecting the activity of 11β-HSD2.[218] Aldosterone increases electrogenic sodium absorption and potassium secretion and inhibits electroneutral absorption.[219] This is in contrast to glucocorticoids, which, at higher concentrations, activate GR to stimulate electroneutral absorption in the proximal and distal colon.[78,220] As in the distal nephron, the aldosterone response can be characterized by an early and late response. The early response gene, *SGK1*, is upregulated by aldosterone via MR.[221] However, in contrast with the kidney, aldosterone and a low-salt diet have been shown to stimulate transcription of β- but not α-ENaC in rat models.[222,223]

Aldosterone stimulates electrogenic potassium secretion from colonic epithelia. The significance of this secretion is evident in anuric patients. Potassium secretion from the colon is much higher in patients undergoing long-term hemodialysis than in patients not undergoing dialysis.[224-226] Indeed, administration of fludrocortisone, a mineralocorticoid agonist, to dialysis patients has been shown to reduce hyperkalemia in small clinical trials.[227] Low doses of the common MR antagonist spironolactone do not result in significant hyperkalemia.[228-230]

LUNG

Vectorial transport of salt and water across the distal airway epithelium (ciliated Clara cells, nonciliated cuboidal cells) and alveoli (type I and type II alveoli) primarily determines fluid clearance from the lung. ENaC is the rate-limiting step in sodium transport in the lung and plays a primary role in several physiologic and pathophysiologic conditions determined by fluid clearance.[231] At birth, the lung assumes a resorptive phenotype, and lack of functional ENaC channels leads to neonatal respiratory distress syndrome in mouse knockout models.[232] In children, lack of functional ENaC (e.g., autosomal recessive pseudohypoaldosteronism type I)[233-235] results in increased rates of recurrent infection due to increased airway liquid.[234] In the mature lung, defective ENaC channels can lead to pulmonary edema and pathologic conditions (e.g., acute respiratory distress syndrome[236] and high-altitude pulmonary edema[237]). Conversely, hyperabsorption through ENaC is emerging as an important mechanism of decreased mucus clearance in cystic fibrosis.[238]

The molecular apparatus for mineralocorticoid-stimulated liquid reabsorption via ENaC (concomitant MR and 11β-HSD2) is present in late gestational and mature adult lung in humans[218,239,240] and rats,[241] and there is some evidence for a significant physiologic role of aldosterone in ENaC-mediated sodium transport,[241] although glucocorticoids acting via GR are likely to play the predominant role in lung.[112,221,242-245] Importantly, glucocorticoids, but not mineralocorticoids, play a critical role in lung maturation in humans, and GR knockout mice, like α-ENaC knockout mice, die of respiratory insufficiency within hours of birth. In contrast, MR knockout mice demonstrate a severe salt-wasting phenotype but no significant lung phenotype.[168,246]

EXOCRINE GLANDS AND SENSORS

ENaC-mediated sodium reabsorption is also measurable in salivary and sweat glands.[247] The importance of these tissues for sodium and water homeostasis is underscored by rare genetic mutations that confer elevated plasma aldosterone levels and pseudohypoaldosteronism with normal renal tubular function but significant sodium loss from salivary or sweat glands.[248,249] ENaC channels also play an important role in transduction of sodium salt taste in the anterior papillae of the tongue.[250,251] The appropriate molecular machinery for mineralocorticoid-responsive sodium reabsorption is expressed in these organs,[218,252,253] and these epithelia are model systems for the study of ENaC regulation.[247,254] As in colonic epithelia, aldosterone stimulates expression of β- and γ-ENaC and sodium transport in glands and taste buds in animal models.[251,255] Moreover, in humans, changes in dietary sodium are inversely proportional to sodium transport across salivary epithelia.[256] As in the aldosterone-responsive distal nephron and distal colon, sodium uptake is coupled with potassium secretion in salivary epithelia. This effect is evident in humans with hyperaldosteronism. Such patients have a salivary $[Na^+]/[K^+]$ ratio significantly lower than that of subjects without the disorder,[257,258] although this has not been accepted as a valid means to screen for hyperaldosteronism.

ROLE OF SERUM- AND GLUCOCORTICOID-REGULATED KINASE IN MEDIATING ALDOSTERONE EFFECTS

INDUCTION OF SGK1 BY ALDOSTERONE

In the early to mid-1960s, primarily from the work of Isidore Edelman and colleagues, it became clear that aldosterone, like cortisol, exerted most, if not all, of its key physiologic effects by altering transcription rates of a specific subset of genes.[259] In particular, hormone-induced changes in gene transcription were shown to be essential for its effects on epithelial Na^+ transport.[69] Attention focused first on enzymes of intermediary metabolism, particularly citrate synthase,[260,261] and after the cloning of the transporters involved in Na^+ translocation (Na^+-K^+-ATPase and ENaC), these were also found to be regulated by aldosterone at the transcriptional level. However, these effects are manifest several hours after most of the change in Na^+ transport has already occurred and hence could not explain the early and greatest proportion of effects of aldosterone.[1] Considerable effort by many groups went into unbiased screening for aldosterone-regulated proteins[262] and later aldosterone-regulated mRNAs (reviewed in Verrey[1]). In 1999, SGK1 was identified as the first early-onset aldosterone-induced gene product, which clearly stimulates ENaC-mediated sodium reabsorption in the distal nephron[221,263] without pleiotropic effects on other cellular processes. The physiologic relevance of SGK1 is now firmly established, and investigations by numerous laboratories into its mechanism of action have revealed critical general features of the mechanism underlying hormone-regulated ion transport: it is therefore addressed in some detail here. SGK1 mRNA levels are increased within 15 minutes, and protein levels within 30 minutes, in cultured cells upon stimulation by aldosterone[264,265] and in the collecting duct by aldosterone or a low-salt diet (a physiologic stimulus for aldosterone secretion) in vivo.[81,221,266] Notably, SGK1 is increased more abundantly in kidney cortex (the connecting tubule and cortical collecting duct) than in medulla, which corresponds to the potency of ENaC activation in these nephron segments.[267] SGK1 is expressed in other nephron segments, including glomeruli, proximal tubule, and papillae[81,221,268]; however, its rapid induction specifically in the ASDN appears to provide most of the basis for its role in aldosterone-regulated sodium and potassium transport. It is of interest that SGK1 is highly expressed in glomeruli and inner medulla and papillae in the absence of aldosterone; recent data are consistent with the idea that its inner medullary induction is related to its role in osmotic responses.[269]

MOLECULAR MECHANISMS OF SGK1 ACTION IN THE ALDOSTERONE-SENSITIVE DISTAL NEPHRON

SGK1 is a serine/threonine kinase of the AGC protein kinase superfamily,[270] and its kinase activity appears to be essential for Na^+ transport regulation. Although it has effects on proliferation and apoptosis in kidney cells, these effects appear to be minor, and the control of ENaC and other transporters[271] predominates. SGK1 transcription is induced by a variety of stimuli in addition to aldosterone. As its name implies, these include serum and glucocorticoids, but also follicle-stimulating hormone, transforming growth factor–β, and hypotonic and hypertonic stress.[272-275] Of these, osmotic regulation is of the clearest physiologic relevance.[276]

SGK1 is interesting as a signaling kinase in that both its expression level and its activity are highly regulated. Regulation of the former occurs primarily through effects on gene transcription, although protein stability is also regulated, whereas regulation of the latter occurs through phosphorylation.[277,278] Like that of its close relative Akt, SGK1 phosphorylation is stimulated by a variety of growth factors including insulin and insulin-like growth factor-1,[277,278-280] which act through PI3K to trigger phosphorylation at two key residues, an activation loop (residue T256) and a hydrophobic motif (S422). Both of these phosphorylation events appear to be PI3K dependent. Specifically, the α-isoform of the p110 subunit of PI3K stimulates PI3K-dependent kinase 1 and mTORC2 (PDK2), respectively.[278,280-283,284] Recent evidence has established that PDK2 is in fact the mammalian target of rapamycin [mTOR] in its complex 2 variant.[284,285] mTORC2 also uses a co-factor, SIN1, to specify activation of SGK1 rather than related family members such as Akt.[286] In turn, the upstream kinases, PI3K-dependent kinase 1 and mTORC2, phosphorylate and thereby activate SGK1 kinase, which is required for its stimulation of ENaC.[283,287,288] Thus, SGK1 serves as a convergence point for different classes of stimuli, which act on the one hand to control its expression (aldosterone) and on the other to control its activity (insulin), which results in the coordinate regulation of ENaC.

In the study of the physiologic and pathophysiologic role of SGK1 in the ASDN, mice lacking SGK1 have provided considerable insight. Unlike MR knockout mice,[168] mice lacking SGK1 survive the neonatal period and appear normal when consuming a diet with normal salt levels, although their aldosterone levels are markedly elevated. When subjected to a low-salt diet, these mice have a profound sodium-wasting phenotype (pseudohypoaldosteronism type I).[289,290] Notably, this is a significantly milder phenotype than in the MR knockout. This comparison suggests that disruption of SGK1 signaling may be insufficient to eliminate aldosterone-mediated sodium transport due to additional aldosterone-induced and aldosterone-repressed proteins that could compensate for the lack of SGK1. Other early aldosterone-induced genes, including K-ras, GILZ, kidney-specific WNK1, Usp45, melanophilin, and promyelocytic leukemia zinc finger,[291-296] have also been implicated in the stimulation of ENaC. Their distinct mechanisms of action have not been studied in vivo and are beyond the scope of this chapter.

Alternatively, SGK1 may play a more significant role in states of aldosterone excess or upregulation of hormonal activators of SGK1 (e.g., insulin). Indeed, SGK1 knockout mice are protected from the development of salt-sensitive hypertension, which accompanies the hyperinsulinemia of the metabolic syndrome.[297,298] Despite its accepted role as a mediator of aldosterone-stimulated sodium reabsorption, the mechanisms by which SGK1 stimulates ENaC are not fully characterized. Several mechanistic studies have demonstrated that SGK1 is rapidly induced but also rapidly degraded.[221,299,300] The N terminus of the kinase, which distinguishes SGK1 from other kinase family members (e.g., Akt), is important for stimulation of sodium transport but is also the target for rapid degradation of the kinase via the ubiquitin-proteasome system.[301-304] In addition, several naturally occurring variants of SGK1 possess distinct N termini that modify the ability to stimulate ENaC and to be degraded.[305-307] The pathophysiologic implications of the N terminus for sodium transport are unclear, but they may involve a negative feedback loop to limit sodium reabsorption in states of hypertension.

The molecular mechanisms of ENaC stimulation by SGK1 can be divided into three known categories (Figure 12.10): (1) posttranslational effects on the E3 ubiquitin ligase Nedd4-2, (2) posttranslational Nedd4-2–independent effects, and (3) transcription of gene products such as α-ENaC.

SGK1 INHIBITS THE UBIQUITIN LIGASE NEDD4-2

Before the discovery of SGK1 as an aldosterone-induced early gene product, the E3 ubiquitin ligase known as *neural developmentally downregulated isoform 4-2* (Nedd4-2) was shown to interact with the C-terminal tails of β-ENaC and γ-ENaC[308] and decrease surface expression of the channel via channel ubiquitination, and hence to inhibit sodium current.[102,309] The genetic defect in Liddle's syndrome (ENaC-mediated hypertension, hypokalemia, and metabolic alkalosis) consists of a gain-of-function mutation in the C-terminal tail of these subunits, which results in decreased inhibition by Nedd4-2 and hence increased ENaC activity.[310] Lack of Nedd4-2 in vivo results in increased ENaC activity and salt-sensitive hypertension,[311,312] recapitulating a Liddle's syndrome–like phenotype. SGK1 interacts with and phosphorylates Nedd4-2[265,287] in an ENaC signaling complex[107] and enhances cell surface expression of ENaC,[264,313] a determinant of ENaC activity (see Figure 12.10A). This interaction coordinates phosphorylation-dependent binding of 14-3-3 proteins to inhibit Nedd4-2 and prevent ubiquitination of ENaC.[314-317] This disinhibition of ENaC parallels a recurring theme in the regulation of ion transport in the kidney seen with the WNK kinases and the NCC, other aldosterone-regulated gene products (e.g., GILZ) and ENaC, and NHERF2 and ROMK.[270,318] Similarly, SGK1 has also been implicated in stimulation of NCC via inhibition of Nedd4-2, but because NCC lacks a PY motif, the mechanism by which SGK1 and Nedd4-2 modify NCC-mediated sodium reabsorption is unknown.[319,320]

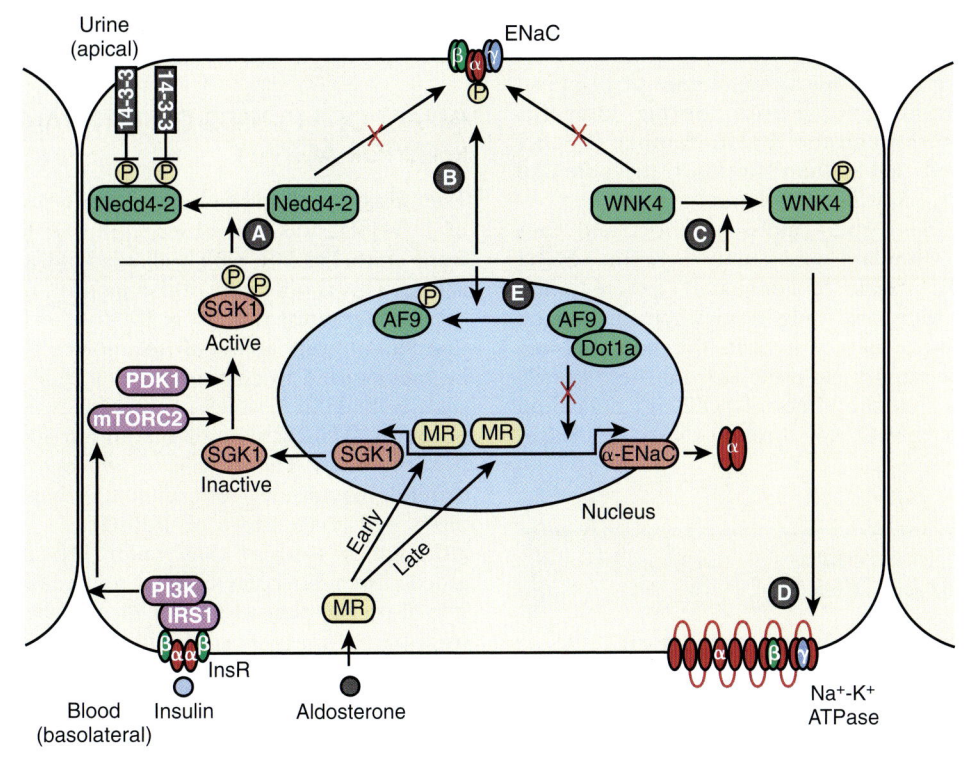

Figure 12.10 Mechanisms of serum- and glucocorticoid-regulated kinase 1 (SGK1)–mediated stimulation of the amiloride-sensitive sodium channel (ENaC). Within principal cells of the mammalian kidney, SGK1 is transcriptionally upregulated as an early aldosterone-induced gene product. SGK1 is then phosphorylated twice via a phosphatidylinositol-3-kinase (PI3K)–dependent cascade of upstream kinases leading to active SGK1. Active SGK1 has multiple effects: it increases apical plasma membrane ENaC by inhibiting Nedd4-2 and Raf-1, and it induces transcription of the α-ENaC (thereby influencing late effects of aldosterone). A to E (clockwise), the individual mechanisms that have been elucidated in principal cells. See text for details. InsR, Insulin receptor; IRS1, insulin receptor substrate 1; MR, mineralocorticoid receptor; mTORC2, mammalian target of rapamycin complex 2; PDK1, 3-phosphoinositide-dependent protein kinase type 1.

SGK1 ENHANCES EPITHELIAL SODIUM CHANNEL ACTIVITY INDEPENDENTLY OF NEDD4-2

In cell culture systems, mutation of SGK1 phosphorylation sites on Nedd4-2 does not completely abolish the ability of SGK1 to stimulate ENaC.[287] Furthermore, SGK1 has been shown to stimulate ENaC channels with Liddle's syndrome mutations, which are unable to bind Nedd4-2.[221,264] Consequently, other Nedd4-2–independent mechanisms of SGK1 stimulation have been proposed. SGK1 directly phosphorylates a serine residue in the intracellular C-terminal tail of α-ENaC, which directly activates channels at the cell surface (see Figure 12.10B).[321,322] SGK1 has been implicated in the stimulation of ENaC via phosphorylation of WNK4, a kinase mutated in pseudohypoaldosteronism type II (see Figure 12.10C).[206] Cell-surface expressed SGK1 may also increase open probability of the channel.[322,323] In addition to showing effects on ENaC, SGK1 has been found to stimulate the activity of basolateral Na$^+$-K$^+$-ATPase, which separately increases ENaC-mediated sodium transport (see Figure 12.10D).[324,325] The time course of these effects and their relative importance compared with Nedd4-2–dependent inhibition have not been explored.[321] The next generation of molecular studies of SGK1 will elucidate the relative importance of each of these pathways.

SGK1 STIMULATES THE COMPONENTS OF SODIUM TRANSPORT MACHINERY

SGK1 also regulates the expression of late aldosterone-responsive genes, primarily α-ENaC.[326,327] Active SGK1 is an important mediator of aldosterone-sensitive α-ENaC transcription in vivo via inhibition of a transcriptional repression element, the disruptor of telomeric silencing alternative splice variant a (Dot1a)–ALL1–fused gene from chromosome 9 (Af9) complex.[327] SGK1 phosphorylates Af9 and reduces interaction between Dot1a and Af9. This releases suppression of ENaC transcription by this complex (see Figure 12.10E). Thus, SGK1 not only acts on ENaC channels to rapidly enhance sodium channel activity through the increase of active channels at the apical surface and increase of the Na$^+$-K$^+$-ATPase at the basolateral surface but also stimulates transcription of elements of the machinery for sodium transport to promote a sustained response to aldosterone. SGK1 is an early-onset gene, but its effects influence both immediate and long-term aldosterone-stimulated sodium reabsorption.

SGK1 STIMULATES POTASSIUM SECRETION IN THE ALDOSTERONE-SENSITIVE DISTAL NEPHRON

Further evidence of a role for SGK1 in the regulation of sodium transport in the ASDN is revealed by the study of potassium secretion. As outlined earlier, sodium reabsorption through ENaC increases the negative charge on the luminal surface of the apical membrane of principal cells, thereby providing an electrical driving force for potassium secretion through the ROMK channel. If SGK1 enhances ENaC-mediated sodium transport, the potential difference across the apical-to-basolateral surface of principal cells should be higher (more negative) and thus should indirectly stimulate potassium secretion. SGK1 knockout mice are unable to adequately secrete potassium in both the short and long term when challenged with a high-potassium diet. Moreover, the potential difference across collecting duct epithelia from these knockout mice indicates that the effect of SGK1 on potassium secretion occurs via ENaC, not through direct regulation of ROMK.[328]

11β-HYDROXYSTEROID DEHYDROGENASE TYPE 2

11β-HSD2: AN ESSENTIAL DETERMINANT OF MINERALOCORTICOID SPECIFICITY

The physiologic glucocorticoid cortisol (corticosterone in rats and mice) has a high affinity for MR, equivalent to that of aldosterone and, as noted earlier, circulates at plasma free concentrations that are 100-fold or more greater than those of aldosterone. Central to the ability of MR to selectively respond to aldosterone in the ASDN is the coexpression of the enzyme 11β-HSD2.[5,6] 11β-HSD2 converts cortisol/corticosterone to receptor-inactive 11-keto steroids (cortisone in humans, 11-dehydrocorticosterone in rats and mice), using nicotinamide adenine dinucleotide (NAD) as a cosubstrate and generating sufficient amounts of the reduced form of NAD (NADH) to alter the redox potential of the cell. This dependence sets it in contrast to 11β-HSD1, which uses the reduced form of nicotinamide adenine dinucleotide phosphate (NADPH), preferentially catalyzes the conversion of the oxidized to the reduced form, and has received substantial attention recently as a target for treatment of metabolic syndrome.[329] Aldosterone has a very reactive aldehyde group at carbon 18 (see Figure 12.1), which forms an 11,18-hemiacetal and is protected from dehydrogenation by 11β-HSD2.[5,6]

SITES OF 11β-HSD2 EXPRESSION

In the kidney, 11β-HSD2 is expressed at high levels throughout the ASDN,[166,177,330] where it is coexpressed with MR and ENaC (see Figure 12.9).[331] Consistent with aldosterone regulation of the NCC, it is also coexpressed in DCT with this transporter as well.[332,333] Interestingly, expression has also been found in the thick ascending limb,[177] although expression levels appear to be substantially lower, and increase progressively in DCT. Expression is by far highest in the connecting tubule and cortical collecting duct.[330,333] It is also expressed in the aldosterone-sensitive segments of the colon, particularly the distal colon, as is the case for MR, although there is species variability.[334] 11β-HSD2 expression has also been described in several nonepithelial tissues, including placenta,[335] the nucleus tractus solitarius in the brain,[336] and the vessel wall,[53] which makes all of these tissues potential aldosterone target tissues.

IMPACT OF 11β-HSD2 ON MINERALOCORTICOID RECEPTOR ACTIVITY

The initial[5,6] and still widely held interpretation of the role of 11β-HSD2 was that of excluding active glucocorticoids from epithelial MR, which allowed aldosterone unfettered access. This is only part of the picture, however; to reduce the signal-to-noise ratio from 100-fold to 10% would require that 999 of every 1000 cortisol molecules entering the cell be metabolized to cortisone, a very tall order in an organ such as the kidney, which commands 20% to 25% of cardiac output. 11β-HSD2 in epithelia (and in other tissues in which it is expressed) clearly reduces glucocorticoid levels by an order of magnitude[337] but still leaves them with intracellular levels well above those of aldosterone. At the same time, although it is clear that when 11β-HSD2 is operative, glucocorticoid-occupied MR is not transcriptionally active, it is also clear that when enzyme activity is insufficient (as in apparent mineralocorticoid excess) or deficient (as in licorice abuse or by genetic mutation), cortisol can activate MR and ion transport. Although the subcellular mechanisms involved have yet to be established, it appears that glucocorticoid-MR complexes are conformationally distinct from aldosterone-MR complexes. One intriguing possibility is that these hormone-receptor complexes, in contrast to aldosterone-MR complexes, are held inactive by the obligate generation of NADH from the cosubstrate NAD, required for the operation of 11β-HSD2.[338] There is direct evidence to support the idea that redox potential affects the activity of the glucocorticoid receptor through effects on thioredoxin.[339]

APPARENT MINERALOCORTICOID EXCESS: A DISEASE OF DEFECTIVE 11β-HSD2

Apparent mineralocorticoid excess was first described by Maria New, and the molecular mechanisms responsible were established after an intense but fruitless search for a novel mineralocorticoid.[340] The condition reflects partial or complete deficiency of 11β-HSD2 activity, is more common in consanguinity, and manifests as severe juvenile hypertension (see also Chapter 47).[341] Confectionery licorice (or that added to chewing tobacco) contains glycyrrhizic and glycyrrhetinic acid, suicide substrates for 11β-HSD2, which thus acts as a potent inhibitor of the enzyme. Lack of functional 11β-HSD2 results in MR activation by cortisol and inappropriate mineralocorticoid-like stimulation of ENaC-mediated Na^+ reabsorption. This causes severe hypertension, often accompanied by hypokalemia. Plasma renin, angiotensin II, and aldosterone are suppressed. Treatment of apparent mineralocorticoid excess is the use of MR antagonists and additional antihypertensives as required. Treatment of licorice abuse is moderation.

ROLE OF 11β-HSD2 IN BLOOD VESSELS

Studies of 11β-HSD2 in the human vascular wall[342] defined the activity of aldosterone and cortisol in this physiologic aldosterone target tissue. Aldosterone at nanomolar concentrations caused a rapid rise in intracellular pH, reflecting nongenomic activation of the Na^+-H^+ exchanger. Cortisol alone over a range of doses produced no effect, but when carbenoxolone was added to inhibit 11β-HSD2, cortisol mimicked aldosterone. Inhibitor studies revealed that the effects of both aldosterone and cortisol were mediated by classical MR. In other studies involving tissue damage, mineralocorticoid antagonists were protective, whereas aldosterone or cortisol worsened injury. The inference from these results was that cortisol becomes an MR agonist in the context of tissue damage (or when 11β-HSD2 is pharmacologically inhibited), with alteration of reactive oxygen species generation and redox potential.[343] It is further notable that aldosterone has been shown to have both vasodilatory and vasoconstricting effects in animals and humans.[344] These contradictory results have not been fully reconciled[345] but may well reflect a combination of direct effects on vascular smooth muscle to stimulate myosin light-chain phosphorylation through ERK activation,[346,347] on the one hand, and stimulatory effects on endothelial cell nitric oxide synthase,[344] on the other. Finally, it is of considerable interest that vascular smooth muscle cells express ENaC, in addition to MR, and that the channel might play a role in vascular tone.[348]

SUMMARY OF 11β-HSD2 ROLES

In summary, the enzyme 11β-HSD2 is crucial for aldosterone-selective activation of epithelial MR and possibly of MR in other tissues, including blood vessels, nucleus of the solitary tract, and placenta. It does this in part by debulking intracellular glucocorticoids by an order of magnitude, which is not sufficient to account for its blockade of cortisol agonist activity. Current evidence supports the possibility that 11β-HSD2–mediated generation of NADH renders glucocorticoid-occupied MR inactive. Partial or complete deficiency of 11β-HSD2 results in the syndrome of apparent mineralocorticoid excess, which is mimicked by licorice abuse.

NONGENOMIC EFFECTS OF ALDOSTERONE

The classical effects of aldosterone on ion transport are genomic, with MR acting at the nuclear level to regulate DNA-directed, RNA-mediated protein synthesis and thereby sodium transport. Such genomic effects are characterized by a lag period of 45 to 60 minutes before changes in ion transport can be measured, commensurate with a homeostatic role for aldosterone action in regulating sodium and potassium status in response to dietary intake. In other circumstances (e.g., orthostasis, acute blood volume depletion), aldosterone secretion rises rapidly, and acute nongenomic effects are an understandable response. Such rapid effects were first demonstrated 25 years ago in the laboratory[349]; in human vascular tissues they have been amply demonstrated both in vitro[342] and in vivo.[350] Although most of these rapid nongenomic effects appear to be mediated via activation of classical MR,[342,349] there is evidence from atomic force microscopy studies for non-MR membrane sites binding aldosterone with high affinity on cultured endothelial cells.[351] Such nongenomic effects are not unique to aldosterone, having been shown for the other recognized classes of steroid hormones[352] and reported for dehydroepiandrosterone (DHEA).[344] Genomic effects commonly have a lag period of 20 minutes or longer and are abrogated by inhibitors of transcription such as actinomycin D. Most nongenomic effects of steroids have time courses from onset to plateau of 5 to 10 minutes and are mediated by a variety of pathways.

MR does not have a myristoylation site (unlike, for example, estrogen receptors[353]), and there is little evidence for membrane-associated classical MR. Most rapid nongenomic effects of aldosterone appear to be mediated by classical MR, in that they are inhibited by the MR antagonist RU 28318. In some instances[342] spironolactone is ineffective as an inhibitor: exclusive reliance on blockade by spironolactone led to the assumption of a widely distributed aldosterone receptor distinct from classical MR and a long and unsuccessful search for such a membrane-bound species.[354] The physiology of nongenomic aldosterone actions has been slow to be accepted, which in part reflects the major emphasis on the clearly genomic actions of aldosterone in the kidney. The most obvious example is the conjunction of rapid secretion of aldosterone in response to orthostasis and its demonstrated rapid vascular effects.[345,355] With the recent interest in the pathophysiologic effects of MR activation, particularly in nonclassical aldosterone target tissues, there has been renewed interest in rapid nongenomic effects of aldosterone (and the physiologic glucocorticoids) via classical MR. Further details of the nongenomic actions of aldosterone can be found in Funder[355] and other sources.[356,357]

DISEASE STATES

PRIMARY ALDOSTERONISM

Clinically, by far the most prevalent disorder directly involving aldosterone is Conn's syndrome, or primary aldosteronism.[358] In this syndrome, aldosterone secretion is elevated and (relatively) autonomous as a result of an adrenal adenoma or, more frequently, bilateral adrenal hyperplasia, and, very rarely, adrenal carcinoma or the inherited disorder glucocorticoid remediable aldosteronism (FH-1). Once considered rare (<1% of all cases of hypertension), necessarily characterized by hypokalemia and relatively benign, primary aldosteronism is now thought to account for approximately 8% to 13% of all hypertension, which reflects improved case detection and diagnosis. In contrast with previous teaching, frank hypokalemia is found in only 25% to 30% of cases, and the incidence of cardiovascular pathology (fibrosis, fibrillation, infarct, stroke) is substantially higher than in age-, sex-, and blood pressure–matched individuals with essential hypertension.[359,360]

Guidelines for the case detection, diagnosis, and management of primary aldosteronism have been published[361] as a first step in addressing what is increasingly recognized as a major public health issue. It has long been thought and taught that the role of aldosterone in blood pressure regulation reflects its epithelial effects leading to retention of sodium, and with it water, which thus increases circulating volume. This increase, in turn, is reflected in an increased cardiac output, which is reflexively normalized by vasoconstriction and thus elevation of blood pressure (in keeping with the Guyton hypothesis[362]). Although the epithelial effects of aldosterone on vascular volume are indisputably homeostatically important, there are compelling experimental and clinical studies to suggest a role for nonepithelial effects in mineralocorticoid-induced hypertension.[363,364] Very recently, in addition to MR-mediated central nervous system and vascular effects in hypertension, roles for macrophages have been demonstrated by two groups using distinct and complementary experimental approaches.[365,366]

Recent data have suggested a role for a mutated K$^+$ channel (KCNJ5) in the pathogenesis of aldosterone-producing adrenal adenomas and in the rare condition of FH type III.[22,23] See section "Aldosterone Synthesis" for additional details.

CONGESTIVE HEART FAILURE

Aldosterone has been implicated in the pathophysiology of congestive heart failure since soon after its discovery in the mid-1950s.[367,368] Until fairly recently, most of the focus has been on the counterproductive effects of aldosterone in epithelia. More recently, the beneficial effects of MR antagonists in congestive heart failure have suggested an additional effect in myocardium itself.[369] In the Randomized Aldactone Evaluation Study (RALES),[369] addition of low-dose (mean 26 mg/day) spironolactone to standard-of-care treatment in patients with progressive heart failure produced a 30% reduction in mortality and 35% fewer hospitalizations. This result is often attributed to spironolactone antagonizing the effect of aldosterone on cardiomyocyte MR, but actually reflects its antagonizing of cortisol acting as an MR agonist under ischemic conditions. Subsequently, the Eplerenone Post-Acute Myocardial Infarction Heart Failure Efficacy and Survival Study (EPHESUS) examined the effect of eplerenone, an MR antagonist with improved specificity relative to spironolactone, on heart failure due to systolic dysfunction complicating acute myocardial infarction. The study showed that adding eplerenone (43 mg/day) on top of conventional therapy significantly decreased mortality due to all causes (31%) and cardiovascular mortality (13%).[370] Potassium concentration was only slightly higher in the eplerenone-treated group than in the placebo-treated group (4.47 mmol/L and 4.54 mmol/L, respectively). Coupled with the recent literature on direct vascular effects of aldosterone addressed earlier, these data suggest that MR antagonists have a beneficial effect that cannot be accounted for by diuretic actions in the kidney alone.[371]

It is also notable that a recent trial (*E*plerenone in *M*ild *P*atients *H*ospitalization *A*nd *S*urv*I*val Study in *H*eart *F*ailure [EMPHASIS-HF]) examining the effect of eplerenone in New York Heart Association (NYHA) class II heart failure (milder than previously examined) was stopped early because a significant benefit was found in the treated group.[372] In summary, the pathophysiologic effects of aldosterone excess on the cardiovascular system in primary aldosteronism are well documented, and MR also plays an important role in essential hypertension and heart failure. Importantly, MR expressed in cardiac and vascular cells may commonly be activated by cortisol rather than aldosterone, which is present in serum at levels that are higher by 100-fold or more and mimics aldosterone in the context of tissue damage.

CHRONIC KIDNEY DISEASE

The role of MR blockade in slowing the progression of chronic kidney disease is considered in a recent study and commentary[373,374] and in Chapter 62. The study, a double-blind, randomized, placebo-controlled trial, examines the anti-albuminuric effect of the aldosterone blocker eplerenone in nondiabetic hypertensive patients with albuminuria.

NONEPITHELIAL ACTIONS OF ALDOSTERONE

In addition to the classical epithelial tissues involved in ion transport (kidney, colon, sweat gland, salivary gland), there are documented effects of aldosterone in the brain, vascular wall, and possibly the placenta, as previously noted. Many other tissues and organs have been postulated as physiologic aldosterone target tissues, largely on the inadequate evidence that they express MR and can be shown in vitro to respond by some measure to aldosterone. What underpins these postulates is the misconception that aldosterone is the cognate ligand for MR, which is true for epithelia but not for cells not expressing 11β-HSD2, coupled with disregard for the role of cortisol. Cortisol was not only the ligand for MR in cartilaginous and bony fish, millions of years before the appearance of aldosterone synthase, but is the overwhelming occupant of MR that is not protected by 11β-HSD2 (primarily nonepithelial MR) throughout the body. It is notable that some nonepithelial MR is also protected by 11β-HSD2, for example, in the nucleus tractus solitarius.

The fact that aldosterone can activate MR under experimental conditions without 11β-HSD2 is illustrated by the work of Gómez-Sánchez and colleagues more than two decades ago.[375] Very low doses of aldosterone that did not affect blood pressure when infused systemically elevated blood pressure when infused into the lateral ventricle of conscious, free-living rats. That this did not reflect a physiologic role for aldosterone, however, was shown by the co-infusion of one, two, and five times the dose of corticosterone, which progressively blocked the blood pressure effect of the infused aldosterone, evidence for the absence of 11β-HSD2 in the hypothalamic nuclei involved, and the overwhelming occupancy of their MR by the physiologic glucocorticoid.

The two established nonepithelial aldosterone target tissues are the vascular wall and the nucleus tractus solitarius in the brain. Both of these tissues express 11β-HSD2, as noted earlier, allowing aldosterone-selective MR activation; both can be reasonably envisaged as having important ancillary roles supporting the primary, epithelial role of aldosterone on fluid and electrolyte homeostasis. Aldosterone vasoconstricts blood vessels, acutely and in the longer term, in response to volume depletion; similarly, it acts on the nucleus tractus solitarius to stimulate salt appetite. Both actions are thus harnessed into the physiologic role of aldosterone in maintaining fluid and electrolyte balance.

It is commonly assumed that in pathophysiologic states of high aldosterone level, such as primary aldosteronism, the deleterious effects are mediated by aldosterone occupying and inappropriately activating nonprotected MR, in cardiomyocytes, for example. It is plausible that instead of the approximately 1% physiologic occupancy (given the approximately 100-fold higher levels of plasma free cortisol), aldosterone occupancy of cardiomyocyte MR might rise to 3% to 5%. Relatively minor degrees of MR occupancy have been shown effective for spironolactone, acting as a protective inverse agonist,[376] so similarly minor degrees of cardiomyocyte MR occupancy by aldosterone could potentially produce the deleterious effects seen.

This explanation, however, is almost certainly incorrect. Plasma aldosterone levels are as high or higher in chronic sodium deficiency (or in the effectively volume-depleted condition of secondary hyperaldosteronism), with no deleterious cardiovascular effects. In primary and secondary aldosteronism, and in chronic sodium deficiency, physiologic target tissues, both renal tubular and coronary vascular, are exposed to (and respond to) maintained high levels of aldosterone; it is thus unlikely that in primary aldosteronism the cardiovascular damage reflects increased MR activation in blood vessels, coronary and peripheral. The key difference between the circumstances is that primary aldosteronism is a state of aldosterone and sodium excess, and the others of sodium/volume depletion.

A plausible but untested mechanism of aldosterone-induced damage is that it is secondary to increased renal sodium reabsorption and the action of endogenous ouabain on blood vessels. Endogenous ouabain is incompletely explored, but its levels are elevated in primary aldosteronism.[377] Like aldosterone, its secretion is elevated by ACTH and angiotensin (the latter via AT_2R); in stark contrast with aldosterone, it is *raised* (not lowered) in states of sodium excess.[378-380] It acts via Na^+-K^+-ATPase in vessel wall as a vasoconstrictor, presumably physiologically to produce a pressure natriuresis as a homeostatic response. It may thus be that the cardiovascular damage in primary aldosteronism reflects a combination of the effects of aldosterone plus endogenous ouabain on the vasculature, and, if this is the case, the *fons et origo* of the nonepithelial effects of aldosterone remain squarely in the renal tubule and the exaggerated sodium retention therein.

ACKNOWLEDGMENT

Our co-author, colleague, and friend John Stokes died in 2012, just before work on this new edition began. John was senior author on the chapter "Aldosterone Regulation of Ion Transport", written as a new chapter for the 9th edition of Brenner and Rector, and was the direct predecessor to the present one. John brought to the writing of that chapter, a profound knowledge of aldosterone action in the renal tubules, a sharp wit, and unsurpassed work ethic; for all these reasons, he was the model co-author. In addition, John made enormous contributions to aldosterone and renal tubule research, which enriched all of us, as did his humor and enthusiasm for life. He will be missed. For those interested in reading more about John's remarkable life and contributions to nephrology and renal research, see the eloquent eulogy at http://www.ncbi.nlm.nih.gov/pmc/articles/PMC3715930/.

Complete reference list available at ExpertConsult.com.

KEY REFERENCES

2. Simpson SA, Tait JF: A quantitative method for the bioassay of the effect of adrenal cortical steroids on mineral metabolism. *Endocrinology* 50(2):150–161, 1952.
3. Simpson SA, Tait JF: Physiochemical methods of detection of a previously unidentified adrenal hormone. *Mem Soc Endocrinol* 2:9–24, 1953.
4. Simpson SA, et al: [Constitution of aldosterone, a new mineralocorticoid]. *Experientia* 10(3):132–133, 1954.
5. Funder JW, et al: Mineralocorticoid action: target tissue specificity is enzyme, not receptor, mediated. *Science* 242(4878):583–585, 1988.
14. Lifton RP, et al: A chimaeric 11β-hydroxylase/aldosterone synthase gene causes glucocorticoid-remediable aldosteronism and human hypertension. *Nature* 355:262–265, 1992.
22. Choi M, et al: K^+ channel mutations in adrenal aldosterone-producing adenomas and hereditary hypertension. *Science* 331:768–772, 2011.
24. Boulkroun S, et al: Prevalence, clinical, and molecular correlates of KCNJ5 mutations in primary aldosteronism. *Hypertension* 59(3):592–598, 2012.
26. Azizan EAB, et al: Somatic mutations in ATP1A1 and CACNA1D underlie a common subtype of adrenal hypertension. *Nat Genet* 45:1055, 2013.
33. Bhargava A, Pearce D: Mechanisms of mineralocorticoid action: determinants of receptor specificity and actions of regulated gene products. *Trends Endocrinol Metab* 15(4):147–153, 2004.
51. Geller DS, et al: Autosomal dominant pseudohypoaldosteronism type 1: mechanisms, evidence for neonatal lethality, and phenotypic expression in adults. *J Am Soc Nephrol* 17(5):1429–1436, 2006.
52. Krozowski ZS, Funder JW: Renal mineralocorticoid receptors and hippocampal corticosterone-binding species have identical intrinsic steroid specificity. *Proc Natl Acad Sci U S A* 80(19):6056–6060, 1983.
56. Pearce D, Yamamoto KR: Mineralocorticoid and glucocorticoid receptor activities distinguished by nonreceptor factors at a composite response element. *Science* 259(5098):1161–1165, 1993.
58. Pascual-Le Tallec L, et al: The elongation factor ELL (eleven-nineteen lysine-rich leukemia) is a selective coregulator for steroid receptor functions. *Mol Endocrinol* 19(5):1158–1169, 2005.
63. Hong H, et al: GRIP1, a novel mouse protein that serves as a transcriptional coactivator in yeast for the hormone binding domains of steroid receptors. *Proc Natl Acad Sci U S A* 93(10):4948–4952, 1996.
64. Onate SA, et al: Sequence and characterization of a coactivator for the steroid hormone receptor superfamily. *Science* 270(5240):1354–1357, 1995.
71. Conn JW, Knopf RF, Nesbit RM: Clinical characteristics of primary aldosteronism from an analysis of 145 cases. *Am J Surg* 107:159–172, 1964.
72. Canessa CM, et al: Amiloride-sensitive epithelial Na^+ channel is made of three homologous subunits. *Nature* 367(6462):463–467, 1994.
74. Garty H, Palmer LG: Epithelial sodium channels: function, structure, and regulation. *Physiol Rev* 77:359–396, 1997.
82. Chen S, et al: Epithelial sodium channel regulated by aldosterone-induced protein sgk. *Proc Natl Acad Sci U S A* 96:2514–2519, 1999.
91. Frindt G, Ergonul Z, Palmer LG: Surface expression of epithelial Na channel protein in rat kidney. *J Gen Physiol* 131(6):617–627, 2008.
124. Wade JB, et al: Morphological and physiological responses to aldosterone: time course and sodium dependence. *Am J Physiol* 259(1 Pt 2):F88–F94, 1990.
132. Knight KK, et al: Liddle's syndrome mutations increase Na^+ transport through dual effects on epithelial Na^+ channel surface expression and proteolytic cleavage. *Proc Natl Acad Sci U S A* 103(8):2805–2808, 2006.
133. Stokes JB: Potassium secretion by cortical collecting tubule: relation to sodium absorption, luminal sodium concentration, and transepithelial voltage. *Am J Physiol Renal Fluid Electrolyte Physiol* 241:F395–F402, 1981.
135. Estilo G, Liu W, Pastor-Soler N, et al: Effect of aldosterone on BK channel expression in mammalian cortical collecting duct. *Am J Physiol Renal Physiol* 295:F780–F788, 2008.

145. McCormick JA, Yang CL, Ellison DH: WNK kinases and renal sodium transport in health and disease: an integrated view. *Hypertension* 51(3):588–596, 2008.
153. Shibata S, et al: Regulated mineralocorticoid receptor phosphorylation controls ligand binding, allowing distinct physiologic responses to aldosterone. *Cell Metab* 18(November 5):660–671, 2013.
167. Farman N, et al: Immunolocalization of gluco- and mineralocorticoid receptors in rabbit kidney. *Am J Physiol* 260(2 Pt 1):C226–C233, 1991.
168. Berger S, et al: Mineralocorticoid receptor knockout mice: pathophysiology of Na+ metabolism. *Proc Natl Acad Sci U S A* 95(16):9424–9429, 1998.
175. Vandewalle A, et al: Aldosterone binding along the rabbit nephron: an autoradiographic study on isolated tubules. *Am J Physiol* 240(3):F172–F179, 1981.
197. Ko B, Mistry AC, Hanson L, et al: Aldosterone acutely stimulates NCC activity via a SPAK-mediated pathway. *Am J Physiol Renal Physiol* 305:F645–F652, 2013.
205. Kim GH, et al: The thiazide-sensitive Na-Cl cotransporter is an aldosterone-induced protein. *Proc Natl Acad Sci U S A* 95(24):14552–14557, 1998.
207. Rozansky DJ, et al: Aldosterone mediates activation of the thiazide-sensitive Na-Cl cotransporter through an SGK1 and WNK4 signaling pathway. *J Clin Invest* 119(9):2601–2612, 2009.
217. Levitan R, Ingelfinger FJ: Effect of d-aldosterone on salt and water absorption from the intact human colon. *J Clin Invest* 44:801–808, 1965.
219. Turnamian SG, Binder HJ: Regulation of active sodium and potassium transport in the distal colon of the rat: role of the aldosterone and glucocorticoid receptors. *J Clin Invest* 84(6):1924–1929, 1989.
225. Hayes CP, Jr, McLeod ME, Robinson RR: An extrarenal mechanism for the maintenance of potassium balance in severe chronic renal failure. *Trans Assoc Am Physicians* 80:207–216, 1967.
226. Sandle GI, et al: Enhanced rectal potassium secretion in chronic renal insufficiency: evidence for large intestinal potassium adaptation in man. *Clin Sci* 71(4):393–401, 1986.
270. Bhalla V, et al: Disinhibitory pathways for control of sodium transport: regulation of ENaC by SGK1 and GILZ. *Am J Physiol Renal Physiol* 291(4):F714–F721, 2006.
287. Debonneville C, et al: Phosphorylation of Nedd4-2 by Sgk1 regulates epithelial Na(+) channel cell surface expression. *EMBO J* 20(24):7052–7059, 2001.
288. Snyder PM, Olson DR, Thomas BC: Serum- and glucocorticoid-regulated kinase modulates Nedd4-2-mediated inhibition of the epithelial Na+ channel. *J Biol Chem* 277(1):5–8, 2002.
289. Wulff P, et al: Impaired renal Na(+) retention in the sgk1-knockout mouse. *J Clin Invest* 110(9):1263–1268, 2002.
296. Soundararajan R, et al: A novel role for glucocorticoid-induced leucine zipper protein in epithelial sodium channel-mediated sodium transport. *J Biol Chem* 280(48):39970–39981, 2005.
308. Staub O, et al: WW domains of Nedd4 bind to the proline-rich PY motifs in the epithelial Na+ channel deleted in Liddle's syndrome. *EMBO J* 15(10):2371–2380, 1996.
336. Geerling JC, Loewy AD: Aldosterone in the brain. *Am J Physiol Renal Physiol* 297(3):F559–F576, 2009.
338. Funder JW: Is aldosterone bad for the heart? *Trends Endocrinol Metab* 15(4):139–142, 2004.
345. Oberleithner H: Is the vascular endothelium under the control of aldosterone? Facts and hypothesis. *Pflugers Arch* 454(2):187–193, 2007.
355. Funder JW: The nongenomic actions of aldosterone. *Endocr Rev* 26(3):313–321, 2005.
358. Young WF: Primary aldosteronism: renaissance of a syndrome. *Clin Endocrinol (Oxf)* 66(5):607–618, 2007.
375. Gómez-Sánchez EP, et al: ICV infusion of corticosterone antagonizes ICV-aldosterone hypertension. *Am J Physiol* 258(4 Pt 1):E649–E653, 1990.
376. Milhailidou AS, et al: Glucocorticoids activate cardiac mineralocorticoid receptors during experimental myocardial infarction. *Hypertension* 54:1306–1312, 2009.
378. Dostanic-Larson I, et al: The highly conserved cardiac glycoside binding site of Na,K-ATPase plays a role in blood pressure regulation. *PNAS* 102(44):15845–15850, 2005.
381. Li Y, et al: Structural and biochemical mechanisms for the specificity of hormone binding and coactivator assembly by mineral corticoid receptor. *Mol Cell* 19:367–380, 2005.
385. Bonvalet JP, et al: Distribution of 11 beta-hydroxysteroid dehydrogenase along the rabbit nephron. *J Clin Invest* 86:832–837, 1990.

Vasoactive Molecules and the Kidney

13

Richard E. Gilbert | Andrew Advani

CHAPTER OUTLINE

RENIN-ANGIOTENSIN-ALDOSTERONE SYSTEM, 325
Classical Renin-Angiotensin-Aldosterone System, 326
Expanded Renin-Angiotensin-Aldosterone System: Enzymes, Angiotensin Peptides, and Receptors, 331
Renin-Angiotensin-Aldosterone System in Kidney Pathophysiology, 334
ENDOTHELIN, 335
Structure, Synthesis, and Secretion of the Endothelins, 335
Endothelin Receptors, 336
Physiologic Actions of Endothelin in the Kidney, 336
Role of Endothelin in Essential Hypertension, 336
Role of Endothelin in Renal Injury, 337
Endothelin System in Chronic Kidney Disease and Diabetic Nephropathy, 337
Endothelin System and Other Kidney Diseases, 338
Safety Profile of Endothelin Receptor Antagonists, 338
NATRIURETIC PEPTIDES, 339
Structure and Synthesis of the Natriuretic Peptides, 339

Natriuretic Peptide Receptors, 341
Neutral Endopeptidase, 341
Actions of the Natriuretic Peptides, 342
Natriuretic Peptides as Biomarkers of Disease, 343
Therapeutic Uses of Natriuretic Peptides, 344
Combination Angiotensin Receptor Blockers and Neutral Endopeptidase Inhibitors, 345
Other Natriuretic Peptides, 346
KALLIKREIN-KININ SYSTEM, 346
Components of the Kallikrein-Kinin System, 346
Plasma and Tissue Kallikrein-Kinin System, 347
Renal Kallikrein-Kinin System, 348
Kallikrein-Kinin System in Renal Disease, 349
UROTENSIN II, 351
Synthesis, Structure, and Secretion of Urotensin II, 351
Physiologic Role of Urotensin II, 351
Urotensin II in the Kidney, 352
Observational Studies of Urotensin II in Renal Disease, 352
Interventional Studies of Urotensin II in the Kidney, 352

Vasoactive peptides, arising from both the systemic circulation and local tissue-based generation, play important roles in kidney physiology, not only in the regulation of renal blood flow but also in electrolyte exchange, acid-base balance, and diuresis. More recent interest has focused on the role of these peptide systems in kidney development and in the pathogenesis of organ injury.

RENIN-ANGIOTENSIN-ALDOSTERONE SYSTEM

In their now seminal 1898 report, *Niere und Kreislauf*, Robert Tigerstedt and Per Bergman, while working at the Karolinska Institute in Sweden, described the prolonged vasopressor effects of crude kidney extracts.[1] Although recognizing the impurity of the extract, Tigerstedt named the unidentified active substance "renin," based on its organ of origin. More than 110 years later, our understanding of the renin-angiotensin-aldosterone system (RAAS) continues to evolve with insights into its pivotal role in pathophysiologic and physiologic processes. Underlying this effort to fully understand the RAAS is not only a desire for knowledge but a profound appreciation of the therapeutic importance of its blockade. Much of this insight is derived from work in 1985 by Anderson and colleagues, who defined the renoprotective effects of angiotensin-converting enzyme (ACE) inhibition in a rodent model of progressive kidney disease.[2]

CLASSICAL RENIN-ANGIOTENSIN-ALDOSTERONE SYSTEM

The classical view of the RAAS focuses on the endocrine aspects of this peptidergic system. Angiotensinogen synthesized by the liver enters the circulation, where it is cleaved to form angiotensin I by renin, a peptidase that is secreted from the juxtaglomerular apparatus (JGA) of the kidney. The terminal two amino acids of angiotensin I are then removed to form angiotensin II, as it traverses through the circulation, exposed to ACE, a peptidase expressed on endothelial cells, particularly in the pulmonary vasculature. Angiotensin II, the principal effector molecule of the RAAS, then binds to its type 1 receptor, resulting in vasoconstriction, sodium retention, thirst, and aldosterone secretion. This traditional view of the RAAS is still valid but has been considerably augmented, not only by the discovery of new enzymes, peptides, and receptors but also by an appreciation that in addition to its endocrine paradigm, the RAAS also has an independently functioning local tissue-based component that acts through paracrine, autocrine, and possibly intracrine mechanisms (Figure 13.1).

ANGIOTENSINOGEN

Angiotensinogen is primarily, though by no means exclusively, synthesized in the liver, particularly the pericentral zone of the hepatic lobules.[3] In humans it is coded by a single gene, composed of five exons and four introns, that spans approximately 13 kb of genomic sequence on chromosome 1 (1q42-q43). It is translated to a 453–amino acid globular glycoprotein with a molecular weight between 45 and 65 kd, depending on the extent of its glycosylation, which then undergoes posttranslational cleavage of a 24- or 33–amino acid signal peptide,[4] giving rise to the mature circulating form of angiotensinogen.[5]

Structurally angiotensinogen bears substantial homology to the serpin superfamily of protease inhibitors and like many members of its family behaves as an acute phase reactant in the inflammatory setting,[6] reflecting the presence of an acute phase response element that binds the transcription factor nuclear factor κ-light-chain-enhancer of activated B cells (NF-κB).[7]

RENIN

Like the gene encoding angiotensinogen, the gene encoding renin is located on the long arm of chromosome 1 (1q32) and contains 10 exons and 9 introns, similar to other aspartyl proteases.[8] Unlike humans and rats, which have only a single renin gene, the mouse has two, *Ren1* and *Ren2*, expressed primarily in the submandibular gland and kidney, respectively.

Following its synthesis as a 406–amino acid preprohormone, the 23–amino acid leader sequence of preprorenin is cleaved in the rough endoplasmic reticulum, giving rise to prorenin (also called inactive renin and "big" renin), which may be then rapidly secreted directly from the Golgi apparatus or from protogranules.[4] Alternatively, and virtually exclusively in the JGA, prorenin may be packaged into mature, dense granules that instead of being immediately secreted, undergo further processing to the active enzyme, renin (active renin). In contrast to the more constitutive secretion of prorenin, release of renin-containing granules is tightly regulated.[8]

Mature, active renin is a variably glycosylated 37- to 40-kd aspartyl protease that is active at neutral pH, and in contrast to the more promiscuous activities of most other proteases in this class, has only a single known substrate, cleaving the decapeptide angiotensin I from the amino-terminal of angiotensinogen. Whereas the kidney produces both renin and prorenin, a range of extrarenal tissues, including the adrenals, gonads, and placenta, produce prorenin and contribute to its presence in plasma. However, as evidenced by the near-total absence of active renin in anephric patients, the kidney, and the JGA in particular, appears to be the only source of circulating renin in humans.

Factors that chronically stimulate renin secretion, such as a low-sodium diet and ACE inhibition, lead to an increase in the number of renin-secreting cells rather than an increase in cell size or the number of granules that each JGA cell contains. This expansion of the renin-secreting

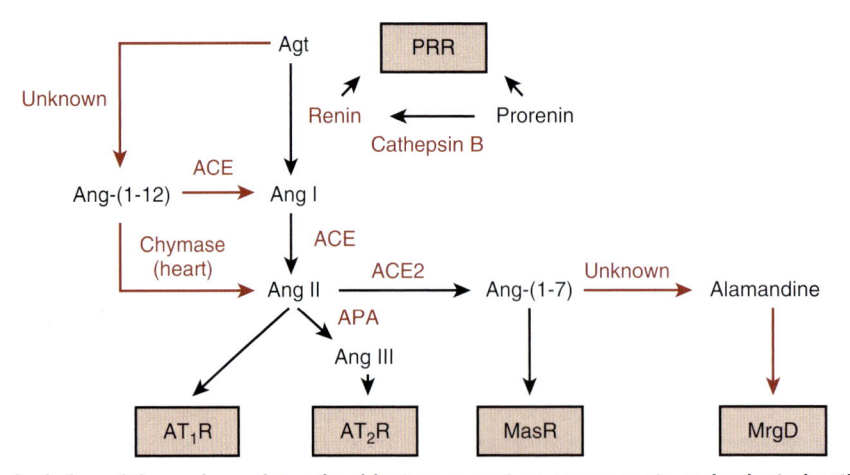

Figure 13.1 Schematic depiction of the renin-angiotensin-aldosterone system components and selected actions. The enzymes of the system are shown in *red*. Newly described enzymatic pathways are shown in *red*. Receptors are shown in the *boxes*. ACE, Angiotensin-converting enzyme; Agt, angiotensinogen; Ang, angiotensin; APA, aminopeptidase A; AT$_1$R, angiotensin type 1 receptor; AT$_2$R, angiotensin type 2 receptor; MasR, Mas receptor; MrgD, Mas-related G protein–coupled receptor; and PRR, (pro)renin receptor. (Reproduced and adapted with permission from Carey RM: Newly discovered components and actions of the renin-angiotensin system. *Hypertension* 62:818-822, 2013.)

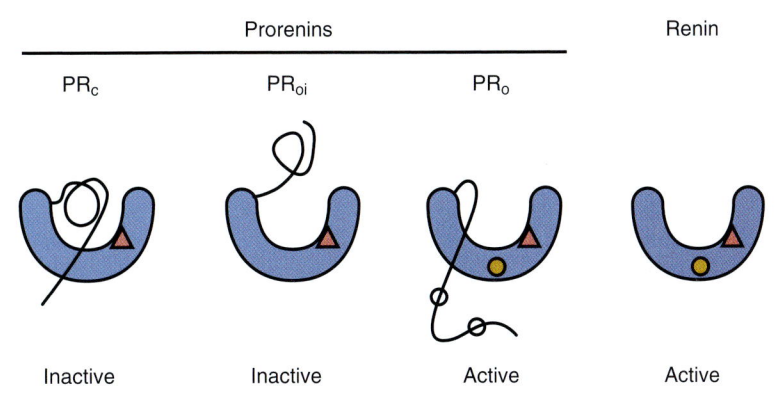

Figure 13.2 Prorenin activation. The conformational changes and the expression of immunoreactive epitopes associated with the activation of prorenin are depicted. The main body of the molecule, the substrate-binding cleft, and the prosegment are shown. The *closed triangle* represents the epitope of the main body expressed by PR_c (prorenin in the inactive closed conformation), PR_{oi} (prorenin in the inactive intermediary open conformation), PR_o (prorenin in the active open conformation), and renin. The *closed circle* represents the epitope of the main body, expressed by PR_o and renin, but not by PR_c and PR_{oi}. The *open circles* represent epitopes of the prosegment expressed by PR_o but not by PR_c and PR_{oi}. (Adapted from Schalekamp MA, Derkx FH, Deinum J, et al: Newly developed renin and prorenin assays and the clinical evaluation of renin inhibitors. *J Hypertens* 26:928-937, 2008.)

mass occurs proximally by metaplastic transformation of smooth muscle cells within the walls of the afferent arteriole. Although sometimes mentioned, ectopic renin expression within the extraglomerular mesangium appears to be an extraordinarily rare event.[9]

PRORENIN ACTIVATION

Prorenin is maintained as an inactive zymogen through the occupation of its catalytic cleft by its prosegment. Removing this prosegment by either proteolytic or nonproteolytic means yields active renin, a term that denotes its enzymatic activity rather than its amino acid sequence (Figure 13.2).

Within the dense core secretory granules of the JGA, acidification by vacuolar adenosine triphosphatases (ATPases) provides the optimal pH for the prosegment-cleaving enzymes: proconvertase 1 and cathepsin B and may also assist the pH-dependent, non-enzymatic activation of prorenin as well.[9-11] Although various peptidases such as trypsin, plasmin, and kallikrein can also cleave the prosegment of prorenin in vitro, these do not appear to contribute to the generation of renin in the in vivo setting. Although traditionally viewed as occurring only in the JGA, cell culture–based studies suggest that proteolytic activation of renin can also occur in cardiac and vascular smooth muscle cells by as-yet-unidentified serine proteases.[12-14] The significance of these findings in the intact organism, however, remains to be established.

In addition to proteolytic cleavage of its prosegment, prorenin can also be reversibly activated nonenzymatically by a conformational change such that the prosegment no longer occupies the enzymatic cleft. Under usual circumstances, less than 2% of prorenin is in this open active conformation. This process can, however, be induced by acid (pH < 4.0)[15,16] and to a lesser extent by cold.[17] In a later study the putative (pro)renin receptor (see later) was also shown to nonproteolytically activate prorenin.[18]

REGULATION OF RENIN SECRETION

Mechanical, neurologic, and chemical factors regulate the activity of the RAAS by modulating renin secretion.

Renal Baroreceptor

The existence of a renal baroreceptor mechanism was first conceptualized by Skinner and associates to explain how renin secretion increases when afferent arteriolar perfusion pressure falls.[19] Studies in conscious dogs show that changes in renal perfusion pressure have only a small effect on renin secretion until a threshold of approximately 90 mm Hg is reached, below which renin secretion abruptly increases, doubling with every 2- to 3–mm Hg fall in pressure.[20] Accordingly, reduction in pressure below this level profoundly stimulates renin secretion, thereby acutely activating the RAAS and resulting in a range of angiotensin II–dependent phenomena that collectively serve to restore systemic pressure. Despite the importance of the baroreceptor function, several decades of research have not identified precisely how the pressure signal is transduced into renin release, though postulated mediators include stretch-activated calcium channels, endothelins (ETs), and prostaglandins.

Neural Control

The JGA is endowed with a rich network of noradrenergic nerve endings and their β_1 receptors. Stimulation of the renal sympathetic nerve activity leads to renin secretion that is independent of changes in renal blood flow, glomerular filtration rate (GFR), or Na^+ resorption. Moreover, this effect can be blocked surgically (by denervation) and pharmacologically (by the administration of β-adrenoreceptor blockers).[20] The role of cholinergic, dopaminergic, and adrenergic activation is controversial, though these agents have also been shown to modulate renin release under certain circumstances.

Tubular Control

Chronic diminution in luminal NaCl delivery to the macula densa is a potent stimulus for renin secretion, reflecting a coordinate interaction between a range of mediators, including adenosine, nitric oxide, and prostaglandins, that affect not only renin release but also its transcription.[21] This mechanism is thought to account for the chronically high plasma renin activity (PRA) in subjects who adhere to a low-salt diet.[22]

Metabolic Control

The tricarboxylic acid cycle provides a final common pathway by which carbohydrates, fatty acids, and amino acids converge in the process of adenosine triphosphate (ATP) generation by aerobic electron transfer. Although the tricarboxylic acid cycle operates within mitochondria, its intermediates can be detected within the extracellular space, increasing in abundance when local energy supply and demand are mismatched or when cells are exposed to hypoxia, toxins, or injury.[23] Succinate, for instance, has been shown to stimulate renin release, and its intravenous administration leads to hypertension, though the mechanisms underlying this effect have only recently been unravelled. In 2004, He and colleagues reported that α-ketoglutarate and succinate are ligands for the previously orphaned G protein–coupled receptors GPR90 and GPR99, respectively, and that succinate-induced hypertension is abolished in GPR91-deficient mice.[24] Notably, in other studies, GPR91 was localized to the apical plasma membrane of macula densa cells, where succinate stimulation was shown to activate p38 and extracellular signal–regulated kinases 1 and 2 (ERK1/2) mitogen-activated protein (MAP) kinases, inducing cyclo-oxygenase-2–dependent synthesis of prostaglandin E_2, a well-established paracrine mediator of renin release.[25] Moreover, the ability of tubular succinate to induce juxtaglomerular renin secretion suggests that this phenomenon is likely an important determinant of JGA function in both physiologic and pathophysiologic settings.

Other Local Factors

In addition to the factors discussed earlier, a large range of locally active factors have also been shown to alter renin secretion. These include peptides (atrial natriuretic peptide, kinins, vasoactive intestinal polypeptide, ET, calcitonin gene–related peptide), amines (dopamine and histamine), and arachidonic acid derivatives.[20]

PLASMA PRORENIN AND RENIN

Under usual circumstances the plasma concentration of prorenin is approximately 10 times greater than renin. In some patients with diabetes, however, the plasma prorenin level is disproportionately increased, where it predicts the development of diabetic nephropathy (including microalbuminuria) and retinopathy.[26,27]

In addition to its role in the research setting, measurement of plasma renin concentration (PRC) is an important clinical assay, providing important information, for example, when evaluating patients with possible hyperaldosteronism, assessing volume status, and in predicting the response to, or monitoring drug adherence to, an ACE inhibitor or angiotensin receptor blocker (ARB). In broad terms, PRC is determined by either activity or immunologic assay methods.[28] The most commonly used method involves the measurement of PRA. With this method the rate at which angiotensin I is produced from plasma angiotensinogen is assayed. To prevent the degradation of angiotensin I or its conversion to angiotensin II, inhibitors of angiotensinase and ACE are added to the assay. Accordingly, PRA is not only dependent on renin and endogenous angiotensinogen concentrations but will also overestimate the extent of inhibition by renin inhibitors because of the displacement of protein-bound drug by the peptidase inhibitors. The latter scenario may be diminished by using an antibody capture method in which anti–angiotensin I antibody, instead of peptidase inhibitors, is used to protect angiotensin I from further catabolism.[28]

The nomenclature of renin assays can be quite confusing in that PRC may be measured by both activity and immunologic assays. With the plasma renin concentration activity assay (PRCa), exogenous angiotensinogen is added to the assay, thereby avoiding the influence that endogenous levels of the substrate might have. However, PRCa may also be affected by the presence of renin inhibitors; as with PRA, this effect may be reduced by antibody capture methodology.[28] In the plasma renin concentration immunologic assay (PRCi), the concentrations of renin and prorenin in its active, open conformation are assessed, so that the PRCi assay, like PRA and PRCa, is time and temperature dependent because lower temperatures will increase the proportion of prorenin in its active conformation. Moreover, renin inhibitors, by binding to the active site of prorenin in its open conformation, prevent the refolding of the prosegment and may therefore lead to an overestimation of PRCi.[28,29]

ANGIOTENSIN-CONVERTING ENZYME

ACE is a zinc-containing dipeptidyl carboxypeptidase that cleaves the terminal histidyl-leucine from angiotensin I to form the octapeptide angiotensin II. In contrast to the single-substrate specificity of renin, ACE is not specific, cleaving the two terminal acids from peptides with the C′-terminal sequence R_1-R_2-R_3-OH, in which R_1 is the protected (noncleaved) amino acid, R_2 is any nonproline L-amino acid, and R_3 is any nondicarboxylic (cysteine, ornithine, lysine, arginine) L-amino acid with a free carboxy-terminal.[4] Importantly, therefore ACE also catalyzes the inactivation of bradykinin. Although encoded by a single ACE gene, two distinct tissue-specific messenger RNAs (mRNAs) are transcribed, each with different initiation and alternative splice sites.[30] The somatic form, present in almost all tissues, is a 1306–amino acid, 140- to 160-kd glycoprotein with two active sites, whereas the 90- to 100-kd testicular or germinal form is found exclusively in postmeiotic male germ cells, contains a single active site, and appears to be involved with spermatogenesis.[4,31,32] The somatic form of ACE is widely distributed with activity present not only in tissues but also in most biologic fluids. In the human kidney, ACE is present to the greatest extent within proximal and distal tubules; however, both the magnitude of expression and its site-specific distribution may be altered by disease.[33]

ANGIOTENSIN TYPE 1 RECEPTOR

The angiotensin type 1 (AT_1) receptor mediates most of the known physiologic effects of angiotensin II. The gene for this widely distributed 359–amino acid, 40-kDa, seven-transmembrane G protein–coupled receptor is located on chromosome 3 in humans.[34]

Within the kidney, AT_1 receptors are widely expressed. In the glomerulus, they are found in both afferent and efferent arterioles as well as in the mesangium, in endothelium, and on podocytes.[35] Consistent with the role of angiotensin II in

Na⁺ resorption, AT_1 receptors are highly abundant on the brush borders of proximal tubular epithelial cells.[36] Prominent expression has also been found in renal medullary interstitial cells, located between the renal tubules and vasa recta, where angiotensin II is purported to have a potential role in the regulation of medullary blood flow.[37]

Angiotensin II binding to the AT_1 receptor initiates cell signaling by several different pathways that have been mostly studied in vascular smooth muscle cells.[38] These include G protein–mediated pathways and the activation of tyrosine kinases, reduced nicotinamide adenine dinucleotide (NADH)/reduced nicotinamide adenine dinucleotide phosphate (NADPH) oxidases, and serine/threonine kinases.[34]

G Protein–Mediated Signaling

In the classical G protein–mediated pathway, AT_1 receptor ligand binding leads to activation of phospholipases C, D, and A_2. Phospholipase C rapidly hydrolyses phosphatidylinositol bisphosphate to inositol trisphosphate and di-acyl glycerol (DAG), initiating calcium release from intracellular stores and protein kinase C (PKC) activation, respectively. Phospholipase D similarly generates DAG and activates PKC, whereas phospholipase A_2 leads to the formation of various vasoactive and proinflammatory arachidonic acid derivatives.

Reactive Oxygen Species

Although reactive oxygen species were previously regarded as toxic waste products, emerging evidence indicates that they may also act as second messengers, activating not only other cell signaling cascades such as p38 MAP kinase but also a number of transcription pathways implicated in the pathogenesis of inflammatory and degenerative disease.[34] Although the mechanisms by which the AT_1 receptor stimulates NADH/NADPH are not well understood, angiotensin II binding to this receptor results in the generation of both superoxide and hydrogen peroxide.

Tyrosine Kinases

Angiotensin II binding to the AT_1 receptor "transactivates" a number of nonreceptor tyrosine kinases (Src, Pyk2, FAK, and JAK), as well as the growth factor receptor tyrosine kinases for epidermal growth factor (EGF)[39,40] and platelet-derived growth factor (PDGF).[41,42] By binding to the AT_1 receptor, angiotensin II initiates the translocation of tumor necrosis factor-α (TNF-α)–converting enzyme (TACE) to the cell surface. TACE then cleaves TNF-α from its membrane-associated precursor (pro–TNF-α), allowing it to bind to EGF receptor (EGFR) on the cell surface. This ligand-receptor interaction then induces EGFR autophosphorylation and activates its downstream signaling pathways that include Akt, ERK1/2, and mammalian target of rapamycin (mTOR) (Figure 13.3). The in vivo relevance of this transactivation pathway has been confirmed. Using mice that express a dominant negative form of EGFR, Lautrette and colleagues showed that despite similar blood pressures, mutant mice infused with angiotensin II had less proteinuria and renal fibrosis than did their wild-type counterparts.[43] Consistent with these findings and the pivotal role of the RAAS in diabetic nephropathy, studies using the specific EGFR tyrosine kinase inhibitor PKI 166 have also shown a reduction in early structural injury in a rat model of diabetic nephropathy.[44]

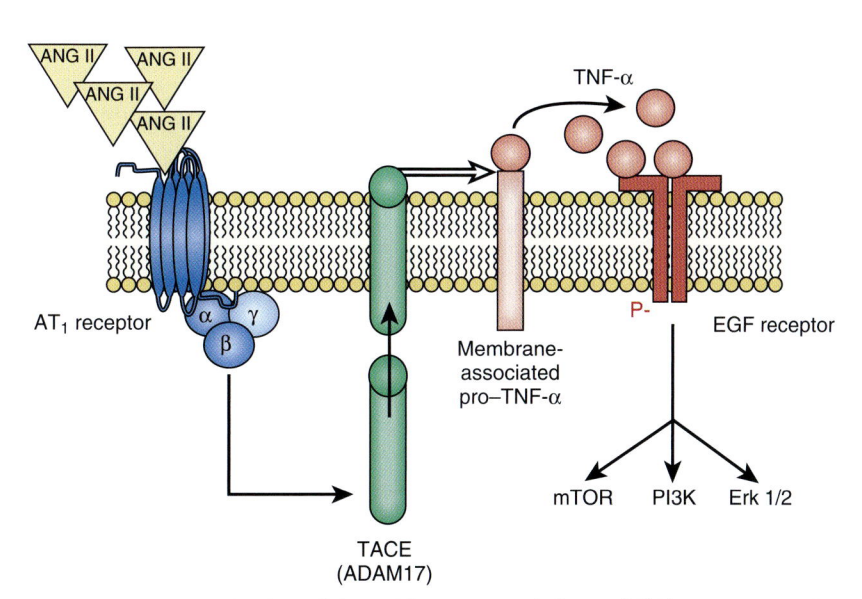

Figure 13.3 Angiotensin II–mediated transactivation of the epidermal growth factor (EGF) receptor. Angiotensin II (Ang II) binds to its angiotensin II type 1 (AT_1) receptor, a G protein–coupled receptor lacking intrinsic tyrosine kinase activity. Through as-yet-undescribed mechanisms, this interaction leads to the translocation of the metalloprotease tumor necrosis factor-α (TNF-α)–converting enzyme (TACE) from the cytosol to the cell surface, where it cleaves TNF-α from its membrane-associated promolecule, allowing it to bind and activate the EGF receptor. Erk 1/2, Extracellular signal–regulated kinases 1 and 2; mTOR, mammalian target of rapamycin; P13K, phosphatidylinositol-3-kinase. (Adapted from Wolf G: "As time goes by": angiotensin II–mediated transactivation of the EGF receptor comes of age. *Nephrol Dial Transplant* 20:2050-2053, 2005.)

Like EGFR, the transactivation of the PDGF receptor (PDGFR) by the AT_1 receptor is also complex, involving the adaptor protein Shc.[41,42] In addition to studies that have explored the angiotensin-PDGFR interaction in cell culture or organ baths,[45] a later report has shown that despite continued hypertension, inhibition of the PDGFR kinase in vivo can also dramatically attenuate angiotensin II–induced vascular remodeling.[46]

Angiotensin Type 1 Receptor Internalization

In addition to the conventional ligand-receptor–mediated pathways, a range of other signaling mechanisms that involve the AT_1 receptor have been described. These include the discovery of receptor-interacting proteins, heterologous receptor dimerization, and ligand-independent activation[47] (Figure 13.4). These new insights, though adding greater complexity to our understanding of the RAAS, also provide the potential for new therapeutic targets in disease prevention and management.

Following ligand binding and the initiation of signal transduction, AT_1 receptors are rapidly internalized, followed by either lysosomal degradation or recycling back to the plasma membrane. Several mechanisms account for AT_1 receptor internalization, including interaction with caveolae, phosphorylation of its carboxy-terminal by G protein–coupled receptor kinases,[34] and association with the newly described AT_1 receptor interacting proteins.[47] To date, two such interacting proteins, AT_1 receptor–associated protein (ATRAP)[48] and AT_1 receptor–associated protein 1 (ARAP1),[49] have been described. ATRAP interacts with the C terminus of AT_1 receptor, downregulating cell surface AT_1 receptor expression and attenuating angiotensin II–mediated effects.[47] ARAP1 though somewhat similar to ATRAP, promotes AT_1 receptor recycling to the plasma membrane such that its kidney-specific overexpression induces hypertension and renal hypertrophy.[49]

Angiotensin Type 1 Receptor Dimerization

In addition to their ability to induce cell signaling in their monomeric state, G protein–coupled receptors such as AT_1 receptor may also associate to form both homodimers and heterodimers.[50] Beyond its constitutive homodimerization,[51] AT_1 receptor may dimerize with angiotensin type 2 (AT_2) receptor and also form hetero-oligomers with receptors for bradykinin (B_2), epinephrine (β_2), dopamine (D1, D3, and D5), endothelin type B, Mas, and EGF that modulate their function.[52-55]

Ligand-Independent Angiotensin Type 1 Receptor Activation

Without involvement of angiotensin II, cell stretch induces a conformational switch that initiates intracellular signaling pathways of the AT_1 receptor.[56,57] As might be expected from an understanding of this mechanism, an AT_1 receptor blocker, acting as an inverse agonist, will abrogate these effects, as described in both cardiac[57] and mesangial cells.[58] A similar means of ligand-independent activation has also been shown to result from the binding of agonist antibodies to AT_1 receptors in some women with preeclampsia[59] and in certain cases of renal allograft rejection.[60]

PHYSIOLOGIC EFFECTS OF ANGIOTENSIN II IN THE KIDNEY

The traditional actions of angiotensin II relate primarily to its effects on vascular tone and fluid balance that are mediated by its actions on the vasculature, heart, kidney, brain, and adrenal glands by the AT_1 receptor. In vascular smooth muscle, stimulation of AT_1 receptors by angiotensin II induces cell contraction and consequent vasoconstriction. In the adrenal cortex, this ligand-receptor interaction stimulates aldosterone release, thereby promoting sodium resorption in the distal nephron. Moreover, angiotensin II will

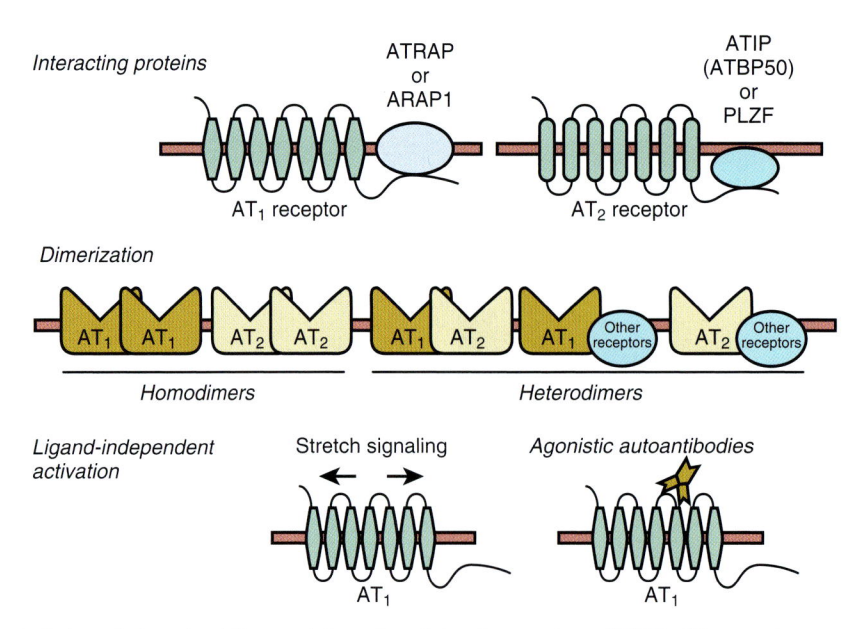

Figure 13.4 Developments in knowledge about the regulation of angiotensin receptors. ARAP1, AT_1 receptor–associated protein 1; ATBP50, AT_2 receptor–binding protein of 50 kDa; ATIP, angiotensin type 2 receptor–interacting protein; ATRAP, AT_1 receptor–associated protein; AT_1 receptor, angiotensin type 1 receptor; AT_2 receptor, angiotensin type 2 receptor; PLZF, promyelocytic leukemia zinc finger. (Adapted from Mogi M, Iwai M, Horiuchi M: New insights into the regulation of angiotensin receptors. *Curr Opin Nephrol Hypertens* 18:138-143, 2009.)

directly enhance sodium retention by the proximal tubule, and in the brain it will stimulate thirst and salt craving. Additional effects include sympathoadrenal stimulation and the augmentation of cardiac contractility. Together these effects serve to maintain extracellular fluid volume and systemic blood pressure. Given the central role that the kidney has in the regulation of these key aspects of mammalian homeostasis, it is not surprising that angiotensin II should have profound effects on renal physiology.

HEMODYNAMIC ACTIONS

The effects of exogenously administered angiotensin II are dose dependent. At low doses, angiotensin II infusion increases renal vascular resistance and lowers renal blood flow without affecting GFR so that the filtration fraction is increased. At higher doses of angiotensin II, renal vascular resistance is further increased, leading to an augmented reduction in renal blood flow and fall in GFR.[61] However, because GFR is reduced to a lesser extent than renal plasma flow, the filtration fraction remains elevated. Such studies are consistent with the view that limited stimulation of the RAAS would mostly serve to enhance tubular sodium levels, as is seen, for instance, in societies unaccustomed to contemporary diets.[22] Greater activation of the RAAS, on the other hand, as might be found in the setting of severe volume depletion, would result in angiotensin II–dependent reduction in renal blood flow that would aid in sustaining systemic blood pressure while further stimulating sodium resorption.

Kidney micropuncture has been used extensively to explore the intrarenal sites of the effects of angiotensin II on vascular resistance. These studies demonstrate that although angiotensin II increases both afferent and efferent arteriolar resistance, glomerular capillary hydraulic pressure (P_{GC}) is consistently elevated,[62] and the glomerular ultrafiltration coefficient (Kf) is reduced.[61] Moreover, as predicted by mathematical modeling, the glomerular hypertension induced by angiotensin II does not lead to acute proteinuria, because the structural barriers to macromolecular passage remain intact.[61] Chronic angiotensin II infusion with sustained intraglomerular hypertension, by contrast, leads to glomerular capillary damage and substantial proteinuria.

TUBULAR TRANSPORT

Sodium

Consistent with its importance in the regulation of volume status, angiotensin II has profound effects on renal Na^+ handling. The proximal tubule is responsible for the resorption of approximately two thirds of the sodium from the glomerular filtrate, and binding sites for angiotensin II are particularly abundant in the proximal tubule with immunohistochemical localization of the AT_1 receptor to both apical and basolateral surfaces.[63] At picomolar concentrations, angiotensin II stimulates the luminal Na^+-H^+-exchanger, the basolateral Na^+-HCO_3^- cotransporter, and sodium-potassium adenosine triphosphatase (Na^+-K^+-ATPase). However, at concentrations higher than 10^{-9} M, angiotensin II inhibits the very same transporters. The mechanisms underlying this dose-dependent effect of angiotensin II on Na^+ transport, which seem to also occur in the loop of Henle,[63] are incompletely understood. In the distal tubule the effects of angiotensin II on Na^+ transport are site dependent. In the early distal tubule, for instance, angiotensin II stimulates apical Na^+-H^+ exchange, whereas in the late distal tubule it stimulates the amiloride-sensitive sodium channel.[63]

Acid-Base Regulation

The kidney has a key role in the maintenance of physiologic pH by regulating the secretion and resorption of acids and bases. As for Na^+, angiotensin II also has substantial effects on acid-base transport in the proximal tubule, distal tubule, and collecting duct. Interest has focused in particular on its actions in the collecting duct. In the collecting duct, angiotensin II not only stimulates Na^+-H^+-exchangers and Na^+-HCO_3^- cotransporters but has also been shown to stimulate the vacuolar hydrogen ion adenosine triphosphatase (H^+-ATPase) in intercalated A cells via its AT_1 receptor.[64] Moreover, elegant and detailed electron microscopic studies have helped to unravel the mechanisms by which angiotensin II exerts its effects at this site, revealing translocation of the H^+-ATPase from the cytoplasm to the apical surface in response to ligand stimulation.[65]

EXPANDED RENIN-ANGIOTENSIN-ALDOSTERONE SYSTEM: ENZYMES, ANGIOTENSIN PEPTIDES, AND RECEPTORS

ANGIOTENSIN TYPE 2 RECEPTOR

In humans the AT_2 receptor is a 363–amino acid protein that maps to the X chromosome and is highly homologous to its rat and mouse counterparts.[66] Like AT_1 receptor, AT_2 receptor is also a seven-transmembrane G protein–coupled receptor, though it shares only 34% homology.

Despite substantial research, the actions of AT_2 receptor are still not well understood and remain somewhat controversial.[67] In general, however, the actions of AT_2 receptor stimulation oppose those of AT_1 receptor. For instance, whereas AT_1 receptor vasoconstricts and promotes Na^+ retention, AT_2 receptor stimulation leads to vasodilation[68] and natriuresis,[69] consistent with its abundance on the epithelium of the proximal tubule.[70] The vasodilatory effects of AT_2 receptor stimulation are mediated by increasing nitric oxide synthesis and cyclic guanosine monophosphate (cGMP) by bradykinin-dependent and bradykinin-independent mechanisms.[71] Its natriuretic effects, however, seem to be dependent on conversion of angiotensin II to angiotensin III by aminopeptidase N.[72]

Like the activity of the AT_1 receptor, the activity of the AT_2 receptor may also be modulated by oligomerization, association with various interacting proteins, and ligand-independent effects.[71]

(PRO)RENIN RECEPTOR

In 2002 an apparently novel, 350–amino acid, single-transmembrane protein that binds both renin and prorenin with high affinity was identified.[18] Ligand binding to this protein was shown to induce a fourfold increase in the catalytic cleavage of angiotensinogen as well as stimulating intracellular signaling with activation of MAP kinases ERK1/2,[18] leading to it being named the (pro)renin receptor ([P]RR). The designation (pro)renin refers to its ability to interact with both renin and prorenin.

Given its localization to the mesangium in initial studies, its actions in augmenting local angiotensin II production, and its ability to increase mesangial transforming growth factor-β (TGF-β) production,[73] the (P)RR has understandably been implicated in the pathogenesis of kidney disease.[74] However, despite the appeal, it has been difficult to reconcile this view of the (P)RR with a number of other experimental findings, regarding not only its potentially pathogenetic role, but also its pattern of distribution within the kidney and its homology to other proteins. For instance, given the purported pathogenetic role of the (P)RR, the increased abundance of renin that follows the use of ACE inhibitors and ARBs would be expected to be adverse, yet these classes of drugs have been repeatedly shown to be renoprotective. Secondly, although the (P)RR was initially localized to the glomerular mesangium, later, highly detailed studies have shown that it is primarily expressed in the collecting duct.[75] Thirdly, although initially reported as having no homology with any known membrane protein,[18] database interrogation shows that the (P)RR is identical to two other proteins: endoplasmic reticulum–localized type 1 transmembrane adaptor precursor (CAPER) and ATPase, H^+ transporting, lysosomal accessory protein 2 (ATP6ap2),[76-80] a protein that associates with the vacuolar H^+-ATPase.[81] Indeed, the predominant expression of the (P)RR at the apex of acid-secreting cells in the collecting duct, in conjunction with its co-localization and homology with an accessory subunit of the vacuolar H^+-ATPase, suggest that the (P)RR may function primarily in urinary acidification.[75] However, the vacuolar H^+-ATPase is not restricted to the kidney but is widely distributed in the plasma membrane and the membranes of organelles in several tissues where it functions, not only in urinary acidification but also in endocytosis, conversion of proinsulin to insulin, and osteoclast bone resorption.[82] Although the prevailing data indicate that (P)RR is an accessory subunit of the vacuolar H^+-ATPase that also binds renin and prorenin, the precise functions of the prorenin- and renin-binding subunit remain to be unravelled in the kidney and elsewhere.

ANGIOTENSIN-CONVERTING ENZYME 2

In 2000, two groups independently reported the existence of the first ACE homolog, angiotensin-converting enzyme 2 (ACE2), an apparently novel zinc metalloprotease but with considerable homology (40% identity and 61% similarity) to ACE.[83,84] The gene encoding ACE2, located on the X chromosome (Xp22) contains 18 exons, several of which bear considerable similarity to the first 17 exons of human ACE. Its transcript is 3.4 kb, generating an 805–amino acid peptide that is most highly expressed in kidney, heart, and testis but is also present in plasma and urine.[85,86] In contrast to ACE, ACE2 functions as a carboxypeptidase, removing the terminal phenylalanine from angiotensin II to yield the vasodilatory heptapeptide angiotensin-(1-7). ACE2 may also indirectly lead to the formation of angiotensin-(1-7) by cleaving the C-terminal leucine from angiotensin I, thereby generating angiotensin-(1-9), which may then give rise to angiotensin-(1-7) under the influence of ACE or neutral endopeptidase (NEP).[86] Thus, ACE2 contributes to both angiotensin II degradation and angiotensin-(1-7) synthesis. Accordingly, ACE and ACE2 were initially viewed as having opposing actions with regard to vascular tone and tissue injury. However, emerging data suggest that the situation is far from clear. For instance, although lentivirus-induced overexpression of ACE2 in the heart exerted a protective influence following experimental myocardial infarction,[87] a later study of cardiac ACE2 overexpression led to cardiac dysfunction and fibrosis, despite lowering systemic blood pressure.[88]

In the kidney, ACE2 co-localizes with ACE and angiotensin receptors in the proximal tubule, whereas in the glomerulus it is predominantly expressed within podocytes and to a lesser extent in mesangial cells, contrasting the endothelial predilection of ACE at that site.[89] Numerous studies have explored changes in ACE2 expression in human kidney disease, as well as in a range of animal models, reporting both increased and decreased levels.[90] Therefore it is uncertain whether increased ACE2 might be detrimental or a beneficial response to injury. With this in mind, the findings of intervention studies are of particular importance.

In experimental diabetic nephropathy, for instance, pharmacologic ACE2 inhibition with MLN-4760 led to worsening albuminuria and glomerular injury[89]; similar findings were obtained in ACE2 knockout mice that were crossed with the Akita model of type 1 diabetes.[91] As might be expected from these findings, augmenting ACE2 activity by the infusion of human recombinant protein (hrACE2) has been shown to attenuate diabetic kidney injury in the Akita mouse. In this study, hrACE2 not only improved kidney structure and function but also showed that the protective effects were likely due to reduction in angiotensin II and an increase in angiotensin-(1-7) signaling.[92] Finally, in addition to its role in the RAAS, ACE2 has also been shown to be the receptor for the severe adult respiratory syndrome coronavirus.[93]

ANGIOTENSIN PEPTIDES

Angiotensin III, or Angiotensin-(2-8)

Formed by the actions of aminopeptidase A, the heptapeptide angiotensin III, also known as angiotensin-(2-8), like angiotensin II, also known as angiotensin-(1-8), exerts its effects by binding to AT_1 receptors and AT_2 receptors.[94] Initially, Angiotensin III was thought to have a predominant role in regulating vasopressin release.[95] However, later studies indicate that while angiotensin III is equipotent to angiotensin II with regard to its effects on blood pressure, aldosterone secretion, and renal function, its metabolic clearance rate is approximately five times as rapid.[96]

Angiotensin IV, or Angiotensin-(3-8)

Angiotensin IV is generated from angiotensin III by the actions of aminopeptidase M. Although some of its actions are mediated by the AT_1 receptor, the majority of the biologic effects of angiotensin IV are thought to result from its binding to insulin-regulated aminopeptidase.[97] Angiotensin IV was previously viewed as inactive, but there has been considerable interest in its actions in the central nervous system (CNS), where it not only enhances learning and memory but also possesses anticonvulsant properties and protects the brain from ischemic injury.[97]

In addition to its CNS effects, angiotensin IV has also been implicated in atherogenesis, principally related to its ability to activate NF-κB and upregulate several proinflammatory factors, which include monocyte chemoattractant protein-1 (MCP-1), intercellular adhesion molecule-1, interleukin-6 (IL-6), and TNF-α, as well as enhancing the synthesis of prothrombotic factor plasminogen activator inhibitor-1.[98,99] In the kidney, angiotensin IV is reported to have variable effects on blood flow and natriuresis.[97]

Angiotensin-(1-7)

The ostensibly vasodilatory and antitrophic angiotensin-(1-7) may be formed by the actions of several endopeptidases, which include removal of the terminal tripeptide of angiotensin I by NEP, cleavage of the C-terminal phenylalanine of angiotensin II by ACE2, and the excision of the dipeptidyl group from the C terminus of angiotensin-(1-9) by ACE. Evolving evidence indicates that the actions of this heptapeptide are mediated by its binding to the previously orphaned G protein–coupled receptor MasR.[100] Angiotensin-(1-7) induces vasodilation by a number of mechanisms, which include the amplification of the effects of bradykinin, stimulating cGMP synthesis, and inhibiting the release of norepinephrine.[101] In addition, angiotensin-(1-7) inhibits vascular smooth muscle proliferation and prevents neointima formation following balloon injury to the carotid arteries.[102] Contrasting these findings, however, is a report that exogenous angiotensin-(1-7), rather than ameliorating diabetic nephropathy, as might have been predicted based on the prevailing paradigm, actually accelerated the progression of the disease.[91]

Angiotensin-(2-10)

In addition to angiotensin II and the other C-terminal cleavage products discussed earlier, angiotensin I, or angiotensin-(1-10), may also give rise to a number of other potentially biologically active peptides that result from removal of amino acids from its N terminus. Of these, angiotensin-(2-10), produced by the actions of aminopeptidase A, has been found to modulate the pressor activity of angiotensin II in rodents.[103]

Angiotensin-(1-12)

Angiotensin-(1-12) is a dodecapeptide, first isolated in rat intestine but also found to be present in the kidney and heart, that is cleaved from angiotensinogen by a heretofore unidentified nonrenin enzyme.[104] Notably, in the kidney, angiotensin-(1-12), akin to other components of the intrarenal RAAS, is primarily localized to the proximal tubular epithelium.[105] Although its biologic activity is incompletely understood, its main mode of action is thought to be mediated by its ability to serve as a precursor to angiotensin II by the site-specific and possibly species-specific actions of ACE and chymase.[106] Other pathways may, however, also contribute to the overall effects of angiotensin-(1-12), which in the rat kidney may also include the formation of angiotensin-(1-7) and angiotensin-(1-4) by neprilysin.[105]

Angiotensin A and Alamandine

Identified by mass spectroscopy, angiotensin A and alamandine are characterized by the decarboxylation of N-terminal aspartic acid to alanine in angiotensin II and angiotensin-(1-7), respectively.[107] Although the extremely low concentrations of angiotensin A suggest that it is unlikely to play a physiologic role, this may not be the case for alamandine, which circulates in human plasma and at increased concentrations in patients with end-stage kidney disease (ESKD).[107] With the ability of alamandine to lower blood pressure and reduce fibrosis, the actions of alamandine resemble those of angiotensin-(1-7). However, rather than exerting its effects via the Mas receptor, the actions of alamandine occur through a related receptor, the Mas-related G protein–coupled receptor (MrgD).[108]

INTRARENAL RENIN-ANGIOTENSIN-ALDOSTERONE SYSTEM

In the traditional view of the RAAS, angiotensin II functions as a hormone that, in classical endocrine fashion, circulates systemically to act at sites distant from those where it was formed. However, since the cloning of its components, it has become increasingly clear that there is an additional local, tissue-based RAAS that functions quasi-independently from its systemic counterpart, acting in paracrine, autocrine, and possibly even intracrine modes.[1] This is most clearly seen in the kidney, where pioneering work of several groups has shown that not only does the kidney possess all the necessary molecular machinery to synthesize angiotensin II and other bioactive angiotensin peptides but that their concentrations in glomerular filtrate, tubule fluid, and the interstitium are frequently between 10- and 1000-fold higher than in plasma.[36,109-112]

Within the kidney, renin-expressing cells have traditionally been considered to be terminally differentiated and confined to the JGA. However, in a series of elegant studies using a fate-mapping Cre-loxP system, Sequeira Lopez and coworkers showed that renin-expressing cells are precursors to a range of other cell types in the kidney, including those of the arteriolar media, mesangium, Bowman's capsule, and proximal tubule.[113] Although normally quiescent, these cells may undergo metaplastic transformation to synthesize renin when homeostasis is challenged.[113] Such threats include not only those related to volume depletion but also tissue injury. For instance, in the setting of single-nephron hyperfiltration and consequent progressive dysfunction that follows renal mass reduction, Gilbert and colleagues noted the de novo expression of renin mRNA and angiotensin II peptide in tubular epithelial cells.[114]

In addition to resident kidney cells, infiltrating mast cells may contribute to activation of the local RAAS in disease. Traditionally associated with allergic reactions and host responses to parasite infestation, mast cells have been increasingly recognized for their role in inflammation, immunomodulation, and chronic disease. In the kidney, interstitial mast cell infiltration accompanies most forms of chronic kidney disease (CKD), in which their abundance correlates with the extent of tubulointerstitial fibrosis and declining GFR, though not proteinuria.[115] Mast cells have been shown to synthesize renin,[116] such that their degranulation will release large quantities of both renin and chymase, accelerating angiotensin II formation in the local environment.

Intracrine Renin-Angiotensin-Aldosterone System

Peptide hormones traditionally bind to their cognate receptors on the plasma membrane and produce their effects through the generation of secondary intermediates. However, emerging evidence suggests that certain peptides may also act directly within the cell's interior, having arrived there by either internalization or intracellular synthesis. For instance, angiotensin II has not only been localized within the cytoplasm and nucleus, but its introduction into the cytoplasm was shown more than a decade ago to have major effects on intracellular calcium currents.[117] Uptake of angiotensin II from the extracellular space likely contributes to its intracellular activity; however, later studies have focused predominantly on its endogenous synthesis. Consistent with the potential role for intracellular angiotensin II, transgenic mice that express an enhanced cyan fluorescent protein–angiotensin II fusion protein that lacks a secretory signal, so that it is retained intracellularly, develop hypertension with microthrombi in glomerular capillaries and small vessels.[118] To date, numerous canonical and noncanonical pathways in the cytoplasm, nucleus, and mitochondria have been implicated in the intracrine RAAS,[119,120] providing a new forefront for the role of the RAAS in physiology, pathophysiology, and therapeutics.

RENIN-ANGIOTENSIN-ALDOSTERONE SYSTEM IN KIDNEY PATHOPHYSIOLOGY

In a critical series of experiments in the 1980s, Brenner, Hostetter, and colleagues studied the hemodynamic effects of renal mass ablation in 5/6 nephrectomized rats, a well-established model of progressive kidney disease.[121] In the setting of nephron loss, those glomeruli that remain undergo compensatory enlargement with increased single nephron GFR (SNGFR) and elevations in P_{GC}, ultimately leading to glomerulosclerosis and loss of function. That this phenomenon might be related to angiotensin II was suggested by previous work in which angiotensin II infusion was demonstrated to also result in elevated P_{GC}.[122] Together these studies suggested that intraglomerular hypertension, as a consequence of the action of angiotensin II, was a pivotal factor underlying the inexorable progression of kidney disease and that strategies that reduce P_{GC} should lead to its amelioration. Indeed, in proof-of-concept studies, blockade of angiotensin II formation with the ACE inhibitor enalapril was shown to dilate the glomerular efferent arteriole and to reduce P_{GC} and disease progression in 5/6 nephrectomized rats.[123] In contrast, combination therapy with hydralazine, reserpine, and hydrochlorothiazide, though equally effective in lowering systemic blood pressure, failed to ameliorate intraglomerular hypertension and disease progression.[123] These studies were soon followed by similar ones in other disease models, particularly diabetes, which, like the 5/6 nephrectomized rat, is also characterized by increased SNGFR and elevated P_{GC}.[124]

FIBROSIS

During the past 20 years considerable research has focused on many of the nonhemodynamic effects of angiotensin II. For instance, in addition to their effects on P_{GC}, ACE inhibitors and ARBs are also highly effective in reducing interstitial fibrosis and tubular atrophy, which are close correlates of progressive kidney dysfunction. Underlying these effects is the ability of angiotensin II to potently induce expression of the profibrotic and proapoptotic growth factor TGF-β in a range of kidney cell types.[125,126] Consistent with these in vitro studies, TGF-β overexpression is seen in both the glomerular and tubulointerstitial compartments in 5/6 nephrectomized and diabetic rats, in which studies also showed that both ACE inhibitors and ARBs were effective at reducing TGF-β and disease progression.[127,128] Similarly, in human diabetic nephropathy, the ACE inhibitor perindopril was found to reduce TGF-β mRNA in a sequential renal biopsy study,[129] and losartan was shown to lower urinary TGF-β excretion.[130]

PROTEINURIA

The development of proteinuria is both a cardinal manifestation of glomerular injury and a pathogenetic factor in the progression of renal dysfunction. Although P_{GC} remains an important factor in determining the transglomerular passage of albumin, later work has focused on the potential contribution of the podocyte. Indeed, podocyte injury is a cardinal manifestation of proteinuric renal disease, in which foot process effacement has been shown to be prevented by both ACE inhibition and angiotensin receptor blockade.[131] Other studies have focused on nephrin, a podocyte slit pore membrane protein, because of its crucial role in the development and function of the glomerular filtration barrier. Of note, podocytes express the AT_1 receptor and respond to the addition of angiotensin II to the cell culture medium by dramatically decreasing their expression of nephrin.[132] Consistent with these findings, the reduction in nephrin expression in patients with diabetic nephropathy was shown to be ameliorated by ACE inhibitor treatment for 2 years.[133]

INFLAMMATION, IMMUNITY, AND THE RENIN–ANGIOTENSIN-ALDOSTERONE SYSTEM

Inflammatory cell infiltration is a long-recognized feature of CKD that is attenuated in rodent models by agents that block the RAAS.[134] In the in vitro setting, angiotensin II activates NF-κB by both AT_1 receptor– and AT_2 receptor–dependent pathways, stimulating the expression of a number of potent chemokines such as MCP-1 and RANTES (regulated on activation, normal T expressed, and secreted), as well as cytokines, such as IL-6.[135] In addition to angiotensin II, angiotensin-(1-7), acting via the Mas receptor, activates NF-κB, inducing proinflammatory effects in the kidney under both basal and disease settings.[136]

In addition to macrophages, mast cells, and other components of the innate immune system, the adaptive immune system also appears to be involved in the pathogenesis of angiotensin II–mediated organ injury. Of note, suppression of the adaptive immune system prevents the development of angiotensin II–dependent hypertension in experimental models,[137] and adoptive transfer of $CD4^+CD25^+$ regulatory T cells is able to ameliorate angiotensin II–dependent injury.[138]

DIABETES PARADOX

Despite the fact that patients with long-standing diabetes characteristically have low plasma renin levels,[139-141] suggesting that the RAAS is not activated by the disease, agents that block the RAAS are the mainstay of therapy in diabetic nephropathy. Compounding this apparent paradox, whereas PRA is normal or low in diabetes, plasma prorenin levels are characteristically elevated. This dichotomy suggests differences in cell-specific responses to diabetes, because the JGA is the primary source of renin secretion, whereas prorenin is secreted by a much wider range of cell types. In a recent commentary, Peti-Peterdi and associates have ventured to explain the (pro)renin paradox of diabetes.[142] Whereas early diabetes would lead to augmented succinate levels and enhanced JGA renin release, elevated angiotensin II levels would thereafter suppress JGA renin secretion. In contrast to this negative feedback at the JGA, angiotensin II has been shown to have the opposite effect in the tubule, with diabetes causing a 3.5-fold increase in collecting duct renin that could be reduced by AT_1 receptor blockade.[143]

ENDOTHELIN

ETs are potent vasoconstrictors that, although expressed primarily in the vascular endothelium, are also notably present within the renal medulla. The biologic effects of the ET system are mediated by two receptors, endothelin types A (ET-A) and B (ET-B). In the kidneys these receptors contribute to the regulation of renal blood flow, salt and water balance, and acid-base homeostasis, as well as potentially mediating tissue inflammation and fibrosis. An important therapeutic role has emerged for ET receptor antagonism in the treatment of pulmonary hypertension[144-147]; ET receptor antagonists have been granted regulatory authority approval for this indication in the United States and in Europe.[148] ET receptor blockade as a therapeutic strategy has been investigated in a range of renal diseases. Clinical trials have demonstrated the antiproteinuric and antihypertensive properties of ET receptor antagonists. However, adverse side effects, most notably fluid retention and hepatotoxicity, and issues related to trial design have impeded the development of ET receptor blockers for these indications.

STRUCTURE, SYNTHESIS, AND SECRETION OF THE ENDOTHELINS

ETs consist of three 21–amino acid isoforms that are structurally and pharmacologically distinct: ET-1, ET-2, and ET-3. The dominant isoform in the cardiovascular system is ET-1. Differences in the amino acid sequence among the isopeptides are minor. All three isoforms share a common structure with a typical hairpin-loop configuration resulting from two disulfide bonds at the amino-terminal and a hydrophobic carboxy-terminal containing an aromatic indol side chain at Trp_{21} (Figure 13.5). Both the carboxy-terminal and the two disulfide bonds are responsible for the biologic activity of the peptide.

ETs are synthesized from preprohormones by posttranslational proteolytic cleavage mediated by furin and other enzymes. Dibasic pair–specific processing endopeptidases, which recognize Arg-Arg or Lys-Arg paired amino acids, cleave preproETs, reducing their size from approximately 203 to 39 amino acids. Subsequent proteolytic cleavage of the largely biologically inactive big ETs is mediated by endothelin-converting enzymes (ECEs), the key enzymes in the ET biosynthetic pathway. ECEs are type II membrane-bound metalloproteases whose amino acid sequence is significantly homologous to that of NEP 24.11.

Secretion of ET-1 is dependent on de novo protein synthesis, which is constitutive. However, a range of stimuli may also increase ET synthesis through both transcriptional and posttranscriptional regulation (Table 13.1). Once it is

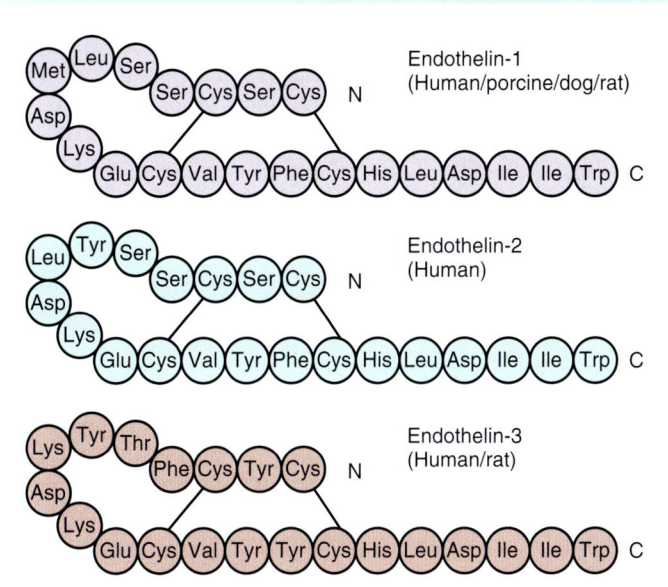

Figure 13.5 Molecular structure of the three endothelin isoforms. (Adapted from Schiffrin EL: Vascular endothelin in hypertension. *Vascul Pharmacol* 43:19-29, 2005.)

Table 13.1 Endothelin Gene and Protein Expression

Stimulation	
Vasoactive peptides	Growth factors
Angiotensin II	Epidermal growth factor
Bradykinin	Insulin-like growth factor
Vasopressin	TGF-β
Endothelin 1	Coagulation
Epinephrine	Thromboxane A_2
Insulin	Tissue plasminogen activator
Glucocorticoids	Other
Prolactin	Calcium
Inflammatory mediators	Hypoxia
Endotoxin	Shear stress
Interleukin-1	Phorbol esters
TNF-α	Oxidized low-density lipoproteins
Interferon-β	
Inhibition	
ANP	Prostacyclin
BNP	Protein kinase A activators
Bradykinin	Nitric oxide
Heparin	ACE inhibitors

ACE, Angiotensin-converting enzyme; ANP, atrial natriuretic peptide; BNP, brain natriuretic peptide; TGF-β, transforming growth factor-β; TNF-α, tumor necrosis factor-α.

synthesized, ET-1 is secreted by endothelial cells into the basolateral compartment, toward the adjacent smooth muscle cells. Because of its abluminal secretion, plasma levels of ET-1 do not necessarily reflect its production.[149]

Within the kidneys, ET-1 expression is most abundant in the inner medulla. In fact, this region possesses the highest concentration of ET-1 of any tissue bed.[150] In addition to the inner medullary collecting ducts (IMCDs), ETs have also been described in glomerular endothelial cells,[151] glomerular epithelial cells,[152] mesangial cells,[153] vasa recta,[154] and tubular epithelial cells.[155] The kidney also synthesizes ET-2 and ET-3, although at much lower levels than ET-1.[156] As with ET-1, ECE mRNA is also more abundant in the renal medulla than in the cortex under normal conditions. However, in disease states such as chronic heart failure, there is upregulation of ECE mRNA primarily within the cortex.[157] In human kidneys, ECE1 has been localized to endothelial and tubular epithelial cells in the cortex and medulla.[158]

ENDOTHELIN RECEPTORS

ETs bind to two seven-transmembrane domain G protein–coupled receptors, ET-A and ET-B. Within the vasculature, ET-A receptors are found on smooth muscle cells, where they mediate vasoconstriction. Although ET-B receptors localized on vascular smooth muscle cells can also mediate vasoconstriction, they are also expressed on endothelial cells, where their activation results in vasodilation through the production of nitric oxide and prostacyclin.[159] In addition to their role in mediating vascular tone, ET-B receptors also act as clearance receptors for ET-1,[160] particularly in the lung, where ET-B receptor–binding accounts for approximately 80% of clearance.[161] In the kidney the ET-B receptor has predominantly renoprotective effects, including natriuresis and vasodilation.

Expression of both ET-A and ET-B receptors in the kidney is most prominent within the IMCDs, although binding of ET-1 also occurs in smooth muscle cells, endothelial cells, renomedullary interstitial cells, thin descending limbs, and medullary thick ascending limbs.[154] ET-A receptors are localized to several renovascular structures, including vascular smooth muscle cells, arcuate arteries, and pericytes of descending vasa recta, as well as glomeruli. ET-B receptors, although prominently represented within the medullary collecting system, have also been demonstrated in proximal convoluted tubules, collecting ducts of the inner cortex, medullary thick ascending limbs, and podocytes.[162]

PHYSIOLOGIC ACTIONS OF ENDOTHELIN IN THE KIDNEY

The ETs have several effects on normal renal function, including regulation of renal blood flow, sodium and water balance, and acid-base homeostasis. Although ET-1 has hemodynamic effects in almost all vessels, sensitivity varies between different vascular beds. The renal vasculature, along with the mesenteric vessels, is the most sensitive, with vasoconstriction occurring at picomolar concentrations of ET-1,[163,164] increasing renal vascular resistance and decreasing renal blood flow. However, long-lasting vasoconstriction, which is mediated by the ET-A receptor, may be preceded by a transient ET-B receptor–mediated vasodilation.[165] Because of the site-specific distribution of ET receptors, ET-1 may exert different vasoconstrictive and vasodilatory effects in different regions of the kidneys. For example, by inducing nitric oxide release from adjacent tubular epithelial cells, ET-1 may actually increase blood flow in the renal medulla, where ET-B receptors predominate.[166]

In addition to effects on renal blood flow, the ET system also plays a direct role in renal sodium and water handling. In the renal medulla, ET is regulated by sodium intake and exerts its natriuretic and diuretic effects through the ET-B receptor.[167-169] In addition to natriuretic and diuretic effects, the ET-B receptor may also contribute to acid-base homeostasis by stimulating proximal tubule Na^+-H^+-exchanger isoform 3.[170] Although the role of ET-B receptor activation in urinary sodium excretion has been appreciated for some time, later evidence suggests that renal medullary ET-A receptors may also mediate natriuresis.[171] This may partly explain the edema that can occur as a side effect of ET-A or dual ET receptor antagonism.

ROLE OF ENDOTHELIN IN ESSENTIAL HYPERTENSION

Given its potent vasoconstrictive properties, it is unsurprising that ET-1 has been implicated in the pathogenesis of hypertension. In preclinical models of hypertension, ET antagonism may ameliorate heart failure, vascular injury, and renal failure, as well as decreasing stroke.[172,173] ET-A receptor antagonism has also been shown to normalize blood pressure in rats exposed to eucapnic intermittent hypoxia, analogous to sleep apnea in humans.[174]

PreproET-1 mRNA is increased in the endothelium of subcutaneous resistance arteries in patients with moderate to severe hypertension.[175] However, plasma ET-1 levels are not universally elevated,[172] with an increase more commonly in the presence of end-organ damage or in salt-depleted, salt-sensitive patients with a blunted renin response.[176] A major component of this increase in disease is often decreased clearance by the kidney. These findings suggest that certain patient subgroups may be more responsive to ET receptor blockade than others. Females appear to be relatively protected from the pressor effects of ET-1 by virtue of both increased ET-B expression and a blunted hemodynamic response to ET-A activation.[177]

Clinical trials of the antihypertensive effects of ET receptor antagonism have been hampered by difficulties with selectivity for the ET-A receptor, study design, dosing regimens, and adverse events.[178] Because the ET-B receptor exerts diuretic and natriuretic effects, induces vasodilation, and clears ET-1, selective ET-A receptor antagonists may be expected to demonstrate a more favorable antihypertensive profile.[178] Mixed ET (ET-A and ET-B) and specific ET-A receptor antagonists are distinguished by their in vitro binding affinities. Mixed ET (ET-A and ET-B) antagonists demonstrate selectivity for ET-A of less than 100-fold, and ET-A selective antagonists have an affinity for the ET-A receptor of 100-fold or greater. However, it has been suggested that an affinity of 1000-fold or higher may be required to induce ET-A receptor–specific effects in vivo.[179,180] In an early study, treatment of patients with essential hypertension with the nonselective ET receptor antagonist bosentan decreased blood pressure as effectively as enalapril, without reflex neurohumoral activation, over a 4-week period.[181] Similarly, in 115 patients with resistant hypertension on three or more agents, the selective ET-A receptor antagonist darusentan significantly reduced blood pressure at 10 weeks.[182] In a subsequent study of 379 individuals with resistant hypertension, darusentan treatment for 14 weeks reduced blood pressure by approximately 18/10 mm Hg with no evidence of dose dependence across a range of 50 to 100 mg/day.[183] However, in a second study of similar design, a large placebo effect meant that darusentan treatment failed to achieve its primary end point of change in office blood pressure, and the development of the drug for this indication was halted.[184] Interestingly, in both of these studies ambulatory blood pressure monitoring revealed a reduction in systolic blood pressure with active treatment.[179,185] However, also in both studies, peripheral edema or fluid retention was more common in patients treated with darusentan than in those receiving placebo.[183,184]

ROLE OF ENDOTHELIN IN RENAL INJURY

Increasing evidence indicates that, beyond its effects on vascular tone, the ET system is also directly involved in the pathogenesis of fibrotic injury in CKD.[186] In patients with CKD, plasma ET-1 concentrations are elevated, due to both increased production and decreased renal clearance,[187] and urinary levels of ET-1 are also increased, indicative of increased renal ET-1 expression.[188] However, as seen in the studies of hypertension, an unfavorable side-effect profile and possibly also dosing issues related to study design have impeded the development of ET receptor antagonists for the treatment of CKD.

One mechanism for increased renal ET-1 in CKD is a direct effect of urinary protein on tubular epithelial ET-1 expression.[189,190] Beyond direct effects of urine protein, a number of proinflammatory factors induce ET-1 expression in the kidney, including hypoxia, angiotensin II, thrombin, thromboxane A_2, TGF-β, and shear stress (see Table 13.1).

Several distinct mechanisms may account for the injurious effects of ET-1 on the kidney. Locally derived ET-1 has direct hemodynamic effects, increasing P_{GC} at high doses and causing vasoconstriction of the vasa recta and peritubular capillaries, with a resultant reduction in tissue oxygen tension. ET-1 also acts as a chemoattractant for inflammatory cells, which may express the peptide themselves, stimulating interstitial fibroblast and mesangial cell proliferation and mediating the production of a number of factors associated with collagenous matrix deposition, including TGF-β, matrix metalloproteinase 1, and tissue inhibitors of metalloproteinases 1 and 2. Finally, ET-1 can induce cytoskeletal remodeling in both mesangial cells and podocytes. ET-1 induces mesangial cell contraction[191] and may promote transformation from a quiescent to an activated state. In podocytes, increased passage of protein across the filtration barrier causes cytoskeletal rearrangements and coincident upregulation of ET-1, which may act in an autocrine manner to further propagate ultrastructural injury in the same cells.[192-194]

ENDOTHELIN SYSTEM IN CHRONIC KIDNEY DISEASE AND DIABETIC NEPHROPATHY

ET receptor antagonists have been employed to study the role of ETs in renal pathophysiology in a range of experimental models, including the rat remnant kidney, lupus nephritis, and diabetes. In the remnant kidney model of progressive renal disease, although beneficial effects have been reported with nonselective ET receptor antagonists,[195] selective ET-A receptor inhibition appears to be superior, with concomitant inhibition of ET-B receptors potentially abrogating any beneficial effects.[196]

Evidence for an effect of glucose itself on ET synthesis and secretion is conflicting. Mesangial cell p38 MAP kinase activation in response to ET-1, angiotensin II, and PDGF is enhanced in the presence of high glucose levels.[197] In contrast, mesangial contraction in response to ET-1 is diminished under high-glucose conditions.[198,199] Circulating ET-1 concentrations are elevated in animal models of both type 1 and type 2 diabetes, although receptor levels are usually not affected. In experimental diabetic nephropathy, increased expression of ET-1 and its receptors has been found in glomeruli and in tubular epithelial cells,[190,200] although increased expression of ET receptors has not been a universal finding.[201] Diabetes also causes an increase in renal ECE1 expression, the effect being synergistic with that of radiocontrast media.[202]

A number of studies have investigated the effect of both nonselective and selective ET-A receptor inhibitors in experimental diabetic nephropathy. In streptozotocin-diabetic rats, the nonselective ET receptor antagonist bosentan has provided conflicting results,[203,204] whereas another nonselective ET receptor inhibitor, PD142893, improved renal function when administered to streptozotocin-diabetic rats that were already proteinuric.[190] In Otsuka Long Evans Tokushima Fatty (OLETF) rats, a model of type 2 diabetes, selective ET-A receptor blockade attenuated albuminuria, without affecting blood pressure, whereas ET-B receptor inhibition had no effect.[205] In a study of streptozotocin-diabetic apolipoprotein E–knockout mice, the renoprotective effects of the predominant ET-A receptor antagonist avosentan were comparable or superior to the ACE inhibitor quinapril.[206] Diabetic ET-B receptor–deficient rats develop severe hypertension and progressive renal failure,[207] supporting a protective role for the ET-B receptor in diabetic nephropathy.

Reactive oxygen species accumulation plays a major role in the pathogenesis of diabetic complications and diabetic nephropathy in particular,[208,209] and several observations suggest that the ET system may contribute to oxidative stress. In low-renin hypertension, ET-1 increases superoxide in carotid arteries,[210] and ET-A receptor blockade decreases vascular superoxide generation.[211,212] Similarly, ET-1 infusion increases urinary 8-isoprostane prostaglandin $F_{2\alpha}$ excretion in rats, indicative of increased generation of reactive oxygen species.[213] In contrast, however, other preclinical studies have suggested a predominantly proinflammatory role for ET-1 in diabetic nephropathy. For instance, the selective ET-A receptor antagonist ABT-627 prevented the development of albuminuria in streptozotocin-diabetic rats without an improvement in markers of oxidative stress but with a reduction in macrophage infiltration and urinary excretion of TGF-β and prostaglandin E_2 metabolites.[214]

Both plasma and urinary ET-1 levels are increased in patients with CKD,[187,215,216] with plasma ET-1 levels correlating inversely with estimated GFR. In a study of hypertensive patients with CKD, both selective ET-A receptor blockade and nonselective ET receptor inhibition lowered blood pressure.[217] However, whereas ET-A receptor blockade increased both renal blood flow and effective filtration fraction and decreased renal vascular resistance, dual blockade had no effect.[217] These observations suggest that, although activation of the ET-B receptor does contribute to systemic vascular tone, its role in mediating renal vasodilation likely predominates.

In a study of 22 persons with CKD who did not have diabetes, intravenous infusion of the ET-A receptor antagonist BQ-123 reduced pulse wave velocity and proteinuria to a greater extent than the calcium channel antagonist nifedipine, which comparably lowered blood pressure.[218] These findings suggest a mechanism of action for the antiproteinuric effect observed that is potentially independent from blood pressure. In a subsequent study by the same investigators, 27 subjects with proteinuric CKD were treated with the ET-A receptor antagonist sitaxsentan for 6 weeks in a three-way crossover study design. Sitaxsentan treatment was associated with a reduction in blood pressure, proteinuria, and pulse wave velocity, whereas nifedipine reduced pulse wave velocity and blood pressure but had no effect on urine protein excretion.[219] A fall in GFR with sitaxsentan therapy observed in this study is analogous to that seen with RAAS blockade.[219] Although no clinically significant adverse effects were seen, sitaxsentan development has subsequently been halted due to hepatotoxicity.

The effect of the ET-A receptor antagonist avosentan was examined in a placebo-controlled trial of 286 patients with diabetic nephropathy and macroalbuminuria in addition to standard treatment with an ACE inhibitor or angiotensin II receptor blocker.[220] At 12 weeks, avosentan was found to decrease urine albumin excretion rate without affecting blood pressure. However, a subsequent large phase III study examining the effects of avosentan, on top of RAAS blockade, in 1392 persons with type 2 diabetes and nephropathy was terminated after a median duration of 4 months due to adverse events.[221] In that study, despite a reduction of greater than 40% in albumin to creatinine ratio with avosentan, adverse events, predominantly fluid overload and congestive heart failure, occurred more frequently in those receiving active therapy than in those receiving placebo.[221] Given the relatively high dose of avosentan used in the study, it remains to be determined whether lower doses of avosentan would attenuate albuminuria without the increase in fluid overload.

ENDOTHELIN SYSTEM AND OTHER KIDNEY DISEASES

In addition to diabetic and nondiabetic CKD, the role of the ET system has also been investigated in a number of other experimental models, including acute renal ischemia, cyclosporine-induced nephrotoxicity, and renal allograft rejection. Overall, these studies have suggested some degree of renoprotection with either selective ET-A or nonselective ET receptor inhibitors.

ENDOTOXEMIA

ET-1 may play a role in sepsis-mediated acute kidney injury,[222] although again experimental findings have been conflicting, dependent to some extent on the ET receptor antagonist employed. For example, in a rat model of early normotensive endotoxemia, neither an ET-A receptor antagonist nor combined ET-A and ET-B receptor blockade improved GFR,[223] whereas ET-B receptor blockade alone resulted in a marked reduction in renal blood flow.[223] In contrast, in a porcine model of endotoxemic shock, the dual ET receptor antagonist tezosentan attenuated the decrease in renal blood flow and increase in plasma creatinine level.[224]

SYSTEMIC LUPUS ERYTHEMATOSUS

Urinary ET-1 excretion is correlated with disease activity in patients with systemic lupus erythematosus (SLE),[225] and serum from patients has been shown to stimulate ET-1 release from endothelial cells in culture.[226] In accordance with a pathogenetic role for the ET system in SLE, the ET-A receptor antagonist FR139317 attenuated renal injury in a murine model of lupus nephritis.[227]

HEPATORENAL SYNDROME

Plasma ET-1 concentrations are increased in individuals with cirrhosis and ascites and in patients with type 2 hepatorenal syndrome (diuretic-resistant or refractory ascites with slowly progressive renal decline), in which there is systemic vasodilation with paradoxical renal vasoconstriction.[228] To investigate the therapeutic potential of ET receptor antagonism in this setting, the combined ET-A and ET-B receptor blocker tezosentan was administered to six patients in an early-phase clinical trial.[229] In this study, treatment was discontinued early in five patients, one because of systemic hypotension and four because of concerns about worsening renal function.[229] These adverse effects are consistent with a dose-dependent decline in renal function in patients with acute heart failure treated with tezosentan, and they highlight the need for caution with the use of ET receptor antagonists in certain patient populations.

PREECLAMPSIA

A role for ET-1 in the development of preeclampsia is suggested by the observations that infusion of fms-like tyrosine kinase 1 and TNF-α into pregnant rats induced ET-A–dependent hypertension,[230-232] whereas ET-A receptor antagonism attenuated placental ischemia-induced hypertension in a rat model.[233] Despite the mechanistic role of ET-1 in the pathogenesis of preeclampsia, however, ET receptor antagonists are very unlikely to be used in this condition given their known teratogenicity.[230]

SAFETY PROFILE OF ENDOTHELIN RECEPTOR ANTAGONISTS

The therapeutic development of ET receptor antagonists has been impeded by the adverse side-effect profile of currently available agents. Most notable has been the development of fluid retention, peripheral edema, and congestive heart failure despite the use of predominant ET-A receptor antagonists. The mechanisms that underlie the fluid retention associated with ET-A receptor antagonism are not fully resolved. It has been suggested that the use of comparatively high doses of ET-A receptor antagonists may have resulted in concurrent ET-B receptor blockade. However, inhibition of nephron ET-A receptors may also be implicated.[165,234] Hepatotoxicity may be a class effect or may be restricted to particular subclasses of ET receptor antagonist. For instance, a rise in hepatic transaminase levels has been observed with both bosentan and sitaxsentan, which are both sulfonamide-based agents, but not with ambrisentan or darusentan, which are propionic acid–based.[179,182,183,235,236] Finally, as discussed earlier, teratogenicity would preclude the use of this class of agents in pregnancy.

NATRIURETIC PEPTIDES

The natriuretic peptides (NPs) are a family of vasoactive hormones that play a role in salt and water homeostasis. The family consists of at least five structurally related but genetically distinct peptides, including atrial natriuretic peptide (ANP), brain natriuretic peptide (BNP), C-type natriuretic peptide (CNP), *Dendroaspis* natriuretic peptide (DNP), and urodilatin. ANP was originally isolated from human and rat atrial tissues in 1984.[237] Since then, the NP family has been expanded to include several other members, all of which share a common 17–amino acid ring structure that is stabilized by a cysteine bridge and that contains several invariant amino acids.[238] BNP[239] and CNP[240] were both originally identified in porcine brain, whereas DNP was first isolated from the venom of the green mamba snake, *Dendroaspis angusticeps*.[241] Urodilatin is an NH_2-terminally extended form of ANP that was initially described in human urine.[242] NP inactivation occurs through at least two distinct pathways, binding to a clearance receptor (natriuretic peptide receptor [NPR]–C) and enzymatic degradation. Other peptides that may be involved in salt and water balance include guanylin, uroguanylin, and adrenomedullin.

ANP and BNP act as endogenous antagonists of the RAAS mediating natriuresis, diuresis, vasodilation, and suppression of sympathetic activity, as well as inhibiting cell growth and decreasing secretion of aldosterone and renin.[243] The role of NPs in cardiovascular and renal disease, particularly BNP, has led to their adoption into clinical practice as indicators of disease states and, to some extent, as therapeutic agents.

STRUCTURE AND SYNTHESIS OF THE NATRIURETIC PEPTIDES

ATRIAL NATRIURETIC PEPTIDE

ANP is a 28–amino acid peptide comprising a 17–amino acid ring linked by a disulfide bond between two cysteine residues and a COOH-terminal extension that confers its biologic activity (Figure 13.6). The gene for ANP, natriuretic peptide precursor type A *(NPPA)*, is found on chromosome 1p36 and encodes the precursor preproANP, which is between 149 and 153 amino acids in length according to the species of origin. Human preproANP consists of 151 amino acids and is rapidly processed to the 126–amino acid proANP. ANP is identical in mammalian species except for a single amino acid substitution at residue 110, which is isoleucine in the rat, rabbit, and mouse, and methionine in the human, pig, dog, sheep, and cow.

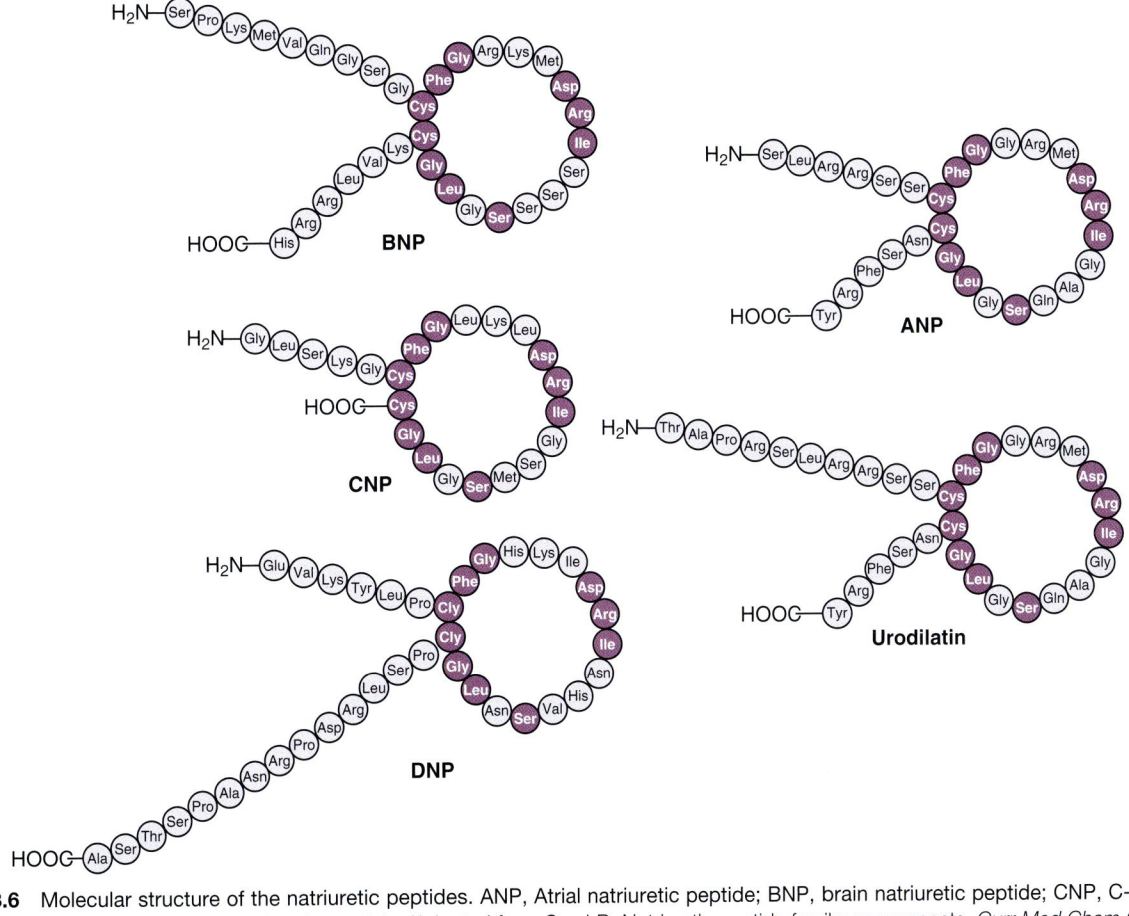

Figure 13.6 Molecular structure of the natriuretic peptides. ANP, Atrial natriuretic peptide; BNP, brain natriuretic peptide; CNP, C-type natriuretic peptide; DNP, *Dendroaspis* natriuretic peptide. (Adapted from Cea LB: Natriuretic peptide family: new aspects. *Curr Med Chem Cardiovasc Hematol Agents* 3:87-98, 2005.)

ANP synthesis occurs primarily within atrial cardiomyocytes, where it is stored as proANP, the main constituent of the atrial secretory granules. The major stimulus to ANP release is mechanical stretch of the atria secondary to increased wall tension. However, ANP synthesis and release may also be stimulated by neurohumoral factors such as glucocorticoids, ET, vasopressin, and angiotensin II, partly through changes in atrial pressure and partly through direct cellular effects. Although ANP mRNA levels are approximately thirty to fiftyfold higher in the cardiac atria than in the ventricles, ventricular expression is dramatically increased in the developing heart and in conditions of hemodynamic overload such as heart failure and hypertension. Beyond the heart, the peptide has also been demonstrated in the kidney, brain, lung, adrenal gland, and liver. In the kidney, alternate processing of proANP adds four amino acids to the NH_2 terminus of the ANP peptide to generate a 32–amino acid peptide, proANP 95-126, or urodilatin.

ANP is stored, primarily as proANP, in the secretory granules of the atrial cardiomyocytes and is released by fusion of the granules with the cell surface. During this process proANP is cleaved to an NH_2-terminal 98–amino acid peptide (ANP 1-98) and the COOH-terminal 28–amino acid biologically active fragment (ANP 99-126). Both fragments circulate in the plasma, with further processing of the NH_2-terminal fragment leading to the generation of peptides ANP 1-30 (long-acting NP), ANP 31-67 (vessel dilator), and ANP 79-98 (kaliuretic peptide), all of whose biologic actions may be similar to those of ANP.[244]

BRAIN NATRIURETIC PEPTIDE

The BNP gene is located approximately only 8 kb upstream of the ANP gene on the short arm of chromosome 1 in humans, which suggests that the two genes may share in common both evolutionary origin and transcriptional regulation. In contrast, CNP is found separately on chromosome 2. CNP is highly conserved across species, indicating that the peptide may represent the evolutionary ancestor of ANP and BNP.

BNP, like ANP, is synthesized as a preprohormone, between 121 and 134 amino acids in length, according to species of origin. Human preproBNP (134 amino acids) is cleaved to produce the 108–amino acid precursor proBNP. Further processing leads to the production of the 32–amino acid, biologically active BNP, which corresponds to the C terminus of the precursor, as well as a 76–amino acid N-terminal fragment (N-terminal proBNP [NT-proBNP]).[245] Active BNP, NT-proBNP, and proBNP all circulate in the plasma. Circulating BNP contains the characteristic 17–amino acid ring structure closed by a disulfide bond between two cysteine residues, along with a 9–amino acid amino-terminal tail and a 6–amino acid carboxy tail (see Figure 13.6).[246]

The term brain natriuretic peptide is somewhat misleading because the primary sites of synthesis of BNP are the cardiac ventricles, with expression also occurring to a lesser extent in atrial cardiomyocytes. Like ANP, expression of BNP is regulated by changes in intracardiac pressure and stretch. However, unlike ANP, which is stored and released from secretory granules, BNP is regulated at the gene expression level and is synthesized and secreted in bursts.

BNP expression is increased in heart failure, hypertension, and renal failure. Its plasma half-life is approximately 20 minutes, in contrast to a circulating half-life of ANP of 2 to 5 minutes and a half-life of the biologically inactive NT-proBNP of 120 minutes. This difference is relevant to the utility of NP measurement as a biologic marker of cardiorenal disease. Changes in pulmonary capillary wedge pressure may be reflected by plasma BNP concentrations every 2 hours and NT-proBNP levels every 12 hours.[247,248] The physiologic actions of BNP are similar to those of ANP, including effects on the kidney (natriuresis and diuresis), vasculature (hypotension), endocrine systems (inhibition of plasma renin and aldosterone secretion), and brain (central vasodepressor activity).

C-TYPE NATRIURETIC PEPTIDE

As is the case for ANP and BNP, CNP is derived from a prepropeptide that undergoes posttranslational proteolytic cleavage. The initial translation product preproCNP is 126 amino acids in length and is cleaved to produce the 103–amino acid prohormone. Cleavage of proCNP yields two mature peptides made up of 22 and 53 amino acids, referred to as CNP and NH_2-terminally extended form of CNP, respectively. Eleven of the 17 amino acids within the CNP ring structure are identical to those in the other NPs, although, uniquely, CNP lacks an amino tail at the carboxy-terminal (see Figure 13.6).

CNP functions in an autocrine/paracrine manner with effects on vascular tone and muscle cell growth.[249] Accordingly, plasma concentrations of CNP are very low, although they are increased in heart failure and renal failure. CNP is present in the heart, kidney, and endothelium, and its receptor is also expressed in abundance in the hypothalamus and pituitary gland, suggesting that the peptide may also play a role as a neuromodulator or neurotransmitter. Because CNP is present in primarily noncardiac tissues, regulation of its expression is distinct from that of ANP and BNP and is controlled by a number of vasoactive mediators, including insulin, vascular endothelial growth factor, TGF-β, TNF-α, and interleukin-1β.[249]

The principal enzymes responsible for the conversion of proANP, proBNP, and proCNP to their active forms are the serine proteases, corin and furin.[250] Corin converts proANP to ANP,[251] furin converts proCNP to CNP,[252] and both corin and furin cleave proBNP.[253] Corin is highly expressed in the heart and to a lesser extent in the kidney.[250] In response to pressure overload, corin-deficient mice develop hypertension together with cardiac hypertrophy and dysfunction.[254,255] In the kidney, corin co-localizes with ANP,[256] and decreased urinary corin excretion has been observed in patients with CKD.[257] Studies combining observations made in organ-specific corin-deficient mice together with human correlative experiments have identified a role for impaired uterine corin/ANP function in the pathogenesis of preeclampsia.[258]

DENDROASPIS NATRIURETIC PEPTIDE

The physiologic role of DNP has been controversial ever since its original identification in the venom of the green mamba snake, *D. angusticeps*, in 1992.[241,259] DNP is a 38–amino acid peptide that shares the 17–amino acid ring structure common to all NPs but that has unique N- and

C-terminal regions (see Figure 13.6).[248] Immunoreactivity for DNP has been reported in human plasma and atrial myocardium, and DNP has also been described in rat[260] and rabbit[261] kidney, rat colon,[262] rat aortic vascular smooth muscle cells,[263] and pig ovarian granulosa cells.[264] DNP binds to natriuretic peptide receptor A (NPR-A)[265] and the clearance receptor NPR-C,[266] which may be of particular relevance given the apparent resistance of the peptide to enzymatic degradation.[267] In dogs, either under normal conditions or in a pacing-induced heart failure model, administration of synthetic DNP decreased cardiac filling pressures and increased GFR, natriuresis, and diuresis, as well as lowering blood pressure, suppressing renin release, and increasing plasma and urine cGMP.[268,269] Despite these propitious findings, several aspects of the biologic role of DNP remain contentious. In particular, the gene for the peptide has not been identified in mammals, nor has it yet been identified in the green mamba. Immunoreactivity experiments can be subject to artifact, and there are no reports of the fractionation of DNP from human samples.[259] These uncertainties have led some authors to question whether DNP is, in fact, expressed at all in humans.[259]

URODILATIN

Urodilatin is a structural homolog of ANP, synthesized in kidney distal tubular cells and differentially processed to a 32–amino acid NH_2-terminally extended form of ANP, sharing the same 17–amino acid ring structure and COOH-terminal tail.[270] The peptide is not found in the plasma, acting in a paracrine manner within the kidney on receptors in the glomeruli and IMCDs to promote natriuresis and diuresis. Urodilatin is upregulated in diabetic animals[271] and in the remnant kidney[272] and is relatively resistant to enzymatic degradation, which may explain its more potent renal effects.

NATRIURETIC PEPTIDE RECEPTORS

NPs mediate their biologic effects by binding to three distinct guanylyl cyclase NPRs. The terminology can be somewhat confusing because NPR-A binds ANP and BNP and natriuretic peptide receptor B (NPR-B) binds CNP, whereas NPR-C acts as a clearance receptor for all three peptides.

NPR-A and NPR-B are structurally similar but share only 44% homology in the extracellular ligand-binding segment, likely responsible for the difference in ligand specificity. Both NPR-A and NPR-B have a molecular weight of approximately 120 kDa and consist of a ligand-binding extracellular domain, a single transmembrane segment, an intracellular kinase domain, and an enzymatically active guanylyl cyclase domain.[238] The kinase homology domain (KHD) of NPR-A and NPR-B shares 30% homology with protein kinases but has no kinase activity. Ligand binding of NPR-A and NPR-B prevents the normal inhibitory action exerted by the KHD on the guanylyl cyclase domain, allowing the generation of cGMP, which acts as a second messenger responsible for most of the biologic effects of the NPs.

NPR-C, in contrast to NPR-A and NPR-B, lacks both the KHD and the catalytic guanylyl cyclase domain and therefore does not signal through a second messenger system. Instead, the receptor contains the extracellular ligand-binding segment, a transmembrane domain, and a 37–amino acid cytoplasmic domain containing a G protein–activating sequence.[273] In NPR-C–knockout mice, blood pressure is reduced and the plasma half-life of ANP is increased, supporting the role of NPR-C as a clearance receptor.[274] NPR-C binds all members of the NP family with high affinity and is the most abundantly expressed of the NPRs, present in the kidney, vascular endothelium, smooth muscle cells, and heart, representing approximately 95% of the total receptor population. Preferential binding of NPR-C to ANP over BNP may explain the relatively increased plasma half-life of BNP.[248] NPR-C clears NPs from the circulation through a process of receptor-mediated endocytosis and lysosomal degradation before rapid recycling of the internalized receptor to the cell surface. Although the primary function of NPR-C is as a clearance receptor, ligand binding may exert biologic effects on the cell through G protein–mediated inhibition of cyclic adenosine monophosphate.[275]

The biologic effects of NPs are largely dependent on the distribution of their receptors. NPR-A mRNA is present mainly in the kidney, especially in the IMCD cells, although the receptor is also notably present within the glomeruli, renal vasculature, and proximal tubules. The distribution of NPR-B overlaps with that of NPR-A, with the receptor found in the kidney, vasculature, and brain. However, consistent with the paracrine effects of CNP on vascular tone, mitogenesis, and cell migration, NPR-B is expressed in greater abundance than NPR-A within the vascular endothelium and smooth muscle, whereas expression levels are relatively lower within the kidney.

NEUTRAL ENDOPEPTIDASE

Receptor-mediated endocytosis probably accounts for approximately 50% of clearance of the NPs from the circulation; catalytic degradation by the enzyme NEP is responsible for the majority of the rest, and only a minor contribution is attributed to direct renal excretion.[248] Receptor clearance probably plays an even smaller role in conditions associated with chronically elevated NP levels, because of increased receptor occupancy and downregulation of NPR-C expression.

NEP is a membrane-bound zinc metalloproteinase, originally termed enkephalinase because of its ability to degrade opioid receptors in the brain. The enzyme has structural and catalytic similarity with other metallopeptidases, including aminopeptidase, ACE, ECE, and carboxypeptidases A, B, and E. ANP, BNP, and CNP are therefore not the only substrates for NEP, with enzymatic activity demonstrated against a number of other vasoactive peptides, including ET-1, angiotensin II, substance P, bradykinin, neurotensin, insulin B chain, calcitonin gene–related peptide, and adrenomedullin. The primary mechanism of action of NEP is to hydrolyze peptide bonds on the NH_2 side of hydrophobic amino acid residues. In the case of ANP, NEP cleaves the Cys^{105}-Phe^{106} bond to disrupt the ring structure and inactivate the peptide. The Cys-Phe bond of BNP is relatively insensitive to enzymatic cleavage.

NEP has a nearly ubiquitous tissue distribution, with expression demonstrated in the kidney, liver, heart, brain, lungs, gut, and adrenal gland. The metallopeptidase is present not only on the surface of endothelial cells, but also on smooth muscle cells, fibroblasts, and cardiac myocytes,[276] although it is most abundant in the brush border of the proximal tubules of the kidneys, where it rapidly degrades filtered ANP, preventing the peptide from reaching more distal luminal receptors.

ACTIONS OF THE NATRIURETIC PEPTIDES

RENAL EFFECTS OF THE NATRIURETIC PEPTIDES

The natriuretic and diuretic actions of the NPs are consequences of both vasomotor and direct tubular effects. Both ANP and BNP cause an increase in glomerular capillary hydrostatic pressure and a rise in GFR by inducing afferent arteriolar vasodilation and efferent arteriolar vasoconstriction. These contrasting effects of the NPs on the afferent and efferent arterioles differ from the actions of classical vasodilators such as bradykinin. In addition to direct effects on vascular tone, ANP can also increase GFR through cGMP-mediated mesangial cell relaxation.

Plasma levels of ANP that do not increase GFR can induce natriuresis, illustrating the potential for direct tubular effects, which may involve either locally produced NPs acting in a paracrine manner, such as urodilatin, or circulating NPs. A number of mechanisms may be responsible for the natriuresis, including direct effects on sodium transport in tubular epithelial cells and indirect effects through inhibition of renin secretion following increased sodium delivery to the macula densa. NPs also antagonize vasopressin in the cortical collecting ducts. It is likely that similar mechanisms underlie the response to ANP, BNP, and urodilatin. In contrast, CNP has little natriuretic or diuretic effect, which may indicate a requirement for the presence of the carboxy-terminal extension of the peptide for renal effects.

The NPs may have antifibrotic effects within the kidney as evidenced by an increase in renal fibrosis in NPR-A–knockout mice after unilateral ureteral obstruction.[277] In cultured proximal tubular cells, ANP attenuates high glucose–induced activation of TGF-β_1, Smad, and collagen synthesis, illustrating the potentially antifibrotic properties of the peptide in the context of diabetic nephropathy.[278]

CARDIOVASCULAR EFFECTS

All NPs have vasodilatory and hypotensive properties. Heterozygous mutant mice with a disrupted proANP gene display evidence of salt-sensitive hypertension,[279] whereas hypotension is a feature of transgenic mice overexpressing ANP.[280] In a patient population, a variant in the ANP promoter was associated with both lower levels of plasma ANP and increased susceptibility to early development of hypertension.[281] However, a caveat to the hypotensive role of ANP is the observation that infusion of high concentrations of ANP can actually induce a rise in blood pressure, suggesting activation of counterregulatory baroreceptors.[282]

There are two major direct mechanisms by which ANP may lower blood pressure. First, it increases vascular permeability with a shift of fluid from the intravascular to extravascular compartments by capillary hydraulic pressure. Second, ANP increases venous capacitance, promoting natriuresis and lowering preload.[283] In addition, ANP and BNP antagonize the vasoconstrictive effects of the RAAS, ET, and the sympathetic nervous system[243] by decreasing sympathetic peripheral vascular tone, suppressing the release of catecholamines and reducing central sympathetic outflow.[245] By lowering the activation threshold of vagal afferents, ANP prevents the vasoconstriction and tachycardia that normally follow a reduction in preload, leading to a sustained drop in blood pressure. CNP is a more potent vasodilator than either ANP or BNP. In fact, CNP relaxes human subcutaneous resistance arteries, whereas ANP and BNP have no effect.[284]

NPs have a number of other effects on the cardiovascular system distinct from their action on vasomotor tone. For example, NPs play a major role in cardiac remodeling. Mice genetically deficient for ANP exhibit an increase in cardiac mass,[279] whereas heart size is diminished in mice transgenically overexpressing ANP.[280] The antimitogenic and antitrophic effects of NPs, which appear to be cGMP-mediated, have also been demonstrated in a range of cultured cell types, including cultured vascular cells, fibroblasts, and myocytes, and in vivo in response to balloon angioplasty. Further evidence for the role of ANP in mediating cardiac hypertrophy comes from population studies, in which variants in either the ANP promoter (associated with reduced circulating ANP) or in the NPR-A gene have both been associated with left ventricular hypertrophy.[285,286] BNP has been shown to have antifibrotic properties within the heart. In vitro BNP antagonizes TGF-β–induced fibrosis in cultured cardiac fibroblasts,[287] and in vivo targeted genetic disruption of BNP in mice is associated with an increase in cardiac fibrosis, in the absence of either hypertension or ventricular hypertrophy.[288]

Cardiac CNP is increased in heart failure, where it may play a role in ventricular remodeling.[289] Comparison of plasma CNP levels in samples taken from the aorta and renal vein at the time of diagnostic heart catheterization has demonstrated that CNP is indeed synthesized and secreted by the kidney.[290] Moreover, this effect was found to be blunted in patients with heart failure, potentially contributing to renal sodium retention.[290]

OTHER EFFECTS OF THE NATRIURETIC PEPTIDES

Even though they do not cross the blood-brain barrier, NPs exert important CNS effects that may augment their peripheral actions. ANP, BNP, and particularly CNP are all expressed within the brain. Circulating NPs may also exert central effects through actions at sites that are outside the blood-brain barrier. The NPR-B receptor is expressed throughout the CNS, reflecting the wide distribution of CNP, whereas the NPR-A receptor is expressed in areas adjacent to the third ventricle, which indicates a role of peripherally circulating ANP and BNP, as well as centrally expressed peptides. Complementing their natriuretic and diuretic effects, NPs inhibit both salt appetite and water drinking. ANP also prevents release of vasopressin and possibly adrenocorticotropic hormone from the pituitary, whereas sympathetic tone is increased by the actions of the NPs on the brainstem.

Clinical and experimental evidence suggests that NPs play a role in mediating metabolism. Circulating levels of NPs are decreased in obese individuals[291] and among patients with the metabolic syndrome,[292,293] correlating inversely with both plasma glucose and fasting insulin levels.[294] In accordance with these epidemiologic observations, infusion of ANP activates hormone-sensitive lipase from fat cells, indicative of lipolysis.[295] In vitro, ANP inhibits preadipocyte proliferation,[296] the lipolytic properties of the peptide being mediated by cGMP phosphorylation.[297,298]

Knockout mouse studies have revealed that CNP plays a predominant role in the regulation of skeletal growth, regulating cartilage homeostasis and endochondral bone formation.[299] In mice genetically deficient in either CNP or its receptor NPR-B, there is lack of growth of longitudinal bones and vertebrae and a shortened life span as a consequence of respiratory insufficiency secondary to abnormal ossification of the skull and vertebrae.[300,301] Mutations in the NPR-B gene have also been reported in patients with the autosomal recessive skeletal dysplasia, Maroteaux type acromesomelic dysplasia, whereas obligate carriers of the mutations have heights that are below predicted levels.[301]

NATRIURETIC PEPTIDES AS BIOMARKERS OF DISEASE

Both ANP and BNP have been studied as clinical biomarkers of heart failure and renal failure. The short half-life of ANP (2 to 5 minutes) restricts its applicability.[302] However, the biologically inactive NH_2-terminal 98–amino acid peptide ANP 1-98 does not bind to NPR-A or NPR-C and so remains in the circulation longer than ANP. In heart failure, levels of ANP 1-98 closely reflect the degree of renal function.[303] Plasma concentrations of the midregional epitopes of the stable prohormones of both ANP and adrenomedullin predict the progression of renal decline in patients with nondiabetic CKD.[304] The prognostic performance of midregional proANP is not superior to that of NT-proBNP or BNP in patients undergoing hemodialysis,[305] and measurement of ANP or one of its prohormone derivatives is currently not part of routine clinical care. Signal peptides from both ANP and BNP are present in venous blood and rise rapidly following myocardial infarction, which suggests that their detection may aid in the diagnosis of cardiac ischemia.[306,307] Commercial assays are widely available for measurement of either BNP or the biologically inactive peptide fragment NT-proBNP. Correspondingly, since 2000, measurement of circulating BNP and NT-proBNP levels has been incorporated into several clinical practice guidelines for the management of heart failure. Important differences distinguish BNP and NT-proBNP from each other as clinical biomarkers. NT-proBNP is not removed from the circulation by binding to the clearance receptor NPR-C, and hence its circulating half-life of approximately 2 hours is significantly longer than that of BNP (approximately 20 minutes). In addition, both BNP and NT-proBNP are affected by renal impairment,[308] with the magnitude of the effect being relatively greater for NT-proBNP.[309]

BRAIN NATRIURETIC PEPTIDE AND N-TERMINAL PRO–BRAIN NATRIURETIC PEPTIDE AS BIOMARKERS OF HEART FAILURE

Measurement of circulating levels of either BNP or NT-proBNP has been demonstrated to be effective in guiding clinical practice in several aspects of the management of heart failure, including diagnosis, screening, prognosis, and monitoring of therapy.[238] The primary role of BNP measurement in the assessment of dyspnea is as a "rule-out" test; a plasma BNP level lower than 100 pg/mL has a negative predictive value for heart failure of 90%.[310] In the ProBNP Investigation of Dyspnea in the Emergency Department (PRIDE) study, an NT-proBNP level lower than 300 pg/mL was optimal in ruling out heart failure, with a negative predictive value of 99%.[311] In interpreting plasma levels of BNP and NT-proBNP a number of other biologic variables should be taken into account. NP levels rise with age and are higher in females, the latter effect possibly secondary to estrogen regulation, because hormone replacement therapy increases BNP levels.[312] Conversely, NP levels fall with increasing obesity.

ROLE OF BRAIN NATRIURETIC PEPTIDE AND N-TERMINAL PRO–BRAIN NATRIURETIC PEPTIDE AS BIOMARKERS IN RENAL DISEASE

The interpretation of NP concentrations in patients with renal disease merits special consideration. NP levels are increased in individuals with impaired renal function. This increase is likely to be the result of multiple factors and not solely the consequence of increased intravascular volume. Other factors that contribute to increased NP levels include decreased NP responsiveness, subclinical ventricular dysfunction, hypertension, left ventricular hypertrophy, subclinical ischemia, myocardial fibrosis, and RAAS activation,[313] as well as decreased filtration and reduced clearance by NPR-C and NEP.[314]

Although, based on observational studies, it has been widely considered that renal clearance plays a greater role in the removal of NT-proBNP from the circulation than BNP, one study has challenged this view. By measuring both NT-proBNP and BNP in the renal arteries and veins of 165 subjects undergoing renal arteriography, investigators found that both NT-proBNP and BNP are equally dependent on renal clearance.[315] However, the NT-proBNP/BNP ratio did increase with declining GFR, which suggests that the two peptides may be differentially cleared at GFRs less than 30 mL/min/1.73 m².[315]

Even though both BNP and NT-proBNP are affected by renal impairment, their clinical utility for the prediction of heart failure persists in CKD patients, in the context of appropriately adjusted reference ranges. For example, in the Breathing Not Properly study, BNP cutpoint values were approximately threefold higher to diagnose heart failure in patients with an estimated GFR below 60 mL/min relative to the conventional cutpoint value of 100 pg/mL.[316] In a cohort of 831 patients with dyspnea and a GFR below 60 mL/min, both BNP and NT-proBNP were effective predictors of heart failure, although NT-proBNP was superior in predicting mortality.[317] In asymptomatic patients with CKD, both BNP and NT-proBNP were equivalent and effective in indicating the presence of left ventricular hypertrophy or coronary artery disease.[318]

In patients with CKD, BNP and NT-proBNP predict progression of renal decline[319,320] and cardiovascular disease and mortality. In a population of patients with CKD who are not undergoing dialysis, NT-proBNP, but not BNP, was an independent predictor of death,[321] whereas in 994 black patients with hypertensive kidney disease (GFR of 20 to 65 mL/min/1.73 m²), NT-proBNP predicted cardiovascular disease and mortality, particularly among individuals with proteinuria.[322] In pediatric patients with CKD, both BNP and proBNP (but not troponins I and T) were indicative of left ventricular hypertrophy or dysfunction.[323]

BNP and NT-proBNP have been studied extensively in dialysis patients both as prognostic indicators and as markers of volume status. The low molecular weight of BNP (3.5 kDa) and NT-proBNP (8.35 kDa) is such that both may be cleared by high-flux dialysis.[324,325] Nevertheless, in contrast to ANP, which falls sharply after either hemodialysis or peritoneal dialysis, levels of BNP and NT-proBNP are less affected.[324,326] The role of NP levels as indicators of volume status in either hemodialysis or peritoneal dialysis recipients is confounded by the common coexistence of left ventricular abnormalities.[308,316,327-330] Both BNP and NT-proBNP levels are predictive of mortality, heart failure, and coronary artery disease in the dialysis population.[331-336] However, no definite cut-point values for diagnosing heart failure in patients undergoing dialysis have been defined.[316]

THERAPEUTIC USES OF NATRIURETIC PEPTIDES

Even though NP levels are increased in heart failure, their biologic effects are blunted. Intravenous administration of recombinant NPs increases their circulating levels several-fold, overcoming this resistance. As such, two recombinant NPs are currently available as therapeutic agents for the treatment of heart failure. Recombinant ANP (carperitide) is available in Japan for the treatment of pulmonary edema. Recombinant BNP (nesiritide) is licensed in several countries, including the United States, for the treatment of acute decompensated heart failure.

RECOMBINANT ATRIAL NATRIURETIC PEPTIDE

ANP has a short half-life and a high total body clearance. Its intravenous administration causes a reduction in blood pressure, diuresis, and natriuresis in healthy individuals, although this response is reduced in the setting of acute heart failure. In a 6-year open-label study of 3777 patients with acute heart failure treated with carperitide, 82% were reported to improve clinically.[337] Early experimental studies also suggested a potential benefit of exogenous ANP in acute renal failure; however, results in patients have generally been disappointing. Nevertheless, the peptide may have a limited role in selected patient populations. For example, low-dose carperitide preserved renal function in patients undergoing abdominal aortic aneurysm repair[338] and reduced the incidence of contrast-induced nephropathy in patients after coronary angiography.[339] However, a meta-analysis suggested that recombinant ANP has no effect on mortality in patients with acute kidney injury, although a trend toward a reduction in the need for renal replacement therapy was shown.[340] In a separate meta-analysis of studies conducted in patients undergoing cardiovascular surgery, ANP infusion decreased peak serum creatinine level, incidence of arrhythmia, and need for renal replacement therapy, whereas both ANP and BNP decreased the length of intensive care unit and hospital stay.[341] Among 367 high-risk individuals undergoing coronary artery bypass graft, recombinant ANP decreased the incidence of major adverse cardiovascular and cerebrovascular events and the need for dialysis, immediately and up to 2 years postoperatively, although survival was unaffected.[342] Similarly, among patients with CKD undergoing coronary artery bypass graft, those receiving recombinant ANP experienced a smaller rise in serum creatinine level, fewer cardiac events, and lower requirement for dialysis, although mortality did not differ from those who did not receive ANP.[343]

RECOMBINANT BRAIN NATRIURETIC PEPTIDE

Nesiritide is recombinant human BNP, manufactured from *Escherichia coli* and identical in structure to native human BNP, with a mean terminal half-life in patients with heart failure of 18 minutes.[344] Intravenous administration of nesiritide lowers pulmonary and systemic vascular resistance, decreases right atrial pressure, and increases cardiac output (presumably through effects on ventricular afterload) in a dose-dependent manner.[345] In the kidney, nesiritide increases renal blood flow and GFR through both direct vasodilatory effects and indirect effects on cardiac output and norepinephrine inhibition.[346] Diuresis and natriuresis may also occur, although these are modest and may not be seen at the approved doses. Additional effects of nesiritide may also include inhibition of renin secretion in the kidney and aldosterone production in the heart and adrenal gland.

In response to meta-analysis data suggesting that nesiritide treatment may be associated with a worsening of renal function and an increase in the rate of early death,[347,348] the Acute Study of Clinical Effectiveness of Nesiritide in Decompensated Heart Failure (ASCEND-HF) trial was initiated.[349] In this study of 7141 patients hospitalized with acute heart failure, nesiritide neither increased nor decreased the rate of death or rehospitalization, rates of worsening renal function were unaffected, and there was a small but nonsignificant improvement in self-reported rates of dyspnea.[349] Based on these results, the investigators concluded that nesiritide cannot be recommended for routine use in the broad population of patients with acute heart failure.[349]

THERAPEUTIC USES OF OTHER NATRIURETIC PEPTIDES

The effects of urodilatin (ularitide) have been assessed in both heart failure and acute renal failure. However, the diuretic effect of urodilatin appears to be attenuated in heart failure patients, reflecting a blunted response as observed for ANP and BNP.[350,351] Similarly, as with ANP and BNP, hypotension appears to be a dose-limiting side effect of ularitide therapy.[351,352] In the Safety and Efficacy of an Intravenous Placebo-Controlled Randomized Infusion of Ularitide in a Prospective Double-blind Study in Patients with Symptomatic, Decompensated Chronic Heart Failure (SIRIUS II) study, a phase II trial of 221 patients hospitalized for decompensated heart failure, a single 24-hour infusion of ularitide preserved short-term renal function.[353] The NP vessel dilator may offer theoretical advantages for the treatment of acute decompensated heart failure in comparison with current NP-based therapies.[354,355] In particular, vessel dilator may produce a greater and more sustained natriuresis than ANP or BNP, without a blunted response in heart failure patients, and may also improve renal function in the setting of experimental acute kidney injury.[356] An alternative therapeutic approach is the development of novel chimeric peptides. For example, researchers have synthesized a peptide (CD-NP) that represents fusion of the 22–amino acid peptide CNP together with the 15–amino acid linear C terminus of DNP.[357] In vitro, this peptide activates cGMP and attenuates cardiac fibroblast proliferation.

In vivo, CD-NP is both natriuretic and diuretic and increases GFR with less hypotension than BNP.[357,358]

NEUTRAL ENDOPEPTIDASE INHIBITION

Notwithstanding concerns regarding the safety, efficacy, and cost-effectiveness of recombinant NP therapy, a major limitation is the requirement for systemic administration, which is unsuitable for chronic treatment. Alternative methods to increase the biologic activity of NPs may offer a more feasible approach for chronic therapy. In particular, inhibition of the enzymatic degradation of NPs by NEP has been the focus of drug discovery efforts for a number of years. NEP is a zinc metallopeptidase with catalytic similarity to ACE and with a wide tissue distribution, although abundant at the proximal tubule brush border. The enzyme has activity against a number of substrates, including the vasodilating peptides ANP, BNP, CNP, substance P, bradykinin, and adrenomedullin and the vasoconstrictors angiotensin II and ET-1. Several pharmacologic NEP inhibitors have been investigated (e.g., candoxatril, thiorphan, and phosphoramidon). Although these agents do in general increase plasma levels of the NPs and, under some experimental conditions, induce natriuresis and diuresis with peripheral vasodilation, clinical trials in hypertension and heart failure have generally been disappointing. Specifically, sustained antihypertensive effects have not been demonstrated, and some studies have reported a paradoxical rise in blood pressure. The biologic actions of the NPs are, however, restored in the presence of an inhibited RAAS, and this has led to the development of compounds that simultaneously inhibit both NEP and ACE, termed *vasopeptidase inhibitors* (VPIs).

VASOPEPTIDASE INHIBITORS

The rational design of metallopeptidase inhibitors (e.g., mixanpril [S21402], CGS30440, aladotril, MDL 100173, sampatrilat, and omapatrilat) is possible because of the similar structural characteristics of the catalytic sites of both ACE and NEP.[276] These VPIs have theoretical advantages over antagonists of either enzyme in isolation, and a number of preclinical studies have demonstrated their efficacy in experimental models of cardiovascular and renal disease. However, phase III clinical studies have not been able to demonstrate superiority of vasopeptidase inhibition over ACE inhibition, and safety concerns exist over an increase in the incidence of angioedema. As a result, development and clinical application of these compounds have been limited.

Although effective against both ACE and NEP, VPIs differ in their relative potencies for each enzyme. For example, the most extensively studied VPI, omapatrilat, has broadly equivalent potency for NEP (affinity constant [K_i] = 8.9 nmol) and for ACE (K_i = 6.0 nmol), whereas the VPI gemopatrilat has an efficacy almost 100 times greater for ACE (K_i = 3.6 nmol) than for NEP (K_i = 305 nmol).[359] The broad substrate specificities of VPIs can also be expected to result in an increase in ET, adrenomedullin, and bradykinin and a reduction in the synthesis of angiotensin-(1-7). Omapatrilat lowers blood pressure and attenuates heart failure in experimental models, associated with dose-dependent increases in ANP and cGMP excretion, diuresis, natriuresis, and decreased plasma renin activity (although a paradoxical increase in plasma renin activity has also been reported).[359] In the remnant kidney model, VPIs have consistently been found to be as effective as or better than ACE inhibitors,[360-362] with similar benefits reported in diabetic apolipoprotein E–knockout mice.[363]

In contrast to the promising findings in preclinical models, trials of VPIs in human disease have, on the whole, been disappointing. In the Inhibition of Metalloproteinase in a Randomized Exercise and Symptoms Study (IMPRESS) in heart failure of patients with New York heart Association classes II to IV congestive heart failure, there was no difference between omapatrilat and lisinopril in the primary end point of maximum exercise tolerance at 12 weeks.[364] The Omapatrilat Cardiovascular Treatment vs. Enalapril (OCTAVE) trial randomly assigned 25,302 hypertensive patients to receive omapatrilat or enalapril.[365] Omapatrilat treatment was associated with a reduction in systolic blood pressure that was 3.6 mm Hg greater than that associated with enalapril. However, angioedema occurred in 2.17% of patients treated with omapatrilat, compared with 0.68% in the group treated with enalapril.[365] This concerning side effect was even more common among black patients.[365] In the Omapatrilat Versus Enalapril Randomized Trial of Utility in Reducing Events (OVERTURE), there was no difference between enalapril and omapatrilat in the primary end point of combined risk for death or hospitalization for heart failure requiring intravenous treatment, although a post hoc analysis showed a significant 9% reduction in cardiovascular death or hospitalization.[366] In this trial the incidence of angioedema was again increased in the omapatrilat group compared to patients treated with enalapril (0.8% vs. 0.5%).[366] In general, the side effects of VPIs are qualitatively similar to those of ACE inhibitors, including cough (in approximately 10% of patients), dizziness, and postural hypotension.[366,367] Flushing appears more commonly with VPIs than with ACE inhibitors, which may be a consequence of increased circulating adrenomedullin concentrations.[368]

COMBINATION ANGIOTENSIN RECEPTOR BLOCKERS AND NEUTRAL ENDOPEPTIDASE INHIBITORS

To circumvent the adverse effects experienced with VPIs, a novel drug class has been developed that combines the action of both an ARB and an NEP inhibitor, termed an angiotensin receptor–neprilysin inhibitor (ARNi).[369] For instance, the compound LCZ696 is a single molecule comprised of molecular moieties of the ARB valsartan and the NEP inhibitor prodrug AHU377 in a 1:1 ratio.[370] In a study of 1328 patients, LCZ696 conferred greater blood pressure lowering than valsartan alone with no cases of angioedema reported.[371] In a phase II study of 149 individuals with heart failure with preserved ejection fraction, LCZ696 lowered NT-proBNP to a greater extent than valsartan and was well tolerated.[372] The efficacy of LCZ696 in comparison to enalapril for the treatment of systolic heart failure was assessed in the Prospective comparison of ARNI with ACEI to Determine Impact on Global Mortality and morbidity in Heart Failure trial (PARADIGM-HF); the study reported that LCZ696 was superior to enalapril in reducing the risks for death and for hospitalization for heart failure.[373] Other molecules combining ARB and NEP inhibition are also currently under development.[374,375]

OTHER NATRIURETIC PEPTIDES

GUANYLIN AND UROGUANYLIN

The existence of intestinal NPs has been suggested by initial observations that sodium excretion is greater after an oral salt load than after an intravenous salt load.[376,377] These intestinal peptides include guanylin and uroguanylin. However, a study of 15 healthy volunteers found that sodium excretion was similar in response to either oral or intravenous sodium load during either a low- or high-sodium–containing diet.[378] Moreover, serum concentrations of either prouroguanylin or proguanylin were unchanged following either oral or intravenous sodium load and showed no correlation with sodium excretion.[378] Collectively, these observations challenge the notion of a gastrointestinal-renal natriuretic axis mediated by the guanylin peptide family.[378,379] It thus appears likely that the natriuretic, kaliuretic, and diuretic effects of guanylin and uroguanylin, which occur without change in GFR or renal blood flow, are mediated by local production of the peptides within the kidney.[379]

ADRENOMEDULLIN

Adrenomedullin is a 52–amino acid peptide originally isolated from human pheochromocytoma cells,[380] although mainly synthesized by vascular smooth muscle cells, endothelial cells, and macrophages[381] and present in the plasma, vasculature, lungs, heart, and adipose tissue. The peptide is upregulated in patients with cardiovascular disease and has positive inotropic and vasodilatory properties. Systemic administration of adrenomedullin induces a nitric oxide–dependent natriuresis and increase in GFR both under normal conditions and in patients with congestive heart failure, also decreasing plasma aldosterone level without affecting renin activity.

KALLIKREIN-KININ SYSTEM

The kallikrein-kinin system (KKS) is a complex network of peptide hormones, receptors, and peptidases that is evolutionarily conserved with homologs in nonmammalian species.[382] Discovery of the KKS is attributed to Abelous and Bardier, who reported in 1909 that experimental injection of urine resulted in an acute fall in systemic blood pressure. Since that time, it has been recognized that the physiologic actions of the KKS also include regulation of tissue blood flow, transepithelial water and electrolyte transport, cellular growth, capillary permeability, and inflammatory responses. The main components of the KKS are the enzyme kallikrein, its substrate kininogen, effector hormones known as *kinins* (including bradykinin and kallidin [also termed lysyl-bradykinin]) and their inactivating enzymes, which include kininases I and II (ACE) and neutral endopeptidase EC 24.11 (NEP, neprilysin).

Kinins exert their biologic effects through binding to two receptors, the type 1 (B1R) and type 2 (B2R) receptors, with B2R being widely expressed and mediating all of the physiologic actions of the kinins under physiologic conditions. The B1R is activated predominantly by des-Arg-bradykinin, a natural degradation product of bradykinin, generated by cleavage of the peptide by kininase I. The KKS may be subdivided into a circulatory (plasma) and tissue (including renal) KKS, which may be distinguished by their principal effector molecules, bradykinin and kallidin, respectively. In the kidney the kinins play a significant role in the modulation of renal hemodynamics and salt and water homeostasis.

COMPONENTS OF THE KALLIKREIN-KININ SYSTEM

KININOGEN

Humans possess a single kininogen gene, which is localized to chromosome 3q26 and encodes both high-molecular-weight (HMW) (626 amino acids, 88 to 120 kDa) and low-molecular-weight (LMW) (409 amino acids, 50 to 68 kDa) kininogens via alternate splicing from 11 exons spread over a 27-kb span. A second kininogen gene has been identified in mice.[383] In humans, kininogen deficiency may be relatively asymptomatic,[384] though the kininogen-deficient Brown Norway Katholiek rat strain shows increased sensitivity to the pressor effects of salt, angiotensin II, and mineralocorticoid.[385,386]

KALLIKREIN

HMW and LMW kininogen are cleaved by the serine protease kallikrein. The name *kallikrein* is derived from the Greek term *kallikreas*, meaning "pancreas," after the work of Frey and others, in the 1930s, who extracted a kinin-producing enzyme from the pancreas of dogs. Since then, 15 tissue kallikreins have been identified, although, in humans, only one (KLK1) is involved in local kinin production. The human kallikrein genes are clustered on chromosome 19 at q13.3-13.4. Plasma kallikrein is found in the circulation and is largely concerned with the coagulation cascade and activation of neutrophils. The tissue kallikreins are acid glycoproteins that are variably and extensively glycosylated. Human renal kallikrein is synthesized as a zymogen (prekallikrein) with a 17–amino acid signal peptide and a 7–amino acid activation sequence, which must be cleaved to activate the enzyme. In most mammals, including humans, tissue kallikrein cleaves kallidin (lysyl-bradykinin) from kininogens, whereas plasma kallikrein releases bradykinin.

Although the physiologic effects of kallikrein have been attributed to increased kinin generation, the enzyme may also have direct effects on the B2R, as well as actions independent of the kinin receptors.[387,388] For example, local injection of kallikrein into the myocardium following coronary artery ligation in kininogen-deficient Brown Norway Katholiek rats had a cardioprotective effect that was abolished by the nitric oxide synthase inhibitor Nω-nitro-L-arginine methylester and the selective B2R inhibitor icatibant (Hoe 140).[387] As a serine protease, kallikrein may also elicit kinin receptor–independent effects on endothelial cell migration and survival through cleavage of growth factors and matrix metalloproteinases.[389] Transgenic mice overexpressing human kallikrein exhibit a sustained reduction in systemic blood pressure throughout their life span, indicating the lack of sufficient compensatory mechanisms to reverse the hypotensive effect of kallikrein.[390] In humans, polymorphisms of the kallikrein gene *KLK1* or its promoter can impair enzymatic activity, potentially affecting both kinin-dependent and kinin-independent effects. Among normotensive men with a common loss-of-function *KLK1* polymorphism (R53H), an increase in wall shear stress and a paradoxical reduction in artery diameter and lumen were noted, although flow-mediated and endothelium-independent vasodilation were unaffected.[391]

KININS

The kinins are bradykinin and kallidin in humans and bradykinin and kallidin-like peptide in rodents.[392] Plasma aminopeptidase can convert kallidin (10 amino acids, Lys-Arg-Pro-Pro-Gly-Phe-Ser-Pro-Phe-Arg) to bradykinin (9 amino acids, Arg-Pro-Pro-Gly-Phe-Ser-Pro-Phe-Arg) by cleavage of the first N-terminal lysine residue. Cleavage of the carboxy-terminal arginine residue by kininase I (carboxypeptidase-N) and carboxypeptidase-M generates their des-Arg derivatives, which are agonists of the B1 receptor.[392] Removal of two carboxy-terminal amino acids (Phe and Arg) by ACE (kininase II), NEP, or ECE is responsible for inactivation of the peptides.[392]

BRADYKININ RECEPTORS

The bradykinin receptors, B1R and B2R, share 36% homology and are both G protein–coupled receptors with seven transmembrane domains. The genes for the two receptors are in tandem on a compact locus (14q23) separated by only 12 kb.[393] The B2R is the principal receptor mediating the actions of both of the kinins, is expressed in abundance by vascular endothelial cells, and is present in most tissues, including kidney, heart, skeletal muscle, CNS, vas deferens, trachea, intestine, uterus, and bladder. In general, B1Rs have a similar distribution and action to B2Rs. The B1R, on the other hand, is expressed at low levels under normal conditions but is upregulated in response to inflammatory stimuli (e.g., lipopolysaccharide, endotoxins, and cytokines such as IL-1β and TNF-α)[394] and in the setting of diabetes[395] and ischemia-reperfusion injury.[396] B2R binds both bradykinin and kallidin, whereas bradykinin has almost no effect at the B1R. The carboxypeptidase required to generate the des-Arg B1R-active kinin fragments is closely associated with the B1R on the cell surface.[397] This association would enable B2R agonists to rapidly activate B1Rs, particularly in response to inflammation.[397]

Ligand binding of both receptor subtypes induces activation of phospholipase C, which results in intracellular calcium mobilization through production of inositol 1,4,5-triphosphate and diacylglycerol via activation of G proteins, including $G\alpha_q$ and $G\alpha_i$. The physiologic effects of bradykinin receptor activation are mediated through generation of both endothelial nitric oxide synthase and prostaglandins. B2R activation leads to a rise in intracellular calcium concentrations in vascular endothelial cells.[392] However, bradykinin-induced vasodilation is not abolished by coadministration of nitric oxide synthase and cyclo-oxygenase inhibitors, indicating that additional effectors are likely to be involved, possibly an endothelium-derived hyperpolarizing factor. In addition, through binding to both B1R[398] and B2R,[399] bradykinin increases the expression of inducible nitric oxide synthase, at least in rodents. It is very difficult to induce the inducible nitric oxide synthase gene in human tissues, especially the vascular endothelium. Mice that have genetic deficiencies of B2R,[400] B1R,[401] or both receptors[402] have been generated; the reported phenotypes of the different knockout strains have been varied, which may be a result of different genetic backgrounds, or, in the case of the single knockouts, differing compensatory effects of the remaining receptor. For example, some studies of B2R-deficient mice report an increase in resting systemic blood pressure, an exaggerated pressor response to angiotensin II,[403] and salt sensitivity,[404] whereas others report no difference in resting blood pressure between mice that are B2R or B1R deficient and wild-type animals.[401,405] Double B2R-/B1R-knockout mice were also reported to have resting blood pressure identical to that of wild-type mice and were resistant to lipopolysaccharide (LPS)-induced hypotension.[402,406] In contrast, transgenic mice expressing the human B2R had a lower resting blood pressure compared to controls.[407] Transgenic mice expressing the rat B1R (as well as their native murine B2R) were normotensive but showed an exaggerated hypotensive response to LPS and, unexpectedly, a hypertensive response to des-Arg bradykinin.[408]

KALLISTATIN

Kallistatin is an endogenous serpin inhibitor of kallikrein that acts by forming a heat-stable complex with the enzyme. Surprisingly, administration of human kallistatin to rodents induced vasodilation and a decline in systemic blood pressure, which was unaltered by either a nitric oxide synthase inhibitor or the B2R antagonist icatibant, suggesting that the vasodilatory properties of kallistatin may be mediated through a smooth muscle mechanism independent of bradykinin receptor activation.[409]

KININASES

With the exception of the metabolites des-Arg-bradykinin and des-Arg-kallidin, kinin-cleavage products are biologically inactive. Kinins are cleaved by a number of enzymes, including carboxypeptidases, ACE, and NEP. ACE also truncates its own reaction product, bradykinin-(1-7) further to form bradykinin-(1-5). NEP, like ACE, cleaves bradykinin at the 7-8 position and has a broad substrate specificity including, not only the kinins, but also the NPs, substance P, angiotensin II, big ET, enkephalins, oxytocin, and gastrin. The amino-terminal of bradykinin possesses two proline residues and is susceptible to cleavage by the proline-specific exopeptidase aminopeptidase P. The resultant peptide, bradykinin-(2-9) may be further cleaved by proteases that include the endothelial enzyme dipeptidyl aminopeptidase IV, which reduces this metabolite to bradykinin-(4-9).

PLASMA AND TISSUE KALLIKREIN-KININ SYSTEM

The two independent KKSs in humans (plasma and tissue) can be distinguished by the specific subtypes of kallikreins, kininogens, and kinins involved. The circulating plasma KKS includes HMW kininogen and plasma prekallikrein, both of which are synthesized in the liver and secreted in the plasma, where kallikrein is generated by the cell matrix–associated prekallikrein activator, prolylcarboxypeptidase.[410] Bradykinin is the effector molecule of the plasma KKS. The tissue-specific KKS, including that of the kidney, consists of locally synthesized or liver-derived kininogen (HMW and LMW), tissue kallikrein, and the effector molecules kallidin

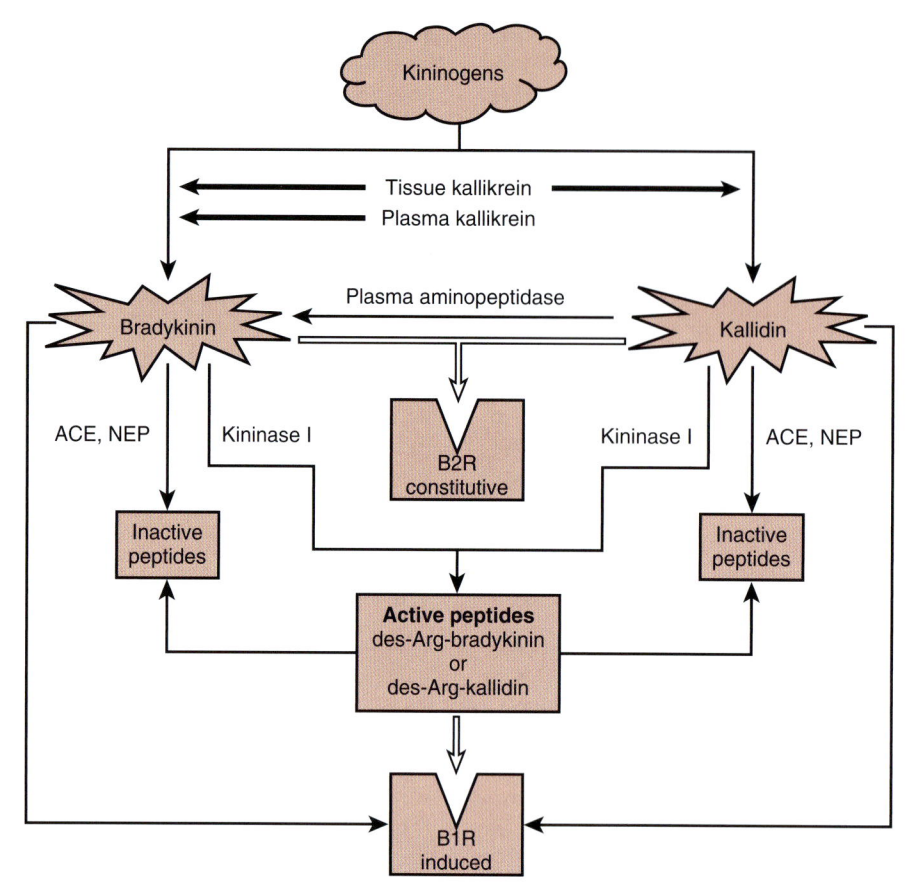

Figure 13.7 Enzymatic cascade of the kallikrein-kinin system. ACE, Angiotensin-converting enzyme; B1R, bradykinin B1 receptor; B2R, bradykinin B2 receptor; NEP, neutral endopeptidase.

in humans and kallidin-like peptide in rodents. The half-life of kinins is 10 to 30 seconds, but in tissues with high kallikrein content, such as the kidney, local and plasma-derived LMW kininogen can be continuously cleaved to produce kallidin.

Figure 13.7 illustrates the enzymatic cascades of the plasma and tissue KKSs.

RENAL KALLIKREIN-KININ SYSTEM

The tissue KKS contributes to the physiologic functions of the kidneys with effects on renal vascular resistance, natriuresis, diuresis, and other vasoactive mediators, including renin and angiotensin, eicosanoids, catecholamines, nitric oxide, vasopressin, and ET. In the kidney, large quantities of kininogen and kallikrein are synthesized by the tubular epithelium and are excreted in the urine. Locally formed kinin is also detectable in the urine, renal interstitial fluid, and renal venous blood.

In the human kidney, kallikrein is localized to the connecting tubules with close anatomic association between the kallikrein-expressing tubules and the afferent arterioles of the JGA. Some studies suggest that renal kallikrein mRNA is also detectable by in situ hybridization at the glomerular vascular pole. This anatomic association highlights the physiologic relationship between the KKS and the RAAS and is consistent with a paracrine function for the KKS in the regulation of renal blood flow, GFR, and renin release. In this regard it has been suggested that, through effects on prostaglandin production, kinins may lower tubuloglomerular feedback sensitivity.

Expression of kallikrein within the kidney is altered during development and is regulated by estrogen and progesterone, salt intake, thyroid hormone, and glucocorticoids.[411-414] The enzyme is not normally filtered at the glomerulus, in the absence of glomerular injury. Kininogens are localized mostly to connecting tubular principal cells in close proximity to kallikrein, which can be found in the connecting tubules of the same nephron. Once activated, renal kallikrein cleaves both HMW and LMW kininogens to release kallidin. The majority of the physiologic effects of kinins are mediated via activation of constitutively expressed B2Rs, with little or no B1R mRNA detectable in normal kidney. In rats, administration of LPS, however, induces expression of B1R throughout the nephron (except the outer medullary collecting ducts), with strong expression in the efferent arteriole, medullary limb, and distal tubule.[415]

The KKS is involved in the regulation of renal hemodynamics and tubular function with diuretic and natriuretic effects playing a pivotal role in the contribution of the renal KKS to fluid and electrolyte balance. Kinins have been reported to increase renal blood flow and papillary blood flow and to mediate the hyperfiltration induced by a high-protein diet. Kinins also inhibit conductive sodium entry in the IMCDs,[416] and B2R-deficient mice demonstrate increased urinary concentration in response to vasopressin, which indicates that, through the B2R, endogenous kinins oppose the antidiuretic effect of vasopressin.[417] Kinins may therefore affect sodium reabsorption through direct effects on sodium transport along the nephron, vasodilatory effects, and changes in the osmotic gradient of the renal medulla. In addition to the effects on renal vascular tone and salt and water homeostasis, evidence, primarily derived from experiments employing the B2R antagonist icatibant, suggests that kinins may also have antihypertrophic and antiproliferative properties in mesangial cells, fibroblasts, and renomedullary interstitial cells. The antiproliferative effect of bradykinin in mesangial cells may be mediated through interaction of the B2R with the protein-tyrosine phosphatase SH2 domain–containing phosphatase-2 (SHP-2).[418]

REGULATION OF TUBULAR TRANSPORT BY TISSUE KALLIKREIN

Independent of its ability to generate kinin, tissue kallikrein also exerts separate effects on tubular solute transport by regulating the activity of the epithelial sodium channel (ENaC), the colonic H^+-K^+-ATPase and the epithelial calcium channel TRPV5 (transient receptor potential cation channel subfamily V member 5).[419] The connecting tubules secrete a large amount of tissue kallikrein, which, through its enzymatic activity, can alter the function of ion transporters expressed on the luminal surface of cells downstream of its site of secretion.[419] For instance, tissue kallikrein may participate in the proteolytic processing of ENaC, increasing its activity, whereas tissue kallikrein–deficient mice have decreased ENaC activity.[420] Despite decreased ENaC activity, however, coincident upregulation of ENaC-independent electroneutral NaCl absorption ensures that tissue kallikrein is not essential for sodium homeostasis.[419,421] The cortical collecting ducts from tissue kallikrein–deficient mice also demonstrate enhanced activity of the colonic H^+-K^+-ATPase in intercalated cells, resulting in net K^+ absorption.[419,422] Finally, tissue kallikrein functions to stabilize the TRPV5 channel at the plasma membrane, promoting Ca^{2+} reabsorption, whereas tissue kallikrein–knockout mice exhibit robust hypercalciuria.[423] Distal tubular defects in potassium[424] and calcium[425] handling have also been reported in humans with the loss-of-function R53H polymorphism in the tissue kallikrein gene.

KALLIKREIN-KININ SYSTEM IN RENAL DISEASE

HYPERTENSION

Although it has been known for many years that kinin infusion results in an acute drop in systemic blood pressure by reducing peripheral resistance, the role of the KKS in mediating primary or secondary hypertension has yet to be fully established. Decreased activity of kallikrein has been reported in the urine of hypertensive patients and hypertensive rats. An inverse relationship between urinary kallikrein excretion and blood pressure in humans may be interpreted as suggesting a role for the renal KKS in protecting against hypertension.[426] However, an alternative interpretation may be that preexisting or hypertension-induced kidney disease may itself lead to a reduction in renal kallikrein excretion. In the Dahl salt-sensitive rat model of hypertension, ACE inhibitors are superior to angiotensin II receptor blockers in attenuating the progression of proteinuria and hypertensive nephrosclerosis.[427] That this difference may be mediated by enhanced kinin activity with ACE inhibition is supported by the observations that infusion of either kallikrein[428] or bradykinin[429] in this model attenuated glomerulosclerosis without affecting blood pressure. Studies in two-kidney–one-clip hypertension have been conflicting. The incidence of two-kidney–one-clip hypertension was increased in B2R-deficient mice, in comparison with wild-type animals.[430] In contrast, when comparing the response between tissue kallikrein–deficient mice and wild-type animals, there was no difference with respect to kidney size, renin release, systemic blood pressure increase, and cardiac remodeling.[431]

Despite the uncertainty about the role of the KKS in mediating the pathogenesis of hypertension, a variety of genetic mutations of the KKS have been associated with hypertension in animal models and in humans.[432] Inactivating mutations in the kallikrein gene have been identified in spontaneously hypertensive rats,[433] and an association between mutations in the regulatory region of the kallikrein gene *KLK1* and hypertension has also been described in African Americans[434] and Chinese Han people.[435] The loss-of-function *KLK1* R53H mutation is found in 5% to 7% of the white population,[436] but this one single-nucleotide polymorphism (SNP) has not in itself been found to markedly alter blood pressure.[437] ACE polymorphisms, responsible for different plasma levels of the enzyme and, accordingly, altered kinin levels, have been identified as independent risk factors for progression of various diseases, including diabetic nephropathy, but they do not affect blood pressure. Finally, a number of SNPs in both the B2R and B1R genes have been associated with hypertension[438,439] and coronary risk in hypertensive individuals.[440]

DIABETIC NEPHROPATHY

Observations in both experimental animal models and in humans indicate a role for altered KKS activity in the pathogenesis of diabetic nephropathy, although results in experimental studies have been conflicting. The KKS is markedly altered in streptozotocin-diabetic rats, with changes correlating with those in renal plasma flow and GFR.[441] Renal and urinary levels of active kallikrein are increased in streptozotocin-diabetic rats with moderate hyperglycemia associated with reduced renal vascular resistance, increased GFR, and increased renal plasma flow. Treatment of diabetic rats with the kallikrein inhibitor aprotinin or with a B2R antagonist reduced renal blood flow and GFR.[441] In contrast, in non–insulin-treated streptozotocin-treated rats with severe hyperglycemia and hypofiltration, kallikrein excretion and expression were reduced.[441,442] In addition to its hemodynamic effects, the KKS may also play a renoprotective role in diabetic nephropathy through its antiinflammatory and antiproliferative properties.[394]

Results of receptor antagonist studies initially suggested that there was a limited role for the KKS in preserving renal structure and function in diabetic nephropathy, in which treatment of diabetic rats with icatibant had no effect on glomerular structure and albuminuria, nor did it alter the attenuating effect of ACE inhibition on either of these parameters.[443] Contrasting this, however, more contemporary work suggests that the beneficial effects of ACE inhibitors in experimental diabetic nephropathy may be attenuated by coadministration of a B2R antagonist.[444-446] For instance, in Akita diabetic mice lacking the B2R, there was a marked increase in mesangial sclerosis and albuminuria,[447] associated with an increase in oxidative stress and mitochondrial damage[448]; however, another study reported that B2R-knockout mice were relatively protected from the renal injury induced by streptozotocin diabetes.[449] Upregulation of B1R occurs in response to B2R knockout and could plausibly contribute to renal pathologic processes or alternatively confer a renoprotective benefit. In support of a renoprotective effect, Akita diabetic mice deficient in both B2R and B1R exhibited augmented renal injury in comparison to those lacking B2R alone.[450]

In further support of a renoprotective effect of the KKS in diabetic nephropathy, one study showed that induction of diabetes by streptozotocin in mice caused a twofold increase in mRNA for kininogen, tissue kallikrein, kinins, and kinin receptors, with a doubling in albumin excretion in kallikrein-knockout mice in comparison with wild-type animals.[451] In another study, gene delivery of human tissue kallikrein with an adeno-associated viral vector attenuated renal injury in diabetes and decreased urinary albumin excretion.[452]

Urinary kallikrein excretion in patients with type 1 diabetes demonstrates a similar association with GFR as observed in streptozotocin-diabetic rats.[453] Active kallikrein excretion is increased in hyperfiltering individuals compared to patients with type 1 diabetes with a normal GFR and normal controls and correlates with both GFR and distal tubular sodium reabsorption.[453] Results of genetic association studies in patients with diabetes have, however, been conflicting. Whereas one study reported an association between B2R polymorphisms and albuminuria in 49 patients with type 1 diabetes and 112 patients with type 2 diabetes,[454] another found no association between either B1R or B2R polymorphisms and incipient or overt nephropathy in 285 patients with type 2 diabetes.[455] Plasma levels of HMW kininogen fragments were observed to be elevated among individuals with type 1 diabetes and progressive renal decline.[456]

ISCHEMIC RENAL INJURY

In models of ischemia-reperfusion injury, ACE inhibitors appear to be superior to ARBs in protecting against tubular necrosis, loss of endothelial function, and excretory dysfunction.[457] This superiority may be due to enhanced kinin activity with ACE inhibition because the effect is negated by B2R antagonists and inhibitors of nitric oxide synthase.[458,459] Bradykinin suppresses the opening of mitochondrial pores,[460] and nitric oxide suppresses oxidative metabolism; both observations indicate that the KKS may exert its protective effects in ischemia-reperfusion injury through attenuation of oxidative damage. In mice genetically deficient in either the B2R alone or both B1R and B2R, ischemic damage was enhanced compared to wild-type mice, with injury being most severe in mice that lacked both receptors.[406] In contrast, tissue kallikrein infusion aggravated renal ischemia-reperfusion injury in rats.[461] Thus, although physiologic kinin levels may be protective in this setting, higher levels may be detrimental, possibly through pathologic reperfusion.[392]

CHRONIC KIDNEY DISEASE

In the remnant kidney model of progressive renal disease, adenovirus-mediated or adeno-associated virus–mediated gene delivery of kallikrein attenuated the decline in renal function.[462] In the model of unilateral ureteric obstruction, both genetic ablation of the B2R and pharmacologic blockade of the B2R increased tubulointerstitial fibrosis.[463] In contrast, expression of the B1R was increased after unilateral ureteric obstruction,[464] and treatment with a nonpeptide B1R antagonist reduced macrophage infiltration and fibrosis.[464] In the same model, B1R-deficient mice similarly showed less upregulation of inflammatory cytokines, reduced albumin excretion, and diminished fibrosis compared with wild-type mice.[465] In an adriamycin-induced mouse model of focal segmental glomerulosclerosis, B1R-antagonist therapy attenuated and B1R-agonist therapy aggravated renal dysfunction.[466] Together, these observations suggest that, although the B2R is renoprotective, under some circumstances (and in contrast to the observations made in Akita diabetic B1R-/B2R-knockout mice) compensatory B1R upregulation may contribute to the pathogenesis of renal fibrosis. In humans, polymorphisms in both the B1R gene[467,468] and B2R gene[467,469] have been associated with the development of ESKD.

LUPUS NEPHRITIS/ANTI–GLOMERULAR BASEMENT MEMBRANE DISEASE

Evidence has linked the KKS to the pathogenesis of the immune-mediated nephritides SLE, Goodpasture's syndrome (anti–glomerular basement membrane [anti-GBM] disease), and spontaneous lupus nephritis. Mice strains differ in their susceptibility to anti-GBM antibody-induced nephritis. Comparison of disease-sensitive and control strains, by microarray analysis of renal cortical tissue, revealed that 360 gene transcripts were differentially expressed.[470] Of the underexpressed genes, one fifth belonged to the kallikrein gene family.[470] Furthermore, in disease-sensitive mice, B2R antagonism augmented proteinuria after anti-GBM challenge, whereas bradykinin administration attenuated disease.[470] In the same study, SNPs in the *KLK1* and *KLK3* promoters were also described in patients with SLE and lupus nephritis.[470] Extending their work further, the same investigators showed that adenoviral delivery of the *KLK1* gene attenuated renal injury in congenic mice possessing a lupus-susceptibility interval on chromosome 7.[471]

ANTINEUTROPHIL CYTOPLASMIC ANTIBODY–ASSOCIATED VASCULITIS

Granulomatosis with polyangiitis (formerly known as Wegener's granulomatosis), antineutrophil cytoplasmic antibody–associated vasculitis (AAV) may be associated with a necrotizing glomerulonephritis. The major antigenic target in granulomatosis with polyangiitis AAV is neutrophil-derived proteinase 3 (PR3). Incubation of PR3 with HMW kininogen resulted in the generation of a novel tridecapeptide kinin, termed *PR3-kinin*.[472] PR3-kinin binds to B1R directly and can also activate B2R after further processing to form bradykinin.[472] These observations suggest that, in granulomatosis with polyangiitis AAV, PR3 may activate the kinin pathway in a kallikrein-independent manner. B1R upregulation has been observed in biopsy specimens from patients with Henoch-Schönlein purpura nephropathy or with AAV.[473] Similarly, B1R upregulation was also observed in a murine serum-induced glomerulonephritis model, whereas treatment with a B1R antagonist attenuated renal decline.[473]

UROTENSIN II

Urotensin II (U-II) is a potent vasoactive cyclic undecapeptide originally isolated from the caudal neurosecretory organ of teleost fish. The two principal regulatory peptides derived from this organ are urotensin I (U-I), which is homologous to mammalian corticotropin-releasing factor, and U-II, which bears sequence similarity to somatostatin[474] and has notable hemodynamic, gastrointestinal, reproductive, osmoregulatory, and metabolic functions in fish. Homologs of U-II have been identified in many species, including humans.

SYNTHESIS, STRUCTURE, AND SECRETION OF UROTENSIN II

Human U-II is derived from two prepropeptide alternate splice variants of 124 and 139 amino acids, differing only in the amino-terminal sequence.[475,476] The C terminus is cleaved by prohormone convertases to yield the mature 11–amino acid U-II peptide. U-II contains a cyclic Cys-Phe-Trp-Lys-Tyr-Cys hexapeptide sequence that is conserved across species and is essential for its biologic activity (Figure 13.8).[477] The N-terminal region of the precursor is highly variable across species.

Prepro–U-II mRNA has been described in a range of cell types, including vascular smooth muscle cells, endothelial cells, neuronal cells, and cardiac fibroblasts. Multiple monobasic and polybasic amino acid sequences have been identified as posttranslational cleavage sites of the prohormone. However, a specific U-II–converting enzyme has not yet been described. With respect to its tissue distribution, immunohistochemical staining has identified U-II protein in the blood vessels of various organs and also within the tubular epithelial cells of the kidney.[474,478,479] A significant arteriovenous gradient exists across the heart, liver, and kidney, indicating that these organs are important sites of U-II production.[480]

In 1999 Ames and colleagues identified U-II to be the ligand for the previously orphan rat receptor GPR14/SENR.[476] The U-II receptor is a seven-transmembrane, G protein–coupled receptor encoded on chromosome 17q25.3 in humans.[481] The U-II receptor bears structural similarity to both somatostatin receptor subtype 4 and the opioid receptors. Ligand binding of the receptor results in G protein–mediated activation of PKC, calmodulin, and phospholipase C with evidence also linking MAP kinases ERK1/2, the Rho kinase pathway, and peroxisome proliferator–activated receptor α in the intracellular signaling cascade.[482-485]

The relationship between U-II and the U-II receptor is not exclusive, with the receptor also binding alternative U-II fragments such as U-II–(4-11) and U-II–(5-11), as well as another peptide termed urotensin-related peptide (URP).[486,487] URP was originally isolated from rat brain and binds with high affinity to the U-II receptor.[487] Although this eight–amino acid peptide retains the cyclic hexapeptide sequence, it is derived from a different precursor to U-II and may have different physiologic properties.[488]

PHYSIOLOGIC ROLE OF UROTENSIN II

U-II is the most potent vasoconstrictor known, being 16 times more potent than ET-1 in the isolated rat thoracic aorta.[476] However, its vasoconstrictive properties are not universal, varying between species and between vascular beds. For example, U-II has little or no effect on venous tone, and it does not cause constriction of rat abdominal aorta, femoral, or renal arteries.[489] It also lacks systemic pressor activity when administered intravenously to anesthetized rats.[476,490] In cynomolgus monkeys, bolus intravenous injection of U-II–induced myocardial depression, circulatory collapse, and death.[476] In contrast to the vasoconstrictive properties of vascular smooth muscle U-II receptor, endothelial U-II receptor may mediate vasodilation in pulmonary and mesenteric vessels.[491] The response to U-II may be dependent on the caliber of the artery, with a small vessel

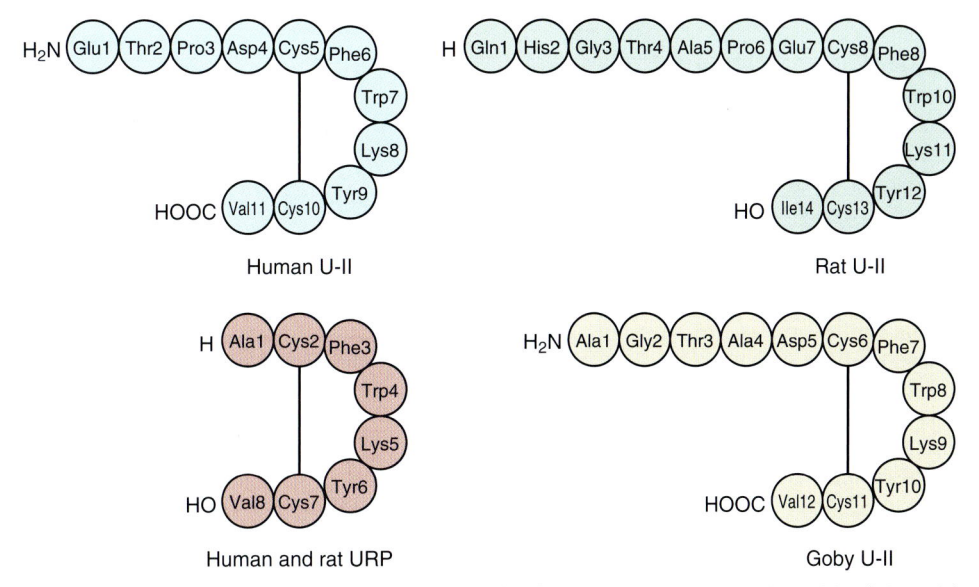

Figure 13.8 Molecular structure of human, rat, and goby urotensin II (U-II). URP, Urotensin-related peptide. (Adapted from Ashton N: Renal and vascular actions of urotensin II, *Kidney Int* 70:624-629, 2006.)

response more endothelium mediated and a large vessel response more dependent on vascular smooth muscle.[474] These disparities are among many examples of how the role of U-II may be influenced by a number of factors, including animal model, vascular bed, method of exogenous U-II administration, and comorbid conditions.

UROTENSIN II IN THE KIDNEY

The kidney is a major site of U-II production, which is indicated by both the arteriovenous gradient of plasma U-II across the kidney and the observation that urinary U-II clearance exceeds urinary creatinine clearance.[474,480] In fact, in humans, urinary concentrations of U-II are approximately three orders of magnitude higher than plasma concentrations.[492] U-II is present in a number of kidney cell types, including the smooth muscle cells and endothelium of arteries, proximal convoluted tubules, and particularly the distal tubules and collecting ducts.[479] U-II receptor mRNA is also present in the kidney, particularly within the renal medulla,[492-494] suggesting that the peptide may have autocrine or paracrine functions at this site. In addition, URP mRNA has also been described in both rat and human kidney.[487,493,494] Studies of the role of U-II in normal renal physiology have been conflicting. In one report, continuous infusion of U-II into the renal artery of anesthetized rats caused a nitric oxide–dependent increase in GFR and urinary water and sodium excretion.[495] In contrast, another study showed that bolus injection of picomolar concentrations of U-II produced a dose-dependent decrease in GFR and a reduction in urine flow and sodium excretion.[494] Still further, a third group of researchers reported that intravenous bolus injection of U-II in nanomolar amounts induced only a minor reduction in GFR and had no effect on sodium excretion.[496] This study also investigated the effect of U-II administration in the context of experimental congestive heart failure, in which the peptide induced an almost 30% increase in GFR.[496]

OBSERVATIONAL STUDIES OF UROTENSIN II IN RENAL DISEASE

Variations in the concentration of U-II in the plasma and urine have been found in a number of diseases with, again, sometimes conflicting results. Plasma U-II levels may be increased in hypertensive individuals compared to normotensive controls and correlate with systolic blood pressure.[497] In one study, U-II concentrations in plasma were increased twofold in patients with renal disease not on hemodialysis and threefold in patients on hemodialysis.[498] In a separate study the same investigators observed U-II levels in both plasma and urine to be higher in patients with type 2 diabetes and renal disease than in such patients with normal renal function.[499] Higher U-II levels in urine have been described in patients with essential hypertension, patients with glomerular disease and hypertension, and patients with renal tubular disorders, but not in normotensive patients with glomerular disease.[492] Increased expression of both U-II and U-II receptor have also been demonstrated in biopsy samples of patients with diabetic nephropathy,[500] with increased U-II also described for glomerulonephritis[501] and in minimal change disease.[502] In contrast, a later study described a reduction in U-II levels with CKD. Here, investigators reported that plasma U-II concentrations were highest in healthy individuals, lower in individuals with ESKD, and lowest in subjects with non-ESKD CKD, while hypothesizing that the discordance with earlier work may reflect the different populations studied or the assays used.[503]

INTERVENTIONAL STUDIES OF UROTENSIN II IN THE KIDNEY

Both peptide and nonpeptide U-II receptor antagonists have been studied. Urantide is a derivative of human U-II.[504] Continuous infusion of urantide into rats induces an increase in GFR and natriuresis,[494] although it is not clear whether the natriuresis is a consequence of altered renal vascular tone or due to a direct effect of U-II on the tubular epithelium. Although urantide is a potent antagonist of the rat U-II receptor,[504] it has been found to have agonist properties in cells expressing the human U-II receptor.[505] An alternative U-II peptide antagonist, UFP-803, has also been shown to have partial agonist properties in human U-II receptor–expressing cells,[506] complicating the interpretation of a peptide-based approach to U-II inhibition. Two compounds in the nonpeptide group of U-II antagonists have been studied: palosuran (ACT-058362) and SB-611812. Intravenous administration of palosuran protected against renal ischemia in a rat model.[507] The same compound was also studied in streptozotocin-diabetic rats, in which it was found to significantly reduce albuminuria.[508] In a study of 19 individuals with type 2 diabetes and macroalbuminuria, palosuran attenuated urine albumin excretion after 2 weeks.[509] However, in a subsequent 4-week study of 54 individuals with type 2 diabetes, hypertension, and nephropathy, palosuran had no effect on albuminuria, blood pressure, GFR, or renal plasma flow,[510] effectively halting the development of this drug for this indication. SB-611812 decreased the carotid intima-to-media ratio in a rat model of balloon angioplasty induced stenosis.[511] The same compound attenuated myocardial remodeling and was associated with a reduced rate of mortality in a rat model of ischemic cardiomyopathy.[512,513] At present, there are no reports of the effect of SB-611812 in renal disease.

Complete reference list available at ExpertConsult.com.

KEY REFERENCES

1. Paul M, Poyan Mehr A, Kreutz R: Physiology of local renin-angiotensin systems. *Physiol Rev* 86:747–803, 2006.
2. Anderson S, Meyer TW, Rennke HG, et al: Control of glomerular hypertension limits glomerular injury in rats with reduced renal mass. *J Clin Invest* 76:612–619, 1985.
4. Griendling KK, Murphy TJ, Alexander RW: Molecular biology of the renin-angiotensin system. *Circulation* 87:1816–1828, 1993.
18. Nguyen G, Delarue F, Burckle C, et al: Pivotal role of the renin/prorenin receptor in angiotensin II production and cellular responses to renin. *J Clin Invest* 109:1417–1427, 2002.
25. Vargas SL, Toma I, Kang JJ, et al: Activation of the succinate receptor GPR91 in macula densa cells causes renin release. *J Am Soc Nephrol* 20:1002–1011, 2009.
28. Campbell DJ, Nussberger J, Stowasser M, et al: Activity assays and immunoassays for plasma renin and prorenin: information provided and precautions necessary for accurate measurement. *Clin Chem* 55:867–877, 2009.

35. Gloy J, Henger A, Fischer KG, et al: Angiotensin II modulates cellular functions of podocytes. *Kidney Int* 54(Suppl 67):S168–S170, 1998.
36. Velez JC: The importance of the intrarenal renin-angiotensin system. *Nat Clin Pract Nephrol* 5:89–100, 2009.
43. Lautrette A, Li S, Alili R, et al: Angiotensin II and EGF receptor cross-talk in chronic kidney diseases: a new therapeutic approach. *Nat Med* 11:867–874, 2005.
46. Kelly DJ, Cox AJ, Gow RM, et al: Platelet-derived growth factor receptor transactivation mediates the trophic effects of angiotensin II in vivo. *Hypertension* 44:195–202, 2004.
63. Kennedy CR, Burns KD: Angiotensin II as a mediator of renal tubular transport. *Contrib Nephrol* 135:47–62, 2001.
75. Advani A, Kelly DJ, Cox AJ, et al: The (Pro)renin receptor: site-specific and functional linkage to the vacuolar H+-ATPase in the kidney. *Hypertension* 54:261–269, 2009.
79. Campbell DJ: Critical review of prorenin and (pro)renin receptor research. *Hypertension* 51:1259–1264, 2008.
84. Donoghue M, Hsieh F, Baronas E, et al: A novel angiotensin-converting enzyme-related carboxypeptidase (ACE2) converts angiotensin I to angiotensin 1-9. *Circ Res* 87:E1–E9, 2000.
89. Soler MJ, Wysocki J, Batlle D: Angiotensin-converting enzyme 2 and the kidney. *Exp Physiol* 93:549–556, 2008.
94. Fyhrquist F, Saijonmaa O: Renin-angiotensin system revisited. *J Intern Med* 264:224–236, 2008.
98. Esteban V, Ruperez M, Sanchez-Lopez E, et al: Angiotensin IV activates the nuclear transcription factor-kappaB and related pro-inflammatory genes in vascular smooth muscle cells. *Circ Res* 96:965–973, 2005.
101. Ferrario CM: Angiotensin-converting enzyme 2 and angiotensin-(1-7): an evolving story in cardiovascular regulation. *Hypertension* 47:515–521, 2006.
106. Dell'Italia LJ, Ferrario CM: The never-ending story of angiotensin peptides: beyond angiotensin I and II. *Circ Res* 112:1086–1087, 2013.
107. Carey RM: Newly discovered components and actions of the renin-angiotensin system. *Hypertension* 62:818–822, 2013.
110. Braam B, Mitchell KD, Fox J, et al: Proximal tubule secretion of angiotensin II in rats. *Am J Physiol* 264:F891–F898, 1993.
116. Silver RB, Reid AC, Mackins CJ, et al: Mast cells: a unique source of renin. *Proc Natl Acad Sci U S A* 101:13607–13612, 2004.
121. Taal MW, Brenner BM: Renoprotective benefits of RAS inhibition: from ACEI to angiotensin II antagonists. *Kidney Int* 57:1803–1817, 2000.
123. Anderson S, Rennke HG, Brenner BM: Therapeutic advantage of converting enzyme inhibitors in arresting progressive renal disease associated with systemic hypertension in the rat. *J Clin Invest* 77:1993–2000, 1986.
125. Kagami S, Border WA, Miller DE, et al: Angiotensin II stimulates extracellular matrix protein synthesis through induction of transforming growth factor-beta expression in rat glomerular mesangial cells. *J Clin Invest* 93:2431–2437, 1994.
128. Gilbert RE, Cox A, Wu LL, et al: Expression of transforming growth factor-β1 and type IV collagen in the renal tubulointerstitium in experimental diabetes: effects of angiotensin converting enzyme inhibition. *Diabetes* 47:414–422, 1998.
129. Langham RG, Kelly DJ, Gow RM, et al: Transforming growth factor-beta in human diabetic nephropathy: effects of ACE inhibition. *Diabetes Care* 29:2670–2675, 2006.
130. Houlihan CA, Akdeniz A, Tsalamandris C, et al: Urinary transforming growth factor-beta excretion in patients with hypertension, type 2 diabetes, and elevated albumin excretion rate: effects of angiotensin receptor blockade and sodium restriction. *Diabetes Care* 25:1072–1077, 2002.
131. Mifsud SA, Allen TJ, Bertram JF, et al: Podocyte foot process broadening in experimental diabetic nephropathy: amelioration with renin-angiotensin blockade. *Diabetologia* 44:870–873, 2001.
133. Langham RG, Kelly DJ, Cox AJ, et al: Proteinuria and the expression of the podocyte slit diaphragm protein, nephrin, in diabetic nephropathy: effects of angiotensin converting enzyme inhibition. *Diabetologia* 45:1572–1576, 2002.

183. Weber MA, Black H, Bakris G, et al: A selective endothelin-receptor antagonist to reduce blood pressure in patients with treatment-resistant hypertension: a randomised, double-blind, placebo-controlled trial. *Lancet* 374:1423–1431, 2009.
218. Dhaun N, Macintyre IM, Melville V, et al: Blood pressure-independent reduction in proteinuria and arterial stiffness after acute endothelin-A receptor antagonism in chronic kidney disease. *Hypertension* 54:113–119, 2009.
219. Dhaun N, MacIntyre IM, Kerr D, et al: Selective endothelin-A receptor antagonism reduces proteinuria, blood pressure, and arterial stiffness in chronic proteinuric kidney disease. *Hypertension* 57:772–779, 2011.
220. Wenzel RR, Littke T, Kuranoff S, et al: Avosentan reduces albumin excretion in diabetics with macroalbuminuria. *J Am Soc Nephrol* 20:655–664, 2009.
221. Mann JF, Green D, Jamerson K, et al: Avosentan for overt diabetic nephropathy. *J Am Soc Nephrol* 21:527–535, 2010.
251. Yan W, Wu F, Morser J, et al: Corin, a transmembrane cardiac serine protease, acts as a pro-atrial natriuretic peptide-converting enzyme. *Proc Natl Acad Sci U S A* 97:8525–8529, 2000.
311. Januzzi JL, Jr, Camargo CA, Anwaruddin S, et al: The N-terminal Pro-BNP investigation of dyspnea in the emergency department (PRIDE) study. *Am J Cardiol* 95:948–954, 2005.
315. van Kimmenade RR, Januzzi JL, Jr, Bakker JA, et al: Renal clearance of B-type natriuretic peptide and amino terminal pro-B-type natriuretic peptide a mechanistic study in hypertensive subjects. *J Am Coll Cardiol* 53:884–890, 2009.
343. Sezai A, Hata M, Niino T, et al: Results of low-dose human atrial natriuretic peptide infusion in nondialysis patients with chronic kidney disease undergoing coronary artery bypass grafting: the NU-HIT (Nihon University working group study of low-dose HANP Infusion Therapy during cardiac surgery) trial for CKD. *J Am Coll Cardiol* 58:897–903, 2011.
349. O'Connor CM, Starling RC, Hernandez AF, et al: Effect of nesiritide in patients with acute decompensated heart failure. *N Engl J Med* 365:32–43, 2011.
371. Ruilope LM, Dukat A, Bohm M, et al: Blood-pressure reduction with LCZ696, a novel dual-acting inhibitor of the angiotensin II receptor and neprilysin: a randomised, double-blind, placebo-controlled, active comparator study. *Lancet* 375:1255–1266, 2010.
372. Solomon SD, Zile M, Pieske B, et al: The angiotensin receptor neprilysin inhibitor LCZ696 in heart failure with preserved ejection fraction: a phase 2 double-blind randomised controlled trial. *Lancet* 380:1387–1395, 2012.
373. McMurray JJ, Packer M, Desai AS, et al: Angiotensin-neprilysin inhibition versus enalapril in heart failure. *N Engl J Med* 371:993–1004, 2014.
378. Preston RA, Afshartous D, Forte LR, et al: Sodium challenge does not support an acute gastrointestinal-renal natriuretic signaling axis in humans. *Kidney Int* 82:1313–1320, 2012.
420. Picard N, Eladari D, El Moghrabi S, et al: Defective ENaC processing and function in tissue kallikrein-deficient mice. *J Biol Chem* 283:4602–4611, 2008.
422. El Moghrabi S, Houillier P, Picard N, et al: Tissue kallikrein permits early renal adaptation to potassium load. *Proc Natl Acad Sci U S A* 107:13526–13531, 2010.
450. Kakoki M, Sullivan KA, Backus C, et al: Lack of both bradykinin B1 and B2 receptors enhances nephropathy, neuropathy, and bone mineral loss in Akita diabetic mice. *Proc Natl Acad Sci U S A* 107:10190–10195, 2010.
470. Liu K, Li QZ, Delgado-Vega AM, et al: Kallikrein genes are associated with lupus and glomerular basement membrane-specific antibody-induced nephritis in mice and humans. *J Clin Invest* 119:911–923, 2009.
473. Klein J, Gonzalez J, Decramer S, et al: Blockade of the kinin B1 receptor ameliorates glomerulonephritis. *J Am Soc Nephrol* 21:1157–1164, 2010.
510. Vogt L, Chiurchiu C, Chadha-Boreham H, et al: Effect of the urotensin receptor antagonist palosuran in hypertensive patients with type 2 diabetic nephropathy. *Hypertension* 55:1206–1209, 2010.

14 Arachidonic Acid Metabolites and the Kidney

Raymond C. Harris | Ming-Zhi Zhang | Richard M. Breyer

CHAPTER OUTLINE

CELLULAR ORIGIN OF EICOSANOIDS, 355
CYCLO-OXYGENASE PATHWAY, 355
Molecular Biology, 355
Regulation of Cyclo-Oxygenase Gene Expression, 357
Regulation of Cyclo-Oxygenase Expression by Antiinflammatory Steroids, 357
Enzymatic Chemistry, 357
RENAL COX-1 AND COX-2 EXPRESSION, 357
COX-2 Expression in the Kidney, 357
COX-2 Expression in the Renal Cortex, 357
COX-1 Expression in the Kidney, 361
RENAL COMPLICATIONS OF NONSTEROIDAL ANTIINFLAMMATORY DRUGS, 361
Na^+ Retention, Edema, and Hypertension, 361
Hyperkalemia, 362
Papillary Necrosis, 362
Acute Kidney Injury, 362
Interstitial Nephritis, 363
Nephrotic Syndrome, 363
Renal Dysgenesis, 363
CARDIOVASCULAR EFFECTS OF COX-2 INHIBITORS, 363
Effects of COX-2 Inhibition on Vascular Tone, 363
Increased Cardiovascular Thrombotic Events, 363
PROSTANOID SYNTHASES, 364
Sources and Nephronal Distribution of Cyclo-Oxygenase Products, 364
PROSTANOID RECEPTORS, 366
TP Receptors, 366
IP Receptors, 369
DP Receptors, 369
FP Receptors, 369
Multiple EP Receptors, 370

EFFECTS OF COX-1 AND COX-2 METABOLITES ON SALT AND WATER TRANSPORT, 373
Proximal Tubule, 373
Loop of Henle, 373
Collecting Duct System, 374
Water Transport, 374
METABOLISM OF PROSTAGLANDINS, 374
15-Ketodehydrogenase, 374
ω/ω-1 Hydroxylation of Prostaglandins, 374
Cyclopentenone Prostaglandins, 374
Nonenzymatic Metabolism of Arachidonic Acid, 375
Prostaglandin Transport and Urinary Excretion, 375
INVOLVEMENT OF CYCLO-OXYGENASE METABOLITES IN RENAL PATHOPHYSIOLOGY, 375
Experimental and Human Glomerular Injury, 375
Acute Kidney Injury, 377
Urinary Tract Obstruction, 377
Allograft Rejection and Cyclosporine Nephrotoxicity, 378
Hepatic Cirrhosis and Hepatorenal Syndrome, 378
Pregnancy, 378
Lithium Nephrotoxicity, 379
Role of Reactive Oxygen Species as Mediators of COX-2 Actions, 379
LIPOXYGENASE PATHWAY, 379
Biologic Activities of Lipoxygenase Products in the Kidney, 381
Involvement of Lipoxygenase Products in Renal Pathophysiology, 381
CYTOCHROME P450 PATHWAY, 382
Vasculature, 383
Tubules, 384
Role in Acute and Chronic Kidney Disease, 385
Role in Hypertension, 385

CELLULAR ORIGIN OF EICOSANOIDS

Eicosanoids comprise a family of biologically active, oxygenated arachidonic acid (AA) metabolites. Arachidonic acid is a polyunsaturated fatty acid possessing 20 carbon atoms and four double bonds (C20:4) and is formed from linoleic acid (C18:2) by the addition of two carbons to the chain and further desaturation. In mammals, linoleic acid is derived strictly from dietary sources. Essential fatty acid (EFA) deficiency occurs when dietary fatty acid precursors, including linoleic acid, are omitted, thereby depleting the hormone-responsive pool of AA. EFA deficiency thereby reduces the intracellular availability of AA in response to hormonal stimulation and abrogates many biologic actions of hormone-induced eicosanoid release.[1]

Of an approximate 10 g of linoleic acid ingested/day, only about 1 mg/day is eliminated as an end product of AA metabolism. Following its formation, AA is esterified into cell membrane phospholipids, principally at the 2 position of the phosphatidylinositol fraction (i.e. sn-2–esterified AA), the major hormone-sensitive pool of AA that is susceptible to release by phospholipases.

Multiple stimuli lead to the release of membrane-bound AA via activation of cellular phospholipases, principally isoforms of phospholipase A_2 (PLA_2).[2] This cleavage step is rate-limiting in the production of biologically relevant arachidonate metabolites. In the case of PLA_2 activation, membrane receptors activate guanine nucleotide–binding (G) proteins, leading to the release of AA directly from membrane phospholipids. Activation of phospholipase C or D, on the other hand, releases AA via the sequential action of the phospholipase-mediated production of diacylglycerol (DAG), with subsequent release of AA from DAG by DAG lipase.[3] This pathway may also lead to the formation of the esterified AA metabolites arachidonoylethanolamide (AEA) and 2-arachidonoylglycerol (2-AG), which are endocannabinoids. These endocannabinoids can subsequently be converted to free AA by the action of monoacylglycerol lipase.[4] When considering eicosanoid formation, the physiologic significance of AA release by these other phospholipases remains uncertain because, at least in the setting of inflammation, PLA_2 action appears essential for the generation of biologically active AA metabolites.[5]

More than 15 proteins with PLA_2 activity are known to exist, including secreted ($sPLA_2$) and cytoplasmic PLA_2 ($cPLA_2$) isoforms.[6,7] A mitogen-activated cytoplasmic PLA_2 has been found to mediate AA release in a calcium-calmodulin–dependent manner. Other hormones and growth factors, including epidermal growth factor (EGF) and platelet-derived growth factors, activate PLA_2 directly through tyrosine residue kinase activity, allowing the recruitment of co-activators to the enzyme without an absolute requirement for the intermediate action of Ca^{2+}-calmodulin or other cellular kinases.

Following de-esterification, AA is rapidly re-esterified into membrane lipids or avidly bound by intracellular proteins, in which case it becomes unavailable to further metabolism. Should it escape re-esterification and protein binding, free AA becomes available as a substrate for one of three major enzymatic transformations, the common result of which is the incorporation of oxygen atoms at various sites of the fatty acid backbone, with accompanying changes in its molecular structure (e.g., ring formation).[8,9] This results in the formation of biologically active molecules, referred to as *eicosanoids*. The specific nature of the products generated is a function of the initial stimuli for AA release, as well as the metabolic enzyme available, which is determined in part by the cell type involved.[9,10]

These products, in turn, mediate or modulate the biologic actions of the agonist in question. AA release may also result from nonspecific stimuli, such as cellular trauma, including ischemia and hypoxia,[11] oxygen free radicals,[12] or osmotic stress.[13] The identity of the specific AA metabolite generated in a particular cell system depends on the proximate stimulus and availability of the downstream AA-metabolizing enzymes present in that cell.

Three major enzymatic pathways of free AA metabolism are present in the kidney: cyclo-oxygenases, lipoxygenases, and cytochrome P450 (Figure 14.1). The cyclo-oxygenase (COX) pathway mediates the formation of prostaglandins (PGs) and thromboxanes, the lipoxygenase (LO) pathway mediates the formation of mono-, di-, and tri-hydroxyeicosatetraenoic acids (HETEs), leukotrienes (LTs), and lipoxins (LXs), and the cytochrome P450–dependent oxygenation of AA mediates the formation of epoxyeicosatrienoic acids (EETs), their corresponding diols, HETEs, and monooxygenated AA derivatives. Fish oil diets, rich in ω-3 polyunsaturated fatty acids,[14] interfere with metabolism via all three pathways by competing with AA oxygenation, resulting in the formation of biologically inactive end products.[15] Interference with the production of proinflammatory lipids has been hypothesized to underlie the beneficial effects of fish oil in immunoglobulin A (IgA) nephropathy and other cardiovascular diseases.[16] The following sections deal with the current understanding of the chemistry, biosynthesis, renal metabolism, mechanisms of release, receptor biology, signal transduction pathways, biologic activities, and functional significance of each of the metabolites generated by the three major routes of AA metabolism in the kidney.

CYCLO-OXYGENASE PATHWAY

MOLECULAR BIOLOGY

The cyclo-oxygenase enzyme system is the major pathway for AA metabolism in the kidney (Figure 14.2). Cyclo-oxygenase (prostaglandin [PG] synthase G_2/H_2) is the enzyme responsible for the initial conversion of arachidonic acid to PGG_2 and subsequently to PGH_2. COX was first purified from ram seminal vesicles and cloned in 1988. The protein is widely expressed, and the level of activity is not dynamically regulated. Other studies supported the presence of a COX that was dynamically regulated and responsible for increased prostanoid production in inflammation. This second inducible COX isoform was identified shortly after the cloning of the initial enzyme and designated COX-2, whereas the initially isolated isoform is now designated COX-1.[8,17,18] COX-1 and COX-2 are encoded by distinct genes located on different chromosomes. The human COX-1 gene (*PTGS1*, PG synthase 1) is on chromosome 9, whereas COX-2 is localized on chromosome 1. The genes are also subject to dramatically different regulatory signals.

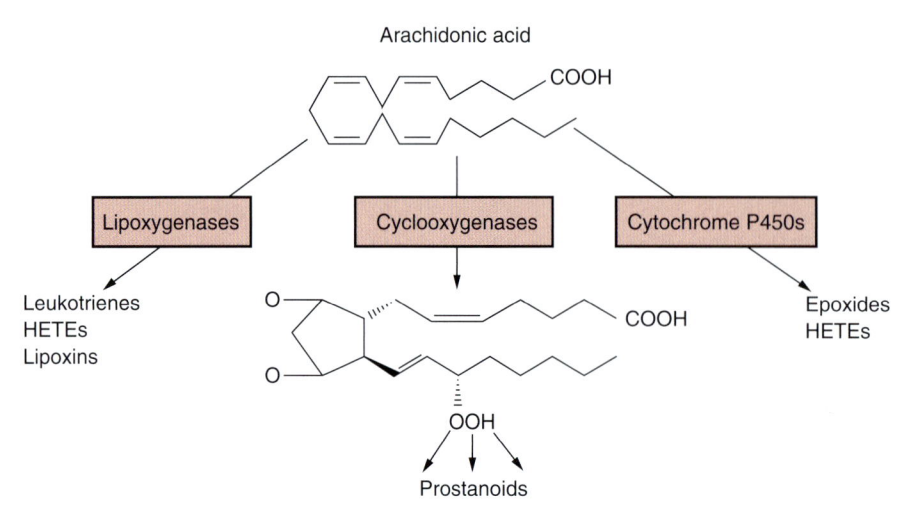

Figure 14.1 Pathways of enzymatically mediated arachidonic acid metabolism. Arachidonic acid can be converted into biologically active compounds by cyclo-oxygenase- (COX), lipoxygenase- (LOX), or cytochrome P450 (CYP450)–mediated metabolism HETE. Hydroxyeicosatetraenoic acid.

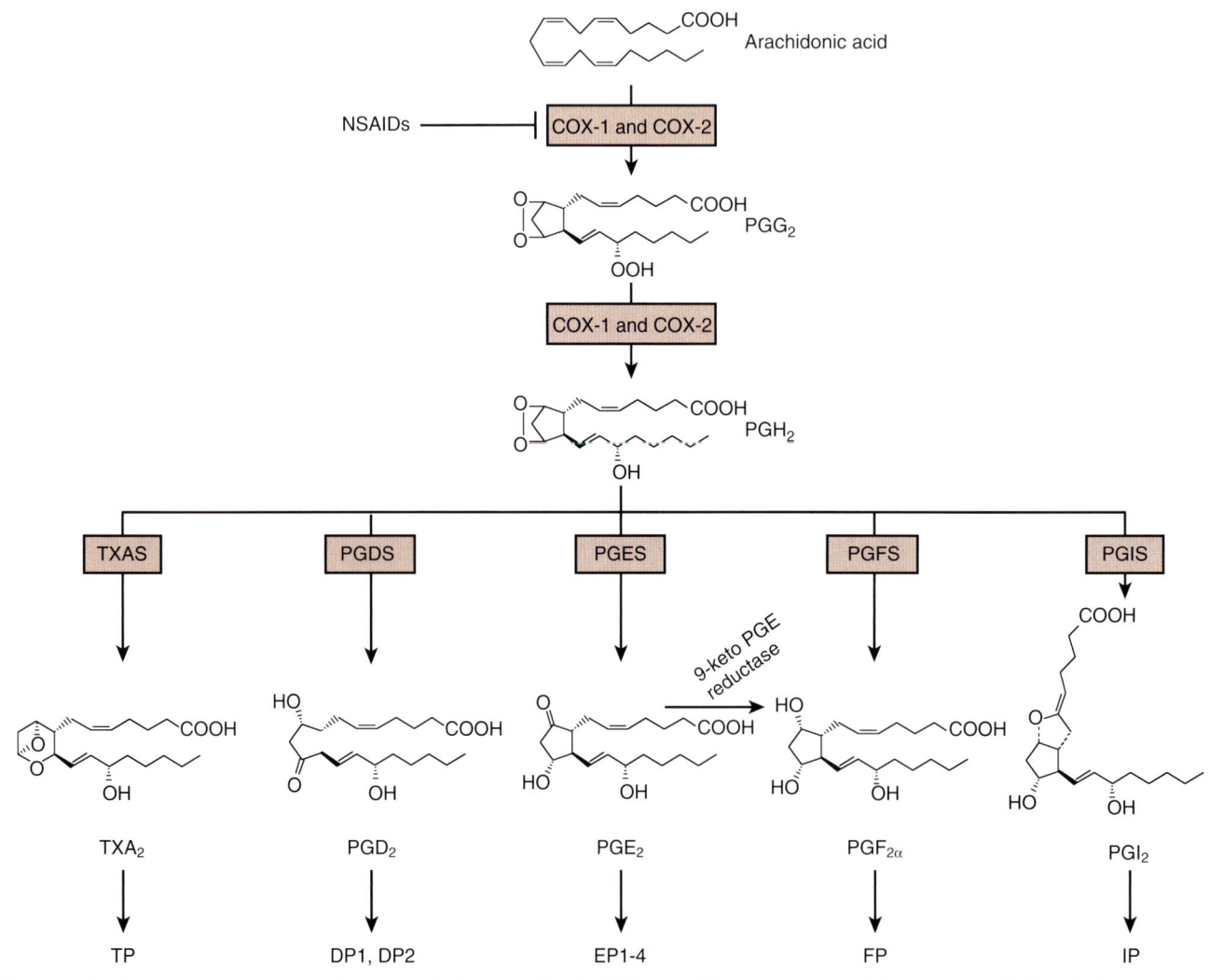

Figure 14.2 Cyclo-oxygenase metabolism of arachidonic acid. Both COX-1 and COX-2 convert arachidonic acid to PGH_2, which is then acted on by specific synthases (TXAS, PGDS, PGES, PGFS, PGIS) to produce prostanoids that act at G protein–coupled receptors (TP. DP1, DP2, EP1-4. FP, IP) that increase or decrease cAMP or increase intracellular calcium levels. cAMP, Cyclic adenosine monophospate; COX, cyclooxygenase; NSAIDs, nonsteroidal antiinflammatory drugs; PGG_2, prostaglandin G_2; PGH_2, prostaglandin H_2.

REGULATION OF CYCLO-OXYGENASE GENE EXPRESSION

At the cellular level, COX-2 expression is highly regulated by several processes that alter its transcription rate, message export from the nucleus, message stability, and efficiency of message translation.[19,20] These processes tightly control the expression of COX-2 in response to many of the same cellular stresses that activate arachidonate release (e.g., cell volume changes, shear stress, hypoxia),[11,21] as well as a variety of cytokines and growth factors, including tumor necrosis factor (TNF), interleukin-1β, EGF, and platelet-derived growth factor (PDGF). Activation of COX-2 gene transcription is mediated via the coordinated activation of several transcription factors that bind to and activate consensus sequences in the 5' flanking region of the COX-2 gene for nuclear factor-kappaB (NF-κB), and NF–interleukin-6 (IL-6)/CCAAT-enhancer binding proteins (C-EBP), and a cyclic adenosine monophosphate (cAMP) response element (CRE).[22] Induction of COX-2 messenger RNA (mRNA) transcription by endotoxin (lipopolysaccharide) may also involve CRE sites[23] and NF-κB sites.[24]

REGULATION OF CYCLO-OXYGENASE EXPRESSION BY ANTIINFLAMMATORY STEROIDS

A molecular basis linking the antiinflammatory effects of COX-inhibiting nonsteroidal antiinflammatory drugs (NSAIDs) and antiinflammatory glucocorticoids has long been sought. A novel mechanism for the suppression of arachidonate metabolism by corticosteroids involving translational inhibition of COX formation had been suggested prior to the molecular recognition of COX-2. With the cloning of COX-2, it became well established that glucocorticoids suppress COX-2 expression and prostaglandin synthesis, an effect now viewed as central to the antiinflammatory effects of glucocorticoids. Posttranscriptional control of COX-2 expression represents another robust mechanism whereby adrenal steroids regulate COX-2 expression.[25] Accumulating evidence has suggested that COX-2 is modulated at multiple steps in addition to transcription rate, including stabilization of the mRNA and enhanced translation.[19,26] Glucocorticoids, including dexamethasone, downregulate COX-2 mRNA in part by destabilizing the mRNA.[26] The 3' untranslated region of COX-2 mRNA contains 22 copies of an AUUUA motif, which are important in destabilizing the COX-2 message in response to dexamethasone, whereas other 3' sequences appear important for COX-2 mRNA stabilization in response to IL-1β.[26] Effects of the 3' untranslated region (UTR), as well as other factors regulating the efficiency of COX-2 translation, have also been suggested.[19] The factors determining the expression of COX-1 are more obscure.

ENZYMATIC CHEMISTRY

Despite these differences, both PG synthases catalyze a similar reaction, resulting in cyclization of carbons 8 to 12 of the AA backbone, forming cyclic endoperoxide, accompanied by the concomitant insertion of two oxygen atoms at carbon 15 to form PGG_2 (a 15-hydroperoxide). In the presence of a reduced glutathione-dependent peroxidase, PGG_2 is converted to the 15-hydroxy derivative, PGH_2. The endoperoxides (PGG_2 and PGH_2) have very short half-lives, about 5 minutes, and are biologically active in inducing aortic contraction and platelet aggregation.[27] However, under some circumstances, the formation of these endoperoxides may be strictly limited via the self-deactivating properties of the enzyme.

The expression of recombinant enzymes and determination of the crystal structure of COX-2 have provided further insight into the observed physiologic and pharmacologic similarities to, and differences from, COX-1. It is now clear that COX-inhibiting NSAIDs work by sterically blocking access of AA to the heme-containing, active enzymatic site.[28] Particularly well-conserved are sequences surrounding the aspirin-sensitive serine residues, at which acetylation by aspirin irreversibly inhibits activity.[29] More recent evidence showed that COX-1 and COX-2 are capable of forming heterodimers and sterically modulating each other's function.[30] The substrate-binding pocket of COX-2 is larger and therefore accepting of bulkier inhibitors and substrates. This difference has allowed the development and marketing of relatively highly selective COX-2 inhibitors for clinical use as analgesics,[31] antipyretics,[32] and antiinflammatory agents.[31] In addition to its central role in inflammation, aberrantly upregulated COX-2 expression has been implicated in the pathogenesis of a number of epithelial cell carcinomas[33] and in Alzheimer's disease and other degenerative neurologic conditions.[34]

RENAL COX-1 AND COX-2 EXPRESSION

COX-2 EXPRESSION IN THE KIDNEY

There is now definitive evidence for significant COX-2 expression in the mammalian kidney (Figure 14.3). COX-2 mRNA and immunoreactive COX-2 are present at low but detectable levels in normal adult mammalian kidney, where in situ hybridization and immunolocalization have demonstrated localized expression of COX-2 mRNA and immunoreactive protein in the cells of the macula densa and a few cells in the cortical thick ascending limb cells immediately adjacent to the macula densa.[35,36] COX-2 expression is also abundant in the lipid-laden medullary interstitial cells in the tip of the papilla.[35,37] Some investigators have reported that COX-2 may be expressed in inner medullary collecting duct cells or intercalated cells in the renal cortex.[38] Nevertheless, COX-1 expression is constitutive and clearly the most abundant isoform in the collecting duct, so the potential existence and physiologic significance of COX-2 coexpression in this segment remains uncertain.

COX-2 EXPRESSION IN THE RENAL CORTEX

It is now well documented that COX-2 is expressed in the macula densa and cortical thick ascending limb (CTAL).[1,36] It is expressed in human kidney, especially in kidneys of older adults,[39,40] and in patients with diabetes mellitus, congestive heart failure,[41] and Bartter-like syndrome.[42]

The presence of COX-2 in the unique group of cells comprising the macula densa points to a potential role

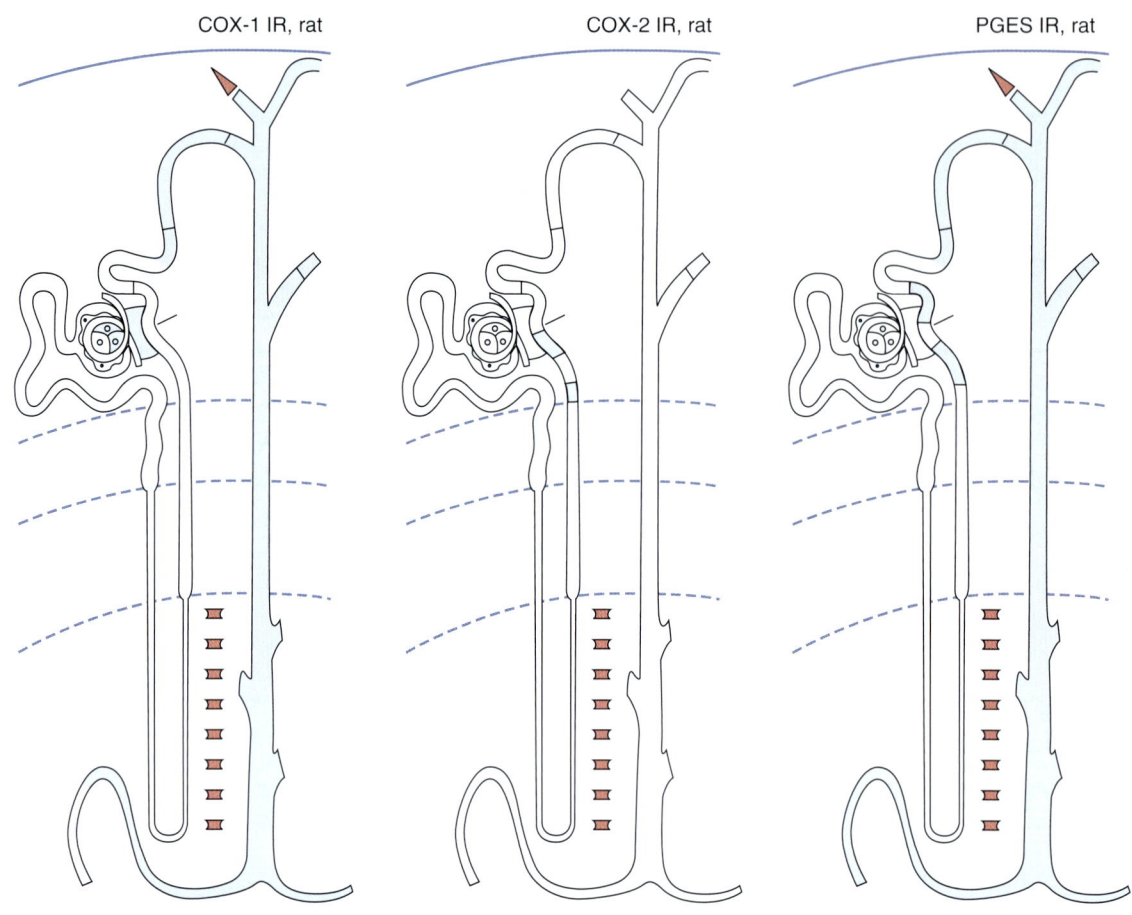

Figure 14.3 Localization of immunoreactive cyclo-oxgenases 1 and 2 (COX-1, COX-2) and microsomal prostaglandin E synthase (PGES) along the rat nephron (*shaded areas*). IR, Immunoreactive. (Courtesy S. Bachmann.)

for COX-2–derived prostanoids in regulating glomerular function.[43] Studies of the prostanoid-dependent control of glomerular filtration rate by the macula densa have suggested effects via vasodilator and vasoconstrictor effects of prostanoids contributing to tubuloglomerular feedback (TGF).[44,45] Some studies have suggested COX-2–derived prostanoids are predominantly vasodilators.[46,47] By inhibiting production of dilator prostanoids contributing to the patency of the adjacent afferent arteriole, COX-2 inhibition may contribute to the decline in glomerular filtration rate (GFR) observed in patients taking NSAIDs or selective COX-2 inhibitors[48] (see later).

The volume-depleted state is typified by low NaCl delivery to the macula densa, and COX-2 expression in the macula densa is also increased in states associated with volume depletion (Figure 14.4).[35] Of note, COX-2 expression in cultured macula densa cells and CTAL cells is also increased in vitro by reducing extracellular Cl^- concentration. Studies in which cortical thick limbs and associated glomeruli were removed and perfused from rabbits pretreated with a low-salt diet to upregulate macula densa COX-2 demonstrated COX-2–dependent release of PGE_2 from the macula densa in response to decreased chloride perfusate.[49] Furthermore the induction of COX-2 by a low Cl^- level can be blocked by a specific p38 mitogen-activated protein (MAP) kinase inhibitor.[50,51] Finally, in vivo, renal cortical immunoreactive pp38 expression (the active form of p38) is predominantly localized to the macula densa and CTAL and increases in response to a low-salt diet.[50] These findings point to a molecular pathway whereby enhanced COX-2 expression occurring in circumstances associated with intracellular volume depletion could result from decreased luminal Cl^- delivery. Some studies have also indicated that the carbonic anhydrase inhibitor acetazolamide and dopamine may both indirectly regulate macula densa COX-2 expression by inhibiting proximal reabsorption and thereby increasing luminal macula densa Cl^- delivery.[52,53] In mice deficient in the Na^+-H^+ exchanger subtype 2 (NHE2), the macula densa is shrunken, accompanied by increased COX-2 expression and juxtaglomerular renin expression, suggesting that NHE2 appears to be the major isoform associated with macula densa cell volume regulation.[54]

In the mammalian kidney, the macula densa is involved in regulating renin release by sensing alterations in luminal chloride via changes in the rate of Na^+-K^+-$2Cl^-$ cotransport (Figure 14.5).[55] In vivo measurements in isolated perfused kidney and isolated perfused juxtaglomerular preparation have all indicated that administration of nonspecific COX inhibitors prevents the increases in renin release mediated by macula densa sensing of decreases in luminal NaCl.[44] Induction of a high renin state by imposition of a salt-deficient diet, angiotensin-converting enzyme (ACE) inhibition, diuretic administration, or experimental renovascular hypertension all significantly increase macula

Control   Low salt

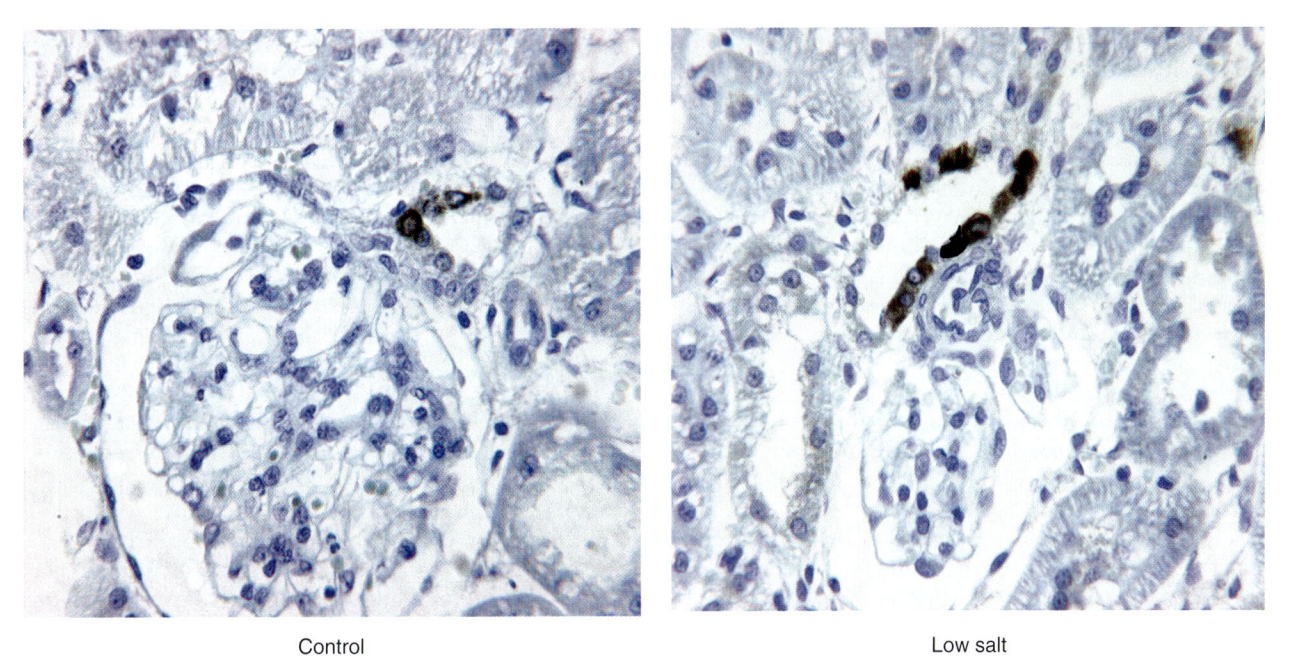

Figure 14.4 COX-2 expression is regulated in renal cortex in rats. Under basal conditions, sparse immunoreactive COX-2 is localized to the macula densa and surrounds the cortical thick ascending limb (CTAL). Following chronic administration of a sodium-deficient diet, macula densa, CTAL, and COX-2 expression increase markedly.

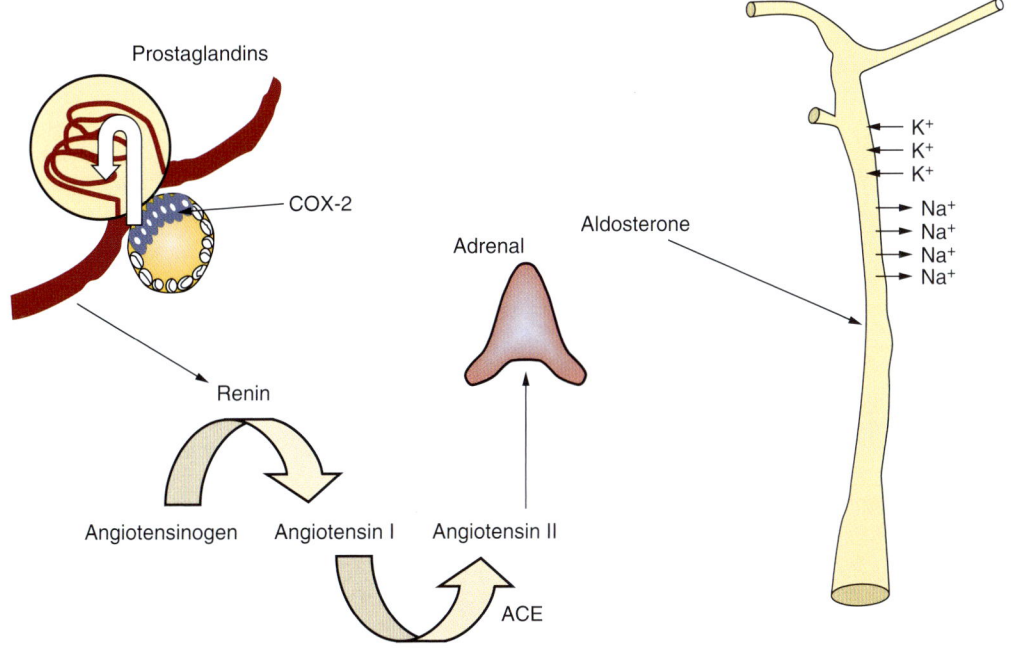

Figure 14.5 Proposed intrarenal roles for vasodilatory prostaglandins to regulate renal function and blood pressure control. Prostaglandins released from the macula densa and/or the afferent arteriole can vasodilate the afferent arteriole and modulate renin release from juxtaglomerular cells. ACE, Angiotensin-converting enzyme; COX-2, cyclo-oxygenase-2.

densa–CTAL COX-2 mRNA and immunoreactive protein.[43] COX-2–selective inhibitors blocked elevations in plasma renin activity, renal renin activity, and renal cortical renin mRNA in response to loop diuretics, ACE inhibitors, or a low-salt diet[43,56-58] and, in an isolated perfused juxtaglomerular preparation, increased renin release in response to lowering the perfusate NaCl concentration was blocked by COX-2 inhibition.[59] In COX-2 knockout mice, increases in renin in response to low salt or ACE inhibitors were significantly blunted[60,61] but were unaffected in COX-1 knockout mice.[62,63] COX-2–derived PGE_2, activating the type 4 (EP4) receptors on juxtaglomerular cells, has been shown to be important for the macula densa regulation of renin release.[49,64] Macula densa COX-2–derived prostanoids appear to be predominantly involved in setting tonic levels of juxtaglomerular renin expression rather than necessarily mediating acute renin release.[65,66] There is evidence that the effect of ACE inhibitors and angiotensin receptor blockers

(ARBs) to increase macula densa COX-2 expression is mediated by feedback of angiotensin II (Ang II) on the macula densa, with Ang II type 1 (AT_1) receptor activation inhibiting and AT_2 receptor activation stimulating COX-2 expression.[56] In addition, prorenin and/or renin may stimulate macula densa COX-2 expression through activation of the prorenin receptor.[67]

COX-2 inhibitors have also been shown to decrease renin production in models of renovascular hypertension,[68] and studies in mice with targeted deletion of the prostacyclin receptor have suggested a predominant role for prostacyclin in mediating renin production and release in these models.[69] In a model of sepsis, COX-2 expression increased in the macula densa and both cortical and medullary TAL. This increased COX-2 expression was mediated by Toll-like receptor 4 (TLR4) and in TLR4$^{-/-}$ mice, juxtaglomerular apparatus renin expression was absent.[70]

In addition to mediating juxtaglomerular renin expression, COX-2 metabolites may also modulate tubuloglomerular feedback (TGF). However, using different methodologies, investigators have reported that COX-2 metabolites predominantly modulate TGF by the production of vasodilatory prostanoids[47,71] or mediate afferent arteriolar vasoconstriction by activating thromboxane receptors through the generation of thromboxane A_2 (TXA_2) and/or PGH_2.[72] Further studies will be required to reconcile these divergent results.

There is evidence that macula densa COX-2 expression is sensitive not only to alterations in intravascular volume, but also to alterations in renal metabolism. Specifically, the G protein–coupled receptor, GPR91, has been shown to be a receptor for succinate, an intermediate of the citric acid cycle.[73] GPR91 is expressed in the macula densa, and GPR91, and intrarenal production of succinate are increased in diabetes. Studies have suggested that succinate activation of GPR91 leads to increased macula densa COX-2 expression.[74,75]

COX-2 EXPRESSION IN THE RENAL MEDULLA

The renal medulla is a major site of prostaglandin synthesis and abundant COX-1 and COX-2 expression (Figure 14.6).[76] COX-1 and COX-2 exhibit differential compartmentalization within the medulla, with COX-1 predominating in the medullary collecting ducts and COX-2 predominating in medullary interstitial cells.[43] In the collecting duct, COX-2 has also been localized to intercalated cells but is absent in principal cells.[77] COX-2 may also be expressed in endothelial cells of the vasa recta supplying the inner medulla.

In medullary interstitial cells, dynamic regulation of COX-2 expression appears to be an important adaptive response to physiologic stresses, including water deprivation, increased dietary sodium, and exposure to endotoxins.[38,76,78,79] In contrast, COX-1 expression is unaffected by water deprivation. Although hormonal factors could also contribute to COX-2 induction, shifting cultured renal medullary interstitial cells to hypertonic media (using NaCl or mannitol) is sufficient to induce COX-2 expression directly. Because prostaglandins play an important role in maintaining renal function during volume depletion or water deprivation, induction of COX-2 by hypertonicity provides an important adaptive response.

As is the case for the macula densa, medullary interstitial cell COX-2 expression is transcriptionally regulated in response to renal extracellular salt and tonicity. Water deprivation and a high-sodium diet both induce COX-2 expression in medullary interstitial cells by activating the NF-κB pathway.[76,79] There is also evidence that nitric oxide may modulate medullary COX-2 expression through MAP

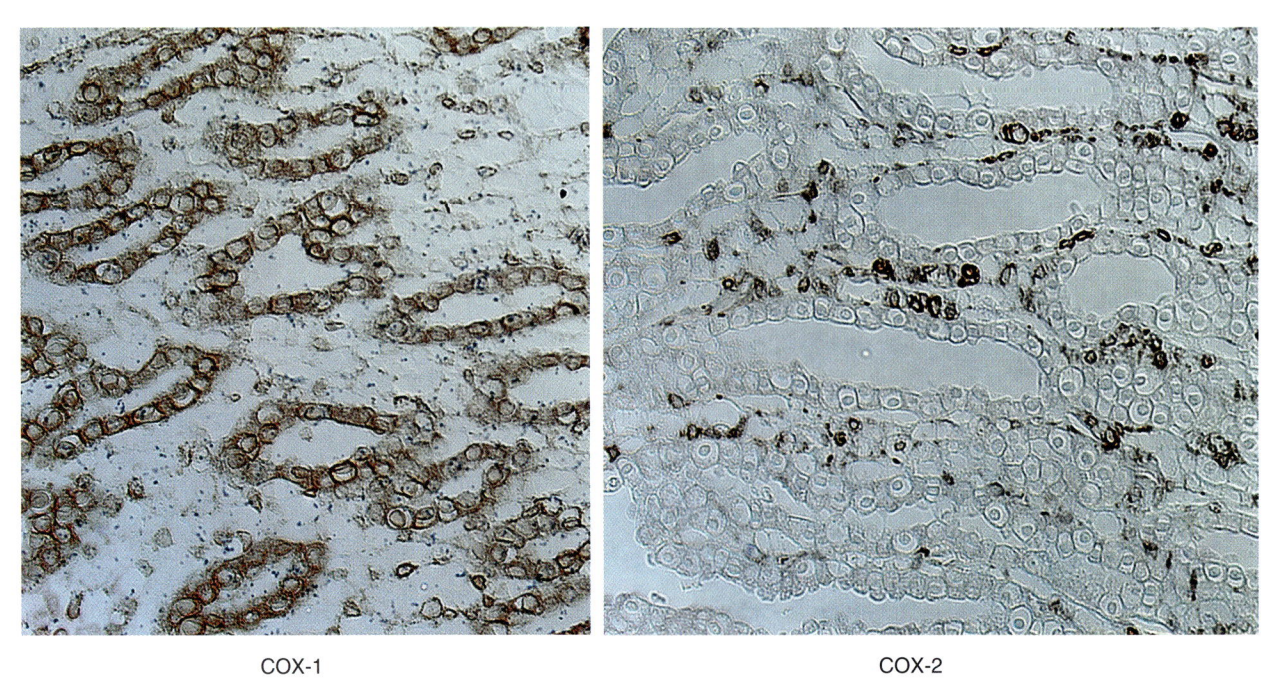

Figure 14.6 Differential immunolocalization of COX-1 and COX-2 in the renal medulla of rodents. COX-1 is predominantly localized to the collecting duct and is also found in a subset of medullary interstitial cells, whereas COX-2 is predominantly localized to a subset of interstitial cells.

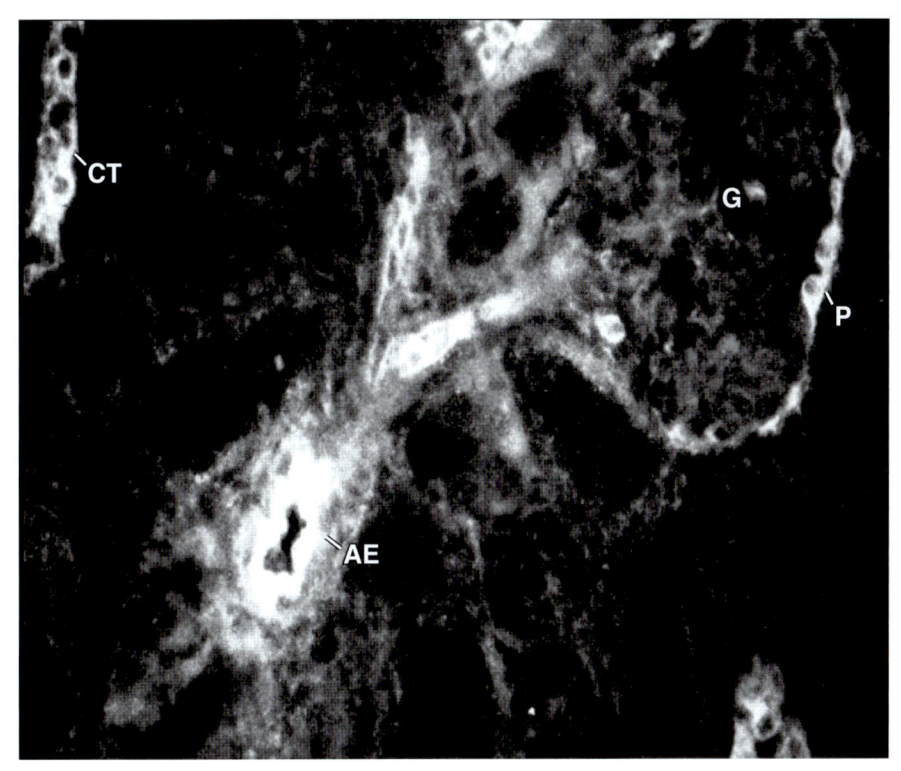

Figure 14.7 Renal cortical COX-1 expression. Immunoreactive COX-1 is predominantly localized to the afferent arteriole (AE), glomerular mesangial cells (G), parietal glomerular epithelial cells (P), and cortical collecting duct (CT). (From Eguchi N, Minami T, Shirafuji N, et al: Lack of tactile pain (allodynia) in lipocalin-type prostaglandin D synthase–deficient mice. *Proc Natl Acad Sci U S A* 96:726-773, 1999.)

kinase–dependent pathways.[80] The mechanisms underlying the upregulation of medullary COX-2 expression in response to volume expansion are probably multifactorial. There is clear evidence that increased medullary tonicity increases medullary COX-2 expression. Different studies have indicated a role for NF-κB,[76] EGF receptor (EGFR) transactivation,[81] and mitochondrial-generated ROS.[82] Whether these represent parallel pathways or are all interrelated is not yet clear; however, it should be noted that the described EGFR transactivation is mediated by cleavage of the EGFR ligand, transforming growth factor-α, by ADAM17 (known as TACE [tumor necrosis factor-α–converting enzyme]). This is known to be activated by src, which can be activated by reactive oxygen species (ROS). In addition to medullary COX-2, cortical COX-2 expression increases in salt-sensitive hypertension, especially in the glomerulus and is inhibited by the superoxide dismutase mimetic, tempol, or an ARB.[83]

COX-1 EXPRESSION IN THE KIDNEY

Although well-defined factors regulating COX-2 and determining the role of COX-2 expression in the kidney are being delineated, the role of renal COX-1 remains more obscure. COX-1 is constitutively expressed in platelets in renal microvasculature and glomerular parietal epithelial cells (Figure 14.7).[84] In addition, COX-1 is abundantly expressed in the collecting duct, but there is little COX-1 expressed in the proximal tubule or TAL.[46,85] Although COX-1 expression levels do not appear to be dynamically regulated and, consistent with this observation, the COX-1 promoter does not possess a TATA box, vasopressin does increase COX-1 expression in collecting duct epithelial cells and in interstitial cells in the inner medulla.[85] The factors accounting for the tissue-specific expression of COX-1 are uncertain but may involve histone acetylation and the presence of two tandem Sp1 sites in the upstream region of the gene.[86]

RENAL COMPLICATIONS OF NONSTEROIDAL ANTIINFLAMMATORY DRUGS

Na+ RETENTION, EDEMA, AND HYPERTENSION

Use of nonselective NSAIDs may be complicated by the development of significant Na+ retention, edema, congestive heart failure and hypertension.[87] These complications are also apparent in patients using COX-2–selective NSAIDs. Studies with celecoxib and rofecoxib have demonstrated that like nonselective NSAIDs, these COX-2–selective NSAIDs reduce urinary Na+ excretion and are associated with modest Na+ retention in otherwise healthy subjects.[88,89] COX-2 inhibition likely promotes salt retention via multiple mechanisms (Figure 14.8). A reduced GFR may limit the filtered Na+ load and salt excretion.[90,91] In addition, PGE_2 directly inhibits Na+ absorption in the thick ascending limb (TAL) and collecting duct.[92] The relative abundance of COX-2 in medullary interstitial cells places this enzyme adjacent to both these nephron segments, allowing for COX-2–derived PGE_2 to modulate salt absorption. COX-2 inhibitors decrease renal PGE_2 production[88,93] and thereby may enhance renal sodium retention. Finally, reduction in renal

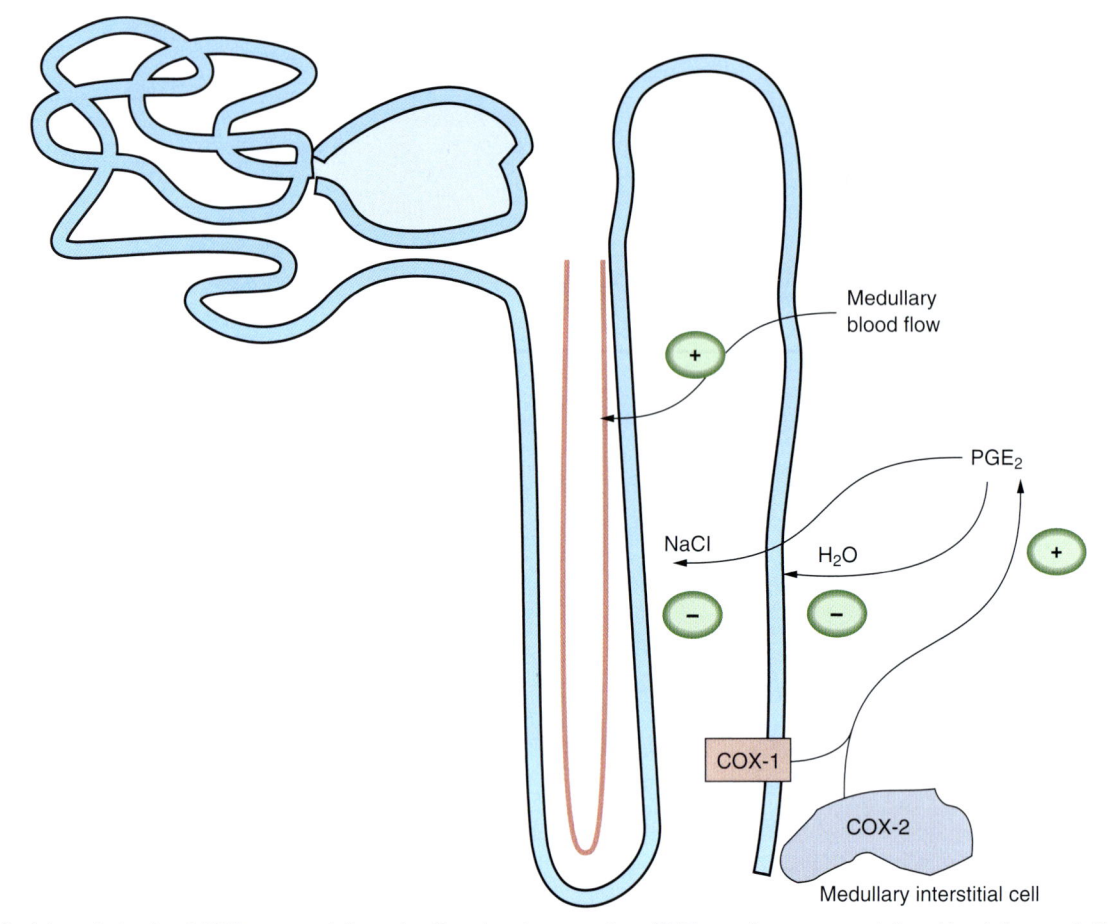

Figure 14.8 Integrated role of PGE_2 on regulation of salt and water excretion. PGE_2 can increase medullary blood flow and directly inhibit NaCl reabsorption in the medullary thick ascending limb and water reabsorption in the collecting duct.

medullary blood flow by the inhibition of vasodilator prostanoids may significantly reduce renal salt excretion and promote the development of edema and hypertension. COX-2–selective NSAIDs have been demonstrated to exacerbate salt-dependent hypertension.[94,95] Similarly, patients with preexisting treated hypertension commonly experience hypertensive exacerbations with COX-2–selective NSAIDs.[89] Taken together, these data suggest that COX-2–selective NSAIDs have effects similar to those of nonselective NSAIDs with respect to salt excretion.

HYPERKALEMIA

Nonselective NSAIDs cause hyperkalemia due to suppression of the renin angiotensin aldosterone axis. Both a decreased GFR and inhibition of renal renin release may compromise renal K^+ excretion. Patients on a salt-restricted diet also have decreased urinary potassium excretion when treated with a COX-2–selective inhibitor,[90,91] and COX-2–selective inhibitors may pose an equal or greater risk as nonselective NSAIDs for the development of hyperkalemia.[96]

PAPILLARY NECROSIS

Acute and subacute forms of papillary necrosis have been observed with NSAID use.[97-99] Acute NSAID-associated renal papillary injury is more likely to occur in the setting of volume depletion, suggesting a critical dependence of renal function on COX metabolism in this setting.[76] Long-term use of NSAIDs has been associated with papillary necrosis and progressive renal structural and functional deterioration, much like the syndrome of analgesic nephropathy observed with an acetaminophen, aspirin, and caffeine combination.[98] Experimental studies have suggested that renal medullary interstitial cells are an early target of injury in analgesic nephropathy.[100] COX-2 has been shown to be an important survival factor for cells exposed to a hypertonic medium.[37,76,101,102] The coincident localized expression of COX-2 in these interstitial cells[37,76] raises the possibility that, like nonselective NSAIDs, long-term use of COX-2–selective NSAIDs may contribute to the development of papillary necrosis.[103]

ACUTE KIDNEY INJURY

Acute kidney injury (AKI) is a well-described complication of NSAID use.[87] This is generally considered to be a result of altered intrarenal microcirculation and glomerular filtration secondary to the inability to produce beneficial endogenous prostanoids when the kidney is dependent on them for normal function. Like the traditional, nonselective NSAIDs, COX-2– selective NSAIDs will also reduce glomerular filtration in susceptible patients.[87] Although generally rare, NSAID-associated renal insufficiency occurs in a significant proportion of patients with underlying volume depletion, renal insufficiency, congestive heart failure, diabetes, and advanced age.[87] These risk factors are additive and rarely are present in patients included in study cohorts used for safety assessment of these drugs. It is therefore relevant that celecoxib and rofecoxib caused a slight but significant fall in the GFR in salt-depleted but otherwise healthy subjects.[90,91] Similar to nonselective NSAIDs, AKI can occur secondary to the use of COX-2–selective NSAIDs.[48,104] Preclinical studies have supported the concept that inhibition of COX-2–derived prostanoids generated in the macula densa contributes to a fall in GFR by reducing the diameter of the afferent arteriole. In vivo video microscopy studies have documented reduced afferent arteriolar diameter following administration of a COX-2 inhibitor.[47] These animal data not only support the concept that COX-2 plays an important role in regulating the GFR, but also the clinical observations that COX-2–selective inhibitors can cause renal insufficiency similar to that reported with nonselective NSAIDs.

INTERSTITIAL NEPHRITIS

The gradual development of renal insufficiency characterized by a subacute inflammatory interstitial infiltrate may occur after several months of continuous NSAID ingestion. Less commonly, the interstitial nephritis and renal failure may be fulminant. The infiltrate is typically accompanied by eosinophils; however, the clinical picture is typically much less dramatic than that of classic drug-induced allergic interstitial nephritis, lacking fever or rash.[105] This syndrome has also been reported with the COX-2–selective drug celecoxib.[106,107] Dysregulation of the immune system is thought to play an important role in the syndrome, which typically abates rapidly following discontinuation of the NSAID or COX-2 inhibitor.

NEPHROTIC SYNDROME

Like interstitial nephritis, nephrotic syndrome typically occurs in patients chronically ingesting any one of a myriad of NSAIDs over a course of months.[105,108] The renal pathology is usually consistent with minimal change disease, with foot process fusion of glomerular podocytes observed on electron microscopy (EM), but membranous nephropathy has also been reported.[109] Typically, the nephrotic syndrome occurs together with the interstitial nephritis.[105] Nephrotic syndrome without interstitial nephritis may occur, as well as immune complex glomerulopathy, in a small subset of patients receiving NSAIDs. It remains uncertain whether this syndrome results from mechanism-based COX inhibition by these drugs, an idiosyncratic immune drug reaction, or a combination of both.

RENAL DYSGENESIS

Reports of renal dysgenesis and oligohydramnios in the offspring of women given nonselective NSAIDs during the third trimester of pregnancy have implicated prostaglandins in the process of normal renal development.[110,111] A similar syndrome of renal dysgenesis has been reported in mice with targeted disruption of the COX-2 gene, as well as mice treated with the specific COX-2 inhibitor SC58236.[112] Because neither COX-1$^{-/-}$ mice nor mice treated with the COX-1– selective inhibitor SC58560 exhibited altered renal development, a specific role for COX-2 in nephrogenesis has been suggested.[113-115] A report of renal dysgenesis in the infant of a woman exposed to the COX-2–selective inhibitor nimesulide suggested that COX-2 also plays a role in renal development in humans.[110]

The intrarenal expression of COX-2 in the developing kidney peaks in the mouse at postnatal day 4 and in the rat in the second postnatal week.[112,116] It has not yet been determined if a similar pattern of COX-2 is seen in humans. Although the most intense staining is observed in a small subset of cells in the nascent macula densa and CTAL, expression in the papilla has also been observed.[112,116] Considering the similar glomerular developmental defects observed in rodents treated with the COX-2 inhibitor and in mice with targeted disruption of the COX-2 gene, it seems likely that prostanoids or other products resulting from COX-2 activity in the CTAL (and macula densa) act in a paracrine manner to influence glomerular development. The identity of the COX-2–derived prostanoids that promote glomerulogenesis remains uncertain. In vitro studies have shown that exogenous PGE_2 promotes renal metanephric development[117] and is a critical growth factor for renal epithelia cells. Nevertheless, none of the prostaglandin receptor knockout mice recapitulated the phenotype of the COX-2 knockout mice.[118]

CARDIOVASCULAR EFFECTS OF COX-2 INHIBITORS

EFFECTS OF COX-2 INHIBITION ON VASCULAR TONE

In addition to their propensity to reduce renal salt excretion and decrease medullary blood flow, NSAIDs and selective COX-2 inhibitors have been shown to exert direct effects on systemic resistance vessels. The acute pressor effect of angiotensin infusion in human subjects was significantly increased by pretreatment with the nonselective NSAID indomethacin at all Ang II doses studied. Administration of selective COX-2 inhibitors or COX-2 gene knockout has been shown to accentuate the pressor effects of angiotensin II in mice.[46] These studies also demonstrated that Ang II–mediated blood pressure increases were markedly reduced by administration of a selective COX-1 inhibitor or in COX-1 gene knockout mice.[46] These findings support the conclusion that COX-1–derived prostaglandins participate in, and are integral to, the pressor activity of Ang II, whereas COX-2–derived prostaglandins are vasodilators that oppose and mitigate the pressor activity of Ang II. Other animal studies have more directly shown that NSAIDs and COX-2 inhibitors blunt arteriolar dilation and decrease flow through resistance vessels.[119]

INCREASED CARDIOVASCULAR THROMBOTIC EVENTS

COX-2 is known to be induced in vascular endothelial cells in response to shear stress,[120] and selective COX-2 inhibition reduces circulating prostacyclin levels in normal human subjects.[121] Therefore, increasing evidence has indicated that COX-2–selective antagonism may carry increased thrombogenic risks due to selective inhibition of the endothelial-derived, antithrombogenic prostacyclin without any inhibition of the prothrombotic, platelet-derived thromboxane generated by COX-1.[122] Although animal studies have provided conflicting results about the role of COX-2 inhibition on development of atherosclerosis, there have been indications that COX-2 inhibition may destabilize atherosclerotic plaques. This has been suggested by studies indicating increased COX-2 expression and colocalization with microsomal PGE synthase 1 and metalloproteinases-2 and -9 in carotid plaques from individuals with symptomatic disease before endarterectomy.[123-129] Because of the concerns about increased cardiovascular risk, two selective COX-2 inhibitors, rofecoxib and valdecoxib, were withdrawn from the market, and remaining coxibs and other NSAIDs have been relabeled to highlight the increased risk for cardiovascular events.

PROSTANOID SYNTHASES

Once PGH_2 is formed in the cell, it can undergo a number of possible transformations, yielding biologically active prostaglandins and TXA_2. As seen in Figure 14.9, in the presence of isomerase and reductase enzymes, PGH_2 is converted to PGE_2 and $PGF_{2\alpha}$, respectively. Thromboxane synthase converts PGH_2 into a bicyclic oxetane-oxane ring metabolite, TXA_2, a prominent reaction product in the platelet and an established synthetic pathway in the glomerulus. Prostacyclin synthase, a 50-kDa protein located in plasma and nuclear membranes and found mostly in vascular endothelial cells, catalyzes the biosynthesis of prostacyclin, PGI_2. PGD_2, the major prostaglandin product in mast cells, is also derived directly from PGH_2, but its role in the kidney is uncertain. The enzymatic machinery and their localization in the kidney are discussed in detail later.

SOURCES AND NEPHRONAL DISTRIBUTION OF CYCLO-OXYGENASE PRODUCTS

COX activity is present in arterial and arteriolar endothelial cells, including glomerular afferent and efferent arterioles.[43] The predominant metabolite from these vascular endothelial cells is PGI_2.[130,131] Whole glomeruli generate PGE_2, PGI_2, $PGF_{2\alpha}$ and TXA_2.[1] The predominant products in rat and rabbit glomeruli are PGE_2, followed by PGI_2 and $PGF_{2\alpha}$ and, finally, TXA_2.

Analysis of individual cultured glomerular cell subpopulations has also provided insight into the localization of prostanoid synthesis. Cultured mesangial cells are capable of generating PGE_2, and, in some cases, $PGF_{2\alpha}$ and PGI_2 have

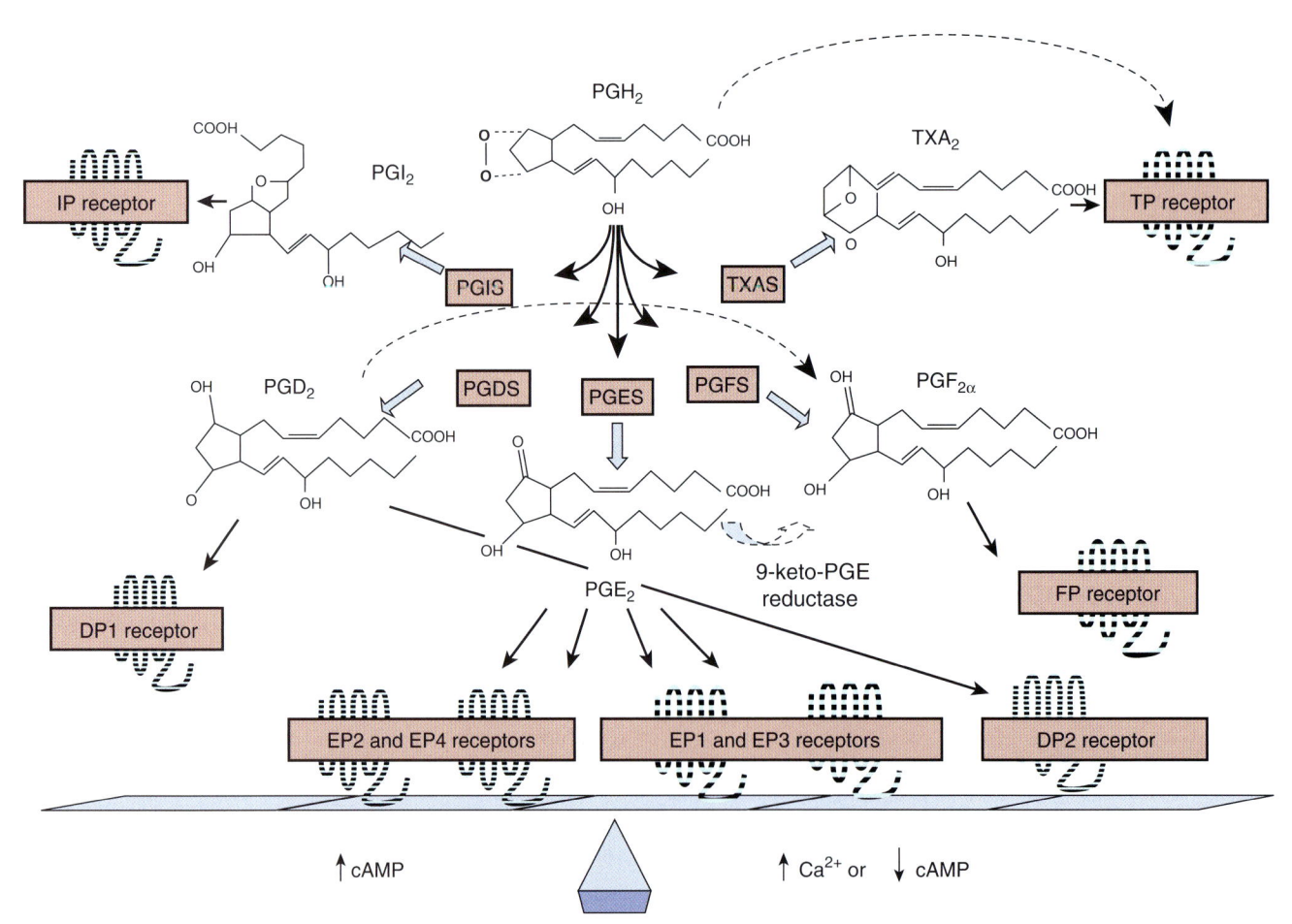

Figure 14.9 Prostaglandin synthases.

also been detected.[132] Other studies have suggested that mesangial cells may produce the endoperoxide PGH_2 as a major COX product.[133] Glomerular epithelial cells also appear to participate in prostaglandin synthesis, but the profile of COX products generated in these cells remains controversial. Immunocytochemical studies of rabbit kidney have demonstrated intense staining for COX-1, predominantly in parietal epithelial cells. Glomerular capillary endothelial cell PG generation profiles remain undefined but may include prostacyclin.

The predominant synthetic site of prostaglandin synthesis along the nephron is the cortical collecting duct (CCD), particularly its medullary portion (MCT).[134] In the presence of exogenous arachidonic acid, PGE_2 is the predominant PG formed in the collecting duct, with variations among the other products being insignificant.[1] PGE_2 is also the major COX metabolite generated in medullary interstitial cells.[135] The role that specific prostanoid synthases may play in the generation of these products is outlined below.

THROMBOXANE SYNTHASE

TXA_2 is produced from PGH_2 by thromboxane synthase (TXAS), a microsomal protein of 533 amino acids with a predicted molecular weight of approximately 60 kDa. The amino acid sequence of the enzyme exhibits homology to the cytochrome P450s and is now classified as CYP5A1.[136] The human gene is localized on chromosome 7q and spans 180 kb. TXAS mRNA is highly expressed in hematopoietic cells, including platelets, macrophages, and leukocytes. TXAS mRNA is expressed in the thymus, kidney, lung, spleen, prostate, and placenta. Immunolocalization of TXAS demonstrates high expression in the dendritic cells of the interstitium, with lower expression in glomerular podocytes of human kidney.[137] TXA_2 synthase expression is regulated by dietary salt intake.[138] Furthermore experimental use of ridogrel, a specific thromboxane synthase inhibitor, reduced blood pressure in spontaneously hypertensive rats.[139] The clinical use of TXA_2 synthase inhibitors is complicated by the fact that its endoperoxide precursors (PGG_2, PGH_2) are also capable of activating its downstream target, the TP receptor.[27]

PROSTACYCLIN SYNTHASE

There are many biologic effects of prostacyclin and include nociception and antithrombotic and vasodilator actions, which have been targeted therapeutically to treat pulmonary hypertension.

Prostacyclin (PGI_2) is derived by the enzymatic conversion of PGH_2 via prostacyclin synthase (PGIS). The cloned cDNA contains a 1500-bp open reading frame that encodes a 500–amino acid protein of approximately 56 kDa. The human prostacyclin synthase gene is present as a single copy per haploid genome and is localized on chromosome 20q. Northern blot analysis shows that prostacyclin synthase mRNA is widely expressed in human tissues and is particularly abundant in the ovary, heart, skeletal muscle, lung, and prostate. PGI synthase expression exhibits segmental expression in the kidney, especially in kidney inner medulla tubules and interstitial cells.

Recently, PGI_2 synthase null mice were generated.[140] PGI_2 levels in the plasma, kidneys, and lungs were reduced, documenting the role of this enzyme as an in vivo source of PGI_2. Blood pressure and blood urea nitrogen and creatinine levels in the PGI_2 synthase knockout mice were significantly increased; renal pathologic findings included surface irregularity, fibrosis, cysts, arterial sclerosis, and hypertrophy of vessel walls. Thickening of the thoracic aortic media and adventitia were observed in aged PGI_2 synthase null mice.[140] Interestingly, this is a phenotype different from that reported for the IP receptor knockout mouse.[141] These differences indicate the presence of additional IP-independent, PGI_2-activated signaling pathways. Regardless, these findings demonstrate the importance of PGI_2 to the maintenance of blood vessels and the kidney.

PROSTAGLANDIN D SYNTHASE

Prostaglandin D_2 is derived from PGH_2 via the action of specific enzymes designated PGD synthases (PGDSs). Two major enzymes are capable of transforming PGH_2 to PGD_2, including a lipocalin-type PGD synthase and a hematopoietic-type PGDS.[142,143] Mice lacking the lipocalin D synthase gene exhibit altered sleep and pain sensation.[144] PGD_2 is the major prostanoid released from mast cells following challenge with immunoglobulin E. The kidney also appears capable of synthesizing PGD_2. RNA for the lipocalin-type PGD synthase has been reported to be widely expressed along the rat nephron, whereas the hematopoietic-type PGD synthase is restricted to the collecting duct.[145] Urinary excretion of lipocalin D synthase has been proposed as a biomarker predictive of renal injury,[146] and lipocalin D synthase knockout mice appear to be more prone to diabetic nephropathy.[147] However, the physiologic roles of these enzymes in the kidney remain less certain. Once synthesized, PGD_2 is available to interact with the DP1 or DP2 receptor (see later) or undergo further metabolism to a PGF_2-like compound.

PROSTAGLANDIN F SYNTHESIS

Prostaglandin $F_{2\alpha}$ is a major urinary COX product. Its synthesis may derive directly from PGH_2 via a PGF synthase or indirectly by metabolism of PGE_2 via a 9-ketoreductase.[148] Another more obscure pathway for PGF formation is by the action of a PGD_2 ketoreductase, yielding a stereoisomer of PGF_2, $9a,11\beta$-PGF_2 (11-epi-$PGF_{2\alpha}$).[148] This reaction, and conversion of PGD_2 into an apparently biologically active metabolite ($9a,11\beta$-$PGF_{2\alpha}$) has been documented in vivo.[149] Interestingly this isomer can also ligate and activate the FP receptor.[150] The physiologically relevant enzymes responsible for renal $PGF_{2\alpha}$ formation remain incompletely characterized.

PROSTAGLANDIN 9-KETOREDUCTASE

Physiologically relevant transformations of COX products occur in the kidney via a reduced nicotinamide adenine dinucleotide phosphate (NADPH)–dependent 9-ketoreductase, which converts PGE_2 into $PGF_{2\alpha}$. This enzymatic activity is typically cytosolic[148] and may be detected in homogenates from the renal cortex, medulla, or papilla. The activity appears to be particularly robust in suspensions from the TALH. Renal PGE_2 9-ketoreductase also exhibits 20α-hydroxysteroid reductase activity that could affect steroid metabolism.[148] This enzyme appears to be a member of the aldo-keto reductase family 1C.[151]

Interestingly, some studies have suggested that activity of a 9-ketoreductase may be modulated by salt intake and Ang

II type 2 (AT$_2$) receptor activation and may play an important role in hypertension.[152] Mice deficient in the AT$_2$ receptor exhibit salt-sensitive hypertension, increased PGE$_2$ production, and reduced production of PGF$_{2\alpha}$,[153] consistent with reduced 9-ketoreductase activity. Other studies have suggested that dietary potassium intake may also enhance the activity of conversion from PGE$_2$ to PGF$_{2\alpha}$.[154] The intrarenal sites of expression of this enzymatic activity remain to be characterized.

PROSTAGLANDIN E SYNTHASES

PGE$_2$ is the other major product of COX-initiated arachidonic acid metabolism in the kidney and is synthesized at high rates along the nephron, particularly in the collecting duct. Two membrane-associated PGE$_2$ synthases have been identified, 33-kDa and 16-kDa membrane-associated enzymes.[155,156] The initial report describing the cloning of a glutathione-dependent microsomal enzyme (the 16-kDa form) that specifically converts PGH$_2$ to PGE$_2$[156] showed that mRNA for this enzyme is highly expressed in reproductive tissues, as well as in the kidney. Genetic disruption confirms that microsomal PGE synthase 1 (mPGES-1)$^{-/-}$ mice exhibit a marked reduction in inflammatory responses compared with mPGES-1$^{+/+}$ mice and indicates that mPGES-1 is also critical for the induction of inflammatory fever.[157,158]

Intrarenal expression of mPGES1 has been demonstrated and mapped to the collecting duct, with lower expression in the medullary interstitial cells and macula densa[134,159] (see Figure 14.3). Thus, in the kidney, this isoform co-localizes with COX-1 and COX-2. In contrast, in inflammatory cells, this PGE synthase is co-induced with COX-2 and appears to be functionally coupled to it.[160] Notably, the kidneys of mPGES-1$^{-/-}$ mice are normal and do not exhibit the renal dysgenesis observed in COX-2$^{-/-}$ mice,[114,161] nor do these mice exhibit perinatal death from patent ductus arteriosus observed with the prostaglandin EP4 receptor knockout mouse.[162]

Another membrane-associated PGE synthase with a relative mass of about 33 kDa was purified from heart. The recombinant enzyme was activated by several sulfhydryl (SH)-reducing reagents, including dithiothreitol, glutathione (GSH), and β-mercaptoethanol. Moreover, the mRNA distribution was high in the heart and brain and was also expressed in the kidney, but the mRNA was not expressed in the seminal vesicles. The intrarenal distribution of this enzyme is, at present, uncharacterized.[155]

Other cytosolic proteins exhibit lower PGE synthase activity, including a 23-kDa glutathione S-transferase (GST) requiring cytoplasmic PGE synthase[163] that is expressed in the kidney and lower genitourinary tract.[164] Some evidence has suggested that this isozyme may constitutively couple to COX-1 in inflammatory cells. In addition, several cytosolic glutathione S-transferases have the capability to convert PGH$_2$ to PGE$_2$; however, their physiologic role in this process remains uncertain[165]

PROSTANOID RECEPTORS

See Figures 14-10 and 14-11.

TP RECEPTORS

The TP receptor was originally purified by chromatography using a high-affinity ligand to capture the receptor.[166] This was the first eicosanoid receptor cloned and is a G protein–coupled transmembrane receptor capable of activating a

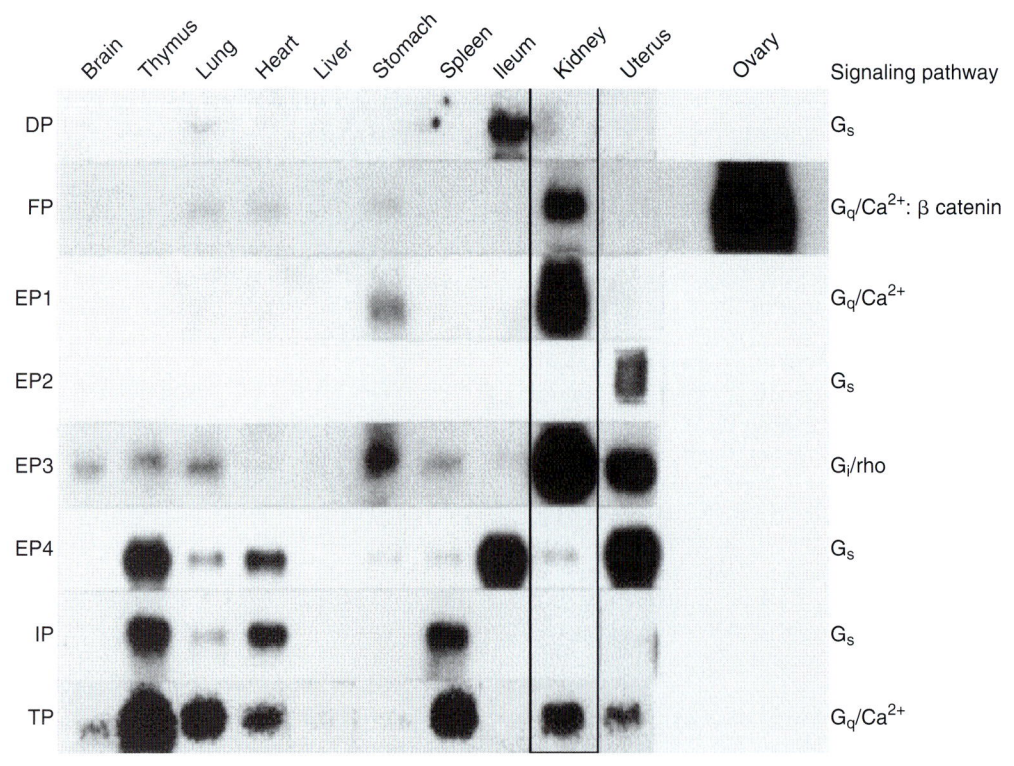

Figure 14.10 Tissue distribution of prostanoid receptor mRNA. (Adapted from Tone Y, Inoue H, Hara S, et al: The regional distribution and cellular localization of mRNA encoding rat prostacyclin synthase. *Eur J Cell Biol* 72:268-277, 1997.)

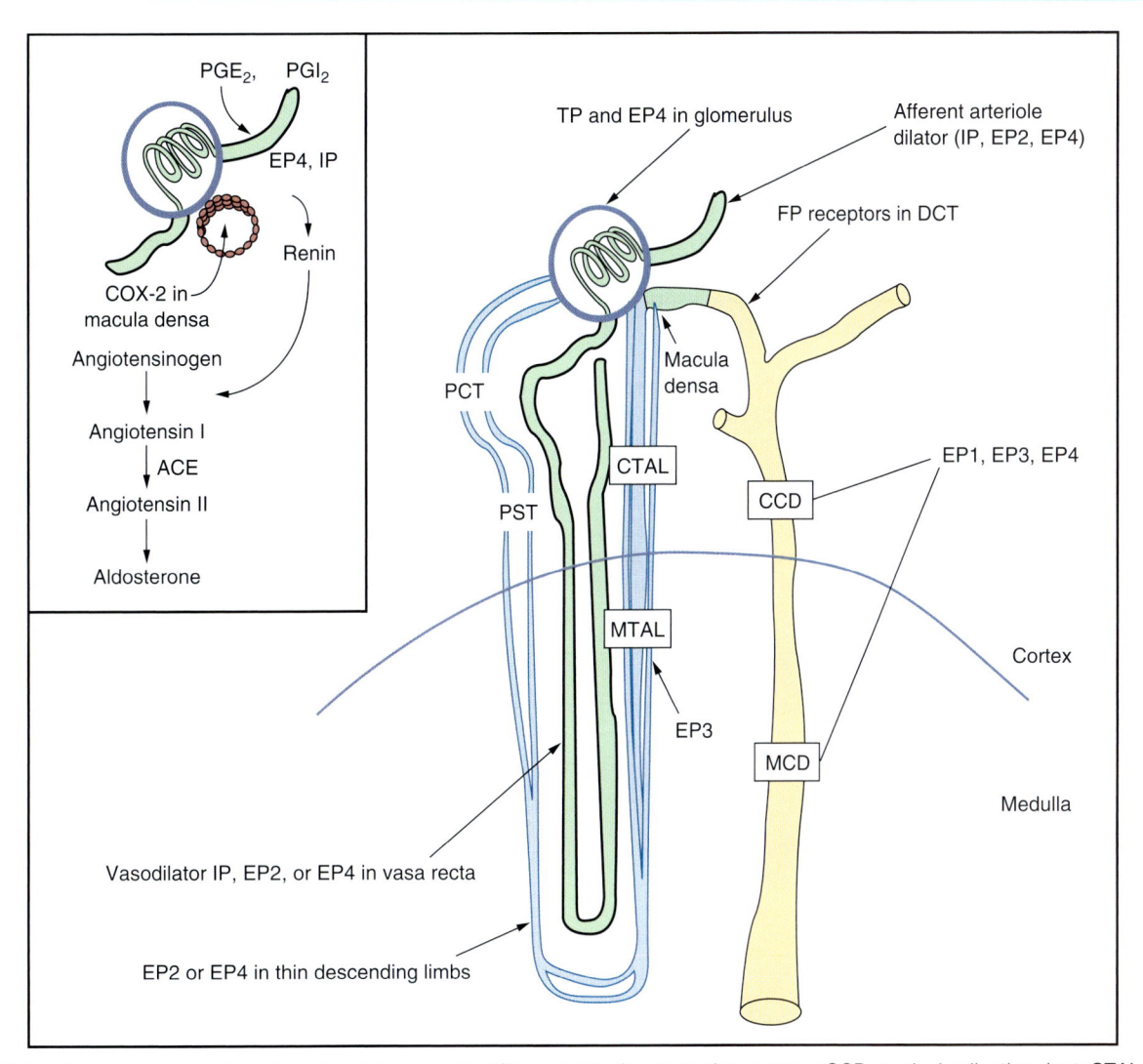

Figure 14.11 Intrarenal localization of prostanoid receptors. ACE, angiotensin-converting enzyme; CCD, cortical collecting duct; CTAL, cortical thick ascending limb; DCT, distal convoluted tubule; MCD, medullary collecting duct; MTAL, medullary thick ascending limb; PCT, proximal convoluted tubule; PST, proximal straight tubule.

calcium-coupled signaling mechanism (Figure 14.12). The cloning of other prostanoid receptors was achieved by finding cDNAs homologous to this TP receptor cDNA. Two alternatively spliced variants of the human thromboxane receptor have been described that differ in their C-terminal tail distal to Arg.[167] Similar patterns of alternative splicing have been described for the EP3 and FP receptors.[168] Heterologous cAMP-mediated signaling of the thromboxane receptor may occur via its heterodimerization with the prostacyclin (IP) receptor.[169]

The endoperoxide PGH_2 or its metabolite, TXA_2, can activate the TP receptor.[27] Competition radioligand binding studies have demonstrated a rank order of potency on the human platelet TP receptor of the ligands I-BOP, S145 > SQ29548 > STA_2 > U-46619.[170,171] Whereas I-BOP, STA_2, and U-46619 are agonists, SQ29548 and S145 are high-affinity TP receptor antagonists.[172] Studies have suggested that the TP receptor may mediate some of the biologic effects of the nonenzymatically derived isoprostanes,[173] including modulation of tubuloglomerular feedback.[174] This latter finding may have significance in pathophysiologic conditions associated with increased oxidative stress.[175] Signal transduction studies have shown that the TP receptor activates phosphatidylinositol bisphosphate (PIP_2) hydrolysis–dependent Ca^{2+} influx.[166,176] Northern blot analysis of mouse tissues has revealed that the highest level of TP mRNA expression is in the thymus,

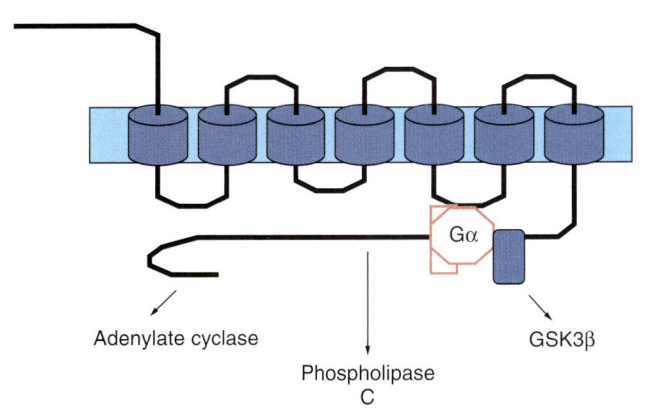

Figure 14.12 Prostaglandin receptors are seven-transmembrane, G protein–coupled receptors.

followed by the spleen, lung, and kidney, with lower levels of expression in the heart, uterus, and brain.[177]

Thromboxane is a potent modulator of platelet shape change and aggregation, as well as smooth muscle contraction and proliferation. Moreover, a point mutation (Arg[60] to Leu) in the first cytoplasmic loop of the TXA_2 receptor was identified in a dominantly inherited bleeding disorder in humans, characterized by a defective platelet response to TXA_2.[178] Targeted gene disruption of the murine TP receptor also resulted in prolonged bleeding times and reduction in collagen-stimulated platelet aggregation (Figure 14.13). Conversely, overexpression of the TP receptor in vascular tissue increases the severity of vascular pathology following injury.[1] Increased thromboxane synthesis has been linked to cardiovascular diseases, including acute myocardial ischemia, heart failure, and inflammatory renal diseases.[1]

In the kidney, TP receptor mRNA has been reported in glomeruli and vasculature. Radioligand autoradiography using ^{125}I-BOP has suggested a similar distribution of binding sites in the mouse renal cortex, but additional renal medullary binding sites were observed.[179] These medullary TXA_2 binding sites are absent following disruption of the TP receptor gene, suggesting that they also represent authentic TP receptors.[180] Glomerular TP receptors may participate in potent vasoconstrictor effects of TXA_2 analogs on the glomerular microcirculation associated with a reduced GFR.[1] Mesangial TP receptors coupled to phosphatidylinositol hydrolysis, protein kinase C activation, and glomerular mesangial cell contraction may contribute to these effects.[181]

An important role for TP receptors in regulating renal hemodynamics and systemic blood pressure has also been suggested. Administration of a TP receptor antagonist reduces blood pressure in spontaneously hypertensive rats (SHRs)[139] and in angiotensin-dependent hypertension.[182] The TP receptor also appears to modulate renal blood flow in Ang II–dependent hypertension[183] and in endotoxemia-induced renal failure.[184] Modulation of renal TP receptor mRNA expression and function by dietary salt intake has also been reported.[185] These studies also suggested an important role for luminal TP receptors in the distal tubule

	Renal Expression	Renal Phenotype	Other Knockout Phenotype
DP1	Minimal?	No	Reduced allergic asthma, reduced niacin flushing
DP2	Minimal?	++ Reduced fibrosis in UUO	Decreased cutaneous inflammatory responses
IP	++ Afferent arterioles	±	Reduced inflammation, increased thrombosis
TP	+ Glomerulus, tubules?	No	Prolonged bleeding time, platelet defect
FP	+++ Distal tubules	No	Failure of parturition
EP1	++++ MCD	No	Decreased Ang II hypertension
EP2	++ interstitial stromal	++ Salt-sensitive hypertension	Impaired female fertility
EP3	++++ TAL, MCD	+	Impaired febrile response
EP4	+++ Glomerulus, + distal tubules	++ Reduced fibrosis in UUO	Perinatal death from persistent patent ductus arteriosus

Figure 14.13 Published phenotypes of prostanoid receptor knockout mice. MCD, Medullary collecting duct; TAL, thick ascending limb; UUO, unilateral ureteral obstruction.

to enhance glomerular vasoconstriction indirectly via effects on the macula densa TGF.[186] However, other studies revealed no significant difference in TGF between wild-type and TP receptor knockout mice.[45]

A major phenotype of TP receptor disruption in mice and humans appears to be reduced platelet aggregation and prolonged bleeding time.[180] Thromboxane may also modulate the glomerular fibrinolytic system by increasing the production of an inhibitor of plasminogen activator (PAI-1) in mesangial cells.[187] Although a specific renal phenotype in the TP receptor knockout mouse has not yet been reported, important pathogenic roles for TXA_2 and glomerular TP receptors in mediating renal dysfunction in glomerulonephritis, diabetes mellitus, and sepsis seem likely.

In an Ang II–dependent mouse model of hypertension, deletion of the TP receptor gene ameliorated hypertension and reduced cardiac hypertrophy, but had no effect on proteinuria.[188] In contrast, although blockade of NO synthase in an L-NAME (N^G-nitro-L-arginine methyl ester) model of hypertension, in which deletion of the TP receptor also ameliorated hypertension and did not decrease GFR, it led to an increased worsening of histopathology and significant renal hypertrophy. This suggests that the TP receptor may play a renal protective role in some settings.[189]

IP RECEPTORS

The cDNA for the IP receptor encodes a transmembrane protein of approximately 41 kDa. The IP receptor is selectively activated by the analog cicaprost.[190] Iloprost and carbaprostacyclin potently activate the IP receptor but also activate the EP1 receptor. Most evidence suggests that the PGI_2 receptor signals via stimulation of cAMP generation; however, at 1000-fold higher concentrations, the cloned mouse PGI_2 receptor also signaled via PIP_2.[191] It remains unclear whether PIP_2 hydrolysis plays any significant role in the physiologic action of PGI_2.

IP receptor mRNA is highly expressed in the mouse thymus, heart, and spleen[191] and in human kidney, liver, and lung.[192] In situ hybridization shows IP receptor mRNA predominantly in neurons of the dorsal root ganglia and vascular tissue, including the aorta, pulmonary artery, and renal interlobular and glomerular afferent arterioles.[193] The expression of IP receptor mRNA in the dorsal root ganglia is consistent with a role for prostacyclin in pain sensation. Mice with IP receptor gene disruption exhibit a predisposition to arterial thrombosis, diminished pain perception, and inflammatory responses.[141]

PGI_2 has been demonstrated to play an important vasodilator role in the kidney,[194] including in the glomerular microvasculature,[195] as well as regulating renin release.[196,197] The capacity of PGI_2 and PGE_2 to stimulate cAMP generation in the glomerular microvasculature is distinct and additive,[198] demonstrating that the effects of these two prostanoids are mediated via separate receptors. IP receptor knockout mice also exhibit salt-sensitive hypertension.[199] Prostacyclin is a potent stimulus of renal renin release, and studies using $IP^{-/-}$ mice have confirmed an important role for the IP receptor in the development of renin-dependent hypertension of renal artery stenosis.[69]

Renal epithelial effects of PGI_2 in the thick ascending limb have also been suggested,[200] and IP receptors have been reported in the collecting duct,[201] but the potential expression and role of prostacyclin in these segments are less well established. Of interest, in situ hybridization also demonstrated significant expression of prostacyclin synthase in medullary collecting ducts,[202] consistent with a role for this metabolite in this region of the kidney. Thus, although IP receptors appear to play an important role regulating renin release and as a vasodilator in the kidney, their role in regulating renal epithelial function remains to be firmly established.

DP RECEPTORS

The DP1 receptor has been cloned and, like the IP and EP2/4 receptors, the DP receptor predominantly signals by increasing cAMP generation. The human DP receptor binds PGD_2 with a high-affinity binding of 300 pM and a lower affinity site of 13.4 nM.[203] DP-selective PGD_2 analogs include the agonist BW 245C.[204] DP receptor mRNA is highly expressed in leptomeninges, retina, and ileum but was not detected in the kidney.[205] Northern blot analysis of the human DP receptor demonstrated mRNA expression in the small intestine and retina,[206] whereas in the mouse the DP receptor mRNA was detected in the ileum and lung.[203] PGD_2 has also been shown to affect the sleep-wake cycle,[207] pain sensation,[144] and body temperature.[208] Peripherally, PGD_2 has been shown to mediate vasodilation as well as possibly inhibiting platelet aggregation. Consistent with this latter finding, the DP receptor knockout displayed reduced inflammation in the ovalbumin model of allergic asthma.[209] Development of the antagonist laropiprant was undertaken to inhibit the niacin-induced vasodilation flushing response.[210] Although the kidney appears capable of synthesizing PGD_2, its role in the kidney remains poorly defined. Intrarenal infusion of PGD_2 resulted in a dose-dependent increase in renal artery flow, urine output, creatinine clearance, and sodium and potassium excretion.[211]

A second G protein–coupled receptor capable of binding and being activated by PGD_2 was cloned as an orphan chemoattractant receptor from eosinophils and T cells (type 2 helper T cell subset) and designated the CRTH2 receptor.[212] This receptor, now referred to as the DP2 receptor, bears no significant sequence homology to the family of prostanoid receptors discussed earlier, and couples to G_i/G_o inhibition of intracellular cAMP. It binds agonists with an order of potency $PGD_2 \gg PGF_{2\alpha}, PGE_2 > PGI_2, TXA_2$. DP2 receptor action is blocked by the antagonist ramatroban, a drug used to treat allergic rhinitis and originally described as a TP receptor antagonist.[213] Deletion of the DP2 receptor gene was protective in a mouse UUO model of fibrosis.[214] The recognition of this molecularly unrelated receptor allows for the possibility of the existence of a distinct and new family of prostanoid-activated membrane receptors.

FP RECEPTORS

The cDNA encoding the $PGF_{2\alpha}$ receptor (FP receptor) was cloned from a human kidney cDNA library and encodes a protein of 359 amino acid residues. The bovine and murine FP receptors, cloned from corpora lutea, similarly encode proteins of 362 and 366 amino acid residues, respectively. Transfection of HEK293 cells with the human FP receptor cDNA conferred preferential ^{3}H-PGF$_{2\alpha}$ binding with a K$_D$ of 4.3 ± 1.0 nM.[172,215] Selective activation of the FP receptor may be achieved using fluprostenol or latanoprost.[172] ^{3}H-PGF$_{2\alpha}$ binding was displaced by a panel of ligands with a rank order potency of PGF$_{2\alpha}$ = fluprostenol > PGD$_2$ > PGE$_2$ > U46619 > iloprost.[190] When expressed in oocytes, PGF$_{2\alpha}$ or fluprostenol induced a Ca^{2+}-dependent Cl$^-$ current. Increased cell calcium has also been observed in fibroblasts expressing an endogenous FP receptor.[216] Other studies have suggested that FP receptors may also activate protein kinase C (PKC)–dependent and Rho-mediated/PKC–independent signaling pathways.[217] An alternatively spliced isoform with a shorter C-terminal tail has been identified that appears to signal via a similar manner as the originally described FP receptor,[218] and other studies have suggested that these two isoforms may exhibit differential desensitization and may also activate a glycogen synthase kinase/β-catenin–coupled signaling pathway.[219]

Tissue distribution of FP receptor mRNA shows highest expression in ovarian corpus luteum followed by kidney, with lower expression in the lung, stomach, and heart.[220] Expression of the FP receptor in corpora lutea is critical for normal birth, and homozygous disruption of the mouse FP receptor gene results in failure of parturition in females, apparently due to failure of the normal preterm decline in progesterone levels.[221] PGF$_{2\alpha}$ is a potent constrictor of smooth muscle in the uterus, bronchi, and blood vessels; however, an endothelial FP receptor may also play a dilator role.[222] The FP receptor is also highly expressed in skin, where it may play an important role in carcinogenesis.[223] A clinically important role for the FP receptor in the eye has been demonstrated to increase uveoscleral outflow and reduce ocular pressure. The FP–selective agonist latanoprost has been used clinically as an effective treatment for glaucoma.[224]

The role of FP receptors in regulating renal function is only partially defined. FP receptor expression has been mapped to the CCD in mouse and rabbit kidney.[225] FP receptor activation in the collecting duct inhibits vasopressin-stimulated water absorption via a pertussis toxin–sensitive (presumably G$_i$) dependent mechanism. Although PGF$_{2\alpha}$ increases cell Ca^{2+} in cortical collecting duct, the FP–selective agonists latanoprost and fluprostenol did not increase calcium.[226] Because PGF$_{2\alpha}$ can also bind to EP1 and EP3 receptors,[190,227,228] these data suggest that the calcium increase activated by PGF$_{2\alpha}$ in the collecting duct may be mediated via an EP receptor. PGF$_{2\alpha}$ also increases Ca^{2+} in cultured glomerular mesangial cells and podocytes,[229,230] suggesting that an FP receptor may modulate glomerular contraction. In contrast to these findings, glomerular FP receptors at the molecular level have not been demonstrated. Other vascular effects of PGF$_{2\alpha}$ have been described, including selective modulation of renal production of PGF$_{2\alpha}$ by sodium or potassium loading and AT$_2$ receptor activation.[152]

Some studies have uncovered a role for the FP receptor in regulating renin expression. Interestingly, FP agonists increased renin mRNA expression in the JGA in a dose-dependent manner but, unlike IP receptor agonists, did not increase intracellular cAMP. Deletion of the FP receptor resulted in decreased renin levels and decreased systemic blood pressure. These data suggest that FP receptor blockade may be a novel target for the treatment of hypertension.[231]

MULTIPLE EP RECEPTORS

Four EP receptor subtypes have been identified.[232] Although these four receptors uniformly bind PGE$_2$ with a higher affinity than other endogenous prostanoids, the amino acid homology of each is more closely related to other prostanoid receptors that signal through similar mechanisms.[171] Thus, the relaxant/cAMP–coupled EP2 receptor is more closely related to other relaxant prostanoid receptors, such as the IP and DP receptors, whereas the constrictor/Ca^{2+}–coupled EP1 receptor is more closely related to the other Ca^{2+}–coupled prostanoid receptors (e.g., TP and FP receptors).[233] These receptors may also be selectively activated or antagonized by different analogs. EP receptor subtypes also exhibit differential expression along the nephron, suggesting distinct functional consequences of activating each EP receptor subtype in the kidney.[234]

EP1 RECEPTORS

The human EP1 receptor cDNA encodes a 402–amino acid polypeptide that signals via inositol 1,4,5-trisphosphate (IP$_3$) generation and increased cell Ca^{2+} with IP$_3$ generation. Studies of EP1 receptors may use one of several relatively selective antagonists, including ONO-871, SC19220, and SC53122. EP1 receptor mRNA has widespread expression, presumably from its vascular expression,[235] and is expressed in the kidney much more than in the gastric muscularis mucosae and more than in the adrenal gland.[236] Renal EP1 mRNA expression determined by in situ hybridization is expressed primarily in the collecting duct and increases from the cortex to the papillae.[236] Activation of the EP1 receptor increases intracellular calcium and inhibits Na$^+$ and water reabsorption in the collecting duct,[236] suggesting that renal EP1 receptor activation might contribute to the natriuretic and diuretic effects of PGE$_2$.

Hemodynamic microvascular effects of EP1 receptors have also been reported. The EP1 receptor was originally described as a smooth muscle constrictor.[237] One report suggested that the EP1 receptor may also be present in cultured glomerular mesangial cells,[238] where it could play a role as a vasoconstrictor and stimulus for mesangial cell proliferation. Although a constrictor PGE$_2$ effect has been reported in the afferent arteriole of rat,[239] apparently produced by EP1 receptor activation,[240] there does not appear to be very high expression of the EP1 receptor mRNA in preglomerular vasculature or other arterial resistance vessels in mice or rabbits.[241] Other reports have suggested that EP1 receptor knockout mice exhibit hypotension and hyperreninemia, supporting a role for this receptor in maintaining blood pressure.[242]

EP2 RECEPTORS

Two cAMP-stimulating EP receptors, designated EP2 and EP4, have been identified. The EP2 receptor can be pharmacologically distinguished from the EP4 receptor by its sensitivity to butaprost.[243] In the literature prior to 1995, the cloned EP4 receptor was designated the EP2 receptor, but then a butaprost-sensitive EP receptor was cloned[244]; the original receptor was reclassified as the EP4 receptor and the newer, butaprost-sensitive protein was designated the EP2 receptor.[245] A pharmacologically defined EP2 receptor has now also been cloned for the mouse, rat, rabbit, dog, and cow.[246] The human EP2 receptor cDNA encodes a 358–amino acid polypeptide, which signals through increased cAMP. The EP2 receptor may also be distinguished from the EP4 receptor, the other major relaxant EP receptor, by its relative insensitivity to the EP4 agonist PGE$_1$-OH and insensitivity to the weak EP4 antagonist AH23848[243] and high-affinity EP4 antagonists ONO-AE3-208 and L-161982.[247] Recently, two EP2 antagonists have been described, PF-04418948 and TG4-155,[248,249] which should greatly facilitate the characterization of EP2 versus EP4 effects in vivo.

The precise distribution of the EP2 receptor mRNA has been partially characterized. This reveals a major mRNA species of about 3.1 kb that is most abundant in the uterus, lung, and spleen, exhibiting only low levels of expression in the kidney.[246] Studies using polymerase chain reaction (PCR) analysis across a range of tissue have demonstrated highest expression in the bone marrow more than in the ovary and more than in the lung, consistent with these earlier findings.[235] EP2 mRNA is expressed at much lower levels than EP4 mRNA in most tissues.[250] There is scant evidence to suggest segmental distribution of the EP2 receptor along the nephron.[246] Interestingly, it is expressed in cultured renal interstitial cells, supporting the possibility that the EP2 receptor is predominantly expressed in this portion of the nephron.[246] Studies in knockout mice have demonstrated a critical role for the EP2 receptor in ovulation and fertilization, and these studies have also suggested a potential role for the EP2 receptor in salt-sensitive hypertension.[251] This latter finding supports an important role for the EP2 receptor in protecting systemic blood pressure, perhaps via its vasodilator effect or effects on renal salt excretion. Evidence for the latter role has been revealed in studies demonstrating that a high-salt diet increases PGE$_2$ production, and infusion of EP-selective agonists identified the EP2 receptor as mediating PGE$_2$-evoked natriuresis. Moreover, deletion of the EP2 receptor ablated the natriuretic effect of PGE$_2$.[252]

EP3 RECEPTORS

The EP3 receptor generally acts as a constrictor of smooth muscle.[253] Nuclease protection and Northern blot analysis demonstrate relatively high levels of EP3 receptor expression in several tissues, including kidney, uterus, adrenal, and stomach, with riboprobes hybridizing to major mRNA species at approximately 2.4 and approximately 7.0 kb.[254] A metabolic pattern of expression was found by PCR testing, with high levels of expression in the pancreas and white and brown fat tissue in addition to expression in the kidney.[235] This receptor is unique in that there are multiple (more than eight) alternatively spliced variants differing only in their C-terminal cytoplasmic tails.[255-257] The EP3 splice variants bind PGE$_2$, and the EP3 agonists MB28767 and sulprostone with similar affinity. Also, although they exhibit common inhibition of cAMP generation via a pertussis toxin–sensitive G$_i$-coupled mechanism, the tails may recruit different signaling pathways, including Ca^{2+}-dependent signaling[171,243] and the small G protein Rho.[258] Recently, a Ptx-insensitive pathway for the inhibition of cAMP generation via guanine nucleotide-binding protein G(z) subunit alpha has also been described.[259] Differences in agonist-independent activity have been observed for several of the splice variants, suggesting that they may play a role in constitutive regulation of cellular events.[260] The physiologic roles of these different C-terminal splice variants and sites of expression within the kidney remain uncertain.

In situ hybridization has demonstrated that EP3 receptor mRNA is abundant in the TAL and collecting duct (CD).[261] This distribution has been confirmed by reverse transcriptase PCR (RT-PCR) testing on microdissected rat and mouse collecting ducts and corresponds to the major binding sites for radioactive PGE$_2$ in the kidney.[262] An important role for a G$_i$-coupled PGE receptor in regulating water and salt transport along the nephron has been recognized for many years. PGE$_2$ directly inhibits salt and water absorption in microperfused TALs and CDs. PGE$_2$ directly inhibits Cl$^-$ absorption in the mouse or rabbit medullary TAL from luminal or basolateral surfaces.[263] PGE$_2$ also inhibits hormone-stimulated cAMP generation in the TAL. Good and George have demonstrated that PGE$_2$ modulates ion transport in the rat TAL by a pertussis toxin–sensitive mechanism.[263] Interestingly, these effects also appear to involve PKC activation,[264] possibly reflecting activation of a novel EP3 receptor signaling pathway, possibly corresponding to alternative signaling pathways, as described earlier.[258] Taken together, these data support a role for the EP3 receptor in regulating transport in both the CCD and TAL.

Blockade of endogenous PGE$_2$ synthesis by NSAIDs enhances urinary concentration. It is likely that PGE$_2$-mediated antagonism of vasopressin-stimulated salt absorption in the TAL and water absorption in the CCD contributes to its diuretic effect. In the in vitro microperfused collecting duct, PGE$_2$ inhibits vasopressin-stimulated osmotic water absorption and vasopressin-stimulated cAMP generation.[226] Furthermore, PGE$_2$ inhibition of water absorption and cAMP generation are both blocked by pertussis toxin, suggesting effects mediated by the inhibitory G protein, G$_i$.[226] When administered in the absence of vasopressin, PGE$_2$ actually stimulates water absorption in the CCD from the luminal or basolateral side.[265] These stimulatory effects of PGE$_2$ on transport in the CCD appear to be related to activation of the EP4 receptor.[265] Despite the presence of this absorption-enhancing EP receptor, in vivo studies have suggested that in the presence of vasopressin, the predominant effects of endogenous PGE$_2$ on water transport are diuretic. Based on the preceding functional considerations, one would expect EP3$^{-/-}$ mice to exhibit inappropriately enhanced urinary concentration. Surprisingly, EP3$^{-/-}$ mice exhibited a comparable urinary concentration following desmopressin (DDAVP) administration, similar 24-hour water intake, and similar maximal and minimal urinary osmolality. The only clear difference was that in mice allowed free access to water, indomethacin increased urinary osmolality in normal mice but not in the knockout animals. These findings raise the possibility that some of the renal actions of PGE$_2$ normally mediated by the EP3 receptor have been co-opted by other receptors (e.g., EP1 or FP receptor) in the EP3 knockout mouse. This remains to be formally tested.

The function of EP3 receptor activation in animal physiology has been significantly advanced by the availability of mice with targeted disruption of this gene. Mice with targeted deletion of the EP3 receptor exhibit an impaired febrile response, suggesting that EP3 receptor antagonists could be effective antipyretic agents.[266] Other studies have suggested that the EP3 receptor plays an important vasopressor role in the peripheral circulation of mice.[241,267] In the intrarenal circulation, PGE$_2$ has variable effects, acting as a vasoconstrictor in the larger, proximal portion of the intralobular arteries and changing to a vasodilator effect in the smaller, distal intralobular arteries and afferent arterioles.[268]

EP4 RECEPTOR

Although the EP4 receptor signals through increased cAMP,[269] like the EP2 receptor, it has been appreciated to signal though a number of other pathways as well.[270] These include arrestin-mediated signaling, phosphatidylinositol-3-kinase, signaling β-catenin and G$_i$ coupling. The human EP4 receptor cDNA encodes a 488–amino acid polypeptide with a predicted molecular mass of about 53 kDa.[271] Note that care must be taken in reviewing the literature prior to 1995, when this receptor was generally referred to as the EP2 receptor.[245] In addition to the human receptor, EP4 receptors for the mouse, rat, rabbit, and dog have been cloned. EP4 receptors can be pharmacologically distinguished from EP1 and EP3 receptors by insensitivity to sulprostone and from EP2 receptors by insensitivity to butaprost and relatively selective activation by PGE$_1$-OH.[172] EP4–selective agonists (ONO-AE1-329, ONO-4819) and antagonists (ONO-AE3-208, L-161,982) have been generated and used to investigate the role of EP4 in vivo. Activation of the EP4 receptor was able to ameliorate the phenotype of a mouse model of nephrogenic diabetes insipidus.[272]

EP4 receptor mRNA is highly expressed relative to the EP2 receptor and is widely distributed, with a major species of approximately 3.8 kb detected by Northern blot analysis in the thymus, ileum, lung, spleen, adrenal, and kidney.[250,273] Dominant vasodilator effects of EP4 receptor activation have been described in venous and arterial beds.[204,253] A critical role for the EP4 receptor in regulating the perinatal closure of the pulmonary ductus arteriosus has also been suggested by studies of mice with targeted disruption of the EP4 receptor gene.[162,274] On a 129- strain background, EP4$^{-/-}$ mice had an almost 100% perinatal mortality due to persistent patent ductus arteriosus.[274] Interestingly, when bred on a mixed genetic background, only 80% of EP4$^{-/-}$ mice died, whereas about 21% underwent closure of the ductus and survived.[162] Preliminary studies in these survivors have supported an important role for the EP4 receptor as a systemic vasodepressor[275]; however, their heterogeneous genetic background complicates the interpretation of these results, because survival may select for modifier genes that not only allow ductus closure, but also alter other hemodynamic responses.

Other roles for the EP4 receptor in controlling blood pressure have been suggested, including the ability to stimulate aldosterone release from zona glomerulosa cells.[276] In the kidney, EP4 receptor mRNA expression is primarily in the glomerulus, where its precise function is uncharacterized[273,277] but might contribute to regulation of the renal microcirculation and renin release.[278] Studies in mice with genetic deletion of selective prostanoid receptors have indicated that EP4$^{-/-}$ mice, as well as IP$^{-/-}$ mice to a lesser extent, failed to increase renin production in response to loop diuretic administration, indicating that macula densa–derived PGE$_2$ increased renin primarily through EP4 activation.[279] This corresponds to studies suggesting that EP4 receptors are expressed in cultured podocytes and JGA cells.[229,278] PGE$_2$ may mediate increased podocyte COX-2 expression through EP4-mediated increased cAMP, which activates P38 through a PKA-independent process.[280] Finally, the EP4 receptor in the renal pelvis may participate in the regulation of salt excretion by altering afferent renal nerve output.[281]

REGULATION OF RENAL FUNCTION BY EP RECEPTORS

PGE$_2$ exerts myriad effects in the kidney, presumably mediated by EP receptors. PGE$_2$ not only dilates the glomerular microcirculation and vasa recta, supplying the renal medulla,[282] but also modulates salt and water transport in the distal tubule (see Figure 14.5).[283] The maintenance of normal renal function during physiologic stress is particularly dependent on endogenous PG synthesis. In this setting, the vasoconstrictor effects of Ang II, catecholamines, and vasopressin are more effectively buffered by prostaglandins in the kidney than in other vascular beds, preserving normal renal blood flow, GFR, and salt excretion. Administration of COX-inhibiting NSAIDs in the setting of volume depletion interferes with these dilator effects and may result in a catastrophic decline in the GFR, resulting in overt renal failure.[284]

Other evidence points to vasoconstrictor and prohypertensive effects of endogenous PGE$_2$. PGE$_2$ stimulates renin release from the JGA,[285] leading to a subsequent increase in the vasoconstrictor Ang II. In conscious dogs, chronic intrarenal PGE$_2$ infusion increases renal renin secretion, resulting in hypertension.[286] Treatment of salt-depleted rats with indomethacin not only decreases plasma renin activity, but also reduces blood pressure, suggesting that PGs support blood pressure during salt depletion via their capacity to increase renin.[287] Direct vasoconstrictor effects of PGE$_2$ on vasculature have also been observed.[241] It is conceivable that these latter effects might predominate in circumstances in which the kidney is exposed to excessively high perfusion pressures. Thus, depending on the setting, the primary effect of PGE$_2$ may be to increase or decrease vascular tone, effects that appear to be mediated by distinct EP receptors.

Renal Cortical Hemodynamics

The expression of the EP4 receptor in the glomerulus suggests that it may play an important role in regulating renal hemodynamics. PGs regulate the renal cortical microcirculation and, as noted, both glomerular constrictor and dilator effects of prostaglandins have been observed.[241,288] In the setting of volume depletion, endogenous PGE$_2$ helps maintain the GFR by dilating the afferent arteriole.[288] Some data have suggested roles for EP and IP receptors coupled to increased cAMP generation in mediating vasodilator effects in the preglomerular circulation.[44,278,289] PGE$_2$ exerts a dilator effect on the afferent arteriole but not the efferent arteriole, consistent with the presence of an EP2 or EP4 receptor in the preglomerular microcirculation.

Renin Release

Other data have suggested that the EP4 receptor may also stimulate renin release. Soon after the introduction of

NSAIDs, it was recognized that endogenous PGs play an important role in stimulating renin release.[44] Treatment of salt-depleted rats with indomethacin not only decreases plasma renin activity, but also causes blood pressure to fall, suggesting that PGs support blood pressure during salt depletion via their capacity to increase renin. Prostanoids also play a central role in the pathogenesis of renovascular hypertension, and administration of NSAIDs lowers blood pressure in animals and humans with renal artery stenosis.[290] PGE_2 induces renin release in isolated preglomerular juxtaglomerular apparatus cells.[285] Like the effect of β-adrenergic agents, this effect appears to be through a cAMP-coupled response, supporting a role for an EP4 or EP2 receptor.[285] EP4 receptor mRNA has been detected in microdissected JGAs,[291] supporting the possibility that renal EP4 receptor activation contributes to enhanced renin release. Finally, regulation of plasma renin activity and intrarenal renin mRNA does not appear to be different in wild-type and EP2 knockout mice,[292] arguing against a major role for the EP2 receptor in regulating renin release. Conversely, one report has suggested that EP3 receptor mRNA is localized to the macula densa, suggesting that this cAMP-inhibiting receptor may also contribute to the control of renin release.[277]

Renal Microcirculation

The EP2 receptor also appears to play an important role in regulating afferent arteriolar tone.[288] In the setting of systemic hypertension, the normal response of the kidney is to increase salt excretion, thereby mitigating the increase in blood pressure. This so-called pressure natriuresis plays a key role in the ability of the kidney to protect against hypertension.[293] Increased blood pressure is accompanied by increased renal perfusion pressure and enhanced urinary PGE_2 excretion.[294] Inhibition of PG synthesis markedly blunts (although it does not eliminate) pressure natriuresis.[295] The mechanism whereby PGE_2 contributes to pressure natriuresis may involve changes in resistance of the renal medullary microcirculation.[296] PGE_2 directly dilates the descending vasa recta, and increased medullary blood flow may contribute to the increased interstitial pressure observed as renal perfusion pressure increases, leading to enhanced salt excretion.[282] The identity of the dilator PGE_2 receptor controlling the contractile properties of the descending vasa recta remains uncertain, but EP2 or EP2 receptors seem likely candidates.[204] Results of studies demonstrating salt-sensitive hypertension in mice with targeted disruption of the EP2 receptor[251] have suggested that the EP2 receptor facilitates the ability of the kidney to increase sodium excretion, thereby protecting systemic blood pressure from a high-salt diet. Given its defined role in vascular smooth muscle,[251] these effects of the EP2 receptor disruption seem more likely to relate to its effects on renal vascular tone. In particular, loss of a vasodilator effect in the renal medulla might modify pressure natriuresis and could contribute to hypertension in EP2 knockout mice. Nonetheless, a role for the EP2 or EP4 receptor in regulating renal medullary blood flow remains to be established. In conclusion, direct vasomotor effects of EP4 receptors, as well as effects on renin release, may play critical roles in regulating systemic blood pressure and renal hemodynamics.

EFFECTS OF COX-1 AND COX-2 METABOLITES ON SALT AND WATER TRANSPORT

COX-1 and COX-2 metabolites of arachidonate have important direct epithelial effects on salt and water transport along the nephron.[297] Thus, functional effects can be observed that are thought to be independent of any hemodynamic changes produced by these compounds. Because biologically active arachidonic acid metabolites are rapidly metabolized, they act predominantly in an autocrine or paracrine fashion and, thus, their locus of action will be quite close to their point of generation. Thus, one can expect that direct epithelial effects of these compounds will result when they are produced by the tubule cells themselves or the neighboring interstitial cells, and the tubules possess an appropriate receptor for the ligand.

PROXIMAL TUBULE

Neither the proximal convoluted tubule nor the proximal straight tubule appears to produce amounts of biologically active COX metabolites of arachidonic acid. As will be discussed in a subsequent section, the dominant arachidonate metabolites produced by proximal convoluted and straight tubules are metabolites of the cytochrome P450 pathway.[298]

Early whole-animal studies suggested that PGE_2 might have an action in the proximal tubule because of its effects on urinary phosphate excretion. PGE_2 blocked the phosphaturic action of calcitonin infusion in thyroparathyroidectomized rats. Nevertheless, studies using in vitro perfused proximal tubules failed to show an effect of PGE_2 on sodium chloride or phosphate transport in the proximal convoluted tubule. More recent studies have suggested that PGE_2 may play a key role in the phosphaturic action of fibroblast growth factor-23[299] because phosphaturia in *hyp* mice with X-linked hyperphosphaturia is associated with markedly increased urine PGE_2 excretion, and phosphaturia was normalized by indomethacin.[300] Nevertheless, there are very little data on the actions of other COX metabolites in proximal tubules and scant molecular evidence for the expression of classic G protein–coupled prostaglandin receptors in this segment of the nephron.

LOOP OF HENLE

The nephron segments making up the loop of Henle also display limited metabolism of exogenous arachidonic acid through the COX pathway although, given the realization that COX-2 is expressed in this segment, it is of note that PGE_2 was uniformly greater in the cortical segment than the medullary thick ascending limb. The TAL has been shown to exhibit high-density PGE_2 receptors.[301] Studies have also demonstrated high expression levels of mRNA for the EP3 receptor in medullary TAL of both rabbit and rat[228] (see earlier, "EP3 Receptors"). Subsequent to the demonstration that PGE_2 inhibits sodium chloride absorption in the medullary TAL of the rabbit perfused in vitro, it was shown that PGE_2 blocks vasopressin (AVP) but not cAMP-stimulated sodium chloride absorption in the medullary TAL of the mouse. It is likely that the mechanism involves activation of

G_i and inhibition of adenyl cyclase by PGE_2, possibly via the EP3 receptors expressed in this segment.

COLLECTING DUCT SYSTEM

In vitro perfusion studies of rabbit cortical collecting tubule have demonstrated that PGE_2 directly inhibits sodium transport in the collecting duct when applied to the basolateral surface of this nephron segment. It is now apparent that PGE_2 uses multiple signal transduction pathways in the cortical collecting duct, including those that modulate intracellular cAMP levels and Ca^{2+}. PGE_2 can stimulate or suppress cAMP accumulation. The latter may also involve stimulation of phosphodiesterase. Although modulation of cAMP levels appears to play an important role in PGE_2 effects on water transport in the CCD (see following section), it is less clear that PGE_2 affects sodium transport via modulation of cAMP levels.[226] PGE_2 has been shown to increase cell calcium, possibly coupled with PKC activation, in in vitro perfused cortical collecting ducts.[302] This effect may be mediated by the EP1 receptor subtype coupled to phosphatidylinositol hydrolysis.[236]

WATER TRANSPORT

AVP-regulated water transport in the collecting duct is markedly influenced by COX products, especially prostaglandins. When COX inhibitors are administered to humans, rat, or dog, the antidiuretic action of AVP is markedly augmented. Because vasopressin also stimulates endogenous PGE_2 production by the collecting duct, these results suggest that PGE_2 participates in a negative feedback loop, whereby endogenous PGE_2 production dampens the action of AVP.[303] In agreement with this model, the early classic studies of Grantham and Orloff directly demonstrated that PGE_1 blunted the water permeability response of the CCD to vasopressin. In these early studies, the action of PGE_1 appeared to be at a pre-cAMP step. Interestingly, when administered by itself, PGE_1 modestly augmented basal water permeability. These earlier studies have been confirmed with respect to PGE_2. PGE_2 also stimulates basal hydraulic conductivity and suppresses the hydraulic conductivity response to AVP in the rabbit cortical collecting duct.[304,305] Inhibition of AVP-stimulated cAMP generation and water permeability appears to be mediated by the EP1 and EP3 receptors, whereas the increase in basal water permeability may be mediated by the EP4 receptor.[265] These data are evidence of consistent functional redundancy between the EP1 and EP3 with respect to their effects on AVP-stimulated water absorption in the collecting duct.

METABOLISM OF PROSTAGLANDINS

15-KETODEHYDROGENASE

The half-life of prostaglandins is 3 to 5 minutes and that of TXA_2 is approximately 30 seconds. Elimination of PGE_2, $PGF_{2\alpha}$, and PGI_2 proceeds through enzymatic and nonenzymatic pathways, whereas that of TXA_2 is nonenzymatic. The end products of all these degradative reactions generally possess minimal biologic activity, although this is not uniformly true (see below). The principal enzyme involved in the transformation of PGE_2, PGI_2, and $PGF_{2\alpha}$ is 15-hydroxyprostaglandin dehydrogenase (15-PGDH), which converts the 15 alcohol group to a ketone.[306]

15-PGDH is an oxidized nicotinamide adenine dinucleotide–oxidized nicotinamide adenine dinucleotide phosphate ($NAD^+/NADP^+$)–dependent enzyme that is 30 to 49 times more active in the kidney of the young rat (3 weeks of age) than in the adult. Its K_m for PGE_2 is 8.4 µmol/L and 22.6 µmol/L for $PGF_{2\alpha}$.[306] It is mainly localized in cortical and juxtamedullary zones,[307] with little activity detected in papillary slices. At baseline, it is found in the proximal tubule, TAL, and CD. However, it was present in the macula densa in COX-2 knockout mice and in the presence of high-salt diet and, in cultured macula densa cells, COX inhibition increased expression.[308] Disruption of the 15-PGDH gene in mice results in persistent patent ductus arteriosus (PDA), thought to be a result of failure of circulating PGE_2 levels to fall in the immediate peripartum period.[309] Thus, administration of COX-inhibiting NSAIDs rescues the knockout mice by decreasing PGs and allowing the animals to survive.

Subsequent catalysis of 15-hydroxy products by a δ-13 reductase leads to the formation of 13,14-dihydro compounds. PGI_2 and TXA_2 undergo rapid degradation to 6-keto-$PGF_{1\alpha}$ and TXB_2, respectively.[306] These stable metabolites are usually measured and their rates of formation taken as representative of those of the parent molecules.

ω/ω-1 HYDROXYLATION OF PROSTAGLANDINS

Both PGA_2 and PGE_2 have been shown to undergo hydroxylation of their terminal or subterminal carbons by a cytochrome P450–dependent mechanism.[310] This reaction may be mediated by CYP4A family members or a CYP4F enzyme. CYP4A[311] and CYP4F members have been mapped along the nephron.[312] Some of these derivatives have been shown to exhibit biologic activity.

CYCLOPENTENONE PROSTAGLANDINS

The cyclopentenone prostaglandins include PGA_2, a PGE_2 derivative, and PGJ_2, a derivative of PGD_2. Although it remains uncertain whether these compounds are actually produced in vivo, this possibility has received increasing attention because some cyclopentenone prostanoids have been shown to be activating ligands for nuclear transcription factors, including peroxisome proliferator–activated receptors δ and γ (PPARδ and PPARγ).[313-315] The realization that the antidiabetic thiazolidinedione drugs act through PPARγ to exert their antihyperglycemic and insulin-sensitizing effects[316] has generated intense interest in the possibility that the cyclopentenone PGs might serve as the endogenous ligands for these receptors. Interestingly, DP2, unlike DP1 or other members of the prostaglandin GPCR family, binds and is activated by PGD_2 metabolites such as 15-deoxy-Δ12,14-PGJ_2, which acts at nanomolar concentrations.[317] An alternative biologic activity of these compounds has been recognized in their capacity to modify thiol groups covalently, forming adducts with cysteine of several intracellular proteins, including thioredoxin 1, vimentin, actin, and tubulin.[318] Studies regarding the biologic activity of cyclopentenone prostanoids abound and the reader is referred to several excellent sources in the literature.[319-321] Although there is evidence supporting the presence of these compounds in vivo,[322] it remains uncertain whether they can form enzymatically or are an unstable spontaneous dehydration product of the E and D ring prostaglandins.[323]

NONENZYMATIC METABOLISM OF ARACHIDONIC ACID

It has long been recognized that oxidant injury can result in peroxidation of lipids. In 1990, Morrow and coworkers reported that a series of prostaglandin-like compounds could be produced by free radical catalyzed peroxidation of arachidonic acid that is independent of COX activity.[324] These compounds, termed *isoprostanes*, have been increasingly used as sensitive markers of oxidant injury in vitro and in vivo.[325] In addition, at least two of these compounds, 8-iso-PGF$_{2\alpha}$ (15-F$_2$-isoprostane) and 8-iso-PGE$_2$ (15-E$_2$-isoprostane) are potent vasoconstrictors when administered exogenously. 8-Iso-PGF$_{2\alpha}$ has been shown to constrict the renal microvasculature and decrease GFR, an effect that is prevented by thromboxane receptor antagonism.[326] However, the role of endogenous isoprostanes as mediators of biologic responses remains unclear.

PROSTAGLANDIN TRANSPORT AND URINARY EXCRETION

It is notable that most of the prostaglandin synthetic enzymes have been localized to the intracellular compartment, yet extracellular prostaglandins are potent autocoids and paracrine factors. Thus, prostanoids must be transported extracellularly to achieve efficient metabolism and termination of their signaling. Similarly, enzymes that metabolize PGE$_2$ to inactive compounds are also intracellular, requiring uptake of the PG for its metabolic inactivation. The molecular basis of these extrusion and uptake processes are now being defined.

As a fatty acid, prostaglandins may be classified as an organic anion at physiologic pH. Early microperfusion studies documented that basolateral PGE$_2$ could be taken up into proximal tubule cells and actively secreted into the lumen. Furthermore this process could be inhibited by a variety of inhibitors of organic anion transport, including *p*-aminohippurate (PAH), probenecid, and indomethacin. Studies of basolateral renal membrane vesicles also supported the notion that this transport process occurs via an electroneutral anion exchanger. These studies are of note because renal prostaglandins enter the urine in Henle's loop, and late proximal tubule secretion could provide an important entry mechanism.[1]

A molecule that mediates PGE$_2$ uptake in exchange for lactate has been cloned and termed *prostaglandin transporter* (PGT).[327] PGT is a member of the SLC21/SLCO organic anion transporting family, and its cDNA encodes a transmembrane protein of 100 amino acids that exhibits broad tissue distribution (heart, placenta, brain, lung, liver, skeletal muscle, pancreas, kidney, spleen, prostate, ovary, small intestine, and colon).[328-330] Immunocytochemical studies of PGT expression in rat kidneys have suggested expression primarily in glomerular endothelial and mesangial cells, arteriolar endothelial and muscularis cells, principal cells of the CD, medullary interstitial cells, medullary vasa recta endothelia, and papillary surface epithelium.[331] PGT appears to mediate PGE$_2$ uptake rather than release,[332] allowing target cells to metabolize this molecule and terminate signaling.[333] PGT expression is decreased with low salt and increased with high salt in the CD, which may allow regulation of PG excretion by taking up more prostaglandins excreted from luminal surface, the site of the PGT, thereby allowing more accumulation at the basolateral surface.[334]

Other members of the organic cation, anion, and zwitterion transporter family SLC22 have also been shown to transport prostaglandins[327] and have been suggested to mediate prostaglandin excretion into the urine. Specifically, OAT1 and OAT3 are localized on the basolateral proximal tubule membrane, where they likely participate in urinary excretion of PGE$_2$.[335,336] Conversely members of the multidrug resistance protein (MRP) have been shown to transport PGs in an adenosine triphosphate–dependent fashion.[337,338] MRP2 (also designated ABBC2) is expressed in kidney proximal tubule brush borders and may contribute to the transport (and urinary excretion) of glutathione-conjugated prostaglandins.[339,340] This transporter has more limited tissue expression, restricted to the kidney, liver, and small intestine, and could contribute not only to renal PAH excretion but also to prostaglandin excretion.[341]

INVOLVEMENT OF CYCLO-OXYGENASE METABOLITES IN RENAL PATHOPHYSIOLOGY

EXPERIMENTAL AND HUMAN GLOMERULAR INJURY

GLOMERULAR INFLAMMATORY INJURY

COX metabolites have been implicated in functional and structural alterations in glomerular and tubulointerstitial inflammatory diseases.[342] Essential fatty acid deficiency totally prevents the structural and functional consequences of the administration of nephrotoxic serum (NTS) to rats, an experimental model of anti–glomerular basement membrane glomerulonephritis.[326] Changes in arteriolar tone during the course of this inflammatory lesion are mediated principally by locally released COX and LO metabolites of AA.[326]

TXA$_2$ release appears to play an essential role in mediating the increased renovascular resistance observed during the early phase of this disease.[1] Subsequently, increasing rates of PGE$_2$ generation may account for the progressive dilation of renal arterioles and increases in renal blood flow at later stages of the disease. Consistent with this hypothesis, TXA$_2$ antagonism ameliorated the falls in renal blood flow (RBF) and GFR 2 hours post-NTS administration, but not after 24 hours. During the latter, heterologous, phase of NTS, COX metabolites mediate the renal vasodilation and reduction in K$_f$ that characterize this phase.[326] The net functional result of COX inhibition during this phase of experimental glomerulonephritis, therefore, would depend on the relative importance of renal perfusion versus the preservation of K$_f$ to the maintenance of the GFR. Evidence has also indicated that COX metabolites are mediators of pathologic lesions and the accompanying proteinuria in this model.[1] COX-2 expression in the kidney increases in experimental anti-GBM (glomerular basement membrane) glomerulonephritis[343,344] and after systemic administration of lipopolysaccharide.[345]

A beneficial effect of fish oil diets (enriched in eicosapentaneoic acid), with an accompanying reduction in the generation of COX products, has been demonstrated on the course of genetic murine lupus (in MRL-lpr mice). In subsequent studies, enhanced renal TXA_2 and PGE_2 generation was demonstrated in this model, as well as in NZB mice, another genetic model of lupus.[1] In addition, studies in humans have demonstrated an inverse relation between TXA_2 biosynthesis and GFR and improvement of renal function following short-term therapy with a thromboxane receptor antagonist in patients with lupus nephritis.[1] Other studies have indicated that in humans, as well as NZB mice, COX-2 expression is upregulated in patients with active lupus nephritis, with co-localization to infiltrating monocytes, suggesting that monocytes infiltrating the glomeruli contribute to the exaggerated local synthesis of TXA_2.[346,347] COX-2 inhibition selectively decreased thromboxane production, and chronic treatment of NZB mice with a COX-2 inhibitor and mycophenolate mofetil significantly prolonged survival.[347] Taken together, these results, as well as others from animal and human studies, support a major role for the intrarenal generation of TXA_2 in mediating renal vasoconstriction during inflammatory and lupus-associated glomerular injury. In contrast, an EP4–selective agonist was shown to reduce glomerular injury in a mouse model of anti-GBM disease.[348]

The demonstration of a functionally significant role for COX metabolites in experimental and human inflammatory glomerular injury has raised the question of the cellular sources of these eicosanoids in the glomerulus. In addition to infiltrating inflammatory cells, resident glomerular macrophages, glomerular mesangial cells, and glomerular epithelial cells represent likely sources for eicosanoid generation. In the anti-Thy1.1 model of mesangioproliferative glomerulonephritis, COX-1 staining was transiently increased in diseased glomeruli at day 6 and was localized mainly to proliferating mesangial cells. COX-2 expression in the macula densa region also transiently increased at day 6.[349,350] Glomerular COX-2 expression in this model has been controversial, with one group reporting increased podocyte COX-2 expression[344] and two other groups reporting minimal, if any, glomerular COX-2 expression.[349,350] However, it is of interest that selective COX-2 inhibitors have been reported to inhibit glomerular repair in the anti-Thy1.1 model.[350] In both anti-Thy1.1 and anti-GBM models of glomerulonephritis, the nonselective COX inhibitor, indomethacin, increased monocyte chemoattractant protein-1 (MCP-1), suggesting that prostaglandins may repress recruitment of monocytes and macrophages in experimental glomerulonephritis.[351]

A variety of cytokines have been reported to stimulate PGE_2 synthesis and COX-2 expression in cultured mesangial cells. Furthermore, complement components, in particular C5b-9, which are known to be involved in the inflammatory models described above, have been implicated in the stimulation of PGE_2 synthesis in glomerular epithelial cells. Cultured glomerular epithelial cells (GECs) express predominantly COX-1, but exposure to C5b-9 significantly increases COX-2 expression.[1]

GLOMERULAR NONINFLAMMATORY INJURY

Studies have suggested that prostanoids may also mediate altered renal function and glomerular damage following subtotal renal ablation, and glomerular prostaglandin production may be altered in such conditions. Glomeruli from remnant kidneys, as well as animals fed a high-protein diet, have increased prostanoid production.[1] These studies have suggested an increase in COX enzyme activity per se rather than, or in addition to, increased substrate availability, because increases in prostanoid production were noted when excess exogenous AA was added.

Following subtotal renal ablation, there are selective increases in renal cortical and glomerular COX-2 mRNA and immunoreactive protein expression, without significant alterations in COX-1 expression.[352] This increased COX-2 expression was most prominent in the macula densa and surrounding TAL. In addition, COX-2 immunoreactivity was also present in podocytes of remnant glomeruli, and increased PG production in isolated glomeruli from remnant kidneys was inhibited by a COX-2–selective inhibitor but was not decreased by a COX-1–selective inhibitor.[352] Of interest, in the fawn-hooded rat, which develops spontaneous glomerulosclerosis, there is increased TAL–macula densa COX-2 and neuronal nitric oxide synthase (nNOS) and juxtaglomerular cell renin expression preceding development of sclerotic lesions.[353] Studies have indicated that selective overexpression of COX-2 in podocytes in mice increases sensitivity to the development of glomerulosclerosis, an effect that is mediated by thromboxane receptor activation.[354-356]

When given 24 hours after subtotal renal ablation, a nonselective NSAID, indomethacin, normalized increases in renal blood flow and single-nephron GFR; similar decreases in hyperfiltration were noted when indomethacin was given acutely to rats 14 days after subtotal nephrectomy although, in this latter study, the increased glomerular capillary pressure (P_{GC}) was not altered because afferent and efferent arteriolar resistances increased.[1] Previous studies also suggested that nonselective COX inhibitors may acutely decrease hyperfiltration in diabetes and inhibit proteinuria and/or structural injury[1]; other studies have indicated that selective COX-2 inhibitors will decrease the hyperfiltration seen in experimental diabetes or increased dietary protein.[357,358] Of note, NSAIDs have also been reported to be effective in reducing proteinuria in patients with refractory nephrotic syndrome.[1] Similarly, selective COX-2 inhibition decreased proteinuria in patients with diabetic or nondiabetic renal disease, without alterations in blood pressure.[359]

The prostanoids involved have not yet been completely characterized, although it is presumed that vasodilatory prostanoids are involved in mediation of the altered renal hemodynamics. Defective autoregulation of renal blood flow due to decreased myogenic tone of the afferent arteriole is seen after subtotal ablation or excessive dietary protein and is corrected by inhibition of COX activity. In these hyperfiltering states, TGF is reset at a higher distal tubular flow rate.[1] Such a resetting dictates that afferent arteriolar vasodilation will be maintained in the presence of increased distal solute delivery. It has previously been shown that alterations in TGF sensitivity after reduction in renal mass are prevented with the nonselective COX inhibitor indomethacin.[1] An important role has been suggested for nNOS, which is localized to the macula densa, in the vasodilatory component of TGF.[360-362] Of interest, studies by Ichihara and colleagues have determined that this nNOS-mediated vasodilation is inhibited by the selective COX-2 inhibitor, NS398, suggesting that COX-2–mediated prostanoids may be essential for arteriolar vasodilation.[47,71]

Administration of COX-2 selective inhibitors decreased proteinuria and inhibited development of glomerular sclerosis in rats with reduced functioning renal mass.[363,364] In addition, COX-2 inhibition decreased mRNA expression of transforming growth factor-β_1 (TGF-β_1) and types III and IV collagen in the remnant kidney.[363] Similar protection was observed with administration of nitroflurbiprofen (NOF), a nitric oxide (NO)–releasing NSAID without gastrointestinal toxicity.[365] Prior studies also demonstrated that thromboxane synthase inhibitors retarded progression of glomerulosclerosis, with decreased proteinuria and glomerulosclerosis in rats with remnant kidneys, and in diabetic nephropathy in association with increased renal prostacyclin production and lower systolic blood pressure.[366] Studies in models of types 1 and 2 diabetes have indicated that COX-2–selective inhibitors retard progression of diabetic nephropathy.[367,368] Schmitz and associates have confirmed increases in TXB_2 excretion in the remnant kidney and correlated decreased arachidonic and linoleic acid levels with increased thromboxane production, because the thromboxane synthase inhibitor U63557A restored fatty acid levels and retarded progressive glomerular destruction.[369]

Enhanced glomerular synthesis and/or urinary excretion of PGE_2 and TXA_2 have been demonstrated in passive Heymann nephritis (PHN) and Adriamycin-induced glomerulopathies in rats. Both COX-1 and COX-2 expression are increased in glomeruli with PHN.[370] Thromboxane synthase inhibitors and selective COX-2 inhibitors also decreased proteinuria in PHN.[1]

In contrast to the putative deleterious effects of thromboxane, the prostacyclin analog cicaprost retarded renal damage in uninephrectomized dogs fed a high-sodium and high-protein diet, an effect that was not mediated by amelioration of systemic hypertension.[371] Similarly, EP2 and EP4 agonists decreased glomerular and tubulointerstitial fibrosis in a model of subtotal renal ablation.[359] Other studies have also indicated that in models of polycystic kidney disease, there is increased COX-2 expression and increased PGE_2 and thromboxane in cyst fluid. Either COX-2 inhibition or EP2 receptor inhibition decreased cyst growth and interstitial fibrosis.[372,373]

Prostanoids have also been shown to alter extracellular matrix production by mesangial cells in culture. TXA_2 stimulates matrix production by both TGF-β–dependent and TGF-β–independent pathways.[374] PGE_2 has been reported to decrease steady-state mRNA levels of alpha 1(I) and alpha 1(III) procollagens, but not alpha 1(IV) procollagen and fibronectin mRNA, and to reduce secretion of all studied collagen types into the cell culture supernatants. Of interest, this effect did not appear to be mediated by cAMP.[375] PGE_2 has also been reported to increase production of matrix metalloproteinase-2 (MMP-2) and to mediate Ang II–induced increases in MMP-2.[376] Whether vasodilatory prostaglandins mediate decrease in fibrillar collagen production and increase in matrix-degrading activity in glomeruli in vivo has not yet been studied; however, there is compelling evidence in nonrenal cells that prostanoids may mediate or modulate matrix production.[377] Cultured lung fibroblasts isolated from patients with idiopathic pulmonary fibrosis exhibit a decreased ability to express COX-2 and synthesize PGE_2.[378]

ACUTE KIDNEY INJURY

When cardiac output is compromised, as in extracellular fluid volume depletion or congestive heart failure, systemic blood pressure is preserved by the action of high circulating levels of systemic vasoconstrictors (e.g., norepinephrine, Ang II, AVP). Amelioration of their effects in the renal vasculature serves to blunt the development of otherwise concomitant marked depression of renal blood flow. Intrarenal generation of vasodilator products of AA, including PGE_2 and PGI_2, is a central part of this protective adaptation. Increased renal vascular resistance induced by exogenously administered Ang II or renal nerve stimulation (increased adrenergic tone) is exaggerated during concomitant inhibition of prostaglandin synthesis. Experiments in animals with volume depletion have demonstrated the existence of intrarenal AVP-prostaglandin interactions, similar to those described earlier for Ang II.[1] Studies in patients with congestive heart failure have confirmed that enhanced prostaglandin synthesis is crucial in protecting the kidneys from various vasoconstrictor influences in this condition.

Renal dysfunction accompanying the acute administration of endotoxin in rats is characterized by progressive reductions in RBF and GFR in the absence of hypotension. Renal histology in such animals is normal, but cortical generation of COX metabolites is markedly elevated. A number of reports have provided evidence for a role for TXA_2-induced renal vasoconstriction in this model of renal dysfunction.[379] In addition, roles for PGs and TXA_2 in modulating or mediating renal injury have been suggested in ischemia and reperfusion[380] and models of toxin-mediated acute tubular injury, including those induced by uranyl nitrate,[381] amphotericin B,[382] aminoglycosides,[383] and glycerol.[384] In experimental acute renal failure, administration of vasodilator PGs has been shown to ameliorate injury.[385] Similarly, administration of nonselective or COX-2–selective NSAIDs exacerbates experimental ischemia-reperfusion injury.[386]

COX-2 expression decreases in the kidney in response to acute ischemic injury.[387] There is some controversy about the role of COX products in ischemia-reperfusion injury. Furthermore, fibrosis resulting from prolonged ischemic injury has been shown to be ameliorated by nonspecific COX inhibition.[388] In contrast, renal injury in response to ischemia-reperfusion is worsened by COX-2–selective inhibitors or in COX-2$^{-/-}$ mice,[386] and administration of vasodilator PGs has been shown to ameliorate injury,[385] possibly through a PPARδ-dependent mechanism.[389]

URINARY TRACT OBSTRUCTION

Following the induction of chronic (>24 hours) ureteral obstruction, renal PG and TXA_2 synthesis is markedly enhanced, particularly in response to stimuli such as endotoxins or bradykinins. Enhanced prostanoid synthesis, especially thromboxane, likely arises from infiltrating mononuclear cells, proliferating fibroblast-like cells, interstitial macrophages, and interstitial medullary cells.[342] Selective COX-2 inhibitors may prevent renal damage in response to unilateral ureteral obstruction (UUO).[390,391] However, PGE_2 acting through the EP4 receptor can limit tubulointerstitial fibrosis resulting from UUO.[392] Prostaglandins derived from medullary COX-2 are mediators of the early phase of diuresis seen after relief of ureteral obstruction, because COX-2 inhibition prevents the acute (24-hour) phase of postobstructive diuresis. However, more persistent, chronic, postobstructive diuresis is not prostaglandin-dependent but results from downregulation of NKCC2 (Na^+-K^+-$2Cl^-$ cotransporter type 2) and decreases aquaporin-2 (AQP2) phosphorylation and translocation to the CCD membrane.[393]

ALLOGRAFT REJECTION AND CYCLOSPORINE NEPHROTOXICITY

ALLOGRAFT REJECTION

Acute administration of a TXA_2 synthesis inhibitor is associated with significant improvement in rat renal allograft function.[394] A number of other experimental and clinical studies have also demonstrated increased TXA_2 synthesis during allograft rejection,[395,396] leading some to suggest that increased urinary TXA_2 excretion may be an early indicator of renal and cardiac allograft rejection.

CALCINEURIN INHIBITOR NEPHROTOXICITY

Numerous investigators have demonstrated effects for cyclosporine A (CsA) on renal prostaglandin-TXA_2 synthesis and provided evidence for a major role for renal and leukocyte TXA_2 synthesis in mediating acute and chronic CsA nephrotoxicity in rats.[397] Fish oil–rich diets, TXA_2 antagonists, or administration of CsA in fish oil as a vehicle have all been shown to reduce renal TXA_2 synthesis and may therefore afford protection against nephrotoxicity. Moreover, CsA has been reported to decrease renal COX-2 expression.[398]

HEPATIC CIRRHOSIS AND HEPATORENAL SYNDROME

Patients with cirrhosis of the liver show an increased renal synthesis of vasodilating PGs, as indicated by the high urinary excretion of PGs and/or their metabolites. Urinary excretion of 2,3-dinor 6-keto-$PGF_{1\alpha}$, an index of systemic PGI_2 synthesis, is increased in patients with cirrhosis and hyperdynamic circulation, thus raising the possibility that systemic synthesis of PGI_2 may contribute to the arterial vasodilatation of these patients. Inhibition of COX activity in these patients may cause a profound reduction in RBF and GFR, a reduction in sodium excretion, and an impairment of free water clearance.[399] The sodium-retaining properties of NSAIDs are particularly exaggerated in patients with cirrhosis of the liver, attesting to the dependence of renal salt excretion on vasodilatory PGs. In the kidneys of rats with cirrhosis, COX-2 expression increases but COX-1 expression is unchanged; however, in these animals, selective inhibition of COX-1 leads to impaired renal hemodynamics and natriuresis, whereas COX-2 inhibition has no effect.[400,401]

Diminished renal PG synthesis has been implicated in the pathogenesis of the severe sodium retention seen in hepatorenal syndrome, as well as in the resistance to diuretic therapy.[402,403] There is reduced renal synthesis of vasodilating PGE_2 when there is activation of endogenous vasoconstrictors and a maintained or increased renal production of TXA_2.[399,404] Therefore, an imbalance between vasoconstricting systems and the renal vasodilator PGE_2 has been proposed as a contributing factor to the renal failure observed in this condition. However, administration of exogenous prostanoids to patients with cirrhosis is not effective for ameliorating renal function or preventing the deleterious effect of NSAIDs.[399]

DIABETES MELLITUS

In the streptozotocin-induced model of diabetes in rats, COX-2 expression is increased in the TAL–macula densa region,[357,367] as well as in podocytes,[405] possibly mediated by epigenetic processes.[406] COX-2 immunoreactivity has also been detected in the macula densa region in human diabetic nephropathy.[407] Studies have suggested that COX-2–dependent vasodilator prostanoids play an important role in the hyperfiltration seen early in diabetes mellitus,[357,408-411] as well as in response to a high-protein diet.[412] The increased COX-2 expression appears to be mediated, at least in part, by increased ROS production in diabetes, because the superoxide dismutase analog, tempol, blocks the increased expression.[413]

Chronic administration of a selective COX-2 inhibitor significantly decreases proteinuria and reduces extracellular matrix deposition, as indicated by decreases in immunoreactive fibronectin expression and mesangial matrix expansion.[367,414] In addition, COX-2 inhibition reduced expression of TGF-β, plasminogen activator inhibitor-1 (PAI-1) and vascular endothelial growth factor (VEGF) in the kidneys of the diabetic hypertensive animals. Increasing intrarenal dopamine production also ameliorates diabetic nephropathy progression, at least in part by inhibiting renal cortical COX-2 expression.[415] The vasoconstrictor TXA_2 may play a role in the development of albuminuria and basement membrane changes with diabetic nephropathy (DN). Also, administration of a selective PGE_2 EP1 receptor antagonist prevented development of experimental diabetic nephropathy,[416] whereas EP4 receptor activation may exacerbate DN.[417]

PREGNANCY

Most, but not all, investigators do not report increases in vasodilator PG synthesis or suggest an essential role for prostanoids in the mediation of the increased GFR and RBF of normal pregnancy[418]; however, diminished synthesis of PGI_2 has been demonstrated in humans and in animal models of pregnancy-induced hypertension,[419] which is associated with decreased expression of COX-2 and PGI_2 synthase in the placental villi.[420] In animal models, inhibition of TXA_2 synthetase has been associated with resolution of the hypertension, suggesting a possible pathophysiologic role.[421] A moderate beneficial effect of reducing TXA_2 generation, while preserving PGI_2 synthesis, by low-dose aspirin therapy (60 to 100 mg/day) has been demonstrated in patients at high risk for pregnancy-induced hypertension and preeclampsia.[422,423]

LITHIUM NEPHROTOXICITY

Lithium chloride is a mainstay of treatment in the psychiatric treatment of bipolar illness. However, it is routinely complicated by polyuria and even frank nephrogenic diabetes insipidus. In vitro and in vivo studies have demonstrated lithium-induced renal medullary interstitial cell COX-2 protein expression via inhibition of glycogen synthase kinase-3β (GSK-3β). COX-2 inhibition prevented lithium-induced polyuria and also resulted in the upregulation of AQP2 and NKCC2.[424,425]

ROLE OF REACTIVE OXYGEN SPECIES AS MEDIATORS OF COX-2 ACTIONS

In addition to NADPH oxidase, nitric oxide synthase, and xanthine oxidase, COX-2 can also be a source of oxygen radicals.[426] COX-2 enzymatic activity is commonly accompanied by associated oxidative mechanisms (co-oxidation) and free radical production.[427] The catalytic activity of COX consists of a series of radical reactions that use molecular oxygen and generate intermediate ROS.[428] Elevated levels of COX-2 protein are associated with increased ROS production and apoptosis in cultured renal cortical cells[429] and human mesangial cells.[430] It has been suggested that COX-2–mediated lipid peroxidation, rather than prostaglandins, can induce DNA damage via adduct formation.[431] A COX-2 specific inhibitor, NS-398, was able to reduce the oxidative activity, with prevention of oxidant stress.[432]

In addition to ROS generated by cyclo-oxygenase per se, prostanoids may also activate intracellular pathways that generate ROS. Locally generated ROS may damage cell membranes, leading to lipid peroxidation and release of arachidonic acid. Prostanoids released during inflammatory reactions cause rapid degenerative changes in some cultured cells, and their potential cytotoxic effect has been suggested to occur by accelerating intracellular oxidative stress. Thromboxane[433] and PGE_2 acting through the EP1 receptor[434] have been reported to induce NADPH oxidase and ROS production. Of interest, PGE_2 acting through the EP4 receptor inhibits macrophage oxidase activity.[435,436] As noted, there is also evidence for cross-talk between COX-2 and ROS, such that ROS may induce COX-2 expression.[431] Interestingly, during aging there is ROS-mediated NF-kB expression, which increases COX-2 expression in the kidney.[437] Furthermore, this appears to induce a vicious cycle, since COX-2 then serves as a source of ROS. This interaction of COX-derived prostaglandin and ROS production has posited to play a role in development of hypertension.[438] The amount of renal ROS resulting from COX activity increases with age, such that up to 25% of total kidney ROS production in aged rat kidneys is inhibited by NSAID administration.

LIPOXYGENASE PATHWAY

The lipoxygenase enzymes metabolize arachidonic acid to form LTs, HETEs), and LXs (Figure 14.14). These lipoxygenase metabolites are primarily produced by leukocytes, mast cells, and macrophages in response to inflammation and injury. There are three lipoxygenase enzymes—5-, 12-, and 15-lipoxygenase (5-LOX, 12-LOX, and 15-LOX)—so-named for the carbon of AA where they insert an oxygen. The lipoxygenases are products of separate genes and have distinct distributions and patterns of regulation. Glomeruli, mesangial cells, cortical tubules, and vessels also produce the 12-LOX product, 12(S)-HETE, and the 15-LOX product,

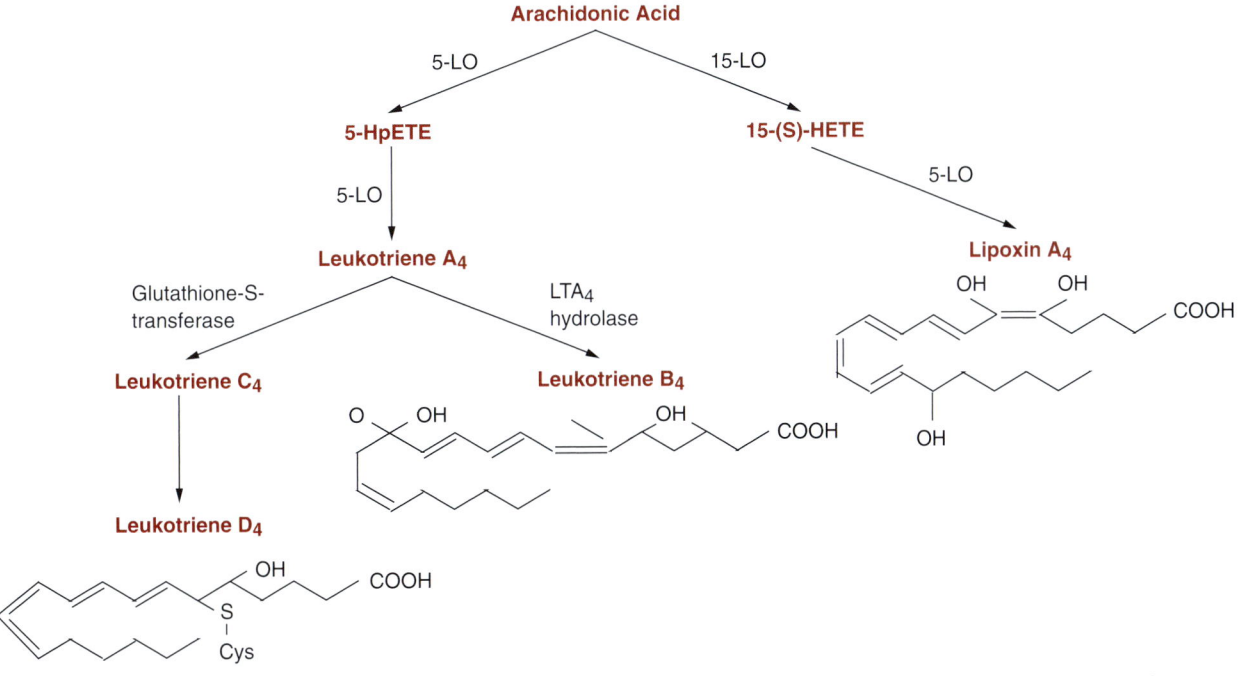

Figure 14.14 Pathways of lipoxygenase (LO) metabolism of arachidonic acid. HETE, Hydroxyeicosatetraenoic acid.

15-HETE. Studies have localized 15-LOX mRNA primarily to the distal nephron and 12-LOX mRNA to the glomerulus. 5-LOX mRNA and 5-lipoxygenase-activating protein (FLAP) mRNA were expressed in the glomerulus and the vasa recta.[439] In polymorphonuclear leukocytes (PMNs), macrophages, and mast cells, 5-LOX mediates the formation of leukotrienes.[440] 5-LOX, which is regulated by FLAP, catalyzes the conversion of arachidonic acid to 5-HPETE, and to leukotriene A_4 (LTA_4).[441] LTA_4 is then further metabolized to the peptidyl leukotrienes (LTC_4 and LTD_4) by glutathione-S-transferase or to LTB_4 by LTA_4 hydrolase. Although glutathione-S-transferase expression is limited to inflammatory cells, LTA_4 hydrolase is also expressed in glomerular mesangial cells and endothelial cells[442]; PCR analysis has actually demonstrated ubiquitous LTA_4 hydrolase mRNA expression throughout the rat nephron.[439] LTC_4 synthase mRNA could not be found in any nephron segment.[439]

Two cysteinyl leukotriene receptors (CysLTRs) have been cloned and identified as members of the G protein–coupled superfamily of receptors. They have been localized to vascular smooth muscle and endothelium of the pulmonary vasculature.[443-445] In the kidney, the cysteinyl leukotriene receptor type 1 is expressed in the glomerulus, whereas cysteinyl receptor type 2 mRNA has not been detected in any nephron segment to date.[439]

The peptidyl leukotrienes are potent mediators of inflammation and vasoconstrictors of vascular, pulmonary, and gastrointestinal smooth muscle. In addition, they increase vascular permeability and promote mucus secretion.[446] Because of the central role that peptidyl leukotrienes play in the inflammatory trigger of asthma exacerbation, effective receptor antagonists have been developed and are now an important component of treatment of asthma.[447]

In the kidney, LTD_4 administration has been shown to decrease renal blood flow and GFR, and peptidyl leukotrienes are thought to be mediators of decreased RBF and GFR associated with acute glomerular inflammation. Micropuncture studies have revealed that the decreases in GFR are the result of afferent and arteriolar vasoconstriction, with more pronounced efferent vasoconstriction and a decrease in K_f.[1] In addition both LTC_4 and LTD_4 increase proliferation of cultured mesangial cells.

The LTB_4 receptor is also a seven-transmembrane, G protein–coupled receptor. On PMNs, receptor activation promotes chemotaxis, aggregation, and attachment to endothelium. In the kidney, LTB_4 mRNA is localized to the glomerulus.[439] A second, low-affinity LTB_4 receptor is also expressed,[448] which may mediate calcium influx into PMNs, thereby leading to activation. LTB_4 receptor blockers lessen acute renal ischemic-reperfusion injury[449] and nephrotoxic nephritis in rats,[450] and PMN infiltration and structural and functional evidence of organ injury by ischemia-reperfusion are magnified in transgenic mice overexpressing the LTB_4 receptor.[451] In addition to activation of cell surface receptors, LTB_4 has also been shown to be a ligand for the nuclear receptor PPARα.[452]

15-LOX leads to the formation of 15(S)-HETE. In addition, dual oxygenation in activated PMNs and macrophages by 5-LOX and 15-LOX leads to the formation of the lipoxins. LX synthesis also can occur via transcellular metabolism of the leukocyte-generated intermediate, LTA_4, by 12-LOX in platelets or adjoining cells, including glomerular endothelial cells.[453,454]

12(S)-HETE is a potent vasoconstrictor in the renal microcirculation[455]; however, 15-LOX–derived metabolites antagonize proinflammatory actions of leukotrienes, both by inhibiting PMN chemotaxis, aggregation, and adherence and by counteracting the vasoconstrictive effects of the peptidyl leukotrienes.[456,457] Administration of 15(S)-HETE reduced LTB_4 production by glomeruli isolated from rats with acute nephrotoxic serum-induced glomerulonephritis; it has been proposed that 15-LOX may regulate 5-LOX activity in chronic glomerular inflammation because it is known that in experimental glomerulonephritis, lipoxin A_4 (LXA_4) administration increases renal blood flow and GFR, mainly by inducing afferent arteriolar vasodilation, an effect mediated in part by release of vasodilator prostaglandins.[1] LXA_4 also antagonizes the effects of LTD_4 to decrease GFR, but not RBF, even though administration of LXA_4 and LXB_4 directly into the renal artery has induced vasoconstriction. Glomerular micropuncture studies have revealed that LXA_4 leads to moderate decreases in K_f.[456] Lipoxins signal through a specific G protein–coupled receptor denoted ALXR. This receptor is related at the nucleotide sequence level to chemokine and chemotactic peptide receptors, such as N-formyl peptide receptor.[458] It is also noteworthy that in isolated perfused canine renal arteries and veins, LTC_4 and LTD_4 were found to be vasodilators, which were partially dependent on an intact endothelium, and were mediated by nitric oxide production.[459]

A potential interaction between COX- and LOX-mediated pathways has been reported. Although aspirin inhibits prostaglandin formation by COX-1 and COX-2, aspirin-induced acetylation converts COX-2 to a selective generator of 15(R)-HETE. This product can then be released, taken up in a transcellular route by PMNs and converted to 15-epilipoxins, which have similar biologic actions as the lipoxins.[460]

Similar to 15-HETE, 12(S)-HETE also potently vasoconstricts glomerular and renal vasculature.[453] 12(S)-HETE increases protein kinase C and depolarizes cultured vascular smooth muscle cells. Afferent arteriolar vasoconstriction and increases in smooth muscle calcium in response to 12(S)-HETE were partially inhibited by voltage-gated, L-type calcium channel inhibitors.[461] 12(S)-HETE has also been proposed to be an angiogenic factor because in cultured endothelial cells, 12-LOX inhibition reduces cell proliferation and 12-LOX overexpression stimulates cell migration and endothelial tube formation.[462] 12/15-LOX inhibitors and elective elimination of the leukocyte 12-LOX enzyme also ameliorate the development of diabetic nephropathy in mice.[463] There is also interaction between 12/15-LOX pathways and TGF-β–mediated pathways in the diabetic kidney[464] 12(S)-HETE has also been proposed to be a mediator of renal vasoconstriction by Ang II, with inhibition of the 12-LOX pathway attenuating Ang II–mediated afferent arteriolar vasoconstriction and decreased renal blood flow.[465] Lipoxygenase inhibition also blunted renal arcuate artery vasoconstriction by norepinephrine and KCl.[466] However, 12-LOX products have also been implicated as inhibitors of renal renin release.[467,468]

Although the major significance of LOX products in the kidney derives from their release from infiltrating leukocytes or resident cells of macrophage or monocyte origin, there is evidence to suggest that intrinsic renal cells are capable of generating LTs and LXs directly or through transcellular metabolism of intermediates.[469] Human and rat glomeruli can generate 12- and 15-HETE, although the cells of origin are unclear. LTB_4 can be detected in supernatants of normal rat glomeruli, and its synthesis could be markedly diminished by maneuvers that deplete glomeruli of resident macrophages, such as irradiation or fatty acid deficiency. In addition, 5-, 12-, and 15-HETEs were detected from pig glomeruli, and their structural identity confirmed by mass spectrometry.[1] 12-LOX products are increased in mesangial cells exposed to hyperglycemia and in diabetic nephropathy.[470] There also appears to be crosstalk between 12/15-LOX and COX-2. Both are increased with diabetes or high glucose levels and, in cultured cells, 12(S)-HETE increases COX-2 whereas PGE_2 increases 12/15-LOX. Knockdown of 12/15-LOX expression with ShRNA decreases COX-2 expression, and 12/15-LOX overexpression increases COX-2 expression.[427]

Glomeruli subjected to immune injury release LTB_4,[471] and LTB_4 generation was suppressed by resident macrophage depletion. Synthesis of peptido-LTs by inflamed glomeruli has also been demonstrated,[472] but leukocytes could not be excluded as its primary source. LXA_4 is generated by immune-injured glomeruli.[473] Rat mesangial cells generate LXA_4 when provided with LTA_4 as substrate, thereby providing a potential intraglomerular source of LXs during inflammatory reactions. In nonglomerular tissue, 12-HETE production has been reported from rat cortical tubules and epithelial cells and 12- and 15-HETE from rabbit medulla.[1]

BIOLOGIC ACTIVITIES OF LIPOXYGENASE PRODUCTS IN THE KIDNEY

In early experiments, systemic administration of LTC_4 in the rat and administration of LTC_4 and LTD_4 in the isolated perfused kidney revealed potent renal vasoconstrictor actions of these eicosanoids. Subsequently, micropuncture measurements revealed that LTD_4 exerts preferential constrictor effects on postglomerular arteriolar resistance and depresses K_f and GFR. The latter is likely due to receptor-mediated contraction of glomerular mesangial cells, which has been demonstrated for LTC_4 and LTD_4 in vitro (see above). These actions of LTD_4 in the kidney are consistent with its known smooth muscle contractile properties. LTB_4, a potent chemotactic and leukocyte-activating agent, is devoid of constrictor action in the normal rat kidney. Lipoxin A_4 dilates afferent arterioles when infused into the renal artery, without affecting efferent arteriolar tone. This results in elevations in intraglomerular pressure and plasma flow rate, thereby augmenting the GFR.[1]

INVOLVEMENT OF LIPOXYGENASE PRODUCTS IN RENAL PATHOPHYSIOLOGY

Increased generation rates of LTC_4 and LTD_4 have been documented in glomeruli from rats with immune complex nephritis and mice with spontaneously developing lupus nephritis.[440,473] Moreover, results from numerous physiologic studies using specific LTD_4 receptor antagonists have provided strong evidence for the release of these eicosanoids during glomerular inflammation. In four animal models of glomerular immune injury—anti-GBM nephritis, anti-Thy1.1 antibody–mediated mesangiolysis, passive Heymann nephritis, and murine lupus nephritis—acute antagonism of LTD_4 by receptor binding competition or inhibition of LTD_4 synthesis led to highly significant increases in GFR in nephritic animals.[474] The principal mechanism underlying the improvement in GFR was reversal of the depressed values of the glomerular ultrafiltration coefficient (K_f), which is characteristically compromised in immune-injured glomeruli. In other studies in PHN, Katoh and colleagues have provided evidence that endogenous LTD_4 not only mediates reductions in K_f and GFR, but that LTD_4-evoked increases in intraglomerular pressure underlie, to a large extent, the accompanying proteinuria.[474] Cysteinyl leukotrienes have been implicated in cyclosporine nephrotoxicity.[475] Of interest, 5-lipoxygenase deficiency accelerates renal allograft rejection.[476]

LTB_4 synthesis, measured in the supernates of isolated glomeruli, is markedly enhanced early in the course of several forms of glomerular immune injury.[477] Cellular sources of LTB_4 in injured glomeruli include PMNs and macrophages. All studies concur as to the transient nature of LTB_4 release. LTB_4 production decreases 24 hours after onset of the inflammation, which coincides with macrophage infiltration, a major source of 15-LOX activity.[478] 15-HPETE incubation decreased lipopolysaccharide-induced tumor necrosis factor (TNF) expression in a human monocytic cell line,[479] and HVJ (hemagglutinating virus of Japan) liposome-mediated glomerular transfection of 15-LOX in rats decreased markers of injury (blood urea nitrogen [BUN,] proteinuria) and accelerated functional (GFR, RBF) recovery in experimental glomerulonephritis.[480] In addition, MK501, a FLAP antagonist, restored size selectivity and decreased glomerular permeability in acute glomerulonephritis (GN).[481]

The suppression of LTB_4 synthesis beyond the first 24 hours of injury is rather surprising, because both PMNs and macrophages are capable of effecting the total synthesis of LTB_4; they contain the two necessary enzymes that convert AA to LTB_4—5-LOX and LTA_4 hydrolase. It has therefore been suggested, based on in vitro evidence, that the major route for LTB_4 synthesis in inflamed glomeruli is through transcellular metabolism of leukocyte-generated LTA_4 to LTB_4 by LTA_4 hydrolase present in glomerular mesangial, endothelial, and epithelial cells. Because the transformation of LTA_4 to LTB_4 is rate-limiting, regulation of the LTB_4 synthetic rate might relate to regulation of LTA_4 hydrolase gene expression or catalytic activity in these parenchymal cells, rather than to the number of infiltrating leukocytes. In any case, leukocytes represent an indispensable source for LTA_4, the initial 5-LOX product and the precursor for LTB_4, since endogenous glomerular cells do not express the 5-LOX gene.[482] Thus, it was demonstrated that the PMN cell-specific activator, N-formyl-Met-Leu-Phe, stimulated LTB_4 production from isolated perfused kidneys harvested from NTS-treated rats to a significantly greater degree than from control animals treated with nonimmune rabbit serum.[483] The renal production of LTB_4 correlated directly with renal myeloperoxidase activity, suggesting interdependence of LTB_4 generation and PMN infiltration.

The acute and long-term significance of LTB$_4$ generation in conditioning the extent of glomerular structural and functional deterioration has been highlighted in studies in which LTB$_4$ was exogenously administered or in which its endogenous synthesis was inhibited. Intrarenal administration of LTB$_4$ to rats with mild NTS-induced injury was associated with an increase in PMN infiltration, reduction in renal plasma flow rate, and marked exacerbation of the fall in GFR, the latter correlating strongly with the number of infiltrating PMNs and glomerulus, whereas inhibition of 5-LOX led to preservation of GFR and abrogation of proteinuria.[483] Similarly, both 5-LOX knockout mice and wild-type mice treated with the 5-LOX inhibitor, zileuton, had reduced renal injury in response to ischemia and reperfusion.[484] Thus, although devoid of vasoconstrictor actions in the normal kidney, increased intrarenal generation of LTB$_4$ during early glomerular injury amplifies leukocyte-dependent reductions in glomerular perfusion and filtration rates and inflammatory injury, likely due to enhancement of PMN recruitment and/or activation.

12(S)-HETE has been reported to increase AT$_1$ receptor (AT$_1$R) mRNA and protein expression in cultured rat mesangial cells by stabilizing AT$_1$R mRNA and enhancing the profibrotic effects of Ang II.[485] Urinary 12(S)- and 15(S)-HETE levels have been shown to correlate positively with elevated serum creatinine levels after kidney transplantation.[486] In the JCR:LA-corpulent rat, a model of the metabolic syndrome, fish oil (ω-3 polyunsaturated fatty acid) supplement markedly reduced albuminuria and glomerulosclerosis in association with decreases in 5(S)-, 12(S)-, and 15(S)-HETE.[487]

CYTOCHROME P450 PATHWAY

Following their elucidation and characterization as endogenous metabolites of arachidonic acid, numerous studies have investigated the possibility that cytochrome P450 (CYP450) AA metabolites subserve physiologic and/or pathophysiologic roles in the kidney (Figure 14.15). In whole-animal physiology, these compounds have been implicated in the mediation of release of peptide hormones, regulation of vascular tone, and regulation of volume homeostasis. On the cellular level, CYP450 AA metabolites have been proposed to regulate ion channels and transporters and to act as mitogens.

CYP450 monooxygenases are mixed-function oxidases that use molecular oxygen and NADPH as co-factors[488,489] and will add an oxygen molecule to AA in a regiospecific and stereospecific geometry. CYP450 monooxygenase pathways metabolize AA to generate HETEs and EETs, the latter of which can be hydrolyzed to dihydroxyeicosatrienoic acids (DHETs).[298,488,490] The kidney displays one of the highest CYP450 activities of any organ and produces CYP450 AA metabolites in significant amounts.[461,488,491] HETEs are formed primarily via CYP450 hydroxylase enzymes; EETs and DHETs are formed primarily via CYP450 epoxygenase enzymes.[491] The CYP450 4A gene family is the major pathway for synthesis of hydroxylase metabolites, especially 20-HETE and 19-HETE,[298,491] whereas the production of epoxygenase metabolites is primarily via the 2C gene family.[461,488] A member of the 2J family that is an active epoxygenase is also expressed in the kidney.[492] CYP450 enzymes have been

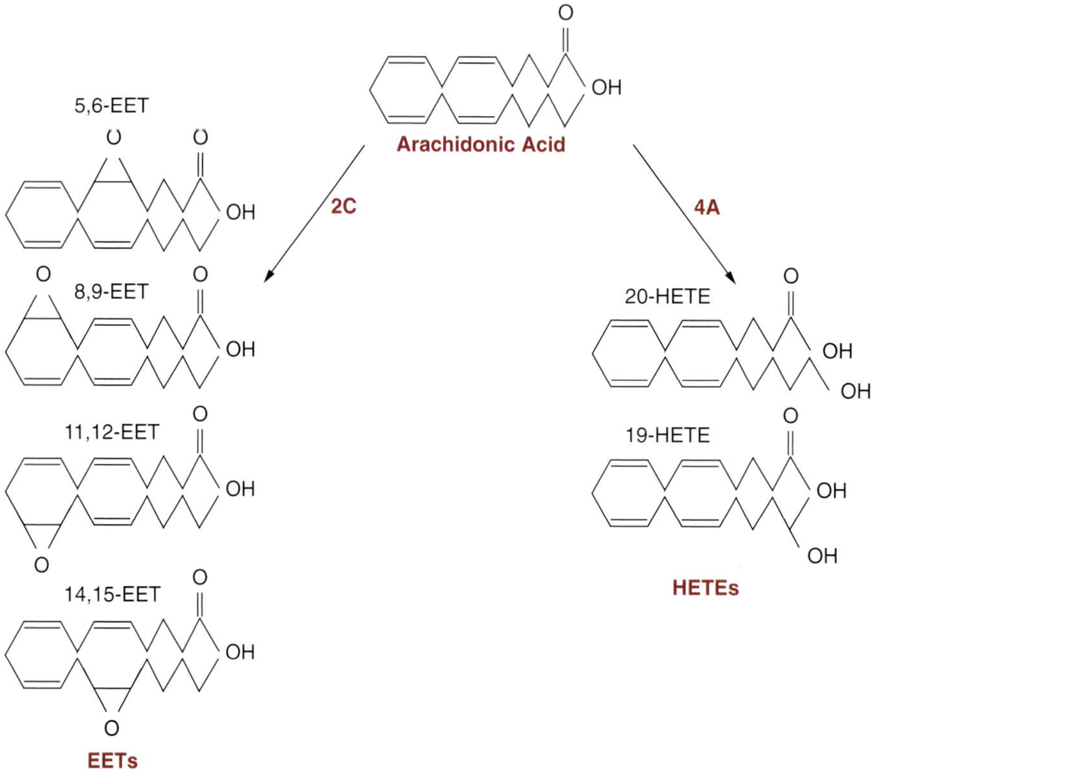

Figure 14.15 Pathways of CYP450 metabolism of arachidonic acid. EET, Epoxyeicosatrienoic acid; HETE, hydroxyeicosatetraenoic acid.

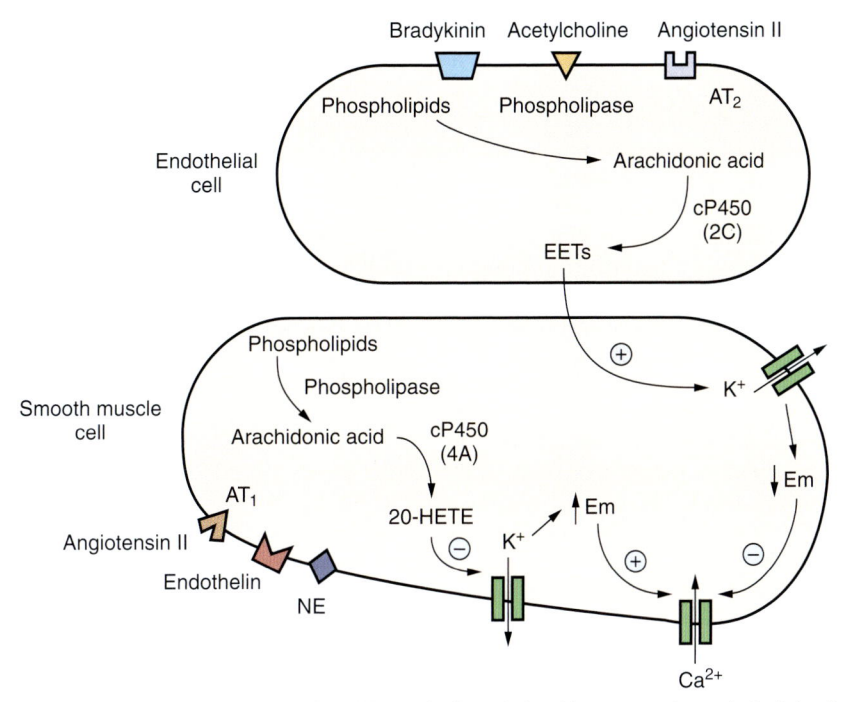

Figure 14.16 Proposed interactions of CYP450 arachidonic acid metabolites derived from vascular endothelial cells and smooth muscle cells to regulate vascular tone. AT_1 and AT_2, Angiotensin II type 1 and 2 receptors; cP450, cytochrome P450 system; EET, epoxyeicosatrienoic acid; HETE, hydroxyeicosatetraenoic acid.

localized to vasculature and tubules.[298] The 4A family of hydroxylases is expressed in preglomerular renal arterioles, glomeruli, proximal tubules, TAL, and macula densa.[493]

The 2C and 2J families of epoxygenases are expressed at their highest levels in the proximal tubule and collecting duct.[492,494] When isolated nephron segments expressing CYP450 protein have been incubated with AA, production of CYP450 AA metabolites can be detected. 20-HETE and EETs are both produced in the afferent arterioles,[495] glomerulus,[496] and proximal tubule.[497] 20-HETE is the predominant CYP450 AA metabolite produced by the TAL and in the pericytes surrounding the vasa recta capillaries,[498,499] whereas EETs are the predominant CYP450 AA metabolites produced by the collecting duct.[500]

Renal production of epoxygenase and hydroxylase metabolites has been shown to be regulated by hormones and growth factors, including Ang II, endothelin, bradykinin, parathyroid hormone (PTH), and epidermal growth factor.[298,461,489] Alterations in dietary salt intake also modulate CYP450 expression and activity.[501] Alterations in the production of CYP450 metabolites have also been reported with uninephrectomy, diabetes mellitus, and hypertension.[298,502] Glycerol-containing epoxygenase metabolites are produced endogenously and serve as high-affinity ligands for cannabinoid receptors, implicating these compounds as endocannabinoids.[503]

VASCULATURE

20-HYDROXYEICOSATETRAENOIC ACID

In rat and dog renal arteries and afferent arterioles, 20-HETE is a potent vasoconstrictor,[495] whereas it is a vasodilator in rabbit renal arteries. The vasoconstriction is associated with membrane depolarization and a sustained rise in intracellular calcium levels. 20-HETE is produced in the smooth muscle cells, and its afferent arteriolar vasoconstrictive effects are mediated by closure of K_{Ca} channels through a tyrosine kinase- and extracellular signal–regulated kinase (ERK)–dependent mechanism (Figure 14.16).

An interaction between CYP450 AA metabolites and NO has also been demonstrated. NO can inhibit the formation of 20-HETE in renal vascular smooth muscle cells; a significant portion of NO's vasodilator effects in the preglomerular vasculature appear to be mediated by the inhibition of tonic 20-HETE vasoconstriction, and inhibition of 20-HETE formation attenuates the pressor response and decrease in renal blood flow seen with NOS inhibition.[504,505]

EPOXIDES

Unlike CYP450 hydroxylase metabolites, epoxygenase metabolites of arachidonic acid increase renal blood flow and glomerular filtration rate.[298,461,489] 11,12-EET and 14,15-EET vasodilate the preglomerular arterioles independently of COX activity, whereas 5,6-EET and 8,9-EET cause COX-dependent vasodilation or vasoconstriction.[506] It is possible that these COX-dependent effects are mediated by COX conversion of 5,6-EET and 8,9-EET to prostaglandin- or thromboxane-like compounds.[507] EETs are produced primarily in the endothelial cells and exert their vasoactive effects on the adjacent smooth muscle cells. In this regard, it has been suggested that EETs, specifically 11,12-EET, may serve as an endothelium-derived hyperpolarizing factor (EDHF) in the renal microcirculation.[461,508] EET-induced vasodilation is mediated by activation of K_{Ca} channels, through cAMP-dependent stimulation of PKC.

CYP450 metabolites may serve as second messengers or modulators of the actions of hormonal and paracrine agents. Vasopressin increases renal production of CYP450 metabolites, and increases in intracellular calcium and proliferation in cultured renal mesangial cells are augmented by EET administration.[509] CYP450 metabolites also may serve to modulate the renal hemodynamic responses of endothelin-1 (ET-1), with 20-HETE as a possible mediator of the vasoconstrictive effects and EETs counteracting the vasoconstriction.[461,510] Formation of 20-HETE does not affect the ability of ET-1 to increase free intracellular calcium transients in renal vascular smooth muscle intracellularly, but appears to enhance the sustained elevations that represent calcium influx through voltage-sensitive channels.

CYP450 metabolites have also been implicated in the mediation of renal vascular responses to Ang II. In the presence of AT_1R blockers, Ang II produces an endothelial-dependent vasodilation in rabbit afferent arterioles that is dependent on CYP450 epoxygenase metabolite production by AT_2Rr activation.[511] With intact AT_1Rs, Ang II increases 20-HETE release from isolated preglomerular microvessels through an endothelium-independent mechanism.[512] Ang II's vasoconstrictive effects are in part the result of 20-HETE-mediated inhibition of K_{Ca}, which enhances sustained increases in intracellular calcium concentration by calcium influx through voltage-sensitive channels. Inhibition of 20-HETE production reduces the vasoconstrictor response to Ang II by more than 50% in rat renal interlobular arteries in which the endothelium has been removed.[512]

AUTOREGULATION

CYP450 metabolites of AA have been shown to be mediators of RBF autoregulatory mechanisms. When prostaglandin production was blocked in canine arcuate arteries, AA administration enhanced myogenic responsiveness, and renal blood flow autoregulation was blocked by CYP450 inhibitors.[298,461] Similarly, in the rat juxtamedullary preparation, selective blockade of 20-HETE formation significantly decreased afferent arteriolar vasoconstrictor responses to elevations in perfusion pressure, and inhibition of epoxygenase activity enhanced vasoconstriction,[513] suggesting that 20-HETE is involved in afferent arteriolar autoregulatory adjustment; however, release of vasodilatory epoxygenase metabolites in response to increases in renal perfusion pressure acts to attenuate the vasoconstriction. In vivo studies have also implicated 20-HETE as a mediator of the autoregulatory response to increased perfusion pressure.[514] Bradykinin-induced efferent arteriolar vasodilation has been shown to be mediated in part by direct release of EETs from this vascular segment. In addition, bradykinin-induced release of 20-HETE from the glomerulus can modulate the EET-mediated vasodilation.[515]

TUBULOGLOMERULAR FEEDBACK

CYP450 metabolites may also be involved in the tubuloglomerular feedback response.[298] As noted, 20-HETE is produced by the afferent arteriole and macula densa, and studies have suggested the possibility that 20-HETE may serve as a vasoconstrictive mediator of TGF released by the macula densa or as a second messenger in the afferent arteriole in response to mediators released by the macula densa, such as adenosine or ATP.[516] 20-HETE may also mediate the regulation of intrarenal distribution of blood flow.[517,518] In addition, there is evidence for connecting TGF, in which increased sodium reabsorption in the connecting segment, which abuts the afferent arteriole, leads to increased AA release, leading to increased production of EETs and vasodilatory prostaglandins. These then diffuse to the adjacent afferent arteriole and dilate it.[519]

TUBULES

20-HETE and EETs both inhibit tubular sodium reabsorption.[298,489] Renal cortical interstitial infusion of the nonselective CYP450 inhibitor 17-octadecynoic acid (17-ODYA) increases papillary blood flow, renal interstitial hydrostatic pressure, and sodium excretion without affecting total RBF or GFR. High dietary salt intake in rats increases expression of the renal epoxygenase 2C23 and production and urinary excretion of EETs while decreasing 20-HETE production in the renal cortex.[488,501] 14,15-EET has also been shown to inhibit renin secretion[520]; however, clotrimazole, which is a relatively selective epoxygenase inhibitor, induced hypertension in rats fed a high-salt diet, suggesting a role in the regulation of blood pressure.[501]

PROXIMAL TUBULE

The proximal tubule contains the highest concentration of CYP450 in the mammalian kidney and expresses minimal COX and LOX activity.[488] The 4A CYP450 family of hydroxylases that produce 19- and 20-HETE is highly expressed in the mammalian proximal tubule.[311] CYP450 enzymes of the 2C and 2J families that catalyze the formation of EETs are also expressed in the proximal tubule.[488] Both EETs and 20-HETE have been shown to be produced in the proximal tubule and have been proposed to be modulators of sodium reabsorption in the proximal tubule.

Studies in isolated perfused proximal tubule have indicated that 20-HETE inhibits sodium transport, whereas 19-HETE stimulates sodium transport, suggesting that 19-HETE may serve as a competitive antagonist of 20-HETE.[497,521] Administration of EETs inhibits amiloride-sensitive sodium transport in primary cultures of proximal tubule cells[522] and in LLC-PK1 cells, a nontransformed immortalized cell line from pig kidney with proximal tubule characteristics.[523,524]

20-HETE has been proposed to be a mediator of hormonal inhibition of proximal tubule reabsorption by PTH, dopamine, Ang II, and EGF. Although the mechanisms of 20-HETE's inhibition have not yet been completely elucidated, there is evidence that it can inhibit Na^+-K^+-ATPase activity by phosphorylation of the Na^+-K^+-ATPase α-subunit through a PKC-dependent pathway.[525,526]

EETs may also serve as second messengers in the proximal tubule for EGF[527] and Ang II.[528] In the proximal tubule, Ang II has been noted to exert a biphasic response on net sodium uptake via AT_1Rs, with low (10^{-10} to 10^{-11}) concentrations stimulating and high (10^{-7}) concentrations inhibiting net uptake.[528] Such high concentrations are not normally seen in plasma but may exist in the proximal tubule lumen as a result of the local production of Ang II by the proximal tubule.[529] The mechanisms whereby CYP450 AA metabolites modulate proximal tubule reabsorption have not been completely elucidated, and may involve luminal (Na^+-H^+ exchanger isoform 3 [NHE3]) and basolateral (Na^+-K^+-ATPase) transporters.[522,525] CYP450 AA metabolites may modulate the proximal tubule component of the pressure-natriuresis response.[530]

THICK ASCENDING LIMB OF THE LOOP OF HENLE

20-HETE also serves as a second messenger to regulation transport in the TAL. It is produced in this nephron segment[493] and can inhibit net Na^+-K^+-$2Cl^-$ cotransport by direct inhibition of the transporter and by blocking the 70-pS apical K^+ channel.[498,531] In addition, 20-HETE has been implicated as a mediator of the inhibitory effects of Ang II[532] and bradykinin[533] on TAL transport.

COLLECTING DUCT

In the collecting duct, EETs and/or their diol metabolites serve as inhibitors of the hydroosmotic effects of vasopressin, as well as inhibitors of sodium transport in this segment.[500,534] Patch clamp studies have indicated that the eNaC sodium channel activity in the CCD is inhibited by 11,12-EET.[535,536] Recent studies using mice with selective deletion of Cyp2c44, the major kidney epoxygenase, have confirmed that EETs modulate eNaC activity and that EET production is mediated in part by activation of CCD EGF receptors.[537-539] There is also an intriguing association of 20-HETE with circadian clock sodium regulation in the CCD.[540]

ROLE IN ACUTE AND CHRONIC KIDNEY DISEASE

In rat mesangial cells, endogenous non-COX metabolites of AA modulate the proliferative responses to phorbol esters, vasopressin, and EGF, and agonist-induced expression of the immediate early response genes *c-fos* and *Egr-1* is inhibited by ketoconazole or nordihydroguaiaretic acid (NDGA), but not specific LOX inhibitors.[541] EET-mediated increases in rat mesangial cell proliferation was the first direct evidence that CYP450 AA metabolites are cellular mitogens.[542] In cultured rabbit proximal tubule cells, CYP450 inhibitors blunted EGF-stimulated proliferation in proximal tubule cells.[527] In LLC-PKcl$_4$ cells, EETs were found to be potent mitogens, cytoprotective agents, and second messengers for EGF signaling. 14,15-EET–mediated signaling and mitogenesis are dependent on EGF receptor transactivation, which is mediated by metalloproteinase-dependent release of heparin-binding EGF.[543] In addition to the EETs, 20-HETE has been shown to increase thymidine incorporation in primary cultures of rat proximal tubule and LLC-PK1 cells[544] and in vascular smooth muscle cells.[545] EETs are also pro-angiogenic factors.[546]

There is increasing evidence that activation of EETs or administration of EET analogs can protect against AKI.[547-549] Conversely, inhibition of 20-HETE is beneficial in AKI.[550] There have also been recent studies suggesting that the EETs may be protective in diabetic nephropathy and in a 5/6 nephrectomy model.[551,552]

ROLE IN HYPERTENSION

There is increasing evidence that the renal production of CYP450 AA metabolites is altered in a variety of models of hypertension, and that blockade of the formation of compounds can alter blood pressure in several of these models. CYP450 AA metabolites may have both pro- and antihypertensive properties. At the level of the renal tubule, 20-HETE and EETs inhibit sodium transport. However, in the vasculature, 20-HETE promotes vasoconstriction and hypertension, whereas EETs are endothelial-derived vasodilators that have antihypertensive properties. Rats fed a high-salt diet increase expression of the CYP450 epoxygenase 2C23[553] and develop hypertension if treated with a relatively selective epoxygenase inhibitor. Because EETs have antihypertensive properties, efforts have been made to develop selective inhibitors of soluble epoxide hydrolase (sEH), which converts active EETs to their inactive metabolites, DHETs, and thereby increases EET levels. Studies in rats have indicated that one such sEH inhibitor, 1-cyclohexyl-3-dodecylurea, lowered blood pressure and reduced glomerular and tubulointerstitial injury in an Ang II–mediated model of hypertension in rats.[554] Furthermore, genetic deletion of Cyp2c44, the major kidney epoxygenase, leads to development of salt-sensitive hypertension.[537]

In deoxycorticosterone acetate–salt hypertension, administration of a CYP450 inhibitor prevented the development of hypertension.[510,555] Ang II stimulated the formation of 20-HETE in the renal circulation,[556] and 20-HETE synthesis inhibition attenuated Ang II–mediated renal vasoconstriction[512] and reduced Ang II–mediated hypertension.[555]

The CYP450 4A2 gene is regulated by salt and overexpressed in SHRs,[557] and production of 20-HETE and di-HETE is increased and production of EETs is reduced.[311,558] CYP450 inhibitors or antisense oligonucleotides directed against CYP4A1 and CYP4A2 lowered blood pressure in SHRs.[505,559] Conversely, studies in humans have indicated that a variant of the human CYP4A11 with reduced 20-HETE synthase activity is associated with hypertension.[560]

In Dahl salt–sensitive rats (Dahl S), pressure-natriuresis in response to salt loading is shifted such that the kidney requires a higher perfusion pressure to excrete the same amount of sodium as normotensive salt-resistant (Dahl R) rats,[298,488,489] which is due at least in part to increased TAL reabsorption. The production of 20-HETE and expression of CYP4A protein are reduced in the outer medulla and TAL of Dahl S rats relative to Dahl R rats, which is consistent with the observed effect of 20-HETE to inhibit TAL transport. In addition, Dahl S rats do not increase EET production in response to salt loading.

Studies have indicated that Ang II acts on AT_2Rs on renal vascular endothelial cells to release EETs that may then counteract AT_1-induced renal vasoconstriction and influence pressure natriuresis.[495,561,562] AT_2R knockout mice develop hypertension, which is associated with blunted pressure natriuresis, reduced renal blood flow and GFR, and defects in kidney 20-HETE production.[563] There is also evidence that the natriuretic effects of dopamine are mediated by EETs and 20-HETE.[564,565]

There has been recent interest in the role of sEH, which is the major enzyme mediating the metabolism of EETs to the inactive dHETEs in the regulation of blood pressure. Progressively more selective sEH inhibitors are being developed and have been shown to be effective in reducing blood pressure in a number of experimental models of hypertension.

ACKNOWLEDGMENTS

The writing of this chapter was supported by grants from the Veterans Administration to Raymond C. Harris and Richard M. Breyer and from the National Institute of Diabetes and Digestive and Kidney Diseases to Raymond C. Harris (DK62794 and DK95785) and Ming-Zhi Zhang (DK95785 and CA122620).

Complete reference list available at ExpertConsult.com.

KEY REFERENCES

2. Murakami M, Kudo I: Phospholipase A2. *J Biochem (Tokyo)* 131:285–292, 2002.
8. Smith WL, Langenbach R: Why there are two cyclooxygenase isozymes. *J Clin Invest* 107:1491–1495, 2001.
24. Tanabe T, Tohnai N: Cyclooxygenase isozymes and their gene structures and expression. *Prostaglandins Other Lipid Mediat* 68-69:95–114, 2002.
31. Crofford LJ: Specific cyclooxygenase-2 inhibitors: what have we learned since they came into widespread clinical use? *Curr Opin Rheumatol* 14:225–230, 2002.
35. Harris RC, McKanna JA, Akai Y, et al: Cyclooxygenase-2 is associated with the macula densa of rat kidney and increases with salt restriction. *J Clin Invest* 94:2504–2510, 1994.
36. Peti-Peterdi J, Harris RC: Macula densa sensing and signaling mechanisms of renin release. *J Am Soc Nephrol* 21:1093–1096, 2010.
49. Peti-Peterdi J, Komlosi P, Fuson AL, et al: Luminal NaCl delivery regulates basolateral PGE2 release from macula densa cells. *J Clin Invest* 112:76–82, 2003.
50. Cheng HF, Wang JL, Zhang MZ, et al: Role of p38 in the regulation of renal cortical cyclooxygenase-2 expression by extracellular chloride. *J Clin Invest* 106:681–688, 2000.
55. Schnermann J, Briggs JP: Tubular control of renin synthesis and secretion. *Pflugers Arch* 465:39–51, 2013.
74. Toma I, Kang JJ, Sipos A, et al: Succinate receptor GPR91 provides a direct link between high glucose levels and renin release in murine and rabbit kidney. *J Clin Invest* 118:2526–2534, 2008.
79. He W, Zhang M, Zhao M, et al: Increased dietary sodium induces COX2 expression by activating NFkappaB in renal medullary interstitial cells. *Pflugers Arch* 466:357–367, 2013. 2014.
112. Komhoff M, Wang JL, Cheng HF, et al: Cyclooxygenase-2-selective inhibitors impair glomerulogenesis and renal cortical development. *Kidney Int* 57:414–422, 2000.
114. Morham SG, Langenbach R, Loftin CD, et al: Prostaglandin synthase 2 gene disruption causes severe renal pathology in the mouse. *Cell* 83:473–482, 1995.
115. Langenbach R, Morham SG, Tiano HF, et al: Prostaglandin synthase 1 gene disruption in mice reduces arachidonic acid-induced inflammation and indomethacin-induced gastric ulceration. *Cell* 83:483–492, 1995.
122. Fitzgerald GA: Coxibs and cardiovascular disease. *N Engl J Med* 351:1709–1711, 2004.
138. Wilcox CS, Welch WJ: Thromboxane synthase and TP receptor mRNA in rat kidney and brain: effects of salt intake and ANG II. *Am J Physiol Renal Physiol* 284:F525–F531, 2003.
141. Murata T, Ushikubi F, Matsuoka T, et al: Altered pain perception and inflammatory response in mice lacking prostacyclin receptor. *Nature* 388:678–682, 1997.
158. Engblom D, Saha S, Engstrom L, et al: Microsomal prostaglandin E synthase-1 is the central switch during immune-induced pyresis. *Nat Neurosci* 6:1137–1138, 2003.
169. Wilson RJ, Rhodes SA, Wood RL, et al: Functional pharmacology of human prostanoid EP2 and EP4 receptors. *Eur J Pharmacol* 501:49–58, 2004.
175. Morrow JD: Quantification of isoprostanes as indices of oxidant stress and the risk of atherosclerosis in humans. *Arterioscler Thromb Vasc Biol* 25:279–286, 2005.
189. Francois H, Makhanova N, Ruiz P, et al: A role for the thromboxane receptor in L-NAME hypertension. *Am J Physiol Renal Physiol* 295:F1096–F1102, 2008.
201. Komhoff M, Lesener B, Nakao K, et al: Localization of the prostacyclin receptor in human kidney. *Kidney Int* 54:1899–1908, 1998.
234. Breyer MD, Breyer RM: G protein-coupled prostanoid receptors and the kidney. *Annu Rev Physiol* 63:579–605, 2001.
251. Kennedy C, Schneider A, Young-Siegler A, et al: Regulation of renin and aldosterone levels in mice lacking the prostaglandin EP2 receptor. *J Am Soc Nephrol* 10:348A, 1999.
261. Breyer MD, Davis L, Jacobson HR, et al: Differential localization of prostaglandin E receptor subtypes in human kidney. *Am J Physiol* 270:F912–F918, 1996.
303. Breyer MD, Jacobson HR, Hebert RL: Cellular mechanisms of prostaglandin E2 and vasopressin interactions in the collecting duct. *Kidney Int* 38:618–624, 1990.
308. Yao B, Xu J, Harris RC, et al: Renal localization and regulation of 15-hydroxyprostaglandin dehydrogenase. *Am J Physiol Renal Physiol* 294:F433–F439, 2008.
319. Straus DS, Glass CK: Cyclopentenone prostaglandins: new insights on biological activities and cellular targets. *Med Res Rev* 21:185–210, 2001.
325. Roberts LJ, 2nd, Morrow JD: Products of the isoprostane pathway: unique bioactive compounds and markers of lipid peroxidation. *Cell Mol Life Sci* 59:808–820, 2002.
327. Schuster VL: Prostaglandin transport. *Prostaglandins Other Lipid Mediat* 68-69:633–647, 2002.
348. Nagamatsu T, Imai H, Yokoi M, et al: Protective effect of prostaglandin EP4-receptor agonist on anti-glomerular basement membrane antibody-associated nephritis. *J Pharmacol Sci* 102:182–188, 2006.
352. Wang JL, Cheng HF, Zhang MZ, et al: Selective increase of cyclooxygenase-2 expression in a model of renal ablation. *Am J Physiol* 275:F613–F622, 1998.
354. Cheng H, Fan X, Guan Y, et al: Distinct roles for basal and induced COX-2 in podocyte injury. *J Am Soc Nephrol* 20:1953–1962, 2009.
357. Komers R, Lindsley JN, Oyama TT, et al: Immunohistochemical and functional correlations of renal cyclooxygenase-2 in experimental diabetes. *J Clin Invest* 107:889–898, 2001.
367. Cheng HF, Wang CJ, Moeckel GW, et al: Cyclooxygenase-2 inhibitor blocks expression of mediators of renal injury in a model of diabetes and hypertension. *Kidney Int* 62:929–939, 2002.
392. Nakagawa N, Yuhki K, Kawabe J, et al: The intrinsic prostaglandin E2-EP4 system of the renal tubular epithelium limits the development of tubulointerstitial fibrosis in mice. *Kidney Int* 82:158–171, 2012.
414. Quilley J, Santos M, Pedraza P: Renal protective effect of chronic inhibition of COX-2 with SC-58236 in streptozotocin-diabetic rats. *Am J Physiol Heart Circ Physiol* 300:H2316–H2322, 2011.
415. Zhang MZ, Yao B, Yang S, et al: Intrarenal dopamine inhibits progression of diabetic nephropathy. *Diabetes* 61:2575–2584, 2012.
424. Rao R, Zhang MZ, Zhao M, et al: Lithium treatment inhibits renal GSK-3 activity and promotes cyclooxygenase 2-dependent polyuria. *Am J Physiol Renal Physiol* 288:F642–F649, 2005.
433. Wilcox CS: Oxidative stress and nitric oxide deficiency in the kidney: a critical link to hypertension? *Am J Physiol Regul Integr Comp Physiol* 289:R913–R935, 2005.
441. Dixon RA, Diehl RE, Opas E, et al: Requirement of a 5-lipoxygenase-activating protein for leukotriene synthesis. *Nature* 343:282–284, 1990.
445. Hui Y, Funk CD: Cysteinyl leukotriene receptors. *Biochem Pharmacol* 64:1549–1557, 2002.
488. Capdevila JH, Harris RC, Falck JR: Microsomal cytochrome P450 and eicosanoid metabolism. *Cell Mol Life Sci* 59:780–789, 2002.
495. Imig J, Gebremedhin D, Zou A, et al: Formation and actions of 20-hydroxyeicosatetraenoic acid in the renal microcirculation. *Am J Physiol* 270:R217–R227, 1996.
537. Capdevila JH, Pidkovka N, Mei S, et al: The Cyp2c44 epoxygenase regulates epithelial sodium channel activity and the blood pressure responses to increased dietary salt. *J Biol Chem* 289:4377–4386, 2014.
539. Pidkovka N, Rao R, Mei S, et al: Epoxyeicosatrienoic acids (EETs) regulate epithelial sodium channel activity by extracellular signal-regulated kinase 1/2 (ERK1/2)-mediated phosphorylation. *J Biol Chem* 288:5223–5231, 2013.
551. Chen G, Xu R, Wang Y, et al: Genetic disruption of soluble epoxide hydrolase is protective against streptozotocin-induced

diabetic nephropathy. *Am J Physiol Endocrinol Metab* 303:E563–E575, 2012.
553. Holla VR, Makita K, Zaphiropoulos PG, et al: The kidney cytochrome P-450 2C23 arachidonic acid epoxygenase is upregulated during dietary salt loading. *J Clin Invest* 104:751–760, 1999.
554. Imig JD: Epoxide hydrolase and epoxygenase metabolites as therapeutic targets for renal diseases. *Am J Physiol Renal Physiol* 289:F496–F503, 2005.
560. Gainer JV, Bellamine A, Dawson EP, et al: Functional variant of CYP4A11 20-hydroxyeicosatetraenoic acid synthase is associated with essential hypertension. *Circulation* 111:63–69, 2005.

SECTION II

DISORDERS OF BODY FLUID VOLUME AND COMPOSITION

15 Disorders of Sodium Balance

Itzchak N. Slotki | Karl L. Skorecki

CHAPTER OUTLINE

PHYSIOLOGY, 390
Sodium Balance, 391
Effective Arterial Blood Volume, 393
Regulation of Effective Arterial Blood Volume, 394
SODIUM BALANCE DISORDERS, 421
Hypovolemia, 421
Hypervolemia, 425
SPECIFIC TREATMENTS BASED ON THE PATHOPHYSIOLOGY OF CONGESTIVE HEART FAILURE, 451
Inhibition of the Renin-Angiotensin-Aldosterone System, 451
β-Blockade, 452
Nitric Oxide Donor and Reactive Oxygen Species/Peroxynitrite Scavengers, 452

Endothelin Antagonists, 452
Natriuretic Peptides, 453
Neutral Endopeptidase Inhibitors and Vasopeptidase Inhibitors, 453
Vasopressin Receptor Antagonists, 454
SPECIFIC TREATMENTS BASED ON THE PATHOPHYSIOLOGY OF SODIUM RETENTION IN CIRRHOSIS, 455
Pharmacologic Treatment, 455
Transjugular Intrahepatic Portosystemic Shunt, 457
Renal Replacement Therapy, 457
Liver Transplantation, 458

Sodium (Na^+) and water balance and their distribution among the various body compartments are essential for the maintenance of fluid homeostasis, particularly intravascular volume. Disturbances of either or both of these components have serious medical consequences, are relatively frequent, and are among the most common conditions encountered in hospital clinical practice. In fact, abnormalities of Na^+ and water balance are responsible for, or associated with, a wide spectrum of medical and surgical admissions or complications. The principal disorders of Na^+ balance are manifested clinically as hypovolemia or hypervolemia, whereas disruption in water balance can be diagnosed only in the laboratory as hyponatremia or hypernatremia. Although disorders of Na^+ and water balance are often interrelated, the latter are considered in a separate chapter. In this chapter, the physiologic and pathophysiologic features of Na^+ balance are discussed. Because Na^+ is restricted predominantly to the extracellular compartment, this chapter also addresses perturbations of extracellular fluid (ECF) volume homeostasis.

PHYSIOLOGY

Approximately 60% of adult body mass is composed of solute-containing fluids that can be divided into extracellular and intracellular compartments. Because water flows freely across cell membranes in accordance with the prevailing osmotic forces on either side of the membrane, the solute/water ratios in the intracellular fluid (ICF) and ECF are almost equal. However, the solute compositions of the ICF and ECF are quite different, as shown in Figure 15.1. The principal ECF cation is sodium; minor cations are potassium (K^+), calcium, and magnesium. In contrast, potassium is the major ICF cation. The accompanying anions in the ECF are chloride, bicarbonate, and plasma proteins (mainly albumin), whereas electroneutrality of the ICF is maintained by phosphate and the negative charges on organic molecules. The difference in cationic composition of the two compartments is maintained by a pump leak mechanism consisting of sodium-potassium adenosine triphosphatase (Na^+-K^+-ATPase), which operates in concert with sodium and potassium conductance pathways in the cell membrane.

The free movement of water across the membrane ensures that the ECF and ICF osmolalities are the same. However, the intracellular volume is greater because the amount of potassium salts inside the cell is larger than that of sodium salts outside the cell. The movement of water is determined by the "effective osmolality," or tonicity, of each compartment, so that if tonicity of the ECF rises—for example, as a result of excess Na^+—water will move from the ICF to ECF to restore tonicity. On the other hand, addition of solute-free water leads to a proportionate decrease in both

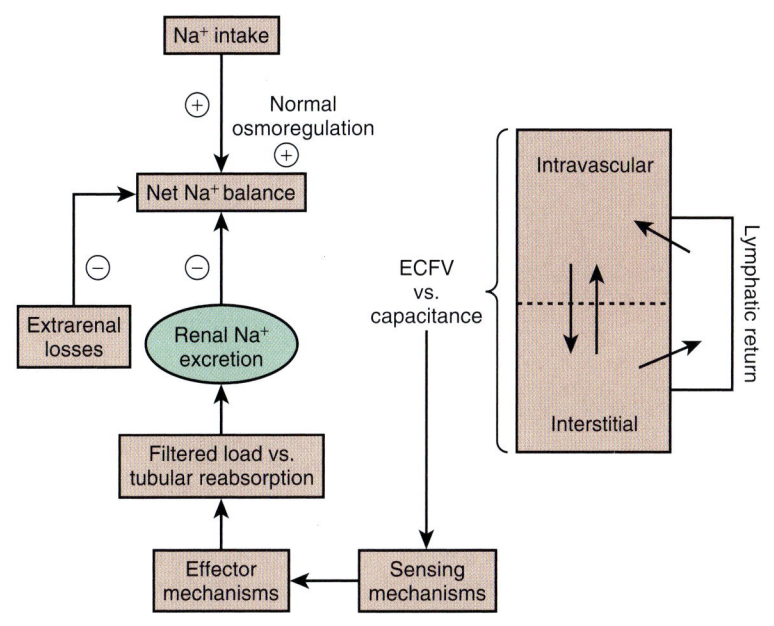

Figure 15.1 Traditional two-compartmental scheme for body sodium balance and partitioning of extracellular fluid volume (ECFV), based on exchangeable and osmotically active Na$^+$. In the setting of normal osmoregulation, extracellular Na$^+$ content is the primary determinant of ECFV. Overall Na$^+$ homeostasis depends on the balance between losses (extrarenal and renal) and intake. Renal Na$^+$ excretion is determined by the balance between filtered load and tubule reabsorption. This latter balance is modulated under the influence of effector mechanisms, which, in turn, are responsive to sensing mechanisms that monitor the relationship between ECFV and capacitance. In rats, a high-salt diet leads to interstitial hypertonic Na$^+$ accumulation in skin, resulting in increased density and hyperplasia of the lymphatic capillary network.

osmolality and tonicity of all body fluid compartments (see Chapter 16 for a detailed discussion). The restriction of Na$^+$ to the ECF compartment by the pump leak mechanism, in combination with maintenance of the osmotic equilibrium between ECF and ICF, ensures that ECF volume is determined mainly by total body Na$^+$ content.

The same mechanisms also govern the partitioning of fluid between the two compartments and are crucial for the preservation of near constancy of ECF and ICF volume in the presence of variations in dietary intake and extrarenal losses of Na$^+$ and water. To maintain constancy of the ECF and ICF and thereby safeguard hemodynamic stability, cell volume, and solute composition, even minute changes in these parameters can be detected by a number of sensing mechanisms. These sensory signals lead to activation of neural and hormonal factors, which, in turn, cause appropriate adjustments in urinary Na$^+$ and water excretion and, hence, restoration of fluid balance (Figure 15.2). Constancy of ECF volume ensures a high degree of circulatory stability, whereas constancy of ICF volume protects against significant brain cell swelling or shrinkage.

SODIUM BALANCE

Na$^+$ balance is the difference between intake (diet or supplementary fluids) and output (renal, gastrointestinal, perspiratory, and respiratory). In healthy humans in steady state, dietary intake is closely matched by urinary output of Na$^+$. Thus, a person consuming a chronically low-Na$^+$ diet (20 mmol/day, or ≈1.2 g/day) excretes, in the steady state, a similar quantity of Na$^+$ in the urine (minus extrarenal losses). Conversely, on a high-Na$^+$ diet (200 mmol/day, or 12 g/day), approximately 200 mmol of Na$^+$ is excreted in the urine. Any perturbation of this balance leads to activation of the sensory and effector mechanisms outlined in the following discussions. In practice, any deviation in ECF volume in relation to its capacitance is sensed and translated, under the influence of neural and hormonal factors, into the appropriate change in Na$^+$ excretion, principally through the kidneys but also, to a much lesser degree, through stool and sweat.

According to the traditional two-compartment model, body sodium balance and partitioning of extracellular fluid volume (ECFV) is based solely on exchangeable and osmotically active Na$^+$. For normal functioning of the afferent sensing and efferent effector mechanisms that regulate ECF volume, the integrity of the intravascular and extravascular subcompartments of the ECF is crucial[1] (see Figure 15.1). Although the composition and concentration of small, noncolloid electrolyte solutes in these two subcompartments are approximately equal (slight differences are due to the Gibbs-Donnan effect), the concentration of colloid osmotic particles (mainly albumin and globulin) is higher in the intravascular compartment. The balance between transcapillary hydraulic and colloid osmotic (oncotic) gradients (Starling forces) favors the net transudation of fluid from the intravascular to interstitial compartment. However, this is countered by movement of lymphatic fluid from the interstitial to intravascular compartment via the thoracic duct. The net effect is to restore and maintain the intravascular subcompartment at 25% of the total ECF volume (corresponding to 3.5 L of plasma); the remaining 75% is contained in the interstitial space (equivalent to 10.5 L in a 70-kg man; see Figure 15.2). The constancy of ECF volume and the appropriate partitioning of the fluid between intravascular and interstitial subcompartments are crucial for maintaining hemodynamic stability. In particular, intravascular volume in relation to overall vascular capacitance is a

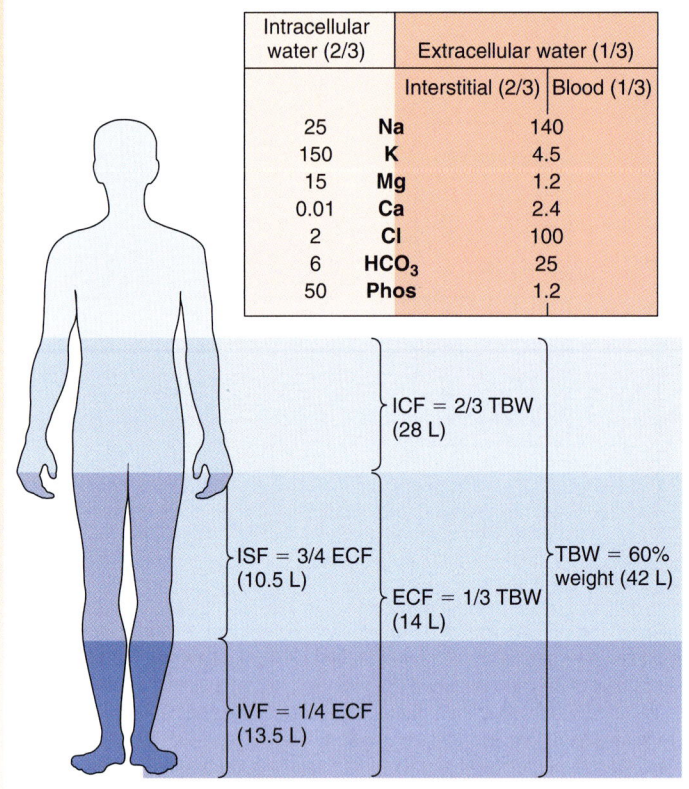

Intracellular water (2/3)	Extracellular water (1/3)	
	Interstitial (2/3)	Blood (1/3)
25	Na	140
150	K	4.5
15	Mg	1.2
0.01	Ca	2.4
2	Cl	100
6	HCO$_3$	25
50	Phos	1.2

ICF = 2/3 TBW (28 L)
ISF = 3/4 ECF (10.5 L)
ECF = 1/3 TBW (14 L)
IVF = 1/4 ECF (13.5 L)
TBW = 60% weight (42 L)

Figure 15.2 Composition of body fluid compartments. This is a schematic representation of electrolyte composition of compartments (**upper panel**) and body fluid compartments in humans (**lower panel**). In the **upper panel**, electrolyte concentrations are in millimoles per liter; intracellular concentrations are typical values obtained from muscle. In the **lower panel**, shaded areas depict the approximate size of each compartment as a function of body weight. In a normally built individual, the total body water content is roughly 60% of body weight. Because adipose tissue has a low concentration of water, the relative water/total body weight ratio is lower in obese individuals. Relative volumes of each compartment are shown as fractions; approximate absolute volumes of the compartments (in liters) in a 70-kg adult are shown in parentheses. ECF, Extracellular fluid; ICF, intracellular fluid; ISF, interstitial fluid; IVF, intravascular fluid; TBW, total body water. (From Verbalis JG: Body water osmolality. In Wilkinson B, Jamison R, editors: Textbook of nephrology, London, 1997, Chapman & Hall, pp 89-94. Reproduced with permission of Hodder Arnold.)

major determinant of left ventricular filling volume and, hence, cardiac output and mean arterial pressure.

The traditional two-compartment model of volume regulation, according to which the intravascular and interstitial spaces are in equilibrium, has been recently challenged. It now appears that Na$^+$ can be bound to and stored on proteoglycans in interstitial sites, where it becomes osmotically inactive; accordingly, a novel mechanism of volume regulation has been elucidated.[2-9] In rats fed a high-salt diet, this uniquely bound Na$^+$ was found to induce a state of subcutaneous interstitial hypertonicity and systemic hypertension.[4] Machnik and colleagues have offered compelling experimental evidence that this hypertonicity is sensed by macrophages,[3] which then produce vascular endothelial growth factor C (VEGF-C), an angiogenic protein. In turn, VEGF-C stimulates increased numbers and density of lymphatic capillaries. In parallel work, using cultured macrophage cell lines subjected to osmotic stress, Go and associates have demonstrated activation of a transcription factor, tonicity-responsive enhancer–binding protein (TonEBP). This factor is known to activate osmoprotective genes in other hypertonic environments, such as the renal medulla.[10] Moreover, analysis of the VEGF-C promoter revealed two TonEBP binding sites and, in subsequent experiments, parallel upregulation of TonEBP and VEGF-C was observed. The effect of TonEBP on VEGF-C was shown to be specific, inasmuch as small interfering RNA for TonEBP and deletion of the murine TonEBP gene, but not nonspecific small interfering RNA, inhibited the VEGF-C upregulation and increased blood pressure. Furthermore, macrophage depletion or inhibition of VEGF-C signaling led to exacerbation of high-salt diet–induced hypertension.[3] Also, an antibody that blocks the lymph-endothelial VEGF-C receptor, VEGFR-3, selectively inhibited macrophage-driven increases in cutaneous lymphatic capillary density, led to skin chloride (Cl$^-$) accumulation, and induced salt-sensitive hypertension. Mice overexpressing soluble VEGFR3 in epidermal keratinocytes exhibited hypoplastic cutaneous lymph capillaries and increased Na$^+$, Cl$^-$, and water retention in skin and salt-sensitive hypertension.[11] A high-salt diet also led to elevated skin osmolality above plasma levels. In addition, in humans with relatively resistant hypertension, elevated levels of VEGF-C were found,[3] which is consistent with a potential role of this growth factor in the redistribution of excess volume to the intravascular space and exacerbation of hypertension.[12]

Interestingly, mice skin arterioles isolated from animals fed a high-salt diet compared to those on a normal salt diet exhibited increased contractile sensitivity to concentrations of angiotensin II (Ang II) from 10^{-10} M upward and to norepinephrine at high doses (10^{-5} to 10^{-4} M). This salt sensitivity was not observed in muscle arterioles. Finally, a unique human study involving astronauts on the Mars expedition, who received diets with fixed salt intake that varied between 6 and 12 g daily, each for 35 days, was recently reported (reviewed in Reference 14). At each level of salt in the diet, the astronauts reached overall equilibrium between intake and output, as measured in 24-hour urine collections, within the expected 6 days. In parallel, there were the expected early changes in body weight, ECF water, and inverse relationship with the urine aldosterone level. However, changes in total body Na$^+$ only occurred after 7 days, and blood pressure reached a new steady state after 3 weeks. Moreover, on the 12-g salt diet, blood pressure continued to rise over a further 4 weeks, with an initial rise and then subsequent fall in body weight and ECF water. During this period, urine aldosterone levels did not change, whereas total body Na$^+$ decreased back to original levels, despite the maintained high salt intake. From these data, it appears that intrinsic rhythms with a periodicity of 30 days or more exist for aldosterone and Na$^+$ retention, independent of salt intake. Taken together, all these results clearly demonstrate that the skin contains a hypertonic interstitial fluid compartment in which macrophages exert homeostatic and blood pressure regulatory control by local organization of interstitial electrolyte clearance via TonEBP and VEGF-C/VEGFR-3–mediated modification of cutaneous lymphatic capillary function.[11] This compartment may be associated with increased vasoreactivity in precapillary arterioles, the major

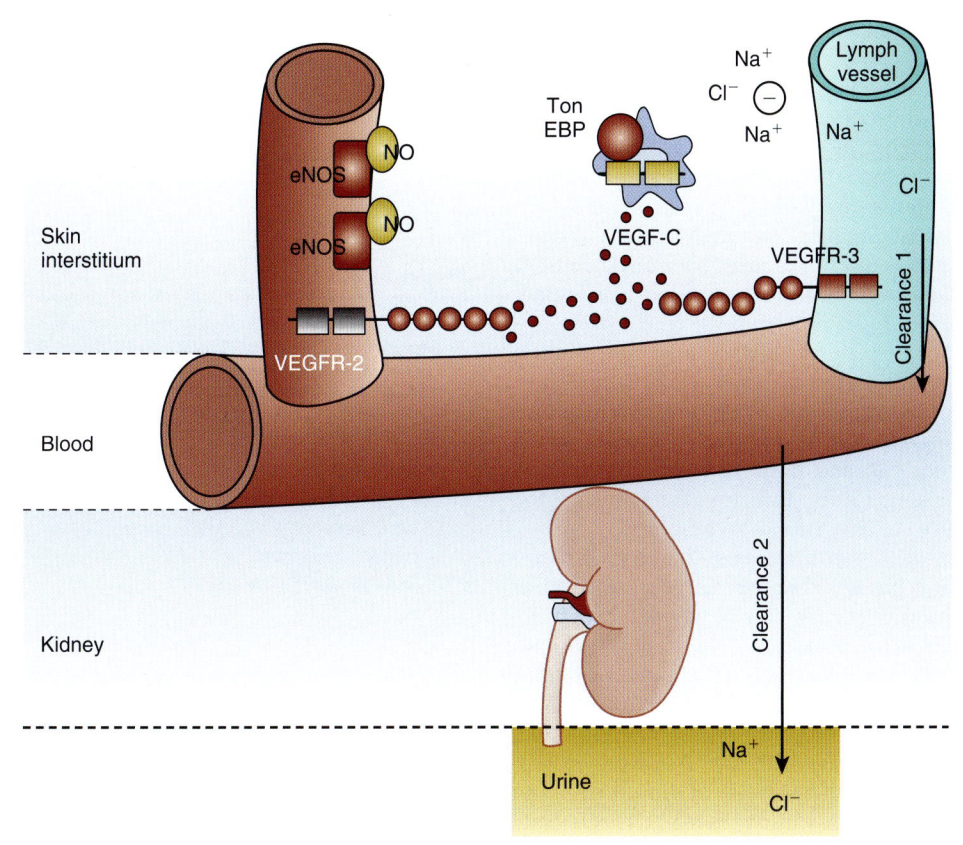

Figure 15.3 New model of body electrolyte balance and blood pressure homeostasis. This is based on the finding that interstitial electrolyte concentrations are higher than in blood (so-called skin Na⁺ storage). Interstitial electrolyte balance is not achieved by renal blood purification alone, but relies on additional extrarenal regulatory mechanisms within the skin interstitium. Macrophages act as local osmosensors that regulate local interstitial electrolyte composition via a tonicity-responsive enhancer–binding protein/vascular endothelial growth factor type C (TonEBP/VEGF-C)–dependent mechanism, enhancing electrolyte clearance via VEGF-C/VEGFR-3–mediated modulation of the lymph capillary network in the skin. eNOS, Endothelial nitric oxide synthase; VEGFR, vascular endothelial growth factor receptor. (Adapted from Titze J, Dahlmann A, Lerchl K, et al: Spooky sodium balance. *Kidney Int* 85:759-767, 2014.)

resistance vessel of rat skin, which could increase peripheral resistance and contribute independently of the kidney to higher blood pressure in salt-sensitive hypertension.[13]

Figure 15.3 summarizes the novel three-compartment model of Na⁺ balance. The reader is also referred to an excellent recent review of this fascinating subject.[14]

EFFECTIVE ARTERIAL BLOOD VOLUME

To understand the mechanisms regulating ECF volume, it is important to appreciate that what is sensed is the effective arterial blood volume (EABV). This can be defined as the part of the ECF in the arterial blood system that effectively perfuses the tissues. More specifically, in physiologic terms, what is sensed is the threat to arterial pressure induced by the EABV[15] that perfuses the arterial baroreceptors in the carotid sinus and glomerular afferent arterioles. Any change in perfusion pressure (or stretch) at these sites evokes appropriate compensatory responses. EABV is often, although not always, correlated with actual ECF volume and is proportional to total body Na⁺. This means that the regulation of Na⁺ balance and the maintenance of EABV are closely related functions. Na⁺ loading generally leads to EABV expansion, whereas loss leads to depletion. However, in several situations, EABV and actual blood volume are not well correlated (see Table 15-5). For example, in heart failure (HF), a primary decrease in cardiac output leads to lowered pressure in the perfusion of the baroceptors; that is, reduced EABV is sensed. This leads to renal Na⁺ retention and ECF volume expansion. The net result is a state of increased plasma and total ECF volume, in association with reduced EABV.

The increase in plasma volume is partially appropriate in that intraventricular filling pressure rises and, by increasing myocardial stretching, leads to improved ventricular contractility, thereby raising cardiac output and restoring systemic blood pressure and baroceptor perfusion. However, this response is also maladaptive in that the elevated intraarterial pressure promotes fluid movement out of the intravascular space and into the tissues, which leads to peripheral and pulmonary edema. In HF, EABV is dependent on cardiac output; in other disease settings, however, these two parameters may be dissociated. Dissociation occurs in the presence of an arteriovenous fistula when cardiac output rises in proportion to the blood flow through the fistula. However, the flow through the fistula shunts blood away from the capillaries perfusing the tissues, and therefore the EABV does not rise in conjunction with the rise in cardiac output. Similarly, a fall in systemic vascular resistance—which, together with cardiac output, is a determinant of blood pressure—leads to reductions in blood pressure and EABV.

Another situation in which cardiac output and EABV change in opposite directions is advanced cirrhosis with ascites. ECF volume expands because of the ascites, and plasma volume is increased as a result of fluid accumulation in the splanchnic venous circulation, in which the vessels are dilated but flow is sluggish. Although cardiac output may increase modestly as a result of arteriovenous shunting, marked peripheral vasodilation leads to a fall in systemic vascular resistance, with reductions in EABV and blood pressure. In the presence of reduced EABV, renal perfusion is impaired; under the influence of hormones, such as renin, norepinephrine, and antidiuretic hormone (or arginine vasopressin [AVP])—released in response to the perceived hypovolemia—further Na^+ and water retention ensue (see later section, "Efferent Limb: Effector Mechanisms for Maintaining Effective Arterial Blood Volume").

To summarize, EABV is an unmeasured index of tissue perfusion that usually, but not always, reflects actual arterial blood volume. Therefore, EABV can be viewed as a functional parameter of organ perfusion. The diagnostic hallmark of reduced EABV is evidence of renal sodium retention, manifested as a urinary sodium (U_{Na}) level less than 15 to 20 mmol/L.

This relationship holds true with the following exceptions. If renal Na^+ wasting occurs because of diuretic therapy or intrinsic tubular disease or injury, then U_{Na} is relatively high, despite low EABV. Conversely, the presence of selective renal or glomerular ischemia (e.g., as a result of bilateral renal artery stenosis or acute glomerular injury) will be misinterpreted as indicative of poor renal perfusion and is associated with renal Na^+ retention (low U_{Na}).

REGULATION OF EFFECTIVE ARTERIAL BLOOD VOLUME

Regulation of EABV can be divided into two stages, afferent sensing and efferent effector mechanisms. A number of mechanisms for sensing low EABV exist, all of them primed to stimulate renal Na^+ retention.

AFFERENT LIMB: SENSING OF EFFECTIVE ARTERIAL BLOOD VOLUME

Volume sensors are strategically situated at critical points in the circulation (Table 15.1). Each sensor reflects a specific characteristic of overall circulatory function so that atrial and ventricular sensors sense cardiac filling, arterial sensors respond to cardiac output, and renal, central nervous system (CNS), and gastrointestinal (GI) tract sensors monitor perfusion of the kidneys, brain, and gut, respectively. The common mechanism whereby volume is monitored is by physical alterations in the vessel wall, such as stretch or tension. How exactly this occurs is still not fully elucidated, but the process of mechanosensing probably is dependent on afferent sensory nerve endings in the vessel wall and activation of endothelial cells. Signal transduction mechanisms in endothelial cells include stretch-activated ion channels, cytoskeleton-associated protein kinases, integrin-cytoskeletal interactions, cytoskeletal-nuclear interactions, and generation of reactive oxygen species.[16,17] In addition, mechanical stretch and tension of blood vessel walls, as well as the frictional forces of the circulation or shear stress, can lead to alterations in gene expression that are mediated by specific recognition sites in the upstream promoter elements of responsive genes.[18,19] These signals induce efferent effector mechanisms that lead to modifications in renal Na^+ excretion, appropriate to the volume status.

Sensors of Cardiac Filling

Atrial Sensors. The pioneering experiments of Henry and associates[20] and Goetz and colleagues[21] in conscious dogs provided a clear demonstration that increased atrial wall tension leads to diuresis and natriuresis. The role of the atria in volume regulation in humans has been elucidated in experiments involving head-out water immersion (HWI) and exposure to head-down tilt or nonhypotensive lower body negative pressure (LBNP). During HWI, the increased hydrostatic pressure of the water on the lower limbs leads to redistribution of the intravascular fluid from the peripheral to central circulation. The resulting increase in central blood volume causes a rise in cardiac output, which in turn produces a brisk increase in Na^+ and water excretion in an attempt to restore euvolemia.[22] In contrast, LBNP results in a redistribution of blood to the lower limbs, thereby reducing central venous and cardiac filling pressures without affecting arterial pressure, heart rate, or atrial diameter. The resulting retention of Na^+ and water occurs without any change in renal plasma flow rate (RPF).[23]

Central hypervolemia may not be the only mechanism of HWI-induced Na^+ and water diuresis. The external hydrostatic pressure of the water also reduces the hydrostatic pressure gradient across the capillary wall in the legs, leading to a net transfer of fluid from the interstitial to intravascular compartment. The resulting hemodilution causes a fall in the colloid osmotic pressure. The hemodilution effect may actually predominate, inasmuch as its abolition by placement of a tight inflated cuff (80 mm Hg) during HWI

Table 15.1 Mechanisms for Sensing Regional Changes in Effective Arterial Blood Volume

Sensors of Cardiac Filling

Atrial
  Neural pathways
  Humoral pathways
Ventricular
Pulmonary

Sensors of Cardiac Output

Carotid and aortic baroceptors

Sensors of Organ Perfusion

Renal sensors
CNS sensors
GI tract sensors
  Hepatic receptors
  Guanylin peptides

CNS, Central nervous system, GI, gastrointestinal.

abrogates the natriuresis.[24,25] Regardless of which effect is dominant, a combination of hemodilution and central hypervolemia, through atrial stretch, induces neural and humoral changes that bring about the subsequent diuresis and natriuresis.

Neural Pathways. Two types of neural receptors in the atrium have been described, type A and type B. They are thought to be branching ends of small medullated fibers running in the vagus nerve. Only type B receptor activity is increased by atrial filling and stretch; type A receptors are not affected.[26] The signal is then thought to travel along cranial nerves IX and X to the hypothalamic and medullary centers, where a series of responses is initiated—inhibition of AVP release (left atrial signal),[27] a selective decrease in renal but not lumbar sympathetic nerve discharge,[28,29] and decreased tone in peripheral precapillary and postcapillary resistance vessels. Conversely, reduction in central venous pressure and atrial volume, as illustrated by LBNP, stimulates renal nerve activity, as assessed by renal norepinephrine spillover and plasma norepinephrine concentration.[30,31]

The effects just described occur in response to acute atrial stretch, whereas chronic atrial stretch leads to adaptation and downregulation of the neural responses. This phenomenon has been described in rhesus monkeys exposed to 10-degree, head-down tilt. In this model, natriuresis after saline infusion occurs at lower central venous and, hence, lower cardiac filling pressures.[31] Cardiac nerves appear to be essential only for the restoration of Na$^+$ balance in states of repletion, but not for the renal response to acute volume depletion.[32] For example, after human cardiac transplantation, a natural model of cardiac denervation, the expected suppression of the renin-angiotensin-aldosterone (RAAS) system in response to chronic volume expansion is not observed.[33]

Humoral Pathways. Cardiac denervation does not abolish the natriuresis and diuresis during atrial distension. This implies that additional factors other than cardiac nerves are involved in the response to volume repletion. The discovery of a factor in atrial extracts with strong natriuretic and vasodilatory activity led to the isolation and characterization of natriuretic peptides of cardiac origin.[34,35] The NP family is comprised of atrial NP (ANP), brain NP (BNP), C-type NP (CNP), *Dendroaspis* NP (DNP), and urodilatin. Although their structures are quite similar, each is encoded by different genes and has distinct, albeit overlapping, functions.[36-39] The actions of NPs and their interaction with other hormone systems are discussed in detail later (see section, "Efferent Limb: Effector Mechanisms for Maintaining Effective Arterial Blood Volume" and Chapters 11 to 14). This section is confined to a discussion of the afferent mechanisms of NP stimulation.

From studies in animals and humans, it has become abundantly clear that any acute increment in atrial stretch or pressure causes a brisk release in ANP. Every 1-mm Hg rise in atrial pressure results in an approximate rise in ANP of 10 to 15 pmol/L. The process involves the cleavage of the prohormone, located in preformed stores in atrial granules, to the mature 28–amino acid C-terminus peptide in a sequence-specific manner by corin, a transmembrane serine protease.[40] Release of the hormone appears to occur in two steps, the first a Ca^{2+}-sensitive K$^+$ channel–dependent release of ANP from myocytes into the intercellular space and then a Ca^{2+}-independent translocation of the hormone into the atrial lumen.[41] The afferent mechanism for ANP release is activated by intravascular volume expansion and by supine posture, HWI, saline administration, exercise, Ang II, tachycardia, and ventricular dysfunction.[42,43] Conversely, volume depletion induced by Na$^+$ restriction, furosemide administration, or LNBP-mediated reduction in central venous pressure causes a fall in plasma ANP concentration.

The signal transduction pathways, whereby atrial stretch is translated into ANP release, are yet to be fully elaborated. However, a study has shown that mice with a mutation in the acid-sensing ion channel 3 gene or in which the channel was pharmacologically inhibited have a blunted response in blood volume expansion–induced urine flow.[19]

In contrast to the effects of acute changes in atrial pressure on ANP release, the role of this peptide in the long-term regulation of plasma volume appears to be modest, at best. For example, although incremental oral salt loading was associated with correspondingly higher baseline plasma ANP levels, only intravenous (not oral) salt loading led to increased ANP levels.[44] Moreover, in humans subjected to intravenous or oral salt loading, no correlation could be found between changes in ANP levels and the degree of natriuresis.[45-47] The contrasting relationships among acute and chronic Na$^+$ loading, plasma ANP levels, and natriuresis have been elegantly demonstrated in ANP gene knockout mice. These mice display a reduced natriuretic response to acute ECFV expansion in comparison with their wild-type counterparts. However, no differences in cumulative Na$^+$ and water excretion were observed between the knockout and wild-type mice after a high- or low-Na$^+$ diet for 1 week. The only difference between the two types of mice was a significant increase in mean arterial pressure. Further experiments using disruptions of the genes for ANP or its receptor, guanylate cyclase A (GC-A), have shown the importance of this system in the maintenance of normal blood pressure and in modulating cardiac hypertrophy.[48]

In contrast to ANP, the other members of the NP family appear not to be involved in the physiologic regulation of Na$^+$ excretion. Thus, results of gene disruption studies involving BNP, CNP, or the guanylate cyclase B (GC-B) receptor[49] indicated that these proteins exert local paracrine-autocrine cyclic guanosine monophosphate (cGMP)–mediated effects on cellular proliferation and differentiation in various tissues.[36,38,50] In summary, of the various NPs, only ANP appears to have a direct role in sensing volume in the atria.

Ventricular and Pulmonary Sensors. Volume sensors have been found in the ventricles, coronary arteries, main pulmonary artery and bifurcation,[51] and juxtapulmonary capillaries in the interstitium of the lungs,[52] but not in the intrapulmonary circulation.[53] These sensors have generally been considered as mediating reflex changes in heart rate and systemic vascular resistance through modulation of the sympathetic nervous system (SNS) and of ANP. This also appears to be true for the coronary baroreceptor reflex described in anesthetized dogs, by which changes in coronary artery pressure lead to alterations in lumbar and renal sympathetic discharge and a coronary artery response much slower than that of the carotid and aortic baroreceptors.[54]

However, some evidence, also in dogs, has suggested that ventricular and pulmonary sensors may also detect changes in blood volume through increased left ventricular pressure, which causes a reflex inhibition of plasma renin activity (PRA).[55,56]

Sensors of Cardiac Output

The sensors described so far are situated in low-pressure sites, where they sense the fullness of the circulation and are probably more important for defending against excessive volume expansion and the consequent congestive manifestations of cardiac failure. The arterial (high-pressure) sensors, on the other hand, are geared more toward detecting low cardiac output or systemic vascular resistance, which manifest as underfilling of the vascular tree (i.e., EABV depletion threatening arterial pressure[15]) and as signaling the kidneys to retain Na^+. These high-pressure sensors are found in the aortic arch, carotid sinus, and renal vessels.

Carotid and Aortic Baroceptors. Histologic and molecular analysis of the carotid baroceptor has revealed a large content of elastic tissue in the tunica media, which makes the vessel wall highly distensible in response to changes in intraluminal pressure, thereby facilitating transmission of the stimulus intensity to sensory nerve terminals. A change in the mean arterial pressure induces depolarization of these sensory endings, which results in action potentials. Transient receptor potential vanilloid receptors may mediate this process.[57] Afferent signals from the baroceptors are integrated in the nucleus tractus solitarius (NTS) of the medulla oblongata,[58] which leads to reflex changes in systemic and renal sympathetic nerve activity (RSNA) and, to a lesser degree, release of AVP. A role for endocannabinoids has been postulated in baroreceptor reflex modulation. In this regard, a significant increase in the endocannabinoid anandamide in the NTS was observed after an increase in blood pressure. Also, anandamide microinjections into the NTS induced prolonged baroreflex inhibition of RSNA. The cannabinoid effect appears to be mediated by activation of 5-hydroxytryptamine type 1A (5-HT1A) receptors.[59] These results, along with other studies,[60] support the hypothesis that endogenous anandamide can modulate the baroreflex through cannabinoid CB(1) receptor activation within the nucleus tractus solitarius.[61] Conversely, hypovolemia-induced activation of NTS (A1) adenosine receptors may serve as a negative feedback regulator of sympathoinhibitory reflexes integrated in the NTS.[62] An important additional function of the carotid baroceptors is maintenance of adequate cerebral perfusion. The aortic baroceptor appears to behave in a way similar to the carotid baroceptor. Finally, there is evidence in dogs for an interaction between pulmonary arterial and carotid sinus baroceptor reflexes.[63]

Sensors of Organ Perfusion

Renal Sensors. The kidney not only is the major effector target responding to signals that indicate the need for adjustments in Na^+ excretion, but also has a central role in the afferent sensing of volume homeostasis by virtue of the local sympathetic innervation. However, despite considerable knowledge concerning the mechanisms of renal sensing of EABV, the molecular identity and exact cellular location of the renal sensor or sensors remain elusive.[64] The integral relationship between afferent and efferent renal sympathetic activities and the central arterial baroceptors was highlighted by Kopp and colleagues.[65] They showed that a high-Na^+ diet increases afferent RSNA, which then decreases efferent RSNA and leads to natriuresis. Using dorsal rhizotomy to induce afferent renal denervation in rats maintained on a high-Na^+ diet, they demonstrated increased mean arterial pressure that was dependent on impaired arterial baroreflex suppression of efferent RSNA activity. Animals fed a normal-Na^+ diet displayed no changes in arterial baroceptor function. Kopp and coworkers concluded that arterial baroreflex function contributes to increased efferent RSNA, which, in the absence of intact afferent RSNA, would eventually lead to Na^+ retention and hypertension. The role of RSNA in Na^+ regulation is discussed further later in this chapter (see section, "Neural Mechanisms: Renal Nerves and Sympathetic Nervous System").

An additional level of renal sensing depends on the close anatomic proximity of the sensor and effector limbs to one another: Volume changes may be sensed through alterations in glomerular hemodynamics and renal interstitial pressure. These alterations result simultaneously in adjustments in the physical forces governing tubular Na^+ handling (see section, "Efferent Limb: Effector Mechanisms for Maintaining Effective Arterial Blood Volume").

The kidneys, along with other organs, have the ability to maintain a constant blood flow and constant glomerular filtration rate (GFR) at varying arterial pressures. This phenomenon, termed *autoregulation*, operates over a wide range of renal perfusion pressures (RPPs). Autoregulation of renal blood flow (RBF) occurs through three mechanisms—the myogenic response, tubuloglomerular feedback (TGF), and a third mechanism. In the myogenic response, changes in RPP are sensed by smooth muscle elements that serve as baroreceptors in the afferent glomerular arteriole and dynamically respond by adjusting transmural pressure and tension across the arteriolar wall.[66] An example of this can be seen in Ang II–infused rats on a high salt intake. These animals show reduced dynamic autoregulation of RBF, an effect mediated, at least in part, by superoxide.[67] The myogenic response is attenuated by endothelial nitric oxide synthase (eNOS)–dependent production of nitric oxide.[68]

The second mechanism, TGF, is operated by the juxtaglomerular apparatus, which is comprised of the afferent arteriole and, to a lesser extent, the cells of the macula densa in the early distal tubule.[66,69,70] The juxtaglomerular apparatus is also important because of its involvement in the synthesis and release of renin.[69] The physiologic release of renin from the cells of the juxtaglomerular apparatus is controlled by three pathways, all of which are driven by EABV status. First, renin release is inversely related to RPP and directly related to intrarenal tissue pressure. When RPP falls below the autoregulatory range, renin release is further enhanced. Second, renin secretion is influenced by solute delivery to the macula densa. Increased NaCl delivery past the macula densa leads to inhibition of renin release, whereas a decrease has the opposite effect. Sensing at the macula densa is mediated by NaCl entry through the Na^+-K^+-$2Cl^-$ cotransporter (NKCC2),[71,72] which leads to alterations in intracellular Ca^{2+} together with the production of prostaglandin E_2 (PGE_2),[73,74] adenosine,[75] and, subsequently, renin release. Third, changes in renal nerve activity influence renin release. Renal nerve stimulation increases renin release through direct activation of β-adrenergic receptors on juxtaglomerular cells. This effect is independent of major changes in renal hemodynamics.[76,77] Sympathetic stimulation also affects intrarenal baroreceptor input, composition of the fluid delivered to the macula densa, and renal actions of Ang II so that renal nerves may serve primarily to potentiate other regulatory signals.[76-78]

The nature of the third mechanism of RBF autoregulation is still unclear, but Seeliger and associates,[79] using a normotensive Ang II clamp in anesthetized rats, were able to abolish the resetting of autoregulation during incremental shaped RPP changes. Under control conditions, the initial TGF response was dilatory after total occlusions but constrictive after partial occlusions. The initial third mechanism response was a mirror image of TGF, it was constrictive after total occlusions but dilatory after partial occlusions. The angiotensin clamp suppressed the TGF and turned the initial third mechanism response after total occlusions into dilation. Seeliger and coworkers reached the following conclusions: (1) pressure-dependent renin angiotensin system (RAS) stimulation was a major factor behind hypotensive resetting of autoregulation; (2) TGF sensitivity depended strongly on pressure-dependent changes in RAS activity; (3) the third mechanism was modulated, but not mediated, by the RAS; and (4) the third mechanism acted as a counterbalance to TGF.[79] They proposed that their findings might be related to feedback between the connecting tubule and glomerulus.[80-82] TGF is discussed later (see section, "Integration of Changes in Glomerular Filtration Rate and Tubular Reabsorption").

Central Nervous System Sensors. Certain areas in the CNS appear to act as sensors to detect alterations in body salt balance. This was suggested originally by results of experiments in rats, in which intracerebral injection of hypertonic saline led to reduced renal nerve activity and natriuresis.[83,84] Subsequently, DiBona[85] showed that administration of Ang II into the cerebral ventricles and changes in dietary Na$^+$ modulate baroreflex regulation of RSNA. Similarly, stimulation of neurons located in the paraventricular nucleus and in a region extending to the anteroventral third ventricle led to ANP release, inducing Ang II blockade and inhibition of salt and water intake. Conversely, disruption of these neurons, as well as of the median eminence or neural lobe, led to decreased ANP release and impaired response to volume expansion.[86] Overall, despite the substantial evidence for CNS sensing of ECF volume status, the exact nature, mode of operation, and relative importance of this aspect of sensing remains unclear.

Gastrointestinal Tract Sensors. Under normal physiologic conditions, Na$^+$ and water reach the ECF by absorption in the GI tract. Therefore, it is not surprising that sensing and regulatory mechanisms of ECF volume have been found in the GI tract itself. The evidence for this phenomenon comes from experiments that showed more rapid natriuresis after an oral salt load than after a similar intravenous load. Moreover, infusions of hypertonic saline into the portal vein led to greater natriuresis than similar infusions into the femoral vein. These findings were consistent with the presence of Na$^+$-sensing mechanisms in the splanchnic or portal circulation, or both.[87] In fact, these mechanisms appear to be located primarily in the portal system and are probably important in the pathogenesis of the hepatorenal syndrome (HRS; see later).

Hepatoportal Receptors. The two main neural reflexes, termed the *hepatorenal* and *hepatointestinal reflexes,* originate from receptors in the hepatoportal region. They transduce portal plasma Na$^+$ concentration into hepatic afferent nerve activity; before a measurable increase in systemic Na$^+$ concentration occurs, the hepatointestinal reflex attenuates intestinal Na$^+$ absorption via the vagus nerve, and the hepatorenal reflex augments Na$^+$ excretion.[88-90] These reflexes have been observed in rats and rabbits, as well as in humans, and have been shown to be impaired in the chronic bile duct ligation model of cirrhosis and portal hypertension.[91] In addition, the hepatic artery shows significant autoregulatory capacity, dilating when perfusion pressure falls and constricting when pressure rises, thereby maintaining hepatic arterial blood flow over a wide range of perfusion pressures. Moreover, there is extensive crosstalk between the portal and systemic circulations. For example, when portal blood flow decreases, the hepatic artery dilates; this is indicative of the presence of a sensor in the hepatic artery, which responds to changes in the contribution of the portal vein to total hepatic blood flow.[92] Clues to the mechanism of hepatic autoregulation come from models of reduced portal venous blood flow and acute hepatic injury, in which reduced Na$^+$ excretion was abolished by administration of an A$_1$ adenosine receptor (A1AR) antagonist; thus, these receptors probably have a role in the hepatorenal reflex.[93,94]

The observation that intraportal infusion of bumetanide or furosemide suppresses the response of hepatic afferent nerve activity to intraportal hypertonic saline suggests that the NKCC2 may be involved in sensing portal Na$^+$ concentration.[95] In addition to hepatoportal Na$^+$-sensing chemoreceptors, the liver also contains mechanoreceptors (baroreceptors). Increased intrahepatic hydrostatic pressure has been shown to be associated with enhanced RSNA and renal Na$^+$ retention in various experimental models.[96,97] For example, when increased intrahepatic pressure was induced by thoracic caval constriction in dogs, raising venous pressure led to a positive Na$^+$ balance, which was inhibited by liver denervation.[96] A clinical model for increased intrahepatic pressure is the Budd-Chiari syndrome,[98] and it is in situations such as this that hepatic volume-sensing mechanisms probably play a role in renal Na$^+$ retention (see section, "Specific Treatments Based on the Pathophysiology of Sodium Retention in Cirrhosis").

Intestinal Natriuretic Hormones: Guanylin Peptides. As described previously, the natriuretic response of the kidneys to a Na$^+$ load is more rapid when the load is delivered orally than when the same load is administered intravenously.[76] The different responses are observed without accompanying differences in plasma aldosterone.[99] This observation led to the idea that the gut produces a substance that signals the kidneys to excrete excess Na$^+$. The discovery of the guanylin family of cGMP-regulating peptides (intestinal natriuretic hormones) has shed light on this phenomenon.[100,101] Of the four currently known guanylin peptides, guanylin and uroguanylin have been best studied. They are small (15 to 16 amino acids), heat-stable peptides with intramolecular disulfide bridges similar to the bacterial heat-stable enterotoxins that cause traveler's diarrhea and are found in mammals, birds, and fish.[100]

Both guanylin and uroguanylin are synthesized as prepropeptides, primarily in the intestine. The former, produced mainly by the ileum through the proximal colon, circulates as proguanylin; the latter, which is expressed principally in the jejunum, circulates in its active form.[101] A physiologically important difference between guanylin and uroguanylin lies in their sensitivity to proteases. Because of a tyrosine residue at the ninth amino acid, guanylin is sensitive to protease digestion in the kidneys, which leads to its inactivation, whereas uroguanylin can be locally activated by the same proteases.[100] After an oral salt load, guanylin and uroguanylin released in the intestine lead to increased intestinal secretion of Cl^-, HCO_3^-, and water and to inhibition of Na^+ absorption.

In the kidneys, Na^+, K^+, and water excretion is increased, without any change in RBF or GFR and independently of RAAS, AVP, or ANPs.[100] The signaling pathway of guanylin peptides in the intestine involves binding to and activation of the receptor guanylate cyclase C (GC-C), one of the eight guanylate cyclases.[101] GC-C is a transmembrane protein, composed of 1050 to 1053 amino acids, that is present in the intestinal brush border. Propagation of the signal occurs through the second messenger cGMP, which inhibits Na^+/H^+ exchange and activates protein kinase G II and protein kinase A. These in turn activate the cystic fibrosis transmembrane conductance regulator (CFTR), leading to Cl^- secretion. CFTR then activates the Cl^-/HCO_3^- exchanger, which leads to HCO_3^- secretion.

The best evidence for a link between the gut and kidneys comes from mice lacking the uroguanylin gene, which display an impaired natriuretic response to oral salt loading but not to intravenous NaCl infusion.[102] However, because plasma pro-uroguanylin levels do not rise but urinary uroguanylin levels do increase after a high-salt meal, locally released peptide by the kidneys could still play a role in uroguanylin-associated natriuresis.[103,104] In the kidneys, both GC-C–dependent and GC-C–independent signaling pathways for guanylin peptides exist, inasmuch as knockout of GC-C in mice does not affect the high-salt diet–induced increase in uroguanylin.[100] From experiments on cell lines and isolated tubules, it appears that uroguanylin acts on the proximal tubule and principal cells of the cortical collecting duct.

In proximal cell lines, guanylin peptides increase cGMP and decrease cyclic adenosine monophosphate (cAMP), which leads to inhibition of Na^+/H^+ exchange and Na^+-K^+-ATPase; such events are consistent with decreased Na^+ reabsorption in this segment.[100] Crosstalk between guanylin peptides and ANPs may also occur in the proximal tubule.[105] In the principal cell, uroguanylin activation of a G protein–coupled receptor results in phospholipase A_2–dependent inhibition of the renal outer medullary potassium (ROMK) channel, which leads to depolarization and a reduced driving force for Na^+ reabsorption.[100] There is also evidence that guanylin may cause cell shrinkage in the inner medullary collecting duct (IMCD), which is suggestive of water secretion from this segment and a role in water diuresis.[100] Together, these data are highly suggestive of a role at least for uroguanylin, as a natriuretic hormone, in adjusting U_{Na} excretion to balance the levels of NaCl absorbed via the GI tract.[100,101] However, recent work has cast substantial doubt on this GI renal signaling axis for Na regulation.[106] The importance of this system in the control of renal Na^+ excretion in humans awaits further clarification.

A final point is that although multiple receptors are clearly involved in the regulation of EABV, their functions appear to be considerably redundant. For example, cardiac or renal denervation in nonhuman primates and chronic aldosterone administration do not significantly affect the maintenance of Na^+ balance.[107,108]

EFFERENT LIMB: EFFECTOR MECHANISMS FOR MAINTAINING EFFECTIVE ARTERIAL BLOOD VOLUME

The maintenance of Na^+ homeostasis is achieved by adjustment of renal Na^+ excretion according to the body's needs. Like the mechanisms sensing changes in EABV, there are a number of pathways that enable the required adjustments in renal Na^+ excretion. The adjustments are made by integrated changes in GFR and tubular reabsorption, so that changes in one component lead to appropriate changes in the other to maintain Na^+ homeostasis. In addition, tubular reabsorption is regulated by local peritubular and luminal factors and by neural and humoral mechanisms (Table 15.2).

INTEGRATION OF CHANGES IN GLOMERULAR FILTRATION RATE AND TUBULAR REABSORPTION

In humans, normal GFR leads to the delivery of approximately 24,000 mmol of Na^+/day for downstream processing by the tubules. More than 99% of the filtrate is reabsorbed; only a tiny amount escapes into the final urine. Therefore, it is clear that even minute changes in the relationship between filtered load and fraction of Na^+ absorbed can exert a profound cumulative influence on net Na^+ balance. However, even marked perturbations in GFR are

Table 15.2 Major Renal Effector Mechanisms for Regulating Effective Arterial Blood Volume

Glomerular Filtration Rate and Tubular Reabsorption

Tubuloglomerular feedback
Glomerulotubular balance
Peritubular capillary Starling forces
Luminal composition
Physical factors beyond proximal tubule
Medullary hemodynamics (pressure natriuresis)

Neural Mechanisms

Sympathetic nervous system
Renal nerves

Humoral Mechanisms

Renin-angiotensin-aldosterone system
Vasopressin
Prostaglandins
Natriuretic peptides
Endothelium-derived factors
    Endothelins
    Nitric oxide
Others (see text)

not necessarily associated with drastic alterations in U_{Na} excretion; thus, overall Na^+ balance is usually preserved. Such preservation results from appropriate adjustments in two important protective mechanisms—TGF, in which changes in tubular fluid Na^+ inversely affect GFR, and glomerulotubular balance, whereby changes in tubular flow rate resulting from changes in GFR directly affect tubular reabsorption.[69,70,109]

Tubuloglomerular Feedback

A remarkable feature of nephron architecture is that after emerging from Bowman's capsule and descending deep into the medulla, each tubule returns to its parent glomerulus. Guyton and associates[110] envisioned a functional relationship between the tubule and glomerulus; this concept led to a wealth of experimental evidence supporting the existence of TGF[111] (see also Chapter 3). TGF operates by changes in tubular fluid Na^+ at the macula densa (the point of contact between the specialized tubular cells of the cortical thick ascending limb of Henle adjacent to the extraglomerular mesangium), which elicit adjustments in glomerular arteriolar resistance. The system is constructed as a negative feedback loop in which an increase in NaCl concentration leads to increases in afferent arteriolar resistance and a consequent fall in the GFR. This, in turn, leads to an increase in proximal reabsorption and a reduction in distal delivery of solute. Thus, NaCl delivery to the distal nephron is maintained within narrow limits.[111]

The complexities of TGF and detailed mechanisms of changes in epithelial function in response to luminal NaCl composition were unraveled initially by elaborate micropuncture studies that clearly established the tubular-glomerular link and, subsequently, by imaging and electrophysiologic techniques in isolated perfused tubule/glomerulus preparations. However, the signaling mechanisms linking changes in tubular composition with altered glomerular arteriolar tone became evident only much later through experiments in gene-manipulated mice.[111] The primary detection mechanism of TGF appears to be uptake of salt by means of the NKCC2, located in the apical membrane of macula densa cells. The evidence comes from TGF inhibition by inhibitors of the cotransporter, furosemide and bumetanide,[112] and by deletions in mice of the A or B isoform of NKCC2, both of which are expressed in macula densa cells.[71,111] In fact, complete inactivation of the NKCC2 gene leads to the severe salt-losing phenotype of antenatal Bartter syndrome.[113] Similarly, inhibition or deletion of the ROMK channel in mice abolishes TGF.[111]

The next step in the juxtaglomerular cascade is less clear. One possibility is direct coupling of NKCC2-dependent NaCl uptake to the mediation step. Results of studies in the isolated perfused rabbit juxtaglomerular apparatus have indicated that depolarization, alkalinization, and various ionic compositional changes occur after increased NaCl uptake; thus, one or more of these changes could trigger the signal.[114] A second possibility is that signal propagation is the consequence of transcellular NaCl transport and Na^+-K^+-ATPase–dependent basolateral extrusion. Experiments using double-knockout mice, in which the α_1-subunit of Na^+-K^+-ATPase was made sensitive and the α_2-subunit resistant to the pump inhibitor, ouabain, clearly indicate an important role for Na^+-K^+-ATPase in supporting TGF and that adenosine triphosphate (ATP) consumption is required for the process.[111]

In contrast, there is strong evidence that ATP release and degradation, rather than consumption, may be the link in the chain connecting NaCl changes in the macula densa with alteration of glomerular arteriolar tone. According to the current working model, after NaCl uptake and transcellular transport, ATP is released from macula densa cells and undergoes stepwise hydrolysis and dephosphorylation by ecto-ATPases and nucleotidases to adenosine diphosphate, adenosine monophosphate, and then adenosine, which, in a paracrine manner, causes A1AR–dependent afferent arteriolar constriction. Although the evidence for ATP breakdown is as yet incomplete, evidence for the effects of adenosine as a mediator of TGF is very strong. For example, isolated perfused mouse afferent arterioles exposed to adenosine display vigorous vasoconstriction, an effect not seen in A1AR–deficient mice.[115,116] As shown by overexpression[117] and conditional knockout of the receptor, this A1AR effect is primarily on afferent arteriolar smooth muscle cells, although A1AR effects on extravascular, perhaps mesangial, cells appear to contribute to the TGF response.[118] The response is mediated by inhibitory G protein (G_i)–dependent activation of phospholipase C, release of Ca^{2+} from intracellular stores, and subsequent entry of Ca^{2+} through L-type Ca^{2+} channels.[115,119] Cellular adenosine uptake is likely to be involved in the TGF response because targeted deletion of the type 1 equilibrative nucleoside transporter (ENT1) led to significant attenuation of the response.[120] Of particular interest is the fact that the vasodilatory adenosine A_2 receptor is more abundant than the A1AR in the renal vasculature, and continuous exogenous application of adenosine to mouse kidneys is indeed vasodilatory.[121] However, the generation of adenosine in the confines of the juxtaglomerular interstitium and its exclusive delivery to the afferent arteriole, where A1AR expression predominates, ensures the appropriate response for TGF.

Other factors, both co-constrictors and modulators, appear to be involved in TGF. Ang II has been shown to act as an important cofactor in the vasoconstrictive action of adenosine. In this regard, deletions of the Ang II receptor or angiotensin-converting enzyme (ACE) in mice were found to abolish TGF. The effect may result from nonresponsiveness to adenosine in the absence of an intact RAS.[11] By contrast, aldosterone has recently been shown to blunt TGF through the activation of mineralocorticoid receptors on macula densa cells.[122] This effect may be mediated by superoxide,[123] which in turn may also be upregulated by Ang II via the NOX2 and NOX4 isoforms of NADPH (nicotinamide adenine dinucleotide phosphate) oxidase.[124] The high levels of neuronal nitric oxide synthase (nNOS) expression in macula densa cells are indicative of a role for nitric oxide in TGF.[125] Nitric oxide is thought to counterbalance Ang II–induced efferent arteriolar vasoconstriction and to modulate renin secretion by the juxtaglomerular apparatus.[126,127] Consistent with this concept is the finding that chronic absence of functional nNOS in macula densa cells is associated with enhanced vasoconstriction in the subnormal flow range, probably as a result of proportional increases in preglomerular and postglomerular tone. In addition, increased delivery of fluid to the macula densa induces nitric oxide release from these cells.[126]

Inhibition of the nitric oxide system by nonselective blockers of nitric oxide synthase (NOS) results in an exaggerated TGF response that leads to even further renal vasoconstriction, Na$^+$ and water retention, and arterial hypertension.[127] Also, TGF responses are absent in mice with concurrent deficiencies in nNOS and the A1AR, which implies that nNOS deficiency does not overcome deficient A1AR signaling. Moreover, nitric oxide modulation of TGF can be mediated by ecto 5′-nucleotidase, the enzyme responsible for adenine formation.[128] Furthermore, nitric oxide, via eNOS, modulates the afferent arteriolar myogenic response.[68] Finally, aldosterone-induced modulation of TGF appears to involve interactions between nitric oxide and superoxide.[129] Together, these data suggest that A1AR signaling is primary and that nNOS and eNOS, as well as superoxide, play modulatory roles in TGF.

Apart from the RAAS, other hormonal systems and secondary messengers appear to be involved in TGF. For example, stimulation of the glucagon-like peptide 1 receptor leads to an increased GFR and reduced proximal tubular reabsorption.[130] Moreover, high salt intake–induced activation of AMP-activated protein kinase leads to an enhanced TGF response and increased delivery of Na$^+$ to the end of the proximal tubule.[67] Furthermore, acute saline expansion leads to an increased single-nephron glomerular filtration rate (SNGFR) and distal nephron flow rate, an effect independent of the Ang II receptor.[131]

The afferent arteriolar A1AR may not be the sole mediator of TGF. Activation by adenosine of the adenosine A$_2$ receptor has been shown to dilate mouse cortical efferent receptors. The effect appeared to be mediated by the low-affinity adenosine A$_{2b}$ receptor[121] via increased levels of eNOS.[132] It is remarkable that this highly specific effect occurs despite the presence of A1AR in the efferent arteriole. Apparently, therefore, the relative abundance of the various adenosine receptor subtypes in afferent and efferent arterioles ultimately allows fine-tuning of TGF by concerted changes in glomerular vascular tone.[133] On the other hand, purine receptors do not seem to affect TGF.[134]

Connexin 40, which plays a predominant role in the formation of gap junctions in the vasculature, also participates in the autoregulation of RBF by the afferent arteriole and, therefore, in TGF.[135] Connexin-40 knockout mice displayed impaired steady-state autoregulation to a sudden step increase in RPP. A marked reduction in TGF in connexin 40 knockout mice was thought to be responsible. Connexin 40–mediated RBF autoregulation occurred by paracrine signaling between tubular and vascular cells to the afferent arteriole,[136] independently of nitric oxide.[137] Other endogenous modulators of TGF include the eicosanoid 20-hydroxyeicosatetraenoic acid (20-HETE), which modifies the myogenic afferent arteriolar and TGF responses,[138] and the heme oxygenase pathway via carbon monoxide and cGAMP generation, which inhibits TGF through inhibition of depolarization and Ca^{2+} entry in macular densa cells.[139,140]

In addition to hormones of the RAAS, sex hormones also appear to regulate TGF. Testosterone in rats leads to upregulation of TGF by generation of superoxide dismutase,[141] whereas enhanced Ang II receptor activity attenuates Ang II–dependent resetting of TGF activity in female rats.[142] A final point in the complexity of TGF is that there is evidence for three sites in addition to the macula densa that are in contact with the efferent arteriole—the terminal cortical thick ascending limb of Henle, the early distal tubule, and the connecting tubule. In particular, perimacular cells and oscillatory cells of the early distal tubule may be involved in the intracellular Ca^{2+} signaling required for adenosine-induced afferent vasoconstriction. On the other hand, the effect of the connecting tubule on the afferent arteriolar tone appears to be modulatory in that elevations in luminal NaCl and cellular Na$^+$ entry via the epithelial sodium channel (ENaC)[143] lead to afferent arteriolar dilation through the release of prostaglandins and epoxyeicosatrienoic acids.[80,144] Moreover, connecting tubule glomerular feedback has been shown to antagonize TGF,[145] at least in the acute setting.[146]

Glomerulotubular Balance

Several factors are involved in the phenomenon of glomerulotubular balance (GTB), which describes the ability of proximal tubular reabsorption to adapt proportionally to the changes in filtered load.

Peritubular Capillary Starling Forces. Researchers have studied the natriuretic response to ECFV expansion by examining the effects of acute infusions of saline or albumin in experimental animals and in humans. Therefore, their relevance to the chronic regulation of ECF sodium balance is questionable. Nevertheless, the findings from these studies led to the notion that alterations in hydraulic and oncotic pressures (Starling forces) in the peritubular capillary play an important role in the regulation of Na$^+$ and water transport, especially in the proximal nephron. The peritubular capillary network is anatomically connected in series with the glomerular capillary bed of cortical glomeruli through the efferent arteriole; thus, changes in the physical determinants of GFR critically influence Starling forces in the peritubular capillaries.

Of importance is that about 10% of glomeruli, mainly those at the corticomedullary junction, are connected in series to the vasa recta of the medulla. In the proximal tubule—whose peritubular capillaries receive 90% of blood flow from glomeruli—the relationship of hydraulic and oncotic driving forces to the transcapillary fluid flux is given by the Starling equation, as follows:

$$\text{Rate}_{abs} = K_r[(\pi_c - \pi_i) - (P_c - P_i)]$$

where Rate$_{abs}$ is the absolute rate of reabsorption of proximal tubule absorbate by the peritubular capillary, K_r is the capillary reabsorption coefficient (the product of capillary hydraulic conductivity and absorptive surface area), π_c and P_c are the local capillary colloid osmotic (oncotic) and hydraulic pressures, respectively, and π_i and P_i are the corresponding interstitial pressures. Whereas π_i and P_c oppose fluid absorption, π_c and P_i tend to favor uptake of the reabsorbate. By simultaneously determining these driving forces, investigators can analyze the net pressure favoring fluid absorption or filtration. As a consequence of the anatomic relationship of the postglomerular efferent arteriole to the peritubular capillary, the hydraulic pressure is significantly lower in the peritubular capillary than in the glomerular capillary. The function of the efferent arteriole as a resistance vessel contributes to a decrease in hydraulic pressure between the glomerulus and peritubular capillary.

Also, because the peritubular capillary receives blood from the glomerulus, the plasma oncotic pressure is high at the outset as a result of prior filtration of protein-free fluid. It follows that the greater the GFR in relation to plasma flow rate, the higher the protein concentration in the efferent arteriolar plasma and the lower the hydraulic pressure in the proximal peritubule capillary. As a consequence, proximal fluid reabsorption is enhanced (Figure 15.4). Therefore, in contradistinction to the glomerular and peripheral capillary, the peritubular capillary is characterized by high values of $\pi_c - \pi_i$ that greatly exceed $P_c - P_i$, which results in net reabsorption of fluid.

The ratio of GFR to RBF defines the filtration fraction. The relationship of proximal reabsorption to filtration fraction may contribute to Na$^+$-retaining and edema-forming states, such as heart failure (see Figure 15.4). A series of in vivo micropuncture and microperfusion studies,[147-150] as well as studies using the isolated perfused tubule model,[151] have yielded compelling experimental evidence for the relationship between proximal peritubular Starling forces and proximal fluid reabsorption. As a result of these studies, the role of peritubular forces in the setting of increased ECF volume can be summarized as follows:

1. Acute saline expansion results in dilution of plasma proteins and reduction in efferent arteriolar oncotic pressure. The SNGFR and peritubular P_c may be increased as well, but the decrease in peritubular π_c by itself results in a decreased net peritubular capillary reabsorptive force and decreased Rate$_{abs}$. GTB is disrupted because Rate$_{abs}$ falls, despite the tendency for SNGFR to rise, and this development allows the excess Na$^+$ to be excreted and plasma volume to be restored.
2. Iso-oncotic plasma infusions tend to raise SNGFR and peritubular P_c but lead to relative constancy of efferent arteriolar oncotic pressure. Rate$_{abs}$ may therefore decrease

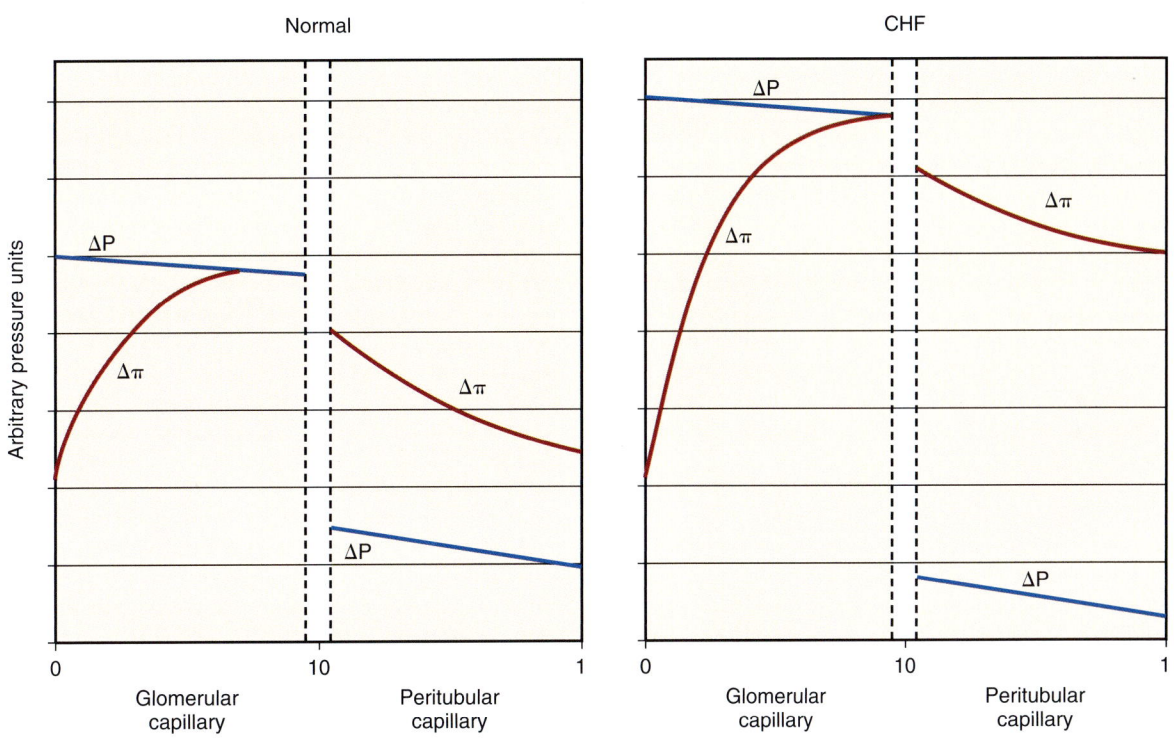

Figure 15.4 The glomerular and peritubular microcirculations. **Left,** Approximate transcapillary pressure profiles for the glomerular and peritubular capillaries in normal humans. Vessel lengths are given in normalized nondimensional terms, with 0 being the most proximal portion of the capillary bed and 1 the most distal portion. Thus, for the glomerulus, 0 corresponds to the afferent arteriolar end of the capillary bed, and 1 corresponds to the efferent arteriolar end. The transcapillary hydraulic pressure difference (ΔP) is relatively constant with distance along the glomerular capillary, and the net driving force for ultrafiltration ($\Delta P - \Delta \pi$) diminishes primarily as a consequence of the increase in the opposing colloid osmotic pressure difference ($\Delta \pi$), the latter resulting from the formation of an essentially protein-free ultrafiltrate. As a result of the drop in pressure along the efferent arteriole, the net driving pressure in the peritubular capillaries ($\Delta P - \Delta \pi$, in which $\Delta \pi$ is the change in transcapillary oncotic pressure) becomes negative, favoring reabsorption. **Right,** Hemodynamic alterations in the renal microcirculation in congestive heart failure (CHF). The fall in renal plasma flow (RPF) rate in heart failure is associated with a compensatory increase in ΔP for the glomerular capillary, which is conducive to a greater than normal rise in the plasma protein concentration and, hence, in $\Delta \pi$ along the glomerular capillary. This increase in $\Delta \pi$ by the distal end of the glomerular capillary also translates to an increase in $\Delta \pi$ in the peritubular capillaries, resulting in an increased net driving pressure for enhanced proximal tubule fluid absorption, believed to take place in heart failure. The increased peritubular capillary absorptive force in heart failure also probably results from the decline in ΔP, a presumed consequence of the rise in renal vascular resistance. (From Humes HD, Gottlieb M, Brenner BM: *The kidney in congestive heart failure: contemporary issues in nephrology*, vol 1, New York, 1978, Churchill Livingstone, pp 51-72.)

slightly, resulting in less disruption of GTB and natriuresis of lesser magnitude than that observed with saline expansion.
3. Hyperoncotic expansion usually increases both SNGFR (because of volume expansion) and efferent arteriolar oncotic pressure. As a result, Rate$_{abs}$ is enhanced. GTB therefore tends to be better preserved than with iso-oncotic plasma or saline expansion.
4. Changes in π_i can directly alter proximal tubular reabsorption, independently of the peritubular capillary bed.

The alterations in proximal peritubular Starling forces that modulate fluid and electrolyte movements across the peritubular basement membrane into the surrounding capillary bed appear to be accompanied by corresponding changes in the structure of the peritubular interstitial compartment. Ultrastructural data from rats have suggested that the peritubular capillary wall is in tight apposition to the tubule basement membrane for about 60% of the tubule basolateral surface. However, irregularly shaped wide portions of peritubular interstitium also exist over about 40% of the tubule basolateral surface; thus, a major portion of reabsorbed fluid has to cross a true interstitial space before entering the peritubular capillaries. Alterations in the physical properties of the interstitial compartment could conceivably modulate passive or active components of net fluid transport in the proximal tubule. Starling forces in the peritubular capillary are thought to regulate the rate of volume entry from the peritubular interstitium into the capillary. Any change in this rate of flux could lead to changes in interstitial pressure that secondarily modify proximal tubule solute transport. This formulation could explain why experimental maneuvers known to raise P_i (e.g., infusion of renal vasodilators, renal venous constriction, renal lymph ligation) were associated with a natriuretic response, whereas the opposite effect was seen with renal decapsulation, which lowers P_i (see section, "Medullary Hemodynamics and Interstitial Pressure in the Control of Sodium Excretion: Pressure Natriuresis").

Because of the relatively high permeability of the proximal tubule, changes in interstitial Starling forces are likely to be transduced mainly through alterations in passive bidirectional paracellular flux through the tight junctions.[152] The claudin family of adhesion molecules has clearly proved that the tight junction is a dynamic, multifunctional complex that may be amenable to physiologic regulation by cellular second messengers or in pathologic states.[153-155] Among the 24 known mammalian claudin family members, at least three—claudin-2, claudin-10, and claudin-11—are located in the proximal nephron of the mouse, and others are located at more distal nephron sites.[154,156] Claudin-2 is selectively expressed in the proximal nephron.[157] However, the exact role of the claudin family members in the influence of Starling forces on fluid reabsorption remains to be elucidated.[158]

Luminal Composition. In addition to peritubular capillary and interstitial Starling forces, luminal factors may also play a role in the regulation of proximal tubule transport. For example, Romano and colleagues[159] have shown that GTB could be fully expressed, even when the native peritubular environment was kept constant while the rate of perfusion of proximal tubular segments with native tubular fluid was changed. Moreover, studies in isolated perfused rabbit proximal tubules have indicated that the presence of a transtubular anion gradient, normally present in the late portion of the proximal nephron, is necessary for the flow dependence to occur.[160] A potential mechanism for the modulation of proximal Na$^+$ reabsorption in response to changes in filtered load depends on the close coupling of Na$^+$ transport with the cotransport of glucose, amino acids, and other organic solutes. The increased delivery of organic solutes that accompanies increases in GFR, together with the preferential reabsorption of Na$^+$ with bicarbonate in the early proximal tubule, would lead to increased delivery of both Cl$^-$ and organic solutes to the late proximal tubule. The resulting transtubular anion gradient would then facilitate the "passive" reabsorption of the organic solutes and NaCl in this segment, but overall net reabsorption would be reduced.

In summary, regardless of the exact mechanism, ECFV expansion impairs the integrity of GTB, thus allowing increased delivery of salt and fluid to more distal parts of the nephron. The major factors acting on the proximal nephron during a decrease in ECF and effective arterial circulating volume are outlined schematically in Figure 15.5.

Physical Factors Beyond the Proximal Tubule. Because the final urinary excretion of Na$^+$, in response to volume expansion or depletion, can be dissociated from the amount delivered out of the superficial proximal nephron, more distal or deeper segments of the nephron contribute to the modulation of Na$^+$ and water excretion. Several sites along the nephron, such as the loop of Henle, distal nephron, and cortical and papillary collecting ducts, were found (by micropuncture and microcatheterization techniques) to increase or decrease the rate of Na$^+$ reabsorption in response to enhanced delivery from early segments of the nephron. However, direct evidence that these transport processes are mediated by changes in Starling forces per se is lacking. Jamison and coworkers[161] have provided a detailed review of these experiments.

In summary, the intrarenal control of Na$^+$ excretion can be generalized as follows. If ECFV is held relatively constant, an increase in GFR leads to little or no increase in salt excretion because of a close coupling between the GFR and intrarenal physical forces acting at the peritubular capillary to control Rate$_{abs}$. In addition, changes in the filtered load of small organic solutes, and perhaps other, as yet uncharacterized, glomerulus-borne substances in tubule fluid may influence Rate$_{abs}$. To the extent that changes, if any, in the load of Na$^+$ delivered to more distal segments also occur, parallel changes in distal reabsorptive rates also occur to ensure a high degree of GTB for the kidneys as a whole. Conversely, ECFV expansion leads to large increases in Na$^+$ excretion, even in the presence of a reduced GFR. Changes in Na$^+$ reabsorption in the proximal tubule alone cannot account for this natriuresis of volume expansion, and a number of mechanisms for suppressing renal Na$^+$ reabsorption at more distal sites has been proposed.

Medullary Hemodynamics and Interstitial Pressure in the Control of Sodium Excretion: Pressure Natriuresis. The idea that changes in renal medullary hemodynamics may be

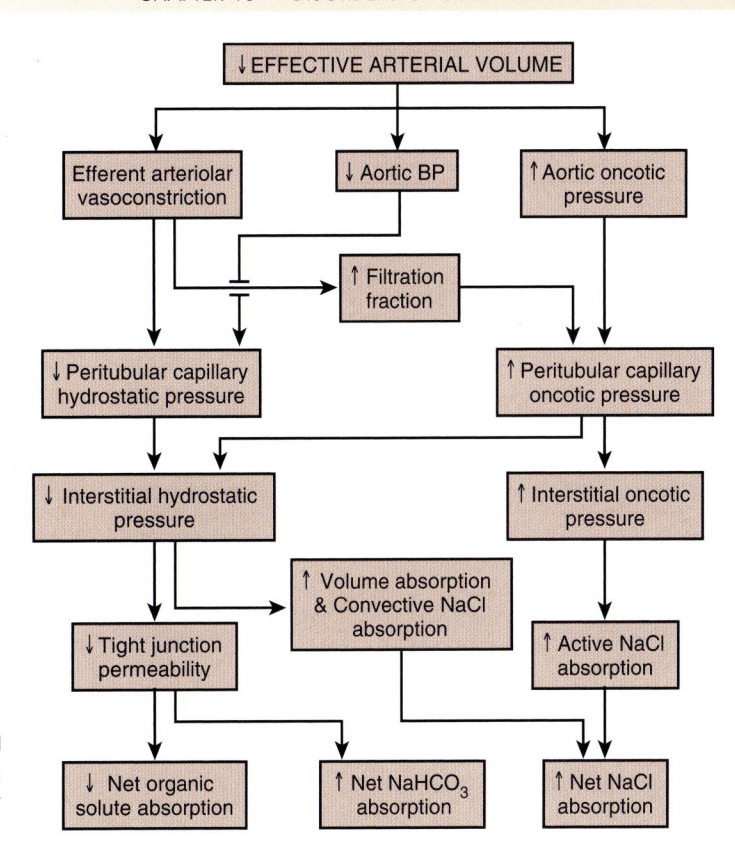

Figure 15.5 Effects of hemodynamic changes on proximal tubule solute transport. BP, Blood pressure. (From Seldin DW, Preisig PA, Alpern RJ: Regulation of proximal reabsorption by effective arterial blood volume, *Semin Nephrol* 11:212-219, 1991.)

involved in the natriuresis evoked by volume expansion was initially proposed in the 1960s by Earley and Friedler and colleagues.[162,163] According to their theory, ECFV expansion results in an increase in RPP that is transmitted as an increase in medullary plasma flow; this leads to a subsequent loss of medullary hypertonicity, elimination of the medullary osmotic gradient ("medullary washout") and, thereby, decreased water reabsorption in the thin descending loop of Henle. The decrease in water reabsorption in the thin descending limb lowers the Na^+ concentration in the fluid entering the ascending loop of Henle, thus decreasing the transepithelial driving force for salt transport in this nephron segment. At the same time, a similar mechanism was proposed to explain the natriuresis after elevations in systemic blood pressure, a phenomenon termed *pressure natriuresis*.

The concept that alterations in the solute composition of the renal medulla and papilla play a key role in the regulation of Na^+ transport gained significant support in the 1970s and 1980s, when results of micropuncture studies suggested that volume expansion, renal vasodilation, and increased RPP produced a greater inhibition of salt reabsorption in the loops of Henle within juxtamedullary nephrons than in those within superficial nephrons. Measurement of medullary plasma flow with laser Doppler flowmetry and videomicroscopy in experimental animals has provided strong evidence for the redistribution of intrarenal blood flow toward the medulla after volume expansion and renal vasodilation. These studies were of particular interest with regard to the role of medullary hemodynamics in the control of Na^+ excretion, especially in the context of pressure natriuresis.[164-168]

The importance of pressure natriuresis in the long-term control of arterial blood pressure and ECFV regulation was first recognized by Hall and associates.[167,168] According to this view, the kidneys alter Na^+ excretion in response to changes in arterial blood pressure. For example, an increase in RPP results in a concomitant increase in Na^+ excretion, thereby decreasing circulating blood volume and restoring arterial pressure. The coupling between arterial pressure and Na^+ excretion was found to occur in the setting of preserved cortical autoregulation (i.e., in the absence of changes in total RBF, GFR, or filtered load of Na^+). This has led to the suggestion that the pressure natriuresis mechanism is triggered by changes in medullary circulation.[162,165,169-171] Laser Doppler flowmetry and servo-null measurements of capillary pressure in volume-expanded rats have revealed that papillary blood flow is directly related to RPP over a wide range of pressures studied.

As mentioned earlier, an increase in medullary plasma flow might lead to medullary washout with a consequent reduction in the driving force for Na^+ reabsorption in the ascending loop of Henle, particularly in the deep nephrons. In addition, the increase in medullary perfusion may be associated with a rise in P_i. In fact, increasing P_i by ECFV expansion by infusion of renal vasodilatory agents, long-term mineralocorticoid escape, or hilar lymph ligation has resulted in a significant increase in Na^+ excretion.[172,173] Moreover, prevention of the increase in P_i by removal of the renal capsule significantly attenuates, but does not completely block, the natriuretic response to elevations in RPP. Thus, as depicted in Figure 15.6, elevation in RPP is associated with an increase in medullary plasma flow and increased vasa recta capillary pressure, which results in an increase in medullary P_i. This increase of P_i is thought to be transmitted to the renal cortex in the encapsulated kidneys and to provide a signal that inhibits Na^+ reabsorption along the

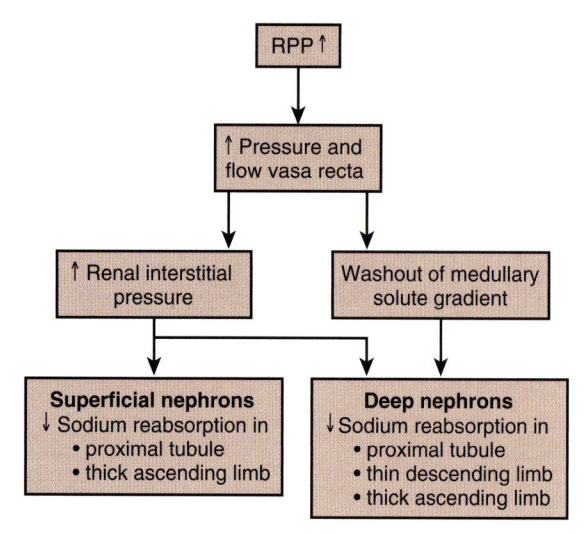

Figure 15.6 Role of the renal medulla in modulating tubular reabsorption of sodium in response to changes in renal perfusion pressure (RPP). (Adapted from Cowley AW, Jr: Role of the renal medulla in volume and arterial pressure regulation, *Am J Physiol* 273:R1-R15, 1997.)

nephron. In that regard, the renal medulla may be viewed as a sensor that can detect changes in RPP and initiate the pressure natriuresis mechanism.

To explain how changes in systemic blood pressure are transmitted to the medulla in the presence of efficient RBF and GFR autoregulation, it has been suggested that shunt pathways connect preglomerular vessels of juxtamedullary nephrons directly to the postglomerular capillaries of the vasa recta.[162] Alternatively, autoregulation of RBF might lead to increased shear stress in the preglomerular vasculature, triggering the release of nitric oxide and perhaps cytochrome P450 products of arachidonic acid metabolism (see later), thereby driving the cascade of events that inhibit Na^+ reabsorption.[174,175] The mechanisms by which changes in P_i and U_{Na} excretion decrease tubular Na^+ reabsorption, as well as the nephron sites responding to the alterations in P_i, have not been fully clarified.[172] As noted earlier, it was postulated that elevations in P_i may increase passive backleak or the paracellular pathway hydraulic conductivity, with a resultant increase in back flux of Na^+ through the paracellular pathways.[173] However, the absolute changes in P_i, in the range of 3 to 8 mm Hg in response to increments of about 50 to 90 mm Hg in RPP, are probably not sufficient to account for the decrease in tubular Na^+ reabsorption, even in the proximal tubule, the nephron segment with the highest transepithelial hydraulic conductivity.[164] Nevertheless, considerable evidence from micropuncture studies has indicated that pressure natriuresis is associated with significant reduction in proximal fluid reabsorption, particularly in deep nephrons, with enhanced delivery to the loop of Henle, inhibition of sodium reabsorption in the thin descending limb and reduced blood flow in the vasa recta.[176]

Pressure-induced changes in tubular reabsorption may also occur in more distal parts of the nephron, such as the ascending loop of Henle, distal nephron, and collecting duct.[177] Therefore, elevations in RPP can affect tubular Na^+ reabsorption by proximal and distal mechanisms. The finding that small changes in P_i are associated with significant alterations in tubular Na^+ reabsorption has led to the hypothesis that the changes in P_i may be amplified by various hemodynamic, hormonal, and paracrine factors.[159,162,165,169,173] Specifically, the phenomenon of pressure natriuresis is demonstrable, particularly in states of volume expansion and renal vasodilation, and is significantly attenuated in states of volume depletion.[173] Among a variety of hormonal and paracrine systems that have been documented to play a role in modulating pressure natriuresis, changes in the activity of the RAAS and local production of prostaglandins within the kidneys have received considerable attention.[173] Removal of the influence of Ang II by ACE inhibitors or Ang II type 1 receptor antagonists potentiates the pressure natriuretic response, and inhibitors of cyclooxygenase attenuate it.[173,178] Moreover, blockade of the Ang II type 2 receptor allows the same amount of Na^+ to be excreted at lower arterial pressure.[179] Of importance, however, is that pharmacologic blockade of these systems only attenuates but does not completely eliminate the pressure natriuresis response, which indicates that they act as modulators and not as mediators of the phenomenon.

The importance of endothelium-derived factors in the regulation of renal circulatory and excretory function has been recognized. Studies have suggested that endothelium-derived nitric oxide and P450 eicosanoids play a role in the mechanism of pressure natriuresis.[164,169,174,175,180-182] Nitric oxide, generated in large amounts in the renal medulla, appears to play a critical role in the regulation of medullary blood flow and Na^+ excretion.[170,171] Several studies have shown that inhibition of intrarenal nitric oxide production can reduce Na^+ excretion and markedly suppress the pressure natriuretic response, whereas administration of a nitric oxide precursor improves transmission of perfusion pressure into the renal interstitium and normalizes the defect in the pressure natriuresis response in Dahl salt-sensitive rats.[164,177,183,184] Similarly, a positive correlation between urinary excretion of nitrites and nitrates (metabolites of nitric oxide) and changes in renal arterial pressure or U_{Na} excretion were observed both in dogs[180,185,186] and in rats.[180] Hydrogen peroxide (H_2O_2) has also been invoked in the mediation of RPP-induced changes in outer medullary blood flow and natriuresis. The response appears to be localized to the medullary thick ascending limb of Henle, in contrast to the nitric oxide effect, which occurs in the vasa recta.[180] Other factors involved in the regulation of medullary blood flow include superoxide and heme oxygenase, both of which are released in the renal medulla in response to increased RPP.[181,186]

The cytochrome P450 eicosanoids, particularly 20-HETE, are additional endothelium-derived factors that may participate in the mechanism of pressure natriuresis.[174,175,187] These agents play an important role in the regulation of renal Na^+ transport and of renal and systemic hemodynamics.[188] These observations support the hypothesis that alterations in the production of renal nitric oxide, reactive oxygen species, and eicosanoids may be involved in mediation of the pressure-induced natriuretic response.

It is tempting to speculate that acute elevations in RPP in the autoregulatory range result in increased blood flow velocity and shear stress, leading to increased endothelial release of nitric oxide and reactive oxygen species. Enhanced renal production of these molecules may increase U_{Na} excretion by acting directly on tubular Na^+ reabsorption or through its vasodilatory effect on renal vasculature. ATP is another paracrine factor involved in pressure natriuresis. ATP is an important regulator of renal salt and water homeostasis. ATP release appears to be mediated by connexin 30 inasmuch as release in response to increased tubular flow or hypotonicity was abolished in connexin 30–deficient mice. Moreover, increased arterial pressure, induced by ligation of the distal aorta, led to diuresis and natriuresis in normal mice, but the response was attenuated in connexin 30 knockout mice. These data imply that mechanosensitive connexin 30 hemichannels play an integral role in pressure natriuresis by releasing ATP into the tubular fluid, thereby inhibiting salt and water reabsorption.[189] Finally, Magyar and colleagues[190] have reported that in response to an increase in RPP, the apical Na^+/H^+ exchanger in the proximal tubules may be redistributed out of the brush border into intracellular compartments. Concomitantly, basolateral Na^+-K^+-ATPase activity decreased significantly. The mechanisms of these cellular events have not been fully elucidated, but they may be related directly to changes in P_i or to changes in the intrarenal paracrine agents described previously.

A major assumption of the pressure natriuresis theory is that changes in systemic and RPP mediate the natriuretic response by the kidneys. As noted in comprehensive reviews, acute regulatory changes in renal salt excretion may occur without measurable elevation in arterial blood pressure.[47,191-193] Of interest is that in many of these studies, the natriuresis was accompanied by a decrease in the activity of the RAAS, without changes in plasma ANP levels.[47,79,192,193] Thus, whereas increases in arterial blood pressure can drive renal Na^+ excretion, other so-called pressure-independent control mechanisms must also operate to mediate the volume natriuresis.[47]

Neural Mechanisms: Renal Nerves and Sympathetic Nervous System

Extensive autonomic innervation of the kidneys makes an important contribution to the physiologic regulation of all aspects of renal function.[76,194] Sympathetic nerves, predominantly adrenergic, have been observed at all segments of the renal vasculature and tubule.[195] Adrenergic nerve endings reach vascular smooth muscle cells and mesangial cells, cells of the juxtaglomerular apparatus, and all segments of the tubule—proximal, loop of Henle, and distal. Only the basolateral membrane separates the nerve endings from the tubular cells. Initial studies have determined that the greatest innervation is found in the renal vasculature, mostly at the level of the afferent arterioles, followed by the efferent arterioles and outer medullary descending vasa recta.[196] However, high-density tubular innervation was found in the ascending limb of the loop of Henle, and the lowest density was observed in the collecting duct, inner medullary vascular elements, and papilla.[78,197] The magnitude of the tubular response to renal nerve activation may thus be proportional to the differential density of innervation. In accordance with these anatomic observations, stimulation of the renal nerve results in vasoconstriction of afferent and efferent arterioles[194,197] mediated by the activation of postjunctional α_1-adrenoceptors.[198]

The presence of high-affinity adrenergic receptors in the nephron is also indicative of a significant role of the renal nerves in tubular function. The α_1-adrenergic receptors and most of the α_2-adrenergic receptors are localized in the basolateral membranes of the proximal tubule.[199] In the rat, β-adrenoreceptors have been found in the cortical thick ascending limb of Henle and are subtyped as β_1-adrenoceptors.[200] The predominant neurotransmitters in renal sympathetic nerves are noradrenaline and, to a lesser extent, dopamine and acetylcholine.[197] There is abundant evidence that changes in the activity of the renal sympathetic nerve play an important role in controlling body fluid homeostasis and blood pressure.[76,194,195] Renal sympathetic nerve activity can influence renal function and Na^+ excretion through several mechanisms: (1) changes in renal and glomerular hemodynamics; (2) effect on renin release from juxtaglomerular cells, with increased formation of Ang II; and (3) direct effect on renal tubular fluid and electrolyte reabsorption.[76] Graded direct electrical stimulation of renal nerves produces frequency-dependent changes in RBF and GFR, reabsorption of renal tubular Na^+ and water, and secretion of renin.[76,195] The lowest frequency (0.5 to 1.0 Hz) stimulates renin secretion, and frequencies of 1.0 to 2.5 Hz increase renal tubule Na^+ and water reabsorption. Increasing the frequency of stimulation to 2.5 Hz and higher results in decreased RBF and GFR.[76,194]

The decrease in SNGFR in response to enhanced renal nerve activity has been attributed to a combination of increases in afferent and efferent glomerular resistance, as well as decreases in glomerular capillary hydrostatic pressure (ΔP) and glomerular ultrafiltration coefficient (Kf).[194,195] In Munich-Wistar rats, micropuncture experiments before and after renal nerve stimulation at different frequencies revealed that the effector loci for vasomotor control by renal nerves were in the afferent and efferent arteriole. In addition, although urine flow and Na^+ excretion declined with renal nerve stimulation, there was no change in absolute proximal fluid reabsorption rate, which suggests that reabsorption is increased in the more distal segments of the nephron.

Studies of the response of the kidneys to reflex activation of renal nerves have also indicated that the SNS has a role in regulating renal hemodynamic function and Na^+ excretion. In rats receiving diets with different Na^+ levels, DiBona and Kopp[194] measured renal nerve activity in response to isotonic saline volume expansion and furosemide-induced volume contraction. A low-Na^+ diet resulted in a reduction in right atrial pressure and an increase in renal nerve activity. The magnitude of the increase in renal nerve activity was approximately 20% for each 1-mm Hg fall in atrial pressure. Conversely, the high-Na^+ diet resulted in increased right atrial pressure and a reduction in renal nerve activity. Other studies in conscious animals in which researchers used maneuvers such as HWI and left atrial balloon inflation[76] have yielded evidence of the importance of reflex regulation of renal nerve activity.

Collectively, these studies demonstrated the reciprocal relationship between ECFV and renal nerve activity, which is consistent with the role of central cardiopulmonary mechanoreceptors governing renal nerve activity. Moreover, the contribution of efferent renal nerve activity is of greater significance during conditions of dietary Na^+ restriction, when the need for renal Na^+ conservation is maximal. When this linkage between the renal SNS and excretory renal function is defective, abnormalities in the regulation of ECF volume and blood pressure may develop.[197,201]

Several studies in which the response of denervated kidneys to various physiologic maneuvers was examined also yielded evidence that renal nerves play a role in regulating renal hemodynamic function and Na^+ excretion. Early studies showed that acute denervation of the kidneys is associated with increased urine flow and Na^+ excretion.[194] Micropuncture techniques showed that in euvolemic animals, elimination of renal innervation does not alter any of the determinants of SNGFR, indicating that renal nerves contribute little to the vasomotor tone of normal animals under baseline physiologic conditions. However, absolute proximal reabsorption was significantly reduced in the absence of changes in peritubular capillary oncotic pressure, hydraulic pressure, and renal interstitial pressure.[194] The decrease in tubular electrolyte and water reabsorption after renal denervation was also observed in the loop of Henle and segments of the distal nephron.[194]

In another micropuncture study in control rats and in rats with experimentally induced heart failure or acute volume depletion, denervation resulted in diuresis and natriuresis in normal rats but failed to alter any of the parameters of renal cortical microcirculation.[194] In rats with heart failure, in contrast, denervation caused both an amelioration of renal vasoconstriction by decreasing afferent and efferent arteriolar resistance and, again, natriuresis. This study indicated that in situations in which efferent neural tone is heightened above baseline level, renal nerve activity may profoundly influence renal circulatory dynamics. However, although the basal level of renal nerve activity in normal rats or conscious animals is apparently insufficient to influence renal hemodynamics, it is sufficient to exert a tonic stimulation on renal tubular epithelial Na^+ reabsorption and renin release.[194] Classic studies, in which guanethidine was given to achieve autonomic blockade or in patients with idiopathic autonomic insufficiency, have revealed that intact adrenergic innervation is required for the normal renal adaptive response to dietary Na^+ restriction.[202]

More direct examination of efferent RSNA in humans has been made possible by the measurement of renal norepinephrine spillover to elucidate the kinetics of norepinephrine release. Friberg and associates[203] have determined that in normal subjects, a low-Na^+ diet results in a fall in U_{Na} excretion and an increase in norepinephrine spillover, with no change in cardiac norepinephrine uptake; these findings support the concept of a true increase of efferent renal nerve activity secondary to Na^+ restriction. Similarly, low-dose infusion of norepinephrine to normal salt-replete volunteers resulted in a physiologic plasma increment of this neurotransmitter in association with antinatriuresis.[204] This reduction in Na^+ excretion occurred without any change in GFR but was associated with a significant decline in lithium (Li^+) clearance, an indication of enhanced proximal tubule reabsorption.

The cellular mechanisms mediating the tubular actions of norepinephrine appear to include stimulation of Na^+-K^+-ATPase activity and Na^+/H^+ exchange in proximal tubular epithelial cells.[194] It is assumed that α_1-adrenoreceptor stimulation, mediated by phospholipase C, causes an increase in intracellular Ca^{2+} that activates the Ca^{2+} calmodulin-dependent calcineurin phosphatase. Calcineurin converts Na^+-K^+-ATPase from its inactive phosphorylated form to its active dephosphorylated form.[205] The stimulatory effect of renal nerves on Na^+/H^+ exchange is mediated through stimulation of the α_2-adrenoreceptor.[194]

In addition to the direct action of Na^+ on epithelial cell transport and renal hemodynamics, interactions of renal nerve input with other effector mechanisms may contribute to the regulation of renal handling of Na^+. Efferent sympathetic nerve activity influences the rate of renin secretion in the kidneys by a variety of mechanisms, either directly or by interacting with the macula densa and vascular baroreceptor mechanisms for renin secretion.[194] The increase in renin secretion is mediated primarily by direct stimulation of β_1-adrenergic receptors located on juxtaglomerular granular cells.[194] Sympathetic activation of renin release is augmented during RPP reduction.[194] Results of studies in the isolated perfused rat kidney have suggested that intrarenal generation of Ang II has an important prejunctional action on renal sympathetic nerve terminals to facilitate norepinephrine release during renal nerve stimulation.[194] However, the physiologic significance of this facilitatory interaction on tubular Na^+ reabsorption remains controversial. Thus, administration of an ACE inhibitor or an angiotensin receptor blocker (ARB) attenuates the antinatriuretic response to electrical renal nerve stimulation in anesthetized rats.[194] In contrast, when nonhypotensive hemorrhage was used to produce a reflex increase in RSNA in conscious dogs, the associated antinatriuresis was unaffected by ACE inhibition or Ang II receptor blockade.[206]

Sympathetic activity is also a stimulus for the production and release of renal prostaglandins, coupled in series to the adrenergic-mediated renal vasoconstriction.[194] Evidence indicates that renal vasodilatory prostaglandins attenuate the renal hemodynamic vasoconstrictive response to activation of the renal adrenergic system in vivo and on isolated renal arterioles.[194] In Munich-Wistar rats, results of micropuncture experiments have indicated that the primary factor responsible for the reduction in the glomerular Kf during renal nerve stimulation may be Ang II rather than norepinephrine, and that endogenously produced prostaglandins neutralize the vasoconstrictive effects of renal nerve stimulation at an intraglomerular locus rather than at the arteriolar level.

Another interaction examined is that between the renal SNS and AVP. Studies in conscious animals have shown that AVP exerts a dose-related effect on the arterial baroreflex. Low doses of AVP might have sensitized the central baroreflex neurons to afferent input, whereas higher doses caused direct excitations of these neurons, which resulted in a reduction in sympathetic outflow.[194] In addition, AVP suppresses renal sympathetic outflow, and this response depends on the number of afferent inputs from baroreceptors.[207] Conversely, renal nerve stimulation resulted in elevations of plasma AVP levels and arterial pressure in conscious, baroreceptor-intact Wistar rats.[208] Many studies have demonstrated in normal and pathologic situations that increased RSNA can antagonize the natriuretic/diuretic response to ANP and that removal of the influence of sympathetic activity enhances the natriuretic action of the peptide.[194] Conversely, renal denervation in Wistar rats increased ANP receptors and cGMP generation in glomeruli, which resulted in an increase in Kf after ANP infusion.[209]

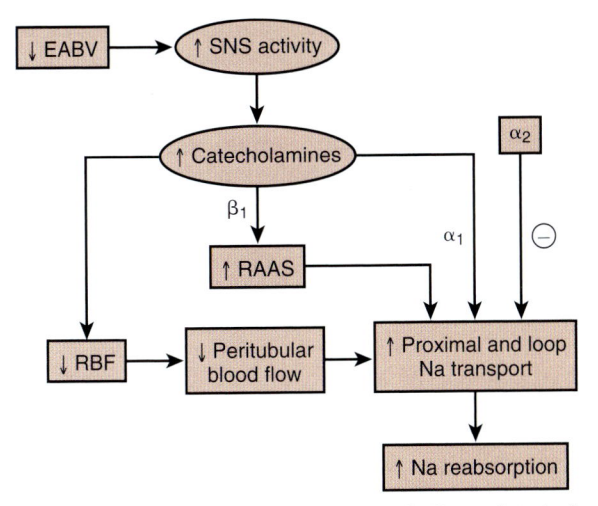

Figure 15.7 Sympathetic nervous system (SNS)–mediated effects of decreased effective arterial blood volume (EABV) on the kidneys. α_1, α_2, β_1, α_1-, α_2-, and β_1-Adrenergic receptors, respectively. RAAS, Renin-angiotensin-aldosterone system; RBF, renal blood flow; –, inhibitory effect.

In summary, renal sympathetic nerves can regulate U_{Na} and water excretion by changing renal vascular resistance, by influencing renin release from the juxtaglomerular granular cells, and through a direct effect on tubular epithelial cells (Figure 15.7). These effects may be modulated through interactions with other hormonal systems, including ANP, prostaglandins, and AVP.

Humoral Mechanisms

Renin-Angiotensin-Aldosterone System. The RAAS plays a central role in the regulation of ECF volume, Na+ homeostasis, and cardiac function.[210] The system is activated in situations that compromise hemodynamic stability, such as blood loss, reduced EABV, low Na+ intake, hypotension, and increase in sympathetic nerve activity. The RAAS is comprised of a coordinated hormonal cascade whose synthesis is initiated by the release of renin from the juxtaglomerular apparatus in response to reduced renal perfusion or decrease in arterial pressure.[211] Messenger RNA for renin exists in juxtaglomerular cells and in renal tubular cells.[212] Renin acts on its circulating substrate, angiotensinogen, which is produced and secreted mainly by the liver, but also by the kidneys.[210] ACE 1 (ACE1), which cleaves Ang I to Ang II, exists in large amounts in the microvasculature of the lungs but also on endothelial cells of other vascular beds and cell membranes of the brush border of the proximal nephron, heart, and brain.[210] Ang II is the principal effector of the RAAS, although other smaller metabolic products of Ang II also have biologic activities.[213,214] Nonrenin (cathepsin G, plasminogen-activating factor, tonin) and non-ACE pathways (chymase, cathepsin G) also exist in these tissues and may contribute to tissue Ang II synthesis.[210]

In addition to its important function as a circulating hormone, Ang II produced locally acts as a paracrine agent in an organ-specific mode.[215] In that regard, the properties of Ang II as a growth-promoting agent in the cardiovascular system and kidneys have been increasingly appreciated.[210,215] For example, local generation of Ang II in the kidneys results in higher intrarenal levels of this peptide in proximal tubular fluid, interstitial fluid, and renal medulla than in the circulation. The epithelial cells of the proximal nephron are an important source for the in situ generation of Ang II because these cells show abundant expression of the messenger RNA for angiotensinogen.[216] Furthermore, Ang II is secreted from tubular epithelial cells into the lumen of the proximal nephron.[217] This may account for the fact that concentrations of Ang II are approximately 1000 times higher in the proximal tubular fluid than in the plasma.[217,218] Moreover, the mechanisms regulating intrarenal levels of Ang II appear to be dissociated from those controlling the systemic concentrations of the peptide.[216]

The biologic actions of Ang II are mediated through activation of at least two receptor subtypes, AT_1 and AT_2, encoded by different genes residing on different chromosomes.[219,220] Both receptors are G protein–coupled, seven-transmembrane polypeptides containing approximately 360 amino acids.[210,220] In the adult organism, the AT_1 receptor mediates most of the biologic activities of Ang II, whereas the AT_2 receptor appears to have a vasodilatory and antiproliferative effect.[213,221] AT_1 is expressed in the vascular poles of glomeruli, juxtaglomerular apparatus, and mesangial cells, whereas the quantitatively lower expression of AT_2 is confined to renal arteries and tubular structures.[219] In addition to their functional distinction, the two receptor types use different downstream pathways. Stimulation of the AT_1 receptor activates phospholipases A_2, C, and D, which results in increased cytosolic Ca^{2+} and inositol triphosphate and inhibition of adenylate cyclase. In contrast, activation of the AT_2 receptor results in increases in nitric oxide and bradykinin levels, which lead to elevation in cGMP concentrations and to vasodilation.[222]

In addition to being an important source of several components of the RAAS, the kidney acts as a major target organ for the principal hormonal mediators of this cascade, Ang II and aldosterone. The direct effect of Ang II is mediated via AT_1 receptors that exert multiple direct intrarenal influences, including renal vasoconstriction, stimulation of tubular epithelial Na+ reabsorption, augmentation of TGF sensitivity, modulation of pressure natriuresis, and stimulation of mitogenic pathways.[210] Moreover, exogenous infusion of Ang II, which results in relatively low circulating levels of Ang II (picomolar range), is highly effective in modulating renal hemodynamic and tubular function, in comparison with the 10- to 100-fold higher concentrations required for its extrarenal effects. Thus, the kidneys appear to be uniquely sensitive to the actions of Ang II.

Furthermore, the synergistic interactions that exist between the renal vascular and tubular actions of Ang II significantly amplify the influence of Ang II on Na+ excretion.[216] Of the direct renal actions of Ang II, its effect on renal hemodynamics appears to be of critical importance. Ang II elicits a dose-dependent decrease in RBF but slightly augments GFR as a result of its preferential vasoconstrictive effect on the efferent arteriole, and therefore increases the filtration fraction. In turn, the increased filtration fraction may further modulate peritubular Starling forces, possibly by decreasing hydraulic pressure and increasing colloid osmotic pressure in the interstitium. These peritubular changes eventually lead to enhanced reabsorption of proximal Na+ and fluid. Of importance, however, is that changes in preglomerular resistance have also been described during

Ang II infusion or blockade.[223] These may be secondary to changes in systemic arterial pressure (myogenic reflex) or to increased sensitivity of TGF because Ang II does not alter preglomerular resistance when RPP is clamped or adjustments in TGF are prevented.[223]

In addition, Ang II may affect GFR by reducing Kf, thereby altering the filtered load of Na^+.[224] This effect is believed to reflect the action of the hormone on mesangial cell contractility and increasing permeability to macromolecules.[223] Finally, Ang II may also influence Na^+ excretion through its action on the medullary circulation. Because Ang II receptors are highly abundant in the renal medulla, this peptide may contribute significantly to the regulation of medullary blood flow.[223,225] In fact, use of fiberoptic probes has revealed that Ang II usually reduces cortical blood flow and medullary blood flow and decreases Na^+ and water excretion.[223,225] As noted earlier, changes in medullary blood flow may affect medullary tonicity, which determines the magnitude of passive salt reabsorption in the loop of Henle, and may also modulate pressure natriuresis through alterations in renal interstitial pressure.[226]

The other well-characterized renal effect of Ang II is a direct action on proximal tubular epithelial transport. Infusions of Ang II to achieve systemic concentrations of 10^{-12} to 10^{-11} mol markedly stimulated Na^+ and water transport, independently of changes in renal or systemic hemodynamics.[210,227] Ang II exerts a dose-dependent biphasic effect on proximal Na^+ reabsorption. Peritubular capillary infusion with solutions containing low concentrations of Ang II (10^{-12} to 10^{-10} mol) stimulated the proximal Na^+ reabsorption rate, whereas perfusion at higher concentrations of Ang II ($>10^{-7}$ mol) inhibited the proximal Na^+ reabsorption rate. Addition of the AT_1 receptor antagonist losartan or the ACE inhibitor enalaprilat directly into the luminal fluid of the proximal nephron resulted in a significant decrease in proximal fluid reabsorption, which is indicative of tonic regulation of proximal tubule transport by endogenous Ang II.[228]

The specific mechanisms by which Ang II influences proximal tubule transport include increases in reabsorption of Na^+ and HCO_3^- by stimulation of the apical Na^+-H^+ antiporter, Na^+/H^+-exchanger isoform 3 (NHE3), basolateral Na^+-$3HCO_3^-$ symporter, and Na^+-K^+-ATPase.[229,230] Thus, Ang II can affect NaCl absorption by two mechanisms:

1. Activation of NHE3 can directly increase NaCl absorption.
2. Conditions that increase the rate of $NaHCO_3$ absorption can stimulate passive NaCl absorption by increasing the concentration gradient for passive Cl^- diffusion.[231]

Na^+ reabsorption is further promoted by the action of Ang II on NHE3 and Na^+-K^+-ATPase in the medullary thick ascending limb of Henle.[210]

In the early and late portions of the distal tubule, as well as the connecting tubule, Ang II regulates Na^+ and HCO_3^- reabsorption by stimulating NHE3 and the amiloride-sensitive Na^+ channel.[232-234] Two additional mechanisms may amplify the antinatriuretic effects of Ang II that are mediated by the direct actions of the peptide on renal hemodynamics and tubular transport. The first concerns the increased sensitivity of the TGF mechanism in the presence of Ang II, and the second is related to the effect of Ang II on pressure natriuresis. The decrease in distal delivery produced by the action of Ang II on renal hemodynamics and proximal fluid reabsorption could elicit afferent arteriolar vasodilation by means of the TGF mechanism, which, in turn, could antagonize the Ang II–mediated increase in proximal reabsorption. This effect, however, is minimized because Ang II increases the responsiveness of the TGF mechanism, thus maintaining GFR at a lower delivery rate to the macula densa.[82] The second mechanism by which the antinatriuretic effects of Ang II may be amplified is blunting of the pressure natriuresis mechanism so that higher pressures are needed to induce a given amount of Na^+ excretion.[174,210] This shift to the right in the pressure natriuresis curve may be viewed as an important Na^+-conserving mechanism in situations of elevated arterial pressure.

The use of ACE inhibitors and highly specific ARBs has provided additional insight into the mechanisms of action of Ang II in the kidneys; the findings have suggested that most of the known intrarenal actions of Ang II, particularly regulation of renal hemodynamics and proximal tubule reabsorption of Na^+ and HCO_3^-, are mediated by the AT_1 receptor.[219] However, functional studies have shown that some of the actions of Ang II at the renal level are mediated by AT_2 receptors.[219] The AT_2 receptor subtype plays a counterregulatory protective role against the AT_1 receptor–mediated antinatriuretic and pressor actions of Ang II. The accepted concept that Ang I was converted solely to Ang II was revised through the demonstration that Ang I is also a substrate for the formation of angiotensin-(1-7).[214] Moreover, a recently discovered homolog of ACE, ACE type 2 (ACE2), is responsible for the formation of angiotensin-(1-7) from Ang II and for the conversion of Ang I to angiotensin-(1-9), which may be converted to angiotensin-(1-7) by ACE.[213,214]

Angiotensin-(1-7), through its G protein–coupled receptor, Mas, may play a significant role as a regulator of cardiovascular and renal function by opposing the effects of Ang II; it does this through vasodilation, diuresis, and an antihypertrophic action.[213] Thus, the RAAS can currently be envisioned as a dual-function system in which the vasoconstrictor/proliferative or vasodilator/antiproliferative actions are driven primarily by the ACE/ACE2 balance. According to this model, an increased ACE/ACE2 activity ratio leads to increased generation of Ang II and increased catabolism of angiotensin-(1-7), which is conducive to vasoconstriction; conversely, a decreased ACE/ACE2 ratio reduces Ang II and increases angiotensin-(1-7) levels, facilitating vasodilation. The additional effect of angiotensin-(1-7)/Mas to antagonize the actions of Ang II directly adds a further level of counterregulation.[213]

The final component of the RAAS, aldosterone, is produced via Ang II stimulation of the adrenal cortex and also plays an important physiologic role in the maintenance of ECFV and Na^+ homeostasis.[235] The primary sites of aldosterone action are the principal cells of the cortical collecting tubule and convoluted distal tubule, in which the hormone promotes the reabsorption of Na^+ and the secretion of K^+ and protons.[235] Aldosterone may also enhance electrogenic Na^+ transport, but not K^+ secretion, in the IMCD[236] and has recently been shown to act also in the proximal tubule.[237] Aldosterone exerts its effects on ionic transport by increasing the number of open Na^+ and K^+ channels in the luminal membrane and the activity of Na^+-K^+-ATPase in the basolateral membrane.[238] The effect of aldosterone on Na^+ permeability appears to be the primary event because blockade of the ENaC with amiloride prevents the initial increase in Na^+ permeability and Na^+-K^+-ATPase activity.[238] This effect on Na^+ permeability is mediated by changes in intracellular Ca^{2+} levels, intracellular pH,[239] trafficking via protein kinase D1-phosphatidylinositol 4-kinaseIIIβ trans Golgi signaling,[240] and methylation of channel proteins, thus increasing the mean open probability of ENaC.[239] However, the long-term effect of aldosterone on Na^+-K^+-ATPase activity involves de novo protein synthesis, which is regulated at the transcriptional level by serum- and glucocorticoid-induced kinase-1.[239]

It has become clear that aldosterone specifically regulates the α-subunit of ENaC and that changes in expression of a variety of genes are important intermediates in this process. Using microarray analysis in a mouse IMCD line, Gumz and associates[241] examined the acute transcriptional effects of aldosterone. They found that the most prominent transcript was period homolog 1 (Per1), an important component of the circadian clock, and that disruption of the Per1 gene leads to attenuated expression of messenger RNA encoding for the α-subunit of ENaC and increased U_{Na} excretion. They also noted that messenger RNA encoded by the α-subunit of ENaC was expressed in an apparent circadian pattern that was dramatically altered in mice lacking functional Per1 genes. These results imply that the circadian clock has a previously unknown role in the control of Na^+ balance. Perhaps of more importance is that it provides molecular insight into how the circadian cycle directly affects Na^+ homeostasis.

The Na^+-retaining effect of aldosterone in the collecting tubule induces an increase in the transepithelial potential difference, which is conducive to K^+ excretion. In terms of overall body fluid homeostasis, the actions of aldosterone in the defense of ECF result from the net loss of an osmotically active particle confined primarily to the intracellular compartment (K^+) and its replacement with a corresponding particle confined primarily to the ECF (Na^+). The effect of a given circulating level of aldosterone on overall Na^+ excretion depends on the volume of filtrate reaching the collecting duct and the composition of luminal and intracellular fluids. As noted earlier, this delivery of filtrate is, in turn, determined by other effector mechanisms (Ang II, sympathetic nerve activity, and peritubular physical forces) acting at more proximal nephron sites.

It is not surprising that Na^+ balance can be regulated over a wide range of intake, even in subjects without adrenal glands and despite fixed low or high supplemental doses of mineralocorticoids. Under these circumstances, other effector mechanisms predominate in controlling urinary Na^+ excretion, although often in a setting of altered ECF volume or K^+ concentration. In this regard, how renal Na^+ reabsorption and K^+ excretion are coordinately regulated by aldosterone has long been a puzzle. In states of EABV depletion, aldosterone release stimulated by Ang II induces maximal Na^+ reabsorption without significantly affecting plasma K^+ levels. Conversely, hyperkalemia-induced aldosterone secretion stimulates maximum K^+ excretion without major effects on renal Na^+ handling.

Elegant studies on the intracellular signaling pathways involved in renal Na^+ and K^+ transport have shed light on this puzzle. The key elements in this transport regulation are the Ste20/SPS1-related proline/alanine-rich kinase (SPAK), oxidative stress-related kinase (OSR1) the with-no-lysine kinases (WNKs) and their effectors, the thiazide-sensitive NaCl cotransporter, and the K^+ secretory channel ROMK. According to the proposed model, when EABV is reduced or dietary salt intake is low, Ang II, mediated by the AT_1 receptor, leads to phosphorylation of WNK4, which stimulates phosphorylation of SPAK and OSR1. In turn, SPAK and OSR1 phosphorylate the NaCl cotransporter, inducing Na^+ transport and conservation. Simultaneous phosphorylation of the full-length isoform of WNK1, WNK1-L, causes endocytosis of the ROMK channel, thereby enabling K^+ conservation, despite high aldosterone levels. In contrast, in the presence of hyperkalemia or low dietary salt, Ang II levels are low so that WNK4 cannot be activated, SPAK, OSR1 and the NaCl cotransporter are not phosphorylated, and NaCl cotransporter trafficking to the apical membrane is inhibited. At the same time, K^+-induced kidney-specific WNK1 leads to suppression of WNK1-L, which allows ROMK trafficking to the apical membrane and maximal K^+ secretion.[242] For further details, the reader is referred to an excellent recent review.[243]

In terms of blood pressure maintenance, systemic vasoconstriction—another major extrarenal action of Ang II—may be considered the appropriate response to perceived ECF volume contraction. As mentioned previously, higher concentrations of Ang II are needed to elicit this response than those that govern the renal antinatriuretic actions of Ang II, a situation analogous to the discrepancy between antidiuretic and pressor actions of vasopressin. Transition from an antinatriuretic to a natriuretic action of Ang II at high infusion rates can be attributed almost entirely to a concomitant rise in blood pressure.[244] There is now clear evidence that in addition to the adrenal glomerulosa, aldosterone may also be produced by the heart and vasculature. It exerts powerful effects on blood vessels,[245] independently of actions that can be attributed to the blood pressure rise through regulation of salt and water balance. As observed with Ang II, aldosterone also possesses significant mitogenic and fibrogenic properties. It directly increases the expression and production of transforming growth factor-β and thus is involved in the development of glomerulosclerosis, hypertension, and cardiac injury/hypertrophy.[210,235,245]

In summary, Ang II, the principal effector of the RAAS, regulates extracellular volume and renal Na^+ excretion through intrarenal and extrarenal mechanisms. The intrarenal hemodynamic and tubular actions of the peptide and its main extrarenal actions (systemic vasoconstriction and aldosterone release) act in concert to adjust U_{Na} excretion under a variety of circumstances associated with alterations in ECF volume. Many of these mechanisms are synergistic and tend to amplify the overall influence of the RAAS. However, additional counterregulatory mechanisms, induced directly or indirectly by Ang II, provide a buffer against the unopposed actions of the primary components of the RAAS.

Vasopressin. AVP is a nonapeptide (nine–amino acid) hormone, synthesized in the brain, that is secreted from the posterior pituitary gland into the circulation in response to an increase in plasma osmolality (through osmoreceptor stimulation) or a decrease in EABV and blood pressure (through baroreceptor stimulation).[246] Thus, AVP plays a major role in the regulation of water balance and the support of blood pressure and EABV. AVP exerts its biologic actions through at least three different G protein–coupled receptors. Two of these receptors, V_{1A} and V_2, are abundantly expressed in the cardiovascular system and the kidneys; V_{1B} receptors are expressed on the surfaces of corticotrophic cells of the anterior pituitary gland, in the pancreas, and in the adrenal medulla. V_{1A} and V_2 receptors mediate the two main biologic actions of the hormone, vasoconstriction and increased water reabsorption by the kidneys, respectively. (V_2 receptor–mediated effects on hemostasis are discussed in Chapter 29.) The V_{1A} and V_{1B} receptors operate through the phosphoinositide signaling pathway, causing release of intracellular Ca^{2+}. The V_{1A} receptor, found in vascular smooth muscle cells, hepatocytes, and platelets, mediates vasoconstriction, glycogenolysis, and platelet aggregation, respectively. The V_2 receptor, found mainly in the renal collecting duct epithelial cells, is linked to the adenylate cyclase pathway, and cAMP is used as its second messenger.

Under physiologic conditions, AVP functions primarily to regulate water content in the body by adjusting water reabsorption in the collecting duct according to plasma tonicity. A change in plasma tonicity by as little as 1% causes a parallel change in AVP release. This change, in turn, alters the water permeability of the collecting duct. The antidiuretic action of AVP results from complex effects of this hormone on principal cells of the collecting duct. First, AVP provokes the insertion of aquaporin-2 (AQP2)[247] water channels into the luminal membrane (short-term response) and increases the synthesis of AQP2 messenger RNA and protein[248]; both responses increase water permeability along the collecting duct. This is considered in detail in Chapter 11. In brief, activation of V_2 receptors localized to the basolateral membrane of the principal cells increases cytosolic cAMP, which stimulates the activity of protein kinase A. The latter triggers a series of phosphorylation events that promotes the translocation of AQP2 from intracellular stores to the apical membrane,[249] which allows the reabsorption of water from the lumen to the cells. The water then exits the cell to the hypertonic interstitium via aquaporin-3 and aquaporin-4, localized at the basolateral membrane.[250]

The second complex effect of AVP on the collecting duct is to increase the permeability of the IMCD to urea through activation of the urea transporter UT-A1, which enables the accumulation of urea in the interstitium; there, along with Na^+, it contributes to the hypertonicity of the medullary interstitium, which is a prerequisite for maximum urine concentration and water reabsorption.[251] AVP exerts several effects on Na^+ handling at different segments of the nephron, in which it increases Na^+ reabsorption through activation of ENaC, mainly in the cortical and outer medullary collecting ducts.[252]

In addition, AVP may influence renal hemodynamics and reduce RBF, especially to the inner medulla.[253] The latter effect is mediated by the V_{1A} receptor and may be modulated by the local release of nitric oxide and prostaglandins. At higher concentrations,[254] AVP may also decrease total RBF and GFR as part of the generalized vasoconstriction induced by the peptide.[248,255]

The role of the V_{1A} receptor in the kidneys has been further elaborated. In V_{1A} receptor–deficient ($V_{1A}R^{-/-}$) mice, plasma volume and blood pressure were decreased.[255] Also, urine volume of $V_{1A}R^{-/-}$ mice was greater than that of wild-type mice, particularly after a water load; however, GFR, U_{Na} excretion, AVP-dependent cAMP generation, levels of V_2 receptor, and AQP2 expression in the kidneys were lower, which indicates that the diminishment of GFR and the V_2 receptor–AQP2 system led to impaired urinary concentration in $V_{1A}R^{-/-}$ mice. This result is interesting because classic models implicate the V_2 receptors in water handling by the nephron. Moreover, plasma renin and Ang II levels were decreased, as was renin expression in granule cells. In addition, the expression of renin stimulators such as nNOS and cyclo-oxygenase-2 (COX-2) in macula densa cells, where $V_{1A}R$ is specifically expressed, was decreased in $V_{1A}R^{-/-}$ mice. Aoyagi and colleagues have concluded that AVP regulates body fluid homeostasis and GFR through the $V_{1A}R$ in macula densa cells by activating the RAAS and subsequently the V_2 receptor–AQP2 system.[255] Recent work from the same group (Yasuoka and associates[256]) has confirmed the importance of the $V_{1A}R$ for the expression of AQP2 in the collecting ducts during control conditions and dehydration.

A third receptor for AVP, V_3,[257] is found predominantly in the anterior pituitary gland and is involved in the regulation of adrenocorticotropic hormone (ACTH) release. In addition to its renal effects, AVP also regulates extrarenal vascular tone through the V_{1A} receptor. Stimulation of this receptor by AVP results in a potent arteriolar vasoconstriction in various vascular beds, with a significant increase in systemic vascular resistance.[258] However, physiologic increases in AVP do not usually cause a significant increase in blood pressure because AVP also potentiates the sinoaortic baroreflexes that subsequently reduce heart rate and cardiac output.[258] Nevertheless, at supraphysiologic concentrations of AVP, such as those that occur when EABV is severely compromised (e.g., in shock or heart failure), AVP plays an important role in supporting arterial pressure and maintaining adequate perfusion to vital organs such as the brain and myocardium. AVP also has a direct, V_1 receptor–mediated, inotropic effect in the isolated heart.[259] In vivo, however, AVP has been reported to decrease myocardial function[260]; this effect is attributed to cardioinhibitory reflexes or coronary vasoconstriction induced by the peptide. Of more importance is that AVP has been shown to stimulate cardiomyocyte hypertrophy and protein synthesis in neonatal rat cardiomyocytes and in intact myocardium through a V_1-dependent mechanism.[261] These effects are very similar to those obtained with exposure of cardiomyocytes to Ang II or catecholamines, although not necessarily through the same cellular mechanisms. By this growth-promoting property, AVP may contribute to the induction of cardiac hypertrophy and remodeling in heart failure.[262]

Until recently, uncertainty existed regarding the effect of AVP on natriuresis; some authors have found a natriuretic response with infusions, and others have found Na^+ retention.[263,264] These variations may have resulted from differences between species or from acute changes in volume status.[265] It is now clear that an increase in Na^+ reabsorption along the distal nephron (connecting tubule and collecting duct), mediated by activation of ENaC by vasopressin, makes an important contribution to maintenance of the axial corticomedullary osmotic gradient necessary for maximal water reabsorption. Thus, the renal action of vasopressin includes not only a direct decrease in free water excretion to dilute plasma, but also Na^+ reabsorption and, consequently, decreased Na^+ excretion via ENaC activated along the distal nephron.[266] In terms of overall volume homeostasis, regardless of the effects of AVP on Na^+ excretion, the predominant influence of the hormone is indirectly through water accumulation or vasoconstriction. In fact, the vasoconstrictive V_1 receptor effect of AVP overrides the osmotically driven effect in the presence of an ECF volume deficit of 20% or more (see Chapters 10, 11, and 16). Nevertheless, in this regard, potential hypertensive effects of AVP are buffered by a concomitant increase in baroreflex-mediated sympathoinhibition or by an increase in PGE_2, which results in a blunting of vasoconstriction, and by a direct vasodepressor action of V_2 receptor activation.[267]

Prostaglandins. Prostaglandins (see also Chapter 14), or cyclo-oxygenase–derived prostanoids, possess complex and diverse regulatory functions in the kidneys, including hemodynamics, renin secretion, growth response, tubular transport processes, and immune response in health and disease (Table 15.3).[268,269] Currently, two known principal isoforms of cyclo-oxygenase (COX-1 and COX-2) catalyze the synthesis of prostaglandin H_2 (PGH_2) from arachidonic acid, released from membrane phospholipids. PGH_2 is then metabolized to the five major prostanoids—PGE_2, prostaglandins I_2, D_2, and $F_2\alpha$ (PGI_2, PGD_2, and $PGF_2\alpha$), and thromboxane A_2 (TXA_2)—through specific synthases (see also Chapter 14).[270] An additional splice variant of the COX-1 gene, COX-3, has been identified, but its function in humans remains unclear.[271]

Prostanoids are rapidly degraded, so their effect is localized strictly to their site of synthesis, which accounts for the predominance of their autocrine and paracrine modes of action. Each prostanoid has a specific cell surface G protein–coupled receptor, distinct for a given location, that determines the specific function of the prostaglandin in the given cell type.[269] COX-1 is constitutively expressed and serves in a housekeeping role in many cell types; it is expressed abundantly and is highly immunoreactive in the kidneys, especially in the collecting duct but also in medullary interstitial, mesangial, and arteriolar endothelial cells of most species.[269] In contrast, the expression of COX-2 is inducible and cell type–specific, and its renal expression is prominent in medullary interstitial cells, cortical cells of the thick ascending limb of Henle, and cells of the macula densa, in which expression is regulated in response to varying amounts of salt intake.[269] Furthermore, the profile of sensitivity to pharmacologic inhibitors differs between the two isoforms.[272] The principal prostanoid in the kidneys is PGE_2; others present are PGI_2, PGF_2, and TXA_2.[269] PGI_2 and PGE_2 are the main products in the cortex of normal kidneys, and PGE_2 predominates in the medulla.[269] The metabolism of arachidonic acid by other pathways (e.g., lipoxygenase, epoxygenase) leads to products that are involved in crosstalk with cyclo-oxygenase.[268] The major sites for prostaglandin production (and hence for local actions) are the renal arteries and arterioles and glomeruli in the cortex and interstitial cells in the medulla, with additional contributions from epithelial cells of the cortical and medullary collecting tubules.[273,274]

The two major roles for prostaglandins in volume homeostasis are (1) their effect on RBF and GFR and (2) their effect on tubular handling of salt and water. Table 15.3 lists target structures, mode of action, and major biologic effects of the active renal prostanoids. PGI_2 and PGE_2 have predominantly vasodilating and natriuretic activities; they also modulate the action of AVP and tend to stimulate renin secretion. TXA_2 has been shown to cause vasoconstriction, although the importance of the physiologic effects of TXA_2 on the kidneys is still controversial. The end results of the stimulation of renal prostaglandin secretion in the kidneys are vasodilation, increased renal perfusion, natriuresis, and facilitation of water excretion.

The role of prostaglandins as vasodilators in the glomerular microcirculation is now well established. The cellular targets for vasoactive hormones in the glomerular microcirculation are vascular smooth muscle cells of the afferent and efferent arterioles and mesangial cells within the glomeruli. Action at these sites governs renal vascular resistance,

Table 15.3 Major Renal Biologic Effects of Prostaglandins and Thromboxane

Agent	Target Structure	Mode of Action	Direct Consequences
PGE_2, PGI_2	Intrarenal arterioles	Vasodilation	Increased renal perfusion (more pronounced in inner cortical and medullary regions)
PGI_2	Glomeruli	Vasodilation	Increased filtration rate
PGE_2, PGI_2	Efferent arterioles	Vasodilation	Increased Na^+ excretion through increased postglomerular perfusion
PGE_2, PGI_2, $PGF_2\alpha$	Distal tubules	Decreased transport	Increased Na^+ excretion, decreased maximum medullary hypertonicity
PGE_2, PGI_2, $PGF_2\alpha$	Distal tubules	Inhibition of cAMP synthesis	Interference with AVP action
PGE_2, PGI_2	Juxtaglomerular apparatus	cAMP stimulation (?)	Increased renin release
TxA_2	Intrarenal arterioles	Vasoconstriction	Decreased renal perfusion

AVP, Arginine vasopressin; cAMP, cyclic adenosine monophosphate; PGE_2, prostaglandin E_2; $PGF_2\alpha$, prostaglandin $F_2\alpha$; PGI_2, prostaglandin I_2; TxA_2, thromboxane A_2.

glomerular function, and downstream microcirculatory function in peritubular capillaries and vasa recta. In vivo studies have shown that intrarenal infusions of PGE_2 and PGI_2 cause vasodilation and increased RBF.[273] In agreement with these findings, in vitro experiments with isolated renal microvessels have shown that PGE_2 and prostaglandin E_1 (PGE_1) attenuate Ang II–induced afferent arteriolar vasoconstriction, and PGI_2 antagonizes Ang II–induced efferent arteriolar vasoconstriction.[275] Similarly, PGE_2 has been shown to counteract Ang II–induced contraction of isolated glomeruli and glomerular mesangial cells in culture and, conversely, cyclo-oxygenase inhibition augments these contractile responses.[276] An inhibitory counterregulatory role of prostaglandins with regard to renal nerve stimulation has also been demonstrated from micropuncture studies.[277] Furthermore, in volume-contracted states, COX-2 expression and PGE_2 release in the macula densa and cortical thick ascending limb of Henle dramatically increase in response to decreased luminal Cl^- delivery. In addition to its direct vasodilator effect on afferent arterioles, PGE_2 leads to increased renin release from the macula densa.[269] The resulting rise in Ang II and consequent efferent arteriolar constriction also ensure maintenance of the GFR.

In the clinical situation, in volume-replete states, the renal vasoconstrictive influences of Ang II and norepinephrine are mitigated by their simultaneous stimulation of vasodilatory renal prostaglandins, so that RBF and GFR are maintained.[278] However, in the setting of heightened vasoconstrictor input from the RAAS, SNS, and AVP, as occurs during states of EABV depletion, the vasorelaxant action of PGE_2 and PGI_2 is overwhelmed, with the concomitant risk for the development of acute kidney injury.[269] Similarly, when this prostaglandin-mediated counterregulatory mechanism is suppressed by nonselective or COX-2–selective inhibitors, the unopposed actions of Ang II and norepinephrine can also lead to a rapid deterioration in renal function.[279] Moreover, COX-2–derived prostanoids also promote natriuresis and stimulate renin secretion.[269] Therefore, during states of volume depletion, low Na^+ intake, or the use of loop diuretics, COX-2 inhibitors (e.g., celecoxib), and the nonselective COX inhibitors diclofenac and naproxen, can cause Na^+ and K^+ retention, edema formation, heart failure, and hypertension.[274]

In addition to the role of prostaglandins in modulating glomerular vasoreactivity in states of varying salt balance, prostaglandins also have direct effects on salt excretion. Clearly, the aforementioned vascular effects of prostaglandins can be expected to have secondary effects on tubular function through the various physical factors described earlier in this chapter. One particular consequence of prostaglandin-induced renal vasodilation may be medullary interstitial solute washout. Such a change in medullary interstitial composition could potentially account for the observed increase in U_{Na} excretion with intrarenal infusion of PGE_2.[273] The natriuretic response to PGE_2 may also be attenuated by preventing an increase in renal interstitial hydraulic pressure, even in the presence of a persistent increase in RBF.[280] In addition, in rats, the natriuresis usually accompanying direct expansion of renal interstitial volume can be significantly attenuated by inhibition of prostaglandin synthesis.[280] These findings are consistent with the proposal that changes in prostaglandins have a significant effect on renal Na^+ excretion.

Results of micropuncture and microcatheterization studies in vivo have suggested that prostaglandins affect U_{Na} excretion independently of hemodynamic changes.[273] Subsequently, direct effects of PGE_2 on epithelial transport processes were demonstrated and found to vary considerably in different nephron segments. In the medullary thick ascending limb of Henle and collecting tubule, PGE_2 caused a decrease in the reabsorption of water, Na^+, and Cl^- that was correlated with reduced Na^+-K^+-ATPase activity. In contrast, in the distal convoluted tubule, PGE_2 caused increased Na^+-K^+-ATPase activity.[281] The net effect of locally produced prostaglandins on tubular Na^+ handling is probably inhibitory because complete blockade of prostaglandin synthesis by indomethacin in rats receiving a normal or salt-loaded diet increased fractional Na^+ reabsorption and enhanced the activity of the renal medullary Na^+-K^+-ATPase.[282] In addition, PGE_2 inhibited AVP-stimulated NaCl reabsorption in the medullary thick ascending limb of Henle and AVP-stimulated water reabsorption in the collecting duct.[283,284] Both these effects tend to antagonize the overall hydroosmotic response to AVP. However, because no such effect is seen in the cortical thick ascending limb of Henle, which is capable of augmenting NaCl reabsorption in response to an increased delivered load, and because the effects of prostaglandins on solute transport in the collecting tubule remain unresolved, no conclusions can be reached from these studies about the contribution of direct epithelial effects of prostaglandins to overall Na^+ excretion.[283]

In whole animal and clinical balance studies, researchers have examined the effects of prostaglandin infusion or prostaglandin synthesis inhibition on urinary Na^+ excretion, or have attempted to correlate changes in urinary prostaglandin excretion with changes in salt balance; these studies have also yielded conflicting and inconclusive results. Nevertheless, as elaborated earlier, prostaglandins have an important role in states of Na^+ imbalance (real or perceived Na^+ depletion) in which they are involved to preserve GFR by countervailing renal vasoconstrictive influences.

The influence of changes in Na^+ intake on renal COX-1 and COX-2 expression has been studied extensively. The expression of COX-2 in the macula densa and thick ascending limb of Henle is increased by a low-salt diet, inhibition of RAAS, and renal hypoperfusion. In contrast, a high-salt diet has been reported to decrease COX-2 expression in the renal cortex.[268,269] None of these changes in Na^+ intake affect the expression of COX-1 in the cortex. In the medulla, whereas a low-salt diet downregulated both COX-1 and COX-2, a high-salt diet enhanced the expression of these cyclo-oxygenase isoforms.[268,269] In vitro studies have shown that high osmolarity of the medium of cultured IMCD cells induces the expression of COX-2.[274] Infusion of nimesulide (a selective COX-2 inhibitor) into anesthetized dogs on a normal Na^+ diet reduced U_{Na} excretion and urine flow rate, despite the lack of effect on renal hemodynamics or systemic blood pressure.[274]

Collectively, the differential regulation of COX-2 in the renal cortex and medulla can be integrated into a physiologically relevant model in which upregulation of COX-2 in the cortical thick ascending limb of Henle and macula densa is induced in a volume-contracted or vasoconstrictor state. In the cortical thick ascending limb of Henle, the effect is by direct inhibition of Na^+ excretion, whereas in the macula densa, COX-2 stimulates renin release, which leads to Ang II–mediated Na^+ retention. In contrast, medullary COX-2 is induced by a high-salt diet, which leads to net Na^+ excretion.[269]

Finally, in addition to the hemodynamically mediated and potential direct epithelial effects of prostaglandins, these agents may mediate the physiologic responses to other hormonal agents. The intermediacy of prostaglandins in renin release responses has already been cited. As another example, some, but not all, of the known physiologic effects of bradykinin and other products of the kallikrein-kinin system are mediated through bradykinin-stimulated prostaglandin production (e.g., inhibition of AVP-stimulated osmotic water permeability in the cortical collecting tubule).[283] In addition, the renal and systemic actions of Ang II appear to be differentially regulated by prostaglandin production that is catalyzed by COX-1 and COX-2. For example, COX-2 deficiency in mice, induced by COX-2 inhibitors or gene knockout, dramatically augmented the systemic pressor effect of Ang II, whereas COX-1 deficiency abolished this pressor effect. Similarly, Ang II infusion reduced medullary blood flow in COX-2–deficient animals, but not in COX-1–deficient animals, which suggests that COX-2–dependent vasodilators are synthesized in the renal medulla. Moreover, the diuretic and natriuretic effects of Ang II were absent in COX-2–deficient animals but remained in COX-1–deficient animals. Thus, COX-1 and COX-2 exert opposite effects on systemic blood pressure and renal function.[285]

Natriuretic Peptides. The physiologic and pathophysiologic roles of the NP family in the regulation of Na^+ and water balance have been extensively investigated since the discovery of ANP by de Bold and colleagues.[34] ANP is an endogenous, 28–amino acid peptide secreted mainly by the right atrium. In addition to ANP, three other NPs have renal effects—BNP, CNP, and DNP.[36] Although encoded by different genes, these peptides are highly similar in chemical structure, gene regulation, and degradation pathways, constituting a hormonal system that exerts various biologic actions on the renal, cardiac, and blood vessel tissues.[286] ANP plays an important role in blood pressure and volume homeostasis through its ability to induce natriuretic/diuretic, and vasodilatory responses.[287,288] BNP has an amino acid sequence similar to that of ANP, with an extended NH_2-terminus. In humans, BNP is produced from pro–brain NP (proBNP), which contains 108 amino acids and, in accordance with a proteolytic process, releases a mature, 32–amino acid molecule and N-terminal fragment into the circulation. Although BNP was originally cloned from the brain, it is now considered a circulating hormone produced mainly in the cardiac ventricles.[287,288] CNP, which is produced mostly by endothelial cells, shares the ring structure common to all NP members; however, it lacks the C-terminal tail. DNP is released by the kidney and is a more effective activator of renal functions than ANP.[289]

The biologic effects of the natriuretic peptides (NPs) are mediated by binding the peptide to specific membrane receptors localized to numerous tissues, including the vasculature, renal arteries, glomerular mesangial and epithelial cells, collecting ducts, adrenal zona glomerulosa, and the CNS.[36] At least three different subtypes of NP receptors have been identified—NP-A, NP-B, and NP-C.[286] NP-A and NP-B, single-transmembrane proteins with molecular weights of approximately 120 to 140 kDa, mediate most of the biologic effects of NPs. Both are coupled to guanylate cyclase in their intracellular portions.[286] After binding to their receptors, all three NP isoforms markedly increase cGMP in target tissues and in plasma. Therefore, analogues of cGMP or inhibitors of degradation of this second messenger mimic the vasorelaxant and renal effects of NPs. The third class of NP-binding receptors, NP-C (molecular weight, 60 to 70 kDa), is believed to serve as a clearance receptor because it is not coupled to any known second-messenger system.[290] ANP-C is the most abundant type of NP receptor in many key target organs of NPs.[290]

Two additional routes for the removal of NPs are worth noting. The first well-established pathway is the enzymatic degradation by neutral endopeptidase (NEP) 24.11, a metalloproteinase located mainly in the lungs and the kidneys.[290] This pathway has undergone extensive research in attempts to find specific inhibitors that would lead to enhanced NP activity in situations of Na^+ retention (see section, "Specific Treatments Based on the Pathophysiology of Congestive Heart Failure"). The second route is entirely novel and involves the negative regulation of ANP by microRNA-425 (miRNA-425). In this context, carriers of the rs5068 minor G allele of the gene encoding ANP, *NPPA*, have a 15% lower risk of hypertension and ANP levels 50% higher than those with two copies of the major A allele. miRNA-425, expressed in human atria and ventricles, is predicted to bind the sequence spanning rs5068 in the 3′ untranslated region of the A, but not G, allele. Only the A allele was silenced by miRNA-425, whereas possession of the G allele conferred resistance to miR-425. The results raise the possibility that miR-425 antagonists could be used to treat disorders of salt overload, such as hypertension and heart failure.[291]

Atrial Natriuretic Peptide. Both in vivo and in vitro studies, in humans and experimental animals, have established the role of ANP in the regulation of ECFV and blood pressure by acting on all organs and tissues involved in the homeostasis of Na^+ and blood pressure (Table 15.4).[288] Therefore, it is not surprising that ANP and NH_2-terminal ANP levels are increased in certain situations: (1) conditions associated with enhanced atrial pressure; (2) systolic or diastolic cardiac dysfunction; (3) cardiac hypertrophy/remodeling; and (4) severe myocardial infarction.[36] In the kidneys, ANP exerts hemodynamic/glomerular effects that increase Na^+ and water delivery to the tubule in combination with inhibitory effects on tubular Na^+ and water reabsorption, which lead to remarkable diuresis and natriuresis.[288]

In addition to its powerful diuretic and natriuretic activities, ANP also relaxes vascular smooth muscle and leads to vasodilation by antagonizing the concomitant vasoconstrictive influences of Ang II, endothelin, AVP, and α_1-adrenergic input.[288] This vasodilation reduces preload, which results in a fall in cardiac output.[288] In addition, ANP reduces cardiac output by shifting fluid from the intravascular to extravascular compartment, an effect mediated by increased capillary hydraulic conductivity for water.[292] Studies in endothelial-restricted, GC-A knockout mice have found that

Table 15.4 Physiologic Actions of the Natriuretic Peptides

Target Organ	Biologic Effects
Kidney	Increased GFR
	Afferent arteriolar vasodilation
	Efferent arteriolar vasoconstriction
	Natriuresis
	Inhibition of Na^+/H^+ exchanger (proximal tubule)
	Inhibition of Na^+-Cl^- cotransporter (distal tubule)
	Inhibition of Na^+ channels (collecting duct)
	Diuresis
	Inhibition of AVP-induced AQP2 incorporation into CD-AM
Cardiac	Reduction in preload, leading to reduced cardiac output
	Inhibition of cardiac remodeling
Hemodynamic	Vasorelaxation
	Elevation of capillary hydraulic conductivity
	Decreased cardiac preload and afterload
Endocrine	Suppression of RAAS
	Suppression of sympathetic outflow
	Suppression of AVP
	Suppression of endothelin
Mitogenesis	Inhibition of mitogenesis in vascular smooth muscle cells
	Inhibition of growth factor–mediated hypertrophy of cardiac fibroblasts

AQP-2, Aquaporin 2; AVP, arginine vasopressin; CD-AM, collecting duct apical membrane; GFR, glomerular filtration rate; RAAS, renin-angiotensin-aldosterone system.

ANP, through GC-A, enhances albumin permeability in the microcirculation of the skin and skeletal muscle. This effect is mediated by caveolae[293] and is critically involved in the endocrine hypovolemic and hypotensive actions of the cardiac hormone in vivo.[294]

ANP has also been shown to exert antiproliferative, growth regulatory properties in cultured glomerular mesangial cells, vascular smooth muscle cells, and endothelial cells.[295] Within the kidneys, ANP causes afferent vasodilation, efferent vasoconstriction, and mesangial relaxation, which lead to increases in glomerular capillary pressure, GFR, and filtration fraction.[288] In combination with increased medullary blood flow, these hemodynamic effects enhance diuresis and natriuresis. However, the overall natriuretic effect of ANP infusion does not require these changes in glomerular function (except in response to larger doses of the peptide). At the tubular level, ANP inhibits the stimulatory effect of Ang II on the luminal Na^+/H^+ exchanger of the proximal tubule.[288] Similarly, ANP, acting through cGMP, inhibits the thiazide-sensitive NaCl cotransporter in the distal tubule and ENaC in the collecting duct, along with inhibition of AVP-induced AQP2 incorporation into the apical membrane of these segments of the nephron (see Table 15.4).[288]

Brain Natriuretic Peptide. BNP is produced by activated satellite cells in ischemic skeletal muscle or by cardiomyocytes in response to pressure load, thereby regulating the regeneration of neighboring endothelia through GC-A. BNP-mediated paracrine communication may be critically involved in coordinating muscle regeneration or hypertrophy and angiogenesis. However, the administration of BNP to human subjects induces natriuretic, endocrine, and hemodynamic responses similar to those induced by ANP.[288]

BNP is produced and secreted mainly by the ventricles but also, in small amounts, by the atrium.[288] Increased volume or pressure overload states such as HF and hypertension enhance the secretion of BNP from the ventricles. Despite the comparable elevation in plasma levels of ANP and BNP in patients with HF and other chronic volume-expanded conditions, acute intravenous saline loading or infusion of pressor doses of Ang II yields different patterns of ANP and BNP secretion.[296,297] Whereas plasma levels of ANP increase rapidly, the changes in plasma BNP of atrial origin are negligible, as expected in view of the minimal atrial content of BNP, in contrast to the abundance of ANP.[288] Moreover, plasma levels of BNP rise with age, from 26 ± 2 pg/mL in subjects aged 55 to 64 years to 31 ± 2 pg/mL in those aged 65 to 74 years and to 64 ± 6 pg/mL in those 75 years of age or older.[298]

Studies in animals and humans have demonstrated the natriuretic effects of pharmacologic doses of BNP. When administered to normal volunteers and hypertensive subjects at low doses, BNP induces a significant increase in U_{Na} excretion and, to a lesser extent, in urinary flow. Significant natriuresis and diuresis were observed after the infusion of ANP or BNP to normal subjects. The combination of ANP and BNP did not produce a synergistic renal effect, which suggests that these peptides share similar mechanisms of action.[288] Moreover, like ANP, BNP exerts a hypotensive effect in animals and humans. For example, transgenic mice that overexpress the BNP gene exhibit significant and life-long hypotension to the same extent as transgenic mice that overexpress the ANP gene.[288] Therefore, it is clear that BNP induces its biologic actions through mechanisms similar to those of ANP.[288]

This notion is supported by several findings: (1) both ANP and BNP act through the same receptors, and both induce similar renal, cardiovascular, and endocrine actions in association with an increase in cGMP production (see Table 15.4); and (2) BNP suppresses ACTH-induced aldosterone generation both in cell culture and when BNP is infused in vivo. The latter action may be attributed to BNP inhibition of renin secretion, at least in dogs, although apparently not in humans.[288] Similar to the hemodynamic effects of ANP, those of BNP vary according to dose and species. When injected as a bolus at high doses, BNP caused a profound fall in systolic blood pressure in humans; however, when infused at low doses, this peptide fails to change blood pressure or heart rate.[288] The effects of BNP have been used in the clinical setting in the diagnosis and treatment of the volume overload state of HF (see section, "Specific Treatments Based on the Pathophysiology of Congestive Heart Failure").

C-Type Natriuretic Peptide. Although CNP is considered a neurotransmitter in the CNS, considerable amounts of this NP are produced by endothelial cells, where it plays a role in the local regulation of vascular tone.[290] Smaller amounts of CNP are produced in the kidneys, heart ventricles, and intestines.[290] In addition, CNP, which could be of endothelial or cardiac origin, has been found in human plasma. The physiologic stimuli for CNP production have not been identified, although enhanced expression of CNP messenger RNA has been reported after volume overload.[290] Intravenous infusion of CNP decreases blood pressure, cardiac output, urinary volume, and Na^+ excretion. Furthermore, the hypotensive effects of CNP are less pronounced compared to those of ANP and BNP, but CNP strongly stimulates cGMP production and inhibits vascular smooth muscle cell proliferation.[299]

All three NPs inhibit the RAAS, although CNP does not induce significant changes in cardiac output, blood pressure, and plasma volume in sheep.[290] This finding supports the widely accepted concept that ANP and BNP are the major circulating NPs, whereas CNP is a local regulator of vascular structure and tone.

D-Type Natriuretic Peptide. DNP infused intravenously into rabbits increased urine volume and urinary excretion of electrolytes. These renal actions, induced by DNP, were more pronounced than those of ANP, possibly because of the degradation resistance of DNP against the endogenous peptidases in plasma or tissues. DNP, specifically via the NP-A receptor, induced the greatest cGMP production in glomeruli compared to other renal structures, including cortical tubules, outer medullary tubules, and inner medullary tubules. Thus, DNP appears to play a pivotal role, at least in sheep, as a renal regulating peptide via specific NP receptors with a guanylate cyclase domain.[289]

Although all forms of NPs exist in the brain, the role and significance of their CNS expression in the regulation of salt and water balance are not understood. Together, the various biologic actions of NPs lead to reduction of EABV, an expected response to perceived overfilling of the central intrathoracic circulation. Furthermore, all NPs counteract the adverse effects of the RAAS, which suggests that the two systems are acting in opposite directions in the regulation of body fluid and cardiovascular homeostasis.

Endothelium-Derived Factors. The endothelium is a major source of active substances that regulate vascular tone in healthy states and disease.[300] The best known representatives are endothelin, nitric oxide, and PGI_2. These vasoconstricting and vasodilating factors regulate the perfusion pressure of multiple organ systems that are strongly involved in water and Na^+ balance, such as the kidneys, heart, and vasculature. This section summarizes some concepts regarding actions of endothelin and nitric oxide that are relevant to volume homeostasis.

Endothelin. The endothelin system consists of three vasoactive peptides—endothelin 1 (ET-1), endothelin 2 (ET-2), and endothelin 3 (ET-3). These peptides are synthesized and released mainly by endothelial cells and act in a paracrine and autocrine manner.[301,302] ET-1, the major representative of the endothelin family, is still the most potent vasoconstrictor known[303] (and see section, "Urotensin"). All endothelins are synthesized by proteolytic cleavage from specific prepro-endothelins that are further cleaved to form 37– to 39–amino acid precursors, called *big endothelin.* Big endothelin is then converted into the biologically active, 21–amino acid peptide by a highly specific endothelin-converting enzyme (ECE), a phosphoramidon-sensitive, membrane-bound metalloprotease. To date, two isoforms of ECE have been identified, ECE-1 and ECE-2. ECE-1 exists as four different isoforms.[304] ECE-2 is localized mainly to vascular smooth muscle cells and is probably an intracellular enzyme. In ECE-1 knockout mice, tissue levels of ET-1 are reduced by about one third, which suggests that ECE-independent pathways are involved in the synthesis of this peptide.[305] In this regard, both chymase[306] and carboxypeptidase A[307] have been shown to be involved in mature endothelin production.

The endothelins bind to two distinct receptors, designated endothelin types A and B (ET-A and ET-B).[303] The ET-A receptor shows a higher affinity for ET-1 than for ET-2 or ET-3. The ET-B receptor shows equal affinity for each of the three endothelins. ET-A receptors are found mainly on vascular smooth muscle cells, on which their activation leads to vasoconstriction through an increase in cytosolic Ca^{2+}. ET-B receptors are also found on vascular smooth muscle cells, on which they can mediate vasoconstriction, but are found predominantly on vascular endothelium, in which their activation results in vasodilation through prostacyclin and nitric oxide.[303] Endothelin is detectable in the plasma of human subjects and many experimental animals, and therefore may also act as a circulating vasoactive hormone.[308]

Selective ET-A receptor antagonism is associated with vasodilation and a reduction in blood pressure, whereas selective ET-B antagonism is accompanied by vasoconstriction and a rise in blood pressure.[303] These data suggest complementary roles for the endothelin receptor subtypes in the maintenance of vascular tone. In addition to its vasoconstrictive action, endothelin has a variety of effects on the kidneys.[301,309-312] The kidney (mainly the inner medulla) is both a source and an important target organ of endothelin. ET-1 is synthesized by the endothelial cells of the renal vessels, whereas ET-1 and ET-3 are produced by various cell types of the nephron. ET-2 and ET-3 are produced at a rate one to two orders of magnitude lower than ET-1, which appears to be the principal subtype involved in renal functional regulation.[301,309]

In relation to volume homeostasis, three major aspects of renal function are affected by ET-1 in a paracrine or autocrine manner: (1) renal and intrarenal blood flow; (2) glomerular hemodynamics; and (3) renal tubular transport of salt and water. Both ET-A and ET-B receptors are present in the glomerulus, renal vessels, and tubular epithelial cells, but most ET-B receptors are found in the medulla.[313] The renal vasculature, in comparison with other vascular beds, appears to be most sensitive to the vasoconstrictor action of ET-1. Infusion of ET-1 into the renal artery of anesthetized rabbits was found to decrease RBF, GFR, natriuresis, and urine volume.[314] Micropuncture studies have demonstrated that ET-1 increases afferent and efferent arteriolar resistance (afferent more than efferent), which results in a reduction in the glomerular plasma flow rate. In addition, Kf is reduced because of mesangial cell contraction, resulting in a diminished SNGFR.

The profound reduction of RBF and concomitant lesser reduction in GFR should result in a rise in filtration fraction, but the effect of ET-1 on the filtration fraction appears to be variable. Some groups, using low doses in a canine model, have reported an increase,[315] and others have reported no significant effect.[316] Infusion of ET-1 for 8 days into conscious dogs increased plasma levels of endothelin by twofold to threefold and resulted in increased renal vascular resistance and decreased GFR and RBF.[254] Interestingly, the effect of endothelin on regional intrarenal blood flow is not homogeneous. Using laser Doppler flowmetry, administration of ET-1 in control rats produced a sustained cortical vasoconstriction and a transient medullary vasodilatory response.[317] These results are in line with the medullary predominance of ET-B receptors and the high density of ET-A–binding sites in the cortex.[318]

The effect of endothelin on Na^+ and water excretion varies and depends on the dose and source of endothelin. Systemic infusion of endothelin in high doses results in profound antinatriuresis and antidiuresis, apparently secondary to the decrease in GFR and RBF. However, in low doses, or when produced locally in tubular epithelial cells, endothelin decreases the reabsorption of salt and water, consistent with ET-1 target sites on renal tubules.[319] Also, administration of the endothelin precursor, big endothelin, has been shown to cause natriuresis, which supports the notion of a direct inhibitory autocrine action of endothelin on tubular salt reabsorption.[320]

The natriuretic and diuretic actions of big ET-1 can be significantly reduced by ET-B–specific blockade given acutely and chronically by osmotic minipump.[321] Furthermore, ET-B knockout rats have salt-sensitive hypertension that is reversed by luminal ENaC blockade with amiloride, which suggests that ET-B in the collecting duct in vivo tonically inhibits ENaC activity, the final regulator of Na^+ balance.[322] Similarly, mice with collecting duct–specific knockout of the ET-1 gene have impaired Na^+ excretion in response to Na^+ load and develop hypertension with a high salt intake.[311] These mice also have heightened sensitivity to AVP and reduced ability to excrete an acute water load. These findings are in line with in vitro observations that ET-B mediates the inhibitory effects of ET-1 on Na^+ and water transport in the collecting duct and thick ascending limb of Henle.[311] Thus, if vascular and mesangial endothelin exerts a greater physiologic effect than tubule-derived endothelin, then RBF is diminished and net fluid retention occurs, whereas if the tubule-derived endothelin effect predominates, salt and water excretion are increased.

The ability of ET-1 to inhibit AVP-stimulated water permeability reversibly was first shown in the isolated perfused IMCD.[323] ET-1 also reduces AVP-stimulated cAMP accumulation and water permeability in the IMCD,[311] and mitigates the hydroosmotic effect of AVP in the cortical and outer medullary collecting ducts.[311] Furthermore, studies of the rabbit cortical collecting duct have demonstrated that ET-1 may inhibit the luminal amiloride-sensitive ENaC by a Ca^{2+}-dependent effect. Moreover, collecting duct–specific ET-1 knockout mice were shown to have an impaired ability to excrete Na^+ and water loads in comparison with their wild-type counterparts. Taking into account the fact that the medulla contains ET-B receptors and the highest endothelin concentrations in the body, and that endothelins also inhibit Na^+-K^+-ATPase in IMCD,[311] these effects may contribute to the diuretic and natriuretic actions of locally produced ET-1. This may also explain the natriuretic effect of ET-1 reported by some investigators, despite the reduction in RBF and GFR.[324]

Endothelin production in the kidneys is regulated differently than in the vasculature. Whereas vascular (and mesangial) endothelin generation is controlled by thrombin, Ang II, and transforming growth factor–β, tubular endothelin production seems to depend on entirely different mechanisms, of which medullary tonicity may be particularly important. Volume expansion in humans increases urinary endothelin excretion, suggestive of an inhibitory action of renal endothelin on water reabsorption, particularly in the collecting duct.[311] Also, a high-salt diet, by raising medullary tonicity, stimulates ET-1 release, which in turn leads to increased eNOS (NOS3) expression and natriuresis.[310] (The NOS-dependent ET-1 effects are discussed further in the "Nitric Oxide" section, below). Therefore, salt and water balance appear to regulate renal endothelin production and collecting duct fluid reabsorption by altering medullary tonicity. The signaling mechanisms for these phenomena, as well other renal actions of ET-1, continue to be a subject of intensive research, and the interested reader is referred to a recent review that summarizes the current state of knowledge.[311]

Nitric Oxide. Nitric oxide (NO) is a diffusible gaseous molecule produced from its precursor L-arginine by the enzyme NOS, which exists in three distinct isoforms—nNOS (NOS1), inducible NOS (iNOS, or NOS2), and eNOS (NOS3).[321] NOS is expressed in endothelial cells of the renal vasculature (mainly eNOS), tubular epithelial and mesangial cells, and macula densa (mainly nNOS). There is controversy regarding the renal expression of iNOS in normal kidneys, but upregulation of this isoform is clearly seen in pathologic conditions such as ischemia-reperfusion injury.[325]

The availability of selective NOS inhibitors and NOS knockout mice has facilitated the investigation of the individual role of the NOS isoforms in the regulation of renal function.[325] However, the role of specific nitric oxide isoforms in a given cell type is still a work in progress. Therefore, this discussion refers to the renal effects of nitric oxide regardless of its isoform, unless otherwise specified.

The action of nitric oxide is mediated by activation of a soluble guanylate cyclase (sGC), thereby increasing intracellular levels of its second messenger, cGMP.[326] In the kidneys, the physiologic roles of nitric oxide include the regulation of glomerular hemodynamics, attenuation of TGF, mediation of pressure natriuresis, maintenance of medullary perfusion, inhibition of tubular Na^+ reabsorption, and modulation of RSNA.[321,327] Renal NOS activity is regulated by several humoral factors, such as Ang II (see earlier section, "Tubuloglomerular Feedback") and salt intake.[126]

The role of nitric oxide in the regulation of renal hemodynamics and excretory function is best illustrated by the fact that inhibition of intrarenal nitric oxide production results in increased blood pressure and impaired renal function.[325] Infusion of the NOS inhibitor, N^G-monomethyl-L-arginine (L-NMMA), into one kidney in anesthetized dogs resulted in a dose-dependent decrease in urinary cGMP levels, decreases in RBF and GFR, Na^+ and water retention, and a decline in fractional Na^+ excretion in the ipsilateral kidney in comparison with the contralateral kidney.[328] In addition, acute nitric oxide blockade amplified the renal vasoconstrictive action of Ang II in isolated microperfused rabbit afferent arterioles and in conscious rats, which suggests that nitric oxide and Ang II interact in the control of renal vasculature.[126,325] This concept is supported by the finding that L-NMMA–induced vasoconstriction leads to decreased RBF and Kf and is prevented by RAAS blockade; thus, some of the major effects of nitric oxide are to counterbalance the vasoconstrictive action of Ang II.

Nitric oxide has also been shown to exert a vasodilatory action on afferent arterioles and to mediate the renal vasorelaxant actions of acetylcholine, but not bradykinin.[329] The counterbalancing effect of nitric oxide on Ang II–induced efferent arteriolar vasoconstriction and its role in regulating TGF and in modulating renin secretion by the juxtaglomerular apparatus have been discussed earlier (see section, "Tubuloglomerular Feedback").[126,127]

The involvement of nitric oxide in the regulation of Na^+ balance is well characterized. In conscious dogs on a normal Na^+ diet, nitric oxide inhibition induces a significant decrease in natriuresis and diuresis without a change in arterial pressure. In dogs receiving a high-Na^+ diet and treatment with the nitric oxide inhibitor, N^G-nitro-L-arginine methyl ester (L-NAME), both arterial pressure and cumulative Na^+ balance were higher than in dogs receiving a comparable diet but no treatment with nitric oxide inhibitors.[330] Exposure of rats to a high salt intake (1% NaCl drinking water) for 2 weeks induced increased serum concentration and urinary excretion of the nitric oxide metabolites, NO_2 and NO_3. Urinary $NO_2 + NO_3$ and Na^+ excretion were significantly correlated. The increase in urinary nitric oxide metabolites is attributed to the enhanced expression of all three NOS isoforms in the renal medulla by high salt intake.[127] These findings suggest that nitric oxide has a role in promoting diuresis and natriuresis in normal and increased salt intake/volume-expanded states.[321]

The action of L-NAME infused directly into the renal medullary interstitium of anesthetized rats to reduce papillary blood flow, in association with decreased Na^+ and water excretion, indicates that nitric oxide exerts a vasodilatory effect on the renal medullary circulation and promotes Na^+ excretion.[170] Consistent with these data are the findings of high levels of eNOS in the renal medulla and the inhibitory effect of nitric oxide on Na^+-K^+-ATPase in the collecting duct.[331] Additional evidence of the involvement of the nitric oxide system in Na^+ homeostasis has been derived from studies in which researchers examined the mechanism of salt-sensitive hypertension. According to these studies, activity of NOS, mainly nNOS, is significantly lower in salt-sensitive rats than in salt-resistant rats maintained on a high-salt diet.[332,333] In another study, intravenous L-arginine increased nitric oxide production and prevented the development of salt-induced hypertension in Dahl salt-sensitive rats.[334] These findings suggest that nNOS plays an important role in Na^+ handling and that decreases in nNOS activity may in part be involved in the mechanism of salt-sensitive hypertension.

The involvement of nitric oxide in the abnormal Na^+ handling in hypertension could result from an inadequate direct effect on tubular Na^+ reabsorption in proximal and distal segments. However, attenuated inhibitory actions of nitric oxide on renin secretion and TGF may also contribute to salt retention and subsequent hypertension. In this context, investigators concluded that nitric oxide originating from the macula densa blunted the TGF-mediated vasoconstriction during high salt intake in salt-resistant rats, whereas in salt-sensitive rats, this response was lost.[335] As noted, there is strong evidence that the medullary and other effects of nitric oxide occur in response to local endothelin production.[321] For example, the inhibition of NOS by L-NAME or the highly selective ET-B antagonist A-192621 abolished the diuretic and natriuretic effects of big ET-1 in the kidneys of anesthetized rats.[336] In addition, ET-1 acutely activated eNOS in the isolated medullary thick ascending limb of Henle and nNOS in isolated IMCD cells, via ET-B activation. Studies in ET-B receptor–deficient rats have shown that this activation of nNOS and eNOS is accompanied by an increase in nNOS protein but no change in messenger RNA expression.[321] These data suggest that nNOS and eNOS activation occur by posttranscriptional pathways. NO also reduces Cl^- absorption in the cortical collecting duct (CCD) through a mechanism that is ENaC dependent.[337]

Activation of eNOS in the IMCD, where the highest renal NOS activity is found,[338] is also associated with inhibition of Na^+ reabsorption in the medullary thick ascending limb of Henle through phosphatidylinositol-3-kinase (PI3K)–stimulated Akt activity, leading to eNOS phosphorylation at Ser1177.[339] Thus, ET-1 has a paracrine effect on eNOS expression in the IMCD. However, the functional corollary of nNOS activation in the IMCD remains to be determined. A further action of nitric oxide is the inhibition of AVP-enhanced Na^+ reabsorption and hydroosmotic water permeability of the cortical collecting duct.[340] A new mouse model of specific collecting duct NOS1 gene deletion should be a valuable tool to study the signaling mechanisms involved in the nitric oxide effects on AVP-enhanced Na^+ reabsorption, as well as salt-dependent blood pressure mechanisms in general.[327] The role of nitric oxide in pressure natriuresis and RSNA is discussed in the relevant sections.

Kinins. The kallikrein-kinin system is a complex cascade responsible for the generation and release of vasoactive kinins. The active peptides bradykinin and kallidin are formed from precursors (kininogens) that are cleaved by tissue and circulatory kinin-forming enzymes.[341] Kinins are produced by many cell types and can be detected in urine, saliva, sweat, interstitial fluid and, in rare cases, venous blood. The levels of bradykinin in the circulation are almost undetectable because of rapid metabolism by kininases, particularly kininase II/ACE1. The renal kallikrein-kinin system can produce local concentrations of bradykinin much higher than those present in blood. In the kidneys, bradykinin is metabolized by NEP.[342]

Kinins play an important role in hemodynamic and excretory processes through their G protein–coupled receptors, BK-B_1 and BK-B_2. The BK-B_2 receptors mediate most of the actions of kinins[342] and are located mainly in the kidneys, although they are also detectable in the heart, lungs, brain, uterus, and testes. Activation of BK-B_2 receptors results in vasodilation, probably through a nitric oxide– or arachidonic acid metabolite–dependent mechanism.[341] For example, bradykinin selectively increases perfusion of the medulla, especially of its inner layer, via activation of the NO system and of Ca^{2+}-activated K^+ channels.[343] Bradykinin is known for its multiple effects on the cardiovascular system, particularly vasodilation and plasma extravasation.[344]

In addition to the vasculature, the kidney is an important target organ of kinins, in which they induce diuresis and natriuresis through activation of BK-B_2 receptors. These effects are attributed to an increase in RBF and to inhibition of Na^+ and water reabsorption via ENaC in the distal nephron.[345] The latter effect is secondary to the observed action of kinins in reducing vascular resistance. Unlike many vasodilators, bradykinin increases RBF without significantly affecting GFR or Na^+ reabsorption at the proximal tubule level, but the accompanying marked decrease in water and salt reabsorption in the distal nephron contributes significantly to increased urine volume and Na^+ excretion.

Studies with transgenic animals have enriched the understanding of the physiologic role of the kinins and the interaction between the kallikrein-kinin system and the RAAS.[344] For example, in the kidneys, Ang II acting through the AT_2 receptor stimulates a vasodilator cascade of bradykinin, nitric oxide, and cGMP during conditions of increased Ang II, such as Na^+ depletion.[328] In the absence of the AT_2 receptor, pressor and antinatriuretic hypersensitivity to Ang II is associated with bradykinin and nitric oxide deficiency.[328] Furthermore, involvement of the renal kinins in pressure natriuresis has been documented.[172] Bradykinin also mediates the biologic actions of angiotensin-(1-7), as shown in rats transgenic for the kallikrein gene, which display significantly augmented angiotensin-(1-7)–mediated diuresis and natriuresis.[346] Because ACE is involved in the degradation of kinins, ACE inhibitors not only attenuate the formation of Ang II but may also lead to the accumulation of kinins. The latter are believed to be responsible in part for the beneficial effects of ACE inhibitors in patients with HF, but also for their troublesome side effect of cough.[347] On the basis of the results of these studies, as well as those in which $BK-B_2$-specific antagonists were used, the kallikrein-kinin system is believed to play a pivotal role in the regulation of fluid and electrolyte balance, mainly by acting as a counterregulatory modulator of vasoconstrictor and Na^+-retaining mechanisms.

Adrenomedullin. Human adrenomedullin (AM) is a 52–amino acid peptide that was discovered in 1993 in extracts of human pheochromocytoma cells.[348] Adrenomedullin is approximately 30% homologous in structure with calcitonin gene–related peptide and amylin.[348,349] Adrenomedullin is produced from a 185–amino acid preprohormone that also contains a unique 20–amino acid sequence in the NH_2-terminus, termed *proadrenomedullin NH_2-terminal 20 peptide*. This sequence exists in vivo and has biologic activity similar to that of AM.

Adrenomedullin messenger RNA is expressed in several tissues, including those of the atria, ventricles, vascular tissue, lungs, kidneys, pancreas, smooth muscle cells, small intestine, and brain. The synthesis and secretion of AM are stimulated by chemical factors and physical stress. Among these stimulants are cytokines, corticosteroids, thyroid hormones, Ang II, norepinephrine, endothelin, bradykinin, and shear stress.[349] AM immunoreactivity has been localized in high concentrations in pheochromocytoma cells, adrenal medulla, atria, pituitary gland and, at lower levels, in cardiac ventricles, vascular smooth muscle cells, endothelial cells, glomeruli, distal and medullary collecting tubules, and digestive, respiratory, reproductive, and endocrine systems.[349]

Adrenomedullin acts through a 395–amino acid membrane receptor that structurally resembles a G protein–coupled receptor and contains seven transmembrane domains. AM receptors constitute the calcitonin receptor-like receptor and a family of receptor activity–modifying proteins.[350] Activation of these receptors increases intracellular cAMP, which probably serves as a second messenger for the peptide.[349] The most impressive biologic effect of AM is long-lasting and dose-dependent vasodilation of the vascular system, including the coronary arteries.[351] Injection of AM into anesthetized rats, cats, or conscious sheep induces a potent and long-lasting hypotensive response associated with reduction in vascular resistance in the kidneys, brain, lungs, hind limbs, and mesentery.[349] The hypotensive action of AM is accompanied by increases in heart rate and cardiac output caused by positive inotropic effects.[349] The vasodilating effect of AM can be blocked by inhibiting NOS, which suggests that nitric oxide partly mediates the decrease in systemic vascular resistance.[352]

In addition to its hypotensive action, AM increases RBF through preglomerular and postglomerular arteriolar vasodilation.[353,354] The AM-induced hyperperfusion is associated with dose-dependent diuresis and natriuresis.[349,353] These effects result from a decrease in tubular Na^+ reabsorption, despite the AM-induced hyperfiltration[354] and may be mediated partially by locally released nitric oxide[355,356] and prostaglandins.[357] In addition, NEP inhibition potentiates exogenous AM-induced natriuresis without affecting GFR.[358] Like NPs, AM suppresses aldosterone secretion in response to Ang II and high potassium levels.[349] Furthermore, in cultured vascular smooth muscle cells, AM inhibits endothelin production induced by various stimuli.[349] AM acts in the CNS to inhibit water and salt intake.[349] In the hypothalamus, AM inhibits the secretion of AVP, an effect that may also contribute to its diuretic and natriuretic actions.[349]

Together, these findings show that AM is a vasoactive peptide that may be involved in the physiologic control of renal, adrenal, vascular, and cardiac function. Furthermore, the existence of AM-like immunoreactivity in the glomerulus and collecting tubule, in association with detectable amounts of AM messenger RNA in the kidneys, suggests that AM plays a renal paracrine role.[359]

Two other members of the AM family, AM-2 (intermedin) and AM-5, have been identified. AM-2 is about 30% homologous with AM and has renal and cardiovascular effects similar to those of AM-1. AM-5 has cardiovascular effects similar to those of AM-1, but no apparent renal effects, in normal animals.[360,361]

Urotensin. Urotensin II is a highly conserved peptide that binds to the human orphan G protein–coupled receptor GPR14, now termed the *urotensin II receptor*. The parent peptide, prepro–urotensin II, is widely expressed in human tissues, including those of the CNS and peripheral nervous system, GI tract, vascular system, and kidneys.[362] In the kidneys, immunoreactive staining for urotensin II was detected in the epithelial cells of the tubules, mostly in the distal tubule, with moderate staining in endothelial cells of the renal capillaries.[362] The C-terminus of the prohormone is cleaved to produce urotensin II, an 11–amino acid residue peptide. The human form of urotensin II includes a cyclic hexapeptide sequence that is fundamental for the action of this compound. The metabolic pathway leading to the production of urotensin II still remains incompletely characterized. Substantial urotensin II arteriovenous gradients (36% to 44%) have been demonstrated in the heart, liver, and kidneys, indicative of local urotensin II production.[363]

In vivo in humans, systemic infusion of urotensin II range leads to local vasoconstriction in the forearm, no effect, or cutaneous vasodilation.[364] These dissimilarities are probably attributable to many factors, including species variation, site and modality of injection, dose, vascular bed, and functional conditions of the experimental model.[364] Because urotensin II has been described as the most potent vasoconstrictor (see earlier section, "Endothelin"), it is reasonable to postulate that the vasoconstrictive action is direct, whereas the vasodilatory response may be mediated by other factors, such as cyclo-oxygenase products and nitric oxide.

The involvement of the urotensin II system in the regulation of renal function in mammals is still unclear, and the data reported to date are as contradictory as those for vascular tone. In normal rats, intravenous boluses in the nanomolar range caused minor reductions in GFR and no effect on Na^+ excretion.[362] However, in another study in which the same model was used, continuous infusion of urotensin II at doses in the picomolar range elicited clear increases in GFR and nitric oxide–dependent diuresis and natriuresis.[362] In contrast, bolus injections in the picomolar range produced a dose-dependent decrease in GFR associated with reduced urine flow and Na^+ excretion.[303] Studies in rats with an aortocaval fistula (a model of chronic volume overload) have shown that urotensin II boluses in the nanomolar range exert favorable, nitric oxide–dependent, renal hemodynamic effects.[362] Thus, the effect of urotensin II on renal function seems dependent on the modality of administration (bolus vs. continuous infusion) and on the experimental condition being investigated (normal rats vs. those with heart failure).

The variability in renal and vascular responses to urotensin II administration may also depend on the fact that the action of this peptide is regulated at the receptor level. The binding density of urotensin II is correlated with vasoconstrictor response in rats, and small changes in receptor density may result in pathophysiologic effects. Under normal conditions, most urotensin II receptors are already occupied by urotensin II. Changes in unoccupied receptor reserve—perhaps in response to alterations in urotensin II levels generated in experimental models or observed in disease states—might explain, at least in part, the observed variability in studies of renal and vascular function.[362]

Selective urotensin II receptor antagonists have been developed, the most potent of which currently is urantide. In normal rats, continuous administration of this compound increases GFR, as well as urine flow and Na^+ excretion.[365] On the basis of experimental results indicating that urotensin II increases epithelial Na^+ transport in fish, it appears likely that urotensin II exerts a direct tubular effect, inasmuch as its receptor is expressed in the distal tubule.[365] In light of the contradictory effects of urotensin II on renal function, the focus on potential clinical applications of urotensin 2 inhibition has moved away from the kidney to the treatment of chronic lung and cardiovascular diseases.[362]

Digitalis-Like Factors. In the early 1960s, Clarkson, de Wardener, and coworkers[366,367] hypothesized the existence of endogenous digitalis-like factors, and an endogenous ouabain-like compound in human and other mammalian plasma was initially reported in the late 1970s. Since 2000, interest in such factors—also known as endogenous cardiotonic steroids—has expanded considerably. In particular, two specific cardiotonic steroids in humans have been characterized extensively, endogenous cardenolide (or ouabain) and bufadienolide (marinobufagenin). An alternative mechanism whereby cardiotonic steroids can signal through the Na^+-K^+-ATPase has also been described.[305] The main site of synthesis of these compounds is the adrenal cortex,[10] and the main consequences of Na^+ pump inhibition are attenuation of renal Na^+ transport and increased cytosolic Ca^{2+} in vascular smooth muscle cells, which lead to increased vascular resistance.[306] The latter mechanism has been implicated in the pathogenesis of hypertension.[368] These hormones also play a role in the regulation of cell growth, differentiation, apoptosis, and fibrosis, in the modulation of immunity and carbohydrate metabolism, and in the control of various central nervous functions, including behavior.[369,370]

Neuropeptide Y. Neuropeptide Y, a 36-residue peptide, is a sympathetic cotransmitter stored and released together with noradrenaline by adrenergic nerve terminals of the SNS. Structurally, neuropeptide Y is highly homologous to two other members of the pancreatic polypeptide family, peptide YY and pancreatic polypeptide. These two closely related peptides are produced and released by the intestinal endocrine and pancreatic islet cells, respectively, and act as hormones.[371,372] Although neuropeptide Y was originally isolated from the brain and is highly expressed in the CNS, the peptide exhibits a wide spectrum of biologic activities in the cardiovascular system, GI tract, and kidneys through multiple $G_{i/o}$ protein–coupled receptors—Y1, Y2, Y4, and Y5.[372,373]

In numerous studies, in vivo and in vitro techniques have demonstrated the capacity of neuropeptide Y to reduce RBF and increase renal vascular resistance in various species, including humans.[372] Despite the potent vasoconstrictor effect of the peptide on renal vasculature, this effect does not appear to be associated with any significant change in GFR. Similarly, neuropeptide Y may exert a natriuretic or antinatriuretic action, depending on the experimental conditions and the species studied.[372] These data suggest that neuropeptide Y is unlikely to have a significant role in the physiologic regulation of renal hemodynamics and electrolyte excretion.

Apelin. Apelin is the endogenous ligand of the angiotensin-like receptor 1, a G protein–coupled receptor found to be involved in various physiologic events, such as water homeostasis, regulation of cardiovascular tone, and cardiac contractility.[374] Apelin and its receptor are widely expressed in the CNS and in peripheral tissues, especially in endothelial cells. Apelin is also expressed in endothelial and vascular smooth muscle cells of glomerular arterioles and, to a lesser extent, in other parts of the nephron.[374]

Angiotensin-like receptor 1 activation leads to inhibition of cAMP production and activation of the Na^+/H^+ exchanger type 1. Through the former pathway, apelin enhances vascular dilation after the induction of eNOS, whereas the burst of Na^+/H^+ exchanger type 1 activity in cardiomyocytes leads to a dose-dependent increase in myocardial contractility.[374] With regard to the renal effects of apelin, direct injection into the hypothalamus of lactating rats inhibited AVP release and reduced circulating AVP. Conversely, water deprivation led to increased systemic AVP and decreased apelin levels.[374] These findings suggest that AVP and apelin have a reciprocal relationship in controlling water diuresis.

Apelin appears to also counterregulate several effects of Ang II. For example, intravenous injection of apelin caused a nitric oxide–dependent fall in arterial pressure. Moreover, apelin receptor knockout mice displayed an enhanced vasopressor response to systemic Ang II.[375] In addition, apelin modulated the abnormal aortic vascular tone in response to Ang II through eNOS phosphorylation in diabetic mice; this finding provided further evidence of a role for apelin in vascular function.[374] Intravenous injection of apelin also induced a significant diuresis and caused vasorelaxation of Ang II–preconstricted efferent and afferent arterioles. Activation of endothelial apelin receptors caused release of nitric oxide, which inhibited the Ang II–induced rise in intracellular Ca^{2+} levels. Furthermore, apelin had a direct receptor-mediated vasoconstrictive effect on vascular smooth muscle.[375] These results indicate that apelin has complex effects on the preglomerular and postglomerular microvasculature regulating renal hemodynamics. A direct role in tubular function remains to be determined but is suggested by collecting duct expression in close proximity to the vasopressin V_2 receptor.[376]

Glucagon-Like Peptide-1

The incretin hormone glucagon-like peptide-1 (GLP-1) is released from the gut in response to fat or carbohydrate and contributes to negative feedback control of blood glucose by stimulating insulin secretion, inhibiting glucagon, and slowing gastric emptying. GLP-1 receptors (GLP-1Rs) are also expressed in the proximal tubule and possibly elsewhere in the kidney. The GLP-1 agonist, exenatide, has natriuretic effects by reducing proximal tubular reabsorption of sodium, an effect that may be mediated by Ang II inhibition. Exenatide also increased SNGFR by 33% to 50%, doubled early distal flow rate, and increased urine flow rate sixfold without altering the efficiency of glomerulotubular balance, TGF responsiveness, or the tonic influence of TGF. This implies that exenatide is a proximal diuretic and a renal vasodilator.[130,377] Because the natural agonist for the GLP-1 receptor is regulated by intake of fat and carbohydrate, but not by salt or fluid, the control of salt excretion by the GLP-1R system departs from the usual negative-feedback paradigm for regulating salt balance.[377]

Novel Factors

A novel intrarenal paracrine mechanism for sodium regulation in mice has been described. Earlier studies showed that changes in dietary acid-base load can reverse the direction of apical transport of the tricarboxylic acid intermediate, α-ketoglutarate (α-KG), in the proximal tubule and loop of Henle from reabsorption following an acid load to secretion following a base load.[378] Recent work on isolated microperfused cortical collecting ducts from $Oxgr1^{-/-}$ mice has indicated that the concentration of α-KG is sensed by the α-KG receptor, OXGR1, expressed in the type B and non-A, non-B intercalated cells of the connecting tubule and cortical collecting duct. Addition of 1 mM α-KG to the tubular lumen strongly stimulated Cl-dependent HCO_3^- secretion and electroneutral NaCl reabsorption in tubules of wild-type but not $Oxgr1^{-/-}$ mice. $Oxgr1^{-/-}$ mice also displayed significantly increased functional activity of ENaC, without changes in plasma aldosterone.[378] In contrast, α-KG has been shown to inhibit amiloride-sensitive sodium reabsorption in principal cells independently of OXGR1 activation. This effect is possibly related to increased ATP production inducing autocrine activation of P2Y2 receptors and, thereby, inhibition of ENaC.[379] It appears that receptor-dependent and receptor-independent effects of α-KG converge to compensate for an alkalosis-induced decrease in proximal tubular reabsorption of NaCl by favoring NaCl reabsorption over Na^+/K^+ exchange along the connecting tubule and cortical collecting duct.[378] Taken together, the data indicate that α-KG acts as a paracrine mediator involved in the functional coordination of proximal and distal parts of the tubule in the adaptive regulation of HCO_3^- secretion and NaCl reabsorption in the presence of acid-base disturbances.[378]

Members of the epidermal growth factor (EGF) family have been shown to be important for maintaining transepithelial Na^+ transport. For example, a high salt diet was shown to decrease cortical EGF levels promoting ENaC-mediated Na^+ reabsorption in the collecting duct and the development of hypertension. Conversely, EGF infused intravenously decreased ENaC activity, prevented the development of hypertension, and attenuated glomerular and renal tubular damage in the Dahl salt-sensitive rat.[380] The implications of these observations are eagerly awaited.

The role of obesity in the pathogenesis of hypertension and renal dysfunction has led to the exploration of appetite-related hormones in salt and water retention. In this context, the orexigenic hormone, ghrelin, secreted by the stomach, has recently been shown to stimulate Na^+ absorption through cAMP-dependent trafficking of ENaC in the cortical collecting duct. The effect appears to be mediated via ghrelin receptors in this nephron segment.[381] Although ghrelin seems to be a physiologic regulator of ENaC, future studies will be needed to clarify its physiologic and pathologic roles in sodium homeostasis.[382]

Another novel development is the growing interest in the circadian rhythmicity of many basic physiologic functions. These functional rhythms are driven, in part, by the circadian clock, a ubiquitous molecular mechanism allowing cells and tissues to anticipate regular environmental events and to prepare for them. This mechanism has been shown to play a role in the regulation and maintenance of RPF, GFR, tubular reabsorption, and secretion of Na^+, Cl^- and K^+.[383] Studies in clock-deficient mice have identified the 20-HETE synthesis pathway as one of the clock's principal renal targets to mediate Na^+ excretion.[384] The researchers suggested that the circadian clock affects blood pressure, at least in part, by exerting dynamic control over renal sodium handling.

Rhythmicity of salt regulation seems to occur not only at the circadian level but also on a longer periodic basis (so-called infradian rhythms). In a fascinating study on men involved in space flight simulations, Rakova and colleagues[385] have shown that even on fixed salt diets (6, 9, or 12 g/day), daily Na^+ excretion exhibited aldosterone-dependent, weekly (circaseptan) rhythms, resulting in periodic Na^+ storage. Changes in total-body Na^+ (±200 to 400 mmol) exhibited monthly or longer period lengths, without parallel changes in body weight and extracellular water. These changes were directly related to urinary aldosterone excretion and inversely to urinary cortisol, suggesting rhythmic hormonal control. These findings suggest the existence of rhythmic Na⁺ excretory and retention patterns independent of blood pressure or body water and irrespective of salt intake.[385]

SODIUM BALANCE DISORDERS

HYPOVOLEMIA

DEFINITION

Hypovolemia is the condition in which the volume of the ECF compartment is reduced in relation to its capacitance. As noted, the reduction may be absolute or relative. In states of absolute hypovolemia, the Na⁺ balance is truly negative, reflecting past or ongoing losses. Hypovolemia is described as *relative* when there is no Na⁺ deficit but the capacitance of the ECF compartment is increased. In this situation, of reduced EABV, the ECF intravascular and extravascular (interstitial) compartments may vary in the same or opposite directions. ICF volume, reflected by measurements of plasma Na⁺ or osmolality, may or may not be concomitantly disturbed; thus, hypovolemia may be classified as normonatremic, hyponatremic, or hypernatremic (see Chapter 16).

ETIOLOGY

The causes of hypovolemia are summarized in Table 15.5. Absolute and relative hypovolemia, in turn, can have extrarenal or renal causes. Absolute hypovolemia results from massive blood loss or from fluid loss from the skin, GI or respiratory system, or kidneys. Relative hypovolemia results from states of vasodilation, generalized edema, or third-space loss. In absolute and relative hypovolemia, the perceived reduction in intravascular volume prompts the compensatory hemodynamic changes and renal responses described earlier (see section, "Physiology").

PATHOPHYSIOLOGY

Absolute Hypovolemia

Extrarenal. The most common causes of absolute hypovolemia include persistent diarrhea, vomiting, and massive bleeding, either gastrointestinal or as a result of trauma. The reduction in ECF volume is isotonic inasmuch as there is a proportionate loss of water and plasma. The consequent fall in systemic blood pressure leads to compensatory tachycardia and vasoconstriction, and the ensuing altered transcapillary Starling hydraulic forces enable a shift of fluid from the interstitial to intravascular compartment. In addition, the neural and hormonal responses to hypovolemia (see section, "Physiology") result in renal Na⁺ and water retention, with the aim of restoring intravascular volume and hemodynamic stability.

Similar compensatory mechanisms become activated after fluid losses from the skin, GI system, and respiratory system. Because of the large surface area of the skin, large amounts of fluid can be lost from this tissue, which can be caused by burns or excessive perspiration. Severe burns allow the loss of large volumes of plasma and interstitial fluid and can lead rapidly to profound hypovolemia. Without medical intervention, hemoconcentration and hypoalbuminemia supervene. As occurs after massive bleeding, the fluid loss is isotonic, so plasma Na⁺ concentration and osmolality remain normal. In contrast, excessive sweating, induced by exertion in a hot environment, leads to hypotonic fluid loss as a result of the relatively low Na⁺ concentration in this fluid (20 to 50 mmol/L). The resulting hypovolemia may therefore be accompanied by hypernatremia and hyperosmolality, and the type of fluid replacement must be tailored accordingly (see Chapter 16).

In addition to oral intake, the GI tract is characterized by the entry of approximately 7 L of isotonic fluid, the overwhelming majority of which is reabsorbed in the large intestine. Hence, in normal conditions, fecal fluid loss is minimal. However, in the presence of pathologic conditions, such as vomiting, diarrhea, colostomy, and ileostomy secretions, especially those caused by infection, considerable or even massive fluid loss may occur. The ionic composition, osmolality, and pH of secretions vary according to the part of the GI tract involved; therefore, the resulting hypovolemia is associated with a large spectrum of electrolyte and acid-base abnormalities (see Chapters 17 and 18 for further discussion).

Table 15.5 Causes of Absolute and Relative Hypovolemia

Absolute
Extrarenal
Gastrointestinal fluid loss
Bleeding
Skin fluid loss
Respiratory fluid loss
Extracorporeal ultrafiltration
Renal
Diuretics
Obstructive uropathy/postobstructive diuresis
Hormone deficiency
Hypoaldosteronism
Adrenal insufficiency
Na+ wasting tubulopathies
Genetic
Acquired tubulointerstitial disease
Relative
Extrarenal
Edematous states
Heart failure
Cirrhosis
Generalized vasodilation
Sepsis
Drugs
Pregnancy
Third-space loss
Renal
Severe nephrotic syndrome

In contrast to the massive losses that can occur from the skin and GI system, fluid loss from the respiratory tract—as occurs in febrile states and in patients who receive mechanical ventilation with inadequate humidification—is usually modest, and hypovolemia ensues only in the presence of accompanying causes. Finally, a special situation in which hypovolemia can occur is after excessive ultrafiltration in dialysis patients (see Chapter 65).

Renal. As described earlier, when the GFR and plasma Na^+ concentration are normal, approximately 24,000 mmol of Na^+ is filtered/day. Even when GFR is markedly impaired, the amount of filtered Na^+ far exceeds the dietary intake. To maintain Na^+ balance, all but 1% of the filtered load is reabsorbed. However, if the integrity of one or more of the tubular reabsorptive mechanisms is impaired, serious Na^+ deficit and absolute volume depletion can occur. The causes of absolute renal Na^+ losses include pharmacologic agents and renal structural, endocrine, and systemic disorders (see Table 15.5). All the diuretics widely used to treat hypervolemic states may induce hypovolemia if administered in excess or inappropriately. In particular, the powerful loop diuretics furosemide, bumetanide, torsemide, and ethacrynic acid are often given in combination with diuretics acting on other tubular segments (e.g., thiazides, aldosterone antagonists, distal ENaC blockers, and carbonic anhydrase inhibitors). Patients receiving these combinations need to be carefully monitored and fluid balance scrupulously adjusted to prevent hypovolemia. Patients commonly at risk are those with HF or underlying hypertension who develop intercurrent infections.

In patients with hypertension, the frequent use of diuretics for treatment appreciably increases the risk of volume depletion. Osmotic diuretics, endogenous or exogenous, may also reduce tubular Na^+ reabsorption. Endogenous agents include urea, the principle molecule involved in the polyuric recovery phase of acute kidney injury and postobstructive diuresis, and glucose in hyperglycemia. In patients with increased intracranial pressure, exogenous agents, such as mannitol or glycerol, may be used to induce translocation of fluid from the ICF to the ECF compartment and decrease brain swelling. The resulting polyuria may be associated with electrolyte and acid-base disturbances, the nature of which depends on the complex interplay between fluid intake and intercompartmental fluid shifts.

Na^+ reabsorption may also be disrupted in inherited and acquired tubular disorders. Inherited disorders of the proximal tubules (e.g., Fanconi syndrome) and distal tubules (e.g., Bartter and Gitelman syndromes) may lead to salt-wasting states in association with other electrolyte or acid-base disturbances. Acquired disorders of Na^+ reabsorption may be acute, as in nonoliguric acute kidney injury, the period immediately after renal transplantation, the polyuric recovery phase of acute kidney injury, and postobstructive diuresis (see relevant chapters for further details), or they may be chronic as a result of tubulointerstitial diseases with a propensity for salt wasting. Chronic kidney disease of any cause is associated with heightened vulnerability to Na^+ losses because the ability to match tubular reabsorption with the sum of filtered load minus dietary intake is impaired.

In addition to intrinsic tubular disorders, endocrine and other systemic disturbances may lead to impaired Na^+ reabsorption. The principal endocrine causes are mineralocorticoid deficiency and resistance states. A controversial cause is the systemic disturbance known as cerebral salt wasting. In this condition, salt wasting is thought to occur in response to an as yet unidentified factor released in the setting of acute head injury or intracranial hemorrhage.[386,387] The condition is usually diagnosed because of concomitant hyponatremia, and some experts doubt its independent existence, regarding cerebral salt wasting as essentially indistinguishable from the syndrome of inappropriate antidiuretic hormone.[387,388]

An underappreciated, but not uncommon, clinical setting for renal Na^+ loss is after the administration of large volumes of intravenous saline to patients over several days after surgery or after trauma. In this situation, tubular reabsorption of Na^+ is downregulated. If intravenous fluids are stopped before full reabsorptive capacity is restored, volume depletion may ensue. The phenomenon can be minimized by graded reduction in the infusion rate, which allows Na^+ reabsorptive pathways to be restored gradually.

In the context of volume depletion, diabetes insipidus should be mentioned. However, because this results from a deficiency of or tubular resistance to AVP, water loss is the main consequence, and the impact on ECF volume is only minor. AVP-related disorders are considered in Chapters 10, 11, and 16.

Relative Hypovolemia

Extrarenal. As outlined previously, the principal causes of relative hypovolemia are edematous states, vasodilation, and third-space loss (see Table 15.5). Vasodilation may be physiologic, as in normal pregnancy, or induced by drugs (hypotensive agents, such as hydralazine or minoxidil, that cause arteriolar vasodilation), or it may occur in sepsis during the phase of peripheral vasodilation and consequent low systemic vascular resistance.[389]

Edematous states in which the EABV and, hence, tissue perfusion are reduced include HF, decompensated cirrhosis with ascites, and nephrotic syndrome. In severe HF, low cardiac output and resulting low systemic blood pressure lead to a fall in RPP. As in absolute hypovolemia, the kidneys respond by retaining Na^+. Because the increased venous return cannot raise the cardiac output, a vicious cycle is created in which edema is further exacerbated and the persistently reduced cardiac output leads to further Na^+ retention. In decompensated cirrhosis, splanchnic venous pooling leads to decreased venous return, a consequent fall in cardiac output, and compensatory renal Na^+ retention. The pathophysiologic features of edematous states are discussed later in more detail (see section, "Hypervolemia"). Third-space loss occurs when fluid is sequestered into compartments not normally perfused with fluids, as in states of GI obstruction, after trauma, with burns, or in pancreatitis, peritonitis, or malignant ascites. The end result is that even though total body Na^+ is markedly increased, the EABV is severely reduced.

Renal. Approximately 10% of patients with the nephrotic syndrome—especially children with minimal change disease, but also any patient with a serum albumin level lower than 2 g/dL—manifest the clinical signs of hypovolemia. The low plasma oncotic pressure is conducive to movement of fluid from the ECF compartment to the interstitial space, thereby leading to reduced EABV.[390,391]

CLINICAL MANIFESTATIONS

The clinical manifestations of hypovolemia depend on the magnitude and rate of volume loss, solute composition of the net fluid loss (i.e., the difference between input and output), and vascular and renal responses. The clinical features can be considered as being related to the underlying pathophysiologic process, hemodynamic consequences, and electrolyte and acid-base disturbances that accompany the renal response to hypovolemia. A detailed history often reveals the cause of volume depletion (bleeding, vomiting, diarrhea, polyuria, diaphoresis, medications).

The symptoms and physical signs of hypovolemia appear only when intravascular volume is decreased by 5% to 15% and are often related to tissue hypoperfusion. Symptoms include generalized weakness, muscle cramps, and postural lightheadedness. Thirst is prominent if concomitant hypertonicity is present (hypertonic hypovolemia). Physical signs are related to the hemodynamic consequences of hypovolemia and include tachycardia, hypotension, which may be postural, absolute, or relative to the usual blood pressure, and low central or jugular venous pressure. Elevation of jugular venous pressure, however, does not rule out hypovolemia, because of the possible confounding effects of underlying heart failure or lung disease. When volume depletion exceeds 10% to 20%, circulatory collapse is liable to occur, with severe supine hypotension, peripheral cyanosis, cold extremities, and impaired consciousness, extending even to coma. This is especially possible if fluid loss is rapid or occurs against a background of comorbid conditions. When the source of volume loss is extrarenal, oliguria also occurs. The traditional signs—reduced skin turgor, sunken eyes, and dry mucous membranes—are inconstant findings, and their absence is not considered useful for ruling out hypovolemia.

DIAGNOSIS

The diagnosis of hypovolemia is based essentially on the clinical findings. Nevertheless, when the clinical findings are equivocal, various laboratory parameters may be helpful for confirming the diagnosis or for elucidating other changes that may be associated with volume depletion.

Laboratory Findings

Hemoglobin. This may decrease if significant bleeding has occurred or is ongoing, but this change, which is caused by hemodilution that results from translocation of fluid from the interstitial to intravascular compartment, may take up to 24 hours. Therefore, stable hemoglobin does not rule out significant bleeding. Moreover, the adaptive response of hemodilution may moderate the severity of hemodynamic compromise and resulting physical signs. In hypovolemic situations that do not arise from bleeding, hemoconcentration is often seen, although this too is not universal, inasmuch as underlying chronic diseases that cause anemia may mask the differential loss of plasma.

Hemoconcentration may also be manifested as a rise in plasma albumin concentration if albumin-free fluid is lost from the skin, GI tract, or kidneys. On the other hand, when albumin is lost, either in parallel with other extracellular fluids (as in proteinuria, hepatic disease, protein-losing enteropathy, or catabolic states) or in protein-rich fluid (third-space sequestration, burns), significant hypoalbuminemia is observed.

Plasma Na^+ Concentration. This may be low, normal, or high, depending on the solute composition of the fluid lost and the replacement solution administered by the patient or the treating physician. For example, the hypovolemic stimulus for AVP release may lead to preferential water retention and hyponatremia, especially if hypotonic replacement fluid is used. In contrast, the fluid content of diarrhea may be hypotonic or hypertonic, resulting in hypernatremia or hyponatremia, respectively. The plasma Na^+ concentration reflects the tonicity of plasma and provides no direct information about volume status, which is a clinical diagnosis.

Plasma K^+ and Acid-Base Parameters. These can also change in hypovolemic conditions. After vomiting, and after some forms of diarrhea, loss of K^+ and Cl^- may lead to alkalosis. More often, the principal anion lost in diarrhea is bicarbonate, which leads to hyperchloremic (non–anion gap) acidosis. When diuretics or Bartter and Gitelman syndromes (the inherited tubulopathies; see Chapter 45) are the cause of hypovolemia, hypokalemic alkalosis is again typically seen. On the other hand, U_{Na} loss that occurs in adrenal insufficiency or is caused by aldosterone hyporesponsiveness is accompanied by a tendency for hyperkalemia and metabolic acidosis. Finally, when hypovolemia is sufficiently severe to impair tissue perfusion, high anion gap acidosis caused by lactic acid accumulation may be observed.

Blood Urea and Creatinine Levels. These frequently rise in hypovolemic states, and this elevation reflects impaired renal perfusion. If tubular integrity is preserved, then the rise in urea level is typically disproportionate to that of creatinine (see Chapter 31). This results mainly because AVP enhances reabsorption of urea in the medullary collecting duct and as an effect of an increased filtration fraction on proximal tubule handling of urea.[392] In the presence of severe hypovolemia, acute kidney injury may ensue, leading to loss of the differential rise in urea level. Proportional rises in urea and creatinine are also observed when hypovolemia occurs against a background of underlying renal functional impairment, as in chronic kidney disease, stages 3 to 5 (see Chapter 52).

Urine Biochemical Parameters. These can be extremely useful in establishing the diagnosis of hypovolemia caused by extrarenal fluid losses if there is no intrinsic renal injury and the patient is oliguric. The expected renal response of Na^+ and water conservation, by enhanced renal tubular reabsorption, results in oliguria, urine specific gravity exceeding 1.020, Na^+ concentration less than 10 mmol/L, and osmolality higher than 400 mOsm/kg. When Na^+ concentration is 20 to 40 mmol/L, the finding of a fractional excretion of Na^+ $\frac{[\text{urine } Na^+ \times \text{plasma creatinine}]}{[\text{plasma } Na^+ \times \text{urine creatinine}]} \times 100$ of less than 1% in the presence of a reduced GFR may be helpful. In a patient who previously had undergone diuretic therapy, especially with loop diuretics, these indices may merely reflect the U_{Na} losses. In that case, fractional excretion of urea from less than 30% to 35% may help in the diagnosis of hypovolemia, although the specificity of this test is rather low.[393-395]

When hypovolemia occurs in the presence of arterial vasodilation, as observed in sepsis, some, but not all, of the clinical manifestations of hypovolemia are observed. Thus, tachycardia and hypotension are usually present, but the extremities are warm, which suggests that perfusion is maintained. This finding is misleading because vital organs, particularly the brain and kidneys, are underperfused as a result of the hypotension. The presence of lactic acidosis helps establish the correct diagnosis. Reduction in the EABV, as manifested by relative hypotension, may be observed in generalized edematous states, even though there is an overall excess of Na^+ and water; however, this excess is maldistributed between the extracellular and interstitial spaces.

TREATMENT
Absolute Hypovolemia

General Principles. The goals of treatment of hypovolemia are to restore normal hemodynamic status and tissue perfusion. These goals are achieved by reversal of the clinical symptoms and signs, described previously. Treatment can be divided into three stages: (1) initial replacement of the immediate fluid deficit; (2) maintenance of the restored ECF volume in the presence of ongoing losses; and (3) treatment of the underlying cause, whenever possible. The main strategies to be addressed by the clinician are the route, volume, rate of administration, and composition of the replacement and maintenance fluids. These are liable to change according to the patient's response.

In general, when hypovolemia is associated with a significant hemodynamic disturbance, intravenous rehydration is required. (The use of oral electrolyte solutions in the management of infants and children is discussed in Chapter 75.) The volume of fluid and rate of administration should be determined on the basis of the urgency of the threat to circulatory integrity, adequacy of the clinical response, and underlying cardiac function. Older patients are especially vulnerable to aggressive fluid challenge, and careful monitoring is required, particularly to prevent acute left ventricular failure and pulmonary edema that result from overzealous correction.

Sometimes the clinical signs do not point unequivocally to the diagnosis of hypovolemia, even though the history is strongly suggestive. Because invasive monitoring of central venous and pulmonary venous pressures has not been shown to improve outcomes in this situation,[396,397] a so-called diagnostic fluid challenge can be performed. If the patient improves clinically, blood pressure and urine output increase, and no overt signs of heart failure appear over the succeeding 6 to 12 hours, then the diagnosis is substantiated and fluid therapy can be cautiously continued. Conversely, if overt signs of fluid overload appear, the fluid challenge can be stopped and diuretic therapy reinstituted.

The initial calculations for replacing the fluid deficit are based on hemodynamic status. It is notoriously difficult to calculate volume deficits; therefore, good clinical judgment is necessary for successful management. Patients with life-threatening circulatory collapse and hypovolemic shock require rapid intravenous replacement through the cannula with the widest bore possible. This replacement should continue until blood pressure is corrected and tissue perfusion is restored. In the second stage of fluid replacement, the rate of administration should be reduced to maintain blood pressure and tissue perfusion. In older patients and those with underlying cardiac dysfunction, the risk of over rapid correction and precipitating pulmonary edema is heightened; therefore, slower treatment is preferable, to allow gradual filling of the ECF volume rather than causing pulmonary edema and the threat of mechanical ventilation associated with adverse outcomes.[398,399]

Composition of Replacement Fluids. The composition of replacement fluid had been thought to be less critical than the rate of infusion. However, recent work has cast serious doubt on this and is discussed here. The two main categories of replacement solution are crystalloid and colloid solutions. Crystalloid solutions are based largely on NaCl of varying tonicity or dextrose. Isotonic (0.9%) saline, containing 154 mmol of Na^+/L, is the mainstay of volume replacement therapy inasmuch as it is confined to the ECF compartment in the absence of deviations in Na^+ concentration. One L of isotonic saline increases plasma volume by approximately 300 mL; the rest is distributed to the interstitial compartment. In contrast, 1 L of 5% dextrose in water (D_5W), which is also isosmotic (277 mOsm/L), is eventually distributed throughout all the body fluid compartments so that only 10% to 15% (100 to 150 mL) remains in the ECF. Therefore, D_5W should not be used for volume replacement.

Administration of 1 L of 0.45% saline (77 mmol of Na^+/L) in D_5W is equivalent to giving 500 mL of isotonic saline and the same volume of solute-free water. The distribution of the solute-free compartment throughout all the fluid compartments would result in plasma dilution and reduction in the plasma Na^+. Therefore, this solution should be reserved for the management of hypernatremic hypovolemia. Even in that situation, it must be remembered that volume replacement is less efficient than with isotonic saline and, early on during the treatment course, may cause plasma tonicity to fall too rapidly.

When hypovolemia is accompanied by severe metabolic acidosis (pH < 7.10; plasma HCO_3^- < 10 mmol/L), bicarbonate supplementation may be indicated. (For a discussion of bicarbonate balance, see Chapter 27.) Because this anion is manufactured as 8.4% sodium bicarbonate (1000 mmol/L) for use in cardiac resuscitation, appropriate dilution is required for the treatment of acidosis associated with hypovolemia. Nephrologists are frequently called on for consultation in these situations, and they should be ready to provide detailed protocols for the preparation of isotonic $NaHCO_3$. Two convenient methods are suggested. Either 75 mL (75 mmol) of 8.4% $NaHCO_3$ can be added to 1 L of 0.45% saline, or 150 mL of concentrated bicarbonate can be added to 1 L of D_5W. Although the latter is hypertonic in the short term, it is unlikely to be harmful.

In the presence of accompanying hypokalemia, especially if metabolic alkalosis is also present, volume replacement solutions must be supplemented with K^+. Commercially available 1-L solutions of isotonic saline supplemented with 10 or 20 mmol of KCl make this option safe and convenient. (For details, see Chapters 18 and 75.) On the other hand, other commercially available crystalloid solutions containing lactate (converted by the liver to bicarbonate) and low concentrations of KCl were traditionally regarded as offering no advantage and less flexibility than isotonic saline. This "dogma" was recently challenged by the findings of a large prospective observational study performed in the intensive care unit setting. In this study, two periods were compared; in the control period, all patients received isotonic saline as fluid replacement, whereas during the intervention period, Hartmann solution (lactate-containing), Plasma-Lyte 148 (a balanced salt solution), or chloride-poor 20% albumin solution was administered. The chloride-poor solutions were associated with a significantly lower risk of all stages of subsequent acute kidney injury, as defined by the RIFLE (Risk, Injury, Failure, Loss, End-stage renal disease) criteria, even after adjustment for covariates.[400] Clearly, these provocative results indicate the need for randomized control trials comparing chloride-rich with more balanced salt solutions for fluid resuscitation.[401]

Colloid solutions include plasma itself, albumin, and high-molecular-weight carbohydrate molecules, such as hydroxyethyl starch and dextrans, at concentrations that exert colloid osmotic pressures equal to or greater than that of plasma. Because the transcapillary barrier is impermeable to these large molecules, in theory they expand the intravascular compartment more rapidly and efficiently than crystalloid solutions. Colloid solutions may be useful in the management of burns and severe trauma when plasma protein losses are substantial, and rapid plasma expansion with relatively small volumes is efficacious. However, when capillary permeability is increased, as in states of multiorgan failure or the systemic inflammatory response syndrome, colloid administration is ineffective. Moreover, randomized controlled studies in which crystalloid solutions were compared with colloid solutions have shown no survival benefit and even harm with some colloid solutions, particularly hydroxyethyl starch.[402-404] Therefore, the much cheaper and more readily available crystalloid solutions should remain the mainstay of therapy pending further studies.

Relative Hypovolemia

Treatment of relative hypovolemia is more difficult than that of absolute hypovolemia because there is no real fluid deficit. If the relative hypovolemia is caused by peripheral vasodilation, as in a septic patient, it may be necessary to administer a crystalloid solution cautiously, such as isotonic saline, to maintain ECF volume until the systemic vascular resistance and venous capacitance return to normal. The excess volume administered can then be excreted by the kidneys. When vasodilation is more severe, vasoconstrictor agents may be needed to maintain systemic blood pressure. In the edematous states of severe HF, advanced cirrhosis with portal hypertension, and severe nephrotic syndrome, when EABV is low but there is an overall excess of Na^+ and water, treatment may be extremely problematic. Administration of crystalloid solution will, in all likelihood, lead to worsening interstitial edema without significantly affecting the EABV. In these situations, prognosis is determined by whether the underlying condition can be reversed.

Table 15.6 Causes of Renal Sodium Retention

Primary
Oliguric acute kidney injury
Chronic kidney disease
Glomerular disease
Severe bilateral renal artery stenosis
Na^+-retaining tubulopathies (genetic)
Mineralocorticoid excess
Secondary
Heart failure
Cirrhosis
Idiopathic edema

HYPERVOLEMIA

DEFINITION

Hypervolemia is the condition in which the volume of the ECF compartment is expanded in relation to its capacitance. In most people, increments in Na^+ intake are matched by corresponding changes in Na^+ excretion as a result of the actions of the compensatory mechanisms detailed earlier (see section, "Physiology"). In these cases, no clinically detectable changes are observed. However, in the approximately 20% of the population who are salt-sensitive, the upward shift in ECF volume induced by high salt intake leads to a persistent rise in systemic arterial pressure, albeit without other overt signs of fluid retention (see Chapter 47 for a detailed discussion). In the following sections, the discussion is confined to the strict definition of hypervolemia, in which Na^+ retention is ongoing and inappropriate for the prevailing ECF volume, with the appearance of clinical signs of volume overload.

ETIOLOGY

The causes of hypervolemia can be conveniently divided into two major categories, primary renal Na^+ retention and secondary retention resulting from compensatory mechanisms activated as a result of disease in other major organs (Table 15.6).

Primary Renal Na^+ Retention

This can be further subclassified as caused by intrinsic kidney disease or primary mineralocorticoid excess. Of the primary renal diseases causing Na^+ retention, oliguric renal failure limits the ability to excrete Na^+ and water, and affected patients are at risk for rapidly developing ECF volume overload (see Chapter 31). In contrast, in chronic kidney disease, renal tubular adaptation to salt intake is usually efficient until late stage 4 and stage 5. However, in some primary glomerular diseases, especially in the presence of nephrotic range proteinuria, significant Na^+ retention may occur, even when GFR is close to normal (see section, "Pathophysiology," and Chapters 52 and 54). Primary mineralocorticoid excess or enhanced activity, in their early phases, lead to transient Na^+ retention. However, because of the phenomenon of "mineralocorticoid escape," the dominant clinical expression of these diseases is hypertension.

Mineralocorticoid excess as a cause of secondary hypertension is discussed in Chapters 12 and 47.

Secondary Renal Na⁺ Retention

This occurs in low- and high-output cardiac failure and in systolic and diastolic dysfunction. Hepatic cirrhosis with portal hypertension and nephrotic syndrome are also accompanied by renal Na⁺ retention. In this chapter, only HF and cirrhosis are considered. Nephrotic syndrome is discussed in detail in Chapter 53.

PATHOPHYSIOLOGY

The cause of primary renal Na⁺ retention is clearly disruption of normal renal function. In contrast, secondary renal Na⁺ retention occurs because of reduced EABV in the presence of total ECF volume expansion or in response to various factors secreted by the heart or liver that signal the kidneys to retain Na⁺. In all conditions associated with secondary Na⁺ retention, the renal effector mechanisms that normally operate to conserve Na⁺ and protect against a Na⁺ deficit are exaggerated, and their actions continue, despite subtle or overt expansion of ECF volume. The pathophysiologic process of hypervolemia is comprised of local mechanisms of edema formation and systemic factors stimulating renal Na⁺ retention; systemic factors can be further subclassified as abnormalities of the afferent sensing limb or efferent effector limb.

Local Mechanisms of Edema Formation

Peripheral interstitial fluid accumulation, which is common to all conditions that cause ECF volume expansion, results from disruption of the normal balance of transcapillary Starling forces. Transcapillary fluid and solute transport can be viewed as consisting of two types of flow, convective and diffusive. Bulk water movement occurs via convective transport induced by hydraulic and osmotic pressure gradients. Capillary hydraulic pressure (P_c) is under the influence of a number of factors, including systemic arterial and venous blood pressures, local blood flow, and the resistances imposed by the precapillary and postcapillary sphincters. Systemic arterial blood pressure, in turn, is determined by cardiac output, intravascular volume, and systemic vascular resistance; systemic venous pressure is determined by right atrial pressure, intravascular volume, and venous capacitance. Na⁺ balance is a key determinant of these latter hemodynamic parameters. Also, massive accumulation of fluid in the peripheral interstitial compartment (anasarca) can itself diminish venous compliance and, hence, alter overall cardiovascular performance.[405]

The balance of Starling forces prevailing at the arteriolar end of the capillary ($\Delta P > \Delta \pi$, in which $\Delta \pi$ is the change in transcapillary oncotic pressure) is favorable for the net filtration of fluid into the interstitium. Net outward movement of fluid along the length of the capillary is associated with an axial decrease in P_c and an increase in π_c. Nevertheless, the local ΔP continues to exceed the opposing $\Delta \pi$ throughout the length of the capillary bed in several tissues; thus, filtration occurs along its entire length.[406] In such capillary beds, a substantial volume of filtered fluid must, therefore, return to the circulation via lymphatic vessels. In view of the importance of lymphatic drainage, the lymphatic vessels must be able to expand and proliferate, and the lymphatic flow must be able to increase in response to increased interstitial fluid formation; these mechanisms help minimize edema formation.

Several other mechanisms for minimizing edema formation have been identified. First, precapillary vasoconstriction tends to lower P_c and diminish the filtering surface area in a given capillary bed. In fact, in the absence of appropriate regulation of microcirculatory myogenic reflex, excessive precapillary vasodilation appears to account for interstitial edema in the lower extremities that is associated with some Ca^{2+} entry blocker vasodilators.[407] Second, increased net filtration itself is associated with dissipation of P_c, dilution of interstitial fluid protein concentration, and a corresponding rise in intracapillary plasma protein concentration. The resulting change in the profile of Starling forces in association with increased filtration, therefore, tends to mitigate further interstitial fluid accumulation.[1,408] Finally, interstitial fluid hydraulic pressure (P_i) is normally subatmospheric; however, even small increases in interstitial fluid volume tend to augment P_i, again opposing further transudation of fluid into the interstitial space.[409] The appearance of generalized edema therefore implies that one or more disturbances in microcirculatory hemodynamics is present in association with expansion of the ECF volume—increased venous pressure transmitted to the capillary, unfavorable adjustments in precapillary and postcapillary resistances, and/or inadequacy of lymphatic flow for draining the interstitial compartment and replenishing the intravascular compartment.

Insofar as the continued net accumulation of interstitial fluid without renal Na⁺ retention might result in prohibitive intravascular volume contraction and cessation of interstitial fluid formation, generalized edema is therefore indicative of substantial renal Na⁺ retention. The volume of accumulated interstitial fluid required for clinical detection of generalized edema (>2 to 3 L) necessitates that all states of generalized edema are associated with expansion of ECF volume and, hence, body exchangeable Na⁺ content. In summary, all states of generalized edema reflect past or ongoing renal Na⁺ retention.

Systemic Factors Stimulating Renal Sodium Retention

Reduced Effective Arterial Blood Volume. Renal Na⁺ (and water retention) in edematous disorders occurs, despite an increase in total blood and ECF volumes. In stark contrast, healthy individuals with the same degree of Na⁺ retention readily increase Na⁺ and water excretion. Moreover, intrinsic renal function, in the absence of underlying renal disease, is normal in edematous states. This fact is dramatically illustrated by the observation that after heart transplantation in patients with HF[410] or liver transplantation in patients with hepatic cirrhosis,[411] Na⁺ excretion is restored to normal. Similarly, when kidneys from patients with end-stage liver disease are transplanted into patients with normal liver function, Na⁺ retention no longer occurs.[411]

The paradox of Na⁺ retention in the presence of expanded total and ECF volume is explained by the concept of EABV (or threat to arterial pressure[15]), described earlier. In brief, because 85% of blood circulates in the venous compartment and only 15% in the arterial compartment, expansion of the venous compartment leads to overall ECF volume excess that could occur concurrently with arterial underfilling. Arterial underfilling could result from low cardiac output, peripheral arterial vasodilation, or a combination of the two. In turn, low cardiac output could result from true ECF volume depletion (see earlier discussion), cardiac failure, or decreased π_c, with or without increased capillary permeability. All these stimuli would cause activation of ventricular and arterial sensors. Similarly, conditions such as high-output cardiac failure, sepsis, cirrhosis, and normal pregnancy lead to peripheral arterial vasodilation and activation of arterial baroceptors. Activation of these afferent mechanisms would then induce the neurohumoral mechanisms that result in renal Na^+ and water retention (Figure 15.8).[412,413]

Although the mechanisms leading to Na^+ retention in HF and cirrhosis are similar, specific differences between the two conditions have been observed, and these findings are discussed separately in the following sections.

Renal Sodium Retention in Heart Failure

Abnormalities of Sensing Mechanisms in Heart Failure. Both the cardiopulmonary and baroceptor reflexes are blunted in HF, so that they cannot exert an adequate tonic inhibitory effect on sympathetic outflow.[414] The resulting activated SNS triggers renal Na^+ retention by the mechanisms already described. With regard to cardiopulmonary receptor reflexes, several researchers, using a variety of models of HF, have shown marked attenuation of atrial receptor firing in HF in response to volume expansion.[414] In addition, loss of nerve ending arborization has been observed directly.[414] Similarly, maneuvers that selectively alter central cardiac filling pressures (e.g., head-up tilt, LBNP) have shown that HF patients, in contrast to normal subjects, usually do not demonstrate significant alterations in limb blood flow, circulating catecholamines, AVP, or renin activity in response to postural stimuli.[415,416] This diminished reflex responsiveness may be most impaired in patients with the greatest ventricular dysfunction.

Arterial baroceptor reflex impairment in HF has been observed in humans and experimental models of HF. High baseline values of muscle sympathetic activity were found in patients with HF who failed to respond to activation and deactivation of arterial baroreceptors by infusion of phenylephrine and Na^+ nitroprusside, respectively.[414] Carotid and aortic baroreceptor function were also depressed in experimental models of cardiac failure.[414] These changes were associated with upward resetting of receptor threshold and a reduced range of pressures over which the receptors functioned.

Multiple abnormalities have been described in cardiopulmonary and arterial baroreceptor control of RSNA in HF. Thus, rats with coronary ligation displayed an increased basal level of efferent RSNA that failed to decrease normally during volume expansion.[76,277] Similarly, in sinoaortic denervated dogs with pacing-induced HF, the cardiopulmonary baroreflex control of efferent RSNA became markedly attenuated in response to cardiopulmonary receptor stimulation by volume expansion. Left atrial baroreceptor stimulation produced by inflation of small balloons at the junction of the left atrial-pulmonary vein produced the same effect.[417] The abnormal regulation of efferent RSNA was caused by impaired function of aortic and cardiopulmonary baroreflexes; the defect in cardiopulmonary baroreceptors was functionally more important.[277]

Several mechanisms have been implicated in the pathogenesis of the abnormal cardiopulmonary and arterial baroreflexes in HF. Zucker and colleagues[414] have suggested that loss of compliance in the dilated hearts, as well as gross changes in the structure of the receptors themselves, were the mechanisms underlying the depressed atrial receptor discharge in dogs with aortocaval fistula. In dogs with pacing-induced HF, the decrease in carotid sinus baroreceptor sensitivity was related to augmented Na^+-K^+-ATPase activity in the baroreceptor membranes.[414] Increased activity of Ang II through the AT_1 receptor has also been proposed to explain depressed baroreflex sensitivity in HF. Specifically, intracerebral or systemic administration of AT_1 receptor antagonists to rats or rabbits with HF significantly improved arterial baroreflex control of RSNA or heart rate, respectively.[417] Moreover, Ang II injected into the vertebral artery of normal rabbits significantly attenuated arterial baroreflex function. This effect of Ang II could be blocked by the central α_1-adrenoreceptor prazosin.[418] In addition, ACE inhibition augmented arterial and cardiopulmonary baroreflex control of sympathetic nerve activity in HF patients.[414]

More recent studies have indicated that Ang II in the paraventricular nucleus potentiates—and AT_1 receptor antisense messenger RNA normalizes—the enhanced cardiac sympathetic afferent reflex in rats with chronic heart failure.[414] AT_1 receptors in the nucleus tractus solitarii are thought to mediate the interaction between the baroreflex and cardiac sympathetic afferent reflex.[419] Consistent with this notion, Ang II generation is enhanced and its degradation reduced in central sympathoregulatory neurons, as shown by upregulation of ACE1 and downregulation of ACE2.[420] AT_2 receptors in the rostral ventrolateral medulla exhibited an inhibitory effect on sympathetic outflow, which was mediated at least partially by an arachidonic acid metabolic pathway.[421] These studies indicated that a downregulation in the AT_2 receptor was a contributory factor in the sympathetic neural excitation in HF.[414]

Together, these data provide evidence of the role of high endogenous levels of Ang II, acting through the AT_1 receptor in concert with downregulation of the AT_2 receptor, in the impaired baroreflex sensitivity observed in HF, both in the afferent limb of the reflex arch and at more central sites. The central effect may be mediated through a central α_1-adrenoreceptor. The blunted cardiopulmonary and arterial baroreceptor sensitivity in HF may also lead to an increase in AVP release and renin secretion.[414]

The disturbances in the sensing mechanisms that initiate and maintain renal Na^+ retention in HF are summarized in Figure 15.7. As indicated, a decrease in cardiac output or a diversion of systemic blood flow diminishes the blood flow to the critical sites of the arterial circuit with pressure- and flow-sensing capabilities. The responses to diminished blood flow culminate in renal Na^+ retention, mediated by the effector mechanisms. An increase in systemic venous pressure promotes the transudation of fluid from the intravascular to interstitial compartment by increasing the peripheral transcapillary ΔP. These processes augment the perceived loss of volume and flow in the arterial circuit. In addition, distortion of the pressure-volume relationships as a result of chronic dilation in the cardiac atria attenuates the normal

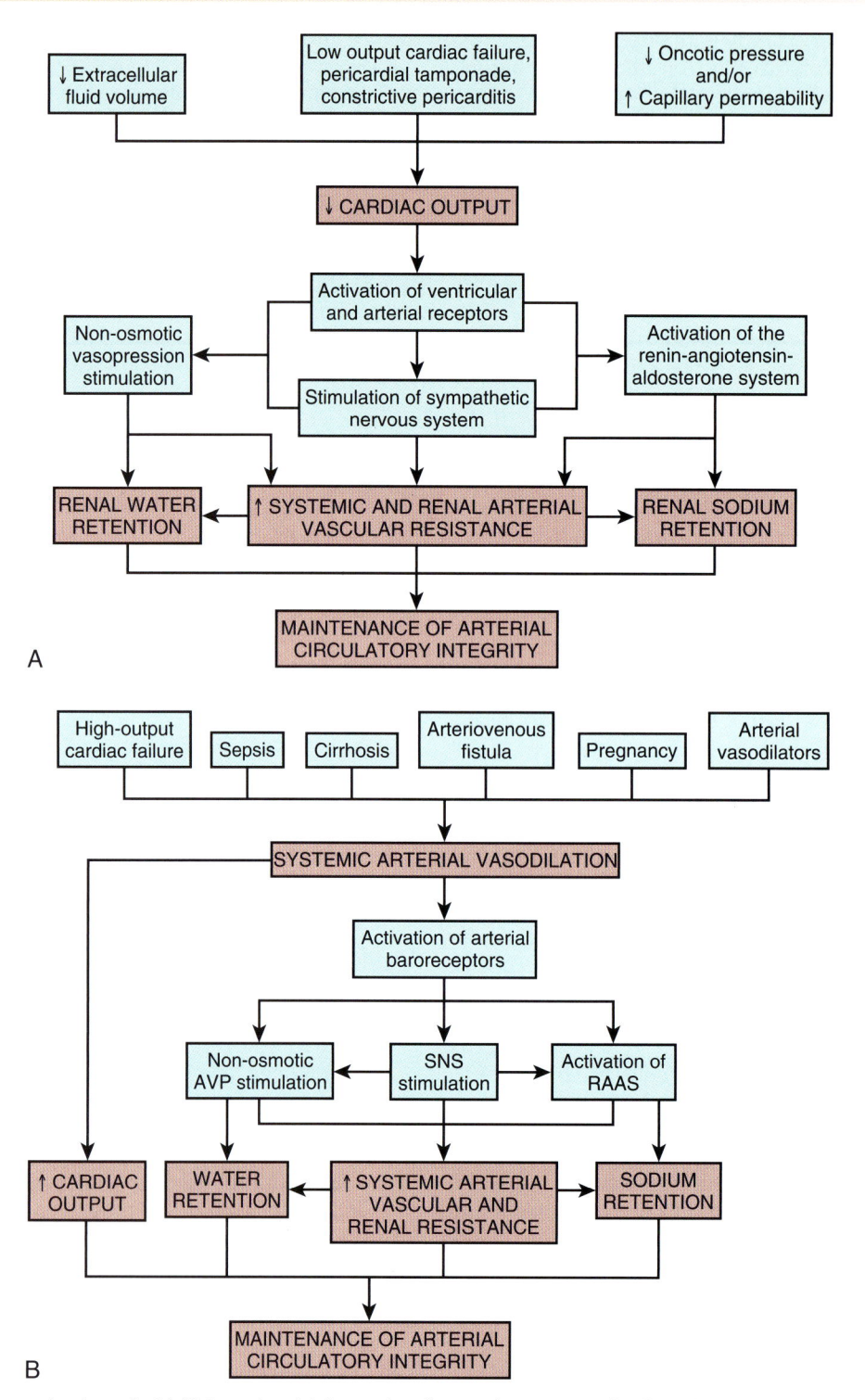

Figure 15.8 Sensing mechanisms that initiate and maintain renal sodium and water retention in various clinical conditions in which arterial underfilling, with resultant neurohumoral activation and renal sodium and water retention, is caused by a decrease in cardiac output (**A**) and by systemic arterial vasodilation (**B**). In addition to activating the neurohumoral axis, adrenergic stimulation causes renal vasoconstriction and enhances sodium and fluid transport by the proximal tubule epithelium. (From Schrier RW: Decreased effective blood volume in edematous disorders: what does this mean? *J Am Soc Nephrol* 18:2028-2031, 2007.)

natriuretic response to central venous congestion. This attenuation is manifested predominantly as a diminished neural suppressive response to atrial stretch, which results in increased sympathetic nerve activity and augmented release of renin and AVP.

Abnormalities of Effector Mechanisms in Heart Failure. HF is also characterized by a series of adaptive changes in the efferent limb of the volume control system, many of which are similar to those that govern renal function in states of true Na^+ depletion. These include adjustments in glomerular hemodynamics and tubular transport, which, in turn, are brought about by alterations in the neural, humoral, and paracrine systems. However, in contrast to true volume depletion, HF is also associated with activation of vasodilatory natriuretic agents, which tend to oppose the effects of the vasoconstrictor/antinatriuretic systems. The final effect on urinary Na^+ excretion is determined by the balance among these antagonistic effector systems, which, in turn, may shift during the evolution of heart failure toward a dominance of Na^+-retaining systems. The abnormal regulation of the efferent limb of the volume control system reflects not only the exaggerated activity of the antinatriuretic systems but also the failure of vasodilatory/natriuretic systems that are activated in the course of the deterioration in cardiac function.

Alterations in Glomerular Hemodynamics. HF in patients and experimental models is characterized by an increase in renal vascular resistance and a reduction in GFR, but also by an even more marked reduction of RPF, so that the filtration fraction is increased.[422] As shown in rat models of HF, these changes seem to result from diminished Kf and elevated afferent and efferent arteriolar resistances, The rise in single-nephron filtration fraction is probably caused by a disproportionate increase in efferent arteriolar resistance.[423,424]

In Figure 15.4, a comparison of the glomerular capillary hemodynamic profile in the normal state versus the HF state is illustrated on the left graph of each panel. First, ΔP declines along the length of the glomerular capillary in normal and HF states, but much more so in HF because of the increased efferent arteriolar resistance. Second, $\Delta \pi$ increases over the length of the glomerular capillary in both states as fluid is filtered into Bowman's space, but again to a greater extent in HF because of the increased filtration fraction. As outlined below (see section, "Renin-Angiotensin-Aldosterone System"), the preferential increase in efferent arteriolar resistance is mediated principally by Ang II and is critical for the preservation of GFR in the presence of reduced RPF. Because of the intense efferent arteriolar vasoconstriction, further compensation is not possible if RPP falls as a result of systemic hypotension, causing a sharp decline in GFR. This phenomenon is dramatically illustrated by HF patients whose Ang II drive is removed by RAAS inhibitors, particularly those with preexisting renal failure, massive diuretic treatment, and limited cardiac reserve.[424] In these patients, blood pressure may fall below the level necessary to maintain renal perfusion.

Enhanced Tubular Reabsorption of Sodium. Enhanced tubular reabsorption of Na^+ in HF is secondary to the altered glomerular function described above and is a direct result of neurohumeral mechanisms. A direct consequence of the glomerular hemodynamic alterations, and of augmented single-nephron filtration fraction, is an increase in the fractional reabsorption of filtered Na^+ at the level of the proximal tubule. In Figure 15.4, the peritubular capillary hemodynamic profile of the normal state is compared with that of HF on the right graph of each panel. In HF, in comparison with the normal state, the average value of $\Delta \pi$ along the peritubular capillary is increased and that of ΔP is decreased. These values are favorable for fluid movement into the capillary and may also help reduce backleak of fluid into the tubule via paracellular pathways, promoting overall net reabsorption.

The peritubular control of proximal fluid reabsorption in normal and HF states is illustrated schematically in Figure 15.9. A critical mediator of the enhanced tubular reabsorption of Na^+ is Ang II, which, by increasing efferent arteriolar resistance, increases the filtration fraction and augments proximal epithelial transporter activities directly, thereby amplifying the overall increase in proximal Na^+ reabsorption. This is clearly illustrated by the favorable effects of RAAS blockers in heart failure to modulate single-nephron filtration fraction and normalize proximal peritubular capillary Starling forces and Na^+ reabsorption.[425]

Distal nephron sites also participate in the enhanced tubule Na^+ reabsorption in HF. Enhanced reabsorption of Na^+ has been shown in the loop of Henle, an effect probably due to altered renal hemodynamics as in the proximal tubule.[162] In the distal tubule and collecting duct, elevated Ang II and aldosterone levels, respectively, enhance activities of the NaCl cotransporter and ENaC.[426]

Neurohumoral Mediators. The primary neurohumoral mediators of Na^+ and water retention in HF include the RAAS, SNS, AVP, and endothelins, which are vasoconstrictor/antinatriuretic (and antidiuretic) systems. In addition, several vasodilator/natriuretic substances, such as nitric oxide, prostaglandins, and AM, are also activated. Upregulation of urotensin II and neuropeptide Y also appears to have a vasodilator/natriuretic effect, in contrast to the physiologic tonic effects of these peptides. In the final analysis, salt and water homeostasis is determined by the fine balance between these opposing systems; the development of positive Na^+ balance and edema formation in HF represents a turning point at which the balance is in favor of the vasoconstrictor/antinatriuretic forces (Figure 15.10). The dominant activity of Na^+-retaining systems in HF is clinically important because impaired renal function is a strong predictor of mortality,[427] and reversal of the neurohumoral impairment is associated with improved outcomes.[428]

VASOCONSTRICTOR/ANTINATRIURETIC (ANTIDIURETIC) SYSTEMS

Renin-Angiotensin-Aldosterone System

The activity of the RAAS is enhanced in most patients with HF in correlation with the severity of cardiac dysfunction[429]; therefore, the activity of this system provides a prognostic index for HF patients. It is now abundantly clear that despite providing initial benefits in hemodynamic support, continued activation of the RAAS also contributes to the progression and worsening of the primary cardiac component of the HF syndrome through maladaptive myocardial remodeling.[429] RAAS activation induces direct systemic vasoconstriction and activates other neurohormonal systems such as AVP, which contribute to maintaining adequate intravascular volume.[429] However, numerous studies in patients and in experimental models of HF have established the deleterious role of the RAAS in the progression of cardiovascular and renal dysfunction.[398]

The kidneys in particular are highly sensitive to the action of vasoconstrictor agents, especially Ang II, and a decrease in RPF is one of the most common pathophysiologic alterations in clinical and experimental HF. Micropuncture techniques have demonstrated that rats with chronic stable HF display depressed RPF and SNGFR, as well as elevations in

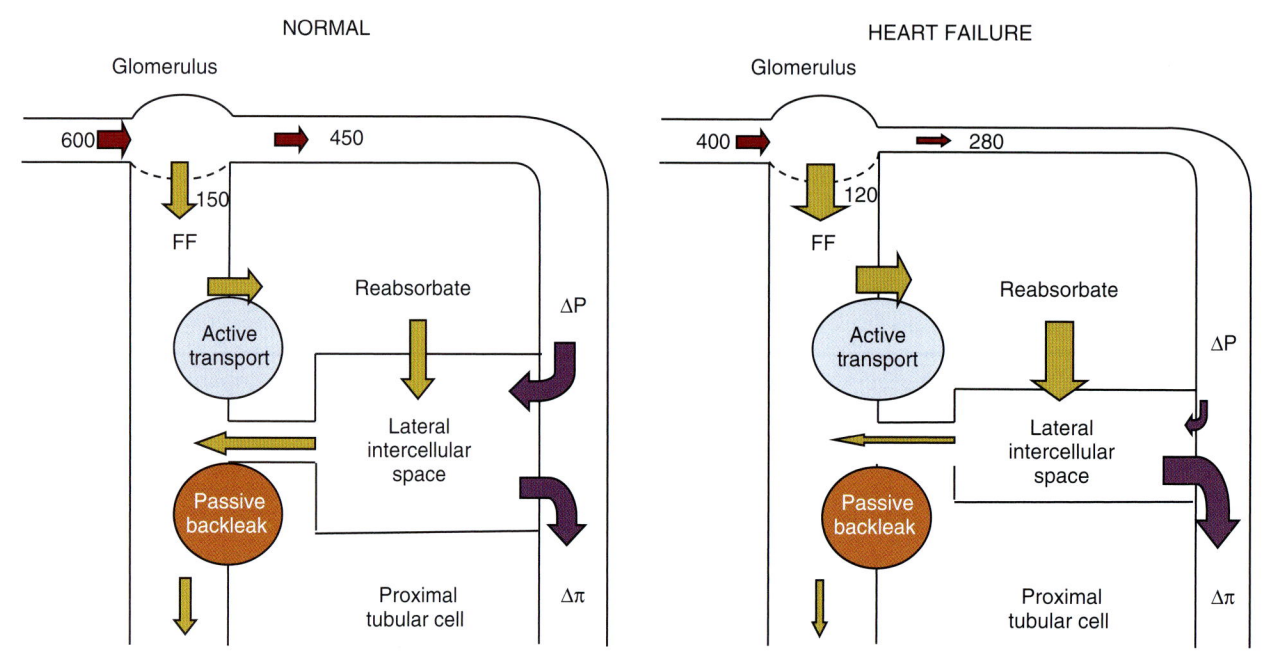

Figure 15.9 Peritubular control of proximal tubule fluid reabsorption. Fluid reabsorption in the normal state (**left**) and in patients with heart failure (**right**) is shown. Increased postglomerular arteriolar resistance in heart failure is depicted as narrowing. The thickness and font size of the *block arrows* depict relative magnitude of effect. The increase in filtration fraction (FF) in heart failure causes $\Delta\pi$ to rise. The increase in renal vascular resistance in heart failure is believed to reduce ΔP. Both the increase in $\Delta\pi$ and the fall in ΔP enhance peritubular capillary uptake of proximal reabsorbate and thus increase absolute Na^+ reabsorption by the proximal tubule. Numbers and *red block arrows* depict blood flow in preglomerular and postglomerular capillaries; ΔP and $\Delta\pi$ are the transcapillary hydraulic and oncotic pressure differences across the peritubular capillary, respectively; *yellow block arrows* indicate transtubular transport; *purple block arrows* represent the effect of peritubular capillary Starling forces on uptake of proximal reabsorbate. (Adapted from Humes HD, Gottlieb M, Brenner BM: *The kidney in congestive heart failure: contemporary issues in nephrology,* vol 1, New York, 1978, Churchill Livingstone, pp 51-72.)

efferent arteriolar resistance and filtration fraction. Direct renal administration of an ACE inhibitor normalized renal function in rats with experimental HF, but not sham-operated control rats. Using the aortocaval fistula model of HF, Winaver and associates[430] have shown that only some animals develop Na^+ retention, whereas the rest maintain Na^+ balance. The former subgroup was characterized by a marked increase in PRA and aldosterone levels. In contrast, levels of these hormones in compensated animals were no different from those in sham-operated controls. Treatment with the ACE inhibitor enalapril resulted in a dramatic natriuretic response in rats with Na^+ retention. Similarly, most patients with HF maintain normal Na^+ balance when placed on a low-salt diet, but about 50% develop a positive Na^+ balance when fed a normal salt diet.[431] A feature common to both animals and patients with Na^+ retention was the activation of the RAAS. In dogs with experimental high-output HF, the initial period of Na^+ retention was associated with a profound activation of the RAAS, and the return to normal Na^+ balance was accompanied by a progressive fall in PRA.[430]

The deleterious effects of the RAAS on renal function are not surprising in view of the previously mentioned actions of Ang II and aldosterone on renal hemodynamics and excretory function. Activation of Ang II in response to the decreased pumping capacity of the failing myocardium promotes systemic vasoconstriction as well as vasoconstriction of efferent and afferent arterioles and mesangial cells.[210,432] In addition, Ang II exerts a negative influence on renal cortical circulation in rats with HF and increases tubular Na^+ reabsorption directly and indirectly by augmenting aldosterone release.[433] In combination, these hemodynamic and tubular actions lead to avid Na^+ and water retention, thus promoting circulatory congestion and edema formation.

There is considerable evidence for the existence of a local RAAS in the heart and kidney. The presence of the system in the kidney likely explains earlier findings of an inconsistent relationship between RAAS and positive Na^+ balance, as well as the maintained efficacy of RAAS inhibition in chronic HF, even when systemic levels of the component hormones were not elevated.[434] To summarize the plethora of data on systemic and local RAAS activation, it appears that systemic RAAS activation is most pronounced in acute and decompensated HF, whereas local renal RAAS activation may dominate in chronic stable HF.

In the heart, local RAAS activation has a number of effects. In addition to the mechanical stress exerted on the myocardium due to systemic Ang II–mediated increased afterload, pressure overload activates the production of local Ang II as a result of upregulation of angiotensinogen and tissue ACE.[432] Local Ang II acts through AT_1 in a paracrine/autocrine manner, leading to cell swelling and cardiac hypertrophy, remodeling and fibrosis (mediated by transforming growth factor-β), and reduced coronary flow, hallmarks of severe HF.[434] These observations help explain the improved cardiac function, prolonged survival, prevention of end-organ damage, and prevention or regression of cardiac hypertrophy in humans and animals with HF treated with ACE inhibitors and ARBs.[211,432] In addition, ACE inhibitors and ARBs may improve endothelial

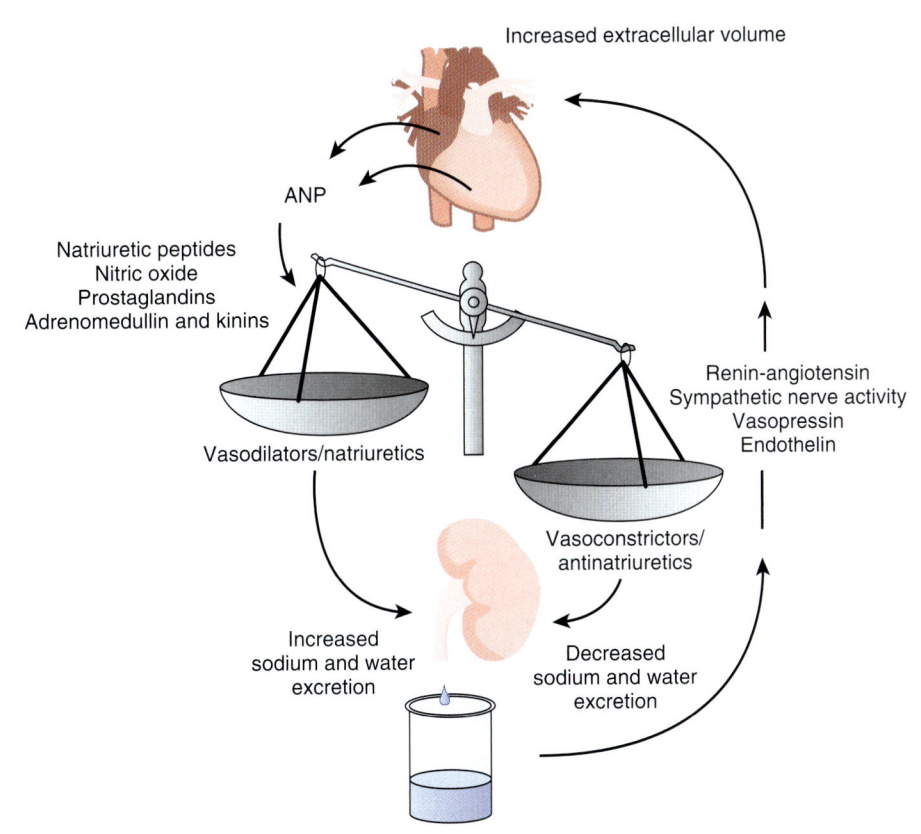

Figure 15.10 Efferent limb of extracellular fluid volume control in heart failure. Volume homeostasis in heart failure is determined by the balance between natriuretic and antinatriuretic forces. In decompensated heart failure, enhanced activities of the Na^+-retaining systems overwhelm the effects of the vasodilatory/natriuretic systems, which leads to a net reduction in Na^+ excretion and an increase in ECF volume. ANP, Atrial natriuretic peptide. (Adapted from Winaver J, Hoffman A, Abassi Z, et al: Does the heart's hormone, ANP, help in congestive heart failure? *News Physiol Sci* 10:247-253, 1995.)

dysfunction, vascular remodeling, and potentiation of the vasodilatory effects of the kinins.[344]

Like Ang II, aldosterone also acts directly on the myocardium, inducing structural remodeling of the interstitial collagen matrix.[435] Moreover, cardiac aldosterone production is increased in patients with HF, especially when caused by systolic dysfunction. Convincing evidence for the local production of aldosterone was provided by the finding that CYP11B2 messenger RNA (aldosterone synthase) is expressed in cultured neonatal rat cardiac myocytes. The adverse contribution of aldosterone to the functional and structural alterations of the failing heart was elegantly proved by the use of eplerenone, a specific aldosterone antagonist, which prevented progressive left ventricular systolic and diastolic dysfunction in association with reduced interstitial fibrosis, cardiomyocyte hypertrophy, and left ventricular chamber sphericity in dogs with HF. Similarly, eplerenone attenuated the development of ventricular remodeling and reactive (but not reparative) fibrosis after myocardial infarction in rats.[436,437] These findings are in agreement with the results of landmark clinical trials (see section, "Specific Treatments Based on the Pathophysiology of Heart Failure").[438,439]

As noted, in addition to its renal and cardiovascular hemodynamic effects, the RAAS is involved directly in the exaggerated Na^+ reabsorption by the tubule in HF. Ang II, produced systemically and locally, has a direct effect on the proximal tubular epithelium that is favorable for active Na^+ reabsorption.[440] The predominant effect of the RAAS in the distal nephron is mediated by aldosterone, which acts on cortical and medullary portions of the collecting duct to enhance Na^+ reabsorption, as outlined previously. Numerous researchers have reported elevations in plasma aldosterone concentration, urinary aldosterone secretion, or natriuretic effects of aldosterone antagonists in animal models and human subjects with HF, despite further activation of other antinatriuretic systems; these findings provide evidence of the pivotal role of this hormone in the mediation of Na^+ retention in HF.[441]

As with Ang II, the relative importance of mineralocorticoid action in the Na^+ retention of HF varies with the stage and severity of disease. Further evidence for the involvement of the RAAS in the development of positive Na^+ balance comes from studies showing that the renal and hemodynamic responses to ANP are impaired in HF and that administration of ARB or ACE inhibition restores the blunted response to ANP (for further details, see later section, "Natriuretic Peptides").[442] Although patients with HF have low plasma osmolality, they display increased thirst, probably because of the high concentrations of Ang II, which stimulates thirst center cells in the hypothalamus.[443] This behavior may contribute to the positive water balance and hyponatremia often seen in these patients (see section, "Arginine Vasopressin").

Sympathetic Nervous System

As mentioned earlier, patients with HF experience progressive activation of the SNS with declining cardiac function.[414,444] Plasma norepinephrine levels are frequently elevated in HF, and a strong consensus exists about the adverse influence of sympathetic overactivity on the progression and outcome of patients with HF.[445,446] Thus, sympathetic neural activity is significantly correlated with intracardiac pressures, cardiac hypertrophy, and left ventricular ejection fraction (LVEF).[447] Direct intraneural recordings in patients with HF have also shown increased neural traffic, which correlated with the increased plasma norepinephrine levels.[445,446] Activation of the SNS not only precedes the appearance of congestive symptoms but also is preferentially directed toward the heart and kidneys. Clinical investigations have revealed that patients with mild HF have higher plasma norepinephrine levels in the coronary sinus than in the renal veins.[446] In the early stages of HF, increased activity of the SNS ameliorates the hemodynamic abnormalities—including hypoperfusion, diminished plasma volume, and impaired cardiac function—by producing vasoconstriction and avid Na^+ reabsorption.[414] However, chronic exposure to this system induces several long-term adverse myocardial effects, including induction of apoptosis and hypertrophy, with an overall reduction in cardiac function, which reduces contractility. Some of these effects may be mediated by activation of the RAAS which, in turn, can augment sympathetic activity and create a vicious cycle.[414,448]

Measurements made with catecholamine spillover techniques have revealed that the basal sympathetic outflow to the kidneys is significantly increased in patients with HF.[449] The activation of the SNS and increased efferent RSNA may be involved in the alterations in renal function in HF. For example, exaggerated RSNA contributes to the increased renal vasoconstriction, avid Na^+ and water retention, renin secretion, and attenuation of the renal actions of ANP.[450] Experimental studies have demonstrated that in rats with experimental HF caused by coronary artery ligation, renal denervation results in an increase in RPF and SNGFR and a decrease in afferent and efferent arteriolar resistance.[445] Similarly, in dogs with low cardiac output induced by vena caval constriction, administration of a ganglionic blocker resulted in a marked increase in Na^+ excretion.[445] In rats with HF induced by coronary ligation, the decrease in RSNA in response to an acute saline load was less than that of control rats.[277] Bilateral renal denervation restored the natriuretic response to volume expansion; this finding implicates increased RSNA in the Na^+ avidity characteristic of HF.[445]

Studies in dogs with high-output HF induced by aortocaval fistula have demonstrated that total postprandial urinary Na^+ excretion is approximately twofold higher in dogs with renal denervation than in control dogs with intact nerves.[445] In line with these observations, administration of the α-adrenoreceptor blocker dibenamine to patients with HF caused an increase in fractional Na^+ excretion, without a change in RPF or GFR. Treatment with ibopamine, an oral dopamine analogue, resulted in vasodilation and positive inotropic and diuretic effects in patients with HF.[451] Moreover, for a given degree of cardiac dysfunction, the concentration of norepinephrine is significantly higher in patients with concomitant abnormal renal function than in patients with preserved renal function.[452] These findings suggest that the association between renal function and prognosis in patients with HF is linked by neurohormonal activation, including that in the CNS.

An additional mechanism by which RSNA may affect renal hemodynamics and Na^+ excretion in HF is through its antagonistic interaction with ANP. On the one hand, ANP has sympathoinhibitory effects[453,454]; on the other, the SNS-induced salt and water retention in HF may reduce renal responsiveness to ANP. For example, the blunted diuretic/natriuretic response to ANP in rats with HF could be restored by prior renal denervation[455] or by administration of clonidine,[456] a centrally acting $α_2$-adrenoreceptor agonist, which decreases RSNA in HF. These examples illustrate the complexity of interactions between the SNS and other humoral factors involved in the pathogenesis of Na^+ retention in HF.

In summary, the SNS plays an important role in the regulation of Na^+ excretion and glomerular hemodynamics in HF, either by a direct renal action or by a complex interplay between the SNS itself and other neurohumeral mechanisms that act on the glomeruli and renal tubules. The recent introduction of renal denervation as a potential therapeutic treatment for HF should facilitate the further elucidation of these neurohumoral interactions.

Vasopressin

Numerous studies have demonstrated elevated plasma levels of AVP in patients with HF, mostly in those with advanced HF and hyponatremia, but also in asymptomatic patients with left ventricular dysfunction.[457] The high plasma levels of AVP in HF are related to nonosmotic factors such as attenuated compliance of the left atrium, hypotension, and activation of the RAAS[458] and are reversed by RAAS inhibition or α-blockade (prazosin). Therefore, improved cardiac function in response to afterload reduction (e.g., pulse pressure, stroke volume) was probably responsible for the removal of the nonosmotic stimulus to AVP release.

The high circulating levels of AVP in HF adversely affect the kidneys and cardiovascular system. In fact, raised levels of the C-terminal portion of the AVP prohormone (copeptin) at the time of diagnosis of acute decompensated heart failure are highly predictive of 1-year mortality.[459,460] The prognostic power of an increased copeptin level in HF is similar to that of BNP levels (see section, "Brain Natriuretic Peptide"). The most recognized renal effect of AVP in HF is the development of hyponatremia, which usually occurs in advanced stages of the disease and most probably results from impaired solute-free water excretion in the presence of sustained release of AVP, irrespective of plasma osmolality. In accordance with this notion, studies in animal models of HF have demonstrated increased collecting duct expression of AQP2.[461] In addition, administration of specific V_2 receptor antagonists (VRAs) has been consistently associated with improvement in plasma Na^+ levels in animals and patients with hyponatremia.[462,463] The improvement is associated with correction of the impaired urinary dilution in response to acute water load,[464] increased plasma osmolarity, and downregulation of renal AQP2 expression, but no effect on RBF, GFR or Na^+ excretion.[465]

The adverse effects of AVP on cardiac function[466] occur through its V_{1A} receptor on systemic vascular resistance (increased cardiac afterload), as well as by V_2-receptor–mediated water retention, which leads to systemic and pulmonary congestion (increased preload). In addition, AVP, through its V_{1A} receptor, acts directly on cardiomyocytes, causing a rise in intracellular Ca^{2+} and activation of mitogen-activated kinases and protein kinase C. These signaling mechanisms appear to mediate the observed cardiac remodeling, dilation, and hypertrophy. The remodeling might be further exacerbated by these abnormalities in preload and afterload.

In summary, the data suggest the following: (1) AVP is involved in the pathogenesis of water retention and hyponatremia that characterize HF; and (2) AVP receptor antagonists result in remarkable diuresis in experimental and clinical models of HF. Treatment of HF with VRA will be discussed further (see section, "Specific Treatments Based on the Pathophysiology of Congestive Heart Failure").

Endothelin

There is considerable evidence that ET-1 is involved in the development and progression of HF. Furthermore, this peptide is probably involved in the reduced renal function that characterizes HF by inducing renal remodeling, interstitial fibrosis, glomerulosclerosis, hypoperfusion and hypofiltration, and positive salt and water balance.[467] The pathophysiologic role of ET-1 in HF is supported by two major lines of evidence: (1) the endothelin system is activated in HF; and (2) ET-1 receptor antagonists modify this pathophysiologic process.[468] The first line of evidence is based on the demonstration that plasma ET-1 and big ET-1 concentrations in clinical HF and experimental models of HF are elevated and correlate with hemodynamic severity and symptoms.[469] Also, a negative correlation between plasma ET-1 concentration and LVEF has been reported.[470] In addition, the degree of pulmonary hypertension was the strongest predictor of plasma ET-1 level in patients with HF.[470] Moreover, plasma levels of big endothelin and ET-1 are especially high in patients with moderate to severe HF and are independent markers of mortality and morbidity.[469]

The increase in plasma levels of ET-1 may be the result of enhanced synthesis in the lungs, heart, and circulation by several stimuli such as Ang II and thrombin or of decreased pulmonary clearance.[470] In parallel to ET-1 levels, ET-A receptors are upregulated, whereas ET-B receptors are downregulated in the failing human heart.[471]

A cause-and-effect relationship between these hemodynamic abnormalities and ET-1 in HF was demonstrated with the development of selective and highly specific endothelin receptor antagonists.[470] In this regard, acute administration of the mixed ET-A/ET-B receptor antagonists, bosentan and tezosentan significantly improved renal cortical perfusion, reversed the profoundly increased renal vascular resistance, and increased RBF and Na^+ excretion in rats with severe decompensated HF.[472] In addition, chronic blockade of ET-A by selective or dual ET-A/ET-B receptor antagonists attenuated the magnitude of Na^+ retention and prevented the decline in GFR in experimental HF.[467] These data are in line with observations that infusion of ET-1 in normal rats produced a sustained cortical vasoconstrictor and transient medullary vasodilatory response.[331] In contrast, rats with decompensated HF displayed severely blunted cortical vasoconstriction but significantly prolonged and preserved medullary vasodilation.[331] These effects could result from activation of vasodilatory systems such as prostaglandins and nitric oxide. The medullary tissue of rats with decompensated HF contains higher eNOS immunoreactive levels than sham-treated controls.[331] Taken together, the data are consistent with a role for endothelin in the altered renal hemodynamics and pathogenesis of cortical vasoconstriction in HF.

VASODILATORY/NATRIURETIC SYSTEMS

Natriuretic Peptides

In decompensated heart failure, renal Na^+ and water retention occurs, despite expansion of the ECF volume, even when the NP system is activated. Results of many clinical and experimental studies have implicated both ANP and BNP in the pathophysiologic process of the deranged cardiorenal axis in HF.

Atrial Natriuretic Peptide. Plasma levels of ANP and NH_2-terminal ANP are frequently elevated in patients with HF and are correlated positively with the severity of cardiac failure, elevated atrial pressure, and parameters of left ventricular dysfunction.[288,473] Hence, the concentration of circulating ANP was proposed as a diagnostic tool in the determination of cardiac dysfunction and as a prognostic marker in the prediction of survival of patients with HF.[42] However, in this context, ANP has since been superseded by BNP. There is also recent evidence that midregional (MR) proANP may perform similarly to BNP as a biomarker of ADHF (see section, "Brain Natriuretic Peptide").[473]

The high levels of plasma ANP are attributed to increased production rather than to decreased clearance. Although volume-induced atrial stretch is the main source for the elevated circulating ANP levels in HF, enhanced synthesis and release of the hormone by the ventricular tissue in response to Ang II and endothelin also contribute to this phenomenon.[288,473] Despite the high levels of this potent natriuretic and diuretic agent, patients and experimental animals with HF retain salt and water because renal responsiveness to NPs is attenuated.[474] However, infusion of ANP to patients with HF does lead to hemodynamic improvement and inhibition of activated neurohumoral systems. These data are in line with findings in patients and animals that ANP is a weak counterregulatory hormone, insufficient to overcome the substantial vasoconstriction mediated by the SNS, RAAS, and AVP.[475] However, despite the blunted renal response to ANP in HF, elimination of ANP production by atrial appendectomy in dogs with HF aggravated the activation of these vasoconstrictive hormones and resulted in marked Na^+ and water retention.[476] These data suggest that ANP plays a critical role as a suppressor of Na^+-retaining systems and as an important adaptive or compensatory mechanism aimed at reducing pulmonary vascular resistance and hypervolemia.

Brain Natriuretic Peptide. As noted, BNP is structurally similar to ANP but is produced mainly by the ventricles in response to stretch and pressure overload.[288,473] As with ANP, plasma levels of BNP and N-terminal (NT)–proBNP are elevated in patients with HF in proportion to the severity of myocardial systolic and diastolic dysfunction and New York Heart Association (NYHA) classification.[288] Plasma levels of BNP are elevated only in severe HF, whereas circulating concentrations of ANP are high in mild and severe cases.[288,477] The extreme elevation of plasma BNP in severe HF probably stems from the increased synthesis of BNP, predominantly by the hypertrophied ventricular tissue, although the contribution of the atria is significant.[288,477]

Although echocardiography remains the gold standard for the evaluation of left ventricular dysfunction, numerous studies have shown that plasma levels of BNP and NT-proBNP are reliable markers and, in fact, are superior to ANP and NT-proANP for the diagnosis and prognosis of HF.[288] The diagnostic capability of NT-proBNP is impressive, with high sensitivity, specificity, and negative predictive value in patients with an ejection fraction less than 35%. Similar high predictive values are found in patients with concomitant left ventricular hypertrophy, either in the absence of or after myocardial infarction.[288] The added presence of renal dysfunction appears to enhance these predictive values,[478,479] and graded increases in mortality throughout each quartile of BNP levels have been shown in several clinical trials.[480] In addition, elevated plasma BNP (or NT-proBNP) levels and LVEF lower than 40% are complementary independent predictors of death, HF, and new myocardial infarction at 3 years after an initial myocardial infarction. Moreover, risk stratification with the combination of LVEF lower than 40% and high levels of NT-proBNP is substantially better than that provided by either alone.[481] However, even though BNP levels tend to be lower in patients with preserved LVEF than in HF patients with reduced LVEF, the prognosis in patients with preserved LVEF is as poor as in those with reduced LVEF for a given BNP level.[482]

In asymptomatic patients with preserved LVEF, elevated BNP levels are correlated with diastolic abnormalities on Doppler studies. Conversely, a reduction in BNP levels with treatment is associated with a reduction in left ventricular filling pressures, lower readmission rates, and a better prognosis; thus, monitoring of BNP levels may provide valuable information regarding treatment efficacy and expected patient outcomes.[483]

Another diagnostic role for BNP is in the distinction of dyspnea caused by HF from that caused by noncardiac entities. This point was dramatically illustrated by the N-terminal Pro-BNP Investigation of Dyspnea in the Emergency Department (PRIDE) study, in which the median NT-proBNP level in 209 patients who had acute HF was 4054 pg/mL in contrast to 131 pg/mL in 390 patients (65%) who did not have acute HF. At cut points of more than 450 pg/mL for patients younger than 50 years and more than 900 pg/mL for patients at least 50 years of age, NT-proBNP levels were highly sensitive and specific for the diagnosis of acute HF. An NT-proBNP level lower than 300 pg/mL was optimal for ruling out acute HF, with a negative predictive value of 99%. An increased level of NT-proBNP was the strongest independent predictor of a final diagnosis of acute HF. NT-proBNP testing alone was superior to clinical judgment alone for diagnosing acute HF; NT-proBNP plus clinical judgment was superior to NT-proBNP or clinical judgment alone.[484] Thus, the predictive accuracy of circulating BNP for distinguishing dyspnea caused by HF from dyspnea with noncardiac causes equals and even exceeds the accuracy of classic examinations, such as radiography and physical examination.[485] Moreover, NT-proBNP levels perform better than the National Health and Nutrition Examination score and Framingham clinical parameters (the most established criteria in use for the diagnosis of HF).

BNP levels were proposed to be helpful in reducing length of hospital stay and costs, but two recent meta-analyses have cast serious doubt on this notion.[486,487] Circulating BNP and NT-proBNP levels have also been used as a guide in determining the therapeutic efficacy of drugs typically prescribed for HF patients, including ACE inhibitors, ARBs, diuretics, digitalis, and β-blockers.[485,488-490] Two meta-analyses have recently confirmed the overall utility of BNP levels for monitoring the success of HF treatment.[491,492] Finally, BNP, but not NT-proBNP, levels at 24 and 48 hours after admission for acute decompensated HF (ADHF) predicted both 30-day and 1-year mortality. Predischarge levels of both peptides were predictive of 30-day and 1-year mortality but not of 1-year readmission due to HF.[492]

Together, these findings suggest that a simple and rapid determination of plasma levels of BNP or NT-proBNP in HF patients can be used to assess cardiac dysfunction, serve as a diagnostic and prognostic marker, and assist in titrating relevant therapy. However, it should be emphasized that plasma levels of ANP and BNP are affected by several factors, including age, salt intake, gender, obesity, hemodynamic status, and renal function, and there is considerable overlap among different diagnostic groups.[480] In this regard, the recent finding that MR-proANP added significant incremental diagnostic value in patients with BNP levels in the grey zone (between 100 and 500 pg/mL) should enhance the ability of biomarkers to distinguish between cardiac and noncardiac causes of dyspnea.[473] Nevertheless, for the present, a combination of conventional parameters such as clinical and echocardiographic measures, assessed together with plasma levels of BNP and MR-proANP, yield better clinical guidelines in HF patients than each tool alone.[493]

C-Type Natriuretic Peptide. As mentioned earlier (see section, "Physiology"), CNP is synthesized mainly by endothelial cells, but small amounts are also produced by cardiac tissue.[494] In contrast to other NPs, CNP is predominantly a vasodilator and has little effect on or may even reduce urinary flow and Na^+ excretion.[494] However, the production of CNP by the endothelium in proximity to its receptors in vascular smooth muscle cells suggests that this peptide may play a role in the control of vascular tone and growth.[494]

Like those of ANP and BNP, plasma CNP levels are increased in HF, and CNP levels are directly correlated with NYHA classification with levels of BNP, ET-1, and AM and with pulmonary capillary wedge pressure, ejection fraction, and left ventricular end-diastolic diameter.[494] Higher levels of CNP have been found in the coronary sinuses than in the adjacent aorta, which is indicative of CNP release from the myocardium. The demonstration of a CNP-induced inhibitory effect on cultured cardiac myocyte hypertrophy suggests that overexpression of CNP in the myocardium during HF may be involved in counteracting cardiac remodeling.[494] In contrast to the diminished physiologic responses to ANP and BNP in animals with HF in comparison with control animals, CNP elicited twice as much sGC activity as ANP, which was shown to result from dramatic reductions in NP receptor A (NPR-A) activity without any change in NP receptor B (NPR-B) activity.[494] These novel findings imply a significant role for NPR-B–mediated NP activity in the failing heart and may explain the modest effects of nesiritide (BNP) treatment in HF, inasmuch as the latter is NPR-A–selective.[495]

Higher CNP levels in the renal vein than in the adjacent aorta have been reported in normal people, and this difference was blunted in patients with HF.[496] The physiologic significance of these data currently remains unexplained. Overall, the evidence available points to a possible peripheral vascular compensatory response to HF by overexpression of CNP. Alternately, CNP may be involved in mitigating the cardiac remodeling characteristic of HF. Elaboration of the exact role of CNP in HF is crucial for the design of more effective NP analogues than those currently available for the management of HF.

Overall Relationship Between Natriuretic and Antinatriuretic Factors in Heart Failure

The maintenance of Na^+ balance in the initial compensated phase of HF has been attributed in part to the elevated levels of ANP and BNP.[288] This notion is supported by the findings that inhibition of NP receptors in experimental HF induces Na^+ retention.[497] In addition, NPs inhibit the Ang II–induced systemic vasoconstriction, proximal tubule Na^+ reabsorption, and secretion of aldosterone and endothelin.[473] Furthermore, in an experimental model of HF, inhibition of the NPs by specific antibodies to their receptors caused further impairment in renal function, as indicated by increased renal vascular resistance and decreased GFR, RBF, urine flow, Na^+ excretion, and activation of the RAAS.[498]

In view of the remarkable activation of the NP system and the ability of NPs to counter the effects of the vasoconstrictor/antinatriuretic neurohormonal systems, why then do salt and water retention occur in overt HF? Several mechanisms could explain this apparent discrepancy:

1. Appearance of abnormal circulating peptides and inadequate secretory reserves in comparison with the degree of HF. Using an extremely sensitive mass spectrometry–based method, altered processing of proBNP1-108 and/or BNP1-32 has been demonstrated in HF, resulting in very low levels of BNP1-32, despite markedly elevated levels of immunoreactive (i.e., total) BNP.[499] Moreover, proBNP1-108 has a lower affinity for the GC-A receptor, which would reduce effector function of BNP.[500]
2. Decreased availability of NPs by downregulation of corin[501] or upregulation of NEP and clearance receptors.[498] Downregulation of corin may explain, at least in part, the decreased availability of NPs in HF. Consistent with this concept, lower levels of corin in parallel with elevated levels of proANP have been observed in the plasma of HF patients. On the other hand, circulating cGMP levels are elevated in HF patients, implying enhanced activity of NPs. In an attempt to reconcile these apparently contradictory findings, intracardiac expression of corin was examined in an experimental model of HF caused by dilated cardiomyopathy. Low levels of corin in cardiac tissue were demonstrated in this model. Moreover, transfection of the gene encoding for corin into these animals led to a reduction in cardiac fibrosis, improvement in contractility, and reduced mortality.[501] With regard to clearance receptors, no convincing evidence to date suggests that upregulation exists in the renal tissue of HF animals or patients, although increased abundance of clearance receptors for NPs in platelets of patients with advanced HF has been reported.[502] In contrast, several studies have demonstrated enhanced expression and activity of NEP in experimental HF.[503,504] Moreover, numerous reports have shown that NEP inhibitors improve the vascular and renal response to NPs in HF (see section, "Specific Treatments Based on the Pathophysiology of Congestive Heart Failure").
3. Activation of vasoconstrictor/antinatriuretic factors and development of renal hyporesponsiveness to ANP. Renal resistance to ANP may be present, even in the early presymptomatic stage of the disease, but it progresses proportionately as HF worsens.[498] In advanced HF, when RPF is markedly impaired, the ability of NPs to antagonize the renal effects of Ang II is limited.[505] This was clearly demonstrated in an animal model of HF, in which chronic blockade by enalapril of the profoundly activated RAAS partially, but significantly, improved the natriuretic response to endogenous and exogenous ANP.[506] The favorable effects of ACE inhibition were especially evident in decompensated heart failure. These findings are in line with the fact that activation of RAAS in HF largely contributes to Na^+ and water retention by antagonizing the renal actions of ANP. The mechanisms underlying the attenuated renal effects of ANP in HF are not completely understood, but they include Ang II–induced afferent and efferent vasoconstriction, mesangial cell contraction, activation of cGMP phosphodiesterases that attenuate the accumulation of the second messenger of NPs in target organs, and stimulation of Na^+-H^+-exchanger and Na^+ channels in the proximal tubule and collecting duct.[506]

Activation of the SNS also can overwhelm the renal effects of ANP. As described earlier, overactivity of the SNS leads to vasoconstriction of the peripheral circulation and of the afferent and efferent arterioles, which causes reduction of RPF and GFR. These actions, together with the direct stimulatory effects of SNS on Na^+ reabsorption in the proximal tubule and loop of Henle, contribute to the attenuated renal responsiveness to ANP in HF. Moreover, the SNS-induced renal hypoperfusion/hypofiltration stimulates renin secretion, thereby aggravating the positive Na^+ and water balance. In rat models of HF, the diuretic and natriuretic responses to ANP were increased after sympathetic inhibition by low-dose clonidine[456] or bilateral renal denervation.[507] The beneficial effects of renal denervation could be attributed to upregulation of NP receptors and cGMP production.[209]

In summary, the development of renal hyporesponsiveness to NPs is paralleled closely by overreactivity of the RAAS and SNS and represents a critical point in the development of positive salt balance and edema formation in advanced HF.

Nitric Oxide

After the discovery that nitric oxide is the prototypic endothelium-derived relaxing factor, this signaling molecule was implicated in the increased vascular resistance and impaired endothelium-dependent vascular responses characteristic of HF.[508,509] Thus, the response to acetylcholine, an endothelium-dependent vasodilator that acts by releasing nitric oxide, was found to be markedly attenuated in HF, both in patients[510] and experimental animals[510] as well as in isolated resistance arteries from patients with HF.[511] Mechanisms mediating the impaired activity of the nitric oxide system in HF include a reduction in shear stress associated with the decreased cardiac output,[512] downregulation or uncoupling of eNOS, decreased availability of the nitric oxide precursor L-arginine caused by increased activity of arginase, increased levels of the endogenous NOS inhibitor asymmetric dimethyl arginine (ADMA), inactivation of NO by superoxide ion, and alteration of the redox state of sGC through oxidative stress, which leads to reduced levels of the NO-sensitive form of sGC and subsequent production of its second messenger cGMP.[509] This oxidative stress may be worsened by excessive activity of counterregulatory neurohumoral systems, such as the RAAS, and by the release of proinflammatory messengers.[509]

Altered activity of the NO-sGC-cGMP system also underlies the regional vasomotor dysregulation of the renal circulation in HF. In line with this idea, rats with HF induced by an aortocaval fistula had attenuated nitric oxide–mediated renal vasodilation, which was reversed by pretreatment with an AT_1 receptor antagonist. This suggests that Ang II may be involved in mediating the impaired nitric oxide–dependent renal vasodilation.[513] The resulting imbalance between nitric oxide and excessive activation of the RAAS and endothelin systems could explain some of the beneficial effects of ACE inhibitors, ARBs, and aldosterone antagonists.[514]

Support for this imbalance concept came from a model of experimental HF in rats, which overexpress eNOS in the renal medulla and, to a lesser extent, in the renal cortex.[331] It was speculated that this eNOS might play a role in the preservation of intact medullary perfusion and could attenuate the severe cortical vasoconstriction. Another explanation for the impaired renal hemodynamics in HF is the accumulation of ADMA. In this context, plasma ADMA concentrations in patients with normotensive HF were significantly higher than in controls and, in a multiple regression analysis, ADMA levels were independently predictive of reduced effective RBF.[515]

An additional issue is that the myocardium contains all three NOS isoforms, and the locally generated nitric oxide is believed to play a modulatory role on cardiac function.[508,509] Thus, alterations in the cardiac nitric oxide system in HF might contribute to the pathogenesis of cardiac dysfunction and, thereby indirectly to the impaired renal function.[509] Alterations in the expression of cardiac NOS isoforms in HF are complex, and the functional consequences of these changes depend on a balance among various factors, including disruption of the unique subcellular localization of each isoform and nitroso-redox imbalance.[508,509]

In summary, endothelium-dependent vasodilation is attenuated in various vascular beds in HF. This attenuation may occur as a result of decreased levels of NO and downregulation or inhibition of downstream NO signal transduction pathways. These effects may occur directly or via counterregulatory vasoconstrictor neurohumoral mechanisms.

Prostaglandins

Although the contribution of prostaglandins to renal function in euvolemic states is minimal, they play an important role in maintaining renal function in the setting of impaired RBF, as occurs in HF. Renal hypoperfusion, directly or by activation of the RAAS, stimulates the release of prostaglandins that exert a vasodilatory effect, predominantly at the level of the afferent arteriole, and promote Na^+ excretion by inhibiting Na^+ transport in the thick ascending limb of Henle and the medullary collecting duct.[516] Evidence of the compensatory role of prostaglandins in experimental and clinical HF comes from two sources. First, plasma levels of PGE_2, PGE_2 metabolites, and 6-keto-PGF_1 were higher in HF patients than in normal subjects.[517] Moreover, studies in experimental and human HF have demonstrated a direct linear relationship between PRA and Ang II concentrations and levels of circulating and urinary PGE_2 and PGI_2 metabolites.[518] This correlation probably reflects both Ang II–induced stimulation of prostaglandin synthesis and prostaglandin-mediated increased renin release.

A similar counterregulatory role of prostaglandins with regard to the other vasoconstrictors (e.g., catecholamines, AVP) may also be inferred. An inverse correlation between plasma Na^+ concentrations and plasma levels of PGE_2 metabolites has also been demonstrated. The second approach, which established the protective role of renal and vascular prostaglandins in HF, was derived from studies of nonsteroidal antiinflammatory drugs (NSAIDs), which inhibit the synthesis of prostaglandins. In various experimental models of HF, inhibition of prostaglandin synthesis by indomethacin was associated with an elevation in urinary excretion of PGE_2, significant increase in body weight, profound increase in renal vascular resistance, and resultant decrease in RBF, related mainly to afferent arteriolar constriction.[517,519] Serum creatinine and urea levels rose, and urine flow rate declined significantly.[519] In accordance with these observations, patients with HF and hyponatremia, in whom extreme activation of the SNS and RAAS occurred, were most susceptible to the adverse glomerular hemodynamic consequences of indomethacin treatment.[517] Such patients developed significant decreases in RBF and GFR accompanied by reduced urinary Na^+ excretion.[520] These effects were prevented by intravenous infusion of PGE_2. Moreover, pretreatment with indomethacin before captopril administration attenuated the captopril-induced increase in RBF. Thus, prostaglandins have a significant role in the regulation of renal function in patients with HF, and ACE inhibitor (ACEI) improvement in renal hemodynamics is mediated in part by increased prostaglandin synthesis.

Renal prostaglandins may also play an important role in mediating the natriuretic effects of ANP. For example, in dogs with experimental HF,[521] indomethacin reduced ANP-induced Na^+ excretion and creatinine clearance by 75% and 35%, respectively. Collectively, the results of human and animal studies have indicated that HF is a so-called prostaglandin-dependent state, in which elevated Ang II levels and enhanced RSNA stimulate renal synthesis of PGE_2 and PGI_2, which would counteract the vasoconstrictor effects of these stimuli to maintain GFR and RBF. Therefore, administration of NSAIDs to patients or animals with HF leaves these vasoconstrictor systems unopposed, leading to hypoperfusion, hypofiltration, and subsequent Na$^+$ and water retention.[522]

Clinical data amply bear out the close relationship between the consumption of NSAIDs, both nonselective COX inhibitors and selective COX-2 inhibitors, and a significant worsening of chronic HF, especially in older patients taking diuretics.[513,523] In fact, the COX-2 inhibitor, rofecoxib, was found to blunt the diuretic effect of furosemide directly.[524] The deleterious effects of selective COX-2 inhibitors on cardiac and renal function are consistent with the relative abundance of COX-2 in renal tissue and, to a lesser extent, in the myocardium in HF patients.[525,526] Moreover, the significant increase in the risk of myocardial infarction and death with the COX-2 inhibitor rofecoxib has raised serious safety problems in the use of these drugs and led to the withdrawal of rofecoxib from the market and a black box warning from the U.S. Food and Drug Administration (FDA) about celecoxib.[523] The adverse cardiovascular effects are thought to be related to an imbalance between platelet COX-1–derived prothrombotic TXA$_2$ and endothelial COX-2–derived antithrombotic PGI$_2$, although maladaptive renal effects cannot be ruled out.[527] This would explain why not only selective COX-2 inhibitors, but also nonselective COX inhibitors, increase cardiovascular morbidity and mortality.[527] However, epidemiologic studies carried out since the withdrawal of rofecoxib have indicated a decrease in the relative risk for hospitalization in HF patients receiving NSAIDs, which suggests that physicians are prescribing these drugs more judiciously than in the past.[528] In addition, there is some evidence that celecoxib is safer than rofecoxib or nonselective COX inhibitors in older HF patients.[529,530] The adverse effects of celecoxib may also be dose-dependent.[531]

In summary, patients with preexisting HF are dependent on adequate local prostaglandin levels to maintain RPF, GFR, and Na$^+$ excretion. Consequently, they are at high risk of volume overload, edema, and deterioration of cardiac function after the use of COX-2 or nonselective COX inhibitors.

Adrenomedullin

Evidence suggests that AM plays a role in the pathophysiology of HF. In comparison with healthy subjects, HF patients have plasma levels of the mature form of AM, as well as of the glycine-extended form, that are elevated up to fivefold in proportion to the severity of cardiac and hemodynamic impairment.[349,532] High levels of midregional pro-AM are also strong predictors of mortality in HF.[533-537] In accordance with the correlation between plasma AM levels and the severity of HF, plasma AM levels are also correlated with pulmonary arterial pressure, pulmonary capillary wedge pressure, norepinephrine level, ANP level, BNP level, and PRA in these patients. Plasma levels of the peptide decreased with effective anti-HF treatment, such as carvedilol.[538]

The origin of the increased amount of circulating AM appears to be the failing myocardium itself, including the ventricles and, to a lesser extent, the atria.[538] Similar findings have been reported for AM-2.[539] Not only cardiac but also renal AM levels were significantly increased in some but not all experimental models of HF, in comparison with normal animals.[540,541] Although the significance of this renal upregulation of AM in HF is unclear, there is evidence that AM has favorable effects on salt and water balance, as well as on hemodynamic abnormalities characterizing HF. Experimental and clinical studies have shown that infusion of AM produced beneficial renal effects in HF-related volume overload. For example, in sheep with HF caused by rapid pacing, brief administration (90 minutes) of AM produced a threefold increase in Na$^+$ excretion, with maintenance of urine output, and a rise in creatinine clearance in comparison with baseline levels in normal sheep.[538] Prolonged administration (for 4 days) of AM in sheep with HF produced a significant and sustained increase in cardiac output in association with enhanced urine volume.[538]

In contrast to the results in experimental HF, acute administration of AM to patients with HF increased forearm blood flow but to a lesser extent than in normal subjects, which suggests that the vascular effects of AM are significantly attenuated in HF.[538] In addition, AM had no significant effect on urine volume and Na$^+$ excretion in patients with HF, but did reduce plasma aldosterone levels.[538] Also, AM infusion led to increased stroke index, dilation of resistance arteries, and urinary Na$^+$ excretion.[538] The improvement in cardiac function after AM infusion is not surprising in view of its beneficial effects on preload and afterload and cardiac contractility.[349] Collectively, the vasodilatory and natriuretic activities of AM, and its origin from the failing heart, suggest that AM acts as a compensatory agent to balance the elevation in systemic vascular resistance and volume expansion in this disease state.

Because the favorable effects of AM alone are rather modest, attempts at combination therapy with other vasodilatory/natriuretic substances have been made. In this regard, AM in combination with other therapies such as BNP, ACEIs, NEP inhibitors, and epinephrine have resulted in hemodynamic and renal benefits greater than those achieved by each agent administered separately.[538,542] A small pilot trial[543] of combined long-term human ANP and AM in patients with acute decompensated HF has demonstrated significant reductions in mean arterial pressure, pulmonary arterial pressure, systemic vascular resistance, and pulmonary vascular resistance without changing heart rate; cardiac output was also increased in comparison with baseline. In addition, the combination of AM and human ANP reduced amounts of aldosterone, BNP, and free radical metabolites, as well as increasing urine volume and Na$^+$ excretion over baseline values.[543]

These promising results should pave the way for larger controlled trials of AM in combination with other vasodilator/natriuretic agents. However, expectation of benefits from AM combined with other natriuretics for HF therapy should be guarded in view of their known propensity to cause compensatory rises in vasoconstrictor/antinatriuretic mechanisms, such as the RAAS, SNS, and endothelin.

Urotensin

A role for urotensin II and its receptor, GPR14, in the pathogenesis of HF has been suggested on the basis of the following findings. First, some but not all studies revealed that plasma levels of urotensin II are elevated in patients with HF in correlation with levels of other markers, such as NT-proBNP and ET-1.[544] Second, strong expression of urotensin II was demonstrated in the myocardium of patients with end-stage HF in correlation with the impairment of cardiac function.[544] This suggests that upregulation of the urotensin II/GPR14 system could play a part in the cardiac dysfunction associated with HF. The upregulated urotensin II/GPR14 system in HF may also have a role in the regulation of renal function in HF. In rat models of HF, urotensin II was shown to act primarily as a renal vasodilator, apparently by a nitric oxide–dependent mechanism.[362] Moreover, human urotensin II increased GFR in rats with HF but did not alter urinary Na^+ excretion in control or HF rats. However, in contrast to the negligible renal vasodilatory effect in control rats, the peptide produced a prominent and prolonged decrease in renal vascular resistance in association with a significant increase in RPF and GFR in rats with HF. On the other hand, infusion of rat urotensin II into normal animals led to intense renal vasoconstriction and, hence, a fall in GFR and Na^+ retention.[362] Thus, under conditions of increased baseline renal vascular tone found in HF, human urotensin II has the capacity to act as a potent vasodilator in the kidneys. In light of the contradictory effects of urotensin II in different conditions and across species, the clinical application of these data remains to be elucidated and is likely to be complicated.

Neuropeptides

In contrast to the enigma surrounding its function in normal physiology, there is abundant evidence that neuropeptide Y has a significant role in the pathophysiologic process of HF. Because neuropeptide Y co-localizes and is released with the adrenergic neurotransmitters, it is not surprising that the activated peripheral SNS, with high circulating norepinephrine levels in HF, is also accompanied by excessive co-release of neuropeptide Y.[373] Numerous studies have demonstrated elevated plasma levels of neuropeptide Y of HF patients, regardless of the cause of the disease. This increase was correlated with the severity of disease, which suggested that neuropeptide Y might serve as an independent prognostic factor for severity and outcome of HF.[373]

Although circulating levels of neuropeptide Y are elevated in patients with HF, local concentrations of neuropeptide Y in the myocardium, like those of norepinephrine, appear to be lower than normal in association with decreased Y1 and increased Y2 receptor expression. Moreover, cardiac Y1 receptor expression decreased in proportion to the severity of cardiac hypertrophy and decompensation.[373] Because Y1 receptor activation is associated with cardiomyocyte hypertrophy and Y2 receptor activation with angiogenesis, the data in this model suggest that neuropeptide Y may simultaneously attenuate the maladaptive cardiac remodeling observed in HF and stimulate angiogenesis in the ischemic heart.[373] Similar patterns of receptor expression change were observed in the kidneys that were proportional to the degree of renal failure and Na^+ retention.[373] In contrast, administration of neuropeptide Y was shown in experimental models of HF to exert diuretic and natriuretic properties, probably by increasing the release of ANP and inhibiting the RAAS,[545] thereby facilitating water and electrolyte clearance and reducing congestion. Therefore, in HF, the higher circulating levels, together with the reduced tissue levels of neuropeptide Y, could be a counterregulatory mechanism to modulate the vasoconstrictive and Na^+ retention, as well as the cardiac remodeling, effects of the RAAS and SNS. In addition, the downregulation of Y1 receptors, by reducing vascular constriction, could contribute to reductions in vascular resistance in the coronary and renal circulations. However, once the stage of decompensated heart failure is reached, the likelihood is that RAAS and SNS effects dominate, thereby overwhelming any favorable effects of neuropeptide Y. This point might explain the notable absence of publications on the subject since 2007.

Another recently described neuropeptide with multiple cardiovascular actions is catestatin, a chromogranin A–derived peptide. In a single, relatively small study, elevated levels of this peptide were found in HF patients but the area under the receiver operating characteristic curve was inferior to that of BNP, and combining the two biomarkers did not improve diagnostic accuracy over BNP alone.[546]

Apelin

The expression of apelin and its receptor in the kidney and heart and the involvement of the system in the maintenance of water balance suggest a potential role in HF. Circulating levels rise in early HF but decline in later stages of the disease.[374,547] However, this decline correlates poorly with severity classification of HF, as indicated by LVEF and peak oxygen consumption during exercise. Therefore, it is unlikely that apelin could be used as a biomarker of HF progression.[374,547]

The fact that activation of the apelin receptor induces aquaresis, vasodilation, and a positive cardiac inotropic effect has paved the way for the receptor as a potential therapeutic target in HF. Along these lines, acute IV injection of apelin to rats with HF following induced myocardial function led to improved systolic and diastolic function. Moreover, more chronic infusion (3 weeks) decreased Ang II–induced cardiac fibrosis and remodeling.[374] In HF patients, acute intravenous apelin led to increased cardiac output, reduced BP, and vascular resistance.[374] No data are yet available on the direct renal effects of apelin in HF, although, by reducing AVP levels and improving the renal microcirculation, apelin might increase aquaresis. In addition, the favorable effects on cardiac function are likely to increase renal perfusion and hence promote diuresis.[374]

Peroxisome Proliferator–Activated Receptors

Peroxisome proliferator–activated receptors (PPARs) are nutrient-sensing nuclear transcription factors, of which PPARγ is of special interest in the context of Na^+ and water retention because of its ligands, the thiazolidinediones. Thiazolidinediones, by virtue of their ability to increase insulin sensitivity, are clinically used for the management of type 2 diabetes mellitus. In addition, thiazolidinediones decrease amounts of circulating free fatty acids and triglycerides, lower blood pressure, reduce levels of inflammatory markers, and reduce atherosclerosis in insulin-resistant patients and animal models. Moreover, they have been shown to be beneficial for cardiac remodeling in models of myocardial ischemia.[548] However, a troubling side effect of thiazolidinediones is fluid retention; therefore, HF is one of the major contraindications to the clinical use of thiazolidinediones.

The site of PPARγ-induced fluid retention appears, in part, to involve the collecting duct, inasmuch as mice with collecting duct knockout of PPARγ were able to excrete salt loads more easily than wild-type controls. Because PPARγ knockout also blocked the effect of thiazolidinediones on messenger RNA expression of the γ-subunit of the ENaC, the Na^+-retaining effect of thiazolidinediones was thought to result from PPARγ stimulation of ENaC-mediated renal salt reabsorption.[549] However, other studies have shown suppression of ENaC by PPARγ stimulation. Alternative mechanisms in the collecting duct include stimulation of non-ENaC sodium channel and inhibition of Cl^- secretion to the tubular lumen. In addition, thiazolidinediones may augment Na^+ reabsorption in the proximal tubule by stimulating the expression and activity of apical NEH3, basolateral Na^+-HCO_3^- cotransporter, and Na^+-K^+-ATPase. These effects are mediated by PPARγ-induced nongenomic transactivation of the epidermal growth factor receptor and downstream extracellular signal-regulated kinases.[549] In clinical terms, the Na^+-retaining effect of thiazolidinediones translates into an increased incidence of HF in patients receiving these drugs in comparison with controls.[550] Because of the Na^+-retaining and fluid-retaining effects, as well as other concerns related to increased cardiovascular events on the one hand and favorable effects on the myocardium on the other, the exact role of thiazolidinediones in HF remains a hotly debated subject.[551]

In summary, the alterations in the efferent limb of volume regulation in HF include enhanced activities of vasoconstrictor/Na^+-retaining systems and activation of counterregulatory vasodilatory/natriuretic systems. The magnitude of Na^+ excretion by the kidneys and, therefore, the disturbance in volume homeostasis in HF are largely determined by the balance between these antagonistic systems. In the early stages of HF, the balancing effect of the vasodilatory/natriuretic systems is of importance in the maintenance of circulatory and renal function. However, with the progression of HF, this balance shifts toward dysfunction of the vasodilatory/natriuretic systems and marked activation of the vasoconstrictor/antinatriuretic systems. These disturbances are translated at the renal circulatory and tubular level to alterations that result in avid retention of salt and water, thereby leading to edema formation.

Renal Sodium Retention in Cirrhosis with Portal Hypertension. Abnormalities in renal Na^+ and water excretion commonly occur with cirrhosis, in human as well as in experimental animal models.[552,553] Avid Na^+ and water retention may lead eventually to ascites, a common complication of cirrhosis and a major cause of morbidity and mortality, with the occurrence of spontaneous bacterial peritonitis, variceal bleeding, and development of the HRS.[553,554] As in HF, the pathogenesis of renal Na^+ and water retention in cirrhosis is related not to an intrinsic abnormality of the kidneys but to extrarenal mechanisms that regulate renal Na^+ and water handling.

Abnormalities of Sensing Mechanisms in Cirrhosis. Several hypotheses have been proposed to explain the mechanisms of Na^+ and water retention in cirrhosis, of which the two major ones are the overflow and underfilling hypotheses. According to the overflow hypothesis, an extrarenal signal, possibly from the abnormal liver, induces primary renal Na^+ and water retention and plasma volume expansion, even before the appearance of clinical signs such as ascites. Conversely, the classic underfilling theory posits that ascites formation causes hypovolemia, which further initiates secondary renal Na^+ and water retention.

In 1988, Schrier and associates[555] proposed the peripheral arterial vasodilation hypothesis as the basis for relative hypovolemia. This concept was promoted in the 1990s as a unifying mechanism to explain renal Na^+ and water retention in such diverse states of edema formation as cirrhosis and pregnancy.[553,556,557] At the same time, the importance of NO, as well as other vasodilatory mechanisms, in the induction of peripheral arterial vasodilation and the generation of the so-called hyperdynamic circulation, which mediates salt and water retention in cirrhosis, became increasingly evident.[558-561] In the following sections, these complementary theories of the disturbance in volume sensing in cirrhosis are briefly presented, followed by a description of the efferent limb of the volume control system.

Overflow Hypothesis. On the basis of findings in patients with cirrhosis, Lieberman and colleagues[562] postulated non–volume-dependent renal Na^+ retention as the primary disturbance in Na^+ homeostasis in cirrhosis. In turn, this type of renal Na^+ retention leads to total plasma volume expansion, and the resulting increased hydrostatic pressure in the portosplanchnic bed promotes so-called overflow ascites. Strong support for the overflow theory came from extensive and carefully designed studies in dogs with experimental cirrhosis.[563] Results of these studies indicated that renal Na^+ retention and volume expansion could precede ascites formation by 10 days. Na^+ retention occurred independently of measurable changes in cardiac output, mean arterial pressure, splanchnic blood volume, hepatic arterial blood flow, GFR, RPF, aldosterone level, and increased RSNA.[563] Also, elimination of ascites with the peritoneojugular LeVeen shunt did not prevent Na^+ retention during liberal salt intake. In additional studies in dogs with cirrhosis induced by common bile duct ligation, Na^+ retention and ascites formation occurred only in dogs with partially or fully occluded portocaval fistulas, but not in animals with a patent portocaval anastomosis and normal intrahepatic pressure. These results suggested that intrahepatic hypertension secondary to hepatic venous outflow obstruction is the primary stimulus for renal salt retention.[563]

In addition to the well-characterized increase in intrahepatic vascular resistance and sinusoidal pressure in cirrhosis, portal venous blood flow is decreased, and hepatic arterial blood flow is increased or normal. Moreover, the lower the portal venous flow, the higher the hepatic arterial flow (Figure 15.11A). Of note, a similar response in portal venous and hepatic arterial flows is observed during hemorrhage-induced hypotension.[92] Therefore, it is abundantly clear that the liver is integrally involved in volume sensing. However, the exact anatomic interactions among hepatic arterioles, presinusoidal portal vein branches, and hepatic sinusoids in the normal liver and cirrhotic liver are still being unraveled.

Afferent Sensing of Intrahepatic Hypertension. The pathway by which intrahepatic hypertension could stimulate renal Na^+ retention, without the intermediary of underfilling, would probably involve the hepatic volume-sensing mechanisms mentioned earlier. These sensing mechanisms would respond specifically to elevated hepatic venous pressure with increased hepatic afferent nerve activity. The relays for these impulses consist of two autonomic nerve

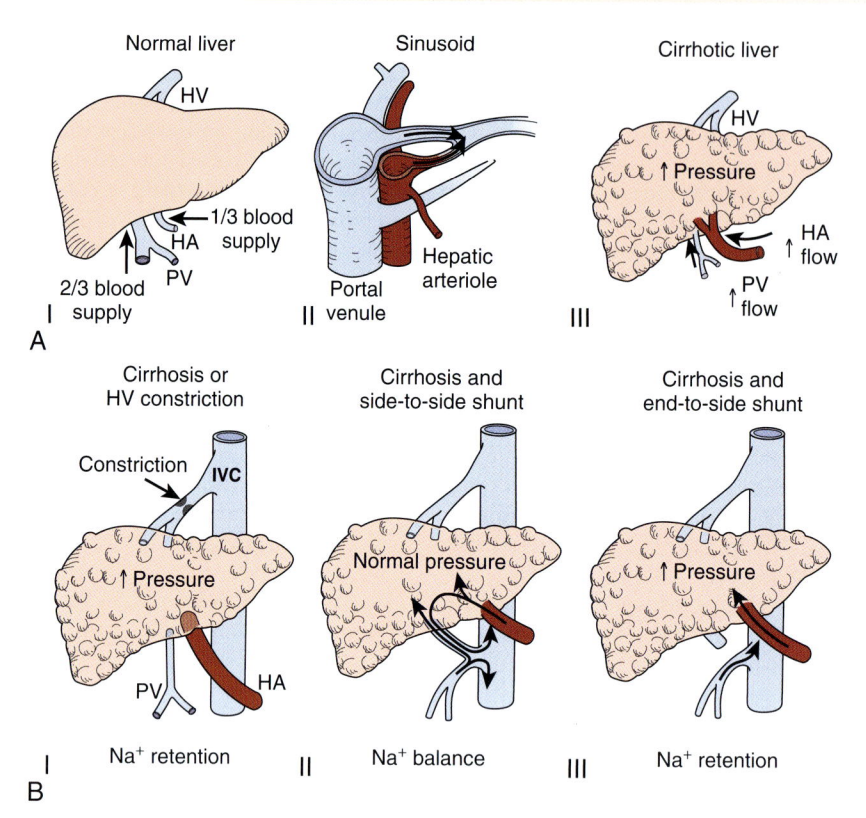

Figure 15.11 Characteristics of hepatic blood flow. **A,** Hepatic circulation. **I,** The normal liver receives two thirds of its blood flow from the portal vein (PV) and the remaining third from the hepatic artery (HA). **II,** Both the portal venules and hepatic arterioles drain into hepatic sinusoids, but the exact arrangement that allows forward flow of the mixed venous and arterial blood remains unclear. **III,** Cirrhosis increases intrahepatic vascular resistance and sinusoidal pressure. In addition, PV flow is markedly decreased, and HA flow is unchanged or increased. **B,** Hepatic vascular hemodynamics and sodium balance. **I,** Cirrhosis or restriction of HV flow increases intrahepatic vascular resistance and sinusoidal pressure, markedly decreasing PV flow and increasing HA flow. Changes in the physical forces or in the composition of the hepatic blood trigger Na⁺ retention and edema formation. **II,** Insertion of a side-to-side portocaval shunt decreases sinusoidal pressure and maintains mixing of PV and HA blood, irrigating the liver. Under these conditions and despite cirrhosis, there is no Na⁺ retention. **III,** Insertion of an end-to-side portocaval shunt only partially decreases the elevated sinusoidal pressure and prevents mixing of PV and HA blood supplies, inasmuch as the PV blood is diverted to the inferior vena cava. Under these conditions and, despite normalization of PV pressure, Na⁺ retention continues unabated. IVC, Inferior vena cava. (Adapted from Oliver JA, Verna EC: Afferent mechanisms of sodium retention in cirrhosis and HRS. *Kidney Int* 77:669-680, 2010.)

plexuses, one surrounding the hepatic artery and the other surrounding the portal vein.[564] These neural networks connect hepatic venous congestion to enhanced renal and cardiopulmonary sympathetic activity.

Occlusion of the inferior vena cava at the diaphragm was associated with increases in hepatic, portal, and renal venous pressures and resulted in markedly increased hepatic afferent nerve traffic and renal and cardiopulmonary sympathetic efferent nerve activity. Section of the anterior hepatic nerves eliminated the reflex increase in renal efferent nerve activity.[564] Similarly, denervation of the liver in dogs with vena caval constriction increased urinary Na⁺ excretion.[96] This effect of hepatic denervation was reproduced by intrahepatic administration of an adenosine receptor antagonist, 8-phenyltheophylline, to cirrhotic rats.[563] Subsequently, the adenosine effect was shown to be mediated by the A_1 receptor, inasmuch as a selective antagonist of the A_1 receptor, but not of the A_2 receptor, inhibited Na⁺ retention. Of importance is that the adenosine-dependent effects were abolished by hepatic denervation.[93]

Apart from the adenosine-mediated hepatorenal reflex, other currently undefined humoral pathways could provide an anatomic or physiologic basis for the primary effects of alterations in intrahepatic hemodynamics on renal function. Only a rapid rise in sinusoidal pressure triggers the hepatorenal reflex and ascites formation (e.g., as in Budd-Chiari syndrome). However, chronically increased sinusoidal pressure, to levels even higher than those induced acutely, is usually not associated with ascites formation.[565] Despite the wealth of information on hepatic volume sensing, the molecular identity, cellular location of the sensor, and what is sensed remain elusive. Therefore, much work remains to unravel the role of overflow in the pathogenesis of Na⁺ retention in cirrhosis completely.

Underfilling Hypothesis. In contrast to the overflow concept, the classic underfilling theory holds that during the development of cirrhosis, transudation of fluid and its accumulation in the peritoneal cavity as ascites result in true intravascular hypovolemia. The reduced EABV, in turn, is sensed by the various components of the afferent volume control system described earlier. Subsequent activation of the efferent limb of the volume control system, including the RAAS, SNS, and nonosmotic release of AVP, results in enhanced renal Na⁺ and water retention, failure to escape from the Na⁺-retaining effect of aldosterone, and impaired excretion of solute-free water. The ultimate consequence of this mechanism is the development of a positive Na⁺ balance and exacerbation of ascites formation.[552]

Several mechanisms have been proposed to account for the development of the hypovolemia. One such mechanism arose as a consequence of the disruption in normal Starling relationships that govern fluid movement in the hepatic sinusoids. These, unlike capillaries elsewhere in the body, are highly permeable for plasma proteins. As a result, partitioning of ECF between the intravascular (intrasinusoidal) and interstitial (space of Disse and lymphatic) compartments of the liver is determined predominantly by the ΔP along the length of the hepatic sinusoids. Obstruction of hepatic venous outflow promotes enhanced efflux of a protein-rich filtrate into the space of Disse and results in augmented hepatic lymph formation. Such augmented hepatic lymph flow, the main mechanism of ascites formation, has been observed in human subjects with cirrhosis and in experimental models of liver disease.[566,567]

Vastly increased hepatic lymph formation is accompanied by increased flow through the thoracic duct.[568] When the rate of enhanced hepatic lymph formation exceeds the capacity for return to the intravascular compartment via the thoracic duct, hepatic lymph accumulates as ascites, and the intravascular compartment is further compromised. As liver disease progresses, a fibrotic process surrounds the Kupffer cells lining the sinusoids, rendering the sinusoids less permeable to serum proteins. Under such circumstances, termed *capillarization of sinusoids,* a decrease in oncotic pressure also promotes transudation of ECF within the hepatic lymph space, much as it does in other vascular beds.[569]

Additional consequences of intrahepatic hypertension have been postulated to contribute to perceived volume contraction. Among these, transmission of elevated intrasinusoidal pressures to the portal vein leads to expansion of the splanchnic venous system, collateral vein formation, and portosystemic shunting. This results in increased vascular capacitance and diversion of blood flow from the arterial circuit.[570] Vasodilation seems to occur not only in the splanchnic circulation, but also in the systemic circulation, and has been attributed to refractoriness to the pressor effects of vasoconstrictor hormones, such as Ang II and catecholamines, although the mechanism remains unknown.[571] Along with diminished hepatic reticuloendothelial cell function, portosystemic shunting allows various products of intestinal metabolism and absorption to bypass the liver and escape hepatic elimination. Among these products, endotoxins are thought to contribute to perturbations in renal function in cirrhosis, either because of intestinal bacterial translocation, stimulating the release of proinflammatory cytokines (e.g., tumor necrosis factor-α [TNF-α] and interleukin-6), secondary to the hemodynamic consequences of endotoxemia, or through direct renal effects.[567]

Levels of conjugated bilirubin and bile acids may become elevated as a result of intrahepatic cholestasis or extrahepatic biliary obstruction. In experimental studies of bile duct ligation, it is difficult to distinguish the effects on renal function of jaundice itself from the effects of cirrhosis that ensue after the bile duct ligation. However, bile acids actually decrease proximal tubular reabsorption of Na⁺, a direct renal action that would tend to promote natriuresis.[572]

Nevertheless, the diuretic-like effect of bile salts may also contribute to the underfilling state in cirrhotic patients.[572,573]

Hypoalbuminemia could also contribute to the development of hypovolemia by diminishing colloid osmotic forces in the systemic capillaries and hepatic sinusoids.[569] Hypoalbuminemia was believed to occur as a result of decreased synthesis of albumin by the liver and dilution caused by ECF volume expansion. The development of hypoalbuminemia is a relatively late event in the course of chronic liver disease. Similarly, a relative impairment of cardiac function could contribute to diminished arterial blood pressure in some cirrhotic patients.[574] In these patients, tense ascites might reduce venous return (preload) to the heart.

Other factors that may also adversely affect cardiac performance include diminished β-adrenergic receptor signal transduction, cardiomyocyte cellular plasma membrane dysfunction, and increased activity or levels of cardiodepressant substances, such as cytokines, endocannabinoids, and nitric oxide. Although the cardiac dysfunction, termed *cirrhotic cardiomyopathy,* usually is clinically mild or silent, overt heart failure can be precipitated by stresses such as liver transplantation or transjugular intrahepatic portosystemic shunt (TIPS) insertion.[574] Finally, volume depletion in cirrhotic patients may be aggravated by vomiting, occult variceal bleeding, and excessive use of diuretics. Therefore, patients with cirrhosis tolerate hemorrhage or fluid loss very poorly and are prone to suffer cardiovascular collapse in the setting of hemodynamic disturbances.

Table 15.7 summarizes the various causative factors contributing to underfilling of the circulation in patients with advanced liver disease. Two major arguments have been provided in support of the underfilling theory. First, the progression of cirrhosis is characterized by increased neurohumoral activity with stimulation of the RAAS, increased sympathetic activity, and elevated plasma AVP levels. These classic markers of hypovolemia cannot be explained by the overflow hypothesis. Second, a salutary improvement in volume homeostasis was observed after volume replenishment in cirrhotic patients. Thus, volume expansion, via reinfusion of ascitic fluid, placement of a LeVeen shunt, or HWI suppresses the RAAS, increases GFR, and causes natriuresis and negative salt balance in cirrhotic patients. Conversely, the main argument against the underfilling theory was that measured plasma volume in most

Table 15.7 Factors Causing Underfilling of the Circulation in Cirrhosis

Peripheral vasodilation and blunted vasoconstrictor response to reflex, chemical, and hormonal influences
Arteriovenous shunts, particularly in portal circulation
Increased vascular capacity of portal and systemic circulation
Hypoalbuminemia
Impaired left ventricular function, so-called cirrhotic cardiomyopathy
Diminished venous return secondary to advanced tense ascites
Occult gastrointestinal bleeding from ulcers, gastritis, or varices
Volume losses caused by vomiting and excessive use of diuretics

patients with compensated cirrhosis was increased, which frequently antedated ascites formation.[575] In addition, the volume repletion–induced natriuresis described above was, at best, temporary and occurred only in 30% to 50% of affected patients. Some of the variability could be a result of inadequate volume replenishment but, nevertheless, underfilling cannot be the entire explanation for the renal Na^+ and water retention seen in cirrhotic patients; however, it may be characteristic of specific stages of the disease.

Peripheral Arterial Vasodilation. Irrespective of the initial trigger, the hallmark of fluid retention in cirrhosis is peripheral arterial vasodilation, in association with renal vasoconstriction. Initially, vasodilation occurs in the splanchnic vascular bed and later in the systemic and pulmonary circulations, leading to relative arterial underfilling[553] or, perhaps, more accurately, threatened arterial pressure.[15] This relative underfilling unloads the arterial high-pressure baroreceptors and other volume receptors, which, in turn, stimulate a compensatory neurohumoral response. This response includes activation of the RAAS and SNS, as well as the nonosmotic release of AVP.[553] Thus, increased hepatic resistance to portal flow causes the gradual development of portal hypertension, collateral vein formation, and shunting of blood to the systemic circulation.

As portal hypertension develops, local production of vasodilators—mainly nitric oxide but also carbon monoxide, glucagon, prostacyclin, AM, and endogenous opiates—increases, leading to splanchnic vasodilation.[576] Other contributing factors to splanchnic vasodilation include intestinal bacterial translocation, proinflammatory cytokines, and mesenteric angiogenesis.[567,577] In the early stages of cirrhosis, arterial pressure is maintained through increases in plasma volume and cardiac output, so-called hyperdynamic circulation. However, as the disease progresses, vasodilation in the splanchnic and, presumably, other vascular beds is so pronounced that EABV decreases markedly, leading to sustained neurohumoral activation, renal, brachial, femoral, and cerebral vasoconstriction, and further Na^+ and fluid retention.[576] This hypothesis could, therefore, potentially explain the increased cardiac output and enhanced neurohumoral changes over the entire spectrum of cirrhosis.[574]

Therefore, decreases in systemic vascular resistance associated with low arterial blood pressure and high cardiac output account for the well-known clinical manifestations of the hyperdynamic circulation commonly seen in patients with cirrhosis, including warm extremities, cutaneous vascular spiders, wide pulse pressure, and capillary pulsations in the nail bed.[578] Pulmonary vasodilation, associated with the hepatopulmonary syndrome, one of the most severe complications of chronic liver disease, is another example of the hyperdynamic circulation caused by increased production of nitric oxide (and possibly also carbon monoxide) in the lungs.[579]

The HRS may also develop when the heart is no longer able to compensate for the progressive decrease in systemic vascular resistance.[574] Thus, the hyperdynamic syndrome of chronic liver disease should be considered as a progressive vasodilatory syndrome that finally leads to multiorgan involvement.[578] As noted earlier, increased production of nitric oxide in the splanchnic vasculature plays a cardinal role in initiating this process.

Nitric Oxide. Considerable evidence has indicated that aberrations in the endothelial vasodilator nitric oxide system are involved in the pathogenesis of the hyperdynamic circulation and Na^+ and water retention in cirrhosis, as well as in hepatic encephalopathy, hepatopulmonary syndrome, and cirrhotic cardiomyopathy.[580] Nitric oxide is produced in excess by the vasculature of different animal models of portal hypertension, as well as in cirrhotic patients.[580] In animal models, the increased production of nitric oxide can be detected at the onset of Na^+ retention and before the appearance of ascites, and nitric oxide has been implicated in the impaired vascular responsiveness to vasoconstrictors.[580] Moreover, removal of the vascular endothelial layer has been demonstrated to abolish the difference in vascular reactivity between cirrhotic and control vessels.[578]

Inhibition of NOS has beneficial effects in experimental models of cirrhosis and in humans with the disease. Thus, low-dose L-NAME treatment for 7 days reversed the high nitric oxide production to control levels and corrected the hyperdynamic circulation in cirrhotic rats with ascites. The normalization of nitric oxide production was accompanied by a marked increase in urinary Na^+ and water excretion, a concomitant decrease of ascites, and decreases in PRA and aldosterone and vasopressin concentrations.[581,582] In patients with cirrhosis, the vascular hyporesponsiveness of the forearm circulation to norepinephrine could be reversed by the NOS inhibitor L-NMMA.[583] Inhibition of nitric oxide production also corrected the hypotension and hyperdynamic circulation, led to improved renal function and Na^+ excretion, and led to a decrease in plasma norepinephrine levels in these patients. However, in patients with established ascites, NOS inhibition did not improve renal function.[584]

The main enzymatic source of the increased systemic vascular nitric oxide generation in cirrhosis has been demonstrated to be eNOS in the arterial and splanchnic circulations.[580] The upregulation of eNOS appears, at least in part, to be caused by increased shear stress as a result of portal venous hypertension with increased flow in the splanchnic circulation.[580] However, in rats with portal vein ligation, eNOS upregulation and increased nitric oxide release in the superior mesenteric arteries were found to precede the development of the hyperdynamic splanchnic circulation.[580] In marked contrast to the increased nitric oxide generation in the splanchnic and systemic circulation, there is evidence for impaired nitric oxide production and endothelial dysfunction in the intrahepatic microcirculation in cirrhotic rats.[580] The mechanism of this paradoxic increase in intrahepatic vascular resistance is likely to be a dynamic process, involving contraction of myofibroblasts and stellate cells and mechanical distortion of the vasculature by fibrosis.[580] The increase in intrahepatic vascular resistance may play a significant role in the pathogenesis of intrahepatic thrombosis and collagen synthesis in cirrhosis.[585]

The decrease in nitric oxide production that results from endothelial dysfunction may shift the balance in favor of vasoconstrictors (e.g., endothelin, leukotrienes, TXA_2, Ang II), thus causing an increase in intrahepatic vascular resistance.[585] In accordance with this concept, upregulation of eNOS or nNOS expression in livers of rats with experimental cirrhosis was associated with a decrease in portal hypertension.[586,587] It has been clearly shown that eNOS protein is increased in animal models of portal hypertension, and that this increase is already detectable in cirrhotic rats without ascites.[580] However, mice with targeted deletion of eNOS alone, or with combined deletions of eNOS and iNOS, may still develop a hyperdynamic circulation in association with portal hypertension.[582] This suggests that activation of other vasodilatory agents may participate in the pathogenesis of the hyperdynamic circulation in experimental cirrhosis, such as PGI_2, endothelium-derived hyperpolarizing factor, carbon monoxide and AM.[580]

There are additional lines of evidence for the involvement of isoforms in addition to eNOS in the generation of the hyperdynamic circulation and fluid retention in experimental cirrhosis. nNOS is preferentially expressed in portal endothelial cells, and increased expression of nNOS in mesenteric nerves has been thought to compensate partially for the endothelial isoform deficiency in the eNOS knockout mouse.[580] Moreover, gene delivery techniques for nNOS (as well as eNOS) can increase expression of these isoforms and reduce intrahepatic venous resistance and portal hypertension.[580] nNOS also appears to promote splanchnic vasodilation, possibly by modulating the neurogenic release of norepinephrine, although this effect is probably modest.[580,588] In contrast, the role of iNOS remains controversial; some researchers have shown increased iNOS in the arteries of animals with experimental biliary cirrhosis but not in other forms of experimental cirrhosis.[580] Increased splanchnic iNOS appears to reside in resident macrophages of the superior mesenteric artery, and administration of a specific inhibitor of iNOS leads to peripheral vasoconstriction, supporting a pathologic role for iNOS in the development of HRS. iNOS is primarily regulated at the transcription level by many proinflammatory factors, principally nuclear factor-kappaB (NF-κB); an important stimulus for NF-κB is lipopolysaccharide (endotoxin), which could be generated from translocated intestinal bacteria. Although nonspecific inhibition of NOS may correct the hyperdynamic circulation, preferential iNOS inhibition was shown to be generally ineffective.[580] Interestingly, there is also an interaction between eNOS and iNOS in the vasculature in cirrhosis. Overexpression of eNOS in large arteries results in systemic hypotension and increased blood flow. These effects can be abrogated by activated iNOS in the small vessels of the splanchnic circulation.[580] Thus, overall, available data indicate a predominant role for eNOS deficiency, with possible modulation by both nNOS and iNOS.

In experimental cirrhosis, several cellular mechanisms have been implicated in the upregulation of splanchnic eNOS activity and in the downregulation of intrahepatic eNOS activity. Elevation in shear stress as a result of the hyperdynamic circulation and portal hypertension has already been mentioned and is generally consistent with this well-documented mechanism for upregulating eNOS gene transcription. However, additional factors related to the hepatic dysfunction could further stimulate this upregulation. For example, eNOS activity is not only regulated transcriptionally, but also posttranscriptionally, by tetrahydrobiopterin and direct phosphorylation of eNOS protein.[580] Furthermore, in rats with experimental cirrhosis, circulating endotoxins may increase the enzymatic production of tetrahydrobiopterin, thereby enhancing eNOS activity in the mesenteric vascular bed.[580]

Conversely, potential contributors to intrahepatic eNOS downregulation include interactions with other proteins such as caveolin, calmodulin, heat shock protein 90, and eNOS trafficking inducer.[580] In addition, disorders of guanylate cyclase activity have been described.[589] Increased levels of the NO inhibitor, ADMA, have been reported, and these levels correlate with the severity of portal hypertension during hepatic inflammation. Moreover, higher ADMA levels have been found in patients with decompensated cirrhosis than in those with compensated disease.[589] The raised ADMA levels have been linked to reduced activity of dimethylarginine dimethylaminohydrolases (DDAHs) that normally metabolize ADMA to citrulline. In this regard, targeted disruption of the DDAH-1 gene in mice or chemical inhibition of DDAH-1 in a model of endotoxin shock was associated with increased plasma and tissue levels of ADMA and decreased nitric oxide–dependent vasodilation.[590] Similarly, patients with alcoholic cirrhosis and superimposed inflammatory alcoholic hepatitis had higher plasma and tissue levels of ADMA, higher portal venous pressures, and decreased DDAH expression.[591]

The therapeutic potential for increasing DDAH activity has been shown in an animal model of traumatic vascular injury. Transgenic overexpression of DDAH in this model led to reduced plasma ADMA levels, enhanced endothelial cell regeneration, and reduced neointima formation.[592] These data raise the possibility of translating the favorable effects of DDAH into the management of decompensated portal hypertension.[589] However, increased DDAH expression, in parallel with high basal NO levels, has recently been shown in isolated mesenteric arteries of two rat models of cirrhosis. These data would be consistent with increased degradation of ADMA, resulting in increased generation of endothelial NO and mesenteric vasodilation, hardly favorable for the improvement of portal hypertension.[593] In the final analysis, the relative importance of the various mechanisms involved in the reduced intrahepatic and increased splanchnic and systemic NOS activity in cirrhosis remains to be determined.

Endocannabinoids. Endogenous cannabinoids are lipid-signaling molecules that mimic the activity of Δ9-tetrahydrocannabinol, the main psychotropic constituent of marijuana. They influence neuroprotection, pain and motor function, energy balance and food intake, cardiovascular function, immune and inflammatory responses, and cell proliferation. *N*-arachidonoylethanolamide (anandamide) and 2-arachidonoylglycerol are the two most widely studied endocannabinoids that bind the two specific receptors, CB_1 and CB_2. CB_1 is expressed mainly in the brain, whereas the CB_2 receptor is found mostly in cells of the immune system; both receptors are also expressed in many peripheral tissues under physiologic and pathologic conditions. Anandamide is also able to interact with the vanilloid receptor.[594] Although both hepatocytes and nonparenchymal liver cells are capable of producing endocannabinoids, the physiologic expression of CB_1 and CB_2 receptors in the adult liver is very low or even absent.

A compelling series of experimental and clinical studies has shown that the hepatic expression of CB_1 and CB_2 receptors and endocannabinoid production are greatly upregulated in chronic and acute liver damage.[594] Of relevance to this discussion is that endocannabinoids have been implicated in portal hypertension and the hyperdynamic circulatory syndrome. In this regard, anandamide caused a dose-dependent increase in intrahepatic vascular resistance in the isolated perfused rat liver. This effect was magnified in cirrhotic livers and appeared to be mediated by enhanced production of COX-derived vasoconstrictive eicosanoids. In addition, chronic antagonism of the CB_1 receptor reversed the upregulation of several vasoconstrictive eicosanoids in rat bile duct ligation–induced cirrhosis. With regard to the splanchnic vasodilation observed in cirrhosis, administration of the CB_1 receptor antagonist rimonabant to cirrhotic rats reversed arterial hypotension and increased vascular resistance, with a concomitant decrease in mesenteric arterial blood flow and portal venous pressure and prevention of ascites formation. The reduction in splanchnic blood flow was enhanced by the vanilloid receptor Capsazepine. These findings indicate that the transient receptor potential vanilloid type 1 protein and the CB_1 receptor have a dual role in the splanchnic vasodilation characteristic of cirrhosis.[594]

In contrast to the effects of CB_1 receptor modulation, pharmacologic or genetic upregulation of the CB_2 receptor leads to reduced hepatic fibrosis in experimental cirrhosis. Conversely, CB_2 knockout mice display more severe hepatic fibrosis in carbon tetrachloride (CCl_4)–induced cirrhosis than wild-type mice.[594]

A role for endotoxin in the endocannabinoid effects was suggested by the demonstration that infusion of monocytes isolated from cirrhotic rats but not from control rats induced marked hypotension in normal animals.[594] Also, the amount of anandamide was significantly higher in monocytes isolated from patients or rats with cirrhosis than in those from healthy subjects or animals. Because endotoxin represents a major stimulus for endocannabinoid generation in monocytes and platelets, it has been hypothesized that these cells are stimulated to produce large amounts of endocannabinoids by the elevated circulating endotoxin levels frequently found in patients with advanced cirrhosis. This production could then trigger splanchnic and peripheral vasodilation, arterial hypotension, and intrahepatic vasoconstriction through activation of the CB_1 receptors located in the vascular wall and in perivascular nerves.[594] The potentially favorable effects of CB_1 receptor blockade on Na^+ excretion and/or of CB_2 receptor upregulation on the reduction in hepatic fibrosis opens up the possibility of pharmacologic modification of human HRS.

In summary, afferent sensing of volume in cirrhosis is characterized by increased intrahepatic vascular resistance and sinusoidal pressure, decreased portal venous blood flow, and increased hepatic arterial flow. Either because of changes in intrahepatic physical forces or in the composition of the mixed intrahepatic blood, abnormal Na^+ retention is initiated, and edema develops (see Figure 15.11A). Cirrhosis alone is not sufficient to induce edema, inasmuch as a side-to-side portocaval shunt prevents (if inserted before induction of cirrhosis) or corrects (if inserted after induction of cirrhosis) renal Na^+ retention. This outcome could result from decreases in sinusoidal pressure or maintenance of the mixing of portal venous and hepatic arterial blood perfusing the liver. In contrast, end-to-side portocaval shunting only partially decreases elevated sinusoidal pressure and prevents mixing of portal venous and arterial hepatic blood supplies, inasmuch as the portal venous blood is diverted to the inferior vena cava. Under these conditions, and despite normalization of portal venous pressure, Na^+ retention continues unabated (see Figure 15.11B).

Available data are most consistent with the view that the putative EABV sensor in the hepatic circulation is pathologically activated in cirrhosis, failing to respond to the expanded ECF volume. Therefore, as the disease advances, edema worsens.[92]

Abnormalities of Effector Mechanisms in Cirrhosis. The efferent limb of volume regulation in cirrhosis is similar to that in HF, consisting of adjustments in glomerular hemodynamics and tubule transport that are mediated by vasoconstrictor/antinatriuretic forces (RAAS, SNS, AVP, and endothelin) and counterbalanced by vasodilator/natriuretic systems (NPs and prostaglandins). Therefore, tilting the balance toward Na^+ retaining forces leads to renal Na^+ and water retention, as in HF.[576,595]

VASOCONSTRICTOR AND ANTINATRIURETIC (ANTIDIURETIC) SYSTEMS

Renin-Angiotensin-Aldosterone System

As in other states of secondary Na^+ retention, the RAAS plays a central role in mediating renal Na^+ retention in cirrhosis, as demonstrated in patients and animal models. Although positive Na^+ balance may already be evident in the pre-ascitic phase of the disease, PRA and aldosterone levels remain within the normal range or may even be depressed at this stage.[596] With progression of the disease, RAAS activation increases in parallel. Results of animal models of cirrhosis, in general, are consistent with this pattern.[597]

As noted, these observations were long believed to be evidence for the role of the overflow theory in the mechanism of ascites formation. However, Bernardi and associates have found elevated aldosterone levels that were inversely correlated with renal Na^+ excretion in pre-ascitic cirrhotic patients, particularly in the upright position.[598] This finding suggests that posture-induced activation of the RAAS could already exist in the pre-ascitic phase. In accordance with this notion, renal Na^+ retention induced by LBNP was associated with a prominent increase in renal renin and Ang II excretion.[599] Moreover, treatment with the ARB, losartan, at a dosage that did not affect systemic and renal hemodynamics or glomerular filtration was associated with a significant natriuretic response.[600] The losartan-induced natriuresis in the presence of normal PRA was attributed to inhibition of the local intrarenal RAAS.[598,600] It has been demonstrated in rats with chronic bile duct ligation that activation of the intrarenal RAAS may precede activation of the circulating system.[601] In addition, losartan has been shown to cause a decrease in portal venous pressure in cirrhotic patients with portal hypertension.[602] The postural-induced activation of the RAAS, and the beneficial effects of low-dose losartan treatment, in patients with pre-ascitic cirrhosis may be explained by compartmentalization of the expanded blood volume within the splanchnic venous bed during standing and translocation toward the central and arterial circulatory beds during recumbence.[598]

In contrast, in Na^+-retaining cirrhotic patients with ascites, Ang II inhibition has deleterious effects. For example, administration of captopril, even in low doses, to such patients resulted in a decrease in GFR and urinary Na⁺ excretion.[603] At this stage of the disease, activation of the RAAS serves to support arterial pressure and maintain adequate circulation. Therefore, blockade of the RAAS by ACE inhibition or an ARB may lead to a profound decrease in RPP. This scenario might be important in the pathogenesis of the HRS, which is regularly preceded by a state of Na⁺ retention and may be precipitated by a hypovolemic insult. Abnormalities of the renal circulation characteristic of this syndrome include marked diminution of RPF with renal cortical ischemia and increased renal vascular resistance, abnormalities consistent with the known actions of Ang II on the renal microcirculation. In this regard, several groups have correlated activation of the RAAS with worsening hepatic hemodynamics and decreased rates of survival in patients with cirrhosis.[604] For this reason, ACEIs and ARBs should be avoided in patients with cirrhosis and ascites.

Evolving knowledge on the so-called alternate ACE2, angiotensin-(1-7) Mas receptor pathway has shed new light on the role of the RAAS in the pathogenesis of Na⁺ retention in cirrhosis. In this regard, in situ perfused cirrhotic rat liver elicited a marked endothelium-dependent vasodilatory effect of exogenous angiotensin-(1-7) on the vasoconstrictive response evoked by Ang II. Moreover, this response was completely abolished by the eNOS inhibitor, L-NAME.[605,606] These findings suggest that in the cirrhotic liver, as in other vascular beds, angiotensin-(1-7) may cause a vasodilatory response, mediated by NO, which antagonizes the increase in portal pressure mediated by Ang II and other local vasoconstrictors.[605,606] The data raise the possibility of reducing intrahepatic resistance and portal pressure by targeted upregulation of the alternate RAAS pathway in the liver.

Sympathetic Nervous System

Activation of the SNS is a common feature in patients with cirrhosis and ascites.[588] Circulating norepinephrine levels, as well as urinary excretion of catecholamines and their metabolites, are elevated in patients with cirrhosis and usually are correlated with the severity of the disease. Moreover, high levels of plasma norepinephrine in patients with decompensated cirrhosis are predictive of increased rate of mortality.[607] The source of the increase in norepinephrine levels is enhanced SNS activity, rather than reduced disposal, with nerve terminal spillover from the liver, heart, kidneys, muscle, and cutaneous innervation.[588] Elevated plasma norepinephrine levels were shown to be correlated closely with Na⁺ and water retention in cirrhotic patients.[608] In addition, increased efferent renal sympathetic tone,[609] perhaps as a result of defective arterial and cardiopulmonary baroreflex control, was observed by direct recordings in experimental cirrhosis.[610] This scenario could explain why volume expansion fails to suppress the enhanced RSNA in cirrhosis.

Concomitantly with the increase in norepinephrine release, cardiovascular responsiveness to reflex autonomic stimulation may be impaired in patients with cirrhosis.[608] This impairment includes impeded vasoconstrictor responses to stimuli, such as mental arithmetic, LBNP, and the Valsalva maneuver. This interference in the peripheral and central autonomic nervous systems in cirrhosis could be explained partially by increased occupancy of endogenous catecholamine receptors, downregulation of adrenergic receptors, or a defect at the level of postreceptor signaling.[588,607] It is also possible that the excessive NO-dependent vasodilation alone could account for the vascular hyporesponsiveness in cirrhosis. This concept is supported by the finding that the hyporesponsiveness to pressor agents is not limited to norepinephrine but may also be observed in response to Ang II in patients and experimental animals.[611,612] Interestingly, NPY, which by itself has no vasoconstrictor effect, has been shown to potentiate norepinephrine-evoked vasoconstriction in the mesenteric vasculature of portal vein ligation–induced cirrhosis in rats. Thus, enhanced release of NPY may be a compensatory mechanism to counteract splanchnic vasodilation by restoring the vasoconstrictor efficacy of endogenous catecholamines.[588]

Metabolic derangements caused by hepatic dysfunction, such as hypoglycemia and hyperinsulinemia, could also elicit sympathetic overactivity in cirrhosis.[607] Although hyperinsulinemia in cirrhotic models has been shown to stimulate Na⁺ retention,[613] overt hypoglycemia is seldom observed in patients with compensated cirrhosis. Hypoxia may stimulate the SNS in patients with cirrhosis, as indicated by a negative correlation between circulating norepinephrine levels and arterial oxygen tension. Moreover, inhalation of oxygen significantly reduced circulating levels of norepinephrine, which suggests that a causal relationship exists between hypoxia and increased SNS activity in these patients.[607]

The increase in renal sympathetic tone and plasma norepinephrine levels could contribute to the antinatriuresis of cirrhosis by decreasing total RBF, or its intrarenal distribution, or by acting directly at the tubular epithelial level to enhance Na⁺ reabsorption. Patients with compensated cirrhosis may have decreased RBF, even in the early stages and, as the disease progresses, RBF tends to decline further, concomitantly with the increase in sympathetic activity.[607] In this regard, activation of the SNS in cirrhotic patients was shown to be associated with a rightward and downward shift of the RBF-RPP autoregulatory curve in such a way that RBF became critically dependent on RPP. Moreover, this phenomenon was found to contribute to the development of the HRS. Furthermore, insertion of TIPS to reduce portal venous pressure in patients with HRS leads to a fall in plasma norepinephrine levels and to an upward shift in the RBF-RPP curve.[614]

The spleen also controls renal microvascular tone through reflex activation of the splenic afferent and renal sympathetic nerves. In portal hypertension, the splenorenal reflex–mediated reduction in renal vascular conductance exacerbates sodium and water retention in the kidneys and may eventually contribute to renal dysfunction. There is recent evidence suggesting that the increased splenic venous outflow pressure, resulting from, but independent of, portal hypertension, reflexly activates adrenergic-angiotensinergic mesenteric nerves, vasodilator mesenteric nerves, and the renin angiotensin system. Finally, the spleen itself may be a source of a vasoactive factor.[615,616]

The centrality of SNS overactivity in cirrhosis has been illustrated by the finding that in patients with cirrhosis and increased SNS activity, addition of clonidine to diuretic treatment induces an earlier diuretic response, with fewer diuretic requirements and complications.[617,618] In parallel with the increase in sympathetic activity, patients with progressive cirrhosis also showed an increase in the activities of the RAAS and AVP.[576] The marked neurohumoral activation that occurs at relatively advanced stages of cirrhosis probably represents a shift toward decompensation, characterized by a severe decrease in EABV and, perhaps, true volume depletion. A correlation also exists between plasma norepinephrine and AVP levels; thus, the increased activity of the SNS may stimulate the release of AVP.[619,620] In addition, a direct relationship exists between plasma norepinephrine and activity of the RAAS. Together, evidence suggests that the three pressor systems might be activated by the same mechanisms and could operate in concert to counteract the low arterial blood pressure and decrease in EABV.[607,620]

Arginine Vasopressin

Patients and experimental animals with advanced hepatic cirrhosis frequently exhibit impaired renal water excretion as a result of nonosmotic release of AVP and, consequently, develop water retention with hyponatremia.[412,576,621] For example, cirrhotic patients unable to excrete a water load normally have high immunoreactive levels of AVP in comparison with cirrhotic patients who exhibited a normal response.[622] Affected patients also have higher plasma renin and aldosterone levels and lower urinary Na^+ excretion, which suggests that the inability to suppress vasopressin is secondary to a decrease in EABV.[619] In rats with experimental cirrhosis, plasma levels of AVP were elevated in association with overexpression of hypothalamic AVP messenger RNA, together with a diminished pituitary AVP content.[623] In addition, the expression of AQP2, the AVP-regulated water channel in the collecting duct, is increased in rat models of cirrhosis and the AVP receptor antagonist, terlipressin, significantly diminished AQP2 overexpression.[624] Upregulation of AQP2 clearly plays an important role in water retention associated with hepatic cirrhosis, as well as in other pathologic states.[624]

As noted earlier in this chapter, AVP supports arterial blood pressure through its action on the V_1 receptors found on vascular smooth muscle cells, whereas the V_2 receptor is responsible for water transport in the collecting duct.[625] The availability of selective blockers of these receptors has provided clear evidence for the dual roles of AVP in pathogenesis of cirrhosis.[463,625] Thus, the administration of a V_2 receptor antagonist to cirrhotic patients, as well as to rats with experimental cirrhosis, increases urine volume, decreases urine osmolality, and corrects hyponatremia.[463,625] Clinical applications of V_2 receptor antagonists are discussed later (see section, "Specific Treatments Based on the Pathophysiology of Congestive Heart Failure").

The V_1 receptor is important for the maintenance of arterial pressure and circulatory integrity in cirrhosis and ascites.[625] After the actions of Ang II were blocked with saralasin, a selective V_1 receptor antagonist produced a pronounced fall in arterial blood pressure.[626] Thus, both V1 and V2 receptors are integrally involved in the pathogenesis of fluid retention in cirrhosis.

AVP also increases the synthesis of the vasodilatory PGE_2 and PGI_2 in several vascular beds, including the kidneys. This increase, in turn, may offset the vasoconstrictor action, as well as the hydroosmotic effect of AVP. Consistent with this concept, urinary PGE_2 was found to be markedly increased in cirrhotic patients with positive free water clearance, despite an impaired ability to suppress AVP directly.[627,628] These data suggest that urinary diluting capacity is enhanced after a water load by increased synthesis of PGE_2 in the collecting duct.[627,628]

Endothelin

Plasma levels of immunoreactive endothelin are markedly elevated in patients with cirrhosis and ascites, as well as in the HRS.[629] Compared to normal controls, blood levels of ET-1 and its precursor, big ET-1, were shown to be increased in the systemic circulation and splanchnic and renal venous beds of cirrhotic patients.[630] Levels correlated positively with portal venous pressure and cardiac output and inversely with central blood volume.[629] The rise in ET-1 levels is accompanied by a reduction in ET-3 levels, and the consequently elevated ET-1/ET-3 ratio is associated with a poor outcome of portal hypertension.[631] In animal models of cirrhosis with portal hypertension, ET-A receptor activation in association with attenuated ET-B receptor depressive effect on the portal vein has recently been reported.[632] ET-B receptor blockade in cirrhotic animals led to sinusoidal constriction and hepatotoxicity,[633] whereas the dual ET-A and B receptor blocker, tezosentan, had no effect on hepatic blood flow.[634]

In humans with HRS, although no change in ET levels occurred immediately following TIPS insertion, ET-1 and big ET-1 levels were significantly reduced in portal and renal veins 1 to 2 months after the procedure, with a parallel increase in creatinine clearance and urinary Na^+ excretion.[630] Similar favorable changes have been observed within 1 week after successful orthotopic liver transplantation.[635] Conversely, temporary occlusion of TIPS by angioplasty balloon inflation led to a transient increase in portal venous pressure, increased plasma ET-1, marked reduction of RPF and increased intrarenal generation of ET-1.[636]

The importance of the intrarenal endothelin system in the pathogenesis of the HRS has been demonstrated in a rat model of acute liver failure induced by galactosamine, in which renal failure also developed, despite normal renal histologic findings.[637] Plasma concentrations of ET-1 were increased twofold after the onset of liver and renal failure, and the ET-A receptor was upregulated significantly in the renal cortex. Administration of bosentan, a nonselective endothelin receptor antagonist, prevented the development of renal failure when given before or 24 hours after the onset of liver injury.[637]

Increased local intrahepatic production of endothelin probably also contributes to the development of portal (and pulmonary) hypertension in cirrhosis through contraction of the stellate cells and a concomitant decrease in sinusoidal blood flow.[638] Taken together, the data are consistent with the hypothesis that the hemodynamic changes occurring in patients with cirrhosis and refractory ascites could be related to local production of ET-1 by the splanchnic and renal vascular beds. Nevertheless, after both TIPS and orthotopic liver transplantation, there are improvements in other vasoconstrictive factors (e.g., RAAS and vasopressin) in addition to ET.[639] Therefore, the exact contribution of activation of the intrarenal endothelin system in the pathogenesis of the HRS remains speculative.

Apelin

As mentioned earlier, apelin is the endogenous ligand of the angiotensin-like receptor 1, found to be involved in Na^+ and water homeostasis and in regulation of cardiovascular tone and cardiac contractility through a reciprocal relationship with Ang II and AVP.[374] Because of these properties, apelin is potentially involved in the pathogenesis of advanced liver disease. Evidence for this hypothesis includes raised plasma apelin levels in patients and experimental animals with cirrhosis,[640] as well as enhanced expression of apelin and its receptor in proliferated arterial capillaries directly connected with sinusoids in human cirrhosis.[641,642] Specifically, apelin receptors appear to localize to stellate cells and may mediate the profibrogenic effects of Ang II and ET-1.[641] In addition, an apelin receptor antagonist led to a reduction in the raised cardiac index, reversal of the increased total peripheral resistance, and improvement in Na^+ and water excretion in rats with experimental cirrhosis.[640] These data raise the possibility for a future therapeutic role of apelin antagonism in the management of severe HRS as in HF. However, in view of the complex effects of apelin on glomerular hemodynamics, caution will be needed in the therapeutic application of apelin antagonists.[376]

VASODILATORS/NATRIURETICS

Apart from their role in the hyperdynamic circulation characteristic of advanced cirrhosis, vasodilators play an important part in the pathogenesis of renal Na^+ retention. The principal vasodilators involved are NPs and PGs.

Natriuretic Peptides

Atrial Natriuretic Peptide. Most of the information relating ANP to various stages of cirrhosis and portal hypertension was obtained in the 1990s and, in recent years, measurements of BNP and NT-proBNP have largely superseded ANP as a biomarker of these conditions. Nevertheless, the role of NPs in the pathogenesis of HRS has been largely elucidated through studies on ANP, and these will be summarized here. Plasma levels of ANP are elevated in patients with cirrhosis at all stages, despite the reduction in effective circulating volume in the late stages of the disease.[643,644] In the pre-ascitic stage of cirrhosis, the increase in plasma ANP may be important for the maintenance of Na^+ homeostasis, but with progression of the disease, patients develop resistance to the natriuretic action of the peptide.[643,644] The high levels of ANP mostly reflect increased cardiac release rather than impaired clearance of the peptide.[645] The stimulus for increased cardiac ANP synthesis and release in early cirrhosis is likely increased left atrial size caused by overfilling of the circulation, secondary to intrahepatic hypertension–related renal Na^+ retention.[646]

In addition to elevated ANP levels, pre-ascitic patients also had significantly elevated left and right pulmonary volumes, despite having normal blood pressure and normal renin, aldosterone, and norepinephrine levels.[647] High Na^+ intake in these patients resulted in weight gain and a positive Na^+ balance for 3 weeks, followed by a return to normal Na^+ balance thereafter. Thus, despite continued high-Na^+ intake, pre-ascitic patients reach a new steady state of Na^+ balance, thereby preventing fluid retention and the development of ascites. These findings also suggest that ANP plays an important role in preventing the transition from the pre-ascitic stage to ascites in these patients.[648] The factors responsible for maintaining relatively high levels of ANP during the later stages of cirrhosis, in association with arterial underfilling, also have not been determined, but may be related to a futile vicious cycle of mutual interactions between vasoconstrictor/Na^+-retaining and vasodilatory/natriuretic forces. The fact that ANP levels do not increase further as patients proceed from early to late decompensated stages of cirrhosis would be consistent with this explanation.

The basis for this apparent resistance to ANP was shown to occur at a stage of cellular signaling beyond cGMP production, because ANP receptors in the collecting duct were not defective.[649] ANP resistance in cirrhosis was ameliorated by endopeptidase inhibitors, bradykinin, kininase II inhibitors, and mannitol, renal sympathetic denervation, peritoneovenous shunting, and orthotopic liver transplantation.[650-655] Furthermore, infusion of Ang II mimicked the nonresponder state by causing patients in the early stages of cirrhosis, who still responded to ANP, to become unresponsive.[656] This Ang II effect occurred at proximal (decreased distal delivery of Na^+) and distal nephron sites to abrogate ANP-induced natriuresis and was reversible. The importance of distal solute delivery was confirmed using mannitol, which also resulted in an improved natriuretic response to ANP in responders but not nonresponders.[650,657]

To summarize, ANP resistance is best explained by an effect of decreased delivery of Na^+ to ANP-responsive distal nephron sites (glomerulotubular imbalance caused by abnormal systemic hemodynamics and activation of the RAAS) combined with an overriding effect of more powerful antinatriuretic factors to overcome the natriuretic action of ANP at its site of action in the medullary collecting tubule (Figure 15.12).[649] The latter effect could result from decreased delivery as well as permissive paracrine/autocrine cofactors, such as PGs and kinins.

Brain Natriuretic Peptide and C-Type Natriuretic Peptide. BNP levels have also been found to be elevated in patients with cirrhosis and ascites and, like that of ANP, its natriuretic effect is also blunted in cirrhotic patients with Na^+ retention and ascites.[658-660] Plasma BNP levels may be correlated with cardiac dysfunction[660,661] and with severity of disease and may be of prognostic value in the progression of cirrhosis.[659,660,662] Plasma CNP levels in cirrhotic pre-ascitic patients, although not elevated in comparison to healthy controls, were found to be directly correlated with 24-hour natriuresis and urine volume[663] and inversely correlated with arterial compliance but not with systemic vascular resistance.[664] These data suggested that compensatory downregulation of CNP occurs in cirrhosis when vasodilation persists, and that regulation of large and small arteries by CNP may differ.

In contrast to the pre-ascitic stage, patients with more advanced disease and impaired renal function had lower plasma and higher urinary CNP levels than those with intact renal function. Moreover, urinary CNP was correlated inversely with urinary Na^+ excretion. In patients with refractory ascites or HRS treated with terlipressin infusion or TIPS (see later section, "Specific Treatments Based on the Pathophysiology of Sodium Retention in Cirrhosis"), urinary CNP declined and urinary Na^+ excretion increased 1 week later.[665] Thus, CNP may have a significant role in renal Na^+ handling in cirrhosis.

Finally, *Dendroaspis* NP levels were found to be increased in cirrhotic patients with ascites, but not in those without, and levels were correlated with disease severity.[666] The significance of these findings remains unknown.

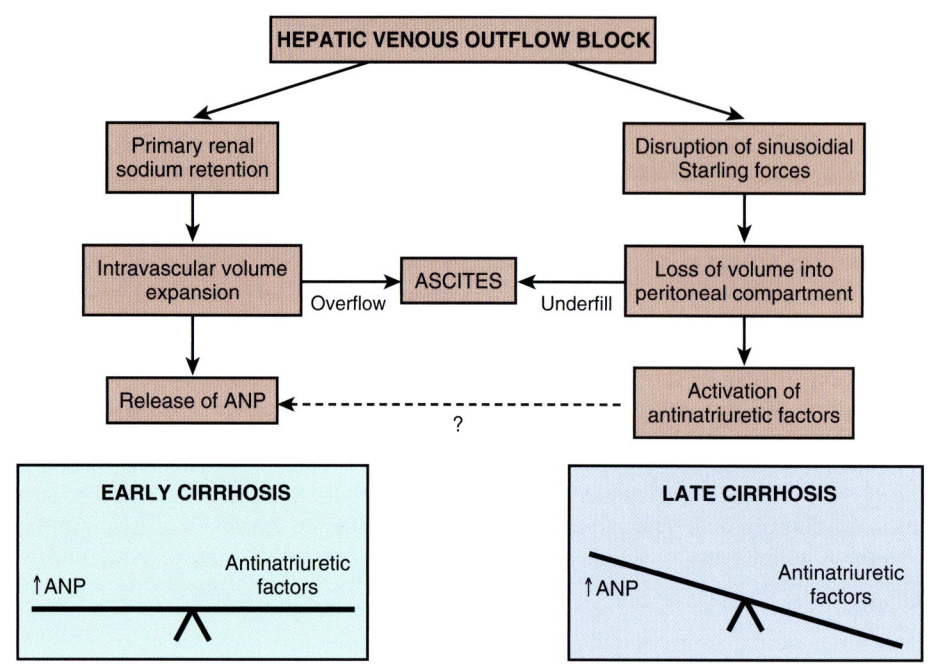

Figure 15.12 Working formulation for the role of atrial natriuretic peptide (ANP) in the renal sodium retention of cirrhosis. The primary hepatic abnormality for renal Na^+ retention is blockade of hepatic venous outflow. In early disease, this signals renal Na^+ retention with consequent intravascular volume expansion and a compensatory rise in plasma ANP. The rise in ANP is sufficient to counterbalance the primary antinatriuretic influences, but the expanded intravascular volume provides the potential for overflow ascites. With progression of disease, intrasinusoidal Starling forces are disrupted and volume is lost from the vascular compartment into the peritoneal compartment. This underfilling of the circulation may attenuate further increases in ANP levels and promote the activation of antinatriuretic factors. Whether the antinatriuretic factors activated by underfilling are the same as or different from those promoting primary renal Na^+ retention in early disease remains to be determined. At this later stage of disease, increased levels of ANP may not be sufficient to counterbalance antinatriuretic forces. (From Warner LC, Leung WM, Campbell P, et al: The role of resistance to atrial natriuretic peptide in the pathogenesis of sodium retention in hepatic cirrhosis. In Brenner BM, Laragh JH [editors]: *Advances in atrial peptide research,* vol 3 of *American Society of Hypertension* series, New York, 1989, Raven Press, pp 185-204.)

Prostaglandins

As noted, prostaglandins make important contributions to the modulation of the hydroosmotic effect of AVP and to the protection of RPF and GFR when the activity of endogenous vasoconstrictor systems is increased. These properties of prostaglandins appear to be critical in patients with decompensated cirrhosis who have ascites but not renal failure. Such patients excrete greater amounts of vasodilatory prostaglandins than healthy subjects, suggesting that renal production of prostaglandins is increased.[278,667] Similarly, in experimental models of cirrhosis, there is evidence for increased synthesis and activity of renal and vascular prostaglandins.[667,668] Recent studies have indicated that PGE_2 upregulation in the thick ascending limb of pre-ascitic cirrhotic rats is mediated via downregulation of calcium-sensing receptors (CaSRs). This maneuver resulted in increased expression of the NKCC2, increased Na^+ reabsorption in this segment, and augmented free water reabsorption in the collecting duct. The effects were reversed by the CaSR agonist poly-L-arginine.[669]

Conversely, it is not surprising that administration of agents that inhibit prostaglandin synthesis results in a clinically important deterioration of renal function in these patients. Administration of nonselective COX inhibitors, such as indomethacin and ibuprofen, resulted in a significant decrease in GFR and RPF in patients with cirrhosis, with or without ascites, in contrast to healthy subjects. The decrement in renal hemodynamics varied directly with the degree of Na^+ retention and neurohumoral activation, so that patients with high plasma renin and norepinephrine levels were particularly sensitive to these adverse effects.[278,667,670]

As in other situations associated with decreased EABV, the COX-2 isoform was strongly upregulated in kidneys from rats with experimental cirrhosis with ascites. Nevertheless, the negative effects of prostaglandin inhibition on renal function appear to be solely COX-2-dependent because studies in human and experimental models of cirrhosis with ascites have shown that administration of selective COX-2 antagonists spares renal function, whereas nonselective cyclooxygenase inhibition leads to a fall in GFR.[667,670] The favorable effect of selective COX-2 antagonists on renal function may be indirect and related to hepatic upregulation of COX-2. This hypothesis is supported by recent data indicating that long-term administration of the selective COX-2 inhibitor, celecoxib, can ameliorate portal hypertension by dual hepatic anti-angiogenic and antifibrotic actions.[669,671,672] These results can lead to studies to establish the safety of selective COX-2 antagonism in patients with advanced cirrhosis.

In contrast to nonazotemic patients with cirrhosis and ascites, it was suggested more than 25 years ago that patients with HRS have reduced renal synthesis of vasodilatory prostaglandins.[673] This situation would exacerbate renal vasoconstriction and Na^+ and fluid retention and may be an important factor in the pathogenesis of HRS.[667] However, treatment with intravenous PGE_2 or its oral analogue, misoprostol, did not improve renal function in HRS patients.[674]

Integrated View of the Pathogenesis of Sodium Retention in Cirrhosis

Two general explanations for Na^+ retention and ascites that complicate cirrhosis have been offered. According to the overflow mechanism, a volume-independent stimulus is responsible for renal Na^+ retention. Possible mediators include adrenergic reflexes activated by hepatic sinusoidal hypertension and increased systemic concentrations of an unidentified antinatriuretic factor as a result of impaired liver metabolism. According to the underfilling theory, in contrast, EABV depletion is responsible for renal Na^+ retention. The peripheral arterial vasodilation hypothesis is that reduced systemic vascular resistance lowers blood pressure and activates arterial baroreceptors, initiating Na^+ retention. The retained fluid extravasates from the hypertensive splanchnic circulation, preventing arterial repletion, and Na^+ retention and ascites formation continue.

It is obvious that neither the underfilling nor overflow theory can account exclusively for all the observed derangements in volume regulation in cirrhosis. Rather, elements of the two concepts may occur simultaneously or sequentially in cirrhotic patients (see Figure 15.12). Thus, there is sufficient evidence that early in cirrhosis, intrahepatic hypertension caused by hepatic venous outflow obstruction signals primary renal Na^+ retention, with consequent intravascular volume expansion. Whether underfilling of the arterial circuit is also a consequence of vasodilation at this stage is not clear. Because of expansion of the intrathoracic venous compartment at this stage, plasma NP levels rise. This increase is sufficient to counterbalance the renal Na^+ retaining forces, but at the expense of an expanded intravascular volume, with the potential for overflow ascites. The propensity for the accumulation of volume in the peritoneal compartment and splanchnic bed results from altered intrahepatic hemodynamics. With progression of disease, intrasinusoidal Starling forces are disrupted, and volume is lost from the vascular compartment into the peritoneal compartment. These events, coupled with other factors, such as portosystemic shunting, hypoalbuminemia, and vascular refractoriness to pressor hormones, lead to underfilling of the arterial circuit without measurably affecting the venous compartment.

This arterial underfilling may attenuate further increases in NP levels and promote the activation of antinatriuretic factors. Whether these factors are the same as, or different from, those that promote primary renal Na^+ retention in early disease remains unclear. At this later stage of disease, elevated levels of NP may be insufficient to counterbalance antinatriuretic influences. In early cirrhosis, salt retention is isotonic, so normonatremia is maintained. However, with advancing cirrhosis, defective water excretion supervenes, resulting in hyponatremia, which reflects combined ECF and ICF space expansion. The impaired water excretion and hyponatremia in cirrhotic patients with ascites is a marker of the severity of the hemodynamic abnormalities that initiate Na^+ retention and eventuate in the HRS. The pathogenesis is related primarily to nonosmotic stimuli for vasopressin release acting together with additional factors, such as impaired distal Na^+ delivery.

CLINICAL MANIFESTATIONS OF HYPERVOLEMIA

Apart from the clinical manifestations of the underlying disease, the symptoms and signs of hypervolemia per se also depend on the amount and relative distribution of the fluid between the intravascular (arterial and venous) and interstitial spaces. Arterial volume overload is manifested as hypertension, whereas venous overload is manifested as raised jugular venous pressure. Interstitial fluid accumulation appears as peripheral edema, effusions in the pleural or peritoneal cavity (ascites) or in the alveolar space (pulmonary edema), or a combination of these. If cardiac and hepatic functions are normal, and transcapillary Starling forces are intact, the excess volume is distributed proportionately throughout the ECF compartments. In this situation, the earliest sign of hypervolemia is hypertension, followed by peripheral edema and raised jugular venous pressure. Peripheral edema appears only when the interstitial volume overload exceeds 3 L and, because plasma volume itself is approximately 3 L, the presence of edema indicates substantial hypervolemia with prior or ongoing renal Na^+ retention.

When cardiac systolic function is impaired, as a result of myocardial, valvular, or pericardial disease, pulmonary and systemic venous hypertension predominate, and systemic blood pressure may be low as a result of disproportionate fluid accumulation in the venous rather than the arterial circulation. Disruption in transcapillary Starling forces, as found in advanced cardiac and hepatic disease, may lead to fluid transudation into the pleural and peritoneal spaces, manifested as pleural effusions and ascites, respectively.

As already mentioned, the constellation of advanced liver cirrhosis or fulminant hepatic failure, ascites, and oliguric renal failure in the absence of significant renal histopathologic disease is the HRS. Two subtypes have been defined. Type 1 is characterized by a rapid decline in renal function (doubling of serum creatinine level to >2.5 mg/dL, or 50% reduction in creatinine clearance to <20 mL/min) over a 2-week period. Typically, an acute precipitating factor can be identified. Type 2 develops spontaneously and progressively over months (serum creatinine level > 1.5 mg/dL, or creatinine clearance < 40 mL/min). HRS is discussed in detail in Chapter 31.

DIAGNOSIS

The diagnosis of hypervolemia is usually evident from the clinical history and physical examination. Any combination of peripheral edema, raised jugular venous pressure, pulmonary crepitations, and pleural effusions is likely to be diagnostic for hypervolemia. In the presence of these findings, the systemic blood pressure is crucial for distinguishing primary renal Na^+ retention from secondary Na^+ retention caused by reduced EABV. For example, in advanced primary renal failure, the blood pressure is high, whereas in severe congestive heart failure or advanced hepatic cirrhosis, blood pressure is likely to be relatively low. In more enigmatic cases, in which dyspnea is the sole complaint and clinical findings are minimal, measurement of plasma BNP, NTproBNP, or MR-proANP may help distinguish between cardiac and pulmonary causes of the dyspnea.[675,676]

Simple laboratory tests may aid in confirming the clinical diagnosis. An elevated cardiac troponin level is consistent with, although not diagnostic of, myocardial damage,[677] and high levels may be observed in acute decompensated HF.[678] Transaminase levels may be raised in hepatic disease, and hypoalbuminemia would be consistent with hepatic cirrhosis or nephrotic-range proteinuria caused by glomerular disease. The latter, of course, would be confirmed by appropriate urine testing.

When blood pressure is low, evidence of prerenal azotemia (increased ratio of blood urea nitrogen to creatinine) may be found, and in advanced cardiac or hepatic failure (the so-called cardiorenal syndrome and HRS respectively), intrinsic renal failure—proportionate increases in blood urea nitrogen and creatinine—may occur (see Chapter 31 for detailed discussion). In the urine, low EABV in the presence of hypervolemia is confirmed by a low Na^+ concentration or low fractional excretion of Na^+, indicative of secondary renal Na^+ retention.

TREATMENT

Therapy for volume overload can be divided broadly into management of the volume overload itself and prevention or minimization of its occurrence and the associated morbidity and mortality. Clearly, recognition and treatment of the underlying disease causing hypervolemia is the critical first step. Thus, when EABV is significantly reduced, as in cardiac and hepatic failure (as well as in severe nephrotic syndrome), hemodynamic parameters should be optimized. Otherwise, therapy to induce negative Na^+ balance is associated with an enhanced risk for worsening hemodynamic compromise.

Once the EABV is adjusted, three basic strategies can be used to induce negative Na^+ balance—dietary Na^+ restriction, diuretics, and extracorporeal ultrafiltration. The degree of hypervolemia and the clinical urgency for Na^+ removal determine which modality should be used. Therefore, in a patient with life-threatening pulmonary edema, immediate intravenous loop diuretics are indicated; if high doses of these drugs do not induce significant diuresis, then extracorporeal ultrafiltration may be life-saving. At the other extreme, a hypertensive patient with mild volume overload and preserved renal function may require only dietary salt restriction and a thiazide diuretic.

Once the acute stage of hypervolemia has been controlled, therapy must be directed toward the prevention or minimization of further acute episodes and improvement in overall prognosis. In addition to maintenance diuretic treatment, several strategies, based on the pathophysiologic process of Na^+ retention, are available clinically or are under experimental development.

Sodium Restriction

Until recently, the prevailing belief has been that effective management of hypervolemia of any cause must include Na^+ restriction. Without this intervention, the success of diuretic therapy was thought to be limited because the relative hypovolemia induced by diuretics leads to compensatory Na^+ retention and the potential creation of a vicious cycle, consisting of increased diuretic dosage, further reduction in EABV, and still more renal Na^+ retention. However, this view has been recently challenged by a randomized controlled trial in patients admitted to hospital with acute decompensated HF. In this study, no difference in weight loss or clinical stability was observed at 3 days between the group restricted to 800 mg sodium/day and those with a more liberal sodium intake. Moreover, those on the severely sodium-restricted diet were significantly thirstier than their less restricted counterparts.[679-681] In light of these new data, a reasonable goal is to restrict Na^+ intake to 50 to 80 mmol (approximately 3 to 5 g of salt)/day.[682] Because of the generally poor palatability of salt-restricted diets, salt substitutes may be used; however, because these preparations usually contain high concentrations of potassium, they must be used with caution by patients with renal impairment or those taking potassium-retaining drugs such as ACEIs, ARBs, or aldosterone antagonists.

In hospitalized patients, extra attention must be paid to amounts and types of intravenous fluids administered. A frequent phenomenon encountered by nephrologists who have been consulted in internal medicine departments is the scenario in which a patient is receiving intravenous saline together with high-dose diuretics. The usual rationale offered for this combination is that the saline will expand the intravascular volume and the diuretic will mobilize the excess interstitial volume. This logic has no sound physiologic or therapeutic basis, inasmuch as both modalities operate principally on the intravascular space. Furthermore, water restriction is also inappropriate, except in the presence of accompanying hyponatremia (plasma Na^+ < 135 mmol/L). In stark contrast to these recommendations, studies have shown that intravenous infusion of small volumes of hypertonic saline during diuretic dosing and liberalizing dietary salt intake while continuing to limit water consumption results in improved fluid removal in HF patients. Furthermore, less deterioration in renal function, shorter hospitalizations, reduced readmission rates, and even reductions in mortality were observed.[682,683]

Diuretics

Diuretics are classified according to their sites of action along the nephron and are discussed in detail in Chapter 51. Bernstein and Ellison have recently presented a comprehensive review.[684] Diuretics are described briefly here in relation to the treatment of hypervolemia.

Proximal Tubule Diuretics. The prototype of a proximal tubular diuretic is acetazolamide, a carbonic anhydrase inhibitor that inhibits the proximal reabsorption of sodium bicarbonate. However, prolonged use may cause hyperchloremic metabolic acidosis. This drug is more typically used in the management of chronic glaucoma rather than for reducing volume overload. Another proximally acting diuretic is metolazone, which, as a member of the thiazide class of diuretics, also inhibits the NaCl cotransporter in the distal tubule. The proximal action of metolazone may be associated with phosphate loss greater than that seen with traditional thiazides.[685] In general, metolazone is used as an adjunct to loop diuretics in resistant heart failure.[686] Mannitol, which also inhibits proximal tubular reabsorption,[687] can be used in combination with furosemide for the management of acute decompensated HF.[688]

Loop Diuretics. This group includes the most powerful diuretics, such as furosemide, bumetanide, torsemide, and ethacrynic acid. Their mode of action is to inhibit transport via the NKCC2 in the apical membrane of the thick ascending limb of the loop of Henle, which is responsible for the reabsorption of about 25% of filtered Na$^+$ (see Chapters 16 and 51).[684] They are used for the treatment of severe hypervolemia and hypertension, especially in stages 4 and 5 of chronic kidney disease. Because of their powerful action, loop diuretics may lead to hypokalemia, intravascular volume depletion, and worsening prerenal azotemia, especially in older patients and in patients with reduced EABV.

Distal Tubule Diuretics. Diuretics in this segment operate by blockade of the apical NaCl cotransporter. The group consists of hydrochlorothiazide, chlorthalidone, and metolazone (see earlier section, "Proximal Tubule Diuretics"). They are typically used as first-line treatment of hypertension and, particularly metolazone, as adjuncts to loop diuretics in resistant heart failure. Thiazides are also useful for reducing hypercalciuria in recurrent nephrolithiasis, in contrast to loop diuretics that are hypercalciuric.[658] Inhibition of Na$^+$ reabsorption by diuretics that work in the proximal tubule (except for carbonic anhydrase inhibitors), loop of Henle, and distal tubule leads to increased solute delivery to the collecting duct. Consequently, rates of potassium and proton secretion are accelerated, which may lead to hypokalemia and metabolic alkalosis.[659]

Collecting Duct Diuretics. Collecting duct (K$^+$-sparing) diuretics operate by competing with aldosterone for occupation of the mineralocorticoid receptor or by direct inhibition of the ENaC (amiloride and triamterene).[684] As their alternative name implies, important side effects of this group are hyperkalemia and metabolic acidosis, which result from concomitant suppression of K$^+$ and proton secretion. Therefore, they are widely used in combination with thiazide and loop diuretics to minimize hypokalemia. The aldosterone antagonists are especially useful in the management of disorders characterized by secondary hyperaldosteronism, such as cirrhosis with ascites. Moreover, aldosterone antagonists have been shown to have cardioprotective and renoprotective effects via nonepithelial mineralocorticoid receptor blockade (see sections, "Pathophysiology" and "Specific Treatments Based on the Pathophysiology of Congestive Heart Failure" in this chapter; also see Chapter 12).

Other Diuretic Agents. Natriuretic peptides are discussed later (see section, "Specific Treatments Based on the Pathophysiology of Congestive Heart Failure"). Patients with cirrhosis and ascites, who typically have little Na$^+$ in their urine, may have a natriuretic response to HWI as a result of effective volume depletion (see earlier section, "Underfilling Hypothesis"), despite elevated plasma volume and cardiac output.[660] This modality has not been used outside the research setting.

Diuretic Resistance. As noted, when Na$^+$ retention is severe and resistant to conventional doses of loop diuretics, combinations of diuretics acting at different nephron sites may produce effective natriuresis. Another method for overcoming diuretic resistance is the administration of a bolus dose of loop diuretic to yield a high plasma level, followed by high-dose continuous infusion. Alternately, high doses given intermittently may be successful in reversing diuretic resistance. As shown in a recent randomized control trial, there appears to be no difference between continuous infusion and repeated bolus administration of high or low doses of furosemide in shortness of breath or volume of diuresis at 72 hours after admission for acute decompensated HF.[661]

Whichever method is used to treat diuretic resistant hypervolemia, it is important to monitor carefully plasma Na$^+$, K$^+$, Mg^{2+}, Ca^{2+}, phosphate, blood urea nitrogen, and creatinine levels and correct any deviations appropriately. Other less common side effects of diuretics include cutaneous allergic reactions, acute interstitial nephritis (see Chapter 36), pancreatitis and, rarely, blood dyscrasias.[662]

Extracorporeal Ultrafiltration

On occasion, extreme resistance to diuretics occurs, often accompanied by renal functional impairment. In such cases, removal of volume excess may be achieved by ultrafiltration through the use of hemofiltration, hemodialysis, peritoneal dialysis (see Chapters 65 and 66), or small devices designed for isolated ultrafiltration (UF). All these modalities are effective for fluid removal in diuretic-resistant HF.[663-665] Chronic ambulatory peritoneal dialysis may also reduce hospitalization rates in patients with resistant HF who are not candidates for surgical intervention.[666]

It is important to emphasize that a recent randomized controlled trial comparing intensive diuretic therapy with UF for the management of acute decompensated HF with worsened renal function (CARRESS-HF) was halted early because of evidence of lack of benefit of UF and an excess of early and late (60 days) adverse events.[689] Moreover, UF was inferior to diuretic therapy in terms of the bivariate primary endpoint of body weight and rise in serum creatinine level at 96 hours after commencement of therapy. Therefore, UF should currently be reserved for those patients with unequivocal diuretic resistance. The exact place of UF in the long-term management of acute decompensated HF remains to be elucidated.[690]

SPECIFIC TREATMENTS BASED ON THE PATHOPHYSIOLOGY OF HEART FAILURE

Because the clinical situation of an HF patient at any given time depends on the delicate balance among vasoconstrictor/antinatriuretic and vasodilator/natriuretic factors, any treatment that can tip the balance in favor of the latter should be efficacious. Thus, increasing the activity of the NPs or reducing the influence of the antinatriuretic mechanisms by pharmacologic means may achieve a shift in the balance in favor of Na$^+$ excretion in HF. In the interplay between the RAAS and ANP in HF, the approaches used in experimental studies and in clinical practice have included reducing the activity of the RAAS by means of ACEIs or ARBs, increasing the activity of ANP or its second messenger, cGMP, or a combination of these.

INHIBITION OF THE RENIN-ANGIOTENSIN-ALDOSTERONE SYSTEM

The maladaptive actions of locally produced or circulatory Ang II have been examined in numerous studies, which have shown unequivocally that ACE inhibition and ARBs improve renal function, cardiac performance, and life expectancy of HF patients.[691,692] A small decline in GFR is occasionally observed as a result of blockade of Ang II–induced preferential efferent arteriolar constriction, which leads to a sharp fall in glomerular capillary pressure, but this is usually not clinically significant. Because patients with HF cannot overcome the Na^+-retaining action of aldosterone and continue to retain Na^+ in response to aldosterone, blockade of the latter by spironolactone or eplerenone induces substantial natriuresis in these patients.[691]

Overall, the effect of Ang II receptor blockade or ACE inhibition on renal function in HF depends on a multiplicity of interacting factors. On the one hand, RBF may improve as a result of lower efferent arteriolar resistance. Systemic vasodilation may be associated with a rise in cardiac output. Under such circumstances, reversal of the hemodynamically mediated effects of Ang II on Na^+ reabsorption would promote natriuresis. Moreover, inhibition of the RAAS could theoretically facilitate the action of NPs to improve GFR and enhance Na^+ excretion. On the other hand, the aim of Ang II–induced elevation of the single-nephron filtration fraction is to preserve GFR in the presence of diminished RPF. In patients with precarious renal hemodynamics, a fall in systemic arterial pressure below the autoregulatory range, combined with removal of the Ang II effect on glomerular hemodynamics, may cause severe deterioration of renal function. The net result depends on the integrated sum of these physiologic effects, which, in turn, depends on the severity and stage of heart disease (Table 15.8).

In addition to their action to promote Na^+ retention, components of the RAAS play a pivotal role in the pathogenesis of HF by contributing to vascular and cardiac remodeling by inducing perivascular and interstitial fibrosis.[691,692] In accordance with this hypothesis, three landmark clinical trials have shown that the addition of small doses of aldosterone inhibitors to standard therapy, including ACEIs or ARBs, substantially reduces the mortality rate and degree of morbidity in HF patients. In the Randomized Aldactone Evaluation Study (RALES), therapy with spironolactone reduced overall mortality among patients with advanced HF by 30% in comparison with placebo.[691] The Eplerenone Post-AMI Heart Failure Efficacy and Survival Study (EPHESUS) has shown that the addition of eplerenone to optimal medical therapy reduces morbidity and mortality in patients with acute myocardial infarction complicated by left ventricular dysfunction and HF.[691] A third trial in patients with mild HF (NYHA class II) and ejection fraction less than 35%, Eplerenone in Mild Patients Hospitalization and Survival Study in Heart Failure (EMPHASIS-HF), was stopped prematurely because of a clearly favorable effect of eplerenone on mortality.[693] As a result, aldosterone inhibitors are now routinely used in the management of HF; the current debate centers on whether eplerenone, with a better side effect profile, should be preferred, particularly in patients at high risk of hyperkalemia, notably those with renal dysfunction.[694]

β-BLOCKADE

Insofar as β-blockade is now the standard of care in the management of HF, this review would not be complete without mention of β-blockers. However, because their effect in HF is not directly related to Na^+ and water, this important therapy is not elaborated further in this chapter. The reader is referred to recent meta-analyses for up-to-date information.[695,696]

NITRIC OXIDE DONOR AND REACTIVE OXYGEN SPECIES/PEROXYNITRITE SCAVENGERS

Because nitric oxide signaling is disrupted in HF, achieving nitric oxide balance by NO donors or selective NOS inhibitors has emerged as an important therapeutic concept in addressing and correcting the pathophysiologic process of HF.[697] In this regard, the beneficial effects of combined isosorbide dinitrate (nitric oxide donor) and hydralazine (reactive oxygen species and peroxynitrite scavenger) therapy, particularly in African American patients, remain noteworthy.[698] However, the question still remains as to the efficacy of this combination in other ethnic groups, given the success of combined RAAS inhibition and β-blockade.[698]

An interesting recent development is the observation in a rat model of HF that increased expression of nNOS within the paraventricular nucleus leads to upregulation of nNOS protein, leading to a reduction in sympathetic outflow. This study raises the potential for nNOS upregulation by ACE2 therapy in HF.[699]

ENDOTHELIN ANTAGONISTS

Initial clinical studies have shown that acute ET nonselective antagonism decreases vascular resistance and increases cardiac index and cardiac output in HF patients, consistent with the role of ET-1 in increasing systemic vascular resistance in HF. However, comprehensive clinical trials have demonstrated, at best, no benefits or, at worst, increased hepatic dysfunction and mortality rate in HF patients treated with ET-A receptor antagonists. These disappointing results

Table 15.8 Renal Effects of RAAS inhibition in Heart Failure

Factors Favoring Improvement in Renal Function

Maintenance of Na^+ balance
    Reduction in diuretic dosage
    Increase in Na^+ intake
    Mean arterial pressure > 80 mm Hg
Minimal neurohumoral activation
Intact counterregulatory mechanisms

Factors Favoring Deterioration in Renal Function

Evidence of Na^+ depletion or poor renal perfusion
    Large doses of diuretics
    Increased urea/creatinine ratio
    Mean arterial pressure < 80 mm Hg
Evidence of maximal neurohumoral activation
    AVP-induced hyponatremia
Interruption of counterregulatory mechanisms
    Coadministration of prostaglandin inhibitors
    Adrenergic dysfunction (e.g., diabetes mellitus)

AVP, Arginine vasopressin; RAAS, renin-angiotensin-aldosterone system.

may be explained by the observation that ET-A receptor antagonism in experimental HF further activates the RAAS in association with sustained Na^+ retention.[472] Moreover, the increased local cardiac, pulmonary, and renal production of ET-1 in HF, together with the marked vasoconstrictor and mitogenic properties of the molecule, suggests that ET-1 contributes directly and indirectly to the enhanced Na^+ retention and edema formation by aggravating renal and cardiac functions, respectively.[472] In addition, nonspecific blockade of ET-B receptors could have exacerbated cardiac remodeling. Given the antiproliferative effect of ET-B receptor signaling through ET-B1–related pathways and the detrimental vasoconstrictor effect of ET-B2 stimulation, combined ET-B1 stimulation and ET-B2 blockade has recently been proposed[471] for control of the remodeling associated with postischemic HF. According to this hypothesis, the vasodilator and antiproliferative effects of an ET-B1 agonist, combined with blockade of the detrimental vasoconstrictor ET-B2 effect, could potentially improve current endothelin modulation therapies. Concomitant ET-A blockade would probably also be required to prevent the undesired effects of unopposed ET-1 activity and exploit the established therapeutic effects of ET-A antagonists.[471] Studies in this direction are eagerly awaited.

NATRIURETIC PEPTIDES

As noted previously, circulating levels of NPs are elevated in HF in proportion to the severity of the disease. However, the renal actions of these peptides are attenuated and even blunted in severe HF. Nevertheless, several studies have demonstrated that elimination of NP action via the use of NPR-A blockers or surgical removal of the atrium disrupts renal function and cardiac performance in experimental models of HF.[480] Conversely, increasing circulating levels of NPs by intravenous administration has been shown to improve general clinical status,[700] reduce pulmonary arterial and capillary wedge pressures, right atrial pressure, and systemic vascular resistance, with improved cardiac output, systemic blood pressure, and diuresis.[701] The hemodynamic and natriuretic effects of exogenous BNP administration were significantly greater than those obtained after similar doses of ANP in HF patients. In parallel, plasma levels of norepinephrine and aldosterone were suppressed.

In view of its beneficial effects, BNP (nesiritide) was approved for the treatment of acute decompensated HF in the United States in 2001. However, more recent controlled studies have shown that the natriuretic effects of nesiritide are minimal in comparison with placebo. Moreover, up to one third of patients did not exhibit increased Na^+ excretion after ANP or BNP infusion.[702] A further limitation of nesiritide treatment was dose-related hypotension,[701] which would be enhanced in combination with other vasodilators, such as RAAS inhibitors. Also, nesiritide led to worsening renal function in more than 20% of patients, which could increase the risk of death as occurs in other situations complicated by renal impairment.[702] Finally, in a recently published randomized controlled trial comparing nesiritide or low-dose dopamine as add-on therapy to intravenous furosemide in patients with HF and renal dysfunction, no improvement in decongestion or renal function was observed with either combination therapy over furosemide alone.[703] Therefore, the therapeutic role of BNP in HF is currently unclear, and different strategies will be required. In this context, a recent pilot study has suggested that subcutaneous administration of BNP might represent a novel, safe, and efficacious therapeutic strategy for HF patients.[704]

Similarly, in light of the excessive levels of NT-proBNP found in HF, strategies to convert the prohormone into its active form might be efficacious. Other possibilities include CNP analogues and, using a more innovative approach, creating so-called designer chimeric peptides.[704] For example, CD-NP is a chimeric peptide consisting of CNP and part of DNP. In a preliminary study in healthy subjects, this peptide was shown to possess cGMP-activating, natriuretic, and aldosterone-suppressing properties, without inducing excessive hypotension.[704] Further clinical trials can be expected.

NEUTRAL ENDOPEPTIDASE INHIBITORS AND VASOPEPTIDASE INHIBITORS

Correcting the imbalance between the RAAS and NP systems could also be achieved by inhibiting the enzymatic degradation of NPs by NEP. Several specific and differently structured NEP inhibitors were developed and tested in experimental models and clinical trials. Most studies revealed enhanced plasma ANP and BNP levels in association with vasodilation, natriuresis, diuresis and, subsequently, reduced cardiac preload and afterload.[499] Given that NEP degrades other peptides (e.g., kinins, AT_1), these may also be involved in the beneficial effects of NEP inhibitors. Candoxatril, the first NEP inhibitor released for clinical trials, produced favorable hemodynamic and neurohormonal effects in patients with HF.[705] In addition, acute NEP inhibition in mild HF resulted in marked increases in RPF and Na^+ excretion, which exceeded the increase observed in control animals or in patients with severe HF.[706] Unfortunately, in later studies of HF, more marked activation of the RAAS, as well as increased ET-1 levels, were observed, thereby attenuating the beneficial renal and hemodynamic actions of NEP inhibitors. Moreover, NEP inhibitors did not reduce afterload.[499] On the basis of these findings, a combination of RAAS and NEP inhibition should be more effective than each treatment alone. This was confirmed in dogs with pacing-induced HF, in which NEP inhibition prevented the ACEI-induced decrease in GFR.[707] These results led to the development of dual NEP and ACE inhibitors, known as vasopeptidase inhibitors.[499]

Of the various vasopeptidase inhibitors, omapatrilat has been the most studied. Results from experimental and clinical HF studies have suggested beneficial hemodynamic and renal effects mediated by the synergistic ACE and NEP inhibition offered by this drug.[499] This was thought to be a potential advantage because deteriorating renal function in acute and chronic HF is one of the most powerful prognostic indicators in patients with HF.[708] However, from the results of definitive clinical trials, it became evident that neither vasopeptidase inhibitors nor NEP inhibitors as add-on therapy to RAAS inhibition were more effective than RAAS inhibitors alone in the treatment of HF.[499] Furthermore, the combination was associated with a significantly increased incidence of severe angioedema. Hence, omapatrilat was not approved by the FDA. Possible reasons for the failure of NEP inhibitors include disproportionate increase in RAAS and endothelin activity over time, the development of tolerance with chronic treatment, and downregulation of NP receptors in response to degradation of NEP inhibitors. The increased incidence of angioedema with vasopeptidase inhibition may result from excessive accumulation of bradykinin or inhibition of aminopeptidase P.[499]

The challenge of preventing angioedema has led to the concept of combined ARB-NEP inhibition in which ARBs, which do not disrupt bradykinin metabolism, are combined with ARBs. Several drugs in this class are at various stages of production; the prototype, LCZ696, which provides a 1:1 ratio of a valsartan moiety and a rapidly metabolized prodrug form of a NEP inhibitor, was the subject of the recently published phase III PARADIGM-HF trial in which LCZ696 was compared with enalapril in patients who had HF with a reduced ejection fraction.[709] The trial was stopped early, after a median follow-up of 27 months, because of an overwhelming benefit of LCZ696. The primary outcome, a composite of death from cardiovascular causes or hospitalization for heart failure had occurred in 914 patients (21.8%) in the LCZ696 group and 1117 patients (26.5%) in the enalapril group (hazard ratio in the LCZ696 group, 0.80; $P < 0.001$). In addition, LCZ696 led to a significant reduction in each of the individual components of the composite endpoint as well as a decrease in symptoms and physical limitations of heart failure. The LCZ696 group had higher proportions of patients with hypotension and nonserious angioedema but lower proportions with renal impairment, hyperkalemia, and cough than the enalapril group. Moreover, in a separate trial, in patients with HF and preserved ejection fraction, therapy with LCZ696 for 36 weeks was associated with preservation of eGFR compared with valsartan therapy, although an increase in urine albumen/creatinine ratio was observed.[709a] Clearly, the results of these trials have the potential to produce a paradigm shift in the management of severe HF.

VASOPRESSIN RECEPTOR ANTAGONISTS

The development of AVP receptor antagonists, known collectively as *vaptans*, has dramatically increased the understanding of the contribution of AVP to the alterations in renal and cardiac function[462,463] and opened the way for their therapeutic use in HF. Vaptans are small, orally active, nonpeptide molecules that lack agonist effects and display high affinity for and specificity to their corresponding receptors.[462,463] Highly selective and potent antagonists for the V_{1A}, V_2, and V_{1B} receptor subtypes and mixed V_{1A}/V_2 receptor antagonists are now available.[463] V_2 receptor–specific vaptans have been clearly shown to produce hemodynamic improvement with transient decrease in systemic vascular resistance, increased cardiac output, and improved water diuresis in experimental models of HF and in clinical trials.[462,463]

These clinical trials have amply demonstrated the efficacy of vaptans in reversing hyponatremia, hemodynamic disturbances, and renal dysfunction in compensated and decompensated HF. In decompensated HF with hyponatremia, three randomized controlled trials involving tolvaptan, a V_2 selective receptor antagonist, and one involving conivaptan, a non-selective V_{1A}/V_2 receptor antagonist (both of which are FDA-approved for use in HF) demonstrated normalization and maintenance of plasma Na^+ levels, decreases in body weight and edema, and increases in urine output after treatment for up to 60 days. There was subjective improvement in dyspnea in some but not all patients. Similar results were reported for tolvaptan in stable class II or III HF.[710,711] In two studies on patients with advanced HF and systolic dysfunction who received a single intravenous dose of conivaptan or placebo, the active drug modestly reduced pulmonary capillary wedge pressure and significantly reduced right atrial pressure in comparison with placebo; cardiac index, pulmonary arterial pressure, systemic and pulmonary vascular resistance, systemic arterial pressure, and heart rate were unaffected. Urine output rose and osmolarity fell significantly.[712,713] However, there was no improvement in functional capacity, exercise tolerance, or overall quality of life.[711]

In contrast to the detrimental effects of aggressive therapy with loop diuretics on renal function, no significant changes in RBF,[710] blood urea nitrogen, and creatinine were reported after vaptan therapy.[462,463] Positive effects were observed, regardless of whether LVEF was less or greater than 40%. In one trial, tolvaptan, but not fluid restriction, corrected hyponatremia.[462,463] Two trials examined the effects of tolvaptan on survival. In one study, patients treated with tolvaptan, and who had an increase in serum Na^+ of 2 mmol/L or more, had half the mortality rate of those with no improvement in serum Na^+ level 2 months after discharge.[714] In contrast, in the other trial, no significant effects of the drug, given for 60 days, were seen on survival after 9 months of follow-up.[711]

Tolvaptan did not adversely affect cardiac remodeling or LVEF after 1 year of treatment in patients receiving optimal, evidence-based background therapies for HF (ACEIs, ARBs, and β-blockers).[715] From these results, it would appear that the highly selective V_2 receptor blockade of tolvaptan does not unmask unopposed V_1 receptor–mediated effects under the influence of raised AVP levels.

Two trials involving the newer V_2 selective lixivaptan have been completed. The first (Treatment of Hyponatremia Based on Lixivaptan in NYHA Class III/IV Cardiac Patient Evaluation [BALANCE]) in decompensated HF was demonstrated a statistically significant but modest rise in serum sodium at day 7 of 2.5 mEq/L versus 1.3 mEq/L in the placebo group. However, the trial was terminated early owing to an excessive mortality rate in the treatment group.[716] The second trial showed that lixivaptan, 100 mg once daily, when added to standard therapy, reduced body weight, improved dyspnea and orthopnea, and was well tolerated.[717] However, the FDA did not approve its use for these indications.[718]

In view of the impressive diuretic effect of vaptans, there is considerable interest in the potential loop diuretic–sparing effect mentioned previously. To date, this idea has been evaluated in one prospective observational and one multicenter, randomized, double-blind, placebo-controlled study. The observational study of 114 patients with acute decompensated HF at high risk for renal functional deterioration showed that tolvaptan use was independently associated with a 72% reduction in the risk for worsening renal function as compared to patients who received furosemide.[719] In the randomized controlled trial, tolvaptan monotherapy, compared to furosemide and the combination of tolvaptan and furosemide in patients with HF and systolic dysfunction, reduced body weight without adverse changes in serum electrolyte levels. All participants received a sodium-restricted diet, ACEIs, and β-blockers.[720] These encouraging data formed the basis for the recently launched Japanese multicenter Clinical Effectiveness of Tolvaptan in Patients with Acute Decompensated Heart Failure and Renal Failure (AQUAMARINE) Study, in which tolvaptan is being compared with standard furosemide therapy in HF patients with renal impairment (University Medical Information Network [UMIN] clinical trial registry number, UMIN000007109).[721]

The adverse effects of vaptans appear to be relatively few and, on the whole, minor. Thirst and dry mouth are not unexpected; hypokalemia occurs in fewer than 10% of recipients, which favorably compares with loop diuretics. In the largest study to date, Efficacy of Vasopressin Antagonism in Heart Failure Outcome Study with Tolvaptan (EVEREST), involving more than 4000 patients, there was a small but significant increase in reported strokes but also a small but significant reduction in myocardial infarction rate.[457]

In summary, AVP receptor antagonists appear to be promising in the treatment of advanced HF, but many unanswered questions remain. These include the potential for long-term efficacy, use in volume overload in the setting of preserved ejection fraction with a nondilated ventricle, role in possible loop diuretic dose sparing, duration of treatment, and dosing over the short and long term. Finally, and perhaps most important, is the question of whether AVP receptor antagonists improve longer term prognosis and reduce the high rate of mortality among HF patients who are already receiving optimal doses of ACEIs, ARBs, and β-blockers.

SPECIFIC TREATMENTS BASED ON THE PATHOPHYSIOLOGY OF SODIUM RETENTION IN CIRRHOSIS

The prognosis of type 1 HRS is dismal; the mortality rate is as high as 80% in the first 2 weeks, and only 10% of patients survive longer than 3 months; therefore, specific aggressive therapy in these patients is usually indicated in preparation for liver transplantation.[553,576,621] Patients with type 2 HRS have a better prognosis; the median length of survival is approximately 6 months.[553,576,621] Aggressive management may be considered for these patients, regardless of transplantation candidacy. There are four major therapeutic interventions for HRS—pharmacologic therapy, TIPS insertion, renal replacement therapy (RRT), and liver transplantation. The management of precipitating factors is beyond the scope of this discussion.

PHARMACOLOGIC TREATMENT

The goals of pharmacologic therapy are to reverse the functional renal failure and prolong survival until suitable candidates can undergo liver transplantation. On the basis of the pathophysiologic features of renal vasoconstriction against a background of systemic and, specifically, splanchnic arterial vasodilation, specific treatments consist broadly of renal vasodilators and systemic vasoconstrictors. The former group includes direct renal vasodilators (e.g., dopamine, fenoldopam, prostaglandins) and antagonists of endogenous renal vasoconstrictors (e.g., ACEIs, ARBs, aldosterone antagonists, endothelin antagonists). Systemic vasoconstrictors are comprised of vasopressin analogues (e.g., ornipressin, terlipressin), the somatostatin analogue octreotide, and the α-adrenergic agonists. In addition, the nonosmotically stimulated rise in plasma AVP levels and resulting impaired water excretion and hyponatremia can be potentially reversed by V_2 receptor antagonists.

RENAL VASODILATORS AND RENAL VASOCONSTRICTOR ANTAGONISTS

Although these agents are theoretically attractive for the management of Na^+ retention in cirrhosis, none of the studies of renal vasodilators have shown improvement in renal perfusion or GFR.[604] Agents tested included low-dose dopamine, the PGE_1 analogue misoprostol given orally or intravenously, an ET-A antagonist, and RAAS blockade. In general, because of adverse effects and lack of benefit, the use of renal vasodilators in HRS has largely been abandoned.[576]

SYSTEMIC VASOCONSTRICTORS

Systemic vasoconstrictors are the mainstay of pharmacologic therapy in HRS by virtue of their predominant action on the vasodilated splanchnic circulation without affecting the renal circulation. Three groups of vasoconstrictors have been studied—vasopressin V_1 receptor analogues (e.g., ornipressin, terlipressin), somatostatin analogue (octreotide), and α-adrenergic agonists.[553,576,621]

Vasopressin V_1 Receptor Analogues

These agents cause marked vasoconstriction through their action on the V_1 receptors present in the smooth muscle of the arterial wall. They are used extensively for the management of acute variceal bleeding in patients with cirrhosis and portal hypertension. Ornipressin infusion in combination with volume expansion or low-dose dopamine was associated with a remarkable improvement in renal function and an increase in RPF, GFR, and Na^+ excretion in almost half of the treated patients.[604] Unfortunately, ornipressin had to be abandoned because of significant ischemic adverse effects that occurred in almost 30% of treated patients.[604]

Terlipressin, on the other hand, has favorable effects similar to those of ornipressin, without the accompanying adverse ischemic reactions. The administration of terlipressin and albumin in type 1 HRS is associated with a significant improvement in GFR, increase in arterial pressure, near-normalization of neurohumoral levels, and reduction of serum creatinine level in 34% to 59% of cases.[553,576,621] Survival is also improved over that of historic cases, but it remains dismal overall (median survival, 25 to 40 days). In nonresponders, who tend to have more severe cirrhosis (Child-Pugh score > 13), length of survival is notably reduced.[553] The rates of response to terlipressin in type 2 HRS are better than those in type 1, with more than 80% survival at 3 months.[553,621] Despite HRS relapses in 50% of cases, reintroduction of therapy produces a further response. However, long-term management of these managements with vasoconstrictors is impractical.

From the results of two randomized controlled trials, it is now clear that terlipressin alone and the combination of terlipressin and albumin are superior to albumin alone in improving renal function and reversing HRS type 1.[722,723] However, these relatively small studies were unable to show a survival benefit for terlipressin. Attempts to prevent relapse of type 2 HRS with midodrine after terlipressin-induced improvement were also unsuccessful.[724] The optimum duration of terlipressin therapy is not clear. In almost all studies, terlipressin was given until serum creatinine levels decreased to less than 1.5 mg/dL or for a maximum of 15 days. Whether extending the therapy beyond 15 days will add any benefit is unknown. So far, only one case series has been reported, in which three patients were maintained on terlipressin for 2 months until liver transplantation.[725] Moreover, the apparent survival advantage of terlipressin, seen in the cohort studies, was unimpressive; 80% of patients who did not receive a transplant died of their liver disease within 3 months of therapy. A key target for predicting prognosis appears to be the response in mean arterial pressure at 3 days after combined terlipressin-albumin therapy. In a small study, patients whose mean arterial pressure rose 10 mm Hg or more from baseline had less requirement for dialysis and greater incidence of liver transplantation than those with smaller responses in mean arterial pressure. More importantly, this response was associated with better short-term and long-term overall survival and transplant-free survival.[726] The importance of V_1 receptor analogues is underscored by the observation that pretransplantation normalization of renal function by this therapy in patients with HRS resulted in similar posttransplantation outcomes to those of patients with normal renal function who received transplants.[727]

A somewhat different approach in patients with HRS already undergoing living related donor liver transplantation has recently been reported.[728] In this study, 80 recipients were randomly allocated to receive terlipressin at the beginning of surgery at a dose of 3 µg/kg/hr, reduced to 1.5 µg/kg/hr after reperfusion and continued for 3 postoperative days or to a control group. All patients received vasoactive agents, as appropriate, and were followed for up to 5 days postoperatively. Compared to the control group, terlipressin infusion was associated throughout the study period with significant increases in mean arterial pressure, systemic vascular resistance and renal function, significantly decreased heart rate, cardiac output, hepatic and renal arterial resistive indices, portal venous blood flow, and use of vasoconstrictor drugs during reperfusion. Further work on this novel approach is eagerly awaited.[729] To summarize, terlipressin and albumin infusion may be appropriate only for patients awaiting or already undergoing liver transplantation, and a favorable hemodynamic response is associated with a better overall prognosis both before and after liver transplantation.

Unfortunately, despite the favorable effects of terlipressin, a major drawback is its unavailability in many countries, including the United States and Canada. In these countries, the α-agonist, midodrine, is generally used.[553]

Somatostatin Analogues and α-Adrenergic Agonists

Octreotide, which inhibits the release of glucagon and other vasodilator peptides, is currently the only available somatostatin analogue. In small cohort studies, octreotide with albumin infusion or midodrine alone had no effect on renal function in HRS. However, both agents in combination with albumin infusion led to a significant improvement in renal function and survival in types 1 and 2 HRS in comparison to controls.[729-731] However, no effect of this combination on outcomes of subsequent liver transplantation was observed.[732] A literature review has concluded that the exact role of combined octreotide-midodrine therapy in HRS management remains to be determined.[730]

Whether vasopressin analogues or combined therapy with octreotide and midodrine are more efficacious in reversing HRS remains an open question. Only one small randomized, controlled trial[553] involving a direct comparison has been reported in abstract form. In this study, terlipressin plus albumin was significantly more effective than octreotide, midodrine, and albumin, both in terms of improved renal function (75% vs. 35%) and complete reversal of HRS (54% vs. 11%). On the other hand, 30-day survival was no different between the two groups. Finally, norepinephrine was compared with terlipressin in the treatment of type 1 HRS in three randomized controlled trials. Responses to both agents were similar in terms of mean arterial pressure and renal function. Cumulative survival and adverse event rates were not significantly different between the two drugs. Norepinephrine is less expensive than terlipressin, but norepinephrine administration requires cardiac monitoring, whereas terlipressin does not. Therefore, total costs might be similar for the two therapies.[553]

Two meta-analyses and a Cochrane review of randomized controlled trials assessing the effects of vasoconstrictors on renal function and outcomes in HRS have been reported. In one meta-analysis, any vasoconstrictor with albumin was superior to albumin alone or no active treatment, both for improvement in renal function and reduced all-cause mortality. A subanalysis of terlipressin trials only showed that terlipressin with albumin led to improved renal function and resolution of HRS compared with albumin alone.[733] In the second meta-analysis, terlipressin with albumin was better than albumin alone or placebo in terms of improved renal function, but not survival.[734] In a Cochrane review published in 2012,[735] the authors concluded that terlipressin may reduce mortality and improve renal function in patients with type 1 HRS, but were concerned about the strength of the evidence to support the intervention for clinical practice due to the results of the trial sequential analysis. However, the outcome measures assessed were objective, which reduced the risk of bias.

VASOPRESSIN V_2 RECEPTOR ANTAGONISTS

As noted, hyponatremia, because of the inability to excrete a free water load caused by persistent nonosmotic stimulation of AVP, is often seen in advanced cirrhosis with ascites and HRS and is a marker of poor prognosis.[736] Therefore, attaining a water diuresis and reversing hyponatremia through the use of V_2 receptor antagonists are potentially important therapeutic goals. To date, several studies performed in animals and patients with cirrhosis have yielded promising results.[462,463] Favorable effects on fluid balance have been demonstrated for lixivaptan, satavaptan, and tolvaptan in comparison with placebo. Two small trials on lixivaptan have been published.[737] In one, a subgroup analysis of 60 cirrhotic patients, who were included in a general trial of lixivaptan in dilutional hyponatremia, showed that a 200-mg but not a 100-mg dose significantly increased the serum Na^+ level compared to no change in the placebo group. Of patients who received the 200-mg dose, 50% achieved a normal serum Na^+ level (136 mmol/L). In the other trial, 33 cirrhotic patients received lixivaptan in doses of 50 to 500 mg, with a dose-response effect; however, even at the highest dose, the overall response was modest (serum Na^+ level increased from 125 ± 1 to 132 ± 1 mmol/L).

Three randomized controlled trials exploring the effects of satavaptan, alone or in combination with diuretics, in a total of 1200 cirrhotics with uncomplicated or difficult to treat ascites have been carried out.[463] Satavaptan (5 to 25 mg) was somewhat more effective than placebo in delaying the onset of ascites and increasing serum Na^+ levels, but a higher mortality was observed in the group that received satavaptan with diuretics, leading to early termination of one study. The specific role of satavaptan in the increased mortality was uncertain, given that most deaths were due to complications of cirrhosis. Tolvaptan compared to placebo was used in the SALT-1 and SALT-2 trials and also demonstrated favorable effects on serum Na^+ levels in cirrhotics, whereas adverse event rates and mortality were similar in both groups. Overall, the effects of vaptans in cirrhotics appear to be modest; this phenomenon may be explained by avid proximal tubular solute reabsorption leading to reduced distal delivery or by V_2 receptor–independent pathways of water retention.[462] Further studies are clearly needed to clarify the exact clinical indications for vaptans in the treatment of cirrhotics with ascites and hyponatremia.

TRANSJUGULAR INTRAHEPATIC PORTOSYSTEMIC SHUNT

The efficacy of TIPS in the reduction of portal venous pressure in patients with cirrhosis and refractory ascites with type 1 or 2 HRS has been demonstrated in several small cohort studies.[553] Significant improvement in renal hemodynamics, GFR, and vasoconstrictive neurohumoral factors were observed in most patients in a study reviewed by Wadei and coworkers.[604] The rates of survival at 3, 6, 12, and 18 months were 81%, 71%, 48%, and 35%, respectively, a marked improvement in comparison with historical controls.[738] Of importance was that among patients who had type 1 HRS and treated with TIPS, 10-week survival was 53%, a significant improvement over that in historical cases and better than that reported after terlipressin and albumin infusion.[739] Four of seven dialysis-dependent patients were able to discontinue this treatment after TIPS insertion. Moreover, liver transplantation was performed in two patients at 7 months and 2 years, respectively, after TIPS insertion, when the medical condition that precluded transplantation had resolved.[738]

TIPS appears to exert its favorable effects by reducing sinusoidal hypertension with suppression of the putative hepatorenal reflex (see earlier), improvement of EABV by shunting portal venous blood into the systemic circulation, or amelioration of cardiac dysfunction.[639] Despite the encouraging beneficial effects of TIPS on reversal of HRS and improvement in patient survival, some unanswered questions remain:

1. The clinical, biochemical, and neurohumoral parameters, although improved, are not normalized after TIPS insertion; thus, other factors in the pathogenetic pathway of HRS may remain active.
2. The maximum renal recovery is delayed for up to 2 to 4 weeks after TIPS insertion, and renal Na^+ excretory capacity is still subnormal. The cause of this delay and the inability to normalize salt excretion are not clear, although one possibility is related to the proportionately greater action of TIPS to reduce presinusoidal pressure, as opposed to postsinusoidal and intrasinusoidal pressures.
3. Patients with advanced cirrhosis are at risk for worsening liver failure, hepatic encephalopathy, or both and are not candidates for TIPS insertion.
4. TIPS has the potential for worsening the existing hyperdynamic circulation or precipitating acute heart failure in at-risk patients; therefore, careful attention to cardiac status is mandatory.
5. TIPS is associated with a high incidence of portosystemic encephalopathy when used for the treatment of refractory ascites. Note that this complication is far less frequent when TIPS is used for treating variceal hemorrhage.[740]

Notwithstanding these unsolved issues, there is clearly a group of HRS patients for whom TIPS might prolong survival long enough to enable liver transplantation or, if they are not candidates, to remain dialysis-independent. The possibility of combination or sequential therapies has also been examined in preliminary studies. For example, treatment with octreotide, midodrine, and albumin infusion, followed by TIPS insertion, in selected type 1 HRS patients with preserved liver function was associated with persistent improvements in serum creatinine, RPF, GFR, natriuresis, PRA, and aldosterone levels.[741] Another group of 11 patients with type 2 HRS showed similar improvement after sequential terlipressin and TIPS insertion. Whether combination therapy can preclude the need for liver transplantation or significantly improve survival remains to be investigated.

RENAL REPLACEMENT THERAPY

Conventional hemodialysis and continuous RRT have been extensively assessed in patients with HRS. The benefits, if any, in terms of prolonging survival, are dubious,[742] and the incidence of morbidity resulting from these therapies is high.[743] In oliguric patients awaiting liver transplantation who do not respond to vasoconstrictors or TIPS and who develop diuretic-resistant volume overload, hyperkalemia, or intractable metabolic acidosis, RRT may be a reasonable option as a bridge to transplantation. In view of the dismal prognosis of HRS, especially type 1, decisions for the use of RRT in patients who are not transplantation candidates should be carefully deliberated on an individual basis.

In contrast to conventional RRT, molecular adsorbent recirculating system (MARS) offers the potential advantage of removing albumin-bound, water-soluble vasoactive agents, toxins, and proinflammatory cytokines. Relevant molecules include bile acids, TNF-α, interleukin-6, and nitric oxide, which are known to be implicated in the pathogenesis of advanced cirrhosis.[576] The uniqueness of MARS lies in its ability to enable partial recovery of hepatic function and provide RRT. Early studies have shown that MARS treatment leads to a decrease in renal vascular resistance and improvement in the splenic resistance index, a parameter related to portal resistance. The hemodynamic effects were thought to be mediated by clearance of vasoactive substances.[744] In another study, MARS led to significantly reduced bilirubin levels, reduced grade of encephalopathy, and decreased serum creatinine and increased serum Na^+ levels.[745] That study also demonstrated a survival benefit; the mortality rate was reduced from 100% in the control group to 62.5% in the MARS-treated patients. At 30 days, 75% of the MARS group had survived.[745] In a recent uncontrolled study of 32 patients with type 1 HRS who underwent MARS treatment, 13 had improved renal function (40%).[746] Among these, 9 (28%) had complete renal recovery. No difference between survivors and nonsurvivors was observed in terms of renal functional response to MARS. The 28-day survival rate was 47%. After diagnosis of HRS, 7 patients received a liver transplant; of these, 4 had complete or partial recovery after transplantation (57%) versus 9 of 25 patients who did not undergo liver transplantation (36%) (difference not significant).[746] Given that all studies to date were small and uncontrolled, MARS, like the pharmacologic therapies described previously, should at present probably be considered only as a bridge to transplantation.

Another novel therapy, known as PROMETHEUS, involves fractional plasma separation, which could be combined with conventional hemodialysis. However, this has yet to be tested in patients with HRS.[743]

LIVER TRANSPLANTATION

Liver transplantation is the treatment of choice for HRS because it offers a cure for the liver disease and renal dysfunction. The outcomes are somewhat worse in transplant recipients with HRS than in those without the syndrome (3-year survival rates of 60% vs. 70% to 80%), but may be improved by the bridging therapies described previously.[621] To date, only small series have been described, and more data are needed to confirm the initial favorable reports.

With respect to renal function after transplantation in patients with HRS, GFR decreases in the first month as a result of the stress of surgery, infections, immunosuppressive therapy, and other factors. Dialysis in the first month is required in 35% of patients with HRS, as opposed to only 5% of patients without HRS. Despite the prompt correction of hemodynamic and neurohumoral parameters, GFR recovers incompletely to 30 to 40 mL/min at 1 to 2 months, and renal functional impairment often persists over the long term. Overall, the rate of posttransplantation reversal of HRS has been estimated to be no greater than 58%. Predictors of renal recovery included younger recipient and donor, nonalcoholic liver disease, and low posttransplantation bilirubin level.[747] Combined simultaneous liver and kidney transplantation apparently offers no greater benefit over liver transplantation alone with respect to posttransplantation kidney function, and dual-organ transplantation should be reserved for patients who have end-stage renal disease (defined as dialysis dependence for 8 weeks or longer pretransplantation) in addition to end-stage hepatic disease.[576,748]

Perhaps surprisingly, duration of dialysis pretransplantation did not influence renal recovery after transplantation. In this regard, the question of combined liver-kidney transplantation becomes critical. Data from the United Network for Organ Sharing have shown better rates of 5-year survival after liver-kidney transplantation than after liver transplantation alone in patients with pretransplantation serum creatinine levels higher than 2.2 mg/dL, irrespective of dialysis requirement. In contrast, single-center results were similar, regardless of pretransplantation renal function.[749] More studies are needed to enable a rational decision to be made about who should receive liver-kidney transplants, as opposed to liver transplants alone.

The introduction of MELD (Model of End-stage Liver Disease) scores for the allocation of livers has increased the number of transplantations in patients with impaired renal function, but more liver-kidney transplantations are also being performed.[750] On the other hand, a favorable response to vasoactive therapy reduces the MELD score and may lead to a paradoxic delay in liver transplantation[750] Therefore, only pretreatment MELD scores should be used to predict potential outcomes of liver transplantation in HRS.[553] A further paradox is that patients with type 2 HRS have lower MELD scores than those with type 1 HRS, resulting in the former being ascribed a lower priority for transplantation and a longer time on the waiting list for transplantation. This delay is associated with higher mortality, despite lower MELD scores, especially in the presence of hyponatremia and persistent ascites. Therefore, the criteria for donor allocation need to be modified to incorporate these factors into the final score for prioritization.[553]

For a general summary of all aspects of liver transplantation, the reader is referred to several excellent recent reviews.[751,752]

Complete reference list available at ExpertConsult.com.

KEY REFERENCES

14. Titze J, Dahlmann A, Lerchl K, et al: Spooky sodium balance. *Kidney Int* 85:759–767, 2014.
15. Anand IS: Cardiorenal syndrome: a cardiologist's perspective of pathophysiology. *Clin J Am Soc Nephrol* 8:1800–1807, 2013.
92. Oliver JA, Verna EC: Afferent mechanisms of sodium retention in cirrhosis and hepatorenal syndrome. *Kidney Int* 77:669–680, 2010.
181. O'Connor PM, Cowley AW, Jr: Modulation of pressure-natriuresis by renal medullary reactive oxygen species and nitric oxide. *Curr Hypertens Rep* 12:86–92, 2010.
243. Welling PA, Chang YP, Delpire E, et al: Multigene kinase network, kidney transport, and salt in essential hypertension. *Kidney Int* 77:1063–1069, 2010.
266. Stockand JD: Vasopressin regulation of renal sodium excretion. *Kidney Int* 78:849–856, 2010.
277. Johns EJ, Kopp UC, Dibona GF: Neural control of renal function. *Compr Physiol* 1:731–767, 2011.
301. Hyndman KA, Pollock JS: Nitric oxide and the A and B of endothelin of sodium homeostasis. *Curr Opin Nephrol Hypertens* 22:26–31, 2013.
384. Nikolaeva S, Pradervand S, Centeno G, et al: The circadian clock modulates renal sodium handling. *J Am Soc Nephrol* 23:1019–1026, 2012.
385. Rakova N, Juttner K, Dahlmann A, et al: Long-term space flight simulation reveals infradian rhythmicity in human Na(+) balance. *Cell Metab* 17:125–131, 2013.
387. Moritz ML: Syndrome of inappropriate antidiuresis and cerebral salt wasting syndrome: are they different and does it matter? *Pediatr Nephrol* 27:689–693, 2012.

390. Siddall EC, Radhakrishnan J: The pathophysiology of edema formation in the nephrotic syndrome. *Kidney Int* 82:635–642, 2012.
397. Rajaram SS, Desai NK, Kalra A, et al: Pulmonary artery catheters for adult patients in intensive care. *Cochrane Database Syst Rev* (2):CD003408, 2013.
398. Sinkeler SJ, Damman K, van Veldhuisen DJ, et al: A re-appraisal of volume status and renal function impairment in chronic heart failure: combined effects of pre-renal failure and venous congestion on renal function. *Heart Fail Rev* 17:263–270, 2012.
400. Yunos NM, Bellomo R, Bailey M: Chloride-restrictive fluid administration and incidence of acute kidney injury—reply. *JAMA* 309:543–544, 2013.
401. Waikar SS, Winkelmayer WC: Saving the kidneys by sparing intravenous chloride? *JAMA* 308:1583–1585, 2012.
403. Mutter TC, Ruth CA, Dart AB: Hydroxyethyl starch (HES) versus other fluid therapies: effects on kidney function. *Cochrane Database Syst Rev* (7):CD007594, 2013.
424. Ronco C, Cicoira M, McCullough PA: Cardiorenal syndrome type 1: pathophysiological crosstalk leading to combined heart and kidney dysfunction in the setting of acutely decompensated heart failure. *J Am Coll Cardiol* 60:1031–1042, 2012.
425. Metra M, Cotter G, Gheorghiade M, et al: The role of the kidney in heart failure. *Eur Heart J* 33:2135–2142, 2012.
446. Parati G, Esler M: The human sympathetic nervous system: its relevance in hypertension and heart failure. *Eur Heart J* 33:1058–1066, 2012.
452. Giamouzis G, Butler J, Triposkiadis F: Renal function in advanced heart failure. *Congest Heart Fail* 17:180–188, 2011.
458. Schrier RW, Sharma S, Shchekochikhin D: Hyponatraemia: more than just a marker of disease severity? *Nat Rev Nephrol* 9:37–50, 2013.
462. Lehrich RW, Ortiz-Melo DI, Patel MB, et al: Role of vaptans in the management of hyponatremia. *Am J Kidney Dis* 62:364–376, 2013.
478. Horii M, Matsumoto T, Uemura S, et al: Prognostic value of B-type natriuretic peptide and its amino-terminal proBNP fragment for cardiovascular events with stratification by renal function. *J Cardiol* 61:410–416, 2013.
482. van Veldhuisen DJ, Linssen GC, Jaarsma T, et al: B-type natriuretic peptide and prognosis in heart failure patients with preserved and reduced ejection fraction. *J Am Coll Cardiol* 61:1498–1506, 2013.
491. Li P, Luo Y, Chen YM: B-type natriuretic peptide-guided chronic heart failure therapy: a meta-analysis of 11 randomised controlled trials. *Heart Lung Circ* 22:852–860, 2013.
537. Alehagen U, Dahlstrom U, Rehfeld JF, et al: Pro-A-type natriuretic peptide, proadrenomedullin, and N-terminal pro-B-type natriuretic peptide used in a multimarker strategy in primary health care in risk assessment of patients with symptoms of heart failure. *J Card Fail* 19:31–39, 2013.
551. Ahmadian M, Suh JM, Hah N, et al: PPARgamma signaling and metabolism: the good, the bad and the future. *Nat Med* 19:557–566, 2013.
553. Wong F: Recent advances in our understanding of hepatorenal syndrome. *Nat Rev Gastroenterol Hepatol* 9:382–391, 2012.
554. Rahimi RS, Rockey DC: End-stage liver disease complications. *Curr Opin Gastroenterol* 29:257–263, 2013.
567. Bellot P, Frances R, Such J: Pathological bacterial translocation in cirrhosis: pathophysiology, diagnosis and clinical implications. *Liver Int* 33:31–39, 2013.
625. Koshimizu TA, Nakamura K, Egashira N, et al: Vasopressin V1a and V1b receptors: from molecules to physiological systems. *Physiol Rev* 92:1813–1864, 2012.
639. Arroyo V, Fernandez J: Management of hepatorenal syndrome in patients with cirrhosis. *Nat Rev Nephrol* 7:517–526, 2011.
659. Palmer BF: Metabolic complications associated with use of diuretics. *Semin Nephrol* 31:542–552, 2011.
661. Felker GM, Lee KL, Bull DA, et al: Diuretic strategies in patients with acute decompensated heart failure. *N Engl J Med* 364:797–805, 2011.
664. Munoz D, Felker GM: Approaches to decongestion in patients with acute decompensated heart failure. *Curr Cardiol Rep* 15:335, 2013.
665. Prosek J, Agarwal A, Parikh SV: Cardiorenal syndrome and the role of ultrafiltration in heart failure. *Curr Heart Fail Rep* 10:81–88, 2013.
679. Rami K: Aggressive salt and water restriction in acutely decompensated heart failure: is it worth its weight in salt? *Expert Rev Cardiovasc Ther* 11:1125–1128, 2013.
681. Aliti GB, Rabelo ER, Clausell N, et al: Aggressive fluid and sodium restriction in acute decompensated heart failure: a randomized clinical trial. *JAMA Intern Med* 173:1058–1064, 2013.
684. Bernstein PL, Ellison DH: Diuretics and salt transport along the nephron. *Semin Nephrol* 31:475–482, 2011.
690. Ronco C, Giomarelli P: Current and future role of ultrafiltration in CRS. *Heart Fail Rev* 16:595–602, 2011.
691. Mentz RJ, Bakris GL, Waeber B, et al: The past, present and future of renin-angiotensin aldosterone system inhibition. *Int J Cardiol* 167:1677–1687, 2013.
703. Chen HH, Anstrom KJ, Givertz MM, et al: Low-dose dopamine or low-dose nesiritide in acute heart failure with renal dysfunction: The ROSE Acute Heart Failure Randomized Trial. *JAMA* 310:2533–2543, 2013.
708. Waldum B, Os I: The cardiorenal syndrome: what the cardiologist needs to know. *Cardiology* 126:175–186, 2013.
718. Borne RT, Krantz MJ: Lixivaptan for hyponatremia—the numbers game. *JAMA* 308:2345–2346, 2012.
727. Sola E, Cardenas A, Gines P: Results of pretransplant treatment of hepatorenal syndrome with terlipressin. *Curr Opin Organ Transplant* 18:265–270, 2013.
735. Gluud LL, Christensen K, Christensen E, et al: Terlipressin for hepatorenal syndrome. *Cochrane Database Syst Rev* (9):CD005162, 2012.
736. Yu C, Sharma N, Saab S: Hyponatremia: clinical associations, prognosis, and treatment in cirrhosis. *Exp Clin Transplant* 11:3–11, 2013.
750. Angeli P, Gines P: Hepatorenal syndrome, MELD score and liver transplantation: an evolving issue with relevant implications for clinical practice. *J Hepatol* 57:1135–1140, 2012.
751. Alqahtani SA, Larson AM: Adult liver transplantation in the USA. *Curr Opin Gastroenterol* 27:240–247, 2011.

16 Disorders of Water Balance

Joseph G. Verbalis

CHAPTER OUTLINE

BODY FLUIDS: COMPARTMENTALIZATION, COMPOSITION, AND TURNOVER, 460
WATER METABOLISM, 462
Vasopressin Synthesis and Secretion, 462
Thirst, 471
Integration of Vasopressin Secretion and Thirst, 472
DISORDERS OF INSUFFICIENT VASOPRESSIN OR VASOPRESSIN EFFECT, 473
Central Diabetes Insipidus, 473
Osmoreceptor Dysfunction, 477
Gestational Diabetes Insipidus, 480
Nephrogenic Diabetes Insipidus, 480
Primary Polydipsia, 482
Clinical Manifestations of Diabetes Insipidus, 483
Differential Diagnosis of Polyuria, 483
Treatment of Diabetes Insipidus, 486
DISORDERS OF EXCESS VASOPRESSIN OR VASOPRESSIN EFFECT, 490
Relationship Between Hypo-Osmolality and Hyponatremia, 490

Variables That Influence Renal Water Excretion, 491
PATHOGENESIS AND CAUSES OF HYPONATREMIA, 491
Hyponatremia with Extracellular Fluid Volume Depletion, 492
Hyponatremia with Excess Extracellular Fluid Volume, 493
Hyponatremia with Normal Extracellular Fluid Volume, 495
Syndrome of Inappropriate Antidiuretic Hormone Secretion, 497
HYPONATREMIA SYMPTOMS, MORBIDITY, AND MORTALITY, 500
HYPONATREMIA TREATMENT, 503
Current Therapies, 503
Treatment Guidelines, 506
Monitoring Serum Sodium Concentration in Hyponatremic Patients, 508
Long-Term Treatment of Chronic Hyponatremia, 508
Future of Hyponatremia Treatment, 508

Disorders of body fluids are among the most commonly encountered problems in clinical medicine. This is in large part because many different disease states can potentially disrupt the finely balanced mechanisms that control the intake and output of water and solute. Because body water is the primary determinant of the osmolality of the extracellular fluid, disorders of water metabolism can be broadly divided into hyperosmolar disorders, in which there is a deficiency of body water relative to body solute, and hypoosmolar disorders, in which there is an excess of body water relative to body solute. Because sodium is the main constituent of plasma osmolality, these disorders are typically characterized by hypernatremia and hyponatremia, respectively. Before discussing specific aspects of these disorders, this chapter will first review the regulatory mechanisms underlying water metabolism, which, in concert with sodium metabolism, maintains body fluid homeostasis.

BODY FLUIDS: COMPARTMENTALIZATION, COMPOSITION, AND TURNOVER

Water constitutes approximately 55% to 65% of body weight, varying with age, gender, and amount of body fat, and therefore constitutes the largest single constituent of the body. Total body water (TBW) is distributed between the intracellular fluid (ICF) and extracellular fluid (ECF) compartments. Estimates of the relative sizes of these two pools differ significantly, depending on the tracer used to measure the ECF volume, but most studies in animals and humans have indicated that 55% to 65% of TBW resides in the ICF and 35% to 45% is in the ECF. Approximately 75% of the ECF compartment is interstitial fluid and only 25% is intravascular fluid (blood volume).[1,2] Figure 16.1 summarizes the estimated body fluid spaces of an average weight adult.

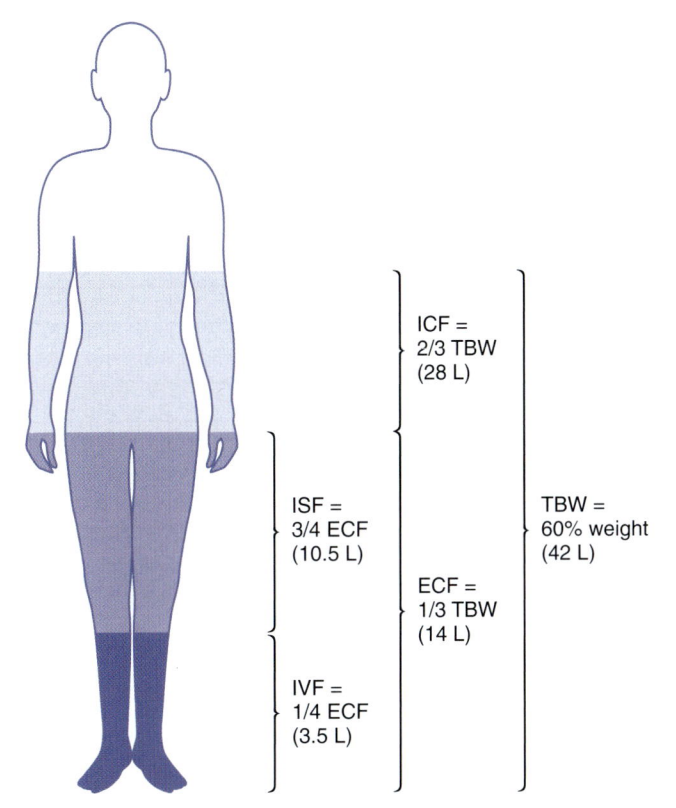

Figure 16.1 Schematic representation of body fluid compartments in humans. The *shaded areas* depict the approximate size of each compartment as a function of body weight. The *numbers* indicate the relative sizes of the various fluid compartments and the approximate absolute volumes of the compartments (in liters) in a 70-kg adult. ECF, Extracellular fluid; ICF, intracellular fluid; ISF, interstitial fluid; IVF, intravascular fluid; TBW, total body water. (From Verbalis JG: Body water and osmolality. In Wilkinson B, Jamison R, editors: *Textbook of nephrology,* London, 1997, Chapman & Hall, pp 89-94.)

The solute composition of the ICF and ECF differs considerably because most cell membranes possess multiple transport systems that actively accumulate or expel specific solutes. Thus, membrane-bound Na^+-K^+-ATPase maintains Na^+ in a primarily extracellular location and K^+ in a primarily intracellular location.[3] Similar transporters effectively result in confining Cl^- largely to the ECF, and Mg^{2+}, organic acids, and phosphates to the ICF. Glucose, which requires an insulin-activated transport system to enter most cells, is present in significant amounts only in the ECF because it is rapidly converted intracellularly to glycogen or metabolites. HCO_3^- is present in both compartments but is approximately three times more concentrated in the ECF. Urea is unique among the major naturally occurring solutes in that it diffuses freely across most cell membranes[4]; therefore, it is present in similar concentrations in almost all body fluids, except in the renal medulla, where it is concentrated by urea transporters (see Chapter 10).

Despite very different solute compositions, both the ICF and ECF have an equivalent osmotic pressure,[5] which is a function of the total concentration of all solutes in a fluid compartment, because most biologic membranes are semipermeable (i.e., freely permeable to water but not to aqueous solutes). Thus, water will flow across membranes into a compartment with a higher solute concentration until a steady state is reached and the osmotic pressures have equalized on both sides of the cell membrane.[6] An important consequence of this thermodynamic law is that the volume of distribution of body Na^+ and K^+ is actually the TBW rather than just the ECF or ICF volume, respectively.[7] For example, any increase in ECF sodium concentration ($[Na^+]$) will cause water to shift from the ICF to ECF until the ICF and ECF osmotic pressures are equal, thereby effectively distributing the Na^+ across extracellular and intracellular water.

Osmolality is defined as the concentration of all of the solutes in a given weight of fluid. The total solute concentration of a fluid can be determined and expressed in several different ways. The most common method is to measure its freezing point or vapor pressure because these are colligative properties of the number of free solute particles in a volume of fluid.[8] The result is expressed relative to a standard solution of known concentration using units of osmolality (milliosmoles of solute per kilogram of water, $mOsm/kg\ H_2O$), or osmolarity (milliosmoles of solute per liter of water, $mOsm/L\ H_2O$). Plasma osmolality (P_{osm}) can be measured directly, as described above, or calculated by summing the concentrations of the major solutes present in the plasma:

$$P_{osm}\ (mOsm/kg\ H_2O) = 2 \times plasma\ [Na^+]\ (mEq/L) \\ + glucose\ (mg/dL)/18 \\ + BUN\ (mg/dL)/2.8$$

Both methods produce comparable results under most conditions (the value obtained using this formula is generally within 1% to 2% of that obtained by direct osmometry), as will simply doubling the plasma $[Na^+]$, because sodium and its accompanying anions are the predominant solutes present in plasma. However, the total osmolality of plasma is not always equivalent to the effective osmolality, often referred to as the tonicity of the plasma, because the latter is a function of the relative solute permeability properties of the membranes separating the two compartments. Solutes that are impermeable to cell membranes (e.g., Na^+, mannitol) are restricted to the ECF compartment. They are effective solutes because they create osmotic pressure gradients across cell membranes, leading to the osmotic movement of water from the ICF to ECF compartments. Solutes that are permeable to cell membranes (e.g., urea, ethanol, methanol) are ineffective solutes because they do not create osmotic pressure gradients across cell membranes and therefore are not associated with such water shifts.[9] Glucose is a unique solute because, at normal physiologic plasma concentrations, it is taken up by cells via active transport mechanisms and therefore acts as an ineffective solute but, under conditions of impaired cellular uptake (e.g., insulin deficiency), it becomes an effective extracellular solute.[10]

The importance of this distinction between total and effective osmolality is that only the effective solutes in plasma are determinants of whether clinically significant hyperosmolality or hypo-osmolality is present. An example of this is uremia; a patient with a blood urea nitrogen (BUN) concentration that has increased by 56 mg/dL will have a corresponding 20-$mOsm/kg\ H_2O$ elevation in plasma osmolality, but the effective osmolality will remain normal because the increased urea is proportionally distributed across the

ECF and ICF. In contrast, a patient whose plasma [Na$^+$] has increased by 10 mEq/L will also have a 20-mOsm/kg H$_2$O elevation of plasma osmolality because the increased cation must be balanced by an equivalent increase in plasma anions. However, in this case the effective osmolality will also be elevated by 20 mOsm/kg H$_2$O because the Na$^+$ and accompanying anions will largely remain restricted to the ECF due to the relative impermeability of cell membranes to Na$^+$ and other ions. Thus, elevations of solutes such as urea, unlike elevations of sodium, do not cause cellular dehydration and consequently do not activate mechanisms that defend body fluid homeostasis by increasing body water stores.

Both body water and solutes are in a state of continuous exchange with the environment. The magnitude of the turnover varies considerably, depending on physical, social, and environmental factors, but in healthy adults it averages 5% to 10% of the total body content each day. For the most part, daily intake of water and electrolytes is not determined by physiologic requirements but is more a function of dietary preferences and cultural influences. Healthy adults have an average daily fluid ingestion of approximately 2 to 3 L, but with considerable individual variation; approximately one third of this is derived from food or the metabolism of fat and the rest from discretionary ingestion of fluids. Similarly, of the 1000 mOsm of solute ingested or generated by the metabolism of nutrients each day, nearly 40% is intrinsic to food, another 35% is added to food as a preservative or flavoring, and the rest is mostly urea. In contrast to the largely unregulated nature of basal intakes, the urinary excretion of water and solute is highly regulated to preserve body fluid homeostasis. Thus, under normal circumstances, almost all ingested Na$^+$, Cl$^-$, and K$^+$, as well as ingested and metabolically generated urea, are excreted in the urine under the control of specific regulatory mechanisms. Other ingested solutes, such as divalent minerals, are excreted primarily by the gastrointestinal tract. Urinary excretion of water is also tightly regulated by the secretion and renal effects of arginine vasopressin (AVP; vasopressin, antidiuretic hormone), discussed in greater detail in Chapters 10 and 11 and in the following section ("Water Metabolism").

WATER METABOLISM

Water metabolism is responsible for the balance between the intake and excretion of water. Each side of this balance equation can be considered to consist of a regulated and unregulated component, the magnitudes of which can vary markedly under different physiologic and pathophysiologic conditions. The unregulated component of water intake consists of the intrinsic water content of ingested foods, consumption of beverages primarily for reasons of palatability or desired secondary effects (e.g., caffeine), or for social or habitual reasons (e.g., alcoholic beverages), whereas the regulated component of water intake consists of fluids consumed in response to a perceived sensation of thirst. Studies of middle-aged subjects have shown mean fluid intakes of 2.1 L/24 hours, and analyses of the fluids consumed have indicated that the vast majority of the fluid ingested is determined by influences such as meal-associated fluid intake, taste, or psychosocial factors rather than true thirst.[11]

The unregulated component of water excretion occurs via insensible water losses from a variety of sources (e.g., cutaneous losses from sweating, evaporative losses in exhaled air, gastrointestinal losses) as well as the obligate amount of water that the kidneys must excrete to eliminate solutes generated by body metabolism, whereas the regulated component of water excretion is comprised of the renal excretion of free water in excess of the obligate amount necessary to excrete metabolic solutes. Unlike solutes, a relatively large proportion of body water is excreted by evaporation from skin and lungs. This amount varies markedly, depending on several factors, including dress, humidity, temperature, and exercise.[12] Under the sedentary and temperature-controlled indoor conditions typical of modern urban life, daily insensible water loss in healthy adults is minimal, approximately 8 to 10 mL/kg body weight (BW; ≈0.5 to 0.7 L in a 70-kg adult man or woman). However, insensible losses can increase to twice this level (20 mL/kg BW) simply under conditions of increased activity and temperature and, if environmental temperature or activity is even higher, such as in an arid environment, the rate of insensible water loss can even approximate the maximal rate of free water excretion by the kidney.[12] Thus, in quantitative terms, insensible loss and the factors that influence it can be just as important to body fluid homeostasis as regulated urine output.

Another major determinant of unregulated water loss is the rate of urine solute excretion, which cannot be reduced below a minimal obligatory level required to excrete the solute load. The volume of urine required depends not only on the solute load, but also on the degree of antidiuresis. At a typical basal level of urinary concentration (urine osmolality = 600 mOsm/kg H$_2$O) and a typical solute load of 900 to 1200 mOsm/day, a 70-kg adult would require a total urine volume of 1.5 to 2.0 L (21 to 29 mL/kg BW) to excrete the solute load. However, under conditions of maximal antidiuresis (urine osmolality = 1200 mOsm/kg H$_2$O), the same solute load would require a minimal obligatory urine output of only 0.75 to 1.0 L/day and, conversely, a decrease in urine concentration to minimal levels (urine osmolality = 60 mOsm/kg H$_2$O) would obligate a proportionately larger urine volume of 15 to 20 L/day to excrete the same solute load.

The above discussion emphasizes that water intake and water excretion have very substantial unregulated components, and these can vary tremendously as a result of factors unrelated to the maintenance of body fluid homeostasis. In effect, the regulated components of water metabolism are those that act to maintain body fluid homeostasis by compensating for whatever perturbations result from unregulated water losses or gains. Within this framework, the major mechanisms responsible for regulating water metabolism are pituitary secretion and the renal effects of vasopressin and thirst, each of which will be discussed in greater detail in the following sections.

VASOPRESSIN SYNTHESIS AND SECRETION

The primary determinant of free water excretion in animals and humans is the regulation of urinary water excretion by circulating levels of AVP in plasma. The renal effects of AVP are covered extensively in Chapters 10 and 11. This chapter will focus on the regulation of AVP synthesis and secretion.

STRUCTURE AND SYNTHESIS

Before AVP was biochemically characterized, early studies used the general term *antidiuretic hormone* (ADH) to describe this substance. Now that AVP is known to be the only naturally occurring antidiuretic substance, it is more appropriate to refer to it by its correct hormonal designation. AVP is a nine–amino acid peptide that is synthesized in the hypothalamus. It is composed of a six–amino acid, ringlike structure formed by a disulfide bridge, with a three–amino acid tail, at the end of which the terminal carboxyl group is amidated. Substitution of lysine for arginine in position 8 yields lysine vasopressin, the antidiuretic hormone found in pigs and other members of the suborder Suina. Substitution of isoleucine for phenylalanine at position 3 and of leucine for arginine at position 8 yields oxytocin (OT), a hormone found in all mammals and in many submammalian species.[13] OT has weak antidiuretic activity[14] but is a potent constrictor of smooth muscle in mammary glands and uterus. As implied by their names, arginine and lysine vasopressin also cause constriction of blood vessels, which was the property that lead to their original discovery in the late nineteenth century,[15] but this pressor effect occurs only at concentrations many times higher than those required to produce antidiuresis. This is probably of little physiologic or pathologic importance in humans except under conditions of severe hypotension and hypovolemia, where it acts to supplement the vasoconstrictive actions of angiotensin II (Ang II) and the sympathetic nervous system.[16] The multiple actions of AVP are mediated by different G protein–coupled receptors, designated V_{1a}, V_{1b}, and V_2.[17] (see Chapter 11).

AVP and OT are produced by the neurohypophysis, often referred to as the posterior pituitary gland, because the neural lobe is located centrally and posterior to the adenohypophysis, or anterior pituitary gland, in the sella turcica. However, it is important to understand that the posterior pituitary gland consists only of the distal axons of the magnocellular neurons that comprise the neurohypophysis. The cell bodies of these axons are located in specialized (magnocellular) neural cells located in two discrete areas of the hypothalamus, the paired supraoptic nuclei (SON) and paraventricular nuclei (PVN; Figure 16.2). In adults, the posterior pituitary is connected to the brain by a short stalk through the diaphragm sellae. The neurohypophysis is supplied with blood by branches of the superior and inferior hypophysial arteries, which arise from the posterior communicating and intracavernous portion of the internal carotid artery. In the posterior pituitary, the arterioles break up into localized capillary networks that drain directly into the jugular vein via the sellar, cavernous, and lateral venous sinuses. Many of the neurosecretory neurons that terminate higher in the infundibulum and median eminence originate in parvicellular neurons in the PVN; they are functionally distinct from the magnocellular neurons that terminate in the posterior pituitary because they primarily enhance secretion of adrenocorticotropic hormone (ACTH) from the anterior pituitary. AVP-containing neurons also project from parvicellular neurons of the PVN to other areas of the brain, including the limbic system, nucleus tractus solitarius, and lateral gray matter of the spinal cord. The full extent of the functions of these extrahypophysial projections are still under study.

The genes encoding the AVP and OT precursors are located in close proximity on chromosome 20, but are expressed in mutually exclusive populations of neurohypophyseal neurons.[18] The AVP gene consists of approximately 2000 base pairs and contains three exons separated by two intervening sequences (Figure 16.3). Each exon encodes one of the three functional domains of the preprohormone, although small parts of the nonconserved sequences of neurophysin are located in the first and third exons that code for AVP and the C-terminal glycoprotein, called copeptin, respectively. The untranslated 5′-flanking region, which regulates expression of the gene, shows extensive sequence homology across several species but is markedly different from the otherwise closely related gene for OT. This promoter region of the AVP gene in the rat contains several putative regulatory elements, including a glucocorticoid response element, cyclic adenosine monophosphate (cAMP) response element, and four activating protein-2 (AP-2) binding sites.[19] Experimental studies have suggested that the DNA sequences between the AVP and OT genes, the intergenic region, may contain critical sites for cell-specific expression of these two hormones.[20]

The gene for AVP is also expressed in a number of other neurons, including but not limited to the parvicellular neurons of the PVN and SON. AVP and OT genes are also expressed in several peripheral tissues, including the adrenal medulla, ovary, testis, thymus, and certain sensory ganglia.[21] However, the AVP mRNA in these tissues appears to be shorter (620 bases) than its hypothalamic counterpart (720 bases), apparently because of tissue-specific differences in the length of the polyA tails. More importantly, the levels of AVP in peripheral tissues are generally two or three orders of magnitude lower than in the neurohypophysis, suggesting that AVP in these tissues likely has paracrine rather than endocrine functions. This is consistent with the observation that destruction of the neurohypophysis essentially eliminates AVP from the plasma, despite the presence of these multiple peripheral sites of AVP synthesis.

Secretion of AVP and its associated neurophysin and copeptin peptide fragments occurs by a calcium-dependent exocytotic process, similar to that described for other neurosecretory systems. Secretion is triggered by propagation of an electrical impulse along the axon that causes depolarization of the cell membrane, an influx of Ca^{2+}, fusion of secretory granules with the cell membrane, and extrusion of their contents. This view is supported by the observation that AVP, neurophysin, and the glycoprotein copeptin are released simultaneously by many stimuli.[22] However, at the physiologic pH of plasma, there is no binding of AVP or OT to their respective neurophysins so, after secretion, each peptide circulates independently in the bloodstream.[23]

Stimuli for secretion of AVP or OT also stimulate transcription and increase the mRNA content of both prohormones in the magnocellular neurons. This has been well documented in rats, in which dehydration, which stimulates secretion of AVP, accelerates transcription and increases the levels of AVP (and OT) mRNA,[24,25] and hypo-osmolality, which inhibits the secretion of AVP, produces a decrease in

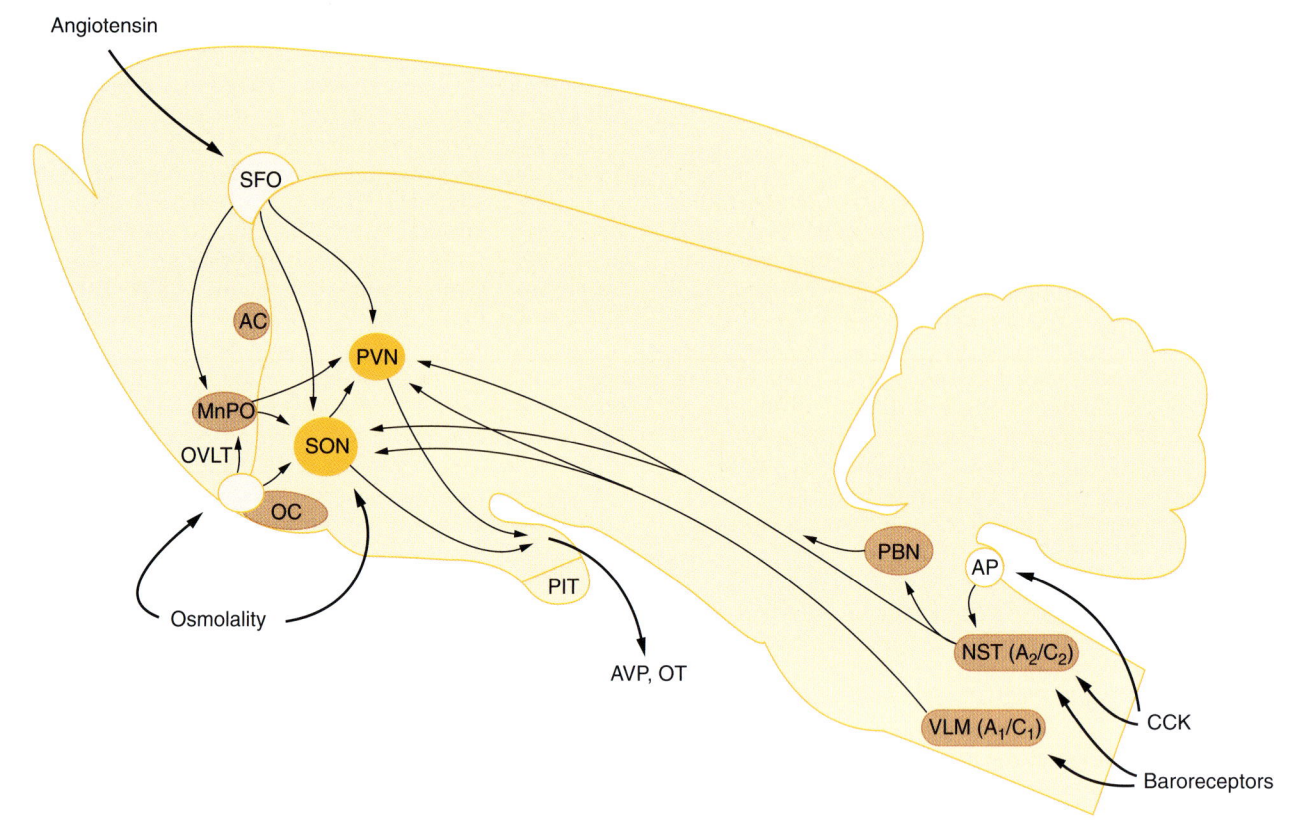

Figure 16.2 Summary of the main anterior hypothalamic pathways that mediate secretion of arginine vasopressin (AVP) and oxytocin (OT). The vascular organ of the lamina terminalis (OVLT) is especially sensitive to hyperosmolality. Hyperosmolality also activates other neurons in the anterior hypothalamus, such as those in the subfornical organ (SFO) and median preoptic nucleus (MnPO), and magnocellular neurons, which are intrinsically osmosensitive. Circulating angiotensin II (Ang II) activates neurons of the SFO, an essential site of Ang II action, as well as cells throughout the lamina terminalis and MnPO. In response to hyperosmolality or Ang II, projections from the SFO and OVLT to the MnPO activate excitatory and inhibitory interneurons that project to the supraoptic nucleus (SON) and paraventricular nucleus (PVN) to modulate direct inputs to these areas from the circumventricular organs. Cholecystokinin (CCK) acts primarily on gastric vagal afferents that terminate in the nucleus of the solitary tract (NST) but, at higher doses, it can also act at the area postrema (AP). Although neurons are apparently activated in the ventrolateral medulla (VLM) and NST, most neurohypophyseal secretion appears to be stimulated by monosynaptic projections from A_2-C_2 cells, and possibly also noncatecholaminergic somatostatin-inhibin B cells, of the NST. Baroreceptor-mediated stimuli, such as hypovolemia and hypotension, are more complex. The major projection to magnocellular AVP neurons appears to arise from A_1 cells of the VLM that are activated by excitatory interneurons from the NST. Other areas, such as the parabrachial nucleus (PBN), may contribute multisynaptic projections. Cranial nerves IX and X, which terminate in the NST, also contribute input to magnocellular AVP neurons. It is unclear whether baroreceptor-mediated secretion of oxytocin results from projections from VLM neurons or from NST neurons. AC, Anterior commissure; OC, optic chiasm; PIT, anterior pituitary. (From Stricker EM, Verbalis JG: Water intake and body fluids. In Squire LR, Bloom FE, McConnell SK, et al, editors: *Fundamental neuroscience,* San Diego, 2003, Academic Press, pp 1011-1029.)

the content of AVP mRNA.[26] These and other studies have indicated that the major control of AVP synthesis most likely resides at the level of transcription.[27]

Antidiuresis occurs via interaction of the circulating hormone with AVP V_2 receptors in the kidney, which results in increased water permeability of the collecting duct through the insertion of the aquaporin-2 (AQP2) water channel into the apical membranes of collecting tubule principal cells (see Chapter 10). The importance of AVP for maintaining water balance is underscored by the fact that the normal pituitary stores of this hormone are very large, allowing more than 1 week's supply of hormone for maximal antidiuresis under conditions of sustained dehydration.[27] Knowledge of the different conditions that stimulate pituitary AVP release in humans is therefore essential for understanding water metabolism.

OSMOTIC REGULATION

AVP secretion is influenced by many different stimuli, but since the pioneering studies of ADH secretion by Ernest Basil Verney, it has been clear that the most important stimulus under physiologic conditions is the osmotic pressure of plasma. With further refinement of radioimmunoassays for AVP, the unique sensitivity of this hormone to small changes in osmolality, as well as the corresponding sensitivity of the kidney to small changes in plasma AVP levels, have become apparent. Although the magnocellular neurons themselves have been found to have intrinsic osmoreceptive properties,[28] research over the last several decades has clearly shown that the most sensitive osmoreceptive cells that can sense small changes in plasma osmolality and transduce these changes into AVP secretion are located in the anterior hypothalamus, likely in or near the circumventricular organ

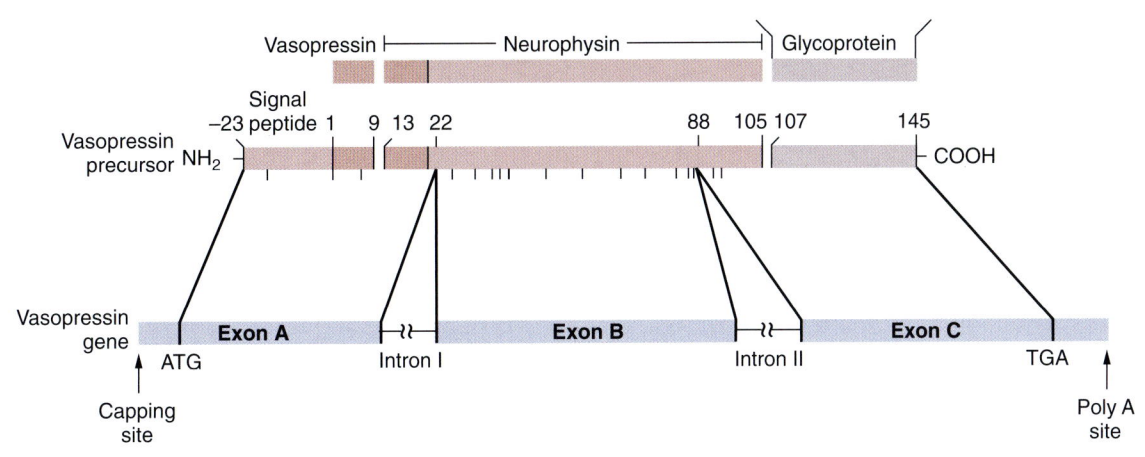

Figure 16.3 The arginine vasopressin (AVP) gene and its protein products. The three exons encode a 145-amino acid prohormone with an NH$_2$-terminal signal peptide. The prohormone is packaged into neurosecretory granules of magnocellular neurons. During axonal transport of the granules from the hypothalamus to the posterior pituitary, enzymatic cleavage of the prohormone generates the final products—AVP, neurophysin, and a COOH-terminal glycoprotein. When afferent stimulation depolarizes the AVP-containing neurons, the three products are released into capillaries of the posterior pituitary. (Adapted from Richter D, Schmale H: The structure of the precursor to arginine vasopressin, a model preprohormone. *Prog Brain Res* 60:227-233, 1983.)

termed the *organum vasculosum of the lamina terminalis* (OVLT; see Figure 16.2).[29] Perhaps the strongest evidence for location of the primary osmoreceptors in this area of the brain are the multiple studies that have demonstrated that destruction of this area disrupts osmotically stimulated AVP secretion and thirst, without affecting the neurohypophysis or its response to nonosmotic stimuli.[30,31]

Although some debate still exists with regard to the exact pattern of osmotically stimulated AVP secretion, most studies to date have supported the concept of a discrete osmotic threshold for AVP secretion, above which there is a linear relationship between plasma osmolality and AVP levels (Figure 16.4).[32] At plasma osmolalities below a threshold level, AVP secretion is suppressed to low or undetectable levels; above this point, AVP secretion increases linearly in direct proportion to plasma osmolality. The slope of the regression line relating AVP secretion to plasma osmolality can vary significantly across individual human subjects, in part because of genetic factors,[33] but also in relation to other factors. In general, each 1-mOsm/kg H$_2$O increase in plasma osmolality causes an increase in the plasma AVP level, ranging from 0.4 to 1.0 pg/mL. The renal response to circulating AVP is similarly linear, with urinary concentration that is directly proportional to AVP levels from 0.5 to 4 to 5 pg/mL, after which urinary osmolality is maximal and cannot increase further, despite additional increases in AVP levels (Figure 16.5). Thus, changes of as little as 1% in plasma osmolality are sufficient to cause significant increases in plasma AVP levels, with proportional increases in urine concentration, and maximal antidiuresis is achieved after increases in plasma osmolality of only 5 to 10 mOsm/kg H$_2$O (2% to 4%) above the threshold for AVP secretion.

However, even this analysis underestimates the sensitivity of this system to regulate free water excretion. Urinary osmolality is directly proportional to plasma AVP levels as a consequence of the fall in urine flow induced by the AVP, but urine volume is inversely related to urine osmolality (see Figure 16.5). An increase in plasma AVP concentration from 0.5 to 2 pg/mL has a much greater relative effect to decrease urine flow than a subsequent increase in AVP concentration

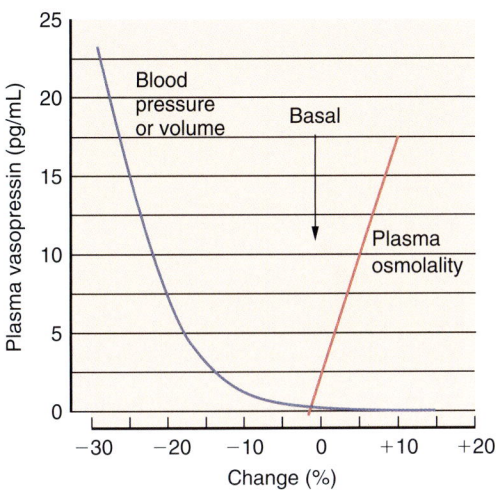

Figure 16.4 Comparative sensitivity of AVP secretion in response to increases in plasma osmolality versus decreases in blood volume or blood pressure in human subjects. The *arrow* indicates the low plasma AVP concentrations found at basal plasma osmolality. Note that AVP secretion is much more sensitive to small changes in blood osmolality than to changes in volume or pressure. (Adapted from Robertson GL: Posterior pituitary. In Felig P, Baxter J, Frohman LA, editors: *Endocrinology and metabolism,* New York, 1986, McGraw Hill, pp 338-386.)

from 2 to 5 pg/mL, thereby magnifying the physiologic effects of small changes in lower plasma AVP levels. Furthermore, the rapid response of AVP secretion to changes in plasma osmolality, coupled with the short half-life of AVP in human plasma (10 to 20 minutes), allows the kidneys to respond to changes in plasma osmolality on a minute-to-minute basis. The net result is a finely tuned osmoregulatory system that adjusts the rate of free water excretion accurately to the ambient plasma osmolality, primarily via changes in pituitary AVP secretion.

The set point of the osmoregulatory system also varies from person to person. In healthy adults, the osmotic threshold for AVP secretion ranges from 275 to 290 mOsm/

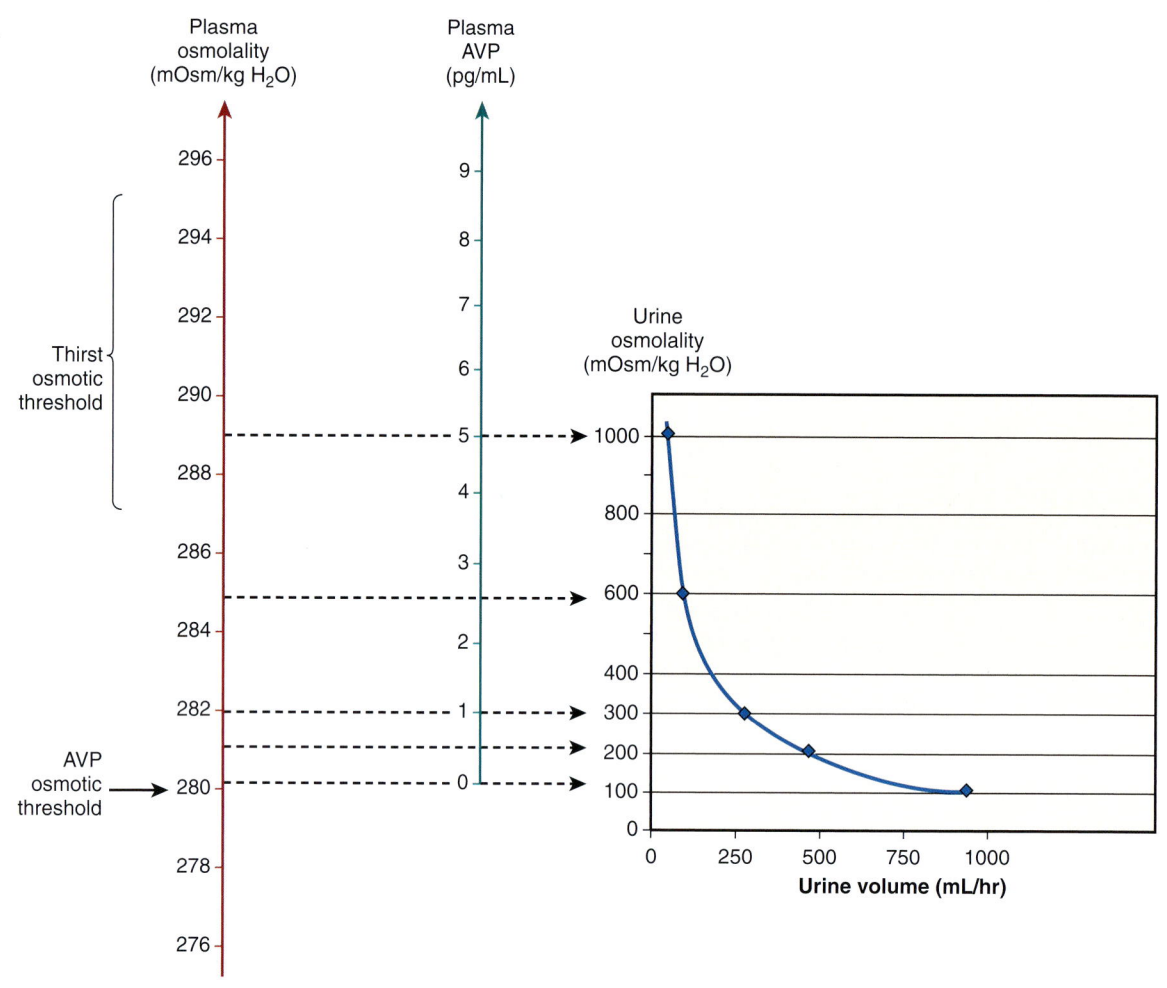

Figure 16.5 Relationship of plasma osmolality, plasma AVP concentrations, urine osmolality, and urine volume in humans. The osmotic threshold for AVP secretion defines the point at which urine concentration begins to increase, but the osmotic threshold for thirst is significantly higher and approximates the point at which maximal urine concentration has already been achieved. Note also that because of the inverse relation between urine osmolality and urine volume, changes in plasma AVP concentrations have much larger effects on urine volume at low plasma AVP concentrations than at high plasma AVP concentrations. (Adapted from Robinson AG: Disorders of antidiuretic hormone secretion. *J Clin Endocrinol Metab* 14:55-88, 1985.)

kg H_2O (averaging ≈280 to 285 mOsm/kg H_2O). Similar to sensitivity, individual differences in the set point of the osmoregulatory system are relatively constant over time and appear to be genetically determined.[33] However, multiple factors can alter the sensitivity and/or set point of the osmoregulatory system for AVP secretion, in addition to genetic influences.[33] Foremost among these are acute changes in blood pressure, effective blood volume, or both (discussed in the following section). Aging has been found to increase the sensitivity of the osmoregulatory system in multiple studies.[34,35] Metabolic factors, such as serum Ca^{2+} levels and various drugs, can alter the slope of the plasma AVP-osmolality relationship as well.[36] Lesser degrees of shifting of the osmosensitivity and set point for AVP secretion have been noted with alterations in gonadal hormones. Some studies have found increased osmosensitivity in women, particularly during the luteal phase of the menstrual cycle,[37] and in estrogen-treated men,[38] but these effects were relatively minor, and others have found no significant gender differences.[33] The set point of the osmoregulatory system is reduced more dramatically and reproducibly during pregnancy.[39] Evidence has suggested the possible involvement of the placental hormone relaxin,[40] rather than gonadal steroids or human chorionic gonadotropin hormone in pregnancy-associated resetting of the osmostat for AVP secretion. Both the changes in volume and in osmolality have been reproduced by infusion of relaxin into virgin female and normal rats and reversed in pregnant rats by immunoneutralization of relaxin.[41] Increased nitric oxide (NO) production by relaxin has been reported to increase vasodilatation, and estrogens also increase NO synthesis.[42] That multiple factors can influence the set point and sensitivity of osmotically regulated AVP secretion is not surprising because AVP secretion reflects a balance of bimodal inputs—inhibitory and stimulatory[43]—from multiple different afferent inputs to the neurohypophysis (Figure 16.6).[44]

Understanding the osmoregulatory mechanism also requires addressing the observation that AVP secretion is not equally sensitive to all plasma solutes. Sodium and its anions, which normally contribute more than 95% of the osmotic pressure of plasma, are the most potent solutes in

CHAPTER 16 — DISORDERS OF WATER BALANCE

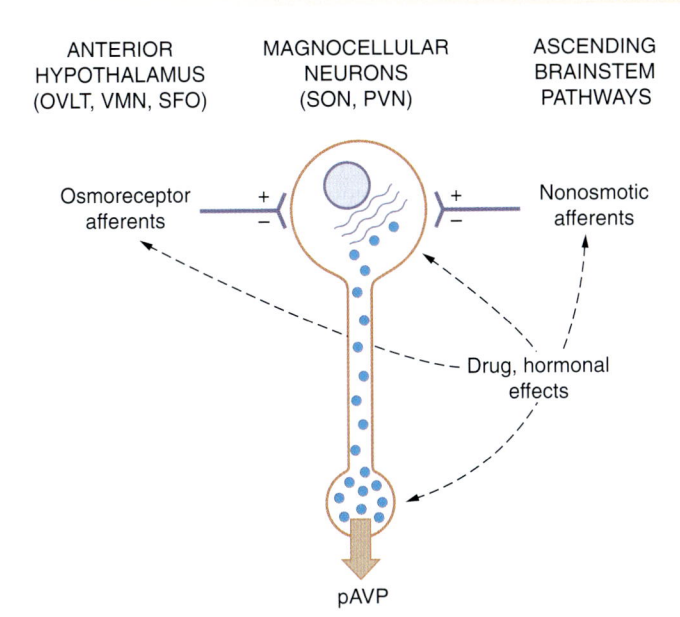

Figure 16.6 Schematic model of the regulatory control of the neurohypophysis. The secretory activity of individual magnocellular neurons is determined by an integration of the activities of excitatory and inhibitory osmotic and nonosmotic afferent inputs. Superimposed on this are the effects of hormones and drugs, which can act at multiple levels to modulate the output of the system. OVLT, Organum vasculosum of the lamina terminalis; PVN, paraventricular nucleus; SFO, subfornical organ; SON, supraoptic nucleus; VMN, ventromedial nucleus. (Adapted from Verbalis JG: Osmotic inhibition of neurohypophyseal secretion. *Ann N Y Acad Sci* 689:227-233, 1983.)

terms of their capacity to stimulate AVP secretion and thirst, although certain sugars such as mannitol and sucrose are also equally effective when infused intravenously.[9] In contrast, increases in plasma osmolality caused by noneffective solutes such as urea or glucose result in little or no increase in plasma AVP levels in humans or animals.[9,45] These differences in response to various plasma solutes are independent of any recognized nonosmotic influence, indicating that they are a property of the osmoregulatory mechanism itself. According to current concepts, the osmoreceptor neuron is stimulated by osmotically induced changes in its water content. In this case, the stimulatory potency of any given solute would be an inverse function of the rate at which it moves from the plasma to the inside of the osmoreceptor neuron. Solutes that penetrate slowly, or not at all, create an osmotic gradient that causes an efflux of water from the osmoreceptor, and the resultant shrinkage of the osmoreceptor neuron activates a stretch-inactivated, noncationic channel that initiates depolarization and firing of the neuron.[46] Conversely, solutes that penetrate the cell readily create no gradient and thus have no effect on the water content and cell volume of the osmoreceptors. This mechanism agrees well with the observed relationship between the effect of certain solutes on AVP secretion, such as Na+, mannitol, and glucose, and the rate at which they penetrate the blood-brain barrier.[29]

Many neurotransmitters have been implicated in mediating the actions of the osmoreceptors on the neurohypophysis. The supraoptic nucleus is richly innervated by multiple pathways, including acetylcholine, catecholamines, glutamate, γ-aminobutyric acid (GABA), histamine, opioids, Ang II, and dopamine.[47] Studies have supported a potential role for all of these and others in the regulation of AVP secretion, as has local secretion of AVP into the hypothalamus from dendrites of the AVP-secreting neurons.[48] Although it remains unclear which of these are involved in the normal physiologic control of AVP secretion, in view of the likelihood that the osmoregulatory system is bimodal and integrated with multiple different afferent pathways (see Figure 16.6), it seems likely that magnocellular AVP neurons are influenced by a very complex mixture of neurotransmitter systems, rather than only a few.

Exactly how cells sense volume changes is a critical step for all the mechanisms activated to achieve osmoregulation. Some of the most exciting new data have come from studies of brain osmoreceptors.[29] The cellular osmosensing mechanism used by the OVLT cells is an intrinsic depolarizing receptor potential. This potential is generated in these cells via a molecular transduction complex. Studies have suggested that this likely includes members of the transient receptor potential vanilloid (TRPV) family of cation channel proteins. These channels are generally activated by cell membrane stretch to cause a nonselective conductance of cations, with a preference for Ca^{2+}. Multiple studies have characterized various members of the TRPV family as cellular mechanoreceptors in different tissues.[49] Both in vitro and in vivo studies of the TRPV family of cation channel proteins has provided evidence supporting the roles of TRPV1, TRPV2, and TRPV4 proteins in the transduction of osmotic stimuli in mammals that are important for sensing cell volume.[50] Moreover, genetic variation in the TRPV4 gene affects TRPV4 function and may influence water balance on a population-wide basis.[51] The details of exactly how and where various members of the TRPV family of cation channel proteins participate in osmoregulation in different species remains to be ascertained by additional studies. However, a strong case can already be made for their involvement in the transduction of osmotic stimuli in the neural cells in the OVLT and surrounding hypothalamus that regulate osmotic homeostasis, which appears to have been highly conserved throughout evolution.[50]

NONOSMOTIC REGULATION

Hemodynamic Stimuli

Not surprisingly, hypovolemia also is a potent stimulus for AVP secretion in humans[32,52] because an appropriate response to volume depletion should include renal water conservation. In humans and many animal species, lowering blood pressure suddenly by any of several methods increases plasma AVP levels by an amount that is proportional to the degree of hypotension achieved.[32,53] This stimulus-response relationship follows an exponential pattern, so that small reductions in blood pressure, of the order of 5% to 10%, usually have little effect on plasma AVP levels, whereas blood pressure decreases of 20% to 30% result in hormone levels many times higher than those required to produce maximal antidiuresis (see Figure 16.4). The AVP response to acute reductions in blood volume appears to be quantitatively and qualitatively similar to the response to blood pressure. In rats, plasma AVP increases as an exponential function of the degree of hypovolemia. Thus, little increase in plasma AVP can be detected until blood volume falls by 5% to 8%;

beyond that point, plasma AVP increases at an exponential rate in relation to the degree of hypovolemia and usually reaches levels 20 to 30 times normal when blood volume is reduced by 20% to 40%.[54,55] The volume-AVP relationship has not been as thoroughly characterized in other species, but it appears to follow a similar pattern to that in humans.[56] Conversely, acute increases in blood volume or pressure suppress AVP secretion. This response has been characterized less well than that of hypotension or hypovolemia, but seems to have a similar quantitative relationship (i.e., relatively large changes, ≈10% to 15%, are required to alter hormone secretion appreciably).[57]

The minimal-to-absent effect of small changes in blood volume and pressure on AVP secretion contrasts sharply with the extraordinary sensitivity of the osmoregulatory system (see Figure 16.4). Recognition of this difference is essential for understanding the relative contribution of each system to control AVP secretion under physiologic and pathologic conditions. Because daily variations of total body water rarely exceed 2% to 3%, their effect on AVP secretion must be mediated largely, if not exclusively, by the osmoregulatory system. Nonetheless, modest changes in blood volume and pressure do, in fact, influence AVP secretion indirectly, even though they are weak stimuli by themselves. This occurs via shifting the sensitivity of AVP secretion to osmotic stimuli so that a given increase in osmolality will cause a greater secretion of AVP during hypovolemic conditions than during euvolemic states (Figure 16.7).[58,59] In the presence of a negative hemodynamic stimulus, plasma AVP continues to respond appropriately to small changes in plasma osmolality and can still be fully suppressed if the osmolality falls below the new (lower) set point. The retention of the threshold function is a vital aspect of the interaction because it ensures that the capability to regulate the osmolality of body fluids is not lost, even in the presence of significant hypovolemia or hypotension. Consequently, it is reasonable to conclude that the major effect of moderate degrees of hypovolemia on AVP secretion and thirst is to modulate the gain of the osmoregulatory responses, with direct effects on thirst and AVP secretion occurring only during more severe degrees of hypovolemia (e.g., >10% to 20% reduction in blood pressure or volume).

These hemodynamic influences on AVP secretion are mediated, at least in part, by neural pathways that originate in stretch-sensitive receptors, generally termed *baroreceptors*, in the cardiac atria, aorta, and carotid sinus (see Figure 16.2; reviewed in detail in Chapter 15). Afferent nerve fibers from these receptors ascend in the vagus and glossopharyngeal nerves to the nuclei of the tractus solitarius (NTS) in the brainstem.[60] A variety of postsynaptic pathways from the NTS then project, directly and indirectly via the ventrolateral medulla and lateral parabrachial nucleus, to the PVN and SON in the hypothalamus.[61] Early studies suggested that the input from these pathways was predominantly inhibitory under basal conditions because interrupting them acutely resulted in large increases in plasma AVP levels as well as in arterial blood pressure.[62] However, as for most neural systems, including the neurohypophysis, innervation is complex and consists of excitatory and inhibitory inputs. Consequently, different effects have been observed under different experimental conditions.

The baroreceptor mechanism also appears to mediate a large number of pharmacologic and pathologic effects on AVP secretion (Table 16.1). Among them are diuretics, isoproterenol, nicotine, prostaglandins, nitroprusside, trimethaphan, histamine, morphine, and bradykinin, all of which stimulate AVP, at least in part by lowering blood volume or pressure,[52] and norepinephrine, which suppresses AVP by raising blood pressure.[63] In addition, an upright posture, sodium depletion, congestive heart failure, cirrhosis, and nephrosis likely stimulate AVP secretion by reducing the effective circulating blood volume.[64,65] Symptomatic orthostatic hypotension, vasovagal reactions, and other forms of syncope stimulate AVP secretion more markedly via greater and more acute decreases in blood pressure, with the exception of orthostatic hypotension associated with loss of afferent baroregulatory function.[66] Almost every hormone, drug, or condition that affects blood volume or pressure will also affect AVP secretion but, in most cases, the degree of change of blood pressure or volume is modest and will result in a shift of the set point and/or sensitivity of the osmoregulatory response, rather than marked stimulation of AVP secretion (see Figure 16.7).

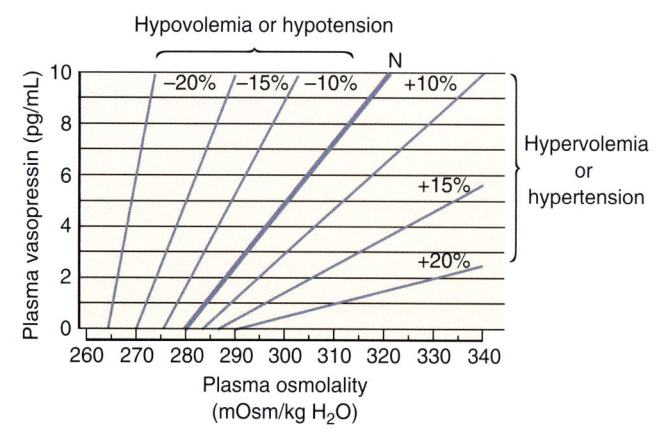

Figure 16.7 The relationship between the osmolality of plasma and concentration of AVP in plasma is modulated by blood volume and pressure. The line labeled N shows plasma AVP concentration across a range of plasma osmolality in an adult with normal intravascular volume (euvolemic) and normal blood pressure (normotensive). The lines to the left of N show the relationship between plasma AVP concentration and plasma osmolality in adults whose low intravascular volume (hypovolemia) or blood pressure (hypotension) is 10%, 15%, and 20% below normal. Lines to the right of N indicate volumes and blood pressures 10%, 15%, and 20% above normal. Note that hemodynamic influences do not disrupt the osmoregulation of AVP but rather raise or lower the set point, and possibly also the sensitivity, of AVP secretion in proportion to the magnitude of the change in blood volume or pressure. (Adapted from Robertson GL, Athar S, Shelton RL: Osmotic control of vasopressin function. In Andreoli TE, Grantham JJ, Rector FC, Jr, editors: *Disturbances in body fluid osmolality,* Bethesda, Md, 1977, American Physiological Society, pp 125.)

Drinking

Peripheral neural sensors other than baroreceptors also can affect AVP secretion. In humans, as well as dogs, drinking lowers plasma AVP before there is any appreciable decrease in plasma osmolality or serum [Na^+]. This is clearly a response to the act of drinking itself because it occurs independently of the composition of the fluid ingested,[67,68] although it may be influenced by the temperature of the fluid because the degree of suppression appears to be greater in response to colder fluids.[69] The pathways responsible for this effect have not been delineated, but likely include sensory afferents originating in the oropharynx and transmitted centrally via the glossopharyngeal nerve.

Nausea

Among other nonosmotic stimuli to AVP secretion in humans, nausea is the most prominent. The sensation of nausea, with or without vomiting, is the most potent stimulus to AVP secretion known in humans. Although 20% increases in osmolality will typically elevate plasma AVP levels to the range of 5 to 20 pg/mL, and 20% decreases in blood pressure to 10 to 100 pg/mL, nausea has been described to cause AVP elevations in excess of 200 to 400 pg/mL.[70] The pathway mediating this effect has been mapped to the chemoreceptor zone in the area postrema of the brainstem in animal studies (see Figure 16.2). It can be activated by a variety of drugs and conditions, including apomorphine, morphine, nicotine, alcohol, and motion sickness. Its effect on AVP is instantaneous and extremely potent (Figure 16.8), even when the nausea is transient and not accompanied by vomiting or changes in blood pressure. Pretreatment with fluphenazine, haloperidol, or promethazine in doses sufficient to prevent nausea completely abolishes the AVP response. The inhibitory effect of these dopamine antagonists is specific for emetic stimuli because they do not alter the AVP response to osmotic and hemodynamic stimuli. Water loading blunts, but does not abolish, the effect of nausea on AVP release, suggesting that osmotic and emetic influences interact in a manner similar to that for osmotic and hemodynamic pathways. Species differences also affect emetic stimuli. Whereas dogs and cats appear to be even more sensitive than humans to emetic stimulation of AVP release, rodents have little or no AVP response but release large amounts of OT instead.[71]

Table 16.1 Drugs and Hormones That Affect Vasopressin Secretion

Stimulatory	Inhibitory
Acetylcholine	Norepinephrine
Nicotine	Fluphenazine
Apomorphine	Haloperidol
Morphine (high doses)	Promethazine
Epinephrine	Oxilorphan
Isoproterenol	Butorphanol
Histamine	Opioid agonists
Bradykinin	Morphine (low doses)
Prostaglandin	Ethanol
β-Endorphin	Carbamazepine
Cyclophosphamide IV	Glucocorticoids
Vincristine	Clonidine
Insulin	Muscimol
2-Deoxyglucose	Phencyclidine
Angiotensin II	Phenytoin
Lithium	
Corticotropin-releasing factor	
Naloxone	
Cholecystokinin	

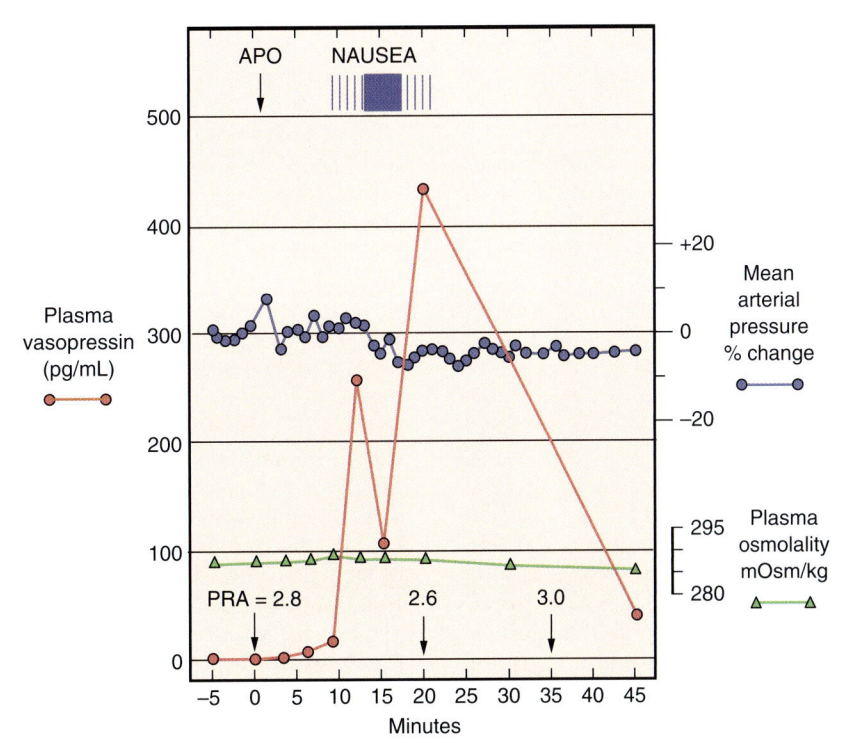

Figure 16.8 Effect of nausea on AVP secretion. Apomorphine (APO) was injected at the point indicated by the *vertical arrow*. Note that the rise in plasma AVP coincided with the occurrence of nausea and was not associated with detectable changes in plasma osmolality or blood pressure. PRA, Plasma renin activity. (Adapted from Robertson GL: The regulation of vasopressin function in health and disease. *Recent Prog Horm Res* 33:333-385, 1977.)

The emetic response probably mediates many pharmacologic and pathologic effects on AVP secretion. In addition to the drugs and conditions already noted, it may be responsible at least in part for the increase in AVP secretion that has been observed with vasovagal reactions, diabetic ketoacidosis, acute hypoxia, and motion sickness. Because nausea and vomiting are frequent side effects of many other drugs and diseases, many additional situations likely occur as well. The reason for this profound stimulation is not known (although it has been speculated that the AVP response assists evacuation of stomach contents via contraction of gastric smooth muscle, AVP is not necessary for vomiting to occur), but it is responsible for the intense vasoconstriction that produces the pallor often associated with this state.

Hypoglycemia

Acute hypoglycemia is a less potent but reasonably consistent stimulus for AVP secretion.[72,73] The receptor and pathway that mediate this effect are unknown; however, they appear separate from those of other recognized stimuli because hypoglycemia stimulates AVP secretion, even in patients who have selectively lost the capacity to respond to hypernatremia, hypotension, or nausea.[73] The factor that actually triggers the release of AVP is likely intracellular deficiency of glucose or ATP because 2-deoxyglucose is also an effective stimulus.[74] Generally, more than 20% decreases in glucose are required to increase plasma AVP levels significantly; the rate of decrease in the glucose level is probably the critical stimulus, however, because the rise in plasma AVP is not sustained with persistent hypoglycemia.[72] However, glucopenic stimuli are of unlikely importance in the physiology or pathology of AVP secretion because there are probably few drugs or conditions that lower plasma glucose rapidly enough to stimulate release of the hormone, and because this effect is transient.

Renin Angiotensin Aldosterone System

The renin angiotensin aldosterone system (RAAS) has also been intimately implicated in the control of AVP secretion.[75] Animal studies have indicated dual sites of action. Blood-borne Ang II stimulates AVP secretion by acting in the brain at the circumventricular subfornical organ (SFO),[76] a small structure located in the dorsal portion of the third cerebral ventricle (see Figure 16.2). Because circumventricular organs lack a blood-brain barrier, the densely expressed Ang II receptor type 1 (AT_1R) of the SFO can detect very small increases in blood levels of Ang II.[77] Neural pathways from the SFO to the hypothalamic SON and PVN mediate AVP secretion, and also appear to use Ang II as a neurotransmitter.[78] This accounts for the observation that the most sensitive site for angiotensin-mediated AVP secretion and thirst is intracerebroventricular injection into the cerebrospinal fluid. Further evidence in support of Ang II as a neurotransmitter is that intraventricular administration of angiotensin receptor antagonists inhibits the AVP response to osmotic and hemodynamic stimuli.[79] The level of plasma Ang II required to stimulate AVP release is quite high, leading some to argue that this stimulus is active only under pharmacologic conditions. This is consistent with observations that even pressor doses of Ang II increase plasma AVP only about two- to fourfold[75] and may account for the failure of some investigators to demonstrate stimulation of thirst by exogenous angiotensin. However, this procedure may underestimate the physiologic effects of angiotensin because the increased blood pressure caused by exogenously administered Ang II appears to blunt the thirst induced via activation of inhibitory baroreceptive pathways.[80]

Stress

Nonspecific stress caused by factors such as pain, emotion, or physical exercise has long been thought to cause AVP secretion, but it has never been determined whether this effect is mediated by a specific pathway or is secondary to the hypotension or nausea that often accompanies stress-induced vasovagal reactions. In rats[81] and humans,[82] a variety of noxious stimuli capable of activating the pituitary-adrenal axis and sympathetic nervous system do not stimulate AVP secretion unless they also lower blood pressure or alter blood volume. The marked rise in plasma AVP levels elicited by manipulation of the abdominal viscera in anesthetized dogs has been attributed to nociceptive influences,[83] but mediation by emetic pathways cannot be excluded in this setting. Endotoxin-induced fever stimulates AVP secretion in rats, and studies have supported the possible mediation of this effect by circulating cytokines, such as interleukin-1 (IL-1) and IL-6.[84] Clarification of the possible role of nociceptive and thermal influences on AVP secretion is particularly important in view of the frequency with which painful or febrile illnesses are associated with osmotically inappropriate secretion of antidiuretic hormone.

Hypoxia and Hypercapnia

Acute hypoxia and hypercapnia also stimulate AVP secretion.[85,86] In conscious humans, however, the stimulatory effect of moderate hypoxia (arterial partial pressure of oxygen [PaO_2] > 35 mm Hg) is inconsistent and seems to occur mainly in subjects who develop nausea or hypotension. In conscious dogs, more severe hypoxia (PaO_2 < 35 mm Hg) consistently increases AVP secretion without reducing arterial pressure.[87] Studies of anesthetized dogs have suggested that the AVP response to acute hypoxia depends on the level of hypoxemia achieved. At a PaO_2 of 35 mm Hg or lower, plasma AVP increases markedly, even though there is no change or even an increase in arterial pressure, but less severe hypoxia (PaO_2 > 40 mm Hg) has no effect on AVP levels.[88] These results indicate that there is likely a hypoxemic threshold for AVP secretion, and suggest that severe hypoxemia alone may also stimulate AVP secretion in humans. If so, it may be responsible, at least in part, for the osmotically inappropriate AVP elevations noted in some patients with acute respiratory failure.[89] In conscious or anesthetized dogs, acute hypercapnia, independent of hypoxia or hypotension, also increases AVP secretion.[87,88] It has not been determined whether this response also exhibits threshold characteristics or otherwise depends on the degree of hypercapnia, nor is it known whether hypercapnia has similar effects on AVP secretion in humans or other animals. The mechanisms whereby hypoxia and hypercapnia release AVP remain undefined, but they likely involve peripheral chemoreceptors and/or baroreceptors because cervical vagotomy abolishes the response to hypoxemia in dogs.[90]

Drugs

As will be discussed more extensively in the section on clinical disorders, a variety of drugs also stimulate AVP secretion, including nicotine (see Table 16.1). Drugs and hormones can potentially affect AVP secretion at many different sites. As already discussed, many excitatory stimulants such as isoproterenol, nicotine, high doses of morphine, and cholecystokinin act, at least in part, by lowering blood pressure and/or producing nausea. Others, such as substance P, prostaglandin, endorphin, and other opioids, have not been studied sufficiently to define their mechanism of action, but they may also work by one or both of the same mechanisms. Inhibitory stimuli similarly have multiple modes of action. Vasopressor drugs such as norepinephrine inhibit AVP secretion indirectly by raising arterial pressure. In low doses, a variety of opioids of all subtypes, including morphine, met-enkephalin and κ-agonists, inhibit AVP secretion in rats and humans.[91] Endogenous opioid peptides interact with the magnocellular neurosecretory system at several levels to inhibit basal and stimulated secretion of AVP and oxytocin. Opioid inhibition of AVP secretion has been found to occur in isolated posterior pituitary tissue, and the action of morphine and of several opioid agonists such as butorphanol and oxilorphan likely occurs via activation of κ-opioid receptors located on nerve terminals of the posterior pituitary.[92] The well-known inhibitory effect of ethanol on AVP secretion may be mediated, at least in part, by endogenous opiates because it is due to an elevation in the osmotic threshold for AVP release[93] and can be partially blocked by treatment with naloxone.[94] Carbamazepine inhibits AVP secretion by diminishing the sensitivity of the osmoregulatory system; this effect occurs independently of changes in blood volume, blood pressure, and/or blood glucose.[95] Other drugs that inhibit AVP secretion include clonidine, which appears to act via central and peripheral adrenoreceptors,[96] muscimol,[97] which acts as a GABA antagonist, and phencyclidine,[98] which probably acts by raising blood pressure. However, despite the importance of these stimuli during pathologic conditions, none of them is a significant determinant of the physiologic regulation of AVP secretion in humans.

DISTRIBUTION AND CLEARANCE

Plasma AVP concentration is determined by the difference between the rates of secretion from the posterior pituitary gland and removal of the hormone from the vascular compartment via metabolism and urinary clearance. In healthy adults, intravenously injected AVP distributes rapidly into a space equivalent in size to the ECF compartment. This initial, or mixing, phase has a half-life of 4 to 8 minutes and is virtually complete in 10 to 15 minutes. The rapid mixing phase is followed by a second, slower decline that corresponds to the metabolic clearance of AVP. Most studies of this phase have yielded mean values of 10 to 20 minutes by steady-state and non–steady-state techniques,[32] consistent with the observed rates of change in urine osmolality after water loading and injection of AVP, which also support a short half-life.[99] In pregnant women, the metabolic clearance rate of AVP increases nearly fourfold,[100] which becomes significant in the pathophysiology of gestational diabetes insipidus (see later discussion). Smaller animals such as rats clear AVP much more rapidly than humans because their cardiac output is higher relative to their body weight and surface area.[99]

Although many tissues have the capacity to inactivate AVP, metabolism in vivo appears to occur largely in the liver and kidney.[99] The enzymatic processes whereby the liver and kidney inactivate AVP involve an initial reduction of the disulfide bridge, followed by aminopeptidase cleavage of the bond between amino acid residues 1 and 2 and cleavage of the C-terminal glycinamide residue. Some AVP is excreted intact in the urine, but there is disagreement about the amount and factors that affect it. For example, in healthy, normally hydrated adults, the urinary clearance of AVP ranges from 0.1 to 0.6 mL/kg/min under basal conditions and has never been found to exceed 2 mL/kg/min, even in the presence of solute diuresis.[32] The mechanisms involved in the excretion of AVP have not been defined with certainty, but the hormone is probably filtered at the glomerulus and variably reabsorbed at sites along the nephron. The latter process may be linked to the reabsorption of Na^+ or other solutes in the proximal nephron because the urinary clearance of AVP has been found to vary by as much as 20-fold in direct relation to the solute clearance.[32] Consequently, measurements of urinary AVP excretion in humans do not provide a consistently reliable index of changes in plasma AVP and should be interpreted cautiously when glomerular filtration or solute clearance are inconstant or abnormal.

THIRST

Thirst is the body's defense mechanism to increase water consumption in response to perceived deficits of body fluids. It can be most easily defined as a consciously perceived desire for water. True thirst must be distinguished from other determinants of fluid intake such as taste, dietary preferences, and social customs, as discussed previously. Thirst can be stimulated in animals and humans by intracellular dehydration caused by increases in the effective osmolality of the ECF or by intravascular hypovolemia caused by losses of ECF.[101,102] As would be expected, these are many of the same variables that provoke AVP secretion. Of these, hypertonicity is clearly the most potent. Similar to AVP secretion, substantial evidence to date has supported mediation of osmotic thirst by osmoreceptors located in the anterior hypothalamus of the brain,[30,31] whereas hypovolemic thirst appears to be stimulated via activation of low- and/or high-pressure baroreceptors[103] and circulating Ang II.[104]

OSMOTIC THIRST

In healthy adults, an increase in effective plasma osmolality of only 2% to 3% above basal levels produces a strong desire to drink.[105] This response is not dependent on changes in ECF or plasma volume because it occurs similarly whether plasma osmolality is raised by infusion of hypertonic solutions or by water deprivation. The absolute level of plasma osmolality at which a person develops a conscious urge to seek and drink water is termed the *osmotic thirst threshold*. It varies appreciably among individuals, likely as a result of genetic factors,[33] but in healthy adults it averages approximately 295 mOsm/kg H_2O. Of physiologic significance is the fact that this level is above the osmotic threshold for AVP release and approximates the plasma osmolality at which maximal concentration of the urine is normally achieved (see Figure 16.5).

The brain pathways that mediate osmotic thirst have not been well defined, but it is clear that initiation of drinking requires osmoreceptors located in the anteroventral hypothalamus in the same area as the osmoreceptors that control osmotic AVP secretion.[30,31] Whether the osmoreceptors for AVP and thirst are the same cells or simply located in the same general area remains unknown.[29] However, the properties of the osmoreceptors are very similar. Ineffective plasma solutes such as urea and glucose, which have little or no effect on AVP secretion, are equally ineffective at stimulating thirst, whereas effective solutes such as NaCl and mannitol can stimulate thirst.[9,106] The sensitivities of the thirst and AVP osmoreceptors cannot be compared precisely, but they are also probably similar. Thus, in healthy adults, the intensity of thirst increases rapidly in direct proportion to serum $[Na^+]$ or plasma osmolality and generally becomes intolerable at levels only 3% to 5% above the threshold level.[107] Water consumption also appears to be proportional to the intensity of thirst in humans and animals and, under conditions of maximal osmotic stimulation, can reach rates as high as 20 to 25 L/day. The dilution of body fluids by ingested water complements the retention of water that occurs during AVP-induced antidiuresis, and both responses occur concurrently when drinking water is available.

As with AVP secretion, the osmoregulation of thirst appears to be bimodal because a modest decline in plasma osmolality induces a sense of satiation and reduces the basal rate of spontaneous fluid intake.[107,108] This effect is sufficient to prevent hypotonic overhydration, even when antidiuresis is fixed at maximal levels for prolonged periods, suggesting that osmotically inappropriate secretion of AVP (syndrome of inappropriate antidiuretic hormone secretion [SIADH]) should not result in the development of hyponatremia unless the satiety mechanism is impaired or fluid intake is inappropriately high for some other reason, such as the unregulated components of fluid intake discussed earlier.[108] Also similar to AVP secretion, thirst can be influenced by oropharyngeal or upper gastrointestinal receptors that respond to the act of drinking itself.[68] In humans, however, the rapid relief provided by this mechanism lasts only a matter of minutes and thirst quickly recurs until enough water is absorbed to lower plasma osmolality to normal. Therefore, although local oropharyngeal sensations may have a significant short-term influence on thirst, it is the hypothalamic osmoreceptors that ultimately determine the volume of water intake in response to dehydration.

HYPOVOLEMIC THIRST

In contrast, the threshold for producing hypovolemic or extracellular thirst is significantly higher in animals and humans. Studies in several species have shown that sustained decreases in plasma volume or blood pressure of at least 4% to 8%, and in some species 10% to 15%, are necessary to stimulate drinking consistently.[109,110] In humans, the degree of hypovolemia or hypotension required to produce thirst has not been precisely defined, but it has been difficult to demonstrate any effects of mild-to-moderate hypovolemia to stimulate thirst independently of osmotic changes occurring with dehydration. This blunted sensitivity to changes in ECF volume or blood pressure in humans probably represents an adaptation that occurred as a result of the erect posture of primates, which predisposes them to wider fluctuations in blood and atrial filling pressures as a result of orthostatic pooling of blood in the lower body. Stimulation of thirst (and AVP secretion) by such transient postural changes in blood pressure might lead to overdrinking and inappropriate antidiuresis in situations in which the ECF volume was actually normal but only transiently maldistributed. Consistent with a blunted response to baroreceptor activation, studies have also shown that systemic infusion of Ang II to pharmacologic levels is a much less potent stimulus to thirst in humans than in animals,[111] in whom it is one of the most potent dipsogens known. Nonetheless, this response is not completely absent in humans, as demonstrated by rare cases of polydipsia in patients with pathologic causes of hyperreninemia.[112] The pathways whereby hypovolemia or hypotension produces thirst have not been well defined, but probably involve the same brainstem baroreceptive pathways that mediate hemodynamic effects on AVP secretion,[103] as well as a likely contribution from circulating levels of Ang II in some species.[113]

INTEGRATION OF VASOPRESSIN SECRETION AND THIRST

A synthesis of what is presently known about the regulation of AVP secretion and thirst in humans leads to a relatively simple but elegant system to maintain water balance. Under normal physiologic conditions, the sensitivity of the osmoregulatory system for AVP secretion accounts for the maintenance of plasma osmolality within narrow limits by adjusting renal water excretion to small changes in osmolality. Stimulated thirst does not represent a major regulatory mechanism under these conditions, and unregulated fluid ingestion supplies adequate water in excess of true "need," which is then excreted in relation to osmoregulated pituitary AVP secretion. However, when unregulated water intake cannot adequately supply body needs in the presence of plasma AVP levels sufficient to produce maximal antidiuresis, then plasma osmolality rises to levels that stimulate thirst (see Figure 16.5), and water intake increases proportional to the elevation of osmolality above this thirst threshold.

In such a system, thirst essentially represents a backup mechanism that becomes active when pituitary and renal mechanisms prove insufficient to maintain plasma osmolality within a few percent of basal levels. This arrangement has the advantage of freeing humans from frequent episodes of thirst. These would require a diversion of activities toward behavior oriented to seeking water when water deficiency is sufficiently mild to be compensated for by renal water conservation, but would stimulate water ingestion once water deficiency reaches potentially harmful levels. Stimulation of AVP secretion at plasma osmolalities below the threshold for subjective thirst acts to maintain an excess of body water sufficient to eliminate the need to drink whenever slight elevations in plasma osmolality occur. This system of differential effective thresholds for thirst and

AVP secretion nicely complements many studies that have demonstrated excess unregulated (or need-free) drinking in humans and animals. Only when this mechanism becomes inadequate to maintain body fluid homeostasis does thirst-induced regulated fluid intake become the predominant defense mechanism for the prevention of severe dehydration.

DISORDERS OF INSUFFICIENT VASOPRESSIN OR VASOPRESSIN EFFECT

Disorders of insufficient AVP or AVP effect are associated with inadequate urine concentration and increased urine output (polyuria). If thirst mechanisms are intact, this is accompanied by compensatory increases in fluid intake (polydipsia) as a result of stimulated thirst to preserve body fluid homeostasis. The net result is polyuria and polydipsia, with preservation of normal plasma osmolality and serum electrolyte concentrations. However, if thirst is impaired, or if fluid intake is insufficient for any reason to compensate for the increased urine excretion, then hyperosmolality and hypernatremia can result, with the consequent complications associated with these disorders. The quintessential disorder of insufficient AVP is diabetes insipidus (DI), which is a clinical syndrome characterized by excretion of abnormally large volumes of urine (diabetes) that is dilute (hypotonic) and devoid of taste from dissolved solutes (e.g., insipid), in contrast to the hypertonic, sweet-tasting urine characteristic of diabetes mellitus (from the Greek, meaning honey).

Several different pathophysiologic mechanisms can cause hypotonic polyuria (Table 16.2). Central DI (also called hypothalamic, neurogenic, or neurohypophyseal DI) is due to inadequate secretion and usually deficient synthesis of AVP in the hypothalamic neurohypophyseal system. Lack of AVP-stimulated activation of the V_2 subtype of AVP receptors in the kidney collecting tubules (see Chapters 10 and 11) causes excretion of large volumes of dilute urine. In most cases, thirst mechanisms are intact, leading to compensatory polydipsia. However, in a variant of central DI, osmoreceptor dysfunction, thirst is also impaired, leading to hypodipsia. DI of pregnancy is a transient disorder due to an accelerated metabolism of AVP as a result of increased activity of the enzyme oxytocinase or vasopressinase in the serum of pregnant women, again leading to polyuria and polydipsia; accelerated metabolism of AVP during pregnancy may also cause a patient with subclinical DI from other causes to shift from a relatively asymptomatic state to a symptomatic state as a result of the more rapid AVP degradation. Nephrogenic DI is due to inappropriate renal responses to AVP. This produces excretion of dilute urine, despite normal pituitary AVP secretion and secondary polydipsia, similar to central DI. The final cause of hypotonic polyuria, primary polydipsia, differs significantly from the other causes because it is not due to deficient AVP secretion or impaired renal responses to AVP, but rather to excessive ingestion of fluids. This can result from an abnormality in the thirst mechanism, in which case it is sometimes called dipsogenic DI, or from psychiatric disorders, in which case it is generally referred to as psychogenic polydipsia.

Table 16.2 Causes of Hypotonic Polyuria

Central (Neurogenic) Diabetes Insipidus

Congenital (congenital malformations, autosomal dominant, arginine vasopressin [AVP] neurophysin gene mutations)
Drug- or toxin-induced (ethanol, diphenylhydantoin, snake venom)
Granulomatous (histiocytosis, sarcoidosis)
Neoplastic (craniopharyngioma, germinoma, lymphoma, leukemia, meningioma, pituitary tumor; metastases)
Infectious (meningitis, tuberculosis, encephalitis)
Inflammatory, autoimmune (lymphocytic infundibuloneurohypophysitis)
Trauma (neurosurgery, deceleration injury)
Vascular (cerebral hemorrhage or infarction, brain death)
Idiopathic

Osmoreceptor Dysfunction

Granulomatous (histiocytosis, sarcoidosis)
Neoplastic (craniopharyngioma, pinealoma, meningioma, metastases)
Vascular (anterior communicating artery aneurysm or ligation, intrahypothalamic hemorrhage)
Other (hydrocephalus, ventricular or suprasellar cyst, trauma, degenerative diseases)
Idiopathic

Increased AVP Metabolism

Pregnancy

Nephrogenic Diabetes Insipidus

Congenital (X-linked recessive, AVP V_2 receptor gene mutations, autosomal recessive or dominant, aquaporin-2 water channel gene mutations)
Drug-induced (demeclocycline, lithium, cisplatin, methoxyflurane)
Hypercalcemia
Hypokalemia
Infiltrating lesions (sarcoidosis, amyloidosis)
Vascular (sickle cell anemia)
Mechanical (polycystic kidney disease, bilateral ureteral obstruction)
Solute diuresis (glucose, mannitol, sodium, radiocontrast dyes)
Idiopathic

Primary Polydipsia

Psychogenic (schizophrenia, obsessive-compulsive behaviors)
Dipsogenic (downward resetting of thirst threshold, idiopathic or similar lesions, as with central DI)

CENTRAL DIABETES INSIPIDUS

CAUSES

Central diabetes insipidus (CDI) is caused by inadequate secretion of AVP from the posterior pituitary in response to osmotic stimulation. In most cases, this is due to destruction of the neurohypophysis by a variety of acquired or congenital anatomic lesions that destroy or damage the neurohypophysis by pressure or infiltration (see Table 16.2). The severity of the resulting hypotonic diuresis depends on the degree of destruction of the neurohypophysis, leading to complete or partial deficiency of AVP secretion.

Despite the wide variety of lesions that can potentially cause CDI, it is much more common not to have CDI in the presence of such lesions than actually to produce the syndrome. This apparent inconsistency can be understood by considering several common principles of neurohypophyseal physiology and pathophysiology that are relevant to all these causes.

First, the synthesis of AVP occurs in the hypothalamus (see Figure 16.2); the posterior pituitary simply represents the site of storage and secretion of the neurosecretory granules that contain AVP. Consequently, lesions contained within the sella turcica that destroy only the posterior pituitary generally do not cause CDI because the cell bodies of the magnocellular neurons that synthesize AVP remain intact, and the site of release of AVP shifts more superiorly, typically into the blood vessels of the median eminence at the base of the brain. Perhaps the best examples of this phenomenon are large pituitary macroadenomas that completely destroy the anterior and posterior pituitary. DI is a distinctly unusual presentation for such pituitary adenomas because destruction of the posterior pituitary by such slowly enlarging intrasellar lesions merely destroys the nerve terminals, but not the cell bodies, of the AVP neurons. As this occurs, the site of release of AVP shifts more superiorly to the pituitary stalk and median eminence. Sometimes this can be detected on noncontrast magnetic resonance imaging (MRI) scans as a shift of the pituitary bright spot more superiorly to the level of the infundibulum or median eminence,[114] but this process is often too diffuse to be detected in this manner. The development of DI from a pituitary adenoma is so uncommon, even with macroadenomas that completely obliterate sellar contents sufficiently to cause panhypopituitarism, that its presence should lead to consideration of alternative diagnoses, such as craniopharyngioma, which often causes damage to the median eminence because of adherence of the capsule to the base of the hypothalamus, more rapidly enlarging sellar or suprasellar masses that do not allow sufficient time for shifting the site of AVP release more superiorly (e.g., metastatic lesions), or granulomatous disease, with more diffuse hypothalamic involvement (e.g., sarcoidosis, histiocytosis). With very large pituitary adenomas that produce adrenocorticotropic hormone (ACTH) deficiency, it is actually more likely that patients will present with hypo-osmolality from an SIADH-like picture as a result of the impaired free water excretion that accompanies hypocortisolism, as will be discussed later.

A second general principle is that the capacity of the neurohypophysis to synthesize AVP is greatly in excess of the body's daily needs for maintenance of water homeostasis. Carefully controlled studies of surgical section of the pituitary stalk in dogs have clearly demonstrated that destruction of 80% to 90% of the magnocellular neurons in the hypothalamus is required to produce polyuria and polydipsia in these species.[115] Thus, even lesions that cause destruction of the AVP magnocellular neuron cell bodies must result in a large degree of destruction to produce DI. The most illustrative example of this is surgical section of the pituitary stalk in humans. Necropsy studies of these patients have revealed atrophy of the posterior pituitary and loss of the magnocellular neurons in the hypothalamus.[116] This loss of magnocellular cells presumably results from retrograde degeneration of neurons whose axons were cut during surgery. As is generally true for all neurons, the likelihood of retrograde neuronal degeneration depends on the proximity of the axotomy, in this case section of the pituitary stalk, to the cell body of the neuron. This was shown clearly in studies of human subjects in whom section of the pituitary stalk at the level of the diaphragm sellae (a low stalk section) produced transient but not permanent DI, whereas section at the level of the infundibulum (a high stalk section) was required to cause permanent DI in most cases.[117]

Several genetic causes of AVP deficiency have also been characterized. Prior to the application of techniques for amplification of genomic DNA, the only experimental model to study the mechanism of hereditary hypothalamic DI was the Brattleboro rat, a strain that was found serendipitously to have CDI.[118] In this animal, the disease demonstrates a classic pattern of autosomal recessive inheritance in which DI is expressed only in the homozygotes. The hereditary basis of the disease has been found to be a single base deletion producing a translational frameshift beginning in the third portion of the neurophysin coding sequence. Because the gene lacks a stop codon, there is a modified neurophysin, no glycopeptides, and a long polylysine tail.[119] Although the mutant prohormone accumulates in the endoplasmic reticulum, sufficient AVP is produced by the normal allele that the heterozygotes are asymptomatic. In contrast, almost all families with genetic CDI in humans that have been described to date demonstrate an autosomal dominant mode of inheritance.[120-122] In these cases, DI is expressed, despite the expression of one normal allele, which is sufficient to prevent the disease in the heterozygous Brattleboro rats. Numerous studies have been directed at understanding this apparent anomaly. Two potentially important clues about the cause of the DI in familial genetic CDI are the following:

1. Severe-to-partial deficiencies of AVP and overt signs of DI do not develop in these patients until several months to several years after birth and then gradually progress over the ensuing decades,[120,123] suggesting adequate initial function of the normal allele, with later decompensation.
2. A limited number of autopsy studies have suggested that some of these cases are associated with gliosis and a marked loss of magnocellular AVP neurons in the hypothalamus,[124] although other studies have shown normal neurons with decreased expression of AVP or no hypothalamic abnormality. In most of these cases, the hyperintense signal normally emitted by the neurohypophysis in T1-weighted MRI scans (see later discussion) is also absent, although some exceptions have been reported.[125]

Another interesting, but as yet unexplained, observation is that some adults in these families have been described in whom DI was clinically apparent during childhood but who went into remission as adults, without evidence that their remissions could be attributed to renal or adrenal insufficiency or to increased AVP synthesis.[126]

The autosomal dominant form of familial CDI is caused by diverse mutations in the gene that codes for the AVP-neurophysin precursor (Figure 16.9). All the mutations identified to date have been in the coding region of the gene and affect only one allele. They are located in all three

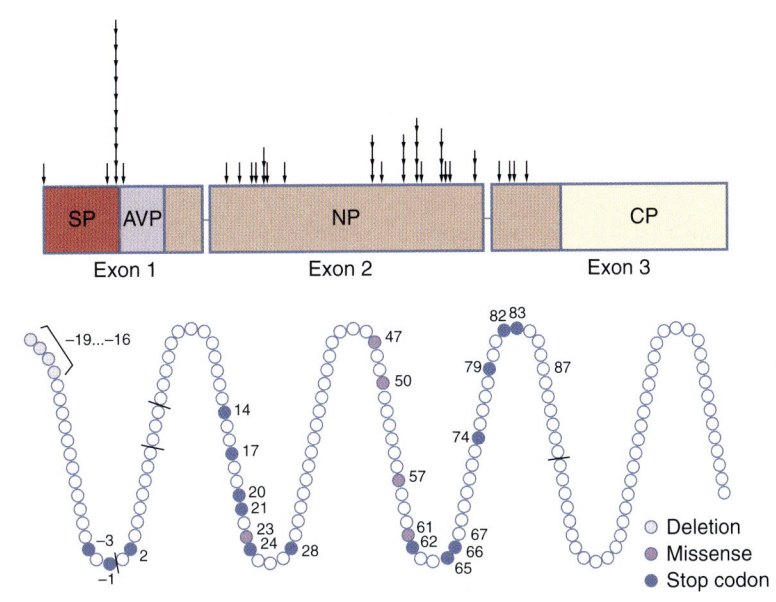

Figure 16.9 Location and type of mutations in the gene that codes for the AVP-neurophysin precursor in kindreds with the autosomal dominant form of familial central diabetes insipidus (CDI). The location of the mutation in a different kindred is indicated by the *arrows*. The various portions of the precursor protein are designated by AVP, vasopressin, CP, copeptin, NP, neurophysin, and SP, signal peptide. Deletion and missense mutations are those expected to remove or replace one or more amino acid residues in the precursor. Those designated stop codons are expected to cause premature termination of the precursor. Note that none of the mutations causes a frameshift or affects the part of the gene that encodes the copeptin moiety, all the stop codons are in the distal part of the neurophysin moiety, and only one of the mutations affects the AVP moiety. All these findings are consistent with the concept that the mutant precursor is produced but cannot be folded properly because of interference with the binding of AVP to neurophysin, formation of intrachain disulfide bonds, or extreme flexibility or rigidity normally required at crucial places in the protein. (Adapted from Rittig S, Robertson GL, Siggaard C, et al: Identification of 13 new mutations in the vasopressin-neurophysin gene in 17 kindreds with familial autosomal dominant neurohypophyseal DI. *Am J Hum Genet* 58:107-117, 1996; and Hansen LK, Rittig S, Robertson GL: Genetic basis of familial neurohypophyseal diabetes insipidus. *Trends Endocrinol Metab* 8:363-372, 1997.)

exons and are predicted to alter or delete amino acid residues in the signal peptide, AVP, and neurophysin moieties of the precursor. Only the C-terminus glycopeptide, or copeptin moiety, has not been found to be affected. Most are missense mutations, but nonsense mutations (premature stop codons) and deletions also occur. One characteristic shared by all the mutations is that they are predicted to alter or delete one or more amino acids known, or reasonably presumed, to be crucial for processing, folding, and oligomerization of the precursor protein in the endoplasmic reticulum.[120,122] Because of the related functional effects of the mutations, the common clinical characteristics of the disease, the dominant-negative mode of transmission, and the autopsy and hormonal evidence of postnatal neurohypophyseal degeneration, it has been postulated that all the mutations act by causing production of an abnormal precursor protein that accumulates and eventually kills the neurons because it cannot be correctly processed, folded, and transported out of the endoplasmic reticulum. Expression studies of mutant DNA from several human mutations in cultured neuroblastoma cells support this misfolding-neurotoxicity hypothesis by demonstrating abnormal trafficking and accumulation of mutant prohormone in the endoplasmic reticulum with low or absent expression in the Golgi apparatus, suggesting difficulty with packaging into neurosecretory granules.[127] However, cell death may not be necessary to decrease available AVP. Normally, proteins retained in the endoplasmic reticulum are selectively degraded, but if excess mutant is produced and the selective normal degradative process is overwhelmed, an alternate, nonselective, degradative system (autophagy) is activated. As more and more mutant precursor builds up in the endoplasmic reticulum, the normal wild-type protein becomes trapped with the mutant protein and degraded by the activated nonspecific degradative system. In this case, the amount of AVP that matures and is packaged would be markedly reduced.[128,129] This explanation is consistent with those cases in which little pathology is found in the magnocellular neurons and also with DI in which a small amount of AVP can still be detected.

Wolfram's syndrome is a rare autosomal recessive disease with DI, diabetes mellitus, optic atrophy, and deafness (DIDMOAD). The genetic defect is the protein wolframin, which is found in the endoplasmic reticulum and is important for folding proteins.[130] Wolframin is involved in β-cell proliferation, intracellular protein processing, and calcium homeostasis, producing a wide spectrum of endocrine and central nervous system (CNS) disorders; DI is usually a late manifestation associated with decreased magnocellular neurons in the paraventricular and supraoptic nuclei.[131]

Idiopathic forms of AVP deficiency represent a large pathogenic category in adults and children. A study in children has revealed that over half (54%) of all cases of CDI were classified as idiopathic.[132] These patients do not have historic or clinical evidence of any injury or disease that can be linked to their DI, and MRI of the pituitary-hypothalamic area generally reveals no abnormality other than the absence of the posterior pituitary bright spot and sometimes varying degrees of thickening of the pituitary stalk. Several lines of evidence have suggested that many of these patients may have had an autoimmune destruction of the neurohypophysis to account for their DI. First, the entity of lymphocytic infundibuloneurohypophysitis has been documented to be present in a subset of patients with idiopathic DI.[133] Lymphocytic infiltration of the anterior pituitary, lymphocytic hypophysitis, has been recognized as a cause of anterior pituitary deficiency for many years, but it was not until an autopsy called attention to a similar finding in the posterior pituitary of a patient with DI that this pathology was recognized to occur in the neurohypophysis as well.[134] Since that initial report, a number of similar cases have been described, including cases in the postpartum period, which is characteristic of lymphocytic hypophysitis.[135] With the advent of MRI, lymphocytic infundibuloneurohypophysitis has been diagnosed based on the appearance of a thickened stalk and/or enlargement of the posterior pituitary, mimicking a pituitary tumor. In these cases, the characteristic bright spot on MRI T1-weighted images is lost. The enlargement of the stalk can mimic a neoplastic process, resulting in some of these patients undergoing surgery based on the suspicion of a pituitary tumor. Since then, a number of patients with a suspicion of infundibuloneurohypophysitis and no other obvious cause of DI have been followed and have shown regression of the thickened pituitary stalk over time.[132,133] Several cases have been reported with the coexistence of CDI and adenohypophysitis; these presumably represent cases of combined lymphocytic infundibuloneurohypophysitis and hypophysitis.[136-138] A second line of evidence supporting an autoimmune cause in many cases of idiopathic DI is based on the finding of AVP antibodies in the serum of as many as one third of patients with idiopathic DI and two thirds of those with Langerhans cell histiocytosis X, but not in patients with DI caused by tumors.[139] A recently recognized form of infundibuloneurohypophysitis occurs in middle-aged to older men and is associated with immunoglobulin G4 (IgG4)–related systemic disease.[140,141] Various organs, especially the pancreas, are infiltrated with IgG4 plasma cells, and neurohypophysitis is only one manifestation of a multiorgan disease that may include other endocrine glands. This cause should be considered as a cause of DI based on age and gender at presentation and evidence of other systemic disease. The diagnosis can be established by elevated serum IgG4 levels and characteristic histology of biopsies. Response to steroids or other immunosuppressive drugs is characteristic.

PATHOPHYSIOLOGY

The normal inverse relationship between urine volume and urine osmolality (see Figure 16.5) means that initial decreases in maximal AVP secretion will not cause an increase in urine volume sufficient to be detected clinically by polyuria. In general, basal AVP secretion must fall to less than 10% to 20% of normal before basal urine osmolality decreases to less than 300 mOsm/kg H_2O and urine flow increases to symptomatic levels (i.e., >50 mL/kg BW/day). This resulting loss of body water produces a slight rise in plasma osmolality that stimulates thirst and induces a compensatory polydipsia. The resultant increase in water intake restores balance with urine output and stabilizes the osmolality of body fluids at a new, slightly higher but still normal level. As the AVP deficit increases, this new steady-state level of plasma osmolality approximates the osmotic threshold for thirst (see Figure 16.5). It is important to recognize that the deficiency of AVP need not be complete for polyuria and polydipsia to occur; it is only necessary that the maximal plasma AVP concentration achievable at or below the osmotic threshold for thirst is inadequate to concentrate the urine.[142] The degree of neurohypophyseal destruction at which such failure occurs varies considerably from person to person, largely because of individual differences in the set point and sensitivity of the osmoregulatory system.[33] In general, functional tests of AVP levels in patients with DI of variable severity, duration, and cause have indicated that AVP secretory capacity must be reduced by at least 75% to 80% for significant polyuria to occur, which also agrees with neuroanatomic studies of cell loss in the supraoptic nuclei of dogs with experimental pituitary stalk section[115] and of patients who had undergone pituitary surgery.[116]

Because renal mechanisms for sodium conservation are unimpaired with impaired or absent AVP secretion, there is no accompanying sodium deficiency. Although untreated DI can lead to hyperosmolality and volume depletion, until the water losses become severe, volume depletion is minimized by osmotic shifts of water from the ICF compartment to the more osmotically concentrated ECF compartment. This phenomenon is not as evident following increases in ECF [Na^+] because such osmotic shifts result in a slower increase in the serum [Na^+] than would otherwise occur. However, when non–sodium solutes such as mannitol are infused, this effect is more obvious due to the progressive dilutional decrease in serum [Na^+] caused by translocation of intracellular water to the ECF compartment. Because patients with DI do not have impaired urine Na^+ conservation, the ECF volume is generally not markedly decreased, and regulatory mechanisms for the maintenance of osmotic homeostasis are primarily activated—stimulation of thirst and AVP secretion (to whatever degree the neurohypophysis is still able to secrete AVP). In cases in which AVP secretion is totally absent (complete DI), patients are dependent entirely on water intake for the maintenance of water balance. However, in cases in which some residual capacity to secrete AVP remains (partial DI), plasma osmolality can eventually reach levels that allow moderate degrees of urinary concentration (Figure 16.10).

The development of DI following surgical or traumatic injury to the neurohypophysis represents a unique situation and can follow any of several different, well-defined patterns. In some patients, polyuria develops 1 to 4 days after injury and resolves spontaneously. Less often, the DI is permanent and continues indefinitely (see previous discussion on the relationship between the level of pituitary stalk section and development of permanent DI). Most interestingly, a triphasic response can occur as a result of pituitary stalk transection (Figure 16.11).[117] The initial DI (first phase) is due to axon shock and lack of function of the damaged neurons. This phase lasts from several hours to several days and is followed by an antidiuretic phase (second phase) that is due to the uncontrolled release of AVP from the disconnected and degenerating posterior pituitary or from the remaining severed neurons.[143] Overly aggressive administration of fluids during this second phase does not suppress the AVP secretion and can lead to hyponatremia. The antidiuresis can last from 2 to 14 days, after which DI recurs following depletion of the AVP from the degenerating posterior pituitary gland (third phase).[144]

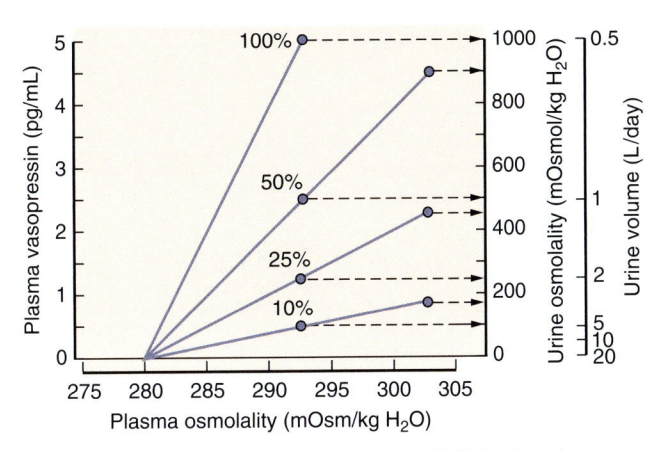

Figure 16.10 Relationship between plasma AVP levels, urine osmolality, and plasma osmolality in subjects with normal posterior pituitary function (100%) compared with patients with graded reductions in AVP-secreting neurons (to 50%, 25%, and 10% of normal). Note that the patient with a 50% secretory capacity can achieve only half the plasma AVP level and half the urine osmolality of normal subjects at a plasma osmolality of 293 mOsm/kg H$_2$O, but with increasing plasma osmolality, this patient can nonetheless eventually stimulate sufficient AVP secretion to reach a near-maximal urine osmolality. In contrast, patients with more severe degrees of AVP-secreting neuron deficits are unable to reach maximal urine osmolalities at any level of plasma osmolality. (Adapted from Robertson GL: Posterior pituitary. In Felig P, Baxter J, Frohman LA, editors: *Endocrinology and metabolism*, New York, 1986, McGraw Hill, pp 338-386.)

Transient hyponatremia without preceding or subsequent DI has been reported following transsphenoidal surgery for pituitary microadenomas,[145] which generally occurs 5 to 10 days postoperatively. The incidence may be as high as 30% when these patients are carefully followed, although most cases are mild and self-limited.[146,147] This is due to inappropriate AVP secretion via the same mechanism as in the triphasic response, except that in these cases only the second phase occurs (isolated second phase) because the initial neural lobe or pituitary stalk damage is not sufficient to impair AVP secretion enough to produce clinical manifestations of DI (see Figure 16.11).[148]

Once a deficiency of AVP secretion has been present for more than a few days or weeks, it rarely improves, even if the underlying cause of the neurohypophyseal destruction is eliminated. The major exception to this is in patients with postoperative DI, for whom spontaneous resolution is the rule. Although recovery from DI that persists more than several weeks postoperatively is less common, well-documented cases of long-term recovery have nonetheless been reported.[144] The reason for amelioration and resolution is apparent from pathologic and histologic examination of neurohypophyseal tissue following pituitary stalk section.[149,150] Neurohypophyseal neurons that have intact perikarya are able to regenerate axons and form new nerve terminal endings capable of releasing AVP into nearby capillaries. In animals, this may be accompanied by a bulbous growth at the end of the severed stalk, which represents a new, albeit small, neural lobe. In humans, the regeneration process appears to proceed more slowly, and formation of a new neural lobe has not been noted. Nonetheless, histologic examination of a severed human stalk from a patient 18 months after hypophysectomy has demonstrated reorganization of neurohypophyseal fibers, with neurosecretory granules in close proximity to nearby blood vessels, closely resembling the histology of a normal posterior pituitary.[150]

Recognition of the fact that almost all patients with CDI retain a limited capacity to secrete some AVP allows an understanding of some otherwise perplexing features of the disorder. For example, in many patients, restricting water intake long enough to raise plasma osmolality by only 1% to 2% induces sufficient AVP secretion to concentrate the urine (Figure 16.12). As the plasma osmolality increases further, some patients with partial DI can even secrete enough AVP to achieve near-maximal urine osmolality (see Figure 16.10). However, this should not cause confusion about the diagnosis of DI because, in these patients, the urine osmolality will still be inappropriately low at plasma osmolality within a normal range, and they will respond to exogenous AVP administration with further increases in urine osmolality. These responses to dehydration illustrate the relative nature of the AVP deficiency in most cases and underscore the importance of the thirst mechanism to restrict the use of residual secretory capacity under basal conditions of ad lib water intake.

CDI is also associated with changes in the renal response to AVP. The most obvious change is a reduction in maximal concentrating capacity, which has been attributed to washout of the medullary concentration gradient caused by the chronic polyuria. The severity of this defect is proportional to the magnitude of the polyuria and is independent of its cause.[142] Because of this, the level of urinary concentration achieved at maximally effective levels of plasma AVP is reduced in all types of DI. In patients with CDI, this concentrating abnormality is offset to some extent by an apparent increase in renal sensitivity to low levels of plasma AVP (Figure 16.13). The cause of this supersensitivity is unknown, but it may reflect upward regulation of AVP V$_2$ receptor expression or function secondary to a chronic deficiency of the hormone.[151]

OSMORECEPTOR DYSFUNCTION

CAUSES

There is an extensive literature in animals indicating that the primary osmoreceptors controlling AVP secretion and thirst are located in the anterior hypothalamus; lesions of this region in animals, called the AV3V area, cause hyperosmolality through a combination of impaired thirst and impaired osmotically stimulated AVP secretion.[30,31] Initial reports in humans described this syndrome as essential hypernatremia,[152] and subsequent studies used the term *adipsic hypernatremia* in recognition of the profound thirst deficits found in most of the patients.[153] Based on the known pathophysiology, all these syndromes can be grouped together as disorders of osmoreceptor dysfunction.[154] Although the pathologies responsible for this condition can be quite varied, all the cases reported to date have been due to various degrees of osmoreceptor destruction associated with a variety of different brain lesions, as summarized in Table 16.2. Many of these are the same types of lesions that can cause CDI but, in contrast to CDI, these lesions usually occur more rostrally in the hypothalamus, consistent with the anterior hypothalamic location of the

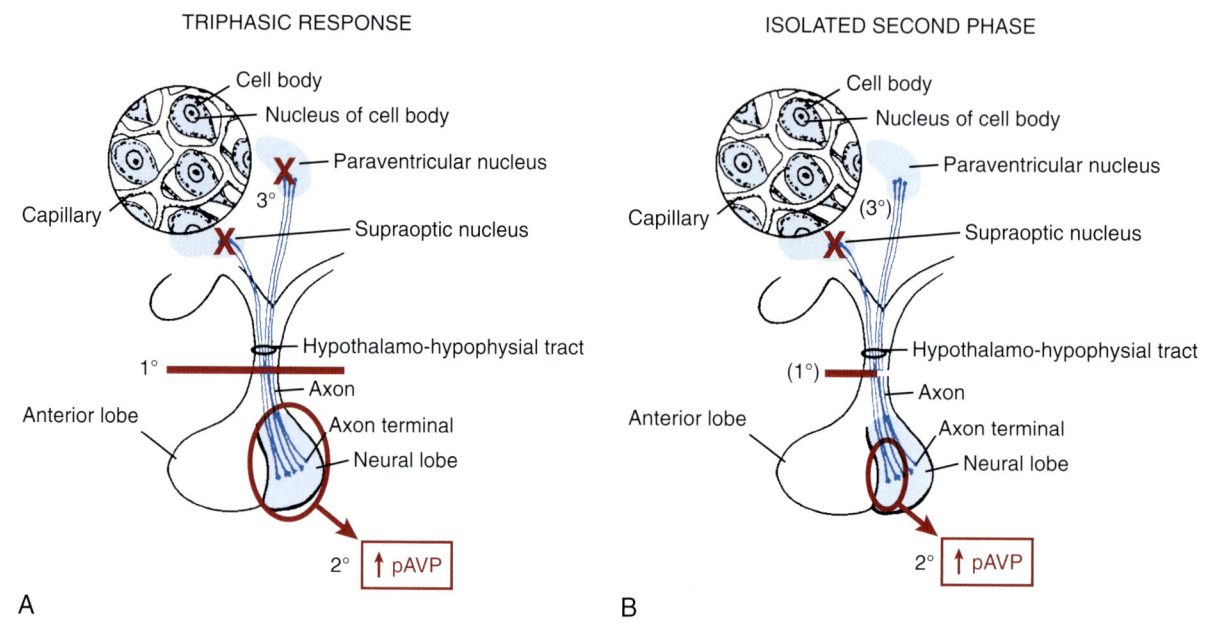

Figure 16.11 Mechanisms underlying the pathophysiology of the triphasic pattern of diabetes insipidus (DI) and the isolated second phase. **A,** In the triphasic response, the first phase of DI is initiated following a partial or complete pituitary stalk section, which severs the connections between the AVP neuronal cell bodies in the hypothalamus and nerve terminals in the posterior pituitary gland, thus preventing stimulated AVP secretion (1 degree). This is followed in several days by the second phase of SIADH, which is caused by uncontrolled release of AVP into the bloodstream from the degenerating nerve terminals in the posterior pituitary (2 degrees). After all of the AVP stored in the posterior pituitary gland has been released, the third phase of DI returns if more than 80% to 90% of the AVP neuronal cell bodies in the hypothalamus have undergone retrograde degeneration (3 degrees). **B,** In the isolated second phase, the pituitary stalk is injured, but not completely cut. Although the maximum AVP secretory response will be diminished as a result of the stalk injury, DI will not result if the injury leaves intact at least 10% to 20% of the nerve fibers connecting the AVP neuronal cell bodies in the hypothalamus to the nerve terminals in the posterior pituitary gland (1 degree). However, this is still followed in several days by the second phase of SIADH, which is caused by uncontrolled release of AVP from the degenerating nerve terminals of the posterior pituitary gland that have been injured or severed (2 degrees). Because a smaller portion of the posterior pituitary is denervated, the magnitude of AVP released as the pituitary degenerates will be smaller and of shorter duration than with a complete triphasic response. After all the AVP stored in the damaged part of the posterior pituitary gland has been released, the second phase ceases, but clinical DI will not occur if less than 80% to 90% of the AVP neuronal cell bodies in the hypothalamus undergo retrograde degeneration (3 degrees). (From Loh JA, Verbalis JG: Disorders of water and salt metabolism associated with pituitary disease. *Endocrinol Metab Clin North Am* 37:213-234, 2008.)

primary osmoreceptor cells (see Figure 16.2). One lesion that is unique to this disorder is an anterior communicating cerebral artery aneurysm. Because the small arterioles that feed the anterior wall of the third ventricle originate from the anterior communicating cerebral artery, an aneurysm in this region[155] (but more often following surgical repair of such an aneurysm that typically involves ligation of the anterior communicating artery[156]) produces infarction of the part of the hypothalamus containing the osmoreceptor cells.

PATHOPHYSIOLOGY

The cardinal defect of patients with this disorder is lack of the osmoreceptors that regulate thirst. With rare exceptions, osmoregulation of AVP is also impaired, although the hormonal response to nonosmotic stimuli remains intact (Figure 16.14).[157,158] Four major patterns of osmoreceptor dysfunction have been described as characterized by defects in thirst and/or AVP secretory responses: (1) upward resetting of the osmostat for both thirst and AVP secretion (normal AVP and thirst responses but at an abnormally high plasma osmolality); (2) partial osmoreceptor destruction (blunted AVP and thirst responses at all plasma osmolalities); (3) total osmoreceptor destruction (absent AVP secretion and thirst, regardless of plasma osmolality); and (4) selective dysfunction of thirst osmoregulation with intact AVP secretion.[154] Regardless of the actual pattern, the hallmark of this disorder is an abnormal thirst response in addition to variable defects in AVP secretion. Thus, such patients fail to drink sufficiently as their plasma osmolality rises and, as a result, the new set point for plasma osmolality rises far above the normal thirst threshold. Unlike patients with CDI, whose polydipsia maintains their plasma osmolality within a normal range, patients with osmoreceptor dysfunction typically have osmolality in the range of 300 to 340 mOsm/kg H_2O. This again underscores the critical role played by normal thirst mechanisms in maintaining body fluid homeostasis; intact renal function alone is insufficient to maintain plasma osmolality within normal limits in such cases.

The rate of development and severity of hyperosmolality and hypertonic dehydration in patients with osmoreceptor dysfunction are influenced by a number of factors. First is the ability to maintain some degree of osmotically stimulated thirst and AVP secretion, which will determine the new set point for plasma osmolality. Second are environmental influences that affect the rate of water output. When physical activity is minimal, and the ambient temperature is not

CHAPTER 16 — DISORDERS OF WATER BALANCE

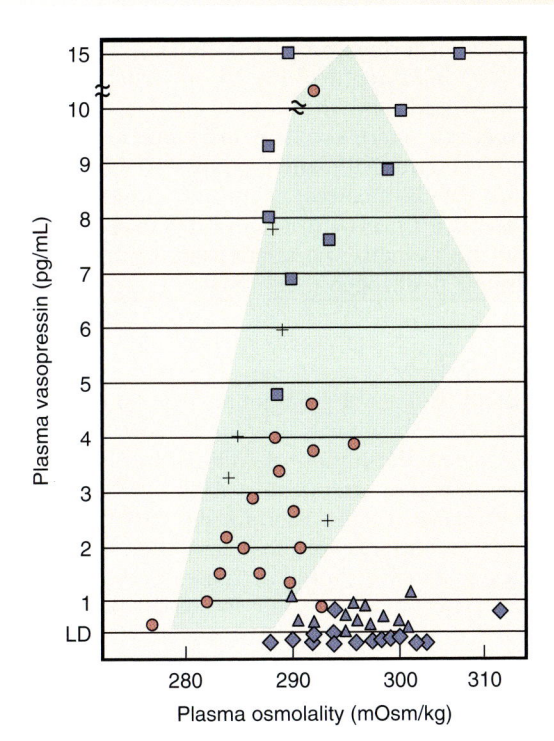

Figure 16.12 Relationship between plasma AVP and concurrent plasma osmolality in patients with polyuria of diverse causes. All measurements were made at the end of a standard dehydration test. *Shaded area,* Range of normal. In patients with severe (♦) or partial (▲) central DI, plasma AVP was almost always subnormal relative to plasma osmolality. In contrast, the values from patients with dipsogenic (●) or nephrogenic (■) DI were consistently within or above the normal range. (From Robertson GL: Diagnosis of diabetes insipidus. In Czernichow AP, Robinson A, editors: *Diabetes insipidus in man: frontiers of hormone research,* Basel, 1985, S Karger, pp 176.)

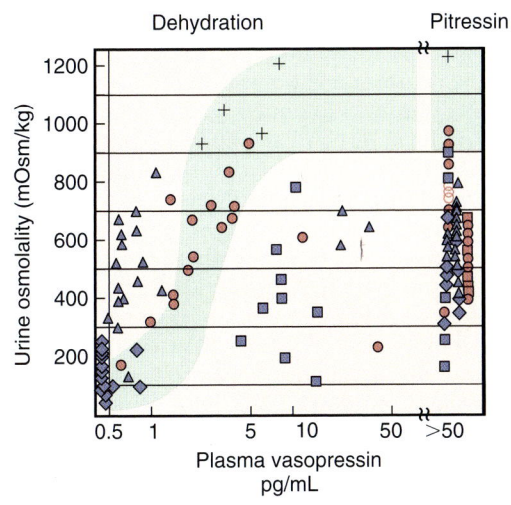

Figure 16.13 Relationship between urine osmolality and concurrent plasma AVP in patients with polyuria of diverse causes. All measurements were made at the end of a standard dehydration test. *Shaded area,* Range of normal. In patients with severe (♦) or partial (▲) central DI, urine osmolality is normal or supranormal relative to plasma AVP when the latter is submaximal. In patients with nephrogenic DI (■), urine osmolality is always subnormal for plasma AVP. In patients with dipsogenic DI (●), the relationship is normal at submaximal levels of plasma AVP but usually subnormal when plasma AVP is high. (From Robertson GL: Diagnosis of diabetes insipidus. In Czernichow AP, Robinson A, editors: *Diabetes insipidus in man: frontiers of hormone research,* Basel, 1985, S Karger, pp 176.)

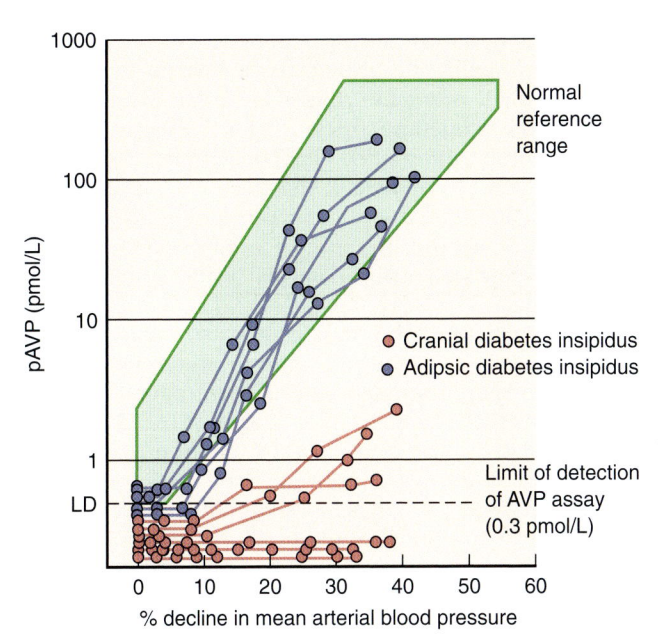

Figure 16.14 Plasma AVP responses to arterial hypotension produced by infusion of trimethephan in patients with central DI (cranial diabetes insipidus) and osmoreceptor dysfunction (adipsic diabetes insipidus). Normal responses in healthy volunteers are shown by the *shaded area.* Note that despite absent or markedly blunted AVP responses to hyperosmolality, patients with osmoreceptor dysfunction respond normally to baroreceptor stimulation induced by hypotension. (From Baylis PH, Thompson CJ: Diabetes insipidus and hyperosmolar syndromes. In Becker KL, editor: *Principles and practice of endocrinology and metabolism,* Philadelphia, 1995, JB Lippincott, pp 257.)

elevated, the overall rates of renal and insensible water loss are low, and the patient's diet may be sufficient to maintain a relatively normal balance for long periods of time. Anything that increases perspiration, respiration, or urine output greatly accelerates the rate of water loss and thereby uncovers the patient's inability to mount an appropriate compensatory increase in water intake.[12] Under these conditions, severe and even fatal hypernatremia can develop relatively quickly. When the dehydration is only moderate (plasma osmolality = 300 to 330 mOsm/kg H$_2$O), the patient is usually asymptomatic and signs of volume depletion are minimal, but if the dehydration becomes severe, the patient can exhibit symptoms and signs of hypovolemia, including weakness, postural dizziness, paralysis, confusion, coma, azotemia, hypokalemia, hyperglycemia, and secondary hyperaldosteronism (see later, "Clinical Manifestations of Diabetes Insipidus"). In severe cases, there may also be rhabdomyolysis, with marked serum elevations in muscle enzyme levels and occasionally acute renal failure.

However, a third factor also influences the degree of hyperosmolality and dehydration present in these patients. For all cases of osmoreceptor dysfunction, it is important to remember that afferent pathways from the brainstem to the hypothalamus remain intact; therefore, these patients will usually have normal AVP and renal concentrating responses to baroreceptor-mediated stimuli, such as hypovolemia and hypotension (see Figure 16.14),[158] or to other nonosmotic stimuli, such as nausea (see Figure 16.8).[153,157] This has the effect of preventing severe dehydration because, as hypovolemia develops, this will stimulate AVP secretion via baroreceptive pathways through the brainstem (see Figure 16.2). Although protective, this effect often causes confusion, because sometimes these patients appear to have DI yet at other times they can concentrate their urine quite normally. Nonetheless, the presence of refractory hyperosmolality with absent or inappropriate thirst should alert clinicians to the presence of osmoreceptor dysfunction, regardless of apparent normal urine concentration occasionally.

In a few patients with osmoreceptor dysfunction, forced hydration has been found to lead to hyponatremia in association with inappropriate urine concentration.[152,153] This paradoxic defect resembles that seen in SIADH and has been postulated to be caused by two different pathogenic mechanisms. One is continuous or fixed secretion of AVP because of loss of the capacity for osmotic inhibition and stimulation of hormone secretion. These observations, as well as electrophysiologic data,[43] have strongly suggested that the osmoregulatory system is bimodal (i.e., it is composed of inhibitory and stimulatory input to the neurohypophysis; see Figure 16.6). The other cause of the diluting defect appears to be hypersensitivity to the antidiuretic effects of AVP because, in some patients, urine osmolality may remain elevated, even when the hormone is undetectable.[153]

Hypodipsia is also a common occurrence in older adults in the absence of any overt hypothalamic lesion.[159] In such cases, it is not clear whether the defect is in the hypothalamic osmoreceptors, in their projections to the cortex, or in some other regulatory mechanism. However, in most cases, the osmoreceptor is likely not involved because basal and stimulated plasma AVP levels have been found to be normal, or even hyperresponsive, in relation to plasma osmolality in older adults, with the exception of only a few studies that showed decreased plasma levels of AVP relative to plasma osmolality.[160]

GESTATIONAL DIABETES INSIPIDUS

CAUSES

A relative deficiency of plasma AVP can also result from an increase in the rate of AVP metabolism.[100,161] This condition has been observed only in pregnancy and therefore it is generally termed *gestational diabetes insipidus*. It is due to the action of a circulating enzyme called cysteine aminopeptidase (oxytocinase or vasopressinase) that is normally produced by the placenta to degrade circulating oxytocin and prevent premature uterine contractions.[162] Because of the close structural similarity between AVP and OT, this enzyme degrades both peptides.[163] There are two types of gestational diabetes insipidus.[162] In the first type, the activity of cysteine aminopeptidase is extremely and abnormally elevated. This syndrome has been referred to as vasopressin-resistant diabetes insipidus of pregnancy.[164] It can occur in association with preeclampsia, acute fatty liver, and coagulopathies (e.g., HELLP syndrome [*h*emolysis, *e*levated *l*iver enzymes, and *l*ow *p*latelet count]). These patients have decreased metabolism of vasopressinase by the liver.[165] Usually, in subsequent pregnancies, these women have neither diabetes insipidus nor acute fatty liver. In the second type, the accelerated metabolic clearance of vasopressin produces DI in a patient with borderline vasopressin function from a specific disease (e.g., mild nephrogenic DI or partial CDI). AVP is rapidly destroyed, and the neurohypophysis is unable to keep up with the increased demand. Labor and parturition usually proceed normally, and patients have no trouble with lactation. There is the threat of chronic and severe dehydration when DI is unrecognized, and this may pose a threat to a pregnant woman. The relationship of this disorder to the transient nephrogenic DI (NDI) of pregnancy is not clear.[164]

PATHOPHYSIOLOGY

The pathophysiology of gestational DI is similar to that of CDI. The only exception is that the polyuria is usually not corrected by administration of AVP because this is rapidly degraded, just as is endogenous AVP, but it can be controlled by treatment with desmopressin, the AVP V_2 receptor agonist that is more resistant to degradation by oxytocinase or vasopressinase.[162] It should be remembered that patients with partial CDI in whom only low levels of AVP can be maintained, or patients with compensated NDI in whom the lack of response of the kidney to AVP may not be absolute, can be relatively asymptomatic with regard to polyuria. However, with accelerated destruction of AVP during pregnancy, the underlying DI may become manifest. Consequently, patients presenting with gestational DI should not be assumed simply to have excess oxytocinase or vasopressinase; rather, these patients should be evaluated for other possible underlying pathologic diagnoses (see Table 16.2).[166]

NEPHROGENIC DIABETES INSIPIDUS

CAUSES

Resistance to the antidiuretic action of AVP is usually due to some defect within the kidney, and is commonly referred to as nephrogenic diabetes insipidus (NDI). It was first recognized in 1945 in several patients with the familial, sex-linked form of the disorder. Subsequently, additional kindreds with the X-linked form of familial NDI were identified. Clinical studies of NDI have indicated that symptomatic polyuria is present from birth, plasma AVP levels are normal or elevated, resistance to the antidiuretic effect of AVP can be partial or almost complete, and the disease affects mostly males and is usually, although not always,[167] mild or absent in carrier females. More than 90% of cases of congenital NDI are caused by mutations of the AVP V_2 receptor[168] (see Chapter 45). Most mutations occur in the part of the receptor that is highly conserved among species and/or is conserved among similar receptors, such as homologies with AVP V_{1A} or OT receptors. The effect of some of these mutations on receptor synthesis, processing, trafficking, and function has been studied by in vitro expression.[169,170] These types of studies have shown that the various mutations cause several different defects in cellular processing and function of the receptor but can be classified into four general categories based on differences in transport to the cell surface and AVP binding and/or stimulation of adenylyl cyclase: (1) the mutant receptor is not inserted in the membrane; (2) the mutant receptor is inserted in the membrane but does not bind or respond to AVP; (3) the mutant receptor is inserted in the membrane and binds AVP but does not activate adenylyl cyclase; or (4) the mutant protein is inserted into the membrane and binds AVP but responds subnormally in terms of adenylyl cyclase activation. Two studies have shown a relationship between the clinical phenotype and genotype and/or cellular phenotype.[169,171] Approximately 10% of the V_2 receptor defects causing congenital NDI are thought to be de novo. This high incidence of de novo cases, coupled with the large number of mutations that have been identified, hinders the clinical use of genetic identification because it is necessary to sequence the entire open reading frame of the receptor gene rather than short sequences of DNA. Nonetheless, the use of automated gene sequencing techniques in selected families has been shown to identify mutations in patients with clinical disease and in asymptomatic carriers.[172] Although most female carriers of the X-linked V_2 receptors defect have no clinical disease, some have been reported with symptomatic NDI.[167] Carriers can have a decreased maximum urine osmolality in response to plasma AVP levels, but are generally asymptomatic because of the absence of overt polyuria. In one study, a girl manifested severe NDI due to a V_2 receptor mutation, which was likely due to skewed inactivation of the normal X chromosome.[173]

Congenital NDI can also result from mutations of the autosomal gene that codes for AQP2, the protein that forms the water channels in renal medullary collecting tubules. When the proband is a girl, it is likely the defect is a mutation of the AQP2 gene on chromosome 12, region q12-q13.[174] More than 20 different mutations of the AQP2 gene have been described[175] (see Chapter 45). The patients may be heterozygous for two different recessive mutations[176] or homozygous for the same abnormality from both parents.[177] Because most of these mutations are recessive, the patients usually do not present with a family history of DI unless consanguinity is present. Functional expression studies of these mutations have shown that all of them result in varying degrees of reduced water transport because the mutant aquaporins are not expressed in normal amounts, are retained in various cellular organelles, or simply do not function as effectively as water channels. Regardless of the type of mutation, the phenotype of NDI from AQP2 mutations is identical to that produced by V_2 receptor mutations. Some of the defects in cellular routing and water transport can be reversed by treatment with chemicals that act like chaperones,[178] suggesting that misfolding of the mutant AQP2 may be responsible for misrouting. Similar salutary effects of chaperones have been found to reverse defects in cell surface expression and function of selected mutations of the AVP V_2 receptor.[179]

NDI can also be caused by a variety of drugs, diseases, and metabolic disturbances, including lithium, hypokalemia, and hypercalcemia (see Table 16.2). Some of these disorders (e.g., polycystic kidney disease) act to distort the normal architecture of the kidney and interfere with the normal urine concentration process. However, experimental studies in animal models have suggested that many have in common a downregulation of AQP2 expression in the renal collecting tubules (Figure 16.15; see also Chapters 10 and 11).[180,181] The polyuria associated with potassium deficiency develops in parallel with decreased expression of kidney AQP2, and repletion of potassium reestablishes the normal urinary concentrating mechanism and normalizes renal expression of AQP2.[182] Similarly, hypercalcemia has also been found to be associated with downregulation of AQP2.[183] A low-protein diet diminishes the ability to concentrate the urine, primarily by a decreased delivery of urea to the inner medulla, thus decreasing the medullary concentration gradient, but rats on a low-protein diet also appear to downregulate AQP2, which could be an additional component of the decreased ability to concentrate the urine.[184] Bilateral urinary tract obstruction causes an inability to produce a maximum concentration of the urine, and rat models have demonstrated a downregulation of AQP2, which persists for several days after release of the obstruction.[185] However, it is not yet clear which of these effects on AQP2 expression are primary or secondary, and which cellular mechanism(s) are responsible for the downregulation of AQP2 expression.

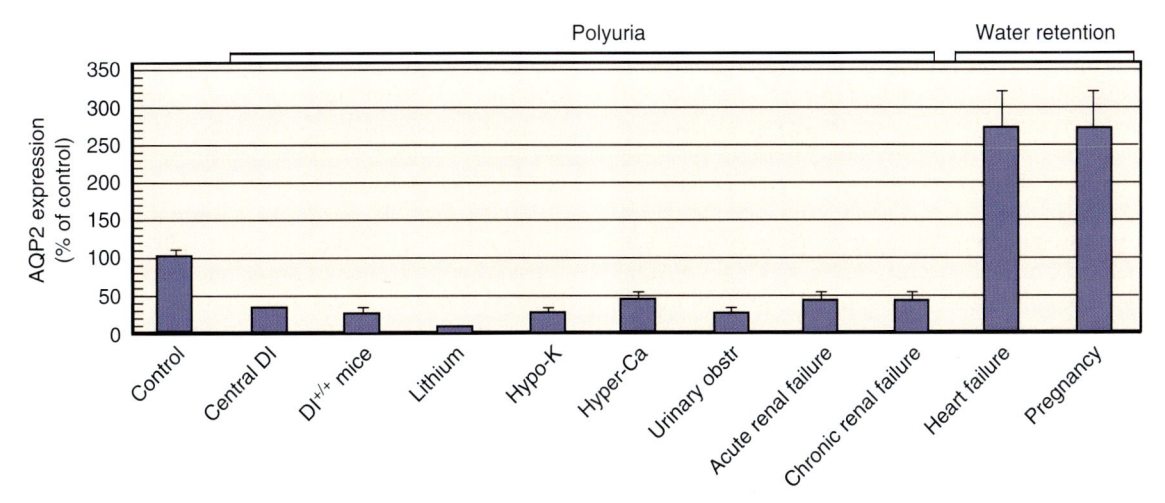

Figure 16.15 Kidney expression of the water channel aquaporin-2 in various animal models of polyuria and water retention. Note that kidney aquaporin-2 expression is uniformly downregulated relative to levels in controls in all animal models of polyuria, but upregulated in animal models of inappropriate antidiuresis. DI$^{+/+}$, Genetic diabetes insipidus; Hyper-Ca, hypercalcemia; Hypo-K, hypokalemia; Urinary obstr, ureteral obstruction. (From Nielsen S, Kwon TH, Christensen BM, et al: Physiology and pathophysiology of renal aquaporins. *J Am Soc Nephrol* 10:647-663, 1999.)

The administration of lithium to treat psychiatric disorders is the most common cause of drug-induced NDI and illustrates the multiple mechanisms likely involved in producing this disorder. As many as 10% to 20% of patients on chronic lithium therapy develop some degree of NDI.[186] Lithium is known to interfere with the production of cAMP[187] and produces a dramatic (95%) reduction in kidney AQP2 levels in animals.[188] The defect of aquaporins is slow to correct in experimental animals and humans and, in some cases, it can be permanent[189] in association with glomerular or tubulointerstitial nephropathy.[190] Several other drugs that are known to induce renal concentrating defects have also been associated with abnormalities of AQP2 synthesis.[191]

PATHOPHYSIOLOGY

Similar to CDI, renal insensitivity to the antidiuretic effect of AVP also results in the excretion of an increased volume of dilute urine, decrease in body water, and rise in plasma osmolality, which by stimulating thirst induces a compensatory increase in water intake. As a consequence, the osmolality of body fluid stabilizes at a slightly higher level, which approximates the osmotic threshold for thirst. As in patients with CDI, the magnitude of polyuria and polydipsia varies greatly depending on a number of factors, including the degree of renal insensitivity to AVP, individual differences in the set points and sensitivity of thirst and AVP secretion, and total solute load. It is important to note that the renal insensitivity to AVP need not be complete for polyuria to occur; it is only necessary that the defect is great enough to prevent concentration of the urine at plasma AVP levels achievable under ordinary conditions of ad lib water intake (i.e., at plasma osmolalities near the osmotic threshold for thirst). Calculations similar to those used for states of AVP deficiency indicate that this requirement is not met until the renal sensitivity to AVP is reduced by more than 10-fold. Because renal insensitivity to the hormone is often incomplete, especially in cases of acquired rather than congenital NDI, many patients with NDI are able to concentrate their urine to varying degrees when they are deprived of water or given large doses of desmopressin.

Information about the renal concentration mechanism from studies of AQP2 expression in experimental animals (see Chapters 10 and 11) has suggested that a form of NDI is likely associated with all types of DI, as well as with primary polydipsia. Brattleboro rats have been found to have low levels of kidney AQP2 expression compared to Long-Evans control rats; AQP2 levels are corrected by treatment with AVP or desmopressin, but this process takes 3 to 5 days, during which time urine concentration remains subnormal, despite pharmacologic concentrations of AVP.[192] Similarly, physiologic suppression of AVP by chronic overadministration of water produces a downregulation of AQP2 in the renal collecting duct.[192] Clinically, it is well known that patients with both CDI and primary polydipsia often fail to achieve maximally concentrated urine when they are given desmopressin during a water deprivation test to differentiate among the various causes of DI. This effect has long been attributed to a washout of the medullary concentration gradient as a result of the high urine flow rates in polyuric patients; however, based on the results of animal studies, it seems certain that at least part of the decreased response to AVP is due to a downregulation of kidney AQP2 expression. This also explains why it takes time, typically several days, to restore normal urinary concentration after patients with primary polydipsia and CDI are treated with water restriction or antidiuretic therapy.[193]

PRIMARY POLYDIPSIA

CAUSES

Excessive fluid intake also causes hypotonic polyuria and, by definition, polydipsia. Consequently, this disorder must be differentiated from the various causes of DI. Furthermore, it is apparent that despite normal pituitary and kidney function, patients with this disorder share many characteristics of both CDI (AVP secretion is suppressed as a result of the decreased plasma osmolality) and NDI (kidney AQP2 expression is decreased as a result of the suppressed plasma AVP levels). Many different names have been used to describe patients with excessive fluid intake, but the term *primary polydipsia* remains the best descriptor because it does not presume any particular cause for the increased fluid intake. Primary polydipsia is often due to a severe mental illness, such as schizophrenia, mania, or an obsessive-compulsive disorder,[194] in which case it is termed *psychogenic polydipsia*. These patients usually deny true thirst and attribute their polydipsia to bizarre motives, such as a need to cleanse their body of poisons. Studies of a series of polydipsic patients in a psychiatric hospital have shown an incidence as high as 42% of patients with some form of polydipsia and, in most reported cases, there was no obvious explanation for the polydipsia.[195]

However, primary polydipsia can also be caused by an abnormality in the osmoregulatory control of thirst, in which case it has been termed *dipsogenic diabetes insipidus*.[196] These patients have no overt psychiatric illness and invariably attribute their polydipsia to a nearly constant thirst. Dipsogenic DI is usually idiopathic but can also be secondary to organic structural lesions in the hypothalamus identical to any of the disorders described as causes of CDI, such as neurosarcoidosis of the hypothalamus, tuberculous meningitis, multiple sclerosis, or trauma. Consequently, all polydipsic patients should be evaluated with an MRI scan of the brain before concluding that excessive water intake has an idiopathic or psychiatric cause. Primary polydipsia can also be produced by drugs that cause a dry mouth or by any peripheral disorder causing pathologic elevations of renin and/or angiotensin levels.[112]

Finally, primary polydipsia is sometimes caused by physicians, nurses, or the lay press who advise a high fluid intake for valid (e.g., recurrent nephrolithiasis) or unsubstantiated reasons of health.[197] These patients lack overt signs of mental illness but also deny thirst and usually attribute their polydipsia to habits acquired from years of adherence to their drinking regimen.

PATHOPHYSIOLOGY

The pathophysiology of primary polydipsia is essentially the reverse of that in CDI—the excessive intake of water expands and slightly dilutes body fluids, suppresses AVP secretion, and dilutes the urine. The resultant increase in the rate of water excretion balances the increase in intake, and the osmolality of body water stabilizes at a new, slightly lower level that approximates the osmotic threshold for AVP secretion. The magnitude of the polyuria and polydipsia vary considerably, depending on the nature or intensity of the stimulus to drink. In patients with abnormal thirst, the polydipsia and polyuria are relatively constant from day to day. However, in patients with psychogenic polydipsia, water intake and urine output tend to fluctuate widely and at times can be quite large.

Occasionally, fluid intake rises to such extraordinary levels that the excretory capacity of the kidneys is exceeded, and dilutional hyponatremia develops.[198] There is little question that excessive water intake alone can sometimes be sufficient to override renal excretory capacity and produce severe hyponatremia. Although the water excretion rate of normal adult kidneys can generally exceed 20 L/day, maximum hourly rates rarely exceed 1000 mL/hr. Because many psychiatric patients drink predominantly during the day or during intense drinking binges,[199] they can transiently achieve symptomatic levels of hyponatremia, with the total daily volume of water intake less than 20 L if ingested rapidly enough. This likely accounts for many of the patients who present with maximally dilute urine, accounting for as many as 50% of patients in some studies, and are corrected quickly via free water diuresis.[200] The prevalence of this disorder, based on hospital admissions for acute symptomatic hyponatremia, may have been underestimated because studies of polydipsic psychiatric patients have shown a marked diurnal variation in serum [Na^+], from 141 mEq/L at 7 AM to 130 mEq/L at 4 PM, suggesting that many such patients drink excessively during the daytime but then correct themselves via water diuresis at night.[201] This and other considerations have led to defining this disorder as the psychosis, intermittent hyponatremia, and polydipsia (PIP) syndrome.[199]

However, many other cases of hyponatremia with psychogenic polydipsia have been found to meet the criteria for a diagnosis of SIADH, suggesting the presence of nonosmotically stimulated AVP secretion. As might be expected, in the presence of much higher than normal water intake, almost any impairment of urinary dilution and water excretion can exacerbate the development of a positive water balance and thereby produce hypo-osmolality. Acute psychosis itself can also cause AVP secretion,[202] which often appears to take the form of a reset osmostat.[194] It is therefore apparent that no single mechanism can completely explain the occurrence of hyponatremia in polydipsic psychiatric patients, but the combination of higher than normal water intake plus modest elevations of plasma AVP levels from a variety of potential sources appears to account for a significant portion of these cases.

CLINICAL MANIFESTATIONS OF DIABETES INSIPIDUS

The characteristic clinical symptoms of DI are the polyuria and polydipsia that result from the underlying impairment of urine-concentrating mechanisms, which have been described earlier in the sections on the pathophysiology of specific types of DI. Interestingly, patients with DI typically describe a craving for cold water, which appears to quench their thirst better.[69] Patients with CDI also typically describe a precipitous onset of their polyuria and polydipsia, which simply reflects the fact that urinary concentration can be maintained fairly well until the number of AVP-producing neurons in the hypothalamus decreases to 10% to 15% of normal, after which plasma AVP levels decrease to the range at which urine output increases dramatically.

However, patients with DI, particularly those with osmoreceptor dysfunction syndromes, can also present with varying degrees of hyperosmolality and dehydration, depending on their overall hydration status. It is therefore also important to be aware of the clinical manifestations of hyperosmolality. These can be divided into the signs and symptoms produced by dehydration, which are largely cardiovascular, and those caused by the hyperosmolality itself, which are predominantly neurologic and reflect brain dehydration as a result of osmotic water shifts out of the CNS. Cardiovascular manifestations of hypertonic dehydration include hypotension, azotemia, acute tubular necrosis secondary to renal hypoperfusion or rhabdomyolysis, and shock.[203,204] Neurologic manifestations range from nonspecific symptoms, such as irritability and cognitive dysfunction, to more severe manifestations of hypertonic encephalopathy, such as disorientation, decreased level of consciousness, obtundation, chorea, seizures, coma, focal neurologic deficits, subarachnoid hemorrhage, and cerebral infarction.[203,205] One study also suggested an increased incidence of deep venous thrombosis in hyperosmolar patients.[206]

The severity of symptoms can be roughly correlated with the degree of hyperosmolality, but individual variability is marked and, for any single patient, the level of serum [Na^+] at which symptoms will appear cannot be accurately predicted. Similar to hypo-osmolar syndromes, the length of time over which hyperosmolality develops can markedly affect the clinical symptomatology. The rapid development of severe hyperosmolality is frequently associated with marked neurologic symptoms, whereas gradual development over several days or weeks generally causes milder symptoms.[203,207] In this case, the brain counteracts osmotic shrinkage by increasing the intracellular content of solutes. These include electrolytes such as potassium and a variety of organic osmolytes, which previously had been termed *idiogenic osmoles;* for the most part, these are the same organic osmolytes that are lost from the brain during adaptation to hypo-osmolality.[208] The net effect of this process is to protect the brain against excessive shrinkage during sustained hyperosmolality. However, once the brain has adapted by increasing its solute content, rapid correction of the hyperosmolality can produce brain edema because it takes a finite length of time (24 to 48 hours in animal studies) to dissipate the accumulated solutes and, until this process has been completed, the brain will accumulate excess water as plasma osmolality is normalized.[209] This effect is usually seen in dehydrated pediatric patients who can develop seizures with rapid rehydration,[210] but has been described only rarely in adults, including the most severely hyperosmolar patients with nonketotic hyperglycemic hyperosmolar coma.

DIFFERENTIAL DIAGNOSIS OF POLYURIA

Before beginning involved diagnostic testing to differentiate among the various forms of DI and primary polydipsia, the presence of true hypotonic polyuria should be established by measurement of a 24-hour urine for volume and osmolality. Generally accepted standards are that the 24-hour urine volume should exceed 50 mL/kg BW, with an osmolality lower than 300 mOsm/kg H_2O.[211] Simultaneously, there should be a determination of whether the polyuria is due to an osmotic agent such as glucose or intrinsic renal disease. Routine laboratory studies and the clinical setting will usually distinguish these disorders; diabetes mellitus and other forms of solute diuresis usually can be excluded by the history, routine urinalysis for glucose, and/or measurement of the solute excretion rate (urine osmolality × 24-hour urine volume [in liters] > 15 mOsm/kg BW/day). There is universal agreement that the diagnosis of DI requires stimulating AVP secretion osmotically and then measuring the adequacy of the secretion by direct measurement of plasma AVP levels or indirect assessment by urine osmolality.

In a patient who is already hyperosmolar, with submaximally concentrated urine (i.e., urine osmolality < 800 mOsm/kg H_2O), the diagnosis is straightforward and simple; primary polydipsia is ruled out by the presence of hyperosmolality,[211] confirming a diagnosis of DI. CDI can then be distinguished from NDI by evaluating the response to the administration of AVP (5 units SC) or, preferably, of the AVP V_2 receptor agonist desmopressin (1-deamino-8-D-arginine vasopressin [DDAVP], 1 to 2 μg subcutaneously or intravenously). A significant increase in urine osmolality within 1 to 2 hours after injection indicates insufficient endogenous AVP secretion, and therefore CDI, whereas an absent response indicates renal resistance to AVP effects, and therefore NDI. Although conceptually simple, interpretational difficulties can arise because the water diuresis produced by AVP deficiency in CDI produces a washout of the renal medullary concentrating gradient and downregulation of kidney AQP2 water channels (see earlier), so that initial increases in urine osmolality in response to administered AVP or desmopressin are not as great as would be expected. Generally, increases of urine osmolality of more than 50% reliably indicate CDI, and responses of less than 10% indicate NDI, but responses between 10% and 50% are indeterminate.[142] Therefore, plasma AVP levels should be measured to aid in this distinction; hyperosmolar patients with NDI will have clearly elevated plasma AVP levels, whereas those with CDI will have absent (complete) or blunted (partial) AVP responses relative to their plasma osmolality (see Figure 16.11). Because it will not be known beforehand which patients will have diagnostic versus indeterminate responses to AVP or desmopressin, a plasma AVP level should be determined prior to AVP or desmopressin administration in patients with hyperosmolality and inadequately concentrated urine without a solute diuresis.

Patients with DI have intact thirst mechanisms, so they usually do not present with hyperosmolality, but rather with a normal plasma osmolality and serum [Na^+] and symptoms of polyuria and polydipsia. In these cases, it is most appropriate to perform a fluid deprivation test. The relative merits of the indirect fluid deprivation test (Miller-Moses test[212]) versus direct measurement of plasma AVP levels after a period of fluid deprivation[142] has been debated in literature, with substantial pros and cons in support of each of these tests. On the one hand, the standard indirect test has a long track record of making an appropriate diagnosis in the large majority of cases, generally yields interpretable results by the end of the test, and does not require sensitive assays for the notoriously difficult measurement of plasma AVP levels.[213,214] However, maximum urine concentrating capacity is well known to be variably reduced in all forms of DI, as well as primary polydipsia,[142] and as a result the absolute levels of urine osmolality achieved during fluid deprivation and after AVP administration are reduced to overlapping degrees in patients with partial CDI, partial NDI, and primary polydipsia.

Measurements of basal plasma osmolality or serum [Na^+] are of little use because they also overlap considerably among these disorders.[211] Although association with certain diseases, surgical procedures, or family history often helps differentiate among these disorders, sometimes the clinical setting may not be helpful because certain disorders (e.g., sarcoidosis, tuberculous meningitis, other hypothalamic pathologies) can cause more than one type of DI (see Table 16.2). Consequently, a simpler approach that has been proposed is to measure plasma or urine AVP before and during a suitable osmotic stimulus, such as fluid restriction or hypertonic NaCl infusion, and plot the results as a function of the concurrent plasma osmolality or plasma [Na^+] (see Figures 16-12 and 16-13).[215,216] Using a highly sensitive and validated research assay for plasma AVP determinations, this approach has been shown to provide a definitive diagnosis in most cases, provided the final level of plasma osmolality or sodium achieved is above the normal range (>295 mOsm/kg H_2O or 145 mmol/L, respectively). The diagnostic effectiveness of this approach derives from the fact that the magnitude of the AVP response to osmotic stimulation is not appreciably diminished by chronic overhydration[194] or dehydration. Hence, the relationship of plasma AVP to plasma osmolality is usually within or above normal limits in NDI and primary polydipsia. In most cases, these two disorders can then be distinguished by measuring urine osmolality before and after the dehydration test and relating these values to the concurrent plasma AVP concentration (see Figure 16.12). However, because maximal concentrating capacity can be severely blunted in patients with primary polydipsia, it is often better to analyze the relationship under basal nondehydrated conditions when the plasma AVP level is not elevated. Because of the solute diuresis that often ensues following infusion of hypertonic NaCl, measurements of urine osmolality or AVP excretion are unreliable indicators of changes in hormone secretion and are of little or no diagnostic value when this procedure is used to increase osmolality to more than 295 mOsm/kg H_2O. Given the proven usefulness of the indirect and direct approaches, a combined fluid deprivation test that synthesizes the crucial aspects of both tests can easily be performed (Table 16.3). In many cases, this will allow interpretation of the plasma AVP levels and response to an AVP challenge.

With use of the fluid deprivation test for plasma AVP determinations, most cases of polyuria and polydipsia can be diagnosed accurately. A useful approach in the remaining indeterminate cases is to conduct a closely monitored trial with standard therapeutic doses of desmopressin. If this treatment abolishes thirst and polydipsia, as well as polyuria, for 48 to 72 hours without producing water intoxication, the patient most likely has uncomplicated CDI. On the other hand, if the treatment abolishes the polyuria but has no or a lesser effect on thirst or polydipsia and results in the

Table 16.3 Fluid Deprivation Test for the Diagnosis of Diabetes Insipidus

Procedure

1. Initiation of the deprivation period depends on the severity of the DI; in routine cases, the patient should be made NPO after dinner, whereas in patients with more severe polyuria and polydipsia, this may be too long a period without fluids, and the water deprivation should be started early on the morning (e.g., 6 AM) of the test.
2. Obtain plasma and urine osmolality and serum electrolyte and plasma AVP levels at the start of the test.
3. Measure urine volume and osmolality hourly or with each voided urine.
4. Stop the test when body weight decreases by ≥3%, the patient develops orthostatic blood pressure changes, the urine osmolality reaches a plateau (i.e., <10% change over two or three consecutive measurements), or the serum Na^+ > 145 mmol/L.
5. Obtain plasma and urine osmolality and serum electrolyte and plasma AVP levels at the end of the test, when the plasma osmolality is elevated, preferably >300 mOsm/kg H_2O.
6. If serum Na^+ < 146 mmol/L or plasma osmolality <300 mOsm/kg H_2O when the test is stopped, then consider a short infusion of hypertonic saline (3% NaCl at a rate of 0.1 mL/kg/min for 1 to 2 hours) to reach these end points.
7. If hypertonic saline infusion is not required to achieve hyperosmolality, administer AVP (5 U) or desmopressin (DDAVP; 1 μg) subcutaneously and continue following urine osmolality and volume for an additional 2 hours.

Interpretation

1. An unequivocal urine concentration after AVP or DDAVP (>50% increase) indicates central diabetes insipidus (CDI); an unequivocal absence of urine concentration (<10%) strongly suggests nephrogenic DI (NDI) or primary polydipsia (PP).
2. Differentiating between NDI and PP, as well as cases in which the increase in urine osmolality after AVP or DDAVP administration is more equivocal (e.g., 10% to 50%), is best done using the relation between plasma AVP levels and plasma osmolality obtained at the end of the dehydration period and/or hypertonic saline infusion and the relation between plasma AVP levels and urine osmolality determined under basal conditions (see Figures 16.12 and 16.13).

development of hyponatremia, it is more likely that the patient has some form of primary polydipsia. If desmopressin has no effect over this time interval, even when given by injection, it is almost certain that the patient has some form of NDI.

As might be expected, most patients with DI will also exhibit a subnormal increase in AVP secretion in response to nonosmotic stimuli, such as hypotension, nausea, and hypoglycemia.[215] For diagnostic purposes, however, these nonosmotic tests of neurohypophyseal function do not provide any advantage over dehydration or hypertonic NaCl infusion because orthostatic, emetic, and glucopenic stimuli are difficult to control or quantitate and generally cause a markedly variable AVP response. A more fundamental disadvantage with all nonosmotic stimuli is the possibility of false-positive or false-negative results because some patients exhibit little or no rise in AVP after hypotension or emesis yet lack polyuria and have a normal response to osmotic stimuli. Conversely, patients with osmoreceptor dysfunction exhibit little or no AVP response to hypertonic NaCl but have a normal increase in response to induced hypotension (see Figure 16.14).[158]

MRI has also proved to be useful for diagnosing DI. In normal subjects, the posterior pituitary produces a characteristic bright signal in the posterior part of the sella turcica that is similar on T1-weighted images, usually best seen in sagittal views.[217] This was originally thought to represent fatty tissue, but more recent evidence indicated that the bright spot was actually due to the stored hormone in neurosecretory granules.[218] An experimental study done in rabbits subjected to dehydration for varying periods of time showed a linear correlation between pituitary AVP content and the signal intensity of the posterior pituitary by MRI.[219] As might be expected from the fact that destruction of more than 85% to 90% of the neurohypophysis is necessary to produce clinical symptomatology of DI, this signal has been found to be almost always absent in patients with CDI in multiple studies.[220] However, as with any diagnostic test, clinical usefulness is dependent on the sensitivity and specificity of the test. Although earlier studies using small numbers of subjects demonstrated the presence of the bright spot in all normal subjects, subsequent larger studies reported an age-related absence of a pituitary bright spot in up to 20% of normal subjects.[221] Conversely, some studies have reported the presence of a bright spot in patients with clinical evidence of DI.[222] This may be because some patients with partial CDI have not yet progressed to the point of depletion of all neurohypophyseal reserves of AVP, or because a persistent bright spot in patients with DI might be due to the pituitary content of OT rather than AVP. In support of this, it is known that oxytocinergic neurons are more resistant to destruction by trauma than vasopressinergic neurons in rats[223] and humans.[22] The presence of a positive posterior pituitary bright spot has been variably reported in other polyuric disorders. In primary polydipsia, the bright spot is usually seen,[220] consistent with studies in animals in which even prolonged lack of secretion of AVP caused by hyponatremia did not cause a decreased content of AVP in the posterior pituitary.[26] In NDI, the bright spot has been reported to be absent in some patients but present in others.[125] Consequently, specificity is lacking in regard to using MRI routinely as a diagnostic screening test for DI. Nonetheless, the sensitivity is sufficient to allow a high probability that a patient with a bright spot on MRI does not have CDI. Thus, MRI is more useful for ruling out than for ruling in a diagnosis of CDI.

Additional useful information can be gained through MRI via assessment of the pituitary stalk. Enlargement of the stalk beyond 2 to 3 mm is generally considered to be pathologic[224] and can be caused by multiple disease processes.[225] Consequently, when MRI scans reveal thickening of the stalk, especially with absence of the posterior pituitary bright spot, systemic diseases should be searched for diligently, including cerebrospinal fluid (CSF), plasma β-human chorionic gonadotropin (β-hCG), and alpha-fetoprotein

Table 16.4	Therapies for the Treatment of Diabetes Insipidus

Water
Antidiuretic agents
    Arginine vasopressin (Pitressin)
    1-Deamino-8-D-arginine vasopressin (desmopressin; DDAVP)
Antidiuresis-enhancing agents
    Chlorpropamide
    Prostaglandin synthetase inhibitors (indomethacin, ibuprofen, tolmetin)
Natriuretic agents
    Thiazide diuretics
    Amiloride

measurements for the evaluation of suprasellar germinoma, chest imaging and CSF and plasma angiotensin-converting enzyme (ACE) levels for the evaluation of sarcoidosis, and bone and skin surveys for the evaluation of histiocytosis. When a diagnosis is still in doubt, the MRI should be repeated every 3 to 6 months. Continued enlargement, especially in children over the first 3 years of follow-up, suggests a germinoma and mandates a biopsy, whereas a decrease in the size of the stalk over time is more indicative of an inflammatory process, such as lymphocytic infundibuloneurohypophysitis.[226]

TREATMENT OF DIABETES INSIPIDUS

The general goals of treatment of all forms of DI are a correction of any preexisting water deficits and a reduction in the ongoing excessive urinary water losses. The specific therapy required (Table 16.4) will vary according to the type of DI present and clinical situation. Awake ambulatory patients with normal thirst have relatively little body water deficit, but benefit greatly by alleviation of the polyuria and polydipsia that disrupt their normal daily activities. In contrast, comatose patients with acute DI after head trauma are unable to drink in response to thirst and, in these patients, progressive hyperosmolality can be life-threatening.

The total body water deficit in a hyperosmolar patient can be estimated using the following formula:

Total body water deficit = $0.6 \times$ premorbid weight $\times (1 - 140/[Na^+])$

where $[Na^+]$ is the serum sodium concentration in mmol/L and weight is in kilograms. This formula is dependent on three assumptions: (1) total body water is approximately 60% of the premorbid body weight; (2) no body solute was lost as the hyperosmolality developed; and (3) the premorbid serum $[Na^+]$ was 140 mEq/L.

To reduce the risk of CNS damage from protracted exposure to severe hyperosmolality, in most cases the plasma osmolality should be rapidly lowered in the first 24 hours to the range of 320 to 330 mOsm/kg H_2O, or by approximately 50%. Plasma osmolality may be most easily estimated as twice the serum $[Na^+]$ if there is no hyperglycemia, and measured osmolality may be substituted if azotemia is not present. As discussed earlier, the brain increases intracellular osmolality by increasing the content of a variety of organic osmolytes as protection against excessive shrinkage during hyperosmolality.[208] Because these osmolytes cannot be immediately dissipated, further correction to a normal plasma osmolality should be spread over the next 24 to 72 hours to avoid producing cerebral edema during treatment.[209] This is especially important in children,[227] in whom several studies have indicated that limiting correction of hypernatremia to a maximal rate of no greater than 0.5 mmol/L/hr prevents the occurrence of symptomatic cerebral edema with seizures.[210,228] In addition, the possibility of associated thyroid or adrenal insufficiency should also be kept in mind, because patients with CDI caused by hypothalamic masses can have associated deficiencies of anterior pituitary function.

The above formula does not take into account ongoing water losses and is, at best, a rough estimate. Frequent serum and urine electrolyte determinations should be made, and the administration rate of oral water, or IV 5% dextrose in water, should be adjusted accordingly. Note, for example, that the estimated deficit of a 70-kg patient whose serum $[Na^+]$ is 160 mEq/L is 5.25 L of water. In such an individual, administration of water at a rate greater than 200 mL/hr would be required simply to correct the established deficit over 24 hours. Additional fluid would be needed to keep up with ongoing losses until a definitive response to treatment has occurred.

THERAPEUTIC AGENTS

The therapeutic agents available for the treatment of DI are shown in Table 16.4. Water should be considered a therapeutic agent because, when ingested or infused in sufficient quantity, there is no abnormality of body fluid volume or composition.

As noted previously, in most patients with DI, thirst remains intact, and the patients will drink sufficient fluid to maintain a relatively normal fluid balance. A patient with known DI should therefore be treated to decrease the polyuria and polydipsia to acceptable levels that allow him or her to maintain a normal lifestyle. Because the major goal of therapy is improvement in symptomatology, the therapeutic regimen prescribed should be individually tailored to each patient to accommodate her or his needs. The safety of the prescribed agent and use of a regimen that avoids potential detrimental effects of overtreatment are primary considerations because of the relatively benign course of DI in most cases and the potential adverse consequences of hyponatremia. Available treatments are summarized below; their use is discussed separately for different types of DI.

Arginine Vasopressin

Arginine vasopressin (Pitressin) is a synthetic form of naturally occurring human AVP. The aqueous solution contains 20 units/mL. Because of the drug's relatively short half-life (2- to 4-hour duration of antidiuretic effect) and propensity to cause acute increases in blood pressure when given as an IV bolus, this route of administration should generally be avoided. This agent is mainly used for acute situations such as postoperative DI. However, repeated dosing is required unless a continuous infusion is used, and the frequency of dosing or infusion rate must be titrated to achieve the desired reduction in urine output (see subsequent discussion of postoperative DI).

Desmopressin

Desmopressin (DDAVP) is an agonist of the AVP V_2 receptor that was developed for therapeutic use because it has a significantly longer half-life than AVP (8- to 20-hour duration of antidiuretic effect) and is devoid of the latter's pressor activity because of the absence of activation of AVP V_{1A} receptors on vascular smooth muscle.[229] As a result of these advantages, it is the drug of choice for acute and chronic administration in patients with CDI.[230] Several different preparations are available. The intranasal form is provided as an aqueous solution containing 100 µg/mL in a bottle with a calibrated rhinal tube, which requires specialized training to use appropriately, or as a nasal spray delivering a metered dose of 10 µg in 0.1 mL. An oral preparation is also available in doses of 0.1 or 0.2 mg. Recently, a sublingual preparation, called Minrin Melt, has been introduced in doses of 60 to 120 µg.[231]

Neither the intranasal or oral preparations should be used in an acute emergency setting, in which it is essential that the patient achieve a therapeutic dose of the drug; in this case, the parenteral form should always be used. This is supplied as a solution containing 4 µg/mL and may be given by the intravenous, intramuscular, or subcutaneous route. The parenteral form is approximately 5 to 10 times more potent than the intranasal preparation, and the recommended dosage is 1 to 2 µg every 8 to 12 hours. For intranasal and parenteral preparations, increasing the dose generally has the effect of prolonging the duration of antidiuresis for several hours rather than increasing its magnitude; consequently, altering the dose can be useful to reduce the required frequency of administration.

Chlorpropamide

Chlorpropamide (Diabinese) is primarily used as an oral hypoglycemic agent; this sulfonylurea also potentiates the hydro-osmotic effect of AVP in the kidney. Chlorpropamide has been reported to reduce polyuria by 25% to 75% in patients with CDI. This effect appears to be independent of the severity of the disease and is associated with a proportional rise in urine osmolality, correction of dehydration, and elimination of the polydipsia, similar to that caused by small doses of AVP or desmopressin.[211] The major site of action of chlorpropamide appears to be at the renal tubule to potentiate the hydro-osmotic action of circulating AVP, but there is also evidence of a pituitary effect to increase the release of AVP; the latter effect may account for the observation that chlorpropamide can produce significant antidiuresis, even in patients with severe CDI and presumed near-total AVP deficiency.[211] The usual dose is 250 to 500 mg/day, with a response noted in 1 or 2 days and a maximum antidiuresis in 4 days. It should be remembered that this is an off-label use of chlorpropamide; it should not be used in pregnant women or in children, it should never be used in an acute emergency setting in which achieving rapid antidiuresis is necessary, and it should be avoided in patients with concurrent hypopituitarism because of the increased risk of hypoglycemia. Other sulfonylureas share chlorpropamide's effect but generally are less potent. In particular, the newer generation of oral hypoglycemic agents, such as glipizide and glyburide, are almost devoid of any AVP-potentiating effects.

Prostaglandin Synthase Inhibitors

Prostaglandins have complex effects in the CNS and kidney, many of which are still incompletely understood due to the variety of different prostaglandins and their multiplicity of cellular effects. In the brain, intracerebroventricular infusion of E prostaglandins stimulates AVP secretion,[232] and administration of prostaglandin synthase inhibitors attenuates osmotically stimulated AVP secretion.[233] However, in the kidney, prostaglandin E_2 (PGE_2) has been reported to inhibit AVP-stimulated generation of cAMP in the cortical collecting tubule by interacting with inhibitory G protein (G_i).[234] Thus, the effect of prostaglandin synthase inhibitors to sensitize AVP effects in the kidney likely result from enhanced cAMP generation on AVP binding to the V_2 receptor. The predominant renal effects of these agents is demonstrated by the fact that clinically these agents successfully reduce urine volume and free water clearance, even in patients with NDI of different causes.[235]

Natriuretic Agents

Thiazide diuretics have a paradoxic antidiuretic effect in patients with CDI.[236] However, given that better antidiuretic agents are available for the treatment of CDI, its main therapeutic use is in NDI. Hydrochlorothiazide at doses of 50 to 100 mg/day usually reduces urine output by approximately 50%, and its efficacy can be further enhanced by restricting sodium intake. Unlike desmopressin or the other antidiuresis-enhancing drugs, these agents are equally effective for treating most forms of NDI (see below).

TREATMENT OF DIFFERENT TYPES OF DIABETES INSIPIDUS

Central Diabetes Insipidus

Patients with CDI should generally be treated with intranasal or oral desmopressin. Unless the hypothalamic thirst center is also affected by the primary lesion causing superimposed osmoreceptor dysfunction, these patients will develop thirst when the plasma osmolality increases by only 2% to 3%.[211] Severe hyperosmolality is therefore not a risk in the patient who is alert, ambulatory, and able to drink in response to perceived thirst. Polyuria and polydipsia are thus inconvenient and disruptive, but not life-threatening. However, hypo-osmolality is largely asymptomatic and may be progressive if water intake continues during a period of continuous antidiuresis. Therefore, treatment must be designed to minimize polyuria and polydipsia but without an undue risk of hyponatremia from overtreatment.

Treatment should be individualized to determine optimal dosage and dosing intervals. Although tablets offer greater convenience and are generally preferred by patients, it is useful to start with the nasal spray initially because of greater consistency of absorption and physiologic effect and then switch to oral tablets only after the patient is comfortable with use of the intranasal preparation to produce antidiuresis. Having tried both preparations, the patient can then choose which they prefer for long-term usage. Because of variability in response among patients, it is desirable to determine the duration of action of individual doses in each patient.[237] A satisfactory schedule can generally be determined using modest doses, and the maximum dose of desmopressin needed is rarely above 0.2 µg orally or 10 µg (one nasal spray) given two or occasionally three times daily.[238] These doses generally produce plasma desmopressin levels many times more than those required to produce maximum antidiuresis but obviate the need for more frequent treatment. Rarely, once-daily dosing suffices. In a few patients, the effect of intranasal or oral desmopressin is erratic, probably as a result of variable interference with absorption from the gastrointestinal tract or nasal mucosa. This variability can be reduced and the duration of action prolonged by administering the drug on an empty stomach[239] or after thorough cleansing of the nostrils. Resistance caused by antibody production has not been reported.

Hyponatremia is a rare complication of desmopressin therapy; however, it only occurs if the patient is continually antidiuretic while maintaining a fluid intake sufficient to become volume expanded and natriuretic.[240] Absence of thirst in this case is protective but, in addition, most patients with CDI on standard therapy are not maximally antidiuretic continuously. There are reports of hyponatremia in patients with normal AVP function, and presumably normal thirst, when they are given desmopressin to treat hemophilia and von Willebrand's disease[241] and in children treated with desmopressin for primary enuresis.[242] In these cases, the hyponatremia can develop rapidly and is often first noted by the onset of convulsions and coma.[243] Severe hyponatremia in patients with DI who are being treated with desmopressin can be avoided by monitoring serum electrolyte levels frequently during the initiation of therapy. Patients who show a tendency to develop a low serum [Na^+] and do not respond to recommended decreases in fluid intake should then be instructed to delay a scheduled dose of desmopressin once or twice weekly so that polyuria recurs, thereby allowing any excess retained fluid to be excreted.[212]

Acute postsurgical DI occurs relatively frequently following surgery that involves the suprasellar hypothalamic area, but several confounding factors must be considered. These patients often receive stress doses of glucocorticoids, and the resulting hyperglycemia with glucosuria may confuse a diagnosis of DI. Thus, the blood glucose level must first be brought under control to eliminate an osmotic diuresis as the cause of the polyuria. In addition, excess fluids administered intravenously may be retained perioperatively but then excreted normally postoperatively. If this large output is matched with continued intravenous input, an incorrect diagnosis of DI may be made based on the resulting polyuria. Therefore, if the serum [Na^+] is not elevated concomitantly with the polyuria, the rate of parenterally administered fluid should be slowed, with careful monitoring of serum [Na^+] and urine output to establish the diagnosis. Once a diagnosis of DI is confirmed, the only acceptable pharmacologic therapy is an antidiuretic agent. However, because many neurosurgeons fear water overload and brain edema after this type of surgery, the patient is sometimes treated only with intravenous fluid replacement for a considerable time before the institution of antidiuretic hormone therapy (see the potential benefits of this approach below). If the patient is awake and able to respond to thirst, he or she can be treated with an antidiuretic hormone, and the patient's thirst can then be the guide for water replacement. However, if the patient is unable to respond to thirst because of a decreased level of consciousness or from hypothalamic damage to the thirst center, fluid balance must be maintained by administering fluid intravenously. The urine osmolality and serum [Na^+] must be checked every several hours during the initial therapy and then at least daily until stabilization or resolution of the DI. Caution must also be exercised regarding the volume of water replacement, because excess water administered during the continued administration of AVP or desmopressin can create a syndrome of inappropriate antidiuresis and potentially severe hyponatremia. Studies in experimental animals have indicated that desmopressin-induced hyponatremia markedly impairs survival of AVP neurons after pituitary stalk compression,[223] suggesting that overhydration with subsequent decreased stimulation of the neurohypophysis may also increase the likelihood of permanent DI.

Postoperatively, desmopressin may be given parenterally in a dose of 1 to 2 µg subcutaneously, intramuscularly, or intravenously. The intravenous route is preferable because it obviates any concern about absorption, is not associated with significant pressor activity, and has the same total duration of action as the other parenteral routes. A prompt reduction in urine output should occur; the duration of the antidiuretic effect is generally 6 to 12 hours. Usually, the patient is hypernatremic with relatively dilute urine when therapy is started. One should monitor the urine osmolality and urine volume to be certain that the dose was effective and check the serum [Na^+] at frequent intervals to ensure some improvement of hypernatremia. It is generally advisable to allow some return of the polyuria before administration of subsequent doses of desmopressin because postoperative DI is often transient, and return of endogenous AVP secretion will become apparent by a lack of return of the polyuria. Also, in some cases, transient postoperative DI is part of a triphasic pattern that has been well described following pituitary stalk transection (see previous discussion and Figure 16.11). Because of this possibility, allowing a return of polyuria before redosing with desmopressin will allow earlier detection of a potential second phase of inappropriate antidiuresis and decrease the likelihood of producing symptomatic hyponatremia by continuing antidiuretic therapy and intravenous fluid administration when it is not required.

Some clinicians have recommended using a continuous intravenous infusion of a dilute solution of AVP to control DI postoperatively. Algorithms for continuous AVP infusion in postoperative and posttraumatic DI in pediatric patients have begun at infusion rates of 0.25 to 1.0 mU/kg/hr and titrated the rate using urine specific gravity (goal of 1.010 to 1.020) and urine volume (goal of 2 to 3 mL/kg/hr) as a guide to adequacy of the antidiuresis.[244] Although pressor effects have not been reported at these infusion rates, and the antidiuretic effects are quickly reversible in 2 to 3 hours, it should be remembered that use of continuous infusions versus intermittent dosing will not allow assessing when the patient has recovered from transient DI or entered the second phase of a triphasic response. If DI persists, the patient should eventually be switched to maintenance therapy with intranasal or oral preparations of desmopressin for the treatment of chronic DI.

Acute traumatic DI can occur after injuries to the head, usually a motor vehicle accident. DI is more common with deceleration injuries that result in a shearing action on the pituitary stalk and/or cause hemorrhagic ischemia of the hypothalamus and/or posterior pituitary.[144] Similar to the onset of postsurgical DI, posttraumatic DI is usually recognized by hypotonic polyuria in the presence of increased plasma osmolality. The clinical management is similar to that of postsurgical DI, as outlined above, except that the possibility of anterior pituitary insufficiency must also be considered in these cases, and the patient should be given stress doses of glucocorticoids (e.g., hydrocortisone, 50-100 mg intravenously every 8 hours) until anterior pituitary function can be definitively evaluated.

Osmoreceptor Dysfunction

Acutely, patients with hypernatremia due to osmoreceptor dysfunction should be treated the same as any hyperosmolar patient by replacing the underlying free water deficit as described at the beginning of this section. The long-term management of osmoreceptor dysfunction syndromes requires a thorough search for potentially treatable causes (see Table 16.2) in conjunction with the use of measures to prevent recurrence of dehydration. Because the hypodipsia cannot be cured, and rarely if ever improves spontaneously, the mainstay of management is education of the patient and family about the importance of continuously regulating his or her fluid intake in accordance with the hydration status. This is never accomplished easily in such patients, but can be done most efficaciously by establishing a daily schedule of water intake based on changes in body weight, regardless of the patient's thirst. In effect, a prescription for daily fluid intake must be written for these patients because they will not drink spontaneously. In addition, if the patient has polyuria, desmopressin should also be given, as for any patient with DI. The success of this regimen should be monitored periodically (weekly at first, later every month, depending on the stability of the patient) by measuring serum [Na^+]. In addition, the target weight (at which hydration status and serum [Na^+] concentration are normal) may need to be recalculated periodically to allow for growth in children or changes in body fat in adults.

Gestational Diabetes Insipidus

The polyuria of gestational DI is usually not corrected by the administration of AVP itself because this is rapidly degraded by high circulating levels of oxytocinase or vasopressinase, just as endogenous AVP is degraded by these enzymes. The treatment of choice is desmopressin because this synthetic AVP V_2 receptor agonist is not destroyed by the cysteine aminopeptidase (oxytocinase-vasopressinase) in the plasma of pregnant women[245] and, to date, appears to be safe for both the mother and child.[246,247] Desmopressin has only 2% to 5% the oxytocic activity of AVP[230] and can be used with minimal stimulation of the OT receptors in the uterus. Doses should be titrated to individual patients because higher doses and more frequent dosing intervals are sometimes required as a result of the increased degradation of the peptide. However, physicians should remember that the naturally occurring volume expansion and reset osmostat that occurs in pregnancy maintains the serum [Na^+] at a lower level during pregnancy.[39] During delivery, these patients can maintain adequate oral intake and continued administration of desmopressin. However, physicians should be cautious about overadministration of fluid parenterally during delivery because these patients will not be able to excrete the fluid and will be susceptible to the development of water intoxication and hyponatremia. After delivery, oxytocinase-vasopressinase levels decrease in plasma within several days and, depending on the cause of the DI, the disorder may disappear or patients may become asymptomatic with regard to fluid intake and urine volume.[248]

Nephrogenic Diabetes Insipidus

By definition, patients with NDI are resistant to the effects of AVP. Some patients with NDI can be treated by eliminating the drug (e.g., lithium) or disease (e.g., hypercalcemia) responsible for the disorder. For many others, however, including those with the genetic forms, the only practical form of treatment at present is to restrict sodium intake and administer a thiazide diuretic alone[236] or in combination with prostaglandin synthetase inhibitors or amiloride.[249-251] The natriuretic effect of the thiazide class of diuretics is conferred by their ability to block sodium absorption in the renal cortical diluting site. When combined with dietary sodium restriction, these drugs cause modest hypovolemia. This stimulates isotonic proximal tubular solute reabsorption and diminishes solute delivery to the more distal diluting site, at which experimental studies have indicated that thiazides also act to enhance water reabsorption in the inner medullary collecting duct independently of AVP.[252] Together, these effects diminish renal diluting ability and free water clearance, also independently of any action of AVP. Thus, agents of this class are the mainstay of therapy for NDI. Monitoring for hypokalemia is recommended, and potassium supplementation is occasionally required. Any drug of the thiazide class may be used with equal potential for benefit, and clinicians should use the one that they are most familiar with from use in other conditions. Care must be exercised when treating patients taking lithium with diuretics because the induced contraction of plasma volume may increase lithium concentrations and worsen potential toxic effects of the therapy. In the acute setting, diuretics are of no use in NDI, and only free water administration can reverse hyperosmolality.

Indomethacin, tolmetin, and ibuprofen have been used in this setting,[249,253,254] although ibuprofen may be less effective than the others. The combination of thiazides and a nonsteroidal antiinflammatory drug (NSAID) will not increase urinary osmolality above that of plasma, but the lessening of polyuria is nonetheless beneficial to patients. In many cases, the combination of thiazides with the potassium-sparing diuretic amiloride is preferred to lessen the potential side effects associated with long-term use of NSAIDs.[250,251] Amiloride also has the advantage of decreasing lithium entrance into cells in the distal tubule and, because of this, may have a preferable action for the treatment of lithium-induced NDI.[255,256]

Although desmopressin is generally not effective in NDI, a few patients may have receptor mutations that allow partial responses to AVP or desmopressin,[257] with increases in urine osmolality following much higher doses of these agents than those typically used to treat CDI (e.g., 6 to 10 μg intravenously). It is generally worth a trial of desmopressin at these doses to ascertain whether this is a potential useful therapy in selected patients in whom the responsivity of other affected family members is not already known. Potential therapies involving the administration of chaperones to bypass defects in cellular routing of misfolded aquaporin[178] and AVP V_2 receptor proteins[179] is an exciting, future possibility.[168]

Primary Polydipsia

At present, there is no completely satisfactory treatment for primary polydipsia. Fluid restriction would seem to be the obvious treatment of choice. However, patients with a reset thirst threshold will be resistant to fluid restriction because of the resulting thirst from stimulation of brain thirst centers at higher plasma osmolalities.[258] In some cases, the use of alternative methods to ameliorate the sensation of thirst (e.g., wetting the mouth with ice chips, using sour candies to increase salivary flow) can help reduce fluid intake. Fluid intake in patients with psychogenic causes of polydipsia is driven by psychiatric factors that have responded variably to behavioral modification and pharmacologic therapy. Several reports have suggested limited efficacy of the antipsychotic drug clozapine as an agent to reduce polydipsia and prevent recurrent hyponatremia in at least a subset of these patients.[259] Administration of any antidiuretic hormone or thiazide to decrease polyuria is hazardous because they invariably produce water intoxication.[211,260] Therefore, if the diagnosis of DI is uncertain, any trial of antidiuretic therapy should be conducted with close monitoring, preferably in the hospital, with frequent evaluation of fluid balance and serum electrolyte levels. If a patient with primary polydipsia is troubled by nocturia, this may be reduced or eliminated by administering a small dose of desmopressin at bedtime; because thirst and fluid intake are reduced during sleep, this treatment is less likely to cause water intoxication, provided the dose is titrated to allow resumption of a water diuresis as soon as the patient awakens the next morning. However, this approach cannot be recommended for patients with psychogenic polydipsia because of the unpredictability of their fluid intake.

DISORDERS OF EXCESS VASOPRESSIN OR VASOPRESSIN EFFECT

The disorders of the renal concentrating mechanism described in the previous section can lead to water depletion, sometimes in association with hyperosmolality and hypernatremia. In contrast, disorders of the renal diluting mechanism usually present as hyponatremia and hypo-osmolality. Hyponatremia is among the most common electrolyte disorders encountered in clinical medicine, with an incidence of 0.97% and a prevalence of 2.48% in hospitalized adult patients when the serum [Na^+] less than 130 mEq/L is the diagnostic criterion[261] and as high as 15% to 30% if the serum [Na^+] less than 135 mEq/L is used.[262] The prevalence may be somewhat lower in the hospitalized pediatric population but, conversely, the prevalence is higher than originally recognized in the geriatric population.[262-264]

RELATIONSHIP BETWEEN HYPO-OSMOLALITY AND HYPONATREMIA

Because plasma osmolality is most often measured to help evaluate hyponatremic disorders, it is useful to bear in mind the basic relationship of plasma osmolality to plasma or serum [Na^+]. As reviewed in the introduction to this chapter, Na^+ and its associated anions account for almost all of the osmotic activity of plasma. Therefore, changes in plasma [Na^+] are usually associated with comparable changes in plasma osmolality. The osmolality calculated from the concentrations of Na^+, urea, and glucose is usually in close agreement with that obtained from a measurement of osmolality.[265] When the measured osmolality exceeds the calculated osmolality by more than 10 mOsm/kg H_2O, an osmolar gap is present.[265] This occurs in two circumstances: (1) with a decrease in the water content of the serum; and (2) with addition of a solute other than urea or glucose to the serum.

A decrease in the water content of serum is usually due to its displacement by excessive amounts of protein or lipids, which can occur in severe hyperlipidemia or hyperglobulinemia. Normally, 92% to 94% plasma volume is water, with the remaining 6% to 8% being lipids and protein. Because of its ionic nature, Na^+ dissolves only in the water phase of plasma. Thus, when a greater than normal proportion of plasma is accounted for by solids, the concentration of Na^+ in plasma water remains normal, but the concentration in the total volume, as measured by flame photometry, is artifactually low. Such a discrepancy can be avoided if [Na^+] is measured with an ion-selective electrode.[266] However, the sample needs to remain undiluted (direct potentiometry) for accurate measurement of the serum [Na^+]. Whereas the flame photometer measures the concentration of Na^+ in the total plasma volume, the ion-selective electrode measures it only in the plasma water. Normally, this difference is only 3 mEq/L but, in the settings under discussion, the difference can be much greater. Because the large lipid and protein molecules contribute only minimally to the total osmolality, the measurement of osmolality by freezing point depression remains normal in these patients.

Hyponatremia associated with normal osmolality has been termed *factitious hyponatremia* or *pseudohyponatremia*. The most common causes of pseudohyponatremia are primary or secondary hyperlipidemic disorders. The serum need not appear lipemic because increments in cholesterol alone can cause the same discrepancy.[266] Plasma protein level elevations above 10 g/dL, as seen in multiple myeloma or macroglobulinemia, can also cause pseudohyponatremia. The administration of intravenous immune globulin was reported to be associated with hyponatremia without hypo-osmolality in several patients.[267]

The second setting in which an osmolar gap occurs is the presence in plasma of an exogenous low-molecular-weight substance such as ethanol, methanol, ethylene glycol, or mannitol.[268] Undialyzed patients with chronic renal failure, as well as critically ill patients,[269] also have an increment in the osmolar gap of unknown cause. Whereas all these exogenous substances, as well as glucose and urea, elevate measured osmolality, the effect they have on the serum [Na^+] and intracellular hydration depends on the solute in question. As noted, in the presence of relative insulin deficiency, glucose does not penetrate cells readily and remains in the ECF. As a consequence, water is drawn osmotically from the ICF compartment, causing cell shrinkage, and this translocation of water commensurately decreases the [Na^+] in the ECF. In this setting, therefore, the serum [Na^+] can be low while plasma osmolality is high. It is generally estimated that

Table 16.5 Relationship Between Serum Tonicity and Sodium Concentration in the Presence of Other Substances

Condition or Substance	Serum Osmolality	Serum Tonicity	Serum [Na+]
Hyperglycemia	↑	↑	↓
Mannitol, maltose, glycine	↑	↑	↓
Azotemia (high blood urea)	↑	↔	↔
Ingestion of ethanol, methanol, ethylene glycol	↑	↔	↔
Elevated serum lipid or protein	↔	↔	↓

↑, Increased; ↓, decreased; ↔, unchanged.

for every 100-mg/dL rise in serum glucose, the osmotic shift of water causes serum [Na+] to fall by 1.6 mEq/L. However, it was suggested that this may represent an underestimate of the decrease caused by hyperglycemia, and a 2.4-mEq/L correction factor was recommended.[270]

Similar "translocational" hyponatremia occurs with mannitol or maltose or with the absorption of glycine during transurethral prostate resection, as well as in gynecologic and orthopedic procedures. A potential toxicity for glycine in this setting also requires consideration.[271] The recent introduction of bipolar retroscopes, which allow for the use of NaCl as an irrigant, should result in disappearance of this clinical entity. When the plasma solute is readily permeable (e.g., urea, ethylene glycol, methanol, ethanol), it enters cells and so does not establish an osmotic gradient for water movement. There is no cellular dehydration, despite the hyperosmolar state, so the serum [Na+] remains unchanged. The relationship among plasma osmolality, plasma tonicity, and serum [Na+] in the presence of various solutes is summarized in Table 16.5.

VARIABLES THAT INFLUENCE RENAL WATER EXCRETION

In considering clinical disorders that result from excessive or inappropriate secretion of AVP, it is helpful to remember the many other variables that also influence renal water excretion. These factors fall into three broad categories.

FLUID DELIVERY FROM THE PROXIMAL TUBULE

In spite of the fact that proximal fluid reabsorption is iso-osmotic and therefore does not contribute directly to urine dilution, the volume of tubular fluid that is delivered to the distal nephron largely determines the volume of dilute urine that can be excreted. Thus, if glomerular filtration is decreased or proximal tubule reabsorption is greatly enhanced, the resulting diminution in the amount of fluid delivered to the distal tubule itself limits the rate of renal water excretion, even if other components of the diluting mechanism are intact.

DILUTION OF TUBULAR FLUID

The excretion of urine that is hypotonic to plasma requires that some segment of the nephron reabsorb solute in excess of water. The water impermeability of the entire ascending limb of Henle, as well as the capacity of its thick segment to reabsorb NaCl, actively endows this segment of the nephron with the characteristics required by the diluting process. Thus, the transport of NaCl by the Na^+-K^+-$2Cl^-$ cotransporter converts the hypertonic tubule fluid delivered from the descending limb of the loop of Henle to a distinctly hypotonic fluid (≈100 mOsm/kg H_2O). Interference with reabsorption of Na^+ and Cl^- in the ascending limb, as occurs with agents that inhibit the Na^+-K^+-$2Cl^-$ cotransporter, such as thiazide diuretics, will therefore impair urine dilution.

WATER IMPERMEABILITY OF THE COLLECTING DUCT

The excretion of urine, which is more dilute than the fluid that is delivered to the distal convoluted tubule, requires continued solute reabsorption and minimal water reabsorption in the terminal segments of the nephron. Because the water permeability of the collecting duct epithelium is primarily dependent on the presence or absence of AVP, this hormone plays a pivotal role in determining the fate of the fluid delivered to the collecting duct and thus the concentration or dilution of the final urine (see Chapter 10). In the absence of AVP, the collecting duct remains essentially impermeable to water, even though some water is still reabsorbed. The continued reabsorption of solute then results in the excretion of a maximally dilute urine (≈50 mOsm/kg H_2O). Because the medullary interstitium is always hypertonic, the absence of circulating AVP, which renders the collecting duct impermeable to water, is critical to the normal diluting process. This diluting mechanism allows for the intake and subsequent excretion of large volumes of water without major alterations in the tonicity of body water.[272] Rarely, this limit can be exceeded, causing water intoxication. Much more commonly, however, hyponatremia occurs at lower rates of water intake because of an intrarenal defect in urine dilution or persistent secretion of AVP in the circulation. Because hypo-osmolality normally suppresses AVP secretion,[273] the hypo-osmolar state frequently reflects the persistent secretion of AVP in response to hemodynamic or other nonosmotic stimuli.[273]

PATHOGENESIS AND CAUSES OF HYPONATREMIA

The plasma or serum [Na+] is determined by the body's total content of sodium, potassium, and water, as shown by the following equation:

$$\text{Serum [Na}^+\text{]} = \frac{\text{Total body exchangeable Na}^+ + \text{total body exchangeable K}^+}{\text{Total body water (TBW)}}$$

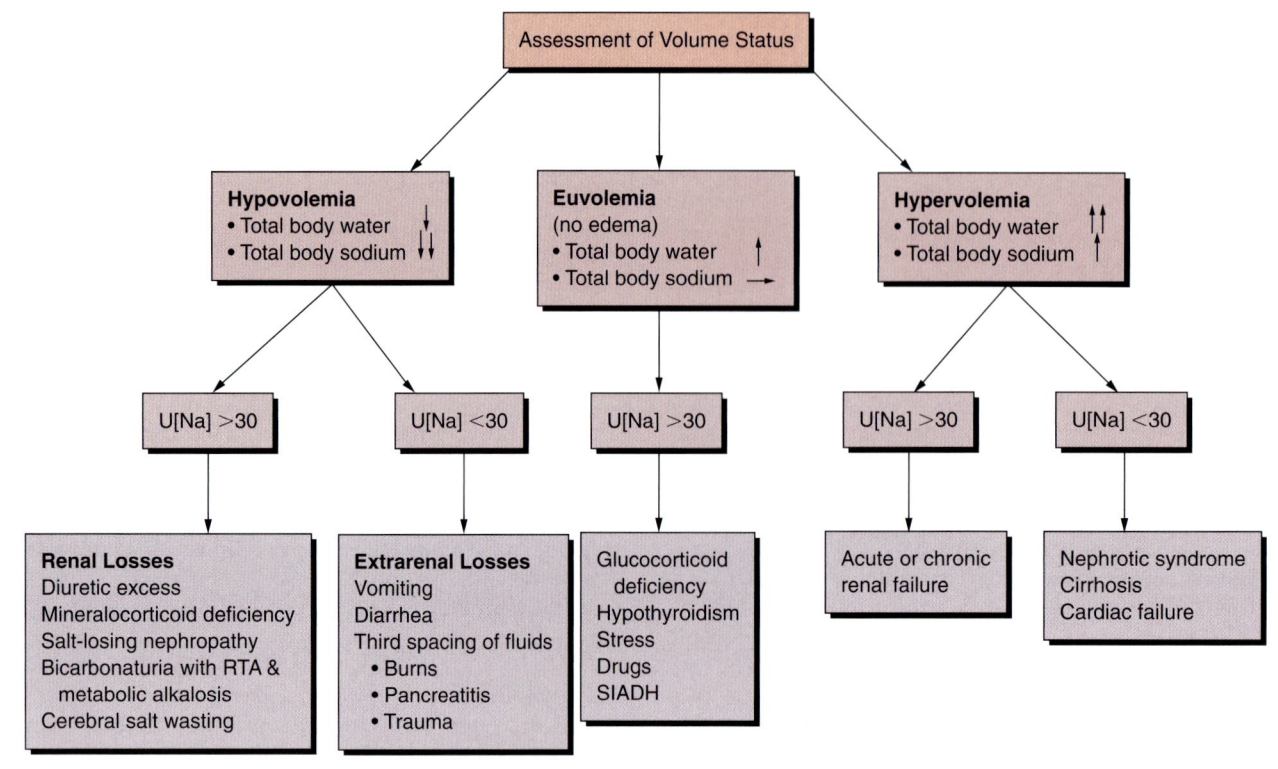

Figure 16.16 Diagnostic approach to the hyponatremic patient. (Modified from Halterman R, Berl T: Therapy of dysnatremic disorders. In Brady H, Wilcox C, editors: *Therapy in nephrology and hypertension,* Philadelphia, 1999, WB Saunders, p 256.)

This formula has been simplified from the observations made by Edelman in the 1950s, which introduced some errors in the prediction of changes in serum [Na^+] and has been subject to reinterpretation by Nguyen and Kurtz.[274] Although this revision of the formula is more accurate, there are so many inaccuracies in the measurements of sodium, potassium, and water losses, as well as intake, that there is no substitute for frequent measurements of serum [Na^+] in rapidly changing clinical settings.[275] As the previous relationship depicts, hyponatremia can therefore occur by an increase in TBW, a decrease in body solutes (Na^+ or K^+), or any combination of these. In most cases, more than one of these mechanisms is operant. Therefore, a classification system to separate the various causes of hyponatremia should be based on factors other than the level of serum [Na^+] itself. In approaching the hyponatremic patient, the physician's first task is to ensure that hyponatremia actually reflects a hypo-osmolar state and is not a consequence of pseudohyponatremia or translocational hyponatremia, as discussed earlier. Thereafter, an assessment of ECF volume (Figure 16.16) provides the most useful working classification of the cause of the hyponatremia, because a low serum [Na^+] can be associated with a decreased, normal, or high total body sodium.[276,277]

HYPONATREMIA WITH EXTRACELLULAR FLUID VOLUME DEPLETION

Patients with hyponatremia who have ECF volume depletion have sustained a deficit in total body Na^+ that exceeds the deficit in TBW. The decrease in ECF volume is manifested by physical findings such as flat neck veins, decreased skin turgor, dry mucous membranes, orthostatic hypotension, and tachycardia. If sufficiently severe, volume depletion is a potent stimulus to AVP secretion. When the osmoreceptors and volume receptors receive opposing stimuli, the former remains active but the set point of the system is lowered (see Figure 16.7). Thus, in the presence of hypovolemia, AVP is secreted and water is retained, despite hypo-osmolality. Whereas the hyponatremia in this setting clearly involves a depletion of body solutes, the concomitant AVP-mediated retention of water is critical to the pathologic process producing hyponatremia.

As depicted in the flow chart in Figure 16.16, measurement of the urine Na^+ concentration is helpful in assessing whether the fluid losses are renal or extrarenal in origin. A urine [Na^+] of less than 30 mEq/L reflects a normal renal response to volume depletion and indicates an extrarenal source of fluid loss. This is usually seen in patients with gastrointestinal disease with vomiting or diarrhea. Other causes include loss of fluid into third spaces, such as the abdominal cavity in pancreatitis or the bowel lumen with ileus. Burns and muscle trauma can also be associated with large fluid and electrolyte losses. Because many of these pathologic states are associated with thirst, an increase in orally ingested or parenterally infused free water can lead to hyponatremia.

Hypovolemic hyponatremia in patients whose urine [Na^+] is greater than 30 mEq/L indicates the kidney as the source of the fluid losses. Diuretic-induced hyponatremia, a commonly observed clinical entity, accounts for a significant proportion of symptomatic hyponatremia in hospitalized patients. It occurs almost exclusively with thiazide rather than loop diuretics, most likely because the latter have no effect on urine-diluting ability but the former do. The hyponatremia is usually evident within 14 days in most patients, but occasionally can occur for up to 2 years.[278] Underweight women appear to be particularly prone to this complication, and advanced age has been found to be a risk factor in some, but not all, studies.[278-280] A careful study of diluting ability in older adults has revealed that thiazide diuretics exaggerate the already slower recovery from hyponatremia induced by water ingestion in this population.[281]

Diuretics can cause hyponatremia by several mechanisms[282]: (1) volume depletion, which results in impaired water excretion by enhanced AVP release and decreased tubular fluid delivery to the diluting segment; (2) a direct effect on the diluting segment in the ascending limb; and (3) K^+ depletion causing a decrease in the water permeability of the collecting duct and an increase in water intake. K^+ depletion leads to hyponatremia independently of the Na^+ depletion that frequently accompanies diuretic use.[283] The concomitant administration of potassium-sparing diuretics does not prevent the development of hyponatremia. Although the diagnosis of diuretic-induced hyponatremia is frequently obvious, surreptitious diuretic abuse should always be considered in patients in whom other electrolyte abnormalities and high urinary Cl^- excretion suggest this possibility.

Salt-losing nephropathy occurs in some patients with advanced renal insufficiency. In most of these patients, the Na^+-wasting tendency is not one that manifests itself at normal rates of sodium intake; however, some patients with interstitial nephropathy, medullary cystic disease, polycystic kidney disease, or partial urinary obstruction develop sufficient Na^+ wasting to exhibit hypovolemic hyponatremia.[284] Patients with proximal renal tubular acidosis exhibit renal Na^+ and K^+ wasting, despite modest renal insufficiency, because bicarbonaturia obligates these cation losses.

It has long been recognized that adrenal insufficiency is associated with impaired renal water excretion and hyponatremia. This diagnosis should be considered in the volume-contracted hyponatremic patient whose urine [Na^+] is not low, particularly when the serum [K^+], BUN, and creatinine levels are elevated. Separate mechanisms for mineralocorticoid and glucocorticoid deficiency have been defined.[285] Observations in glucocorticoid-replete adrenalectomized experimental animals have provided evidence to support a role of mineralocorticoid deficiency in the abnormal water excretion. Conscious adrenalectomized dogs given physiologic doses of glucocorticoids develop hyponatremia. Saline or physiologic doses of mineralocorticoids corrected the defect in association with ECF volume repletion and improvement in renal hemodynamics. Immunoassayable AVP levels were elevated in a similarly treated group of mineralocorticoid-deficient dogs, despite hypo-osmolality.[286] The decreased ECF volume thus provides a nonosmotic stimulus of AVP release. More direct evidence for the role of AVP was provided in studies using an AVP receptor antagonist. When glucocorticoid-replete, adrenally insufficient rats were given an AVP antagonist, minimal urine osmolality was significantly lowered but urine dilution was not fully corrected, in contrast to the mineralocorticoid-replete rats, thereby supporting a role for an AVP-independent mechanism.[287] This is in agreement with studies of adrenalectomized homozygous Brattleboro rats, which also have a defect in water excretion that can be partially corrected by mineralocorticoids or by normalization of volume. In summary, therefore, the mechanism of the defect in water excretion associated with mineralocorticoid deficiency is mediated by AVP and by AVP-independent intrarenal factors, both of which are activated by decrements of ECF volume, rather than by deficiency of the hormone per se.

The presence in the urine of an osmotically active nonreabsorbable or poorly reabsorbable solute causes renal excretion of Na^+ and culminates in volume depletion. Glycosuria secondary to uncontrolled diabetes mellitus, mannitol infusion, or urea diuresis after relief of obstruction is a common setting for this disorder. In patients with diabetes, the Na^+ wasting caused by the glycosuria can be aggravated by ketonuria because hydroxybutyrate and acetoacetate also cause urinary electrolyte losses. In fact, ketonuria can contribute to the renal Na^+ wasting and hyponatremia seen in states of starvation and alcoholic ketoacidosis. Na^+ and water excretion are also increased when a nonreabsorbable anion appears in the urine. This is observed principally with the metabolic alkalosis and bicarbonaturia that accompany severe vomiting or nasogastric suction. In these patients, the excretion of HCO_3 requires concomitant excretion of cations, including Na^+ and K^+, to maintain electroneutrality. Whereas the renal losses in such clinical settings is often hypotonic, the volume contraction–stimulated thirst and water intake can result in the development of hyponatremia.

Cerebral salt wasting is a rare syndrome described primarily in patients with subarachnoid hemorrhage, but also with other types of CNS lesions, which can lead to renal salt wasting and volume contraction.[288] Although hyponatremia is frequently reported in these patients, true cerebral salt wasting is probably less common than reported.[289] One critical review found no conclusive evidence for volume contraction or renal salt wasting in any of these patients,[290] as has a more recent study of patients with subarachnoid hemorrhage.[291] The mechanism of this natriuresis is unknown, but an increased release of brain natriuretic peptides has been suggested.[292]

HYPONATREMIA WITH EXCESS EXTRACELLULAR FLUID VOLUME

In advanced stages, the edematous states listed in Figure 16.16 are associated with a decrease in serum [Na^+]. Patients generally have an increase in total body Na^+ content, but the rise in TBW exceeds that of Na^+. With the exception of renal failure, these states are characterized by avid Na^+ retention (urine Na^+ concentration often < 10 mEq/L). This avid retention may be obscured by the concomitant use of diuretics, which are frequently used in treating these patients. These agents can further contribute to the abnormal water excretion seen in these states.

CONGESTIVE HEART FAILURE

The common association between congestive heart failure and Na^+ and water retention is well established. A mechanism mediated by decreased delivery of tubule fluid to the distal nephron or increased release of AVP has been proposed. In an experimental model of low cardiac output, both AVP and diminished delivery to the diluting segment were found to be important in mediating the abnormality in water excretion. It thus appears that the decrement in effective blood volume and decrease in arterial filling are sensed by aortic and carotid sinus baroreceptors that stimulate AVP secretion.[293]

This stimulation must supersede the inhibition of AVP release that accompanies acute distention of the left atrium. In fact, there is evidence that chronic distention of the atria blunts the sensitivity of this baroreceptor, so high-pressure baroreceptors can act in an uninhibited manner to stimulate AVP release. The importance of AVP in the abnormal dilution in experimental models of heart failure has been underscored by correction of the water excretory defect by an AVP antagonist in rats with inferior vena cava constriction.[294]

High plasma AVP levels have been demonstrated in patients with congestive heart failure in the presence and absence of diuretics.[295] Similarly, the hypothalamic mRNA message for the AVP preprohormone is elevated in rats with chronic cardiac failure.[296] Although these studies did not exclude a role for intrarenal factors in the pathogenesis of the abnormal water retention, they complement the experimental observations that demonstrate a critical role for AVP in the pathologic process. It is most likely that nonosmotic pathways, whose activation is suggested by the increase in sympathetic activity seen in congestive heart failure,[297] are the mediators of AVP secretion in edema-forming states. These neurohumoral factors further contribute to the hyponatremia by decreasing the glomerular filtration rate (GFR) and enhancing tubular Na^+ reabsorption, thereby decreasing fluid delivery to the distal diluting segments of the nephron. The degree of neurohumoral activation correlates with the clinical severity of left ventricular dysfunction.[298] Hyponatremia is a powerful prognostic factor in these patients.[299] The role of the AVP-regulated water channel (AQP2) has also been examined in heart failure. Two studies have described an upregulation of this water channel in rats with heart failure.[300,301] In the latter study, the nonpeptide V_2 receptor antagonist OPC31260 reversed the upregulation, suggesting that a receptor-mediated function, most likely enhanced cAMP generation, is responsible for the process.[300] Consistent with these observations, a selective V_2 antagonist decreased AQP2 excretion and increased urine flow in patients with heart failure.[302]

HEPATIC FAILURE

Patients with advanced cirrhosis and ascites frequently present with hyponatremia as a consequence of their inability to excrete a water load.[303] The classic view suggests that a decrement in effective arterial blood volume leads to avid Na^+ and water retention in an attempt to restore volume toward normal. In this regard, a number of the pathologic derangements in cirrhosis, including splanchnic venous pooling, diminished plasma oncotic pressure secondary to hypoalbuminemia, and decrease in peripheral resistance, could all contribute to a decrease in effective arterial blood volume.[304] This classic theory was challenged by observations that suggested primary renal Na^+ retention, termed the *overflow hypothesis*.[305] A proposal that unifies these views has been presented—Na^+ retention occurs early in the process, but is a consequence of the severe vasodilation-mediated arterial underfilling.[306]

As with cardiac failure, the relative roles of intrarenal versus extrarenal factors in impaired water excretion has been a matter of some controversy. The observation that expansion of intravascular volume with saline, mannitol, ascites fluid, water immersion, or peritoneovenous shunting improves water excretion in cirrhosis could be interpreted as implicating an intrarenal mechanism in the impaired water excretion. This is because these maneuvers increase the GFR and improve distal delivery. Such maneuvers could also suppress baroreceptor-mediated AVP release and cause an osmotic diuresis, which would also improve water excretion.[302] Experimental models of deranged liver function, including acute portal hypertension by vein constriction, bile duct ligation, and chronic cirrhosis produced by administration of carbon tetrachloride have demonstrated a predominant role for AVP secretion in the pathogenesis of the disorder. In this latter model, an increment in hypothalamic AVP mRNA has also been demonstrated.[307] A study using an AVP antagonist also indicates a central role for AVP in the process.[308] As was the case in heart failure, increased expression of AQP2 has also been reported in the cirrhotic rat,[309] but dysregulation of AQP1 and AQP3 is also present in carbon tetrachloride (CCl_4)–induced cirrhosis.[310] In contrast, in the common bile duct model of cirrhosis, no increase in AQP2 was observed.[311]

Although patients with cirrhosis who have no edema or ascites excrete a water load normally, those with ascites usually do not. Several studies have demonstrated elevated AVP levels in these patients.[303] Patients who had a defect in water excretion had higher levels of AVP, plasma renin activity, plasma aldosterone, and norepinephrine,[312] as well as lower rates of PGE_2 production. Similarly, their serum albumin level was lower, as was their urinary excretion of Na^+, all suggesting a decrease in effective arterial blood volume. As is the case in heart failure, sympathetic tone is high in cirrhosis.[313] In fact, the plasma concentration of norepinephrine, a good index of baroreceptor activity in humans, appears to correlate well with the levels of AVP and excretion of water. These studies, therefore, offer strong support for the view that effective arterial blood volume is contracted, rather than expanded, in decompensated cirrhosis.[306] This concept is further strengthened by observations of subjects during head-out water immersion. This maneuver, which translocates fluid to the central blood volume, caused a decrease in AVP levels and improved water excretion[314] but, in this study, peripheral resistance decreased further. By combining head-out water immersion with norepinephrine administration in an effort to increase systemic pressure and peripheral resistance, water excretion was completely normalized.[315] Such observations underline the critical role of peripheral vasodilation in the pathologic process. The observation that inhibition of nitric oxide corrects the arterial hyporesponsiveness to vasodilators and the abnormal water excretion in cirrhotic rats provides strong evidence of a role for nitric oxide in the vasodilation.[316-318]

NEPHROTIC SYNDROME

The incidence of hyponatremia in the nephrotic syndrome is lower than in congestive heart failure or cirrhosis, most likely as a consequence of the higher blood pressure, higher GFR, and more modest impairments in Na^+ and water excretion than in the other groups of patients.[319] Because lipid levels are frequently elevated, a direct measurement of plasma osmolality should always be done. Diminished excretion of free water was first noted in children with the nephrotic syndrome, and since then other investigators[320] have noted elevated plasma levels of AVP in these patients. In view of the alterations in Starling forces that accompany hypoalbuminemia and allow transudation of salt and water across capillary membranes to the interstitial space, patients with the nephrotic syndrome are thought to have intravascular volume contraction. Increased levels of neurohumoral markers of decreased effective arterial blood volume also support this underfilling theory.[321] The possibility that this nonosmotic pathway stimulates AVP release was suggested by studies in which head-out water immersion and blood volume expansion[321] increased water excretion in nephrotic subjects. However, these pathogenic events may not be applicable to all patients with the disorder. Some patients with the nephrotic syndrome have increased plasma volumes with suppressed plasma renin activity and aldosterone levels.[322] The cause of these discrepancies is not immediately evident, but this overfill view has been subject to some criticism.[323] It is most likely that the underfilling mechanism is operant in patients with a normal GFR and with the histologic lesion of minimal change disease, and that hypervolemia may be more prevalent in patients with underlying glomerular pathology and decreased renal function. In such patients, an intrarenal mechanism probably causes Na^+ retention, as has been described in an experimental model of nephrotic syndrome.[324] Also, in contrast to the increase in AQP2 found in the previously described Na^+- and water-retaining states, the expression of AQP2 was decreased in two models of nephrotic syndrome induced with puromycin aminonucleoside[325] or doxorubicin.[326] The animals were not hyponatremic and most likely had expanded ECF volumes to explain the discrepancy.

RENAL FAILURE

Hyponatremia with edema can occur with acute or chronic renal failure. It is clear that in the setting of experimental or human renal disease, the ability to excrete free water is maintained better than the ability to reabsorb water. Nonetheless, the patient's GFR still determines the maximal rate of free water formation. Thus, whenever minimal urine osmolality is reduced to 150 to 250 mOsm/kg H_2O and fractional water excretion approaches 20% to 30% of the filtered load, the uremic patient with a GFR of 2 mL/min can excrete only 300 mL/day. Intake of more fluid than this will result in hyponatremia. Thus, in most cases, a decrement in GFR with an increase in thirst underlies the hyponatremia of patients with renal insufficiency.[327]

HYPONATREMIA WITH NORMAL EXTRACELLULAR FLUID VOLUME

Figure 16.16 lists the clinical entities that have to be considered in patients with hyponatremia whose volume is neither contracted nor expanded and who are, at least by clinical assessment, euvolemic. These are considered individually here.

GLUCOCORTICOID DEFICIENCY

Considerable evidence exists for an important role for glucocorticoids in the abnormal water excretion of adrenal insufficiency.[328] The water excretory defect of anterior pituitary insufficiency, and particularly ACTH deficiency, is associated with elevated AVP levels[329,330] and corrected by physiologic doses of glucocorticoids. Similarly, adrenalectomized dogs receiving replacement of mineralocorticoids still have abnormal water excretion. The relative importance of intrarenal factors and AVP in defective water excretion has been a matter of controversy. Studies using a sensitive radioimmunoassay for plasma AVP and the Brattleboro rat with hypothalamic DI have provided evidence that both factors are involved. Support for a role for AVP has been obtained in studies of conscious adrenalectomized, mineralocorticoid-replaced dogs[331] and rats[332] and with the use of an inhibitor of the hydro-osmotic effect of AVP.[287] Because the plasma AVP level was elevated despite a fall in plasma osmolality, the hormone's release was likely nonosmotically mediated. Although ECF volume was normal in both these studies, a decrease in systemic pressure and cardiac function[331,332] could have provided the hemodynamic stimulus for AVP release. In addition, there may be a direct effect of glucocorticoids that inhibits AVP secretion. In this regard, AVP gene expression is increased in glucocorticoid-deficient rats.[333] The presence of a glucocorticoid-responsive element on the AVP gene promoter may be responsible for the inhibition of AVP gene transcription by glucocorticoids.[334] Also, glucocorticoid receptors are present in magnocellular neurons and are increased during hypo-osmolality.[335]

A role for AVP-independent intrarenal factors was defined in the antidiuretic-deficient, adrenalectomized Brattleboro rat[332] and with use of AVP receptor antagonists.[287] It appears that prolonged glucocorticoid deficiency (14 to 17 days) is accompanied by decreases in renal hemodynamics that impair water excretion. A direct effect of glucocorticoid deficiency that enhances water permeability of the collecting duct has been proposed, but such a concept has not been supported by studies of anuran membranes suggesting that glucocorticoids enhance rather than inhibit water transport. Also, in vitro perfusion studies of the collecting duct of adrenalectomized rabbits have shown an impaired rather than enhanced AVP response,[336] a defect that may be related to enhanced cAMP metabolism.[337] AQP2 and AQP3 abundance appears not to be sensitive to glucocorticoids.[338]

In summary, the defect in glucocorticoid deficiency is primarily AVP-dependent, but an AVP-independent mechanism becomes evident with more prolonged hormone deficiency. It appears likely that alterations in systemic hemodynamics account for the nonosmotic release of AVP, but a direct effect of glucocorticoid hormone on AVP release has not been entirely excluded. The AVP-independent renal mechanism is probably caused by alterations in renal hemodynamics and not by a direct increase in collecting duct permeability. It should be remembered that secondary hypoadrenalism, as occurs in hypopituitarism, can also be associated with hyponatremia.[339,340]

HYPOTHYROIDISM

Patients and experimental animals with hypothyroidism often have impaired water excretion and sometimes develop hyponatremia.[328,341] The dilution defect is reversed by treatment with thyroid hormone. Both decreased delivery of filtrate to the diluting segment and persistent secretion of AVP, alone or in combination, have been proposed as mechanisms responsible for the defect.

Hypothyroidism has been shown to be associated with decreases in GFR and renal plasma flow.[341] In the AVP-deficient Brattleboro rat, the decrement in maximal free water excretion can be entirely accounted for by the decrease in GFR. The osmotic threshold for AVP release appears not to be altered in hypothyroidism.[342] The normal suppression of AVP release with water loading and the normal response to hypertonic saline,[343] coupled with the failure to observe upregulation of hypothalamic AVP gene expression in hypothyroid rats,[344] supports an AVP-independent mechanism. There is, however, also evidence for a role of AVP in impairing water excretion in hypothyroidism. In experimental animals[345] and humans with advanced hypothyroidism,[341] elevated AVP levels were measured in the basal state and after a water load. Although increased sensitivity to AVP in hypothyroidism has been proposed, experimental evidence suggests the contrary, because urine osmolality is relatively low for the circulating levels of the hormone[345] and AVP-stimulated cyclase is impaired in the renal medulla of hypothyroid rats,[346] possibly leading to decreased AQP2 expression.[347] However, the predominant defect is one of water excretion with increased AQP2 expression and reversal with a V_2 receptor antagonist.[348] It appears, therefore, that diminished distal fluid delivery and persistent AVP release mediate the impaired water excretion in this disorder, but the relative contributions of these two factors remain undefined and may depend on the severity of the endocrine disorder.

PRIMARY POLYDIPSIA

It has long been recognized that patients with psychiatric disease demonstrate increased water intake. Although such polydipsia is normally not associated with hyponatremia, it has been observed that these patients are at increased risk of developing hyponatremia when they are acutely psychotic.[349] Most of these patients have schizophrenia, but some have psychotic depression. The frequency of hyponatremia in this population of patients is unknown, but in a survey conducted in one large psychiatric hospital, 20 polydipsic patients with a serum $[Na^+]$ lower than 124 mEq/L were reported,[350] and another survey found hyponatremia in 8 of 239 patients.[351] Elucidation of the mechanism of the impaired water excretion has been confounded by antipsychotic drug treatment (see later). The relative contributions of the pharmacologic agent and the psychosis are therefore difficult to define, because thiazides and carbamazepine are also frequently implicated.[352] Nonetheless, there have been reports of psychotic patients who suffered water intoxication, even when free of medication.[353]

The mechanism responsible for the hyponatremia in psychosis appears to be multifactorial. In a comprehensive study of water metabolism in eight psychotic hyponatremic patients and seven psychotic, normonatremic control subjects, no unifying defect emerged. The investigators found a small defect in osmoregulation that caused AVP to be secreted at plasma osmolalities somewhat lower than those of the control group, but they did not observe a true resetting of the osmostat. Also, the hyponatremic patients had a mild urine dilution defect, even in the absence of AVP. When AVP was present, the renal response was somewhat enhanced, suggesting increased renal sensitivity to the hormone. Psychotic exacerbations appear to be associated with increased AVP levels in schizophrenic patients with hyponatremia.[354] Finally, thirst perception is also increased, because excessive water intake that exceeds excretory capacity is responsible for most episodes of hyponatremia in these patients. However, concurrent nausea caused increased AVP levels in some of the subjects.[355] Although each of these derangements by itself would remain clinically unimportant, it is possible that during exacerbation of the psychosis the defects are more pronounced, and that in combination they can culminate in hyponatremia.[356]

Hyponatremia also occurs in beer drinkers (so-called beer potomania). Although this has been ascribed to an increase in fluid intake in the setting of very low solute intake,[357] such patients may also have sustained significant solute losses.[358]

POSTOPERATIVE HYPONATREMIA

The incidence of hospital-acquired hyponatremia is high in adults[206] and children[359] and is particularly prevalent in the postoperative stage[360,361] (incidence $\cong$ 4%). Most affected patients appear clinically euvolemic and have measurable levels of AVP in their circulation.[360,362] Although this occurs primarily as a consequence of administration of hypotonic fluids,[363] a decrease in serum $[Na^+]$ can occur in this high-AVP state, even when isotonic fluids are given.[364] Hyponatremia has also been reported following cardiac catheterization in patients receiving hypotonic fluids.[365] Although the presence of hyponatremia is a marker for poor outcomes, this is likely a consequence not of the hyponatremia per se but of the severe underlying disease associated with it. There is, however, a subgroup of postoperative hyponatremic patients, almost always premenstrual women, who develop catastrophic neurologic events, frequently accompanied by seizures and hypoxia.[366,367]

ENDURANCE EXERCISE

There has been increasing recognition that strenuous endurance exercise, such as military training[368] and marathons and triathlons,[369] can cause hyponatremia that is frequently symptomatic. A review of 57 such patients found a mean serum $[Na^+]$ of 121 mEq/L.[370] A prospective study of 488 runners in the Boston Marathon revealed that 13% of the runners had a serum $[Na^+]$ lower than 130 mEq/L. A multivariate analysis revealed that weight gain related to excessive fluid intake was the strongest single predictor of the hyponatremia. Longer racing times and a very low body mass index (BMI) were also predictors.[371] Composition of the fluids consumed and use of NSAIDs was not predictive. Symptomatic hyponatremia is even more frequent in ultraendurance events.[372]

PHARMACOLOGIC AGENTS

Many drugs have been associated with water retention. Some of the more clinically important ones are discussed here.

Desmopressin

Because desmopressin is a selective agonist of the AVP V_2 receptors, it would be expected that patients treated with desmopressin are at increased risk of developing hyponatremia. The reported incidence of patients treated with desmopressin for DI is actually low because they generally do not drink excessive amounts of fluid. However, patients who receive desmopressin at higher doses for indications such as von Willebrand's disease,[373] or older patients with decreased renal function who receive desmopressin for nocturnal enuresis,[374,375] can develop symptomatic hyponatremia.

Chlorpropamide

The incidence of mild hyponatremia in patients taking chlorpropamide may be as high as 7%, but severe hyponatremia (<130 mEq/L) occurs in 2% of patients so treated.[376] As noted earlier, the drug exerts its action primarily by potentiating the renal action of AVP.[377] Studies of toad urinary bladder have demonstrated that although chlorpropamide alone has no effect, it enhances AVP- and theophylline-stimulated water flow but decreases cAMP-mediated flow. The enhanced response may be due to upregulation of the AVP V_2 receptor.[378] Alternatively, studies of chlorpropamide-treated animals have suggested that the drug enhances solute reabsorption in the medullary ascending limb (thereby increasing interstitial tonicity and the osmotic drive for water reabsorption) rather than a cAMP-mediated alteration in collecting duct water permeability.[379]

Carbamazepine and Oxcarbazepine

The anticonvulsant drug carbamazepine is well known to have antidiuretic properties. The incidence of hyponatremia in carbamazepine-treated patients was believed to be as high as 21%, but a survey of patients with mental retardation reported a lower incidence of 5%.[380] Cases continue to be reported.[381] The antiepileptic oxcarbazepine, of the same class as carbamazepine, has also been reported to cause hyponatremia.[382] Evidence exists for a mechanism mediated by AVP secretion and for renal enhancement of the hormone's action[383] to explain carbamazepine's antidiuretic effect. The drug also appears to decrease the sensitivity of the AVP response to osmotic stimulation.[384]

Psychotropic Drugs

An increasing number of psychotropic drugs have been associated with hyponatremia, and they are frequently implicated to explain the water intoxication in psychotic patients. Among the agents implicated are the phenothiazines, the butyrophenone haloperidol, and the tricyclic antidepressants.[385-387] An increasing number of cases of amphetamine (ecstasy)-related hyponatremia have been described.[388,389] Similarly, the widely used antidepressants fluoxetine,[390] sertraline,[391] and paroxetine[392] have been associated with hyponatremia. In this latter study, involving 75 patients, 12% developed hyponatremia (serum [Na⁺] < 135 mmol/L). Older adults appear to be particularly susceptible, with an incidence as high as 22% to 28%.[393-396] The tendency for these drugs to cause hyponatremia is further compounded by their anticholinergic effects. By drying the mucous membranes, they can stimulate water intake. The role of these drugs in impaired water excretion has not, in most cases, been dissociated from the role of the underlying disorder for which the drug was given. Furthermore, evaluation of the effect of the drugs on AVP secretion has frequently revealed a failure to increase levels of the hormone, particularly if mean arterial pressure remained unaltered. Therefore, although a clinical association between antipsychotic drugs and hyponatremia is frequently encountered, the pharmacologic agents themselves may not be the principal factors responsible for the water retention.

Antineoplastic Drugs

Several drugs used in cancer therapy cause antidiuresis. The effect of vincristine may be mediated by the drug's neurotoxic effect on the hypothalamic microtubule system, which then alters normal osmoreceptor control of AVP release.[397] A retrospective survey has suggested that this may be more common in Asians who were given the drug.[398] The mechanism of the diluting defect that results from cyclophosphamide administration is not fully understood. It may act, at least in part, to enhance action, because the drug does not increase hormone levels.[399] It is known that the antidiuresis has its onset 4 to 12 hours after injection of the drug, lasts as long as 12 hours, and seems to be temporally related to excretion of a metabolite. The importance of anticipating potentially severe hyponatremia in cyclophosphamide-treated patients who are vigorously hydrated to prevent urologic complications cannot be overstated. The synthetic analogue of cyclophosphamide, ifosfamide, has also been associated with hyponatremia and AVP secretion.[400]

Narcotics

Since the 1940s, it has been known that the administration of opioid agonists, such as morphine, reduces urine flow by causing the release of an antidiuretic substance. The possibility that endogenous opioids could serve as potential neurotransmitters has been suggested by the finding of enkephalins in nerve fibers projecting from the hypothalamus to the pars nervosa. However, the reported effects vary; they range from stimulation to no change and even to inhibition of AVP secretion. The reasons for these diverse observations may be that the opiates and their receptors are widely distributed in the brain, implying that the site of action of the opiate can differ markedly, depending on the route of administration. Also, there are multiple opiate peptides and receptor types. It has now been determined that agonists of μ-receptors have antidiuretic properties, whereas δ-receptors have the opposite effect.

Miscellaneous Agents

Several case reports have suggested an association between the use of ACE inhibitors and hyponatremia.[401-403] Of interest is that all three reported patients were women in their 60s. The use of ACE inhibition was also a concomitant risk factor for the development of hyponatremia in a survey of veterans who received chlorpropamide.[376] However, given the widespread use of these agents, the true incidence of hyponatremia must be vanishingly low. Similarly, an association with angiotensin receptor blockers has not been reported to date. Rare patients have been reported to develop hyponatremia during amiodarone loading.[404]

SYNDROME OF INAPPROPRIATE ANTIDIURETIC HORMONE SECRETION

The syndrome of inappropriate antidiuretic hormone secretion (SIADH) is the most common cause of hyponatremia in hospitalized patients.[261] As first described by Schwartz and associates[405] in two patients with bronchogenic carcinoma, and later characterized further by Bartter and Schwartz,[406] patients with this syndrome have serum hypo-osmolality when excreting urine that is less than maximally dilute (>100 mOsm/kg H_2O). Thus, a diagnostic criterion for this syndrome is the presence of inappropriate urine concentration. The development of hyponatremia with a dilute urine (<100 mOsm/kg H_2O) should raise suspicion of a primary polydipsic disorder. Although large volumes of fluid need to be ingested to overwhelm the normal water excretory ability, this volume need not be excessively high if there are concomitant decreases in solute intake.[407] In SIADH, the urinary Na^+ is dependent on intake, because Na^+ balance is well maintained. As such, urinary Na^+ concentration is usually high, but it may be low in patients with the syndrome who are receiving a low-sodium diet. The presence of Na^+ in the urine is helpful in excluding extrarenal causes of hypovolemic hyponatremia, but a low urinary Na^+ concentration does not exclude SIADH. Before the diagnosis of SIADH is made, other causes for a decreased diluting capacity, such as renal, pituitary, adrenal, thyroid, cardiac, or hepatic disease, must be excluded. In addition, nonosmotic stimuli for AVP release, particularly hemodynamic derangements (e.g., caused by hypotension, nausea, or drugs), need to be ruled out.

Another clue to the presence of SIADH is the finding of hypouricemia. In one study, 16 of 17 patients had levels below 4 mg/dL, whereas in 13 patients with hyponatremia of other causes the level was higher than 5 mg/dL. Hypouricemia appears to occur as a consequence of increased urate clearance.[408] Measurement of an elevated level of AVP can confirm the clinical diagnosis, but is not necessary. It should be noted that most patients with SIADH have AVP levels in the normal range (≤10 pg/mL); the presence of any measurable AVP is, however, abnormal in the hypoosmolar state. Because the presence of hyponatremia is itself evidence for abnormal dilution, a formal urine-diluting test need not be performed in most cases. The water loading test is helpful in determining whether an abnormality remains in a patient whose serum [Na^+] has been corrected by water restriction. Because Brattleboro rats receiving AVP,[409] and an animal model of SIADH, have displayed upregulation of AQP2 expression, the excretion of AQP2 has been investigated as a marker for the persistent secretion of AVP. The excretion of the water channel remains elevated in patients with SIADH but this is not specific to this entity because a similar pattern was observed in patients with hyponatremia due to hypopituitarism.[410]

PATHOPHYSIOLOGY

In 1953, Leaf and associates[411] described the effects of chronic AVP administration on Na^+ and water balance. They noted that high-volume water intake was required for the development of hyponatremia. Concomitant with the water retention, an increment in urinary Na^+ excretion was noted. The relative contributions of the water retention and Na^+ loss to the development of hyponatremia were subsequently investigated. Acute water loading causes transient natriuresis but, when water intake is increased more slowly, no significant negative Na^+ loss can be documented. These studies have clearly demonstrated that the hyponatremia is mainly a consequence of water retention; however, it must be noted that the net increase in water balance fails to account entirely for the decrement in serum [Na^+].[411] In a carefully studied model of SIADH in rats, the retained water was found to be distributed in the intracellular space and in equilibrium with the tonicity of ECF.[412] The natriuresis and kaliuresis that occur early in the development of this model contribute to a decrement of body solutes and, in part, account for the observed hyponatremia.[413] Studies involving analysis of whole-body water and electrolyte content have demonstrated that the relative contributions of water retention and solute losses vary with the duration of induced hyponatremia; the former is central to the process but, with more prolonged hyponatremia, Na^+ depletion becomes predominant.[414] In this regard, it has even been suggested that the natriuresis and volume contraction are important components of the syndrome that maintains the secretion of AVP,[415] with atrial natriuretic peptide as a mediator of the Na^+ loss.[416] Therefore, although natriuresis frequently accompanies the syndrome, nonosmotically stimulated AVP secretion is essential. Finally, patients with the syndrome must also have abnormal thirst regulation, whereby the osmotic inhibition of water intake is not operant. The mechanism of this failure to suppress thirst is not fully understood, but may simply reflect the continued ingestion of beverages for reasons other than true thirst.

After the initial retention of water, loss of Na^+, and development of hyponatremia, continued administration of AVP is accompanied by reestablishment of Na^+ balance and a decline in the hydro-osmotic effect of the hormone. The integrity of renal regulation of Na^+ balance is manifested by the ability to conserve Na^+ during Na^+ restriction and by the normal excretion of a Na^+ load. Thus, the mechanisms that regulate Na^+ excretion are intact. Loss of the hydro-osmotic effect of AVP, albeit to varying degrees, has been evident in many studies[411,413] because urine flow increases and urine osmolality decreases, despite continued administration of the hormone. This effect has been termed *vasopressin escape*.[417] Several studies have demonstrated that hypotonic ECF volume expansion, rather than chronic administration of AVP per se, is needed for escape to occur because the escape phenomenon is seen only when positive water balance is achieved.[417]

The cellular mechanisms responsible for vasopressin escape have been the subject of some investigation. Studies of broken epithelial cell preparations of the toad urinary bladder have revealed downregulation of AVP receptors,[418] as well as vasopressin binding in the inner medulla.[419] Post-cAMP mechanisms are probably also operant. In this regard, a decrease in expression of AQP2 has been reported in the process of escape from desmopressin-induced antidiuresis, without a concomitant change in basolateral AQP3 and AQP4.[420,421] The decrement in AQP2 was associated with decreased V_2 responsiveness.[420] The distal tubule also has an increase in sodium transporters, including the α- and γ-subunits of the epithelial sodium channel and the thiazide-sensitive Na^+-Cl^- cotransporter.[422] In addition to a renal mechanism, it appears that chronic hyponatremia causes a decrement in hypothalamic mRNA production, a process that could ameliorate the syndrome in the clinical setting.[27]

CLINICAL SETTINGS

It is now apparent that the previously described pathophysiologic sequence occurs in a variety of clinical settings

Table 16.6 Disorders Associated with Syndrome of Inappropriate Antidiuretic Hormone Secretion

Carcinomas	Pulmonary Disorders	Central Nervous System Disorders	Other Disorders
Bronchogenic carcinoma	Viral pneumonia	Encephalitis (viral or bacterial)	AIDS
Carcinoma of the duodenum	Bacterial pneumonia	Meningitis (viral, bacterial, tuberculous, fungal)	Prolonged exercise
Carcinoma of the ureter	Pulmonary abscess	Head trauma	Idiopathic (in older individuals)
Carcinoma of the pancreas	Tuberculosis	Brain abscess	Nephrogenic
Thymoma	Aspergillosis	Guillain-Barré syndrome	Acute intermittent porphyria
Carcinoma of the stomach	Positive pressure breathing	Subarachnoid hemorrhage or subdural hematoma	
Lymphoma	Asthma	Cerebellar and cerebral atrophy	
Ewing's sarcoma	Pneumothorax	Cavernous sinus thrombosis	
Carcinoma of the bladder	Mesothelioma	Neonatal hypoxia	
Prostatic carcinoma	Cystic fibrosis	Shy-Drager syndrome	
Oropharyngeal tumor		Rocky Mountain spotted fever	
		Delirium tremens	
		Cerebrovascular accident (cerebral thrombosis or hemorrhage)	
		Acute psychosis	
		Peripheral neuropathy	
		Multiple sclerosis	

Adapted from Berl T, Schrier RW: Disorders of water metabolism. In Schrier RW, editor: *Renal and electrolyte disorders*, ed 6, Philadelphia, 2003, Lippincott Williams & Wilkins.

characterized by persistent AVP secretion. Since the original report of Schwartz and coworkers,[405] the syndrome has been described in an increasing number of clinical settings (Table 16.6). These fall into four general categories[423]: (1) malignancies; (2) pulmonary disease; (3) CNS disorders; and (4) drug effects. In addition, an increasing number of patients with acquired immunodeficiency syndrome have been reported to have hyponatremia. The frequency may be as high as 35% of hospitalized patients with the disease and, in as many as two thirds, SIADH may be the underlying cause.[424] As was noted previously, hyponatremia caused by excessive water repletion can occur after moderate and severe exercise.[369,370,425,426] Finally, it is increasingly recognized that an idiopathic form is common in older adults.[427-430] As many as 25% of older patients admitted to a rehabilitation center had a serum [Na$^+$] lower than 135 mEq/L.[428] In a significant proportion of these patients, no underlying cause was discovered. This may be related to an increase in AQP2 production and excretion in this age group.[431]

A material with antidiuretic properties has been extracted from some of the tumors or metastases of patients with malignancy-associated SIADH. However, not all patients with the syndrome have AVP in their tumors. Of the tumors that cause SIADH secretion, bronchogenic carcinoma, and particularly small cell lung cancer, is the most common, with a reported incidence of 11%.[432] It appears that patients with bronchogenic carcinoma have higher plasma AVP levels in relation to plasma osmolality, even if they do not manifest full-blown SIADH; however, in patients with the syndrome, the levels of the hormone are higher. The possibility that the hormone could serve as a marker of bronchogenic carcinoma has been suggested, and SIADH has been reported occasionally to precede diagnosis of the tumor by several months.[433] In view of the potential to treat patients with this tumor, it is important that patients with unexplained SIADH be fully investigated and evaluated for the presence of this malignancy. Head and neck malignancies are the second most common tumors associated with SIADH, which occurs in approximately 3% of such patients.

The mechanism whereby AVP is produced in other pulmonary disorders is not known, but the associated abnormalities in blood gases could act as mediators of the effect. Antidiuretic activity has also been assayed in tuberculous lung tissue. The syndrome can also occur in the setting of miliary rather than only lung-limited tuberculosis.[434] In CNS disorders, AVP is most likely released from the neurohypophysis. Studies of monkeys have shown that elevations of intracranial pressure cause AVP secretion, which may be the mechanism that mediates the syndrome in at least some CNS disorders. The magnocellular AVP-secreting cells in the hypothalamus are subject to numerous excitatory inputs (see Figure 16.6), and therefore it is conceivable that a large variety of neurologic disorders can stimulate the secretion of AVP.

Although SIADH as typically described is associated with inappropriate secretion of AVP, hyponatremia has been described in two infants who met all the criteria for a diagnosis of SIADH but had undetectable AVP levels. Genetic analysis revealed a gain-of-function mutation at the X-linked AVP V$_2$ receptor, where in codon 137 a missense mutation resulted in the change from arginine to cysteine or leucine. The authors termed this *nephrogenic syndrome of inappropriate antidiuresis* (NSIAD).[435]

Zerbe and colleagues have studied osmoregulation of AVP secretion in a large group of patients with SIADH.[436] In

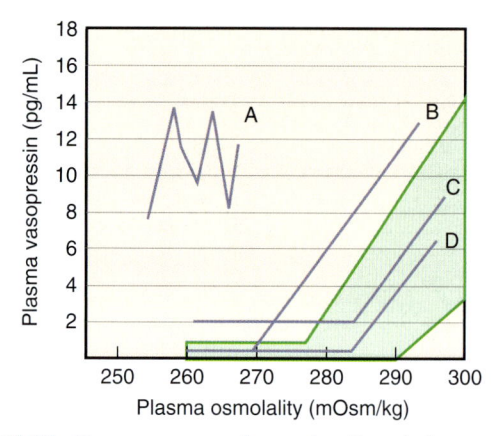

Figure 16.17 Plasma vasopressin as a function of plasma osmolality during the infusion of hypertonic saline in four groups of patients with clinical syndrome of inappropriate antidiuretic hormone (SIADH). *Shaded area,* Range of normal values. See text for description of each group. (From Zerbe R, Stropes L, Robertson G: Vasopressin function in the syndrome of inappropriate antidiuresis. *Annu Rev Med* 31:315, 1980.)

the great majority, the plasma AVP concentration was inadequately suppressed relative to the hypotonicity present. In most patients, the plasma AVP concentration ranged from 1 to 10 pg/mL, the same range as in normally hydrated healthy adults. Inappropriate secretion, therefore, can often be demonstrated only by measuring AVP under hypotonic conditions. Even with this approach, however, abnormalities in plasma AVP were not apparent in almost 10% of patients with clinical evidence of SIADH. To define the nature of the osmoregulatory defect in these patients better, plasma AVP was measured during infusion of hypertonic saline. When this method of analysis was applied to 25 patients with SIADH, four different types of osmoregulatory defects were identified.

As shown in Figure 16.17, infusion of hypertonic saline in the type A osmoregulatory defect was associated with large and erratic fluctuations in plasma AVP, which bore no relation to the rise in plasma osmolality. This pattern was found in 6 of 25 patients studied who had acute respiratory failure, bronchogenic carcinoma, pulmonary tuberculosis, schizophrenia, or rheumatoid arthritis. This pattern indicates that the secretion of AVP had been totally divorced from osmoreceptor control or was responding to some periodic nonosmotic stimulus.

A completely different type of osmoregulatory defect is exemplified by the type B response (see Figure 16.17). The infusion of hypertonic saline resulted in prompt and progressive rises in plasma osmolality. Regression analyses have shown that the precision and sensitivity of this response are essentially the same as those in healthy subjects, except that the intercept or threshold value at 253 mOsm/kg is well below the normal range. This pattern, which reflects the resetting of the osmoreceptor, was found in 9 of 25 patients who had a diagnosis of bronchogenic carcinoma, cerebrovascular disease, tuberculous meningitis, acute respiratory disease, or carcinoma of the pharynx. Another patient was reported with hyponatremia and acute idiopathic polyneuritis who reacted in an identical manner to the hypertonic saline infusion and was determined to have resetting of the osmoreceptor. Because their threshold function is retained when they receive a water load, this patient and others with reset osmostats have been able to dilute their urine maximally and sustain a urine flow sufficient to prevent a further increase in body water. Thus, an abnormality in AVP regulation can exist in spite of the ability to dilute the urine maximally and excrete a water load at some lower level of plasma osmolality.

In the type C response (see Figure 16.17), plasma AVP was elevated initially but did not change during the infusion of hypertonic saline until plasma osmolality reached the normal range. At that point, plasma AVP began to rise appropriately, indicating a normally functioning osmoreceptor mechanism. This response was found in 8 of 25 patients with the diagnosis of CNS disease, bronchogenic carcinoma, carcinoma of the pharynx, pulmonary tuberculosis, or schizophrenia. Its pathogenesis is unknown, but the authors speculated that it may be due to a constant, nonsuppressible leak of AVP, despite otherwise normal osmoregulatory function.[436] Unlike type B, the resetting type of defect, the type C response results in impaired urine dilution and water excretion at all levels of plasma osmolality.

In the type D response (see Figure 16.17), the osmoregulation of AVP appears to be completely normal, despite a marked inability to excrete a water load. The plasma AVP is appropriately suppressed under hypotonic conditions and does not rise until plasma osmolality reaches the normal threshold level. When this procedure is reversed by water loading, plasma osmolality and plasma AVP again fall normally, but urine dilution does not occur, and the water load is not excreted. This defect was present in 2 of 25 patients diagnosed with bronchogenic carcinoma, indicating that in these patients, the antidiuretic defect is caused by some abnormality other than SIADH. It could be due to increased renal tubule sensitivity to AVP or the presence of an antidiuretic substance other than AVP. Alternatively, it is possible that currently available assays are not sensitive enough to detect significant levels of AVP. It is intriguing to speculate that some of these subjects have NSIAD, as described previously,[435] but only a small number of adult kindreds with this diagnosis have been described.[437]

It is of interest that patients with bronchogenic carcinoma, which has generally been believed to be associated with ectopic production of AVP, manifested every category of osmoregulatory defect, including the reset osmostat. It has been suggested that many of these tumors probably cause SIADH secretion not by producing the hormone ectopically, but by interfering with the normal osmoregulation of AVP secretion from the neurohypophysis through direct invasion of the vagus nerve, metastatic implants in the hypothalamus, or some other more generalized neuropathic change.

HYPONATREMIA SYMPTOMS, MORBIDITY, AND MORTALITY

Symptoms of hyponatremia correlate with the degree of decrease in the serum [Na$^+$] and with the chronicity of the hyponatremia. Most clinical manifestations of hyponatremia usually begin at a serum [Na$^+$] lower than 130 mEq/L, although mild neurocognitive symptoms can

Table 16.7 Classification of Hyponatremia According to Severity of Presenting Symptoms

Severity	Serum Sodium Level	Neurologic Symptoms	Typical Duration of Hyponatremia
Severe	<125 mmol/L	Vomiting, seizures, obtundation, respiratory distress, coma	Acute (<24-48 hours)
Moderate	<130 mmol/L	Nausea, confusion, disorientation, altered mental status, unstable gait, falls	Intermediate or chronic (>24-48 hours)
Mild	<135 mmol/L	Headache, irritability, difficulty concentrating, altered mood, depression	Chronic (several days to many weeks or months)

(From Verbalis JG: Emergency management of acute and chronic hyponatremia. In Matfin G, editor: *Endocrine and metabolic emergencies*, Washington DC, 2014, Endocrine Press, p 352.)

begin at any sodium level that is low (Table 16.7). Although gastrointestinal complaints often occur early, most of the manifestations of hyponatremia are neurologic, including lethargy, confusion, disorientation, obtundation, and seizures, designated as hyponatremic encephalopathy.[438] Many of the symptoms of hyponatremic encephalopathy are caused by cerebral edema, which may, at least in part, be mediated by AQP4.[439] In its most severe form, the cerebral edema can lead to tentorial herniation; in such cases, death can occur as a result of brainstem compression with respiratory arrest. The cerebral edema can also cause a neurogenic pulmonary edema and hypoxemia,[440] which can in turn increase the severity of brain swelling.[441] In a retrospective study of 168 hyponatremic patients, most of them acute, there was a strong (13-fold) association between the development of hypoxemia and the risk of mortality.[442] The most severe life-threatening clinical features of hyponatremic encephalopathy are generally seen in cases of acute hyponatremia, defined as shorter than 48 hours in duration. These symptoms can occur abruptly, sometimes with little warning.[438] A number of acutely hyponatremic patients have been reported to develop rhabdomyolysis also.[415]

The development of neurologic symptoms also depends on the age, gender, and magnitude and acuteness of the process. Older persons and young children with hyponatremia are most likely to develop symptoms. It has also become apparent that neurologic complications occur more frequently in menstruating women. In a case-control study, Ayus and colleagues noted that despite an approximately equal incidence of postoperative hyponatremia in males and females, 97% of those with permanent brain damage were women, and 75% of them were menstruating.[367] However, this view is not universally held, because others have not found increased postoperative hyponatremia in this population,[443] and Ayus and associates' retrospective study[367] did not reveal a gender or age association with mortality.[442]

The degree of clinical impairment is related not to the absolute measured level of lowered serum [Na$^+$], but to the rate and extent of the decrease in ECF osmolality. In a survey of hospitalized hyponatremic patients (serum [Na$^+$] < 128 mEq/L), 46% had CNS symptoms and 54% were asymptomatic.[444] It is notable, however, that the authors thought that the hyponatremia was the cause of the symptoms in only 31% of the symptomatic patients. In this subgroup of symptomatic patients, the mortality was no different from that of asymptomatic patients (9% to 10%). In contrast, the mortality of patients whose CNS symptoms were not caused by hyponatremia was high (64%), suggesting that the mortality of these patients is more often due to the associated disease than to the electrolyte disorder itself. This is in agreement with Anderson's study,[261] who noted a 60-fold increase in mortality in hyponatremic patients over that of normonatremic control subjects. In the hyponatremic patients, death frequently occurred after the plasma [Na$^+$] was returned to normal and was generally thought to be due to the progression of severe underlying disease; this suggests that the hyponatremia is an indicator of severe disease and poor prognosis. In fact, a number of studies have further indicated that even mild hyponatremia is an independent predictor of higher mortality across a wide variety of disorders, including patients with acute ST-elevation myocardial infarction, heart failure, and liver disease.[445,446]

The mortality of acute symptomatic hyponatremia has been noted to be as high as 55% and as low as 5%.[447,448] The former reflects the observation of few symptomatic hyponatremic patients in a consultative setting; the latter is the estimate from a broad-based literature survey. Equally controversial is the mortality rate associated with hyponatremia in children. One series found no in-hospital deaths attributable to hyponatremia, but others described an 8.4% mortality in postoperative children and estimated that more than 600 U.S. children die annually as a result of hyponatremia.[263] The mortality associated with chronic hyponatremia has been reported to be between 14% and 27%.[449,450]

The observed central nervous system symptoms are most likely related to the cellular swelling and cerebral edema that result from acute lowering of ECF osmolality, which leads to movement of water into cells. In fact, such cerebral edema occasionally causes herniation, as has been noted in postmortem examination of both humans and experimental animals. The increase in brain water is, however, much less marked than would be predicted from the decrease in tonicity were the brain to operate as a passive osmometer. The volume regulatory responses that protect against cerebral edema, and which probably occur throughout the body, have been extensively studied and reviewed.[450a] Studies of rats demonstrate a prompt loss of both electrolyte and organic osmolytes after the onset of hyponatremia.[450b] Some of the osmolyte losses occur very quickly within 24 hours,[450c]

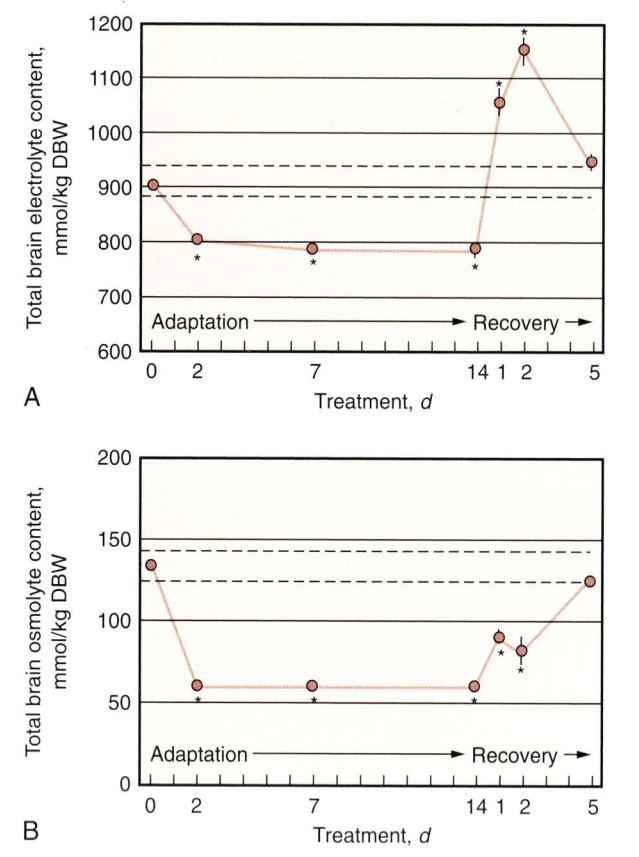

Figure 16.18 Comparison of changes in brain electrolyte (**A**) and organic osmolyte (**B**) content during adaptation to hyponatremia and after rapid correction of hyponatremia in rats. Electrolytes and organic osmolytes are lost quickly after the induction of hyponatremia, beginning on day (*d*) 0. Brain content of both solutes remains depressed during maintenance of hyponatremia from days 2 through 14. After rapid correction of the hyponatremia on day 14, electrolytes reaccumulate rapidly and overshoot normal brain contents on the first 2 days after correction, before returning to normal levels by the fifth day after correction. In contrast, brain organic osmolytes recover much more slowly and do not return to normal brain contents until the fifth day after correction. The *dashed lines* indicate ± SEM (standard error of mean) from the mean values of normonatremic rats on day 0; $P < 0.01$ compared with brain contents of normonatremic rats. DBW, Dry brain weight. (Data from Verbalis JG, Gullans SR: Hyponatremia causes large sustained reductions in brain content of multiple organic osmolytes in rats. *Brain Res* 567:274-282, 1991; and Verbalis JG, Gullans SR: Rapid correction of hyponatremia produces differential effects on brain osmolyte and electrolyte reaccumulation in rats. *Brain Res* 606:19-27, 1993.)

and in experimental animals most of the brain solute loss is completed by 48 hours (Figure 16.18).

The rate at which the brain restores the lost electrolytes and osmolytes when hyponatremia is corrected is also of pathophysiologic importance. Na^+ and Cl^- recover quickly and even overshoot normal brain contents.[450d] However, the reaccumulation of osmolytes is considerably delayed (see Figure 16.18). This process is likely to account for the more marked cerebral dehydration that accompanies the correction in previously adapted animals.[450e] It has been observed that urea may prevent the myelinosis associated with this pathology. This may be due to the more rapid reac-cumulation of organic osmolytes, and particularly myoinositol in the azotemic state.[450f]

In contrast to acute hyponatremia, chronic hyponatremia is much less symptomatic. The reason for the profound differences between the symptoms of acute and chronic hyponatremia is now well understood to be caused by the process of brain volume regulation described above.[451] Despite this powerful adaptation process, chronic hyponatremia is frequently associated with neurologic symptomatology, albeit milder and more subtle in nature (see Table 16.7). One report found a fairly high incidence of symptoms in 223 patients with chronic hyponatremia as a result of thiazide administration—49% had malaise-lethargy, 47% had dizzy spells, 35% had vomiting, 17% had confusion-obtundation, 17% experienced falls, 6% had headaches, and 0.9% had seizures.[452] Although dizziness can potentially be attributed to a diuretic-induced hypovolemia, symptoms such as confusion, obtundation, and seizures are more consistent with hyponatremic symptomatology. Because thiazide-induced hyponatremia can be readily corrected by stopping the thiazide and/or administering sodium, this represents an ideal situation in which to assess improvement in hyponatremia symptomatology with normalization of the serum $[Na^+]$; in this study, all these symptoms improved with correction of the hyponatremia. This represents one of the best examples demonstrating reversal of the symptoms associated with chronic hyponatremia by correction of the hyponatremia, because the patients in this study did not in general have severe underlying comorbidities that might complicate interpretation of their symptoms, as is often the case in patients with SIADH.

Even in patients adjudged to be "asymptomatic" by virtue of a normal neurologic examination, accumulating evidence suggests that there may be previously unrecognized adverse effects as a result of chronic hyponatremia. In one study, 16 patients with hyponatremia secondary to SIADH, in the range of 124 to 130 mmol/L demonstrated a significant gait instability that normalized after correction of the hyponatremia to a normal range.[453] The functional significance of the gait instability was illustrated in a study of 122 Belgian patients with a variety of levels of hyponatremia, all judged to be asymptomatic at the time of visit to an emergency department (ED). These patients were compared with 244 age-, gender-, and disease-matched controls also presenting to the ED during the same time period. Researchers found that 21% of the hyponatremic patients came to the ED because of a recent fall, compared to only 5% of the controls; this difference was highly significant and remained so after multivariable adjustment.[453] Consequently, this study clearly documented an increased incidence of falls in so-called asymptomatic hyponatremic patients.

The clinical significance of the gait instability and fall data have been indicated by multiple independent studies that demonstrated increased rates of bone fractures in patients with hyponatremia.[454-457] Other studies have shown that hyponatremia is associated with increased bone loss in experimental animals and a significantly increased odds ratio for osteoporosis of the femoral neck in those older than 50 years in the Third National Health and Nutrition Examination Survey (NHANES III) database.[458] Thus, the major clinical significance of chronic hyponatremia may lie in the increased morbidity and mortality associated with falls and fractures in our older population.

HYPONATREMIA TREATMENT

Correction of hyponatremia is associated with markedly improved neurologic outcomes in patients with severely symptomatic hyponatremia. In a retrospective review of patients who presented with severe neurologic symptoms and serum [Na$^+$] lower than 125 mmol/L, prompt therapy with isotonic or hypertonic saline resulted in a correction of about 20 mEq/L over several days and neurologic recovery in almost all cases; in contrast, in patients who were treated with fluid restriction alone, there was very little correction over the study period (<5 mEq/L over 72 hours), and the neurologic outcomes were much worse, with most of these patients dying or entering a persistent vegetative state.[459] Consequently, based on this and many similar retrospective analyses, prompt therapy to increase the serum [Na$^+$] rapidly represents the standard of care for treatment of patients presenting with severe life-threatening symptoms of hyponatremia.

Brain herniation, the most dreaded complication of hyponatremia, is seen almost exclusively in patients with acute hyponatremia (usually <24 hours) or in patients with intracranial pathology.[460-462] In postoperative patients and in patients with self-induced water intoxication associated with marathon running, psychosis, or use of ecstasy (3,4-methylenedioxy-methamphetamine [MDMA]), nonspecific symptoms such as headache, nausea and vomiting, or confusion can rapidly progress to seizures, respiratory arrest, and ultimately death or to a permanent vegetative state as a complication of severe cerebral edema.[463] Hypoxia from noncardiogenic pulmonary edema and/or hypoventilation can exacerbate brain swelling caused by the low serum [Na$^+$].[440,441] Seizures can complicate severe chronic hyponatremia and acute hyponatremia. Although usually self-limited, hyponatremic seizures may be refractory to anticonvulsants.

As discussed earlier, chronic hyponatremia is much less symptomatic as a result of the process of brain volume regulation. Because of this adaptation process, chronic hyponatremia is arguably a condition that clinicians think they may not need to be as concerned about, which has been reinforced by common usage of the descriptor *asymptomatic hyponatremia* for many of these patients. However, as discussed previously, it is clear that many such patients very often do have neurologic symptoms, even if milder and more subtle in nature, including headaches, nausea, mood disturbances, depression, difficulty concentrating, slowed reaction times, unstable gait, increased falls, confusion, and disorientation.[453] Consequently, all patients with hyponatremia who manifest any neurologic symptoms that could possibly be related to the hyponatremia should be considered candidates for treatment, regardless of the chronicity of the hyponatremia or the level of serum [Na$^+$]. An additional reason to treat even asymptomatic hyponatremia effectively is to prevent a lowering of the serum [Na$^+$] to more symptomatic and dangerous levels during treatment of underlying conditions (e.g., increased fluid administration via parenteral nutrition, treatment of heart failure with loop diuretics).

CURRENT THERAPIES

Conventional management strategies for hyponatremia range from saline infusion and fluid restriction to pharmacologic measures to adjust fluid balance. Although the number of available treatments for hyponatremia is large, some are not appropriate for correction of symptomatic hyponatremia because they work too slowly or inconsistently to be effective in hospitalized patients (e.g., demeclocycline, mineralocorticoids). Consideration of treatment options should always include an evaluation of the benefits and potential toxicities of any therapy and must be individualized for each patient.[464] It should always be remembered that sometimes simply stopping treatment with an agent associated with hyponatremia is sufficient to correct a low serum [Na$^+$].

HYPERTONIC SALINE

Acute hyponatremia presenting with severe neurologic symptoms is life-threatening and should be treated promptly with hypertonic solutions, typically 3% NaCl ([Na$^+$] = 513 mmol/L), because this represents the most reliable method to raise the serum [Na$^+$] quickly. A continuous infusion of hypertonic NaCl is generally used in inpatient settings. Various formulas have been suggested for calculating the initial rate of infusion of hypertonic solutions,[460] but there has been no consensus regarding optimal infusion rates of 3% NaCl. One of the simplest methods to estimate an initial 3% NaCl infusion rate uses the following relationship[464]:

$$\text{Patient's weight (kg)} \times \text{desired correction rate (mEq/L/hr)} = \text{infusion rate of 3% NaCl (mL/hr)}$$

Depending on individual hospital policies, the administration of a hypertonic solution may require special considerations (e.g., placement in the intensive care unit [ICU], sign-off by a consultant), which each clinician needs to be aware of to optimize patient care.

An alternative option for more emergent situations is administration of a 100-mL bolus of 3% NaCl, repeated once if there is no clinical improvement in 30 minutes. This was recommended by a consensus conference organized to develop guidelines for prevention and treatment of exercise-induced hyponatremia, an acute and potentially lethal condition,[465] and adopted as a general recommendation by an expert panel.[466] Injecting this amount of hypertonic saline intravenously raises the serum [Na$^+$] by an average of 2 to 4 mmol/L, which is well below the recommended maximal daily rate of change of 10 to 12 mmol/24 hours or 18 mmol/48 hours.[467] Because the brain can only accommodate an average increase of approximately 8% in brain volume before herniation occurs, quickly increasing the serum [Na$^+$] by as little as 2 to 4 mmol/L in acute hyponatremia can effectively reduce brain swelling and intracranial pressure.[468]

ISOTONIC SALINE

The treatment of choice for depletional hyponatremia (hypovolemic hyponatremia) is isotonic saline ([Na$^+$] = 154 mmol/L) to restore ECF volume and ensure adequate organ perfusion. This initial therapy is appropriate for

> **Table 16.8** General Recommendations for Using Fluid Restriction and Predictors of Its Increased Likelihood of Failure
>
> **General Recommendations**
> - Restrict *all* intake that is consumed by drinking, not just water.
> - Aim for a fluid restriction that is 500 mL/day *below* the 24-hour urine volume.
> - Do not restrict sodium or protein intake unless indicated.
>
> **Predictors of Likely Failure of Fluid Restriction**
> - High urine osmolality (>500 mOsm/kg H$_2$O).
> - Sum of the urine Na$^+$ and K$^+$ concentrations exceeds the serum Na$^+$ concentration
> - 24-hour urine volume < 1500 mL/day.
> - Increase in serum Na$^+$ sodium concentration < 2 mmol/L/day in 24 hours on fluid restriction ≤ 1 L/day.
>
> From Verbalis JG, Goldsmith SR, Greenberg A, et al: Diagnosis, evaluation, and treatment of hyponatremia: expert panel recommendations. Am J Med 126(Suppl 1):S1-S42, 2013.

patients who have clinical signs of hypovolemia or in whom a spot urine [Na$^+$] is lower than 20 to 30 mEq/L.[466] However, this therapy is ineffective for dilutional hyponatremias such as SIADH,[469] and continued inappropriate administration of isotonic saline to a euvolemic patient may worsen the hyponatremia[470] and/or cause fluid overload. Although isotonic saline may improve the serum [Na$^+$] in some patients with hypervolemic hyponatremia, their volume status will generally worsen with this therapy, so unless the hyponatremia is profound, isotonic saline should be avoided.

FLUID RESTRICTION

For patients with chronic hyponatremia, fluid restriction has been the most popular and most widely accepted treatment. When SIADH is present, fluids should generally be limited to 500 to 1000 mL/24 hours. Because fluid restriction increases the serum [Na$^+$] largely by underreplacing the excretion of fluid by the kidneys, some have advocated an initial restriction to 500 mL less than the 24-hour urine output.[471] When instituting a fluid restriction, it is important for the nursing staff and patient to understand that this includes all fluids that are consumed, not just water (Table 16.8). Generally, the water content of ingested food is not included in the restriction because this is balanced by insensible water losses (e.g., perspiration, exhaled air, feces), but caution should be exercised with foods that have a high fluid concentration (e.g., fruit, soup). Restricting fluid intake can be effective when properly applied and managed in select patients, but serum [Na$^+$] is generally increased only slowly (1 to 2 mmol/L/day), even with severe fluid restriction.[469] In addition, this therapy is often poorly tolerated because of an associated increase in thirst, leading to poor compliance with long-term therapy. However, it is economically favorable, and some patients do respond well to this option.

Fluid restriction should not be used with hypovolemic patients and is particularly difficult to maintain in hospitalized patients with very elevated urine osmolalities secondary to high AVP levels; if the sum of the urine Na$^+$ and K$^+$ concentrations exceeds the serum [Na$^+$], most patients will not respond to a fluid restriction because an electrolyte-free water clearance will be difficult to achieve.[472-474] This and other known predictors of failure of fluid restriction are summarized in Table 16.8; the presence of any of these factors in hospitalized patients with symptomatic hyponatremia make this less than ideal as an initial therapy. In addition, fluid restriction is not practical for some patients, particularly patients in an ICU setting who often require administration of significant volumes of fluids as part of their therapy. Consequently, such patients are candidates for more effective pharmacologic or saline treatment strategies.

ARGININE VASOPRESSIN RECEPTOR ANTAGONISTS

Conventional therapies for hyponatremia, although effective in specific circumstances, are suboptimal for many different reasons, including variable efficacy, slow responses, intolerable side effects, and serious toxicities. However, perhaps the most striking deficiency of most conventional therapies is that most of these therapies do not directly target the underlying cause of most dilutional hyponatremias—namely, inappropriately elevated plasma AVP levels. A newer class of pharmacologic agents, vasopressin receptor antagonists, also known as vaptans, which directly block AVP-mediated receptor activation, have been approved for the treatment of euvolemic hyponatremia (in the United States and European Union) and hypervolemic hyponatremia (in the United States).[475]

Conivaptan has been approved by the U.S. Food and Drug Administration (FDA) for euvolemic and hypervolemic hyponatremia in hospitalized patients. It is available only as an intravenous preparation and is given as a 20-mg loading dose over 30 minutes, followed by a continuous infusion of 20 or 40 mg/day.[476] Generally, the 20-mg continuous infusion is used for the first 24 hours to gauge the initial response. If the correction of serum [Na$^+$] is thought to be inadequate (e.g., <5 mmol/L), the infusion rate can be increased to 40 mg/day. Therapy is limited to a maximum duration of 4 days because of drug interaction effects with other agents metabolized by the CYP3A4 hepatic isoenzyme. Importantly, for conivaptan and all other vaptans, it is critical that the serum [Na$^+$] be measured frequently during the active phase of correction of the hyponatremia—a minimum of every 6 to 8 hours for conivaptan but more frequently in patients with risk factors for what is termed the *osmotic demyelination syndrome* (ODS).[464] If the correction exceeds 8 to 12 mmol/L in the first 24 hours, the infusion should be stopped and the patient monitored closely. Consideration should be given to administering sufficient water, orally or as intravenous 5% dextrose in water, to avoid a correction of more than 12 mmol/L/day. The maximum correction limit should be reduced to 8 mmol/L over the first 24 hours in patients with risk factors for ODS[466] (Figure 16.19 and Table 16.9). The most common side effects of conivaptan include headache, thirst, and hypokalemia.[477]

Tolvaptan, an oral vasopressin receptor antagonist, is also FDA-approved for the treatment of euvolemic and hypervolemic hyponatremia. In contrast to conivaptan, the availability of tolvaptan in tablet form allows short- and long-term use.[478] Similar to conivaptan, tolvaptan treatment must be

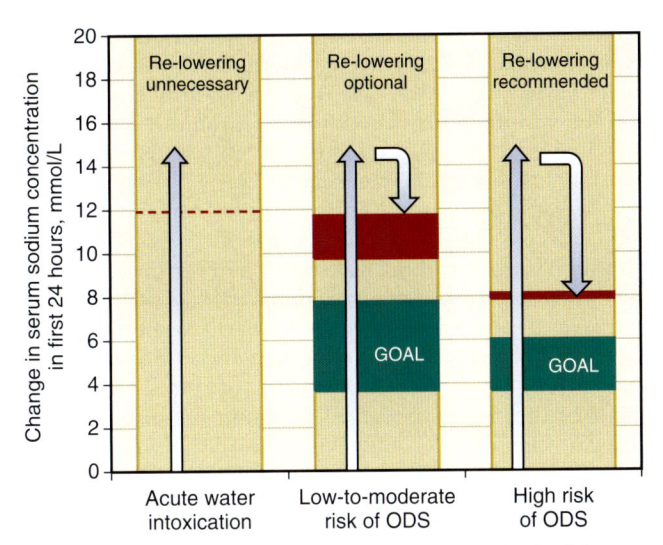

Figure 16.19 Recommended goals (*green*) and limits (*red*) for correction of hyponatremia based on the risk of producing osmotic demyelination syndrome (ODS). Also shown are recommendations for re-lowering of the serum [Na⁺] to goals for patients presenting with serum [Na⁺] < 120 mmol/L who exceed the recommended limits of correction in the first 24 hours. (From Verbalis JG, Goldsmith SR, Greenberg A, et al: Diagnosis, evaluation, and treatment of hyponatremia: expert panel recommendations. *Am J Med* 126(Suppl 1):S1-S42, 2013.)

Table 16.9 Factors Increasing Risk of Osmotic Demyelination Syndrome*

- Serum sodium concentration ≤ 105 mmol/L
- Hypokalemia†
- Alcoholism†
- Malnutrition†
- Advanced liver disease†

*Requiring slower correction of chronic hyponatremia.
†Unlike the rate of increase in serum [Na⁺], neither the precise level of the serum potassium concentration nor the degree of alcoholism, malnutrition, or liver disease that alters the brain's tolerance to an acute osmotic stress have been rigorously defined.

From Verbalis JG, Goldsmith SR, Greenberg A, et al: Diagnosis, evaluation, and treatment of hyponatremia: expert panel recommendations. *Am J Med* 126(Suppl 1):S1-S42, 2013.

initiated in the hospital so that the rate of correction can be monitored carefully. In the United States, patients with a serum [Na⁺] lower than 125 mmol/L are eligible for therapy with tolvaptan as primary therapy; if the serum [Na⁺] is 125 mmol/L or higher, tolvaptan therapy is only indicated if the patient has symptoms that could be attributable to the hyponatremia, and the patient is resistant to attempts at fluid restriction.[479] In the European Union, tolvaptan is approved only for the treatment of euvolemic hyponatremia, but any symptomatic euvolemic patient is eligible for tolvaptan therapy, regardless of the level of hyponatremia or response to previous fluid restriction. The starting dose of tolvaptan is 15 mg on the first day, and the dose can be titrated to 30 and 60 mg at 24-hour intervals if the serum [Na⁺] remains lower than 135 mmol/L or the increase in serum [Na⁺] has been less than 5 mmol/L in the previous 24 hours. As with conivaptan, it is essential that the serum [Na⁺] be measured frequently during the active phase of correction of the hyponatremia at a minimum of every 6 to 8 hours, particularly in patients with risk factors for ODS. Goals and limits for the safe correction of hyponatremia and methods to compensate for overly rapid corrections are the same as described previously for conivaptan (see Figure 16.19). One additional factor that helps avoid overly rapid correction with tolvaptan is the recommendation that fluid restriction not be used during the active phase of correction, thereby allowing the patient's thirst to compensate for an overly vigorous aquaresis. Common side effects of tolvaptan include dry mouth, thirst, increased urinary frequency, dizziness, nausea, and orthostatic hypotension.[478,479]

Vaptans are not needed for the treatment of hypovolemic hyponatremia because simple volume expansion would be expected to abolish the nonosmotic stimulus to AVP secretion and lead to a prompt aquaresis. Furthermore, inducing increased renal fluid excretion via diuresis or aquaresis can cause or worsen hypotension in such patients. This possibility has resulted in the labeling of these drugs as contraindicated for hypovolemic hyponatremia.[464] Importantly, clinically significant hypotension was not observed in the conivaptan or tolvaptan clinical trials in euvolemic and hypervolemic hyponatremic patients. Although vaptans are not contraindicated with decreased renal function, these agents generally will not be effective if the serum creatinine level is more than 3.0 mg/dL.

The FDA recently issued a caution about hepatic injury[480] that was noted in patients who received tolvaptan in a 3-year clinical trial examining the effect of tolvaptan on autosomal dominant polycystic kidney disease, the Tolvaptan Efficacy and Safety in Management of Autosomal Dominant Polycystic Kidney Disease and Its Outcomes (TEMPO) study.[481] An external panel of liver experts found that three cases of reversible jaundice and increased transaminase levels in this trial were probably or highly likely to be caused by tolvaptan. Additionally, 4.4% of autosomal dominant polycystic kidney disease (ADPKD) patients on tolvaptan (42 of 958) exhibited elevations of alanine aminotransferase (ALT) greater than three times that of the upper limit of normal (ULN) compared to 1.0% of patients (5 of 484) on placebo. These findings indicate that tolvaptan has the potential to cause irreversible and potentially fatal liver injury. The doses used in the TEMPO study were up to twice the maximum dose approved for hyponatremia (tolvaptan, 120 mg/day). Also, in clinical trials of tolvaptan at doses approved by the FDA for treatment of clinically significant euvolemic or hypervolemic hyponatremia, liver damage was not reported, including long-term trials longer than 30 days (e.g., SALT-WATER, EVEREST [Efficacy of Vasopressin Antagonism in Heart Failure: Outcome Study with Tolvaptan]).[482,483]

Based largely on the hepatic injury noted in the TEMPO trial, the FDA, on April 30, 2013, recommended that "Samsca treatment should be stopped if the patient develops signs of liver disease. Treatment duration should be limited to 30 days or less, and use should be avoided in patients with underlying liver disease, including cirrhosis."[480] The European Medicines Agency (EMA) has approved the use of tolvaptan for SIADH but not for hyponatremia due to heart failure or cirrhosis. Based on the TEMPO trial results, the EMO also issued a warning about the possible occurrence of hepatic injury in patients treated with tolvaptan, but did not recommend any restriction on the duration of treatment of SIADH patients with tolvaptan.[484]

Accordingly, appropriate caution should be exercised in patients treated with tolvaptan for hyponatremia for extended periods (e.g., >30 days), but this decision should be based on the clinical judgment of the treating physician. Patients who are refractory to or unable to tolerate or obtain other therapies for hyponatremia, and for whom the benefit of tolvaptan treatment outweighs the risks, remain candidates for long-term therapy with tolvaptan. In these patients, liver function tests should be monitored carefully and serially (i.e., every 3 months) and the drug discontinued in the event of significant changes in liver function test results (i.e., twice the ULN of ALT).[465] With rare exceptions, tolvaptan should not be used in patients with underlying liver disease, given the difficulty of attributing causation to any observed deterioration of hepatic function. Such an exception may be hyponatremic patients with end-stage liver disease awaiting imminent liver transplantation who are at little risk of added hepatic injury and will benefit from correction of hyponatremia prior to surgery to decrease the risk of ODS postoperatively.[485]

UREA

Urea has been described as an alternative oral treatment for SIADH and other hyponatremic disorders. The mode of action is to correct hypo-osmolality not only by increasing solute-free water excretion but also by decreasing urinary sodium excretion. Dosages of 15 to 60 g/day are generally effective; the dose can be titrated in increments of 15 g/day at weekly intervals as necessary to achieve normalization of the serum [Na^+]. It is advisable to dissolve the urea in orange juice or some other strongly flavored liquid to camouflage the bitter taste. Even if completely normal water balance is not achieved, it is often possible to allow the patient to maintain a less strict regimen of fluid restriction while receiving urea. The disadvantages associated with the use of urea include poor palatability (although some clinicians believe that this has been exaggerated), the development of azotemia at higher doses, and the unavailability of a convenient or FDA-approved form of the agent. Evidence has suggested that blood urea concentrations may double during treatment,[486] but it is important to remember that this does not represent renal impairment.

Reports from retrospective uncontrolled studies have suggested that the use of urea has been effective in treating SIADH in patients with hyponatremia due to subarachnoid hemorrhage and in critical care patients,[487] and case reports have documented success in infants with chronic SIADH[488] and NSIAD.[489] More recent evidence from a short study in a small cohort of SIADH patients has suggested that urea may have a comparable efficacy to vaptans in reversing hyponatremia due to chronic SIADH.[490]

FUROSEMIDE AND NACL

The use of furosemide (20 to 40 mg/day) coupled with a high salt intake (200 mEq/day), which represents an extension of the treatment of acute symptomatic hyponatremia[491] to the chronic management of euvolemic hyponatremia, has also been reported to be successful in select cases.[492] However, the efficacy of this approach to correct symptomatic hyponatremia promptly and within accepted goals limits (see Figure 16.19) is unknown.

TREATMENT GUIDELINES

Although various authors have published recommendations on the treatment of hyponatremia,[460,462,464,466,493,494] no standardized treatment algorithms have yet been universally accepted. For all treatment recommendations, the initial evaluation includes an assessment of the ECF volume status of the patient because treatment recommendations differ for hypovolemic, euvolemic, and hypervolemic hyponatremic patients. Recommendations for hypovolemic and hypervolemic patients have been updated recently.[466] Euvolemic patients, mainly including those with SIADH, represent a unique challenge because of the multiplicity of causes and presentations of patients with SIADH. A synthesis of existing recommendations for the treatment of hyponatremia is illustrated in Figure 16.20. This algorithm is based primarily on the neurologic symptomatology of hyponatremic patients rather than the serum [Na^+] or the chronicity of the hyponatremia; the latter is often difficult to ascertain.

LEVELS OF SYMPTOMS

A careful neurologic history and assessment should always be done to identify potential causes for the patient's symptoms other than hyponatremia, although it will not always be possible to exclude an additive contribution from the hyponatremia to an underlying neurologic condition. In this algorithm, patients are divided into three major groups based on their presenting symptoms (see Table 16.7).

Severe Symptoms

Coma, obtundation, seizures, respiratory distress or arrest, and unexplained vomiting usually imply a more acute onset or worsening of hyponatremia requiring immediate active treatment. Therapies that will quickly raise serum [Na^+] are required to reduce cerebral edema and decrease the risk of potentially fatal brain herniation.

Moderate Symptoms

Altered mental status, disorientation, confusion, unexplained nausea, gait instability, and falls generally indicate some degree of brain volume regulation and absence of clinically significant cerebral edema. These symptoms can be chronic or acute but allow more time to elaborate a deliberate approach to choice of treatment.

Mild or Absent Symptoms

Minimal symptoms, such as difficulty concentrating, irritability, altered mood, depression, or unexplained headache, or a virtual absence of discernible symptoms, indicate that the patient may have chronic or slowly evolving hyponatremia. These symptoms necessitate a cautious approach, especially when patients have underlying comorbidities.

Patients with severe symptoms should be treated with hypertonic (3%) NaCl as first-line therapy, followed by fluid restriction, with or without vaptan therapy. Because overly

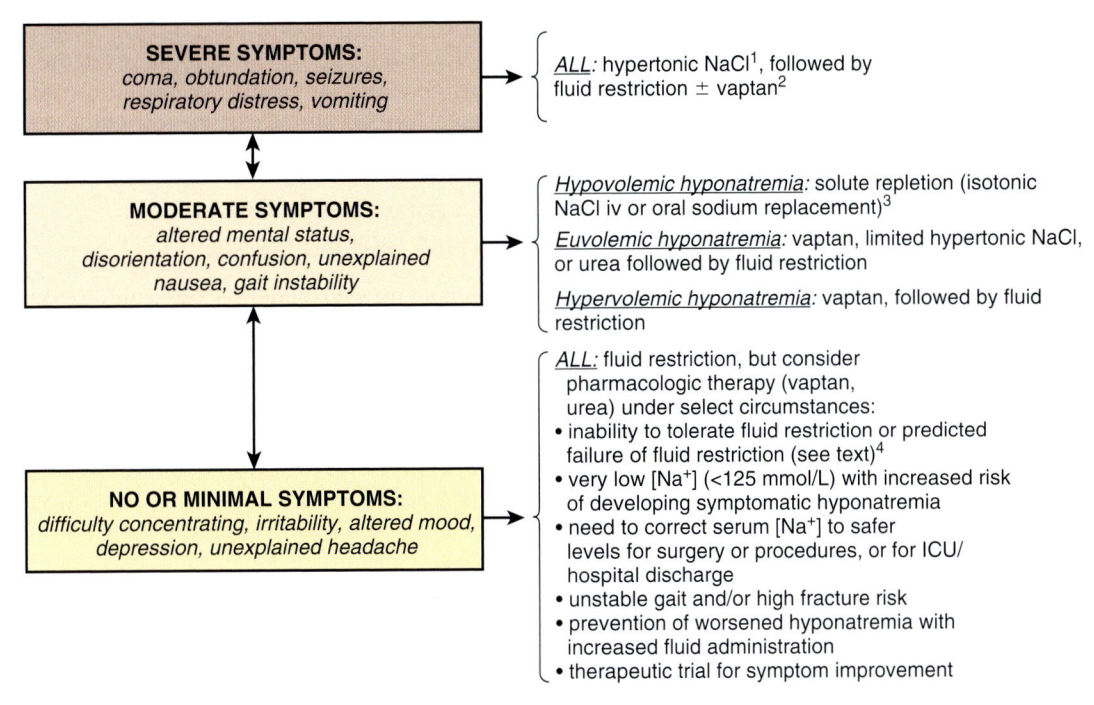

```
┌─────────────────────────┐
│    SEVERE SYMPTOMS:     │──► ALL: hypertonic NaCl¹, followed by
│  coma, obtundation,     │    fluid restriction ± vaptan²
│    seizures,            │
│ respiratory distress,   │
│      vomiting           │
└─────────────────────────┘
          ↕
┌─────────────────────────┐    Hypovolemic hyponatremia: solute repletion (isotonic
│   MODERATE SYMPTOMS:    │──► NaCl iv or oral sodium replacement)³
│  altered mental status, │    Euvolemic hyponatremia: vaptan, limited hypertonic NaCl,
│ disorientation,         │    or urea followed by fluid restriction
│ confusion, unexplained  │    Hypervolemic hyponatremia: vaptan, followed by fluid
│ nausea, gait instability│    restriction
└─────────────────────────┘
          ↕
┌─────────────────────────┐    ALL: fluid restriction, but consider
│                         │       pharmacologic therapy (vaptan,
│                         │       urea) under select circumstances:
│                         │    • inability to tolerate fluid restriction or predicted
│                         │       failure of fluid restriction (see text)⁴
│  NO OR MINIMAL SYMPTOMS:│──► • very low [Na⁺] (<125 mmol/L) with increased risk
│ difficulty concentrating,│       of developing symptomatic hyponatremia
│ irritability, altered mood,│  • need to correct serum [Na⁺] to safer
│ depression, unexplained │       levels for surgery or procedures, or for ICU/
│ headache                │       hospital discharge
│                         │    • unstable gait and/or high fracture risk
│                         │    • prevention of worsened hyponatremia with
│                         │       increased fluid administration
│                         │    • therapeutic trial for symptom improvement
└─────────────────────────┘
```

1. Some authors recommend simultaneous treatment with desmopressin to limit speed of correction.
2. No active therapy should be started within 24 hours of hypertonic saline to decrease the risk of overly rapid correction of [Na⁺] and risk of ODS.
3. With isotonic NaCl infusion, serum [Na⁺] must be followed closely to prevent overly rapid correction and risk of ODS due to secondary water diuresis.
4. See Table 16.8 for predictors of failure of fluid restriction.

Figure 16.20 Algorithm for treatment of patients with euvolemic hyponatremia based on their presenting symptoms. The *arrows* between the symptom boxes indicate movement of patients between different symptom levels. ALL, All types of hypotonic hyponatremia. (Modified from Verbalis JG: Emergency management of acute and chronic hyponatremia. In Matfin G, editor: *Endocrine and metabolic emergencies,* Washington, DC, 2014, Endocrine Press, pp 359.)

rapid correction of serum [Na⁺] occurs in more than 10% of patients treated with hypertonic NaCl,[495] such patients are at risk for ODS unless carefully monitored. For this reason, some authors have proposed simultaneous treatment with desmopressin to reduce the rate of correction to only that produced by the hypertonic NaCl infusion itself.[496,497] Whether sufficient clinical data eventually prove that this approach is effective and safe in larger numbers of patients remains to be determined. Only one case of ODS has been reported in a patient receiving vaptan monotherapy,[498] and two abstracts have reported ODS when vaptans were used directly following hypertonic saline administration within the same 24-hour period.[466] Consequently, no active hyponatremia therapy should be administered until at least 24 hours following successful increases in serum [Na⁺] using hypertonic NaCl.

The choice of treatment for patients with moderate symptoms will depend on their ECF volume status (see Figure 16.20). Hypovolemic patients should be treated with solute repletion via isotonic NaCl infusion or oral sodium replacement.[466] Euvolemic patients, typically with SIADH, will benefit from vaptan therapy, limited hypertonic saline administration or, in some cases, urea, where available. This can be followed by fluid restriction or long-term vaptan therapy when the cause of the SIADH is expected to be chronic.[466] In hypervolemic patients with heart failure, vaptans are usually the best choice because fluid restriction is rarely successful in this group, saline administration can cause fluid retention with increased edema, and urea can lead to ammonia buildup in the gastrointestinal tract if hepatic function is impaired. Although moderate neurologic symptoms can indicate that a patient is in an early stage of acute hyponatremia, they more often indicate a chronically hyponatremic state with sufficient brain volume adaptation to prevent marked symptomatology from cerebral edema. Most patients with moderate hyponatremic symptoms have a more chronic form of hyponatremia, so guidelines for goals and limits of correction should be followed closely (see Figure 16.19), and close monitoring of these patients in a hospital setting is warranted until the symptoms improve or stabilize.

Patients with no or minimal symptoms should be managed initially with fluid restriction, although treatment with pharmacologic therapy, such as vaptans or urea, may be appropriate for a wide range of specific clinical conditions (see Figure 16.20). Foremost of these is a failure to improve the serum [Na⁺], despite reasonable attempts at fluid restriction, or the presence of clinical characteristics associated with poor responses to fluid restriction (see Table 16.8).

A special case is when spontaneous correction of hyponatremia occurs at an undesirably rapid rate because of the onset of water diuresis. This can occur following cessation of desmopressin therapy in a patient who has become hyponatremic, replacement of glucocorticoids in a patient with adrenal insufficiency, replacement of solutes in a patient with diuretic-induced hyponatremia, or spontaneous resolution of transient SIADH. Brain damage from ODS can clearly ensue in this setting if the preceding period of hyponatremia has been long enough (usually, ≥48 hours) to allow brain volume regulation to occur. If the correction parameters discussed above have been exceeded, and the correction is proceeding more rapidly than planned (usually because of continued excretion of hypotonic urine), the pathologic events leading to demyelination can be reversed by administration of hypotonic fluids, with or without desmopressin. The efficacy of this approach has been suggested from animal studies[499] and case reports in humans,[462,500] even when patients are overtly symptomatic.[501] However, relowering the serum [Na^+] after an initial, overly rapid correction is only strongly recommended for patients at high risk of ODS (see Table 16.9); it is considered optional for patients with a low-to-moderate risk of ODS and unnecessary for patients with acute water intoxication (see Figure 16.19).

Although this classification is based on presenting symptoms at the time of initial evaluation, it should be remembered that in some cases, patients initially exhibit more moderate symptoms because they are in the early stages of hyponatremia. In addition, some patients with minimal symptoms are prone to develop more symptomatic hyponatremia during periods of increased fluid ingestion. In support of this, approximately 70% of 31 patients presenting to a university hospital with symptomatic hyponatremia and a mean serum [Na^+] of 119 mmol/L had preexisting asymptomatic hyponatremia as the most common risk factor identified.[502] Consequently, hyponatremia therapy should also be considered to prevent progression from a lower to higher level of symptomatic hyponatremia, particularly in patients with a past history of repeated presentations for symptomatic hyponatremia.

MONITORING SERUM SODIUM CONCENTRATION IN HYPONATREMIC PATIENTS

The frequency of serum [Na^+] monitoring is dependent on the severity of the hyponatremia and therapy chosen. In all hyponatremic patients, neurologic symptomatology should be carefully assessed very early in the diagnostic evaluation to assess the symptomatic severity of the hyponatremia and determine whether the patient requires more urgent therapy. All patients undergoing active treatment with hypertonic saline for symptomatic hyponatremia should have frequent monitoring of their serum [Na^+] and ECF volume status (every 2 to 4 hours) to ensure that the serum [Na^+] does not exceed the limits of safe correction during the active phase of correction,[464] because overly rapid correction of serum sodium will increase the risk of ODS.[503] Patients treated with vaptans for mild-to-moderate symptoms should have their serum [Na^+] monitored every 6 to 8 hours during the active phase of correction, which will generally be the first 24 to 48 hours of therapy. Active treatment with hypertonic saline or vaptans should be stopped when the patient's symptoms are no longer present, a safe serum [Na^+] (usually, >120 mmol/L) has been achieved, or the rate of correction has reached maximum limits of 12 mmol/L within 24 hours or 18 mmol/L within 48 hours,[464,467] or 8 mmol/L over any 24-hour period in patients at high risk of ODS (see Table 16.9). In patients with a stable level of serum [Na^+] treated with fluid restriction or therapy other than hypertonic saline, measurement of the serum [Na^+] daily is generally sufficient because levels will not change that quickly in the absence of active therapy or large changes in fluid intake or administration.

LONG-TERM TREATMENT OF CHRONIC HYPONATREMIA

Some patients will benefit from continued treatment of hyponatremia following discharge from the hospital. In many cases, this will consist of a continued fluid restriction. However, as discussed, long-term compliance with this therapy is poor because of the increased thirst that occurs with more severe degrees of fluid restriction. Thus, for select patients who have responded to tolvaptan in the hospital, consideration should be given to continuing the treatment as an outpatient after discharge. In patients with established chronic hyponatremia, tolvaptan has shown to be effective for maintaining a normal [Na^+] for as long as 3 years of continued daily therapy.[504] However, many patients with inpatient hyponatremia have a transient form of SIADH, without the need for long-term therapy. In the conivaptan open-label study, approximately 70% of patients treated as an inpatient for 4 days had normal serum [Na^+] concentrations 7 and 30 days after cessation of the vaptan therapy in the absence of chronic therapy for hyponatremia. Selection of which patients with inpatient hyponatremia are candidates for long-term therapy should be based on the cause of the SIADH. Figure 16.21 shows estimates of the relative probability that patients with different causes of SIADH will have persistent hyponatremia that may benefit from long-term treatment with tolvaptan following hospital discharge. Nonetheless, for any individual patient, this simply represents an estimate of the likelihood of requiring long-term therapy. In all cases, consideration should be given to a trial of stopping the drug 2 to 4 weeks after discharge to determine if hyponatremia is still present. A reasonable period of tolvaptan cessation to evaluate the presence of continued SIADH is 7 days, because this period was found to be sufficient for demonstration of a recurrence of hyponatremia in the tolvaptan SALT trials.[504,505] Serum [Na^+] should be monitored every 2 to 3 days following cessation of tolvaptan so that the drug can be resumed as quickly as possible in patients with recurrent hyponatremia; the longer the patient is hyponatremic, the greater the risk of subsequent ODS with overly rapid correction of the low serum [Na^+].

Findings of hepatotoxicity in a small number of patients on high doses of tolvaptan in a clinical trial of polycystic kidney disease led to a recent FDA recommendation that tolvaptan not be used for longer than 30 days.[480] This decision should be based on a risk/benefit analysis individualized for specific patients; if tolvaptan is used for longer than 30 days, liver function should be assessed at regular intervals (e.g., every 3 months).[466]

FUTURE OF HYPONATREMIA TREATMENT

Despite the many advances made in understanding the manifestations and consequences of hyponatremia, and the availability of effective pharmacologic therapies for

Etiology of SIADH	Likely duration of SIADH*	Relative risk of chronic SIADH
Tumors producing vasopressin ectopically (small cell lung carcinoma, head and neck carcinoma)	Indefinite	High
Drug-induced, with continuation of offending agent (carbamazepine, SSRI)	Duration of drug therapy	
Brain tumors	Indefinite	
Idiopathic (senile)	Indefinite	
Subarachnoid hemorrhage	1-4 weeks	
Stroke	1-2 weeks	
Inflammatory brain lesions	Dependent on response to therapy	Medium
Respiratory failure (chronic obstructive lung disease)	Dependent on response to therapy	
HIV infection	Dependent on response to therapy	
Traumatic brain injury	2-7 days to indefinite	
Drug-induced, with cessation of offending agent	Duration of drug therapy	
Pneumonia	2-5 days	
Nausea, pain, prolonged exercise	Variable depending on cause	
Postoperative hyponatremia	2-3 days postoperatively	Low

*Time frames are based on clinical experience.

Figure 16.21 Estimated probablity of need for long-term treatment of SIADH, depending on underlying cause.

treatment of hyponatremia, it is obvious that we do not yet have a uniformly accepted consensus on how and when this disorder should be treated. In particular, the indications for the use of vasopressin receptor antagonists by regulatory agencies differ substantially worldwide, and various treatment guidelines published to date also differ substantially in regard to appropriate hyponatremia management.[466,506,507] There are many reasons for this failure to achieve consensus and, until this is achieved via further clinical research studies, physicians must recognize the primary role that clinical judgment must continue to play in making decisions about the management of hyponatremia in individual patients. Their recommendations should take into account appropriate appraisals of evidence by authoritative experts in the field, the decisions of regulatory agencies based on critical reviews of the efficacy and safety data for approved treatments for hyponatremia and, most importantly, the specialized needs of individual hyponatremic patients.[507]

In the meantime, clinical trials using vasopressin receptor antagonists will enable investigators to answer some long-standing questions about the role of vasopressin V_2 receptor activation in producing antidiuresis in various physiologic conditions (e.g., regulation of sweat production),[508] pathophysiologic states (e.g., hyponatremic patients without measurable vasopressin levels), and especially the potential reversibility of long-term adverse effects of hyponatremia. This may account for the increased mortality and bone fracture rates in hyponatremic patients across multiple different comorbidities, as well as in older, community-dwelling subjects without known underlying disease.

Complete reference list available at ExpertConsult.com.

KEY REFERENCES

1. Edelman IS, Leibman J: Anatomy of body water and electrolytes. *Am J Med* 27:256–277, 1959.
17. Thibonnier M, Conarty DM, Preston JA, et al: Molecular pharmacology of human vasopressin receptors. *Adv Exp Med Biol* 449:251–276, 1998.
26. Robinson AG, Roberts MM, Evron WA, et al: Hyponatremia in rats induces downregulation of vasopressin synthesis. *J Clin Invest* 86:1023–1029, 1990.
32. Robertson GL: The regulation of vasopressin function in health and disease. *Rec Prog Horm Res* 33:333–385, 1976.
43. Leng G, Brown CH, Bull PM, et al: Responses of magnocellular neurons to osmotic stimulation involves coactivation of excitatory and inhibitory input: an experimental and theoretical analysis. *J Neurosci* 21:6967–6977, 2001.
46. Bourque CW, Voisin DL, Chakfe Y: Stretch-inactivated cation channels: cellular targets for modulation of osmosensitivity in supraoptic neurons. *Prog Brain Res* 139:85–94, 2002.
50. Liedtke W: Role of TRPV ion channels in sensory transduction of osmotic stimuli in mammals. *Exp Physiol* 92:507–512, 2007.
54. Dunn FL, Brennan TJ, Nelson AE, et al: The role of blood osmolality and volume in regulating vasopressin secretion in the rat. *J Clin Invest* 52:3212–3219, 1973.
64. Schrier RW: Pathogenesis of sodium and water retention in high-output and low-output cardiac failure, nephrotic syndrome, cirrhosis, and pregnancy. *N Eng J Med* 319:1065–1072, 1988.

105. Phillips PA, Rolls BJ, Ledingham JG, et al: Osmotic thirst and vasopressin release in humans: a double-blind crossover study. *Am J Physiol* 248(Pt 2):R645–R650, 1985.
132. Maghnie M, Cosi G, Genovese E, et al: Central diabetes insipidus in children and young adults. *N Engl J Med* 343:998–1007, 2000.
133. Imura H, Nakao K, Shimatsu A, et al: Lymphocytic infundibulo-neurohypophysitis as a cause of central diabetes insipidus. *N Engl J Med* 329:683–689, 1993.
142. Zerbe RL, Robertson GL: A comparison of plasma vasopressin measurements with a standard indirect test in the differential diagnosis of polyuria. *N Eng J Med* 305:1539–1546, 1981.
147. Olson BR, Gumowski J, Rubino D, et al: Pathophysiology of hyponatremia after transsphenoidal pituitary surgery. *J Neurosurg* 87:499–507, 1997.
157. DeRubertis FR, Michelis MF, Beck N, et al: "Essential" hypernatremia due to ineffective osmotic and intact volume regulation of vasopressin secretion. *J Clin Invest* 50:97–111, 1971.
161. Durr JA, Hoggard JG, Hunt JM, et al: Diabetes insipidus in pregnancy associated with abnormally high circulating vasopressinase activity. *N Engl J Med* 316:1070–1074, 1987.
168. Morello JP, Bichet DG: Nephrogenic diabetes insipidus. *Annu Rev Physiol* 63:607–630, 2001.
174. Deen PM, Knoers NV: Vasopressin type-2 receptor and aquaporin-2 water channel mutants in nephrogenic diabetes insipidus. *Am J Med Sci* 316:300–309, 1998.
181. Nielsen S, Kwon TH, Christensen BM, et al: Physiology and pathophysiology of renal aquaporins. *J Am Soc Nephrol* 10:647–663, 1999.
208. Gullans SR, Verbalis JG: Control of brain volume during hyperosmolar and hypoosmolar conditions. *Annu Rev Med* 44:289–301, 1993.
211. Robertson GL: Diabetes insipidus. *Endocrinol Metab Clin North Am* 24:549–572, 1995.
231. Oiso Y, Robertson GL, Norgaard JP, et al: Clinical review: treatment of neurohypophyseal diabetes insipidus. *J Clin Endocrinol Metab* 98:3958–3967, 2013.
237. Richardson DW, Robinson AG: Desmopressin. *Ann Intern Med* 103:228–239, 1985.
262. Hawkins RC: Age and gender as risk factors for hyponatremia and hypernatremia. *Clin Chim Acta* 337:169–172, 2003.
277. Androgue HJ, Madias NE: Hyponatremia. *N Engl J Med* 342:1581–1589, 2000.
330. Oelkers W: Hyponatremia and inappropriate secretion of vasopressin in patients with hypopituitarism. *N Engl J Med* 321:492–496, 1989.
354. Goldman MB, Robertson GL, Luchins DJ, et al: Psychotic exacerbations and enhanced vasopressin secretion in schizophrenic patients with hyponatremia and polydipsia. *Arch Gen Psychiatry* 54:443–449, 1997.
362. Anderson RJ, Chung H-M, Kluge R, et al: Hyponatremia: a prospective analysis of its epidemiology and the pathogenetic role of vasopressin. *Ann Intern Med* 102:164–168, 1985.
371. Almond CS, Shin AY, Fortescue EB, et al: Hyponatremia among runners in the Boston Marathon. *N Engl J Med* 352:1550–1556, 2005.
405. Schwartz WB, Bennett W, Curelop S, et al: A syndrome of renal sodium loss and hyponatremia probably resulting from inappropriate secretion of antidiuretic hormone. *Am J Med* 23:529–542, 1957.
406. Bartter FE, Schwartz WB: The syndrome of inappropriate secretion of antidiuretic hormone. *Am J Med* 42:790–806, 1967.
411. Leaf A, Bartter FC, Santos RF, et al: Evidence in humans that urine electrolyte loss induced by pitressin is a function of water retention. *J Clin Invest* 32:868–878, 1953.
413. Verbalis JG, Drutarosky M: Adaptation to chronic hypo-osmolality in rats. *Kidney Int* 34:351–360, 1988.
421. Ecelbarger C, Nielsen S, Olson BR, et al: Role of renal aquaporins in escape from vasopressin antidiuresis in rat. *J Clin Invest* 99:1852–1863, 1997.
429. Hirshberg B, Ben-Yehuda A: The syndrome of inappropriate antidiuretic hormone secretion in the elderly. *Am J Med* 103:270–273, 1997.
435. Feldman BJ, Rosenthal SM, Vargas GA, et al: Nephrogenic syndrome of inappropriate antidiuresis. *N Engl J Med* 352:1884–1890, 2005.
445. Upadhyay A, Jaber BL, Madias NE: Incidence and prevalence of hyponatremia. *Am J Med* 119(Suppl 1):S30–S35, 2006.
453. Renneboog B, Musch W, Vandemergel X, et al: Mild chronic hyponatremia is associated with falls, unsteadiness, and attention deficits. *Am J Med* 119:71, 2006.
456. Kinsella S, Moran S, Sullivan MO, et al: Hyponatremia independent of osteoporosis is associated with fracture occurrence. *Clin J Am Soc Nephrol* 5:275–280, 2010.
457. Hoorn EJ, Rivadeneira F, van Meurs JB, et al: Mild hyponatremia as a risk factor for fractures: the Rotterdam Study. *J Bone Miner Res* 26:1822–1828, 2011.
458. Verbalis JG, Barsony J, Sugimura Y, et al: Hyponatremia-induced osteoporosis. *J Bone Miner Res* 25:554–563, 2010.
466. Verbalis JG, Goldsmith SR, Greenberg A, et al: Diagnosis, evaluation, and treatment of hyponatremia: expert panel recommendations. *Am J Med* 126(Suppl 1):S1–S42, 2013.
472. Furst H, Hallows KR, Post J, et al: The urine/plasma electrolyte ratio: a predictive guide to water restriction. *Am J Med Sci* 319:240–244, 2000.
475. Greenberg A, Verbalis JG: Vasopressin receptor antagonists. *Kidney Int* 69:2124–2130, 2006.
478. Schrier RW, Gross P, Gheorghiade M, et al: Tolvaptan, a selective oral vasopressin V2-receptor antagonist, for hyponatremia. *N Engl J Med* 355:2099–2112, 2006.
482. Berl T, Quittnat-Pelletier F, Verbalis JG, et al: Oral tolvaptan is safe and effective in chronic hyponatremia. *J Am Soc Nephrol* 21:705–712, 2010.
483. Konstam MA, Gheorghiade M, Burnett JC, Jr, et al: Effects of oral tolvaptan in patients hospitalized for worsening heart failure: the EVEREST Outcome Trial. *JAMA* 297:1319–1331, 2007.
493. Ellison DH, Berl T: Clinical practice. The syndrome of inappropriate antidiuresis. *N Engl J Med* 356:2064–2072, 2007.
497. Sterns RH, Hix JK, Silver S: Treating profound hyponatremia: a strategy for controlled correction. *Am J Kidney Dis* 56:774–779, 2010.
503. Sterns RH, Riggs JE, Schochet SS, Jr: Osmotic demyelination syndrome following correction of hyponatremia. *N Eng J Med* 314:1535–1542, 1986.

17

Disorders of Acid-Base Balance

Thomas D. DuBose, Jr.

CHAPTER OUTLINE

ACID-BASE HOMEOSTASIS, 512
Buffer Systems, 512
Mechanisms of pH Buffering, 512
Chemical Equilibria of Physicochemical Buffer Systems, 512
Chemical Equilibria for the Carbon Dioxide–Bicarbonate System, 513
Physiologic Advantage of an Open Buffer System, 513
Regulation of Buffers, 513
Integration of Regulatory Processes, 514
RENAL REGULATION, 514
SYSTEMIC RESPONSE TO CHANGES IN CARBON DIOXIDE TENSION, 515
Acute Response: Generation of Respiratory Acidosis or Alkalosis, 515
Chronic Response, 516
SYSTEMIC RESPONSE TO ADDITION OF NONVOLATILE ACIDS, 516
Sources of Endogenous Acids, 516
Hepatic and Renal Roles in Acid-Base Homeostasis, 517
Neurorespiratory Response to Acidemia, 518
Renal Excretion, 518

SYSTEMIC RESPONSE TO GAIN OF ALKALI, 519
Distribution and Cellular Buffering, 519
Respiratory Compensation, 519
Renal Excretion, 519
STEPWISE APPROACH TO THE DIAGNOSIS OF ACID-BASE DISORDERS, 520
Step 1: Measure Arterial Blood Gas and Electrolyte Values Simultaneously, 521
Step 2: Verify Acid-Base Laboratory Values, 521
Step 3: Define the Limits of Compensation to Distinguish Simple from Mixed Acid-Base Disorders, 521
Step 4: Calculate the Anion Gap, 523
Step 5 and 6: Recognize Conditions Causing Acid-Base Abnormalities with High or Normal Anion Gap, 524
RESPIRATORY DISORDERS, 525
Respiratory Acidosis, 525
Respiratory Alkalosis, 527
METABOLIC DISORDERS, 528
Metabolic Acidosis, 528
Metabolic Alkalosis, 550

The appropriate diagnosis and management of acid-base disorders requires accurate interpretation of the specific acid-base disorder, as well as consideration of the clinical setting in which these disorders occur as indicated by the patient's history and physical examination. Accuracy requires simultaneous measurement of plasma electrolyte levels and arterial blood gas (ABG) values, as well as an appreciation by the clinician of the physiologic adaptations and compensatory responses that occur with specific acid-base disturbances. In most circumstances, these compensatory responses can be predicted through an analysis of the prevailing disorder in a stepwise manner. This chapter reviews acid-base homeostasis as a consequence of the integration of physiologic and compensatory responses. The approach in this chapter, sometimes referred to as the Boston method, uses measurements of arterial pH, CO_2 pressure (PCO_2), and [HCO_3^-] plus an analysis of the anion gap (corrected for a normal plasma albumin level of 4.5 g/dL), referring to the pathophysiologically established range of compensatory responses for simple disorders. This is the most widely used and generally accepted approach used clinically by nephrologists, and the easiest model to understand.[1] Other methods, such as one requiring calculation and consideration of "base excess" (the Copenhagen method), or a physicochemical method (Stewart method), requiring calculation of the "strong ion difference," the "strong ion gap," and the total concentration of plasma weak acids, are not discussed here.

ACID-BASE HOMEOSTASIS

Acid-base homeostasis operates to maintain systemic arterial pH within a narrow range. Although clinical laboratories consider the normal range to be between 7.35 and 7.45 pH units, pH in vivo in an individual is maintained within a much narrower range. This degree of tight regulation is accomplished through (1) chemical buffering in the extracellular fluid (ECF) and the intracellular fluid and (2) regulatory responses that are under the control of the respiratory and renal systems. Those chemical buffers, respiration, and renal processes efficiently dispose of the physiologic daily load of carbonic acid (as volatile CO_2) and nonvolatile acids, mainly derived from dietary protein intake, and defend against the occasional addition of pathologic quantities of acid and alkali. Therefore chemical buffers within the extracellular and intracellular compartments serve to blunt changes in pH that would occur with retention of either acids or bases. In addition, the control of P_{CO_2} by the central nervous system and respiratory system and the control of the plasma HCO_3^- by the kidneys constitute the regulatory processes that act in concert to stabilize the arterial pH.

The major buffer system in the body comprises a base (H^+ acceptor), which is predominantly HCO_3^-, and an acid (H^+ donor), which is predominantly carbonic acid (H_2CO_3):

$$H^+ + HCO_3^- \Leftrightarrow H_2CO_3 \tag{1}$$

Extracellular H^+ concentration ($[H^+]_e$) throughout the body is constant in the steady state. The HCO_3^-/H_2CO_3 ratio is proportional to the ratio of all the other extracellular buffers such as PO_4^{3-} and plasma proteins:

$$[H^+]_e \propto \frac{HCO_3^-}{H_2CO_3} \propto \frac{B^-}{HB} \tag{2}$$

The intracellular H^+ concentration ($[H^+]_i$), or pH_i, is also relatively stable. Both cellular ion exchange mechanisms and intracellular buffers (hemoglobin, tissue proteins, organophosphate complexes, and bone apatite) participate in the blunting of changes in both $[H^+]_i$ and $[H^+]_e$. Extracellular and intracellular buffers provide the *first line of defense* against the addition of acid or base to the body (see "Mechanisms of pH Buffering" section later).

The second line of defense is the respiratory system. Pulmonary participation in acid-base homeostasis relies on the excretion of CO_2 by the lungs. The reaction is catalyzed by the enzyme carbonic anhydrase:

$$H^+ + HCO_3^- \leftrightarrow H_2CO_3 \xleftrightarrow{\text{Carbonic anhydrase}} H_2O + CO_2 \tag{3}$$

Large amounts of CO_2 (10 to 12 mol/day) accumulate as metabolic end products of tissue metabolism. This CO_2 load is transported in the blood to the lungs as hemoglobin-generated HCO_3^- and hemoglobin-bound carbamino groups[2]:

$$\text{Metabolism} \rightarrow CO_2 \xleftrightarrow{\text{Blood transport}} \text{Lungs} \tag{4}$$

Conventionally H^+ concentration is expressed in two different ways, either directly as $[H^+]$ or indirectly as pH. The relationship between these two factors can be written in mathematically equivalent forms:

$$pH = -\log_{10}[H^+] \tag{5}$$

$$[H^+](Eq/L) = 10^{-pH} \tag{6}$$

When $[H^+]$ is expressed (for numeric convenience) in nanomoles per liter (nmol/L) or nanomolar (nM), then:

$$[H^+] = 10^{9-pH} \tag{7}$$

BUFFER SYSTEMS

Acid-base chemistry deals with molecular interactions that involve the transfer of H^+. A large variety of molecules, both inorganic and organic, contain hydrogen atoms that can dissociate to yield H^+. The relationship between an undissociated acid (HA) and its conjugate, disassociated base (A^-) may be represented as follows:

$$HA \Leftrightarrow H^+ + A^- \tag{8}$$

In addition to the many inorganic and organic acid-base substances encountered in biologic systems, many protein molecules (e.g., hemoglobin) contain acidic groups that may dissociate, yielding a corresponding conjugate base.

MECHANISMS OF pH BUFFERING

Buffer systems are critical to the physiology and pathophysiology of acid-base homeostasis because they attenuate the pH change in a solution or tissue by reversibly combining with or releasing H^+. Thus the pH change of a solution during the addition of acid or base equivalents is smaller in the presence of a buffer system than would have occurred if no buffer systems were present. The acid or base load can be *extrinsic*, such as during systemic acid or base infusion, or *intrinsic*, resulting from net generation of new acid or base equivalents that are added to the extracellular or intracellular compartments.

CHEMICAL EQUILIBRIA OF PHYSICOCHEMICAL BUFFER SYSTEMS

As an example of a physicochemical buffer pair, consider a neutral weak acid (HA) and its conjugate weak base (A^-). Examples of such buffer pairs are acetic acid and acetate and the carboxyl groups on proteins. Another example of a physicochemical buffer pair is a neutral weak base (B) and its conjugate weak acid (BH^+):

$$BH^+ \Leftrightarrow B + H^+ \tag{9}$$

Examples of such buffer pairs are NH_3 and NH_4^+ and the imidazole group in proteins. A rigorous analysis of the kinetics of reversible reactions in solution yields the law of mass action, which states that at equilibrium (i.e., when the velocities of the forward and backward reactions are equal) the ratio of the concentration products of opposing reactions is a constant:

$$K'_a = \frac{[H^+][A^-]}{HA} \tag{10}$$

$$K'_b = \frac{[H^+][B^-]}{BH} \quad (11)$$

K'_a and K'_b are the equilibrium or dissociation constants for equations 10 and 11, respectively.

Taking logarithms of both sides of equations 10 and 11 and defining $pK'_a = -\log_{10}(K'_a)$ and $pK'_b = -\log_{10}(K'_b)$ yields:

$$pH = pK'_a + \log_{10}\frac{[A^-]}{[HA]} \quad (12)$$

$$pH = pK'_b + \log_{10}\frac{[B^-]}{[BH]} \quad (13)$$

The dissociation constants K'_a and K'_b provide an estimate of the strength of the acid and base, respectively. From equations 12 and 13, it can be seen that the buffer pairs are half dissociated at pH = pK'. In other words, pK' of a buffer pair is defined as the pH at which 50% of the buffer pair exists as the weak acid (HA) and 50% as the anion (A^-).

CHEMICAL EQUILIBRIA FOR THE CARBON DIOXIDE–BICARBONATE SYSTEM

When CO_2 is dissolved in water, H_2CO_3 is formed according to the reaction

$$CO_2 + H_2O \Leftrightarrow H_2CO_3 \quad (14)$$

The rate of this reaction, in the absence of the enzyme carbonic anhydrase, is slow, with a half-time of approximately 8 seconds at 37°C. The major portion of CO_2 remains as dissolved CO_2; only approximately 1 part in 1000 forms H_2CO_3, a nonvolatile acid. Because H_2CO_3 is a weak acid, it dissociates to yield H^+ and HCO_3^-:

$$H_2CO_3 \Leftrightarrow H^+ + HCO_3^- \quad (15)$$

The concentration of dissolved CO_2 is given by Henry's law:

$$[CO_2]_{dis} = \alpha_{CO_2} PCO_2 \quad (16)$$

where α_{CO_2} is the physical solubility coefficient for CO_2, which has a value of 0.0301 mmol/L in most body fluids, including plasma. Because the concentration of H_2CO_3 is low and proportional to the concentration of dissolved CO_2, equations 14 and 15 can be combined and treated as a single reaction:

$$CO_2 + H_2O \Leftrightarrow H^+ + HCO_3^- \quad (17)$$

The equilibrium constant for this reaction is given by:

$$K = \frac{[H^+][HCO_3^-]}{[CO_2][H_2O]} \quad (18)$$

Defining $K' = K[H_2O]$ as the apparent equilibrium constant and using equation 17:

$$K' = \frac{[H^+][HCO_3^-]}{\alpha_{CO_2} PCO_2} \quad (19)$$

Taking logarithms of both sides of equation 19 and recognizing that $pK' = \log_{10}(K')$ allows the familiar Henderson-Hasselbalch equation to be derived:

$$pH = pK' + \log_{10}\frac{[HCO_3^-]}{(\alpha_{CO_2} PCO_2)} \quad (20)$$

When pK' = 6.1 is used in equation 20, the Henderson equation is derived, which may be used in clinical interpretation of acid-base data:

$$[H^+](nmol/L) = 24 \frac{PCO_2 (mm\ Hg)}{[HCO_3^-](mmol/L)} \quad (21)$$

PHYSIOLOGIC ADVANTAGE OF AN OPEN BUFFER SYSTEM

The quantitative behavior of an open system buffer pair differs considerably from that of a buffer pair confined to a closed system. In an open system the buffer pair may be envisioned as occurring in two separate but communicating compartments (internal and external). The external compartment provides an effective infinite reservoir of the uncharged buffer pair component, to which the barrier between the internal and the external compartments (e.g., plasma cell membrane, vascular capillary endothelium) is freely permeable.

Physiologically, the most important open system buffer is the CO_2-HCO_3^- system.

Adjustments in alveolar ventilation serve to maintain a constant arterial CO_2 pressure ($PaCO_2$):

$$\begin{array}{ccc} \text{Acid } (H^+) & & \text{(Expired gas)} \\ \downarrow & & \uparrow\uparrow \\ H^+ + HCO_3^- & \to H_2CO_3 \to & H_2O + CO_2 \end{array} \quad (22)$$

The CO_2-HCO_3^- buffer system has an apparent pK' of 6.1 and a base/acid ($[HCO_3^-]/[H_2CO_3]$) ratio of 20:1 at pH 7.4. Because buffer efficiency is greatest in the pH range near pK'_a, it appears at first glance that the CO_2-HCO_3^- system would not function as an effective buffer in the physiologic pH range. The potency and efficacy of the CO_2-HCO_3^- buffer system are due largely to the augmentation of buffer capacity that accompanies operation in an open system. Because CO_2 is freely diffusible across biologic barriers and cell membranes, its concentration in biologic fluids can be modulated rapidly through participation of the respiratory system. When acid (H^+) is added to an HCO_3^--containing fluid, H^+ combines with HCO_3^- to generate H_2CO_3, which, in the presence of the enzyme carbonic anhydrase, is rapidly dehydrated to CO_2 (equation 22). The CO_2 produced can escape rapidly from the fluid and be excreted in the lung, which prevents accumulation of CO_2 concentrations in biologic fluids.

REGULATION OF BUFFERS

The plasma HCO_3^- concentration is protected by both metabolic and renal regulatory mechanisms. In addition, the pH of blood can be affected by respiratory adjustments in $PaCO_2$. Primary changes in $PaCO_2$ may result in acidosis or alkalosis, depending on whether CO_2 is elevated above or depressed below the normal value: 40 mm Hg. Such disorders are termed *respiratory acidosis* and *respiratory alkalosis*, respectively. A primary change in the plasma HCO_3^- concentration owing to metabolic or renal factors triggers commensurate changes in ventilation. The respiratory response to acidemia or alkalemia blunts the change in blood pH that would occur otherwise. Such respiratory alterations that adjust blood pH toward normal are referred to as *secondary* or *compensatory* alterations, because they occur in response to primary metabolic changes.

Humans are confronted, under most physiologic circumstances, with an acid challenge. "Acid production" in biologic systems is represented by the milliequivalents (mEq) of protons (H^+) added to body fluids. Conversely, proton removal is equivalent to equimolar addition of base, OH^- (generation of HCO_3^- from dissolved CO_2). Metabolism generates a daily load of relatively strong acids (lactate, citrate, acetate, and pyruvate), which must be removed by other metabolic reactions. The oxidation of these organic acids in the Krebs cycle, for example, generates CO_2, which must be excreted by the lungs. The oxidation of carbon-containing fuels produces as much as 16,000 to 20,000 mmol of CO_2 gas daily. Nevertheless, the complete combustion of carbon involves the intermediate generation and metabolism of 2000 to 3000 mmol of relatively strong organic acids, such as lactic acids, tricarboxylic acids, ketoacids, or other acids, depending on the type of fuel consumed. These organic acids do not accumulate in the body under most circumstances, with concentrations remaining in the low millimolar range. If production and consumption rates become mismatched, however, these organic acids can accumulate (e.g., lactic acid accumulation with strenuous exertion). Correspondingly, the HCO_3^- in the ECF will decline as the organic acid concentration increases. During recovery, the organic acids reenter metabolic pathways to CO_2 production, removal of H^+, and generation of HCO_3^-. Nevertheless, if the organic anions are excreted (e.g., ketonuria), these entities are no longer available for regeneration of HCO_3^-. Considered in this way, organic anions that can be metabolized may be viewed as "potential bicarbonate." The metabolism of some body constituents such as proteins, nucleic acids, and small fractions of lipids and certain carbohydrates generates specific organic acids that cannot be burned to CO_2 (e.g., uric, oxalic, glucuronic, hippuric acids). In addition, the inorganic acids H_2SO_4 and H_3PO_4, derived respectively, from sulfur-containing dietary amino acids and organophosphates, must be excreted by the kidneys or the gastrointestinal tract.

In summary, in the steady state, as a result of the buffering power of the HCO_3^-/H_2CO_3 buffer system and its preeminence over other body buffer systems, addition or removal of H^+ results in equimolar changes in the HCO_3^- concentration according to the relationship outlined in equation 3. Moreover, because this buffer system is open to air, the concentration of CO_2 remains essentially fixed. Therefore the evidence for H^+ addition or removal can be found in reciprocal changes in the numerator of the Henderson-Hasselbalch equation (equation 20), or the $[HCO_3^-]$.

INTEGRATION OF REGULATORY PROCESSES

Three physiologic processes work against changes in the HCO_3^-/CO_2 ratio: (1) metabolic regulation, (2) respiratory regulation, and (3) renal regulation. Metabolic regulation is of minor importance in terms of overall physiologic regulation of acid-base balance. Nevertheless, regulatory enzymes, whose activity may be pH sensitive, may catalyze metabolic reactions that either generate or consume organic acids. Such a process constitutes a negative feedback regulatory system. The best example is phosphofructokinase, the pivotal enzyme in the glycolytic pathway. Phosphofructokinase is a kinase enzyme that phosphorylates fructose 6-phosphate in glycolysis. The activity of phosphofructokinase is inhibited by low pH and enhanced by high pH. Thus an increase in pH_i accelerates glycolysis and generates pyruvate and lactate. It follows therefore that the generation of lactic acid in patients with lactic acidosis and the generation of ketoacids in patients with ketoacidosis are impeded by acidemia.

Because, under most circumstances, CO_2 excretion and CO_2 production are matched, the usual steady-state $Paco_2$ is maintained at 40 mm Hg. Underexcretion of CO_2 produces hypercapnia, and overexcretion produces hypocapnia. Production and excretion are again matched, but at a new steady-state Pco_2. Therefore the $Paco_2$ is regulated primarily by neurorespiratory factors and is not subject to regulation by the rate of metabolic CO_2 production. Hypercapnia is primarily the result of hypoventilation, not increased CO_2 production. Increases or decreases in Pco_2 represent derangements of control of neurorespiratory regulation or can result from compensatory changes in response to a primary alteration in the plasma HCO_3^- concentration.

RENAL REGULATION

Although temporary relief from changes in the pH of body fluids may be accomplished by chemical buffering or respiratory compensation, the ultimate defense against the addition of nonvolatile acid or of alkali is the responsibility of the kidneys. The addition of a strong acid (HA) to the ECF titrates plasma HCO_3^-:

$$HA + NaHCO_3 \Leftrightarrow NaA + H_2O + CO_2 \qquad (23)$$

The CO_2 is expired by the lungs, and body HCO_3^- buffer stores are diminished. This process occurs constantly as endogenous metabolic acids are generated. In order to maintain a normal plasma HCO_3^- in the face of constant accession of metabolic acids, predominantly as a result of dietary protein metabolism, the kidneys must (1) conserve the HCO_3^- present in glomerular filtrate and (2) regenerate the HCO_3^- decomposed by reaction with metabolic acids (equation 23). The first process (HCO_3^- reclamation) is accomplished predominantly in the proximal tubule, with an additional contribution by the loop of Henle and a minor contribution by more distal nephron segments. Under most circumstances, the filtered load of HCO_3^- is absorbed almost completely, especially during an acid load. "Acid production" in biologic systems is represented by the milliequivalents (mEq) of protons (H^+) added to body fluids. Humans eating a typical Western diet are confronted with a daily acid challenge. The amount of nonvolatile acid produced by metabolism is defined as *endogenous acid production*. Net endogenous acid production is therefore dependent on diet. For example, the inorganic acids H_2SO_4 and H_3PO_4, are derived respectively, from sulfur-containing

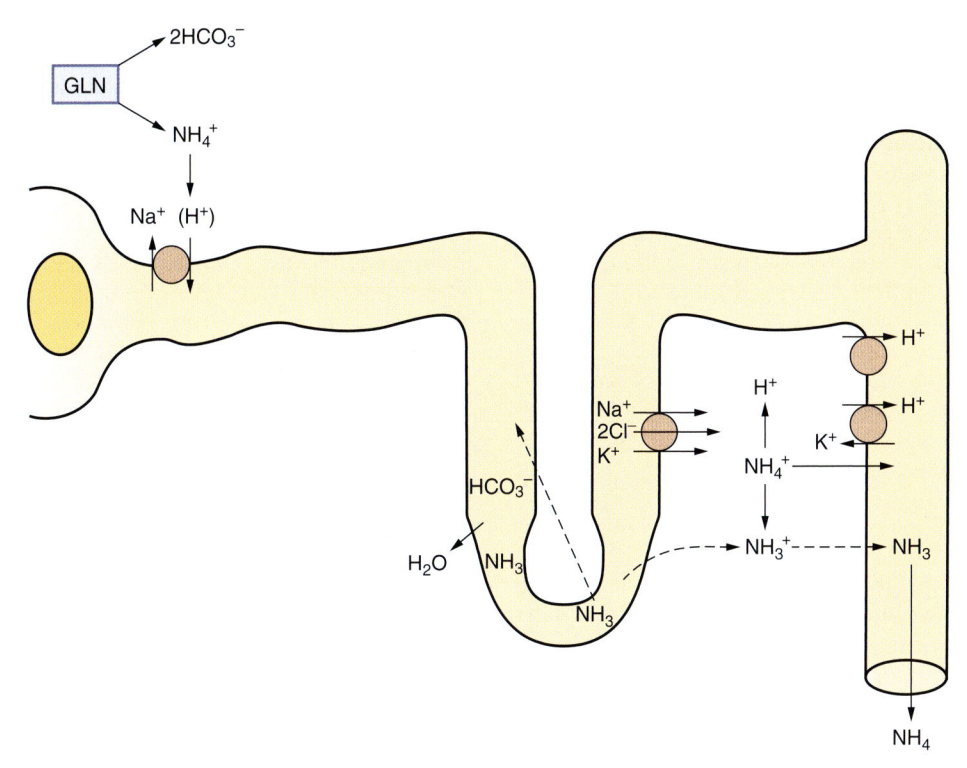

Figure 17.1 Synchrony of regulation of ammonium production (from glutamine [GLN] precursors and excretion). Process allows generation of "new" HCO_3^- by the kidney. NH_4^+ excretion is regulated in response to changes in systemic acid-base and K^+ balance. Contributing segments include the proximal convoluted tubule, proximal straight tubule, thin descending limb, thick ascending limb, and medullary collecting duct. Upregulated by acidosis and hypokalemia. Inhibited by hyperkalemia.

amino acids, such as methionine and cysteine. Conversely, base addition to the ECF via the gastrointestinal tract is derived primarily from dietary fruits and vegetables. If less acid is generated or when, in the face of an alkali load, the plasma HCO_3^- concentration increases above the normal value of 25 mEq/L, HCO_3^- will be excreted efficiently into the urine. Therefore the kidney must efficiently excrete any excess in alkali added to the ECF as well as regenerate the bicarbonate lost when net endogenous acid production is significant. The difference between endogenous acid production and the input of alkali absorbed by the gastrointestinal system (i.e., the difference in acid production and base generation) is known as *net endogenous acid production*. Because a Western diet is high in protein, net endogenous production is positive and consumes bicarbonate; therefore the kidney must regenerate the bicarbonate consumed by dietary protein intake.

The second process, HCO_3^- regeneration, is represented by the renal output of acid or net acid excretion (Figure 17.1):

Net acid excretion = NH_4^+ + Titratable acid − HCO_3^- (24)

On balance, each milliequivalent of net acid excreted corresponds to 1 mEq of HCO_3^- returned to the ECF. This process of HCO_3^- regeneration is necessary to replace the HCO_3^- lost by the entry of fixed acids into the ECF or, less commonly, the HCO_3^- excreted in stool or urine. Because a typical Western diet generates fixed acids at 50 to 70 mEq/day, net acid excretion must be augmented to maintain acid-base balance, avoiding metabolic acidosis. Therefore net acid excretion approximates 50 to 70 mEq/day to match net acid production. Daily acid-base balance can be estimated therefore by subtracting net acid excretion plus any base absorbed from the gut from the amount of net acid produced daily. The daily production of acid is representative of the amount of H_2SO_4 and noncombustible organic acids generated and is synonymous with the milliequivalents of SO_4^{2-} and organic acid anions (A^-) excreted in the urine.

SYSTEMIC RESPONSE TO CHANGES IN CARBON DIOXIDE TENSION

ACUTE RESPONSE: GENERATION OF RESPIRATORY ACIDOSIS OR ALKALOSIS

Intrinsic disturbances in the respiratory system can alter the relationship of CO_2 production and excretion and give rise to abnormal values of $PaCO_2$. Some stimuli evoke a primary increase in ventilation, which lowers systemic $PaCO_2$. These stimuli include hypoxemia, fever, anxiety, central nervous system disease, acute cardiopulmonary processes, septicemia, liver failure, pregnancy, and drugs (e.g., salicylates).[3] Conversely, $PaCO_2$ increases if the respiratory system is depressed by suppression of the respiratory control center or of the respiratory apparatus itself (neuromuscular, parenchymal, and airway components).[4] In both kinds of acute respiratory disorders, CO_2 is added to or subtracted from the body until the $PaCO_2$ assumes a new steady state so that pulmonary CO_2 excretion equals CO_2 production. The accumulation or loss of CO_2 causes changes in blood pH within minutes. The plasma HCO_3^- decreases slightly as the $PaCO_2$ is reduced in acute respiratory alkalosis and increases slightly in acute respiratory acidosis.[2-5] The small changes in HCO_3^- concentration are due to buffering by nonbicarbonate buffers.[2-5] The estimated change in blood HCO_3^- concentration is approximately equal to 0.1 mEq/L of $[HCO_3^-]$ for each millimeter of mercury increase in PCO_2 and 0.25 mEq/L for each millimeter of mercury decrease in PCO_2.[4] Acute alterations in PCO_2 in either direction within the physiologic range do not change the blood HCO_3^- concentration by more than a total of approximately 4 to 5 mEq/L from normal. Organic acid production, especially of lactic and citric acids, increases modestly during acute hypocapnia, decreasing the blood HCO_3^- concentration and blunting the respiratory response to metabolic alkalosis.[2-5]

CHRONIC RESPONSE

Although the blood pH is relatively poorly defended during acute changes in $PaCO_2$, during chronic changes, the kidneys are recruited to excrete or retain HCO_3^- and return blood pH toward normal. The persistence of hypocapnia reduces renal bicarbonate absorption to achieve a further decrease in the plasma HCO_3^- concentration. Hypocapnia decreases renal HCO_3^- reabsorption[3] by inhibiting acidification in both the proximal[5] and the distal nephrons. The resulting decrease in plasma HCO_3^- concentration is equal to approximately 0.4 to 0.5 mEq/L for each millimeter of mercury decrease in PCO_2.[5] Thus the arterial pH falls toward, but not completely back to, normal.

Several hours to days are required for full expression of the renal response to chronic hypocapnia,[4,5] which includes a reduction in the rate of H^+ secretion, an increase in urine pH, a decrease in NH_4^+ and titratable acid excretion, and a modest bicarbonaturia. An increase in blood Cl^- concentration occurs simultaneously by means of several mechanisms: a shift of Cl^- out of red blood cells, ECF volume contraction, and enhanced Cl^- reabsorption. An overshoot in HCO_3^- generation and sustained reabsorption may occur on occasion, so that blood pH may become alkaline with severe chronic hypercapnia (values of $\leq$ 70 mm Hg).[4,5] One example of this phenomenon is the increment in renal HCO_3^- generation caused by nocturnal CO_2 retention in patients with obstructive sleep apnea. Both blood PCO_2 and HCO_3^- concentration increase during the night. Later in the morning, alkalotic blood gas values are often obtained, because $PaCO_2$ has declined more rapidly than HCO_3^- concentration to values characteristic of wakefulness. In chronic hypercapnia, the blood HCO_3^- concentration increases approximately 0.25 to 0.50 mEq/L for each millimeter of mercury elevation in $PaCO_2$.[4,5]

The increase in generation of HCO_3^- by the kidney during chronic hypercapnia takes several days for completion. The mechanism of HCO_3^- retention involves increased H^+ secretion by both proximal and distal nephron segments, regardless of sodium bicarbonate or sodium chloride intake, mineralocorticoid levels, or K^+ depletion.[2,4-6]

Chronic hypercapnia results in sustained increases in renal cortical PCO_2, and the increase in renal cortical PCO_2 that occurs with chronic hypercapnia stimulates acidification.[5] The increased PCO_2 enhances distal H^+ secretion so that increased NH_4^+ excretion occurs even with a low-salt diet or with hypoxemia. However, if hyperkalemia ensues or is present initially, the renal adaptation to chronic hypercapnia is blunted significantly. Hyperkalemia decreases NH_4^+ production and excretion even in the face of acidemia.[6] The effect of an elevated PCO_2 to augment tubule HCO_3^- reabsorption may also be mediated by hemodynamic changes, especially by systemic vasodilation, so that a decreased effective ECF status is sensed by the kidney. Hypercapnia also decreases proximal sodium chloride reabsorption and causes chloruresis, which can further compromise ECF.[5,6] If the hemodynamic alterations induced by hypercapnia are corrected, the direct effect of acute hypercapnia to increase net renal HCO_3^- transport is abated. Thus with time an adaptation occurs in the proximal nephron: HCO_3^- reabsorption is stimulated after several days of hypercapnia.[7]

In summary, although primary alterations in systemic $PaCO_2$ cause relatively marked changes in blood pH, renal homeostatic mechanisms allow the blood pH to return toward normal over a sufficient period. The renal response to chronic hypercapnia is manifest primarily by an increase in net acid excretion and HCO_3^- absorption, which is accomplished by augmented H^+ secretion in both proximal and distal nephron segments.[8]

SYSTEMIC RESPONSE TO ADDITION OF NONVOLATILE ACIDS

In addition to generating large quantities of CO_2, the metabolic processes of the body produce a smaller quantity of nonvolatile acids. The lungs readily excrete CO_2, and this process can respond rapidly to changes in production. In contrast, the kidneys must excrete nonvolatile acids through a much slower adaptive response. The time course of compensation for addition of acid or alkali to the body is displayed schematically in Figure 17.2. The hypothetical completion of each process is plotted as a function of time and progresses in the following sequence: (1) distribution and buffering in the ECF, (2) cellular buffering, (3) respiratory compensation, and (4) renal acid or base excretion.

SOURCES OF ENDOGENOUS ACIDS

Pathologically, acid loads may be derived from endogenous acid production (e.g., generation of ketoacids and lactic acids) or loss of base (e.g., diarrhea) or from exogenous sources (e.g., ammonium chloride or toxin ingestion). Under normal physiologic circumstances, a daily input of acid derived from the diet and metabolism confronts the body with an acid challenge. The net result of these processes amounts to the entry of approximately 1.0 mEq of new H^+ per kilogram per day into the ECF.[2,5]

Sulfuric acid is formed when organic sulfur from methionine and cysteine residues of proteins are oxidized to SO_4^{2-}. The metabolism of sulfur-containing amino acids is the primary source of acid in the usual Western diet, accounting for approximately 50%. The quantity of sulfuric acid generated is equal to the SO_4^{2-} excreted in the urine.

Organic acids are derived from intermediary metabolites formed by partial combustion of dietary carbohydrates, fats,

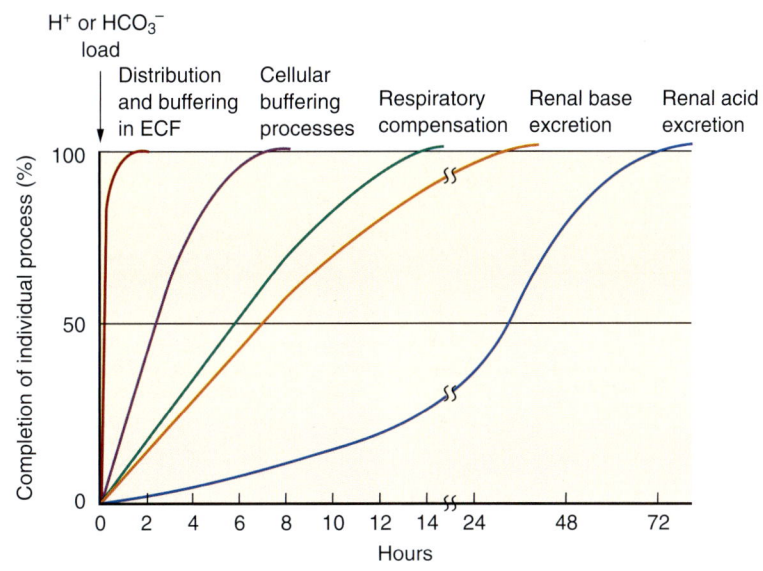

Figure 17.2 Time course of acid-base compensatory mechanisms in response to a metabolic acid or alkaline load. Component processes in completion of the distribution and extracellular buffering mechanisms, cellular buffering events, and respiratory and renal regulatory processes are presented as a function of time. *ECF,* Extracellular fluid.

and proteins as well as from nucleic acids (uric acid). Organic acid generation contributes to net endogenous acid production when the conjugate bases are excreted in the urine as organic anions. If full oxidation of these acids can occur, however, H^+ is reclaimed and eliminated as CO_2 and water. The net amount of H^+ added to the body from this source can be estimated by the amount of organic anions excreted in the urine.

Phosphoric acid can be derived from hydrolysis of PO_4^{3-} esters in proteins and nucleic acids if it is not neutralized by mineral cations (e.g., Na^+, K^+, and Mg^{2+}). The contribution of dietary phosphates to acid production is dependent on the kind of protein ingested. Some proteins generate phosphoric acid, whereas others generate only neutral phosphate salts.[2,5] Hydrochloric acid is generated by metabolism of cationic amino acids (lysine, arginine, and some histidine residues) into neutral products. Other potential acid or base sources in the diet can be estimated from the amount of unidentified cations and anions ingested.

Potential sources of bases are also found in the diet (e.g., acetate, lactate, citrate), primarily from fruits and vegetables, and can be absorbed to neutralize partially the H^+ loads from the three sources just mentioned. These potential base equivalents may be estimated by subtracting the unmeasured anions in the stool ($Na^+ + K^+ + Ca^{2+} + Mg^{2+} - Cl^- = 1.8$ P) from those measured in the diet. The net base absorbed by the gastrointestinal tract is derived from the anion gap (AG) of the diet minus that of the stool. Acid production is partially offset by HCO_3^- produced when organic anions combine with H^+ and are oxidized to CO_2 and H_2O or when dibasic phosphoesters combine with H^+ during hydrolysis. The gastrointestinal tract may modify the amount of these potential bases reabsorbed under particular circumstances of acidosis or growth. It has been confirmed in patients ingesting an artificial diet that urinary (NH_4^+ + titratable acid [TA] – HCO_3^-) is equal to urinary (SO_4^{2-} + organic A^- + dietary phosphoester-derived H^+).[2,5,9]

In summary, dietary foodstuffs contain many sources of acids and bases. These can be estimated by the urinary excretion of SO_4^{2-} and organic anions minus the unmeasured anions. The usual North American diet represents a daily source of acid generation for which the body must compensate constantly.

HEPATIC AND RENAL ROLES IN ACID-BASE HOMEOSTASIS

The generation of acid by protein catabolism is balanced by the generation of new HCO_3^- through renal NH_4^+ and titratable acid excretion (or, in sum, net acid excretion). Hepatic catabolism of proteins, with the exception of sulfur- and PO_4^{3-}-containing amino acids, can be considered a neutral process. The products of these neutral reactions are HCO_3^- and NH_4^+. Most of the NH_4^+ produced by metabolism of amino acids reacts with HCO_3^- or forms urea and thus has no impact on acid-base balance. A portion of this NH_4^+ is diverted to glutamine synthesis, the amount of which is regulated by pH. Acidemia promotes and alkalemia inhibits glutamine synthesis. Glutamine enters the circulation and reaches the kidney, where it is deaminated to form glutamate. Renal glutamine deamination results in NH_4^+ production and initiates a metabolic process that generates new HCO_3^- through α-ketoglutarate. Glutamine deamination in the kidney is also highly regulated by systemic pH, so that acidemia augments and alkalemia inhibits NH_4^+ and HCO_3^- production. The ultimate control, however, resides in the renal excretion of NH_4^+, because the NH_4^+ must be excreted to escape entry into the hepatic urea synthetic pool. Hepatic urea synthesis would negate the new HCO_3^- realized from α-ketoglutarate in the kidney. Hepatic regulation of NH_4^+ metabolic pathways appears to facilitate glutamine production when NH_4^+ excretion is stimulated by acidemia or, conversely, blunts glutamine production when excretion is inhibited by alkalemia.[9]

Table 17.1 Acid-Base Abnormalities and Appropriate Compensatory Responses for Simple Disorders

Primary Acid-Base Disorders	Primary Defect	Effect on pH	Compensatory Response	Expected Range of Compensation	Limits of Compensation
Respiratory acidosis	Alveolar hypoventilation (↑ Pco_2)	↓	↑ Renal HCO_3^- reabsorption (HCO_3^- ↑)	Acute Δ $[HCO_3^-]$ = +1 mEq/L for each ↑ ΔPco_2 of 10 mm Hg Chronic Δ $[HCO_3^-]$ = +4 mEq/L for each ↑ ΔPco_2 of 10 mm Hg	$[HCO_3^-]$ = 38 mEq/L $[HCO_3^-]$ = 45 mEq/L
Respiratory alkalosis	Alveolar hyperventilation (↓ Pco_2)	↑	↓ Renal HCO_3^- reabsorption (HCO_3^- ↓)	Acute Δ $[HCO_3^-]$ = −2 mEq/L for each ↓ ΔPco_2 of 10 mm Hg Chronic Δ $[HCO_3^-]$ = −5 mEq/L for each ↓ ΔPco_2 of 10 mm Hg	$[HCO_3^-]$ = 18 mEq/L $[HCO_3^-]$ = 15 mEq/L
Metabolic acidosis	Loss of HCO_3^- or gain of H^+ (↓ HCO_3^-)	↓	Alveolar hyperventilation to ↑ pulmonary CO_2 excretion (↓ Pco_2)	Pco_2 = 1.5$[HCO_3^-]$ + 8 ± 2 Pco_2 = last 2 digits of pH × 100 Pco_2 = 15 + $[HCO_3^-]$	Pco_2 = 15 mm Hg
Metabolic alkalosis	Gain of $HCO_3Δ$ or loss of H^+ (↑ HCO_3^-)	↑	Alveolar hypoventilation to ↓ pulmonary CO_2 excretion (↑ Pco_2)	Pco_2 = +0.6 mm Hg for Δ $[HCO_3^-]$ of 1 mEq/L Pco_2 = 15 + $[HCO_3^-]$	Pco_2 = 55 mm Hg

Pco_2, Carbon dioxide pressure.
Adapted from Bidani A, Tauzon DM, Heming TA: Regulation of whole body acid-base balance. In DuBose TD, Hamm LL, editors: Acid-base and electrolyte disorders: a companion to Brenner and Rector's the kidney, Philadelphia, 2002, Saunders, pp 1-2.

NEURORESPIRATORY RESPONSE TO ACIDEMIA

A critically important response to an acid load is the neurorespiratory control of ventilation. Although the precise mechanism for this response is debated,[2,4,5,9] the prevailing view is that a fall in systemic arterial pH is sensed by the chemoreceptors that stimulate ventilation and therefore reduce $PaCO_2$. The fall in blood pH that would otherwise occur in uncompensated metabolic acidosis is therefore blunted. The pH is not restored to normal; however, $PaCO_2$ declines by an average of 1.25 mm Hg for each 1.0 mEq/L drop in HCO_3^- concentration. The appropriate $PaCO_2$ in steady-state metabolic acidosis can be estimated from the prevailing HCO_3^- concentration according to the following expression[10]:

$$PaCO_2 = 1.5\,[HCO_3^-] + 8\ (\pm 2\ \text{mm Hg}) \qquad (25)$$

It is convenient to remember that the predicted (or compensatory) $PaCO_2$ can be approximated by adding to the patient's $[HCO_3^-]$ the number 15 (valid in the pH range of 7.2 to 7.5). Because the $PaCO_2$ cannot fall below approximately 10 to 12 mm Hg, the blood pH is less well defended by respiration after very large reductions in the plasma HCO_3^- concentration (Table 17.1).

Approximately 12 to 24 hours is required to achieve full respiratory compensation for metabolic acidosis (see Figure 17.2).

RENAL EXCRETION

As already discussed, the kidneys eliminate the acid that is produced daily by metabolism and diet and have the capacity to increase urinary net acid excretion (and hence HCO_3^- generation) in response to endogenous or exogenous acid loads. Renal excretion of acid is usually matched to the net production of metabolic and dietary acids, approximately 55 to 70 mEq/day, so little disturbance in systemic pH or HCO_3^- concentration occurs. The widely accepted rate of net acid production has been based traditionally on data derived from metabolic studies accomplished many years ago. Later studies involving measurement or estimation of net acid production and net acid excretion have been higher and reflect the changes in our culture with "supersizing" and higher average dietary protein intake. Nevertheless, the key point is that if acid production remains high and unabated by net acid excretion, metabolic acidosis will ensue.

As an acid load is incurred, the kidneys respond to restore balance by increasing NH_4^+ excretion (titratable acid excretion has limited capacity for regulation). With continued acid loading, renal net acid excretion increases over the course of 3 to 5 days (see Figure 17.2) but does not quite achieve the level of acid production. Progressive positive acid balance ensues, buffered presumably by bone carbonate.

Thus the renal response to an acid load requires (1) reclamation of the filtered HCO_3^- by the proximal tubule and (2) augmentation of NH_4^+ production and excretion by the distal nephron. In this way the kidneys efficiently retain all filtered base and attempt to generate enough new base to restore the arterial pH toward normal. There is growing evidence that, because of relatively higher net endogenous acid production due to high dietary protein intake, this adaptive process, augmentation of ammonium production and excretion, can, in and of itself, be harmful and in the face of chronic kidney disease (CKD) may even contribute independently to progression of CKD. Thus recommendations that the plasma [HCO_3^-] be maintained above 22 mEq/L in patients with CKD may be too conservative. Even a normal [HCO_3^-] may become subject to alkali treatment in CKD patients in the near future.[11,12]

In summary, acidosis enhances proximal HCO_3^- absorption, decreasing delivery of HCO_3^- out of the proximal tubule, and enhances distal acidification. Net acid excretion is increased by stimulation of NH_4^+ production and excretion.

SYSTEMIC RESPONSE TO GAIN OF ALKALI

Whereas the major goal of the body in defense of an acid challenge is to conserve body buffer stores and to generate new base, the response to an alkali load is to eliminate base as rapidly as possible. The response is dependent on the same three responses outlined for defense of an acid challenge, namely, cellular buffering and distribution within the ECF, respiratory compensation, and renal excretion.

DISTRIBUTION AND CELLULAR BUFFERING

Ninety-five percent of a base load in the form of HCO_3^- is distributed in the ECF within approximately 25 minutes[2,5,9,13] (see Figure 17.2). Simultaneously, the various processes of cellular buffering serve to dissipate this HCO_3^- load. Cellular buffering of the HCO_3^- load has a half-time of 3.3 hours. The apparent distribution volume for the administered HCO_3^- is inversely proportional to the preexisting plasma HCO_3^- concentration. A lesser fraction of base is buffered via cellular processes than occurs when a comparable amount of acid is administered (see Figure 17.2). Two-thirds of the administered HCO_3^- is retained in the ECF; a third is buffered in cells, principally by Na^+-H^+ exchange, and a small amount is buffered by increased lactate production and Cl^--HCO_3^- exchange.[1] Modest hypokalemia occurs as a result of K^+ shifts into cells and is approximately equal to 0.4 to 0.5 mEq/L of K^+ per 0.1 unit pH increase above 7.40.

In summary, the cellular defense against an alkaline load is somewhat less effective than the defense against an acid load. There is also poorer stabilization of intracellular pH in the alkaline than in the acid range.[2,13]

RESPIRATORY COMPENSATION

The pulmonary response to an acute increase in HCO_3^- concentration is biphasic. Neutralization of sodium bicarbonate by buffers (H^+ buffer$^-$) results in CO_2 liberation and an increase in PCO_2:

$$Na^+HCO_3^- + H^+buffer^- \Leftrightarrow Na^+buffer^- + H_2CO_3 \Leftrightarrow H_2O + CO_2 \quad (26)$$

The increased PCO_2 stimulates ventilation acutely to return PCO_2 toward normal. If the pulmonary system is compromised or the ventilation rate is controlled artificially, increased CO_2 production from infused sodium bicarbonate can lead to hazardous hypercapnia.[2,5,13]

Approximately an hour after an abrupt increment in the HCO_3^- concentration, when the increased generation of CO_2 subsides, stimulation of respiration is transformed into suppression of respiration, and PCO_2 increases. This secondary hypercapnic response takes several hours and partially compensates for the elevated HCO_3^- concentration so that arterial pH is returned toward (although not completely to) normal (see Figure 17.2).

The hypercapnic response to metabolic alkalosis is difficult to reliably predict. Attempts to substantiate a role for K^+ deficiency in preventing hypoventilation have not been illuminating.[9,13,14] Moreover, studies of alkalotic patients taking diuretics demonstrate a predictable hypoventilatory response and cast doubt on a significant role of K^+ deficiency in blunting alkalosis-induced hypoventilation.[13] Most studies have found that an increase in PCO_2 regularly occurs in response to alkalosis. The hypoventilatory response can lead to borderline or even frank hypoxemia in patients with chronic lung disease.[13] In general, the increase in $PaCO_2$ can be predicted to equal 0.75 mm Hg per 1.0 mEq/L increase in plasma HCO_3^-; or more simply, add the value of 15 to the measured plasma [HCO_3^-][14] to predict the expected $PaCO_2$ (see Table 17.1).

RENAL EXCRETION

WITH EXTRACELLULAR VOLUME EXPANSION

The addition of sodium bicarbonate to the body results in prompt cellular buffering and respiratory compensation. However, as with an acid load, the kidneys have the ultimate responsibility for the disposal of base and restoration of base stores to normal. The renal response is more rapid with HCO_3^- addition than with acid ingestion (see Figure 17.2). The speed and efficiency with which HCO_3^- can be excreted by the kidneys are such that it is difficult to render a patient with normal renal function more than mildly alkalotic on a long-term basis, even when as much as 24 mEq/kg/day of sodium bicarbonate is ingested for several weeks.[13]

The type B intercalated cell in the collecting tubule also secretes HCO_3^- through the activity of the HCO_3^--Cl^- exchanger pendrin. In the face of an alkaline systemic pH this exchanger is responsible for net bicarbonate secretion. Accordingly, HCO_3^- secretion by the type B intercalated cell prevents a more severe alkalosis and participates in the HCO_3^- excretory response.

The proximal tubule is responsible principally for HCO_3^- excretion when the blood HCO_3^- concentration increases. Absolute proximal HCO_3^- reabsorption does not increase in proportion to HCO_3^- load in the rat kidney because of suppression of proximal acidification by alkalemia[6] so that HCO_3^- delivery to the distal nephron increases. The limited capacity of the distal nephron to secrete H^+ can be overwhelmed easily, and bicarbonaturia increases progressively. NH_4^+ and titratable acid excretion decline in response to the increasing urine pH.[6,14]

In summary, when kidney function and ECF volume are both normal, an acute base load is excreted entirely, and the blood HCO_3^- concentration is returned to normal within 12 to 24 hours because of depression of fractional proximal HCO_3^- reabsorption. In addition to suppression of reabsorption of the filtered HCO_3^- load, direct HCO_3^- secretion in the cortical collecting tubule (CCT) has been proposed as another mechanism for mediating HCO_3^- disposal during metabolic alkalosis.[14]

The increased delivery of HCO_3^- out of the proximal tubule in response to an increased blood HCO_3^- concentration (and, hence, filtered HCO_3^- load) in the setting of ECF expansion facilitates HCO_3^- excretion and the return of blood pH toward normal. However, other factors may independently enhance distal H^+ secretion sufficiently to prevent HCO_3^- excretion and thus counterbalance the suppressed fractional proximal HCO_3^- reabsorptive capacity. Under these circumstances, the alkalosis is maintained. For example, in the setting of primary hyperaldosteronism, despite the expanded ECF, a stable mild alkalotic condition persists in most experimental models owing to augmented collecting duct H^+ secretion.[14] In such cases, concurrent hypokalemia facilitates the generation and maintenance of metabolic alkalosis by enhancing NH_4^+ production and excretion.[6,14] Moreover, chronic hypokalemia dramatically enhances the abundance and functionality of the H^+-K^+–adenosine triphosphatase (H^+-K^+-ATPase) in the medullary collecting tubule, thus increasing rather than decreasing bicarbonate absorption.[14-17] Enhanced nonreabsorbable anion delivery, as with drug anions such as penicillins, also increases net collecting tubule H^+ secretion by increasing the effective luminal negative potential difference or by suppressing HCO_3^- secretion in the cortical collecting duct (CCD).

WITH EXTRACELLULAR VOLUME CONTRACTION AND POTASSIUM ION DEFICIENCY

The renal response to an increase in plasma HCO_3^- concentration can be modified significantly in the presence of ECF contraction and K^+ depletion.[17,18] Because the volume of distribution of Cl^- is approximately equal to the ECF, the depletion of the ECF is roughly equivalent to the depletion of Cl^-. The critical role of effective ECF and K^+ stores in modifying net HCO_3^- reabsorption has been demonstrated in numerous experimental models.

Deficiency of both Cl^- and K^+ is common in metabolic alkalosis because of renal and/or gastrointestinal losses that occur concurrently with the generation of the alkalosis.[16,18] With Cl^- depletion alone, the normal bicarbonaturic response to an increase in plasma HCO_3^- is prevented, and metabolic alkalosis can develop. K^+ depletion, even without mineralocorticoid administration, can cause metabolic alkalosis in rats and humans. When Cl^- and K^+ depletion coexist, severe metabolic alkalosis may develop in all species studied.

Two general mechanisms exist by which the bicarbonaturic response to hyperbicarbonatemia can be prevented by Cl^- and/or K^+ depletion: (1) As the plasma HCO_3^- concentration increases, there is a reciprocal fall in the glomerular filtration rate (GFR). If the fall in GFR were inversely proportional to the rise in the plasma HCO_3^- concentration, the filtered HCO_3^- load would not exceed the normal level. In this case, normal rates of proximal and distal HCO_3^- reabsorption would suffice to prevent bicarbonaturia. (2) Cl^- deficiency or K^+ deficiency increases overall renal HCO_3^- reabsorption in the setting of a normal GFR and high filtered HCO_3^- load. In this case, overall renal HCO_3^- reabsorption and therefore acidification would be increased. An increase in renal acidification might occur as a result of an increase in H^+ secretion by the proximal or the distal nephron or by both nephron segments.[14-16] The possibility that Cl^- or K^+ depletion might decrease GFR or increase proximal HCO_3^- reabsorption has been evaluated in experimental animals. That extracellular and plasma volume depletion decreases GFR is well described. GFR can also be decreased by K^+ depletion in rats and dogs. The reduction in GFR by K^+ depletion is assumed to be the result of increased production of the vasoconstrictors angiotensin II and thromboxane B_2.[15,17] These results, taken together, provide support for the first mechanism: that metabolic alkalosis can be maintained by a depression in GFR.[14-18]

The combination of an elevated and stable plasma HCO_3^- concentration, negligible urinary HCO_3^- excretion, and normal or only slightly depressed GFR suggests that renal HCO_3^- reabsorption is enhanced. An increase in renal acidification appears to be a major mechanism by which metabolic alkalosis is maintained in models of the chronic disorder. Animals with experimental forms of chronic metabolic alkalosis display increased HCO_3^- reabsorption in both the proximal and the distal tubules. The increase in HCO_3^- absorption in the proximal tubule is due, at least in part, to an increase in the delivered load of HCO_3^-. The augmented HCO_3^- absorption in distal nephron segments appears to be due to a primary increase in H^+ secretion that is independent of the HCO_3^- load delivered. Chronic hypokalemia dramatically enhances the abundance and function of the H^+-K^+-ATPase in the medullary collecting tubule. Therefore upregulation of the H^+-K^+-ATPase by hypokalemia may be a significant factor in the maintenance of chronic metabolic alkalosis.[15,19,20]

The maintenance of a high plasma HCO_3^- concentration by the kidney can be repaired by repletion of Cl^-.[21] The mechanism by which Cl^- repairs metabolic alkalosis could include normalization of the low GFR that was induced by ECF repletion. In addition, Cl^- repletion results in a decrease in proximal HCO_3^- reabsorption and an increase in HCO_3^- secretion by the distal nephron.

Repletion of K^+ alone (without Cl^- repletion) only partially corrects metabolic alkalosis. Indeed, several experimental studies have shown that Cl^- repletion can repair the alkalosis despite persisting K^+ deficiency. Full correction of metabolic alkalosis by Cl^- but not K^+ supplementation does not necessarily prove that K^+ deficiency has no role in maintaining the alkalosis. In fact, in most studies of repair of hyperbicarbonatemia by Cl^- repletion alone (without K^+ repletion), normalization of blood pH occurred only after significant volume expansion occurred. There is complete agreement that, with simultaneous repair of K^+ and Cl^- deficiencies in metabolic alkalosis, correction of the alteration in renal HCO_3^- reabsorption ensues as a result of normalization of GFR, which allows increased HCO_3^- delivery from the proximal tubule and thus excretion of the excess HCO_3^-.

In summary, the physiologic response by the kidney to a base load associated with volume expansion is to excrete the base. Base is retained, however, if there is enhanced distal HCO_3^- reabsorption as a result of K^+ and/or Cl^- deficiency.

STEPWISE APPROACH TO THE DIAGNOSIS OF ACID-BASE DISORDERS

The four cardinal acid-base disorders reviewed thus far, and the predicted compensatory responses and their limits, are summarized in Table 17.1.

> **Table 17.2 Systematic Method for Diagnosis of Simple and Mixed Acid-Base Disorders**
>
> 1. Measure arterial blood gas and electrolyte concentrations simultaneously.
> 2. Compare the [HCO$_3^-$] measured on the electrolyte panel with the calculated value from the arterial blood gas analysis. Agreement of the two values rules out laboratory error or error due to time discrepancy between the drawing of samples.
> 3. Estimate the compensatory response for either Pco$_2$ or HCO$_3^-$ (see Table 17.1).
> 4. Calculate the AG (correct for low albumin level if necessary; see text).
> 5. Appreciate the four major categories of high AG acidoses:
>   Ketoacidosis
>   Lactic acidosis
>   Renal failure acidosis
>   Toxin- or poison-induced acidosis
> 6. Appreciate the two major causes of non-AG acidoses:
>   Gastrointestinal loss of HCO$_3^-$
>   Renal loss of HCO$_3^-$
> 7. Look for a mixed disorder by comparing the delta values.
>   Compare the ΔAG and the ΔHCO$_3^-$ (see text).
>   Compare the Δ[Cl$^-$] and the ΔNa$^+$ (see text).
>
> AG, Anion gap; Pco$_2$, carbon dioxide pressure.

ABG values. In the determination of ABG concentrations by the clinical laboratory, both pH and Paco$_2$ are measured, but the reported HCO$_3^-$ concentration is calculated from the Henderson-Hasselbalch equation (equation 20) by the blood gas analyzer. The calculated value for HCO$_3^-$ or (total CO$_2$) reported with the blood gas results should be compared with the measured HCO$_3^-$ concentration (total CO$_2$) obtained on the electrolyte panel. The two values should agree within ±2 mEq/L. If these values do not agree, the clinician should suspect that the samples were not obtained simultaneously or that a laboratory error is present.

On occasion it may be necessary to compute the third value (pH, Pco$_2$, or HCO$_3^-$) when only two are available. From the Henderson equation, derived previously in this chapter (equation 21), several caveats of clinical significance are apparent. First, the normal H$^+$ concentration in blood is 40 nmol/L (conveniently remembered as the last two digits of the normal blood pH, 7.40), and the corresponding H$^+$ concentration at a pH of 7.00 is 100 nmol/L. Second, the H$^+$ concentration increases by approximately 10 nmol/L for each decrease in the blood pH of 0.10 unit (in the range of 7.20 to 7.50). An acidotic patient with a pH of 7.30 (a reduction of 0.10 pH unit, or an increase of 10 nmol/L H$^+$ concentration to 50 nmol/L) and a Pco$_2$ of 25 mm Hg would have a HCO$_3^-$ concentration of 12 mEq/L:

$$[HCO_3^-] = 24 \times \frac{Paco_2}{[H^+]} = 24 \times \frac{25}{50} = 12 \text{ mEq/L} \quad (27)$$

Although the Henderson equation and H$^+$ concentration have been suggested as the most physiologic way to portray acid-base equilibrium, the logarithmic transformation of the Henderson equation to the familiar Henderson-Hasselbalch equation is used more commonly (see equation 20). This equation is useful because acidity is measured in the clinical laboratory as pH rather than H$^+$ concentration.

Implicit in equations 20 and 21 is the concept that the final pH, or H$^+$ concentration, is determined by the ratio of HCO$_3^-$ and Paco$_2$, not by the absolute value of either. Thus a normal concentration of HCO$_3^-$ does not necessarily mean that the pH is normal, nor does a normal Paco$_2$ denote a normal pH. Conversely, a normal pH does not imply that either HCO$_3^-$ or Paco$_2$ is normal.

Suspicion that an acid-base disorder exists is usually based on clinical judgment or on the finding of an abnormal blood pH, Paco$_2$, or HCO$_3^-$ concentration. It is important to remember that determination of blood pH, Paco$_2$, and HCO$_3^-$ concentration is vital in the management of critically ill patients, especially because a normal value for transcutaneous oxygen saturation does not exclude serious perturbations in blood pH and Paco$_2$. Obviously, acid-base disorders require careful analysis of laboratory parameters along with the clinical processes occurring in the patient as revealed in the history and physical examination. The precise diagnosis is determined by proceeding in a stepwise fashion (Table 17.2).

STEP 1: MEASURE ARTERIAL BLOOD GAS AND ELECTROLYTE VALUES SIMULTANEOUSLY

To avoid errors in diagnosis, ABG values should be measured simultaneously with the plasma electrolyte levels in all patients with component acid-base abnormalities. This is necessary because consideration of changes in plasma HCO$_3^-$, Na$^+$, K$^+$, and Cl$^-$ only does not allow precise diagnosis of specific acid-base disturbances. When drawing a specimen for ABG analysis, care should be taken to obtain the arterial blood sample without excessive heparin.

STEP 2: VERIFY ACID-BASE LABORATORY VALUES

A careful analysis of the blood gas indices (pH, Paco$_2$) should begin with a check to determine whether the concomitantly measured plasma HCO$_3^-$ (total CO$_2$ concentration from the electrolyte panel) is consistent with the

STEP 3: DEFINE THE LIMITS OF COMPENSATION TO DISTINGUISH SIMPLE FROM MIXED ACID-BASE DISORDERS

After verifying the blood acid-base values by either the Henderson equation (equation 21) or the Henderson-Hasselbalch equation (equation 20), one can define the precise acid-base disorder. If the HCO$_3^-$ concentration is low and the Cl$^-$ concentration is high, either chronic respiratory alkalosis or hyperchloremic metabolic acidosis is present. The ABG determination serves to differentiate the two conditions. Although both have a decreased Paco$_2$, the pH is high with a primary respiratory disorder and low in a metabolic disorder. Chronic respiratory acidosis and metabolic alkalosis are both associated with high HCO$_3^-$ and low Cl$^-$ concentration in plasma. Again, a pH measurement distinguishes the two conditions. In many clinical situations,

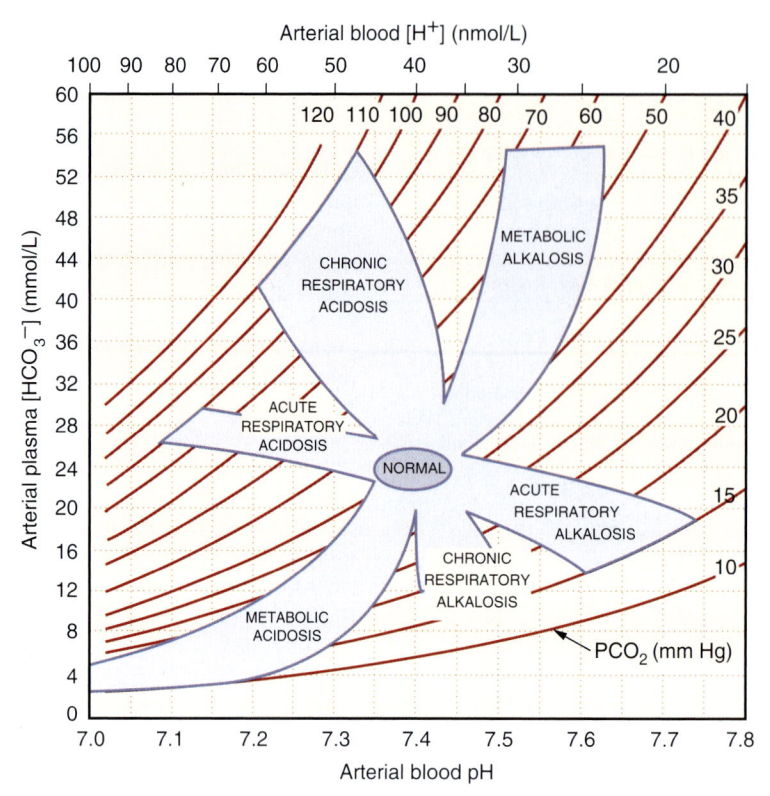

Figure 17.3 Acid-base nomogram (map). *Blue shaded areas* represent the 95% confidence limits of the normal respiratory and metabolic compensations for primary acid-base disturbances. Data falling *outside the blue shaded areas* denote a mixed disorder if a laboratory error is not present (see text).

however, a mixture of acid-base disorders may exist. Diagnosis of these disturbances requires additional information and a more complex analysis of data.

A convenient, but not always reliable, approach is an acid-base map, such as the one displayed in Figure 17.3, which defines the 95% confidence limits of simple acid-base disorders.[2,5,22] If the arterial acid-base values fall within one of the blue shaded areas in Figure 17.3, one may assume that a simple acid-base disturbance is present, and a tentative diagnostic category can be assigned. Values that fall outside the blue shaded areas imply, but do not prove, that a mixed disorder exists.

The two broad types of acid-base disorders are metabolic and respiratory. Metabolic acidosis and alkalosis are disorders characterized by primary disturbances in the concentration of HCO_3^- in plasma (numerator of equation 20), whereas respiratory disorders involve primarily alteration of $Paco_2$ (denominator of equation 20). The most commonly encountered clinical disturbances are simple acid-base disorders, that is, one of the four cardinal acid-base disturbances—metabolic acidosis, metabolic alkalosis, respiratory acidosis, or respiratory alkalosis—occurring in a pure or simple form. More complicated clinical situations, especially in severely ill patients, may give rise to *mixed acid-base disturbances*.[22] The possible combinations of mixed acid-base disturbances include: metabolic acidosis and respiratory acidosis or alkalosis, metabolic acidosis and metabolic alkalosis, metabolic alkalosis and respiratory acidosis or alkalosis. *Triple acid base disturbances* usually include: high anion gap metabolic acidosis, metabolic alkalosis and respiratory alkalosis or acidosis.

To appreciate and recognize a mixed acid-base disturbance, it is important to understand the physiologic compensatory responses that occur in the simple acid-base disorders. Primary respiratory disturbances (denominator of equation 20) invoke secondary metabolic responses (numerator of equation 20), and primary metabolic disturbances evoke a predictable respiratory response (see Table 17.1). To illustrate, metabolic acidosis as a result of gain of endogenous acids (e.g., lactic acid or ketoacidosis) lowers the concentration of HCO_3^- in the ECF and thus extracellular pH. As a result of *acidemia,* the medullary chemoreceptors are stimulated and invoke an increase in ventilation. As a result of the hypocapnic response, the ratio of HCO_3 to $Paco_2$ and the subsequent pH are returned toward, but not completely to, normal. The degree of compensation expected in a simple form of metabolic acidosis can be predicted from the relationship depicted in equation 26. Thus a patient with metabolic acidosis and a plasma HCO_3^- concentration of 12 mEq/L would be expected to have a $Paco_2$ between 24 and 28 mm Hg. Values of $Paco_2$ below 24 or higher than 28 mm Hg define a *mixed metabolic-respiratory disturbance* (metabolic acidosis and respiratory alkalosis or metabolic acidosis and respiratory acidosis, respectively). Therefore, by definition, mixed acid-base disturbances exceed the physiologic limits of compensation.

Similar considerations are examined for each type of acid-base disturbance as these disorders are discussed in detail separately. It should be emphasized that compensation is a predictable physiologic consequence of the primary disturbance and does not represent a secondary acidosis or alkalosis (see Figure 17.3 and Table 17.1). As emphasized in the following sections, the recognition of mixed disturbances demands of the alert physician consideration of additional clinical disorders that may require immediate attention or additional therapy.

CLINICAL AND LABORATORY PARAMETERS IN ACID-BASE DISORDERS

For correct diagnosis of a simple or mixed acid-base disorder, it is imperative that a careful history be obtained. Patients with pneumonia, sepsis, or cardiac failure frequently have a respiratory alkalosis, and patients with chronic obstructive pulmonary disease or a sedative drug overdose often display respiratory acidosis. The patient's drug history assumes importance because patients taking loop or thiazide diuretics may have metabolic alkalosis and patients receiving acetazolamide frequently have metabolic acidosis. Physical findings are often helpful as well. Tetany may occur with alkalemia, cyanosis with respiratory acidosis, and volume contraction with metabolic alkalosis. For example, the plasma HCO_3^- concentration rarely falls below 12 to 15 mEq/L as a result of compensation for respiratory alkalosis and rarely exceeds 45 mEq/L as a result of compensation for respiratory acidosis.[22]

The plasma K^+ value is often useful but should be considered only in conjunction with the HCO_3^- concentration and blood pH. It is generally appreciated that the serum K^+ value can be altered by primary acid-base disturbances as a result of shifts of K^+ either into the extracellular compartment or into the intracellular compartment. Metabolic acidosis leads to hyperkalemia. It has been reported that for each decrease in blood pH of 0.10 pH unit, the K^+ concentration should increase by 0.6 mEq/L. Thus a patient with a pH of 7.20 would be expected to have a plasma K^+ value of 5.2 mEq/L. However, considerable variation in this relationship has been reported in several conditions due to endogenous acid production, especially diabetic ketoacidosis (DKA) and lactic acidosis, which are often associated with K^+ depletion. The lack of correlation between the degree of acidemia and the plasma K^+ level is a result of several factors, including the nature and cellular permeability of the accompanying anion, the magnitude of the osmotic diuresis, the level of renal function, the presence or absence of preexisting changes in K^+ homeostasis, and the degree of catabolism. It is important to appreciate that the relationship between arterial blood pH and plasma K^+ is complex and therefore often variable. Nevertheless, the failure of a patient with severe acidosis to exhibit hyperkalemia or, conversely, the failure of a patient with severe metabolic alkalosis to exhibit hypokalemia suggests a significant derangement of body K^+ homeostasis. The combination of a low plasma K^+ level and elevated HCO_3^- level suggests metabolic alkalosis, whereas the combination of an elevated plasma K^+ value and low HCO_3^- value suggests metabolic acidosis.

It is helpful to compare the serum Cl^- concentration with the Na^+ concentration. The serum Na^+ concentration changes only as a result of changes in hydration. The Cl^- concentration changes for two reasons: (1) changes in hydration and (2) changes in acid-base balance. Thus changes in Cl^- value not reflected by proportional changes in Na^+ value suggest the presence of an acid-base disorder. For example, consider a patient with a history of vomiting, volume depletion, a Cl^- concentration of 85 mEq/L, and a Na^+ concentration of 130 mEq/L. In this case, both Na^+ and Cl^- concentrations are reduced, but the reduction in Cl^- concentrations is proportionally greater (15% versus 7%). A disproportionate decrease in Cl^- concentration suggests metabolic alkalosis or respiratory acidosis, and a disproportionate increase in Cl^- concentration suggests metabolic acidosis or respiratory alkalosis.

STEP 4: CALCULATE THE ANION GAP

All evaluations of acid-base disorders should include a simple calculation of the AG. The AG is calculated from the serum electrolyte levels and is defined as follows:

$$AG = Na^+ - (Cl^- + HCO_3^-) = 10 \pm 2 \text{ mEq/L} \qquad (28)$$

The AG represents the unmeasured anions normally present in plasma and unaccounted for by the serum electrolyte levels exclusive of K^+ that are measured on the electrolyte panel. Normal values for AG vary as to laboratory and analyte measurement techniques but in general have declined with more precise measurement of serum electrolyte levels by ion-selective electrodes. The normal value for AG ranges from 8 to 12 mEq/L, but the clinician should know the normal value for the AG in clinical laboratories used in his or her practice. In the author's hospital the normal value for AG has declined from 11 to 8 mEq/L. Because of this range of normal values for the AG and for convenience, the following computations will use the value of 10 mEq/L as the "normal" AG. The unmeasured anions that contribute to this value are normally present in serum and include anionic proteins (principally albumin and, to lesser extent, α- and β-globulins), PO_4^{3-}, SO_4^{2-}, and organic anions. As already emphasized, interpretation of the AG requires either a normal serum albumin level, or correction of the AG to a normal plasma albumin level. In general, reduction in the serum albumin level by 1 g/dL from the normal value of 4.5 g/dL decreases the AG by 2.5 mEq/L. When acid anions, such as acetoacetate and lactate, are produced endogenously in excess and accumulate in ECF, the AG increases above the normal value. This is referred to as a *high anion gap* acidosis.[22,23] In addition, for each milliequivalent per liter increase in the corrected AG, there should be an equal decrease in the plasma HCO_3^- concentration.

An increase in the AG may be due to a decrease in unmeasured cations or an increase in unmeasured anions. Combined severe hypocalcemia and hypomagnesemia represent a decrease in the contribution of unmeasured cations (Table 17.3). In addition, the AG may increase secondary to an increase in anionic albumin, as a consequence of either an increased albumin concentration or alkalemia.[22,23] The increased AG in severe alkalemia can be explained in part by the effect of alkaline pH on the electrical charge of albumin.

A decrease in the AG can be generated by an increase in unmeasured cations or a decrease in unmeasured anions (see Table 17.3). A decrease in the AG can result from (1) an increase in unmeasured cations (Ca^{2+}, Mg^{2+}, K^+), or (2) the addition to the blood of abnormal cations, such as Li^+ (Li^+ intoxication) or cationic immunoglobulins (immunoglobulin G as in plasma cell dyscrasias). Because albumin is the major unmeasured anion, the AG will also decrease if the quantity of albumin is low (e.g., nephrotic syndrome,

Table 17.3 The Anion Gap

Anion Gap = $Na^+ - (Cl^- + HCO_3^-) = 9 \pm 3$ mEq/L
(Assumes Normal [Albumin])*

Decreased Anion Gap	Increased Anion Gap
Increased Cations (Not Na⁺)	**Increased Anions (Not Cl⁻ or HCO₃⁻)**
↑ Ca^{2+}, Mg^{2+}	↑ Albumin
↑ Li^+	Alkalosis
↑ Immunoglobulin G	↑ Inorganic anions
	Phosphate
Decreased Anions (Not Cl⁻ or HCO₃⁻)	Sulfate
	↑ Organic anions
Hypoalbuminemia*	L-Lactate
Acidosis	D-Lactate
	Ketones
Laboratory Error	Uremic
Hyperviscosity	↑ Exogenously supplied anions
Bromism	Toxins
	Salicylate
	Paraldehyde
	Ethylene glycol
	Propylene glycol
	Methanol
	Toluene
	Pyroglutamic acid (5-oxoprolene)
	↑ Unidentified anions
	Other toxins
	Uremic
	Hyperosmolar, nonketotic states
	Myoglobinuric acute kidney injury
	Decreased Cations (Not Na⁺)
	↓ Ca^{2+}, Mg^{2+}

*For each decline in albumin by 1 g/dL from normal (4.5 g/dL), the anion gap decreases by 2.5 mEq/L.

---

protein malnutrition, capillary leak in patients in intensive care units).[24] Because with each decline in the serum albumin level by 1 g/dL from the normal value of 4.5 g/dL the AG will decline by 2.5 mEq/L, when hypoalbuminemia exists, it is possible to underestimate the AG and even miss an increased AG unless correction for the low albumin level and its effect on the AG is taken into account. For example, in a patient with an albumin level of 1.5 g/dL and an uncorrected AG of 10 mEq/L, the corrected AG is 17.5 mEq/L.

Laboratory errors can create a falsely low AG. Hyperviscosity and hyperlipidemia lead to an underestimation of the true Na^+ concentration, and bromide (Br^-) intoxication causes an overestimation of the true Cl^- concentration.[22]

In the presence of a normal serum albumin level, elevation of unmeasured anions is usually due to addition to the blood of non–Cl⁻-containing acids. Thus in most clinical circumstances a high AG indicates that a metabolic acidosis is present. The anions accompanying such acids include inorganic (PO_4^{3-}, SO_4^{2-}), organic (ketoacids, lactate, uremic organic anions), exogenous (salicylate or ingested toxins with organic acid production), or unidentified anions.[22] When these non–Cl⁻-containing acids are added to the blood in excess of the rate of removal, HCO_3^- is titrated (consumed), and the accompanying anion is retained to balance the preexisting cationic (Na^+) charge:

$$H^+anion^- + NaHCO_3 \Leftrightarrow H_2O + CO_2 + Na^+anion^- \quad (29)$$

The preexisting Cl⁻ concentration is unchanged when the new acid anion is added to the blood. Therefore the high AG acidoses exhibit normochloremia as well as a high gap. If the kidney does not excrete the anion, the magnitude of the decrement in HCO_3^- concentration will match the increment in the AG. If the retained anion can be metabolized to HCO_3^- directly or indirectly (e.g., ketones or lactate, after successful treatment), normal acid-base balance is restored as the AG returns toward the normal value. Alternatively, if the anion can be excreted, ECF contraction occurs, which leads to renal sodium chloride retention. Cl⁻ replaces the excreted anion, effectively bicarbonate is lost, and hyperchloremic acidosis emerges as the anion is excreted and the AG disappears.

In summary, after the titration of HCO_3^-, the ability of the kidney to excrete the anion of an administered acid determines the type of acidosis that develops. If the anion is filtered and is nonreabsorbable (e.g., SO_4^{2-}), ECF contraction, Cl⁻ retention, and hyperchloremic acidosis with a normal AG develops (non-AG acidosis). Conversely, if the anion is poorly filtered (e.g., uremic anions) or is produced endogenously, filtered, and reabsorbed (e.g., lactate and other organic anions), no change in Cl⁻ concentration occurs. The retained anion replaces the HCO_3^- lost when titrated by acid, which creates a high AG acidosis.

STEP 5 AND 6: RECOGNIZE CONDITIONS CAUSING ACID-BASE ABNORMALITIES WITH HIGH OR NORMAL ANION GAP

Appreciation that the AG is elevated requires knowledge of the four causes of a high AG acidosis: (1) ketoacidosis, (2) lactic acidosis, (3) renal failure acidosis, and (4) toxin-induced metabolic acidosis (Table 17.4). Accordingly, if the AG is normal in the face of metabolic acidosis, a hyperchloremic or non-AG acidosis exists. The specific causes of hyperchloremic acidosis that must be appreciated are outlined in a later section. Table 17.1 displays the directional changes in pH, PCO_2, and HCO_3^- for the four simple acid-base disorders. With this stepwise approach, in the next sections the specific causes of the major types of acid-base disorders are reviewed in detail.

STEP 7: COMPARE DELTA VALUES

By definition, a high AG acidosis has two identifying features: a low HCO_3^- concentration and an elevated AG. This means therefore that the elevated AG will remain evident even if another disorder coincides to modify the HCO_3^- concentration independently. Simultaneous metabolic acidosis of the high AG variety plus either metabolic alkalosis or chronic respiratory acidosis is an example of such a situation. The HCO_3^- concentration may be normal or even high in such a setting. However, the AG will be normal, and the Cl⁻ concentration relatively depressed. Consider a patient with chronic obstructive pulmonary disease with compensated respiratory acidosis ($PaCO_2$ of 65 mm Hg and

HCO_3^- concentration of 40 mEq/L) in whom acute bronchopneumonia and respiratory decompensation develop. If this patient has an HCO_3^- concentration of 24 mEq/L, Na^+ concentration of 145 mEq/L, K^+ concentration of 4.8 mEq/L, and Cl^- concentration of 96 mEq/L, it would be incorrect to assume that this "normal" HCO_3^- concentration represents improvement in acid-base status toward normal. Indeed, the arterial pH would probably be low (7.19), as a result of a more serious degree of hypercapnia than observed previously (e.g., if the PCO_2 increased from 65 to 80 mm Hg as a result of pneumonia). Even without blood gas measurements, prompt recognition that the AG was elevated to 25 mEq/L should suggest that a life-threatening lactic acidosis is superimposed on a preexisting chronic respiratory acidosis, which necessitates immediate therapy. In this example, the ΔAG is computed as 25 − 10, or patient's computed AG minus the normal value, and is equal to 15 mEq/L.

Similarly, a normal arterial HCO_3^- concentration, $PaCO_2$, and pH do not ensure the absence of an acid-base disturbance. For example, an alcoholic patient who has been vomiting may develop a metabolic alkalosis with a pH of 7.55, HCO_3^- concentration of 40 mEq/L, PCO_2 of 48 mm Hg, Na^+ concentration of 135 mEq/L, Cl^- of 80 mEq/L, and K^+ concentration of 2.8 mEq/L. If such a patient were then to develop a superimposed alcoholic ketoacidosis (AKA) with a β-hydroxybutyrate concentration of 15 mmol/L, the arterial pH would fall to 7.40, HCO_3^- concentration to 25 mEq/L, and PCO_2 to 40 mm Hg. Although the blood gas values are normal, the AG (assuming no change in Na^+ or Cl^-) is elevated (25 mEq/L), and the ΔAG is 15 mEq/L, which indicates the existence of a mixed metabolic acid-base disorder (mixed metabolic alkalosis and metabolic acidosis). The combination of metabolic acidosis and metabolic alkalosis is not uncommon and is most easily recognized, as in this case, when the ΔAG is elevated, but the HCO_3^- concentration and pH are near normal ($\Delta AG > \Delta HCO_3^-$, or 15 versus 0 mEq/L).

MIXED ACID-BASE DISORDERS

Mixed acid-base disorders—defined as independently coexisting disorders, not merely compensatory responses—are often seen in patients in critical care units and can lead to dangerous extremes of pH. A patient with DKA (metabolic acidosis) may develop an independent respiratory problem, leading to respiratory acidosis or alkalosis. Patients with underlying pulmonary disease may not respond to metabolic acidosis with an appropriate ventilatory response because of insufficient respiratory reserve. Such imposition of respiratory acidosis on metabolic acidosis can lead to severe acidemia and a poor outcome. When metabolic acidosis and metabolic alkalosis coexist in the same patient, the pH may be normal or near normal. When the pH is normal, an elevated AG denotes the presence of a metabolic acidosis. A discrepancy in the ΔAG (prevailing minus normal AG of 10 mEq/L) and the ΔHCO_3^- (normal, 25 mEq/L, minus prevailing HCO_3^-) indicates the presence of a mixed high gap acidosis–metabolic alkalosis (see example later). A diabetic patient with ketoacidosis may have renal dysfunction resulting in simultaneous metabolic acidosis. Patients who have ingested an overdose of drug combinations such as sedatives and salicylates may have mixed disturbances as a result of the acid-base response to the individual drugs (metabolic acidosis mixed with respiratory acidosis or respiratory alkalosis, respectively).

Even more complex are triple acid-base disturbances. For example, patients with metabolic acidosis due to AKA may develop metabolic alkalosis due to vomiting and superimposed respiratory alkalosis due to the hyperventilation of hepatic dysfunction or alcohol withdrawal. Conversely, when hyperchloremic acidosis and metabolic alkalosis occur concomitantly, the increase in Cl^- is out of proportion to the change in HCO_3^- concentration ($\Delta Cl^- > \Delta HCO_3^-$).[22]

In summary, an AG exceeding that expected for a patient's albumin concentration (i.e., >10 mEq/L), denotes the existence of either a simple high AG metabolic acidosis or a complex acid-base disorder in which an organic acidosis is superimposed on another acid-base disorder.

RESPIRATORY DISORDERS

RESPIRATORY ACIDOSIS

Respiratory acidosis occurs as the result of severe pulmonary disease, respiratory muscle fatigue, or depression in ventilatory control. An increase in $PaCO_2$ owing to reduced alveolar

Table 17.4 Clinical Causes of High Anion Gap and Normal Anion Gap Acidosis

High Anion Gap Acidosis

Ketoacidosis
  Diabetic ketoacidosis (acetoacetate)
  Alcoholic ketoacidosis (hydroxybutyrate)
  Starvation ketoacidosis
Lactic acidosis
  L-Lactic acidosis (types A and B)
  D-Lactic acidosis
Toxin-induced acidosis
  Ethylene glycol
  Methyl alcohol
  Salicylate
  Propylene glycol
  Pyroglutamic acid (5-oxoprolene)

Non–Anion Gap Acidosis

Gastrointestinal loss of HCO_3^- (negative urine anion gap)
  Diarrhea
  External fistula
Renal loss of HCO_3^- or failure to excrete NH_4^+
  Positive urine anion gap = low net acid excretion
  Proximal RTA (low serum K^+)
  Classical distal renal tubular acidosis (low serum K^+)
  Generalized distal renal tubular defect (high serum K^+)
  Drugs that cause RTA
    Carbonic anhydrase inhibitors (mixed proximal-distal RTA)
    Amphotericin B ("gradient" classical distal RTA)
Miscellaneous
  NH_4Cl ingestion
  Sulfur ingestion
  Dilutional acidosis

RTA, Renal tubular acidosis.

ventilation is the primary abnormality leading to acidemia. In acute respiratory acidosis, there is an immediate compensatory elevation in HCO_3^- (due to cellular buffering mechanisms), which increases 1 mEq/L for every 10 mm Hg increase in $PaCO_2$. In chronic respiratory acidosis (>24 hours), renal adaption is achieved and the HCO_3^- increases by 4 mEq/L for every 10 mm Hg increase in $PaCO_2$. The serum bicarbonate concentration usually does not increase above 38 mEq/L, however.

The clinical features of respiratory acidosis vary according to the severity, duration, underlying disease, and presence or absence of accompanying hypoxemia. A rapid increase in $PaCO_2$ may result in anxiety, dyspnea, confusion, psychosis, and hallucinations and may progress to coma. Lesser degrees of dysfunction in chronic hypercapnia include sleep disturbances, loss of memory, daytime somnolence, and personality changes. Coordination may be impaired, and motor disturbances such as tremor, myoclonic jerks, and asterixis may develop. The sensitivity of the cerebral vasculature to the vasodilating effects of CO_2 can cause headaches and other signs that mimic increased intracranial pressure, such as papilledema, abnormal reflexes, and focal muscle weakness.

The causes of respiratory acidosis are displayed in Table 17.5 *(right column)*. A reduction in ventilatory drive from depression of the respiratory center by a variety of drugs, injury, or disease can produce respiratory acidosis. Acutely, this may occur with general anesthetics, sedatives, narcotics, alcohol, and head trauma. Chronic causes of respiratory center depression include sedatives, alcohol, intracranial tumors, and the syndromes of sleep-disordered breathing, including the primary alveolar and obesity-hypoventilation syndromes. Neuromuscular disorders involving abnormalities or disease in the motor neurons, neuromuscular junction, and skeletal muscle can cause hypoventilation. Although a number of diseases should be considered in the differential diagnosis, drugs and electrolyte disorders should always be ruled out.

Mechanical ventilation may result in respiratory acidosis when not properly adjusted and supervised or when complicated by barotrauma or displacement of the endotracheal tube. This occurs if carbon dioxide production suddenly rises (because of fever, agitation, sepsis, or overfeeding) or if alveolar ventilation falls because of worsening pulmonary function. High levels of positive end-expiratory pressure in the presence of reduced cardiac output may cause hypercapnia as a result of large increases in alveolar dead space. Permissive hypercapnia may be used because lower tidal volumes may reduce the incidence of the barotrauma associated with high airway pressures and peak airway pressures in mechanically ventilated patients with respiratory distress syndrome.[25] Acute hypercapnia of any cause can lead to severe acidemia, neurologic dysfunction, and death. However, when CO_2 levels are allowed to increase gradually, the resulting acidosis is less severe, and the elevation in arterial PCO_2 is tolerated more readily. The resulting hypercapnia, which is secondary to the attempt to limit airway pressures, causes the arterial pH to decline, and the degree of acidemia may be evident. The magnitude of the acidemia associated with permissive hypercapnia may be augmented if superimposed on metabolic acidosis, such as lactic acidosis. This combination is not uncommon in the setting of the

Table 17.5 Respiratory Acid-Base Disorders

Alkalosis	Acidosis
Central nervous system stimulation	Central nervous system depression
Pain	Drugs (anesthetics, morphine, sedatives)
Anxiety, psychosis	
Fever	Stroke
Cerebrovascular accident	Infection
Meningitis, encephalitis	Airway
Tumor	Obstruction
Trauma	Asthma
Hypoxemia or tissue hypoxia	Parenchyma
High-altitude acclimatization	Emphysema/chronic obstructive pulmonary disease
Pneumonia, pulmonary edema	
Aspiration	Pneumoconiosis
Severe anemia	Bronchitis
Drugs or hormones	Adult respiratory distress syndrome
Pregnancy (progesterone)	
Salicylates	Barotrauma
Nikethamide	Mechanical ventilation
Stimulation of chest receptors	Hypoventilation
Hemothorax	Permissive hypercapnia
Flail chest	Neuromuscular
Cardiac failure	Poliomyelitis
Pulmonary embolism	Kyphoscoliosis
Miscellaneous	Myasthenia
Septicemia	Muscular dystrophies
Hepatic failure	Multiple sclerosis
Mechanical hyperventilation	Miscellaneous
Heat exposure	Obesity
Recovery from metabolic acidosis	Hypoventilation

critical care unit. Bicarbonate infusion may be indicated with mixed metabolic acidosis–respiratory acidosis, but the goal of therapy with alkali is to not increase the bicarbonate and pH to normal. With low tidal volume ventilation, a reasonable therapeutic target for arterial pH is approximately 7.30.[25] Moreover, with hypercapnia in the range of 60 mm Hg, a larger amount of bicarbonate will be necessary to achieve this goal. Bicarbonate administration will further increase the PCO_2, especially in patients with fixed rates of ventilation, and will add to the magnitude of the hypercapnia. Use of a continuous bicarbonate infusion in this setting may be necessary, but frequent monitoring of ABG levels, electrolytes, and the volume status of the patient is necessary.

Disease and obstruction of the airways, when severe or long-standing, causes respiratory acidosis. Acute hypercapnia follows sudden occlusion of the upper airway or the more generalized bronchospasm that occurs with severe asthma, anaphylaxis, and inhalational burn or toxin injury. Chronic hypercapnia and respiratory acidosis occur in end-stage obstructive lung disease.[4] Restrictive disorders involving both the chest wall and the lungs can cause acute and chronic hypercapnia. Rapidly progressing restrictive processes in the lung can lead to respiratory acidosis, because the high cost of breathing causes ventilatory muscle fatigue. Intrapulmonary and extrapulmonary restrictive defects present as chronic respiratory acidosis in their most advanced stages.

The diagnosis of respiratory acidosis requires, by definition, the measurement of arterial $Paco_2$ and pH. Detailed history and physical examination often provide important diagnostic clues to the nature and duration of the acidosis. When a diagnosis of respiratory acidosis is made, its cause should be investigated. Chest radiography is an initial step. Pulmonary function studies, including spirometry, diffusing capacity for carbon monoxide, lung volumes, and arterial $Paco_2$ and oxygen saturation usually provide adequate assessment of whether respiratory acidosis is secondary to lung disease. Workup for nonpulmonary causes should include a detailed drug history, measurement of hematocrit, and assessment of upper airway, chest wall, pleura, and neuromuscular function.[3,4]

The treatment of respiratory acidosis depends on its severity and rate of onset. Acute respiratory acidosis can be life-threatening, and measures to reverse the underlying cause should be undertaken simultaneously with restoration of adequate alveolar ventilation to relieve severe hypoxemia and acidemia. Temporarily, this may necessitate tracheal intubation and assisted mechanical ventilation. Oxygen level should be carefully titrated in patients with severe chronic obstructive pulmonary disease and chronic CO_2 retention who are breathing spontaneously. When oxygen is used injudiciously, these patients may experience progression of the respiratory acidosis when ventilation is driven by oxygen pressure (Pao_2) and not the normal parameters of $Paco_2$ and pH. Aggressive and rapid correction of hypercapnia should be avoided, because the falling $Paco_2$ may provoke the same complications noted with acute respiratory alkalosis (i.e., cardiac arrhythmias, reduced cerebral perfusion, and seizures). It is advisable to lower the $Paco_2$ gradually in chronic respiratory acidosis, with the aim of restoring the $Paco_2$ to baseline levels while at the same time providing sufficient chloride and potassium to enhance the renal excretion of bicarbonate.[4]

Chronic respiratory acidosis is frequently difficult to correct, but general measures aimed at maximizing lung function, including cessation of smoking; use of oxygen, bronchodilators, corticosteroids, and/or diuretics; and physiotherapy can help some patients and can forestall further deterioration. The use of respiratory stimulants may prove useful in selected cases, particularly if the patient appears to have hypercapnia out of proportion to his or her level of lung function.

RESPIRATORY ALKALOSIS

Alveolar hyperventilation decreases $Paco_2$ and increases the $HCO_3^-/Paco_2$ ratio, thus increasing pH (alkalemia). Nonbicarbonate cellular buffers respond by consuming HCO_3^-. Hypocapnia develops whenever a sufficiently strong ventilatory stimulus causes CO_2 output in the lungs to exceed its metabolic production by tissues. Plasma pH and HCO_3^- concentration appear to vary proportionately with $Paco_2$ over a range from 40 to 15 mm Hg. The relationship between arterial hydrogen ion concentration and $Paco_2$ is approximately 0.7 nmol/L/mm Hg (or 0.01 pH unit/mm Hg) and that for plasma $[HCO_3^-]$ is 0.2 mEq/L/mm Hg, or the $[HCO_3^-]$ will decrease approximately 2 mEq/L for each 10 mm Hg.[3]

Beyond 2 to 6 hours, sustained hypocapnia is further compensated by a decrease in renal ammonium and titratable acid excretion and a reduction in filtered HCO_3^- reabsorption. The full expression of renal adaptation may take several days and depends on a normal volume status and renal function. The kidneys appear to respond directly to the lowered $Paco_2$ rather than to the alkalemia per se. A fall of 1 mm Hg in $Paco_2$ causes a drop of 0.4 to 0.5 mEq/L in HCO_3^- and a 0.3-nmol/L fall (or 0.003-unit rise in pH) in hydrogen ion concentration, or the $[HCO_3^-]$ will decrease 4 mEq/L for each 10 mm Hg decrease in $Paco_2$.[3] Chronic respiratory alkalosis is an exception to the general rule that physiologic compensation is never 100% efficient, because patients with this acid-base disorder may exhibit a normal arterial pH and are therefore fully compensated.

The effects of respiratory alkalosis vary according to its duration and severity but, in general, are primarily those of the underlying disease. A rapid decline in $Paco_2$ may cause dizziness, mental confusion, and seizures, even in the absence of hypoxemia, as a consequence of reduced cerebral blood flow. The cardiovascular effects of acute hypocapnia in the awake human are generally minimal, but in the anesthetized or mechanically ventilated patient, cardiac output and blood pressure may fall because of the depressant effects of anesthesia and positive-pressure ventilation on heart rate, systemic resistance, and venous return. Cardiac rhythm disturbances may occur in patients with coronary artery disease as a result of changes in oxygen unloading by blood from a left shift in the hemoglobin-oxygen dissociation curve (Bohr effect). Acute respiratory alkalosis causes minor intracellular shifts of sodium, potassium, and phosphate and reduces serum free calcium by increasing the protein-bound fraction. Hypocapnia-induced hypokalemia is usually minor.[3]

Respiratory alkalosis is among the most common acid-base disturbances encountered in critically ill patients (often as a component of a mixed disorder) and, when severe, portends a poor prognosis. Many cardiopulmonary disorders manifest respiratory alkalosis in the early to intermediate stages. Hyperventilation usually results in hypocapnia. The finding of normocapnia and hypoxemia may herald the onset of rapid respiratory failure and should prompt an assessment to determine whether the patient is becoming fatigued. Respiratory alkalosis is a common occurrence during mechanical ventilation.

The causes of respiratory alkalosis are summarized in Table 17.5 *(left column)*. The hyperventilation syndrome may mimic a number of serious conditions and may be disabling. Paresthesias, circumoral numbness, chest wall tightness or pain, dizziness, inability to take an adequate breath, and, rarely, tetany may be themselves sufficiently stressful to perpetuate a vicious circle. ABG analysis demonstrates an acute or chronic respiratory alkalosis, often with hypocapnia in the range of 15 to 30 mm Hg and no hypoxemia. Central nervous system diseases or injury can produce several patterns of hyperventilation with sustained arterial $Paco_2$ levels of 20 to 30 mm Hg. Conditions such as hyperthyroidism, high caloric loads, and exercise raise the basal metabolic rate, but usually ventilation rises in proportion so that ABG levels are unchanged and respiratory alkalosis does not develop. Salicylates, the most common cause of drug-induced respiratory alkalosis, stimulate the medullary chemoreceptor directly. The methylxanthine drugs theophylline and aminophylline stimulate ventilation and increase the ventilatory response to CO_2. High progesterone levels increase ventilation and decrease the arterial $Paco_2$ by as much as 5 to 10 mm Hg. Thus chronic respiratory alkalosis is an expected feature of pregnancy. Respiratory alkalosis is a prominent feature in liver failure, and its severity correlates well with the degree of hepatic insufficiency and mortality. Respiratory alkalosis is common in patients with gram-negative septicemia, and it is often an early finding, before fever, hypoxemia, and hypotension develop. It is presumed that some bacterial product or toxin acts as a respiratory center stimulant, but the precise mechanism remains unknown.

The diagnosis of respiratory alkalosis requires measurement of arterial pH and $Paco_2$ (higher and lower than normal, respectively). The plasma K^+ concentration is often reduced and the serum Cl^- concentration increased. In the acute phase, respiratory alkalosis is not associated with increased renal HCO_3^- excretion, but within hours, net acid excretion is reduced. In general, the HCO_3^- concentration falls by 2.0 mEq/L for each 10 mm Hg decrease in $Paco_2$. Chronic hypocapnia reduces the serum bicarbonate concentration by 5.0 mEq/L for each 10 mm Hg decrease in $Paco_2$. It is unusual to observe a plasma bicarbonate concentration below 12 mEq/L as a result of a pure respiratory alkalosis. When a diagnosis of hyperventilation or respiratory alkalosis is made, its cause should be investigated. The diagnosis of hyperventilation syndrome is made by exclusion. In difficult cases it may be important to rule out other conditions such as pulmonary embolism, coronary artery disease, and hyperthyroidism.

The treatment of respiratory alkalosis is primarily directed toward alleviation of the underlying disorder. Because respiratory alkalosis is rarely life-threatening, direct measures to correct it will be unsuccessful if the stimulus remains unchecked. If respiratory alkalosis complicates ventilator management, changes in dead space, tidal volume, and frequency can minimize the hypocapnia. Patients with hyperventilation syndrome may benefit from reassurance, rebreathing from a paper bag during symptomatic attacks, and attention to underlying psychologic stress. Antidepressants and sedatives are not recommended, although in a few patients, β-adrenergic blockers may help to ameliorate distressing peripheral manifestations of the hyperadrenergic state.

METABOLIC DISORDERS

METABOLIC ACIDOSIS

Metabolic acidosis occurs as a result of a marked increase in endogenous production of acid (such as L-lactic acid and ketoacids), loss of HCO_3^- or potential HCO_3^- salts (diarrhea or renal tubular acidosis [RTA]), or progressive accumulation of endogenous acids.

The AG, which should be corrected for the prevailing albumin concentration (equation 28),[22] serves a useful role in the initial differentiation of the metabolic acidoses and should always be considered. Metabolic acidosis with a normal AG (hyperchloremic or non-AG acidosis) suggests that HCO_3^- has been effectively replaced by Cl^-. Thus the AG does not change.

In contrast, metabolic acidosis with a high AG (see Table 17.3) indicates addition of an acid other than hydrochloric acid or its equivalent to the ECF. If the attendant non–Cl^- acid anion cannot be readily excreted and is retained after HCO_3^- titration, the anion replaces titrated HCO_3^- without disturbing the Cl^- concentration (equation 29). Hence the acidosis is normochloremic, and the AG increases. The relationship between the rate of addition to the blood of a non–Cl^--containing acid and the rate of excretion of the accompanying anion with secondary Cl^- retention determines whether the resultant metabolic acidosis is expressed as a high AG or non-AG variety.[21,23]

NON–ANION GAP (HYPERCHLOREMIC) METABOLIC ACIDOSES

The diverse clinical disorders that may result in non-AG metabolic acidosis are outlined in Table 17.6. Because a reduced plasma HCO_3^- concentration and elevated Cl^- concentration may also occur in chronic respiratory alkalosis, it is important to confirm the acidemia by measuring arterial pH. Normal AG metabolic acidosis occurs most often as a result of loss of HCO_3^- from the gastrointestinal tract or as a result of a renal acidification defect. The majority of disorders in this category can be attributed to one of two major causes: (1) loss of bicarbonate from the gastrointestinal tract (diarrhea) or from the kidney (proximal RTA) or (2) inappropriately low renal acid excretion (classical distal RTA [cDRTA], type 4 RTA, or renal failure). Hypokalemia may accompany both gastrointestinal loss of HCO_3^- and proximal RTA and cDRTA. Therefore the major challenge in distinguishing these causes is to be able to define whether the response of renal tubular function to the prevailing acidosis is appropriate (gastrointestinal origin) or inappropriate (renal origin).

Diarrhea results in the loss of large quantities of HCO_3^- decomposed by reaction with organic acids. Because diarrheal stools contain a higher concentration of HCO_3^- and decomposed HCO_3^- than plasma, volume depletion and metabolic acidosis develop. Hypokalemia exists because large quantities of K^+ are lost from stool and because volume depletion causes secondary hyperaldosteronism, which enhances renal K^+ secretion by the collecting duct. Instead of an acid urine pH as might be anticipated with chronic diarrhea, a pH of 6.0 or more may be found. This occurs because chronic metabolic acidosis and hypokalemia increase renal NH_4^+ synthesis and excretion, which thus provides more urinary buffer that accommodates an increase in urine pH. Therefore the urine pH, when 6.0 or higher, may erroneously suggest a nonrenal cause. Nevertheless, metabolic acidosis caused by gastrointestinal losses with a high urine pH can be differentiated from RTA. Because urinary NH_4^+ excretion is typically low in patients with RTA and high in patients with diarrhea,[26,27] the level of urinary NH_4^+ excretion (not usually measured by clinical laboratories) in metabolic acidosis can be assessed indirectly[6] by calculating the urine anion gap (UAG):

$$UAG = [Na^+ + K^+]_u - [Cl^-]_u \qquad (30)$$

Table 17.6 Differential Diagnosis of Non–Anion Gap (Hyperchloremic) Metabolic Acidosis

Gastrointestinal Bicarbonate Loss

Diarrhea
External pancreatic or small bowel drainage
Uterosigmoidostomy, jejunal loop
Drugs
    Calcium chloride (acidifying agent)
    Magnesium sulfate (diarrhea)
    Cholestyramine (bile acid diarrhea)

Renal Acidosis

Hypokalemia

Proximal RTA (type 2)
Distal (classical) RTA (type 1)
Drug-induced acidosis
    Acetazolamide and topiramate (proximal RTA)
    Amphotericin B (distal RTA), ifosfamide

Hyperkalemia

Generalized distal nephron dysfunction (type 4 RTA)
    Mineralocorticoid deficiency
    Mineralocorticoid resistance (PHA I autosomal dominant)
    Voltage defects (PHA I, autosomal recessive)
    PHA II
    ↓ Na⁺ delivery to distal nephron
    Tubulointerstitial disease
Drug-induced acidosis
    Potassium-sparing diuretics (amiloride, triamterene, spironolactone)
    Trimethoprim
    Pentamidine
    Angiotensin-converting enzyme inhibitors, angiotensin II receptor blockers
    Nonsteroidal antiinflammatory drugs
    Cyclosporine, tacrolimus

Normokalemia

Chronic kidney disease (stage 3-4)

Other

Acid loads (ammonium chloride, hyperalimentation)
Loss of potential bicarbonate: ketosis with ketone excretion
Dilution acidosis (rapid saline administration)
Hippurate
Cation exchange resins

PHA, Pseudohypoaldosteronism; RTA, renal tubular acidosis.

---

of the major cations ($Na^+ + K^+$) is less than the concentration of Cl^- in urine. A negative UAG (more than –20 mEq/L) implies that sufficient NH_4^+ is present in the urine, as might occur with an extrarenal origin of the hyperchloremic acidosis. Conversely, urine estimated to contain little or no NH_4^+ has more $Na^+ + K^+$ than Cl^- (UAG is positive),[7,26,27] which indicates a renal mechanism for the hyperchloremic acidosis, such as in cDRTA (with hypokalemia) or hypoaldosteronism with hyperkalemia. Note that this qualitative test is useful only in the differential diagnosis of a non-AG metabolic acidosis. If the patient has ketonuria, drug anions (penicillins or aspirin), or toluene metabolites in the urine, the test is not reliable and should not be used.

The urinary ammonium (U_{NH4^+}) may be estimated more reliably from the urine osmolal gap, which is the difference in measured urine osmolality (U_{osm}), and the urine osmolality calculated from the urine [$Na^+ + K^+$] and the urine urea and glucose (all expressed in mmol/L):

$$U_{NH_4^+} = 0.5\left(U_{osm} - [2\,Na^+ + K^+]_u + urea_u + glucose_u\right) \quad (31)$$

Urinary ammonium concentrations of 75 mEq/L or more would be anticipated if renal tubular function is intact and the kidney is responding to the prevailing metabolic acidosis by increasing ammonium production and excretion. Conversely, values below 25 mEq/L denote inappropriately low urinary ammonium concentrations. In addition to the UAG, the fractional excretion of Na^+ may be helpful and would be expected to be low (<1% to 2%) in patients with HCO_3^- loss from the gastrointestinal tract but usually exceeds 2% to 3% in patients with RTA.[27,28]

Gastrointestinal HCO_3^- loss, as well as proximal RTA (type 2) and cDRTA (type 1), results in ECF contraction and stimulation of the renin angiotensin aldosterone system, which leads typically to hypokalemia. The serum K^+ concentration therefore serves to distinguish the previous disorders, which have a low K^+, from either generalized distal nephron dysfunction (e.g., type 4 RTA), in which the renin angiotensin aldosterone system–distal nephron axis is abnormal and hyperkalemia exists, or the acidosis of progressive CKD, in which normokalemia is common (see later).

In addition to gastrointestinal tract HCO_3^- loss, external loss of pancreatic and biliary secretions, as well as cholestyramine, calcium chloride, and magnesium sulfate ingestion can all cause a non-AG acidosis (see Table 17.6), especially in patients with renal insufficiency. Coexistent L-lactic acidosis is common in severe diarrheal illnesses but increases the AG.

Severe non-AG or hyperchloremic metabolic acidosis with hypokalemia may occur in patients with ureteral diversion procedures. Because the ileum and the colon are both endowed with Cl^--HCO_3^--exchangers, when the Cl^- from the urine enters the gut, or pouch, the HCO_3^- concentration increases as a result of the exchange process.[21] Moreover, K^+ secretion is stimulated, which, together with HCO_3^- loss, can result in a hyperchloremic hypokalemic metabolic acidosis. This defect is particularly common in patients with ureterosigmoidostomies and is more common with this type of diversion because of the prolonged transit time of urine caused by stasis in the colonic segment.

Dilutional acidosis, acidosis caused by exogenous acid loads and the posthypocapnic state, can usually be excluded

---

where u denotes the urine concentration of these electrolytes. The rationale for using the UAG as a surrogate for ammonium excretion is that, in chronic metabolic acidosis, ammonium excretion should be elevated if renal tubular function is intact. Because ammonium is a cation, it should balance part of the negative charge of chloride in the previous expression, assuming there is not a lot of HCO_3^- in the urine as in an alkaline urine. Therefore the UAG should become progressively negative as the rate of ammonium excretion increases in response to acidosis or to acid loading.[21,26] NH_4^+ can be assumed to be present if the sum by the history. When isotonic saline is infused rapidly, particularly in patients with temporary or permanent renal functional impairment, the serum HCO_3^- declines reciprocally in relation to Cl^-.[21] Addition of acid or acid equivalents to blood results in metabolic acidosis. Examples include infusion of arginine or lysine hydrochloride during parenteral hyperalimentation or ingestion of ammonium chloride.[29] A similar situation may arise from endogenous addition of ketoacids during recovery from ketoacidosis when the sodium salts of ketones may be excreted by the kidneys and lost as potential HCO_3^-.[30]

This sequence may also occur in mild, chronic ketoacidosis if GFR is maintained with sodium replenishment and renal ketone excretion is high. This may be accentuated by a defect in tubule ketone reabsorption.[30] The plasma ketone concentration is maintained at low levels. Continued titration of HCO_3^- with Cl^- retention and excretion of potential base (ketones) may result in hyperchloremic acidosis. Metabolism of sulfur to sulfuric acid and excretion of SO_4^{2-} with Cl^- retention represents another example of a hyperchloremic acidosis resulting from increased acid loading and anion excretion.[29]

Loss of functioning renal parenchyma in progressive kidney disease is known to be associated with metabolic acidosis. Typically the acidosis is a non-AG type when the GFR is between 20 and 50 mL/min but may convert to the typical high AG acidosis of uremia with more advanced renal failure, that is, when the GFR is less than 20 mL/min.[31] It is generally assumed that such progression is observed more commonly in patients with tubulointerstitial forms of renal disease, but non-AG metabolic acidosis can also occur with advanced glomerular disease. The principal defect in acidification of advanced renal failure is that ammoniagenesis is reduced in proportion to the loss of functional renal mass. In addition, medullary NH_4^+ accumulation and trapping in the outer medullary collecting tubule may be impaired.[31] Because of adaptive increases in K^+ secretion by the collecting duct and colon, the acidosis of chronic renal insufficiency is typically normokalemic.[31] Non-AG metabolic acidosis accompanied by hyperkalemia is almost always associated with a generalized dysfunction of the distal nephron.[27,28] However, K^+-sparing diuretics (amiloride, triamterene), as well as pentamidine, cyclosporine, tacrolimus, nonsteroidal antiinflammatory drugs (NSAIDs), angiotensin-converting enzyme (ACE) inhibitors, angiotensin receptor blockers (ARBs), β-blockers, and heparin may mimic or cause this disorder, resulting in hyperkalemia and a non-AG metabolic acidosis.[27,28] Because hyperkalemia augments the development of acidosis by suppressing urinary net acid excretion, discontinuing these agents while reducing the serum K^+ allows ammonium production and excretion to increase, which will help repair the acidosis.

DISORDERS OF IMPAIRED RENAL BICARBONATE RECLAMATION: PROXIMAL RENAL TUBULAR ACIDOSIS

Physiology

Because the first phase of acidification by the nephron involves reabsorption of the filtered HCO_3^-, 80% of the filtered HCO_3^- is normally returned to the blood by the proximal convoluted tubule.[5] If the capacity of the proximal tubule is reduced, less of the filtered HCO_3^- is reabsorbed in this segment, and more is delivered to the more distal segments. This increased HCO_3^- delivery overwhelms the limited capacity for bicarbonate reabsorption by the distal nephron, and bicarbonaturia ensues, net acid excretion ceases, and metabolic acidosis follows. Enhanced Cl^- reabsorption, stimulated by ECF volume contraction, results in a hyperchloremic (non-AG) chronic metabolic acidosis. With progressive metabolic acidosis and decreased serum HCO_3^- levels, the filtered HCO_3^- load declines progressively. As the plasma HCO_3^- concentration decreases, the absolute amount of HCO_3^- entering the distal nephron eventually reaches the low level approximating the distal HCO_3^- delivery in normal individuals (at the normal threshold). At this point the quantity of HCO_3^- entering the distal nephron can be reabsorbed completely (Figure 17.4), and the urine pH declines. A new steady state in which acid excretion equals acid production is then reached. As a consequence, the serum HCO_3^- concentration usually reaches a nadir of 15 to 18 mEq/L, so that systemic acidosis is not progressive. Therefore in proximal RTA in the steady state the serum HCO_3^- is usually low and the urine pH acid (<5.5). With bicarbonate administration, the amount of bicarbonate in the urine increases the fractional excretion of bicarbonate ($FE_{HCO_3^-}$) to 10% to 15%, and the urine pH becomes alkaline.[27]

Pathogenesis—Inherited and Acquired Forms

Proximal RTA can present in one of three ways: one in which acidification is the only defective function, one in which proximal tubule dysfunction is more generalized with multiple transporter abnormalities, and as a part of a mixed variety of RTA (type 3). Inheritance patterns for isolated proximal RTA include autosomal recessive and autosomal dominant. Isolated pure bicarbonate wasting is typical of autosomal recessive proximal RTA with accompanying ocular abnormalities and has been defined as a number of missense mutations of the gene *SLC4A4*, which encodes for the basolateral transporter NBCe1. A rare variant, inherited as an autosomal dominant trait, has been described and appears to be a mutation of the gene that encodes the apical Na^+-H^+-exchanger, NHE3. This rare disorder has been reported to be associated with short stature. Familial disorders associated with proximal RTA include cystinosis, tyrosinemia, hereditary fructose intolerance, galactosemia, glycogen storage disease type I, Wilson's disease, and Lowe's syndrome.

In addition, features of both proximal RTA (bicarbonate wasting) and distal acidification abnormalities are evident in patients with autosomal recessive RTA (mixed proximal and distal, or type 3 RTA) that has been attributed to a defect in *CA2*, which encodes for carbonic anhydrase II, an intracellular form of the enzyme distributed to the proximal tubule, thick ascending limb of Henle's loop (TAL), distal convoluted tubule, CCD, and medullary collecting duct (MCD).[27] The phenotype includes osteopetrosis and ocular abnormalities (Guibaud-Vainsel syndrome).

The majority of cases of proximal RTA fit into the category of generalized proximal tubule dysfunction with multiple transport abnormalities manifest as glycosuria, aminoaciduria, hypercitraturia, and phosphaturia, and referred to as *Fanconi's syndrome*. Numerous experimental

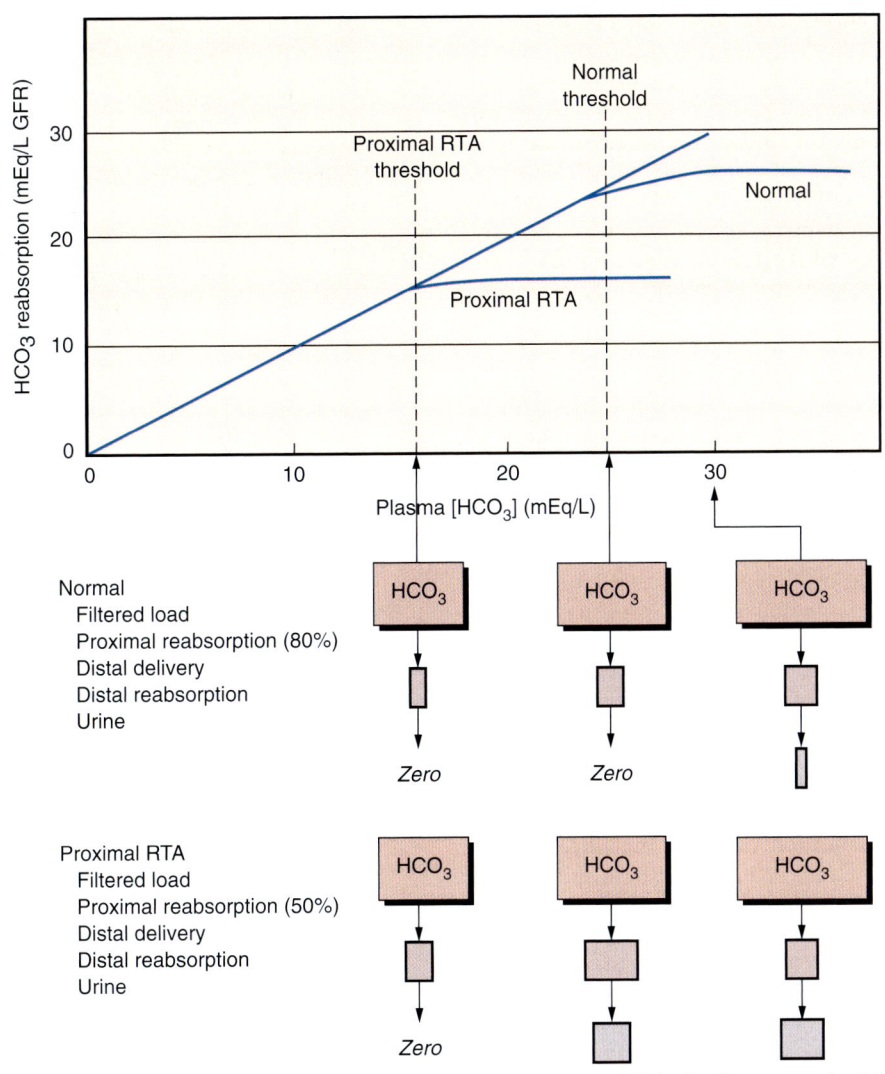

Figure 17.4 Schematic representation of the single-nephron correlates of whole-kidney HCO_3 titration curves **(top)** in normal subjects and in patients with proximal renal tubular acidosis (proximal RTA). The impact of these relationships on bicarbonaturia is displayed below the graph **(bottom)**. Bicarbonate will not appear in the urine when reabsorption is complete at the plasma HCO_3 concentration threshold, and distal H^+ secretory processes are capable of reabsorbing the HCO_3^- delivered out of the proximal nephron. The relationship shows that the fractional proximal HCO_3 reabsorptive capacity is reduced in patients with proximal RTA (50% versus the normal 80%), so the new steady state is achieved at the expense of systemic metabolic acidosis. *GFR*, Glomerular filtration rate.

studies in animal models demonstrate that the nephropathies induced by maleic acid and cystine involve disruption of active transcellular absorption of HCO_3^-, amino acids, and other solutes. Such a defect could be due to a generalized disorder of the Na^+-coupled apical membrane transporters, a selective disorder of the basolateral Na^+-K^+-ATPase, or a specific metabolic disorder that lowers intracellular adenosine triphosphate (ATP) concentration.

Development of Fanconi's syndrome by intracellular PO_4^{3-} depletion has also been proposed in hereditary fructose intolerance, in which ingestion of fructose leads to accumulation of fructose 1-phosphate in the proximal tubule. Because these patients lack the enzyme fructose 1-phosphate aldolase, fructose 1-phosphate cannot be further metabolized, and intracellular PO_4^{3-} is sequestered in this form. The renal lesion is confined to the proximal tubule because this is the only segment in the kidney that possesses the enzyme fructokinase. Administration of large parenteral loads of fructose to rats leads to high intracellular concentrations of fructose 1-phosphate and low concentrations of ATP and guanosine triphosphate, as well as of total adenine nucleotides. Prior PO_4^{3-} loading prevents reductions in intracellular ATP, PO_4^{3-}, and total adenine nucleotides.[27,32]

Numerous investigators have noted an association between vitamin D deficiency and a proximal RTA with aminoaciduria and hyperphosphaturia. In these studies, correction of the vitamin D deficiency has allowed correction of the proximal tubule dysfunction.[26,28] Similar results have been obtained in patients with vitamin D–dependent and vitamin D–resistant rickets treated with dihydrotachysterol.[27] The mechanisms involved in the proximal tubule dysfunction are not yet clear.

Another model for isolated proximal tubule acidosis is inherited carbonic anhydrase deficiency and is discussed earlier. Sly and associates[33] reported an inherited syndrome with osteopetrosis, cerebral calcification, and RTA caused by an inherited deficiency of carbonic anhydrase II. These patients appear to have combined or mixed proximal and distal RTA (type 3 RTA) but have no other evidence for proximal tubule dysfunction, and carbonic anhydrase IV is intact.[33] As already discussed, carbonic anhydrase II is present in the cytoplasm of renal cells, and thus an acidification defect occurring in association with its deficiency is not unexpected. A defect of carbonic anhydrase IV (the membrane-bound form) has not been reported.

Clinical Spectrum

In general, proximal RTA is more common in children. The most common causes of acquired proximal RTA in adults are multiple myeloma, in which increased excretion of immunoglobulin light chains injures the proximal tubule epithelium, and chemotherapeutic drug injury of the proximal tubule (e.g., ifosfamide, a nitrogen mustard alkylating agent used in cancer therapeutics). The light chains that cause injury in multiple myeloma may have a biochemical characteristic in the variable domain that is resistant to degradation by proteases in lysosomes in proximal tubule cells. Accumulation of the variable domain fragments may be responsible for the impairment in tubular function. In contrast, idiopathic RTA and RTA due to ifosfamide toxicity, lead intoxication, and cystinosis are more common in children. Carbonic anhydrase inhibitors cause pure bicarbonate wasting but not Fanconi's syndrome. A comprehensive list of the disorders associated with proximal RTA is presented in Table 17.7.[27] Some of the entities on this list are no longer seen and are of only historic interest. For example, application of sulfanilamide to the skin of patients with large-surface-area burns is no longer practiced in most centers, but sulfanilamide, a carbonic anhydrase inhibitor, is absorbed from burned skin. Topiramate, widely used in the prevention of migraine headaches or for treatment of a seizure disorder, is a potent carbonic anhydrase inhibitor and is an important cause of non-AG metabolic acidosis. As many as 15% to 25% of patients on topiramate will manifest a stable non-AG metabolic acidosis. Because the enzyme carbonic anhydrase II is present in both the proximal and distal tubules, topiramate appears to cause a mixed form of RTA having features of both proximal and distal RTA (type 3 RTA). This manifestation subsides when topiramate is discontinued. Pharmaceutical manufacturing techniques have improved, and outdated tetracycline is no longer associated with proximal RTA. Some of the agents and disorders on this list—such as ifosfamide, Sjögren's syndrome, renal transplantation, and amyloidosis—also appear as causes of distal RTA (see Table 17.7).

Diagnosis

The diagnosis of proximal RTA relies initially on the documentation of a chronic hyperchloremic metabolic acidosis. In the steady state these patients generally show chronic metabolic acidosis, an acid urine pH (<5.5), and a low fractional excretion of HCO_3^-. With alkali therapy or slow infusion of sodium bicarbonate intravenously, when the plasma HCO_3^- level increases above the threshold in these patients, bicarbonaturia ensues, and the urine becomes alkaline (Figure 17.4). When the plasma bicarbonate concentration is increased with an intravenous infusion of sodium bicarbonate at a rate of 0.5 to 1.0 mEq/kg/hr, the urine pH, even if initially acid, will increase once the reabsorptive threshold for bicarbonate has been exceeded. Thus the urine pH may exceed 7.5, and $FE_{HCO_3^-}$ will increase to 15% to 20%. Therefore it is very difficult to increase serum HCO_3^- levels to the normal range.

Table 17.7 Disorders with Dysfunction of Renal Acidification—Defective HCO_3^- Reclamation: Proximal Renal Tubular Acidosis

Isolated Pure Bicarbonate Wasting (Unassociated with Fanconi's Syndrome)

Primary
Inherited autosomal recessive with ocular abnormalities (missense mutations of *SLC4A4*)
Autosomal dominant with short stature (mutation of *SLC9A3*/NHE3)
Carbonic anhydrase deficiency, inhibition, or alteration
   Drugs
      Acetazolamide
      Topiramate
      Sulfanilamide
      Mafenide acetate
   Carbonic anhydrase II deficiency with osteopetrosis (mixed proximal and distal RTA type 3)

Generalized (Associated with Fanconi's Syndrome)

Primary (without associated systemic disease)
   Genetic
   Sporadic
Genetically transmitted systemic diseases
   Cystinosis
   Lowe's syndrome
   Wilson's syndrome
   Tyrosinemia
   Galactosemia
   Hereditary fructose intolerance (during fructose ingestion)
   Metachromatic leukodystrophy
   Pyruvate carboxylase deficiency
   Methylmalonic acidemia
Dysproteinemic states
   Multiple myeloma
   Monoclonal gammopathy
Secondary hyperparathyroidism with chronic hypocalcemia
   Vitamin D deficiency or resistance
   Vitamin D dependency
Drugs or toxins
   Ifosfamide
   Outdated tetracycline
   3-Methylchromone
   Streptozotocin
   Lead
   Mercury
   Amphotericin B (historical)
Tubulointerstitial diseases
   Sjögren's syndrome
   Medullary cystic disease
   Renal transplantation
Other renal and miscellaneous diseases
   Nephrotic syndrome
   Amyloidosis
   Paroxysmal nocturnal hemoglobinuria

The hypercholoremic metabolic acidosis of the steady state is usually seen in association with hypokalemia. If bicarbonate administration has been high in an attempt to repair the acidosis, the bicarbonaturia will drive kaliuresis, and the hypokalemia may be severe.[27] Patients with proximal tubule dysfunction exhibit intact distal nephron function (generate steep urine pH gradients and titrate luminal buffers) when the serum HCO_3^- concentration and hence distal HCO_3^- delivery are sufficiently reduced. A low HCO_3^- threshold exists. Below this plasma HCO_3^- concentration, distal acidification can compensate for defective proximal acidification, although at the expense of systemic metabolic acidosis. When the plasma HCO_3^- concentration is raised to normal values, a large fraction of the filtered HCO_3^- is inappropriately excreted because the limited reabsorptive capacity of the distal nephron cannot compensate for the reduced proximal nephron reabsorption.

Associated Clinical Features

K^+ excretion is typically high in patients with proximal RTA, especially during $NaHCO_3$ administration.[27] Kaliuresis is promoted by the increased delivery of a relatively impermeable anion, HCO_3^-, to the distal nephron in the setting of secondary hyperaldosteronism, which is due to mild volume depletion. Therefore correction of acidosis in such patients leads to an exaggeration of the kaliuresis and K^+ deficiency.

If the acidification defect is part of a generalized proximal tubule dysfunction (Fanconi's syndrome), such patients will have hypophosphatemia, hyperphosphaturia, hypouricemia, hyperuricosuria, glycosuria, aminoaciduria, hypercitraturia, hypercalciuria, and proteinuria.

Although Ca^{2+} excretion may be high in patients with proximal RTA, nephrocalcinosis and renal calculi are rare. This may be related to the high rate of citrate excretion in patients with proximal RTA compared with that of most patients with acidosis from other causes. Osteomalacia, rickets, abnormal gut Ca^{2+} and phosphorus absorption, and abnormal vitamin D metabolism in children are common, although not invariantly present. Adults tend to have osteopenia without pseudofractures.[27]

The proximal reabsorption of filtered low-molecular-weight proteins may also be abnormal in proximal RTA. Lysozymuria and increased urinary excretion of immunoglobulin light chains can occur.[27]

Treatment

The magnitude of the bicarbonaturia (>10% of the filtered load) at a normal HCO_3^- concentration requires that large amounts of HCO_3^- be administered. At least 10 to 30 mEq/kg/day of HCO_3^- or its metabolic equivalent (citrate) is required to maintain plasma HCO_3^- concentration at normal levels. Correcting the HCO_3^- to near-normal values (22 to 24 mEq/L) is desirable in children to reestablish normal growth. Correction to this level is less desirable in adults. Large supplements of K^+ are often necessary because of the kaliuresis induced by high distal HCO_3^- delivery when the plasma HCO_3^- concentration is normalized. Thiazides have proved useful in diminishing therapeutic requirements for HCO_3^- supplementation by causing ECF contraction to stimulate proximal absorption. However, K^+ wasting continues to be a problem, often requiring the addition of a K^+-sparing diuretic.[27] Vitamin D and PO_4^{3-} may be supplemented and in some patients even improve the acidification defect. Fructose should be restricted in patients with fructose intolerance.[32]

DISORDERS OF IMPAIRED NET ACID EXCRETION WITH HYPOKALEMIA: CLASSICAL DISTAL RENAL TUBULAR ACIDOSIS

Pathophysiology

The mechanisms involved in the pathogenesis of hypokalemic cDRTA (type 1 RTA) have been more clearly elucidated by appreciation of the genetic and molecular bases of the inherited forms of this disease in the last 2 decades. The observation that these patients tend to be hypokalemic (rather than hyperkalemic) demonstrates that generalized CCT dysfunction or aldosterone deficiency is not causative. Most studies suggest that the inherited forms of cDRTA are due to defects in the basolateral HCO_3^--Cl^--exchanger (*SLC4A1*) or subunits of the H^+-ATPase (*ATP6V1B1* and *ATP6V0A4*).

Defects in these transport pathways and an increase in apical membrane permeability are displayed in Figure 17.5, which depicts acid-base transporters of a type A intercalated cell in the medullary collecting duct and the possible abnormalities causing cDRTA. Although the classical feature of this entity is an inability to acidify the urine maximally (to a pH of <5.5) in the face of systemic acidosis, attention to urine ammonium excretion rather than urine pH alone is necessary to diagnose this disorder.[26,27] The pathogenesis of the acidification defect in most patients is evident by the response of the urine P_{CO_2} to sodium bicarbonate infusion. When normal subjects are given large infusions of sodium bicarbonate to produce a high HCO_3^- excretion, distal nephron H^+ secretion leads to the generation of a high P_{CO_2} in the renal medulla and final urine.[34,35] The magnitude of the urinary P_{CO_2} (often referred to as the *urine minus blood P_{CO_2}* or $U-B\,P_{CO_2}$) can be used as an index of distal nephron H^+ secretory capacity.[33-36] The $U-B\,P_{CO_2}$ is generally

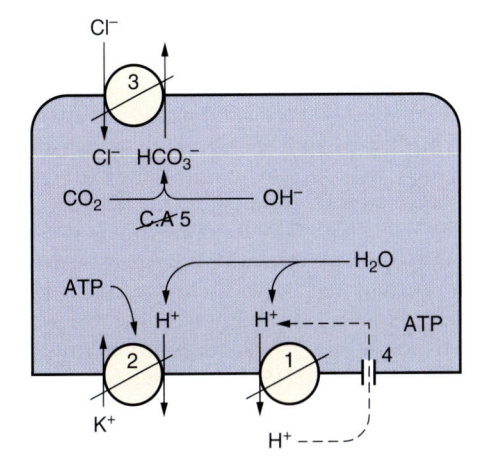

Figure 17.5 Type A intercalated cell of the collecting duct displaying five pathophysiologic defects that could result in classical distal renal tubular acidosis: (1) defective H^+–adenosine triphosphatase (H^+-ATPase), (2) defective H^+-K^+-ATPase, (3) defective HCO_3^--Cl^--exchanger, (4) H^+ leak pathway, and (5) defective intracellular carbonic anhydrase (type II). ATP, Adenosine triphosphate.

subnormal in classical hypokalemic distal RTA, with the notable exception of amphotericin B–induced distal RTA, which remains the most common example of the "gradient" defect.[35-37]

Inherited and Acquired Defects in Type A Intercalated Cell Acid-Base Transporters Responsible for Classical Distal Renal Tubular Acidosis. Recessive cDRTA with deafness is caused by loss-of-function mutations in either of two subunits of the H^+-ATPase of type A intercalated cells (the B1 subunit of the V1 cytoplasmic ATPase and the a4 subunit of the V0 transmembrane complex). Dominant and recessive forms of cDRTA are also caused by loss-of-function mutations in the basolateral membrane AE1 Cl^--HCO_3^--exchanger of type A intercalated cells. The dominant *SLC4A4* gene mutations causing cDRTA are accompanied by mild or asymptomatic erythroid changes, whereas the erythroid dyscrasias accompanying recessive *SLC4A4* cDRTA mutations can be mild or severe.[38,39]

Acquired defects of H^+-ATPase have been demonstrated in renal biopsy specimens of patients with Sjögren's syndrome with evidence of classical hypokalemic distal RTA.[27] These biopsy specimens revealed an absence of H^+-ATPase protein in the apical membrane of type A intercalated cells. Karet and colleagues[40] have described two different mutations in the *ATP6V1B1* gene encoding the B1 subunit of H^+-ATPase. One defect is associated with sensorineural deafness *(rdRTA1)* and the other with normal hearing *(rdRTA2)*.[41] The former recessive disorder is manifest in the first year of life as a failure to thrive; bilateral sensorineural hearing deficits; hyperchloremic, hypokalemic metabolic acidosis; severe nephrolithiasis; nephrocalcinosis; and osteodystrophy. The H^+-ATPase is critical for maintaining pH in the cochlea and endolymph, and its loss in this disorder explains the hearing deficit as well as the renal tubule acidification defect. An autosomal recessive form that is much less commonly associated with deafness is due to a defect in the *ATP6V0A4* gene that encodes for the vacuolar H^+-ATPase a4 subunit.[42,43] The genetic and molecular basis of distal RTA is outlined in Table 17.8.

Alternatively, abnormalities in H^+-K^+-ATPase could result in both hypokalemia and metabolic acidosis. A role for H^+-K^+-ATPase involvement in cDRTA was suggested by the observation that long-term administration of vanadate in rats decreased H^+-K^+-ATPase activity and was associated with metabolic acidosis, hypokalemia, and an inappropriately alkaline urine.[44] In addition, an unusually high incidence of hypokalemic distal RTA (endemic RTA) has been observed in northeastern Thailand. To date, no genetic linkages between H^+-K^+-ATPase genes and inherited forms of cDRTA have been documented. Nevertheless, such an abnormality has been suggested in an infant with severe metabolic acidosis and hypokalemia.[27] Patients with impaired collecting duct H^+ secretion and cDRTA also exhibit uniformly low excretory rates of NH_4^+ when the degree of systemic acidosis is taken into account.[6,26,27] Low NH_4^+ excretion equates with inappropriately low renal regeneration of HCO_3^-, which indicates that the kidney is responsible for causing or perpetuating the chronic metabolic acidosis. Low NH_4^+ excretion in classical hypokalemic distal RTA occurs because of the failure to trap NH_4^+ in the medullary collecting duct as a result of higher-than-normal tubule fluid pH in this segment and loss of the disequilibrium pH (pH > 6.0).[45] The high urine pH indicates impaired H^+ secretion.

In summary, hypokalemic distal RTA is characterized by the inability to acidify the urine below pH 5.5. In some patients this is attributable to an enhanced leakage pathway caused by an amphotericin B lesion; in rare patients, supposedly, this same mechanism occurs without exposure to the antibiotic but has never been documented unequivocally.[46]

Clinical Spectrum and Associated Features

The phenotypic hallmark of classical hypokalemic distal RTA when fully expressed has been recognized widely as the inability to acidify the urine appropriately during spontaneous or chemically induced metabolic acidosis; this is a disease of type A intercalated cells of the collecting duct. The defect in acidification by the collecting duct secondarily impairs NH_4^+ and titratable acid excretion and results in positive acid balance, hyperchloremic metabolic acidosis, and volume depletion.[27,47-49] Moreover, medullary interstitial

Table 17.8 Genetic and Molecular Bases of Distal Renal Tubular Acidoses

Classical Distal RTA	
Inherited	
Autosomal dominant	Defect in *AE1* gene encodes for missense mutation in the HCO_3^--Cl^--exchanger (band 3 protein)
	Transporter may be mistargeted to apical membrane
Autosomal recessive	
With deafness	Mutations in *ATP6V1B1* encoding B1 subunit of the apical H^+-ATPase in distal tubule *(rdRTA1)*
With normal hearing	Mutations in *ATP6V0A4* *(rdRTA2)*
Carbonic anhydrase II	Defect in carbonic anhydrase II in red blood cells, bone, kidney
Endemic (Northeastern Thailand)	Possible abnormality in H^+-K^+-ATPase
Acquired	Reduced apical expression of H^+-ATPase (Sjögren's syndrome)
Generalized Distal Nephron Dysfunction	
Pseudohypoaldosteronism type I	
Autosomal recessive	Loss-of-function mutation of ENaC; four known mutations of genes encoding three subunits of ENaC
Autosomal dominant	Heterozygous mutations of mineralocorticoid receptor gene
Pseudohypoaldosteronism type II	WNK1 and WNK4 constitutively activate NCCT, increasing NaCl absorption in distal convoluted tubule

ATPase, Adenosine triphosphatase; ENaC, epithelial sodium channel; NCCT, Na^+-Cl^--cotransporter in the connecting tubule; WNK1, WNK4, with no lysine (K) isoforms 1 and 4.

disease, which commonly occurs in conjunction with distal RTA, may impair NH_4^+ excretion by interrupting the medullary countercurrent system for NH_4^+.[26,27,47,48] The complete form of classical distal RTA is manifest by a non-AG acidosis without treatment. The clinical spectrum of complete cDRTA may include stunted growth, hypercalciuria, hypocitraturia, osteopenia, nephrolithiasis, and nephrocalcinosis, all a direct consequence of the chronic non-AG metabolic acidosis. The dissolution of bone is due to calcium resorption and mobilization from bone in response to the acidosis[27] and through activation of the pH-sensitive G protein–coupled receptor, OGR1, which resides in bone.[50] Other common electrolyte abnormalities not due to acidosis include hypokalemia, hypernatremia and salt wasting, and polyuria due to nephrogenic diabetes insipidus. The hypokalemia, previously attributed to volume depletion and activation of the renin angiotensin aldosterone system, may be due to a signaling pathway involving activation and release of prostaglandin E_2 by β-intercalated cells that directly communicate to enhance sodium absorption and potassium secretion by activation of the epithelial sodium channel (ENaC) in collecting duct principal cells. Because chronic metabolic acidosis also decreases the production of citrate,[6,26,27] the resulting hypocitraturia in combination with hypercalciuria creates an environment favorable for urinary stone formation and nephrocalcinosis. Nephrocalcinosis appears to be a reliable marker for cDRTA, in some cases, because nephrocalcinosis does not occur in proximal RTA or with generalized dysfunction of the nephron associated with hyperkalemia.[26,27] Nephrocalcinosis probably aggravates further the reduction in net acid excretion by impairing the transfer of ammonia from the loop of Henle into the collecting duct. Pyelonephritis is a common complication of distal RTA, especially in the presence of nephrocalcinosis, and eradication of the causative organism may be difficult.[27] Distal RTA occurs frequently in patients with Sjögren's syndrome.[51]

The clinical spectrum of cDRTA is outlined in detail in Table 17.9.[26,27,49,51]

Treatment

Correction of chronic metabolic acidosis can usually be achieved readily in patients with cDRTA by administration of alkali in an amount sufficient to neutralize the production of metabolic acids derived from the diet.[27] The goal is to correct the plasma HCO_3^- concentration to normal (25 mEq/L), and the concentration should be monitored frequently. In adult patients with distal RTA, the amount of bicarbonate administered may be equal to no more than 1 to 3 mEq/kg/day.[52] In growing children, endogenous acid production is usually between 2 and 3 mEq/kg/day but may on occasion exceed 5 mEq/kg/day. Larger amounts of bicarbonate must be administered to fully correct the acidosis and maintain normal growth.[26,27] The various forms of alkali replacement are outlined in Table 17.10.

In adult patients with distal RTA, correction of acidosis with alkali therapy reduces urinary K^+ excretion and typically corrects the hypokalemia and Na^+ depletion.[27] Therefore in most adult patients with distal RTA, K^+ supplementation is usually not necessary once the potassium level has been corrected initially. Frank wasting of K^+ may occur in a minority of adult patients and in some children in association with

Table 17.9 Disorders with Dysfunction of Renal Acidification—Selective Defect in Net Acid Excretion: Classical Distal Renal Tubular Acidosis

Primary

Familial
  Autosomal dominant
    AE1 gene
  Autosomal recessive
    With deafness (*rdRTA1* or *ATP6V1B1* gene)
    Without deafness (*rdRTA2* or *ATP6V0A4*)
Sporadic

Endemic

Northeastern Thailand

Secondary to Systemic Disorders

Autoimmune Diseases

Hyperglobulinemic purpura	Fibrosing alveolitis
Cryoglobulinemia	Chronic active hepatitis
Sjögren's syndrome	Primary biliary cirrhosis
Thyroiditis	Polyarteritis nodosa
Human immunodeficiency syndrome nephropathy	

Hypercalciuria and Nephrocalcinosis

Primary hyperparathyroidism	Vitamin D intoxication
Hyperthyroidism	Idiopathic hypercalciuria
Medullary sponge kidney	Wilson's disease
Fabry's disease	Hereditary fructose intolerance
X-linked hypophosphatemia	

Drug- and Toxin-Induced Disease

Amphotericin B	Toluene
Cyclamate	Mercury
Hepatic cirrhosis	Vanadate
Ifosfamide	Lithium
Foscarnet	Classical analgesic nephropathy

Tubulointerstitial Diseases

Balkan nephropathy	Kidney transplantation
Chronic pyelonephritis	Leprosy
Obstructive uropathy	Jejunoileal bypass with hyperoxaluria
Vesicoureteral reflux	

Associated with Genetically Transmitted Diseases

Ehlers-Danlos syndrome	Hereditary elliptocytosis
Sickle cell anemia	Marfan's syndrome
Medullary cystic disease	Jejunal bypass with hyperoxaluria
Hereditary sensorineural deafness	Carnitine palmitoyltransferase deficiency
Osteopetrosis with carbonic anhydrase II deficiency (mixed proximal and distal RTA type 3)	

Table 17.10 Forms of Alkali Replacement

Shohl's solution	
Na⁺ citrate 500 mg	Each 1 mL contains 1 mEq
Citric acid 334 mg/5 mL	sodium and is equivalent to 1 mEq of bicarbonate
NaHCO$_3$ tablets	3.9 mEq/tablet (325 mg)
	7.8 mEq/tablet (650 mg)
Baking soda	60 mEq/teaspoon
K-Lyte	25–50 mEq/tablet
Na⁺ citrate and K⁺ citrate (Virtrate-3 or Cytra-3)	
Na⁺ citrate 500 mg, and K⁺ citrate 550 mg/5 mL	Each 1 mL contains 1 mEq potassium and 1 mEq sodium and is equivalent to 2 mEq bicarbonate
K⁺ citrate 550 mg Citric acid 334 mg/5 mL	
Polycitra-K crystals	
K⁺ citrate 3300 mg Citric acid 1002 mg/packet	Each packet contains 30 mEq potassium and is equivalent to 30 mEq bicarbonate
Urocit-K tablets	
K⁺ citrate	5 or 10 mEq/tablet

Table 17.11 Disorders with Dysfunction of Renal Acidification—Generalized Abnormality of Distal Nephron with Hyperkalemia

Mineralocorticoid Deficiency

Primary Mineralocorticoid Deficiency

Combined deficiency of aldosterone, desoxycorticosterone, and cortisol
  Addison's disease
  Bilateral adrenalectomy
  Bilateral adrenal destruction
  Hemorrhage or carcinoma
Congenital enzymatic defects
  21-Hydroxylase deficiency
  3β-Hydroxydehydrogenase deficiency
  Desmolase deficiency
Isolated (selective) aldosterone deficiency
  Chronic idiopathic hypoaldosteronism
  Heparin (low molecular weight or unfractionated) administration in critically ill patient
  Familial hypoaldosteronism
  Corticosterone methyl oxidase deficiency types 1 and 2
  Primary zona glomerulosa defect
  Transient hypoaldosteronism of infancy
  Persistent hypotension and/or hypoxemia
Angiotensin-converting enzyme inhibition
  Endogenous
  Angiotensin-converting enzyme inhibitors and angiotensin receptor blockers

Secondary Mineralocorticoid Deficiency

Hyporeninemic hypoaldosteronism
  Diabetic nephropathy
  Tubulointerstitial nephropathies
  Nephrosclerosis
  Nonsteroidal antiinflammatory agents
  Acquired immunodeficiency syndrome
  Immunoglobulin M monoclonal gammopathy
  Obstructive uropathy

Mineralocorticoid Resistance

PHA I—autosomal dominant (human mineralocorticoid receptor defect)

Renal Tubular Dysfunction (Voltage Defect)

PHA I—autosomal recessive
PHA II—autosomal dominant
Drugs that interfere with Na⁺ channel function in the CCT
  Amiloride
  Triamterene
  Trimethoprim
  Pentamidine
Drugs that interfere with Na⁺-K⁺-ATPase in the CCT
  Cyclosporine, tacrolimus
Drugs that inhibit aldosterone effect on the CCT
  Spironolactone
Disorders associated with tubulointerstitial nephritis and renal insufficiency
  Lupus nephritis
  Methicillin nephrotoxicity
  Obstructive nephropathy
  Kidney transplant rejection
  Sickle cell disease
  Williams' syndrome with uric acid nephrolithiasis

ATPase, Adenosine triphosphatase; CCT, cortical collecting tubule; PHA I, PHA II, pseudohypoaldosteronism types 1 and 2.

---

secondary hyperaldosteronism despite correction of the acidosis by alkali therapy, so that K⁺ supplementation is needed. If required, potassium can be administered as potassium bicarbonate (K-Lyte 25 or 50 mEq), potassium citrate (Urocit-K), or potassium citrate combination products sodium citrate and potassium citrate (Virtrate-3), and Polycitra-K crystals (Cytra-3).[26,27] Maintenance of a normal serum bicarbonate concentration with alkali therapy also raises urinary citrate level, reduces urinary calcium excretion, lowers the frequency of nephrolithiasis, and tends to correct bone disease and restore normal growth in children.[52,53] Therefore every attempt should be made to correct and maintain a near-normal serum [HCO$_3^-$] in all patients with cDRTA.

Severe hypokalemia with flaccid paralysis, metabolic acidosis, and hypocalcemia may occur in some patients under extreme circumstances and require immediate therapy. Because the hypokalemia may result in respiratory depression, increasing systemic pH with alkali therapy may worsen the hypokalemia. Therefore immediate intravenous potassium replacement should be achieved before alkali administration.

DISORDERS OF IMPAIRED NET ACID EXCRETION WITH HYPERKALEMIA: GENERALIZED DISTAL NEPHRON DYSFUNCTION (TYPE 4 RENAL TUBULAR ACIDOSIS)

The coexistence of hyperkalemia and a non-AG metabolic acidosis indicates a generalized dysfunction in the cortical and medullary collecting tubules. In the differential diagnosis it is important to evaluate the functional status of the renin angiotensin aldosterone system and of ECF volume. The specific disorders causing hyperkalemic hyperchloremic metabolic acidosis are outlined in detail in Table 17.11.[26,27]

The regulation of potassium excretion is primarily the result of regulation of potassium secretion, which responds to hyperkalemia, aldosterone, sodium delivery, and

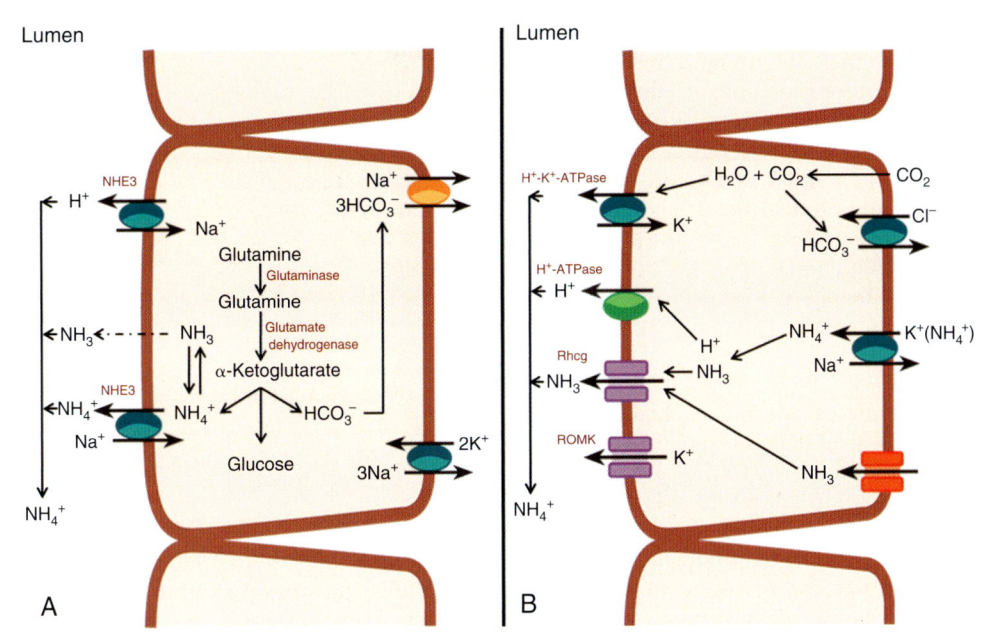

Figure 17.6 Cell models of ammonia synthesis and excretion pathways. **A,** Proximal convoluted tubule. Ammonia is derived from glutamine precursors to produce two NH_4^+ and two HCO_3^- molecules through an enzymatic pathway activated by acidemia and hypokalemia and inhibited by alkalemia and hyperkalemia. **B,** Type A intercalated cell in collecting tubule. Ammonium entry across basolateral membrane through substitution of NH_4^+ for K^+ on K^+ conductance and secreted across apical membrane via ROMK or RhCG (see the text). In both **A** and **B**, NH_3 diffusion coupled with H^+ secretion traps NH_4^+ in the tubule lumen. NHE3, Na^+-H^+-exchanger isoform 3; Rhcg, Rh c glycoprotein; ROMK, renal outer medullary potassium.

nonreabsorbable anions in the CCD. Therefore a clinical estimate of K^+ transfer into that segment could be helpful to recognize hyperkalemia of renal origin. An abnormally low fractional excretion of potassium (FE_{K^+}) or transtubular potassium gradient (TTKG) in the face of hyperkalemia defines hyperkalemia of renal origin. When the TTKG is low (<5) or the FE_{K^+} is less than 25% in a hyperkalemic patient, it reveals that the collecting tubule is not responding appropriately to the prevailing hyperkalemia and that potassium secretion is impaired. In contrast, in hyperkalemia of nonrenal origin the kidney should respond by increasing K^+ secretion, as evidenced by a sharp increase in the TTKG. The TTKG calculation assumes that there is no significant net addition or absorption of K^+ between the CCD and the final urine, that CCD tubule fluid osmolality is approximately the same as plasma osmolality, that "osmoles" are not extracted between the CCD and the final urine, and that plasma $[K^+]$ approximates peritubule fluid $[K^+]$. It is important to note that under certain clinical conditions, some or none of these assumptions may be entirely correct. With high urine flow rates, for example, the TTKG underestimates K^+ secretory capacity in the hyperkalemic patient.

Hyperkalemia should also be regarded as an important mediator of the renal response to acid-base balance. Potassium status can affect distal nephron acidification by both direct and indirect mechanisms. First, the level of potassium in systemic blood is an important determinant of aldosterone elaboration, which is also an important determinant of distal H^+ secretion. Chronic potassium deficiency was demonstrated in studies in the author's laboratory to stimulate ammonium production, whereas chronic hyperkalemia suppressed ammoniagenesis.[54,55] These changes in

Table 17.12 Effects of Hyperkalemia on Ammonium Excretion

Decrease in NH_4^+ production
Decrease in NH_4^+ absorption in thick ascending limb of Henle's loop
Decrease in interstitial NH_4^+ concentration
Impaired countercurrent multiplication
Decrease in NH_3/NH_4^+ secretion into outer and inner medullary collecting ducts

ammonium production may also affect medullary interstitial ammonium concentration and buffer availability.[55] Hyperkalemia has no effect on ammonium transport in the superficial proximal tubule but markedly impairs ammonium absorption in the TAL, reducing inner medullary concentrations of total ammonia and decreasing secretion of NH_3 into the inner medullary collecting duct. It is important to remember that the luminal membrane of the medullary thick ascending limb is very impermeable to both H_2O and NH_3. The mechanism for impaired absorption of NH_4^+ in the TAL is competition between K^+ and NH_4^+ for the K^+-secretory site on the Na^+-K^+-$2Cl^-$-cotransporter on the apical membrane.[56,57] Hyperkalemia may also decrease entry of NH_4^+ into the medullary collecting duct through competition of NH_4^+ and K^+ for the K^+-secretory site on the basolateral membrane sodium pump (Figure 17.6).[57]

In summary, hyperkalemia may have a dramatic impact on ammonium production and excretion (Table 17.12). Chronic hyperkalemia decreases ammonium production in the proximal tubule and whole kidney, inhibits absorption of NH_4^+ in the medullary thick ascending limb of Henle's loop, reduces medullary interstitial concentrations of NH_4^+ and NH_3, and decreases entry of NH_4^+ and NH_3 into the medullary collecting duct. This same series of events leads, in the final analysis, to a marked reduction in urinary ammonium excretion. The potential for development of a hyperchloremic metabolic acidosis is greatly augmented when a reduction in functional renal mass (GFR of <60 mL/min) coexists with hyperkalemia or when aldosterone deficiency or resistance is present.

Clinical Disorders

Generalized distal nephron dysfunction is manifest as a hyperchloremic (non-AG), hyperkalemic metabolic acidosis in which urinary ammonium excretion is invariably depressed (positive UAG) and renal function is often compromised. Although hyperchloremic metabolic acidosis and hyperkalemia occur with regularity in advanced renal insufficiency, patients selected because of severe hyperkalemia (>5.5 mEq/L) with, for example, diabetic nephropathy and tubulointerstitial disease have hyperkalemia that is disproportionate to the reduction in the GFR. The TTKG and/or the FE_{K^+} is usually low in patients with this disorder. In such patients, a unique dysfunction of potassium and acid secretion by the collecting tubule coexists and can be attributed to either mineralocorticoid deficiency, resistance to mineralocorticoid, or a specific type of renal tubular dysfunction (voltage defects). The clinical spectrum of generalized abnormalities in the distal nephron is summarized in Table 17.11.

Primary Mineralocorticoid Deficiency

Although a number of factors modulate aldosterone elaboration, including angiotensin II, adrenocorticotropic hormone, endothelin, dopamine, acetylcholine, epinephrine, plasma K^+, and Mg^{2+}, angiotensin II and plasma K^+ remain the principal modulators of production and secretion. Destruction of the adrenal cortex by hemorrhage, infection, invasion by tumors, or autoimmune processes results in Addison's disease. This disorder is manifest by combined glucocorticoid and mineralocorticoid deficiency and is recognized clinically by hypoglycemia, anorexia, weakness, hyperpigmentation, and a failure to respond to stress. These defects can occur in association with renal salt wasting and hyponatremia, hyperkalemia, and metabolic acidosis. The most common congenital adrenal defect in steroid biosynthesis is 21-hydroxylase deficiency, which is associated with salt wasting, hyperkalemia, and metabolic acidosis in a fraction of patients. Causes of Addison's disease include tuberculosis, autoimmune adrenal failure, fungal infections, adrenal hemorrhage, metastasis, lymphoma, acquired immunodeficiency syndrome (AIDS), amyloidosis, and drug toxicity (ketoconazole, fluconazole, phenytoin, rifampin, and barbiturates). These disorders are associated with low plasma aldosterone levels and high levels of plasma renin activity.[27] The metabolic acidosis of mineralocorticoid deficiency results from a decrease in hydrogen ion secretion in the collecting duct secondary to decreased H^+-ATPase number and function. The accompanying hyperkalemia of mineralocorticoid deficiency decreases ammonium production and excretion.

Table 17.13 Hyporeninemic Hypoaldosteronism: Typical Clinical Features

Mean age 65 yr
Asymptomatic hyperkalemia (75%)
　Weakness (25%)
　Arrhythmia (25%)
Hyperchloremic metabolic acidosis (>50%)
Renal insufficiency (70%)
Diabetes mellitus (50%)
Cardiac disorders
　Arrhythmia (25%)
　Hypertension (75%)
　Congestive heart failure (50%)

Hyporeninemic Hypoaldosteronism

In contrast to patients with the primary adrenal disorder, patients in this group exhibit low plasma renin activity, are usually older (mean age 65 years), and frequently have mild to moderate renal insufficiency (70%) and acidosis (50%) in association with chronic hyperkalemia in the range of 5.5 to 6.5 mEq/L (Table 17.13).[27] Although the hyperkalemia may be asymptomatic, it is important to recognize that both the metabolic acidosis and the hyperkalemia are out of proportion to the level of reduction in GFR. The most frequently associated renal diseases are diabetic nephropathy and tubulointerstitial disease. Additional disorders associated with hyporeninemic hypoaldosteronism include obstructive uropathy, systemic lupus erythematosus, and human immunodeficiency virus (HIV) infection. For 80% to 85% of such patients there is a reduction in plasma renin activity that does not respond to the usual physiologic maneuvers. Because approximately 30% of patients with hyporeninemic hypoaldosteronism are hypertensive, the finding of a low plasma renin activity in such patients suggests a volume-dependent form of hypertension with physiologic suppression of renin elaboration.

Impaired ammonium excretion is the combined result of hyperkalemia, impaired ammoniagenesis, a reduction in nephron mass, reduced proton secretion, and impaired transport of ammonium by nephron segments in the inner medulla.[26,27,58] Hyperchloremic metabolic acidosis occurs in approximately 50% of patients with hyporeninemic hypoaldosteronism. Drugs that may result in similar manifestations are reviewed later.

Isolated Hypoaldosteronism in Critically Ill Patients

Isolated hypoaldosteronism, which may occur in critically ill patients, particularly in the setting of severe sepsis or cardiogenic shock, is manifest by markedly elevated adrenocorticotropic hormone and cortisol levels in concert with a decrease in aldosterone elaboration in response to angiotensin II. This may be secondary to selective inhibition of aldosterone synthase as a result of hypoxia or in response to cytokines such as tumor necrosis factor-α or interleukin-1 or, alternatively, as a result of high circulating levels of atrial natriuretic peptide.[26,27,59] Levels of atrial natriuretic peptide, a powerful suppressor of aldosterone secretion, may be elevated in congestive heart failure (CHF), with

Table 17.14 Isolated Hypoaldosteronism in the Critically Ill Patient

Elevated adrenocorticotropic hormone and cortisol levels in association with a decrease in aldosterone elaboration
Inhibition of aldosterone synthase
    Heparin (low molecular weight and unfractionated)
    Hypoxia
    Cytokines
Atrial natriuretic peptide
Manifestations of hypoaldosteronism
    Hyperkalemia
    Metabolic acidosis
Potentiated by K^+-sparing diuretics, K^+ loads, or heparin

atrial arrhythmias, in subclinical cardiac disease, and in volume expansion. The tendency to manifest the features of hypoaldosteronism, including hyperkalemia and metabolic acidosis, is often potentiated by the administration of potassium-sparing diuretics, potassium loads in parenteral nutrition solutions, or heparin. Both low-molecular-weight and unfractionated heparin suppress aldosterone synthesis in the critically ill patient (Table 17.14).

Resistance to Mineralocorticoid and Voltage Defects

Autosomal dominant pseudohypoaldosteronism type I (PHA I) is an example of a voltage defect in the collecting tubule and is due to aldosterone resistance. This disorder, which is clinically less severe than the autosomal recessive form discussed later, is associated with hyperkalemia (which can be attributed to impaired potassium secretion), renal salt wasting, elevated levels of renin and aldosterone, and hypotension. Physiologic mineralocorticoid replacement therapy does not correct the hyperkalemia. The autosomal dominant disorder has been shown to be the result of a mutation in the intracellular mineralocorticoid receptor in the collecting tubule.[60] In contrast to the autosomal recessive disorder, this defect is not expressed in organs other than the kidney and becomes less severe with advancing age. Because the decrease in mineralocorticoid reduces the activity of the ENaC, transepithelial potential difference declines and K^+ secretion is secondarily impaired. Four hours after administration of fludrocortisone (0.1 mg orally) to patients with autosomal dominant PHA I, the TTKG will *not* increase, which reveals that resistance to mineralocorticoid causes the hyperkalemia.

Autosomal recessive PHA I (Figure 17.7) is a prototypical voltage defect in the CCT. This disorder is the result of a loss-of-function mutation of the gene that encodes one of the α-, β-, or γ-subunits of the ENaC.[61-65] Children with this disorder have severe hyperkalemia and renal salt wasting because of impaired sodium absorption in principal cells of the CCT. In addition, the hyperchloremic metabolic acidosis may be severe and is associated with hypotension and marked elevations of plasma renin and aldosterone levels. These children also manifest vomiting, hyponatremia, failure to thrive, and respiratory distress. The respiratory distress is due to involvement of ENaC in the alveolus, which prevents Na^+ and water absorption in the lungs.[64,66] Patients with this disease respond to a high salt intake and correction

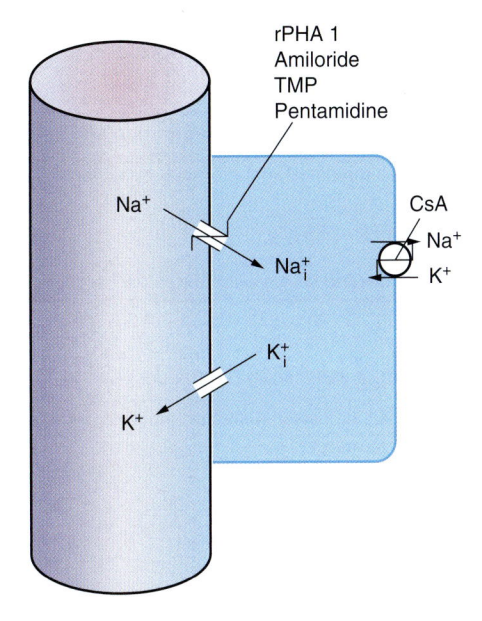

Figure 17.7 Examples of "voltage" defects in the cortical collecting tubule (CCT) causing abnormal Na^+ transport (and K^+ secretion) across the apical membrane of a principal cell: (1) the sodium channel (ENaC) is blocked or occupied by amiloride, trimethoprim (TMP), or pentamidine or is inoperative (autosomal recessive pseudohypoaldosteronism type I [rPHA I]), and (2) basolateral Na^+-K^+–adenosine triphosphatase (Na^+-K^+-ATPase) activity is inhibited by calcineurin inhibitors cyclosporine (CsA) and tacrolimus. As a consequence of impaired Na^+ uptake, transepithelial K^+ secretion is compromised, which leads to hyperkalemia. The pathogenesis of metabolic acidosis, when present, is the unfavorable voltage (which impairs H^+ secretion by the type A intercalated cell, not shown) or the inhibition of NH_4^+ production and transport as a consequence of hyperkalemia.

of the hyperkalemia. Unlike the autosomal dominant form, autosomal recessive PHA I persists throughout life.

A number of additional adult patients have been reported with a rare form of autosomal dominant low-renin hypertension that is invariably associated with hyperkalemia, hyperchloremic metabolic acidosis, mild volume expansion, normal renal function, and low aldosterone levels. This syndrome has been designated *familial hypertension with hyperkalemia* but is also known as *pseudohypoaldosteronism type II* (PHA II) or *Gordon's syndrome*.[67] Wilson and colleagues identified two genes causing PHA II.[68,69] Both genes encode members of the WNK (*w*ith *n*o lysine [*K*]) family of serine-threonine kinases. WNK1 and WNK4 localize to the CCT. WNK4 negatively regulates surface expression of the Na^+-Cl^--cotransporter (NCC) in the connecting tubule.[69] Loss of regulation of NCC by WNK4 results in a gain in NCC function, which, through enhanced absorption of Na and Cl, causes volume expansion, shunting of voltage, and therefore reduced K^+ secretion in the CCT.[69-71] PHA II may be distinguished from selective hypoaldosteronism by the presence of normal renal function and hypertension, the absence of diabetes mellitus and salt wasting, and a kaliuretic response to mineralocorticoids. The acidosis in these patients is mild and can be accounted for by the magnitude of hyperkalemia; the acidosis and renal potassium excretion are resistant to mineralocorticoid administration. Thiazide diuretics consistently correct the hyperkalemia

> **Table 17.15 Causes of Drug-Induced Hyperkalemia**
>
> **Impaired Renin or Aldosterone Elaboration or Function**
>
> Cyclo-oxygenase inhibitors (nonsteroidal antiinflammatory agents)
> β-Adrenergic antagonists
> Spironolactone
> Angiotensin-converting enzyme inhibitors and angiotensin receptor blockers
> Heparin
>
> **Inhibition of Renal Potassium Secretion**
>
> Potassium-sparing diuretics (amiloride, spironolactone, eplerenone, triamterene)
> Trimethoprim
> Pentamidine
> Cyclosporine
> Digitalis overdose
> Lithium
>
> **Altered Potassium Distribution**
>
> Insulin antagonists (somatostatin, diazoxide)
> β-Adrenergic antagonists
> α-Adrenergic agonists
> Hypertonic solutions
> Digitalis
> Succinylcholine
> Arginine hydrochloride, lysine hydrochloride

and metabolic acidosis, as well as the hypertension, plasma aldosterone level, and plasma renin level.

Secondary Renal Diseases Associated with Acquired Voltage Defects

In addition to the inherited voltage defects discussed earlier, there are a number of acquired renal disorders caused by drugs or tubulointerstitial diseases that are often associated with hyperkalemia (Table 17.15).[27] Examples of the former include amiloride and the structurally related compounds trimethoprim (TMP) and pentamidine. This explains the occurrence of hyperkalemic hyperchloremic acidosis in patients receiving higher doses of these agents. TMP and pentamidine occupy the Na^+ channel, as does amiloride, resulting in a reduction in K^+ secretion and thus hyperkalemia, which contributes to the acidosis. Additional drugs not related to amiloride that are associated with hyperkalemia include cyclo-oxygenase-2 (COX-2) inhibitors, the calcineurin inhibitors cyclosporine and tacrolimus, and NSAIDs.[72,73] In these disorders the frequency with which hyperkalemia is associated with metabolic acidosis and decreased net acid excretion as a result of impaired ammonium production or excretion cannot be presumed to be a result of the severity of impairment in renal function. Hyperkalemia that is out of proportion to the degree of renal insufficiency is typically observed in the nephropathies associated with sickle cell disease, HIV infection, systemic lupus erythematosus, obstructive uropathy, acute and chronic renal allograph rejection, hypoaldosteronism, multiple myeloma, and amyloidosis.[27,74] Tubulointerstitial disease with hyperkalemia and hyperchloremic metabolic acidosis with or without salt wasting may be associated with analgesic abuse, sickle cell disease, obstructive uropathy, nephrolithiasis, nephrocalcinosis, and hyperuricemia.[27]

Hyperkalemic Distal Renal Tubular Acidosis

A generalized defect in CCD secretory function that results in hyperkalemic hyperchloremic metabolic acidosis has been designated as *hyperkalemic distal RTA* because of the coexistence of hyperkalemia and an inability to acidify the urine (urine pH of >5.5) during spontaneous acidosis or following an acid load. The hyperkalemia is the result of impaired renal K^+ secretion, and the TTKG or FE_{K^+} is invariably lower than expected for nonrenal hyperkalemia (>5). Urine ammonium excretion is reduced, but aldosterone levels may be low, normal, or even increased.

Hyperkalemic distal RTA can be distinguished from selective hypoaldosteronism because plasma renin and aldosterone levels are usually high or normal. Typically in selective hypoaldosteronism the urine pH is low and the defect in urinary acidification can be attributed to the decrease in ammonium excretion.

Drug-Induced Renal Tubular Secretory Defects

Impaired Renin or Aldosterone Elaboration. Drugs may impair renin or aldosterone elaboration or cause mineralocorticoid resistance and produce effects that mimic the clinical manifestations of the acidification defect seen in the generalized form of distal RTA with hyperkalemia (see Table 17.15). COX inhibitors (NSAIDs or COX-2 inhibitors) can generate hyperkalemia and metabolic acidosis as a result of inhibition of renin release.[73] β-Adrenergic antagonists cause hyperkalemia by altering potassium distribution and by interfering with the renin angiotensin aldosterone system. Heparin impairs aldosterone synthesis as a result of direct toxicity to the zona glomerulosa and inhibition of aldosterone synthase. ACE inhibitors and ARBs interrupt the renin angiotensin aldosterone system and result in hypoaldosteronism with hyperkalemia and acidosis, particularly in patients with advanced renal insufficiency or in patients with a tendency to develop hyporeninemic hypoaldosteronism (diabetic nephropathy). The combination of potassium-sparing diuretics and ACE inhibitors should be avoided in patients with diabetes.

Inhibitors of Potassium Secretion in the Collecting Duct. Spironolactone and eplerenone act as competitive inhibitors of aldosterone and inhibit aldosterone biosynthesis. These drugs may cause hyperkalemia and metabolic acidosis when administered to patients with significant renal insufficiency, patients with advanced liver disease, or patients with unrecognized renal hemodynamic compromise. Similarly, amiloride and triamterene may be associated with hyperkalemia, but through an entirely different mechanism. Both potassium-sparing diuretics occupy and thus block the apical Na^+-selective channel (ENaC) in the collecting duct principal cell (see Figure 17.7). Occupation of ENaC inhibits Na^+ absorption and reduces the negative transepithelial voltage, which alters the driving force for K^+ secretion.

TMP and pentamidine are related structurally to amiloride and triamterene. The protonated forms of both TMP and pentamidine have been demonstrated[75,76] to inhibit ENaC in A6 distal nephron cells. This effect in A6 cells has been verified in rat late distal tubules perfused in vivo.[77] Hyperkalemia has been observed in 20% to 50% of HIV-infected patients receiving high-dose trimethoprim-sulfamethoxazole (TMP-SMX) or TMP-dapsone for the treatment of opportunistic infections and as many as 100% of patients with AIDS-associated infections (due to *Pneumocystis jirovecii*) receiving pentamidine for longer than 6 days.[76] Because both TMP and pentamidine decrease the electrochemical driving force for both K^+ and H^+ secretion in the CCT, metabolic acidosis may accompany the hyperkalemia even in the absence of severe renal failure, adrenal insufficiency, tubulointerstitial disease, or hypoaldosteronism. Whereas it has been assumed that such a "voltage" defect could explain the decrease in H^+ secretion, it is likely that, in addition, hyperkalemia plays a significant role in the development of metabolic acidosis by direct inhibition of ammonium production and excretion (see Figure 17.6 and Table 17.12).

The calcineurin inhibitors cyclosporine and tacrolimus may be associated with hyperkalemia in the transplant recipient as a result of inhibition of the basolateral Na^+-K^+-ATPase and the consequent decrease in $[K^+]_i$ and the transepithelial potential, which together reduce the driving force for K^+ secretion (see Figure 17.7).[73] Additional studies indicate that calcineurin inhibitors may also inhibit K^+ secretion by directly interfering with the renal outer medullary potassium (ROMK) channel.[78] An additional explanation for the association of hyperkalemia, volume expansion, and hypertension, a syndrome that resembles the phenotype of familial hypertension with hyperkalemia, or PHA II, is enhanced activity of NCC in the distal convoluted tubule.[79]

Treatment

In hyperkalemic hyperchloremic metabolic acidosis, documentation of the underlying disorder is necessary, and therapy should be based on a precise diagnosis if possible. Of particular importance is obtaining a thorough drug and dietary history. Contributing or precipitating factors should be considered, including low urine flow or decreased distal Na^+ delivery, a rapid decline in GFR (especially in acute superimposed on CKD), hyperglycemia or hyperosmolality, and unsuspected sources of exogenous K^+ intake.[25] The workup should include evaluation of the TTKG or the FE_{K^+}, an estimate of renal ammonium excretion (UAG, osmolar gap, and urine pH), and evaluation of plasma renin activity and aldosterone secretion. The latter may be assessed under stimulated conditions with dietary salt restriction and furosemide-induced volume depletion, and measurement of the response of potassium excretion to furosemide and fludrocortisone. An increase in the TTKG to a value of more than 6 measured 4 hours after a single oral dose of fludrocortisone (0.1 mg) suggests that mineralocorticoid deficiency, but not resistance, is causative.

The decision to treat is often based on the severity of the hyperkalemia. Reduction in the serum potassium level will often improve the metabolic acidosis by increasing ammonium excretion as potassium levels return to the normal range. Correction of hyperkalemia with sodium polystyrene can correct the metabolic acidosis as the serum potassium level declines.[26,27] Patients with combined glucocorticoid and mineralocorticoid deficiency should receive both adrenal steroids in replacement dosages. Additional measures may include use of laxatives, alkali therapy, or treatment with a loop diuretic to induce renal potassium and salt excretion (Table 17.16). Volume depletion should be avoided unless the patient is volume overexpanded or hypertensive. Suprphysiologic doses of mineralocorticoids are rarely necessary and, if administered, should be given cautiously in combination with a loop diuretic to avoid volume overexpansion or aggravation of hypertension and to increase potassium excretion.[27] Infants with autosomal recessive or dominant PHA I should receive salt supplements in amounts sufficient to correct the volume depletion, hypotension, and other features of the syndrome and to allow normal growth. In contrast, patients with PHA II should receive thiazide diuretics along with dietary salt restriction.

Although it may be prudent to discontinue drugs that are identified as the most likely cause of the hyperkalemia, this may not always be feasible in patients with life-threatening disorders, for example, during TMP-SMX or pentamidine therapy in AIDS patients with *P. jirovecii* pneumonia. Based on the previous analysis of the mechanism by which TMP and pentamidine cause hyperkalemia (voltage defect), it might also be reasoned that the delivery to the CCD of a poorly reabsorbed anion might improve the electrochemical driving force favoring K^+ and H^+ secretion. The combined use of acetazolamide along with sufficient sodium bicarbonate to deliver HCO_3^- to the CCT and thereby increase the negative transepithelial voltage could theoretically increase K^+ and H^+ secretion. Obviously with such an approach, aggravation of metabolic acidosis by excessive acetazolamide or insufficient $NaHCO_3$ administration must be avoided.

Distinguishing the Types of Renal Tubular Acidosis

The contrasting findings and diagnostic features of the three types of RTA discussed in this chapter are summarized in Table 17.17.

DISORDERS OF IMPAIRED NET ACID EXCRETION AND IMPAIRED BICARBONATE RECLAMATION WITH NORMOKALEMIA: ACIDOSIS OF PROGRESSIVE RENAL FAILURE

A reduction in functional renal mass by disease has long been known to be associated with acidosis.[28] The metabolic

---

Table 17.16 Treatment of Generalized Dysfunction of the Nephron with Hyperkalemia

Alkali therapy (Shohl's solution or $NaHCO_3$ tablets)
Loop diuretic (furosemide, bumetanide)
Sodium polystyrene sulfonate (Kayexalate) (without sorbitol) (15 g in H_2O three times weekly)
Low-potassium diet
Fludrocortisone (0.1-0.3 mg/day)
    Avoid in hypertension, volume expansion, heart failure
    Combine with loop diuretic
Avoid drugs associated with hyperkalemia, herbs, and OTC preparations containing potassium (e.g., Noni juice)
In pseudohypoaldosteronism type I, add NaCl tablets

OTC, Over-the-counter.

Table 17.17 Contrasting Features and Diagnostic Studies in Renal Tubular Acidosis

Finding	Proximal	Classical Distal	Generalized Distal Dysfunction
Plasma [K⁺]	Low	Low	High
Urine pH with acidosis	<5.5	>5.5	<5.5 or >5.5
Urine net charge	Positive	Positive	Positive
Fanconi's lesion	Present with acquired PRTA	Absent	Absent
Fractional bicarbonate excretion	>10%-15% during alkali therapy	2%-5%	5%-10%
U − B P_{CO_2}	Normal	Low*	Low
H⁺-ATPase defect		Low	
HCO_3^-/Cl^- defect		High	
Amphotericin B		Normal	
Response to therapy	Least responsive	Responsive	Less responsive
Associated features	Fanconi's syndrome	Nephrocalcinosis/hyperglobulinemia	Renal insufficiency

*See specific defects below.
ATPase, Adenosine triphosphatase; PRTA, proximal renal tubular acidosis; U − B P_{CO_2}, urine minus blood CO_2 pressure.

acidosis is initially hyperchloremic (GFR in the range of 20 to 30 mL/min) but may convert to the high AG variety as renal insufficiency progresses and GFR falls below 15 mL/min.[31,80] Unlike patients with distal RTA, patients with primary renal disease have a normal ability to lower the urine pH during acidosis.[31] The net distal H⁺ secretory capacity is qualitatively normal and can be increased by buffer availability in the form of PO_4^{3-} or by nonreabsorbable anions. Also in contrast to distal RTA, the U − B P_{CO_2} gradient is normal in patients with reduced GFR, which reflects intact distal H⁺ secretory capacity.

The principal defect in net acid excretion in patients with reduced GFR is thus not an inability to secrete H⁺ in the distal nephron, but rather an inability to produce or to excrete NH_4^+ sufficient to match net endogenous acid production. Consequently, the kidneys cannot quantitatively excrete all the metabolic acids produced daily, and metabolic acidosis supervenes.[31]

Studies indicate that higher net endogenous acid production due to higher dietary acid intake, as is typical of the Western-type diet, is associated with a reduction in serum bicarbonate even in the general U.S. population (without evidence of CKD). This association is most significant among middle-aged and older persons.[81] Such findings indicate that the adaptive increase in net acid excretion by the kidney to defend against metabolic acidosis may have deleterious consequences. In this regard, evidence continues to indicate that chronic acidosis in patients with CKD is deleterious. Nevertheless, it is both less well appreciated and less aggressively treated with alkali than indicated by the literature. The numerous consequences of chronic positive acid balance in CKD include progression of CKD at a faster rate,[82] dissolution of bone,[28] impaired hydroxylation of 25-hydroxycholecalciferol,[28,79] renal osteodystrophy, sarcopenia from enhanced skeletal muscle protein degradation, loss of muscle strength, and insulin resistance.

Interestingly, patients with stage 2 and 3 CKD even without overt clinical metabolic acidosis, when given oral alkali progress more slowly and exhibit a significant reduction in net acid excretion. This latter finding suggests that patients progressing with CKD have a higher dietary intake of protein and subsequently higher net endogenous acid production, which evokes a higher rate of net acid excretion, than appropriate for the degree of renal insufficiency.[12,82] Moreover, a study in patients with stage 4 CKD found that a diet emphasizing fruits and vegetables had as beneficial an effect on slowing progression of CKD and compared favorably to $NaHCO_3$ therapy.[83] Note that neither approach, alkali supplementation or additional fruits and vegetables in the diet, requires dietary protein restriction.

The clinical guidelines endorsed by the National Kidney Foundation Kidney Disease Outcomes Quality Initiative recommend monitoring of total CO_2 in patients with CKD with a goal of maintaining the [HCO_3^-] above 22 mEq/L.[84]

In addition, findings indicate that sufficient alkali therapy helps to reverse the deleterious effects of chronic acidosis on bone and skeletal muscle and also slows progression of CKD significantly.[12] An amount of alkali slightly in excess (1 to 2 mEq/kg/day) of dietary metabolic acid production, typically restores the [HCO_3^-] to this level (>22 mEq/L).[28] Alkali therapy may consist of $NaHCO_3$ tablets or modified Shohl's (citric acid–sodium citrate) solution. Fear of Na⁺ retention in CKD as a result of sodium bicarbonate administration appears ill founded. Unlike the case with sodium chloride therapy, patients with CKD retain administered sodium bicarbonate only as long as acidosis is present. Further sodium bicarbonate administration exceeds the reabsorptive threshold and is excreted without causing an increase in weight or in blood pressure unless very large amounts are administered.

Also of concern in chronic progressive kidney disease is the use of sevelamer hydrochloride, which has been shown in patients receiving long-term hemodialysis to result in significantly lower [HCO_3^-] than do Ca^{2+}-containing phosphate binders.[85] Although it is associated with a lower intake of potential alkali, sevelamer may also provide an acid load.[86]

A number of potential mechanisms exist for the acidosis associated with sevelamer. This agent binds monovalent phosphate in exchange for chloride in the gastrointestinal tract. For each molecule of monovalent phosphate bound, one molecule of HCl is liberated. Upon entry of the polymer into the small intestine, exposure to bicarbonate secreted by the pancreas would result in the binding of bicarbonate by the polymer in exchange for chloride—much like the mechanism in chloride diarrhea. Therefore the clinician should be alert for changes in the [HCO_3^-] when the patient is treated with sevelamer.[82] Sevelamer carbonate, the contemporary formulation of sevelamer in a buffered form, is preferred because it compares favorably to sevelamer hydrochloride in terms of serum phosphorus control but without causing a decline in serum [HCO_3^-].

As kidney disease progresses below a GFR of 15 mL/min, the non-AG acidosis typically evolves into the usual high AG acidosis of end-stage kidney disease.[85]

HIGH ANION GAP ACIDOSES

The addition to the body of an acid load in which the attendant non-Cl^- anion is not excreted rapidly results in the development of a high AG acidosis. The normochloremic acidosis is maintained as long as the anion that was part of the original acid load remains in the blood. AG acidosis is caused by the accumulation of organic acids. This may occur if the anion does not undergo glomerular filtration (e.g., uremic acid anions), if the anion is filtered but is readily reabsorbed, or if, because of alteration in metabolic pathways (ketoacidosis, L-lactic acidosis), the anion cannot be used in the body. Theoretically, with a pure AG acidosis the increment in the AG (ΔAG) above the normal value of 10 mEq/L should equal the decrease in bicarbonate concentration (ΔHCO_3^-) below the normal value of 25 mEq/L. When this relationship is considered, circumstances in which the increment in the AG exceeds the decrement in bicarbonate ($\Delta AG > \Delta HCO_3^-$) suggest the coexistence of a metabolic alkalosis. Such findings are not unusual when uremia or ketoacidosis leads to vomiting, for example.

Identification of the underlying cause of a high AG acidosis is facilitated by consideration of the clinical setting and associated laboratory values. The common causes are outlined in Table 17.18 and include (1) lactic acidosis (e.g., L-lactic acidosis and D-lactic acidosis), (2) ketoacidosis (e.g., diabetic, alcoholic, and starvation ketoacidoses), (3) toxin- or poison-induced acidosis (e.g., ethylene glycol, methyl alcohol, propylene glycol, or pyroglutamic acidosis), and (4) uremic acidosis.

Initial screening to differentiate the high AG acidoses should focus on (1) a history or other evidence of drug or toxin ingestion and ABG measurement to detect coexistent respiratory alkalosis (as with salicylates), (2) historical evidence of diabetes mellitus (DKA), (3) evidence of alcoholism or increased levels of β-hydroxybutyrate (AKA), (4) observation for clinical signs of uremia and determination of the blood urea and creatinine levels (uremic acidosis), (5) inspection of the urine for oxalate crystals (ethylene glycol), and, finally, (6) recognition of the numerous settings in which lactic acid levels may be increased (hypotension, cardiac failure, ischemic bowel, intestinal obstruction and bacterial overgrowth, leukemia, cancer, and exposure to certain drugs).

Table 17.18 Metabolic Acidosis with High Anion Gap

Conditions Associated with Type A Lactic Acidosis

Hypovolemic shock
Cholera
Septic shock
Cardiogenic shock
    Low-output heart failure
    High-output heart failure
Regional hypoperfusion
Severe hypoxia
    Severe asthma
    Carbon monoxide poisoning
    Severe anemia

Conditions Associated with Type B Lactic Acidosis

Liver disease
Diabetes mellitus
Catecholamine excess
    Endogenous
    Exogenous
Thiamine deficiency
Intracellular inorganic phosphate depletion
    Intravenous fructose
    Intravenous xylose
    Intravenous sorbitol
Alcohols and other ingested compounds metabolized by alcohol dehydrogenase
    Ethanol
    Methanol
    Ethylene glycol
    Propylene glycol
Mitochondrial toxins
    Salicylates
    Cyanide
    2,4-dinitrophenol
    Nonnucleoside reverse transcriptase drugs
Other drugs
Metastatic tumors (large tumors with regional hypoxemia or liver metastasis)
Seizure
Inborn errors of metabolism

D-Lactic Acidosis

Short bowel syndrome
Ischemic bowel
Small-bowel obstruction

Ketoacidosis

Diabetic
Alcoholic
Starvation

Other Toxins

Salicylates
Paraldehyde
Pyroglutamic acid

Uremia (Late Renal Failure)

LACTIC ACIDOSIS
Physiology

Lactic acid can exist in two forms: L-lactic acid and D-lactic acid. In mammals, only the levorotatory form is a product of mammalian metabolism. D-Lactate can accumulate in humans as a by-product of metabolism by bacteria, which accumulate and overgrow in the gastrointestinal tract with jejunal bypass or short bowel syndrome. Thus D-lactic acidosis is a rare cause of high AG acidosis. Hospital chemical laboratories routinely measure L-lactic acid levels, not D-lactic acid levels. Thus most of the remarks that follow apply to L-lactic acid metabolism and acidosis except as noted. L-Lactic acidosis is one of the most common forms of a high AG acidosis.

Although lactate metabolism bears a close relationship to that of pyruvate,[87] lactic acid is in a metabolic cul-de-sac with pyruvate as its only outlet. In most cells the major metabolic pathway for pyruvate is oxidation in the mitochondria to acetyl coenzyme A (acetyl CoA) by the enzyme pyruvate dehydrogenase within the mitochondria. The overall reaction is usually expressed as

$$\text{Pyruvate}^- + \text{NADH} \leftrightarrow \text{Lactate}^- + \text{NAD} + \text{H}^+ \quad (32)$$

Normally this cytosolic reaction catalyzed by the enzyme lactate dehydrogenase is close to equilibrium, so that the law of mass action applies and the equation is rearranged as

$$[\text{Lactate}^-] = K_{eq}[\text{Pyruvate}^-][\text{H}^+]\frac{[\text{NADH}]}{[\text{NAD}^+]} \quad (33)$$

The lactate concentration is a function of the equilibrium constant (K_{eq}), the pyruvate concentration, the cytosolic pH, and the intracellular redox state represented by the concentration ratio of reduced to oxidized nicotinamide adenine dinucleotide or [NADH]/[NAD$^+$].[87]

After rearranging the mass action equation, the ratio of lactate concentration to pyruvate concentration may be expressed as

$$\frac{[\text{Lactate}^-]}{[\text{Pyruvate}^-]} = K_{eq}[\text{H}^+]\frac{[\text{NADH}]}{[\text{NAD}^+]} \quad (34)$$

Because K_{eq} and [H$^+$]$_i$ are relatively constant, the normal lactate/pyruvate concentration ratio (1.0/0.1 mEq/L) is proportional to the NADH/NAD$^+$ concentration ratio. Therefore the lactate/pyruvate ratio is regulated by the oxidation-reduction potential of the cell.

NADH/NAD$^+$ is also involved in many other metabolic redox reactions.[87] Moreover, the steady-state concentrations of all these redox reactants are related to one another. Important in considerations of acid-base pathophysiology are the redox pairs β-hydroxybutyrate–acetoacetate and ethanol-acetaldehyde. The ratio of the reduced to the oxidized forms of these molecules is thus a function of the cellular redox potential:

$$\frac{[\text{NADH}]}{[\text{NAD}^+]} \propto \frac{[\text{Lactate}]}{[\text{Pyruvate}]} \propto \frac{[\beta\text{-Hydroxybutyrate}]}{[\text{Acetoacetate}]} \propto \frac{[\text{Ethanol}]}{[\text{Acetaldehyde}]} \quad (35)$$

If the lactate concentration is high compared with that of pyruvate, NAD$^+$ will be depleted, and the NADH/NAD$^+$ ratio will increase. Likewise, all the other related redox ratios previously listed would be similarly affected; that is, both the β-hydroxybutyrate/acetoacetate and the ethanol/acetaldehyde ratios would increase. In clinical practice these considerations are of practical importance. If lactate levels are increased as a result of lactic acidosis concurrently with ketone overproduction as a result of diabetic acidosis, the ketones exist primarily in the form of β-hydroxybutyrate. The results of tests for ketones that measure only acetoacetate (such as the nitroprusside reaction, e.g., Acetest tablets and reagent sticks) therefore may be misleadingly low or even negative despite high total ketone concentrations. Some hospital laboratories no longer use the nitroprusside reaction to estimate total ketones, and measurement of β-hydroxybutyrate and acetoacetate are the preferred tests. This assumes importance because high levels of alcohol plus ketones shift the redox ratio, so that the NADH/NAD$^+$ ratio is increased. Again, ketones would then be principally in the form of β-hydroxybutyrate. This situation is commonly found in AKA, in which the results of qualitative ketone tests that are more sensitive to acetoacetate are frequently only trace positive or negative, despite markedly increased β-hydroxybutyrate levels.

The L-lactate concentration can be increased in two ways relative to the pyruvate concentration. First, when pyruvate production is increased at a constant intracellular pH and redox stage, the lactate concentration increases at a constant lactate/pyruvate ratio of 10. In contrast, in states in which the production of lactate exceeds the ability to convert to pyruvate, so that the NADH/NAD$^+$ redox ratio is increased, an increased L-lactic acid concentration is observed, but with a lactate/pyruvate ratio greater than 10. This defines an *excess lactate* state. Therefore the concentration of lactate must be viewed in terms of cellular determinants (e.g., the intracellular pH and redox state) as well as the total body production and removal rates. Normally the rates of lactate entry and exit from the blood are in balance, so that net lactate accumulation is zero. This dynamic aspect of lactate metabolism is termed the *Cori cycle*:

$$2\text{Lactate}^+ + 2\text{H}^+ \underset{\text{Muscle, brain, skin, red blood cells, gut}}{\overset{\text{Liver, kidney, heart}}{\longleftrightarrow}} \text{Glucose} \quad (36)$$

As can be envisioned from this relationship, either net overproduction of lactic acid from glucose by some tissues or underutilization by others results in net addition of L-lactic acid to the blood and lactic acidosis. However, ischemia accelerates lactate production and simultaneously decreases lactate utilization.

The production of lactic acid has been estimated to be approximately 15 to 20 mEq/kg/day in normal humans.[28] This enormous quantity contrasts with total ECF buffer base stores of approximately 10 to 15 mEq/kg, and with enhanced production lactic acid can accumulate. The rate of lactic acid production can be increased by ischemia, seizures, extreme exercise, leukemia, and alkalosis.[87] The increase in production occurs principally through enhanced phosphofructokinase activity.

Decreased lactate consumption may also lead to L-lactic acidosis. The principal organs for lactate removal during rest are the liver and kidneys. Both the liver and the kidneys and perhaps muscle have the capacity for increased lactate removal under the stress of increased lactate loads.[83] Hepatic utilization of lactate can be impeded by several factors: poor perfusion of the liver; defective active transport of lactate into cells; and inadequate metabolic conversion of lactate into pyruvate because of altered intracellular pH, redox state, or enzyme activity. Examples of states causing impaired hepatic lactate removal include primary diseases of the liver, enzymatic defects, tissue anoxia or ischemia, severe acidosis, and altered redox states, as occurs with alcohol intoxication, fructose consumption by fructose-intolerant individuals, or administration of nucleoside (analog) reverse transcriptase inhibitors (NRTIs) such as zidovudine and stavudine in patients with HIV infection,[87-89] or biguanides such as metformin.[87,90,91] Deaths have been reported due to refractory lactic acidosis secondary to thiamine deficiency in patients receiving parenteral nutrition formulations without thiamine.[92] Thiamine is a cofactor for pyruvate dehydrogenase that catalyzes the oxidative decarboxylation of pyruvate to acetyl CoA under aerobic conditions. Pyruvate cannot be metabolized in this manner in the presence of thiamine deficiency, so that excess pyruvate is converted to hydrogen ions and lactate.

The quantitative aspects of normal lactate production and consumption in the Cori cycle demonstrate how the development of lactic acidosis can be the most rapid and devastating form of metabolic acidosis.[87,93]

Diagnosis

Because lactic acid has a pK'a of 3.8, addition of lactic acid to the blood leads to a reduction in blood HCO_3^- concentration and an equivalent elevation in lactate concentration, which is associated with an increase in the AG. Lactate concentrations are mildly increased in various nonpathologic states (e.g., exercise), but the magnitude of the elevation is generally small. In practical terms, a lactate concentration greater than 4 mmol/L (normal is 0.67 to 1.8 mmol/L) is generally accepted as evidence that the metabolic acidosis is ascribable to net lactic acid accumulation.

Clinical Spectrum

In the classical classification of the L-lactic acidoses (see Table 17.18), type A L-lactic acidosis is due to tissue hypoperfusion or acute hypoxia, whereas type B L-lactic acidosis is associated with common diseases, drugs and toxins, and hereditary and miscellaneous disorders.[87]

Tissue underperfusion and acute underoxygenation at the tissue level (tissue hypoxia) are the most common causes of type A lactic acidosis. Severe arterial hypoxemia even in the absence of decreased perfusion can generate L-lactic acidosis. Inadequate cardiac output, of either the low-output or the high-output variety, is the usual pathogenetic factor. The prognosis is related directly to the increment in plasma L-lactate and the severity of the acidemia.[87,91,93]

Numerous medical conditions (without tissue hypoxia) predispose to type B L-lactic acidosis (see Table 17.18). Hepatic failure reduces hepatic lactate metabolism, and leukemia increases lactate production. Severe anemia, especially as a result of iron deficiency or methemoglobinemia, may cause lactic acidosis. Among the most common causes of L-lactic acidosis is bowel ischemia and infarction in patients in the medical intensive care unit. Malignant cells produce more lactate than normal cells even under aerobic conditions. This phenomenon is magnified if the tumor expands rapidly and outstrips the blood supply. Therefore exceptionally large tumors may be associated with severe L-lactic acidosis. Seizures, extreme exertion, heat stroke, and tumor lysis syndrome may all cause L-lactic acidosis.

Several drugs and toxins predispose to L-lactic acidosis (see Table 17.18). Of these, metformin and other biguanides (such as phenformin) are the most widely reported to have this effect.[87,90,91] The occurrence of phenformin-induced lactic acidosis prompted the withdrawal of the drug from U.S. markets in 1977. Although much less frequent than phenformin-induced lactic acidosis, metformin-induced lactic acidosis is a higher risk in patients with CKD (and is contraindicated when the serum creatinine level exceeds 1.4 mg/dL) and whenever there is hypoperfusion or hypotension, including severe volume depletion, shock, CHF, septicemia, acute myocardial infarction, or with chronic metabolic acidosis. Metformin should be discontinued several days before contrast dye administration. Although rare, metformin-induced lactic acidosis is the most frequent cause of lactic acidosis in patients with diabetes and is associated with a mortality of up to 50%. Fructose causes intracellular ATP depletion and lactate accumulation.[87] Inborn errors of metabolism may also cause lactic acidosis, primarily by blocking gluconeogenesis or by inhibiting the oxidation of pyruvate.[87] Carbon monoxide poisoning produces lactic acidosis frequently by reduction of the oxygen-carrying capacity of hemoglobin. Cyanide binds cytochrome a and a_3 and blocks the flow of electrons to oxygen. In patients with HIV infection, nucleoside analogs can induce toxic effects on mitochondria by inhibiting DNA polymerase-γ. Hyperlactatemia is common with NRTI therapy, especially stavudine and zidovudine, but the serum L-lactate level is usually only mildly elevated and compensated.[87-89,94] Nevertheless, with severe concurrent illness, pronounced lactic acidosis may occur in association with hepatic steatosis.[87,89] This combination carries a high mortality. Chronic low-grade hyperlactatemia is also associated with osteopenia and osteodystrophy, possibly due to the effect of chronic acidosis on bone calcium mobilization

Associated Clinical Features

Hyperventilation, abdominal pain, and disturbances in consciousness are frequently present, as are signs of inadequate cardiopulmonary function in type A L-lactic acidosis. Leukocytosis, hyperphosphatemia, hyperuricemia, and hyperaminoacidemia (especially excess of alanine) are common, and hypoglycemia may occur.[87] Hyperkalemia may or may not accompany acute lactic acidosis.

Treatment of L-Lactic Acidosis

General Supportive Care. The overall mortality of patients with L-lactic acidosis is approximately 60% but approaches 100% in those with coexisting hypotension.[87] Therapy for this condition has not advanced substantively in the last 2 decades. The basic principle and only effective form of therapy for L-lactic acidosis is first to correct the underlying condition initiating the disruption in normal lactate metabolism. In type A L-lactic acidosis, cessation of acid production by improvement of tissue oxygenation, restoration of the circulating fluid volume, improvement or augmentation of cardiac function, resection of ischemic tissue, and amelioration of sepsis are necessary in many cases. Septic shock requires control of the underlying infection and volume resuscitation in hypovolemic shock. High L-lactate levels portend a poor prognosis almost uniformly, and sodium bicarbonate administration is of little value in this setting. Use of vasoconstricting agents is problematic because they may potentiate the hypoperfused state. Dopamine is preferred to epinephrine if pressure support is required, but the vasodilator nitroprusside has been suggested because it may enhance cardiac output and hepatic and renal blood flow to augment lactate removal.[87] Nevertheless, nitroprusside therapy may result in cyanide toxicity and has no proven efficacy in the treatment of this disorder.

Alkali Therapy. Alkali therapy is generally advocated for acute, severe acidemia (pH of <7.1) to improve inotropy and lactate utilization. However, in experimental models and clinical examples of lactic acidosis, it has been shown that $NaHCO_3$ therapy in large amounts can depress cardiac performance and exacerbate the acidemia. Paradoxically, bicarbonate therapy activates phosphofructokinase, which is regulated by intracellular pH, thereby increasing lactate production. The use of alkali in states of moderate L-lactic acidemia is therefore controversial, and it is generally agreed that attempts to normalize the pH or HCO_3^- concentration by intravenous $NaHCO_3$ therapy is both potentially deleterious and practically impossible. Thus raising the plasma HCO_3^- to approximately 15 mEq/L (not to the normal value) and the pH to only 7.2 to 7.25 is a reasonable goal to improve tissue pH. Constant infusion of hypertonic bicarbonate has many disadvantages and is discouraged. Fluid overload occurs rapidly with $NaHCO_3$ administration because of the massive amounts required in some cases. In addition, central venoconstriction and decreased cardiac output are common. The accumulation of lactic acid may be relentless and may necessitate administration of diuretics, ultrafiltration, or dialysis. Hemodialysis can simultaneously deliver HCO_3^-, remove lactate, remove excess ECF volume, and correct electrolyte abnormalities. The use of continuous renal replacement therapy as a means of lactate removal and simultaneous alkali addition is a promising adjunctive treatment in critically ill patients with L-lactic acidosis.

If the underlying cause of the L-lactic acidosis can be remedied, blood lactate will be reconverted to HCO_3^-. HCO_3^- derived from lactate conversion and any new HCO_3^- generated by renal mechanisms during acidosis and from exogenous alkali therapy are additive and may result in an overshoot alkalosis.

Other Agents. Dichloroacetate, an activator of pyruvate dehydrogenase, was once advanced as a potentially useful therapeutic agent. In experimental L-lactic acidosis, dichloroacetate stimulated lactate consumption in muscle, decreased lactate production, and improved survival. In nonacidotic patients with diabetes, it successfully lowered lactate as well as glucose, lipid, and amino acid levels. Despite encouraging results of its short-term clinical use in acute lactic acidosis, a prospective multicenter trial failed to substantiate any beneficial effect of dichloroacetate therapy.[95] Administration of methylene blue was once advocated as a means of reversing the altered redox state to enhance lactate metabolism. There is no evidence from controlled studies to support its use. THAM (0.3 mol/L tromethamine) and other preparations of this type are not effective.[87] Tribonat, a mixture of THAM, acetate, $NaHCO_3$, and phosphate, although apparently an effective clinical buffer, has produced no survival advantage in limited clinical trials.[96] Lactated Ringer's solution and lactate-containing peritoneal dialysis solutions should be avoided.

D-Lactic Acidosis

The manifestations of D-lactic acidosis are typically episodic encephalopathy and high AG acidosis in association with short bowel syndrome. Features include slurred speech, confusion, cognitive impairment, clumsiness, ataxia, hallucinations, and behavioral disturbances. D-Lactic acidosis has been described in patients with bowel obstruction, jejunal bypass, short bowel, or ischemic bowel disease. These disorders have in common ileus or stasis associated with overgrowth of flora in the gastrointestinal tract, which is exacerbated by a high-carbohydrate diet.[87] D-Lactic acidosis occurs when fermentation by colonic bacteria in the intestine causes D-lactate to accumulate so that it can be absorbed into the circulation. D-Lactate is not measured by the typical clinical laboratory, which reports the L-isomer. The disorder should be suspected in patients with an unexplained AG acidosis and some of the typical features noted previously. While results of specific testing are awaited, the patient should be under orders to receive nothing by mouth. Serum D-lactate levels of greater than 3 mmol/L confirm the diagnosis. Treatment with a low-carbohydrate diet and antibiotics (neomycin, vancomycin, or metronidazole) is often effective.[97-100]

KETOACIDOSIS

Diabetic Ketoacidosis

DKA is due to increased fatty acid metabolism and the accumulation of ketoacids (acetoacetate and β-hydroxybutyrate) as a result of insulin deficiency or resistance, in association with elevated glucagon levels. DKA is usually seen in insulin-dependent diabetes mellitus upon cessation of insulin therapy or during an intercurrent illness, such as an infection, gastroenteritis, pancreatitis, or myocardial infarction, which increases insulin requirements temporarily and acutely. The accumulation of ketoacids accounts for the increment in the AG, which is accompanied, most often, by evidence of hyperglycemia (glucose level of >300 mg/dL). In comparison to patients with AKA, described later, patients with DKA have metabolic profiles characterized by a higher plasma glucose level and lower β-hydroxybutyrate/acetoacetate and lactate/pyruvate ratios.[30,100,101]

Treatment. Most, if not all, patients with DKA require correction of the volume depletion that almost invariably accompanies the osmotic diuresis of DKA. In general, it seems prudent to initiate therapy with intravenous isotonic saline at a rate of 1000 mL/hr, especially in the severely volume-depleted patient. When the pulse and blood pressure have stabilized and the corrected serum Na^+ concentration is in the range of 130 to 135 mEq/L, switch to 0.45% sodium chloride and slow the infusion rate. When the blood glucose level falls below 300 mg/dL, 0.45% sodium chloride with 5% dextrose should be administered.[30,100]

Low-dose intravenous regular insulin therapy administered as a bolus (0.1 U/kg), and then a continuous infusion (0.1 U/kg/hr), smoothly corrects the biochemical abnormalities and minimizes hypoglycemia and hypokalemia.[30,100] Intramuscular insulin is not effective in patients with volume depletion, which often occurs in ketoacidosis.

Total body K^+ depletion is usually present, although the K^+ level on admission may be elevated or normal. A normal or reduced K^+ value on admission indicates severe K^+ depletion and should be approached with caution. Administration of fluid, insulin, and alkali may cause the K^+ level to plummet. When urine output has been established, 20 mEq of potassium chloride should be administered in each liter of fluid as long as the K^+ value is less than 4.0 mEq/L. Equal caution should be exercised in the presence of hyperkalemia, especially if the patient has renal insufficiency, because the usual therapy does not always correct hyperkalemia. Never administer potassium chloride empirically.

The AG should be followed closely during therapy because it is expected to decline as ketones are cleared from the plasma and projects an increase in plasma HCO_3^- as the acidosis is repaired. Therefore it is not necessary to monitor blood ketone levels continuously. Young patients with a pure AG acidosis ($\Delta AG = \Delta HCO_3^-$) usually do not require exogenous alkali administration because the metabolic acidosis should be entirely reversible. Older patients, patients with severe high AG acidosis (pH of <7.15), or patients with a superimposed hyperchloremic component may receive small amounts of sodium bicarbonate by slow intravenous infusion (no more than 44 to 88 mEq in 60 minutes). Thirty minutes after this infusion is completed, ABG measurement should be repeated. Alkali administration can be repeated only if the pH remains at 7.20 or less or if the patient exhibits a significant hyperchloremic component, but additional $NaHCO_3$ is rarely necessary. Hypokalemia and other complications of alkali therapy dramatically increase when amounts of sodium bicarbonate exceeding 400 mEq are administered. However, the effect of alkali therapy on arterial blood pH needs to be reassessed regularly and the total administered kept at a minimum, if alkali therapy is necessary.[30,100,101] Routine administration of PO_4^{3-} (usually as potassium phosphate) is not advised because of the potential for hyperphosphatemia and hypocalcemia.[30,100] A significant proportion of patients with DKA have significant hyperphosphatemia before initiation of therapy. In the volume-depleted, malnourished patient, however, a normal or elevated PO_4^{3-} concentration on admission may be followed by a rapid fall in plasma PO_4^{3-} levels within 2 to 6 hours after initiation of therapy.

Alcoholic Ketoacidosis

Some patients with chronic alcoholism, especially binge drinkers, who discontinue solid food intake while continuing alcohol consumption develop the alcoholic form of ketoacidosis when alcohol ingestion is curtailed abruptly.[27,97,98] Usually the onset of vomiting and abdominal pain with dehydration leads to cessation of alcohol consumption before the patient comes to the hospital.[30,101] The metabolic acidosis may be severe but is accompanied by only modestly deranged glucose levels, which are usually low but may be slightly elevated.[27,100] Typically insulin levels are low and levels of triglyceride, cortisol, glucagon, and growth hormone are increased. The net result of this deranged metabolic state is ketosis. The acidosis is primarily due to elevated levels of ketones, which exist predominantly in the form of β-hydroxybutyrate because of the altered redox state induced by the metabolism of alcohol. Compared with patients with DKA, patients with AKA have lower plasma glucose concentrations and higher β-hydroxybutyrate/acetoacetate and lactate/pyruvate ratios.[30,101] The clinical presentation in AKA may be complex and is often underdiagnosed. The typical high AG acidosis is often mixed with metabolic alkalosis (vomiting), respiratory alkalosis (alcoholic liver disease), lactic acidosis (hypoperfusion), and/or hyperchloremic acidosis (renal excretion of ketoacids). Finally, the elevation in the osmolar gap is usually accounted for by an increased blood alcohol level, but the differential diagnosis should always include ethylene glycol and/or methanol intoxication.

Treatment. Therapy includes intravenous glucose and saline administration, but insulin should be avoided. K^+, PO_4^{3-}, Mg^{2+}, and vitamin supplementation (especially thiamine) are frequently necessary. Glucose in isotonic saline, not saline alone, is the mainstay of therapy. Because of superimposed starvation, patients with AKA often develop hypophosphatemia within 12 to 18 hours of admission. Treatment with glucose-containing intravenous fluids increases the risk for severe hypophosphatemia. Levels should be checked on admission and at 4, 6, 12, and 18 hours. Profound hypophosphatemia may provoke aspiration, platelet dysfunction, hemolysis, and rhabdomyolysis. Therefore phosphate replacement should be provided promptly when indicated. Hypokalemia and hypomagnesemia are also common and should not be overlooked.[30,101]

Starvation Ketoacidosis

Ketoacidosis occurs within the first 24 to 48 hours of fasting, is accentuated by exercise and pregnancy, and is rapidly reversible by glucose or insulin administration. Starvation-induced hypoinsulinemia and accentuated hepatic ketone production have been implicated pathogenetically.[30,101] Fasting alone can increase ketoacid levels, although not usually above 10 mEq/L. High-protein weight-loss diets typically cause mild ketosis but not ketoacidosis. Patients typically respond to glucose and saline infusion.

DRUG- AND TOXIN-INDUCED ACIDOSIS

Salicylate

Intoxication with salicylates, although more common in children than in adults, may result in the development of a high AG metabolic acidosis, but the acid-base abnormality most commonly associated with salicylate intoxication in adults is respiratory alkalosis due to direct stimulation of the respiratory center by salicylates.[100] Adult patients with salicylate intoxication usually have pure respiratory alkalosis or mixed respiratory alkalosis–metabolic acidosis.[100] Metabolic acidosis occurs because of uncoupling of oxidative phosphorylation and enhances the transit of salicylates into the central nervous system. Only part of the increase in the AG is due to the increase in plasma salicylate concentration, because a toxic salicylate level of 100 mg/dL would account for an increase in the AG of only 7 mEq/L. High ketone concentrations have been reported to be present in as many as 40% of adult salicylate-intoxicated patients, sometimes as a result of salicylate-induced hypoglycemia.[102] L-Lactic acid production is also often increased, partly as a direct drug effect[100] and partly as a result of the decrease in P_{CO_2} induced by salicylate. Proteinuria and pulmonary edema may occur.

Treatment. General treatment should always consist of initial vigorous gastric lavage with isotonic saline followed by administration of activated charcoal via nasogastric tube. Treatment of the metabolic acidosis may be necessary, because acidosis can enhance the entry of salicylate into the central nervous system. Alkali should be given cautiously, and frank alkalemia should be avoided. Coexisting respiratory alkalosis can make this form of therapy hazardous. The renal excretion of salicylate is enhanced by an alkaline diuresis accomplished with intravenous administration of $NaHCO_3$. Caution is urged if the patient exhibits concomitant respiratory alkalosis with frank alkalemia, because $NaHCO_3$ may cause severe alkalosis, and hypokalemia may result from alkalinization of the urine. To minimize the administration of $NaHCO_3$, acetazolamide may be administered to the alkalemic patient, but this can cause acidosis through enhanced bicarbonate excretion and impair salicylate elimination. Hemodialysis may be necessary in severe poisoning, especially if renal failure coexists; it is preferred in cases of severe intoxication (>700 mg/L) and is superior to hemofiltration, which does not correct the acid-base abnormality.[100,102]

Toxins

The Osmolar Gap in Toxin-Induced Acidosis. Under most physiologic conditions, Na^+, urea, and glucose generate the osmotic pressure of blood. Serum osmolality is calculated according to the following expression:

$$\text{Osmolality} = 2[Na^+] + \frac{BUN}{2.8} + \frac{\text{Glucose (mg/dL)}}{18} \quad (37)$$

where BUN is the blood urea nitrogen level. The calculated osmolality and determined osmolality should agree within 10 mOsm/kg. When the measured osmolality exceeds the calculated osmolality by more than 10 mOsm/kg, one of two circumstances prevails. First, the serum Na^+ level may be spuriously low, as occurs with hyperlipidemia or hyperproteinemia (pseudohyponatremia). Second, osmolytes other than sodium salts, glucose, or urea may have accumulated in plasma. Examples are infused mannitol, radiocontrast media, or other solutes, including the alcohols, ethylene glycol, and acetone, which can increase the osmolality in plasma. For these examples, the difference between the osmolality calculated from equation 37 and the measured osmolality is proportional to the concentration of the unmeasured solute. Such differences in these clinical circumstances have been referred to as the *osmolar gap*. In the presence of an appropriate clinical history and index of suspicion, the osmolar gap becomes a very reliable and helpful screening tool in assessing for toxin-associated high AG acidosis.

Ethanol. Ethanol, after absorption from the gastrointestinal tract, is oxidized to acetaldehyde, acetyl CoA, and CO_2. A blood ethanol level over 500 mg/dL is associated with high mortality. Acetaldehyde levels do not increase appreciably unless the load is exceptionally high or if the acetaldehyde dehydrogenase step is inhibited by compounds such as disulfiram, insecticides, or sulfonylurea hypoglycemia agents. In the presence of ethanol such agents result in severe toxicity. The association of ethanol with the development of AKA and lactic acidosis has been discussed in the previous section, but in general, ethanol intoxication does not cause a high AG acidosis.

Ethylene Glycol. Ingestion of ethylene glycol, used in antifreeze, leads to a high AG metabolic[100,103,104] acidosis in addition to severe central nervous system, cardiopulmonary, and renal damage. Disparity between the measured and calculated blood osmolality (high osmolar gap) is often present, especially in the first few hours after ingestion. Typically over time, as the ethylene glycol is metabolized, the osmolar gap begins to fall and the AG begins to rise so that in advanced ethylene glycol intoxication, the AG will be very high but the osmolar gap will close. The high AG is attributable to ethylene glycol metabolites, especially oxalic acid, glycolic acid, and other incompletely identified organic acids.[104] L-Lactic acid production also increases as a result of a toxic depression in the reaction rates of the citric acid cycle and altered intracellular redox state.[104] Recognition of oxalate crystals in the urine facilitates diagnosis. Fluorescence of the urine detected by the Wood lamp (if the ingested ethylene glycol contains a fluorescent vehicle) has been suggested as a diagnostic indicator but is neither specific nor sensitive.[103,104] A colleague of the author with considerable experience treating ethylene glycol toxicity has commented that the Wood lamp almost invariably detects the fluorescent vehicle on the shirt or blouse of the patient who has ingested the agent. Treatment includes prompt institution of osmotic diuresis, thiamine and pyridoxine supplementation, administration of 4-methylpyrazole (fomepizole),[105] or ethyl alcohol administration and dialysis.[100,103,105] Do not induce vomiting. Fomepizole is the drug of choice and should be given intravenously. Fomepizole is a competitive inhibitor of alcohol dehydrogenase. Competitive inhibition of alcohol dehydrogenase with either fomepizole or ethyl alcohol is absolutely necessary in all patients to lessen toxicity, because ethanol and fomepizole compete for metabolic conversion of ethylene glycol and alter the cellular redox state. Fomepizole (initiated as a loading dose of 15 mg/kg, followed by 10 mg/kg every 12 hours), offers the advantages of a predictable decline in ethylene glycol levels without the adverse effect of excessive obtundation, as seen with ethyl alcohol infusion. When these measures have been accomplished, hemodialysis may be initiated to remove the ethylene glycol metabolites. If intravenous ethanol is the only inhibitor of alcohol dehydrogenase available, its infusion should be increased during hemodialysis to allow maintenance of the blood alcohol level in the range of 100 to 150 mg/dL or more than 22 mmol/L. The indications for hemodialysis include (1) arterial pH of less than 7.3, (2) ethylene glycol concentration of more than 20 mEq/L (3.2 mmol/L), (3) osmolal gap of more than 10 mOsm/kg, and (4) oxalate crystalluria.[103]

Methanol. Methanol has wide application in commercially available solvents and is used for industrial and automotive purposes. Sources include windshield wiper fluid, paint remover or thinner, deicing fluid, canned heating sources, varnish, and shellac. Ingestion of methanol (wood alcohol) causes metabolic acidosis in addition to severe optic nerve and central nervous system manifestations resulting from its metabolism to formic acid from formaldehyde.[100,103] Lactic acids and ketoacids as well as other unidentified organic acids may contribute to the acidosis. Because of the low molecular mass of methanol (32 Da), an osmolar gap is usually present early in the course but declines as the AG increases, the latter reflecting the metabolism of methanol. Therapy is generally similar to that for ethylene glycol intoxication, including general supportive measures, fomepizole administration, and usually hemodialysis.[105] The indications for hemodialysis include (1) arterial pH of less than 7.3, (2) methanol concentration of more than 20 mEq/L (6.2 mmol/L), and (3) osmolal gap of more than 10 mOsm/kg.[103]

Isopropyl Alcohol. Rubbing alcohol poisoning is usually the result of accidental oral ingestion (adults) or absorption through the skin (infants and small children). Although isopropyl alcohol is metabolized by the enzyme alcohol dehydrogenase, as are methanol and ethanol, isopropyl alcohol is *not metabolized to a strong acid* and *does not elevate the AG*. Isopropyl alcohol is metabolized to acetone, and the osmolar gap increases as the result of accumulation of both acetone and isopropyl alcohol. Despite a positive nitroprusside reaction from acetone, the AG, as well as the blood glucose level, are typically normal, and the plasma HCO_3^- concentration is not depressed. Thus isopropyl alcohol intoxication does not typically cause metabolic acidosis. Treatment is supportive, with attention to removal of unabsorbed alcohol from the gastrointestinal tract and administration of intravenous fluids. Although patients with significant isopropyl alcohol intoxication (blood levels of >100 mg/dL) may develop cardiovascular collapse and lactic acidosis, watchful waiting with a conservative approach (intravenous fluids, electrolyte replacement, and tracheal intubation) is often sufficient. Only severe intoxication (>400 mg/dL) is an indication for hemodialysis.[100]

Paraldehyde. Intoxication with paraldehyde is very rare but is of historic interest. It is a central nervous system depressant previously used as a sedative or anticonvulsant. Paraldehyde is a cyclic trimer of acetaldehyde. The metabolic acidosis is a result of the accumulation of acetic acid, the metabolic product of the drug from acetaldehyde, and other organic acids. Unmetabolized paraldehyde is exhaled through the respiratory system.

Pyroglutamic Acid. Pyroglutamic acid, or 5-oxoproline, is an intermediate in the γ-glutamyl cycle for the synthesis of glutathione. Acetaminophen ingestion can, in rare cases, deplete glutathione, which results in increased formation of γ-glutamyl cysteine, which is metabolized to pyroglutamic acid.[106] Accumulation of this intermediate, first appreciated in the rare patients with congenital glutathione synthetase deficiency, has been reported in critically ill patients taking acetaminophen, usually with sepsis. Such patients have severe high AG acidosis and alterations in mental status.[106] Many were receiving full therapeutic dosages of acetaminophen. All had elevated blood levels of pyroglutamic acid, which increased in proportion to the increase in the AG. It is conceivable that the heterozygote state for glutathione synthetase deficiency could predispose to pyroglutamic acidosis, because only a minority of critically ill patients receiving acetaminophen develop this newly appreciated form of metabolic acidosis.[106]

Propylene Glycol

Propylene glycol is used as a vehicle for intravenous medications and some cosmetics and is metabolized to lactic acid in the liver by alcohol dehydrogenase. A prospective study of nine patients receiving high-dose lorazepam infusions[90] showed elevated plasma propylene levels and an elevated osmolar gap. Six of nine patients had moderate degrees of metabolic acidosis.[107,108]

Numerous intravenous preparations contain propylene glycol as the vehicle (lorazepam, diazepam, pentobarbital, phenytoin, nitroglycerin, and TMP-SMX). Propylene glycol may accumulate and cause a high AG, high osmolar gap acidosis in patients receiving continuous infusion or higher dosages of these agents, especially in the presence of CKD, chronic liver disease, alcohol abuse, or pregnancy. The acidosis is the result of accumulation of L-lactic acid, D-lactic acid, and L-acetaldehyde. The acidosis typically abates with cessation of the offending agent, and fomepizole administration is necessary only if the acidosis is severe.[12]

Uremia

Advanced renal insufficiency eventually converts the non-AG metabolic acidosis discussed earlier to the typical high AG acidosis, or "uremic acidosis."[31] Poor filtration plus continued reabsorption of poorly identified uremic organic anions contributes to the pathogenesis of this metabolic disturbance.

Classical uremic acidosis is characterized by a reduced rate of NH_4^+ production and excretion because of cumulative and significant loss of renal mass.[5,21,31] Usually acidosis does not occur until a major portion of the total functional nephron population (>75%) has been compromised, because of the adaptation by surviving nephrons to increase ammoniagenesis. Eventually, however, there is a decrease in total renal ammonia excretion as renal mass is reduced to a level at which the GFR is 20 mL/min or less. PO_4^{3-} balance is maintained as a result of both hyperparathyroidism, which decreases proximal PO_4^{3-} absorption, and an increase in plasma PO_4^{3-} as GFR declines. Protein restriction and the administration of phosphate binders reduce the availability of PO_4^{3-}.

Treatment of Acidosis of Chronic Kidney Disease. The uremic acidosis of renal failure requires oral alkali replacement to maintain the HCO_3^- concentration above 20 to 22 mEq/L. This can be accomplished with relatively modest amounts of alkali (1.0 to 1.5 mEq/kg/day). Shohl's solution or sodium bicarbonate tablets (650-mg tablets) are equally effective. It is assumed that alkali replacement serves to prevent the harmful effects of prolonged positive H^+ balance, especially progressive catabolism of muscle and loss of bone. Because sodium citrate (Shohl's solution) has been shown to enhance the absorption of aluminum from the gastrointestinal tract, it should never be administered to patients receiving aluminum-containing antacids because of the risk for aluminum intoxication. When hyperkalemia is present, furosemide (60 to 80 mg/day) should be added. Occasionally a patient may require long-term oral sodium polystyrene sulfonate (Kayexalate) therapy (15 to 30 g/day). The pure powder preparation is better tolerated long term than the commercially available premixed preparation and avoids sorbitol (which has been reported to cause bowel necrosis). Administration by rectal instillation should be avoided. Several newer and novel potassium binding agents for oral administration that are in advanced clinical trials and appear both more effective and much better tolerated that Kayexalate, offer considerable promise for safe and effective administration chronically to both reduce [K^+] significantly and prevent hyperkalemia in susceptible patients. These agents include patiromer and ZS-9. Another unique agent, RDX713, is not yet in clinical trials.

METABOLIC ALKALOSIS

DIAGNOSIS OF SIMPLE AND MIXED FORMS OF METABOLIC ALKALOSIS

Metabolic alkalosis is a primary acid-base disturbance that is manifest in the most pure or simple form as alkalemia (elevated arterial pH) and an increase in $PaCO_2$ as a result of compensatory alveolar hypoventilation. Metabolic alkalosis is one of the more common acid-base disturbances in hospitalized patients and is manifest as both a simple and a mixed acid-base disorder.[13,108] A patient with a high plasma HCO_3^- concentration and a low plasma Cl^- concentration has either metabolic alkalosis or chronic respiratory acidosis. The arterial pH establishes the diagnosis, because it is increased in metabolic alkalosis and is typically decreased in respiratory acidosis. Modest increases in the $PaCO_2$ are expected in metabolic alkalosis. A combination of the two disorders is not unusual, because many patients with chronic obstructive lung disease are treated with diuretics, which promote ECF contraction, hypokalemia, and metabolic alkalosis. Metabolic alkalosis is also frequently observed not as a pure or simple acid-base disturbance, but in association with other disorders such as respiratory acidosis, respiratory alkalosis, and metabolic acidosis *(mixed disorders)*. *Mixed metabolic alkalosis–metabolic acidosis can be appreciated only if the accompanying metabolic acidosis is a high AG acidosis.* The mixed disorder can be appreciated by comparison of the increment in the AG above the normal value of 10 mEq/L (ΔAG = Patient's AG − 10) with the decrement in the [HCO_3^-] below the normal value of 25 mEq/L ($^-HCO_3^-$ = 25 − Patient's HCO_3^-). A mixed metabolic alkalosis–high AG metabolic acidosis is recognized because the delta values are not similar. Often, there is no bicarbonate deficit, yet the AG is significantly elevated. Thus, in a patient with an AG of 20 but a near-normal bicarbonate concentration, mixed metabolic alkalosis–metabolic acidosis should be considered. Common examples include renal failure acidosis (uremic) with vomiting or DKA with vomiting.

Respiratory compensation for metabolic alkalosis is less predictable than that for metabolic acidosis. In general the anticipated PCO_2 can be estimated by adding 15 to the patient's serum [HCO_3^-] in the range of HCO_3^- from 25 to 40 mEq/L. Further elevation in PCO_2 is limited by hypoxemia and, to some extent, hypokalemia, which accompanies metabolic alkalosis with regularity. Nevertheless, if a patient has a PCO_2 of only 40 mm Hg while the [HCO_3^-] is frankly elevated (e.g., 35 mEq/L) and the pH is in the alkalemic range, then respiratory compensation is inadequate and a mixed metabolic alkalosis–respiratory alkalosis exists.

In assessing a patient with metabolic alkalosis, two questions must be considered: (1) What is the source of alkali gain (or acid loss) that *generated* the alkalosis? (2) What renal mechanisms are operating to prevent excretion of excess HCO_3^-, thereby *maintaining*, rather than correcting, the alkalosis? In the following discussion, the entities responsible for generating alkalosis are discussed individually and reference is made to the mechanisms necessary to sustain the increase in blood HCO_3^- concentration in each case. The general mechanisms responsible for the *maintenance of alkalosis* have been discussed in detail earlier in this chapter and are a result of the combined effects of a reduction in GFR and chloride, ECF volume, and potassium depletion (Figure 17.8).

Hypokalemia is an important participant in the maintenance phase of metabolic alkalosis and has selective effects on (1) H^+ secretion and (2) ammonium excretion. The former is a result, in part, of stimulation of the H^+-K^+-ATPase in type A intercalated cells of the collecting duct by hypokalemia. The latter is a direct result of enhanced ammoniagenesis and ammonium transport (proximal convoluted tubule, TAL, medullary collecting duct) in response to hypokalemia. Finally, hyperaldosteronism (primary or secondary) participates in sustaining the alkalosis by increasing activity of the H^+-ATPase and H^+-K^+-ATPase in type A

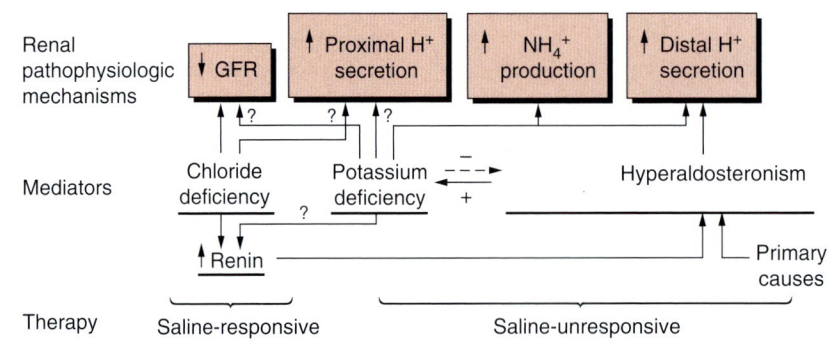

Figure 17.8 Pathophysiologic basis and approach to treatment of the maintenance phase of chronic metabolic alkalosis. Paradoxical stimulation of bicarbonate absorption (H^+ secretion) and NH_4^+ production and excretion is the combined result of Cl^- deficiency (with reduction in GFR), K^+ deficiency, and secondary hyperaldosteronism. *GFR*, Glomerular filtration rate.

intercalated cells as well as the ENaC and the Na$^+$-K$^+$-ATPase in collecting duct principal cells. The net result of the latter process is to stimulate K$^+$ secretion through K$^+$-selective channels in this same cell, which thus maintains the alkalosis.[14]

Under normal circumstances, the kidneys display an impressive capacity to excrete HCO_3^-. For HCO_3^- to be added to the ECF, HCO_3^- must be administered exogenously or retained in some manner. Thus *the development of metabolic alkalosis represents a failure of the kidneys to eliminate HCO_3^- at the normal capacity.* The kidneys retain, rather than excrete, the excess alkali and maintain the alkalosis if one of several mechanisms is operative (see Figure 17.8):

1. Cl$^-$ deficiency (ECF contraction) exists concurrently with K$^+$ deficiency to decrease GFR and/or enhance proximal and distal HCO_3^- absorption. This combination of disorders evokes secondary hyperreninemic hyperaldosteronism and stimulates H$^+$ secretion in the collecting duct. Hypokalemia independently stimulates ammoniagenesis and net acid excretion, thereby adding additional or "new" bicarbonate to the systemic circulation. Repair of the alkalosis may be accomplished by saline and K$^+$ administration.
2. Hypermineralocorticoidism and hypokalemia are induced by autonomous factors unresponsive to increased ECF. The stimulation of distal H$^+$ secretion is then sufficient to reabsorb the increased filtered HCO_3^- load and to overcome the decreased proximal HCO_3^- reabsorption caused by ECF expansion. Repair of the alkalosis in this case rests with removal of the excess autonomous mineralocorticoid and potassium repletion; saline administration is ineffective.

The various causes of metabolic alkalosis are summarized in Table 17.19. In attempting to establish the cause of metabolic alkalosis, one must assess the status of the ECF, blood pressure, serum K$^+$ concentration, and renin angiotensin aldosterone system. For example, the presence of hypertension and hypokalemia in an alkalotic patient suggests that either the patient has some form of primary mineralocorticoid excess (see Table 17.19) or the patient is hypertensive and is taking diuretics. Low plasma renin activity and normal urinary Na$^+$ and Cl$^-$ values in a patient not taking diuretics would also indicate a primary mineralocorticoid excess syndrome. The combination of hypokalemia and alkalosis in a normotensive, nonedematous patient can pose a difficult diagnostic problem. The possible causes to be considered include Bartter's or Gitelman's syndrome, Mg^{2+} deficiency, surreptitious vomiting, exogenous alkali, and diuretic ingestion. Urine electrolyte determinations and urine screening for diuretics are helpful diagnostic tools (Table 17.20). If the urine is alkaline, with high values for Na$^+$ and K$^+$ concentrations but low values for Cl$^-$ concentration, the diagnosis is usually either active (continuous) vomiting (overt or surreptitious) or alkali ingestion. On the one hand, if the urine is relatively acid, with low concentrations of Na$^+$, K$^+$, and Cl$^-$, the most likely possibilities are prior (discontinuous) vomiting, a posthypercapnic state, or prior diuretic ingestion. If, on the other hand, the urinary Na$^+$, K$^+$, and Cl$^-$ concentrations are not depressed, one must consider Mg^{2+} deficiency, Bartter's or Gitelman's syndrome, or

Table 17.19 Causes of Metabolic Alkalosis

Exogenous HCO_3^- Loads

Acute alkali administration
Milk-alkali syndrome

Effective ECV Contraction, Normotension, K$^+$ Deficiency, and Secondary Hyperreninemic Hyperaldosteronism

Gastrointestinal origin
  Vomiting
  Gastric aspiration
  Congenital chloridorrhea
  Villous adenoma
    Combined administration of sodium polystyrene sulfonate (Kayexalate) and aluminum hydroxide
Renal origin
  Diuretics (especially thiazides and loop diuretics)
  Edematous states
  Posthypercapnic state
  Hypercalcemia-hypoparathyroidism
  Recovery from lactic acidosis or ketoacidosis
  Nonreabsorbable anions such as penicillin, carbenicillin
  Mg^{2+} deficiency
  K$^+$ depletion
  Bartter's syndrome (loss-of-function mutations in thick ascending limb of Henle's loop)
  Gitelman's syndrome (loss of function of Na$^+$-Cl$^-$-cotransporter—DCT)
  Carbohydrate refeeding after starvation

ECV Expansion, Hypertension, K$^+$ Deficiency, and Hypermineralocorticoidism

Associated with high renin level
  Renal artery stenosis
  Accelerated hypertension
  Renin-secreting tumor
  Estrogen therapy
Associated with low renin level
  Primary aldosteronism
    Adenoma
    Hyperplasia
    Carcinoma
    Glucocorticoid suppressible
  Adrenal enzymatic defects
    11β-Hydroxylase deficiency
    17α-Hydroxylase deficiency
  Cushing's syndrome or disease
    Ectopic corticotropin
    Adrenal carcinoma
    Adrenal adenoma
    Primary pituitary
  Other
    Licorice
    Carbenoxolone
    Smokeless tobacco
    Lydia Pinkham tablets

Gain-of-Function Mutation of ENaC with ECV Expansion, Hypertension, K$^+$ Deficiency, and Hyporeninemic Hypoaldosteronism

Liddle's syndrome

DCT, Distal convoluted tubule; *ECV*, extracellular fluid volume; *ENaC*, epithelial sodium channel.

current diuretic ingestion. In most patients, Gitelman's syndrome is characterized by a low urine Ca^{2+} concentration in addition to a low serum Mg^{2+} level. In contrast, the urine calcium level is elevated in Bartter's syndrome. The diagnostic approach to metabolic alkalosis is summarized in the flow diagram in Figure 17.9.

Table 17.20 Diagnosis of Metabolic Alkalosis

Saline-Responsive Alkalosis	Saline-Unresponsive Alkalosis
Low Urinary [Cl⁻] (<10 mEq/L)	High or Normal Urinary [Cl⁻] (>15-20 mEq/L)
Normotensive	Hypertensive
Vomiting	Primary aldosteronism
Nasogastric aspiration	Cushing's syndrome
Diuretic use (distant)	Renal artery stenosis
Posthypercapnia	Renal failure plus alkali therapy
Villous adenoma	Normotensive
Bicarbonate treatment of organic acidosis	Mg^{2+} deficiency
	Severe K^+ deficiency
K^+ deficiency	Bartter's syndrome
Hypertensive	Gitelman's syndrome
Liddle's syndrome	Diuretic use (recent)

EXOGENOUS BICARBONATE LOADS

Long-term administration of alkali to individuals with normal renal function results in minimal, if any, alkalosis. In patients with chronic renal insufficiency, however, overt alkalosis can develop after alkali administration, presumably because the capacity to excrete HCO_3^- is exceeded or because coexistent hemodynamic disturbances have caused enhanced fractional HCO_3^- reabsorption.

Bicarbonate and Bicarbonate-Precursor Administration

The propensity of patients who have ECF contraction or renal disease plus alkali loads to develop alkalosis is exemplified by patients who receive oral or intravenous HCO_3^-, acetate loads in parenteral hyperalimentation solutions, sodium citrate loads (via regional anticoagulation, systemic anticoagulation during plasmapheresis, transfusions, or infant formula), or antacids plus cation exchange resins. The use of trisodium citrate solution for regional anticoagulation has been reported to be a cause of metabolic alkalosis in patients receiving continuous renal replacement therapy.[109,110] Citrate metabolism consumes a hydrogen ion and thereby generates HCO_3^- in liver and skeletal muscle. Dilute (0.1 normal) HCl is often required for correction in this setting.[110] The risk for alkalosis is reduced when

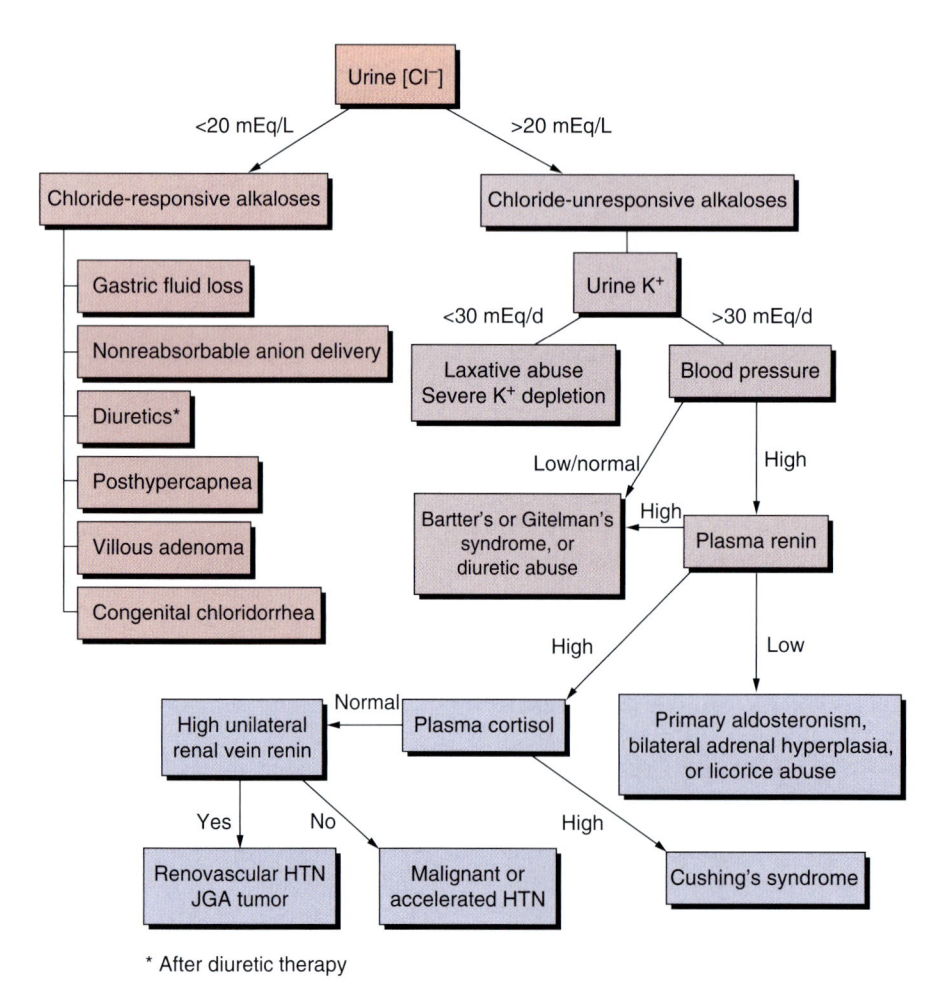

Figure 17.9 Diagnostic algorithm for metabolic alkalosis, based on the spot urine Cl⁻ and K⁺ concentrations. HTN, Hypertension; JGA, juxtaglomerular apparatus.

anticoagulant citrate dextrose formula A is used, because less bicarbonate is generated than with hypertonic trisodium citrate administration.

Milk-Alkali Syndrome

Another cause of metabolic alkalosis is long-standing excessive ingestion of milk and antacids. The incidence of milk-alkali syndrome is now increasing because of the use of calcium supplementation (e.g., calcium carbonate) by women for osteoporosis treatment or prevention. Older women with poor dietary intake ("tea and toasters") are especially prone. In Asia, betel nut chewing is a cause because the erosive nut is often wrapped in calcium hydroxide. Both hypercalcemia and vitamin D excess have been suggested to increase renal HCO_3^- reabsorption. Patients with these disorders are prone to developing nephrocalcinosis, renal insufficiency, and metabolic alkalosis.[14] Discontinuation of alkali ingestion or administration is usually sufficient to repair the alkalosis.

NORMAL BLOOD PRESSURE, EXTRACELLULAR VOLUME CONTRACTION, POTASSIUM DEPLETION, AND HYPERRENINEMIC HYPERALDOSTERONISM

Gastrointestinal Origin

Vomiting and Gastric Aspiration. Gastrointestinal loss of H^+ results in retention of HCO_3^- in the body fluids. Increased H^+ loss through gastric secretions can be caused by vomiting due to physical or psychiatric reasons, nasogastric tube aspiration, or a gastric fistula (see Table 17.19).[14]

The fluid and sodium chloride loss in vomitus or in nasogastric suction results in ECF contraction with an increase in plasma renin activity and aldosterone.[14] These factors decrease GFR and enhance the capacity of the renal tubule to reabsorb HCO_3^-.[13] During the active phase of vomiting, there is continued addition of HCO_3^- to plasma in exchange for Cl^-. The plasma HCO_3^- concentration increases to a level that exceeds the reabsorptive capacity of the proximal tubule. The excess sodium bicarbonate enters the distal tubule, where, under the influence of the increased level of aldosterone, K^+ and H^+ secretion is stimulated. Because of ECF contraction and hypochloremia, the kidney avidly conserves Cl^-. Consequently, in this disequilibrium state generated by active vomiting, the urine contains large quantities of Na^+, K^+, and HCO_3^- but has a low concentration of Cl^-. On cessation of vomiting, the plasma HCO_3^- concentration falls to the HCO_3^- threshold, which is markedly elevated by the continued effects of ECF contraction, hypokalemia, and hyperaldosteronism. The alkalosis is maintained at a slightly lower level than during the phase of active vomiting, and the urine is now relatively acidic with low concentrations of Na^+, HCO_3^-, and Cl^-.

Correction of the ECF contraction with sodium chloride may be sufficient to reverse these events, with restoration of normal blood pH even without repair of K^+ deficits.[13] Good clinical practice, however, dictates K^+ repletion as well.[14]

Congenital Chloridorrhea

Congenital chloridorrhea is a rare autosomal recessive disorder associated with severe diarrhea, fecal acid loss, and HCO_3^- retention. The pathogenesis is loss of the normal ileal HCO_3^-/Cl^- anion exchange mechanism so that Cl^- cannot be reabsorbed. The parallel Na^+-H^+-exchanger remains functional, which allows Na^+ to be reabsorbed and H^+ to be secreted. Subsequently, net H^+ and Cl^- exit in the stool, which causes Na^+ and HCO_3^- retention in the ECF.[13,14] Alkalosis results and is sustained by concomitant ECF contraction with hyperaldosteronism and K^+ deficiency. Therapy consists of oral supplements of sodium and potassium chloride. The use of proton pump inhibitors has been advanced as a means of reducing chloride secretion by the parietal cells and thus reducing the diarrhea.[111]

Villous Adenoma

Metabolic alkalosis has been described in cases of villous adenoma and is ascribed to high adenoma-derived K^+ secretory rates. K^+ and volume depletion likely cause the alkalosis, because colonic secretion is alkaline.

RENAL ORIGIN

Diuretics

Drugs that induce chloruresis without bicarbonaturia, such as thiazides and loop diuretics (furosemide, bumetanide, and torsemide), acutely diminish ECF volume without altering the total body HCO_3^- content. The HCO_3^- concentration in the blood and ECF increases. The P_{CO_2} does not increase commensurately, and a "contraction" alkalosis results.[14] The degree of alkalosis is usually small, however, because of cellular and non-HCO_3^- ECF buffering processes.[13,14] Long-term administration of diuretics tends to generate an alkalosis by increasing distal salt delivery, so that both K^+ and H^+ secretion are stimulated. Diuretics, by blocking Cl^- reabsorption in the distal tubule or by increasing H^+ pump activity, may also stimulate distal H^+ secretion and increase net acid excretion. Maintenance of alkalosis is ensured by the persistence of ECF contraction, secondary hyperaldosteronism, K^+ deficiency, enhanced ammonium production, and stimulation of the apical H^+- and H^+-K^+-ATPases, which persists for as long as diuretic administration continues. Repair of the alkalosis is achieved by cessation of diuretic administration and by providing Cl^- to normalize the ECF deficit.

Edematous States

In diseases associated with edema formation (CHF, nephrotic syndrome, cirrhosis), effective arterial blood volume is diminished, although total ECF is increased. Common to these diseases is diminished renal plasma flow and GFR with limited distal Na^+ delivery. Net acid excretion is usually normal, and alkalosis does not develop, even with an enhanced proximal HCO_3^- reabsorptive capacity. However, the distal H^+ secretory mechanism is primed by hyperaldosteronism to excrete excessive net acid if GFR can be increased to enhance distal Na^+ delivery or if K^+ deficiency or diuretic administration supervenes.

Posthypercapnia

Prolonged CO_2 retention with chronic respiratory acidosis enhances renal HCO_3^- absorption and the generation of new HCO_3^- (increased net acid excretion). If the P_{CO_2} is returned to normal, metabolic alkalosis, caused by the persistently elevated HCO_3^- concentration, emerges. Alkalosis develops immediately if the elevated P_{CO_2} is abruptly returned toward normal by a change in mechanically controlled ventilation. There is a brisk bicarbonaturic response proportional to the change in PCO_2. The accompanying cation is predominantly K^+, especially if dietary potassium is not limited. Secondary hyperaldosteronism in states of chronic hypercapnia may be responsible for this pattern of response. Associated ECF contraction does not allow complete repair of the alkalosis by normalization of the PCO_2 alone. Alkalosis persists until Cl^- supplementation is provided. Enhanced proximal acidification as a result of conditioning induced by the previous hypercapnic state may also contribute to the maintenance of the posthypercapnic alkalosis.[5]

Bartter's Syndrome

Both classical Bartter's syndrome and antenatal Bartter's syndrome are inherited as autosomal recessive disorders and involve impaired TAL salt absorption, which results in salt wasting, volume depletion, and activation of the renin angiotensin aldosterone system.[112] These manifestations are the result of loss-of-function mutations of one of the genes that encode three transporters involved in vectorial NaCl absorption in the TAL. The most prevalent disorder is the inheritance from both parents of mutations of the gene *SLC12A1*, which encodes the bumetanide-sensitive Na^+-$2Cl^-$-K^+-cotransporter on the apical membrane. Other mutations have also been described in rare families. For example, a mutation has been discovered in the gene *KCNJ1*, which encodes the ATP-sensitive apical K^+ conductance channel (ROMK) that operates in parallel with the Na^+-$2Cl^-$-K^+ transporter to recycle K^+. Both defects can be associated with classical Bartter's syndrome. A third mutation of the *CLCNKB* gene encoding the voltage-gated basolateral chloride channel (ClC-Kb) is associated only with classical Bartter's syndrome and is milder and rarely associated with nephrocalcinosis. All three defects have the same net effect, loss of Cl^- transport in the TAL.[113] Antenatal Bartter's syndrome has been observed in consanguineous families in association with sensorineural deafness. The responsible gene, *BSND*, encodes the associated subunit, barttin, which co-localizes with the ClC-Kb channel in both the TAL and K-secreting epithelial cells in the inner ear. Barttin appears to be necessary for the function of the voltage-gated chloride channel. Expression of ClC-Kb is lost when coexpressed with mutant barttins. Thus mutations in *BSND* represent a fourth category of patients with Bartter's syndrome.[112] With the exception of the deafness, the electrolyte and acid-base abnormalities are identical to the other forms of Bartter's syndrome.

Two groups of investigators have reported features of Bartter's syndrome in patients with tetany who inherit autosomal dominant hypocalcemia as a result of activating mutations in the calcium-sensing receptor (CaSR). Gain-of-function mutations of the gene encoding CaSR on the basolateral surface of the TAL cell inhibit the function of ROMK. Thus mutations in CaSR appear to represent a fifth gene associated with Bartter's syndrome.[94] Acquired forms of Bartter's syndrome, usually characterized by hypokalemic metabolic alkalosis, hypomagnesemia, hypocalcemia, and normal kidney function, have been reported in children and adults in association with aminoglycoside toxicity including gentamicin, amikacin, netilmicin, capreomycin, viomycin, colistin, and neomycin. Similarly, cisplatin and cyclosporine have also been implicated. Although the cellular mechanism of this association has not been clearly elucidated, in vitro studies suggest an effect on the CaSR.

Therefore these defects, when considered collectively, lead to ECF contraction, hyperreninemic hyperaldosteronism, and increased delivery of Na^+ to the distal nephron and thus alkalosis and renal K^+ wasting and hypokalemia. Secondary overproduction of prostaglandins, juxtaglomerular apparatus hypertrophy, and vascular pressor unresponsiveness then ensue. Most patients have hypercalciuria and normal serum magnesium levels, which distinguishes this disorder from Gitelman's syndrome.

Distinction from surreptitious vomiting, diuretic administration, and laxative abuse is necessary to make the diagnosis of Bartter's syndrome. The finding of a low urinary Cl^- concentration is helpful in identifying the vomiting patient. The urinary Cl^- concentration in Bartter's syndrome would be expected to be normal or increased, rather than depressed. Bartter-like manifestations have been reported in sporadic cases associated with chronic intermittent diuretic and laxative abuse, cystic fibrosis, and congenital chloride diarrhea.

The treatment of Bartter's syndrome is generally focused on repair of the hypokalemia by inhibition of the renin angiotensin aldosterone or prostaglandin-kinin system. K^+ supplementation, Mg^{2+} repletion, and administration of propranolol, spironolactone, amiloride, prostaglandin inhibitors, or ACE inhibitors have been used with limited success.

Gitelman's Syndrome

Patients with Gitelman's syndrome have a phenotype resembling that of Bartter's syndrome in that an autosomal recessive chloride-resistant metabolic alkalosis is associated with hypokalemia, a normal to low blood pressure, volume depletion with secondary hyperreninemic hyperaldosteronism, and juxtaglomerular hyperplasia.[113,114] However, hypocalciuria and symptomatic hypomagnesemia are consistently useful in distinguishing Gitelman's syndrome from Bartter's syndrome on clinical grounds.[114] These unique features mimic the effect of long-term thiazide diuretic administration. A number of missense mutations in the gene *SLC12A3*, which encodes the thiazide-sensitive sodium-chloride cotransporter in the distal convoluted tubule, have been described and account for the spectrum of clinical features, including the classical finding of hypocalciuria.[115] It is not clear, however, why these patients have pronounced hypomagnesemia.

A large study of adults with proven Gitelman's syndrome and *SLC12A3* mutations showed that salt craving, nocturia, cramps, and fatigue were more common than in sex- and age-matched controls.[115] Women experienced exacerbation of symptoms during menses, and many had complicated pregnancies. Salt craving seems to be a near universal feature and aggravates renal K^+ wasting.

Treatment of Gitelman's syndrome, as of Bartter's syndrome, consists of potassium supplementation (KCl 40 mEq, three or four times daily, or more), but also magnesium supplementation in most patients. Amiloride (5 to 10 mg twice daily) is more effective than spironolactone. ACE inhibitors or ARBs in very low dose have been suggested as helpful in selected patients but may cause symptomatic hypotension. Discouraging *excessive* dietary salt intake requires dietary counseling and may be a challenging component of management.

After Treatment of Lactic Acidosis or Ketoacidosis

When an underlying stimulus for the generation of lactic acid or ketoacid is removed rapidly, as occurs with repair of circulatory insufficiency or with insulin administration, the lactate or ketones can be metabolized to yield an equivalent amount of HCO_3^-. Thus the initial process of HCO_3^- titration that induced the metabolic acidosis is effectively reversed. In the oxidative metabolism of ketones or lactate, HCO_3^- is not directly produced; rather, H^+ is consumed by metabolism of the organic anions, with the liberation of an equivalent amount of HCO_3^-. This process regenerates HCO_3^- if the organic acids can be metabolized to HCO_3^- before their renal excretion. Other sources of new HCO_3^- are additive with the original amount of HCO_3^- regenerated by organic anion metabolism to create a surfeit of HCO_3^-. Such sources include (1) new HCO_3^- added to the blood by the kidneys as a result of enhanced net acid excretion during the preexisting acidotic period and (2) alkali therapy during the treatment phase of the acidosis. The coexistence of acidosis-induced ECF contraction and K^+ deficiency acts to sustain the alkalosis.[13,14]

Nonreabsorbable Anions and Magnesium Ion Deficiency

Administration of large amounts of nonreabsorbable anions, such as penicillin or carbenicillin, can enhance distal acidification and K^+ excretion by increasing the luminal potential difference attained or possibly by allowing Na^+ delivery to the CCT without Cl^-, which favors H^+ secretion without Cl^--dependent HCO_3^- secretion.[14] Mg^{2+} deficiency also results in hypokalemic alkalosis by enhancing distal acidification through stimulation of renin and hence aldosterone secretion.

Potassium Ion Depletion

Pure K^+ depletion causes metabolic alkalosis, although generally of only modest severity. One reason that the alkalosis is usually mild is that K^+ depletion also causes positive sodium chloride balance with or without mineralocorticoid administration. The salt retention, in turn, antagonizes the degree of alkalemia. When access to salt as well as to K^+ is restricted, more severe alkalosis develops. Activation of the renal H^+-K^+-ATPase in the collecting duct by chronic hypokalemia likely plays a role in maintenance of the alkalosis. The alkalosis is maintained in part by reduction in GFR without a change in tubule HCO_3^- transport. The pathophysiologic basis of the alkalosis has not been well defined in humans, but the alkalosis associated with severe K^+ depletion is resistant to salt administration. Repair of the K^+ deficiency is necessary to correct the alkalosis.

EXTRACELLULAR VOLUME EXPANSION, HYPERTENSION, AND HYPERMINERALOCORTICOIDISM (see Table 17.17)

As previously discussed, mineralocorticoid administration increases net acid excretion and tends to create metabolic alkalosis. The degree of alkalosis is augmented by the simultaneous increase in K^+ excretion, which leads to K^+ deficiency and hypokalemia. Salt intake for sufficient distal Na^+ delivery is also a prerequisite for the development of both the hypokalemia and the alkalosis. Hypertension develops partly as a result of ECF expansion from salt retention. The alkalosis is not progressive and is generally mild. Volume expansion tends to antagonize the decrease in GFR and/or increase in tubule acidification induced by hypermineralocorticoidism and K^+ deficiency. Increased mineralocorticoid hormone levels may be the result of autonomous primary adrenal overproduction of mineralocorticoid or of secondary aldosterone release by primary renal overproduction of renin. In both cases the normal feedback by ECF on net mineralocorticoid production is disrupted, and volume retention results in hypertension.

High Renin Levels

States accompanied by inappropriately high renin levels may be associated with hyperaldosteronism and alkalosis. Renin levels are elevated because of primary elaboration of renin or, secondarily, by diminished effective circulating blood volume. Total ECF may not be diminished. Examples of high-renin hypertension include renovascular, accelerated, and malignant hypertension. Estrogens increase renin substrate and hence angiotensin II formation. Primary tumor overproduction of renin is another rare cause of hyperreninemic hyperaldosteronism–induced metabolic alkalosis.[14]

Low Renin Levels

In some disorders, primary adrenal overproduction of mineralocorticoid suppresses renin elaboration. Hypertension occurs as the result of mineralocorticoid excess with volume overexpansion.

Primary Aldosteronism. Tumor involvement (adenoma or, rarely, carcinoma) or hyperplasia of the adrenal gland is associated with aldosterone overproduction. Mineralocorticoid administration or excess production (primary aldosteronism of Cushing's syndrome and adrenal cortical enzyme defects) increases net acid excretion and may result in metabolic alkalosis, which may be worsened by associated K^+ deficiency. ECF volume expansion from salt retention causes hypertension and antagonizes the reduction in GFR and/ or increases tubule acidification induced by aldosterone and by K^+ deficiency. The kaliuresis persists and causes continued K^+ depletion with polydipsia, inability to concentrate the urine, and polyuria. Increased aldosterone levels may be the result of autonomous primary adrenal overproduction or of secondary aldosterone release due to renal overproduction of renin. In both situations, the normal feedback of ECF volume on net aldosterone production is disrupted, and hypertension from volume retention can result.

Glucocorticoid-Remediable Hyperaldosteronism. Glucocorticoid-remediable hyperaldosteronism is an autosomal dominant form of hypertension, the features of which resemble those of primary aldosteronism (hypokalemic metabolic alkalosis and volume-dependent hypertension). In this disorder, however, glucocorticoid administration corrects the hypertension as well as the excessive excretion of 18-hydroxysteroid in the urine. Dluhy and associates have demonstrated that this disorder results from unequal crossing over between two genes located in close proximity on chromosome 8.[116] This region contains the glucocorticoid-responsive promoter region of the gene encoding 11β-hydroxylase *(CYP11B1)* where it is joined to the structural portion of the *CYP11B2* gene encoding aldosterone synthase.[116] The chimeric gene produces excess amounts of aldosterone synthase, unresponsive to serum potassium or renin levels, but it is suppressed by glucocorticoid administration. Although a rare cause of primary aldosteronism, the syndrome is important to distinguish because treatment differs and it can be associated with severe hypertension, stroke, and accelerated hypertension during pregnancy.

Cushing's Disease or Syndrome. Abnormally high glucocorticoid production caused by adrenal adenoma or carcinoma or ectopic corticotropin production causes metabolic alkalosis. The alkalosis may be ascribed to coexisting mineralocorticoid (deoxycorticosterone and corticosterone) hypersecretion. Glucocorticoids also have the ability to enhance net acid secretion and NH_4^+ production by occupancy of mineralocorticoid receptors.

Liddle's Syndrome. Liddle's syndrome is associated with severe hypertension presenting in childhood, accompanied by hypokalemic metabolic alkalosis. These features resemble those of primary hyperaldosteronism, but the renin and aldosterone levels are suppressed (pseudohyperaldosteronism).[117] The defect is constitutive activation of the ENaC at the apical membrane of principal cells in the CCD. Liddle originally described patients with low renin and low aldosterone levels that did not respond to spironolactone. The defect in Liddle's syndrome is inherited as an autosomal dominant form of monogenic hypertension. This disorder has been attributed to an inherited abnormality in the gene that encodes the β- or the γ-subunit of renal ENaC. Either mutation results in deletion of the cytoplasmic tails of the β- or γ-subunit. The C termini contain PY amino acid motifs that are highly conserved, and essentially all mutations in patients with Liddle's syndrome involve disruption or deletion of this motif. These PY motifs are important in regulating the number of sodium channels in the luminal membrane by binding to the WW domains of the Nedd4 (neural developmentally downregulated isoform 4)–like family of ubiquitin-protein ligases.[117] Disruption of the PY motif dramatically increases the surface localization of ENaC complex, because these channels are not internalized or degraded (Nedd4 pathway) but remain activated on the cell surface.[117] Persistent Na^+ absorption eventuates in volume expansion, hypertension, hypokalemia, and metabolic alkalosis.[117]

Miscellaneous Conditions. Ingestion of licorice, carbenoxolone, smokeless tobacco, or nasal spray can cause a typical pattern of hypermineralocorticoidism. These substances inhibit 11β-hydroxysteroid dehydrogenase (which normally metabolizes cortisol to an inactive metabolite), so that cortisol is allowed to occupy type I renal mineralocorticoid receptors, mimicking aldosterone. Apparent mineralocorticoid excess syndrome resembles excessive ingestion of licorice: volume expansion, low renin level, low aldosterone level, and a salt-sensitive form of hypertension, which may include metabolic alkalosis and hypokalemia. The hypertension responds to thiazides and spironolactone but without abnormal steroid products in the urine. Licorice and carbenoxolone contain glycyrrhetinic acid, which inhibits 11β-hydroxysteroid dehydrogenase. This enzyme is responsible for converting cortisol to cortisone, an essential step in protecting the mineralocorticoid receptor from cortisol, and protects normal individuals from exhibiting apparent mineralocorticoid excess. Without the renal-specific form of this enzyme, monogenic hypertension develops.

SYMPTOMS

Symptoms of metabolic alkalosis include changes in central and peripheral nervous system function similar to those in hypocalcemia: mental confusion, obtundation, and a predisposition to seizures, as well as paresthesias, muscular cramping, and even tetany. Aggravation of arrhythmias and hypoxemia in chronic obstructive pulmonary disease is also a problem. Related electrolyte abnormalities, including hypokalemia and hypophosphatemia, are common, and patients may show symptoms of these deficiencies.

TREATMENT

The maintenance of metabolic alkalosis represents a failure of the kidney to excrete bicarbonate efficiently because of chloride or potassium deficiency or continuous mineralocorticoid elaboration, or both. Treatment is primarily directed at correcting the underlying stimulus for HCO_3^- generation and at restoring the ability of the kidney to excrete the excess bicarbonate. Assistance is gained in the diagnosis and treatment of metabolic alkalosis by paying attention to the urinary chloride concentration, systemic blood pressure, and the volume status of the patient (particularly the presence or absence of orthostasis) (see Figure 17.9). Particularly helpful in the history is the presence or absence of vomiting, diuretic use, or alkali therapy. A high urine chloride level and hypertension suggest that mineralocorticoid excess is present. If primary aldosteronism is present, correction of the underlying cause (adenoma, bilateral hyperplasia, Cushing's syndrome) will reverse the alkalosis. Patients with bilateral adrenal hyperplasia may respond to spironolactone. Normotensive patients with a high urine chloride concentration may have Bartter's or Gitelman's syndrome if diuretic use or vomiting can be excluded. A low urine chloride level and relative hypotension suggests a chloride-responsive metabolic alkalosis such as vomiting or nasogastric suction. $[H^+]$ loss by the stomach or kidneys can be mitigated by the use of proton pump inhibitors or the discontinuation of diuretics. The second aspect of treatment is to remove the factors that sustain HCO_3^- reabsorption, such as ECF volume contraction or K^+ deficiency. Although K^+ deficits should be corrected, NaCl therapy is usually sufficient to reverse the alkalosis if ECF volume contraction is present, as indicated by a low urine $[Cl^-]$.

Patients with CHF or unexplained volume overexpansion represent special challenges in the critical care setting. Patients with a low urine chloride concentration, usually indicative of a "chloride-responsive" form of metabolic alkalosis, may not tolerate normal saline infusion. Renal HCO_3^- loss can be accelerated by administration of acetazolamide (250 to 500 mg intravenously), a carbonic anhydrase inhibitor, if associated conditions that preclude infusion of saline (e.g., elevated pulmonary capillary wedge pressure, or evidence of CHF) are present.[14] Acetazolamide is usually very effective in patients with adequate renal function but can exacerbate urinary K⁺ losses. Hypokalemia should be expected in alkalotic patients following intravenous acetazolamide and should be treated promptly. Dilute hydrochloric acid (0.1 Normal HCl) is also effective but must be infused slowly in a central line because it may cause severe hemolysis and is difficult to titrate. If 0.1 normal HCl is used, the goal should not be to restore the pH to normal, but to reduce the pH to approximately 7.50. Patients receiving continuous renal replacement therapy in the intensive care unit typically develop metabolic alkalosis when high-bicarbonate dialysate is used or when citrate regional anticoagulation is employed. Therapy should include reduction of alkali loads via dialysis by reducing the bicarbonate concentration in the dialysate when possible. If not effective, intravenous 0.1 normal HCl may be necessary in this setting.

Complete reference list available at ExpertConsult.com.

KEY REFERENCES

1. Adrogue HJ, Gennan FJ, Galla JH, et al: Assessing acid-base disorders. *Kidney Int* 76:1239–1247, 2009.
3. Madias NE, Adrogue HJ: Respiratory alkalosis. In DuBose TD, Hamm LL, editors: *Acid-base and electrolyte disorders: a companion to Brenner and Rector's the kidney*, Philadelphia, 2002, Saunders, pp 147–164.
4. Madias NE: Renal acidification responses to respiratory acid-base disorders. *J Nephrol* 23(Suppl 16):S85–S91, 2010.
8. Schwartz GJ, Al-Awqati Q: Carbon dioxide causes exocytosis of vesicles containing H⁺ pumps in isolated perfused proximal and collecting tubules. *J Clin Invest* 75:1638–1644, 1985.
11. Goraya N, Wesson DE: Dietary management of chronic kidney disease: protein restriction and beyond. *Curr Opin Nephrol Hypertens* 21:635–640, 2012.
12. Loniewski I, Wesson DE: Bicarbonate therapy for prevention of chronic kidney disease progression. *Kidney Int* 85:529–535, 2014.
13. Gennari FJ: Pathophysiology of metabolic alkalosis: a new classification based on the centrality of stimulated collecting duct ion transport. *Am J Kidney Dis* 58:626–636, 2011.
14. DuBose TD: Metabolic alkalosis. In Gilbert S, Weiner DE, editors: *National Kidney Foundation's primer on kidney diseases*, ed 6, Philadelphia, 2014, Elsevier, pp 137–143.
21. Krapf R, Alpern RJ, Seldin DW: Clinical syndromes of metabolic acidosis. In Alpern RJ, Orson W, Moe OW, et al, editors: *Seldin and Giebisch's the kidney*, ed 5, Philadelphia, 2013, Academic Press, pp 2055–2072.
22. Emmett M: Diagnosis of simple and mixed disorders. In DuBose TD, Hamm LL, editors: *Acid-base and electrolyte disorders: a companion to Brenner and Rector's the kidney*, Philadelphia, 2002, Saunders, pp 41–54.
31. Kraut JA, Kurtz I: Metabolic acidosis of CKD: diagnosis, clinical characteristics, and treatment. *Am J Kidney Dis* 45:978–993, 2005.
32. Morris RC, Jr, Nigon K, Reed EB: Evidence that the severity of depletion of inorganic phosphate determines the severity of the disturbance of adenine nucleotide metabolism in the liver and renal cortex of the fructose-loaded rat. *J Clin Invest* 61:209–220, 1978.
34. DuBose TD, Jr: Hydrogen ion secretion by the collecting duct as a determinant of the urine to blood P_{CO_2} gradient in alkaline urine. *J Clin Invest* 69:145–156, 1982.
36. DuBose TD, Jr, Caflisch CR: Validation of the difference in urine and blood carbon dioxide tension during bicarbonate loading as an index of distal nephron acidification in experimental models of distal renal tubular acidosis. *J Clin Invest* 75:1116–1123, 1985.
39. Jarolim P, Shayakul C, Prabakaran D, et al: Autosomal dominant distal renal tubular acidosis is associated in three families with heterozygosity for the R589H mutation in the AE1 (band 3) Cl-/HCO3-exchanger. *J Biol Chem* 273:6380–6388, 1998.
40. Karet FE, Finberg KE, Nelson RD, et al: Mutations in the gene encoding B1 subunit of H⁺ATPase cause renal tubular acidosis with sensorineural deafness. *Nat Genet* 21:84–90, 1999.
41. Karet FE, Finberg KE, Nayir A, et al: Localization of a gene for autosomal recessive distal renal tubular acidosis with normal hearing (rdRTA2) to 7q33-34. *Am J Hum Genet* 65:1656–1665, 1999.
42. Smith AN, Finberg KE, Wagner CA, et al: Molecular cloning and characterization of Atp6n1b: a novel fourth murine vacuolar H⁺-ATPase a-subunit gene. *J Biol Chem* 276:42382–42388, 2001.
48. DuBose TD, Jr, Good DW, Hamm LL, et al: Ammonium transport in the kidney: new physiological concepts and their clinical implications. *J Am Soc Nephrol* 1:1193–1203, 1991.
50. Frick KK, Krieger NS, Nehrke K, et al: Metabolic acidosis increases intracellular calcium in bone cells through activation of the proton receptor OGR1. *J Bone Miner Res* 24:305–313, 2009.
52. Morris RC, Jr, Sebastian A: Alkali therapy in renal tubular acidosis: who needs it? *J Am Soc Nephrol* 13:2186–2188, 2002.
53. Wrong O, Henderson JE, Kaye M: Distal renal tubular acidosis: alkali heals osteomalacia and increases net production of 1,25-dihydroxyvitamin D. *Nephron Physiol* 101:72–76, 2005.
55. DuBose TD, Jr, Good DW: Chronic hyperkalemia impairs ammonium transport and accumulation in the inner medulla of the rat. *J Clin Invest* 90:1443–1449, 1992.
56. Good DW: Ammonium transport by the thick ascending limb of Henle's loop. *Annu Rev Physiol* 56:623–647, 1994.
57. Watts BA, III, Good DW: Effects of ammonium on intracellular pH in rat medullary thick ascending limb: mechanisms of apical membrane NH4+ transport. *J Gen Physiol* 103:917–936, 1994.
58. DuBose TD, Jr, Caflisch CR: Effect of selective aldosterone deficiency on acidification in nephron segments of the rat inner medulla. *J Clin Invest* 82:1624–1632, 1988.
63. Viemann M, Peter M, Lopez-Siguero JP, et al: Evidence for genetic heterogeneity of pseudohypoaldosteronism type 1: identification of a novel mutation in the human mineralocorticoid receptor in one sporadic case and no mutations in two autosomal dominant kindreds. *J Clin Endocrinol Metab* 86:2056–2059, 2001.
66. Barker PM, Nguyen MS, Gatzy JT, et al: Role of gamma ENaC subunit in lung liquid clearance and electrolyte balance in newborn mice: insights into perinatal adaptation and pseudohypoaldosteronism. *J Clin Invest* 102:1634–1640, 1998.
69. Wilson FH, Kahle KT, Sabath E, et al: Molecular pathogenesis of inherited hypertension with hyperkalemia: the Na-Cl cotransporter is inhibited by wild-type but not mutant WNK4. *Proc Natl Acad Sci U S A* 100:680–684, 2003.
71. Kahle KT, Wilson FH, Leng Q, et al: WNK4 regulates the balance between renal NaCl reabsorption and K+ secretion. *Nat Genet* 35:372–376, 2003.
73. Caliskan Y, Kalayoglu-Besisik S, Sargin D, et al: Cyclosporine-associated hyperkalemia: report of four allogeneic blood stem-cell transplant cases. *Transplantation* 75:1069–1072, 2003.
74. Caramelo C, Bello E, Ruiz E, et al: Hyperkalemia in patients infected with the human immunodeficiency virus: involvement of a systemic mechanism. *Kidney Int* 56:198–205, 1999.
76. Kleyman TR, Roberts C, Ling BN: A mechanism for pentamidine-induced hyperkalemia: inhibition of distal nephron sodium transport. *Ann Intern Med* 122:103–106, 1995.
77. Velazquez H, Perazella MA, Wright FS, et al: Renal mechanism of trimethoprim-induced hyperkalemia. *Ann Intern Med* 119:296–301, 1993.
79. Hoorn EJ, Walsh SB, McCormick JA, et al: The calcineurin inhibitor tacrolimus activates the renal sodium chloride cotransporter to cause hypertension. *Nat Med* 17:1304–1309, 2011.
80. Abramowitz MK, Melamed ML, Bauer C, et al: Effects of oral sodium bicarbonate in patients with CKD. *Clin J Am Soc Nephrol* 8:714–720, 2013.
85. Qunibi WY, Hootkins RE, McDowell LL, et al: Treatment of hyperphosphatemia in hemodialysis patients: the Calcium Acetate Renagel Evaluation (CARE Study). *Kidney Int* 65:1914–1926, 2004.
93. Luft FC: Lactic acidosis update for critical care clinicians. *J Am Soc Nephrol* 12(Suppl 17):S15–S19, 2001.
95. Stacpoole PW, Wright EC, Baumgartner TG, et al: A controlled clinical trial of dichloroacetate for treatment of lactic acidosis in adults. The Dichloroacetate-Lactic Acidosis Study Group. *N Engl J Med* 327:1564–1569, 1992.

101. Umpierrez GE, DiGirolamo M, Tuvlin JA, et al: Differences in metabolic and hormonal milieu in diabetic- and alcohol-induced ketoacidosis. *J Crit Care* 15:52–59, 2000.
103. Brent J: Fomepizole for ethylene glycol and methanol poisoning. *N Engl J Med* 360:2216–2223, 2009.
106. Mizock BA, Belyaev S, Mecher C: Unexplained metabolic acidosis in critically ill patients: the role of pyroglutamic acid. *Intensive Care Med* 30:502–505, 2004.
107. Wilson KC, Reardon C, Farber HW: Propylene glycol toxicity in a patient receiving intravenous diazepam. *N Engl J Med* 343:815, 2000.
108. Zar T, Yusufzai I, Sullivan A, et al: Acute kidney injury, hyperosmolality and metabolic acidosis associated with lorazepam. *Nat Clin Pract Nephrol* 3:515–520, 2007.
109. Gupta M, Wadhwa NK, Bukovsky R: Regional citrate anticoagulation for continuous venovenous hemodiafiltration using calcium-containing dialysate. *Am J Kidney Dis* 43:67–73, 2004.
112. Simon DB, Karet FE, Rodriguez-Soriano J, et al: Genetic heterogeneity of Bartter's syndrome revealed by mutations in the K+ channel, ROMK. *Nat Genet* 14:152–156, 1996.
115. Monkawa T, Kurihara I, Kobayashi K, et al: Novel mutations in thiazide-sensitive Na-Cl cotransporter gene of patients with Gitelman's syndrome. *J Am Soc Nephrol* 11:65–70, 2000.
116. Dluhy RG, Anderson B, Harlin B, et al: Glucocorticoid-remediable aldosteronism is associated with severe hypertension in early childhood. *J Pediatr* 138:715–720, 2001.
117. Kamynina E, Staub O: Concerted action of ENaC, Nedd4-2, and Sgk1 in transepithelial Na(+) transport. *Am J Physiol Renal Physiol* 283:F377–F387, 2002.

Disorders of Potassium Balance

18

David B. Mount

CHAPTER OUTLINE

NORMAL POTASSIUM BALANCE, 559
Potassium Transport Mechanisms, 560
Factors Affecting Internal Distribution of Potassium, 562
RENAL POTASSIUM EXCRETION, 563
Potassium Transport in the Distal Nephron, 563
Control of Potassium Secretion, 565
Integrated Regulation of Distal Sodium Absorption and Potassium Secretion, 566
Regulation of Renal Renin and Adrenal Aldosterone, 568
Urinary Indices of Potassium Excretion, 569
CONSEQUENCES OF HYPOKALEMIA AND HYPERKALEMIA, 569
Consequences of Hypokalemia, 569
Consequences of Hyperkalemia, 570
HYPOKALEMIA, 572
Epidemiology, 572

Spurious Hypokalemia, 572
Redistribution and Hypokalemia, 572
Hypokalemic Periodic Paralysis, 573
Potassium Loss, 574
Clinical Approach to Hypokalemia, 581
Treatment of Hypokalemia, 583
HYPERKALEMIA, 585
Epidemiology, 585
Pseudohyperkalemia, 585
Excess Intake of Potassium and Tissue Necrosis, 586
Redistribution and Hyperkalemia, 586
Reduced Renal Potassium Excretion, 588
Medication-Related Hyperkalemia, 590
Clinical Approach to Hyperkalemia, 592
Treatment of Hyperkalemia, 592

The diagnosis and management of potassium disorders are central skills in clinical nephrology, relevant not only to consultative nephrology but also to dialysis and renal transplantation. An understanding of the underlying physiology is critical to the diagnostic and management approach to hyperkalemic and hypokalemic patients. This chapter reviews those aspects of the physiology of potassium homeostasis judged to be relevant to the understanding of potassium disorders; a more detailed review of renal potassium transport is provided in Chapter 6.

The pathophysiology of potassium disorders continues to evolve. The expanding list of drugs with a potential to affect plasma potassium concentration (K^+) has complicated clinical management and provided new insights. In addition, the evolving molecular understanding of rare disorders affecting plasma K^+ has uncovered novel pathways of regulation[1-6]; whereas none of these disorders constitutes a public health menace,[7] they are experiments of nature that have provided new windows on critical aspects of potassium homeostasis. These advances can be incorporated into an increasingly mechanistic, molecular understanding of potassium disorders.

NORMAL POTASSIUM BALANCE

The dietary intake of potassium ranges from less than 35 to more than 110 mmol/day in U.S. adults. Despite this widespread variation in intake, homeostatic mechanisms serve to maintain plasma K^+ precisely between 3.5 and 5.0 mmol/L. In a healthy individual at steady state, the entire daily intake of potassium is excreted, approximately 90% in the urine and 10% in the stool. More than 98% of total body potassium is intracellular, chiefly in muscle (Figure 18.1). Buffering of extracellular K^+ by this large intracellular pool plays a crucial role in the regulation of plasma K^+.[8] Thus, within 60 minutes of an intravenous load of 0.5 mmol/kg of K^+-Cl^-, only 41% appears in the urine, yet serum K^+ rises by no more than 0.6 mmol/L[9]; adding the equivalent 35 mmol exclusively to the extracellular space of a 70-kg man would be expected to raise serum K^+ by ~2.5 mmol/L.[10] Changes in cellular distribution also serve to defend plasma K^+ during K^+ depletion. For example, military recruits have been shown to maintain a normal serum K^+ after 11 days of basic training, despite a profound K^+ deficit generated by renal

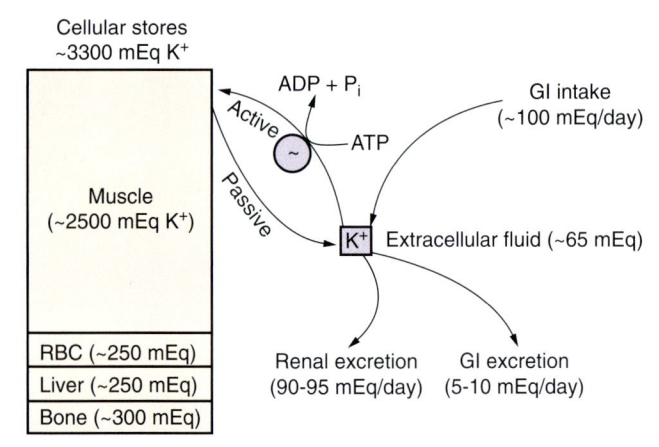

Figure 18.1 Body K⁺ distribution and cellular K⁺ flux. ADP, Adenosine diphosphate; ATP, adenosine triphosphate; GI, gastrointestinal; P_i, inorganic phosphorus; RBC, red blood cells. (From Wingo CS, Weiner ID: Disorders of potassium balance. In Brenner BM, editor: *The kidney,* vol 1, Philadelphia, 2000, WB Saunders, pp 998-1035.)

and extrarenal loss.[11] The rapid exchange of intracellular K⁺ with extracellular K⁺ plays a crucial role in maintaining plasma K⁺ within such a narrow range; this is accomplished by overlapping and synergistic[12] regulation of a number of renal and extrarenal transport pathways.

POTASSIUM TRANSPORT MECHANISMS

The intracellular accumulation of K⁺ against its electrochemical gradient is an energy-consuming process, mediated by the ubiquitous Na⁺-K⁺-ATPase enzyme. The Na⁺-K⁺-ATPase functions as an electrogenic pump, since the stoichiometry of transport is three intracellular Na⁺ ions to two extracellular K⁺ ions. The enzyme complex is made up of a tissue-specific combination of multiple α-, β-, and γ-subunits, which are further subject to tissue-specific patterns of regulation.[13] The Na⁺-K⁺-ATPase proteins share significant homology with the corresponding subunits of the H⁺-K⁺-ATPase enzymes (see "Potassium Transport in the Distal Nephron"). Cardiac glycosides—digoxin and ouabain—bind to the α-subunits of Na⁺-K⁺-ATPase at an exposed extracellular hairpin loop that also contains the major binding sites for extracellular K⁺.[14] The binding of digoxin and K⁺ to the Na⁺-K⁺-ATPase complex is thus mutually antagonistic, explaining in part the potentiation of digoxin toxicity by hypokalemia.[15] Although the four α-subunits have equivalent affinity for ouabain, they differ significantly in intrinsic K⁺-ouabain antagonism.[16] Ouabain binding to isozymes containing the ubiquitous $α_1$-subunit is relatively insensitive to K⁺ concentrations within the physiologic range, such that this isozyme is protected from digoxin under conditions wherein cardiac $α_2$- and $α_3$-subunits, the probable therapeutic targets,[17] are inhibited.[16] Genetic reduction in cardiac $α_1$-subunit content has a negative ionotropic effect,[17] such that the relative resistance of this subunit to digoxin at physiologic plasma K⁺ has an additional cardioprotective effect. Notably, the digoxin-ouabain binding site of α-subunits is highly conserved, suggesting a potential role in the physiologic response to endogenous ouabain and digoxin-like compounds. Novel knock-in mice have been generated that express $α_2$-subunits with engineered resistance to ouabain. These mice are strikingly resistant to ouabain-induced hypertension and to adrenocorticotropic hormone (ACTH)–dependent hypertension,[18] the latter known to involve an increase in circulating ouabain-like glycosides. This provocative data have given more credence to the controversial role of such ouabain-like molecules in hypertension and cardiovascular disease. Furthermore, modulation of the K⁺-dependent binding of circulating ouabain-like compounds to Na⁺-K⁺-ATPase may underlie at least some of cardiovascular complications of hypokalemia[19] (see "Consequences of Hypokalemia").

Skeletal muscle contains as much as 75% of body potassium (see Figure 18.1), and exerts considerable influence on extracellular K⁺. Exercise is thus a well-described cause of transient hyperkalemia; interstitial K⁺ in human muscle can reach levels as high as 10 mmol/L after fatiguing exercise.[20] Not surprisingly, therefore, changes in skeletal muscle Na⁺-K⁺-ATPase activity and abundance are major determinants of the capacity for extrarenal K⁺ homeostasis. Hypokalemia induces a marked decrease in muscle K⁺ content and Na⁺-K⁺-ATPase activity,[21] an apparently altruistic[8] mechanism to regulate plasma K⁺. This is primarily due to dramatic decreases in the protein abundance of the $α_2$-subunit of Na⁺/K⁺-ATPase.[22] In contrast, hyperkalemia due to potassium loading is associated with adaptive increases in muscle K⁺ content and Na⁺-K⁺-ATPase activity.[23] These interactions are reflected in the relationship between physical activity and the ability to regulate extracellular K⁺ during exercise.[24] For example, exercise training is associated with increases in muscle Na⁺-K⁺-ATPase concentration and activity, with reduced interstitial K⁺ in trained muscles[25] and an enhanced recovery of plasma K⁺ after defined amounts of exercise.[24]

Potassium can also accumulate in cells by coupling to the gradient for Na⁺ entry, entering via the electroneutral Na⁺-K⁺-2Cl⁻ cotransporters NKCC1 and NKCC2. The NKCC2 protein is found only at the apical membrane of the thick ascending limb (TAL) and macula densa cells (Figure 18.2; see Figure 18.10), where it functions in transepithelial salt transport and tubular regulation of renin release.[26] In contrast, NKCC1 is widely expressed in multiple tissues,[26] including muscle.[27] The cotransport of K⁺-Cl⁻ by the four K⁺-Cl⁻ cotransporters (KCC1-4) can also function in the transfer of K⁺ across membranes; although the KCCs typically function as efflux pathways, they can mediate influx when extracellular K⁺ increases.[26]

The efflux of K⁺ out of cells is largely accomplished by K⁺ channels, which comprise the largest family of ion channels in the human genome. There are three major subclasses of mammalian K⁺ channels: the six-transmembrane domain (TMD) family, which encompasses the voltage-sensitive and Ca^{2+}-activated K⁺ channels; the two-pore, four-TMD family; and the two-TMD family of inward rectifying K⁺ (Kir) channels.[28] There is tremendous genomic variety in human K⁺ channels, with at least 26 separate genes encoding principal subunits of the voltage-gated Kv channels and 16 genes encoding the principal Kir subunits. Further complexity is generated by the presence of multiple accessory subunits and alternative patterns of messenger RNA (mRNA) splicing. Not surprisingly, an increasing number and variety of K⁺ channels have been implicated in the control of K⁺ homeostasis and the membrane potential of excitable cells,

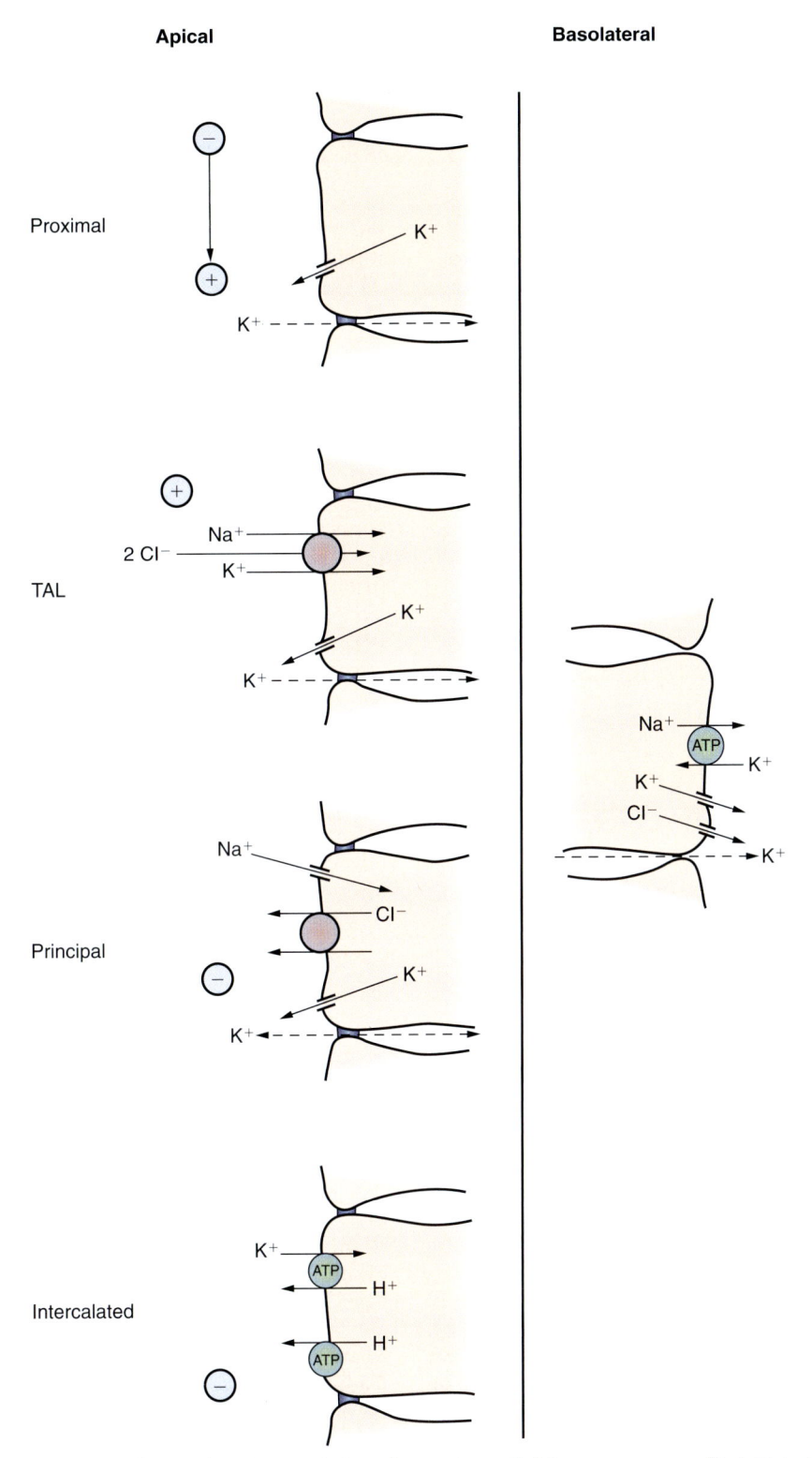

Figure 18.2 Schematic cell models of potassium transport along the nephron. Cell types are as specified. Note the differences in luminal potential difference along the nephron. TAL, Thick ascending limb. (From Giebisch G: Renal potassium transport: mechanisms and regulation. *Am J Physiol* 274:F817-F833, 1998.)

Table 18.1 Factors Affecting Distribution of Potassium between Intracellular and Extracellular Compartments

Factor	Effect
Acute: Effect on Potassium	
Insulin	Enhanced cell uptake
β-Catecholamines	Enhanced cell uptake
α-Catecholamines	Impaired cell uptake
Acidosis	Impaired cell uptake
Alkalosis	Enhanced cell uptake
External potassium balance	Loose correlation
Cell damage	Impaired cell uptake
Hyperosmolality	Enhanced cell efflux
Chronic: Effect on ATP Pump Density	
Thyroid	Enhanced
Adrenal steroids	Enhanced
Exercise (training)	Enhanced
Growth	Enhanced
Diabetes	Impaired
Potassium deficiency	Impaired
Chronic renal failure	Impaired

From Giebisch G: Renal potassium transport: mechanisms and regulation. Am J Physiol 274:F817-F833, 1998.

such as muscle and heart, with important and evolving roles in the pathophysiology of potassium disorders.[1,29,30]

FACTORS AFFECTING INTERNAL DISTRIBUTION OF POTASSIUM

A number of hormones and physiologic conditions have acute effects on the distribution of K^+ between the intracellular and extracellular spaces (Table 18.1). Some of these factors are of particular clinical relevance and are therefore reviewed here in detail.

INSULIN

The hypokalemic effect of insulin has been known since the early twentieth century.[31] The impact of insulin on plasma K^+ and plasma glucose is separable at multiple levels, suggesting independent mechanisms.[21,32,33] For example, despite impaired glucose uptake, peripheral K^+ uptake is not impaired in humans with type 2 diabetes.[33] Notably, the hypokalemic effect of insulin is not renal-dependent.[34] Insulin and K^+ appear to form a feedback loop of sorts, in that increases in plasma K^+ have a marked stimulatory effect on insulin levels.[21,35] Insulin-stimulated K^+ uptake, measured in rats using a K^+ clamp technique, is rapidly reduced by 2 days of K^+ depletion, prior to a modest drop in plasma K^+,[36] and in the absence of a change in plasma K^+ in rats subject to a lesser K^+ restriction for 14 days.[12] Insulin-mediated K^+ uptake is thus modulated by the factors that serve to preserve plasma K^+ in the setting of K^+ deprivation (see also "Control of Potassium Secretion: Effect of Potassium Intake"). Inhibition of basal insulin secretion in normal subjects by somatostatin infusion increases serum K^+ by up to 0.5 mmol/L in the absence of a change in urinary excretion, emphasizing the crucial role of circulating insulin in the regulation of plasma K^+.[37] Clinically, inhibition of insulin secretion by the somatostatin agonist octreotide can cause significant hyperkalemia in anephric patients[38] and patients with normal renal function.[39]

Insulin stimulates the uptake of K^+ by several tissues, most prominently liver, skeletal muscle, cardiac muscle, and fat.[21,40] It does so by activating several K^+ transport pathways, with particularly well-documented effects on the Na^+-K^+-ATPase.[41] Insulin activates Na^+-H^+ exchange and/or Na^+-K^+-$2Cl^-$ cotransport in several tissues; although the ensuing increase in intracellular Na^+ was postulated to have a secondary activating effect on Na^+-K^+-ATPase,[28] it is clear that this is not the primary mechanism in most cell types.[42] Insulin induces translocation of the Na^+-K^+-ATPase α_2-subunit to the plasma membrane of skeletal muscle cells, with a lesser effect on the α_1-subunit.[43] This translocation is dependent on the activity of phosphatidylinositol-3-kinase (PI3K),[43] which itself also binds to a proline-rich motif in the N terminus of the α-subunit.[44] The activation of PI3K by insulin thus induces phosphatase enzymes to dephosphorylate a specific serine residue adjacent to the PI3K binding domain. Trafficking of Na^+-K^+-ATPase to the cell surface also appears to require the phosphorylation of an adjacent tyrosine residue, perhaps catalyzed by the tyrosine kinase activity of the insulin receptor itself.[45] Finally, the serum- and glucocorticoid-regulated kinase-1 (SGK1) plays a critical role in insulin-stimulated K^+ uptake, presumably via the known stimulatory effects of this kinase on Na^+-K^+-ATPase activity and/or Na^+-K^+-$2Cl^-$ cotransport.[46] The hypokalemic effect of insulin plus glucose is blunted in SGK1 knockout mice, with a marked reduction in hepatic insulin-stimulated K^+ uptake.[46]

SYMPATHETIC NERVOUS SYSTEM

The sympathetic nervous system plays a prominent role in regulating the balance between extracellular and intracellular K^+. Again, as is the case for insulin, the effect of catecholamines on plasma K^+ has been known since the 1930s[47]; however, a complicating issue is the differential effect of stimulating α- and β-adrenergic receptors (Table 18.2). Uptake of K^+ by liver and muscle, with resultant hypokalemia, is stimulated via β_2-receptors.[28] The hypokalemic effect of catecholamines appears to be largely independent of changes in circulating insulin[28] and has been reported in nephrectomized animals.[48] The cellular mechanisms whereby catecholamines induce K^+ uptake in muscle include an activation of the Na^+-K^+-ATPase,[49] likely via increases in cyclic adenosine monophosphate (cAMP).[50] However, β-adrenergic receptors in skeletal muscle also activate the inwardly directed Na^+-K^+-$2Cl^-$ cotransporter NKCC1, which may account for as much as one third of the uptake response to catecholamines.[21,27]

In contrast to β-adrenergic stimulation, α-adrenergic agonists impair the ability to buffer increases in K^+ induced via intravenous loading or by exercise[51]; the cellular mechanisms whereby this occurs are not known. It is thought that β-adrenergic stimulation increases K^+ uptake during exercise to avoid hyperkalemia, whereas α-adrenergic mechanisms help blunt the ensuing postexercise nadir.[51] The clinical consequences of the sympathetic control of extrarenal K^+ homeostasis are reviewed elsewhere in this chapter.

Table 18.2 Sustained Effects of β- and α-Adrenergic Agonists and Antagonists on Serum Potassium Concentration

Catecholamine Specificity	Sustained Effect on Serum K$^+$
β$_1$- + β$_2$-Agonist (epinephrine, isoproterenol)	Decreased
Pure β$_1$-agonist (ITP)	None
Pure β$_2$-agonist (salbutamol, soterenol, terbutaline)	Decreased
β$_1$- + β$_2$-Antagonist (propranolol, sotalol)	Increased; blocks the effect of β-agonists
β$_1$-Antagonist (practolol, metoprolol, atenolol)	None; does not block effect of β-agonists
β$_2$-Antagonist (butoxamine, H 35/25)	Blocks hypokalemic effect of β-agonists
α-Agonist (phenylephrine)	Increased
α-Antagonist (phenoxybenzamine)	None; blocks effect of α-agonists

ITP, Isopropylamino-3-(2-thiazoloxy)-2-propanol.
From Giebisch G: Renal potassium transport: mechanisms and regulation. Am J Physiol 274:F817-F833, 1998.

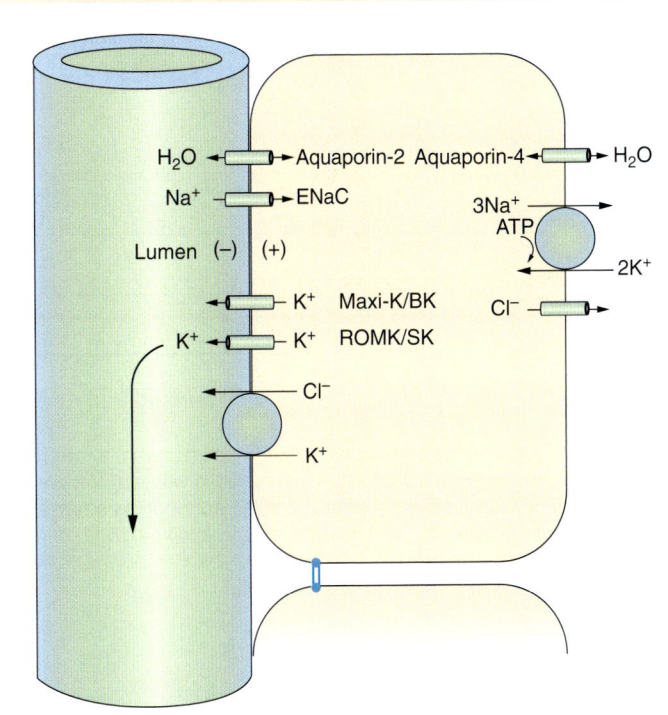

Figure 18.3 K$^+$ secretory pathways in principal cells of the connecting segment (CNT) and cortical collecting duct (CCD). The absorption of Na$^+$ via the amiloride-sensitive epithelial sodium channel (ENaC) generates a lumen-negative potential difference, which drives K$^+$ excretion through the apical secretory K$^+$ channel ROMK. Flow-dependent K$^+$ secretion is mediated by an apical voltage-gated, calcium-sensitive BK channel. Chloride-dependent, electroneutral K$^+$ secretion is likely mediated by a K$^+$-Cl$^-$ cotransporter.

ACID-BASE STATUS

The association between changes in pH and plasma K$^+$ was observed in 1934.[52] It has long been thought that acute disturbances in acid-base equilibrium result in changes in serum K$^+$, such that alkalemia shifts K$^+$ into cells, whereas acidemia is associated with K$^+$ release.[53,54] It is thought that this effective K$^+$-H$^+$ exchange serves to help maintain extracellular pH. Rather limited data exist for the durable concept that a change of 0.1 unit in serum pH will result in a 0.6-mmol/L change in serum K$^+$ in the opposite direction.[55] However, despite the complexities of changes in K$^+$ homeostasis associated with various acid-base disorders, a few general observations can be made. The induction of metabolic acidosis by the infusion of mineral acids (NH$_4^+$-Cl$^-$ or H$^+$-Cl$^-$) consistently increases serum K$^+$,[53-57] whereas organic acidosis generally fails to increase serum K$^+$.[54,56,58,59] Notably, another study failed to detect an increase in serum K$^+$ in normal human subjects with acute acidosis secondary to duodenal NH$_4^+$-Cl$^-$ infusion, in which a modest acidosis was accompanied by an increase in circulating insulin.[60] However, as noted by Adrogué and Madias,[61] the concomitant infusion of 350 mL of 5% dextrose in water (D$_5$W) in these fasting subjects may have served to increase circulating insulin, thus blunting the potential hyperkalemic response to NH$_4^+$-Cl$^-$. Clinically, use of the oral phosphate binder sevelamer hydrochloride in patients with end-stage kidney disease (ESKD) is associated with acidosis due to effective gastrointestinal absorption of H$^+$-Cl$^-$; in hemodialysis patients, this acidosis has been associated with an increase in serum K$^+$, which is ameliorated by an increase in dialysis bicarbonate concentration.[62] Of note, hyperkalemia is not an expected complication of sevelamer carbonate, which has supplanted sevelamer hydrochloride as a phosphate binder. Metabolic alkalosis induced by sodium bicarbonate infusion usually results in a modest reduction in serum K$^+$.[53-55,57,63] Respiratory alkalosis reduces plasma K$^+$ by a magnitude comparable to that of metabolic alkalosis.[53-55,64] Finally, acute respiratory acidosis increases plasma K$^+$; the absolute increase is smaller than that induced by metabolic acidosis secondary to inorganic acids.[53-55] Again, however, some studies have failed to show a change in serum K$^+$ following acute respiratory acidosis.[54,65]

RENAL POTASSIUM EXCRETION

POTASSIUM TRANSPORT IN THE DISTAL NEPHRON

The proximal tubule and loop of Henle mediate the bulk of potassium reabsorption, such that a considerable fraction of filtered potassium is reabsorbed prior to entry into the superficial distal tubules.[66] Renal potassium excretion is primarily determined by regulated secretion in the distal nephron, specifically within the connecting segment (CNT) and cortical collecting duct (CCD). The principal cells of the CNT and CCD play a dominant role in K$^+$ secretion; the relevant transport pathways are shown in Figures 18-2 and 18-3. Apical Na$^+$ entry via the amiloride-sensitive epithelial Na$^+$ channel (ENaC)[67] results in the generation of a lumen-negative potential difference in the CNT and CCD, which drives passive K$^+$ exit through apical K$^+$ channels. A critical,

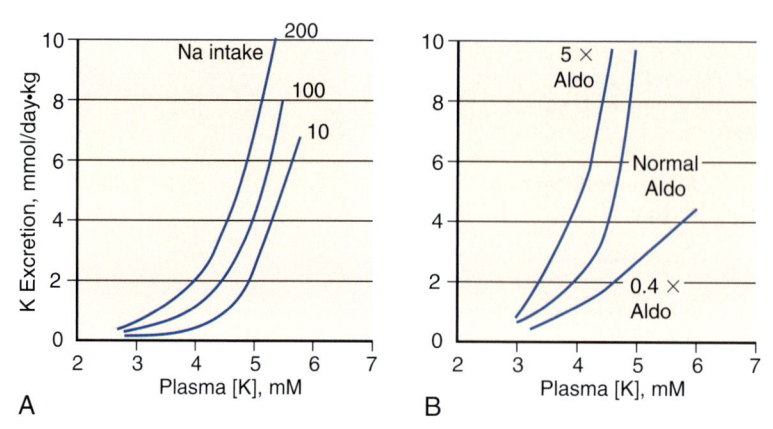

Figure 18.4 **A,** Relationship between steady-state serum K⁺ and urinary K⁺ excretion in the dog as a function of dietary Na⁺ intake (mmol/day). Animals were adrenalectomized and replaced with aldosterone (Aldo); dietary K⁺ and Na⁺ content were varied as specified. **B,** Relationship between steady-state serum K⁺ and urinary K⁺ excretion as a function of circulating aldosterone. Animals were adrenalectomized and variably replaced with aldosterone; dietary K⁺ content was varied. (**A** from Young DB, Jackson TE, Tipayamontri U, Scott RC: Effects of sodium intake on steady-state potassium excretion. *Am J Physiol* 246:F772-F778, 1984; **B** from Young DB: Quantitative analysis of aldosterone's role in potassium regulation. *Am J Physiol* 255:F811-F822, 1988.)

clinically relevant consequence of this relationship is that K^+ secretion is dependent on delivery of adequate luminal Na^+ to the CNT and CCD[68,69]; K^+ secretion by the CCD essentially ceases as luminal Na^+ drops below 8 mmol/L.[70] Selective increases in thiazide-sensitive Na^+-Cl^- cotransport in the distal convoluted tubule (DCT), as seen in familial hyperkalemia with hypertension (FHHt; see "Hyperkalemia: Hereditary Tubular Defects and Potassium Excretion"), reduce Na^+ delivery to principal cells in the downstream CNT and CCD, leading to hyperkalemia.[71] Dietary Na^+ intake also influences K^+ excretion, such that excretion is enhanced by excess Na^+ intake and reduced by Na^+ restriction (Figure 18.4).[68,69] Basolateral exchange of Na^+ and K^+ is mediated by the Na^+-K^+-ATPase, providing the driving force for Na^+ entry and K^+ exit at the apical membrane (see Figures 18-2 and 18-3).

Under basal conditions of high Na^+-Cl^- and low K^+ intake, the bulk of aldosterone-stimulated Na^+ and K^+ transport occurs in the CNT, prior to the entry of tubular fluid into the CCD.[72] The density of Na^+ and K^+ channels is thus considerably greater in the CNT than in the CCD[73,74]; the capacity of the CNT for Na^+ reabsorption may be as much as 10 times greater than that of the CCD.[74] The recruitment of ENaC subunits in response to dietary Na^+ restriction begins in the CNT, with progressive recruitment of subunits to the apical membrane of the CCD at lower levels of dietary Na^+.[75] The activity of secretory K^+ channels in the CNT is also influenced by changes in dietary K^+; again, this is consistent with progressive axial recruitment of transport capacity for the absorption of Na^+ and secretion of K^+ along the distal nephron.[76]

Electrophysiologic characterization has documented the presence of several subpopulations of apical K^+ channels in the CCD and CNT, most prominently a small-conductance (SK), 30-picosiemens (pS) channel[73,77] and a large-conductance, Ca^{2+}-activated 150-pS (BK) channel[73,78] (see Figure 18.3). The SK channel is thought to mediate K^+ secretion under baseline conditions, hence its designation as the secretory K^+ channel. SK channel activity is mediated by the ROMK (renal outer medullary K^+) channel protein, encoded by the *Kcnj1* gene; targeted deletion of this gene in mice results in complete loss of SK activity within the CCD.[78] Increased distal flow has a significant stimulatory effect on K^+ secretion, due in part to enhanced delivery and absorption of Na^+ and to increased removal of secreted K^+.[68,69] The apical Ca^{2+}-activated BK channel plays a critical role in flow-dependent K^+ secretion by the CNT and CCD.[77] BK channels have a heteromeric structure, with α-subunits that form the ion channel pore and modulatory β-subunits.[77] The $β_1$-subunits of BK channels are restricted to principal cells within the CNT,[77,79] whereas $β_4$-subunits are detectable at the apical membranes of TAL, DCT, and intercalated cells.[79] Flow-dependent K^+ secretion is reduced in mice with targeted deletion of the $α_1$- and $β_1$-subunits,[77,80,81] consistent with a dominant role for BK channels.

In addition to apical K^+ channels, considerable evidence implicates apical K^+-Cl^- cotransport in distal K^+ secretion.[68,82,83] Pharmacologic studies of perfused tubules are consistent with K^+-Cl^- cotransport mediated by the KCC proteins.[82] A provocative study has underlined the importance of ENaC-independent K^+ excretion, whether it is mediated by apical K^+-Cl^- cotransport and/or by other mechanisms.[84] Rats were infused with amiloride via osmotic minipumps, generating urinary concentrations considered sufficient to inhibit more than 98% of ENaC activity. Whereas amiloride almost abolished K^+ excretion in rats with normal K^+ intake, acute and long-term high K^+ diets led to an increasing fraction of K^+ excretion that was independent of ENaC activity (~50% after 7 to 9 days on a high-K^+ diet).[84]

In addition to secretion, the distal nephron is capable of considerable reabsorption of K^+, particularly during restriction of dietary K^+.[21,66,85,86] This reabsorption is accomplished primarily by intercalated cells in the outer medullary collecting duct (OMCD) via the activity of apical H^+-K^+-ATPase pumps (see Figure 18.2). The molecular physiology of H^+-K^+-ATPase–mediated K^+ reabsorption is reviewed in Chapter 6.

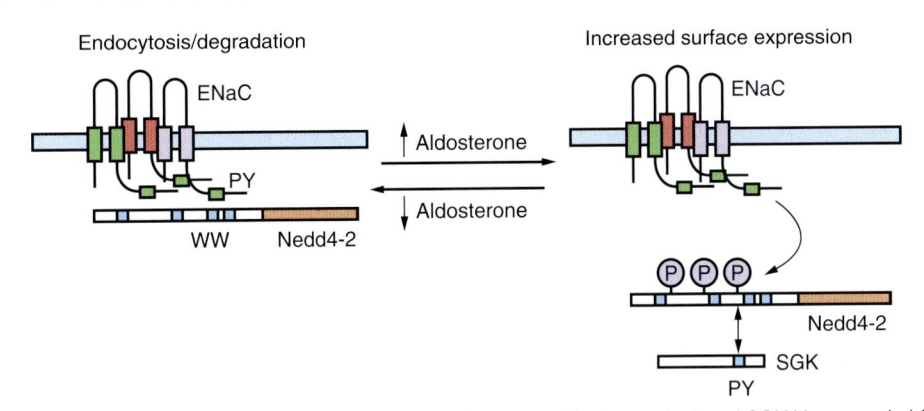

Figure 18.5 Coordinated regulation of the epithelial Na⁺ channel (ENaC) by the aldosterone-induced SGK kinase and ubiquitin ligase Nedd4-2. Nedd4-2 binds via its WW domains to ENaC subunits via their PPXY domains (denoted PY here), ubiquitinating the channel subunits and targeting them for removal from the cell membrane and destruction in the proteasome. Aldosterone induces the SGK kinase, which phosphorylates and inactivates Nedd4-2, thus increasing surface expression of ENaC channels. Mutations that cause Liddle's syndrome affect the interaction between ENaC and Nedd4-2. (From Snyder PM, Olson DR, Thomas BC: Serum and glucocorticoid-regulated kinase modulates Nedd4-2-mediated inhibition of the epithelial Na⁺ channel. *J Biol Chem* 277:5-8, 2002.)

CONTROL OF POTASSIUM SECRETION

ALDOSTERONE

Aldosterone is well established as an important regulatory factor in K^+ excretion, and increases in plasma K^+ are an important stimulus for aldosterone secretion (see also "Regulation of Renal Renin and Adrenal Aldosterone"). However, an increasingly dominant theme is that aldosterone plays a permissive and synergistic role in K^+ homeostasis.[87-89] This is reflected clinically in the frequent absence of hyperkalemia or hypokalemia in disorders associated with a deficiency or an overabundance of circulating aldosterone, respectively (see "Hyperaldosteronism" and "Hypoaldosteronism"). Regardless, it is clear that aldosterone and downstream effectors of this hormone have clinically relevant effects on plasma K^+ levels and that the ability to excrete K^+ is modulated by systemic aldosterone levels (see Figure 18.4).

Aldosterone has no effect on the density of apical SK channels in the CCD or CNT; rather, the hormone induces a marked increase in the density of apical Na⁺ channels,[90] thus increasing the driving force for apical K^+ excretion. The apical, amiloride-sensitive ENaC is comprised of three subunits, α-, β-, and γ-, that assemble together to traffic synergistically to the cell membrane and mediate Na⁺ transport. Aldosterone activates ENaC channel complexes by multiple mechanisms. First, it induces transcription of the α-ENaC subunit,[91,92] increasing the availability for co-assembly with the more abundant β- and γ-subunits.[93] Second, aldosterone and dietary Na⁺-Cl⁻ restriction stimulate a significant redistribution of ENaC subunits in the CNT and early CCD, from a largely cytoplasmic location during dietary Na⁺-Cl⁻ excess to a purely apical distribution after aldosterone or Na⁺-Cl⁻ restriction.[75,94,95] Third, aldosterone induces the expression of a serine-threonine kinase called SGK-1 (serum and glucocorticoid-induced kinase-1)[96]; coexpression of SGK-1 with ENaC subunits results in increased expression at the plasma membrane.[94] SGK-1 modulates membrane expression of ENaC by interfering with regulated endocytosis of its channel subunits. Specifically, the kinase interferes with interactions between ENaC subunits and the ubiquitin ligase Nedd4-2.[93] The so-called PPxY domains in the C termini of all three ENaC subunits bind to WW domains of Nedd4-2[97]; these PPxY domains are deleted, truncated, or mutated in patients with Liddle's syndrome[98] (see later, "Liddle's Syndrome"), leading to a gain of function in channel activity.[99] Nedd4-2 ubiquitinates ENaC subunits, thus inducing removal of channel subunits from the cell membrane, followed by degradation in lysosomes and the proteasome.[93] A PPxY domain in SGK-1 also binds to Nedd4-2, which is a phosphorylation substrate for the kinase; phosphorylation of Nedd4-2 by SGK-1 abrogates the inhibitory effect of this ubiquitin ligase on ENaC subunits[2] (Figure 18.5).

The importance of SGK-1 in K^+ and Na^+ homeostasis is illustrated by the phenotype of SGK-1 knockout mice.[100,101] On a normal diet, homozygous SGK-1$^{-/-}$ mice exhibit normal blood pressure and a normal plasma K^+, with only a mild elevation of circulating aldosterone. However, dietary Na⁺-Cl⁻ restriction of these mice results in relative Na⁺ wasting and hypotension, marked weight loss, and a drop in the glomerular filtration rate (GFR), despite considerable increases in circulating aldosterone.[101] In addition, dietary K^+ loading over 6 days leads to a 1.5-mmol/L increase in serum K^+, also accompanied by a considerable increase in circulating aldosterone (~fivefold greater than that of wild-type littermate controls).[100] This hyperkalemia occurs despite evident increases in apical ROMK expression, compared to the normokalemic littermate controls. The amiloride-sensitive, lumen-negative potential difference generated by ENaC is reduced in these SGK-1 knockout mice,[100] resulting in a decreased driving force for distal K^+ secretion and the observed susceptibility to hyperkalemia.

Another mechanism whereby aldosterone activates ENaC involves proteolytic cleavage of the channel proteins by serine proteases. A channel-activating protease that increases channel activity of ENaC was initially identified in *Xenopus laevis* A6 cells.[102] The mammalian ortholog, denoted CAP1 (channel-activating protease-1), or prostasin, is an aldosterone-induced protein in principal cells.[103] Urinary excretion of CAP1 is increased in hyperaldosteronism, with a reduction after adrenalectomy.[103] CAP1 is membrane-associated via a glycosylphosphatidylinositol (GPI) linkage[102];

mammalian principal cells also express two transmembrane proteases, denoted CAP2 and CAP3, with homology to CAP1.[104] These and other proteases (e.g., furin, plasmin) activate ENaC by excising extracellular inhibitory domains from the α- and γ-subunits, increasing the open probability of channels at the plasma membrane.[104,105] This proteolytic cleavage of ENaC appears to activate the channel by removing the so-called self-inhibitory effect of external Na^+; in the case of furin-mediated proteolysis of α-ENaC, this appears to involve the removal of an inhibitory domain from within the extracellular loop.[106,107] Extracellular Na^+ appears to interact with a specific acidic cleft in the cleaved extracellular loop of α-ENaC, causing inhibition of the channel.[108] Since SGK-1 increases channel expression at the cell surface,[94] one would expect synergistic activation by coexpressed CAP1-3 and SGK, and this is indeed the case.[104] Therefore, aldosterone activates ENaC by at least three separate synergistic mechanisms—induction of α-ENaC, induction of SGK-1 and repression of Nedd4-2, and induction of channel-activating proteases. Clinically, the inhibition of channel-activating proteases by the protease inhibitor nafamostat causes hyperkalemia due to inhibition of ENaC activity.[109,110]

EFFECT OF POTASSIUM INTAKE

Changes in K^+ intake strongly modulate K^+ channel activity in the CNT and CCD (secretory capacity), in addition to H^+-K^+-ATPase activity in the OMCD (reabsorptive capacity). Increased dietary K^+ rapidly increases the activity of SK channels in the CCD and CNT,[76,111] along with a modest increase in Na^+ channel (ENaC) activity[90]; this is associated with an increase in apical expression of the ROMK channel protein.[112] The increase in ENaC and SK channel density in the CCD occurs within hours of intake of a high-K^+ diet, with a minimal associated increase in circulating aldosterone.[111] BK channels in the CNT and CCD are also activated by dietary K^+ loading. Trafficking of BK subunits is thus affected by dietary K^+, with largely intracellular distribution of α-subunits in K^+-restricted rats and prominent apical expression in K^+-loaded rats.[113] Again, aldosterone does not contribute to the regulation of BK channel activity or expression in response to a high-K^+ diet.[114]

A complex synergistic mix of signaling pathways regulates K^+ channel activity in response to changes in dietary K^+ (see also Chapter 6). In particular, the WNK (*with no lysine*) kinases play a critical role in modulating distal K^+ secretion. WNK1 and WNK4 were initially identified as the causative genes for FHHt (see also "Hyperkalemia: and Potassium Excretion"). ROMK expression at the membrane of *Xenopus* oocytes is reduced by coexpression of WNK4; FHHt-associated mutations increase this effect, suggesting a direction inhibition of SK channels in FHHt.[115] Transcription of the WNK1 gene generates several different isoforms; the predominant intrarenal WNK1 isoform is generated by a distal nephron transcriptional site that bypasses the N-terminal exons that encode the kinase domain, yielding a kinase-deficient short isoform[116] ("WNK1-S"). Full-length WNK1 (WNK1-L) inhibits ROMK by inducing endocytosis of the channel protein; the shorter, kinase-deficient WNK1-S isoform inhibits this effect of WNK1-L.[117,118] The ratio of WNK1-S to WNK1-L transcripts is reduced by K^+ restriction (greater endocytosis of ROMK)[118,119] and increased by K^+ loading (reduced endocytosis of ROMK),[117,119] suggesting that this ratio between WNK1-S and WNK1-L functions as a molecular switch to regulate distal K^+ secretion. The BK channel is also regulated by the WNK kinases.[120-122]

The membrane trafficking of ROMK is also modulated by tyrosine phosphorylation of the channel protein, such that tyrosine phosphorylation stimulates endocytosis, and tyrosine dephosphorylation induces exocytosis.[123,124] Intrarenal activity of the cytoplasmic tyrosine kinases c-src and c-yes is inversely related to dietary K^+ intake, with a decrease under high K^+ conditions and a marked increase after several days of K^+ restriction.[125,126] Several studies have implicated the intrarenal generation of superoxide anions in the activation of cytoplasmic tyrosine kinases by K^+ depletion.[127-129] Potential candidates for the upstream hormonal signals include angiotensin II (Ang II) and growth factors such as insulin-like growth factor-1 (IGF-1).[127] In particular, Ang II inhibits ROMK activity in K^+-restricted rats, but not rats on a normal K^+ diet.[130] This inhibition by Ang II involves downstream activation of superoxide production and c-src activity, such that the induction of Ang II by a low-K^+ diet appears to play a major role in reducing distal tubular K^+ secretion.[131]

INTEGRATED REGULATION OF DISTAL SODIUM ABSORPTION AND POTASSIUM SECRETION

Under certain physiologic conditions associated with marked induction of aldosterone, such as dietary sodium restriction, Na^+ balance can be maintained without significant effects on K^+ excretion. However, by activating ENaC and generating a more lumen-negative potential difference, increases in aldosterone should lead to an obligatory kaliuresis. How is this physiologic consequence avoided? The mechanisms that underlie this aldosterone paradox, the independent regulation of Na^+ and K^+ handling by the aldosterone-sensitive distal nephron, have been delineated. The major factors that allow for integrated but independent control of Na^+ and K^+ transport appear to include electroneutral thiazide-sensitive Na^+-Cl^- transport within the CCD,[132-134] ENaC-independent K^+ excretion within the distal nephron,[84] and differential regulation of various signaling pathways by aldosterone, Ang II, and dietary K^+[135,136] (see also Chapter 6).

Electroneutral Na^+-Cl^- transport in the CCD and ENaC-independent K^+ secretion may play important roles in disconnecting Na^+ and K^+ transport within the distal nephron. Electroneutral, thiazide-sensitive, and amiloride-resistant Na^+-Cl^- transport within the CCD[132-134] is mediated by the combined activity of the Na^+-dependent Cl^--HCO_3^- SLC4A8 Cl^--HCO_3^- exchanger and the SLC26A4 Cl^--HCO_3^- exchanger[134] (see also Chapter 6). This transport mechanism is apparently responsible for as much as 50% of Na^+-Cl^- transport in mineralocorticoid-stimulated rat CCD,[132,133] allowing for ENaC-independent, electroneutral Na^+ absorption that will not directly affect K^+ secretion. The converse effect emerges after dietary K^+ loading, which increases the fraction of ENaC-independent, amiloride-resistant K^+ excretion to approximately 50%.[84]

Studies have indicated a key role in K^+ homeostasis for NCC, the thiazide-sensitive Na^+-Cl^- cotransporter in the DCT. Selective increases in DCT and NCC activity, as seen in FHHt, reduce Na^+ delivery to principal cells in the

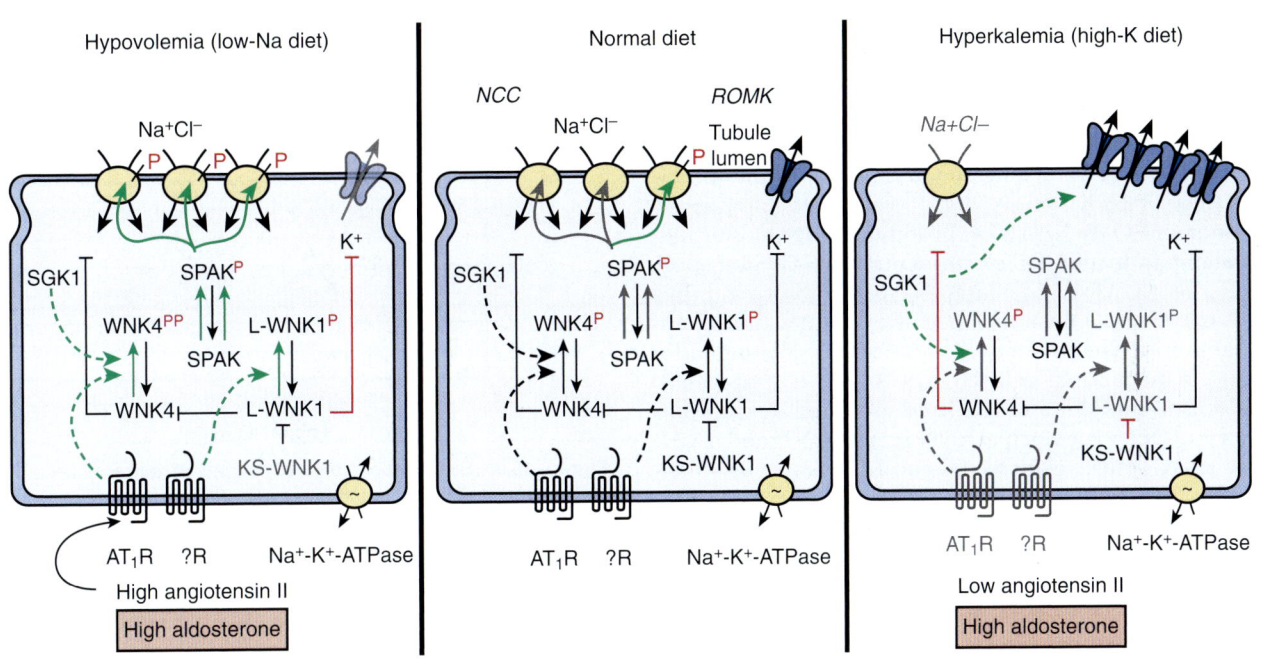

Figure 18.6 Integrated regulation of Na$^+$-Cl$^-$ and K$^+$ transport in the DCT, CNT, and CCD. Activating pathways are shown by *green arrowheads* and the inhibitory pathway is indicated by the *red blunt end*. **Left panel,** Pathway in the setting of a low-Na$^+$ diet, wherein angiotensin II (Ang II) and SGK-1 signaling lead to phosphorylation of WNK4. This stimulates phosphorylation of SPAK, which in turn phosphorylates and activates thiazide-sensitive Na$^+$-Cl$^-$ cotransport in the DCT via NCC. Stimulation of unknown receptors is hypothesized to cause phosphorylation of L-WNK1, which can also stimulate SPAK phosphorylation. L-WNK1 has other functions: (1) it blocks the NCC inhibitory form of WNK4, thus activating NCC; (2) it inhibits secretion of K$^+$ via ROMK channels. **Right panel,** Pathway in the setting of high dietary K$^+$ intake, wherein aldosterone is stimulated and Ang II is low. In the absence of sufficient Ang II, its type 1 receptor (AT$_1$R) cannot activate WNK4. This reduces SPAK activation and NCC phosphorylation. Dietary potassium loading also increases the level of the KS-WNK1 isoform to suppress the activity of L-WNK1. In consequence, the inhibitory effect of WNK4 on NCC dominates, blocking traffic of NCC to the apical membrane and thereby reducing NCC activity. KS-WNK1 also blocks the effect of L-WNK1 on ROMK endocytosis, causing ROMK to increase at the apical membrane. The net effect is that K$^+$ secretion in the DCT and CNT-CCD is maximized, whereas NCC is suppressed. Aldosterone stimulation of the epithelial sodium channel (ENaC; not shown) offsets the decreased Na$^+$ reabsorption by NCC, allowing robust potassium secretion without changes in sodium balance. The roles of WNK3, SGK1, and c-src cytoplasmic tyrosine kinases are not shown in the interest of clarity; see text for further details. NCC, NaCl cotransporter; ROMK, renal outer medullary K channel; SPAK, STE20/SPS1-related proline/alanine-rich kinase; WNK, *w*ith *n*o *K* (lysine) kinase. (From Welling PA, Chang YP, Delpire E, Wade JB: Multigene kinase network, kidney transport, and salt in essential hypertension. *Kidney Int* 77:1063-1069, 2010.)

downstream CNT and CCD, leading to hyperkalemia.[71] The DCT also clearly functions as a potassium sensor, directly responding to changes in circulating potassium. Reduction in potassium intake and/or hypokalemia thus lead to reduced basolateral [K$^+$] in the DCT; the subsequent hyperpolarization is dependent on basolateral KIR4.1-containing K$^+$ channels.[3] Hyperpolarization leads to chloride exit via basolateral CLC-NKB chloride channels and a reduction in intracellular chloride; the reduction in intracellular chloride activates the WNK cascade, resulting in phosphorylation of NCC and activation of the transporter.[3] Ang II also activates NCC via WNK-dependent activation of the SPAK kinase and phosphorylation of the transporter protein,[137,138] reducing delivery of Na$^+$ to the CNT and limiting K$^+$ secretion. In contrast, Ang II inhibits ROMK activity via several mechanisms, including downstream activation of c-src tyrosine kinases (see earlier).[129-131] Whereas K$^+$ restriction induces renin and circulating angiotensin-II (see "Consequences of Hypokalemia"), increases in dietary K$^+$ are suppressive.[131,139] A high-K$^+$ diet also inactivates NCC[140] due to the associated decrease in Ang II in addition to the increase in the ratio of WNK1-S to WNK1-L isoforms that occurs with increased K$^+$ intake.[117-119] WNK1-S antagonizes the effect of WNK1-L on NCC, leading to inhibition of NCC in conditions with a relative excess of WNK1-S.[135]

Finally, within principal cells, increases in aldosterone induce the SGK1 kinase, which phosphorylates WNK4 and attenuates the effect of WNK4 on ROMK[141] while activating ENaC.[93,94,96] However, when dietary K$^+$ intake is reduced, c-src tyrosine kinase activity increases under the influence of increased Ang II, causing direction inhibition of ROMK activity via tyrosine phosphorylation of the channel.[123,142,143] The increase in c-src tyrosine kinase activity also abrogates the inhibitory effect of SGK1 on WNK4.[136] Again, Ang II appears to mediate part of its inhibitory effect on ROMK through activation of c-src,[131] such that c-src serves as an important component of the switch that regulates K$^+$ secretion in response to changes in dietary K$^+$.

To summarize this important physiology, the differential effects of K$^+$ intake on Ang II versus aldosterone appear to be critical in resolving the aldosterone paradox; so too are the differential effects of K$^+$ intake on NCC-dependent Na$^+$-Cl$^-$ transport in the DCT and on secretory K$^+$ channels within the downstream CNT and CCD (Figure 18.6). Under conditions of low Na$^+$ intake but moderate K$^+$ intake, Ang II and aldosterone are both strongly induced, leading to enhanced Na$^+$-Cl$^-$ transport via NCC, increased ENaC activity, and decreased secretory K$^+$ channel activity. Although ENaC is activated, the relative inhibition of ROMK by the increased Ang II prevents excessive kaliuresis. Ang II–dependent activation of c-src kinases has direct inhibitory effects on ROMK trafficking and also abrogates the inhibitory effect of SGK1 on WNK4,[136] leading to unopposed inhibition of ROMK by WNK4. In addition, the aldosterone-dependent induction of electroneutral Na$^+$-Cl$^-$ transport within the CCD[132-134] increases Na$^+$-Cl$^-$ reabsorption but blunts the effect on the lumen-negative potential, thus limiting kaliuresis. When dietary K$^+$ increases, circulating aldosterone is moderately induced, but Ang II is suppressed. This leads to inhibition of NCC and increased downstream delivery of Na$^+$ to principal cells in the CNT and CCD, where ENaC activity is increased and ROMK and BK channels are significantly activated. ENaC-independent K$^+$ secretion is also strongly induced by increased dietary K$^+$ intake,[84] contributing significantly to the ability to excrete K$^+$ in the urine.

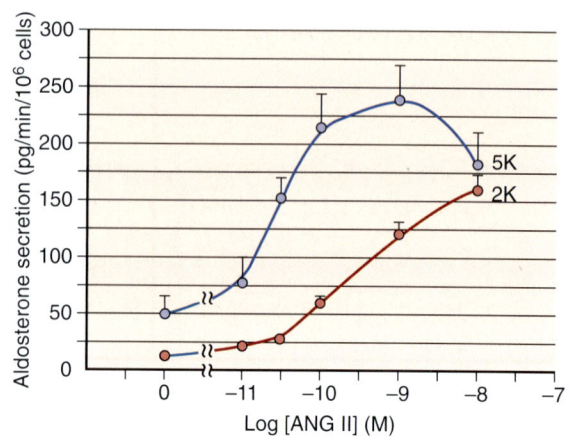

Figure 18.7 Synergistic effect of increased extracellular K$^+$ and angiotensin II (ANG II) in inducing aldosterone release from bovine adrenal glomerulosa cells. Dose response curves for ANG II were performed at an extracellular K$^+$ of 2 mmol/L (*blue circles*) and 5 mmol/L (*red circles*). (From Chen XL, Bayliss DA, Fern RJ, Barrett PQ: A role for T-type Ca^{2+} channels in the synergistic control of aldosterone production by ANG II and K$^+$. *Am J Physiol* 276: F674-F683, 1999.)

REGULATION OF RENAL RENIN AND ADRENAL ALDOSTERONE

Modulation of the renin angiotensin aldosterone (RAAS) axis has profound clinical effects on K$^+$ homeostasis. Although multiple tissues are capable of renin secretion, renin of renal origin has a dominant physiologic impact. Renin secretion by juxtaglomerular cells within the afferent arteriole is initiated in response to a signal from the macula densa,[144] specifically a decrease in luminal chloride[145] transported through the Na$^+$-K$^+$-2Cl$^-$ cotransporter (NKCC2) at the apical membrane of macula densa cells.[26] In addition to this macula densa signal, decreased renal perfusion pressure and renal sympathetic tone stimulate renal renin secretion.[21,146] The various inhibitors of renin release include Ang II, endothelin,[147] adenosine,[148] atrial natriuretic peptide (ANP),[149] tumor necrosis factor-α (TNF-α),[150] and active vitamin D.[151] The cyclic guanosine monophosphate (cGMP)–dependent protein kinase type II (cGKII) tonically inhibits renin secretion in that renin secretion in response to several stimuli is exaggerated in homozygous *cGKII* knockout mice.[152] Activation of cGKII by ANP and/or nitric oxide has a marked inhibitory effect on the release of renin from juxtaglomerular cells.[149] Local factors that stimulate renin release from juxtaglomerular cells include prostaglandins,[153] adrenomedullin,[154] catecholamines (β$_1$-receptors),[155] and succinate (GPR91 receptor).[156]

The relationship between renal renin release, the RAAS, and cyclo-oxygenase-2 (COX-2) is particularly complex.[153] COX-2 is heavily expressed in the macula densa,[153] with a significant recruitment of COX-2$^{(+)}$ cells seen with salt restriction or furosemide treatment.[21,153] Reduced intracellular chloride in macula densa cells appears to stimulate COX-2 expression via p38 MAP kinase,[157] whereas both aldosterone and Ang II reduce its expression.[153] Prostaglandins derived from COX-2 in the macula densa play a dominant role in the stimulation of renal renin release by salt restriction, furosemide, renal artery occlusion, or angiotensin-converting enzyme (ACE) inhibition.[21,158] Specifically, COX-2–derived prostaglandins appear to play a role in tonic expression of renin in juxtaglomerular (JG) cells via modulation of intracellular cAMP and calcium, rather than functioning in the acute regulation of renin release.[153] Prostaglandins generated by the macula densa also participate in the recruitment of CD44$^+$ mesenchymal stromal cells during salt restriction, which differentiate into renin-producing cells.[159]

Renin released from the kidney ultimately stimulates aldosterone release from the adrenal via Ang II. Hyperkalemia per se is also an independent and synergistic stimulus (Figure 18.7) for aldosterone release from the adrenal gland,[21,160] although dietary K$^+$ loading is less potent than dietary Na$^+$-Cl$^-$ restriction in increasing circulating aldosterone.[87] The resting membrane potential of adrenal glomerulosa cells is hyperpolarized due to the activity of the leak K$^+$ channels TASK-1 and TASK-3; combined deletion of genes encoding these channels leads to baseline depolarization of adrenal glomerulosa cells and an increase in serum aldosterone that is resistant to dietary sodium loading.[161] Ang II and K$^+$ both activate Ca^{2+} entry in glomerulosa cells via voltage-sensitive, T-type Ca^{2+} channels,[21,162] primarily Cav3.2.[163] Elevations in extracellular K$^+$ thus depolarize glomerulosa cells and activate these Ca^{2+} channels, which are independently and synergistically activated by Ang II.[162] Calcium-dependent activation of calcium-calmodulin (CaM)–dependent protein kinase in turn activates the synthesis and release of aldosterone via induction of aldosterone synthase.[164] K$^+$ and Ang II also enhance transcription of the Cav3.2 Ca^{2+} channel by abrogating repression of this gene by the neuron-restrictive silencing factor (NRS); this ultimately amplifies the induction of aldosterone synthase.[163]

The role of adrenal K$^+$ sensing in aldosterone release has been dramatically underlined by the reports of germline and somatic mutations in aldosterone-producing adenomas of transport proteins that control membrane excitability of adrenal zona glomerulosa cells (see also "Hyperaldosteronism"). For example, somatic mutations in the adrenal K$^+$ channel KCNJ5 (GIRK4) can be detected in about 40% of aldosterone-producing adrenal adenomas[165]; these mutations endow the channel with a novel Na^+ conductance, leading to adrenal glomerulosa cell depolarization, Ca^{2+} influx, and aldosterone release.

The adrenal release of aldosterone due to increased K^+ is dependent on an intact adrenal renin angiotensin system,[166] particularly during Na^+ restriction. ACE inhibitors and angiotensin-receptor blockers (ARBs) thus completely abrogate the effect of high K^+ on salt-restricted adrenals.[167] Direct, G protein–dependent activation of the TASK-1 and/or TASK-3 K^+ channels by Ang II receptor type 1A ($AT_{1A}R$) or Ang II receptor type 1B ($AT_{1B}R$) is thought to underlie the effect of Ang II on adrenal aldosterone release,[161] with abrogation of this effect by ARBs or ACE inhibitors. Other clinically relevant activators of adrenal aldosterone release include prostaglandins[168] and catecholamines[169] via increases in cAMP.[170,171] Finally, ANP exerts a potent negative effect on aldosterone release induced by K^+ and other stimuli,[172] at least in part by inhibiting early events in aldosterone synthesis.[173] ANP is therefore capable of inhibiting renal renin release and adrenal aldosterone release, functions that may be central to the pathophysiology of hyporeninemic hypoaldosteronism.

URINARY INDICES OF POTASSIUM EXCRETION

A bedside test to measure distal tubular K^+ secretion directly in humans would be ideal; however, for obvious reasons, this not technically feasible. A widely used surrogate is the transtubular K^+ gradient (TTKG), which is defined as follows:

$$TTKG = ([K^+]_{urine} \times osmality_{blood})/([K^+]_{blood} \times osmality_{urine})$$

The expected values of the TTKG are largely based on historical data, and are less than 3 to 4 in the presence of hypokalemia and more than 6 to 7 in the presence of hyperkalemia; the shifting opinions regarding the physiologically appropriate TTKG in hyperkalemia have been reviewed multiple times.[174] Clearly, water absorption in the CCD and medullary collecting duct is an important determinant of the absolute K^+ concentration in the final urine—hence, the use of a ratio of urine/plasma osmolality. Indeed, water absorption may in large part determine the TTKG, such that it far exceeds the limiting K^+ gradient.[175] The TTKG may be less useful in patients ingesting diets of changing K^+ and mineralocorticoid intake.[176] There is, however, a linear relationship between plasma aldosterone and the TTKG, suggesting that it provides a rough approximation of the ability to respond to aldosterone with a kaliuresis.[177] The response of the TTKG to mineralocorticoid administration, typically fludrocortisone, can thus be used in the diagnostic approach to hyperkalemia[174] (see also Figures 18-11 and 18-15). In hypokalemic patients, a TTKG of less than 2 to 3 separates patients with redistributive hypokalemia from those with hypokalemia due to renal potassium wasting, who will have TTKG values that are more than 4.[178]

An alternative to the TTKG in hypokalemic patients is measurement of the urine K^+/creatinine ratio. The urine K^+/creatinine ratio is usually less than 13 mEq/g creatinine (1.5 mEq/mmol creatinine) when hypokalemia is caused by poor dietary intake, transcellular potassium shifts, gastrointestinal losses, or previous use of diuretics.[178] Higher values are indicative of ongoing renal potassium wasting. The utility of the K^+/creatinine ratio was evaluated in a study of 43 patients with severe hypokalemia (range, 1.5 to 2.6 mmol/L) associated with paralysis.[178] The urine K^+/creatinine ratio reliably distinguished between the 30 patients with hypokalemic periodic paralysis and the 13 patients with hypokalemia due mostly to renal potassium wasting. The K^+/creatinine ratio was thus significantly lower in the patients with periodic paralysis (11 versus 36 mEq/g creatinine; 1.3 versus 4.1 mEq/mmol creatinine). The cutoff value was approximately 22 mEq/g creatinine (2.5 mEq/mmol).

The determination of urinary electrolytes for calculation of the TTKG or urine K^+/creatinine ratio provides the opportunity for the measurement of urinary Na^+, which will determine whether significant prerenal stimuli are limiting distal Na^+ delivery and thus K^+ excretion (see also Figure 18.4). Urinary electrolytes also afford the opportunity to calculate the urinary anion gap, an indirect index of urinary NH_4^+ content. and thus the ability to respond to an acidemia.[179]

CONSEQUENCES OF HYPOKALEMIA AND HYPERKALEMIA

CONSEQUENCES OF HYPOKALEMIA

EXCITABLE TISSUES: MUSCLE AND HEART

Hypokalemia is a well-described risk factor for ventricular and atrial arrhythmias.[28,180,181] For example, in patients undergoing cardiac surgery, a serum K^+ of less than 3.5 mmol/L is a predictor of serious intraoperative arrhythmia, perioperative arrhythmia, and postoperative atrial fibrillation.[182] Moderate hypokalemia does not, however, appear to increase the risk of serious arrhythmia during exercise stress testing.[183] Electrocardiographic changes in hypokalemia include broad flat T waves, ST depression, and QT prolongation; these are most marked when serum K^+ is less than 2.7 mmol/L.[184] Hypokalemia, often accompanied by hypomagnesemia, is an important cause of the long QT syndrome (LQTS) and torsades de pointes, either alone[185] or in combination with drug toxicity,[186] or with LQTS-associated mutations in cardiac K^+ and Na^+ channels.[187] Hypokalemia accelerates the clathrin-dependent internalization and degradation of the cardiac hERG (human ether-à-go-go–related gene) K^+ channel protein.[30] hERG encodes pore-forming subunits of the cardiac rapidly activating delayed rectifier K^+ channel (I_{Kr}); I_{Kr} is largely responsible for potassium efflux during phases 2 and 3 of the cardiac action potential.[188] Loss-of-function mutations in hERG reduce I_{Kr} and cause type II LQTS[30]; downregulation of hERG and I_{Kr} by hypokalemia provides an elegant explanation for the association with LQTS and torsades de pointes.

In accordance with the Nernst equation, the resting membrane potential is related to the ratio of the intracellular to extracellular potassium concentration. In skeletal muscle, a reduction in plasma K^+ will increase this ratio and therefore hyperpolarize the cell membrane (i.e., make the resting potential more electronegative); this impairs the ability of the muscle to depolarize and contract, leading to weakness. However, in some human cardiac cells, particularly Purkinje fibers in the conducting system, hypokalemia results in a paradoxic depolarization[189]; this paradoxic depolarization plays an important role in the genesis of hypokalemic cardiac arrhythmias.[189,190] Resting membrane potential in excitable cells is largely determined by a large family of K2P1 K$^+$ channels, so-named due to the presence of two pore-forming (P) loop domains in each subunit. Hypokalemia causes K2P1 channels, which are normally selective for potassium, to transport sodium into cells suddenly, causing the paradoxic depolarization.[191] Notably, rodent cardiac cells respond to hypokalemia with a Nernst equation–predicted hyperpolarization and, unlike human cardiomyocytes, do not express the K2P1 channel TWIK-1; genetic manipulation indicates that TWIK-1 expression confers this paradoxic depolarization behavior on human and mouse cardiomyocytes.[191]

In skeletal muscle, hypokalemia causes hyperpolarization, thus impairing the capacity to depolarize and contract. Weakness and paralysis is therefore a not infrequent consequence of hypokalemia of diverse causes.[192,193] On a historical note, the realization in 1946 that K$^+$ replacement reversed the hypokalemic diaphragmatic paralysis induced by treatment of diabetic ketoacidosis (DKA) was a milestone in diabetes care.[194] Pathologically, muscle biopsies in hypokalemic myopathy demonstrate phagocytosis of degenerating muscle fibers, fiber regeneration, and atrophy of type 2 fibers.[195] Most patients with significant myopathy will have elevations in creatine kinase, and hypokalemia of diverse causes predisposes to rhabdomyolysis, with acute renal failure.

RENAL CONSEQUENCES

Hypokalemia causes a host of structural and functional changes in the kidney, which are reviewed in detail elsewhere.[196] In humans, the renal pathology includes a relatively specific proximal tubular vacuolization,[196,197] interstitial nephritis,[198] and renal cysts.[199] Hypokalemic nephropathy can cause ESKD, mostly in patients with long-standing hypokalemia due to eating disorders and/or laxative abuse[200]; acute renal failure with proximal tubular vasculopathy has also been described.[201] In animal models, hypokalemia increases susceptibility to acute renal failure induced by ischemia, gentamicin, and amphotericin.[21] Potassium restriction in rats induces cortical AT-II and medullary endothelin-1 expression, with an ischemic pattern of renal injury.[202]

The prominent functional changes in renal physiology that are induced by hypokalemia include Na$^+$-Cl$^-$ retention, polyuria,[197] phosphaturia,[28] hypocitraturia,[203] and increased ammoniagenesis.[196] K$^+$ depletion in rats causes proximal tubular hyperabsorption of Na$^+$-Cl$^-$ in association with an upregulation of Ang II,[202] AT$_1$ receptor,[28] and α$_2$-adrenergic receptor[28] in this nephron segment. NHE3, the dominant apical Na$^+$ entry site in the proximal tubule, is massively (>700%) upregulated in K$^+$-deficient rats,[204] which is consistent with the observed hyperabsorption of Na$^+$-Cl$^-$ and bicarbonate.[196] Polyuria in hypokalemia is due to polydipsia[205] and to a vasopressin-resistant defect in urine-concentrating ability.[196] This renal concentrating defect is multifactorial, with evidence for a reduced hydroosmotic response to vasopressin in the collecting duct[196] and for decreased Na$^+$-Cl$^-$ absorption by the TAL.[28] K$^+$ restriction has been shown to result in a rapid, reversible decrease in the expression of aquaporin-2 in the collecting duct,[206] beginning in the CCD and extending to the medullary collecting duct within the first 24 hours.[207] In the TAL, the marked reductions seen during K$^+$ restriction in the apical K$^+$ channel ROMK and apical Na$^+$-K$^+$-2Cl$^-$ cotransporter NKCC2[204] reduce Na$^+$-Cl$^-$ absorption, thus inhibiting countercurrent multiplication and the driving force for water absorption by the collecting duct.

CARDIOVASCULAR CONSEQUENCES

A large body of experimental and epidemiologic evidence has implicated hypokalemia and/or reduced dietary K$^+$ in the genesis or worsening of hypertension, heart failure, and stroke.[208] K$^+$ depletion in young rats induces hypertension,[209] with a salt sensitivity that persists after K$^+$ levels are normalized; presumably this salt sensitivity is due to the significant tubulointerstitial injury induced by K$^+$ restriction.[202] Short-term K$^+$ restriction in healthy humans and patients with essential hypertension also induces Na$^+$-Cl$^-$ retention and hypertension,[28] and abundant epidemiologic data have linked dietary K$^+$ deficiency and/or hypokalemia with hypertension.[181,208] Correction of hypokalemia is particularly important in hypertensive patients treated with diuretics; blood pressure in this setting is improved with the establishment of normokalemia,[210] and the cardiovascular benefits of diuretic agents are blunted by hypokalemia.[28,211] Hypokalemia reduces insulin secretion; this mechanism may play an important role in thiazide-associated diabetes.[212] Finally, K$^+$ depletion may play important roles in the pathophysiology and progression of heart failure.[208]

CONSEQUENCES OF HYPERKALEMIA
EXCITABLE TISSUES: MUSCLE AND HEART

Hyperkalemia constitutes a medical emergency, primarily due to its effect on the heart. Hyperkalemia depolarizes cardiac myocytes, reducing the membrane potential from −90 mV to approximately −80 mV. This brings the membrane potential closer to the threshold for generation of an action potential; mild and/or rapid-onset hyperkalemia will initially increase cardiac excitability, since a lesser depolarizing stimulus is required to generate an action potential. Mild increases in extracellular K$^+$ also affect the repolarization phase of the cardiac action potential, via increases in I$_{Kr}$; as discussed earlier (see "Consequences of Hypokalemia"), I$_{Kr}$ is highly sensitive to changes in extracellular K$^+$.[30] This effect on repolarization is thought to underlie the early signs of hyperkalemia,[213] including ST-T segment depression, peaked T waves, and Q-T interval shortening.[188] Persistent and increasing depolarization inactivates cardiac sodium channels, thus reducing the rate of phase 0 of the action potential (V$_{max}$); the decrease in V$_{max}$ results in a reduction in myocardial conduction, with progressive prolongation of the P wave, PR interval, and QRS complex.[188] Severe hyperkalemia results in loss of the P wave and a progressive widening of the QRS complex; fusion with T waves causes a sine wave sinoventricular rhythm.

Cardiac arrhythmias associated with hyperkalemia include sinus bradycardia, sinus arrest, slow idioventricular rhythms, ventricular tachycardia, ventricular fibrillation, and asystole.[213,214] The differential diagnosis and treatment

Table 18.3 Approximate Relationship between Hyperkalemic Electrocardiographic Changes and Serum Potassium Concentration

Serum K^+ Concentration (mmol/L)	Electrocardiographic Abnormality
5.5-6.5	Tall peaked T waves with narrow base, best seen in precordial leads
6.5-8.0	Peaked T waves
	Prolonged PR interval
	Decreased amplitude of P waves
	Widening of QRS complex
>8.0	Absence of P waves
	Intraventricular blocks, fascicular blocks, bundle branch blocks, QRS axis shift
	Progressive widening of the QRS complex
	Sine wave pattern (sinoventricular rhythm), ventricular fibrillation, asystole

From Mattu A, Brady WJ, Robinson DA: Electrocardiographic manifestations of hyperkalemia. Am J Emerg Med 18:721-729, 2000.

of a wide-complex tachycardia in hyperkalemia can be particularly problematic; moreover, hyperkalemia potentiates the blocking effect of lidocaine on the cardiac Na^+ channel, such that use of this agent may precipitate asystole or ventricular fibrillation in this setting.[215] Hyperkalemia can also cause a type I Brugada pattern in the electrocardiogram, with a pseudo–right bundle branch block (RBBB) and persistent coved ST segment elevation in at least two precordial leads. This hyperkalemic Brugada sign occurs in critically ill patients with significant hyperkalemia (serum K^+ > 7 mmol/L) and can be differentiated from genetic Brugada syndrome by an absence of P waves, marked QRS widening, and an abnormal QRS axis.[216]

Classically, the electrocardiographic manifestations in hyperkalemia progress as shown in Table 18.3. However, these changes are notoriously insensitive, such that only 55% of patients with serum K^+ more than 6.8 mmol/L in one case series manifested peaked T waves.[217] There is large interpatient variability in the absolute potassium level, leading to electrocardiographic changes and cardiac toxicity of hyperkalemia. Relevant variables include the rapidity of the onset of hyperkalemia[218,219] and the presence or absence of concomitant hypocalcemia, acidemia, and/or hyponatremia.[220,221] Hemodialysis patients[221] and patients with chronic renal failure[222] in particular may not demonstrate electrocardiographic changes. Care should also be taken to adequately distinguish the symmetrically peaked, church steeple T waves induced by hyperkalemia from T wave changes of other causes.[223] The ratio of precordial T wave to R wave amplitude (T/R ratio) may be a more specific sign of hyperkalemia than T wave tenting.[224]

Hyperkalemia can also rarely present with ascending paralysis,[21] termed *secondary hyperkalemic paralysis* to differentiate it from familial hyperkalemic periodic paralysis (HYPP). This presentation of hyperkalemia can mimic Guillain-Barré syndrome and may include diaphragmatic paralysis and respiratory failure.[225] Hyperkalemia from a diversity of causes can cause paralysis, as reviewed by Evers and colleagues.[226] The mechanism is not entirely clear; however, nerve conduction studies in one case suggested a neurogenic mechanism, rather than a direct effect on muscle excitability.[226]

In contrast to secondary hyperkalemic paralysis, HYPP is a primary myopathy. Patients with HYPP develop myopathic weakness during hyperkalemia induced by increased K^+ intake or rest after heavy exercise.[227] The hyperkalemic trigger in HYPP serves to differentiate this syndrome from hypokalemic periodic paralysis (HOKP); a further distinguishing feature is the presence of myotonia in HYPP.[227] Depolarization of skeletal muscle by hyperkalemia unmasks an inactivation defect in a tetrodotoxin-sensitive Na^+ channel in patients with HYPP, and autosomal dominant mutations in the *SCN4A* gene encoding this channel cause most forms of the disease.[228] Mild muscle depolarization (5 to 10 mV) in HYPP results in a persistent inward Na^+ current through the mutant channel; the normal, allelic SCN4 channels quickly recover from inactivation and can then be reactivated, resulting in myotonia. When muscle depolarization is more marked (20 to 30 mV), all the Na^+ channels are inactivated, rendering the muscle inexcitable and causing weakness (Figure 18.8). Related disorders due to mutations within the large SCN4A channel protein include HOKP type II,[229] paramyotonia congenita,[228] and K^+-aggravated myopathy.[228] American quarter horses have a high incidence (4.4%) of HYPP due to a mutation in equine *SCN4A* traced to the sire named *Impressive* (see Figure 18.8).[228] Finally, loss-of-function mutations in the muscle-specific K^+ channel subunit MinK-related peptide 2 (MiRP2) have also been shown to cause HYPP; MiRP2 and the associated Kv3.4 K^+ channel play a role in setting the resting membrane potential of skeletal muscle.[230]

RENAL CONSEQUENCES

Hyperkalemia has a significant effect on the ability to excrete an acid urine due to interference with the urinary excretion of ammonium (NH_4^+). Potassium loading in humans results in modest reduction in urinary NH_4^+ excretion and an impaired response to acid loading.[231] In rats, chronic potassium loading leads to hyperkalemia and a metabolic acidosis due to a 40% reduction in urinary NH_4^+ excretion.[232] Proximal tubular ammonia generation falls, but without a significant effect on proximal tubular secretion of NH_4^+.[232] The TAL absorbs NH_4^+ from the tubular lumen, followed by countercurrent multiplication and ultimately excretion from the medullary interstitium[233]; hyperkalemia appears to inhibit renal acid excretion by competing with NH_4^+ for reabsorption by the TAL.[234]

The NH_4^+ ion has the same ionic radius as K^+ and can be transported in lieu of K^+ by NKCC2,[235] the apical Na^+-K^+-NH_4^+-$2Cl^-$ cotransporter of the TAL; NH_4^+ exits the TAL via the basolateral Na^+-H^+ exchanger NHE4.[236] As is the case for other cations, countercurrent multiplication of NH_4^+ by the TAL greatly increases the concentration of NH_4^+-NH_3

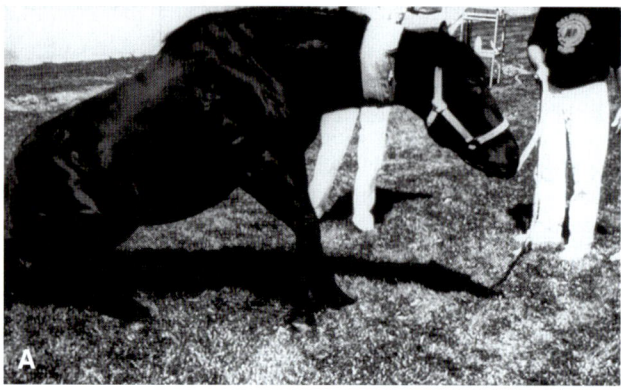

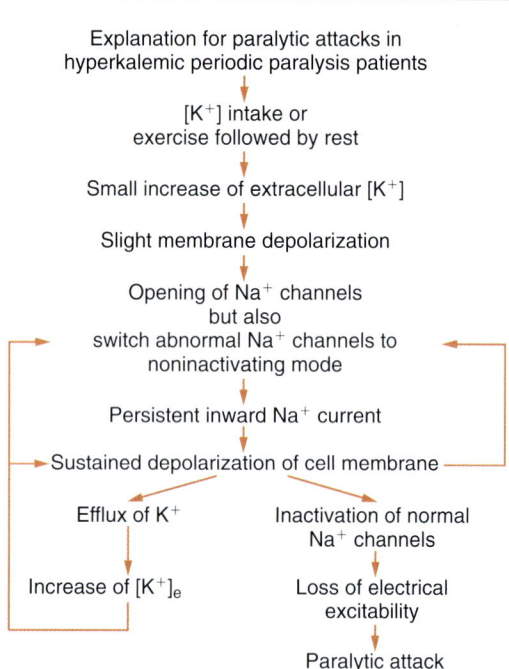

Figure 18.8 Hyperkalemic periodic paralysis (HYPP) due to mutations in the voltage-gated Na⁺ channel of skeletal muscle. **A,** This disorder is particularly common in thoroughbred quarter horses; an affected horse is shown during a paralytic attack, triggered by rest after heavy exercise. **B,** Mechanistic explanation for muscle paralysis in HYPP. (From Lehmann-Horn F, Jurkat-Rott K: Voltage-gated ion channels and hereditary disease. *Physiol Rev* 79:1317–1372, 1999; **A** courtesy Dr. Eric Hoffman).

available for secretion in the collecting duct. The NH_4^+ produced by the proximal tubule in response to acidosis is thus reabsorbed across the TAL, concentrated by countercurrent multiplication in the medullary interstitium, and secreted in the collecting duct. The capacity of the TAL to reabsorb NH_4^+ is increased during acidosis due to an induction of NKCC2[235] and NHE4 expression.[236] Hyperkalemia induces acidosis in rats by reducing the NH_4^+ between the vasa recta (surrogate for interstitial fluid) and collecting duct[234] due to interference with absorption of NH_4^+ by the TAL.

Clinically, patients with hyperkalemic acidosis due to hyporeninemic hypoaldosteronism demonstrate an increase in urinary NH_4^+ excretion in response to normalization of plasma K^+ with cation exchange resins,[237,238] indicating a significant role for hyperkalemia in generation of the acidosis.

HYPOKALEMIA

EPIDEMIOLOGY

Hypokalemia is a relatively common finding in outpatients and inpatients, perhaps the most common electrolyte abnormality encountered in clinical practice.[239] When defined as a serum K^+ less than 3.6 mmol/L, it is found in up to 20% of hospitalized patients[240]; defined as a serum K^+ less than 3.4 mmol/L, it occurs in 16.8% of first-time hospital admissions.[241] Hypokalemia is usually mild, with K^+ levels in the 3.0- to 3.5-mmol/L range, but in up to 25% of hypokalemic patients it can be moderate to severe (<3.0 mmol/L).[240,242] The most common causative factors in hospitalized patients with hypokalemia are gastrointestinal losses of potassium, diuretic therapy, and hypomagnesemia.[243] It is a particularly prominent problem in patients receiving thiazide diuretics for hypertension, with an incidence of up to 48% (average, 15% to 30%).[28,244] The thiazide-type diuretic metolazone is frequently used in the management of heart failure refractory to loop diuretics alone, causing moderate ($K^+ \leq 3.0$ mmol/L) or severe ($K^+ \leq 2.5$ mmol/L) hypokalemia in approximately 40% and 10% of patients, respectively.[245] Hypokalemia is also a common finding in patients receiving peritoneal dialysis, with 10% to 20% requiring potassium supplementation.[246] Hypokalemia per se can increase in-hospital mortality rate up to 10-fold,[241,242] likely due to the profound effects on arrhythmogenesis, blood pressure, and cardiovascular morbidity.[208,247]

SPURIOUS HYPOKALEMIA

Delayed sample analysis is a well-recognized cause of spurious hypokalemia due to increased cellular uptake; this may become clinically relevant if the ambient temperature is increased.[28,248,249] Very rarely, patients with profound leukocytosis due to acute leukemia present with artifactual hypokalemia caused by time-dependent uptake of K^+ by the large white cell mass.[248] Such patients do not develop clinical or electrocardiographic complications of hypokalemia, and plasma K^+ is normal if measured immediately after venipuncture.

REDISTRIBUTION AND HYPOKALEMIA

Manipulation of the factors affecting internal distribution of K^+ (see "Factors Affecting Internal Distribution of Potassium") can cause hypokalemia due to redistribution of K^+ between the extracellular and intracellular compartments. Endogenous insulin is rarely a cause of hypokalemia, but administered insulin is a frequent cause of iatrogenic hypokalemia[240] and may be a factor in what has been termed the *dead in bed syndrome* associated with aggressive glycemic control.[250] Insulin also may play a significant role in the hypokalemia associated with refeeding syndrome.[251] Alterations in the activity of the endogenous sympathetic nervous system can cause hypokalemia in several settings, including alcohol withdrawal,[252] acute myocardial infarction,[208,253] and head injury.[254,255] Redistributive hypokalemia after severe head injury can be truly profound, with reported serum K^+ of 1.2 mmol/L[254] and 1.9 mmol/L[255] and marked rebound hyperkalemia after repletion.

Due to their ability to activate Na^+-K^+-ATPase[49] and the Na^+-K^+-$2Cl^-$ cotransporter NKCC1,[21,27] β_2-agonists are powerful activators of cellular K^+ uptake. These agents are chiefly encountered in the therapy of asthma, but tocolytics such as ritodrine can induce hypokalemia and arrhythmias during maternal labor.[256] The long-acting β_2-agonist clenbuterol, not approved for medical use in the United States, has caused hypokalemia in poisonings, including an outbreak of toxicity from clenbuterol-adulterated heroin in the East Coast of the United States.[257] Occult sources of sympathomimetics, such as pseudoephedrine and ephedrine in cough syrup[193] or dieting agents,[258] can be an overlooked cause of hypokalemia. Finally, downstream activation of cAMP by xanthines such as theophylline[21,259] and dietary caffeine[260] may induce hypokalemia and may synergize in this respect with β_2-agonists.[261]

Whereas β_2-agonists activate K^+ uptake via Na^+-K^+-ATPase, one would expect that inhibition of passive K^+ efflux would also lead to hypokalemia; this is accomplished by barium, a potent inhibitor of inward-rectifying K^+ channels.[262] This rare cause of hypokalemia is usually due to ingestion of the rodenticide barium carbonate, either unintentionally or during a suicide attempt.[263] Suicidal ingestion of barium-containing shaving powder[264] and hair remover[265] has also been described. Barium salts are widely used in industry, and poisoning has been described by various mechanisms in industrial accidents.[21,266] Patients have a particularly prominent U wave, likely due to direct inhibition of cardiac inward-rectifying K^+ channels.[262] Muscle paralysis can also occur[262] due to inhibition of muscle Kir channels. Treatment of barium poisoning with K^+ serves to increase plasma K^+ and displace barium from affected K^+ channels[263]; hemodialysis is also an effective treatment.[267] Hypokalemia is also common with chloroquine toxicity or overdose,[268] although the mechanism is not entirely clear.

HYPOKALEMIC PERIODIC PARALYSIS

The periodic paralyses have genetic and acquired causes and are further subdivided into hyperkalemic and hypokalemic forms.[21,227-229] The genetic and secondary forms of hyperkalemic paralysis are discussed earlier (see "Consequences of Hyperkalemia"). Autosomal dominant mutations in the CACNA1S gene encoding the α_1-subunit of L-type calcium channels are the most common genetic cause of hypokalemic periodic paralysis (HOKP type I), whereas type II HOKP is due to mutations in the SCN4A gene encoding the skeletal Na^+ channel.[269] In Andersen's syndrome, autosomal dominant mutations in the KCNJ2 gene encoding the inwardly rectifying K^+ channel Kir2.1 cause periodic paralysis, cardiac arrhythmias, and dysmorphic features.[270] Paralysis in Andersen's syndrome can be normokalemic, hypokalemic, or hyperkalemic; however, the symptomatic trigger is consistent within individual kindreds.[270]

The pathophysiology of HOKP is complex. Structurally, about 90% of the HOKP-associated mutations result in loss of positively charged arginine residues in the S4, voltage sensor domains of L-type calcium channels and the skeletal Na^+ channel.[229] This generates a so-called gating current generated by a cation leak through an aberrant pore; this abnormal cation leak may directly lead to K^+-dependent paradoxic depolarization and hypokalemic weakness.[271] Muscles of a Na^+ channel knock-in mutant mouse ($Na_v1.4$-R669H) also exhibit an anomalous inward current at hyperpolarized potentials, attributed to this gating pore current.[272]

Abnormalities in insulin-sensitive transport events may also contribute to the hypokalemic weakness in HOKP. Reversible attacks of paralysis with hypokalemia in HOKP are typically precipitated by rest after exercise and/or meals rich in carbohydrate.[229] Although the induction of endogenous insulin by carbohydrate meals is thought to reduce plasma K^+, thus triggering weakness, insulin can precipitate paralysis in HOKP in the absence of significant hypokalemia.[273] The generation of action potentials and muscle contraction are reduced in types I and II HOKP muscle fibers exposed to insulin in vitro[269,274]; this effect is seen at an extracellular K^+ of 4.0 mmol/L and is potentiated as K^+ decreases.[274] Type I HOKP muscles have a reduced activity of ATP-sensitive, inward-rectifying K^+ channels (K_{ATP}),[275,276] which likely contributes to hypokalemia due to the resultant unopposed activity of muscle Na^+-K^+-ATPase.[277] Insulin inhibits the remaining K_{ATP} activity in muscle fibers of type I HOKP patients[274] and hypokalemic rats,[278] resulting in a depolarizing shift toward the equilibrium potential for the Cl^- ion (≈ 50 mV); at this potential, voltage-dependent Na^+ channels are largely inactivated, resulting in paralysis.

Paralysis is associated with multiple other causes of hypokalemia, acquired and genetic.[192,193,279] Renal causes of hypokalemia with paralysis include Fanconi's syndrome,[280] Gitelman's syndrome,[279] and the various causes of hypokalemic distal renal tubular acidosis.[28,281] The activity and regulation of skeletal muscle K_{ATP} channels are aberrant in animal models of hypokalemia, suggesting a parallel muscle physiology to that of genetic HOKP (see earlier). However, the pathophysiology of thyrotoxic periodic paralysis (TPP), a particularly important cause of hypokalemic paralysis, is distinctly different from that of HOKP; for example, despite the clinical similarities between the two syndromes, thyroxine has no effect on HOKP.

TPP is classically seen in patients of Asian origin, but also occurs at higher frequencies in Hispanic patients[282]; this shared predisposition has been linked to genetic variation in Kir2.6, a muscle-specific, thyroid hormone–responsive K^+ channel.[29] Patients typically present with weakness of the extremities and limb girdles, with attacks occurring most frequently between 1 and 6 AM. As in HOKP, paralytic attacks in TPP may be precipitated by rest and/or by carbohydrate-rich meals. Clinical signs and symptoms of hyperthyroidism are not invariably present.[282,283] Hypokalemia is profound, with K^+ ranging between 1.1 and 3.4 mol/L, and is frequently accompanied by hypophosphatemia and hypomagnesemia[282]; all three abnormalities presumably contribute to the associated weakness. Diagnostically, a TTKG of less than 2 to 3 separates patients with TPP from those with hypokalemia due to renal potassium wasting, who will have TTKG values that are more than 4.[178] This distinction is of considerable therapeutic relevance; patients with large potassium deficits require aggressive repletion with

K^+-Cl^-, which has a significant risk of rebound hyperkalemia in TPP and related disorders.[284]

The hypokalemia in TPP is most likely due to direct and indirect activation of Na^+-K^+-ATPase, given the evidence for increased activity in erythrocytes and platelets in TPP patients.[28,285] Thyroid hormone clearly induces expression of multiple subunits of Na^+-K^+-ATPase in skeletal muscle.[286] Increases in β-adrenergic responses due to hyperthyroidism also play an important role, since high-dose propranolol (3 mg/kg) rapidly reverses the hypokalemia, hypophosphatemia, and paralysis seen in acute attacks.[287,288] Of particular importance, no rebound hyperkalemia is associated with this treatment, whereas aggressive K^+ replacement in TPP is associated with an incidence of about 25%[284]; repletion-associated rebound hyperkalemia in TPP can be fatal.[289]

Outward-directed, inward-rectifying K^+ current, mediated by Kir channels (particularly Kir2.6 and Kir2.1), is also reduced in skeletal muscles of patients with TPP,[276] providing an additional mechanism for hypokalemia. In patients with Kir2.6 mutations, this reduction is at least in part hereditary.[29] Together with increased Na^+-K^+-ATPase activity and increased circulating insulin, this reduced Kir current may trigger a feed-forward cycle of hypokalemia, leading to inactivation of muscle Na^+ channels, paradoxic depolarization, and paralysis.[290]

POTASSIUM LOSS

NONRENAL POTASSIUM LOSS

The loss of K^+ from skin is typically low, with the exception of extremes in physical exertion.[11] Direct gastric loss of K^+ due to vomiting or nasogastric suctioning is also typically minimal; however, the ensuing hypochloremic alkalosis results in persistent kaliuresis due to secondary hyperaldosteronism and bicarbonaturia.[291,292] Intestinal loss of K^+ due to diarrhea is a quantitatively important cause of hypokalemia, given the worldwide prevalence of diarrheal disease, and may be associated with acute complications, such as myopathy and flaccid paralysis.[293] The presence of a non–anion gap metabolic acidosis with a negative urinary anion gap[179] (consistent with an intact ability to increase NH_4^+ excretion) should strongly suggest diarrhea as a cause of hypokalemia. Polyethylene glycol–based bowel preparation regimens for colonoscopy can also lead to hypokalemia in older patients.[294] Noninfectious gastrointestinal processes such as celiac disease,[295] ileostomy,[296] and chronic laxative abuse can present with acute hypokalemic syndromes or with chronic complications, such as ESKD.[21]

Three reports initially identified a novel association between colonic pseudo-obstruction (Ogilvie's syndrome) and hypokalemia due to secretory diarrhea with an abnormally high K^+ content.[297-299] In one patient with concomitant ESKD, immunohistochemistry revealed massive upregulation of the apical BK channel throughout the surface crypt axes[297]; colonic BK channels may play a significant role in intestinal K^+ secretion in a variety of pathologies, including ESKD.[300] Several hypotheses for the association between Ogilvie's syndrome and enhanced intestinal K^+ secretion have been postulated, including active stimulation by catecholamines induced by colonic pseudo-obstruction[299]; BK channels appear to mediate adrenaline-induced colonic K^+ secretion.[301]

Increased fecal loss of K^+ may play a broader role in hypokalemia associated with diarrhea.[300] Recruitment of colonic BK channels along intestinal crypts, similar to that seen in Ogilvie's syndrome, has thus been demonstrated as a consistent feature of colonic biopsies in ulcerative colitis.[302] Direct enhancement of intestinal K^+ excretion has also been demonstrated in a hypokalemic patient with Crohn's disease following treatment with budesonide.[303]

RENAL POTASSIUM LOSS

Drugs

Diuretics are an especially important cause of hypokalemia due to their ability to increase distal flow rate and distal delivery of Na^+. For a given degree of natriuresis, thiazides generally cause more profound degrees of hypokalemia[21,210,244] than loop diuretics, despite their lower natriuretic efficacy. One potential explanation is the differential effect of loop diuretics and thiazides on calcium excretion. Whereas thiazides and loss-of-function mutations in the Na^+-Cl^- cotransporter decrease Ca^{2+} excretion,[304] loop diuretics cause a significant calciuresis.[305] Increases in luminal Ca^{2+} in the distal nephron serve to reduce the lumen-negative driving force for K^+ excretion,[306] perhaps by direct inhibition of ENaC in principal cells. A mechanistic explanation is provided by the presence of an apical calcium-sensing receptor (CaSR) in the collecting duct[307]; analogous to the evident decrease in the apical trafficking of aquaporin-2 induced by luminal Ca^{2+}, tubular Ca^{2+} may stimulate endocytosis of ENaC via the CaSR and thus limit generation of the lumen-negative potential difference that is so critical for distal K^+ excretion. Regardless of the underlying mechanism, the increase in distal delivery of Ca^{2+} induced by loop diuretics may serve to blunt kaliuresis; such a mechanism would not occur with thiazides, which reduce distal delivery of Ca^{2+}, with unopposed activity of ENaC and increased kaliuresis.

Some studies have also indicated a key role in K^+ homeostasis for NCC, the thiazide-sensitive Na^+-Cl^- cotransporter in the DCT, so it is not surprising that thiazide treatment has such potent effects on serum K^+. Selective increases in DCT and NCC activity, as seen in FHHt, reduce Na^+ delivery to principal cells in the downstream CNT and CCD, leading to hyperkalemia.[71] The DCT also clearly functions as a potassium sensor, directly responding to changes in circulating potassium.[3] A high-K^+ diet also inactivates NCC, whereas NCC is activated in hypokalemia.[140]

Other drugs associated with hypokalemia due to kaliuresis include toxic levels of acetaminophen, which causes dose-dependent hypokalemia.[308,309] High doses of penicillin-related antibiotics are another important cause of hypokalemia, increasing obligatory K^+ excretion by acting as nonreabsorbable anions in the distal nephron; in addition to penicillin, implicated antibiotics include nafcillin, dicloxacillin, ticarcillin, oxacillin, and carbenecillin.[310] Increased distal delivery of other anions such as SO_4^{2-} and HCO_3^- also induces a kaliuresis. The usual explanation is that K^+ excretion increases so as to balance the negative charge of these nonreabsorbable anions. However, increased delivery of such anions will also increase the electrochemical gradient for K^+-Cl^- exit via apical K^+-Cl^- cotransport or parallel K^+-H^+ and Cl^--HCO_3^- exchange[68,82,83] (see also "Potassium

Transport in the Distal Nephron"). Drugs are also an important cause of Fanconi's syndrome,[311] which is often associated with significant hypokalemia (see "Renal Tubular Acidosis").

Several tubular toxins result in K[+] and magnesium wasting. These include gentamicin, which can cause tubular toxicity with hypokalemia that can masquerade as Bartter's syndrome.[312] Other drugs that can cause mixed magnesium and K[+] wasting include amphotericin, foscarnet,[313] cisplatin,[21,314] and ifosfamide.[315] One intriguing cause of hypomagnesemia and hypokalemia is cetuximab, a humanized monoclonal antibody specific for the receptor for epidermal growth factor (EGF)[316]; paracrine EGF stimulates magnesium transport via the apical TRPM6 cation channel in the DCT, with magnesium wasting and hypomagnesemia in patients treated with cetuximab.[317] Aggressive replacement of magnesium is obligatory in the treatment of combined hypokalemia and hypomagnesemia, since successful K[+] replacement depends on treatment of the hypomagnesemia.

Hyperaldosteronism

Increases in circulating aldosterone (hyperaldosteronism) may be primary or secondary. Increased levels of circulating renin in secondary forms of hyperaldosteronism lead to increased levels of Ang II, and thus aldosterone, and can be associated with hypokalemia; causes include renal artery stenosis,[318] Page kidney (renal compression by a subcapsular mass or hematoma, with hyperreninemia),[319] a paraneoplastic process,[320] or renin-secreting renal tumors.[321] The incidence of hypokalemia in renal artery stenosis is thought to be less than 20%.[318] An unusual presentation of renal artery stenosis and renal ischemia is what has been termed the *hyponatremic hypertensive syndrome,* in which concurrent hypokalemia may be profound.[322]

Primary hyperaldosteronism may be genetic or acquired. Hypertension and hypokalemia, generally attributed to increases in circulating 11-deoxycorticosterone,[323] are seen in patients with congenital adrenal hyperplasia due to defects in steroid 11β-hydroxylase[323] or steroid 17α-hydroxylase[324]; deficient 11β-hydroxylase results in virilization and other signs of androgen excess,[323] whereas reduced sex steroids in 17α-hydroxylase deficiency result in hypogonadism.[324] The two major forms of isolated PA are denoted familial hyperaldosteronism type I (FH-I, also known as glucocorticoid-remediable hyperaldosteronism [GRA])[325] and familial hyperaldosteronism type II (FH-II), in which aldosterone production is not repressible by exogenous glucocorticoids. Patients with FH-II are clinically indistinguishable from sporadic forms of PA due to bilateral adrenal hyperplasia; a gene has been localized to chromosome 7p22 by linkage analysis, but has yet to be characterized.[326] A third form of familial hyperaldosteronism (FH-III) was initially described in 2008, with hyporeninemia, hyperaldosteronism resistant to dexamethasone, and very high levels of 18-oxocortisol and 18-hydroxycortisol.[327] FH-III is due to somatic mutations in the adrenal K[+] channel KCNJ5, which endow the channel with a novel Na[+] conductance and activate adrenal glomerulosa proliferation and aldosterone release[1]; somatic mutations in KCNJ5 are also found in spontaneous adrenal adenomas (see later).

Patients with FH-I (GRA) are generally hypertensive, typically presenting at an early age; the severity of hypertension is variable, however, such that some affected individuals are normotensive.[325] Aldosterone levels are modestly elevated and regulated solely by ACTH. The diagnosis can be biochemically confirmed by a dexamethasone suppression test, with a suppression of aldosterone to less than 4 ng/dL consistent with the diagnosis.[328] Patients also have high levels of abnormal hybrid 18-hydroxylated steroids, generated by transformation of steroids typically formed in the zona fasciculata by aldosterone synthase, an enzyme that is normally expressed in the zona glomerulosa.[329,330] FH-I has been shown to be caused by a chimeric gene duplication between the homologous 11β-hydroxylase gene (*CYP11B1*) and aldosterone synthase gene (*CYP11B2*), fusing the ACTH-responsive 11β-hydroxylase promoter to the coding region of aldosterone synthase. This chimeric gene is thus under the control of ACTH and is expressed in a glucocorticoid-repressible fashion.[329] Ectopic expression of the hybrid *CYP11B1-CYP11B1* gene in the zona fasciculata has been reported in a single case in which adrenal tissue became available for molecular analysis.[331] Direct genetic testing for the hybrid *CYP11B1-CYP11B2* has largely supplanted biochemical screening for FH-I; genetic testing for FH-I should be pursued in patients with PA and a family history of PA and/or of strokes at a young age, or in younger patients with PA (age < 20 years).[332]

Although the initial patients reported with FH-I were hypokalemic, most are normokalemic,[330,333] albeit perhaps with a propensity to develop hypokalemia while on thiazide diuretics.[330] Patients with FH-I are able to increase K[+] excretion appropriately in response to K[+] loading or fludrocortisone, but fail to increase plasma aldosterone in response to hyperkalemia.[334] This may reflect the ectopic expression of the chimeric aldosterone synthase in the adrenal fasciculata, which likely lacks the appropriate constellation of ion channels to respond to increases in extracellular K[+] with an increase in aldosterone secretion.

Acquired causes of PA include aldosterone-producing adenomas (APAs; 35% of cases), primary (or unilateral) adrenal hyperplasia (PAH; 2% of cases), idiopathic hyperaldosteronism (IHA) due to bilateral adrenal hyperplasia (60% of cases), and adrenal carcinoma (<1% of cases).[335] A rare case involving paraneoplastic overexpression of aldosterone synthase in lymphoma has also been described.[336]

The molecular characterization of adrenal adenomas with whole-genome sequencing and related techniques has been remarkably fruitful. In particular, acquired mutations in the adrenal K[+] channel KCNJ5 can be detected in about 40% of aldosterone-producing adrenal adenomas.[165] As in FH-III (see earlier), these somatic mutations endow the channel with a novel Na[+] conductance, leading to adrenal glomerulosa cell depolarization, Ca[2+] influx, and aldosterone release. Clinically, patients with adrenal KCNJ5 mutations have a higher preoperative aldosterone level[165] and higher lateralization index in adrenal vein sampling,[337] without affecting the surgical response to adrenalectomy.[165] Less frequently, somatic mutations in adrenal adenomas can be detected in the calcium channel CACNA1D[338] or in a subunit (ATP2B3) of the Ca[2+]-ATPase pump,[339] predicted also to lead to increased Ca[2+] influx and aldosterone release.[338] Acquired mutations in the ATP1A α1-subunit of

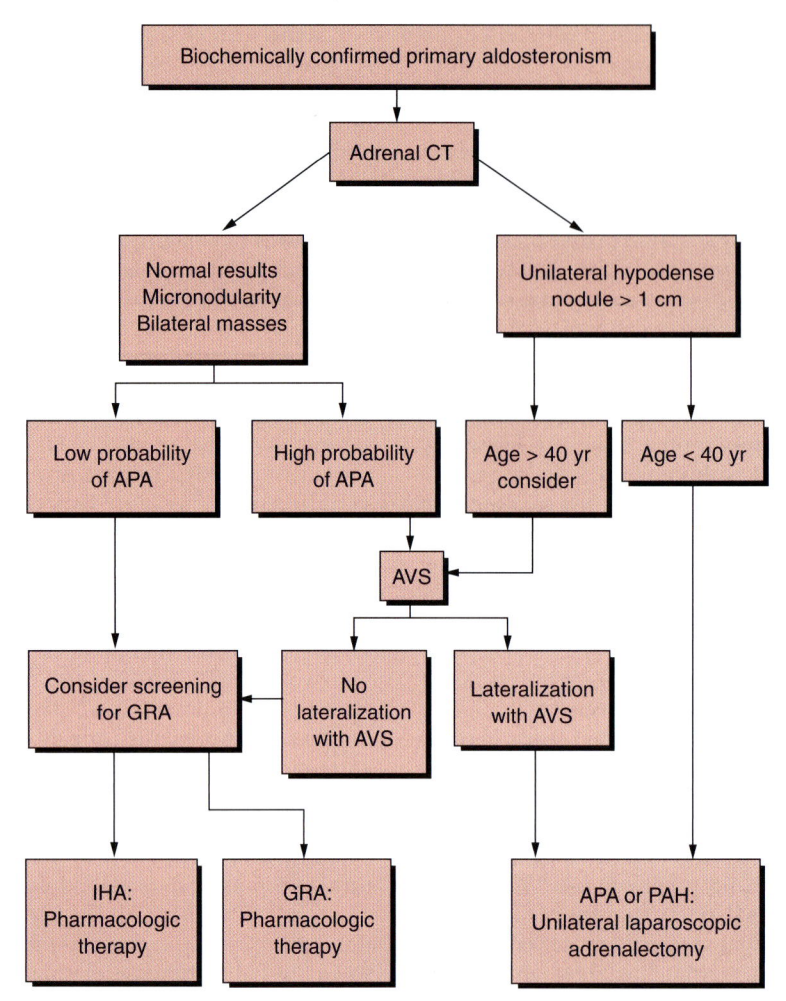

Figure 18.9 Diagnostic algorithm for patients with primary hyperaldosteronism. Adrenal adenoma (APA) must be distinguished from glucocorticoid remediable hyperaldosteronism (FH-I [GRA]), primary or unilateral adrenal hyperplasia (PAH), and idiopathic hyperaldosteronism (IHA). This requires computed tomography (CT), adrenal venous sampling (AVS), and the relevant diagnostic biochemical and hormonal assays (see text). (From Young WF Jr: Adrenalectomy for primary aldosteronism. *Ann Intern Med* 138:157-159, 2003.)

Na+-K+-ATPase are in turn thought to generate chronic depolarization, leading also to exaggerated aldosterone release.[339]

Increasing use of the plasma aldosterone concentration (PAC)/plasma renin activity (PRA) ratio in hypertension clinics has led to reports of a much higher incidence of PA than previously appreciated, with incidence rates in hypertension ranging from 0% to 72%[340]; however, the prevalence was 3.2% in a large multicenter study of patients with mild to moderate hypertension without hypokalemia.[341] Regardless, the PAC/PRA ratio is a screening tool, which typically must be confirmed by aldosterone suppression testing, which measures PAC or aldosterone secretion after loading with salt or intravenous saline.[332,335] After controlling hypertension and hypokalemia, oral salt loading over 3 days is followed by measurement of 24-hour urine aldosterone, sodium, and creatinine excretion. The 24-hour sodium excretion should exceed 200 mmol/day for adequate suppression, and a urinary aldosterone of more than 33 nmol/day (12 μm/day) is consistent with PA. Alternatively, in the saline infusion test, recumbent patients are infused with 2 L of isotonic saline over 4 hours, followed by measurement of PAC. In patients without PA, the measured PAC after saline infusion should decrease to less than 139 pmol/L. The measured PAC in patients with PA usually does not decrease to less than 277 pmol/L; indeterminate values between 139 and 277 pmol/L can been seen in patients with IHA.[335] It should be noted, however, that patients with high-probability factors (hypokalemia, hypertension, high PAC/PRA ratio, abnormalities) may not necessarily require confirmatory testing, proceeding instead directly to adrenal venous sampling.[342]

Since surgery can be curative in APA, adequate differentiation of APA from IHA is critical; this requires adrenal imaging and adrenal venous sampling (Figure 18.9). Contemporary reports and recommendations have thus emphasized the continued importance of adrenal vein sampling in subtype differentiation.[332] Laparoscopic adrenalectomy has increasingly been the preferred surgical management for APA or PAH.[332,335] Mineralocorticoid receptor antagonists are indicated for medical therapy of PA, with carefully monitored use of glucocorticoid to suppress ACTH in some patients with FH-I.[332,335]

The true incidence of hypokalemia in patients with acquired forms of PA remains difficult to evaluate due to a variety of factors. First, historically, patients have only been screened for hyperaldosteronism when hypokalemia is present, so even case series from clinics with such a referral pattern may suffer from a selection bias; other series have concentrated on hypertensive patients, also with a selection bias. Second, the incidence of hypokalemia is higher in adrenal adenomas than in IHA, likely due to higher average levels of aldosterone.[343] Third, since increased kaliuresis in hyperaldosteronism can be induced by dietary Na^+-Cl^- loading or diuretics, dietary factors and/or medications may play a role in the incidence of hypokalemia at presentation. Regardless, it is clear that hypokalemia is not a universal feature of PA; this is perhaps not unexpected, since aldosterone does not appear to affect the hypokalemic response of H^+-K^+-ATPase,[344] the major reabsorptive pathway for K^+ in the distal nephron (see also Chapter 6). A related issue is whether PA is underdiagnosed when hypokalemia is used as a criterion for further investigation; the utility of the PAC/PRA ratio in screening for hyperaldosteronism is an active issue in hypertension research.[340,341]

Finally, hypokalemia may also occur with systemic increases in glucocorticoids.[345,346] In bona fide Cushing's syndrome caused by increases in pituitary ACTH, the incidence of hypokalemia is only 10%,[345] whereas it is 57%[346] to 100%[345] in patients with ectopic ACTH, despite a similar incidence of hypertension. Ectopic ACTH expression is associated primarily with neuroendocrine malignancies, most commonly bronchial carcinoid tumors, small lung cancer, and other neuroendocrine tumors.[347] Indirect evidence suggests that the activity of renal 11β-hydroxysteroid dehydrogenase-2 (11βHSD-2) is reduced in patients with ectopic ACTH compared with Cushing's syndrome,[348] resulting in a syndrome of apparent mineralocorticoid excess (see later). Whether this reflects a greater degree of saturation of the enzyme by circulating cortisol or direct inhibition of 11βHSD-2 by ACTH is not entirely clear, and there is evidence for both mechanisms[346]; however, indirect indices of 11βHSD-2 activity in patients with ectopic ACTH expression correlate with hypokalemia and other measures of mineralocorticoid activity.[349] Similar mechanisms likely underlie the severe hypokalemia reported in patients with familial glucocorticoid resistance, in which loss-of-function mutations in the glucocorticoid receptor result in marked hypercortisolism without cushingoid features, accompanied by very high ACTH levels.[350]

Syndromes of Apparent Mineralocorticoid Excess

The syndromes of apparent mineralocorticoid excess (AME) have a self-explanatory label. In the classic form of AME, recessive loss-of-function mutations in the 11β-hydroxysteroid dehydrogenase-2 gene (*11βHSD-2*) cause a defect in the peripheral conversion of cortisol to the inactive glucocorticoid cortisone; the resulting increase in the half-life of cortisol is associated with a marked decrease in synthesis, such that plasma levels of cortisol are normal and patients are not cushingoid.[351] The 11βHSD-2 protein is expressed in epithelial cells that are targets for aldosterone; in the kidney, these include cells of the DCT, CNT, and CCD.[352] Since the mineralocorticoid receptor (MR) has equivalent affinity for aldosterone and cortisol, generation of cortisone by 11βHSD-2 serves to protect mineralocorticoid-responsive cells from illicit activation by cortisol.[353] In patients with AME, the unregulated mineralocorticoid effect of glucocorticoids results in hypertension, hypokalemia, and metabolic alkalosis, with suppressed PRA and aldosterone levels.[351] Biochemical diagnosis entails measuring the urinary free cortisol to urinary free cortisone ratio on a 24-hour urine collection. Biochemical studies of mutant enzymes usually indicate a complete loss of function; lesser enzymatic defects in patients with AME are associated with altered ratios of urinary cortisone-cortisol metabolites,[354] lesser impairment in the peripheral conversion of cortisol to cortisone,[355] and/or older age at presentation.[356]

Mice with a homozygous targeted deletion of *11βHsd-2* exhibit hypertension, hypokalemia, and polyuria; the polyuria is likely secondary to the hypokalemia (see "Consequences of Hypokalemia: Renal Consequences"), which reaches 2.4 mmol/mL in *11βHsd-2* null mice.[357] As expected, PRA and plasma aldosterone levels in the *11βHsd-2*-null mice are profoundly suppressed, with a decreased urinary Na^+/K^+ ratio that is increased by dexamethasone (given to suppress endogenous cortisol). These knockout mice have significant nephromegaly, due to a massive hypertrophy and hyperplasia of distal convoluted tubules. The relative effect of genotype on the morphology of cells in the DCT, CNT, and CCD was not determined by appropriate phenotypic studies[358]; however, it is known that the DCT and CCD are target cells for aldosterone,[359,360] and both cell types express 11βHSD-2. The induction of ENaC activity by unregulated glucocorticoid likely causes the Na^+ retention and marked increase in K^+ excretion in *11βHsd-2* null mice; distal tubular micropuncture studies in rats treated with a systemic inhibitor of 11βHSD-2 are consistent with such a mechanism.[361] In addition, the cellular gain of function in the DCT would be expected to be associated with hypercalciuria, given the phenotype of pseudohypoaldosteronism type II and Gitelman's syndrome (see "Hereditary Tubular Causes of Hyperkalemia" and later, "Gitelman's Syndrome"); indeed, patients with AME are reported to exhibit nephrocalcinosis.[351]

Pharmacologic inhibition of 11βHSD-2 is also associated with hypokalemia and AME. The most infamous offender is licorice, in its multiple guises (e.g., licorice root, tea, candies, herbal remedies). The early observations that licorice required small amounts of cortisol to exert its kaliuretic effect, in the addisonian absence of endogenous glucocorticoid,[362] presaged the observations that its active ingredients (glycyrrhetinic acid or glycyrrhizinic acid and carbenoxolone) inhibit 11βHSD-2 and related enzymes.[351] Licorice intake remains considerable in European countries, particularly Iceland, the Netherlands, and Scandinavia[363]; Pontefract cakes, eaten as sweets and as a laxative, are a continued source of licorice in the United Kingdom,[363] whereas it is an ingredient in several popular sweeteners and preservatives in Malaysia.[364] Glycyrrhizinic acid is used in Japan to treat hepatitis and has been under evaluation elsewhere for the management of hepatitis C; AME has been reported with its use for this indication.[365] Glycyrrhizinic acid is also a component of Chinese herbal remedies, prescribed for disorders such as allergic rhinitis.[366] Pharmacologic inhibition of 11βHSD-2 has also been tested in patients with ESKD as a novel mechanism to control hyperkalemia (see "Treatment of Hyperkalemia").[367] Carbenoxolone is, in turn, used in some countries in the management of peptic ulcer disease.[351]

Finally, a mechanistically distinct form of AME has been reported due to a gain-of-function mutation in the MR.[368] A single kindred has been described with autosomal dominant inheritance of severe hypertension and hypokalemia; the causative mutation involves a serine residue that is conserved in the MR from multiple species, yet differs in other nuclear steroid receptors. This mutation results in constitutive activation of the MR in the absence of ligand and induces significant affinity for progesterone.[368] The MR is thus constitutively "on" in these patients, with a marked stimulation by progesterone; of interest, pregnancies in the affected female members of the family were all complicated by severe hypertension due to marked increases in plasma progesterone induced by the gravid state.[368]

Liddle's Syndrome

Liddle's syndrome constitutes an autosomal dominant gain in function of ENaC, the amiloride-sensitive Na$^+$ channel of the CNT and CCD.[369] Patients manifest severe hypertension with hypokalemia, unresponsive to spironolactone yet sensitive to triamterene and amiloride. Liddle's syndrome could therefore also be classified as a syndrome of apparent mineralocorticoid excess. Both hypertension and hypokalemia are variable aspects of the Liddle's phenotype; consistent features include a blunted aldosterone response to ACTH and reduced urinary aldosterone excretion.[98,370] The differential diagnosis for Liddle's syndrome, as a cause of hereditary hypertension with hypokalemia and suppressed aldosterone, includes AME due to deficient 11βHSD-2; however, whereas the Liddle's syndrome phenotype is resistant to blockade of the MR with spironolactone and sensitive to amiloride, AME patients are sensitive to both drugs. Commercial genetic testing for both syndromes is available in the United States.

The vast majority of mutations target the C terminus of the β- or γ-ENaC subunit. ENaC channels containing Liddle's syndrome mutations are constitutively overexpressed at the cell membrane[99,371]; unlike wild-type ENaC channels, they are not sensitive to inhibition by intracellular Na$^+$,[372] an important regulator of endogenous channel activity in the CCD.[373] The mechanism whereby mutations in the C terminus of ENaC subunits lead to this channel phenotype have been discussed earlier in this chapter (see Figure 18.5 and "Control of Potassium Secretion: Aldosterone"). In addition to effects on interaction with Nedd4-2–dependent retrieval from the plasma membrane, Liddle's syndrome–associated mutations increase proteolytic cleavage of ENaC at the cell membrane[374]; aldosterone-induced channel-activating proteases activate ENaC channels at the plasma membrane. This important result provides a mechanistic explanation for the long-standing observation that Liddle's syndrome–associated mutations in ENaC appear to have a dual activating effect on both the open probability of the channel (i.e., on channel activity) and on expression at the cell membrane.[99]

Given the overlapping and synergistic mechanisms that regulate ENaC activity, it stands to reason that mutations in ENaC that give rise to Liddle's syndrome might do so by a variety of means. Indeed, mutation of a residue within the extracellular domain of ENaC increases open probability of the channel without changing surface expression; the patient with this mutation has a typical Liddle's syndrome phenotype.[375] Extensive searches for more common mutations and polymorphisms in ENaC subunits that correlate with blood pressure in the general population have essentially been negative. However, there are a handful of genetic studies that correlate specific variants in ENaC subunits with biochemical evidence of greater in vivo activity of the channel—that is, a suppressed PRA and aldosterone and/or increased ratios of the urinary K$^+$ level to aldosterone or to PRA.[376,377]

Familial Hypokalemic Alkalosis

Bartter's Syndrome. Bartter's and Gitelman's syndromes are the two major variants of familial hypokalemic alkalosis; Gitelman's syndrome is a much more common cause of hypokalemia than Bartter's syndrome.[378] Whereas a clinical subdivision of these syndromes has been used in the past, a genetic classification is increasingly in use, due in part to phenotypic overlap. Patients with classic Bartter's syndrome (BS) typically suffer from polyuria and polydipsia and manifest a hypokalemic, hypochloremic alkalosis. They may have an increase in urinary calcium (Ca^{2+}) excretion, and 20% are hypomagnesemic.[379] Other features include marked elevation of plasma Ang II, plasma aldosterone, and plasma renin levels. Patients with antenatal BS present earlier in life with a severe systemic disorder characterized by marked electrolyte wasting, polyhydramnios, and significant hypercalciuria with nephrocalcinosis. Prostaglandin synthesis and excretion is significantly increased and may account for many of the systemic symptoms. Decreasing prostaglandin synthesis by COX inhibition can improve polyuria in patients with BS by reducing the amplifying inhibition of urine-concentrating mechanisms by prostaglandins. Indomethacin also increases plasma K$^+$ and decreases plasma renin activity, but does not correct the basic tubular defect; it does, however, appear to help increase the growth of BS patients.[380] Of interest, COX-2 immunoreactivity is increased in the TAL and macula densa of patients with BS,[381] and studies have indicated a clinical benefit of COX-2 inhibitors.[382]

Early studies in BS have suggested that these patients have a defect in the function of the TAL.[383] Many of the clinical features are mimicked by the administration of loop diuretics, to which at least a subset of patients with antenatal BS do not respond.[384] The apical Na$^+$-K$^+$-2Cl$^-$ cotransporter (NKCC2, SLC12A1) of the mammalian TAL[26] (Figure 18.10) was thus an early candidate gene. In 1996, disease-associated mutations were found in the human NKCC2 gene in four kindreds with antenatal BS[385]; in the genetic classification of BS, these patients are considered to have BS type I. Although the functional consequences of disease-associated NKCC2 mutations have not been comprehensively studied, the first[385] and subsequent reports[28] included patients with frameshift mutations and premature stop codons that predicted the absence of a functional NKCC2 protein.

BS is a genetically heterogeneous disease. Given the role of apical K$^+$ permeability in the TAL, encoded at least in part by ROMK,[78,386] this K$^+$ channel was another early candidate gene. K$^+$ recycling via the Na$^+$-K$^+$-2Cl$^-$ cotransporter and apical K$^+$ channels generates a lumen-positive potential difference in the TAL, which drives the paracellular transport of Na$^+$ and other cations[387] (see also Figure 18.10). Multiple disease-associated mutations in ROMK have been reported in patients with BS type II, most of whom exhibited the

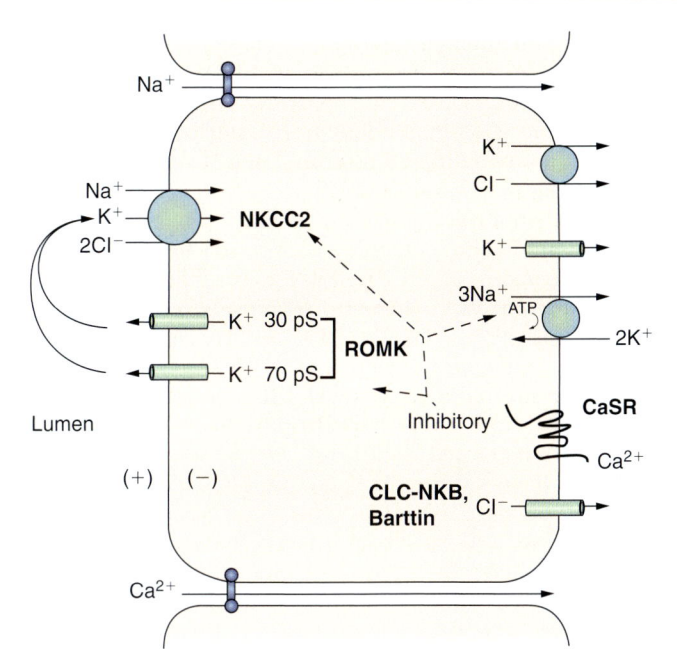

Figure 18.10 Bartter's syndrome and the thick ascending limb. Bartter's syndrome can result from loss-of-function mutations in the Na$^+$-K$^+$-2Cl$^-$ cotransporter NKCC2, the K$^+$ channel subunit ROMK, or the Cl$^-$ channel subunits CLC-NKB and Barttin (Bartter's syndrome types I to IV, respectively). Gain-of-function mutations in the calcium-sensing receptor (CaSR) can also cause a Bartter's syndrome phenotype (type V); the CaSR has an inhibitory effect on salt transport by the thick ascending limb, targeting several transport pathways. ROMK encodes the low-conductance, 30-pS K$^+$ channel in the apical membrane and also appears to function as a critical subunit of the higher conductance 70-pS channel. The loss of K$^+$ channel activity in Bartter's syndrome type II leads to reduced apical K$^+$ recycling and reduced Na$^+$-K$^+$-2Cl$^-$ cotransport. Decreased apical K$^+$ channels also lead to a decrease in the lumen-positive potential difference, which drives paracellular Na$^+$, Ca^{2+}, and Mg^{2+} transport.

antenatal phenotype.[380,388] Finally, mutations in BS type III have been reported in the chloride channel CLC-NKB,[389] which is expressed at the basolateral membrane of at least the TAL and DCT.[390] Patients with mutations in CLC-NKB typically have the classic Bartter's phenotype, with a relative absence of nephrocalcinosis. In a significant fraction of patients with BS, the NKCC2, ROMK, and CLC-NKB genes are not involved.[389] For example, a subset of patients with associated sensorineural deafness exhibit linkage to chromosome 1p31[28]; the gene for this syndrome, denoted Barttin, is an obligatory subunit for the CLC-NKB chloride channel.[391] The occurrence of deafness in these patients suggests that Barttin functions in the regulation or function of Cl$^-$ channels in the inner ear. Notably, the CLC-NKB gene is immediately adjacent to that for another epithelial Cl$^-$ channel, denoted CLC-NKA; digenic inactivation was described in two siblings with deafness and BS,[392] suggesting that CLC-NKA plays an important role in Barttin-dependent Cl$^-$ transport in the inner ear.

Patients with activating mutations in the CaSR have been described with autosomal dominant hypocalcemia and hypokalemic alkalosis.[393,394] The CaSR is heavily expressed at the basolateral membrane of the TAL,[395] where it is thought to play an important inhibitory role in regulating the transcellular transport of both Na$^+$-Cl$^-$ and Ca^{2+}. For example, activation of the basolateral CaSR in the TAL is known to reduce apical K$^+$ channel activity,[396] which would induce a Bartter-like syndrome (see Figure 18.10). Coexpression of NKCC2 with a Bartter's syndrome gain-of-function mutant in the CaSR reveals reduced phosphorylation and reduced activity of NKCC2, dependent on the generation of inhibitory arachidonic acid–derived metabolites known to inhibit TAL function.[397] Genetic activation of the CaSR by these mutations is also expected to increase urinary Ca^{2+} excretion by inhibiting generation of the lumen-positive potential difference that drives paracellular Ca^{2+} transport in the TAL. In addition, the set point of the CaSR response to Ca^{2+} in the parathyroid is shifted to the left, inhibiting parathyroid hormone (PTH) secretion by this gland. It is very likely that the positional cloning of other BS genes will have a considerable impact on the mechanistic understanding of the TAL.

Despite the reasonable correlation between the disease gene involved and the associated subtype of familial alkalosis, there is significant phenotypic overlap and phenotypic variability in hereditary hypokalemic alkalosis. For example, patients with mutations in CLC-NKB usually exhibit classic BS, but can present with a more severe antenatal phenotype, or even with a phenotype similar to Gitelman's syndrome.[28,398] With respect to BS due to mutations in NKCC2, a number of patients have been described with variant presentations, including an absence of hypokalemia.[28] Two brothers were described with a late onset of mild BS; these patients were found to be compound heterozygotes for a mutant form of NKCC2 that exhibits partial function, with a loss-of-function mutation on the other NKCC2 allele.[399]

BS type II is particularly relevant to K$^+$ homeostasis, given that ROMK is the SK secretory channel of the CNT and CCD (see Chapter 6, "K$^+$ Secretion by the Distal Convoluted Tubule, Connecting Tubule, and Cortical Collecting Duct"). Patients with BS type II typically have slightly higher serum K$^+$ than the other genetic forms of BS[388,398]; patients with severe (9.0 mmol/L), transient, neonatal hyperkalemia have also been described.[400] It is likely that this reflects a transient developmental deficit in the other K$^+$ channels involved in distal K$^+$ secretion, including the apical maxi-K channel responsible for flow-dependent K$^+$ secretion in the distal nephron.[77,401] Distal K$^+$ secretion in ROMK knockout mice is primarily mediated by maxi-K–BK channel activity,[402] such that developmental deficits in this channel would lead to hyperkalemia in BS type II. The mammalian TAL has two major apical K$^+$ conductances, the 30-pS channel corresponding to ROMK and a 70-pS channel[403]; both are thought to play a role in transepithelial salt transport by the TAL. ROMK is evidently a subunit of the 70-pS channel, given the absence of this conductance in TAL segments of ROMK knockout mice.[404] The identity of the other putative subunit of this 70-pS channel is not as yet known; one would assume that deficiencies in this gene would also be a cause of BS.

Finally, BS must be clinically differentiated from the various causes of pseudo–Bartter's syndrome; these commonly include laxative abuse, furosemide abuse, and bulimia (see "Clinical Approach to Hypokalemia"). Other reported causes include gentamicin nephrotoxicity,[312] Sjögren's syndrome,[28] and cystic fibrosis (CF).[28,405] Fixed loss of Na$^+$-Cl$^-$ in sweat is likely the dominant predisposing factor for hypokalemic alkalosis in patients with CF; patients with this presentation generally respond promptly to intravenous fluids and electrolyte replacement. However, the cystic fibrosis transmembrane conductance regularor (CFTR) protein coassociates with ROMK in the TAL and confers sensitivity to ATP and glibenclamide to apical K+ channels in this nephron segment.[406] Lu and associates have proposed that this interaction serves to modulate the response of ROMK to cAMP and vasopressin, such that K+ excretion in CFTR deficiency would not be appropriately reduced during water diuresis, therefore predisposing these patients to the development of hypokalemic alkalosis.[406]

Gitelman's Syndrome. A major advance in the understanding of hereditary alkaloses was the realization that a subset of patients exhibit marked hypocalciuria, rather than the hypercalciuria typically seen in BS; patients in this hypocalciuric subset are universally hypomagnesemic.[304] Such patients are now clinically classified as suffering from Gitelman's syndrome (GS). Although plasma renin activity may be increased, renal prostaglandin excretion is not elevated in these hypocalciuric patients,[407] another distinguishing feature between BS and GS. GS is a milder disorder than BS; however, patients do report significant morbidity, mostly related to muscular symptoms and fatigue.[408] The QT interval is frequently prolonged in GS, suggesting an increased risk of cardiac arrhythmia[409]; however, a more exhaustive cardiac evaluation of a large group of patients failed to detect significant abnormalities of cardiac structure or rhythm.[410] However, presyncope and/or ventricular tachycardia has been observed in at least two patients with GS,[28,187] one with concomitant long QT syndrome due to a mutation in the cardiac KCNQ1 K+ channel.[187]

The hypocalciuria detected in GS was an expected consequence of inactivating the thiazide-sensitive Na+-Cl- cotransporter NCC (SLC12A2), and loss-of-function mutations in the human gene have been reported.[411] Many of these mutations lead to a defect in cellular trafficking when introduced into the human NCC protein.[412] GS is genetically homogeneous, except for the occasional patient with mutations in CLC-NKB and an overlapping phenotype.[28,187,398] However, genetic analysis is not generally available, given the significant number of exons in SLC12A2 and the absence of hot spot mutations in this disorder. One diagnostic alternative is to assess the physiologic response to thiazides; patients with GS have a blunted excretion of chloride after the administration of hydrochlorothiazide.[413]

The NCC protein has been localized to the apical membrane of epithelial cells in the DCT and connecting segment. A mouse strain with targeted deletion of the *Slc12a2* gene encoding NCC exhibits hypocalciuria and hypomagnesemia, with a mild alkalosis and marked increase in circulating aldosterone.[414] These knockout mice exhibit marked morphologic defects in the early DCT,[414] with a reduction in absolute number of DCT cells and changes in ultrastructural appearance. That GS is a disorder of cellular development and/or cellular apoptosis should perhaps not be a surprise, given the observation that thiazide treatment promotes marked apoptosis of this nephron segment.[415] This cellular deficit leads to downregulation of the DCT magnesium channel TRPM6,[416] resulting in the magnesium wasting and hypomagnesemia seen in GS. The downstream CNT tubules are hypertrophied in NCC-deficient mice,[414] reminiscent of the hypertrophic DCT and CNT segments seen in furosemide-treated animals.[28] These CNT cells also exhibit an increased expression of ENaC at their apical membranes versus littermate controls[414]; this is likely due to activation of SGK1-dependent trafficking of ENaC by the increase in circulating aldosterone (see "Control of Potassium Secretion: Aldosterone").

Hypokalemia does not occur in NCC$^{-/-}$ mice on a standard rodent diet but emerges on a K+-restricted diet; plasma K+ of these mice is about 1 mmol/L lower than K+-restricted littermate controls.[417] Several mechanisms account for the hypokalemia seen in GS and NCC$^{-/-}$ mice. The distal delivery of Na+ and fluid is decreased in NCC$^{-/-}$ mice, at least those on a normal diet; however, the increased circulating aldosterone and CNT hypertrophy likely compensate, leading to increased kaliuresis. As discussed earlier for thiazides, decreased luminal Ca^{2+} in NCC deficiency may augment baseline ENaC activity,[306] further exacerbating the kaliuresis. Of particular interest, NCC-deficient mice develop considerable polydipsia and polyuria on a K+-restricted diet[417]; this is reminiscent perhaps of the polydipsia that has been implicated in thiazide-associated hyponatremia.[418]

Hypocalciuria in GS is not accompanied by changes in plasma calcium, phosphate, vitamin D, or PTH levels,[419] suggesting a direct effect on renal calcium transport. The late DCT is morphologically intact in NCC-deficient mice, with preserved expression of the epithelial calcium channel (ECAC1, or TRPV5) and the basolateral Na+-Ca^{2+} exchanger.[414] Furthermore, the hypocalciuric effect of thiazides persists in mice deficient in TRPV5,[416] arguing against the putative effects of this drug on distal Ca^{2+} absorption. Rather, several lines of evidence have argued that the hypocalciuria of GS and thiazide treatment is due to increased absorption of Na+ by the proximal tubule,[414,416] with secondary increases in proximal Ca^{2+} absorption. Regardless, reminiscent of the clinical effect of thiazides on bone, there are clear differences in bone density between affected and unaffected members of specific Gitelman kindreds. Thus, homozygous patients have much higher bone densities than unaffected wild-type family members, whereas heterozygotes have intermediate values for bone density and calcium excretion.[419] An interesting association has repeatedly been described between chondrocalcinosis, the abnormal deposition of calcium pyrophosphate dihydrate (CPPD) in joint cartilage, and GS.[420] Patients have also been reported with ocular choroidal calcification.[421]

Finally, as in BS, there have been reports of acquired tubular defects that mimic those of GS. These include patients with hypokalemic alkalosis, hypomagnesemia, and hypocalciuria after chemotherapy with cisplatin.[422] Patients have also been described with acquired GS due to Sjögren's syndrome and tubulointerstitial nephritis,[28,423] with a documented absence of coding sequence mutations in NCC.[423]

RENAL TUBULAR ACIDOSIS

Renal tubular acidosis (RTA) and related tubular defects can be associated with hypokalemia. Proximal RTA is characterized by a reduction in proximal bicarbonate absorption, with a reduced plasma bicarbonate concentration. Isolated proximal RTA is rare; genetic causes include loss of function by mutations in the basolateral Na+-HCO$_3^-$ transporter. More commonly, proximal RTA occurs in the context of multiple proximal tubular transport defects, encompassing Fanconi's syndrome (FS).[311] The cardinal features of FS include hyperaminoaciduria, glycosuria with a normal plasma glucose concentration, and phosphate wasting; associated defects include the proximal RTA, hypouricemia, hypercalciuria, hypokalemia, salt wasting, and increased excretion of low-molecular-weight proteins. FS is usually drug-associated; important causes include aristolochic acid, ifosfamide, and the acyclic nucleoside phosphonates (e.g., tenofovir, cidofovir, adefovir).[311] Prior to treatment with bicarbonate, patients with a proximal RTA will typically demonstrate mild hypokalemia, due primarily to baseline hyperaldosteronism[424]; however, prior to treatment, patients have been described with profound hypokalemia on presentation.[425] Regardless, treatment with oral sodium bicarbonate will markedly increase distal tubular Na^+ and HCO_3^- delivery, causing a marked increase in renal potassium wasting.[424] Patients will often require mixed base replacement with oral citrate and bicarbonate in addition to aggressive K^+-Cl^- supplementation.

Hypokalemia is also associated with distal RTA, the so-called type 1 RTA. Hypokalemic distal RTA is most commonly due to a secretory defect, with reduced H^+-ATPase activity and decreased ability to acidify the urine. For example, hereditary defects in subunits of H^+-ATPase are associated with profound hypokalemia in addition to acidosis and hypercalciuria.[426] Pathophysiology of the associated hypokalemia is multifactorial due to the loss of electrogenic H^+ secretion (with enhanced K^+ secretion to maintain electroneutrality in the distal nephron), loss of H^+-K^+-ATPase activity, and increases in aldosterone.[427,428] Sjögren's syndrome is perhaps the most common cause of hypokalemic distal RTA in adults; the associated hypokalemia can be truly profound, often resulting in marked weakness and respiratory arrest.[428]

MAGNESIUM DEFICIENCY

Magnesium deficiency results in refractory hypokalemia, particularly if the plasma Mg^{2+} level is less than 0.5 mmol/L[240]; hypomagnesemic patients are thus refractory to K^+ replacement in the absence of Mg^{2+} repletion.[429,430] Magnesium deficiency is also a common concomitant of hypokalemia, in part because associated tubular disorders (e.g., aminoglycoside nephrotoxicity) may cause kaliuresis and magnesium wasting. Plasma Mg^{2+} levels must therefore be checked on a routine basis in hypokalemia.[239,431]

Several mechanisms appear to contribute to the effect of magnesium depletion on plasma K^+. Magnesium depletion has inhibitory effects on muscle Na^+-K^+-ATPase activity,[432] resulting in significant efflux from muscle and a secondary kaliuresis. Distal K^+ secretion also appears to be enhanced due to a reduction in the normal physiologic inward rectification of ROMK secretory K^+ channels, with a subsequent increase in outward conductance.[433] ROMK and other Kir channels are inward-rectifying—that is, K^+ flows inward more readily than outward; even though outward conductance is usually less than inward conductance, K^+ efflux predominates in the CNT and CCD since the membrane potential is more positive than the equilibrium potential for K^+. Intracellular Mg^{2+} plays a key role in inward rectification, binding and blocking the pore of the channel from the cytoplasmic side.[433] The hypomagnesemia-associated reduction in cytoplasmic Mg^{2+} in principal cells reduces inward rectification of ROMK, increasing outward conductance and increasing K^+ secretion; this has been confirmed in vivo.[434] Finally, it has been suggested that the repletion of intracellular K^+ is impaired in hypomagnesemia, even in normokalemic patients.[431] Decreased intracellular Mg^{2+} enhances K^+ efflux from the cytoplasm of cardiac and perhaps skeletal myocytes, likely due to reduced intracellular blockade of inward rectifying K^+ channels (increased efflux) and inhibition of Na^+-K^+-ATPase (decreased influx); plasma K^+ levels thus remain normal at the expense of intracellular K^+.[21,431,435] This phenomenon is particularly important in patients with cardiac disease who are taking both diuretics and digoxin. In such patients, hypokalemia and arrhythmias will respond to a correction of the magnesium deficiency and potassium supplementation.[21,431]

CLINICAL APPROACH TO HYPOKALEMIA

The initial priority in the evaluation of hypokalemia is an assessment for signs and/or symptoms (e.g., muscle weakness, changes in the electrocardiogram [ECG]) suggestive of an impending emergency that requires immediate treatment. The cause of hypokalemia is usually obvious from the history, physical examination, and/or basic laboratory tests. However, persistent hypokalemia, despite appropriate initial intervention, requires a more rigorous workup; in most cases, a systematic approach reveals the underlying cause (Figure 18.11).

The history should focus on medications (e.g., diuretics, laxatives, antibiotics, herbal medications), diet and dietary supplements (e.g., licorice), and associated symptoms (e.g., diarrhea). During the physical examination, particular attention should be paid to blood pressure, volume status, and signs suggestive of specific disorders associated with hypokalemia (e.g., hyperthyroidism, Cushing's syndrome). Initial laboratory tests should include electrolytes, blood urea nitrogen (BUN), creatinine, plasma osmolality, Mg^{2+}, Ca^{2+}, complete blood count, and urinary pH, creatinine, electrolytes, and osmolality. Plasma and urine osmolality are required for calculation of the TTKG[174] and urinary K^+/creatinine ratio (see "Urinary Indices of Potassium Excretion"). A TTKG less than 2 to 3 separates patients with redistributive hypokalemia from those with hypokalemia due to renal potassium wasting, who will have TTKG values that are higher than 4.[178] Further tests, such as urinary Mg^{2+} and Ca^{2+} and plasma renin and aldosterone levels, may be necessary in specific cases (see Figure 18.11). The timing and evolution of hypokalemia are also helpful in differentiating the cause, particularly in hospitalized patients; for example, hypokalemia due to transcellular shift usually occurs in a matter of hours.[436]

The most common causes of chronic, diagnosis-resistant hypokalemia are GS, surreptitious vomiting, and diuretic abuse.[437] Alternatively, an associated acidosis would suggest the diagnosis of hypokalemic distal or proximal renal tubular acidosis. Hypokalemia occurred in 5.5% of patients with eating disorders in a U.S. study from the mid-1990s,[438] mostly in those with surreptitious vomiting (bulimia) or laxative abuse (the purging subtype of anorexia nervosa[292]). These patients may have a constellation of associated symptoms and signs, including dental erosion and depression.[439]

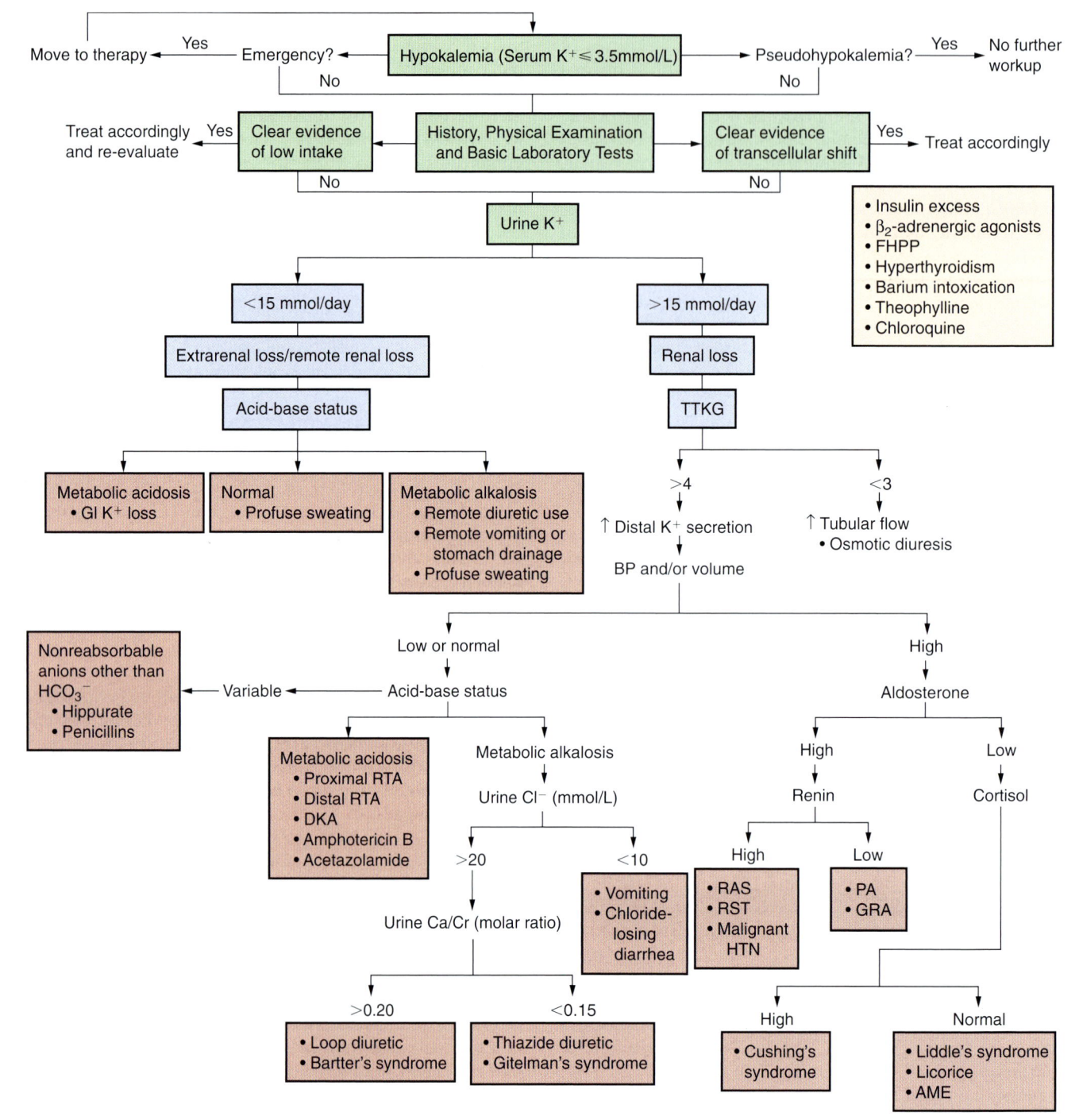

Figure 18.11 The clinical approach to hypokalemia. See text for details. AME, Apparent mineralocorticoid excess; BP, blood pressure; CCD, cortical collecting duct; DKA, diabetic ketoacidosis; FHPP, familial hypokalemic periodic paralysis; GI, gastrointestinal; GRA, glucocorticoid-remediable aldosteronism; HTN, hypertension; PA, primary aldosteronism; RAS, renal artery stenosis; RST, renin-secreting tumor; RTA, renal tubular acidosis; TTKG, transtubular potassium gradient.

Hypokalemic patients with bulimia will have an associated metabolic alkalosis, with an obligatory natriuresis accompanying the loss of bicarbonate; urinary Cl⁻ is typically less than 10 mmol/L, and this clue can often yield the diagnosis.[437,440] Urinary electrolytes are, however, generally unremarkable in unselected, mostly normokalemic patients with bulimia.[439] Urinary excretion of Na^+, K^+, and Cl^- is high in patients who abuse diuretics, albeit not to the levels seen in GS. Marked variability in urinary electrolyte levels is an important clue for diuretic abuse, which can be verified with urinary drug screens. Clinically, nephrocalcinosis is very common in furosemide abuse due to the increase in urinary calcium excretion.[441] Differentiation of GS from BS requires a 24-hour urine to assess calcium excretion, since hypocalciuria is a distinguishing feature for the former[304]; patients with GS are also invariably hypomagnesemic. BS must be differentiated from pseudo–Bartter's syndrome due to gentamicin toxicity,[312,442] mutations in *CFTR*, the cystic fibrosis gene,[405,443] or Sjögren's syndrome with tubulointerstitial nephritis.[444] Acquired forms of GS have in turn been reported after cisplatin therapy[422] and in patients with Sjögren's syndrome.[28,423] Finally, although laxative abuse is perhaps a less common cause of chronic hypokalemia, an accompanying metabolic acidosis with a negative urinary anion gap should raise the diagnostic suspicion of this cause.[179]

TREATMENT OF HYPOKALEMIA

The goals of therapy in hypokalemia are to prevent life-threatening conditions (e.g., diaphragmatic weakness, rhabdomyolysis, cardiac arrhythmias), replace any K+ deficit, and diagnose and correct the underlying cause. The urgency of therapy depends on the severity of hypokalemia, associated conditions and settings (e.g., a patient with heart failure on digoxin or a patient with hepatic encephalopathy), and the rate of decline in plasma K+. A rapid drop to less than 2.5 mmol/L poses a high risk of cardiac arrhythmias and calls for urgent replacement.[445] Although replacement is usually limited to patients with a true deficit, it should be considered in patients with hypokalemia due to redistribution (e.g., HYPP) when serious complications such as muscle weakness, rhabdomyolysis, and cardiac arrhythmias are present or imminent.[446] The risk of arrhythmia from hypokalemia is highest in older patients, patients with evidence of organic heart disease, and patients on digoxin or antiarrhythmic drugs.[239] In these high-risk patients, an increased incidence of arrhythmias may occur at even mild to modest degrees of hypokalemia. The American Heart Association guidelines on the use of hospital telemetry recommend monitoring for patients with hypokalemia and a prolonged QT interval.[447]

It is also crucial to diagnose and eliminate the underlying cause so as to tailor therapy to the pathophysiology involved. For example, the risk of overcorrection or rebound hyperkalemia in hypokalemia caused by redistribution is particularly high, with the potential for fatal hyperkalemic arrhythmias.[240,254,289,446,448] When increased sympathetic tone or increased sympathetic response is thought to play a dominant role, the use of nonspecific β-adrenergic blockade with propranolol generally avoids this complication and should be considered; the relevant causes of hypokalemia include thyrotoxic periodic paralysis,[287] theophylline overdose,[449] and acute head injury.[254]

K+ replacement is the mainstay of therapy in hypokalemia. However, hypomagnesemic patients can be refractory to K+ replacement alone,[430] such that concomitant Mg^{2+} deficiency should always be addressed with oral or parenteral repletion. To prevent hyperkalemia due to excessive supplementation, the deficit and rate of correction should be estimated as accurately as possible. Renal function, medications, and comorbid conditions such as diabetes (with a risk of both insulinopenia and autonomic neuropathy) should also be considered so as to gauge the risk of overcorrection. Arbitrary adjustments in the dose of administered K+-Cl− replacement based on the estimated GFR can potentially reduce the risk of hyperkalemia.[450] The goal is to raise the plasma K+ rapidly to a safe range and then replace the remaining deficit at a slower rate over days to weeks.[239,240,446] In the absence of abnormal K+ redistribution, the total deficit correlates with serum K+,[240,446,451] such that serum K+ drops by approximately 0.27 mmol/L for every 100-mmol reduction in total body stores. Loss of 400 to 800 mmol of body K+ results in a reduction in serum K+ by approximately 2.0 mmol/L[451]; these parameters can be used to estimate replacement goals. However, such estimates are just an approximation of the amount of K+ replacement required to normalize plasma K+, with as much as a 1 in 6 risk of overreplacement[243]; serum K+ should also be closely monitored during replacement, withdrawing or adjusting K+ replacement if necessary.

Although the treatment of asymptomatic patients with borderline or low-normal serum K+ remains controversial, supplementation is recommended for patients with a serum K+ lower than 3 mmol/L. In high-risk patients (e.g., those with heart failure, cardiac arrhythmias, myocardial infarction, ischemic heart disease, taking digoxin), serum K+ should be maintained at 4.0 mmol/L or higher[239] or even 4.5 mmol/L or higher.[247] Patients with severe hepatic disease may not be able to tolerate mild to moderate hypokalemia due to the associated augmentation in ammoniagenesis, and thus serum K+ should be maintained at approximately 4.0 mmol/L.[452,453] In asymptomatic patients with mild to moderate hypertension, an attempt should be made to maintain serum K+ above 4.0 mmol/L,[239] and potassium supplementation should be considered when serum K+ falls below 3.5 mmol/L.[239] Notably, prospective studies have shown an inverse relationship between dietary potassium intake and fatal and nonfatal stroke, independently of the associated antihypertensive effect.[239,454,455]

Potassium is available in the form of potassium chloride, potassium phosphate, potassium bicarbonate or its precursors (potassium citrate, potassium acetate), and potassium gluconate.[239,240,446] Potassium phosphate is indicated when phosphate deficit accompanies K+ depletion (e.g., in diabetic ketoacidosis).[446] Potassium bicarbonate (or its precursors) should be considered for patients with hypokalemia and metabolic acidosis.[239,446] Potassium chloride should otherwise be the default salt of choice for most patients for several reasons. First, metabolic alkalosis typically accompanies chloride loss from renal (e.g., diuretics) or upper gastrointestinal routes (e.g., vomiting) and contributes significantly to renal K+ wasting.[240] In this setting, replacing chloride along with K+ is essential in treating the alkalosis and preventing further kaliuresis; because dietary K+ is mainly in the form of potassium phosphate or potassium citrate, it usually does not suffice. Second, potassium bicarbonate may offset the benefits of K+ administration by aggravating concomitant alkalosis. Third, potassium chloride raises serum K+ at a faster rate than potassium bicarbonate, a factor that is crucial in patients with marked hypokalemia and related symptoms. In all likelihood, this faster rise in plasma K+ occurs because Cl− is mainly an extracellular fluid anion that does not enter cells to the same extent as bicarbonate, keeping the K+ in the extracellular fluid compartment.[456]

Parenteral (intravenous) K+ administration should be limited to patients unable to use the enteral route or when the patient is experiencing associated signs and symptoms. However, rapid correction of hypokalemia through oral supplementation is possible and may be faster than intravenous K^+ supplementation due to limitations in the rapidity of intravenous K^+ infusion. For example, serum K^+ can be increased by 1 to 1.4 mmol/L in 60 to 90 minutes following the oral intake of 75 mmol of K^+[457]; the ingestion of approximately 125 to 165 mmol of K^+ as a single oral dose can increase serum K^+ by approximately 2.5 to 3.5 mmol/L in 60 to 120 minutes.[458] The oral route is therefore effective and appropriate in patients with asymptomatic severe hypokalemia. If the patient is experiencing life-threatening signs and symptoms of hypokalemia, however, the maximum possible IV infusion of K^+ should be administered acutely for symptom control, followed by rapid oral supplementation.

The usual intravenous dose is 20 to 40 mmol of K^+-Cl^- in 1 L of vehicle solution.[446] The vehicle solution should be dextrose-free to prevent a transient reduction in the serum K^+ level of 0.2 to 1.4 mmol/L due to an enhanced endogenous insulin secretion induced by the dextrose.[459] Higher concentrations of K^+-Cl^- (up to 400 mmol/L—40 mmol in 100 mL of normal saline) have been used in life-threatening situations.[460,461] In these cases, the amount of K^+ per intravenous bag should be limited (e.g., 20 mmol in 100 ml of saline solution) to prevent inadvertent infusion of a large dose.[461,462] These solutions are best given through a large central vein to avoid painful peripheral vein irritation. Femoral veins are preferable since infusion through upper body central lines can acutely increase the local intracardiac concentration of K^+, with life-threatening deleterious effects on cardiac conduction.[461,462] As a general rule, and to avoid venous pain, irritation, and sclerosis, concentrations of more than 60 mmol/L should not be given through a peripheral vein.[446] Although the recommended rate of administration is 10 to 20 mmol/hour, rates of 40 to 100 mmol/hour or even higher (for a short period) have been used in patients with life-threatening conditions.[460,462-464] However, a rapid increase in serum K^+ associated with electrocardiographic changes may occur with higher rates of infusion (e.g., ≥80 mmol/hour).[465] Intravenous administration of K^+ at a rate of more than 10 mmol/hour requires continuous electrocardiographic monitoring.[446] In patients receiving such high infusion rates, close monitoring of the appropriate physiologic consequences of hypokalemia is essential; after these effects have abated, the rate of infusion should be decreased to the standard dose of 10 to 20 mmol/hour.[462]

It is important to remember that volume expansion in patients with moderate to severe hypokalemia and Cl^--responsive metabolic alkalosis should be performed cautiously and with close follow-up of serum K^+ since bicarbonaturia associated with volume expansion may aggravate renal K^+ wasting and hypokalemia.[445] In patients with combined severe hypokalemia and hypophosphatemia (e.g., diabetic ketoacidosis), intravenous K^+ phosphate can be used. However, this solution should be infused at a rate of less than 50 mmol over 8 hours to prevent the risk of hypocalcemia and metastatic calcification.[445] A combination of potassium phosphate and potassium chloride may be necessary to correct hypokalemia effectively in these patients.

The easiest and most straightforward method of oral K^+ supplementation is to increase dietary intake of potassium-rich foods[240] (see Table 18.4). One study compared the effectiveness of diet versus medication supplementation in cardiac surgery patients receiving diuretics in the hospital and found no difference between the two groups in respect to maintenance of serum K^+. However, limitations of this study included a small number of subjects, relatively short duration, and lack of information on acid-base status, making it less than conclusive and not generalizable.[466] Regardless, dietary K^+ is mainly in the form of potassium phosphate or potassium citrate and is inadequate in most patients who have concomitant K^+ and Cl^- deficiency. Most patients will therefore need to combine a high-K^+ diet with a prescribed dose of K^+-Cl^-.[240] Salt substitutes are an inexpensive and potent source of K^+-Cl^-; 1 g contains 10 to 13 mmol of K^+.[467] However, these patients, particularly those with an impaired ability to excrete potassium, need to be counseled regarding the appropriate amount and potential for hyperkalemia.[468] Potassium chloride is also available in liquid or tablet form (Table 18.5).[239] In general, the available preparations are well absorbed.[240] Liquid forms are less expensive but are less well tolerated. Slow-release forms are more palatable and better tolerated; however, they have been associated with gastrointestinal ulceration and bleeding, ascribed to local accumulation of high concentrations of K^+.[240,462] Notably, this risk is rather low, and it is lower still with the microencapsulated forms.[240] The chance of

Table 18.4 Foods with High Potassium Content

Highest content (>1000 mg [25 mmol]/100 g)
    Dried figs
    Molasses
    Seaweed
Very high content (>500 mg [12.5 mmol]/100 g)
    Dried fruits (dates, prunes)
    Nuts
    Avocados
    Bran cereals
    Wheat germ
    Lima beans
High content (>250 mg [6.2 mmol]/100 g)
    Vegetables
        Spinach
        Tomatoes
        Broccoli
        Winter squash
        Beets
        Carrots
        Cauliflower
        Potatoes
    Fruits
        Bananas
        Cantaloupe
        Kiwis
        Oranges
        Mangos
    Meats
        Ground beef
        Steak
        Pork
        Veal
        Lamb

From Gennari FJ: Hypokalemia. N Engl J Med 339:451-458, 1998.

Table 18.5 Oral Preparations of Potassium Chloride

Supplement	Characteristics
Controlled-release microencapsulated tablets	Disintegrate better in stomach than encapsulated microparticles; less adherent and less cohesive
Encapsulated, controlled-release microencapsulated particles	Fewer gastrointestinal tract erosions than with wax matrix tablets
Potassium chloride elixir	Inexpensive, tastes bad, poor patient adherence; few gastrointestinal tract erosions; immediate effect
Potassium chloride (effervescent tablets) for solution	Convenient, but more expensive than elixir; immediate effect
Wax matrix extended-release tablets	Easier to swallow; more gastrointestinal tract erosions than with microencapsulated formulas

From Cohn JN, Kowey PR, Whelton PK, et al: New guidelines for potassium replacement in clinical practice: a contemporary review by the National Council on Potassium in Clinical Practice. Arch Intern Med 160:2429-2436, 2000.

overdose and hyperkalemia is higher with slow-release formulations; unlike the immediate-release forms, these tablets are less irritating to the stomach and less likely to induce vomiting.[469] The usual dose is 40 to 100 mmol of K^+ (as K^+-Cl^-)/day, divided into two or three doses, in patients taking diuretics[240] (K^+-Cl^- can be toxic in doses > 2 mmol/kg[469]). This dose is effective in maintaining serum K^+ in up to 90% of patients; however, in the 10% of patients who remain hypokalemic, increasing the oral dose or adding a K^+-sparing diuretic is an appropriate choice.[240]

In addition to potassium supplementation, strategies to minimize K^+ losses should be considered. These measures may include minimizing the dose of non-K^+–sparing diuretics, restricting Na^+ intake, and using a combination of non-K^+–sparing and K^+-sparing medications (e.g., ACE inhibitors, ARBs, K^+-sparing diuretics, β-blockers).[210,239] The use of a K^+-sparing diuretic is of particular importance in hypokalemia resulting from primary hyperaldosteronism and related disorders, such as Liddle's syndrome and AME; K^+ supplementation alone may be ineffective in these settings.[470-472] In patients with hypokalemia due to loss through upper gastrointestinal secretion (e.g., continuous nasogastric tube suction, continuous or self-induced vomiting), proton pump inhibitors are reportedly useful in helping correct the metabolic alkalosis and reduce hypokalemia.[473]

HYPERKALEMIA

EPIDEMIOLOGY

Hyperkalemia is usually defined as a potassium level of 5.5 mmol/L or higher although, in some studies, 5.0 to 5.4 mmol/L qualified for the diagnosis.[474-476] Hyperkalemia has been reported in 1.1% to 10% of all hospitalized patients,[217,474-477] with approximately 1.0% of patients (8% to 10% of hyperkalemic patients) having significant hyperkalemia (≥6.0 mmol/L).[474] Hyperkalemia has been associated with a higher mortality rate (14.3% to 41%),[28,474,475] accounting for approximately 1 death per 1000 patients in one case series from the mid-1980's.[478] In most hospitalized patients, the pathophysiology of hyperkalemia is multifactorial, with reduced renal function, medications, older age (≥60 years), and hyperglycemia being the most common contributing factors.[217,474,475]

In patients with ESKD, the prevalence of hyperkalemia is 5% to 10%.[479-481] The prevalence increases from 2% to 42% as GFR decreases from 60 to 90 mL/min/1.73 m^2; the risk of hyperkalemia is increased in males with chronic kidney disease (CKD) and tripled by treatment with ACE inhibitors or ARBs.[482] Hyperkalemia accounts for or contributes to 1.9% to 5% of deaths among patients with ESKD.[217,481] Notably, however, the risk of death from hyperkalemia is reduced as CKD progresses, presumably due to as yet uncharacterized cardiac adaptation to chronic hyperkalemia.[483] Hyperkalemia is the reason for emergency hemodialysis in 24% of patients with ESKD on hemodialysis,[481] and renal failure is the most common cause of hyperkalemia diagnosed in the emergency room.[479] The prevalence of marked hyperkalemia (K^+ ≥ 5.8 mmol/L) is approximately 1% in a general medicine outpatient setting. Alarmingly, the management of outpatient hyperkalemia is often suboptimal, with approximately 25% of patients lacking any follow-up, ECGs performed in only 36% of cases, and frequent delays in repeating measurement of serum K^+.[484]

PSEUDOHYPERKALEMIA

Factitious or pseudohyperkalemia is an artifactual increase in serum K^+ due to the release of K^+ during or after venipuncture. There are several potential causes for pseudohyperkalemia[485]:

1. Forearm contraction,[486] fist clenching,[21] or tourniquet use[485] may increase K^+ efflux from local muscle and thus raise the measured serum K^+.
2. Thrombocytosis,[487] leukocytosis,[488] and/or erythrocytosis[489] may cause pseudohyperkalemia due to release from these cellular elements.
3. Acute anxiety during venipuncture may provoke a respiratory alkalosis and hyperkalemia due to redistribution.[53-55,64]
4. Sample contamination with K^+-EDTA (ethylenediaminetetraacetic acid), used as a sample anticoagulant for some laboratory assays, can cause spurious hyperkalemia.[490]

There are several mechanisms for sample contamination with K^+-EDTA during blood draws or sample handling.[490] Gross contamination with K^+-EDTA usually results in spurious hypocalcemia and hypomagnesemia; lesser contamination is less obvious, leading to the practice in some laboratories to perform EDTA assays on samples with a plasma K^+ more than 6 mmol/L with K^+-EDTA. Finally, mechanical and physical factors may induce pseudohyperkalemia after blood has been drawn. For example, pneumatic tube transport has been shown to induce pseudohyperkalemia in one patient with leukemia and massive leukocytosis.[491] Cooling of blood prior to the separation of cells from serum or plasma is also a well-recognized cause of artifactual hyperkalemia.[492] The converse is the risk of increased uptake of K^+ by cells at high ambient temperatures, leading to normal values for hyperkalemic patients and/or to spurious hypokalemia in patients who are normokalemic.[28,249] This issue is particularly important for outpatient primary practice samples that are transported off site and analyzed at a central facility[28]; this leads to so-called seasonal pseudohyperkalemia and hypokalemia,[28,493] with fluctuations of outpatient samples as a function of season and ambient temperature.

Finally, there are several hereditary subtypes of pseudohyperkalemia, caused by increases in passive K^+ permeability of erythrocytes. Abnormal red cell morphology, varying degrees of hemolysis, and/or perinatal edema can accompany hereditary pseudohyperkalemia, whereas in many kindreds there are no overt hematologic consequences. Serum K^+ increases in pseudohyperkalemia patient samples that have been left at room temperature due to abnormal K^+ permeability of erythrocytes. Several subtypes have been defined, based on differences in the temperature dependence curve of this red cell leak pathway.[28,494] The disorder is genetically heterogeneous, with a characterized gene on chromosome 17q21 and uncharacterized loci on chromosomes 16q23-ter and 2q35-36.[28] Of particular interest, 11 pedigrees of patients with autosomal dominant hemolysis, pseudohyperkalemia, and temperature-dependent loss of red cell K^+ were found to have heterozygous mutations in the *SLC4A1* gene on chromosome 17q21, which encodes the band 3 anion exchanger, AE1.[494] The mutations that were detected all cluster within exon 17 of the gene,[494] between transmembrane domains 8 and 10 of the AE1 protein. These mutations reduce anion transport in red cells and *Xenopus* oocytes injected with AE1, with the novel acquisition of a nonselective transport pathway for Na^+ and K^+. Pseudohyperkalemia in these patients thus results from a genetic event that endows AE1 with the ability to transport K^+; the fact that single point mutations can convert an anion exchanger to a nonselective cation channel serves to underline the narrow boundaries that separate exchangers and transporters from ion channels.[494]

More recently, mutations in the red cell Rh-associated glycoprotein (RhAG) were linked to the monovalent cation leak associated with overhydrated hereditary stomatocytosis.[495] These mutations cause an exaggerated cation leak in the RhAG, thought to function as an NH_3 or NH_4^+ transporter RhAG. Exaggerated red cell cation leaks are also implicated in stomatocytosis due to mutations in the mechanically activated cation channel PIEZO1[496]; disease-associated mutations give rise to mechanically activated currents that inactivate more slowly than wild-type channels.

EXCESS INTAKE OF POTASSIUM AND TISSUE NECROSIS

Increased intake of even small amounts of K^+ may provoke severe hyperkalemia in patients with predisposing factors. For example, the oral administration of 32 mmol to a diabetic patient with hyporeninemic hypoaldosteronism resulted in an increase in serum K^+ from 4.9 mmol/L to a peak of 7.3 mmol/L, within 3 hours.[497] Increased intake or changes in intake of dietary sources rich in K^+ (see Table 18.4) may also provoke hyperkalemia in susceptible patients. Very rarely, marked intake of K^+—for example, in sports beverages[498]—may provoke severe hyperkalemia in individuals free of predisposing factors. Other occult sources of K^+ must also be considered, including salt substitutes,[467] alternative medicines,[499] and alternative diets.[500] Geophagia with ingestion of K^+-rich clay[28] and cautopyreiophagia[501] (ingestion of burnt matchsticks) are two forms of pica that have been reported to cause hyperkalemia in dialysis patients. Sustained-release K^+-Cl^- tablets can cause hyperkalemia in suicidal overdoses.[469] Such pills are radiopaque and may thus be seen on radiographs; whole-bowel irrigation should be used for gastrointestinal decontamination.[469] Iatrogenic causes include simple overreplacement with K^+-Cl^-, as can occur commonly in hypokalemic patients,[243] or administration of a potassium-containing medication, such as K^+-penicillin,[502] to a susceptible patient.

Red cell transfusion is a well-described cause of hyperkalemia, typically seen in children or in those receiving massive transfusions. Risk factors for transfusion-related hyperkalemia include the rate and volume of the transfusion, use of a central venous infusion and/or pressure pumping, use of irradiated blood, and age of the blood infused.[21,503] Whereas 7-day-old blood has a free K^+ concentration of about 23 mmol/L, this rises to the 50-mmol/L range in 42-day-old blood.[504] Hyperkalemia is a common occurrence in patients with severe trauma, with a period prevalence of 29% in massively traumatized patients at a U.S. military combat support hospital in Iraq.[505] Although red cell and/or blood product transfusion plays an important role, this and other studies have indicated a complex pathophysiology for resuscitative hyperkalemia, with low cardiac output, acidosis, hypocalcemia, and other factors contributing to the risk of hyperkalemia in patients with severe trauma.[503,505]

Tissue necrosis is an important cause of hyperkalemia. Hyperkalemia due to rhabdomyolysis is particularly common because of the enormous store of K^+ in muscle (see Figure 18.1). In many cases, volume depletion, medications (statins in particular), and metabolic predisposition contribute to the genesis of rhabdomyolysis. Hypokalemia is an important metabolic predisposing factor in rhabdomyolysis (see "Consequences of Hypokalemia"); others include hypophosphatemia, hyper- and hyponatremia, and hyperglycemia. Patients with hypokalemia-associated rhabdomyolysis in whom redistribution is the cause of hypokalemia are at particular risk of subsequent hyperkalemia, as rhabdomyolysis evolves and renal function worsens.[21,265] Finally, massive release of K^+ and other intracellular contents may occur as a result of acute tumor lysis.[497]

REDISTRIBUTION AND HYPERKALEMIA

Several different mechanisms can induce an efflux of intracellular K^+, resulting in hyperkalemia. The infusion of hypertonic mannitol or saline, but not hypertonic bicarbonate, generates an increase in serum K^+.[506] Potential mechanisms include a dilutional acidosis with subsequent shift in K^+, increased passive exit of K^+ due to an increase in intracellular K^+ activity from intracellular water loss, acute hemolysis, and a solvent drag effect as water exits cells.[507,508] Regardless, severe hyperkalemia, typically with an acute dilutional hyponatremia, is a well-described complication of mannitol for the treatment or prevention of cerebral edema.[508-510] Diabetics are prone to severe hyperkalemia in response to intravenous hypertonic glucose in the absence of adequate coadministered insulin due to a similar osmotic effect.[511,512] Finally, a retrospective report has documented considerable increases in serum K$^+$ after IV contrast dye in five patients with chronic kidney disease, four on dialysis and one with stage 4 CKD[513]; again, the acute osmolar load was the likely cause of the acute hyperkalemia in these patients. The implications of this provocative study are not entirely clear; however, one would expect the development or worsening of hyperkalemia in dialysis patients exposed to large volumes of hyperosmolar contrast dye.

Several reports have appeared regarding the risk of hyperkalemia with ε-aminocaproic acid (Amicar),[514-516] a cationic amino acid that is structurally similar to lysine and arginine. Cationic but not anionic amino acids induce efflux of K$^+$ from cells, although the transport pathways involved are unknown.[21]

Muscle plays a dominant role in extrarenal K$^+$ homeostasis, primarily via regulated uptake by Na$^+$-K$^+$-ATPase. Although exercise is a well-described cause of acute hyperkalemia, this effect is usually transient, and its clinical relevance is difficult to judge. ESKD patients on dialysis do not have an exaggerated increase in plasma K$^+$ with maximal exercise, perhaps due to greater insulin, catecholamine, and aldosterone responses to exercise and/or to their preexisting hyperkalemia.[517] The results and design of this and other studies of exercise-associated hyperkalemia in ESKD were criticized by a more recent report, which linked abnormal extrarenal K$^+$ homeostasis to increased fatigue in ESKD.[518] Nonetheless, exercise-associated hyperkalemia is not a major clinical cause of hyperkalemia. Dialysis patients are, however, susceptible to modest increases in plasma K$^+$ after prolonged fasting due to the relative insulinopenia in this setting.[519] This may be clinically relevant in preoperative ESKD patients, for whom intravenous glucose infusions with or without insulin are appropriate preventive measures for the development of hyperkalemia.[519]

Insulin stimulates the uptake of K$^+$ by several tissues, primarily via stimulation of Na$^+$-K$^+$-ATPase activity.[28,41,43,46] Reduction in circulating insulin is thus an important factor or co-factor in the generation of hyperkalemia in diabetic patients. Patients with DKA typically present with serum K$^+$ levels that are within normal limits or moderately elevated, but with profound, whole-body potassium deficits. However, significant hyperkalemia (serum K$^+$ > 6 to 6.5 mmol/L) is not uncommon in DKA[520,521] due to a variety of potential factors, such as insulinopenia, renal dysfunction, and the hyperosmolar effect of severe hyperglycemia.[520-522] Inhibition of insulin secretion by the somatostatin agonist octreotide can also cause significant hyperkalemia in anephric patients[38] and in patients with normal renal function.[39]

Digoxin inhibits Na$^+$-K$^+$-ATPase and thus impairs the uptake of K$^+$ by skeletal muscle (see "Factors Affecting Internal Distribution of Potassium"), such that a digoxin overdose can result in hyperkalemia. The skin and venom gland of the cane toad *Bufo marinus* contains high concentrations of bufadienolide, a structurally similar glycoside. The direct

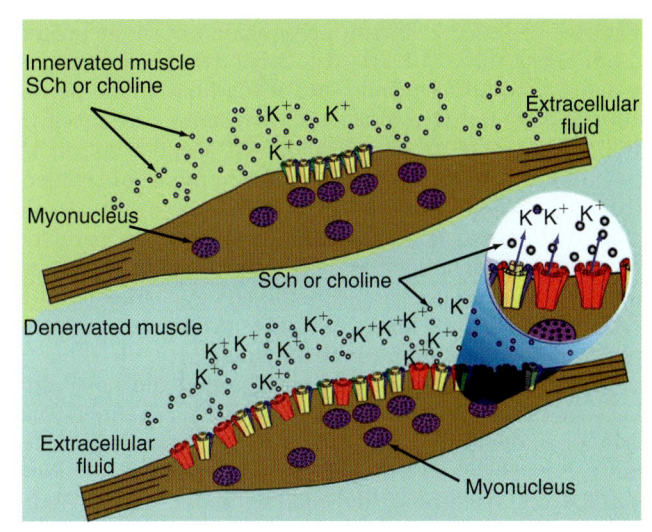

Figure 18.12 Succinylcholine-induced efflux of potassium is increased in denervated muscle. In innervated muscle, succinylcholine (SCh) interacts with the entire plasma membrane, but depolarizes only the junctional ($α_1$, $β_1$, $δ$, and $ε$ [*multicolored*]) acetylcholine receptors (AChRs); this leads to a modest transient hyperkalemia. With denervation, there is a considerable upregulation of muscle AChRs, with increased extrajunctional AChRs ($α_1$, $β_1$, $δ$, and $γ$ [*multicolored*]) and acquisition of homomeric, neuronal-type $α_7$-AChRs. Depolarization of denervated muscle leads to an exaggerated K$^+$ efflux due to the upregulation and redistribution of these AChRs. In addition, choline generated from metabolism of succinylcholine maintains the depolarization mediated via $α_7$-AChRs, thus enhancing and prolonging the K$^+$ efflux after paralysis has subsided. (From Martyn JA, Richtsfeld M: Succinylcholine-induced hyperkalemia in acquired pathologic states: etiologic factors and molecular mechanisms. *Anesthesiology* 104:158-169, 2006.)

ingestion of these toads[523] or of toad extracts can result in fatal hyperkalemia. In particular, certain herbal aphrodisiac pills contain appreciable amounts of toad venom and have led to several case reports in the United States.[21,524] Patients may have detectable plasma levels using standard digoxin assays, since bufadienolide is immunologically similar to digoxin. Moreover, treatment with a digoxin-specific Fab fragment, indicated for treatment of digoxin overdoses, may be effective and life-saving in bufadienolide toxicity.[21,524] Finally, fluoride ions also inhibit Na$^+$-K$^+$-ATPase, such that fluoride poisoning is typically associated with hyperkalemia.[525]

Succinylcholine depolarizes muscle cells, resulting in the efflux of K$^+$ through acetylcholine receptors (AChRs) and a rapid, but usually transient, hyperkalemia. The use of this agent is contraindicated in patients who have sustained thermal trauma, neuromuscular injury (upper or lower motor neuron), disuse atrophy, mucositis, or prolonged immobilization in an intensive care unit (ICU) setting; the efflux of K$^+$ induced by succinylcholine is enhanced in these patients and can result in significant hyperkalemia.[526] These disorders share a two- to 100-fold upregulation of AChRs at the plasma membrane of muscle cells, with loss of the normal clustering at the neuromuscular junction.[526] Depolarization of these upregulated AChRs by succinylcholine results in an exaggerated efflux of K$^+$ through the receptor-associated cation channels that are spread throughout the muscle cell membrane

(Figure 18.12). Concomitant upregulation of the neuronal α_7-subunit of the AChR (α_7-AChR) has also been observed in denervated muscle; the α_7-AChR is a homomeric pentameric channel that depolarizes in response to succinylcholine and choline, its metabolite.[526] Depolarization of α_7-AChRs in response to choline is furthermore not subject to desensitization and may explain in part the hyperkalemic effect that persists in some patients well after the paralytic effect of succinylcholine has subsided.[526] Perhaps consistent with this neuromuscular pathophysiology, patients with renal failure do not appear to have an increased risk of succinylcholine-associated hyperkalemia.[527]

A report of three patients has suggested the possibility that drugs that share the ability to open K_{ATP} channels may have an underappreciated propensity to cause hyperkalemia in critically ill patients. The drugs implicated included cyclosporine, isoflurane, and nicorandil.[528] These patients exhibited hyperkalemia that resisted usual therapies (insulin-dextrose ± hemofiltration), with a temporal hypokalemic response to the K_{ATP} inhibitor glibenclamide (glyburide). The daring, off-label use of glybenclamide was presumably instigated by the senior author's observation that cyclosporine activates K_{ATP} channels in vascular smooth muscle.[529] K_{ATP} channels are widely distributed, including in skeletal muscle, so that activation of these channels is a plausible cause of acute hyperkalemia. Other case reports have emerged of nicorandil-associated hyperkalemia.[530,531] However, it still remains to be seen whether this is a common or important mechanism for acute hyperkalemia.

Finally, β-blockers cause hyperkalemia in part by inhibiting cellular uptake, but also through hyporeninemic hypoaldosteronism induced by the effects of these drugs on renal renin release and adrenal aldosterone release (see "Regulation of Renal Renin and Adrenal Aldosterone Release"). Labetalol, a broadly reactive sympathetic blocker, is a particularly common cause of hyperkalemia in susceptible patients.[21,532] However, nonspecific and cardiospecific β-blockers have been shown to reduce PRA, Ang II, and aldosterone,[533] such that β-blockade in general will increase susceptibility to hyperkalemia.

REDUCED RENAL POTASSIUM EXCRETION

HYPOALDOSTERONISM

Aldosterone promotes kaliuresis by activating apical amiloride-sensitive Na^+ currents in the CNT and CCD and thus increasing the lumen-negative driving force for K^+ excretion (see Chapter 6, "Aldosterone and K^+ Loading"). Aldosterone release from the adrenal may be reduced by hyporeninemic hypoaldosteronism and its multiple causes, medications, or isolated deficiency of ACTH. The isolated loss in pituitary secretion of ACTH leads to a deficit in circulating cortisol; variable defects in other pituitary hormones are likely secondary to this reduction in cortisol.[534] Concomitant hyporeninemic hypoaldosteronism is frequent,[28] but hyperkalemia is perhaps less common in secondary hypoaldosteronism than in Addison's disease.[534]

Primary hypoaldosteronism may be genetic or acquired.[535] The X-linked disorder adrenal hypoplasia congenita (AHC) is caused by loss-of-function mutations in the transcriptional repressor Dax-1. Patients with AHC present with primary adrenal failure and hyperkalemia shortly after birth or much later in childhood.[536] This bimodal presentation pattern does not appear to be influenced by *Dax-1* genotype; rather, if patients survive the early neonatal period, they will then miss being diagnosed until much later in life, presenting with delayed puberty (see later) or with an adrenal crisis. The steroidogenic factor-1 (SF-1), a functional partner for Dax-1, is also required for adrenal development in mice and humans. Both genes are involved in gonadal development, with *Dax-1* deficiency leading to hypogonadotropic hypogonadism[536] and *SF-1* deficiency causing male to female sex reversal in addition to adrenal insufficiency.

Reduced steroidogenesis causes two other important forms of primary hypoaldosteronism.[535] Congenital lipoid adrenal hyperplasia (lipoid CAH) is a severe autosomal recessive syndrome characterized by impaired synthesis of mineralocorticoids, glucocorticoids, and gonadal steroids.[21] Patients present in early infancy with adrenal crisis, including severe hyperkalemia.[537] Genotypically male 46,XY patients with lipoid CAH have female external genitalia due to the developmental absence of testosterone. Lipoid CAH is caused by loss-of-function mutations in steroidogenic acute regulatory protein, a small mitochondrial protein that helps shuttle cholesterol from the outer to inner mitochondrial membrane, thus initiating steroidogenesis[538]; some patients may alternatively have mutations in the side-chain cleavage P450 enzyme.[539] The classic, salt-wasting form of CAH due to 21-hydroxylase deficiency is associated with marked reductions in cortisol and aldosterone, leading to adrenal insufficiency.[540] Concomitant overproduction of androgenic steroids results in virilization in female patients with this form of CAH.

Isolated deficits in aldosterone synthesis with hyperreninemia are caused by loss-of-function mutations in aldosterone synthase, although genetic heterogeneity has been reported.[541] Patients typically present in childhood with volume depletion and hyperkalemia.[542] Much like pseudohypoaldosteronism due to loss-of-function mutations in the MR (see later), patients tend to become asymptomatic in adulthood. Acquired hyperreninemic hypoaldosteronism has been described in critical illness,[21] type 2 diabetes,[543] amyloidosis due to familial Mediterranean fever,[544] and after metastasis of carcinoma to the adrenal gland.[21] Finally, aldosterone synthesis is selectively reduced by heparin, with a 7% incidence of hyperkalemia associated with heparin therapy.[545] Both unfractionated[545] and low-molecular-weight[21,546] heparin can cause hyperkalemia. Hyperkalemia due to prophylactic subcutaneous unfractionated heparin (5000 units twice daily) has also been reported.[547] Heparin reduces the adrenal aldosterone response to Ang II and hyperkalemia, resulting in hyperreninemic hypoaldosteronism. Histologic findings in experimental animals include a marked diminution in the size of the zona glomerulosa and an attenuated hyperplastic response to salt depletion.[545]

Most primary adrenal insufficiency is due to autoimmunity in Addison's disease or in the context of a polyglandular endocrinopathy.[535,548] Adrenal insufficiency can be seen following adrenalectomy for primary hyperaldosteronism, with 14% of patients developing postoperative hyperkalemia and 5% developing long-term insufficiency requiring fludrocortisone.[549] The antiphospholipid syndrome may also cause bilateral adrenal hemorrhage and adrenal insufficiency.[550]

Another renal syndrome in which there should be a high index of suspicion for adrenal insufficiency is renal amyloidosis.[551] Finally, human immunodeficiency virus (HIV) infection has surpassed tuberculosis as the most important infectious cause of adrenal insufficiency. The most common cause of adrenalitis in HIV disease is cytomegalovirus (CMV), but a long list of infectious, degenerative, and infiltrative processes may involve the adrenal glands in these patients.[552] Although the adrenal involvement in HIV is usually subclinical, adrenal insufficiency may be precipitated by stress, drugs such as ketoconazole that inhibit steroidogenesis, or acute withdrawal of steroid agents such as megestrol.

Current estimates of the risk of hyperkalemia with Addison's disease are lacking, but the incidence is likely 50% to 60%.[21] The absence of hyperkalemia in such a high percentage of hypoadrenal patients underscores the importance of aldosterone-independent modulation of K^+ excretion by the distal nephron. A high-K^+ diet and high peritubular K^+ serves to increase apical Na^+ reabsorption and K^+ secretion in the CNT and CCD (see Chapter 6 "Aldosterone and K^+ Loading"); in most patients with reductions in circulating aldosterone, this homeostatic mechanism would appear to be sufficient to regulate plasma K^+ to within normal limits.

HYPORENINEMIC HYPOALDOSTERONISM

Hyporeninemic hypoaldosteronism[553] is a very common predisposing factor in several large, overlapping subsets of hyperkalemic patients—diabetics,[554] older patients,[21,172,555] and patients with renal insufficiency.[21] Hyporeninemic hypoaldosteronism has also been described in systemic lupus erythematosus (SLE),[21,556] multiple myeloma,[28] and acute glomerulonephritis.[28] Classically, patients should have suppressed PRA and aldosterone, which cannot be activated by typical modalities such as furosemide or sodium restriction.[553] Approximately 50% have an associated acidosis, with a reduced renal excretion of NH_4^+, a positive urinary anion gap, and urine pH lower than 5.5.[179,238] Although the generation of this acidosis is clearly multifactorial,[557] strong clinical[237,238,558] and experimental[234] evidence has suggested that hyperkalemia per se is the dominant factor, due to competitive inhibition of NH_4^+ transport in the thick ascending limb and reduced distal excretion of NH_4^+ (see also "Consequences of Hyperkalemia").[559]

Several factors account for the reduced PRA in diabetic patients with hyporeninemic hypoaldosteronism.[554] First, many patients have an associated autonomic neuropathy, with impaired release of renin during orthostatic challenges.[21] Failure to respond to isoproterenol with an increase in PRA, despite an adequate cardiovascular response, suggests a postreceptor defect in the ability of the juxtaglomerular apparatus to respond to β-adrenergic stimuli[21] (see also "Regulation of Renal Renin and Adrenal Aldosterone"). Second, the conversion of prorenin to active renin is impaired in some diabetics,[554] despite adequate release of the prorenin in response to furosemide[21]; this suggests a defect in the normal processing of prorenin. Third, as is the case with perhaps all patients with hyporeninemic hypoaldosteronism (see later), many diabetic patients appear to be volume-expanded, with subsequent suppression of PRA.

The most attractive current hypothesis for the suppression of PRA in hyporeninemic hypoaldosteronism is that primary volume expansion increases circulating ANP, which then exerts a negative effect on renal renin release and adrenal aldosterone release (see also "Regulation of Renal Renin and Adrenal Aldosterone"). There is evidence that these patients are volume-expanded, and many will respond to Na^+-Cl^- restriction or furosemide with an increased PRA—that is, renin is physiologically rather than pathologically suppressed.[560-562] Patients with hyporeninemic hypoaldosteronism due to a diversity of underlying causes have elevated ANP levels,[21,28,172,561,563] which is also an indicator of their underlying volume expansion. Patients who respond to furosemide with an increase in PRA exhibit a concomitant decrease in ANP.[561] Furthermore, the infusion of exogenous ANP can suppress the adrenal aldosterone response to hyperkalemia[172] and dietary Na^+-Cl^- depletion.[564]

ACQUIRED TUBULAR DEFECTS AND POTASSIUM EXCRETION

Unlike hyporeninemic hypoaldosteronism, hyperkalemic distal renal tubular acidosis is associated with a normal or increased aldosterone and/or PRA. Urine pH in these patients is higher than 5.5, and they are unable to increase acid or K^+ excretion in response to furosemide, Na^+-SO_4^{2-} or fludrocortisone.[565-567] Classic causes include SLE,[565] sickle cell anemia,[21,567] and amyloidosis.[21]

HEREDITARY TUBULAR DEFECTS AND POTASSIUM EXCRETION

Hereditary tubular causes of hyperkalemia have overlapping clinical features with hypoaldosteronism—hence, the shared label *pseudohypoaldosteronism* (PHA). PHA-I has an autosomal recessive and autosomal dominant form. The autosomal dominant form is due to loss-of-function mutations in the mineralocorticoid receptor.[568] These patients require aggressive salt supplementation during early childhood; however, similar to the hypoaldosteronism caused by mutations in aldosterone synthase, they typically become asymptomatic in adulthood.[369] Of interest, the lifelong increases in circulating aldosterone, Ang II, and renin seen in this syndrome do not appear to have untoward cardiovascular consequences.[568]

The recessive form of PHA-I is caused by various combinations of mutations in all three subunits of ENaC, resulting in impairment in its channel activity.[369] Patients with this syndrome present with severe neonatal salt wasting, hypotension, and hyperkalemia; in contrast to the autosomal dominant form of PHA-I, the syndrome does not improve in adulthood.[369] One unexpected result in the physiologic characterization of ENaC was that mice with a targeted deletion of the α-ENaC subunit were found to die within 40 hours of birth due to pulmonary edema.[28] Patients with recessive PHA-I may have pulmonary symptoms, which can occasionally be very severe[569]; however, it appears that unlike in ENaC-deficient mice, the modest residual activity associated with heteromeric PHA-I channels is generally sufficient to mediate pulmonary Na^+ and fluid clearance in humans with loss-of-function mutations in ENaC.[570]

Pseudohypoaldosteronism type II (PHA-II) (also known as Gordon's syndrome and, more recently, as FHHt) is in every respect the mirror image of Gitelman's syndrome; the clinical phenotype includes hypertension, hyperkalemia, hyperchloremic metabolic acidosis, suppressed PRA and aldosterone, hypercalciuria, and reduced bone density.[571]

FHHt behaves like a gain of function in the thiazide-sensitive Na+-Cl− cotransporter NCC, and treatment with thiazides typically results in resolution of the entire clinical picture.[571] FHHt is an extreme form of hyporeninemic hypoaldosteronism due to volume expansion; aggressive salt restriction decreases ANP levels and increases PRA, with resolution of the hypertension, hyperkalemia, and metabolic acidosis.[563]

FHHt is an autosomal dominant syndrome, with as many as four genetic loci.[21] In a landmark paper, mutations in two related serine-threonine kinases were detected in various kindreds with FHHt.[572] The catalytic sites of these kinases lack specific catalytic lysines conserved in other kinases—hence the designation WNK (*w*ith *n*o *l*ysine, as noted earlier). Whereas FHHt mutations in WNK4 affect the C terminus of the coding sequence, large intronic deletions in the WNK1 gene result in increased expression. Both kinases are expressed within the distal nephron in DCT and CCD cells; whereas WNK1 localizes to the cytoplasm and basolateral membrane, WNK4 protein is found at the apical tight junctions.[572] WNK-dependent phosphorylation and activation of the downstream SPAK (STE20/SPS1-related proline/alanine-rich kinase) and OSR1 (oxidative stress-responsive kinase 1) kinases lead to phosphorylation of a cluster of N-terminal threonines in NCC, resulting in an activation of Na+-Cl− cotransport[135] (see also Figure 18.6). However, coexpression of WNK4 with NCC reveals an additional inhibitory influence of the kinase on NCC, effects that are blocked by FHHt-associated point mutations in the kinase.[573] In particular, the inhibitory effects of WNK4 appear to dominate in mouse models with overexpression of wild-type versus FHHt mutant WNK4.[71] Competing divergent mechanisms can be reconciled by the likelihood that the physiologic context determines whether WNK4 will have an activating or inhibitory effect on NCC.[135,573] For example, the activation of NCC by the Ang II receptor appears to require the downstream activation of SPAK by WNK4.[137]

A key insight from the mechanistic study of FHHt is that activation of NCC in the DCT in this syndrome serves to reduce Na+ delivery to principal cells in the downstream CNT and CCD, leading to hyperkalemia.[71] This and other effects of the WNK pathways on distal K+ secretion are discussed earlier in this chapter (see "Control of Potassium Secretion: Effect of Potassium Intake").

MEDICATION-RELATED HYPERKALEMIA

CYCLO-OXYGENASE INHIBITORS

Hyperkalemia is a well-recognized complication of nonsteroidal antiinflammatory drugs (NSAIDs) that inhibit cyclo-oxygenases. NSAIDs cause hyperkalemia by a variety of mechanisms, as would be predicted from the relevant physiology. By decreasing the GFR and increasing sodium retention, they decrease distal delivery of Na+ and reduce distal flow rate. Moreover, the flow-activated apical maxi-K channel in the CNT and CCD is activated by prostaglandins[574]; hence, NSAIDs will reduce its activity and the flow-dependent component of K+ excretion.[77,401] NSAIDs are also a classic cause of hyporeninemic hypoaldosteronism.[575,576] The administration of indomethacin to normal volunteers was found to attenuate furosemide-induced increases in PRA.[158,577] Finally, NSAIDs would not cause hyperkalemia with such regularity if they did not also blunt the adrenal response to hyperkalemia, which is at least partially dependent on prostaglandins acting through prostaglandin EP2 receptors and cAMP.[171]

The physiology reviewed earlier in this chapter (see "Regulation of Renal Renin and Adrenal Aldosterone") would suggest that COX-2 inhibitors are equally likely to cause hyperkalemia. Indeed, COX-2 inhibitors can clearly cause sodium retention and a decrease in glomerular filtration rate,[578,579] suggesting NSAID-like effects on renal pathophysiology. COX-2–derived prostaglandins stimulate renal renin release,[21] and COX-2 inhibitors reduce PRA in dogs[28] and humans.[158] Salt restriction potentiates the hyperkalemia seen in dogs treated with COX-2 inhibitors,[28] such that hypovolemic patients may be particularly prone to hyperkalemia in this setting. The COX-2 inhibitor celecoxib and the nonselective NSAID ibuprofen have equivalent negative effects on K+ excretion after a defined oral load.[580] Not surprisingly, clinical reports have noted hyperkalemia and acute kidney injury associated with COX-2 inhibitors.[21,581,582] Where the data have been reported, circulating PRA and/or aldosterone have been reduced in hyperkalemia associated with COX-2 inhibitors.[28,582]

CYCLOSPORINE AND TACROLIMUS

Both cyclosporine[583] (CsA) and tacrolimus[584] cause hyperkalemia; the risk of sustained hyperkalemia may be higher in renal transplantation patients treated with tacrolimus than in those treated with CsA.[585] CsA is perhaps the most versatile of all drugs in regard to the variety of mechanisms whereby it causes hyperkalemia. It causes hyporeninemic hypoaldosteronism[586] due in part to its inhibitory effect on COX-2 expression in the macula densa.[587] CsA inhibits apical SK secretory K+ channels in the distal nephron[588] in addition to basolateral Na+-K+-ATPase.[21] Finally, CsA causes redistribution of K+ and hyperkalemia, particularly when used in combination with β-blockers.[589] A provocative preliminary report has linked acute hyperkalemia secondary to CsA to indirect activation of K_{ATP} channels (also see earlier)[528]; this is particularly intriguing given the reported response to K_{ATP} inhibition with glibenclamide infusion.

EPITHELIAL SODIUM CHANNEL INHIBITION

Inhibition of apical ENaC activity in the distal nephron by amiloride and other K+-sparing diuretics predictably results in hyperkalemia. Amiloride is structurally similar to the antibiotics trimethoprim (TMP) and pentamidine, which can also inhibit ENaC.[590-592] Trimethoprim thus inhibits Na+ reabsorption and K+ secretion in perfused CCDs.[593] Both TMP-sulfamethoxazole (SMX; Bactrim) and pentamidine were reported to cause hyperkalemia during high-dose treatment of *Pneumocystis* pneumonia in HIV patients,[21,592] who are otherwise predisposed to hyperkalemia. However, this side effect is not restricted to high-dose intravenous therapy; in a study of hospitalized patients treated with standard doses of TMP, significant hyperkalemia occurred in more than 50%, with severe hyperkalemia (>5.5 mmol/L) in 21%.[594] Risk factors for hyperkalemia due to normal-dose TMP include renal insufficiency,[594] hyporeninemic hypoaldosteronism,[595] and concomitant use of ACE inhibitors and ARBs.[596] This is not a trivial association, in that TMP-SMX administration increases the risk of sudden death in patients treated with ACE inhibitors, ARBs, or spironolactone.[597,598]

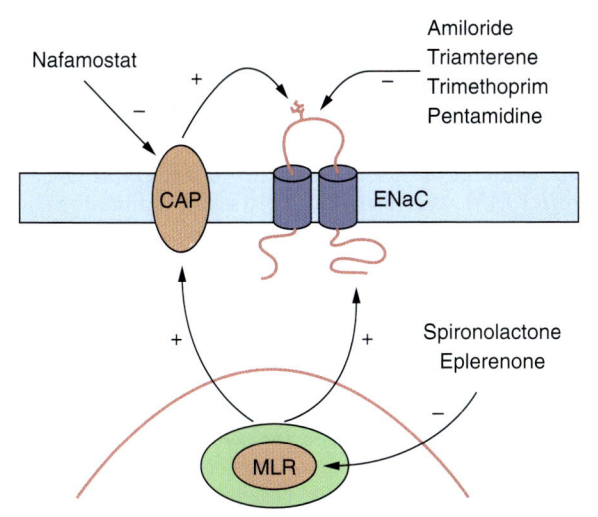

Figure 18.13 Pharmacologic inhibition of the epithelial Na+ channel (ENaC). Whereas amiloride and related compounds directly inhibit the channel, the protease inhibitor nafamostat inhibits membrane-associated proteases such as CAP1 (channel-activating protease 1), thus indirectly inhibiting the channel. Spironolactone and related drugs inhibit the mineralocorticoid receptor (MLR), thus reducing transcription of the α-subunit of ENaC, ENaC-activating kinase SGK, and several other target genes (see text for details).

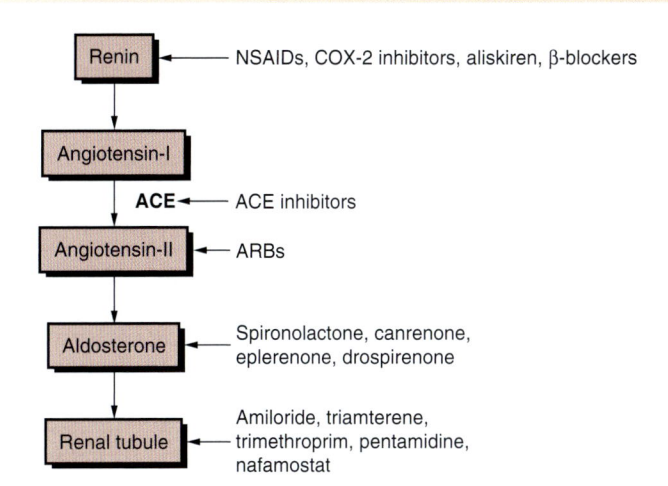

Figure 18.14 Medications that target the renin-angiotensin-aldosterone axis are common causes of hyperkalemia, as are drugs that inhibit epithelial Na+ channels (ENaCs) in the renal tubule (CNT or CCD).

Whereas TMP and pentamidine directly inhibit ENaC, a novel, indirect mechanism for ENaC inhibition-associated hyperkalemia has been reported.[21,109] Aldosterone induces expression of the membrane-associated proteases CAP1 to CAP3 (see "Control of Potassium Secretion: Aldosterone"). Nafamostat, a protease inhibitor widely used in Japan for pancreatitis and other indications, is known to cause hyperkalemia[109]; indirect evidence has suggested that the mechanism involves inhibition of amiloride-sensitive Na+ channels in the CCD.[21] Treatment of rats with nafamostat was also shown to reduce the urinary excretion of CAP1 prostasin, in contrast to the reported effect of aldosterone.[103] Thus inhibition of the protease activity of CAP1 by nafamostat appears to abrogate its activating effect on ENaC (Figure 18.13), and may reduce expression of the protein in the CCD.[110]

ANGIOTENSIN-CONVERTING ENZYME INHIBITORS AND MINERALOCORTICOID AND ANGIOTENSIN ANTAGONISTS

Hyperkalemia is a predictable and common effect of ACE inhibition, direct renin inhibition, and antagonism of the mineralocorticoid and angiotensin receptors[599] (Figure 18.14). The oral contraceptive agent Yasmin 28 and related products contain the progestin drospirenone, which inhibits the MR[600] and can potentially cause hyperkalemia in susceptible patients. As with many other causes of hyperkalemia, that induced by pharmacologic targeting of the RAAS axis depends on concomitant inhibition of adrenal aldosterone release by hyperkalemia; the adrenal release of aldosterone due to increased K+ is clearly dependent on an intact adrenal renal-angiotensin system, such that this response is abrogated by systemic ACE inhibitors and ARBs[166] (see "Regulation of Renal Renin and Adrenal Aldosterone Release"). Dual treatment with lisinopril and spironolactone in subjects with CKD is also associated with a reduction in extrarenal potassium disposition, given that reduced K+ excretion alone does not explain the substantial increase in serum K+ after a defined oral potassium load.[601] Similarly, the addition of spironolactone to losartan in the treatment of diabetic nephropathy causes a significant increase in serum K+ without significant change in urinary K+ excretion.[602] ACE inhibitors and ARBs have the additional potential to cause acute renal failure and acute hyperkalemia in patients with an angiotensin-dependent GFR; the renin inhibitor aliskiren has also been reported to cause acute renal failure with acute hyperkalemia, albeit in conjunction with spironolactone.[603]

RAAS inhibitors are an increasingly important cause of hyperkalemia, given the increasing indications to combine spironolactone or aliskiren with ACE inhibitors and/or ARBs in renal and cardiac disease,[604,605] in addition to the emergence of MR antagonists with perhaps a greater potential for hyperkalemia.[606] Hyperkalemia can evidently occur within 1 week of starting angiotensin receptor blockade.[607] Heart failure, diabetes, and CKD increase the risk of hyperkalemia from these agents.[599,608,609] The prevalence of hyperkalemia associated with the combined use of MR antagonists and ACE inhibitors and ARBs appears to be much higher in clinical practice (≈10%)[610] than what has been reported in large clinical trials,[599] in part due to the use of higher than recommended doses.[21] Notably, Pitt and colleagues studied the correlation between the rate of spironolactone prescription for Canadian patients with heart failure on ACE inhibitors following the publication of the Randomized Aldactone Evaluation Study (RALES),[611] with hyperkalemia and associated morbidity.[612] This provocative study found an abrupt increase in the rate of prescription for spironolactone after release of RALES, with a temporal correlation to increases in the rate of admissions with hyperkalemia[612]; the association remained statistically significant for admissions when hyperkalemia was the primary diagnosis.[613] However, a study from the United Kingdom found a similar increase in spironolactone use after the publication of RALES, but without an increase in hyperkalemia or hyperkalemia-associated admissions to hospital.[614] It should also be emphasized that the development of hyperkalemia, or the presence of predisposing factors for hyperkalemia, does not appear to mitigate the mortality benefits of eplerenone in heart failure.[609]

Given the mounting evidence supporting the combined use of ACE inhibitors, ARBs, and/or MR antagonists, it is prudent to adhere to measures systematically that will minimize the chance of associated hyperkalemia, therefore allowing patients to benefit from the cardiovascular and renal effects of these agents. The patients at risk for the development of hyperkalemia in response to drugs that target the RAAS axis, singly or in combination therapy, are those for whom the ability of kidneys to excrete the potassium load is markedly diminished due to one or more of the following factors: (1) decreased delivery of sodium to the cortical collecting duct (e.g., as in congestive heart failure, volume depletion); (2) decreased circulating aldosterone (e.g., hyporeninemic hypoaldosteronism, drugs such as heparin or ketoconazole); (3) inhibition of amiloride-sensitive Na^+ channels in the CNT and CCD by coadministration of TMP-SMX, pentamidine, or amiloride; (4) chronic tubulointerstitial disease, with associated dysfunction of the distal nephron; and (5) increased potassium intake (e.g., salt substitutes, diet). Overall, patients with diabetes, heart failure, and/or CKD are at particular risk for hyperkalemia from RAAS inhibition.[599,608,609] In these susceptible patients, the following approach is recommended to prevent or minimize the occurrence of hyperkalemia in response to medications that interfere with the RAAS[28,615]:

1. Estimate the GFR using the Modification of Diet in Renal Disease (MDRD) equation, Cockcroft-Gault equation, and/or 24-hour creatinine clearance.
2. Inquire about diet and dietary supplements (e.g., salt substitutes, licorice) and prescribe a low-potassium diet.
3. Inquire about medications, particularly those that can interfere with renal K^+ excretion (e.g., NSAIDs, COX-2 inhibitors, K^+-sparing diuretics) and, if appropriate, discontinue these agents.
4. Continue or initiate loop or thiazide-like diuretics.
5. Correct acidosis with sodium bicarbonate.
6. Initiate treatment with a low dose of only one of the agents—ACE inhibitor, ARB, or MR antagonists.
7. Check serum K^+ 3 to 5 days after initiation of the therapy and each dose increment, at most within 1 week,[607] followed by another measurement 1 week later.
8. If the serum K^+ is more than 5.6, ACE inhibitors, ARBs, and/or MR blockers should be stopped and the patient treated for hyperkalemia.
9. If serum K^+ is increased but lower than 5.6 mmol/L, reduce the dose and reassess the possible contributing factors. If the patient is on a combination of ACE inhibitors, ARBs, and/or MR blockers, all but one should be stopped and the K^+ rechecked.
10. A combination of an MR blocker and an ACE inhibitor or ARB should not be prescribed to patients with stage 4 or 5 CKD (estimated GFR < 30 mL/min).
11. The dosage of spironolactone in combination with ACE inhibitors or ARBs should be no more than 25 mg/day.

CLINICAL APPROACH TO HYPERKALEMIA

The first priority in the management of hyperkalemia is to assess the need for emergency treatment (electrocardiographic changes; $K^+ \geq 6.5$ mmol/L). This should be followed by a comprehensive workup to determine the cause (Figure 18.15). The history and physical examination should focus on medications (e.g., ACE inhibitors, NSAIDs, TMP-SMX), diet and dietary supplements (e.g., salt substitute), risk factors for kidney failure, reduction in urine output, blood pressure, and volume status. Initial laboratory tests should include electrolytes, BUN, creatinine, plasma osmolality, Mg^{2+}, and Ca^{2+}, and complete blood count and urinary pH, osmolality, creatinine, and electrolytes. Plasma and urine osmolality are required for calculation of the transtubular K^+ gradient (see "Urinary Indices of Potassium Excretion"). Plasma renin activity, plasma aldosterone, and the response in TTKG to fludrocortisone may be necessary to determine the specific cause of an inappropriately low TTKG in hyperkalemia.

TREATMENT OF HYPERKALEMIA

Indications for the hospitalization of patients with hyperkalemia are poorly defined, in part because there is no universally accepted definition for mild, moderate, or severe hyperkalemia. The clinical sequelae of hyperkalemia, which are primarily cardiac and neuromuscular, depend on many other variables (e.g., plasma calcium level, acid-base status, and rate of change in plasma K^+), in addition to the absolute value of the serum K^+; these issues are likely to influence management decisions.[218-221,477,616] Severe hyperkalemia (serum $K^+ \geq 8.0$ mmol/L), electrocardiographic changes other than peaked T waves, acute deterioration of renal function, and presence of additional medical problems have been suggested as appropriate criteria for hospitalization.[477] However, hyperkalemia in patients with any electrocardiographic manifestation should be considered a true medical emergency and treated urgently[214,476,617,618]; adequate management and serial monitoring of serum K^+ will generally require admission. Given the limitations of electrocardiographic changes as a predictor of cardiac toxicity (see "Consequences of Hyperkalemia"), patients with severe hyperkalemia ($K^+ \geq 6.5$ to 7.0 mmol/L) in the absence of electrocardiographic changes should be aggressively managed.[188,214,476,618-620]

Urgent management of hyperkalemia constitutes a 12-lead ECG, admission to the hospital, continuous electrocardiographic monitoring, and immediate treatment. The treatment of hyperkalemia is generally divided into three categories: (1) antagonism of the cardiac effects of hyperkalemia; (2) rapid reduction in K^+ by redistribution into cells; and (3) removal of K^+ from the body. The necessary measures to treat the underlying conditions causing hyperkalemia should be undertaken to minimize factors that are contributing to hyperkalemia and to prevent future episodes.[214] Dietary restriction (usually, 60 mEq/day) with emphasis on K^+ content of total parenteral nutrition (TPN) solutions and enteral feeding products (typically, 25 to 50 mmol/L) and adjustment of medications and intravenous fluids are necessary; hidden sources of K^+, such as intravenous antibiotics,[502] should not be overlooked.

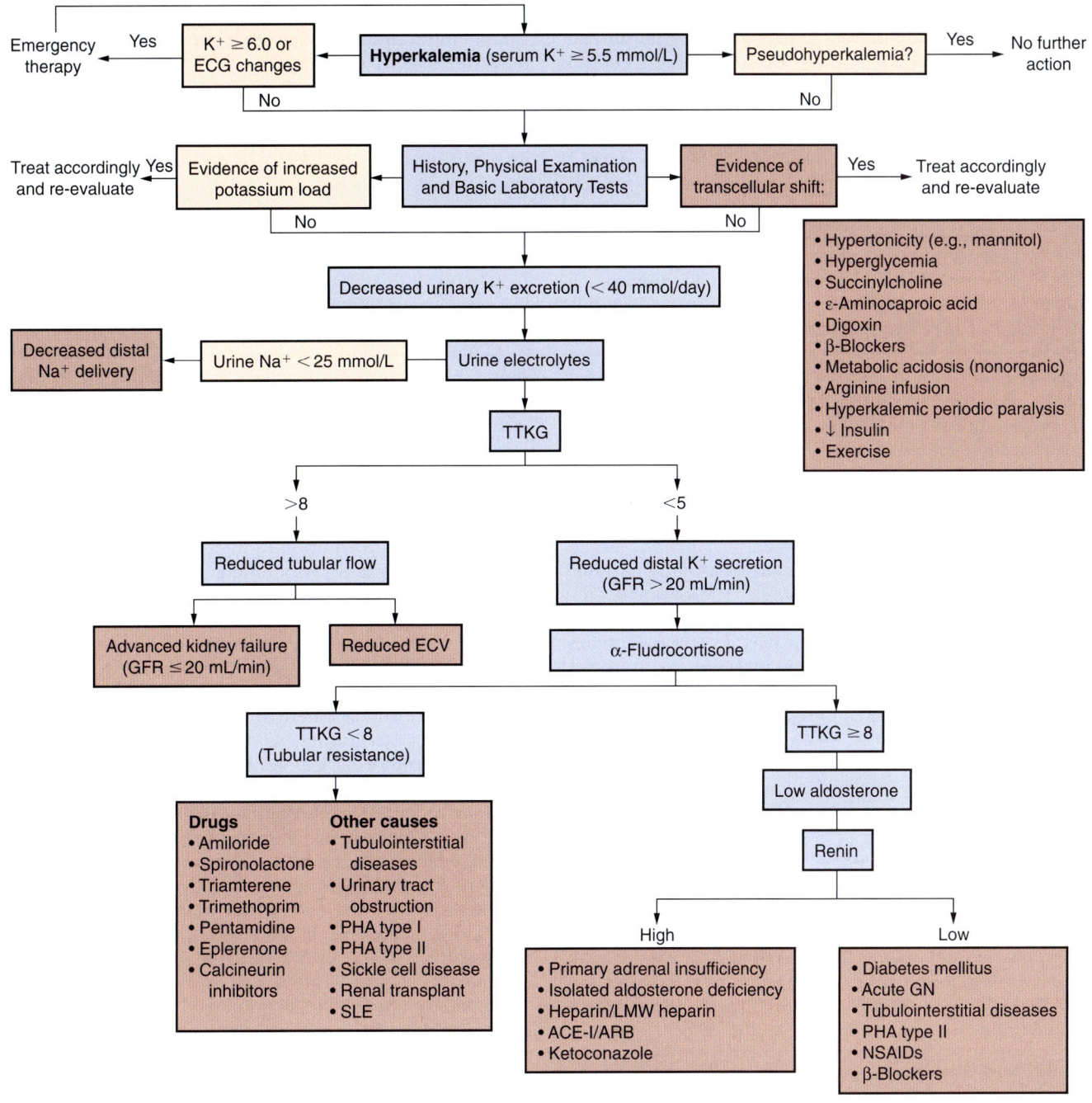

Figure 18.15 Clinical approach to hyperkalemia. See text for details. ACE-I, Angiotensin-converting enzyme inhibitor; ECG, electrocardiogram; GN, glomerulonephritis; ARB, angiotensin II receptor blocker; CCD, cortical collecting duct; ECV, effective circulatory volume; GFR, glomerular filtration rate; HIV, human immunodeficiency virus; LMW heparin, low-molecular-weight heparin; NSAIDs, nonsteroidal antiinflammatory drugs; PHA, pseudohypoaldosteronism; SLE, systemic lupus erythematosus; TTKG, transtubular potassium gradient.

ANTAGONISM OF CARDIAC EFFECTS

Intravenous calcium is the first-line drug in the emergency management of hyperkalemia, even in patients with normal calcium levels. The mutually antagonistic effects of calcium and K+ on the myocardium and protective role of Ca^{2+} in hyperkalemia have long been known.[621] Calcium raises the action potential threshold to a less negative value, without changing the resting membrane potential; by restoring the usual 15-mV difference between resting and threshold potentials, myocyte excitability is reduced.[188,622] Administration of calcium also alters the relationship between V_{max} and the resting membrane potential, maintaining a more normal V_{max} at less negative resting membrane potentials and thus restoring myocardial conduction.[188]

Calcium is available as calcium chloride or calcium gluconate (10-mL ampules of 10% solutions) for intravenous infusion. Each milliliter of 10% calcium gluconate or calcium chloride has 8.9 mg (0.22 mmol) and 27.2 mg (0.68 mmol) of elemental calcium, respectively.[623] Calcium gluconate[624] is less irritating to the veins and can be used through a peripheral intravenous line; calcium chloride can cause tissue necrosis if it extravasates and requires a central line. A study of patients undergoing cardiac surgery with extracorporeal perfusion (with concomitant high gluconate infusion) has suggested that the increase in the ionized calcium level is significantly lower with calcium gluconate.[625] This finding was attributed to a requirement for hepatic metabolism in the release of ionized calcium from calcium gluconate, such that less ionized calcium would be bioavailable in cases of liver failure or diminished hepatic perfusion.[625] However, further studies in vitro in animals, in humans with normal hepatic function, and during the anhepatic stage of liver transplantation have shown equal and rapid dissociation of ionized calcium from equal doses of calcium chloride and calcium gluconate, indicating that release of ionized calcium from calcium gluconate is independent of hepatic metabolism.[28]

The recommended dose is 10 mL of 10% calcium gluconate (3 to 4 mL of calcium chloride), infused intravenously over 2 to 3 minutes and under continuous electrocardiographic monitoring. The effect of the infusion starts in 1 to 3 minutes and lasts 30 to 60 minutes.[481,620] The dose should be repeated if there is no change in electrocardiographic findings or if they recur after initial improvement.[481,620] However, calcium should be used with extreme caution in patients taking digitalis because hypercalcemia potentiates the toxic effects of digitalis on the myocardium.[624] In this case, 10 mL of 10% calcium gluconate should be added to 100 mL of D_5W and infused over 20 to 30 minutes to avoid hypercalcemia and allow for an even distribution of calcium in the extracellular compartment.[479,619,622] To prevent the precipitation of calcium carbonate, calcium should not be administered in solutions containing bicarbonate.

REDISTRIBUTION OF POTASSIUM INTO CELLS

Sodium bicarbonate, β_2-agonists, and insulin with glucose are all used in the treatment of hyperkalemia to induce a redistribution of K^+. Of these, insulin with glucose is the most constant and reliable, whereas bicarbonate is the most controversial. However, they are all temporary measures and should not be substituted for the definitive therapy of hyperkalemia, which is removal of K^+ from the body.

Insulin and Glucose

Insulin has the ability to lower plasma K^+ level by shifting K^+ into cells, particularly into skeletal myocytes and hepatocytes (see "Factors Affecting Internal Distribution of Potassium"). This effect is reliable, reproducible, dose-dependent,[481] and effective, even in patients with chronic kidney disease and ESKD[626-628] and those in the anhepatic stage of liver transplantation.[629] The effect of insulin on plasma K^+ levels is independent of age, adrenergic activity,[630] and its hypoglycemic effect, which may be impaired in patients with CKD and/or ESKD.[28]

Insulin can be administered with glucose as a constant infusion or as a bolus injection.[627,628] The recommended dose for insulin with glucose infusion is 10 units of regular insulin in 500 mL of 10% dextrose, given over 60 minutes (there is no further drop in plasma K^+ after 90 minutes of insulin infusion[622,630]). However, a bolus injection is easier to administer, particularly under emergency conditions.[214] The recommended dose is 10 units of regular insulin administered intravenously followed immediately by 50 mL of 50% dextrose (25 g of glucose).[617,627,631,632] The effect of insulin on the K^+ level begins in 10 to 20 minutes, peaks at 30 to 60 minutes, and lasts for 4 to 6 hours.[481,619,627,633] In almost all patients, the serum K^+ drops by 0.5 to 1.2 mmol/L after this treatment.[628,629,632,633] The dose can be repeated as necessary.

Despite glucose administration, hypoglycemia may occur in up to 75% of patients treated with the bolus regimen described earlier, typically 1 hour after the infusion.[627] The likelihood of hypoglycemia is greater when the dose of glucose given is less than 30 g.[479] To prevent this, infusion of 10% dextrose at 50 to 75 mL/hour and close monitoring of blood glucose levels is recommended.[617,631] Administration of glucose without insulin is not recommended, since the endogenous insulin release may be variable.[519] Glucose in the absence of insulin may in fact increase plasma K^+ by increasing plasma osmolality.[511,512,631] In hyperglycemic patients with glucose levels of 200 to 250 mg/dL or higher, insulin should be administered without glucose and with close monitoring of plasma glucose.[622] Combined treatment with β_2-agonists, in addition to their synergism with insulin in lowering plasma K^+, may reduce the level of hypoglycemia.[627] Of note, the combined regimen may increase the heart rate by 15.1 ± 6.0 beats per minute (beats/min).[627]

β_2-Adrenergic Agonists

β_2-agonists are an important but underused group of agents for the acute management of hyperkalemia. They exert their effect by activating Na^+-K^+-ATPase and the NKCC1 Na^+-K^+-$2Cl^-$ cotransporter, shifting K^+ into hepatocytes and skeletal myocytes (see also "Factors Affecting Internal Distribution of Potassium"). Albuterol (Salbutamol), a selective β_2-agonist, is the most widely studied and used. It is available in oral, inhaled, and intravenous forms; the intravenous and inhaled or nebulized forms are effective.[634]

The recommended dose for intravenous administration, which is not available in the United States, is 0.5 mg of albuterol in 100 mL of 5% dextrose, given over 10 to 15 minutes.[622,634,635] Its K^+-lowering effect starts in a few minutes, is maximal at about 30 to 40 minutes,[634,635] and lasts for 2 to 6 hours.[479] It reduces serum K^+ levels by approximately 0.9 to 1.4 mmol/L.[479]

The recommended dose for inhaled albuterol is 10 to 20 mg of nebulized albuterol in 4 mL of normal saline, inhaled over 10 minutes[627] (nebulized levalbuterol is as effective as albuterol[636]). Its kaliopenic effect starts at about 30 minutes, reaches its peak at about 90 minutes,[627,634] and lasts for 2 to 6 hours.[479,634] Inhaled albuterol reduces serum K^+ levels by approximately 0.5 to 1.0 mmol/L[479]; albuterol administered by a metered-dose inhaler with a spacer has reduced serum K^+ by approximately 0.4 mmol/L.[637] Albuterol (in inhaled or parenteral form) and insulin with glucose have an additive effect on reducing serum K^+ levels by approximately 1.2 to 1.5 mmol/L in total.[479,627,633] However, a subset of patients with ESKD (≈20% to 40%) are not responsive to the K^+-lowering effect of albuterol ($\Delta K \leq 0.4$ mmol/L); albuterol (or some other β_2-agonist) should not be used as a single agent in the treatment of hyperkalemia.[481,519] In an attempt to reduce pharmacokinetic variability, one study tested the effects of weight-based dosing on serum K⁺ levels, using 7 μg/kg of subcutaneous terbutaline (a β_2-agonist) in a group of ESKD patients.[638] The results showed a significant decline in serum K⁺ levels in almost all patients (mean, 1.31 ± 0.5 mmol/L; range, 0.5 to 2.3 mmol/L) in 30 to 90 minutes; of note, the heart rate increased by an average of 25.8 ± 10.5 beats/min (range, 6.5 to 48 beats/min).[638]

Treatment with albuterol may result in an increase in plasma glucose (≈2 to 3 mmol/L) and heart rate. The increase in heart rate is more pronounced with the intravenous form (≈20 beats/min) than with inhaled form (≈6 to 10 beats/min).[519,634] There is no significant increase in systolic or diastolic blood pressure with nebulized or intravenous administration of albuterol.[634] However, it is prudent to use these agents with caution in patients with ischemic heart disease.[479]

Sodium Bicarbonate

Bicarbonate prevailed as a preferred treatment modality of hyperkalemia for decades. For example, in a survey of nephrology-training program directors in 1989, it was ranked as the second-line treatment, after Ca^{2+}.[639] Its use to treat acute hyperkalemia was mainly based on small, older, uncontrolled clinical studies with a very limited number of patients,[55,63,640] in whom bicarbonate was typically administered as a long infusion over many hours (contrary to intravenous push, which later became the routine).[641] One of these studies, which is frequently quoted, concluded that the K⁺-lowering effect of bicarbonate is independent of changes in pH.[63] However, confounding variables included the duration of infusion, use of glucose-containing solutions, and infrequent monitoring of serum K⁺.[63,642]

The role of bicarbonate in the acute treatment of hyperkalemia has been challenged.[628,641,643] Blumberg and associates compared different K⁺-lowering modalities (Figure 18.16) and showed that bicarbonate infusion (isotonic or hypertonic) for up to 60 minutes had no effect on serum K⁺ in their cohort of ESKD patients on hemodialysis[628]; there is, however, an effect of isotonic bicarbonate at 4 to 6 hours.[641] These observations were later confirmed by others, who failed to show any acute (60 to 120 minutes) K⁺-lowering effects for bicarbonate.[641-643] A few studies have shown that metabolic acidosis may attenuate the physiologic responses to insulin and β_2-agonists.[481,643] The combined effect of bicarbonate and insulin with glucose has been studied, with conflicting results.[643] In addition, bicarbonate and albuterol coadministration failed to show any additional benefit over albuterol alone.[643]

In summary, bicarbonate administration, especially as a single agent, has no role in the current treatment of acute hyperkalemia. Prolonged infusion of isotonic bicarbonate in ESKD patients does, however, reduce serum K⁺ at 5 to 6 hours, by up to 0.7 mmol/L; approximately half of this effect is due to volume expansion.[641] Regardless of the mechanism, bicarbonate infusion may thus have a limited role in the subacute control of hyperkalemia—for example, in the nondialytic management of patients with severe hyperkalemia.[644] The acute effect of bicarbonate infusion on serum K⁺ in severely acidemic patients is not clear; however, it may be of some benefit in this setting.[214,617] Of note, the infusion of sodium bicarbonate may reduce serum ionized calcium levels and cause volume overload, issues of relevance in acidemic patients with renal failure.[481,619] When bicarbonate administration is used for hyperkalemia, we recommend isotonic infusion of sodium bicarbonate; although hypertonic sodium bicarbonate does not increase serum K⁺, it has been reported to cause hypernatremia.[506,628]

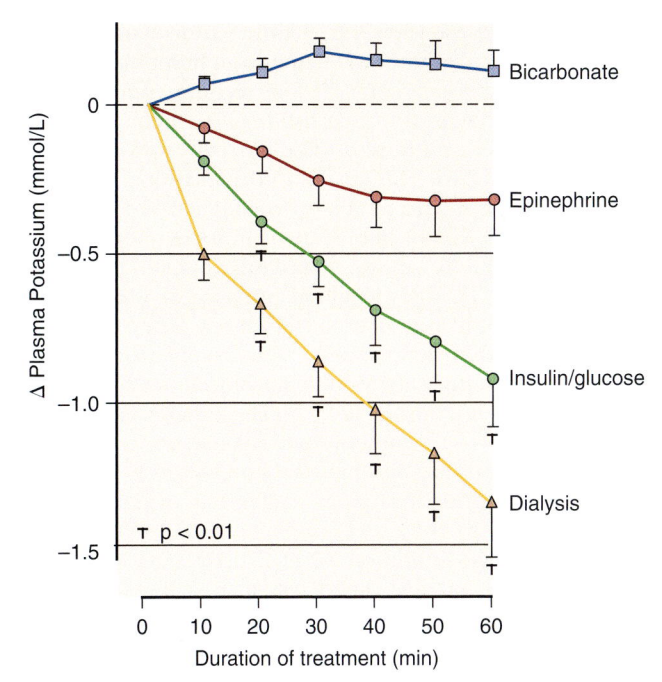

Figure 18.16 Changes in serum K⁺ during intravenous infusion of bicarbonate, epinephrine, or insulin in glucose and during hemodialysis. (From Blumberg A, Weidmann P, Shaw S, Gnadinger M: Effect of various therapeutic approaches on plasma potassium and major regulating factors in terminal renal failure. Am J Med 85:507-512, 1988.)

REMOVAL OF POTASSIUM

Diuretics

Diuretics have a relatively modest effect on urinary K⁺ excretion in patients with CKD,[645] particularly in an acute setting.[620] However, these medications are useful in correcting hyperkalemia in patients with the syndrome of hyporeninemic hypoaldosteronism[646] and selective renal K⁺ secretory problems (e.g., after transplantation or administration of TMP).[647,648] In patients with impaired renal function, use of the following agents is recommended: (1) oral diuretics with the highest bioavailability (e.g., torsemide) and the least renal metabolism (e.g., torsemide, bumetanide) to minimize the chance of accumulation and toxicity; (2) intravenous agents (short-term treatment) with the least hepatic metabolism (e.g., furosemide rather than bumetanide); (3) combinations of loop and thiazide-like diuretics for better efficacy (although this may decrease the GFR due to activation of tubuloglomerular feedback[649]); and (4) maximal effective ceiling dose.[645,649]

Mineralocorticoids

Limited data are available on the role of mineralocorticoids in the management of acute hyperkalemia.[28,650] However, these agents have been used for treating chronic hyperkalemia in patients with hypoaldosteronism, with or without hyporeninism, those with SLE,[651] kidney transplant patients on cyclosporine,[652] and ESKD patients on hemodialysis with interdialytic hyperkalemia.[653,654] The recommended dose is 0.1 to 0.3 mg/day of fludrocortisone, a synthetic glucocorticoid with potent mineralocorticoid activity and moderate glucocorticoid activity (0.3 mg of fludrocortisone = 1 mg of prednisone with regard to glucocorticoid activity).[28,652-654] In patients with ESKD on hemodialysis, this regimen reduces serum K^+ by 0.5 to 0.7 mmol/L and has not been associated with significant changes in blood pressure or weight (as a surrogate for fluid retention).[653] However, other studies of 0.1 mg/day of fludrocortisone in patients on chronic hemodialysis found statistically significant but clinically inconsequential effects on serum K^+.[655,656] The long-term safety of fludrocortisone for treatment of ESKD has not been established and, given the minimal effect on serum K^+, I do not recommend its use for the management of interdialytic hyperkalemia.

Pharmacologic inhibition of 11βHSD-2 with glycyrrhetinic acid (GA) has also been tested as a mechanism to control hyperkalemia in ESKD.[367] As in other aldosterone-sensitive epithelia, the 11βHSD-2 enzyme protects colonic epithelial cells from illicit activation of the MR by cortisol. Hypothesizing that GA would activate extrarenal potassium secretion by the colon and other tissues, Farese and coworkers tested the effect of the drug in a double-blind, placebo-controlled trial in 10 ESKD patients.[367] Treatment with GA significantly increased the serum ratio of cortisol/cortisone, consistent with successful inhibition of 11βHSD-2. This effect was associated with a significant reduction in mean serum K^+, with 70% of predialysis values in the normal range (3.5 to 4.7 mmol/L) in the GA phase of the trial versus 24% in the placebo phase. Plasma renin activity and aldosterone levels also dropped, perhaps due to the lower median plasma K^+ level. Glycyrrhetinic acid is thus a promising agent for long-term management of plasma K^+ in ESKD; clearly, however, more extensive clinical testing is required before widespread utilization.

CATION EXCHANGE RESINS

Ion exchange resins are cross-linked polymers containing acidic or basic structural units that can exchange anions or cations on contact with a solution. They are capable of binding to a variety of monovalent and divalent cations. Cation exchange resins are classified based on the cation (e.g., hydrogen, ammonium, sodium, potassium, calcium) that is cycled during synthesis of the resin to saturate sulfonic or carboxylic groups. In 1950, Elkinton and colleagues successfully used a carboxylic resin in the ammonium cycle in three patients with hyperkalemia.[657] However, hydrogen- or ammonium-cycled resins were associated with metabolic acidosis[658] and mouth ulcers,[659] making the sodium-cycled resins preferable.[660] Calcium-cycled resins may have other potential benefits, including a phosphate-lowering effect; however, this requires large, potentially toxic doses of resin[661]; moreover, these resins have been associated with hypercalcemia.[662] The dominant resin clinically available in the United States is sodium polystyrene sulfonate (SPS).

SPS exchanges Na^+ for K^+ in the gastrointestinal tract, mainly in the colon,[617,659,663] and has been shown to increase the fecal excretion of K^+.[659] Occasional constipation that is easily controlled with enema or cathartics has been reported with oral administration of SPS in water.[659] To prevent constipation and facilitate the passage of the resin through the gastrointestinal tract, Flinn and associates added sorbitol to the resin,[664] despite an absence of prior constipation or impaction in a prior study.[660] It has since become routine to administer SPS with sorbitol, with approximately 5 million annual doses administered in the United States alone.[665] Notably, although we utilize SPS herein to denote sodium polystyrene sulfonate, SPS is actually a brand name for sodium polystyrene sulfonate in sorbitol, illustrating the frequency in which these agents are administered together.[618]

The effect of ingested SPS on serum K^+ is slow; it may take from 4 to 24 hours to see a significant effect on serum K^+.[619,620,659] The oral dose is usually 15 to 30 g, which can be repeated every 4 to 6 hours. Each gram of resin binds 0.5 to 1.2 mEq of K^+ in exchange for 2 to 3 mEq of Na^+.[620,659,666,667] The discrepancy is caused in part by the binding of small amounts of other cations.[659] The hypokalemic effect may be due in part to the coadministered laxative. One study of healthy subjects compared the rate of fecal excretion of K^+ by different laxatives, with or without SPS, and found that the combination of phenolphthalein and docusate with resin produced greater fecal excretion of K^+ (49 mmol in 12 hours) than phenolphthalein or docusate alone (37 mmol in 12 hours) or other laxative-resin combinations.[666]

Earlier studies with SPS, mostly before the era of chronic hemodialysis, used multiple doses of the exchange resin orally or rectally as an enema and were associated with declines in serum K^+ of 1 and 0.8 mmol/L in 24 hours, respectively.[659] However, with the advent of routine hemodialysis, it has become common to order only a single dose of resin-cathartic in the management of acute hyperkalemia. One study addressed the efficacy of this practice, evaluating the effect of four single-dose, resin-cathartic regimens on serum K^+ levels of six patients with CKD on maintenance hemodialysis; none of the regimens used reduced the serum K^+ below the initial baseline.[667] Notably, the subjects in this study were normokalemic. Nevertheless, if SPS is judged to be appropriate for the management of hyperkalemia (see later), repeated doses are usually required for an adequate effect.

SPS can be administered rectally as a retention enema in patients unable to take or tolerate the oral form. The recommended dose is 30 to 50 g of resin as an emulsion in 100 mL of an aqueous vehicle (e.g., 20% dextrose in water) every 6 hours. It should be administered warm (body temperature) after a cleansing enema with body temperature tap water through a rubber tube placed at about 20 cm from the rectum, with the tip well into the sigmoid colon. The emulsion should be introduced by gravity, flushed with an additional 50 to 100 mL of non–sodium-containing fluid, retained for at least 30 to 60 minutes and followed by a cleansing enema (250 to 1000 mL of body temperature tap water).[668] SPS in sorbitol should not be used for enemas, given the risk of colonic necrosis.[620,669]

An increasing concern with SPS in sorbitol has been intestinal necrosis due to the administration of this preparation; this is frequently a fatal complication.[665,669-672] Studies in experimental animals have suggested that sorbitol is required for the intestinal injury[669]; however, SPS crystals can often be detected in human pathologic specimens, adherent to the injured mucosa.[671,672] Several cases of colonic necrosis following oral SPS alone, without sorbitol, have also been reported,[673,674] directly implicating SPS in the intestinal injury. The risk of intestinal necrosis appears to be greatest when SPS is given with sorbitol within the first week after surgery. For example, out of 117 patients who received SPS with sorbitol within 1 week of surgery, two patients developed intestinal necrosis.[670] Notably, however, in a case series of SPS in sorbitol-associated intestinal necrosis, only 2 of 11 confirmed cases occurred in the postoperative setting.[671] Although most cases of intestinal necrosis occurred in patients receiving SPS in 70% sorbitol, this has also been reported in patients receiving SPS in 33% sorbitol.[665]

In response to these findings, the U.S. Food and Drug Administration (FDA) removed recommendations for concomitant or postdosing use of sorbitol from the labeling of SPS in 2005.[665] However, the FDA allowed continuous marketing of the most frequently used ready-made SPS in sorbitol suspension, given that it contained only 33% sorbitol. Since that time, more cases of intestinal necrosis have been reported, some reportedly associated with SPS in 33% sorbitol.[665] As a result, in September 2009, the FDA changed safety labeling for SPS powder, stating that concomitant administration of sorbitol is no longer recommended.[665]

Given these serious concerns, clinicians must carefully consider whether emergency treatment with SPS is actually necessary for the treatment of hyperkalemia.[618,665,675] There are minimal data on the efficacy of SPS within the first 24 hours of administration for hyperkalemia[665]; at best, the effect occurs within 4 to 6 hours of administration.[619,620,659] This temporal limitation should be taken into consideration when deciding whether to administer SPS in acute hyperkalemia. In patients with intact renal function, alternative measures such as hydration to increase distal tubular delivery of Na^+ and distal tubular flow rate, and/or diuretics are often sufficient for potassium removal. In patients with advanced renal failure, the use of SPS is reasonable as a temporizing maneuver while awaiting hemodialysis, but if hemodialysis is available within 1 to 4 hours, I question the need for SPS, given the delayed hypokalemic response and risk of potentially fatal intestinal necrosis. Furthermore, if a patient has an existing vascular access for hemodialysis, the risk of intestinal necrosis outweighs that of the dialysis procedure.

If SPS is administered, the preparation should ideally not contain sorbitol; SPS without sorbitol is typically available as a powder, which must be reconstituted with water. If a laxative other than sorbitol is coadministered, it should not contain potassium or other cations, such as magnesium or calcium, which can compete with potassium for binding to the resin. In patients with renal insufficiency, the laxative should not contain phosphorus. Reasonable laxatives for this purpose include lactulose and some preparations of polyethylene glycol 3350. However, data demonstrating the efficacy and safety of these laxatives with SPS are not available.[618] We should also note that administering SPS without sorbitol might not eliminate the risk of intestinal necrosis, given the role for the SPS resin itself in this complication.[671-674] Notably, SPS without sorbitol is rarely available in the United States; many pharmacies and hospitals only stock SPS premixed with sorbitol.[665] Although there are indications that SPS preparations with 33% sorbitol have a lesser risk, cases of intestinal necrosis have also been described with this preparation; clinicians will have to weigh the relative risk of using this preparation in the management of acute hyperkalemia.[665] Regardless, SPS with sorbitol should not be used in patients at higher risk for intestinal necrosis, including postoperative patients, patients with a history of bowel obstruction, patients with slow intestinal transit, patients with ischemic bowel disease, and renal transplant recipients.

Finally, oral SPS with sorbitol can also injure the upper gastrointestinal tract, although the clinical significance of these findings is not known.[676] Other potential complications include reduction of serum calcium,[677] volume overload,[658] interference with lithium absorption,[678] and iatrogenic hypokalemia.[668]

NOVEL INTESTINAL POTASSIUM BINDERS

Recent reports have detailed the effect of two novel potassium binders, patiromer and ZS-9, on patients with hyperkalemia. Given the clinical need and serious limitations of SPS, there is considerable interest in these drugs, which hopefully will be clinically available within the next few years.

Patiromer is a nonabsorbed polymer, provided as a powder for suspension, that binds K^+ in exchange for Ca^{2+}. In a study of 237 patients with CKD and hyperkalemia, the mean change in serum K^+ after treatment with patiromer was 1.01 ± 0.03 mmol/L.[679] Approximately 75% of patients achieved the target serum K^+ of 3.8 to 5.0 mEq/L. The 107 patients whose baseline serum potassium was 5.5 mEq/L or higher and who achieved the target serum K^+ during the initial 4-week treatment period were randomly assigned to patiromer or placebo for another 8 weeks. Serum K^+ remained the same in patients continuing patiromer and increased by 0.7 mEq/L in those assigned placebo. The incidence of hyperkalemia (≥ 5.5 mEq/L) was significantly higher in the placebo group (60% vs. 15%). Serious adverse events were rare. However, a serum magnesium level lower than 1.4 mg/dL occurred in eight patients (3%) during the initial phase, and nine patients were initiated on magnesium replacement, suggesting that impaired intestinal absorption of magnesium may be a limitation in long-term use.

Sodium zirconium cyclosilicate (ZS-9) is an inorganic, nonabsorbable crystalline compound that exchanges sodium and hydrogen ions for K^+ and NH_4^+ in the intestine. The binding of K^+ to ZS-9 has some similarity to the selectivity filter of K^+ channels, with more than 25-fold selectivity for K^+ over Ca^{2+} and Mg^{2+}.[680] The efficacy of ZS-9 in hyperkalemic outpatients was evaluated in two nearly identical phase III randomized placebo-controlled trials.

In the Hyperkalemia Randomized Intervention Multidose ZS-9 Maintenance (HARMONIZE) study, 258 adult patients with persistent hyperkalemia entered a 48-hour, open-label run-in during which they received 10 g of ZS-9 three times daily.[681] Of the 258 patients who entered the open-label run-in, 237 (92%) achieved a normal serum K^+ (3.5 to 5.0 mEq/L) at 48 hours and were then randomly assigned to placebo or 5, 10, or 15 g of ZS-9 once daily for 4 weeks. During randomized therapy, the mean serum K^+ was significantly lower with ZS-9 (4.8, 4.5, and 4.4 mEq/L with 5-, 10-, and 15-g dosing, respectively) as compared with placebo (5.1 mEq/L). Similarly, the proportion of normokalemic patients at the end of the study was significantly higher with ZS-9 (71% to 85% vs. 48% with placebo). Serious adverse events were uncommon and were not significantly increased with ZS-9. However, edema was more common with the 10- and 15-g doses compared with placebo, as was hypokalemia.

In the second ZS-9 trial, 682 753 adult patients with a serum K^+ of 5.0 to 6.5 mmol/L were randomly assigned to receive 1.25, 2.5, 5, or 10 g of ZS-9 three times daily for 48 hours. A normal serum K^+ (3.5 to 4.9 mEq/L) at 48 hours was attained by 543 patients (72%), and they were then reassigned to receive placebo or 1.25, 2.5, 5, or 10 g of ZS-9 once daily for 2 weeks. The serum potassium at 2 weeks was significantly lower in patients receiving 5- and 10-g doses of ZS-9 as compared with placebo (by ≈0.3 and 0.5 mEq/L, respectively), but not with 1.25- and 2.5-g doses. Adverse events were similar with placebo and ZS-9.

In these trials, the steepest decline in serum potassium with ZS-9 occurred during the first 4 hours of therapy.[681,682] This suggests an acute effect on intestinal potassium secretion, rather than simply a reduction in intestinal potassium absorption.

DIALYSIS

All modes of acute renal replacement therapies are effective in removing K^+. Continuous hemodiafiltration has been increasingly used in the management of critically ill and hemodynamically unstable patients.[683] Peritoneal dialysis, although not very effective in an acute setting, has been used effectively in cardiac arrest complicating acute hyperkalemia.[684] Peritoneal dialysis is capable of removing significant amounts of K^+ (5 mmol/hour or 240 mmol in 48 hours) using 2-L exchanges, with each exchange taking almost 1 hour.[622] However, hemodialysis is the preferred mode when rapid correction of a hyperkalemic episode is desired.[685]

An average 3- to 5-hour hemodialysis session removes approximately 40 to 120 mmol of K^+.[28,685-692] Approximately 15% of the total K^+ removal results from ultrafiltration, with the remaining clearance from dialysis.[689,693] Of the total K^+ removed, about 40% is from extracellular space, and the remainder is from intracellular compartments.[687,689,690] In most patients, the greatest decline in serum K^+ (1.2 to 1.5 mmol/L) and the largest amount of K^+ removed occur during the first hour; the serum K^+ usually reaches its nadir at about 3 hours. Despite a relatively constant serum K^+, removal of K^+ continues until the end of the hemodialysis session, although at a significantly lower rate.[28,688,689]

The amount of K^+ removed depends primarily on the type and surface area of the dialyzer used, blood flow rate, dialysate flow rate, dialysis duration, and serum/dialysate K^+ gradient. However, about 40% of the difference in removal cannot be explained by these factors and may instead be related to the relative distribution of K^+ between intracellular and extracellular spaces.[687] Glucose-free dialysates are more efficient in removing K^+.[687,690] This effect may be caused by alterations in endogenous insulin levels, with concomitant intracellular shift of K^+; the insulin level is 50% lower when glucose-free dialysates are used.[687] Furthermore, these findings imply that K^+ removal may be greater if hemodialysis is performed with the patient in a fasting state.[693] Treatment with β_2-agonists also reduces the total K^+ removal by approximately 40%.[685] The change in pH during dialysis was thought to have no significant effect on K^+ removal.[685,693] One study evaluated this issue in detail, examining the effect of dialysate bicarbonate concentration on both serum K^+ and K^+ removal. Dialysates with bicarbonate concentration of 39 mmol/L (high), 35 mmol/L (standard), and 27 mmol/L (low) were used. The use of a high concentration of bicarbonate was associated with a more rapid decline in serum K^+; this was statistically significant for high versus both standard- and low-bicarbonate dialysates, at 60 and 240 minutes. However, the total amount of K^+ removed was higher with the low-bicarbonate dialysate (116.4 ± 21.6 mmol/dialysis) in comparison to standard- (73.2 ± 12.8 mmol/dialysis) and high- (80.9 ± 15.4 mmol/dialysis) bicarbonate dialysates, all statistically not significant.[694] Therefore, whereas high-bicarbonate dialysis may acutely have a more rapid effect on serum K^+, this advantage is potentially mitigated by a lesser total removal of the ion over the course of a typical treatment session.

One of the major determinants of total K^+ removal is the K^+ gradient between the plasma and dialysate. Dialysates with a lower K^+ concentration are more effective at reducing plasma K^+.[688,692] Many nephrologists use the "rule of 7s" to set the dialysate K^+ concentration; the plasma K^+ plus the dialysate K^+ should equal approximately 7. However, this then entails dialysis with 0 or 1.0 mEq/L K^+ dialysate (0 K or 1 K bath) in patients with serum K^+ that exceeds 6 to 7 mmol/L. However, a rapid decline in plasma K^+ due to 0 K or 1 K dialysates can be deleterious via several mechanisms. First, an acute decrease in plasma K^+ can be associated with rebound hypertension (i.e., a significant increase in blood pressure 1 hour after dialysis),[686] which is attributed in part to the peripheral vasoconstriction that is a direct result of the change in plasma K^+.[686] Second, a low plasma K^+ can alter the rate of tissue metabolism, the so-called Solandt effect,[695] and decrease tissue oxygen consumption, promoting arteriolar constriction.[686] This vasoconstriction, in turn, may reduce the efficiency of dialysis[28]; a randomized prospective study did not, however, confirm this finding.[688] The difference may have been due to the glucose content of the dialysate (200 mg/dL in the former and 0 mg/dL in the latter study); differences in circulating insulin may have had additional unrelated effects on muscle blood flow.[696] Finally, dialysates with a very low K^+ concentration may increase the risk of significant arrhythmia.[692,697]

Several studies have found an increased incidence of significant arrhythmia with hemodialysis, occurring during and immediately after treatment[697-699]; an incidence of up to 76% has been reported.[700] However, many investigators do not consider the hemodialysis procedure to be significantly arrhythmogenic.[701-703] Some have suggested that a relationship exists between decreases in K^+, dialysate K^+, and incidence of significant arrhythmias.[697] Despite the controversy, it seems prudent to recommend that dialysates with a very low K^+ (0 or 1 mmol/L) be used cautiously, particularly in high-risk patients. This definition includes patients receiving digitalis, those with a history of arrhythmia, coronary artery disease, left ventricular hypertrophy, or high systolic blood pressure, and those of advanced age. Continuous cardiac monitoring for all patients dialyzed against a 0- or 1-mmol/L K^+ bath is strongly recommended.[481]

Given the risk of inducing arrhythmias with very low potassium dialysates, an alternative approach has been proposed for the treatment of significant hyperkalemia.[481,704] In this regimen, dialysis is initiated with a 3- to 4-mEq/L potassium bath, which will immediately lower the plasma potassium concentration in a slower and perhaps safer manner.[697] The potassium concentration in the dialysate may then be lowered stepwise with each subsequent hour. A more sophisticated approach uses potassium profiling to maintain a constant potassium gradient during dialysis.[704-706] Potassium profiling results in a more sustained, even removal of potassium[705] than dialysis against a fixed potassium bath (2.5 mEq/L), with less effect on ventricular ectopy.[704-706]

For the management of severe hyperkalemia (serum K$^+$ ≥ 7.0 mEq/L) we favor the use of stepped reduction or potassium profiling of dialysate potassium concentrations. We rarely encounter the need to use 1 K or 0 K dialysis baths, which we also avoid at the beginning of dialysis sessions for acute hyperkalemia. We recommend restricting the upfront use of these low-potassium baths to patients with life-threatening hyperkalemic arrhythmias and/or life-threatening conduction abnormalities.

A rebound increase in plasma K$^+$ can occur after hemodialysis. This can be especially marked in cases of massive release from devitalized tissues (e.g., tumor lysis, rhabdomyolysis), requiring frequent monitoring of serum K$^+$ and further hemodialysis. However, a rebound increase may also occur in ESKD patients during regular maintenance hemodialysis, despite technically adequate treatment,[689] particularly in those patients with a high predialysis K$^+$. Factors attenuating K$^+$ removal and thus increasing the risk and magnitude of postdialysis rebound include pretreatment with β$_2$-agonists, pretreatment with insulin and glucose, eating early during the dialysis treatment, a high predialysis plasma K$^+$, and higher dialysate Na$^+$ concentrations.[685,689,691,693]

Complete reference list available at ExpertConsult.com.

KEY REFERENCES

1. Choi M, et al: K$^+$ channel mutations in adrenal aldosterone-producing adenomas and hereditary hypertension. *Science* 331:768–772, 2011.
2. Snyder PM, Olson DR, Thomas BC: Serum and glucocorticoid-regulated kinase modulates Nedd4-2-mediated inhibition of the epithelial Na+ channel. *J Biol Chem* 277:5–8, 2002.
3. Terker AS, et al: Potassium modulates electrolyte balance and blood pressure through effects on distal cell voltage and chloride. *Cell Metab* 21:39–50, 2015.
4. Shibata S, et al: Angiotensin II signaling via protein kinase C phosphorylates Kelch-like 3, preventing WNK4 degradation. *Proc Natl Acad Sci U S A* 111:15556–15561, 2014.
5. Shibata S, Zhang J, Puthumana J, et al: Kelch-like 3 and Cullin 3 regulate electrolyte homeostasis via ubiquitination and degradation of WNK4. *Proc Natl Acad Sci U S A* 110:7838–7843, 2013.
6. Boyden LM, et al: Mutations in kelch-like 3 and cullin 3 cause hypertension and electrolyte abnormalities. *Nature* 482:98–102, 2012.
8. McDonough AA, Thompson CB, Youn JH: Skeletal muscle regulates extracellular potassium. *Am J Physiol Renal Physiol* 282:F967–F974, 2002.
9. Williams ME, Rosa RM, Silva P, et al: Impairment of extrarenal potassium disposal by alpha-adrenergic stimulation. *N Engl J Med* 311:145–149, 1984.
12. Chen P, et al: Modest dietary K$^+$ restriction provokes insulin resistance of cellular K$^+$ uptake and phosphorylation of renal outer medulla K$^+$ channel without fall in plasma K$^+$ concentration. *Am J Physiol Cell Physiol* 290:C1355–C1363, 2006.
40. DeFronzo RA, Felig P, Ferrannini E, et al: Effect of graded doses of insulin on splanchnic and peripheral potassium metabolism in man. *Am J Physiol* 238:E421–E427, 1980.
61. Adrogué HJ, Madias NE: PCO2 and [K+]p in metabolic acidosis: certainty for the first and uncertainty for the other. *J Am Soc Nephrol* 15:1667–1668, 2004.
68. Giebisch G: Renal potassium transport: mechanisms and regulation. *Am J Physiol* 274:F817–F833, 1998.
73. Frindt G, Palmer LG: Apical potassium channels in the rat connecting tubule. *Am J Physiol Renal Physiol* 287:F1030–F1037, 2004.
84. Frindt G, Palmer LG: K+ secretion in the rat kidney: Na+ channel-dependent and -independent mechanisms. *Am J Physiol Renal Physiol* 297:F389–F396, 2009.
111. Palmer LG, Frindt G: Regulation of apical K channels in rat cortical collecting tubule during changes in dietary K intake. *Am J Physiol* 277:F805–F812, 1999.
115. Kahle KT, et al: WNK4 regulates the balance between renal NaCl reabsorption and K+ secretion. *Nat Genet* 35:372–376, 2003.
157. Cheng HF, Wang JL, Zhang MZ, et al: Role of p38 in the regulation of renal cortical cyclooxygenase-2 expression by extracellular chloride. *J Clin Invest* 106:681–688, 2000.
194. Tattersall RB: A paper which changed clinical practice (slowly). Jacob Holler on potassium deficiency in diabetic acidosis (1946). *Diabet Med* 16:978–984, 1999.
199. Torres VE, Young WF, Jr, Offord KP, et al: Association of hypokalemia, aldosteronism, and renal cysts. *N Engl J Med* 322:345–351, 1990.
205. Berl T, Linas SL, Aisenbrey GA, et al: On the mechanism of polyuria in potassium depletion. The role of polydipsia. *J Clin Invest* 60:620–625, 1977.
208. Coca SG, Perazella MA, Buller GK: The cardiovascular implications of hypokalemia. *Am J Kidney Dis* 45:233–247, 2005.
216. Littmann L, Monroe MH, Taylor L, 3rd, et al: The hyperkalemic Brugada sign. *J Electrocardiol* 40:53–59, 2007.
234. DuBose TD, Jr, Good DW: Chronic hyperkalemia impairs ammonium transport and accumulation in the inner medulla of the rat. *J Clin Invest* 90:1443–1449, 1992.
297. Simon M, et al: Over-expression of colonic K+ channels associated with severe potassium secretory diarrhoea after haemorrhagic shock. *Nephrol Dial Transplant* 23:3350–3352, 2008.
298. Blondon H, Bechade D, Desrame J, et al: Secretory diarrhoea with high faecal potassium concentrations: a new mechanism of diarrhoea associated with colonic pseudo-obstruction? Report of five patients. *Gastroenterol Clin Biol* 32:401–404, 2008.
299. van Dinter TG, Jr, et al: Stimulated active potassium secretion in a patient with colonic pseudo-obstruction: a new mechanism of secretory diarrhea. *Gastroenterology* 129:1268–1273, 2005.
402. Bailey MA, et al: Maxi-K channels contribute to urinary potassium excretion in the ROMK-deficient mouse model of type II Bartter's syndrome and in adaptation to a high-K diet. *Kidney Int* 70:51–59, 2006.
434. Yang L, Frindt G, Palmer LG: Magnesium modulates ROMK channel-mediated potassium secretion. *J Am Soc Nephrol* 21:2109–2116, 2010.
494. Bruce LJ, et al: Monovalent cation leaks in human red cells caused by single amino-acid substitutions in the transport domain of the band 3 chloride-bicarbonate exchanger, AE1. *Nat Genet* 37:1258–1263, 2005.
515. Nzerue CM, Falana B: Refractory hyperkalaemia associated with use of epsilon-aminocaproic acid during coronary bypass in a dialysis patient. *Nephrol Dial Transplant* 17:1150–1151, 2002.
516. Banerjee A, Stoica C, Walia A: Acute hyperkalemia as a complication of intravenous therapy with epsilon-aminocaproic acid. *J Clin Anesth* 23:565–568, 2011.
563. Klemm SA, Gordon RD, Tunny TJ, et al: Biochemical correction in the syndrome of hypertension and hyperkalaemia by severe dietary salt restriction suggests renin-aldosterone suppression critical in pathophysiology. *Clin Exp Pharmacol Physiol* 17:191–195, 1990.
571. Mayan H, et al: Pseudohypoaldosteronism type II: marked sensitivity to thiazides, hypercalciuria, normomagnesemia, and low bone mineral density. *J Clin Endocrinol Metab* 87:3248–3254, 2002.
572. Wilson FH, et al: Human hypertension caused by mutations in WNK kinases. *Science* 293:1107–1112, 2001.

576. Tan SY, Shapiro R, Franco R, et al: Indomethacin-induced prostaglandin inhibition with hyperkalemia. A reversible cause of hyporeninemic hypoaldosteronism. *Ann Intern Med* 90:783–785, 1979.
590. Choi MJ, et al: Brief report: trimethoprim-induced hyperkalemia in a patient with AIDS. *N Engl J Med* 328:703–706, 1993.
592. Velazquez H, Perazella MA, Wright FS, et al: Renal mechanism of trimethoprim-induced hyperkalemia. *Ann Intern Med* 119:296–301, 1993.
593. Muto S, Tsuruoka S, Miyata Y, et al: Effect of trimethoprim-sulfamethoxazole on Na and K+ transport properties in the rabbit cortical collecting duct perfused in vitro. *Nephron Physiol* 102:p51–p60, 2006.
594. Alappan R, Perazella MA, Buller GK: Hyperkalemia in hospitalized patients treated with trimethoprim-sulfamethoxazole. *Ann Intern Med* 124:316–320, 1996.
597. Antoniou T, et al: Trimethoprim-sulfamethoxazole and risk of sudden death among patients taking spironolactone. *CMAJ* 187:E138–E143, 2015.
598. Fralick M, et al: Co-trimoxazole and sudden death in patients receiving inhibitors of renin-angiotensin system: population based study. *BMJ* 349:g6196, 2014.
599. Weir MR, Rolfe M: Potassium homeostasis and renin-angiotensin-aldosterone system inhibitors. *Clin J Am Soc Nephrol* 5:531–548, 2010.
612. Juurlink DN, et al: Rates of hyperkalemia after publication of the Randomized Aldactone Evaluation Study. *N Engl J Med* 351:543–551, 2004.
628. Blumberg A, Weidmann P, Shaw S, et al: Effect of various therapeutic approaches on plasma potassium and major regulating factors in terminal renal failure. *Am J Med* 85:507–512, 1988.
641. Blumberg A, Weidmann P, Ferrari P: Effect of prolonged bicarbonate administration on plasma potassium in terminal renal failure. *Kidney Int* 41:369–374, 1992.
665. Sterns RH, Rojas M, Bernstein P, et al: Ion-exchange resins for the treatment of hyperkalemia: are they safe and effective? *J Am Soc Nephrol* 21:733–735, 2010.
671. McGowan CE, Saha S, Chu G, et al: Intestinal necrosis due to sodium polystyrene sulfonate (Kayexalate) in sorbitol. *South Med J* 102:493–497, 2009.
679. Weir MR, et al: Patiromer in patients with kidney disease and hyperkalemia receiving RAAS inhibitors. *N Engl J Med* 372:211–221, 2015.
682. Packham DK, et al: Sodium zirconium cyclosilicate in hyperkalemia. *N Engl J Med* 15:372, 222–231, 2015.
704. Redaelli B, et al: Effect of a new model of hemodialysis potassium removal on the control of ventricular arrhythmias. *Kidney Int* 50:609–617, 1996.
705. Santoro A, et al: Patients with complex arrhythmias during and after haemodialysis suffer from different regimens of potassium removal. *Nephrol Dial Transplant* 23:1415–1421, 2008.

Disorders of Calcium, Magnesium, and Phosphate Balance

Miroslaw J. Smogorzewski | Jason R. Stubbs | Alan S.L. Yu

CHAPTER OUTLINE

DISORDERS OF CALCIUM HOMEOSTASIS, 601
Whole-Body Calcium Homeostasis, 601
Hypercalcemia, 602
Hypocalcemia, 612
DISORDERS OF MAGNESIUM HOMEOSTASIS, 618
Hypomagnesemia and Magnesium Deficiency, 618

Hypermagnesemia, 625
DISORDERS OF PHOSPHATE HOMEOSTASIS, 626
Hyperphosphatemia, 626
Hypophosphatemia, 629

DISORDERS OF CALCIUM HOMEOSTASIS

The extracellular fluid (ECF) calcium concentration in the human body is tightly regulated by a complex process. Three organs—skeleton, kidney, and intestine—are involved in this process through their direct or indirect interaction with parathyroid hormone (PTH), parathyroid hormone–related peptide (PTHrP), vitamin D, and calcitonin. Phosphatonins such as fibroblast growth factor 23 (FGF-23), although they participate in phosphate and vitamin D homeostasis, do not directly modify extracellular calcium.

This homeostatic system is modulated by dietary and environmental factors, including vitamins, hormones, medications, and mobility. Disorders of extracellular calcium homeostasis may be regarded as perturbations of this homeostatic system, either at the level of the genes controlling this system (e.g., as in familial hypocalciuric hypercalcemia, pseudohypoparathyroidism, or vitamin D–dependent rickets) or perturbations of this system induced by nongenetic means (e.g., as in lithium toxicity or postsurgical hypoparathyroidism).

Calcium fluxes between the ECF and one of the organs (skeleton, kidney, and intestine) or their combination, as well as abnormal binding of the calcium to serum protein, can cause hypercalcemia. PTH directly protects against hypocalcemia by augmenting calcium mobilization from bone, increasing renal tubular reabsorption of calcium, and enhancing intestinal absorption of calcium. PTH indirectly protects against hypocalcemia through its effect on vitamin D metabolism. States with excess PTH may cause hypercalcemia, whereas PTH deficiency is associated with hypocalcemia. Similarly, PTHrP promotes bone resorption, enhances renal reabsorption of calcium, and decreases renal tubular reabsorption of phosphate. Excess of this hormone is responsible for the hypercalcemia of malignancy. Vitamin D and its metabolites increase intestinal absorption of calcium and cause bone resorption; therefore, excess vitamin D would induce hypercalcemia. Calcitonin inhibits bone resorption, but its physiologic role in the protection against hypercalcemia in humans is not proven.

WHOLE-BODY CALCIUM HOMEOSTASIS

An adult human body contains approximately 1000 to 1300 g of calcium, with 99.3% in bone and teeth as hydroxyapatite crystal, 0.6% in soft tissues, and 0.1% in ECF, including 0.03% in plasma.[1] Maintenance of normal calcium balance and serum calcium levels depends on the integrated regulation of calcium absorption and secretion by the intestinal tract, excretion of calcium by the kidney, and calcium release from and deposition into bone. In young adults, calcium balance is neutral. Approximately 1000 mg of calcium is ingested per day, 200 mg absorbed by gut, mainly duodenum and 800 mg excreted via the gut. Out of 10 g of calcium filtered by the kidney daily, only approximately 200 mg is excreted in the urine. At the same time, 0.5 g of calcium is released from bone, and the same amount is deposited with new bone formation. PTH, by stimulating bone resorption and distal tubular calcium reabsorption in the kidney, and activating renal hydroxylation of $25(OH)D_3$ to $1,25(OH)D_3$, increases serum calcium levels. Depression in serum levels of calcium, by itself, stimulates, through the calcium-sensing receptor (CaSR) in the parathyroid gland, the secretion of preformed PTH from the parathyroid gland within seconds. Subsequently, PTH biosynthesis by the parathyroid gland increases over 24 to 48 hours and is followed by parathyroid gland hypertrophy and hyperplasia. Vitamin D metabolites, serum phosphorus, and FGF-23 levels also regulate PTH levels in blood.

The values for total serum calcium concentration in adults vary among clinical laboratories, depending on the methods of measurement, with the normal range being between 8.6 and 10.3 mg/dL (2.15 to 2.57 mmol/L).[2,3] Variation in serum calcium levels occur, depending on age and gender, with a general trend for lower serum calcium level with aging.[4]

Calcium in blood exists in three distinct fractions—protein-bound calcium (40%), free (ionized) calcium (48%), and calcium to complexed various anions, such as phosphate, lactate, citrate, and bicarbonate (12%).[5] The latter two forms, complexed calcium and free calcium ion, together comprise the fraction of plasma calcium that can be filtered. Plasma albumin is responsible for 90% and globulins for 10% of protein-bound calcium. Free calcium is the physiologically active component of extracellular calcium with regard to cardiac myocyte contractility, neuromuscular activity, bone mineralization, and other calcium-dependent processes. It is measured in most hospitals using ion-selective electrodes; values in adults range from 4.65 to 5.28 mg/dL (1.16 to 1.32 mmol/L).[4,6] Total calcium reflects the levels of free calcium if plasma levels of protein, pH, and anions are normal.

The relationship between calcium ion and the concentration of protein in the serum is represented by a simple mass action expression:

$$([Ionized\ Ca^{2+}] \times [protein])/[calcium\ proteinate] = K$$

where [protein] equals the concentration of serum proteins, primarily albumin. Because K is a constant, the numerator and denominator must change proportionately in any physiologic or pathologic state. A change in the concentration of total serum calcium will occur after a change in the concentration of serum proteins or alterations in their binding properties and after a primary change in the concentration of calcium ion. A fall in the serum albumin level reduces the protein and calcium proteinate levels proportionately, resulting in a fall in the total serum calcium level, with the free calcium ion concentration remaining normal. If plasma levels of albumin are low, an adjustment of the measured serum levels of calcium should be made (commonly but erroneously referred to as a "correction"). For the routine clinical interpretation of serum calcium needed for appropriate care of patients, a simple formula for adjustment of total serum calcium concentration for changes in plasma albumin concentration is used by clinicians.

In conventional units:

Adjusted total calcium (mg/dL)
= total calcium (mg/dL) + 0.8(4 − albumin [g/dL])

In SI units:

Adjusted total calcium (mmol/L)
= total calcium (mmol/L) + 0.02[40 − albumin (g/L)]

This formula was endorsed in 1977 by an editorial in the *British Medical Journal*[7]; the correction factor of 0.02 (in SI units) was chosen arbitrarily for simplicity from the range available in the literature at that time (0.018 to 0.025). This adjustment can also correct for errors in measurement of total calcium related to hemoconcentration of a blood sample because of the prolonged use of a tourniquet or because of hemodilution when blood is drawn in a supine position in hospitalized patients.[3] Other formulas have been developed, particularly for chronic kidney disease (CKD) patients, that have a slightly better (although not statistically significant) discriminatory ability to make the diagnosis of hypocalcemia or hypercalcemia, as established from measurement of free calcium.[8,9] Also, a fall in pH of 0.1 unit will cause approximately a 0.1 mEq/L rise in the concentration of ionized calcium, because hydrogen ion displaces calcium from albumin, whereas alkalosis decreases free calcium by enhancing the binding of calcium to albumin.[4] There is no correction for this effect of pH in the above formula, which also limits its accuracy.

Calcium binding to globulin is small (1.0 g of globulin binds 0.2 to 0.3 mg of calcium), and it is unusual to see a change in the total concentration of serum calcium as a result of alterations in the levels of globulin in blood. However, in cases in which the globulin concentration in serum is extremely high (>8.0 g/dL), such as in multiple myeloma, a mild to moderate hypercalcemia may be seen because of an elevation of the globulin-bound calcium. In addition, immunoglobulin G (IgG) myeloma proteins may have increased calcium-binding properties, and an elevation in the total level of serum calcium could occur, even with a moderate increase in serum levels of globulins. In these cases, the ionized calcium in serum is normal; therefore, this type of hypercalcemia would not require treatment.

Unfortunately, calcium status will be incorrectly predicted by this formula in 20% to 30% of subjects,[10] and the agreement between corrected and free calcium is only fair.[11] Thus, free calcium should be assessed, particularly in critically ill patients with acid-base disturbances, in patients exposed to large amounts of citrated blood, and in those with severe blood protein disorders. Patients with CKD and those treated with dialysis may also benefit from free calcium measurements in an evaluation of their mineral bone metabolism status.[12] It is important to recognize that free calcium results in blood are affected by factors related to the handling of specimens, including duration of cellular metabolism, loss of CO_2, and use of anticoagulants.[2]

HYPERCALCEMIA

Hypercalcemia is relatively common and frequently overlooked, with an annual incidence estimated to be about 0.1% to 0.2% and a prevalence of 0.17% to 2.92% in a hospital population and 1.07% to 3.9% in a normal population.[13]

Hypercalcemia results from an alteration in the net fluxes of calcium to and from four compartments—bone, gut, kidney, and serum binding proteins (Table 19.1). Usually, the hypercalcemia is caused by net calcium movement from the skeleton into ECF through increased osteoclastic bone resorption, as in hyperparathyroidism (HPT) or excess PTHrP production in malignancy. PTH acts via the PTH receptor 1 on the osteoblasts. PTH receptor 1 is encoded by the *PTH1R* gene. It activates cyclic adenosine monophosphate (cAMP) signalling in osteoblasts and upregulates their expression of receptor activator for nuclear factor-kappaB (RANK) ligand (RANKL). RANKL binds to RANK on osteoclasts. RANK activation on osteoclasts through the RANK/RANKL interaction causes recruitment, proliferation, and activation of osteoclasts for bone resorption. Increase in bone resorption rate without increase in bone formation rate will cause hypercalcemia.

Myeloma cells may induce multiple osteoclastogenic factors such as RANKL in nonosteoblastic stromal cells or decrease production of osteoprotegerin, a decoy receptor for RANKL. Excess circulating 1,25-dihydroxyvitamin D (1,25[OH]$_2$D) from various causes also activates osteoclastic bone resorption indirectly through osteoblasts. Increased intestinal calcium absorption may lead to the development of hypercalcemia, as in vitamin D overdose or milk-alkali syndrome. In general, the kidney does not contribute to hypercalcemia; rather, it defends against the development of hypercalcemia. Typically, hypercalciuria precedes hypercalcemia. Extracellular calcium itself appears to have a calciuric effect on the renal tubule by its direct action on the CaSR of the thick ascending limb (TAL). Thus, in most hypercalcemic states, renal calcium handling is subject to competing influences; excess PTH or PTHrP acts on the PTH/PTHrP receptor to promote renal calcium reabsorption, and excess calcium acts on the calcium receptor to promote calcium excretion.[14]

In rare cases, the kidney can actively contribute to the development of hypercalcemia. As opposed to primary HPT and humoral hypercalcemia of malignancy, in which increases in renal calcium excretion are observed, renal calcium excretion is not elevated in familial hypocalciuric hypercalcemia because of a defective renal response to calcium itself. The hypercalcemia associated with thiazide use is also mediated by the kidney: in both thiazide use and its genetic counterpart, Gitelman's syndrome, renal calcium excretion is decreased.

SIGNS AND SYMPTOMS

Hypercalcemia adversely affects the function of almost all organ systems, but in particular the kidney, central nervous system, and cardiovascular system. The clinical manifestations of hypercalcemia relate more to the degree of hypercalcemia and rate of increase than the underlying cause. Hypercalcemia may be classified based on the level of total serum calcium[15]:

Mild: [Ca] = 10.4 to 11.9 mg/dL
Moderate: [Ca] = 12.0 to 13.9 mg/dL
Severe (hypercalcemic crisis): [Ca] = 14.0 to 16 mg/dL
(Much higher levels are occasionally observed.)

Signs and symptoms and complications of hypercalcemia are summarized in Table 19.2.

As many as 10% of patients with elevated levels of serum calcium are detected by a routine screening test of blood chemistry and are considered to have so-called asymptomatic hypercalcemia. However, even very mild hypercalcemia may be of clinical significance inasmuch as some studies have suggested an increased cardiovascular risk from mild but prolonged calcium level elevations.[16]

In symptomatic patients, the spectrum of the clinical presentation is varied and could be nonspecific. Mild hypercalcemia may present with malaise, weakness, minor joint pain,

Table 19.1 Causes of Hypercalcemia

Malignancy-associated hypercalcemia
    Humoral hypercalcemia of malignancy (HHM) with secretion of PTH-related protein by the tumor
    Local osteolytic hypercalcemia (LOH)
    Tumor (lymphoma, germinoma) generation of 1,25(OH)$_2$D
    Ectopic PTH secretion from tumor
Primary hyperparathyroidism
    Adenoma, hyperplasia, carcinoma
    Multiple endocrine neoplasia types 1 and 2a
Familial hypocalciuric hypercalcemia
Neonatal severe hyperparathyroidism
Other endocrine disorders
    Hyperthyroidism
    Acromegaly
    Pheochromocytoma
    Acute adrenal insufficiency
Granulomatous disorders
    Sarcoidosis
    Tuberculosis
    Berylliosis
    Disseminated coccidioidomycosis or candidiasis
    Histoplasmosis
    Leprosy
    Granulomatous lipoid pneumonia
    Silicone-induced granuloma
    Eosinophilic granuloma
    Farmer's lung
Vitamin overdoses
    Vitamin D
    Vitamin A
Immobilization
Renal failure
    Diuretic phase of acute renal failure, especially resulting from rhabdomyolysis
    Chronic renal failure
    After renal transplantation
Medications
    Milk-alkali syndrome
    Thiazide diuretics
    Lithium
    Foscarnet
    Growth hormone
    Recombinant human PTH (1-34; teriparatide)
    Theophylline and aminophylline toxicity
    Estrogen and selective estrogen receptor modulators (SERMs)
    Vasoactive intestinal polypeptide
    Hyperalimentation regimens
Idiopathic hypercalcemia of infancy
Increased serum protein level
    Hemoconcentration
    Hyperglobulinemia due to multiple myeloma

Table 19.2 Clinical Features of Hypercalcemia
General
Malaise, tiredness, weakness
Neuropsychiatric
Impaired concentration, loss of memory, headache, drowsiness, lethargy, disorientation, confusion, irritability, depression, paranoia, hallucinations, ataxia, speech defects, visual disturbances, deafness (calcification of eardrum), pruritus, mental retardation (infants), stupor, coma
Neuromuscular
Muscle weakness, hyporeflexia or absent reflexes, hypotonia, myalgia, arthralgia, bone pain, joint effusion, chondrocalcinosis, dwarfism (infants)
Gastrointestinal
Loss of appetite, dry mouth, thirst, polydipsia, nausea, vomiting, constipation, abdominal pain, weight loss, acute pancreatitis (calcifying), peptic ulcer, acute gastric dilation
Renal
Polyuria, nocturia, nephrocalcinosis, nephrolithiasis, interstitial nephritis, acute and chronic renal failure
Cardiovascular
Arrhythmia, bradycardia, first-degree heart block, short Q-T interval, bundle branch block, arrest (rare), hypertension, vascular calcification
Metastatic Calcification
Band keratopathy, red eye syndrome, conjunctival calcification nephrocalcinosis, vascular calcification, pruritus

and other vague symptoms. In patients with severe hypercalcemia, the major symptoms are more likely to be nausea, vomiting, constipation, polyuria, and mental disturbances, ranging from headache and lethargy to coma. Recent loss of memory could be prominent and be a presenting symptom.

Hypercalciuria induced by hypercalcemia causes nephrogenic diabetes insipidus, with polyuria and polydipsia leading to ECF volume depletion, decreased glomerular filtration rate (GFR), and further increases in the serum calcium level. The effect of hypercalcemia on urinary concentration is mediated through CaSR activation, which decreases vasopressin-dependent aquaporin-2 (AQP2) water channels trafficking in the inner medullary collecting duct.[17] Nephrolithiasis and nephrocalcinosis are common complications of hypercalcemia, seen in 15% to 20% of cases of primary HPT.

LABORATORY FINDINGS

Laboratory findings in patients with hypercalcemia include abnormalities related to the underlying disease causing the hypercalcemia, which are beyond the scope of this chapter. Alterations in the electrocardiogram (ECG) and electroencephalogram (EEG) occur in hypercalcemic patients, independent of the cause of the hypercalcemia. The ECG shows a shortened ST segment and therefore a reduced QT interval as a result of an increased rate of cardiac repolarization. In patients with severe hypercalcemia (>16 mg/dL), there is a widening of the T waves, resulting in an increase in the QT interval. Bradycardia and first-degree heart block may be present in the ECGs of patients with acute and severe hypercalcemia. The EEG displays slowing and other nonspecific changes.

DIAGNOSIS

A careful history, physical examination, and routine laboratory tests will, in most patients, lead to the correct diagnosis in hypercalcemia. A flow diagram for the evaluation of hypercalcemia is shown in Figure 19.1. Primary HPT (PHPT) and malignancy-associated hypercalcemia together are responsible for 90% of cases of hypercalcemia, with malignancy being the most common cause in hospitalized patients and PHPT being the most common cause in the outpatient clinic.[15,18-20]

It is generally easy to differentiate these two entities. Hypercalcemia is only rarely an early finding in occult malignancy. PTH levels are essential in the diagnosis of hypercalcemia. There are two types of assay for PTH, depending on which epitopes of 1-84 PTH are recognized by the antibodies in the assay. Second-generation assays, the immunoradiometric assay (IRMA) and immunochemiluminometric assay (IMCA), use antibodies against 7-34 and 39-84 epitopes of 1-84 PTH. Despite their being called intact PTH assays, implying that they measure only the biologically active PTH, they also detect large carboxy-terminal fragments of PTH, such as PTH (7-84). Thus, they may overestimate the amount of bioactive hormone in serum, especially in CKD patients. The third-generation, whole or biointact PTH assays, use antibodies against 1-5 and C-terminal epitopes and detect biologically active intact PTH. The normal levels of PTH measured by various assays range from 8 to 80 ng/L (1 to 9 pmol/L).[2,21] Intraoperative PTH measurements are frequently used to assess the adequacy of parathyroidectomy. There is no cross reactivity between PTH and PTHrP assays. In PHPT, levels of PTH can be frankly elevated but can also be in the middle or upper range of normal, particularly in young individuals (Figure 19.2).

The differential diagnosis of patients with hypercalcemia and elevated PTH level includes HPT due to thiazide diuretics or lithium, familial hypocalciuric hypercalcemia (FHH), and the tertiary HPT associated with renal failure and kidney transplantation. Patients with FHH have a positive family history, onset of hypercalcemia at a young age, very low urinary calcium excretion, and specific gene abnormalities. In malignancy-associated hypercalcemia and in hypercalcemia of most other causes, PTH levels are low. The diagnosis of humoral hypercalcemia of malignancy (HHM) frequently can be made on clinical grounds. In addition, PTHrP can now be assayed by commercial clinical laboratories to support HHM or when the cause of hypercalcemia is obscure.

Approximately 10% of cases of hypercalcemia are due to other causes. Of particular importance in the evaluation of a hypercalcemic patient are the family history (because of familial syndromes, including multiple endocrine neoplasia type 1 [MEN1], MEN2, and familial hypocalciuric hypercalcemia), medication history (because of the several medication-induced forms of hypercalcemia), and presence

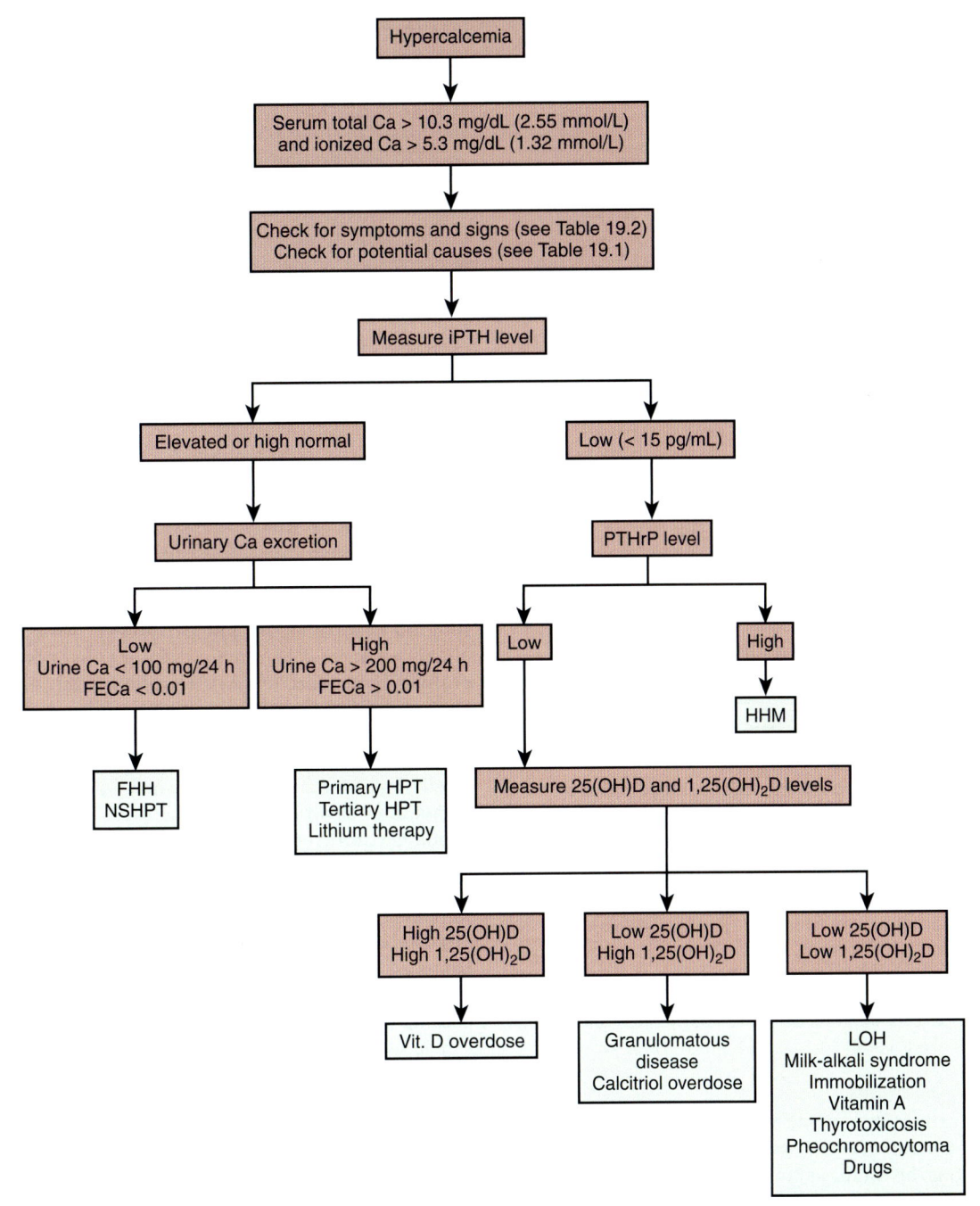

Figure 19.1 Algorithm for evaluation of hypercalcemia. FECa, Fractional excretion of calcium; FHH, familial hypocalciuric hypercalcemia; HHM, humoral hypercalcemia of malignancy; HPT, hyperparathyroidism; iPTH, intact parathyroid hormone; LOH, localized osteolytic hypercalcemia; NSHPT, neonatal severe hyperparathyroidism; PTHrP, parathyroid hormone–related peptide.

of other disease (e.g., granulomatous or malignant disease). Plasma 1,25(OH)$_2$D levels should be measured when granulomatous disorders or 1,25(OH)$_2$D lymphoma syndrome is considered. High 25(OH)$_2$D levels may suggest vitamin D intoxication as a cause of hypercalcemia.

CAUSES

Primary Hyperparathyroidism

PHPT is caused by excessive and incompletely regulated secretion of PTH, with consequent hypercalcemia and hypophosphatemia (see Table 19.1). It is the underlying cause of approximately 50% of hypercalcemic cases in the general population. The estimated prevalence of PHPT is about 1%, but may be as high as 2% in postmenopausal women.[22,23] The annual incidence is approximately 0.03% to 0.04%.[22-24] A single enlarged parathyroid gland (adenoma) is the cause of PHPT in 80% to 85% of cases. These adenomas are benign clonal neoplasms of parathyroid chief cells, which lose their normal sensitivity to calcium. In about 15% to 20% of patients with PHPT, all four parathyroid glands are hyperplastic. This occurs in sporadic PHPT or in

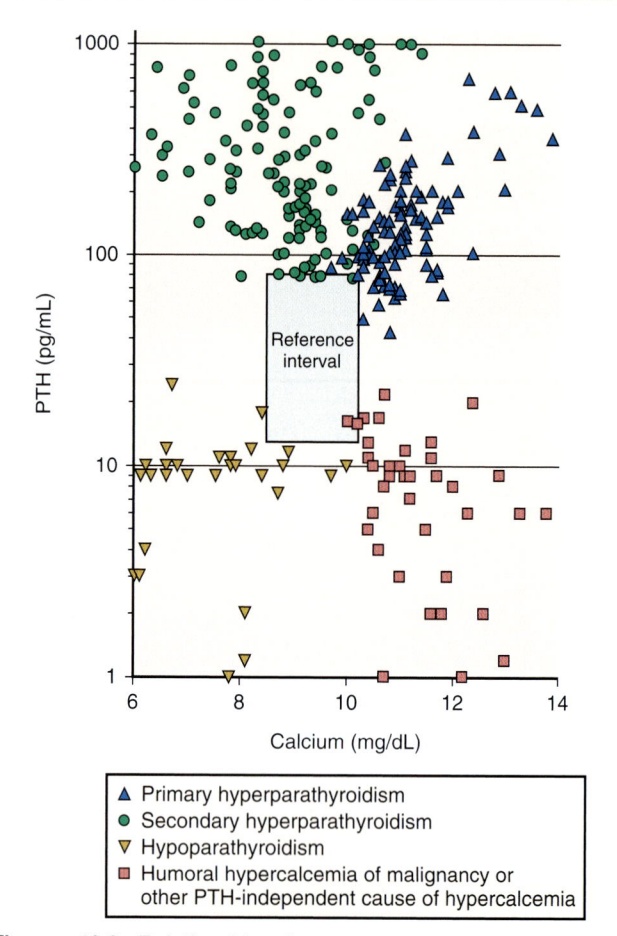

Figure 19.2 Relationship between total serum calcium and intact PTH concentrations. Values for patients with known primary hyperparathyroidism, secondary hyperparathyroidism, humoral hypercalcemia of malignancy or other PTH-independent cause of hypercalcemia, and hypoparathyroidism are plotted. The *rectangle* represents the normal reference range for the assays. (Reproduced with permission from O'Neill S, Gordon C, Guo R, et al: Multivariate analysis of clinical, demographic, and laboratory data for classification of patients with disorders of calcium homeostasis. *Am J Clin Pathol* 135:100-107, 2011.)

conjunction with MEN1 or MEN2.[19] In diffuse hyperplasia, the set point for calcium is not changed in any given parathyroid cell, but the increased number of cells causes excess PTH production and hypercalcemia. Parathyroid carcinoma is seen in no more than 0.5% to 1% of patients with PHPT.[25]

PHPT occurs at all ages but is most common in older individuals; peak incidence is in the sixth decade of life. After age 50 years, women are about three times more frequently affected than men. Sporadic PHPT is the most common. External neck irradiation during childhood is recognized as a risk factor for PHPT. The genetic alterations underlying parathyroid adenomas are being partially elucidated.[26] Rearrangements and overexpression of the PRAD-1/cyclin D1 oncogene have been observed in about 20% of parathyroid adenomas.[27,28] The MEN1 tumor suppressor gene is inactivated in about 15% of adenomas.[29,30] Other chromosomal regions may also harbor parathyroid tumor suppressor genes.

PHPT typically presents in one of three ways. In 60% to 80% of cases, there are minimal or no symptoms, and mild hypercalcemia is usually discovered during routine laboratory examination. Another 20% to 25% of patients have a chronic course manifested by mild or intermittent hypercalcemia, recurrent renal stones, and complications of nephrolithiasis; in these patients, the parathyroid tumor is small (<1.0 g) and slow-growing. In 5% to 10% of patients, there is severe and symptomatic hypercalcemia and overt osteitis fibrosa cystica; in these patients, the parathyroid tumor is usually large (>5.0 g). Patients with parathyroid carcinoma typically have severe hypercalcemia, with classic renal and bone involvement.[26]

The diagnosis of PHPT is now usually suggested by the incidental finding of hypercalcemia rather than by any of the sequelae of PTH excess, such as skeletal and renal complications or symptomatic hypercalcemia.[18] Hypercalcemia may be mild and intermittent. Hypercalciuria was noted in 40% of PHPT, nephrolithiasis in 19%, and classic bone disease and osteitis fibrosa cystica only in 2% of studies performed between 1984 and 2000 in the United States.[16] However, even in individuals with mild PHPT, there is also progressive bone loss as measured by bone mineral densitometry over 15 years of observation.[31]

The diagnosis of PHPT is established by laboratory tests showing hypercalcemia, inappropriately normal or elevated blood levels of PTH, hypercalciuria, hypophosphatemia, phosphaturia, and increased urinary excretion of cAMP. Hyperchloremic acidosis may be present, and the ratio of serum chloride to phosphorus is elevated. The serum levels of alkaline phosphatase and of uric acid may be also elevated. The serum concentration of magnesium is usually normal but may be low or high.

Some controversy surrounds the potential relationship between primary HPT and increased mortality.[15] A number of studies have shown that primary HPT may be associated with hypertension, dyslipidemia, diabetes, increased thickness of the carotid artery,[3] and increased mortality, primarily from cardiovascular disease.[20,32] The morbidity from primary HPT can also be substantial, especially in symptomatic patients with severe hypercalcemia and a late diagnosis.

The classic bone lesion in primary HPT, osteitis fibrosa cystica, is now rarely seen. Diffuse osteopenia is more common.[20,32] Even in asymptomatic patients, increased rates of bone turnover are always present.[20,32]

Surgery is still standard therapy for PHPT.[18,32,33] It is generally agreed that parathyroidectomy is indicated in all patients with biochemically confirmed PHPT who have specific symptoms or signs of disease, such as a history of life-threatening hypercalcemia, renal insufficiency, and/or kidney stones. In 2008, a Third International Workshop on Hyperparathyroidism updated 2002 National Institutes of Health guidelines for the management of asymptomatic HPT.[33] Surgery is advised for asymptomatic disease in patients with serum calcium levels greater than 1 mg/dL above normal, reduced bone mass (T-score < −2.5 at any site), GFR less than 60 mL/min, or age younger 50 years. Hypercalciuria (>400 mg calcium/24 hours) is no longer regarded as an indication for parathyroid surgery because hypercalciuria in PHPT has not been established as a risk factor for stone formation. Patients older than 50 years with no obvious symptoms should receive close follow-up, including measurements of bone density every 1 to 2 years and serum creatinine and calcium levels annually. All monitored patients should be repleted with vitamin D to achieve a 25-hydroxyvitamin D (25[OH])D level above 20 ng/dL and should maintain calcium intake the same as individuals without PHPT.

Preoperative localization of the parathyroid glands has generally been considered unnecessary in uncomplicated patients undergoing surgery for the first time with bilateral neck exploration. However, imaging studies are recommended to be used in complicated cases and if minimally invasive surgery is planned.[34] Sestamibi scanning is the most popular and sensitive technique to localize PTH glands, with accuracy rates up to 94%, followed by ultrasound of the neck.[32,35] If a single adenoma is visualized, minimally invasive parathyroidectomy may be an option, with a cure rate of 95% to 98%: this procedure requires the surgeon to visualize only one gland as long as resection results in a substantial intraoperative decline in PTH level. Otherwise, all four parathyroid glands should be surgically identified. Recurrence of HPT is rare after identification and removal of one enlarged gland.[36] If the initial exploration fails, and hypercalcemia persists or recurs, more extensive preoperative parathyroid localization should be performed.[18,32,35] Complications are greater with re-exploration of the neck than after the initial operation.

Although parathyroidectomy remains the definitive treatment of PHPT, patients refusing surgery, those with contraindications for surgery, or those who do not meet current operative guidelines can be treated pharmacologically. There are four classes of medications that can be useful—calcimimetics, bisphosphonates, estrogens, and selective estrogen receptor modulators.[32,37] There are insufficient long-term data to recommend any of these medications as alternatives to surgery. The CaSR agonist, cinacalcet, is approved in some European countries for PHPT and in the United States for severe hypercalcemia in adult patients with PHPT who are unable to undergo parathyroidectomy. Cinacalcet therapy in PHPT patients reduced plasma PTH levels, normalized serum calcium levels in the short and long terms, and preserved bone mineral density (BMD).[37-40] Bisphosphonates and hormone replacement therapy decreased bone turnover and increased BMD in PHPT patients without change in serum calcium levels.[37]

Parathyroid carcinoma probably accounts for less than 1% of PHPT cases.[25] The diagnosis of parathyroid carcinoma may be difficult to make in the absence of metastases because the histologic appearance may be similar to that of atypical adenomas.[41] In general, parathyroid carcinomas are typically large (3 cm), irregular, hard tumors with a low degree of aggressive growth, and survival is common if the entire gland can be removed.[25,42] Cinacalcet is approved for patients with inoperable parathyroid cancer to control hypercalcemia.

Malignancy

Hypercalcemia occurs in approximately 10% to 25% of patients with some cancer, especially during the last 4 to 6 weeks of their life. It can be classified into four categories—HHM, local osteolytic hypercalcemia (LOH), 1,25 $(OH)_2$ vitamin D–induced hypercalcemia, and ectopic secretion of authentic PTH.[43,44]

HHM from secretion of PTHrP by a malignant tumor accounts for approximately 80% of cases. Numerous types of malignancies are associated with HHM, including squamous cell cancer (e.g., head and neck, esophagus, cervix, lung) and renal cell, breast, and ovarian carcinomas. Lymphomas associated with human T-lymphotropic virus type 1 (HTLV-1) infection may cause PTHrP-mediated HHM, and other non-Hodgkin lymphomas may also be associated with PTHrP-mediated hypercalcemia.[44,45] PTHrP is a large protein encoded by a gene on chromosome 12; it is similar to PTH only at the NH_2 terminus, where the initial eight amino acids are identical.[45] PTHrP is widely expressed in a variety of tissues, including keratinocytes, mammary gland, placenta, cartilage, nervous system, vascular smooth muscle, and various endocrine sites.[46] Injection of PTHrP produces hypercalcemia in rats[47] and essentially reproduces the entire clinical syndrome of HHM, but other circulating factors such as cytokines may also be important. Normal circulating levels of PTHrP are negligible; these are probably unimportant in normal calcium homeostasis. However, mice with a targeted disruption in the PTHrP gene have shown a lethal defect in bone development,[48-50] thus demonstrating its importance in normal development.

Circulating PTHrP interacts with the PTH/PTHrP receptor in bone and the renal tubule. It activates bone resorption and suppresses osteoblastic bone formation, thus causing flux of calcium (up to 700 to 1000 mg/day) from bone into ECF. The reason for this uncoupling of bone formation from bone resorption remains unclear.[45] One possible explanation is a difference in the affinity of PTH versus that of PTHrP for the PTH receptor on osteoblasts.[49] PTHrP mimics the anticalciuric effect of PTH on the kidney, which exacerbates hypercalcemia. Other effects of PTHrP include phosphaturia, hypophosphatemia, and increased cAMP excretion by the kidney.

HHM is associated with a reduction in $1,25(OH)_2D$ levels (in contrast to PHPT), which may limit intestinal calcium absorption. Patients are hypercalcemic and hypophosphatemic and demonstrate increased osteoclastic bone resorption, increased urinary cAMP, and hypercalciuria.

LOH accounts for 20% of patients with malignancy-associated hypercalcemia. LOH-producing tumors include breast and prostate cancers and hematologic neoplasms (e.g., multiple myeloma, lymphoma, leukemia). LOH is caused by locally produced osteoclast-activating cytokines, which include PTHrP, interleukin-1 (IL-1), IL-6, and IL-8. PTHrP increases RANKL expression on osteoblast and RANK-mediated osteoclast bone resorption. The resorbing bone releases transforming growth factor-β (TGF-β), which in turn stimulates PTHrP expression on tumor cells.[50,51] The bone metastases can be classified as osteolytic, osteoblastic, or mixed. Osteolytic lesions are caused by osteoclast activation by malignant cells and appear as areas of increased radiolucency on radiographs. LOH leads to predictable pathophysiologic events, which include hypercalcemia, suppression of circulating PTH and $1,25(OH)_2D$, hyperphosphatemia, and hypercalciuria. Bone metastases may produce severe pain and pathologic fractures.

Hypercalcemia in breast cancer is associated with the presence of extensive osteolytic metastases and HHM.[50,51] Extensive osteolytic bone destruction is seen in multiple myeloma.[52] Although bone lesions develop in all patients with myeloma, hypercalcemia occurs only in 15% to 20% of patients in later stages of disease and with impaired kidney function. The degree of hypercalcemia and bone destruction is not well correlated.[53] Treatment with bisphosphonates appears to protect against the development of skeletal complications (including hypercalcemia) in patients with myeloma and lytic bone lesions.[54]

Hypercalcemia caused by 1,25 $(OH)_2$ vitamin D production by malignant lymphomas has been reported.[55,56] All types of lymphoma can cause this syndrome. The malignant cells or adjacent cells overexpress the enzyme 1α-hydroxylase, which converts $25(OH)D$ to $1,25(OH)_2D$. Hypercalcemia is mainly secondary to increased intestinal calcium, although decreased renal clearance and bone resorption may also develop. In addition, increased osteoclastic activity mediated through activation of the RANKL pathway by $1,25(OH)2D$ augment hypercalcemia. Ectopic production of authentic PTH by a nonparathyroid tumor may occur, but is very rare.[57]

Familial Primary Hyperparathyroidism Syndromes

Familial primary HPT syndromes are defined by a combination of hypercalcemia and elevated or nonsuppressed serum PTH levels.

Familial Hypocalciuric Hypercalcemia and Neonatal Severe Hyperparathyroidism. FHH (benign) is a rare disease (estimated prevalence, 1/78,000), with autosomal dominant inheritance, high penetrance for hypercalcemia, and relative hypocalciuria.[58-60] FHH was first described in 1966 by Jackson and Boonstra and in 1972 by Foley and colleagues.[61,62] The hypercalcemia is typically mild to moderate (10.5 to 12 mg/dL), and affected patients do not exhibit the typical complications associated with elevated serum calcium concentrations. Both total and ionized calcium concentrations are elevated, but the PTH level is generally inappropriately normal, although mild elevations in approximately 15% to 20% of cases have been reported. Urinary calcium excretion is not elevated, as would be expected in hypercalcemia of other causes. The fractional excretion of calcium is usually less than 1%.[59] The serum magnesium level is commonly mildly elevated, and the serum phosphate level is decreased. Bone mineral density is normal, as are vitamin D levels. The finding of a right-shifted set point for Ca^{2+}-regulated PTH release in FHH has indicated the role of CaSR in FHH.[63]

Most families have FHH type 1, which is caused by autosomal dominant loss-of-function mutations in the CaSR gene located on chromosome 3q, which encodes for the CaSR. FHH types 2 and 3 are much rarer and are caused by heterozygous mutations in the GNA11 (guanidine nucleotide-binding protein alpha-11) gene or the AP2S1 (adaptor-related protein complex 2, sigma 1 subunit) gene, respectively.[64,65] Both genes localize on chromosome 19q13, and their mutations render the CaSR less sensitive to extracellular calcium.

The fact that relative hypocalciuria persists even after parathyroidectomy in FHH patients confirms the role of CaSR in regulating renal calcium handling.[66] More than 257 mutations have been described for the CaSR, most of which are inactivating and missense and found throughout the large predicted structure of the CaSR protein.[63,67,68] Expression studies of mutant CaSRs have shown great variability in their effect on calcium responsiveness. In some cases, CaSR mutations only slightly shift the set point for calcium; other mutations appear to render the receptor largely inactive.[69-71] CaSR mutation analysis has an occasional role in the diagnosis of FHH in cases in which biochemical test results remain inconclusive, and the distinction of FHH from mild primary HPT is unclear. It is critically important to make an accurate diagnosis because the hypercalcemia in FHH is benign and does not respond to subtotal parathyroidectomy.

Hypercalcemia in FHH has a generally benign course and is resistant to medications, except it is successfully treated with cinacalcet in some patients.[72] Potential benefit of calcimimetic agents in FHH has been supported by in vitro studies with human CaSR mutants, which have shown that the calcimimetic agent R-568 enhances the potency of extracellular calcium toward the mutants.[73]

Patients who inherit two copies of CaSR alleles bearing inactivating mutations develop neonatal severe HPT (NSHPT). NSHPT is an extremely rare disorder that is often reported in the offspring of consanguineous FHH parents; it is characterized by severe hyperparathyroid hyperplasia, PTH elevation, severe hyperparathyroid bone disease, and elevated extracellular calcium levels.[58,63,74,75] In a few affected infants, only one defective allele has been found, but it is unclear whether this finding is due to the presence of an undetected defect in the other CaSR allele. Treatment is total parathyroidectomy, followed by vitamin D and calcium supplementation. This disease is usually lethal without surgical intervention.

Multiple Endocrine Neoplasia. MEN1 is a rare, autosomal dominant disorder with an estimated prevalence of two to three cases/100,000, characterized by endocrine tumors in at least two of three main tissues—parathyroid gland, pituitary gland, and enteropancreatic tissue. It is the most common form of familial PHPT. PHPT is present in 87% to 97% of patients, whereas pancreatic and pituitary tumors are more likely to be absent.[18,76] The responsible gene, MEN1,[77] encodes a nuclear protein, menin, of 610 amino acids, which functions in cell division, genome stability, and transcription regulation.[78]

MEN2A is a syndrome of heritable predisposition to medullary thyroid carcinoma, pheochromocytoma, and PHPT. Mutations in the RET proto-oncogene, which encodes a tyrosine kinase receptor, are responsible for MEN2A.[79] The biochemical diagnosis and indications for surgery for patients with PHPT in association with MEN1 or MEN2A are similar to those for sporadic PHPT.[80]

Hyperparathyroidism–Jaw Tumor Syndrome. Hyperparathyroidism–jaw tumor (HPT-JT) syndrome is a rare autosomal dominant disorder characterized by severe hypercalcemia, parathyroid adenoma, and fibro-osseous tumors of mandible or maxilla.[81] Renal manifestations include cysts, hamartomas, and Wilms' tumors. Mutations in the HRPT2 (hyperparathyroidism 2) gene, and elimination of its product, parafibromin, which has tumor suppressor activity, are responsible for HPT-JT.[82] If biochemical changes consistent with PHPT are present, parathyroidectomy is indicated.

Nonparathyroid Endocrinopathies

Hypercalcemia may occur in patients with other endocrine diseases. Mild hypercalcemia is present in up to 20% of the patients with hyperthyroidism, but severe hypercalcemia is uncommon.[83,84] Thyroid hormones (thyroxine, triiodothyronine) increase bone resorption and lead to hypercalcemia and/or hypercalciuria when bone resorption exceeds bone formation significantly.[85] Because of a possible increased association between hyperthyroidism and parathyroid adenoma, the latter must be ruled out in patients with thyrotoxicosis and hypercalcemia. Furthermore, the hypercalcemia in a patient with thyrotoxicosis should be attributed to this disease only if it resolves after achieving an euthyroid state.

Pheochromocytoma may be associated with hypercalcemia[86]; it is usually caused by coincident PHPT and MEN2A. In some patients, hypercalcemia disappears after removal of the adrenal tumor, and some of these tumors produce PTHrP.[87] Acute adrenal insufficiency is a rare cause of hypercalcemia.[88] Because these patients may be dehydrated and have hemoconcentration, a rise in the serum albumin concentration and increased binding of calcium to serum albumin secondary to hyponatremia may contribute to the increase in serum calcium levels. In addition, isolated adrenocorticotropic hormone (ACTH) deficiency can result in hypercalcemia.[89]

Growth hormone administration[90] and acromegaly[91] have both been associated with hypercalcemia. Acromegaly is often (15% to 20% of cases) accompanied by mild hypercalcemia, which results from enhanced intestinal calcium absorption and augmented bone resorption.[92,93] In acromegalic patients with hypercalcemia, the serum levels of PTH are normal but may be inappropriately high for the levels of serum calcium.

Vitamin D–Mediated Hypercalcemia

Vitamin D is naturally generated in skin under exposure to ultraviolet B (UVB) light or is acquired from the diet and medical supplements. Excess of vitamin D or its metabolites can cause hypercalcemia and hypercalciuria. The mechanism of hypercalcemia is a combination of increased intestinal calcium absorption and bone resorption induced by vitamin D and decreased renal calcium clearance resulting from dehydration. The effect of toxic amounts of vitamin D is due to an increase in plasma total 25(OH)D, well in excess of 80 ng/mL, which exceeds the binding capacity of vitamin D–binding protein (DBP) for 25(OH)D. The resulting increase in free circulating 25(OH)D may activate the vitamin D nuclear receptor (VDR). Vitamin D metabolites may also displace $1\alpha,25(OH)_2D$ from DBP, increasing free $1\alpha,25(OH)_2D$ levels and thus increasing signal transduction.[94]

Hypercalcemia has been reported in accidental overdoses of vitamin D from fortified cow's milk,[95,96] consumption by children of a fish oil with manufacturing error that caused an excess of vitamin D, and over-the-counter supplements.[97] Serum 25(OH)D levels were elevated, $1,25(OH)_2D$ levels were normal, and PTH levels were depressed or normal in these settings. However, vitamin D well in excess of the tolerable upper intake of 2000 IU/day is required for this form of hypercalcemia to develop.[98] Polymorphism in genes that regulate vitamin D metabolism may predispose certain individuals to develop toxicity, even with exposure to small vitamin D doses.[96] The diagnosis is made by the history and detection of elevated 25(OH)D levels. In the syndrome of idiopathic infantile hypercalcemia, a defect in degradation of $1,25(OH)_2D$ to $24,25(OH)_2D$ caused by a CYP24A1 loss-of-function mutation is responsible for extremely high levels of $1,25(OH)_2D$ and hypercalcemia. Vitamin D analogues, including $1,25(OH)_2D$ used in the treatment of HPT and metabolic bone disease in CKD patients, can also cause hypercalcemia.[99]

Medications

Hypercalcemia and HPT is a long-recognized, well-described consequence of lithium therapy.[100-103] The prevalence of lithium-associated hypercalcemia is estimated to be 4% to 6%.[101,104] Lithium probably interferes with signal transduction elicited by the CaSR, which increases the set point for extracellular calcium to inhibit PTH secretion.[103-105] This leads to parathyroid hyperplasia or adenoma.[106] The spectrum of lithium-induced calcium disorders is wide and includes patients with overt HPT and mild or severe hypercalcemia, with or without elevated PTH levels. Hypocalciuria is common, although hypercalciuria was reported in a few case series. Hypercalcemia can be reversible after a few weeks of discontinuing lithium in most patients with short lithium treatment (<5 years). The CaSR agonist cinacalcet was also used with good results in those patients when cessation of lithium therapy was not an option.[107] Symptomatic patients with HPT should be treated with parathyroidectomy.[102,103]

Vitamin A intake in doses exceeding the recommended daily allowance over prolonged periods, especially in older adults and patients with impaired kidney function, may cause hypercalcemia, with increased alkaline phosphatase levels, presumably from increased osteoclast-mediated bone resorption.[108-110] The hypercalcemia is accompanied by high retinol plasma levels, and discontinuation of vitamin A caused normalization of plasma calcium levels. Vitamin A analogues, used in the management of dermatologic and hematologic malignant diseases, have also been reported to cause hypercalcemia.[111,112]

Estrogens and selective estrogen receptor modifiers (e.g., tamoxifen) used in the management of breast cancer may cause hypercalcemia early during treatment, even in the presence of bone metastasis.[113]

Thiazide diuretic–associated hypercalcemia was noted in approximately 0.4% to 1.9% of treated subjects, with an annual incidence rate of 7.7/100,000 in the population of Olmsted County, Minnesota.[114,115] A reduction in urinary calcium excretion, volume contraction, and metabolic alkalosis are the major reasons for thiazide-induced hypercalcemia. Also, thiazides may increase intestinal calcium absorption and reveal primary HPT.[115-117] Hypercalcemia is usually mild, asymptomatic, and nonprogressive. Subjects with unsuppressed PTH levels, despite hypercalcemia or with severe and continued hypercalcemia, may have primary HPT.

Many other medications occasionally cause hypercalcemia, including theophylline, foscarnet, growth hormone, parenteral nutrition, manganese in toxic doses, and 8-chloro-cAMP.

Milk-Alkali Syndrome

Milk-alkali syndrome was originally described in patients with duodenal ulcers receiving therapy with sodium bicarbonate and large amounts of milk. These patients have hypercalcemia, hyperphosphatemia, hypocalciuria, and renal insufficiency, together with kidney and other soft tissue calcifications.[118] During the last 20 years, calcium supplements in the form of calcium carbonate for the prevention and treatment of osteoporosis have become the main cause of this syndrome.[119,120] In the most recent literature, the name *calcium-alkali syndrome* was proposed.[121] In some studies, milk-alkali syndrome was the third most common cause of hypercalcemia in non–end-stage kidney disease (ESKD) hospitalized patients.[122] The pathogenesis of milk-alkali syndrome can be divided into two phases, the generation of hypercalcemia by intake of calcium and the maintenance phase. Usually, oral intake of more than 4 g of elemental calcium/day has been reported, but even 2 g of calcium/day, especially if taken together with vitamin D, may induce this syndrome. Hypercalcemia activates the renal CaSR, causing natriuresis and water diuresis, with volume depletion and a decrease in the GFR. Increased tubular reabsorption of calcium as a result of metabolic alkalosis and volume depletion contribute to the maintenance of hypercalcemia.[120] The diagnosis is made largely by the history and may not be obvious because of atypical dietary sources of calcium and alkali. Hypercalcemia can be corrected, but renal damage may be permanent.

Immobilization

Immobilization, especially in high bone turnover states (e.g., in young people, hyperparathyroidism, breast cancer with bone involvement, Paget's disease), suppresses osteoblastic bone formation and increases osteoclastic bone resorption, leading to uncoupling of these two processes, with subsequent release of calcium from the bone and hypercalcemia.[123,124] Typically, it takes from 10 days to a few weeks for the development of immobilization hypercalcemia. Increased sclerostin production by osteocytes during mechanical unloading and disuse of the bone is implicated in the pathogenesis of hypercalcemia.[125] Sclerostin is a glycoprotein that inhibits Wnt/β catenin signaling in the osteoblast and decreases bone formation.[126] It is of interest that antisclerostin antibodies are being studied for the treatment of osteoporosis. Bisphosphonates may help decrease hypercalcemia and osteopenia in the setting of immobilization-induced hypercalcemia.[127] There are case reports showing that denosumab also can correct hypercalcemia of immobilization. Mobilization remains the ultimate cure for this condition.

Granulomatous Disease

A variety of granulomatous diseases are associated with hypercalcemia. The most common is sarcoidosis (prevalence of hypercalcemia and hypercalciuria of 10% and 20%, respectively), but tuberculosis, berylliosis, histoplasmosis, coccidioidomycosis, pneumocystosis, leprosy, histiocytosis X, eosinophilic granulomatosis, and inflammatory bowel disease may present with hypercalcemia.[89,128-130] Hypercalcemia is more common in chronic and disseminated granulomatous diseases. Sun exposure, or even small doses of vitamin D supplementation, may precipitate or worsen this syndrome. The hypercalcemia, which has been best studied in sarcoidosis, is caused by inappropriate extrarenal production of $1,25(OH)_2D$ by activated macrophages with increased 1α-hydroxylase activity.[131,132] Elevated circulating $1,25(OH)_2D$ levels have been described in most granulomatous diseases during hypercalcemia, except in coccidioidomycosis. The $1,25(OH)_2D$ in turn leads to intestinal hyperabsorption of calcium, hypercalciuria, and hypercalcemia. Osteopontin, highly expressed by histiocytes in granulomas, may contribute to hypercalcemia via osteoclast activation and bone resorption. Bone mineral content tends to be reduced in these patients. Hypercalciuria may precede hypercalcemia and may be an early indicator of this complication.

Standard treatment consists of administration of glucocorticoids, which decreases the abnormal $1,25(OH)_2D$ production.[133] Chloroquine and ketoconazole, which also decrease $1,25(OH)_2D$ production by competitive inhibition of CYP450-dependent 1α-hydroxylase, have also been shown to be efficacious.[134,135]

Liver Disease

Hypercalcemia has been reported in patients with end-stage liver disease with hyperbilirubinemia awaiting liver transplantation in the absence of HPT or hypervitaminosis D.[136]

Acute and Chronic Kidney Disease

Hypercalcemia may be observed in patients with certain forms of acute and chronic kidney disease and in kidney transplant recipients. These conditions are discussed in detail in Chapter 55.

MANAGEMENT OF HYPERCALCEMIA

The optimal therapy for hypercalcemia must be tailored to the degree of hypercalcemia, clinical condition, and underlying cause (Table 19.3).[15] Theoretically, a decrease in serum calcium levels can be achieved by enhancing its urinary excretion, augmenting net movement of calcium into bone, inhibiting bone resorption, reducing intestinal absorption of calcium, and/or removing calcium from the ECF by other means. Patients with mild hypercalcemia (<12 mg/dL) do not require immediate treatment. They should discontinue any medications implicated in causing hypercalcemia, avoid volume depletion and physical inactivity, and maintain adequate hydration. Moderate hypercalcemia (12 to 14 mg/dL), especially if acute and symptomatic, requires more aggressive therapy. Patients with severe hypercalcemia (>14 mg/dL), even without symptoms, should be treated intensively.

Volume Repletion and Loop Diuretics

Correction of the ECF volume is the first and most important step in the treatment of severe hypercalcemia from any causes. It can be achieved with a normal isotonic saline infusion at 200 to 500 mL/hour, adjusted to obtain a urine output of 150 to 200 ml/hour and with appropriate hemodynamic monitoring.[15,137,138] Volume repletion can lower the calcium concentration by approximately 1 to 3 mg/dL by increasing GFR and decreasing sodium and calcium reabsorption in the proximal and distal tubules.

Once volume expansion is achieved, loop diuretics can be given concurrently with saline to increase the calciuresis by blocking the Na-K-2Cl cotransporter in the TAL.[137] Usually, furosemide is given at a dose of 40 to 80 mg every 6 hours and this, together with saline therapy, may decrease the serum calcium concentration by 2 to 4 mg/dL. Urinary losses of fluid, potassium, and magnesium should be

Table 19.3 Pharmacologic Therapy for Hypercalcemia*

Intervention	Dose	Adverse Effect
Hydration or Calciuresis		
Intravenous saline	200-500 mL/hr, depending on patient's cardiovascular and renal status	Congestive heart failure
Furosemide	20-40 mg IV (after rehydration has been achieved)	Dehydration, hypokalemia, hypomagnesemia
First-Line Medications		
IV bisphosphonates[†]		
Pamidronate	60-90 mg IV over 2 hr in 50-200 mL saline solution or 5% dextrose in water[§]	Renal failure, transient flulike syndrome with aches, chills, and fever
Zoledronate	4 mg IV over 15 min in 50 mL of saline solution or 5% dextrose in water	Renal failure, transient flulike syndrome with aches, chills, and fever
Second-Line Medications		
Glucocorticoids[‡]	Example: prednisone, 60 mg orally daily, for 10 days	Potential interference with chemotherapy; hypokalemia, hyperglycemia, hypertension, Cushing's syndrome, immunosuppression
Mithramycin	Single dose of 25 μg/kg of body weight over 4-6 hr in saline	Thrombocytopenia, platelet aggregation defect, anemia, leukopenia, hepatitis, renal failure[‖]
Calcitonin	4-8 IU/kg subcutaneously or intramuscularly every 12 hr	Flushing, nausea, escape phenomenon
Gallium nitrate	100-200 mg/m² of body surface area IV given continuously over 24 hr for 5 days	Renal failure
Denosumab[¶]	120 mg on days 1, 8, 15, and 29 and every 4 wk	Hypocalcemia, hypophosphatemia, osteonecrosis of the jaw, atypical femoral fractures

*Many recommendations in this table are based on historical precedent and common practice rather than on randomized clinical trials. There are data from randomized trials comparing bisphosphonates to the other agents listed and to one another.
[†]Pamidronate and zoledronate are approved by the FDA. Ibandronate and clodronate are available in continental Europe, United Kingdom, and elsewhere. Bisphosphonates should be used with caution, if at all, when the serum creatinine level exceeds 2.5 to 3.0 mg/dL (221.0 to 265.2 μmol/L).
[‡]Pamidronate is generally used at a dose of 90 mg, but the 60-mg dose may be used to treat patients of small stature or those with renal impairment or mild hypercalcemia.
[§]These drugs have a slow onset of action, as compared with bisphosphonates; approximately 4 to 10 days are required for a response.
[‖]These effects have been reported in association with higher dose regimens used to treat testicular cancer (50 μg/kg body weight/day over a period of 5 days) and in patients receiving multiple doses of 25 μg/kg; they are not expected to occur with a single dose of 25 μg/kg unless preexisting liver, kidney, or hematologic disease is present.
[¶]Approved by the FDA for the prevention of skeletal-related events in patients with bone metastasis from solid tumor; used in an open label fashion as a rescue therapy if bisphosphonates are not effective.
Modified with permission from Stewart AF: Clinical practice. Hypercalcemia associated with cancer. N Engl J Med 352:373-379, 2005.

evaluated at intervals of 2 to 4 hours and quantitatively replaced to prevent dehydration, hypokalemia, and hypomagnesemia. Usually, 20 to 40 mEq of KCl and 15 to 30 mg of magnesium ion/L of saline infusate are adequate to replenish the urinary losses of these electrolytes. Care must be taken to monitor the patient's volume status closely during the administration of large amounts of saline and diuretic, particularly in hospitalized patients with cardiac or pulmonary disease. It must be noted that the use of loop diuretics for hypercalcemia is not supported by any randomized controlled studies and has been criticized for this reason.[138] However, in our opinion, loop diuretics still remain an important tool in the management of hypercalcemia, especially for patients at risk of volume overload.

Inhibition of Bone Resorption

The increase in bone resorption, as the most common pathology leading to hypercalcemia, must be addressed concurrently with volume expansion and hydration. Bisphosphonates are currently the agents of choice in the treatment of mild to severe hypercalcemia, especially that associated with cancer and vitamin D toxicity.[96] They are pyrophosphate analogues with a high affinity for hydroxyapatite and inhibit osteoclast function in areas of high bone turnover.[15] The U.S. Food and Drug Administration (FDA) has approved two bisphosphonates for the treatment of hypercalcemia, zoledronate (4 mg intravenous [IV] over 15 minutes or longer) and pamidronate (60 to 90 mg IV over 2 to 24 hours). The clinical response takes 48 to 96 hours and is sustained for up to 3 weeks. Doses can be repeated no sooner than every 7 days. Both agents are effective in lowering calcium levels. Zoledronate was slightly more efficacious than pamidronate in a randomized clinical trial.[139] In Europe, other bisphosphonates, such as clodronate and ibandronate, have also been approved.

Fever is observed in about 20% of patients taking bisphosphonates; rare side effects include acute renal failure, collapsing glomerulopathy, and osteonecrosis of the jaw.

Ibandronate seems to have minimal to no renal toxicity. The dose of bisphosphonates should be adjusted in patients with preexisting kidney disease.[140] The renal component of hypercalcemia, which includes increased distal tubular calcium reabsorption driven by PTH-PTHrP, does not respond to bisphosphonates.

Calcitonin is also an effective inhibitor of osteoclast bone resorption. It has a rapid onset (within 12 hours), its effect is transient, and it has minimal toxicity.[141-145] Calcitonin is usually given as 4 to 8 U/kg subcutaneously every 6 to 12 hours.[141,142] Its role is mainly in the initial treatment of severe hypercalcemia while waiting for the more sustained effect of bisphosphonates.

Gallium nitrate inhibits bone resorption by increasing the solubility of hydroxyapatite crystals. The usual dose is 200 mg/m^2 IV over 24 hours, with adequate hydration for 5 consecutive days; the hypocalcemic effect is not generally observed until the end of this period. Gallium nitrate is effective, but can be nephrotoxic.[143,144]

Denosumab, a fully humanized monoclonal antibody that binds to RANKL and inhibits osteoclasts. Denosumab inhibits the maturation of preosteoclasts to osteoclasts by binding to and inhibiting RANKL. In 2010, denosumab was approved by the FDA for use in postmenopausal women at risk for osteoporosis.[145] It was also approved for the prevention of skeleton-related events in patients with bone metastasis from a solid tumor. It has also been used for the treatment of hypercalcemia of malignancy not corrected by bisphosphonates in an open label study.[145,146]

Plicamycin (Mithramycin), 25 μg/kg IV, every 5 to 7 days, may be used in patients with severe renal failure. Other therapies for hypercalcemia, such as chelation with ethylenediaminetetraacetic acid (EDTA) and IV phosphate, have adverse side effect profiles and are no longer recommended.

Glucocorticoids are useful therapy for hypercalcemia in a specific subset of causes. They are most effective in hematologic malignancies (e.g., multiple myeloma, Hodgkin's disease) and disorders of vitamin D metabolism (e.g., granulomatous disease, vitamin D toxicity).[128,133]

In severely hypercalcemic patients who are comatose with changes in the ECG, in severe renal failure, or who cannot receive aggressive hydration, hemodialysis with a low- or no-calcium dialysate is an effective treatment.[147] Continuous renal replacement therapy can also be used to treat severe hypercalcemia.[148] The effect of dialysis is transitory and needs to be followed by other measures.

As discussed above, cinacalcet, an allosteric activator of CaSR, is approved for patients with inoperable parathyroid cancer to control hypercalcemia. The off-label use of cinacalcet has been reported in patients with PHPT who have mild disease, failed parathyroid surgery, or contraindications to surgery.[32,37,39,40] Other hypercalcemic disorders, such as FHH[72] and lithium-induced HPT, have also been treated with cinacalcet.[104,107]

HYPOCALCEMIA

Hypocalcemia is usually defined as a total serum calcium concentration, corrected for protein, of less than 8.4 mg/dL and/or an ionized calcium level less 1.16 mmol/L, although these values may vary slightly, depending on the laboratory. Estimation of the ionized calcium concentration based on the total serum calcium corrected for albumin is encumbered with errors, as discussed in the introduction. Thus, ionized calcium should be directly measured before a major workup for the causes of hypocalcemia is undertaken.

Hypocalcemia is highly prevalent in hospitalized patients (10% to 18%) and is particularly common in the intensive care unit (70% to 80%).[149,150]

SIGNS AND SYMPTOMS

Acute hypocalcemia can result in severe clinical symptoms that need rapid correction, whereas chronic hypocalcemia may be an asymptomatic laboratory finding. The clinical features of hypocalcemia are summarized in Table 19.4. Their presentation reflects the absolute calcium concentration and the rapidity of its fall. The threshold for overt symptoms depends also on serum pH and the severity of any concurrent hypomagnesemia, hyponatremia, or hypokalemia. The classic symptoms of hypocalcemia include neuromuscular excitability in the form of numbness, circumoral tingling, feeling of pins and needles in the feet and hands, muscle cramps, carpopedal spasms, laryngeal stridor, and frank tetany. Tapping over the facial nerve anterior to the ear can induce facial muscle spasm (Chvostek's sign). However, Chvostek's sign may occur in 10% of normal people, and it was negative in 29% of patients with mild hypocalcemia. Trousseau's sign of *main d'accoucheur*, elicited by inflation of a sphygmomanometer cuff placed on the upper arm to 10 mm Hg above systolic blood pressure for 3 minutes, has greater than 90% sensitivity and specificity.[151] Patients with hypocalcemia may experience emotional disturbances, irritability, impairment of memory, confusion, delusion, hallucination, paranoia, and depression. Epileptic

Table 19.4 Clinical Features of Hypocalcemia

Neuromuscular Irritability

General fatigability and muscle weakness
Paresthesias, numbness
Circumoral and peripheral extremity tingling
Muscle twitching and cramping
Tetany, carpopedal spasms
Chvostek's sign, Trousseau's sign
Laryngeal and bronchial spasms

Altered Central Nervous System Function

Emotional disturbances—irritability, depression
Altered mental status, coma
Tonic-clonic seizures
Papilledema, pseudotumor cerebri
Cerebral calcifications

Cardiovascular

Lengthening of the QTc interval
Dysrhythmias
Hypotension
Congestive heart failure

Dermatologic and Ocular

Dry skin, coarse hair, brittle nails
Cataracts

seizures, often Jacksonian, may occur but are usually not associated with aura, loss of consciousness, and incontinence. Patients with chronic hypocalcemia, including those with idiopathic and postsurgical hypoparathyroidism and those with pseudohypoparathyroidism, may have papilledema, elevated cerebrospinal fluid pressure, and neurologic signs simulating those of a cerebral tumor.

Bilateral cataracts affecting the anterior and posterior subcapsular areas of the cortical portions of the lens may develop after 1 year of hypocalcemia. The cataracts do not resolve after correction of the hypocalcemia. In patients with idiopathic hypoparathyroidism, the skin could be dry and scaly, eczema and psoriasis may worsen, and candidiasis can occur. The eyelashes and eyebrows may be scanty, and axillary and pubic hair may be absent. Because some forms of this disease have an autoimmune cause, manifestations of other autoimmune diseases, such as adrenal, thyroid, and gonadal insufficiency, diabetes mellitus, pernicious anemia, vitiligo, and alopecia areata may be present and should be sought.

Long-lasting hypocalcemia in children and adults can cause congestive heart failure caused by cardiomyopathy, which is reversible with correction of the calcium.[152-154] Prolongation of the QTc interval on the ECG is a well-known effect of hypocalcemia on heart conduction.

Hypoparathyroidism in children often causes teeth abnormalities, such as defective enamel and root formation, dental hypoplasia, or failure of adult teeth to erupt. Severe skeletal mineralization may occur in the fetus of untreated pregnant women with hypoparathyroidism and hypocalcemia.

LABORATORY FINDINGS

It is important to establish the diagnosis of hypocalcemia, based not only on the measurement of total calcium with proper adjustment to albumin and pH levels, but with evidence that ionized calcium is low. The alterations in serum PTH and serum and urinary electrolyte levels in various hypocalcemic states depend on the mechanisms responsible for the hypocalcemia (see Figure 19.2), and knowledge of these changes aids in the differential diagnosis of these disorders.

X-ray examination of the skull or computed axial tomography scanning of the brain may reveal intracranial calcifications, especially of the basal ganglia.[155] These have been noted in up to 20% of hypocalcemic patients with idiopathic hypoparathyroidism but are less common in postsurgical hypoparathyroidism unless the disease is long-standing. Such calcifications are also encountered in patients with pseudohypoparathyroidism. Bone disease may be observed, but its findings differ in the various causes of hypocalcemia (see later).

DIAGNOSIS

The most common causes of hypocalcemia in the nonacute setting are hypoparathyroidism, hypomagnesemia, renal failure, and vitamin D deficiencies (Table 19.5). These entities should be considered early in the diagnosis of hypocalcemic individuals. It is conceptually and clinically useful to subclassify hypocalcemic individuals into those with elevated PTH levels and those with subnormal or inappropriately normal PTH concentrations, as in

Table 19.5 Causes of Hypocalcemia

Inherited and genetic syndromes with hypoparathyroidism
  PTH gene mutations, isolated congenital hypoparathyroidism
  Autosomal dominant hypoparathyroidism with activating mutation of the CaSR (OMIM #146200)
  DiGeorge syndrome (OMIM #188400)
  Other forms of familial hypoparathyroidism
Inherited and genetic syndromes with resistance to PTH action
  Pseudohypoparathyroidism, types 1a, 1b, and 2
  Hypomagnesemic syndromes
Acquired hypoparathyroidism, inadequate PTH production
  Damage or destruction of the parathyroid glands
    Postsurgical
    Autoimmune—isolated or with multiple endocrine dysfunction
      Acquired antibodies against CaSR
      Polyglandular failure syndrome type I (OMIM #240300 and #607358)
    Irradiation
    Metastatic and infiltrative diseases
    Deposition of heavy metals—iron overload, copper overload
  Reversible impairment of PTH secretion
    Severe hypomagnesemia
    Hypermagnesemia
Inadequate vitamin D production
  Vitamin D deficiency—nutritional, lack of sunlight exposure
  Malabsorption
  End-stage liver disease and cirrhosis
  Chronic kidney disease
Vitamin D resistance
  Pseudovitamin D deficiency rickets (vitamin D–dependent rickets type 1)
  Vitamin D–resistant rickets (vitamin D–dependent rickets type 2)
Miscellaneous causes
  Hyperphosphatemia
  Phosphate retention caused by acute or chronic renal failure
  Excess phosphate absorption caused by enemas, oral supplements
  Massive phosphate release caused by tumor lysis or crush injury
Drugs
  Foscarnet
  Bisphosphonate therapy (especially in patients with vitamin D deficiency)
  Denosumab
Rapid transfusion of large volumes of citrate-containing blood
Acute critical illness (multiple contributing causes)
Hungry bone syndrome, recalcification tetany
  Postthyroidectomy for Graves' disease
  Postparathyroidectomy
Osteoblastic metastases
Acute pancreatitis
Rhabdomyolysis
Substances interfering with the laboratory assay for total calcium
  Gadolinium salts in contrast agents given during MRI, MRA

CaSR, Calcium-sensing receptor; OMIM, Online Mendelian Inheritance in Man; MRI, magnetic resonance imaging; MRA, magnetic resonance angiography; PTH, parathyroid hormone.

primary hypoparathyroidism (Figure 19.3). A thorough medical history and physical examination are diagnostically important because hypocalcemia can be caused by postsurgical, pharmacologic, inherited, developmental, and nutritional problems, in addition to being part of complex syndromes.

CAUSES

The causes of hypocalcemia are summarized in Table 19.5. They can be broadly classified into one of three categories—PTH-related (hypoparathyroidism and pseudohypoparathyroidism), vitamin D–related (low production, vitamin D resistance), and miscellaneous causes.

Parathyroid Hormone–Related Disorders: Hypoparathyroidism and Pseudohypoparathyroidism

This group of disorders presents with hypocalcemia and hyperphosphatemia caused by failure of the parathyroid gland to secrete adequate amounts of biologically active PTH or resistance to PTH action at the tissue level. Both can be inherited or acquired. The levels of PTH are low or absent in hypoparathyroidism (HP) due to lack of PTH production, but elevated in pseudohypoparathyroidism (PHP) due to a secondary or adaptive increase in PTH secretion. The fractional calcium excretion is elevated in HP and low in PHP. Insufficient $1,25(OH)_2D$ is generated for efficient intestinal calcium absorption because of decreased activity of 1α-hydroxylase in the proximal tubules. Skeletal response in both categories is appropriate to the levels of circulating PTH, with low bone turnover in HP and excessive bone remodeling in PHP.[156,157] Hypoparathyroidism is a rare disorder. One study from Japan found the prevalence to be 7.2/million people.[158]

Genetic Causes of Hypoparathyroidism. At least four different mutations affecting the PTH gene(s) involved in parathyroid development have been identified as a cause of familial isolated HP (Table 19.6). All these conditions present during the neonatal period with severe hypocalcemia without any other organ involvement and respond well to therapy with vitamin D analogues.

Heterozygous gain-of-function mutations in the CaSR can activate CaSR or cause CaSR to be hyperresponsive to extracellular calcium.[159] The phenotype seen is essentially the opposite of FHH and has been termed *autosomal dominant*

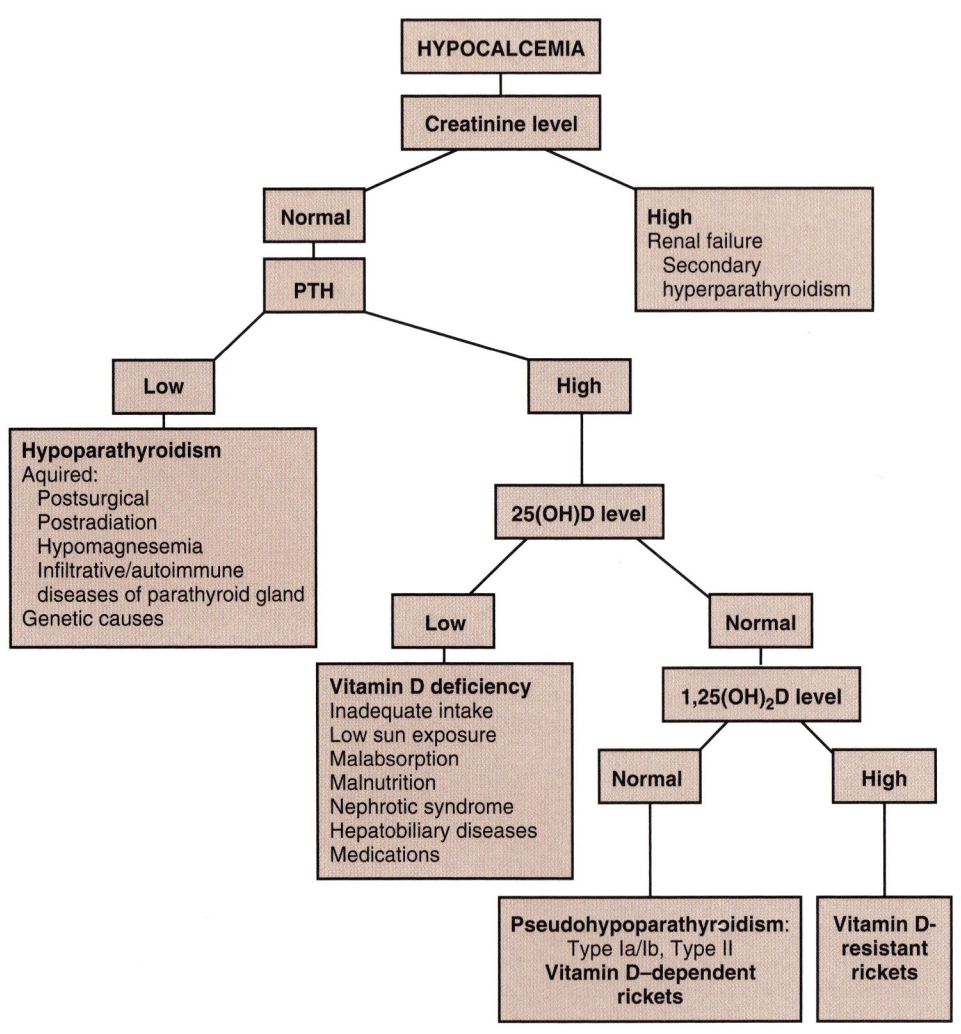

Figure 19.3 Algorithm for evaluation of hypocalcemia.

Table 19.6 Genetic Syndromes with Hypoparathyroidism

Reference	Syndrome	Other Clinical Features	Process Affected	Inheritance	Gene Mutated	Syndrome OMIM No.
Ding et al[466]	Familial isolated hypoparathyroidism	None	Parathyroid gland development	AR	GCM2	146200
Bowl et al[467]				X-linked	SOX3?	307700
Parkinson and Thakker[468]			PTH gene mutation affecting its synthesis	AR	Prepro-PTH splice site	
Arnold et al[469]				AD	Prepro-PTH signal peptide	
Pollak et al[159]	Autosomal dominant hypoparathyroidism	Hypocalcemia, hypomagnesemia, hypercalciuria	Calcium sensing	AD	CaSR	146200 601298
Yagi et al[470]	DiGeorge, CATCH22	Cardiac anomalies, abnormal facies, thymic aplasia, cleft palate	Defective third and fourth branchial pouch development	Sporadic or AD	Chromosome 22q11 deletions (including TBX1)	188400
Van Esch et al[471]	HDR	Hypoparathyroidism, deafness, renal anomalies	Parathyroid development	AD	GATA3 transcription factor	146255
Parvari et al[472]	Kenny-Caffey, Sanjad-Sakati	Microcephaly, mental retardation, growth failure ± osteosclerosis		AR	TBCE (chaperone for tubulin folding)	241410 244460
Neufeld et al[473]	Autoimmune polyendocrinopathy—candidiasis—ectodermal dystrophy (APECED)	Chronic mucocutaneous candidiasis, Addison's disease	Immune tolerance	AR	AIRE (autoimmune transcriptional regulator)	240300

AD, Autosomal dominant; AR, autosomal recessive; CaSR, calcium-sensing receptor; OMIM, Online Mendelian Inheritance in Man; PTH, parathyroid hormone.

hypoparathyroidism or *familiar hypocalcemia with hypercalciuria.* Patients present with mild hypocalcemia, hypomagnesemia and hypercalciuria, with low or inappropriately normal PTH levels. The set point for PTH secretion is shifted to the left. Treatment with calcium supplements and vitamin D is warranted only for patients with severe symptomatic hypocalcemia. The goal should be to increase the calcium level to render the patient asymptomatic, not necessarily to a normocalcemic level. Renal calcium excretion requires monitoring because these patients may develop frank hypercalciuria and nephrocalcinosis.[160,161] Thiazide diuretics or injectable PTH can be used to decrease calciuria at any given level of serum calcium.[162,163]

A number of rare congenital syndromes with multiple developmental abnormalities can also be associated with familial hypoparathyroidism, including DiGeorge syndrome, hypoparathyroid, deafness, and renal anomalies (HDR), autoimmune polyendocrinopathy—candidiasis—ectodermal dystrophy (APECED), and mitochondrial disorders (see Table 19.6).

Genetic Syndromes with Resistance to Parathyroid Hormone Action. Individuals with PHP are hypocalcemic and hyperphosphatemic but have elevated PTH levels. This condition, reported in 1942 by Albright, was the first described example of a hormone resistance disease.[164] The patients exhibited a pattern of features of Albright's hereditary osteodystrophy (AHO) that included short stature, round face, mental retardation, brachydactyly, and the lack of a phosphaturic response to parathyroid extract. PHP is now recognized as a heterogeneous group of related disorders.[165,166] It may be inherited or sporadic.

PHP is subdivided into two types dependent on the renal tubular response to infused exogenous PTH. PHP type 1 (PHP-1) refers to complete resistance to the effects of PTH, as demonstrated by the failure of patients to increase serum calcium, urinary cAMP, and phosphate levels in response to PTH infusion.[167,168] PHP-1 is subdivided into PHP type 1a (PHP-1a), with AHO, and PHP type1b (PHP-1b), without AHO. The presence of AHO without hypocalcemia and endocrine dysfunction is termed *pseudopseudohypoparathyroidism* (PPHP).

PHP-1a and PPHP result from loss-of-function mutations of the GNAS1 gene, which encodes the stimulatory G protein α-subunit ($G_{\alpha s}$) that couples the type 1 PTH/PTHrP receptor (PTH1R) to the adenylyl cyclase pathway.[169] Patients with the GNAS1 gene mutation also have resistance to thyroid-stimulating hormone (TSH), gonadotropins, glucagons, calcitonin, and gonadotropin-releasing hormone (GnRH) because the same $G_{\alpha s}$ pathway is used by these hormones. Promoter-specific genomic imprinting of GNAS1 has been established and provides the probable explanation for the complex phenotypic expression of the dominantly inherited genetic defect. Maternal transmission of the mutation causes PHP-1a; paternal transmission leads to PPHP.[170]

PHP-1b appears to be caused by mutations that affect the regulatory elements of GNAS1, mainly in the proximal tubules.[171,172] Patients with PHP-1c exhibit the features of PHP-1, but without defective $G_{\alpha s}$ activity.

PHP-2 is a heterogeneous group of disorders characterized by a reduced phosphaturic response to PTH but a normal increase in urinary cAMP.[173] The cause is unclear but may be caused by a defect in the intracellular response to cAMP or some other component of the PTH signaling pathway. It does not appear to follow a clear familial pattern.

Hypomagnesemic Syndromes

Impaired PTH secretion and inadequate PTH response to hypocalcemia are typically observed in hypomagnesemic patients. This is corrected by magnesium replacement. Congenital defects leading to hypomagnesemia and hypocalcemia are discussed later (see "Magnesium Disorders") and in Chapters 43 and 75.

Acquired Hypoparathyroidism and Inadequate Parathyroid Hormone Production

Postsurgical Causes. The most common cause of acquired hypoparathyroidism in adults is surgical removal of or damage to the parathyroid glands. Transient hypocalcemia after thyroid surgery was observed in 2% to 23% of cases, whereas permanent hypocalcemia occurred in approximately 1% to 2%.[163,174-176] Hypocalcemia was more likely to occur after total thyroidectomy for cancer, Graves' disease, radical neck dissection for other cancers, and repeated operations for parathyroid adenoma removal. Hypoparathyroidism may result from inadvertent removal of the parathyroids, damage from bleeding, or devascularization. Removal of a single hyperfunctioning parathyroid adenoma can result in transient hypocalcemia because of hypercalcemia-induced suppression of PTH secretion from the normal glands. Surgical experience and use of appropriate surgical technique may reduce the frequency of hypothyroidism.[176]

The so-called hungry bone or recalcification syndrome represents an important cause of prolonged hypocalcemia after parathyroidectomy or thyroidectomy for any form of HPT or hyperthyroidism, respectively.[177] Postoperative withdrawal of PTH decreases osteoclastic bone resorption without affecting osteoblastic activity and leads to increased bone uptake of calcium, phosphate, and magnesium. Risk factors for the development of the so-called hungry bone syndrome include large parathyroid adenomas, age older than 60 years, and high preoperative levels of serum PTH, calcium, and alkaline phosphatase. There are reports that bisphosphonate therapy for Paget's disease and cinacalcet use for secondary HPT can also cause hungry bone syndrome.[178,179]

Acquired HP from nonsurgical causes is rare, with the exception of autoimmune disorders and magnesium deficiency. Although metal overload diseases (e.g., hemochromatosis, Wilson's disease),[180,181] granulomatous diseases, miliary tuberculosis, amyloidosis, or neoplastic infiltrate are often mentioned as causes of hypoparathyroidism, these entities are rare. Alcohol consumption has been reported to cause transient hypocalcemia.[182]

Magnesium Disorders. Both magnesium excess and deficiency can produce generally mild hypocalcemia and reversible HP. Acute infusion of magnesium or hypermagnesemia inhibits PTH secretion.[183] Magnesium is an extracellular CaSR agonist, although less potent than calcium. Hypermagnesemia, when severe enough, as observed in patients with chronic renal failure or who have received acute high doses of IV magnesium sulfate (used in obstetrics), can activate the CaSR and inhibit PTH secretion.[184]

Hypomagnesemic patients typically have low or inappropriately normal PTH levels for the degree of hypocalcemia observed.[185] Moderate hypomagnesemia (serum magnesium levels = 0.8 to 1 mg/dL) primarily causes PTH resistance at the level of target organ,[186] whereas severe hypomagnesemia, in addition, decreases PTH secretion.[187] The effect of chronic severe hypomagnesemia is not from an extracellular effect on CaSR but from intracellular magnesium depletion, which leads to $G_{\alpha s}$ activation, enhanced CaSR signaling and, hence, blunted PTH secretion.[187] The appropriate therapy is magnesium repletion; in the absence of adequate magnesium repletion, the hypocalcemia is resistant to PTH and vitamin D therapy.

Autoimmune Disease. Autoimmune HP can present as an isolated finding or as part of the polyendocrinopathy type 1 syndrome (APS1). APS1 can be sporadic or familial (also referred to as APECED; see Table 19.6).[188] Autoantibodies against parathyroid tissue have been reported in a significant percentage of cases of hypoparathyroidism, but the causative role of these antibodies is unclear. The CaSR has been identified as a possible autoantigen in some cases of autoimmune HP (isolated or polyglandular).[189]

Vitamin D–Related Disorders

Low Vitamin D Production. Inherited and acquired disorders of vitamin D and its metabolites can be associated with hypocalcemia.[190] Vitamin D is a fat-soluble vitamin that is produced in the skin under UVB radiation from 7-dehydrocholesterol or absorbed in the gastrointestinal tract from external sources. Vitamin D is present naturally in a few foods, is artificially added to others, and is available as a food supplement or drug.[191]

Despite routine dietary supplementation in milk and other foods, vitamin D deficiency is common in certain populations,[190,191] such as breast-feeding infants, older adults, people with dark skin and limited sun exposure, people with fat malabsorption,[191] and patients after gastric bypass surgery.[192] A study of hospitalized patients found a high prevalence of vitamin D deficiency, even in younger patients without risk factors who were consuming the recommended daily allowance of vitamin D_3.[193] Fat malabsorption syndromes, common in liver diseases, sprue, and Whipple's and Crohn's diseases may result in malabsorption of vitamin D.[194,195] Liver diseases may impair the hydroxylation of vitamin D to 25(OH)D (calcidiol), and drugs such as phenytoin and barbiturates stimulate the conversion of 25(OH)D to inactive metabolites.[196] Therapy of hepatic osteodystrophy with vitamin D and calcium is not fully effective.[197]

Deficiency of 1α-hydroxylase, as observed in advanced CKD, leads to deficiency of $1,25(OH)_2D$ (calcitriol), the most important biologic form for maintaining calcium and phosphorus homeostasis. Vitamin D deficiency with hypocalcemia is commonly seen in patients with renal insufficiency (see Chapter 55). Patients with nephrotic syndrome may also have decreased 25(OH)D levels as a result of urinary loss, leading to hypocalcemia and secondary HPT.[198]

The serum level of 25(OH)D is the best indicator of vitamin D status. Levels of $1,25(OH)_2D$ do not decrease until vitamin D deficiency is severe. Prolonged vitamin D deficiency causes rickets in children (a disorder of mineralization of growing bone) and osteomalacia in adults (a disorder of mineralization of formed bone). The combination of calcium deficiency and vitamin D deficiency accelerates skeletal abnormalities and the development of hypocalcemia. The diagnosis of vitamin D deficiency is confirmed by measurement of serum 25(OH)D levels. Hypocalcemia is usually observed only in severe vitamin D deficiency—25(OH)D levels less than 10 ng/mL—and when skeletal stores of calcium are depleted; otherwise, the compensatory rise of PTH would be able to mobilize calcium from bone.[190,191,199,200] The 24-hour urinary calcium excretion is low to very low. Hypophosphatemia and increased alkaline phosphatase and normal FGF-23 levels are typically seen with vitamin D deficiency.[190]

Vitamin D Resistance. The observation that some forms of rickets cannot be cured by regular doses of vitamin D led to the discovery of rare inherited abnormalities in vitamin D metabolism or the vitamin D receptor. Vitamin D–dependent rickets type 1 (VDDR-1; Online Mendelian Inheritance in Man [OMIM database] #264700) is characterized by autosomal recessive, childhood-onset rickets, hypocalcemia, secondary HPT, and aminoaciduria. The biochemical abnormality is defective 1α-hydroxylation of 25(OH)D, caused by mutations in the gene for the 25(OH)D–1α-hydroxylase.[201] Therapy with calcitriol or 1α(OH)D (alfacalcidol) restores serum $1,25(OH)_2D$ and must be continued for life.

VDDR-2 (also called hereditary vitamin D–resistant rickets) is an autosomal recessive disorder (OMIM #277440). Affected patients have extreme elevations in $1,25(OH)_2D$ levels in addition to alopecia and the abnormalities seen in VDDR-1.[202] Biochemically, the disorder results from end-organ resistance to $1,25(OH)_2D$. A number of different mutations have been found in the vitamin D receptor gene of affected individuals.[203] High-dose calcium intake and calcium infusion may be the only way to treat hypocalcemia and rickets in these children.

Miscellaneous Causes

Medications. Medication-induced hypocalcemia is a relatively common cause of hypocalcemia, particularly in hospitalized patients.[204,205] Some of the gadolinium-based contrast agents (e.g., gadodiamide, gadoversetamide) used in magnetic resonance imaging (MRI) studies cause pseudohypocalcemia by interference with colorimetric assays for calcium. Calcium readings can be as low as 6 mg/dL, but with no symptoms or signs of hypocalcemia.[204,205] Propofol and IV contrast agents may also complex calcium.

Drug-induced hypomagnesemia (e.g., cisplatin, aminoglycoside, amphotericin, diuretics) and hypermagnesemia (e.g., magnesium sulfate infusion, magnesium-containing antacids) can cause hypocalcemia. Inhibitors of bone resorption (e.g., bisphosphonates, denosumab, calcimimetics, mithramycin, calcitonin) may depress serum calcium to subnormal levels.[204] Proton pump inhibitors and histamine-2 antagonists may reduce calcium absorption, provoke hypocalcemia, and/or inhibit bone resorption.[206] Regional citrate anticoagulation for continuous renal replacement therapy (CRRT) and for plasmapheresis can chelate calcium and cause hypocalcemia.[207,208] Transfusions of citrated blood rarely cause significant hypocalcemia, but it may occur in the course of massive transfusion.[209]

Foscarnet (trisodium phosphonoformate), an antiviral medication used to treat herpes viruses, is a structural mimic of the pyrophosphate anion. Foscarnet can cause hypocalcemia through the chelation of extracellular calcium ions, so normal total calcium measurements may not reflect ionized hypocalcemia.[210] Magnesium losses by the kidney may exaggerate hypocalcemia. Patients treated with foscarnet should undergo total calcium and ionized calcium measurements. As noted, anticonvulsants, particularly phenytoin and phenobarbital, can induce the hepatic CYP3A4 enzyme, which shortens vitamin D half-life and causes vitamin D deficiency.[205] Fluoride overdose is an exceedingly rare cause of hypocalcemia. Oral sodium phosphate–induced hyperphosphatemia may cause hypocalcemia, particularly in patients with renal failure.[204,211] Other drugs associated with hypocalcemia include antiinfectious (e.g., pentamidine, ketoconazole) and chemotherapeutic agents (e.g., asparaginase, cisplatin, doxorubicin).

Critical Illness. In complicated, critically ill patients, total calcium measurements may be poor indicators of the ionized calcium concentration because many factors that could interfere with or alter calcium and protein binding may be present (e.g., albumin infusion, citrate, IV fluids, acid-base disturbances, dialysis therapy, propofol infusion). Thus, it is particularly important to measure ionized calcium in this setting. Hypocalcemia is frequently noted in gram-negative sepsis and toxic shock syndrome.[150,212] This entity is multifactorial; the primary cause is unclear, but a direct effect of interleukin-1 on parathyroid function may be partly responsible.[213]

Other Causes. Hypocalcemia is common in acute pancreatitis and is a poor prognostic indicator. It is probably due to calcium chelation by free fatty acids generated by the action of pancreatic lipase, although some animal studies have challenged this hypothesis.[214] Massive tumor lysis, particularly from rapidly growing hematologic malignancies, may cause hyperphosphatemia, hyperuricemia, and hypocalcemia.[215] The early phase of rhabdomyolysis may include severe hyperphosphatemia and associated hypocalcemia, in contrast to the recovery phase, when hypercalcemia is common. In hemodialysis patients, hypocalcemia is common and may result, at least in part, from reduced renal phosphate clearance and consequent hyperphosphatemia and reduced $1,25(OH)_2D$ production (see Chapter 55).

MANAGEMENT OF HYPOCALCEMIA

The optimal management of hypocalcemia has not been examined in clinical trials, but accepted practices exist. The treatment depends on speed of onset and the severity of clinical and laboratory features. Oral calcium supplementation may be sufficient treatment for mild hypocalcemia. Patients with acute, severe symptomatic hypocalcemia (Ca level < 7 to 7.5 mg/dL; ionized Ca^{2+} < 0.8 mmol/L), such as after parathyroidectomy, with evidence of neuromuscular effects or tetany, should be treated promptly with IV calcium. The preferred calcium salt is calcium gluconate (10 mL of 10% calcium gluconate contains 93 mg of elemental calcium). Initially, 1 to 2 g (93 to 186 mg of elemental Ca) of IV calcium gluconate in 50 mL of 5% dextrose is given over a period of 10 to 20 minutes, followed by slow infusion at a rate of 0.3 to 1.0 mg elemental Ca/kg/hr.[186] The dose can be adjusted to maintain the serum calcium level at the lower end of normal values.

Moderate asymptomatic hypocalcemia (ionized Ca^{2+} > 0.8 mmol/L) can be treated by repeated doses of 1 to 2 g calcium gluconate IV every 4 hours, without continuous infusion. Ionized Ca should be measured every 4 to 6 hours initially.

The infusion solution should not contain phosphates or bicarbonates. IV infusion may be needed until the patient is stabilized and oral calcium and calcitriol therapy begin to take effect. Correction of hypomagnesemia and hyperphosphatemia should also be undertaken, when present. Dialysis may be appropriate if hyperphosphatemia is also present.

Treatment of chronic hypocalcemia depends on the underlying cause. For example, underlying hypomagnesemia or vitamin D deficiency should be corrected. The principal therapy for primary parathyroid dysfunction or PTH resistance is dietary calcium supplementation and vitamin D therapy. Oral calcium supplementation, beginning with 500 to 1000 mg of elemental calcium daily and increasing up to a maximum of 2000 mg daily, is a good strategy. Correction of serum calcium to the low-normal range is generally advised; correction to normal levels may lead to frank hypercalciuria. Several preparations of vitamin D are available for the treatment of hypocalcemia. The role of vitamin D therapy in CKDs is discussed separately.

Replacement therapy using synthetic human parathyroid hormone, PTH (1-34) (teriparatide in a dosage of 20 mcg SQ once daily) has been FDA-approved for treatment of osteoporosis. Teriparatide has also been used as hormone replacement in patients with hypoparathyroidism in a dose of 20 μg subcutaneously, twice daily.[216] More recently, PTH (1-84) (100 μg every other day) was studied in 30 hypoparathyroid patients for 24 months.[217] Improvement or normalization of the serum calcium level was observed with both hormonal preparations.

DISORDERS OF MAGNESIUM HOMEOSTASIS

HYPOMAGNESEMIA AND MAGNESIUM DEFICIENCY

The terms *hypomagnesemia* and *magnesium deficiency* tend to be used interchangeably. However, extracellular fluid magnesium accounts for only 1% of total body magnesium, so serum magnesium concentrations have been found to correlate poorly with overall magnesium status. In patients with magnesium deficiency, serum magnesium concentrations may be normal or may seriously underestimate the severity of the magnesium deficit.[218] Approximately 50% to 60% of magnesium is in the skeleton and most of the remaining 40% to 50% is intracellular. No satisfactory clinical test to assay body magnesium stores is available.[219]

The magnesium tolerance test has been proposed to be the best test of overall magnesium status.[219] It is based on the observation that magnesium-deficient patients tend to retain a greater proportion of a parenterally administered magnesium load and excrete less in the urine than normal individuals.[220] Clinical studies have indicated that the results of a magnesium tolerance test correlate well with magnesium status, as assessed by skeletal muscle magnesium content and exchangeable magnesium pools. However, the test is invalid in patients who have impaired renal function or a renal magnesium-wasting syndrome or in patients taking diuretics or other medications that induce renal magnesium wasting. Thus, and also because of the time and effort required to perform the magnesium tolerance test, it is used primarily as a research tool.

The serum magnesium concentration, although an insensitive measure of magnesium deficit, remains the only practical test of magnesium status in widespread use. Surveys of serum magnesium levels in hospitalized patients have indicated a high incidence of hypomagnesemia (presumably an underestimate of the true incidence of magnesium deficiency), ranging from 11% in general inpatients[221] to 60% in patients admitted to intensive care units (ICUs).[222,223] Furthermore, in ICU patients, hypomagnesemia was associated with increased mortality when compared with normomagnesemic patients.[222]

The functionally important value is believed to be the ionized Mg^{2+} concentration, which is less than total serum magnesium due to protein binding. Measurements with ion-selective electrodes have found ionized Mg^{2+} concentrations that are approximately 70% of the total serum magnesium, a proportion that is fairly constant among the general population.[219] However, in critically ill patients, there is a poor correlation between total and ionized serum magnesium levels.[223]

CAUSES

Magnesium deficiency may be caused by decreased intake or intestinal absorption, increased losses via the gastrointestinal tract, kidneys, or skin, or, rarely, sequestration in the bone compartment (Figure 19.4). It is often helpful to distinguish between renal magnesium wasting and extrarenal causes of magnesium deficiency by assessing urinary magnesium excretion. In the setting of magnesium deficiency, a urine magnesium excretion rate greater than 24 mg/day is abnormal and usually suggestive of renal magnesium wasting.[224] If a 24-hour urine collection is unavailable, the fractional excretion of magnesium (F_EMg) can be calculated from a random urine specimen as follows:

$$F_EMg = \frac{\text{urine Mg concentration} \times \text{plasma Cr}}{(0.7 \times \text{plasma total Mg concentration}) \times \text{urine Cr concentration}}$$

where Cr is creatinine. Note that a correction factor of 0.7 is applied to the plasma total magnesium concentration to estimate the free magnesium concentration. In general, a

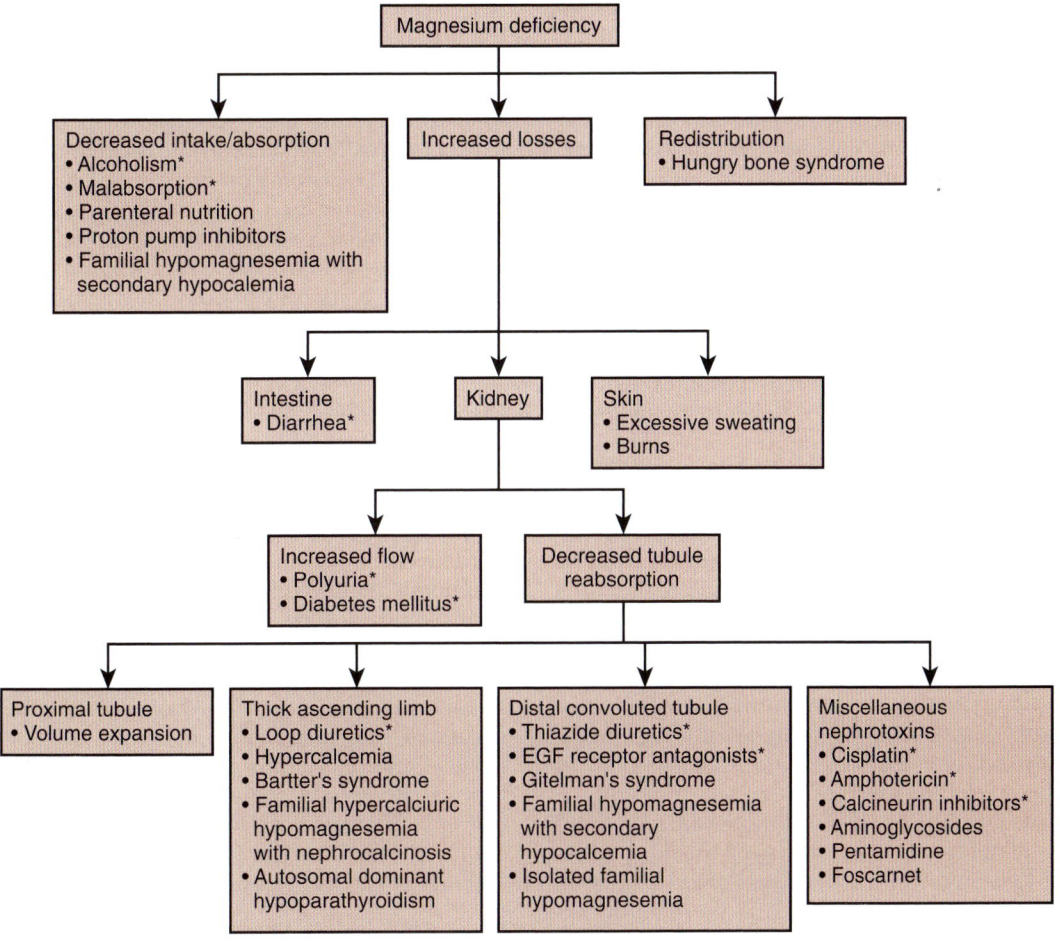

Figure 19.4 Causes of magnesium deficiency.

*Common causes.

F_EMg of more than 3% to 4% in an individual with normal GFR is indicative of inappropriate urinary magnesium loss.[185] If renal magnesium wasting has been excluded, the losses must be extrarenal in origin, and the underlying cause can usually be identified from the case history.

Extrarenal Causes

Nutritional Deficiency. Development of magnesium deficiency due to dietary deficiency in normal individuals is unusual because almost all foods contain significant amounts of magnesium, and renal adaptation to conserve magnesium is very efficient. Thus, magnesium deficiency of nutritional origin is observed primarily in two clinical settings—alcoholism and parenteral feeding.

In chronic alcoholics, the intake of ethanol substitutes for the intake of important nutrients.[225] Approximately 20% to 25% of alcoholics are frankly hypomagnesemic, and most can be shown to be magnesium-deficient with the magnesium tolerance test.[220] Alcohol also impairs renal magnesium reabsorption.[226]

Patients receiving parenteral nutrition may also develop hypomagnesemia.[227] In general, these patients are sicker than the average inpatient and are more likely to have other conditions associated with a magnesium deficit and ongoing magnesium losses. Hypomagnesemia may also be a consequence of the refeeding syndrome.[228] In this condition, overzealous parenteral feeding of severely malnourished patients causes hyperinsulinemia, as well as rapid cellular uptake of glucose and water, together with phosphorus, potassium, and magnesium.

Intestinal Malabsorption. Generalized malabsorption syndromes caused by conditions such as celiac disease, Whipple's disease, and inflammatory bowel disease are frequently associated with intestinal magnesium wasting and magnesium deficiency.[229] In fat malabsorption with concomitant steatorrhea, free fatty acids in the intestinal lumen may combine with magnesium to form nonabsorbable soaps, a process termed *saponification,* thus contributing to impaired magnesium absorption. The severity of hypomagnesemia in patients with malabsorption syndrome correlates with the fecal fat excretion rate and, in rare patients, reduction of dietary fat intake alone, which reduces steatorrhea, can correct the hypomagnesemia. Previous intestinal resection, particularly of the distal part of the small intestine, is also an important cause of magnesium malabsorption.[230] Magnesium deficiency was a common complication of bariatric surgery by jejunoileal bypass,[231] but fortunately does not occur with the modern technique of gastric bypass.[232]

Proton pump inhibitors (PPIs) have been reported to cause hypomagnesemia due to intestinal magnesium malabsorption.[233] Among patients admitted to an ICU, concurrent use of PPIs with diuretics was associated with a significant increase of hypomagnesemia (odds ratio [OR], 1.54) and a 0.03-mg/dL lower serum magnesium concentration compared to patients taking diuretics alone, whereas patients taking PPI alone did not have an increased risk of hypomagnesemia.[234] Interestingly, in a recent case-control study of hospitalized patients, hypomagnesemia at the time of hospital admission was not associated with out-of-hospital use of PPI.[235] However, most of these patients were not taking diuretics. A rare mutation of the TRPM6 magnesium transport channel can also lead to intestinal magnesium malabsorption, along with renal magnesium wasting, causing hypomagnesemia with secondary hypocalcemia.[236]

Diarrhea and Gastrointestinal Fistula. The magnesium concentration of diarrheal fluid is high and ranges from 1 to 16 mg/dL,[230] so magnesium deficiency may occur in patients with chronic diarrhea of any cause, even in the absence of concomitant malabsorption,[218] and in patients who abuse laxatives. By contrast, secretions from the upper gastrointestinal tract are low in magnesium content, and significant magnesium deficiency is, therefore, rarely observed in patients with an intestinal, biliary, or pancreatic fistula, ileostomy, or prolonged gastric drainage (except as a consequence of malnutrition).[230]

Cutaneous Losses. Hypomagnesemia may be observed after prolonged intense exertion. For example, serum magnesium concentrations fall 20% on average after a marathon run.[237] About 25% of the decrease in the serum magnesium level can be accounted for by losses in sweat, which can contain up to 0.5 mg/dL of magnesium; the remainder is most likely due to transient redistribution into the intracellular space. Magnesium supplements may be indicated in a number of sports, especially if the athlete is on a suboptimal magnesium diet.[238] Hypomagnesemia occurs in 40% of patients with severe burn injuries during the early period of recovery. The major cause is loss of magnesium in the cutaneous exudate, which can exceed 1 g/day.[239]

Redistribution to Bone Compartment. Hypomagnesemia may occasionally accompany the profound hypocalcemia of hungry bone syndrome observed in some patients with HPT and severe bone disease immediately after parathyroidectomy.[240] In such cases, there is high bone turnover, and sudden removal of excess PTH is believed to result in virtual cessation of bone resorption, with a continued high rate of bone formation and consequent sequestration of calcium and magnesium into bone mineral.

Diabetes Mellitus. Hypomagnesemia is common in patients with diabetes mellitus, and has been reported to occur in 13.5% to 47.7% of nonhospitalized patients with type 2 diabetes.[241] The cause is thought to be multifactorial; contributing factors include decreased oral intake of magnesium-rich foods, poor intestinal absorption due to diabetic autonomic neuropathy, and increased renal excretion. The latter could, in turn, be caused by glomerular hyperfiltration, osmotic diuresis, or decreased thick ascending limb and distal tubule magnesium reabsorption caused by functional insulin deficiency.[242,243] In addition, some studies have suggested that magnesium deficiency might itself impair glucose tolerance, thus partly explaining the association. Conversely, genetic variants in the magnesium transport channels, TRPM6 and TRPM7, may increase the risk of type 2 diabetes mellitus in women on a diet with less than 250 mg/day of magnesium.[244]

Renal Magnesium Wasting

The diagnosis of renal magnesium wasting is made by demonstrating an inappropriately high rate of renal magnesium excretion in the face of hypomagnesemia, as described above. The causes are summarized in Figure 19.4.

Polyuria. Increased urine output from any cause is often accompanied by increased renal losses of magnesium. Renal magnesium wasting occurs with osmotic diuresis—for example, in hyperglycemic crises in diabetics.[245,246] Hypermagnesuria also occurs during the polyuric phase of recovery from acute renal failure in a native kidney, during recovery from ischemic injury in a transplanted kidney, and in postobstructive diuresis. In such cases, it is likely that residual tubule reabsorptive defects persisting from the primary renal injury play as important a role as polyuria itself in inducing renal magnesium wasting.[247]

Extracellular Fluid Volume Expansion. In the proximal tubule, magnesium reabsorption is passive and driven by the reabsorption of sodium and water in this segment. Extracellular volume expansion, which decreases proximal sodium and water reabsorption, also increases urinary magnesium excretion. Thus, chronic therapy with magnesium-free parenteral fluids, crystalloid or hyperalimentation,[248] can cause renal magnesium wasting, as can hyperaldosteronism.[249]

Diuretics. Loop diuretics inhibit the apical membrane Na-K-2Cl cotransporter of the TAL and abolish the transepithelial potential difference, thereby inhibiting paracellular magnesium reabsorption. Hypomagnesemia is, therefore, a frequent finding in patients receiving chronic loop diuretic therapy.[250] Chronic treatment with thiazide diuretics, which inhibit the NaCl cotransporter (NCC), also causes renal magnesium wasting. Thiazide diuretics or knockout of NCC in mice causes down-regulation of expression of the apical magnesium entry channel in the distal convoluted tubule, TRPM6, which may explain the mechanism of the magnesuria.[251]

Epidermal Growth Factor Receptor Blockers. Hypomagnesemia is common in patients receiving cetuximab[252] and panitumumab,[253] which are monoclonal blocking antibodies of the epidermal growth factor (EGF) receptor that are used in the treatment of metastatic colorectal cancer. The incidence of hypomagnesemia increases with increasing duration of therapy, reaching almost 50% in patients treated for longer than 6 months.[254] The median time to onset of hypomagnesemia after beginning treatment is 99 days, and it generally reverses 1 to 3 months after discontinuing therapy.[255] $F_E Mg$ is inappropriately elevated, suggesting a defect in renal magnesium reabsorption.[256] Studies have suggested that the EGF receptor is located basolaterally in the distal convoluted tubule (DCT).[256] Autocrine or paracrine activation of the receptor stimulates redistribution of TRPM6 to the apical membrane via a Rac1-dependent signaling pathway[257] and presumably increases transepithelial magnesium reabsorption. Thus, EGF receptor blockade likely causes renal magnesium wasting by antagonizing this pathway.

Hypercalcemia. Elevated serum ionized Ca^{2+} levels—for example, in patients with malignant bone metastases—directly induce renal magnesium wasting and hypomagnesemia,[258] probably by stimulating the basolateral CaSR in the thick ascending limb of Henle. In HPT, the situation is more complicated because the hypercalcemia-induced tendency to Mg wasting is counteracted by the action of PTH to stimulate magnesium reabsorption; thus, renal magnesium handling is usually normal and magnesium deficiency is rare.[259]

Tubule Nephrotoxins. Cisplatin, a widely used chemotherapeutic agent for solid tumors, frequently causes renal magnesium wasting. Hypomagnesemia is almost universal at a monthly dose of 50 mg/m^2.[260] The occurrence of Mg wasting does not appear to correlate with the incidence of cisplatin-induced acute renal failure.[261] Renal magnesuria continues after cessation of the drug for a mean of 4 to 5 months, but can persist for years.[261] Although the nephrotoxic effects of cisplatin are manifested histologically as acute tubular necrosis confined to the S3 segment of the proximal tubule, the magnesuria does not correlate temporally with the clinical development of acute renal failure secondary to acute tubular necrosis. Furthermore, patients who become hypomagnesemic are also subject to the development of hypocalciuria, thus suggesting that the reabsorption defect may actually be in the DCT. Mouse studies have also suggested that cisplatin may reduce expression of transport proteins in the DCT.[262] Cisplatin may also impair intestinal magnesium absorption.[263] Carboplatin, an analogue of cisplatin, is considerably less nephrotoxic and only rarely causes acute renal failure or hypomagnesemia.[264]

Amphotericin B is a well-recognized tubule nephrotoxin that can cause renal potassium wasting, distal renal tubular acidosis, and acute renal failure, with tubule necrosis and calcium deposition noted in the DCT and TAL on renal biopsy.[265] Amphotericin B causes renal magnesium wasting and hypomagnesemia related to the cumulative dose administered, but these effects may be observed after as little as a 200-mg total dose.[266] Interestingly, the amphotericin-induced magnesuria is accompanied by the reciprocal development of hypocalciuria so, as with cisplatin, the serum calcium concentration is usually preserved, again suggesting that the functional tubule defect resides in the DCT.

Aminoglycosides cause a syndrome of renal magnesium and potassium wasting with hypomagnesemia, hypokalemia, hypocalcemia, and tetany. Hypomagnesemia may occur despite levels in the appropriate therapeutic range.[267] Most patients reported that they had delayed onset of hypomagnesemia occurring after at least 2 weeks of therapy, and received total doses in excess of 8 g, thus suggesting that it is the cumulative dose of aminoglycoside that is the key predictor of toxicity. In addition, no correlation was found between the occurrence of aminoglycoside-induced acute tubular necrosis and hypomagnesemia. Magnesium wasting persists after cessation of the aminoglycoside, often for several months. All aminoglycosides in clinical use have been implicated, including gentamicin, tobramycin, and amikacin, as well as neomycin when administered topically for extensive burn injuries. This form of symptomatic aminoglycoside-induced renal magnesium wasting is now relatively uncommon because of heightened general awareness of its toxicity. However, asymptomatic hypomagnesemia can be observed in one third of those treated with a single course of an aminoglycoside at standard doses (3 to 5 mg/kg/day, for a mean of 10 days). In these cases, the hypomagnesemia occurs on average 3 to 4 days after the start of therapy and readily reverses after cessation of therapy.[268]

IV pentamidine causes hypomagnesemia as a result of renal magnesium wasting in most patients, typically in association with hypocalcemia.[269] The average onset of symptomatic hypomagnesemia occurs after 9 days of therapy, and the defect persists for at least 1 to 2 months after discontinuation of pentamidine. Hypomagnesemia is also observed in two thirds of AIDS patients with cytomegalovirus retinitis treated intravenously with the pyrophosphate analogue foscarnet.[270] As with aminoglycosides and pentamidine, foscarnet-induced hypomagnesemia is often associated with significant hypocalcemia.

The calcineurin inhibitors cyclosporine and tacrolimus cause renal magnesium wasting and hypomagnesemia in patients after organ transplantation.[271] The mechanism is thought to be downregulation of the distal tubule magnesium channel, TRPM6.[272]

Tubulointerstitial Nephropathies. Renal Mg wasting has occasionally been reported in patients with acute or chronic tubulointerstitial nephritis not caused by nephrotoxic drugs—for example, in chronic pyelonephritis and acute renal allograft rejection. Other manifestations of tubule dysfunction, such as salt wasting, hypokalemia, renal tubular acidosis, and Fanconi's syndrome, may also be present and provide clues to the diagnosis.[247]

Inherited Renal Magnesium-Wasting Disorders

Primary Magnesium-Wasting Disorders. Primary magnesium-wasting disorders are rare. Patients can be broadly classified into distinct clinical syndromes depending on whether the hypomagnesemia is isolated, occurs together with hypocalcemia, or is associated with hypercalciuria and nephrocalcinosis.[273] The pathogenesis and clinical features of these syndromes, which generally present in childhood, are discussed in detail in Chapter 75.

Bartter's and Gitelman's Syndromes. (See also Chapter 44.) Bartter's syndrome is an autosomal recessive disorder characterized by Na wasting, hypokalemic metabolic alkalosis, and hypercalciuria, and it usually occurs in infancy or early childhood.[274] All Bartter's syndrome patients are by definition hypercalciuric and, in addition, one third have hypomagnesemia with inappropriate magnesuria, consistent with loss of the TAL transepithelial potential difference that drives paracellular divalent cation reabsorption. Thus, the physiology of Bartter's syndrome is essentially identical to that of chronic loop diuretic therapy. Gitelman's syndrome is a variant of Bartter's syndrome distinguished primarily by hypocalciuria.[275] Patients with Gitelman's syndrome are identified later in life, usually after the age of 6 years, and have milder symptoms. The genetic defect in these families is caused by inactivating mutations in the DCT electroneutral thiazide-sensitive NCC, and therefore resembles chronic thiazide diuretic therapy. Renal magnesium wasting and hypomagnesemia are universally found in patients with Gitelman's syndrome.

Calcium-Sensing Disorders. In FHH, the hypercalcemia is due to inactivating mutations in CaSR (discussed earlier). As a consequence of the inactivated CaSR, the normal magnesuric response to hypercalcemia is impaired,[276] so these patients are paradoxically mildly hypermagnesemic. Activating mutations in CaSR cause the opposite syndrome, autosomal dominant hypoparathyroidism. As might be expected, most such patients are mildly hypomagnesemic, presumably because of TAL magnesium wasting.[160]

CLINICAL MANIFESTATIONS

Hypomagnesemia may cause symptoms and signs of disordered cardiac, neuromuscular, and central nervous system function. It is also associated with an imbalance of other electrolytes, such as potassium and calcium. Many of the cardiac and neurologic manifestations attributed to magnesium deficiency may be explained by the frequent coexistence of hypokalemia and hypocalcemia in the same patient. Patients with mild hypomagnesemia or who are magnesium-deficient with normal serum magnesium levels may be completely asymptomatic.[277] Thus, the clinical importance of mild-to-moderate magnesium depletion remains controversial, although it has been associated with a number of disorders, such as hypertension and osteoporosis (see below).

Cardiovascular System

Magnesium has protean and complex effects on myocardial ion fluxes. Because magnesium is an obligate cofactor in all reactions that require ATP, it is essential for the activity of Na^+-K^+-ATPase.[278] During magnesium deficiency, Na^+-K^+-ATPase function is impaired. The intracellular potassium concentration falls, which may potentially result in a relatively depolarized resting membrane potential and predispose to ectopic excitation and tachyarrhythmias.[279] Furthermore, the magnitude of the outward potassium gradient is decreased, thereby reducing the driving force for the potassium efflux needed to terminate the cardiac action potential and, as a result, repolarization is delayed. Changes in the ECG may be observed with isolated hypomagnesemia and usually reflect abnormal cardiac repolarization, including bifid T waves and other nonspecific abnormalities in T wave morphology, U waves, prolongation of the QT or QU interval and, rarely, electrical alternation of the T or U wave.[280]

Numerous anecdotal reports have indicated that hypomagnesemia alone can predispose to cardiac tachyarrhythmias, particularly of ventricular origin, including torsades de pointes, monomorphic ventricular tachycardia, and ventricular fibrillation, which may be resistant to standard therapy and respond only to magnesium repletion.[280] Many of the reported patients also had a prolonged QT interval, an abnormality known to predispose to torsades de pointes, and may also increase the period of vulnerability to the R-on-T phenomenon. In the setting of exaggerated cardiac excitability, hypomagnesemia may be the trigger for other types of ventricular tachyarrhythmias.[280] In addition, hypomagnesemia facilitates the development of digoxin cardiotoxicity.[281] Because cardiac glycosides and magnesium depletion inhibit Na^+-K^+-ATPase, their additive effects on intracellular potassium depletion may account for their enhanced toxicity in combination.

It is clear that patients with underlying cardiac disease who have severe hypomagnesemia, particularly in combination with hypokalemia, may develop arrhythmias. The issue of whether mild isolated hypomagnesemia and magnesium depletion in individuals without overt heart disease carries the same risk has been controversial.[282] In one small prospective study, low dietary magnesium appeared to increase the risk for supraventricular and ventricular ectopy, despite the absence of frank hypomagnesemia, hypokalemia, and hypocalcemia.[283] In the Framingham Offspring Study, lower levels of serum magnesium were associated with a higher prevalence of ventricular premature complexes.[284] A low serum magnesium level is also associated with the development of atrial fibrillation.[285] In the Framingham Offspring Study, individuals in the lowest quartile of serum magnesium were, after up to 20 years of follow-up, approximately 50% more likely to develop atrial fibrillation compared with those in the upper quartiles.

Several large population-based studies have shown a strong association between low serum magnesium levels and increased cardiovascular and all-cause mortality.[286-288] Higher magnesium intake is associated with reduced risk of coronary heart disease and cardiac death,[289-292] stroke,[289,293] and coronary calcification.[294]

An inverse relationship between dietary magnesium intake and blood pressure has also been observed.[295-298] Hypomagnesemia and/or reduction of intracellular magnesium have also been inversely correlated with blood pressure. This may be especially important in diabetes mellitus.[299] Patients with essential hypertension were found to have reduced free magnesium concentrations in red blood cells. The magnesium levels were inversely related to systolic and diastolic blood pressures. Intervention studies with magnesium therapy in hypertension have led to conflicting results. Several have shown a positive blood pressure–lowering effect of supplements, but others have not. Other dietary factors may also play a role. In the DASH study, a diet rich in fruits and vegetables, which increased magnesium intake from 176 to 423 mg/day (along with an increase in potassium), significantly lowered blood pressure.[300] The mechanism whereby magnesium deficit may affect blood pressure is not clear, but magnesium does regulate vascular tone and reactivity and attenuates agonist-induced vasoconstriction. Magnesium depletion may involve decreased production of prostacyclin, increased production of thromboxane A_2, and enhanced vasoconstrictive effects of angiotensin II and norepinephrine. Importantly, in none of these studies has magnesium therapy been rigorously studied, whether as a therapy for blood pressure reduction or prophylaxis against cardiovascular disease, arrhythmias, or stroke.

The only setting in which the role of magnesium deficiency and clinical utility of adjunctive magnesium therapy has been studied extensively is in acute myocardial infarction (AMI). Magnesium deficiency may be a risk factor because it has been shown to play a role in systemic and coronary vascular tone, in cardiac dysrhythmias (see earlier), and in the inhibition of steps in the coagulation process and platelet aggregation. Although several small controlled trials have suggested that adjunctive magnesium therapy reduces mortality from AMI by 50%, three major trials have defined our understanding of magnesium therapy in AMI.[301] The LIMIT-2 study was the first study involving large numbers of participants. Magnesium treatment showed an approximately 25% lower mortality rate. In the Fourth International Study of Infarct, unlike LIMIT-2, the mortality rate in the magnesium-treated group was not significantly different from that in the control group. The most recently published Magnesium in Coronaries (MAGIC) trial was designed to address early intervention in higher risk patients.[301] Over a 3-year period, 6213 participants were studied. The magnesium-treated group mortality at 30 days was not significantly different from that of those given placebo. The overall evidence from clinical trials does not support the routine application of adjunctive magnesium therapy in patients with AMI at this time.

Neuromuscular System

Symptoms and signs of neuromuscular irritability, including tremor, muscle twitching, Trousseau's and Chvostek's signs, and frank tetany, may develop in patients with isolated hypomagnesemia[302] and in patients with concomitant hypocalcemia. Hypomagnesemia is also frequently manifested as seizures, which may be generalized and tonic-clonic in nature or multifocal motor seizures, and they are sometimes triggered by loud noises.[302] Interestingly, noise-induced seizures and sudden death are also characteristic of mice made hypomagnesemic by dietary magnesium deprivation. The effects of magnesium deficiency on brain neuronal excitability are thought to be mediated by N-methyl-D-aspartate (NMDA)–type glutamate receptors.[303] Glutamate is the principal excitatory neurotransmitter in the brain; it acts as an agonist at NMDA receptors and opens a cation conductance channel that depolarizes the postsynaptic membrane. Extracellular magnesium normally blocks NMDA receptors, so hypomagnesemia may release the inhibition of glutamate-activated depolarization of the postsynaptic membrane and thereby trigger epileptiform electrical activity.[304] Vertical nystagmus is a rare but diagnostically useful neurologic sign of severe hypomagnesemia.[305] In the absence of a structural lesion of the cerebellar or vestibular pathways, the only recognized metabolic causes are Wernicke's encephalopathy and severe magnesium deficiency.[305]

Skeletal System

Dietary magnesium depletion in animals has been shown to lead to a decrease in skeletal growth and increased skeletal fragility.[306] A decrease in osteoblastic bone formation and an increase in osteoclastic bone resorption are implicated as the cause of decreased bone mass. In humans, epidemiologic studies have suggested a correlation between bone mass and dietary magnesium intake.[307] Few studies have been conducted assessing magnesium status in patients with osteoporosis. Low serum and red blood cell (RBC) magnesium concentrations, as well as high retention of parenterally administered magnesium, have suggested a deficit. Low skeletal magnesium content has been observed in some, but not all, studies. The effect of supplements on bone mass has generally led to an increase in bone mineral density, although study design limits useful information. Larger long-term, placebo-controlled, double-blind investigations are required.

There are several potential mechanisms that may account for a decrease in bone mass in magnesium deficiency. Magnesium is mitogenic for bone cell growth, which may directly result in a decrease in bone formation. It also affects crystal formation; a lack results in a larger, more perfect crystal, which may affect bone strength. Magnesium deficiency may result in a fall in serum PTH and 1,25 $(OH)_2$ vitamin D levels (see earlier). Because both hormones are trophic for bone, impaired secretion or skeletal resistance may result in osteoporosis. A low serum 1,25 (OH)$_2$ vitamin D level may also result in decreased intestinal calcium absorption. An observed increased release of inflammatory cytokines in bone may result in activation of osteoclasts and increased bone resorption in rodent.[306,308]

Electrolyte Homeostasis

Patients with hypomagnesemia are frequently also hypokalemic. Many of the conditions associated with hypomagnesemia that have been outlined earlier can cause simultaneous magnesium and potassium loss. However, hypomagnesemia by itself can induce hypokalemia in humans and experimental animals, and such patients are often refractory to potassium repletion until their magnesium deficit is corrected.[309] The cause of the hypokalemia appears to be increased secretion in the distal nephron.[310] The mechanism has been attributed to cytosolic magnesium depletion, which would release intracellular block of the apical secretory potassium channel, ROMK.[311]

Hypocalcemia is present in approximately 50% of patients with hypomagnesemia.[277] The major cause is impairment of PTH secretion by magnesium deficiency, which is reversed within 24 hours by magnesium repletion.[186] In addition, hypomagnesemic patients also have low circulating 1,25(OH)$_2$D levels and end-organ resistance to PTH and vitamin D.[186]

Other Disorders

Magnesium depletion has also been associated with several other disorders, such as insulin resistance and the metabolic syndrome in type 2 diabetes mellitus.[299,312] Magnesium deficiency has been associated with migraine headache, and magnesium therapy has been reported to be effective in the treatment of migraine.[313] Because magnesium deficiency results in smooth muscle spasm, it has also been implicated in asthma, and magnesium therapy has been effective in asthma in some studies.[314,315] Finally, a high dietary magnesium intake has been associated with a reduced risk of colon cancer.[316,317]

TREATMENT

Magnesium deficiency can sometimes be prevented. Individuals whose dietary intake has been reduced or who are being maintained by parenteral nutrition should receive magnesium supplementation. The recommended daily allowance of magnesium for adults is 420 mg (35 mEq) for men and 320 mg (27 mEq) for women.[318] Thus, in the absence of dietary magnesium intake, an appropriate supplement would therefore be one 140-mg tablet of magnesium oxide four to five times daily or the equivalent dose of an alternative oral magnesium-containing salt. Because the oral bioavailability of magnesium is approximately 33% in patients with normal intestinal function, the equivalent parenteral maintenance requirement of magnesium would be 10 mEq daily.

Once symptomatic magnesium deficiency develops, patients should clearly be repleted with magnesium. However, the importance of treating asymptomatic magnesium deficiency remains controversial. Given the clinical manifestations outlined earlier, it seems prudent to replete all magnesium-deficient patients with a significant underlying cardiac or seizure disorder, patients with concurrent severe hypocalcemia or hypokalemia, and patients with isolated asymptomatic hypomagnesemia, if it is severe (<1.4 mg/dL).

Intravenous Replacement

In the inpatient setting, the IV route of administration of magnesium is favored because it is highly effective, inexpensive, and usually well tolerated. The standard preparation is $MgSO_4 \cdot 7H_2O$. The initial rate of repletion depends on the urgency of the clinical situation. In a patient who is actively seizing or who has a cardiac arrhythmia, 8 to 16 mEq (1 to 2 g) may be administered IV over a 2- to 4-minute period; otherwise, a slower rate of repletion is safer. Because the added extracellular magnesium equilibrates slowly with the intracellular compartment, and because renal excretion of extracellular magnesium exhibits a threshold effect, approximately 50% of parenterally administered magnesium is excreted into urine.[319] A slower rate and prolonged course of repletion would be expected to decrease these urinary losses and therefore be much more efficient and effective at repleting body magnesium stores. The magnitude of the magnesium deficit is difficult to gauge clinically and cannot be readily deduced from the serum magnesium concentration. In general, however, the average deficit can be assumed to be 1 to 2 mEq/kg body weight.[319] A simple regimen for nonemergency magnesium repletion is to administer 64 mEq (8 g) of $MgSO_4$ over the first 24 hours and then 32 mEq (4 g) daily for the next 2 to 6 days. It is important to remember that serum magnesium levels rise early, whereas intracellular stores take longer to replete, so magnesium repletion should continue for at least 1 to 2 days after the serum magnesium level normalizes. In patients with renal magnesium wasting, additional magnesium may be needed to replace ongoing losses. In patients with a reduced GFR, the rate of repletion should be reduced by 25% to 50%,[319] the patient should be carefully monitored for signs of hypermagnesemia, and the serum magnesium level should be checked frequently.

The main adverse effects of magnesium repletion are due to hypermagnesemia as a consequence of an excessive rate or amount of magnesium administered. These effects include facial flushing, loss of deep tendon reflexes, hypotension, and atrioventricular block. Monitoring the tendon reflexes is a useful bedside test to detect magnesium overdose. In addition, IV administration of large amounts of $MgSO_4$ results in an acute decrease in the serum ionized Ca^{2+} level,[320] which is related to increased urinary calcium excretion and complexing of calcium by sulfate. Thus, in an asymptomatic patient who is already hypocalcemic, administration of $MgSO_4$ may further lower the ionized Ca^{2+} level and thereby precipitate tetany.[321]

Oral Replacement

Oral magnesium administration is used initially for repletion of mild cases of hypomagnesemia or for continued replacement of ongoing losses in the outpatient setting after an initial course of IV repletion. A number of oral magnesium salts are available that vary in their content of elemental magnesium and their oral bioavailability, and little is known about their relative efficacy. Importantly, all of them cause diarrhea, which limits the dose that can be used. Magnesium hydroxide and magnesium oxide are alkalinizing salts with the potential to cause systemic alkalosis, whereas the sulfate and gluconate salts, which present nonreabsorbable anions to the collecting duct, may potentially exacerbate renal potassium wasting.

A typical daily dose in a patient with normal renal function and severe hypomagnesemia is 10 to 40 mmol of elemental magnesium in divided doses. Half of this may be sufficient in mild hypomagnesemia, whereas in patients with intestinal magnesium malabsorption, the dose may need to be increased twofold to fourfold. Sustained-release preparations, such as magnesium chloride (Mag-Delay, Slow-Mag) and magnesium L-lactate sustained release (Mag-Tab SR) have the advantage that they are slowly absorbed and thereby minimize renal excretion of the administered magnesium. By allowing the use of lower doses, these preparations minimize diarrhea.

Potassium-Sparing Diuretics

In patients with inappropriate renal magnesium wasting, potassium-sparing diuretics that block the distal tubule epithelial sodium channel, such as amiloride and triamterene, may reduce renal magnesium losses.[322] These drugs may be particularly useful in patients who are refractory to oral repletion or require such high doses of oral magnesium that diarrhea develops. In rats, amiloride and triamterene have been demonstrated to reduce renal magnesium clearance at baseline and after induction of magnesium diuresis by furosemide, but the mechanism is unknown. One possibility is that these drugs, by reducing luminal sodium uptake and inhibiting the development of a negative luminal transepithelial potential difference, may favor passive reabsorption of magnesium in the late distal tubule or collecting duct.[323]

HYPERMAGNESEMIA

CAUSES

In states of body magnesium excess, the kidney has a very large capacity for magnesium excretion. Once the apparent renal threshold is exceeded, most of the excess filtered magnesium is excreted unchanged into the final urine; the serum magnesium concentration is then determined by the GFR. Thus, hypermagnesemia generally occurs only in two clinical settings, compromised renal function and excessive magnesium intake.

Renal Insufficiency

In chronic renal failure, the remaining nephrons adapt to the decreased filtered load of magnesium by markedly increasing their fractional excretion of magnesium.[324] As a consequence, serum magnesium levels are usually well maintained until the creatinine clearance falls below about 20 mL/min.[324] Even in advanced renal insufficiency, significant hypermagnesemia is rare unless the patient has received exogenous magnesium in the form of antacids, cathartics, or enemas. Increasing age is an important risk factor for hypermagnesemia in individuals with apparently normal renal function; it presumably reflects the decline in GFR that normally accompanies old age.[325]

Excessive Magnesium Intake

Hypermagnesemia can occur in individuals with a normal GFR when the rate of magnesium intake exceeds the renal excretory capacity. It has been reported with excessive oral ingestion of magnesium-containing antacids[326] and cathartics,[327] with the use of rectal magnesium sulfate enemas,[328] and is common with large parenteral doses of magnesium, such as those given for preeclampsia. Toxicity from enterally administered magnesium salts is particularly common in patients with inflammatory disease, obstruction,[326] or perforation of the gastrointestinal tract, presumably because magnesium absorption is enhanced.

Miscellaneous

Modest elevations in serum magnesium levels have occasionally been described in patients receiving lithium therapy, as well as in postoperative patients and in those with bone metastases, milk-alkali syndrome, FHH,[276] hypothyroidism, pituitary dwarfism, and Addison's disease. In most cases, the mechanism is unknown.

CLINICAL MANIFESTATIONS

Magnesium toxicity is a serious and potentially fatal condition. Progressive hypermagnesemia is usually associated with a predictable sequence of symptoms and signs.[329] Initial manifestations, observed once the serum magnesium level exceeds 4 to 6 mg/dL, are hypotension, nausea, vomiting, facial flushing, urinary retention, and ileus. If untreated, it may progress to flaccid skeletal muscular paralysis and hyporeflexia, bradycardia and bradyarrhythmias, respiratory depression, coma, and cardiac arrest. An abnormally low (or even negative) serum anion gap may be a clue to hypermagnesemia,[325] but it is not consistently observed and probably depends on the nature of the anion that accompanies the excess body magnesium.

Cardiovascular System

Hypotension is one of the earliest manifestations of hypermagnesemia,[330] is often accompanied by cutaneous flushing, and is thought to be due to vasodilation of vascular smooth muscle and inhibition of norepinephrine release by sympathetic postganglionic nerves. Electrocardiographic changes are common but nonspecific.[330] Sinus or junctional bradycardia may develop, as well as varying degrees of sinoatrial, atrioventricular, and His bundle conduction block. Cardiac arrest as a result of asystole is often the terminal event.

Nervous System

High levels of extracellular magnesium inhibit acetylcholine release from the neuromuscular end plate,[331] leading to the development of flaccid skeletal muscle paralysis and hyporeflexia when the serum magnesium level exceeds 8 to 12 mg/dL. Respiratory depression is a serious complication of advanced magnesium toxicity.[330] Smooth muscle paralysis also occurs and is manifested as urinary retention, intestinal ileus, and pupillary dilation. Signs of central nervous system depression, including lethargy, drowsiness, and eventually coma, are well described in severe hypermagnesemia, but may also be entirely absent.

Treatment

Mild cases of magnesium toxicity in individuals with good renal function may require no treatment other than cessation of magnesium supplements because renal magnesium clearance is usually quite rapid. The normal half-life of serum magnesium is approximately 28 hours. In the event of serious toxicity, particularly cardiac toxicity, temporary antagonism of the effect of magnesium may be achieved by the administration of IV calcium (1 g of calcium chloride infused into a central vein over a period of 2 to 5 minutes, or calcium gluconate infused through a peripheral vein, repeated after 5 minutes if necessary).[329] Renal excretion of magnesium can be enhanced by saline diuresis and by the administration of furosemide, which inhibits tubular reabsorption of magnesium in the medullary TAL.

In patients with renal failure, the only way to clear the excess magnesium may be by dialysis or hemofiltration. The typical dialysate for hemodialysis contains 0.6 to 1.2 mg/dL of magnesium, but magnesium-free dialysate can also be used and is generally well tolerated, except for muscle cramps.[332] Hemodialysis is extremely effective at removing excess magnesium and can achieve clearances of up to 100 mL/min.[332] As a rough rule of thumb, the expected change in the serum magnesium level after a 3- to 4-hour dialysis session with a high-efficiency membrane is approximately one third to one half the difference between the dialysate Mg^{2+} concentration and predialysis serum ultrafilterable magnesium (estimated at 70% of total serum magnesium).[332] Note that when hemodialysis is performed using a bath with the same total concentration of magnesium as in serum, the net transfer of magnesium into the patient occurs because the ultrafilterable (and therefore free) magnesium concentration in serum is less than the total concentration; thus, the gradient of free Mg^{2+} is directed from the dialysate to blood.

DISORDERS OF PHOSPHATE HOMEOSTASIS

Body phosphate metabolism is regulated through plasma inorganic phosphorus (Pi) concentration. Of the total body phosphorus content (500 to 800 g), 85% is in the skeleton, 14% in soft tissues, and the rest is distributed between other tissues and ECF. Of the Pi contained in bone, roughly 200 mg is recycled daily.[1] Two thirds of the phosphorus in blood exists as organic phosphates (mainly phospholipids) and one third as Pi. Inorganic phosphorus in blood, for practical purposes, involves two orthophosphates, $H_2PO_4^-$ and HPO_4^{2-}. At a plasma pH of 7.4, there are four divalent HPO_4^{2-} ions for every one monovalent $H_2PO_4^-$ ion, so the composite valence is 1.8 (i.e., 1 mmol Pi = 1.8 mEq). Thus, Pi in plasma circulates as phosphates, but is measured in the laboratory as phosphorus (normal values, 2.5 to 4.5 mg/dL). There are great variations in the normal range of plasma Pi levels with age, from up to 7.4 mg/dL in infants and up to 5.8 mg/dL in children between 1 and 2 years of age.[4,333] Even in adults, there is a gradual decline in plasma Pi with age, although postmenopausal women, in general, tend to have slightly higher plasma Pi levels compared to their male counterparts.[334] Between 85% and 90% of plasma phosphorus is filterable by the kidneys (50% as ionized Pi and 40% complexed with cations), and the remainder is bound to plasma proteins.

The average daily phosphorus intake varies from 800 to 1500 mg, mostly as Pi. Approximately 60% of this is absorbed by the intestine through active transport and paracellular diffusion. The active transport of intestinal phosphate is primarily through type IIb sodium-phosphate cotransporters (NaPi-IIb) and, to a lesser extent, type III transporters (Pit1 and Pit2).[335] Systemic $1,25(OH)_2D$ levels and dietary phosphorus are important physiologic regulators of intestinal phosphate absorption, with high $1,25(OH)_2D$ and low dietary phosphate levels promoting the intestinal uptake of phosphate. However, the discovery of several novel phosphatonins, combined with other studies suggesting the existence of a poorly defined intestine-kidney signalling axis,[336] implies that this process may be more complex than originally appreciated. In addition to its absorption from the small intestine, approximately 150 to 200 mg of phosphorus is secreted daily by the colon.[1]

As discussed in detail in Chapter 7, the kidney is the major organ regulating phosphate homeostasis. The net renal excretion of Pi under steady-state conditions is the same as Pi absorbed by the gastrointestinal tract. Up to 80% of renal reabsorption of phosphate occurs in the proximal tubule by means of the NaPi cotransporter family of proteins, type IIa (NaPi-IIa) and type IIc (NaPi-IIc) in the luminal brush border membrane.[337] The rest of the urinary phosphate is reabsorbed in the distal tubules or excreted in the urine. PTH increases Pi excretion by decreasing the abundance of NaPi-IIa and NaPi-IIc in the brush border membrane. FGF-23 possesses similar actions to those of PTH to limit phosphate reabsorption in the proximal tubule; however, unlike PTH, FGF-23 blocks renal $1,25(OH)_2D$ production by suppressing 1α-hydroxylase activity and stimulating 24-hydroxylation. A low serum phosphate level stimulates renal NaPi cotransporters and hence phosphate reabsorption.[337] Urinary phosphate excretion can be quantified directly from a 24-hour urine collection or can be estimated by calculating the fractional excretion of filtered phosphate (FE_{Pi}) or the renal tubular maximum reabsorption of phosphate (TmP) to GFR ratio[338] (in mg/dL):

$$TmP/GFR_{Cr} = \text{serum Pi} - (\text{urine Pi} \times [\text{serum Cr}/\text{urine Cr}])$$

The latter method is preferred because the TmP/GFR ratio is independent of kidney function. The normal range for TmP/GFR is 2.6 to 4.4 mg/dL[339]; lower values indicate a decreased maximum renal phosphate reabsorption threshold and hence excessive urinary phosphate loss. Of note, similar to plasma phosphate levels, TmP/GFR appears to steadily decline with age but, again, slightly increases in women around the time of menopause.[334]

HYPERPHOSPHATEMIA

Hyperphosphatemia is generally defined as a serum phosphate level elevated above 5 mg/dL. For children, the upper range of normal is 6 mg/dL. In infants, phosphorus levels as high as 7.4 mg/dL are considered normal.[333] The serum phosphorus level usually exhibits diurnal variation, with the lowest levels typically being observed in the later morning and peak levels occurring in the first morning hours.[340]

The clinical causes of hyperphosphatemia[341] can be broadly classified into one of four groups—reduced renal excretion of phosphate, exogenous phosphate load, acute

Table 19.7 Causes of Hyperphosphatemia
Decreased Renal Excretion of Phosphorus
CKD stages 3 to 5
Acute kidney injury
Hypoparathyroidism, pseudohypoparathyroidism
Acromegaly
Tumoral calcinosis
FGF-23 inactivating gene mutation
GALNT3 mutation with aberrant FGF-23 glycosylation
KLOTHO inactivating mutation with FGF-23 resistance
Bisphosphonates
Exogenous Phosphorus Administration
Ingestion of phosphate, phosphate-containing enemas
Intravenous phosphate delivery
Redistribution of Phosphorus (Intracellular to Extracellular Shift)
Respiratory acidosis, metabolic acidosis
Tumor lysis syndrome
Rhabdomyolysis
Hemolytic anemia
Catabolic state
Pseudohyperphosphatemia
Hyperglobulinemia
Hyperlipidemia
Hyperbilirubinemia
Medications:
Liposomal amphotericin B
Rec tissue plasm activator
Heparin
Hemolysis of blood specimen

extracellular shift of phosphorus, or pseudohyperphosphatemia (Table 19.7).

CAUSES

Decreased Renal Phosphate Excretion

Reduced Glomerular Filtration Rate. Both acute kidney injury (AKI) and CKD can lead to hyperphosphatemia. In the early stages of kidney injury, elevations in PTH and FGF-23 levels increase the urinary fractional excretion of phosphate to compensate for the declining GFR, thus maintaining plasma Pi levels in the normal range. With further decrements in GFR (as in severe AKI or CKD, stage 4 or 5), the reduced functional nephron mass is insufficient to maintain maximal Pi excretion, resulting in hyperphosphatemia. A detailed discussion of hyperphosphatemia caused by decreased renal function is not provided here; this topic is extensively reviewed in Chapter 55 in the context of chronic kidney disease-mineral bone disorder.

Hypoparathyroidism and Pseudohypoparathyroidism. Deficient secretion of PTH (hypoparathyroidism) or renal resistance to PTH (pseudohypoparathyroidism) decrease the renal excretion of phosphate, leading to hyperphosphatemia. In these entities, circulating phosphorus generally reaches a higher than normal steady-state level (6 to 7 mg/dL) and is accompanied by hypocalcemia due to decreased bone resorption and urine calcium losses. Hypoparathyroidism and pseudohypoparathyroidism have been discussed extensively (see earlier).

Acromegaly. Some patients with acromegaly demonstrate hyperphosphatemia. Parathyroid function is usually normal or slightly increased in acromegaly.[91] The hyperphosphatemia observed appears to result from increased proximal tubule phosphate reabsorption. Growth hormone and insulin-like growth factor-1 directly stimulate proximal tubule phosphorus reabsorption and increase the TmP/GFR.[342]

Familial Tumoral Calcinosis. Familial tumoral calcinosis (FTC; OMIM #211900) is a rare autosomal recessive disorder characterized by hyperphosphatemia and the progressive deposition of calcium phosphate crystals in periarticular and soft tissues. The hyperphosphatemia in this disease results from increased proximal tubular reabsorption of phosphate, usually due to loss-of-function mutations in the UDP-N-acetyl-α-D-galactosamine gene *(GALNT3)*,[343] which encodes a glycosyltransferase that is thought to prevent the degradation of intact FGF-23.[344,345] Additional gene mutations have been linked to tumoral calcinosis, including deactivating mutations in the FGF-23 gene[346,347] and in the *KLOTHO* gene, which encodes a co-factor necessary for FGF-23 binding to its receptor.[348] FTC has been described mainly in families of African and Mediterranean descent.

The unifying pathogenic mechanism in FTC is abrogation of the phosphaturic effect of FGF-23. As such, missense mutations in FGF-23 inhibit its secretion, mutations in *GALNT3* cause aberrant glycosylation and premature degradation of FGF-23,[344] and mutations in *KLOTHO* lead to end-organ resistance to FGF-23. Similar to humans, mice lacking FGF-23 or *KLOTHO* expression exhibit severe hyperphosphatemia associated with extensive soft tissue calcification.[349] Thus, FTC may be the phenotypic opposite of X-linked and autosomal dominant hypophosphatemic rickets (see later discussion).

PTH, alkaline phosphatase, and calcium levels in FTC are commonly within the normal range. On the other hand, serum $1,25(OH)_2D$ levels are often increased.[350] Together, a normal serum calcium concentration and increased serum phosphorus level lead to an elevated calcium-phosphate product and the slow tissue deposition of calcium phosphate crystals. Decreasing the intestinal absorption of phosphate, either by decreasing dietary phosphorus intake or adding phosphate binders such as sevelamer, is standard therapy for FTC. Additional studies have indicated that the chronic use of acetazolamide may increase urinary phosphate wasting and reduce calcium-phosphate deposits in these patients.[351]

Bisphosphonates. Bisphosphonates generally cause mild hyperphosphatemia by altering systemic phosphate distribution and decreasing urinary phosphate excretion.[352,353] The levels of PTH and response with urinary excretion of cAMP to exogenous PTH are normal in patients receiving bisphosphonates.

Exogenous Phosphate Load

Severe hyperphosphatemia has been recognized for at least a half-century as a complication of sodium phosphate taken orally as a cathartic agent or a sodium phosphate monobasic/dibasic rectal enema (Fleet enema).[341] Acute renal failure, hypocalcemia, severe electrolyte disturbances, and death have been described in response to high-dose sodium phosphate administration. Despite these reports, sodium phosphate preparations remain widely used for bowel preparation prior to colonoscopy. Although the risk for hyperphosphatemia is most pronounced in patients with underlying CKD, even healthy individuals can experience a substantial rise in serum Pi levels (up to 9.6 mg/dL in one prospective study) following sodium phosphate therapy.[354] Over the last 10 years, numerous case reports and case series have described an association between use of oral sodium phosphate for bowel cleansing and phosphate nephropathy. The typical presentation of phosphate nephropathy involves an acute deterioration in kidney function days to weeks following a colonoscopy. Kidney biopsy shows acute and chronic tubular injury, with calcium phosphate deposits (tubular calcifications).[355,356] Most patients will not recover kidney function fully, and some progress to end-stage disease. Overall, such adverse renal effects are uncommon in patients treated with sodium phosphate, but for those select few who are affected, consequences may be serious. The risk factors for developing phosphate nephropathy are advanced age, female gender, impaired kidney function, volume contraction, ulceration of bowel mucosa, bowel obstruction or ileus, hypertension, and use of angiotensin-converting enzyme inhibitors (ACEIs), angiotensin receptor blockers (ARBs), and nonsteroidal antiinflammatory drugs (NSAIDs).[355,357] Alternative methods of bowel preparation should be considered for patients with these risk factors.

Less commonly, hyperphosphatemia can be observed in the ICU setting when an excessive amount of IV phosphate is given for hyperalimentation, particularly in patients with renal failure. Similarly, the administration of high-dose fosphenytoin for seizure treatment in the setting of kidney dysfunction has been associated with hyperphosphatemia because phosphate is one of the major metabolites of this drug.[358] Finally, vitamin D intoxication can result in hyperphosphatemia, largely because of the simultaneous suppression of PTH production and stimulation of intestinal absorption of phosphate.

Intracellular to Extracellular Shift of Phosphorus

Respiratory Acidosis and Metabolic Acidosis. Respiratory acidosis can lead to hyperphosphatemia, renal resistance to the effect of PTH, and hypocalcemia.[359] The effect is more pronounced in acute respiratory acidosis than in the chronic form. Respiratory acidosis does not appear to significantly alter the renal handling of phosphorus. Rather, efflux of phosphate from cells into the extracellular space is probably responsible for the hyperphosphatemia of respiratory acidosis.[360]

Lactic acidosis and, to lesser extent, diabetic ketoacidosis also cause hyperphosphatemia.[361,362] Metabolic acidosis in general reduces glycolysis and Pi utilization. In lactic acidosis, this effect is intensified by tissue hypoxia and intracellular Pi release. Patients with uncontrolled diabetes mellitus are intracellularly phosphate-depleted, despite hyperphosphatemia, an abnormality that becomes unmasked once insulin therapy is initiated.

Tumor Lysis and Rhabdomyolysis. Because phosphate is predominantly stored intracellularly, clinical conditions associated with increased catabolism and tissue destruction, such as rhabdomyolysis, fulminant hepatitis, hemolytic anemia, severe hyperthermia, and tumor lysis syndrome, often result in hyperphosphatemia. The severity of the hyperphosphatemia may be exacerbated by the development of AKI.

Tumor lysis syndrome is a constellation of metabolic abnormalities such as hyperuricemia, hyperkalemia, and hyperphosphatemia that is caused by rapid and massive breakdown of tumor cells.[363,364] Clinical consequences may include AKI, pulmonary edema, cardiac arrhythmia, and seizures. The syndrome typically occurs from 3 days before to 7 days after the initiation of chemotherapy. Hyperphosphatemia is an extremely common clinical finding following treatment for Burkitt's lymphoma, especially in patients with preexisting kidney disease; it is also seen in other forms of lymphoma, lymphoblastic and myelogenous leukemias, and in patients with solid cancers characterized by a high tumor burden. Malignant lymphoid cells may contain up to four times more intracellular phosphorus compared to mature lymphoid cells, which explains the high prevalence of hyperphosphatemia following chemotherapy in patients with lymphoid malignancies. The lactate dehydrogenase level before the initiation of therapy appears to correlate with the development of hyperphosphatemia and azotemia in these patients.[365] Phosphate nephropathy with tubular calcifications has been reported in tumor lysis syndrome cases exhibiting extremely high serum Pi levels.[363]

To prevent tumor lysis syndrome, intensive volume expansion is generally recommended before chemotherapy to induce a high urine output (120 to 150 mL/hour) and phosphate and uric acid excretion.[366] The usefulness of urine alkalinization (pH > 7.0) with bicarbonate infusion and/or acetazolamide is unclear, and its practice is controversial. Alkalinization may increase uric acid solubility in the tubules but requires caution; nephrocalcinosis can occur with aggressive alkalinization of the urine because calcium phosphate crystals usually precipitate in alkaline urine. Phosphate binders can be used to decrease the intestinal absorption of phosphate in patients who maintain their oral intake during chemotherapy, but the utility of these drugs is limited in this setting. In severe cases of tumor lysis syndrome, hemodialysis may be necessary to control severe hyperphosphatemia and associated metabolic derangements, with CRRT being most efficacious for maintaining phosphate homeostasis.

Pseudohyperphosphatemia

Spurious measurements of high plasma phosphorus levels may occur under certain conditions as a result of interference with the analytic method used. This problem is most common in the case of paraproteinemia (as occurs in multiple myeloma or Waldenström's macroglobulinemia).[367] This phenomenon can also be observed in patients being treated with liposomal amphotericin B,[368] recombinant tissue plasminogen activator,[369] or heparin therapy.[370] Spurious phosphate readings can also occur in hemolyzed specimens or in samples from patients with severe hyperlipidemia or hyperbilirubinemia.

CLINICAL MANIFESTATIONS AND TREATMENT

Most of the acute clinical manifestations of hyperphosphatemia stem from hypocalcemia, discussed earlier in this chapter. Chronic hyperphosphatemia of CKD and its metabolic consequences are discussed in Chapter 55. Little is known about the effects of chronic hyperphosphatemia in the absence of CKD because this is very rarely observed.

Treatment of chronic hyperphosphatemia is generally accomplished through dietary phosphate restriction, oral phosphate binders, and renal replacement therapy. Acute hyperphosphatemia in association with hypocalcemia requires rapid attention. Discontinuation of supplemental phosphates and initiation of hydration are indicated for patients with acute exogenous Pi overload and intact renal function. Volume expansion can significantly increase urinary phosphate excretion, but plasma calcium levels must be followed closely because further hypocalcemia may occur due to hemodilution. Acetazolamide administration may also increase urinary phosphate excretion.[371-373] Severe hyperphosphatemia in patients with reduced renal function or AKI, particularly in those with tumor lysis syndrome, may require renal replacement therapy. In patients with respiratory or metabolic acidosis, treatment of the underlying acidosis corrects the phosphate derangement. Similarly, in diabetic ketoacidosis, treatment with insulin and correction of metabolic acidosis rapidly reverses the hyperphosphatemia.

HYPOPHOSPHATEMIA

Hypophosphatemia is a decrease in the concentration of Pi in plasma, and phosphate depletion is a decrease in the total body content of phosphorus. Hypophosphatemia can occur in the presence of a low, normal, or high total body phosphorus content. Similarly, total body phosphate depletion may exist with low, normal, or high plasma Pi levels. The incidence of hypophosphatemia is from 0.2% to 2.2% in hospitalized population but may be present in up to 30% of chronic alcoholics, 28% to 34% of ICU patients, and 65% to 80% of patients with sepsis.[374,375] There is an association between hypophosphatemia and in-hospital mortality among hospitalized patients[376] and all-cause mortality in the dialysis population.[377] It is unclear if hypophosphatemia is a direct contributor to these outcomes.

CLINICAL MANIFESTATIONS

Moderate hypophosphatemia (plasma Pi from 1.0 to 2.5 mg/dL) usually occurs without significant phosphate depletion and without specific signs or symptoms. In severe hypophosphatemia (plasma Pi below 1.0 mg/dL), phosphate depletion is typically present and can have significant clinical consequences.

The clinical manifestations of hypophosphatemia and phosphate depletion generally result from a decrease in intracellular ATP levels. In addition, erythrocytes experience a decrease in 2,3-diphosphoglycerate levels, which increases hemoglobin-oxygen affinity and prevents efficient oxygen delivery to tissues.[378] Hypophosphatemia causes a rise in intracellular cytosolic calcium in cells such as leukocytes, pancreatic islets, and synaptosomes isolated from phosphate-depleted animals. These elevated cytosolic calcium levels were associated with decreased ATP levels and impaired cell response to stimuli.[379]

Hematologic consequences include a predisposition to hemolysis, thought to result from increased red cell rigidity.[380,381] Spontaneous hemolysis is rarely observed with hypophosphatemia alone, but hypophosphatemia can predispose to red cell lysis in the presence of other risk factors. Phagocytosis and chemotaxis of polymorphonuclear cells are diminished because impaired ATP production decreases the phagocytic capability of these cells.[382]

Severe hypophosphatemia can result in numerous neuromuscular and skeletal abnormalities, including proximal myopathy, bone pain,[374,383] and rhabdomyolysis.[384] Because cell breakdown may lead to the release of intracellular phosphate, normophosphatemia or hyperphosphatemia in this setting may mask the existence of true phosphate depletion. Overt heart failure and respiratory failure as a result of decreased muscle performance may also be observed.[385,386] Correction of the Pi level leads to improvement of myocardial and pulmonary function.[387,388] Neurologic manifestations of severe hypophosphatemia include paresthesias, tremor, and encephalopathy; these also improve with phosphate replacement.[374] Chronic phosphate depletion alters bone metabolism, leading to increased bone resorption and severe mineralization defects that impair bone structure and strength (e.g., osteomalacia, rickets).

Chronic hypophosphatemia can also lead to proximal and distal renal tubule defects resulting in water diuresis, glucosuria, bicarbonaturia, hypercalciuria, and hypermagnesuria.[389] The hypercalciuria is not solely the result of altered renal calcium handling but also reflects increased calcium release from bone, consequent to phosphate mobilization, and increased intestinal calcium absorption in response to the accompanying elevation in plasma $1,25(OH)_2D$ levels.[390] Metabolic consequences of hypophosphatemia include insulin resistance, diminished gluconeogenesis, hypoparathyroidism, and metabolic acidosis with reduced H^+ excretion and ammonia generation. Hypophosphatemia is also a potent stimulator of 1α-hydroxylation to convert $25(OH)D$ to $1,25(OH)_2D$.

DIAGNOSIS

The cause of hypophosphatemia can often be delineated from the clinical history or physical examination alone. Shifts of phosphorus from the extracellular to intracellular space usually occur in the setting of an acute illness or treatment (e.g., respiratory alkalosis, treatment of diabetic ketoacidosis); thus, hypophosphatemia in hospitalized patients typically results from shifts of phosphorus into the intracellular compartment as opposed to renal losses of phosphorus.[391]

In situations in which the underlying diagnosis is not immediately apparent, it can be clinically useful to determine the rate of urine phosphate excretion by quantification in a 24-hour urine collection or by calculation of the FE_{Pi} or TmP/GFR. A 24-hour urine phosphate greater than 100 mg, FE_{Pi} greater than 5%, or TmP/GFR less than 2.5 mg/100 mL indicates inappropriate urinary phosphate wasting.[339] A high urine phosphate level in the presence of hypophosphatemia results from an acquired defect (e.g., primary HPT) or genetic defect (e.g., X-linked hypophosphatemic rickets) in phosphate reabsorption by the proximal tubule.

CAUSES

Hypophosphatemia may be due to increased renal phosphate excretion, decreased intestinal absorption, shift of

Table 19.8 Causes of Hypophosphatemia

Increased Urinary Phosphate Excretion

Increased production or activity of FGF-23
  Inherited disorders
    X-linked hypophosphatemia (*PHEX* mutations)
    Autosomal dominant hypophosphatemic rickets (*FGF-23* mutations)
    Autosomal recessive hypophosphatemic rickets (*DMP1* and *ENPP1* mutations)
  Acquired disorder
    Tumor-induced osteomalacia
Disorders of proximal tubule Pi reabsorption
  Hereditary hypophosphatemic rickets with hypercalciuria (*SLC34A3* mutations)
  Autosomal recessive renal phosphate wasting (*SLC34A1* mutations)
  NHERF1 mutations
  KLOTHO mutations
  Fanconi's syndrome
  Primary and secondary hyperparathyroidism
  Post–renal transplantation
  Medications—acetazolamide, calcitonin, glucocorticoids, diuretics, bicarbonate, acetaminophen, iron (IV), antineoplastics, antiretrovirals, aminoglycosides, anticonvulsants
  Acute tubular necrosis recovery, post–urinary obstruction
  Miscellaneous—post-hepatectomy, colorectal surgery, volume expansion, osmotic diuresis

Decreased Intestinal Absorption of Phosphate

Malnutrition with low phosphate intake, anorexia, starvation
Malabsorption of phosphate—chronic diarrhea, gastrointestinal tract diseases
Intake of phosphate-binding agents
Vitamin D deficiency or vitamin D resistance
  Nutritional deficiency—low dietary intake, low sun exposure
  Malabsorption
  Chronic kidney disease
  Chronic liver disease
  Vitamin D synthesis and vitamin D receptor defects

Altered Phosphorus Distribution, Intracellular Shift

Acute respiratory alkalosis
Refeeding of malnourished patients, alcoholics
Hungry bone syndrome (postparathyroidectomy)

Hypophosphatemia Resulting from Multiple Mechanisms

Alcoholism
Diabetic ketoacidosis, insulin therapy
Miscellaneous
  Tumor consumption of phosphate—leukemia blast crisis, lymphoma
  Sepsis
  Heat stroke and hyperthermia

---

phosphate from extracellular to intracellular fluid, or a combination of these mechanisms (Table 19.8).

Increased Renal Phosphate Excretion

Hypophosphatemia caused by increased urinary phosphate excretion is generally the result of excess PTH, increased production or activity of FGF-23 from normal or dysplastic bone, or a disorder of renal phosphate handling in the proximal tubule. The recent discovery of several inherited disorders of renal wasting has contributed to the elucidation of the underlying mechanisms (Figure 19.5).

Hyperparathyroidism. Both primary and secondary HPT may lead to hyperphosphaturia and hypophosphatemia. Primary HPT is discussed earlier in this chapter. The degree of hypophosphatemia observed is usually mild to moderate in severity; increased urinary phosphate excretion is balanced by mobilization of Pi from the bone and enhanced intestinal absorption of Pi. Secondary HPT resulting from vitamin D deficiency causes hypophosphatemia, not only through the promotion of urinary phosphate wasting by PTH, but also through decreased intestinal absorption of phosphate from low vitamin D levels. The secondary HPT observed in patients with CKD is typically associated with hyperphosphatemia because of a decreased ability of the kidney to excrete phosphorus.

Increased Production or Activity of Phosphatonins. There are several rare syndromes of renal phosphate wasting associated with rickets or osteomalacia that result from increased production or activity of FGF-23 or other phosphatonins (see Figure 19.4).[392]

X-Linked Hypophosphatemia. X-linked hypophosphatemia (XLH; OMIM #307800) is a rare X-linked dominant disorder characterized by hypophosphatemia, rickets and osteomalacia, growth retardation, decreased intestinal calcium and phosphate absorption, and decreased renal phosphate reabsorption. Serum 1,25(OH)D levels are inappropriately normal or low, and calcium and PTH levels are normal in patients with XLH. The prevalence of the disease is 1:20,000, penetrance is high, and both females and males are affected.[393]

The gene responsible for this disorder, a phosphate-regulating gene with homology to endopeptidases on the X chromosome (*PHEX*), was identified by positional cloning.[394] Binding of *PHEX* to another bone-derived protein, dentin matrix protein 1 (DMP1), appears critical for the suppression of osteocyte production of FGF-23 in bone.[395] Inactivating mutations in—*PHEX* or DMP1 result in higher circulating levels of FGF-23 and resultant phosphate wasting.[394,396,397] Abnormal synthesis of $1,25(OH)_2D$ in XLH can be explained by increased levels of FGF-23, which suppress renal 1α-hydroxylase activity.[398]

Treatment of XLH patients with oral phosphate and calcitriol improves their growth rate; however, these therapies do not reduce renal phosphate excretion. As a result, the major goal of therapy in these patients has been to allow normal growth and reduce bone pain.[399] More recently, an FGF23-neutralizing antibody has been developed as a potential treatment for XLH patients and initial evidence from a phase I study suggests this therapy can effectively reduce renal phosphate excretion.[399a] Thus, FGF23-neutralizing antibodies hold considerable promise as a future treatment for XLH patients.

Autosomal Dominant Hypophosphatemic Rickets. Autosomal dominant hypophosphatemic rickets (ADHR, OMIM #193100) is an extremely rare disorder of phosphate wasting, with a clinical phenotype similar to that of XLH. Some individuals initially present in childhood with

Inherited Disorders of Urinary Phosphate Wasting

Primary defect in endocrine regulation of phosphate homeostasis

Resistance of intact FGF23 to cleavage
- Primary FGF23 protein mutation (ADHR)

Mutation in regulators of FGF23 cleavage
- PHEX inactivation (XLH)
- DMP1 inactivation ⎫
- ENPP1 inactivation ⎬ (ARHR)

Primary defect in renal phosphate transport

Primary defect in phosphate transporter
- Na/Pi-IIa mutation (SLC34A1 gene)
- Na/Pi-IIc mutation (SLC34A3 gene)

Mutation in regulator of phosphate transporters
- NHERF1 inactivation
- KLOTHO overexpression (?)

↓

Elevated plasma FGF23 levels → Decreased proximal tubule expression of Na/Pi cotransporters

↓ ↓

Decreased 1,25(OH)$_2$D production | Increased urinary phosphate excretion

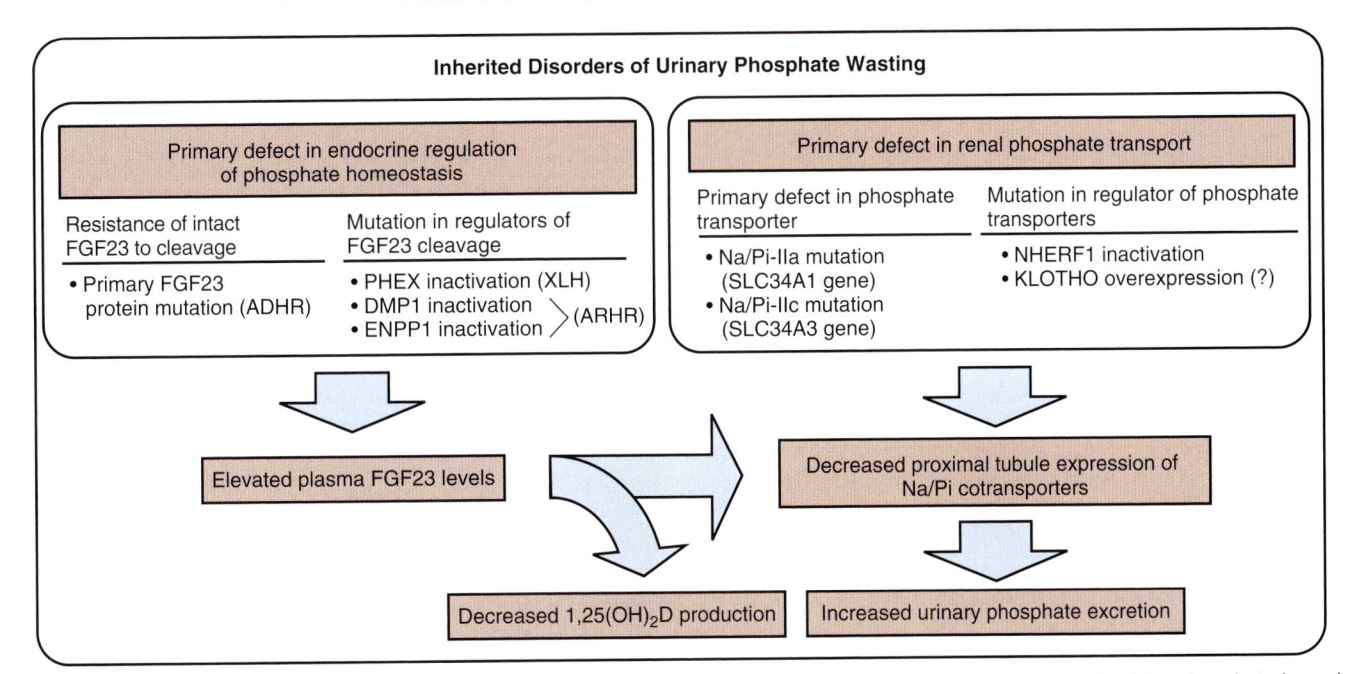

Figure 19.5 Summary of the inherited disorders of urinary phosphate wasting. Inherited diseases characterized by phosphaturia and hypophosphatemia can occur from a defect in endocrine pathways involved in the systemic regulation of phosphate homeostasis or from a direct mutation in local regulators of renal phosphate transport. ADHR, Autosomal dominant hypophosphatemic rickets; ARHR, autosomal recessive hypophosphatemic rickets; DMP1, dentin matrix protein 1; ENPP1, ectonucleotide pyrophosphatase/phosphodiesterase 1; FGF23, fibroblast growth factor 23; Na/Pi-IIa, type IIa sodium-phosphate cotransporter; Na/Pi-IIc, type IIc sodium-phosphate cotransporter; NHERF1, sodium-hydrogen exchanger regulatory factor; 1 PHEX, phosphate-regulating gene with homology to endopeptidases on the X chromosome; XLH, X-linked hypophosphatemic rickets.

hypophosphatemia associated with lower extremity deformities, whereas others present in adolescence or adulthood with bone pain, weakness, and phosphate wasting. In some individuals with early-onset disease, the phosphate wasting returns to normal after puberty.

The ADHR locus was mapped to chromosome 12p13.3 and identified as FGF-23.[400] Missense mutations of FGF-23 appear to interfere with its proteolytic cleavage by furin or other subtilisin-like proprotein convertases,[401-403] causing prolonged or enhanced FGF-23 action on the kidney. Treatment is with phosphate replacement and calcitriol, similar to that for patients with XLH.

Autosomal Recessive Hypophosphatemic Rickets. Reports describing families with autosomal recessive forms of hypophosphatemic rickets have also emerged. As mentioned previously, inactivating mutations in the gene encoding DMP1 lead to a hypophosphatemic syndrome in humans.[404] Similarly, a more recently described mutation in ectonucleotide pyrophosphatase/phosphodiesterase 1 (ENPP1), a protein responsible for the conversion of extracellular ATP into inorganic pyrophosphate,[405] has also been demonstrated to result in a phosphate-wasting syndrome in humans.[406] Interestingly, the deletion of ENPP1 in mice not only leads to increased FGF-23 production by bone and associated urinary phosphate wasting, but also defective bone mineralization and soft tissue calcification.[407] To date, no studies have elucidated how ENPP1 or pyrophosphate may regulate FGF-23 production.

Tumor-Induced Osteomalacia. Tumor-induced osteomalacia (TIO), or oncogenic osteomalacia, is an acquired paraneoplastic syndrome of renal phosphate wasting. Usually this syndrome presents in older adults, with a protracted course. Hypophosphatemia with normal serum calcium and PTH levels, renal Pi wasting, low calcitriol levels, and decreased bone mineralization are the hallmarks of TIO.[408] It is caused by mesenchymal tumors that express and secrete FGF-23.[409] In addition to FGF-23, other phosphaturic factors are often secreted by these tumors, including matrix extracellular phosphoglycoprotein (MEPE), frizzled-related protein 4 (FRP-4), and FGF-7.[410]

The definitive treatment of TIO is complete resection of the inciting tumor; however, these mesenchymal tumors are often small and difficult to localize. Medical treatment with phosphate supplementation and calcitriol is frequently necessary to improve bone healing in patients for whom tumor localization or resection is unsuccessful. Cinacalcet has also been used to induce hypoparathyroidism and decrease phosphate wasting, with good response,[411] although hypocalcemia is always a concern when using this therapy in patients with normal renal function.

Disorders of Proximal Tubule Inorganic Phosphorus Reabsorption

Hereditary Hypophosphatemic Rickets with Hypercalciuria. Hereditary hypophosphatemic rickets with hypercalciuria (HHRH; OMIM #241530) is a rare autosomal recessive syndrome characterized by rickets, short stature, renal phosphate wasting, and hypercalciuria. HHRH is caused by mutations in *SLC34A3*, the gene encoding the renal sodium-phosphate cotransporter NaPi-2c.[412] Patients have an appropriate elevation in 1,25(OH)$_2$D, which results in hypercalciuria. They are treated with phosphorus supplementation.

A similar autosomal recessive disorder has been described in two patients with loss-of-function mutations in the *SLC34A1* gene, which encodes the NaPi-IIa sodium phosphate cotransporter. However, unlike HHRH, these patients also had Fanconi's syndrome (see later).[413]

More recently, gene mutations in the sodium-hydrogen exchanger regulatory factor 1 (NHERF1) have been described in patients with hypophosphatemia and nephrolithiasis from renal phosphate wasting.[414] NHERF1 is a protein that plays an essential role in delivery of sodium phosphate cotransporters to the apical membrane in the proximal tubule.[415] Similarly, a de novo translocation mutation in the *KLOTHO* gene has also been linked to a syndrome characterized by elevated plasma α-klotho levels, hypophosphatemia, and HPT.[416] The membrane-bound form of klotho is expressed locally in the kidney in the proximal and distal tubules, and prior studies have suggested that klotho has an independent role in renal phosphate transport.[417] However, the exact mechanisms responsible for the clinical phenotype in this patient exhibiting a translocation mutation of the *KLOTHO* gene remain undetermined.

Fanconi's Syndrome. Fanconi's syndrome is a disorder characterized by generalized proximal tubule dysfunction leading to defects in the reabsorption of glucose, phosphate, calcium, amino acids, bicarbonate, uric acid, and other organic compounds.[418] This syndrome can be genetic or acquired. Inherited causes of Fanconi's syndrome include cystinosis, tyrosinemia, and Wilson's disease. Acquired causes include monoclonal gammopathies, amyloidosis, collagen vascular diseases, kidney transplant rejection, and many drugs or toxins, such as heavy metals, antineoplastic agents, antiretroviral agents, aminoglycosides, and anticonvulsants.[419,420] Over time, severe hypophosphatemia in Fanconi's syndrome can lead to defective bone mineralization, with increased fracture risk. Of interest, a recessive loss of function mutation in the *SLC34A1* gene encoding the NaPi-IIa proximal tubule transporter was shown to cause Fanconi's syndrome, including phosphaturia and hypophosphatemia and other perturbations in proximal tubule transport, perhaps arising from the accumulation of the misfolded gene product and consequent endoplasmic reticulum–associated stress response.[421]

Kidney Transplantation. Hypophosphatemia is observed in up to 90% of patients after kidney transplantation.[422,423] It is typically mild to moderate, and mostly occurs during the first weeks after surgery but may persist for months to years.[422] These patients have phosphaturia and decreased TmP/GFR, with a well-preserved GFR. The causes of posttransplantation hypophosphatemia include persistent (tertiary) HPT,[422] excess of FGF-23 in the posttransplantation period,[424] 25(OH)D and 1,25(OH)$_2$D deficiency, and immunosuppressive medication.[425] Pretransplantation levels of PTH and FGF-23 predict the severity of hypophosphatemia, and both hormones may act synergistically to increase phosphaturia in this setting.[426] Cinacalcet has been shown to correct urinary phosphate wasting and normalize plasma Pi in posttransplantation patients by decreasing PTH levels without an impact on high levels of FGF-23.[427] The major consequence of posttransplantation hypophosphatemia is progressive bone loss and osteomalacia. Management of posttransplantation hypophosphatemia concentrates on replacement of phosphate, correction of vitamin D deficiency, and treatment of HPT.

Drug-Induced Hypophosphatemia. There is an extensive and growing list of medications that can cause hypophosphatemia and phosphate urinary losses as part of Fanconi's syndrome, as discussed above, or by affecting only NaPi transporters in the kidney. Diuretics, including acetazolamide, loop diuretics, and some thiazides with carbonic anhydrase activity, such as metolazone, can increase phosphaturia. The volume contraction that accompanies the use of diuretics usually stimulates proximal tubular NaPi reabsorption and prevents the development of severe hypophosphatemia. Conversely, volume expansion with saline can cause phosphaturia and hypophosphatemia.[428] Corticosteroids decrease intestinal phosphorus absorption and increase renal phosphorus excretion and thus may cause mild-to-moderate hypophosphatemia.[429] Hypophosphatemia has been reported in patients treated for malignancies with many of the novel tyrosine kinase inhibitors, including imatinib (50%),[430] sorafenib (13%),[431] and nilotinib.[432] The mechanism is thought to be due to inhibition of calcium and Pi resorption from bone, together with secondary HPT, leading to phosphaturia,[433] or may be caused by development of a partial Fanconi's syndrome.[434] Administration of parenteral iron formulations containing carbohydrate moieties has been associated with hypophosphatemia, phosphate wasting, and inhibition of 1α-hydroxylation of vitamin D,[435,436] which was found to be mediated by an increase in circulating levels of intact FGF-23.[437] Hypophosphatemia has also been reported in acetaminophen toxicity; the mechanism for this association is likely multifactorial, but appears at least partially to result from urinary phosphate wasting.[438] Finally, the administration of large doses of estrogens in patients with metastatic prostate carcinoma can also produce hypophosphatemia.[439]

Miscellaneous Causes. Significant urinary losses of phosphate may lead to hypophosphatemia during recovery from acute tubular necrosis and from obstructive uropathy. Postoperative hypophosphatemia has been reported after liver resection, colorectal surgery, aortic bypass, and cardiothoracic surgery.[440-442] Posthepatectomy hypophosphatemia appears to be due to a transient increase in renal fractional excretion of phosphate rather than to increased metabolic demand by the regenerative liver.[443]

Decreased Intestinal Absorption

Malnutrition. Malnutrition from low phosphate intake is not a common cause of hypophosphatemia. Increased renal reabsorption of phosphorus can compensate for all but the most severe decreases in oral phosphate intake. However, if phosphate deprivation is prolonged and severe (<100 mg/day), or if it coexists with diarrhea, the continued colonic secretion of phosphate can lead to hypophosphatemia. Hypophosphatemia seen in children with protein malnutrition and kwashiorkor correlates with increased mortality.[444]

Malabsorption. More common is hypophosphatemia resulting from malabsorption. Most phosphorus absorption occurs in the duodenum and jejunum, and intestinal disorders affecting the small intestine may lead to hypophosphatemia.[445] Phosphate-binding cations such as aluminum, calcium, magnesium, and iron form complexes with phosphorus in the gastrointestinal tract, resulting in decreased phosphate absorption. Hypophosphatemia can develop quickly, even in patients given a relatively moderate but sustained dosage of phosphate binders. When combined with poor nutritional intake or extensive dialysis, this therapy may result in so-called overshoot hypophosphatemia. Prolonged use of phosphate-binding antacids can lead to clinically significant osteomalacia.[446]

Vitamin D–Mediated Disorders. Vitamin D is critical for normal control of phosphorus. Deficiency of vitamin D leads to decreased intestinal absorption of phosphorus and to hypocalcemia, HPT, and a consequent PTH-mediated increase in renal phosphorus excretion. Syndromes of vitamin D deficiency or resistance characterized by hypophosphatemia, hypocalcemia, and bone disease are discussed in an earlier section of this chapter that discusses hypocalcemia.

Redistribution of Phosphate. Redistribution of phosphate from the extracellular space into cells is a common cause of hypophosphatemia in hospitalized patients. This shift of phosphate occurs by various mechanisms, including elevated levels of insulin, glucose, and catecholamines, respiratory alkalosis, increased cell proliferation (leukemia blast crisis, lymphoma), and rapid bone mineralization (hungry bone syndrome).

Respiratory Alkalosis. The fall in carbon dioxide during acute respiratory alkalosis causes carbon dioxide diffusion from the intracellular space, increases intracellular pH, and stimulates glycolysis. The consequent increase in the formation of phosphorylated carbohydrates leads to a decrease in extracellular phosphorus levels.[447] When the alkalosis is prolonged and severe, phosphorus levels can drop below 1 mg/dL.[448] Mild hypophosphatemia may occur during the increased ventilation after treatment of asthma attack[449] and in patients with panic disorders with intermittent hypocapnia. Hypophosphatemia is common in mechanically ventilated patients, particularly if they are also receiving glucose infusions. The urinary phosphate excretion can drop to undetectable levels, indicating maximal urinary Pi reabsorption.

Refeeding Syndrome. In chronically malnourished individuals, rapid refeeding can result in significant hypophosphatemia. The incidence of refeeding-related hypophosphatemia is high in hospitalized patients receiving parenteral nutrition, as high as one in three in one series.[450,451] Risk factors for refeeding syndrome include eating disorders, chronic alcoholism, kwashiorkor, cancer, and diabetes mellitus.[450] Refeeding after even very short periods of starvation can lead to hypophosphatemia.[451] The mechanism is related to an insulin-induced increase in cellular phosphate uptake and utilization. The maintenance of serum Pi in the normal range is essential in the management of refeeding syndrome. Adequate phosphate (20-30 mmol of Pi/L) in the parenteral nutrition formulation generally prevents this complication. Even higher amounts may be required for patients with diabetes or chronic alcoholism.

Hypophosphatemia Resulting from Multiple Mechanisms

Alcoholism. Hypophosphatemia and phosphate depletion are particularly common and often a severe problem in alcoholic patients with poor intake, vitamin D deficiency, and heavy use of phosphate-binding antacids.[452] Alcohol-induced proximal tubule dysfunction also contributes to phosphate depletion.[226] Alcoholics frequently develop acute respiratory alkalosis due to alcohol withdrawal, sepsis, or cirrhosis. Phosphorus deficiency is often not manifested as hypophosphatemia at the initial evaluation for medical care. Typically, refeeding or administration of IV glucose (or both) in this patient population stimulates shifts of phosphorus into cells and thereby uncovers severe hypophosphatemia. Hypophosphatemic alcoholics are at high risk for the development of rhabdomyolysis.[384]

Diabetic Ketoacidosis. In uncontrolled diabetes, phosphate is released from cells and ultimately appears in the urine because of concomitant glycosuria, ketonuria, acidosis, and osmotic diuresis. which all increase urinary phosphate excretion.[453] Although serum phosphate levels may be normal, total phosphate stores are usually low. During treatment of diabetic ketoacidosis, the development of hypophosphatemia is extremely common.[454] Administration of insulin stimulates the cellular uptake of phosphorus, and thus the serum phosphate level can fall dramatically with treatment.[362] However, routine administration of phosphate in this setting, before the development of hypophosphatemia, is discouraged because it may lead to significant hypocalcemia.[455] Phosphate depletion can itself be a cause of insulin resistance, and a decrease in insulin requirements has been observed after phosphate replacement therapy.[456,457]

Miscellaneous Disorders. Moderate, and at times severe, hypophosphatemia may be observed in acute leukemia in the leukemic phase of lymphomas[458] and during hematopoietic reconstitution after stem cell transplantation.[459] Rapid cell growth, with consequent phosphorus utilization, is very likely responsible for the decrease in extracellular phosphorus. Hypophosphatemia has been observed in a woman with toxic shock syndrome[460] and is commonly observed in sepsis,[461] but the complicated clinical picture in septic patients makes it difficult to delineate a specific mechanism. Rapid volume expansion diminishes proximal tubule sodium phosphate reabsorption and may lead to transient hypophosphatemia.[428] Hypophosphatemia is seen in patients with heat stroke, as well as hyperthermia, mainly due to increased renal phosphorus excretion.

TREATMENT

The first step in the management of hypophosphatemia is to establish the cause of the low Pi, followed by a determination of whether Pi replacement is necessary. There is little evidence that mild hypophosphatemia (Pi = 2.0 to 2.5 mg/dL) has significant clinical consequences in humans or that aggressive Pi replacement is needed. This is particularly true when Pi shift is the major cause of the hypophosphatemia.

Patients with symptomatic hypophosphatemia and phosphate depletion do require replacement therapy. Those with severe hypophosphatemia, with a plasma Pi level less than 1 mg/dL, even in the absence of phosphate depletion, will need IV phosphate therapy. Because the serum level of phosphorus may not be an accurate reflection of total body stores, it is essentially impossible to predict the amount of phosphorus necessary to correct phosphorus deficiency and hypophosphatemia.⁴⁶² In chronically malnourished patients (e.g., anorectics, alcoholics), significant phosphorus repletion will be necessary, whereas in patients who are hypophosphatemic from other causes (e.g., antacid ingestion, acetazolamide use), correction of the underlying problem may be sufficient.

Phosphate can be administered orally or parenterally. In mild or moderate hypophosphatemia, oral repletion with low-fat milk (containing 0.9 mg Pi/mL) is well tolerated and effective. Alternatively, oral tablets containing 250 mg (8 mmol) of phosphorus from a combination of sodium-phosphate and potassium-phosphate salts can be prescribed. A typical patient with moderate to severe hypophosphatemia would probably need 1000 to 2000 mg (32 to 64 mmol) of phosphorus/day to have body stores repleted within 7 to 10 days. Side effects include diarrhea, hyperkalemia, and volume overload.

IV phosphorus repletion is generally reserved for individuals with severe hypophosphatemia (Pi < 1 mg/dL). Various regimens are used in clinical practice, all based on uncontrolled observational studies. Some are more conservative in the amount of phosphate delivered to avoid side effects, which may include renal failure, hypocalcemic tetany, and hyperphosphatemia. One standard regimen is to administer 2.5 mg/kg body mass of elemental phosphorus (0.08 mmol/kg of phosphate over a 6-hour period for severe asymptomatic hypophosphatemia; 5 mg/kg body mass of elemental phosphorus [0.16 mmol/kg of phosphate] over a 6-hour period for severe symptomatic hypophosphatemia).⁴⁶³ Others have used a more intensive regimen of 10 mg/kg body mass (0.32 mmol/kg of phosphate) administered over 12 hours.⁴⁶⁴ However, even with these higher doses, only 58% of treated patients achieved serum Pi levels above 2 mg/dL. A graded dosing scheme for IV phosphate replacement (0.16 mmol/kg over 4 to 6 hours, 0.32 mmol/kg over 4 to 6 hours, and 0.64 mmol/kg over 6 to 8 hours for serum Pi levels of 2.3 to 3.0, 1.6 to 2.2, and <1.5 mg/dL, respectively) was used effectively in ICU patients without renal dysfunction and hypercalcemia.⁴⁶⁵ Other intensive phosphate replacement regimens have been reported and found to be effective and safe in the ICU for select patients with severe hypophosphatemia.³⁷⁶

Complete reference list available at ExpertConsult.com.

KEY REFERENCES

4. Portale AA: Blood calcium, phosphorus, and magnesium. In Favus MJ, editor: *Primer on the metabolic bone diseases and disorders of mineral metabolism*, Philadelphia, 1999, Lippincott, Williams & Wilkins, pp 115–118.
5. Moore EW: Ionized calcium in normal serum, ultrafiltrates, and whole blood determined by ion-exchange electrodes. *J Clin Invest* 49:318–334, 1970.
11. Gauci C, Moranne O, Fouqueray B, et al: Pitfalls of measuring total blood calcium in patients with CKD. *J Am Soc Nephrol* 19:1592–1598, 2008.
31. Rubin MR, Bilezikian JP, McMahon DJ, et al: The natural history of primary hyperparathyroidism with or without parathyroid surgery after 15 years. *J Clin Endocrinol Metab* 93:3462–3470, 2008.
45. Mundy GR, Edwards JR: PTH-related peptide (PTHrP) in hypercalcemia. *J Am Soc Nephrol* 19:672–675, 2008.
52. Edwards CM, Zhuang J, Mundy GR: The pathogenesis of the bone disease of multiple myeloma. *Bone* 42:1007–1013, 2008.
57. Nussbaum SR, Gaz RD, Arnold A: Hypercalcemia and ectopic secretion of parathyroid hormone by an ovarian carcinoma with rearrangement of the gene for parathyroid hormone. *N Engl J Med* 323:1324–1328, 1990.
59. Marx SJ, Attie MF, Levine MA, et al: The hypocalciuric or benign variant of familial hypercalcemia: clinical and biochemical features in fifteen kindreds. *Medicine (Baltimore)* 60:397–412, 1981.
63. Egbuna OI, Brown EM: Hypercalcaemic and hypocalcaemic conditions due to calcium-sensing receptor mutations. *Best Pract Res Clin Rheumatol* 22:129–148, 2008.
64. Nesbit MA, Hannan FM, Howles SA, et al: Mutations affecting G-protein subunit alpha11 in hypercalcemia and hypocalcemia. *N Engl J Med* 368:2476–2486, 2013.
74. Pollak MR, Brown EM, Chou YH, et al: Mutations in the human Ca(2+)-sensing receptor gene cause familial hypocalciuric hypercalcemia and neonatal severe hyperparathyroidism. *Cell* 75:1297–1303, 1993.
89. Jacobs TP, Bilezikian JP: Clinical review: Rare causes of hypercalcemia. *J Clin Endocrinol Metab* 90:6316–6322, 2005.
96. Vagiatzi MG, Jackobson-Dickman E, DeBoer MD, et al: Vitamin D supplementation and risk of toxicity in pediatrics: a review of current literature. *J Clin Endocrinol Metab* 99:1132–1141, 2014.
103. Khairallah W, Fawaz A, Brown EM, et al: Hypercalcemia and diabetes insipidus in a patient previously treated with lithium. *Nat Clin Pract Nephrol* 3:397–404, 2007.
119. Felsenfeld AJ, Levine BS: Milk alkali syndrome and the dynamics of calcium homeostasis. *Clin J Am Soc Nephrol* 1:641–654, 2006.
123. Stewart AF, Adler M, Byers CM, et al: Calcium homeostasis in immobilization: an example of resorptive hypercalciuria. *N Engl J Med* 306:1136–1140, 1982.
125. Gaudio A, Pennisi P, Bratengeier C, et al: Increased sclerostin serum levels associated with bone formation and resorption markers in patients with immobilization-induced bone loss. *J Clin Endocrinol Metab* 95:2248–2253, 2010.
137. Suki WN, Yium JJ, Von Minden M, et al: Acute treatment of hypercalcemia with furosemide. *N Engl J Med* 283:836–840, 1970.
146. Hu MI, Glezerman I, Leboulleux S, et al: Denosumab for patients with persistent or relapsed hypercalcemia of malignancy despite recent bisphosphonate treatment. *J Natl Cancer Inst* 105:1417–1420, 2013.
147. Camus C, Charasse C, Jouannic-Montier I, et al: Calcium-free hemodialysis: experience in the treatment of 33 patients with severe hypercalcemia. *Intensive Care Med* 22:116–121, 1996.
159. Pollak MR, Brown EM, Estep HL, et al: Autosomal dominant hypocalcaemia caused by a Ca(2+)-sensing receptor gene mutation. *Nat Genet* 8:303–307, 1994.
163. Bilezikian JP, Khan A, Potts JT, Jr, et al: Hypoparathyroidism in the adult: epidemiology, diagnosis, pathophysiology, target-organ involvement, treatment, and challenges for future research. *J Bone Miner Res* 26:2317–2337, 2011.
166. Ringel MD, Schwindinger WF, Levine MA: Clinical implications of genetic defects in G proteins. The molecular basis of McCune-Albright syndrome and Albright hereditary osteodystrophy. *Medicine (Baltimore)* 75:171–184, 1996.
183. Cholst IN, Steinberg SF, Tropper PJ, et al: The influence of hypermagnesemia on serum calcium and parathyroid hormone levels in human subjects. *N Engl J Med* 310:1221–1225, 1984.
201. Kitanaka S, Takeyama K, Murayama A, et al: Inactivating mutations in the 25-hydroxyvitamin D3 1alpha-hydroxylase gene in patients with pseudovitamin D-deficiency rickets. *N Engl J Med* 338:653–661, 1998.
204. Liamis G, Milionis HJ, Elisaf M: A review of drug-induced hypocalcemia. *J Bone Miner Metab* 27:635–642, 2009.
205. Kelly A, Levine MA: Hypocalcemia in the critically ill patient. *J Intensive Care Med* 28:166–177, 2013.
222. Tong GM, Rude RK: Magnesium deficiency in critical illness. *J Intensive Care Med* 20:3–17, 2005.
233. Cundy T, Dissanayake A: Severe hypomagnesaemia in long-term users of proton-pump inhibitors. *Clin Endocrinol (Oxf)* 69:338–341, 2008.
234. Danziger J, William JH, Scott DJ, et al: Proton-pump inhibitor use is associated with low serum magnesium concentrations. *Kidney Int* 83:692–699, 2013.
236. Schlingmann KP, Weber S, Peters M, et al: Hypomagnesemia with secondary hypocalcemia is caused by mutations in TRPM6,

241. Pham PC, Pham PM, Pham SV, et al: Hypomagnesemia in patients with type 2 diabetes. *Clin J Am Soc Nephrol* 2:366–373, 2007.
251. Nijenhuis T, Vallon V, van der Kemp AW, et al: Enhanced passive Ca^{2+} reabsorption and reduced Mg^{2+} channel abundance explains thiazide-induced hypocalciuria and hypomagnesemia. *J Clin Invest* 115:1651–1658, 2005.
252. Schrag D, Chung KY, Flombaum C, et al: Cetuximab therapy and symptomatic hypomagnesemia. *J Natl Cancer Inst* 97:1221–1224, 2005.
256. Groenestege WM, Thebault S, van der Wijst J, et al: Impaired basolateral sorting of pro-EGF causes isolated recessive renal hypomagnesemia. *J Clin Invest* 117:2260–2267, 2007.
262. van Angelen AA, Glaudemans B, van der Kemp AW, et al: Cisplatin-induced injury of the renal distal convoluted tubule is associated with hypomagnesaemia in mice. *Nephrol Dial Transplant* 28:879–889, 2013.
272. Nijenhuis T, Hoenderop JG, Bindels RJ: Downregulation of Ca(2+) and Mg(2+) transport proteins in the kidney explains tacrolimus (FK506)-induced hypercalciuria and hypomagnesemia. *J Am Soc Nephrol* 15:549–557, 2004.
285. Khan AM, Lubitz SA, Sullivan LM, et al: Low serum magnesium and the development of atrial fibrillation in the community: the Framingham Heart Study. *Circulation* 127:33–38, 2013.
291. Chiuve SE, Sun Q, Curhan GC, et al: Dietary and plasma magnesium and risk of coronary heart disease among women. *J Am Heart Assoc* 2:e000114, 2013.
301. Magnesium in Coronaries (MAGIC) Trial Investigators: Early administration of intravenous magnesium to high-risk patients with acute myocardial infarction in the Magnesium in Coronaries (MAGIC) trial: a randomised controlled trial. *Lancet* 360:1189–1196, 2002.
334. Cirillo M, Ciacci C, De Santo NG: Age, renal tubular phosphate reabsorption, and serum phosphate levels in adults. *N Engl J Med* 359:864–866, 2008.
335. Marks J, Debnam ES, Unwin RJ: Phosphate homeostasis and the renal-gastrointestinal axis. *Am J Physiol Renal Physiol* 299:F285–F296, 2010.
337. Murer H, Hernando N, Forster I, et al: Proximal tubular phosphate reabsorption: Molecular mechanisms. *Physiol Rev* 80:1373–1409, 2000.
345. Ichikawa S, Sorenson AH, Austin AM, et al: Ablation of the Galnt3 gene leads to low-circulating intact fibroblast growth factor 23 (Fgf23) concentrations and hyperphosphatemia despite increased Fgf23 expression. *Endocrinology* 150:2543–2550, 2009.
349. Shimada T, Kakitani M, Yamazaki Y, et al: Targeted ablation of FGF23 demonstrates an essential physiological role of FGF23 in phosphate and vitamin D metabolism. *J Clin Invest* 113:561–568, 2004.
376. Brunelli SM, Goldfarb S: Hypophosphatemia: clinical consequences and management. *J Am Soc Nephrol* 18:1999–2003, 2007.
394. A gene (PEX) with homologies to endopeptidases is mutated in patients with X-linked hypophosphatemic rickets. The HYP Consortium. *Nat Genet* 11:130–136, 1995.
398. Shimada T, Hasegawa H, Yamazaki Y, et al: FGF-23 is a potent regulator of vitamin D metabolism and phosphate homeostasis. *J Bone Miner Res* 19:429–435, 2004.
409. Shimada T, Mizutani S, Muto T, et al: Cloning and characterization of FGF23 as a causative factor of tumor-induced osteomalacia. *Proc Natl Acad Sci U S A* 98:6500–6505, 2001.
418. Roth KS, Foreman JW, Segal S: The Fanconi syndrome and mechanisms of tubular transport dysfunction. *Kidney Int* 20:705–716, 1981.

EPIDEMIOLOGY AND RISK FACTORS IN KIDNEY DISEASE

SECTION III

20 Epidemiology of Kidney Disease

Raymond K. Hsu | Chi-yuan Hsu

CHAPTER OUTLINE

EPIDEMIOLOGY OF END-STAGE KIDNEY DISEASE, 638
Incidence, 638
Prevalence, 641
Kidney Transplantation, 642
International Comparisons, 643
EPIDEMIOLOGY OF CHRONIC KIDNEY DISEASE, 643
Prevalence, 645
Incidence, 645

Outcome by Stages, 645
International Comparisons, 647
Relationship Between CKD Epidemiology and ESKD Epidemiology, 647
EPIDEMIOLOGY OF ACUTE KIDNEY INJURY, 647
Incidence, 648
Prevalence, 648
LINKING ACUTE, CHRONIC, AND END-STAGE KIDNEY DISEASE, 652

Epidemiology is defined by the *Oxford English Dictionary* as "the study of the incidence and distribution of diseases." This chapter focuses on the epidemiology of end-stage kidney disease (ESKD), chronic kidney disease (CKD), and acute kidney injury (AKI), the three most important clinical problems in nephrology, measured either by number of patients affected or by rates of associated morbidity and mortality. Some initial definitions are useful. The *incidence rate* of a disease is typically defined as number of new cases per person-year from longitudinal studies that enrolled patients without disease at baseline. The *prevalence rate* of a disease is typically defined as number of persons with disease per population at any one point in time in cross-sectional studies. Disease prevalence thus depends not only on disease incidence but also how long the condition persists. Both incidence rates and prevalence rates are typically normalized to some underlying population (e.g., the total U.S. population). Hence, if the underlying population size were to increase, as the U.S. population has, absolute incidence (and prevalence) *count* could increase over time even if the incidence (or prevalence) *rate* were unchanged.

This chapter also touches upon risk factors for kidney disease, which are discussed in greater detail in Chapters 21 and 22.

EPIDEMIOLOGY OF END-STAGE KIDNEY DISEASE

In the study of kidney disease epidemiology, the traditional focus has been on end-stage kidney disease (ESKD), usually defined operationally as kidney failure being treated with long-term dialysis or kidney transplantation. ESKD is the most serious and dramatic manifestation of kidney disease and naturally was the focus of much clinical attention in the early decades of nephrology, the 1950s and 1960s. During this time, with pioneering work in renal transplantation and dialysis, nephrology became recognized as a separate discipline. Several decades' worth of very strong data exist with regard to the epidemiology of ESKD, in large part because of the existence of ESKD registries such as the Michigan Kidney Registry[1] and United States Renal Data System (USRDS).[2] USRDS provides powerful epidemiology data because it has nationally comprehensive patient-level data and tracks outcomes after the diagnosis of ESKD.

INCIDENCE

The USRDS *Annual Data Report* for 2013 showed for the first time that not only had the incidence rate of ESKD fallen (by 3.8% to 357 cases per million people in 2011, the most recent year for which data were available), the incident count also fell from 117,390 (in 2010) to 115,643 (in 2011) (Figure 20.1).[2] This was the first time since 1980 that USRDS ever documented a fall in the absolute number of new (incident) ESKD cases in the United States.

This secular trend is quite different from that observed in the 1980s and 1990s, when the incidence rate of ESKD rose rapidly (Figure 20.2). It is, however, a continuation of the trend reported by USRDS that the incidence rate of ESKD has more or less reached a plateau in the past decade (see Figure 20.2).[2]

Similar encouraging observations have been reported from other countries. For example, the 2014 *Canadian Organ Replacement Register (CORR) Report*,[3] the 2013 UK Renal Registry's *Annual Report*,[4] and the 2013 *Australia and New Zealand Dialysis and Transplant Registry (ANZDATA) Report*[5] all show stable or declining incidence of ESKD in their respective countries (Figure 20.3).

The reasons for these encouraging trends are not entirely clear but may involve successes in retarding the progression of CKD resulting from more aggressive control of blood pressure with drugs such as those that block the renin angiotensin aldosterone system (RAAS). For example, when the landmark United Kingdom Prospective Diabetes Study (UKPDS) trial was conducted in the 1980s, it was thought acceptable to allow patients with type 2 diabetes in the control arm to have blood pressures as high as 200 mm Hg systolic/105 mm Hg diastolic (this value was lowered to 180/105 mm Hg in 1992).[6] The first large, randomized controlled trial to demonstrate the renoprotective effect of RAAS blockade was not published until 1993.[7] In addition, improved glycemic control among patients with diabetes mellitus may have an important role. The impact of such treatment is illustrated by a Finnish study that tracked outcome among young patients with type 1 diabetes over several decades. In that study, patients with type 1 diabetes diagnosed from 1980 through 1999 had less than half the risk for development of ESKD of those diagnosed from 1965 through 1969.[8] Similar results have been reported in the United States for patients with type 2 diabetes, with one paper reporting a 28% drop in rates of ESKD between 1990 and 2010.[9]

There remains considerable variation in the incidence of ESKD across patient subgroups. In the United States, the incidence of ESKD among African Americans is strikingly higher than the incidence among whites (by more than threefold after adjustments for gender and age) (Table 20.1). Incidence rates are also higher among those of Asian descent and Hispanic ethnicity (see Table 20.1). Men (compared with women) and older (compared with younger) people have higher rates of ESKD (see Table 20.1).

The most common listed etiology of ESKD in the United States is diabetes (156.8 per million population; 44%), followed by hypertension (100.6 per million population; 28%).

However, these are "primary diagnoses" for ESKD assigned by the treating physician at the start of dialysis, when the original etiology of disease may be difficult to discern. For

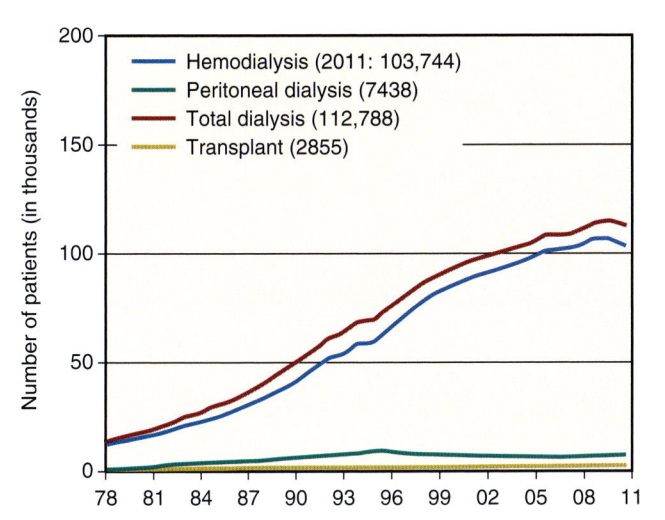

Figure 20.1 Incident counts of end-stage kidney disease in the United States by initial renal replacement therapy modality by calendar year. Hemodialysis is by far the most common. (From U.S. Renal Data System: *USRDS 2013 annual data report: atlas of chronic kidney disease and end-stage renal disease in the United States,* vol 2, 2013, Bethesda, MD, National Institutes of Health, National Institute of Diabetes and Digestive and Kidney Diseases, p 174, figure 1.1.)

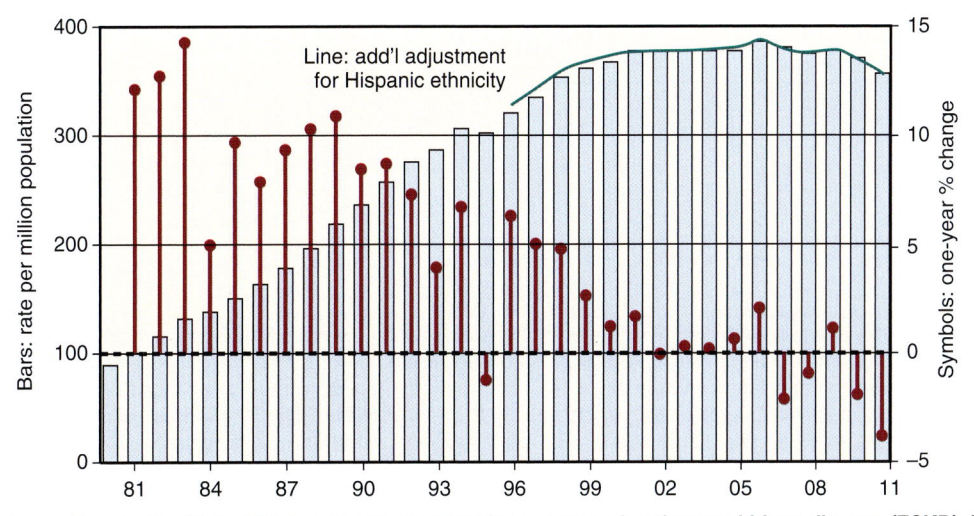

Figure 20.2 Trend over time in the United States in adjusted incidence rates of end-stage kidney disease (ESKD). This rate (adjusted for age, gender, and race) had been relatively stable from 2000 to 2011 and has even declined in the most recent years. (From U.S. Renal Data System: *USRDS 2013 annual data report: atlas of chronic kidney disease and end-stage renal disease in the United States,* vol 2, 2013, Bethesda, MD, National Institutes of Health, National Institute of Diabetes and Digestive and Kidney Diseases, 174, figure 1.2.)

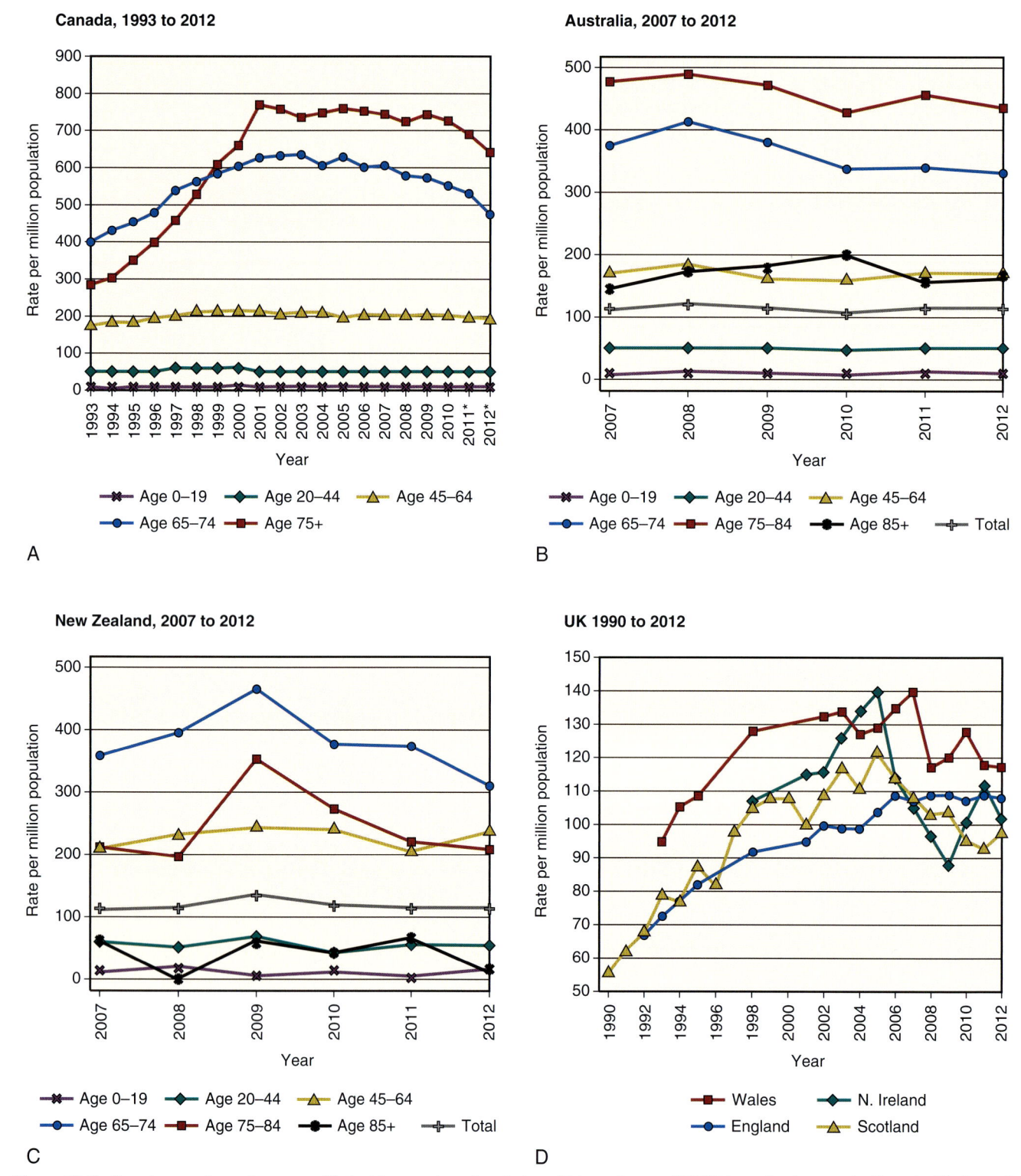

Figure 20.3 Trends over time of age-specific incidence rates of end-stage kidney disease (ESKD) by calendar year in Canada (**A**), Australia (**B**), and New Zealand (**C**). **D**, Overall incidence rates of ESKD in the United Kingdom. In the most recent 5 to 10 years, rates have been stable or declining. RPMP, rate per million population. (**A** from the 2014 *Canadian Organ Replacement Register annual report*, p14, figure 1, available at https://secure.cihi.ca/free_products/2014_CORR_Annual_Report_EN.pdf; **B** and **C** from the *36th* (2013) *Annual Australia and New Zealand Dialysis and Transplant Registry report*, p2-2, figures 2.2 & 2.3, available at http://www.anzdata.org.au/anzdata/AnzdataReport/36thReport/2013c02_newpatients_v1.7.pdf; **D** from the *UK Renal Registry sixteenth annual report* (2013), p11, figure 1.1, available at https://www.renalreg.org/wp-content/uploads/2014/09/01-Chap-01.pdf.)

Table 20.1	Adjusted Incidence Rates of End-Stage Kidney Disease (ESKD) in Different Subgroups in the United States*	
Subgroup		Adjusted Incidence (per million population)
By Race		
White		279.8
Asian		398.5
Native American		452.5
Black/African American		939.8
By Ethnicity		
Non-Hispanic		342.7
Hispanic		517.5
By Age (yr)		
0-19		15.6
20-44		126.5
45-64		571.1
65-74		1306.8
75+		1706.9
By Gender		
Female		281.3
Male		451.2

*Overall incidence (adjusted for age, gender, and race) is 357.0 per million population. Rates by race or ethnicity are adjusted for age and gender; rates by age are adjusted for gender and race; rates by gender are adjusted for age and race.

Modified from U.S. Renal Data System: USRDS 2013 annual data report: atlas of chronic kidney disease and end-stage renal disease in the United States, vol 2, 2013, Bethesda, MD, National Institutes of Health, National Institute of Diabetes and Digestive and Kidney Diseases.

example, it has been documented that numerous cases of ESKD ascribed to hypertension have preceding clinical features highly suggestive of other renal parenchymal diseases (e.g., nephrotic range proteinuria).[10,11] Also, genetic studies have demonstrated that variants in the gene encoding apolipoprotein L1 *(APOL1)* appear to account for much of the higher incidence of "hypertensive nephrosclerosis" observed among African Americans.[12-15] These novel advances will undoubtedly force a rethinking of how we currently assign etiologies for ESKD—specifically the question, "Should we accept hypertension as being the cause of ESKD in a large number of cases?"

Furthermore, the convention of ascribing only one primary cause to any ESKD case may be inherently limited. For example, prospective studies have shown that patients with diabetes mellitus appear to be at several-fold higher risk for ESKD ascribed to nondiabetic causes.[16] This convention also cannot reflect the contribution of multiple disease processes to the final ESKD outcome (e.g., nonrecovery of renal function after acute tubular necrosis in a patient with underlying diabetic nephropathy).

PREVALENCE

According to the *2013 USRDS Annual Report*, the annual prevalence of ESKD in the United States was 1901 per million population (adjusted for age, gender, and race).[2] As alluded to previously, the prevalence of disease depends not only on the number of new cases but also on the survival of existing patients. Better survival of patients on both dialysis and transplant will therefore increase the prevalence of disease (and "burden of ESKD") but actually reflects improvement in care. Indeed, the adjusted mortality rates for patients undergoing dialysis and transplantation have improved over the past three decades (Figure 20.4).

Another reflection of the difference between incidence and prevalence is that although only 3% of patients with incident ESKD are treated by kidney transplantation as the initial modality, 30% of patients with prevalent (existing) ESKD are maintained with kidney transplants. This is due not only to the fact that numerous patients undergoing dialysis subsequently undergo kidney transplantation but also because patients with kidney transplants survive longer. Similarly, the black-white disparity in ESKD is even more pronounced when ESKD prevalence is used as the metric rather than ESKD incidence, because on average, black patients survive longer with ESKD than their white counterparts.[2,17]

Mortality rates among patients with ESKD, especially those undergoing dialysis, remain alarmingly high—in excess of 20% per year (see Figure 20.4). This high mortality rate is paralleled by high rates of hospitalization and health care utilization.[2] Several studies have shown that death rates are particularly high in the first weeks to months immediately after patients start hemodialysis,[18-20] and there is concern that this problem is underestimated by some national registry data because patients die prior to being registered.[21]

Many epidemiology studies have sought to account for the high mortality rates among patients undergoing dialysis. The burden of medical conditions already present at the start of dialysis appears to be a key problem. This possibility is consistent with the observation that interventions to manipulate dialysis-related parameters, such as dose of dialysis[22,23] and use of more recombinant erythropoietin,[24] have not succeeded in reducing mortality.

Notably, many papers have reported that numerous risk factors for mortality in the general population, such as higher blood pressure, higher cholesterol level, and higher body mass index, appear to be paradoxically associated with lower risk of mortality among patients receiving maintenance hemodialysis.[25] The reasons for these reverse "J-shaped" or "U-shaped" associations are not entirely clear. Part of the explanation may be confounding factors such as malnutrition and inflammation.[26] Another factor may be the unique physiology of patients undergoing hemodialysis, such as hemodynamics related to interdialytic fluid accumulation, because several studies have shown that higher blood pressure measured outside the dialysis unit (in contrast to measured just before a hemodialysis session[27-29]) was associated with a linear increase in the risk of adverse outcomes.[30-32]

Results of interventional studies are mixed, with some[33] but not other studies showing benefits of treating conventional "Framingham" cardiovascular disease risk factors *after*

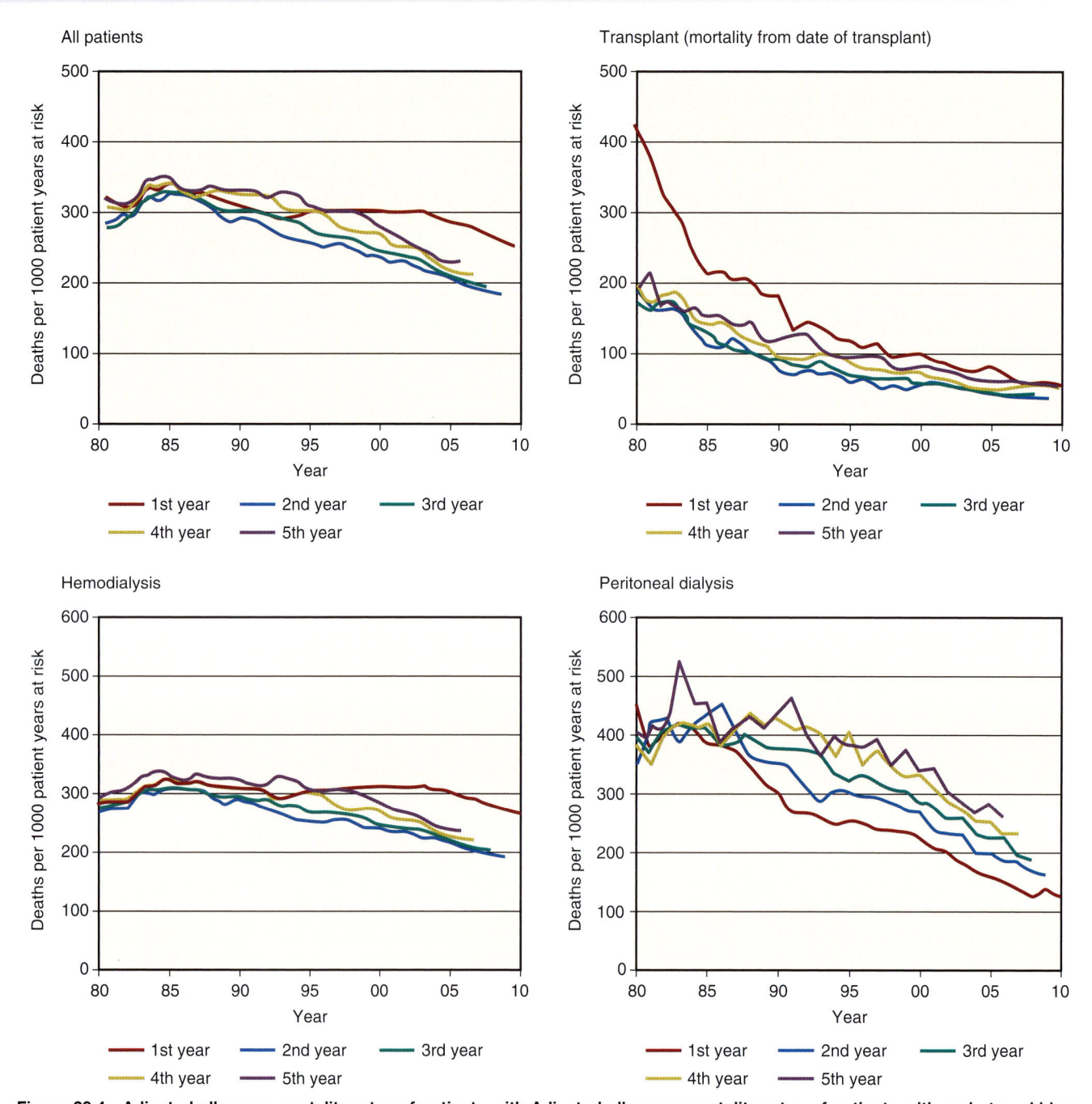

Figure 20.4 Adjusted all-cause mortality rates of patients with Adjusted all-cause mortality rates of patients with end-stage kidney disease (ESKD) over time, by different modalities of renal replacement therapy. From 1980 to 2010, the first-year mortality rate among all incident patients with ESKD has fallen 30.5%, from 321.8 to 254.4 per 1000 patient years. All mortality rates are adjusted for age, gender, race, and primary diagnosis. (From U.S. Renal Data System: *USRDS 2013 annual data report: atlas of chronic kidney disease and end-stage renal disease in the United States,* vol 2, 2013, Bethesda, MD, National Institutes of Health, National Institute of Diabetes and Digestive and Kidney Diseases, p 265, figure 5.1.)

onset of ESKD, such as lipid lowering.[34,35] And there is some evidence (but not strong) in favor of blood pressure lowering in the dialysis population.[36,37]

KIDNEY TRANSPLANTATION

Although no randomized controlled clinical trials have been performed, the best evidence from observational data indicate that, all else being equal, receipt of a kidney transplant confers mortality benefit[38] in addition to improved quality of life in comparison with maintenance dialysis.[39] Currently, 1-year survival with a functioning allograft is 92% for recipients of deceased donor kidneys and 97% for recipients of living donor kidneys.[2]

In 2011, the number of kidney transplantations performed in the United States was 17,671.[2] Figure 20.5 shows the trend over time according to donor type. Shortage of transplant organs, however, remains a major problem that

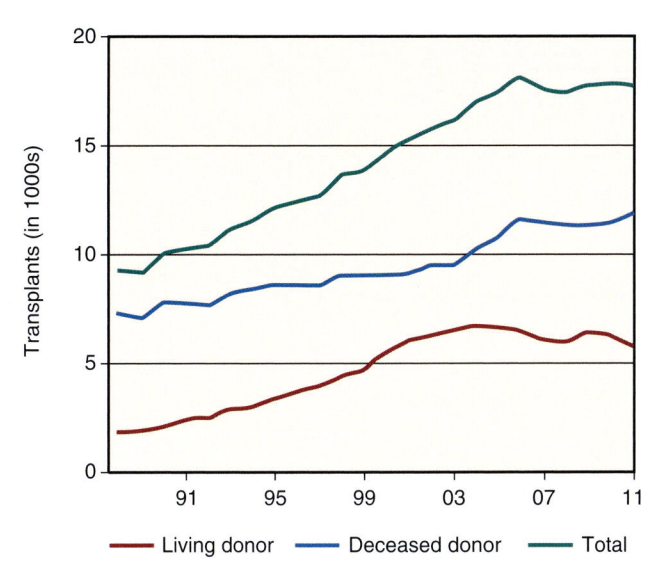

Figure 20.5 Number of transplantations in the United States (limited to patients with end-stage kidney disease aged 20 years and older). Shown are total number and breakdown by donor type. (From U.S. Renal Data System: *USRDS 2013 annual data report: atlas of chronic kidney disease and end-stage renal disease in the United States,* vol 2, 2013, Bethesda, MD, National Institutes of Health, National Institute of Diabetes and Digestive and Kidney Diseases, p 285, figure 7.1.)

Table 20.2 Classification and Staging of Chronic Kidney Disease (CKD) by the National Kidney Foundation*

Stage	Description	GFR (mL/min/1.73 m^2)
1	Kidney damage with normal or ↑ GFR	≥90
2	Kidney damage with mild ↓ GFR	60-89
3	Moderate ↓ GFR	30-59
4	Severe ↓ GFR	15-29
5	Kidney failure	<15 or dialysis

*This widely adopted classification required evidence of kidney damage (such as increased proteinuria) above a glomerular filtration rate (GFR) level of 60 mL/min/1.73 m^2 for the diagnosis of CKD but not below this threshold. *Chronic kidney disease* is defined as either kidney damage or GFR < 60 mL/min/1.73 m^2 for ≥ 3 months. *Kidney damage* is defined as pathologic abnormalities or markers of damage, including abnormalities in blood or urine test results, or imaging studies.
From K/DOQI clinical practice guidelines for chronic kidney disease: evaluation, classification, and stratification. *Am J Kidney Dis* 39(Suppl 1):S1-S266, 2002.

has resulted in longer waiting times. The pressure to increase number of organs has led to numerous contentious discussions regarding proposed schemes to pay donors and use of living donors who have medical conditions that were previously considered contraindications to donation, such as hypertension.

INTERNATIONAL COMPARISONS

Incidence and prevalence rates of ESKD vary considerably across different regions and countries. In 2011, Jalisco (Mexico), the United States, and Taiwan (2010 figure) reported the highest rates of incident ESKD at 527, 362, and 361 per million population, respectively (Figure 20.6).[2] Interpreting incidence rates of ESKD across countries however, is complicated by lack of uniform data collection methods. Furthermore, because only treated ESKD cases are counted, differences in access to renal replacement therapy due to economics, public policy, or local practice patterns greatly influence incidence and prevalence rates.[40,41]

Despite these limitations, it is clear that there is considerable variation in the practice of renal replacement therapy around the world. For example, in Hong Kong, the great majority of patients undergoing dialysis are treated with peritoneal dialysis (74% of prevalent patients [those continuing dialysis] vs. 33% in New Zealand, 20% in Iceland, and 7% in the United States). Home hemodialysis use also varies greatly (18% in New Zealand, 9% in Australia, and 1% in the United States). In terms of transplantation, the reported rates in 2010 were 57 per million person-years in the United States, 37 in Israel, 29 in Argentina, and 8 in Romania.[2]

Finally, the economic models of delivery of dialysis also vary. In the United States currently, about two thirds of patients with ESKD are dialyzed at facilities owned by large dialysis companies. In other countries (such as Germany), the system is much more decentralized.

Beyond registry data, international observational studies such as the Dialysis Outcomes and Practice Patterns Study (DOPPS) have documented noticeable practice variations. For example, in the late 1990s, arteriovenous fistula was used as the dialysis access in 80% of European but only 24% of U.S. prevalent patients. For patients who were new to hemodialysis, the rates of fistula use were 66% in Europe and 15% in the United States.[42] This and other differences may explain the much higher mortality among U.S. patients than patients elsewhere in the world.[43] For further international comparisons, see Chapters 77-82.

EPIDEMIOLOGY OF CHRONIC KIDNEY DISEASE

The past dozen years have seen an explosion of research into CKD. This field was codified in large part following the publication in 2002 of the National Kidney Foundation (NKF) Kidney Disease Outcomes Quality Initiative (KDOQI) definition and classification of chronic kidney disease.[44] Prior to this, there had been no consensus definition of CKD, a lack that made defining disease incidence and prevalence difficult. The NKF CKD definition and classification have been very influential, widely disseminated, and widely adopted (Table 20.2). Although a newer classification of CKD—building on the KDOQI definition but with additional emphasis on the role of albuminuria—has since been

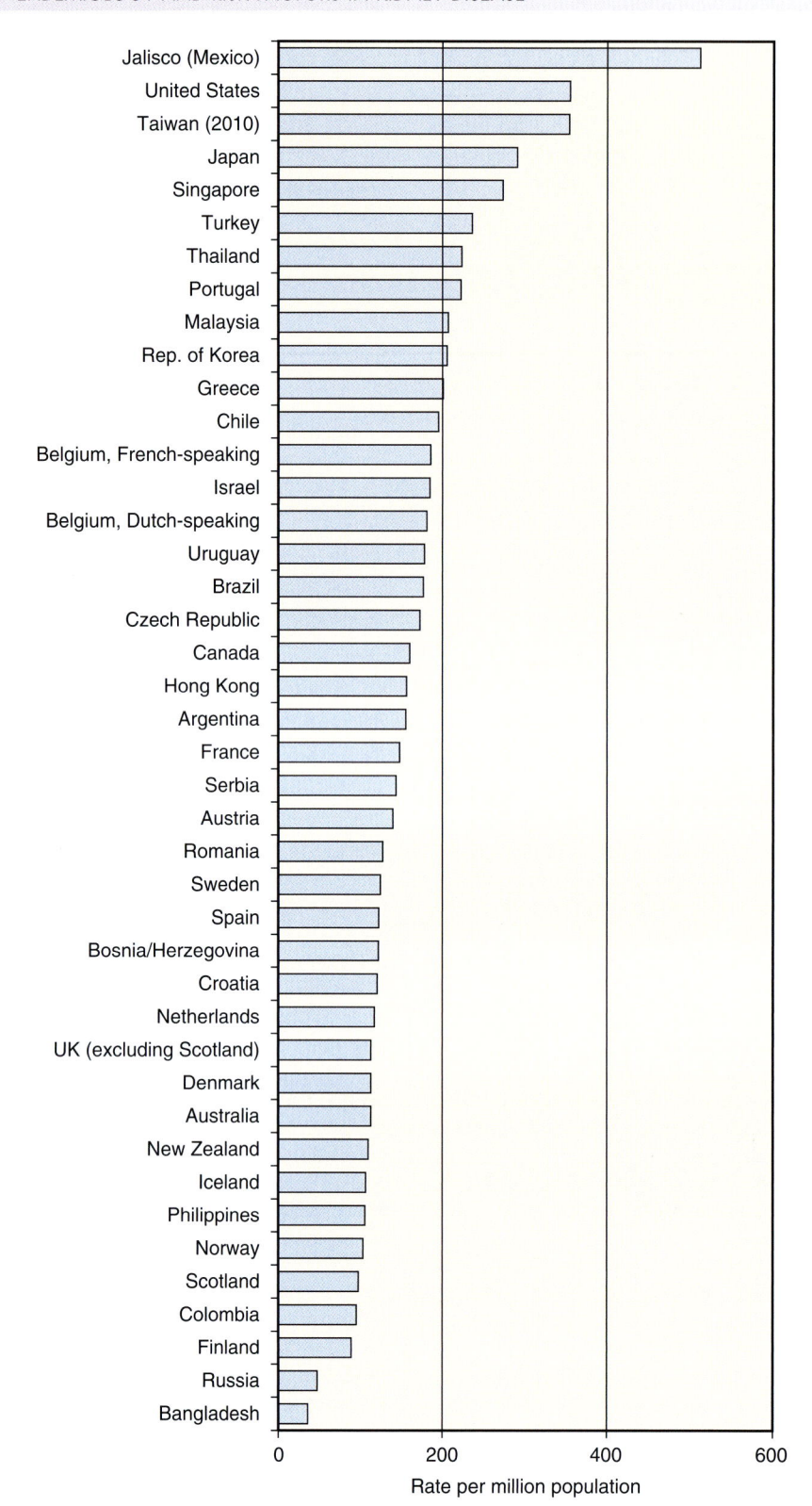

Figure 20.6 Reported incidence of end-stage kidney disease (ESKD) in different countries in 2011. Incidence rates of reported ESKD in 2011 were greatest in Jalisco (Mexico), at 527 per million population, followed by the United States (362), Taiwan (2010 figure: 361), Japan (295), and Singapore (279). Rates of less than 100 per million were reported by Scotland, Colombia, Finland, Russia, and Bangladesh. (From U.S. Renal Data System: *USRDS 2013 annual data report: atlas of chronic kidney disease and end-stage renal disease in the United States,* vol 2, 2013, Bethesda, MD, National Institutes of Health, National Institute of Diabetes and Digestive and Kidney Diseases, p 338, figure 12.3.)

put forth by the NKF program Kidney Disease/Improving Global Outcomes (KDIGO), in 2011[45] it has not yet influenced studies of the population epidemiology of CKD.

Since the publication of the NKF CKD guidelines, the most common method used to estimate renal function is the simplified 4-variable Modification of Diet in Renal Disease (MDRD) equation.[46] An important advance in the field has been improved standardization in serum creatinine calibration among different laboratories, specifically the adoption of assays traceable to an isotope-dilution mass spectrometry method.[47] This development is important for epidemiology studies because even relatively small calibration differences in serum creatinine assays can translate into rather large differences for estimated disease prevalence. A newer equation has been proposed and is increasingly being adopted. The Chronic Kidney Disease Epidemiology Collaboration (CKD-EPI) equation has the same data input elements (serum creatinine, age, sex, and race) but is derived from a more broad-based set of studies and in general results in lower estimates of CKD prevalence in the general population than the MDRD equation.[48] There are now also equations based on alternate filtration markers such as cystatin C, which can be used alone or in combination with serum creatinine[49] (see Chapter 26).

PREVALENCE

Most of the population epidemiology of CKD has focused on the prevalence of CKD. Probably the best longitudinal data source for determining the prevalence of CKD over time in the population of an entire country has been the National Health and Nutrition Examination Survey (NHANES) in the United States. Sponsored by the U.S. Centers for Disease Control and Prevention (CDC), NHANES is a series of surveys encompassing interviews and physical examinations on a nationally representative sample of participants. The second NHANES (NHANES II) was conducted from 1976 through 1980, and the third NHANES (NHANES III) from 1988 through 1994; the latest NHANES was launched in 1999 as a continuous survey.

Table 20.3 summarizes findings of a number of studies published over the last decade that have examined temporal trends in CKD prevalence in the United States on the basis of NHANES.[50] Most of the studies have shown an increase in the crude prevalence of CKD over time (unadjusted for important secular trends such as aging of the population over time). As Table 20.3 illustrates, differences in choice and calibration of filtration marker and choice of estimating equation result in different estimates of CKD prevalence as well as differences in rates of change of disease burden over time. Regardless of the exact figure, it is clear that the number of individuals with CKD is two orders of magnitude larger than the absolute number of incident ESKD cases, underscoring the public health burden of the disease and how ESKD can truly be considered only the "tip of the iceberg."

INCIDENCE

Less is known about incidence of CKD because there are few truly representative longitudinal cohorts available to track and quantify the development of new cases of CKD.

One paper based on the Atherosclerosis Risk in Communities (ARIC) Study reported an incidence rate of 10,380 per million person-years when incident CKD was defined as MDRD equation–estimated GFR (eGFR) less than 60 mL/min/1.73 m^2.[51] This reported incidence is similar to that based on another analysis of data from ARIC as well as the Cardiovascular Health Study (CHS): 13,000 per million person-years.[52] A separate analysis using the Framingham Offspring Study—a cohort of younger persons compared with ARIC and CHS cohorts and using a slightly different definition for CKD—found an incidence rate of 5102 per million person-years.[53] Naturally the reported rate was higher if the presence of new-onset albuminuria was also counted as a new CKD case.[54]

A common limitation of these studies is that only one observed low GFR is used to define new cases of CKD. (The KDOQI definition requires two low GFR readings taken at least 3 months apart.) This is also a problem with the prevalence data. Because some patients may only have a transient drop in GFR, prevalence and incidence estimates would be lower if case definition required documentation of chronically low GFR levels.

OUTCOME BY STAGES

Although there is great interest in knowing outcomes (such as incidence of dialysis vs. death) by CKD stage, it is clear that within the same stage of CKD, different subgroups have rather different outcomes.

In one study of patients enrolled in an integrated health care organization in the United States, rates of renal replacement therapy over a 5-year observation period were 1.3% and 19.9%; for those with stages 3 and 4 CKD, the corresponding rates of death were 24.3% and 45.7%.[55] This and other studies of CKD patients receiving usual medical care[56] show that in general, risk of death is much greater than risk of ESKD. The same must be true for the population as a whole, given the small number of incident ESKD cases compared with the much larger number of prevalent CKD cases (about two orders of magnitude difference).

However, this ratio between death and ESKD varies greatly with age. In a large study of U.S. male veterans with CKD stages 3 to 5 followed for a mean of 3.2 years, rates of both death and ESKD were inversely related to eGFR at baseline among patients of all ages. However, in those with comparable levels of eGFR, older patients had higher rates of death and lower rates of ESKD than younger patients. Consequently, the level of eGFR below which the risk of ESKD exceeded the risk of death varied by age, ranging from 45 mL/min/1.73 m^2 for patients 18 to 44 years old to 15 mL/min/1.73 m^2 for patients 65 to 84 years old. Among those 85 years or older, the risk of death always exceeded the risk of ESKD (Figure 20.7).[57]

Furthermore, it should be noted that among patients enrolled in randomized clinical trials of interventions to retard renal disease progression—such as the MDRD study,[58] the Reduction of Endpoints in NIDDM with the Angiotensin II Antagonist Losartan (RENAAL) study,[59] and the Irbesartan in Diabetic Nephropathy Trial (IDNT)[60]—risk of ESKD was higher than risk of death. The reason is that trial enrollees are not representative of the general population with CKD.

Table 20.3 Studies of Temporal Trends in the U.S. Population Prevalence of Chronic Kidney Disease Derived from the National Health and Nutrition Examination Surveys (NHANESs)

Study	CKD Definition	Disease Prevalence During Time Period (%)			Change in Prevalence per Year	GFR Estimating Equation	Filtration Marker Calibration and Alignment
		1976-1980	1988-1994	1999-2004			
Hsu et al, 2004[106]	eGFRcr < 60	2.0*	2.5*		+1.7% per year[†]	4-variable MDRD Study Equation[46]	For both time periods, Cleveland Clinic calibrated Cr = Cr − 0.23
Coresh et al, 2005[107]	CKD stages 1-4 (eGFRcr and ACR)		8.8	9.4 (1999-2000)	+0.8% per year	4-variable MDRD Study Equation[46]	1988-1994: Cleveland Clinic calibrated Cr = Cr − 0.23; 1999-2000: Cleveland Clinic calibrated Cr = Cr + 0.13
	eGFRcr < 60		4.4	3.8 (1999-2000)	−1.7% per year		
Coresh et al, 2007[108]	CKD stages 1-4 (eGFRcr and ACR)		10.0	13.1	+2.6% per year[†]	IDMS-traceable MDRD Study Equation[109]	1998-1994: standardized Cr = −0.184 + 0.960 × Cr; 1999-2000: standardized Cr = 0.147+1.013 × Cr; After 2000: did not require calibration Conservative trend analysis added 0.04 mg/dL to 1988-1994 creatinine values
	eGFRcr < 60 (primary analysis)		5.6	8.1	+3.5% per year[†]		
	eGFRcr < 60 (conservative trend analysis)		Data not shown	Data not shown	+1.4% per year[†]		
Foley et al, 2009[110]	CKD stages 1-5 (eGFRcyc and ACR)		15.1	14.9 (1999-2002)	−0.1% per year	CKD-EPI cystatin C 2008[111]	No calibration performed for cystatin C
	eGFRcys < 60		6.4	6.9 (1999-2002)	+0.8% per year		
Grams et al, 2013[112]	eGFRcys < 60		5.5	8.7 (1999-2002)	+4.9% per year[†]	CKD-EPI Cystatin C 2012[49]	1988-1994: standardized cystatin C = 1.12 × [0.022 + 0.80 × (cystatin C)]; 1999-2002: standardized cystatin C = 1.12 × [cystatin C − 0.12]
	eGFRcr-cys < 60		4.4	7.1 (1999-2002)	+5.0% per year[†]	CKD-EPI Cr-cystatin C 2012[49]	

ACR, albumin-to-creatinine ratio; CKD-EPI, Chronic Kidney Disease Epidemiology Collaboration; Cr, creatinine (mg/dL); eGFRcr, creatinine-based estimated glomerular filtration rate (mL/min/1.73 m²); eGFRcr-cys, creatinine and cystatin C-based estimated glomerular filtration rate (mL/min/1.73 m²); eGFRcys, cystatin C-based estimated glomerular filtration rate (mL/min/1.73 m²); IDMS, isotope dilution mass spectrometry; MDRD, Modification of Diet in Renal Disease.

*For age 20 yr-74 yr blacks and whites only.
[†]Represents statistically significant change in the original study.

From Hsu RK, Hsu CY: *Temporal trends in prevalence of CKD: the glass is half full and not half empty.* Am J Kidney Dis 62:214-216, 2013.

Table 20.4 Estimated Prevalence of Chronic Kidney Disease (CKD) Stages 1 through 4 in Norway versus the United States*

CKD Stage	Prevalence in Norway, 1995 to 1997[†] White (n = 65,181)	Prevalence in United States, 1988 to 1994[†]		
		White (n = 6635)	Black (n = 4163)	Overall (n = 15,625)
1	2.7 (0.3)	2.8 (0.3)	5.8 (0.3)	3.3 (0.3)
2	3.2 (0.4)	3.2 (0.3)	2.5 (0.3)	3.0 (0.3)
3	4.2 (0.1)	4.8 (0.3)	3.1 (0.2)	4.3 (0.3)
4	0.16 (0.01)	0.21 (0.03)	0.25 (0.08)	0.20 (0.03)
Total	10.2 (0.5)	11.0 (0.6)	11.6 (0.5)	11.0 (0.5)

*Total CKD prevalence in Norway was 10.2%, which closely approximates reported U.S. CKD prevalence. Thus, lower progression to end-stage kidney disease (ESKD) rather than a smaller pool of individuals at risk appears to explain the much lower incidence of ESKD in Norway than in the United States.
[†]Prevalence expressed as % of population; standard error in parentheses.
From Hallan SI, Coresh J, Astor BC, et al: International comparison of the relationship of chronic kidney disease prevalence and ESRD risk. J Am Soc Nephrol 17:2275-2284, 2006.

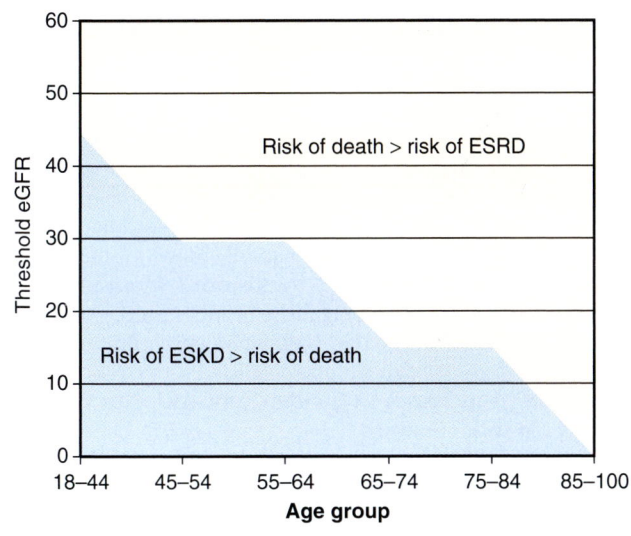

Figure 20.7 Relative risk of death versus end-stage kidney disease (ESKD) by age and estimated glomerular filtration rate (eGFR) threshold among U.S. male veterans. Among patients who were younger than 45 years, the incidence of treated ESKD was greater than that of death at all estimated GFR (eGFR) levels < 45 mL/min/1.73 m². Conversely, among those aged 65 to 84, only at eGFR levels < 15 mL/min/1.73 m² did risk for ESKD exceed risk for death. Among those aged 85 to 100, risk for death exceeded risk for ESKD even at eGFR levels < 15 mL/min/1.73 m². (From O'Hare AM, Choi AI, Bertenthal D, et al: Age affects outcomes in chronic kidney disease. J Am Soc Nephrol 18:2758-2765, 2007.)

INTERNATIONAL COMPARISONS

The NHANES-based studies from the United States discussed previously are the most reliable and sophisticated analyses regarding the longitudinal estimates of CKD prevalence in the general population. Direct international comparison is problematic owing to lack of uniformity in calibration of serum creatinine or lack of a representative community-based sample—two critical elements needed to obtain reliable estimates of disease prevalence in the population. As summarized in the previous edition of this chapter, prevalence of GFR values 60 mL/min/1.73 m² or lower has been reported to vary from less than 2% (20,000 per million persons) to more than 40% (400,000 per million persons) in different studies from different countries.[61]

One study using data from the population-based Health Survey of Nord-Trondelag County (HUNT II) in Norway did show that the prevalence of CKD was similar in the United States and Norway (Table 20.4).[62] This study explicitly analyzed data using the same methods as NHANES and involved calibration of creatinine measurements.

RELATIONSHIP BETWEEN CKD EPIDEMIOLOGY AND ESKD EPIDEMIOLOGY

The HUNT II study is also interesting because it highlighted another notable epidemiologic feature. Although the prevalence of CKD is similar, the incidence of ESKD in Norway is much lower than that in the United States (see Table 20.4).[62]

Similar dissociations between CKD epidemiology and ESKD epidemiology have been noted in the United States For example, an analysis which juxtaposed CKD prevalence with ESKD incidence using data from NHANES and U.S. Renal Data System found that although African Americans in the United States have a much higher incidence of ESKD than white persons, African Americans do not appear to have a higher prevalence of CKD.[63] The lack of higher prevalence of stage 3 and 4 CKD in African Americans than in white persons has also been observed in other population-based studies.[64,65] Presumably the much higher incidence rate of ESKD among African Americans is due to more rapid progression from CKD to ESKD.[15,63]

EPIDEMIOLOGY OF ACUTE KIDNEY INJURY

The systematic study of population epidemiology of AKI is a relatively new development.

One limiting factor in the past has been the lack of a consensus definition for acute kidney injury (or acute renal failure). Because different studies used different acute increases in serum creatinine to define cases, it is difficult to compare disease incidence among different clinical settings, patient populations, and calendar years because it is not known how much of the observed variation is due to differences in definition versus differences in frequency of true underlying disease. This may be less of a problem when the outcome is dialysis-requiring acute kidney injury. But in those cases, an additional layer of complexity is that the threshold for initiating acute dialysis may vary by place and time.

The proposed consensus definitions of acute renal failure or acute kidney injury in the last 10 years have improved the situation. In 2004, the Acute Dialysis Quality Initiative (ADQI) Group proposed the RIFLE classification schema for acute renal failure.[66] Three years later, the Acute Kidney Injury Network (AKIN) put forth its own system, which included replacing "acute renal failure" with "acute kidney injury" and defining "abrupt" changes in renal function as being within 48 hours.[67] Most recently, in 2012, the Kidney Disease Improving Global Outcomes (KDIGO) Acute Kidney Injury Work Group proposed a third definition with slightly differing time intervals and definition of "baseline renal function."[68] Table 20.5 compares and contrasts the three definitions. It should be emphasized that many published studies of AKI have not used the exact definitions of baseline or time interval outlined here.

All three definitions also allow for changes in urine output to identify and stage severity of AKI. However, reliable information on urine output is often not available in large epidemiology datasets, so this information has rarely been used to define incidence of AKI in a population.

A second limiting factor in the past has been that most studies have been based on hospitalized patients or on the subgroup of hospitalized patients in the intensive care unit (ICU).[69-73] The denominator in these studies is often hospitalization or ICU admission, which is suboptimal because rates of hospitalization (or ICU admission) per population are not defined and also vary in different countries and across time. For example, one much cited study found, among medical and surgical patients from Tufts–New England Medical Center in Boston from 1978 to 1979, that the incidence of AKI was 4.9% per hospitalization.[69] Applying the identical criteria to patients admitted to Rush Presbyterian–St Luke's Medical Center in Chicago in 1996, the same investigative team found the incidence of AKI to be 7.2% per hospitalization.[70] However, it not possible to determine how much of this change is accounted for by variation in threshold for hospital admission and how much by true underlying changes in the incidence of AKI. This bias is minimized by studies that have used the underlying population as the denominator.

INCIDENCE

A population-based study from the Grampian region of Scotland reported that during the first 6 months of 2003, the incidence of AKI using the RIFLE classification was 2147 per million person-years[74] (among which 336 per million person-years was considered acute-on-chronic renal failure). Overall, 8.5% of the cases required dialysis (183 per million person-years). Sepsis was a precipitating factor in 47% of patients.

One study based on a large integrated health care delivery system in Northern California (Kaiser Permanente) estimated that the community-based incidence of non–dialysis-requiring AKI increased from 3227 to 5224 per million person-years from 1996 to 2003.[75] This is one of the few studies that have quantified temporal changes in AKI incidence on the basis of the documented abrupt changes in serum creatinine levels (albeit using an older definition of acute renal failure[69]). This study also documented that a parallel increase in incidence of dialysis-requiring AKI over the same period (from 195 to 295 per million person-years).

A number of other studies have reported that the incidence rate of AKI has increased considerably over the last decade,[76] including a 2013 study concluding that the incidence of dialysis-requiring AKI had risen by 10% per year in the United States from 2000 to 2009, with higher incidences seen in the elderly, in men, and in African Americans.[77] Other studies are outlined in Table 20.6.[78] Comparing findings among studies is not straightforward. In addition to heterogeneity in disease subtype, population, and calendar year period, studies also differ by the unit of disease frequency, which has been expressed as cases per infant delivery,[7,8] per surgical procedure,[4,5] and per hospitalization.[3,6] A large fraction of the U.S. literature turns out to be based on the same data source—the Nationwide Inpatient Sample. All but two studies relied on administrative billing codes to identify cases.[75,79] These codes, however, have been shown to be specific but quite insensitive.[80] More problematically, there is almost certainly "code creep," whereby patients are more likely to be diagnosed with milder degrees of AKI as awareness of this condition increases over time.[78,80] The reported increases in incidence of AKI thus must be interpreted with caution.

Changes in the performance characteristics of diagnostic codes may be less of a problem when the outcome is dialysis-requiring AKI, because under-ascertainment is less likely (*dialysis* here refers both to acute intermittent hemodialysis and continuous renal replacement therapy).[76,80] Figure 20.8 summarizes a number of studies from North America, Western Europe, and Australia.[77,81-90] An additional factor in the complexity of interpretation is that the threshold for initiating acute renal replacement therapy may vary by place and time. There is no strong evidence, however, that the rising incidence of AKI requiring dialysis is more liberal application of acute renal replacement therapy.[76]

The exact reasons for the increasing incidence of AKI are unclear. It may be due to an increase in the incidence of sepsis,[72,91] a dominant risk factor for AKI.[92] In addition, there may also have been more widespread use of nephrotoxic drugs or high-risk procedures, although few studies have rigorously quantified this situation.[76]

PREVALENCE

Given the relatively short duration of AKI, defining prevalence of disease is likely not a very meaningful parameter, and there are no reliable data on the population prevalence of AKI.

Table 20.5 Three Proposed Consensus Definitions for Acute Renal Failure/Acute Kidney Injury

Criteria	RIFLE	AKIN	KDIGO
Date of Release	2004	2007	2012
Baseline	Not specifically defined. If not available, serum creatinine should be back-calculated using an eGFR of 75 mL/min/1.73 m² and the MDRD equation	48-h window	Not specifically defined. If not available, lowest serum creatinine during hospitalization should be used, or SCr should be calculated using MDRD equation, assuming baseline eGFR 75 mL/min/1.73 m² when there is no evidence of CKD
Time Interval	Diagnosis and staging: within 1-7 days and sustained more than 24 h	Diagnosis within 48 h Staging: 1 week	Diagnosis: 50% increase in SCr within 7 days OR 0.3 mg/dL (26.5 µmol/L) within 48 h
Stages and Criteria	**RISK:** *Creatinine:* SCr increased to 1.5-1.9 times baseline OR GFR *Urine Output:* <0.5 mL/kg/h for 6-12 h **INJURY:** *Creatinine:* 2.0-2.9 times baseline OR GFR decreased >50% 3.0 times baseline, GFR decreased >75% OR SCr ≥4.0 mg/dL (354 µmol/L) with an acute rise of ≥0.5 mg/dL (44 µmol/L) *Urine Output:* <0.5 mL/kg/h for ≥12 h 0.3 mL/kg/h for ≥12 h OR anuria for ≥12 h	**STAGE 1:** *Creatinine:* SCr increased to 1.5-1.9 times baseline OR ≥0.3 mg/dL (≥26.5 µmol/L) increase *Urine Output:* Same as for RIFLE "Risk" category **STAGE 2:** *Creatinine:* Same as for RIFLE "Injury" category minus eGFR criteria *Urine Output:* Same as for RIFLE "Injury" category **STAGE 3:** *Creatinine:* Same as for RIFLE "Failure" category OR patient receiving RRT; eGFR criteria removed *Urine Output:* Same as for RIFLE "Failure" category	**STAGE 1:** *Creatinine:* SCr increased to 1.5-1.9 times baseline (over 7 days) OR by ≥0.3 mg/dL (≥26.5 µmol/L) increase (48 h) *Urine Output:* Same as for RIFLE "Risk" category **STAGE 2:** *Creatinine:* Same as for RIFLE "Injury" category minus eGFR criteria *Urine Output:* Same as for RIFLE "Injury" category **STAGE 3:** *Creatinine:* SCr increased to 3.0 times baseline OR by ≥4.0 mg/dL (354 µmol/L) OR initiation of RRT OR for patients <18 years, decrease in eGFR to <35 mL/min/1.73 m² *Urine Output:* Same as for RIFLE "Failure" category
	Loss Persistent ARF = complete loss of kidney function (need for dialysis >4 weeks) **ESKD** End-stage kidney disease (> 3 months)	**Loss** Notable differences: (1) Addition of 0.3 mg/dl absolute change in SCr to increase diagnostic sensitivity (2) eGFR criteria removed (3) 48-h time window to ensure acuity (also allows for inpatient baseline values) (4) Exclusion of Loss/ESKD categories as diagnostic criteria	**Loss** Notable differences: (1) Time frame differences for absolute versus relative changes in serum creatinine (2) 0.5 mg/dl increase for those with SCr ≥4.0 mg/dl (354 µmol/l) no longer required if minimum AKI threshold met (3) Inclusion of eGFR criteria for children

AKI, Acute kidney injury, AKIN, Acute Kidney injury Network; ARF, acute renal failure, eGFR, estimated glomerular filtration rate; ESKD, end-stage kidney disease; ESRD, end-stage renal disease; GFR, glomerular filtration rate; KDIGO, Kidney Disease: Improving Global Outcomes; MDRD, Modification of Diet in Renal Disease; RIFLE, Risk, Injury, Failure, Loss, and End-stage Kidney Disease; RRT, renal replacement therapy; SCr, serum creatinine.

Table 20.6 Selected Studies of Temporal Trends in Incidence of Acute Kidney Injury

Study	Population	Dataset	AKI Definition	Calendar Years	Incidence Unit	Finding	Calculated Annual Incidence Change*
Xue et al, 2006[72]	Representative sample of elderly patients in the U.S.	Medicare 5% sample	ICD-9-CM diagnosis codes	1992-2001	Per 1000 hospital discharges	AKI increased from 14.6 cases per 1000 discharges in 1992 to 36.4 cases per 1000 discharges in 2001	Increase of ≈11% annually
Waikar et al, 2006[80]	Nationally representative sample of U.S. hospitalized patients	Nationwide Inpatient Sample	ICD-9-CM diagnosis codes for AKI and with ICD-9-CM procedure code for AKI-D	1988-2002	Per 100,000 people (general population)	AKI incidence rose from 61 cases per 100,000 people in 1988 to 288 cases per 100,000 people; AKI-D incidence increased from 4 cases per 100,000 people to 27 cases per 100,000 people	Increase of ≈12% annually for AKI Increase of ≈15% annually for AKI-D
Hsu et al, 2007[75]	All patients aged at least 20 years who are members of an integrated health care delivery system	Kaiser Permanente of Northern California clinical data	Hou et al[69] serum creatinine change criteria for AKI Patients who were not undergoing maintenance dialysis on admission but who received dialysis during hospitalization were considered to have AKI-D	1996-2003	Per 100,000 person-years (general population)	AKI incidence increased from 322.7 cases per 100,000 person-years to 522.4 cases per 100,000 person-years; AKI-D incidence increased from 19.5 cases per 100,000 person-years to 29.5 cases per 100,000 person-years	Increase of ≈7% annually for AKI Increase of ≈6% annually for AKI-D
Swaminathan et al, 2007[113]	Nationally representative sample of U.S. patients who underwent CABG	Nationwide Inpatient Sample	ICD-9-CM diagnosis codes for AKI	1988-2003	Per hospital discharge post-CABG	AKI incidence increased from 1.5% to 7.2%	Increase of ≈11% annually
Liu et al, 2010[114]	All in-hospital infant deliveries in Canada (except Québec)	Discharge Abstract Database, Canadian Institute for Health Information	ICD-10CA diagnosis codes and CCI procedure codes	2003-2007	Per 10,000 deliveries	AKI incidence increased from 1.6 cases per 10,000 deliveries in 2003 to 2.3 cases per 10,000 deliveries in 2007; AKI-D incidence was 0.4 cases per 10,000 deliveries in 2003 and 0.4 cases per 10,000 deliveries in 2007	Increase of ≈10% annually for AKI No change in AKI-D incidence

Study	Population	Data Source	Case-Finding Method	Period	Unit	Incidence	Trend
Amin et al, 2012[79]	Patients admitted with AMI to 56 hospitals across the U.S.	Cerner Corporation's Health Facts database	AKIN serum creatinine change criteria[67]	2000-2008	Per AMI hospitalization	AKI incidence declined from 26.6% in 2000 to 19.7% in 2008	Decrease of ≈4% annually
Callaghan et al, 2012[115]	Nationally representative sample of U.S. infant deliveries and postpartum hospitalizations	Nationwide Inpatient Sample	ICD-9-CM diagnostic codes	1998-2009	Per 10,000 deliveries	AKI incidence increased from 2.29 cases during delivery hospitalizations per 10,000 deliveries in 1998-1999 to 4.52 cases during delivery hospitalizations per 10,000 deliveries in 2008-2009	Increase of ≈6% annually
Hsu et al, 2013[77]	Nationally representative sample of U.S. hospitalized patients	Nationwide Inpatient Sample	ICD-9-CM diagnostic and procedure codes for AKI-D	2000-2009	Per 1,000,000 person-years (general population)	AKI-D incidence increased from 222 cases per 1,000,000 person-years in 2000 to 533 cases per 1,000,000 person-years in 2009	Increase of ≈10% annually
Lenihan et al, 2013[116]	Nationally representative sample of U.S. patients who underwent either CABG using a bypass machine or open-chamber valve repair or replacement	Nationwide Inpatient Sample	ICD-9 diagnostic codes for AKI and procedure codes for AKI-D	1999-2008	Per hospital discharge for CABG or open-heart valve procedure	AKI incidence increased from 4.5% in 1999 to 12.8% in 2008; AKI-D incidence increased from 0.45% in 1999 to 1.28% in 2008	Increase of ≈12% annually for AKI Increase of ≈12% annually for AKI-D
Mehrabadi et al, 2014[117]	All in-hospital infant deliveries in Canada (except Québec)	Discharge Abstract Database, Canadian Institute for Health Information	ICD-10CA diagnostic codes for AKI	2003-2010	Per 10,000 deliveries	AKI incidence increased from 1.66 cases per 10,000 deliveries in 2003-2004 to 2.68 cases per 10,000 deliveries in 2009-2010	Increase of ≈5% annually

*Incidence calculated from unadjusted rates reported in each publication and assuming a constant rate of change over the study period.
AKI, Acute kidney injury; AKI-D, AKI requiring dialysis; AMI, acute myocardial infarction; AKIN, AKI Network; CABG, coronary artery bypass grafting; CCI, Canadian Classification of Health Interventions; ICD-9, International Classification of Diseases, 9th Revision; ICD-9-CM, International Classification of Diseases, 9th Revision, Clinical Modification; ICD-10CA, International Statistical Classification of Diseases and Related Health Problems, 10th Revision, Canada.
Modified slightly from Lunn MR, Obedin-Maliver J, Hsu CY: Increasing incidence of AKI: also a problem in pregnancy? Am J Kidney Dis 2015 Jan 7. pii: S0272-6386(14)01443-7.

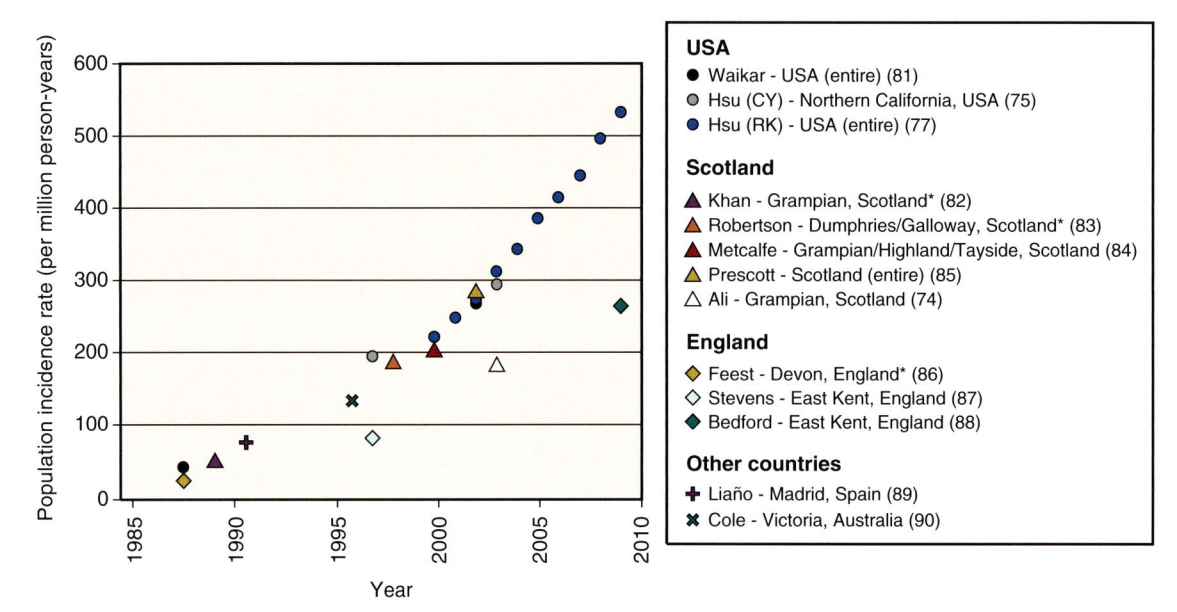

Figure 20.8 Population incidence rate of dialysis-requiring acute kidney injury over time and in different regions around the world. *For studies that estimated a single incidence rate for a multiyear period, only a single point is shown (at the midpoint of the study period). (Data are from references 74, 75, 77, and 81-90, as indicated in list.)

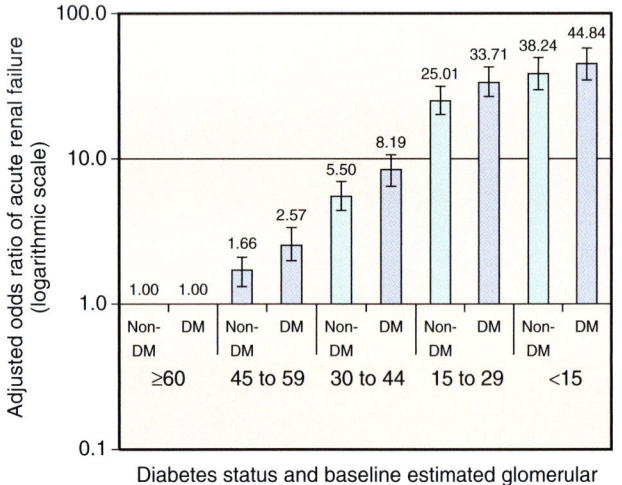

Figure 20.9 Baseline severity of chronic kidney disease (CKD) and risk of dialysis-requiring acute kidney injury (AKI). Among both patients with and patients without diabetes, there was a strong association between level of pre-admission estimated glomerular filtration rate (eGFR) and risk of AKI, which was evident at an eGFR as high as 60 mL/min/1.73 m². Each model was adjusted for age, sex, race/ethnicity, diagnosed hypertension, and documented proteinuria. (From Hsu CY, Ordonez JD, Chertow GM, et al: The risk of acute renal failure in patients with chronic kidney disease. *Kidney Int* 74:101-107, 2008.)

LINKING ACUTE, CHRONIC, AND END-STAGE KIDNEY DISEASE

A number of studies have defined linkages among the epidemiologic patterns of AKI, CKD, and ESKD.

First, although it has been well known that CKD is a strong (probably the strongest) risk factor for AKI, this relationship has only lately been quantified rigorously. It turns out that even patients with only stage "3a" CKD (eGFR 45-59 mL/min/1.73 m²) are at nearly twice the risk for AKI compared with patients with eGFR 60 mL/min/1.73 m² or greater.[93] And at every GFR value, patients with diabetes had higher risk than those without it (Figure 20.9).[93] Furthermore, it appears that even low-grade proteinuria (in the microalbuminuria range or below)[94] is a risk factor for AKI.[95]

Second, data have now shown that episodes of severe AKI accelerate development or progression of CKD.[96] For example, one study demonstrated that among patients with dialysis-requiring AKI who had baseline Stage 3b or worse CKD (preadmission eGFR 15-44 mL/min/1.73 m²) approximately half of the survivors went on to have ESKD because they did not recover sufficient renal function to stop dialysis.[97] For patients with baseline preadmission GFR values of 45 mL/min/1.73 m² or higher, dialysis-requiring AKI was independently associated with a 28-fold increase in the risk for development of stage 4 or 5 CKD in the subsequent months to years.[98] A number of epidemiology studies have also shown that even milder degrees of AKI are associated with more rapid subsequent loss of renal function.[99-102] Although there are plausible animal models demonstrating pathophysiologic pathways for this association,[103] some of it is likely due to confounding by shared risk factors for AKI and CKD, such as diabetes mellitus.[104] Analysis of a 2014 randomized trial showed that reduction of mild to moderate AKI after cardiac surgery failed to reduce loss of kidney function at 1 year.[105]

CONCLUSION

Much progress has been made in the past decade and a half with regard to defining the epidemiology of kidney disease. Although the field was traditionally dominated by ESKD epidemiology, a large amount of attention is now being paid to the prevalence and distribution of CKD, and ongoing investigations into the population epidemiology of AKI will fill important gaps in our knowledge.

Complete reference list available at ExpertConsult.com.

KEY REFERENCES

2. US Renal Data System: *USRDS 2013 annual data report: atlas of chronic kidney disease and end-stage renal disease in the United States*, Bethesda, MD, 2013, National Institutes of Health, National Institute of Diabetes and Digestive and Kidney Diseases. Available at http://www.usrds.org. Accessed May 31, 2014.
7. Lewis EJ, Hunsicker LG, Bain RP, et al: The effect of angiotensin-converting-enzyme inhibition on diabetic nephropathy. *N Engl J Med* 329:1456–1462, 1993.
8. Finne P, Reunanen A, Stenman S, et al: Incidence of end-stage renal disease in patients with type 1 diabetes. *JAMA* 294:1782–1787, 2005.
11. Hsu CY: Does non-malignant hypertension cause renal insufficiency? Evidence-based perspective. *Curr Opin Nephrol Hypertens* 11:267–272, 2002.
13. Genovese G, Friedman DJ, Ross MD, et al: Association of trypanolytic ApoL1 variants with kidney disease in African Americans. *Science* 329:841–845, 2010.
15. Parsa A, Kao WH, Xie D, et al: APOL1 risk variants, race, and progression of chronic kidney disease. *N Engl J Med* 369:2183–2196, 2013.
16. Brancati FL, Whelton PK, Randall BL, et al: Risk of end-stage renal disease in diabetes mellitus: a prospective cohort study of men screened for MRFIT. *JAMA* 278:2069–2074, 1997.
17. Robinson BM, Joffe MM, Pisoni RL, et al: Revisiting survival differences by race and ethnicity among hemodialysis patients: the Dialysis Outcomes and Practice Patterns Study. *J Am Soc Nephrol* 17:2910–2918, 2006.
20. Robinson BM, Zhang J, Morgenstern H, et al: Worldwide, mortality risk is high soon after initiation of hemodialysis. *Kidney Int* 85:158–165, 2014.
21. Foley RN, Chen SC, Solid CA, et al: Early mortality in patients starting dialysis appears to go unregistered. *Kidney Int* 86:392–398, 2014.
22. Eknoyan G, Beck GJ, Cheung AK, et al: Effect of dialysis dose and membrane flux in maintenance hemodialysis. *N Engl J Med* 347:2010–2019, 2002.
25. Kalantar-Zadeh K, Block G, Humphreys MH, et al: Reverse epidemiology of cardiovascular risk factors in maintenance dialysis patients. *Kidney Int* 63:793–808, 2003.
26. Liu Y, Coresh J, Eustace JA, et al: Association between cholesterol level and mortality in dialysis patients: role of inflammation and malnutrition. *JAMA* 291:451–459, 2004.
29. Li Z, Lacson E, Jr, Lowrie EG, et al: The epidemiology of systolic blood pressure and death risk in hemodialysis patients. *Am J Kidney Dis* 48:606–615, 2006.
30. Alborzi P, Patel N, Agarwal R: Home blood pressures are of greater prognostic value than hemodialysis unit recordings. *Clin J Am Soc Nephro* 2:1228–1234, 2007.
32. Bansal N, McCulloch CE, Rahman M, et al: Blood pressure and risk of all-cause mortality in advanced chronic kidney disease and hemodialysis: the Chronic Renal Insufficiency Cohort study. *Hypertension* 65:93–100, 2015.
33. Baigent C, Landray MJ, Reith C, et al: The effects of lowering LDL cholesterol with simvastatin plus ezetimibe in patients with chronic kidney disease (Study of Heart and Renal Protection): a randomised placebo-controlled trial. *Lancet* 377:2181–2192, 2011.
34. Wanner C, Krane V, Marz W, et al: Atorvastatin in patients with type 2 diabetes mellitus undergoing hemodialysis. *N Engl J Med* 353:238–248, 2005.
35. Fellstrom BC, Jardine AG, Schmieder RE, et al: Rosuvastatin and cardiovascular events in patients undergoing hemodialysis. *N Engl J Med* 360:1395–1407, 2009.
37. Tomson CRV: Blood pressure and outcome in patients on dialysis. *The Lancet* 373:981–982, 2009.
38. Wolfe RA, Ashby VB, Milford EL, et al: Comparison of mortality in all patients on dialysis, patients on dialysis awaiting transplantation, and recipients of a first cadaveric transplant. *N Engl J Med* 341:1725–1730, 1999.
43. Foley RN, Hakim RM: Why is the mortality of dialysis patients in the United States much higher than the rest of the world? *J Am Soc Nephrol* 20:1432–1435, 2009.
44. National Kidney Foundation: K/DOQI clinical practice guidelines for chronic kidney disease: evaluation, classification, and stratification. *Am J Kidney Dis* 39:S1–S266, 2002.
45. Levey AS, de Jong PE, Coresh J, et al: The definition, classification, and prognosis of chronic kidney disease: a KDIGO Controversies Conference report. *Kidney Int* 80:17–28, 2011.
47. Levey AS, Coresh J, Greene T, et al: Using standardized serum creatinine values in the Modification of Diet in Renal Disease study equation for estimating glomerular filtration rate. *Ann Intern Med* 145:247–254, 2006.
48. Levey AS, Stevens LA, Schmid CH, et al: A new equation to estimate glomerular filtration rate. *Ann Intern Med* 150:604–612, 2009.
49. Inker LA, Schmid CH, Tighiouart H, et al: Estimating glomerular filtration rate from serum creatinine and cystatin C. *N Engl J Med* 367:20–29, 2012.
50. Hsu RK, Hsu CY: Temporal trends in prevalence of CKD: the glass is half full and not half empty. *Am J Kidney Dis* 62:214–216, 2013.
56. Go AS, Chertow GM, Fan D, et al: Chronic kidney disease and the risks of death, cardiovascular events, and hospitalization. *N Engl J Med* 351:1296–1305, 2004.
59. Brenner BM, Cooper ME, de Zeeuw D, et al: Effects of losartan on renal and cardiovascular outcomes in patients with type 2 diabetes and nephropathy. *N Engl J Med* 345:861–869, 2001.
60. Lewis EJ, Hunsicker LG, Clarke WR, et al: Renoprotective effect of the angiotensin-receptor antagonist irbesartan in patients with nephropathy due to type 2 diabetes. *N Engl J Med* 345:851–860, 2001.
63. Hsu CY, Lin F, Vittinghoff E, et al: Racial differences in the progression from chronic renal insufficiency to end-stage renal disease in the United States. *J Am Soc Nephrol* 14:2902–2907, 2003.
68. Kidney Disease Improving Global Outcomes (KDIGO) Acute Kidney Injury Work Group: KDIGO clinical practice guideline for acute kidney injury. *Kidney Int Suppl* 2:1–138, 2012.
69. Hou SH, Bushinsky DA, Wish JB, et al: Hospital-acquired renal insufficiency: a prospective study. *Am J Med* 74:243–248, 1983.
75. Hsu CY, McCulloch CE, Fan D, et al: Community-based incidence of acute renal failure. *Kidney Int* 72:208–212, 2007.
76. Siew ED, Davenport A: The growth of acute kidney injury: a rising tide or just closer attention to detail? *Kidney Int* 87:46–61, 2015.
77. Hsu RK, McCulloch CE, Dudley RA, et al: Temporal changes in incidence of dialysis-requiring AKI. *J Am Soc Nephrol* 24:37–42, 2013.
81. Waikar S, Curhan G, Wald R, et al: Declining mortality in patients with acute renal failure, 1988 to 2002. *J Am Soc Nephrol* 17:1143–1150, 2006.
93. Hsu CY, Ordonez JD, Chertow GM, et al: The risk of acute renal failure in patients with chronic kidney disease. *Kidney Int* 74:101–107, 2008.
94. Grams ME, Astor BC, Bash LD, et al: Albuminuria and estimated glomerular filtration rate independently associate with acute kidney injury. *J Am Soc Nephrol* 21:1757–1764, 2010.
95. Hsu RK, Hsu CY: Proteinuria and reduced glomerular filtration rate as risk factors for acute kidney injury. *Curr Opin Nephrol Hypertens* 20:211–217, 2011.
96. Wald R, Quinn RR, Luo J, et al: Chronic dialysis and death among survivors of acute kidney injury requiring dialysis. *JAMA* 302:1179–1185, 2009.
97. Hsu CY, Chertow GM, McCulloch CE, et al: Non-recovery of kidney function and death after acute on chronic renal failure. *Clin J Am Soc Nephrol* 4:891–898, 2009.
98. Lo LJ, Go AS, Chertow GM, et al: Dialysis-requiring acute renal failure increases the risk of progressive chronic kidney disease. *Kidney Int* 76:893–899, 2009.
99. Coca SG, Singanamala S, Parikh CR: Chronic kidney disease after acute kidney injury: a systematic review and meta-analysis. *Kidney Int* 81:442–448, 2012.

101. Ishani A, Xue JL, Himmelfarb J, et al: Acute kidney injury increases risk of ESRD among elderly. *J Am Soc Nephrol* 20:223–228, 2009.
105. Garg AX, Devereaux PJ, Yusuf S, et al: Kidney function after off-pump or on-pump coronary artery bypass graft surgery: a randomized clinical trial. *JAMA* 311:2191–2198, 2014.
106. Hsu CY, Vittinghoff E, Lin F, et al: The incidence of end-stage renal disease is increasing faster than the prevalence of chronic renal insufficiency. *Ann Intern Med* 141:95–101, 2004.
108. Coresh J, Selvin E, Stevens L, et al: Prevalence of chronic kidney disease in the United States. *JAMA* 298:2038–2047, 2007.
110. Foley RN, Wang C, Snydbber JJ, et al: Cystatin C levels in U.S. adults, 1988-1994 versus 1999-2002: NHANES. *Clin J Am Soc Nephrol: CJASN* 4:965–972, 2009.

Demographics of Kidney Disease

21

Amanda Hyre Anderson | Jeffrey S. Berns |
F. Perry Wilson | Harold I. Feldman

CHAPTER OUTLINE

SEX AND CHRONIC KIDNEY
DISEASE, 655
  Factors Related to Sex Differences, 657
  Oral Contraceptives, Hormone Replacement
  Therapy, and Kidney Disease, 659
  Summary, 660
RACE, ETHNICITY, AND CHRONIC KIDNEY
DISEASE, 660
  Defining Race and Ethnicity, 660
  Factors Related to Race and Ethnicity, 660

  Potential Mechanisms of Racial and Ethnic
  Disparities, 662
  Summary, 663
SOCIOECONOMIC FACTORS AND
CHRONIC KIDNEY DISEASE, 663
  Socioeconomic Exposures, 663
  Relationship to Socioeconomic Factors, 664
  Summary, 666
CONCLUSION, 666

Chronic kidney disease (CKD) prevalence in the United States has increased over the past decade, with 10% of the population having CKD stages 1 to 4 in 1994 compared to 13.1% in 2004, a trend only partly accounted for by the increased prevalence of diabetes and obesity.[1] In addition, this increased prevalence of CKD has translated into a 32.4% increase in years of life lost between 1990 and 2010 on a U.S. population basis.[2] Worldwide, the incidence of CKD has risen as well. A recent sampling of Chinese individuals found that 1.7% had an estimated glomerular filtration rate (eGFR) lower than 60 mL/min/1.73 m^2 and 9.4% had albuminuria, translating into an estimated 119.5 million individuals with CKD in that country alone.[3] Worldwide incidence and prevalence estimates are presented in Figure 21.1 and reflect generally higher rates of CKD in industrialized nations.[4] Patterns in the prevalence, incidence, and progression of chronic kidney disease vary by certain demographic characteristics, including sex, race and ethnicity, and socioeconomic status. This chapter will summarize what is known of these patterns, highlight consistent findings across sociodemographic groups, speculate on the genesis of variations across demographic groups, and highlight questions that still remain pertaining to kidney outcomes among these populations.

SEX AND CHRONIC KIDNEY DISEASE

Differences between men and women in the incidence and prevalence of various kidney diseases and rate of kidney disease progression may be influenced by sex differences in glomerular mass, responses to hormones, cytokines, apoptosis, vasoactive, and other soluble circulating factors, and differences in the responses to aging and reductions in nephron mass. Women have been reported, on average, to have approximately 10% to 15% fewer glomeruli than men, but this is thought to be a function primarily of birth weight and body surface area (BSA) rather than sex.[5-8] Glomerular volume tends to be similar in men and women.[5,7] The glomerular filtration rate (GFR) is also similar in men and women when corrected for BSA and muscle mass.[9-14] However, some have reported a somewhat lower BSA-adjusted GFR in women.[15] Thus, although some subtle differences in renal mass and structure have been reported in men compared to women, these are probably of little or no clinical significance and are more likely related to factors other than sex.

Experimental animal models and human studies have described sex differences and sex hormone influences in the synthesis and plasma levels of, and biologic responses to, a variety of circulating factors involved in the regulation of normal renal function. These same factors may also be involved in responses to renal injury and susceptibility to kidney disease. Some of these include angiotensinogen, angiotensin II, prorenin, renin, angiotensin-converting enzyme (ACE), and angiotensin receptor expression. Sex differences have also been reported in nitric oxide and prostaglandin synthesis and responsiveness, lipid oxidation and oxidative stress, mesangial cell collagen synthesis and degradation, responses to transforming growth factor-β (TGF-β) and tumor necrosis factor-α (TNF-α), as well as in apoptotic and profibrotic signaling pathways.[16-18] High

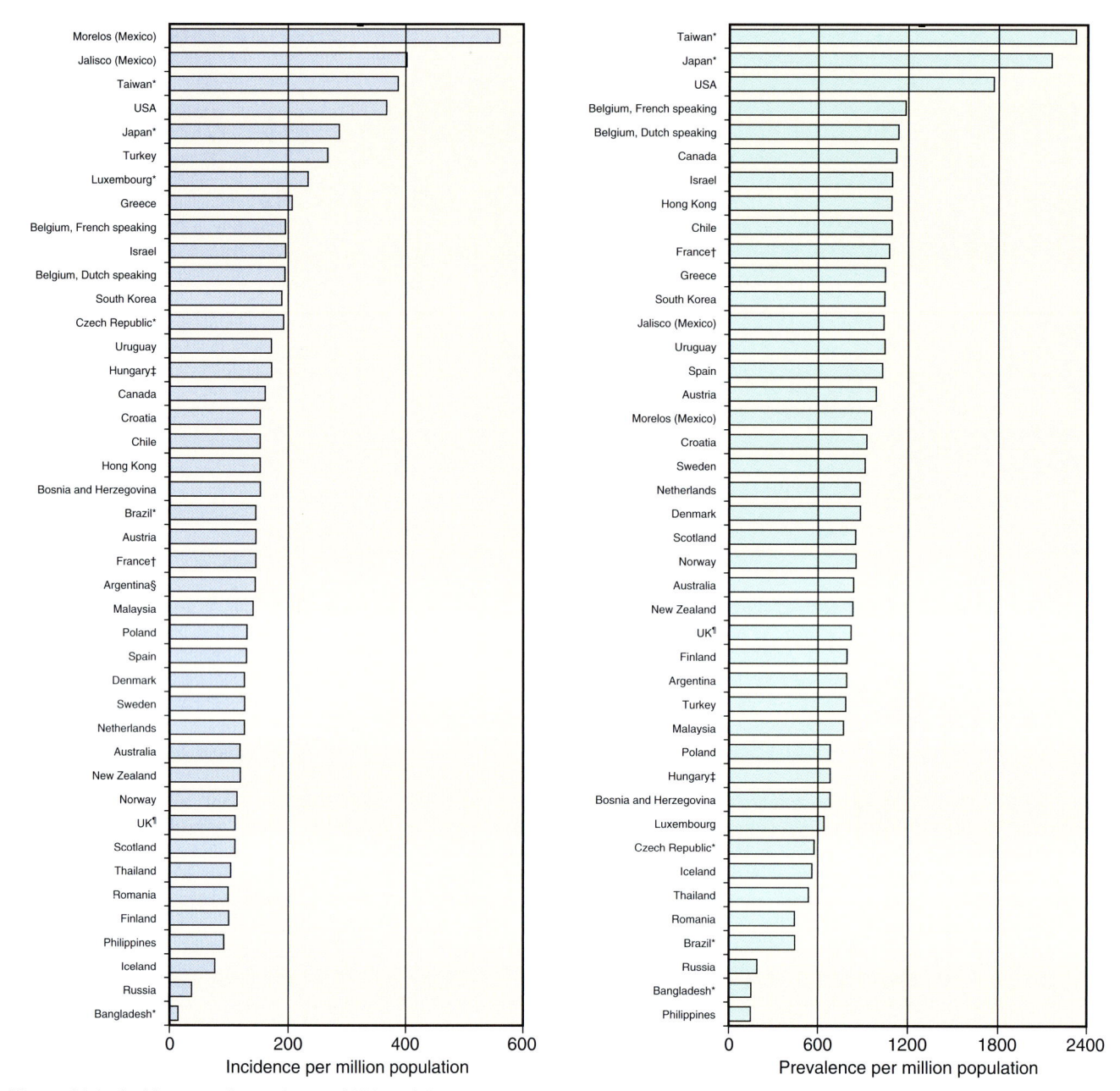

Figure 21.1 Incidence and prevalence of kidney failure treated by dialysis or transplantation (end-stage kidney disease) in 2008. Data are only for countries for which relevant information was available. All rates are unadjusted. Average survival with treated kidney failure in each country can be computed from the ratio of prevalence to incidence. *Data from Bangladesh, Brazil, Czech Republic, Japan, Luxembourg, and Taiwan are dialysis-only. †Data for France are from 13 regions in 2005, 15 in 2006, 18 in 2007, and 20 in 2008. ‡Latest data for Hungary are from 2007. §Data for Argentina from before 2008 are dialysis only. ¶UK—England, Wales, and Northern Ireland. (Reprinted with permission from Levery AS, Coresh J: Chronic kidney disease. *Lancet* 379:165-180, 2012.)

adiponectin levels have also been reported to predict CKD progression in men, but not in women.[19] Estradiol has been identified as having various effects on mesangial cells.[20-23] Neither androgens nor estrogens directly influence GFR or renal blood flow in humans.[24,25] The extent to which any of these factors are specifically and causally related to sex differences in kidney function or kidney disease incidence and progression is still uncertain.

The incidence rate of end-stage kidney disease (ESKD) in the United States is approximately 60% higher among men compared to women,[26] whereas the estimated prevalence of moderate (i.e., stages 3 and 4) CKD is higher among women (8.0% in women vs. 5.4% in men).[12] A recent Canadian study demonstrated similar rates of CKD by sex, however.[27] A large international meta-analysis of more than 2 million individuals with CKD revealed that men with CKD had higher absolute risks of death and cardiovascular disease than women, whereas women had a steeper relationship of these outcomes with levels of eGFR.[28]

FACTORS RELATED TO SEX DIFFERENCES

GLOMERULAR DISEASE INCIDENCE AND PREVALENCE

Research assessments of glomerular disease incidence and prevalence in adults are made difficult because of uncertainty about the population base from which these figures are derived, variations in study participants' ages, and varying indications for kidney biopsy. The overall incidence of primary glomerular diseases among residents of Olmsted County, Minnesota, a primarily white population, has been estimated based on kidney biopsy records to be 7.9/100,000 person-years in men and 5.4/100,000 person-years in women.[29] A study from France reported a prevalence of primary glomerular disease of 8.2/1000 men and 5.1/1000 women during a 27-year period ending in 2002.[30] Men tend to predominate in many series of adult patients with focal segmental glomerulosclerosis (FSGS) and immunoglobulin A (IgA) nephropathy, with a more variable sex mix for adults with minimal change disease and membranous nephropathy.[31-37]

PROGRESSION OF CHRONIC KIDNEY DISEASE

There is a paucity of data examining the effects of sex on CKD progression at the population level. A study by Eriksen and Ingebretsen examined a total of 3047 patients from a municipality in Norway and found that the rate of CKD progression was significantly slower among women.[38] This study, which also reported a lower aggregate rate of kidney disease progression than is commonly seen in other industrialized nations, also revealed that women had better renal and patient survival. A study that modeled CKD incidence based on prevalence data also found lower rates of progression to ESKD among U.S. women.[39]

Several more recent meta-analyses have also considered sex influences on kidney disease progression from a variety of underlying causes. Jafar and associates performed a patient-level meta-analysis using a pooled database for patients with nondiabetic kidney disease from 11 prospective randomized controlled trials of ACE inhibitors for slowing progression.[40] Using doubling of serum creatinine levels or onset of ESKD as a composite primary end point, they concluded that the risk of kidney disease progression was not different in men and women in an unadjusted analysis, but that the risk was actually higher in women than men after adjustment for baseline variables, including urine protein excretion and treatment assignment (relative risk [RR], 1.30 to 1.36, depending on the model). They noted that most of the women in these trials were of postmenopausal age, limiting their applicability to younger premenopausal women.

Several additional studies considering sex influences on kidney disease progression have also been published. Two large population-based studies reported a more favorable prognosis for women compared to men with CKD in Norway and Sweden.[38,41] The Modification of Diet in Renal Disease (MDRD) study, which enrolled patients with autosomal dominant polycystic kidney disease (ADPKD), glomerulonephritis, or other nondiabetic kidney diseases, reported the rate of kidney disease progression to be slower in women compared to men, particularly among younger premenopausal women.[42] This difference was markedly diminished and no longer statistically significant after adjustment for level of proteinuria and blood pressure. A more recent report of the MDRD study participants' long-term outcomes also found similar kidney failure event rates for men and women.[43]

PROGRESSION OF PRIMARY GLOMERULAR DISEASE

The prognosis—that is, the rate of progression of the underlying kidney disease—is generally considered to be worse in men than in women with membranous nephropathy, IgA nephropathy, FSGS, and lupus nephritis.[31,32,38,41,44-49] However, studies using multivariable analysis to evaluate the effect of sex on kidney disease progression have produced variable findings.[44,45,50-54] Although none have found female gender to be associated with more rapid kidney disease progression, the often cited association of male gender with more rapid disease progression has been inconsistent. Much of this literature was analyzed in a recent meta-analysis by Neugarten and coworkers.[44] This meta-analysis considered eight studies, including over 2000 patients with nondiabetic "chronic kidney disease" for which no specific cause was identified, and concluded that kidney disease progression was statistically significantly associated with male gender (Figure 21.2).[44,45,50-52,55-57] Among five studies excluded from this analysis because of incomplete reporting of effect size,[53,58-61] two found that kidney disease progression was more rapid in men, whereas three found no sex difference. Although not assessed in this meta-analysis, other studies have reported that the more favorable rate of progression in women is limited to the premenopausal period.[42,45]

An association between male gender and progression of IgA nephropathy was demonstrated in the meta-analysis by Neugarten and colleagues, with 25 studies and over 3000 patients (Figure 21.3).[44,62-83] Of these 25 studies, 21 found more rapid progression in men. In all but a few of the studies in this meta-analysis, however, the association was not statistically significant. In addition, several studies suggested that men had better outcomes. Of 13 studies that were excluded from this meta-analysis because of the inability to calculate effect size, 12 found no sex differences.[84-95] Combined, these data suggest that any association between sex and IgA nephropathy progression is likely to be weak.

Among 21 studies of almost 1900 patients with membranous nephropathy considered in the Neugarten and associates' meta-analysis,[44,96-115] male gender was significantly associated with disease progression (Figure 21.4). However, five excluded studies (because of inability to calculate effect sizes) reported no sex association with progression.[116-120] Other older, pooled analyses have also reported an association of male gender with poorer renal outcomes for membranous nephropathy.[121,122]

Cattran and coworkers analyzed outcomes from over 1300 patients enrolled in the Toronto Glomerulonephritis Registry with membranous nephropathy, FSGS, and IgA nephropathy.[48] After adjusting for blood pressure and proteinuria, disease progression and renal survival rates were not different between men and women, except among those with levels of proteinuria more than 7 g/day in which men had more rapid loss of GFR than women. Disease progression has also been found to be similar for men and women with IgA nephropathy in most other studies.[62,63,83,89,91,92,95,123]

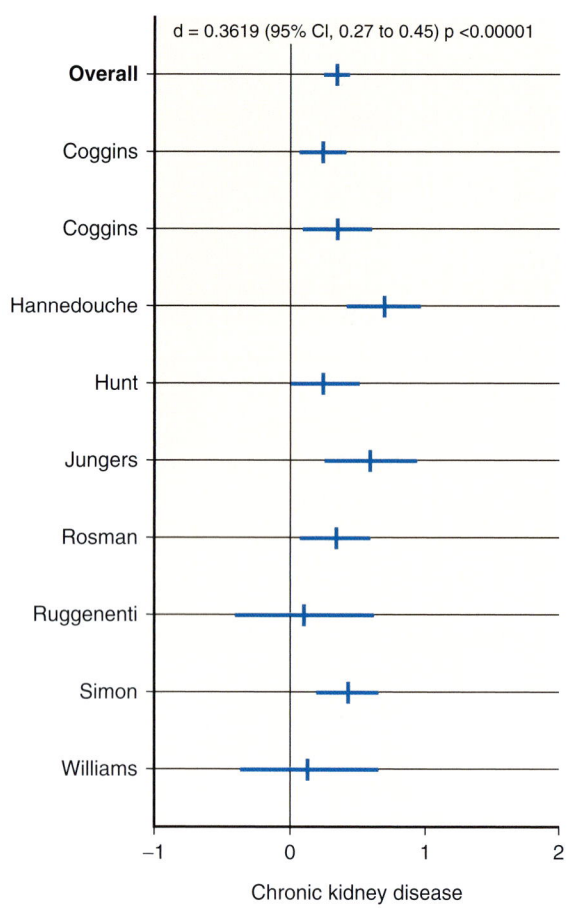

Figure 21.2 Effect size and 95% confidence interval (CI) for individual studies of the effect of sex on the progression of chronic kidney disease of mixed causes. **Top,** Overall mean effect size and 95% CI. A positive value indicates that male gender is associated with an adverse renal outcome. (Reprinted with permission from Neugarten J, Acharya A, Silbiger SR: Effect of gender on the progression of nondiabetic renal disease: a meta-analysis. J Am Soc Nephrol 11:319-329, 2000.)

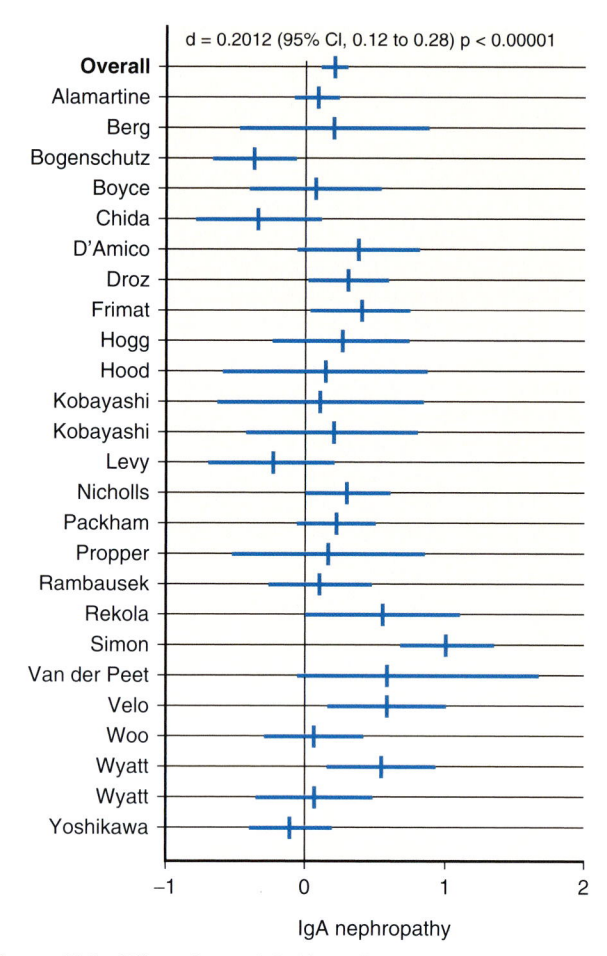

Figure 21.3 Effect size and 95% confidence interval (CI) for individual studies of the effect of sex on the progression of IgA nephropathy. **Top,** Overall mean effect size and 95% CI. A positive value indicates that male gender is associated with an adverse renal outcome. (Reprinted with permission from Neugarten J, Acharya A, Silbiger SR: Effect of gender on the progression of nondiabetic renal disease: a meta-analysis. J Am Soc Nephrol 11:319-329, 2000.)

LUPUS NEPHRITIS PROGRESSION

Recent studies of sex influences on lupus nephritis outcomes in adults have reported discrepant findings[124-129] but were limited by small numbers of patients, variable outcome measures, and varying assessment of other covariates such as histopathologic disease class, proteinuria, blood pressure, and immunosuppressive treatment.

AUTOSOMAL DOMINANT POLYCYSTIC KIDNEY DISEASE PROGRESSION

In the meta-analysis by Neugarten and colleagues mentioned above,[44] of 12 studies with over 3000 patients with ADPKD,[130-141] there was an apparent small protective effect of male gender on disease progression (Figure 21.5). However, this conclusion was largely the result of inclusion of a single Italian study that reported a highly statistically significant favorable association with male gender and disease progression.[140] Excluding this study resulted in the finding of a statistically significant association of male gender and more rapid progression, an effect seen in 10 of 12 studies (although all four excluded studies found no sex association with disease progression).[142-145] More recent studies published since this meta-analysis have suggested that male gender is likely a risk factor for progression of CKD and ESKD in patients with ADPKD.[146-150] Among two recent reports of magnetic resonance imaging of kidney and cyst growth, only one found male gender to be associated with more rapid growth.[151,152]

It is worth noting that the association between ADPKD genotype and progression of kidney disease appears to interact with sex. Sex does not appear to influence renal outcomes significantly in the more common variant of ADPKD caused by mutation in the polycystin 1 gene.[150,153,154] In contrast, women with ADPKD caused by mutations in the polycystin 2 gene tend to have more favorable renal outcomes compared to men.[154,155] The biologic basis for this difference is not presently known.

DIABETIC NEPHROPATHY PROGRESSION

Influences of sex hormones on diabetes and diabetic nephropathy have been reviewed in detail.[156] There are relatively few data on the association of sex with rate of

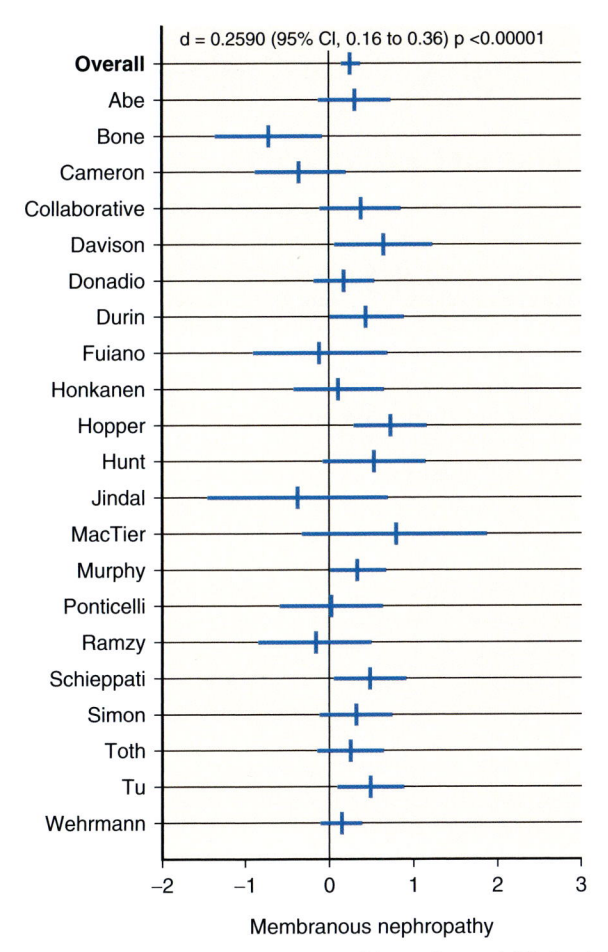

Figure 21.4 Effect size and 95% confidence interval (CI) for individual studies of the effect of sex on the progression of membranous nephropathy. **Top,** Overall mean effect size and 95% CI. A positive value indicates that male gender is associated with an adverse renal outcome. (Reprinted with permission from Neugarten J, Acharya A, Silbiger SR: Effect of gender on the progression of nondiabetic renal disease: a meta-analysis. *J Am Soc Nephrol* 11:319-329, 2000.)

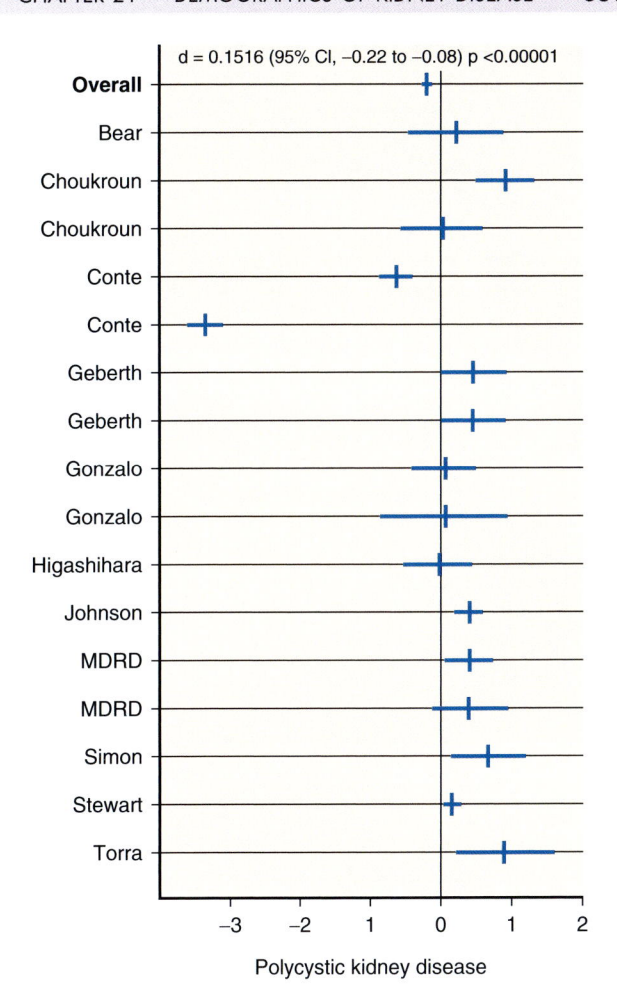

Figure 21.5 Effect size and 95% confidence interval (CI) for individual studies of the effect of sex on the progression of autosomal dominant polycystic kidney disease. **Top,** Overall mean effect size and 95% CI. A negative value indicates that female gender is associated with an adverse renal outcome. (Reprinted with permission from Neugarten J, Acharya A, Silbiger SR: Effect of gender on the progression of nondiabetic renal disease: a meta-analysis. *J Am Soc Nephrol* 11:319-329, 2000.)

progression of diabetic nephropathy, and the studies that have been performed reported inconsistent findings.[157-168] Girls with type 1 diabetes are more likely to develop moderately increased albuminuria during puberty than boys, and there tends to be a more rapid loss of GFR following puberty in women compared to men.[158,164,167] Among adults with childhood-onset type 1 diabetes mellitus (T1DM), several studies have suggested that males have a greater likelihood of developing albuminuria and, among those with diabetic nephropathy, the rate of decline in GFR is faster.[157,160,168-173] One study found that compared to men, women with T1DM are more likely to develop diabetic nephropathy while under good metabolic control, a sex effect that was attenuated in the setting of poor metabolic control.[165] Other studies have not found an independent adverse influence of male gender on rate of progression of diabetic kidney disease.[157,158,164,165,167,174]

A large U.S. study of 10,290 patients with type 2 diabetes mellitus (T2DM) has shown that male gender is associated with a greater risk of progression than female gender in those with microalbuminuria but not in those who had macroalbuminuria or no albuminuria.[175] The percentage of men and women with diabetic nephropathy starting dialysis is similar, although recent data from the U.S. Renal Data System (USRDS) have indicated that the incidence of ESKD is slightly higher among white men with T2DM compared to white women.[26] Studies have also suggested a greater incidence and prevalence of microalbuminuria and macroalbuminuria in white men compared to white women, with the opposite sex predilection among blacks.[156,176-179] Some studies have reported similar rates of disease progression and risk for development of renal end points, including ESKD across sexes.[156,176-185]

ORAL CONTRACEPTIVES, HORMONE REPLACEMENT THERAPY, AND KIDNEY DISEASE

Few studies have examined the influence of oral contraceptives and hormone replacement therapy (HRT) on kidney function in women, with and without recognized kidney disease. Oral contraceptives have been associated with a higher prevalence of microalbuminuria in women with diabetic nephropathy in some[186,187] but not other studies.[188] One study found a greater risk associated with higher estrogen strength and longer term use (>5 years).[187] Oral contraceptives have also been associated with a higher risk of microalbuminuria and decline of GFR in premenopausal women without CKD.[189]

In a small, short-term prospective study, administration of a combination of estradiol and norgestrel for 3.5 months to 16 postmenopausal women with diabetes mellitus and hypertension was associated with a statistically significant reduction in mean level of proteinuria from 452 to 370 mg/day and increase in creatinine clearance from 100.8 to 106.2 mL/min.[190] In a community-based case-control study, postmenopausal HRT was associated with a twofold higher odds ratio (OR) for microalbuminuria after adjustment for several clinical variables.[187] The OR for microalbuminuria was similar among women receiving HRT with and without progestins. The association between HRT use and microalbuminuria was limited to women using HRT for longer than 5 years. In contrast, in another study, postmenopausal HRT was associated with a lower mean urine albumin-to-creatinine ratio and a lower prevalence of microalbuminuria at a baseline examination and after 5 years of follow-up.[191]

More recently, Ahmed and colleagues studied almost 6000 postmenopausal women for over 2 years to examine the effect of HRT on the eGFR using the abbreviated MDRD equation.[192] After adjustment for age, diabetes, other comorbidities, and baseline eGFR, it was found that HRT use is associated with a more rapid decline in eGFR and a 19% greater risk for eGFR to fall by 4 mL/min/1.73 m^2/yr or more. The higher rate of eGFR decline and risk of rapid GFR loss were limited to users of estrogen-only HRT; use of combined or progestin-only HRT was not associated with a decline in eGFR. There was also a linear relationship between cumulative dose of estrogen and decline in mean eGFR. In contrast, a smaller study of 443 patients with 10 years of follow-up demonstrated no association between postmenopausal estrogen use and decline in GFR.[193] Thus, although women are considered to be at less risk for development and progression of many types of kidney disease, the influences of menopausal status and hormonal replacement have not been thoroughly investigated. The findings of Ahmed and associates[192] need to be further explored with consideration of factors not evaluated in that study, such as blood pressure, level of proteinuria, and obesity, before concluding with any certainty that oral estrogen-based HRT accelerates the progression of CKD.

SUMMARY

Patterns of the incidence of kidney disease across sexes are generally consistent, with higher rates occurring in men compared to women. Similarly, men are reported to have greater rates of progression of nondiabetic CKD for some specific types of kidney disease, especially compared to premenopausal women. More investigation into rates of progression of IgA nephropathy, lupus nephritis, and ADPKD across sexes and of overall progression rates in postmenopausal women is warranted. Additional study of the effects of HRT in women on the incidence and progression of kidney disease is also needed.

RACE, ETHNICITY, AND CHRONIC KIDNEY DISEASE

DEFINING RACE AND ETHNICITY

Population genetics studies have refuted the existence of biologic races in human populations; nevertheless, the term is still used widely in medicine in relation to continental population ancestry.[194,195] The use of race classifications in medicine and epidemiology has been the subject of much debate, mainly because of the many ways this information can be captured and interpreted. Nonetheless, classifying race and ethnicity in biomedical research facilitates several important activities, including the characterization of health statistics, risk of adverse health outcomes, and examination of delivery of health care services across subpopulations. Also, these classifications can be used as a proxy for unmeasured biologic and social factors.[196]

The utility of describing race and ethnicity and relating it to outcomes of interest lies in the ability to capture information about differences in genetics and biology, behavior, exposure to environmental factors, and social and physical environments. However, the imperfect nature of the relationship between race and these factors highlights the importance of supplementing race and ethnicity data, when possible, with those on individual-level factors that are often meant to be represented by race. To reflect factors related to social, cultural, and physical environments and exposures most accurately, individual race and ethnicity is often self-designated. This approach to classification was first adopted by the U.S. Census Bureau in 1960, followed by the opportunity to self-designate Hispanic ethnicity in 1970 and finally, in 2000, the ability to designate more than one race category.[197,198] The increasing percentage of the U.S. population that can trace its roots to multiracial or multiethnic sources has motivated researchers and demographers to collect and analyze self-designated racial and ethnic data so as to reflect this racial and ethnic admixture. However, limited knowledge of ancestry, and the large and increasing frequency of migration, creates additional challenges for valid race classification. Despite these limitations, when race is used as an explanatory factor to represent genetic and biologic determinants of disease, self-designated race may be informative as long as there is enough additional information on important socioeconomic, behavioral, and physical environment factors. Finally, it has been suggested that ethnic groups that share a unique history, language, customs, ancestry, geography, religion, and/or specific genetic markers should replace traditional race classifications in biomedical research.[199-201] However, these approaches may limit the usefulness of race as an explanatory factor in research and may not be suitable across all types of investigations.

FACTORS RELATED TO RACE AND ETHNICITY

INCIDENCE OF CHRONIC KIDNEY DISEASE

An emphasis on defining and investigating CKD prior to dependence on dialysis has only emerged in more recent years. National guidelines were first established in 2002 to define and stage prevalent CKD.[202] To date, no such guidance has been provided to define and capture information on the incidence of CKD nationally or in the research setting. To address the lack of national data on the burden, awareness, risk factors, and health consequences of CKD, the National Chronic Kidney Disease Surveillance System has been under development after a pilot and feasibility phase as part of the CKD Initiative of the Centers for Disease Control and Prevention.[203] This system uses passive surveillance strategies that incorporate a broad network of data sources and aims to disseminate information through fact sheets, reports, and a website. To date, the only U.S. CKD data on incidence available in the surveillance system come from the Department of Veterans Affairs, documenting an incidence of CKD stages 3 to 5 of 46.55 (95% confidence interval [CI], 46.35 to 46.75)/1000 person-years.[204]

In research, large longitudinal studies are necessary to provide reliable estimates of the incidence of disease. International guidelines have suggested that incidence be defined by a combination of eGFR, proteinuria, and cause of kidney disease (e.g., allowing for individuals with polycystic kidney disease but normal GFR and no proteinuria to be included in CKD incidence data).[205] Other published definitions include data on serum creatinine, International Classification of Diseases (ICD) codes, and/or death records, but do so in varied ways.[206-212] Variations in the definition of incident CKD can modify the relationship between race and CKD occurrence. For example, incident CKD among participants aged 45 to 64 years at baseline in the Atherosclerosis Risk in Communities (ARIC) study occurred at a higher rate among blacks than whites using a definition of CKD based on a rise in serum creatinine levels (8.0 vs. 3.2/1000 person-years, respectively) and ICD codes (2.0 vs. 1.0/1000 person-years), but at a lower rate when CKD was defined as a low eGFR (8.9 vs. 10.8/1000 person-years).[213] A composite definition requiring a low eGFR and at least a 25% drop in eGFR resulted in similar incidence rates for blacks and whites (6.9 vs. 6.6/1000 person-years, respectively).

Despite the lack of consistency in defining incident CKD, several estimates of CKD incidence rates across different racial and ethnic groups have been reported. The 2009 USRDS Annual Data Report cited the incidence of CKD, based on diagnostic codes, among the general Medicare population (mean age, 75.5 years) at 5.6% in African Americans compared to 3.8% in whites in 2007.[26] A 1999 publication that included ARIC participants reported a CKD incidence of 28.4/1000 person-years among black participants with diabetes compared to 9.6/1000 person-years among whites with diabetes, and an age-, sex-, and baseline serum creatinine level–adjusted odds ratio of early kidney function decline among blacks compared to whites of 3.2 (95% CI, 1.9 to 5.3).[212] After further adjustment for potentially modifiable risk factors related to socioeconomic status and health behaviors, including education, household income, health insurance, fasting glucose level, mean systolic blood pressure, smoking history, and physical activity level, the odds ratio (95% CI) decreased to 1.4 (0.7 to 2.7), an 82% reduction in excess risk.[212] Although this and other studies have attributed a substantial proportion of the excess risk for kidney disease in black Americans to these nonracial factors, a difference in risk across race still remains in adjusted analyses. A more recent study, which modeled CKD incidence based on published prevalence data, has suggested that 59.1% of U.S. individuals would suffer from CKD stage 3A or worse in their lifetime, with blacks of both sexes experiencing higher rates of CKD stages 4 or 5 and ESKD.[39]

PREVALENCE OF CHRONIC KIDNEY DISEASE

Estimates of CKD prevalence are much more frequently reported than estimates of incidence because of the ability to do so with a single assessment of renal function. These estimates are associated with certain limitations (see Chapter 20). Racial disparities in CKD were examined at entry into the Reasons for Geographic and Racial Differences in Stroke (REGARDS) study, a population-based cohort study of adults older than 45 years. An eGFR of less than 60 mL/min/1.73 m^2 (i.e., CKD stages 3 to 5) was found in 43.3% overall and was more prevalent among whites compared to blacks (49.9% vs. 33.7%, respectively; Table 21-1).[214] However, although blacks were less likely than whites to have

Table 21.1 Racial Differences in Renal Function*

eGFR (mL/min/1.73 m^2)	N (%) Black (n = 8139)	N (%) White (n = 11,620)	OR (95% CI)	aOR† (95% CI)
>60	5394 (66.3)	5817 (50.1)	Reference	Reference
50-59	1541 (18.9)	3611 (31.1)	0.46 (0.43-0.49)	0.42 (0.40-0.46)
40-49	693 (8.5)	1506 (13.0)	0.50 (0.45-0.55)	0.37 (0.33-0.41)
30-39	287 (3.5)	521 (4.5)	0.59 (0.51-0.67)	0.38 (0.32-0.45)
20-29	116 (1.4)	131 (1.1)	0.95 (0.74-1.22)	0.48 (0.36-0.64)
10-19	60 (0.7)	25 (0.2)	2.56 (1.62-4.13)	1.73 (1.02-2.94)
<10	48 (0.6)	9 (0.08)	5.75 (2.82-11.7)	4.19 (1.90-9.24)

*By level of MDRD eGFR and odds of a low GFR in blacks compared with whites. A total of 2029 participants were excluded from analyses because of missing values for MDRD components.
†aOR controlling for age, sex, hypertension, diabetes, previous stroke or myocardial infarction, region, and smoking status.
aOR, Adjusted odds ratio; eGFR, estimated GFR; OR, odds ratio; MDRD, Modification of Diet in Renal Disease study.
Reprinted with permission from McClellan W, Warnock DG, McClure L, et al: Racial differences in the prevalence of chronic kidney disease among participants in the Reasons for Geographic and Racial Differences in Stroke (REGARDS) Cohort Study. J Am Soc Nephrol 17:1710-1715, 2006.

an eGFR between 30 and 60 mL/min/1.73 m², the reverse was true in the eGFR range of less than 30 mL/min/1.73 m². Using data from the National Health and Nutrition Examination Surveys (NHANES) from 1988 to 1994 and 1999 to 2004, and the MDRD GFR estimating equation, the prevalence of CKD increased from 10.5% to 13.8% among non-Hispanic whites, from 10.2% to 11.7% among non-Hispanic blacks, and from 6.3% to 8.0% among Mexican Americans over this time period.[215] Emphasizing the impact of the tool used to assess kidney function, the 1999 to 2004 estimates of the prevalence of CKD stages 1 to 4 among non-Hispanic whites and blacks in the United States were no longer significantly different when made using the more accurate Chronic Kidney Disease Epidemiology Collaboration (CKD-EPI) equation to estimate GFR.[12] However, a racial difference persists in the prevalence of CKD stages 3 to 4; estimates shifted from 9.6% and 5.2% using the MDRD GFR estimating equation to 7.8% and 5.4% using the CKD-EPI equation among whites and blacks, respectively. Another analysis of NHANES 1988 to 1994 data revealed a higher likelihood, even after multivariable adjustment, of U.S. blacks and Mexican Americans with and without diabetes to have albuminuria compared to U.S. whites with or without diabetes (odds ratio [OR], 1.8 to 2.8).[216] Finally, in a study of adult Navajo Indians, 3% to 6% of nondiabetics and 10% to 11% of diabetics had an elevated serum creatinine level consistent with a creatinine clearance of 65 mL/min or higher for men and 53 mL/min or higher for women.[217]

Hispanic ethnicity is often aggregated into one group, despite a wide variety of national origins and races represented by this classification. Rodriguez and coworkers[218] examined data from the Hispanic Health and Nutrition Examination Survey (HHANES) on differences in serum creatinine levels and estimated creatinine clearances across Hispanic subgroups, including Mexican Americans, mainland Puerto Ricans, and Cuban Americans. Cuban Americans had the highest mean serum creatinine levels, and both Puerto Ricans (OR 1.7; 95% CI, 1.2 to 2.6) and Cuban Americans (OR 4.6; 95% CI, 2.5 to 8.3) were more likely than Mexican Americans to have estimated creatinine clearances lower than 60 mL/min/1.73 m².[218] These observations further highlight the heterogeneity of physiology within currently used race and ethnicity categorizations.

PROGRESSION OF CHRONIC KIDNEY DISEASE

Rates of progression of CKD to ESKD are higher among African American, Hispanic, and American Indian adults compared to white U.S. adults, as described in Chapter 20.[26,219,220] For example, Hispanic ethnicity was associated with a significantly increased risk (hazard ratio [HR] 1.33; 95% CI, 1.17 to 1.52) for ESKD among individuals with CKD compared to non-Hispanic whites in large study of Kaiser Permanente of Northern California health plan enrollees.[221] Among African Americans, the rate of decline of GFR is greater (i.e., 1.4 to 1.5 mL/min/yr greater decline in blacks compared to whites), and the risk of developing ESKD was twofold higher (RR [95% CI], 2.0 [1.1 to 3.6]) compared with whites.[222,223] This finding was reinforced by a longitudinal study of Medicare recipients aged 65 years or older followed for up to 10 years.[224] After adjustment for age and sex, black patients with diabetes were 2.4 to 2.7 times and other races and ethnicities were 1.6 to 1.7 times more likely to develop ESKD compared to whites. Similar elevations in risk were noted among black and other racial and ethnic minorities with hypertension. Finally, among patients with neither diabetes nor hypertension, black patients were still 3.5 times more likely, and those with "other" designated race, were twice as likely to develop ESKD than whites.

POTENTIAL MECHANISMS OF RACIAL AND ETHNIC DISPARITIES

Racial disparities in kidney disease may partially be explained by a higher prevalence and lower levels of control of hypertension among African American adults (Figure 21.6).[225-230] The onset of hypertension appears to occur earlier and with more severity in African Americans, leading to greater end-organ damage.[229] Additional potential causes of kidney disease disparities between whites and blacks may be differences in the prevalence and control of diabetes,[226,231] prevalence and severity of obesity,[232,233] physiologic differences in cytokine production,[234,235] renal hemodynamics,[236,237] and

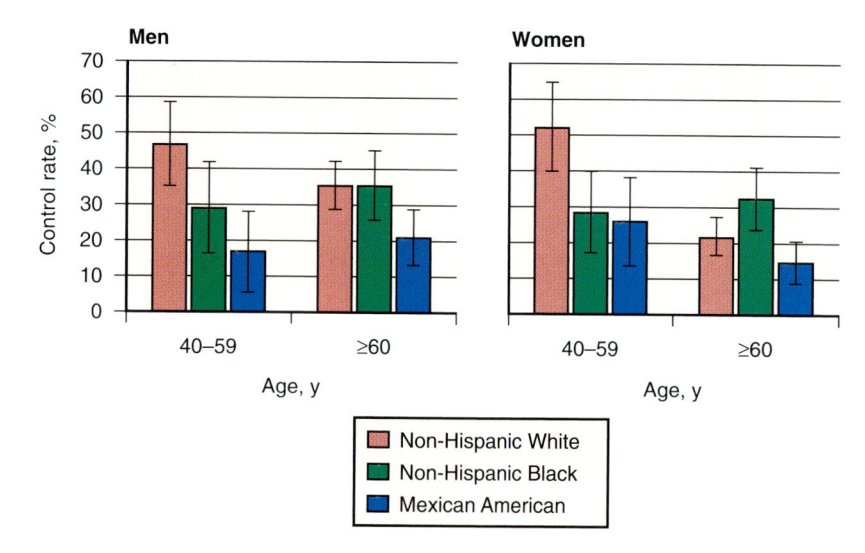

Figure 21.6 Overall hypertension control rates in 1999 to 2000 by age and race and ethnicity in men and women. Error bars indicate 95% CIs. Data are weighted to the U.S. population. For comparisons between racial and ethnic groups (with non-Hispanic whites as the referent), P values are as follows (by age): for Mexican Americans, men, 40 to 59 years, $P < 0.001$; men, at least 60 years, $P = 0.003$; women, 40 to 59 years, $P = 0.002$; women, at least 60 years, $P = 0.04$; for non-Hispanic blacks, men, 40 to 59 years, $P = 0.02$; men, at least 60 years, $P = 0.51$; women, 40 to 59 years, $P = 0.003$; women, at least 60 years, $P = 0.98$. (Reprinted with permission from Hajjar I, Kotchen TA: Trends in prevalence, awareness, treatment, and control of hypertension in the United States, 1988-2000. *JAMA* 290:199-206, 2003.)

electrolyte regulation,[238] genetic factors, and differences in socioeconomic status, access to health care, behavioral factors, and physical environments. One such explanation was provided in a publication in which Hung and colleagues reported a higher risk for CKD progression among participants of the African American Study of Kidney Disease and Hypertension (AASK) with certain C-reactive protein polymorphisms.[239] Similar disparities exist between Hispanic adults compared to whites that may be partially explained by a higher prevalence, earlier onset, and increased severity of diabetes in this ethnic minority population,[240-243] lower rates of awareness, treatment, and control of hypertension,[228] and higher prevalence of obesity,[244,245] among other biologic, social, behavioral, and communication factors.

Several studies have also identified factors related to access to health care as being strongly predictive of the development of ESKD.[212,246] One ecologic study comparing regions in California defined by zip codes reported a higher incidence of ESKD caused by diabetes in areas with a higher proportion of hospitalizations of those with no insurance or with Medicaid, and a lower incidence in areas with more hospitalizations for those with managed care insurance plans.[247] Surprisingly, the unadjusted incidence rates were lower in zip codes with known shortages of health professionals compared to zip codes with ample health professional populations (adjusted rates were not presented). Also, incidences of ESKD were higher in areas with more hospitalizations for hyperglycemic complications, suggesting a role for ineffective or poor access to treatment in the development of ESRD caused by diabetes. Similarly, a report cited more abnormal laboratory values at the onset of ESKD treatment in those without medical insurance.[247]

The persistence of variations in risk of CKD progression by race after adjustment for many of these factors has motivated investigation of previously unexplained genetic variation using new investigative tools. Two independent groups performed genome-wide analyses for ESKD risk loci within incident African American ESKD patients. Both used admixture linkage dysequilibrium analysis, which is based on the premise that when two genetically diverse populations mix, the admixed population receives chromosomal regions from either ancestry that can be identified by genotyping markers with different allelic frequencies between the ancestral populations. The groups screened the genome of African Americans with ESKD to identify ESKD susceptibility loci, regions of the genome where individuals with ESKD have more or less African ancestry than their nondiseased counterparts. The results from the Family Investigation of Nephropathy and Diabetes Research Group identified an association between excess African ancestry and nondiabetic ESKD on chromosome 22q12, but not with diabetic ESKD.[248] In contrast, the presence of an allele of European origin at this locus was found to be protective, with a relative risk of 0.5 compared with an allele of African origin. In this study, most of the excess ESKD risk in those of African ancestry was correlated with a number of common single-nucleotide polymorphisms (SNPs) in the gene encoding nonmuscle myosin heavy chain type II isoform A (MYH9). Similarly, Kopp and associates found this same gene to be associated with biopsy-proven, idiopathic FSGS and human immunodeficiency virus type 1 (HIV-1)–associated FSGS in African Americans.[249] In this study, the OR associated with the recessive E-1 haplotype for MYH9 SNPs in African Americans was 4.7 (95% CI, 3.1 to 7.0) in idiopathic FSGS and 5.9 (95% CI, 2.9 to 12.9) in HIV-associated FSGS. However, subsequent studies have suggested that certain polymorphisms of an adjacent gene, *APOL1*, are responsible for different rates of renal progression across races. This gene, which codes for apolipoprotein L-1 (apo L-1), is in linkage disequilibrium with MYH9, which likely accounts for the findings of prior studies. In 2010, Genovese and coworkers and Tzur and colleagues demonstrated two sequence variants in apo L-1 that were strongly associated with the development of FSGS and hypertensive nephrosclerosis in African Americans.[250,251] These variants were also considered to have risen in allele frequency under positive evolutionary selection and were shown to have an increased ability to lyse the human pathogen *Trypanosoma brucei rhodesiense*, suggesting that positive-selection pressure may account for the increased prevalence of these isoforms among African Americans.[252]

In a study of 2955 participants in the Chronic Renal Insufficiency Cohort, black individuals homozygous for a high-risk apo L-1 allele had an increased risk of doubling of creatinine level or progression to ESKD compared to nonhomozygous blacks or whites. Among diabetics, the HR for adverse renal outcomes was 3.1 (2.1 to 4.5) times higher among high-risk blacks compared to whites. Among nondiabetics, the risk was 2.5 (1.8 to 3.4) times higher.[253] Similarly, among AASK participants, those with a high-risk, apo L-1 genotype had a rate of doubling of creatinine level or ESKD 1.9 times higher than in those without a high-risk genotype.[253]

The ARIC study of 3067 African Americans without CKD at baseline revealed a significantly elevated risk of developing incident CKD (HR 1.5; 95% CI, 1.0 to 2.2) and progressing to ESKD (HR 2.2; 95% CI, 1.0 to 4.8) among those homozygous for the apo L-1 risk alleles compared to heterozygotes and those with the wild-type alleles.[254] The mechanisms through which *APOL1* mutations accelerate kidney disease progression remain unclear, but are an area of very active research.[255,256]

SUMMARY

There is little variation in reports of the patterns of incidence, prevalence, and progression of kidney disease across race and ethnicity. In general, despite a lower prevalence of CKD among African Americans and Hispanics compared to whites, the incidence of CKD is higher in African Americans and rates of progression are faster in African Americans, Hispanics, and American Indians compared to non-Hispanic whites.

SOCIOECONOMIC FACTORS AND CHRONIC KIDNEY DISEASE

SOCIOECONOMIC EXPOSURES

Earlier in this chapter, we discussed racial disparities in the incidence and progression of CKD. Racial differences in kidney disease risk are partially mediated by factors related to socioeconomic status and social deprivation (see also Chapter 84). This portion of the excess risk is potentially modifiable and, therefore, of particular interest for targeting prevention strategies. Socioeconomic status has been described as a distal risk factor for kidney disease that acts through several proximal factors, including poverty and low income, lack of nutrition, low educational levels, exposure to heavy metals, substance abuse, and limited access to health care.[246] These factors can be examined at the individual and neighborhood level at any given point in time. As a result, several analyses have accounted for both individual- and area-level socioeconomic status.[210,257] A framework for considering the numerous social and cultural determinants of disparities in CKD is shown in Figure 21.7. In addition, as in many disease processes that develop over protracted periods of time, past and present exposures are responsible for increases in risk. For this reason, life course (i.e., the cumulative effect of social environments over the course of a lifetime) and parental socioeconomic factors have also been investigated as contributors to the incidence and progression of kidney disease.[258] Full evaluation of these individual- and area-level factors in biomedical research studies is key to explaining the observed racial and ethnic disparities in kidney disease.

RELATIONSHIP TO SOCIOECONOMIC FACTORS

INCIDENCE OF CHRONIC KIDNEY DISEASE

Very few studies have examined risk factors for the incidence of CKD and fewer yet have investigated socioeconomic factors. Krop and associates observed that blacks with diabetes mellitus were three times more likely than whites with diabetes mellitus to develop CKD in unadjusted analyses.[212] Subsequent adjustment for additional covariates revealed that 6% of the excess risk for development of CKD in black adults compared to white adults with diabetes was explained by income and education level. Suboptimal health behaviors and poor control for glucose level and blood pressure accounted for a substantial proportion of the remaining risk. Given the strong relationship among socioeconomic status, health behaviors, and glycemic and hypertensive control,[226,259,260] the overall effect of socioeconomic factors on the incidence of CKD is understated in the aforementioned 6% excess risk.

A similar constellation of risk factors has been described in conjunction with renal involvement in systemic lupus erythematosus (SLE). A higher incidence of lupus nephritis has been noted among minority populations. One report, which included participants with recently diagnosed SLE from the Lupus in Minorities: Nature vs. Nurture (LUMINA) study, noted the development of lupus nephritis among 44.6% of Texas Hispanics, 11.3% of Puerto Rican Hispanics, 45.8% of African Americans, and 18.3% of whites.[261] When examined further, a composite socioeconomic status factor, including information on education, insurance, and poverty status, accounted for 14.5% of the variance because of ethnicity after adjustment; socioeconomic status and genetic

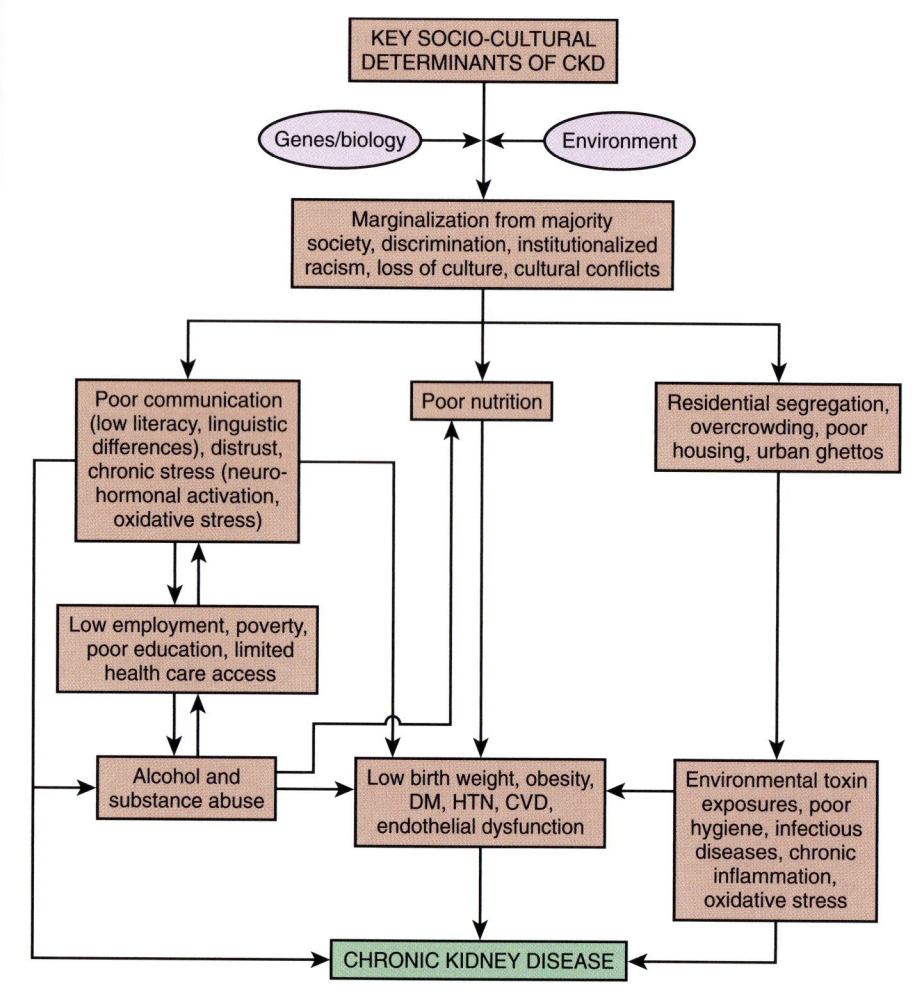

Figure 21.7 A framework for integrating key sociocultural determinants of CKD. CVD, Cardiovascular disease; DM, diabetes mellitus; HTN, hypertension. (Reprinted with permission from Norris K, Nissenson AR: Race, gender, and socioeconomic disparities in CKD in the United States. *J Am Soc Nephrol* 19:1261-1270, 2008.)

admixture together accounted for an additional 12.2% of the variance. Of note, an additional 36.8% of the variance in this model could be attributed to genetic admixture, underscoring the importance of genetic factors over socioeconomic factors in explaining the racial disparities in renal involvement in SLE.

A population-based case-control study in Sweden has provided additional evidence of the risk of incident CKD with low socioeconomic status. ORs of incident CKD associated with families of solely unskilled workers were 2.1 (95% CI, 1.1 to 4.0) and 1.6 (95% CI, 1.0 to 2.6) among women and men, respectively, compared to families with at least one professional worker.[262] In addition, Swedish adults with 9 years or less of education were 30% more likely (OR, 1.3; 95% CI, 1.0 to 1.7) to develop CKD than adults with a college education.

Finally, in parts of the United Kingdom, an approximate 50% increase in the incidence of CKD was reported among those in the highest quintile of social deprivation (i.e., living in an electoral ward with a high proportion of households without a car, unemployed, overcrowded, and not owner-occupied) compared to the lowest quintile.[263] A more recent analysis of the ARIC study demonstrated an increased incidence of CKD among blacks compared to whites (14.7 vs. 12.0 cases/1000 person years). Demographic, socioeconomic, lifestyle, clinical factors, and access to health care accounted for 74% of this increased risk.[264]

PREVALENCE OF CHRONIC KIDNEY DISEASE

The relationship of measures of socioeconomic status and social deprivation with the prevalence of CKD has been better characterized than with the incidence of CKD. Using data from the ARIC study, Shoham and coworkers found that being a member of the working class across some or all of their life course was associated with an increased OR of CKD among whites and blacks (OR [95% CI], 1.4 [0.9 to 2.0] and 1.9 [1.3 to 2.9], respectively).[265] Martins and colleagues have cited a significant association (OR 1.2; 95% CI, 1.1 to 1.3) between living at less than 200% of the federal poverty level and microalbuminuria using data from NHANES III after multivariable adjustment.[266] Another analysis of data from NHANES III has confirmed these findings; it also revealed a higher prevalence of CKD in those with less than 12 years of education among non-Hispanic whites and blacks and with an income equivalence level (i.e., total household income divided by the square root of the number of people dependent on that income) less than $12,000 compared to $28,000 or more among non-Hispanic whites only.[267] An even stronger relationship was observed between unemployment and prevalent CKD, but only among non-Hispanic blacks and Mexican Americans. Interestingly, these same associations could not be detected using similar surveys of adults in Australia and Thailand.[267]

Some effects of socioeconomic status on CKD are mediated through more proximal factors, such as nutritional status, health behaviors, and environmental exposures. Nutritional deprivation or physiologic insults in utero cause intrauterine growth restriction (IUGR). Building on the developmental origins of health and disease hypothesis proposed by Barker,[268] Brenner and Chertow hypothesized that IUGR causes a decrease in nephron number, leading to a susceptibility to hypertension and reduced kidney function later in life.[269] A systematic review and meta-analysis of observational studies evaluating the relationship between birth weight and CKD, assessed at age older than 12 months, included 32 studies.[270] Combined weighted estimates of effect provided an OR for CKD associated with low birth weight of 1.7 (95% CI, 1.4 to 2.1). These results were consistent across multiple definitions of CKD, including albuminuria, ESKD, and low eGFR. (For further discussion, see Chapter 23.)

Finally, numerous environmental exposures that affect kidney health occur disproportionately among certain populations, including those of low socioeconomic status. Exposure to cadmium and lead, even at low levels, is associated with a significantly increased prevalence of kidney disease.[271-279] Data on the renal effects of drinking water or residential environmental exposure to uranium are scarce, and very few studies have found a significant association between this type of exposure to uranium and renal outcomes, including kidney stones, chronic nephritis, and microalbuminuria.[280-282] Overcrowding in housing poses more risk for streptococcal infections, which may lead to poststreptococcal glomerulonephritis. Reductions in renal functional reserve, chronic kidney disease, and development of ESKD have been reported in patients who have recovered from poststreptococcal glomerulonephritis.[283-285]

The effect of income on CKD prevalence may vary by country. An analysis of individuals who participated in NHANES (1999 to 2002) demonstrated that low income was strongly associated with CKD prevalence. Applying the same analysis to a Dutch cohort, low income was only weakly associated with CKD prevalence.[286] This may be a result of the fact that access to health care is more income-dependent in the United States than in the Netherlands. A study of an English cohort revealed significant associations between low income and CKD prevalence, but these disappeared after adjustment for lifestyle and clinical factors.[287]

The impact of income on CKD prevalence may differ by sex and race in U.S. studies, but evidence is sparse. In the Jackson Heart Study, an all–African American cohort, high socioeconomic status was statistically significantly protective against CKD among men (OR 0.5; 95% CI, 0.2 to 1.0), but of only borderline significance among women (OR 0.6; 95% CI, 0.4 to 1.0).[288] A study of 2375 community-living adults in Baltimore, Maryland, has demonstrated that low socioeconomic status is associated with CKD in blacks (OR 1.9; 95% CI, 1.5 to 2.4), but not in whites (OR 1.0; 95% CI, 0.6 to 1.6).[289]

PROGRESSION OF CHRONIC KIDNEY DISEASE

The association between race and ethnicity and the progression of CKD was discussed earlier in this chapter. As noted, socioeconomic factors highly correlated with race and ethnicity account for a proportion of this excess risk. In particular, Tarver-Carr and colleagues reported a 2.7-fold increased risk of ESKD among African Americans compared with whites.[222] Of the excess risk of developing ESLD among African Americans, 12% was explained by sociodemographic factors, including education, poverty status, and marital status. A large longitudinal study of over 170,000 members of Kaiser Permanente of Northern California reported a significant risk of developing ESKD among members who never attended college (HR 1.6; 95% CI, 1.2

to 2.0) or who completed some college (HR 1.5; 95% CI, 1.1 to 1.9) compared to college graduates after multivariable adjustment.[290]

Further studies have integrated neighborhood-level socioeconomic factors in the examination of the progression of CKD. One study, using data on the incidence of ESKD in Georgia, North Carolina, and South Carolina, defined neighborhood poverty using the percentage of the census tract population living below the poverty level.[291] Unadjusted incidence rate ratios of ESKD increased from 1.5 to 4.5 in a dose-response manner for census tracts with 5% to 9.9%, 10% to 14.9%, 15% to 19.9%, 20% to 24.9%, and 25% or more of the population below the poverty level, respectively, compared to tracts with fewer than 5% below the poverty level. This marker of neighborhood poverty was significantly associated with a higher incidence of ESKD among blacks and whites. However, there was a stronger relationship between the incidence of ESKD and census tract poverty among blacks compared to whites. Finally, Merkin and associates[210] analyzed data from the ARIC and Cardiovascular Health Studies separately to assess the relationship between individual- and neighborhood-level socioeconomic status and progressive CKD. In the ARIC study, age- and center-adjusted incidence rates of progressive CKD increased with declining area-level socioeconomic scores for African American women and white men, but not for African American men and white women.[210] Living in the lowest quartile of area-level socioeconomic status was significantly associated with a 60% greater risk (HR 1.6; 95% CI, 1.0% to 2.5) for progressive CKD only among white men after multivariable adjustment, including individual-level socioeconomic status. Among participants in the Cardiovascular Health Study, age- and center-adjusted incidence rates of progressive CKD were inversely related to area-level socioeconomic scores and to individual levels of income and education.[257] After multivariable adjustment, including individual-level socioeconomic status, living in the lowest quartile of area-level socioeconomic status was associated with an HR for progressive CKD of 1.5 (95% CI, 1.0 to 2.0) compared to the highest quartile. The association with individual-level socioeconomic status no longer remained significant after adjustment in this older population.

A study of 4735 older Cardiovascular Health Study participants demonstrated that the risk of progressive CKD was 50% higher among those living in an area with low socioeconomic status, even after adjustment for personal socioeconomic status.[292] These findings suggest that local factors may be more important than individual income in the relationship between low socioeconomic status and progression of CKD in older adults.

SUMMARY

Socioeconomic factors, especially income, education, and environmental factors, appear to explain a large proportion of the excess incidence and progression of CKD among African American and other racial and ethnic groups compared to whites. Additional studies are needed to clarify the influence of access to health care and early-life socioeconomic status on kidney health.

CONCLUSION

Although there are several studies and data sets reporting the incidence of CKD in the United States, more consistency in the definition of incident CKD is needed to facilitate the assessment of differences and disparities across sociodemographic groups. Also, there is no single way to capture information on the progression of CKD, which poses a challenge to researchers and clinicians trying to review and interpret findings across studies systematically. Examination of the pattern of kidney disease across sexes has not yielded a consistent relationship. With the exception of the prevalence of CKD, which appears to be higher among women, men are reported to have a higher incidence of glomerular disease and greater progression of nondiabetic CKD, especially compared to premenopausal women.

Results are less consistent across sexes, however, regarding the progression of IgA nephropathy and with progression overall in postmenopausal women. More studies are needed to elucidate any sex differences in the progression of lupus nephritis. Similarly, the reported relationships between sex and ADPKD progression, and sex and the development of microalbuminuria and macroalbuminuria and progression of diabetic nephropathy, are not consistent and may be modified by age and race.

Reported patterns of kidney disease across race and ethnic groups have been more consistent than those reported across sex. A lower prevalence of CKD has been observed among African Americans and Hispanics compared to whites. As GFR levels decline, however, African Americans seem to have a higher prevalence of CKD and albuminuria compared to non-Hispanic whites, consistent with the long-observed pattern of higher rates of ESKD among African Americans. The incidence of CKD is higher in African Americans, and rates of progression are faster in African Americans, Hispanics, and Native Americans compared to non-Hispanic whites. A substantial proportion of the excess incidence and progression of CKD among African Americans and other racial and ethnic groups compared to whites is associated with socioeconomic determinants, but an increasing body of literature supports a significant role for specific apo L-1 genotypes as a causative factor for African Americans in particular.[253] Evidence of the impact of income, education, and environmental factors on kidney outcomes is consistent; however, the association between access to care and these same outcomes is less clearly documented. There is some suggestion of interactions between socioeconomic status and race with kidney outcomes, but these need further study.

Complete reference list available at ExpertConsult.com.

KEY REFERENCES

1. Coresh J, Selvin E, Stevens LA, et al: Prevalence of chronic kidney disease in the United States. *JAMA* 298:2038–2047, 2007.
5. Hughson M, Farris AB 3rd, Douglas-Denton R, et al: Glomerular number and size in autopsy kidneys: the relationship to birth weight. *Kidney Int* 63:2113–2122, 2003.
8. Nyengaard JR, Bendtsen TF: Glomerular number and size in relation to age, kidney weight, and body surface in normal man. *Anat Rec* 232:194–201, 1992.

12. Levey AS, Stevens LA, Schmid CH, et al: A new equation to estimate glomerular filtration rate. *Ann Intern Med* 150:604–612, 2009.
13. Levey AS, Bosch JP, Lewis JB, et al: A more accurate method to estimate glomerular filtration rate from serum creatinine: a new prediction equation. Modification of Diet in Renal Disease Study Group. *Ann Intern Med* 130:461–470, 1999.
19. Kollerits B, Fliser D, Heid IM, et al: Gender-specific association of adiponectin as a predictor of progression of chronic kidney disease: the Mild to Moderate Kidney Disease Study. *Kidney Int* 71:1279–1286, 2007.
20. Lei J, Silbiger S, Ziyadeh FN, et al: Serum-stimulated alpha 1 type IV collagen gene transcription is mediated by TGF-beta and inhibited by estradiol. *Am J Physiol* 274:F252–F258, 1998.
26. U.S. Renal Data System: *USRDS 2009 annual data report: atlas of end-stage renal disease in the United States,* Bethesda, Md, 2009, National Institutes of Health, National Institute of Diabetes and Digestive and Kidney Diseases.
28. Nitsch D, Grams M, Sang Y, et al: Associations of estimated glomerular filtration rate and albuminuria with mortality and renal failure by sex: a meta-analysis. *BMJ* 346:f324, 2013.
29. Swaminathan S, Leung N, Lager DJ, et al: Changing incidence of glomerular disease in Olmsted County, Minnesota: a 30-year renal biopsy study. *Clin J Am Soc Nephrol* 1:483–487, 2006.
33. Korbet SM, Genchi RM, Borok RZ, et al: The racial prevalence of glomerular lesions in nephrotic adults. *Am J Kidney Dis* 27:647–651, 1996.
39. Grams ME, Chow EK, Segev DL, et al: Lifetime incidence of CKD stages 3-5 in the United States. *Am J Kidney Dis* 62:245–252, 2013.
41. Evans M, Fryzek JP, Elinder CG, et al: The natural history of chronic renal failure: results from an unselected, population-based, inception cohort in Sweden. *Am J Kidney Dis* 46:863–870, 2005.
44. Neugarten J, Acharya A, Silbiger SR: Effect of gender on the progression of nondiabetic renal disease: a meta-analysis. *J Am Soc Nephrol* 11:319–329, 2000.
54. D'Amico G, Gentile MG, Fellin G, et al: Effect of dietary protein restriction on the progression of renal failure: a prospective randomized trial. *Nephrol Dial Transplant* 9:1590–1594, 1994.
55. Rosman JB, Langer K, Brandl M, et al: Protein-restricted diets in chronic renal failure: a four-year follow-up shows limited indications. *Kidney Int Suppl* 27:S96–S102, 1989.
56. Ruggenenti P, Gaspari F, Perna A, et al: Cross-sectional longitudinal study of spot morning urine protein:creatinine ratio, 24-hour urine protein excretion rate, glomerular filtration rate, and end-stage renal failure in chronic renal disease in patients without diabetes. *BMJ* 316:504–509, 1998.
61. Hannedouche T, Chauveau P, Fehrat A, et al: Effect of moderate protein restriction on the rate of progression of chronic renal failure. *Kidney Int Suppl* 27:S91–S95, 1989.
72. Velo M, Lozano L, Egido J, et al: Natural history of IgA nephropathy in patients followed-up for more than ten years in Spain. *Semin Nephrol* 7:346–350, 1987.
82. Yoshikawa N, Ito H, Nakamura H: Prognostic indicators in childhood IgA nephropathy. *Nephron* 60:60–67, 1992.
88. Cattran DC, Greenwood C, Ritchie S: Long-term benefits of angiotensin-converting enzyme-inhibitor therapy in patients with severe immunoglobulin a nephropathy–a comparison to patients receiving treatment with other antihypertensive agents and to patients receiving no therapy. *Am J Kidney Dis* 23:247–254, 1994.
99. A controlled study of short-term prednisone treatment in adults with membranous nephropathy. Collaborative Study of the Adult Idiopathic Nephrotic Syndrome. *N Engl J Med* 301:1301–1306, 1979.
101. Fuiano G, Stanziale P, Balletta M, et al: Effectiveness of steroid therapy in different stages of membranous nephropathy. *Nephrol Dial Transplant* 4:1022–1029, 1989.
106. Ponticelli C, Zucchelli P, Imbasciati E, et al: Controlled trial of methylprednisolone and chlorambucil in idiopathic membranous nephropathy. *N Engl J Med* 310:946–950, 1984.
108. Schieppati A, Mosconi L, Perna A, et al: Prognosis of untreated patients with idiopathic membranous nephropathy. *N Engl J Med* 329:85–89, 1993.
116. Cattran DC, Pei Y, Greenwood CM, et al: Validation of a predictive model of idiopathic membranous nephropathy: its clinical and research implications. *Kidney Int* 51:901–907, 1997.
119. Ponticelli C, Zucchelli P, Passerini P, et al: A randomized trial of methylprednisolone and chlorambucil in idiopathic membranous nephropathy. *N Engl J Med* 320:8–13, 1989.
132. Johnson AM, Gabow PA: Identification of patients with autosomal dominant polycystic kidney disease at highest risk for end-stage renal disease. *J Am Soc Nephrol* 8:1560–1567, 1997.
149. Dicks E, Ravani P, Langman D, et al: Incident renal events and risk factors in autosomal dominant polycystic kidney disease: a population and family-based cohort followed for 22 years. *Clin J Am Soc Nephrol* 1:710–717, 2006.
151. Harris PC, Bae KT, Rossetti S, et al: Cyst number but not the rate of cystic growth is associated with the mutated gene in autosomal dominant polycystic kidney disease. *J Am Soc Nephrol* 17:3013–3019, 2006.
187. Monster TBM, Janssen WMT, de Jong PE, et al: Oral contraceptive use and hormone replacement therapy are associated with microalbuminuria. *Arch Intern Med* 161:2000–2005, 2001.
188. Garg SK, Chase HP, Marshall G, et al: Oral contraceptives and renal and retinal complications in young women with insulin-dependent diabetes mellitus. *JAMA* 271:1099–1102, 1994.
191. Agarwal M, Selvan V, Freedman BI, et al: The relationship between albuminuria and hormone therapy in postmenopausal women. *Am J Kidney Dis* 45:1019–1025, 2005.
199. Institute of Medicine: *The unequal burden of cancer: an assessment of NIH research and programs for ethnic minorities and the medically underserved,* Washington, DC, 1999, Institute of Medicine.
202. National Kidney Foundation: KDOQI clinical practice guidelines for chronic kidney disease: evaluation, classification, and stratification. *Am J Kidney Dis* 39:S1–S266, 2002.
205. Improving Glocal Outcomes (KDIGO) CKD Work Group: KDIGO 2012 clinical practice guideline for the evaluation and management of chronic kidney disease. *Kidney Int Suppl* 3:1–150, 2012.
206. Hsu CC, Kao WH, Coresh J, et al: Apolipoprotein E and progression of chronic kidney disease. *JAMA* 293:2892–2899, 2005.
211. Hsu CC, Bray MS, Kao WH, et al: Genetic variation of the renin-angiotensin system and chronic kidney disease progression in black individuals in the atherosclerosis risk in communities study. *J Am Soc Nephrol* 17:504–512, 2006.
213. Bash LD, Coresh J, Kottgen A, et al: Defining incident chronic kidney disease in the research setting: The ARIC Study. *Am J Epidemiol* 170:414–424, 2009.
214. McClellan W, Warnock DG, McClure L, et al: Racial differences in the prevalence of chronic kidney disease among participants in the Reasons for Geographic and Racial Differences in Stroke (REGARDS) Cohort Study. *J Am Soc Nephrol* 17:1710–1715, 2006.
221. Peralta CA, Shlipak MG, Fan D, et al: Risks for end-stage renal disease, cardiovascular events, and death in Hispanic versus non-Hispanic white adults with chronic kidney disease. *J Am Soc Nephrol* 17:2892–2899, 2006.
224. Xue JL, Eggers PW, Agodoa LY, et al: Longitudinal study of racial and ethnic differences in developing end-stage renal disease among aged Medicare beneficiaries. *J Am Soc Nephrol* 18:1299–1306, 2007.
229. Chobanian AV, Bakris GL, Black HR, et al: Seventh report of the Joint National Committee on Prevention, Detection, Evaluation, and Treatment of High Blood Pressure. *Hypertension* 42:1206–1252, 2003.
249. Kopp JB, Smith MW, Nelson GW, et al: MYH9 is a major effect risk gene for focal segmental glomerulosclerosis. *Nat Genet* 40:1175–1184, 2008.
250. Genovese G, Friedman DJ, Ross MD, et al: Association of trypanolytic ApoL1 variants with kidney disease in African Americans. *Science* 329:841–845, 2010.

253. Parsa A, Kao WH, Xie D, et al: APOL1 risk variants, race, and progression of chronic kidney disease. *N Engl J Med* 369:2183–2196, 2013.
254. Foster MC, Coresh J, Fornage M, et al: APOL1 variants associated with increased risk of CKD among African Americans. *J Am Soc Nephrol* 24:1484–1491, 2013.
264. Evans K, Coresh J, Bash LD, et al: Race differences in access to health care and disparities in incident chronic kidney disease in the US. *Nephrol Dialysis Transplant* 26:899–908, 2011.
286. Vart P, Gansevoort RT, Coresh J, et al: Socioeconomic measures and CKD in the United States and the Netherlands. *Clin J Am Soc Nephrol* 8:1685–1693, 2013.
287. Fraser S, Roderick P, Aitken G, et al: PP55 socioeconomic status and chronic kidney disease: further findings from the health surveys for England 2009 and 2010. *J Epidemiol Community Health* 67:A71, 2013.

Risk Factors and Chronic Kidney Disease

Maarten W. Taal

CHAPTER OUTLINE

THE NEED TO DEFINE RISK IN CHRONIC KIDNEY DISEASE, 669
Definition of a Risk Factor, 670
Epidemiologic Methods for Identifying Risk Factors, 670
RISK FACTORS AND MECHANISMS OF CHRONIC KIDNEY DISEASE PROGRESSION, 671
Susceptibility Factors, 671
Initiation Factors, 673
Progression Factors, 673
DEMOGRAPHIC VARIABLES, 673
Age, 673
Gender, 673
Ethnicity, 674
HEREDITARY FACTORS, 674
HEMODYNAMIC FACTORS, 676
Decreased Nephron Number, 676
Blood Pressure, 679
Obesity and Metabolic Syndrome, 679
High Dietary Protein Intake, 680
Pregnancy and Preeclampsia, 680
MULTISYSTEM DISORDERS, 681
Diabetes Mellitus, 681
PRIMARY RENAL DISEASE, 681
CARDIOVASCULAR DISEASE, 681
BIOMARKERS, 682
Urinary Protein Excretion, 682
Serum Albumin, 683
Anemia, 683
Dyslipidemia, 683
Serum Uric Acid, 684
Serum Bicarbonate, 684
Plasma Asymmetric Dimethylarginine, 685
Serum Phosphate, 685
Other Biomarkers, 685
NEPHROTOXINS, 685
Smoking, 685
Alcohol, 685
Recreational Drugs, 686
Analgesics, 686
Heavy Metals, 686
RENAL RISK SCORES, 687
General Population Renal Risk Scores, 687
Risk Scores for Patients with Diagnosed Chronic Kidney Disease, 689
Risk Scores for Predicting Chronic Kidney Disease After Acute Kidney Injury, 691
FUTURE CONSIDERATIONS, 691

THE NEED TO DEFINE RISK IN CHRONIC KIDNEY DISEASE

The proposal in 2002 of a simple definition for chronic kidney disease (CKD)[1] and its subsequent worldwide adoption, coupled with the development of the four-variable Modification of Diet in Renal Disease (MDRD) formula that facilitated automated estimation of glomerular filtration rate (GFR) from a measurement of serum creatinine, has brought about an increase in awareness of CKD. Population-based studies from around the world have reported a prevalence of 8% to 16%,[2,3] values substantially higher than anticipated. The large number of people known to be affected by CKD has major implications for the provision of health care—in particular, nephrology services. In the past decade, nephrology has moved from a position where it provided highly specialized services to a relatively small number of patients, with specific and relatively rare kidney disease or advanced CKD, to one where it must concern itself with the care of less advanced CKD in a substantial proportion of the general population. Furthermore, early-stage CKD is largely asymptomatic, and detection therefore requires a screening process. Studies have indicated that screening whole populations is not cost effective,[4] and a means of identifying high-risk subgroups for targeted screening is therefore required. Successful screening programs are likely to identify large numbers of patients with previously undiagnosed CKD but, in most countries, nephrology services are unable to provide long-term care to all CKD patients, and the associated costs would be prohibitive. A solution to this problem was suggested by studies showing that there is substantial heterogeneity among patients who meet the diagnostic criteria for CKD, with most being at relatively low risk of ever progressing to end-stage kidney disease (ESKD). The Kidney Disease Outcomes and Quality Initiative (K/DOQI) classification system for CKD was widely adopted and proved valuable, particularly for identifying the prevalence of different stages of CKD in epidemiologic studies.[5] It was noted, however, that the classification provided little information on the future risk of decline in renal function.[6] The Kidney Disease Improving Global Outcomes (KDIGO) classification system therefore modified the K/DOQI system so that categories defined by GFR and albuminuria do correlate with risk,[7] but this does not provide accurate, individual risk prediction. Previous studies identified a wide range of rates of decline in GFR among patients with CKD, and up to 15% may even show an increase over time.[8] There is thus a need to develop methods for risk stratification within CKD to identify the relatively small subgroup of patients who are at risk of progression to ESKD and who may benefit from specialist intervention to slow or halt disease progression. Such risk stratification would be equally important for identifying individuals who are at low risk for progression who could be reassured and spared unnecessary referral to a nephrologist.

Another important aspect of CKD is its association with a substantially increased risk of future cardiovascular events (CVEs) that in most patients with mild CKD substantially exceeds the risk of ESKD.[9] Whereas CKD is associated with a high prevalence of many traditional risk factors for cardiovascular disease, such as hypertension and dyslipidemia, risk prediction tools such as the Framingham risk score substantially underestimate cardiovascular risk in patients with CKD.[10] It has been proposed that this observation is due to the role of several nontraditional cardiovascular risk factors that are specific to CKD.

From the above discussion, it is clear that there is a need to identify and understand factors associated with an increased risk of developing CKD and, once diagnosed, factors associated with an increased risk of progression to ESKD and CVE. In this chapter, we will review current knowledge of these risk factors and the methods being applied to predict risk in CKD patients. Risk factors for cardiovascular disease in patients with CKD, many of which overlap with risk factors for CKD progression, are discussed in Chapter 56.

DEFINITION OF A RISK FACTOR

A risk factor is a variable that has a causal association with a disease or disease process such that the presence of the variable in an individual or population is associated with an increased risk of the disease being present or developing in the future. Thus, risk factors may be useful for identifying subjects at increased risk for a disease or particular outcome due to a disease process. In the course of epidemiologic research, many variables may show associations with a disease of interest but these may be chance associations, noncausal associations, or causal associations (true risk factors). The Bradford Hill criteria provide minimum requirements to be fulfilled to identify a causal relationship between a putative risk factor (exposure) and a disease (outcome; Table 22.1). In complex diseases such as CKD that result from the combined effects of multiple factors, it is likely that many risk factors will not fulfill all the criteria. Nevertheless, they do provide a useful framework for assessing the strength of a proposed causal relationship between risk factor and disease.

Table 22.1 Bradford-Hill Criteria of Causality

Parameter	Explanation
Strength of association	The stronger the association, the more likely the relationship is causal.
Consistency	A causal association is consistent when replicated in different populations and studies.
Specificity	A single putative cause produces a single effect.
Temporality	Exposure precedes outcome (i.e., risk factor predates disease).
Biological gradient	Increasing exposure to risk factor increases risk of disease, and reduction in exposure reduces risk.
Plausibility	The observed association is consistent with biologic mechanisms of disease processes.
Coherence	The observed association is compatible with existing theory and knowledge in a given field.
Experimental evidence	The factor under investigation is amenable to modification by an appropriate experimental approach.
Analogy	An established cause and effect relationship exists for a similar exposure or disease.

Modified from Hill AB: The environment and disease: association or causation? Proc R Soc Med 58:295-300, 1965.

EPIDEMIOLOGIC METHODS FOR IDENTIFYING RISK FACTORS

Studies to investigate associations between putative risk factors and a disease may be classified as observational or experimental. Observational studies include cross-sectional, case-control, and cohort studies, whereas the randomized controlled trial is the main experimental study.

CROSS-SECTIONAL STUDIES

In this study type, associations between putative risk factors and a disease are investigated in a study population at a single time point. Cross-sectional studies therefore have the advantage of being relatively quick and simple to perform but, because they are limited to a single point in time, they are unable to fulfill the Bradford Hill criterion for temporality. Thus, associations may be identified but inference regarding causality cannot be made. Nevertheless, these studies are useful as an initial search for putative risk factors and hypothesis generation.

CASE-CONTROL STUDIES

These studies also examine subjects at a single point in time but, in this design, cases with a particular disease are identified according to specific criteria and are compared to controls similar to the cases with respect to age, gender, and other variables but who do not have the disease. Cases and controls are then compared with respect to the prevalence of a particular exposure or putative risk factor. One weakness of case-control studies is that they often rely on recollection of past exposure to the putative risk factor. A further challenge is to achieve adequate matching of cases and controls with respect to variables other than the putative risk factor(s).

COHORT STUDIES

Cohort studies are prospective studies in which a population of subjects with and without exposure to a putative risk factor (or variable exposure to a putative risk factor) are followed into the future, and the rate of disease occurrence is compared between the two groups. Advantages are that the temporality criterion for causality may be fulfilled and a direct measure of the incidence of disease obtained. Nevertheless, one weakness of cohort studies is the potential for confounding. This may occur when a variable is associated with both the putative risk factor (exposure) and the disease (outcome). Thus, the presence of a confounder may alter (strengthen, weaken, or mask) the association between exposure and outcome. Multivariable regression analysis may be used to adjust or control for potential confounding but may not completely eliminate the effects of confounding, and incomplete adjustment may result in residual confounding.

Another technique to assist in differentiating causality from association is mendelian randomization. This approach tests whether genetically determined variation in a particular biomarker (which is not affected by nongenetic confounding) is associated with outcomes in a similar manner to that observed in other observational studies. If the biomarker is directly involved in the pathogenesis of a disease, then inherited variation that changes the plasma concentration of the biomarker should be associated with the outcome in the manner predicted by the plasma concentration.[11]

RANDOMIZED CONTROLLED TRIALS

In this study design, a randomized controlled trial (RCT), subjects in a population are randomly assigned to one of two or more treatments or interventions. After a fixed period of follow-up, the randomized groups are compared with respect to the rate of a predefined outcome. To reduce the potential for bias, subjects and/or investigators are often blinded to the treatment. In a single-blinded study, only subjects are unaware of what treatment they receive, whereas in a double-blinded study, subjects and investigators are blinded, usually by the use of a matching placebo. Randomization, if successful, will produce close matching of the groups with respect to a wide range of known and unknown variables at baseline to reduce the possibility of confounding. Furthermore, the RCT is the only study design capable of fulfilling the causality criterion for experimental evidence. Nevertheless, although the RCT constitutes the gold standard for investigating the effect of a therapeutic intervention, it is not as definitive for evaluating putative risk factors. This is because a particular intervention may modify more than one risk factor, and it is therefore not possible to attribute a change in the outcome to the change in a single risk factor. Perhaps the best example of this in CKD is treatment with an angiotensin-converting enzyme (ACE) inhibitor that modifies blood pressure and proteinuria. It is therefore not possible to attribute the subsequent slowing of GFR decline to lowering of blood pressure or to reduction of proteinuria alone.

Data from RCTs may also be used to perform subgroup or post hoc analyses. Subgroup analyses may be prespecified in the trial design (preferable) or be performed post hoc. Although subgroup and post hoc analyses may be useful for exploratory analyses and hypothesis generation, they are prone to several weaknesses. First, they may be underpowered and therefore prone to type 2 errors (incorrect failure to reject the null hypothesis). Second, if too many hypotheses are tested, they may be prone to type 1 errors (incorrect rejection of a true null hypothesis).

RISK FACTORS AND MECHANISMS OF CHRONIC KIDNEY DISEASE PROGRESSION

It has been appreciated for several decades that once GFR has decreased to below a critical level, CKD tends to progress relentlessly toward ESKD. This observation suggests that loss of a critical number of nephrons provokes a vicious cycle of further nephron loss. Detailed studies have elucidated a number of interrelated mechanisms that together contribute to CKD progression, including glomerular hemodynamic responses to nephron loss (raised glomerular capillary hydraulic pressure and single-nephron GFR [SNGFR]), proteinuria, and proinflammatory responses. A generally good prognosis after unilateral nephrectomy[12] attests to the fact that a single pathogenic factor may be insufficient to initiate progressive CKD, but the multihit hypothesis proposes that multiple factors interact to overcome renal reserve and provoke progressive nephron loss.[13] To meet the Bradford Hill criteria of plausibility and coherence, a putative risk factor should therefore somehow affect known mechanisms of CKD progression (see Chapter 52 for further details). Figure 22.1 shows how risk factors may interact with pathophysiologic mechanisms to initiate or accelerate CKD progression. Based on our understanding of the mechanisms underlying the pathogenesis of CKD and its progression, risk factors may be divided into susceptibility factors, initiation factors, and progression factors (Table 22.2). Nevertheless, distinguishing among these categories may in some cases be difficult because some factors (e.g., diabetes mellitus) may act in all three ways and, in some studies, it may be impossible to separate susceptibility factors from progression factors due to inadequate characterization of participants at study entry.

SUSCEPTIBILITY FACTORS

These are risk factors associated with an increased risk of an individual developing CKD after exposure to a factor that has potential to cause renal damage. An example is a reduced nephron number after uninephrectomy, which is

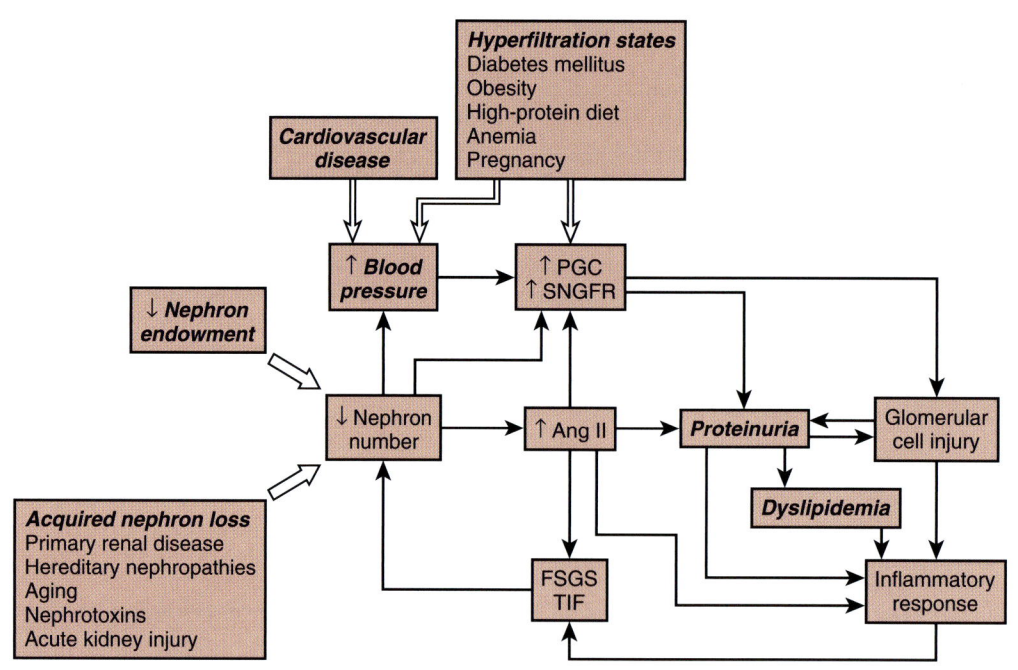

Figure 22.1 Schematic representation showing the interaction of risk factors for chronic kidney disease (CKD) progression with pathophysiologic mechanisms that contribute to a vicious cycle of progressive nephron loss. Ang II, Angiotensin II; FSGS, focal segmental glomerulosclerosis; PGC, glomerular capillary hydraulic pressure; SNGFR, single-nephron glomerular filtration rate; TIF, tubulointerstitial fibrosis. (Adapted from Taal MW, Brenner BM: Predicting initiation and progression of chronic kidney disease: developing renal risk scores. *Kidney Int* 70:1694-1705, 2006.)

Table 22.2 Risk Factors for Chronic Kidney Disease (CKD)			
Risk Factor	**Susceptibility**	**Initiating**	**Progression**
Older age	+		
Gender	+		
Ethnicity	+		+
Family history of CKD	+		
Metabolic syndrome	+		
Hemodynamic factors			
Low nephron number	+		+
Diabetes mellitus	+	+	+
Hypertension	+		+
Obesity	+		+
High protein intake	+		+
Pregnancy		+	+
Primary renal disease		+	
Genetic renal disease		+	
Urologic disorders		+	
Acute kidney injury		+	+
Cardiovascular disease	+		+
Albuminuria			+
Hypoalbuminemia			+
Anemia	+		+
Dyslipidemia	+		+
Hyperuricemia	+		+
↑ ADMA			+
Hyperphosphatemia			+
Low serum bicarbonate			+
Smoking	+		+
Nephrotoxins		+	+

ADMA, Asymmetric dimethylarginine.

associated with an increased risk of developing diabetic nephropathy if the individual develops diabetes.[14] Studies to identify susceptibility factors should recruit subjects free of CKD at baseline who have been exposed to an initiating factor and followed over a prolonged period to allow ascertainment of outcomes. This could be achieved through a cohort study or subgroup analysis of an RCT.

INITIATION FACTORS

Initiation factors directly cause or initiate kidney damage in a susceptible individual. Examples include exposure to nephrotoxic drugs, urinary tract obstruction, or primary glomerulopathies that may provoke CKD in some (but not all) exposed individuals. Studies investigating initiation factors should aim to recruit subjects without CKD at entry or known susceptibility factors, with variable exposure to a putative initiating factor. A cohort study design is best suited to investigate outcomes in subjects exposed versus not exposed to the factor of interest, or an RCT design could be used to assess the potential nephrotoxicity of a new drug.

PROGRESSION FACTORS

These are factors that contribute to the progression of kidney damage once CKD has developed. An example is hypertension, which exacerbates raised intraglomerular hydraulic pressure and therefore accelerates glomerular damage. Studies investigating progression factors should recruit subjects with relatively early-stage CKD in a cohort study design. RCTs may also be used to study progression factors if the intervention being investigated modifies a putative progression factor. Outcomes may therefore be compared between the group in whom the risk factor was modified versus a control group. Unfortunately, however, many interventions alter several risk factors, and it may therefore not be possible to attribute an improved outcome to changes in a single risk factor.

DEMOGRAPHIC VARIABLES

AGE

The prevalence of CKD increases with age and is reported to be as high as 56% in those 75 years of age or older.[15] Longitudinal studies of subjects without kidney disease have observed a decline in GFR with increasing age in some subjects, implying that nephron loss may be regarded as part of normal aging.[16] On the other hand, aging is associated with an increase in several other risk factors for CKD, including hypertension, obesity, and cardiovascular disease, which may contribute to the rise in CKD prevalence. Several population-based studies have found a higher incidence of proteinuria and CKD[17-19] as well as ESKD with increasing age.[20] Similarly, the incidence of a decline in renal function over 5 years was greater among older patients with hypertension.[21] One study reported that advanced age is a negative predictor of ESKD among patients with CKD, although older age was associated with a greater rate of decline in GFR.[22] This apparent contradiction is most likely explained by the competing risks of death and ESKD in older patients,

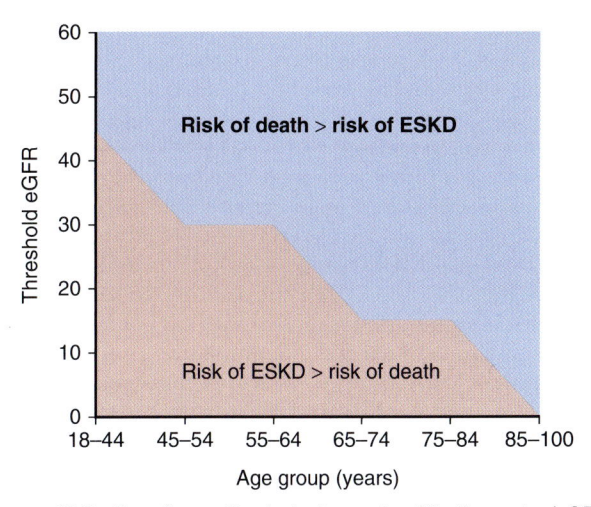

Figure 22.2 Baseline estimated glomerular filtration rate (eGFR) threshold. Below this the risk for end-stage kidney disease (ESKD) exceeded the risk for death in each age group among 209,622 U.S. veterans with chronic kidney disease stages 3 to 5 followed for a mean of 3.2 years. (From O'Hare AM, Choi AI, Bertenthal D, et al: Age affects outcomes in chronic kidney disease. *J Am Soc Nephrol* 18:2758-2765, 2007.)

illustrated by the observation from one longitudinal study that for patients 65 years and older, the risk of ESKD exceeded the risk of death only when the GFR was 15 mL/min/1.73 m^2 or less (Figure 22.2).[23] On the other hand, another study found that in patients with CKD stage 4 or 5, renal function in those 65 years or older was associated with a slower decline than in those younger than 45 years.[24]

A large individual-level meta-analysis that included data from 2,051,244 participants in 46 cohort studies has provided robust data regarding the effect of age on the risks associated with CKD. In general population and high cardiovascular risk cohorts, the increase in relative risk of mortality associated with lower GFR declined with increasing age but the increase in absolute risk of death was higher in older age groups. Similar trends were observed for the mortality risks associated with albuminuria. On the other hand, the relative increase in risk of mortality did not decrease with increasing age in data from CKD cohorts. Furthermore, there was no attenuation of the risk of ESKD with increasing age in any of the cohort categories.[25] Thus, older age is a susceptibility factor for CKD, and the associated increase in risk of death and ESKD is observed at all ages. These observations suggest that targeted screening for CKD in older subjects would be a cost-effective strategy, but further studies are required to investigate the extent to which the risks associated with CKD in older adults may be attenuated by intervention. For further discussion of CKD in older age groups, see Chapters 24 and 85.

GENDER

In experimental studies, male rodents were more susceptible to age-related glomerulosclerosis than females, an observation that was independent of glomerular hemodynamics or hypertrophy and was attributable to a specific androgen effect.[26] Data regarding the effect of gender on the risk of CKD and progression in humans are, however, somewhat contradictory. Many reports have indicated that male gender is associated with worse renal outcomes. Studies have reported a higher incidence of proteinuria and CKD among men in the general population and an increased risk of ESKD or death associated with CKD,[17,20,27] a higher risk of decline in renal function in male hypertensive patients,[21] a lower risk of ESKD in female patients with CKD stage 3,[22] and a shorter time to renal replacement therapy (RRT) in male patients with CKD stage 4 or 5.[24] In addition, most national registries, including the U.S. Renal Data Service (USRDS), have reported a substantially higher incidence of ESKD in males (413 per million population [pmp] in 2003) versus females (280 pmp).[28] Previous meta-analyses have, however, yielded conflicting results, with one reporting a higher rate of decline in GFR in men[29] and another reporting a higher risk of doubling of the serum creatinine level or ESKD in women after adjustment for baseline variables, including blood pressure and urinary protein excretion.[30]

The largest meta-analysis to date included data from studies of 2,051,158 participants investigating the impact of gender on CKD-related outcomes. Whereas the risk of all-cause and cardiovascular mortality was higher in men than women, the relative risk of mortality increased with lower GFR and higher albuminuria in both, and the slope of increase in risk was steeper in women than men. Importantly, the relative risk of ESKD increased with lower GFR and higher albuminuria in both sexes and there was no evidence of a difference in the increase in risk between men and women (Figure 22.3).[31] One limitation of many of the studies quoted is that menopausal status of the women was not documented. Nevertheless, it is clear from the most robust data published that CKD is associated with at least the same relative increase in risk of death and ESKD in women as in men. The reasons for the higher absolute incidence of renal replacement therapy in men versus women require further investigation. For further discussion of the impact of gender on CKD, see Chapters 20, 21, and 52.

ETHNICITY

African Americans are overrepresented in the U.S. dialysis population, suggesting that ethnicity is a strong risk factor for the progression of CKD to ESKD. Population-based studies have found a higher incidence of ESKD among African Americans that was attributable only in part to socioeconomic and other known risk factors.[5,20,32,33] Similarly, the risk of early renal function decline (increase in serum creatinine ≥ 0.4 mg/dL) was approximately threefold higher (odds ratio [OR], 3.15; 95% confidence interval [CI], 1.86 to 5.33) among black versus white diabetic adults, but 82% of this excess risk was attributable to socioeconomic and other known risk factors.[34] The risk of renal function decline over 5 years among hypertensive patients was greater in African Americans,[21] and African ancestry was independently associated with a greater rate of GFR decline in the MDRD study.[8] Interestingly, data from the Reasons for Geographic and Racial Differences in Stroke (REGARDS) Cohort Study have shown a lower prevalence of estimated GFR (50 to 59 mL/min/1.73 m^2) among African American versus white subjects but a higher prevalence of estimated GFR (10 to 19 mL/min/1.73 m^2),[35] suggesting that African American ethnicity acts as a progression factor but not as a susceptibility factor. A 2012 report from the USRDS showed a substantially higher incidence of ESKD in African Americans (3.3 times higher than whites), Hispanics (1.5 times higher than non-Hispanics), and Native Americans (1.5 times higher than whites).[36] Similarly, the prevalence of ESKD in 2012 was higher among minority groups: African Americans, 5671 pmp; Native Americans, 2600 pmp; Hispanics, 2932 pmp; Asians, 2272 pmp; and whites, 1432 pmp.[36] CKD and ESKD have also been reported to be more prevalent in other ethnic groups, including Asians,[37] Hispanics[38] Native Americans,[39] Mexican Americans,[40] and Aboriginal Australians.[41]

A large meta-analysis that included data from 940,366 participants in 25 general population cohort studies investigated the impact of ethnicity on the risks associated with CKD in blacks, whites, and Asians. The absolute risk of all-cause or cardiovascular mortality (after adjustment for age) and ESKD was higher in black versus white versus Asian participants. However, the relative risk of all-cause or cardiovascular mortality and ESKD increased to a similar degree with lower GFR or greater albuminuria in all the ethnic groups.[42] Thus, the risk between lower GFR or greater albuminuria and mortality or ESKD was not modified by ethnicity. The mechanisms underlying the associations between ethnicity and CKD remain to be elucidated, but possible explanations include genetic factors (see below, "Hereditary Factors"), increased prevalence of diabetes mellitus, lower nephron endowment, increased susceptibility to salt-sensitive hypertension, and environmental, lifestyle, and socioeconomic differences. Ethnicity and CKD are discussed further in Chapters 20, 21, and 52.

HEREDITARY FACTORS

Hereditary renal diseases resulting from a single gene defect, such as autosomal dominant polycystic kidney disease, Alport's disease, Fabry's disease, and congenital nephrotic syndrome, account for a relatively small yet clinically important proportion of all patients with CKD. Nevertheless, evidence is rapidly accumulating that genetic factors account for familial clustering of many other forms of CKD with multifactorial causes. Among 25,883 incident ESKD patients, 22.8% reported a family history of ESKD,[43] and screening of the relatives of patients with ESKD revealed evidence of CKD in 49.3%.[44] In another case-control study, including 689 patients with ESKD and 361 controls, having one first-degree relative with CKD increased the risk of ESKD by 1.3 (95% CI, 0.7 to 2.6) and having two such relatives increased it by 10.4 (95% CI, 2.7 to 40.2) after controlling for multiple known risk factors, including diabetes and hypertension.[45] Similarly, a case-control study of 103 U.S. white patients with ESKD reported a 3.5-fold increase in risk of ESKD (95% CI, 1.5 to 8.4) with the presence of a first-, second-, or third-degree relative with ESKD.[46]

A genetic explanation for the high incidence of ESKD observed in African Americans was provided by groundbreaking research that identified strong associations between ESKD and two coding variants in the *APOL1* gene. These gene variants confer resistance to infection with *Trypanosoma brucei rhodesiense,* which causes sleeping sickness.

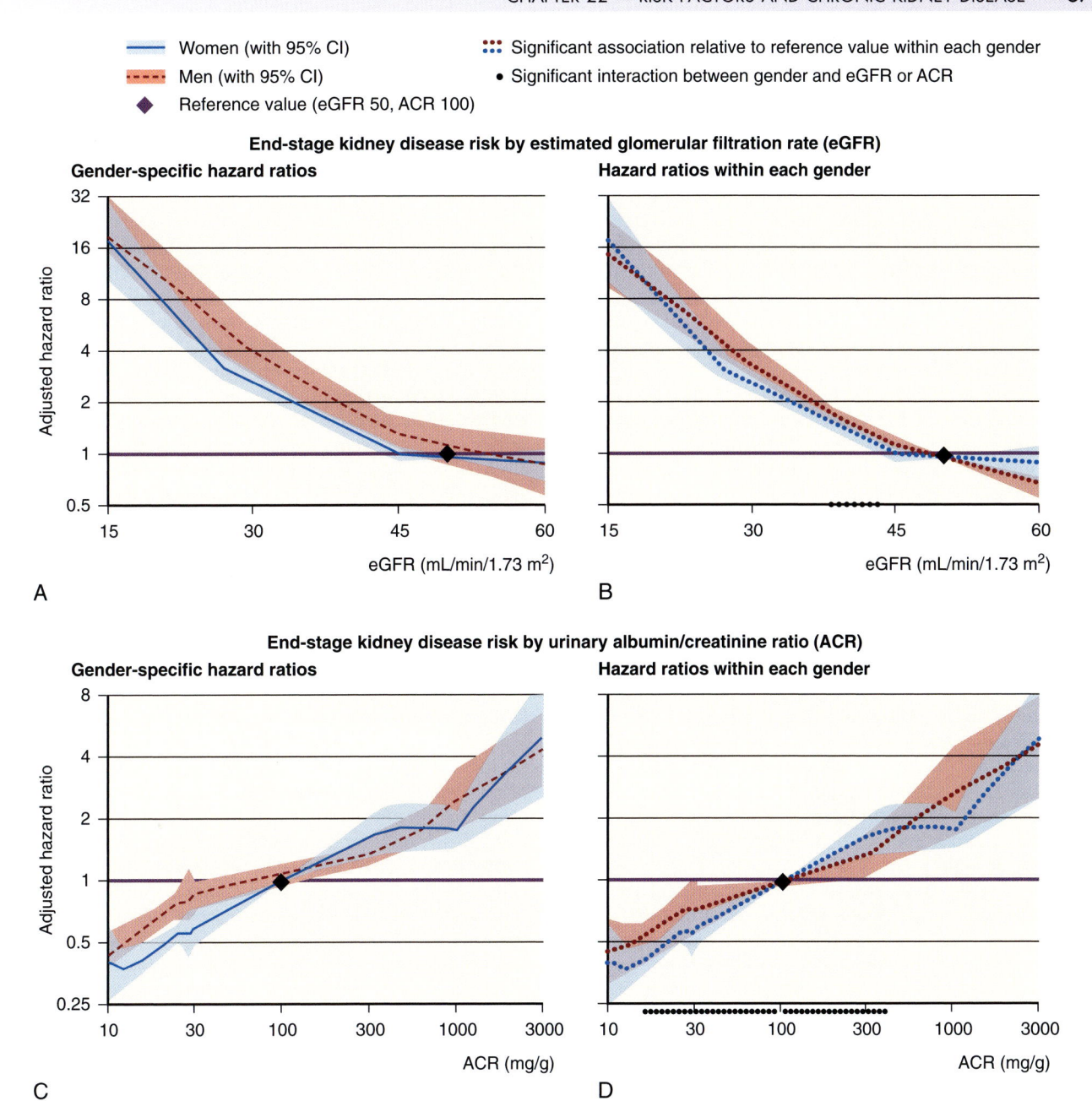

Figure 22.3 **A, B,** Hazard ratios of end-stage kidney disease according to estimated glomerular filtration rate. **C, D,** Urinary albumin/creatinine ratio in men versus women in chronic kidney disease cohorts. **A, C,** Gender-specific hazard ratios, including a main effect for male gender at the reference point. **B, D,** Hazard ratios in each gender, thus visually removing the baseline difference between men and women. Hazard ratios were adjusted for age, gender, race, smoking status, systolic blood pressure, history of cardiovascular disease, diabetes, serum total cholesterol concentration, body mass index, and estimated glomerular filtration rate splines or albuminuria. (Adapted from Nitsch D, Grams M, Sang Y, et al: Associations of estimated glomerular filtration rate and albuminuria with mortality and renal failure by sex: a meta-analysis. *BMJ* 346:f324, 2013.)

This observation explains how selection likely resulted in a high prevalence of these variants in the population. Subsequent studies have identified associations between *APOL1* risk variants and several renal pathologies, including focal segmental glomerulosclerosis (FSGS), HIV-associated nephropathy (HIVAN), sickle cell kidney disease, and severe lupus nephritis.[47] Moreover, cohort studies have reported associations between *APOL1* risk variants and risk of progression to ESKD. Risk of progression was the lowest in European Americans (with no risk variants), intermediate in African Americans, with no or one risk variant, and highest in African Americans, with two risk variants.[48] It is estimated that *APOL1* variants account for 40% of disease burden due to CKD in African Americans.

Despite the strong association between inheritance of two *APOL1* risk variants and ESKD, only a minority of people with this genotype actually develop kidney disease, suggesting that the action of a second factor is required to cause disease in genetically susceptible individuals. HIV is one example of such a second hit, but it has been proposed that other viruses and other gene variants may also be important.[47]

Other studies have suggested that genetic factors also increase susceptibility to early manifestations of CKD. In a study of 169 families with one type 2 diabetic proband, the diabetic siblings of probands with microalbuminuria had a significantly increased risk of also having microalbuminuria, after adjustment for confounding risk factors (OR, 3.94; 95% CI, 1.93 to 9.01) than the diabetic siblings of probands without microalbuminuria.[49] Furthermore, the nondiabetic siblings of diabetic probands with microalbuminuria had a significantly higher urinary albumin excretion rate (within the normal range) than the nondiabetic siblings of normoalbuminuric diabetic probands.

Genomewide association studies (GWAS) have identified multiple novel loci that are significantly associated with serum creatinine levels or CKD.[50-52] Furthermore, a recent GWAS meta-analysis conducted in 63,558 participants of European descent identified significant associations between GFR decline over time and three gene loci—*UMOD* (previously associated with CKD and ESKD), *GALNTL5/GALNT11*, and *CDH23*. It was estimated that the heritability of GFR decline in this population was 38%.[53] Further studies have investigated the role of epigenetic factors (heritable changes in the pattern of gene expression not attributable to changes in the primary nucleotide sequence) that may affect the risk of CKD progression. One study compared the genomewide DNA methylation profile in 20 people from the Chronic Renal Insufficiency Cohort (CRIC) study with the most rapid decline in GFR and 20 with the most stable GFR. Results identified differences in the methylation of several genes associated with epithelial to mesenchymal transition and inflammation that may be involved in the mechanisms of CKD progression.[54]

From this discussion, it is clear that genetic factors may act as susceptibility factors in some subjects, initiating factors in those with CKD due to a single gene defect, or progression factors in others. The rapid growth in knowledge of genetic aspects of CKD will likely result in genetic risk factors becoming increasingly important in risk prediction for patients with CKD. For a more detailed discussion of genetic aspects of kidney disease, see Chapters 43 to 46.

HEMODYNAMIC FACTORS

Experimental studies have shown that glomerular hemodynamic responses (e.g., glomerular capillary hypertension and hyperfiltration) to nephron loss[55] and chronic hyperglycemia[56] are critical factors in establishing the vicious cycle of nephron loss characteristic of CKD. In addition, any factor that further increases glomerular hypertension and/or hyperfiltration may be expected to exacerbate glomerular damage and accelerate the progression of CKD (see Figure 22.1).

DECREASED NEPHRON NUMBER

NEPHRON ENDOWMENT

Autopsy studies have revealed that the number of nephrons per kidney varies widely in humans, from 210,332 to 2,702,079 in one series.[57] Multiple factors have been shown to influence nephron endowment, including those that affect the fetomaternal environment as well as genetic factors.[58] A substantial body of evidence supports the hypothesis that low nephron endowment predisposes individuals to CKD by provoking an increase in SNGFR and, therefore, a reduction in renal reserve. The ascertainment of nephron number in living human subjects is currently not possible, but autopsy studies have shown an association between reduced nephron number and hypertension,[59] as well as glomerulosclerosis.[60] In human autopsy studies, low birth weight is directly associated with reduced nephron number,[61,62] and birth weight may therefore serve as a marker of nephron endowment. Low birth weight is also a risk factor for later life hypertension and diabetes mellitus, both of which further increase the risk of CKD.[63] One meta-analysis of 32 studies, which included data from over 2 million subjects, reported a significantly increased risk of albuminuria (OR, 1.81; 95% CI, 1.19 to 2.77) and ESKD (OR, 1.58; 95% CI, 1.33 to 1.88) associated with low birth weight.[64] Thus low birth weight, acting as a marker of reduced nephron endowment, may be regarded as a susceptibility and progression risk factor for CKD. Factors affecting nephron endowment and the consequences of reduced nephron endowment are discussed in more detail in Chapter 23.

ACQUIRED NEPHRON DEFICIT

In experimental models of acquired nephron deficit, severe nephron loss (5/6 nephrectomy) alone initiates a cycle of progressive injury in the remaining glomeruli, mediated primarily through glomerular hypertension and hyperfiltration.[55] In 14 patients subjected to similarly large reductions in nephron number following partial resection of a single kidney, 2 developed ESKD and 9 developed proteinuria, the extent of which was inversely correlated with the amount of renal tissue remaining.[65] Lesser degrees of acquired nephron loss, such as removal of one of two previously normal kidneys (uninephrectomy), may not be sufficient to cause CKD in most subjects.[12,66,67] However, nephrectomy for renal cell carcinoma is associated with an increased risk of developing CKD that is greater after radical nephrectomy than partial nephrectomy, suggesting that in the presence of subclinical kidney damage, acquired nephron loss may provoke CKD, and that the risk is proportional to the number of nephrons removed.[68]

Nephron loss may also predispose individuals to CKD if they are also exposed to other risk factors. This is perhaps best illustrated by the observation that uninephrectomy exacerbates renal injury in experimental diabetic nephropathy[69] and, in diabetics, uninephrectomy increases the risk of developing diabetic nephropathy.[14]

The interaction between nephron loss and other risk factors is further illustrated by the observation that in a study of 488 people who had surgery for renal cell carcinoma, radical nephrectomy (compared to partial nephrectomy), diabetes, and increased age were each independently associated with an increased risk of developing CKD at least 6 months after surgery. In those who had a partial nephrectomy but no additional risk factors, only 7% developed CKD, but this increased to 24%, 30%, and 42% in those 60 years of age or older, those with hypertension, and diabetics, respectively.[70]

In most forms of human CKD, initial nephron loss due to primary renal disease, multisystem disorders that involve the kidney or exposure to nephrotoxins is focal, but hemodynamic adaptations in the remaining glomeruli are thought to contribute to nephron loss by provoking further glomerulosclerosis (see Chapter 52). Several epidemiologic studies have supported this hypothesis by showing that patients with a reduced GFR are at increased risk of a further decline in renal function. Two large meta-analyses of cohort studies identified baseline GFR as a strong predictor of ESKD. Among 845,125 participants from the general population, the estimated GFR (eGFR) was independently associated with an increased risk of developing ESKD when it fell below 75 mL/min/1.73 m^2. For groups of patients with average eGFRs of 60, 45, and 15 mL/min/1.73 m^2, the hazard ratios for developing ESKD were 4, 29, and 454, respectively, when compared to a reference group with an eGFR of 95 mL/min/1.73 m^2. Similar findings were reported in a further 173,892 participants selected for being at increased risk of developing CKD (Figure 22.4).[71] Among 21,688 patients selected for having CKD, a lower eGFR was an independent risk factor for ESKD, such that a fall of 15 mL/min/1.73 m^2 below a threshold of 45 mL/min/1.73 m^2 was associated with a pooled hazard ratio of 6.24.[72] Further analyses by the CKD Prognosis Consortium have confirmed that the association between reduced GFR and increased risk of ESKD persists independently of gender,[31] age,[25] ethnicity,[42] diabetes,[73] and hypertension.[74] Additionally, analysis of data from 1,530,648 participants has shown that change in GFR over time is strongly predictive of future risk of ESKD (and mortality), suggesting that a GFR decline of 30% may be useful as a surrogate marker of CKD progression in clinical trials.[75] Thus, in different contexts, acquired nephron deficit may be regarded as a susceptibility factor (e.g., after donor nephrectomy in a healthy kidney donor), initiation factor (when severe nephron loss provokes glomerulosclerosis in remaining previously normal glomeruli), or progression factor (when nephron loss accelerates pre-existing damage in remaining glomeruli).

The importance of GFR as a risk factor has emphasized the need for more accurate methods to estimate it. Adoption of the MDRD equation improved detection of CKD and made possible much of the epidemiologic research on CKD, but it was recognized from the outset that the MDRD equation was imperfect and, in particular, tended to underestimate true GFR at values above 60 mL/min/1.73 m^2. This is important because this is the threshold below which CKD may be diagnosed without other evidence of kidney damage.

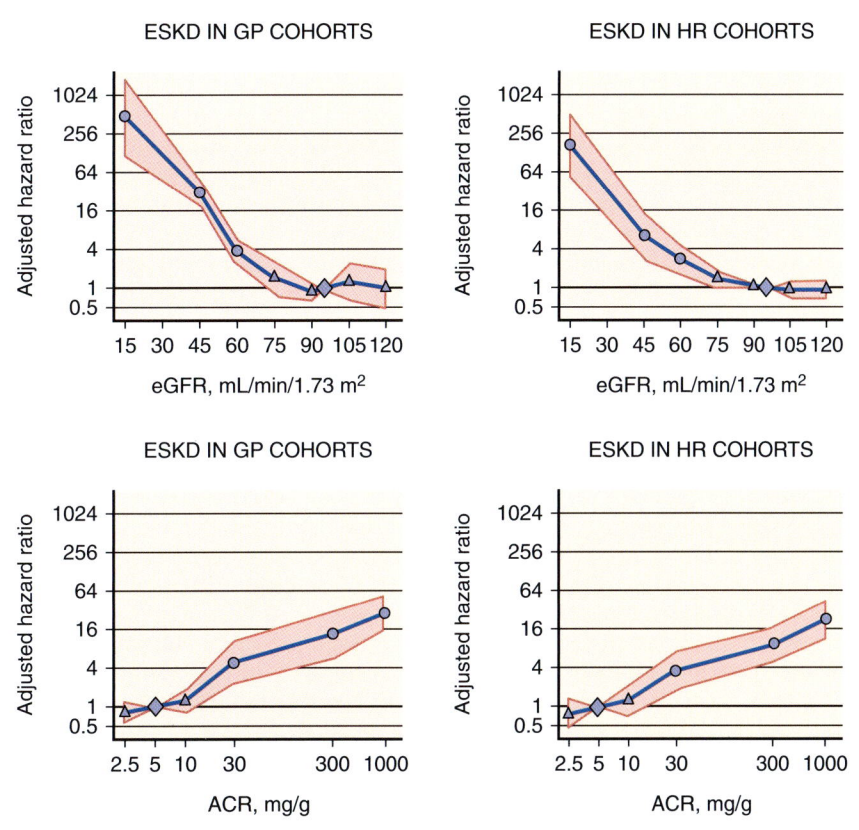

Figure 22.4 Pooled hazard ratios (95% CI) for end-stage kidney disease (ESKD) according to spline estimated glomerular filtration rate (eGFR) **(upper panels)** and albumin/creatinine ratio **(lower panels)**, adjusted for each other and for age, gender, and cardiovascular risk factors (continuous analyses). Reference categories are eGFR of 95 mL/min/1.73 m^2 and albumin/creatinine ratio of 5 mg/g or dipstick-negative or trace. **Left panels,** Results for general population cohorts. **Right panels,** High-risk cohorts. *Dots* represent statistical significance, *triangles* represent nonsignificance, and *shaded areas* are 95% confidence interval. ACR, Albumin/creatinine ratio; GP, general population; HR, high risk. (From Gansevoort RT, Matsushita K, van der Velde M, et al; Chronic Kidney Disease Prognosis Consortium: lower estimated GFR and higher albuminuria are associated with adverse kidney outcomes in both general and high-risk populations. A collaborative meta-analysis of general and high-risk population cohorts. *Kidney Int* 79:1341-1352, 2011.)

Several other equations have been developed to estimate GFR from serum creatinine concentration, culminating in a recommendation by KDIGO that the MDRD equation should be replaced by the Chronic Kidney Disease Epidemiology Collaboration (CKD-EPI) equation, which is more accurate than the MDRD equation and results in less bias, particularly at GFR values above 60 mL/min/1.73 m^2. Further analysis by the CKD Prognosis Consortium found that the eGFR determined by the CKD-EPI equation results in a lower prevalence of CKD stages 3 to 5 (8.7% vs. 6.3%) and affords better risk prediction than the MDRD equation. Among those classified as having an eGFR of 59 to 45 mL/min/1.73 m^2 by the MDRD equation, 34.7% were reclassified by the CKD-EPI as having an eGFR of 89 to 60 mL/min/1.73 m^2, and those reclassified had a lower incidence of adverse outcomes versus those not reclassified (e.g., incidence of all-cause mortality 9.9 vs. 34.5/1000 person-years).[76]

The limitations of creatinine as a marker of GFR due to nonrenal factors that affect serum creatinine concentration, including muscle mass and diet, have prompted a search for alternatives. Cystatin C, a peptide produced by all nucleated cells and therefore not affected by muscle mass, has emerged as the most promising alternative. The production of reference material to standardize cystatin C assays has greatly improved the potential for clinical application, and equations have been developed to estimate the GFR from the serum cystatin C concentration or from creatinine and cystatin C levels together. The combined equation and CKD-EPI (creatinine) equation have similar bias, but the combined equation yields better precision and accuracy.[77] Further work by the CKD Prognosis Consortium has reported that when cystatin C is used to estimate GFR, reclassification to a higher GFR category (higher than that assigned by eGFR creatinine) is associated with a lower risk of all-cause mortality, cardiovascular mortality, and ESKD.[78] It should be noted, however, that in this analysis, CKD was defined by a single eGFR value. It therefore remains to be established whether the use of cystatin C will improve risk prediction in those with CKD defined by two eGFR values determined at least 90 days apart, as required by the KDIGO definition.

ACUTE KIDNEY INJURY

Despite previous perceptions that patients who recover from acute kidney injury (AKI) regain normal renal function and have a good prognosis, several cohort studies have reported that recovery from AKI is associated with a substantially increased risk of CKD and death. Among 3769 adults who required dialysis for AKI and survived dialysis free for at least 30 days, the incidence rate for chronic dialysis was 2.63/100 versus 0.91/100-person years in 13,598 matched controls (adjusted hazard ratio [HR], 3.23; 95% CI, 2.70 to 3.86).[79] The relative risk was particularly high for those with no previous diagnosis of CKD (adjusted HR, 15.54; 95% CI, 9.65 to 25.03). There was no difference in survival between the groups. In another study of similar design, outcomes were investigated in 343 patients with a preadmission eGFR more than 45 mL/min/1.73 m^2 who required dialysis for AKI but survived for at least 30 days after discharge without dialysis. After controlling for potential confounders, AKI that required dialysis was associated with a 28-fold increase in the risk of developing CKD stage 4 or 5 (adjusted HR, 28.1; 95% CI, 21.1 to 37.6) and more than double the risk of death (adjusted HR, 2.3; 95% CI, 1.8 to 3.0) versus 555,660 adult patients hospitalized during the same period but without AKI.[80]

Analysis of data from a cohort of 233,803 Medicare beneficiaries 67 years or older who were hospitalized in 2000 reported a substantially increased risk of developing ESKD in those who developed AKI on a background of CKD (HR, 41.2; 95% CI, 34.6 to 49.1) or without previous CKD (HR, 13.0; 95% CI, 10.6 to 16.0) versus those who did not develop AKI. The importance of AKI as a risk factor for CKD initiation was further illustrated by the observation that among patients who had AKI without preexisting CKD ($N = 4730$), 72.1% developed CKD within 2 years of the AKI episode. Furthermore, 25.2% of those who developed ESKD had a history of AKI.[81] In a similar study, a cohort of 113,272 patients hospitalized with a primary diagnosis of acute tubular necrosis (ATN), AKI, pneumonia, or myocardial infarction (control group) was studied. Overall, 11.4% progressed to CKD stage 4 during follow-up, including 20.0% of those with ATN, 13.2% of those with AKI, 24.7% of those with preexisting CKD, and 3.3% of the control patients. After controlling for other variables, having a diagnosis of AKI, ATN, or CKD increased the risk of developing CKD stage 4 by 303%, 564%, and 550%, respectively, versus controls. After controlling for covariates, AKI and CKD were associated with an increased risk of death of 12% and 20%, respectively, versus controls.[82]

The multiplicative effect of AKI on CKD progression is further illustrated by a study of 39,805 patients with an eGFR less than 45 mL/min/1.73 m^2 prior to hospitalization. Those who survived an episode of dialysis-requiring AKI had a very high risk of developing ESKD within 30 days of hospital discharge (i.e., nonrecovery of AKI) that was related to the preadmission eGFR. For an eGFR of 30 to 44 mL/min/1.73 m^2, the incidence of ESKD was 42% and, for an eGFR of 15 to 29 mL/min/1.73 m^2, it was as high as 63%, whereas the incidence of ESKD was only 1.5% in those who did not have dialysis-requiring AKI. In patients who survived longer than 30 days after hospital discharge without ESKD, the incidence of ESKD and death at 6 months was 12.7% and 19.7%, respectively, versus 1.7% and 7.4% in the comparator group with CKD but no AKI. After adjustment for multiple risk factors, AKI was associated with a 30% increase in long-term risk for death or ESKD (adjusted HR, 1.30; 95% CI, 1.04 to 1.64).[83]

Consistent with the findings of individual studies, a meta-analysis of 13 cohort studies reported a significantly increased risk of developing CKD and ESKD in patients who had survived an episode of AKI versus participants without AKI (pooled adjusted HR for CKD, 8.8; 95% CI, 3.1 to 25.5; pooled HR for ESKD, 3.1; 95% CI, 1.9 to 5.0).[84] Taken together, these data show that AKI should be regarded as an important risk factor for CKD initiation and progression. The mechanisms responsible for these observations require further elucidation but have been proposed to include nephron loss, loss of peritubular capillaries, cell cycle arrest, cell senescence, pericyte and myofibroblast activation, fibrogenic cytokine production, and interstitial fibrosis.[85,86] The incidence of AKI has increased, and it is likely to become an increasingly important risk factor for CKD among older patients.

BLOOD PRESSURE

Hypertension is an almost universal consequence of reduced renal function but is also an important factor in the progression of CKD. In the hypothesis of CKD progression presented in Figure 22.1, it is clear that elevated systemic blood pressure transmitted to the glomerulus would contribute to glomerular hypertension and thus accelerate glomerular damage. Hypertension has been shown to be predictive of ESKD risk in several large population-based studies.[17,18,27,87] Furthermore, a close association between the magnitude of increased risk and level of blood pressure has been reported in several studies, so that even elevations in blood pressure below the threshold for the diagnosis of hypertension were associated with increased risk of ESKD.[17,27,88]

Among patients with CKD in the MDRD study, higher baseline mean arterial pressure (MAP) independently predicted a greater rate of GFR decline.[8] These observations have led to the suggestion that blood pressure be viewed as a continuous rather than dichotomous risk factor for CKD, with less emphasis on traditional definitions of hypertension and normotension.[89] Despite these close associations, the causality criterion for a risk factor requires evidence from an RCT. Three large RCTs have sought to investigate the effect on CKD progression of intensive versus standard blood pressure lowering. Whereas the primary analysis of data from the MDRD study found no significant difference between the rate of decline in GFR between patients randomized to intensive blood pressure control (target MAP < 92 mm Hg, equivalent to <125/75 mm Hg) versus standard blood pressure control (target MAP < 107 mm Hg, equivalent to 140/90 mm Hg), a secondary analysis did show benefit associated with the low blood pressure target in patients with higher levels of baseline proteinuria.[90] Further secondary analysis showed that the lower achieved blood pressure was also associated with a slower GFR decline, an effect that was more marked in patients with higher baseline proteinuria.[91] Furthermore, long-term follow-up (mean, 6.6 years) of patients from the MDRD study reported a significant reduction in the risk of ESKD (adjusted HR, 0.68; 95% CI, 0.57 to 0.82) or a combined end point of ESKD or death (adjusted HR 0.77; 95% CI, 0.65 to 0.91) in patients randomized to low blood pressure targets, even though treatment and blood pressure data were not available beyond the 2.2 years of the original trial.[92]

In the African American Study of Kidney Disease and Hypertension (AASK), no significant difference in the rate of GFR decline was observed between subjects randomized to MAP goals of ≤92 mm Hg or lower versus 102 to 107 mm Hg. It should be noted, however, that patients in AASK generally had low levels of baseline proteinuria (mean urine protein, 0.38 to 0.63 g/day).[93] Furthermore, prolonged follow-up of the AASK cohort after completion of the randomized trial found no significant differences in the primary outcome for the whole cohort; however, it did show a significantly reduced risk of creatinine doubling, ESKD, or death in subjects with a baseline urine protein/creatinine ratio more than 0.22 g/g who were initially randomized to intensive blood pressure control.[94] Thus, the MDRD and AASK study results suggest a significant interaction between blood pressure and proteinuria as risk factors for CKD progression.

In a third study, additional blood pressure reduction with a calcium channel blocker in patients with nondiabetic CKD on ACE inhibitor (ACEI) treatment failed to produce additional renoprotection, but the degree of additional blood pressure reduction was modest (4.1/2.8 mm Hg) and may have been insufficient to improve outcomes in patients already receiving optimal ACEI therapy.[95] A recent RCT has reported significant benefit associated with a lower blood pressure target in young people with autosomal dominant polycystic kidney disease (age < 50 years) and GFR higher than 60 mL/min/1.73 m². Participants randomized to a low blood pressure target (110/75 to 95/60 mm Hg) evidenced a slower rate of increase in kidney volume and a greater decrease in albuminuria and left ventricular mass index than those randomized to usual blood pressure control (120/70 to 130/80 mm Hg).[96] Interestingly blood pressure was not an independent predictor of ESKD in diabetic patients in the RENAAL study[97] or in predominantly nondiabetic subjects in the Chronic Renal Insufficiency in Birmingham (CRIB) study.[98] This is likely due to the fact that blood pressure was well controlled in all subjects (in the RENAAL study) and illustrates how risk factors may vary in importance, depending on the population studied.

Taken together, there is convincing evidence that elevated blood pressure is an important risk factor for progression of CKD, although unequivocal evidence from RCTs is lacking, and some uncertainty remains regarding optimal treatment targets. It is hoped that the ongoing Systolic Blood Pressure Intervention Trial (SPRINT; NCT01206062 at www.clinicaltrials.gov), which randomized more than 9000 subjects, including about one third with nondiabetic CKD, to systolic blood pressure targets of less than 120 or 140 mm Hg, will yield new data to guide future recommendations.[99]

OBESITY AND METABOLIC SYNDROME

In experimental models, obesity is associated with hypertension, proteinuria, and progressive renal disease. Micropuncture studies have confirmed that obesity is another cause of glomerular hyperfiltration and glomerular hypertension that can be predicted to exacerbate the progression of CKD.[100,101] Furthermore, several other factors associated with obesity and the metabolic syndrome may contribute to renal damage, including hormones and proinflammatory molecules produced by adipocytes,[102] increased mineralocorticoid levels and/or mineralocorticoid receptor activation by cortisol,[103] and reduced adiponectin levels.[104] In humans, severe obesity is associated with increased renal plasma flow, glomerular hyperfiltration, and albuminuria, abnormalities that are reversed by weight loss.[105] Obesity, as defined by increased body mass index (BMI), has been associated with increased risk of developing CKD in several large population-based studies.[18,106,107] Furthermore, one study has found a progressive increase in relative risk of developing ESKD associated with increasing BMI (RR, 3.57; 95% CI, 3.05 to 4.18 for BMI of 30.0 to 34.9 kg/m² vs. BMI of 18.5 to 24.9 kg/m²) among 320,252 subjects confirmed to have no evidence of CKD at initial screening.[108]

There is evidence that obesity may directly cause a specific form of glomerulopathy characterized by proteinuria and histologic features of focal and segmental glomerulosclerosis,[109,110] but it is likely that it also acts as a risk factor in the development of several other forms of renal disease. One study has identified childhood obesity as a risk factor for CKD in adulthood. Among 4340 participants born in one week in 1946, pubertal-onset obesity and obesity throughout childhood were associated with an increased risk of CKD (defined by eGFR < 60 mL/min/1.73 m^2 or albuminuria) at age 60 to 64 years.[111] Interest has also focused on the role of the metabolic syndrome (insulin resistance), as defined by the presence of abdominal obesity, dyslipidemia, hypertension, and fasting hyperglycemia, in the development of CKD. An analysis of data from the Third National Health and Nutrition Examination Survey (NHANES III) data found a significantly increased risk of CKD and microalbuminuria in subjects with the metabolic syndrome as well as a progressive increase in risk associated with the number of components of the metabolic syndrome present.[112] Furthermore, a large longitudinal study of 10,096 patients without diabetes or CKD at baseline identified metabolic syndrome as an independent risk factor for the development of CKD over 9 years (adjusted OR, 1.43; 95% CI, 1.18 to 1.73). Again, there was a progressive increase in risk associated with the number of traits of the metabolic syndrome present (OR, 1.13; 95% CI, 0.89 to 1.45 for one trait vs. OR, 2.45; 95% CI, 1.32 to 4.54 for five traits).[113] In another study, patient hip/waist ratio, a marker of insulin resistance, was independently associated with impaired renal function, even in lean individuals (BMI < 25 kg/m^2), among a population-based cohort of 7676 subjects.[114]

The effect of obesity on the progression of established CKD is less well documented. Increased BMI has been identified as a risk factor for CKD progression among subjects with immunoglobulin A (IgA) nephropathy,[115] renal mass reduction surgery or renal agenesis,[116] and renal transplants.[117] On the other hand, BMI was unrelated to the risk of ESKD among a cohort of patients with CKD stage 4 or 5.[24] It is widely recognized that weight loss is difficult to achieve in obese individuals, but surgical intervention in the form of gastric banding or bypass appears to offer the most effective long-term outcomes. Two large cohort studies have shown significant survival benefit in subjects who underwent bariatric surgery,[118,119] but unfortunately renal end points were not reported in these studies. Beneficial renoprotective effects of weight loss have been reported in a meta-analysis of observational studies that found an association between weight loss and reduction in proteinuria independent of blood pressure,[120] as well as smaller studies that reported improvement or stabilization of renal function[121] or reduction in proteinuria[122] following bariatric surgery in subjects with CKD.

The best method for assessing obesity in CKD remains to be determined. A further systematic review analyzed the effects of weight loss achieved by bariatric surgery, medication, or diet in 31 studies and found that in most studies, weight loss was associated with reductions in proteinuria. In people with glomerular hyperfiltration, the GFR tended to decrease with weight loss, and in those with a reduced GFR, it tended to increase.[123] BMI is the most widely applied method but does not take body composition into account. One study has reported a high sensitivity but relatively low specificity of BMI to detect obesity in subjects with CKD.[124]

HIGH DIETARY PROTEIN INTAKE

Protein feeding provokes an increase in GFR in rodents[125] and humans.[126] Consistent with the hypothesis that the glomerular hemodynamic changes associated with hyperfiltration accelerate glomerular injury, experimental studies have reported that a high-protein diet accelerates renal disease progression, whereas dietary protein restriction[127,128] results in normalization of glomerular capillary hydraulic pressure as well as SNGFR and marked attenuation of glomerular damage.[55] Observational studies in humans have reported an increased risk of microalbuminuria associated with higher dietary protein intake in subjects with diabetes and hypertension (OR, 3.3; 95% CI, 1.4 to 7.8) but not in healthy subjects or those with isolated diabetes or hypertension,[129] again illustrating the interaction between risk factors for CKD. In another study, high intake of protein, particularly nondairy animal protein, was associated with a greater rate of GFR decline among women with an eGFR of 80 to 55 mL/min/1.73 m^2 but not in those with an eGFR of more than 80 mL/min/1.73 m^2.[130] Randomized trials investigating the effects of high protein are lacking, but several studies have sought to examine the potential renoprotective effects of dietary protein restriction. In the MDRD study, primary analysis revealed no significant difference in the mean rate of GFR decline in subjects randomized to low- or very low-protein diets,[90] but secondary analysis of outcomes according to achieved dietary protein intake indicated that a reduction in protein intake of 0.2 g/kg/day correlated with a 1.15-mL/min/year reduction in the rate of GFR decline, equivalent to a 29% reduction in the mean rate of GFR decline.[131] On the other hand, long-term follow-up of participants in study 2 of the MDRD trial found no renoprotective benefit among those randomized to very low-protein diet in the original study, but did report a higher risk of death in this group (HR, 1.92; 95% CI 1.15 to 3.20).[132] Nevertheless, three meta-analyses of smaller studies have all reported a significant renoprotective benefit associated with dietary protein restriction.[133-135] The role of dietary protein restriction in the management of CKD is discussed further in Chapters 52 and 61.

PREGNANCY AND PREECLAMPSIA

Physiologic adaptations during pregnancy provoke glomerular hyperfiltration that usually does not cause renal damage. In the context of preexisting CKD, however, the glomerular hyperfiltration of pregnancy can be predicted to exacerbate proteinuria and glomerular injury. Several studies have shown an increased risk of CKD progression during pregnancy, particularly when the pregestational serum creatinine is 1.4 mg/dL or higher (≥124 µmol/L). In one study of 82 pregnancies in 67 women with primary renal disease and serum creatinine level of 1.4 mg/dL or more, blood pressure, serum creatinine, and proteinuria increased during pregnancy. In 70 pregnancies with postpartum data available, persistent loss of maternal renal function at 6 months was reported in 31%, and by 12 months 8 women had progressed to ESKD. Adverse obstetric outcomes included preterm delivery in 59% and low birth weight in 37%, although fetal survival was 93%.[136]

In a more recent series of 49 women with CKD stage 3 to 5 before pregnancy, the mean GFR declined during pregnancy (from 35 ± 12.2 to 30 ± 13.8 mL/min/1.73 m^2), but there was no change in the mean postpartum rate of GFR decline. Nevertheless, a pregestational GFR less than 40 mL/min/1.73 m^2, combined with proteinuria of more than 1 g/day, was associated with a more rapid postpartum GFR decline and a shorter time to ESKD or halving of GFR and low birth weight.[137] Although earlier reports suggested good outcomes, one recent study has reported adverse effects associated even with early-stage CKD. In 91 pregnancies with predominantly CKD stages 1 and 2, modest increases in hypertension, serum creatinine, and proteinuria were observed.[138] An increase in adverse obstetric outcomes, including preterm delivery, lower birth weight, and admission to a neonatal intensive care unit versus low-risk pregnancy controls was also reported; this remained true, even when only those with CKD stage 1 were considered, although there were no perinatal deaths. On the other hand, pregnancy was not associated with a more rapid decline in the GFR over 5 years in a cohort of 245 women of childbearing age with IgA nephropathy and serum creatinine level of 1.2 mg/dL or lower (in the majority).[139]

Complications of pregnancy and, in particular, hypertension and preeclampsia, may also cause renal damage. In one large population-based study, renal outcomes were assessed in 570,433 women who had had at least one singleton pregnancy. Only 477 women developed ESKD at a mean of 17 ± 9 years after the first pregnancy (overall rate, 3.7/100,000/women/year), but preeclampsia was associated with a significant increase in the risk of ESKD, ranging from a relative risk of 4.7 for preeclampsia in a single pregnancy (95% CI, 3.6 to 6.1) to a relative risk of 15.5 for preeclampsia in two or three pregnancies (95% CI, 7.8 to 30.8). The risk was further increased if the pregnancy resulted in a low-birth weight or preterm infant. Causes of ESKD were glomerulonephritis in 35%, hereditary or congenital disease in 21%, diabetic nephropathy in 14%, and interstitial nephritis in 12%.[140] Similarly, in women with diabetes prior to pregnancy, preeclampsia and preterm birth were associated with significantly increased risks of ESKD and death, illustrating how different risk factors for CKD may interact to increase risk.[141]

A large cohort study reported an increased risk of multiple adverse health outcomes after hypertension during pregnancy, including cardiovascular disease, diabetes mellitus, and CKD (HR, 1.91; 95% CI, 1.18 to 3.09).[142] Similarly, a very large case-control study found that hypertension during pregnancy was associated with a substantially increased risk of subsequent CKD (HR, 9.38; 95% CI, 7.09 to 12.4) or ESKD (HR, 12.4; 95% CI, 8.53 to 18.0).[143] In both these studies, the risks of CKD were substantially higher if preeclampsia developed during the pregnancy. Possible explanations for these observations include the presence of pathogenic factors common to CKD and preeclampsia, including obesity, hypertension, insulin resistance, and endothelial dysfunction, exacerbation by preeclampsia of preexisting subclinical CKD, and effects of preeclampsia on the kidney that increase the risk of CKD later in life.[144] That preeclampsia may provoke renal damage has been suggested by several studies showing an increased incidence of microalbuminuria after preeclampsia. A meta-analysis of seven of these studies reported a 31% prevalence of microalbuminuria at a weighted mean of 7.1 years after preeclampsia versus 7% in a control group with uncomplicated pregnancies.[145] Further research is required to identify which mechanisms are most relevant but, even without further information, preeclampsia should be regarded as a risk factor for the development and progression of CKD.

MULTISYSTEM DISORDERS

DIABETES MELLITUS

Diabetic nephropathy has rapidly become the single most common cause of ESKD worldwide. Diabetes was associated with a substantially increased risk of ESKD or death associated with CKD in one population-based study of 23,534 subjects (HR, 7.5; 95% CI, 4.8 to 11.7),[27] as well as an increased risk of moderate CKD (estimated creatinine clearance < 50 mL/min) in another study of 1428 subjects with an estimated creatinine clearance of more than 70 mL/min at baseline.[146] Evidence that glycemic control is a key risk factor for the development of diabetic nephropathy has been shown in randomized trials that found a reduced risk of developing nephropathy in subjects with type 1[147] and type 2[148] diabetes randomized to tight glycemic control. The pathogenesis of diabetic nephropathy is complex and involves multiple mechanisms, including glomerular hemodynamic factors,[56,149] advanced glycation end product formation, generation of reactive oxygen species, and upregulation of profibrotic growth factors and cytokines.[150,151] In at least one study, diabetic nephropathy was associated with more rapid progression to ESKD than other causes of CKD.[24,152,153] Thus, diabetes may be regarded as a susceptibility, initiation, and progression risk factor for CKD. For further discussion of the pathogenesis of diabetic nephropathy, see Chapter 39.

PRIMARY RENAL DISEASE

Whereas substantial variation in the rate of GFR decline has been observed among subjects with a common cause of CKD, there is also evidence that some forms of CKD may provoke more rapid progression than others. In the MDRD study[8] and the Chronic Renal Insufficiency Standards Implementation Study (CRISIS),[152] a diagnosis of adult polycystic kidney disease was an independent predictor of a greater rate of GFR decline. In several cohort studies, diabetic nephropathy was associated with shorter time to ESKD[24] or a more rapid GFR decline than other diagnoses.[152,153]

CARDIOVASCULAR DISEASE

Multiple studies have reported that CKD is associated with a substantial increase in the risk of cardiovascular disease (CVD),[154] and it is therefore not surprising that CVD is also associated with an increased risk of CKD. Among hospitalized Medicare beneficiaries, the prevalence of CKD stage 3 or worse was 60.4% for those with heart failure and 51.7% for those with myocardial infarction. The presence of CKD in addition to heart disease was associated with a significantly increased risk of death and progression to ESKD.[155] These observations may in part be explained by the fact that CVD and CKD share many risk factors, including obesity, metabolic syndrome, hypertension, diabetes mellitus, dyslipidemia, and smoking. In addition, CVD may exert effects on the kidneys that promote the initiation and progression of CKD, including decreased renal perfusion in heart failure and atherosclerosis of the renal arteries. For example, renal atherosclerosis was detected in 39% of patients (≥70% stenosis in 7.3%) undergoing elective coronary angiography.[156] Furthermore, arterial stiffness may result in greater transmission of an elevated systemic blood pressure to glomerular capillaries and exacerbate glomerular hypertension. In one study, pulse wave velocity (PWV) and augmentation index (AI), markers of arterial stiffness, were identified as independent risk factors for progression to ESKD among subjects with CKD stage 4 or 5[157]; in another study, AI was an independent determinant of rate of creatinine clearance decline among subjects with CKD stage 3.[158] On the other hand, neither PWV nor AI were predictors of the rate of GFR decline in a cohort of subjects with CKD stages 2 to 4.[159] In two relatively small cohort studies of those with CKD, a diagnosis of CVD was associated with an increased risk of progression to ESKD[160,161] but, in the CRIC study, a history of any CVD at baseline was not associated with an increased risk of the primary end point of ESKD or 50% GFR reduction among 3939 participants. Conversely, in the same study, a history of heart failure was independently associated with a 29% higher risk of the primary outcome.[162] For further discussion of cardiovascular disease in patients with CKD, see Chapter 56.

BIOMARKERS

URINARY PROTEIN EXCRETION

Abnormal excretion of protein in the urine indicates dysfunction of the glomerular filtration barrier and is therefore a marker of glomerulopathy and an index of disease severity. Experimental evidence has suggested that proteinuria may also contribute to progressive renal damage in CKD (see Chapter 53). A large body of evidence attests to a strong association between proteinuria and the risk of CKD progression, as well as cardiovascular and all-cause mortality. Mass screening of a general population of 107,192 participants by dipstick urinalysis identified proteinuria as the most powerful predictor of ESKD risk over 10 years (OR, 14.9; 95% CI, 10.9 to 20.2).[17] Similarly, among 12,866 middle-aged men enrolled in the multiple risk factor intervention trial (MRFIT), proteinuria detected by dipstick test was associated with a significantly increased risk of developing ESKD over 25 years (HR for 1+ proteinuria, 3.1; 95% CI, 1.8 to 3.8; HR for ≥2+ proteinuria, 15.7; 95% CI, 10.3 to 23.9). Furthermore, detection of 2+ proteinuria or more increased the hazard ratio for ESKD associated with an eGFR less than 60 mL/min/1.73 m^2 from 2.4 without proteinuria (95% CI, 1.5 to 3.8) to 41 with proteinuria (95% CI 15.2 to 71.1).[163]

Similar associations have been reported for measurements of urinary albumin in the general population. In the Nord-Trøndelag Health (HUNT 2) study, which included 65,589 adults, micro- and macroalbuminuria were independent predictors of ESKD after 10.3 years (HR, 13.0 and 47.2, respectively) and combining reduced eGFR with albuminuria substantially improved the prediction of ESKD.[164] In the Prevention of Renal and Vascular End-stage Disease (PREVEND) study, albuminuria was an independent predictor of a decline in eGFR to less than 60 mL/min/1.73 m^2.[165,166]

Among patients selected for having CKD from a wide variety of causes, baseline proteinuria has consistently predicted renal outcomes.[167-169] In three large prospective studies that included patients with nondiabetic CKD (MDRD study, Ramipril Efficacy In Nephropathy [REIN] study, and AASK), higher baseline proteinuria was strongly associated with a more rapid decline in GFR.[8,91,170,171] Similarly, among patients with diabetic nephropathy, the baseline urinary albumin/creatinine ratio was a strong independent predictor of ESKD in the RENAAL study and Irbesartan in Diabetic Nephropathy Trial (IDNT).[97,172] The findings of these individual studies have been confirmed by two large meta-analyses. In one analysis, which included nine general population cohorts ($N = 845,125$) and eight cohorts with increased risk of developing CKD ($N = 173,892$), urine albumin/creatinine ratios of more than 30, 300, and 1000 mg/g were independently associated with progressive increases in the risk of ESKD, progressive CKD, and AKI, respectively (see Figure 22.4).[71] Among 21,688 patients known to have CKD from 13 studies, an eightfold higher urine albumin/creatinine or protein/creatinine ratio was associated with increased all-cause mortality (pooled HR, 1.40) and risk of ESKD (pooled HR, 3.04).[72] Further meta-analyses by the CKD Prognosis Consortium have shown that the magnitude of proteinuria remains a risk factor for ESKD independent of gender,[31] ethnicity,[42] age,[25] diabetes,[73] or hypertension.[74]

Secondary analyses of prospective RCTs have found that the extent of residual proteinuria that persists, despite optimal treatment with an ACEI or angiotensin receptor blocker (ARB), also predicts renal prognosis. In the REIN study, percentage reduction in proteinuria over the first 3 months and the absolute level of proteinuria at 3 months were strong independent predictors of the subsequent rate of decline in GFR.[173] In the IDNT, a greater reduction in proteinuria at 12 months was associated with a greater reduction in the risk of ESKD (HR, 0.44; 95% CI, 0.40 to 0.49 for each halving of baseline proteinuria).[172] In the AASK study, a change in proteinuria from baseline to 6 months predicted subsequent progression.[171] Similarly, a meta-analysis of data from 1860 patients with nondiabetic CKD showed that during antihypertensive treatment, the current level of proteinuria was a powerful predictor of the combined end point of doubling of the baseline serum creatinine level or onset of ESKD (relative risk [RR], 5.56; 95% CI, 3.87 to 7.98 for each 1.0-g/day increase in proteinuria).[30] Furthermore, a meta-analysis of 21 randomized trials of drug treatment in CKD, which included 78,342 participants, found that for each 30% initial reduction in albuminuria on treatment, the risk of ESKD decreased by 23.7% (95% CI, 11.4% to 34.2%) independent of the class of drug used for treatment.[174] These data support the proposal that proteinuria, like blood pressure, should be regarded as a continuous risk factor for CKD progression.[89] Proteinuria thus appears to be a powerful predictor of renal risk in the general population, in patients with CKD prior to treatment, and in CKD patients on treatment. Recognition of the importance of proteinuria as a risk factor in CKD prompted the addition of an albuminuria category (A1 to A3) to the CKD classification proposed by KDIGO.[7]

These important observations raise the question of how best to measure proteinuria. As discussed, all measurements of proteinuria have been reported to predict renal outcomes, including dipstick urinalysis, urine albumin/creatinine ratio or protein/creatinine ratio (ACR and PCR) and 24-hour urinary albumin or protein excretion. A secondary analysis of data from the RENAAL trial found that urine ACR measured on the first morning void was better than 24-hour urinary protein or albumin concentration as a predictor of time to doubling of the serum creatinine level or ESKD among patients with diabetes and CKD.[175] On the other hand, retrospective analysis of data from 5586 patients with CKD reported similar HRs associated with urinary ACR and PCR for the outcomes of all-cause mortality, start of renal replacement therapy, or doubling of serum creatinine.[176] Further analysis of these data identified a cohort of patients with a normal urine ACR but elevated urine PCR in whom the risk of ESKD or death was intermediate between the groups with both urine ACR and PCR abnormal or normal.[177] Analysis of data from the CRIC study also reported that urine ACR and PCR had similar associations with complications of CKD.[178] Together, these data imply that any measure of proteinuria is better than no measurement. If the goal is to detect and monitor low levels of albuminuria (category A1 and A2), the urine ACR measured on the first morning void is best. For patients with CKD, urine ACR or PCR may be used, and there is some evidence that there may be added information gained by requesting both.[179]

SERUM ALBUMIN

Serum albumin levels are widely regarded as a marker of nutritional status but may also be reduced due to proteinuria or inflammation. Several studies have identified lower serum albumin levels as a risk factor for CKD progression. In the MDRD study, higher baseline serum albumin was associated with slower subsequent rate of GFR decline but, in a multivariable analysis, this was displaced by a similar correlation with baseline serum transferrin levels, another marker of protein nutrition.[8] Three studies have found associations between serum albumin and renal outcomes in patients with type 2 diabetes and CKD. Among 182 patients with a mean serum creatinine of 1.5 mg/dL at baseline, hypoalbuminemia was an independent risk factor for ESKD.[180] In a long-term follow-up of 343 patients, lower baseline serum albumin was an independent predictor of CKD progression[181] and, in the RENAAL study, lower serum albumin was an independent predictor of ESKD.[97] Similar observations have been reported in other forms of CKD. In a large cohort of patients with IgA nephropathy ($N = 2269$), lower serum total protein (composed largely of albumin) was an independent risk factor for ESKD.[182] In a cohort of 3449 patients with CKD referred to a nephrology service, lower serum albumin was an independent risk factor for ESKD.[183] In these studies, the predictive value of serum albumin was independent of and additional to that of proteinuria, indicating that it was not merely acting as a marker of albuminuria.

ANEMIA

Chronic anemia due to inherited hemoglobinopathy is associated with increased renal plasma flow, glomerular hyperfiltration, and subsequent development of proteinuria, hypertension, and ESKD.[184,185] Anemia is a common complication of CKD from any cause, and several studies have shown that it is also an independent predictor of CKD progression. In the RENAAL study, baseline hemoglobin was a significant independent predictor of ESKD among diabetic patients—each 1-g/dL decrease in hemoglobin was associated with an 11% increase in the risk of ESKD.[186] Baseline hemoglobin was also one of four variables included in the renal risk score developed from the RENAAL data.[97] Similarly, a higher hemoglobin level was independently associated with lower risk of progression to ESKD (halving of GFR or need for dialysis) or death among 131 patients with all forms of CKD (HR, 0.778; 95% CI, 0.639 to 0.948 for each 1-g/dL increase).[169] Furthermore, time-averaged hemoglobin of less than 12 g/dL was associated with a significantly increased risk of ESKD among 853 male veterans with CKD stages 3 to 5 (HR, 0.74; 95% CI, 0.65 to 0.84 for each 1-g/dL increase in hemoglobin).[187]

Two other cohort studies have identified lower hemoglobin as an independent risk factor for a more rapid decline in GFR in patients with CKD stage 4[188] and ESKD in patients with CKD stage 3 or 4.[189] Consistent with the hypothesis that anemia contributes directly to CKD progression, two small randomized studies have reported a renoprotective benefit associated with erythropoietin therapy. Among patients with serum creatinine of 2 to 4 mg/dL and hematocrit less than 30%, erythropoietin treatment was associated with significantly improved renal survival.[190] In nondiabetic patients with serum creatinine of 2 to 6 mg/dL, early treatment (started when hemoglobin < 11.6 g/dL) with erythropoietin alpha was associated with a 60% reduction in the risk of doubling the serum creatinine level, ESKD, or death versus delayed treatment (started when hemoglobin < 9.0 g/dL).[191]

On the other hand, two other studies that had left ventricular mass as their primary end point[192,193] and the Trial to Reduce Cardiovascular Events with Aranesp Therapy (TREAT)[194] found no effect of a high versus low hemoglobin target on the rate of decline in the GFR. Several studies have, however, reported adverse outcomes associated with normalization of hemoglobin in patients with CKD. In the Cardiovascular Risk Reduction by Early Anemia Treatment with Epoetin Beta (CREATE) study, randomization to a higher hemoglobin target (13 to 15 mg/dL) was associated with a shorter time to initiation of dialysis than a lower target (10.5 to 11.5 mg/dL).[195] In TREAT, randomization to a higher hemoglobin target was associated with an increased risk of stroke[194] and, in the Correction of Hemoglobin and Outcomes in Renal Insufficiency (CHOIR) study, a higher hemoglobin target was associated with an increased incidence of the combined end point of all-cause mortality, myocardial infarction, or hospitalization for congestive cardiac failure.[196]

DYSLIPIDEMIA

Lipid abnormalities are common in patients with CKD, and several studies have identified dyslipidemia as a susceptibility and progression factor for CKD. In population-based studies, several lipid profile abnormalities have been associated with an increased risk of developing CKD, including an elevated low-density lipoprotein (LDL) to high-density lipoprotein (HDL) cholesterol ratio,[197] higher triglyceride and lower HDL cholesterol levels,[198] lower HDL cholesterol levels[18] and elevated total cholesterol, low HDL cholesterol, and elevated total to HDL cholesterol.[199] Several observational studies have reported dyslipidemia as a risk factor for CKD progression. In the MDRD study, lower HDL cholesterol levels independently predicted a more rapid decline in GFR[8]; in a smaller study of patients with CKD, total cholesterol, LDL cholesterol, and apolipoprotein B levels were all associated with a more rapid decline in the GFR.[200] Among 223 patients with IgA nephropathy, hypertriglyceridemia was independently predictive of CKD progression.[201] Hypercholesterolemia was reported to predict loss of renal function in patients with type 1 or 2 diabetes[202,203] and, among nondiabetic patients, CKD advanced more rapidly in those with hypercholesterolemia and hypertriglyceridemia.[204]

RCTs of lipid lowering have produced mixed results with respect to renal outcomes. Subgroup analysis of a prospective randomized trial of pravastatin treatment in patients with previous myocardial infarction found that pravastatin slowed the rate of decline in patients with an eGFR less than 40 mL/min/1.73 m^2, an effect that was also more pronounced in those with proteinuria.[205] Similarly, in the Heart Protection Study, patients with previous cardiovascular disease or diabetes randomized to simvastatin treatment had a smaller increase in serum creatinine than those who received placebo.[206] In a placebo-controlled, open-label study, atorvastatin treatment in patients with CKD, proteinuria, and hypercholesterolemia was associated with preservation of creatinine clearance, whereas it declined in those receiving placebo.[207] On the other hand, lipid lowering with fibrates was not associated with renoprotection in two studies,[197,208] although one study did show a reduced incidence of microalbuminuria in patients with type 2 diabetes receiving fenofibrate.[209]

One meta-analysis of 13 small controlled trials found that lipid-lowering therapy was associated with a significantly slower rate of GFR decline (0.156 mL/min/month; 95% CI, 0.026 to 0.285; $P = 0.008$) among patients with CKD.[210] On the other hand, several other studies found no association between dyslipidemia and risk of CKD progression. Analysis of data from a relatively small subgroup of studies with renal end points recorded in a meta-analysis found that statin therapy was associated with a reduction in proteinuria but with no improvement in creatinine clearance in participants with CKD.[211] Furthermore, analysis of data from 3939 participants in the CRIC study found no association between total or LDL cholesterol and the risk of ESKD or 50% reduction in eGFR. Indeed, among participants with proteinuria of less than 0.2 g/day, higher LDL and total cholesterol were associated with a lower risk of reaching this end point.[212] The Study of Heart and Renal Protection (SHARP) is the largest RCT to investigate the cardiovascular and renoprotective effects of lipid lowering in CKD. Patients with CKD or undergoing dialysis were randomized to treatment with simvastatin and ezetimibe or placebo. In 6245 participants with CKD not requiring dialysis, treatment resulted in an average reduction in LDL cholesterol of 0.96 mmol/L but was not associated with a reduction in the primary outcome of ESKD or secondary outcome of ESKD or creatinine doubling.[213] Similarly, a meta-analysis of 38 studies, which included 37,274 participants with CKD, found that statin therapy was associated with a reduction in mortality and cardiovascular events but no clear effect on CKD progression.[214] Together, evidence that dyslipidemia is a risk factor for CKD progression remains mixed, with the most recent studies indicating no association. Mechanisms whereby dyslipidemia may contribute to CKD progression are discussed in Chapter 52.

SERUM URIC ACID

Hyperuricemia is a common consequence of chronic renal failure and may also contribute to CKD progression. Several cohort studies have investigated uric acid as a risk factor in CKD and were summarized in a recent review.[215] Most but not all population-based studies have identified hyperuricemia as an independent risk factor for the development of incident CKD. Similarly, most cohort studies that included people with CKD have identified a higher serum uric acid level as a risk factor for CKD progression. Possible mechanisms whereby hyperuricemia may contribute to CKD progression are exacerbation of glomerular hypertension,[216,217] endothelial dysfunction,[218,219] and proinflammatory effects.[220] On the other hand, it is possible that an elevated uric acid concentration is acting as a marker of reduced kidney function or oxidative stress—uric acid is produced by xanthine oxidase, which also generates reactive oxygen species.

To date, only small studies investigating the effect of uric acid–lowering therapy on CKD progression have been published. A meta-analysis of eight trials found no difference in the eGFR among participants treated with allopurinol versus those with no treatment or placebo in five trials, whereas three trials that reported only serum creatinine reported benefit in favor of allopurinol. In five trials that measured proteinuria, no benefit was observed.[221] Together, published evidence suggests that an elevated serum uric acid level may act as a susceptibility and progression risk factor in CKD, but large randomized trials are still required to determine whether treatment of hyperuricemia is beneficial for slowing CKD progression.

SERUM BICARBONATE

Studies in animal models have shown that acidosis may promote the progression of CKD through several mechanisms, including activation of the alternative complement pathway by elevated cortical ammonia levels,[222] increased production of endothelin and aldosterone,[223] and calcium deposition.[224] At least five studies have investigated serum bicarbonate as a risk factor in human CKD. In all except the MDRD study,[225] lower serum bicarbonate levels, even within the normal range, were independently associated with an increased risk of CKD progression.[183,226-228] Two small randomized trials have reported slowing of CKD progression with bicarbonate supplementation,[229,230] and another trial found that correction of acidosis with oral sodium bicarbonate or a diet rich in fruits and vegetables was associated with a lower rate of GFR decline.[231] Bicarbonate supplementation is already recommended for patients with levels below 22 mEq/L, but several studies are underway to investigate further whether it is beneficial in the setting of less severe acidosis.[232]

PLASMA ASYMMETRIC DIMETHYLARGININE

Asymmetric dimethylarginine (ADMA) is formed by the breakdown of arginine methylated proteins and acts as an endogenous inhibitor of nitric oxide synthase to reduce nitric oxide production. The increased ADMA levels observed with a reduced GFR have been proposed as one mechanism for the endothelial dysfunction associated with CKD. Elevated ADMA levels are associated with CVD and cardiovascular mortality in patients with CKD.[233] In animal models, administration of ADMA was associated with the development of hypertension, increased deposition of collagen I and III and fibronectin in glomeruli and blood vessels, and rarefaction of peritubular capillaries.[234] Conversely, the overexpression of dimethylarginine dimethylaminohydrolase (DDAH), the enzyme responsible for degradation of ADMA, was associated with reduced ADMA levels and amelioration of renal injury in rats after 5/6 nephrectomy, implying that ADMA may also promote CKD progression.[235]

Several relatively small studies have identified increased ADMA levels as a risk factor for CKD progression. Among 131 patients with CKD, a higher plasma ADMA level was an independent risk factor for ESKD or death (HR, 1.20; 95% CI, 1.07 to 1.35 for each 0.1-μmol/L increase).[169] In 227 relatively young patients with mild-to-moderate nondiabetic CKD, higher ADMA levels predicted progression to the combined end point of creatinine doubling or ESKD (HR, 1.47; 95% CI, 1.12 to 1.93 for each 0.1-μmol/L increase).[236] Finally, retrospective analysis of data from 109 patients with IgA nephropathy showed associations between ADMA levels and glomerular and tubulointerstitial injury. Furthermore, the plasma ADMA level was an independent determinant of annual GFR reduction rate.[237]

SERUM PHOSPHATE

When rats were fed a high-phosphate diet after uninephrectomy, renal calcium and phosphate deposition, as well as tubulointerstitial injury, were observed within 5 weeks.[238] Furthermore, in animals and humans with CKD, dietary phosphate restriction or treatment with oral phosphate binders was associated with reductions in proteinuria and glomerulosclerosis and attenuation of CKD progression.[239-242] Together, these data suggest that phosphate loading and/or hyperphosphatemia exacerbate renal injury in CKD. In addition, higher levels of the phosphatonin fibroblast growth factor 23 (FGF23) have been identified as an independent predictor of CKD progression.[243,244] Three cohort studies of patients with CKD have identified higher serum phosphate levels as an independent risk factor for progression.[98,183,188] On the other hand, the largest study to date, which included 10,672 participants with CKD, found no independent association between higher serum phosphate and risk of progression.[245] It should be noted, however, that the number of ESKD events was low, and the study therefore had limited power to detect a moderate association between serum phosphate levels and CKD progression.[246]

OTHER BIOMARKERS

A number of other biomarkers are currently being investigated as risk factors in CKD. Although many have been reported to be associated with adverse outcomes, the challenge is to identify biomarkers that add to the predictive power of established risk factors. For a comprehensive discussion of novel biomarkers, see Chapter 30.

NEPHROTOXINS

SMOKING

Population-based studies have identified cigarette smoking as an independent risk factor for various manifestations of CKD, including proteinuria,[247] elevated serum creatinine levels,[248] decreased eGFR,[18,249] and development of ESKD or death associated with CKD (HR, 2.6; 95% CI, 1.8 to 3.7).[27] In the latter study, 31% of the attributable risk of CKD was associated with smoking. In a longitudinal study of 10,118 middle-aged Japanese workers, smoking was associated with an increased risk of developing glomerular hyperfiltration (eGFR ≥ 117 mL/min/1.73 m^2; OR, 1.32 vs. nonsmokers) as well as proteinuria (OR, 1.51 vs. nonsmokers).[250] Two other similar longitudinal studies from Japan have confirmed that smoking is associated with an increased risk of developing proteinuria but with a higher mean eGFR than in nonsmokers.[251,252] In one study, smoking was associated with a reduced risk of developing CKD stage 3.[252] Smoking has been shown to increase the risk of progression of CKD due to diabetes,[253,254] hypertensive nephropathy,[255] glomerulonephritis,[256] lupus nephritis,[257] IgA nephropathy,[258] and adult polycystic kidney disease.[258] Randomized trials of the effect of smoking cessation on CKD progression are lacking but, in one observational study, smoking cessation was associated with less progression to macroalbuminuria and a slower rate of GFR decline than continued smoking in patients with diabetes.[259] Similarly, in the CRIC study, nonsmoking was associated with a reduced risk of CKD progression (HR, 0.68; 95% CI, 0.55 to 0.84), atherosclerotic cardiovascular events (HR, 0.55; 95% CI, 0.40 to 0.75) and mortality (HR, 0.45; 95% CI, 0.34 to 0.60).[260] Possible mechanisms whereby cigarette smoking may contribute to renal damage include sympathetic nervous system activation, glomerular capillary hypertension, endothelial cell injury, and direct tubulotoxocity.[261]

ALCOHOL

The role of alcohol consumption as a potential risk factor for CKD remains unclear. One case-control study found a significant association between ESKD and consumption of more than two alcoholic drinks daily,[262] whereas another similar study found no association (with the exception of moonshine).[263] Some population-based studies have found that alcohol consumption is not related to CKD risk,[264-266] but one study found a significant association of heavy alcohol intake (more than four drinks daily) and prevalent CKD, as well as the risk of developing CKD in participants with a normal GFR.[249] Furthermore, heavy alcohol intake substantially increased the risk of CKD progression associated with smoking, such that participants who smoked and drank heavily had an almost fivefold increased risk of developing CKD.[249]

Conversely, several large cohort studies have reported an inverse relationship between alcohol consumption and the risk of developing CKD[267,268] or ESKD.[269] Another study found that moderate-to-heavy alcohol consumption was associated with an increased risk of developing albuminuria but decreased risk of eGFR less than 60 mL/min/1.73 m^2.[270] The most rigorous study published to date investigated the incidence of CKD defined by an eGFR determined using the combined cystatin C and creatinine equation or albuminuria more than 30 mg/day based on two consecutive 24-hour urine collections. The risk of developing CKD over a mean of 10.2 years decreased progressively with increasing alcohol consumption: HR of 0.85 (95% CI, 0.69 to 1.04) for occasional alcohol consumption (<10 g/week), HR of 0.82 (95% CI, 0.69 to 0.98) for light alcohol consumption (10 to 69.9 g/week), HR of 0.71 (95% CI, 0.58 to 0.88) for moderate alcohol consumption (70 to 210 g/week), and HR of 0.60 (95% CI, 0.42 to 0.86) for heavier alcohol consumption (>210 g/week).[271]

RECREATIONAL DRUGS

The role of recreational drugs as a risk factor for CKD has not been widely studied, but one case-control study reported a positive association between heroin, cocaine, or psychedelic drug use and ESKD.[272] Following reports of a specific renal lesion characterized by proteinuria and FSGS, termed *heroin nephropathy*, other investigators reported a wide range of renal lesions in patients with a history of heroin abuse. It is unclear whether the observed renal lesions resulted from direct effects of heroin or were attributable to impurities in the drug or associated blood-borne virus infections and endocarditis. An association with renal amyloidosis, possibly due to chronic skin infections, has also been reported.[273] Interestingly, heroin abuse was not associated with an increased risk of mild CKD in 647 hypertensive patients who showed an association between illicit drug abuse and CKD.[274] Cocaine exerts several adverse effects that may induce renal injury, including rhabdomyolysis, vasoconstriction, activation of the renin angiotensin aldosterone system, oxidative stress, and increased collagen synthesis.[273] Furthermore, chronic administration of cocaine to rats resulted in multiple renal lesions, including glomerular atrophy and sclerosis, tubule cell necrosis, and areas of interstitial necrosis.[275] Among 647 patients attending a hypertension clinic, a history of any illicit drug use was independently associated with a relative risk of 2.3 (95% CI, 1.0 to 5.1) for mild CKD, whereas cocaine and psychedelic drug use were associated with relative risks of 3.0 (95% CI, 1.1 to 8.0) and 3.9 (95% CI, 1.1 to 14.4), respectively.[274] On the other hand, analysis of population-based data from NHANES, 2005 to 2008, found no association between a self-reported history of illicit drug use and CKD (defined by eGFR < 60 mL/min/1.73 m^2 or albuminuria) but did report an association between cocaine use and blood pressure of 130/85 mm Hg or higher.[276]

ANALGESICS

Analgesic nephropathy has been well described as a cause of CKD and ESKD resulting from abuse of combination analgesics containing aspirin and phenacetin; this was prevalent in Australia and Switzerland until the sale of these products was restricted[277] (see Chapter 82). Cohort studies of participants without CKD at baseline have, however, not reported strong associations between analgesic use and the development of CKD. Among 1697 women in the Nurses Health Study, consumption of more than 3000 g of acetaminophen was associated with an increased risk of a GFR decline of more than 30 mL/min/1.73 m^2 over 11 years (HR, 2.04; 95% CI, 1.28 to 3.24), but greater use of aspirin or nonsteroidal antiinflammatory drugs (NSAIDs) was not associated with increased risk.[278] Among 4494 male physicians, there was no association between occasional-to-moderate use of aspirin, acetaminophen, and NSAIDs and GFR decline over 14 years.[279] Similarly, in NHANES, there were no significant associations between habitual use of aspirin, acetaminophen, or ibuprofen and a prevalently low GFR or albuminuria.[280]

On the other hand, analgesic use may exacerbate the progression of established CKD. In one large study of 19,163 patients with newly diagnosed CKD, use of aspirin, acetaminophen, or NSAIDs was associated with an increased risk of progression to ESKD in a dose-dependent manner. Among cyclo-oxygenase 2 (COX-2) inhibitors, use of rofecoxib but not celecoxib was associated with increased risk of ESKD.[281] In a cohort study of 4101 people with rheumatoid arthritis, chronic use of NSAIDs was not associated with a more rapid GFR decline in the entire study population, but NSAID use was independently associated with more rapid GFR decline in a small minority of patients with CKD stage 4 or 5 ($N = 17$).[282] A meta-analysis of three studies that included data from 54,663 participants with CKD stages 3 to 5 found no association between regular NSAID use and accelerated GFR decline (defined as ≥15 mL/min over 2 years) but did report an association with high-dose NSAID use (defined as 90th percentile or above in one study and not defined in the other) in two studies.[283] The use of single-compound acetaminophen or aspirin was reported not to accelerate progression among patients with CKD stage 4 or 5,[284] but a systematic review of the safety of paracetamol treatment reported an increased risk of renal adverse events in three of four observational studies—in addition to an increased risk of all-cause mortality and cardiovascular and gastrointestinal adverse events in other studies.[285] As the authors noted, these results must be interpreted with some caution due to the possibility of "confounding by indication" resulting from associations between the indication for prescribing analgesia and adverse outcomes.

HEAVY METALS

LEAD

Overt lead toxicity results in the well-recognized entity of lead nephropathy, characterized by chronic interstitial nephritis and an association with gout. In addition, epidemiologic studies have reported that mild elevations in blood lead levels are associated with moderate reductions in GFR and/or hypertension in the general population.[286,287] Furthermore, a prospective study has identified elevations in blood lead levels and body lead burden (BLB) within the normal range as important risk factors for progression in patients with CKD.[288] Similarly, BLB was a risk factor for progression among 108 patients with low-normal BLB values and no history of lead exposure.[289] Furthermore, randomization to chelation therapy was associated with a modest improvement in GFR over 24 months versus a small decline in those randomized to control (+6.6 ± 10.7 versus −4.6 ± 4.3 mL/min/1.73 m^2; $P < 0.001$).[289]

On the other hand, a case-control study of patients with incident advanced CKD in Sweden found no association between incident CKD or rate of GFR decline and occupational exposure to lead.[290] In one NHANES study, the use of cystatin C, a multivariable equation, and/or a combined creatinine–cystatin C equation to estimate GFR identified greater reductions in GFR associated with doubling of blood lead levels than creatinine-based estimates of GFR using the MDRD or CKD-EPI equation.[291]

CADMIUM

Chronic exposure to cadmium is also associated with a distinctive nephropathy characterized by proximal tubule damage and low-molecular-weight proteinuria.[292] Furthermore, low-level cadmium exposure resulting from environmental contamination was associated with tubular proteinuria[293]; and analysis of data from 14,778 participants in NHANES showed an independent increased risk of albuminuria, reduced GFR, or both between the highest and lowest quartiles of blood cadmium levels.[294] Comparison of the lowest and highest quartiles for blood cadmium and lead levels showed an even greater increased risk of albuminuria, reduced GFR, or both.[294] In another NHANES study, blood and urine cadmium levels were positively correlated with the urine albumin/creatinine ratio and negatively associated with GFR. Higher blood and urine cadmium levels were independently associated with albuminuria, and higher blood cadmium levels were associated with albuminuria and a reduced GFR.[292] Occupational or low-level environmental exposure to cadmium was associated with an increased risk of ESKD in a population-based study from Sweden.[295]

Some studies have investigated associations between CKD and exposure to several heavy metals. In a case-control study from Sweden, higher erythrocyte lead levels were independently associated with an increased risk of ESKD, but higher mercury levels were associated with a lower risk. Higher cadmium levels were associated with an increased risk of ESKD, but this did not persist after adjustment for the other two metals, smoking, BMI, diabetes, and hypertension.[296] In a population-based study in Korea, higher lead and cadmium but not mercury levels were associated with an increased risk of CKD in a univariate analysis, but these associations did not persist after multivariable analysis. Nevertheless, subgroup analyses have found that higher cadmium levels are independently associated with a higher risk of CKD in people with hypertension or diabetes.[297]

RENAL RISK SCORES

The focus on investigating risk factors that predict the development and/or progression of CKD in diverse populations has led to the observation that a relatively small group of risk factors appears to be common to different forms of CKD. This supports the notion of a common pathway of mechanisms that underlie the progression of CKD. It has also led to the proposal that these common risk factors could be combined to develop a renal risk score to predict the development and future risk of progression of CKD in a manner analogous to the Framingham risk score for predicting cardiovascular risk in the general population.[298] The revised classification system for CKD proposed by KDIGO has in part addressed this need by incorporating the evidence that a reduced GFR and albuminuria are powerful risk factors to incorporate into a system in which CKD categories correspond to risk categories.[7]

In addition, considerable progress has been made in developing renal risk scores to facilitate more accurate risk prediction. These may conveniently be divided into two groups—those that apply to the general population (i.e., without CKD as baseline) and those that predict the risk of progression in patients already diagnosed with CKD. In addition, one study has developed a risk score to predict the development of CKD after an episode of AKI.

GENERAL POPULATION RENAL RISK SCORES

Risk scores have been proposed to assess the risk of developing CKD in the general population and, in some cases, its subsequent progression. These are summarized in Table 22.3 and have been assessed in a recent systematic review.[299] In the first study, data from 8530 adults included in NHANES were used to identify risk factors for prevalent CKD (defined as eGFR < 60 mL/min/1.73 m^2). The authors proposed a risk score that included age, female gender, hypertension, anemia, diabetes, peripheral vascular disease, history of CVD, congestive heart failure; and proteinuria. The area under the receiver operator curve (AUC) was high at 0.88, and a score of 4 or higher resulted in a sensitivity of 92% and specificity of 68%. The positive predictive value was low at 18%, but the negative predictive value was 99%. External validation using data from the Atherosclerosis Risk in Communities (ARIC) study gave an AUC value of 0.71.[300] This was a cross-sectional study, and the risk score therefore did not predict the risk of future CKD. Rather, it identified individuals at increased risk of having current undiagnosed CKD. As such, it would be useful for guiding efforts to screen populations for CKD, but gives no information about the future risk of CKD progression. The applicability of the score to general populations is somewhat weakened by the inclusion of two variables that require prior laboratory testing—namely, anemia and proteinuria. Furthermore, the presence of significant proteinuria is sufficient to diagnose CKD in the absence of any reduction in GFR.

Another risk score was developed to predict the risk of incident CKD using combined data from 14,155 participants in the ARIC study and Cardiovascular Health Study (CHS; ≥45 years) with baseline eGFR more than 60 mL/min/1.73 m^2. After identifying 10 predictors of incident CKD (defined as eGFR < 60 mL/min/1.73 m^2 during follow-up for up to 9 years), they proposed a simplified model based on eight variables: age, anemia, female gender, hypertension, diabetes mellitus, peripheral vascular disease, and history of congestive heart failure or CVD. This gave an AUC value of 0.69, and a score of 3 or higher resulted in a sensitivity of 69% and specificity of 58% but the positive predictive value was low, only 17%.[301] A similar study used data from 2490 participants in the Framingham Heart Study to produce a risk score for incident CKD, defined as eGFR

Table 22.3 Renal Risk Scores for the General Population

Parameter	SCORED[300]	SCORED2[301]	Chinese[303]	Framingham[302]	QKIDNEY[304]	PREVEND[165]
			Study			
Population	NHANES	CHS + ARIC	General population	FHS	QResearch	eGFR > 45
Outcome	eGFR < 60 (prevalent)	eGFR < 60 (incident)	eGFR < 60 (incident)	eGFR < 60 (incident)	CKD, ESKD	Rapid ↓ GFR
Factor	Age	Age	Age	Age	Age	Age
	Female	Female				
					Ethnicity	
					Deprivation	
					Family history	
					Smoking	
			BMI			
	HT	HT		HT	HT	HT
	DM	DM	Type 2 DM	DM	DM	
	PVD	PVD			PVD	
	CVD	CVD	Stroke		CVD	
	CCF	CCF			CCF	
					RA	
	Anemia	Anemia				
			DBP		SBP	SBP
					BMI	
				eGFR		eGFR
	Proteinuria		Proteinuria	Albuminuria		Albuminuria
						CRP
			Uric acid			
			HbA$_{1c}$			
			Glucose			
					NSAIDs	
AUC	0.88	0.69	0.77	0.81	0.88	0.84
Validation	ARIC	CHS + ARIC	General population	ARIC	THIN	Internal

AUC, Area under the concentration-time curve; ARIC, Atherosclerosis Risk in Communities; CCF, congestive cardiac failure; CHS, Cardiovascular Health Study; CRP, C-reactive protein; CVD, cardiovascular disease; DBP, diastolic blood pressure; DM, diabetes mellitus; eGFR, estimated glomerular filtration rate; FHS, Framingham Heart Study; HbA$_{1c}$, hemoglobin A$_{1c}$; HT, hypertension; NHANES, National Health and Nutrition Examination Survey; NSAIDs, nonsteroidal antiinflammatory drugs; PVD, peripheral vascular disease; RA, rheumatoid arthritis; SBP, systolic blood pressure; THIN, the Health Improvement Network.

less than 60 mL/min/1.73 m^2. The final model included age, diabetes, hypertension, baseline eGFR, and albuminuria and gave an AUC value of 0.813. External validation was performed with data from the ARIC study (AUC = 0.79 and 0.75 in whites and blacks, respectively).[302] One further study developed a risk score for incident CKD (eGFR < 60 mL/min/1.73 m^2) in 5168 Chinese participants. Age, BMI, diastolic blood pressure, type 2 diabetes, previous stroke, serum uric acid, postprandial blood glucose, and hemoglobin A$_{1c}$ levels and proteinuria more than 100 mg/dL were included in two risk scores (one using clinical variables only and a second with all variables) that gave an AUC value of 0.77. The study was limited by relatively short follow-up (median, 2.2 years) and a low AUC value of 0.67 for external validation data.[303]

These scores are useful to identify individuals at higher risk of developing CKD for monitoring or intervention to reduce risk, but do not distinguish the minority who are at risk of progressing to ESKD from the majority, who are at low risk. In an attempt to identify only high-risk individuals, another group used data from patients (775,091 women and 799,658 men aged 35 to 74 years, without a recorded diagnosis of CKD) in 368 primary care practices in the United Kingdom to develop a risk score. Two outcomes were studied over a period of up to 7 years—moderate-to-severe CKD (defined as kidney transplantation, dialysis, diagnosis of nephropathy, proteinuria, or eGFR < 45 mL/min/1.73 m^2) and ESKD (defined as kidney transplantation, dialysis, or eGFR < 15 mL/min/1.73 m^2); separate risk scores were developed for men and women. The final model for moderate-to-severe CKD included age, ethnicity, social deprivation, smoking, BMI, systolic blood pressure, diabetes, rheumatoid arthritis, CVD, treated hypertension, congestive cardiac failure, peripheral vascular disease, use of NSAIDs, and family history of kidney disease. In women, it also included systemic lupus erythematosus (SLE) and history of kidney stones. The model for ESKD was similar but did not include NSAID use. Internal and external validation was performed, giving AUC values of 0.818 to 0.878.[304]

One important limitation of this study is that it was observational and therefore likely to be subject to significant bias. Furthermore, only 56% of participants had a serum creatinine level recorded at inclusion, and it is therefore probable that several had undiagnosed CKD. The composite outcome of moderate-to-severe CKD was comprised of several disparate variables and is therefore not clinically useful, but the

ESKD outcome is relevant because it identified only the minority at increased risk of severe progression. This study also illustrates the utility of a risk score that could be programmed into primary care computer systems to alert family practitioners to patients who are at risk of progression to ESKD.

Another study used data from 6809 participants in the PREVEND study to develop a risk score with the primary outcome of progressive CKD over 6.4 years, defined as the 20% of participants with the most rapid decline in GFR and eGFR less than 60 mL/min/1.73 m². The final risk score included baseline eGFR, age, albuminuria, systolic blood pressure, C-reactive protein, and known hypertension. The AUC value was 0.84, and internal validation was performed using a bootstrapping procedure.[165] Despite this, the risk score has a relatively low sensitivity and positive predictive value. The proposed threshold score of 27 or higher identified 2.1% of the population as high risk, but with a sensitivity of only 15.7% and a positive predictive value of 28.1%. The specificity and negative predictive value were high at 98.4% and 96.7%, respectively. Thus, a low score is useful to identify low-risk individuals but a high score does not identify most high-risk individuals. Selecting a lower threshold would improve sensitivity with some reduction in specificity and could be used to identify a group at intermediate risk for closer monitoring. Limitations of this study are that it was performed in a white population and was not validated externally. External validation in other populations is therefore required before it can be considered for clinical use.

RISK SCORES FOR PATIENTS WITH DIAGNOSED CHRONIC KIDNEY DISEASE

Several risk scores have been developed for patients with diagnosed CKD in a variety of study populations and are summarized in Table 22.4 and in recent systematic reviews.[299,305] Analysis of data from 1513 patients with diabetic nephropathy included in the RENAAL study identified urine albumin/creatinine ratio, serum albumin, serum creatinine, and hemoglobin as independent risk factors for ESKD. A risk score was derived from the coefficients of these variables in the Cox proportional hazards model, which successfully separated the participants into quartiles of ESKD risk (Figure 22.5), with a marked difference in risk between the first and last quartiles (6.7 versus 257.2/1000 patient-years).[97]

Among 1860 patients with nondiabetic CKD from a combined database of 11 clinical trials, Cox proportional hazards analysis identified age, serum creatinine, proteinuria, and systolic blood pressure as independent risk factors for the combined end point of time to ESKD or creatinine doubling. Using similar methodology as the previous study, a risk model based on these variables was developed to stratify patients into quartiles of risk. The annual incidence of the combined end point was 0.4% versus 28.7% in the lowest versus highest quartile for patients in the control group and 0.2% versus 19.7% in those randomized to ACEI treatment.[306] Analysis of data from 2269 patients with IgA nephropathy identified systolic blood pressure, proteinuria

Table 22.4 Renal Risk Scores for Patients with Chronic Kidney Disease (CKD)

Parameter	RENAAL[97]	AIPRD[306]	IGAN[182]	KPC[189]	CRIB[98]	SHC[183]
Disease studied	DN	CKD	IgAN	CKD, stage 3 or 4	CKD, stages 3 to 5	CKD, stages 3 to 5
Variables		Age	Age	Age		Age
			Male	Male	Female	Male
	Creatinine	Creatinine	1/creatinine	eGFR	Creatinine	eGFR
	UACR	UPE	Proteinuria	NA	UACR	UACR
		SBP	SBP	HT		
				DM		
	Alb		TP			Alb
	Hb			Anemia		
						Calcium
					Phos	Phos
						Bicarb
			Histol Hematuria			
Outcome	ESKD	ESKD or doubling of serum creatinine level	ESKD	RRT	ESKD	ESKD
AUC			0.939	0.89	0.873	0.917
Validation	No	No	No	No	Yes	Yes

AIPRD, ACE Inhibition in Progressive Renal Disease study; Alb, serum albumin; AUC, area under the concentration-time curve; Bicarb, serum bicarbonate; CRIB, Chronic Renal Impairment in Birmingham study; DM, diabetes mellitus; DN, diabetic nephropathy; Hb, hemoglobin; Histol, histologic grade; HT, hypertension; IgAN, IgA nephropathy; KPC, Kaiser Permanente Cohort; Phos, serum phosphate; Proteinuria, urine dipstick proteinuria; RENAAL, Reduction of Endpoints in NIDDM with the Angiotensin II Antagonist Losartan study; RRT, renal replacement therapy; SBP, systolic blood pressure; SHC, Sunnybrook Hospital cohort; TP, serum total protein; UACR, urine albumin/creatinine ratio; UPE, 24-hour urinary protein excretion.

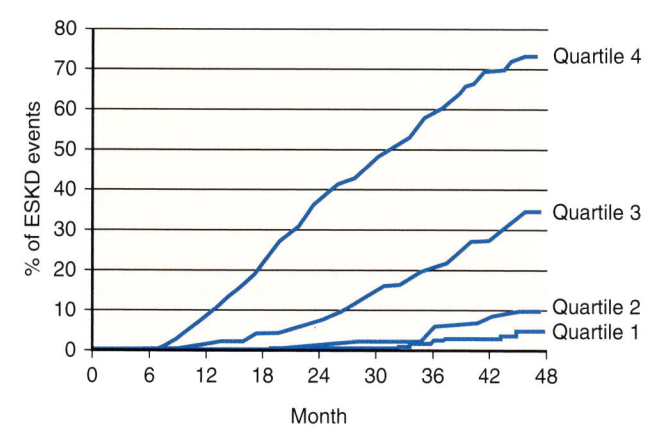

Figure 22.5 Kaplan-Meier curve for the end-stage kidney disease (ESKD) end point stratified by quartile of risk score in 1513 patients with diabetic nephropathy from the Reduction of Endpoints in NIDDM with the Angiotensin II Antagonist Losartan (RENAAL) study. NIDDM, Non–insulin-dependent diabetes mellitus. (From Keane WF, Zhang Z, Lyle PA, et al: Risk scores for predicting outcomes in patients with type 2 diabetes and nephropathy: the RENAAL study. *Clin J Am Soc Nephrol* 1:761-767, 2006.)

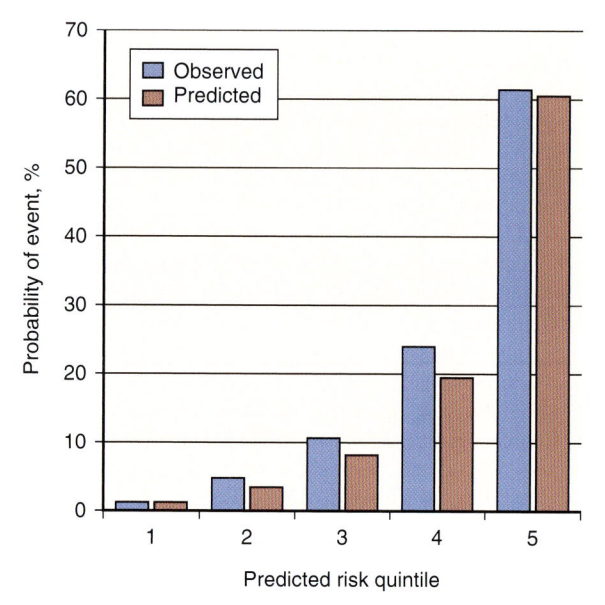

Figure 22.6 Renal risk score predicted versus observed risk of developing end-stage kidney disease at 3 years in a validation cohort of patients with chronic kidney disease stages 3 to 5. (From Tangri N, Stevens LA, Griffith J, et al: A predictive model for progression of chronic kidney disease to kidney failure. *JAMA* 305:1553-1559, 2011.)

(assessed with urine dipstick test), serum total protein, 1/ serum creatinine, and histologic grade at initial biopsy as predictors of time to ESKD. Age, gender, and severity of hematuria were added to these variables to develop a scoring system for estimating 4- and 7-year cumulative incidence of ESKD. There was close agreement between estimated and observed risks (AUC value = 0.939).[182]

In a retrospective study, data from 9782 patients with CKD stages 3 to 4 were analyzed with regard to a primary outcome of onset of RRT (dialysis or transplantation). Six independent risk factors were identified—age, male gender, eGFR, hypertension, diabetes, and anemia—and were incorporated into a risk score that stratified participants into quintiles of risk. The risk of progression to RRT was 19% in the highest risk quintile versus 0.2% in the lowest. The AUC value was 0.89, and observed risk differed from predicted by less than 1%.[189] One limitation of this study, apart from its retrospective design, was the lack of data regarding proteinuria.

Among 382 patients with CKD stages 3 to 5 from the CRIB study, independent risk factors for progression to ESKD during a mean of 4.1 years' follow-up were female gender, serum creatinine, serum phosphate, and urine albumin/creatinine ratio. A risk score was derived from these variables (AUC value = 0.873) and externally validated in a similar cohort of patients with CKD stages 3 to 5 (East Kent cohort), giving an AUC value of 0.91, even though the urine albumin/creatinine ratio was not available in the validation cohort.[98]

Finally, a risk score for predicting ESKD was developed by Tangri and colleagues using data from a cohort of 3449 Canadian patients with CKD stages 3 to 5 (Sunnybrook Hospital cohort).[183] It included age, male gender, eGFR, albuminuria, serum calcium, serum phosphate, serum bicarbonate, and serum albumin (AUC value = 0.917). External validation was performed with data from a separate cohort of 4942 patients with CKD stages 3 to 5 (British Columbia CKD Registry), giving an AUC value of 0.841.

There was close agreement between predicted and observed risk in the validation cohort (Figure 22.6). Simpler three-variable (age, gender, eGFR) and four-variable models (age, gender, eGFR, and albuminuria) also performed well (C statistic [equivalent to AUC] of 0.89 and 0.91, respectively, in the development cohort), but the eight-variable equation performed better in the validation cohort with respect to discrimination (C statistic, 0.79 and 0.83, respectively, for the three- and four-variable equations), calibration, and reclassification. The authors facilitated clinical application of this risk score by producing an electronic risk calculator and smartphone app (available for no charge at www.qxmd.com/calculate-online/nephrology/kidney-failure-risk-equation) that reports an estimated risk of ESKD at 2 and 5 years. Further external validation of this risk equation has been reported by independent investigators from the MASTERPLAN (Multifactorial Approach and Superior Treatment Efficacy in Renal Patients with the Aid of Nurse practitioners) study, a cohort of 595 people from the Netherlands with CKD stages 3 to 5. The model again performed well with the eight-variable equation, giving an AUC value of 0.89.[307] A further advantage of the Tangri risk score is that it includes variables that are all available to a biochemistry laboratory, making it possible for laboratories to automate reporting of a risk score with each eGFR. Nevertheless, it should be noted that this risk score has been validated only in white populations treated by secondary care. Further validation work is therefore required in different ethnic groups and in those with milder forms of CKD treated by primary care.

One group of investigators has developed a risk score to predict the risk of progressive GFR decline, defined as more than 7.5 mL/min/1.73 m^2, in primary care. The study included 803 people with CKD or at high risk of developing

CKD due to hypertension and/or diabetes. The risk model variables included hypertension, eGFR less than 60 mL/min/1.73 m^2, severe obesity, proteinuria, congestive heart failure (CHF), C-reactive protein level more than 10 mg/L, and use of an ACEI or ARB, and had good discrimination (AUC value = 0.85) and calibration.[308] Despite significant limitations due to lack of external validation and the relatively small decline in GFR used to define progressive CKD, this study has made important progress in developing risk scores applicable to most people with CKD who are never referred to a nephrologist.

An attempt has also been made to develop a risk score to predict the risk of ESKD within 1 year in older patients with advanced CKD to guide decisions related to preparation for RRT. The development cohort included 1866 people 65 years or older with CKD stage 4 (eGFR, 29 to 15 mL/min/1.73 m^2) who were treated by a Veterans Administration (VA) health center. The final model included eGFR, age, history of CHF, average systolic blood pressure, serum potassium and albumin levels, and interactions between age and eGFR and between eGFR and CHF. The model achieved excellent discrimination (C statistic = 0.85) that persisted in a separate validation cohort of 819 people (C statistic = 0.82).[309] Interestingly, the Tangri equation also performed well in the development and validation cohorts (C statistic = 0.78 for both). Nevertheless, the VA equation may be helpful in identifying older people who are at low risk of ESKD in the following year to support a delay in preparation for RRT and avoid potentially unnecessary surgery for vascular access.

RISK SCORES FOR PREDICTING CHRONIC KIDNEY DISEASE AFTER ACUTE KIDNEY INJURY

A growing appreciation of the risk of CKD and progression to ESKD following an episode of AKI has prompted efforts to develop a risk score for identifying those at highest risk. Three risk prediction models were developed in one study population of 5351 predominantly male veterans with a primary admission diagnosis of AKI to predict the risk of progression to CKD stage 4. Risk factors that entered the models included increased age, low serum albumin, diabetes, lower baseline eGFR, higher mean serum creatinine levels during hospitalization, and severity of AKI as assessed by the RIFLE score (*r*isk, *i*njury, *f*ailure, *l*oss, and *e*nd-stage kidney disease) or need for dialysis, non–African American ethnicity, and time at risk. The AUC value was 0.77 to 0.82 for the three models. Sensitivity at the optimal cutpoint was 0.71 to 0.77, and specificity was 0.64 to 0.74. External validation was performed on a control population of 11,589 patients admitted for pneumonia or myocardial infarction and yielded good prediction accuracy (AUC value = 0.81 to 0.82). Sensitivity at the optimal cutpoint was 0.66 to 0.71, and specificity was 0.61 to 0.70).[310] Further validation in other populations that include a more representative proportion of women is required before these risk models can be applied. A validated risk score for patients recovering from AKI may prove very important for identifying high-risk patients for closer follow-up and interventions to reduce the risk of progressive CKD, although further trials are required to evaluate the impact of renoprotective interventions in this setting.

FUTURE CONSIDERATIONS

Considerable progress has been made since 2000 in identifying risk factors that predict the progression of CKD in diverse cohorts from the general population and nephrology clinics. There is some variation among studies, likely due to differences in the populations and variables studied. Remarkably, a relatively small group of risk factors appears common to many studies, and much progress has been made in developing risk scores based on these variables to predict CKD progression. Further evaluation of proposed risk scores is required to determine their applicability to unselected populations.

It seems likely that separate risk scores will be required for patients without CKD to predict the future risk of developing CKD and those already diagnosed with CKD, although some variables included would be common to both. It would be an advantage if a risk score applicable to the general population did not depend on laboratory variables, whereas for the CKD population, a score based entirely on laboratory variables would facilitate automated reporting of a risk score.

Future studies will likely focus on the use of novel biomarkers and genetic factors as risk factors (see Chapter 30) and variables in risk scores, although measurement of such markers is likely to be associated with greater cost than the simple risk factors used to date. Further studies are also required to develop risk scores to predict cardiovascular risk in patients with CKD that take into account the close association between CKD and CVD.

Complete reference list available at ExpertConsult.com.

KEY REFERENCES

2. Jha V, Garcia-Garcia G, Iseki K, et al: Chronic kidney disease: global dimension and perspectives. *Lancet* 382:260–272, 2013.
7. Stevens PE, Levin A: Evaluation and management of chronic kidney disease: synopsis of the kidney disease: improving global outcomes 2012 clinical practice guideline. *Ann Intern Med* 158:825–830, 2013.
11. Voight BF, Peloso GM, Orho-Melander M, et al: Plasma HDL cholesterol and risk of myocardial infarction: a mendelian randomisation study. *Lancet* 380:572–580, 2012.
25. Hallan SI, Matsushita K, Sang Y, et al: Age and association of kidney measures with mortality and end-stage renal disease. *JAMA* 308:2349–2360, 2012.
31. Nitsch D, Grams M, Sang Y, et al: Associations of estimated glomerular filtration rate and albuminuria with mortality and renal failure by sex: a meta-analysis. *BMJ* 346:f324, 2013.
42. Wen CP, Matsushita K, Coresh J, et al: Relative risks of chronic kidney disease for mortality and end-stage renal disease across races are similar. *Kidney Int* 86:819–827, 2014.
47. Freedman BI, Skorecki K: Gene-gene and gene-environment interactions in apolipoprotein L1 gene-associated nephropathy. *Clin J Am Soc Nephrol* 9:2006–2013, 2014.
48. Parsa A, Kao WH, Xie D, et al: APOL1 risk variants, race, and progression of chronic kidney disease. *N Engl J Med* 369:2183–2196, 2013.
53. Gorski M, Tin A, Garnaas M, et al: Genome-wide association study of kidney function decline in individuals of European descent. *Kidney Int* 87:1017–1029, 2015.
54. Wing MR, Devaney JM, Joffe MM, et al: DNA methylation profile associated with rapid decline in kidney function: findings from the CRIC study. *Nephrol Dial Transplant* 29:864–872, 2014.
68. Kim SP, Murad MH, Thompson RH, et al: Comparative effectiveness for survival and renal function of partial and radical

nephrectomy for localized renal tumors: a systematic review and meta-analysis. *J Urol* (12)05254–05258, 2012. Epub October 18, 2012.
70. Satasivam P, Reeves F, Rao K, et al: Patients with medical risk factors for chronic kidney disease are at increased risk of renal impairment despite the use of nephron-sparing surgery. *BJU Int*, 2015. Epub February 13, 2015.
71. Gansevoort RT, Matsushita K, van der Velde M, et al: Lower estimated GFR and higher albuminuria are associated with adverse kidney outcomes in both general and high-risk populations. A collaborative meta-analysis of general and high-risk population cohorts. *Kidney Int* 80:93–104, 2011.
73. Fox CS, Matsushita K, Woodward M, et al: Associations of kidney disease measures with mortality and end-stage renal disease in individuals with and without diabetes: a meta-analysis. *Lancet* 380:1662–1673, 2012.
74. Mahmoodi BK, Matsushita K, Woodward M, et al: Associations of kidney disease measures with mortality and end-stage renal disease in individuals with and without hypertension: a meta-analysis. *Lancet* 380:1649–1661, 2012.
75. Coresh J, Turin TC, Matsushita K, et al: Decline in estimated glomerular filtration rate and subsequent risk of end-stage renal disease and mortality. *JAMA* 311:2518–2531, 2014.
76. Matsushita K, Mahmoodi BK, Woodward M, et al: Comparison of risk prediction using the CKD-EPI equation and the MDRD study equation for estimated glomerular filtration rate. *JAMA* 307:1941–1951, 2012.
77. Inker LA, Schmid CH, Tighiouart H, et al: Estimating glomerular filtration rate from serum creatinine and cystatin C. *N Engl J Med* 367:20–29, 2012.
78. Shlipak MG, Matsushita K, Arnlov J, et al: Cystatin C versus creatinine in determining risk based on kidney function. *N Engl J Med* 369:932–943, 2013.
84. Coca SG, Singanamala S, Parikh CR: Chronic kidney disease after acute kidney injury: a systematic review and meta-analysis. *Kidney Int* 81:442–448, 2012.
85. Ferenbach DA, Bonventre JV: Mechanisms of maladaptive repair after AKI leading to accelerated kidney ageing and CKD. *Nat Rev Nephrol* 11:264–276, 2015.
96. Schrier RW, Abebe KZ, Perrone RD, et al: Blood pressure in early autosomal dominant polycystic kidney disease. *N Engl J Med* 371:2255–2266, 2014.
111. Silverwood RJ, Pierce M, Hardy R, et al: Early-life overweight trajectory and CKD in the 1946 British birth cohort study. *Am J Kidney Dis* 62:276–284, 2013.
123. Bolignano D, Zoccali C: Effects of weight loss on renal function in obese CKD patients: a systematic review. *Nephrol Dial Transplant* 28(Suppl 4):iv82–iv98, 2013.
142. Mannisto T, Mendola P, Vaarasmaki M, et al: Elevated blood pressure in pregnancy and subsequent chronic disease risk. *Circulation* 127:681–690, 2013.
152. Hoefield RA, Kalra PA, Lane B, et al: Associations of baseline characteristics with evolution of eGFR in a referred chronic kidney disease cohort. *QJM* 106:915–924, 2013.
153. Vejakama P, Ingsathit A, Attia J, et al: Epidemiological study of chronic kidney disease progression: a large-scale population-based cohort study. *Medicine* 94:e475, 2015.
162. Rahman M, Xie D, Feldman HI, et al: Association between chronic kidney disease progression and cardiovascular disease: results from the CRIC study. *Am J Nephrol* 40:399–407, 2014.
174. Lambers Heerspink HJ, Kropelin TF, Hoekman J, et al: Drug-induced reduction in albuminuria is associated with subsequent renoprotection: a meta-analysis. *J Am Soc Nephrol*, 2014. Epub November 24, 2014.
183. Tangri N, Stevens LA, Griffith J, et al: A predictive model for progression of chronic kidney disease to kidney failure. *JAMA* 305:1553–1559, 2011.
194. Pfeffer MA, Burdmann EA, Chen CY, et al: A trial of darbepoetin alfa in type 2 diabetes and chronic kidney disease. *N Engl J Med* 361:2019–2032, 2009.
213. Haynes R, Lewis D, Emberson J, et al: Effects of lowering LDL cholesterol on progression of kidney disease. *J Am Soc Nephrol* 25:1825–1833, 2014.
214. Palmer SC, Navaneethan SD, Craig JC, et al: HMG CoA reductase inhibitors (statins) for people with chronic kidney disease not requiring dialysis. *Cochrane Database Syst Rev* (5):CD007784, 2014.
221. Bose B, Badve SV, Hiremath SS, et al: Effects of uric acid-lowering therapy on renal outcomes: a systematic review and meta-analysis. *Nephrol Dial Transplant* 29:406–413, 2014.
226. Dobre M, Yang W, Chen J, et al: Association of serum bicarbonate with risk of renal and cardiovascular outcomes in CKD: a report from the Chronic Renal Insufficiency Cohort (CRIC) study. *Am J Kidney Dis* 62:670–678, 2013.
231. Goraya N, Simoni J, Jo CH, et al: Treatment of metabolic acidosis in patients with stage 3 chronic kidney disease with fruits and vegetables or oral bicarbonate reduces urine angiotensinogen and preserves glomerular filtration rate. *Kidney Int* 86:1031–1038, 2014.
232. Dobre M, Rahman M, Hostetter TH: Current status of bicarbonate in CKD. *J Am Soc Nephrol* 26:515–523, 2015.
245. Mehrotra R, Peralta CA, Chen SC, et al: No independent association of serum phosphorus with risk for death or progression to end-stage renal disease in a large screen for chronic kidney disease. *Kidney Int* 84:989–997, 2013.
252. Noborisaka Y, Ishizaki M, Yamada Y, et al: The effects of continuing and discontinuing smoking on the development of chronic kidney disease (CKD) in the healthy middle-aged working population in Japan. *Environ Health Prev Med* 18:24–32, 2013.
271. Koning SH, Gansevoort RT, Mukamal KJ, et al: Alcohol consumption is inversely associated with the risk of developing chronic kidney disease. *Kidney Int* 87:1009–1016, 2015.
276. Akkina SK, Ricardo AC, Patel A, et al: Illicit drug use, hypertension, and chronic kidney disease in the US adult population. *Transl Res* 160:391–398, 2012.
285. Roberts E, Delgado Nunes V, Buckner S, et al: Paracetamol: not as safe as we thought? A systematic literature review of observational studies. *Ann Rheum Dis*, 2015. Epub March 2, 2015.
296. Sommar JN, Svensson MK, Bjor BM, et al: End-stage renal disease and low level exposure to lead, cadmium and mercury; a population-based, prospective nested case-referent study in Sweden. *Environ Health* 12:9, 2013.
297. Kim NH, Hyun YY, Lee KB, et al: Environmental heavy metal exposure and chronic kidney disease in the general population. *J Korean Med Sci* 30:272–277, 2015.
299. Echouffo-Tcheugui JB, Kengne AP: Risk models to predict chronic kidney disease and its progression: a systematic review. *PLoS Med* 9:e1001344, 2012.
305. Tangri N, Kitsios GD, Inker LA, et al: Risk prediction models for patients with chronic kidney disease: a systematic review. *Ann Intern Med* 158:596–603, 2013.
307. Peeters MJ, van Zuilen AD, van den Brand JA, et al: Validation of the kidney failure risk equation in European CKD patients. *Nephrol Dial Transplant* 28:1773–1779, 2013.
308. Herget-Rosenthal S, Dehnen D, Kribben A, et al: Progressive chronic kidney disease in primary care: modifiable risk factors and predictive model. *Prev Med* 57:357–362, 2013.
309. Drawz PE, Goswami P, Azem R, et al: A simple tool to predict end-stage renal disease within 1 year in elderly adults with advanced chronic kidney disease. *J Am Geriatr Soc* 61:762–768, 2013.
310. Chawla LS, Amdur RL, Amodeo S, et al: The severity of acute kidney injury predicts progression to chronic kidney disease. *Kidney Int* 79:1361–1369, 2011.

23

Nephron Endowment and Developmental Programming of Blood Pressure and Renal Function

Valerie A. Luyckx | Paul Goodyer | John F. Bertram

CHAPTER OUTLINE

DEVELOPMENTAL PROGRAMMING, 694
DEVELOPMENTAL PROGRAMMING IN THE KIDNEY, 694
Plausibility of the Nephron Number Hypothesis, 695
Evidence for Programming in the Kidney, 696
PROGRAMMING OF RENAL FUNCTION AND DISEASE, 703
Experimental Evidence, 705
Human Evidence, 706
PROPOSED MECHANISMS FOR DEVELOPMENTAL PROGRAMMING IN THE KIDNEY, 713
Genetic Variants Associated with Kidney Size and Nephron Number in Humans, 713
Maternal Nutrient Restriction, 715
Fetal Exposure to Glucocorticoids, 717

Fetal Exposure to Hyperglycemia and the Role of Insulin-like Growth Factors and Their Receptors, 717
Apoptosis, 718
Glial Cell Line–Derived Neurotrophic Factor and c-Ret Receptor Function, 719
Fetal Drug Exposure, 719
Obstruction of the Developing Kidney, 719
Impact of Sex, 720
Potential for Rescue of Nephron Number, 720
Catch-up Growth, 721
IMPACT OF NEPHRON ENDOWMENT IN TRANSPLANTATION, 723
Implications of Nephron Endowment for the Donor, 723
Implications of Nephron Endowment for the Recipient, 723
CONCLUSION, 724

Genetic factors are important determinants of the development and function of major organ systems as well as of susceptibility to disease. Rare genetic and congenital abnormalities leading to abnormal kidney development are associated with the occurrence of subsequent renal dysfunction, often manifest very early in life.[1,2] Most renal disease in the general population, however, is not ascribable to genetic mutations, with the most common etiologic associations with end-stage kidney disease (ESKD) worldwide being the polygenic disorders diabetes and hypertension. Hypertension and renal disease prevalences vary among populations from different ethnic backgrounds, with very high rates being observed in Aboriginal Australians, Native Americans, and people of African descent.[3-5] It is well established that lifestyle factors pose significant risk for the development and persistence of hypertension and diabetes in the general population, with obesity becoming an increasing concern, especially in the developing world.[6] Of note there is evidence linking mutations in the apolipoprotein-1 (APOL1) gene in people of African descent with increased predisposition to the development of human immunodeficiency virus (HIV)–associated nephropathy and focal and segmental glomerulosclerosis (FSGS) in African Americans. Searches for specific gene polymorphisms or mutations have not implicated global culprit genes, however, but instead point to a likely complex interplay between polygenic predisposition and environmental factors in the development of hypertension, diabetes, and renal disease.[6-11] Furthermore, evidence highlighting the far-reaching effects of the intrauterine environment and early postnatal growth on organ development, organ function, and subsequent susceptibility to adult disease is quite compelling.[12-14] These data suggest that stresses experienced during early development (for which low birth weight or prematurity may be a surrogate marker), "program" long-term organ function and may be the first in a succession of "hits" that ultimately manifest in overt disease. This chapter outlines the effects of fetal and early-life programming on renal development (particularly nephrogenesis), nephron endowment, and the risks of hypertension and kidney disease in later life. Major congenital renal anomalies are discussed elsewhere in this book. In addition, it must be borne in mind that low birth weight and prematurity also predict later-life diabetes, cardiovascular disease, and metabolic syndrome, so renal function may be additionally impacted through developmental programming of these organ systems and, in turn, affect outcomes of these diseases, the discussion of which is beyond the scope of the current chapter.[14-18]

DEVELOPMENTAL PROGRAMMING

The process through which an environmental insult experienced early in life can predispose to adult disease is known as *developmental programming*, which refers to the observation that an environmental stimulus experienced during a critical period of development in utero or early after birth can induce long-term structural and functional effects in the organism.[13,19] This phenomenon, nowadays often termed *developmental origins of health and disease* or DOHaD, can have far-reaching implications in that the effects can be perpetuated across generations.[20,21] The association between adverse intrauterine events and subsequent cardiovascular disease has long been recognized.[13,19,22,23] In early studies, adults of low birth weight were found to have higher cardiovascular morbidity and mortality than those of normal birth weight.[24] Subsequently, evidence from diverse populations has confirmed these findings and expanded them to include other conditions, such as hypertension, impaired glucose tolerance, type 2 diabetes, obesity, preeclampsia, and chronic kidney disease (CKD).[19,25-31] Of these, the associations between low birth weight and prematurity and subsequent hypertension have been the most studied.[32-35] Attention had largely focused on prematurity and low birth weight as markers for developmental programming of hypertension and renal disease, but high birth weight, often the result of a diabetic pregnancy or maternal obesity, is also emerging as a risk factor.[36-38] Currently birth weight and prematurity are the best available surrogates for an adverse intrauterine environment, but some intrauterine stresses may not manifest as such and therefore may not be recognized. Ongoing work is required to develop more sensitive measures of developmental stress. Table 23.1 outlines the definitions of birth weight and gestational age categories that are referred to throughout this chapter. Globally, the respective incidences of low birth weight and prematurity are around 15% and 9.6%.[12,39] The global incidence of high birth weight, which ranges from 5% to 20%, is rising.[38] A significant number of infants born yearly therefore likely undergo developmental programming and are at risk for chronic disease later in life.

Table 23.1 Definitions of Birth Weight and Prematurity Categories

Category	Definition
Birth Weight Categories	
Normal birth weight	>2500 g and <4000 g (usually)
Large for gestational age	>2 standard deviations above the mean birth weight for gestational age
Low birth weight	<2500 g
Very low birth weight	<1500 g
Appropriate for gestational age	Within ±2 standard deviations of the mean birth weight for gestational age
Small for gestational age	>2 standard deviations below the mean birth weight for gestational age
Intrauterine growth restriction	Evidence of fetal malnutrition and growth restriction at any time during gestation
Gestational Categories	
Extremely preterm	<28 weeks of gestation
Very preterm	<32 and >28 weeks of gestation
Moderately preterm	<34 and >32 weeks of gestation
Late preterm	<37 and >34 weeks of gestation
Full term	>37 weeks of gestation

From Abitbol CL, Rodriguez MM: The long-term renal and cardiovascular consequences of prematurity. Nat Rev Nephrol 8:265-274, 2012.

DEVELOPMENTAL PROGRAMMING IN THE KIDNEY

The kidney is the organ central to the development of hypertension. The relationship between renal sodium handling, intravascular volume homeostasis, and hypertension is well accepted.[40,41] That factors intrinsic to the kidney itself affect blood pressure has been demonstrated clinically in kidney transplantation, in which the blood pressure in the recipient after transplantation has been shown to be related to the blood pressure or hypertension risk factors of the donor; that is, hypertension "follows" the kidney.[42] In 1988 Brenner and colleagues proposed that a congenital (programmed) reduction in nephron number may be a factor explaining why some individuals are susceptible to hypertension and renal injury whereas others may seem relatively resistant under similar circumstances (e.g., sodium excess or diabetes mellitus).[43] Reductions in nephron number and whole kidney glomerular surface area would result in lower sodium excretory capacity, enhancing susceptibility to hypertension, and a reduced renal reserve, limiting compensation for renal injury. This hypothesis was attractive in that an association between a reduced nephron number and low birth weight, for example, could explain differences in hypertension and renal disease prevalence observed in populations of different ethnicity, among whom those who tend to have lower birth weights often have a greater prevalence of hypertension and renal disease.[44-47]

Table 23.2 Variability of Nephron Number in Humans

Reference	Population	Sample Size	Mean	Range	Fold
Nyengaard et al[9]	Danish	37	617,000	331,000-1,424,000	4.3
Merlet-Benichou et al[368]*	French	28	1,107,000	655,000-1,554,000	2.4
Keller et al[55]	German	20	1,074,414	531,140-1,959,914	3.7
	Hypertensive	10	702,379	531,140-954,893	1.8
	Normotensive	10	1,429,200	884,458-1,959,914	2.2
Douglas-Denton et al[369]	African Americans	105	884,938	210,332-2,026,541	9.6
	White Americans	84	843,106	227,327-1,660,232	7.3
Hoy et al[370]	non-Aboriginal Australians	24	861,541	380,517-1,493,665	3.9
	Aboriginal Australians	19	713,209	364,161-1,129,223	3.1
McNamara et al[371,372]†	Senegalese	47	992,353	536,171-1,764,421	3.3
Hoy et al[373]	African and white Americans, Australian Aborigines and non-Aborigines non-Aboriginal Australians, and Senegalese	420	901,902	210,232-2,702,079	12.8

*Used acid maceration technique. All other studies used unbiased stereology.
†Values for 47 participants were combined from two publications.
From Puelles VG, Hoy WE, Hughson MD, et al: Glomerular number and size variability and risk for kidney disease. Curr Opin Nephrol Hypertens 20:7-15, 2011.

PLAUSIBILITY OF THE NEPHRON NUMBER HYPOTHESIS

An obstacle to investigation of the nephron number hypothesis has been the difficulty of accurately counting or estimating the total number of nephrons in a kidney.[48] Review of early studies shows that humans were believed to have an average of approximately one million nephrons per kidney.[49] Such studies, however, were performed using techniques such as acid maceration or traditional model-based stereologic approaches, which are prone to bias because of required assumptions, extrapolations, and operator sensitivity.[48-50] Over the past 20 years, the "unbiased" dissector (counting method)/fractionator (sampling method) has emerged as the "gold standard" for counting glomeruli, and it generates accurate and precise estimates.[48-50] Importantly, all reported glomerular counting techniques have been performed on autopsy samples. To date, no validated technique permits determination of nephron number in vivo, although a magnetic resonance imaging (MRI) technique using cationic ferritin shows promise.[51,52]

In one study using the dissector/fractionator combination method in 37 normal Danish adults, the average glomerular (nephron) number was reported to be 617,000 per kidney (range 331,000-1,424,000).[49] A positive correlation was noted between glomerular number and kidney weight, which has subsequently been used as a surrogate marker for nephron number. In general, numbers of viable glomeruli are reduced in kidneys from older subjects, owing to age-related glomerulosclerosis and obsolescence.[49,53] Later studies among patients of varying ethnicities have reported an up to 13-fold variation in total nephron number, with values ranging from 210,332 to 2,702,079 per kidney (Table 23.2).[54] This large variability in total nephron number in subjects without kidney disease may influence susceptibility to hypertension and kidney disease.[49,54,55]

In support of the nephron number hypothesis, it is known that progressive proteinuria, glomerulosclerosis, and renal dysfunction develop with time in persons born with severe nephron deficits, for example, unilateral renal agenesis, bilateral renal hypoplasia, and oligomeganephronia.[2,56] Analogously, therefore, people born with nephron numbers at or below the median level may be more susceptible to superimposed postnatal factors that act as subsequent "hits"; thus, a significant proportion of the population may be at risk for the development of hypertension and renal disease,[12] given that some 30% of the world's adult population is hypertensive.[6]

The counter-argument to the nephron number hypothesis is that in experimental animals and in humans, removal of one kidney (presumed reduction in nephron number by 50%) under varying circumstances may be associated with higher blood pressures or low-grade proteinuria but does not always lead to hypertension and renal disease.[50,57,58] It is of interest, however, that uninephrectomy on postnatal day 1 in rats or fetal uninephrectomy in sheep—that is, loss of nephrons at a time when nephrogenesis is not yet completed—does lead to adult hypertension prior to any evidence of renal injury.[59-61] These data support the hypothesis that intrauterine or congenital reduction in nephron number may be associated with compensatory mechanisms or a reduced compensatory capacity that are different from those associated with later nephron loss, resulting in increased risk of hypertension. Consistent with this notion, kidneys from rats that underwent unilateral nephrectomy at 3 days of age showed a similar total glomerular number but a significantly smaller number of mature glomeruli in the remaining kidney than kidneys from those that underwent nephrectomy at 120 days of age.[62] Furthermore, after unilateral nephrectomy in the neonatal period, the mean glomerular volume in the remaining kidney of rats increased by 59% in comparison with 20% in adult rats, likely indicating a greater burden of compensatory hypertrophy and hyperfiltration in response to neonatal nephrectomy.

In potential contrast, however, a study of 97 subjects aged 2.5 to 25 years who had radiologically normal single kidneys, found that renal function declined faster over time in those with acquired single kidneys (surgical removal of other kidney) than in those with congenital single kidneys, although blood pressures and proteinuria were not

Table 23.3 Glomerular Characteristics by Birth Weight in Humans

Mean Birth Weight (Range)	N	Mean Number of Glomeruli (Range)*	Mean Glomerular Tuft Volume ($\mu m^3 \times 10^6$)	Total Glomerular Tuft Volume (cm^3)
2.65 kg (1.81-3.12)	29	770,860 (658,757-882,963)	9.2	6.7
3.27 kg (3.18-3.38)	28	965,729 (885,714-1,075,744)	7.2	6.8
3.93 kg (3.41-4.94)	30	1,005,356 (900,094-1,110,599)	6.9	6.6

*Adjusted for age, gender, race, body surface area.
From Hoy WE, Hughson MD, Bertram JF, et al: Nephron number, hypertension, renal disease, and renal failure. J Am Soc Nephrol 16:2557-2564, 2005.

different.[63] However, these findings may be confounded by indication for nephrectomy, because approximately 25% of the nephrectomies were performed for obstruction, which may affect contralateral kidney development, as discussed later.[64,65] In addition, unilateral in utero nephrectomy in sheep was associated with significant hypertrophy and a 45% increase in nephron number in the remaining kidney; therefore, a congenital solitary kidney may have a higher-than-normal nephron endowment and therefore may be relatively protected in comparison with an acquired single kidney.[66,67] Timing of nephron loss is likely a crucial factor in determining the compensatory capacity of remaining nephrons.

NEPHRON NUMBER AND GLOMERULAR VOLUME

Human glomeruli have been reported to increase in size up to sevenfold from infancy to adulthood.[68,69] Glomerular size also increases in adulthood in people without overt renal disease, and the increase is associated with rising age, increasing body size, and lower birth weight.[70] Mean glomerular volume has also been consistently noted to vary inversely with total glomerular number although the correlation appears stronger among whites and Aboriginal Australians than in people of African origin.[55,71-73] This relationship suggests that larger glomeruli may reflect compensatory hyperfiltration and hypertrophy in subjects with fewer nephrons and may therefore be a surrogate marker for reduced nephron number.[53,72] In fact, Hoy and coworkers found that, although mean glomerular volume was increased in subjects with reduced nephron number, total glomerular tuft volume (a surrogate for total filtration surface area) was no different among groups with different nephron numbers (Table 23.3).[71] This observation suggests that total filtration surface area may initially be maintained in the setting of reduced nephron number but at the expense of glomerular hypertension and hypertrophy, which are maladaptive and predict poor outcomes.[74-76] Consistent with this possibility, glomerulomegaly is common in renal biopsy specimens from Aboriginal Australians, a population with high rates of low birth weight and renal disease, and has also been associated with faster rate of decline of glomerular filtration rate (GFR) in Pima Indians.[77-79] Furthermore, in a study of donor kidneys, maximal planar area of glomeruli was found to be higher in kidneys from African Americans than in those from whites and to be a predictor of poorer transplant function.[75] Among 111 adult males from four ethnic groups, mean glomerular volume and variability were highest among African Americans and Aboriginal Australians, likely associated with susceptibility to hypertension and renal disease.[80] In populations at high risk for kidney failure, therefore, large glomeruli are a common finding at early stages of renal disease and may reflect programmed reductions in nephron number in these populations, in which access to prenatal and subsequent health care is often suboptimal.[81-83] An increase in glomerular volume, however, is not always associated with lower glomerular number, and individual glomerular volume varies considerably within kidneys.[73] Nevertheless, overall, glomerulomegaly and greater intrasubject variability in glomerular volume have been found to be associated with older age, fewer nephrons, lower birth weight, hypertension, obesity, and severity of cardiovascular disease.[80]

EVIDENCE FOR PROGRAMMING IN THE KIDNEY

DEVELOPMENTAL PROGRAMMING OF NEPHRON ENDOWMENT

Experimental Evidence for Programming of Nephron Endowment

Developmental programming of nephron number has been the most rigorously studied link to later-life hypertension and kidney disease so far. Numerous animal models have demonstrated the association of low birth weight (induced by gestational exposure to low-protein or low-calorie diets, uterine ischemia, dexamethasone, or vitamin A deprivation) with subsequent hypertension.[84-91] The link between adult hypertension and low birth weight in these animal models appears to be mediated, at least in part, by an associated congenital nephron deficit.[84,88,89] Corresponding blood pressures and nephron numbers associated with various programming models are outlined in Table 23.4. As shown, the association between birth weight, nephron numbers, and blood pressures varies among models, underscoring the complexity of developmental programming and the need for better markers than birth weight.

Vehaskari and colleagues demonstrated an almost 30% reduction in glomerular number in offspring of pregnant rats fed a low-protein diet in comparison with those fed a normal-protein diet during pregnancy.[89] As shown in

Table 23.4 Associations of Nephron Number and Renal Size with Blood Pressure and Renal Function

Experimental Model	Animal	Experimental Evidence Glomerular Number (%)	Birth Weight	Blood Pressure	Renal Function
Reduction in Nephron Number					
Maternal calorie restriction[148,374,375]	Rat	↓ 20-40	↓	↑	↓ GFR Proteinuria
Uterine artery ligation[93,227,276]	Rat	↓ 20-30	↓	↑	Impaired proteinuria
Low-protein diet during gestation[89,376-378]	Rat	↓ 25 ↓ 17 ↓ 16	↓/↔	↑	↓ GFR Proteinuria ↓ longevity
Postnatal nutrient restriction[379]	Rat	↓ 27	Normal	↑	NA
Iron deficiency[242]	Rat	↓ 22	↓	↑	NA
Vitamin A deficiency[245]	Rat	↓ 20	↔	NA	NA
Zinc deficiency[244]	Rat	↓ 25	NA	↑	↓ GFR Proteinuria
Ethanol[247]	Sheep	↓ 11	↔	NA	NA
Hypoxia[380]	Rat	↓ 26-52	↓	NA	NA
Cigarette smoke[381]	Mouse	NA	↓	NA	↓ kidney mass
Ureteral obstruction—neonatal[65]	Rat	↓ 50	NA	↑	↓ GFR ↓ renal growth after relief of obstruction
Prematurity[94]	Mouse	↓ 17-24	↓	↑	↓ GFR ↑ albuminuria
Glucocorticoids[84,88,254,382]	Rat Sheep	↓ 20 ↓ 38	↓/↔ ↔	↑ ↑	Glomerulosclerosis ↑ collagen deposition
Maternal diabetes[124,261]	Rat	↓ 10-35	↔	↑	Salt sensitivity
Gentamicin[280,282]	Rat	↓ 10-20	↓	NA	NA
β-lactams[284]	Rat	↓ 5-10	↔	NA	Tubular dilatation Interstitial inflammation
Cyclosporine[150,383]	Rabbit	↓ 25-33	↓/↔	↑	↓ GFR ↑ RVR Proteinuria
Dahl salt-sensitive[43]	Rat	↓ 15		↑ with Na intake	Accelerated FSGS
Munich-Wistar-Fromter[43,384]	Rat	↓ 40		↑ with age	↑ Single-nephron GFR FSGS
Milan hypertensive[43]	Rat	↓ 17		↑	NA
PVG/c[43]	Rat	↑ 122		Resistant	Resistant to FSGS
PAX2 mutations[230,270,274]	Mouse Human	↓ 22		NA	Renal coloboma syndrome in humans Small kidneys
GDNF heterozygote[277,385]	Mouse	↓ 30	↔	↑	Normal GFR Enlarged glomeruli
c-Ret null mutant[222]	Mouse	↓	NA	NA	Severe renal dysplasia
hIGFBP-1 overexpression[267]	Mouse	↓18-25	↓	NA	Glomerulo-sclerosis
Bcl-2 deficiency[271]	Mouse	↓	NA	NA	↑ blood urea nitrogen and creatinine
p53 transgenic[275]	Mouse	↓ 50	NA	NA	Glomerular hypertrophy Renal failure
COX2 null mutant[386]	Mouse	NA	↔	↔	↓ GFR
Augmentation of Nephron Number					
Vitamin A supplementation (with low-protein diet)[297]	Rat	Normalized	NA	NA	NA
Amino acid (glycine, urea, or alanine) supplementation to maternal low-protein diet[387]	Rat	Normalized	NA	Normalized with glycine only	NA
Restoration of post-natal nutrition post-intrauterine growth restriction[93]	Rat	Normalized	↓	Normalized	NA
Iron supplementation to iron-deficient mothers[243]	Rat	Partial rescue	NA	NA	NA

Continued on following page

Table 23.4 Associations of Nephron Number and Renal Size with Blood Pressure and Renal Function (Continued)

Experimental Evidence

Experimental Model	Animal	Glomerular Number (%)	Birth Weight	Blood Pressure	Renal Function
Ouabain administration (with low-protein diet)[293]	Mouse	Prevented ↓	NA	NA	NA
Maternal uninephrectomy prior to gestation[298]	Rat	↑	NA	NA	NA
Post-natal overfeeding, normal birthweight[114]	Rat	↑ 20	↔	↑	Glomerulosclerosis

Human Evidence

Clinical Circumstance	Population	Glomerular Number/ Kidney Volume (%)*	Birth Weight	Blood Pressure	Renal Function
Low birth weight[72,102]	Human 0-1 yr	↓ 13-35	↓	NA	NA
Prematurity[100]	Human	↓ correlated with gestational age	↓	NA	NA
Females vs. males	Human	↓ 12	NA	Variable	Variable
Hypertensive vs. normotensive Caucasians[55,99]	Human 35-59 yr	↓ 19-50	NA	↑	No ↑ Glomerulo-sclerosis
Hypertensive vs. normotensive African Americans[99]	Human 35-59 yr	NS ↓	NA	↑	No ↑ Glomerulosclerosis
Aboriginal Australians vs. Caucasian Australians[50]	Human 0-85 yr	↓ 23%	↓	NA	
Senegalese Africans[372,388]	Human 5-70 yr	NA	NA	NA	↑ variability of glomerular size ↓ glomerular numbers
Maternal vitamin A deficiency[389]	Indian vs. Canadian newborns	↓ newborn renal volume	NA	NA	NA
Genetic polymorphisms:					
RET(1476A) polymorphism[105]	Newborns	↓ 10*	NA	NA	NA
PAX2 AAA haplotype[230]	Newborns	↓ 10*	NA	NA	NA
Combined RET(1476A) polymorphism and PAX2 AAA haplotype[105]	Newborns	↓ 23*	NA	NA	NA
I/D ACE polymorphism[390]	Newborns	↓ 8	NA	NA	NA
BMPR1A rs7922846 polymorphism[231]	Newborns	↓ 13*	NA	NA	NA
OSR1 rs12329305(T) polymorphism[234]	Newborns	↓ 12*	NA	NA	NA
Combined OSR1 and RET polymorphisms[234]	Newborns	↓ 22*	NA	NA	NA
Combined OSR1 and PAX2 polymorphisms[234]	Newborns	↓ 27*	NA	NA	NA
ALDH1A2 rs7169289(G) polymorphism[232]	Newborns	↑ 22*	NA	NA	NA

FSGS, Focal segmental glomerulosclerosis; GFR, glomerular filtration rate; NA, not assessed; NS, nonsignificant; RVR, renal vascular resistance; ↑, increase/increased; ↓, decrease/decreased; ↔, no change/unchanged.
*Kidney volume.
Adapted from references 12, 43, 50, 222, and 225.

Figure 23.1, tail-cuff systolic blood pressures in the low-protein offspring were 20 to 25 mm Hg higher by 8 weeks of age.[89] Similarly, prenatal administration of dexamethasone was associated with low birth weight and fewer glomeruli in the offspring.[84] In these nephron-deficient rats, GFR was reduced, albuminuria was increased, and urinary sodium excretion was lower than in those with a greater nephron complement.[84] Uteroplacental insufficiency, induced by maternal uterine artery ligation late in gestation, has also been found to result in low nephron number and was associated with increased profibrotic renal gene expression with age, although hypertension developed only in males.[92,93] Conversely, adequate postnatal nutrition, achieved by cross-fostering of the offspring of mothers with uteroplacental insufficiency onto normal lactating females at birth, restored nephron number and prevented subsequent hypertension in the males.[93] In a later study of the impact of prematurity, mice delivered 1 to 2 days early (normal mouse gestation 21 days) had reduced nephron numbers, lower GFR, and higher blood pressures than mice born at term, as well as albuminuria.[94] Interestingly, nephron numbers were lower in mice delivered 2 days early than in those delivered 1 day early, suggesting the degree of prematurity is important in determining final nephron endowment, even though

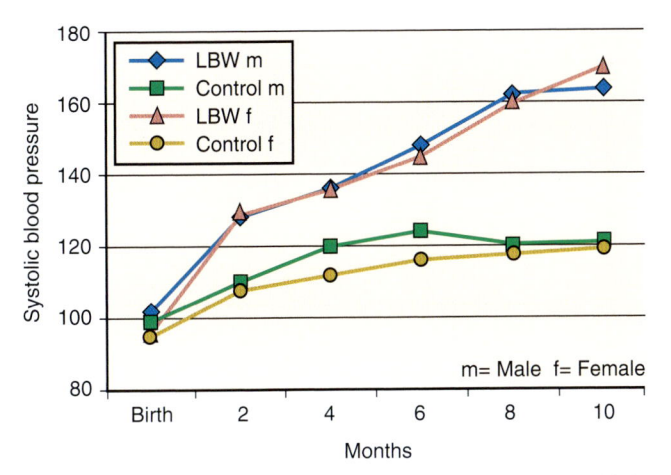

Figure 23.1 Fetal programming of hypertension in low-birth-weight (LBW) rats. (Adapted from Vehaskari VM, Aviles DH, Manning J: Prenatal programming of adult hypertension in the rat. *Kidney Int* 59:238-245, 2001.)

nephrogenesis continues after birth in the normal mouse. Not surprisingly, in animal studies, timing of the gestational insult has been found to be crucial in renal programming, with the greatest impact on nephron number occurring during periods of most active nephrogenesis.[95]

Programming of Nephron Number in Humans

As noted previously, total nephron number varies widely in the normal human population (see Table 23.2).[54,96] A significant proportion of the interindividual variability in nephron number appears to be already present perinatally, demonstrating a strong developmental effect.[97,98] Overall, the data support a direct relationship between nephron number and birth weight and an inverse relationship between nephron number and glomerular volume.[69,72,99] Hughson and colleagues reported a linear relationship between glomerular number and birth weight and calculated a regression coefficient predicting an increase of 257,426 glomeruli per kilogram increase in birth weight, although the generalizability of the regression coefficient to populations in which the distribution of nephron number appears bimodal, such as among African Americans, may not be valid.[69] It has also been calculated that in the normal population without renal disease, approximately 4500 glomeruli are lost per kidney per year after age 18.[71] Glomerular numbers tend to be lower in females than in males. A kidney starting with a lower nephron number, therefore, would conceivably reach a critical reduction of nephron mass, either with age or in response to a renal insult, earlier than a kidney with a greater nephron complement, predisposing to hypertension and/or renal dysfunction.

Nephrogenesis in humans begins during the 9th week of gestation and continues until the 34th to 36th week.[71] Nephron number at birth therefore largely depends on the intrauterine environment and gestational age. It is generally believed that no new nephrons are formed in humans after term birth. To investigate whether glomerulogenesis does continue postnatally in premature infants, Rodriguez and colleagues studied kidneys at autopsy from 56 extremely premature infants and compared them with kidneys of 10 full-term infants as controls.[100] The radial glomerular counts (an estimate of glomerular number based on the number of layers of glomeruli in the cortex) were lower in premature than in full-term infants and correlated with gestational age. Furthermore, evidence of active glomerulogenesis, indicated by the presence of S-shaped bodies immediately under the renal capsule, was seen in premature infants who died before 40 days but was absent in those who died after 40 days of life, suggesting that nephrogenesis may continue for up to 40 days after premature birth. These investigators also stratified their cases by presence or absence of renal failure.[100] Among infants surviving longer than 40 days, those with renal failure (serum creatinine > 2.0 mg/dL) had significantly fewer glomeruli than those without renal failure. This cross-sectional observation may suggest that renal failure inhibited glomerulogenesis or, conversely, that the presence of fewer glomeruli lowered the threshold for development of renal failure in these infants. Those premature infants surviving longer than 40 days without renal failure exhibited glomerulomegaly, which may reflect, at least in the short term, a compensatory renoprotective response.

Faa and colleagues also reported evidence of active glomerulogenesis in kidneys of premature infants and two term infants who died at birth, but not in a child who died at age 3 months, suggesting that glomerular maturation may continue for a short period even after term birth.[97] In contrast, Hinchliffe and associates studied nephron number in premature and full-term stillbirths and in infants who died at 1 year of age and who were born either with appropriate weight for gestational age or small for gestational age.[101,102] At both time points, growth-restricted infants had fewer nephrons than controls. In addition, the number of nephrons in growth-restricted infants dying at 1 year of age had not increased in comparison with that in the growth-restricted stillbirths, demonstrating a lack of postnatal nephrogenesis (Figure 23.2A). Manalich and coworkers examined the kidneys of neonates dying within 2 weeks of birth in relation to their birth weights (Figure 23.2B).[75] A significant direct correlation was found between glomerular number and birth weight, and a strong inverse correlation between glomerular volume and glomerular number, independent of sex and race. These studies all support the hypothesis that an adverse intrauterine environment, which may manifest as low birth weight or prematurity, is associated with a congenital reduction in nephron endowment and an early, compensatory increase in glomerular volume.

In a population of 140 adults aged 18 to 65 years who died of various causes, a significant correlation was also observed between birth weight and glomerular number.[99] Glomerular volume was inversely correlated with glomerular number. Total glomerular number did not differ statistically among African American and white subjects, although the distribution among African Americans appeared bimodal. The range of nephron number was greatest among African Americans. Significantly, however, none of the subjects in this study had been of low birth weight; therefore, no conclusion can be drawn as to whether an association between low birth weight and nephron number existed in either population group.[99] It may be argued that because low birth weight is more prevalent among African Americans, this cohort was more representative of the general white population than the general black population, having

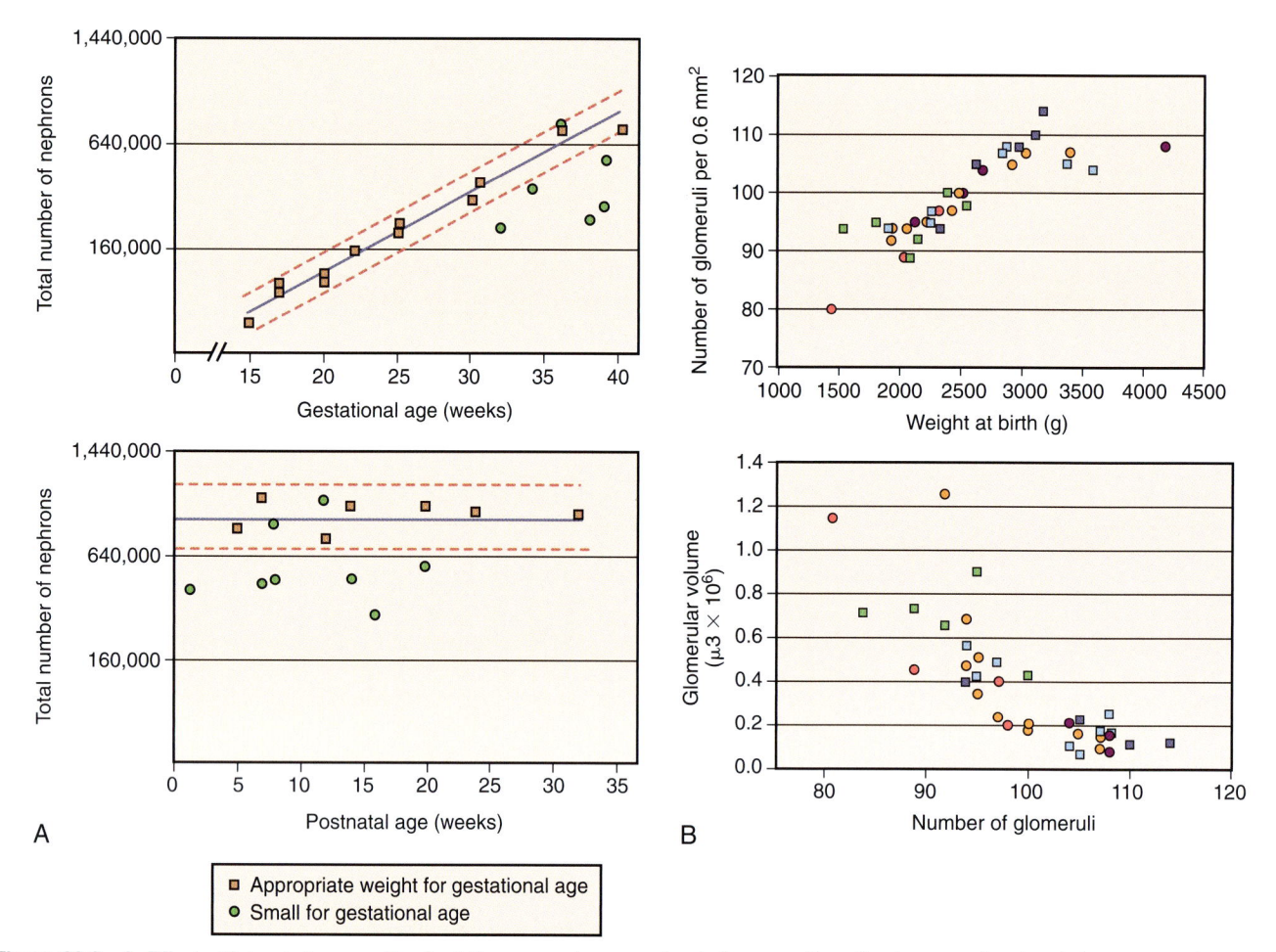

Figure 23.2 **A,** Effect of intrauterine growth retardation on nephron number in humans. **Top,** Nephron number in relation to gestational age. **Bottom,** Lack of postnatal catch-up in nephron number. **B,** Birth weight **(top)** and glomerular volume **(bottom)** plotted against glomerular number in neonates. (**A** from Hinchliffe SA, Lynch MR, Sargent PH, et al: The effect of intrauterine growth retardation on the development of renal nephrons. *Br J Obstet Gynaecol* 99:296-301, 1992; **B** from Manalich R, Reyes L, Herrera M, et al: Relationship between weight at birth and the number and size of renal glomeruli in humans: a histomorphometric study. *Kidney Int* 58:770-773, 2000.)

included only subjects of normal birth weight.[103] In a European study comparing 26 subjects with non–insulin-dependent diabetes compared with 19 age-matched nondiabetic controls, no difference in glomerular number was found, but again, all subjects had birth weights above 3000 g, and, therefore, the impact of low birth weight on nephron number could not be assessed.[104]

Kidney Size as a Correlate for Nephron Number. Analysis of the relationship between kidney weight and nephron number in infants less than 3 months of age (a time at which compensatory hypertrophy has likely not yet occurred) revealed a direct relationship (Figure 23.3).[105] Regression analysis predicted an increase of 23,459 nephrons per gram of kidney weight.[105] Renal mass is therefore proportional to nephron number, and renal volume is proportional to renal mass; for that reason, renal volume has been analyzed as a surrogate for nephron endowment in infants in vivo.[49] Ultrasonographic evaluation of fetal renal function in utero revealed a reduction in hourly urine volume, higher prevalence of oligohydramnios, reduced renal perfusion, and reduced renal volume in growth-restricted fetuses.[106-108] These findings may represent reduced fetal perfusion in

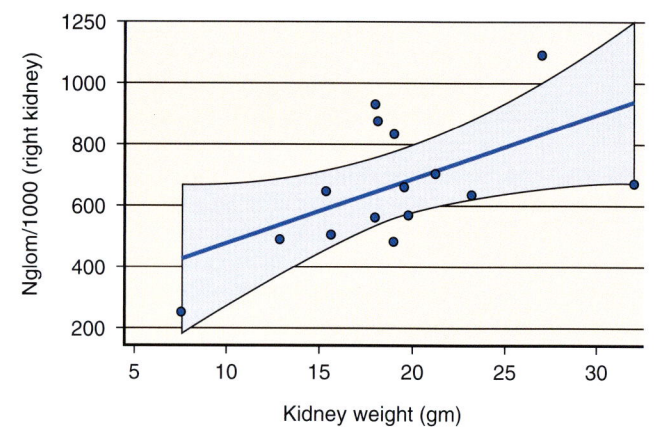

Figure 23.3 Relationship between nephron number and mass of the right kidney in white infants who died within the first 3 months of life. (From Zhang Z, Quinlan J, Hoy WE, et al: A common RET variant is associated with reduced newborn kidney size and function. *J Am Soc Nephrol* 19:2027-2034, 2008.)

situations of uterine compromise, however, and do not necessarily reflect altered renal development. Similarly, among premature infants, another study found that kidney volume at a corrected age of 38 weeks was significantly lower than that in term infants and was associated with a significantly lower GFR estimated from serum cystatin C.[109]

Analysis of kidney size and postnatal growth measured by ultrasonography in 178 children born premature or small for gestational age in comparison with 717 mature children with appropriate weight for gestational age at 0, 3, and 18 months found that weight for gestational age was positively associated with kidney volume at all three time points.[110] Slight catch-up in kidney growth was observed in growth-restricted infants but not in premature infants. Among term neonates, renal parenchymal thickness, proposed as a more accurate screening tool than renal volume estimation, was significantly reduced in those with low compared to normal birth weights.[111] In Australian Aboriginal children, low birth weight was also found to be associated with lower renal volumes on ultrasonography.[112] Comparison of renal volume between children aged 9 to 12 years who were born premature, either small or at appropriate weight for gestational age and controls found that kidneys were smallest in those who had been preterm and small for gestational age, but when findings were adjusted for body surface area (BSA), there were no significant differences between the groups.[113] A smaller kidney size, therefore, may be a surrogate marker for reduced nephron endowment, but importantly, growth in kidney size on ultrasonography cannot distinguish between normal growth with age and renal hypertrophy.

EVIDENCE OF ADDITIONAL PROGRAMMING EFFECTS IN THE KIDNEY

Taken together, the findings in animals and humans lend credence to the hypothesis that a congenital deficit in nephron number can be programmed during development and is likely to be an independent factor determining susceptibility to essential hypertension and subsequent renal injury. Low nephron number alone, however, does not account for all observed programmed hypertension (see Table 23.4). In one study, supplementation of a low-protein diet during gestation with glycine, urea, or alanine resulted in a normalization of nephron number in rat offspring, but blood pressure normalized only in those supplemented with glycine.[32] Likewise, augmentation of nephron number by postnatal hypernutrition in another study resulted in a 20% increase in nephron number but also in development of obesity, hypertension, and glomerulosclerosis with age.[114] These findings suggest that additional factors contribute to the developmental programming of hypertension. Later evidence has shown alterations in renal tubular sodium handling and vascular function in developmentally programmed kidneys that likely also contribute to later-life blood pressure and renal function changes as listed in Table 23.5.[95]

Altered Sodium Handling by the Kidney

The pressure-natriuresis curve is shifted to the right in most forms of hypertension. A reduction in filtration surface area associated with a reduction in nephron number is one plausible hypothesis to explain the associated higher blood pressures. Consistent with this association, salt sensitivity has been reported in several animal models to be associated with low birth weight and reduced nephron number.[33,115-119] Some investigators have reported the presence of salt-sensitive hypertension in rats in which low birth weight was induced by maternal uterine artery ligation, whereas others report no salt sensitivity in rats in which low birth weight was induced by maternal protein restriction, although timing of dietary intervention and age at study appear to play a role.[116,120,121] Elevations in blood pressure in response to high-salt diet have been more consistently observed in aging than in young rats, suggesting either an early adaptive mechanism that may decline with age or worsening salt sensitivity as nephron number declines with age.[122] In young rats, however, despite no change in blood pressure, an increase in plasma volume was observed, consistent with sodium retention.[123] Similar salt sensitivity was observed in adult rat offspring exposed to maternal gestational diabetes, a model also associated with reduced nephron number.[124]

The effect of nephron "dose" and filtration surface area on salt sensitivity was examined in glial cell line–derived neurotrophic factor (GDNF) heterozygous mice that have either one kidney and a 65% reduction in total nephron number (HET1K) or two kidneys and a 25% reduction in total nephron number (HET2K).[125] Given the accompanying glomerular hypertrophy, total glomerular surface area was normal in HET2K but remained reduced in HET1K mice. At baseline the mice did not have elevated blood pressures, but both groups became hypertensive in response to high-sodium feeding. A gradient of increasing blood pressure was observed from wild-type to HET2K to HET1K, suggesting dependence on nephron number and filtration surface area, given that no change in expression of tubular sodium transporters was observed.[125] In the converse experiment transforming growth factor-β_2 heterozygous (Tgf$\beta 2^{+/-}$) mice, which have 30% higher nephron number, were relatively protected against development of high blood pressure on a chronic high salt diet compared with wild-type mice.[126] Surprisingly, however, the Tgf$\beta 2^{+/-}$ mice did develop increased blood pressures in response to an acute sodium load, suggesting that the benefit conferred by the higher nephron number requires time for adaptation to occur. Early change in sodium diet in itself has been found to have a long-term impact on programming of hypertension in low-birth-weight (LBW) rats. Two studies have found that short-term feeding of a low-salt diet from weaning to 6 weeks of age abrogated, whereas high-salt feeding

Table 23.5 Developmentally Programmed Changes Observed in the Kidney

- Nephron number
- Glomerular volume
- Accelerated maturation of glomeruli
- Tubular sodium transporter expression and/or activity
- Altered renal vascular reactivity
- Alterations in renin angiotensin aldosterone system
- Alterations in sympathetic nervous system activity
- Accelerated senescence, especially after catch-up growth
- Predisposition to inflammation and fibrosis
- Kidney size

exacerbated, hypertension at 10 and 51 weeks despite re-institution of normal-salt diet at 6 weeks.[115,127] The role of sodium intake on long-term renal programming requires further study.

Salt sensitivity therefore does appear to be developmentally programmed. From the GDNF mouse data, filtration surface area may be crucial in determining salt sensitivity but, as discussed previously, is often not reduced initially in the setting of low nephron number. Expression and activity of renal tubule sodium transporters has therefore been investigated. Expression of the Na-K-2Cl (NKCC2) and Na-Cl (NCC) cotransporters was significantly higher in prehypertensive offspring of rats fed a protein-restricted diet during gestation than in controls, although expression of the sodium-hydrogen exchanger isoform 3 (NHE3) and epithelial sodium channel (ENaC) was not changed (Figure 23.4A).[128] Higher activity of NKCC2 was shown by increases in chloride transport and lumen-positive transepithelial potential difference in the medullary thick ascending limb in offspring of protein-restricted or dexamethasone-treated mothers (Figure 23.4B).[129] Furthermore, after development of hypertension, furosemide administration reduced the blood pressure, supporting increased NKCC2 activity as a mediator of hypertension in the protein restriction model.[129] Expression of the glucocorticoid receptor and the glucocorticoid-responsive α_1- and β_1-subunits of Na$^+$-K$^+$-adenosine triphosphatase (ATPase) were increased in offspring of pregnant rats fed a low-protein diet.[130] In rats who were suckled by mothers given low-protein feedings during lactation, expression of Na$^+$-K$^+$-ATPase was increased by 40%, but its activity was increased by 300%, demonstrating that expression levels may not fully reflect activity levels.[131] Prenatal dexamethasone administration was associated with increased expression of proximal tubular NHE3

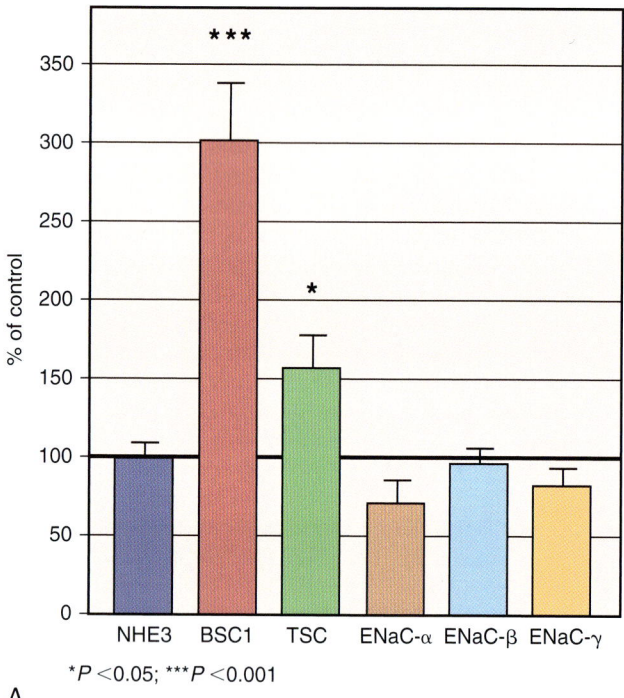

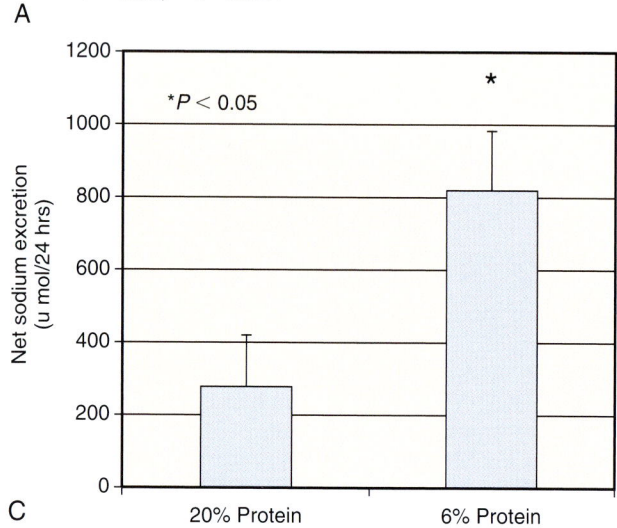

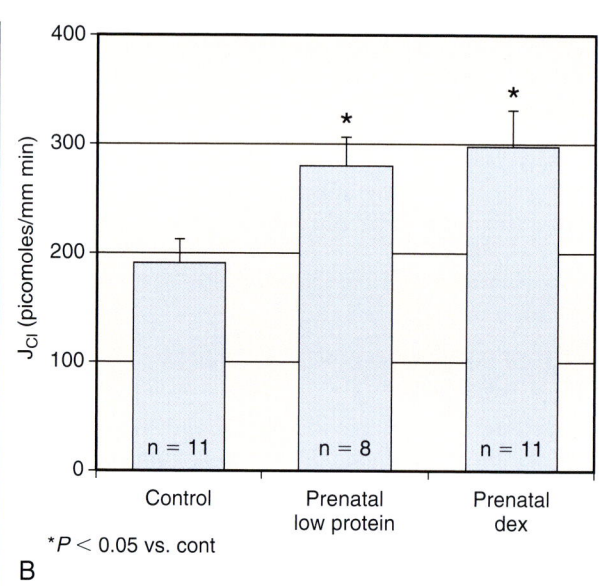

Figure 23.4 **A,** Apical renal sodium transporter expression, quantified by immunoblotting, in 4-week-old rat offspring of mothers fed a low-protein diet. BSC, Bumetanide-sensitive cotransporter (NKCC2); ENac, epithelial sodium channel; NHE3, Na$^+$-H$^+$ exchanger isoform 3; TSC, thiazide-sensitive cotransporter (NCC). **B,** Increased rate of medullary thick ascending limb (mTAL) chloride transport (J$_{Cl}$) in in vitro perfused mTAL from 6-week-old rat offspring of mothers fed a prenatal low-protein diet or given prenatal dexamethasone (dex). **C,** Net increase in urine sodium excretion after administration of ENaC inhibitor benzamil in adult rat offspring of mothers fed a low-protein (6%) or normal (20%) diet during gestation. Data are expressed as means ± standard error. (**A** from Vehaskari VM, Woods LL: Prenatal programming of hypertension: lessons from experimental models. *J Am Soc Nephrol* 16:2545-2556, 2005; **B** from Dagan A, Habib S, Gattineni J, et al: Prenatal programming of rat thick ascending limb chloride transport by low-protein diet and dexamethasone. *Am J Physiol Regul Integr Comp Physiol* 297:R93-R99, 2009; **C** from Cheng CJ, Lozano G, Baum M: Prenatal programming of rat cortical collecting tubule sodium transport. *Am J Physiol Renal Physiol* 302:F674-F678, 2012.)

as well as of the more distal NKCC2 and NCC, but there was no change in ENaC expression.[132] Interestingly, renal denervation reduced systolic blood pressure and sodium transporter expression in this model, suggesting indirect regulation of these genes via sympathetic nerve activity.[132] In another study, baseline expression of β– and γ-ENaC, but not α-ENaC, as well as of Na$^+$-K$^+$-ATPase was significantly higher in rats subjected to maternal diabetes than in controls.[124] Despite several studies showing no change in ENaC expression in programmed animals, an enhanced natriuretic response to the ENaC inhibitor benzamil demonstrated increased ENaC activity in offspring of mothers fed a low-protein diet (Figure 23.4C).[133] Taken together, despite differences among models, the data suggest increased sodium transport in all segments of the renal tubule. Whether a reduced nephron number may contribute indirectly to increased sodium transport through increased single-nephron GFR (SNGFR), necessitating glomerulotubular balance or sodium transporter activity is independently programmed has not yet been elucidated.

Renin Angiotensin Aldosterone System

All components of the renin angiotensin aldosterone system (RAAS) are expressed in the developing kidney.[134] Alterations in the RAAS have been studied in various programming models, but a consistent pattern of upregulation or downregulation of RAAS components has not been found. For example, expression of angiotensinogen and renin messenger RNA (mRNA) was decreased in neonatal kidneys of rats subjected to uterine ischemia but increased in the kidneys of mouse offspring of diabetic mothers.[135,136] Such differences likely also reflect species differences, differences in timing of intervention, timing of study, and so on, as summarized in Table 23.6.[67] The importance of angiotensin II (Ang II) in nephrogenesis was demonstrated by the administration of the Ang II subtype 1 receptor (AT$_1$R) blocker losartan to normal rats during the first 12 days of life (while nephrogenesis is proceeding), which resulted in a reduction in final nephron number and subsequent development of hypertension.[137] Ang II can stimulate the expression of Pax-2 (an anti-apoptotic factor) through AT$_2$R.[138] AT$_2$R expression, therefore, is likely to affect nephrogenesis and kidney development, but its role in programming is still unclear. Administration of an angiotensin-converting enzyme inhibitor (ACEI), captopril, or losartan to LBW rats from 2 to 4 weeks of age, abrogated the development of adult hypertension in these animals.[19,93,135,139] Similarly, administration of Ang II or an ACEI to adult rats subjected to a low-protein diet in utero resulted in a more exaggerated hypertensive or hypotensive response, respectively, than in control rats.[19,140-142] Differential regulation of the RAAS by sex hormones during development is thought to contribute to the observation that the effects of developmental programming are often less severe in young females.[143,144] Overall, programmed suppression of the intrarenal RAAS during nephrogenesis is likely to contribute to the reduction in nephron number under adverse circumstances, and postnatal upregulation of the AT$_1$R, possibly mediated by an increase in glucocorticoid activity or sensitivity, may contribute to the subsequent development of hypertension and glomerular hyperfiltration, as reviewed in detail elsewhere.[67,143]

Underscoring the relevance of the RAAS in developmental programming of blood pressure, Ajala and colleagues found that ACE activity was significantly higher in children of low birth weight than in those with normal birth weight and that there was a greater frequency of the *ACE* gene DD genotype among LBW children with the highest blood pressures.[145] The latter finding suggests that the programming effect of blood pressure may be modulated in part by *ACE* gene polymorphisms.

The Sympathetic Nervous System and Renal Vascular Reactivity

Within the kidney, the sympathetic nervous system modulates activity of the RAAS, sodium transport and vascular function, and thereby contributes to blood pressure through regulation of vascular tone and volume status.[67] Development of the renal sympathetic nervous system, and how it may be programmed during nephrogenesis and modulated by the RAAS, is expertly reviewed by Kett and Denton.[67] Renal denervation has been shown to abrogate development of adult hypertension as well as alter sodium transporter expression in the prenatal dexamethasone and uterine ischemia programming models, and the age-associated hypertension that develops in growth-restricted female rats.[132,146,147] Consistent with the findings in whole animals, an increase in baseline renal vascular resistance within the kidney has been described in different programming models.[148-150] For example, Sanders and colleagues reported that renal arterial responses to β-adrenergic stimulation and sensitivity to adenylyl cyclase were increased in 21-day-old growth-restricted offspring subjected to placental insufficiency.[151] Although the renal expression of β$_2$-adrenoreceptor mRNA was increased in these pups, there was also evidence of adaptations to the signal transduction pathway that contributed to the β-adrenergic hyperresponsiveness.[151] Intriguingly, these findings were much more marked in the right than in the left kidney, an observation that remains unexplained but that is not without precedent: Asymmetry of renal blood flow was found in 51% of a cohort of hypertensive patients without renovascular disease.[152] In the Sanders study, growth-restricted rats had reduced glomerular numbers, exhibited glomerular hyperfiltration and hyperperfusion, and had significantly increased proteinuria in comparison with the controls, suggesting alteration in glomerular pressures that likely were mediated by renal vasoreactivity. Interestingly, in a cohort of white and black U.S. subjects, the effect of birth weight on subsequent blood pressures was significantly modified by β-adrenergic receptor genotype, further underscoring a relationship among birth weight, sympathetic activity, and blood pressure.[153]

PROGRAMMING OF RENAL FUNCTION AND DISEASE

In contrast to premature infants or those of low birth weight, in whom nephron numbers have been shown to be reduced, there are no data on nephron numbers in adults who were known to be of low birth weight. The association between nephron number and birth weight and prematurity, however, is a consistent finding in infants, so it seems reasonable to extrapolate that nephron numbers would remain reduced in

Table 23.6 Programming Effects on the Renin Angiotensin Aldosterone System

Model	Species	Timing of Insult	Age and Sex of Offspring at Study	mRNA or Protein Expression	Physiologic Response	Reference(s)
Glucocorticoids	Sheep	Early gestation	40 mo ♀	↔ Plasma renin, Ang II or aogen	↑ Basal MAP, females only	394
	Rat		6-7 mo ♂♀	↔ Renal aogen ↑ PRA, plasma aogen in females only	↑ Basal TBP, females only	395
	Rat	Mid- to late gestation	6 mo	↑ Renal ACE and renin in males and females	ND	396
	Rat	Mid- to late gestation	4 and 8 wk ♂	↔ PRA, plasma Ang II, and renal Ang II levels ↑ Urine Ang II at 4 and 8 wk	↑ Basal TBP at 8 but not 4 wk of age	397
Maternal nutrient restriction or low-protein diet	Sheep	Early to mid-gestation	9 mo	↑ Renal cortical ACE protein ↔ AT_1R in the renal cortex and medulla ↔ Renal cortical but ↑ renal medulla AT_2R	↑ Basal MAP	398
	Rat	Mid- to late gestation	4-12 wk ♂♀	↑ PRA	↑ Basal TBP from 8 wk of age	399
	Rat	Throughout gestation	1-5 days and 22 wk ♂	↓ Renal renin mRNA and Ang II levels at 1 to 5 days of age	↑ Basal MAP at 22 wk of age ↔ No change GFR or RBF	400, 401
	Rat	Throughout gestation	16 wk ♂	↓ Renal AT_1R and AT_2R protein	↑ Basal TBP, ↓ sodium excretion, ↔ GFR	402
	Rat	Throughout gestation	4 wk ♂	↑ Renal AT_1R protein ↓ Renal AT_2R protein ↑ Ang II receptor binding ↔ Renal renin and Ang II tissue levels	↑ Basal MAP (anesthetized) ↑ Basal renal vascular resistance ↔ No change GFR or RBF	403, 404
	Rat	Mid- to late gestation	1-11 mo ♂♀		↑ Basal TBP at 8 wk of age	405-408
			1-2 mo	↓PRA ↓ Renal AT_1R protein and mRNA ↓ Renal AT_2R protein, ↑ AT_2R mRNA	Salt-sensitive TBP TBP normalized by ACE inhibition and low-salt diet Urinary protein/creatinine ratio increased in males only	
			6 to 11 mo	↑ PRA ↔ Plasma or renal Ang I and Ang II ↑ AT_1R protein and mRNA ↑ AT_2R protein, ↔ AT_2R mRNA		
Placental insufficiency	Rat	Late gestation	0-16 wk ♂			409, 410
			Newborn	↓ renal renin and aogen	↑ Basal MAP that was abolished by ACEi treatment	

Table 23.6 Programming Effects on the Renin Angiotensin Aldosterone System (Continued)

Model	Species	Timing of Insult	Age and Sex of Offspring at Study	mRNA or Protein Expression	Physiologic Response	Reference(s)
			16 wk	↑ Renal renin and aogen mRNA, ↑ ACE activity ↔ Renal AT$_1$R and Ang II, ↔ PRA and plasma ACE	↑ Pressor response to ANG II in presence of ACEi ↓ GFR	
Maternal renal hypertension	Rabbit	Throughout gestation	10-45 wk ♂♀	↓ PRA 5 and 10 wk ↔ PRA 30 and 45 wk	↑ Basal MAP at 30 and 45 wk	411-413

ACE, Angiotensin-converting enzyme; ACEi, ACE inhibition; aogen, angiotensinogen; Ang, angiotensin; AT$_{1/2}$R, angiotensin receptor type 1/2; GFR, glomerular filtration rate; MAP, mean arterial pressure; mRNA, messenger RNA; ND, not done; PRA, plasma renin activity; RBF, renal blood flow; TBP, tail artery pressure; ↑, increase in; ↓, decrease in; ↔, unchanged.
From Kett MM, Denton KM: Renal programming: cause for concern? Am J Physiol Regul Integr Comp Physiol 300:R791-R803, 2011.

adults of low birth weight.[69] The determination of nephron number in vivo is not yet reliable enough; therefore, the most utilized in vivo surrogate markers at present are birth weight and prematurity. Importantly, however, in some animal models, low nephron numbers have been observed also in the setting of normal birth weight (see Table 23.4); therefore, among humans, if birth weight is the only surrogate marker used, the impact of renal programming on any outcome is likely to be underestimated.[154] Other clinical surrogates for an adverse intrauterine environment and low nephron numbers are outlined in Table 23.7.

EXPERIMENTAL EVIDENCE

Glomerulomegaly is consistently observed in the setting of low nephron number (see Figure 23.2B). In rats in which low birth weight was induced by maternal protein restriction, GFR was reduced by 10%, although nephron number was reduced by 25%, implying some degree of compensatory hyperfunction per nephron.[33] Although the hyperfunction may be a compensatory mechanism to restore filtration surface area, it is conceivable that renal reserve in these kidneys is reduced.[71] If so, these kidneys may be expected to be less able to compensate further in the setting of additional renal insults and to begin to manifest signs of renal dysfunction (i.e., proteinuria, elevations in serum creatinine, and hypertension). To investigate this hypothesis, diabetes was induced by streptozotocin injection in subgroups of LBW (induced by maternal protein restriction) and normal-birth-weight (NBW) rats.[155] LBW rats had reduced nephron numbers and higher blood pressures compared to NBW rats. Among those rendered diabetic, there was a greater proportional increase in renal size and glomerular hypertrophy in the LBW rats than in NBW controls after 1 week (Figure 23.5).[155] This study demonstrates that the renal response to injury in the setting of a reduced nephron number may be exaggerated and could lead to accelerated loss of renal function.

Subsequently, the same researchers reported outcomes in LBW and NBW diabetic rats at 40 weeks.[156] Histologically,

Table 23.7 Clinical Surrogates for Programmed Low Nephron Number in Humans

- Low birth weight[72,100,102]
- Prematurity[100,102]
- Low kidney mass[49,105]
- Reduced kidney volume[110,112]
- Glomerulomegaly[69,72,102]
- Female sex[391]
- ? Ethnicity—Aboriginal Australian[391]

the podocyte density was reduced and the average area covered by each podocyte was greater in the LBW diabetic rats than in the NBW controls. These findings correlated with urine albumin excretion rate, which was higher in LBW diabetic rats, although the difference did not reach statistical significance. In support of the role of altered podocyte physiology in renal disease progression, similar findings were observed in the Munich Wistar Frömter rat, a strain that has congenitally reduced nephron numbers and demonstrates spontaneous renal disease.[157] Whether these podocyte changes are secondary to an increase in glomerular pressure in the setting of reduced nephron numbers or constitute a primary programmed structural change leading to glomerular injury is not yet known. The role of podocyte depletion, either absolute (loss of podocytes) or relative (podocyte density), in disease progression deserves more research focus, and currently nothing is known about the possible effects of developmental programming on podocyte endowment.

Of interest, in contrast, in low-birth-weight rats exposed to prenatal dexamethasone and subsequently fed a high-protein diet, GFR was similar to that in NBW controls.[158] Nephron numbers were reduced by 13% in only male LBW rats. This study may suggest that there is a threshold reduction in nephron number above which compensation is adequate or that the high-protein diet induced supranormal GFRs in both groups, masking subtle differences in baseline

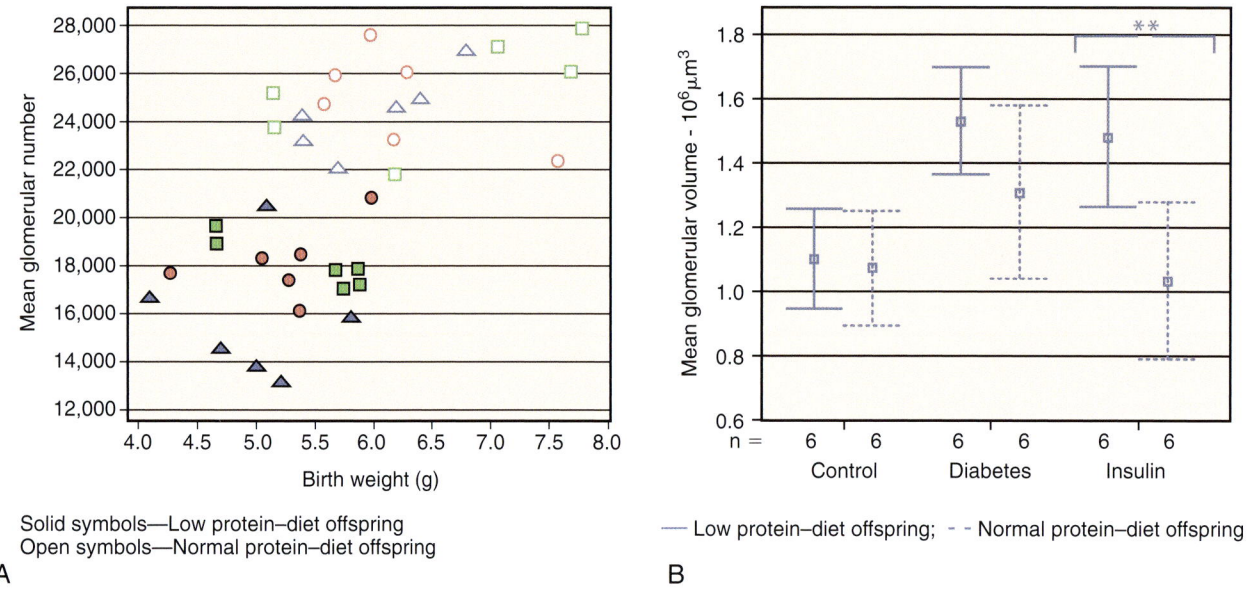

Figure 23.5 A, Scatter plot of mean glomerular number and birth weight in low protein diet rats *(solid symbols)* and normal protein diet rats *(open symbols)*. Control groups *(triangles)*; diabetes groups *(circles)*; diabetes+insulin group *(squares)*. (From Jones SE, Bilous RW, Flyvbjerg A, et al: Intra-uterine environment influences glomerular number and the acute renal adaptation to experimental diabetes. *Diabetologia* 44:721-728, 2001.)

GFR. Another study that measured GFR in LBW rats, induced by placental insufficiency, also failed to demonstrate lower GFRs in LBW rats, but they were significantly hypertensive compared with NBW controls.[91] Conceivably, in this study, the higher intra-glomerular pressure due to elevated blood pressure and reduced nephron mass in LBW rats may have led to a compensatory increase in SNGFR and, thus, normalization of whole-kidney GFR.

The definitive pathophysiologic impact of a reduction in nephron number on the development of renal dysfunction is difficult to elucidate from the existing literature, which comprises studies using very varied experimental conditions. Overall, however, it is possible that, although whole-kidney GFR may not change, SNGFR is likely to be increased in the setting of a reduced nephron number and exacerbated in the presence of renal injury. Interestingly, SNGFR was found to be significantly higher in the Munich Wistar Frömter rat, which has reduced nephron numbers and is known to demonstrate spontaneous progressive glomerular injury, than in the control Wistar rat strain.[157] Renal dysfunction may also result from a programmed predisposition to inflammation and scarring that may be independent of glomerular pressures. In a glomerulonephritis model, injection of anti–Thy-1 antibody in LBW rats resulted in significant upregulation of inflammatory markers and development of sclerotic lesions by day 14, but with no difference in blood pressure or proteinuria, in comparison with NBW controls.[159]

HUMAN EVIDENCE

Most human data rely on the surrogates birth weight, prematurity, renal size, and so on to reflect the risk of renal programming. Although there is no direct proven relationship with nephron number, the consistency of the data is strongly suggestive of a programming effect.

BIRTH WEIGHT, PREMATURITY, AND BLOOD PRESSURE

Two meta-analyses and systematic reviews have shown consistent associations of lower birth weight and prematurity with higher blood pressures in later life.[34,35] Meta-analysis of 27 studies investigating the relationship between birth weight and blood pressure found that systolic blood pressures were 2.28 mm Hg (95% confidence interval [CI], 1.24 to 3.33 mm Hg) higher in subjects with birth weights lower than 2.5 kg than in subjects with birth weights higher than 2.5 kg (Figure 23.6A).[35] Many studies do not discriminate between low birth weight occurring as a result of growth restriction (a marker of intrauterine stress) at any gestational age and that occurring as a result of prematurity with an appropriate (low) weight for that gestational age. Therefore, the relative effect of growth restriction and prematurity on subsequent blood pressures is not always easy to dissect.[160] To investigate this question, a study of 232 50-year-old subjects all born at term, one group with and one group without growth restriction, reported an odds ratio (OR) of 1.9 (95% CI, 1.1 to 3.3) for hypertension among those who had experienced growth restriction in comparison with those who had normal birth weights.[161] Growth restriction before birth per se therefore is associated with subsequent higher blood pressure.

A systematic review of 10 studies comparing premature subjects with those born at term found that in premature subjects, having a mean gestational age of 30.2 weeks and a mean birth weight of 1280 g, systolic blood pressures in later life were 2.5 mm Hg higher (95% CI, 1.7 to 3.3 mm Hg) than in those born at term (Figure 23.6B).[34] Prematurity therefore is also independently associated with higher blood pressure, which in some studies meets the definition of hypertension by 1 to 2 years of age.[162-164] Whether the risk of higher blood pressure is greater among premature subjects who were born small for gestational age (growth restricted) than in those born appropriate for gestational age is not yet clear, however, with some studies suggesting an additional effect of growth restriction and others not.[165-168]

Ultimately, the importance of dissecting the risk from low birth weight and that from prematurity may lie in the future potential for prevention. Given that effect estimates for risk of higher blood pressures were similar in the meta-analyses and systematic reviews cited previously, however, at present both conditions must be deemed important risk factors for subsequent high blood pressure.

Importantly, blood pressures of LBW and NBW subjects, although different, may be still within the normal range in childhood, but differences become amplified with age, such that adults who had been of low birth weight often experience overt hypertension that increases with age.[169] Although the majority of studies have been conducted in white populations, generally consistent data are accumulating in other populations.[170] An association of higher blood pressure with lower birth weight in African American children has been reported in some studies, but not all, suggesting that additional factors may contribute to the greater severity of blood pressure in those of African origin.[170-175] An important effect modifier of the association with low birth weight or prematurity and blood pressure, noted in diverse populations, is current body mass index, which may override an effect of birth weight, especially in children at different stages of growth.[170,176] Furthermore, in most populations, blood pressures are highest in those born premature or of low birth weight who "catch up" fastest in postnatal weight (i.e. rapid upward crossing of weight percentiles), highlighting the importance of early postnatal nutrition in developmental programming.[177-181]

Associations between blood pressure and other markers of potential developmental stresses have also been reported. A meta-analysis of 31 studies found that blood pressures were higher in children who had high birth weights but interestingly tended to be lower in high-birth-weight adults, suggesting that age may modify this risk differently from how it does in LBW subjects.[37,182] Additionally, a systematic review and meta-analysis investigating the impact of a diabetic pregnancy on blood pressure found an overall association with higher blood pressure in offspring aged 2 to 20 years after exposure to diabetes during gestation, but this effect was seen only in males.[183] The researchers did not discuss the potential impact of birth weight in this study, however, and whether these effects may have been modified by high birth weight in offspring is not reported. Another potential risk factor for higher offspring blood pressure is maternal gestational hypertension or preeclampsia.[184,185] Whether this effect is mediated by the often accompanying fetal growth restriction or prematurity, or whether it is associated with circulating anti-angiogenic factors or other humoral changes in preeclampsia, requires further investigation.[11] Having been born small for gestational age is in turn a risk factor for subsequent development of preeclampsia, emphasizing the far-reaching effects of developmental programming.[31]

Gender differences in programming effects on blood pressure have been inconsistently reported. In some studies

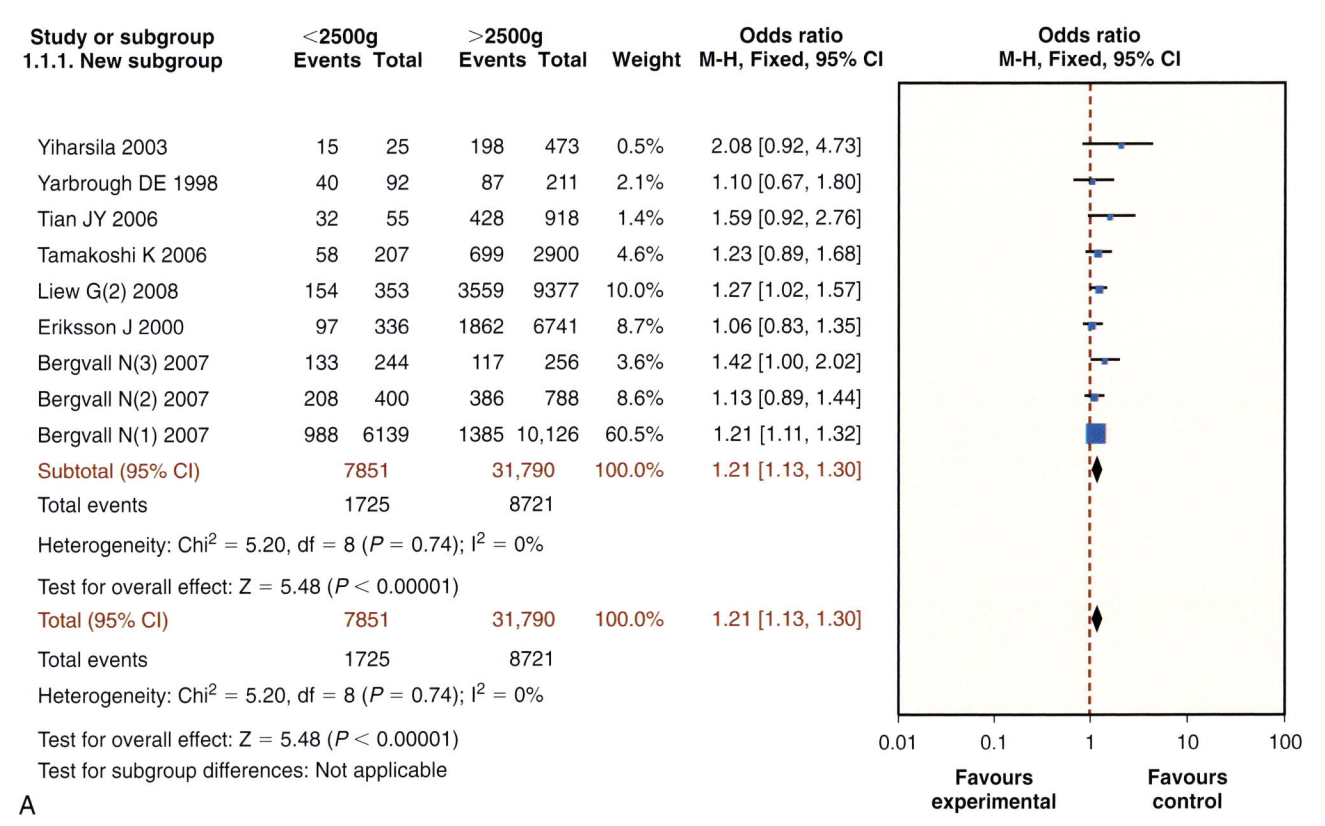

Study or subgroup 1.1.1. New subgroup	<2500g Events	Total	>2500g Events	Total	Weight	Odds ratio M-H, Fixed, 95% CI
Yiharsila 2003	15	25	198	473	0.5%	2.08 [0.92, 4.73]
Yarbrough DE 1998	40	92	87	211	2.1%	1.10 [0.67, 1.80]
Tian JY 2006	32	55	428	918	1.4%	1.59 [0.92, 2.76]
Tamakoshi K 2006	58	207	699	2900	4.6%	1.23 [0.89, 1.68]
Liew G(2) 2008	154	353	3559	9377	10.0%	1.27 [1.02, 1.57]
Eriksson J 2000	97	336	1862	6741	8.7%	1.06 [0.83, 1.35]
Bergvall N(3) 2007	133	244	117	256	3.6%	1.42 [1.00, 2.02]
Bergvall N(2) 2007	208	400	386	788	8.6%	1.13 [0.89, 1.44]
Bergvall N(1) 2007	988	6139	1385	10,126	60.5%	1.21 [1.11, 1.32]
Subtotal (95% CI)		7851		31,790	100.0%	1.21 [1.13, 1.30]
Total events	1725		8721			

Heterogeneity: Chi² = 5.20, df = 8 (P = 0.74); I² = 0%

Test for overall effect: Z = 5.48 (P < 0.00001)

Total (95% CI)		7851		31,790	100.0%	1.21 [1.13, 1.30]
Total events	1725		8721			

Heterogeneity: Chi² = 5.20, df = 8 (P = 0.74); I² = 0%

Test for overall effect: Z = 5.48 (P < 0.00001)
Test for subgroup differences: Not applicable

A

Figure 23.6 **A**, Odds ratios for hypertension with birth weights below 2500 g (low birth weight) compared with those with birth weights above 2500 g in a meta-analysis. The pooled odds ratios are shown as *diamonds*; 95% confidence intervals are in *rackets*.

Continued

Study	SBP difference (95% CI)	Weight %
UK	−2.30 (−4.50, −0.10)	17.19
Netherlands	15.00 (8.80, 21.20)	2.16
Finland	4.80 (2.20, 7.40)	12.31
Sweden	2.60 (0.60, 4.60)	20.80
US	3.50 (1.40, 5.60)	18.87
Australia	10.60 (5.70, 15.50)	3.47
UK	4.40 (1.80, 7.00)	12.31
Australia	−1.01 (−3.55, 1.53)	12.90
Overall (I-squared = 87.9%, p = 0.000)	2.50 (1.59, 3.41)	100.00

Study	SBP difference (95% CI)	Weight %
Netherlands	15.00 (8.80, 21.20)	2.00
Finland	4.80 (2.40, 7.20)	13.37
Sweden	2.60 (0.60, 4.60)	19.25
New Zealand	3.30 (0.90, 5.70)	13.37
US	3.50 (1.40, 5.60)	17.46
Australia	10.60 (5.70, 15.50)	3.21
Brazil	1.09 (−2.01, 4.19)	8.01
UK	4.40 (1.80, 7.00)	11.39
Australia	−1.01 (−3.55, 1.53)	11.94
Overall (I-squared = 78.9%, p = 0.000)	3.30 (2.43, 4.18)	100.00

Study	SBP difference (95% CI)	Weight %
Finland	4.80 (2.20, 7.40)	21.32
New Zealand	3.30 (0.90, 5.70)	25.02
US	3.50 (1.40, 5.60)	32.67
Australia	10.60 (5.70, 15.50)	6.00
Brazil	1.10 (−2.00, 4.20)	14.99
Overall (I-squared = 64.0%, p = 0.025)	3.79 (2.59, 4.99)	100.00

Systolic blood pressure difference (mm Hg)

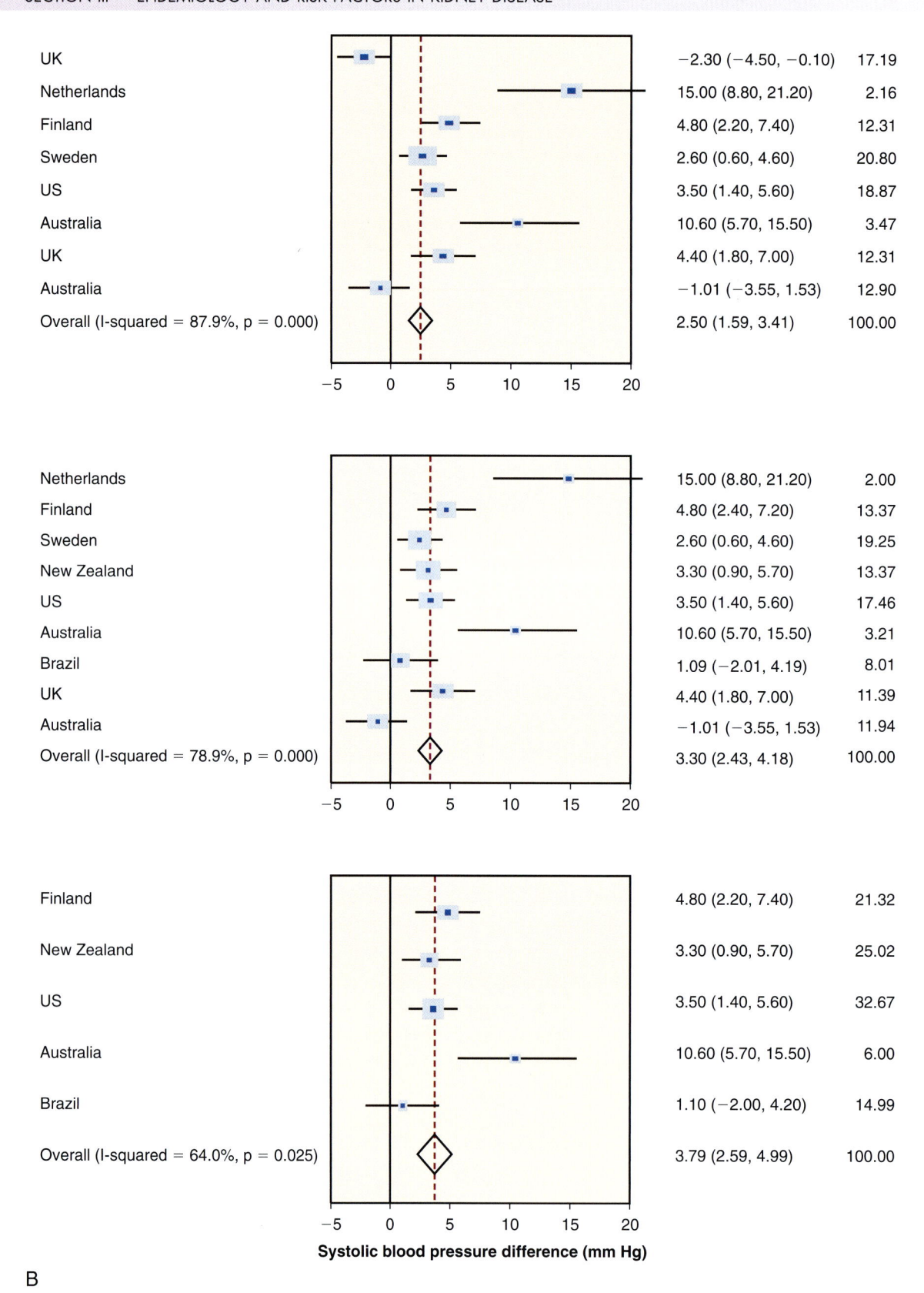

B

Figure 23.6, cont'd B, Meta-analysis of differences in systolic blood pressure (SBP) between subjects born preterm or very preterm and those born at term. Pooled SBP differences are indicated by the *open diamonds* and *dashed vertical lines; solid vertical lines* represent the null hypothesis. **Top,** Studies that adjusted for attained size; **middle,** Studies of only very preterm or very low-birth-weight subjects; **bottom,** higher-quality studies. (**A** from Mu M, Wang SF, Sheng J, et al: Birth weight and subsequent blood pressure: a meta-analysis. *Arch Cardiovasc Dis* 105:99-113, 2012; **B** from de Jong F, Monuteaux MC, van Elburg RM, et al: Systematic review and meta-analysis of preterm birth and later systolic blood pressure. *Hypertension* 59:226-234, 2012. See original papers for full references.)

programming effects appear more pronounced in males, and in others the differential effects of gender are modified by age of study, ethnicity, and body mass index.[170] In a meta-regression of 20 Nordic cohorts including 183,026 males and 14,928 women, a linear inverse association between birth weight and systolic blood pressure was present across all birth weights in males, which strengthened with age, whereas the relationship was U-shaped in women, with increasing risk also observed with birth weights above 4 kg.[186] Potential mechanisms whereby developmental programming may be expressed differently in males and females are discussed later in this chapter and are reviewed in detail elsewhere.[143,144]

The relative importance of genetics and environmental factors in programming of blood pressure has been studied in twins.[187-189] In a large Swedish cohort of 16,265 twins, the overall adjusted OR for hypertension was 1.42 (95% CI, 1.25 to 1.62) for each 500-g decrease in birth weight. Consistently, within like-sexed twin pairs, the ORs were 1.43 (95% CI, 1.07 to 1.69) and 1.74 (95% CI, 1.13 to 2.70) for dizygotic and monozygotic pairs, respectively, suggesting that environmental factors that contributed to differences in birth weight had a greater impact than genetics in this cohort, a suggestion consistent with a developmental programming effect.[187]

Nephron Number and Blood Pressure

In support of the potential association of nephron number and hypertension, a study of whites aged 35 to 59 years who died in accidents found that in 10 subjects with a history of essential hypertension the number of glomeruli per kidney was significantly lower, and glomerular volume significantly higher, than in 10 normotensive matched controls (Figure 23.7).[55] Birth weights were not reported in this study, but the investigators concluded that a reduced nephron number is associated with susceptibility to essential hypertension. Similarly, among a subset of 63 subjects in whom mean arterial pressures and birth weights were available, Hughson and coworkers reported a significant correlation between birth weight and glomerular number, mean arterial pressure and glomerular number as well as mean arterial pressure and birth weight among the white but not African American subjects.[99] Among African Americans having nephron numbers below the mean, however, twice as many were hypertensive as normotensive, suggesting a possible contribution of lower nephron number in this group as well.[99] The relationship of low birth weight and nephron number was similar in a study of black and white Cuban neonates[72]; therefore, it is expected that a similar relationship between low birth weight and low nephron number exists in the black population. Glomerular volumes were found to be higher among the hypertensive African American subjects than in the hypertensive whites.[99] The consistent finding of larger glomeruli among African Americans suggests either a greater prevalence of low nephron number in this population as a result of higher prevalence of low birth weight or independent or additional programming of glomerular size. This topic warrants further research attention, especially in light of the discovery of the *APOL1* gene association with kidney disease among African Americans.[7,11]

Consistent with an association between nephron number and blood pressure in humans, salt sensitivity has been

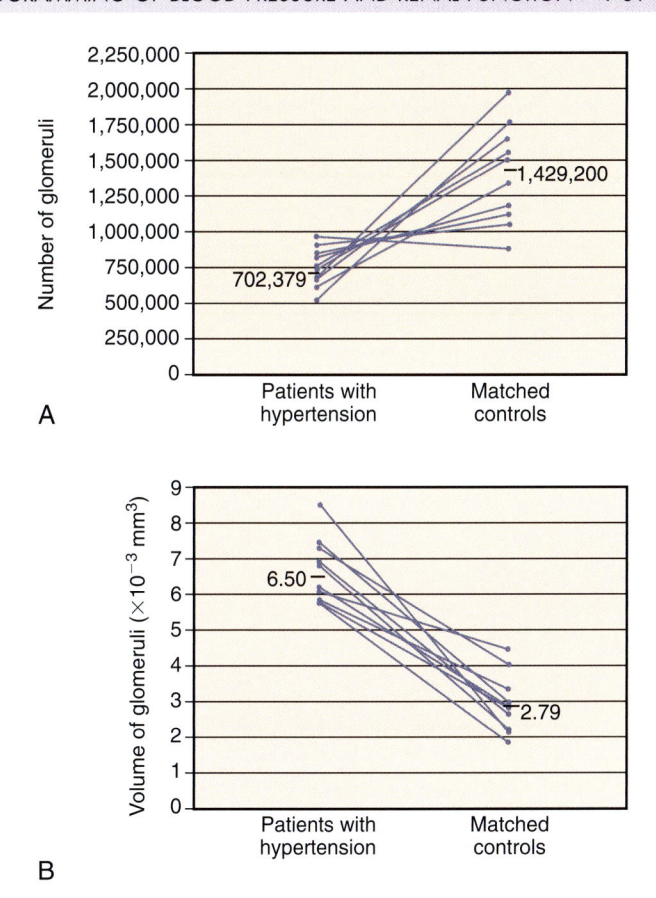

Figure 23.7 Nephron number **(A)** and glomerular volume **(B)** in white subjects with primary hypertension in comparison with those in controls. (From Keller G, Zimmer G, Mall G, et al: Nephron number in patients with primary hypertension. *N Engl J Med* 348:101-108, 2003.)

found to correlate inversely with birth weight and inversely with kidney size in adults and children (Figure 23.8).[118,119] In both studies salt-induced changes were independent of GFR, excluding confounding by renal function. Among 1512 subjects aged 62 years, investigators found an inverse association between birth weight and blood pressure among those with birth weights less than 3050 g, with a progressive 2.48–mm Hg (95% CI, 0.4 to 4.52 mm Hg) increase in blood pressure for every 1-g rise in daily salt intake up to 10 g a day.[190] Interestingly, above this threshold birth weight there was no association between blood pressure and salt intake, potentially suggesting protection against salt-sensitivity with higher birth weights.

BIRTH WEIGHT, PREMATURITY, KIDNEY SIZE, AND RENAL FUNCTION

As with blood pressure, programmed changes in renal function that occur, at least in the early stages, may not be outside normal limits. With time or exposure to additional insults, however, these changes may manifest as kidney disease.

Glomerular Filtration Rate

The GFR, in the absence of compensatory hyperfiltration, should reflect the filtration surface area and, therefore, nephron number. Compensatory hyperfiltration is thought

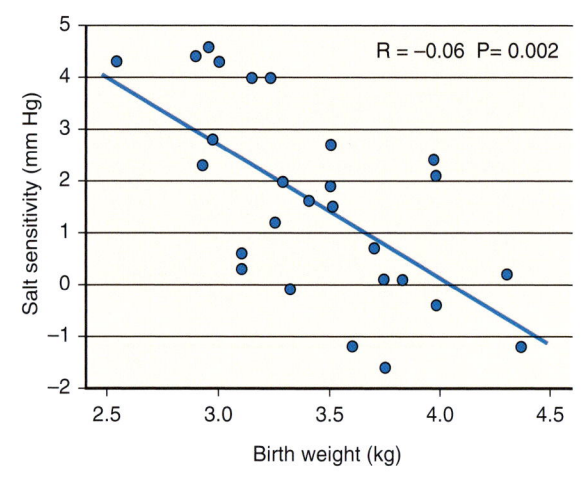

Figure 23.8 Correlation between birth weight and salt sensitivity in 27 normotensive adults. (From de Boer MP, Ijzerman RP, de Jongh RT, et al: Birth weight relates to salt sensitivity of blood pressure in healthy adults. *Hypertension* 51:928-932, 2008.)

not to occur in the immediate neonatal period, so measurement of neonatal GFR may be a good proxy for nephron endowment. Consistent with this idea, amikacin clearance on day 1 of life, measured as a correlate for neonatal GFR, was found to be significantly lower in LBW and premature neonates than in term controls.[191] Similarly, in a cohort of very premature children aged 7.6 years, GFR measured by inulin clearance, although still within the normal range, was significantly lower among those who had been growth restricted perinatally than in those who had not.[192] Importantly, the GFR was lower among children who had been growth restricted before (in utero) or in the first weeks after birth (in intensive care), pointing to the role of postnatal nutrition in renal programming. Several studies in children found similar associations of decreased GFR in LBW or premature children; however, studies using creatinine-based formulas may underestimate the impact of birth weight on GFR, suggesting a need to validate measures of renal function in LBW and premature subjects, whose body composition may remain different over time.[191,193-199] Overall a meta-analysis found an OR of 1.79 (95% CI, 1.31 to 2.45) for a reduced GFR with low birth weight (Figure 23.9).[30] Linear regression analysis in a cohort of 2192 British adults aged 60 to 64 years revealed that for each 1-kg decrease in birth weight, GFR estimated using cystatin C was reduced by 2.25 mL/min/1.73 m^2 (95% CI, 0.69 to 3.58 mL/min/1.73 m^2).[200] Taken together, these findings are consistent with the hypothesis that low birth weight and prematurity are risk factors for a reduced GFR. The relative contributions of genetics and the fetal environment on programming of renal function were investigated in 653 twins.[201] Creatinine clearance was significantly lower in LBW than in NBW twins. Furthermore, intrapair birth weight differences were positively correlated with GFR in both monozygotic and dizygotic twin pairs, suggesting that fetoplacental factors have a greater impact than genetic factors on adult renal function.

To approach an understanding of the mechanism of reduced GFR in LBW and premature individuals, renal functional reserve, determined by measuring GFR and effective renal plasma flow (ERPF) before and after low-dose dopamine infusion or an oral amino acid load, was studied in 20-year-old subjects who had been premature and either small or appropriate for gestational age, and compared with that in controls, who had been born at full term and normal birth weight.[165] After renal stimulation, the relative increase in GFR tended to be lower in small-for-gestational-age than in appropriate-for-gestational-age and control subjects, and ERPF was lower in both groups of premature subjects, although the differences did not reach statistical significance, likely because of small numbers. Reduced renal functional reserve was also observed among young adults with type 1 diabetic mothers, who had been exposed to diabetes during gestation, but not those with diabetic fathers, again suggesting a programming rather than genetic effect.[64] A reduced renal reserve capacity in these subjects may be consistent with a programmed reduction in nephron number.

Proteinuria

One of the earliest signs of hyperfiltration, which would be expected in the setting of reduced nephron number and filtration surface area, is microalbuminuria, which may progress to overt proteinuria with ongoing renal injury and worsening hyperfiltration. Consistent with this hypothesis, in Aboriginal Australians who had low birth weights, the odds ratio for macroalbuminuria was 2.8 (95% CI, 1.26 to 6.31) in comparison with those who had normal birth weights and increased with age.[202] Importantly, proteinuria was also associated with a higher rate of cardiovascular and renal deaths, underscoring its clinical relevance.[78] Subsequently, a meta-analysis including eight additional studies reported an OR of 1.81 (95% CI, 1.19 to 2.77) for albuminuria with low birth weight (see Figure 23.9.)[30] As with blood pressure, whether prematurity modifies the association of birth weight with proteinuria is not always easy to dissect, although studies of premature children and adolescents show consistent findings. Among children aged 4 years who had been premature, albuminuria was higher in both boys and girls who had reached normal height (presumably caught up in growth), and among 19-year-olds who had been very preterm, albuminuria was higher among those who had been growth restricted, again showing the interplay between prematurity, growth restriction, and catch-up growth and later risk of disease.[198,203]

Analysis of 724 subjects aged 48 to 53 years who had been subjected to malnutrition in midgestation during the Dutch famine of 1944 revealed a higher prevalence of microalbuminuria (12%) than those subjected to malnutrition during early gestation (9%) or late gestation (7%), or who had not been exposed to the famine (4%-8%).[204] Size at birth was not associated with the observed increase in microalbuminuria, however, suggesting that renal development may have been irreversibly affected in midgestation, although later gestation whole-body growth was able to catch up with restoration of more normal nutrition. This observation emphasizes the need for surrogate markers in addition to birth weight, in order to identify individuals at risk for renal programming.

A U-shaped association between birth weight and proteinuria was described among Pima Indians, showing that the risk increased for birth weights less than 2.5 kg and more than 4.5 kg.[5] The strongest predictor of proteinuria among

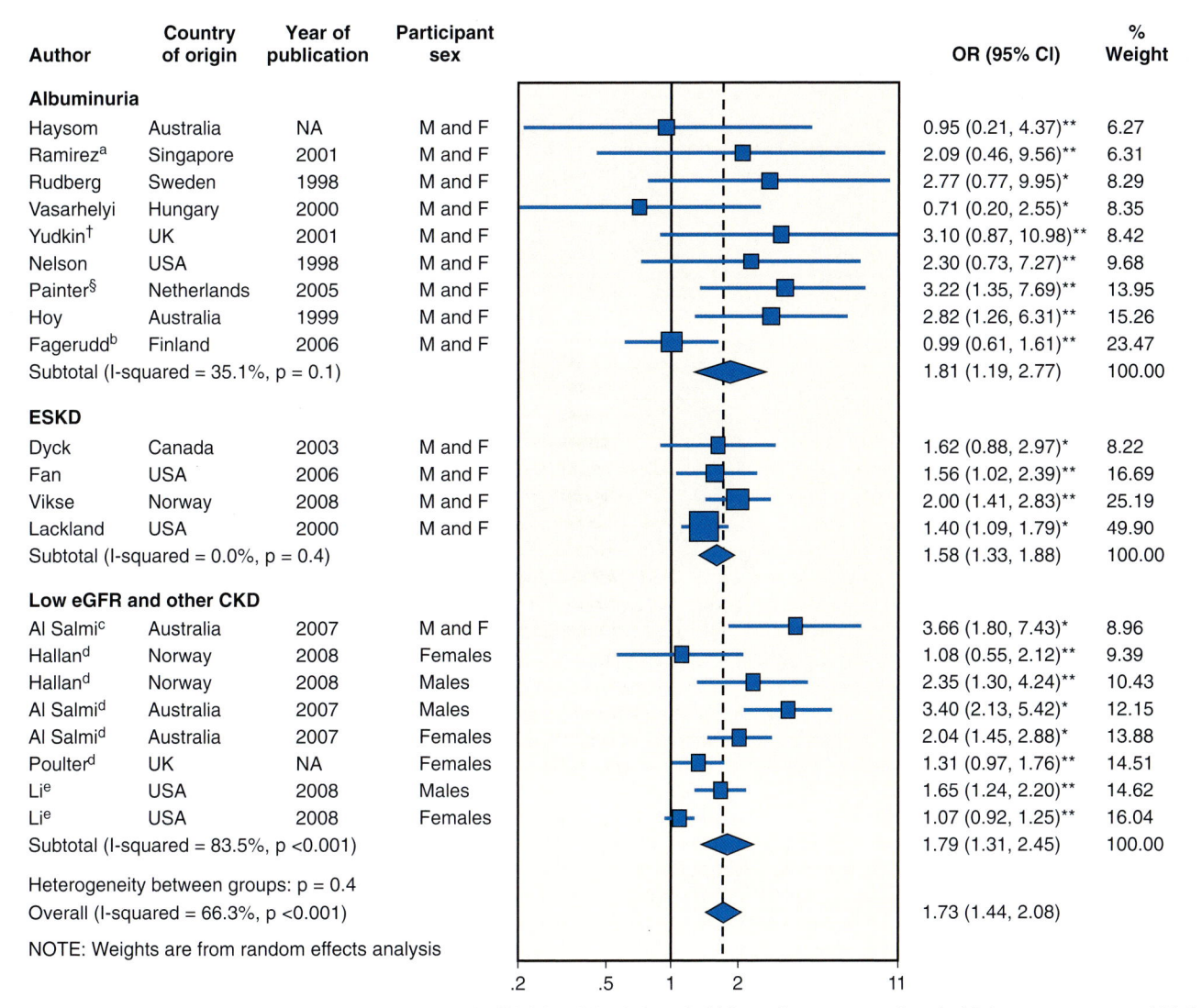

Author	Country of origin	Year of publication	Participant sex		OR (95% CI)	% Weight
Albuminuria						
Haysom	Australia	NA	M and F		0.95 (0.21, 4.37)**	6.27
Ramirez[a]	Singapore	2001	M and F		2.09 (0.46, 9.56)**	6.31
Rudberg	Sweden	1998	M and F		2.77 (0.77, 9.95)*	8.29
Vasarhelyi	Hungary	2000	M and F		0.71 (0.20, 2.55)*	8.35
Yudkin[†]	UK	2001	M and F		3.10 (0.87, 10.98)**	8.42
Nelson	USA	1998	M and F		2.30 (0.73, 7.27)**	9.68
Painter[§]	Netherlands	2005	M and F		3.22 (1.35, 7.69)**	13.95
Hoy	Australia	1999	M and F		2.82 (1.26, 6.31)**	15.26
Fagerudd[b]	Finland	2006	M and F		0.99 (0.61, 1.61)**	23.47
Subtotal (I-squared = 35.1%, p = 0.1)					1.81 (1.19, 2.77)	100.00
ESKD						
Dyck	Canada	2003	M and F		1.62 (0.88, 2.97)*	8.22
Fan	USA	2006	M and F		1.56 (1.02, 2.39)**	16.69
Vikse	Norway	2008	M and F		2.00 (1.41, 2.83)**	25.19
Lackland	USA	2000	M and F		1.40 (1.09, 1.79)*	49.90
Subtotal (I-squared = 0.0%, p = 0.4)					1.58 (1.33, 1.88)	100.00
Low eGFR and other CKD						
Al Salmi[c]	Australia	2007	M and F		3.66 (1.80, 7.43)*	8.96
Hallan[d]	Norway	2008	Females		1.08 (0.55, 2.12)**	9.39
Hallan[d]	Norway	2008	Males		2.35 (1.30, 4.24)**	10.43
Al Salmi[d]	Australia	2007	Males		3.40 (2.13, 5.42)*	12.15
Al Salmi[d]	Australia	2007	Females		2.04 (1.45, 2.88)*	13.88
Poulter[d]	UK	NA	Females		1.31 (0.97, 1.76)**	14.51
Li[e]	USA	2008	Males		1.65 (1.24, 2.20)**	14.62
Li[e]	USA	2008	Females		1.07 (0.92, 1.25)**	16.04
Subtotal (I-squared = 83.5%, p <0.001)					1.79 (1.31, 2.45)	100.00
Heterogeneity between groups: p = 0.4						
Overall (I-squared = 66.3%, p <0.001)					1.73 (1.44, 2.08)	

NOTE: Weights are from random effects analysis

Figure 23.9 Odds ratios and 95% confidence intervals (CIs) for risk of chronic kidney disease associated with low versus normal birth weight. The statistical size of the study was defined in terms of the inverse of the variance of the regression coefficient, indicated by grey squares. Dashed vertical line, the inverse variance-weighted regression through the overall point estimate. *Individual study estimates not adjusted for confounders or estimate are adjusted/controlled for age and/or sex only. **Estimates adjusted for additional factors. Outcome is [a]proteinuria; [b]diabetic nephropathy (albuminuria or end-stage renal disease); [c]CKD stages 2 to 5: estimated glomerular filtration rate (eGFR) of 60 to 90 mL/min/1.73 m² with proteinuria ± hematuria or eGFR less than 60 mL/min/1.73 m² or on dialysis therapy; [d]eGFR less than 10th percentile for sex; and [e]albuminuria or eGFR less than 60 mL/min/1.73 m². Exposure measured as [§]exposure to famine midgestation (versus not exposed) and [†]ponderal index in the lower 3rd percentile (versus highest 3rd). (From White SL, Perkovic V, Cass AM, et al: Is low birth weight an antecedent of CKD in later life? A systematic review of observational studies. Am J Kidney Dis 54:248-261, 2009.)

high-birth-weight subjects in this study was exposure to gestational diabetes, raising the question whether gestational diabetes exposure, rather than birth weight per se, was the predominant programming risk factor.[5] In a Canadian study, urine albumin-to-creatinine ratios were lower in infants of diabetic mothers than in those of nondiabetic mothers at 1 year of age, but were higher at 3 years, although independent of birth weight.[205] The researchers interpret these findings to reflect abnormal renal programming in offspring of diabetic mothers, but the effects of gestational diabetes and high birth weight on renal programming require much more study.

Acute Kidney Injury

Prematurity is emerging as an important risk factor for acute kidney injury (AKI) in neonates, estimated to occur in between 12.5% and 71% depending on the population studied.[206] In turn, AKI in very LBW infants is an independent predictor of mortality and subsequent CKD.[160] Neonates in intensive care are particularly susceptible to renal dysfunction, not only because of potentially programmed risk and reduced nephron number, but also because of frequent exposure to nephrotoxins, which may injure the kidney directly and interfere with healing or nephrogenesis.[207] A retrospective analysis of preoperative renal volume in neonates undergoing congenital heart surgery found higher peak postoperative creatinine values, and therefore potentially increased risk of AKI, in infants with a preoperative renal volume of 17 cm³ or less.[208] Neonatologists are working to raise awareness of the renal risk, but at present there is no accepted definition of renal failure in this population. Cutoff values according to gestational age have been

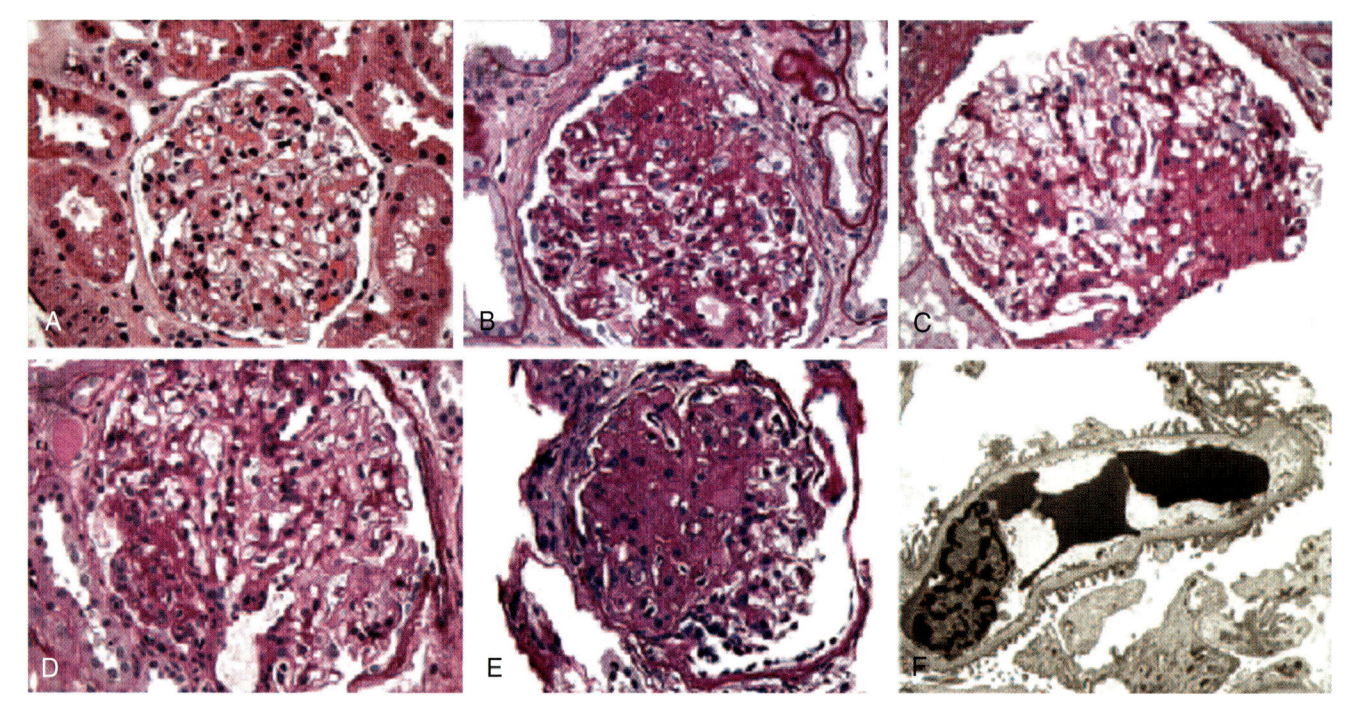

Figure 23.10 Renal biopsy findings associated with low birth weight and prematurity. **A**, Normal-sized control glomerulus (hematoxylin & eosin stain). **B** through **E**, Representative glomeruli from four patients who had been premature and of very low birth weight, demonstrating glomerulomegaly and segmental occlusion of glomerular capillaries by matrix accumulation and hyalinosis (PAS stain). **F**, Ultrastructural examination of glomerular capillary demonstrating podocyte foot process effacement (electron micrograph). (From Hodgin JB, Rasoulpour M, Markowitz GS, et al: Very low birth weight is a risk factor for secondary focal segmental glomerulosclerosis. *Clin J Am Soc Nephrol* 4:71-76, 2009.)

proposed.[195] High creatinine values were associated with lower gestational age and lower birth weight Z-score. The risk and significant adverse consequences of AKI associated with prematurity therefore highlight the need for long-term follow-up of premature babies.[206] To our knowledge, such studies have not been conducted in term neonates or adults with low birth weight; therefore, an association with AKI is unknown. AKI may emerge as an area of divergent risk between prematurity and term low birth weight, because nephrogenesis can continue for several weeks after birth in premature infants, and their kidneys may be especially vulnerable during this period.

Chronic Kidney Disease and End-Stage Kidney Disease

A case series of six patients, aged 15 to 52 years, who had been born prematurely with low birth weight described findings consistent with secondary focal and segmental glomerulosclerosis, associated with glomerulomegaly in all biopsy specimens (Figure 23.10).[209] The investigators suggest a susceptibility to hyperfiltration and glomerulosclerosis associated with prematurity and low birth weight. Consistent with this suggestion, a variety of generally small studies have reported a greater severity of renal disease and more rapid progression of diverse renal diseases, including immunoglobulin A (IgA) nephropathy, membranous nephropathy, minimal change disease, chronic pyelonephritis, Alport's syndrome, and polycystic kidney disease, among children and adults who were of low birth weight.[210-218] A handful of studies have examined the relationship between birth weight and diabetic nephropathy and found an increased susceptibility among subjects who had been growth restricted, although not invariably.[5,213,219,220] Taken together, most of these observations suggest that low birth weight is a risk factor for renal disease. Consistently, a meta-analysis of 18 studies reported an OR for CKD of 1.73 (95% CI, 1.44 to 2.08) with low birth weight (see Figure 23.9).[30] Similarly, in a retrospective analysis of a cohort of more than 2 million white children, the relative risk for development of ESKD was 1.7 in those with birth weights lower than the 10th percentile (Figure 23.11).[29] In a dialysis-based study, low birth weight was also associated with increased risk of ESKD, but the OR for diabetic ESKD was also increased among those with birth weights higher than 4000 g (OR 2.4; 95% CI, 1.3 to 4.2) (Figure 23.12).[45] The relevance of high birth weight was also highlighted by the finding of a U-shaped association of renal disease with birth weight in two large population-based studies, although effects differed between males and females in both studies, again reflecting potential effect modification by gender under conditions as yet not fully elucidated.[28,29]

It is likely too simplistic to assume that altered kidney development associated with low birth weight, prematurity, or other developmental stresses of themselves are enough to cause renal disease, but exposure to additional "hits"—nephrotoxin exposure, AKI, glomerulonephritis—or superimposed developmental programming of conditions that are themselves risk factors for kidney disease—diabetes, cardiovascular disease, metabolic syndrome, obesity—all likely exacerbate risk of renal disease.[14,17,160,221] Overall, combined meta-analysis of 31 studies, involving more than 2 million subjects, concluded that individuals of low birth weight have a 70% increased risk for development of CKD, including albuminuria, reduced GFR, and renal failure in later life (see Figure 23.9).[30] Clinical associations of developmental programming in the kidney are outlined in Table 23.8.

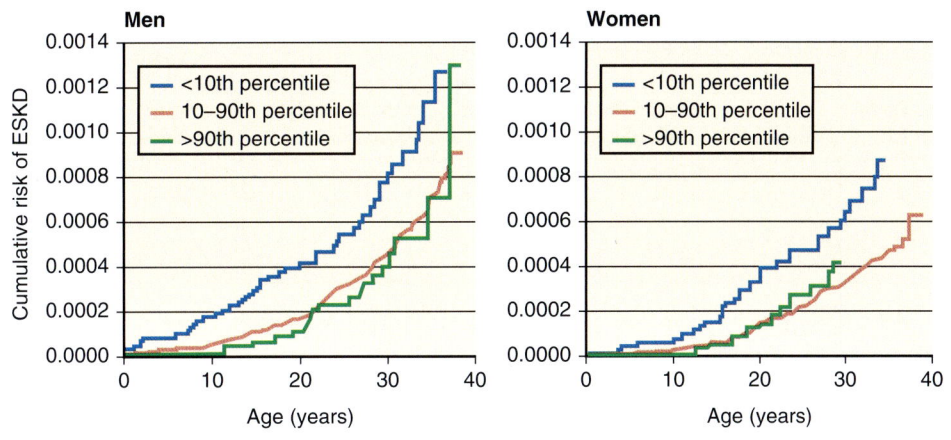

Figure 23.11 Cumulative risk of end-stage kidney disease (ESKD) by age and birth weight (shown as percentiles). (From Vikse BE, Irgens LM, Leivestad T, et al: Low birth weight increases risk for end-stage renal disease. *J Am Soc Nephrol* 19:151-157, 2008.)

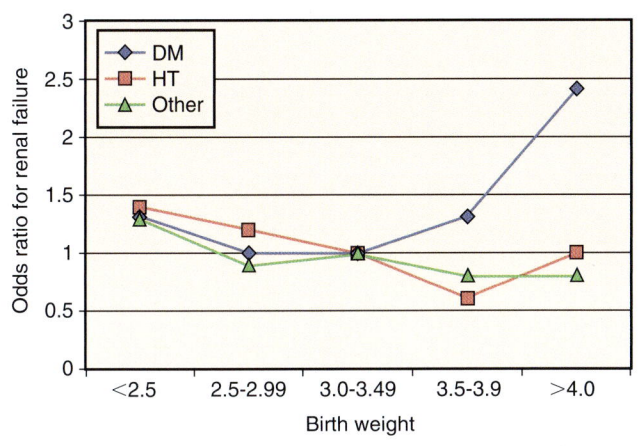

Figure 23.12 Birth weight (kg) and risk of end-stage kidney disease due to diabetes mellitus (DM), hypertension (HT), or other causes. (From Lackland DT, Bendall HE, Osmond C, et al: Low birth weights contribute to high rates of early-onset chronic renal failure in the Southeastern United States. *Arch Intern Med* 160:1472-1476, 2000.)

PROPOSED MECHANISMS FOR DEVELOPMENTAL PROGRAMMING IN THE KIDNEY

Kidney development is a complex process involving tightly controlled expression of many genes and constant remodeling.[92,222-226] The molecular regulation of kidney development is exhaustively reviewed elsewhere.[223-226] Many experimental models, as outlined in Table 23.4, have been shown to result in a reduced nephron number. In many of the experimental models of programming, reduced nephron number has been shown to be associated with low birth weight and subsequent hypertension and renal injury. Interestingly, in normal rat litters, those pups with naturally occurring low birth weight (i.e., birth weights < −2 SD from the mean) were found to have a 13% reduction in nephron number, which was associated with glomerulomegaly and proteinuria.[227] Low birth weight in rodents, therefore, may be associated with a low nephron number even in nonexperimental conditions. Maternal factors that affect birth weight and prematurity in humans may therefore also affect nephrogenesis.[71] In humans, nephrogenesis begins in week 9 of gestation and continues until about 36 weeks. Approximately two thirds of the nephrons develop during the last trimester, making this the time of greatest susceptibility to adverse effects, although earlier insults can also affect nephrogenesis.[101,228] In rodents, nephrogenesis continues for up to 10 days after birth but is most active in mid- to late gestation, when studies show the most impact from manipulation of environmental factors.[228]

In general terms, three processes are considered to play critical roles in determining nephron endowment at the conclusion of nephrogenesis: branching of the ureteric tree, condensation of metanephric mesenchymal cells at the ureteric branch tips, and conversion of these mesenchymal condensates into nephron epithelium.[223-226] It has been estimated that a 2% decrease in ureteric tree branching efficiency would result in a 50% reduction in final nephron complement after 20 generations of branching.[229] The specific molecular mechanisms whereby nephron numbers may be affected and/or their function altered, however, are not yet completely understood. Perturbations to the fetomaternal environment that result in reduced nephron endowment are summarized in Table 23.9 and discussed later.

GENETIC VARIANTS ASSOCIATED WITH KIDNEY SIZE AND NEPHRON NUMBER IN HUMANS

Rare genetic and congenital abnormalities of the kidney and urinary tract (CAKUT) contribute to about 40% of all childhood ESKD (NAPRTCS Report 2011).[229a] The common pathology linking these malformations involves a disturbance of the normal interaction between the ureteric bud and the pool of renal progenitor cells. Of the more than 25 mutant genes associated with monogenic forms of CAKUT, most encode transcription factors (e.g., *PAX2*, *GATA3*) and growth factor receptors (e.g., RET) expressed in ureteric bud/tree cells during branching morphogenesis or in intermediate mesoderm (e.g., *SIX2*, *EYA1*, *ROBO*), where they set the fate of renal progenitor cells and regulate interactions with the ureteric bud.

Completely dysfunctional alleles for crucial developmental genes are rare, because they produce malformations with

Table 23.8 Clinical Associations of Renal Programming

	Low Birth Weight	Prematurity	High Birth Weight	Gestational Diabetes Exposure	Rapid Catch-Up Growth/ Overweight	Low Nephron Number	Smaller Kidney Size/ Weight	Increased Glomerular Volume
Increased blood pressure	✓	✓	✓	✓	✓	✓	✓	✓
Salt sensitivity	✓			a		a	✓	
Reduced glomerular filtration rate	✓	✓		a	✓	a	✓	
Reduced renal functional reserve		✓		✓				
Proteinuria	✓	✓	✓	✓		a	✓	
Acute kidney injury (neonates)		✓				✓	✓	
Chronic kidney disease	✓	✓		✓	✓	a	✓	✓
End-stage kidney disease	✓		✓					
Transplant outcomes							✓	✓
Death	✓							
Increased glomerular volume	✓	✓		a	✓	✓		
Smaller kidney size/ weight	✓	✓				✓		

✓, From human studies; a, evidence only from animal studies.

a major disadvantage. However, there is some evidence that mild mutations of these same genes exert subtler effects on renal mesenchyme/ureteric bud interactions and may be fairly common in the normal population (see Table 23.4). For example, heterozygous null alleles of the *PAX2* gene cause the rare autosomal dominant renal coloboma syndrome, characterized by decreased ureteric branching during fetal life, sharply reduced nephron number at birth, and progressive renal failure in childhood. *PAX2* is highly expressed in the ureteric bud, where it suppresses apoptosis and optimizes the extent of branching. Interestingly, an intronic *PAX2* polymorphism, which reduces PAX transcript levels from the mutant allele by only 50%, is found in 18.5% of Canadians and is associated with a subtle (10%) reduction in newborn kidney size.[230] Ureteric bud branching is also highly dependent on GDNF signaling from the metanephric mesenchyme to the ureteric bud, via the RET tyrosine kinase receptor on ureteric bud cells. Although no common hypomorphic variants of the human *GDNF* gene have been shown to affect kidney size, a polymorphic variant of the GDNF receptor, *RET(1476A)*, was associated with a 10% reduction in kidney volume at birth compared to the wild-type *(RET 1476G)* allele.[105] In this study, newborn kidney volume was shown to be proportional to nephron number, suggesting that the modest renal hypoplasia seen with somewhat dysfunctional *PAX2* and *RET* polymorphisms represents a reduction in congenital nephron number.[105] Newborn kidney size was reduced by 13% among Polish babies with a common variant of the *BMPR1A* gene, which encodes a bone morphogenetic protein receptor on ureteric bud cells.[231] Conversely, 22% of Canadian newborns inherit a variant of the *ALHD1A2* gene [*rs7169289(G)*] associated with increased production of all-trans retinoic acid metabolism in fetal tissues; this retinoid is known to enhance *RET* expression in the ureteric bud, and newborns with the G allele were shown to have a 22% greater kidney size than those with the wild-type allele.[232]

Although final nephron number is clearly affected by genes regulating the extent of ureteric branching, animal studies also indicate that the size of the renal progenitor cell pool may also be rate limiting. One of the earliest transcription factors marking the nephron progenitor cells of intermediate mesoderm is OSR1; Osr1 knockout mice lack nephrogenic mesenchyme and are anephric at birth.[233] A variant of the human *OSR1* gene that interferes with mRNA splicing was identified in about 6% of normal whites.[234] This OSR1rs12329305(T) variant was associated with a 12% reduction in newborn kidney size. Taken together, these

Table 23.9 Proposed Mechanisms of Developmental Programming in the Kidney

Experimental Model	Possible Mechanism of Nephron Number Reduction	Reference(s)
Maternal low-protein diet	↑ apoptosis in metanephros and postnatal kidney Altered gene expression in developing kidney Altered gene methylation ↓ placental 11-βHSD2 expression → increased fetal exposure to glucocorticoids	236, 237, 240, 327
Maternal vitamin A restriction	↓ branching of ureteric bud ? maintenance of spatial orientation of vascular development ↓ c-Ret expression	245
Maternal iron restriction	? reduced oxygen delivery ? altered glucocorticoid responsiveness ? altered micronutrient availability ↑ inflammation ? tissue hypoxia	242, 243
Maternal Zn deficiency	↑ apoptosis ↓ antioxidant activity	244
Gestational glucocorticoid exposure	↑ fetal glucocorticoid exposure ? enhanced tissue maturation ↑ glucocorticoid receptor expression ↑ 1α– and 1β–ATPase expression ↓ renal and adrenal 11-βHSD2 expression	130, 254, 258, 392
Uterine artery ligation/embolization	↑ pro-apoptotic gene expression in developing kidney: caspase-3, Bax, p53 ↓ anti-apoptotic gene expression: PAX2, bcl-2 Altered gene methylation Altered renin angiotensin gene expression	135, 276
Maternal diabetes/hyperglycemia	↓ IGF-II/mannose-6-phosphate receptor expression Altered IGF-II activity/bioavailability Activation of NF-κB Altered ureteric branching morphogenesis	130, 252, 255, 256

Gestational drug exposure:
  Gentamicin
  β-Lactams
  Cyclosporine
  Ethanol
  COX-2 inhibitors
	
	↓ branching morphogenesis
	↑ mesenchymal apoptosis
	Arrest of nephron formation
	? via reduced vitamin A levels
	Affects prostaglandins
		150, 282, 284, 286

Maternal hypoxia	? affects expression of retinoid receptors ? increased expression of glucocorticoid receptors ? increased expression of angiopoietin-2 Accelerated aging	380
Ureteral obstruction—postnatal	↓ cell proliferation ↑ apoptosis of tubular cells Delayed maturation of interstitial fibroblasts → interstitial fibrosis ? alteration of post-induction processes	65
Prematurity	Abnormal maturation of glomeruli ? factors associated with shift from intrauterine to extrauterine environment ? loss of progenitor cell populations	94, 393

11β–HSD2, 11β-hydroxysteroid dehydrogenase type 2; ATPase, adenosine triphosphatase; COX-2, cyclo-oxygenase-2; IGF, insulin-like growth factor; NF-κB, nuclear factor kappaB; ↑, increased; ↓, decreased; →, leads to.

observations suggest that final nephron endowment may represent a complex polygenic trait determined by the additive effects of multiple genes regulating either the extent of ureteric branching or the renal progenitor cell pool during fetal life. As reviewed by Walker and Bertram, full or partial deletion of more than 25 genes has been shown to result in kidney hypoplasia, and deletion of several of these genes results in low nephron endowment.[226] Not all have been studied in humans, so the impact of genetic variation on nephron endowment alone and in the context of developmental stresses and the risk of later-life hypertension and renal disease requires further study.

MATERNAL NUTRIENT RESTRICTION

In humans, maternal malnutrition, as measured by hemoglobin, triceps skinfold thickness, or lower weight gain during later pregnancy, have all been found to be associated with higher offspring blood pressures, suggesting a programming effect.[235] Experimental alterations in rat maternal dietary composition at different stages of gestation have been shown to program kidney gene expression early in the course of gestation, which later affects nephron number (Table 23.9).[236] Fetal nutrient supply is also affected by alterations in placental blood flow. Maternal *protein and calorie restriction* during all or the later stages of pregnancy have been the most widely studied models of low birth weight and reduced nephron number. Not all low-protein diets have the same programming effects, however. It has been proposed that relative deficiencies of specific amino acids—methionine or glycine, for example—may have a greater impact on organ development than total protein restriction per se, potentially through epigenetic modulation of gene expression.[32,237] Use of the model of uterine ischemia in the rat showed that restoration of good fetal nutrition postnatally, during ongoing nephrogenesis, resulted in restoration of nephron number, further emphasizing the critical importance of nutrition during renal development.[93] Greater fetal exposure to glucocorticoids has been proposed as a mechanism whereby low-protein diet reduces nephron number, which is discussed later.[238] Other potential mechanisms include: reduced renal angiogenesis, associated with reduced expression of vascular endothelial growth factor (VEGF), observed in offspring of mothers exposed to 50% calorie restriction during gestation[239]; global downregulation of gene expression in fetal kidneys of microswine exposed to low-protein diet in late gestation/early lactation[240]; and altered epigenetic DNA methylation, which may affect gene expression, which has been described in the livers of offspring of protein-restricted mothers.[241] Taken together, findings of these studies suggest that many of the processes that occur during kidney development are likely affected by maternal diet.

In terms of micronutrients, maternal *iron restriction* during pregnancy has also been found to lead to reductions in birth weight and nephron number and to the development of hypertension in rat offspring.[242] In another study, offspring of iron-deficient dams had reduced radial glomerular counts and increased tubulointerstitial fibrosis, which were reversed with iron supplementation during gestation.[243] Conceivably, fetal anemia may result in reduced tissue oxygen delivery, altered fetal kidney glucocorticoid sensitivity, or altered availability of other micronutrients that may affect nephrogenesis.[242] Similarly, pre- or post-weaning *zinc deficiency* was also found to be associated with decreased nephron number, reduced GFR, and higher blood pressures in rats, effects that were potentially mediated by reduction in the antioxidant, anti-apoptotic effects of zinc.[244]

Maternal *vitamin A restriction* has also been associated with a reduction in nephron number in offspring.[87,245] Severe vitamin A deficiency during pregnancy is associated with congenital malformations and renal defects in offspring. Vitamin A and all-*trans* retinoic acid have been shown to stimulate nephrogenesis through modulation of ureteric branching capacity in ureteric epithelial cell culture, and participate in maintenance of spatial organization of blood vessel development in cultured renal cortical explants.[245] Analysis of 21-day-old fetal rats (just before birth) revealed a direct correlation between plasma retinol concentration and nephron number, as shown in Figure 23.13.[245] The

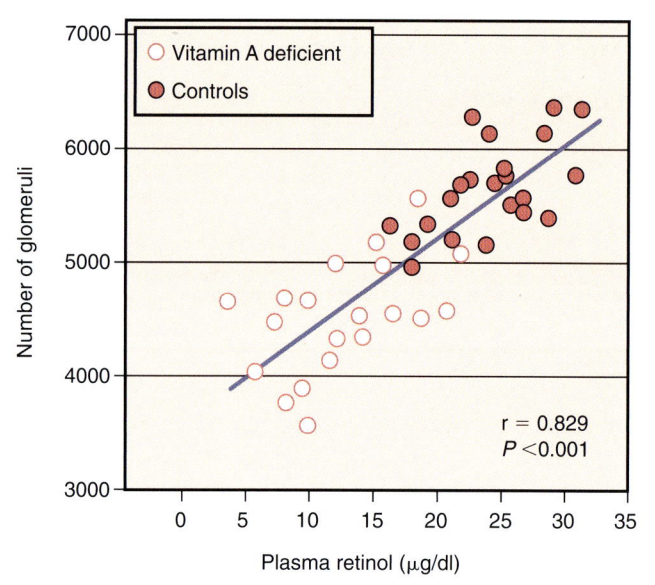

Figure 23.13 Nephron number and plasma retinol concentration in term rat fetuses. (From Merlet-Benichou C: Influence of fetal environment on kidney development. *Int J Dev Biol* 43:453-456, 1999.)

reduction in nephron number in the setting of vitamin A deficiency is likely mediated at least in part by modulation of genes regulating branching morphogenesis.[245] In vivo, a vitamin A–deficient diet sufficient to reduce circulating vitamin A levels by 50% in pregnant rats resulted in a 25% reduction in nephron endowment in the offspring, whereas supplementation of vitamin A increased nephron endowment.[245] In contrast, supplemental retinoic acid was examined in another study as a means to stimulate nephrogenesis in postnatal preterm baboons, but no effect was observed, suggesting a more proximal period in which vitamin A may be most critical.[246]

It is interesting to note that smoking and alcohol intake may be associated with reduced levels of circulating vitamin A, and both, in pregnancy, are associated with low birth weight. In sheep, repeated *ethanol* exposure during the second half of pregnancy resulted in an 11% reduction in nephron number.[247] There has been a single abstract suggesting the effect of maternal alcohol ingestion on kidney development in children, but whether the effects are mediated by associated vitamin A deficiency or other mechanisms is not known.[71] Subtle differences in vitamin A level during pregnancy, therefore, may be a significant factor contributing to the wide distribution of nephron number in the general population.[71]

With recognition of the importance of nutrition during pregnancy and after birth, maternal and neonatal replacement of micronutrients has been implemented as a public health policy in several countries.[248] From a global review, the incidence of low birth weight was reduced by 19% with iron and folate supplementation and by 11% to 13% with multi-micronutrient supplements, and balanced energy supplementation increased birth weights by a mean of 73 g and reduced the risk of being small for gestational age by 34%.[248,249] Vitamin A supplementation did not affect birth weight but did improve child mortality.[248,250] Interestingly, children of mothers who received folate or a preparation containing folate + iron + zinc during pregnancy in addition to vitamin A supplementation in the early postpartum period in Nepal showed no change in blood pressure but had less microalbuminuria, suggesting a potential programming effect of these micronutrients.[251] Very high doses of vitamin A, however have been shown to be teratogenic and to reduce nephrogenesis; therefore, vitamin A supplementation as a strategy to "rescue nephron number should target normalization of vitamin A levels and avoid excess."[252] Folate is not known to impact renal development, but it does affect gene methylation, and folate deficiencies may program epigenetic effects.[241] Diastolic blood pressures appeared marginally lower (0.78 mm Hg; 95% CI, 0.16 to 1.28) in 4.5-year-old children whose mothers had received early prenatal food supplements at the usual time in Bangladesh, but were marginally higher (0.87 mm Hg; 95% CI, 0.18 to 1.56) among those whose mothers had received a multimicronutrient supplement during pregnancy.[253] GFRs were 4.98 mL/min/1.73 m² higher in children whose mothers had received higher-dose iron supplementation, however.[253] Potential confounding factors or effect modifiers in these cohorts include baseline vitamin A supplementation, which may have an overriding renal programming effect in all subjects, as well as frequent persistent malnutrition and stunting. Long-term follow-up of children of mothers who receive supplements during pregnancy is sparse and, thus far, does not consistently suggest a positive effect on renal programming. The effects should become clearer as cohorts of children age and more data emerge.[248,253]

FETAL EXPOSURE TO GLUCOCORTICOIDS

Under normal circumstances, the fetus is protected from exposure to excess maternal corticosteroids by the placental enzyme 11β-hydroxysteroid dehydrogenase type 2 (11β-HSD2), which metabolizes corticosterone to the inert 11-dehydrocorticosterone.[19] Prenatal administration of dexamethasone, a steroid not metabolized by 11β-HSD2, leads to fetal growth restriction, a 20% to 60% reduction in nephron number, glomerulomegaly, and subsequent hypertension in rats and sheep.[84,88,158,254] Similar effects have been seen with lower levels of placental 11β-HSD2 in rats and humans with mutations in the 11β-HSD2 gene, in whom birth weights are low and hypertension develops prematurely.[255,256] Maternal low-protein diet during gestation has been shown to result in decreased placental expression of 11β-HSD2, therefore likely increasing exposure of the fetus to maternal corticosteroids.[32,130] Treatment of pregnant rats fed a low-protein diet with an inhibitor of steroid synthesis ameliorates the programming of hypertension and increases nephron numbers in the offspring.[19,32,257] Although reversal of effects was not complete, these data strongly implicate glucocorticoids as modulators of nephrogenesis in the setting of maternal low-protein diet.[257] Excessive fetal steroid exposure may then drive inappropriate gene expression and affect growth and nephrogenesis, potentially through more rapid maturation of tissues.[32] Furthermore, expression of steroid-responsive receptors, including the corticosteroid-responsive renal Na^+-K^+-ATPase α_1- and β_1-subunits, was found to be significantly greater in offspring of rats fed a low-protein diet during gestation.[130] In another study, prenatal dexamethasone was associated with increased proximal tubule sodium transport, in part related to higher activity of tubular NHE3.[258] These changes may contribute to hypertension.

In humans there has been concern about perinatal exposure to corticosteroids; however, follow-up of subjects whose mothers participated in a randomized placebo-controlled study of antenatal betamethasone did not find any difference in blood pressure or other cardiovascular risk factors at age 30 years between exposed and unexposed individuals.[259] Similarly, no effect on blood pressure or renal function was noted within the first 2 years of life among premature infants who had received antenatal steroids in comparison with those who had not.[164,260] The short-term use of perinatal corticosteroid administration therefore does not appear to have major long-term consequences in humans, although the effects of long-term use (e.g., throughout pregnancy) has not been studied.

FETAL EXPOSURE TO HYPERGLYCEMIA AND THE ROLE OF INSULIN-LIKE GROWTH FACTORS AND THEIR RECEPTORS

As discussed previously, in some populations high birth weight is associated with an increased susceptibility to proteinuria and renal disease (see Figure 23.12).[5,36,45] High birth weight is a complication of gestational hyperglycemia and diabetes and may therefore also be a surrogate marker of abnormal intrauterine programming. In offspring of rats rendered hyperglycemic during pregnancy either by induction of diabetes mellitus with streptozotocin or by infusion of glucose from gestational days 12 to 16, nephron numbers were reduced by 10% to 35%, correlating with the degree of maternal hyperglycemia (Figure 23.14).[261] Furthermore, culture of metanephroi in varying glucose concentrations demonstrated that tight glucose control is necessary for optimal metanephric growth and differentiation. In mice, offspring of diabetic mothers had fewer nephrons, a finding associated with increased evidence of apoptosis in tubules and podocytes, potentially mediated via increased renal angiotensinogen and renin mRNA expression and nuclear

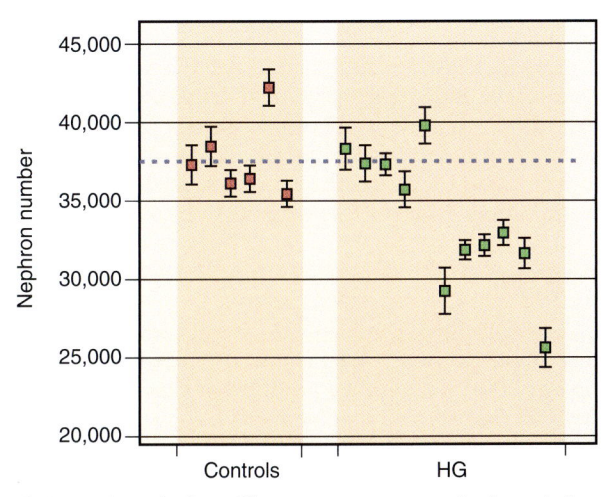

Figure 23.14 Effects of maternal hyperglycemia (HG) on nephron number in rat offspring. (From Amri K, Freund N, Vilar J, et al: Adverse effects of hyperglycemia on kidney development in rats: in vivo and in vitro studies. *Diabetes* 48:2240-2245, 1999.)

factor-kappaB (NF-κB) activation.[136] Other researchers suggest altered branching morphogenesis, increased asymmetric dimethylarginine,[11] and reduced nitric oxide levels as potential mediators of reduced nephron numbers in offspring of diabetic mothers.[262,263] These offspring demonstrated higher blood pressures and renal hypertrophy and had greater tubulointerstitial injury than controls, and these changes were abrogated by normalization of asymmetric dimethylarginine (ADMA) levels through maternal supplementation with L-citrulline.[263] Multiple pathways are therefore likely implicated in hyperglycemia-induced renal programming. In terms of effects on renal function, studies of adult rat offspring of diabetic mothers revealed glomerular hypertrophy, reductions in GFR and renal plasma flow, hypertension, and decreased endothelium-mediated vasodilation, suggesting that programming of hypertension in offspring of diabetic mothers may be multifactorial.[264,265]

Human offspring of diabetic pregnancies have a higher incidence of congenital malformations, resulting from defects in early organogenesis.[266] Furthermore, it is known that expression and bioavailability of the insulin-like growth factors (IGFs) are altered in diabetic pregnancies and that IGFs and their binding proteins are important regulators of fetal development.[266] The impact of maternal diabetes on metanephric expression of IGFs and their receptors was studied in rats in which diabetes was induced by streptozotocin in comparison with gestational age–matched normal controls.[266] There was no significant difference in IGF-1 or IGF-II or insulin receptor expression at any stage, but in offspring of diabetic mothers, there was a significantly increased expression of the IGF-II/mannose-6-phosphate receptor. This receptor tightly regulates the action of IGF-II, and an increase in expression would lead to reduced IGF-II bioavailability.[266] IGF-II is a critical player in renal development. The same investigators examined the role of IGF binding protein-1 (IGFBP-1) on nephrogenesis in genetically modified mice.[267] Offspring of females overexpressing human IGFBP-1 were growth restricted and had an 18% to 25% reduction in nephron number, depending on whether human IGFBP-1 was overexpressed in the mother only, the fetus only, or both. When metanephroi from these mice were cultured in the presence of IGF-I or IGF-II, only IGF-II increased nephron numbers by 25% to 40% in a concentration-dependent manner.[267] Interestingly, in a cohort of preterm infants, diastolic blood pressure at age 4 years was found to correlate positively with IGFBP-1 levels measured at postnatal weeks 32.6 through 34.6, suggesting a programming effect of this pathway in humans.[268]

APOPTOSIS

To evaluate at which stage of development a low-protein diet affects nephrogenesis, Welham and colleagues studied embryonic rat metanephroi at different time points.[236] At embryonic day 13, the metanephros has just formed, the ureteric bud has branched once, branch tips were surrounded by condensed mesenchyme that later transforms into tubule epithelium, and the ureteric stalk is surrounded by loose stromal mesenchyme.[236] By day 15, multiple branching cycles have occurred and primitive nephrons begin to be form.[236] At embryonic day 13, there is no difference in the number of cells in metanephroi between embryos whose mothers receive low-protein diets and those whose mothers receive normal-protein diets, but by day 15, there are significantly fewer cells per metanephros in the low-protein group. In contrast, a significant increase in the number of apoptotic cells was observed in the low-protein group at day 13 but not at day 15, suggesting that increased apoptosis on day 13 likely contributed to the reduced cell numbers on day 15.[236] On postnatal day 1 in kidneys from offspring of mothers exposed to 50% calorie restriction, apoptosis was most evident in the nephrogenic zone and co-localized to the mesenchyme and peritubular aggregates, suggesting a role in modulation of nephrogenesis.[269] In 8-week-old hypertensive LBW rat offspring of mothers subjected to a low-protein diet, the kidneys were histologically normal but also showed evidence of increased apoptosis, without an increase in proliferation, in comparison with NBW controls.[89] The increase in apoptotic activity observed in the kidney in these studies suggests possible successive waves of apoptosis at different stages of nephrogenesis in programmed rats that may impact nephron endowment.

Several studies have suggested that altered regulation of apoptosis in the developing kidney may be due to down-regulation of anti-apoptotic factors (e.g., Pax-2, Bcl-2) and/or upregulation of pro-apoptotic factors (e.g., Bax, p53, Fas receptor, caspases 3 and 9) in response to environmental or other stimuli.[269-273] Humans with haploinsufficiency of *PAX2* have renal coloboma syndrome, and those with certain *PAX2* polymorphisms have smaller neonatal kidney size, as discussed above.[230,270,274] PAX2 is an anti-apoptotic transcriptional regulator that is highly expressed in the branching ureteric tree as well as in foci of induced nephrogenic mesenchyme during kidney development.[270] Porteous and colleagues reported that heterozygous mice with *Pax2* mutations were very small at birth and had significant reductions in nephron number. In addition, there was a significant increase in apoptotic cell death in the developing kidneys. Subsequently, the same group demonstrated that loss of Pax2 anti-apoptotic activity reduced ureteric branching and increased ureteric apoptosis.[274] Similarly, loss of the anti-apoptotic factor Bcl-2 and gain of function of the pro-apoptotic factor p53 are both associated with a significant reduction in nephron number, which is also associated with increased apoptosis in metanephric blastemas, in Bcl-2 knockout mice and p53 transgenic mice.[271,275]

Mutant mouse models, although providing evidence that an increase in apoptosis results in reduced nephron numbers, do not address the impact of environmental factors on renal development. Pham and associates examined gene expression in the kidneys of offspring of rats subjected to uterine artery ligation during gestation.[276] These researchers found a 25% reduction in glomerular number associated with evidence of increases in both apoptosis and pro-apoptotic caspase-3 activity in the kidney at birth. Furthermore, they found evidence of increased mRNA expression of the pro-apoptotic genes *Bax* and *p53* and decreased expression of the anti-apoptotic gene *Bcl-2*. They also found evidence of hypomethylation of the *p53* gene, which in addition to a decrease in *Bcl-2* expression would lead to an increase in p53 activity, suggesting programming of a pro-apoptotic milieu as a potential modulator of nephron endowment.

GLIAL CELL LINE–DERIVED NEUROTROPHIC FACTOR AND C-RET RECEPTOR FUNCTION

GDNF signaling through its receptor-tyrosine kinase Ret is a key ligand-receptor interaction driving ureteric budding and branching. C-Ret is expressed on the tips of the ureteric bud branches, and knockout of this receptor in mice leads to severe renal dysplasia and reduction in nephron number.[222] Homozygous GDNF null mutant mice have complete renal agenesis and die shortly after birth.[277] Heterozygous GDNF mice, as described previously, have reduced nephron numbers, demonstrate glomerulomegaly, and are susceptible to hypertension.[125] Polymorphisms in *RET* but not *GDNF* are associated with newborn renal size in humans.[105,278] As described previously, maternal dietary vitamin A has a significant impact on nephrogenesis (see Figure 23.13). In cultured metanephroi, the expression of c-Ret has been found to be regulated by retinoic acid supplementation in a dose-dependent manner.[245] GDNF expression was not affected by vitamin A fluctuations. Modulation of c-Ret expression is therefore likely to be a significant pathway through which vitamin A availability regulates nephrogenesis and nephron endowment.

FETAL DRUG EXPOSURE

Among 397 pregnant women in one study, antibiotic use was associated with a 138-g lower offspring birth weight in comparison with no antibiotic use.[279] Furthermore, analysis of methylation levels of imprinted genes showed antibiotic use to be associated with methylation at five differentially mediated regions, although methylation at only one region was associated with birth weight.[279] Although the study was small and the data on antibiotic use were self-reported, these findings suggest a programming effect of antenatal antibiotic use. Several medications commonly used during pregnancy or early postnatally have been studied for their effects on nephrogenesis. The aminoglycoside antibiotic *gentamicin*, administered to pregnant rats, results in a permanent nephron deficit in offspring.[280] A significant reduction in nephron number has been observed in metanephric explants cultured in the presence of gentamicin.[281] In cultured metanephroi in one study, within 8 hours of administration, gentamicin was localized to the growing tips of ureteric buds and the surrounding blastema, and within 24 hours, gentamicin exposure was associated with a significant reduction in the number of branch points.[282] In contrast, however, another study did not find a reduction in nephron number in rat pups administered gentamicin intraperitoneally from birth to 14 days of age.[283] Taken together, these studies suggest an early window of action for gentamicin that may be relevant for premature infants.

The *β-lactams* have also been shown to result in impaired nephrogenesis.[284] Administration of ampicillin to pregnant rats led to an 11% average reduction in nephron endowment in offspring as well as evidence of focal cystic tubule dilation and interstitial inflammation. Administration of ceftriaxone in vivo did not result in a nephron deficit, but there was histologic evidence of renal interstitial inflammation. The penicillins were also found to inhibit nephrogenesis in cultured metanephroi in a dose-dependent fashion, an effect that was less evident with ceftriaxone. Importantly, nephrogenesis was affected even at therapeutic doses of penicillins in the rat, a finding that warrants further research on these antibiotics, which are frequently used in human pregnancy. The mechanism whereby the *β-lactams* reduce nephron endowment is likely through an increase in apoptosis in the induced mesenchyme.[87]

The immunosuppressive medication *cyclosporine* is a known nephrotoxin in humans that crosses the placenta. Women treated with this medication may have successful pregnancies, although their infants tend to have birth weights in the low range, and its effect on the fetal kidney is not well described.[285] Cyclosporine administration in varying doses and at different stages of gestation was compared in pregnant rabbits and rabbits receiving either vehicle or no drug.[285] Cyclosporine administration in the later, but not the earlier, period of gestation resulted in smaller litters and growth-restricted pups. All pups exposed to cyclosporine in utero had a 25% to 33% reduction in nephron number compared with controls. The reduction in nephron number was accompanied by glomerulomegaly and was independent of birth weight. At 1 month of age, the kidneys of the exposed pups also demonstrated foci of glomerulosclerosis. Subsequent functional evaluation of the kidneys of rabbits exposed to cyclosporine in utero demonstrated a reduction in GFR at 18 and 35 weeks of age and an increase in proteinuria at 11, 18, and 35 weeks of age.[150] Spontaneous hypertension developed by 11 weeks of age in rabbits exposed to cyclosporine in utero and worsened with time.[150] In the presence of cyclosporine, nephron formation was found to be arrested, potentially owing to inhibition of conversion of metanephric mesenchyme to epithelium.[87]

Nonsteroidal antiinflammatory drugs are sometimes used in premature neonates. Administration of a cyclo-oxygenase-2 (COX-2) inhibitor but not a cyclo-oxygenase-1 inhibitor postnatally in rats and mice resulted in reduced cortical volume, impairment of nephrogenesis, and smaller glomerular diameter.[286] Administration of indomethacin or ibuprofen postnatally did not affect nephron number in rats.[283] In the preterm baboon kidney, early postnatal administration of five doses of ibuprofen (consistent with recommended dosing in premature infants with patent ductus arteriosus) was associated with a reduction in width of the nephrogenic zone, suggesting premature termination of nephrogenesis.[287] The impact of these medications on human nephrogenesis is not known.

OBSTRUCTION OF THE DEVELOPING KIDNEY

Congenital urinary tract obstruction and vesicoureteric reflux may be associated with poor long-term renal outcomes in humans, and perinatal obstruction may lead to reduced nephron numbers.[288] To explore this issue, normal rats underwent unilateral ureteral obstruction or sham operation either on postnatal day 1 with relief on day 5, or on postnatal day 14 with relief on day 19.[65] Renal growth after 3 months was reduced by 50% in the day 14 group and by 30% in the day 5 group, although nephron number was reduced by 50% in both groups. Similar intervention in adult rats did not affect nephron number. This study demonstrated that urinary obstruction in a normal developing kidney can impact nephrogenesis. Importantly, temporary neonatal obstruction was also associated with histologic

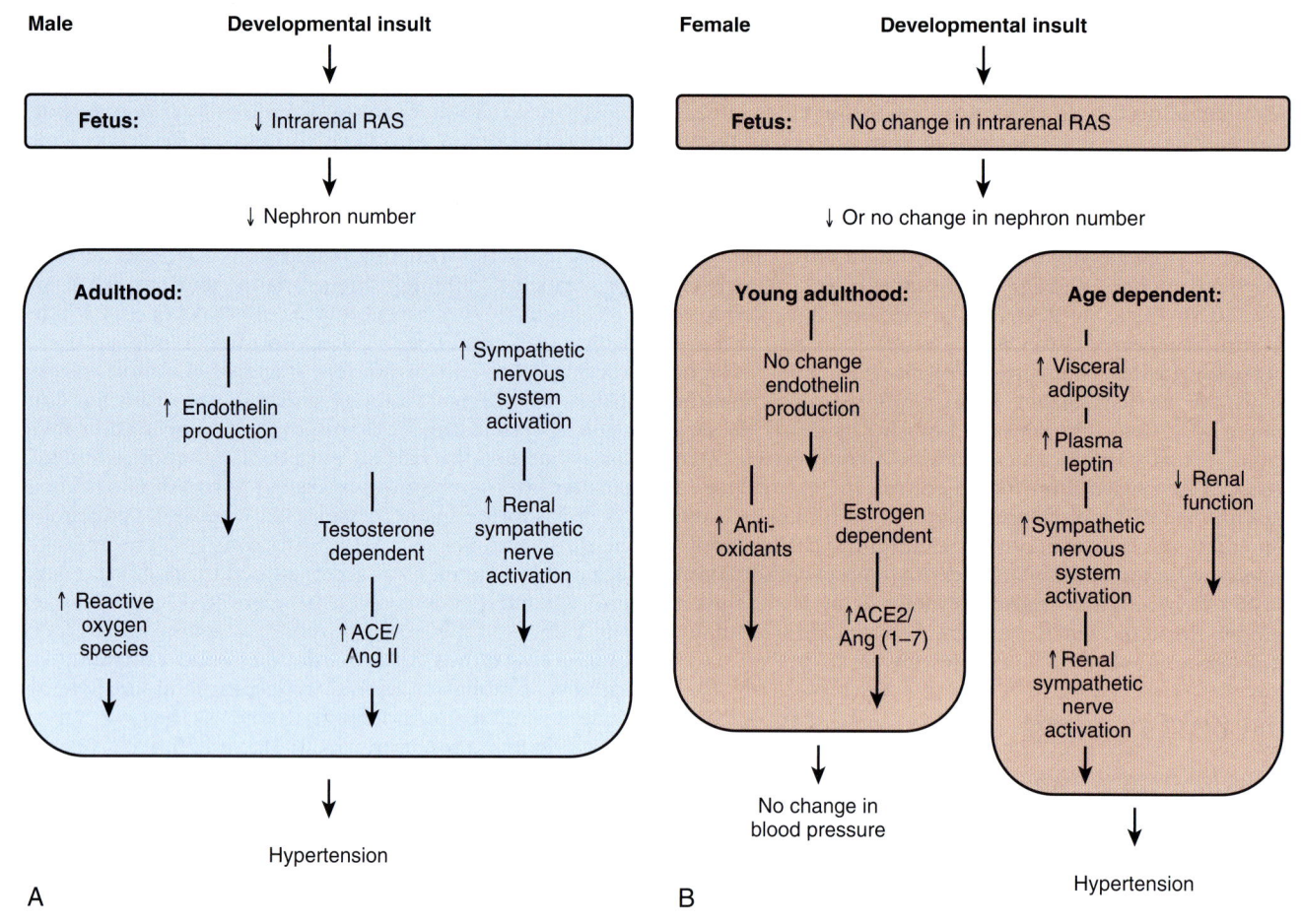

Figure 23.15 Potential differing mechanisms affecting developmental programming of blood pressure in males **(A)** and females **(B)**. ACE, Angiotensin-converting enzyme; Ang, angiotensin; RAS, renin angiotensin (aldosterone) system. (From Ojeda NB, Intapad S, Alexander BT: Sex differences in the developmental programming of hypertension. *Acta Physiol (Oxf)* 210:307-316, 2014; reviews mechanisms detail.)

scarring and loss of function of the contralateral kidney in 1-year-old rats, suggesting consequent programming in the contralateral kidney as well.[289]

IMPACT OF SEX

In some experimental models and human studies, although not all, programming effects on blood pressure and kidney function appear different in males and females, especially at young ages. In female rats with similar programmed reductions in nephron numbers, blood pressures are often not as high as in males, or they increase much later.[89,290] Sex hormones have been implicated as contributing to these differences. Growth-restricted males (induced by uterine artery ligation) have higher testosterone levels than controls, and hypertension can be abrogated by castration.[290] Such changes are not observed in male offspring of protein-restricted mothers, however, pointing to the intricacies of the programming models. In female rats growth restricted by placental insufficiency, hypertension develops only late but onset can be accelerated by ovariectomy.[290] These data suggest that in the uterine ischemia programming model, testosterone exacerbates and estrogen protects against hypertension. Sex differences in relative expression of components of the RAAS appear to participate in programming of hypertension, possibly differentially altering the balance between vasoconstriction and vasodilation and sodium handling.[143,290] Furthermore, growth-restricted male rats exhibit higher levels of markers of renal oxidative stress than controls, findings that are absent in similarly programmed females, and antioxidant treatment normalized blood pressure in the male rats.[144,291] Multiple other suggested mechanisms underlying these gender differences have been expertly reviewed by Ojeda and colleagues and as summarized in Figure 23.15.[144,290]

POTENTIAL FOR RESCUE OF NEPHRON NUMBER

Given the evidence for developmental programming of hypertension and kidney disease, and the associations with birth weight, prematurity, other intrauterine exposures and the impact of nutrition in early childhood, it is possible that interventions could be designed to modulate developmentally programmed changes in the kidney and reduce long-term disease risk. Optimization of maternal health and nutrition prior to and during pregnancy to attenuate any risk factors for low birth weight and prematurity is the most obvious intervention, as it has been estimated that intrauterine factors determine around 60% of the variation in birth weight.[292] In addition, minimization of nephrotoxin exposure and attention to neonatal nutrition in premature infants are important to permit optimal nephrogenesis after birth. Specific interventions that may augment nephron number per se have been investigated, some clinically feasible and others still in research stages (see Table 23.4). Interventions to modulate other aspects of developmental programming in the kidney have not yet been reported, but it could be assumed that the effects may be similar to those affecting nephrogenesis.

Prevention is likely more realistic than rescue of low nephron number. Ouabain is a highly specific ligand for Na^+-K^+-ATPase, the activity of which is known to be reduced in erythrocytes of LBW young men.[293,294] Na^+-K^+-ATPase is a ubiquitously expressed plasma membrane protein that regulates the release of calcium waves and thereby is an important regulator of early development.[293] In vitro, addition of ouabain to the medium of metanephroi in culture was found to abrogate the effect of serum starvation on ureteric branching.[293] Similarly, in vivo, ouabain administration throughout pregnancy prevented the reduction in nephron number in rats subjected to maternal low-protein diet.[293] Whether ouabain can rescue nephron number if given late in pregnancy was not addressed in this study. Supplementation of glycine, urea, or alanine to a maternal low-protein diet prevented development of low nephron numbers in rat offspring, but only glycine supplementation prevented subsequent hypertension.[32] Intriguingly, water restriction of rat mothers during gestation resulted in augmentation of normal nephron number but also induced hypertension in the offspring. The researchers implicated vasopressin as a mediator of this programming effect.[295]

Vitamin A deficiency is common among women in poorer nations, and in animals is associated with reduced nephron number, as discussed previously.[245,296] In rats exposed to maternal low-protein diet, nephron numbers were restored to normal by one dose of retinoic acid given to the pregnant dams during early nephrogenesis.[297] In preterm baboons, however, postnatal administration of retinoic acid did not rescue nephron number, suggesting that vitamin A is likely necessary earlier in gestation.[246] These baboons also received postnatal antibiotics, which may have confounded the effect of the vitamin A.

Postnatal nutrition is an important modulator of kidney development, especially in premature infants. Restoration of normal protein intake by cross-fostering growth-restricted pups onto normal mothers after birth rescued nephron number and prevented hypertension, compared to those fed by protein-deficient mothers.[93]

A *maternal single kidney* may affect fetal kidney development. In offspring of rats that had undergone nephrectomy prior to pregnancy, nephron numbers were increased at birth, although not at 6 weeks.[298,299] A circulating renotrophic factor in the mother may therefore accelerate nephrogenesis but does not appear to affect final nephron number. How these observations would apply in humans is difficult to extrapolate, because outcomes may differ according to the mother's age, whether she has a congenital or acquired single kidney, and whether the kidney is a transplant, with the attendant required medications that in turn may affect nephrogenesis.

Modulation of regression of nephron number, although still hypothetical, has been suggested by the researchers of one study as a potential pathway to augment final nephron number.[300] They evaluated glomerular number from postnatal day 7 to day 28 in normal mice. Maximal nephron number was seen at day 7, with a subsequent regression and plateau at day 18. Such a time course would need to be studied in growth-restricted animals before any potential intervention to inhibit this regression could be tested.

CATCH-UP GROWTH

Postnatal nutrition is important for infant growth, especially in the setting of prematurity or growth restriction, and can affect nephron number and long-term renal function, as discussed previously.[160,192] In one study already described, cross-fostering of growth-restricted newborn rats (induced by placental insufficiency) on normal mothers permitted restoration of normal nephron number and prevented subsequent hypertension, demonstrating the potential "rescue" effect of adequate postnatal nutrition.[93] Postnatal overfeeding of LBW rats, induced by reduction of litter size to three pups, however, did not augment low nephron numbers, and with aging, rats became obese and hypertensive and demonstrated renal injury.[301] In this model, even though the mother is switched to a normal-protein diet at time of delivery, the pups may remain somewhat protein deficient despite consuming larger quantities of milk—unlike with cross-fostering, which provides normal milk immediately—a difference that may explain why nephron number remained low and underscores the importance of diet composition. In contrast, overfeeding of NBW rats led to higher-than-normal nephron numbers, despite which high blood pressure and renal injury developed over time.[114] These animal data suggest that restoration of normal dietary components after growth restriction may permit some reversal of programmed changes but that overfeeding is harmful.

In diverse populations worldwide, rapid "catch-up" growth (defined as upward crossing of weight centiles) or an increase in body mass index, even in children of normal birth weight, is associated with higher blood pressures and increased cardiovascular risk.[302-304] On the other hand, catch-up growth has been advocated in poorer countries to improve child survival from infectious diseases and reduce stunting and malnutrition.[305] The timing of catch-up growth in early infancy and childhood, which tends to occur rapidly in LBW children when adequate nutrition is available, appears to be a crucial factor in determining this long-term risk.[304-307] The importance of birth weight and catch-up growth was examined in a cohort of 22-year-old subjects, in whom systolic blood pressure was observed to increase by 1.3 mm Hg (95% CI, 0.3 to 2.3 mm Hg) for each standard deviation decrease in birth weight, and to increase by 1.6 mm Hg (95% CI, 0.6 to 2.7 mm Hg) for each standard deviation increase in weight gain between the ages of 1 and 10 years.[308] Such observations have been reproduced in several populations, together with evidence of increased arterial stiffness and greater prevalence of cardiovascular risk factors in early childhood after rapid growth, with children who had been of low birth weight but became overweight being at highest risk.[181,302,306] Low birth weight independently predicted both proteinuria and obesity in a rural Canadian cohort, demonstrating likely simultaneous programming of multiple risk factors for kidney disease.[309]

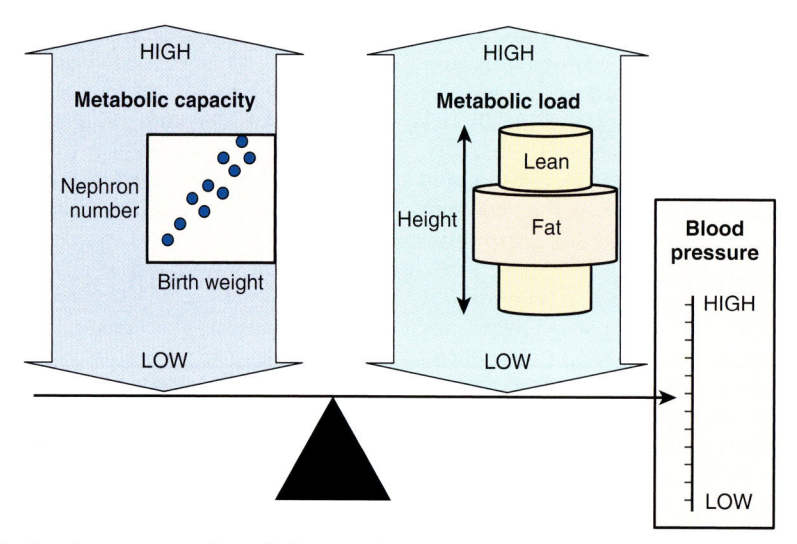

Figure 23.16 Diagram illustrating the concepts of metabolic capacity and metabolic load in relation to blood pressure. A high load and low capacity are each predicted to increase blood pressure. (From Grijalva-Eternod CS, Lawlor DA, Wells JC: Testing a capacity-load model for hypertension: disentangling early and late growth effects on childhood blood pressure in a prospective birth cohort. *PLoS One* 8:e56078, 2013.)

Risk factors for childhood overweight and obesity also include high birth weight and exposure to gestational diabetes.[310] Obesity, in turn, is a risk factor for renal disease.[311] Finding the balance at which postnatal nutrition is optimized to improve short-term survival and reduce long-term risk of chronic disease requires further study. In general, avoidance of overweight through diet and exercise are likely safe principles.[312,313]

IMPACT OF EARLY GROWTH ON KIDNEY FUNCTION

Grijalva-Eternod and colleagues developed a model to test whether "mismatch" between a small kidney and a (relatively) larger body, as would occur with catch-up growth and overweight in a person who had been born small, is associated with hypertension.[314] Birth weight was presumed to reflect the homeostatic metabolic capacity of the kidney and childhood body composition to reflect the metabolic load. When the model was applied to a birth cohort of children, a high metabolic load, relative to innate metabolic capacity, was found to be associated with higher blood pressures (Figure 23.16). Consistent with this hypothesis, proteinuric renal disease progressed faster in children who had been born prematurely and became obese than in those who were not obese.[315] In this study, all obese children, whether born at term or prematurely, were found to have glomerulomegaly, although kidney size remained small in all those born prematurely, even among the obese. Similarly, excessive weight gain was a predictor of worse renal function at age 7.5 years in a cohort of very LBW premature infants who had experienced acute kidney injury as neonates.[316]

Accelerated senescence has been proposed as a potential mechanism whereby catch-up growth may increase the risk of cardiovascular and renal disease.[317] Senescence is a state of cellular growth arrest that naturally occurs with age but may be accelerated in the presence of stress, an acceleration mediated by upregulation of the cell cycle inhibitors (p53, p21, and p16INK4a) and progressive shortening of telomeres.[318] Increased expression of senescence markers has been observed in diseased human kidneys.[319] In animals, rapid weight gain in growth-restricted animals has been found to be associated with evidence of accelerated senescence in the kidney and cardiovascular system and with premature death, consistent with accelerated aging.[317,320,321] Senescence markers are not more highly expressed at birth in growth-restricted than in NBW animals, but they do increase more rapidly as the growth-restricted animals age.[320] Hyperfiltration in a small kidney, exacerbated by high metabolic demand from increasing body size, likely contributes to ongoing injury and progressive senescence.[319,320] Senescence markers have not been studied in LBW human kidneys, but leukocyte telomere length was found to be significantly shorter among 5-year-old Bangladeshi children who had been of low birth weight than in those of normal birth weight, lending support to this hypothesis.[322,323] Oxidative stress is a driver of senescence, and in small-for-gestational-age children, markers of oxidative stress were higher in those who experienced catch-up growth than in controls, suggesting oxidative stress as a possible initiator of accelerated senescence.[324] A programmed link between low nephron number, catch-up growth, and accelerated senescence as a potential mediator of hypertension and renal disease in humans has yet to be proven.[325,326]

TRANSGENERATIONAL EFFECTS OF PROGRAMMING

In a population-based cohort of women, the odds of pregnancy-associated gestational diabetes or gestational hypertension (including preeclampsia and eclampsia) among those who had been born premature were significantly increased and were higher with lower gestational age at birth.[163] Gestational hypertension and preeclampsia are risk factors for low birth weight and prematurity, and gestational diabetes is a risk factor for high birth weight; therefore, the offspring of pregnancies affected by these conditions were likely at risk for programmed hypertension and renal dysfunction, including gestational hypertension. The cycle could therefore continue.

In rats, maternal protein restriction results in persistence of transgenerational programming into the F2 generation.[327] These effects have been proposed to be mediated largely by changes in DNA methylation, determined by amino acid availability and resulting in epigenetic changes in gene expression.[19] Whether these epigenetic changes can be transmitted through the germline and persist in the offspring, or whether a mother who had been subjected to adverse intrauterine events may experience changes in renal function and blood pressure during pregnancy that may in turn, *de novo*, impact the development of her offspring is still a point of debate.[328-330] The latter hypothesis seems more likely.

IMPACT OF NEPHRON ENDOWMENT IN TRANSPLANTATION

Nephron endowment in transplantation is relevant for both the donor and the recipient. Removal of a kidney in a healthy donor implies loss of 50% of original nephron endowment, and gain of a kidney in a recipient may provide more or less than half of the recipient's original nephron endowment, depending on relative sizes of donor and recipient, periprocedural nephron loss, and other factors. Consideration of nephron endowment prior to transplantation could affect long-term renal health in both donors and recipients.

IMPLICATIONS OF NEPHRON ENDOWMENT FOR THE DONOR

Living donation after appropriate donor screening is generally presumed to be safe, although there are donor groups, including the young and obese, the older donor, and some ethnic groups, who may be at increased risk of long-term renal dysfunction but are not well represented in the current literature.[331] In predominantly white cohorts, hypertension and proteinuria do increase over time in living donors, but renal function remains generally well preserved over the first decades.[58,332] In a cross-sectional retrospective study of donors followed for up to 40 years, however, donor GFRs were found to decline after 15 to 17 years after donation; therefore, duration of follow-up is important to fully understand potential associations with risk.[333] Furthermore, Aboriginal Australian donors were found to have a significantly higher risk of hypertension, renal dysfunction, and ESKD at a median of 16 years after donation than whites.[334] Similarly, hypertension and proteinuria were found to be much more prevalent among Aboriginal than among white Canadian donors at 20 years of follow-up, and African Americans as well as Hispanics were reported to have more hypertension and CKD after donation than white Americans.[335-337] These data are troubling because the donors were screened prior to donation, so donor nephrectomy can be implicated in the disease process. Importantly, African Americans and Aboriginal Australian populations have lower birth weights than their white counterparts, and Aboriginal Canadians have higher birth weights; therefore, developmental programming of the kidney may be a risk factor contributing to poorer outcomes after donation.[338] Given the growing need for donors worldwide, better understanding of renal risk in these populations is urgently needed.[325,326]

IMPLICATIONS OF NEPHRON ENDOWMENT FOR THE RECIPIENT

Prescription of donor kidneys is largely based on immunologic matching. In animal experiments of renal transplantation, however, the impact of transplanted nephron mass, independent of immunologic factors, on the subsequent development of chronic allograft nephropathy has been demonstrated.[339-343] Despite such evidence, prescription of kidneys on the basis of the physiologic capacity of the donor organ to meet the metabolic needs of the recipient has not generally been considered.[344] More and more data are accumulating, however, that suggest a significant impact of transplanted renal mass on long-term post-transplantation outcomes.

Demographic and anthropomorphic factors associated with late renal allograft loss include donor age, sex, and race, as well as recipient BSA.[345-347] In general, kidneys from older, female, and African American donors fare worse.[49,76,348,349] Indirectly, these observations suggest that the intrinsic nephron endowment of the transplanted kidney is likely to play a role in the development of chronic allograft nephropathy. Because nephron numbers are not yet measurable in vivo, several investigators have compared recipient and donor BSAs as surrogates for metabolic demand and kidney size; others have used kidney weights or renal volumetric measurements made by ultrasonography as surrogates for nephron mass.[350-354] Importantly, although kidney mass and kidney volume may be proportional to nephron number and measures of body size tend to be proportional to kidney size, these relationships do vary in strength of association, so these data should be interpreted cautiously. In general, however, the preponderance of evidence does support the hypothesis that small kidneys perform less well when transplanted into larger recipients.[350-354]

A retrospective analysis of 32,083 patients who received a first cadaver kidney found that large recipients of kidneys from small donors had a 43% higher risk of late allograft failure than medium-sized recipients receiving kidneys from medium-sized donors.[353] Outcomes were best in small recipients receiving kidneys from large donors. Subsequently, among 69,737 deceased donor kidney transplantations, a severe recipient/donor size mismatch (>1.38) was associated with higher 10-year graft loss in comparison with closer matches, and the risk was doubled in the case of extended-criteria donors with severe mismatches (22% and 10%, respectively).[355] Similar findings were seen among recipients of older (>60 years) compared with younger kidneys.[356] These data suggest that donor and recipient size should be considered in organ allocation decisions, especially if the donor kidney is known to be "suboptimal." Smaller studies have not consistently found similar results, however, potentially reflecting lack of statistical power.[352,353]

Kidney size, however, may not always be directly proportional to BSA; therefore, ratios of donor BSA to recipient BSA may not be an ideal method of estimating mismatch between nephron mass and recipient. Kidney weight may be a better surrogate for nephron mass.[49,357] Using this parameter, Kim and associates analyzed the ratio of donor kidney

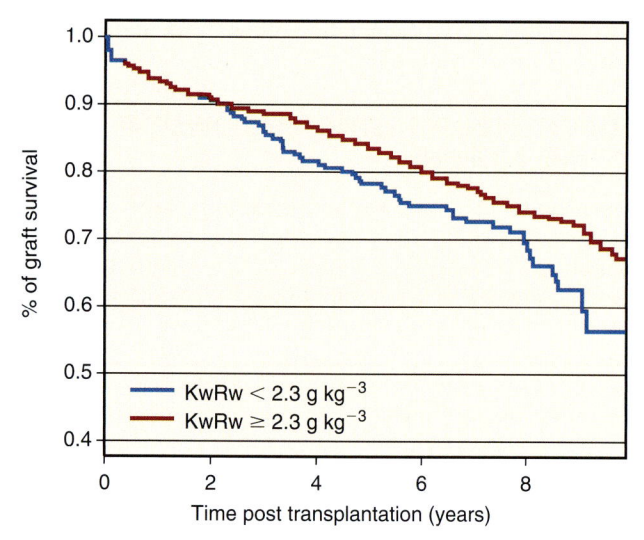

Figure 23.17 Correlation between kidney weight/recipient weight (KwRw) ratio and long-term graft survival in renal transplantation. Graft survival declines faster with a KwRw < 2.3 g/kg ($P = 0.016$). (From Giral M, Foucher Y, Karam G, et al: Kidney and recipient weight incompatibility reduces long-term graft survival. *J Am Soc Nephrol* 21:1022-1029, 2010.)

weight to recipient body weight (DKW/RBW) in 259 live-donor transplants.[358] These investigators found that a higher DKW/RBW—greater than 4.5 g/kg—was significantly associated with improved allograft function at 3 years in comparison with a ratio of less than 3.0 g/kg. A similar study involving 964 recipients of cadaveric kidneys, in whom proteinuria severity and Cockroft-Gault creatinine clearances were also calculated, found that 10% of the subjects were "strongly" mismatched, having a DKW/RBW ratio of less than 2 g/kg.[349] The DKW/RBW ratio was lowest when male recipients received kidneys from female donors. The risk of having proteinuria higher than 0.5 g/24 hr was significantly greater, and developed earlier, in those with DKW/RBW ratios less than 2 g/kg than in those with higher ratios. Proteinuria was present in 50% of those with DKW/RBW ratios less than 2 g/kg, 33% of those with DKW/RBW ratios of 2 to 4 g/kg, and 23% in those with DKW/RBW ratios of 4 g/kg or greater. At 5-year follow-up, however, there was no difference in graft survival among the three DKW/RBW groups, but the investigators conceded that longer follow-up was needed.[349] Subsequent analysis of the same cohort 5 years later showed that GFR declined more rapidly after 7 years in the low than in the high DKW/RBW group, suggesting that the smaller kidneys were likely hyperfiltering early on, initiating the cycle of progressive nephron loss (Figure 23.17).[359]

In an attempt to more accurately reflect transplanted nephron mass, another group used renal ultrasonography to measure cadaveric transplant kidney (Tx) cross-sectional area in relation to recipient body weight (W) to calculate a "nephron dose index," Tx/W.[360] The group found that during the first 5 years after transplantation, serum creatinine was significantly lower in patients with a high Tx/W than in those with lower values, with a ratio of better graft survival. A similar analysis, using renal volume determined by computed tomography angiographic volumetry (performed pretransplantation in living donors) to recipient BSA, found that GFRs during the first year after transplantation correlated with transplanted renal volume, and GFRs were lower among those with a donor/recipient BSA ratio of 1 or less.[361] A small kidney transplanted into a large recipient may not have an adequate capacity to meet the metabolic needs of the recipient without imposing glomerular hyperfiltration, which ultimately leads to nephron loss and eventual allograft failure.[362,363]

Transplanted nephron mass may be a function of congenital endowment and attrition of nephrons with age but is also affected by peritransplantation renal injury (i.e., donor hypotension, prolonged cold or warm ischemia, nephrotoxic immunosuppressive drugs). All of these factors must be closely considered, in addition to immunologic matching, in the selection of appropriate recipients in whom the allograft is likely to function for the longest time and therefore provide best possible improvement in quality of life.

CONCLUSION

The association between an adverse fetal environment and subsequent hypertension as well as kidney disease in later life is now quite compelling and appears to be mediated, at least in part, by impaired nephrogenesis and suboptimal nephron endowment (Figure 23.18). Concomitant glomerular hypertrophy and altered expression of sodium transporters in the programmed kidney also contribute to the vicious circle of glomerular hypertension, glomerular injury, and sclerosis leading to worsening hypertension and ongoing renal injury. In addition, multiple other factors, such as increased oxidative stress, renal inflammation, accelerated senescence, and catch-up body growth, are all likely contributors to ongoing nephron loss and eventual renal disease.[364-367] The number of nephrons in humans without kidney disease varies widely, suggesting that a significant proportion of the general population, especially in areas where high or low birth weights are prevalent, may be at increased risk for development of later-life hypertension and renal dysfunction. Measurement of nephron number in vivo remains an obstacle, with the best surrogate markers thus far being low birth weight, high birth weight, prematurity, and, in the absence of other known renal diseases, reduced kidney volume on ultrasonography, especially in children, and glomerular enlargement on kidney biopsy. A kidney with a reduced complement of nephrons would have less renal reserve to adapt to dietary excesses or to compensate for renal injury. The molecular mechanisms through which fetal programming exerts its effects on nephrogenesis are varied and likely complementary and intertwined. Although in some animal studies nephron number and blood pressure can be "rescued" by good postnatal nutrition or vitamin A supplementation, applicability of these findings to humans requires further study. The fact that even seemingly minor influences, such as composition of maternal diet during fetal life, can have major consequences on renal development in the offspring underscores the critical importance of optimization of perinatal care and early nutrition, which could have a major impact on population health in the future.

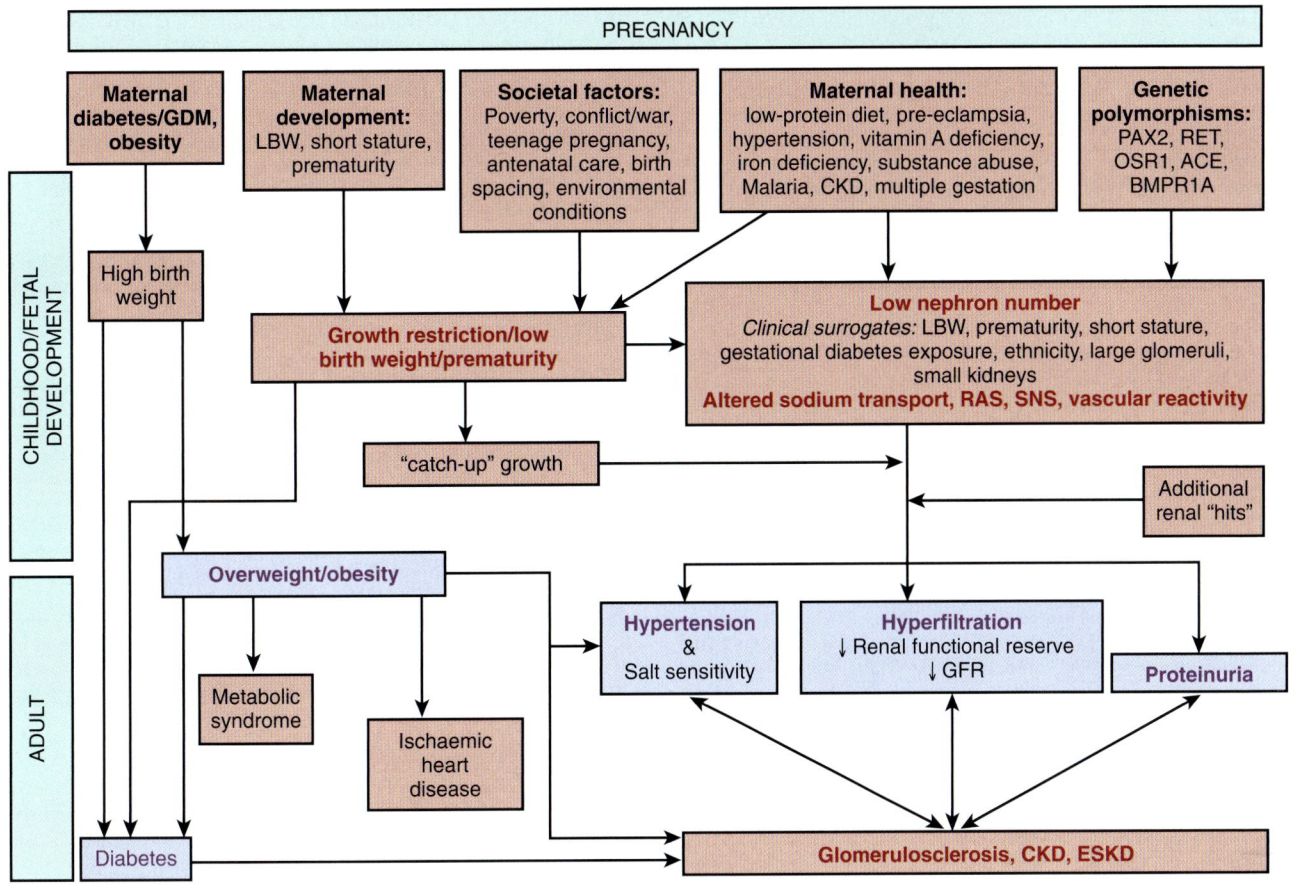

Figure 23.18 Proposed mechanism of fetal programming of hypertension and renal disease. CKD, Chronic kidney disease; ESKD, end-stage kidney disease; GDM, gestational diabetes mellitus; GFR, glomerular filtration rate; LBW, low birth weight; RAS, renin angiotensin (aldosterone) system; SNS, sympathetic nervous system. (Adapted from Luyckx VA, Bertram JF, Brenner BM, et al: Effect of fetal and child health on kidney development and long-term risk of hypertension and kidney disease. *Lancet* 382:273-283, 2013.)

Complete reference list available at ExpertConsult.com.

KEY REFERENCES

3. Hoy WE, Rees M, Kile E, et al: Low birthweight and renal disease in Australian aborigines. *Lancet* 352:1826–1827, 1998.
12. Luyckx VA, Bertram JF, Brenner BM, et al: Effect of fetal and child health on kidney development and long-term risk of hypertension and kidney disease. *Lancet* 382:273–283, 2013.
13. Barker DJ: Developmental origins of adult health and disease. *J Epidemiol Community Health* 58:114–115, 2004.
29. Vikse BE, Irgens LM, Leivestad T, et al: Low birth weight increases risk for end-stage renal disease. *J Am Soc Nephrol* 19:151–157, 2008.
30. White SL, Perkovic V, Cass A, et al: Is low birth weight an antecedent of CKD in later life? A systematic review of observational studies. *Am J Kidney Dis* 54:248–261, 2009.
32. Langley-Evans S, Langley-Evans A, Marchand M: Nutritional programming of blood pressure and renal morphology. *Arch Physiol Biochem* 111:8–16, 2003.
34. de Jong F, Monteaux MC, van Elburg RM, et al: Systematic review and meta-analysis of preterm birth and later systolic blood pressure. *Hypertension* 59:226–234, 2012.
35. Mu M, Wang SF, Sheng J, et al: Birth weight and subsequent blood pressure: a meta-analysis. *Arch Cardiovasc Dis* 105:99–113, 2012.
36. Nelson RG, Morgenstern H, Bennett PH: Intrauterine diabetes exposure and the risk of renal disease in diabetic Pima Indians. *Diabetes* 47:1489–1493, 1998.
43. Brenner BM, Garcia DL, Anderson S: Glomeruli and blood pressure: less of one, more the other? *Am J Hypertens* 1:335–347, 1988.
45. Lackland DT, Bendall HE, Osmond C, et al: Low birth weights contribute to high rates of early-onset chronic renal failure in the Southeastern United States. *Arch Intern Med* 160:1472–1476, 2000.
49. Nyengaard JR, Bendtsen TF: Glomerular number and size in relation to age, kidney weight, and body surface in normal man. *Anat Rec* 232:194–201, 1992.
53. Hoy WE, Douglas-Denton RN, Hughson MD, et al: A stereological study of glomerular number and volume: preliminary findings in a multiracial study of kidneys at autopsy. *Kidney Int Suppl* (83):S31–S37, 2003.
54. Puelles VG, Hoy WE, Hughson MD, et al: Glomerular number and size variability and risk for kidney disease. *Curr Opin Nephrol Hypertens* 20:7–15, 2011.
55. Keller G, Zimmer G, Mall G, et al: Nephron number in patients with primary hypertension. *N Engl J Med* 348:101–108, 2003.
67. Kett MM, Denton KM: Renal programming: cause for concern? *Am J Physiol Regul Integr Comp Physiol* 300:R791–R803, 2011.
69. Hughson M, Farris AB, Douglas-Denton R, et al: Glomerular number and size in autopsy kidneys: The relationship to birth weight. *Kidney Int* 63:2113–2122, 2003.
72. Manalich R, Reyes L, Herrera M, et al: Relationship between weight at birth and the number and size of renal glomeruli in humans: a histomorphometric study. *Kidney Int* 58:770–773, 2000.
77. Hoy WE, Wang Z, VanBuynder P, et al: The natural history of renal disease in Australian Aborigines. Part 1. Changes in albuminuria and glomerular filtration rate over time. *Kidney Int* 60:243–248, 2001.
80. Hoy WE, Hughson MD, Diouf B, et al: Distribution of volumes of individual glomeruli in kidneys at autopsy: association with physical and clinical characteristics and with ethnic group. *Am J Nephrol* 33(Suppl 1):15–20, 2011.

86. Langley-Evans SC: Intrauterine programming of hypertension in the rat: nutrient interactions. *Comp Biochem Physiol A Physiol* 114:327–333, 1996.
89. Vehaskari VM, Aviles DH, Manning J: Prenatal programming of adult hypertension in the rat. *Kidney Int* 59:238–245, 2001.
93. Wlodek ME, Mibus A, Tan A, et al: Normal lactational environment restores nephron endowment and prevents hypertension after placental restriction in the rat. *J Am Soc Nephrol* 18:1688–1696, 2007.
95. Baum M: Role of the kidney in the prenatal and early postnatal programming of hypertension. *Am J Physiol Renal Physiol* 298:F235–F247, 2010.
96. Bertram JF, Douglas-Denton RN, Diouf B, et al: Human nephron number: implications for health and disease. *Pediatr Nephrol* 26:1529–1533, 2011.
99. Hughson MD, Douglas-Denton R, Bertram JF, et al: Hypertension, glomerular number, and birth weight in African Americans and white subjects in the southeastern United States. *Kidney Int* 69:671–678, 2006.
100. Rodriguez MM, Gomez AH, Abitbol CL, et al: Histomorphometric analysis of postnatal glomerulogenesis in extremely preterm infants. *Pediatr Dev Pathol* 7:17–25, 2004.
102. Hinchliffe SA, Lynch MR, Sargent PH, et al: The effect of intrauterine growth retardation on the development of renal nephrons. *Br J Obstet Gynaecol* 99:296–301, 1992.
105. Zhang Z, Quinlan J, Hoy W, et al: A common RET variant is associated with reduced newborn kidney size and function. *J Am Soc Nephrol* 19:2027–2034, 2008.
121. Gilbert JS: Sex, salt, and senescence: sorting out mechanisms of the developmental origins of hypertension. *Hypertension* 51:997–999, 2008.
143. Moritz KM, Cuffe JS, Wilson LB, et al: Review: Sex specific programming: a critical role for the renal renin-angiotensin system. *Placenta* 31(Suppl):S40–S46, 2010.
144. Ojeda NB, Intapad S, Alexander BT: Sex differences in the developmental programming of hypertension. *Acta Physiol (Oxf)* 210:307–316, 2014.
155. Jones SE, Bilous RW, Flyvbjerg A, et al: Intra-uterine environment influences glomerular number and the acute renal adaptation to experimental diabetes. *Diabetologia* 44:721–728, 2001.
160. Abitbol CL, Rodriguez MM: The long-term renal and cardiovascular consequences of prematurity. *Nat Rev Nephrol* 8:265–274, 2012.
163. Boivin A, Luo ZC, Audibert F, et al: Pregnancy complications among women born preterm. *CMAJ* 184:1777–1784, 2012.
165. Keijzer-Veen MG, Kleinveld HA, Lequin MH, et al: Renal function and size at young adult age after intrauterine growth restriction and very premature birth. *Am J Kidney Dis* 50:542–551, 2007.
170. Richardson LJ, Hussey JM, Strutz KL: Origins of disparities in cardiovascular disease: birth weight, body mass index, and young adult systolic blood pressure in the National Longitudinal Study of Adolescent Health. *Ann Epidemiol* 21:598–607, 2011.
209. Hodgin JB, Rasoulpour M, Markowitz GS, et al: Very low birth weight is a risk factor for secondary focal segmental glomerulosclerosis. *Clin J Am Soc Nephrol* 4:71–76, 2009.
225. Moritz KM, Wintour EM, Black MJ, et al: Factors influencing mammalian kidney development: implications for health in adult life. *Adv Anat Embryol Cell Biol* 196:1–78, 2008.
226. Walker KA, Bertram JF: Kidney development: core curriculum 2011. *Am J Kidney Dis* 57:948–958, 2011.
245. Merlet-Benichou C, Vilar J, Lelievre-Pegorier M, et al: Role of retinoids in renal development: pathophysiological implication. *Curr Opin Nephrol Hypertens* 8:39–43, 1999.
261. Amri K, Freund N, Vilar J, et al: Adverse effects of hyperglycemia on kidney development in rats: in vivo and in vitro studies. *Diabetes* 48:2240–2245, 1999.
314. Grijalva-Eternod CS, Lawlor DA, Wells JC: Testing a capacity-load model for hypertension: disentangling early and late growth effects on childhood blood pressure in a prospective birth cohort. *PLoS ONE* 8:e56078, 2013.
315. Abitbol CL, Chandar J, Rodriguez MM, et al: Obesity and preterm birth: additive risks in the progression of kidney disease in children. *Pediatr Nephrol* 24:1363–1370, 2009.
317. Ozanne SE, Hales CN: Lifespan: catch-up growth and obesity in male mice. *Nature* 427:411–412, 2004.
343. Szabo AJ, Muller V, Chen GF, et al: Nephron number determines susceptibility to renal mass reduction-induced CKD in Lewis and Fisher 344 rats: implications for development of experimentally induced chronic allograft nephropathy. *Nephrol Dial Transplant* 23:2492–2495, 2008.
359. Giral M, Foucher Y, Karam G, et al: Kidney and recipient weight incompatibility reduces long-term graft survival. *J Am Soc Nephrol* 21:1022–1029, 2010.
364. Luyckx VA, Brenner BM: The clinical importance of nephron mass. *J Am Soc Nephrol* 21:898–910, 2010.
389. Goodyer P, Kurpad A, Rekha S, et al: Effects of maternal vitamin A status on kidney development: a pilot study. *Pediatr Nephrol* 22:209–214, 2007.
391. Hoy WE, Bertram JF, Denton RD, et al: Nephron number, glomerular volume, renal disease and hypertension. *Curr Opin Nephrol Hypertens* 17:258–265, 2008.

Aging and Kidney Disease

24

Devasmita Choudhury | Moshe Levi

CHAPTER OUTLINE

STRUCTURAL CHANGES IN THE AGING KIDNEY, 727
Gross, 727
Microscopic, 727
Biologic Mediators and Potential Modulators of Age-Related Renal Fibrosis, 728
FUNCTIONAL CHANGES IN THE AGING KIDNEY, 735
Renal Plasma Flow, 735
Glomerular Filtration Rate, 736
Sodium Conservation, 737
Sodium Excretion, 738
Urinary Concentration, 739
Urinary Dilution, 740
Acid-Base Balance, 740

Potassium Balance, 741
Calcium Balance, 741
Phosphate Balance, 742
RENAL DISEASE IN THE AGING KIDNEY, 742
Disorders of Osmoregulation, 742
Acute Kidney Injury, 742
Hypertension, 744
Renovascular Disease, 746
Glomerular Disease, 746
Chronic Kidney Disease, 747
Renal Replacement Therapy, 747
Renal Transplantation, 748
Urinary Tract Infection, 749
Renal Cysts, 750

Though the kidneys undergo change in structure and function with age, they are remarkable in maintaining the internal milieu unless renal reserve is challenged. Older kidneys adapt less well and recover more slowly after acute ischemic injury, infections, exposure to toxins, or immunologic processes, or in the presence of other organ dysfunction. For example, transplanted kidneys from older healthy donors are more prone to allograft dysfunction than younger donor kidneys.[1-5] In addition, subtle changes in function with age are associated with greater cardiovascular mortality in older adults.[6] With growing numbers of aging adults and increased longevity,[7] a greater number of elderly are more likely to experience chronic kidney disease[8] and progress to end-stage kidney disease (ESKD). Renal failure is present or develops in an estimated 30% of older hospitalized adults.[9] Therefore a careful study of the changes in kidney structure, function, and its ability to adapt to the short- and long-term physiologic changes with age becomes relevant to avoid unwanted outcomes in aging individuals.

STRUCTURAL CHANGES IN THE AGING KIDNEY

GROSS

Renal mass, size, weight, and volume decrease with normal aging. Kidney weight is found to decrease by as much as 15% to 20% with age, to 180 to 200 g (both kidneys) in those 90 years of age in comparison to 245 to 290 g in young adults, according to both radiologic and postmortem findings. These changes appear to be age appropriate in conjunction with a concurrent loss in body surface area.[10-14]

MICROSCOPIC

A gross decrease in kidney size and weight is accompanied by microscopic findings of glomerulosclerosis and tubulointerstitial fibrosis. A greater number of sclerotic glomeruli are present in donor kidney biopsy specimens from patients older than 55 years.[15] Intervening insults and comorbid conditions hasten the gradual and progressive senescence of the renal vasculature, glomeruli, tubules, and interstitium. Hypertension worsens sclerotic changes in the renal arteries. An increase in fibrointimal and medial sclerosis is present in cortical arteries of humans at age 70.[16] Interlobular and arcuate arteries of older donor kidneys demonstrate greater arteriolosclerosis than younger healthy donor kidneys. By age 70, ischemic changes, including lobulation of the glomerular tuft, increased mesangial volume, and capillary collapse and obliteration, are present in the cortical nephrons. Little cellular response is evident, with hyaline deposition in the residual glomeruli (Figure 24.1).[17,18] Peritubular capillary density is decreased, offering a reason for the lower concentrations of pro-angiogenic vascular endothelial growth factors and increased expression of

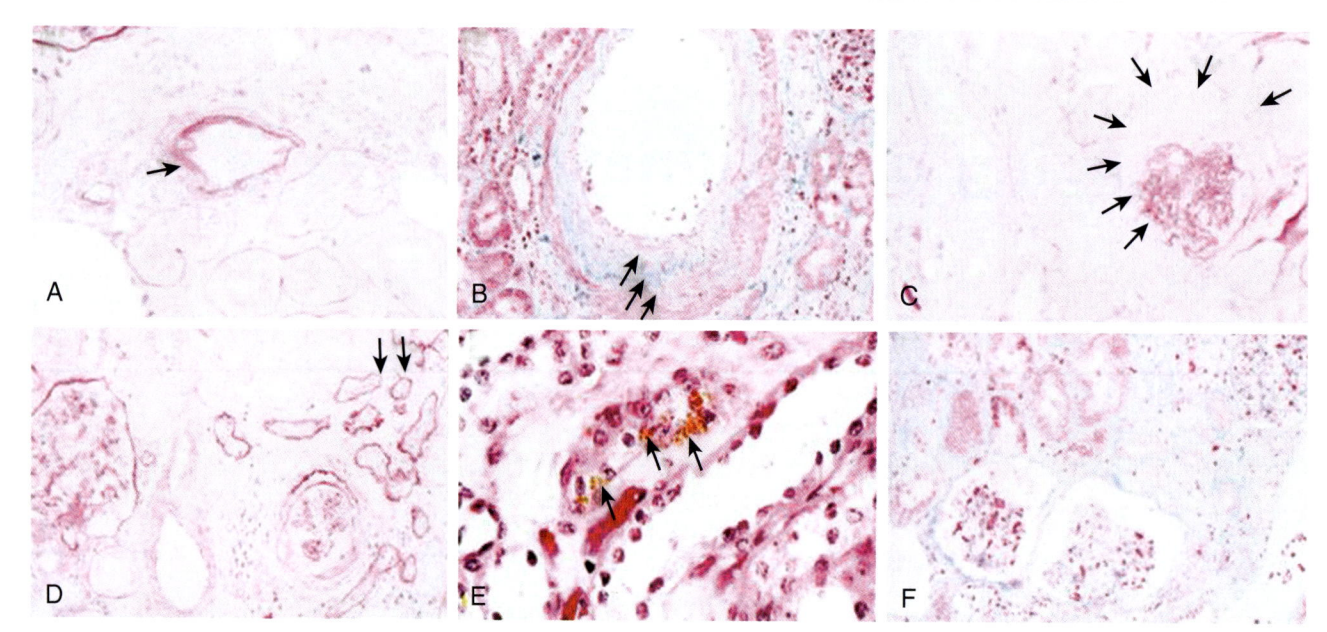

Figure 24.1 Histologic features of renal senescence. **A,** Arteriohyalinosis. **B,** Fibrous intimal thickening. **C,** Glomerulosclerosis. **D,** Tubular atrophy. **E,** Lipofuscin pigment. **F,** Interstitial fibrosis. (Courtesy Dr. Marjan Afrouzian, Edmonton, Alberta, Canada.)

anti-angiogenic thrombospondin in aging rats.[19] Basement membrane thickening and wrinkling in both glomeruli and tubules along with changes in the renal vasculature lead to progressive reduction and simplification of vascular channels, shunting blood from afferent to efferent arterioles of the juxtamedullary glomeruli.[20,21] Intact arteriolar vasa rectae continue to deliver adequate blood flow to the renal medulla.

As glomeruli sclerose, tubular atrophy follows, with a decrease in size and number. Tubules atrophy to form distal diverticula that may lead to early renal cysts frequently seen in older kidneys.[22] Debris and bacterial accumulation in these structures may account for the increased incidence of infection in aging individuals.

Animal studies indicate that tubulointerstitial fibrosis may precede the development of focal glomerulosclerosis and tubular atrophy.[23,24] Morphometry in aging mice suggests greater tubulointerstitial fibrosis in males than females.[25] Aging rodents with accelerated apoptosis demonstrate interstitial inflammation with fibroblast activation. Immunostaining showing adhesive proteins osteopontin and intracellular adhesion molecule-1 (ICAM-1) as well as deposition of collagen IV are associated with focal tubular proliferation, myofibroblast activation, and macrophage infiltration in aged rat kidneys. The trigger for inflammation leading to focal glomerulosclerosis and tubular atrophy may be altered endothelial nitric oxide synthase (eNOS) expression in the presence of peritubular atrophy.[26] Increased collagen-1 protein accumulation with age correlates with the extent of interstitial fibrosis,[27,28] highlighting perhaps the importance of collagen-1 in age-associated interstitial fibrosis. Further molecular probing of aged kidneys reveals increased levels of the cell cycle inhibitor p16INK4a with age, glomerulosclerosis, and interstitial fibrosis.[29] Because glomerulosclerosis can result from podocyte damage and loss, various mechanisms—adrenergic activation, increased free cytosolic calcium, low nitric oxide bioavailability, elevated endothelin-1 levels, and increases in oxidative stress and telomere shortening—are pathogenic processes that lead to podocyte dysfunction with subsequent age-related glomerulosclerosis.[30] Critical telomere shortening, a marker of replicative senescence, is evident in aging renal cortical tissue. Telomere DNA repeats shorten with each cell replication, acting as a mitotic clock. However stress may also induce premature structural changes and lead to early senescence.[31,32]

BIOLOGIC MEDIATORS AND POTENTIAL MODULATORS OF AGE-RELATED RENAL FIBROSIS

The finding that nearly a third of healthy elderly have little functional decline in renal clearance with age while two thirds show a gradual decline of renal function[33,34] prompts the need to understand the factors mediating and modulating fibrosis (Figure 24.2). Kidneys of aging animals have demonstrated changes in both level and function of various mediators of fibrosis, such as angiotensin II (Ang II), transforming growth factor-β (TGF-β), nitric oxide (NO), advanced glycosylation end products (AGEs), oxidative stress, inflammation, and lipids. Similarly, factors and processes have been identified that oppose fibrosis, such as Klotho, vitamin D and its receptor, the farnesoid X receptor (FXR), and autophagy. These may be potential and feasible targets for modulating progressive sclerosis in aging.

ANGIOTENSIN II

Effects of Ang II on filtration, growth modulation, oxidative stress, apoptosis, and extracellular matrix accumulation influence the rate of glomerulosclerosis and tubulointerstitial fibrosis in kidney aging.[35-39] Intraglomerular hypertension with efferent vasoconstriction in aging glomeruli increases sclerosis.[40] Angiotensin-converting enzyme (ACE) inhibition in aged rats decreases intrarenal vascular resistance and intracapillary protein leak[41] as well

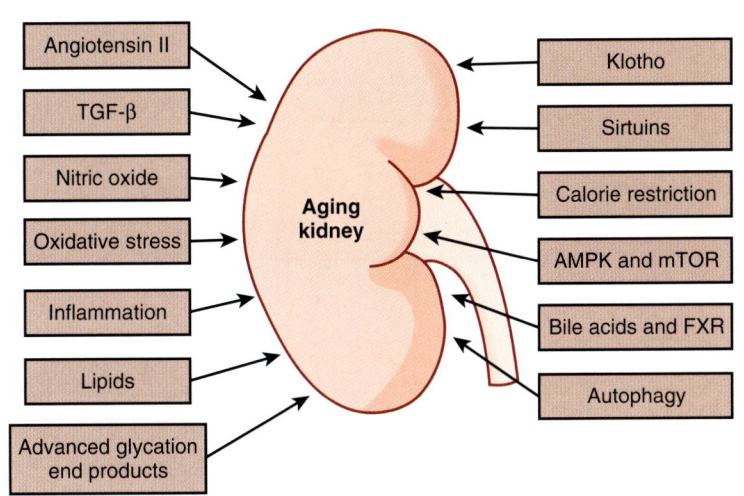

Figure 24.2 Factors that increase and decrease age-related renal glomerulosclerosis and tubulointerstitial fibrosis. AMPK, Adenosine monophosphate–activated protein kinase; FXR, farnesoid X receptor; mTOR, mammalian target of rapamycin; TGF-β, transforming growth factor-β.

as postprandial hyperfiltration.[42] An overall decrease in glomerulosclerosis is also observed in aged mice treated with ACE inhibitors (ACEIs) in comparison with untreated age- and sex-matched mice.[43-47] Although measured renin and angiotensin levels seem not to decrease with age, intrarenal downregulation of renin messenger RNA (mRNA) and ACE levels occur in aged rats.

Profibrotic effects of Ang II—inducing TGF-β to promote collagen IV, promoting influx of monocytes/macrophages, stimulating mRNA and protein expression of the chemokine RANTES (regulated on activation, normal T cell expressed and secreted) in endothelial cells, and also inducing transcription of the pro-inflammatory chemokine monocyte chemoattractant protein-1 (MCP-1) via NO inhibition—are significantly reduced with ACEI treatment.[48-51] Use of enalapril in aged rats showed marked reduction in tubulointerstitial fibrosis and smooth muscle actin in comparison with rats either treated with nifedipine or untreated, independent of blood pressure control.[51] Matrix accumulation via Ang II's effect on plasminogen activator inhibitor-1 (PAI-1) was also decreased with angiotensin antagonists,[41,52,53] as were vascular sclerosis and collagen content.[54] Ang II antagonists were found to prevent increases in age-related mitochondrial oxidants and dysfunction in aged rats.[55] Furthermore, mouse Klotho gene transfer to Sprague-Dawley rats ameliorated Ang II–mediated renal damage.[56]

Renal protective effects of ACEI and angiotensin receptor blockers (ARBs) in aging kidneys are mediated by many complementary mechanisms, including prevention of age-related increases in oxidative stress and glycation end products, and decreases in eNOS and Klotho.[57-63] Furthermore, disruption of type 1 angiotensin II receptor (AT1R) in mice increases longevity and prevents cardiovascular and renal pathology mediated in part via increased oxidative stress and increased mitochondrial upregulation of survival genes nicotinamide phosphoribosyltransferase (Nampt) and Sirtuin 3 (Sirt3) in the kidney.[64] Angiotensin II, via its diverse AT_{1A} receptor signaling pathways in the kidney and cardiovascular system,[65] appears to play a crucial role in kidney aging, although data specific to humans have yet to be generated.

TRANSFORMING GROWTH FACTOR-β

TGF-β, an active modulator of tissue repair, is associated with age-related renal scarring. Gradual renal fibrosis with age likely results from normal and/or pathologic wound healing with tissue repair after injury. Persistent or repeated renal injury or insult may hasten tissue fibrosis. Various factors can stimulate TGF-β, including Ang II, abnormal glucose metabolism, platelet-derived growth factors (PDGFs), hypoxia, oxidative stress, mesangial stretch, and high AGE levels. TGF-β promotes gene transcription with matrix protein production and accumulation of collagens III, IV, and I, fibronectin, tenascin, osteonectin, osteopontin, thrombospondin, and matrix glycosaminoglycans,[66,67] with subsequent glomerulosclerosis and tubulointerstitial fibrosis.[68-71] Haplotype association mapping of genetic loci of chromosome 6 in aged mice reveals increased expression of *Far2* in those mice that have increased mesangial matrix expansion. Overexpression of *Far2* in mice mesangial cells leads to upregulation of PDGF and TGF-β.[72] The renal interstitium in aged rats has increased TGF-β mRNA.[24,73] Signaling by TGF-β and the protein SMAD3 adds to microRNA 21 (miR-21) production. Renal fibrosis secondary to injury depends on miR-21. MicroRNA-21 content is noted to be increased in the renal cortex of older mice than in that of both young and middle-aged mice, suggesting that age-specific regulation of matrix protein synthesis involves matrix protein–specific transcription and posttranscription mechanisms (Figure 24.3).[67] Angiotensin II inhibition downregulates TGF-β, resulting in decreased interstitial fibrosis.[73] Although increased TGF-β expression may contribute in part to age-related sclerosis, direct evidence to implicate TGF-β needs further investigation. Decorin antisense oligonucleotides inhibit TGF-β expression and function and may provide better understanding of the role TGF-β plays in age-related sclerosis. The peptide hormone relaxin, produced by the prostate and the pregnant ovary, has antifibrotic properties. Use of relaxin in relaxin-deficient 12-month male knockout mice improved established interstitial fibrosis, glomerulosclerosis, and cortical thickening, with a decrease in collagen content via direct action on TGF-β–stimulated fibroblasts to decrease collagen I and

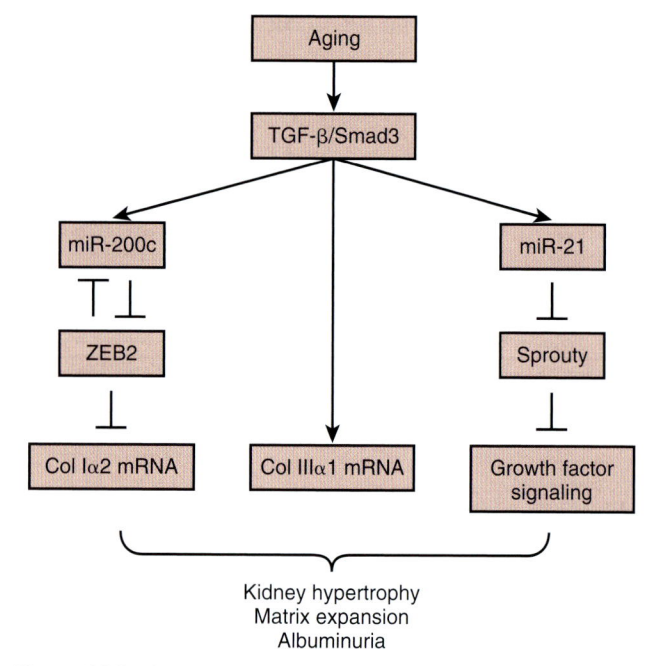

Figure 24.3 Suggested pathway of microRNA's effect on matrix protein and expansion in aged mice, including the products of genes *Sprouty, Smad3,* and *ZEB2*. Col, Collagen; miR, micro-RNA; mRNA, messenger RNA;TGF-β, transforming growth factor-β. (From Wolf G: Link between angiotensin II and TGF-beta in the kidney. *Miner Electrolyte Metab.* 24:174-180, 1998.)

III.[74,75] Relaxin, via its primary receptor, RXFP1, and NO pathway, inhibits Smad2 phosphorylation. Smad2 inhibition prevents TGF-β signaling, which is responsible for myofibroblast differentiation as well as collagen and fibronectin production, thereby regulating matrix synthesis.[76] Studies in relaxin knockout mice indicate that relaxin and castration may decrease the renal fibrosis seen with age.[77]

NITRIC OXIDE

Although nitric oxide is found to moderate fibrosis, low NO levels in the aging renal vasculature is thought to mediate renal fibrosis with age. Vascular reactivity is an immediate response to nitric oxide, but its paracrine effects—to decrease fibrosis by inhibiting the nuclear factor κ light chain enhancer of activated B cells (NF-κB) family of transcription factors—can be important for the aging kidney. NF-κB promotes monocyte/macrophage influx in the presence of reactive oxygen species (ROS), with progression to injury and inflammation.[78,79] Aging vessels have lower levels of NO.[80,81] Oxidation stress also induces nicotinamide adenine dinucleotide phosphate oxidase (NADPH oxidase)–mediated NO scavenging and NO depletion in aged kidneys.[82] Peritubular capillaries of aged rats express less eNOS,[26] a change that can lead to chronic tubulointerstitial ischemia and fibrosis. Treatment with dietary L-arginine supplementation in older rats improves renal plasma flow (RPF) and glomerular filtration (GFR) and decreases proteinuria and glomerulosclerosis.[83] L-arginine supplementation also reduces kidney collagen and Nε-(carboxymethyl) lysine accumulation.[84] Hypoxia, oxidative stress, increased dietary protein intake, insulin resistance, as well as increased angiotensin II activity are factors thought to decrease eNOS with age, so that use of angiotensin inhibitors and or dietary protein restriction seem to increase and normalize urinary NO excretion.[81-89] Lower eNOS levels in males than in females are also thought to be the reason behind the sexual dimorphism seen in the aging kidney.[90] Lower glomerular arginine transport is noted in male than in female rodents.[91] Changes in estrogen and androgen activity may in part mediate the sex-dependent effects.

With aging, there is a noted decrease in eNOS phosphorylation and activity in endothelial cells from human umbilical veins.[92] The eNOS phosphorylation induced at serine 1177 by Akt (protein kinase B) is critical in regulation of eNOS activity.[89] Age-related decreases in eNOS activity are reversed by inhibition of (1) oxidative stress with use of α-lipoic acid,[93] (2) the generation of ceramide levels,[94] or (3) arginase.[95] Studies examining endothelial cells from brachial arteries and peripheral veins from subjects with vascular endothelial dysfunction suggest that increased endothelin-1 activity and not decreased eNOS activity is more to blame for endothelial dysfunction with age.[96,97]

ADVANCED GLYCOSYLATION END PRODUCTS

Cross-links between proteins, lipids, and nucleic acids (AGEs) accumulate over time with age to produce vascular and tissue damage.[98,99] Hyperglycemia accelerates the rate of end product accumulation and tissue damage.[100] Glycated proteins decrease vascular elasticity, induce endothelial cell permeability, and increase monocyte chemotactic activity via AGE–receptor ligand binding, which stimulates activation of macrophages and secretion of cytokines and growth factors. Disturbance of NO-induced vascular endothelial vasodilation, thought to be secondary to chemical inactivation of endothelium-relaxing factor, occurs with endothelial and basement membrane AGE deposition.[101-104] Diabetic patients display perturbations of the vascular endothelium similar to those in persons with age-related vasculopathy. Older animal kidneys demonstrate increased AGE and AGE receptor (RAGE) levels.[98] Accumulation of AGEs in the kidney increases mesangial matrix, basement membrane thickening, and vascular permeability and induces PDGF and TGF-β, leading to glomerulosclerosis and tubulointerstitial fibrosis.[101] Gradual age-related GFR loss—in addition to an increase in oxidative stress that modifies glycated proteins, as well as accumulation of Nε-(carboxymethyl) lysine—contributes to increased AGE and RAGE in aged kidneys. Furthermore, abnormal glucose metabolism with age-related insulin resistance adds to protein glycation. Lifelong consumption of AGE-enriched foods as well as smoking also increase AGE load and tissue accumulation.[105,106]

The mesangial AGE receptor 1 (AGER1) has been shown to counter the proinflammatory mesangial cell response to AGE accumulation. Supersaturation and possible receptor downregulation under increased AGE burden may prevent AGER1 control.[107] Studies in embryonic kidney cells indicate that AGER1 counteracts AGE-induced cellular oxidant stress via prevention of p66shc-dependent FKHRL1 phosphorylation, thus inactivating FKHRL1 and MnSOD suppression.[108] P66shc knockout mice are protected against oxidative stress and oxidant-dependent injury, highlighting the importance of this pathway.[109] AGER1 provides protection also against AGE-induced generation of ROS via

NADPH.[110] Mice eating low-AGE diet over time have lower RAGE and higher AGER1 levels (Figure 24.4) and demonstrate less glomerulosclerosis and proteinuria (Figure 24.5).[111] Interestingly, AGER1 is suppressed in human subjects with chronic kidney disease. However, dietary decrease in AGE restores AGER1 levels.[112]

Results of aminoguanidine treatment and calorie restriction in aged animals suggest some possible treatment options for AGE-mediated aging and sclerosis. Prolonged aminoguanidine treatment of aged rats and rabbits caused decreases in proteinuria and glomerulosclerosis[113] in addition to age-related arterial stiffening and cardiac hypertrophy.[114] Furthermore, AGE-associated changes in vascular permeability and abnormal vasodilatory responses to acetylcholine and nitroglycerin reversed with aminoguanidine treatment.[115] Mononuclear cell activity was also prevented in aminoguanidine-treated animals. Similarly, 60% calorie restriction (CR) of the ad libitum diet of control rats decreased AGE burden with lowering of other glycated proteins, including Nε-(carboxymethyl)lysine and pentosidine, and increases life span.[116,117] Even a 30% calorie restriction in comparison with control diet produced a decrease in AGE accumulation in the renal glomeruli and abdominal aorta.[118] Therefore measures that can decrease AGE burden

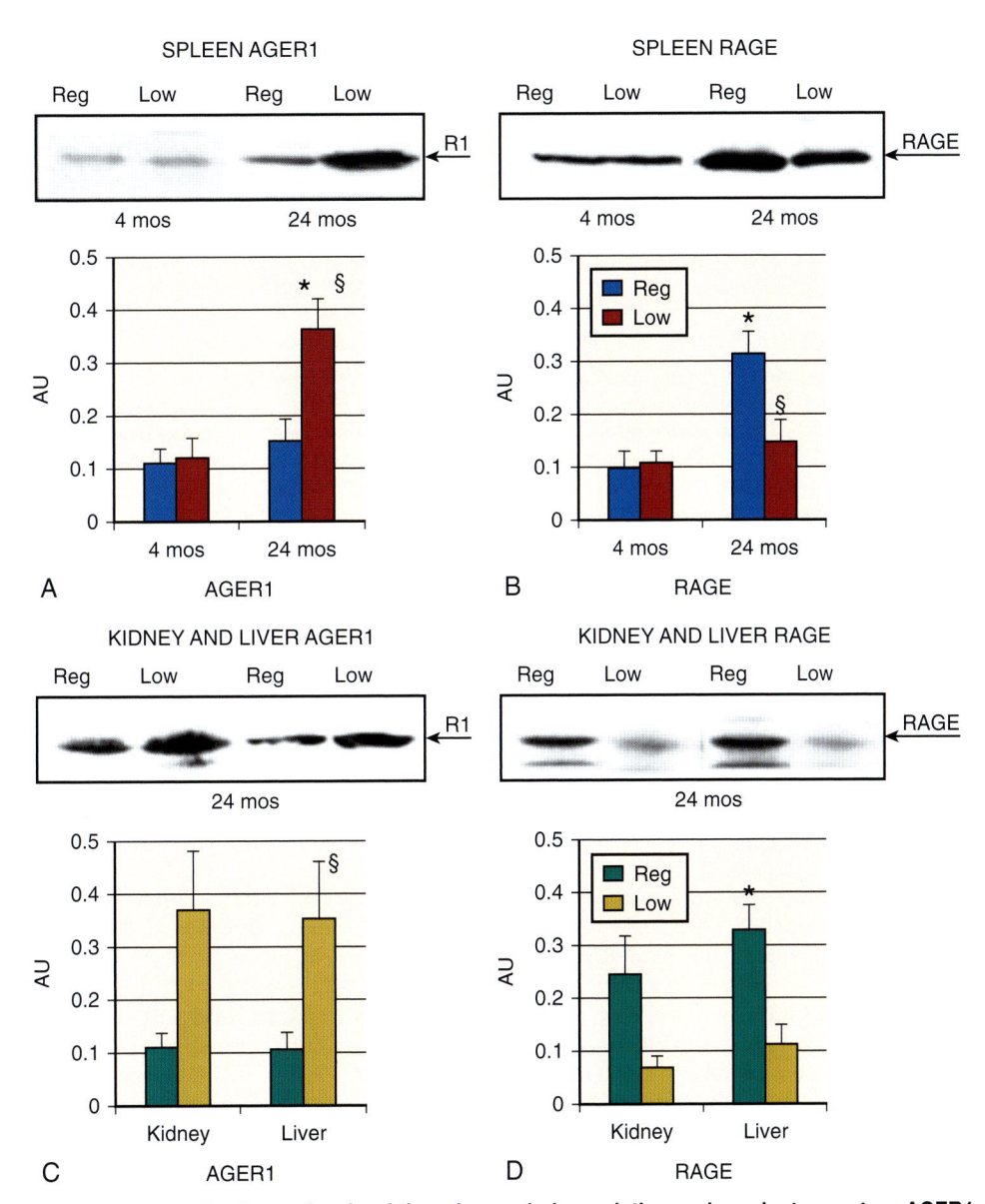

Figure 24.4 **Effect of a low-glycotoxin diet on levels of the advanced glycosylation end-product receptors AGER1 and RAGE.** Levels of the proteins AGER1 (**A**) and RAGE (**B**) were assessed in spleen tissues from mice consuming either a diet with normal high levels of advanced glycation end products (AGEs) (Reg$_{AGE}$) or a low-AGE diet (Low$_{AGE}$) ($n = 6$ per group) at 4 and 24 months. AGER1 expression (**C**) in kidney and liver and RAGE expression (**D**) in kidney and liver of the same mouse groups were also assessed at 24 months by Western blotting and densitometric analysis. Data are shown as mean ± standard error for three independent experiments. *Statistically significant difference compared with 4-month Reg$_{AGE}$ at the $P < 0.01$ level. §Statistically significant difference compared with 24-month Reg$_{AGE}$ at the $P < 0.01$ level. (From Cai W, et al: Reduced oxidant stress and extended lifespan in mice exposed to a low glycotoxin diet: association with increased AGER1 expression, *Am J Pathol* 170[6]:1893-1902, 2007.)

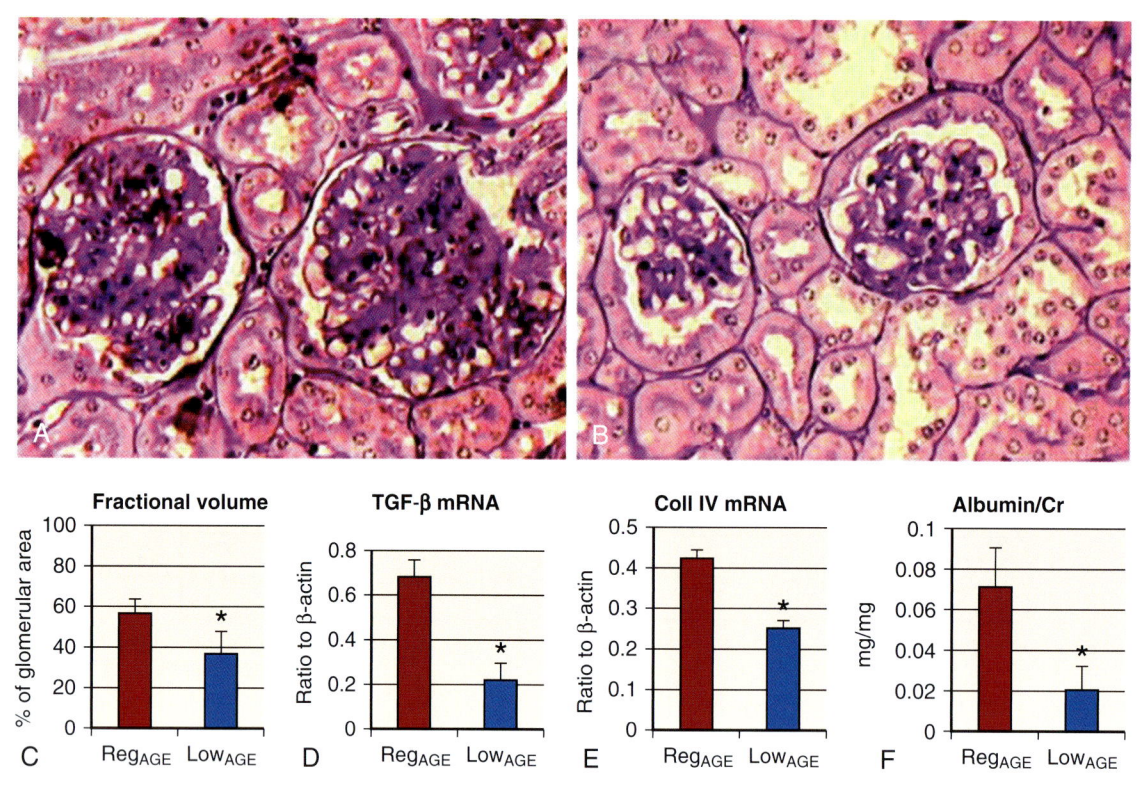

Figure 24.5 **Effect of a low-glycotoxin diet on glomeruli and renal function in mice.** Morphology of renal cortex (**A**) with consumption of a diet containing normal high levels of advanced glycosylation end products (AGEs) (Reg$_{AGE}$), and (**B**) after consumption of a low-AGE diet (Low$_{AGE}$) (n = 6 per group). (Periodic acid–Schiff stain, original magnification ×200.) **C,** Fractional mesangial volume (*$P < 0.05$) in Reg$_{AGE}$ versus Low$_{AGE}$ mice. **D,** Transforming growth factor-β (TGF-β) levels (*$P < 0.05$). **E,** Collagen type IV (Coll IV) messenger RNA (mRNA) levels (*$P < 0.05$). **F,** Albumin-to-creatinine ratio (*$P < 0.05$). Data are shown as mean ± standard error of triplicate values. (From Cai W, et al: Reduced oxidant stress and extended lifespan in mice exposed to a low glycotoxin diet: association with increased AGER1 expression. *Am J Pathol* 170:1893-1902, 2007.)

in aging individuals may be important in slowing age-related renal disease.

OXIDATIVE STRESS

Free radical generation and/or antioxidant enzyme deficiency leads to lipid peroxidation and oxidative stress, inducing tissue injury that can be seen with aging.[119-122] High levels of oxidized amino acids in the urine of older rats signify higher levels of oxidized skeletal muscle proteins.[123] Both thiobarbituric acid–reactive substances and levels of ROS are higher in aged kidneys and are associated with lipid peroxidative damage.[124] Isoprostanes, AGE, and RAGE as well as heme oxygenase, other markers of oxidative stress, and lipid peroxidation are also increased in aged rats.[125] *Klotho* gene expression in the distal inner medullary collecting duct (IMCD3) is reduced with oxidative stress in mouse cells,[126] implying other possible reasons for renal aging. Use of a diet enriched in the antioxidant vitamin E in aged rats lowers markers of oxidative stress, decreases glomerulosclerosis, and improves RPF and GFR.[125] ACEI use increases antioxidant enzyme activity and blocks TGF-β induction by ROS.[127,128] Antioxidant taurine also blocks ROS in cultured mesangial cells.[129] Tempol, a superoxide scavenger, restored the ability of ARBs to suppress oxygen consumption mediated via NO in renal cortical tissue.[82] These findings suggest angiotensin antagonists and antioxidants as possible therapeutic options to decrease age-related renal scarring.

Calorie restriction also reduces age-related oxidative stress, suppressing activation of mitogen-activated protein kinase cellular signaling pathways. Calorie restriction also decreases mitochondrial lipid peroxidation and membrane damage with concomitant decrease in apoptosis.[130,131] Thus dietary discrimination may be important in preventing age-associated renal sclerosis. Mitochondrial generation of ROS may also be contributing to age-associated diseases.[132,133] In several genetic mouse models of longevity, including Ames and Snell dwarf mice, p66sch knockout mice, and mice heterozygous for insulin-like growth factor receptor, longer life span correlates with increased resistance to oxidative stress.[134-138] Under-expression and over-expression of genes encoding for antioxidant enzymes show that superoxide dismutase 1 (copper-zinc superoxide dismutase or SOD1) knockout mice had decreased life span and greater oxidative stress. However transgenic SOD1 mice did not have a longer life span.[139] Effects of superoxide dismutase deletion or over-expression in age-related renal disease continue to be of interest, given the possible therapeutic targets.

CALORIE RESTRICTION: SIRTUINS, ADENOSINE MONOPHOSPHATE–ACTIVATED PROTEIN KINASE, MAMMALIAN TARGET OF RAPAMYCIN, AND RIBOSOMAL PROTEIN S6 KINASE 1A

Reducing calorie intake by 25% to 45% while maintaining intake of all essential nutrients increases longevity in many rodent strains as well as in fruit flies, worms, and yeasts.[140-145] In addition, disease related to older age, including insulin resistance, atherosclerosis, oxidative damage, and immune dysfunction, are also decreased in calorie-restricted rhesus monkeys.[146-153] Furthermore, mortality is decreased in these monkeys as the incidence of diabetes, cancer, cardiovascular disease, and brain atrophy lessens.[154] A similar benefit is seen in human health, although the effect of longevity is yet to be reported.[155,156] Rats and mice have also shown a decrease in age-related proteinuria and glomerulosclerosis with calorie restriction.[157,158]

The potential mechanisms and proposed benefits of calorie restriction are numerous, including reduced body fat content, decreased metabolic rate, attenuation of oxidative stress and inflammation, modulation of mitochondrial function, and increases in sirtuin activity, and adenosine monophosphate (AMP)–activated protein kinase (AMPK) signaling, and decreases in mTOR (mammalian target of rapamycin) and S6K1 (ribosomal protein S6 kinase 1) signaling.[159-161] Sir2 (silent information regulator 2), first identified in yeast, mediates nicotinamide adenine dinucleotide (NAD)–dependent histone deacetylase enzyme activity. At least seven mammalian homologs have been identified, sirtuins SIRT1 through SIRT7. Present in different subcellular compartments, these enzymes cause histone deacetylation, thereby controlling activity of various proteins and genes regulating cell survival, differentiation, and metabolism, DNA repair, inflammation, and longevity.[162-164] Calorie restriction seems to increase SIRT1 activity in most tissues, including kidneys.[165-170] Further support is seen in SIRT1 knockout mouse, which show resistance to effects of calorie restriction[171]; in contrast, SIRT1 transgenic mice show a phenotype similar to that of mice given a calorie-restricted diet.[172-174] Mice treated with resveratrol, a synthetic activator of SIRT1, behave similarly to calorie-restricted mice, including being protected against age-related renal disease.[175-179] Calorie restriction also increases SIRT1-induced FOXO3 (forkhead Box3) deacetylation, resulting in increases in Bnip3 (BCL2/adenovirus E1B 19 kDa protein–interacting protein3) and mitochondrial autophagy as well as prevention of age-dependent decreases in kidney function.[180] Sirtuins thus have diverse physiologic functions extending beyond their important role in the process of aging.

A complex regulation of metabolic pathways in response to calorie restriction integrates the effects of the restriction on insulin release, AMPK, SIRT1, and FOXO activation as well as mTOR inhibition.[181-183] Exercise and fasting have similar metabolic effects, regulating AMPK, SIRT1, peroxisome proliferator–activated receptor γ coactivator 1α (PGC-1α), and FOXO activity. Because aging is associated with decreased SIRT1 activity secondary to decreased systemic NAD$^+$ synthesis[184] as well as reduced AMPK activity and mitochondrial biogenesis,[185] these findings are very important. Thus activation of SIRT1 and AMPK activity holds promise for the prevention of age-related metabolic defects and disease.[186]

In addition, SIRT1 deacetylates and positively regulates the oxysterol-activated nuclear receptor LXR (liver X receptor),[187] which plays an important role in mediating reverse cholesterol efflux and inhibiting inflammation, adding further complexity to metabolic regulation. SIRT1 also deacetylates the bile acid–activated nuclear receptor FXR (farnesoid X receptor),[188] a bile acid activated nuclear hormone receptor that plays an important role in inhibiting fatty acid synthesis mediated by sterol regulatory element binding protein-1 (SREBP-1) and also inflammation, oxidative stress, and fibrosis. Although the effects of LXR on renal disease and aging remain to be determined, LXR activation prevents progression of diabetic kidney disease.[186] Activation of FXR using both natural and synthetic bile acid analogs modulates lipid metabolism, preventing development and progression of proteinuria in mouse models of type 2 diabetes mellitus, diet-induced obesity, and insulin resistance.[189-191] Whether FXR agonists would have similar effects on aged rodent and human kidneys needs to be determined.

Studies also suggest potential important roles for mTOR and S6K1 in regulating mammalian life span. Treatment with rapamycin, an mTOR inhibitor, of older male and female mice extended their life span.[192] In fact, long-lived Ames dwarf mice have reduced mTOR signaling.[193,194] Mechanistic studies in yeast indicate that deletion or inhibition of TOR upregulates mitochondrial gene expression and prevents cellular accumulation of ROS.[195] Deletion of S6K1, a component of the nutrient-responsive mTOR signaling pathway, results in longer life span and reductions in resistance to insulin and to diverse age-related pathologies.[196] Intriguingly, S6K1-induced gene expression patterns are similar to those seen with calorie restriction and activation of AMPK.

LIPID METABOLISM

Various studies have found altered expression of a number of transcriptional factors and nuclear hormone receptors regulating lipid metabolism in both chronic kidney disease (CKD)[197-199] and aging.[157] Expression of both SREBP-1 and SREBP-2 is increased in the liver and adipose tissue of animal models of CKD.[197-200] As master regulators of fatty acid, triglyceride, and cholesterol synthesis, these transcription factors are associated with increased serum lipid levels and insulin resistance.[197-199] In addition, decreased peroxisome proliferator–activated receptor-α (PPARα) results in impaired fatty acid oxidation.[200] These changes mimic those seen in kidneys of animals with nephritic syndrome and with aging.[158,201-205]

Activity and expression of FXR are also decreased in livers of aging mice.[206] FXR plays an important role in regulation of bile acid, fatty acid, cholesterol, and glucose metabolism in the liver and kidney.[189,207] Decreased FXR activity may mediate increased SREBP-1 activity and decreased PPARα expression and activity in aging. Calorie restriction can prevent age-related changes in metabolic function, and studies indicate that it also prevents age-related increases in SREBP-1 expression and decreases in PPARα.[140,208-210]

The expression of SIRT1 is increased with calorie restriction. Sirtuin analogs seem to replicate several beneficial effects of such restriction, including adipogenesis, insulin sensitivity and signaling, and lipid metabolism.[173,175,211,212] Likewise, SIRT1 transgenic mice show phenotypes resembling the phenotype found in mice given calorie-restricted diets.[172,203]

Experimental data in animals[213,214] and observational data in humans suggest that dyslipidemia adds to the burden of disease progression in those with kidney disease.[129,215-221] Low high-density lipoprotein (HDL) cholesterol levels in aging adults appear to be associated with a greater decline in GFR.[222,223] This finding suggests that lipid lowering may be beneficial in those with CKD. Post hoc subgroup analysis of several prospective trials showed that subjects given 3-hydroxy-3 methylglutaryl-coenzyme A reductase (HMG-CoA) inhibitors (statins) had slower decrease in renal function and proteinuria than subjects not given statins. Pooled data from 3402 patients with CKD stage 3 from three large randomized double-blind trials comparing pravastatin 40 mg/day with placebo showed a 34% reduction in the slope of estimated GFR (eGFR), based on the Modification of Diet in Renal Disease (MDRD) study equation, with an absolute reduction of 0.22 mL/min/1.73 m^2 per year (95% confidence interval [CI] 0.07 to 0.37) in patients using statins in comparison with those given placebo.[224] Meta-analysis of other randomized trials also noted a slower decline, by 1.2 mL/min/1.73 m^2 per year, and lower protein excretion in statin-treated subjects in comparison with subjects given placebo.[225,226] Post hoc analysis in the Stroke Prevention by Aggressive Reduction in Cholesterol Levels (SPARCL) trial, which involved 4719 patients with 5-year follow-up, showed that of the 1600 patients who had eGFR levels lower than 60 mL/min and mean age of 68 years, those who were randomly assigned to receive 80 mg daily of atorvastatin had an increase in eGFR of 3.46 ± 0.33 mL/min, compared with 1.42 ± 0.34 mL/min in the placebo group, independent of baseline function.[227] A decrease in protein excretion has not been seen in all trials with statins. Favorable effects of statins on protein excretion were noted on meta-analysis when protein excretion was greater than 30 mg/day.[228] However, statins might also exert their beneficial effects by suppressing inflammation and improving endothelial function and vessel stiffness.[229] In the substudy of the Lescol Intervention Prevention Study, creatinine clearance as calculated with the Cockcroft-Gault equation remained stable for both fluvastatin-treated and placebo groups regardless of baseline renal function.[230] Comparison of serum creatinine levels at baseline and end of treatment for pooled data of 10,000 patients using rosuvastatin (5-40 mg) in comparison with those using other statins and those receiving placebo for mean of 8 weeks showed no change in serum creatinine in either statin-treated or the placebo group. However, for those patients who continued to take rosuvastatin over 96 weeks, MDRD-estimated GFR either remained unchanged or increased but did not decrease from baseline.[231] Post hoc analysis and meta-analysis randomized studies using statins on primary cardiovascular outcomes suggest either stability of GFR or possible improvement in renal function and/or proteinuria with treatment, but there are no primary prevention trials examining the effect of statins on the outcome of renal function in the elderly. Therefore, with no clear-cut evidence of the effectiveness of statins for primary renoprotection, use of these agents for renoprotection alone in the elderly remains premature.

BILE ACID METABOLISM AND THE FARNESOID X RECEPTOR

Studies in a long-lived dwarf mutant mouse, the little mouse ($Ghrhr^{lit/lit}$), which does not secrete growth hormone (GH) and therefore has very low circulating levels of GH and insulin-like growth factor-1 (IGF-1), have identified a potential role for alterations in xenobiotic metabolism mediated by FXR in association with longevity in these mice.[232] A possible role for bile acids as endocrine regulators of aging has also been found in *Caenorhabditis elegans*, in which bile acid–like steroids influence life span via the DAF-12 nuclear receptor.[233] Although the age-related renal pathology in long-lived dwarf mutant mice has not been well studied, research involving diet-induced obesity in diabetic mice treated with FXR agonists indicates that these agents decrease proteinuria and glomerulosclerosis by modulating renal lipid metabolism, oxidative stress, inflammation, and fibrosis.[189,190] Whether FXR can also modulate age-related renal disease remains to be determined.

KLOTHO

The *Klotho* gene can be identified as an "aging gene" that has multiple effects regulating the aging process, mineral metabolism, and other endocrine functions.[234,235] Mice with defects in *Klotho* gene expression exhibit multiple aging-like phenotypes and die prematurely, whereas transgenic mice that overexpress the *Klotho* gene live longer than wild-type mice.[236,237] The mechanisms of the anti-aging effects of Klotho are still being determined, but potential mechanisms include effects on antioxidative stress as well as modulation of insulin and IGF-1 signaling processes.[234,235] *Klotho* is strongly expressed in the kidney and plays an important role in the regulation of fibroblast growth factor 23 signaling, phosphate transport activity, TRPV5 (transient receptor potential cation channel subfamily V member 5) activity, and ROMK1 (regulation of Kir 1.1 potassium channel) activity.[234,235] Specific deletion of *Klotho* in the mouse kidney resulted in a phenotype similar to that observed in *Klotho* knockout mice, suggesting that the kidney may be a primary organ for *Klotho*'s effects.[238,239] Studies suggest that Klotho protein may endogenously block Wnt/β-catenin signaling, which promotes fibrogenesis. Secreted Klotho suppressed myofibroblast activation, reduced matrix expression, and ameliorated renal fibrosis. Klotho inhibited expression of its target genes in tubular epithelial cells in addition to blocking Wnt-triggered activation and nuclear translocation of β-catenin. TGF-β$_1$ suppresses *Klotho* expression, with concomitant β-catenin activation; however, *Klotho* overexpression abrogates the fibrogenic effects of TGF-β1. Further, in vivo expression of secreted Klotho in both Adriamycin and ureteral obstruction mouse models of CKD inhibited the activation of renal β-catenin and expression of its target genes. Thus because *Klotho* is an antagonist of endogenous Wnt/β-catenin activity, its loss may contribute to kidney injury by removing the repression of pathogenic Wnt/β-catenin signaling.[240]

Other studies also indicate that renal actions of Ang II are mediated via modulation of renal *Klotho* expression.[56] In addition, the effects of the PPARγ agonists,[241] including their beneficial effects in age-related renal disease,[242] are mediated by regulation of intrarenal *Klotho* expression.

AUTOPHAGY

Phagolysosomal degradation of cytosolic debris, including organelles and proteins, known as *autophagy*, is noted to decrease with age. Accumulation of cellular waste leads to progressive cellular aging as seen from altered mitochondrial morphology and accumulation of age-related proteins

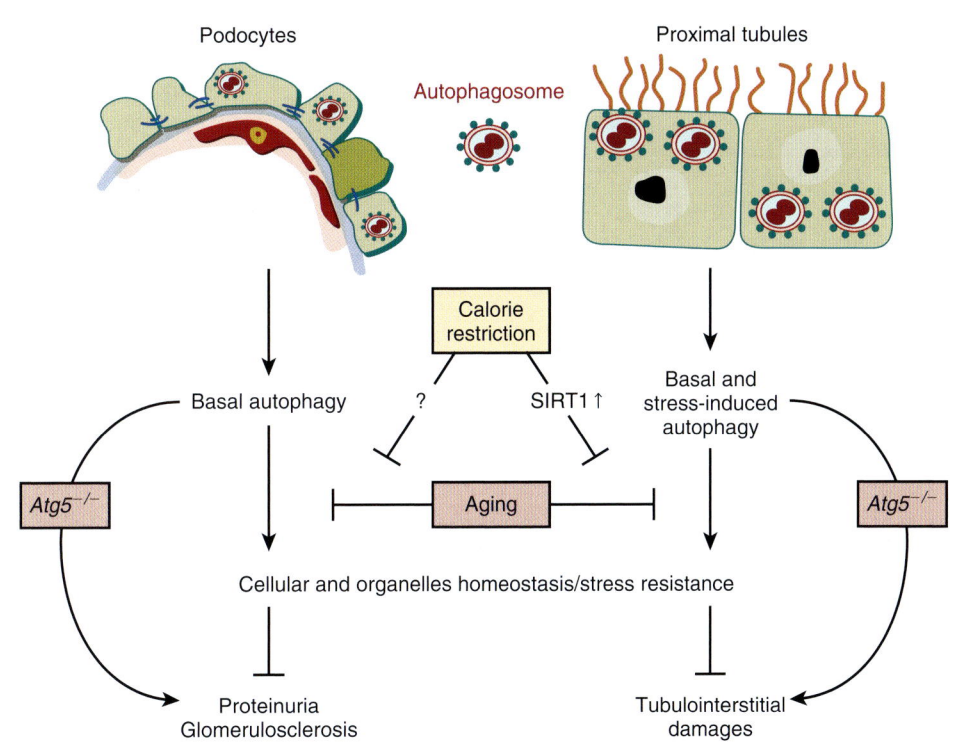

Figure 24.6 Autophagy in kidney aging. In both podocytes and proximal tubular cells, autophagy maintains cellular and organelles homeostasis under both basal and stress conditions. Normal aging process or a deletion of *Atg5* gene alters autophagy in podocytes and proximal tubular cells, leading to kidney aging. Calorie restriction prevents the progression of kidney aging in part through *SIRT1*-dependent autophagy. (From Huber TB, et al: Emerging role of autophagy in kidney function, diseases and aging. *Autophagy* 8:1009-1031, 2012; © 2012 Landes Bioscience.)

such as SQSTM1 in kidneys of aging rats and mice.[243,244] Renal tubular epithelial cells and podocytes process a high filtrate burden and therefore have an abundance of cellular cytoplasmic organelles, including mitochondria and endoplasmic reticulum, that are reprocessed via autophagy to maintain cellular integrity and conserve nutrient and energy. How this process prevents aging in podocytes and proximal tubular cells is becoming evident.[243,245] Gene deletion of *Atg5* gene in podocytes results in damaged mitochondrial debris and ubiquinated proteins in podocytes, leading to age-dependent albuminuria and glomerulosclerosis.[244,245] Similarly *Atg5* gene deletion in proximal renal tubular cells leads to accumulation of damaged mitochondria, ubiquinated proteins, and SQSTM1, thereby increasing proximal tubule cell apoptosis.[244,246] Calorie restriction physiologically induces autophagy via SIRT1-mediated deacetylation of FOXO3/FOXO3A and continues to be investigated as a possible mechanism in the intervention to decrease renal aging[244] (Figure 24.6).

FUNCTIONAL CHANGES IN THE AGING KIDNEY

RENAL PLASMA FLOW

Effective renal plasma flow decreases by 10% per decade in healthy aging adults, the rate of decline being greater in men than in women (Figure 24.7).[247] Cortical blood flow decreases in parallel with observed histologic changes but medullary blood flow remains preserved. A fractional decrease in the cardiac output to the kidneys in addition to structural changes in the vessels and vascular responsiveness are also thought to decrease renal blood flow.[248,249] Use of potent vasodilators, such as intraarterial acetylcholine,[250] intravenous pyrogen, and atrial natriuretic peptide (ANP), results in a blunted vasodilatory response in older individuals in comparison with the response in younger individuals.[251] Similarly, although increases in GFR and RPF are seen with amino acid infusion and low-dose dopamine in healthy older subjects, the degree of vasodilation is less than in younger subjects.[252,253] Higher levels of the eNOS inhibitor asymmetric dimethyl arginine (ADMA) are found with rising age, which has an inverse association with effective renal plasma flow rate (ERPF) in healthy and hypertensive elderly.[254] Whether tubular cell senescence and the inability to degrade ADMA lead to higher levels of ADMA with aging is not clear. One study reported that an overexpression of dimethylaminohydrolase, the enzyme that hydrolyzes ADMA to dimethylamine and citrulline, in five of six nephrectomized rats ameliorated sclerotic glomerular changes.[255] Cell senescence thus may contribute to the vascular changes in response seen with age.

An imbalance in the vasodilatory and vasoconstrictive mediators can also alter intrarenal signaling and affect renal vasculature and RPF. NO production in isolated conduit arteries decreases with age,[256-258] and levels of NOS and L-arginine are low.[258,259] However, gene expression for substrate synthesis remains unaffected.[260] Prostacyclin (prostaglandin I$_2$ [PGI$_2$]) is decreased in aging human vascular

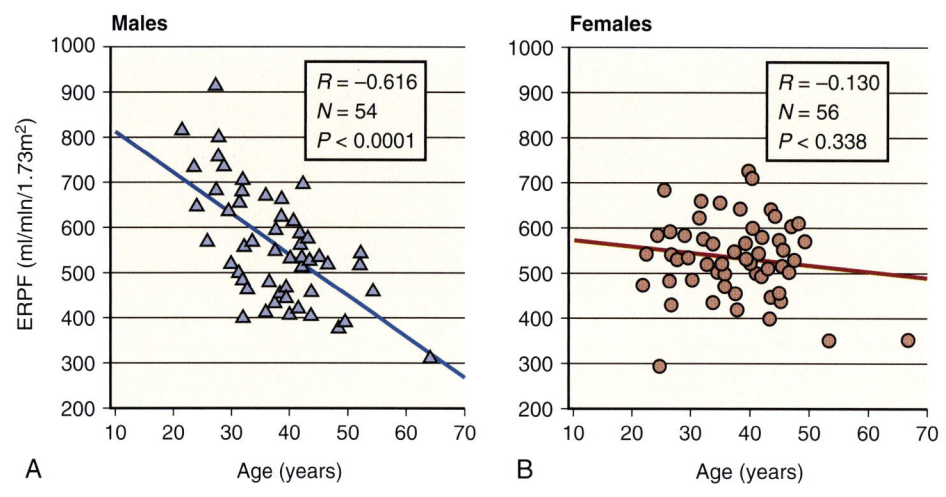

Figure 24.7 Relationship between age and relative effective renal plasma flow (ERPF, in milliliters per minute per 1.73 m² body surface area [BSA]) in males (**A**) and females (**B**). (From Berg UB: Differences in decline in GFR with age between males and females: reference data on clearances of inulin and PAH in potential kidney donors. *Nephrol Dial Transplant* 21:2577-2582, 2006.)

cells and older rat kidneys in comparison with vasoconstrictive thromboxane.[261,262] Excretion of vasodilatory natriuretic hormones is also lower in older subjects. Forearm vasodilation in response to PGI_2 infusion was also lower in older than younger healthy individuals, a difference that appeared to be due to reduced contribution of endothelium-derived NO.[263] Older and younger subjects have similar vasoconstrictive responses to intraarterial angiotensin infusion. Inhibition of angiotensin II–mediated vasoconstriction with ACEIs leads to less vasodilation in older individuals[264] than in younger subjects.[265] ACE inhibition also led to renal vasodilation in aged rats with an increase in RPF.[266] Glycine infusion in older rats, however, causes a decreased vasodilation response.[267] Competitive NO inhibition leads to increased vasoconstriction, increased vascular resistance, and decreased RPF in older than in younger rats.[268] Maximal vasodilation was applied with dopamine and amino acid in young (27-37 years), middle-aged (44-74 years), and elderly (81-96 years) subjects; the increase in NO levels and RPF seen in young and middle-aged subjects did not occur in elderly subjects, who also had a reduction in renal functional reserve that paralleled the number of sclerotic glomeruli found in elderly kidney biopsy specimens.[269] These findings suggest that in order to preserve renal plasma flow, the aged renal vasculature may be in a state of renal vasodilation to compensate for underlying glomerular sclerotic damage. Renal function is thereby maintained despite a decrease in renal functional reserve.[269]

GLOMERULAR FILTRATION RATE

A progressive decline in GFR is seen with aging, though the rate of change can vary depending on whether inulin, iothalamate, urea or creatinine clearance measurements are used.[270] Annual decline in creatinine clearance averages 0.8 mL/min/1.73 m², whereas iohexol clearance decreases by 1.0 mL/min/1.73 m² per year.[271,272] Various factors, including race, gender, genetic variation, and underlying renal and cardiovascular risks, affect the rate of decline for a given individual. Some writers have suggested that healthy older men have a slightly faster rate of decline in renal function than healthy older women,[247] although the difference is relatively small.[273] However, when the rate is scaled to body surface area, women appear to show a slightly greater decline in GFR (Figure 24.8).[274] Elderly African American or Japanese individuals seem to have a higher rate of decline in renal function than white individuals.[12,275] A longitudinal 5-year evaluation of baseline factors in healthy elderly subjects noted that higher eGFR at baseline, higher systolic blood pressures, higher low-density lipoprotein (LDL) cholesterol and lower transferrin levels were associated with a greater decline in eGFR.[34] The presence of hypertension, impaired glucose tolerance, diabetes, systemic and/or renal atherosclerosis, and lipid abnormalities are associated with higher rate of GFR loss in the elderly.[276-278] Higher pulse pressure, often seen in aging individuals and indicating increased arterial stiffness, correlates inversely with GFR. Older participants in a cardiovascular study who had evidence of systemic microvascular disease on retinal examination had a greater decrease in GFR over time.[272]

In micropuncture studies, Ang II increases both preglomerular and efferent arteriolar resistances, decreases renal and glomerular plasma flow, and increases glomerular hydraulic pressure and filtration fraction in both young and old rats. However, Ang II infusion lowers single-nephron GFR and whole kidney GFR in older rats by decreasing single nephron ultrafiltration coefficient (SNKf), parameters that remain unchanged in younger rats.[279] Ang II decreases SNKf likely by causing mesangial cell contraction and smaller filtration surface. These parameters can be estimated in recipients of transplanted kidneys from older and younger donors. In one study, the nonsclerotic glomeruli in transplants from deceased older donors actually had larger filtration surface and *higher* SNKf than those from young donors. Overall GFR was 32% lower, a difference that was attributable to a reduction in allograft ultrafiltration coefficient, which in turn was explained by a significantly lower number of functioning glomeruli than in organs from younger donors.[15] In healthy volunteers who had not received transplants, similar results were found, except that

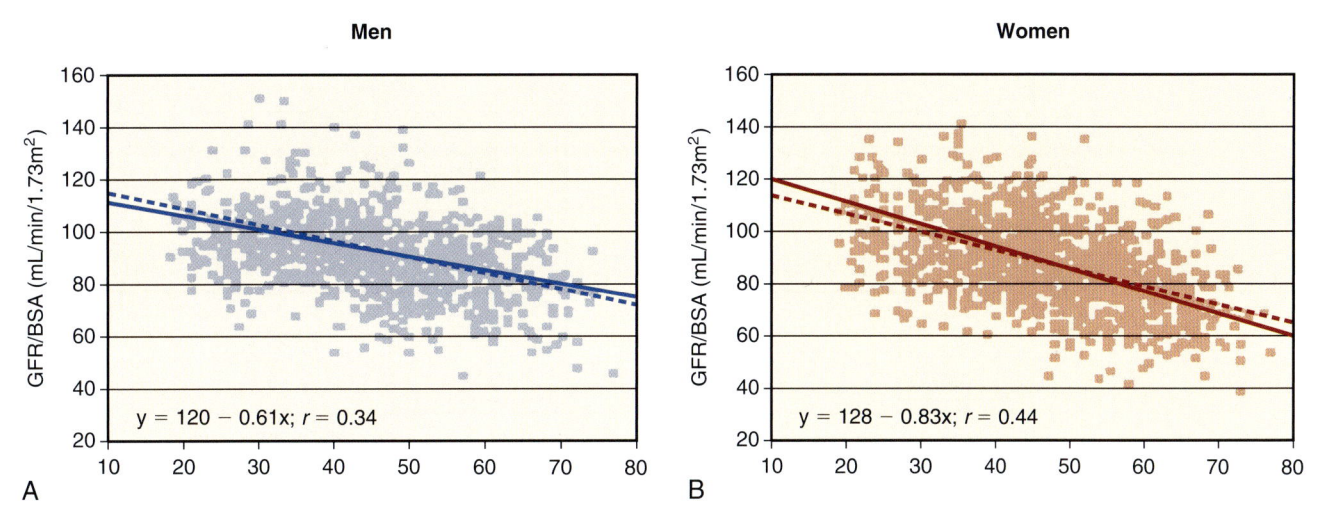

Figure 24.8 Relations between glomerular filtration rate and age in all subjects. **A,** In men; **B,** in women. Glomerular filtration rate (GFR) scaled to body surface area (BSA); *broken* and *continuous lines* are the least squares regressions fitted to data from age 30 to 40 years, respectively. The regression equations are from age 40 years. Note the more rapid age-dependent decline in GFR in women. (Adapted from Esposito C, et al: Renal function and functional reserve in healthy elderly individuals. *J Nephrol* 20:617-625, 2007.)

SNKf was reduced in older individuals.[270] Despite a linear decrease in RPF with age, the filtration fraction appears to be increased. This may be explained by a higher filtration fraction in juxtamedullary nephrons than cortical nephrons in light of relatively preserved medullary flow and decreased cortical RPF (Figure 24.9).[269,270,280,281] In summary, the age-related reduction in GFR may be explained by decreases in functioning nephrons, in RPF, and in SNKf at baseline, as well as a response to Ang II. This reduction is only partially ameliorated by the increase in filtration fraction and by an increase in SNKf that occurs in remnant glomeruli exclusively in a transplanted kidney.

Although a gradual decrease in GFR is noted with age, a parallel increase in serum creatinine may not be evident because muscle mass also decreases with age, frequently leading to an overestimation of GFR. GFR estimation can therefore be tricky in the older patient. Steady-state 24-hour urine creatinine clearances depend on collected volume and diet. Appropriate collection times are cumbersome for the older individual. Clearance studies using a radionuclide such as technetium Tc 99m–labeled diethylenetriaminepentaacetic acid, iothalamate, or iohexol are more accurate;[282] the expense, radioactivity exposure, and/or test variability limit their use for routine GFR measurements. Formulas commonly used to calculate GFR either overestimate or underestimate actual GFR in older individuals. The MDRD study and Chronic Kidney Disease–Epidemiology Collaboration (CKD-EPI) equations may provide closer estimations of GFR than the Cockroft-Gault equation.[283,284] Other endogenous markers of GFR, such as cystatin C, a cysteine proteinase inhibitor continuously produced by all nucleated cells that is freely filtered, internalized, and catabolized by proximal renal tubular cells, has been found to be comparable to the MDRD equation in estimating GFR in the elderly; however, body mass index may contribute to the discrepancies between cystatin-based and MDRD equation estimates of GFR.[285-287] Comparison of the first MDRD equation (incoporating BUN, serum albumin, age, creatinie) MDRD1 and second MDRD equation (incorporating serum creatinine and age only) MDRD2, the 2009 CKD-EPI (creatinine) equation, and the 2012 CKD-EPI (creatinine [cr]–cystatin [cys]) equation for approximating GFR with GFR values measured by radionuclide studies in the elderly indicates that the CKD-EPI equations may be more accurate than the MDRD equations.[288-290] Validation studies seem to confirm that CKD-EPI (cr) is comparable in estimating GFR in both the young and the elderly.[291] In the healthy elderly patient, use of other factors, including the presence of albuminuria and other comorbid conditions, may be more helpful in determining the presence or absence of CKD than an estimation of GFR alone.[292]

SODIUM CONSERVATION

Tubular efficiency in reabsorbing filtered sodium decreases with age. Healthy subjects more than 60 years old take nearly twice as long to decrease urine sodium as those 30 years and younger (31 hours vs. 17.6 hours, respectively) after the initiation of sodium restriction.[293] This difference may be secondary to decreased distal tubular sodium reabsorption.[294] Age-related interstitial scarring, fewer nephrons, and increased medullary blood flow leading to a greater solute burden per nephron may contribute to decreased tubular sodium reabsorption in the elderly. However, one study found that use of indomethacin to reduce medullary flow in older individuals did not decrease distal tubular sodium clearance, suggesting that increased medullary blood flow may not contribute to decreased sodium conservation in the elderly.[295]

Changes in both levels and response of hormones regulating sodium conservation with age also influence sodium conservation. Plasma renin and aldosterone levels are lower in the healthy elderly. A 30% to 50% decrease in basal renin activity is found, although renin substrate levels remain normal. Maneuvers that increase renin activity, such as upright position, sodium restriction to 10 mEq/day, furosemide administration, and air jet stress, further amplify age-related differences in renin activity.[296] Plasma renin levels

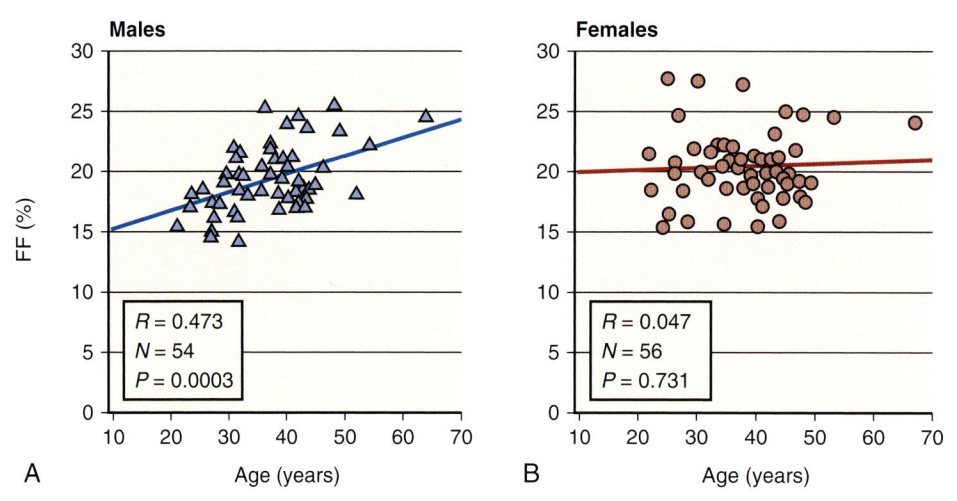

Figure 24.9 Relationship between age and filtration fraction (FF, in percentage) in males (**A**) and females (**B**). (From Berg UB: Differences in decline in GFR with age between males and females: reference data on clearances of inulin and PAH in potential kidney donors. *Nephrol Dial Transplant* 2:2577-2582, 2006.)

both before and after hemorrhage were lower in 15-month-old rats than in 3-month-old rats, reflecting age-related differences in plasma renin even prior to the stress event.[297] Renin mRNA abundance is downregulated and juxtamedullary single-nephron renin activity decreased in older rats.[298] With sodium deprivation and a drop in mean arterial pressure, older rats demonstrate a blunted plasma renin activity with delayed decrease in urinary sodium excretion. Plasma renin substrate measurements in healthy older adults suggest decreased conversion of inactive to active renin.[299]

Plasma aldosterone changes with age parallel the change in plasma renin activity with a 30% to 50% decrease in older adults. An intrinsic adrenal defect appears less likely because both aldosterone and cortisol responses to adrenocorticotropic hormone remain appropriate with age, suggesting a renin-angiotensin deficiency.[300] The sluggish response to dietary sodium restriction seen in the elderly can be reproduced by ACE inhibition and blockade of the renin angiotensin aldosterone system (RAAS).[301] With aldosterone infusion, tubular sensitivity to appropriate sodium reabsorption appears preserved in the elderly, further supporting an abnormal RAAS response to delayed sodium reabsorption in the elderly.

SODIUM EXCRETION

Older individuals have a blunted natriuretic response to sodium or volume loading. Sodium excretion after a 2-liter saline load is slower and occurs relatively more during the night in subjects older than 40 years than gender-, size-, and race-matched younger control subjects (Figure 24.10).[275,302] Nocturia is more prevalent and evident in older individuals. The natriuretic response to saline loading normally decreases after uninephrectomy for kidney donation, and this decrease is greater in older kidney donors than in younger donors (Figure 24.11).[301]

The tubule response to ANP, an important controller of sodium excretion, is decreased with aging. ANP induces hyperfiltration, inhibits luminal membrane sodium channels and reabsorption, and suppresses renin release via specific cell surface receptors on renal vasculature and tubular epithelium. ANP is rapidly degraded; however, selective blockade of degradative enzymes or clearance can prolong serum ANP half-life.[303] Serum ANP levels are three to five times higher in healthy older adults than in younger adults. ANP levels rise in response to greater salt load and head-out water immersion in older subjects to a greater extent than in younger ones,[304-306] although decreased salt intake results in similar ANP levels in the old and young. ANP secretion

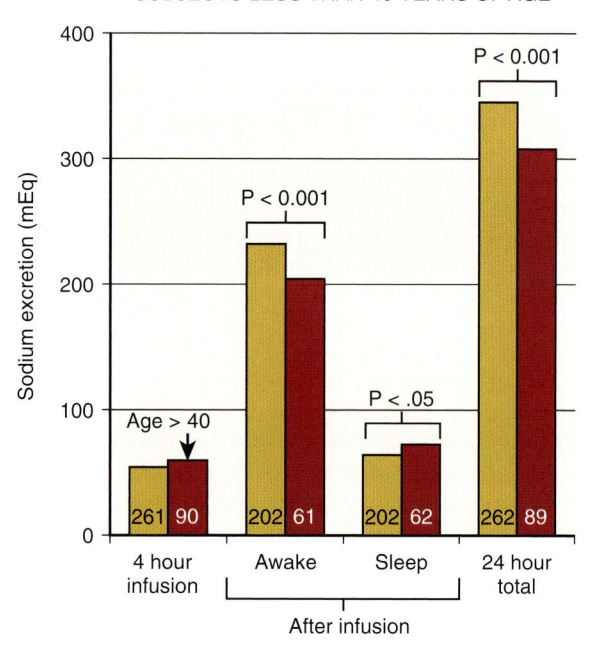

Figure 24.10 Comparison of urinary sodium excretion in younger (*gold bars*) and older (*red bars*) subjects after administration of 2 L of intravenous normal saline. Numbers at the bottoms of *bars* are the number of subjects in each group. (From Luft FC, et al: Effects of volume expansion and contraction in normotensive whites, blacks, and subjects of different ages, *Circulation* 59[4]:643-650, 1979.)

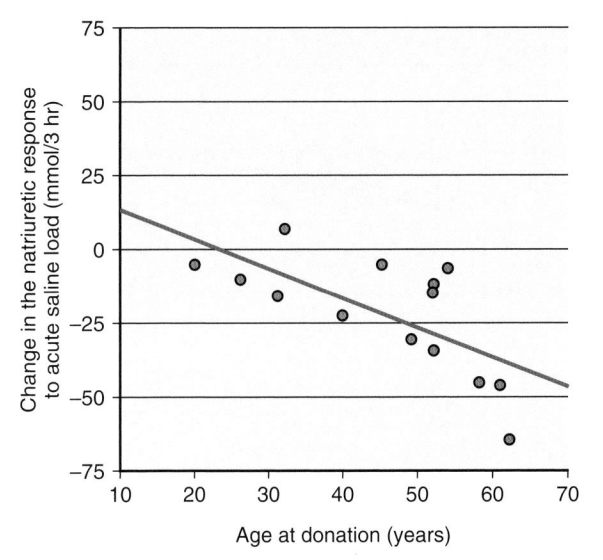

Figure 24.11 Influence of age at donation on change in natriuretic response to acute saline load in kidney donors after uninephrectomy. *Red circles* indicate normotensive. (Adapted from Mimran A, et al: Aging and sodium homeostasis. *Kidney Int Suppl* 37:S107-S113, 1992.)

remains intact with aging, higher basal levels resulting from decreased metabolic clearance.[307,308] An age-related decrease in GFR does not appear to contribute, because patients with CKD and low GFR do not have high ANP levels.[309]

Decreased metabolic clearance of ANP in aged subjects also suggests the possibility of lower proximal brush border endopeptidase levels that break down ANP.[310] This possibility is supported by the observation that endopeptidase inhibitors restored vagal reflex bradycardia in old rats to levels similar to those seen in young rats.[311]

Some writers have proposed that higher ANP levels are a homeostatic response to reduced ANP renal sensitivity with age. In support of this idea, urinary sodium excretion reaches a plateau after a 2 ng/kg/min ANP infusion in older adults,[312,313] whereas younger subjects continue to have increased urinary sodium excretion with incremental increases in ANP.[312] Although cGMP and ANP levels are similar at baseline, low-dose ANP increases urinary excretion of cyclic guanosine monophosphate (cGMP) but not sodium in older subjects.[307,314] This finding suggests that the problem is downstream of cGMP. ANP can suppress the RAAS and inhibit sodium reabsorption. Simultaneous measurements of plasma renin activity and plasma aldosterone concentration during ANP infusion imply that the natriuretic effects of ANP are different from those of RAAS suppression. Age seems to affect each ANP action differently.[307,312,313]

URINARY CONCENTRATION

Older individuals are frequently unable to achieve maximal urinary concentrating capacity.[271,315] A combination of processes leads to impairment of water reabsorption with aging. The presence of an intact osmoreceptor and volume receptor sensitivity to arginine vasopressin (AVP) release, in addition to an intact collecting tubule response to AVP under maximal medullary tonicity, is necessary for appropriate urinary concentration. A study found urinary osmolality to be lower in aged than in young rats and to persist after a 5-day water restriction, although plasma AVP levels increased equivalently in young and old rats.[315] Both volume and osmotic stimulation of AVP remain intact with age, with actually enhanced osmoreceptor sensitivity for AVP in the elderly.[316-318] A concentration defect remains after AVP infusion, suggesting an impaired AVP response.[319] One study found that AVP receptor type 2 (V_2R) mRNA expression decreased similarly in 8-week-old and 7-month-old rats at baseline and with dehydration. Although aquaporin-2 (AQP2) mRNA increased, the increase was smaller in older rats.[320] In another study, no difference in V_2R mRNA was seen between older and younger female nondehydrated WAG/Rij rats.[321] Some investigators have noted lower V_2R mRNA expression and decreased AQP2 protein levels in older than in younger hybrid F344/BN rats under baseline conditions.[315] Previous studies in renal medullary cells from 6-month-old and 30-month-old mice found little difference in maximum AVP receptor binding, suggesting a postreceptor defect.[322] Higher AVP levels are required to increase cyclic adenosine monophosphate (cAMP), because older animals have decreased cAMP levels.[323,324]

Postreceptor guanine nucleotide–binding protein (G_s protein) levels are also lower in older kidneys.[325] Stimulation of G protein with cholera toxin and of adenylate cyclase with forskolin at the level of the catalytic unit and G protein interaction evoked a significantly reduced response in hydraulic conductivity of older rabbit collecting tubules, suggesting that the age-associated decrease in the cortical collecting tubule response to AVP may occur at the level of the G_s catalytic subunit of adenylate cyclase.[326] In the previously mentioned study in female WAG/Rij rats, however, expression of both AQP2 and AQP3 was markedly lower in older than in younger rats. AQP2 was noted to also redistribute into the intracellular compartment in the inner medulla and not in the renal cortex in the presence of low papillary osmolality and unchanged papillary cAMP in the older rats, suggesting that AQP2 and AQP3 expression may be independent of vasopressin-mediated cAMP accumulation.[321] These data suggest that although vasopressin response appears to be preserved with age, the extent of this response may be affected by mechanistic factors, leading to actual aquaporin insertion and urinary concentration.

It has been proposed that older individuals have medullary "washout" on the basis of the observation that solute and osmolar clearances are increased and urine osmolality decreased after 12 hours of water deprivation.[271] Evaluation of proximal and distal nephron clearance of sodium in comparison with free water clearance after water load followed by 0.45% saline load resulted in 29% lower distal tubular sodium reabsorption in older healthy versus younger healthy subjects, suggesting impaired distal sodium transport in the older subjects. Very old (31 months) rats have decreased Na-K-2CL cotransporter type 2 (NKCC2).[327] However, renal cortical to medullary non-urea solute concentration and solute-free water clearance as a measure of loop salt transport (CH_2O/GFR) in aged rats were not significantly different from those in younger rats at comparable rates of distal solute delivery; medullary washout is therefore less likely to be a contributing factor to the decrease in urinary concentrating ability with age.[328]

Decreased urinary concentration with age may also be affected by reduced expression of urea transporters UT-A1 and UT-B1 in the renal medulla; one study found a decrease in papillary osmolality in senescent female WAG/Rij rats whether they received food restriction or ad libitum feeding.[329] Other investigators report that papillary urea accumulation as well as urine osmolality and flow rates improved with upregulation of urea transporters when 1-desamino-8-D-rginine vasopressin (desmopressin; DDAVP) was given.[330,331]

URINARY DILUTION

Renal diluting capacity in the elderly may be affected by an underlying decrease in GFR with age as well as a decrease in distal sodium resorption.[294] Maximum urinary dilution depends on appropriate solute extraction, adequate AVP suppression, and distal delivery of the filtered load. In one study, water loading of 20 mL/kg in healthy older adults resulted in excretion of only 41% of the water load over 2 hours, compared with excretion of 100% of the water load in young water-repleted individuals and 70% excretion of the water load in young water-depleted individuals; the lower excretion is partly attributable to an age-related decline in glomerular filtration.[332] In another study, peak free water clearance after overnight fast and oral water loading of 20 mL/kg was 6 ± 0.6 mL/min in healthy elderly volunteers, compared with 10.1 ± 0.8 mL/min in young volunteers.[317] However, total free water clearance over time was comparable in both older and younger groups in the two studies.[317,332] Minimum urinary osmolality for subjects older than 70 years is 92 mOsm/kg H_2O, compared with 52 mOsm/kg H_2O in subjects younger than 40 years.

ACID-BASE BALANCE

Acid-base homeostasis with usual daily acid or alkali intake remains well maintained in the elderly. Only during acid loading is the impaired ability to excrete an acid load evident. Although age-related decreases in renal mass and GFR contribute, endogenous acid production from acid diets can lower serum bicarbonate levels in older individuals. Healthy elderly demonstrated a lower net acid excretion capacity when compared in cross-sectional observational analysis with that of younger healthy adults.[333] In the same group of elderly subjects, net acid excretion correlated positively with calcium and magnesium excretion. In older, cross-sectional studies, plasma bicarbonate and blood pH appear to decrease with age, concomitant with decreases in GFR (Figure 24.12).[334] There is a reciprocal increase in plasma chloride, as seen with renal tubular acidosis or early renal disease.[335]

Ammonium excretion is found to decrease with age. Whereas ammonium excretion increased similarly with glutamine intake in both young and old in one study, ammonium loading resulted in lower ammonium excretion and inability to achieve minimal urine pH despite correction for GFR in older patients,[336] suggesting a possible intrinsic tubular defect. Sodium-hydrogen exchanger activity, however, increased similarly in both older and younger rats, with phosphate transport also decreasing to the same extent in both groups.[336a]

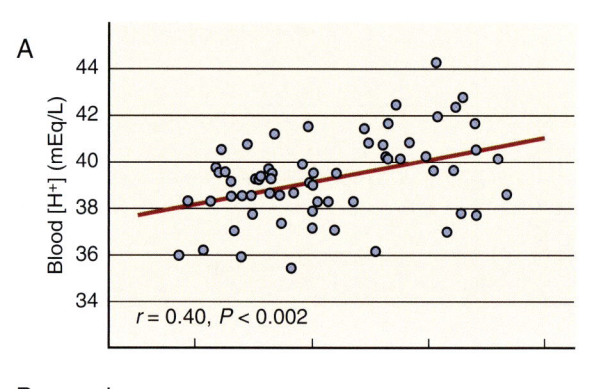

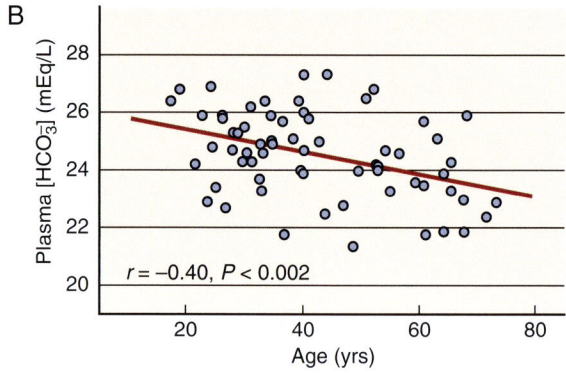

Figure 24.12 Relation between blood pH [$(H^+)b$] and age (**A**) and between plasma bicarbonate concentration [$(HCO_3^-)p$] and age (**B**) in normal adult humans ($n = 64$). Each data point represents the mean steady-state value in a subject eating a constant diet. Regression equation: $(H^+)b = 0.045 \times age + 37.2$ $(HCO_3^-)p = -0.038 \times age + 26.0$. (From Frassetto LA, et al: Effect of age on blood acid-base composition in adult humans: role of age-related renal functional decline. *Am J Physiol* 271:F1114-F1122, 1996.)

Although the degree of acidosis observed in the elderly in these older studies is subtle, complications of chronic acidosis including bone demineralization and muscle wasting can be seen in the elderly. Higher protein intake results in endogenous acid production. In a population study in Pakistan, net endogenous acid production was reported to be higher in the elderly compared to younger cohorts owing to intake of protein rich foods.[337] Increased dietary acid load would be expected to result in lower serum bicarbonate levels, which would be more evident in those over 40 years of age.[338] This may not, however, be generalizable to populations elsewhere. Additionally, changes in net acid excretion can be seen in patients with small decreases in estimated GFR without overt changes in acid base parameters.[339]

Muscle breakdown mediated by activation of the adenosine triphosphate (ATP)–dependent ubiquitin and proteasome pathway is induced by acidosis.[340] Net acid excretion correlates positively with changes in parathyroid hormone (PTH) and urinary calcium excretion.[341] Acidemia regulates calcium and alkali mobilization from bone and inhibits renal calcium reabsorption. Higher protein intake in Western diets, in conjunction with age-related impairment in acid excretion, negatively affects calcium balance and predisposes to osteoporosis, increased incidence of muscle wasting, and fractures despite normal bicarbonate levels.[342]

In one study, 24-hour net acid excretion in healthy elderly subjects also correlated with magnesuria irrespective of magnesium intake and when adjusted for potassium intake.[330] In another, elderly men and women with increased potassium excretion, a marker of greater potassium intake due to consumption of potassium-rich alkaline fruits and vegetables, did not exhibit the mild metabolic acidosis noted with protein-rich diets, and this finding was associated with higher percentage of lean body mass.[343] Bicarbonate supplementation in elderly patients with chronic kidney failure was reported to correct metabolic acidosis, improve serum albumin and prealbumin levels, and decrease whole-body protein degradation as evaluated by a decrease in normalized protein catabolic rate.[344] Postmenopausal women were found to have improved nitrogen and calcium balance with potassium bicarbonate supplementation,[345] which also was reported to have favorable effects on bone resorption and calcium excretion in older men and women.[346] In a randomized double-blind placebo-controlled study of healthy elderly men and women, potassium citrate supplementation at both 60 and 90 mmol/day neutralized net acid excretion, with the further benefit of decreased 24-hour urinary calcium level even though calcium absorption was not affected.[347]

POTASSIUM BALANCE

Total-body potassium decreases with age as muscle mass declines, and this decrease is more evident in women. Lower plasma levels of renin and aldosterone could explain this decrease, with presence of relative hypoaldosteronism in the elderly.[348] Potassium infusion results in decreased aldosterone response in older individuals (Figure 24.13).[349] There is a relative decrease in fractional potassium excretion in relation to GFR in healthy older individuals.[350] Aged rats given high-potassium diet demonstrate lower efficiency in potassium excretion.[351] KCl infusion results in higher plasma potassium levels and inability to shift potassium into cells. After bilateral nephrectomy, sodium pump (Na^+/K^+-ATPase) activity is 38% lower in older than in younger rats with high-potassium feedings.[351] Age, however, does not appear to affect insulin-mediated potassium uptake in humans.[352] Exercise-induced increases in potassium levels in the elderly suggests an impaired β-adrenergic–induced increase in adenylate cyclase system resulting in decreased activity of the Na^+/K^+-ATPase pump in the skeletal muscle.[256] Older individuals are more prone to development of hyporeninemic hypoaldosteronism (type 4 renal tubular acidosis) with abnormalities in both RAAS and renal acidification. Thus, medications that further impair long-term potassium adaptation, including RAAS inhibitors (ACEI, ARBs, heparin, calcineurin inhibitors, spironolactone, eplerenone), β-blockers, nonsteroidal antiinflammatory agents (NSAIDs), and sodium channel blockers (trimethoprim, pentamidine, amiloride, triamterene) can lead to significant hyperkalemia in the elderly and require close monitoring.

CALCIUM BALANCE

Both renal calcium excretion and reabsorption in response to decreased or increased calcium intake are reported to be appropriate, as are the filtered load of calcium and proximal tubular calcium reabsorption per nephron, in both old and young rats.[352,353] An age-related decrease in distal tubular epithelial calcium channel protein TRPV5 abundance is noted that corresponds to a decrease in TRPV5 mRNA and slight increases in 2-hour urine calcium excretion in older mice.[354] It is possible that age-related deficiency in β-glucuronidase klotho is contributing to inadequate Na^+-K^+-ATPase sensing of low extracellular calcium.[354-357] Healthy older males are found to have a higher calcium set point for PTH release as well as a greater number of parathyroid cells, not attributable to either lower ionized calcium or 1,25-hydroxyvitamin D levels.[358] How the G protein–coupled calcium sensing receptor plays a role in this changed set point is yet to be clarified.[359] However, fractional calcium excretion in the healthy older individuals with GFR values similar to those with stage 3 chronic kidney disease (CKD3) suggests greater calcium loss in those with CKD3.[360]

Intestinal calcium reabsorption, however, is decreased with aging, in association with decreases in 1-α-hydroxylase activity and 1,25-dihydroxycholecalciferol (1,25$[OH]_2D_3$) levels and increased basal PTH levels. Levels of vitamin

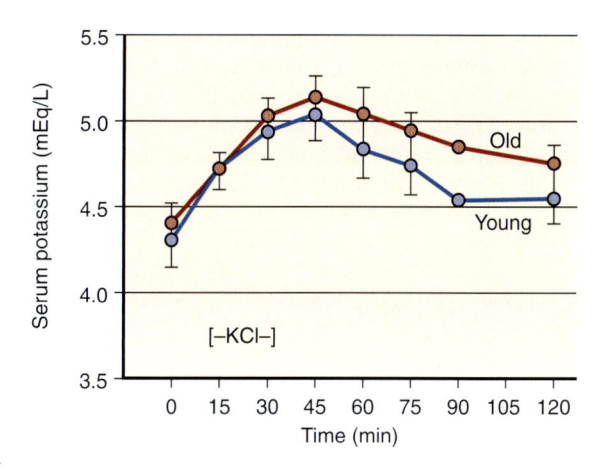

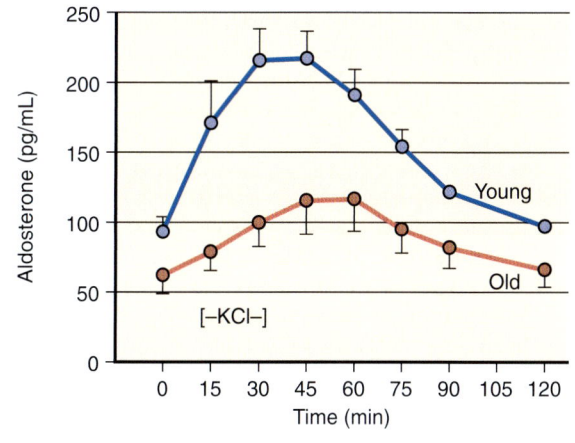

Figure 24.13 Serum potassium and aldosterone levels before, during, and after infusion of potassium chloride (0.05 mEq/kg body weight over 45 minutes) in six healthy young and six healthy elderly men. Changes in serum potassium levels were similar, but elderly subjects have a lower aldosterone response ($P < 0.005$) by analysis of variance. (From Mulkerrin E, et al: Aldosterone responses to hyperkalemia in healthy elderly humans. *J Am Soc Nephrol* 6:1459-1462, 1995.)

D–dependent calcium-binding proteins also diminish with age in association with the change in intestinal calcium absorption.[351,361] Although renal vitamin D production is lower with PTH stimulation, final concentrations of vitamin D are similar in both old and young. Urinary cAMP and fractional phosphorus levels also increase with PTH infusion as expected in both young and old, suggesting an intact renal response to PTH with aging.[362]

PHOSPHATE BALANCE

Intrinsic renal tubular capacity for phosphate reabsorption decreases with age.[358,363] Older kidneys adapt less well to phosphate restriction.[364,365] Intestinal phosphate absorption is also lower in the elderly. The lower maximal inorganic phosphate (Pi) transport capacity (TmPi) observed in older parathyroidectomized rats infused with graded levels of Pi suggests a significantly lower TmPi with age. Although TmPi decreased further with PTH infusion in these rats, the magnitude of the response was less with age.[363]

Primary cultures of renal tubular cells from young and aged rats show a similar age-related impaired response in phosphate transport as seen in vivo studies.[366] Decreases in maximum sodium-dependent phosphate transport velocity (Na/Pi cotransport) and the ability to adapt to low-phosphate culture media are found in cultured cells from older rats, accompanied by a decrease in type IIa Na/Pi cotransporter cortical mRNA levels and apical brush border membrane protein abundance.[365,367]

Increase in membrane cholesterol content may further act to decrease Na/Pi cotransport with aging.[368] In vitro cholesterol enrichment of isolated brush border membranes from young adult rats reproduces the age-related impairment in maximum velocity of Na/Pi cotransport activity.[368] Direct changes in opossum kidney cell cholesterol content seem to affect Na/Pi cotransport activity by changing expression of the apical membrane type II Na/Pi cotransport protein.[369] Thus, changes in membrane cholesterol content with age may contribute to changes in phosphate transport.

The effect of age-related changes in $1,25(OH)_2D_3$ metabolism on intestinal phosphate transport should be considered, given that vitamin D replacement improves renal and intestinal phosphate transport in vitamin D–deficient animals.[370-372] Interestingly, changes in phosphate transport resulting from vitamin D administration parallel significant changes in brush border membrane lipid composition and fluidity.[373] Thus, age-related effects of $1,25(OH)_2D_3$ may possibly be mediated by lipid-modulating properties that improve renal and intestinal transport of phosphate (and calcium).

RENAL DISEASE IN THE AGING KIDNEY

DISORDERS OF OSMOREGULATION

HYPONATREMIA

Hyponatremia can be a common finding in geriatric adults, given their enhanced osmotic AVP release and impaired ability to dilute urine.[374,375] Many older ambulatory patients are also found to have an idiopathic form of the syndrome of inappropriate antidiuretic hormone.[376] This predisposition to hyponatremia can be further exacerbated by medications that can affect AVP action or release (see Chapter 16). In addition, thiazide-type diuretics with distal tubular effects on solute reabsorption further impair urinary dilution in the elderly and can be implicated in nearly 20% to 30% of cases of hyponatremia.[377] Aging-associated decreases in prostaglandin synthesis also inhibit water diuresis and increase susceptibility to hyponatremia with thiazide use.[377] Acute or significant hyponatremia can manifest subtly as apathy, disorientation, lethargy, muscle cramps, anorexia, or nausea, which can progress to more devastating signs such as agitation, depressed deep tendon reflexes, pseudobulbar palsy, and seizures resulting from osmotic water shifts from the extracellular to the intracellular space. Thus early recognition with prompt appropriate therapy is indicated to avoid severe neurologic sequelae, including central pontine myelinolysis.

HYPERNATREMIA

Both a concentrating defect and a decreased thirst response with aging[378] predispose older individuals to dehydration and hypernatremia. Certainly the inability to access free water because of altered level of consciousness or immobility in the elderly can lead to a marked rise in serum sodium and osmolality, with associated mortality reported as high as 46% to 70%, particularly with sodium levels higher than 160 mEq/L.[379] Medications that cloud sensorium and inhibit thirst, such as tranquilizers and sedatives, or that decrease AVP action in the renal tubules, such as lithium and demeclocycline, should be used with caution in older adults. In addition, osmotic diuretics, high-protein or high-glucose parenteral feedings, and bowel cathartics need to be used carefully in older adults to avoid dehydration. The presence of systemic illness, infection, fever, or neurologic impairment may add to impaired AVP secretion and increase the underlying predisposition for hypernatremia. Symptomatic severe cellular dehydration can be associated with obtundation, stupor, coma, seizures, and death. Thus, particular care in use of medications and medication review are necessary in the older debilitated patient to avoid hypernatremia.

ACUTE KIDNEY INJURY

Susceptibility to both ischemic and nephrotoxic acute kidney injury (AKI), as well as time for recovery from injury, increases with age.[380,381] Acute kidney injury is 3.5 times more prevalent in those older than 70 years and is associated with greater morbidity and mortality in older hospitalized patients.[9,382,383] An estimated 28% of those older than 65 years are unlikely to recover kidney function after AKI.[384]

Renal artery occlusion in older rats produced a larger increase in renal vascular resistance and a greater fall in glomerular filtration, and it took these rats longer to recover from ischemic injury than younger rats. Renal cortical slices from aged rats that were exposed to anoxia were less able to take up paraaminohippurate and tetraethylammonium than renal cortical slices from younger rats.[380] Reduced antioxidant potential and increased oxidative stress predisposed older rats to more severe reperfusion injury.[385] Expression of candidate genes, including claudin-7 (*Cldn7*), kidney injury molecule-1 (Kim-1), and matrix metalloproteinase (MMP-7), was increased during ischemic injury in slices of kidney from older rats in comparison with younger rats; interestingly, gene expression was attenuated in calorie-restricted older rats.[386] Hemoglobin infusion to induce heme protein nephrotoxic injury to older rats resulted in significantly greater increase in blood urea nitrogen and creatinine as well as histologic evidence of acute tubular necrosis with tubular cast formation in older (16 months) mice but not in younger (6 months) mice. Older mice failed to increase protective heme oxygenase 2 (HO-2) mRNA but did increase the nephrotoxic cytokine interleukin-6 (IL-6) 30-fold, compared with a 10-fold increase in younger rats.[387]

Transcriptomic analysis of murine kidney tissue in experimental AKI suggested that tumor necrosis factor–like weak inducer of apoptosis (TWEAK) activation of its receptor, fibroblast growth factor–inducible 14 (Fn14), via secretion of chemokine CXCL16 decreased both mRNA and protein expression of the anti-aging hormone Klotho.[388] Klotho reduction persisted after recovery from nephrotoxic injury and may add to the progression of CKD,[388] which is more common in the elderly after AKI. In addition, critical telomere shortening with increased cell cycle inhibitor p21 and greater numbers of apoptotic cells in relation to significantly reduced tubular, glomerular, and interstitial cell proliferative capacity were noted in older telomerase-deficient mice in comparison with younger mice.[389] Evaluation of renal progenitor cells with bromodeoxyuridine before and after ischemia reperfusion noted decreases in progenitor cells with age, with no significant difference in the ratio of label retaining cell division after injury among rats tested of different ages. Higher numbers of renal progenitor cells were noted in cells co-cultured with human umbilical vein endothelial cells (HUVECs) than in cells cultured without HUVECs, suggesting that tubular regeneration with age may be affected by access to surrounding peritubular capillary network.[390] Proximal tubular cells also failed to induce autophagy during ischemic stress, and this feature seemed to correlate with the development of age-related AKI.[391] Data also show more decreased autophagy in older than in younger mice after ischemic and nephrotoxic injury.[392]

Thus, decreased regenerative capacity in relation to injury appears to add to prolonged recovery from AKI with age.

Data from older humans reflect similar findings. Euvolemic older men consuming a constant sodium diet have higher renal vascular resistance with a blunted response to orthostatic change. Also, unlike younger adults, older adults are unable to improve medullary oxygenation with water diuresis (Figure 24.14).[362] In patients without kidney dysfunction who underwent cardiopulmonary bypass, postoperative excretion of kidney-specific proteins (N-acetyl-β-glucosaminidase, α₁-microglobulin, π-glutathione-S-transferase, α-glutathione-S-transferase) and fractional sodium excretion were higher in the older patients than in the younger patients.[393] Similarly, increasing donor age significantly correlated with higher expression of the enzyme poly (ADP-ribose) polymerase 1 (PARP-1) in kidney biopsy specimens from aged donors, suggesting a greater susceptibility to cold ischemia and ischemia reperfusion in older kidneys.[394]

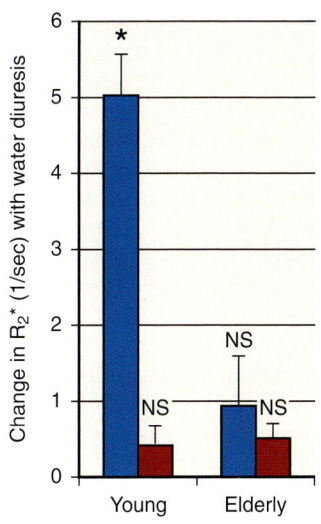

Figure 24.14 Comparison of changes in R_2^* (1/sec) in response to water load in nine young and nine elderly subjects. R_2^* reflects the apparent spin-spin relaxation of deoxygenated hemoglobin by magnetic resonance and is equal to the slope or equivalent to the concentration of deoxyhemoglobin or blood oxygen pressure (PO_2) or tissue PO_2. Because blood PO_2 is thought to be in rapid equilibrium with tissue PO_2, changes in blood oxygen level–dependent magnetic resonance imaging signal intensity, or R_2^*, should reflect changes in the PO_2 of the tissue. *Blue bars* indicate medulla; *red bars* indicate cortex. Bar heights represent mean values with standard error indicated. NS, Not significant. *Statistically significant at the $P < 0.01$ level. (From Prasad PV, Epstein FH: Changes in renal medullary pO₂ during water diuresis as evaluated by blood oxygenation level–dependent magnetic resonance imaging: effects of aging and cyclooxygenase inhibition, *Kidney Int* 55:294-298, 1999.)

Multifactorial and iatrogenic insults, whether prerenal, intrinsic, or postrenal, that lead to AKI are poorly tolerated as age increases and renal reserve decreases. The common presence of comorbid diabetes, hypertension, heart failure, liver disease, or malignancies in older individuals adds to the poor tolerability of an acute renal insult. Generalized atherosclerosis in older patients predisposes to renal ischemic events and spontaneous or procedure-related cholesterol renal atheroemboli. In addition, acute vasculitis and rapidly progressive glomerulonephritis can be devastating in older individuals.

Approximately half of the AKI events in the elderly result from prerenal processes. Vomiting, diarrhea, bleeding, and use of excessive diuretics are common causes of dehydration and volume depletion in this population. Impaired thirst, decreased urinary concentration ability, and diminished sodium conservation capacity predispose to these processes. Blunted autoregulation, decreased RPF, and reduced renal reserve in the older kidney allow volume changes to be less well tolerated. Renal hypoperfusion from decreased cardiac output, sepsis, and use of medications that interfere with renal autoregulatory mechanisms, such as angiotensin antagonists (ACEIs, ARBs) and prostaglandin inhibitors (NSAIDs), can cause and exacerbate prerenal processes, leading to AKI in older adults. NSAID use increases the risk of AKI in those 65 years and older by 58%.[395] Because tubular defects in older individuals may lead to a higher urine sodium excretion despite underlying hypoperfusion, the usual renal indices used to differentiate prerenal from intrinsic causes—urine sodium excretion, fractional sodium excretion, and urine osmolality—need careful interpretation in the elderly.[396] Although prerenal processes are often reversible with careful volume management, discontinuation of the exacerbating factor, or improvement in cardiac output, the evolution from prerenal azotemia to acute tubular necrosis (ATN) occurs more commonly in older (23%) than younger (15%) patients.[397]

Intrinsic AKI results in acute structural insults that prolong recovery of renal clearance in the elderly. ATN from ischemic and nephrotoxic tubular injury affects approximately 50% of hospitalized older patients with intrinsic AKI.[398] Lower levels of the NO substrate, L-arginine, in the elderly are associated with decreased NO synthesis in aging vasculature[258,399] and higher ADMA levels,[400,401] impairing vasodilation and predisposing older kidneys to ischemia. Data from aged rats support these findings. Feeding L-arginine to older rats prior to renal artery occlusion improved GFR, RFP, and renal vascular resistance (RVR), whereas administration of the NO inhibitor L-NAME (N^G-nitro-L-arginine methyl ester) abolished these effects.[401a] With an increase in eNOS mRNA and protein, NO availability was improved when RhoA protein activation was partially inhibited by statins.[401b] This increases NO availability therefore renal vasoconstriction and significantly attenuates ischemic lesions in older animals with ischemic acute renal failure, suggesting the vulnerability of aging kidneys to AKI.

Hypotension, either before or after surgery, sepsis, and nephrotoxins are poorly tolerated by aging kidneys and are major culprits in hospital-acquired AKI in the elderly. A prospective evaluation of all patients admitted to one hospital over a 12-month period, of whom 4176 were older than 60 years, noted that the incidence of treatment-related in-hospital AKI in the elderly was 1.4%. Nephrotoxins contributed to AKI in 66% of the elderly patients, sepsis and hypotension in 45.7%, contrast-induced nephropathy in 16.9%, and postoperative renal failure in 25.4%, with various combinations of these factors leading to AKI. Sepsis, oliguria, and hypotension were independent predictors of poor outcome in this older population.[402]

Both decreased clearance and tubular changes in older kidneys predispose to the toxic effects of antibiotics, chemotherapeutics, and diagnostic agents such as those using iodinated contrast. Therefore careful estimation of renal clearance is crucial in the elderly prior to antibiotic and chemotherapy dosing with continued close monitoring and drug dose adjustment as necessary. Drug-induced interstitial nephritis is more common in the elderly, particularly with commonly used drugs such as penicillins and proton pump inhibitors.[403] Careful assessment of renal clearance should be considered before infusion of contrast agents in the elderly. Use of concurrent medications such as NSAIDs, ACEIs, and ARBs as well as metformin for underlying comorbidities in the elderly should be carefully evaluated and appropriately discontinued before an intravenous injection of a contrast agent. Whenever possible, diuretic agents should also be discontinued several days prior to contrast agent injection in the elderly to prevent an added prerenal process. Furthermore, intravenous saline infusion should be considered to avoid prerenal process in the elderly before and after contrast infusion. Dose and duration of saline infusion should be individualized through clinical evaluation of volume status and other underlying comorbidities for each elderly patient.

Atheroembolic AKI is of greater risk in elderly patients who have generalized atherosclerosis, particularly with intraarterial cannulation and the use of anticoagulation.[404,405] In one study, approximately 7.1% of renal biopsy specimens obtained for acute kidney failure in patients older than 60 years were found to have atheroemboli.[406] Subtle increases in blood urea nitrogen and creatinine with or without complaints of dysuria, hesitancy, or dribbling should prompt an evaluation for underlying urinary tract obstruction. Careful investigation for urogenital tumors, pelvic prolapse, and papillary sloughing, as well as medication review for anticholinergic drugs, sedatives and hypnotics, narcotic and opioid analgesics, antipsychotics, and histamine-1 receptor antagonists, should be considered, with prompt urologic intervention as necessary.

AKI also increases the risk of ESKD in the elderly. In a cohort of nearly 234,000 Medicare beneficiaries 67 years and older discharged from the hospital, the incidence of AKI was 3.1%, and ESKD developed in 5.3 per 1000.[407] Therefore early recognition of a greater susceptibility of elderly patients to AKI is crucial, with the aim of preventing the disease by avoiding nephrotoxic medications and interventions that increase the risk. Early nephrology referral and management are prudent if these exposures cannot be avoided.

Although aging individuals have both greater risks for AKI and prolonged recovery from it, therapeutic intervention should not be based on age alone, because factors other than age can contribute to overall survival in the elderly.[408-410] Response to dialysis therapy for AKI in the elderly is frequently good, providing relief of uremic symptoms and complications such as volume overload, bleeding, disorientation, catabolic state, and electrolyte disturbances. Therefore, as in any patient, it is important to consider the overall assessment of the elderly patient in the decision about renal replacement therapy (RRT), including illness severity, comorbidities, and projected cognitive and/or physical recovery in addition to patient and family wishes.

HYPERTENSION

Hypertension leading to kidney disease is a common problem in the elderly in most developed nations. NHANES data from 1999 to 2004 indicate the presence of hypertension in 67% of U.S. adults 60 years and older.[411] Overall there is a progressive increase in the incidence of coronary disease, stroke, and cardiovascular mortality as blood pressure rises above 115 mm Hg systolic/75 mm Hg diastolic, with some notable differences in risk based on age and underlying comorbid conditions. Between the ages of 40 and 69 years, a 20-mm Hg systolic blood pressure (SBP) change is associated with a twofold difference in the death rates from ischemic heart disease and other vascular causes, with an even greater difference noted in the stroke death rate.[412] As age increases, SBP and pulse pressure become better predictors of cardiovascular disease (CVD).[413] Elastic senescence, altered extracellular matrix cross-linking, and calcium deposition lead to fibrotic changes with medial elastocalcinosis and stiffness in the larger elastic aging vasculature, which decrease vascular capacitance and propagation of the pulse wave velocity, clinically evident as widened pulse pressure.[414] Impaired endothelial function and relaxation from low NO production with age are also noted to increase vascular stiffness.[415] With greater arterial stiffness in aging as diastolic blood pressure (DBP) decreases and pulse pressure increases, studies suggest that evaluating a combination of parameters such as SBP + DBP or pulse pressure + mean arterial pressure may be more useful in predicting mortality outcomes.[416] Isolated systolic hypertension (ISH), with SBP more than 160 mm Hg and DBP less than 90 mm Hg, is evident in nearly 75% of U.S. hypertensive elderly patients.[417] Although hypertension independently increases the risk of ESKD, elevated SBP appears to be associated with greater risk of ESKD.[418] ISH is a strong independent risk factor for a decline in kidney function in older individuals (Figure 24.15).[419]

Measurement of blood pressure in the elderly should follow standard guidelines in the American Heart Association recommendations,[420] although standing blood pressure should also be measured periodically in the elderly, given the increased risk for postural hypotension. A thorough examination to assess underlying causes and end-organ involvement, including laboratory evaluation of renal function (serum creatinine level or eGFR), is important in those elderly diagnosed with hypertension.[421] Although treatment of elevated blood pressure in the elderly, including those older than 80 years, is clearly beneficial,[422-424] the goal of SBP less than 140 mm Hg that was developed for the general population needs to be adjusted for those with ISH and for patients 80 years and older. Blood pressure therapy that decreases DBP to 60 mm Hg or less in the elderly with ISH can impair tissue perfusion, increase cardiovascular risk, and reduce survival. Thus SBP goals should not be reached at the expense of excessive DBP reduction. The intention-to-treat Hypertension in the Very Elderly Trial (HYVET) supports a target blood pressure of 150/80 mm Hg in patients 80 years or older, reporting a 21% reduction in all-cause mortality and a marked reduction in other cardiovascular morbidity, such as stroke and heart failure.[423] The Eighth Joint National Committee (JNC8) guidelines, based on a review of a number of randomized trials—including HYVET, the Systolic Hypertension in Europe Trial (Sys-Euro), the Japanese trial to assess optimal systolic blood pressure in elderly hypertensive patients (JATOS), the Valsartan in Elderly Isolated Systolic Hypertension (VALISH) Study, and the usual versus tight control of systolic blood pressure in non-diabetic patients with hypertension trial (CARDIO-SIS)—recommend blood pressure goals of less than 150/90 mm Hg for people older than 60 years.[425-431]

Lifestyle modification with appropriate dietary salt restriction, exercise, and weight loss when necessary remains the primary treatment, with medications added as required and tailored to each patient. Various medications have been used and are tolerated in the elderly, including chlorthalidone, hydrochlorothiazide, ACEIs, ARBs, and calcium channel blockers.[432-435] These drugs should be initiated at lower dosages and titrated carefully, with awareness of the greater risk of postural and postprandial hypertension in the elderly given the exaggerated response in those with ISH.[436] In a random sample of individuals 75 years or older, SBP was found to drop by more than 50% with the rise from a supine to a standing position. The total prevalence of orthostatic hypotension was 34% in this cohort,[437] which emphasizes the need to monitor and initiate antihypertensive therapy carefully in the elderly. Furthermore, given that many elderly persons are taking a variety of medications, it is important to be wary of drug-drug interactions, which may either potentiate antihypertensive therapy, as do the α_1-blockers frequently used to treat benign prostatic

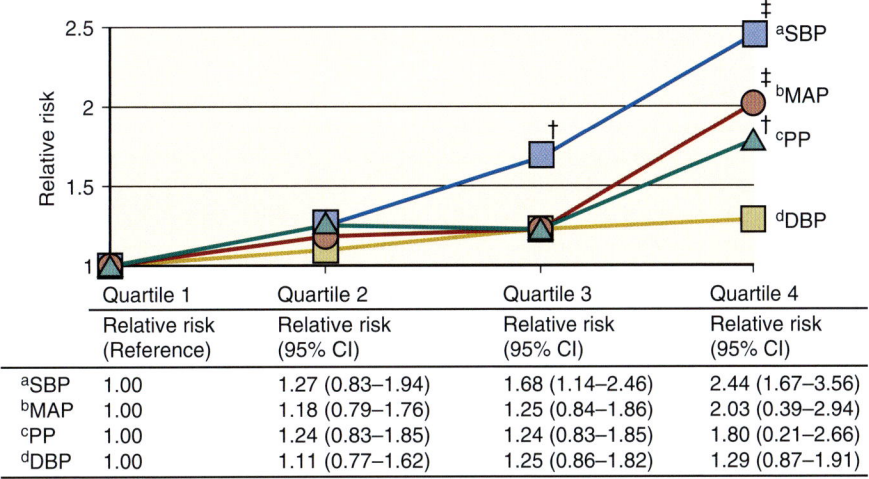

	Quartile 1 Relative risk (Reference)	Quartile 2 Relative risk (95% CI)	Quartile 3 Relative risk (95% CI)	Quartile 4 Relative risk (95% CI)
aSBP	1.00	1.27 (0.83–1.94)	1.68 (1.14–2.46)	2.44 (1.67–3.56)
bMAP	1.00	1.18 (0.79–1.76)	1.25 (0.84–1.86)	2.03 (0.39–2.94)
cPP	1.00	1.24 (0.83–1.85)	1.24 (0.83–1.85)	1.80 (0.21–2.66)
dDBP	1.00	1.11 (0.77–1.62)	1.25 (0.86–1.82)	1.29 (0.87–1.91)

*Each model adjusted for age, gender, ethnicity, history of diabetes, history of cardiovascular disease, and current smoking.
†P value <0.01 for comparison with Quartile 1.
‡P value <0.001 for comparison with Quartile 1.

Figure 24.15 Adjusted relative risk of a decline in kidney function according to quartiles of blood pressure (BP) component in 2181 participants in the Systolic Hypertension in the Elderly Program (SHEP). CI, confidence interval; DBP, diastolic blood pressure; MAP, mean arterial pressure; PP, pulse pressure; SBP, systolic blood pressure. (From Young JH, et al: Blood pressure and decline in kidney function: findings from the Systolic Hypertension in the Elderly Program (SHEP). *J Am Soc Nephrol* 13:2776-2782, 2002.)

hypertrophy, or inhibit antihypertensive therapy, as do the NSAIDs frequently used to manage antiinflammatory processes in the elderly.[438]

RENOVASCULAR DISEASE

Renovascular disease is an important cause of resistant hypertension and progressive renal insufficiency, often manifesting in the elderly as part of a generalized atherosclerotic process rather than an isolated syndrome. USRDS data report incidence and prevalence rates of 1.3% and 0.7% respectively of ESKD in those diagnosed with atherosclerotic renovascular disease (ARVD).[439] The prevalence of renovascular disease has been estimated to be 6.8% in unselected community-dwelling African American and white men and women older than 65 years.[440] Angiographically determined stenosis of 75% or greater in the renal arteries is more likely to progress to occlusion.[441] Unexplained progressive azotemia, worsening or new-onset hypertension, and/or development of AKI with antihypertensive therapy should raise suspicion of renovascular disease in an elderly patient. These signs may be more evident when ACEIs and ARBs are used. Patients also may experience recurrent episodes of acute (flash) pulmonary edema or otherwise unexplained heart failure.[441,442] Patients with ARVD are at increased risk of death from CVD[443]; therefore, aggressive control of atherosclerotic risk factors is recommended. Screening and diagnostic tests should be performed in patients with moderate to high probability of ARVD (see Chapter 48 for complete discussion).[444]

Treatment options for hemodynamically significant lesions, including medical therapy with antihypertensive drugs, revascularization with angioplasty with or without stenting, and surgery, should be individualized for each patient with consideration of the benefits and risks of each procedure. A randomized trial comparing endovascular revascularization plus medical therapy with medical therapy alone in 806 older patients with ARVD found no clinical benefit for revascularization when the end points of renal function, blood pressure, time to renal and cardiovascular events, and mortality were assessed over 34 months of follow-up. Serious complications associated with revascularization occurred in 23 patients, including two deaths and three amputations of toes or limbs.[445] A later study comparing stenting and medical therapy for atherosclerotic renal artery stenosis similarly determined that renal artery stenting did not confer a significant benefit with respect to the prevention of clinical events when added to comprehensive, multifactorial medical therapy in people with atherosclerotic renal artery stenosis and hypertension or CKD.[446,447]

Revascularization also carries the risk of atheroemboli, although the reported incidence is low. There is no evidence that revascularization improves any outcomes in asymptomatic patients.[448]

GLOMERULAR DISEASE

Renal biopsy findings in the elderly suggest that acute and chronic glomerular disease is common in this patient population.[449-457] As in younger patients, AKI and/or nephrotic syndrome often is the reason for renal biopsy in the elderly.[455,456,458]

Nephritic presentations with acute or rapidly progressive renal failure can be devastating in the elderly. Several small case series suggest that pauci-immune glomerulonephritis (GN) is more common in older adults more than 60 years of age.[454,456,459,460] Greater age is associated with increased risk of death from therapy as well as from all causes in older patients with pauci-immune GN.[461] Of the pauci-immune GN biopsy specimens evaluated at a large referral center, 79% of cases were noted in those older than 60 years.[462] Although fewer cases of anti–glomerular basement membrane GN and immune complex crescentic GN were noted in these reports, diagnostic workup for these processes must be included. Similarly, although the incidence of postinfectious or poststreptococcal diffuse proliferative GN has decreased in most developed nations, the disease is becoming more evident in the elderly in underdeveloped regions and in those elderly living in poor socioeconomic or debilitating conditions.[463,464] Therefore a careful history should be taken to identify possible exposure, and a history and/or physical examination findings suggesting the possibility of infection should prompt early diagnosis and supportive treatment in the elderly.

Paraproteinemia, particularly multiple myeloma, can also manifest as AKI in the elderly with or without overt hypercalcemia.[465] Thus quantification of urine protein, serum free monoclonal light-chain analysis immunoelectrophoresis, and immunofixation can be important early on, particularly if the cause of AKI remains unclear. A test result positive for monoclonal proteins should also be followed by further evaluation for the presence of amyloidosis or light-chain deposition disease. In addition, minimal change disease can manifest as AKI in the elderly with significant proteinuria and hypertension. Renal biopsy findings frequently suggest acute tubular injury in the presence of minimal change disease, but the cause remains speculative.[466,467]

Primary glomerular diseases appear to be more prevalent in the elderly than secondary diseases, although diabetic glomerulopathy may be underrepresented because biopsies often are not performed in cases of presumed diabetic renal disease.[458] Relative frequencies of various glomerular diseases are different in older and younger patients. Membranous nephropathy is the most common histologic finding in numerous case series,[453,464,468,469] with 36% of 317 renal biopsy specimens from patients older than 60 years showing nephrotic syndrome.[469a] Anti-PLA2R antibodies may be detected by ELISA in 75% of patients with idiopathic membranous nephropathy with higher levels associated with both greater chance of partial or complete remission as well as greater risk for decreased renal function on follow-up.[470]

Minimal change disease (11%) and amyloidosis (10.7%) also were noted and were more frequent than other diagnoses in this large series.[453] In the very elderly (≥80 years), focal sclerosis from hypertension and hypertensive nephrosclerosis seemed to be more prevalent, followed by immunoglobulin A and membranous nephropathy.[460]

Nephrotic syndrome can coexist with or precede malignancy in up to 30% of elderly diagnosed with malignancy. An immune response to tumor antigens is considered the possible pathologic cause. Solid tumors of the lung, breast, colon or rectum, kidney, and stomach have been commonly reported in association with membranous lesions in renal biopsy specimens, with resolution of the nephrosis after tumor treatment.[471,472] The presence of anti–phospholipase A_2 receptor (PLA_2R) antibodies may be helpful in differentiating idiopathic from secondary malignancy–associated membranous nephropathy.[473] Minimal change lesions in renal biopsy specimens have also been noted in conjunction with Hodgkin's and non-Hodgkin's lymphoma in the elderly.[474,475] Given this association, a thorough history taking, physical examination, and basic screening to rule out a secondary malignant cause should be considered in elderly patients with new-onset nephrosis.

Retrospective studies and meta-analysis of randomized trials as well as pooled analysis of randomized prospective and case series suggest that use of steroids alone for the treatment of membranous lesions has little impact on the rate of renal functional decline in the elderly, although the incidence of CKD is noted to be greater in the elderly,[476-479] likely owing to decreased functional reserve. Although treatment with steroids and cytotoxic agents may lead to partial or complete remission, individual risk/benefit assessment is important given the high risk of infection in the elderly. Case series of minimal change lesions in the elderly suggest that such lesions may respond to steroid use alone; however, the response to both steroids and cytotoxic agents is less than for younger patients. Older patients with minimal change disease seem to experience relapse less frequently and have more stable remissions after cyclophosphamide treatment.[480,481]

Evaluation for primary and secondary amyloidosis should be included in the elderly patient presenting with nephrotic syndrome; Congo red staining of renal or other tissue signifies the presence of amyloid fibrils, confirming the diagnosis. In a small number of elderly patients, generalized global sclerosis can also manifest as nephrotic proteinuria caused by undiagnosed processes that lead to renal scarring, with hypertension hastening this process.

Based on limited data, recommendations for treatment of glomerular diseases are to select and tailor therapy for the elderly using the same criteria as for younger individuals. Treatment with medications requires cautious dosing and careful follow-up because drug metabolism and renal excretion are altered in the elderly, raising the risk of drug toxicity.[482]

CHRONIC KIDNEY DISEASE

CKD increases in prevalence with age and heralds a poor outcome.[483-485] Recognized as a global public health problem, CKD with eGFR less than 60 mL/min/1.73 m^2 is present in approximately 38% of U.S. adults 70 years and older.[486] CKD in the elderly is associated with a greater risk of kidney failure and CVD, including ischemic stroke and death.[485,487,488] A high risk for all-cause and CVD mortality has been described in community-dwelling elderly individuals with CKD, particularly those with an eGFR of less than 45 mL/min/1.73 m^2 and in men.[6] Frailty is also more prevalent among older patients with CKD than among those with normal renal function,[489] and cognitive impairment increases in older CKD patients independently of other confounding factors,[490,491] although the full extent of the burden of CKD in the elderly is yet to be known.

AKI can hasten the progression of CKD secondary to medical disease such as diabetes, hypertension, chronic GN, and renovascular and obstructive nephropathy. In addition, prolonged use of analgesics, frequently seen in the elderly, may be associated with papillary necrosis and progression to CKD.[492,493] Similarly, decompensated medical illness can result from gradual CKD progression even though frank uremic symptoms are absent. Older individuals may experience episodes of volume overload and symptoms of heart failure, gastrointestinal bleeding, hypertension, or gradual confusion that indicate progression of renal loss. Interestingly, the most common cause of death in elderly patients with CKD is CVD rather than the progression of kidney disease to kidney failure,[488,494] whereas in patients younger than 65, renal replacement is more common.[495]

Therefore, cardiovascular risk management remains important in elderly patients with CKD. Estimates of renal function from serum creatinine levels alone may be inadequate in the elderly, given the changes in muscle mass with age. Although the accuracy of available formulas for estimating GFR in the elderly continues to be investigated,[496-499] the MDRD and CKD-EPI equations may be useful.[283] Validation studies suggest comparable accuracy for the CKD-EPI (cr) equation in both young and elderly patients.[291]

RENAL REPLACEMENT THERAPY

A significant number of elderly diagnosed with ESKD initiate RRT.[500,501] The number of octogenarians and nonagenarians starting dialysis has nearly doubled, rising from 7054 persons in 1996 to 13,577 persons in 2003, with the 2013 report of initiation of dialysis in a centenerian.[502,503] In a retrospective analysis of patient survival among those older than 75 years who had stage 5 CKD, the 1- and 2-year survival rates were 84% and 76%, respectively, in the group receiving dialysis compared with 68% and 47%, respectively, in the group treated conservatively. This survival advantage was lost in patients with multiple comorbid conditions, particularly in those with ischemic heart disease.[504] In-center hemodialysis is the modality of choice for 96% of those older than 75 years.[505] Approximately 19% of the elderly undergo peritoneal dialysis.[505] Although no clear modality advantage exists in the elderly,[506-508] some studies suggest a higher mortality in elderly patients receiving peritoneal dialysis, particularly in those with diabetes.[509,510] For either modality, overall survival for the elderly is shorter than that for younger patients, as would be expected.[505,511] Thus, the choice between hemodialysis and peritoneal dialysis should remain individualized in the elderly, with consideration given to medical and psychosocial factors.

For maintenance hemodialysis, an arteriovenous fistula (AVF) is the preferred access, particularly in the elderly, because it is associated with a lower incidence of infectious complications.[512] Concern for fistula maturation is not unique to older patients, and thus age should not be a limiting factor in AVF creation given the equivalent procedural and fistula survival rates in younger and older patients.[512] Factors limiting fistula creation such as significant vascular disease and cardiovascular instability may be more prevalent in the elderly. Retrospective analysis or United States Renal Data System (USRDS) data adjusted for vascular disease, diabetes, nutritional status, gender, and race suggest little difference in mortality benefit between AVF and arteriovenous graft (AVG) placement.[513] The prevalence of central venous catheter use for maintenance hemodialysis is reported to be as high as 24% in Europe and 28% in North America.[514] Although AVF remains an optimal choice for hemodialysis access in the elderly, AVG and central venous catheters continue to be prevalent access options in the elderly. Similarly, peritoneal dialysis may be an option for elderly patients who experience hemodynamic instability during hemodialysis.[515,516] There is little difference between older and younger patients in the likelihood of technique failure, number of peritonitis episodes, and types of infections, and fewer peritoneal catheter replacements are actually required in older patients.[516,517]

RRT in the elderly patient heralds important problems requiring careful medical management. Clearance levels of numerous concurrent medications required for comorbid conditions in the elderly change with ESKD and dialysis. Elderly patients undergoing dialysis may be more prone to hypoglycemia because of prolonged insulin clearance, poor intake, and decreased sympathetic response due to other medications. Therefore, close monitoring of medications and careful attention to detect subtle changes in the clinical condition of the elderly patient undergoing dialysis are essential.[518] Despite limited survival of some patients, many elderly patients have a high quality of life while undergoing dialysis, and they should not be denied treatment on the basis of chronologic age alone.[519-521] On the other hand, among 3702 nursing home residents in the United States for whom dialysis treatment was started between June 1998 and October 2000, initiation of dialysis was associated with a substantial and sustained decline in functional status.[522] Prospective data from the Australian and New Zealand Dialysis and Transplant Registry show that patients 75 years or older at dialysis initiation with median follow-up between 2 and 3 years have a 1.24 hazard ratio for death for every 5-year increase in age. The presence of low body mass index (<18.5), the number of comorbidities, and late referral added further to higher mortality in this population.[523] Dialysis should not be used only to prolong the dying process. Symptom relief and maintenance of independence should be considered the main goals of treatment.

RENAL TRANSPLANTATION

Age alone does not necessarily preclude candidacy for renal transplantation for those medically eligible. As the subset of older patients with ESKD grows, there is a shift toward older renal transplant candidates while kidney allocation remains skewed toward younger recipients.[524] The 2013 Scientific Registry of Transplant Recipients reports that approximately 40% of all candidates waiting for transplant are between 50 and 64 years old and 18% are 65 years or older. In 2011, 60% of kidney transplant recipients were older than 50 years, of whom 18% were older than 65 years.[525] The proportion of older patients receiving kidney transplants in relation to the number of older patients wait-listed to receive transplants are similar to the proportion of younger recipients of kidney transplants compared with younger wait-listed patients.[526] Although younger transplant recipients experience a higher number of healthy life-years, older patients undergoing transplantation have a significant survival advantage over those remaining on dialysis.[527-529] The overall risk of death is 41% lower for older kidney transplant recipients than for wait-listed candidates, with survival advantage also noted for recipients of extended criteria donor (ECD) kidneys.[530]

In one study, patients 60 years and older who did not undergo transplantation had an overall 2.54 times higher adjusted risk of death than patients of the same age who did receive transplants, regardless of the type of graft; when data were stratified by donor graft type, risk of death was 3.78 times higher for patients receiving non-ECD donor grafts and 2.31 times higher for those receiving ECD grafts.[531] Allograft type affects recipient survival in recipients 65 years and older, with 2009 registry data suggesting better survival rates for living donor grafts than for both deceased non-ECD grafts and deceased ECD donor grafts (Table 24.1) at 3 months, 1 year, and 5 years. Allograft survival is similarly excellent after 3 months, 1 year, and 5 years for recipients 65 years and older, with living donor allografts faring best, followed by deceased non-ECD grafts and deceased ECD grafts (see Table 24.1).[532]

Increasing the kidney transplant donor pool for a growing number of wait-listed candidates forces consideration of graft procurement from older donors. Delayed graft function and some decrease in allograft survival, as well as in patient survival, can be associated with increasing donor age.[533,534] Graft survival at 3 and 5 years for living donor grafts from donors 55 years of age and older was noted to be 85% and 76%, respectively, compared with 89% and 82%, respectively, for grafts from living donors younger than 55 years, and 82% and 73%, respectively, for grafts from deceased donors younger than 55 years.[535]

As the upper age limit for kidney transplant recipients has shifted over time, twice as many patients 65 years and

Table 24.1 Adjusted Patient and Allograft Survival Rates for Transplant Recipients 65 Years of Age and Older

	3 Months		1 Year		5 Years	
	Patient Survival (%)	Allograft Survival (%)	Patient Survival (%)	Allograft Survival (%)	Patient Survival (%)	Allograft Survival (%)
Living donor	99.2	98	96.9	95.4	79.2	73.9
Deceased non–extended criteria donor	97.5	95.2	93.3	89.4	69.6	61.6
Deceased extended criteria donor	95.5	90.3	90.1	83.2	61.3	52.5

Data from U.S. Organ Procurement and Transplantation Network and the Scientific Registry of Transplant Recipients: 2009 annual report. Available at http://optn.transplant.hrsa.gov/ar2009/survival rates.htm. Accessed April 2011.

older are receiving kidney transplants now than in the year 2000. Nearly half the patients age 60 or older die waiting for deceased donor transplants. In a study comparing retrospective cohorts of patients 65 years or older with those between 50 and 64 years and those younger than 50 years over 15 years, cohorts older than 50 years were found to have a higher risk of death over time. Time to death was significantly shorter for those 65 years or older who had coronary artery disease or congestive heart failure.[536]

Although risk of acute rejection can be lower in older recipients, the impact of acute rejection on overall long-term allograft function may be more significant.[537] Nevertheless, transplant graft loss in older recipients occurs primarily from patient death secondary to infection and CVD.[538-540] Thus a careful, thorough preoperative evaluation in the prospective elderly transplant recipient is necessary.[541,542]

The use of immunosuppressive agents in elderly patients can be challenging because of the increased incidence of associated comorbid conditions and altered pharmacokinetics in this age group.[537,538,543] Data from which to evaluate induction regimens and the optimal combination of medications for maintenance immunosuppression among the elderly remain limited at this time. In conclusion, with careful screening and the absence of contraindications to transplant candidacy, recipient performance status as well as discussions regarding life expectancy with and without transplantation may be more useful than age alone in the consideration of renal transplantation in the elderly patient.

URINARY TRACT INFECTION

Urinary tract infection (UTI), whether symptomatic or asymptomatic, is relatively common and a frequent reason for hospital admission in the elderly as various comorbid conditions, anatomic abnormalities, and weakened host defense mechanisms become evident.[544] Age-related mechanical and hormonal changes in the urinary tract often lead to urinary tract obstruction or urine stasis. Coexisting illnesses in the elderly, including cerebrovascular accidents, dementia, impaired mobility, and incontinence of bladder and bowel, often are associated with poor hygiene. Bladder dystonia, changes in the pelvic musculature, prostatic enlargement, and urethral stricture can contribute to obstructive uropathy. Decreased prostatic secretions in older men may predispose to infections of the lower urinary tract. Prostatic microcalculi can harbor bacteria and become a nidus for infection in an elderly man. Decreased vaginal estrogen levels in postmenopausal women may lead to increased vaginal pH by causing relative depletion of lactobacilli and may raise the risk for bacterial colonization and infection.[545] Data are conflicting, however, on the role of systemic and topical estrogen therapy to decrease the incidence of UTI.

Classic signs and symptoms of UTI are urinary frequency, urinary urgency, dysuria, nocturia, and suprapubic discomfort as well as occasional hematuria with cystitis. Pyelonephritis usually manifests as costovertebral angle tenderness, fever, and variable lower urinary tract symptoms. However, a wide spectrum of nonspecific clinical symptoms is interpreted inappropriately as UTI in the elderly, leading to a tendency to both overdiagnosis and overtreatment.[546] Even typical symptoms require cautious interpretation, because they are common in elderly people without infection.[547] A retrospective case series from one hospital suggests that in approximately 40% of cases, UTI is incorrectly diagnosed in hospitalized older people.[544] There has also been a tendency to manage all clinical deterioration in long-term care facility residents who have positive urine culture results as UTIs, which again contributes to excess antimicrobial use, heightens the problem of antimicrobial resistance, and exposes older patients to unnecessary antibiotic side effects.[548] On the other hand, cognitively impaired older patients may not recall or report symptoms and do not have classic genitourinary symptoms, making the diagnosis more problematic. A prospective cohort study of women and men in nursing homes addressed the question of clinical presentation of UTI in residents of long-term care facilities. Dysuria, change in the character of the urine, and altered mental status were the only clinical features significantly associated with bacteriuria plus pyuria. Of these features, dysuria most effectively discriminated between those with and those without bacteriuria plus pyuria.[549]

Atypical clinical manifestations can make diagnosis, prevention, and treatment of UTI in the older patient challenging. The incidence of asymptomatic bacteriuria increases with rising age. Although community-dwelling older women experience symptomatic UTI more often than older men, gender differences are less pronounced in older age groups than in younger age groups.[550] Estimated prevalence of asymptomatic bacteriuria in women older than 80 years living in the community is 20%, whereas 5% to 10% of similarly aged men are bacteriuric without symptoms. Nearly 25% to 50% of institutionalized elderly women and 15% to 40% of institutionalized elderly men, however, are found to have asymptomatic bacteriuria.[550] Because asymptomatic bacteriuria does not necessarily predict poor outcome or treatment effect on morbidity or mortality in the elderly,[551] routine screening for and treatment of asymptomatic bacteriuria, whether or not accompanied by pyuria, is not recommended for either community-dwelling or institutionalized elderly individuals.[547,551-554] Use of indwelling urinary catheters, although common in the elderly, raises concerns about bacterial colonization and biofilm formation on both external and internal catheter surfaces and is associated with a 5% per day rate of asymptomatic bacteriuria (see also Chapter 37). Asymptomatic catheter-associated bacteriuria does not require antimicrobials. UTI most commonly manifests as fever without localized genitourinary signs and symptoms in these patients and requires treatment.

For elderly patients without indwelling catheters, the minimum criterion for initiating antibiotic therapy according to consensus guidelines is acute dysuria alone or fever in the presence of at least one of the following: new or worsening urgency, frequency, suprapubic pain, gross hematuria, costovertebral angle tenderness, and urinary incontinence.[555] For treatment of symptomatic infection, selection of an antimicrobial should be delayed, wherever possible, until culture results are available. For symptomatic infection in the patient with an indwelling catheter, the catheter should be removed and replaced with a new catheter before initiation of antimicrobial treatment.[556]

Escherichia coli remains the most common cause of symptomatic UTI in older men and women.[557] Nevertheless, a wide spectrum of organisms has been isolated from individuals with long-term indwelling catheters, including yeast species.[556] A urine culture should be performed before initiation of antimicrobial therapy in older individuals with suspected UTI. In relatively healthy women living in the community, however, a short course of empiric antimicrobial therapy can be effective if the patient shows typical symptoms. A 3-day course of antibiotic therapy for uncomplicated symptomatic UTI in older women seems to offer efficacy similar to that of the more standard 7-day therapy, with significantly fewer adverse events.[558] Duration of therapy in men is usually 7 days for cystitis. Treatment is continued for 10 to 14 days for pyelonephritis in both men and women.

Chronic bacterial prostatitis is characterized by positive results on cultures of expressed prostatic fluid and is usually associated with recurrent UTIs. The initial treatment for chronic bacterial prostatitis is the use of a prostate-penetrating antimicrobial agent (e.g., a fluoroquinolone or trimethoprim-sulfamethoxazole) that is effective against the pathogen identified by prostatic localization cultures. The usual course of therapy is 4 weeks.[559]

Long-term (6- to 12-month) low-dose prophylactic antimicrobial therapy can be used for prevention of recurrent uncomplicated UTI in older women in the community who are experiencing two or more UTI episodes in a 6-month period. A first-line regimen is nitrofurantoin 50 or 100 mg or trimethoprim-sulfamethoxazole, one half a regular-strength tablet daily or every other day at bedtime.[550] The optimal duration of UTI therapy for residents of long-term care facilities is not known. In general, the diagnosis of UTI in frail elderly people should be made only after a careful clinical evaluation and thorough review of laboratory data.

RENAL CYSTS

Simple renal cysts occur commonly in aging kidneys.[560,561] One study reported prevalence of 11.5% in individuals aged 50 to 70 years and 22.1% in those aged 70 years and older,[562] whereas another found rates as high as 36.1% in the eighth decade of life, with a relative frequency of 2:1 in men compared with women.[563]

Simple cysts are benign and asymptomatic and usually are incidental findings in patients undergoing abdominal imaging for other causes. They may be solitary, or multiple and bilateral and generally have little clinical significance.[563] Rarely, however, they may be associated with pain, infection, rupture, hematuria, and hypertension.[564-567] Cysts that have smooth clear walls and are fluid filled without internal echoes on ultrasonography usually require no further workup.[568-570] However, a cyst that is filled with debris and/or internal echoes, is thick walled, or occurs in association with a possible renal mass is considered complicated and needs careful follow-up and investigation with further imaging,[569,571,572] cyst puncture, angiography, or surgical exploration as indicated.

ACKNOWLEDGMENTS

The authors would like to acknowledge S. Nicole Akers, for her excellent secretarial assistance, and Melissa McElroy-Elve and Jean Kennedy of the Salem VA Medical Center Library, for their prompt assistance in making papers available for review in the preparation of this chapter.

Complete reference list available at ExpertConsult.com.

KEY REFERENCES

6. Roderick PJ, et al: CKD and mortality risk in older people: a community-based population study in the United Kingdom. *Am J Kidney Dis* 53:950–960, 2009.
15. Tan JC, et al: Glomerular function, structure, and number in renal allografts from older deceased donors. *J Am Soc Nephrol* 20:181–188, 2009.
17. Melk A, Halloran PF: Cell senescence and its implications for nephrology. *J Am Soc Nephrol* 12:385–393, 2001.
18. Hill GS, Heudes D, Bariety J: Morphometric study of arterioles and glomeruli in the aging kidney suggests focal loss of autoregulation. *Kidney Int* 63:1027–1036, 2003.
21. Takazakura E, et al: Intrarenal vascular changes with age and disease. *Kidney Int* 2:224–230, 1972.
30. Camici M, et al: Podocyte dysfunction in aging-related glomerulosclerosis. *Front Biosci (Schol Ed)* 3:995–1006, 2011.
33. Lindeman RD, Tobin J, Shock NW: Longitudinal studies on the rate of decline in renal function with age. *J Am Geriatr Soc* 33:278–285, 1985.
64. Benigni A, et al: Disruption of the Ang II type 1 receptor promotes longevity in mice. *J Clin Invest* 119:524–530, 2009.
67. Sataranatarajan K, et al: Molecular events in matrix protein metabolism in the aging kidney. *Aging Cell* 11:1065–1073, 2012.
72. Noordmans GA, et al: Genetic analysis of mesangial matrix expansion in aging mice and identification of Far2 as a candidate gene. *J Am Soc Nephrol* 24:1995–2001, 2013.
77. Hewitson TD, et al: Relaxin and castration in male mice protect from, but testosterone exacerbates, age-related cardiac and renal fibrosis, whereas estrogens are an independent determinant of organ size. *Endocrinology* 153:188–199, 2012.
89. Huang PL: eNOS, metabolic syndrome and cardiovascular disease. *Trends Endocrinol Metab* 20:295–302, 2009.
96. Donato AJ, et al: Direct evidence of endothelial oxidative stress with aging in humans: relation to impaired endothelium-dependent dilation and upregulation of nuclear factor-kappaB. *Circ Res* 100:1659–1666, 2007.
97. Donato AJ, et al: Vascular endothelial dysfunction with aging: endothelin-1 and endothelial nitric oxide synthase. *Am J Physiol Heart Circ Physiol* 297:H425–H432, 2009.
100. Raj DS, et al: Advanced glycation end products: a nephrologist's perspective. *Am J Kidney Dis* 35:365–380, 2000.
131. Lee JH, et al: Suppression of apoptosis by calorie restriction in aged kidney. *Exp Gerontol* 39:1361–1368, 2004.
132. Storz P: Reactive oxygen species-mediated mitochondria-to-nucleus signaling: a key to aging and radical-caused diseases. *Sci STKE*, 2006.
142. Masoro EJ: Overview of caloric restriction and ageing. *Mech Ageing Dev* 126:913–922, 2005.
154. Colman RJ, et al: Caloric restriction delays disease onset and mortality in rhesus monkeys. *Science* 325:201–204, 2009.
156. Holloszy JO, Fontana L: Caloric restriction in humans. *Exp Gerontol* 42:709–712, 2007.
159. Russell SJ, Kahn CR: Endocrine regulation of ageing. *Nat Rev Mol Cell Biol* 8:681–691, 2007.
165. Imai S: SIRT1 and caloric restriction: an insight into possible trade-offs between robustness and frailty. *Curr Opin Clin Nutr Metab Care* 12:350–356, 2009.
179. Pearson KJ, et al: Resveratrol delays age-related deterioration and mimics transcriptional aspects of dietary restriction without extending life span. *Cell Metab* 8:157–168, 2008.
180. Kume S, et al: Calorie restriction enhances cell adaptation to hypoxia through Sirt1-dependent mitochondrial autophagy in mouse aged kidney. *J Clin Invest* 120:1043–1055, 2010.
192. Harrison DE, et al: Rapamycin fed late in life extends lifespan in genetically heterogeneous mice. *Nature* 460:392–395, 2009.
212. Lavu S, et al: Sirtuins—novel therapeutic targets to treat age-associated diseases. *Nat Rev Drug Discov* 7:841–853, 2008.
220. Chen SC, et al: Association of dyslipidemia with renal outcomes in chronic kidney disease. *PLoS ONE* 8:e55643, 2013.
234. Kuro-o M: Klotho and aging. *Biochim Biophys Acta* 1790:1049–1058, 2009.

244. Huber TB, et al: Emerging role of autophagy in kidney function, diseases and aging. *Autophagy* 8:1009–1031, 2012.
271. Rowe JW, Shock NW, DeFronzo RA: The influence of age on the renal response to water deprivation in man. *Nephron* 17:270–278, 1976.
281. Fliser D, et al: Renal functional reserve in healthy elderly subjects. *J Am Soc Nephrol* 3:1371–1377, 1993.
283. Levey AS, et al: A new equation to estimate glomerular filtration rate. *Ann Intern Med* 150:604–612, 2009.
289. Kilbride HS, et al: Accuracy of the MDRD (Modification of Diet in Renal Disease) study and CKD-EPI (CKD Epidemiology Collaboration) equations for estimation of GFR in the elderly. *Am J Kidney Dis* 61:57–66, 2013.
290. Zhu Y, et al: Comparisons between the 2012 new CKD-EPI (Chronic Kidney Disease Epidemiology Collaboration) equations and other four approved equations. *PLoS ONE* (9):e84688, 2014.
293. Epstein M, Hollenberg NK: Age as a determinant of renal sodium conservation in normal man. *J Lab Clin Med* 87:411–417, 1976.
315. Tian Y, Serino R, Verbalis JG: Downregulation of renal vasopressin V2 receptor and aquaporin-2 expression parallels age-associated defects in urine concentration. *Am J Physiol Renal Physiol* 287:F797–F805, 2004.
332. Crowe MJ, et al: Altered water excretion in healthy elderly men. *Age Ageing* 16:285–293, 1987.
334. Frassetto LA, et al: Effect of age on blood acid-base composition in adult humans: role of age-related renal functional decline. *Am J Physiol* 271:F1114–F1122, 1996.
338. Amodu A, Abramowitz MK: Dietary acid, age, and serum bicarbonate levels among adults in the United States. *Clin J Am Soc Nephrol* 8:2034–2042, 2013.
346. Dawson-Hughes B, et al: Treatment with potassium bicarbonate lowers calcium excretion and bone resorption in older men and women. *J Clin Endocrinol Metab* 94:96–102, 2009.
347. Moseley KF, et al: Potassium citrate supplementation results in sustained improvement in calcium balance in older men and women. *J Bone Miner Res* 28:497–504, 2013.
349. Mulkerrin E, et al: Aldosterone responses to hyperkalemia in healthy elderly humans. *J Am Soc Nephrol* 6:1459–1462, 1995.
356. Kuro-o M: Klotho as a regulator of fibroblast growth factor signaling and phosphate/calcium metabolism. *Curr Opin Nephrol Hypertens* 15:437–441, 2006.
358. Portale AA, et al: Aging alters calcium regulation of serum concentration of parathyroid hormone in healthy men. *Am J Physiol* 272:E139–E146, 1997.
390. Miya M, et al: Age-related decline in label-retaining tubular cells: implication for reduced regenerative capacity after injury in the aging kidney. *Am J Physiol Renal Physiol* 302:F694–F702, 2012.
391. Cui J, et al: Age-related changes in the function of autophagy in rat kidneys. *Age (Dordr)* 34:329–339, 2012.
407. Ishani A, et al: Acute kidney injury increases risk of ESRD among elderly. *J Am Soc Nephrol* 20:223–228, 2009.
498. Poggio ED, Rule AD: A critical evaluation of chronic kidney disease—should isolated reduced estimated glomerular filtration rate be considered a "disease"? *Nephrol Dial Transplant* 24:698–700, 2009.
522. Kurella Tamura M, et al: Functional status of elderly adults before and after initiation of dialysis. *N Engl J Med* 361:1539–1547, 2009.
526. Abecassis M, et al: Solid-organ transplantation in older adults: current status and future research. *Am J Transplant* 12:2608–2622, 2012.

SECTION IV

EVALUATION OF THE PATIENT WITH KIDNEY DISEASE

25 Approach to the Patient with Kidney Disease

Michael Emmett | Andrew Z. Fenves | John C. Schwartz

CHAPTER OUTLINE

HEMATURIA, 754
 History and Review of Systems, 755
 Physical Examination, 756
 Laboratory Tests, 756
 Imaging, 757
NEPHRITIC SYNDROME, 757
 History and Review of Systems, 757
 Physical Examination, 758
 Laboratory Tests, 758
 Imaging, 760
 Kidney Biopsy, 760
NEPHROTIC SYNDROME, 760
 History and Review of Systems, 761
 Physical Examination, 761
 Laboratory Tests, 762
 Imaging, 763
 Kidney Biopsy, 763
OBSTRUCTIVE UROPATHY, 764
 History and Review of Systems, 764
 Physical Examination, 764
 Laboratory Tests, 764
 Imaging, 765
HYPERTENSION, 765
 History and Review of Systems, 765
 Physical Examination, 766
 Laboratory Tests, 766

Imaging, 767
 Other Studies, 767
NEPHROLITHIASIS, 767
 History and Review of Systems, 767
 Physical Examination, 768
 Laboratory Tests, 768
 Imaging, 768
 Differential Diagnosis, 769
 Initial Treatment, 769
ACUTE KIDNEY INJURY, 769
 History and Review of Systems, 771
 Physical Examination, 771
 Laboratory Tests, 771
 Imaging, 772
 Kidney Biopsy, 772
CHRONIC KIDNEY DISEASE, 773
 History and Review of Systems, 774
 Physical Examination, 775
 Laboratory Tests, 776
 Imaging, 776
URINARY TRACT INFECTION, 777
 History and Review of Systems, 777
 Physical Examination, 777
 Laboratory Tests, 777
 Imaging, 778

Readers of this chapter are assumed already to be competent medical historians and to be very familiar with the essentials of the general physical examination. Furthermore, many of the topics that are briefly reviewed in this chapter are addressed in much greater detail in other parts of this textbook. Consequently, the focus here is on certain features of the history, physical examination, and laboratory testing that might be of specific utility to nephrologists and nephrology trainees. The chapter is divided into nine broad areas of kidney disorder and addresses those features of greatest importance to the early diagnostic and therapeutic phases of the patient's workup.

HEMATURIA

Hematuria is the excretion of an abnormal number of red blood cells (RBCs) into the urine. Normal individuals excrete about 1 million RBCs per day in their urine. Extrapolated to the microscopic examination of the sediment of a spun urine specimen, this equates to about 1 to 3 RBCs per high-power field (HPF). Therefore, excretion of more than 3 RBC/HPF is abnormal and may warrant further evaluation. The excretion of more than 3 RBC/HPF, but not enough RBCs to make the urine visibly red, defines microscopic hematuria. Asymptomatic microscopic hematuria is very common; it may be detected in up to 13% of adults.[1] Although it is most often of no consequence, hematuria can be a sign of serious disease and should never be ignored. Gross hematuria occurs when the quantity of urine blood is large enough to color the specimen red or brown. Although microscopic and gross hematuria are generally caused by the same conditions, there are marked differences in the relative frequencies with which various pathologic conditions generate these two presentations. Therefore, the diagnostic approaches to these two conditions are different. Although routine screening of healthy individuals for the presence of hematuria is currently not recommended by the U.S. Preventive Services Task Force, more recent studies have suggested that screening urinalysis may be a strong indicator of subsequent renal disease.[2,3] In addition, asymptomatic microscopic hematuria is still often detected when a urinalysis is performed during the evaluation of a patient for nonurinary complaints. Furthermore, when a urinalysis reveals hematuria, the person's age, gender, population ancestry, medical history, and physical findings must be considered to determine if further evaluation is indicated.[4]

A diagnosis of asymptomatic hematuria requires microscopic examination showing more than 3 RBC/HPF in at least two of three freshly voided, midstream, clean-catch (in women not during menstruation) urine specimens.[5,6]

If microscopic hematuria spontaneously resolves, evaluation decisions are strongly influenced by the clinician's index of suspicion. Microscopic hematuria associated with symptoms such as urinary frequency or pain is more worrisome and mandates further evaluation. Gross hematuria, especially if clots are passed, usually indicates a urologic source of bleeding. Even a single episode of gross hematuria mandates further evaluation. The most common cause of gross hematuria in young women (<40 years) is urinary tract infection (UTI). Malignancy must be strongly considered and ruled out by appropriate studies in older patients.[4,7] Brown, cola–colored, or smoky urine with RBCs present on microscopy is very suggestive of a glomerular source of bleeding.

HISTORY AND REVIEW OF SYSTEMS

Three major factors influencing the workup are the patient's age, gender, and ancestry. The common causes of hematuria in children and young adults are much different than those in older individuals. Hematuria in adults older than 40 years (some propose an age cutoff of >50 years) must be considered a sign of malignancy (of the bladder, upper urinary tract, or kidney) until proven otherwise.[4] Although malignancy is much less frequent in young patients with hematuria, a Wilms' tumor should be considered. Bladder cancer is much more common in men and in whites. Hypercalciuria, and less commonly hyperuricosuria, are frequently the cause of hematuria in children but a less common cause in adults. Hematuria due to UTI is much more common in women, whereas older men may bleed from the prostate. In women, cyclic gross hematuria concurrent with the menses raises the strong possibility of genitourinary (GU) tract endometriosis. The combination of hematuria with fever, dysuria, or flank pain, or a prior history of these symptoms, suggests infection, stones, or malignancy. Colicky pain suggests ureteral obstruction from a stone, blood clot, or sloughed renal papilla. This is especially the case if the pain radiates to the testicle or labia.

A family history of renal dysfunction or renal stones should be sought. When a patient with hematuria has family members with renal failure, diagnoses such as polycystic kidney disease or Alport's disease should be considered. Familial hearing loss, especially in male relatives, suggests Alport's disease. A very common cause of otherwise unexplained asymptomatic familial hematuria is thin basement membrane disease.[8] Sickle cell trait or anemia are very common causes of hematuria in African Americans.[9]

Hematuria sometimes occurs after vigorous exercise or participation in contact or noncontact sports.[10] Mechanisms include direct recurrent trauma to the bladder or kidneys and pathologic renal hemodynamic effects. However, the fact that hematuria occurs after completing a long bicycle ride or running a marathon does not exclude the possibility of other potentially serious pathologic conditions, and generally a complete evaluation is necessary. Exercise-related hemoglobinuria, such as march hemoglobinuria, and postexercise myoglobinuria result in excretion of globin pigments and positive results on dipstick testing without RBCs in the urine.

Travel history may be very important as, for example, when hematuria develops in patients who have traveled to areas where *Schistosoma haematobium* infection or tuberculosis is endemic. Although otherwise unexplained bleeding into the urine can occur in patients with hereditary or acquired coagulation disorders or in patients who require therapeutic anticoagulation, these conditions and drugs should not preclude consideration of other underlying causes. Bleeding disorders and anticoagulants will cause any pathologic GU structures such as malignancies to bleed more readily. This is especially common in older patients.[11] A history of cigarette smoking (or second-hand smoke exposure) increases the risk of bladder cancer twofold to fourfold.[12] Occupational exposure to aniline dyes and aromatic amines and amides, treatment with some chemotherapeutic agents (e.g., cyclophosphamide, mitotane), and radiation to the pelvis increase the risk for uroepithelial cancers. In the past, long-term use of analgesics did increase the risk of bladder cancer, but this was probably due to the presence of phenacetin, which has now been removed from these medications. Indeed, the use of aspirin and other nonsteroidal antiinflammatory drugs (NSAIDs) has been shown to reduce the likelihood of bladder cancer in some epidemiologic studies.[13] Over the past decade, it has become apparent that ingestion or occupational exposure to Chinese herbals containing aristolochic acid markedly increases the risk of urothelial carcinoma.[14,15]

A recent history of pharyngitis followed by hematuria raises the possibility of glomerulonephritis with synpharyngitic bleeding. Chronic glomerulonephritis, usually immunoglobulin A (IgA) nephropathy, is often exacerbated by an upper respiratory tract infection and may result in gross hematuria. This is distinct from poststreptococcal glomerulonephritis, which occurs 2 to 6 weeks following the infection.

With gross hematuria, it is useful to determine if the bleeding is more pronounced at the very beginning or at the termination of voiding. Although formal three-glass urine collections are now rarely performed, a history of initiation hematuria suggests a urethral source, whereas termination hematuria is suggestive of bladder neck or prostatic urethral pathology. Blood clots in the urine usually denote structural urologic pathology.

PHYSICAL EXAMINATION

Evaluation of blood pressure and volume status is especially important when glomerulonephritis is a consideration. If palpation of the abdomen reveals a mass, a renal tumor or hydronephrosis may exist. A palpable bladder after voiding indicates obstruction or retention. Atrial fibrillation raises the possibility of renal embolic infarction, especially if the patient has flank pain. Costovertebral angle tenderness is also suggestive of pyelonephritis, nephrolithiasis, or ureteropelvic junction obstruction. A bruit over the kidney suggests a vascular cause. A careful genital and rectal examination is necessary to help rule out disorders such as prostatitis, prostate cancer, epididymitis, and meatal stenosis.

LABORATORY TESTS

A diagnosis of gross hematuria is suggested by red or brown urine. It requires only about 1 mL of blood to make urine turn red. However, many substances other than RBCs can produce red or brown urine. They include chemicals, medications, and food metabolites. A chemical test for hemoglobin is very helpful in distinguishing among these possibilities. The most commonly used method of testing the urine for blood is the urine test strip or dipstick, which uses the peroxidase-like activity of hemoglobin to generate a color change in a chromogen (dark green to blue). These test strips do not react with most nonhemoglobin pigments that can color the urine.

In addition to detecting the hemoglobin in RBCs, the reaction also yields a positive result with any free hemoglobin and/or myoglobin in the urine. A false-positive hemoglobin test can be produced by hypochlorite solutions, which are sometimes used to clean urine collection containers, and by some urine bacteria that produce peroxidases.[16] Therefore, any positive dipstick test for hemoglobin must be followed by a microscopic examination of the urine to confirm the presence of RBCs.[17] Some of the causes of red or brown urine are shown in Table 25.1. It is also important to separate hematuria caused by glomerular abnormalities from bleeding due to other pathologic kidney conditions (e.g., tumors, cysts) or pathologic processes distal to the glomerulus (e.g., interstitial disease, stones, tumors, other processes affecting the renal pelvis, ureters, bladder, urethra, or prostate. When blood originates from glomeruli, the RBCs pass through the length of the renal tubules, where they are subjected to marked changes in osmolality, ionic strength, pH, and other forces. Compression of the RBCs, together with urine proteins, creates RBC casts (Fig. 25.1), and the identification of these casts on microscopic examination provides excellent evidence for glomerular bleeding. Although quite specific, RBC casts often are not seen, even when definite glomerular bleeding exists. A more common helpful sign of glomerular bleeding is the identification of dysmorphic RBCs of varying shape and sizes with blebs,

Table 25.1 Causes of Red or Brown Urine

Endogenous Substances	Foods	Drugs
Red blood cells	Artificial food coloring	Adriamycin
Hemoglobin	Beets	Chloroquine
Myoglobin	Blackberries	Deferoxamine
Bilirubin	Blueberries	Levodopa
Porphyrins	Fava beans	Methyldopa
Melanin	Paprika	Metronidazole
	Rhubarb	Nitrofurantoin
		Phenazopyridine (Pyridium)
		Phenolphthalein
		Phenytoin
		Prochlorperazine
		Quinine
		Rifampin
		Sulfonamides

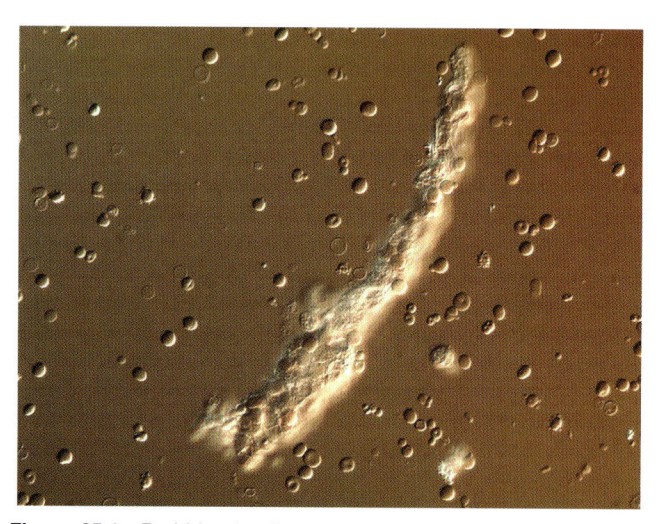

Figure 25.1 Red blood cell cast and acanthocytes consistent with glomerular bleeding (diffusion interference contrast optics). (Courtesy Dr. Rajiv Agarwal, Nephrology Division, Indiana University School of Medicine, Indianapolis.)

budding and, especially, the vesicle-shaped protrusions that characterize acanthocytes (i.e., so-called Mickey Mouse ears; see Fig. 25.1). Dysmorphic RBCs are an excellent indicator of glomerular bleeding when most of the urine RBCs are affected.[18] Acanthocytes are quite specific when they represent more than 5% of the urinary RBCs; this is a very good sign of glomerular bleeding. These distinct RBC anatomic alterations are most readily seen with phase-contrast microscopy. Another indication that bleeding is more likely of glomerular origin is coexistent significant proteinuria (>0.5 g/day or >0.5 protein/g of creatinine). The presence of pyuria together with hematuria suggests inflammation or infection and warrants a urine culture.

Table 25.2 highlights the features that can be used to differentiate glomerular and nonglomerular, or urologic, hematuria. Urine cytologic analysis is indicated when otherwise unexplained hematuria is documented. It has good

Table 25.2 Differentiation of Glomerular from Urologic Bleeding

Feature	Glomerular Hematuria	Urothelial Hematuria
Urine color	Dark red, brown, cola-colored, smoky	Bright red
Clots	−	+
Proteinuria	+	−
Red blood cell morphology	Dysmorphic (especially acanthocytes)	Isomorphic
Hypertension	+	−
Edema	+	−
Urinary voiding symptoms	−	+
Back pain, flank pain	+	+
Renal function	Reduced	Normal
Family history	+	+
Trauma	−	+
Upper respiratory tract infection	+	−
Fever, rash	+	−

specificity and a sensitivity of about 80% for bladder cancer but a much lower sensitivity for upper tract malignancy.[19]

IMAGING

When hematuria is not believed to be of glomerular origin, computed tomography (CT) with and without intravenous (IV) contrast is currently the preferred initial imaging modality to evaluate microscopic and gross hematuria and has largely replaced intravenous pyelography (IVP). CT urography has excellent sensitivity for stones, identifies most kidney tumors, and reveals other non–GU tract abdominal pathologic processes. The major disadvantage of a CT scan is the need for IV radiocontrast and the significant quantity of radiation exposure.[20] If CT cannot be done, renal ultrasonography is the next best initial imaging test. If the explanation for hematuria is not evident on the initial study, the next diagnostic imaging test to perform is cystoscopy. Direct visualization of the bladder requires cystoscopy. Abnormal areas or lesions can be biopsied. Performing cystoscopy at the time of bleeding may localize the bleeding site. If no abnormality is noted and there is any suspicion of upper tract disease, retrograde pyelography may be performed.

One diagnostic approach is illustrated in Figure 25.2. A major decision branch is based on the patient's age and other risk factors for bladder cancer. There is controversy about the specific age to be used for diagnostic stratification. Some experts believe it should be 40 years, and others argue for 50 years. Figure 25.3 shows the frequency of renal, uroepithelial, and bladder cancers stratified by gender and age in 1930 patients evaluated for hematuria.[3]

NEPHRITIC SYNDROME

Classic nephritic syndrome is characterized by glomerular hematuria and an active urine sediment, manifested by dysmorphic RBCs (especially acanthocytes) and RBC casts and often white blood cells (WBCs) and WBC casts. In general, these are the result of an inflammatory process in the glomerulus. Usually, the glomerular filtration rate (GFR) is reduced, and variable degrees of hypertension, oliguria, and edema occur. Proteinuria is common but often of relatively low magnitude. In many cases, the degree of proteinuria is limited by the accompanying reduction in GFR. However, high-grade proteinuria and even full-blown nephrotic syndrome can coexist with nephritic syndrome in some patients. The hematuria can be sporadic, intermittent, or persistent. It can be microscopic or gross. Isolated glomerular hematuria without inflammation (e.g., that which occurs with thin basement membrane disease) is generally not considered to be the result of a nephritic process. The character of the glomerular hematuria does not always predict the underlying cause of the disorder, nor does it predict the long-term renal outcome of the process. Nephritic syndrome can occur as an isolated renal process or as a feature of a systemic disease or a hereditary disorder.

Glomerular hematuria due to nephritic syndrome must be distinguished from bleeding caused by other kidney, interstitial, or lower GU tract pathology, including stones, benign or malignant mass lesions, and infections. The features that help differentiate these classes of hematuria have been discussed earlier (see "Hematuria") and are listed in Table 25.2. When nephritic hematuria is identified, additional renal evaluation is required.

HISTORY AND REVIEW OF SYSTEMS

The patient's history often helps distinguish glomerular hematuria from urothelial hematuria. Glomerular hematuria, when visible, is often described as dark brown, tea- or cola-colored, or smoky as opposed to the overtly red color often seen with urologic pathology. Clots are almost never formed with glomerular hematuria. The patient may also note that the urine has become foamy as a result of the excretion of albumin, which has a soaplike action and reduces the surface tension of urine. Urinary voiding symptoms are distinctly uncommon. Back, flank, or abdominal pain does not distinguish glomerular hematuria from urothelial hematuria. There may be a history of an antecedent upper respiratory tract or skin infection in patients with poststreptococcal glomerulonephritis (e.g., postpharyngitic hematuria).[21] A recent episode of staphylococcal infection particularly in older diabetic patients raises the issue of IgA-dominant postinfectious glomerulonephritis.[22-24]

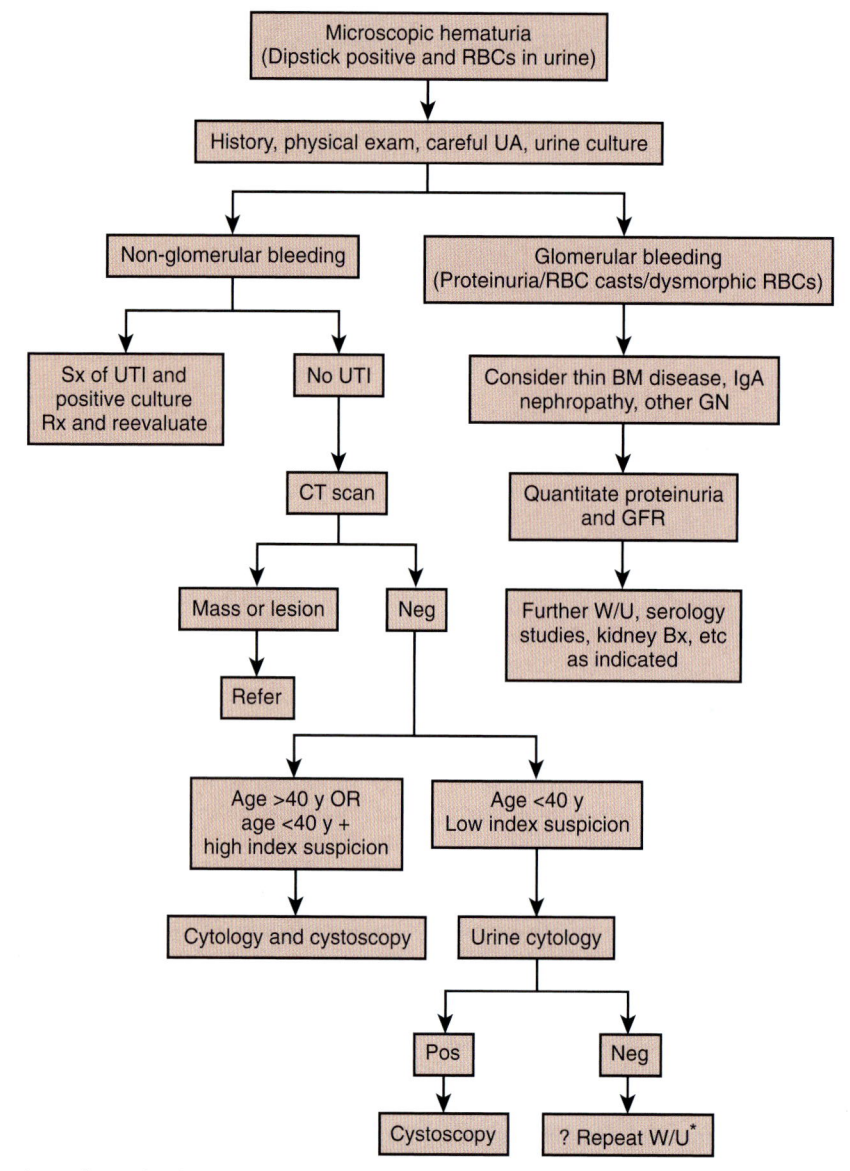

Figure 25.2 Diagnostic scheme for evaluation of microscopic hematuria. *Workup should be repeated if the patient develops new symptoms of gross hematuria.

In other patients with an underlying form of chronic glomerulonephritis, such as IgA nephropathy, gross hematuria may occur simultaneously with, or immediately after, an episode of pharyngitis (synpharyngitic hematuria). There may be a family history of glomerular disease. A history of hypertension, fluid retention, and/or edema formation suggests glomerular hematuria, particularly if renal function is reduced. Fever, skin rash, and joint symptoms raise the possibility of a systemic disease causing glomerular hematuria. Hearing loss and visual symptoms related to lens abnormalities can be seen with Alport's disease. Hemoptysis raises the possibility of vasculitis or anti–glomerular basement membrane (anti-GBM) disease.

PHYSICAL EXAMINATION

Hypertension is very frequent with glomerular hematuria. Most often this is caused by renal salt retention and volume expansion. The salt retention is caused by enhanced reabsorption in the distal nephron, especially the cortical collecting tubule.[25] The renin-angiotensin-aldosterone system in most patients with nephritic syndrome is functioning normally.[26] Malignant hypertension with vital organ injury occurs in some patients. A careful retinal examination may yield a specific diagnosis. High-frequency sensorineural hearing loss strongly suggests Alport's disease. Typical skin findings can be seen in systemic lupus erythematosus, vasculitis, Fabry's disease, and Henoch-Schönlein purpura. Joint findings may suggest a rheumatologic-collagen vascular disease or vasculitis. Examination of the suprapubic area, back, and the flanks is generally unrevealing.

LABORATORY TESTS

URINE STUDIES

The hallmark of nephritic syndrome is glomerular hematuria. Hematuria is most easily recognized by a positive result

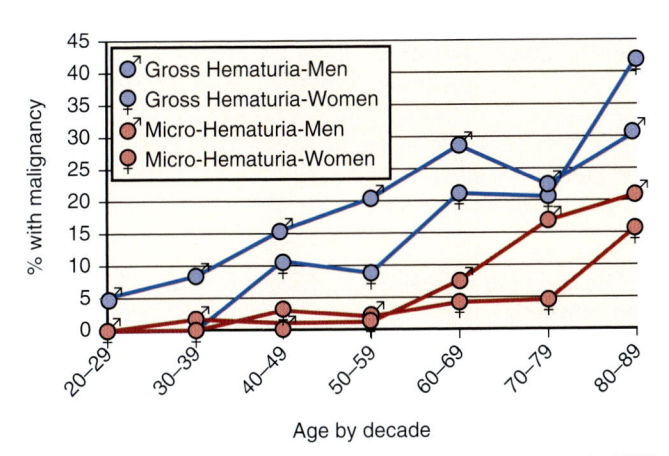

Figure 25.3 Prospective analysis of the risk of malignancy in 1930 patients undergoing workup for hematuria. (Adapted from Khadra MH, Pickard RS, Charlton M, et al: A prospective analysis of 1,930 patients with hematuria to evaluate current diagnostic practice, *J Urol* 163:524-527, 2000.)

on a urine dipstick test for blood (see earlier, "Hematuria," for further discussion). Proteinuria is a frequent accompaniment to hematuria in patients with nephritic syndrome but is usually absent in patients with urothelial hematuria. The proteinuria can range from low-grade (<500 to 1000 mg/day) to overt nephrotic levels (>3000 mg/day). Protein excretion can be quantitated with 24-hour urine collection. Alternatively, a spot urine protein/creatinine ratio can be determined, which gives a reasonable estimate of the magnitude of proteinuria.[27] Microscopic examination of the urine in the nephritic state reveals a variable number of free RBCs. Often, a small pellet of RBCs can be noted at the bottom of a test tube of centrifuged urine. RBC casts are the definitive finding in the nephritic syndrome but very often cannot be seen. A more commonly identified characteristic of glomerular bleeding is dysmorphic urine RBCs with blebs, budding, and vesicle-shaped protrusions[10] (see Fig. 25.1). Examination of the urine sediment with phase-contrast microscopy can be especially helpful. Kidney inflammation also generates pyuria and WBC casts. Hyaline casts can be seen, especially with marked proteinuria.

BLOOD STUDIES

Routine laboratory studies should include a complete blood count (CBC), electrolyte levels, determination of blood urea nitrogen (BUN) and creatinine concentrations, and liver panel. Sedimentation rate and C-reactive protein level are often elevated, regardless of the cause of nephritic syndrome. A determination of the GFR is required. Usually, this is accomplished with a quantitative urine collection for the measurement of creatinine clearance. Iothalamate clearance, if available, provides the most accurate measurement. Various formulas have been developed to estimate the GFR based on a single and presumably stable serum creatinine measurement and are reviewed in Chapter 26. The most accurate formula currently in use is that developed by the Chronic Kidney Disease Epidemiology Collaboration (CKD-EPI). However, all methods that rely on a single serum creatinine measurement will give erroneous results when renal function is rapidly changing, and the serum creatinine concentration is not relatively stable.

Table 25.3 Complement Levels in Acute Nephritic Syndromes

Low Serum Complement Levels
Systemic Diseases (Low C3 and C4)
Systemic lupus erythematosus Cryoglobulinemia (hepatitis C) Bacterial endocarditis Shunt nephritis
Renal Localized Diseases

Acute poststreptococcal glomerulonephritis (low C3, normal C4)
Membranoproliferative glomerulonephritis
  Type I (low C3 and C4)
  Type II (dense deposit disease) (low C3, normal C4)

Normal Serum Complement Levels
Systemic Diseases
Polyarteritis nodosa Antineutrophil cytoplasmic antibody–positive granulomatosis with polyangiitis (Wegener's granulomatosis) Hypersensitivity vasculitis Henoch-Schönlein purpura Goodpasture's syndrome
Renal Localized Diseases
Immunoglobulin A nephropathy Rapidly progressive glomerulonephritis Anti–glomerular basement membrane disease isolated to kidney Pauci-immune glomerulonephritis (kidney-localized)

Measurements of complement levels can be very helpful in patients with nephritic syndrome.[28] It is generally best to begin with a measure of total hemolytic complement (CH_{50}) and then proceed to measurement of C3 (a component of both the classic and alternative complement pathways) and C4 (a component of the classic pathway only). Table 25.3 separates the various forms of acute nephritic glomerulonephritis into those with normal and those with reduced complement levels. A low C3 with normal C4 levels suggests poststreptococcal glomerulonephritis or membranoproliferative glomerulonephritis, whereas low C3 and C4 levels are more consistent with postinfectious glomerulonephritis, systemic lupus erythematosus, hepatitis C–associated membranoproliferative glomerulonephritis (type I), or mixed cryoglobulinemia. Complement levels are extremely variable in poststaphylococcal IgA glomerulonephritis. Other serologic studies, mainly to measure various autoantibodies, are ordered when specific underlying systemic diseases are considered the possible cause. The antinuclear antibody (ANA) and anti-DNA, anti-Smith, and anti-Rho antibodies help confirm the diagnosis of systemic lupus erythematosus and other collagen vascular diseases. The perinuclear antineutrophil cytoplasmic antibody (P-ANCA) and cytoplasmic antineutrophil cytoplasmic antibody (C-ANCA) tests help establish a diagnosis of vasculitis. Anti-GBM antibodies are seen in patients with Goodpasture's syndrome. A number of infectious diseases can produce an acute nephritic

Table 25.4	Blood Studies for Acute Nephritic Syndrome

Routine

Complete blood count
Electrolyte levels
Blood urea nitrogen and creatinine concentrations
Liver function studies
Complement levels (total hemolytic complement [CH_{50}], C3, C4)

As Clinical Findings Suggest

Anti-DNA antibody test
Antineutrophil cytoplasmic antibody (ANCA) titer
Anti–glomerular basement membrane antibody test
Antistreptolysin O titer or streptozyme test
Cryoglobulin titer
Hepatitis B and C antibody assay and viral load determination
Human immunodeficiency virus test
Blood cultures

Table 25.5	Causes of Secondary Nephrotic Syndrome

Systemic Diseases

Diabetes mellitus
Systemic lupus erythematosus
Amyloidosis
Carcinoma
Lymphoma and myeloma
Preeclampsia
Drugs
Gold
Antibiotics
Nonsteroidal antiinflammatory drugs
Penicillamine
Heroin
Infections
Human immunodeficiency virus infection
Hepatitis B and C
Malaria
Syphilis

Congenital or Inherited Disorders

Alport's syndrome
Congenital nephrotic syndrome
Nail-patella syndrome

syndrome. It is also important to consider viral hepatitis, both B and C, as well as human immunodeficiency virus (HIV) infection and syphilis. Other infectious diseases that must always be considered are infectious endocarditis or another persistent bacterial infection, such as an abscess or infected vascular access. Blood cultures must be ordered for all patients with otherwise unexplained fever, heart murmurs, or leukocytosis. The commonly ordered laboratory studies for patients with nephritic syndrome are shown in Table 25.4.

IMAGING

Renal size is a very important parameter to define in patients with nephritic syndrome and is most easily accomplished with renal ultrasonography. Although normal-sized kidneys do not definitively predict reversibility (even irreversible end-stage kidneys can be of normal size as a result of swelling or infiltration in patients with diabetes mellitus or amyloidosis), small kidneys do indicate that irreversible fibrosis and atrophy are probably present. The assessment of renal size is therefore especially important for determining renal prognosis and making decisions regarding renal biopsy. If the kidneys are small (<9 cm in a normal-sized adult), the likelihood of reversible disease decreases markedly, and the difficulty and risk of the biopsy procedure increase.

KIDNEY BIOPSY

Patients with glomerular hematuria who have normal blood pressure, normal renal function, and minimal proteinuria rarely require a renal biopsy unless the clinical presentation suggests an underlying systemic illness causing secondary glomerular disease. Kidney biopsy may be helpful when glomerular hematuria is associated with abnormal renal function and is especially valuable when it is important to establish the specific diagnosis to guide therapy.[29] When renal function is decreasing rapidly (rapidly progressive glomerulonephritis), and a nephritic picture exists, the biopsy may need to be obtained very rapidly for potential preservation of renal function.

NEPHROTIC SYNDROME

Nephrotic syndrome has historically been considered to include five principal clinical or biochemical findings:

1. High-grade, albumin-dominant proteinuria (generally >3000 mg/day or spot urine protein/creatinine ratio of >3000 mg of protein/gm of creatinine)
2. Hypoalbuminemia
3. Edema
4. Hyperlipidemia
5. Lipiduria

However, milder and earlier forms of many clinical disorders that can generate the full nephrotic syndrome may produce lower degrees of albuminuria in the range from 30 to 3000 mg/day, with or without the other features. Also, the full spectrum of nephrotic syndrome may not develop in some patients, despite high-grade albuminuria. The principal underlying abnormality responsible for all the clinical features of nephrotic syndrome is increased permeability of the glomerular capillaries. Nephrotic syndrome may occur as an idiopathic and isolated condition, may be an inherited disorder, or may be a complication of an underlying systemic disease or allergic or immunologic disorder. It is always imperative to identify any underlying cause, when one exists (Table 25.5). This is accomplished by recognizing clues from the history and physical examination, reviewing a routine set of laboratory studies, and performing more specific tests suggested by the initial findings.

HISTORY AND REVIEW OF SYSTEMS

The patient's history often helps elucidate the cause of nephrotic syndrome. The most common underlying systemic disease causing nephrotic syndrome is diabetes mellitus. Nephrotic syndrome can develop with all subtypes of this disorder. Other nondiabetic glomerulopathies can also occur in patients with diabetes. Usually, an atypical history and physical and laboratory findings suggest that another cause for nephrotic syndrome may exist.[30,31]

The history may point to other disorders that can generate nephrotic syndrome. These include systemic lupus erythematosus and the various forms of systemic amyloidosis (primary, secondary or reactive, and familial-hereditary). Infectious causes of nephrotic syndrome include viral hepatitis, HIV infection, parvovirus, *Mycoplasma* infection, and syphilis, as well as parasitic diseases such as malaria, schistosomiasis, filariasis, and toxoplasmosis. Many drugs can cause the syndrome, so it is extremely important to obtain a complete list of medications, including prescribed and over-the-counter (OTC) medications, herbal or natural products, and illicit drugs. Drugs and drug classes that have been linked to nephrotic syndrome include NSAIDs, penicillamine, antibiotics and, much more rarely, angiotensin-converting enzyme inhibitors (ACEIs), tamoxifen, and lithium. Paraneoplastic nephrotic syndrome can be the presenting complaint of a variety of solid malignancies, lymphomas, and leukemias or can develop during treatment, sometimes as a complication of the treatment medications. Recently, the use of drugs that target the vascular endothelial growth factor (VEGF) or its receptor (VEGFR) has markedly increased. These drugs often produce proteinuria and hypertension. Less commonly, they generate nephrotic syndrome.[32,33] Rarely, the nephrotic syndrome may be a prominent feature in patients with Alport's syndrome and nail-patella syndrome. Some patients can date the onset of major proteinuria because they have noted when their urine became foamy. This phenomenon, which **is** most readily observed by men, occurs because albumin has a soaplike effect that reduces the surface tension of urine. This can be a very useful sign in patients with recurring episodes of nephrotic syndrome.

PHYSICAL EXAMINATION

Edema is a major characteristic of nephrotic syndrome. The development of hypoalbuminemia reduces the oncotic pressure within the capillaries, which favors the net translocation of fluid into the interstitial spaces. To the extent that this occurs, intravascular volume and blood pressure fall, which triggers the sympathetic nervous system, activates the renin angiotensin aldosterone axis, elevates vasopressin levels, and modulates many other control systems that act together to promote net renal salt and water retention. This pathogenic sequence has been termed the underfill mechanism of salt and water retention in nephrotic syndrome. However, edema formation in many, perhaps most, nephrotic patients cannot be fully explained by underfill mechanisms. Although reduced intravascular oncotic pressures certainly exist in nephrotic patients, the net hydrostatic gradient for water movement across capillary beds is also influenced by the interstitial oncotic pressure, and this generally falls in parallel with reductions in plasma oncotic pressure. Consequently, the net hydrostatic pressure gradient from the intravascular compartment to the interstitial space may not significantly increase. Edema formation under these conditions may be the consequence of a primary form of renal salt and water retention. This pathogenic sequence for edema formation is called the overfill mechanism.

Undoubtedly, each of these mechanisms plays a role in various phases and forms of nephrotic syndrome. The mechanism that predominates is probably related to the specific renal lesion causing the nephrotic syndrome.[34,35] Also, these mechanisms may evolve from one form to the other. (For a more detailed discussion of the mechanisms contributing to edema formation in nephrotic syndrome, see Chapter 53). Regardless of which mechanism occurs initially, either will likely progress to a steady-state condition in which the effective arterial volume status that initiated the disorder is difficult or impossible to discern. Whether the initiating event is underfill of the effective arterial space, leading to renal salt and water retention, or overfill of this compartment, causing excess salt and water to enter the interstitial spaces, the development of clinically apparent edema in an adult requires the net retention of about 4 to 5 kg of fluid, which is equivalent to 4 to 5 L of normal saline. Nephrotic edema is a form of pitting edema. When the thumb is pushed against a bony structure such as the tibia or sacrum, the resulting pit remains visible for a short period of time. Pitting edema is graded on a scale of 1 to 4 (from very slight to more apparent to deep pitting that persists for >2 minutes). Nephrotic edema is diffuse and, to some degree, probably affects almost all tissues, but it is not equally distributed.

The interstitial pressure in various locations has a major impact on edema formation. Thus, the low ambient interstitial pressure often results in prominent periorbital edema. Gravitational forces also cause nephrotic edema to accumulate in dependent body parts. Edema is generally worse in the lower legs and feet at the end of the day and becomes more prominent in the face after nocturnal recumbency. Bedridden patients accumulate edema fluid in their back and sacral areas. The diurnal variation of edema formation becomes less prominent when the degree of edema worsens. Edema that is massive and generalized is termed anasarca. Dropsy is a historical term for generalized edema. Nephrotic edema is usually symmetric (after adjustment for gravitational dependency), and unilateral edema should raise the possibility of local anatomic abnormalities, such as venous thromboses, varicosities, or lymphatic obstruction. However, asymmetric nephrotic edema can result from an anatomic condition that generates greater local or asymmetric edema. Severe edema can cause skin breakdown, blisters, weeping, and superinfection. Chronic (months to years) severe edema of any cause, including nephrotic syndrome, can produce fibrosis of the skin and subcutaneous tissues. The resulting brawny edema is usually pigmented, is very firm, and often will not pit.

Physical clues to other disorders that produce generalized edema should be sought during physical examination. The neck veins must be carefully evaluated to determine whether right-sided cardiac pressures are increased due to cardiac, pulmonary, or pericardial abnormalities. Elevated jugular venous pressures, pericardial knock, Kussmaul's sign (absence of inspiratory decline in jugular pressure), and prominent *x* and *y* descents suggest pericardial disease.

Pulsus paradoxus (an exaggerated fall in systemic blood pressure ≥ 10 mm Hg with inspiration) suggests pericardial or pulmonary disease. Although prominent ascites often indicates liver disease, and pulmonary congestion and pleural effusions suggest cardiac or pulmonary pathology, fluid may accumulate in each of these locations in patients with severe nephrotic syndrome in the absence of cardiac or hepatic abnormalities.

Many skin findings other than edema are also associated with nephrotic syndrome. Some may suggest certain underlying primary diseases. Xanthelasma palpebrarum (periorbital-eyelid xanthomas) is often associated with hypercholesterolemia and may become very prominent in nephrotic patients. Much rarer are eruptive xanthomas, usually associated with extreme hypertriglyceridemia, which may also occur with nephrotic syndrome. A number of relatively specific skin, nail, and scalp abnormalities are associated with various rheumatologic conditions that may cause the nephrotic syndrome. These include a malar facial rash, scarring alopecia, mat telangiectasia, nail bed telangiectasia and nail fold capillary loops and vascular infarcts, and erythema nodosum. Sarcoidosis, which occasionally causes nephrotic syndrome, is associated with erythema nodosum and skin papules. Jaundice, angiomata, telangiectasia, and palmar erythema raise the likelihood of hepatic disorders. The vasculitides produce a number of skin manifestations, including leukocytoclastic rashes and skin infarctions. Several distinct nail findings occur in nephrotic patients. Transverse white lines, or leukonychia (sometimes called Muehrcke's lines), can develop during periods of marked hypoalbuminemia. Chronic hypoalbuminemia may also cause more diffuse white nails (Terry's or half-and-half nails) or yellow nails.[36] None of these nail findings is specific, however, and they can also have other causes, such as another debilitating disease or after chemotherapy.

Nail-patella syndrome—characterized by dystrophic nails, hypoplastic patellae, and iliac horns—may present with nephrotic syndrome. The eyes, in addition to being swollen, may be inflamed or show evidence of scleritis with systemic vasculitic disease. The heart and liver must be carefully examined. The extremities must be carefully evaluated for evidence of arthritis and for deep vein thrombi, which occur with increased frequency in these patients.[37]

LABORATORY TESTS (see also Chapter 26)

URINE STUDIES

Proteinuria is readily detected using a semiquantitative urine dipstick test. The protein-detecting pad is impregnated with a protein-sensitive pH indicator dye and a strong pH buffer, which keeps the pH of the wetted pad constant and independent of the urine pH. These pH indicators change color when moistened with urine containing dissolved proteins, a phenomenon called the protein error of pH indicators. Dipstick protein tests are most sensitive to albumin and react much less with urine globulins and immunoglobulin light chains (Bence Jones protein).

Dipstick results have the following approximate correlations with protein concentration:

- Negative: <15 mg/dL
- Trace: 15-30 mg/dL
- 1+: 30-100 mg/dL
- 2+: 100-300 mg/dL
- 3+: 300-1000 mg/dL
- 4+: >1000 mg/dL

Extremely alkaline urine (i.e., urine infected with urease-generating bacteria) can overwhelm the dipstick buffers, change its local pH, and thereby produce a false-positive dipstick protein test result. More recently, albumin-specific urine dipstick tests have been marketed specifically to detect low-grade albuminuria (i.e., microalbuminuria). Some also simultaneously measure creatinine concentrations (semiquantitatively) so that the urine albumin/creatinine ratio can be estimated. Albumin-specific dipstick tests are generally not used to diagnose or follow patients with overt albuminuria (macroalbuminuria) or nephrotic syndrome. Another method for urine protein determination is its reaction with sulfosalicylic acid, which precipitates most urine proteins. The resulting turbidity is proportional to the protein concentration. The sulfosalicylic acid turbidity test detects albumin, globulins, and Bence Jones proteins. Although it was a very useful test, environmental safety concerns have led to the removal of sulfosalicylic acid from most physicians' offices.

If a high urine protein concentration is documented, a quantitative measurement of protein excretion will be required. This is usually achieved with a 24-hour urine collection. Alternatively, the protein/creatinine concentration ratio (protein/creatinine) in a morning specimen may be used.[26,38] If the creatinine excretion rate is assumed to be about 1 g/day, then the ratio of g protein to 1 g of creatinine will approximate the 24-hour protein excretion. Approximate corrections can be made on the basis of the patient's gender and body habitus. A timed quantitative urine collection has the advantage of permitting a simultaneous measurement of creatinine clearance.

Urine dipstick protein tests, sulfosalicylic acid turbidity, 24-hour protein excretion, and protein/creatinine ratio are all measures of protein concentration or excretion. None of these tests will characterize the specific urine proteins (except that the urine dipstick tests are more sensitive to albumin, and the albumin dipsticks are specific to that protein). Agarose gel protein electrophoresis of the urine separates the urine protein classes (albumin, α_1-globulin, α_2-globulin, β-globulin, γ-globulin), and permits identification of monoclonal immunoglobulins and light chains. Electrophoresis results also allow stratification of nephrotic patients into those with selective proteinuria (mainly albumin) and those with nonselective proteinuria (high-grade albuminuria and globulinuria). This differentiation may have prognostic implications. Characterization of intact immunoglobulins, heavy chains, and light chains is accomplished with immunoelectrophoresis or immunofixation. Hyaline casts are common in patients with nephrotic syndrome and are composed mainly of precipitated Tamm-Horsfall protein, with a small fraction of some abnormally filtered and excreted serum proteins.[39,40] Cellular casts can be indicative of renal infection and/or interstitial inflammation (WBC casts) or glomerular inflammation, proliferation, and/or necrosis (RBC casts; see Fig. 25.1). Such disorders may be idiopathic and isolated to the kidney or may be related to a systemic inflammatory disease process,

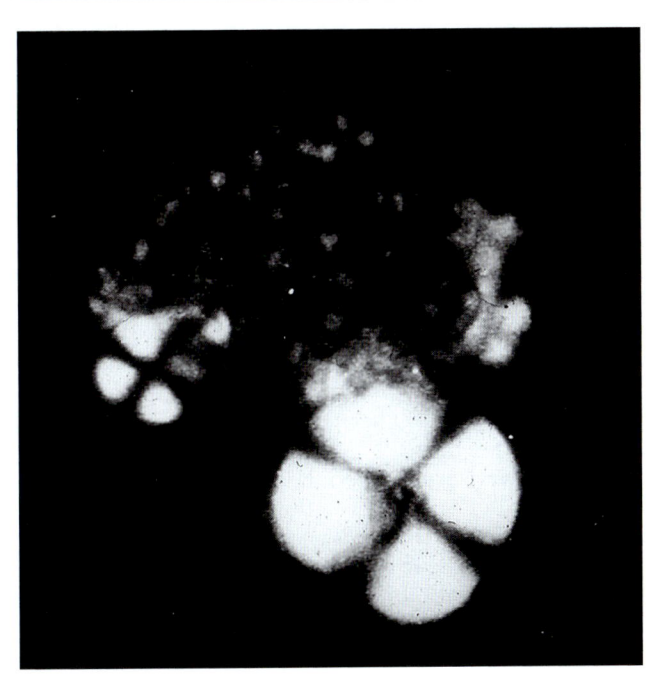

Figure 25.4 Lipiduria. Shown are birefringent cholesterol crystals seen with polarizing light microscopy.

such as systemic lupus erythematosus. Lipiduria is a characteristic feature of nephrotic syndrome. Visible lipids in the urine sediment can be seen in excreted tubule cells (oval fat bodies), within fatty casts, and/or as free-floating lipid globules. Most urine lipid is esterified cholesterol, and this component is birefringent. It can best be seen by examining the urine with a polarizing microscope, which demonstrates the deposit's characteristic bright cross like appearance[41] (Fig. 25.4). Some of the urine fat originates from filtered high-density lipoprotein, which is small enough to be filtered by leaky glomeruli and is then partially reabsorbed by renal tubule epithelial cells. These fat-laden cells subsequently degenerate and slough into the urine.[42]

BLOOD STUDIES

Initial studies should include a routine chemical profile (electrolytes, glucose, BUN, creatinine, total protein, albumin, calcium, phosphate, liver enzymes), lipid panel (total cholesterol, triglycerides, high-density lipoprotein cholesterol, low-density lipoprotein cholesterol), and CBC. The sodium concentration may be artifactually reduced (pseudohyponatremia) as a result of a displacement error caused by hyperlipidemia. This error occurs when the sodium concentration is measured by flame photometry or indirect potentiometry but not by analyzers using direct potentiometry. The calcium concentration must be corrected for the low albumin concentration, and direct measurement of the ionized calcium concentration may be helpful.

Additional testing is then directed by the patient's clinical presentation and findings and the suspicions of the physician. Testing for syphilis, HIV infection, and viral hepatitis (hepatitis B and C) is generally done. If a collagen vascular disease is suspected, testing for ANA, anti–double-stranded DNA antibody, and complement levels is indicated, as are other, more specific studies for autoimmune disorders. Although determination of the sedimentation rate is sometimes helpful, it is usually elevated in all patients with nephrotic syndrome, regardless of cause.[43] If a paraproteinemia disorder (including primary amyloidosis) is suspected, a serum immunoelectrophoresis or immunofixation study should be performed (in addition to qualitative and quantitative urine protein studies). When clinical and historical features are suggestive, cryoglobulin and antistreptolysin O titers should be obtained. Assessment of the GFR is mandatory and is usually accomplished with a timed urine collection for calculation of the creatinine clearance. Although the GFR calculated from the serum creatinine concentration with one of several estimation equations can be helpful, collection of a timed urine specimen for quantitative measurement of protein and creatinine excretion is indicated for all nephrotic patients who are considered to be compliant and who can understand the instructions for accurate collection of such a specimen. If an iothalamate clearance measurement of GFR is available, this may be very helpful and remains the gold standard for determining the GFR.

IMAGING

A chest x-ray study may be required to assess cardiac size and evaluate for pericardial disease or pleural effusions although, if readily accessible, an echocardiographic examination and bedside chest ultrasonography may provide the information, without ionizing irradiation. A renal sonogram with Doppler study is required to determine the renal anatomy and status of the collection system and renal vasculature. Special attention is directed to the possibility of renal vein thrombosis. The finding of a single kidney, asymmetric kidney size, or bilaterally small kidneys will direct the subsequent evaluation. Large kidneys are suggestive of diabetes mellitus, amyloidosis, HIV, or renal vein thrombosis. Patients should have routine age-indicated screening studies for malignancy, such as mammography and colonoscopy. However, extensive studies to rule out occult malignancy are not indicated.

KIDNEY BIOPSY

Kidney biopsy is not always indicated in patients with nephrotic syndrome. If the cause seems apparent from the history and laboratory studies, treatment can be initiated without histologic confirmation. For example, biopsy is rarely required in a patient with long-standing diabetes mellitus who develops nephrotic syndrome after the expected time period. However, if atypical features exist, such as a very active urine sediment with RBC casts, a very short time course (diabetic nephrotic syndrome usually evolves over 15 to 20 years), paraproteinemia or paraproteinuria, hypocomplementemia, and/or the absence of retinopathy and other end-organ involvement, a biopsy may be indicated to rule out other causes of the nephrotic syndrome. In young children with a classic clinical and biochemical presentation, the diagnosis of minimal change disease can usually be assumed and therapy initiated without histologic confirmation. This particular diagnosis is much less frequent in adults, so empirical therapy is less commonly initiated in these patients. Nonetheless, empirical therapy may be appropriate when there are contraindications to performing a biopsy, or the patient is very reluctant to undergo an invasive procedure, and the clinical features are consistent with minimal change nephropathy. In most adults with nephrotic syndrome, however, a biopsy is indicated to define the disease, improve prognostication, and direct therapeutic intervention.

OBSTRUCTIVE UROPATHY

Obstructive uropathy (see also Chapter 38) refers to structural or functional interference with normal urine flow. It can develop anywhere from the renal pelvis to the urethra. The resultant increase in pressure within the urinary tract proximal to the obstruction leads to a number of structural and physiologic changes. The anatomic outcome of an obstructive process often includes dilation of the renal calyces and renal pelvis, termed *hydronephrosis*, and, if the obstruction is distal to the ureteropelvic junction, it is termed *hydroureter*. Obstructive uropathy is a common cause of acute or subacute renal failure. Early recognition of obstruction guides therapy, which is different than that used to treat other forms of acute kidney injury (AKI), and improves prognosis. Untreated obstructive uropathy can result in a progressive and irreversible loss of renal function and eventually end-stage kidney disease (ESKD). However, early recognition and treatment can allow a potentially full renal recovery. Obstructive uropathy may be categorized as acute (hours to days), subacute (days to weeks), and chronic (months to years). Obstruction may be unilateral or bilateral, partial or complete. The clinician should establish the severity and chronicity of the condition so that appropriate therapy can be instituted. This is accomplished by means of careful history taking and physical examination, appropriate laboratory tests, and selected imaging studies.

HISTORY AND REVIEW OF SYSTEMS

Patients with acute obstructive uropathy may report an abrupt onset of severe flank pain (if the obstruction is at the level of the ureter or above) or suprapubic pain and fullness (if there is lower level obstruction). The pain is often colicky when the intraluminal process is due to nephrolithiasis or papillary necrosis. The pain may be accompanied by urinary frequency and urgency if there is partial urinary tract obstruction. Occasionally, nausea and even vomiting may occur when severe pain is present. A history of complete anuria should always alert the physician to the possibility of obstruction, especially in the appropriate clinical setting—for example, in an older man with a history of prostate cancer or prostatic hypertrophy. Gross hematuria may occur when obstructive uropathy is caused by nephrolithiasis, papillary necrosis, or neoplasms of the urinary tract. Rarely, patients may report the passage of renal calculi or small pieces of tissue with the sudden cessation of pain after such an event. The history with subacute or chronic obstruction is often negative or vague, but symptoms can include suprapubic fullness, frequency, polyuria, and/or nocturia. Patients may also complain of difficulty with initiating or stopping micturition if bladder outlet obstruction is present. Occasionally, urinary tract obstruction leads to infection, such as pyelonephritis, with accompanying high fever, flank pain, and dysuria.

PHYSICAL EXAMINATION

The physical examination can be very informative when bladder obstruction exists. The enlarged bladder may be detected with palpation and percussion. In rare cases, a flank mass may be palpable from a hydronephrotic kidney. Prostatic enlargement and other prostate pathology, such as malignancy or infection, can be detected via rectal examination. In an older woman, a careful pelvic examination should be performed to identify severe uterine prolapse, which has been reported to cause severe hydroureteronephrosis.[44,45]

The physical examination is usually of limited value, however, for detecting obstruction of the ureters or pelvis of the kidney. Hypertension is occasionally caused by urinary tract obstruction. Several mechanisms have been proposed for this development. In acute unilateral obstruction, there can be activation of the renin angiotensin aldosterone system, with increased renin secretion by the obstructed kidney.[46,47] The plasma renin activity is typically normal with bilateral or chronic unilateral obstruction. The hypertension that may occur in this setting has been attributed to renal failure with extracellular fluid (ECF) volume expansion.[48] In these cases, the diuresis that follows the relief of the obstruction often, but not always, eliminates the hypertension. Fever may be present if infection complicates the obstruction.

LABORATORY TESTS

The initial laboratory evaluation may provide clues to the presence of obstructive uropathy. The urinalysis may reveal a few RBCs and WBCs. There may be evidence of impaired renal function in patients with complete or severe partial bilateral obstruction or in those with obstruction of a solitary kidney. The plasma creatinine concentration is usually normal in patients with unilateral obstruction due to the presence of the normal contralateral kidney. However, unilateral renal obstruction can, very rarely, lead to anuria and AKI. This has been attributed to vascular or ureteral spasm.[49] Renal tubular acidosis with hyperkalemia has been well described with obstructive uropathy.[50] Multiple defects in renin, aldosterone, and distal tubule function have been described. In some patients, the renin and aldosterone levels are reduced, and the electrolyte abnormalities resolve in response to exogenous mineralocorticoids. In other patients, distal tubule injury diminishes sodium reabsorption and potassium secretion. The hyperchloremic acidosis is caused by hyperkalemia-induced suppression of ammoniagenesis and by directly impaired proton secretion. Consequently, obstructive uropathy is a common cause of hyperkalemia and type 4 renal tubular acidosis.[50,51] Often, the maximal urine concentrating capacity is also reduced.[51]

Acute obstruction causes an initial increase in renal blood flow, but this is soon followed by a reduction, which is attributed to vasoconstriction.[51] This can sometimes increase the BUN/creatinine ratio, similar to that seen in prerenal azotemia.

IMAGING

Renal ultrasonography is the test of choice to diagnose obstructive uropathy. This modality avoids IV radiocontrast exposure and ionizing irradiation. It has an extremely high sensitivity (>95%) and very good specificity (75%) for the diagnosis of hydronephrosis.[52,53] In early obstruction (first 1 to 3 days), however, the collecting system can be relatively noncompliant, and therefore overt hydronephrosis may not occur. Furthermore, when there is extrinsic compression of the ureter, obstructive uropathy can develop without overt dilation of the ureter or the renal pelvis. This usually occurs in older men with malignancy involving the retroperitoneum or prostate or when retroperitoneal fibrosis exists.[54] Furthermore, hydronephrosis or hydroureter should not be equated with obstruction. Nonobstructive hydronephrosis can occur as a result of neuromuscular abnormalities of the bladder and/or ureters (megacystis-megaureter syndrome) and in other conditions, such as vesicoureteral reflux and pregnancy.[55] Examination of the resistive index of the renal vasculature (vasoconstriction occurring with obstruction) and the response of the resistive index to a diuretic challenge can be a helpful differentiator.[55] As Ellenbogen and colleagues have stated, "It should be clear that the degree of hydronephrosis does not always correspond with the degree of obstruction."[53] When ultrasonographic results are inconclusive, or the suspicion of obstruction is very high despite a nondiagnostic sonogram, CT scanning should be performed. The combination of renal ultrasonography and CT of the kidneys will establish the diagnosis of obstructive uropathy in the overwhelming majority of cases.[52,55] CT scans have generally replaced IVP. In some cases, a retrograde study or percutaneous nephrostomy is necessary. These two procedures are much more invasive but do not require IV contrast material, have a very high diagnostic yield, and often treat the obstruction. Whenever a high degree of clinical suspicion of bladder obstruction exists, bladder catheterization, as both a diagnostic and therapeutic procedure, should be performed.

HYPERTENSION (see also Chapter 47)

Systemic hypertension is one of the most common disorders seen in clinical practice. In the United States, it affects about 20% of white adults, 40% of African American adults, and more than 80% of those older than 80 years. In addition, it is extremely common in patients with almost any type of renal disease. The nephrologist must be an expert in the diagnosis and treatment of this disease and should have a rigorous and systematic approach for the diagnosis and treatment of hypertension.

Over time, the definition and classification of adult hypertension has been a moving target. The most recent diagnostic classification and therapeutic guidelines were published in the *Eighth Report of the Joint National Committee on Prevention, Detection, Evaluation, and Treatment of High Blood Pressure*.[56] Table 25.6 shows how this report classifies blood pressure, but these guidelines should always be viewed in the context of the individual patient's history and clinical circumstances. Also, these blood pressure levels are for patients who are not acutely ill and are not taking antihypertensive medications. A patient with a consistently elevated blood pressure and no comorbid conditions is obviously treated differently than an individual with a similar degree of hypertension but with coexistent diabetes mellitus or other cardiovascular or renal disease. Chronic systemic hypertension is also associated with the development of cardiovascular disease, congestive heart failure, stroke, and chronic kidney disease (CKD). Appropriate treatment of the hypertension clearly reduces the risk of development of these complications, and it is therefore imperative to carefully evaluate and classify hypertensive patients so that appropriate therapy can be rendered.

Table 25.6 Classification of Blood Pressure in Adults

Hypertension Classification	Systolic Pressure (mm Hg)	Diastolic Pressure (mm Hg)
Normal	<120	and <80
Prehypertension	120-139	or 80-89
Stage 1 hypertension	140-159	or 90-99
Stage 2 hypertension	≥160	or ≥100

HISTORY AND REVIEW OF SYSTEMS

The evaluation of patients with hypertension should include an assessment of target organ function and/or damage Concomitant risk factors, and comorbid conditions. Search for secondary forms of hypertension, especially reversible conditions.[57] Obviously, a complete and detailed medical history is the first step in the evaluation. Particular attention should be paid to the presence of other cardiovascular risk factors, such as age, African American ethnicity, underlying CKD, dyslipidemia, history of smoking, obesity, microalbuminuria, left ventricular hypertrophy, family history of a myocardial infarction before age 50, and coincident arterial disease. The clinician should determine the duration and degree of hypertension and assess for any symptoms of severe hypertension, such as blurry vision, visual loss, headache, encephalopathy, and nausea. A thorough dietary history is also essential and should include an estimate of sodium, potassium, calcium, and fat intake.

Other important factors to identify include tobacco use, alcohol consumption, all prescribed and OTC medications, illicit drug use, efficacy of previous antihypertensive drug therapy and any adverse effects, and the presence or absence of sexual dysfunction. It is remarkable that patients and many physicians remain unaware of the potential hypertensive effects of many OTC medications, particularly NSAIDs. A family history of hypertension is also very important for the diagnosis of familial monogenetic forms of hypertension and essential hypertension. Nephrologists are often asked to evaluate and treat hypertensive patients who are referred for a second opinion, particularly those with poor blood pressure control. It is particularly important to identify any potentially reversible cause of secondary hypertension in these patients (Table 25.7). In this regard, symptoms

Table 25.7 Causes of Secondary Hypertension

Renal parenchymal disease
Renovascular hypertension
Fibromuscular dysplasia
Atherosclerotic renal artery disease
Renal vasculitis
Renal infarction
Primary hyperaldosteronism
Renin-secreting tumor
Pheochromocytoma
Cushing's syndrome
Liddle's syndrome
Apparent mineralocorticoid excess
Geller's syndrome
Aortic coarctation
Thyroid disease
Drugs (e.g., corticosteroids, cocaine, amphetamines, oral contraceptives)
Sleep apnea

characteristic of certain underlying causes of hypertension should be sought, such as paroxysmal hypertension, sweating, palpitations, and severe headache for pheochromocytomas; sweating, palpitations, and weight loss for thyrotoxicosis; and weight gain, edema, and polyuria for Cushing's syndrome. A common form of secondary hypertension is that caused by atherosclerotic renal artery stenosis. These patients may relate a history of recent worsening of their blood pressure control, despite adherence to the antihypertensive medication regimen. Also, they frequently have a history of generalized vascular disease. Primary hyperaldosteronism is now recognized as a common condition, especially in patients with difficult-to-control or severe hypertension. The prevalence among hypertensive patients may be as high as 10%. Spontaneous or diuretic-related hypokalemia suggests this diagnosis, but hyperaldosteronism can present with normal electrolyte levels.

A worldwide obesity epidemic has been the subject of numerous studies. Sleep-disordered breathing in general, and obstructive sleep apnea in particular, are associated with obesity, and its incidence is accordingly on the rise. The association of sleep-disordered breathing and development of hypertension have been validated in prospective studies and is an important modifiable hypertension risk factor.[58] When sleep apnea is suspected, the patient may complain of snoring, daytime sleepiness, or morning headaches. Of note, obstructive sleep apnea and associated hypertension is becoming more common among young adults.[59]

PHYSICAL EXAMINATION

The physical examination begins with a careful blood pressure measurement. Patients should not smoke or ingest caffeine for at least 30 minutes prior to the examination. They should be comfortably seated in a chair with back support, with the arm resting at heart level. An appropriately sized cuff must be used. Its width should be at least 40% of arm circumference and its length at least 80% of arm circumference.[60] Two or more readings should be taken 2 to 5 minutes apart and averaged. When orthostatic hypotension is a consideration, blood pressure should be measured in the supine and standing positions. When a coarctation is considered, blood pressure should be measured in each arm and leg. Use of incorrect cuff size in obese individuals causes an overestimation of blood pressure. Because of environmental toxicity concerns, mercury manometers have been replaced by regularly calibrated aneroid or electronic devices. Overestimation of systolic blood pressure is common in older patients who have calcified and stiff arteries that cannot be compressed. This condition, termed *pseudohypertension,* is suspected when the radial artery remains palpable after the cuff has been inflated above systolic blood pressure.

An important aspect of the physical examination is the patient's general appearance. Consider the possibility of sleep apnea if the body habitus and/or neck circumference are large. A careful funduscopic evaluation is essential. The presence and severity of hypertensive retinopathy provides important evidence of the duration and severity of the hypertension. Special note should be made of hemorrhage, arteriolar narrowing, papilledema, and/or cotton-wool spots. The cardiovascular and pulmonary examination may reveal carotid and/or peripheral vascular disease, left ventricular hypertrophy (e.g., hyperdynamic precordium and the presence of a fourth heart sound), or congestive heart failure (e.g., jugular venous distension, rales, third heart sound, and/or peripheral edema). Coarctation of the aorta is suggested by differences in the intensity of the radial pulses or a radial-femoral arterial pulsation difference or temporal delay. The abdominal and flank examination may reveal abdominal bruits suggesting renal artery stenosis. The neurologic examination in severely hypertensive patients may reveal findings consistent with encephalopathy. The neck examination may suggest otherwise occult thyroid disease. The presence of hyperpigmentation and striae raises the possibility of Cushing's syndrome. Neurofibroma and café au lait spots suggest the possibility of neurofibromatosis (and pheochromocytoma or renal vascular disease).

LABORATORY TESTS

The extent of the laboratory evaluation depends on the clinical circumstances of the individual patient. The initial evaluation of a person with stage 1 hypertension includes measurement of a CBC, serum electrolyte, BUN, creatinine, calcium, and glucose levels, lipid profile, and urinalysis. If warranted by the clinical history and physical examination findings, additional testing, such as thyroid studies, urine albumin/creatinine ratio, and quantitation of GFR with a creatinine or iothalamate clearance. When a pheochromocytoma is suspected, catecholamine and fractionated metanephrine levels in urine and/or blood should be measured. A plasma aldosterone/plasma renin activity ratio is a reasonable screening test for the detection of primary hyperaldosteronism if this condition is clinically suspected. This test probably should be performed if patients have unprovoked hypokalemia, develop severe diuretic-induced hypokalemia, or develop hypokalemia after having taken a stable dose of diuretics over a long period. It is also a reasonable consideration if unexpected metabolic alkalosis, severe or resistant hypertension, or an incidentally discovered adrenal mass (incidentaloma) in a patient with hypertension is found. When obstructive sleep apnea is suspected, home sleep testing or formal 12-channel, in-laboratory polysomnography can confirm this diagnosis.[61]

IMAGING

A baseline chest x-ray is indicated for all hypertensive patients to rule out some rare secondary causes (e.g., coarctation, as evidenced by rib notching) and for assessment of left ventricular size. However, other more advanced imaging modalities are required when the history, physical examination, and laboratory results suggest secondary hypertension due to anatomic abnormalities or to document pathologic end-organ changes caused by the hypertension. Renal sonography is an excellent noninvasive test for assessing renal size, identifying cysts, and detecting hydronephrosis. It is obviously indicated whenever enlarged kidneys or a mass can be palpated. When there is clinical suspicion of renovascular hypertension, several diagnostic options are available to help establish the diagnosis, including spiral CT angiography, magnetic resonance angiography (MRA), and duplex Doppler ultrasonography.

The best screening test is a function of the specific features of each patient and skill of the imaging center that is used. Renal artery Doppler studies are very operator-dependent and difficult to perform in large patients. CT angiography of the renal arteries is an excellent diagnostic tool but carries the risk of radiocontrast-related kidney injury in susceptible patients, as well as considerable radiation exposure. Gadolinium-enhanced MRA can also yield excellent results but is contraindicated if kidney function is reduced because of the risk of nephrogenic systemic fibrosis. Also, this modality cannot be used when patients are claustrophobic or have metal implants. Captopril renal perfusion scans, once popular, are no longer recommended as a screening test because of their relatively low predictive value. Catheter angiography should be the first study performed if clinical suspicion of renal artery stenosis is very high. If angiography is clearly indicated then screening tests are not appropriate.

OTHER STUDIES

Electrocardiography is useful for accessing left ventricular hypertrophy, cardiac arrhythmias, and to provide a baseline for future comparison. Cardiac echocardiography provides excellent noninvasive assessment and serial monitoring and documentation.

NEPHROLITHIASIS (see also Chapter 40)

Kidney stones are an increasingly prevalent medical problem. Over 5% of the U.S. population is affected, and the lifetime risk of developing a stone is 10% to 15%.[62] Patients who develop a first stone are very likely to have a second one (50% within 5 years and 80% within 20 years).[62] Therefore, every nephrologist is likely to encounter patients with this problem.

HISTORY AND REVIEW OF SYSTEMS

Kidney stones are strongly suspected when patients present with classic signs and symptoms, such as gross hematuria associated with waves of flank and/or lower abdominal pain (colic), which may radiate into the genital region. However, symptoms are sometimes vague. Hematuria is usually but not always present, and its absence does not exclude a diagnosis of nephrolithiasis.[63] Poorly localized abdominal pain, nausea, vomiting, and urinary frequency may occur. Often, patients are entirely asymptomatic, and the stones are noted incidentally when an imaging study is done for a different reason. When painful symptoms do develop, they generally indicate that an asymptomatic stone has passed from the renal pelvis into the ureter, where it has caused obstruction, inflammation, and/or bleeding.

These symptoms often occur first during the night or in the early morning, beginning abruptly with rapidly worsening pain. The paroxysms of pain probably reflect hyperperistalsis of the renal calyces, pelvis, and ureter. The site of pain and its referral pattern are clues to the stone's location. Upper ureteral obstruction usually produces flank pain and tenderness and anterior abdominal radiation of pain. Lower ureteral obstruction produces lower abdominal pain, which frequently radiates into the testicle or labia. Very often, stones lodge near the ureterovesical junction, where they irritate the bladder, producing urinary frequency, urinary urgency, suprapubic tenderness, and dysuria. If the stone enters the bladder and then obstructs its outlet, suprapubic pain and anuria may develop.

Potential kidney stone risk factors should be identified. The patient should be questioned about unusual dietary habits. Large amounts of oxalate-rich foods such as spinach, rhubarb, beets, or black tea can predispose to calcium oxalate stones. Excessive intake of animal protein, which reduces urine citrate excretion, predisposes to calcium stones. High salt ingestion increases urine calcium excretion. Sardines, anchovies, and organ meat are rich sources of purines and thereby increase urine uric acid excretion. The medication history may reveal other important clues to stone pathogenesis. Some medications increase the risk of stones by reducing urine citrate excretion; carbonic anhydrase inhibitors such as acetazolamide and topiramate are important examples. Dietary supplements, vitamins, and minerals such as calcium salts and vitamin D can produce hypercalciuria.[64] Other medications may precipitate to form stones, such as triamterene, some sulfonamides, ceftriaxone, and the protease inhibitor indinavir.[65]

A number of underlying medical conditions can predispose patients to the development of kidney stones. These include most chronic disorders associated with hypercalciuria, such as hyperparathyroidism and sarcoidosis. Hypercalcemia-hypercalciuria of malignancy usually does not result in kidney stones, most likely as a result of its acute presentation and relatively short course. Any medical or surgical condition associated with significant steatorrhea (e.g., short gut disorders, cystic fibrosis, bile salt depletion from ileal disease, gastrointestinal bypass) may generate stones as a result of hyperoxaluria (from intestinal hyperabsorption) and reduced urine volume. Chronic diarrhea without steatorrhea often causes chronic metabolic acidosis and persistent aciduria. This is a risk factor for the development of uric acid stones. Strong epidemiologic associations with calcium and uric acid kidney stones have been demonstrated for obesity, weight gain, diabetes mellitus, and the metabolic syndrome.[66] The impact of occupations associated with reduced fluid intake and/or excessive sweating should be considered because low urine volume is a major risk factor for stone formation. A history of recurrent urinary tract infections raises concern for infection (struvite) stones. The age at which the first kidney stone developed is also a clue to the diagnosis of causative factors. Kidney stones associated with inherited disorders such as cystinuria and congenital hyperoxaluria often present at a young age. Ethnicity has a major impact on risk. Over a 6-year period (1988 to 1994) in the United States, whites had the highest risk of kidney stones (5.9%), African Americans the lowest risk (1.7%), and Mexican Americans an intermediate risk (2.6%).[62] The family history also may be helpful; first-degree relatives of patients with stones very often also have had stones.[67]

PHYSICAL EXAMINATION

Fever is a sign of possible infection, which must be rapidly addressed. It is of critical importance to recognize a bacterial infection proximal to an obstructing stone. This is a medical and urologic emergency requiring urgent drainage of the renal pelvis (surgically or via percutaneous intervention) and appropriate antibiotic therapy. Fever and/or leukocytosis do not usually occur with uncomplicated kidney stones and are therefore red flags for infection. The skin may be pale, cool, and often clammy. Costovertebral angle tenderness is often present. Hypoactive bowel sounds and ileus may develop in patients with nephrolithiasis but abdominal tenderness is unusual. If rebound tenderness exists, a cause other than an uncomplicated kidney stone should be sought. Bruits over the abdominal aorta and/or iliac vessels may be indicative of a leaking aortic abdominal aneurysm, which can mimic the symptoms of renal colic. In men, a rectal examination may reveal prostatitis and, in women, a pelvic examination may suggest ovarian pathology or an ectopic pregnancy.

LABORATORY TESTS

The WBC count may be slightly increased with an uncomplicated stone, but leukocytosis greater than 15,000 cells/mm^3 and a left shift suggests an infection. The BUN and creatinine levels may increase if renal function is reduced, severe obstruction exists, or the patient is volume-depleted. An electrolyte panel may provide clues that distal renal tubular acidosis exists (hyperchloremic acidosis and hypokalemia). The serum calcium, phosphate, and uric acid levels can indicate the existence of a hypercalcemic-hypercalciuric condition, renal phosphate wasting, or hyperuricosuric condition. In women of childbearing age, a pregnancy test must be performed prior to radiation exposure.

URINE STUDIES

Hematuria with isomorphic RBCs is very common, but not universal.[60] RBC casts should not be seen. Proteinuria should be absent or of low grade. Although pyuria may occur without infection, it should always raise suspicion, and a urine culture should be performed. The urine pH may provide a helpful clue. A very high pH of freshly voided urine (>7.5) almost always indicates the existence of a UTI. Chronic UTIs may lead to the development of struvite stones, also called triple phosphate, urease-related, or infection stones. When infecting bacteria produce the enzyme urease, the urea in urine is split into two molecules of NH_3 and one of CO_2. The CO_2 escapes from the urine, whereas each NH_3 molecule binds a proton and thereby elevates the urine pH above levels that exist under physiologic conditions. Abundant ammonium in an alkaline urine tends to precipitate with magnesium and phosphate to form struvite ($MgNH_4PO_4$). Note that struvite is really a double-phosphate crystal. The term *triple phosphate* derives from the fact that carbonate-apatite ($Ca_{10}[PO_4]_6 \cdot CO_3$) commonly coprecipitates with struvite, which results in three cations—calcium, magnesium, and ammonium—precipitating with the phosphate anion. Struvite stones often grow to large staghorn shapes. Urease-producing bacteria include *Ureaplasma urealyticum,* most *Proteus* species, and many *Staphylococcus, Klebsiella,* and *Pseudomonas* species. *Escherichia coli* does not generate urease. A urine pH that is not appropriately acidic (<5.5) in a patient with hyperchloremic acidosis suggests distal renal tubular acidosis, a disorder often associated with calcium phosphate stones. Conversely, persistently acidic urine is associated with uric acid stones (because uric acid becomes increasingly insoluble as the pH falls below 6.5). When bacteriuria is identified, a urine sample must be sent for culture. If overt signs of infection exist, hospital admission for additional evaluation and treatment is generally required.

Identification of crystals in the urine sediment can be helpful and sometimes diagnostic. Recognition of benzene ring–shaped cysteine crystals is almost diagnostic of cystinuria. The so-called coffin lid crystals of struvite are also very characteristic and indicate that an infection-related stone is likely. Although uric acid and calcium oxalate crystals commonly occur and are relatively nonspecific, when a kidney stone exists these crystals may be very helpful etiologic clues.[68] Also, a 24-hour urine collection for quantitation of nephrolithiasis-relevant solutes can be helpful. Several commercial laboratories offer a metabolic stone risk profile. These studies may identify abnormally high (e.g., calcium, oxalate, urate) and/or low (e.g., citrate) solute concentrations and excretion rates. The saturation-supersaturation state of the urine for various stone-forming crystals is also routinely calculated. In general, at least two 24-hour samples should be collected because of significant daily variation in excretion rates. Urine metabolic stone risk testing should be done whenever recurrent stones develop or when a first stone is documented in a patient with a higher than usual risk for recurrence (e.g., those with a family history of stones or patients with gastrointestinal disorders). Some experts believe that 24-hour urine studies should be performed after the first kidney stone in all patients, but this approach may not be practical.

IMAGING

The imaging procedure of choice is a noncontrast helical CT scan with relatively thin (3 to 5-mm) cuts.[20] This study has replaced IVP as the preferred imaging procedure for kidney stones. Although a plain radiograph of the abdomen KUB (kidneys, ureters, and bladder) is very inexpensive and may be diagnostic, it has generally also been replaced by CT as the initial screening test.[20,69] The CT scan can detect radiopaque calculi as small as 1 mm in diameter. Calcium stones are radiopaque, cysteine stones are slightly radiopaque, and pure uric acid stones are radiolucent. Struvite stones have variable radiopacity, depending on the calcium content. Stones comprised of indinavir or triamterene are radiolucent. The CT scan will also reveal renal anatomy, presence of hydronephrosis, other abdominal and pelvic pathology, and other potential causes of the patient's symptoms. Although a renal-abdominal sonogram will demonstrate renal anatomy and detect hydronephrosis and most stones in the renal pelvis, it will miss most ureteral stones. Therefore, sonography is generally used to follow the progress of known stone disease, but not as an initial study. However, sonography is indicated as the initial procedure in pregnant women or whenever radiation exposure must be minimized. Magnetic resonance imaging (MRI) is generally not very helpful for the diagnosis of kidney stones.

DIFFERENTIAL DIAGNOSIS

Many conditions can mimic nephrolithiasis. Any form of renal bleeding associated with blood clots can cause ureteral obstruction and produce symptoms identical to those of a kidney stone. Other clinical mimics of kidney stones are an abdominal aortic aneurysm, pyelonephritis, renal cancer, renal tuberculosis, papillary necrosis, renal infarction, and renal vein thrombosis. Papillary necrosis, which is more likely in patients with diabetes or sickle cell disease, can cause true renal colic when sloughed papillae obstruct the ureter. Ectopic pregnancy, appendicitis, and bowel obstruction must be considered. Some patients seeking analgesic drugs complain of kidney stone symptoms. Table 25.8 presents the differential diagnosis of urolithiasis-like pain.

Table 25.8 Differential Diagnosis of Urolithiasis-Like Pain

Category	Disorders
Renal	Pyelonephritis
	Blood clot
	Renal infarction
	Tumor (kidney or pelvis)
	Papillary necrosis
Ureteral	Tumor
	Blood clot
	Stricture
Bladder	Tumor
	Blood clot
	Urinary retention
Intraabdominal	Peritonitis
	Appendicitis
	Biliary disease
	Bowel obstruction
	Vascular disorder
	Aortic aneurysm
	Mesenteric insufficiency
Retroperitoneal	Lymphadenopathy
	Fibrosis
	Tumor
Gynecologic	Ectopic or tubal pregnancy
	Ovarian torsion, cyst rupture
	Pelvic inflammatory disease
	Cervical cancer
	Endometriosis
	Ovarian vein syndrome
Neuromuscular	Muscle pain
	Rib fracture
	Radiculitis
Infectious	Herpes zoster
	Pleuritis, pneumonia
	Fungal bezoar

INITIAL TREATMENT

Patients with renal colic can often be managed conservatively as outpatients with analgesics and fluids. However, admission and urgent urologic consultation is required if the patient is septic, has an infection proximal to an obstruction, or has obstruction of a solitary kidney (including a renal transplant). Bilateral kidney obstruction, high-grade obstruction with a large (>7 mm) stone, acute kidney injury, urine extravasation, or unrelenting pain despite analgesics also requires urologic consultation. The most important determinant of the likelihood that a stone will pass is its size. Most kidney stones smaller than 4 mm in diameter will pass spontaneously. As stone size increases the chance of its passing falls progressively. Passage of the stone is very unlikely at a diameter of 10 mm or more. Consequently, conservative outpatient therapy becomes less likely to be successful as the stone size increases beyond 4 to 5 mm.[70,71]

Narcotics and/or NSAIDs are used for analgesia. If the patient is to be managed as an outpatient, NSAIDs are the preferred agents. If nausea and vomiting are prominent, a parenteral NSAID such as ketorolac can be used. For severe pain, IV morphine is generally given.[72-74] If the stone has a reasonable chance of passing without urologic intervention, glucocorticoids, calcium channel blockers (usually nifedipine), and/or α_1-adrenergic antagonists (usually tamsulosin, which is used to treat benign prostatic hyperplasia) may be used to relax ureteral muscles and thereby assist stone passage. Although aggressive volume expansion with or without diuretics is often used, and would seem to be an appropriate treatment, several trials have not found evidence that such an intervention is effective.[75] Patients should always attempt to retrieve the passed stone for analysis. This can be accomplished by urinating through a filter or fine screen—an aquarium net is a good option. If none is available, the patient can urinate through a fine gauze pad or simply void into a glass jar so that the calculus will be visible.

ACUTE KIDNEY INJURY
(see also Chapter 31)

AKI is a clinical syndrome broadly defined as an abrupt decline in renal function occurring over a period of hours to days, resulting in the retention of nitrogenous and other

Table 25.9	RIFLE Criteria for Acute Kidney Injury (AKI)	
Class	GFR	Urine Output
Risk	Creatinine increase × 1.5 or GFR decrease > 25%	<0.5 mL/kg/hr for >6 hr
Injury	Creatinine increase × 2 or GFR decrease > 50%	<0.5 mL/kg/hr for >12 hr
Failure	Creatinine increase × 3 or GFR decrease > 75% or Creatinine ≥ 4 mg% (acute increase ≥ 0.5 mg%)	<0.3 mL/kg/hr for >24 hr or Anuria > 12 hr
Loss	Persistent AKI = complete loss of renal function >4 wk	
End stage	End-stage renal disease > 3 mo	

GFR, Glomerular filtration rate.

Table 25.10	Acute Kidney Injury Network (AKIN) Criteria	
Stage	Creatinine Criteria	Urine Output Criteria
1	Increase in serum creatinine ≥ 3 mg/dL (≥26.4 μmol/L) or increase ≥ 150%-200% (1.5-2 fold) above baseline	<0.5 mL/kg/hr for >6 hr
2	Increase in serum creatinine > 200%-300% (>twofold or threefold) above baseline	<0.5 mL/kg/hr for >12 hr
3	Increase in serum creatinine > 300% (>threefold) above baseline or serum creatinine ≥ 4 mg/dL (≥354 μmol/L) with an acute rise ≥ 0.5mg/dL (≥44 μmol/L)	<0.3 mL/kg/hr ×24 hr or Anuria ×12 hr

metabolic waste products and usually ECF volume expansion. Very often, electrolyte and acid-base disorders also develop (e.g., hyperkalemia, hyponatremia, metabolic acidosis). AKI develops as a result of various pathophysiologic disturbances that may lead to varying degrees of damage to one or more anatomic divisions of the nephron, with subsequent adverse functional consequences. Although the initial clinical manifestation of AKI is often oliguria, urine volume can remain normal or even increase, and patients can remain completely asymptomatic. The diagnosis is often established as a result of routine biochemical screening that reveals a recent increase in serum creatinine and/or BUN concentrations.

There is no universally accepted operational definition of AKI, and more than 30 different diagnostic criteria have been used in various clinical studies.[76] Commonly used definitions include an absolute increase in serum creatinine concentration of 0.5 to 1.0 mg/dL and/or relative increases of 25% to 100% over a period of 1 to several days. Although not optimal, these approaches have nonetheless been proven to be useful in identifying patients with AKI in clinical practice. Two new classification and diagnostic systems have been introduced—the RIFLE (*r*isk, *i*njury, *f*ailure, *l*oss, *e*nd-stage) criteria and AKIN (*A*cute *K*idney *I*njury *N*etwork) criteria[52,76,77] (Tables 25.9 and 25.10). These systems have been successfully adopted by investigators worldwide. All agree that it would be very helpful to compare different clinical studies by using the same definition for AKI.

The incidence of AKI varies greatly, depending on the patient population studied and the specific criteria used to identify the disorder. Among ambulatory patients, the incidence of AKI is very low, but AKI develops in up to 7% of hospitalized patients, and about 30% of those admitted to intensive care units.[78,79]

A population study conducted in the United Kingdom in 2003 reported the incidence of AKI as 1811 per million population.[79] Outcomes associated with AKI have changed little over the last 60 years. The in-hospital mortality rate of critically ill patients with AKI exceeds 50%. Older age, female gender, respiratory failure, liver failure, sepsis, and impaired consciousness all correlate with higher in-hospital mortality rates.[80]

Table 25.11 Causes of Acute Kidney Injury
Prerenal
Gastrointestinal or other severe hemorrhage
Burns
Pancreatitis
Capillary leak
Diarrhea, vomiting, nasogastric suction, fistula fluid loss
Excessive sweating
Diuretics, nonsteroidal antiinflammatory drugs
Congestive heart failure
Cirrhosis
Intrinsic
Ischemia (e.g., postoperative acute tubular necrosis)
Nephrotoxins (e.g., radiocontrast agents, aminoglycosides)
Sepsis
Acute interstitial nephritis
Acute glomerulonephritis
Acute vascular syndrome (e.g., bilateral renal artery thromboembolism or dissection)
Atheroembolic disease
Postrenal
Bilateral upper tract obstruction (e.g., nephrolithiasis, papillary necrosis) or obstruction of solitary functioning kidney
Lower tract obstruction (e.g., prostatic hypertrophy, urethral stricture, bladder mass or stone, obstructed urinary catheter)

The causes of AKI can be broadly divided into three categories (Table 25.11):

1. Prerenal azotemia (a disorder characterized by renal hypoperfusion, in which renal parenchymal tissue integrity is preserved)
2. Intrinsic renal failure, with parenchymal tissue injury
3. Postrenal failure (dysfunction caused by acute obstruction of the urinary tract)

Categorization of AKI requires the clinician to integrate the findings and results from a careful history, physical examination, and appropriate laboratory and imaging studies.

HISTORY AND REVIEW OF SYSTEMS

The initial goal of history taking is to seek information to help establish whether the patient actually has AKI. In this regard, a careful review of clinical, pharmacy, nursing, laboratory and radiologic records is necessary. A relatively recent serum creatinine determination is invaluable but not always available. In some cases, the clinician must make a presumptive diagnosis of AKI pending further data collection and investigation. A diagnosis of AKI can usually be more readily established when it occurs during a hospitalization because serial laboratory values are frequently available, and urine outputs may also be available. Complete anuria is unusual with AKI and raises the possibility of obstructive uropathy. Some of the features that assist in the differentiation of AKI into various categories are shown in Table 25.11.

One risk factor that most strongly predicts the development of AKI is the presence of CKD.[81] Often, such patients develop superimposed AKI because of a variety of renal insults. A history of salt and fluid losses, as may occur with diarrhea or vomiting, or ECF loss into a third space in response to extensive burns, pancreatitis, or leaky capillaries suggests a prerenal cause. A medication review may disclose ingestion of NSAIDs, ACEIs, or angiotensin receptor blockers, which can generate a renal hypoperfusion state and AKI, especially when combined with diuretics. It is also essential to identify any other potential nephrotoxic agents such as phosphate loads given as cathartics. A history of heart failure or liver disease increases the likelihood that AKI is the result of reduced effective arterial volume.

Often, the cause of AKI is multifactorial (e.g., a patient with a gastrointestinal hemorrhage may undergo a radiologic study with IV contrast). Although a history of decreased urine output or anuria is important, many patients with AKI have normal urine output.

A history of voiding symptoms such as urinary frequency, hesitancy, or incontinence suggests the possibility of obstructive uropathy. Patients with renal artery emboli and some with renal vein thrombosis may present with flank pain and a history of hematuria. It is also important to elicit any history of a recent interventional radiologic procedure, which raises the possibility of AKI caused by intravenous (IV) or intraarterial contrast infusion or atheroembolic disease. A history of fever, skin rash, arthralgias, sinusitis, and/or hemoptysis raises the possibility of glomerulonephritis related to infection, collagen vascular disease, or vasculitis.

PHYSICAL EXAMINATION

An extremely important aspect of the physical examination in every patient with AKI is an assessment of ECF and effective arterial volume status. Overt hypotension is the strongest indicator of potential renal underperfusion. Less severe volume depletion is suggested by an orthostatic pulse increase of more than 30 beats/min (measured 1 minute after standing). Orthostatic hypotension, defined as a drop in systolic blood pressure of more than 20 mm Hg after standing, is less helpful because it occurs in 10% of normal subjects.[82] Dry axillae and dry mucous membranes with a furrowed tongue are useful signs of volume depletion. However, poor skin turgor and slow capillary refill have not been shown to be helpful signs in adults.[82] The neck veins are usually flat when volume contraction exists. Renal perfusion may be reduced as a result of heart failure or hepatic cirrhosis. Signs of the former condition include distended neck veins, pulmonary rales, an S_3 gallop, and pitting peripheral edema. Stigmata of chronic liver disease, including jaundice, hepatosplenomegaly, ascites, gynecomastia, nail clubbing, palmar erythema, vascular spiders, and testicular atrophy should be sought. The presence of true ECF volume depletion or reduced effective arterial volume raises the very strong possibility of a prerenal (and potentially readily reversible) cause of the AKI.

The physical examination may suggest a systemic disease associated with an intrinsic AKI, such as vasculitis, endocarditis, thrombotic thrombocytopenic purpura, and hemolytic uremic syndrome. An important cause of AKI in the hospitalized or recently hospitalized patient is atheroembolic disease. This often overlooked condition generally occurs following an invasive procedure that requires intraarterial catheterization (e.g., cardiac catheterization, angiography) or cardiac or vascular surgeries. Skin findings include livedo reticularis, ulcers, purpura, petechiae, painful erythematous nodules, cyanosis, and gangrene. A retinal examination may reveal arterial atheroemboli (Hollenhorst plaques). Flank tenderness or an enlarged palpable bladder indicates a possible postrenal cause for AKI. A digital examination of the prostate should be performed in all men with AKI, and a bimanual pelvic examination to detect pelvic masses should be considered in women. If lower tract obstruction is a serious consideration, a diagnostic postvoiding bladder scan or catheterization should be done. The normal postvoiding residual urine volume is less than 50 mL. If urine is collected, a sample should be saved for potential additional studies.

LABORATORY TESTS

Initial testing in AKI must include urinalysis and an estimate of the GFR. Prerenal AKI associated with ECF volume contraction usually causes marked urine concentration. This increases the urine specific gravity and may generate positive dipstick protein results. Microscopy often reveals hyaline casts, but in general there should be few cells and no cellular casts. Quantitative protein excretion is relatively low (<1000 mg/day). However, a bland urinalysis is also consistent with an obstructive or postrenal cause for AKI unless a complicating infection has produced pyuria and bacteriuria, or stone disease has generated hematuria. AKI due to intrinsic damage such as tubular necrosis will typically generate a so-called dirty urinalysis, with many epithelial cells and muddy brown granular and epithelial cell casts. The urine is generally isosthenuric (specific gravity of about 1.010). Rhabdomyolysis causes myoglobinuria, and pigmented granular casts are seen. Acute glomerulonephritis produces proteinuria, hematuria, and RBC casts. Acute interstitial nephritis causes pyuria and white cell casts. If AKI is caused by an allergic reaction, urine eosinophils may be seen, but this is not a specific finding.[83] A recent retrospective study has found that identification of urine eosinophils, using the relatively specific Hansel stain, is a poor marker for acute interstitial nephritis, and some have suggested that this diagnostic test be eliminated.[84,85]

Table 25.12 Tests to Differentiate Prerenal from Intrinsic Kidney Damage

Parameter	Prerenal Acute Kidney Injury	Intrinsic Kidney Damage (e.g., ATN)
Urine Na (mEq/L)	<20	>40
Urine osmolality (mOsm/kg H$_2$O)	>500	<350
Serum BUN/creatinine (Cr) ratio	>20	10-15*
Fractional excretion of Na $\dfrac{[U_{Na} \times P_{Cr}]}{[P_{Na} \times U_{Cr}]} \times 100$	<1†	>2
Fractional excretion of urea $\dfrac{[U_{Urea} \times P_{Cr}]}{[P_{Urea} \times U_{Cr}]} \times 100$	<30†	>50

*A BUN/Cr ratio of <10 may occur with rhabdomyolysis because the Cr concentration increases sharply as a result of increased release from necrotic muscle. A low BUN/Cr ratio can also develop in malnourished individuals because of a very low BUN level.

†The fractional excretion of Na and fractional excretion of urea are often also very low with contrast nephropathy, rhabdomyolysis, acute myeloma kidney, and acute urate nephropathy.

ATN, Acute tubular necrosis; BUN, blood urea nitrogen; P, plasma; U, urinary.

Estimation of the GFR gives an approximate measure of the number of functioning nephrons. In the setting of AKI, the GFR is, by definition, not in a steady state. This makes GFR estimates, especially those based on the plasma creatinine level, unreliable. However, a rising creatinine concentration indicates that the renal injury is stable or worsening, whereas a falling creatinine concentration is generally indicative of improvement. A daily increase in the creatinine concentration of more than 1 mg/dL is usually associated with a GFR of less than 10 mL/min. A timed urine collection for determination of creatinine clearance can be very helpful, but even this measurement can overestimate the GFR as a result of tubular secretion of creatinine. When available, the renal clearance of radioisotopes such as iothalamate will provide the most accurate measurement of GFR.

In general, serum electrolyte, BUN, calcium, phosphorus, and uric acid levels should be measured. Potentially life-threatening hyperkalemia and severe metabolic acidosis must be identified and treated. Table 25.12 lists a number of urine and plasma chemical measurements and various calculations that can help differentiate prerenal AKI from intrinsic renal injury. Although a measurement of the urine sodium concentration can be helpful in distinguishing these disorders, the fractional excretion of sodium and/or urea are better indicators. It is important to note that several disorders that generate AKI may be associated with urine studies suggesting prerenal AKI. They include AKI caused by contrast nephropathy, rhabdomyolysis, acute myeloma kidney, and acute urate nephropathy.

Although the traditional diagnosis of AKI requires a measurable increase in the plasma creatinine level, it is clear that this is an insensitive and delayed biomarker. Renal injury may have been present for hours to days before a noticeable rise in plasma creatinine concentration is detected. An ideal biomarker would be a substance that can be easily obtained and readily and rapidly measured, with a high sensitivity and specificity for AKI and able to predict clinical outcomes. A number of urinary biomarkers of tubular injury have been recognized over the past decade (see also Chapter 30), although they are far from ideal.[86-88] These substances are normal constituents of renal tubular cells that are upregulated and released into the urine in response to renal injury. Early measurement of these biomarkers might allow the detection of renal injury within hours of the insult. Kidney injury molecule-1 (KIM-1), one of the first urinary biomarkers, was characterized over a decade ago.[89] Renal biopsies in patients with ischemic AKI have shown that KIM-1 expression in proximal tubular cells is markedly upregulated, and urinary KIM-1 levels have been used to identify AKI in children and adults after heart surgery.[90]

Neutrophil gelatinase-associated lipocalin (NGAL) is a protein expressed primarily in immune cells, but also by renal tubular cells. Its production markedly increases in response to ischemic renal injury. Urinary NGAL levels rapidly rise in response to renal ischemia and return to baseline following the resolution of the renal injury. Increased urinary NGAL levels have been noted within 6 hours of injury in children and adults following heart surgery and radiocontrast exposure.[90] Although these urinary biomarkers are very promising, they have relatively low (70% to 75%) sensitivity and specificity and have not yet been adopted by most nephrologists or intensivists.[91] For a detailed discussion of biomarkers for the assessment of kidney disease, see Chapter 30.

IMAGING

Imaging of the urinary tract by ultrasonography is an extremely helpful and important test in the setting of AKI. It will generally diagnose obstruction. However, it is not 100% sensitive nor specific; ultrasonography can have a false-negative result immediately following obstruction or in patients with ureteric encasement. Renal ultrasonography also provides an excellent measurement of kidney size, which helps distinguish chronic renal failure (in which the kidneys are often small and echogenic) from AKI (in which renal size is expected to be normal). If contrast nephropathy is suspected, a radiograph of the abdomen (KUB) may reveal a persistent nephrogram because of retained IV contrast material. Doppler ultrasonography can also be used to assess renal arterial and venous patency when vascular obstruction is suspected. Although CT, MRI, and angiography can be used when ultrasonography results are insufficient, the use of these modalities in this setting is limited because renal injury restricts the use of contrast agents.

KIDNEY BIOPSY

A kidney biopsy is generally not necessary in the setting of AKI. However, kidney biopsy can be useful when vasculitis, glomerulonephritis, or allergic interstitial nephritis is considered a possible cause of the AKI.[92] Accordingly, a kidney biopsy is often performed when a noninvasive evaluation has not been able to establish a definite cause for the AKI, especially if an acute nephritic syndrome or nephrotic-range proteinuria is present.

CHRONIC KIDNEY DISEASE

CKD, regardless of the specific cause, is defined as an irreversible and usually progressive decline in renal function and is generally measured by a reduction in GFR. As GFR falls from 90 to approximately 30 mL/min, retention in the plasma of substances that are handled primarily by glomerular filtration develops. The plasma concentrations of urea nitrogen and creatinine, two such substances that are routinely measured, increase. As the GFR falls from 30 to 15 mL/min, additional alterations in plasma composition develop, and other pathophysiologic disturbances, including anemia, altered calcium and phosphate metabolism, and nutritional changes, occur. Although overt symptoms may be absent, careful evaluation generally reveals a wide spectrum of abnormalities in these patients. Then, generally when the GFR falls below 10 mL/min, overt uremic signs and symptoms develop and, if the decline is irreversible, the patient will have reached ESKD. Uremic syndrome is the result of severely reduced excretory function, with retention of metabolic products, fluid and acid-base derangements, hormonal abnormalities, and other consequences of the loss of renal function.

In 2002, the National Kidney Foundation proposed a new classification system for CKD based on the severity of GFR reduction and made recommendations for appropriate actions to be taken at each disease stage.[93] This system, known as the Kidney Disease Outcomes Quality Initiative (KDOQI) classification, is presented in Table 25.13.[93] Also shown in Table 25.13 are the number of U.S. adults at each stage of CKD. Most individuals with CKD have stage 1 or 2 disease. Patients with stage 3 CKD, numbering almost 8 million, comprise the most rapidly expanding group. The Kidney Disease Improving Global Outcomes (KDIGO) group has proposed a modification of the KDOQI classification that divides stage 3 into stages 3A and 3B and also takes account of the magnitude of albuminuria (Table 25.14).[94] Recent studies have suggested that the lifetime risk of developing stage 3 CKD is in excess of 50% and the ultimate risk of ESKD is 4%. The risk is higher in men, African Americans, and patients older than 70 years.[95] The most recent information from the U.S. Renal Data System at the end of 2011 found that the incidence of ESKD in the United States had fallen, for the first time in over a decade, to approximately 357 per million. In late 2011, the prevalence had risen to 1901 per million population (this number includes dialysis patients and those with a functioning renal transplant).[96]

These findings suggest that better implementation of CKD management may be having a favorable impact on slowing the progression of kidney disease. However, prevalence data are also affected by the improved longevity of patients with CKD, including better kidney transplantation outcomes.

A number of risk factors for the development of CKD have been identified (Table 25.15). These include diabetes, hypertension, male gender, African-American or Hispanic race, increased age, and prior AKI.[93]

Mortality in patients with CKD is high and, in patients with stage 3 CKD, the risk of death (usually from cardiovascular disease) is at least 10 times higher than the risk of progression to ESKD. Patients with ESKD have a mortality rate of about 50% after 3 years and 65% to 75% at 5 years. At least 60% of these deaths are also related to cardiovascular disease.

CKD has manifestations and complications affecting almost every organ system, including the central and peripheral nervous, neuropsychiatric, endocrine, hematologic, cardiovascular, gastrointestinal, peripheral vascular, and skeletal systems. Consequently, the diagnosis and treatment of CKD require a broad multifaceted approach. The most common renal diseases that progress to ESKD (in order of incidence and prevalence) are diabetic nephropathy, hypertensive nephrosclerosis, polycystic kidney disease,

Table 25.13 National Kidney Foundation Kidney Disease Outcomes Quality Initiative (KDOQI) Classification System, Disease Prevalence, and Action Plan

Stage	Description	GFR (mL/min/1.73 m^2)	Prevalence (in millions)*	Action
—	At increased risk	≥90 (with CKD risk factors)		Reduction of CKD risk factors
1	Kidney damage with normal or ↑ GFR	≥90	3.6	Treatment of comorbid conditions and reduction of cardiovascular disease risks
2	Kidney damage with mild ↓ GFR	60-89	6.5	Estimation of progression rate
3	Moderate ↓ GFR	30-59	15.5	Evaluation and treatment of complications
4	Severe ↓ GFR	15-29	0.7	Preparation for kidney replacement therapy
5	Kidney failure (end-stage kidney disease)	<15 (or dialysis)	0.6	Kidney replacement therapy (if uremic)

*Prevalence data from National Kidney Foundation,[93] U.S. Renal Data System,[96] and Coresh J, Selvin E, Stevens LA, et al: Prevalence of chronic kidney disease in the United States. *JAMA* 298:2038-2047, 2007.
CKD, Chronic kidney disease; GFR, glomerular filtration rate.
Data are for adults aged ≥20 years.

Table 25.14 Kidney Disease Improving Global Outcome (KDIGO) Classification of Chronic Kidney Disease (CKD)

			Persistent Albuminuria Categories Description and Range		
			A1	A2	A3
			Normal to mildly increased <30 mg/g <3 mg/mmol	Moderately increased 30–300 mg/g 3–30 mg/mmol	Severely increased >300 mg/g >30 mg/mmol
GFR Categories (mL/min/1.73 m^2) Description and Range					
G1	Normal or high	≥90			
G2	Mildly decreased	60–89			
G3a	Mildly to moderately decreased	45–59			
G3b	Moderately to severely decreased	30–44			
G4	Severely decreased	15–29			
G5	Kidney failure	<15			

Gradations of dark to light shades correspond to increasing risk and progression of CKD.
GFR, Glomerular filtration rate.
Reproduced with permission from Kidney Int Suppl 3:5-14, 2013.

Table 25.15 Prevalence of Individuals at Increased Risk for Chronic Kidney Disease

Risk Factor	Estimated Percentage	Estimated Total No.
Diabetes mellitus	Diagnosed: 5.1% of adults ≥ 20 yr	10.2 million
	Undiagnosed: 2.7% of adults age ≥20	5.4 million
Hypertension	14.0% of adults ≥ 18 yr	43.1 million
Systemic lupus erythematosus	~0.05% definite or suspected	~239,000
Functioning kidney graft	~0.03%	88,311*
African American	12.3%	34.7 million
Hispanic or Latino (of any race)	12.5%	35.3 million
American Indian and Alaska Native	0.9%	2.5 million
Age 60-70 yr	7.3%	20.3 million
Age ≥ 70 yr	9.2%	25.5 million
Acute kidney failure	~0.14%	~363,000 non–federal hospital stays in 1997
Daily NSAID use	~5.2% with rheumatoid arthritis or osteoarthritis (assumed daily use)	~13 million assumed daily use
	~30% annual use	~75 million annual use

*As of December 31, 1998.
NSAID, Nonsteroidal antiinflammatory drug.

and chronic glomerulonephritis. The focus of the history, physical examination, and laboratory studies in these patients is to establish the specific diagnosis, determine the severity of kidney dysfunction, identify any reversible component, identify and quantitate any comorbid conditions and complications, assess the risk for continued loss of kidney function, and assess the risk for cardiovascular disease.

HISTORY AND REVIEW OF SYSTEMS

Patients are often referred to a nephrologist for evaluation of CKD when the BUN and creatinine concentrations are noted to be elevated on routine laboratory testing. The patient may have no knowledge of any kidney disorder or abnormal kidney function. Other patients may have had an extensive prior renal evaluation. In some, the kidney disease is an isolated abnormality; in others, an underlying disease known to be associated with kidney involvement such as diabetes, systemic lupus erythematosus, hepatitis B or C, scleroderma, or vasculitis may exist. The duration of the kidney disease and rate of progression must be established whenever possible. The patient might know about a specific diagnosis, severity or stage of the kidney disease, and its pace. Any prior laboratory data, biopsy reports, imaging results, and urologic interventions should be reviewed. Any previous discussions regarding treatment or renal replacement therapy should be reviewed, and the patient's adherence to prior medical recommendations should be determined.

A detailed family history of kidney disease can be extremely informative. Monogenic familial kidney diseases include polycystic kidney disease, Alport's disease, medullary cystic disease, certain forms of membranoproliferative glomerulonephritis, and Fabry's disease. Polygenic familial disorders include diabetes mellitus, hypertension, obesity, hyperlipidemia, and premature vascular disease.

The patient's general health, ability to perform activities of daily living, energy level, appetite, and recent weight changes should be assessed. Mental acuity, memory, mood, and change in sleep pattern must be evaluated. Sometimes, family members can provide a more accurate assessment of these parameters than the patient. Many symptoms do not become apparent until very late in the disease course. Patients with CKD may exhibit an amazing adaptive ability. Urinary voiding symptomatology should be identified, including voiding symptoms such as polyuria, nocturia, hesitancy, frequency, and any history of urinary tract infections, back, flank, abdominal, or pelvic pain, renal calculi, or urologic manipulation. A prior history of GU malignancy, including cancer of the bladder, prostate, kidney, or cervix should be obtained. A cardiovascular, peripheral vascular, and cerebrovascular disease history should be elicited. Coronary artery disease is the most important vascular complication in patients with CKD.[97] Any history of myocardial infarction and/or congestive heart failure should be documented and left ventricular function assessed. A history of coronary artery interventions, significant arrhythmias, or insertion of a pacemaker or defibrillator should be identified.

It is imperative that any history of resting or exertional chest pain and/or shortness of breath be recognized. Peripheral vascular disease is also very common in patients with CKD. A history of claudication, peripheral ulcers, revascularization, gangrenous extremities, or extremity amputation must be documented. Symptoms secondary to autonomic and sensorimotor neuropathy should be identified. Nutritional status, appetite, and weight changes should be determined. The interpretation of weight change is complicated, however, because loss of body mass may be masked by fluid accumulation. Food may taste bad and a foul breath may develop. Anorexia, nausea, and vomiting are symptoms of uremia. Occasionally, diarrhea develops. In the diabetic patient with ESKD, it may be difficult to distinguish between uremic symptoms and those of diabetic neuropathy and enteropathy.

Musculoskeletal complaints occur frequently with CKD. Muscle cramps are often related to diuretic use. Muscle wasting and loss of muscle strength occur. Bone and joint pain may be caused by osteodystrophy. Spontaneous fractures can occur. All medications should be carefully reviewed and documented. The review should include current and prior medications, OTC, and nonprescription medications. Medications should be reviewed for potential nephrotoxic effects and for appropriate dosing for renal function.[98] Calcineurin inhibitors (e.g., cyclosporine, tacrolimus), lithium, pamidronate, chemotherapy agents (e.g., cisplatin, gemcitabine, mitomycin C), and various analgesics are some drugs that can damage the kidneys.[99] Sodium phosphate–based bowel preparations administered prior to colonoscopy or GI surgical procedures have been found to cause irreversible renal disease.[100] Therefore, medication toxicity is a critically important consideration whenever otherwise unexplained CKD occurs.

Ophthalmic complications, largely related to diabetes and hypertension, are common in CKD. Lens abnormalities may occur in patients with Alport's disease. When diabetes exists, its duration, specific medications, adequacy of control, hemoglobin A_{1C} levels, and results of microalbuminuria studies should be ascertained. In general, the onset of type 2 diabetes is difficult to determine because this disease may be clinically silent for years. Hypertensive nephrosclerosis is the second leading cause of CKD resulting in ESKD, and hypertension is also a very common complication of almost all forms of CKD. Differentiating primary hypertension that has caused CKD from a kidney disease complicated by hypertension is frequently very difficult. The duration of hypertension may also be difficult to establish. A history of high or low blood pressure extremes, as well as response to and adherence to antihypertensive medication regimens, should be documented.

A history of gross or microscopic hematuria, proteinuria, or foamy urine suggests the possibility of glomerulonephritis, the third most common cause of CKD progressing to ESKD. Back or flank pain may be presenting or prominent complaints. Fever, skin rash, inflammation of the eyes or sinuses, and joint pains raise the possibility of secondary forms of glomerulonephritis. Occasionally, a family history of glomerulonephritis can be elicited. Although polycystic kidney disease is often diagnosed from the family history, it is occasionally first recognized after an abdominal imaging procedure reveals the diagnosis. These patients frequently develop shoulder, back, flank, and/or pelvic pain. Abdominal fullness, bloating, and episodes of hematuria are often described. Sometimes, the patient feels the enlarged kidneys. The multiple extrarenal manifestations of polycystic kidney disease include cerebral aneurysms, which are the most life-threatening extrarenal complication. Because these aneurysms occur more commonly within families, a history of cerebral aneurysms, stroke, or sudden death at a young age among relatives should be sought. Colonic diverticula and abdominal wall or inguinal hernias are also common in these patients.

PHYSICAL EXAMINATION

Assessment of vital signs should include supine and upright pulse and blood pressure measurements. One primary focus of the physical examination in patients with CKD is the assessment of ECF and effective intraarterial volume status, but this is not always straightforward. Physical findings that indicate volume depletion were also discussed earlier (see "Acute Kidney Disease: Physical Examination").

Although overt hypotension is the strongest indicator of possible renal underperfusion, an orthostatic pulse increase of more than 30 beats/min (measured 1 minute after standing) is indicative of less severe volume depletion.[82] Orthostatic hypotension, defined as a drop in systolic blood pressure of more than 20 mm Hg after standing, is less helpful because it is seen in 10% of normal subjects. Autonomic neuropathy also complicates the assessment of orthostatic hypotension. Dry axillae and dry mucous membranes with a furrowed tongue are useful signs of volume depletion. However, poor skin turgor and slow capillary refill have not been shown to be helpful signs in adults.[82] The neck veins are usually flat in the volume-contracted patient. If volume depletion is possible, a trial of ECF expansion with crystalloid solutions is indicated to determine if there is a reversible component of kidney dysfunction.

At the other extreme, hypertension, peripheral edema, pleural effusions, and pulmonary rales may indicate volume overload and require treatment with diuretics or ultrafiltration. However, edema and effusions may also be the result of nephrotic syndrome. Heart failure and cirrhosis also generate total body salt and water expansion, with effective intraarterial volume contraction. Advanced CKD produces a sallow appearance. Generalized muscle wasting may be observed. Current body weight should be noted and compared with prior known weights. A thorough evaluation of the cardiovascular system is mandatory. A retinal examination may reveal hypertensive or diabetic retinopathy. The carotid pulse should be evaluated and the presence of bruits identified. The cardiac examination may reveal left ventricular hypertrophy or decompensation. Flank or abdominal bruits may suggest renovascular disease. Palpation of the abdomen may reveal an enlarged bladder or large kidneys. Costovertebral tenderness indicates possible inflammatory or infectious kidney disease. Motor and/or sensory neuropathy can occur with CKD, as well as diabetes. Muscle wasting is common. Neuromuscular irritability with tremor and myoclonic jerks can be seen when CKD is advanced or is complicated by hypocalcemia or hypomagnesemia. Skin changes common in CKD include pallor related to anemia, hyperpigmentation, and scratch marks and excoriations produced as a result of pruritus. Uremic frost, representing residue from evaporated urea-rich sweat, occurs in severe untreated ESKD. Skin necrosis caused by calcific arteriopathy and calciphylaxis is a dreaded complication.

LABORATORY TESTS

The urinalysis can provide important clues to the diagnosis. Hematuria with high-grade proteinuria suggests a glomerular process, whereas low-grade proteinuria is consistent with nephrosclerosis, an interstitial disease, or polycystic disease. When the urine sediment reveals RBCs, their appearance as acanthocytes (see Fig. 25.1) or RBC casts supports a glomerular origin. The urine protein/creatinine ratio provides an estimate of protein excretion. With the assumption that urine creatinine excretion is about 1 g/day, this ratio, expressed as grams of protein per gram of creatinine, represents the daily protein excretion in grams per day. Adjustments can be made for very small or very large patients. Excretion of more than 3000 mg/day of protein (primarily albumin) is most consistent with a glomerular process. Quantitative measurement of protein and creatinine excretion may be very helpful in selected patients.

Blood studies should include a CBC, BUN and creatinine concentrations, electrolyte panel, calcium and phosphate levels, liver function studies, and a lipid panel. Sedimentation rate and C-reactive protein level provide information about the patient's inflammatory state. Based on the results of these tests and the patient's underlying conditions, the iron storage status, vitamin B_{12} and folate levels, and hemoglobin A_{1C} levels are often measured. When diseases such as systemic lupus erythematosus or other collagen vascular diseases, HIV infection, hepatitis B or C, or multiple myeloma are suspected, appropriate serologic and protein studies are done. Evaluation of complement levels may be helpful with certain types of glomerulonephritis. An assessment of the GFR is an essential component of the evaluation of the patient with CKD. The GFR can be estimated from the serum creatinine concentration using one of several standard formulas. However, these formulas are inaccurate in patients with extremes in age and size. Patients with a relatively high GFR (normal serum creatinine concentration) may have a relatively low estimated GFR, although the more recently published Chronic Kidney Disease Epidemiology Collaboration (CKD-EPI) formula has improved accuracy and performs better in people with normal GFR.[101] In addition, these estimating equations are only useful when the serum creatinine concentration is relatively stable. In general, a timed urine collection to measure creatinine clearance is the standard method for documenting renal glomerular function. A timed urine collection for urea nitrogen can be obtained to judge nutritional status by estimating a protein catabolic rate. Fractional urea (and sodium) clearance can be calculated to assess if a renal hypoperfusion state exists in addition to underlying CKD. A radioisotope clearance study (usually iothalamate) is the most accurate, gold standard method for determining GFR. The serum cystatin C level has been proposed as a better marker of renal function, but this test is not routinely done in most facilities. Although it may have some advantage relative to creatinine concentration, this remains unproven.

Important goals of laboratory investigations in patients with CKD are to assess the risks of progression to ESKD and the cardiovascular risk to guide management. The KDIGO classification system combines the estimated GFR (eGFR) and albuminuria results to improve stratification as shown in Table 25.14.

IMAGING

Renal ultrasonography should be done for all patients being evaluated for CKD. The sonogram provides a kidney size assessment, supplies information on cortical width and echogenicity, and demonstrates the presence or absence of scars and hydronephrosis, as well as renal stones or masses. Renal Doppler ultrasound imaging is used to assess renovascular flow. If there is any suspicion of coexistent heart disease, echocardiography can be done to assess cardiac size, left ventricular function, regional wall motion abnormalities, pulmonary pressures, valvular function, and pericardial fluid.

URINARY TRACT INFECTION
(see also Chapter 37)

UTIs are one of the most frequent infectious illnesses occurring in humans and are probably the most common bacterial infection.[102] UTIs account for almost 9 million outpatient visits yearly in the United States. Although urinary tract infections usually affect women, hospitalizations from UTIs with complications occur more often in men.[103] A UTI can occur at all ages, from the very young to the very old, but most often affects women in the reproductive age group. UTI presents in a number of ways, from asymptomatic bacteriuria to bothersome local symptoms of pelvic pain and dysuria to severe local symptoms of back or flank pain and fever to overwhelming infection with septic shock and multiorgan failure. It is useful to separate UTIs on an anatomic basis. Pyelonephritis represents an upper UTI of the kidney itself. Lower UTIs may be separated into those of the bladder (cystitis), prostate, and urethra.

HISTORY AND REVIEW OF SYSTEMS

The most common complaint of a patient with an acute UTI is urinary frequency and dysuria. Other voiding symptoms such as difficulty voiding, polyuria, halting voiding symptoms, or frequent small voids also occur. Sometimes, a change in the appearance of the urine is the presenting complaint. The patient may complain of grossly purulent, foul-smelling, and/or blood-tinged or frankly bloody urine. Passage of a stone or tissue debris may be reported. Patients with UTIs (other than asymptomatic bacteriuria) also often present with some localizing symptom. Back, flank, abdominal, and/or pelvic pain may be the presenting complaint. Fever, with or without chills, suggests a more serious illness. A past history of similar symptoms associated with a documented UTI can often be elicited.

The frequency of prior UTIs should be established. The patient's report of specific antibiotics used for treatment of previous UTIs is helpful. Some patients can describe prior infecting organisms as demonstrated on urine culture. In addition to localizing symptoms of pain, with or without fever, some patients have constitutional symptoms of fatigue, malaise, and weight loss. Gastrointestinal symptoms of nausea and vomiting, constipation, or diarrhea may be present. With severe UTIs, symptoms of hypotension with orthostatic dizziness may occur.

Asymptomatic bacteriuria can be the initial presentation. It must be distinguished from urinary contamination at the time of urine culture. It is often identified in patients with a history of UTIs and is sometimes noted when urine cultures are performed during follow-up of previously treated symptomatic UTIs. Usually, it is detected in patients at high risk for UTIs for whom surveillance urine cultures are performed. High-risk groups include pregnant women, sexually active young women, older adults, particularly in a nursing home setting, patients with indwelling urinary catheters or other drainage devices, patients with diabetes, and patients with spinal cord injury. Current recommendations are that only pregnant women should be screened (and treated) for asymptomatic bacteriuria.[104-106] There is no evidence that the benefits of screening outweigh its potential negative impact in any other adult patient group.[104]

It is important to identify underlying risk factors for the development of the current UTI, as well as previous episodes of UTIs. Most young and middle-aged women have no apparent anatomic abnormality that might predispose them to UTIs. Recurrent UTIs in this group should prompt a discussion regarding the timing of the UTI with respect to sexual activity. The use of diaphragms and spermicides, as well as delayed postcoital micturition, has been associated with UTIs. Vaginitis is an important risk factor for UTIs in women, so a history of associated symptoms should be elicited. There is little evidence that tampon use or the method (direction of wiping) of cleansing after defecation have a significant impact on the risk of developing UTIs. The frequency of UTIs increases during pregnancy and is probably related to a combination of physiologic and anatomic changes, frequent glucosuria, and hormonal effects.

UTIs in men raise concern for an anatomic abnormality. The most common abnormalities that predispose men to UTIs are prostatic enlargement and prostatitis. Sexual history regarding homosexual activity, and specifically anal intercourse, which increases UTI risk in men, is also important. Other anatomic abnormalities that predispose patients to UTIs include bladder pathology (e.g., neurogenic bladder, especially in the setting of spinal cord injury, bladder cancer with disruption of the urothelium, bladder diverticula), enterovesical fistula, polycystic kidney disease, prostate cancer, urinary drainage devices and procedures (e.g., indwelling transurethral or suprapubic bladder catheters, percutaneous nephrostomy, ureteral stent, ileal conduit), renal calculi with or without urinary obstruction, vesicoureteral reflux, and urinary obstruction at any level. Certain medical conditions also increase the risk for developing UTIs and complications of these infections. These include pregnancy, diabetes, renal transplantation, and long-term immunosuppression.

PHYSICAL EXAMINATION

Physical examination findings in the setting of UTI are often nonspecific.[105,106] Fever may indicate a more serious or complicated UTI, as does hypotension and tachycardia. The patient with a severe systemic infection of urinary origin may have a toxic appearance and altered mentation. Careful attention should be given to the back, flank, abdomen, and pelvic areas to detect localized tenderness or a palpable mass. The patient should be inspected for urinary drainage devices. In men a rectal examination for assessment of the prostate is important.

LABORATORY TESTS

The urinalysis results often confirm the presence of an active UTI.[105-107] Gross visual inspection of the urine may reveal turbidity or blood, and the urine often has a foul smell. On the urine dipstick test, the pH can be markedly alkaline (supraphysiologic level; i.e., >7.5) when the urine is infected with urea-splitting bacteria (see earlier, "Nephrolithiasis: Laboratory Tests"). The dipstick result is often positive for occult blood. The nitrite test result is positive when the urine is infected with Enterobacteriaceae.

These gram-negative bacilli have an enzyme that reduces urinary nitrate to nitrite. A false-negative nitrite test result can be the result of very dilute urine (e.g., the patient is taking a diuretic) or infecting bacteria that do not produce the nitrate reductase enzyme (*Staphylococcus* or *Enterococcus* species or *Pseudomonas aeruginosa*). Urine granulocytes generally indicate inflammation, which may or may not be due to infection. They can be detected by a dipstick test for leukocyte esterase, an enzyme contained in the granules of neutrophils. More than five WBCs/HPF is needed for a positive test finding. In rare cases, false-positive results are produced by strong oxidants in the urine collection container. High-grade proteinuria or glucosuria, some antibiotics, and high levels of ascorbic acid can produce false-negative results.

Simultaneous positive test results for nitrite and leukocyte esterase are almost always diagnostic of a UTI. A finding of marked proteinuria raises the possibility of reflux nephropathy complicated by focal glomerulosclerosis, whereas moderate proteinuria (in the range of 1000 to 1500 mg/day or less) can occur with chronic interstitial nephritis. The spun urine sediment shows neutrophils, often in clumps, and occasionally neutrophil casts. RBCs are also usually seen. Bacteria are generally easily observed when significant bacteriuria exists. A Gram-stained smear of unspun urine or spun sediment can aid in identification of the bacteria and help target empirical therapy.

Urine culture will verify an active UTI. Good urine collection and culture techniques are necessary to avoid contamination. Midstream urine should be collected after careful washing of external genitalia followed by voiding into a sterile container. Bladder catheterization, suprapubic needle bladder aspiration, or sterile aspiration of urine from the tube of a closed catheter drainage system is sometimes required. Most true UTIs are caused by a single organism. Therefore, demonstration of multiple organisms on urine culture strongly suggests contamination. A colony count of more than 10^5 organisms/mL (from voided specimens) correlates with active infection. However, colony counts of less than 10^5/mL may be significant in a symptomatic patient.[106,107]

The vast majority (80% to 90%) of positive urine cultures in the outpatient setting grow *Escherichia coli*. The presence of other gram-negative bacteria on urine culture suggests a complicated UTI possibly related to renal calculi or obstruction. *Proteus* infections occur in patients with staghorn calculi. Urine culture findings for hospitalized patients are much more diverse. UTIs caused by gram-positive cocci (usually *Enterococcus*) are uncommon, and those caused by *Staphylococcus* species are extremely rare. *Staphylococcus aureus* UTIs may suggest staphylococcal bacteremia, whereas coagulase-negative staphylococci UTI can occur after instrumentation in older men. Mycobacterial and fungal UTIs are very rare. *Candida* infections may develop in immunocompromised patients or in those with long-standing catheters. Anaerobic bacteria almost never cause UTIs.

An assessment of baseline renal function should be done. This is usually accomplished using a serum creatinine measurement and one of several estimating equations. A decline in renal function may be due to an acute or chronic process. AKI occurs in patients with volume depletion and sepsis syndromes with hypotension. Infection with bilateral urinary obstruction or obstruction in a solitary functional kidney can present with AKI. A chronic reduction in the GFR can occur with vesicoureteral reflux, chronic pyelonephritis, or chronic urinary obstruction. If estimates of kidney function are persistently reduced, formal GFR measurements should be obtained with a timed urine collection to assess creatinine clearance or an isotopic measurement of GFR.

A number of acid-base and potassium abnormalities may occur in patients with UTIs. If the UTI causes nausea and vomiting, metabolic alkalosis and hypokalemia ensue. Hyperkalemia can be caused by a reduced GFR or may be a component of type 4 renal tubular acidosis because of chronic renal interstitial disease or urinary obstruction. Metabolic acidosis can be caused by lactic acidosis associated with sepsis, renal tubular acidosis, or low GFR.

IMAGING

Kidney and GU tract imaging are usually done to diagnose vesicoureteral reflux, renal calculi, and other lesions that obstruct urine flow or otherwise cause stasis. In general, imaging studies are not required in adult women with an uncomplicated UTI that responds rapidly to antibiotic treatment. Imaging is generally recommended for all men with their first UTI. Imaging should also be done when patients have a complicated UTI, bacteremia has developed, the UTI has failed to respond to appropriate antibiotic therapy, and urinary obstruction or stones are suspected. Women with unexplained recurrent UTIs and all patients with pyelonephritis serious enough to warrant hospitalization should undergo imaging. Also, if hematuria persists following resolution of a UTI, imaging is indicated. Renal ultrasonography has replaced IV urography as the standard renal imaging procedure in patients with UTIs. Renal size, cortical width and echogenicity, obstruction, and presence of stones can be readily determined with ultrasonography. Bladder and prostate anatomy can be assessed. CT imaging with contrast infusion permits further assessment of renal and ureteral anatomy and pathology. Pyelonephritis in an obstructed kidney requires emergent intervention for drainage, and detection of a perinephric abscess usually also calls for surgical intervention. Some patients require cystoscopy, retrograde pyelography, and/or voiding cystography to detect vesicoureteral reflux.

Complete reference list available at ExpertConsult.com.

KEY REFERENCES

1. Mohr DN, Offord KP, Owen RA, et al: Asymptomatic microhematuria and urologic disease. A population-based study. *JAMA* 256:224–229, 1986.
2. U.S. Preventive Services Task Force: *Screening for bladder cancer in adults: recommendation statement.* June 2004. Available at: http://www.uspreventiveservicestaskforce.org/ 3rduspstf/ bladder/blacanrs.htm Accessed March 12, 2011.
4. Loo RK, Lieberman SF, Slezak JM, et al: Stratifying risk of urinary tract malignant tumors in patients with asymptomatic microscopic hematuria. *Mayo Clin Proc* 88:129–138, 2013.
5. Grossfeld GD, Litwin MS, Wolf S, et al: Evaluation of asymptomatic microscopic hematuria in adults: the American Urological Association best practice policy. Part I: definition, detection, prevalence and etiology. *Urology* 57:599–603, 2001.
6. Grossfeld GD, Litwin MS, Wolf S, et al: Evaluation of asymptomatic microscopic hematuria in adults: the American Urological

7. Khadra MH, Pickard RS, Charlton M, et al: A prospective analysis of 1,930 patients with hematuria to evaluate current diagnostic practice. *J Urol* 163:524–527, 2000.
11. Culclasure TF, Bray VJ, Hasbaragen JA: The significance of hematuria in the anticoagulated patient. *Arch Intern Med* 154:649–652, 1994.
15. Yang HY, Wang JD, Lo TC, et al: Occupational exposure to herbs containing aristolochic acids increases the risk of urothelial carcinoma in Chinese herbalists. *J Urol* 189:48–52, 2013.
18. Pollock C, Liu PL, Gyory AZ, et al: Dysmorphism of urinary RBCs-value in diagnosis. *Kidney Int* 36:1045–1049, 1989.
20. Cowan NC: CT urography for hematuria. *Nat Rev Urol* 9:218–226, 2012.
29. Madalio MP, Harrington JT: Current concepts: the diagnosis of acute glomerulonephritis. *N Engl J Med* 309:1299–1302, 1983.
31. Sharma SG, Bomback AS, Radhakrishnan J, et al: The modern spectrum of renal biopsy findings in patients with diabetes. *Clin J Am Soc Nephrol* 8:1718–1724, 2013.
34. Schrier RW, Fassett RG: A critique of the overfill hypothesis of sodium and water retention in the nephrotic syndrome. *Kidney Int* 53:1111–1117, 1998.
37. Llach F: Hypercoagulability, renal vein thrombosis, and other thrombotic complications of nephrotic syndrome. *Kidney Int* 28:429–439, 1985.
38. Ginsberg JM, Chang BS, Matarese RA, et al: Use of single voided urine samples to estimate quantitative proteinuria. *N Engl J Med* 309:1543–1546, 1983.
46. Weidmann P, Beretta-Piccoli C, Hirsch D, et al: Curable hypertension with unilateral hydronephrosis. Studies on the role of circulating renin. *Ann Intern Med* 87:437–440, 1977.
49. Maletz R, Beman D, Peelle K, et al: Reflex anuria and uremia from unilateral ureteral obstruction. *Am J Kidney Dis* 22:870–873, 1993.
50. Batlle DC, Arruda JA, Kurtzman NA: Hyperkalemic distal renal tubular acidosis associated with obstructive uropathy. *N Engl J Med* 304:373–380, 1981.
52. Webb JA: Ultrasonography and Doppler studies in the diagnosis of renal obstruction. *BJU Int* 86(Suppl 1):25–32, 2000.
54. Spital A, Valvo JR, Segal AJ: Nondilated obstructive uropathy. *Urology* 31:478–482, 1988.
56. James PA, Oparil S, Carter BL, et al: 2014 Evidence-based guideline for the management of high blood pressure in adults. report from the panel members appointed to the Eighth Joint National Committee (JNC 8). *JAMA* 311:507–520, 2014.
58. Peppard PE, Young T, Palta M, et al: Prospective study of the association between sleep-disordered breathing and hypertension. *N Engl J Med* 342:1378–1384, 2000.
62. Stamatelou KK, Francis ME, Jones CA, et al: Time trends in reported prevalence of kidney stones in the United States. *Kidney Int* 63:1951–1952, 2003.
65. Daudon M, Jungers P: Drug-induced renal calculi: epidemiology, prevention and management. *Drugs* 64:245–275, 2004.
66. Taylor EN, Stampler MJ, Curhan GC: Obesity, weight gain, and the risk of kidney stones. *JAMA* 293:455–462, 2005.
70. Consensus conference: Prevention and treatment of kidney stones. *JAMA* 260:977–981, 1988.
71. Preminger GM, Tiselius HG, Assimos DG, et al: EAU/AUA Nephrolithiasis Guideline Panel: 2007 guideline for the management of ureteral calculi. *J Urol* 178:2418–2434, 2007.
74. Carter MR, Green BR: Renal calculi: emergency department diagnosis and treatment. *Emerg Med Pract* 13:1–170, 2011.
76. Bellomo R, Ronco C, Kellum JA, et al: Acute Dialysis Quality Initiative workgroup: Acute renal failure—definition, outcome measures, animal models, fluid therapy and information technology needs: the Second International Consensus Conference of the Acute Dialysis Quality Initiative (ADQI) Group. *Crit Care* 8:R204–R212, 2004.
77. Levin A, Warnock DG, Mehta RL, et al: Improving outcomes from acute kidney injury: report of an initiative. *Am J Kidney Dis* 50:1–4, 2007.
78. Nash K, Hafeez A, Hon S: Hospital-acquired renal insufficiency. *Am J Kidney Dis* 39:930–936, 2002.
80. Liaño F, Gallego A, Pascual J, et al: Prognosis of acute tubular necrosis: an extended prospectively contrasted study. *Nephron* 63:21–31, 1993.
81. Hsu CY, Ordoñez JD, Chertow GM, et al: The risk of acute renal failure in patients with chronic kidney disease. *Kidney Int* 74:101–107, 2008.
82. McGee S, Abernethy WB, 3rd, Simel DL: The rational clinical examination. Is this patient hypovolemic? *JAMA* 281:1022–1029, 1999.
85. Perazella MA, Bomback AS: Urinary eosinophils in AIN: farewell to an old biomarker? *Clin J Am Soc Nephrol* 8:1841–1843, 2013.
87. McMahon GM, Waikar SS: Biomarkers in nephrology: core curriculum 2013. *Am J Kidney Dis* 62:165–178, 2013.
91. Honore PM, Jacobs R, Johannes-Boyau O, et al: Biomarkers for early diagnosis of AKI in the ICU: ready for prime time use at the bedside? *Ann Intensive Care* 2:24–28, 2012.
92. Solez K, Racusen LC: Role of the renal biopsy in acute renal failure. *Contrib Nephrol* 132:68–75, 2001.
94. Levin A, Stevens PE: Summary of KDIGO 2012 CKD Guideline: behind the scenes, need for guidance, and a framework for moving forward. *Kidney Int* 85:49–61, 2013.
95. Grams ME, Chow EK, Segev DL: Lifetime incidence of CKD stages 3-5 in the United States. *Am J Kidney Dis* 62:245–252, 2013.
96. U.S. Renal Data System, USRDS 2013 annual data report: atlas of chronic kidney disease and end-stage renal disease in the United States, National Institutes of Health, National Institute of Diabetes and Digestive and Kidney Diseases, Bethesda, MD, 2013. Available at: http://www.usrds.org/adr.aspx. Accessed 12/24/2013.
99. Perazella M: Onco-nephrology: renal toxicities of chemotherapeutic agents. *Clin J Am Soc Nephrol* 7:1713–1721, 2012.
102. Foxman B: Epidemiology of urinary tract infections: incidence, morbidity, and economic costs. *Am J Med* 113(Suppl 1A):5S–13S, 2002.
104. Lin K, Fajardo K, U.S. Preventive Services Task Force: Screening for asymptomatic bacteriuria in adults: evidence for the U.S. Preventive Services Task Force reaffirmation recommendation statement. *Ann Intern Med* 149:W20–W24, 2008.
106. Young JL, Soper DE: Urinalysis and urinary tract infection: update for clinicians. *Infect Dis Obstet Gynecol* 9:249–255, 2001.
107. Hooton TM, Roberts PL, Cox ME, et al: Voided midstream urine culture and acute cystitis in premenopausal women. *N Engl J Med* 369:1883–1891, 2013.

26 Laboratory Assessment of Kidney Disease: Glomerular Filtration Rate, Urinalysis, and Proteinuria

Katrina Chau | Holly Hutton | Adeera Levin

CHAPTER OUTLINE

GLOMERULAR FILTRATION RATE, 781
Normal Physiology, 781
Measurement of Glomerular Filtration Rate, 781
Filtration Markers, 781
Specific Circumstances or Populations, 787
URINALYSIS, 788
Color, 788
Odor, 789
Relative Density, 789
Urine pH, 789
Bilirubin and Urobilinogen, 790
Leukocyte Esterase and Nitrites, 790
Glucose, 790
Ketones, 790
Hemoglobin and Myoglobin, 790
PROTEINURIA, 790
Normal Physiology, 791
Types of Proteinuria, 791
Normal Levels of Proteinuria, 791
Categorization of Proteinuria, 791
Sources of Error in Measurement, 792
Advantages of Urinary Albumin Over Total Protein Measurements, 793
Issues with Measuring Albumin Rather than Total Protein, 793
Diagnostic Utility of Protein Type, 793
Methods to Measure Urinary Total Protein, 793
Methods to Measure Urinary Albumin, 793
Timed versus Random Collection for Proteinuria Assessment, 795
Translating Protein- and Albumin-to-Creatinine Ratios into Total Daily Protein Measurements, 795
Correlation Between Ratios and 24-Hour Urine Protein, 795
Variability in Creatinine Excretion, 796
Fluctuations in Protein Excretion, 796
Urinary ACR versus PCR, 796
Reagent Strip Testing, 796
Proteinuria Measurement in Specific Populations, 798
URINE MICROSCOPY, 798
Preparation and Method, 798
Cells of the Urinary Sediment, 798
Other Elements, 800
Limitations, 802

An appreciation of the components of laboratory assessment of kidney disease is essential to the practicing clinician. This chapter describes three key aspects of laboratory assessment: the glomerular filtration rate, urinalysis, and proteinuria. Issues related to measurement tools, precision, bias, and interpretation are addressed for each of these variables, so that the reader may better appreciate the role of the laboratory in the diagnosis, follow-up, and management of kidney disease. Understanding the physiology of kidney function is essential to the interpretation of laboratory measurements and is highlighted within each section.

Glomerular filtration rate (GFR) is the single best measure of kidney function. Large studies consistently demonstrate the relationship of GFR to outcomes in general and renal populations, and the Kidney Disease Improving Global Outcomes (KDIGO) classification system uses GFR as one of the key dimensions in the diagnosis of chronic kidney disease (CKD). Abnormalities of urinalysis results may indicate acute or chronic conditions and isolated kidney or systemic diseases, and can be used to monitor both kidney and systemic diseases. Proteinuria is similarly an important marker of kidney disease and can also be seen in acute or chronic kidney conditions. In patients with CKD, the presence of proteinuria is proposed as a second dimension for the classification of severity in the KDIGO classification system, because it affects prognosis.

The laboratory assessment of kidney disease can be used to diagnose, prognosticate, and measure progression of disease or response to therapy. CKD is increasingly recognized as an important public health problem, so accurate and appropriate use of laboratory testing is important. This chapter facilitates understanding and interpretation of key tests used in the assessment of kidney disease, both acute and chronic.

GLOMERULAR FILTRATION RATE

Glomerular filtration rate describes one of the key roles of the kidney: to filter plasma so as to excrete waste products and produce urine (an ultrafiltrate of plasma). In clinical practice, estimates of GFR are obtained using equations, and direct measurement is reserved for specific circumstances. This section reviews normal physiology, use of various filtration markers, the development and use of equations, and special circumstances in which GFR interpretation needs to be contextualized.

NORMAL PHYSIOLOGY

Separation of an ultrafiltrate of plasma across the barrier comprising the capillary wall, glomerular basement membrane, and epithelial cell of Bowman's space (or capsule) is the first step in the production of urine and multiple functions of the kidney. The amount of fluid filtered in to the Bowman's space per unit of time is the glomerular filtration rate. Fluid movement is governed by Starling's forces and so the glomerular filtrate that is produced is dependent on the following determinants:

- Porosity of the membrane (p)
- Surface area of the membrane (K)
- Hydraulic pressure and oncotic pressure on the capillary side (P_{GC} and π_{GC})
- Hydraulic pressure and oncotic pressure in Bowman's space (P_{BS} and π_{BS})

GFR can be calculated using the following equation

$$GFR = p \times [(P_{GC} - P_{BS}) - K(\pi_{GC} - \pi_{BS})]$$

Factors that tend to alter the magnitude of each of these determinants are as follows:

p	Generally less important than other factors
K	↑ by relaxation of mesangial cells ↓ in glomerulonephritis and glomerulosclerosis
P_{GC}	↑ by afferent arteriole dilatation and efferent arteriole constriction
P_{BS}	↑ by raised intratubular pressure due to obstruction
π_{GC}	↑ by raised systemic oncotic pressure or decreased renal plasma flow
π_{BS}	Minimal impact

For further discussion of factors that determine glomerular ultrafiltration, please see Chapter 3.

The kidney filters approximately 180 L of plasma per day, which is equivalent to 125 mL/min. Kidney function is proportional to kidney size, which in turn is proportional to body surface area. Normal GFR is more than 90 mL/min/1.73 m². In young adults GFR is approximately 120 to 130 mL/min/1.73 m². There is a gradual decline in GFR with age, but the effect of age is variable, in that some elderly patients have no change in renal function (see Chapter 85).

Protein intake and hyperglycemia can raise GFR by increasing renal plasma flow; the mechanism by which this occurs is unclear but may be activation of the intrarenal renin-angiotensin system.

MEASUREMENT OF GFR

Because GFR is defined as the volume of ultrafiltrate filtered from the glomerular capillaries into Bowman's capsule per unit time, GFR can be measured provided that the concentration of a substance that is freely filtered and neither reabsorbed nor secreted in the plasma and the urine is known. GFR is equivalent to the "clearance rate" of this substance or filtration marker, which can be calculated as follows:

$$GFR = \frac{\text{Urine concentration} \times \text{urine volume}}{\text{Plasma concentration} \times \text{time}}$$

GFR can be measured by direct measurement of the clearance of a filtration marker or can be estimated with use of an equation based on a filtration marker. Filtration markers may be endogenous (e.g., creatinine, cystatin C) or exogenous (e.g., inulin, iohexol).

GFR can be expressed as normalized to body surface area as a result of physiologic matching of GFR to kidney size and in turn to body surface area (mL/min/1.73 m²) or as an absolute value (mL/min). An absolute value of GFR is useful in the setting of drug dosing, which is discussed further later.

The most appropriate method for measurement of GFR depends on the purpose for which kidney function is being monitored. Direct measurement of GFR is time-consuming and may require medical supervision or the patient's presence at the hospital, so it is not usually performed as part of everyday practice. An exact value of the GFR is not required for most clinical settings. Understanding the trend within an individual patient's renal function is often what is needed. As a result, plasma urea and creatinine and estimated GFR calculations based on creatinine are most often used. Alternatively, accuracy in the measurement of GFR is important for drug dosing of medications with narrow therapeutic windows (e.g., chemotherapy drugs) and is vital for appropriate selection and approval of live donors for kidney transplantation.

FILTRATION MARKERS

The ideal filtration marker probably does not exist. Such a marker would have the following characteristics:

- Distributed freely and instantaneously throughout the extracellular space

- Not bound to plasma proteins
- Freely filtered at the glomerulus
- Not secreted or reabsorbed at the tubules
- Eliminated wholly by the kidney
- Resistant to degradation
- Easy and inexpensive to measure

An understanding of the limitations of each filtration marker is important to be able to interpret results. Given that kidney disease is often asymptomatic and dependent on the accuracy of laboratory tests, it is imperative that the clinician know the advantages and disadvantages of each specific test before making clinical decisions.

ENDOGENOUS FILTRATION MARKERS

Urea

Urea is not an accurate filtration marker because it is subject to a number of influences in addition to glomerular filtration. The liver produces urea in the urea cycle as a waste product of the digestion of protein. Therefore, increased plasma levels may be due to factors independent of renal function, such as increased production in high protein intake, gastrointestinal bleeding due to absorption of amino acids in the gastrointestinal tract, and high catabolic states such as those associated with glucocorticoid therapy.

Low urea levels are seen in decreased protein intake and chronic liver disease due to reduced synthesis of urea.

Urea is readily reabsorbed in the proximal tubule, particularly at low urinary flow rates. As a filtration marker, urea has limited use because, although it is freely filtered, significant reabsorption means that the amount that is excreted is not what was filtered. High levels of urea may indicate not poor renal function but, rather, hypovolemia or renal hypoperfusion.

Creatinine

Creatinine is a product of muscle metabolism. Phosphocreatine is a source for replenishment of phosphate when adenosine triphosphate (ATP) is used by muscle cells. Creatine and phosphocreatine are nonenzymatically converted at an almost steady rate (approximately 2% of total creatine per day) to creatinine. Creatinine is not bound to plasma proteins, being freely filtered by the kidney, but it is unfortunately secreted by the tubules, making it an imperfect filtration marker. Despite its many limitations, however, its measurement is still the test most widely used by physicians to gauge renal function.

Serum creatinine level does not measure GFR but varies inversely with GFR and so is an indirect marker of GFR. The serum creatinine level can be used in estimation equations for GFR, and urinary creatinine clearance can be used to approximate GFR.

Factors affecting creatinine levels unrelated to renal function include muscle mass and/or injury and consumption of meat or creatine. Factors affecting muscle mass, such as age, sex, race, and physical activity, can in turn affect creatinine levels, with women, for example, having lower creatinine levels than men but obviously not more renal failure. Rhabdomyolysis has also been suggested to cause a greater rise in serum creatinine than other causes of acute kidney injury, because of the release of preformed creatine and phosphocreatine that is converted into creatinine.

Secretion of creatinine from the renal tubule is affected by:

Drugs: e.g., trimethoprim, cimetidine, pyrimethamine, dapsone.

Decreased renal function: Each tubule excretes a higher proportion of creatinine as renal function declines. This secretory process is saturated when the serum creatinine level exceeds 1.5 to 2 mg/dL (132-176 μmol/L).

Extrarenal degradation of creatinine in the gut also rises as renal function declines. This extrarenal clearance may be as much as two thirds of total daily creatinine excretion.

Sources of Error in Measurement of Creatinine. Clinicians may be unaware of the intricacies and complexities of creatinine measurement and how they may be relevant to day-to-day practice.

Laboratory methods to measure serum creatinine include:

- Alkaline picrate (Jaffe method)
- Enzymatic methods
- Isotope dilution mass spectrometry (IDMS)
- High-performance liquid chromatography (HPLC)

There is wide variation in measured creatinine concentration, depending on the laboratory method and the instruments used. In 2003, the College of American Pathologists conducted a survey of 5624 participating laboratories that showed a bias from the reference value of between −0.06 to 0.31 mg/dL or −7% to 34%.[1] This bias was thought to be predominantly due to differences in instrument calibration among manufacturers. As a result a creatinine standard reference material was prepared by the National Institute of Standards and Technology, which is currently being used by almost all major manufacturers for calibration. The method of analysis (Jaffe or enzymatic) should also have minimal bias in comparison to IDMS reference methodology.

Measurement of creatinine obviously affects measured creatinine clearance and calculation of estimated creatinine clearance or GFR, and therefore it has been recommended as part of the KDIGO initiative guidelines that all creatinine results be traceable to reference materials and methods listed on the Joint Committee for Traceability in Laboratory Medicine database.

The Jaffe method measures creatinine by complexing creatinine with alkaline picrate, followed by measurement with a colorimetric technique. This colorimetric assay may falsely measure normal plasma constituents such as glucose and plasma proteins as creatinine. As a result, the measured creatinine result may be falsely high. The Jaffe method may also report falsely low creatinine levels if there are very high serum bilirubin levels. Modified Jaffe methods attempt to take this into account by removing these interfering chromogens before analysis. This inference is sometimes corrected for by some manufacturers by deducting an estimated value based on average bias from measured results. Currently, the techniques used in most laboratories are modified alkaline picrate and enzymatic methods, but it is recommended that the enzymatic method be adopted because this is more specific.

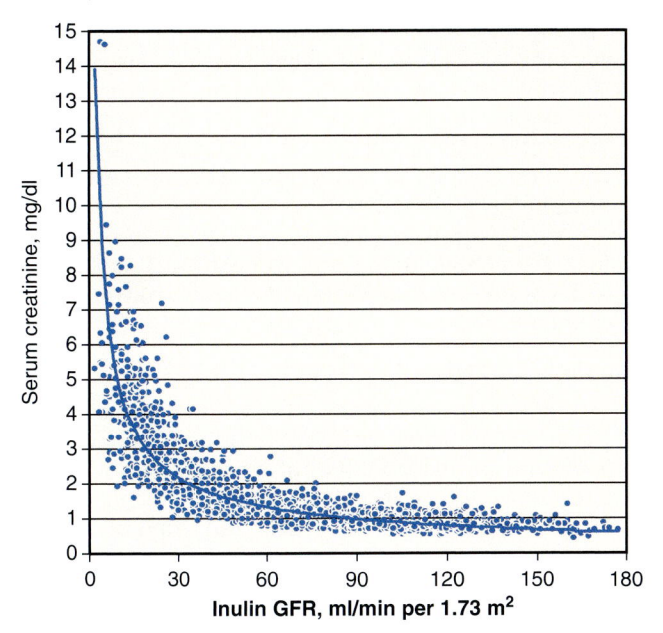

Figure 26.1 Relationship between plasma creatinine and glomerular filtration rate (GFR). (From Botev R, Mallie JP, Couchoud C, et al: Estimating glomerular filtration rate: Cockcroft-Gault and Modification of Diet in Renal Disease Formulas compared to renal inulin clearance. *Clin J Am Soc* 4:899-906, 2009.)

Although serum creatinine value is widely used as a marker of renal function, it is insensitive to even significant declines in GFR at the upper limit of normal due to the nonlinear relationship between creatinine and GFR (Figure 26.1). This is due to compensatory hyperfiltration of remaining functioning nephrons, secretion of creatinine, and extrarenal elimination of creatinine as the GFR declines. It is consequently a poor screening tool for early kidney disease. Within-person variability of creatinine is also significant, at 8%; therefore, significant change in serum creatinine is generally defined as at least 10%, which at early stages of kidney disease may represent a significant decline in GFR.

Serum creatinine results should be interpreted in the clinical context. Creatinine of the same value may correspond to a vastly different GFR in patients of different body composition. Volume status should be taken into account because dilution of creatinine leads to an apparently low result.

Creatinine Clearance. Creatinine clearance (CrCl) is measured by collecting the patient's urine for 24 hours and measuring the total amount of excreted creatinine and the volume of urine. With the equation discussed earlier to calculate clearance of a filtration marker, CrCl is calculated as follows:

$$CrCl = \frac{\text{Urine concentration} \times \text{urine volume}}{\text{Plasma concentration} \times \text{time}}$$

For example, for a patient with a serum creatinine value of 100 μmol/L, a urine creatinine value of 10,000 μmol/L, and a urine volume of 1.44 L, creatinine clearance would be calculated as follows:

$$CrCl = \frac{10,000\ \mu mol/L \times 1440\ mL}{100\ \mu mol/mL \times 1440\ min}$$

$$= 100\ mL/min$$

If this result is adjusted for a small person (height = 160 cm, weight = 50 kg) with a body surface area of 1.5 m, then the creatinine clearance would be:

$$\frac{CrCl \times 1.73}{BSA} = \frac{100 \times 1.73}{1.5} = \frac{115\ mL/min}{1.73\ m^2}$$

For a larger person with a body surface area of 2.0 (height = 180 cm, weight = 80 kg), the adjusted CrCl would be 86.5 mL/min/1.73 m².

Although the clearance of an ideal substance would be equivalent to GFR, creatinine clearance tends to exceed true GFR by approximately 10% to 20% because of the secretion of creatinine by the tubules. This error was previously compensated for by errors in the Jaffe assay that would overestimate serum creatinine value. Now that creatinine measurement has been standardized CrCl will consistently overestimate true GFR.

The main problem with creatinine clearance is its reliance on timed urine collection, which is often inaccurate. Furthermore, tubular secretion of creatinine increases with decreased renal function, thus masking a true drop in GFR.

Cystatin C

Cystatin C is a low-molecular-weight (LMW) (13-kD) basic protein that is produced at a constant rate by all nucleated cells. It is freely filtered by the kidney and is not secreted; proximal tubule cells reabsorb and catabolize the filtered cystatin C so that little is normally excreted in the urine. Therefore, although plasma cystatin C levels are used in estimating GFR, cystatin C measurement cannot be used as a conventional urinary excretory marker for GFR. Rather, urinary cystatin C has been regarded as one of several available markers of kidney injury and may be found in the urine during glomerular injury with heavy proteinuria.

Plasma cystatin C levels are highest in the first days of life and stabilize after age 1 year, with levels approximating those of adults. Polymorphic variants in the *CST3* gene encoding cystatin C appear to affect production, and interindividual variations in cystatin C values account for 25% of its biologic variability, in comparison with 93% for creatinine. Within-person variation of cystatin C values is 6.8%.[2]

Cystatin C levels were reported to be independent of sex, muscle mass, and age after 12 months of age, but there is a growing body of evidence that this may not be the case. Cystatin C levels may be affected by factors independent of renal function, such as corticosteroids, thyroid dysfunction, obesity, diabetes, smoking, and high C-reactive protein (CRP) value. This is problematic as, for example, cystatin C may not be useful in renal transplant patients because they have subclinical inflammation and commonly use long-term corticosteroids.

A meta-analysis published in 2002 showed that serum cystatin C measured with an immunonephelometric assay is more accurate than serum creatinine as a marker of GFR.[3,4] However, as noted previously, the cystatin C value, like the creatinine value, may be affected by a number of factors other than the GFR.

Laboratory techniques to measure cystatin C include latex immunoassays such as automated particle-enhanced turbidimetric immunoassay (PETIA) and nephelometric immunoassay (PENIA). Other techniques are radioimmunoassay, fluorescent techniques, and enzymatic immunoassays.

At the writing of this chapter, the measurement of serum cystatin C is not internationally standardized. A reference material was produced in 2010, and manufacturers are in the process of recalibrating their assays against this standard.

The adoption of serum cystatin C in place of serum creatinine at present is made difficult predominantly by the expense of the assay, variation in production, and absence of universal assay standardization. Furthermore estimated GFR equations using cystatin C only have not been shown to be superior to estimated GFR equations using creatinine, and with the default reporting of estimated GFR (eGFR) along with creatinine results—thereby improving the interpretation of serum creatinine values—there may be no immediate advantage to replacing this well-known filtration marker with cystatin C.

Novel Endogenous Filtration Markers

Several alternative novel endogenous substances are under investigation as potential markers that could be used aside from urea, creatinine and cystatin C. They are: Beta trace protein, β_2-microglobulin, and symmetrical dimethylarginine. These filtration markers will undoubtedly also have determinants unrelated to GFR.

Equations for Estimating GFR

Because direct measurement of GFR is not practical in clinical practice, estimation equations have been developed to aid clinicians in interpretation of serum creatinine, given the limitations previously cited.

A multitude of equations (Table 26.1) derived for the estimation of GFR are available. They all attempt to transform a laboratory measurement of a filtration marker into a value approximating the GFR, usually with the addition of

Table 26.1 Most Commonly Used Equations for Estimating Glomerular Filtration Rate

Equation Name	Equation	Derivation Population
Cockcroft-Gault (1976)	[140 − age] × wt (kg)/creatinine (µmol/L) × 0.81 Female: × 0.85 (140 − age) × lean body weight (kg)/Cr [mg/dL] × 72	249 male veterans Median GFR 34
MDRD equation (1999) MDRD equation without ethnicity factor*	$175 \times SCr^{-1.154} \times age^{-0.203} \times 0.742$ (if female) × 1.212 (if black) $175 \times SCr^{-1.154} \times age^{-0.203} \times 0.742$ (if female)	1628 patients enrolled in the MDRD Study (mean age, 50.6 yr) Mean GFR 39.8 mL/min/1.73 m²
CKD-EPI equation (2009)	$141 \times \min(SCr/\kappa, 1)^\alpha \times \max(SCr/\kappa, 1)^{-1.209} \times 0.993^{age} \times 1.018$ (if female) × 1.159 (if black) where: κ is 0.7 for females and 0.9 for males α is −0.329 for females and −0.411 for males min indicates the minimum of SCr/κ or 1 max indicates the maximum of SCr/κ or 1	8254 participants from 6 research studies and 4 clinical populations (mean age, 47 yr) Mean GFR 68 mL/min/1.73 m²
CKD-EPI cystatin C (2012)	$133 \times \min(SCysC/0.8, 1)^{-0.499} \times \max(SCysC/0.8, 1)^{-1.328} \times 0.996^{Age} \times 0.932$ [if female] where: min indicates the minimum of SCysC/0.8 or 1 max indicates the maximum of SCysC/0.8 or 1	5352 participants from 13 studies (mean age, 47 yr) Mean GFR 68 mL/min/1.73 m²
CKD-EPI creatinine–cystatin C (2012)	$135 \times \min(SCr/\kappa, 1)^\alpha \times \max(SCr/\kappa, 1)^{-0.601} \times \min(SCysC/0.8, 1)^{-0.375} \times \max(SCysC/0.8, 1)^{-0.711} \times 0.995^{Age} \times 0.969$ [if female] × 1.08 [if black] where: α is −0.248 for females and −0.207 for males κ is 0.7 for females and 0.9 for males min(SCr/κ,1) indicates the minimum of SCr/k or 1 and max(SCr/κ,1) indicates the maximum of SCr/k or 1 min(SCysC/0.8,1) indicates the minimum of SCysC/0.8 or 1 and max(SCysC/0.8,1) indicates the maximum of SCysC/0.8 or 1	

*African-American coefficient of the MDRD study equation.
CKD-EPI, Chronic Kidney Disease Epidemiology Collaboration; Cr, creatinine; GFR, glomerular filtration rate; IDMS, isotope-dilution mass spectrometry; IFCC, International Federation for Clinical Chemists; MDRD, Modification of Diet in Renal Disease; SCr, serum creatinine; SCysC, serum cystatin C; wt, weight.
Adapted from Kidney Disease: Improving Global Outcomes (KDIGO) CKD Work Group: KDIGO 2012 clinical practice guideline for the evaluation and management of chronic kidney disease. Kidney Int Suppl 3:1-150, 2013, Table 12 and 16.

other factors, such as age, sex, weight, and height, in part because the main filtration marker that is used is creatinine, which is known to be affected by these factors.

The main use of eGFR equations is in the detection, monitoring, and prognostication of CKD, which is largely asymptomatic. These equations have been derived from populations with stable CKD and are therefore not useful in the acute setting. Translating creatinine values especially at the upper limit of normal (which as previously discussed do not reflect significant declines in GFR) into an estimated GFR has heightened the awareness of CKD. Estimation equations also appear to be reasonably accurate for following changes in GFR over time.[5,6]

Bias, Precision, and Accuracy. The performance of estimation equations is assessed by measurements of bias, precision, and accuracy.

- *Bias* results from the systematic under- or over-estimation of the GFR in a population due to an error within the equation itself. It is calculated as the mean or median difference between the measured and estimated GFR values.
- *Precision* refers to the reliability and reproducibility of repeated measurements with one another. In the case of eGFR, it is the range of differences between estimated and measured GFR values.
- *Accuracy* combines bias and precision and is the most useful assessment of an estimation equation. It is measured as the percentage of GFR estimations within a particular percentage range from their respective GFR measurements.

The problem of bias with eGFR equations can potentially be overcome with derivation of the equation from larger sample sizes and use of filtration markers such as cystatin C, which are less subject to interference by other factors.

Accuracy, however, is difficult to achieve in a heterogeneous population. Even the latest Chronic Kidney Disease Epidemiology Collaboration (CKD-EPI) equation using creatinine, which is being adopted widely, has accuracy such that 80.6% of estimated GFR values are within 30% of measured GFR (Figure 26.2). This means that one in five values of eGFR in the general population is incorrect. Again, in day-to-day clinical practice, accuracy may not be necessary, and establishing an eGFR trend within an individual patient with CKD is probably more important.

Modification of Diet in Renal Disease and Chronic Kidney Disease Epidemiology Collaboration Equations. Although a number of GFR estimation equations have been developed, two equations are most widely used in clinical practice.

The Modification of Diet in Renal Disease (MDRD) study equation was initially derived in 1999 from a population of 1628 subjects who had participated in the MDRD study, using creatinine measured by a modified Jaffe method.[7] A new MDRD equation was expressed in 2004 for IDMS-traceable creatinine values. The MDRD equation was compared against a gold standard, urinary clearance of iothalamate. The performance of the MDRD equation was evaluated in a number of populations because it was initially derived from a primarily Caucasian American population. A number of coefficients have been derived to compensate for differences in body mass and diet in populations of different ethnicity with varying degrees of performance.

The MDRD equation has been widely adopted in the United States, Europe, and Australia, where eGFR is routinely reported with serum creatinine results. It is gradually being replaced by the CKD-EPI equation.

The limitations of the MDRD equation are mainly its tendency to underestimate the GFR and its relatively low accuracy at higher GFR values.

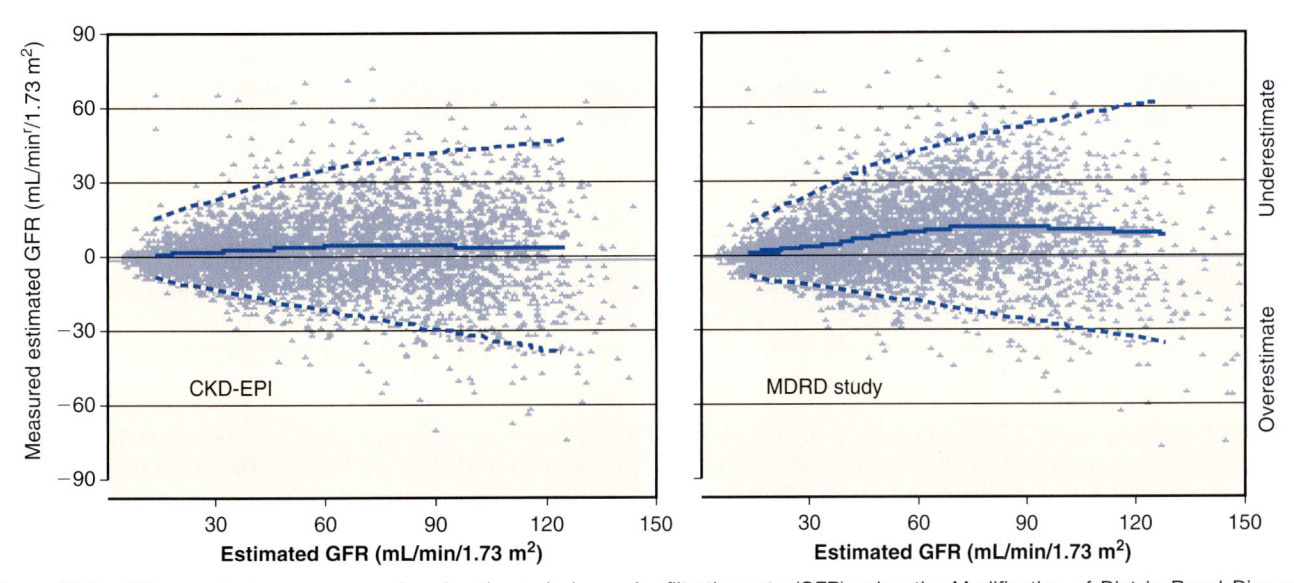

Figure 26.2 Difference between measured and estimated glomerular filtration rate (GFR) using the Modification of Diet in Renal Disease (MDRD) and Chronic Kidney Disease Epidemiology Collaboration (CKD-EPI) estimation equations. Shown are smoothed regression lines and hashed 95% confidence interval (CI) lines. Although both the MDRD and CKD-EPI equations tend to underestimate the GFR, the CKD-EPI equation does so to a lesser degree, particularly at higher GFR. Therefore, the CKD-EPI equation has less bias. (From Levey AS, Stevens LA, Schmid CH, et al: A new equation to estimate glomerular filtration rate. *Ann Intern Med* 150:604-612, 2009.)

The CKD-EPI equation was derived in 2009 in 8254 subjects (a further 3896 subjects pooled from 16 studies were used for validation), with urinary clearance of iothalamate again used as the gold standard.[8] It has less bias and greater accuracy than the MDRD equation, especially at higher GFR. A meta-analysis involving 1.1 million adults showed that the CKD-EPI equation reclassified a significant number of patients (24.4%) into a higher GFR range[9]; 34.7% of patients who were classified as having stage 3A CKD (eGFR 45-59 mL/min/1.73m^2) with the MDRD equation did not have GFRs less than 60 mL/min/1.73m^2 with the CKD-EPI equation and were therefore no longer regarded as having CKD according to the newest definition. The precision of the CKD-EPI and MDRD equations is still suboptimal, however, because eGFR and measured GFR values varied by at least 16.6 and 18.3 mL/min/1.73 m^2 (the interquartile range of differences for patients across the range of GFR), respectively.

CKD-EPI equations have also been derived for cystatin C and a combination of cystatin C and creatinine. Cystatin C measurement in the derivation of these equations was traceable to the standard reference material for cystatin C, although cystatin C measurement is not uniformly standardized, as noted previously. GFR estimation using cystatin C and creatinine has been shown to be more accurate than either marker alone, but eGFR using cystatin C is not superior to eGFR using creatinine.[10] Widespread application of these equations is limited mainly by the availability of cystatin C assay. The KDIGO guideline recommends that eGFR derived from serum creatinine should be used for most patients but that the detection of a reduced eGFR in the range 45 to 59 mL/min/1.73m^2 derived from creatinine should be confirmed with an eGFR derived from cystatin C

Risk Stratification of CKD with eGFR. Estimated GFR equations transform the creatinine or cystatin C measurement into a value that approximates the measured GFR. This value can also be used to classify the patient as having a stage of CKD. Decreasing ranges of GFR in patients with CKD have been associated with increasing risk for metabolic complications of CKD, end-stage kidney disease (ESKD), cardiovascular disease, and death. The many eGFR equations have performed variably in their ability to predict certain outcomes in different populations. This difference in ability to risk-stratify is due to the different degrees of importance placed on factors such as age and sex, which also affect prognosis, in these equations. The importance of accuracy in measuring GFR versus stratification of risk as a result of decreased GFR is a matter of ongoing debate and beyond the scope of this text. For further discussion of risk factors in CKD please see Chapter 22.

Cockcroft-Gault Equation. The Cockcroft-Gault (CG) equation estimates creatinine clearance rather than the GFR. This equation was developed in 1976 from a cohort of 249 men, and the creatinine assay method that was used to derive this equation was not standardized.[11] The CG equation also has not been re-expressed since the adoption of new assay methods. For these reasons, the CG equation systematically overestimates GFR and should not be used, although it is currently still often used to guide drug dosing. The equation is:

$$\mathrm{CrCl\,(mL/min)} = \frac{(140 - \mathrm{age}) \times \mathrm{lean\ body\ weight\ (kg)}}{\mathrm{Cr\,(mg/dL)} \times 72}$$

EXOGENOUS FILTRATION MARKERS

Inulin

Inulin remains the gold standard filtration marker but its use is impractical for routine clinical purposes. Inulin is a polymer of fructose found in tubers such as the Jerusalem artichoke and chicory. It distributes in extracellular fluid, does not bind to plasma proteins, is freely filtered at the glomerulus, and is neither reabsorbed nor secreted by the renal tubules.

Inulin is intravenously infused at a constant rate while blood and urine are sampled frequently over several hours, ideally following insertion of a bladder catheter. The patient takes an oral water load and must continue consuming water throughout the test to ensure a high urine output.

Clearance Methods for Other Exogenous Filtration Markers

Owing to the difficulty and expense of using inulin, new reference standard filtration markers have been introduced as alternatives and have been widely used since the 1990s. Urinary iothalamate and iohexol clearance has now been adopted as the reference standard for measurement of GFR. Clearance of these filtration markers can be measured in the urine or in blood or with nuclear imaging in the case of radiolabeled markers to avoid problems with urine collection.[12]

GFR is calculated from plasma clearance after a bolus intravenous injection of an exogenous filtration marker, with clearance being calculated from the amount of the marker administered divided by the area under the curve of plasma concentration over time. The decline in serum levels is due initially to the disappearance of the marker from the plasma into its volume of distribution (fast component) and then subsequently to renal excretion (slow component). It is best estimated using a two-compartment model that requires blood sampling early (usually two or three time points until 60 minutes) and late (one to three time points from 120 minutes onward). GFR can also be measured by counting a radioactive exogenous filtration marker over the kidneys and bladder areas; however, this technique is thought to be generally less accurate.

These methods are not perfect and are subject to imprecision, albeit at a much lower level than that of equations that estimate GFR. Urinary clearance of inulin may vary by up to 4.9 to 9 mL/min over 2 days, a variation that may represent normal variation in healthy individuals.

Radiolabeled Markers

Radiolabeled iothalamate, EDTA (ethylenediaminetetraacetic acid), and DTPA (diethylenetriaminepentaacetic acid) are all used as filtration markers.

Iothalamate may be labelled with iodide I 125 (^{125}I) or used unlabeled. EDTA is commonly used in Europe, whereas DTPA is widely used in the United States. EDTA is usually labeled with chromium Cr 51 (^{51}Cr), but EDTA may be reabsorbed by the tubules, leading to underestimation of GFR. DTPA is labeled with technetium Tc 9m (^{99m}Tc), and the major limitation of its use is the potential for an unpredictable dissociation of ^{99m}Tc from DTPA and binding to plasma proteins, resulting in underestimation of GFR.

Unlabeled Radiocontrast Agents

Because of concerns about exposure to radiation, storage and disposal of radionuclide marker techniques have been developed to measure low levels of iodine in urine and plasma. Iothalamate and iohexol levels have been measured using HPLC, but the main disadvantage of this approach is the complexity of the HPLC assay. X-ray fluorescence of samples may also be used to measure iodine levels but requires a higher dose of contrast agent.

Iohexol is a non-ionic, low osmolar contrast agent. It is not reabsorbed, metabolized, or secreted by the kidney and is excreted completely nonmetabolized in the urine. It has low toxicity and is usually used in doses 10 to 50 times higher in radiologic procedures than those used for GFR determination.

Urinary clearances of iothalamate and iohexol closely correlate with urinary inulin clearance, and there is a high correlation among the methods.

SPECIFIC CIRCUMSTANCES OR POPULATIONS

CHILDREN

Adult GFR equations such as the MDRD have been shown to be inappropriate in children 9 and under (see also Chapter 74). Multiple equations (Table 26.2) have been derived for estimation of GFR in children, but the most popular is the Schwarz equation, which was devised in 1976 to measure GFR in children[13]:

$$eGFR = \frac{k \times L}{SCr}$$

where k depends on the age of the child, L is length or height, and SCr is serum creatinine. Like the CG equation, the Schwarz equation has now been shown to systematically overestimate GFR. The reasons are the assay technique and measurement factors specific to children. As previously mentioned, the Jaffe method can be interfered with by plasma proteins, and the correction factor that is deducted to account for this interference is estimated by taking an average bias from measured results. In children, who have lower levels of plasma proteins, this correction factor may be too high, resulting in an erroneously low creatinine value. Because of the low muscle mass of children, the influence of a measurement error is also proportionately larger than an error of the same magnitude in an adult sample.

The simple bedside Schwartz equation—eGFR = 0.413 × (height [cm]/serum creatinine [mg/dL])—was developed using standardized creatinine methods in 2009.[14] This equation provides good approximation of the more complicated Schwartz eGFR formula, using creatinine, urea, and cystatin C as well as height. Cystatin C has been suggested to be more accurate than creatinine as an indirect marker of renal function in children.[15]

A limitation is that the equation was derived from a cohort of 600 children with CKD who had abnormal growth. Therefore, this GFR estimation equation may not be accurate for children who have less impairment of renal function and normal skeletal growth (see Table 26.2).

Table 26.2 Equations Using Serum Biomarkers for Estimating GFR in Children and Adolescents

Equation Name	Equation	Derivation Population		
		No. Children	Age (yr)	GFR Range or Median (mL/min)
Creatinine Based				
Schwartz, 1976	0.55 × Ht/Scr	77	1-21	3-220
Counahan, 1976	0.43 × Ht/Scr	103	0.2-14	4-200
Leger, 2002	(0.641 × Wt)/Scr + (0.00131 × Ht^2)/Scr	97	1-21	97
Schwartz, 2009	0.413 × Ht/Scr 40.7 × (HT/Scr)$^{0.640}$ × (30/BUN)$^{0.202}$	349	1-17	41
Cystatin C Based				
Filler, 2003	91.62 × (cysC)$^{-1.123}$	85	1-18	103
Grubb, 2005	84.69 × (cysC)$^{-1.680}$ × 1.384 if < 14 yrs	85	3-17	108
Zappitelli, 2006	75.94 × (cysC)$^{-1.17}$ × 1.2 if Tx	103	1-18	74
Creatinine and Cystatin C Based				
Bouvet, 2006	63.2 × (Scr/1.086)$^{-0.35}$ × (cysC/1.2)$^{-0.56}$ × (Wt/45)$^{0.30}$ × (years/14)$^{0.40}$	100	1-23	92
Zappitelli, 2006	43.82 × e$^{0.003}$ × Ht × (cysC)$^{-0.635}$ × (Scr)$^{-0.547}$	103	1-18	74
Schwartz, 2009	39.1 × (HT/Scr)$^{0.516}$ × (1.8/cysC)$^{0.294}$ × (30/BUN)$^{0.169}$ × (1.099) if male × (HT/1.4)$^{0.188}$	349	1-17	41

BUN, blood urea nitrogen; cysC, cystatin C; GFR, glomerular filtration rate; Ht/HT, height; Scr, serum creatinine; Tx, transplant: Wt, weight.
Adapted from Schwartz GJ, Work DF: Measurement and estimation of GFR in children and adolescents. Clin J Am Soc Nephrol 4:1832-1843, 2009, Table 3.

PREGNANCY

It is well known that there is a physiologic increase in GFR and a drop in serum creatinine in pregnancy. Serum creatinine decreases because of a real increase in GFR but also because of physiologic hemodilution.

Estimation equations are inappropriate for measuring GFR in pregnant women because they were not derived from this population. Most pregnant women have GFRs higher than 60 mL/min, which is above the range at which the MDRD or CKD-EPI equations are known to be accurate in any case. Twenty-four–hour urine collection for creatinine clearance therefore remains the best method in pregnancy.[16]

ACUTE KIDNEY INJURY

Measurement of GFR in patients with acute kidney injury (AKI) is difficult as it is constantly changing, and measurements and estimates that depend on a steady state are not readily applicable. Serum creatinine is the most commonly used marker of GFR in this setting, but creatinine is slow to rise in response to a decrease in GFR and is subject to the influence of dilution by fluid given as part of treatment for AKI.[17,18] As previously mentioned, creatinine is also insensitive to substantial decreases in GFR. Estimation equations for GFR in patients with AKI are inaccurate because these equations have been derived from stable patients, in whom the creatinine is at a steady state, and are not applicable to the diverse AKI patient population. A kinetic estimation GFR equation has been developed but has not yet been validated.[19]

Accurate measurement of GFR in this population can be achieved by calculation of the elimination kinetics after a single bolus injection of a filtration marker. Alternatively, brief-duration measurements of GFR, such as short-duration urinary creatinine clearance, can be performed, assuming that a patient's creatinine does not increase rapidly over the period of 2 to 8 hours.[20] These tests are not widely performed and are probably impractical in many centers. This situation has led to extensive research into a biomarker that is more sensitive in demonstrating early stages of AKI so as to lead to more timely intervention.

DRUG DOSING

The CG equation, despite its limitations, is still used regularly in many jurisdictions, for drug dose adjustment in patients with renal impairment. Historically this equation has been used to enroll subjects in renal impairment categories for pharmacokinetic studies. The U.S. Food and Drug Administration (FDA) has now suggested using the MDRD equation or the CG equation for this purpose in new drug development.

A large simulation study comparing drug dosages administered to patients through the use of the MDRD and CG equations showed that the concordance figures of the two equations' kidney function estimates with measured GFR were similar.[21] Because the majority of FDA-approved drug dosing labels use the CG equation, which expresses creatinine clearance in mL/min, the eGFR value must be converted to units of mL/min by multiplying by the individual's body surface area and dividing by 1.73 m^2.

The stimulation study concluded that either equation can be used for drug dosing but that caution should be exercised in patients in whom the creatinine value may be inaccurate. This caution is particularly relevant in sick or hospitalized patients, in whom low body weight or changes in body weight are present, in the elderly, and in amputees. The CG equation tends to give a lower estimate of renal function,[22] leading to a dose reduction.[23] The lower estimate results from the greater effect of age and weight on the CG equation. In the elderly, the MDRD and CKD-EPI equations have been shown to overestimate the GFR in some studies but to be reliable in others.[24,25] The use of the CG equation leads to drug dosing errors that are due to "under-dosing," thus minimizing exposure to toxicity. The elderly are more likely to experience side effects and to be subject to the dangers of polypharmacy, so using the CG equation in these patients may be more appropriate.[22]

Ultimately the importance of drug dosage adjustment depends on the purpose of the medication as well as the therapeutic range and toxicity of the drug. In cases in which a medication has a narrow therapeutic window, such as chemotherapy, all estimation equations may have an unacceptable degree of error, and accurate measurement of GFR using an exogenous filtration marker should be performed.

The CG equation should not be completely abandoned in favor of the MDRD equation, especially because recommendations for drug dosages of existing medications were based on the CG equation. The CKD-EPI equation has not yet been considered in this context.

URINALYSIS

Urinalysis may be used in the assessment of acute or chronic kidney disease, the workup for kidney stones, or the evaluation of systemic conditions with potential renal involvement, such as systemic lupus erythematosus. There are three ways to obtain a urine specimen: spontaneous voiding, ureteral catheterization, and percutaneous bladder puncture. Technique is important in collecting a sample to avoid contamination. For spontaneously voided urine, a midstream sample should be collected after cleaning of the external genitalia. If a patient has an indwelling catheter, a fresh specimen should be submitted for analysis; samples that have been stagnant in the catheter tubing or bag may have undergone degradation. Suprapubic needle aspiration of the bladder is used when urine cannot easily be obtained by other means, most commonly in infants. Whatever the collection method, it is recommended that a sample be analyzed within 2 to 4 hours of the time of collection to prevent cell lysis and precipitation of solutes.[26] There are numerous techniques for examining urine; this section focuses on methods commonly used for assessment of chemical content and microscopy.

COLOR (Table 26.3)

The color of urine is determined by chemical content, concentration, and pH. Urine may be almost colorless if the output is high and the concentration is low. Abnormal color changes can be due to drugs, foods, and pathologic conditions. Cloudy urine is most commonly due to leukocytes and bacteria. The most common cause of red urine is

Table 26.3 Main Causes of Abnormal Color Changes in Urine

	Cause	Color
Pathologic conditions	Gross hematuria, hemoglobinuria, myoglobinuria	Pink, red, brown, black
	Jaundice	Yellow to brown
	Chyluria	White milky urine
	Massive uric acid crystalluria	Pink
	Porphyrinuria, alkaptonuria	Red to black; increases after urine left to stand
Medications	Rifampin	Yellow-orange to red
	Propofol	White
	Phenytoin, phenazopyridine	Red
	Chloroquine, nitrofurantoin	Brown
	Triamterene, blue dyes of enteral feeds	Green
	Metronidazole, methyldopa, imipenem-cilastatin	Darkening after urine left to stand
Foods	Beetroot	Red
	Senna rhubarb	Yellow to brown red

From Fogazzi GB, Verdesca S, Garigali G: Urinalysis: core curriculum 2008. Am J Kidney Dis 51:1052-1067, 2008; and Davsion, A: Urinalysis, ed 3, Oxford, 2005, Oxford University Press.

---

hemoglobin. Red urine in the absence of red blood cells in the sediment usually indicates either free hemoglobin or myoglobin. In the latter case, the patient's serum is not pink. Red urine with red sediment indicates hemoglobin. In contrast, red urine with clear sediment is most often the result of myoglobin but may also be seen in some porphyrias, or with the use of some medications or the ingestion of beets in some individuals.[27]

ODOR

Infection, the most common cause of abnormal urine odor, is caused by the production of ammonia by bacteria. Ketones may cause a fruity or sweet odor. Some rare pathologic conditions may confer a specific odor to the urine. Examples are maple syrup urine disease (maple syrup odor), phenylketonuria (mousy odor), isovaleric acidemia (sweaty feet odor), and hypermethioninemia (fishy odor).[26]

RELATIVE DENSITY

The concentration, or relative density, of urine can be assessed by either specific gravity or osmolality. *Specific gravity* is defined as the weight of a solution relative to that of an equal volume of water. It is determined by the number and size of particles in the urine. Specific gravity is traditionally measured by a urinometer, which is a weighted float marked with a scale from 1.000 to 1.060. This method is simple but outdated owing to the need for a larger volume of urine than with other methods and the potential for inaccuracy in reading the device. Today, specific gravity is commonly measured by refractometry or dry chemistry methods. Refractometry measures specific gravity using the refractive index of a solution, which is a function of the weight of solute per unit volume. It requires only a drop of urine.

Dry chemistry techniques are used in reagent strips. An indirect method is used to determine specific gravity, relying on the fact that there is generally a linear relationship between urine's ionic strength and its specific gravity. The reagent strip contains a polyionic polymer that has binding sites that are saturated with hydrogen ions, and an indicator substance. The release of hydrogen ions when they are competitively replaced with urinary cations causes a change in the pH-sensitive indicator dye. Specific gravity values measured by dipstick tend to be falsely high if the urine pH is less than 6 and falsely low if the pH is higher than 7. The effects of non-ionized molecules such as glucose and urea on osmolality are not reflected by changes in the dipstick specific gravity. Dry chemistry measurements of specific gravity therefore tend to correlate poorly with refractometry and osmolality.[26]

Osmolality, the gold standard for relative density, is defined as the number of osmoles of solute per kilogram of solvent. It is measured directly with an osmometer. It depends on the number of particles in solution and is not influenced by their size or temperature. High-glucose solutions significantly increase osmolality (10 g/L glucose = 55.5 mOsmol/L).[26] Urine specific gravity is generally proportional to the osmolality and rises by approximately 0.001 for every 35- to 40-mOsmol/kg increase in urine osmolality.[28] A urine osmolality of 280 mOsmol/kg (which is isosmotic to normal plasma) is usually associated with a urine specific gravity of 1.008 or 1.009. Specific gravity is affected by protein, mannitol, dextrans, and radiographic contrast media. In these settings, specific gravity can be increased disproportionately to the osmolality, falsely suggesting highly concentrated urine. There are no causes of a falsely low urine specific gravity value, and thus, a specific gravity of 1.003 or less measured by refractometry always indicates a maximally dilute urine (≤100 mOsmol/kg).

URINE pH

Urine pH is usually measured with a reagent test strip. Most commonly, the double indicators methyl red and bromthymol blue are used in the reagent strips to give a broad range of colors at different pH values. The normal range for urine pH is 4.5 to 7.8. Significant deviations from true pH occur with values less than 5.5 or greater than 7.5 with reagent strip methods.[21,25] Urine pH can be useful in diagnosing systemic acid-base disorders when used in conjunction with other investigations, although in isolation it provides little useful diagnostic information. A very alkaline urine (pH > 7.0) is suggestive of infection with a urea-splitting organism, such as *Proteus mirabilis*. Prolonged storage can lead to overgrowth of urea-splitting bacteria and the laboratory measurement of a high urine pH. Diuretic therapy, vomiting, gastric suction, and alkali therapy can also cause a high urine pH. Acidic urine (pH < 5.0) is seen most commonly in metabolic acidosis. A urine pH greater than 5 in the setting of metabolic acidosis may indicate one of the forms of renal tubular acidosis, though there are forms of renal acidosis in which the urine pH is low despite a defect in the total kidney ability to excrete acid and generate bicarbonate (see also Chapters 17 and 27).[27]

BILIRUBIN AND UROBILINOGEN

Only conjugated bilirubin is passed into the urine. Thus, the result of a reagent test for bilirubin is typically positive in patients with obstructive or hepatocellular jaundice, whereas it is usually negative in patients with jaundice due to hemolysis. In patients with hemolysis, the urine urobilinogen result is often positive. Reagent test strips are very sensitive to bilirubin, detecting as little as 0.05 mg/dL. However, the measurement of bilirubin in the urine is not very sensitive for detecting liver disease. Prolonged storage and exposure to light can lead to false-negative results.[27] False-positive test results for urine bilirubin can occur if the urine is contaminated with stool.

LEUKOCYTE ESTERASE AND NITRITES

The esterase method relies on the fact that esterases are released from lysed urine granulocytes. These esterases liberate 3-hydroxy-5-phenylpyrrole after substrate hydrolysis. The pyrrole reacts with a diazonium salt, yielding a pink to purple color. The result is usually interpreted as negative, trace, small, moderate, or large. Factors that may increase leukocyte lysis include allowing urine to stand for long periods, low pH, and low relative density. In these settings, there may be a positive dipstick result for leukocyte esterase with no leukocytes seen on microscopy. High levels of glucose, albumin, ascorbic acid, tetracycline, cephalexin, or cephalothin or large amounts of oxalic acid may inhibit the reaction and cause false-negative results.[29]

Urinary nitrites indicate the presence of nitrate-reducing bacteria. In the reagent strip test, nitrite reacts with a p-arsanilic acid to form a diazonium compound; further reaction with 1,2,3,4-tetrahydrobenzo(h)quinolin-3-ol results in a pink color end point. Results are usually interpreted as positive or negative. High specific gravity and ascorbic acid may interfere with the test. False-negative results are common and may be due to prolonged sample storage or low dietary intake. It may take up to 4 hours to convert nitrate to nitrite, so inadequate bladder retention time can also give false-negative results.[29]

GLUCOSE

Glycosuria due to hyperglycemia may occur at blood glucose levels greater than 10 mmol/L (180 mg/dL) in subjects with normal renal function. Less commonly, glycosuria indicates failure of proximal renal tubular reabsorption in tubular disorders such as Fanconi's syndrome. Most reagent strips use an oxidase-peroxidase method to measure glucose. Glucose is first oxidized to form glucuronic acid and hydrogen peroxide. Hydrogen peroxide then reacts via a peroxidase with a reduced chromogen to form a colored product.[26] This test is sensitive to glucose concentrations between 0.5 and 20 g/L.[26] Large quantities of ketones, ascorbate, and phenazopyridine hydrochloride (Pyridium) metabolites may interfere with the color reaction, causing false-negative results. Oxidizing agents and hydrochloric acid may cause false-positive results.[29] Enzymatic methods such as a hexokinase give more precise quantification of urinary glucose levels.[26]

KETONES

Ketones (acetoacetate and acetone) are generally detected with the nitroprusside reaction.[29] Ascorbic acid and phenazopyridine can give false-positive reactions. β-Hydroxybutyrate (often 80% of total serum ketones in ketosis) is not normally detected by the nitroprusside reaction. Ketones may appear in the urine, but not in serum, with prolonged fasting or starvation. Ketones may also be measured in the urine in alcoholic or diabetic ketoacidosis.

HEMOGLOBIN AND MYOGLOBIN

Reagent strips use the peroxidase-like activity of the heme moiety of hemoglobin to catalyze the reaction between a peroxide and a chromogen, giving a colored product. This test is very sensitive for the presence of heme in the urine. False-negative results are uncommon but may be caused by ascorbic acid, a strong reducing agent. False-positive results may occur because of oxidizing contaminants, povidone-iodine, semen, or a high concentration of bacteria with pseudoperoxidase activity (such as Enterobacteriaceae, staphylococci, and *Streptococcus* spp).[26] Normally, haptoglobin binds circulating heme-containing substances, such as hemoglobin and myoglobin. When these substances are produced in large quantities, as occurs in hemolysis or rhabdomyolysis, the capacity for binding is overwhelmed and they appear in the urine. A positive dipstick test result for hemoglobin in the absence of red blood cells in the urine sediment therefore suggests either hemolysis or rhabdomyolysis.

PROTEINURIA (see also Chapter 53)

Proteinuria is an important sign of kidney disease, imparting powerful diagnostic and prognostic information. It is a cornerstone of the workup for CKD, AKI, hematuria, and preeclampsia. It is often the earliest marker of glomerular diseases, occurring before a reduction in GFR. Proteinuria is associated with hypertension, obesity, and vascular disease. It can be used to predict risks of CKD progression, cardiovascular disease, and all-cause mortality in general population[30] cohorts and patients with diabetes[31] and CKD.[32] Proteinuria-lowering therapies may be renoprotective,[33] and monitoring proteinuria is a key aspect of assessing treatment response in a variety of kidney diseases, including diabetes[34] and nondiabetic glomerulopathies.[35] Additionally, filtered protein probably contributes to the pathogenesis of renal injury and disease progression rather than just being a marker of it.[36] Although measurement of urinary protein has long been recommended in clinical practice guidelines, recommendations regarding this practice vary substantially.[37] This section reviews the normal physiology of proteinuria as well as strengths, limitations, and applications of the different measurement techniques.

NORMAL PHYSIOLOGY

In humans, on the basis of a GFR of 100 mL/min, 180 L of primary urine is produced per day from plasma that contains about 10 kg of protein. However, only about 0.01% or 1 gram of protein passes through the glomerular filtration barrier into the filtrate.[38] The glomerular filtration barrier acts as a size-, shape-, and charge-dependent permselective molecular sieve the unique properties of which are still incompletely understood. It restricts the passage of macromolecules, such as albumin and globulin, and enables the excretion of an almost protein-free ultrafiltrate containing water and small solvents.[39]

The glomerular filtration barrier acts to minimize diffusion of large molecules (with a Stokes-Einstein radius greater than 1.5 nm)[40] that would otherwise occur down a concentration gradient from the plasma to the filtrate (see also Chapter 3). It is composed of three major layers—endothelial cells, the glomerular basement membrane, and podocytes, which cover the basement membrane on the side of the urinary space. Podocytes are highly specialized epithelial cells with long, interdigitated foot processes that wrap around the glomerular capillaries, forming 40 nm–wide gaps, known as filtration slits, between adjacent processes (see also Chapter 4).[41] The slit diaphragm is a cell-to-cell contact that inserts laterally into the podocyte cell membrane, bridging the filtration slit. The podocyte plays a central role in integrating the components of the glomerular filtration barrier by interacting with the glomerular basement membrane and signaling at the slit diaphragm.[42] To date, at least 26 podocyte-specific gene defects, such as those encoding for the podocyte proteins nephrin and podocin, have been identified in hereditary causes of nephrotic syndrome.[43-45] In response to signals from the podocytes and mesangium, the endothelial cells acquire a highly fenestrated phenotype, with small pores covering about 20% of their surfaces.[41] This phenotype facilitates high-flux transport of fluid and small solutes. Normally, large quantities of high-molecular-weight (HMW) plasma proteins traverse the glomerular capillaries, mesangium, or both without entering the urinary space. Damage to any one of the three layers of the glomerular filtration barrier allows proteins through, resulting in abnormal, "glomerular" proteinuria.

Albumin, the dominant HMW protein in plasma, is a negatively charged, approximately 67-kDa protein.[39] Size selectivity restricts the passage of albumin through the glomerular filtration barrier. Charge selectivity, in which the negatively charged proteoglycans and heparan sulfates in the glomerular basement membrane repel albumin molecules, is a theory seeking to explain the low glomerular sieving coefficient of albumin in relation to other molecules of its size.[46] However, experimental data have called the role of basement membrane charge in permselectivity into question.[47-49] Some albumin filtration across the capillary wall does occur, after which it is resorbed by the proximal tubule cells.[50,51]

Low-molecular-weight proteins (<20,000 Da) pass readily across the capillary wall. Because the plasma concentration of these proteins is much lower than that of albumin and globulins, however, the filtered load is small. Moreover, LMW proteins are normally reabsorbed by the proximal tubule. Thus, proteins such as α_2-microglobulin, apoproteins, enzymes, and peptide hormones are normally excreted in only very small amounts in the urine.[27]

A small amount of protein that normally appears in the urine is the result of normal tubular secretion. Tamm-Horsfall protein is an HMW glycoprotein (23×10^6 Da) that is formed on the epithelial surfaces of the thick ascending limb of the loop of Henle and early distal convoluted tubule. Immunoglobulin A (IgA) and urokinase are also secreted by the renal tubule and appear in the urine in small amounts.[27]

TYPES OF PROTEINURIA

The types of proteinuria are as follows:

Glomerular: Increased filtration of macromolecules across the glomerular filtration barrier may occur from a loss of charge and size selectivity. Unlike the other types listed here, glomerular proteinuria often results in urinary protein loss of more than 1 g per day.

Tubular: Tubular damage or dysfunction may inhibit the normal resorptive capacity of the proximal tubule, resulting in higher amounts of mostly LMW proteins in the urine. A degree of tubular proteinuria often occurs with glomerular proteinuria. Classic causes of tubular proteinuria in isolation are Fanconi's syndrome and Dent's disease.

Overflow: Normal or abnormal plasma proteins produced in increased amounts may be filtered at the glomerulus and may overwhelm the resorptive capacity of the proximal tubule. This occurs particularly with small or positively charged proteins and is of clinical importance principally in plasma cell dyscrasias (e.g., myeloma). It may also occur with myoglobin in rhabdomyolysis and with hemoglobin in severe intravascular hemolysis.

Postrenal: Small amounts of protein, usually non-albumin IgG or IgA, may be excreted in the urinary tract in the setting of infection or stones. Leukocytes are also commonly present in the urine sediment.

NORMAL LEVELS OF PROTEINURIA

As previously described, two main groups of proteins are present in the urine: plasma proteins, predominately albumin, that crosses the filtration barrier, and nonplasma proteins, predominantly Tamm-Horsfall protein, that originates in renal tubules or the urinary tract. In normal physiologic conditions, about half of the excreted protein is Tamm-Horsfall protein, and less than 30 mg of albumin is excreted per day.[37] At normal levels of protein loss, albumin accounts for approximately 20% of total protein. As protein loss increases, albumin becomes the most significant single protein present.[52]

CATEGORIZATION OF PROTEINURIA

The persistent excretion of abnormal levels of urinary albumin, equivalent to between 30 and 300 mg/day, is below the level that can be detected by a standard urine protein dipstick and has historically been termed *microalbuminuria*. Albumin excretion of more than 300 mg/day, or *macroalbuminuria*, is overt proteinuria and can be detected by a

Table 26.4 Kidney Disease: Improving Global Outcomes (KDIGO) Guideline: Categories of Proteinuria*

	Normal to Mildly Increased (KDIGO A1)	Moderately Increased (KDIGO A2)	Severely Increased (KDIGO A3)
AER (mg/24 hours)	<30	30-300	>300
PER (mg/24 hours)	<150	150-500	>500
ACR:			
mg/mmol	<3	3-30	>30
mg/g	<30	30-300	>300
PCR:			
Mg/mmol	<15	15-50	>50
Mg/g	<150	150-500	>500
Protein reagent strip	Negative to trace	Trace to +	+ or greater

*Relationships between AER and ACR and between PER and PCR are based on the assumption that average creatinine excretion rate is 1.0g/d or 10 mmol/day (conversions are rounded for pragmatic reasons).
ACR, albumin-to-creatinine ratio; AER, albumin excretion rate; PCR, protein-to-creatinine ratio; PER, protein excretion rate.
From Kidney Disease: Improving Global Outcomes (KDIGO) CKD Work Group: KDIGO 2012 clinical practice guideline for the evaluation and management of chronic kidney disease. Kidney Int Suppl 3:1-150, 2013.

Table 26.5 Patient Factors That May Increase Urinary Protein or Albumin

Posture (postural proteinuria)
Urinary tract infection
Hematuria
High dietary protein intake
High-intensity exercise
Congestive cardiac failure
Menstruation or vaginal discharge
Drugs (e.g., nonsteroidal antiinflammatory drugs)

Adapted from Johnson DW, Jones GR, Mathew TH, et al: Chronic kidney disease and measurement of albuminuria or proteinuria: a position statement. Med J Aust 197:224-225, 2012; and Miller WG, Bruns DE, Hortin GL, et al: [Current issues in measurement and reporting of urinary albumin excretion]. Ann Biol Clin (Paris) 68:9-25, 2010.

Table 26.6 Factors Influencing Accuracy of Proteinuria Measurement

Preanalysis Phase	Analysis Phase

Collection type
  timed or random
  timing of random measurement
	Total protein or albumin measurement

Degradation of protein or albumin
  during storage
  adsorption to plastic
Storage temperature
	Assay type

Adapted from Miller WG, Bruns DE, Hortin GL, et al: [Current issues in measurement and reporting of urinary albumin excretion]. Ann Biol Clin (Paris) 68:9-25, 2010; and Martin H: Laboratory measurement of urine albumin and urine total protein in screening for proteinuria in chronic kidney disease. Clin Biochem Rev 32:97-102, 2011.

standard urine dipstick. *Nephrotic-range proteinuria* is protein excretion of more than 3.5 g/24 hours and is usually indicative of glomerular pathology. The 2012 KDIGO guidelines discourage the use of the term 'microalbuminuria,' instead suggesting that the term *albuminuria* be used and the level subsequently quantified (Table 26.4).[35] This recommendation has been sanctioned by the Association of Laboratory Physicians and Clinical Chemists in different jurisdictions. The presence of proteinuria or albuminuria strongly predicts outcomes of CKD progression as well as of cardiovascular and all-cause mortality in the population with CKD. The risk rises continuously as albuminuria increases.[53] The 2012 KDIGO guidelines suggest the addition of an albuminuria category for risk stratification of patients with CKD.

SOURCES OF ERROR IN MEASUREMENT
(Tables 26.5 and 26.6)

Twenty-four–hour urine collection for protein measurement is considered the gold standard for measuring protein or albumin. Methods such as reagent strips, random measurement of protein or albumin concentrations, and albumin- or protein-to-creatinine ratios (ACRs or PCRs) aim to estimate a 24-hour protein measure. A positive result from a semiquantitative test, such as a urinary dipstick test, should prompt further evaluation with a quantitative test. Both preanalytical factors and factors intrinsic to the analysis itself can be sources of error in protein measurement. In the assessment of the quality of a test, both accuracy and precision need to be taken into account. Although a test may give reproducible results, it may not accurately measure all clinically significant types of proteinuria. The heterogeneous types of protein and the different molecular forms of proteins (such as albumin) that may be present in urine make for a challenge to both accuracy and precision of measurement. Using a consistent form of measurement with a consistent assay to monitor proteinuria, and using multiple measurements to confirm findings, is therefore advisable.

ADVANTAGES OF URINARY ALBUMIN OVER TOTAL PROTEIN MEASUREMENTS

Either albumin or total protein can be measured in urine. Many current guidelines recommend the measurement of urine albumin on the basis of a need to detect lower levels of protein than were previously thought to be clinically significant. Multiple studies have shown that the presence of small amounts of albumin in the urine—between 30 and 300 mg per day—have prognostic significance; increasing amounts of albuminuria are associated with continuous increases in risk of all-cause and cardiovascular mortality, AKI, and ESKD in the general population,[54] with decline in eGFR,[55,56] and with adverse outcomes in CKD.[57] Measures of total protein are imprecise at low levels of protein and are insensitive at detecting clinically important changes in albuminuria.[37] Relatively large increases in urinary albumin excretion can occur without causing a measurable increase in urinary total protein.[58] Urine albumin measurements are more specific and more sensitive for changes in glomerular permeability than are measures of urinary total protein.[35,37,58-60] Additionally, because a single protein is being measured, standardization of albumin measurement is simpler than standardization of total protein measurements.[61]

ISSUES WITH MEASURING ALBUMIN RATHER THAN TOTAL PROTEIN

EVIDENCE FOR CKD PROGRESSION RISK AND INTERVENTIONS

Much evidence on the natural history and progression of CKD has centered on measurement of 24-hour total protein.[61] In general, studies on diabetic patients have used measurements of urinary albumin, but studies of interventions and outcomes for glomerular diseases, for preeclampsia, and in children have used proteinuria measurements. One difficulty with the implementation of albumin as a replacement for total protein is the lack of a constant numerical relationship between the two that would enable clinicians to translate the existing evidence base from one to the other.[37]

MISSED TUBULAR PROTEINURIA

Relying on measurement of urinary albumin risks missing "tubular" and "overflow" proteinuria, in which non-albumin proteins predominate. However, total protein assays are generally more sensitive to albumin than to LMW proteins, and many have poor sensitivity for detecting tubular proteinuria.[62] Although "tubular" disorders are characterized by a relative increase in the proportion of LMW protein to albumin, albumin generally still constitutes a significant portion of total protein, probably because of failure of tubular resorption of protein.[63] In the AusDiab study, random urine samples from more than 10,000 people in the Australian adult population were tested, using cutoff values of 3.45 mg/mmol for ACR and 22.6 mg/mmol for PCR. Of patients who screened positive for albuminuria, 68% had negative results for proteinuria. Albuminuria performed well as a screening test for proteinuria: Sensitivity was 91.7%, specificity 95.3%, and negative predictive value 99.8%. However, among those with proteinuria, 8% excreted albumin within the normal range. The investigators postulated that these individuals may have had light-chain proteinuria or interstitial nephropathies.[52] In a study of 23 patients with Dent's disease, a rare but classic tubular disorder, only 2 patients had no significant urinary albumin loss in addition to losses of LMW proteins. In these 2 patients, the levels of LMW proteinuria were low enough that they would probably also have been missed by a total protein measurement approach.[64]

Overall, the significance of this issue in both the CKD and general populations is difficult to estimate with the current available data. If tubular proteinuria is suspected, it is best assessed with immunoassays directed at a specific tubular proteins, such as α_1-microglobulin or monoclonal heavy or light chains.[35,37] One study that attempted to identify the proteins composing tubular proteinuria in elderly people with mild proteinuria was unable to consistently identify proteins using electrophoresis, and the researchers suggested that the elevated urinary protein measurements were due to artifact.[65]

DIAGNOSTIC UTILITY OF PROTEIN TYPE

Simultaneous measurement of different types of urinary protein may be a useful tool in differentiating between glomerular and tubulointerstitial diseases. Several studies using gel electrophoretic techniques to separate proteins on the basis of molecular size have shown that larger proteins such as albumin predominate in glomerular disease and that the ratio of LMW proteins is increased in tubulointerstitial disorders.[66] Higher albumin-to-total protein ratios, obtained from simultaneous measurement of ACR and PCR, have been shown to be significantly associated with glomerular rather than nonglomerular pathology on renal biopsy in patients with kidney disease.[67]

METHODS TO MEASURE URINARY TOTAL PROTEIN (Table 26.7)

Total protein in urine has been measured by chemical, turbidimetric, and dye-binding (colorimetric) methods. These methods are prone to interference by inorganic ions and nonprotein substances in the urine.[37] Falsely high results may occur as result of interference by aminoglycoside antibiotics[68] plasma expanders,[69] and other substances. There is large sample-to-sample variation in the type and composition of proteins present, making accurate measurement difficult. Turbidimetric methods, which are commonly used, are imprecise, with a coefficient of variation as high as 20%.[70] Currently there is no reference measurement procedure or standardized reference material for urinary protein. Each of the different methods in use has differing sensitivity and specificity for the diverse range of proteins found in urine, potentially leading to divergent results. The range of methods and calibrants in use means that between-laboratory variation is unavoidable. Most laboratories currently use turbidimetric or colorimetric measures, which tend to react more strongly with albumin than with globulin and other nonalbumin proteins.[71]

METHODS TO MEASURE URINARY ALBUMIN

Urinary albumin can be measured in a number of ways. Antibody binding methods are most commonly used, and

Table 26.7 Methods of Proteinuria Measurement

Method	Description	Detection Limit (mg/L)	Protein Types	Causes of Falsely Increased Results	Causes of Falsely Decreased Results
Chemical: Biuret	Copper reagent, measures peptide bonds	50	—	—	Tubular/LMW proteins
Kjeldahl	Precipitated nitrogen				
Turbidimetric (sulfosalicylic acid, trichloracetic acid)	Addition of precipitant denatures protein; suspension's turbidity is read in a densitometer	50-100	Many, including γ-globulin light chains and albumin. More sensitive to albumin than to globulins and nonalbumin proteins	Tolmetin sodium (Tolectin), tolbutamide, antibiotics (penicillin, nafcillin, oxacillin), radiocontrast agents	Tubular/LMW proteins
Dye-binding (e.g., Coomassie Brilliant Blue, pyrogallol red)	Indicator changes color in presence of protein	50-100	More sensitive to albumin than to globulins and nonalbumin proteins (pyrogallol red improves this shortcoming)	Pyrogallol red: aminoglycoside, gelatin solutions such as plasma expanders	Tubular/LMW proteins

LMW, low-molecular-weight.
Adapted from Cameron JS: The patient with proteinuria and or hematuria. In Davison A, editor: Oxford textbook of clinical nephrology, ed 3, Oxford, 2005, Oxford University Press, pp 389-411.

immunoturbidimetry is the most commonly used of the antibody binding methods in diagnostic laboratories.[37,71] Because a single protein is being measured, performance of albumin assays tend to be superior to total protein assays, at least at low concentrations of protein.[71] However, the urine of healthy individuals contains a range of albumin molecules. Albumin may be immunoreactive, nonimmunoreactive, fragmented, or biochemically modified.[72] The proportions of these different types of albumin molecules in normal urine are variable and subject to debate.

Albumin fragments may be generated during proteolysis of albumin in renal tubules or plasma and may account for a significant proportion of total urinary albumin. A study in subjects with type 1 diabetes found that 99% of albumin was excreted as fragments less than 10 kDa. Another study showed that albumin fragments constituted up to 30% of total urinary protein in patients with nephrotic syndrome.[73] Intact albumin has at least five antigenic sites.[74] Routine clinical methods use both polyclonal and monoclonal antibodies, which have different sensitivities for the detection of altered forms of albumin.[61] Nonimmunoreactive forms of albumin also exist; these are either fragments that do not contain the binding sites for the antibody in use in a particular assay or intact albumin in which the epitopes have undergone conformational change.[75]

HPLC detects both immunoreactive and nonimmunoreactive albumin. Higher values for urinary albumin are generally seen in HPLC than in immunologic detection methods. This observation led to a hypothesis that there are clinically significant amounts of nonimmunoreactive albumin in urine. In a study exploring this issue, differences in urinary albumin were detected by four immunoassays and HPLC. However, the higher values seen in HPLC techniques may represent the detection of non-albumin macromolecules.[76] Conformational change in albumin molecules may be induced by changes in urinary pH, urea, glucose, and ascorbate concentrations. Bilirubin usually occupies a small proportion of albumin molecules, but in severe hyperbilirubinemia it may bind to more than 50% of albumin.[61]

DIFFERENT LABORATORY METHODS TO MEASURE ALBUMIN IN THE URINE

The laboratory methods for measuring urinary albumin are as follows:

Immunoturbidimetric technique: Albumin in a sample of urine reacts with a specific antibody. The turbidity is measured with a spectrophotometer, and the absorbency is proportional to the albumin concentration.[77]

Double-antibody radioimmunoassay: Albumin in a urine sample competes with a known amount of radiolabeled albumin for fixed binding sites of anti-albumin antibodies. Free albumin can be separated from bound albumin by immunoabsorption of the (albumin-bound) antibody. Albumin concentration in the resulting sample of albumin-bound antibody is inversely proportional to its radioactivity, which is measured against a standard curve.[78] This is a sensitive assay but its use is limited by its expense and the need that it be performed in a laboratory that can manage radioactive substances.[72]

Nephelometry: Albumin in the urine sample reacts with a specific anti-albumin antibody, forming light-scattering antigen-antibody complexes that can be measured with a laser nephelometer. The amount of albumin is directly proportional to scatter in the signal.[79]

Competitive enzyme-linked immunosorbent assay (ELISA).[80]

Size-exclusion HPLC (SE-HPLC): Chromatographic techniques are used to measure both immunoreactive and nonimmunoreactive albumin. Proteins of different sizes are separated as they pass at different speeds through a column containing size-selective gel.[81] SE-HPLC is more sensitive for the detection of albumin than the immune-based methods, but its specificity is limited by an inability to discriminate between albumin and other proteins of the same size, such as globulins.[72]

Although the correlation among results obtained using most of these quantitative assays is very good,[59] a good correlation indicates only precision, a strong linear relationship, but not accuracy in quantifying all clinically significant proteins present. Results obtained by radioimmunoassay, immunoturbidimetry, nephelometry, and HPLC may vary significantly.[72] Therefore, ideally, the same assay should be used when albuminuria results are compared over time for a given patient. The choice of assay used to measure albuminuria is largely determined by issues of accuracy, cost, and convenience. Currently, there is no standardized procedure for measuring urine albumin and reporting results in standardized units; however, considering the recommendations for using ACRs as the standard measure for urinary protein, a number of professional bodies have moved toward establishing standard laboratory collection, measuring, and reporting procedures.[61] Standardization for measurement of albumin requires a reference material and reference measurement procedure. Using purified albumin as the reference material would not reflect the various molecular forms that may be present in the urine but may be the most practical approach to standardization. Most routine methods for urinary albumin measurement are currently calibrated against dilutions of CRM 470, a higher-order serum protein reference material with an albumin concentration of 39.7g/L.[61,71] Other issues that would need to be addressed to standardize the measurement of urinary albumin include clarification of the molecular forms of albumin in freshly voided urine, the degree of degradation that occurs during storage and freezing, and the appropriate upper limits of normal in different age, sex, and gender groups.[61]

TIMED VERSUS RANDOM COLLECTION FOR PROTEINURIA ASSESSMENT

Random "spot" specimens for urinary protein, expressed as a concentration, are often inaccurate for estimation of 24-hour levels because of the impact of patient hydration status on urine concentration. There is also variation in protein excretion, which can occur throughout the day (especially resulting from exercise and posture) and from day to day.[82] Methods to improve the accuracy of spot urine testing include corrections for urine creatinine and specific gravity.[83]

Protein or albumin measurement in 24-hour urine collection is generally considered the gold standard for measuring protein excretion. However, it can also be inaccurate, primarily through inaccurate urine collection. Urine creatinine can be measured to judge the adequacy of the 24-hour collection. If creatinine excretion is similar to that in previous 24-hour samples, the collection is likely to be reasonably accurate. If no other collections are available for comparison, the adequacy of collection can be judged from the expected normal range of creatinine excretion. For hospitalized men aged 20 to 50 years, this range was found to be 18.5 to 25.0 mg per kg of body weight per day, and for women of the same age, 16.5 to 22.4 mg/kg/day. These values declined with age, so that for men aged 50 to 70 years, creatinine excretion was 15.7 to 20.2 mg/kg/day, and for women, 11.8 to 16.1 mg/kg/day.[27] Factors influencing the daily creatinine excretion include determinants of muscle mass, such as gender, race, age, and body surface area.[60]

TRANSLATING PCR AND ACR VALUES INTO TOTAL DAILY PROTEIN MEASUREMENTS

ACR and PCR are obtained by dividing the urine protein concentrations by the urine creatinine concentration and expressing the result as mg/mmol or mg/g. Both enzymatic and Jaffe assays are used for the measurement of creatinine in urine.[35] The ratio-based tests aim to correct for the effects of urine concentration on protein measurements. Overall, these tests have shown greater accuracy and less intraindividual variability than concentrations measured in random samples[61,83,84] and are more acceptable to patients than 24-hour protein measurements. Intra-individual variability is further reduced by using a first void rather than a daytime collection specimen to measure ACR. However, there remains substantial day-to-day variability in both PCR and ACR.[61] A positive result should be followed with a second measurement, ideally in an early morning sample, to confirm the result.[35,60]

Clinicians commonly use these tests as estimations of the 24-hour protein in mg by multiplying the PCR in mg/mmol or ACR in mg/mmol by 10 (given an average daily creatinine excretion of 10 mmol) or using the value as given if measured in mg/g. (Although the PCR or ACR in mg/g should be multiplied by 8.8 to get an exact measurement in mg/mmol, these are estimates of 24-hour levels only.) Despite the reasonable performance of the ratio-based tests to estimate 24-hour protein measurements, their ability to predict the true 24-hour protein for an individual is limited by two major factors. The first is variability in the total daily creatinine excretion, in and between individuals, which affects the ratio. The second is the fluctuations in protein excretion that occur throughout the day. An understanding of the factors that may make an ACR or PCR value inaccurate is important for clinicians using these tests.

CORRELATION BETWEEN RATIOS AND 24-HOUR URINE PROTEIN

Summary tables of studies comparing ACR and PCR with timed collections for urinary albumin and protein can be found in the 2002 KDIGO-CKD 2012 guideline. There is a relatively high degree of correlation between 24-hour urine protein excretion and PCRs in random, single-voided urine samples in healthy controls[85] and in patients with a variety of kidney diseases.[86-89] The correlation has been shown in studies in patients with glomerulonephritis[90] and with type 1 diabetes mellitus (DM),[91] and in renal transplant recipients.[92,93] In some studies, the correlation between PCR and 24-hour protein measurements was less robust when proteinuria was in the nephrotic range and above.[88,91]

The ACR has been shown to correlate well with 24-hour urinary albumin measurements in a number of studies in people with diabetes.[94] However, a large study evaluating the correlation between ACR and 24-hour albumin excretion in 1186 subjects with type 1 DM enrolled in the Diabetes Control and Complications Trial and its follow-up study Epidemiology of Diabetes Interventions and Complications (DCCT/EDIC) showed that ACR systematically underestimated albumin excretion, particularly in men.[95] Another study in the diabetic population showed that ACR increased relative to 24-hour albumin excretion with increasing age.[96] These studies highlight the fact that variability in creatinine excretion in certain groups alters the ratio. Individuals with lower muscle mass, such as females and elderly patients, would be expected to have higher ACRs than those with higher muscle mass for the same level of urinary albumin excretion.

VARIABILITY IN CREATININE EXCRETION

Under normal circumstances, a steady rate of creatinine excretion occurs throughout the day.[97] The accuracy of the ratio-based tests depends on a constant excretion rate. This drawback limits their usefulness in the setting of rapidly changing renal function such as AKI, in which creatinine excretion is reduced, increasing the ratio for the same amount of protein excretion.

Creatinine excretion rises with increasing muscle mass, so ACR and PCR are reduced for a given level of protein excretion in groups with higher muscle mass, such as men, younger people, and certain population ancestry groups.[98,99] The fact that the average urinary creatinine excretion is 40% to 50% higher in men than in women[95,96] has led some guidelines to recommend gender-specific cutoff values for ACRs, with lower thresholds for men than women. Commonly used ACR thresholds for diabetic nephropathy are 25 mg/g (2.5 mg/mmol) for males and 35 mg/g (3.5 mg/mmol) for females.[60] However, the 2012 KDIGO guidelines recommend an ACR threshold of 3.0 mg/mmol for both sexes, reflecting that the ACR is an estimation with a variety of other variables, such as age and population ancestry, that are not corrected for.[35]

FLUCTUATIONS IN PROTEIN EXCRETION

Factors that may cause transient increases in urinary protein excretion include exercise, urinary tract infections, and upright posture. High-intensity exercise may cause transient proteinuria lasting for 24 to 48 hours in healthy subjects.[100,101] Patients with CKD or diabetes have been shown to have higher levels of urinary protein or albumin excretion after exercise than control subjects.[102-104] Some guidelines have recommended screening for urinary tract infection if proteinuria is detected. However, a review of available studies suggested that asymptomatic urinary tract infection was unlikely to cause proteinuria and that screening may be unnecessary.[105]

Upright posture can cause an increase in urine protein excretion in otherwise healthy young adults.[106] Postural proteinuria is usually diagnosed by detecting proteinuria in a random sample taken while that subject has been upright that is absent in a first morning void specimen. It usually does not exceed 1 g in 24 hours. Kidney histologic examination in patients with postural proteinuria generally yields normal or nonspecific findings,[106,107] and patients with postural proteinuria have been shown to have an excellent long-term prognosis.[108] An increased urine protein excretion found on a random sample in a young person should prompt a testing of an early morning specimen to exclude postural proteinuria.[61]

Diurnal variation in protein excretion occurs in healthy individuals and patients with CKD. Overnight urinary protein excretion is lower, and the amount less variable, than in the daytime.[109,110] Thus, timing of urine collection is likely to influence the sensitivity and specificity of screening tests for urine protein or albumin excretion. Samples taken at first void are most likely to accurately quantify 24-hour protein or albumin excretion,[111,112] and first void specimens are therefore regarded as preferable by a number of guidelines.[34,35,60]

URINARY ACR VERSUS PCR

Because the relationship between albumin excretion and total protein excretion is nonlinear,[113] an ACR cannot be derived from a PCR, and vice versa. The ACR, rather than PCR, has been recommended by a number of guidelines because of an improved ability to standardize urinary albumin versus total protein measurement and the fact that albumin is the predominant protein lost in the urine.[35,60] These advantages have already been outlined. ACR has not been shown to be superior to PCR in determining prognosis or detecting CKD in nondiabetic subjects.[60] A retrospective cohort study comparing urine PCR, ACR, and 24-hour protein at a single center showed that the three were equal in predictive utility for doubling of serum creatinine, commencement of renal replacement therapy, and all-cause mortality.[113]

REAGENT STRIP TESTING

Multireagent dipstick urinalysis has been used widely as an initial screening tool for the evaluation of proteinuria because of its low cost, availability, and ability to provide rapid point-of-care information to clinicians. Most dipstick reagents are semiquantitative, containing a pH-sensitive colorimetric indicator that changes color when negatively charged proteins bind to it. Dipstick testing for protein has limited sensitivity for non-albumin and positively charged proteins[26,114-116] and therefore often has false-negative results in the presence of predominantly LMW (tubular or overflow) proteinuria.[72] Albumin-specific dipsticks may also be used.

The dipstick tests protein or albumin concentration, rather than an excretion rate, so it is strongly affected by changes in urine concentration. Very dilute urine may give false-negative results, and concentrated urine may give false-positive results. Measuring specific gravity concurrently with urinary protein on a dipstick can thus help with interpretation of a urine dipstick result.[117] A very high urine pH (>7.0) can give false-positive results, as can contamination of the urine with blood. Operator-dependent differences may also occur with manual reading of dipsticks, decreasing reproducibility.[111,115] The use of automated reader devices improves inter-operator variability.

ALBUMIN-SPECIFIC DIPSTICKS

In addition to dipsticks that are designed to measure total protein, albumin-specific dipsticks are in use. Many of these use dye-binding methods.[118-120] Antibody-based detection methods are also in use.[121] Several studies have examined the sensitivity and specificity of the newer reagent strips that measure very low concentrations of urine albumin. Most of these investigations studied patients with diabetes, and most examined the Micral-Test[119,122-125] (Boehringer Mannheim, Mannheim, Germany) the Micro-Bumintest[119,126] (Ames Division, Miles Laboratories, Elkhart, Indiana) or both. In general, these albumin reagent strip tests are more sensitive than standard dipstick tests, but they also have a relatively high rate of false-positive results.

NEW DEVICES FOR POINT-OF-CARE PROTEIN TESTING

New systems with a creatinine test pad can report albumin-to-creatinine ratios in the range previously classified as "microalbuminuric" (corresponding to < 300 mg/g) or total protein-to-creatinine ratios. They overcome some of the error inherent in measuring urinary protein concentrations rather than protein excretion rates. The CLINITEK system (CLINITEK microalbumin, Siemens Medical Solutions Diagnostics, Mishawaka, Indiana) uses a reagent strip with two pads, using a dye-binding method for albumin measurement and a creatinine assay based on the peroxidase-like activity of a copper creatinine complex. The reagent strips are used in combination with an analyzer to give a semiquantitative assessment of ACR.[127,128]

ROLE OF POINT-OF-CARE AND REAGENT STRIP TESTING

The role of urinary reagent strip testing, using either protein or albumin-specific dipsticks, in the general and high-risk population is the subject of debate. Most guidelines do not recommend the use of the urine dipstick as an initial screening test for proteinuria.[37] However, reagent strip testing may be of particular use in settings where laboratory access is limited. Newer point-of-care devices that can measure low levels of albuminuria and provide ACRs may have a role to play in population screening, but this role has not yet been defined by large studies.[35]

General Population

Observational studies have shown that reagent strip–proven proteinuria is associated with progression to ESKD and mortality in the general population.[30,32] However, general population screening could lead to unnecessary investigations, possible harm, and excess costs.[129-132] As with all diagnostic tests, the positive and negative predictive values of the urinary reagent strips and point-of-care devices depend on the setting in which they are used as well as their sensitivity and specificity.[133,134] A study comparing urinary ACRs with protein dipsticks (Bayer Multistix) using data from the previously mentioned AusDiab study showed that positive predictive values varied greatly across low- and high-risk subgroups. The dipstick test showed a good ability to rule out proteinuria, with a reagent strip result of less than trace having a negative predictive value of 97.6% for ACR values of 30 mg/g or higher and a negative predictive value of 100% for ACR values of 300 mg/g or higher.[135] The investigators concluded that urine reagent strip testing is a reasonable "rule-out" test for proteinuria. However, an analysis by Samal and Linder argues that the rate of false-positive results, which was as high as 53% using an ACR cut-off of 30 mg/g or higher, makes urinary reagent strip testing unacceptable in the general population owing to the cost, anxiety, and workload generated by false-positive results.[132] Because of the high rate of false-positive results, a positive reagent strip test result mandates confirmation with a quantitive test. This is a factor that significantly limits the cost-effectiveness of reagent strip testing for population screening.[130,132]

Screening of schoolchildren with urinary reagent strips in Japan, Taiwan, and Korea, can detect asymptomatic renal disease at an early stage.[136-138] However, there are no data to show that this policy results in improved outcomes or has benefits from a health economics perspective. Several studies have used models to assess the benefits of general population screening with urinary reagent strips, followed by ACEI or ARB use in the proteinuric population. One such study, assessing the utility of general practitioner–led general population screening for proteinuria in Australia in 2002, concluded that there was insufficient evidence to support this practice.[130] A study that assessed this practice in a nondiabetic, nonhypertensive U.S. population using cost per quality-adjusted life-year concluded that it was cost-effective only if selectively directed toward high-risk groups (aged more than 60 years or with hypertension) or conducted at long intervals (10 years).[131]

High-Risk Populations

In contrast to general population screening, there are several studies showing the cost effectiveness of high-risk population screening for proteinuria with urinary dipstick testing[131,139,140] and subsequent antiproteinuric therapy. A model based on screening of a hypertensive, diabetic U.S. population cohort with Micral-II semiquantitative reagent strips for albumin and initiating irbesartan treatment in patients who had microalbuminuria (estimated 24-hour urinary albumin excretion >20 μg/min) or higher levels of urinary albumin showed a 44% reduced incidence in the cumulative incidence of ESKD and was likely to be cost effective.[139] Screening high-risk populations, such as patients with diabetes, hypertension, or known vascular disease, for microalbuminuria is recommended in most guidelines,[35,141,142] although the frequency at which testing should occur is either not specified or inconsistent. Guidelines generally advise the use of laboratory rather than reagent strip testing in the high-risk population.[143] Studies using newer devices such as the CLINITEK system have shown good negative predictive values, making it an effective rule-out test.[144-146] The CLINITEK system has shown good performance in diabetic, general population,[127] and CKD cohorts.[147] However, the usefulness and cost-effectiveness of these newer devices is yet to be confirmed by large studies.

PROTEINURIA MEASUREMENT IN SPECIFIC POPULATIONS

PREGNANT PATIENTS

Proteinuria is generally defined as 300 mg/24 hours for the diagnosis of preeclampsia. The roughly equivalent PCR of 300 mg/g (30 mg/mmol) showed reasonable performance in estimating 24-hour protein excretion and as a rule-out test in two systematic reviews of studies in this setting, although there was no data on PCR for predicting outcomes. Currently, there is insufficient evidence to substitute urine albumin measurement for total protein in pregnant women with hypertension or suspected preeclampsia.[148,149]

CHILDREN

Normal levels of protein excretion in children are less than 10 mg/m^2/d, or less than 4 mg/m^2/hr.[150] Nephrotic-range proteinuria is defined as 1000 mg/m^2/d, or 40 mg/m^2/hr, or higher. PCR has been shown to have reasonable accuracy in reflecting 24-hour levels of protein excretion in a small study of 15 children.[151] PCR has been shown to predict an increased rate of GFR decline in children.[152-154] There is currently insufficient evidence linking elevated ACRs with adverse outcomes to recommend the use of ACR in a pediatric population.[155]

KIDNEY TRANSPLANT RECIPIENTS

Proteinuria predicts allograft loss, cardiovascular risk, and death in kidney transplant recipients.[156] One study showed that 24-hour urinary albumin measurement was superior to total protein measurement in predicting graft loss[157]; another using ACR and PCR showed equivalent performances.[158]

URINE MICROSCOPY

Examination of the urine by microscopy has been performed systematically at least since the 19th century[159] and remains a vital investigation that is often considered a component of the physical examination of a patient in whom kidney disease is suspected.

PREPARATION AND METHOD

Elements in urine degrade rapidly and so urine microscopy is best performed on a fresh urine sample within 2 hours of collection. Urine preservation is not a routinely applied technique but has been performed successfully by some institutions. Traditionally, ethanol is used to preserve uroepithelial cells for cytology but this does not prevent lysis of red and white blood cells.[160] Formaldehyde-based solutions have been used to preserve urine sediment for up to 3 months, and commercial preservatives such as buffered boric acid are also available.

The first urine of the morning specimen has been recommended in the past for urine microscopy because it is acidic and concentrated, but a midstream specimen of the second urine of the morning is favored owing to the lysis of urine particles after prolonged standing of urine in the bladder overnight. Specimens should preferably not be refrigerated because of precipitation of crystals. High urine pH and dilute urine lead to more degradation of formed elements.

A guideline provided by the European Confederation of Laboratory Medicine suggests standardization of preparation of the urine sediment for microscopy.[161] A sample of 5 to 12 mL of urine should be centrifuged at 400 g or 2000 rpm for 5 minutes, a defined volume of supernatant removed by suction rather than arbitrary decanting, and the pellet resuspended by gentle agitation. A drop of urine should be placed on a slide under a coverslip, and it should be examined ideally with phase-contrast microscopy rather than usual brightfield microscopy, at low power (×160) then at high power (×400). Staining or polarized light may also be useful to identify certain substances.

CELLS OF THE URINARY SEDIMENT

ERYTHROCYTES

Hematuria is defined as three or more erythrocytes per high-power field. Transient hematuria is common and may be due to strenuous exercise. Persistent hematuria on three repeated urine samples warrants investigation. Studies show great variation in the prevalence of microscopic hematuria from as low as 0.18% to as high as 16.1%.[162] A study of more than a million Israeli military recruits showed an incidence of persistent hematuria of 0.3%.[163] This finding was associated with an increased risk of subsequent ESKD (hazard ratio = 19.5) although the absolute risk of ESKD was low, at 34.0 per 100,000 person-years.

Even when the urine appears red the sediment should be examined to determine whether red blood cells are present because a red appearance may be due to other causes, such as hemoglobinuria and myoglobinuria. Macroscopic hematuria is much more likely to be due to malignancy. Isomorphic red blood cells, which look similar to the erythrocytes found in the bloodstream, are thought to be nonglomerular in origin. Dysmorphic red blood cells (Figure 26.3) are erythrocytes from the glomerular capillary, and their irregular appearance is a consequence of damage due to pH and osmolality changes as the cells travel through the tubule. Glomerular hematuria is defined by some institutions in terms of percentage of dysmorphic red blood cells, but the threshold at which this value is believed to be significant is not standardized. Glomerular hematuria is variously defined as more than 10% to 80% dysmorphic red blood cells or more than 2% to 5% acanthocytes, which are a subtype of dysmorphic red blood cells with protruding blebs.

Automated methods of examining for glomerular or nonglomerular hematuria have been developed in an attempt to overcome the problems with reliability and reproducibility of urine microscopy. These methods function by measuring the mean corpuscular volume (MCV) of the red cells. An MCV smaller or larger than the normal range (50-80 femtoliters [fL]) is recorded as dysmorphic. The role of urinary red blood cell MCV in diagnosis was reviewed in a meta-analysis,[164] which concluded that the diagnostic value of this test is limited and that the urinary MCV test was not reliable in cases of low-grade hematuria because of interfering debris.

Causes of hematuria are listed in Table 26.8. Although anticoagulation often unmasks another underlying etiology for hematuria, over-anticoagulation itself may cause

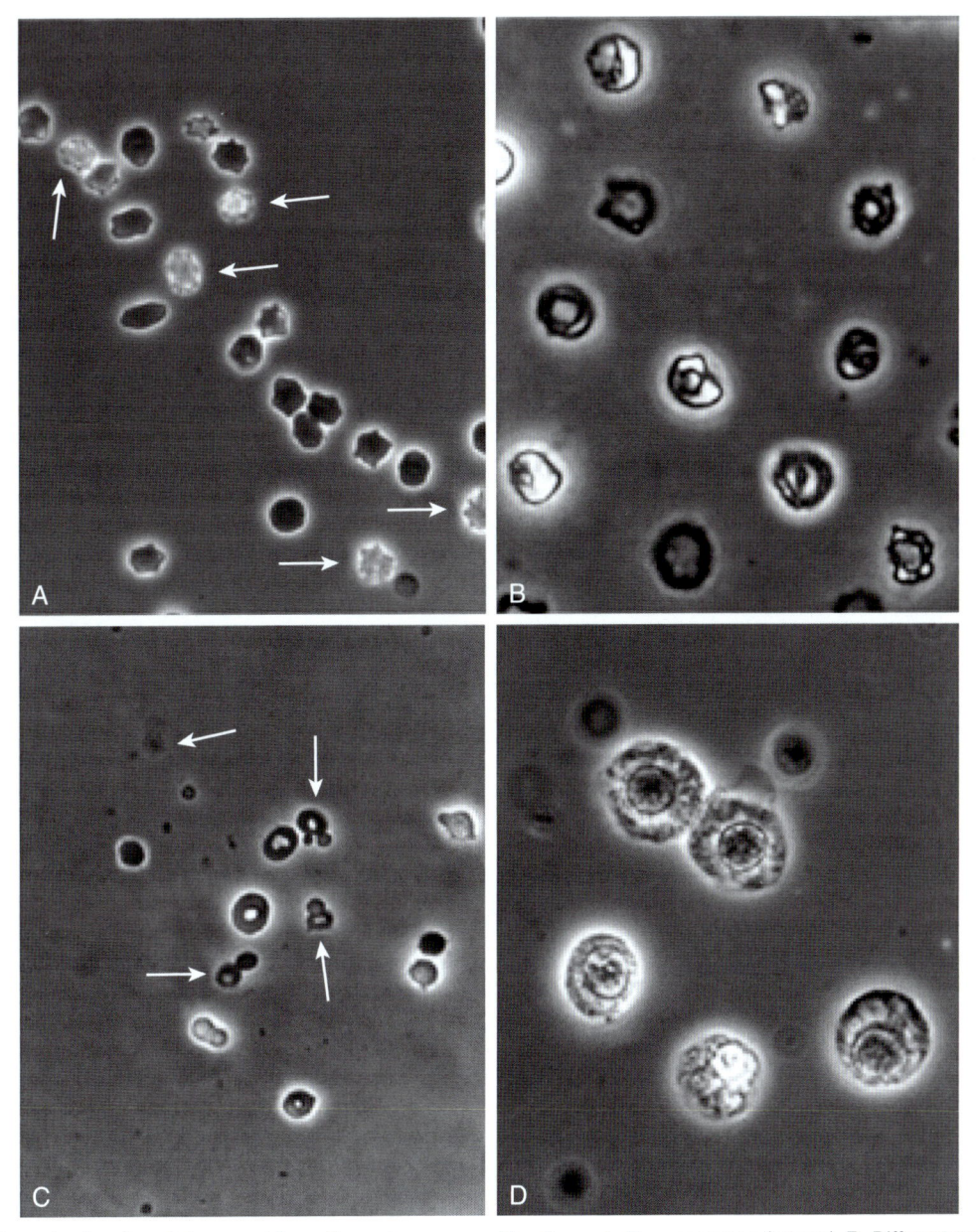

Figure 26.3 Erythrocytes in urine. **A,** Isomorphic erythrocytes, some with a "crenated" appearance *(arrows).* **B,** Different types of dysmorphic erythrocytes. **C,** Acanthocytes *(arrows).* **D,** Proximal renal tubule cells. (From Fogazzi GB, Verdesca S, Garigali G: Urinalysis: core curriculum 2008. *Am J Kidney Dis* 51:1052-1067, 2008.)

glomerular bleeding, as in the case of the relatively newly recognized condition, warfarin-induced nephropathy, in which obstruction of tubules by red blood cell casts may cause AKI.[165]

URINE CYTOLOGY

Cytology is usually performed and is recommended as part of the investigation for nonglomerular hematuria. Although it is the realm of urologists, nephrologists may frequently encounter patients with nonglomerular hematuria as part of the investigative process for asymptomatic microscopic hematuria. A number of studies have suggested that the value of routine urine cytology as part of the workup for nonglomerular hematuria is limited if other investigations such as imaging and flexible cystoscopy are performed. For example, in a study of 2778 patients[166] who presented to a hospital hematuria clinic in the United Kingdom, 974 patients had "non-visible" or microscopic hematuria. Of the patients with microscopic hematuria, 4.6% had a urothelial malignancy, which in 93% of these patients was a bladder tumor. Urothelial cancer cytology demonstrated only 45.5% sensitivity and 89.5% specificity. Only 2 patients with abnormal urine cytology as the only positive finding, had urothelial malignancy on further investigation.

LEUKOCYTES

The most common leukocytes found in the urine, neutrophils are usually an indication of infection or contamination. Eosinophils are detectable with Wright's stain or Hansel's stain. Hansel's stain has improved sensitivity,

Table 26.8 Causes of Hematuria*

Glomerular Hematuria
Glomerular Lesions

Thin basement membrane nephropathy
Mesangial immunoglobulin A (IgA) glomerulonephritis
Focal and segmental hyalinosis and sclerosis (focal glomerulosclerosis)
Lupus glomerulonephritis
Crescentic glomerulonephritis, including Wegener's granulomatosis, microscopic polyangiitis, and Goodpasture's syndrome
Membranous glomerulonephritis
Mesangiocapillary glomerulonephritis
Dense deposit disease
Poststreptococcal glomerulonephritis

Nonglomerular Disease

Autosomal dominant polycystic kidney disease
Exercise hematuria
Bleeding diathesis
Drugs, including anticoagulants

Nonglomerular Hematuria

Urinary tract infection
Urinary tract calculi
Hypercalciuria and hyperuricosuria
Autosomal dominant polycystic kidney disease
Benign prostatic hypertrophy
Transitional cell carcinoma
Renal cell carcinoma
Prostatic carcinoma
Exercise hematuria
Trauma
Bleeding diathesis and anticoagulants
Drugs
Renal papillary necrosis
Sickle cell disease

*Unknown whether glomerular or nonglomerular hematuria after percutaneous coronary artery angioplasty.
From Kincaid Smith P, Fairley K: The investigation of haematuria. Semin Nephrol 25:127-135, 2005.

Table 26.9 Common Casts

Cast	Main Clinical Association(s)
Hyaline	Normal and in renal disease
Granular	Renal disease of any cause
Waxy	Renal disease of any cause
Fatty	Heavy proteinuria
Red blood cell	Proliferative glomerulonephritis, glomerular bleeding
White blood cell	Acute interstitial nephritis, acute pyelonephritis
Tubular epithelial cell	Acute tubular necrosis ("muddy brown" casts), acute interstitial nephritis, proliferative glomerulonephritis

From Fogazzi GB, Verdesca S, Garigali G: Urinalysis: core curriculum 2008. Am J Kidney Dis 51:1052-1067, 2008.

especially because a urine pH of less than 7 inhibits Wright's stain. Although eosinophiluria was initially associated with drug-induced hypersensitivity, the list of diseases that may be associated with eosinophiluria is diverse and includes renal cholesterol embolism, rapidly progressive glomerulonephritis, and prostatitis.

The diagnostic value of the presence of other leukocytes, such as lymphocytes and macrophages, is currently limited, although lymphocytes have been indicative of transplant rejection, and macrophages may be found in glomerulonephritis.

OTHER CELLS

Squamous cells, the largest cells of the urinary sediment, derive from the urethra or external genitalia. *Renal tubule epithelial cells* may be present in tubular injury.

Urothelial cells may be seen in urologic diseases such as malignancy.

OTHER ELEMENTS

LIPIDS

Lipids appear as spherical, translucent drops of varying size. They may also be within the cytoplasm of cells as "oval fat bodies." Under polarized light, lipid droplets look like Maltese crosses. Lipiduria is usually associated with heavy proteinuria but may also be present in Fabry's disease.

CASTS (Figure 26.4)

Casts are cylindrical bodies of renal origin that form from the aggregation of fibrils of Tamm-Horsfall glycoprotein (uromodulin), which is secreted by cells of the thick ascending limb of the loop of Henle. Trapping of various particles within the cast matrix, as well as degenerative processes, result in casts with different appearances and clinical significance (Table 26.9). Hyaline casts are nonspecific and may be present normally. Granular casts are nonspecific and contain protein aggregates or degenerated cellular elements. Waxy casts are also nonspecific and result from degeneration of other casts. Broad casts are wider waxy casts that are seen in chronic renal failure in which there is dilation of the tubule. Renal tubule epithelial cell casts are formed from the aggregation of desquamated cells of the tubule lining. Because the epithelial cells still appear intact, this finding is usually the result of an acute disease process such as acute tubular necrosis. Red blood cell casts are always pathologic and indicate significant glomerular bleeding, which is often due to rapidly progressive glomerulonephritis.

CRYSTALS

A large variety of crystals can be seen in the urine that may be of diagnostic value (Table 26.10). However, uric acid, calcium oxalate, and calcium phosphate crystals are common and may have little clinical significance because they may precipitate as a result of transient supersaturation of urine due to dehydration or cooling of the sample. Of course, depending on the clinical setting, uric acid crystals may be highly significant because they are present in acute uric acid nephropathy as part of tumor lysis syndrome, and

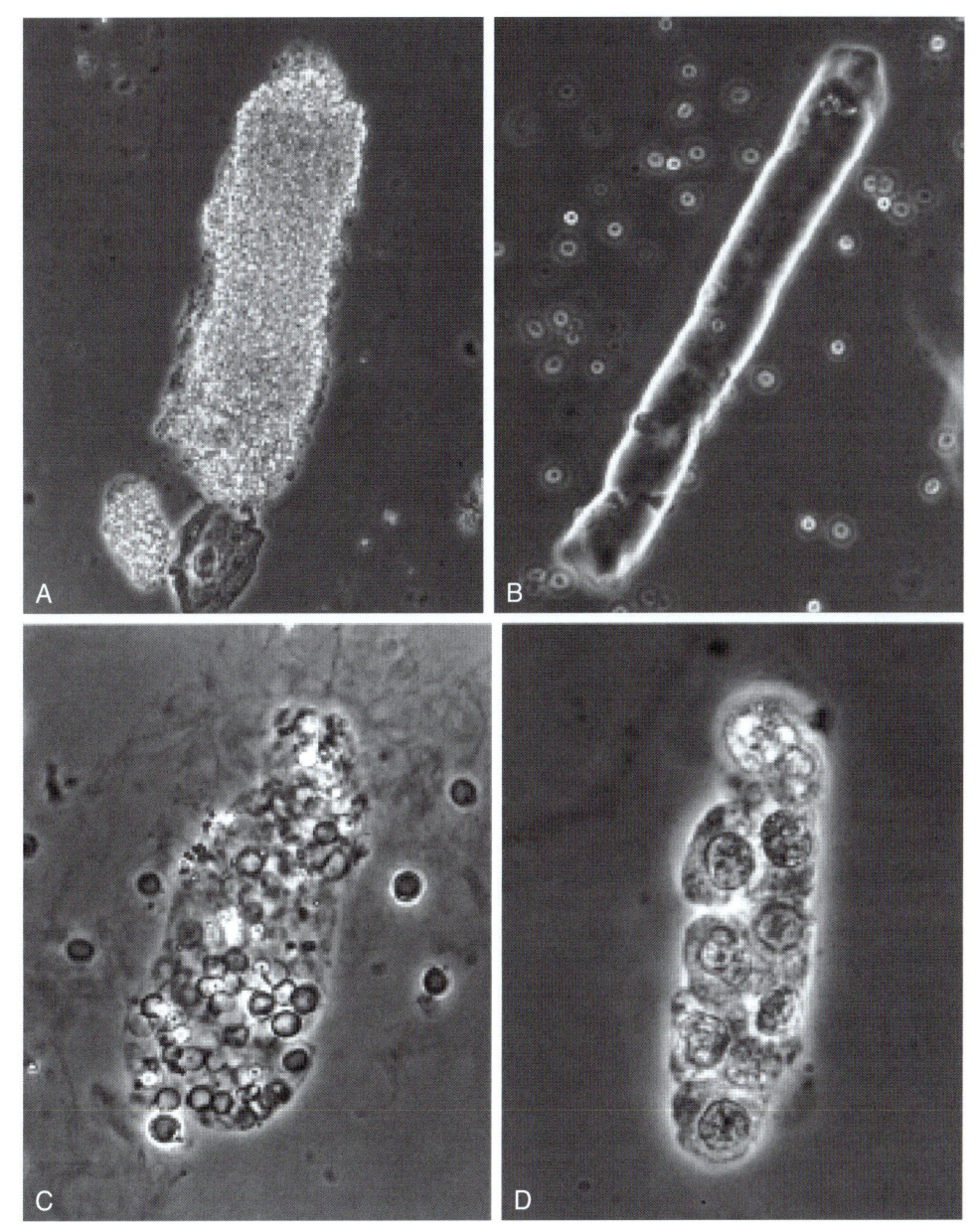

Figure 26.4 Urinary casts. **A,** A finely granular cast. **B,** Waxy cast with the typical "melted wax" appearance. **C,** A red blood cell cast. **D,** A renal tubule epithelial cell cast. (From Stevens LA, Nolin TD, Richardson MM, et al: Comparison of drug dosing recommendations based on measured GFR and kidney function estimating equations. *Am J Kidney Dis* 54:33-42, 2009.)

Table 26.10 Common Crystals and Their Appearance

Crystal	Appearance
Uric acid	Usually lozenges but varying shape, yellow-tinged
Calcium oxalate	Monohydrate: ovoid or dumbbell-shaped, biconcave discs
	Dihydrate: bipyramidal
Calcium phosphate	Prisms, starlike particles or needles of various sizes
Triple phosphate (struvite)	Coffin lids
Cholesterol	Transparent thin plates
Cystine	Hexagonal plates with irregular sides

From Fogazzi GB, Verdesca S, Garigali G: Urinalysis: core curriculum 2008. *Am J Kidney Dis 51:1052-1067, 2008.*

calcium oxalate crystals may indicate ethylene glycol poisoning or hyperoxaluria.

A growing list of drugs, beginning with acyclovir and indinavir, may cause crystals in the urine that commonly have unusual shapes.

MICROORGANISMS

Bacteria are commonly seen because of contamination or infection. Fungi such as *Candida*, protozoa such as *Trichomonas*, and parasites such as *Schistosoma* may also be seen.

LIMITATIONS

Urine microscopy depends on expertise and has poor interobserver reliability. In a study involving ten nephrologists, agreement for various elements in urine microscopy ranged from 31.4% to 79.1% and interobserver agreement was not associated with seniority.[167] Despite this limitation, urinary microscopy is still a vital component of the laboratory assessment of renal disease because its findings may crucially influence management of a patient. For example, identification of dysmorphic red blood cells and red blood cell casts in a patient with AKI may prompt empirical treatment with immunosuppressive therapy well in advance of results of serology or renal biopsy.

Complete reference list available at ExpertConsult.com.

KEY REFERENCES

1. Miller WG, Myers GL, Ashwood ER, et al: Creatinine measurement: state of the art in accuracy and interlaboratory harmonization. *Arch Pathol Lab Med* 129(3):297–304, 2005.
4. Dharnidharka VR, Kwon C, Stevens G: Serum cystatin C is superior to serum creatinine as a marker of kidney function: a meta-analysis. *Am J Kidney Dis* 40(2):221–226, 2002.
7. Levey AS, Stevens LA, Schmid CH, et al: A new equation to estimate glomerular filtration rate. *Ann Intern Med* 150:604–612, 2009.
8. Levey AS, Bosch JP, Lewis JB, et al: A more accurate method to estimate glomerular filtration rate from serum creatinine: a new prediction equation. Modification of Diet in Renal Disease Study Group. *Ann Intern Med* 130(6):461–470, 2009.
9. Matsushita K, Mahmoodi BK, Woodward M, et al: Comparison of risk prediction using the CKD-EPI equation and the MDRD study equation for estimated glomerular filtration rate. *JAMA* 307(18):1941–1951, 2012.
10. Eriksen BO, Mathisen UD, Melsom T, et al: The role of cystatin C in improving GFR estimation in the general population. *Am J Kidney Dis* 59(1):32–40, 2012.
11. Cockcroft DW, Gault MH: Prediction of creatinine clearance from serum creatinine. *Nephron* 16(1):31–41, 2012.
13. Schwartz GJ, Haycock GB, Edelmann CM, et al: A simple estimate of glomerular filtration rate in children derived from body length and plasma creatinine. *Pediatrics* 58(2):259–263, 1976.
14. Schwartz GJ, Muñoz A, Schneider MF, et al: New equations to estimate GFR in children with CKD. *J Am Soc Nephrol* 20(3):629–637, 1976.
15. Schwartz GJ, Work DF: Measurement and estimation of GFR in children and adolescents. *Clin J Am Soc Nephrol* 4(11):1832–1843, 2009.
19. Chen S: Retooling the creatinine clearance equation to estimate kinetic GFR when the plasma creatinine is changing acutely. *J Am Soc Nephrol* 24(6):877–888, 2013.
20. Endre ZH, Pickering JW, Walker RJ: Clearance and beyond: the complementary roles of GFR measurement and injury biomarkers in acute kidney injury (AKI). *Am J Physiol Renal Physiol* 301(4):F697–F707, 2013.
21. Stevens LA, Nolin TD, Richardson MM, et al: Comparison of drug dosing recommendations based on measured GFR and kidney function estimating equations. *Am J Kidney Dis* 54(1):33–42, 2009.
24. Kilbride HS, Stevens PE, Eaglestone G, et al: Accuracy of the MDRD (Modification of Diet in Renal Disease) study and CKD-EPI (CKD Epidemiology Collaboration) equations for estimation of GFR in the elderly. *Am J Kidney Dis* 61(1):57–66, 2013.
26. Fogazzi GB, Verdesca S, Garigali G: Urinalysis: core curriculum 2008. *Am J Kidney Dis* 51(6):1052–1067, 2008.
27. Israni A, Kasiske B: Laboratory Assessment of kidney disease: glomerular filtration rate, urinalysis, and proteinuria. In Taal M, Chertow G, Marsden P, et al, editors: *Brenner and Rector's The Kidney*, ed 9, Philadelphia, 2011, Saunders, pp 868–892.
29. Jacobs D, De Mott WR, Willie GR: Urinalysis and clinical microscopy. In Jacobs D, Kasten BL, De Mott WR, et al, editors: *Laboratory test handbook*, Baltimore, 1990, Williams & Wilkins, pp 906–909.
30. Kannel WB, Stampfer MJ, Castelli WP, et al: The prognostic significance of proteinuria: the Framingham study. *Am Heart J* 108(5):1347–1352, 1984.
34. KDOQI: KDOQI clinical practice guidelines and clinical practice recommendations for diabetes and chronic kidney disease. *Am J Kidney Dis* 49(2 Suppl 2):S12–S154, 2007.
35. Kidney Disease: Improving Global Outcomes (KDIGO) CKD Work Group: KDIGO 2012 clinical practice guideline for the evaluation and management of chronic kidney disease. *Kidney Int* (Suppl 3):1–150, 2013.
37. Lamb EJ, MacKenzie F, Stevens PE: How should proteinuria be detected and measured? *Ann Clin Biochem* 46(Pt 3):205–217, 2009.
40. Cameron JS: The patient with proteinuria and or hematuria. In Davison A, editor: *Oxford textbook of clinical nephrology*, ed 3, 2005, Oxford University Press, pp 389–411.
41. Brinkkoetter PT, Ising C, Benzing T: The role of the podocyte in albumin filtration. *Nat Rev Nephrol* 9(6):328–336, 2013.
50. Russo LM, Bakris GL, Comper WD: Renal handling of albumin: a critical review of basic concepts and perspective. *Am J Kidney Dis* 39(5):899–919, 2002.
52. Atkins RC, Briganti EM, Zimmet PZ, et al: Association between albuminuria and proteinuria in the general population: the AusDiab Study. *Nephrol Dial Transplant* 18(10):2170–2174, 2003.
54. Hillege HL, Fidler V, Diercks GF, et al: Urinary albumin excretion predicts cardiovascular and noncardiovascular mortality in general population. *Circulation* 106(14):1777–1782, 2002.
60. Johnson DW, Jones GR, Mathew TH, et al: Chronic kidney disease and measurement of albuminuria or proteinuria: a position statement. *Med J Aust* 197(4):224–225, 2012.
61. Miller WG, Bruns DE, Hortin GL, et al: Current issues in measurement and reporting of urinary albumin excretion. *Ann Biol Clin (Paris)* 68(1):9–25, 2010.
71. Martin H: Laboratory measurement of urine albumin and urine total protein in screening for proteinuria in chronic kidney disease. *Clin Biochem Rev* 32(2):97–102, 2011.
72. Viswanathan G, Upadhyay A: Assessment of proteinuria. *Adv Chronic Kidney Dis* 18(4):243–248, 2011.
74. Sviridov D, Drake SK, Hortin GL: Reactivity of urinary albumin (microalbumin) assays with fragmented or modified albumin. *Clin Chem* 54(1):61–68, 2008.
82. Naresh CN, Hayen A, Craig JC, et al: Day-to-day variability in spot urine protein-creatinine ratio measurements. *Am J Kidney Dis* 60(4):561–566, 2012.
83. Newman DJ, Pugia MJ, Lott JA, et al: Urinary protein and albumin excretion corrected by creatinine and specific gravity. *Clin Chim Acta* 294(1–2):139–155, 2000.
88. Ruggenenti P, Gaspari F, Perna A, et al: Cross sectional longitudinal study of spot morning urine protein:creatinine ratio, 24 hour urine protein excretion rate, glomerular filtration rate, and end stage renal failure in chronic renal disease in patients without diabetes. *BMJ* 316(7130):504–509, 1998.
89. Price CP, Newall RG, Boyd JC: Use of protein:creatinine ratio measurements on random urine samples for prediction of significant proteinuria: a systematic review. *Clin Chem* 51(9):1577–1586, 2005.
106. Robinson RR: Isolated proteinuria in asymptomatic patients. *Nephrology Forum* 18:395–406, 1980.
112. Witte EC, Lambers Heerspink HJ, de Zeeuw D, et al: First morning voids are more reliable than spot urine samples to assess microalbuminuria. *J Am Soc Nephrol* 20(2):436–443, 2009.

113. Methven S, Macgregor MS, Traynor JP, et al: Comparison of urinary albumin and urinary total protein as predictors of patient outcomes in CKD. *Am J Kidney Dis* 57(1):21–28, 2011.
129. Iseki K, Kinjo K, Iseki C, et al: Relationship between predicted creatinine clearance and proteinuria and the risk of developing ESRD in Okinawa, Japan. *Am J Kidney Dis* 44(5):806–814, 2004.
130. Craig JC, Barratt A, Cumming R, et al: Feasibility study of the early detection and treatment of renal disease by mass screening. *Intern Med J* 32(1–2):6–14, 2002.
131. Boulware LE, Jaar BG, Tarver-Carr ME, et al: Screening for proteinuria in US adults: a cost-effectiveness analysis. *JAMA* 290(23):3101–3114, 2003.
132. Samal L, Linder JA: The primary care perspective on routine urine dipstick screening to identify patients with albuminuria. *Clin J Am Soc Nephrol* 8(1):131–135, 2013.
150. Hogg RJ, Portman RJ, Milliner D, et al: Evaluation and management of proteinuria and nephrotic syndrome in children: recommendations from a pediatric nephrology panel established at the National Kidney Foundation conference on proteinuria, albuminuria, risk, assessment, detection, and elimination (PARADE). *Pediatrics* 105(6):1242–1249, 2000.
158. Panek R, Lawen T, Kiberd BA: Screening for proteinuria in kidney transplant recipients. *Nephrol Dial Transplant* 26(4):1385–1387, 2011.
163. Vivante A, Afek A, Frenkel-Nir Y, et al: Persistent asymptomatic isolated microscopic hematuria in Israeli adolescents and young adults and risk for end-stage renal disease. *JAMA* 306(7):729–736, 2011.
164. Offringa M, Benbassat J: The value of urinary red cell shape in the diagnosis of glomerular and post-glomerular haematuria. A meta-analysis. *Postgrad Med J* 68(802):648–654, 1992.
166. Mishriki SF, Aboumarzouk O, Vint R, et al: Routine urine cytology has no role in hematuria investigations. *J Urol* 189(4):1255–1258, 2013.
167. Wald R, Bell CM, Nisenbaum R, et al: Interobserver reliability of urine sediment interpretation. *Clin J Am Soc Nephrol* 4(3):567–571, 2009.

27 Interpretation of Electrolyte and Acid-Base Parameters in Blood and Urine

Kamel S. Kamel | Mogamet R. Davids | Shih-Hua Lin | Mitchell L. Halperin

CHAPTER OUTLINE

WATER AND SODIUM, 804
Polyuria, 804
Water Diuresis, 805
Osmotic Diuresis, 811
Decreased Effective Arterial Blood Volume, 813
Hyponatremia, 815
POTASSIUM, 818
Transcellular Distribution of Potassium, 818

METABOLIC ALKALOSIS, 830
METABOLIC ACIDOSIS, 833
Clinical Approach: Intial Steps, 835
Metabolic Acidosis Due to Added Acids, 835
Clinical Approach to the Patient with Metabolic Acidosis Due to Added Acids, 838
Hyperchloremic Metabolic Acidosis, 840
Clinical Approach to the Patient with Hyperchloremic Metabolic Acidosis, 841

An analysis of laboratory data from samples of blood and urine is essential to make accurate diagnoses and to design optimal therapy for patients with disturbances of water, sodium (Na^+), potassium (K^+), and acid-base homeostasis.[1] Our clinical approach and interpretation of these tests rely heavily on an understanding of concepts in renal physiology. Hence each section begins with a discussion of physiologic concepts that help focus on the important factor(s) in the regulation of the homeostasis of the substances in question. This discussion is followed by a discussion of the clinical tools that utilize the laboratory data to help determine the underlying pathophysiology of the disturbance. This information is then used to construct our approach to patients with each of these disorders. At the end of each section, Consults are presented succinctly to illustrate how this approach is used at the bedside.

We emphasize that there are no normal values for the urinary excretion of water and electrolytes, because subjects in steady state excrete all ions that are consumed and not lost by nonrenal routes. Hence data should be interpreted in the context of the prevailing stimulus and the "expected" renal response.

WATER AND SODIUM

In this section, we illustrate how we use information about the volume and composition of the urine in the differential diagnosis and treatment of disorders causing polyuria, those causing decreased effective arterial blood volume (EABV), and those causing hyponatremia.

POLYURIA

There are two definitions of polyuria.

Conventional Definition: Polyuria is defined as a urine volume that is more than 2.5 L/day. This is an arbitrary definition based on comparing the 24-hour urine volume with usual values observed in individuals who consume a typical Western diet.

Physiology-Based Definition: Polyuria is defined as a urine flow rate that is higher than what is expected in a specific setting. Polyuria is present if the urine volume is higher than what is expected for the rate of excretion of effective osmoles in the presence of actions of vasopressin even if the urine volume does not exceed 2.5 L/day. In contrast, if the concentration of Na^+ in plasma (P_{Na}) is less than 136 mmol/L, the release of vasopressin should be inhibited and the urine flow rate should be as high as 10 to 15 mL/min in an adult subject (which extrapolates to 14 to 21 L/day). A lower urine volume in this setting, even if higher than 2.5 L/day, represents oliguria rather than polyuria.

CLASSIFICATION

There are two categories of polyuria, a water diuresis and an osmotic diuresis.

WATER DIURESIS

CONCEPT 1

To move water across a membrane, there must be a channel that allows water to cross that membrane (an aquaporin [AQP]) and a driving force for the movement of water (a difference in the concentrations of effective osmoles or a difference in the hydrostatic pressures across that membrane).

WATER CHANNELS

There are two critically important aquaporin water channels in the luminal membranes of cells in the kidney, AQP1 and AQP2. With regard to water excretion, we divide the nephron into three functional units on the basis of the presence of AQP1 or AQP2. AQP1 channels are nonregulated water channels that are present in the proximal convoluted tubule (PCT) cells (the first functional nephron unit) (Figure 27.1). AQP1 channels are also present in the descending thin limbs of the loop of Henle (DtLs) of the juxtamedullary nephrons, which constitute about 15% of the total nephrons (the second functional nephron unit). Of note, AQP1 channels are not present in the DtLs of the superficial nephrons, making the entire loop of Henle of the superficial nephrons (i.e., 85% of all the nephrons) relatively impermeable to water.[2]

Vasopressin causes the insertion of AQP2 channels into the luminal membrane of principal cells in the late distal convoluted tubule (DCT), the connecting segment, the cortical collecting duct (CCD), and the medullary collecting duct (MCD) (together, these nephron segments constitute the final or third functional unit). AQP2 channels permit water to be reabsorbed in the presence of an osmotic driving force. Notwithstanding, even in the absence of vasopressin, there seems to be a small degree of water permeability in the inner MCD, called basal or residual water permeability.

DRIVING FORCE

Water is drawn from a compartment with a lower effective osmolality to one with a higher effective osmolality. The magnitude of this force is enormous, in that a difference of 1 mOsm/kg H_2O generates a pressure of about 19.3 mm Hg. The osmolality of fluid that reaches the late DCT is close to 100 mOsm/L. Hence, the effective osmotic pressure difference is about 200 mOsm/L; interstitial effective osmolality is ≈ 300 mOsm/L, because it is equal to the effective plasma osmolality (P_{osm}), which is double the concentration of sodium (Na^+) in plasma water (P_{Na}), which is ≈ 150 mmol/L). Hence the osmotic driving force is almost 4000 mm Hg (19.3 mm Hg × 200 mOsm/L). Because AQP2 channels are present in the luminal membranes of cells of the late cortical distal nephron (CDN) when vasopressin acts, two thirds of the water delivered to the late CDN is reabsorbed here. It follows that in patients with a severe degree of chronic hyponatremia and thereby a lower effective cortical interstitial osmolality, more water is delivered to and reabsorbed in the MCD. Hence in this setting, there is washout of the medullary interstitial fluid compartment, and hence the urine effective osmolality falls.

CONCEPT 2

The maximum volume of urine during a water diuresis is equal to the volume of distal delivery of filtrate minus the small volume of filtrate reabsorbed in the inner MCD via its residual water permeability (RWP).[3]

DISTAL DELIVERY OF FILTRATE

The volume of distal delivery of filtrate is the volume of glomerular filtration minus the volume of filtrate that is reabsorbed in the nephron segments prior to the late CDN. Findings now suggest that AQP1 channels are not present in the luminal membranes of the DtLs in the superficial nephrons (i.e., 85% of all the nephrons).[2] Therefore, the entire loop of Henle of the majority of these nephrons is impermeable to water. Hence, the volume of distal delivery of filtrate should be equal to the volume of glomerular filtration minus the volume that is reabsorbed by PCT (including its pars recta segment).

It was thought that about 66% of the glomerular filtration rate (GFR) is reabsorbed along the entire PCT. This idea was based on the measured ratio of inulin concentrations in fluid from the PCT (TF) in comparison with that in plasma (P)—(TF/P)inulin—in micropuncture studies in rats. Because inulin is freely filtered at the glomerulus and is not reabsorbed or secreted in the tubules, a (TF/P)inulin value of around 3 suggests that approximately 66% of the filtrate was reabsorbed in the PCT. However, these micropuncture measurements underestimate the volume of fluid reabsorbed in the PCT, because measurements were made

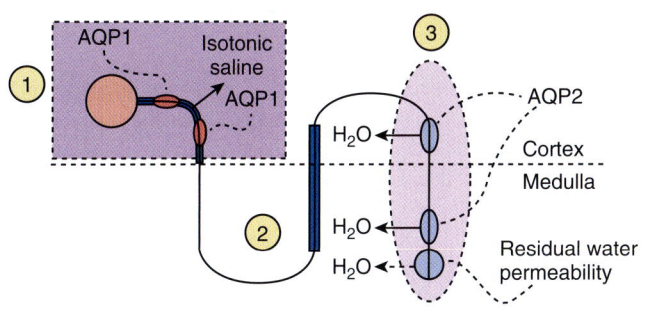

Figure 27.1 Functional units of the nephron based on presence of aquaporins AQP1 and AQP2. The stylized structure represents a nephron; AQP1 is represented as a *small pink oval*, and AQP2 as *blue ovals*. The *solid line* represents the descending thin limb of the loop of Henle (DtL). With regard to water excretion, we divide the nephron into three functional units on the basis of the presence of AQP1 or AQP2. AQP1 is always present in the proximal convoluted tubule (PCT) cells—the first functional nephron unit **(1)**, shown within the *rectangle*). AQP1 is also present in DtLs of the juxtamedullary nephrons, which constitute about 15% of the total nephrons—the second functional nephron unit **(2)**, shown as a *blue rectangle*. AQP1 is not present in the DtLs of the superficial nephrons, making the entire loop of Henle of the superficial nephrons (i.e., 85% of all the nephrons) impermeable to water. Vasopressin causes the insertion of AQP2 into the luminal membrane of principal cells in the late distal convoluted tubule (DCT), the connecting segment, the cortical collecting duct (CCD), and the medullary collecting duct (MCD); together, these nephron segments constitute the final or third functional unit **(3)**, shown within the *large oval*). Notwithstanding, even in the absence of vasopressin, there seems to be a small degree of water permeability in the inner MCD (called basal or residual water permeability). (Reproduced with the permission of the author and the publisher from Halperin ML: *The ACID truth and BASIC facts—with a sweet touch, an enLYTEnment,* 6th ed, Toronto, 2015, RossMark Medical Publishers.)

at the last portion of the PCT at the surface of the renal cortex and hence did not take into account that additional volume may have been reabsorbed in the deeper part of the PCT, including its pars recta portion.

If the majority of nephrons in the entire loop of Henle lack AQP1 and thereby should mainly be impermeable to water, the volume of filtrate that enters their loops of Henle can be deduced through the use of the minimum value for the (TF/P)inulin obtained using the micropuncture technique from the early DCT, which has been done in rats. Because this value is around 6, a reasonable estimate of the proportion of filtrate that is reabsorbed in the rat PCTs is close to five sixths (83%). This value is close to the estimate of fractional reabsorption in PCTs obtained with measurement of lithium clearance (which is thought to be a marker for fractional reabsorption in PCT) in human subjects.

When these findings are extrapolated to humans with GFR values of 180 L/day, only about 30 L of filtrate per day (180 ÷ 6) would be delivered to the DCT if all nephrons were superficial. This number needs to be adjusted downward because juxtamedullary nephrons have AQP1 along their DtLs. If these nephrons are 15% of the total and receive 27 L of glomerular filtrate per day (15% of 180 L/day), and if five sixths of the glomerular filtrate of these nephrons is reabsorbed along their PCTs, 4.5 L/day reach their DtLs. Because the interstitial osmolality rises threefold (from 300 to 900 mOsmol/kg H_2O) in the outer medulla, two thirds, or 3 L of the 4.5 L/day, are reabsorbed in the DtLs of these nephrons. Therefore, the volume of filtrate delivered to DCTs is likely to be 27 L/day (30 L/day exit the PCTs minus 3 L/day that are reabsorbed in DtLs of the juxtamedullary nephrons).

RESIDUAL WATER PERMEABILITY

There are two pathways for transport of water in the inner MCD, a vasopressin-responsive system via AQP2 and a vasopressin-independent system called residual water permeability. Two factors may affect the volume of water reabsorbed by RWP. The driving force is the enormous difference in osmotic pressure between the luminal and interstitial fluid compartments in the inner MCD during a water diuresis, which should drive the reabsorption of water via RWP. The second factor is contraction of the renal pelvis. Each time the renal pelvis contracts, some of the fluid in the renal pelvis travels in a retrograde direction up toward the inner MCD; some of that fluid may be reabsorbed via RWP after it enters the inner MCD for a second (or a third) time, especially if there is some turbulence, which aids diffusion and prolongs contact time.

As calculated previously, 27 L/day are delivered to the distal nephron in a normal subject, and the urine flow rate during maximum water diuresis is around 10 to 15 mL/min (≈14 to 22 L/day). If this maximum water diuresis could be maintained for 24 hours, somewhat more than 5 L of water would be reabsorbed per day in the inner MCD by RWP during water diuresis.

CONCEPT 3

Another component of the physiology of water diuresis is "desalination" of luminal fluid in nephron segments that can reabsorb Na^+ but lack water channel.

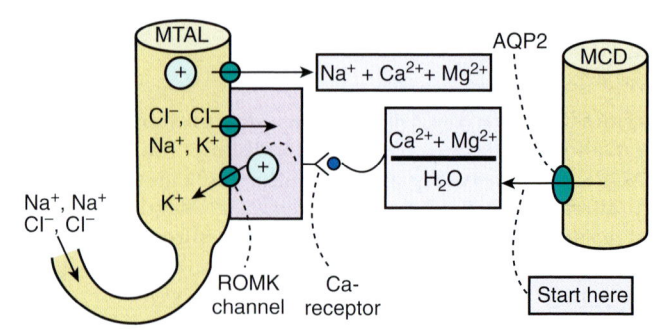

Figure 27.2 Regulation of the concentrating process in the renal medulla by the concentration of ionized calcium in the medullary interstitial compartment. To reabsorb Na^+ and Cl^- in the medullary thick ascending limb (mTAL) of the loop of Henle, K^+ must enter its lumen via renal outer medullary K^+ (ROMK) channels to be a substrate for the Na-K-2Cl cotransporter. This creates a lumen-positive voltage that drives the passive reabsorption of Na^+ and Ca^{2+} via the paracellular pathway (tight junction protein: claudins 16 and 19). Once the activity of Ca^{2+} rises sufficiently in the medullary interstitial compartment, a signal is generated to inhibit flux of K^+ through luminal ROMK and, hence, further reabsorption of Na^+ and Cl^- in this nephron unit. When water is reabsorbed from the medullary collecting duct (MCD), the concentration of ionized Ca^{2+} in the medullary interstitial compartment falls. This drop removes the inhibition on the flux of K^+ through luminal ROMK, leading to reabsorption of more Na^+ and Ca^{2+} until the activity of Ca^{2+} rises sufficiently in the medullary interstitial compartment to reestablish the cycle of inhibitory control. (Reproduced with the permission of the author and the publisher from Halperin ML: *The ACID truth and BASIC facts—with a sweet touch, an enLYTEnment*, 6th ed, Toronto, 2015, RossMark Medical Publishers.)

The desalination process occurs in the cortical and medullary thick ascending limbs (TALs) of the loop of Henle and the early DCT (the middle functional nephron unit).

Regulation of the reabsorption of Na^+ and Cl^- in the medullary TAL (mTAL) seems to occur via dilution of the concentration of an inhibitor of this process in the medullary interstitial compartment (possibly ionized calcium, Figure 27.2), by water reabsorption from the water-permeable nephron segments in the renal medulla (i.e., the MCD and the DtLs of the juxtamedullary nephrons).[4]

TOOLS FOR ASSESSING WATER DIURESIS

Urine Flow Rate

The maximum volume of urine during water diuresis is equal to the volume of distal delivery of filtrate minus the small volume of filtrate reabsorbed in the inner MCD via RWP. Hence, the peak urine flow rate is about 10 to 15 mL/min (about 14 to 22 L/day). If the urine volume is considerably less than 10 L/day, one should look for a reason for decreased distal delivery of filtrate. Notwithstanding, the distal delivery of filtrate will ultimately fall, and this high urine flow rate is not likely to be sustained.

The urine flow rate declines when desmopressin (dDAVP) is given to a patient with central diabetes insipidus (DI). The urine flow rate, however, will be higher than that observed in response to dDAVP in a normal subject who consumes a typical Western diet. The reason is that the medullary interstitial osmolality is likely to be lower owing to a prior medullary washout during the water diuresis.

Osmole Excretion Rate

The osmole excretion rate is equal to the product of the urine osmolality (U_{osm}) and the urine flow rate (see Equation 1). In subjects eating a typical Western diet, the rate of excretion of osmoles is 600 to 900 mOsm/day, with electrolytes and urea each accounting for close to half of the urine osmoles. During a water diuresis, a change in the rate of excretion of osmoles does not directly affect the urine volume, because AQP2 should not be present in the luminal membrane of principal cells in the final functional unit of the nephron. Nevertheless, the rate of excretion of osmoles must be calculated in the patient with a water diuresis because if high, it will lead to polyuria due to an osmotic diuresis, once there is a renal response to the administration of dDAVP.

$$\text{Osmole excretion rate} = U_{osm} \times \text{Urine flow rate} \quad (1)$$

Urine Osmolality

The U_{osm} is equal to the number of excreted osmoles divided by the urine volume. Therefore during a water diuresis, a change in the U_{osm} could reflect a change in the osmole excretion rate and/or in the volume of filtrate delivered to the distal nephron (which largely determines the urine volume in this setting). For example, if the rate of excretion of osmoles is 800 mOsm/day, the U_{osm} is 50 mOsm/L if the 24-hour urine volume is 16 L, and 100 mOsm/L if the 24-hour urine volume is 8 L. A note of caution is needed—a rise in the U_{osm} following the administration of dDAVP may reflect a fall in the distal delivery of filtrate due to a fall in blood pressure and the GFR rather than a renal response to dDAVP with the insertion of AQP2 in the luminal membrane of principal cells.

Electrolyte-Free Water Balance

Calculation of the electrolyte-free water balance is based on how much water is needed to make all of the $Na^+ + K^+$ into a solution with a tonicity equal to the normal plasma tonicity (i.e., 150 mmol in 1 L of water). To perform this calculation, one must know the volume of and the concentrations of $Na^+ + K^+$ in the input and in the urine.

For example, a patient received 3 L of 0.9% saline (Na^+ concentration = 150 mmol/L) and excreted 3 L of urine with a concentration of ($Na^+ + K^+$) of 50 mmol/L. There is no electrolyte-free water in the input. With regard to the output, this patient excreted 1 L of isotonic salt solution and 2 L of electrolyte-free water. Hence, the patient has a negative electrolyte-free water balance of 2 L and the P_{Na} will rise. Another patient received 3 L of 0.9% saline but excreted 3 L of urine, each of which has a concentration of ($Na^+ + K^+$) of 200 mmol/L. As in the first example, there is no electrolyte-free water in the input. With regard to the output, because this patient would have needed to excrete 4 L (and not 3 L) of urine to make this total of 600 mmol of $Na^+ + K^+$ into an isotonic solution, the patient has a positive electrolyte-free water balance of 1 L and hence the P_{Na} will fall (i.e., a deficit of $Na^+ + K^+$ of 150 mmol resulted in making 1 L of body water into 1 L of electrolyte-free water). As shown in Table 27.1, although the balances for $Na^+ + K^+$ and for water are very different in three examples used, calculation of electrolyte-free water balance provided the same answer, a negative balance of 2 L of electrolyte-free water. Therefore, although calculation of electrolyte-free water balance correctly predicts the change in P_{Na}, it does not reveal whether its basis is a change in water balance or, in fact, a change in $Na^+ + K^+$ balance. Hence, this calculation is not helpful to design the therapy needed to return the volume and composition of the extracellular fluid (ECF) and intracellular fluid (ICF) compartments to their normal values.

Tonicity Balance

To decide what the basis is for a change in the P_{Na} and to define the proper therapy to return the volume and composition of the ECF and ICF compartments to their normal values, separate balances for water and $Na^+ + K^+$ must be calculated.[5] To perform a tonicity balance, one must examine the input and output volumes and the quantity of Na^+ and K^+ infused and excreted over the period when the P_{Na} changed (Figure 27.3). In practical terms, a tonicity balance can be performed only in a hospital setting, where inputs and outputs are accurately recorded. In a febrile patient, balance calculations will not be as accurate because sweat losses are not measured. Nevertheless, restricting the analysis of the output to the urine data would be sufficient in an acute setting.

Even if measurements of the concentrations of Na^+ and K^+ in the urine are not available, if the P_{Na} at the beginning and the end of a certain period, the volume of the urine,

Table 27.1 Comparison of a Tonicity Balance and an Electrolyte-Free Water Balance in a Patient with Hypernatremia

	$Na^+ + K^+$ (mmol)	Water (L)	Electrolyte-Free Water (L)
Infusion of 3 L of isotonic saline:			
Input	450	3	0
Output	150	3	2
Balance	**+300**	**0**	**−2**
Infusion of 4 L of isotonic saline:			
Input	600	4	0
Output	150	3	2
Balance	**+450**	**+1**	**−2**
No intravenous fluid infusion:			
Input	0	0	0
Output	150	3	2
Balance	**−150**	**−3**	**−2**

Three settings are described, in which the P_{Na} rises from 140 to 150 mmol/L. The only difference is the volume of isotonic saline infused in each setting. Note that although the balances for $Na^+ + K^+$ and for water are very different in these three examples, calculation of electrolyte-free water shows a negative balance of 2 L of electrolyte-free water in all of them. The goals for therapy—to correct the hypernatremia and to return the volume and the composition of the extracellular and intracellular fluid compartments to their normal values—are clear only after a tonicity balance is calculated.

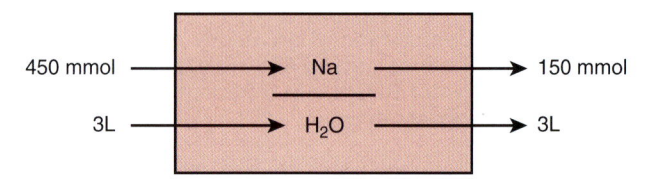

Figure 27.3 Tonicity balance to determine the basis for a rise in the P_{Na}. Performing a tonicity balance requires the input and output volumes and the quantity of Na^+ and K^+ infused and excreted in the urine. The values in this figure are from the patient discussed in Consult 2. The patient had an acute rise in P_{Na} from 140 mmol/L to 150 mmol/L. The tonicity balance illustrated here indicates that the basis for the rise in her P_{Na} was due to a positive balance of 300 mmol of Na^+, and not a negative balance of water. Therefore, the goal of therapy is to induce a negative balance of 300 mmol of Na^+ while maintaining water balance. (Reproduced with the permission of the author and the publisher from Halperin ML: The ACID truth and BASIC facts—with a sweet touch, an enLYTEnment, 6th ed, Toronto, Ross-Mark Medical Publishers, 2015.)

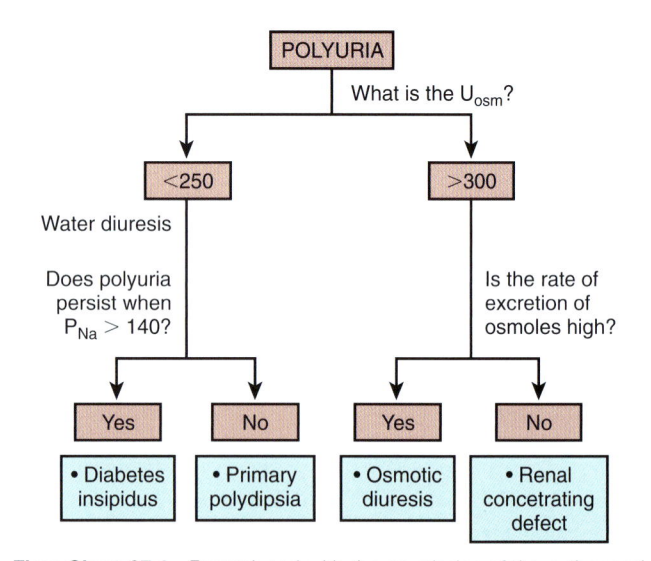

Flow Chart 27.1 Reproduced with the permission of the author and the publisher from Halperin ML: *The ACID truth and BASIC facts—with a sweet touch, an enLYTEnment*, 6th ed, Toronto, 2015, RossMark Medical Publishers.

and the volume and amount of $Na^+ + K^+$ in the fluid infused during that period are known, the clinician can use these data to calculate the quantity of $Na^+ + K^+$ in the urine so as to determine why the P_{Na} changed.

CLINICAL APPROACH TO THE PATIENT WITH A WATER DIURESIS

The steps to take to determine the diagnosis in a patient with a water diuresis are outlined in Flow Charts 27.1 and 27.2.

Step 1: What Is the U_{osm}?

A value of the U_{osm} that is less than 250 mOsm/kg H_2O suggests that the basis of polyuria is a water diuresis. A large water diuresis is the expected physiologic response to a water intake that is large enough to cause the arterial P_{Na} to fall below 136 mmol/L. In this case, the diagnosis is primary polydipsia. Once the P_{Na} has returned to the normal range, the urine flow rate should decrease and the U_{osm} should rise appropriately, although one must keep in mind that the prior water diuresis may have caused a lower medullary interstitial osmolality due to medullary washout. In contrast, diabetes insipidus is present if a water diuresis persists when the P_{Na} is higher than 140 mmol/L.

Calculate the osmole excretion rate (Equation 1)—the usual value is close to 0.6 mOsm/min (600-900 mOsm/day) in subjects consuming a typical Western diet. If the osmole excretion rate is more than double this rate, an osmotic diuresis will ensue once the patient has a renal response to the administration of vasopressin or its dDAVP analog. This response may lead to significant changes in the P_{Na} and hence brain cell volume, depending on the concentrations of Na^+ and K^+ in the urine and the tonicity of administered fluids.

Step 2: Examine the Renal Response to Vasopressin or dDAVP (see Flow Chart 27.2)

Diabetes insipidus could be due to a lesion in the hypothalamic–posterior pituitary axis, which controls the production and/or release of vasopressin (central DI),

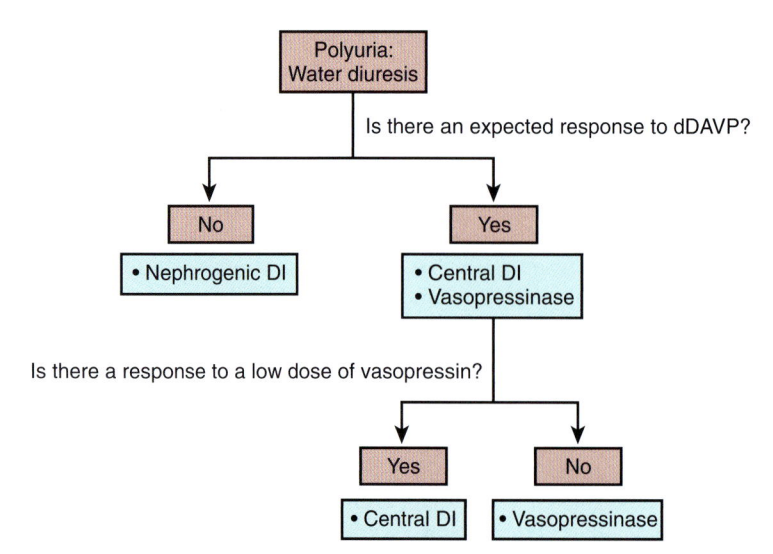

Flow Chart 27.2 Reproduced with the permission of the author and the publisher from Halperin ML: *The ACID truth and BASIC facts—with a sweet touch, an enLYTEnment*, 6th ed, Toronto, 2015, RossMark Medical Publishers.

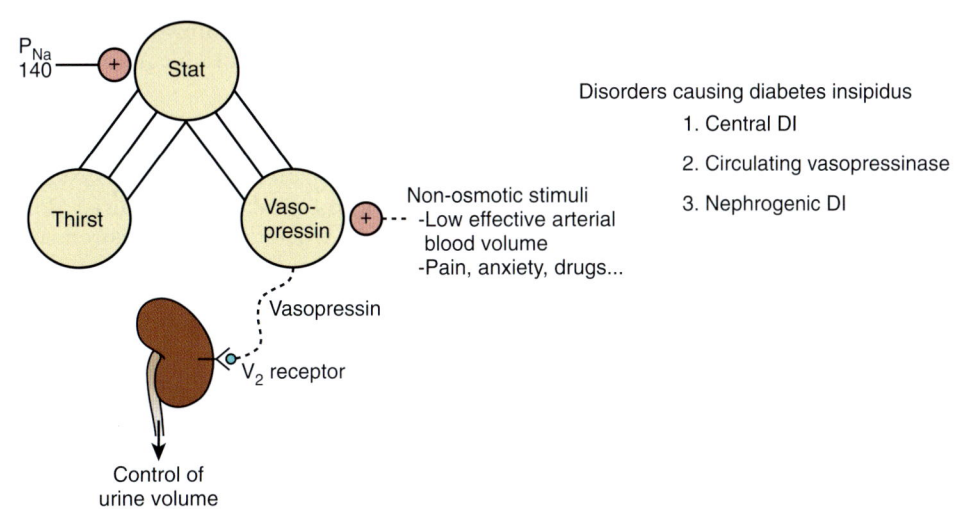

Figure 27.4 Water control system. Left, The sensor is the osmostat or tonicity stat *(top circle)*, which detects a change in P_{Na} via an effect on the volume of its cells. The tonicity stat is linked to the thirst center *(left circle)* and to the vasopressin release center *(right circle)*. Nonosmotic stimuli (e.g., certain drugs, nausea, pain, anxiety) also influence the release of vasopressin. Vasopressin release is also stimulated when there is a large decrease in the effective arterial blood volume (EABV); a lower P_{Na} is needed to suppress the release of vasopressin in this setting. When vasopressin acts, the urine flow rate is directly proportional to the number of effective osmoles in the inner medullary collecting duct and indirectly proportional to the effective osmolality in the inner medullary interstitial compartment. The clinical disorders associated with polyuria due to a water diuresis (i.e., diabetes insipidus [DI]) and the sites of these lesions are listed on the **right**. (Reproduced with the permission of the author and the publisher from Halperin ML: *The ACID truth and BASIC facts—with a sweet touch, an enLYTEnment,* 6th ed, Toronto, 2015, RossMark Medical Publishers.)

the presence of a circulating vasopressinase that breaks down vasopressin, or a renal lesion that prevents the binding of vasopressin to its V_2 receptor (V_2R) and/or causes the insertion of AQP2 in the luminal membrane of principal cells in the final functional unit of the nephron (nephrogenic DI) (see Figure 27.1).

If the water diuresis is curtailed by the administration of dDAVP, the diagnosis is central DI or the release of an enzyme that hydrolyzes vasopressin in plasma (a vasopressinase). If there is a reason to suspect the latter, one should examine the response to the administration of vasopressin after the effect of dDAVP has worn off and the patient is having a water diuresis again. In contrast to the response to the administration of dDAVP, a patient in whom a vasopressinase has been released will not show response to the administration of a small dose of vasopressin.

Step 3: Establish the Basis for Central Diabetes Insipidus

The central water control system (Figure 27.4) should be examined for a lesion that has caused the defect in vasopressin biosynthesis or release. An important part of this workup is to determine in a patient with hypernatremia whether thirst is present; its absence suggests that the defect involves the hypothalamic osmostat (*tonicity stat* is a better term because it refers only to effective osmoles; i.e., it ignores the osmotic contribution of urea, because cell membranes of most organs have transporters for urea and thus they are permeable to urea).

Step 4: Establish the Basis for Nephrogenic Diabetes Insipidus

If dDAVP fails to cause an appropriate decrease in the urine flow rate (depending on the rate of excretion of effective osmoles) and the appropriate rise in the effective U_{osm} (depending on the value of medullary interstitial effective osmolality, which is usually lower from a prior water diuresis), the diagnosis is the AQP2 deficiency type of nephrogenic DI. Hereditary nephrogenic DI could be due to an X-linked recessive, V_2R mutation (more common), or autosomal recessive or dominant AQP2 mutations. In the noninherited disorders, the most common cause of nephrogenic DI in an adult is the ingestion of lithium.

CONSULT 1: WHAT IS "PARTIAL" ABOUT PARTIAL CENTRAL DIABETES INSIPIDUS?

A 32-year-old healthy man had a recent basal skull fracture. Since his head injury, his urine output had been consistently about 4 L/day and his U_{osm} around 200 mOsm/kg H_2O in multiple 24-hour urine collections. In blood samples drawn early in the morning, his P_{Na} was around 143 mmol/L, and vasopressin was not detectable in his plasma. During the daytime, his U_{osm} was consistently around 90 mOsm/kg H_2O and his P_{Na} 137 mmol/L. When he was given dDAVP, his urine flow rate decreased to 0.5 mL/min and the U_{osm} rose to 900 mOsm/kg H_2O. He noted that if he stopped drinking water after supper, his sleep was not interrupted by a need to void. In fact, his U_{osm} was around 425 mOsm/kg H_2O in several overnight urine samples. Of interest, his urine flow rate fell to 0.5 mL/min and his U_{osm} rose to 900 mOsm/kg H_2O after an infusion of hypertonic saline.

Questions

- Is this a water diuresis?
- What are the best options for therapy in this patient?

Discussion of Questions

Is This a Water Diuresis? Because the patient's U_{osm} was 200 mOsm/kg H_2O and the urine volume was 4 L/day, this was a water diuresis with the usual total osmole excretion

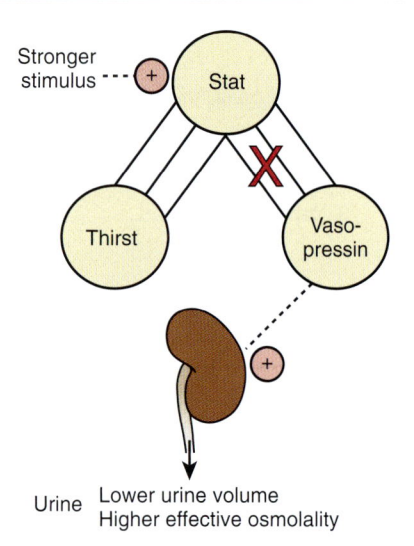

Figure 27.5 Lesion causing "partial" central diabetes insipidus. The *top circle* represents the osmostat or tonicity stat, which is the sensor, the *left circle* the thirst center, and the *right circle* the vasopressin release center. The *X* symbol represents a hypothetical lesion that causes severing of some but not all of the fibers connecting the tonicity stat to the vasopressin release center. (Reproduced with the permission of the author and the publisher from Halperin ML: *The ACID truth and BASIC facts—with a sweet touch, an enLYTEnment,* 6th ed, Toronto, 2015, RossMark Medical Publishers.)

rate for a subject consuming a typical Western diet (800 mOsm/day) (see Flow Chart 27.1). The patient had an adequate renal response to dDAVP because his U_{osm} rose to 900 mOsm/kg H_2O. Hence he had central DI. Because his urine volume was only 4 L/day and not 10 to 15 L/day, the diagnosis was "partial" central DI.

Central Diabetes Insipidus: Although the diagnosis of central DI was straightforward, there were two facts that have not yet been interpreted. First, because he complained of thirst, the patient's "tonicity stat" and thirst center, as well as the fibers connecting them, appeared to be functionally intact (see Figure 27.4). Similarly, because the U_{osm} was greater than the P_{osm} in the first-voided morning urine (U_{osm} was 425 mOsm/kg H_2O) when the P_{Na} was 143 mmol/L, the vasopressin release center seemed to function but only when there was a "relatively strong stimulus" for the release of this hormone (P_{Na} of 143 mmol/L). In keeping with this hypothesis is the fact that the urine flow rate fell to 0.5 mL/min and the U_{osm} rose to 900 mOsm/kg H_2O after an infusion of hypertonic saline. Therefore a possible site for the lesion is destruction of some but not of all of the fibers linking the tonicity stat to the vasopressin release center (Figure 27.5). Such a lesion might explain why polyuria was not present overnight if the patient stopped water intake several hours prior to going to sleep. This example provides insights into the pathophysiology of partial central DI.[6]

Primary Polydipsia: The patient's P_{Na} was high enough early in the morning (143 mmol/L) to stimulate the release of vasopressin. In contrast, during the daytime, his P_{Na} was 137 mmol/L and his U_{osm} was consistently around 90 mOsm/kg H_2O, which suggest that primary polydipsia was present while he was awake. Its basis probably was a "learned behavior" to avoid the uncomfortable feeling of thirst. This interpretation provides a rationale to understand the pathophysiology and, importantly, the options for treatment of his partial central DI.

What Are the Best Options for Therapy? The major point here is that a higher P_{Na} could stimulate the release of vasopressin. The patient selected oral NaCl tablets to raise his P_{Na} to control his daytime polyuria. Moreover, this therapy avoided the risk of acute hyponatremia, which might occur if he were given dDAVP and drank an excessive quantity of water by habit. In contrast, he selected water deprivation to raise his P_{Na} overnight, which seemed to permit him to have undisturbed sleep.

CONSULT 2: IN A PATIENT WITH CENTRAL DIABETES INSIPIDUS, WHY DID POLYURIA PERSIST AFTER THE ADMINISTRATION OF dDAVP?

A 16-year-old male (weight 50 kg, total body water 30 L) underwent craniopharyngioma resection in the morning. Over the next 5 hours his urine output was 3 L (urine flow rate 10 mL/min). The P_{Na} rose from 140 to 150 mmol/L. During this time, he received 3 L of isotonic saline. The U_{osm} was 120 mOsm/kg H_2O and the urine $Na^+ + K^+$ concentration was 50 mmol/L. To confirm the diagnosis of central DI, he was given dDAVP, and the urine flow rate fell to 6 mL/min, the U_{osm} rose to 375 mOsm/kg H_2O, and the urine $Na^+ + K^+$ concentration rose to 175 mmol/L.

Additional Questions
- Does the drop in the patient's urine flow rate to 6 mL/min represent a partial response to dDAVP?
- Why did the P_{Na} rise from 140 to 150 mmol/L during the large water diuresis?

Discussion of Additional Questions

Does the Drop in the Patient's Urine Flow Rate to 6 mL/min Represent a Partial Response to dDAVP? When dDAVP acts, the urine flow rate is directly proportional to the osmole excretion rate and inversely proportional to the medullary interstitial osmolality. The expected urine flow rate in response to dDAVP in a subject who consumes a typical Western diet (≈900 osmoles/day, of which half is electrolyte osmoles and the other half is urea osmoles) and has a medullary interstitial osmolality of 900 mOsm/kg H_2O (half of which is electrolyte osmoles and the other half is urea osmoles) is about 0.7 mL/min. The osmole excretion rate in this patient before the administration of dDAVP was 1.2 mOsm/min—U_{osm} (120 mOsm/kg H_2O) × urine flow rate (10 mL/min). This value was double the usual osmole excretion rate (0.6 mOsm/min) in subjects consuming a typical Western diet. Another point merits emphasis with regard to the nature of excreted osmoles. Prior to the administration of dDAVP, five sixths of the osmoles in the urine were $Na^+ + K^+$ salts—$2(U_{Na} + U_K) = 100$ mmol/L; $U_{osm} = 120$ mOsm/kg H_2O. Because electrolytes are effective osmoles in the urine but urea is not usually an effective osmole in the urine when vasopressin acts, most of osmoles in the patient's urine were effective osmoles, which obligate the excretion of water after dDAVP acts.

It is also important to recognize that because of a prior water diuresis, there would be a degree of washout of the renal medulla. Hence the maximum U_{osm} in response to the administration of dDAVP would be significantly lower than that observed in normal subjects. That fact may explain why this patient's U_{osm} rose to only 375 mOsm/kg H_2O following the administration of dDAVP.

On the basis of the preceding findings and discussion, the drop in the patient's urine flow rate to only about 6 mL/min represented not a partial response to dDAVP but, rather, the expected response because of the high rate of excretion of effective osmoles (osmotic diuresis) and the low medullary interstitial osmolality (urinary concentrating defect due to medullary washout).

Why Did the P_{Na} Rise from 140 to 150 mmol/L During the Large Water Diuresis? Although the tendency here is to assume that this patient's hypernatremia was due to a water deficit because he had a large water diuresis, the basis of the rise in his P_{Na} can be revealed with calculation of tonicity balance.

Calculate the tonicity balance:

Water Balance: The patient received 3 L of isotonic saline, and hence had an input of 3 L of water. He excreted 3 L of urine, so there is a nil balance of water.

Na^+ + K^+ Balance: The patient received 450 mmol (3 L × 150 mmol Na^+/L) and excreted only 150 mmol (3 L urine × 50 mmol Na^+/L). Hence he had a positive balance of 300 mmol of Na^+. When one divides this surplus of Na^+ by the total body water (30 L), the rise in P_{Na} is 10 mmol/L, a value equal to the actual rise in P_{Na}. Therefore the basis for the rise in P_{Na} was a positive balance of Na^+ rather than a deficit of water. The proper treatment to restore body tonicity and the volume and composition of the ECF and ICF compartments in this patient was to induce a negative balance of 300 mmol of Na^+ + K^+.

OSMOTIC DIURESIS

CONCEPT 4

The volume of the urine during an osmotic diuresis is directly proportional to the rate of excretion of effective osmoles and indirectly proportional to the medullary interstitial effective osmolality.

When vasopressin acts, AQP2 channels are present in the luminal membrane of the late distal nephron, so the U_{osm} should be equal to the medullary interstitial osmolality. Not all osmoles, however, are equal in their ability to increase the urine volume. Only osmoles that do not achieve equal concentrations in the lumen of the MCD and in the medullary interstitial compartment are effective osmoles; they determine what the urine flow rate will be.

Because cells in the inner MCD have urea transporters in their luminal membranes when vasopressin acts, urea is usually an "ineffective" osmole (the concentration of urea is equal on the two sides of that membrane) so it does not cause water to be excreted. The net result of excreting some extra urea is a higher U_{osm} but not a higher urine flow rate. Therefore, it is more correct to say that the urine flow rate is directly proportional to the number of non-urea or effective urine osmoles and inversely proportional to their concentration in the medullary interstitial compartment (Equation 2).

$$\text{Urine flow rate} = \text{\# effective urine osmoles} / \text{effective } U_{osm} \quad (2)$$

Urea, however, may be an effective urine osmole in some circumstances. When the rate of excretion of urea rises by a large amount, urea might not be absorbed fast enough to achieve equal concentrations in the lumen of the inner MCD and in the interstitium in the inner medulla. Hence, urea may become an effective osmole in the inner MCD and thereby obligate the excretion of water. Urea may be also an effective urine osmole if the rate of excretion of electrolytes is low.

CONCEPT 5

The medullary interstitial osmolality falls during an osmotic diuresis because of medullary washout.

During an osmotic diuresis, a larger number of liters of fluid is delivered to and reabsorbed in the MCD. Hence, medullary washout occurs and medullary interstitial osmolality falls. The "expected" medullary interstitial osmolality is about 600 mOsm/kg H_2O at somewhat high osmole excretion rates, and values closer to the P_{osm} are observed at much higher osmole excretion rates.

TOOLS FOR EVALUATION OF OSMOTIC DIURESIS

U_{osm}

The U_{osm} should be higher than the P_{osm}.

Osmole Excretion Rate

In an adult during an osmotic diuresis, the rate of excretion of osmoles should be much greater than 1000 mOsm/day (more than 0.7 mOsm/min).

Nature of the Urine Osmoles

The nature of the urine osmoles should be determined by measuring the rate of excretion of the individual osmoles in the urine. One can deduce which solute is likely to be responsible for the osmotic diuresis by measuring their concentrations in plasma (e.g., glucose, urea). A large amount of mannitol is rarely given; hence it is unlikely to be the sole cause of a large and sustained osmotic diuresis. A saline-induced osmotic diuresis may occur if there was a large infusion of saline or in a patient who has cerebral or renal salt wasting. For diagnosis of a state of salt wasting, there must be an appreciable excretion of Na^+ at a time when the EABV is definitely contracted.

Sources of the Urine Osmoles

In a patient with a glucose- or a urea-induced osmotic diuresis, it is important to decide whether these osmoles were derived from an exogenous source or from catabolism of endogenous proteins.

Sources of Urea

Urea Appearance Rate. The rate of appearance of urea can be determined from the amount of urea that is retained in the body plus the amount that is excreted in the urine over a given period. The former can be calculated from the rise in the concentration of urea in plasma (P_{urea}) and assuming a volume of distribution of urea equal to total body water ($\approx$60% of body weight in the absence of obesity).

One can use the following calculation to determine whether the source of urea was the breakdown of exogenous or endogenous proteins, if the intake of proteins is known.

Close to 16% of the weight of protein is nitrogen. Therefore if 100 g of protein were oxidized, 16 g of nitrogen would be formed. The molecular weight of nitrogen is 14, so about 1140 mmol of nitrogen would be produced. Because each mmol of urea contains two atoms of nitrogen, about 570 mmol of urea would be produced from the oxidation of 100 g of protein. In terms of lean body mass: Water is the main constituent in the body (80% of weight): each kg has 800 g of water and 180 g of protein. Therefore, breakdown of 1 kg of lean mass will produce about 1026 mmol of urea.

Sources of Glucose. The production of glucose from endogenous sources is relatively small. In more detail, only 60% of the weight of protein can be converted to glucose. Hence, to produce enough glucose from protein to induce 1 L of osmotic diuresis (≈300 mmol of glucose), one would need the catabolism of 90 g of protein (equivalent to the catabolism of 1 lb of lean body mass). Therefore, if there is a large glucose-induced osmotic diuresis, the glucose must be from an exogenous source (e.g., the ingestion of fruit juice or sugar-containing soft drinks).

CLINICAL APPROACH TO THE PATIENT WITH AN OSMOTIC DIURESIS

The steps in the clinical approach to the patient with osmotic diuresis are illustrated in Flow Charts 27.1 and 27.3.

Step 1: Calculate the Osmole Excretion Rate

If the U_{osm} is greater than the P_{osm} and the osmole excretion rate exceeds 1000 mOsm/day (or 0.7 mOsm/min), an osmotic diuresis is likely to be present. The caveat here, however, is that the U_{osm} from a spot urine sample may not be representative of the value of the U_{osm} throughout the 24-hour period if there are intermittent periods of water diuresis.

Step 2: Define the Nature of the Excreted Osmoles

One can make a reasonable assessment of the likelihood that a solute will cause polyuria if its concentration in plasma is measured, the GFR is estimated, and the renal handling of that solute is known. One should also determine whether enough mannitol was administered to cause the observed degree of polyuria. Osmotic diuresis could be due to a saline diuresis if Na^+ and Cl^- are excreted at high rates and represent the majority of the urine osmoles.

Step 3: Identify the Source of the Osmoles in the Urine

In a patient with a glucose- or urea-induced osmotic diuresis, it is important to decide whether these osmoles were derived from an endogenous source or from catabolism of exogenous proteins. The clinician should be aware of hidden glucose in the lumen of the gastrointestinal tract, because it may soon be absorbed and contribute to the osmotic diuresis.

In a patient with a saline-induced osmotic diuresis, one must determine why so much NaCl is being excreted. Some potential causes are prior excessive saline administration (a common situation in a hospital setting), administration of a loop diuretic in a patient with significant edema, cerebral salt wasting, and renal salt wasting.

CONSULT 3: AN UNUSUALLY LARGE OSMOTIC DIURESIS IN A PATIENT WITH DIABETES MELLITUS

A 50-kg, 14-year-old female had a long history of type 1 diabetes mellitus, which was poorly controlled because she did not take insulin regularly. In the past 48 hours, she was thirsty, drank large volumes of fruit juice, and noted that her urine volume was very high. On physical examination, her EABV was not appreciably contracted. The urine flow rate was 10 mL/min over this 100-min period. Other laboratory data included: pH = 7.33, plasma bicarbonate (HCO_3^-) concentration (P_{HCO3}) = 24 mmol/L, plasma anion gap (P_{AG}) = 16 mEq/L, plasma K^+ concentration (P_K) = 4.8 mmol/L, plasma creatinine concentration (P_{Cr}) = was close to her usual values of 1.0 mg/dL (88 µmol/L), blood urea nitrogen (BUN) = 22 mg/dL (P_{urea} 8 mmol/L), and hematocrit = 0.50. Of note, there was no decrease in her plasma glucose concentration (P_{Glu}) over that period, despite the excretion of a large amount of glucose in urine; the following results were also reported:

	Admission		After 100 min	
	Plasma	Urine	Plasma	Urine
Glucose, mg/dL (mmol/L)	1260 (70)	5400 (300)	1260 (70)	5400 (300)
Na^+, mmol/L	125	50	123	50
Osmolality, mOsm/L	320	450	316	450

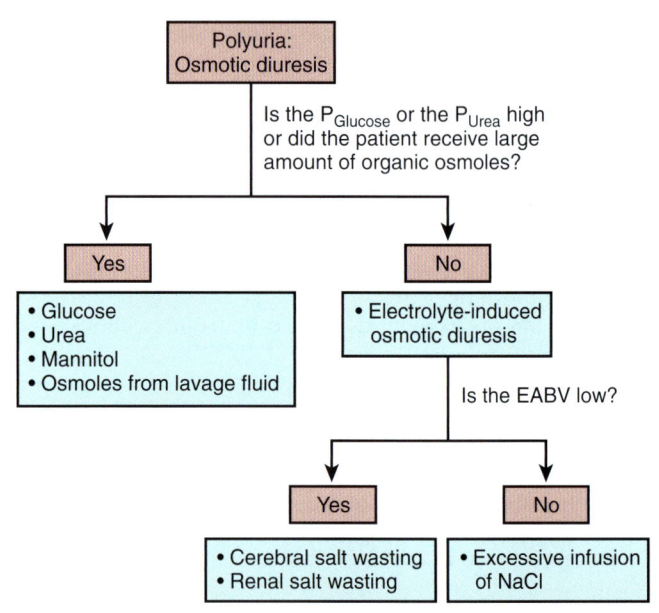

Flow Chart 27.3 Reproduced with the permission of the author and the publisher from Halperin ML: *The ACID truth and BASIC facts—with a sweet touch, an enLYTEnment,* 6th ed, Toronto, 2015, RossMark Medical Publishers.

Questions

- What is the basis of the polyuria?
- What dangers do you anticipate for this patient?

Discussion of Questions

What Is the Basis of the Polyuria?

U_{osm}: The U_{osm} of 450 mOsm/kg H_2O indicates that this polyuria was due to an osmotic diuresis. The U_{osm} was lower than the expected value during an osmotic diuresis, probably reflecting the very high osmole excretion rate, which caused a larger fall in the patient's medullary interstitial osmolality owing to a large volume of water reabsorption in her MCD.

Osmole Excretion Rate: The product of her U_{osm} (450 mOsm/L) and urine flow rate (10 mL/min) yielded an osmole excretion rate of 4.5 mOsm/min, a value that is sevenfold higher than the usual value in an adult (≈0.6 mOsm/min).

Nature of the Urine Osmoles: Because the patient's GFR was not low and her P_{Glu} was extremely high (1260 mg/dL, 70 mmol/L), the filtered load of glucose was markedly higher than the maximum tubular capacity for its reabsorption; hence this was a glucose-induced osmotic diuresis (confirmed by the finding of a urine glucose concentration [U_{Glu}] of about 300 mmol/L).

Sources of the Urine Osmoles: Of special emphasis, this patient's P_{Glu} did not decline despite such a high rate of excretion of glucose. In quantitative terms, the total content of glucose in her ECF compartment was 126 g—(1260 mg/dL × 10 to convert to mg/L) × 10 L ECFV ÷ 1000. During this 100-minute period, she excreted 54 g of glucose—(5400 mg/dL × 10 to convert to mg/L) × 1 L ÷1000. Therefore, although she excreted close to half of the content of glucose in her entire ECF compartment, there was no change in her P_{Glu}. Accordingly, to maintain this degree of hyperglycemia, she needed a large input of glucose in a short time. The only likely source of such a large amount of glucose was glucose that was retained in her stomach. As a reference, 1 L of apple juice contains about 135 g of glucose. Although the usual effect of hyperglycemia is to slow gastric emptying, it did *not* occur in this patient, because a rapid rate of exit of fluid from the stomach and absorption in the intestine are needed for this degree of osmotic diuresis to occur.[7]

What Dangers Do You Anticipate in this Patient?

Cerebral Edema: Brain cell swelling might occur if there were a significant fall in her effective P_{osm} (Equation 3).[8] This could occur if glucose and water entered the body and glucose was metabolized (rather than be excreted in the urine), causing a gain of electrolyte-free water in the body. This risk would be even greater if she had changed her intake to water rather than sugar-containing beverages.

$$\text{Effective } P_{osm} = 2\, P_{Na} + P_{Glu} \text{ (all values in mmol/L)} \quad (3)$$

DECREASED EFFECTIVE ARTERIAL BLOOD VOLUME

CONCEPT 6

Water crosses cell membranes rapidly through AQP channels to achieve osmotic equilibrium. Hence, the numbers of effective osmoles in the ECF and ICF compartments determine their respective volumes.

The effective osmoles in the ECF compartment are Na^+ and its attendant anions (Cl^- plus HCO_3^-); their content in the ECF compartment determines its volume.

CONCEPT 7

The hydrostatic pressure and the oncotic pressure across the capillary membrane are the major forces that determine the distribution of the ECF compartment between its intravascular and interstitial spaces.

The major driving force for outward movement of an ultrafiltrate across the capillary membrane is the hydrostatic pressure difference. The hydrostatic pressure at the venous end of the capillary is higher under conditions that lead to venous hypertension (e.g., venous obstruction, congestive heart failure).

The major driving force for inward fluid movement from the interstitial space to the intravascular space is the colloidal osmotic pressure difference. This is largely due to the higher concentration of albumin in the intravascular space (40 g/L) in comparison with the interstitial space (10 g/L). Fluid accumulates in the interstitial space in patients with hypoalbuminemia (e.g., patients with nephrotic syndrome). Thus the ECF volume (ECFV) in these patients may be increased but their EABV may be decreased.

CONCEPT 8

The signal for the regulation of the ECF volume is related to the pressure rather than to the volume in the large blood vessels.

Control mechanisms are set to defend the EABV rather than the ECF volume. The expected renal response to decreased EABV is the excretion of very little Na^+ and Cl^- in the urine.

TOOLS FOR EVALUATION OF DECREASED EABV

Quantitative Assessment of the Extracellular Fluid Volume

The physical examination, the plasma concentrations of K^+, HCO_3^-, creatinine, urea, and urate, as well as the fractional excretions of urea and urate are useful at times to suggest that the EABV is contracted. Nevertheless, they do not provide a quantitative estimate of the ECFV. A quantitative assessment of the ECFV can be obtained using the hematocrit (Table 27.2) or the total plasma proteins (if their values were normal to begin with).[9]

Sample Calculation. In a normal adult at sea level, the usual hematocrit is 0.40 and the blood volume is about 5 L (2 L of red blood cells [RBCs] and 3 L of plasma; Equation 4). Therefore, when the hematocrit is 0.50, and because there are still 2 L of RBCs, the current blood volume is 4 L, and the plasma volume is 2 L (Equation 5). Hence the plasma volume is reduced by 1 L from its normal value of 3 L. If one ignores changes in Starling forces for simplicity, the ECFV should have declined to approximately two thirds of its normal volume.

$$\text{Hematocrit } (0.40) = 2\text{ L RBCs}/5\text{ L Blood volume} \atop (2\text{ L RBCs} + 3\text{ L plasma}) \quad (4)$$

$$\text{Hematocrit } (0.50) = 2\text{ L RBCs}/4\text{ L Blood volume} \quad (5)$$

Table 27.2 Use of the Hematocrit to Estimate the Extracellular Fluid Volume (ECFV)

Hematocrit	% Change ECFV
0.40	0
0.50	−33
0.60	−60

The assumptions made when using this calculation are that the patient does not have anemia or erythrocytosis, that the red blood cell (RBC) volume is 2 L, and that the plasma volume is 3 L (blood volume 5 L). The formula is: Hematocrit = RBC volume/(RBC volume + plasma volume). Values between those listed can be deduced by iteration.

Table 27.3 Urine Electrolyte Values in a Patient with a Contracted Effective Arterial Blood Volume

Condition	Urine Na⁺	Urine Cl⁻
Vomiting:		
Recent	High	Low
Remote	Low	Low
Diuretics:		
Recent	High	High
Remote	Low	Low
Diarrhea or laxative abuse	Low	High
Bartter's syndrome or Gitelman's syndrome	High	High

Values of the urine electrolyte concentration must be adjusted when polyuria is present. Urine Cl⁻ is high in patients with diarrhea or laxative abuse if they have a high rate of excretion of NH_4^+. *High* = urine concentration more than 15 mmol/L; *low* = urine concentration less than 15 mmol/L.

Basis for the Low EABV

The expected response to a low EABV is to excrete as little Na^+ and Cl^- as possible. Because timed and complete urine collections to calculate rates of excretion of Na^+ and Cl^- are usually not obtained, clinicians use the urinary concentrations of Na^+ (U_{Na}) and Cl^- (U_{Cl}) in a spot urine sample (Table 27.3) to assess the renal response to the presence of a low EABV. These, however, are concentration terms, which do not necessarily indicate low rates of excretion if the urine flow rate is high. To avoid this type of error, the U_{Na} and U_{Cl} should be related to the concentration of creatinine in the urine (U_{Cr}), because the rate of excretion of creatinine is relatively constant throughout the day and its total excretion can be predicted according to the estimate of muscle mass. Notwithstanding, there are some caveats about the use of urine Na^+ and Cl^- excretion rates to assess EABV (see later).[10]

A Low Rate of Excretion of Sodium and Chloride. A low rate of excretion of Na^+ and Cl^- in a patient with a decreased EABV suggests either a loss of NaCl via nonrenal routes (e.g., sweat or the intestinal tract) or that there was a prior renal loss of Na^+ and Cl^- (e.g., remote use of diuretics). In the absence of a low EABV, a low rate of excretion of Na^+ and Cl^- may reflect a low intake of NaCl.

A High Rate of Excretion of Sodium But Little Excretion of Chloride. In a patient with a low EABV, there is an anion other than Cl^- being excreted with Na^+. If the anion is HCO_3^- (the urine pH is alkaline), suspect recent vomiting. The anion could also be one that was ingested or administered (e.g., penicillin) in which case, the urine pH would be close to 6.

A High Rate of Excretion of Chloride But Little Excretion of Sodium. In a patient with a low EABV, a cation other than Na^+ is being excreted with Cl^-. Most often the cation is NH_4^+, and the setting is diarrhea or laxative abuse. The cation could also be K^+ in a patient with chronic hypokalemia who is given KCl.

The Excretions of Sodium and Chloride Are Not Low. In a patient who has a low EABV, a high rate of excretion of both Na^+ and Cl^- suggests the absence of a stimulator of the reabsorption of Na^+ and Cl^- (e.g., aldosterone deficiency), the presence of an inhibitor of the reabsorption of NaCl (e.g., a diuretic), or an intrinsic renal lesion that has effects similar to those of a diuretic (e.g., Bartter's syndrome or Gitelman's syndrome). The pattern of excretion of electrolytes throughout the day can also be very important. For example, the use of diuretics is suspected if U_{Na} and U_{Cl} in a spot urine sample are both very low at times, but high at others.

Fractional Excretion of Sodium or Chloride

Calculation of the fraction excretion of Na^+ (FE_{Na}) or Cl^- (FE_{Cl}) expresses the amount of Na^+ or Cl^- that is excreted in the urine as a percentage of the amount that is filtered. For example, adults consuming a typical Western diet, excrete about 150 mmol/day of each of Na^+ and Cl^-, because a normal GFR is about 180 L/day, and the kidney filters about 27,000 mmol of Na^+ and about 20,000 mmol of Cl^- per day (P_{Na} or $P_{Cl} \times$ GFR); hence FE_{Na} is about 0.5%, and FE_{Cl} about 0.75%. (The formula to use for this calculation is shown in Equation 6.

$$FE_{Na} = 100 \times (U_{Na}/P_{Na})/(U_{Cr}/P_{Cr}) \quad (6)$$

The three practical points one should bear in mind when using the FE_{Na} or FE_{Cl} are (1) the excretions of Na^+ and Cl^- are directly related to the dietary intake of NaCl. Hence a low FE_{Na} or FE_{Cl} may represent a low intake of NaCl rather than a low EABV; (2) the numeric values for FE_{Na} and FE_{Cl} will be twice as high in a euvolemic subject who consumes 150 mmol of NaCl daily whose GFR is reduced by 50% as in another subject who consumes the same amount of NaCl and has a normal GFR. Hence FE_{Na} and FE_{Cl} numeric values must be interpreted in the context of the GFR at the time the measurements are made; and (3) as is the case with the use of U_{Na} or U_{Cl}, the FE_{Na} may be high in a patient with a low EABV when there is an unusually large excretion of another anion (e.g., HCO_3^-) in the urine, and the FE_{Cl} may be high in a patient with a low EABV when there is an unusually large excretion of another cation (e.g., NH_4^+) in the urine.

Calculations of FE_{Na} and FE_{Cl} are commonly used in patients with acute kidney injury in the differential diagnosis of prerenal azotemia versus acute tubular necrosis (in the absence of diuretics).[11] The advantage of using fraction excretion in this setting over the urinary Na^+ and Cl^- concentrations is that the use of FE_{Na} and FE_{Cl} adjusts these concentration terms for water reabsorption in the nephron.

Determine the Nephron Site Where There Is a Defect in Reabsorption of Sodium

If another compound or an ion that should have been reabsorbed in a given nephron segment is being excreted, one has presumptive evidence for a reabsorptive defect in that nephron segment. For example, if the defect is in the PCT, one might find glucosuria in the absence of hyperglycemia (e.g., Fanconi's syndrome).

The presence of hypokalemia may suggest a defect in the TAL of the loop of Henle or in the DCT with enhanced rate of K^+ secretion in the cortical distal nephron due to increased delivery of Na^+ and the presence of aldosterone due to decreased EABV. The presence of hypocalciuria would suggest that the site of the lesion is in the DCT (e.g., Gitelman's syndrome). The presence of hyperkalemia suggests a lesion in the CDN (e.g., Addison's disease, use of potassium-sparing diuretics such as spironolactone).

CONSULT 4: ASSESSMENT OF THE EABV

A 25-year-old woman was assessed by her family physician because of feeling weak. Although she admitted to being concerned about her body image, she reported no vomiting or intake of diuretics. Her blood pressure was 90 mm Hg systolic/60 mm Hg diastolic, her pulse rate was 110 beats/min, and her jugular venous pressure was low. Measurements in a venous blood sample showed P_{HCO_3} = 24 mmol/L, P_{AG} = 17 mEq/L, P_K = 2.9 mmol/L, hematocrit = 0.50, and plasma albumin concentration P_{Alb} = 5.0 g/dL (50 g/L). The urine electrolyte values were U_{Na} < 5 mmol/L, U_{Cl} = 42 mmol/L, urinary K^+ concentration (U_K) = 10 mmol/L, and U_{Cr} = 7 mmol/L.

Questions

- How severe is this patient's ECFV contraction?
- What is the cause of her low EABV?

Discussion of Questions

How Severe Is this Patient's EABV Contraction? The elevated value for the hematocrit (0.50) provides quantitative information about her ECF volume (see Table 27.2); her ECF volume was reduced by 33%. If she had anemia, the degree of her ECFV contraction would be even greater.

What Is the Cause of Her Low EABV? The low U_{Na} implies that her EABV was low. The high U_{Cl} (42 mmol/L), which exceeded the sum of her U_{Na} + U_K, indicates that there was another cation in that urine, most likely NH_4^+.

Interpretation: Calculating the content of HCO_3^- in this patient's ECF compartment revealed that she had a deficit of $NaHCO_3$. Loss of NaCl plus $NaHCO_3$ via the gastrointestinal (GI) tract was suspected as the cause of contracted EABV. The patient later admitted to the frequent use of a laxative. Hypokalemia could be explained by the loss of K^+ via the GI tract because her low U_K and U_{Cr} values suggest that the loss of K^+ was extrarenal (see section on potassium). Hypokalemia is associated with acidosis in PCT cells, which stimulates ammoniagenesis. The increased rate of excretion of the cation NH_4^+ obligates the excretion of Cl^- despite the presence of a low EABV.

HYPONATREMIA

Hyponatremia is defined as a P_{Na} less than 135 mmol/L.

CONCEPT 9

Because water moves across cell membranes to achieve osmotic equilibrium, acute hyponatremia is associated with swelling of brain cells. Brain cells adapt by exporting effective osmoles, mainly K^+ (and an anion from their ICF) and a number of organic solutes (e.g., taurine, myoinositol).

If hyponatremia is present for more than 48 hours, these adaptive changes have proceeded sufficiently to shrink brain cells back close to their normal volume. In this setting, a rapid increase in the P_{Na} shrinks cerebral vascular endothelial cells, leading to opening of the blood-brain barrier, allowing lymphocytes, complement, and cytokines to enter the brain, damage oligodendrocytes, and cause demyelination. Microglial activation also plays a role in this process.

From a clinical perspective, hyponatremia should be divided into the following three categories: acute, chronic, and chronic with an acute component; this classification has important implications for the design of therapy:

1. When hyponatremia is *acute* (i.e., <48 hours): The major risk is an increase in intracranial pressure, which may lead to brain herniation. Urgent therapy with hypertonic saline is needed to draw water out of the cranium.
2. When hyponatremia is *chronic* (i.e., >48 hours) and there is no acute element: The major risk related to hyponatremia is the development of osmotic demyelination from too rapid a rise in the P_{Na}.
3. When an acute element of hyponatremia is present in a patient with chronic hyponatremia: The P_{Na} must be raised quickly to lower intracranial pressure, but this rise should not exceed the maximum upper limit for the rise in P_{Na} over a 24-hour period to avoid causing osmotic demyelination.

CONCEPT 10

Chronic hyponatremia is usually due to a defect in the renal excretion of water. There are two causes for diminished renal excretion of water: low distal delivery of filtrate and the actions of vasopressin.

Hyponatremia is not a specific disease; rather it is a diagnostic category with many different causes. The traditional approach to the pathophysiology of hyponatremia centers on a reduced electrolyte-free water excretion due to actions of vasopressin. In some clinical settings, release of vasopressin is thought to be due to a diminished EABV. Notwithstanding, at least in some patients the decrease in EABV does not seem to be large enough to cause the release of vasopressin. We suggest that hyponatremia may develop in some patients in the absence of vasopressin's actions. Two factors are important in this context: the volume of filtrate that is delivered to the distal nephron and the volume of water that is reabsorbed in the inner MCD through its RWP.[3]

The volume of distal delivery of filtrate is reduced if the GFR is decreased or the fractional reabsorption of NaCl in the PCT is increased.

The fractional reabsorption of NaCl in the PCT is increased in response to a decreased EABV. Decreased EABV can be due to a total body deficit of NaCl (e.g., diuretic use in a patient who consumes little salt, NaCl loss in diarrhea fluid or in sweat) or to a disorder that causes a low cardiac output. Because there is an obligatory minimal loss of Na^+ in each liter of urine during a large water diuresis, a deficit of Na^+ can be created during the polyuria induced by a large intake of water in a subject who consumes little NaCl (e.g., a patient with beer potomania).

The driving force for water reabsorption via RWP is the osmotic pressure gradient generated by the difference in osmolality between the luminal fluid in the inner MCD and that in the medullary interstitium. As discussed previously, we estimate that somewhat more than 5 L of water is reabsorbed per day in the inner MCD by RWP during water diuresis.

In some patients, hyponatremia is caused by reduced electrolyte-free water excretion due to actions of vasopressin, but the release of vasopressin is not caused by a decreased EABV. This category is called the *syndrome of the inappropriate secretion of antidiuretic hormone* (SIADH). SIADH, however, is a diagnosis of exclusion; it cannot be made if the patient has a condition that may lead to a low distal delivery of filtrate.

LABORATORY TESTS IN PATIENT WITH HYPONATREMIA

Measurement of Plasma Sodium Concentration

Pseudohyponatremia is present when the P_{Na} measured by the laboratory is lower than the actual ratio of Na^+ to plasma water in the patient. In fact, it is always present when P_{Na} is measured in a diluted plasma sample, because close to 7% of the plasma volume is a nonaqueous volume (lipids or proteins). Hence, although the actual P_{Na} is about 150 mmol/L, the measured laboratory value of P_{Na} using flame photometry is 140 mmol/L. A large nonaqueous volume in plasma (e.g., hypertriglyceridemia or hyperproteinemia) can lead to underestimation of the value of P_{Na} with this method. With the use of an ion-selective electrode, the activity of Na^+ in the aqueous plasma volume is measured; nevertheless, because of the use of automatic aspirators and dilutors to prepare the plasma samples, the P_{Na} in plasma with a large nonaqueous volume may still be incorrectly reported as low. This error in measurement of P_{Na} is detected by the finding of a normal P_{osm} value (in the absence of high concentration of other osmoles, e.g., urea, glucose, alcohol).[12]

Tools to Detect a Low Effective Arterial Blood Volume

A difficulty with the diagnosis of the syndrome of inappropriate secretion of antidiuretic hormone (SIADH) is that patients may have a mild to modest degree of EABV contraction that cannot always be detected by the physical examination. The following laboratory tests may provide helpful clues to detect the presence of a low distal delivery of filtrate. At times, however, EABV expansion with infusion of saline may be required to rule out low distal delivery of filtrate as the cause of hyponatremia. Absence of water diuresis confirms the diagnosis of SIADH.

Concentrations of Sodium and Chloride in Urine. Assessment of U_{Na} and U_{Cl} are helpful to detect the presence of a low EABV, and they may also provide clues about its cause. This was discussed in detail earlier.

Concentrations of Urea and Urate in Plasma. Patients with a low EABV tend to have a high P_{urea} and plasma urate concentration (P_{urate}) because reabsorption of urea and urate is increased in the PCT.[13] The converse is also true in patients with chronic hyponatremia due to SIADH, because this subgroup has some EABV expansion. Because the reabsorption of urea is influenced by the EABV but that of creatinine is not, the rise in the P_{urea} is more pronounced than the rise in P_{Cr} in patients with low EABV. Therefore, the ratio of urea to creatinine in plasma is likely to be high in patients with hyponatremia as a result of a deficit of Na^+ that causes a low distal delivery of filtrate. This, however, may not be the case if protein intake is low.

Other Tests. A low or a high P_K, a rise in the P_{Cr}, and a low or a high P_{HCO3} may suggest that the EABV is low.

CONSULT 5: HYPONATREMIA WITH BROWN SPOTS

A 22-year-old woman had myasthenia gravis. In the previous 6 months, she noted a marked decline in her energy, and her weight was down from 50 kg to 47 kg. She often felt faint when standing up quickly. She reported no large recent intake of water. On physical examination, her blood pressure was 80/50 mm Hg, pulse rate was 126 beats/min, jugular venous pressure was below the level of the sternal angle, and there was no peripheral edema. Brown pigmented spots were evident in her buccal mucosa. The electrocardiogram (ECG) findings were unremarkable. The biochemistry data are as follows:

	Plasma	Urine
Na^+, mmol/L	112	130
K^+, mmol/L	5.5	24
Urea	BUN: 28 mg/dL (10 mmol/L)	Urea concentration: 130 mmol/L
Creatinine	1.7 mg/dL (150 µmol/L)	6.0 mmol/L
Osmolality, mOsm/kg H_2O	240	325

Questions

- What is the most likely basis for the very low EABV?
- Are emergency situations present on admission?
- What dangers should be anticipated during therapy, and how can they be avoided?

Discussion of Questions

What Is the Most Likely Basis for the Very Low EABV? In this case, the very contracted EABV (manifested by the low blood pressure and tachycardia), the low P_{Na}, the high P_K of 5.5 mmol/L, and the renal salt wasting strongly suggested that the most likely diagnosis was adrenal insufficiency. It was likely due to autoimmune adrenalitis because the patient also had myasthenia gravis. The basis for the renal salt wasting is a lack of aldosterone. The low EABV was also caused in part by a lower degree of contraction of venous capacitance vessels because of glucocorticoid deficiency.

Are Emergency Situations Present on Admission? Two potential emergencies dominate the initial management: a very contracted EABV and the lack of cortisol. To deal with the former requires an infusion of a solution that is isotonic to the patient to reexpand her EABV without changing the P_{Na}. We would infuse this saline solution quickly at the outset and then at a slower rate once the hemodynamic state improved. The second potential emergency is not life threatening at the moment, and it can be dealt with by administering cortisol. There is one other possible emergency to consider: brain swelling due to the presence of an acute element to her hyponatremia. Such an acute element did not seem to be present because the patient did not have significant symptoms that could be related to an increased intracranial pressure and she also did not report a recent large water intake.

What Dangers Should Be Anticipated During Therapy, and How Can They Be Avoided? Reexpansion of the patient's EABV could lead to an increased excretion of water due to an increased distal delivery of filtrate and, possibly, suppression of the release of vasopressin. In addition, the administration of cortisol would improve her hemodynamic state and inhibit the release of corticotrophin-releasing factor and, hence, of vasopressin. The net result of this therapy would be to cause water diuresis and thereby a dangerous rise in the P_{Na}. Because the patient had a small muscle mass (and therefore a small total body water volume), the excretion of a relatively small volume of electrolyte-free water could lead to too rapid a rise in P_{Na}. In addition, because of her poor nutritional state, which becomes even more evident if one interprets her weight loss in conjunction with a large gain of water in her cells (her loss of muscle mass was larger than revealed by her weight loss), she was at high risk for osmotic demyelination if her P_{Na} were to rise rapidly. The rise in her P_{Na} should not exceed a maximum of 4 mmol/L per 24 hours. Accordingly, we would administer dDAVP early on in therapy to prevent water diuresis.

CONSULT 6: HYPONATREMIA IN A PATIENT ON THIAZIDE DIURETIC THERAPY

A 71-year-old woman was prescribed a thiazide diuretic for treatment of hypertension. She had ischemic renal disease with an estimated GFR of 28 mL/min (40 L/day). She consumed a low-salt, low-protein diet and drank several large cups of tea a day to remain hydrated. A month later, she presented to her family doctor feeling unwell. Her blood pressure was 130/80 mm Hg, her heart rate was 80 beats/min, there were no postural changes in her blood pressure or heart rate and her jugular venous pressure was about 1 cm below the level of the sternal angle. Her P_{Na} was 112 mmol/L with a U_{osm} of 325 mOsm/kg H_2O. Other laboratory results are as follows:

	Plasma	Urine
Na^+, mmol/L	112	22
K^+, mmol/L	3.6	10
HCO_3^-, mmol/L	28	0
Urea, mmol/L	8	241
Creatinine, μmol/L (mg/dL)	145 (1.3)	6.1 (0.7)

Questions

- What is the most likely basis for the chronic hyponatremia in this patient?
- What dangers should be anticipated during therapy, and how can they be avoided?

Discussion of the Questions

What is the Most Likely Basis for the Chronic Hyponatremia in this Patient? Although the patient was taking a thiazide diuretic, the degree of decrease in her EABV did not seem to be large enough to cause the release of vasopressin. The patient had a low baseline GFR of 40 L/day. The use of diuretics and the low-salt diet led to a deficit of Na^+ and a mild reduction in EABV. Even a relatively small decrease in EABV leads to sympathetic activation, and β-adrenergic stimulation activates the rein angiotensin aldosterone system (RAAS), both of which increase the reabsorption of sodium and water in the PCT. If the patient were to reabsorb 90% of her glomerular filtrate (which may be even lower because of the mild reduction in her EABV) in the PCT instead of 83% (as discussed previously, this is the percentage of the filtrate that is usually reabsorbed in the PCT in the absence of low EABV), less than 4 L/day of filtrate would be delivered distally; this is the maximum volume of urine she could excrete. This volume exceeds the usual daily intake of water, but hyponatremia might still develop in such a patient because there is water reabsorption by RWP along the inner MCD even in the absence of vasopressin action.

Because of the low rate of excretion of osmoles, and because the volume of filtrate delivered to the inner MCD in the absence of vasopressin is larger than during antidiuresis, the osmolality of fluid in the lumen of the inner MCD will be low. If the osmole excretion rate in this patient is 300 mOsm/day, and if 4 L are delivered to the inner MCD, the osmolality of the luminal fluid in the inner MCD would be 75 mOsm/L. Even if the medullary interstitial osmolality is substantially lower than normal, for instance, 375 mOsm/L, there is still an enormous osmotic driving force for water reabsorption along the inner MCD, because a difference of 1 mOsm/kg H_2O generates a pressure of about 19.3 mm Hg.

What Dangers Should Be Anticipated During Therapy, and How Can They Be Avoided? Understanding this pathophysiology has clinical implications for the management of the patient with hyponatremia. Initially, this patient's hyponatremia was thought to be caused by stimulation of vasopressin release due to decreased EABV owing to her intake of a thiazide diuretic; hence she was given isotonic saline to reexpand her EABV. Even a relatively small volume of saline (especially, if it were given as a bolus) might be sufficient to reduce the fractional reabsorption of filtrate in the PCT and increase its distal delivery. If the fractional reabsorption in PCT were decreased to 83% of the GFR of 40 L/day, distal delivery of filtrate would increase to about 7 L/day. This exceeds the capacity for water reabsorption by RWP (estimated to be ≈5 L/day), so water diuresis would ensue. Because of the patient's small muscle mass, even a modest water diuresis might be large enough to cause a rapid rise in P_{Na} and increase the risk of osmotic demyelination syndrome, especially if she were malnourished or potassium depleted.

POTASSIUM

Hypokalemia and hyperkalemia are common electrolyte disorders in clinical practice that may be associated with life-threatening cardiac arrhythmias. The analysis of the urine composition provides essential information to establish the underlying pathophysiology and to plan therapy.

Regulation of K^+ homeostasis has two main aspects:

1. Control of the transcellular distribution of K^+, which is vital for survival because it limits acute changes in the P_K.
2. The regulation of K^+ excretion by the kidney, which maintains whole-body K^+ balance; this is, however, a much slower process.

CONCEPT 11

Three factors regulate the movement of K^+ across cell membranes: the concentration difference for K^+, the electrical voltage across cell membranes, and the presence of open K^+ channels in cell membranes.

TRANSCELLULAR DISTRIBUTION OF POTASSIUM

Approximately 98% of K^+ in the body is in cells, retained there by the cell interior negative voltage owing primarily to negatively charged nucleic acids (i.e., RNA). In resting cells, K^+ ions are relatively free to cross the membrane via some K^+ channels as the concentration difference for K^+ favors its movement out of cells. The diffusion and electrical forces eventually come into balance, and the equilibrium potential for K^+ (E_K) is achieved. Because cell membranes have much higher permeability to K^+ than to Na^+, the resting membrane potential (RMP) of cells is close to E_K.

The normal RMP of active cells relies on the activity of Na^+–K^+–adenosine triphosphatase (Na^+-K^+-ATPase), an electrogenic pump that creates intracellular negative potential by exporting three Na^+ ions while importing only two K^+ ions. There are three ways to acutely increase ion pumping by the Na^+-K^+-ATPase: (1) a rise in the concentration of its limiting substrate—intracellular Na^+; (2) an increase in the affinity (lower K_m [concentration for half-maximal activation]) for Na^+ and K^+ or an increase in the V_{max} (maximal pump turnover rate) of the Na^+-K^+-ATPase units in cell membranes; and (3) an increase in the number of active Na^+-K^+-ATPase pump units in the cell membrane through recruitment of new units. A long-term increase in Na^+-K^+-ATPase pump activity requires the synthesis of new pump units, as occurs with exercise training, excess thyroid hormones, or high dietary K^+ intake.

Insulin causes a shift of K^+ into cells as it promotes the translocation of Na^+-K^+-ATPase units from an intracellular pool to the cell membrane. Insulin causes phosphorylation of FXYD1 (phospholamen) via atypical protein kinase C, which increase the V_{max} of Na^+-K^+-ATPase. Insulin also activates the Na^+-H^+ exchanger isoform 1 (NHE1) and hence increases the electroneutral entry of Na^+ into cells. β_2-adrenergic agonists induce phosphorylation of the FXYD1 via cyclic adenosine monophosphate mediated activation of protein kinase A. Another activator of NHE1 is a rise in intracellular H^+ concentration. Monocarboxylic acids (e.g., L-lactic acid, ketoacids) enter cells on the monocarboxylic acid cotransporter (MCT). The release of H^+ near NHE1 may cause its activation, which leads to an increase in the electroneutral entry of Na^+ into cells and, in the presence of insulin, a shift of K^+ into cells (Figure 27.6).[14]

A shift of K^+ out of cells may occur in patients with metabolic acidosis due to acids that are not transported on MCT (e.g., metabolic acidosis due to loss of $NaHCO_3$ [gain of HCl] in a patient with diarrhea or the ingestion of citric acid, a tricarboxylic acid).

RENAL K^+ EXCRETION.

Control of K^+ secretion occurs primarily in the late CDN, namely the late DCT, the connecting segment, and the CCD. Two factors influence the rate of excretion of K^+, the net secretion of K^+ by principal cells in the CDN and the flow rate in the terminal CCD.

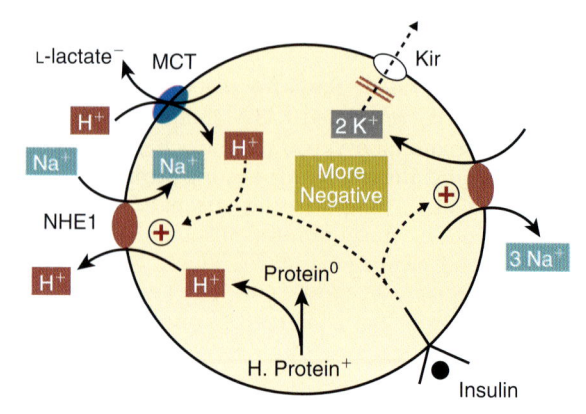

Figure 27.6 Possible mechanism for how monocarboxylic acids cause a shift of K^+ into cells. The *circle* represents a cell. Na^+-H^+ exchanger isoform 1 (NHE1) in cell membranes is activated by insulin and by a high concentration of H^+ in the cell interior, because H^+ binds to the modifier site of NHE1. The concentration of H^+ near NHE1 could rise when monocarboxylic acids (lactic acid in this example) enter cells on the monocarboxylic acid cotransporter (MCT) and their H^+ ions are released close to NHE1. In the presence of insulin, which activates the Na^+-K^+-ATPase and NHE1 in cell membranes, electroneutral entry of Na^+ into cells is increased. The subsequent transport of Na^+ out of cells via the electrogenic Na^+-K^+-ATPase increases the cell interior negative voltage and causes the retention of K^+ in cells. (Reproduced with the permission of the author and the publisher from Halperin ML: *The ACID truth and BASIC facts—with a sweet touch, an enLYTEnment*, 6th ed, Toronto, 2015, RossMark Medical Publishers.)

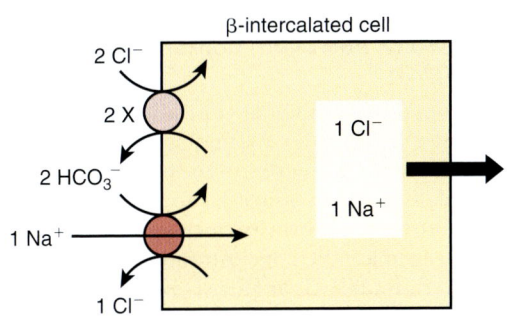

Figure 27.7 Electroneutral reabsorption of Na⁺ in the cortical distal nephron (CDN). The *pink circle* represents pendrin, and the *red circle* the Na⁺-dependent Cl⁻/HCO₃⁻ exchanger (NDCBE). The exchange of 2 Cl⁻ for 2 HCO₃⁻, via two cycles *(2X)* of pendrin with the subsequent uptake of 2 HCO₃⁻ and 1 Na⁺ in exchange for 1 Cl⁻ via one cycle of NDCBE, results in net electroneutral transport of 1 Na⁺ and 1 Cl⁻ across the luminal membrane of each β-intercalated cell in the CDN. (Reproduced with the permission of the author and the publisher from Halperin ML: *The ACID truth and BASIC facts—with a sweet touch, an enLYTEnment*, 6th ed, Toronto, 2015, RossMark Medical Publishers.)

K⁺ Secretion in the Cortical Distal Nephron

The process for secretion of K⁺ by principal cells in the CDN has two elements.[15] First, a lumen-negative transepithelial voltage must be generated by electrogenic reabsorption of Na⁺ (i.e., reabsorption of Na⁺ via the amiloride-sensitive sodium channel [ENaC] without its accompanying anion, which is largely Cl⁻). Second, open renal outer medullary K⁺ (ROMK) channels must be present in the luminal membranes of principal cells. Aldosterone actions lead to an increase in the number of open ENaC units in the luminal membranes of principal cells in the CDN. Aldosterone binds to its receptor in the cytoplasm of principal cells, and the hormone-receptor complex then enters the nucleus, leading to the synthesis of new proteins including the serum and glucocorticoid regulated kinase-1 (SGK-1). SGK-1 increases the number of open ENaCs in the apical membrane of principal cells via phosphorylation and inactivation of the ubiquitin ligase, neural developmentally downregulated isoform 4-2 (Nedd 4-2).

It was thought that the paracellular pathway plays an important role in the reabsorption of Cl⁻ in the CDN, but the large peritubular/luminal concentration difference for Cl⁻ and the relatively small luminal/peritubular electrical driving force make this mechanism an unlikely one. An electroneutral, thiazide-sensitive, and amiloride-resistant NaCl transport process has been identified in the β-intercalated cells of the CCD in mice. This seems to be mediated by the parallel activity of the Na⁺-independent Cl⁻/HCO₃⁻ exchanger (pendrin) and the Na⁺-dependent Cl⁻/HCO₃⁻ exchanger (NDCBE), resulting in electroneutral NaCl reabsorption (Figure 27.7).[16]

An increase in luminal fluid concentration of HCO₃⁻ and/or an alkaline luminal fluid pH seem to increase the amount of K⁺ secreted in the late CDN.[17] It was suggested that this effect might be due to a decrease in the paracellular permeability of Cl⁻. A different mechanism for the effect of luminal HCO₃⁻ may be that because the HCO₃⁻ gradient is needed to increase flux through pendrin, an increase in luminal HCO₃⁻ concentration may inhibit flux through pendrin, and hence NDCBE, and thereby decrease the electroneutral NaCl reabsorption, in turn increasing the electrogenic reabsorption of Na⁺ and the secretion of K⁺.

ROMK channels are the most important K⁺ channels for the secretion of K⁺ in the CDN. Large-K⁺ conductance—BK or maxi-K⁺—channels seem to play an important role in flow-dependent K⁺ secretion, but their role in physiologic regulation of renal excretion of K⁺ and its disorders is not clear.[18]

A complex network of "with-no-lysine kinases" (WNKs), WNK4 and WNK1, via effects on the thiazide-sensitive NaCl cotransporter (NCC) in the DCT and ROMK in the CDN, may function as a switch to change the aldosterone response of the kidney to either conserve Na⁺ or excrete K⁺.[19] Increased activity of NCC diminishes the delivery of NaCl to the CDN and hence the rate of electrogenic reabsorption of Na⁺ and the ability to generate large negative luminal voltage. WNKs also affect K⁺ secretion via induction of endocytosis/exocytosis of ROMK channels.[20]

CONCEPT 12

When vasopressin acts, the flow rate in the terminal CCD is determined by the number of effective osmoles present in luminal fluid.

When vasopressin acts, the late CDN is permeable to water owing to the insertion of AQP2 channels in the luminal membranes of principal cells. The osmolality of fluid in the terminal CCD becomes equal to the P_{osm} and hence is relatively fixed. Therefore the number of osmoles present in the luminal fluid in the terminal CCD determines its flow rate. These osmoles are largely urea, Na⁺, Cl⁻, and K⁺ with an accompanying anion. Owing to the process of intrarenal urea recycling, the largest fraction of the osmoles delivered to the terminal CCD is urea osmoles. In subjects eating a typical Western diet, the amount of urea that recycles would be approximately 600 mmol/day. This process of urea recycling adds an extra 2 L to the flow rate in the terminal CCD (600 mOsm divided by a luminal fluid osmolality that is equal to plasma osmolality, i.e., ≈300 mOsm/L).

In a quantitative analysis, Kamel and Halperin illustrated that even in patients with a large defect in the ability to generate a lumen-negative voltage in the CDN, a significant degree of hyperkalemia is not likely to develop with a usual K⁺ intake, unless there is decreased flow rate in the terminal CCD. Restricting protein intake may decrease the amount of urea that recycles and hence the rate of flow in the terminal CCD.[21]

CONCEPT 13

There is no normal rate of K⁺ excretion in the urine because normal subjects in steady state excrete all the K⁺ they eat and absorb from the GI tract.

To assess the renal response in a patient with a disorder in K⁺ homeostasis, we use the expected rate of excretion of K⁺ in patients in whom hypokalemia was present because of nonrenal causes and in subjects with normal renal function who were given a large K⁺ load. In patients who become K⁺ depleted with low dietary K⁺ intake, the excretion of K⁺ falls to 10 to 15 mmol/day. On the other hand, in subjects who consume a large quantity of K⁺ (in excess of 200 mmol/day) on a long-term basis, the rate of excretion of K⁺ matches their intake, with only a minor rise in P_K.

TOOLS FOR EVALUATION OF A PATIENT WITH A DYSKALEMIA

Assess the Rate of Excretion of Potassium in the Urine

A 24-hour urine collection is not necessary to assess the daily rate of excretion of K^+. Taking advantage of the fact that creatinine is excreted at a near-constant rate throughout the day, we use the ratio of the concentration of K^+ in the urine (U_K) to the concentration of creatinine in the urine (U_{Cr}) (i.e., the U_K/U_{Cr}). This approach has the following advantages: The data are available quickly and more relevant information is gathered because one knows the stimulus, the P_K, that influences the rate of excretion of K^+ at that time. The limitation is the diurnal variation in K^+ excretion, but it does not negate the advantages. The expected U_K/U_{Cr} in patients with hypokalemia due to an intracellular shift of K^+ and in those with chronic hypokalemia due to extrarenal loss of K^+ is less than 15 (mmol K^+ per gram creatinine when creatinine measured in grams; mmol/g) or less than 1.5 (mmol K^+ per mmol creatinine when creatinine is measured in moles; mmol/mmol). The expected ratio in a patient with hyperkalemia and a normal renal response is greater than 200 (mmol/g) (or more than 20 [mmol/mmol]). Patients with chronic hyperkalemia, however, must have a defect in renal excretion of K^+ and so are expected to have a low U_K/U_{Cr}. A 24-hour urine collection may be needed in such patients to assess the contribution of the dietary K^+ intake to the degree of hyperkalemia.

The Transtubular Potassium Concentration Gradient (TTKG)

The transtubular potassium concentration gradient (TTKG) was developed to provide a semiquantitative reflection of the driving force for K^+ secretion in the late CDN. The goal in this calculation was to adjust U_K for the amount of water that was reabsorbed in downstream nephron segments (i.e., the MCD) to estimate the concentration of K^+ in the luminal fluid in the terminal CCD, or $[K_{CCD}]$. To calculate the $[K_{CCD}]$, we suggested dividing the U_K by the ratio of U_{osm} to the P_{osm} (i.e., U_{osm}/P_{osm}), because the P_{osm} should be equal to the osmolality in the luminal fluid in the terminal CCD when AQP2 channels are present in the luminal membranes of principal cells in the CCD.

The assumption made with use of the U_{osm}/P_{osm} ratio to adjust for the amount of water that is reabsorbed in the MCD is that the majority of the osmoles delivered to the MCD were not reabsorbed in this nephron segment. Although the amount of electrolytes reabsorbed in the MCD should not pose a problem, this is not true for urea because of intrarenal urea recycling. We estimated that in subjects eating a typical Western diet, close to 600 mmol of urea is reabsorbed downstream from the CCD per day (Figure 27.8). It follows that the calculated KCCD obtained from $U_K \div (U_{osm}/P_{osm})$ is likely to be appreciably higher than the actual value in vivo.[21] Therefore we no longer use the TTKG in the clinical assessment of patients with dyskalemia. Rather

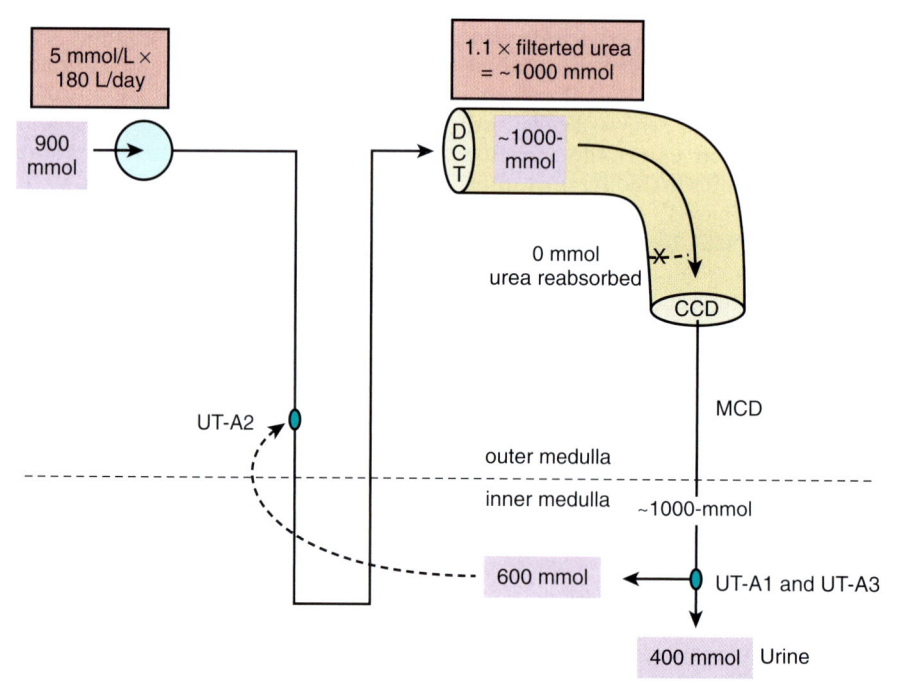

Figure 27.8 Intrarenal recycling of urea increases flow in the cortical distal nephron (CDN). Vasopressin phosphorylates and causes the insertion of urea transporters (UTs) UT-A3 in the luminal membranes of cells in the inner medullary collecting duct (MCD) and UT-A1 in the basolateral membranes of cells in the inner MCD. The bulk of the urea that is reabsorbed in the inner MCD leaves the inner medulla via ascending vasa recta, because it has UT-A2. Most of these urea molecules enter the luminal fluid of the descending thin limbs of the loop of Henle (DtLs) in superficial nephrons, which have their bends deep in the outer medulla, because they possess UT-A2. The estimated increase in delivery of urea to the CDN of about 600 mmol/day results in a rise in flow rate in the terminal cortical collecting duct (CCD) by 2 L. This calculation does not take into account the relatively small amount of urea that exits the medulla via the ascending vasa recta. (Reproduced with the permission of the author and the publisher from Halperin ML: *The ACID truth and BASIC facts—with a sweet touch, an enLYTEnment*, 6th ed, Toronto, 2015, RossMark Medical Publishers.)

Table 27.4 Use of Plasma Renin and Plasma Aldosterone Values to Assess the Basis of Hypokalemia or Hyperkalemia

	Renin	Aldosterone
Lesions That Cause Hypokalemia		
Adrenal gland:		
Primary hyperaldosteronism	Low	High
Glucocorticoid-remediable hyperaldosteronism	Low	High
Kidney:		
Renal artery stenosis	High	High
Malignant hypertension	High	High
Renin-secreting tumor	High	High
Liddle's syndrome	Low	Low
Disorders involving 11β-hydroxysteroid dehydrogenase (HSDH)	Low	Low
Lesions That Cause Hyperkalemia		
Adrenal gland:		
Addison's disease	High	Low
Kidney:		
Pseudohypoaldosteronism type 1	High	High
Hyporeninemic hypoaldosteronism	Low	Low

we rely on the U_K/U_{Cr} to provide the information needed to assess the renal response in these patients.

Establish the Basis for the Abnormal Rate of Excretion of Potassium. In a patient with hypokalemia, a higher than expected rate of excretion of K^+ implies that the lumen-negative voltage is abnormally more negative and that open ROMK channels are present in the luminal membranes of principal cells in the CDN. The greater lumen-negative voltage is due to more electrogenic versus electroneutral Na^+ reabsorption in the CDN. The converse is true in a patient with hyperkalemia where there is a lower than expected rate of excretion of K^+.

The clinical indices that help in the differential diagnosis of the pathophysiology of the abnormal rate of electrogenic reabsorption of Na^+ in CDN are an assessment of the EABV and the presence or absence of hypertension. The measurement of plasma renin mass ($P_{renin\ mass}$) and the level of aldosterone in plasma (P_{Ald}) are helpful in in this differential diagnosis (Table 27.4).

CLINICAL APPROACH TO THE PATIENT WITH HYPOKALEMIA

Table 27.5 lists causes of hypokalemia.

Step 1. Deal with Medical Emergencies That May Be Present on Presentation and Anticipate and Prevent Risks That May Arise During Therapy

The major emergencies related to hypokalemia are cardiac arrhythmias and respiratory muscle weakness leading to respiratory failure. Patients with chronic hyponatremia and hypokalemia are at a high risk for development of osmotic demyelination with a rapid rise in P_{Na}. Administration of KCl may lead to a rapid rise in P_{Na}[22] because K^+ ions enter and Na^+ ions leave muscle cells. This movement of Na^+ ions into the ECF compartment may also expand the EABV, leading to an increase in distal delivery of filtrate and resulting in water diuresis.

Step 2. Determine Whether the Basis for Hypokalemia Is an Acute Shift of Potassium into Cells

The basis for hypokalemia is likely to be an acute shift of K^+ into cells if the duration of illness is known to be short, if there is a minimum rate of excretion of K^+ (<15 mmol K^+/g creatinine (or <1.5 mmol K^+/mmol creatinine), and there is no significant degree of metabolic acidosis or metabolic alkalosis (Flow Chart 27.4).[23]

Having established that there is an acute shift of K^+ into cells, the next step is to determine whether an adrenergic surge may have caused this shift. In these settings, tachycardia, a wide pulse pressure, and systolic hypertension are often present. It is very important to recognize patients with these features because the administration of nonspecific β-blockers can lead to a very rapid recovery without administration of a large amount of KCl and hence avoid the risk of development of rebound hyperkalemia when the stimulus for shift of K^+ ions abates.[24]

Step 3. Examine the Acid-Basis Status in the Patient with Chronic Hypokalemia

If the patient has chronic hypokalemia, the first step is to examine the acid-base status in plasma.

Subgroup with Metabolic Acidosis. The group of patients with metabolic acidosis can be divided into two categories according to the rate of excretion of NH_4^+ in the urine (Flow Chart 27.5). The rate of excretion of NH_4^+ can be estimated with use of the urine osmolal gap (see discussion of metabolic acidosis).

Subgroup with Metabolic Alkalosis. The first step in the patient with metabolic alkalosis is to determine whether the site of loss of K^+ is renal or extrarenal on the basis of the assessment of the rate of renal excretion of K^+ using the U_K/U_{Cr} (Flow Chart 27.6). Patients with a low value for this ratio (i.e., <15 mmol/g or 1.5 mmol/mmol) have conditions with loss of K^+ via nonrenal routes such as in sweat (e.g., patients with cystic fibrosis) and via the GI tract (e.g., patients with diarrhea associated with decreased activity of the colonic luminal anion exchanger [Cl^-/HCO_3^-], a condition called downregulated in adenoma [DRA]). On the other hand, patients in whom the U_K/U_{Cr} that is higher than these values have a condition associated with a renal loss of K^+. The steps to take to determine the underlying pathophysiology in this latter group of patients are outlined in Flow Chart 27.7.

In essence, we are trying to determine the cause of a higher rate of electrogenic reabsorption of Na^+ in the CDN. The primary reason is an increased number of open ENaC units in the luminal membranes of principal cells in the late CDN. This increase could be due to two groups of disorders. The first group involves secondary increase in ENaC activity due to the release of aldosterone in response to a low EABV. Hence, patients with these disorders are not likely to have

Table 27.5 Causes of Hypokalemia*

Shift of K⁺ into cells	
Associated with an adrenergic surge	β_2-adrenergic surge due to stress conditions (e.g., head trauma, subarachnoid hemorrhage, myocardial infarction), drugs (e.g., amphetamines, theophylline, albuterol, clenbutrol), large dose of caffeine, pheochromocytoma
	High insulin levels causing hypoglycemia
	Thyrotoxic periodic paralysis
Not associated with an adrenergic surge	Familial periodic paralysis
	Sporadic periodic paralysis
	K⁺ channel blockers (e.g., barium sulfide)
	Anabolic state (e.g., recovery from diabetic ketoacidosis)
Increased K⁺ loss associated with hyperchloremic metabolic acidosis	Gastrointestinal loss of $NaHCO_3$ (e.g., diarrhea, laxative abuse, fistula, ileus, ureteral diversion)
	Overproduction of an acid with high rate of excretion of its anion in the urine (e.g., hippuric acid in glue sniffers)
	Reduced reabsorption of $NaHCO_3$ in the proximal convoluted tubule (e.g., patients with proximal renal tubular acidosis treated with large amounts of $NaHCO_3$, long-term use of acetazolamide)
	Distal renal tubular acidosis:
	Low distal H⁺ secretion subtype (e.g., Sjögren's syndrome)
	High distal secretion of HCO_3^- (e.g., Southeast Asian ovalocytosis with second mutation involving the Cl^-/HCO_3^- anion exchanger
Increased K⁺ loss associated with metabolic alkalosis	
Extrarenal loss of K⁺	Skin (e.g., patients with cystic fibrosis)
	Colonic loss of K⁺ (patients with diarrhea due to diminished activity of the Cl^-/HCO_3^- exchanger; down regulated in adenoma [DRA])
Renal loss of K⁺	Increased amiloride-sensitive sodium channel (ENaC) activity due to release of aldosterone in response to low effective arterial blood volume:
	Vomiting, diuretic use or abuse
	Bartter's syndrome, Gitelman's syndrome
	Pseudo-Bartter's syndrome due to ligand binding to calcium-sensing receptor) in the thick ascending limb of the loop of Henle (e.g., Ca^{2+} in a patient with hypercalcemia), drugs (e.g., gentamicin, cisplatin), cationic proteins (e.g., cationic monoclonal immunoglobulins in a patient with multiple myeloma)
	Primary increased ENaC activity:
	Primary hyperreninemic hyperaldosteronism (e.g., renal artery stenosis, malignant hypertension, renin-secreting tumor)
	Primary hyperaldosteronism (e.g., adrenal adenoma, bilateral adrenal hyperplasia, glucocorticoid-remediable aldosteronism)
	Disorders in which cortisol acts as a mineralocorticoid (e.g., apparent mineralocorticoid excess syndrome, inhibition of 11β-hydroxysteroid dehydrogenase by glycyrrhizic acid, adrenocorticotropic hormone–producing tumor)
	Constitutively active ENaC (e.g., Liddle's syndrome)

*A decreased intake of K⁺ is rarely a sole cause of chronic hypokalemia unless the intake of K⁺ is very low and the duration of this low intake of K⁺ is prolonged. Nevertheless, a low intake of K⁺ can lead to a more severe degree of the hypokalemia if there is an ongoing K⁺ loss.

---

high blood pressure. The most common causes are protracted vomiting and the use of diuretic agents. The diuretic effect may also be due to an inherited disorder affecting NaCl reabsorption in the medullary TAL (i.e., Bartter's syndrome) or in the DCT (i.e., Gitelman's syndrome). Ligands that occupy the calcium-sensing receptor in the medullary TAL (e.g., ionized calcium in a patient with hypercalcemia), drugs (e.g., gentamicin, cisplatin), and possibly cationic proteins (e.g., cationic monoclonal immunoglobulins in a patient with multiple myeloma) may result in a clinical picture that mimics Bartter's syndrome. The use of urine electrolyte values in the differential diagnosis of hypokalemia in a patient with a contracted EABV is summarized in Table 27.3.

The second group of disorders involves a condition that is associated with a primary increase in ENaC activity (e.g., primary hyperreninemic hyperaldosteronism, primary hyperaldosteronism, disorders in which cortisol acts as a mineralocorticoid in CDN, constitutively active ENaC in the luminal membrane of principal cells in CDN). Patients with these disorders are expected to have hypertension and not to have low EABV.

In some patients a decreased rate of electroneutral Na⁺ reabsorption may contribute to the increased rate of electrogenic Na⁺ reabsorption and enhanced kaliuresis. This may be the case when Na⁺ is delivered to the CDN with little Cl⁻ (e.g., delivery of Na⁺ with HCO_3^- in a patient with recent vomiting or with an anion of a drug such as penicillin).

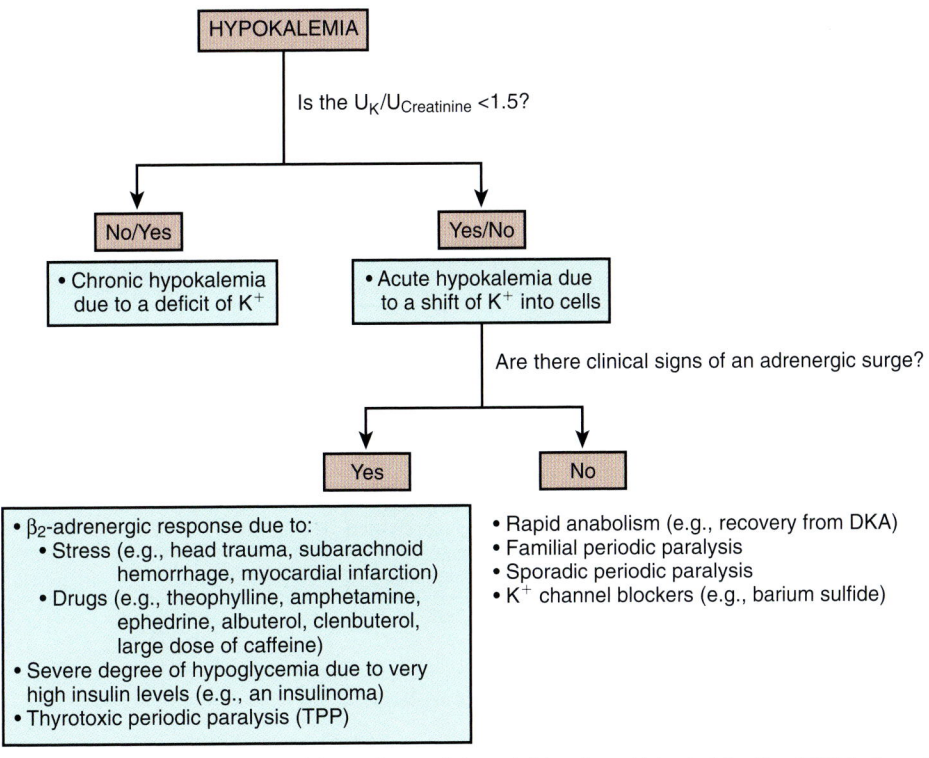

Flow Chart 27.4

```
                    HYPOKALEMIA
                         |
              Is the $U_K/U_{Creatinine}$ <1.5?
                    /         \
                No/Yes        Yes/No
                   |             |
        • Chronic hypokalemia   • Acute hypokalemia due
          due to a deficit of    to a shift of $K^+$ into cells
          $K^+$                          |
                          Are there clinical signs of an adrenergic surge?
                                    /        \
                                  Yes         No
```

- β_2-adrenergic response due to:
  - Stress (e.g., head trauma, subarachnoid hemorrhage, myocardial infarction)
  - Drugs (e.g., theophylline, amphetamine, ephedrine, albuterol, clenbuterol, large dose of caffeine)
- Severe degree of hypoglycemia due to very high insulin levels (e.g., an insulinoma)
- Thyrotoxic periodic paralysis (TPP)

- Rapid anabolism (e.g., recovery from DKA)
- Familial periodic paralysis
- Sporadic periodic paralysis
- K^+ channel blockers (e.g., barium sulfide)

Flow Chart 27.4 Reproduced with the permission of the author and the publisher from Halperin ML: *The ACID truth and BASIC facts—with a sweet touch, an enLYTEnment*, 6th ed, Toronto, 2015, RossMark Medical Publishers.

Flow Chart 27.5

Chronic hypokalemia and metabolic acidosis → What is the rate of excretion of NH_4^+ (mmol/day)?

<40:
- Distal RTA
  - Low H^+ secretion
  - High HCO_3^- secretion
- Proximal RTA treated with large dose of $NaHCO_3$

>100:
- Diarrhea, laxative abuse
- Acetazolamide (chronic use)
- Overproduction of acids and high excretion of their anions with NH_4^+, Na^+, and K^+ (e.g., glue sniffer and some patients with DKA)

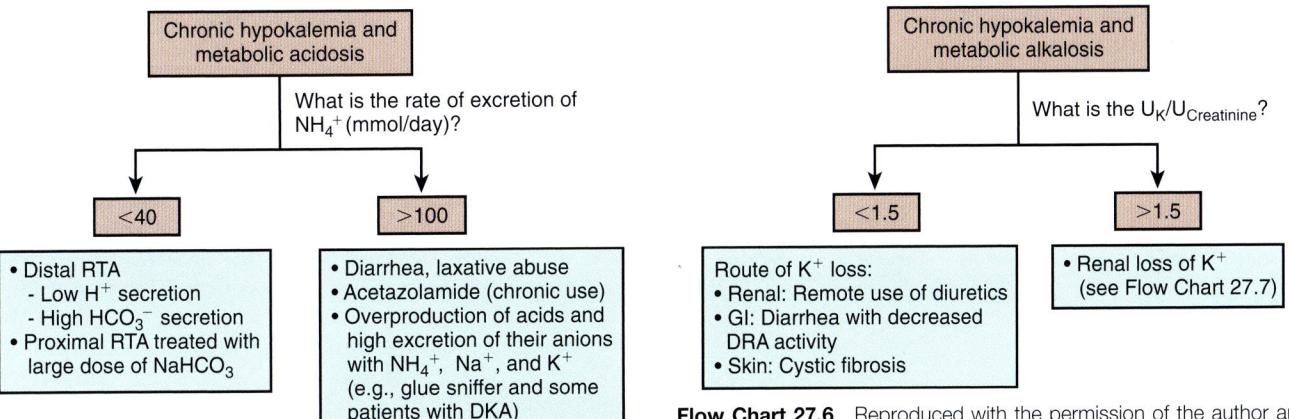

Flow Chart 27.5 Reproduced with the permission of the author and the publisher from Halperin ML: *The ACID truth and BASIC facts—with a sweet touch, an enLYTEnment*, 6th ed, Toronto, 2015, RossMark Medical Publishers.

Flow Chart 27.6

Chronic hypokalemia and metabolic alkalosis → What is the $U_K/U_{Creatinine}$?

<1.5:
- Route of K^+ loss:
  - Renal: Remote use of diuretics
  - GI: Diarrhea with decreased DRA activity
  - Skin: Cystic fibrosis

>1.5:
- Renal loss of K^+ (see Flow Chart 27.7)

Flow Chart 27.6 Reproduced with the permission of the author and the publisher from Halperin ML: *The ACID truth and BASIC facts—with a sweet touch, an enLYTEnment*, 6th ed, Toronto, 2015, RossMark Medical Publishers.

Magnesium (Mg^{2+}) deficiency is frequently associated with hypokalemia. This relationship is likely due to the underlying disorders that cause losses of both Mg^{2+} and K^+ (e.g., diarrhea, diuretic therapy, Gitelman's syndrome). K^+ secretion in the CDN is mediated by ROMK, a process that is inhibited by intracellular Mg^{2+}. A decrease in intracellular Mg^{2+}, caused by Mg^{2+} deficiency, releases the Mg^{2+}-mediated inhibition of ROMK. Mg^{2+} deficiency alone, however, does not necessarily cause hypokalemia, because an increase in the rate of electrogenic reabsorption of Na^+ is required to enhance the rate of secretion of K^+.

CONSULT 7: HYPOKALEMIA AND A LOW RATE OF POTASSIUM EXCRETION

A 28-year-old Asian woman presented with sudden onset of generalized muscle weakness and inability to ambulate upon awakening this morning. She had lost 7 kg of body weight in the last 2 months but did not report nausea, vomiting, diarrhea, or the use of diuretics, laxatives, exogenous thyroid hormone, herbal medications, or illicit drugs. The attack was not preceded by strenuous exercise or the consumption of a carbohydrate-rich meal. She had no family history of hypokalemia, paralysis, or hyperthyroidism. On physical examination, she was alert and oriented; blood pressure was 150/70 mm Hg, heart rate was 116 beats/min,

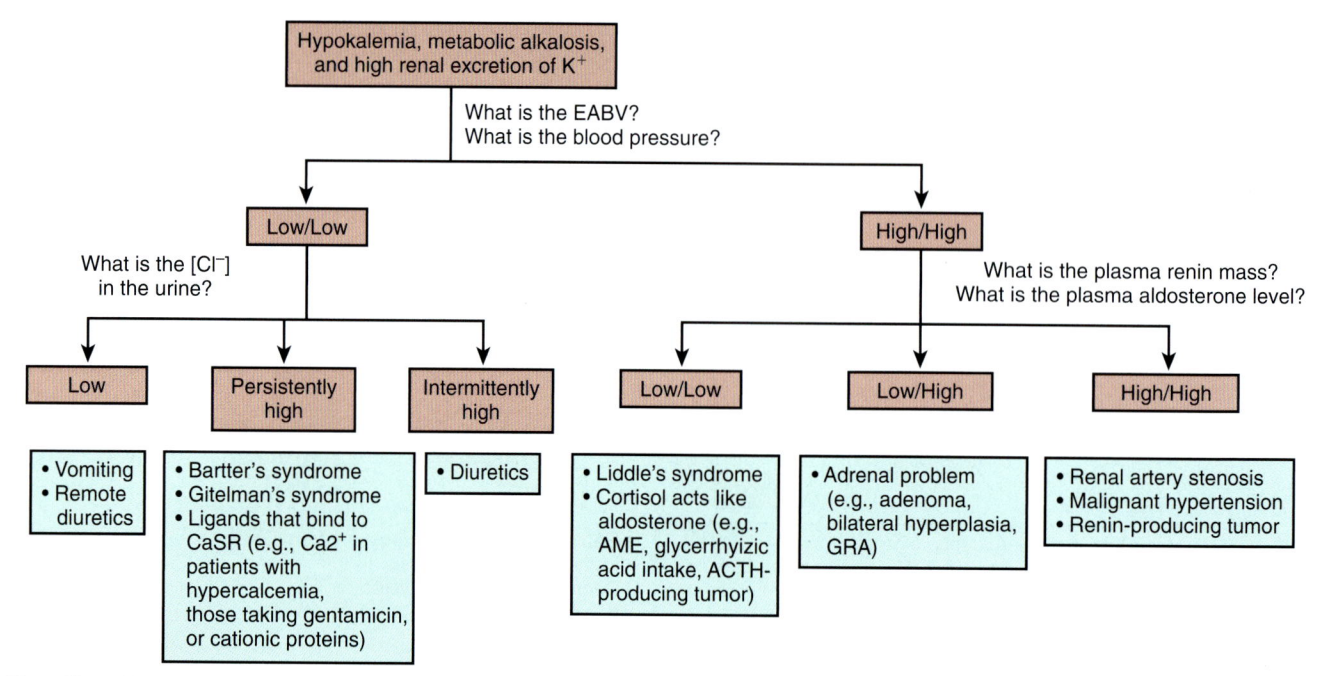

```
                    ┌─────────────────────────────┐
                    │ Hypokalemia, metabolic alkalosis, │
                    │ and high renal excretion of K⁺   │
                    └─────────────────────────────┘
                              What is the EABV?
                              What is the blood pressure?
```

Flow Chart 27.7 Reproduced with the permission of the author and the publisher from Halperin ML: *The ACID truth and BASIC facts—with a sweet touch, an enLYTEnment*, 6th ed, Toronto, 2015, RossMark Medical Publishers.

---

and respiratory rate was 18 breaths/min. The thyroid gland was not obviously enlarged, and there was no exophthalmos. Symmetric flaccid paralysis with areflexia was present in all four limbs. The remainder of the physical findings was unremarkable. The pH and P_{CO_2} shown in the following table of laboratory findings were from arterial blood sample, whereas all other blood data were from the venous blood sample. The ECG showed sinus tachycardia and prominent U waves.

	Blood	Urine
K^+, mmol/L	1.8	12
Creatinine	0.7 mg/dL	1.9 g/L
Na^+, mmol/L	140	179
Cl^-, mmol/L	108	184
pH	7.41	—
P_{CO_2}, mm Hg	36	—
HCO_3^-, mmol/L	23	—
Glucose, mg/dL	112	0

Questions

- Is there a medical emergency?
- What is the basis of the hypokalemia?
- What are the options for therapy?

Discussion of Questions

Is there a Medical Emergency? Because the ECG did not show significant changes that could be due to hypokalemia and because respiratory muscle weakness causing hypoventilation was not present as assessed from the arterial P_{CO_2}, there were no serious emergencies related to hypokalemia at this time.

What Is the Basis of the Hypokalemia? A U_K/U_{Cr} ratio less than 1 (mmol/mmol) and the absence of a metabolic acid-base disorder on presentation suggest that the basis of severe hypokalemia in this patient was an acute shift of K^+ into cells.

Possible Reasons for Potassium Shift into Cells: The presence of tachycardia, systolic hypertension, and wide pulse pressure suggest that an adrenergic surge was the cause of the acute shift of K^+ into cells. On further laboratory testing she was found to have hyperthyroidism, so the diagnosis was thyrotoxic periodic paralysis (TPP). Patients with TPP often have subtle signs and symptoms of thyrotoxicosis. In contrast to standard teaching, most patients with TTP do not have clear precipitating factors such as strenuous exercise or the consumption of a carbohydrate-rich meal. Increased Na^+-K^+-ATPase activity has traditionally been implicated in the pathogenesis of TPP. Later studies have shown, however, that susceptibility to TPP can be conferred by loss-of-function mutations in the skeletal muscle–specific inward-rectifying K^+ (Kir) channel, Kir2.1, and loci on 17q24.3 involved in *KCNJ2* gene expression. The dual hits of increased intracellular K^+ influx via activated Na^+-K^+-ATPase and decreased K^+ efflux due to defective Kir channels lead to hypokalemia with decreased muscle excitability in patients with TPP.

What are the Options for Therapy? The patient received intravenous KCl at a rate of 10 mmol/hour in a normal saline solution. In a patient with severe hypokalemia, one should not use a dextrose-containing solution, because the release of insulin may induce a further shift of K^+ into cells and aggravate the severity of hypokalemia. Although she received only 80 mmol of KCl, rebound hyperkalemia (P_K 5.7 mmol/L) developed; the P_K returned to normal 6 hours later. Data suggest that hypokalemia in patients with TPP can be rapidly corrected without the risk of rebound hyperkalemia by the administration of a nonselective β-blocker and only a small dose of KCl.

CONSULT 8: HYPOKALEMIA AND A HIGH RATE OF EXCRETION OF POTASSIUM

Progressive muscle weakness developed over the last 6 hours in a 76-year-old Asian man that became so severe that he was unable to move. He had no other neurologic symptoms. He reported no nausea, vomiting, or diarrhea, or the use of diuretics or laxatives. Hypokalemia (P_K 3.3 mmol/L) and hypertension had been noted 1 year ago but had not been investigated further. On this admission, his blood pressure was 160/96 mm Hg and his heart rate was 70 beats/min. Neurologic examination revealed symmetric flaccid paralysis with areflexia but no other findings. The laboratory data prior to therapy are shown in the following table. The pH and P_{CO_2} values are from an arterial blood sample. Subsequent measurements indicated that the $P_{renin\,mass}$ and P_{Ald} were low. The plasma cortisol value was in the normal range.

	Blood	Urine
K^+, mmol/L	1.8	26
Na^+, mmol/L	147	132
Cl^-, mmol/L	90	138
Creatinine	0.8 mg/dL	0.6 g/L
pH	7.55	
P_{CO_2}, mm Hg	40	—
HCO_3^-, mmol/L	45	0
Osmolality, mOsm/L	302	482

Question
- What is the cause of hypokalemia in this patient?

Discussion of the Question

What Is the Cause of Hypokalemia in this Patient? In the presence of hypokalemia, the U_K/U_{Cr} was 5 (mmol/mmol), and metabolic alkalosis was also present. Hence the hypokalemia was largely due to a disorder that caused excessive loss of K^+ in the urine. Notwithstanding, that acute presentation with extreme weakness was likely due to an acute shift of K^+ into cells in conjunction with a chronic disorder that caused loss of K^+. This component of an acute shift of K^+ into cells was attributed to vigorous exercise and a large carbohydrate intake during breakfast prior to the onset of symptoms.

On clinical assessment, the patient's EABV volume was thought not to be contracted and he had hypertension. Therefore, the increased electrogenic reabsorption of Na^+ in the CDN was due to a primary increase in ENaC activity. The differential diagnosis is guided by measurements of the $P_{renin\,mass}$ and P_{Ald} (see Table 27.4). Because both P_{Ald} and $P_{renin\,mass}$ were suppressed, the differential diagnosis was between disorders in which cortisol acts as mineralocorticoid and those with constitutively active ENaCs in the luminal membranes of principal cells in the CDN. Inherited disorders in which ENaC is constitutively active (Liddle's syndrome) seemed unlikely, considering the patient's age. Plasma cortisol values were not elevated. Computed tomography (CT) of the chest showed no lung mass. Although the patient denied consuming licorice or chewing tobacco, it turned out that he used an herbal preparation containing large amounts of glycyrrhizic acid (the active ingredient in licorice) to sweeten his tea. The patient was treated initially with intravenous KCl; the weakness improved when the P_K reached 2.5 mmol/L. Oral KCl supplementation was continued. Two weeks later, P_K and blood pressure values had returned to normal levels, and his body weight had decreased from 78 kg to 74 kg.

CLINICAL APPROACH TO THE PATIENT WITH HYPERKALEMIA

A list of causes of hyperkalemia is provided in Table 27.6.

Step 1. Address Emergencies

Hyperkalemia constitutes a medical emergency, primarily because of its effect on the heart, which may lead to cardiac conduction abnormalities, arrhythmias, and, ultimately, asystole.

Step 2. Determine Whether the Cause of the Hyperkalemia Is an Acute Shift of Potassium Out of Cells in Vivo or Pseudohyperkalemia

Flow Chart 27.8 illustrates the procedure for determining the cause of the hyperkalemia.

Is the time short and/or has the intake of K^+ been low? If the answer is yes, the following three options should be considered:

There Is Destruction of Cells in the Body. Cell destruction could be due to, for example, crush injury, rhabdomyolysis, or tumor lysis syndrome.

There Is a Shift of K^+ Out of Cells in the Body. Shift of K^+ out of cells in the body may occur in conditions in which there is a less negative voltage in cells. Such conditions include tissue hypoxia affecting the Na^+-K^+-ATPase (those causing hypoxic lactic acidosis), lack of a stimulus for Na^+-K^+-ATPase (e.g., lack of insulin in patients with diabetic ketoacidosis [DKA], β_2-adrenergic blockade), and conditions in which there is an α-adrenergic surge (e.g., marked decrease in EABV causing inhibition of the release of insulin or directly causing a shift of K^+ out of cells). A shift of K^+ may also occur in conditions with metabolic acidosis due to non-monocarboxylic acids, that is, acids that cannot be transported on the MCT (e.g., metabolic acidosis due to a gain of HCl acid from loss of $NaHCO_3$ in a patient with diarrhea, ingestion of citric acid). Digoxin inhibits the Na^+-K^+-ATPase, so digoxin overdose can result in hyperkalemia. Acute hyperkalemia may occur during exhaustive exercise or in patients with status epilepticus. Severe hyperkalemia has been described as a complication of the administration of mannitol for the treatment or prevention of cerebral edema, because a rise in effective osmolality in the interstitial fluid causes the movement of water out of cells via AQP channels in cell membranes, which raises the concentration of K^+ in the ICF and provides a chemical driving force for the movement of K^+ out of cells. Succinylcholine depolarizes muscle cells, resulting in the efflux of K^+ through acetylcholine receptors in conditions that may lead to upregulation of acetylcholine receptors (e.g., burns, neuromuscular

Table 27.6 Causes of Hyperkalemia

High intake of K^+	Only if combined with low excretion of K^+
Shift of K^+ out of cells	Tissue breakdown (e.g., crush trauma, rhabdomyolysis, tumor lysis), exhaustive exercise:
	Na^+-K^+-ATPase problem
	Tissue hypoxia
	Lack of a stimulus (e.g., inhibition of insulin release by α-adrenergic surge, use of nonselective β-blockers [small effect if only factor])
	Inhibition of Na^+-K^+-ATPase (e.g., by drugs such as digoxin)
	Hyperosmolality (e.g., administration of mannitol)
	Metabolic acidosis due to acids that cannot be transported on the monocarboxylic acid cotransporter (e.g., HCl, citric acid)
	Increased K^+ efflux from cells (due to cell depolarizers such as succinylcholine, fluoride intoxication)
	Hyperkalemic periodic paralysis
Diminished K^+ loss in the urine	Advanced chronic renal failure
	Drugs that interfere with renal K^+ excretion:
	Drugs that cause acute renal failure or interstitial nephritis
	Drugs that interfere with the renin angiotensin aldosterone axis (e.g., nonsteroidal anti-inflammatory drugs, direct renin blockers, angiotensin-converting enzyme inhibitors, and angiotensin receptor blockers)
	Drugs that inhibit aldosterone synthesis (e.g., heparin)
	Aldosterone receptor blockers (e.g., spironolactone)
	Drugs that block amiloride-sensitive sodium channels (ENaCs) in the cortical distal nephron (CDN) (e.g., amiloride, trimethoprim)
	Drugs that interfere with activation of ENaC via proteolytic cleavage (e.g. nafamostat mesylate)
	Diminished electrogenic reabsorption of Na^+ in the CDN:
	Very low delivery of Na^+ to the CDN
	In some patients with hyporeninemic hypoaldosteronism due to destruction of or biosynthetic defect in the juxtaglomerular apparatus
	Low levels of aldosterone (e.g., Addison's disease)
	Genetic disorders involving the aldosterone receptor or ENaC (type I pseudohypoaldosteronism)
	Increased electroneutral reabsorption of Na^+:
	Increased reabsorption of Na^+ and Cl^- in the distal convoluted tubule (e.g., familial hypertension with hyperkalemia [*WNK4* or *WNK1* mutation], drugs [e.g., calcineurin inhibitors], in some patients with diabetic nephropathy and hyporeninemic hypoaldosteronism)
	Enhanced electroneutral reabsorption of Na^+ and Cl^- in the CDN due to increased parallel activity of pendrin and the sodium-driven Cl^-/HCO_3^- (e.g., in some patients with diabetic nephropathy and hyporeninemic hypoaldosteronism)

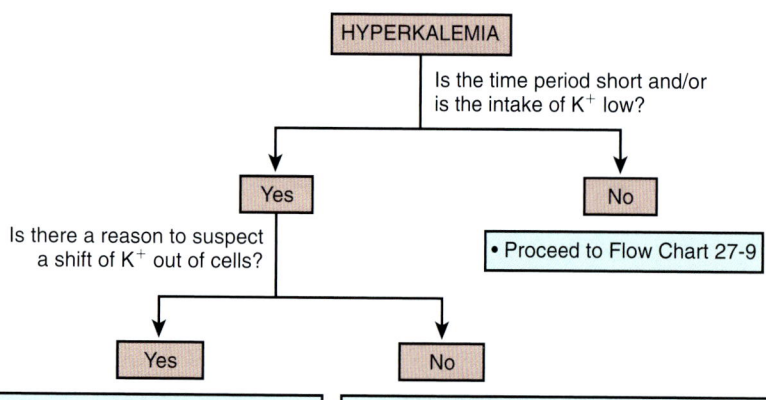

HYPERKALEMIA

Is the time period short and/or is the intake of K^+ low?

- **Yes** → Is there a reason to suspect a shift of K^+ out of cells?
  - **Yes**:
    - Tissue trauma or crush injury
    - Na^+/K^+-ATPase problem
      - Hypoxia
      - Lack of a stimulator (e.g., insulin lack, $β_2$-blockers)
      - Presence of an inhibitor (e.g., digoxin toxicity)
    - Hyperosmolality
    - α-adrenergic release
    - Depolarizing agents (e.g., succinylcholine)
    - Metabolic acidosis due to non-monocarboxylic acids
  - **No**:
    - Pseudohyperkalemia
      - Fist clenching, especially in a cachexic patient
      - Blood cell lysis in test tube (e.g., hemolysis thrombocytosis with megakaryocytes, leukocytosis with fragile WBCs)
      - Leak of K^+ across RBC membranes in vitro
- **No** → Proceed to Flow Chart 27-9

Flow Chart 27.8 Reproduced with the permission of the author and the publisher from Halperin ML: *The ACID truth and BASIC facts—with a sweet touch, an enLY-TEnment,* 6th ed, Toronto, 2015, RossMark Medical Publishers.

injury [upper or lower motor neuron], disuse atrophy, or prolonged immobilization). Fluoride can open the Ca^{2+}-sensitive K^+ channels, and fluoride intoxication can lead to fatal hyperkalemia. A positive family history for acute hyperkalemia suggests that there may be a molecular basis for this disorder (e.g., hyperkalemic periodic paralysis).

Pseudohyperkalemia May Be Present. The presence of ECG changes related to hyperkalemia rules out pseudohyperkalemia as the sole cause of the hyperkalemia. Pseudohyperkalemia is caused by the release of K^+ during or after venipuncture. Excessive fist clenching during blood sampling may increase K^+ release from local muscle and thus raise the measured P_K. Pseudohyperkalemia can be present in cachectic patients, in whom the normal T-tubule architecture in skeletal muscle may be disturbed. Thrombocytosis (especially megakaryocytosis), leukocytosis (especially due to fragile leukemia cells), and erythrocytosis may cause pseudohyperkalemia through the release of K^+ from cells. Cooling of blood prior to the separation of cells from plasma is a recognized cause of pseudohyperkalemia. There are several hereditary subtypes of pseudohyperkalemia, caused by increase in passive K^+ permeability of erythrocytes. The P_K increases in blood samples from patients with these subtypes that have been left at room temperature.

Step 3. What Is the Rate of Potassium Excretion?

In a patient with chronic hyperkalemia, pseudohyperkalemia should be ruled out first. In normal subjects, a K^+ load can augment the rate of excretion of K^+ to more than 200 mmol/day with only a minor increase in P_K. Patients with chronic hyperkalemia often have a defect in renal K^+ excretion. In a steady state, they excrete what they eat (minus the amount of K^+ lost in stool), but at the expense of maintaining hyperkalemia. Therefore, the value of assessing the rate of K^+ excretion is to determine the contribution of K^+ intake to the degree of hyperkalemia. A 24-hour urine collection is necessary for this purpose, rather than determination of U_K/U_{Cr} in a spot urine sample, because of the diurnal variation in K^+ excretion.

Step 4. What Is the Basis for the Defect in Renal Potassium Excretion?

Does the Patient Have Advanced Chronic Renal Failure? The first subgroup consists of patients who have very low delivery of Na^+ to the CDN resulting from a marked decrease in EABV.

Is the Patient Taking Drugs That Interfere with the Renal Excretion of Potassium? A list of drugs that may interfere with the renal excretion of K^+ is provided in Table 27.6.

Does the Patient Have a Disorder That Leads to Diminished Reabsorption of Sodium via ENACs in the Cortical Distal Nephron? The second subgroup consists of patients who have lesions that lead to a diminished number of open ENaC units in the luminal membranes of principal cells in the CDN. This includes patients who have hypoaldosteronism (e.g., adrenal insufficiency) and those with molecular defects that involve the aldosterone receptor or ENaC. Patients in this subgroup have a low EABV and higher than expected rates of excretion of Na^+ and Cl^- in a setting of low EABV and a high $P_{renin\ mass}$. The P_{Ald} is helpful to determine the reason for this diminished Na^+ reabsorption via ENaC in the CDN.

A subset of patients with hypoaldosteronism has low $P_{renin\ mass}$ (hyporeninemic hypoaldosteronism) and a low EABV. Their lesions may be destruction of or a biosynthetic defect in the juxtaglomerular apparatus, leading to a low $P_{renin\ mass}$ and thereby a low P_{Ald}. Patients with such disorders are expected to have a significant rise in U_K/U_{Cr} with the administration of exogenous mineralocorticoids.

Does the Patient Have a Disorder That Increases Electroneutral Sodium Reabsorption in the Distal Convoluted Tubule? In the subgroup of patients with disorders that increase electroneutral Na^+ reabsorption in the DCT, the site of the lesion is the early DCT, where there is enhanced electroneutral reabsorption of Na^+ and Cl^- via NCC mediated by an increase in the NCC-activating form of WNK4 or an increase in the long form of WNK1 (L-WNK1). Suppression of release of aldosterone by an expanded EABV leads to a diminished number of open ENaC units in the luminal membranes of principal cells in CDN. These kinases also cause endocytosis of ROMKs from the luminal membranes of principal cells in CDN. Such patients tend to have expanded EABV, hypertension, and suppressed $P_{renin\ mass}$ and P_{Ald} (hyporeninemic hypoaldosteronism). Patients with this pathophysiology are expected to show a good response to the administration of thiazide diuretics, in terms of lowering of blood pressure and correction of hyperkalemia.

The clinical picture in patients with the syndrome of familial hyperkalemia with hypertension (also known as pseudohypoaldosteronism type II or Gordon's syndrome) resembles that of a gain-of-function in the thiazide-sensitive NCC. Major deletions in the gene encoding for WNK1 and missense mutations in the gene encoding for WNK4 have been reported in these patients.[25] A set of clinical findings similar to those in patients with familial hyperkalemia with hypertension may occur in other patients, most commonly those with diabetic nephropathy.[20] Support for the hypothesis that suppression of renin release in these patients is the result of EABV expansion are the findings that circulating atrial natriuretic peptide blood values are elevated in these patients, and many show response to either NaCl restriction or furosemide therapy with an increased $P_{renin\ mass}$. Another example of this pathophysiology is the hyperkalemia in patients treated with calcineurin inhibitors.[26]

Does the Patient Have a Disorder that Increases Electroneutral Reabsorption of Sodium in the Cortical Collecting Duct? The pathophysiology in patients with disorders that increase electroneutral Na^+ reabsorption in the CCD may consist of increased parallel transport activity of pendrin and Na^+-dependent Cl^-/HCO_3^- exchanger (NDBC). This may be the pathophysiology for what used to be thought of as "chloride shunt disorder."[27] These patients will also have an expanded EABV and suppressed $P_{renin\ mass}$ and P_{Ald} (hyporeninemic hypoaldosteronism). The disorders in these patients may be more responsive, in terms of increasing K^+ excretion, to the induction of bicarbonaturia by the administration of the carbonic anhydrase inhibitor acetazolamide than to the administration of thiazide diuretics. This possibility, however, needs to be examined in a clinical study.

Step 5. Is a Low Flow Rate in the Terminal Cortical Collecting Duct Contributing to Hyperkalemia?

Because of the process of intrarenal urea recycling, a large fraction of the osmoles delivered to the terminal CCD is urea osmoles. A low protein intake may decrease the amount of urea that recycles and hence the rate of flow in the terminal CCD. The usual rate of excretion of urea in subjects consuming typical Western diet is about 400 mmol/day. If the rate of excretion of urea is appreciably lower than that, a low flow rate in the terminal CCD may be a contributing factor in hyperkalemia.

CONSULT 8: HYPERKALEMIA IN A PATIENT TAKING TRIMETHOPRIM

Pneumocystis jiroveci pneumonia (PJP) developed in a 35-year-old cachectic male with the human immune deficiency virus (HIV) infection. On admission, he was febrile, there were no physical findings indicating contraction of EABV volume, and all plasma electrolyte values were in normal ranges. He was treated with co-trimoxazole (sulfamethoxazole and trimethoprim). Three days later, he was noted to have low blood pressure, his EABV was low, and his P_K rose to 6.8 mmol/L. An ECG shows tall, peaked, narrow-based T waves. The urine volume was 0.8 L/day, and the U_{osm} value was 350 mOsm/kg H_2O; other laboratory findings were as follows:

	Blood	Urine
K^+, mmol/L	6.8	14
Na^+, mmol/L	130	60
Cl^-, mmol/L	105	43
Creatinine	0.9 mg/dL	0.8 g/L
pH	7.30	—
P_{CO_2}, mm Hg	30	—
HCO_3^-, mmol/L	15	0
Urea	BUN: 14 mg/dL	Urea concentration: 280 mmol/L

Questions

- Why is hyperkalemia present?
- What are the implications of the pathophysiology of hyperkalemia for the choice of treatment in this patient?

Discussion of the Questions

Why Is Hyperkalemia Present? The steps to follow are provided in Flow Chart 27.8. Although an element of pseudohyperkalemia could have been present in this cachectic patient, the ECG changes indicated that he had true hyperkalemia.

Is the Time Short and/or Has the Intake of Potassium Been Low? The U_K was 14 mmol/L and his rate of excretion of K^+ was extremely low in the presence of hyperkalemia (U_K/U_{Cr} 17.5 [mmol/g]), so one might conclude that the major basis for the hyperkalemia is the low rate of K^+ excretion. This severe degree of hyperkalemia developed over a relatively short time, however, and while the patient was consuming very little K^+. Therefore, a shift of K^+ from cells rather than a large positive external balance for K^+ is likely the major cause of hyperkalemia. The cause of this exit of K^+ from cells could be cell necrosis or the α-adrenergic effect of adrenaline released in response to the low EABV to suppress the release of insulin or to directly cause a shift of K^+ out of cells. Nevertheless, he also had a large defect in renal K^+ excretion. Because EABV was low and U_{Na} and U_{Cl} were inappropriately high in the presence of a contracted EABV, the low U_K/U_{Cr} was due to diminished reabsorption of Na^+ in the CDN (Flow Chart 27.9). The presumptive diagnosis was adrenal insufficiency due to an infection in a patient with HIV. The plasma cortisol value, however, was appropriately high, and moreover, he did not show a response to exogenous mineralocorticoids with an increase in U_K/U_{Cr}. It was thought that diminished Na^+ reabsorption in the CDN was due to inhibition of ENaCs by the trimethoprim that was used to treat the PJP. Both the $P_{renin\ mass}$ and P_{Ald} (which became available later) were high, as expected in this setting (see Table 27.4).

Interpretation: Renal salt wasting due to blockade of ENaCs by trimethoprim led to the development of a contracted EABV. As a result, there was a shift of K^+ out of cells probably because of inhibition of insulin release by binding of catecholamines to pancreatic islet cells α-adrenergic receptors. Because of the low EABV and the low intake of proteins, there was a low rate of flow in the CCD. This, in addition to diminishing the rate of K^+ excretion, caused the concentration of trimethoprim to be higher in the lumen of the CCD (same amount of trimethoprim in a smaller volume); hence trimethoprim became a more effective blocker of ENaCs.

What Are the Implications of the Pathophysiology of Hyperkalemia for the Choice of Treatment in this Patient? The basis of hyperkalemia is a shift of K^+ from cells, so it would be an error to induce a large loss of K^+ when there is likely no total body K^+ surplus. The appropriate treatment would be to expand the EABV with an infusion of saline to suppress the release of catecholamines, removing the inhibition of the release of insulin by their binding to pancreatic islet cells α-adrenergic receptors, which could result in a shift of K^+ into cells.

The question arose as to whether trimethoprim should be discontinued. Because the drug was needed to treat the PJP, a means to remove its renal ENaC-blocking effect was sought. The concentration of trimethoprim would fall in the lumen of the CDN if flow in CDN were to rise through an increase in the number of osmoles delivered to this nephron segment. To achieve this aim, one could increase the delivery of urea to the CDN by increasing the intake of protein or one could inhibit the reabsorption of Na^+ and Cl^- in the TAL of the loop of Henle using a loop diuretic plus the infusion of enough NaCl to reexpand the EABV. Because it is the cationic form of trimethoprim that blocks ENaC, inducing bicarbonaturia could also be considered to lower the concentration of H^+ in the luminal fluid in the CDN and thereby the concentration of the cationic form of the drug.

CONSULT 9: CHRONIC HYPERKALEMIA IN A PATIENT WITH TYPE 2 DIABETES MELLITUS

A 50-year-old man was referred for investigation of hyperkalemia; his P_K ranged from 5.5 to 6 mmol/L in a number of measurements that were done over the last several weeks. He

Flow Chart 27.9

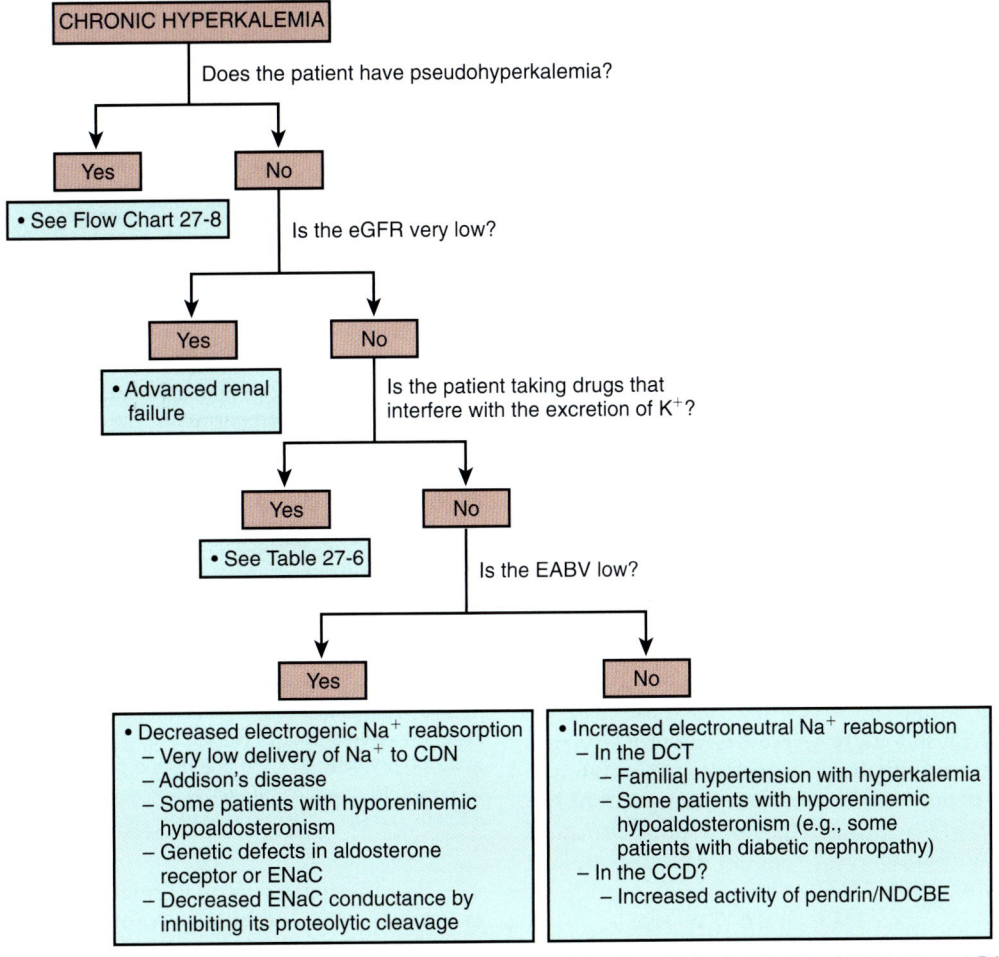

```
CHRONIC HYPERKALEMIA
         │
         ▼
Does the patient have pseudohyperkalemia?
   ├── Yes → • See Flow Chart 27-8
   └── No
         │
         ▼
   Is the eGFR very low?
      ├── Yes → • Advanced renal failure
      └── No
            │
            ▼
      Is the patient taking drugs that interfere with the excretion of K⁺?
         ├── Yes → • See Table 27-6
         └── No
               │
               ▼
         Is the EABV low?
```

Yes:
- Decreased electrogenic Na^+ reabsorption
  - Very low delivery of Na^+ to CDN
  - Addison's disease
  - Some patients with hyporeninemic hypoaldosteronism
  - Genetic defects in aldosterone receptor or ENaC
  - Decreased ENaC conductance by inhibiting its proteolytic cleavage

No:
- Increased electroneutral Na^+ reabsorption
  - In the DCT
    - Familial hypertension with hyperkalemia
    - Some patients with hyporeninemic hypoaldosteronism (e.g., some patients with diabetic nephropathy)
  - In the CCD?
    - Increased activity of pendrin/NDCBE

Flow Chart 27.9 Reproduced with the permission of the author and the publisher from Halperin ML: *The ACID truth and BASIC facts—with a sweet touch, an enLYTEnment*, 6th ed, Toronto, 2015, RossMark Medical Publishers.

---

was on an angiotensin-converting enzyme (ACE) inhibitor for treatment of hypertension, but hyperkalemia persisted after this medication was discontinued. He was currently on amlodipine 10 mg once a day. He was noted to have microalbuminuria, but no other history of macrovascular or microvascular disease related to diabetes mellitus. On physical examination, his blood pressure was 160/90 mm Hg, his jugular venous pressure was about 2 cm above the level of the sternal angle, and he had pitting edema of the ankles bilaterally. Results of laboratory investigations were as follows:

P_{Na}, mmol/L	140
P_K, mmol/L	5.7
P_{Cl}, mmol/L	108
$P_{renin\ mass}$, ng/L	4.50 (range 9.30-43.4)
P_{Ald}, pmol/L	321 (range 111-860)
P_{HCO3}, mmol/L	19
P_{Alb}, g/L (mg/dL)	40 (4.0)
P_{Cr}, μmol/L (mg/dL)	100 (1.2)

Question
- What is the cause of hyperkalemia in this patient?

Discussion of the Question

What Is the Cause of Hyperkalemia in this Patient? The first step is to rule out pseudohyperkalemia. The presence of hyperchloremic metabolic acidosis (HCMA) would suggest true hyperkalemia. Hyperkalemia is associated with an alkaline PCT cell pH, which leads to inhibition of ammoniagenesis. K^+ ions compete with NH_4^+ for transport on the Na^+-K^+-$2Cl^-$ cotransporter in the TAL of the loop of Henle, which leads to decreased medullary interstitial availability of NH_3. Both effects result in a low rate of excretion of NH_4^+.

The patient did not have advanced renal dysfunction and was not currently taking drugs that may interfere with renal excretion of K^+. The $P_{renin\ mass}$ was decreased and P_{Ald} was suppressed if one considers the presence of hyperkalemia. He was then thought to have hyporeninemic hypoaldosteronism, commonly labeled as type IV renal tubular acidosis (RTA). This disorder is traditionally thought to be the result of destruction of, or a biosynthetic defect in, the juxtaglomerular apparatus (JGA) leading to low $P_{renin\ mass}$ and thereby to low P_{Ald}. If type IV RTA were present, one would expect the patient to have renal salt wasting with decreased EABV and the absence of hypertension—although such features are not found in many patients with this disorder. Another hypothesis is that suppression of renin release in patients with this disorder is the result of EABV expansion because circulating values of atrial natriuretic peptide blood are elevated, and many cases respond to either NaCl restriction or furosemide with an increased $P_{renin\ mass}$. The basis of the disorder remains to be established. It is possible that the reabsorption of Na^+ and Cl^- may be augmented in the DCT as in patients with familial hyperkalemia with hypertension. Interesting in regard to patients with type 2 diabetes mellitus, who may have hyperinsulinemia and the metabolic syndrome, is the finding that long-term insulin infusion in rats is associated with the retention of NaCl owing to its enhanced reabsorption in different nephron segments, including the DCT, and with less *WNK4* expression in the renal cortex.[20] Studies in hyperinsulinemic db/db mice suggested that the phosphatidylinositol-3-kinase (PI3K)/Akt signaling pathway activates the WNK1-NCC phosphorylation cascade, possibly leading to active NCCs in the luminal membranes of DCT cells.[28]

Differentiation between these two groups of patients with hyporeninemic hypoaldosteronism has implications for therapy, those with JGA defect or destruction, and those with excessive Na^+ and Cl^- reabsorption in the DCT. The use of exogenous mineralocorticoids (9α-fludrocortisone) is of benefit for the first group, as it results in both a kaliuresis and reexpansion of the EABV owing to retention of Na^+. Diuretic therapy would pose a threat to these patients because it would cause a more severe degree of EABV contraction. In contrast, mineralocorticoids may aggravate the hypertension in patients with excessive reabsorption of Na^+ and Cl^- in the DCT. In this group, the administration of thiazide diuretics to inhibit NCCs should lead to both kaliuresis and lowering of the blood pressure.

METABOLIC ALKALOSIS

Metabolic alkalosis is an electrolyte disorder that is accompanied by an elevated P_{HCO3} and a high plasma pH. Most patients with metabolic alkalosis have a deficit of NaCl, KCl, and/or HCl, any of which may lead to a higher P_{HCO3}.

CONCEPT 14

The concentration of HCO_3^- is the ratio of the content of HCO_3^- in the ECF compartment (numerator) and the ECFV (denominator), as shown in Equation 7.

$$[HCO_3^-]\ in\ plasma = Quantity\ HCO_3^-\ in\ ECF/ECFV \quad (7)$$

A rise in the concentration of HCO_3^- might be due to an increase in its numerator (positive balance of HCO_3^-) and/or a decrease in its denominator (diminished ECFV) (Figure 27.9; Equation 7). A quantitative assessment of the ECFV is critical to estimate the quantity of HCO_3^- in the ECF compartment and thereby to determine the basis of the metabolic alkalosis.

CONCEPT 15

Electroneutrality must be present in every body compartment and in the urine.

Terms such as "Cl^--depletion alkalosis" do not take into account the need for electroneutrality. Hence, in our opinion, a deficit must be defined as to whether it is a deficit of HCl, KCl, and/or NaCl.[29] Knowing the balances for Na^+, K^+, and Cl^- would make it possible for one to decide why the P_{HCO3} is higher than normal and what changes have occurred in the composition of the ECF and ICF compartments. Balance data are not available in most patients. Nevertheless, with a quantitative assessment of the ECFV, tentative conclusions about the contribution of deficits of each of the different Cl^--containing compounds to the development of metabolic alkalosis can be deduced (Flow Chart 27.10).

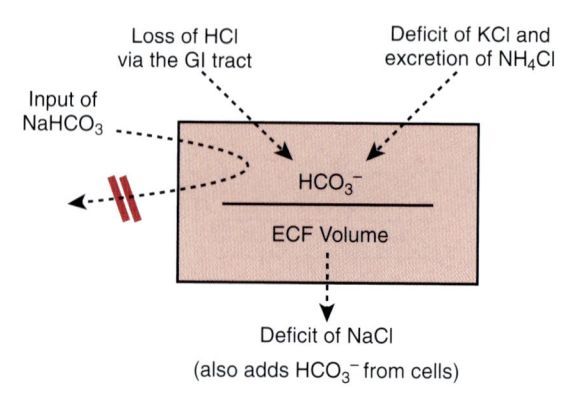

Figure 27.9 **Basis for a high concentration of HCO_3^- in the extracellular fluid (ECF) compartment.** The *rectangle* represents the ECF compartment. The concentration of HCO_3^- is the ratio of the content of HCO_3^- in the ECF compartment (numerator) and the ECF volume (ECFV) (denominator). The major causes for a rise in the content of HCO_3^- in the ECF compartment are a deficit of HCl and a deficit of KCl (*upper portion* of the figure). The major cause for a fall in the ECFV is a deficit of NaCl. An intake of $NaHCO_3$ is not sufficient on its own to cause a sustained increase in the content of HCO_3^- in the ECF compartment, unless there also is a marked reduction in the glomerular filtration rate (GFR) or there is another lesion that leads to a stimulus for the reabsorption of $NaHCO_3$ in the proximal convoluted tubule. *Double red lines* on the left portion of the figure indicate the reduced renal output of $NaHCO_3$. GI, Gastrointestinal. (Reproduced with the permission of the author and the publisher from Halperin ML: *The ACID truth and BASIC facts—with a sweet touch, an enLYTEnment*, 6th ed, Toronto, 2015, RossMark Medical Publishers.)

CONCEPT 16

There is no tubular maximum for renal HCO_3^- reabsorption.

Contrary to the widely held view, there is no renal tubular maximum for the reabsorption of $NaHCO_3$.[30,31] Filtered HCO_3^- ions are reabsorbed and retained in the ECF compartment unless their reabsorption in the PCT is inhibited. Angiotensin II (Ang II) and the usual pH in PCT cells are the two major physiologic stimuli for $NaHCO_3$ reabsorption in the PCT. Both of these stimuli must be removed for filtered $NaHCO_3$ to be excreted. Ingesting a large amount of $NaHCO_3$ will not cause chronic metabolic alkalosis because it results in expansion of the EABV, which lowers Ang II, and raises the pH in cells of the PCT. On the other hand, $NaHCO_3$ may be retained when there is a large decrease in its filtered load owing to a marked reduction in the GFR.

A deficit of NaCl or HCl may cause a higher P_{HCO3} and may also lead to a secondary deficit of K^+ and hypokalemia. A deficit of K^+ may be associated with an acidified PCT cell pH, which can then both initiate and sustain a high P_{HCO3} as a result of renal new HCO_3^- generation (higher excretion of NH_4^+) and enhanced reabsorption of HCO_3^- and organic anions (potential HCO_3^-) in the PCT (see Flow Chart 27.10).

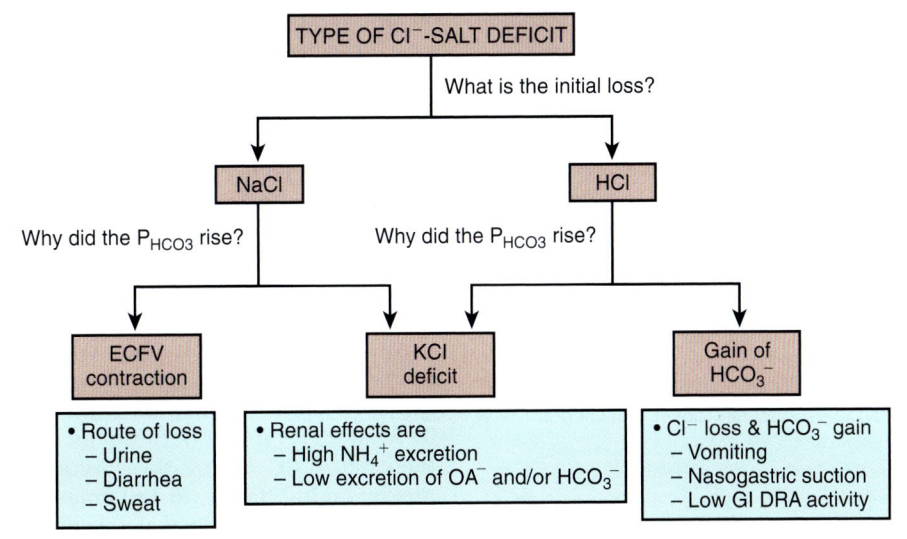

CHAPTER 27 — INTERPRETATION OF ELECTROLYTE AND ACID-BASE PARAMETERS IN BLOOD AND URINE

Flow Chart 27.10 Reproduced with the permission of the author and the publisher from Halperin ML: *The ACID truth and BASIC facts—with a sweet touch, an enLYTEnment,* 6th ed, Toronto, 2015, RossMark Medical Publishers.

TOOLS FOR ASSESSMENT OF METABOLIC ALKALOSIS

Quantitative Estimate of the Extracellular Fluid Volume

It is critical to have a quantitative estimate of the ECFV to determine its content of HCO_3^- and thereby why the P_{HCO3} rose. As discussed earlier in this chapter, we use the hematocrit for this purpose provided that anemia or polycythemia is not present (see Table 27.2).

Balance Data for Sodium, Potassium, and Chloride

Balance data for Na^+, K^+, and Cl^- are essential to describe deficits in electroneutral terms, but they are rarely available in clinical medicine. Nevertheless, they can be deduced if one has a quantitative estimate of the ECFV and measurements of the P_{Na}, P_{Cl}, and P_{HCO3}. One cannot know the balances for K^+ from these calculations, but its rough magnitude can be deduced by comparing the differences in the content of Na^+ versus that of Cl^- and HCO_3^- in the ECF compartment (see Consult 10).

CLINICAL APPROACH TO THE PATIENT WITH METABOLIC AKALOSIS

A list of causes of metabolic alkalosis is provided in Table 27.7. Our clinical approach to a patient with metabolic alkalosis is outlined in Flow Chart 27.11. The first step is to rule out the common causes of metabolic alkalosis, namely vomiting and the use of diuretics. Some patients may deny vomiting or the use of diuretics; measuring urine electrolyte levels is particularly helpful for suspicion of one of these diagnoses (see Table 27.3).

The most important test is to examine the U_{Cl}. A very low U_{Cl} is expected when there is a deficit of HCl and/or NaCl. The U_{Na} may be high if there is a recent episode of vomiting (see Table 27.3). If the U_{Cl} is not low, assessment of EABV and blood pressure helps identify patients with disorders of primary high ENaC activity in the late CDN (see Table 27.5) (the EABV is not low, hypertension is present) from patients with recent use of diuretics and those with Bartter's or Gitelman's syndrome (EABV is low, hypertension is absent).

Measurements of U_{Cl} in multiple spot urine samples are helpful to separate patients with Bartter's or Gitelman's syndrome (persistent high U_{Cl}) from those with diuretic abuse (U_{Cl} is high only while the diuretic is acting).

CONSULT 10: METABOLIC ALKALOSIS WITHOUT VOMITING OR USE OF DIURETICS

After a forced 6-hour intense training exercise in the desert in the heat of the day, an elite corps soldier was the only one in his squad who collapsed. He perspired profusely during the training exercise and drank a large volume of water and glucose-containing fluids. He did not vomit and reported he did not take any medications. Physical examination revealed a markedly contracted EABV. Initial laboratory data are shown in the table. The pH and $P{CO_2}$ values are from an arterial blood sample, whereas all other data are from a venous blood sample.

P_{Na}, mmol/L	125
P_K, mmol/L	2.7
P_{Cl}, mmol/L	70
Hematocrit	0.50
pH	7.50
P_{HCO3}, mmol/L	38
$P{CO_2}$, mm Hg	47

Questions

- What are the major threats to the patient and how should they dictate therapy?
- What is the basis for metabolic alkalosis?
- What is the therapy for metabolic alkalosis in this patient?

Discussion of Questions

What Are the Major Threats to the Patient and How Should They Dictate Therapy?

Acute Hyponatremia: The danger is brain herniation due to increased intracranial pressure from swelling of brain cells.

Table 27.7 Causes of Metabolic Alkalosis

Causes associated with a contracted effective arterial blood volume (EABV)	**Low urine chloride concentration:** Loss of gastric secretions (e.g., vomiting, nasogastric suction) Remote use of diuretics Delivery of Na$^+$ to the cortical distal nephron with anions that cannot be absorbed plus a reason for Na$^+$ avidity Posthypercapnic states Loss of NaCl via lower gastrointestinal tract (e.g., congenital disorder with Na$^+$ and Cl$^-$ loss in diarrhea, acquired forms of diminished activity of the Cl$^-$/HCO$_3^-$ exchanger; down regulated in adenoma [DRA]) **High urine chloride concentration:** Current diuretic use Ligand binding to calcium-sensing receptor in the thick ascending limb of the loop of Henle (e.g., Ca^{2+} in patients with hypercalcemia, drugs [e.g., gentamicin, cisplatin], cationic proteins [e.g., cationic monoclonal immunoglobulins in a patient with multiple myeloma]) Inborn error affecting transporters of Na$^+$ and/or Cl$^-$ in the nephron (e.g., Bartter's syndrome, Gitelman's syndrome)
Causes associated with an expanded EABV and hypertension	Disorders with enhanced mineralocorticoid activity that may cause hypokalemia Primary hyperaldosteronism (e.g., adrenal adenoma, bilateral adrenal hyperplasia, glucocorticoid-remediable aldosteronism) Primary hyperreninemic hyperaldosteronism (e.g., renal artery stenosis, malignant hypertension, renin-producing tumor) Disorders with cortisol acting as a mineralocorticoid (e.g., apparent mineralocorticoid excess syndrome [AME], inhibition of 11β-hydroxysteroid dehydrogenase by glycyrrhizic acid, adrenocorticotropic hormone–producing tumor) Disorders with constitutively active amiloride-sensitive sodium channels in the cortical collecting duct (e.g., Liddle's syndrome) Large reduction in glomerular filtration rate plus a source of NaHCO$_3$

Basis of Hyponatremia: Because he weighed 80 kg and had a muscular build, the patient's initial total body water (TBW) was about 50 L (ECFV was 15 L, ICF volume 35 L). Because the patient had hyponatremia, his ICF volume was expanded because of a water gain. The percentage expansion of ICF volume is close to the percentage fall in P$_{Na}$, around 11%. Hence, he had a water gain in the ICF, of about 4 L. With a hematocrit of 0.50, the ECFV volume decreased by one third, from its normal value of about 15 L to about 10 L; accordingly, he lost 5 L of ECFV. This represents the loss of 5 L of water and 700 mmol of Na$^+$. In addition, as the P$_{Na}$ decreased from 140 mmol/L to 125 mmol/L, each of the remaining 10 L of ECVF volume had a loss of 15 mmol of Na$^+$. Hence, the total Na$^+$ loss was 850 mmol. In total body balance terms, he had a loss of 850 mmol of Na$^+$ and 1 L of water (a loss of 5 L of water from the ECF and again of 4 L of water in the ICF). Therefore, the primary basis of his hyponatremia was Na$^+$ loss.

Hemodynamic Instability: An infusion of isotonic saline was started in the field, and the patient was hemodynamically stable on arrival at the emergency department.

After it was recognized that his P$_{Na}$ was 125 mmol/L, intravenous therapy was changed from isotonic saline to 3% hypertonic saline. The goal of therapy was to raise the P$_{Na}$ by 5 mmol/L rapidly. Because the hyponatremia was acute, there was little if any risk of osmotic demyelination from rapidly raising the P$_{Na}$ to 130 mmol/L.

Hypokalemia: The hypokalemia did not represent an emergency, as he did not have a cardiac arrhythmia or respiratory muscle weakness. As discussed later, the basis of the hypokalemia seemed to be largely an acute shift of K$^+$ into the ICF. An intravenous infusion of isotonic saline supplemented with 40 mmol/L of KCl was started. The P$_K$ was followed closely.

What Is the Basis for Metabolic Alkalosis? To distinguish between HCl, KCl, and NaCl deficits, a quantitative analysis of the degree of contraction of the ECFV is needed. As mentioned previously, with a hematocrit of 0.50, this patient's ECFV was decreased by a third, from its normal value of 15 L to about 10 L, so he had lost 5 L of ECFV.

Balance Data for Sodium, Potassium, and Chloride
Deficit of HCl: There was no history of vomiting so an HCL deficit is a very unlikely basis for the metabolic alkalosis.
Deficit of NaCl: The decrease in his ECF volume was about 5 L. One can now calculate how much this degree of ECFV contraction would raise the P$_{HCO3}$ (divide the normal content of HCO$_3^-$ in the ECF compartment (15 L × 25 mmol/L, or 375 mmol) by the new ECFV (10 L) and the result is 37.5 mmol/L. This value is remarkably close to the measured P$_{HCO3}$, 38 mmol/L, suggesting that a major reason for the rise in the P$_{HCO3}$ is the fall in his ECFV.
Balance for Sodium: Multiplying the P$_{Na}$ (140 mmol/L) before the training exercise by the normal ECFV (15 L) yields an Na$^+$ content of about 2100 mmol. After the training exercise, the P$_{Na}$ was 125 mmol/L and the ECFV was 10 L, so the ECF Na$^+$ content was 1250 mmol. Accordingly, the deficit of Na$^+$ in the ECF compartment was about 850 mmol.
Balance for Chloride: Multiplying the P$_{Cl}$ before the training exercise (103 mmol/L) by the normal ECFV (15 L) yields a Cl$^-$ content of about 1545 mmol. After the training exercise, the P$_{Cl}$ was 70 mmol/L and the ECF volume was 10 L, so ECF Cl$^-$ content was 700 mmol. Accordingly, the deficit of Cl$^-$ was about 840 mmol, a value close to the deficit of Na$^+$.
Balance for Potassium: There was little difference between the deficits of Na$^+$ and Cl$^-$, so there was no appreciable deficit of KCl to account for a drop in P$_K$ to 2.7 mmol/L. Especially in this muscular elite soldier, the loss of K$^+$ would

Flow Chart 27.11

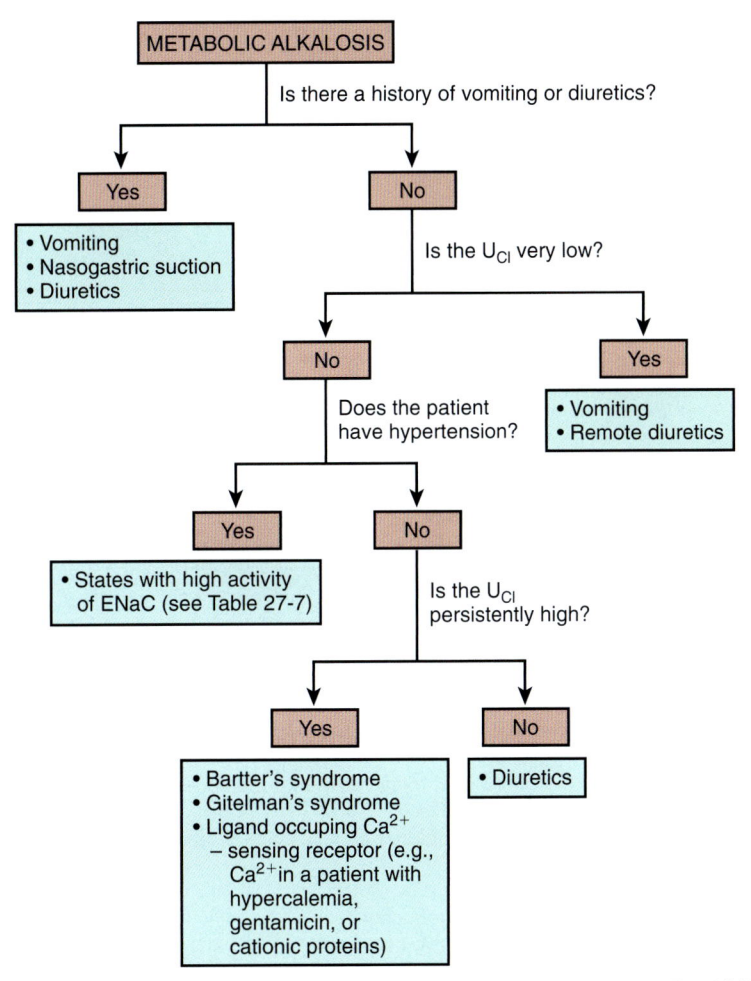

```
METABOLIC ALKALOSIS
         │
Is there a history of vomiting or diuretics?
    ┌────┴────┐
   Yes        No
    │          │
• Vomiting    Is the U_Cl very low?
• Nasogastric      ┌────┴────┐
  suction         No         Yes
• Diuretics       │           │
                  │         • Vomiting
         Does the patient    • Remote diuretics
         have hypertension?
         ┌────┴────┐
        Yes        No
         │          │
• States with     Is the U_Cl
  high activity   persistently high?
  of ENaC          ┌────┴────┐
  (see Table      Yes        No
  27-7)            │          │
              • Bartter's   • Diuretics
                syndrome
              • Gitelman's
                syndrome
              • Ligand occupying Ca²⁺
                – sensing receptor (e.g.,
                  Ca²⁺ in a patient with
                  hypercalemia,
                  gentamicin, or
                  cationic proteins)
```

Flow Chart 27.11 Reproduced with the permission of the author and the publisher from Halperin ML: *The ACID truth and BASIC facts—with a sweet touch, an enLYTEnment,* 6th ed, Toronto, 2015, RossMark Medical Publishers.

have to have been very large to account for this degree of hypokalemia. Accordingly, the major mechanism for the hypokalemia is likely to be a shift of K^+ into cells (due to a β-adrenergic surge and possibly the alkalemia).

Routes for NaCl Loss: The next issue is to examine possible routes for a large loss of NaCl in such a short time. Because diarrhea and polyuria were not present, the only route for a large NaCl loss was via sweat. To have a high electrolyte concentration in sweat and a large sweat volume, the likely underlying lesion would be cystic fibrosis. The diagnosis of cystic fibrosis was confirmed later by molecular studies.

What Is the Therapy for Metabolic Alkalosis in this Patient? Because the basis for the metabolic alkalosis was largely an acute deficit of NaCl, the patient required a positive balance of about 850 mmol of NaCl to replace the deficit. He was initially given hypertonic saline to deal with the danger of acute hyponatremia. If all of this deficit were replaced with 3% hypertonic saline (which would also give him about 1.5 L of H_2O), the P_{Na} would rise to about 140 mmol/L, assuming that a water diuresis does not occur following expansion of the EABV. He likely had nonosmotic stimuli (e.g., pain, anxiety) for the release of vasopressin, and hence may not have had a water diuresis with expansion of his EABV. On the other hand, he might still have had a large volume of water in the GI tract that could have been absorbed later and cause the P_{Na} to drop. Hence P_{Na} needed to be followed closely, and the tonicity of administered fluid modified accordingly. After the administration of only 40 mmol of KCl, the patient's P_K rose to 3.8 mmol/L, adding support to our speculation that the major cause of the hypokalemia was an acute shift of K^+ into cells.

METABOLIC ACIDOSIS

Metabolic acidosis is a process that causes a drop in the P_{HCO3} and a rise in the concentration of H^+ in plasma. Metabolic acidosis represents a diagnostic category with many different causes (Table 27.8). The risks for the patient depend on the underlying disorder that caused the metabolic acidosis, the ill effects of the binding of H^+ to intracellular proteins in vital organs (e.g., the brain and the heart), and possible dangers associated with the anions that accompanied the H^+ load (e.g., chelation of ionized calcium by citrate in a patient with metabolic acidosis due to ingestion of citric acid)[32] (Table 27.9).

CONCEPT 17

The P_{HCO3} is the ratio of the content of HCO_3^- in the ECF compartment to the ECFV.

Table 27.8 Causes of Metabolic Acidosis

Acid Gain

With retention of anions in plasma	L-Lactic acidosis:
	  Due predominantly to overproduction of L-lactic acid
	    Hypoxic lactic acidosis:
	      Inadequate delivery of O_2 (cardiogenic shock, shunting of blood past organs (e.g., sepsis), or excessive demand for oxygen (e.g., seizures)
	    Increased production of L-lactic acid in absence of hypoxia
	    Overproduction of reduced nicotinamide adenine dinucleotide (NADH) and accumulation of pyruvate in the liver (e.g., metabolism of ethanol plus thiamine deficiency)
	    Decreased pyruvate dehydrogenase activity (e.g., thiamine deficiency, inborn errors of metabolism)
	    Compromised mitochondrial electron transport system (e.g., riboflavin deficiency, inborn errors affecting the electron transport system)
	    Excessive degree of uncoupling of oxidative phosphorylation (e.g., phenformin, accumulation of metformin in patients with acute renal failure)
	  Due predominantly to reduced removal of L-lactate:
	    Liver failure (e.g., severe acute viral hepatitis, shock liver)
	  Due to a combination of reduced removal and overproduction of L-lactic acid:
	    Antiretroviral drugs (inhibition of mitochondrial electron transport plus hepatic steatosis)
	    Metastatic tumors (especially large tumors with hypoxic areas plus liver involvement)
	Ketoacidosis (diabetic ketoacidosis, alcoholic ketoacidosis, hypoglycemic ketoacidosis including starvation, ketoacidosis due to a large supply of short-chain fatty acids [e.g., acetic acid from fermentation of poorly absorbed carbohydrate in the colon plus a cause for inhibition of fatty acids synthesis in the liver owing to diminished activity of acetyl-coenzyme A carboxylase])
	Renal insufficiency (metabolism of dietary sulfur-containing amino acids and decreased renal excretion of NH_4^+)
	Metabolism of toxic alcohols (e.g., formic acid from metabolism of methanol, glycolic acid, and oxalic acid from metabolism of ethylene glycol)
	D-Lactic acidosis (and presence of other organic acids produced by metabolism of carbohydrates by colonic bacteria)
	Pyroglutamic acidosis

With a high rate of excretion of anions in urine	Glue-sniffing (hippuric acid overproduction) Diabetic ketoacidosis with excessive ketonuria

$NaHCO_3$ Loss

Direct loss of $NaHCO_3$	Via the gastrointestinal tract (e.g., diarrhea, ileus, fistula) Via the urine (e.g., patients in the early phase of a disease causing proximal renal tubular acidosis)

Indirect loss of $NaHCO_3$	Low glomerular filtration rate
	Renal tubular acidosis:
	  Low availability of NH_3 owing to a defect in ammoniagenesis in cells of the proximal collecting tubule (PCT) (urine pH ≈ 5) (e.g., hyperkalemia, alkaline pH in PCT cells)
	  Defect in net distal H^+ secretion (urine pH often ≈ 7):
	    H^+-ATPase defect or alkaline α-intercalated cells (e.g., autoimmune diseases and hypergammaglobulinemic states such as Sjögren's disease and systemic lupus erythematosus)
	    H^+ backleak (e.g., amphotericin B)
	    HCO_3^- secretion in the collecting ducts (e.g., some patients with Southeast Asian ovalocytosis with a second mutation in the gene encoding for anion exchanger 1, which causes it to be mistargeted to the luminal membrane of α-intercalated cells)
	  Problem with both distal H^+ secretion and NH_3 availability (urine pH ≈ 6):
	  Diseases involving the renal medullary interstitial compartment (a long list including infections, drugs, infiltrations, precipitations, inflammatory disorders, and sickle cell anemia)

It is important to distinguish between acidemia and acidosis. *Acidemia* simply describes the concentration of H^+ in plasma. Acidemia may not be present in a patient who has metabolic acidosis if there is, for example, a large decrease in the ECFV, which may sufficiently raise the P_{HCO3} even though there is a decreased content of HCO_3^- in the ECF compartment (e.g., in the patient with severe diarrhea[33] and in some patients with DKA). For a diagnosis of metabolic acidosis to be made in this setting, a quantitative estimate of the ECFV is needed to assess its content of HCO_3^-.

CONCEPT 18

H^+ ions must be removed by the bicarbonate buffer system (BBS) to avoid their binding to intracellular proteins.

Binding of H^+ to proteins could change their charge, shape, and possibly their functions. To minimize binding of

CHAPTER 27 — INTERPRETATION OF ELECTROLYTE AND ACID-BASE PARAMETERS IN BLOOD AND URINE

Table 27.9 Threats to Life Associated with the Cause of Metabolic Acidosis

On Admission

Hemodynamic instability:
  Marked decrease in myocardial contractility (e.g., cardiogenic shock)
  Very low intravascular volume (e.g., NaCl loss, hemorrhage)
  Decreased peripheral vascular resistance (e.g., sepsis)
Cardiac arrhythmia:
  Most frequently seen in patients with hyperkalemia or hypokalemia
Failure of ventilation (e.g., respiratory muscle weakness due to hypokalemia)
Presence of toxins (e.g., methanol, ethylene glycol)
Presence of reactive oxygen species (e.g., pyroglutamic acidosis)
Nutritional deficiency (especially B vitamins)

During Therapy

Development of cerebral edema during therapy of diabetic ketoacidosis in children:
  Overly rapid infusion of isotonic saline
  Failure to prevent a fall in the effective plasma osmolality during the first 15 hours of therapy (the period in which most cases of cerebral edema occur)
Pulmonary edema (e.g., in patients with severe diarrhea if the extracellular fluid volume is expanded, but $NaHCO_3$ [or Na^+ with an anion that can be metabolized to produce HCO_3^- such as L-lactate] is not given)
Too rapid a rise in P_{Na} in patients with chronic hyponatremia
Acute shift of K^+ into cells (e.g., administration of glucose to patients with hypokalemia, administration of insulin to patients with diabetic ketoacidosis and hypokalemia, administration of $NaHCO_3$ to patients with hypokalemia)
Wernicke's encephalopathy due to failure to give thiamin (vitamin B_1) to a chronic alcoholic with alcoholic ketoacidosis

---

H^+ to proteins, H^+ removal should be carried out by the BBS, the bulk of which is in the ICF compartment and the interstitial spaces of skeletal muscles.[34]

TOOLS FOR ASSESSMENT OF METABOLIC ACIDOSIS

The tools for assessing metabolic acidosis are listed in Table 27.10.

Quantitative Assessment of the Extracellular Fluid Volume

To assess the ECF, we use the hematocrit or the concentration of total proteins in plasma. The assumption is that the patient did not have a preexisting anemia, polycythemia, or a low total plasma protein concentration.

Tools to Assess the Removal of Hydrogen by the Bicarbonate Buffer System

As shown in Equation 8, the BBS is driven by "pull" (i.e., by a lower P_{CO_2}). Effective buffering of H^+ by the BBS requires a low P_{CO_2} primarily in the interstitial space and ICF of skeletal muscles.

$$H^+ + HCO_3^- \leftrightarrow H_2CO_3 \leftrightarrow H_2O + CO_2 \quad (8)$$

Acidemia stimulates the respiratory center, leading to a fall in arterial P_{CO_2}. While the arterial P_{CO_2} sets the lower limit on the P_{CO_2} in capillaries, it does not guarantee that the capillary P_{CO_2} in skeletal muscles will be low enough to ensure effective buffering of H^+ by the BBS. Because the free-flowing brachial venous P_{CO_2} reflects the P_{CO_2} in capillary blood of skeletal muscles in its drainage pool, it should provide a means of assessing the effectiveness of the BBS in patients with metabolic acidosis. The capillary P_{CO_2} in skeletal muscles will be higher if the rate of blood flow to muscles is low, for example, as a result of decreased EABV. If muscle oxygen consumption in this setting remains unchanged, more oxygen will be extracted from, and more CO_2 will be added to, each liter of blood. The higher P_{CO_2} in muscle capillaries will diminish the effectiveness of the BBS to remove extra H^+. Hence, acidemia may become more pronounced, with the risk that more H^+ will be titrated by intracellular proteins in vital organs (Figure 27.10).[35] At usual rates of blood flow and metabolic work at rest, the brachial venous P_{CO_2} is about 6 mm Hg greater than arterial P_{CO_2}. If the blood flow rate to muscles is low, their venous P_{CO_2} will be more than 6 mm Hg greater than the arterial P_{CO_2}. Enough saline should be administered to increase this blood flow rate to muscle to achieve a brachial venous P_{CO_2} that is close to 6 mm Hg more than the arterial P_{CO_2}.

CLINICAL APPROACH: INTIAL STEPS

The initial steps in the clinical approach to a patient with metabolic acidosis are summarized in Flow Chart 27.12.

1. Identify threats for that patient, anticipate and prevent dangers that may arise during therapy (see Table 27.9).
2. Determine whether H^+ ions were buffered appropriately by the BBS.

METABOLIC ACIDOSIS DUE TO ADDED ACIDS

CONCEPT 19

When addition of acids is the cause of metabolic acidosis, one can detect the addition of H^+ by the appearance of new anions. These new anions may remain in the body or be excreted (e.g., in the urine or diarrhea fluid).

TOOLS FOR ASSESSING METABOLIC ACIDOSIS DUE TO ADDED ACIDS

Tools for assessment of metabolic acidosis due to added acids are shown in Table 27.10.

Detect New Anions in Plasma

The accumulation of new anions in plasma can be detected from a calculation of the P_{AG}.[36,37] The major cation in plasma is Na^+, and the major anions are Cl^- and HCO_3^-. In quantitative terms (and ignoring K^+), the difference between P_{Na} and $(P_{Cl} + P_{HCO3})$ is usually 12 ± 2 mEq/L. Nevertheless, because of different laboratory methods, the mean value of a normal P_{AG} varies greatly among clinical laboratories, and the range of normal values is wide. This difference reflects the other negative charges in plasma, which are due primarily to the

Table 27.10 Laboratory Tests for Diagnosis of Metabolic Acidosis

Question	Parameter(s) Assessed	Tool(s) to Use
Is the content of HCO_3^- low in the extracellular fluid (ECF)?	ECF volume	Hematocrit or total plasma proteins
Is metabolic acidosis due to overproduction of acids?	Appearance of new anions in the body or the urine	Plasma anion gap Urine anion gap
Is metabolic acidosis due to ingestion of alcohol?	Presence of alcohols as unmeasured osmoles	Plasma osmolal gap
Is buffering of H^+ by bicarbonate buffer system in skeletal muscle?	Buffering of H^+ by HCO_3^- in interstitial fluid and intracellular fluid compartment of muscle	Brachial venous P_{CO_2}
Is the renal response to chronic acidemia adequate?	Examine the rate of excretion of NH_4^+	Urine osmolal gap
If NH_4^+ excretion is high, which anion is excreted with NH_4^+?	Gastrointestinal loss of $NaHCO_3$ Acid added, but the anion is excreted in the urine	Urine Cl^- Urine anion gap
What is the basis for a low excretion of NH_4^+?	Low distal H^+ secretion Low NH_3 availability Both defects	Urine pH > 7.0 Urine pH ≈ 5.0 Urine pH ≈ 6.0
Where is the defect in H^+ secretion?	Distal H^+ secretion Proximal H^+ secretion	P_{CO_2} in alkaline urine Fractional excretion of HCO_3, urine citrate concentration

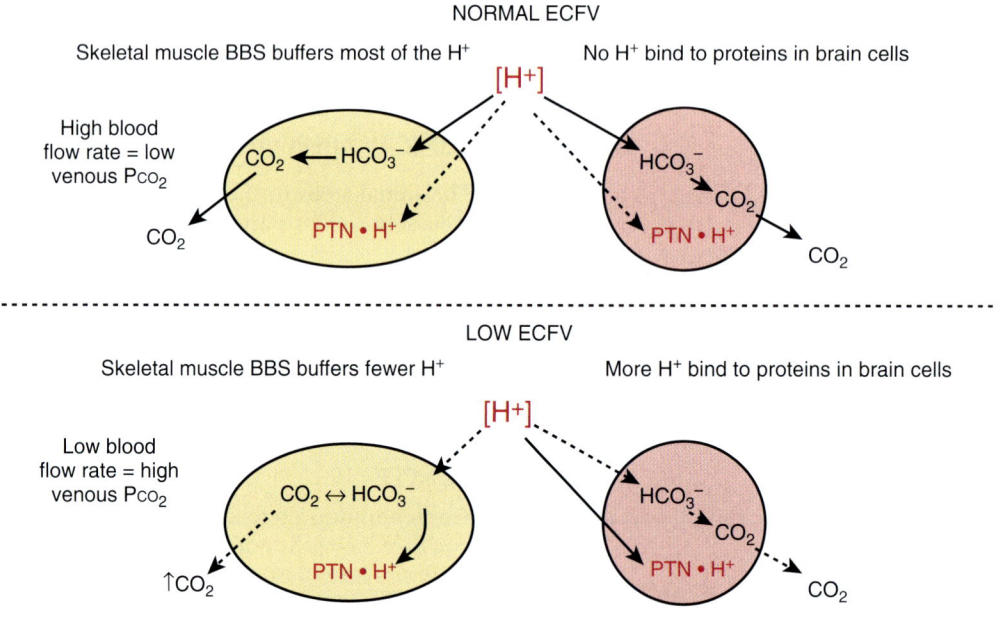

Figure 27.10 Buffering of H^+ in the brain in a patient with a contracted effective arterial blood volume (EABV). *Top,* Buffering of H^+ in a patient with a normal EABV and thereby a low muscle venous P_{CO_2}. The vast majority of H^+ removal occurs by the bicarbonate buffer system (BBS) in the interstitial space and in cells of skeletal muscles. *Bottom,* Buffering of a H^+ load in a patient with a contracted EABV and thereby high venous and capillary P_{CO_2} values. A high muscle venous P_{CO_2} prevents H^+ removal by its BBS. As a result, the degree of acidemia may become more pronounced, and more H^+ may bind to proteins (PTN·H^+) in the extracellular and intracellular fluids in other organs, including the brain. Notwithstanding, owing to autoregulation of cerebral blood flow, it is likely that the P_{CO_2} in brain capillary blood will change minimally unless there is severe contraction of the EABV and failure of autoregulation of cerebral blood flow. Considering the limited content of HCO_3^- in the brain, however, and that the brain receives a relatively larger proportion of the cardiac output, there is a risk that more H^+ will bind to proteins within the brain cells, further compromising their functions. (Reproduced with the permission of the author and the publisher from Halperin ML: *The ACID truth and BASIC facts—with a sweet touch, an enLYTEnment*, 6th ed, Toronto, 2015, RossMark Medical Publishers.)

negative valence on albumin. Therefore, when using this calculation to detect the presence of new anions in plasma, one must adjust the baseline value of the P_{AG} for the P_{Alb}. As a rough estimate, the baseline value for the P_{AG} falls (or rises) by 2.5 mEq/L for every 10-g/L or 1-g/dL fall (or rise) in the P_{Alb}.[38] Even with this adjustment, it seems that net negative valence on albumin is increased if there is an appreciable decrease in the EABV.[39]

Stewart recommended another approach to detect new anions in plasma, the *strong ion difference* (SID).[40] This

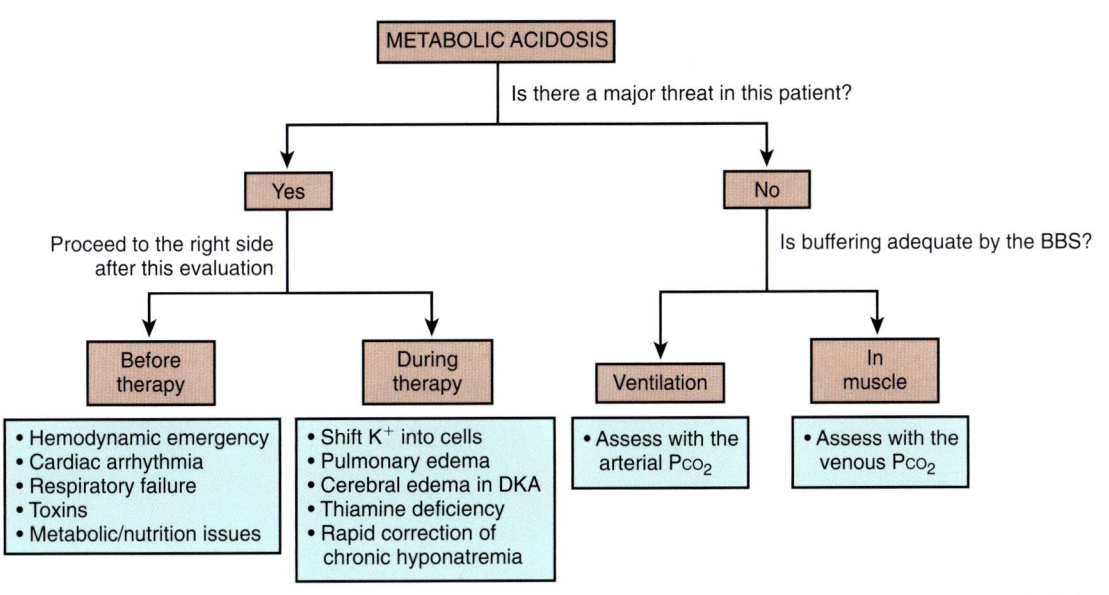

```
                        METABOLIC ACIDOSIS
                                │
                   Is there a major threat in this patient?
                    ┌───────────┴───────────┐
                   Yes                      No
         Proceed to the right side    Is buffering adequate by the BBS?
          after this evaluation
          ┌──────────┴──────────┐      ┌──────────┴──────────┐
        Before               During                        In
       therapy              therapy        Ventilation    muscle
```

Before therapy	During therapy	Ventilation	In muscle
• Hemodynamic emergency • Cardiac arrhythmia • Respiratory failure • Toxins • Metabolic/nutrition issues	• Shift K$^+$ into cells • Pulmonary edema • Cerebral edema in DKA • Thiamine deficiency • Rapid correction of chronic hyponatremia	• Assess with the arterial P$_{CO_2}$	• Assess with the venous P$_{CO_2}$

Flow Chart 27.12 Reproduced with the permission of the author and the publisher from Halperin ML: *The ACID truth and BASIC facts—with a sweet touch, an enLYTEnment*, 6th ed, Toronto, 2015, RossMark Medical Publishers.

approach is rather complex and offers only a minor advantage over the P_{AG} in that it includes a correction for the net negative charge on P_{Alb}.[41]

Use of the Delta Gap. The relationship between the rise in P_{AG} and the fall in P_{HCO3}, or the delta gap (delta AG/delta HCO_3^-), is used to detect the presence of coexisting metabolic alkalosis (the rise in P_{AG} is larger than the fall in P_{HCO3}) and/or the presence of both an "acid over production" type and a "NaHCO$_3$ loss" type of metabolic acidosis (the rise in P_{AG} is smaller than the fall in P_{HCO3}).

There are several pitfalls in using this relationship that must be recognized. One is failure to adjust for changes in the ECFV.[42] Consider, for example, a patient with DKA who has a P_{HCO3} of 10 mmol/L, and the "expected" 1:1 relationship between the rise in P_{AG} and the fall in the P_{HCO3}. The patient had a normal ECFV of 10 L before DKA developed, but as a result of the glucose-induced osmotic diuresis and natriuresis, the current ECFV is only 8 L. Although the fall in the P_{HCO3} and the rise in the concentration of ketoacid anions are equal, the deficit of HCO_3^- and the amount of ketoacids added to the ECF compartment are not. The sum of the content of HCO_3^- and ketoacid anions in the ECF compartment prior to the development of DKA is 250 mmol (25 + 0 mmol/L × 10 L). Their sum in ECFV after the DKA developed, however, is only 200 mmol (10 + 15 mmol/L × 8 L). The deficit of HCO_3^- in this example is 150 mmol, but the quantity of new anions in the ECF is only 120 mmol. The reason is that another component of the loss of HCO_3^- occurred when ketoacids were added, and some of the ketoacid anions were excreted in the urine with Na$^+$ and/or K$^+$, an indirect form of NaHCO$_3$ loss that would not be reflected in an increase in the P_{AG}. Hence the rise in the P_{AG} did not reveal the actual quantity of ketoacids that were added and the fall in P_{HCO3} did not reflect the actual magnitude of the deficit of HCO_3^-. When the ECFV is expanded with saline, the degree of deficit of HCO_3^- will become evident. In addition, the fall in the P_{AG} will not be matched by a rise in the P_{HCO3}, because some ketoacid anions will be lost in urine when their filtered load is increased with the rise in GFR.

Another pitfall in the use of the delta AG/delta HCO_3^- is the failure to correct for the net negative valence attributable to P_{Alb}. When calculating the P_{AG}, one must adjust the base value for changes in the charge on the most abundant unmeasured anion, P_{Alb}. We emphasize that adjustments should be made for a fall or an increase in P_{Alb}.

Detect New Anions in the Urine

New anions can be detected with the calculation of the urine anion gap (U_{AG}) (Equation 9). The concentration of NH_4^+ in the urine (U_{NH4}) is estimated from the urine osmolal gap (U_{OG}), as discussed in the next section. The nature of these new anions may sometimes be deduced by comparing their filtered load with their excretion rate. For example, when there is a very large quantity of the new anion in the urine in comparison with the rise in the P_{AG}, one should suspect that this anion is secreted in the PCT (e.g., hippurate anion from the metabolism of toluene) or freely filtered and poorly reabsorbed by the PCT (e.g., reabsorption of ketoacid anions may be inhibited by salicylate anions). On the other hand, a very low excretion of new anions suggests that they were avidly reabsorbed in the PCT (e.g. L-lactate anions).

$$U_{AG} = (U_{Na} + U_K + U_{NH4}) - U_{Cl} \qquad (9)$$

Detect Toxic Alcohols

Alcohols in plasma can be detected by calculating the plasma osmolal gap (P_{OG}) (Equation 10); a large increase in P_{OG} signifies the presence of alcohols. They occur because they are uncharged and have a low molecular weight, and because large quantities have been ingested.

$$P_{OG} = \text{Measured } P_{osm} - (2\,P_{Na} + P_{Glu} + P_{urea}), \qquad (10)$$
$$\text{(all in mmol/L terms)}$$

CLINICAL APPROACH TO THE PATIENT WITH METABOLIC ACIDOSIS DUE TO ADDED ACIDS

The steps in the clinical approach to the patient with metabolic acidosis due to added acids are shown in Flow Chart 27.13. If metabolic acidosis develops over a short period, the likely causes are overproduction of L-lactic acid (e.g., shock, ingestion of alcohol in a patient with thiamine deficiency) or ingestion of acids (e.g., metabolic acidosis due to ingestion of citric acid).

CONSULT 11

A 52-year-old man presented to the emergency department with abdominal pain, visual disturbances, and shortness of breath.[43] He had a history of drinking excessive amounts of alcohol on a regular basis. He admitted to drinking approximately 1 L of vodka the day before hospital admission but denied ingesting any other substances. During the 24 hours before admission he had not eaten at all. In the 5 hours before his admission, he had had several bouts of vomiting and did not drink any alcohol. His dietary intake had been generally very poor over the last several months, because he had diminished appetite.

On physical examination, he was fully conscious and oriented. His respiration rate was rapid (40 breaths/min). His pulse rate was also rapid (150 beats/min), and his blood pressure was 120/58 mm Hg. Neurologic findings were unremarkable.

The patient's urine tested strongly positive for ketones. His initial laboratory results on admission to the emergency

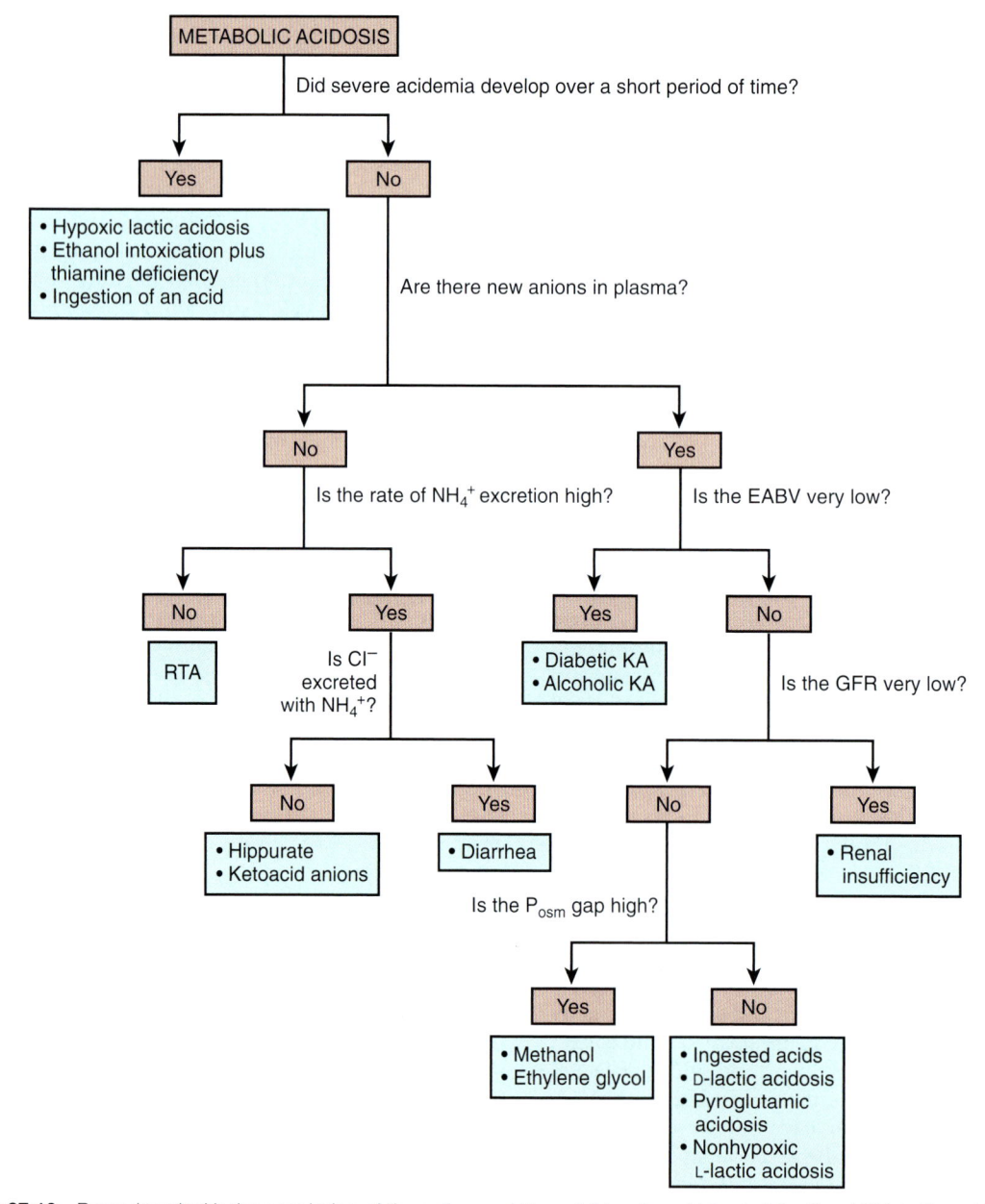

Flow Chart 27.13 Reproduced with the permission of the author and the publisher from Halperin ML: *The ACID truth and BASIC facts—with a sweet touch, an enLYTEnment*, 6th ed, Toronto, 2015, RossMark Medical Publishers.

department are shown in the following table. The pH and P_{CO_2} are from an arterial blood sample, whereas all other data are from a venous blood sample.

P_{Na}, mmol/L	132
P_K, mmol/L	5.4
P_{Cl}, mmol/L	85
P_{HCO3}, mmol/L	3.3
P_{AG} mEq/L	44
P_{osm}, mOsm/L	325
Hematocrit	0.46
pH	6.78
P_{CO_2}, mm Hg	23
Glucose, mmol/L	3.0
Albumin, g/L	36
P_{OG}, mOsm/L	42

Questions

- What dangers may be present on admission or may arise during therapy?
- What is the cause of the severe degree of L-lactic acidosis in this patient?

Discussion of the Questions

What Dangers May Be Present on Admission or May Arise During Therapy?

Severe Acidemia: The patient had a severe degree of acidemia with a large increase in the P_{AG}, indicating overproduction of acids. Although he was hemodynamically stable, a quantitatively small additional H^+ load would produce a proportionately larger fall in the P_{HCO3} and plasma pH. For instance, a halving of the P_{HCO3} would cause the arterial pH to drop by 0.30 unit if the arterial P_{CO_2} has not changed. By the same token, doubling of the P_{HCO3} would raise the plasma pH by 0.30 unit. A large dose of $NaHCO_3$ would be needed to achieve this, because the administered $NaHCO_3$ might lead to back-titration of some of the large H^+ load that is bound to the patient's intracellular proteins, and in addition he might have ongoing production of acids.

Toxic Alcohol Ingestion: Because the patient had a severe degree of metabolic acidemia with a large plasma osmolal gap, ingestion of methanol or ethylene glycol was suspected. Aldehydes produced from the metabolism of these alcohols by the enzyme alcohol dehydrogenase in the liver are the major cause of toxicity because they rapidly bind to tissue proteins. Although the patient ingested a large amount of ethanol, which could have caused the large plasma osmolal gap, and his urine was strongly positive for ketones, such a severe degree of acidemia is not usual in patients with alcoholic ketoacidosis. Because of the strong clinical suspicion of toxic alcohol ingestion, the patient was started on fomepizole (an inhibitor of alcohol dehydrogenase) during the wait for results of the measurements of the level of these toxic alcohols in his blood.

Thiamine Deficiency: Malnourished patients who present with alcoholic ketoacidosis are at risk for development of encephalopathy due to thiamine deficiency. When available, ketoacids are the preferred brain fuel because they are derived from storage fat, and hence, proteins from lean body mass are spared as a source of glucose for the brain during prolonged starvation. After successful treatment of alcoholic ketoacidosis, ketoacids are no longer an important brain fuel, so the brain must regenerate most of its ATP from oxidation of glucose. Thiamine (vitamin B_1) is a key co-factor for pyruvate dehydrogenase (PDH). The activity of PDH will be diminished by the lack of thiamine, so the rate of regeneration of ATP in brain cells will not be sufficient for their biologic work. Probably of greater significance is the likelihood of an increased demand for ATP regeneration in this setting (e.g., due to delirium tremens or the use of salicylates that may uncouple oxidative phosphorylation in the brain). Therefore anaerobic glycolysis will be stimulated in the brain to make ATP. As a result, there will be a sudden rise in the production of H^+ and L-lactate anions in areas of the brain where the metabolic rate is the most rapid and/or areas that had the lowest reserve of thiamine. Thiamine must be administered early in therapy in such patients.

More Information: The patient's plasma lactate was 23 mmol/L; results of blood assays for methanol and ethylene glycol were negative.

What is the Cause of the Severe Degree of L-Lactic Acidosis in this Patient? A rise in the concentration of L-lactate and H^+ can be caused by an increased rate of production and/or a decreased rate of removal of L-lactic acid. The rapid development and the severity of L-lactic acidosis in this patient suggest that the L-lactic acidosis is largely due to overproduction of L-lactic acid.

The degree of L-lactic acidosis in patients presenting with alcohol intoxication is usually mild (≈ 5 mmol/L) because it reflects the increased $NADH/NAD^+$ ratio owing to the ongoing production of NADH through ethanol metabolism, which is largely restricted to metabolic events in the liver (Equation 11). Other organs in the body are capable of oxidizing the L-lactate, because they lack the enzyme alcohol dehydrogenase and hence do not have a high $NADH/NAD^+$ ratio in this setting.

$$Pyruvate^- + NADH + H^+ \leftrightarrow \text{L-lactate-} + NAD^+ \qquad (11)$$

A severe degree of lactic acidosis may develop rapidly if there is a large intake of alcohol in a patient who is thiamine deficient. The site of L-lactic acid production is likely to be the liver, which has accumulation of pyruvate (owing to diminished activity of PDH) and a high $NADH/NAD^+$ ratio (due to metabolism of ethanol).

Nevertheless, for a severe degree of L-lactic acidosis to develop, there must be high flux in glycolysis, which results from the hydrolysis of ATP to adenosine diphosphate (ADP) and inorganic phosphate to perform work (H^+ are produced in this process) at a rate that exceeds the rate of regeneration of ATP from ADP in oxidative phosphorylation. Perhaps, the conversion of NADH to NAD^+ in the cytosol limits its availability for mitochondrial oxidative phosphorylation and the regeneration of ATP. Hence the concentration of ADP will rise and anaerobic glycolysis will be stimulated in the liver to make ATP.

Riboflavin deficiency may be also present in this malnourished patient with chronic alcoholism. The active metabolites formed from vitamin B_2 (riboflavin), flavin mononucleotide (FMN), and flavin adenine dinucleotide (FAD) are components of the mitochondrial electron transport system, which is the principal pathway in mitochondria to regenerate ATP.

HYPERCHLOREMIC METABOLIC ACIDOSIS

In hyperchloremic metabolic acidosis, almost no new anions are present in plasma. There are two major groups of causes for this type of metabolic acidosis, direct loss of $NaHCO_3$ and indirect loss of $NaHCO_3$. The direct loss of $NaHCO_3$ may occur via the GI tract, for instance, in patients with diarrhea, or through the urine in patients at the start of a disease process that causes proximal renal tubular acidosis (pRTA). The indirect loss of $NaHCO_3$ may be due to a low rate of excretion of NH_4^+ that is insufficient to match the daily rate of production of sulfuric acid from the metabolism of sulfur-containing amino acids (e.g., in patients with chronic renal failure or distal renal tubular acidosis [dRTA]). Indirect loss of $NaHCO_3$ may also be due to an overproduction of an acid (e.g., hippuric acid formed during the metabolism of toluene) with the excretion of its conjugate base (hippurate anions) in the urine at a rate that exceeds the rate of excretion of NH_4^+.

CONCEPT 20

The expected renal response to chronic metabolic acidosis is a high rate of excretion of NH_4^+.

In a patient with chronic metabolic acidosis, the expected rate of excretion of NH_4^+ should be more than 200 mmol/day.[44] There is a lag period of a few days before very high rates of excretion of NH_4^+ can be achieved.

CONCEPT 21

A low rate of excretion of NH_4^+ could be due to a decreased medullary interstitial availability of NH_3 or a decreased net H^+ secretion in the distal nephron.[45]

A low rate of ammoniagenesis has several possible causes. One is alkaline PCT cells due to hyperkalemia or a genetic and/or acquired disorder that compromises proximal H^+ secretion. The other involves a reduction in GFR, which produces a low filtered load of Na^+; in this situation, less work can be performed in PCT cells so the availability of ADP is decreased. Another cause of a low rate of excretion of NH_4^+ is a low net secretion of H^+ in the distal nephron; this could be due to an H^+-ATPase defect (e.g., autoimmune and hypergammaglobulinemic disorders, including Sjögren's syndrome), backleak of H^+ (e.g., due to drugs such as amphotericin B), or a disorder associated with the distal secretion of HCO_3^- (e.g., in certain patients with Southeast Asian ovalocytosis [SAO]). Patients with medullary interstitial disease (e.g., sickle cell disease) may have a low rate of excretion of NH_4^+ because of diminished accumulation of NH_4^+ in the medullary interstitium and a decreased rate of H^+ secretion in the MCD.

TOOLS FOR ASSESSING HYPERCHLOREMIC METABOLIC ACIDOSIS

Table 27.10 summarizes the steps for assessment of hyperchloremic metabolic acidosis.

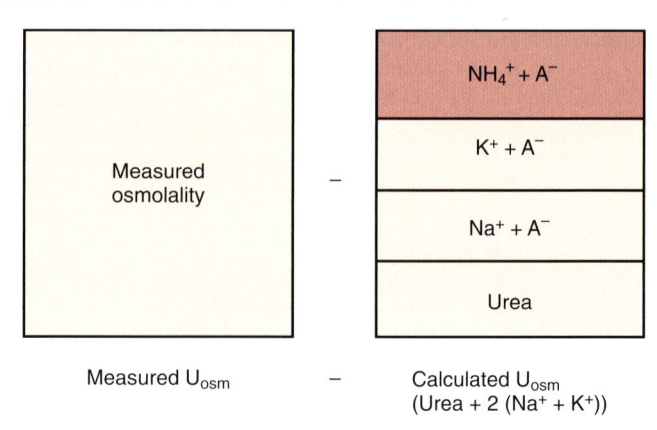

Figure 27.11 Indirect assessment of the concentration of NH_4^+ in the urine using the urine osmolal gap. The essence of the test is that a high concentration of NH_4^+ (shown in the *shaded region* on the *right*) is detected in the urine from its contribution to the urine osmolality. The *urine osmolal gap* is the difference between the measured urine osmolality and the urine osmolality calculated from the concentrations of the principal usual urine osmoles, urea, double the concentrations of $Na^+ + K^+$ (to account for the concentrations of the usual monovalent anions in the urine) and glucose in a patient with hyperglycemia. The concentration of NH_4^+ in the urine = $U_{OG}/2$. A^-, Anion. (Reproduced with the permission of the author and the publisher from Halperin ML: *The ACID truth and BASIC facts—with a sweet touch, an enLYTEnment*, 6th ed, Toronto, 2015, RossMark Medical Publishers.)

Assess the Rate of Excretion of NH_4^+ in the Urine

Urine Osmolal Gap. If a direct assay for urine NH_4^+ is not available, calculation of the U_{OG} provides the best indirect estimate of the U_{NH4} (Equation 12), because it detects all NH_4^+ salts in the urine (Figure 27.11).[46,47] We no longer use the urine net charge (or U_{AG}) for this purpose.

$$U_{OG} = \text{Measured } U_{osm} - \text{calculated } U_{osm}$$
$$\text{Calculated } U_{osm} = 2(U_{Na} + U_K) + U_{urea} + U_{Glu} \quad (12)$$
$$\text{(all in mmol/L)}$$
$$\text{Concentration of } NH_4^+ \text{ in the urine} = U_{OG}/2$$

We use the U_{NH4}/U_{Cr} ratio in a spot urine sample to assess the rate of excretion of NH_4^+. The rationale is that the rate of excretion of creatinine is relatively constant over the 24-hour period. In a patient with chronic metabolic acidosis, the expected renal response is a U_{NH4}/U_{Cr} ratio higher than 150 mmol NH_4^+ per g creatinine (more than 15 if creatinine is measured in mmol).

Determine Why the Rate of Excretion of NH_4^+ Is Low

Urine pH. The urine pH is not a reliable indicator for the rate of excretion of NH_4^+.[48] For example, at a urine pH of 6.0, the U_{NH4} can be 20 or 200 mmol/L (Figure 27.12). On the other hand, the basis for the low rate of excretion of NH_4^+ may be deduced from the urine pH. A urine pH around 5 suggests that the primary basis for a low rate of excretion of NH_4^+ is decreased availability of NH_3 in the medullary interstitial compartment due to a defect in ammoniagenesis. A urine pH higher than 7.0 suggests that NH_4^+ excretion is low because there is a defect in net H^+

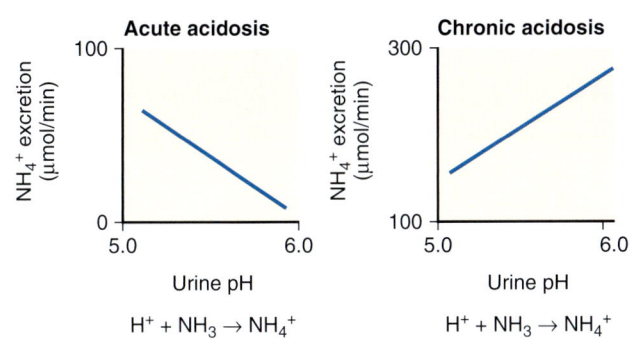

Figure 27.12 Urine pH is not a reliable indicator for the rate of excretion of NH_4^+. Left, During acute metabolic acidosis, the NH_4^+ is only modestly higher and the urine pH is low. This is because distal H^+ secretion is enhanced, and there is a time lag before the rate of renal production of NH_4^+ is augmented. Right, In contrast, during chronic metabolic acidosis, the rate of renal production of NH_4^+ is so high that the availability of NH_3 in the medullary interstitial compartment provides more NH_3 in the lumen of the medullary collecting duct (MCD) than H^+ secretion in this nephron segment. Note the much higher NH_4^+ excretion rate at a urine pH of 6. Note also the different scales on the y-axes. (Reproduced with the permission of the author and the publisher from Halperin ML: *The ACID truth and BASIC facts—with a sweet touch, an enLYTEnment*, 6th ed, Toronto, 2015, RossMark Medical Publishers.)

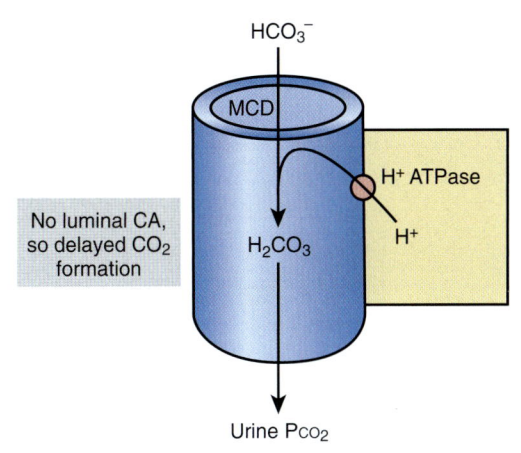

Figure 27.13 Use of the P_{CO_2} in alkaline urine to assess the distal secretion of H^+. The *cylinder* represents the medullary collecting duct (MCD) and the rectangle on its right side represents an β-intercalated cell, which contains a hydrogen–adenosine triphosphatase (H^+-ATPase pump). There are two requirements for using the urine P_{CO_2} in alkaline urine to reflect the capacity to secrete H^+ *(gray box)*. First, the patient is given an oral load of $NaHCO_3$ to increase both the filtered load of HCO_3^- and its delivery to the distal nephron. Second, because the luminal membranes of the MCD lack carbonic anhydrase (CA), the carbonic acid formed is delivered to the lower urinary tract, where it decomposes to CO_2 and H_2O and thereby elevates the urine P_{CO_2}. A high P_{CO_2} in alkaline urine (usually to ≈70 mm Hg) suggests that there is no major defect in H^+ secretory capacity in this nephron segment. (Reproduced with the permission of the author and the publisher from Halperin ML: *The ACID truth and BASIC facts—with a sweet touch, an enLYTEnment*, 6th ed, Toronto, 2015, RossMark Medical Publishers.)

secretion in the distal nephron. On the other hand, a urine pH around 6 would suggest a medullary interstitial disease that diminishes both accumulation of NH_4^+ in the medullary interstitium and H^+ secretion in the MCD.[49]

Assess Distal Hydrogen Secretion. H^+ secretion in the distal nephron can be evaluated with use of the P_{CO_2} in alkaline urine (U_{PCO_2}) during bicarbonate loading (Figure 27.13).[50] A U_{PCO_2} that is about 70 mm Hg in a second-voided alkaline urine implies that H^+ secretion in the distal nephron is likely to be normal, whereas much lower U_{PCO_2} values suggest that distal H^+ secretion is impaired. In patients with low net distal H^+ secretion, the U_{PCO_2} can be high if there is a lesion causing a backleak of H^+ from the lumen of the collecting ducts (e.g., from use of amphotericin B)[51] or distal secretion of HCO_3^- (as in some patients with SAO who also have a second mutation in HCO_3^-/Cl^- anion exchangers that leads to mistargeting of the exchangers to the luminal membranes of the α-intercalated cells).[52]

Assess Proximal Cell pH

Fractional Excretion of HCO_3^-. In patients with metabolic acidosis associated with a low capacity to reabsorb filtered HCO_3^- (e.g., with disorders involving defects in H^+ secretion in the PCT [pRTA]), some clinicians would measure the fractional excretion of HCO_3^- after infusing $NaHCO_3$ to confirm this diagnosis. This evaluation is rarely needed, in our opinion. Often the results are far from clear (e.g., in a patient with an abnormal ECFV or P_K) and, in addition, the test can impose a danger (e.g., in a patient with a low P_K). These disorders are signified clinically by failure to correct metabolic acidosis after administration of large amounts of $NaHCO_3$.

Rate of Citrate Excretion. The rate of excretion of citrate is a marker of pH in cells of the PCT.[53] The rate of excretion of citrate in children and adults consuming their usual diet is around 400 mg/day (≈2.1 mmol/day). Although the rate of excretion of citrate is very low during most forms of metabolic acidosis, a notable exception is in patients with disorders causing an alkaline PCT cell.

CLINICAL APPROACH TO THE PATIENT WITH HYPERCHLOREMIC METABOLIC ACIDOSIS

The steps in the clinical approach to the patient with hyperchloremic metabolic acidosis on the basis of the laboratory data detailed previously are shown in Flow Chart 27.14.

CONSULT 12

A 28-year-old man had been sniffing glue on a long-term, but intermittent basis. Over the past 3 days, he became profoundly weak and had a very unsteady gait. On physical examination, his blood pressure was 100/60 mm Hg and his pulse rate was 110 beats/min when he was lying flat. When he sat up, his blood pressure fell to 80/50 mm Hg and his pulse rate rose to 130 beats/min. Arterial blood pH was 7.20 and arterial P_{CO_2} was 25 mm Hg. Venous blood and urine laboratory values were as follows:

Flow Chart 27.14

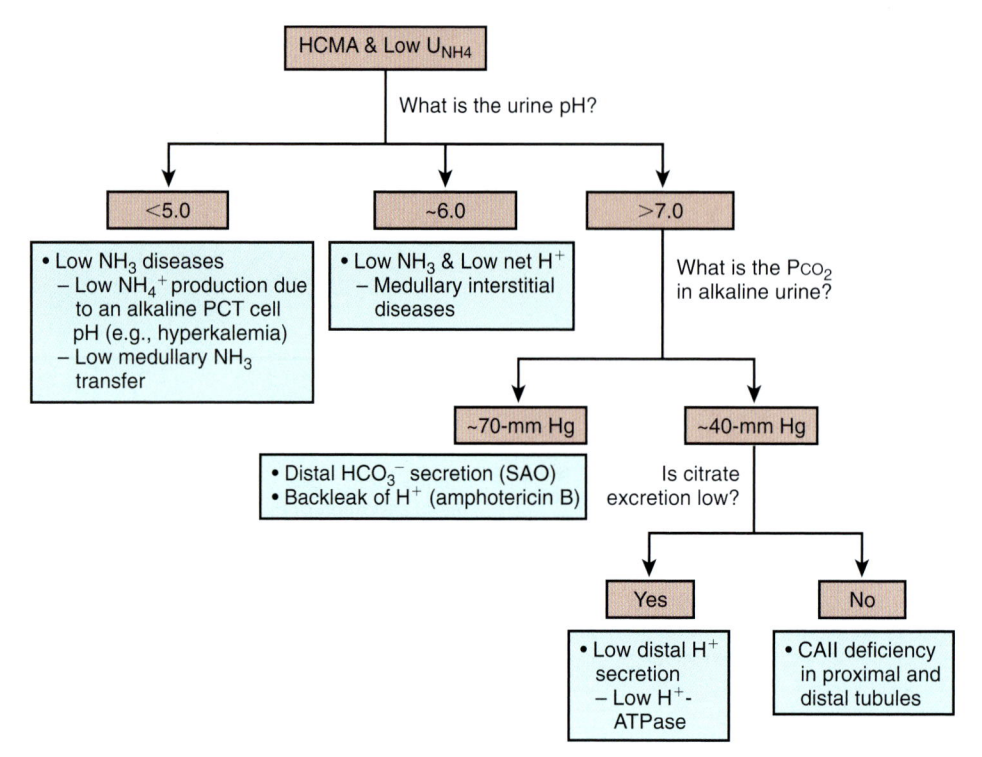

```
                    HCMA & Low U_NH4
                            │
                   What is the urine pH?
          ┌─────────────────┼─────────────────┐
        <5.0              ~6.0              >7.0
          │                 │                 │
  • Low NH3 diseases   • Low NH3 & Low    What is the Pco2
    – Low NH4+           net H+           in alkaline urine?
      production due   – Medullary            │
      to an alkaline     interstitial    ┌────┴────┐
      PCT cell pH        diseases      ~70-mm Hg  ~40-mm Hg
      (e.g.,                              │           │
      hyperkalemia)                 • Distal HCO3−   Is citrate
    – Low medullary                   secretion      excretion
      NH3 transfer                    (SAO)          low?
                                    • Backleak of  ┌──┴──┐
                                      H+ (ampho-  Yes    No
                                      tericin B)   │      │
                                              • Low     • CAII
                                                distal    deficiency
                                                H+        in proximal
                                                secretion and distal
                                                – Low     tubules
                                                  H+-
                                                  ATPase
```

Flow Chart 27.14 Reproduced with the permission of the author and the publisher from Halperin ML: *The ACID truth and BASIC facts—with a sweet touch, an enLYTEnment*, 6th ed, Toronto, 2015, RossMark Medical Publishers.

	Venous Blood	Urine
pH	7.0	6.0
P_{CO_2}, mm Hg	60	—
HCO_3^-, mmol/L	12	—
Na^+, mmol/L	120	50
K^+, mmol/L	2.3	30
Cl^-, mmol/L	90	5
Creatinine	1.7 mg/dL (150 μmol/L)	3.0 mmol/L
Glucose, mmol/L	3.5 (63 mg/dL)	0
Urea	BUN: 14 mg/dL (5.0 mmol/L)	Urea concentration: 150 mmol/L
Albumin, g/L (mg/dL)	60 (6)	—
Osmolality, mOsm/kg H_2O	260	400

Questions

- What dangers are present on admission?
- What dangers should be anticipated during therapy?
- What is the basis for the metabolic acidosis?

Discussion of the Questions

What Dangers Were Present on Admission?

Marked Degree of Contraction of the EABV

Severe Degree of Hypokalemia: The dangers of a severe degree of hypokalemia are cardiac arrhythmias and respiratory muscle weakness. However, this patient's ECG demonstrated only prominent U waves. Analysis of arterial blood gases showed only a mild degree of respiratory acidosis. Therefore, although he had a severe degree of hypokalemia that would require aggressive K^+ therapy, he did not have an emergency related to hypokalemia on admission.

Hyponatremia: Hyponatremia was likely chronic, because there were no symptoms that would strongly suggest an appreciable acute component to the hyponatremia or a history of a large recent water intake.

Binding of H^+ to Proteins in Cells: Because the brachial venous P_{CO_2} (60 mm Hg) was considerably higher than the arterial P_{CO_2} (25 mm Hg), buffering of H^+ by the BBS in muscle was compromised and there was a risk of binding of more H^+ to proteins in cells of vital organs (e.g., the heart and the brain) (see Figure 27.10).

What Dangers Should Be Anticipated During Therapy?

A More Severe Degree of Hypokalemia: Reexpansion of the EABV with the administration of saline can lead to the release of catecholamines, removing the inhibition of the release of insulin by their binding to pancreatic islet cells α-adrenergic receptors, which could result in a shift of K^+ into cells. A shift of K^+ into cells with worsening hypokalemia may also occur if $NaHCO_3$ is administered to correct the metabolic acidosis.

Rapid Rise in P_{Na}: P_{Na} may rise rapidly if water diuresis occurs with reexpansion of the EABV. As K^+ is administered, there will be a shift of K^+ into muscle cells in exchange for Na^+, which will also lead to a rise in P_{Na}. Patients who are malnourished and/or hypokalemic are at high risk of osmotic demyelination with a rapid rise in P_{Na}. It is our opinion that the maximum rise in P_{Na} in high-risk patients should not exceed 4 mmol/L in the first 24 hours.

Further Fall in P_{HCO3}: Expansion of the EABV with rapid administration of saline may also lead to a further fall in P_{HCO3}. First, there is a dilution effect. Second, with improved blood flow to muscles and the fall in capillary

P_{CO_2}, there will be titration of HCO_3^- by H^+ bound to intracellular proteins. The need to give $NaHCO_3$, however, must be balanced by the danger of creating more severe hypokalemia. We would not administer $NaHCO_3$ unless there is hemodynamic instability that is not responsive to the usual maneuvers to restore blood pressure, and with a central line in place to give KCl if cardiac arrhythmia develops.

Plan for Initial Therapy: On arrival to the emergency department, the patient was given 1 L of intravenous isotonic saline. To correct hypokalemia and prevent a rapid rise in P_{Na}, the intravenous solution was changed to a saline solution with 40 mEq of KCl, which was designed to have a tonicity similar to that in the plasma of the patient. To prevent water diuresis, dDAVP was administered at initiation of therapy, and water restriction was imposed. Hemodynamic status, P_K, P_{Na}, arterial pH, arterial P_{CO_2}, brachial venous P_{CO_2}, and P_{HCO3} were monitored closely.

What Is the Basis for the Metabolic Acidosis? Because the P_{AG} was not increased despite the high value for the P_{Alb}, the metabolic acidosis was judged not to be due to a gain of acids. In fact, the initial diagnosis was dRTA to explain the metabolic acidemia, urine pH of 6.0, and hypokalemia. Calculation of the U_{OG} (90 mOsm/kg H_2O), however, revealed a high urinary concentration of NH_4^+ (45 mmol/L). Furthermore, the rate of excretion of NH_4^+, as assessed by the U_{NH4}/U_{Cr}, was about 15 (mmol/mmol). Therefore, the basis for the patient's findings was not solely dRTA.

The anion that was excreted with NH_4^+ was not Cl^-, so diarrhea was not the cause of the metabolic acidosis. Hence the patient had an acid gain type of metabolic acidosis with a high rate of excretion of its anion in the urine. Because the P_{AG} was not elevated, very few of the new anions could enter the urine by filtration at the glomerulus. Therefore, clinicians deduced that these new anions were more likely to have entered the urine via secretion in the PCT, such as *p*-aminohippurate anions. The major chemical in glue is toluene; it is converted to benzoic acid by cytochrome P450, and benzoic acid is in turn conjugated to the amino acid glycine to form hippuric acid in the liver.[54] After hippuric acid is formed, the PCT actively secretes these hippurate anions, so their concentration is very low in plasma and very high in the urine. In fact, the rate of excretion of hippurate anions exceeds the rate of excretion of NH_4^+ in the urine because a limited amount of NH_4^+ can be made in the PCT. The remaining hippurate anions are excreted along with Na^+, resulting in the indirect loss of $NaHCO_3$ and contraction of the EABV. The low EABV, via the renin angiotensin aldosterone system, leads to high levels of aldosterone in plasma, causing electrogenic reabsorption of Na^+ in the CDN and thereby a high concentration of K^+ in the luminal fluid in the terminal CCD. In this patient, the high rate of excretion of hippurate and its accompanying cations caused a high flow rate in the late CDN and thereby a high rate of excretion of K^+ (Figure 27.14).

CONSULT 13: DETERMINE THE CAUSE OF HYPERCHLOREMIC METABOLIC ACIDOSIS

A 23-year-old woman with Southeast Asian ovalocytosis was referred for assessment of hypokalemia. Her physical examination was unremarkable. The laboratory results in plasma

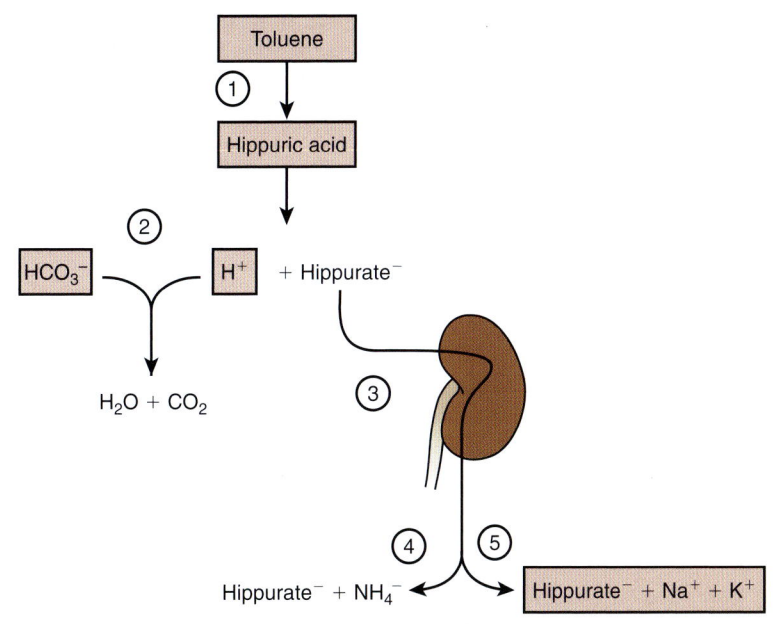

Figure 27.14 Metabolic acidosis due to the metabolism of toluene. The metabolism of toluene occurs in the liver, where benzoic acid is produced via cytochrome P450, alcohol, and aldehyde dehydrogenases. Conjugating benzoic acid with glycine produces hippuric acid. The H^+ are titrated by HCO_3^- for the most part. The hippurate anions are filtered and also secreted in the proximal convoluted tubule (PCT). Therefore, instead of accumulating in blood and increasing the plasma anion gap, the anions are excreted in the urine. The hippurate anions are excreted in the urine with NH_4^+ if the kidneys can produce enough of this cation, and when the capacity to excrete NH_4^+ is exceeded, the remaining hippurate anions are excreted with Na^+ and K^+. The excretion of hippurate anions with Na^+ and/or K^+ (but not NH_4^+) leads to the development of HCMA, contraction of the extracellular fluid volume, and hypokalemia. (Reproduced with the permission of the author and the publisher from Halperin ML: *The ACID truth and BASIC facts—with a sweet touch, an enLYTEnment*, 6th ed, Toronto, 2015, RossMark Medical Publishers.)

and a spot urine sample are summarized in the following table. The pH and P_{CO_2} are from an arterial blood sample, whereas all other blood data are from a venous blood sample. The urine urea concentration was 220 mmol/L and the urine was glucose-free.

	Plasma	Urine
pH	7.35	6.8
HCO_3^-, mmol/L	15	10
Na^+, mmol/L	140	75
Anion gap, mEq/L	12	5
Osmolality, mOsm/L	290	450
P_{CO_2}, mm Hg	30	—
K^+, mmol/L	3.1	35
Cl^-, mmol/L	113	95
Creatinine, mg/dL	0.7	60
Citrate, mg/dL	—	Low

Questions

- What is the basis for the hyperchloremic metabolic acidosis?
- What is the cause of the low rate of excretion of NH_4^+?

Discussion of the Questions

What Is the Basis for the Hyperchloremic Metabolic Acidosis? The patient had a low U_{NH_4} because the measured U_{osm} (450 mOsm/kg H_2O) was very similar to the calculated U_{osm}, 440 mOsm/kg H_2O—that is, 2 (U_{Na} [75 mmol/L] + U_K [35 mmol/L]) + U_{urea} (220 mOsm/kg H_2O) + U_{Glu} (0). In addition, the rate of excretion of NH_4^+ was low because the U_{NH_4}/U_{Cr} was very low. Because the GFR was not very low, the diagnosis was RTA.

What Is the Cause of the Low Rate of Excretion of NH_4^+?
Urine pH: Because the urine pH is 6.8, the basis for the low rate of NH_4^+ excretion is a low net secretion of H^+ in the distal nephron (see Flow Charts 27.14).
Assessment of Distal H^+ Secretion: After hypokalemia was corrected, H^+ secretion in the distal nephron could be evaluated using U_{PCO_2} during bicarbonate loading. The U_{PCO_2} in alkaline urine was 70 mm Hg (see Flow Charts 27.14). Because the U_{PCO_2} was unexpectedly high and a backleak of H^+ type of defect was unlikely, the patient's mutant Cl^-/HCO_3^- anion exchangers might have been targeted abnormally to the luminal membranes of α-intercalated cells. The U_{PCO_2} would be high due to distal secretion of HCO_3^- by alkaline intercalated cells. The secretion of HCO_3^- caused the luminal pH to increase, liberating H^+ from $H_2PO_4^-$, which raised the P_{CO_2} in alkaline urine to or above 70 mm Hg.

Complete reference list available at ExpertConsult.com.

KEY REFERENCES

1. Halperin ML, Kamel KS, Goldstein MB: *Fluid, Electrolyte and acid-base physiology; a problem-based approach*, Philadelphia, 2010, W.B. Saunders.
2. Zhai XY, Fenton RA, Andreasen A, et al: Aquaporin-1 is not expressed in descending thin limbs of short-loop nephrons. *J Am Soc Nephrol* 18:2937–2944, 2007.
3. Kamel KS, Halperin ML: The importance of distal delivery of filtrate and residual water permeability in the pathophysiology of hyponatremia. *Nephrol Dial Transplant* 27:872–875, 2012.
4. Halperin ML, Kamel KS, Oh MS: Mechanisms to concentrate the urine: an opinion. *Curr Opin Nephrol Hypert* 17:416–422, 2008.
5. Carlotti AP, Bohn D, Mallie JP, et al: Tonicity balance, and not electrolyte-free water calculations, more accurately guides therapy for acute changes in natremia. *Intensive Care Med* 27:921–924, 2001.
6. Kamel KS, Bichet DG, Halperin ML: Studies to clarify the pathophysiology of partial central diabetes insipidus. *Am J Nephrol* 37:1290–1293, 2001.
7. Carlotti ACP, St George-Hyslop C, Guerguerian AM, et al: Occult risk factor for the development of cerebral edema in children with diabetic ketoacidosis: possible role for stomach emptying. *Ped Diabetes* 10:522–533, 2009.
8. Hoorn EJ, Carlotti AP, Costa LA, et al: Preventing a drop in effective plasma osmolality to minimize the likelihood of cerebral edema during treatment of children with diabetic ketoacidosis. *J Pediatr* 150:467–473, 2007.
9. Napolova O, Urbach S, Davids MR, et al: Assessing the degree of extracellular fluid volume contraction in a patient with a severe degree of hyperglycaemia. *Nephrol Dial Transplant* 18:2674–2677, 2003.
10. Kamel KS, Magner PO, Ethier JH, et al: Urine electrolytes in the assessment of extracellular fluid volume contraction. *Am J Nephrol* 9:344–347, 1989.
11. Miller TR, Anderson RJ, Linas SL, et al: Urinary diagnostic indices in acute renal failure: a prospective study. *Ann Intern Med* 89:47–50, 1978.
12. Weisberg LS: Pseudohyponatremia: a reappraisal. *Am J Med* 86:315–318, 1989.
13. Decaux G, Schlesser M, Coffernils M, et al: Uric acid, anion gap and urea concentration in the diagnostic approach to hyponatremia. *Clin Nephrol* 42:102–108, 1994.
14. Cheema-Dhadli S, Chong CK, Kamel KS, et al: An acute infusion of lactic acid lowers the concentration of potassium in arterial plasma by inducing a shift of potassium into cells of the liver in fed rats. *Nephron Physiol* 120:p7–p15, 2012.
15. Wang WH, Giebisch G: Regulation of potassium (K) handling in the renal collecting duct. *Pflügers Arch* 458:157–168, 2009.
16. Leviel F, Hubner CA, Houillier P, et al: The Na^+-dependent chloride-bicarbonate exchanger SLC4A8 mediates an electroneutral Na^+ reabsorption process in the renal cortical collecting ducts of mice. *J Clin Invest* 120:1627–1635, 2010.
17. Carlisle E, Donnelly S, Ethier J, et al: Modulation of the secretion of potassium by accompanying anions in humans. *Kidney Int* 39:1206–1212, 1991.
18. Sansom SC, Welling PA: Two channels for one job. *Kidney Int* 72:529–530, 2007.
19. Welling PA, Chang YP, Delpire E, et al: Multigene kinase network, kidney transport, and salt in essential hypertension. *Kidney Int* 77:1063–1069, 2010.
20. Kamel KS, Schreiber M, Halperin ML: Integration of the response to a dietary potassium load: a Paleolithic perspective. *Nephrol Dial Transplant* 29:982–989, 2014.
21. Kamel KS, Halperin ML: Intrarenal urea recycling leads to a higher rate of renal excretion of potassium: an hypothesis with clinical implications. *Curr Opin Nephrol Hypertens* 20:547–554, 2011.
22. Berl T, Rastegar A: A patient with severe hyponatremia and hypokalemia: osmotic demyelination following potassium repletion. *Am J Kidney Dis* 55:742–748, 2010.
23. Lin SH, Lin YF, Halperin ML: Hypokalaemia and paralysis. *QJM* 94:133–139, 2001.
24. Lin SH, Lin YF: Propranolol rapidly reverses paralysis, hypokalemia and hypophosphatemia in thyrotoxic periodic paralysis. *Am J Kidney Dis* 37:620–624, 2001.
25. Wilson FH, Disse-Nicodeme S, Choate KA, et al: Human hypertension caused by mutations in WNK kinases. *Science* 293:1107–1112, 2001.
26. Hoorn EJ, Walsh SB, McCormick JA, et al: The calcineurin inhibitor tacrolimus activates the renal sodium chloride cotransporter to cause hypertension. *Nat Med* 17:1304–1309, 2011.
27. Schambelan M, Sebastian A, Rector FC, Jr: Mineralocorticoid-resistant renal hyperkalemia without salt wasting (type II pseudohypoaldosteronism): role of increased renal chloride reabsorption. *Kidney Int* 19:716–727, 1981.

28. Nishida H, Sohara E, Nomura N, et al: Phosphatidylinositol 3-kinase/Akt signaling pathway activates the WNK-OSR1/SPAK-NCC phosphorylation cascade in hyperinsulinemic db/db mice. *Hypertension* 60:981–990, 2012.
29. Halperin ML, Scheich A: Should we continue to recommend that a deficit of KCl be treated with NaCl? A fresh look at chloride-depletion metabolic alkalosis. *Nephron* 67:263–269, 1994.
30. Scheich A, Donnelly S, Cheema-Dhadli S, et al: Does saline "correct" the abnormal mass balance in metabolic alkalosis associated with chloride depletion in the rat? *Clin Invest Med* 17:448–460, 1994.
31. Rubin SI, Sonnenberg B, Zettle R, et al: Metabolic alkalosis mimicking the acute sequestration of HCl in rats: bucking the alkaline tide. *Clin Invest Med* 17:515–521, 1994.
32. DeMars C, Hollister K, Tomassoni A, et al: Citric acidosis: a life-threatening cause of metabolic acidosis. *Ann Emerg Med* 38:588–591, 2001.
33. Zalunardo N, Lemaire M, Davids MR, et al: Acidosis in a patient with cholera: a need to redefine concepts. *QJM* 97:681–696, 2004.
34. Gowrishankar M, Kamel KS, Halperin ML: Buffering of a H^+ load: a "brain-protein-centered" view. *J Amer Soc Nephrol* 18:2278–2280, 2007.
35. Halperin ML, Kamel KS: Some observations on the clinical approach to metabolic acidosis. *J Am Soc Nephrol* 21:894–897, 2010.
36. Kraut JA, Madias NE: Serum anion gap: its uses and limitations in clinical medicine. *Clin J Am Soc Nephrol* 2:162–174, 2007.
37. Emmett M: Anion-gap interpretation: the old and the new. *Nat Clin Pract Nephrol* 2:4–5, 2006.
38. Feldman M, Soni N, Dickson B: Influence of hypoalbuminemia or hyperalbuminemia on the serum anion gap. *J Lab Clin Med* 146:317–320, 2005.
39. Kamel KS, Cheema-Dhadli S, Halperin FA, et al: Anion gap: may the anions restricted to the intravascular space undergo modification in their valence? *Nephron* 73:382–389, 1996.
40. Stewart PA: Modern quantitative acid-base chemistry. *Can J Physiol Pharmacol* 61:1444–1461, 1983.
41. Rastegar A: Clinical utility of Stewart's method in diagnosis and management of acid-base disorders. *Clin J Am Soc Nephrol* 4:1267–1274, 2009.
42. Kamel KS, Halperin ML: Acid-base problems in diabetic ketoacidosis. *NEJM* 372:546–554, 2015.
43. Shull PD, Rapoport J: Life-threatening reversible acidosis caused by alcohol abuse. *Nat Rev Nephrol* 6:555–559, 2010.
44. Simpson DP: Control of hydrogen ion homeostasis and renal acidosis. *Medicine* 50:503–541, 1971.
45. Weiner ID, Verlander JW: Renal ammonia metabolism and transport. *Compr Physiol* 3:201–220, 2013.
46. Dyck R, Asthana S, Kalra J, et al: A modification of the urine osmolal gap: an improved method for estimating urine ammonium. *Am J Nephrol* 10:359–362, 1990.
47. Kamel KS, Halperin ML: An improved approach to the patient with metabolic acidosis: a need for four amendments. *J Nephrol* 65:S76–S85, 2006.
48. Richardson RMA, Halperin ML: The urine pH: a potentially misleading diagnostic test in patients with hyperchloremic metabolic acidosis. *Am J Kidney Dis* 10:140–143, 1987.
49. Kamel KS, Briceno LF, Santos MI, et al: A new classification for renal defects in net acid excretion. *Am J Kidney Dis* 29:136–146, 1997.
50. Halperin ML, Goldstein MB, Haig A, et al: Studies on the pathogenesis of type I (distal) renal tubular acidosis as revealed by the urinary PCO2 tensions. *J Clin Invest* 53:669–677, 1974.
51. Roscoe JM, Goldstein MB, Halperin ML, et al: Effect of amphotericin B on urine acidification in rats: implications for the pathogenesis of distal renal tubular acidosis. *J Lab Clin Med* 89:463–470, 1977.
52. Kaitwatcharachai C, Vasuvattakul S, Yenchitsomanus P, et al: Distal renal tubular acidosis in a patient with Southeast Asian ovalocytosis: possible interpretations of a high urine PCO2. *Am J Kidney Dis* 33:1147–1152, 1999.
53. Simpson DP: Citrate excretion: a window on renal metabolism. *Am J Physiol* 244:F223–F234, 1983.
54. Carlisle EJF, Donnelly SM, Vasuvattakul S, et al: Glue-sniffing and distal renal tubular acidosis: sticking to the facts. *J Am Soc Nephrol* 1:1019–1027, 1991.

28 Diagnostic Kidney Imaging

Vinay A. Duddalwar | Hossein Jadvar | Suzanne L. Palmer | William D. Boswell, Jr.

CHAPTER OUTLINE

IMAGING TECHNIQUES, 846
Plain Radiograph of the Abdomen, 846
Intravenous Urography, 846
Iodinated Contrast Media, 847
Ultrasonography, 848
Computed Tomography, 851
Magnetic Resonance Imaging, 856
Nuclear Medicine, 864
IMAGING IN CLINICAL NEPHROLOGY, 865
Normal Renal Function, 865
Kidney Injury: Acute and Chronic, 866
Unilateral Obstruction, 871

Renal Calcifications and Renal Stone Disease, 871
Renal Infection, 878
Renal Mass: Cysts to Renal Cell Carcinoma, 883
Renal Cancer: Positron Emission Tomography and Positron Emission Tomography–Computed Tomography, 899
Renal Vascular Disease, 903
Nuclear Imaging and Renovascular Disease, 907
Renal Vein Thrombosis, 908
Assessment for Renal Transplantation, 909
Assessment of Transplanted Kidneys, 910

Medical imaging has made major strides over the past century since the discovery of x-rays by Wilhelm Roentgen. Imaging tools now include sophisticated systems that can noninvasively interrogate structure, function, and metabolism in health and disease states of all organ systems, including the urinary system. X-ray studies primarily provide anatomic information and include plain radiography, intravenous urography (IVU), antegrade and retrograde pyelography, and computed tomography (CT). Ultrasonography (US), which does not have ionizing radiation, involves the use of high-frequency sound waves. The development of additional techniques in US such as Doppler US, elastography, and contrast-enhanced US has led to an expansion of the role of US in the evaluation of the kidney. Magnetic resonance imaging (MRI) uses the phenomenon of nuclear magnetic resonance and yields primarily anatomic information but also can provide some functional information. Nuclear medicine studies, including planar and single-photon computed tomography (SPECT) techniques, contribute primarily functional information; positron emission tomography (PET) and integrated PET-CT and PET-MRI in conjunction with a number of current and novel radiotracers provide means for quantitative assessment of a variety of physiologic parameters. In addition, there have been significant changes in image processing and visualization technology that have led to an increase in the imaging applications for the kidney. Understanding the diagnostic utility and limitation of each imaging modality facilitates the proper evaluation of patients in various specific clinical settings.

IMAGING TECHNIQUES

PLAIN RADIOGRAPH OF THE ABDOMEN

Historically, plain radiography of the abdomen was used as the starting point in the evaluation of the kidneys, as well as the rest of the abdomen. Relative to more advanced technology, radiography of the kidneys, ureters, and bladder (KUB) (Figure 28.1) yields little significant information on its own and if used at all, should be the starting point for further evaluation of the kidneys, such as the scout film for IVU.

INTRAVENOUS UROGRAPHY

In the past, IVU (also known as intravenous pyelography) was used as the primary means of evaluating the kidneys and urinary tract[1,2]; however, CT has supplanted IVU for routine imaging. IVU may be appropriate if CT is not readily available[3] or when a specific clinical question needs to be answered. A scout film (KUB) is performed before any contrast material is injected intravenously. Subsequently, iodinated contrast material is injected intravenously as a

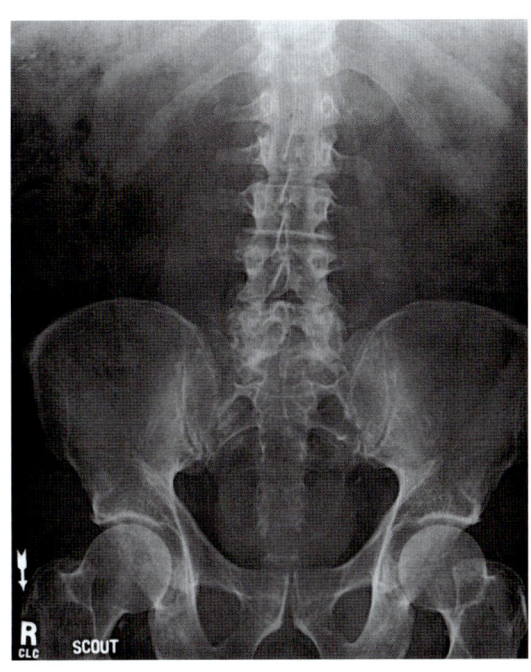

Figure 28.1 Plain radiograph of the abdomen: kidneys, ureters, and bladder. The kidneys lie posteriorly in the retroperitoneum in the upper abdomen. They are surrounded by fat. The ribs overlie the kidney, and bowel gas is visible in the right upper quadrant. The psoas muscles are also well viewed because retroperitoneal fat abuts them.

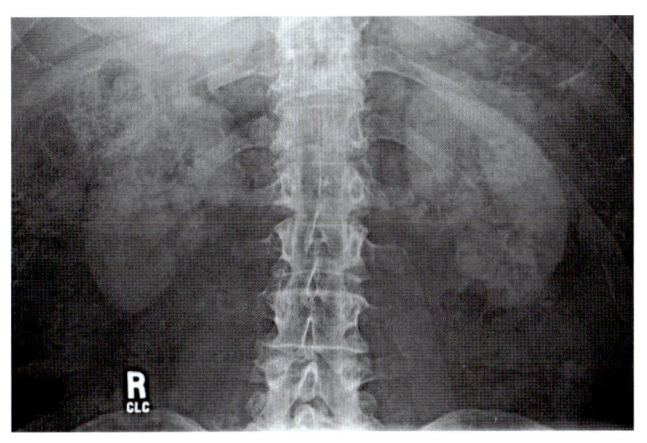

Figure 28.2 Intravenous urography: nephrogram. This image is obtained within 60 seconds after injection of contrast material. The kidneys are visible with smooth borders and the overlying bowel gas.

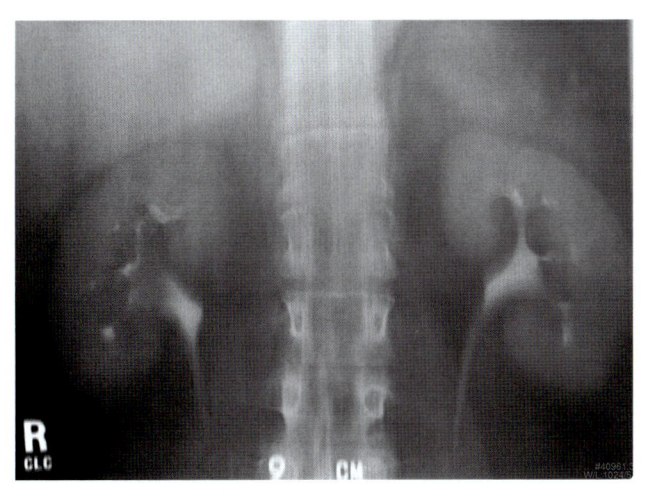

Figure 28.3 Intravenous urography: nephrotomogram. This image is obtained 5 to 7 minutes after the injection of contrast material. The overall outline of kidney is well depicted; the calyces, renal pelvis, and proximal ureter are opacified with the excreted contrast material.

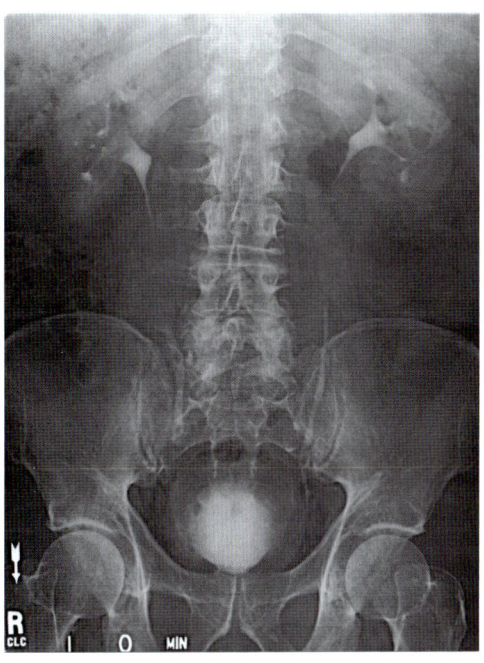

Figure 28.4 Intravenous urography: excretory phase. This image is obtained 10 minutes after the injection of the contrast material. The kidneys are well visualized; contrast material outlines the calyces, pelvis, ureters, and bladder.

bolus for the study. Timed sequential images of the kidneys and the remainder of the genitourinary system are then obtained.[4,5] The first image obtained in IVU is taken within 30 to 60 seconds after the injection of the contrast medium is completed. The nephrogram, or image of the kidneys, reflects the iodine concentration within the tubular system of the kidneys (Figure 28.2).[6] This nephrogram may be used to evaluate the size, shape, and contour of the kidneys. The overall appearance and density of the kidneys should be symmetric. The outlines of the kidneys are usually well depicted against the darker appearance of perirenal fat. Normal kidneys are typically homogeneous in appearance throughout. The excretion of the contrast medium by the kidneys should be symmetric. The anatomic depiction of the calyces, infundibula, and pelvis is best displayed by 5 to 10 minutes after injection (Figure 28.3). Imaging of the ureters is usually accomplished 10 to 15 minutes after injection (Figure 28.4). The total number of images needed for the complete study depends on the clinical question to be answered.[2-4]

IODINATED CONTRAST MEDIA

Over the years, many different intravascular contrast media have been employed.[7] These agents are divided into categories based on their osmolality relative to plasma: *high osmolar contrast media* (HOCM), *low osmolar contrast media* (LOCM), or *isotonic contrast media* (IOCM). HOCM was used successfully from the 1960s through the 1990s for most intravascular applications. Since the introduction of LOCM in the mid-1980s and IOCM in the 1990s, there has been a gradual shift to these agents. Since the mid-2000s, virtually all studies involving intravascular injection of contrast material have been performed with LOCM or IOCM.

All the HOCM agents are ionic, water-soluble salt solutions, and all are hyperosmolar in relation to plasma. Virtually all of the contrast material injected is filtered by the glomerulus; in patients with normal renal function, there is no tubular reabsorption of excreted material.[7]

Most LOCM agents are non-ionic compounds that do not dissociate in solution.[8] LOCM are less hyperosmolar (compared to HOCM) in relation to plasma. These agents, like HOCM, are filtered by the glomerulus but have a higher concentration within the tubular system because less water is reabsorbed. The osmotic effect of LOCM is less than HOCM in the tubular system; therefore within the urine there is a higher concentration, which generally improves the quality of imaging studies.[9] IOCM agents are isotonic in relation to plasma. They, like HOCM and LOCM, are filtered by the glomerulus with no tubular reabsorption or excretion.

Contrast material has a plasma half-life of 1 to 2 hours in patients with normal renal function. Virtually all contrast material is excreted by the kidneys within 24 hours. In patients with renal failure, contrast media may be excreted via other routes, including the biliary system or gastrointestinal tract. All iodinated contrast agents are dialyzable.

Reactions to the injection of any of the contrast agents may occur; however, these reactions are not "allergic" responses in the sense of an antigen-antibody reaction.[10] Although the majority of these reactions are mild or minor, severe reactions and deaths do occur. With ionic HOCM agents the reaction rate in the general population is 5% to 6%.[11] The rates of reactions to LOCM and IOCM agents are much lower, in the range of 1% to 2%.[12-14] Most reactions are mild, consisting of flushing, nausea, and vomiting, and treatment is not required. Mild dermal reactions, primarily urticaria, do occur and may or may not necessitate treatment. Moderate and severe reactions, which occur with considerably less frequency, include bronchospasm, laryngeal edema, seizures, arrhythmias, syncope, shock, and cardiac arrest. All moderate and severe reactions necessitate treatment.

Because the reaction that occurs in patients after injection of contrast material is not antigen-antibody mediated, pretesting plays no role.[15] Neither the rate of injection nor the dose of contrast material has been clearly established as a determinant in the occurrence of contrast material–related reactions.[12,16] The only regimen that has proven to reduce the incidence of contrast-induced reactions is the modified Greenberger protocol[17]:

Two frequently used regimens are as follows: (1) Prednisone—50 mg orally at 13 hours, 7 hours, and 1 hour before contrast injection, plus diphenhydramine 50 mg intravenously, intramuscularly, or orally 1 hour before contrast medium.[16] (2) Methylprednisolone—32 mg orally 12 hours and 2 hours before contrast media injection. An antihistamine (as in option 1) can also be added to this regimen (see "Contrast Media–Induced Nephropathy" section).

ULTRASONOGRAPHY

US is the most frequently used diagnostic examination for the evaluation of the kidneys and urinary tract.[18] It is non-invasive, uses no ionizing radiation, and requires minimal patient preparation. It is the first-line examination in azotemic patients for assessing renal size and the presence or absence of hydronephrosis and obstruction. It is used to assess the vasculature of native and transplanted kidneys. US is also used to evaluate renal structure and to characterize renal masses. It is the primary modality of imaging for evaluation of a transplanted kidney. It is also the most commonly used modality for imaging guidance for a kidney biopsy.

Diagnostic US is an outgrowth of sound navigation and ranging (sonar) technology, used first during World War II for the detection of objects under water. In medical US, high-frequency sound waves are used to evaluate various organs. In the abdomen and, more particularly, the kidneys, 2.5- to 4.0-mHz sound waves are generally employed.

The US unit consists of a transducer, which sends and receives the sound waves; a microprocessor or computer, which obtains and processes the returning signal; and an image display system or monitor, which displays the processed images. The piezoelectric transducer converts electrical energy into high-frequency sound waves that are transmitted through the patient's body. It converts the returning reflected sound waves back into electrical energy that can be processed by a computer. Sound travels as a waveform through the tissues being imaged. The speed of the sound wave depends on the tissue through which it is traveling.

Different tissues and the interface between these tissues have different acoustic impedance. As the sound wave travels through different tissues, part of the wave is reflected back to the transducer. The depth of the tissue interface is measured by the time the sound wave takes to return to the transducer. A gray-scale image is produced by the measured reflected sound, in which the intensity of the pixels (picture elements) is proportional to the intensities of the reflected sound (Figure 28.5). When the acoustic interfaces are quite large, strong echoes result. These are known as *specular reflectors* and are visible from the renal capsule and bladder wall. Nonspecular reflectors generate echoes of lower amplitude and are visible in the renal parenchyma. Strong reflection of sound by bone and air results in little or no information from the tissues beneath; this appearance is known as *shadowing*. Lack of acoustic impedance as observed in fluid-filled structures, such as the urinary bladder and renal cysts, allows the sound waves to penetrate further, which results in a relative increase in intensity distal to the structures; this is known as *increased through-transmission*. All of these features are used to help characterize various lesions. Real-time US, which provides sequential images at a rapid frame rate, allows the demonstration of motion of organs and pulsation of vessels.

Doppler US, based on the Doppler frequency shift of the sound wave caused by moving objects, can be used to assess venous and arterial blood flow.[19,20] The movement of blood cells in blood vessels is used to generate Doppler information, and this is used to derive diagnostic information. In a technique called pulsed wave Doppler US, quantification of this flow and assessment of the waveforms can be used in evaluating various organ systems (Figure 28.6A). With Doppler color-flow US, the image is encoded with colors assigned to the pixels representing the direction and volume of flow within vessels (Figure 28.7). In power Doppler US the amplitude of the signal, without any directional information, is used to produce a color map of the intrarenal vasculature and flow within the kidneys (Figure 28.8).

Resistive index is a measure of the resistance to blood flow caused by the microvascular bed distally. This serves as a nonspecific indicator of disease in both native and transplanted kidneys. In general, a normal resistive index is 0.70 or less (see Figure 28.6B). An increased resistive index is a nonspecific indicator of disease and a sign of increased peripheral vascular resistance.[19-21]

Elastography is another technique by which the mechanical properties of a target tissue are assessed. It is a measure of the stiffness in a tissue, and its role in the evaluation of chronic parenchymal disease is being evaluated. The change in the elasticity of a particular tissue is assessed by changes in the propagation velocity of ultrasound waves.[22]

There has been an increase in the use of intravenous contrast agents with dynamic US for the evaluation of the kidneys and renal masses.[23] The advantage of these agents is that they are excreted by pulmonary ventilation, and therefore they can be used in patients with very poor renal function. The contrast agents are microbubbles of a high-molecular-weight gas such as perfluorocarbons that are stabilized by a thin capsule of lipid or protein. They are of the same size as blood cells and therefore are not filtered out in the lungs or the kidneys. These remain in the vascular system (acting as blood pool agents) and can provide another method of providing information on organ perfusion and vascularity. This has expanded the role of US and has given an additional option in the imaging of patients with compromised renal function. The development of these contrast agents enables the display of microvasculature and dynamic enhancement patterns.

Imaging after injection of these contrast agents is performed using contrast-specific ultrasonographic modes. These are based on the cancellation of linear ultrasound signals from tissue and using a nonlinear response from microbubbles. The techniques for contrast-enhanced US (CEUS) evaluation use a low mechanical index technique

Uses for CEUS in the kidney include the following: (1) Characterization of focal renal lesions. This includes characterization of complex renal cysts accurately into different Bosniak groups. CEUS also enables an increase in diagnostic confidence in the evaluation of focal renal masses. It also permits differentiation of variant normal anatomy, including conditions such as a hypertrophied column of Bertin.[24] (2) Evaluation of transplanted kidney. CEUS can help identify vascular complications such as arterial and venous thrombosis and ischemia. It can also

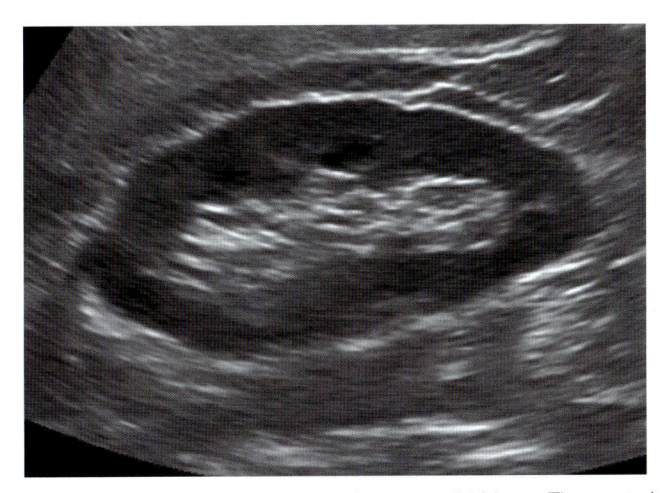

Figure 28.5 Renal ultrasonography: normal kidney. The central echogenic structure represents the vascular elements, calyces, and renal sinus fat. The peripheral cortex is noted to be smooth and regular. Renal pyramids may be depicted as hypoechoic structures between the central echo complex and the cortex.

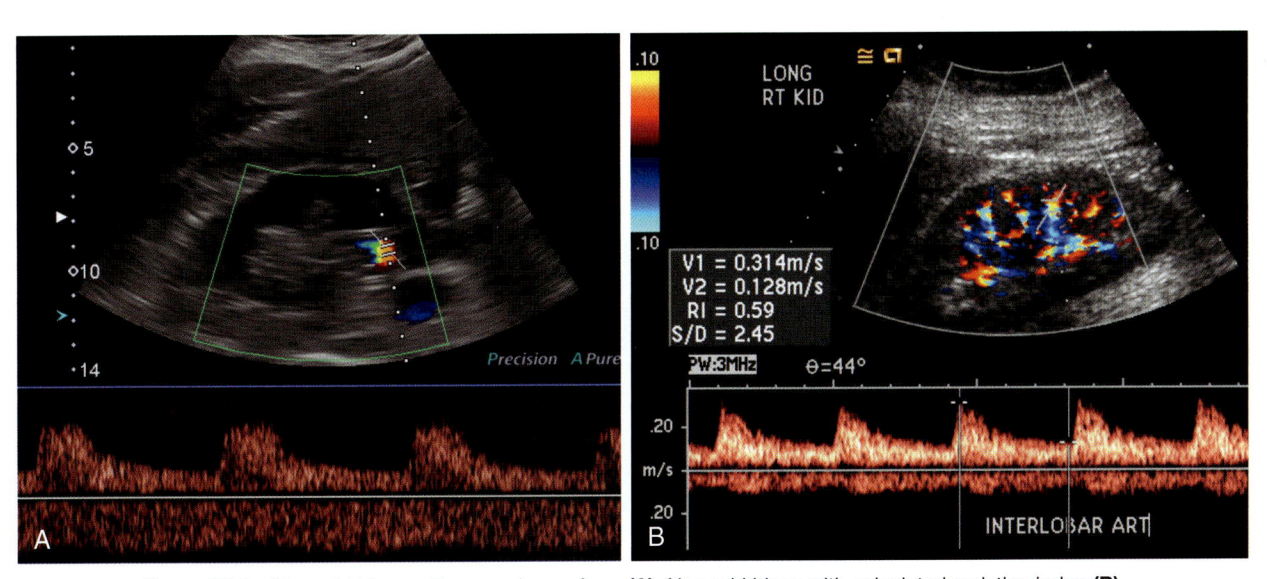

Figure 28.6 Normal kidney with normal waveform **(A)**. Normal kidney with calculated resistive index **(B)**.

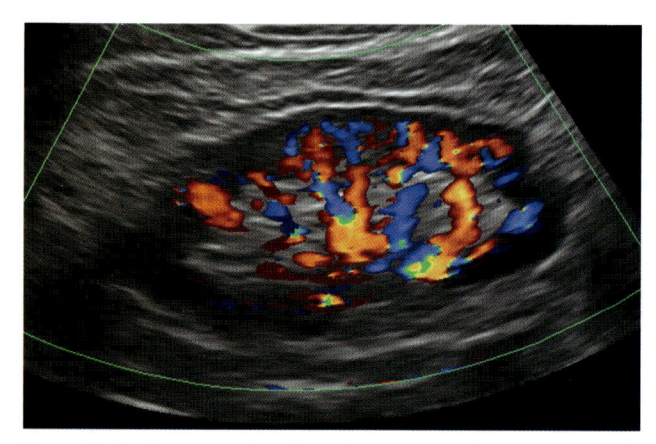

Figure 28.7 Doppler color-flow ultrasonography: normal kidney. The red echogenic areas represent arterial flow (flow toward the transducer), and blue echogenic areas represent venous flow (flow away from the transducer).

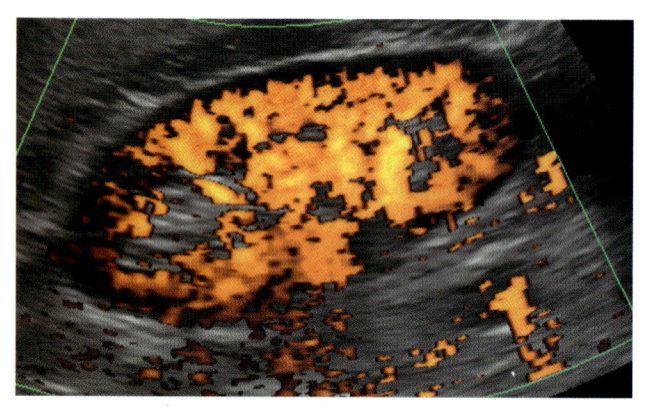

Figure 28.8 Power Doppler ultrasonography: normal kidney. The color image represents a summation of all flow—arterial and venous—within the kidney.

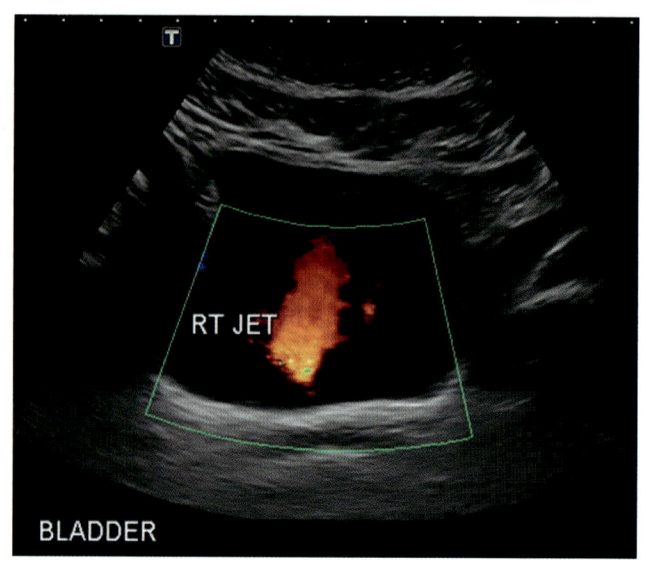

Figure 28.9 Ureteral jet. Color-flow image of urine entering the bladder.

identify and characterize postintervention complications.[25]
3. Follow-up of renal trauma.[26]

US is very useful in directing kidney biopsy. The use of US has decreased both the procedure time and rates of morbidity and mortality. US guidance is also used for other interventional procedures such as percutaneous nephrostomy and renal mass ablations.

ULTRASONOGRAPHY: NORMAL ANATOMY

US images of the kidneys are generally obtained in the longitudinal, transverse, and parasagittal planes.[27] The appearance of the perinephric fat varies from slightly less echogenic to highly echogenic in comparison with the renal cortex. The renal capsule is visible as an echogenic line surrounding the kidney. The centrally located renal sinus and hilum, containing renal sinus fat, vessels, and the collecting system, are usually echogenic because of the presence of fat (see Figure 28.5). The amount of renal sinus fat generally increases with age. Tubular structures corresponding to vessels and the collecting system may be visible in the renal hilum. Doppler color-flow US may be used to differentiate the vessels from the collecting system.

The normal renal cortex is less echogenic than the liver and spleen. The renal medullary pyramids are hypoechoic, and their triangular shape points to the renal hilum. The renal cortex lies peripherally, and the separation from the medulla is usually demarcated by an echogenic focus attributable to the arcuate arteries along the corticomedullary junction. Columns of Bertin have the same echogenicity as the renal cortex and separate the renal pyramids. On occasion, a large column of Bertin may simulate a mass. Even when a column of Bertin is large or prominent, its echogenicity is the same as the remainder of the cortex, and the vascular pattern observed on power Doppler images is also the same.

Renal size is accurately measured by US. Normal kidneys range from 8.5 to 13 cm, depending on the age, sex, and body habitus of the patient. The contours of the kidneys should be smooth; occasionally some slight nodularity is present as a result of developmental fetal lobulation. The renal arteries and veins may be visible extending from the renal hilum to the aorta and inferior vena cava (IVC). The veins lie anterior to the arteries. The renal arterial branching pattern within the kidneys may be visible on Doppler color-flow US (see Figure 28.7).[28] The resistive indices of the main, intralobar, and arcuate vessels may be calculated (see Figure 28.6). With power Doppler US, the intrarenal vasculature may be assessed; it demonstrates an overall increased pattern in the cortex in relation to the medulla, which corresponds to the normal arterial flow to the kidney (see Figure 28.8).[29,30] The renal calyces and collecting systems are not typically visible with US unless distension caused by diuresis or obstruction is present. When visible, the collecting systems are anechoic structures in the renal sinus fat, connecting together at the renal pelvis. The urinary bladder is visible in the pelvis as a fluid-filled anechoic structure. The entrance of the ureters into the bladder at the trigone may be visualized on Doppler color-flow US as ureteral jets (Figure 28.9).

When a kidney is not identified in its normal location, the remainder of the abdomen and pelvis should be assessed. Ectopic kidneys may lie lower in the abdomen or within the pelvis and may also be located on the opposite side; the kidneys may even be fused (e.g., horseshoe kidneys).

Horseshoe kidneys tend to lie lower in the retroperitoneum, and their axes may be different from those of normal kidneys.

COMPUTED TOMOGRAPHY

CT has become an essential imaging tool for diagnosis in all areas of the body. In the genitourinary tract, it has supplanted IVU, especially for the evaluation of flank pain, hematuria, renal masses, and trauma. Even in areas in which US is the first-line imaging modality, CT offers a complementary and sometimes superior means of imaging. CT is now the first examination to be performed in patients with renal colic, renal stone disease, renal trauma, renal infection and abscess, renal mass, hematuria, and urothelial abnormalities.

Computed tomography has been heralded as the greatest improvement in diagnostic radiology since Roentgen discovered x-rays in 1895. Sir Godfrey Hounsfield developed the first CT scanner in 1970.[31] The first clinical applications in 1971 were in the head. The first body CT scanner was installed in Georgetown University Medical Center in 1974. The field has grown rapidly since that time with new technical innovations, image processing, and visualization methods. For his outstanding work in the field and for demonstrating the unique and remarkable clinical capabilities of CT, Sir Godfrey Hounsfield was awarded the Nobel Prize in Physiology or Medicine in 1979.

CT is the computer reconstruction of a radiographically generated image that typically depicts a slice through the area being studied in the body. The x-ray tube produces a highly collimated fan beam and is mounted opposite an array of electronic detectors. This system rotates in tandem around the patient. The detector system collects hundreds of thousands of samples representing the attenuation of the x-ray along the line formed from the x-ray source to the detector as the rotation occurs. This data set is transferred to a computer, where the image is reconstructed. The CT image is made up of pixels (picture elements), each corresponding to a CT density number (*Hounsfield unit*) that represents the amount of x-rays absorbed by the patient at a particular point in the cross-sectional image. These pixels represent a two-dimensional display of a three-dimensional object or volume element (voxel). The third dimension is the slice thickness or depth. Thus the Hounsfield unit (HU) is the average attenuation of x-rays of all the tissues within a specific voxel, which is then used to create the individual image. The images are then displayed on a computer monitor for reviewing and analysis.

The HU of water is 0. Tissues that attenuate more x-rays than water have positive HU, and those with less x-ray attenuation than water have negative HU. Different shades of gray on a scale of white to black are assigned to HU (the highest number is depicted as white, the lowest as black). The image of each slice is thus created on a display monitor, and this image may be manipulated to accentuate the regions being imaged. The advantage of this digital image set is that by using various tools such as window levels and widths and different summation and reconstruction techniques, images can be optimized to evaluate a particular organ or region.

The initial CT scanners were relatively slow because the technology required a point-and-shoot process. One slice was obtained, the patient moved, and the next slice obtained. This initial generation of body CT scanner led to a scan of the abdomen that took up to 2 to 4 minutes or more to complete. In 1990, helical/spiral technology was introduced in which the x-ray tube and detector system continuously rotated around the patient, and the patient moved continuously through the gantry. Scan time through the abdomen was significantly reduced. After helical/spiral CT, a two-detector system was introduced that produced two slices for every 360-degree rotation of the x-ray tube and detector system. Today, multidetector CT (MDCT) systems with 640 detectors are in use, primarily for advanced applications, such as computed tomographic angiography (CTA) for the coronary arteries. Most commonly today, MDCT systems varying from 64 to 320 detectors are used in abdominal and pelvic scanning. With MDCT each 360-degree rotation results in the number of slices equal to the number of detectors (i.e., a 64-detector system produces 64 slices in one 360-degree rotation). These technologic advances have led to dramatic increase in the speed of scans (4 to 10 seconds), routine use of thin slices or collimation (1 to 2 mm thick), and marked improvement in spatial resolution (ability to display small objects clearly).[32]

As a result of the faster scanning times, the use of enhancement by intravenous contrast material has improved and become more widely used.[33] For example, the kidneys can be scanned in the arterial, venous, nephrographic, and delayed phases, which allows for a more complete assessment. Current, state-of-the-art MDCT acquires data as a volumetric study, and the slice thickness has been reduced to the point that sagittal, coronal, oblique, and off-axis images may be displayed with no loss of resolution. The data acquisition may also be displayed as a three-dimensional volumetric display with the regions of interest highlighted.[32] The kidneys are well suited for assessment with MDCT.[33-37]

Technical developments include dual-energy and spectral-energy scanners that offer the ability to image an organ at different energy strengths.[38] Tissues behave differently at different energies, and this fact is used in techniques such as characterization of calculi and obtaining virtual unenhanced images and iodine maps in different organs (Figure 28.10).

COMPUTED TOMOGRAPHY TECHNIQUE, INCLUDING UROGRAPHY

Most clinical questions require the use of intravenous contrast; tailored CT urography (CTU) is a way to provide a comprehensive examination of the genitourinary tract. CTU may be used to assess the kidney as a whole (anatomic), the vascular tree (function and perfusion), and the excretory (urothelial) patterns.[39] Noncontrast scans enable assessment of renal calculi, high-density cysts, and contour abnormalities.[40] Early-phase scans (12 to 15 seconds) enable arterial assessment, for example, the evaluation for renal artery stenosis (RAS). Scanning at 25 to 30 seconds yields a combined arterial-venous–phase image with clear corticomedullary differentiation, recommended for renal mass evaluation. At 90 to 100 seconds, true nephrographic-phase imaging of the kidneys is obtained.[33] Delayed imaging, typically at 3 to 7 minutes and up to 10 minutes, enables the evaluation of the urothelium (calyces, renal pelvis, ureters, and bladder) in the excretory phase.[41] Axial images,

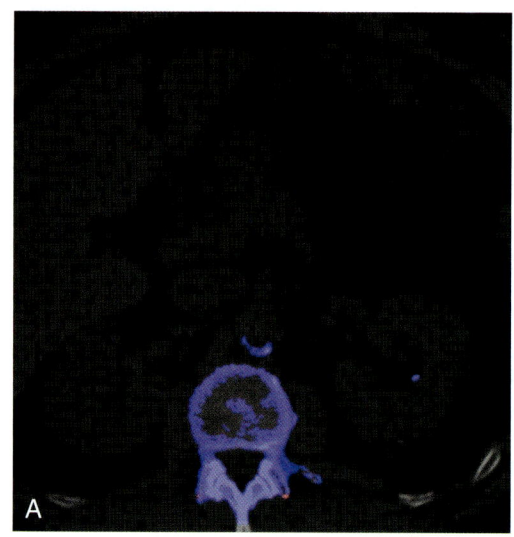

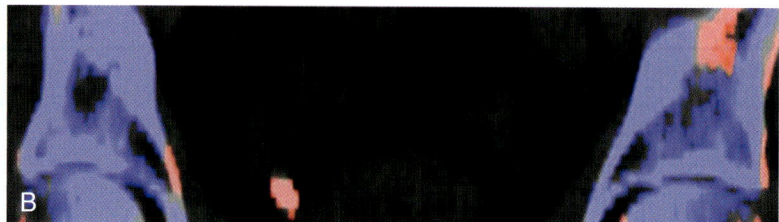

Figure 28.10 Dual-energy computed tomography (CT) for stone characterization in two different patients. **A,** Postprocessed color-coded axial CT image in a 54-year-old patient obtained after dual-energy CT scanning demonstrates a left renal calculus coded blue, indicating a non–uric acid stone. **B,** Postprocessed color-coded coronal CT image in a 66-year-old patient obtained after dual-energy CT scanning demonstrates right distal ureteric calculus color-coded red, indicating a uric acid stone. **Technique:** An initial routine stone protocol multidetector CT scan is performed for detection and localization of the calculi along the renal pelvicalyceal system. Subsequently a focused dual-source CT scan is performed in the region of the stone. Dual-energy CT is performed on the dual-source CT scanner (Somatom Definition) with the following technique: 80 kV/350-380 mAs and 140 kV/80-98 mAs, 14 × 1.2 mm/64 × 0.6 mm. The postprocessing is performed using a three-material decomposition algorithm on the dual-energy software on the scanner console (Syngo.via). (Image courtesy Avinash Kambadakone, MD, Massachusetts General Hospital, Boston, Mass.)

multiplanar reconstructions, maximum-intensity projection images, and three-dimensional volumetric displays complement each other in CTU. CTU is superior to IVU.[42-45] Not all the phases are required for all clinical situations; therefore the examination should be tailored to a specific clinical question. Urothelial lesions can often be evaluated by combining the nephrographic and delayed phases into a single phase by using a split–contrast bolus technique. This involves giving the iodinated contrast intravenously in two separate boluses, but scanning only once.

Another technical innovation is the development of spectral CT or multienergy CT.[38] This involves the ability to scan a particular tissue with two or more different energies. Knowing how a target tissue attenuates at different energies can provide further details of the tissue composition. For example, spectral CT can help in differentiating types of renal calculi and characterizing renal masses. It also provides the ability to generate virtual unenhanced data sets, as well as increasing detection rates of iodine-containing tissues.

Work on reducing radiation exposure is also being aggressively pursued. Because of the development of new reconstruction algorithms such as iterative reconstruction and model-based reconstruction, there has been a significant (50% to 70%) reduction in the resultant radiation dose without any change in the quality of the study. Further advances in technology will result in incremental reductions of dose.

COMPUTED TOMOGRAPHY: NORMAL ANATOMY

The retroperitoneal anatomy is easily viewed with CT (Figures 28.11 to 28.16). The kidneys lie in the retroperitoneum, surrounded by Gerota's fascia in the perinephric

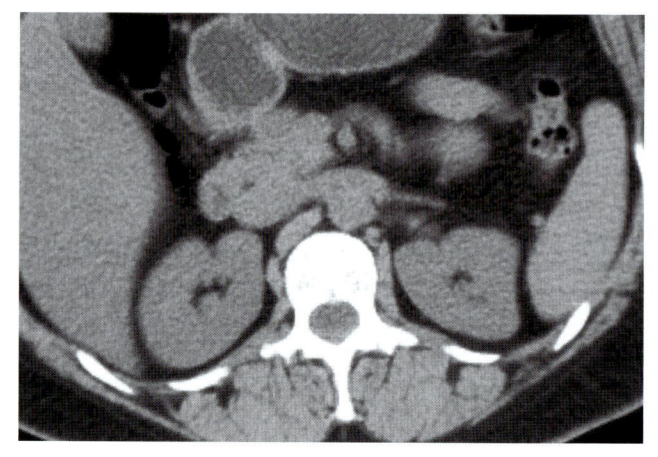

Figure 28.11 Noncontrast computed tomographic scan through the midportion of normal kidneys. The kidneys lie in the retroperitoneum with the lumbar spine and psoas muscles more centrally. The liver is anterolateral to the right kidney, and the spleen anterolateral to the left kidney.

space. Fat will generally outline the kidneys with the liver anterior-superior on the right, the spleen superior on the left, and the spine, aorta, and IVC central to each kidney. The abdominal contents lie anteriorly. The renal arteries are easily seen on both arterial and venous phases, generally located posterior to the venous structures. The adrenal glands are found in a location superior to the upper poles of the kidneys. In venous phase imaging, it is easy to distinguish the renal cortex from the medulla. Cortical thickness and medullary appearance may be readily assessed. The nephrographic phase should demonstrate the symmetric

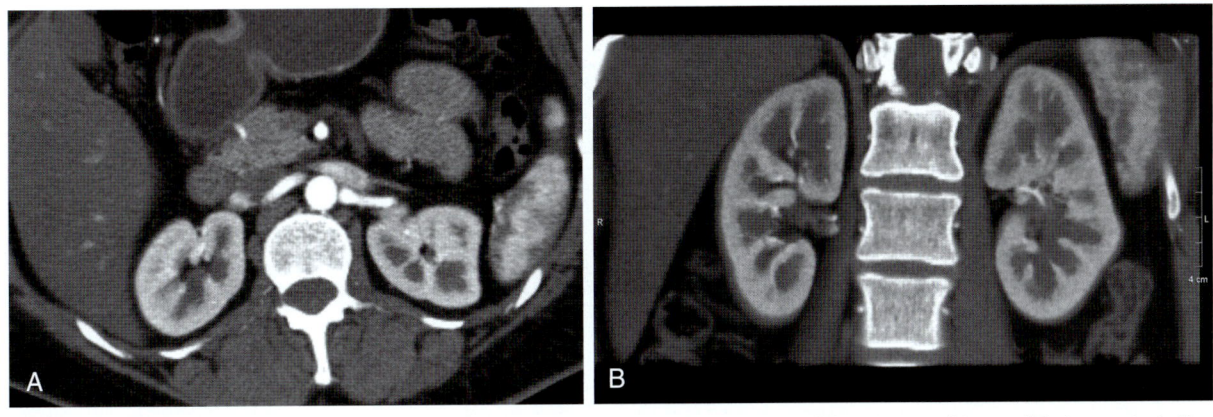

Figure 28.12 Computed tomographic scan: normal corticomedullary phase. Axial slice **(A)** and coronal image **(B)** demonstrate the dense enhancement of the cortex in relation to the medulla containing the renal pyramids.

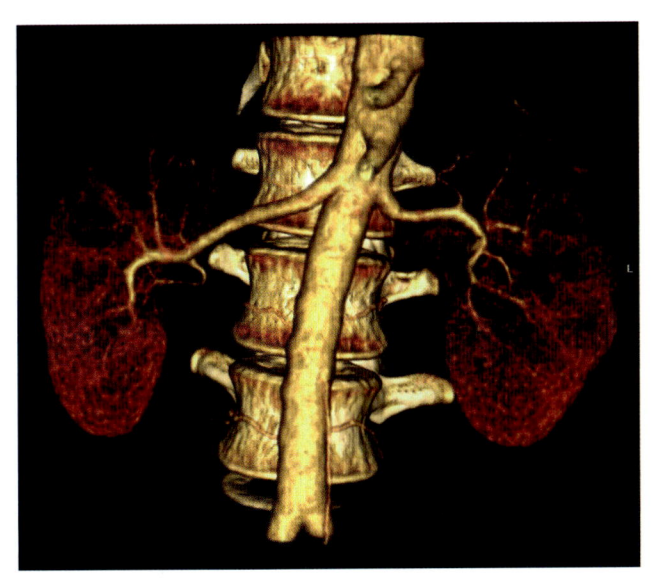

Figure 28.13 Renal computed tomographic angiogram: normal findings. The aorta and the exiting renal arteries on the right and left are visible. The kidneys are visible peripherally with the branching renal arteries.

enhancement for each of the kidneys.[33] At 7 to 10 minutes in the excretory phase, the calyces should be well depicted with sharp fornices, a cupped central section, and a narrow, smooth infundibulum leading to the renal pelvis.[41] Coronal images in slab maximum-intensity projection three-dimensional volumetric reformations also may display the anatomic details.[44] The excretory phase images delineate the ureters from the renal pelvis to the bladder. A curved reformatted series of images or three-dimensional display is needed to display the ureters in their entirety. Proper tailoring of the examination to the diagnostic problem provides guidance for the correct imaging acquisition.[34,36,45]

CONTRAST MEDIA–INDUCED NEPHROPATHY: BACKGROUND

Shortly after the invention of the first modern ionic contrast agent, the potential for nephrotoxicity of contrast agents was proposed.[46] Contrast media–induced nephropathy (CIN) is most often qualitatively defined as acute kidney injury (AKI) occurring within 48 hours of exposure to intravascular radiographic contrast material that is not attributable to other causes. However, there is no universally accepted quantitative definition of CIN. The most commonly used definition is a 25% increase in serum creatinine from baseline value or an absolute increase of at least 0.5 mg/dL that appears within 48 hours after contrast administration and is maintained for 2 to 5 days.[47] Importantly, these definitions do not follow the Acute Kidney Injury Network (AKIN)[48] or Kidney Disease: Improving Global Outcomes (KDIGO)[49] definitions of AKI. We therefore propose using AKIN/KDIGO criteria for a definition of AKI related to intravascular CIN:

1. Absolute increase in serum creatinine level of 0.3 mg/dL or more or
2. A percentage increase in serum creatinine level of 50% or higher (1.5-fold above baseline) or
3. Urine output reduced to 0.5 mL/kg/hr or less for at least 6 hours

The concept that contrast agents pose serious risks has become a dogma with far-reaching consequences. Yet this belief stems from clinical studies with significant limitations. Inclusion of highly selected patient populations (e.g., those undergoing angiography), poor study design (i.e., uncontrolled case studies), and use of inconsistent definitions of CIN call into question to what extent the risk for CIN is applicable to the vast majority of people undergoing diagnostic radiology studies.

Of the approximately 13 published studies that included a control group, just 1 found possible evidence of CIN. Although these studies are a significant improvement over noncontrolled studies, bias in control group selection within the studies may also have introduced error. Articles by Davenport and colleagues and McDonald and associates used propensity matching to correct for potential bias introduced by assigning patients to either group on the basis of factors other than those whose effects the experiment is designed to test.[50,51] Davenport and colleagues found that patients with creatinine levels less than 1.5 mg/dL before CT scan were not at risk for nephropathy. As creatinine levels increased, the risk for nephropathy after CT scan increased for both groups (contrast group and noncontrast group),

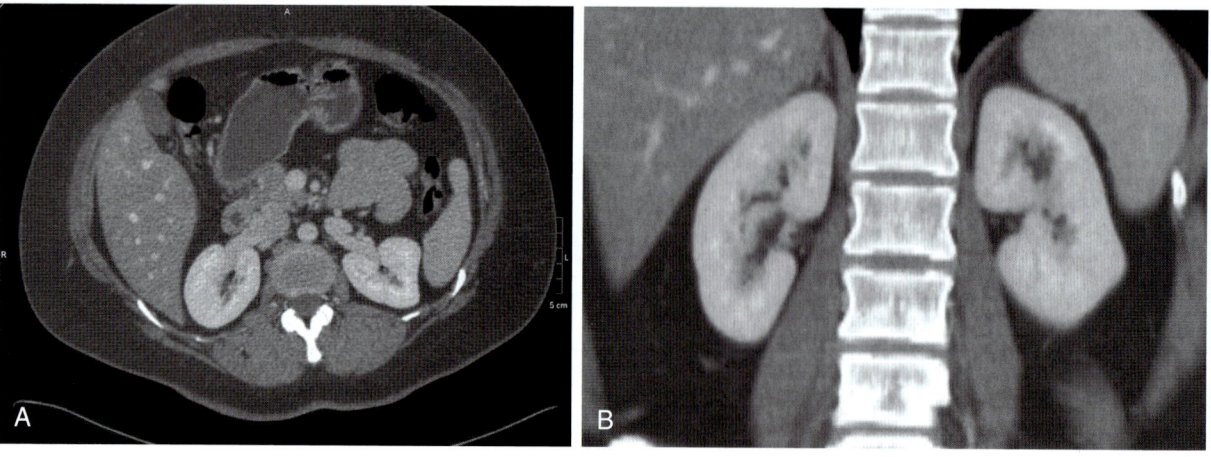

Figure 28.14 Computed tomographic scan: normal nephrographic phase. The axial image **(A)** and the coronal image **(B)** demonstrate the homogeneous appearance of the kidneys, with the cortex and medulla no longer differentially enhanced. These images are typically obtained 80 to 120 seconds after the injection of contrast material.

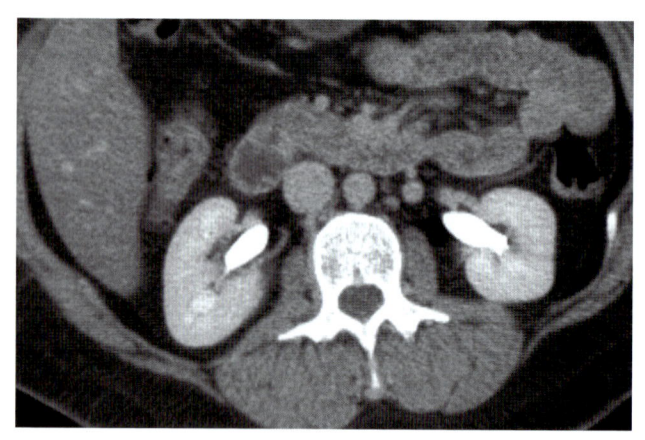

Figure 28.15 Computed tomographic scan: normal excretory phase. The calyces and renal pelvis are now easily noted because they are opacified by the excreted contrast material. This scan is obtained 5 to 10 minutes after the injection of contrast material.

but contrast medium administration remained an independent risk factor. Contrary to this, McDonald and associates concluded that intravenous contrast medium was not associated with increased risk for nephrotoxicity and that it may not pose any long-term threat to renal function, even in those with preexisting chronic kidney disease (CKD).

The contradicting results between these similarly designed studies calls into question whether a causal relationship between intravenous contrast administration and AKI truly exists. Other studies have reported similar results and further challenge this conceptual status quo.[52-56] It is important to note that both the Davenport and colleagues and McDonald and associates studies agree that true CIN in patients with mild renal failure is much less common than previously believed. Furthermore, the most common course of nephropathy after contrast medium administration is a transient asymptomatic increase in serum creatinine level of doubtful long-term clinical significance. No convincing data exist to support increased morbidity or mortality in patients who do not require dialysis for the treatment of contrast nephropathy. In many cases the risk for diagnostic error caused by withholding intravenous contrast may be greater than the risk for CIN.

Because current data cannot definitely refute the existence of CIN, many professional society guidelines advise a conservative approach. The American College of Radiology's *Manual on Contrast Media* states that available data are insufficient to permit a specific recommended threshold level but suggests that contrast medium is safe at creatinine levels below 2.0 mg/dL.[100] The guidelines on contrast media of the European Society of Urogenital Radiology identify an estimated glomerular filtration rate (eGFR) of 45 mL/min/1.7 m^2 as a threshold below which contrast medium poses a risk.[57,58] The Canadian Association of Radiologists suggests that nephropathy risk begins to appear at an eGFR of 45 mL/min/1.7 m^2 and increases when the eGFR reaches 30 mL/min/1.7 m^2.[59]

The following section provides our recommended *guidelines* for administration of intravenous contrast in adults, including references to current literature and society guidelines. Each patient referral should be considered on an individual basis within the context of this background information, and strict adherence to these guidelines in all cases is discouraged. Physician judgment is paramount.

CONTRAST ADMINISTRATION IN PATIENTS WITH ELEVATED CREATININE LEVEL

The decision to proceed with contrast administration in patients with an eGFR below 45 mL/min/1.7 m^2 should always be a matter of clinical judgment. If contrast administration is considered essential, the following options should be considered. (These are suggested protocols that are used at the University of Southern California Keck School of Medicine.)

HYDRATION: This is one of the most important methods for decreasing the incidence of CIN. Broad consensus exists that volume expansion reduces the risk for CIN. Adequate volume expansion improves renal blood flow, induces diuresis with dilution of contrast material within the tubules, reduces the activation of the renin angiotensin aldosterone system, suppresses the secretion of antidiuretic hormone, and minimizes reductions in the renal

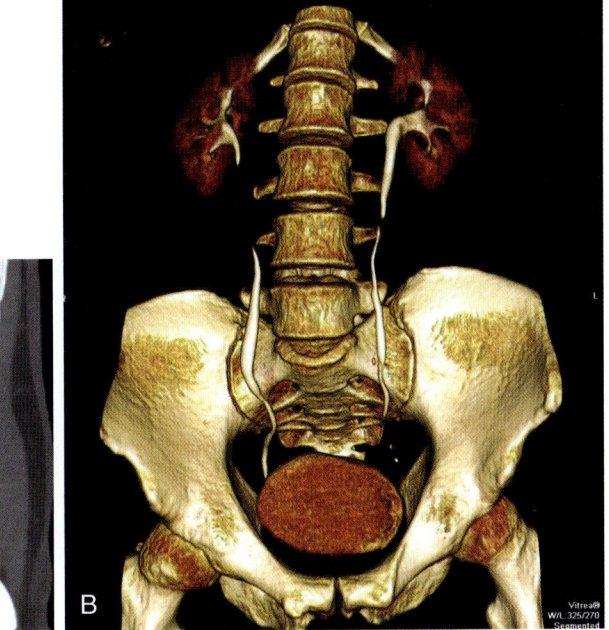

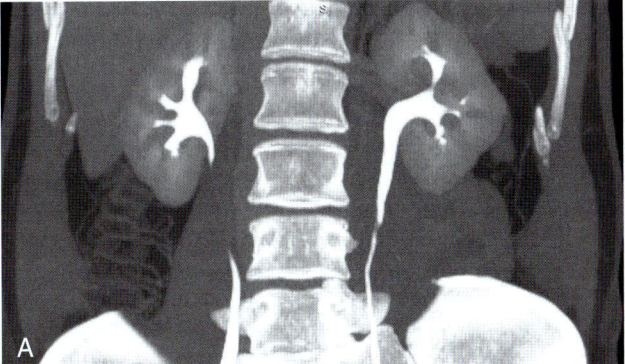

Figure 28.16 Computed tomographic urogram: normal findings. The maximum-intensity projection (MIP) image **(A)** and the volume-rendered image **(B)** demonstrate the calyces, renal pelvis, ureters, and bladder. The MIP image is a slab, 15-mm thick, in the coronal plane. The volume-rendered image was taken as the extraneous tissues adjacent to the kidneys were removed, and it highlights the genitourinary tract.

production of endogenous vasodilators such as nitric oxide and prostacyclin. However, the optimal hydration protocol is unclear. For example, intravenous hydration has not been proven superior to oral hydration. The hydration protocol is not as important as the fact that some form of hydration is administered.

ORAL VERSUS INTRAVENOUS HYDRATION: Studies directly comparing intravenous with oral hydration are sparse because most of the hydration studies are with intravenous hydration and include forms of therapy for prevention of CIN. One study, Preparation for Angiography in Renal Dysfunction (PREPARED), showed no significant difference between outpatient oral hydration and inpatient intravenous hydration.[60] However, another study by Trivedi and coworkers favored intravenous hydration over oral hydration.[61] This study was limited by lack of an objective measurement of oral volume intake in the unrestricted oral hydration group. A study comparing oral fluids (1100 mL) versus intravenous fluids showed no difference in the incidence of CIN in patients with mild CKD.[62] KDIGO 2012 recommends volume expansion with intravenous fluids because there are currently not many studies showing oral volume expansion is as effective as intravenous volume expansion.[63] Because intravenous administration allows us to confirm the volume of hydration, we propose using intravenous hydration.

SODIUM BICARBONATE VERSUS SALINE: The use of sodium bicarbonate instead of sodium chloride has been advocated. It is suggested that the resulting urine alkalinization reduces the generation of free radicals and may also increase urine flow. Several clinical trials and meta-analyses suggest that sodium bicarbonate provides equal or superior protection to isotonic saline.[64-67] However, these results have been subsequently challenged, and the 2013 American College of Radiology (ACR) guidelines do not consider this finding definitive. The most widely used sodium bicarbonate regimen is 3 mL/kg/hr for 1 hour before contrast medium followed by 1 mL/kg/hr for 6 hours after, limited to patients who do not have congestive heart failure (CHF). Studies have recommended that optimal hydration with intravenous normal saline is 1 to 1.5 mL/kg/hr for at least 6 hours before and after contrast medium administration in patients who do not have CHF. Although these protocols are impractical in the outpatient setting, they should be implemented for inpatients after discussion with the referring clinician, with particular attention to volume load and cardiac function. A proposed intravenous volume expansion protocol (using either isotonic saline or sodium bicarbonate) is 3 mL/kg/hr for 1 hour or 1 mL/kg/hr for 6 hours before the procedure followed by 1 mL/kg/hr for 6 hours after the procedure. Additional studies are required to assess whether a single bolus of sodium bicarbonate administered just before contrast medium administration is effective, as Tamura and coworkers suggested, because this protocol would be extremely useful in daily practice.[68] Due to the logistical complications of performing hydration protocols in an outpatient setting, the following regimen is suggested for outpatients with an eGFR of less than 45 mL/min/1.7 m^2. Oral hydration should be strongly encouraged in all such patients. If the patient can tolerate a hydration bolus, a total intravenous bolus of 500 to 1000 mL of isotonic saline should be administered before and after the examination. This should be adjusted according to cardiac status. Blood urea nitrogen

(BUN) determination may be useful as a reflection of hydration but should not be relied on solely in evaluating renal dysfunction. A BUN/creatinine (Cr) ratio above 20 suggests a prerenal state, which could be due to volume depletion or CHF, for example. In outpatients with BUN/Cr ratio above 20 and no evidence of CHF, at least 500 mL isotonic saline as an intravenous bolus should be administered before the examination, regardless of the eGFR.

USE LOW OSMOLAR CONTRAST MEDIA: Iopamidol (Isovue) and iohexol (Omnipaque) are LOCM. Most centers no longer use intravascular HOCM because of the greater incidence of various adverse effects associated with their use.

Studies have failed, however, to show a clear advantage of the intravenous isoosmolar agent, iodixanol, over intravenous LOCM with regard to CIN.

DECREASE TOTAL AMOUNT OF CONTRAST ADMINISTERED: It should be noted that robust data supporting a dose-toxicity relationship for intravenous iodinated contrast media administration are lacking.

DISCONTINUE NEPHROTOXIC DRUGS, IF POSSIBLE

INCREASE THE AMOUNT OF TIME BETWEEN CONTRAST-ENHANCED STUDIES: It takes approximately 24 hours for the entire administered dose of contrast media to be excreted by the kidneys (if the GFR is normal), so it has long been recommended to avoid intervals of less than 24 hours between studies except in urgent situations. For example, it has been recommended that patients should not receive more than 300 mL of contrast media within 24 hours unless the benefits clearly outweigh the risks. Little solid data support this recommendation. A 2009 paper from Massachusetts General Hospital, although criticized by some authorities for methodologic issues, supports checking a repeat creatinine level before performing a second contrast media–enhanced CT (CE-CT) examination within 24 hours of a prior CE-CT scan.[69] The 2013 ACR guidelines, however, find there is insufficient evidence to justify this recommendation.[100]

N-ACETYLCYSTEINE (Mucomyst): Multiple randomized controlled trials and meta-analyses have shown conflicting results regarding the utility of acetylcysteine to prevent CIN. It is controversial whether it is truly nephroprotective or simply lowers the serum creatinine level without preventing renal damage. Given the heterogeneity of data, it is difficult to support the administration of acetylcysteine as a proven and effective means by which to prevent CIN.[70,71]

MAGNETIC RESONANCE IMAGING

Like CT, MRI is a computer-based, multiplanar imaging modality. Instead of ionizing radiation, however, electromagnetic radiation is used in MRI. MRI is an alternative to CE-CT, especially in patients with allergy to iodinated contrast material and in patients for whom reduction of radiation exposure is desired, such as pregnant women and children. MRI routinely allows detailed tissue characterization of the kidney and surrounding structures. The properties of physics underlying MRI are complex and are addressed only briefly.

Clinical MRI is based on the interaction of hydrogen ions (protons) and radiofrequency waves in the presence of a strong magnetic field.[72-74] The strong magnetic field, called the *external magnetic field*, is generated by a large-bore, high–field strength magnet. Most magnets in clinical use are superconducting magnets. The magnet strength is measured in teslas (T) and can range from 0.2 to 3 T for clinical imaging and up to 15 T for animal research. Renal imaging is performed best on high-field magnets (1.5 to 3 T) that allow for higher spatial resolution and faster imaging.

Images of the patient are obtained through a multistep process of energy transfer and signal transmission. When a patient is placed in the magnet, the mobile protons associated with fat and water molecules align longitudinal to the external magnetic field. No signal is obtained unless a resonant radiofrequency pulse is applied to the patient. The radiofrequency pulse causes the mobile protons within the patient to move from a lower, stable energy state to a higher, unstable energy state *(excitation)*. When the radiofrequency pulse is removed, the protons return to the lower-energy steady state while emitting frequency transmissions or signals *(relaxation)*. In radiologic terms, an external radiofrequency pulse "excites" the protons, causing them to "flip" to a higher energy state. When the radiofrequency pulse is removed, the protons "relax" with emission of a "radio signal." The signals produced during proton relaxation are separated from one another with applied magnetic field gradients. The emitted signals are captured by a receiving coil and reconstructed into images through a complex computerized algorithm: the Fourier transform.[72-74]

Different tissues have different relaxation rates that lead to different levels of signal production or signal intensity. The signal intensity of each tissue is determined by three characteristics:

1. *Proton density of the tissue.* The greater the number of mobile protons, the greater the signal produced by the tissue. For example, a volume of urine has more mobile protons than does the same volume of renal tissue; therefore urine produces more signal than do the kidneys. Stones have far fewer mobile protons per unit volume and therefore produce little signal.
2. *T1 relaxation time.* The T1 time is how quickly a proton returns to the preexcitation energy state. The shortest T1 times (rapid relaxation) produce the strongest signal.
3. *T2 relaxation time.* The T2 time is how quickly the proton signal decays as a result of non-uniformity of the magnetic field. A non-uniform field accelerates signal decay and leads to signal loss.[72-74]

In MRI, multiple pulse sequences are obtained. A pulse sequence is a set of defined radiofrequency pulses and timing parameters used to obtain image data. These sequences include, but are not limited to, spin echo, gradient echo, inversion recovery, and steady-state free precession. The data are obtained in volumes (voxels), reconstructed as two-dimensional pixels, and displayed in relation to variations in tissue signal intensity (tissue contrast). Tissue contrast, like signal intensity, is determined by proton density and relaxation times. T1 weighting is related to the rate of T1 relaxation and the time allowed for relaxation, also known as the *pulse repetition time* (TR). T2 weighting is

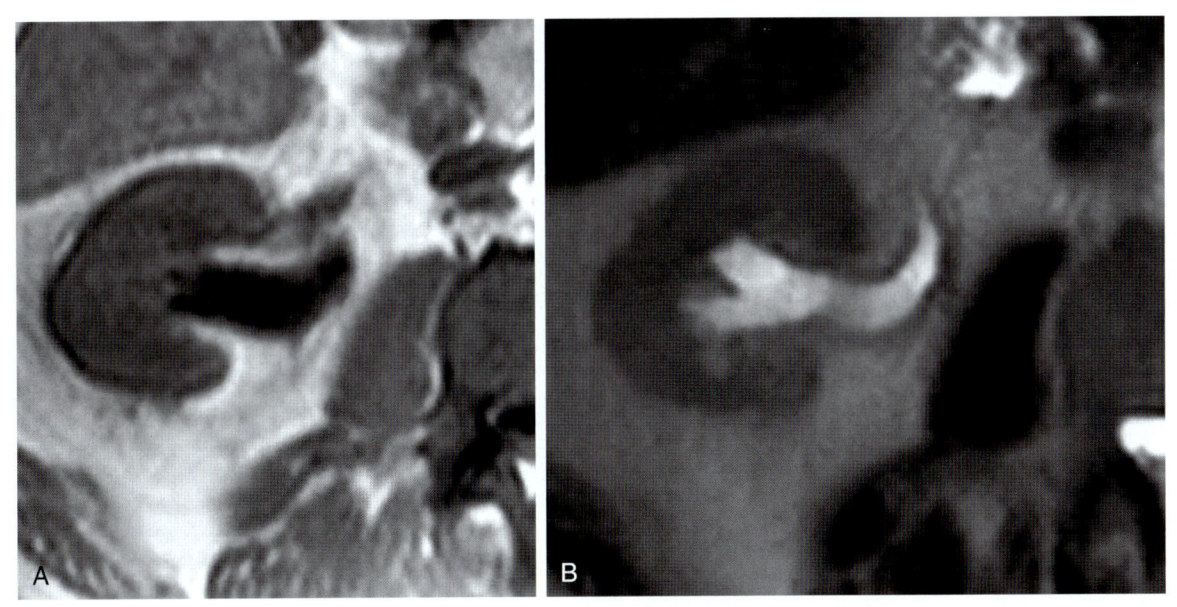

Figure 28.17 Normal signal characteristics of simple fluids on magnetic resonance imaging. Urine appears dark on T1-weighted sequences **(A)** and bright on T2-weighted sequences **(B)**.

related to the rate of T2 relaxation and the time at which the "radio signal" is sampled by the receiver coil, also known as the *echo time* (TE). TR and TE are programmable parameters that can be altered to accentuate T1 and T2 weighting with contrast media.[72-74] For the general observer, T1-weighted sequences have short TR and TE and show simple fluid as black. T2-weighted sequences have long TR and TE and show simple fluid as white (Figure 28.17).

Many programmable parameters other than TR and TE are used to optimize imaging. These include, but are not limited to, choice of pulse sequence, coil types and gradients, slice orientation and thickness, field of view and matrix, gating to reduce motion, and use of intravenous contrast material. Although many pulse sequences are used in clinical MRI, ultrafast sequences are preferred for renal imaging. These fast sequences can be obtained in less than 30 seconds while the patients hold their breath. The benefits of rapid acquisition include improvement in image quality, as a result of reduction of motion artifact; reduction of total scan time; and the ability to perform dynamic imaging.[75]

MRI is not indicated for patients who have certain implanted medical devices, such as most pacemakers, ferromagnetic aneurysm clips, and ferromagnetic stapedial implants. Not all implants or devices cause problems, but knowledge of the type of device is crucial for determining whether the patient can safely enter the magnet.[76] Regularly updated information regarding patient safety and the compatibility of a medical device in the MRI environment may be found at Shellock's MRIsafety.com.[77]

GADOLINIUM CHELATE CONTRAST MEDIA AND NEPHROGENIC SYSTEMIC FIBROSIS

Intravenous contrast material is used routinely in renal imaging because it improves lesion detection and diagnostic accuracy. Gadolinium is a paramagnetic substance that shortens the T1 and T2 relaxation times, resulting in increased signal intensity on T1-weighted images and decreased signal intensity on T2-weighted sequences (Figure 28.18). The pharmacokinetics and enhancement patterns of intravenous gadolinium chelate (Gd-C) agents used in renal imaging are similar to those of iodinated contrast agents used for IVU and CT examinations. Unlike iodinated contrast agents, the dose response to Gd-C is nonlinear; the signal intensity increases at low concentrations and then decreases at higher concentrations. Hence the collecting systems, ureters, and bladder first brighten and then darken on T1-weighted sequences as the gadolinium concentration within the urine increases.

Gd-C agents have been approved for parenteral use since the 1980s and are generally well tolerated with a good safety profile. Although most Gd-C agents are clinically interchangeable, they can be differentiated on the basis of molecular stability, viscosity, and osmolality. Gd-C agents can be divided into three categories based on molecular configuration: non-ionic linear, ionic linear, and macrocyclic (Figure 28.19). Macrocyclic agents have the greatest kinetic stability. Adverse reactions occur in approximately 0.07% to 2.4% of cases.[78] Minor reactions include coldness, warmth, or pain at the injection site; nausea; vomiting; headache; paresthesias; dizziness; and itching. Rash, hives, or urticaria occurs in 0.004% to 0.07% of cases; and severe, life-threatening reactions occur in approximately 0.001% to 0.01%. Risk factors for adverse reactions include a history of prior reaction to Gd-C and/or iodinated contrast agents, where rates are at an eight-fold higher risk; and asthma, as well as other allergies, where rates are reported as high as 3.7%.[52] If a patient has had a prior adverse reaction to Gd-C, premedication with antihistamines and corticosteroids is recommended (same as the premedication regimen discussed for iodinated contrast media). Because adverse reactions may occur more frequently with ionic Gd-C agents, the use of a non-ionic agent should be considered, if available.

Gd-C agents are considered to have no nephrotoxicity at the approved doses used for clinical MRI.[79-82] Because there have been some case reports of nephrotoxicity with high

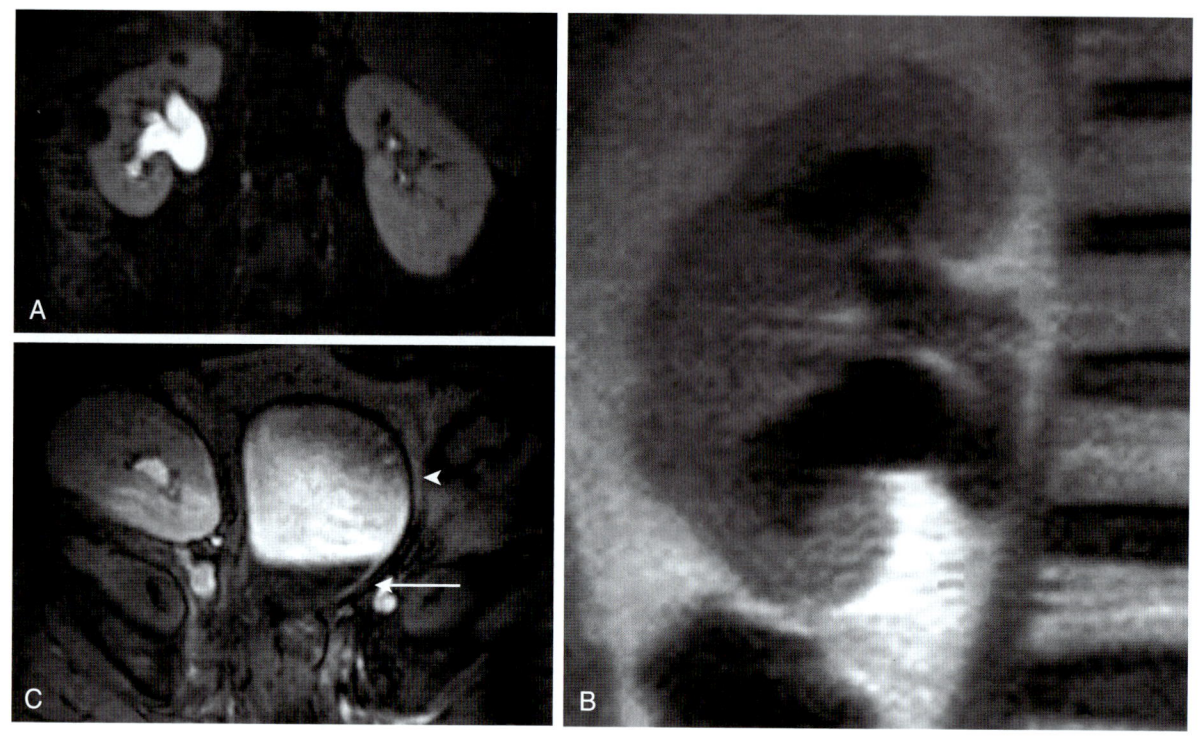

Figure 28.18 Paramagnetic effects of gadolinium on urine. **A,** Coronal T1-weighted image from a magnetic resonance urogram (MRU) demonstrates enhancement of the urine in the collection system. **B,** Coronal T2-weighted image from an MRU demonstrates low signal intensity of urine in the collecting system secondary to effects of gadolinium. **C,** Axial T1-weighted, delayed image after contrast medium enhancement demonstrates layering of contrast material. The denser, more concentrated gadolinium is dark (*arrow*). The less concentrated gadolinium is brighter and layers above (*arrowhead*).

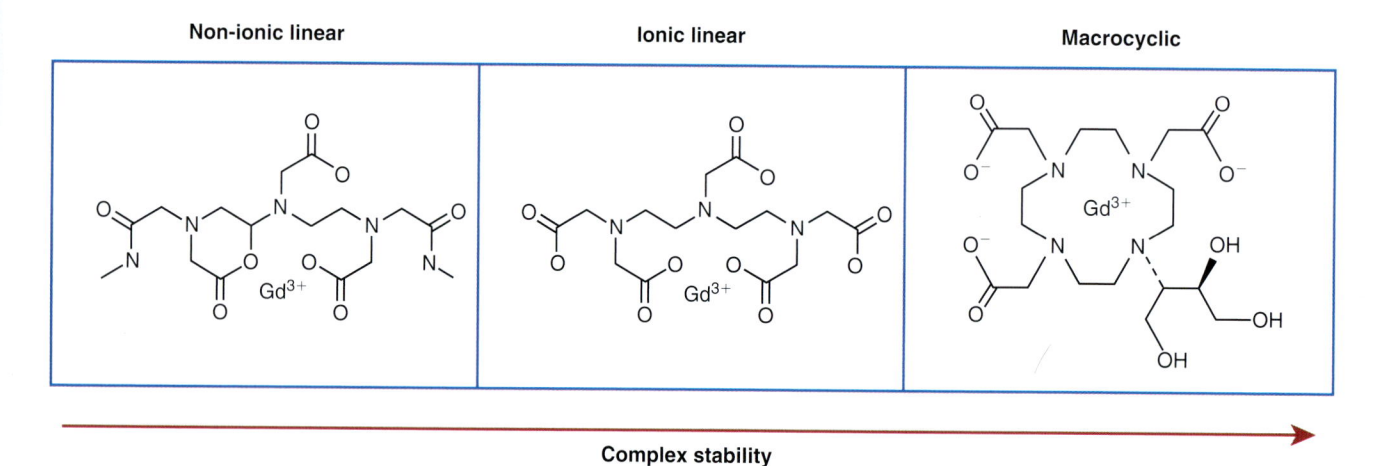

Figure 28.19 Gadolinium molecular configurations.

doses of intravenous Gd-C in populations at high risk (moderate to severe kidney injury), the use of Gd-C in conventional angiography is not recommended.[83,84] Gd-C may interfere with serum calcium and magnesium measurements, especially in patients with renal insufficiency.[85] Gd-C does not cause an actual reduction in serum calcium level; Gd-C interferes with standard colorimetric methods of measuring serum calcium. As with iodinated contrast material, hemodialysis filters Gd-C effectively, and dialysis is therefore recommended immediately after use of contrast material in patients already on hemodialysis.[86]

Although Gd-C agents were once considered the safest intravenous contrast agents in clinical imaging, they are now thought to carry significant risk in patients with moderate to severe renal disease.[87-92] Gd-C agents have been associated with nephrogenic systemic fibrosis (NSF), a rare, multiorgan, fibrosing condition for which there is no known effective treatment.[93] Patients with NSF typically present with symmetric, dark red patches or papules on the skin, swelling of extremities, and thickening of skin that sometimes is described as "woody" and like an "orange peel." The skin thickening can inhibit motion of joints, leading to contractures and immobility. Burning, itching, or severe pain in involved areas or "deep bone pain" in hips and ribs has been described, as has rapid, new-onset fluctuating hypertension. Other structures affected include the lungs, esophagus, skeletal muscles, and heart. These structures may become scarred, which leads to restriction of function; and although NSF is not by itself a cause of death, the resulting restriction of function may contribute to death.[94] Symptoms may develop over a period of days to months; however, in approximately 5% of patients, the course may be rapidly progressive.[94] Diagnosis is confirmed by full-thickness skin biopsy, which reveals thickened collagen bundles, mucin deposition, and proliferation of fibroblasts and elastic fibers without signs of inflammation. NSF tends to affect middle-aged patients without predilection for gender or ethnicity. Although no treatment is known to be consistently successful, improving renal function appears to slow or stop the progression of NSF.[94]

NSF was first described in 1997, and the description was first published in 2000.[95] It was not until January 2006 that a possible causal relationship between Gd-C and NSF was presented in the literature by Grobner.[89] The U.S. Food and Drug Administration (FDA), European Medicines Agency (EMA), and the ACR began publishing warnings and recommendations in 2006 with an almost immediate drop in the number of new cases of NSF; no new cases occurring after 2008 have been reported. To date, almost 100 million patients have been exposed to Gd-C agents; however less than 600 cases of NSF have been reported in the literature. The patients at highest risk are those with severely impaired renal function, both acute and chronic, for whom the risk for developing NSF is 1% to 7%. The duration and underlying cause of the kidney disease is irrelevant. No cases of NSF have been documented in patients with normal renal function. The FDA, EMA, and ACR continue to update recommendations for the use of all classes of Gd-C agents in high-risk patients as new information and products become available.[57,94-96,100]

All patients should be screened for renal disease before the use of a Gd-C agent, and those who may be high risk should have an eGFR calculated. Patients who may be at high risk include those over 60 years of age and those with a history of renal disease, diabetes treated with prescribed medications, and/or hypertension. The eGFR should be obtained within 6 weeks of the anticipated Gd-C study in otherwise stable patients; however, for those with severe liver disease, acute kidney disease, or those who are hospitalized, an eGFR should be calculated nearly simultaneously with the anticipated Gd-C study. The most current 2013 recommendations for the use of Gd-C are as follows:

1. The use of Gd-C is not contraindicated in patients when the eGFR is greater than 40 mL/min/1.73 m^2.
2. The use of Gd-C is not contraindicated when the eGFR is between 30 and 40 mL/min/1.73 m^2; however, this is a "gray zone" because the eGFR may fluctuate to lower levels depending on the health of the patient. Physician discretion should be used to determine the risk of Gd-C use in this patient population. High Gd-C doses and repeated exposure should be avoided in these patients.
3. The use of Gd-C should be avoided when the eGFR is less than 30 mL/min/1.73 m^2. This is not an absolute contraindication; however, the use of Gd-C should be at the discretion and judgment of the ordering physician. If possible, alternative imaging should be considered. If contrast media–enhanced MRI (CE-MRI) is necessary, this should be documented in the record, and if the patient is on hemodialysis, the CE-MRI should be scheduled immediately before dialysis. Although Gd-C agents are effectively removed with hemodialysis, no published report has proved that early dialysis prevents the development of NSF.[96] Specific agents are contraindicated in patients with an eGFR of less than 30 mL/min/1.73 m^2, including non-ionic linear (gadodiamide, gadoversetamide) and gadopentetate dimeglumine, so other Gd-C agents should be used.
4. All contrast material should be avoided in patients with AKI; Gd-C should be administered only if absolutely necessary.

Suspected cases of NSF should be confirmed by skin biopsy and reported to the International Center for Nephrogenic Systemic Fibrosis Research (ICNSFR) to help further the understanding of NSF and its association with Gd-C. For further reading on the different FDA-approved Gd-C agents, including their properties, how these properties may affect safety profiles, and a complete discussion on the relationship of NSF and Gd-C agents, please refer to "Update on Nephrogenic Systemic Fibrosis"[101] and the "ACR Guidance Document for Safe MR Practices."[95]

DIAGNOSTIC MAGNETIC RESONANCE IMAGING TECHNIQUE

Routine MRI evaluation of the kidneys includes axial and coronal T1-weighted and T2-weighted sequences. Dynamic contrast media–enhanced T1-weighted sequences with fat suppression are also routinely obtained. Due to excellent tissue differentiation provided by MRI, the renal cortex and medullary pyramids are easily differentiated on sequences that are not enhanced by contrast media. On T1-weighted sequences the renal cortex has higher signal intensity than do the medullary pyramids. On T2-weighted sequences the renal cortex has lower signal intensity than do the medullary pyramids (Figure 28.20). With kidney injury, this corticomedullary differentiation disappears (Figure 28.21).[100,101] Urine, like water, normally appears black on T1-weighted sequences and white on T2-weighted sequences (see Figure 28.17).

CE-MRI allows for dynamic evaluation of the kidneys and surrounding structures. Serial acquisitions are obtained after bolus injection of Gd-C (0.1 to 0.2 mmol per kilogram of body weight) at 2 mL/sec.[102,103] The injection should be administered by means of an automatic, MRI-compatible power injector to ensure accuracy of the timed bolus, including volume and rate of injection.[103,104] The corticomedullary-arterial phase (approximately 20 seconds after injection) is best for evaluating the arterial structures and corticomedullary differentiation. In the nephrographic phase (70 to 90 seconds after injection), tumor detection is maximized, and the renal veins and surrounding structures are best demonstrated (Figure 28.22). Imaging can be performed in any plane, but the coronal plane is used most frequently for dynamic imaging because it allows imaging of the kidneys, ureters, vessels, and surrounding structures in the fewest number of images. The characteristics of parenchymal enhancement are similar to those observed on CE-CT.

The blood vessels can be variable in signal intensity on routine MRI that is not enhanced by contrast media, ranging

Figure 28.20 Normal appearance of corticomedullary differentiation on magnetic resonance imaging. Coronal (A) and axial (B) T2-weighted images demonstrate decreased signal intensity of the renal cortex in relation to the medullary pyramids. Axial T1-weighted image (C) demonstrates increased signal intensity of the renal cortex in relation to the medullary pyramids.

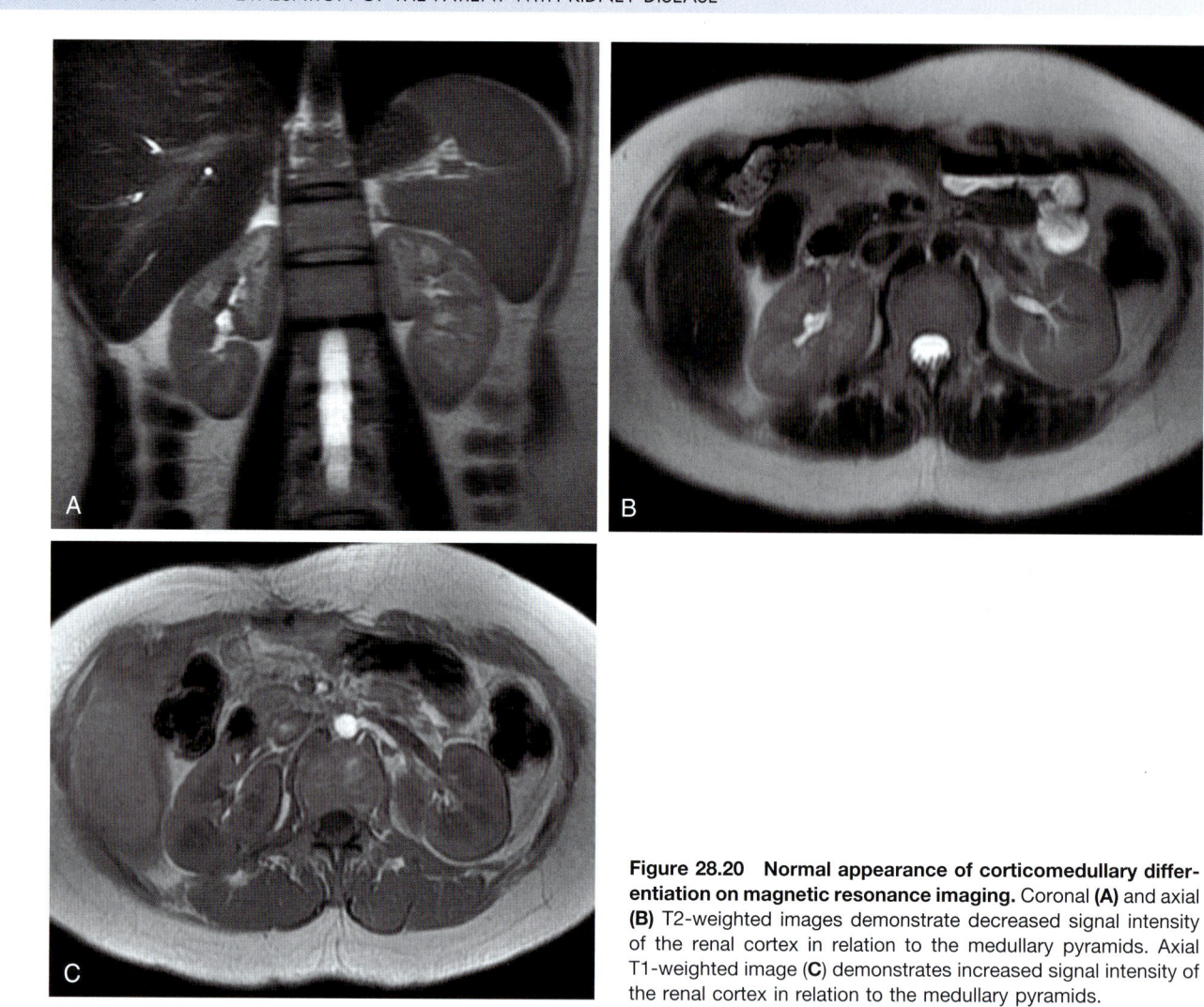

Figure 28.21 Coronal T2-weighted image demonstrates loss of corticomedullary differentiation in patient with elevated creatinine level. Also, the renal sizes are asymmetric.

from white to black. This is due to many factors, including, but not limited to, flow-related parameters, location and orientation of the imaged vessel, and choice of pulse sequence. By taking advantage of some of these factors, diagnostic angiography and venography may be performed without the use of intravenous contrast; these sequences are sometimes called "bright-blood" sequences. Although contrast media–enhanced magnetic resonance angiography (CE-MRA) remains the preferred method of vascular imaging, high-quality MRA that is not enhanced by contrast media has regained popularity because of the advancement in MR hardware and imaging sequences, as well as the risk of NSF in patients with poor renal function. MRA that is not enhanced by contrast media is particularly attractive for evaluating the renal arteries in patients with severe renal dysfunction or those with a relative contraindication for CE-CMA. The most robust sequences are based on inversion recovery, balanced steady-state free precession techniques.[105,106] Older, less robust techniques include time-of-flight MRA, which is based on flow-related enhancement, and phase-contrast MRA, which is based on velocity and direction of flow. Phase-contrast MRA can be used in conjunction with CE-MRA to detect turbulent flow and high velocities associated with stenoses. Unlike MRA that is not

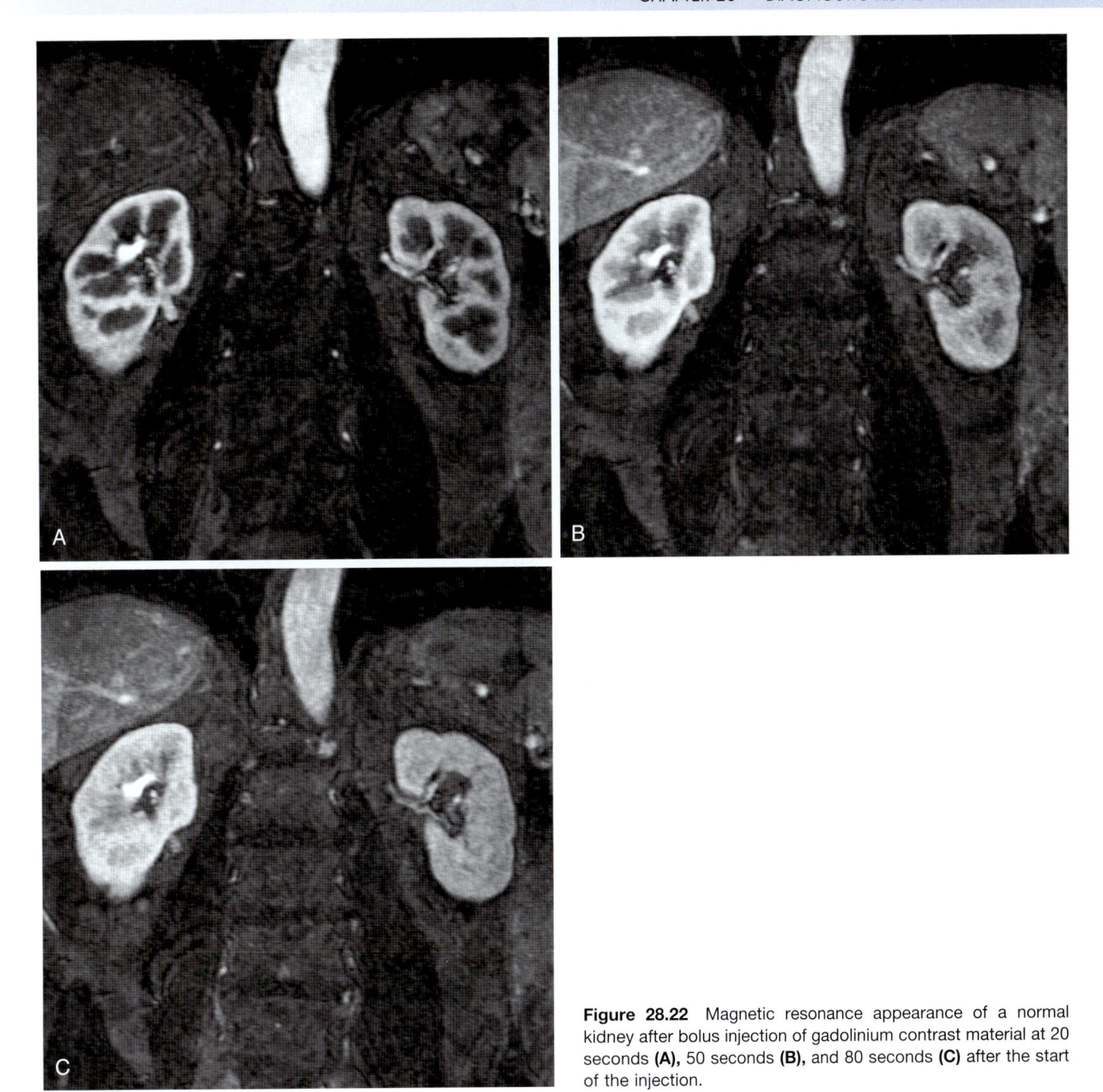

Figure 28.22 Magnetic resonance appearance of a normal kidney after bolus injection of gadolinium contrast material at 20 seconds **(A)**, 50 seconds **(B)**, and 80 seconds **(C)** after the start of the injection.

enhanced by contrast media, CE-MRA minimizes flow-related enhancement and motion. The success of CE-MRA depends on the T1-shortening properties of gadolinium, which allow for faster imaging, increased coverage, and improved resolution.[72,107] Accurate timing of the bolus injection is critical in CE-MRA. The time at which the bolus arrives at the renal arteries may be determined with a bolus injection of 1 mL of Gd-C, followed by a saline flush. A three-dimensional T1-weighted gradient-echo MRI pulse sequence is then obtained in the coronal plane during the injection of approximately 15 to 20 mL of Gd-C at 2 mL/sec, timed to capture the arterial phase.[102,103] Sequential three-dimensional sequences are obtained to capture the venous phase (magnetic resonance venography). The data sets can be postprocessed into multiple formats, improving ease and accuracy of interpretation (Figure 28.23).[108-110]

Magnetic resonance urography (MRU) consists of protocols tailored to the evaluation of the renal collecting system and the disease found there. MRU can be performed with heavily T2-weighted sequences, in which urine provides the intrinsic contrast, or with contrast media–enhanced T1-weighted sequences, which mimic conventional IVU and CTU. Heavily T2-weighted sequences are most useful in patients with dilated collecting systems, in whom all water-filled structures are bright (Figure 28.24), and in patients with impaired renal excretion, in whom contrast media–enhanced urography is most limited. Unfortunately, without adequate distension of the collecting system, T2-weighted evaluation is limited. Although a good morphologic examination, T2-weighted urography is ultimately limited by a lack of functional information. For example, T2-weighted urography cannot reliably differentiate between an

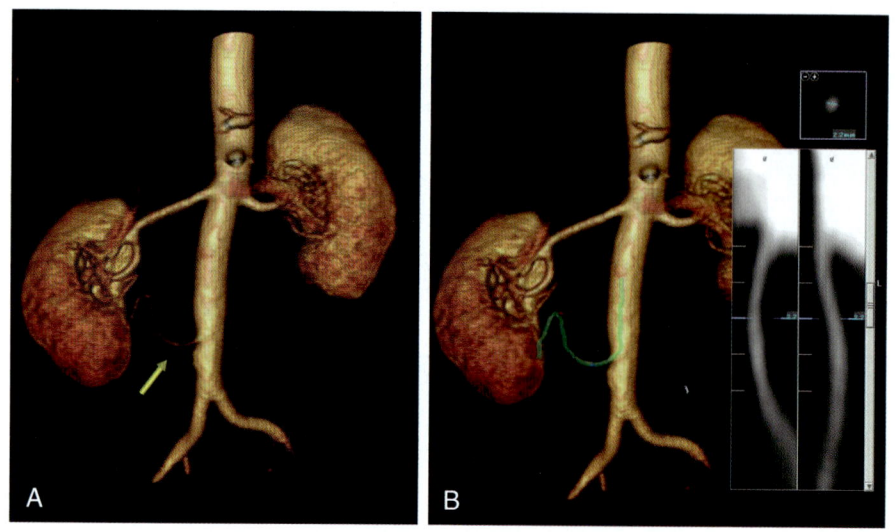

862 SECTION IV — EVALUATION OF THE PATIENT WITH KIDNEY DISEASE

Figure 28.23 Magnetic resonance angiogram reconstructed with three-dimensional software. **A,** Visualization of a small accessory right renal artery (*arrow*) is excellent. **B,** The accessory artery is depicted in a way to make more accurate luminal measurements.

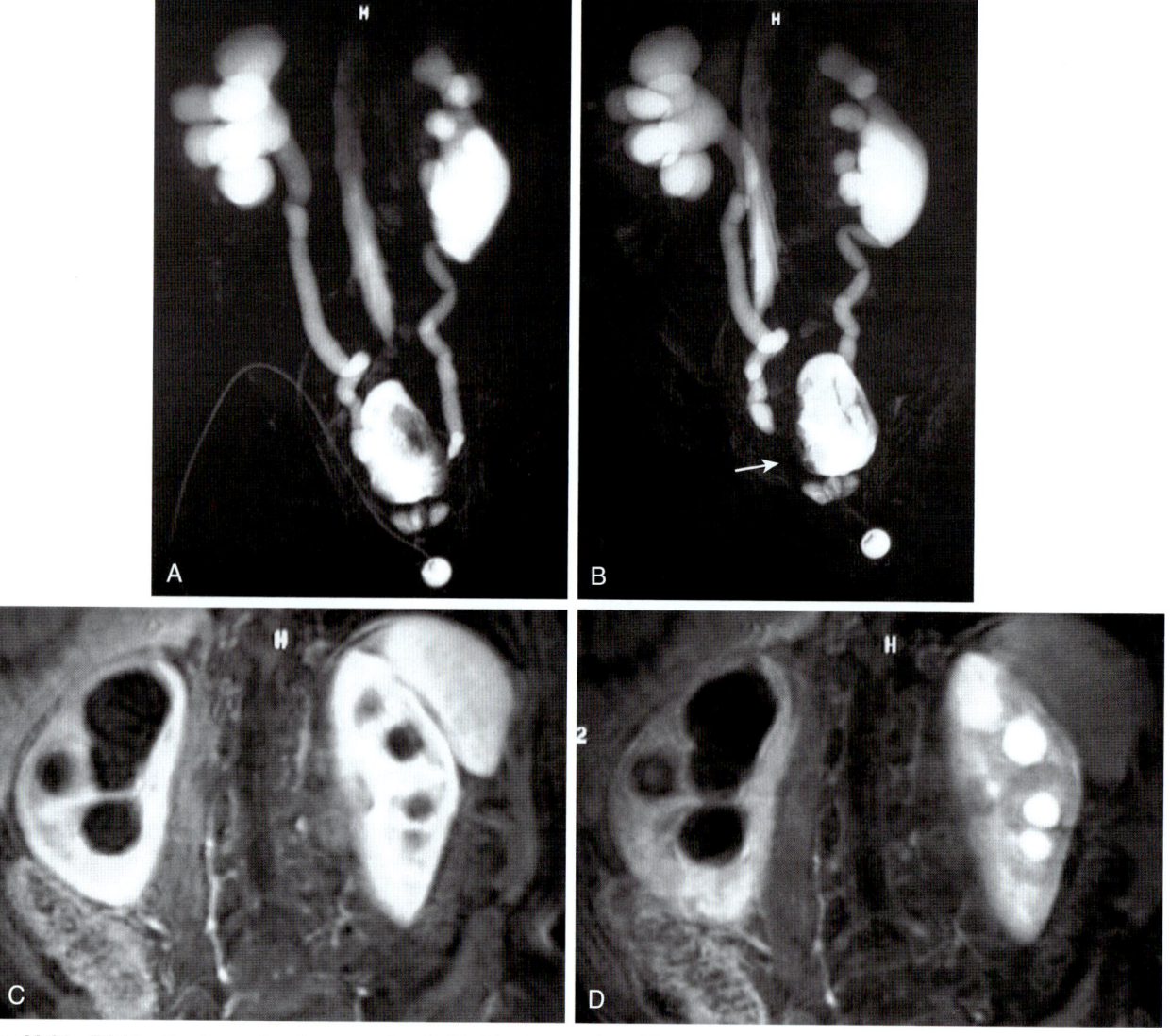

Figure 28.24 Bilateral hydronephrosis secondary to bladder tumor. **A** and **B,** Heavily T2-weighted magnetic resonance urograms (MRUs) demonstrate bilateral hydronephrosis and hydroureter caused by bladder mass (*arrow*). **C,** Contrast medium–enhanced MRU in the nephrographic phase demonstrates asymmetric enhancement of the kidneys. **D,** MRU in the excretory phase demonstrates asymmetric excretion of gadolinium. There is no excretion on the right as demonstrated by unenhanced (dark) urine within the collecting system.

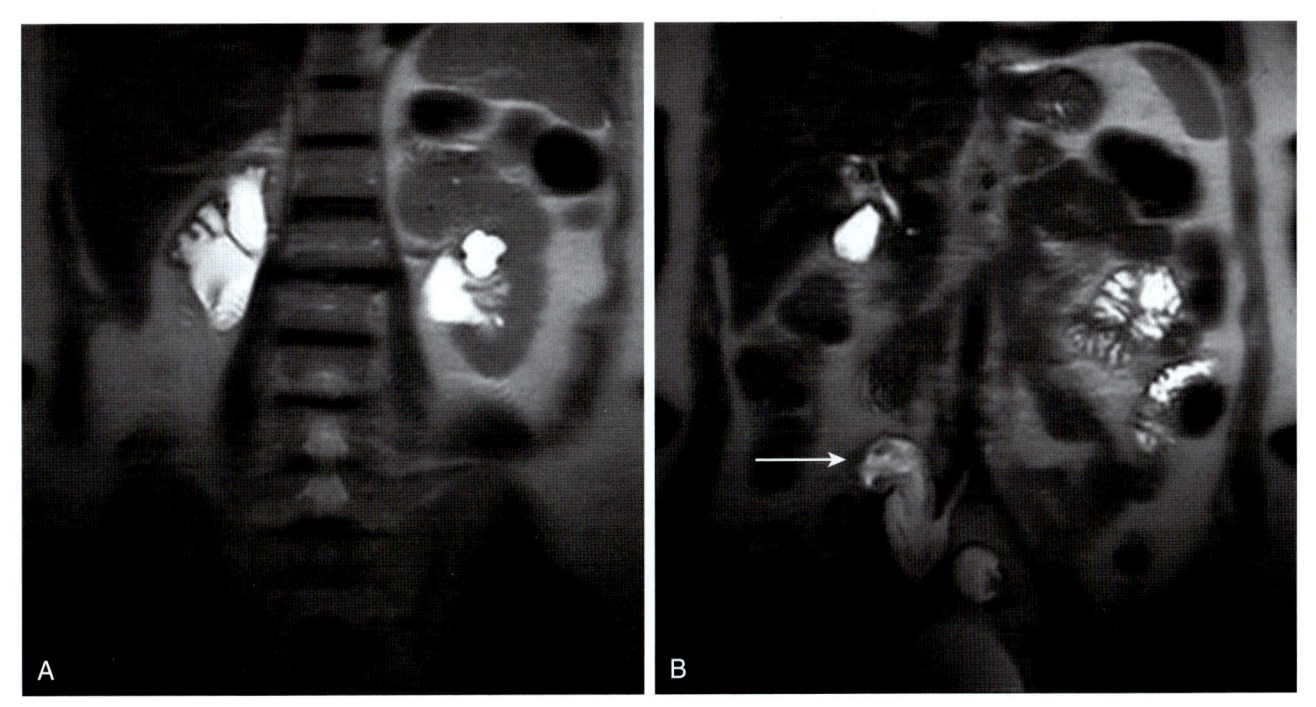

Figure 28.25 **A** and **B**, Coronal T2-weighted images demonstrate right renal atrophy and dilation of the right collecting system in a patient who had undergone bladder resection and ilioconduit reconstruction (*arrow*). On these static images, it is difficult to differentiate between an obstructed system and a nonobstructed system. The patient had pelvocaliectasis without obstruction, demonstrated on the contrast medium–enhanced portion of the examination.

obstructed system and an ectatic collecting system (Figure 28.25).[111] Contrast media–enhanced T1-weighted urography in the excretory phase is superior to T2-weighted urography because both structure and function can be evaluated.[111-113]

T2-weighted and contrast media–enhanced T1-weighted sequences are complementary and are frequently obtained together as part of a complete MRU examination. In patients with nondilated systems, both techniques require hydration and furosemide for adequate distension of the renal collecting system.[111,114] Typical MRU starts with a coronal, heavily T2-weighted sequence in which simple fluid (urine, cerebrospinal fluid, ascites) is bright and all other tissues are dark (see Figure 28.24). This rapid breath-hold sequence takes less than 5 seconds to obtain and is presented as a urogram-like image. The T2-weighted sequence is used as an initial survey of fluid within the collecting system. Low-dose furosemide (0.1 mg per kilogram of body weight; maximum dose, 10 mg) is administered intravenously, 30 to 60 seconds before the intravenous administration of Gd-C (0.1 mmol/kg).[112,113] Furosemide is given to increase urine volume and dilute the Gd-C within the collecting system.[112,114] Coronal, three-dimensional, contrast media–enhanced T1-weighted sequences are obtained with the same technique as in renal CE-MRA, in the corticomedullary-arterial phase, nephrographic phase, and excretory phase (see Figure 28.24).[113] Additional sequences may be obtained in any plane to better evaluate suspected pathologic conditions.

By combining renal MRI and MRU, the clinician can obtain a comprehensive morphologic and functional evaluation of the urinary tract. MRU helps accurately evaluate the upper urinary tract and is useful in the evaluation of anatomic anomalies, including duplications, ureteropelvic obstruction, anomalous crossing vessels, and ureteroceles[114,115] (Figure 28.26). Obstructive disease is well evaluated regardless of whether the cause is intrinsic or extrinsic to the collecting system.

FUNCTIONAL MAGNETIC RESONANCE IMAGING OF THE KIDNEY

MRI is suited for measurement of various aspects of renal function, given the role of the kidney in fluid regulation. Techniques for the evaluation of renal function include dynamic contrast media–enhanced MR renography, diffusion-weighted imaging (DWI), and blood oxygen level–dependent (BOLD) MRI. Dynamic contrast media–enhanced MR renography is a contrast media–enhanced sequence in which dynamic images are obtained during the 7 to 10 minutes after administration of intravenous contrast material; tissue signal intensities are converted to tissue gadolinium concentrations, and these values are plotted against time. Current clinical applications include the evaluation of the renal artery stenosis, both with and without the use of angiotensin-converting enzyme (ACE) inhibitors, functional urinary obstruction, and the evaluation of early postoperative renal transplant dysfunction, to distinguish acute rejection from acute tubular necrosis. What prevents widespread clinical use, however, is the lack of consensus on optimal imaging technique and methods of data analysis.[116]

DWI is based on the brownian motion of water molecules in tissue and is a noncontrast MRI technique that is used for both structural and functional imaging. Initial experience with DWI has yielded reproducible information on renal function, with the possibility of determining the degree of dysfunction.[117] No large studies have been

Figure 28.26 Duplicated collecting system. A and **B,** Contrast material–enhanced magnetic resonance urograms demonstrate a duplicated collecting system on the right with delayed excretion of the upper pole moiety. **C,** Obstruction of the upper pole moiety is confirmed on intravenous urogram.

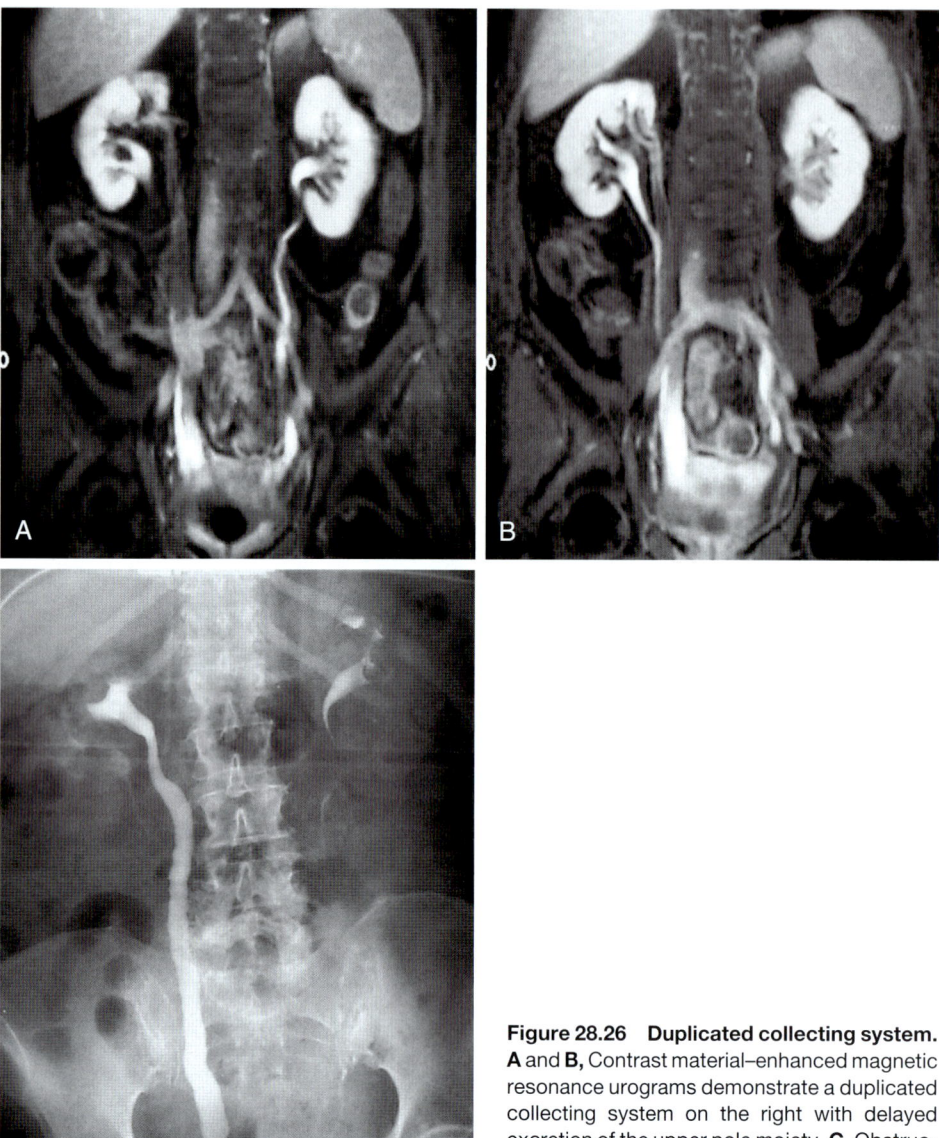

performed, and further research is required before the usefulness of DWI is confirmed. Animal research is being performed with the hope of using noninvasive DWI as a tool for monitoring early renal graft rejection after transplantation.[118]

BOLD MRI is a noninvasive technique to estimate intrarenal oxygenation.[116] Various researchers use this technique to explore renal artery stenosis, renal transplant dysfunction, and diabetic nephropathy. Sadowski and colleagues[121] demonstrated the feasibility of using BOLD MRI to evaluate the oxygen status of renal transplants and to detect the presence of acute rejection. They concluded that BOLD MRI may differentiate acute rejection from normal function and acute tubular necrosis, but further research is required.

NUCLEAR MEDICINE

Scintigraphy offers imaging-based diagnostic information on renal structure and function.[120] Many single-photon radiotracers have long been in routine clinical use in renal scintigraphy; they are tailored to provide physiologic information complementing the primarily anatomic and structural-based imaging modalities, such as US, CT, and MRI. With the rapid expansion of PET and hybrid structural-functional imaging systems such as PET-CT, additional unprecedented opportunities have developed for quantitative imaging evaluation of renal diseases in clinical medicine and in research.[121] Scintigraphy, including PET, makes a unique contribution to the imaging evaluation of renal structure and function. The common radiopharmaceuticals used in renal scintigraphy are described first.

RADIOPHARMACEUTICALS

Technetium 99m–Labeled Diethylenetriaminepentaacetic Acid

Technetium 99m–labeled diethylenetriaminepentaacetic acid (^{99m}Tc-DTPA) is the common agent for assessing GFR.

The ideal agent for measuring GFR would be cleared only by glomerular filtration and would not be secreted or reabsorbed. ^{99m}Tc-DTPA satisfies the first requirement but has variable degrees of protein binding, which deviates its kinetics from the ideal agent such as inulin. For a 20-mCi (740-MBq) dose, the radiation exposures of the kidneys and the urinary bladder are 1.8 and 2.3 rad, respectively.[122]

Iodine 131–Labeled Ortho-iodohippurate

The mechanisms underlying renal clearance of iodine 131–labeled ortho-iodohippurate (^{131}I-ortho-iodohippurate) are GFR (approximately 20%) and tubular secretion (approximately 80%). ^{131}I-ortho-iodohippurate is an acceptable alternative to *p*-aminohippuric acid (PAH) for determining renal plasma flow (RPF), although the amount cleared is 15% lower than that of PAH. PAH is not entirely cleared by the kidneys; approximately 10% of arterial PAH remains in the renal venous blood. Therefore ^{131}I-ortho-iodohippurate helps measure *effective* RPF. The efficiency of tubular extraction of ^{131}I-ortho-iodohippurate is 90%, and there is no hepatobiliary excretion. Ortho-iodohippurate may also be labeled with iodine 123, which not only provides urinary kinetics equivalent to those provided by iodine 131 but also enables improved image quality because the administered dose is typically larger, in view of its more favorable profile of radiation exposure. For a 300-µCi (11.1-MBq) dose of ^{131}I-ortho-iodohippurate, the radiation exposures of the kidneys and the urinary bladder are 0.02 and 1.4 rad, respectively. A few drops of nonradioactive iodine (e.g., saturated solution of potassium iodide) administered orally help minimize the thyroid uptake of free iodine 131.[122]

Technetium 99m–Labeled Mercaptoacetyltriglycine

Technetium 99m–labeled mercaptoacetyltriglycine (^{99m}Tc-MAG3) has properties similar to those of ^{131}I-ortho-iodohippurate but has significant advantages of better image quality and less radiation exposure. The tubular extraction fraction of ^{99m}Tc-MAG3 is lower than that of ^{131}I-ortho-iodohippurate, at approximately 60% to 70%. Also, hepatobiliary excretion is approximately 3%, which increases with renal insufficiency. Despite these features, however, ^{99m}Tc-MAG3 is commonly used in scintigraphic evaluation of renal function. For a 10-mCi (370-MBq) dose, the radiation exposures of the kidneys and the urinary bladder are 0.15 and 4.4 rad, respectively.[122]

Technetium 99m–Labeled Dimercaptosuccinic Acid

Technetium 99m–labeled dimercaptosuccinic acid (^{99m}Tc-DMSA) localizes to the renal cortex at high concentration and has a slow urinary excretion rate. Approximately 50% of the injected dose accumulates in the renal cortex in 1 hour. The tracer is bound to the renal proximal tubular cells. In view of the high retention of ^{99m}Tc-DMSA in the renal cortex, it has become useful for imaging of the renal parenchyma. For a 6-mCi (222-MBq) dose, the radiation exposures of the kidneys and the urinary bladder are 3.78 and 0.42 rad, respectively.[122]

Fluorine 18 2-Fluoro-2-deoxy-D-glucose

Fluorine 18 2-fluoro-2-deoxy-D-glucose (FDG) is the most common positron-labeled radiotracer in PET. FDG is a modified form of glucose in which the hydroxyl group in the 2′ position is replaced by the fluorine 18 positron emitter. FDG accumulates in cells in proportion to glucose metabolism. Cell membrane glucose transporters facilitate the transport of glucose and FDG across the cell membrane. Both glucose and FDG are phosphorylated in the 6′ position by the hexokinase. The conversion of glucose-6-phosphate or FDG-6-phosphate back to glucose or FDG, respectively, is effected by the enzyme phosphatase. In most tissues, including cancer cells, there is little phosphatase activity. FDG-6-phosphate cannot undergo further conversions and is therefore trapped in the cell.

FDG is excreted in the urine. The typical FDG dose is 0.144 mCi/kg (minimum, 1 mCi; maximum, 20 mCi). The urinary bladder wall receives the highest radiation dose from FDG.[123,124] The radiation dose depends on the excretion rate, the varying size of the bladder, the bladder volume at the time of FDG administration, and an activity curve of estimated bladder time. For a typical 15-mCi dose of FDG and voiding at 1 hour after tracer injection, the average estimated radiation dose absorbed by the adult bladder wall is 3.3 rad (0.22 rad/mCi).[125] The doses absorbed by other organs are between 0.75 and 1.28 rad (0.050 to 0.085 rad/mCi); the average dose absorbed is 1.0 rad.[126] Renal failure may alter the FDG biodistribution, which may necessitate reduction of dose or image acquisition time after tracer administration, or both.[127] Specifically, in patients with suspected renal failure (blood serum creatinine level in excess of 1.1 mg/dL), the FDG accumulation in the brain may decrease, whereas the blood pool activity is increased.[128]

IMAGING IN CLINICAL NEPHROLOGY

NORMAL RENAL FUNCTION

GFR and effective RPF may be assessed by means of dynamic quantitative nuclear imaging techniques. The GFR quantifies the amount of filtrate formed per minute (normal, 125 mL/min in adults). Only 20% of RPF is filtered through the semipermeable membrane of the glomerulus. The filtrate is protein free and almost completely reabsorbed in the tubules. Filtration is maintained over a range of arterial pressures with autoregulation. The ideal agent for the determination of GFR is inulin, which is only filtered but is neither secreted nor reabsorbed.[123,129]

In these studies ^{99m}Tc-DTPA is often used to demonstrate renal perfusion and assess glomerular filtration, although 5% to 10% of injected ^{99m}Tc-DTPA is protein bound and 5% remains in the kidneys after 4 hours. A typical imaging protocol includes posterior 5-second flow images for 1 minute, followed by 1-minute-per-frame images for 20 minutes. The GFR may be obtained through the Gates method, in which images of renal uptake are obtained during the second and third minutes after ^{99m}Tc-DTPA administration. Regions of interest are drawn over the kidneys, and background activity correction is applied. A standard dose is counted by the gamma camera for normalization. Depth photon attenuation is corrected according to a formula relating body weight and height. A split GFR can be obtained for each kidney, which is not possible with the creatinine clearance method.[123,129]

The effective RPF (normal, 585 mL/min in adults) can be obtained with ^{131}I-ortho-iodohippurate and ^{99m}Tc-MAG3 imaging.[130] However, ^{131}I-ortho-iodohippurate has been largely replaced by ^{99m}Tc-MAG3 because MAG3 has better imaging characteristics and dosimetry (when radiolabeled with ^{99m}Tc). Currently ^{99m}Tc-MAG3 is the renal imaging agent of choice primarily because of the combined renal clearance of ^{99m}Tc-MAG3 by both filtration and tubular extraction, which enables clinicians to obtain relatively high-quality images even in patients with impaired renal function. The imaging protocol includes posterior 1-second images for 60 seconds (flow study), followed by 1-minute images for 5 minutes and then 5-minute images for 30 minutes. The relative tubular function may be obtained by drawing renal regions of interest, corrected for background activity.[131,132] A renogram is constructed to depict the renal tracer uptake over time. The first portion of the renogram has a sharp upward slope occurring approximately 6 seconds after peak aortic activity (phase I); the upward slope represents perfusion. This is followed by extension to the peak value, which represents both renal perfusion and early renal clearance (phase II), which can be dependent on body position.[133] The next phase (phase III) is depicted by a downward slope, which represents excretion. Normal perfusion of the kidneys is symmetric (50% ± 5%). The peak of the renogram occurs at approximately 2 to 3 minutes (versus 3 to 5 minutes with DTPA) in normal adults, and by 30 minutes, more than 70% of the tracer is cleared and present in the urinary bladder (Figure 28.27).[123,129,134]

Renal cortical structure can be imaged with ^{99m}Tc-DMSA; the appearance of these images is correlated strongly with differential GFR and differential renal blood flow. Imaging is started 90 to 120 minutes after administration of the tracer and can be obtained up to 4 hours later. Planar images are obtained in the anterior, posterior, left anterior oblique/right anterior oblique, and right posterior oblique/left posterior oblique projections. SPECT is also often performed. In a scan with normal results, renal cortical uptake is evenly distributed. Normal variations include dromedary hump (splenic impression on the left kidney), fetal lobulation, horseshoe kidney, crossed fused ectopy, and hypertrophied column of Bertin. The renal images also allow accurate assessment of the relative renal size, position, and axis.[123,129]

KIDNEY INJURY: ACUTE AND CHRONIC

When a patient presents with previously undiagnosed renal failure, the question is whether the kidney disease is acute or chronic. US is the most helpful initial imaging study for

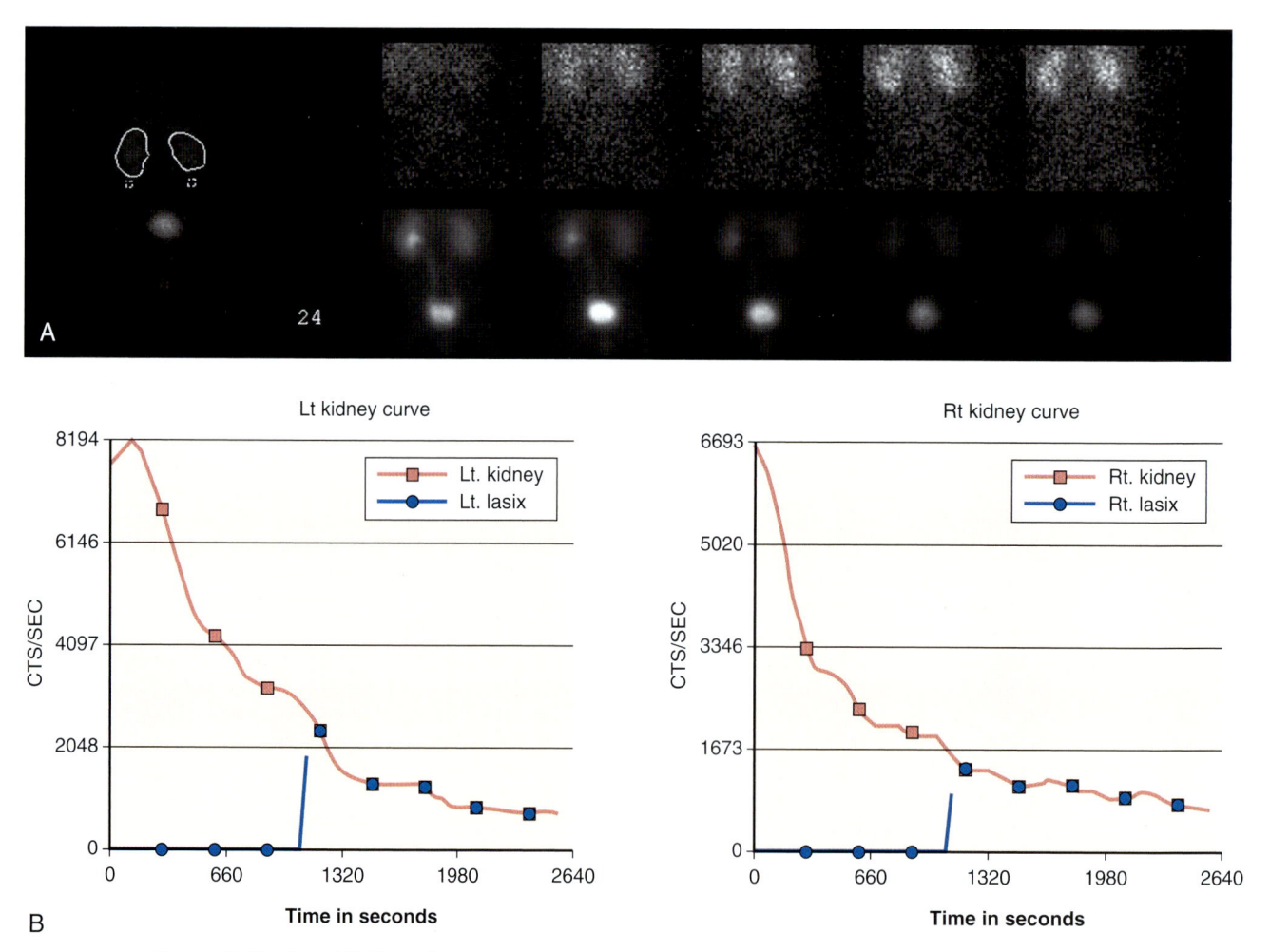

Figure 28.27 A and B, Normal-appearing renogram with technetium 99m–labeled mercaptoacetyltriglycine.

evaluating the patient with an elevated creatinine level of unknown duration. US can help separate chronic, end-stage kidney disease (ESKD) from potentially reversible AKI or CKD by defining renal size, echogenicity, and presence or absence of hydronephrosis and cystic disease. This is easily achieved using gray-scale US.[135] A thin rim of decreased echogenicity may surround the kidneys in patients experiencing kidney injury, also known as renal sweat.[136] Small, echogenic kidneys indicate preexisting CKD; however, acute reversible components must still be searched for. Acute, reversible components that can be diagnosed on imaging are few but include hydronephrosis and hypertension caused by renal artery stenosis. If no acute process is found on US, no further imaging workup is necessary (according to the ACR appropriateness criteria for elevated Cr of unknown duration).[139] Normal renal size, with or without increased echogenicity, typically requires more extensive evaluation for acute causes because gray-scale US may not be accurate in the minimally dilated obstructive situation.

Many causes of AKI are encountered in the hospital setting. Prerenal and renal causes include hypotension or dehydration resulting in hypoperfusion of the kidneys and nephrotoxic drugs[138] and account for more than 90% of all cases. Typically prerenal and renal causes are diagnosed clinically, not with imaging. Although postrenal causes for AKI are less common, when they are identified and treated, the AKI is often rapidly reversible.

US is more than 95% accurate in detecting hydronephrosis (i.e., dilation of the collecting systems and renal pelvis)[139,140]; however, the cause of the hydronephrosis may not be seen. If US cannot determine the cause of obstruction, CT or MRI that is not enhanced by contrast media is the appropriate next imaging study.[137] The typical US findings of hydronephrosis are a dilated, anechoic, fluid-filled renal pelvis and calyces. Hydronephrosis is generally graded according to the extent of calyceal dilation and the degree of cortical thinning.[126,139,141] In mild (grade I) hydronephrosis the pelvicalyceal system is filled with fluid, which causes slight separation of the central renal sinus fat (Figure 28.28). The calyces are not distorted, and the thickness of the renal cortex appears normal. In moderate (grade II) hydronephrosis the pelvicalyceal system appears more distended with greater separation of the central echo complex. The contour of the calyces is rounded, but the cortical thickness is unaltered (Figure 28.29). With moderate-to-severe (grade III) hydronephrosis the calyces are more distended, and cortical thinning is recognized. In severe (grade IV) hydronephrosis the calyceal system is markedly dilated (Figure 28.30). The calyces appear as large, ballooned, fluid-filled structures with a dilated renal pelvis of variable size. Cortical loss is evident, with the dilated calyces approaching or reaching the renal capsule. In general, the length and overall size of a hydronephrotic kidney is increased. Long-standing obstruction may, however, result

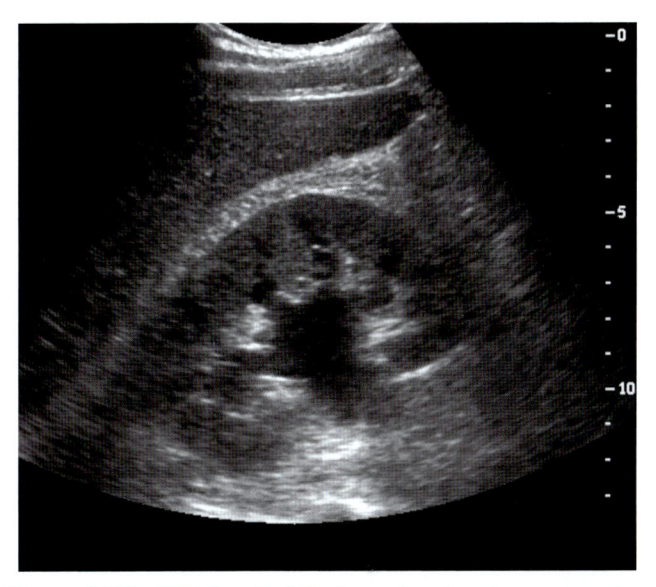

Figure 28.28 Mild (grade I) hydronephrosis: ultrasonography. The central echo complex is separated by the mildly distended calyces and renal pelvis. Notice the connection between the calyces and the renal pelvis. The thickness of the cortex is preserved, and the renal border remains smooth.

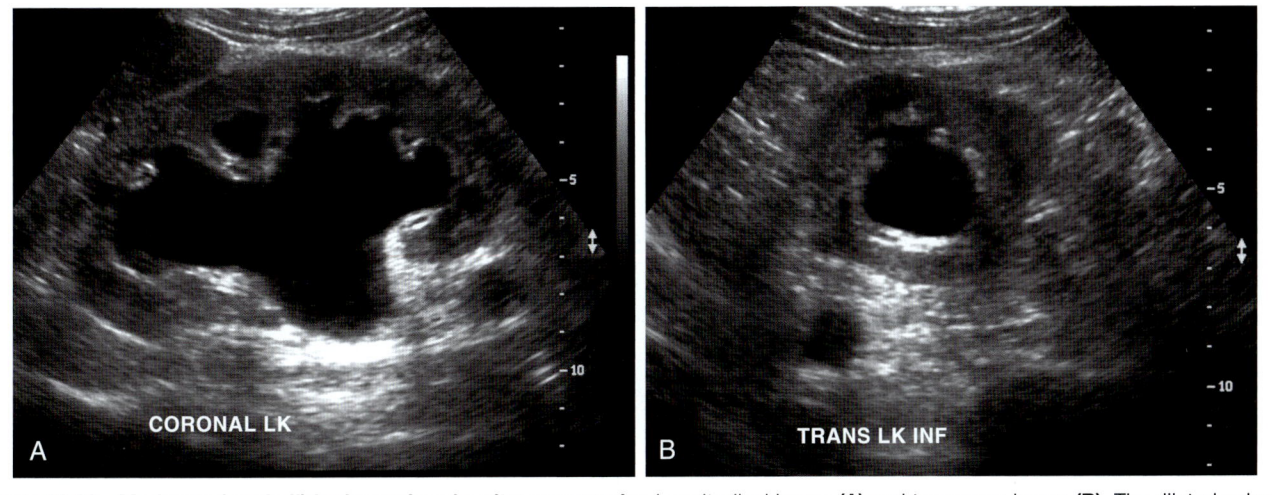

Figure 28.29 Moderate (grade II) hydronephrosis: ultrasonography. Longitudinal image **(A)** and transverse image **(B)**. The dilated calyces are rounded and filled with urine. The renal pelvis is dilated as well. Again, note the connection between the calyces and the renal pelvis. The cortex remains relatively normal in thickness, and the renal border is smooth.

in renal parenchymal atrophy, and the kidney may be somewhat small, with marked cortical thinning. The degree of hydronephrosis is not always correlated with the amount of obstruction.

Although hydronephrosis is usually easily diagnosed with US, it must not be confused with renal cystic disease. In hydronephrosis the dilated calyces have a visibly direct communication with the renal pelvis, which is also dilated.[27] In cystic disease the round fluid-filled cysts have walls, and no direct communication is evident between each calyx and the renal pelvis. Cases of peripelvic cysts are frequently misdiagnosed as a dilated renal pelvis. Renal artery aneurysm may also be confused with a dilated renal pelvis but can be diagnosed correctly with added Doppler color-flow US.

The presence of hydronephrosis on US does not always indicate obstruction.[142,143] Grade I hydronephrosis and possibly more severe grades may be observed in patients in whom no obstructive cause is found. Nonobstructive causes of hydronephrosis include increased urine production and flow, acute and chronic infection, vesicoureteral reflux, papillary necrosis, congenital megacalyces, overdistended bladder, and postobstructive dilation.[144] In patients with repeated episodes of intermittent or partial obstruction, the calyces become quite distensible or compliant, which causes the appearance of hydronephrosis to vary, depending on the state of hydration and urine production. Patients with vesicoureteral reflux also demonstrate distensible pelvicalyceal systems. Doppler color-flow US has been suggested as an additive means of differentiating obstructive from nonobstructive hydronephrosis.[145,146] The measurement of resistive indices has been investigated as a means of diagnosing acute renal obstruction, as well; the acutely obstructed kidney has an elevated resistive index, and the nonobstructed kidney has a normal resistive index of less than 0.70.[147,148] The results have been variable, and thus no consistent recommendation is available.[148,149]

US is also used in patients with CKD. Cortical echogenicity may be increased in both acute and chronic renal parenchymal disease (Figure 28.31).[150] The pattern should be bilateral in CKD, and the degree of cortical echogenicity is correlated with the severity of the interstitial fibrosis, global sclerosis, focal tubular atrophy, and number of hyaline casts per glomerulus.[21] Similar correlation is observed with decreasing renal size. These findings, however, are nonspecific, and kidney biopsy may be required for diagnosis. The normal corticomedullary differentiation is lost with increasing cortical echogenicity.[151] Cortical echogenicity may also be increased in some patients with AKI, as in glomerulonephritis and lupus nephritis. Sequential studies over time may be used to assess the progression of disease by monitoring the renal size and cortical echogenicity.

The key to the diagnosis of renal parenchymal disease is renal core biopsy and resulting histopathologic study.[150] US facilitates the performance of kidney biopsy by demonstrating the kidney and the proper location for biopsy. US may also be used to evaluate for complications associated with kidney biopsy, such as perirenal hematoma and arteriovenous fistula.

When US evaluation demonstrates hydronephrosis, but not the cause, it is usually followed by CT. Noncontrast CT will demonstrate the dilated pelvicalyceal systems in the

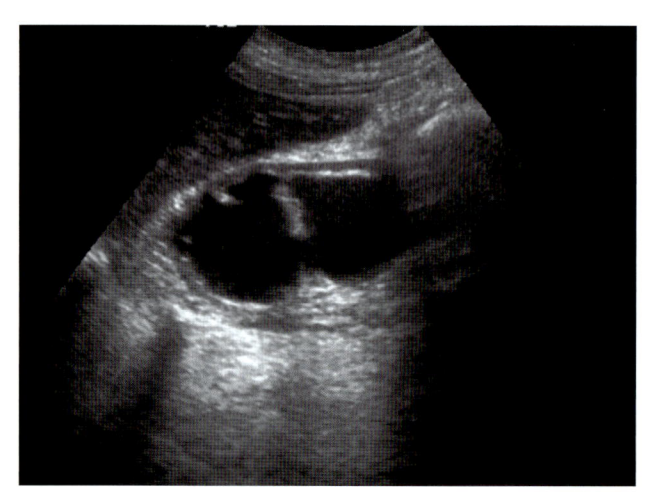

Figure 28.30 Severe (grade IV) hydronephrosis: ultrasonography. Longitudinal image of the right kidney demonstrates a large fluid-filled sac; no normal elements of the kidney remain visible. The cortex is almost gone, but the outer border of the kidney remains smooth.

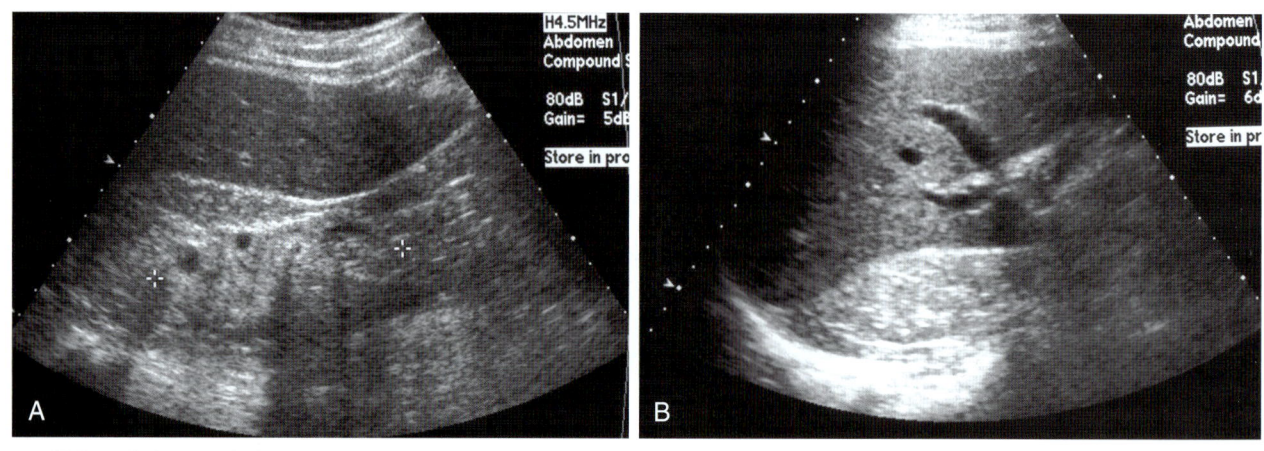

Figure 28.31 End-stage kidney disease: ultrasonography. A and **B,** The kidneys are highly echogenic in relation to the adjacent liver. No normal renal structures are visible, but the kidneys remain smooth in overall contour. Note the two small hypoechoic renal cysts in the surface in **A.**

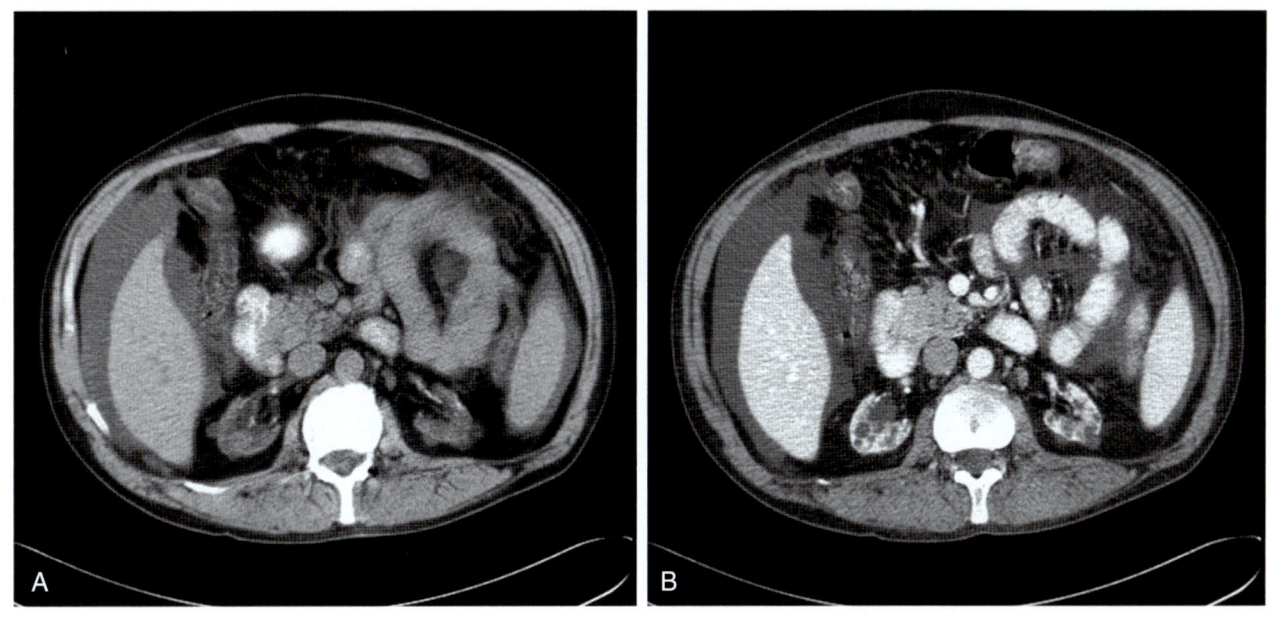

Figure 28.32 Adulthood-acquired polycystic kidney disease: computed tomographic scan, axial image without contrast material **(A)** and axial image after administration of contrast material **(B)**. The kidneys are small bilaterally with multiple 1-cm cysts primarily in the cortex.

kidney. The parenchymal thickness can be visualized in relation to the dilated collecting systems; the urine-filled calyces and pelvis are less dense than the surrounding parenchyma. The course of the dilated ureters may be followed distally to establish the site of obstruction. The cause of obstruction is frequently visible and may include pelvic tumors, distal ureteral stones, and retroperitoneal adenopathy or mass. For patients in whom chronic long-standing obstruction is the cause of kidney injury, CT generally demonstrates large, fluid-containing kidneys with little or no cortex remaining. If obstruction is not the cause, other potential causes such as cirrhosis and ascites with accompanying hepatic failure may be evident.

In CKD without obstruction, CT typically demonstrates small, contracted kidneys, which may also show evidence of adulthood-acquired polycystic disease if the patient is on dialysis (Figure 28.32). In general, the overall size and thickness of the renal parenchyma appear to decrease with age.[152] Other causes for CKD may be demonstrated on imaging, including autosomal dominant polycystic kidney disease (Figure 28.33); the kidneys are enlarged and contain innumerable cysts. Frequently some of the cyst walls may contain thin rims of calcification. The density of the internal contents of the cysts may also vary as a result of hemorrhage or proteinaceous debris. For patients undergoing regular dialysis, iodinated contrast may be given if necessary for CT scans because the material is dialyzable.

Like CT, MRI is accurate in demonstrating renal structure, as well as prerenal and postrenal causes of kidney injury. MRI is sensitive for the detection of renal parenchymal disease, but the renal parenchymal causes of injury have nonspecific features, and biopsy is generally required (Figures 28.34 and 28.35).[153] Noncontrast MRI routinely allows for detailed tissue characterization of the kidney and surrounding structures. Both iodinated contrast and Gd-C should be avoided in patients with AKI and CKD stage 4 and 5. Newer MRI sequences, such as diffusion-weighted and bright blood techniques, provide a way to increase the conspicuity of neoplastic and vascular causes of renal failure without the use of intravenous contrast agents (Figure 28.36).[96,154]

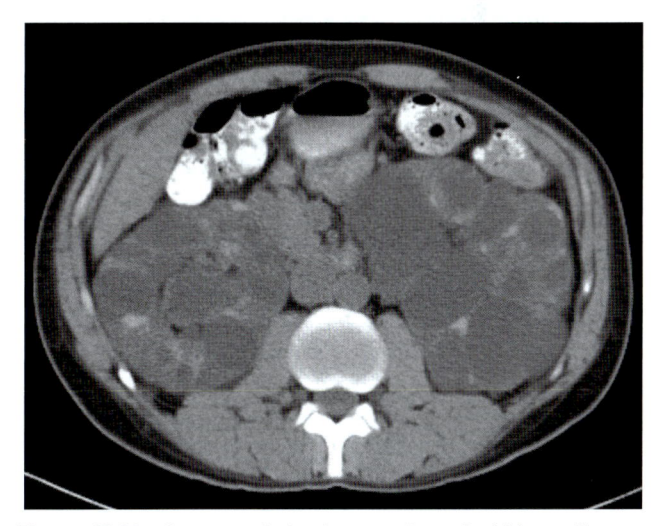

Figure 28.33 Autosomal dominant polycystic kidney disease: computed tomographic (CT) scan without contrast material. This CT image demonstrates the markedly enlarged kidney bilaterally with multiple low-density cysts throughout both kidneys. The little remaining renal parenchyma is noted by the sparse, higher density material squeezed by the cysts.

In kidney injury, glomerular and tubular dysfunctions are reflected by abnormal findings on renal scintigraphy and renography. Renal uptake of ^{99m}Tc-MAG3 is prolonged, with tubular tracer stasis and little or no excretion. In patients with AKI, if ^{99m}Tc-MAG3 has more renal activity than hepatic activity 1 to 3 minutes after injection, recovery is likely, whereas when renal uptake is less than the hepatic uptake, dialysis may be needed.[155] In CKD, renal perfusion, cortical

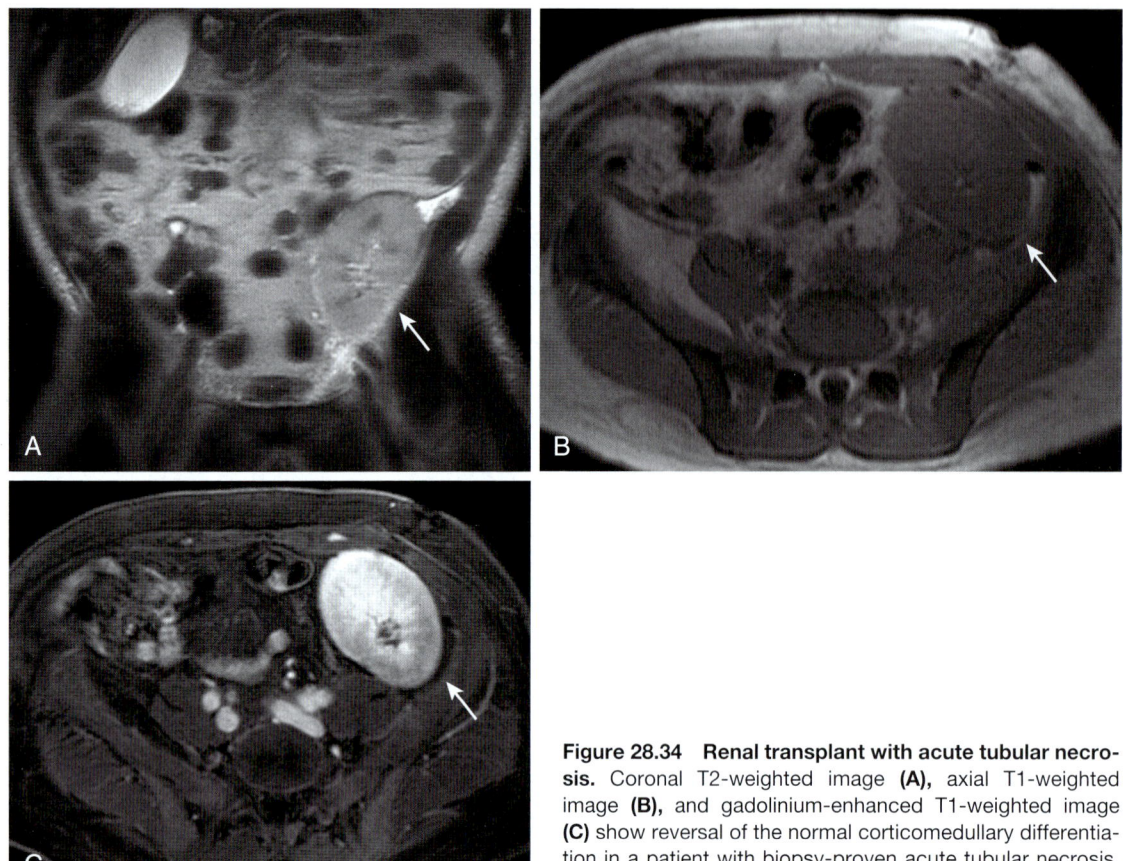

870 SECTION IV — EVALUATION OF THE PATIENT WITH KIDNEY DISEASE

Figure 28.34 **Renal transplant with acute tubular necrosis.** Coronal T2-weighted image **(A)**, axial T1-weighted image **(B)**, and gadolinium-enhanced T1-weighted image **(C)** show reversal of the normal corticomedullary differentiation in a patient with biopsy-proven acute tubular necrosis. *Arrows* point to the transplanted kidney.

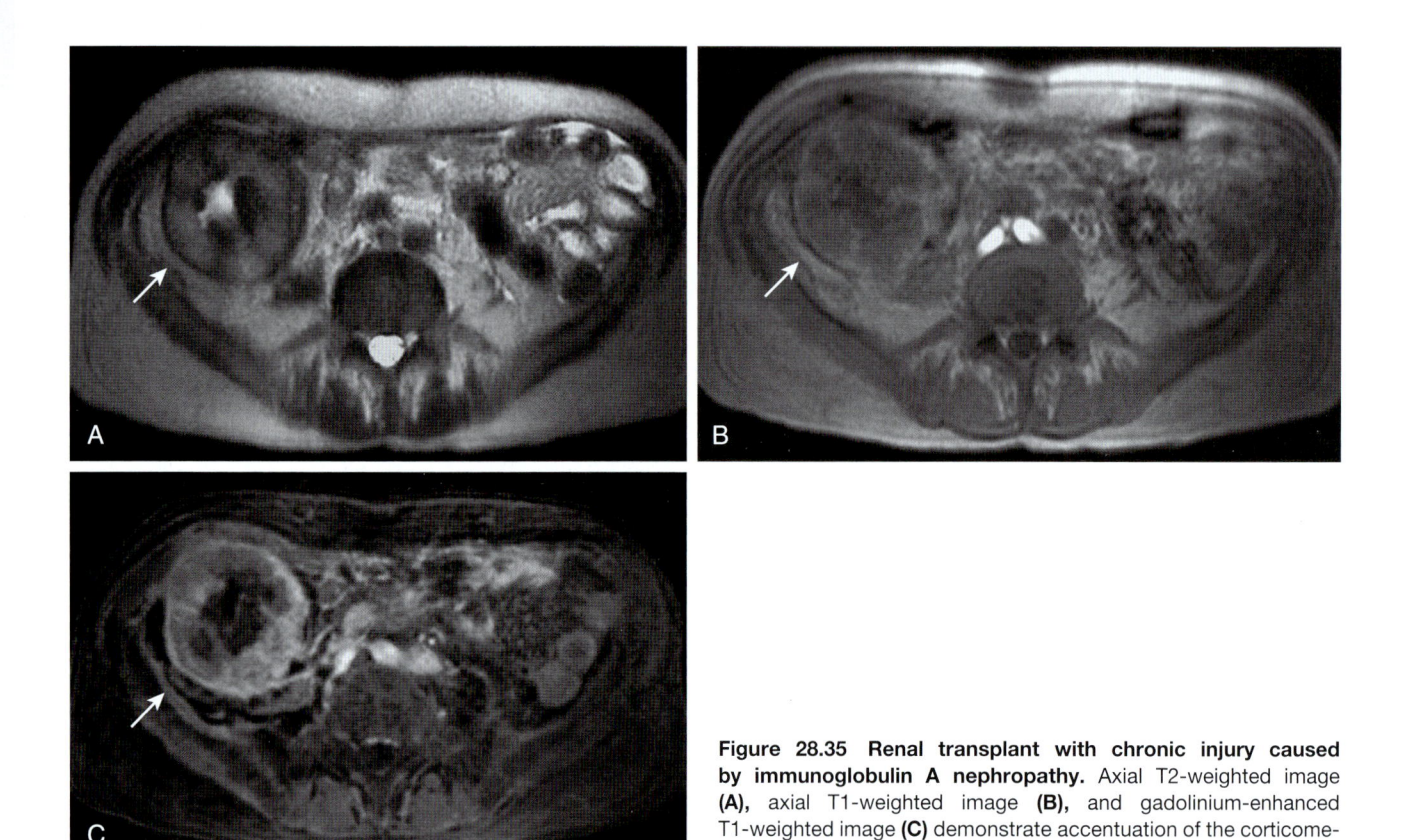

Figure 28.35 **Renal transplant with chronic injury caused by immunoglobulin A nephropathy.** Axial T2-weighted image **(A)**, axial T1-weighted image **(B)**, and gadolinium-enhanced T1-weighted image **(C)** demonstrate accentuation of the corticomedullary differentiation. *Arrows* point to the transplanted kidney.

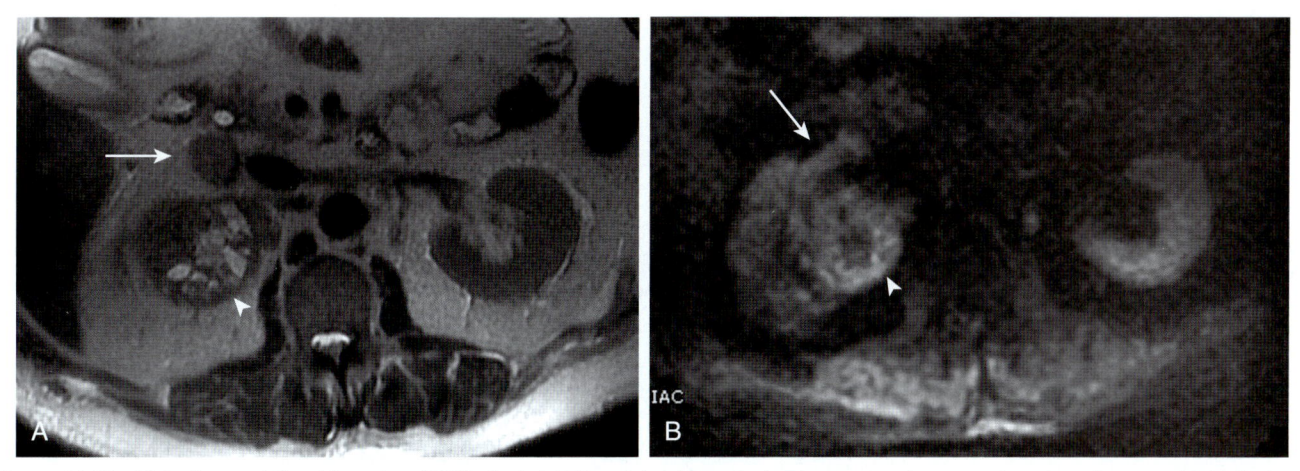

Figure 28.36 Diffusion-weighted imaging (DWI). **A,** Axial T2-weighted image demonstrates a heterogeneous renal mass with high signal intensity (*arrowhead*) and a structure of intermediate signal intensity adjacent to the inferior vena cava that is suspect for vascular invasion (*arrow*). **B,** Axial DWI demonstrates the renal mass (*arrowhead*) and increased signal intensity within the renal vein, which confirms renal vein invasion (*arrow*).

tracer extraction, and tracer excretion are diminished. However, this imaging pattern is nonspecific and must be interpreted in the clinical context.[123]

UNILATERAL OBSTRUCTION

Although US is frequently the first imaging method used to detect obstruction, it may not establish the cause. If US cannot determine the cause of obstruction, CT is the next imaging modality of choice due to rapid speed of acquisition and accuracy.[137] IVU and antegrade or retrograde pyelography may be used if CT is not available.[139] With IVU the site of obstruction may be visible, but the cause may be only inferred; this is also true with antegrade and retrograde pyelography.

CE-CT and, more specifically, CTU are most useful in assessing the patient with unilateral obstruction.[37] Small differences in the enhancement pattern of the kidneys are well demonstrated with CE-CT (Figure 28.37). Differences in the excretion patterns by the kidneys are also sensitively depicted on CE-CT.[36,37] The urine-filled or contrast material–filled ureters point to the obstruction with demonstration of both intraureteral and extraureteral causes of the obstruction (Figure 28.38). MRI demonstrates similar findings and may be used when CE-CT is contraindicated.

Nuclear medicine assessment by means of diuretic renography may also be used to evaluate for obstructive uropathy. Scintigraphy with ^{99m}Tc-MAG3 is often employed. Furosemide (Lasix) is administered intravenously (1 mg/kg; higher dose in cases of renal insufficiency) when the renal pelvis and ureter are maximally distended.[156] Regions of interest are drawn around each renal pelvis, with the background regions as crescent shapes lateral to each kidney. After furosemide administration, in cases of dilation without obstruction, the collecting system empties rapidly, with a subsequent steep decline in the renogram curve. Obstruction can be ruled out if the clearance half-time of the renal pelvic emptying is less than 10 minutes. A curve that reaches a plateau or continues to rise after administration of furosemide is indicative of obstruction, with a clearance half-time of more than 20 minutes (Figure 28.39). A slow downward slope after furosemide administration may be indicative of partial obstruction. An apparent poor response to furosemide may also occur in patients with severe pelvic dilation (reservoir effect). Other pitfalls include poor injection technique of either the diuretic or the radiotracer, impaired renal function, and dehydration, in which delayed tracer transit and excretion may not be overcome by the effect of a diuretic. Kidneys in neonates (<1 month of age) may be too immature to respond to furosemide, and neonates are thus not suitable candidates for diuretic renal scintigraphy.[123,157]

Various protocols in relation to the timing of furosemide administration have also been reported. In the F0 method, furosemide is injected simultaneously with ^{99m}Tc-MAG3 administration. A 17-year clinical experience at one institution proved that this protocol is useful for patients of all ages and for all indications.[158] Taghavi and associates compared diuresis renographic protocols with injection of furosemide 15 minutes before (F−15) and 20 minutes after (F+20) administration of ^{99m}Tc-MAG3.[161] In this comparative study of 21 patients with dilation of the pelvicalyceal system, the F−15 protocol produced fewer equivocal results than did the F+20 method and therefore was considered the preferable protocol. Further experience is needed to determine the most optimal timing interval between furosemide and ^{99m}Tc-MAG3 injections in diuresis renography.

RENAL CALCIFICATIONS AND RENAL STONE DISEASE

Calcifications may occur in many regions of the kidney.[160] Nephrolithiasis or renal calculi are the most common and occur in the pelvicalyceal system. Nephrocalcinosis refers to diffuse or punctate renal parenchymal calcification occurring in either the medulla or cortex, usually bilaterally. Some patients with nephrocalcinosis may also develop nephrolithiasis. Calcifications also occur in vascular structures, particularly in patients with diabetes and advanced atherosclerotic disease. Rimlike calcifications may occur in simple renal cysts and polycystic disease. Patients with renal carcinomas may exhibit variable calcifications as well. All

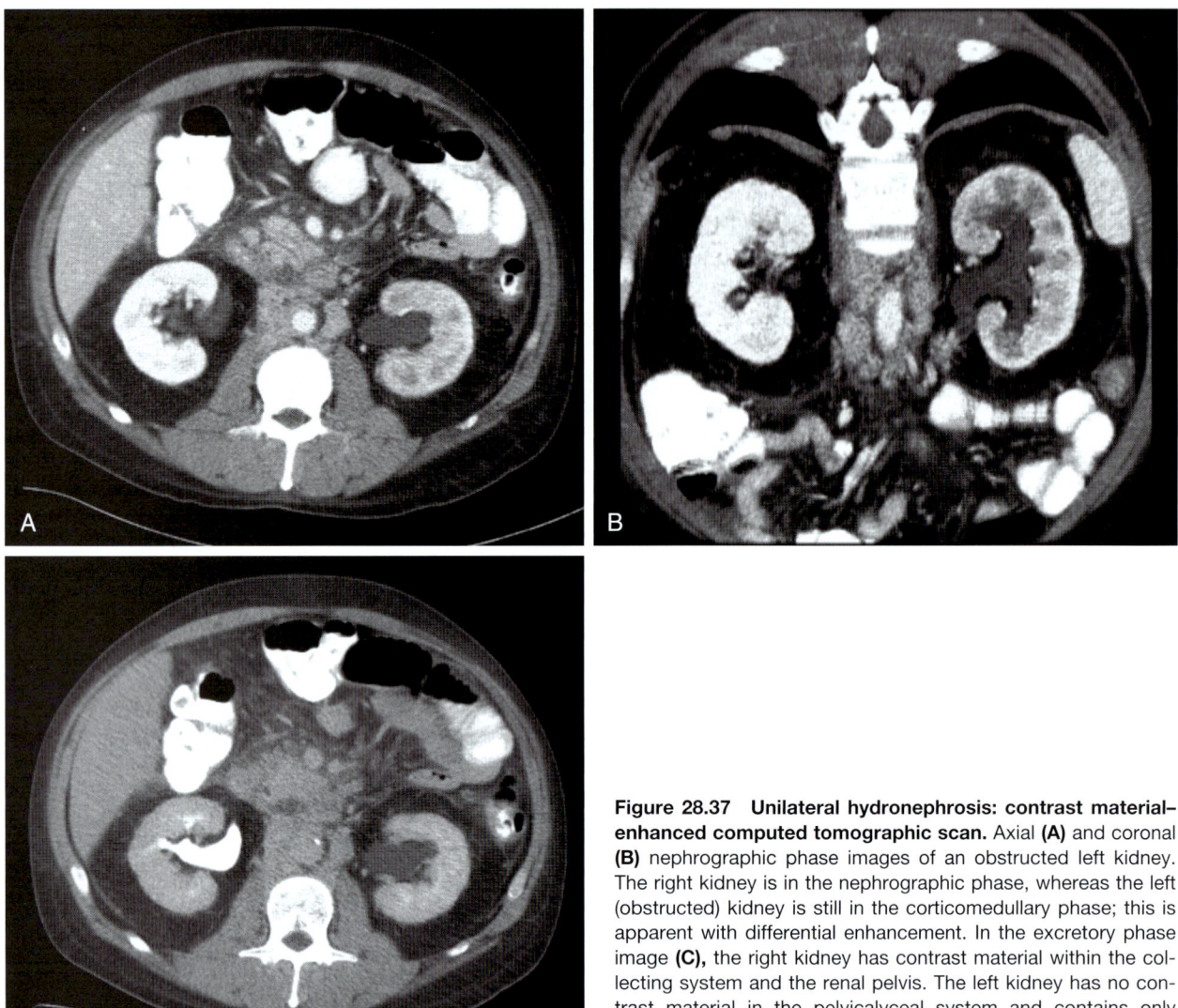

Figure 28.37 **Unilateral hydronephrosis: contrast material–enhanced computed tomographic scan.** Axial **(A)** and coronal **(B)** nephrographic phase images of an obstructed left kidney. The right kidney is in the nephrographic phase, whereas the left (obstructed) kidney is still in the corticomedullary phase; this is apparent with differential enhancement. In the excretory phase image **(C)**, the right kidney has contrast material within the collecting system and the renal pelvis. The left kidney has no contrast material in the pelvicalyceal system and contains only nonopacified urine. The patient had lymphoma with retroperitoneal lymph nodes, which caused the obstruction more distally.

types of calcification are best demonstrated on noncontrast CT (see Figure 28.42).

Cortical calcification is most often associated with cortical necrosis from any cause.[160] The calcifications are dystrophic and tend to resemble tram tracks and to be circumferential. Other entities in which cortical calcification are found include hyperoxaluria, Alport's syndrome, and, in rare cases, chronic glomerulonephritis. The stippled calcifications of hyperoxaluria may be found in both the cortex and the medulla, as well as in other organs, such as the heart. In Alport's syndrome, only cortical calcifications are found.

Calcifications in the medulla are much more common than cortical calcifications.[160] The most common cause of medullary nephrocalcinosis is primary hyperparathyroidism. The distribution appears to be within the renal pyramid and may be either focal or diffuse and either unilateral or bilateral. Nephrocalcinosis occurs in other diseases in which hypercalcemia or hypercalciuria occur, such as hyperthyroidism, sarcoidosis, hypervitaminosis D, immobilization, multiple myeloma, and metastatic neoplasms. These calcifications are nonspecific and punctate in appearance and are usually medullary in location.

In 70% to 75% of cases of renal tubular acidosis, there is evidence of nephrocalcinosis. The calcifications tend to be uniform and distributed throughout the renal pyramids bilaterally. With medullary sponge kidney and renal tubular ectasia, small calculi form in the distal collecting tubules, probably because of stasis. The appearance varies from involvement of only a single calyx to involvement of both kidneys throughout. The calcifications are small, round, and within the peak of the pyramid adjacent to the calyx. Medullary sponge kidney is also associated with nephrolithiasis, because the small calculi in the distal collecting tubules may pass into the collecting systems and ureters, resulting in renal colic.[161]

The calcifications that occur in renal tuberculosis are typically medullary in location and may mimic other forms of nephrocalcinosis.[162] Calcification occurs in the pyramids as part of the healing process. With overwhelming involvement of the kidney, the entire kidney may be destroyed; this

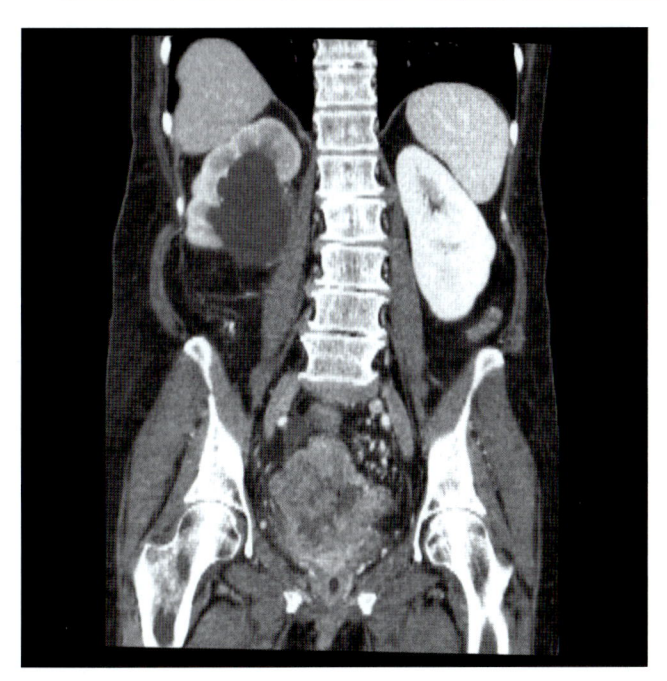

Figure 28.38 Unilateral obstruction: contrast material–enhanced computed tomographic scan. The coronal image demonstrates the difference in enhancement between the two kidneys, with the moderately dilated renal pelvis and calyces on the right. The large heterogeneous pelvis mass is the source of the obstruction: recurrent rectal carcinoma.

results in diffuse, heavy calcification throughout the entire kidney, which becomes small and scarred. Medullary calcifications are also visible in patients with renal papillary necrosis. With necrosis of the papilla, the material is sloughed into the calyces. Retained tissue fragments may calcify and have the appearance of medullary nephrocalcinosis.

Nephrolithiasis is a common clinical entity. The lifetime risk for developing renal calculi is 12%, with males being two to three times more at risk than females.[163] Most urinary tract stones are composed of calcium salts of either oxalate or phosphate or a combination of the two.[164-167] This composition accounts for the dense appearance on imaging. Stasis contributes to the formation of stones in the urinary tract. Renal colic or flank pain is the most common presenting symptom. Most patients also have hematuria, although it may be absent if a ureter is completely obstructed by the stone. The pain that occurs with a passing renal stone is probably caused by the distension of the tubular system and renal capsule of the kidney and by the peristalsis associated with ureteral contractions as the stone moves distally.

Most urinary calculi that are 4 mm or smaller pass with conservative treatment.[168] The larger the stone, the more likely other measures will be necessary to treat the stone and associated obstruction.

Plain radiograph of the abdomen yields little significant information on its own and should not be used to diagnose stone disease.[169] The KUB is useful for following stone disease only when a stone is densely calcified and large enough to be visible (Figure 28.40). For years, IVU has been the method of choice for the assessment of patients with renal colic[170,171]; however it has been supplanted by CT that is not enhanced by contrast media, which is a more rapid examination and more accurate than IVU.[169] IVU remains the best examination if CT is not available. However, IVU can be time consuming, requiring delayed images up to 24 hours after injection, in some, to visualize the contrast-filled, dilated collecting systems, pelvis, and ureter. Also, if an obstructing stone is not visualized, alternate diagnoses are difficult to confirm.

Ultrasonographic assessment has also been used in the evaluation of renal colic.[172] This is a quick and usually easily performed examination. Unilateral hydronephrosis may be observed, although the examination results may be normal early in the passage of a renal stone. Renal stones may be visualized within the kidney as hyperechoic foci with distal acoustic shadowing or reverberation artifacts (Figure 28.41).[172] Ureteral stones are rarely seen because of overlying bowel gas. Distal ureteral stones near the ureterovesical junction may be visualized through the urine-filled bladder transabdominally. US may demonstrate an absent ureteral jet in the bladder on the side in which a stone is being passed. Doppler US and assessment of the peripheral vasculature resistance may occasionally be helpful in pointing to the affected kidney, but the study results have been variable.[147]

Noncontrast CT scanning of the abdomen and pelvis has emerged as the standard evaluation in patients with renal colic.[173-177] The sensitivities for CT are 96% to 100%; the specificities are 95% to 100%; and the accuracy rates are 96% to 98%; for this reason, nonenhanced CT has supplanted plain radiography, IVU, and US.[174,178-180] In comparisons of nonenhanced CT and IVU, CT is much more useful, with 94% to 100% sensitivity and 92% to 100% specificity; IVU has 64% to 97% sensitivity and 92% to 94% specificity.[174] Also, when noncontrast CT was used as the reference standard in comparison with US, 24% sensitivity and 90% specificity were found for US.[181,182] An alternative diagnosis is made in patients with "renal colic" in 9% to 29% of cases in which noncontrast CT is used for evaluation.[183]

Nonenhanced CT is performed from the top of the kidneys to below the pubic symphysis. No preparation is needed. Intravenous contrast material is rarely needed. The studies are performed with 3-mm collimation or less, and the slices are reconstructed to be contiguous or slightly overlapping.[184-186] Virtually all renal stones are denser than the adjacent soft tissues (Figure 28.42)[187]; exceptions are renal stones associated with indinavir (a protease inhibitor used in the management of acquired immunodeficiency syndrome (AIDS) and very small uric acid stones (<1 to 2 mm in diameter).[188,189] As expected, calcium oxalate and calcium phosphate stones are the most dense.[165,166] Matrix stones, which are rare, may also be relatively low in density, but they usually contain calcium impurities that make them visible.[164,167]

For detecting stones, low-dose scanning has been shown to be as effective as CT with standard techniques.[190,191] The radiation dose is usually 20% to 25% of the standard dose. The development of iterative reconstruction techniques has also reduced radiation doses. Dual-energy imaging with CT has demonstrated the ability to distinguish different types of stones[192,193] (see Figure 28.10).

Calculi may be visible in all parts of the collecting system and the urinary tract. Small punctate calcifications (≈1 mm)

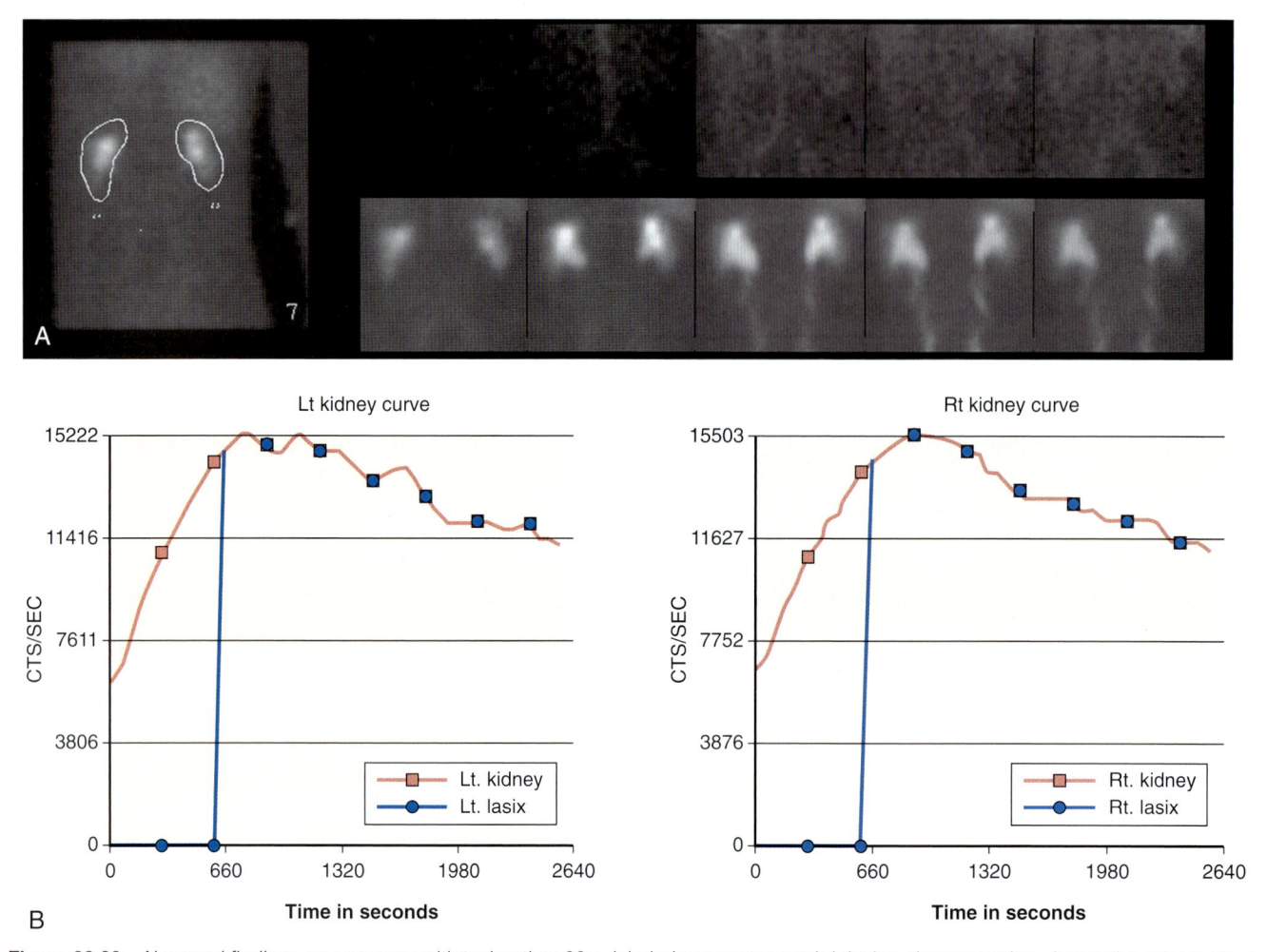

Figure 28.39 Abnormal findings on renogram with technetium 99m–labeled mercaptoacetyltriglycine, demonstrating obstructive urinary kinetics with a poor response to furosemide. **A,** Static and timed images. **B,** Individual curves for each kidney.

are occasionally observed just at the tip of the renal pyramid. These may represent the calcification noted in Randall plaques.[194] Obstruction occurs most commonly at the ureteropelvic junction; at the pelvic brim, where the ureters cross over the iliac vessels; and at the ureterovesical junction. The diagnosis is made on the noncontrast CT scan by demonstrating the calcified stone within the urine-filled ureters (Figure 28.43).[184] Secondary signs may be present to assist in the diagnosis.[178] Hydronephrosis and hydroureter to the point of the stone may be visible. Asymmetric perinephric and periureteral stranding may also be related to forniceal rupture and urine leak (Figure 28.44).[195] The involved kidney may be less dense than the normal kidney because of increased interstitial fluid and edema.[196,197] The affected kidney may also be larger than the normal kidney. At the point of obstruction the stone may be visible within the ureter, with soft tissue thickening of the ureteral wall at that level. This thickening is probably caused by edema and inflammation associated with the passage of the stone.

Noncontrast CT has the additional advantage of assessing the overall stone burden of the patient, not just the passing stone. Also, the size may be accurately measured, which enables clinicians to make treatment decisions.[169,198,199] Distal ureteral stones are occasionally confused with phleboliths, which are common in the pelvis (see Figure 28.44).

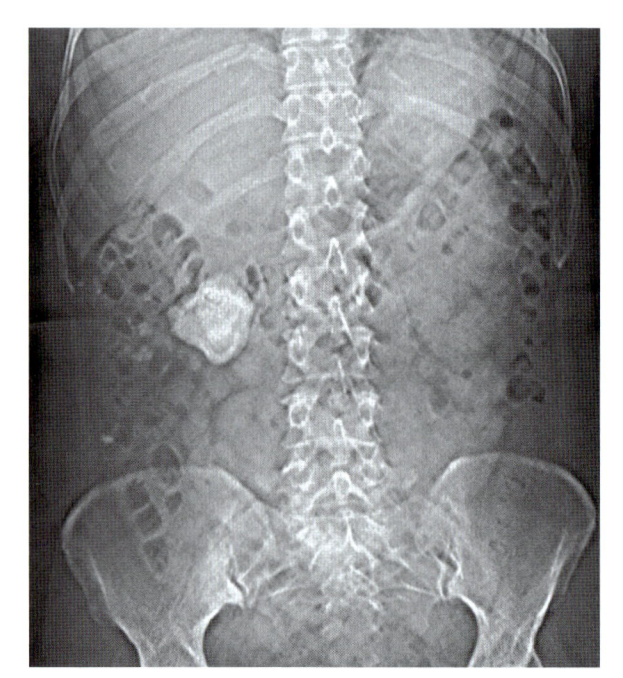

Figure 28.40 Renal stone: plain radiograph of the kidneys, ureters, and bladder. A large laminated stone is visible in the renal pelvis of the right kidney. The outline of the normal left kidney can be seen with no calcifications overlying it. The right kidney outline cannot be seen.

CHAPTER 28 — DIAGNOSTIC KIDNEY IMAGING   875

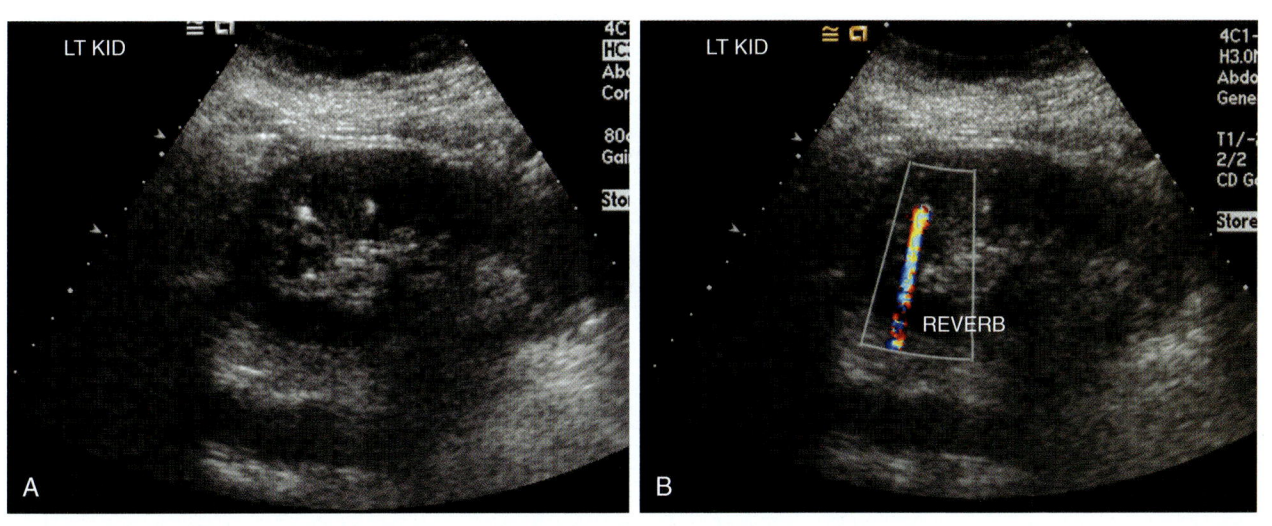

Figure 28.41 Renal stone: ultrasonography. Longitudinal image **(A)** and Doppler color-flow image **(B)** demonstrate an echogenic focus at the corticomedullary junction. Not all stones show shadowing, but in this case, reverberation artifact is visible on the Doppler color-flow image, which helps establish the diagnosis.

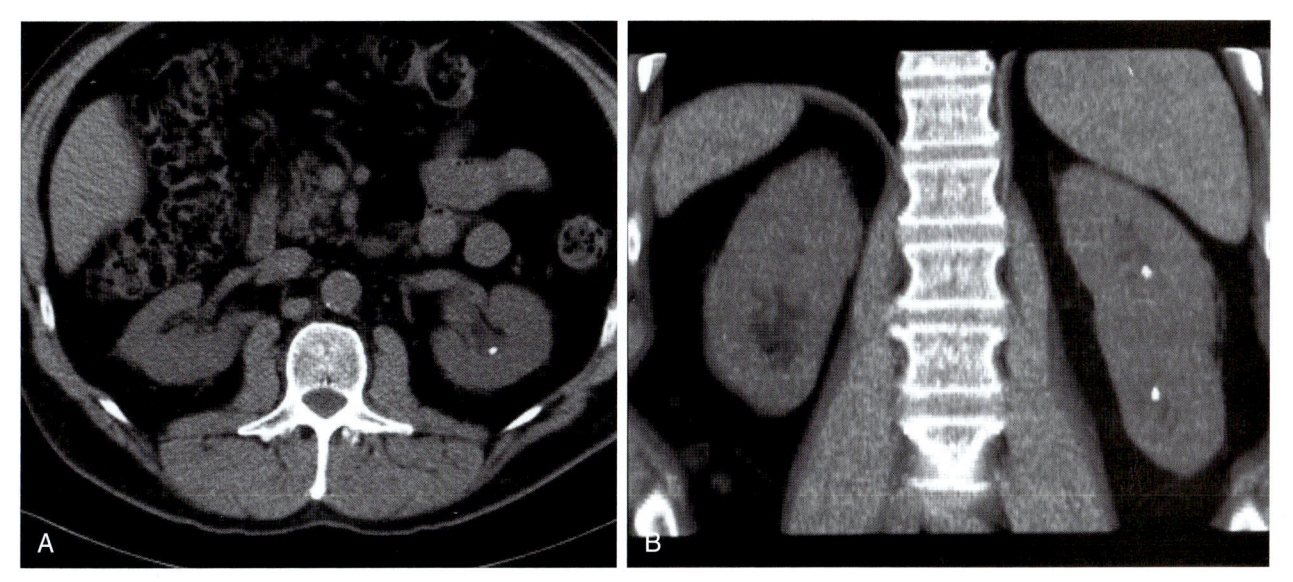

Figure 28.42 Renal stones: noncontrast computed tomographic scan. Axial image **(A)** and coronal image **(B)** demonstrate 4- to 5-mm stones in the upper and lower poles of the left kidney. There are no signs of obstruction.

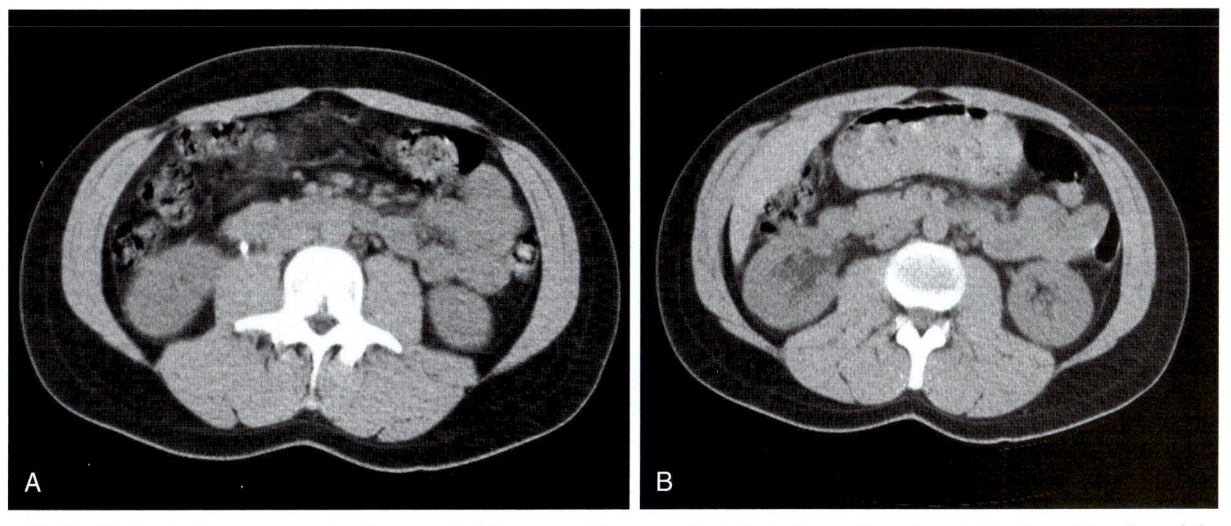

Figure 28.43 Ureteral stone: noncontrast computed tomographic scan. A, A 5- to 6-mm stone is noted in the midportion of the right ureter. **B,** Axial image of the midportion of the kidneys reveals the urine-filled right renal pelvis and a right kidney that is slightly less dense than the left. These are signs of obstruction.

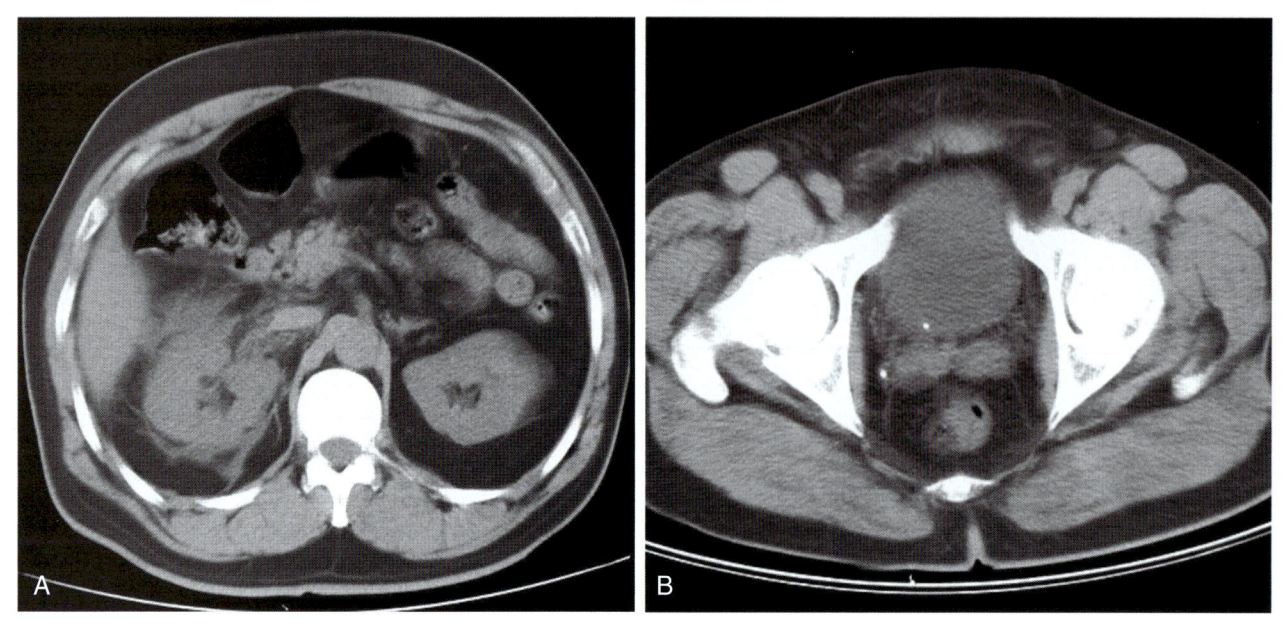

Figure 28.44 Ureteral stone: noncontrast computed tomographic scan. Axial images of the kidneys show perinephric and peripelvic stranding and fluid on the right **(A)** caused by forniceal rupture and leakage of urine as a result of the distal obstructing stone at the right ureterovesical junction **(B)**. Note the phlebolith on the right posterior to the bladder and lateral to the seminal vesicle; phleboliths are commonly confused with distal ureteral stones.

Images reconstructed in the coronal plane along the course of the ureters down to the level of the stone may be helpful.[200] Also, close inspection of phleboliths frequently reveals a small, soft tissue tag leading to the calcification: the "comet tail" sign.[201] Enhancement with contrast material is occasionally necessary in confusing or difficult cases. Also, CE-CT may be used in complicated cases in which the patient is febrile and pyelonephritis or pyohydronephrosis is suspected.[177]

In the evaluation of acute stone disease, MRI or MRU is not the examination of first choice, but it is a suitable alternative for selected patients, especially those in whom reduction of radiation exposure is desired (pediatric and pregnant patients).[202] Stones are difficult to identify in nondilated systems, even in retrospect. When stones are observed on MRI, they are visible as black foci on both T1- and T2-weighted sequences. Stones become more conspicuous in a dilated collecting system (Figure 28.45); however, a nonenhanced filling defect is a nonspecific finding. Blood, air, or debris may have the same appearance. If stones or other calcifications are a concern, noncontrast CT is the examination of choice for improved conspicuity (Figure 28.46).

When the use of iodinated contrast material is contraindicated, or when reduction of radiation exposure is desired, MRU can be used to determine the cause and location of an obstructing process (Figure 28.47). MRU is highly accurate in demonstrating obstruction, regardless of whether the process is acute or chronic.[202] Acute obstruction may be associated with perinephric fluid, which is well demonstrated on T2-weighted sequences.[202,203] However, perinephric fluid is a nonspecific finding and can be found in association with other renal disease. MRI is useful in evaluating the patient who has recently undergone surgery for renal stone disease. MRI has been reported as being more accurate than CT in differentiating perirenal and intrarenal

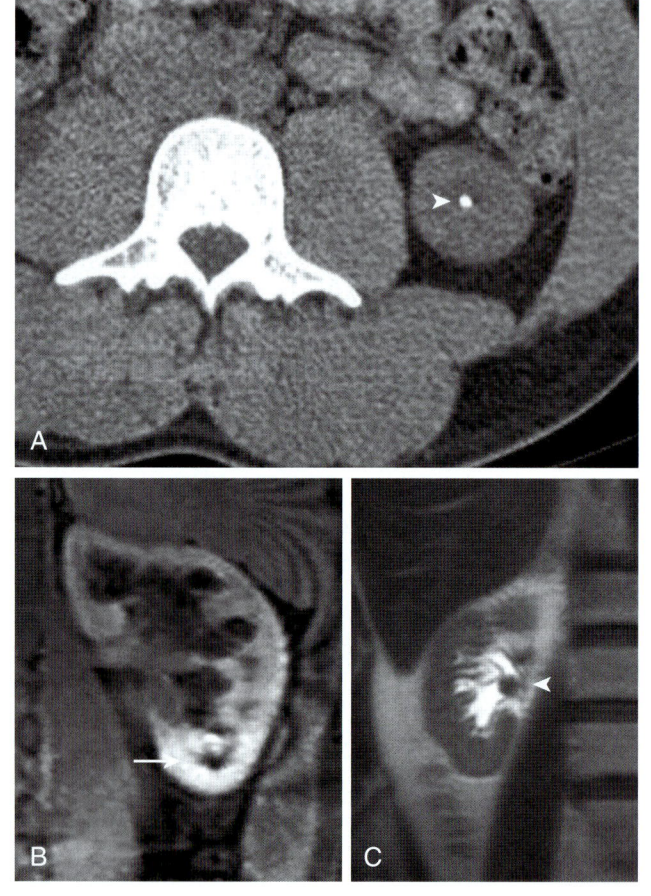

Figure 28.45 Renal stones. Calcification (*arrowhead*) well viewed on computed tomography **(A)** is difficult to demonstrate on magnetic resonance imaging **(B)** (*arrow*), even in retrospect. **C,** A stone (*arrowhead*) is more conspicuous when it is located within a mildly dilated collection system.

CHAPTER 28 — DIAGNOSTIC KIDNEY IMAGING   877

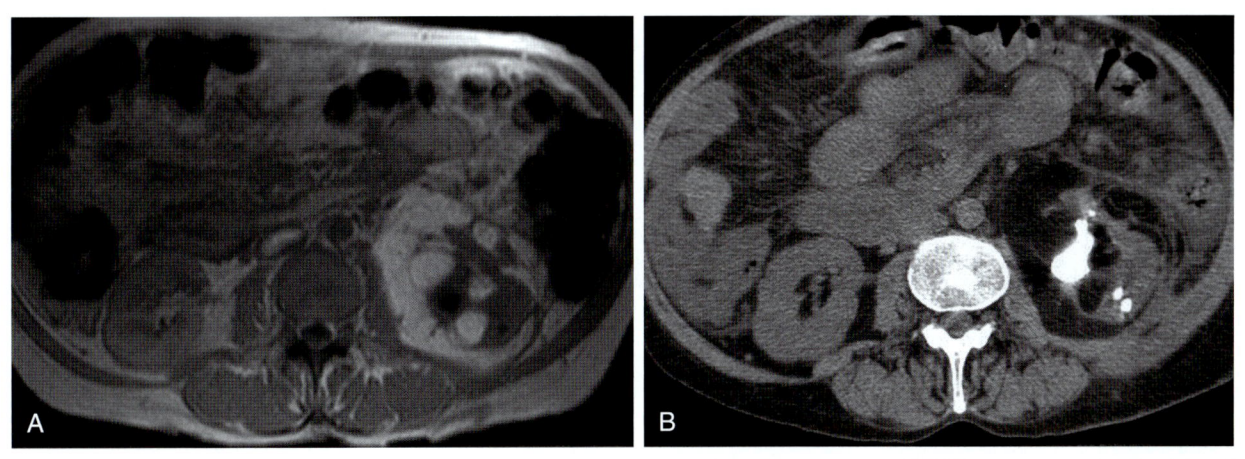

Figure 28.46 Staghorn calculus. Magnetic resonance imaging (MRI) **(A)** and computed tomography (CT) **(B)** demonstrate large pelvic calculus with associated left renal atrophy. Even large stones may be difficult to recognize on MRI. Calcifications are more conspicuous on CT.

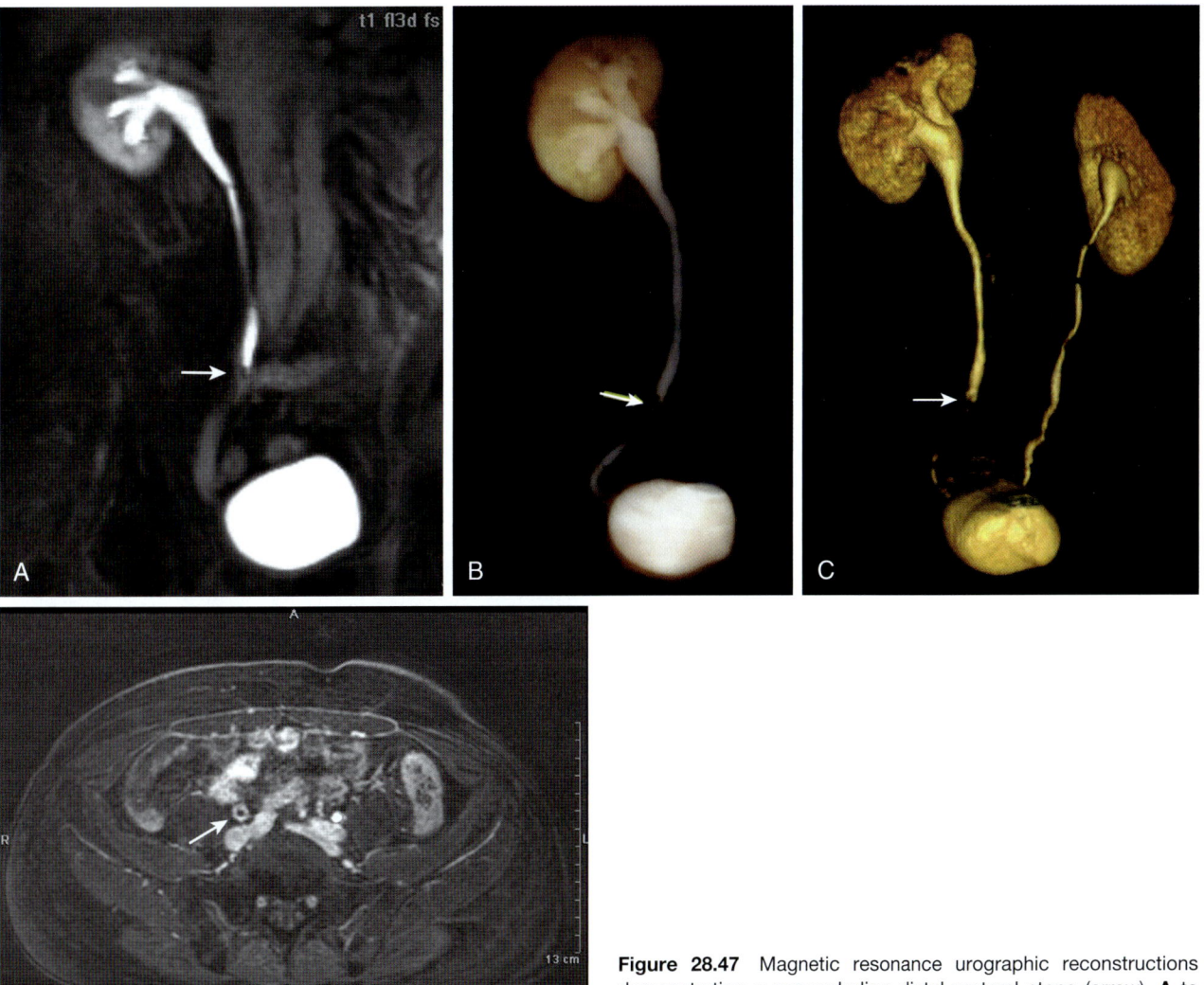

Figure 28.47 Magnetic resonance urographic reconstructions demonstrating a nonoccluding distal ureteral stone (*arrow*). **A** to **C**, Three-dimensional postrenal processing techniques are used to mimic intravenous urography. **D**, Postcontrast axial imaging demonstrates a stone within the lumen of the distal ureters.

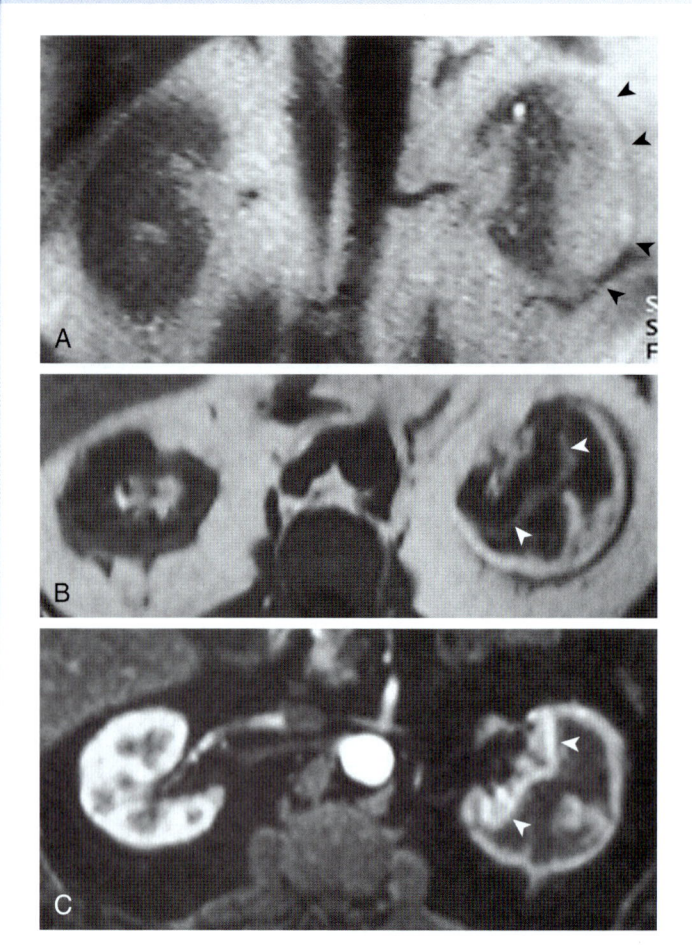

Figure 28.48 Subcapsular hematoma after lithotripsy. Coronal T2-weighted sequence **(A)** demonstrates high–signal intensity blood contained by left renal capsule (*arrowheads*). Axial T1-weighted image **(B)** and gadolinium-enhanced T1-weighted image **(C)** show mass effect on left kidney (*arrowheads*) caused by a subcapsular hematoma. The signal intensity is consistent with the presence of intracellular methemoglobin.

hematomas (Figures 28.48 to 28.50).[204] CE-MRI can also demonstrate damage to the collecting system and areas of ischemia without the risk for nephrotoxicity.

RENAL INFECTION

Acute pyelonephritis is typically a diagnosis made clinically.[205] Most cases of acute pyelonephritis occur by the ascending route from the bladder and are caused by gram-negative bacteria.[206] Vesicoureteral reflux may contribute, although the ascent of the bacteria up the ureter also occurs in its absence. This is due to the presence of the adhesin P fimbriae and powerful endotoxins that appear to inhibit ureteral peristalsis creating a functional obstruction.[207] The bacteria are transported to the renal pelvis, where intrarenal reflux occurs and the bacteria traverse the calyceal system to the ducts and tubules within the renal pyramid. Enzyme release results in destruction of tubular cells with subsequent bacterial invasion of the interstitium. As the infection progresses, it spreads throughout the pyramid and to the adjacent parenchyma. The inflammatory response leads to focal or more diffuse swelling of the kidney. Without adequate treatment, necrosis of the involved regions and microabscess formation occur. These microabscesses may coalesce into larger macroabscesses, which tend to be surrounded by a rim of granulation tissue.[208] Perinephric abscess results from the rupture of an intrarenal abscess through the renal capsule or the leak from an infected and obstructed kidney (pyonephrosis). The overall distribution in the kidney is usually patchy or lobar, but sometimes it is diffuse.[206] Subsequent scarring of the kidney after treatment reflects the magnitude of the infection and tissue destruction that occurred.

Pyelonephritis may also occur by hematogenous spread of bacteria to the cortex of the kidney and eventual involvement of the medulla. The pattern of involvement is usually round, peripheral, and frequently multiple. Blood-borne infection is less common than ascending infection and is usually observed in intravenous drug abusers, immunocompromised patients, or patients with a source of infection outside the kidney, such as heart valves or teeth.

Imaging is rarely used or needed in uncomplicated pyelonephritis, and most patients respond to therapy within 72 hours. Imaging should be reserved for patients who are not responding to conventional antibiotic treatment, patients with an unclear diagnosis, patients with coexisting stone disease and possible obstruction, patients with diabetes and poor antibiotic response, and patients who are immunocompromised. Imaging is used to assess complications of acute pyelonephritis, including renal and perinephric abscess, emphysematous pyelonephritis, and xanthogranulomatous pyelonephritis.[209-211] All of these entities are imaged best with cross-sectional imaging techniques, specifically CT.

US results are normal in the majority of patients with acute pyelonephritis. When the examination results are abnormal, the findings are often nonspecific. US is performed to look for a cause for acute pyelonephritis, such as obstruction or renal calculi, and to search for complications. Altered parenchymal echogenicity is the most frequent finding with loss of the normal corticomedullary differentiation. The echogenicity is usually decreased or heterogeneous in the affected area (Figure 28.51). There may be focal or generalized swelling of the kidney. Power Doppler imaging may improve sensitivity in demonstrating focal hypoperfusion, but this is nonspecific. Tissue harmonic US imaging may be more sensitive in demonstrating focal or segmental, patchy, hypoechoic areas extending from the medulla to the renal capsule.[212]

CE-CT is the most sensitive and specific imaging study in the patient with acute pyelonephritis.[213,214] The nephrographic phase of CT is best for imaging in patients with acute pyelonephritis (Figure 28.52). Wedge-shaped areas of decreased density extending from the renal pyramid to the cortex are most characteristic.[213] The nephrogram may be streaky or striated in either a focal or global manner (Figure 28.53).[215] There may be focal or diffuse swelling of the kidney.[216] The areas of involvement may appear almost masslike (see Figure 28.52). The changes in the nephrogram are related to decreased concentration of contrast media in the tubules with focal ischemia. Tubular destruction and obstruction with debris are also present. There is usually a sharp demarcation between diseased tissue and the normal parenchyma, which continues to enhance normally in the nephrographic phase. Soft tissue stranding and thickening of Gerota's fascia are caused by the adjacent inflammatory

CHAPTER 28 — DIAGNOSTIC KIDNEY IMAGING 879

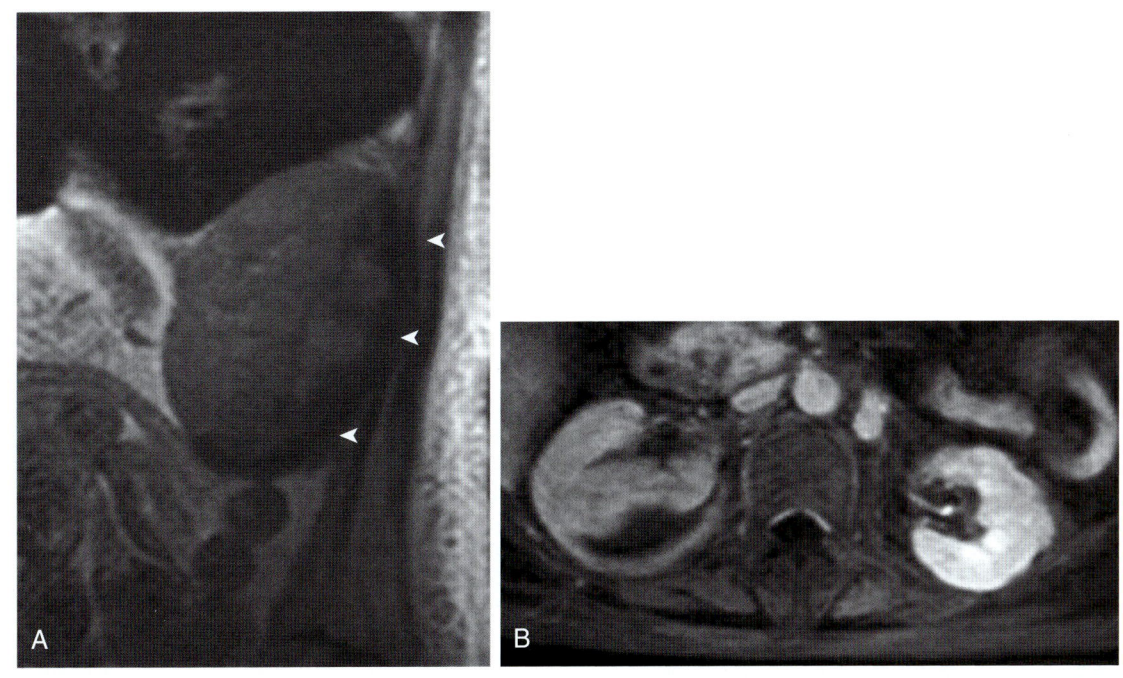

Figure 28.49 Posttraumatic subcapsular hematoma. Sagittal T2-weighted image **(A)** and postcontrast T1-weighted image **(B)** show a subcapsular hematoma (*arrowheads*) in which signal intensity is consistent with the presence of extracellular methemoglobin. This hematoma is older than the one shown in Figure 28.48.

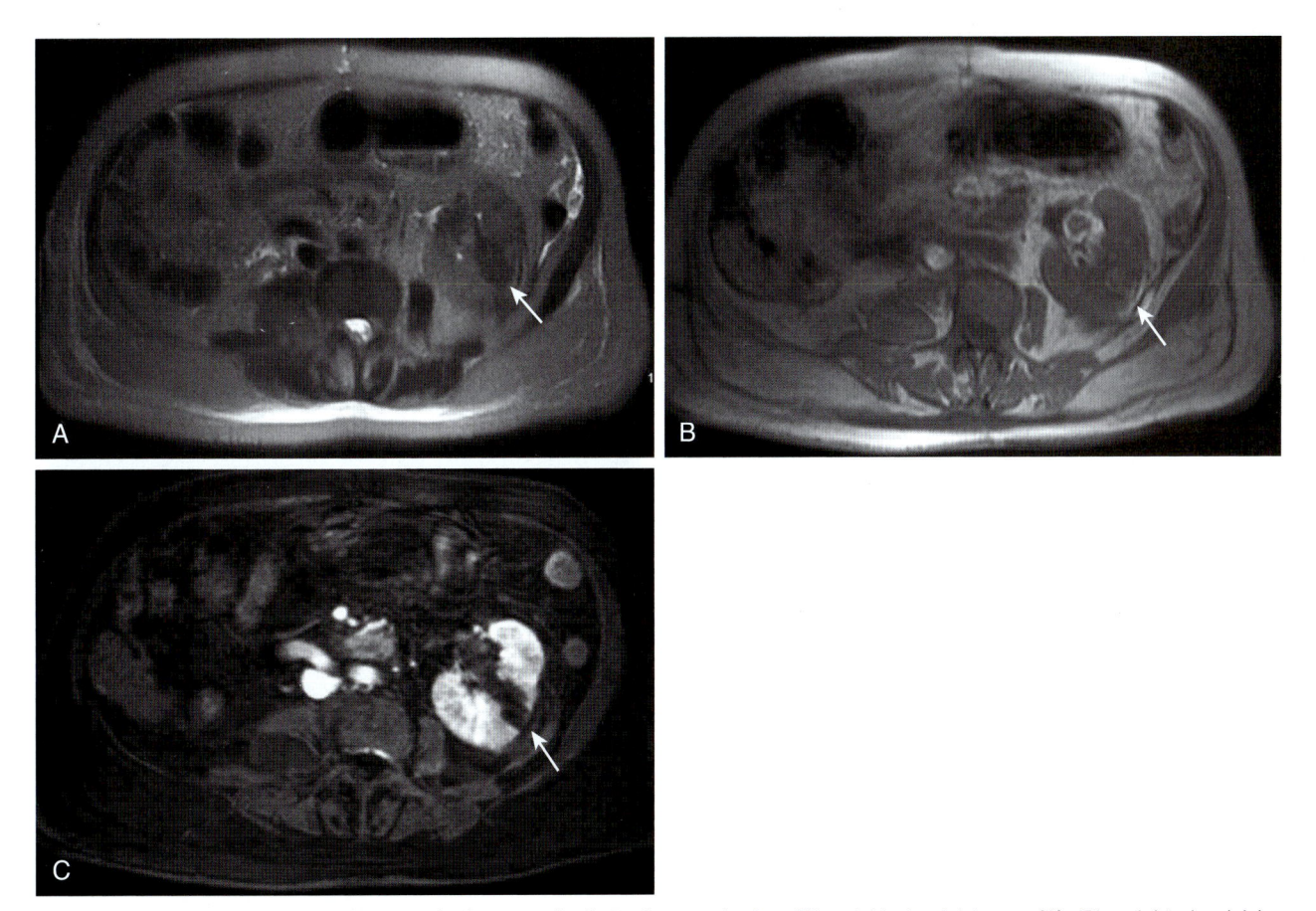

Figure 28.50 Hematoma status after surgical removal of staghorn calculus. T2-weighted axial image **(A)**, T1-weighted axial image **(B)**, and postcontrast T1-weighted axial image **(C)** show an intrarenal hematoma (*arrows*) at the site of incision plane. This extends into the renal pelvis. No urine extravasation was demonstrated.

process (see Figure 28.53).[208] The walls of the renal pelvis and proximal ureter may be thickened. The calyces and renal pelvis may be effaced. Mild dilation is also occasionally noted. With hematogenous-related pyelonephritis, the early findings tend to be multiple, round cortical regions of hypodensity that become more confluent and involve the medulla with time.[216] These findings may persist for weeks despite successful treatment with antibiotics.

MRI is comparable with CE-CT for the evaluation of pyelonephritis.[217] The enhancement characteristics of acute pyelonephritis on MRI are similar to those on CT. On noncontrast sequences, the affected area has increased T2 signal intensity and decreased T1 signal intensity in relation to the normal renal parenchyma.

Other modalities do not have a significant role in evaluating acute pyelonephritis, unless CT is unavailable. IVU findings may appear normal in up to 75% of cases[208,213]; IVU has been shown to be noncontributory to clinical care in 90% of patients with pyelonephritis.[206,214] Radiolabeled leukocyte scans (e.g., indium 111–labeled white blood cells) and gallium 67 citrate scans can identify acute pyelonephritis. However, these methods have the drawbacks of extended imaging time (more than 24 hours) and higher radiation exposure. Cortical imaging with ^{99m}Tc-DMSA has been shown to be highly sensitive for detecting acute pyelonephritis in the appropriate clinical setting.[218,219] In acute pyelonephritis, segmental regions of decreased tracer uptake are demonstrated in oval, round, or wedge patterns. There may also be diffuse generalized decrease in renal uptake, which, in association with a normal or slightly enlarged kidney, is suggestive of an acute infectious process. The pathophysiologic basis for decline in ^{99m}Tc-DMSA cortical uptake in infection is related to diminished delivery of the tracer to the infected area and to direct infectious injury to the tubular cells, which compromises their function and tracer uptake. A wedge-shaped cortical defect with regional decrease in renal size is compatible with postinfectious scarring. Renal infarcts may also have similar appearance.[123,129] Attention to ^{99m}Tc-DMSA image processing and quality is paramount to achieving high interreader agreement.[220,221] There may also be a role for FDG PET-CT in the imaging evaluation of renal infection.[222]

Renal abscess results from severe pyelonephritis and occurs two to three times more frequently in patients with diabetes.[210] Abscesses are more common with hematogenous infection than with ascending infection.[205] CE-CT characteristics of renal abscess include a reasonably well-defined mass with a low-density central region and a thick, irregular wall or pseudocapsule (Figure 28.54).[213] Enhancement adjacent to the abscess is variable, depending on the amount of inflammation. Mature abscesses may demonstrate a more sharply demarcated border with peripheral rim enhancement. Gas may be visible within the abscess. MRI is comparable with CE-CT for the evaluation of renal abscess.[217] The central region of the abscess can have a variable appearance, but generally it is of decreased T1 and increased T2 signal intensity. The wall enhancement characteristics are also similar to those on CE-CT (Figure 28.55).

Renal parenchymal infections can extend into the perinephric space with resulting abscess formation.[216] CT and MRI best reveal the involvement of the perinephric and

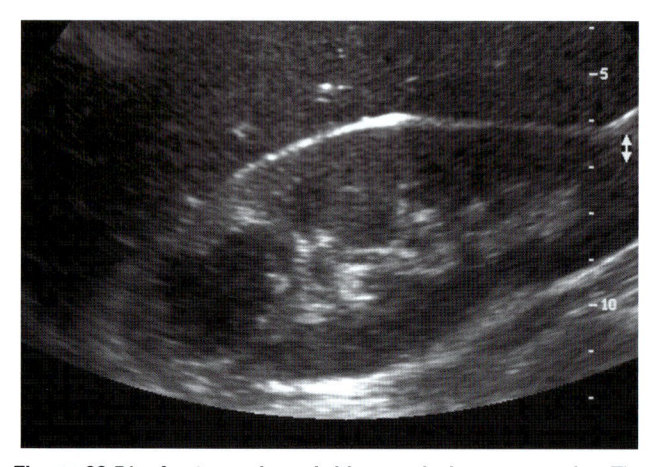

Figure 28.51 Acute pyelonephritis: renal ultrasonography. The hypoechoic region in the upper pole represents an area affected by acute pyelonephritis. The surrounding parenchyma is somewhat distorted, with loss of the normal corticomedullary junction.

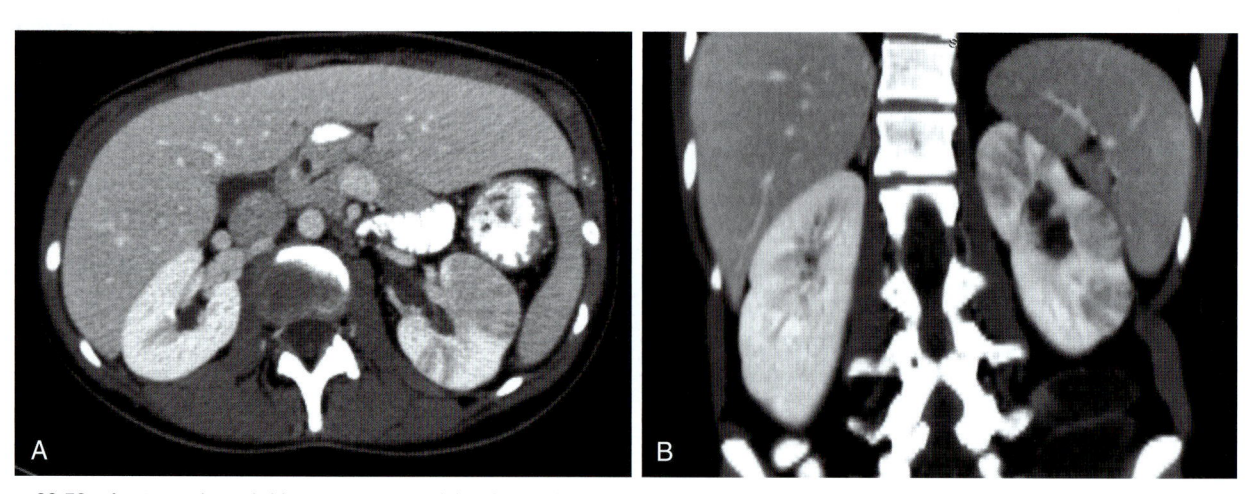

Figure 28.52 Acute pyelonephritis: contrast material–enhanced computed tomographic scan, axial (**A**) and coronal (**B**) images. The left kidney shows multiple areas of involvement. The hypodense region in the midportion of the kidney appears almost masslike (**A** and **B**). A nephrogram is striated in the region of involvement in the upper pole (**B**).

paranephric spaces within the retroperitoneum. In general, inflammatory changes and heterogeneous fluid-density or signal intensity collections may be identified. Associated gas is best identified on CT.

Emphysematous pyelonephritis is a severe necrotizing infection of the renal parenchyma, usually caused by gram-negative bacteria (*Escherichia coli*, *Klebsiella pneumoniae*, *Proteus mirabilis*).[209] Of patients with emphysematous pyelonephritis, 90% have uncontrolled diabetes.[210] Emphysematous pyelonephritis is characterized by severe acute pyelonephritis, urosepsis, and hypotension. The gas found in the renal parenchyma is believed to form as a result of the high levels of glucose in the tissue by fermentation with the production of CO_2. The gas may also be observed in the pelvicalyceal system or perinephric space (or both). If the gas is extensive enough, it may be visible on plain radiographs or KUB images. The gas is usually mottled, bubbly, or streaky in appearance and may be observed in the areas over the kidneys. US may suggest the diagnosis of emphysematous pyelonephritis by demonstrating gas within the kidney.[223] With gas present, there is acoustic shadowing in the involved region. CT is the most specific and sensitive modality for the identification of renal gas.[224] The gas dissects through the parenchyma in a linear focal or global manner, radiating along the pyramid to the cortex. It may extend into the perinephric space. There is generally extensive parenchymal destruction with streaks or mottled collections of gas within the kidney (Figure 28.56). Little or no fluid is seen. Emphysematous pyelitis represents gas within the pelvicalyceal system without parenchymal gas.[225] The distinction is important because emphysematous pyelitis carries a less grave prognosis.

Xanthogranulomatous pyelonephritis is an end-stage condition resulting from chronic obstruction with long-standing infection, usually with *Proteus* species or *E. coli*.[211] The renal parenchyma is destroyed and replaced by vast amounts of lipid-laden macrophages. The kidney is usually barely functional or nonfunctional. The destruction is typically global, but it may involve only a portion of the kidney. A staghorn calculus may be seen on KUB. On US the kidney appears enlarged with loss of identifiable landmarks. A large calculus or staghorn calculus usually fills the renal pelvis, with debris filling adjacent hypoechoic regions (Figure 28.57). CT defines the extent and adjacent organ involvement best. The findings on CT include an enlarged but generally reniform mass filling the perinephric space.[211,226] Calcification is found in 75% of cases, excretion is absent or markedly decreased in 85% of cases, and the involved region appears as a mass in more than 85% of cases.[211] The process is focal in fewer than 15% of cases. There is frequent perinephric extension. Fistulas may occur in adjacent structures, with adenopathy noted in the retroperitoneum. MRI may show many similar findings when compared with CT, although calcifications are less conspicuous (Figure 28.58).

Malacoplakia is a rare inflammatory condition that most commonly involves the bladder but may also involve the ureter and kidney. Typically the kidney is affected by obstruction from the lower urinary tract. When the kidney is directly

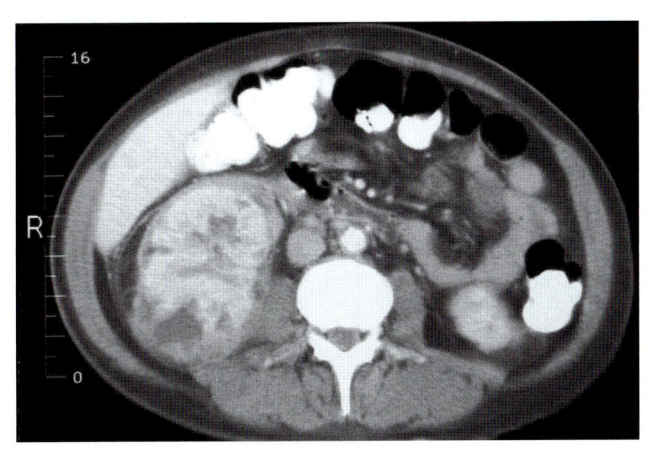

Figure 28.53 Acute pyelonephritis: contrast material–enhanced computed tomographic (CT) scan. The heterogeneous CT nephrogram shows the diffuse involvement of the right kidney. Stranding and some fluid are visible in the perinephritic space with thickening of Gerota's fascia.

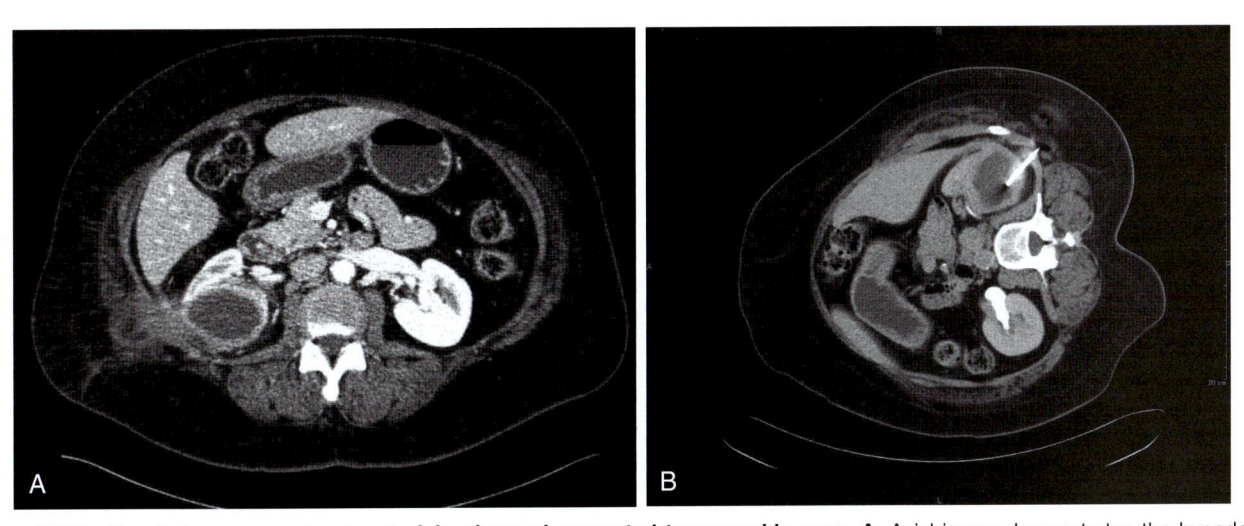

Figure 28.54 Renal abscess: contrast material–enhanced computed tomographic scan. A, Axial image demonstrates the hypodense abscess in the right kidney with extension into the perinephritic space and the right flank. **B,** Axial image with the patient in the decubitus position reveals the method of diagnosis: needle aspiration. A drainage catheter was subsequently placed for treatment.

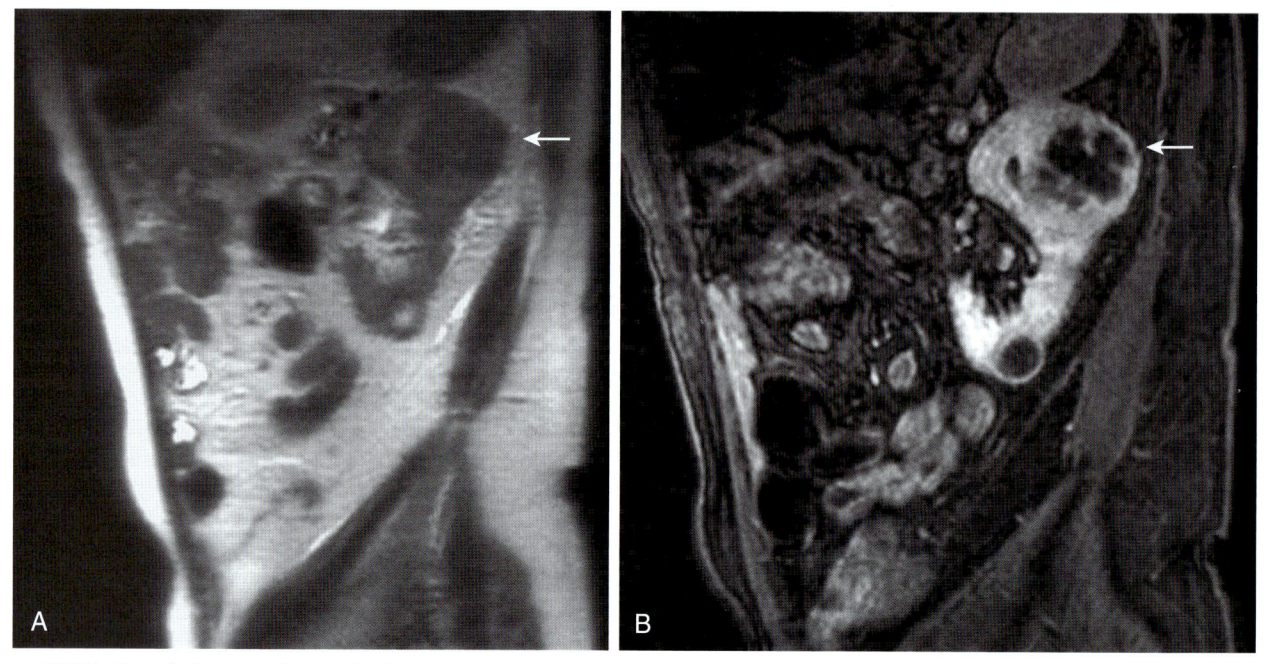

Figure 28.55 Renal abscess. A mass in the upper pole of the left kidney demonstrates intermediate to low signal intensity (*arrow*) on the sagittal T2-weighted image **(A)** and heterogeneous but predominantly peripheral enhancement (*arrow*) on the sagittal postcontrast T1-weighted image **(B)**. On biopsy, this mass was found to be *Aspergillus* infection.

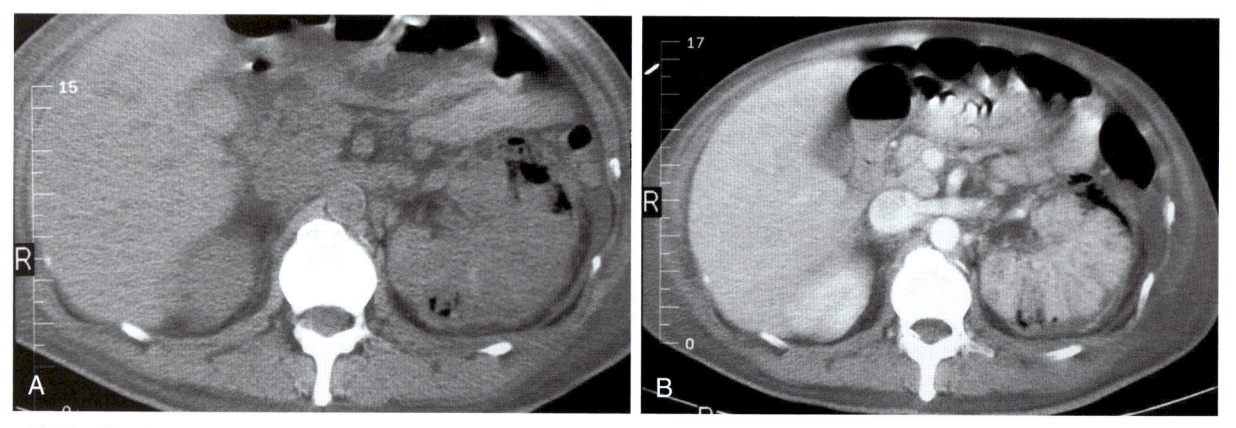

Figure 28.56 Emphysematous pyelonephritis: contrast material–enhanced computed tomographic scan. A noncontrast image **(A)** and a contrast material–enhanced image **(B)** demonstrate gas in the renal parenchyma with extension into the perinephritic space. The nephrogram is striated throughout. Global involvement of the kidney is frequent.

involved, it is a multifocal process that may appear similar to xanthogranulomatous pyelonephritis on imaging.

Renal tuberculosis occurs by hematogenous spread. The genitourinary tract is the second most common site of involvement. Evidence of previous pulmonary tuberculosis is found in fewer than 50% of patients with genitourinary tuberculosis. Only 5% may have active tuberculosis. Renal involvement is bilateral; the findings are determined by the extent of the infection, the stage of the infection, and the host's response. Calcified granuloma may be found within the cortex or medulla; papillary necrosis may be visible (Figure 28.59); and hydrocalyx with infundibular strictures may develop (Figure 28.60). The kidney may become focally or globally scarred as the disease progresses. There may be areas of nonfunction with dystrophic calcifications. In the end stage, the kidney may be small and scarred with bizarre calcifications; this condition is the so-called autonephrectomy.[162,227]

Chronic pyelonephritis is usually associated with vesicoureteral reflux that occurs in childhood.[227] One or both kidneys may be involved. An affected kidney has focal scars that are associated with calyceal dilation. The scarring is often separated by normal regions of the kidney and normal-appearing calyces. When involvement is global, the kidney may be small. IVU demonstrates dilated or ballooned calyces that extend to the cortical surface, which is thinned. The outline of the affected kidney is distorted. With US the kidneys have irregular outlines with regions of cortical loss. Underlying dilated calyces may be visible. The regions of scarring may be echogenic in comparison with the adjacent normal kidney. CT and MRI demonstrate the abnormal architecture of the affected kidney.[216,217] Nephrographic phase images reveal the regions of cortical loss; the involved dilated calyces extend to the capsular surface. Dilation of the calyces is variable. Chronic pyelonephritis may be unilateral or bilateral. Excretory phase images best delineate the extent of involvement, especially in the coronal format.

In the patient with AIDS, urinary tract infections are quite common.[228,229] The infections are frequently hematogenous with unusual organisms such as *Pneumocystis jiroveci*, cytomegalovirus, and *Mycobacterium avium-intracellulare*. The infections may also be seen in other abdominal organs—liver, spleen, and adrenals.[230,231] In patients with AIDS, renal involvement may be detected in US demonstrating increased cortical echogenicity and loss of the corticomedullary differentiation (Figure 28.61).[231] Renal size is also increased, and it is a bilateral process.

RENAL MASS: CYSTS TO RENAL CELL CARCINOMA

Most renal masses are simple cysts, frequently found incidentally on US, CT, and MRI. They rarely occur in individuals younger than 25 years, but are found in more than 50% of patients older than 50 years. Typically, renal cysts are asymptomatic and cortical in location; they may be single or multiple. Their cause is unknown, although tubular obstruction has been postulated to be a necessary element.

Renal masses produce variable findings on imaging studies, depending on their location. For years IVU was the imaging modality of choice for detection of renal masses; however, the findings on IVU are frequently nonspecific, and further imaging is necessary to characterize most abnormalities found (Figure 28.62). Studies have shown that IVU has low sensitivity for detection of renal masses, especially those smaller than 3 cm in diameter.[232] With CT as the gold standard, IVU detected 10% of masses smaller than 1 cm in diameter, 21% of masses 1 to 2 cm in diameter, 52% of masses 2 to 3 cm in diameter, and 85% of masses larger than 3 cm in diameter.[232] US fared better than IVU but detected only 26% of masses smaller than 1 cm, 60% of those 1 to 2 cm, 82% of those 2 to 3 cm, and 85% of those larger than 3 cm.[232]

The findings on IVU are nonspecific, and US, CT, and MRI are used to characterize the renal mass, differentiating solid from cystic.

US is an excellent means of diagnosing a simple renal cyst if all imaging criteria are met.[27] The lesion in the kidney must be round or oval and anechoic (Figure 28.63); it must be well circumscribed with a smooth wall; and there must be enhanced through-transmission with a sharp interface between the wall and adjacent renal parenchyma. Thin septa may be visible within the cyst, but no nodules should be visible (Figure 28.64). If all these criteria are met, the diagnosis of cyst is established. If there is any deviation from these criteria, further imaging with CT or MRI is necessary.

CE-CT is the method of choice for characterizing and differentiating renal masses.[233-235] A simple renal cyst appears as a well-circumscribed, round, water-density lesion with no measurable wall (Figure 28.65). The contents should not enhance after the injection of contrast media. The contents may vary slightly from water density, but no more than 10 to 15 HU. The interface with the adjacent parenchyma is sharp. The margins are smooth with no perceptible nodules. Thin rimlike calcification may be visible. "High-density"

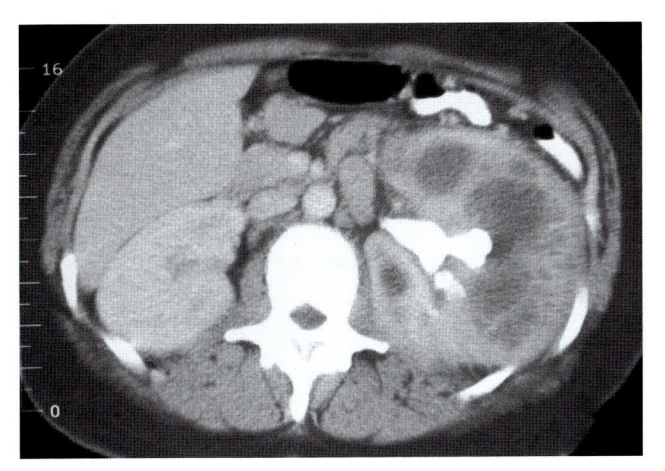

Figure 28.57 Xanthogranulomatous pyelonephritis: contrast material–enhanced computed tomographic scan. A large staghorn calculus fills the renal pelvis and collecting systems in the left kidney. Much of the remainder of the kidney is replaced by hypodense material—the xanthogranulomatous infection—within the calyces and parenchyma; some minimal enhancement of the cortex remains.

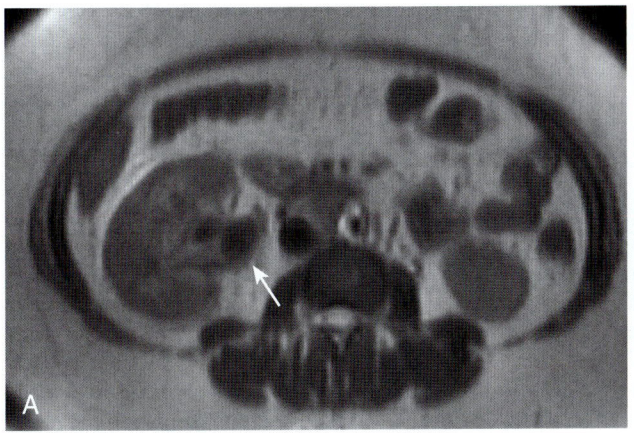

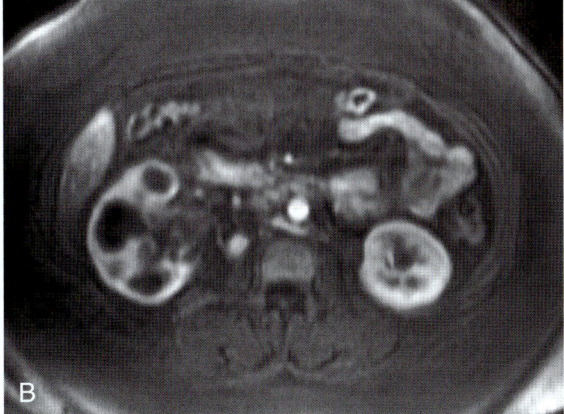

Figure 28.58 Xanthogranulomatous pyelonephritis with staghorn calculus. A, Axial T2-weighted image demonstrates a stone of low signal intensity within the right renal pelvis (*arrow*) that is associated with increased renal size and replacement of the medullary pyramids and calyces with material of high signal intensity. **B,** Axial postcontrast T1-weighted image demonstrates asymmetric enhancement and hydronephrosis.

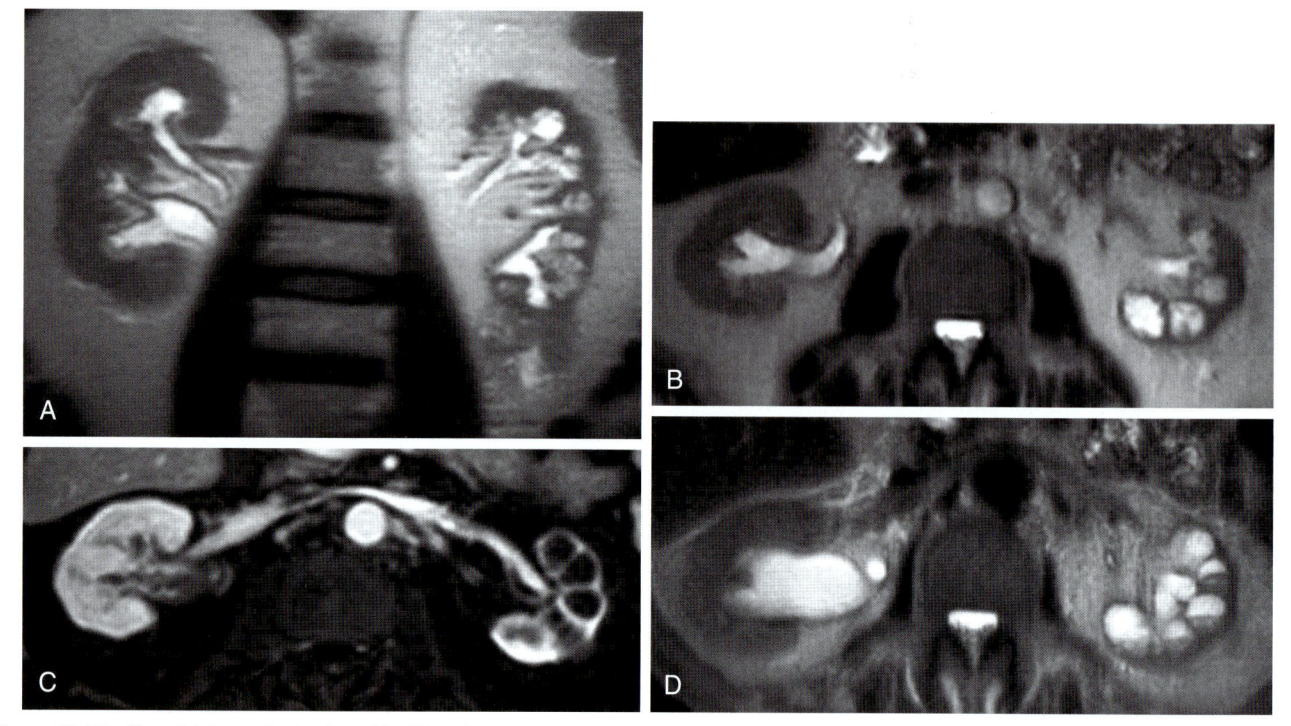

Figure 28.59 Renal tuberculosis. A and **B,** T2-weighted images demonstrate asymmetric cortical thinning and focal areas of increased signal intensity in the distribution of the medullary pyramids. **C,** Postcontrast T1-weighted image shows absence of enhancement, which is consistent with the presence of granulomas with caseous necrosis. **D,** T2-weighted image after treatment shows distorted, dilated calyces containing debris. Right-sided hydronephrosis is present as a result of a distal ureteral stricture.

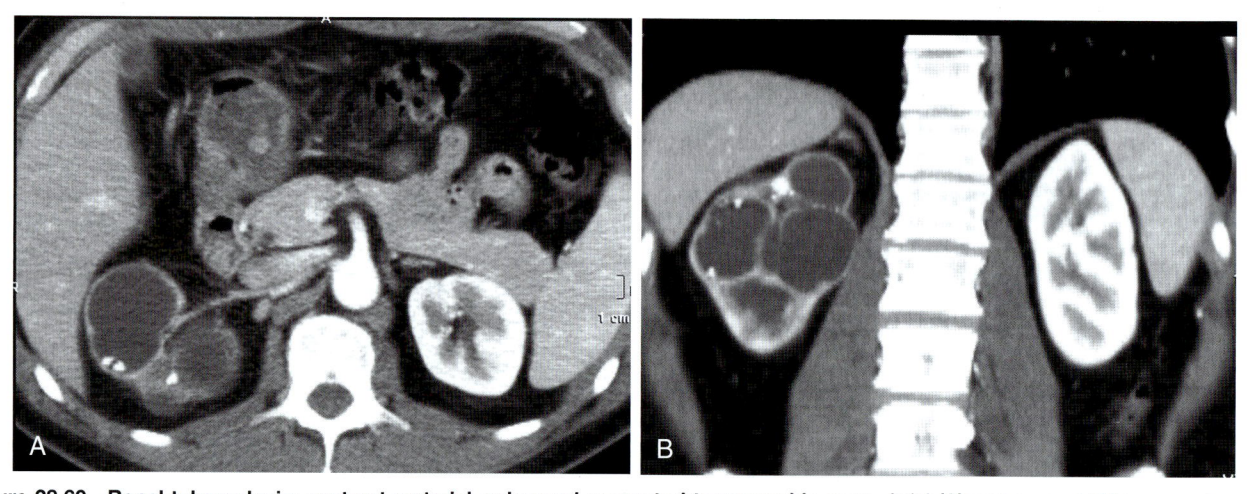

Figure 28.60 Renal tuberculosis: contrast material–enhanced computed tomographic scan. Axial **(A)** and coronal **(B)** images show the destruction of the right kidney as a result of renal tuberculosis. Parenchymal calcifications are present with dilated calyces as a result of the attenuation and truncation of the renal pelvis and ureter.

cysts may be encountered with density ranging from 50 to 80 HU; these are cysts containing hemorrhagic or proteinaceous debris. Like simple cysts, they should demonstrate no wall nodularity and have no significant enhancement after injection of contrast material. High-density cysts are common in polycystic or multicystic kidneys. Cysts are well demonstrated on MRI because of excellent soft tissue contrast. On MRI, simple cysts are well-circumscribed, thin-walled structures containing fluid that appears dark on T1-weighted sequences and bright on T2-weighted sequences (Figure 28.66). Complex cysts contain proteinaceous or hemorrhagic fluid and may have septations and calcification. The T1 signal intensity of the fluid is higher than expected for simple fluid, ranging from isointense to hyperintense. T2 signal intensity is lower than expected for simple fluid and may be black, depending on the blood content. Cysts do not enhance. In comparison with CE-CT, CE-MRI has been found to have higher contrast material resolution, which allows for better visualization of septa.[236,237] MRI also better characterizes blood products and is more sensitive to subtle enhancement, especially when subtraction techniques are used. This makes MRI superior to CT

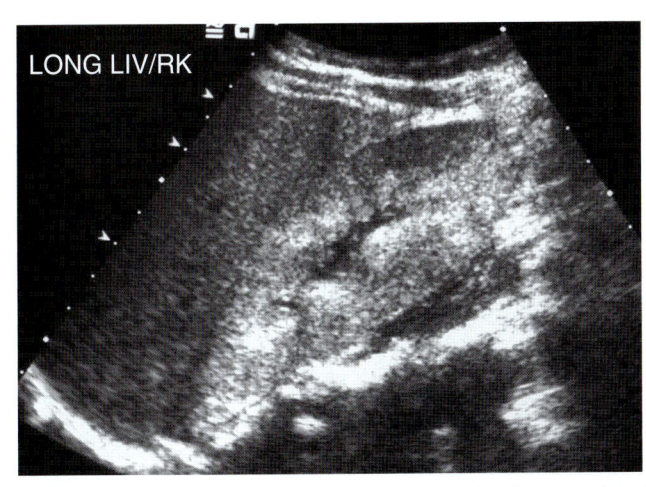

Figure 28.61 Acquired immunodeficiency syndrome–related nephropathy: ultrasonography. Longitudinal image of the right kidney. The size of the kidney is normal to slightly increased. The corticomedullary distinction is lost with diffuse increased cortical echogenicity.

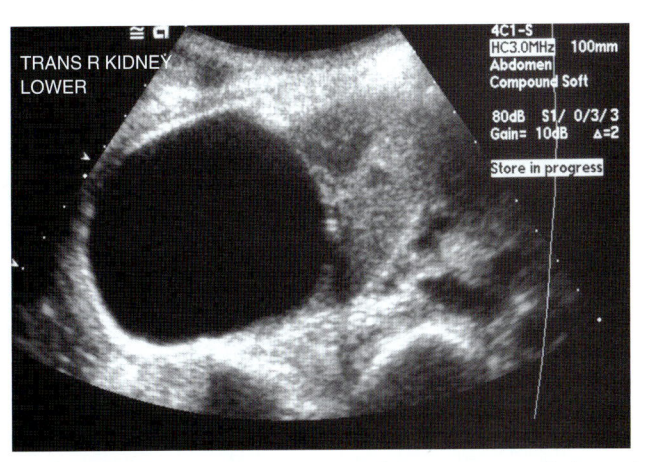

Figure 28.63 Renal cyst: ultrasonography. A large, anechoic renal mass projects off the lateral border of the right kidney. The features of the cyst include a well-circumscribed lesion with a sharp back wall and increased through-transmission. There are no internal echoes or nodularity, and the wall is smooth. There is a clear interface with the kidney.

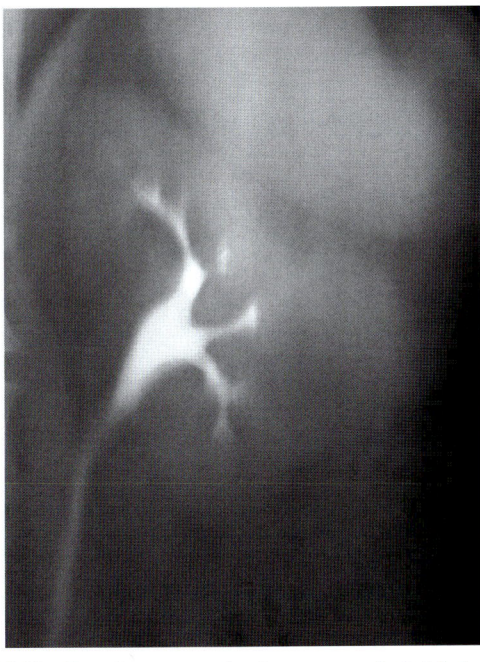

Figure 28.62 Renal mass: nephrotomogram. A slightly hypodense mass projects off the lateral border of the left kidney. Subsequent imaging proved this to be a renal cyst.

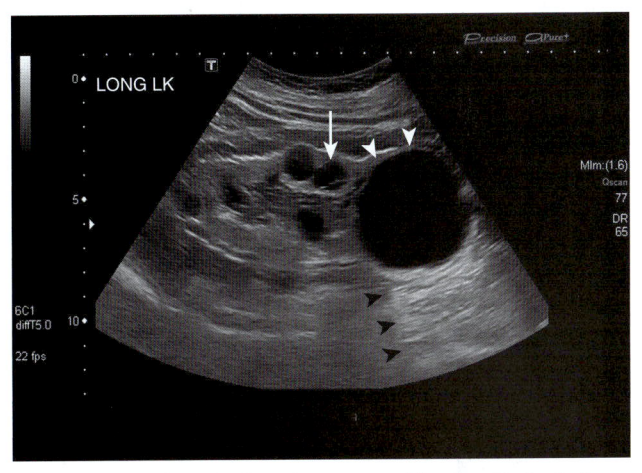

Figure 28.64 Gray-scale ultrasonographic longitudinal image reveals a cyst (*white arrowheads*) that is completely anechoic, and there are no septations in it. The appearance of posterior acoustic enhancement (*black arrowheads*) further confirms that the lesion is a cyst. The small, more superficial lesion (*small white arrow*) has a single thin septation, thus representing a Bosniak category II cyst.

in differentiating a complex cyst from a cystic neoplasm[236-238] (Figures 28.67 and 28.68).

Polycystic renal disease is classified as infantile, adult, or acquired. The infantile form is inherited as an autosomal recessive disorder.[239] It has a variable manifestation: severe kidney injury is found in the neonatal period, and CHF and hepatic failure manifest in older children. Organomegaly is common, with bilateral symmetric renal enlargement. IVU yields poor visualization of the kidneys because of renal impairment, and the nephrogram is prolonged and mottled with a striated or streaky appearance. US reveals enlarged, diffusely hyperechoic kidneys as a result of dilated, ectatic collecting tubules.[240] There is loss of the corticomedullary differentiation as well. Because the diagnosis is made clinically with the associated US findings, CT and MRI are rarely used in this condition.

Autosomal dominant polycystic kidney disease (ADPKD) is the adult form.[241] There is no role for KUB or IVU in the evaluation for ADPKD. US reveals bilateral enlargement of the kidneys, which are markedly lobulated and contain multiple anechoic areas of varying size throughout.[242]

CT and MRI in ADPKD depict enlarged, lobulated kidneys with cysts of varying size throughout (Figure 28.69). One kidney may be more involved than the other. The cysts may have calcifications with the wall. It is not uncommon to encounter cysts with varying density or signal intensity as a result of episodes of hemorrhage that occur within the cysts (Figure 28.70). A fluid level may be visible as a result of the presence of debris or hemorrhage within some of the cysts. In the excretory phase, there is marked distortion of the calyces. The extent of renal involvement by ADPKD is better

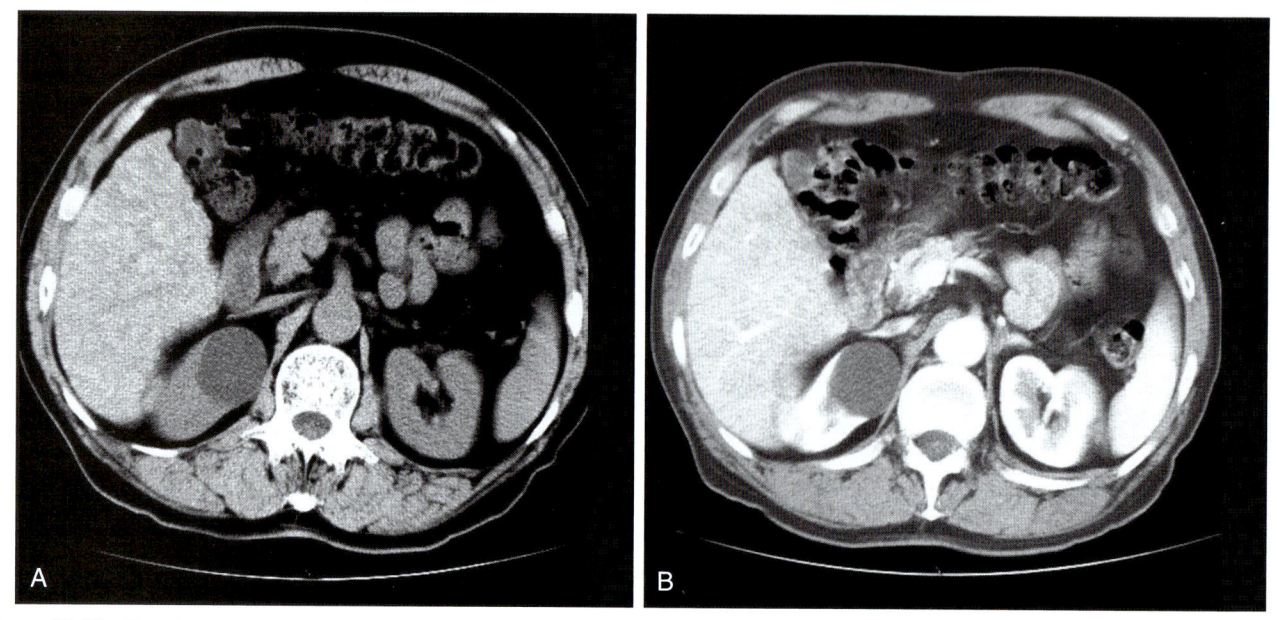

Figure 28.65 Renal cyst: computed tomographic (CT) scan. Noncontrast **(A)** and postcontrast **(B)** axial images. The cyst is well circumscribed with no enhancement. It displays water density with CT numbers of 0 to 5. There is a sharp interface with the kidney and no perceptible wall. No nodules are visible, and the cyst is uniform throughout.

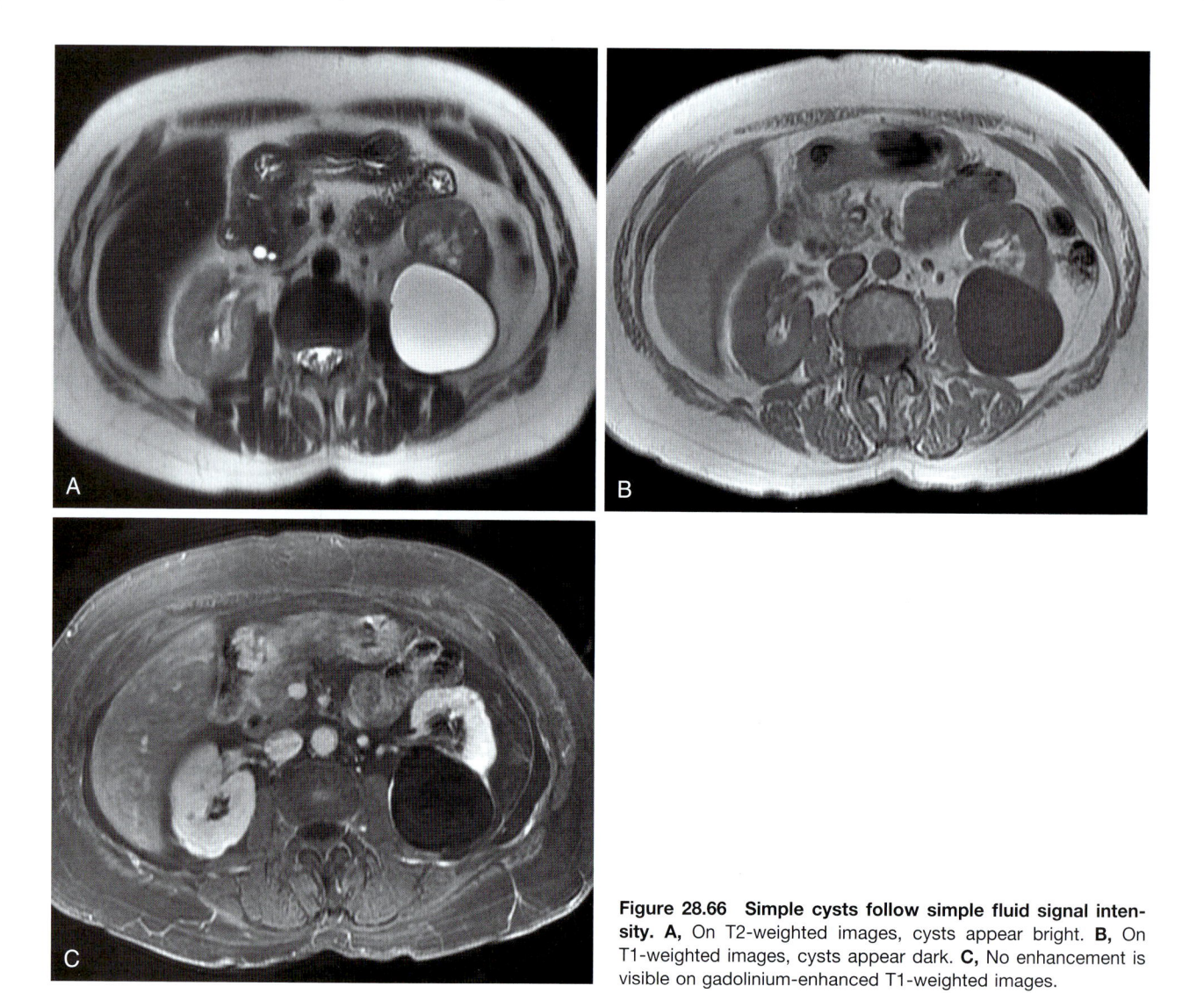

Figure 28.66 Simple cysts follow simple fluid signal intensity. A, On T2-weighted images, cysts appear bright. **B,** On T1-weighted images, cysts appear dark. **C,** No enhancement is visible on gadolinium-enhanced T1-weighted images.

CHAPTER 28 — DIAGNOSTIC KIDNEY IMAGING 887

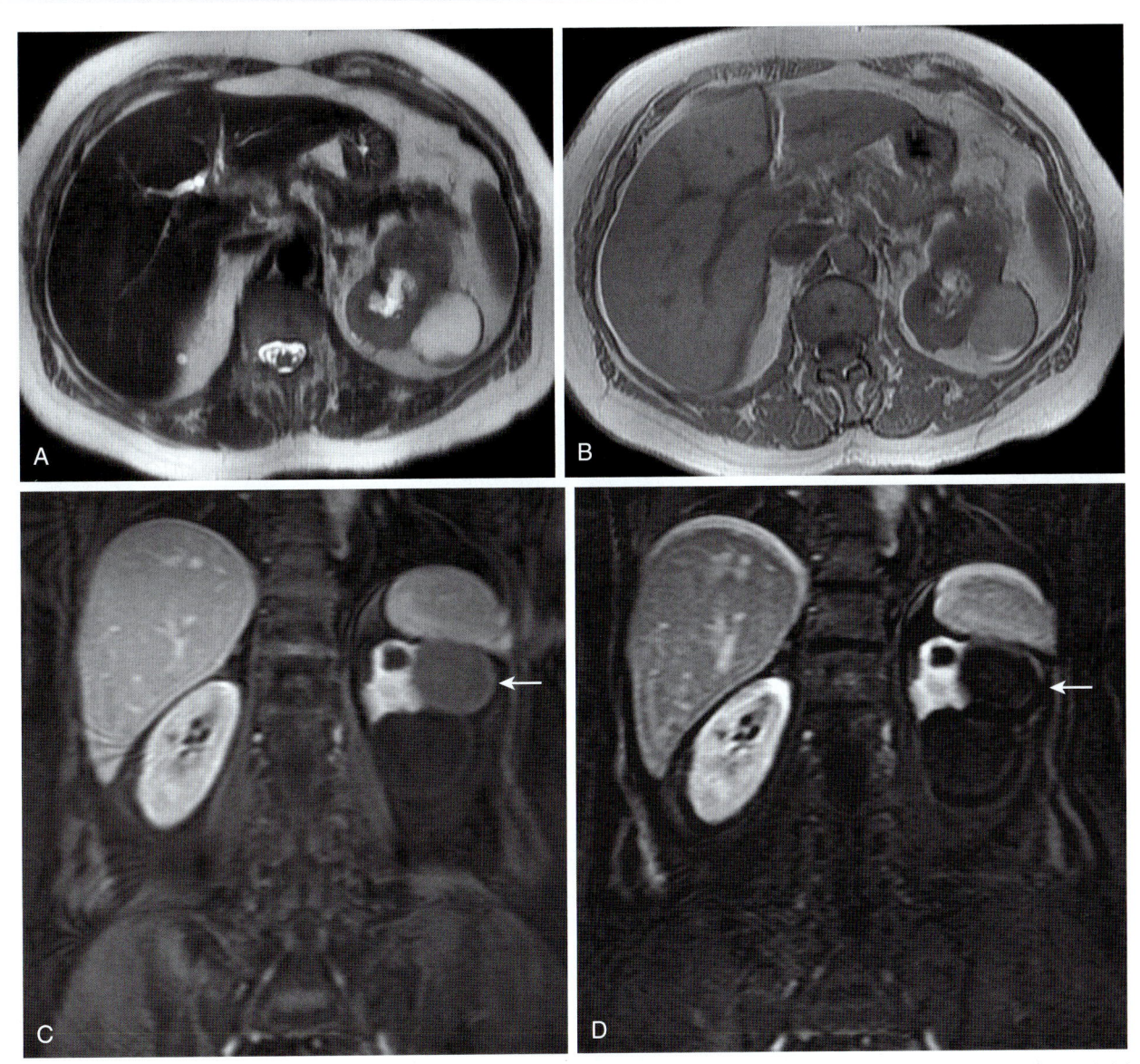

Figure 28.67 Complex cyst confirmed by computed tomography with image subtraction. A, T2-weighted axial image shows a bright left upper pole structure. **B,** T1-weighted axial image shows the same structure as intermediate in signal intensity. The cyst has internal debris that is visible on both sequences. Because the postcontrast T1-weighted coronal image **(C)** shows higher signal intensity than expected for a cyst (*arrow*), postcontrast subtraction images **(D)** are needed to confirm absence of enhancement (*arrow*).

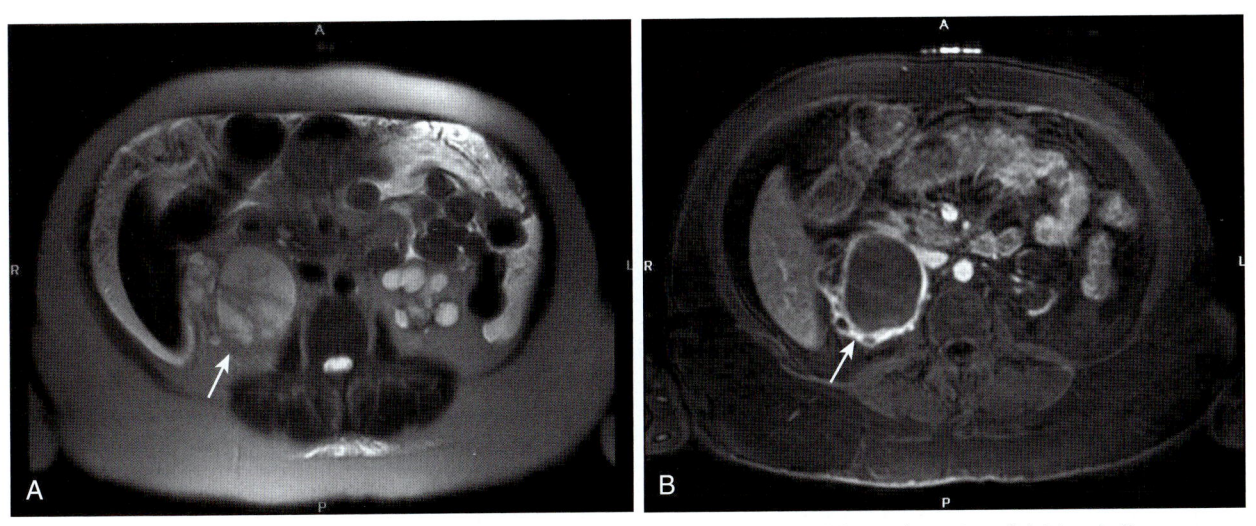

Figure 28.68 Complex hemorrhagic cyst. A, T1-weighted axial images show a complex right renal structure, bright on both sequences and with internal septations (*arrow*). **B,** Gadolinium on T1-weighted images produced no enhancement (*arrow*). This structure was diagnosed on fine-needle aspiration as a hemorrhagic cyst.

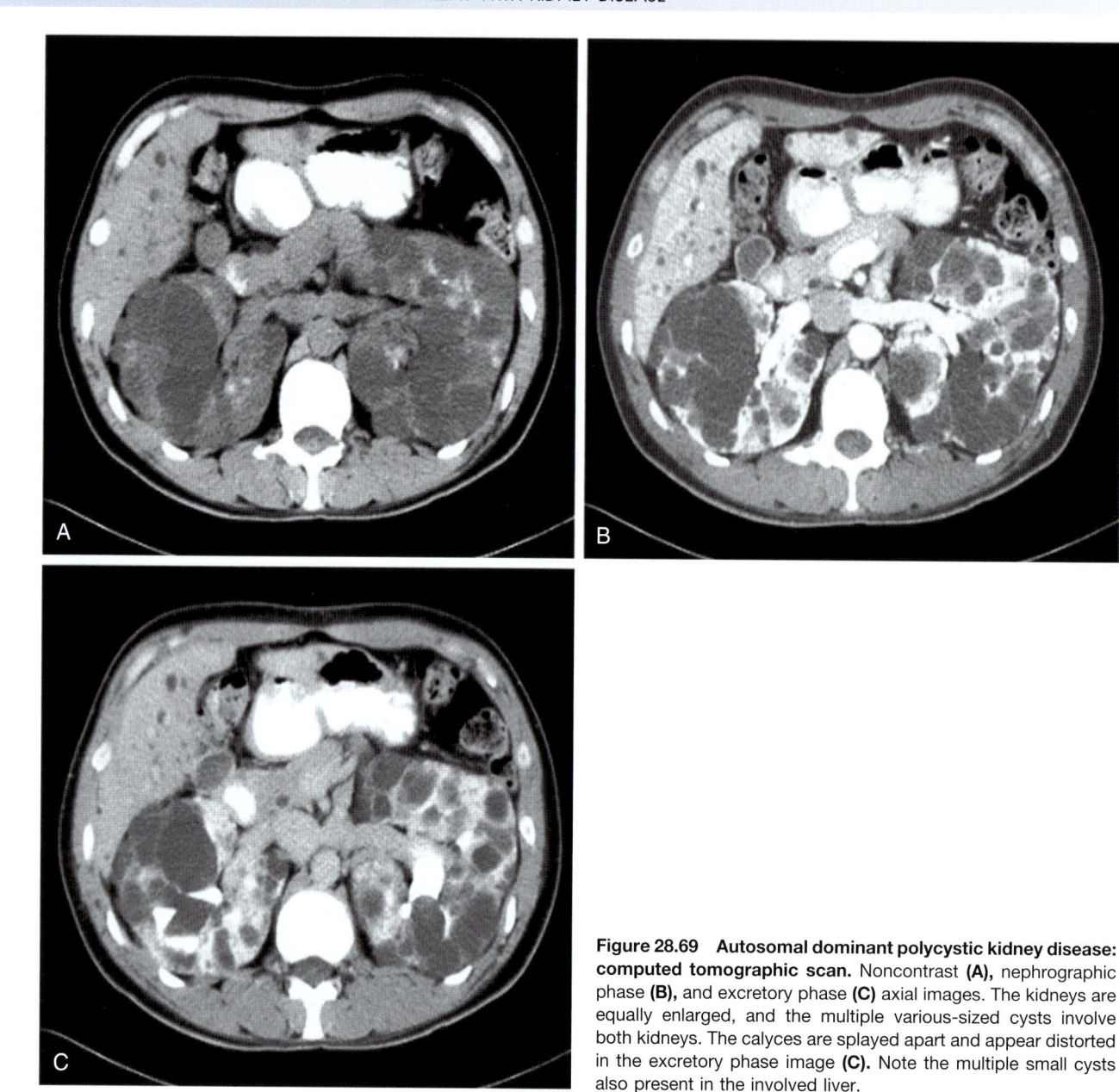

Figure 28.69 Autosomal dominant polycystic kidney disease: computed tomographic scan. Noncontrast **(A)**, nephrographic phase **(B)**, and excretory phase **(C)** axial images. The kidneys are equally enlarged, and the multiple various-sized cysts involve both kidneys. The calyces are splayed apart and appear distorted in the excretory phase image **(C)**. Note the multiple small cysts also present in the involved liver.

appreciated on CT and MRI than on US. Cysts may be found in the liver, spleen, and pancreas as well.

Adult-acquired polycystic kidney disease occurs in patients with kidney injury who are undergoing continuous peritoneal dialysis or hemodialysis.[243] The longer the patient has undergone dialysis, the more likely the patient is to develop adult-acquired polycystic kidney disease.[244,245] The cysts are generally quite small (0.5 to 2 cm in most patients). Calcification may occur in the wall. Plain radiographs and IVU play no role in evaluation because renal function is impaired. US reveals small, shrunken kidneys with anechoic or hypoechoic regions that represent the cysts. The findings are usually bilateral. CT or MRI shows the small bilateral kidneys with cysts of size that varies, but usually in the range of 1 to 2 cm (Figure 28.71; see Figure 28.32).[246,247] These cysts must be closely evaluated for solid components because carcinomas and adenomas occur with increased frequency in these patients. Solid lesions smaller than 3 cm in diameter may represent either adenomas or renal cell carcinomas, whereas most lesions larger than 3 cm are renal cell carcinomas.[248,249] Screening for adult-acquired polycystic kidney disease is usually done with US every 6 months; CT or MRI is reserved for patients with questionable or solid lesions.[250]

Medullary sponge kidney, or renal tubular ectasia, is a nonhereditary developmental disorder with ectasia and cystic dilation of the distal collecting tubules. The cystic spaces predispose to stasis, which leads to stone formation and potential infection. Involvement is usually bilateral, although not always symmetric, with as few as one calyx involved. The kidneys are typically normal sized with an appearance of medullary nephrocalcinosis when small stones are present.[161] IVU reveals linear or round collections of contrast material extending from the calyceal border, forming parallel brushlike striations. With more severe involvement, the cystic dilations may appear grapelike or beadlike. CT is an excellent method for demonstrating the

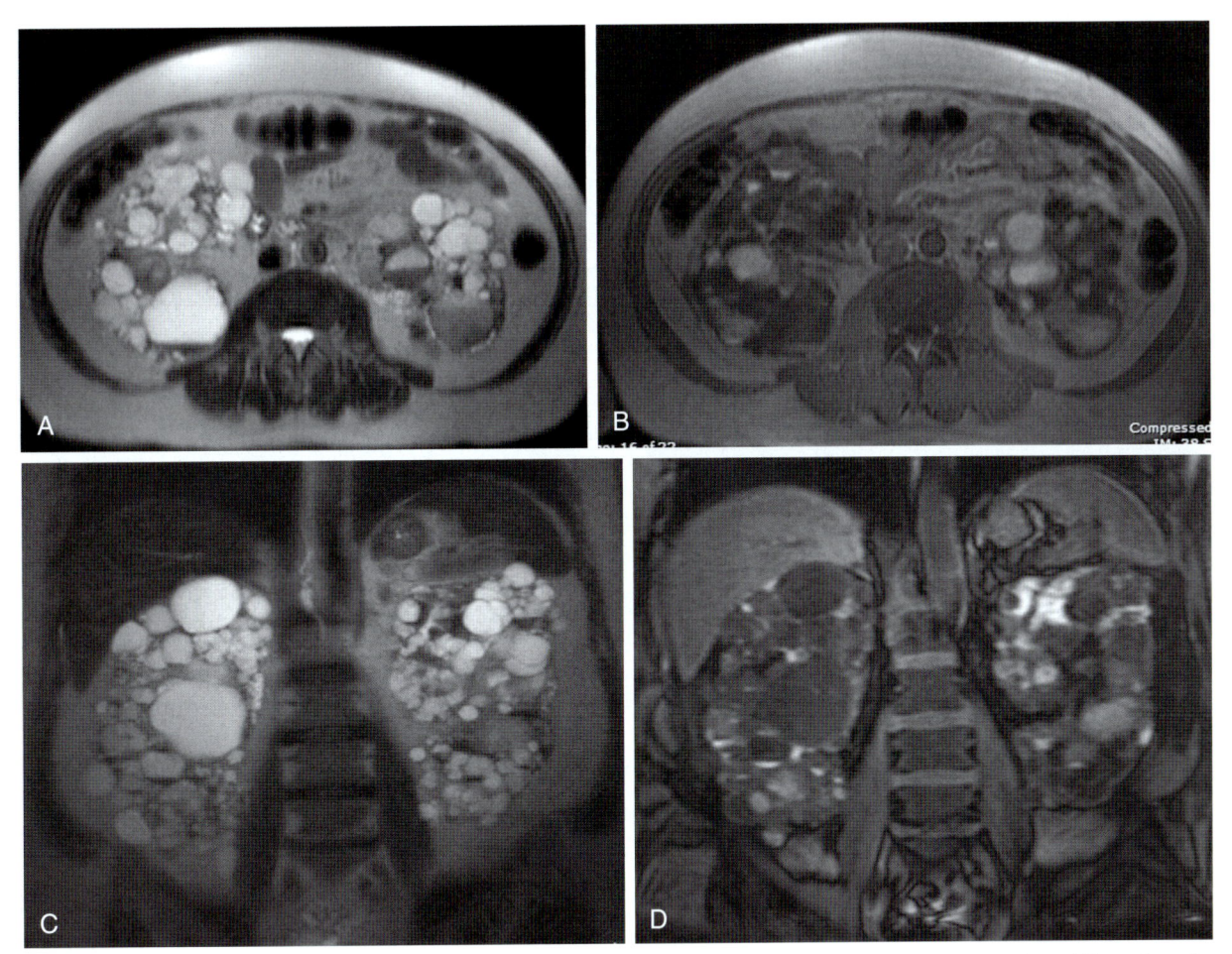

Figure 28.70 Autosomal dominant polycystic kidney disease. Axial **(A)** and coronal **(C)** T2-weighted images show bilateral renal cortical atrophy and multiple cysts, most of which are bright. Axial T1-weighted image **(B)** shows multiple bright and dark structures that are not enhanced after gadolinium injection; this appearance was confirmed with subtraction image **(D)** and is therefore consistent with cysts.

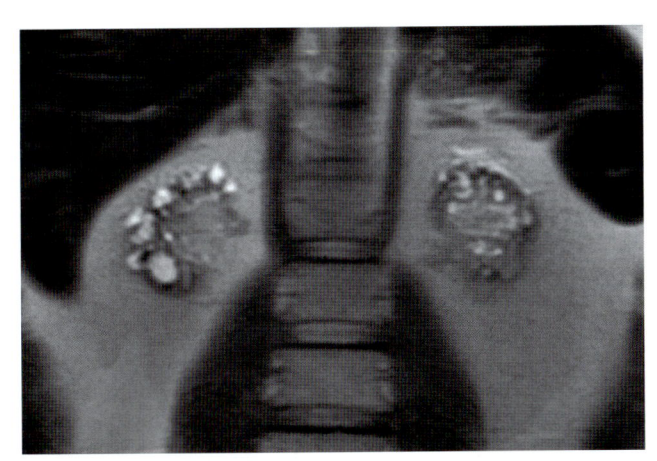

Figure 28.71 End-stage kidney disease. T2-weighted coronal image shows diffuse atrophy and multiple cysts in a patient on chronic dialysis.

calculi, although the striations or cystic dilation may be difficult to visualize even with thin-section excretory phase imaging.

Multicystic dysplastic kidney is an uncommon, congenital, nonhereditary condition. It is usually unilateral and affects the entire kidney. In rare cases only a portion of the kidney is involved. US reveals multiple anechoic cystic structures of varying size replacing the kidney, with no normal parenchyma. Calcification in the wall of the cystic spaces may be visible. CT demonstrates multiple fluid-filled structures filling the renal fossa. Septa and some rimlike calcifications may be visible. The density of the fluid is usually the same as or slightly higher than water. The kidney does not enhance after the injection of intravenous contrast material, and the renal artery on the affected side is not visible. It may be difficult to differentiate this condition from severe hydronephrosis if no cyst walls or septa are visible.

Small cortical cysts may occur in some hereditary syndromes (e.g., tuberous sclerosis) and in acquired conditions (e.g., lithium nephropathy; Figure 28.72). These cysts are typically multiple and very small (millimeters). They are viewed best with MRI but may also be viewed on CT if the cysts are slightly larger.[251] Cortical cysts may be larger in hereditary disorders, such as von Hippel–Lindau disease (Figure 28.73).[252] Pyelogenic cysts or calyceal diverticula are small cystic structures that connect with a portion of the pelvicalyceal system. On contrast material–enhanced studies a calyceal diverticulum appears as a small round or oval collection of contrast material connected to the fornix of the calyx. As stasis occurs within the diverticulum, renal stone formation may occur.

Cystic renal masses present a diagnostic problem in that not all are benign.[253] In 1986 Bosniak developed a classification system based on CT imaging characteristics to help guide the clinical management of cystic renal masses.[254-256] Category I lesions are simple, benign cysts (see Figure 28.65). Category II cysts are benign with thin septa, fine rimlike calcification, or they are uniform high-density cysts less than 3 cm in diameter that do not enhance (Figure 28.74). Category IIF represents more indeterminate category II lesions that necessitate follow-up, usually at 6 to 12 months, to prove benignity (Figure 28.75).[257] These cystic lesions may have multiple septa, or an area of thick or nodular calcification, or they may be high-density cysts larger than 3 cm in diameter. Category III cystic lesions have thickened, irregular walls, which demonstrate some enhancement. Dense irregular calcification may also be visible. In these cases, clinical history may be helpful in determining whether they are renal abscesses or infected cysts. Although some of these lesions are benign, surgery may be necessary for diagnosis and treatment.[258] Biopsy has been advocated by some authorities[259-262] (see Figure 28.54). Category IV cystic masses are clearly malignant and demonstrate distinct enhanced soft tissue masses or nodules within the cyst (Figure 28.76).[263] Nephrectomy is required for these lesions, although if they are not larger than 5 to 6 cm and are in proper locations, a nephron-sparing procedure may be performed.

CE-CT is the imaging modality of choice for the characterization of all solid masses, suspected solid masses, or masses that do not meet US criteria for a true renal cyst.[254,264,265] MRI has sensitivities and specificities similar to those of CT but is generally reserved for cases in which the patient has a contraindication to iodinated contrast medium or in which radiation dose must be limited. MRI may be helpful in cases of renal masses for which CT yielded indeterminate findings; in cases with venous involvement; and in distinguishing vessels from retroperitoneal lymph nodes. CEUS is now an additional technique that can be used especially in patients with compromised renal function (Figure 28.77).

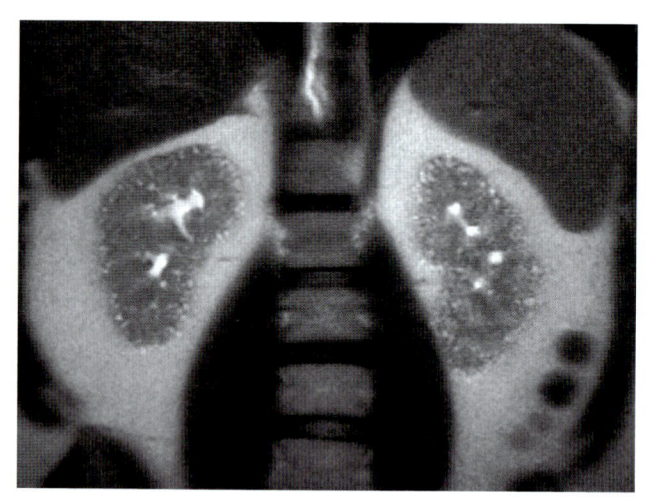

Figure 28.72 Lithium toxicity. Coronal T2-weighted image demonstrates innumerable small renal cortical cysts, characteristic of lithium toxicity.

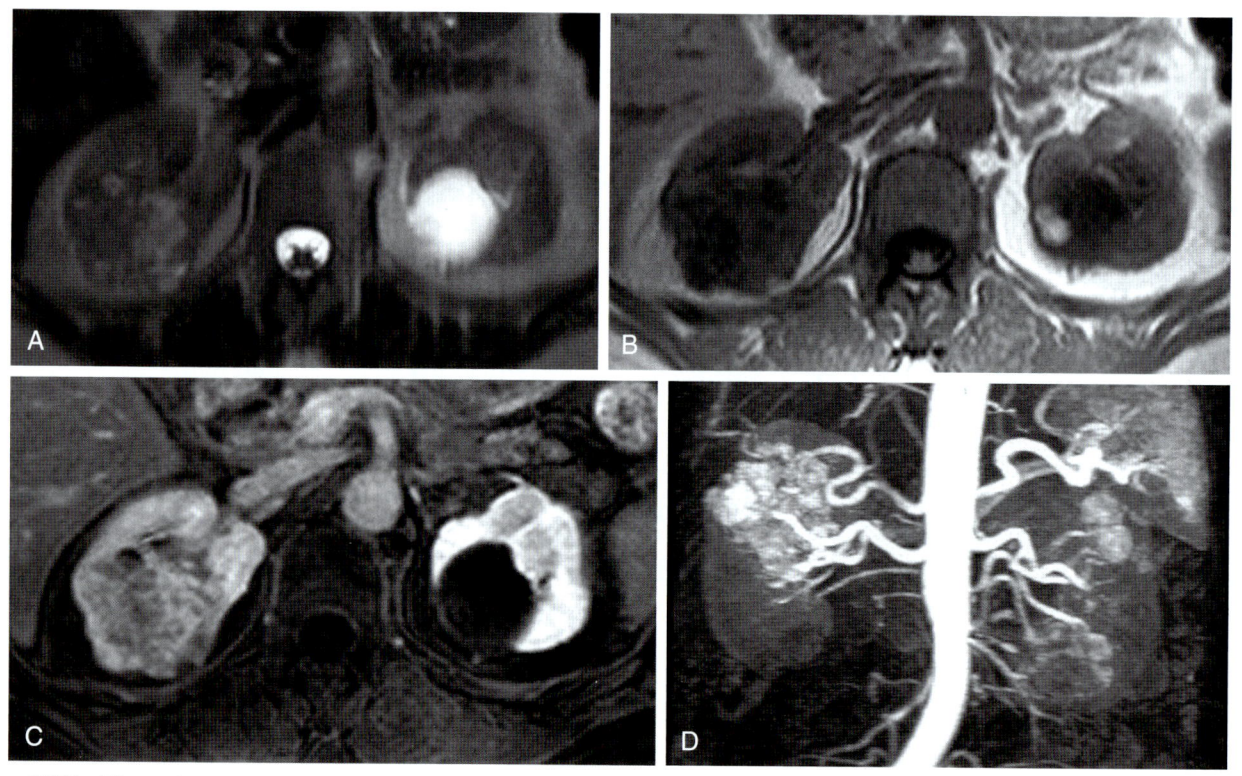

Figure 28.73 Bilateral clear cell carcinoma in von Hippel–Lindau syndrome. Bilateral heterogeneous renal masses and left renal cyst are visible on T2-weighted image **(A)** and T1-weighted image **(B)**. **C,** The larger right renal mass demonstrates heterogeneous enhancement, and two smaller left renal masses demonstrate more homogeneous enhancement. **D,** Maximum-intensity projection depicts the multiple renal masses in angiographic format.

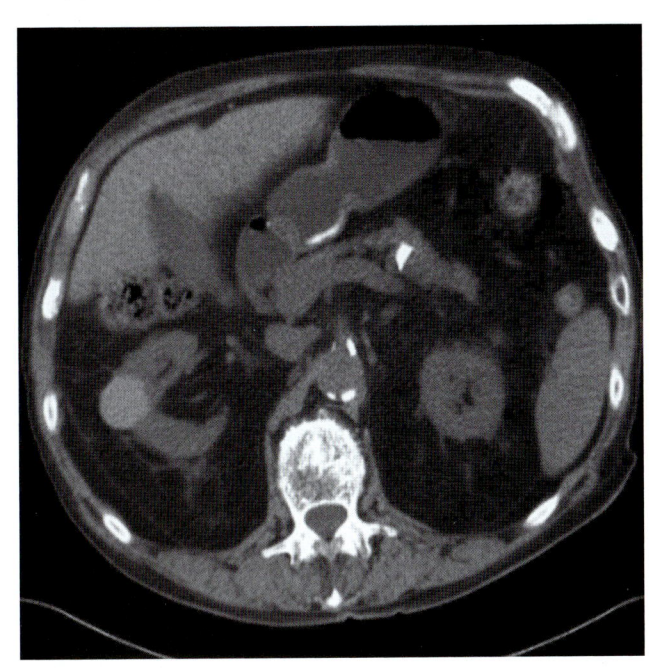

Figure 28.74 Hyperdense renal cyst: computed tomographic scan, axial noncontrast image. A single well-circumscribed hyperdense mass is visible in the right kidney. This represents a Bosniak category II renal cyst. It is sharply defined and less than 3 cm in diameter, and it will demonstrate no enhancement on the contrast material–enhanced scan.

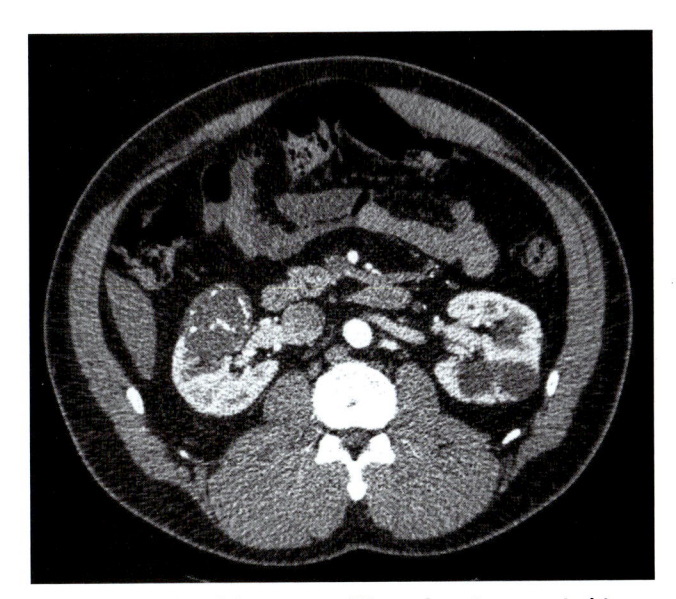

Figure 28.75 Bosniak category IIF renal cyst: computed tomographic (CT) scan, axial nephrographic phase image. A cystic lesion in the right kidney also demonstrates large clumps of calcification on the outer wall and on internal septa. There was no change in the CT numbers between the noncontrast scan and the enhanced images. This cyst necessitates follow-up. Note the Bosniak category I cysts in the left kidney.

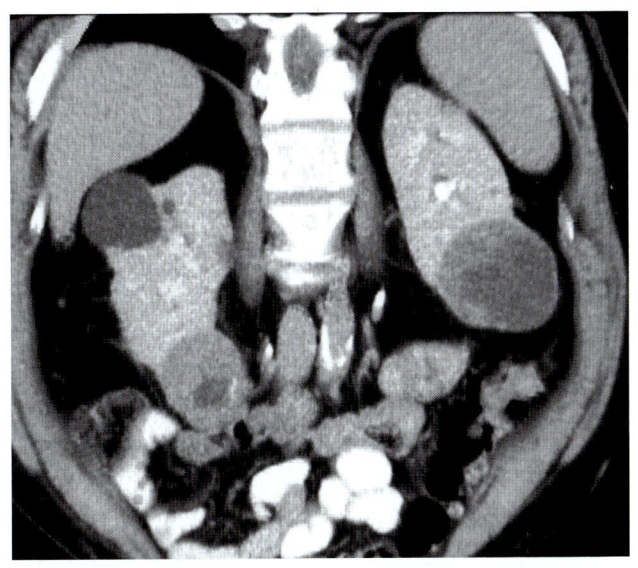

Figure 28.76 Bosniak category IV renal cyst: computed tomographic scan, coronal nephrographic phase image. A cystic mass is visible in the left kidney with an internal solid component in the lower pole. In the lower pole of the right kidney, there is a solid mass with central necrosis, which represents a renal cell carcinoma. Note the Bosniak category I cysts in the upper pole of the right kidney. A renal calculus is also present in the midportion of the left kidney. The left lower pole cystic lesion proved to be a renal cell carcinoma, papillary type.

Renal neoplasms may arise from either the renal parenchyma or the urothelium of the pelvicalyceal system. With the increased use of cross-sectional imaging techniques, more small neoplasms are discovered incidentally.[266,267] Renal adenoma is the most common benign neoplasm; it almost always is less than 2 to 3 cm in size and has no characteristic radiologic features to distinguish it from other solid tumors. Typically, renal adenomas are corticomedullary in location, appear solid on US, and demonstrate uniform enhancement on CE-CT.

Renal hamartomas, known as angiomyolipomas (AMLs), are benign renal tumors composed of different tissues, including fat, muscle, vascular elements, and even cartilage. It is the fat component that makes AML distinguishable radiologically (Figure 28.78).[268,269] On US the mass is solid and hyperechoic due to the presence of fat.[270,271] On CT the diagnosis of AML can be made with ease, because most AML have a large amount of fat. In uncommon cases, only a minimal amount of fat is present, and it must be searched for diligently.[272-275] MRI with fat-suppressed and opposed-phase chemical shift sequences can be used to make an accurate diagnosis.[276] Signal intensity of fat is high on both T1- and T2-weighted sequences. Macroscopic fat in AML has decreased signal intensity with fat-suppression sequences. Opposed-phase chemical shift sequences cause an "India ink" outline of the tumor at its interface with normal renal parenchyma. The enhancement pattern of AML may be variable, depending on the composition of the lesion. Fat should be searched for in all solid lesions in the kidney; if present, the diagnosis of AML is virtually ensured.[277-279] Most AMLs measuring 4 cm in diameter or smaller are monitored; surgery is reserved for larger ones, especially with hemorrhage.[280,281] Multiple, bilateral AMLs may be found in patients with tuberous sclerosis.

Oncocytoma is an uncommon benign tumor originating in the epithelium of the proximal collecting tubule. Radiologically, its features include a solid mass with homogeneous enhancement; a central stellate scar that may be visible on US, CE-CT, or MRI; and a spoked-wheel pattern on angiography.[282-284] These findings are nonspecific,

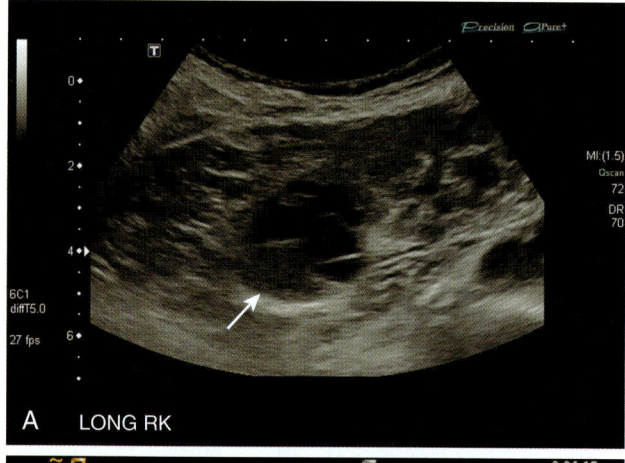

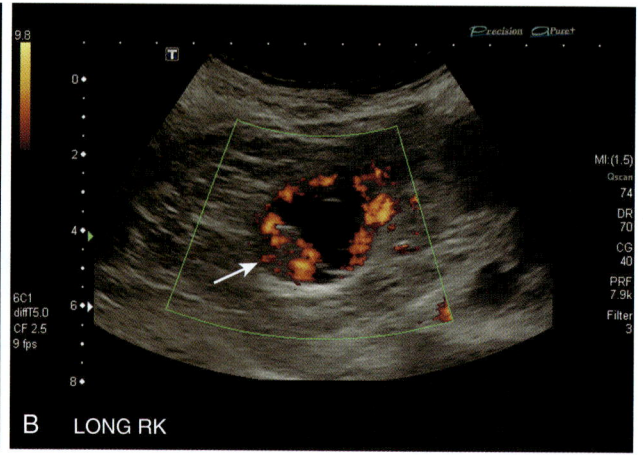

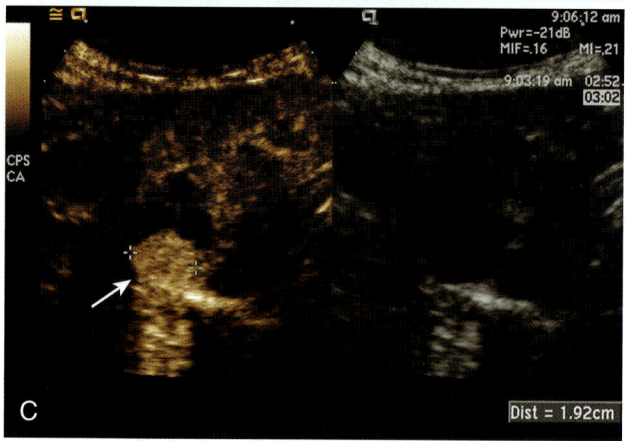

Figure 28.77 A Bosniak category IV cyst in a 58-year-old woman. **A,** Gray-scale ultrasonogram reveals a complex cyst with a solid nodular component (*arrow*). **B,** Power Doppler image reveals flow within the nodular component of the lesion (*arrow*), confirming its vascularized nature. **C,** Composite image including a contrast material–enhanced image on the left and a gray-scale image on the right. The nodule (*arrow*) reveals dense arterial phase enhancement with heterogeneous washout. The findings were consistent with a neoplastic cyst. The lesion was subsequently resected and was found to be a clear cell carcinoma, Fuhrman grade 2.

however, and histologic confirmation is needed.[285,286] Oncocytic renal cell carcinomas also occur, and surgery is generally needed for the correct diagnosis.

Renal cell carcinoma is the third most common tumor of the genitourinary tract after carcinoma of the prostate and bladder. CE-CT is the modality of choice for imaging renal cell carcinoma because it has proved to be effective in detection, diagnosis, characterization, and staging, with accuracy exceeding 90%.[287,288] On noncontrast CT, renal cell carcinoma appears as an ill-defined area in the kidney with HU close to that of the renal parenchyma (Figure 28.79). After the injection of intravenous contrast material, most renal cell carcinomas show enhancement. The best phase for depiction of the mass is the nephrographic phase (see Figure 28.79).[289-291] The corticomedullary phase is most helpful for showing the relationship of the tumor to the vascular structures because there is maximal enhancement of the arteries and veins (Figure 28.80).[292,293] The excretory phase is most helpful for showing the relationship of the tumor to the pelvicalyceal system and in preoperative planning for nephron-sparing partial nephrectomy (see Figure 28.79).[294,295] Clear cell renal cell carcinoma tends to have greater and more heterogenous enhancement than the papillary types (see Figures 28.79 and 28.80).[296,297] Chromophobe tumors typically have a homogeneous enhancement pattern (see Figure 28.79).[296] Chromophobe and papillary types more often contain calcification than does the clear cell type, and they demonstrate only mild enhancement of 25 to 30 HU.[298]

The appearance of renal cell carcinoma on MRI can vary with the histologic type. For example, the clear cell type tends to be larger and is associated more frequently with hemorrhage and necrosis (Figures 28.81 and 28.82) than is the papillary type (Figure 28.83) and chromophobe renal cell carcinoma. The feasibility of differentiating histologic types of renal cell carcinoma by means of advanced MRI techniques such as diffusion weighting is being evaluated, but further research is required.[299] Renal cell carcinoma is most commonly heterogeneously hyperintense on T2-weighted sequences and hypointense to isointense on T1-weighted sequences (Figure 28.84). Renal cell carcinoma enhances less than normal renal cortex tissue. The heterogeneity increases with increasing size as a result of variable amounts of necrosis and intraluminal lipid. The intraluminal lipid may make areas of the mass drop in signal intensity on opposed-phase T1-weighted sequences.

The staging of renal cell carcinoma is important in predicting survival rates and planning the proper surgical approach to the mass. Both the World Health Organization and the Robson classifications are used in the staging of renal cell carcinoma.[287] In the Robson classification of renal cell carcinoma, a stage I tumor is confined to the renal parenchyma by the renal capsule (see Figure 28.79). In stage II renal cell carcinoma, the tumor extends through the renal capsule into the perinephric fat but is still within Gerota's fascia (see Figure 28.80). Stage III lesions are subdivided: IIIA tumors extend into the renal vein or IVC

Text continued on p. 898

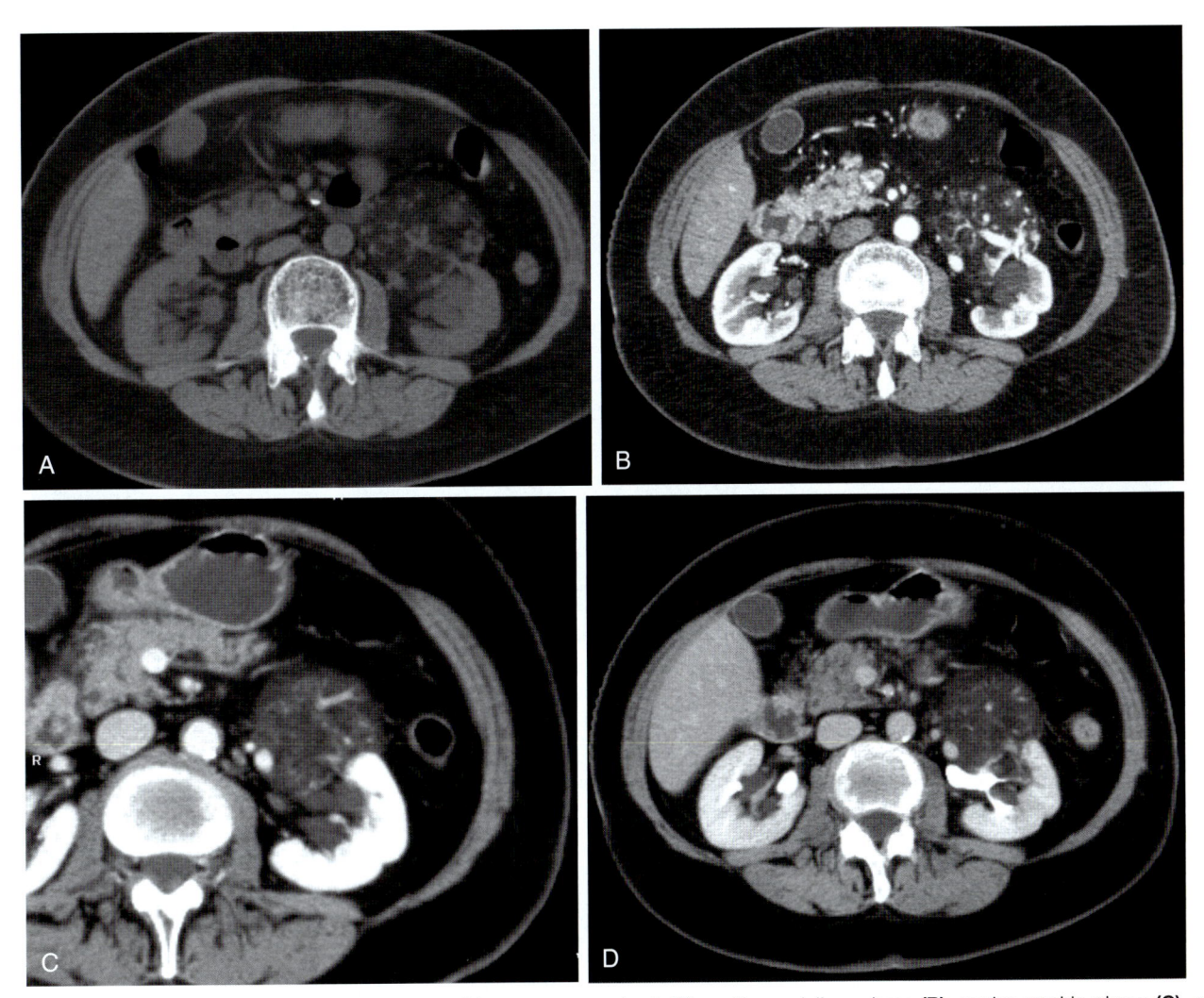

Figure 28.78 Angiomyolipoma: computed tomographic scan, noncontrast **(A)**, corticomedullary phase **(B)**, nephrographic phase **(C)**, and excretory phase **(D)** axial images. The fat-containing mass is visible projecting anteriorly from the left kidney. The internal structure in this very vascular benign tumor demonstrates enhancement.

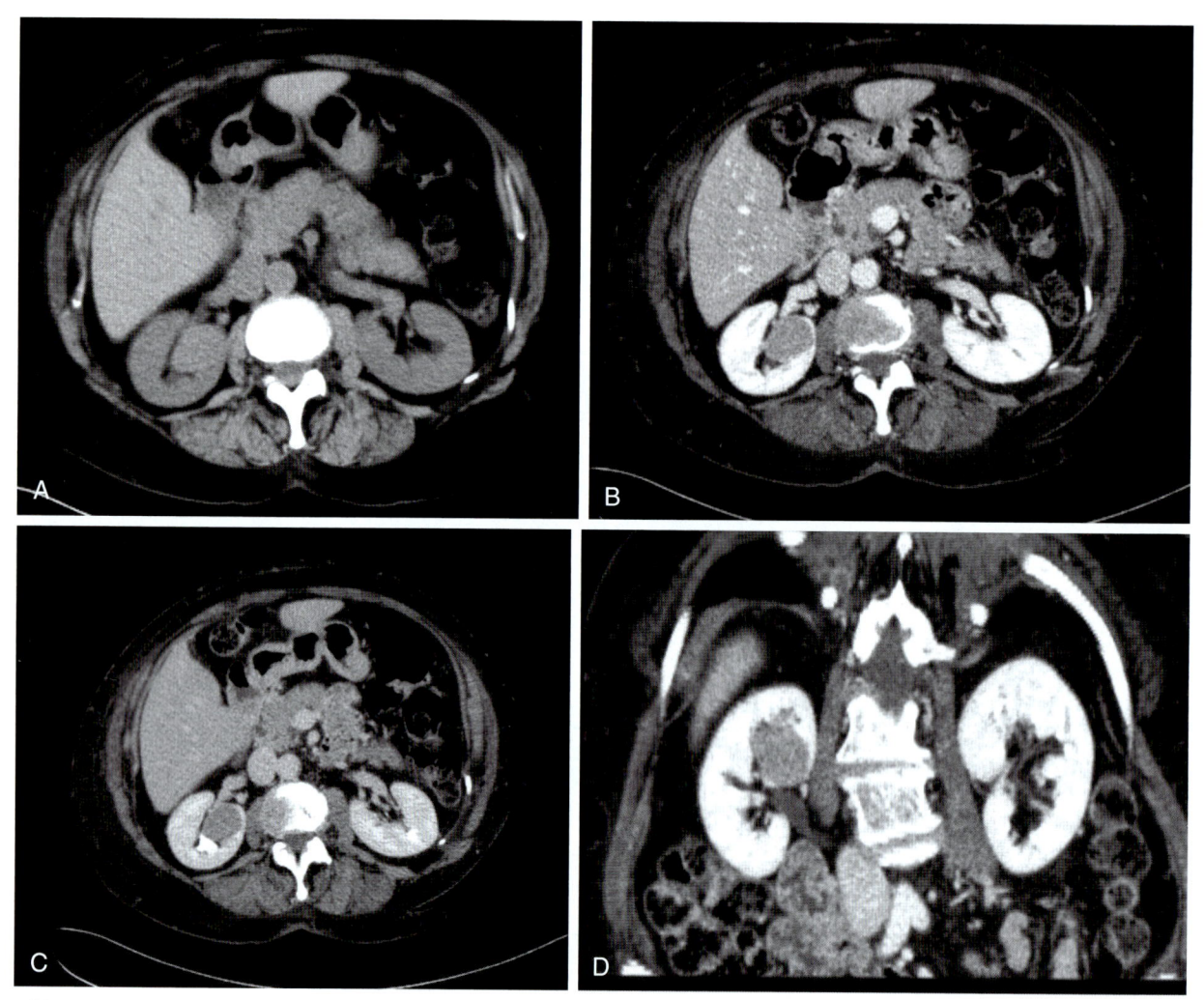

Figure 28.79 Renal cell carcinoma: computed tomographic scan. Noncontrast **(A)**, nephrographic phase **(B)**, and excretory phase **(C)** axial images combined with a coronal nephrographic phase image **(D)**. On the noncontrast scan **(A)**, the right renal mass appears slightly hyperdense in relation to the rest of the kidney. Contrast material–enhanced scans **(B, C,** and **D)** show the enhanced structure surrounded by the normal renal parenchyma. This proved to be a renal cell carcinoma, chromophobe type.

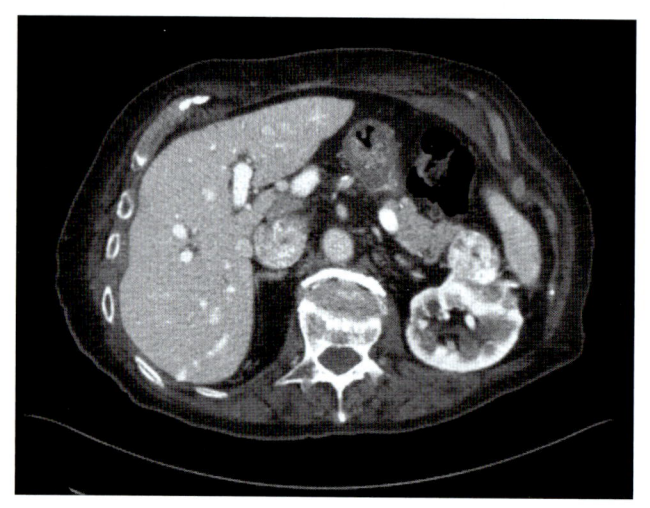

Figure 28.80 Renal cell carcinoma: computed tomographic scan. Contrast material–enhanced axial image in the corticomedullary phase. Note the heterogeneously enhanced mass in the anterior aspect of the left kidney. This is a stage II renal cell carcinoma, inasmuch as it has extended through the renal capsule into Gerota's fascia. This proved to be a renal cell carcinoma, clear cell type.

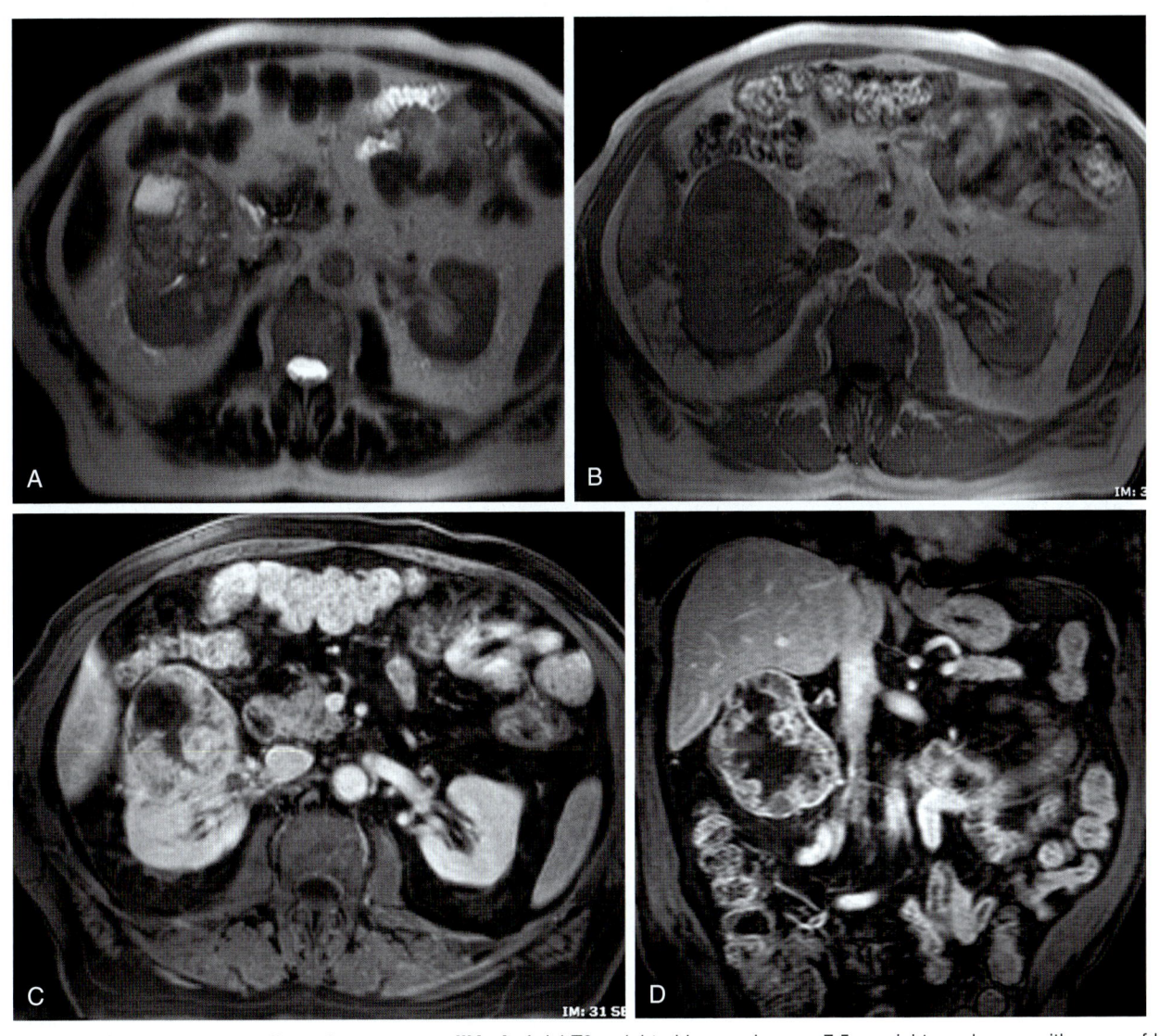

Figure 28.81 Clear cell renal cell carcinoma, stage IIIA. A, Axial T2-weighted image shows a 7.5-cm right renal mass with areas of high signal intensity, consistent with necrosis and cystic degeneration. **B,** Axial T1-weighted image shows a heterogeneous, isointense mass with increased perinephric fat stranding. Axial **(C)** and coronal **(D)** gadolinium-enhanced images confirm central areas of necrosis. No venous invasion is visible. Focal microinvasion of the perinephric fat was found at surgery.

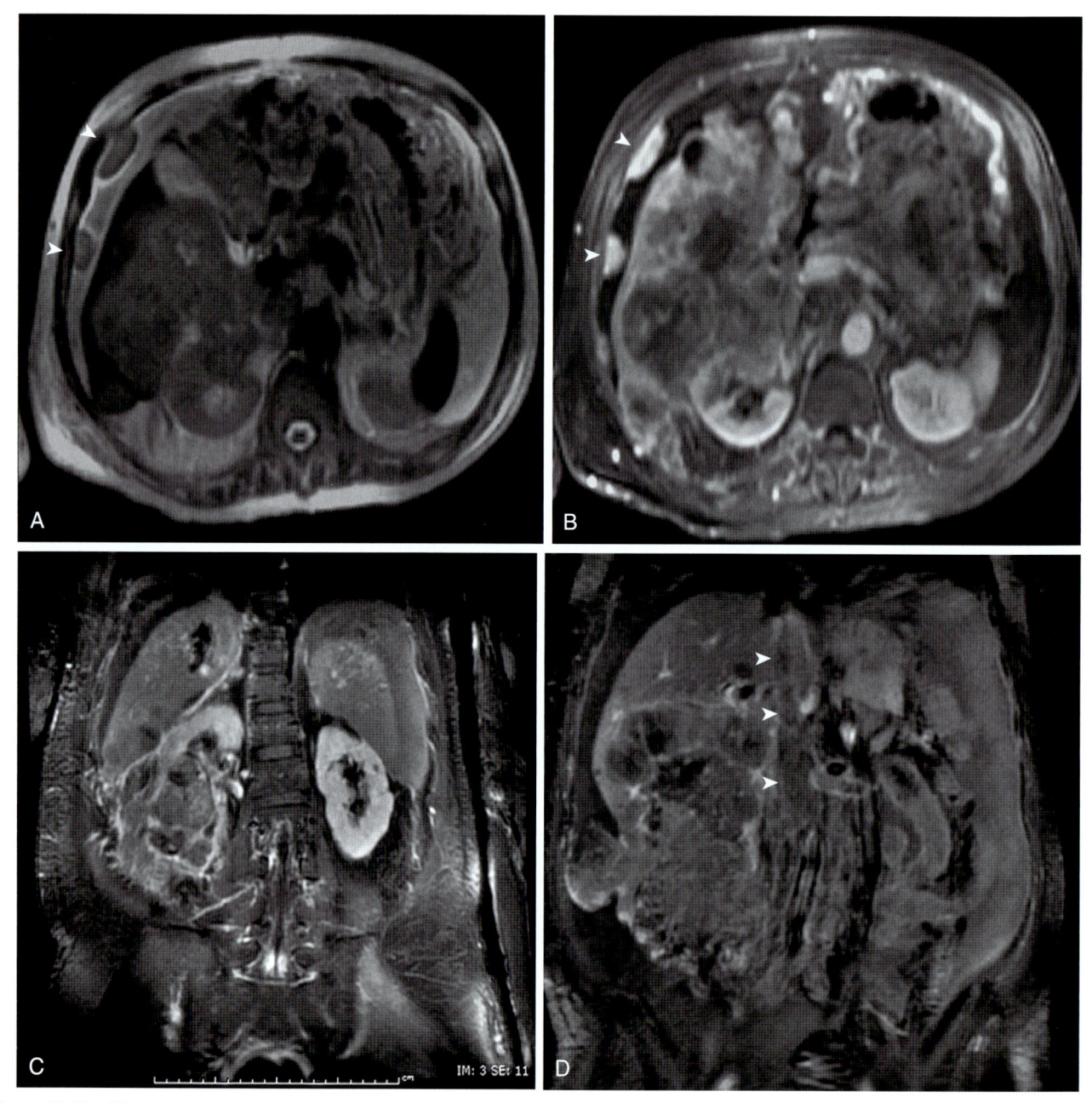

Figure 28.82 Metastatic clear cell renal cell carcinoma, stage IV. T2-weighted **(A)** and gadolinium-enhanced T1-weighted **(B)** axial images show a large, heterogeneous mass with invasion of the adjacent liver and peritoneal metastases (*arrowheads*). **C** and **D,** Coronal gadolinium-enhanced T1-weighted images show the large mass extending inferiorly and medially, with invasion of the inferior vena cava to the level of the hepatic veins (*arrowheads*).

CHAPTER 28 — DIAGNOSTIC KIDNEY IMAGING   897

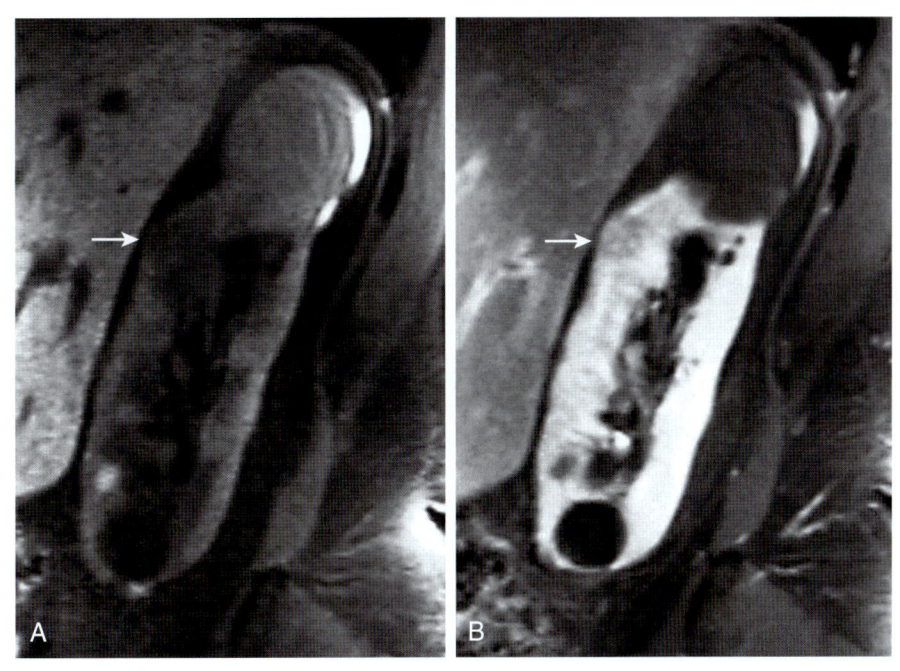

Figure 28.83 **Papillary renal cell carcinoma, stage I.** Sagittal T1-weighted images before **(A)** and after **(B)** the administration of gadolinium show a subtle mass (*arrow*) in the anterior cortex and multiple nonenhanced cysts. No perinephric invasion was found at surgery.

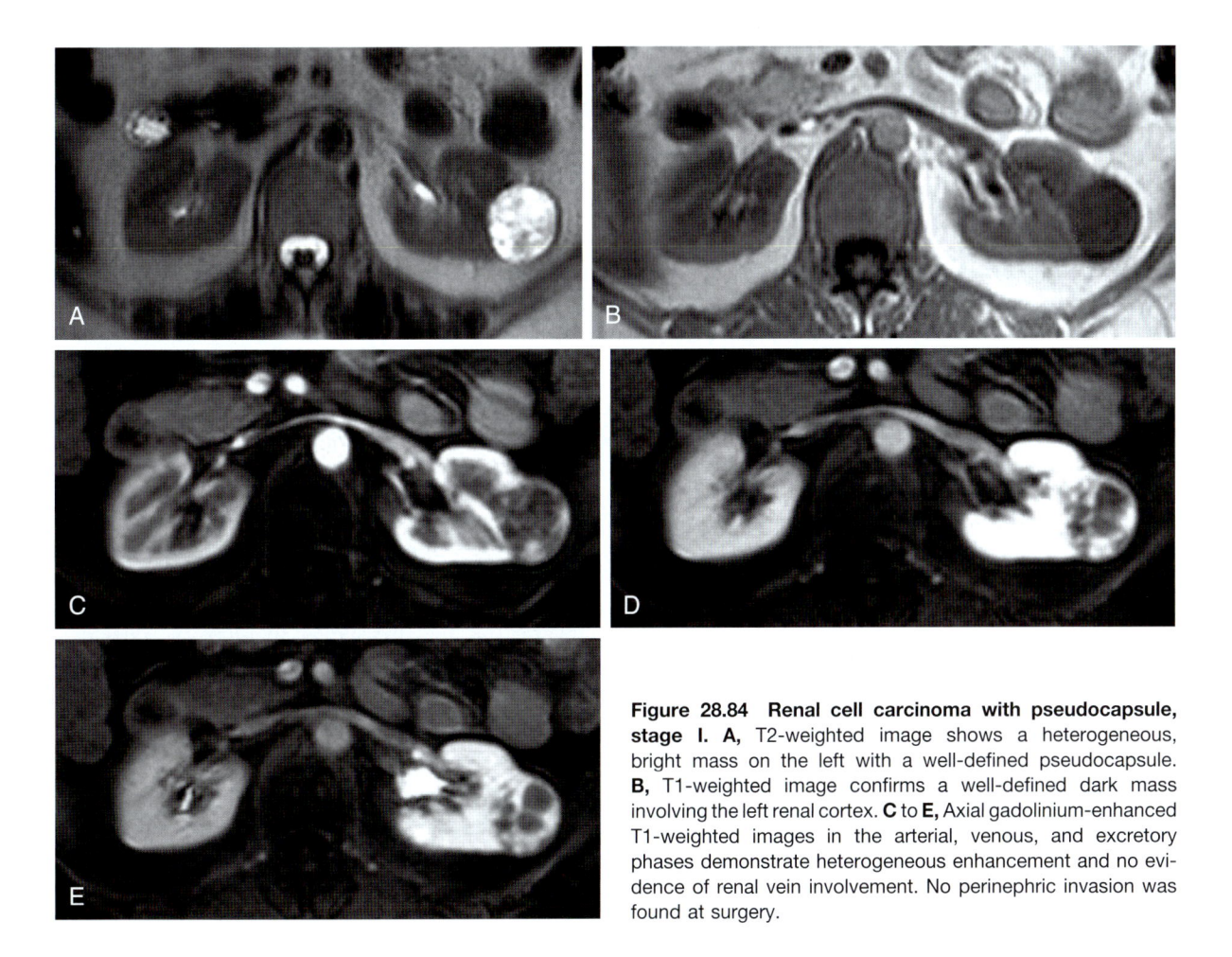

Figure 28.84 **Renal cell carcinoma with pseudocapsule, stage I. A,** T2-weighted image shows a heterogeneous, bright mass on the left with a well-defined pseudocapsule. **B,** T1-weighted image confirms a well-defined dark mass involving the left renal cortex. **C** to **E,** Axial gadolinium-enhanced T1-weighted images in the arterial, venous, and excretory phases demonstrate heterogeneous enhancement and no evidence of renal vein involvement. No perinephric invasion was found at surgery.

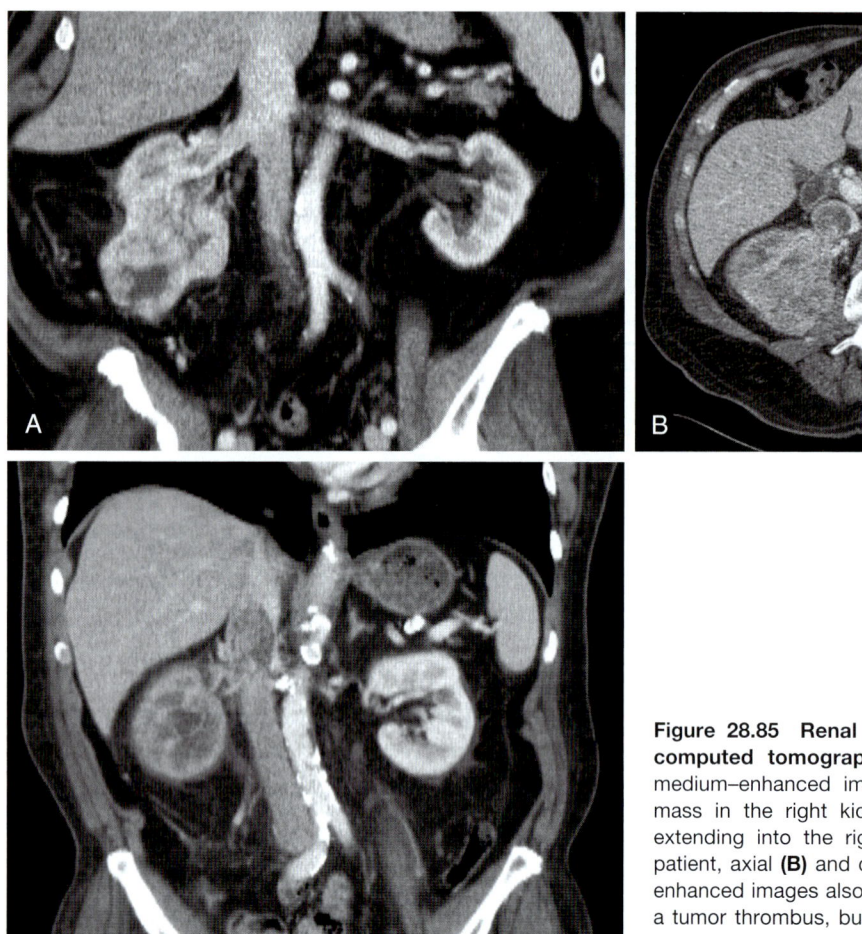

Figure 28.85 Renal cell carcinoma, stage IIIA: computed tomographic scan. Coronal contrast medium–enhanced image **(A)** shows a stage IIIA mass in the right kidney and a tumor thrombus extending into the right renal vein. In a different patient, axial **(B)** and coronal **(C)** contrast medium–enhanced images also show a right renal mass with a tumor thrombus, but the thrombus has extended into the inferior vena cava. Both these tumors proved to be of the clear cell type.

(Figure 28.85); IIIB tumors involve regional retroperitoneal lymph nodes; and IIIC tumors involve the veins and nodes (see Figure 28.85). In stage IVA renal cell carcinoma, the tumor extends outside Gerota's fascia with involvement of adjacent organs or muscles other than the ipsilateral adrenal gland. Stage IVB renal cell carcinoma represents tumor with distant metastases, the most common sites being the lungs, mediastinum, liver, and bone.

MRI has been found to be highly accurate in staging renal cell carcinoma; however, as with CT, the areas of greatest challenge remain the evaluation for local invasion of the perinephric fat and direct invasion of adjacent organs, especially with large tumors.[300] The presence of an intact pseudocapsule aids in ruling out local invasion. A pseudocapsule is a hypointense rim around the tumor, viewed best on T2-weighted images (see Figure 28.84A) and most frequently observed in association with small or slow-growing tumors. When the tumor extends beyond the confines of the kidney, the pseudocapsule is made of fibrous tissue; otherwise it is made up of compressed normal renal tissue.[301] If the pseudocapsule is intact, the perinephric fat is unlikely to have been invaded.[301]

Detecting and assessing vascular thrombosis in patients with renal cell carcinoma is highly accurate and reliable with MRI.[300,302] Coronal imaging in the venous and delayed phases demonstrates the presence or absence of venous invasion; determines the extent of venous invasion, if present; and differentiates enhancing intravascular tumor from nonenhanced bland thrombus (Figure 28.86). Accurate determination of renal vein, IVC, and right atrial involvement is important for deciding the surgical approach.[303]

Although renal cell carcinoma is the most common primary malignancy in the kidney, transitional cell carcinoma also occurs within the kidneys.[304] Most transitional cell carcinomas involve the urothelium and project into the lumen of the renal pelvis or ureter. As a result, IVU images show a filling defect within the renal pelvis or ureter that can be confused with a renal stone, blood clot, or debris (Figure 28.87). Transitional cell carcinoma of the bladder is much more common than that of the kidney or ureter.[305] The neoplasm may extend into the renal parenchyma and, on imaging, appears as a mass within the kidney. The imaging findings are similar to those of renal cell carcinoma, except the lesions tend not to enhance as much on postcontrast imaging. Renal vein involvement is rare. CTU and MRU show similar findings: transitional cell carcinoma in the upper collecting system can be either a focal or irregular mass within the collecting system (Figure 28.88) or an ill-defined mass infiltrating the renal parenchyma. When small, they may be difficult to identify on both CT and MRI. Evaluation of the entire collecting system is required because synchronous lesions may be present. Both CTU and MRU are valuable for complete evaluation of the

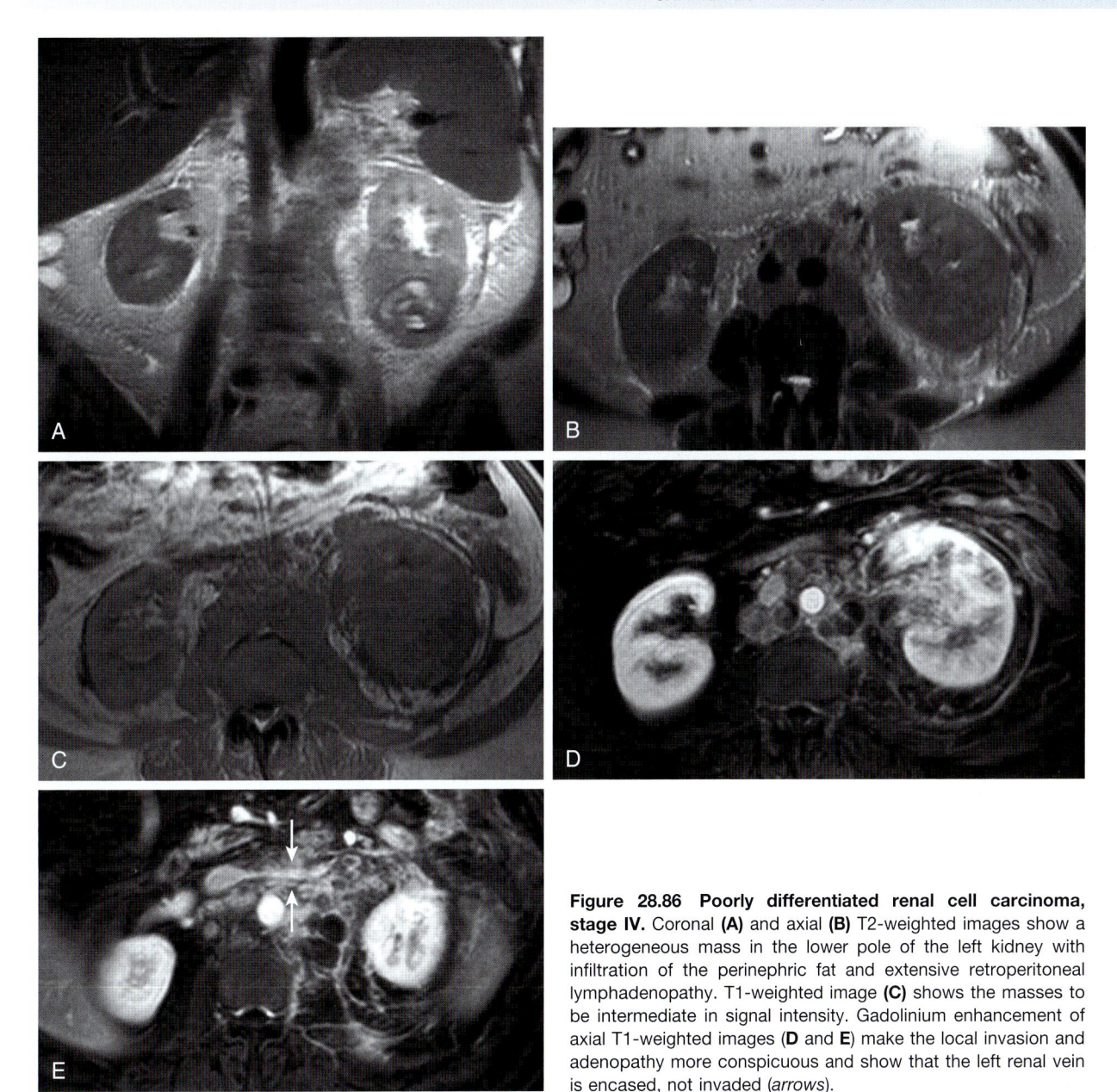

Figure 28.86 Poorly differentiated renal cell carcinoma, stage IV. Coronal **(A)** and axial **(B)** T2-weighted images show a heterogeneous mass in the lower pole of the left kidney with infiltration of the perinephric fat and extensive retroperitoneal lymphadenopathy. T1-weighted image **(C)** shows the masses to be intermediate in signal intensity. Gadolinium enhancement of axial T1-weighted images **(D** and **E)** make the local invasion and adenopathy more conspicuous and show that the left renal vein is encased, not invaded (*arrows*).

collecting system; however, retrograde pyelography with ureteroscopy and biopsy will make the diagnosis.

Lymphoma may involve the kidney as part of multiorgan involvement or, in rare cases, as a primary neoplasm.[306] Lymphoma may be solitary or multifocal, within one or both kidneys. Perirenal extension may be visible as well. An infiltrative picture with lymphomatous replacement of the kidney may also be observed. This form is usually accompanied by adjacent retroperitoneal adenopathy. CE-CT is the imaging method of choice in these patients. MRI findings are similar to those on CE-CT. Lymphoma typically appears hypointense on T1-weighted sequences and heterogeneous to slightly hypointense on T2-weighted sequences. Enhancement is minimal on postcontrast sequences[307] (Figure 28.89). Vessels are usually encased, not invaded, and necrosis is usually not observed. Treated lymphoma may vary in signal intensity, as a result of the effects of therapy.[307]

Metastatic disease may also involve the kidney. Metastases are most commonly hematogenous and usually result in multiple foci of involvement, although single lesions do occur (Figure 28.90). They are observed most frequently with CE-CT, inasmuch as CT is used in the regular follow-up of most patients with cancer. Hypodense round masses, usually in the periphery, are the typical finding. When present as a single lesion, a metastasis cannot be differentiated from a primary renal neoplasm without biopsy.

RENAL CANCER: POSITRON EMISSION TOMOGRAPHY AND POSITRON EMISSION TOMOGRAPHY–COMPUTED TOMOGRAPHY

Preliminary studies of PET imaging of renal cell carcinoma have revealed a promising role in the evaluation of indeterminate renal masses; preoperative staging and assessment of tumor burden; detection of osseous and nonosseous

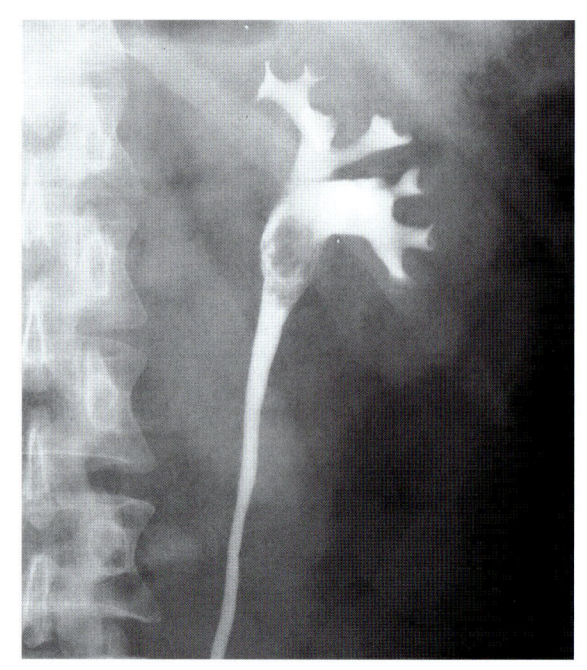

Figure 28.87 Transitional cell carcinoma: intravenous urogram. The irregular filling defect in the left renal pelvis represents a transitional cell carcinoma. Note that there is no significant obstruction of the left kidney, and the calyces appear normal.

metastases (including vascular invasion); restaging after therapy; treatment evaluation; and the determination of effect of imaging findings on clinical management.[308-320] However, other PET studies have demonstrated less encouraging results and no advantage over standard imaging methods.[321-323]

A relatively high false-negative rate (23%) has been reported with FDG-PET in the preoperative staging of renal cell carcinoma in comparison with histologic analysis of surgical specimens. In one study, PET exhibited 60% sensitivity (versus 91.7% for CT) and 100% specificity (versus 100% for CT) for primary renal cell carcinoma tumors. For retroperitoneal lymph node metastases or renal bed recurrence, PET had 75.0% sensitivity (versus 92.6% for CT) and 100% specificity (versus 98.1% for CT). For metastases to the lung parenchyma, PET had 75% sensitivity (versus 91.1% for chest CT) and 97.1% specificity (versus 73.1% for chest CT). For bone metastases, PET had 77.3% sensitivity and 100% specificity (in comparison with 93.8% and 87.2% for combined CT and bone scan).[324] For restaging renal cell carcinoma, 87% sensitivity and 100% specificity have been reported.[325] A comparative investigation of bone scan and FDG-PET for detecting osseous metastases in renal cell carcinoma revealed that PET had 100% sensitivity (versus 77.5% for bone scan) and 100% specificity (versus 59.6% for bone scan).[313] Another report revealed a negative predictive value of 33% and a positive predictive value of 94% for restaging renal cell carcinoma.[309] Other studies have revealed high accuracy in characterizing indeterminate renal masses, with a mean tumor-to-kidney uptake ratio of 3.0 for malignancy.[308]

These mixed observations are probably related to the heterogeneous expression of glucose transporter 1 in renal cell carcinoma, which may not be correlated with the tumor grade or extent.[326,327] Negative study findings may not rule out disease, whereas a positive result is highly suspect for malignancy.[328] If the tumor binds FDG avidly, then PET can be a reasonable imaging modality for follow-up after treatment and for surveillance (Figure 28.91). In fact, it has been shown that FDG-PET can alter clinical management in up to 40% of patients with suspected locally recurrent and metastatic renal cancer.[311] A meta-analysis of 14 published studies on the diagnostic utility of FDG-PET (FDG PET-CT) in renal cell carcinoma reported a pooled sensitivity of 62% and a pooled specificity of 88% for renal lesions.[329]

Because FDG is excreted in the urine, the intense urine activity may confound lesion detection in and near the renal bed. Intravenous administration of furosemide has been proposed to improve urine clearance from the renal collecting system, although the exact benefit of such intervention in improving lesion detection remains undefined.

Many investigators since have reported on the unique diagnostic synergism of the combined PET-CT imaging systems.[330] Studies have demonstrated that FDG PET-CT has a sensitivity of 46.6% and specificity of 66.6% for primary renal cell carcinoma in the imaging evaluation of indeterminate renal masses.[331] In a study by Park and colleagues in South Korea, 63 patients with renal cell carcinoma underwent both FDG PET-CT and conventional imaging evaluation during follow-up after surgical treatment.[334] FDG PET-CT demonstrated 89.5% sensitivity, 83.3% specificity, a positive predictive value of 77.3%, and a negative predictive value of 92.6% in detecting recurrent and metastatic disease; these values were not significantly different from the diagnostic performance of conventional imaging studies. Park and colleagues concluded that FDG PET-CT can replace multiple conventional imaging studies without the need for contrast agents. The role of PET-CT in renal cancer imaging and its effect on both short- and long-term clinical management and decision making also must be investigated.

Studies have demonstrated that PET-CT might be potentially useful in treatment response evaluation and prognostication. One Japanese group of investigators reported on the use of FDG PET-CT in early assessment of therapy response to tyrosine kinase inhibitors in 35 patients with advanced renal cell carcinoma.[333] These authors found that improved progression-free survival and overall survival were both associated with favorable response to therapy (defined as decline in tumor maximum standardized uptake value by 20% or more from pretreatment scan to the scan obtained 1 month after completion of therapy). Similar findings have been reported by other investigators.[334-338] One study reported that although FDG PET-CT may be helpful in assessing treatment response to chemotherapy, it may not be useful in monitoring response to immunotherapy, such as with interferon alfa monotherapy or in combination with interleukin-2 and 5-fluorouracil.[339] Moreover, other studies have shown that the higher the FDG uptake in the renal cancer lesions, the higher the mortality.[340,341]

Other tracers used in PET (e.g., carbon 11–labeled acetate [^{11}C-acetate], ^{18}F labeled fluoromisonidazole [^{18}F-FMISO], ^{18}F–labeled sodium fluoride) have been investigated in the imaging evaluation of patients with renal cell carcinoma, but further studies are needed to establish the exact role of these and other non-FDG tracers in this clinical setting.[342-345] For example, one study revealed high accumulation of ^{11}C-acetate

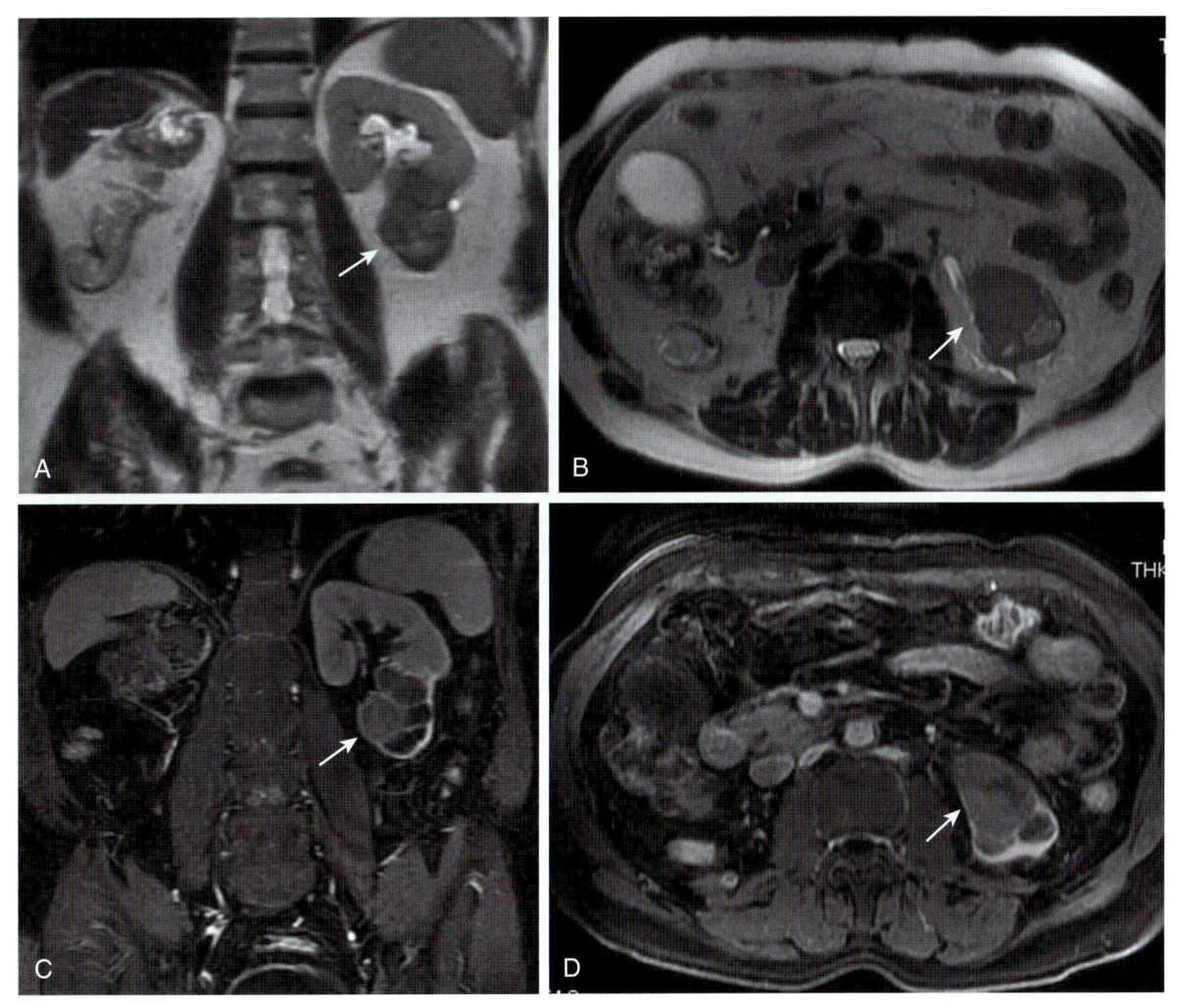

Figure 28.88 Transitional cell carcinoma. Coronal **(A)** and axial **(B)** T2-weighted images show intermediate signal intensity and an infiltrating mass (*arrow*) within the atrophic lower pole moiety of a duplicated left kidney. Coronal **(C)** and axial **(D)** gadolinium-enhanced T1-weighted images show enhancing material within dilated calyces and pelvis of the lower pole moiety (*arrow*). The cortical atrophy is well demonstrated.

in 70% of renal cell carcinomas.[346] However, an earlier similar study had demonstrated that in most kidney tumors, accumulation of ^{11}C-acetate was not higher than in normal renal parenchyma.[347] Aside from renal cell carcinoma, ^{11}C-acetate has also been demonstrated to be useful in the imaging-based assessment of renal oxygen consumption and tubular sodium reabsorption.[348] Another investigation using a dual-tracer (^{11}C-acetate and FDG) method showed that AMLs are highly avid for ^{11}C-acetate but not at all for FDG. The uptake of ^{11}C-acetate in renal cell cancer was lower than that in AML. In fact this study suggested that ^{11}C-acetate may be useful in differentiating "fat-poor angiomyolipoma" from renal cell cancer with a sensitivity of 93.8% and specificity of 98%.[349] ^{11}C-acetate has also been found to be potentially useful in early prediction of response to the tyrosine kinase inhibitor, sunitinib, in patients with metastatic renal cell carcinoma.[350]

Murakami and associates used the hypoxia imaging probe ^{18}F-FMISO in preclinical models of renal cell carcinoma to show that ^{18}F-FMISO hypoxia imaging can confirm "tumor starvation" as the mechanistic explanation for tumor response to anti-angiogenic therapy.[353] A pilot clinical study with ^{18}F-FMISO also showed that patients with hypoxic metastatic tumors have shorter progression-free survival than those with nonhypoxic tumors.[352]

Other tracers that have been investigated include iodine 124 (^{124}I)– and zirconium 89–labeled anti–carbonic anhydrase IX monoclonal antibody that is avid to clear cell renal cell carcinoma.[353] An early trial of the ^{124}I-labeled compound for detection of clear cell renal cell carcinoma (with histopathology as reference standard) showed an average sensitivity and specificity of 86.2% and 85.9%, respectively, for PET-CT, which were statistically higher than sensitivity and specificity of 75.5% and 46.8%, respectively, for CE-CT.[354]

Schuster and coworkers reported on their initial experience with anti-1-amino-3-^{18}F-fluorocyclobutane-1-carboxylic acid, which is a nonmetabolized synthetic L-leucine analog with low urinary excretion, in the imaging evaluation of renal cell carcinoma.[357] Their preliminary results in six patients showed that the uptake of this amino acid–based radiotracer may be elevated in renal papillary cell carcinoma but not in clear cell carcinoma.

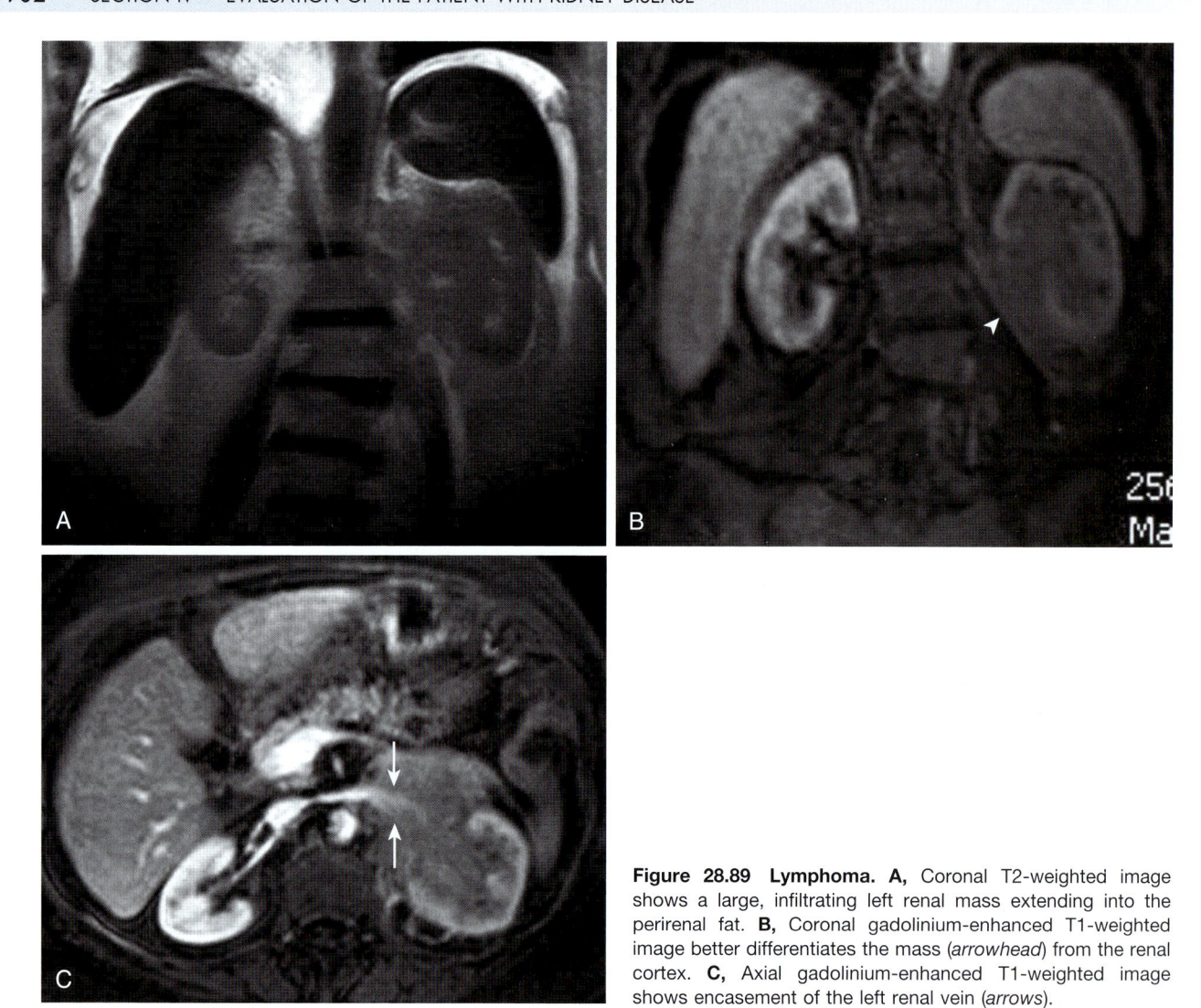

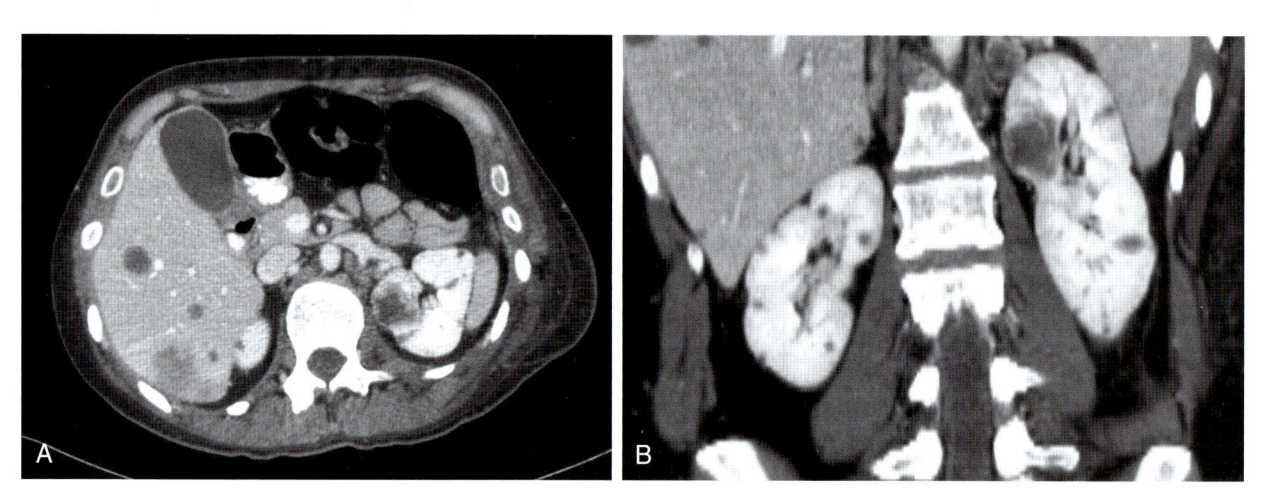

Figure 28.89 Lymphoma. A, Coronal T2-weighted image shows a large, infiltrating left renal mass extending into the perirenal fat. **B,** Coronal gadolinium-enhanced T1-weighted image better differentiates the mass (*arrowhead*) from the renal cortex. **C,** Axial gadolinium-enhanced T1-weighted image shows encasement of the left renal vein (*arrows*).

Figure 28.90 Metastases to the kidney: computed tomographic scan. Axial **(A)** and coronal **(B)** contrast material–enhanced images in the nephrographic phase. Multiple heterogeneous but hypodense lesions are visible in the kidneys bilaterally; the largest is in the left upper pole. These appeared in a 2-month period in a patient with metastatic lung carcinoma. Note the metastases also present in the liver.

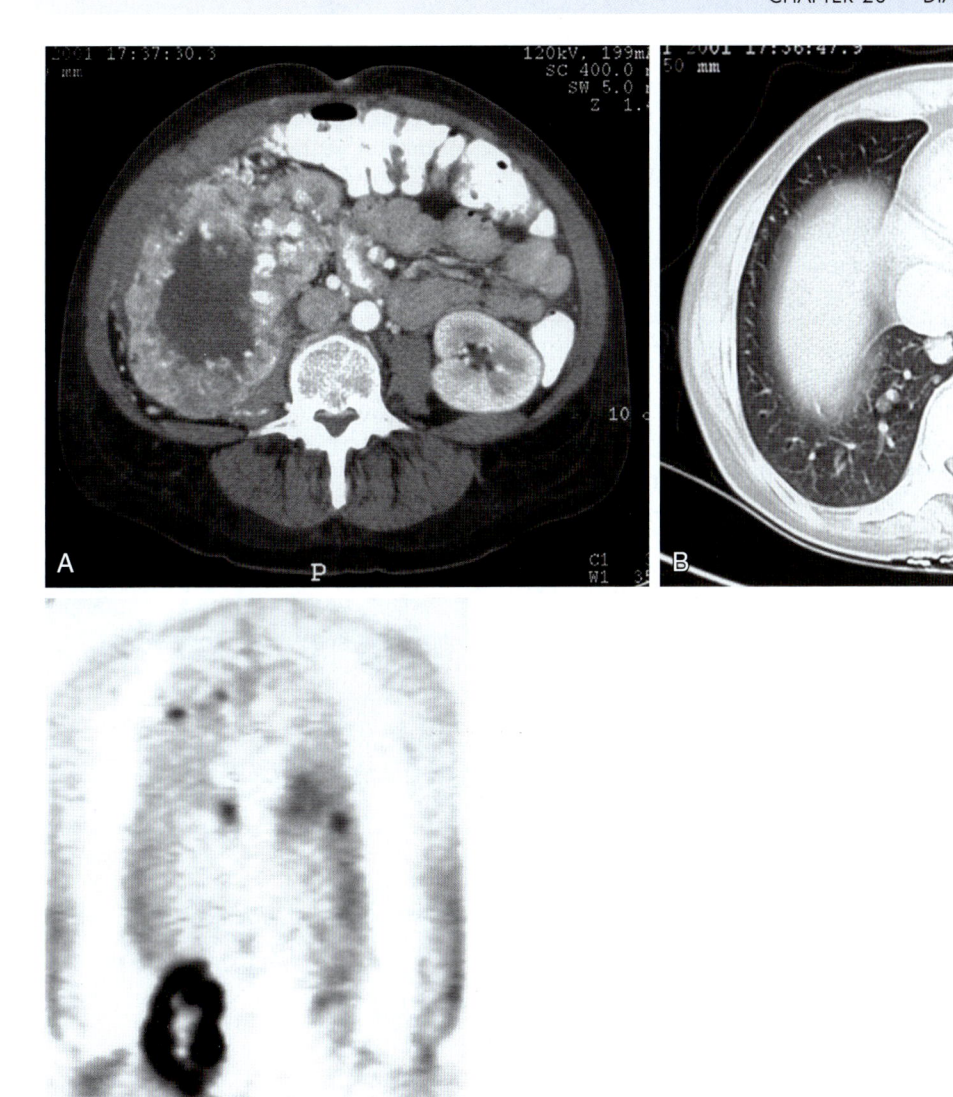

Figure 28.91 Renal cell carcinoma. Computed tomography shows a large necrotic renal mass **(A)** with several bilateral pulmonary nodules **(B)**. The positron emission tomographic scan **(C)** shows hypermetabolism at the periphery of the large renal mass and within the pulmonary nodules. The interior hypometabolism of the renal mass is compatible with central tumor necrosis.

Other uses of PET in the imaging evaluation of renal perfusion, function, and metabolism have also been investigated.[356] In addition, there is some effort to evaluate the role of radiolabeled antibodies as therapeutic agents in the treatment of renal cell carcinoma.[357]

RENAL VASCULAR DISEASE

Diagnostic imaging for hypertension depends on the clinical index of suspicion for renovascular hypertension, which is found in less than 5% of the hypertensive population, but the percentage is higher in those with severe hypertension and ESKD.[358] The most common cause of renovascular hypertension is renal artery stenosis (RAS), with approximately 90% of cases due to atherosclerosis and approximately 10% due to fibromuscular dysplasia. The diagnosis of RAS at the time of screening has been problematic, because the preintervention definition of significant RAS has varied. Significant RAS is best defined as a fall in blood pressure *after intervention*. According to the ACR, in patients with normal renal function in whom RAS is suspected, MRA or CTA is usually appropriate. Doppler US or ACE-inhibitor scintigraphy is appropriate if MRA is not desired or contraindicated, and conventional angiography is reserved for confirmation of RAS and definitive therapy. IVU has no role in the evaluation for RAS.[359]

Doppler US is a noninvasive screening test that can be used independent of the patient's renal function. In experienced hands, US has been reported to have high sensitivity and specificity; however, sensitivities have been reported as low as 0%. US screening can be technically challenging and therefore should be performed only in centers where US screening has been proven to be reliable and where there are dedicated technologists and physicians. In such centers 75% to 80% of scans are technically adequate.

Doppler US has been used with variable success to assess the main renal arteries for RAS and the intrarenal vasculature for secondary effects.[360,361] The success of Doppler US is highly operator dependent, and results may be inadequate or incomplete because of overlying bowel gas, body habitus, or aortic pulsatility.[360] A stable Doppler signal may be difficult to reproduce in some patients with renovascular hypertension. A complete examination has been possible in 50% to 90% of affected patients. Variant anatomy may also be a challenge; accessory renal arteries, which occur in 15% to 20% of affected patients, may not be imaged.[362]

The criteria used for evaluation of the main renal artery include an increase in the peak systolic velocity to more than 180 cm/sec, a renal/aortic ratio of peak systolic velocity of more than 3.0, and turbulent flow beyond the region of the stenosis.[363] Visualization of the main renal artery with no detectable Doppler signal is suggestive of renal artery occlusion. Intrarenal vascular assessment with Doppler US has depicted the shape and character of the waveform. A dampened appearance of the waveform, with a slowed systolic upstroke and delay to peak velocity (tardus-parvus), has been shown in varying degrees in RAS.[364] Using resistive indices, a difference between the kidneys of more than 5% has also been suggestive of RAS. Sensitivity and specificity for the techniques have generally been in the range of 50% to 70%. CEUS has been suggested as a means of improving the accuracy of Doppler US.[365,366]

CTA performed with MDCT has sensitivity and specificity at or near 100% (Figure 28.92).[367-369] CTA is an effective alternative to Doppler US and MRA. When compared to MRA, CTA has higher spatial resolution and shorter examination times. CTA evaluates calcified and noncalcified atherosclerotic plaques and may be used to assess stent grafts (Figure 28.93).[370,371] A normal result should rule out RAS[372] (Figures 28.94 and 28.95). The main renal artery, as well as its segmental branches, can be viewed and evaluated. Accessory renal arteries as small as 1 mm in diameter can be seen.[373] CTA and MRA are of equivalent quality in the detection of hemodynamically significant RAS.[374] Both CTA and MRA can demonstrate renal cortical volume and thickness as well as secondary signs of RAS, including poststenotic dilation, renal atrophy, and decreased cortical enhancement.

Because CTA is sensitive, accurate, fast, and reproducible, MRA is reserved for patients for whom iodinated contrast material is contraindicated. Renal insufficiency is not uncommon in the population clinically at high risk for RAS. For this reason, MRA has been widely accepted as a reliable and accurate examination in the evaluation of RAS in this population.[109,374-376] CE-MRA is being used more selectively, given the risk for NSF in patients with CKD stage 4 and 5. Noncontrast MRA techniques are being used more frequently to reduce the amount of Gd-C needed. Like CTA, MRA is noninvasive and provides excellent visualization of the aortoiliac and renal arteries.[374]

CE-MRA is more than 95% sensitive in demonstrating the main renal arteries and has a high negative predictive value. A normal CE-MRA finding almost completely rules out a stenosis in the visualized vessels.[377] CE-MRA is a reliable examination but has been limited by incomplete visualization of segmental and small accessory vessels.[378] Whereas

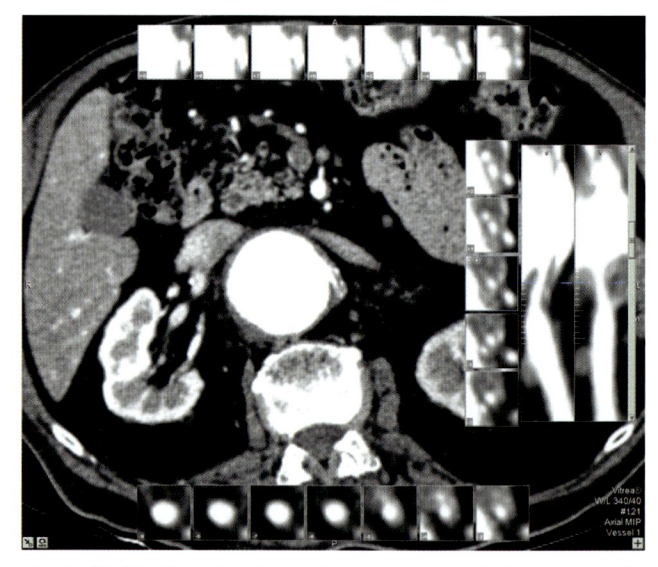

Figure 28.92 Renal artery stenosis: computed tomographic angiogram, axial image with vessel analysis. The origin of the left renal artery is markedly narrowed by calcified and noncalcified atherosclerotic plaque. The vessel analysis demonstrates the renal artery in cross section for accurate calculation of the degree of stenosis, which in this case was greater than 70%.

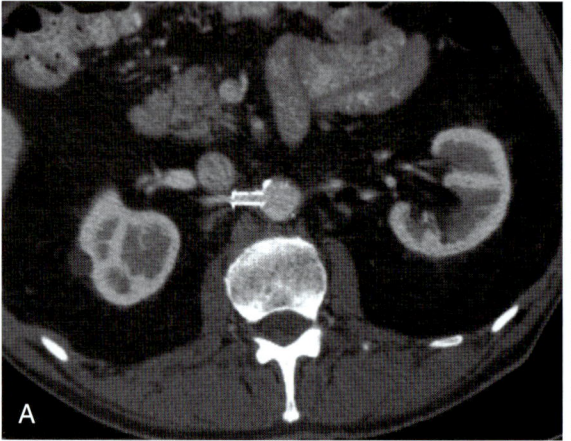

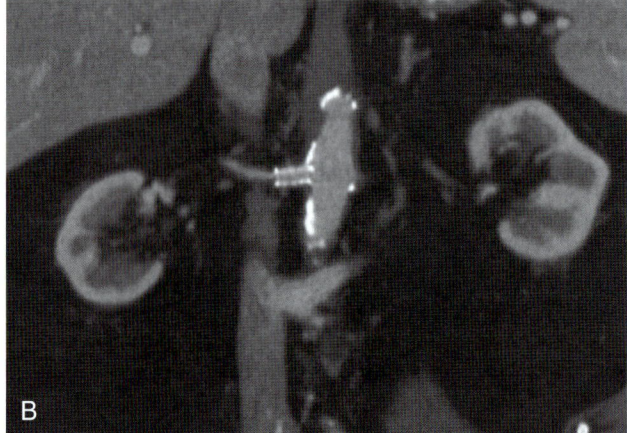

Figure 28.93 Renal artery stent: computed tomographic scan. Axial **(A)** and coronal **(B)** images of a contrast material–enhanced scan in the corticomedullary phase. The metallic stent is visible at the origin of the right renal artery. It had been placed for treatment of renal artery stenosis that was caused by atherosclerosis. Good flow through the stent is observed as contrast material fills the lumen.

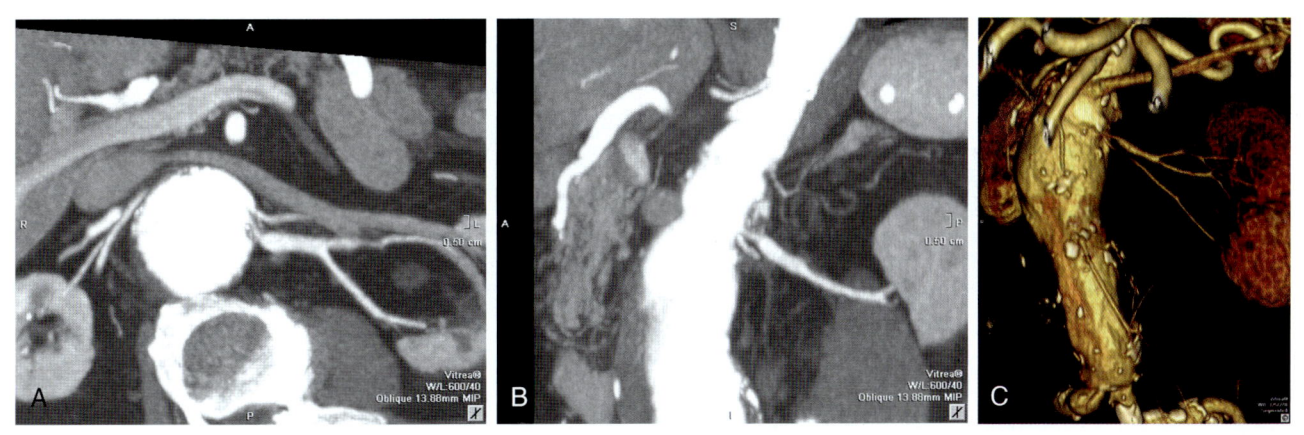

Figure 28.94 Renal artery stenosis: computed tomographic angiography (CTA). Image processing was applied to the case depicted in Figure 28.92. Axial **(A)** and coronal **(B)** slab maximum-intensity projection images demonstrate the atherosclerotic stenosis of the proximal renal artery. Note the accessory renal artery arising adjacent to the left main renal artery. Volume rendering of the CTA produced a three-dimensional display **(C)**, which may be rotated for best viewing and analysis.

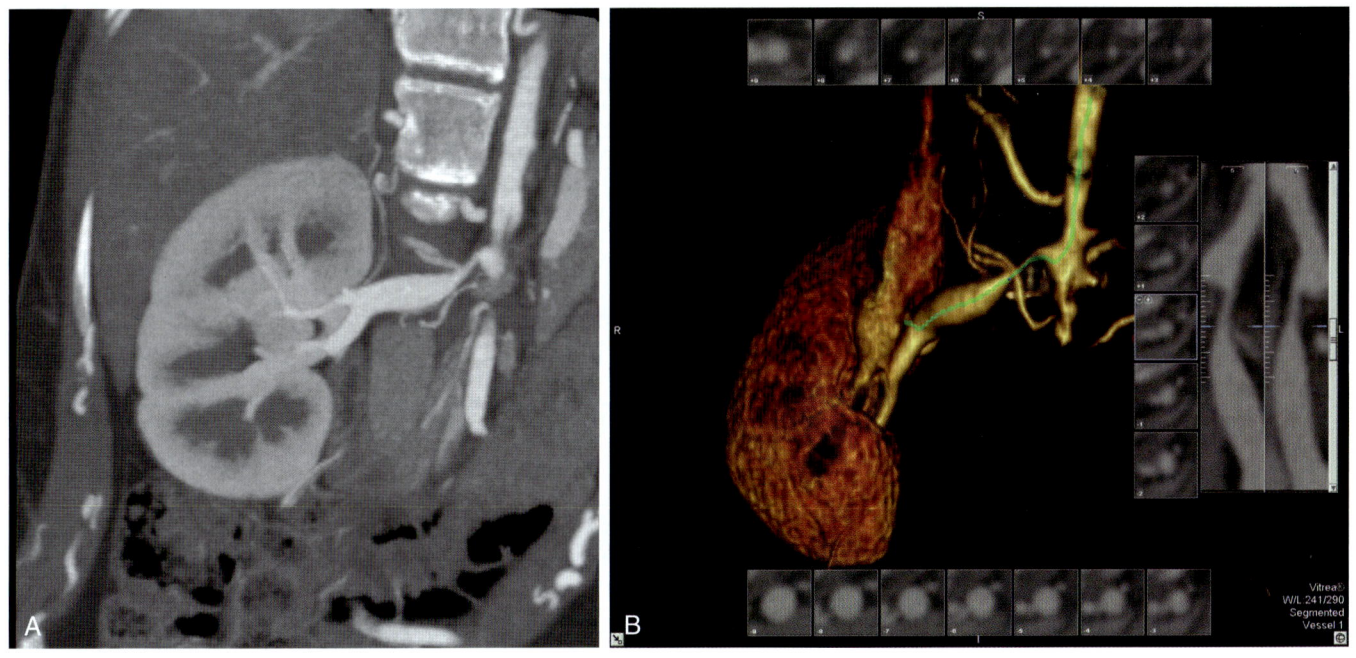

Figure 28.95 Renal artery stenosis: abdominal computed tomographic angiography (CTA) with image processing. A, Coronal slab maximum-intensity projection demonstrates the smooth narrowing of the proximal right renal artery in a patient with Takayasu's arteritis. Note the markedly abnormal aorta with occlusion distal to the origin of the renal artery. **B,** Volume rendering of the CTA with vessel analysis reveals the 80% stenosis of the right renal artery. The left renal artery had been occluded previously, and the kidney was supplied by collateral vessels.

visualization of all accessory vessels is desired, Bude and colleagues found isolated hemodynamically significant stenosis of an accessory artery in only 1 (1.5%) of their 68 patients.[381] Bude and colleagues concluded that this limitation does not substantially reduce the rate of detection of renovascular hypertension by MRI. With the use of three-dimensional reconstruction, studies have demonstrated no significant difference between CE-MRA and CTA in the detection of hemodynamically significant RAS.[374] Volume rendering and multiplanar reformatting improve accuracy in depicting RAS.[108] Volume rendering increases the positive predictive value of CE-MRA by reducing the overestimation of stenosis yielded by earlier reconstruction techniques (Figure 28.96).[109,377] Volume rendering has better correlation with digital subtraction angiography and improves delineation of the renal arteries.[109]

The usefulness of MRA is restricted in part by limitations in spatial resolution and by motion artifacts.[380,381] Advancements in magnetic resonance gradient strengths and newer MRA techniques have improved image resolution and reduced motion artifacts, while reducing imaging times.[381] Higher magnetic field strength (3 T) can result in higher spatial and temporal resolution when compared to imaging at 1.5 T. This higher resolution was found to improve the evaluation of smaller structures.[382,383] As MRI hardware and software improve, so will noncontrast MRA. Noncontrast

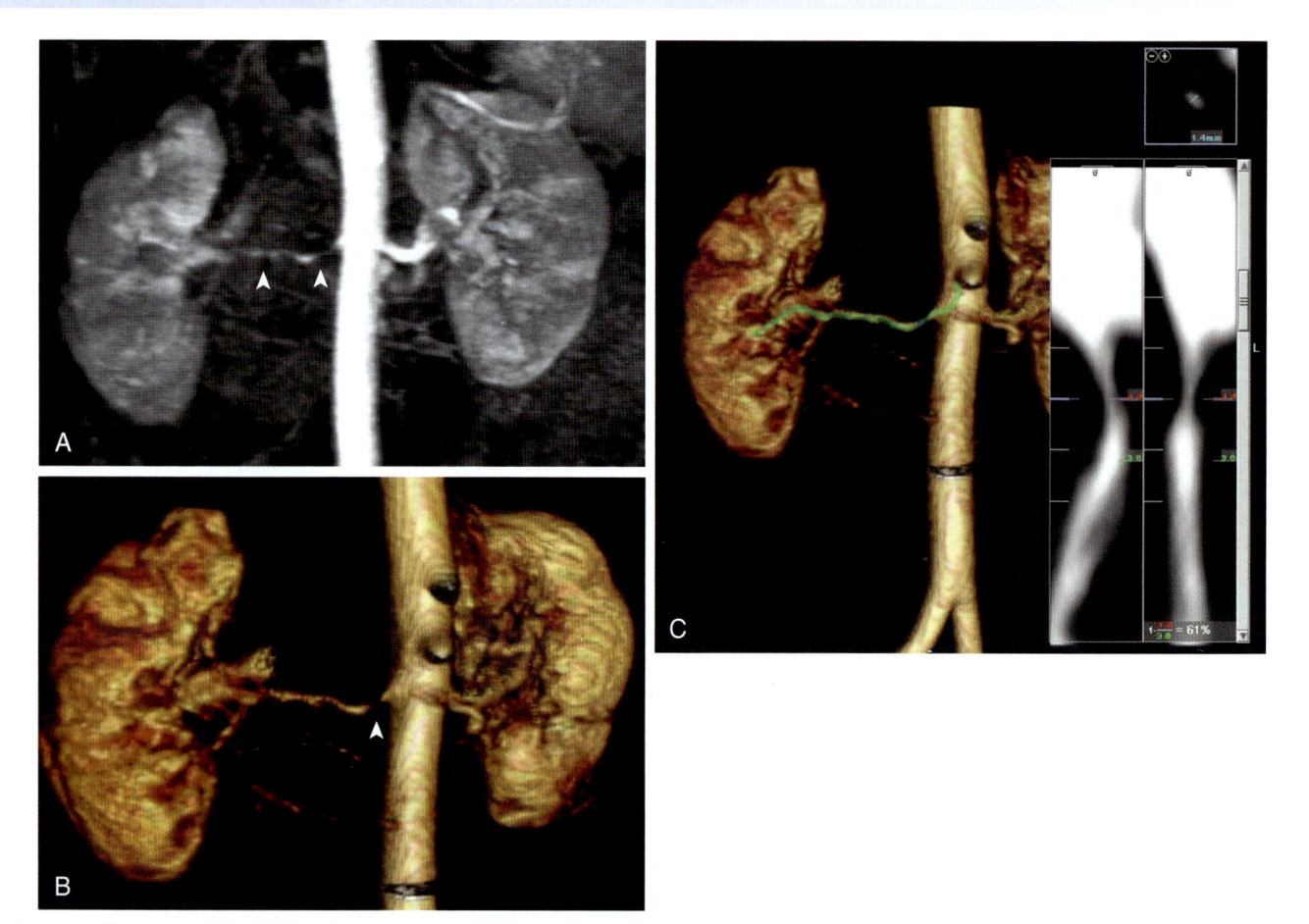

Figure 28.96 Renal artery stenosis. Advancements in postprocessing allow for more accurate evaluation of stenosis with magnetic resonance angiography. **A,** Maximum-intensity projection displays a high-grade stenosis near the origin of the renal artery with areas of apparent narrowing in the midportion of the renal artery (*arrowheads*), mimicking fibromuscular dysplasia. **B,** Volume rendering shows the proximal stenosis (*arrowhead*), but the midportion of the artery is more normal in appearance. **C,** A view of the artery in two dimensions allowed measurement of the proximal stenosis and demonstrated a normal midportion of the artery. This stenosis was confirmed with angiography.

MRA may be performed independent of renal function, and small studies have shown good results for the diagnosis of RAS.

Phase-contrast MRA can be used to calculate blood flow through the renal artery.[384] Phase-contrast flow curves can be generated, and the severity of the hemodynamic abnormalities can be graded as normal, low-grade, moderate, and high-grade stenosis. This is similar to the Doppler US method. Grading can be used to evaluate the hemodynamic significance of a detected stenosis.[385] The significance of a stenosis on parenchymal function, however, is not currently evaluated by conventional MRA. Renal MRI perfusion studies are being performed to grade the effect of RAS on parenchymal perfusion; initial results show that MRI perfusion measurements with high spatial and temporal resolution reflect renal function as measured with serum creatinine level.[386] Volumetric analysis of functional renal cortical tissue may also yield clinically useful information in patients with RAS.[387] Further research is required before this will be known, however.

MRA is currently of limited value in the evaluation of restenosis in patients with renal artery stents. Although stent technology is rapidly changing, metal artifact still obscures the stent lumen to varying degrees as a result of susceptibility artifacts (Figure 28.97). Phase-contrast MRA may be used

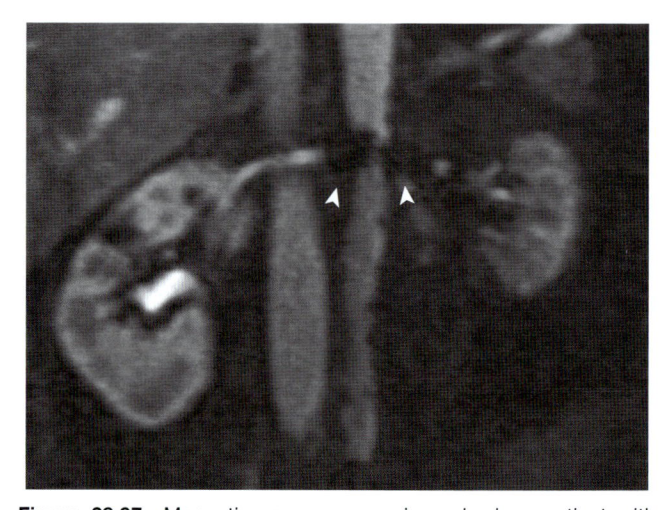

Figure 28.97 Magnetic resonance angiography in a patient with bilateral renal artery stents (*arrowheads*). The metal in the stent causes artifact that obscures the vessel lumen. Contrast material is visible beyond the stent, which indicates that no complete occlusion is present.

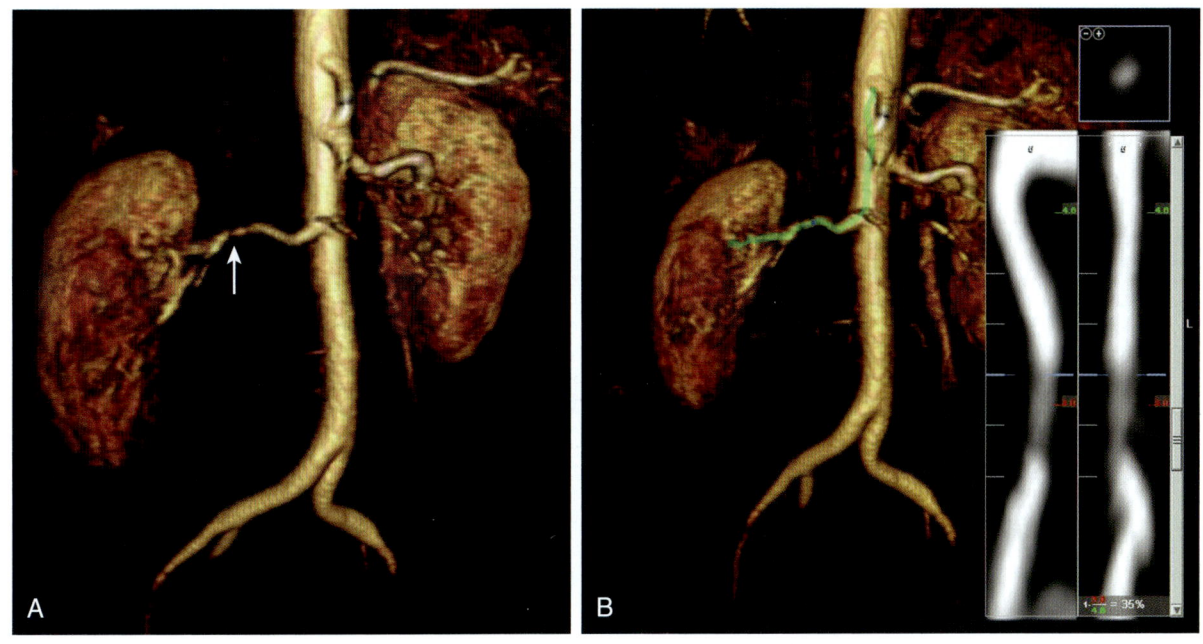

Figure 28.98 **A** and **B,** Magnetic resonance angiography with volume reconstruction demonstrates a subtle irregularity in the midportion of the right renal artery (*arrow*). Fibromuscular dysplasia was confirmed with conventional angiography.

to measure velocities proximal and distal to the stent, but this is an indirect approach to evaluating for stenosis. Work is being done to develop a metallic renal artery stent that will allow for lumen visualization on MRI; however, this is not currently available clinically.[388]

Fibromuscular dysplasia has a characteristic appearance of focal narrowing and dilation ("string of beads"; Figure 28.98). Because fibromuscular dysplasia frequently involves the middle to distal portions of the renal artery and segmental branches, resolution limits MRA evaluation. For this reason, MRA is not as reliable for diagnosis of fibromuscular dysplasia as it is for atherosclerotic RAS. Renal infarctions are well demonstrated on MRA as wedge-shaped areas of decreased parenchymal enhancement. These areas are most conspicuous in the nephrographic phase. Evaluation of the arterial and venous structures may demonstrate the origin of the emboli or thrombosis (Figure 28.99).

NUCLEAR IMAGING AND RENOVASCULAR DISEASE

ACE inhibition prevents conversion of angiotensin I to angiotensin II. In RAS, angiotensin II constricts the efferent arterioles as a compensatory mechanism to maintain GFR despite diminished afferent renal blood flow. Therefore ACE inhibition in RAS reduces GFR by interfering with the compensatory mechanism. Captopril-enhanced renography has been successful in evaluating patients with RAS.

Before the study the patient should be well hydrated, and ACE inhibitors should be discontinued (captopril for 2 days; enalapril or lisinopril for 4 to 5 days) because diagnostic sensitivity may otherwise be reduced. Diuretics should also be discontinued before the study, preferably for 1 week. Dehydration resulting from diuretics may potentiate the effect of captopril and contribute to hypotension. Captopril (25 to 50 mg) crushed and dissolved in 250 mL water is

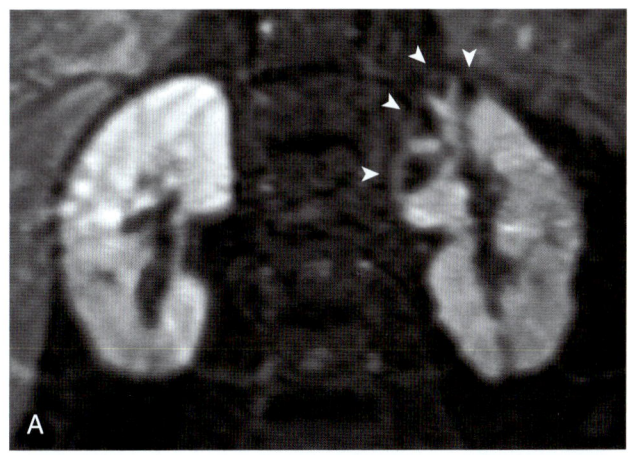

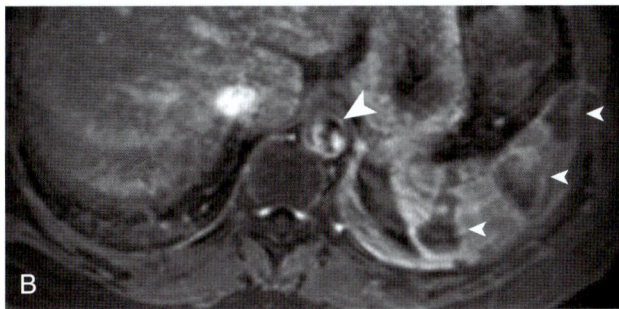

Figure 28.99 Renal infarcts caused by embolic disease. **A,** Coronal gadolinium-enhanced T1-weighted image shows wedge-shaped cortical areas without enhancement (*arrowheads*). **B,** Axial gadolinium-enhanced T1-weighted image shows an irregular filling defect in the aorta (*large arrowhead*), which is consistent with thrombus, and three focal defects in the spleen (*small arrowheads*), which are consistent with splenic infarcts.

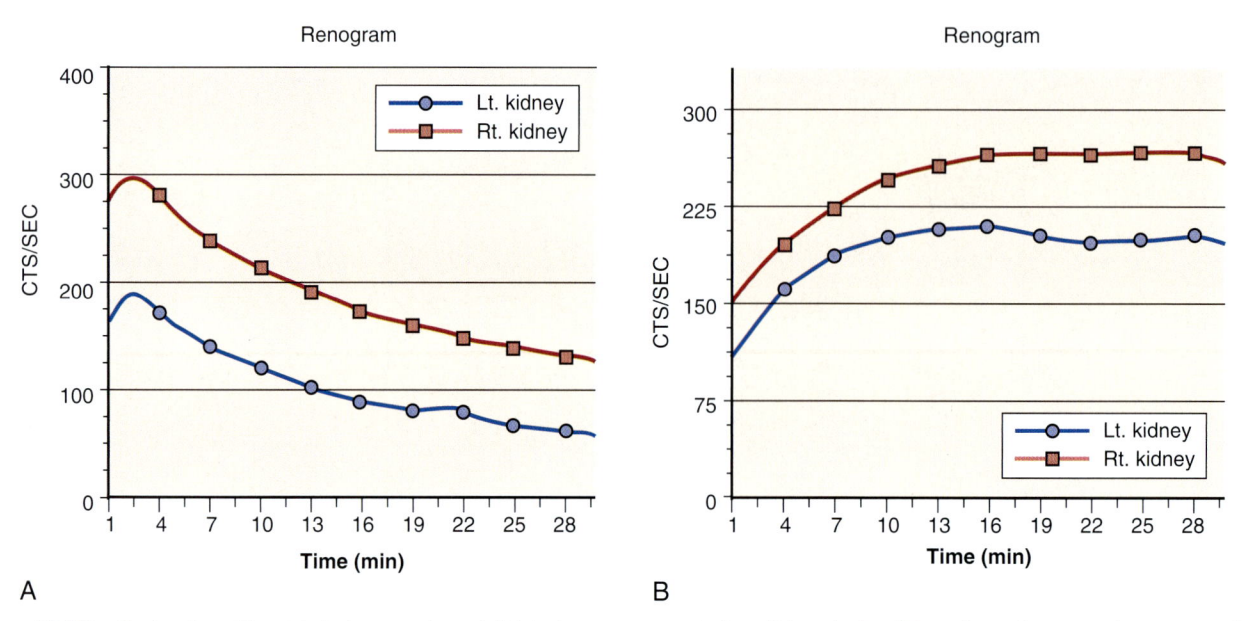

Figure 28.100 Technetium 99m–labeled mercaptoacetyltriglycine renograms before **(A)** and after **(B)** angiotensin-converting enzyme (ACE) inhibition with captopril. Note the relatively normal renograms **(A)** and the reduced initial slope, delayed time to peak activity, and plateau compatible with captopril-induced cortical tracer retention **(B)**. These findings suggest a high probability of hemodynamically significant bilateral renal artery stenosis that is more severe on the left side (*connected circles*) than the right side (*connected squares*). Bilateral renal artery stenosis was later confirmed with angiography. (Adapted from Saremi F, Jadvar H, Siegel M: Pharmacologic interventions in nuclear radiology: indications, imaging protocols, and clinical results. *Radiographics* 22:447-490, 2002.)

administered orally, followed by blood pressure monitoring every 15 minutes for 1 hour. Alternatively, enalaprilat (40 μg/kg with total dose not exceeding 2.5 mg) is administered intravenously over 3 to 5 minutes. A baseline scan can be performed before captopril-enhanced renography (1-day protocol) or the next day, only if captopril-enhanced study findings are abnormal (2-day protocol).

The affected kidney in renovascular hypertension often has a renogram curve with reduced initial slope, a delayed time to peak activity, prolonged cortical retention, and a slow downward slope after the peak (Figure 28.100). These findings are caused by the slowing of renal tracer transit as a result of increased retention of solute and water in response to ACE inhibition. Reduced urine flow causes delayed and decreased washout of tracer into the collecting system in ^{99m}Tc-MAG3 and ^{131}I-ortho-iodohippurate studies. ^{99m}Tc-DTPA demonstrates reduced uptake on the affected side.[389]

Consensus reports regarding methods and interpretation of ACE-enhanced renograms elaborate on a scoring system of renographic curves.[390-392] It has been recommended that high (>90%), intermediate (10% to 90%), and low (<10%) probability categories be applied to captopril-enhanced renography on the basis of the change of renographic curve score between baseline values and those after captopril-enhanced renograms. Among quantitative measurements, relative renal function, the time to peak activity, and the ratio of 20-minute renal activity to peak activity (20/peak) are used more commonly than other parameters. For ^{99m}Tc-MAG3 renal scintigraphy, a 10% change in relative renal function, peak activity increase of 2 minutes or more, and a parenchymal increase by 0.15 in 20/peak after captopril-enhanced study represent a high probability of renovascular hypertension.[393]

Captopril-enhanced renography has 80% to 95% sensitivity and 50% specificity for detecting impaired GFR; the detection of stenosis by captopril-enhanced renography may be more complicated.[389] With bilateral renovascular stenosis, it is more the exception than the rule for findings to be symmetric on captopril-enhanced renography. Studies in canine models with bilateral RAS demonstrated that captopril produced striking changes in the time-activity curve of each kidney, which are even more pronounced in the more severely stenotic kidney.[389] In practice, captopril-enhanced renography has largely been replaced by CTA or MRA for the investigation of renovascular disease.

RENAL VEIN THROMBOSIS

Renal vein thrombosis is usually clinically unsuspected. It is found in patients with a hypercoagulable state, underlying renal disease, or both.[389] The classic manifestation of acute renal vein thrombosis with gross hematuria, flank pain, and decreasing renal function is uncommon.[394] It may present clinically as nephrotic syndrome.[394] Other causes include collagen vascular diseases, diabetic nephropathy, trauma, and tumor thrombus. It can be diagnosed by Doppler US, CT, and MRI.

IVU yields nonspecific findings in renal vein thrombosis and is no longer used for diagnosis. It may yield normal findings in more than 25% of cases. On gray-scale and Doppler US, the involved kidney appears enlarged and swollen with relative hypoechogenicity in comparison with the normal kidney.[395] The finding of a filling defect in the renal vein is both sensitive and specific for diagnosis and is the only convincing sign of renal vein thrombosis. The lack of flow on Doppler US, however, is a nonspecific finding and may be observed because of technical limitations of the

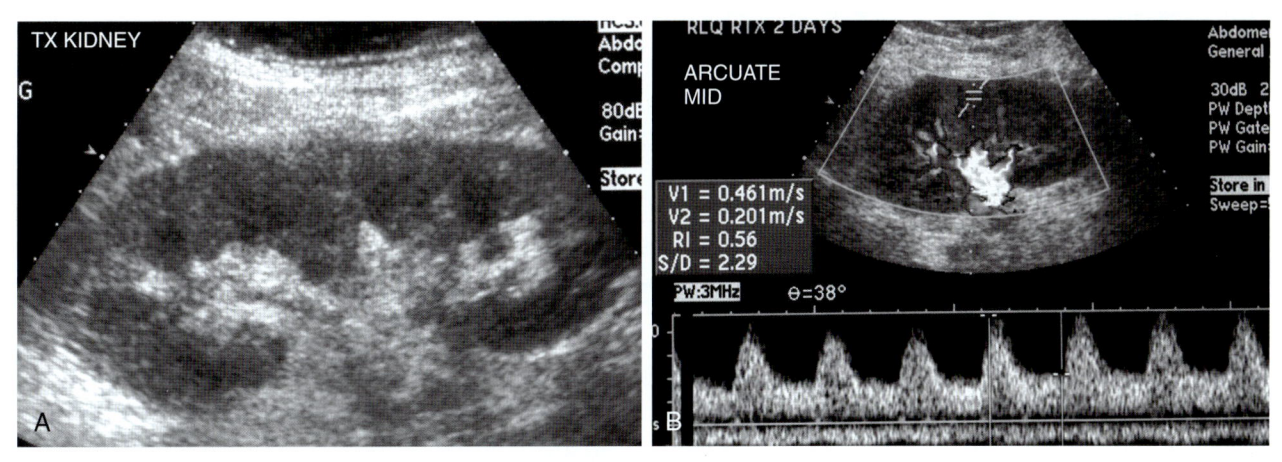

Figure 28.101 Normal renal transplant: ultrasonography. Coronal image **(A)** of a recently transplanted kidney in the right lower quadrant. The central echo complex, medullary pyramids, and cortex are well depicted. The duplex Doppler image **(B)** demonstrates normal flow to the transplanted kidney with a normal resistive index of 0.56.

study. Other findings include an absence or reversal of the diastolic waveform on Doppler US, but this may also be seen in other conditions.

CE-CT is needed to properly assess the patient with suspected renal vein thrombosis. If renal function is impaired, MRI can be used. Findings on CT include an enlarged renal vein with a low signal-attenuating filling defect that represents the clot within the renal vein.[396] Parenchymal enhancement may be abnormal, with prolonged corticomedullary differentiation and a delayed or persistent nephrogram. The kidney appears enlarged, with edema in the renal sinus leading to a striated nephrogram and attenuation of the pelvicalyceal system, and in extreme cases the pelvicalyceal system is completely compressed. Stranding and thickening of Gerota's fascia may be observed. Within chronic renal vein thrombosis, the renal vein may be narrowed because of clot retraction, and pericapsular collateral veins may be noted. Affected patients have an increased risk for pulmonary emboli as well. With renal tumors and, in rare cases, adrenal tumors, thrombus may develop in the renal vein with extension to the IVC. Imaging appearances suggesting tumor thrombus rather than bland thrombus include arterial enhancement in the thrombus, significant expansion of the vein, and continuity of the thrombus with a mass.

The appearance of renal vein thrombosis on noncontrast MRI is variable. If the thrombosis is acute, the renal vein appears distended, no normal flow void is visible, and the affected kidney appears enlarged. Renal infarction may also be present. If the thrombosis is chronic, the renal vein is small and difficult to see. A nonenhanced filling defect in the vein is visible on contrast-enhanced magnetic resonance venography, which is consistent with thrombus.

ASSESSMENT FOR RENAL TRANSPLANTATION

The treatment of choice for patients with ESKD is renal transplantation. Although there have been significant improvements in continuous peritoneal dialysis and hemodialysis, patient survival is longer and overall quality of life is better after renal transplantation. Radiologic evaluation is performed on the potential renal transplant donor and in the postoperative assessment of the transplant recipient. Although IVU and angiography were used in the past, US, CT, MRI, and renal scintigraphy are the current methods used in evaluation of these patients (Figure 28.101).[397-399]

A comprehensive radiologic assessment of the living renal transplant donor is crucial.[400] The anatomic information that is necessary is vascular, parenchymal, and pelvicalyceal. The renal artery must be visualized for number, length, location, and branching pattern. The parenchyma must be evaluated for scars, overall volume, renal masses, and calculi. The venous anatomy must be viewed, and the number of veins, anatomic variants, and significant systemic tributaries noted. The pelvicalyceal system must be scrutinized for anomalies such as duplication and papillary necrosis. The detailed anatomy and mapping techniques now possible have led to the increased use of laparoscopic techniques for donor kidney harvesting.[401-404]

With the development of MDCT, the complete evaluation of the living renal transplant donor is possible.[401,405,406] Noncontrast CT is performed with a low dose of radiation just to search for renal stones, locate the kidneys, and identify renal masses (see Figure 28.11). Arterial phase scanning is generally performed at 15 to 25 seconds to demonstrate the main renal artery, branching pattern of the artery, and abnormalities such as atherosclerotic plaques or fibromuscular dysplasia (see Figure 28.13); 25% to 40% of donors have accessory renal arteries, and 10% have early branching patterns in the main renal artery.[402,404] For transplantation the main renal artery should be free of branching for the first 15 to 20 mm. Because of the rapid transit of contrast material through the kidney, most renal veins are also well viewed in this phase (see Figure 28.12). Venous variants occur in 15% to 28% of donors, with multiple renal veins being most common, especially on the right. On the left side, 8% to 15% have a circumaortic renal vein, and 1% to 3% have a retroaortic vein.[404,407] It is also important to visualize venous tributaries, including the gonadal, left adrenal, and lumbar veins. These are best viewed on the nephrographic phase.[402,403] Imaging in this phase is performed 80 to 120 seconds after injection of contrast material and is used to evaluate the cortex and medulla for scars and masses (see Figure 28.14). Excretory phase imaging is performed with CT, CT digital radiography, or plain radiography to note anomalies or abnormalities in the pelvicalyceal system (see Figure 28.15). CT has a demonstrated accuracy of 91%

to 97% for arterial phase imaging, 93% to 100% for the venous phase, and 99% for the pelvicalyceal system.[406,408,409] Similar results have been noted for MRI; the biggest discrepancy is found in imaging accessory renal arteries.[410,411] Most centers today use CT in the evaluation of living renal transplant donors.

MRI, MRA, and MRU can be combined into one examination for the evaluation of the renal transplant donor.[412] MRI and CT are comparable for the evaluation of renal vasculature, structure, and function. To avoid radiation exposure and nephrotoxicity, MRI may be preferred over CT for preoperative evaluation.

In healthy renal donors it is possible to quantify functional renal volume with MRA by determining only the cortical volume. The hypothesis supported by Van den Dool and associates was that glomerular filtration is an important component of renal function, and because the majority of glomeruli are in the cortex, renal function should be well correlated with cortical volume.[414]

ASSESSMENT OF TRANSPLANTED KIDNEYS

After surgically successful renal transplantation, radiologic evaluation is frequently necessary. Conventional US, Doppler US, CT, MRI, and renal scintigraphy are used in various settings. US assumes the primary role for assessing patients with changes in serum creatinine level, urine output, pain, or hematuria.[414] It is also used to direct kidney biopsy. Doppler US is used to evaluate renal perfusion, the patency of the renal artery and vein, and the integrity of the vascular anastomoses.[415] CT, MRI, and renal scintigraphy are adjunctive studies.

Conventional gray-scale US is essential in assessing for transplant obstruction and fluid collections around the transplanted kidney.[399] Conventional US yields nonspecific findings in acute tubular necrosis and acute rejection, including obliteration of the corticomedullary junction, prominent swollen pyramids, and loss of the renal sinus echoes.[398,400] All these findings are indicative of edema of the transplanted kidney, which leads to increased peripheral vascular resistance, decreased diastolic perfusion, and elevation of the resistive index (>0.80) (Figure 28.102).[402] Chronic rejection may lead to diffusely increased echogenicity throughout the kidney.

Doppler US adds valuable information pertaining to the integrity of the vascular elements. Despite early enthusiasm with the ability of Doppler US to differentiate acute transplant rejection from acute tubular necrosis, it is now known that the findings are nonspecific and cannot obviate the need for kidney biopsy in these cases.[416] Both acute tubular necrosis and acute rejection can cause an increase in peripheral vascular resistance.[417,418] A significant number of patients with acute rejection have a normal resistive index (<0.80). It is now known that vascular rejection is no more likely to cause increases in peripheral vascular resistance than is cellular rejection.[416] Neither the timing nor clinical symptoms of the renal dysfunction can be used to differentiate acute rejection from acute tubular necrosis.[416] Doppler US is most helpful in detecting acute arterial thrombosis when signal in the artery is absent or renal vein thrombosis when the waveform is plateau-like and diastolic flow is retrograde. An abnormal Doppler waveform in the allograft indicates compromise of the transplanted kidney.[419] Sequential examinations may be used to show improvement or deterioration in the condition affecting the kidney and to note the progress of treatment.

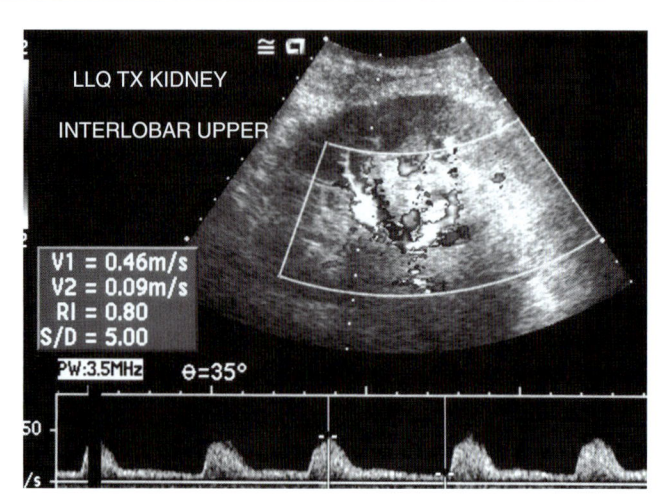

Figure 28.102 Renal transplant with acute tubular necrosis: ultrasonography. Duplex Doppler image of the transplanted kidney shows normal size and normal appearance with a high resistive index of 0.80 in the interlobar artery. The patient recovered with return of normal renal function in 5 days.

MRI and CE-CT are useful in patients in whom the transplanted kidney is obscured by overlying bowel gas or in patients with large body habitus in whom US may be limited by the depth of the transplanted kidney. If any doubt exists after a thorough US evaluation, MRI or CT may be performed to clarify or confirm the US findings.

Fluid collections around a transplanted kidney are very common, occurring in up to 50% of cases.[414] These fluid collections may represent urinoma, hematoma, lymphocele, abscess, or seroma. The effects of the collection depend on the size and location. Urinomas and hematomas are found early, usually immediately after surgery. Lymphoceles generally are not found until 3 to 6 weeks after surgery. Abscesses are usually associated with transplant infection.

On US evaluation, extrarenal or subcapsular hematomas usually have a complex echogenic appearance, which becomes less echogenic with time (Figure 28.103).[414] On CT they appear as high signal-attenuating fluid collections early. Such collections are usually too complex to be successfully drained percutaneously. Urine leaks and the associated urinoma are also found in the immediate postoperative period (Figure 28.104).[414] On US these appear as anechoic fluid collection with no septations. They may rapidly increase in size. Drainage may be performed under guidance by either US or CT.[420] Antegrade pyelography via a percutaneous nephrostomy is needed to detect the site of leak, usually the ureteral anastomoses. Stent placement for treatment is necessary.

Lymphoceles are recognized weeks to years after transplantation and occur in up to 20% of cases.[414] They form from the leakage of lymph fluid from the interrupted lymphatic vessels at surgery. Lymphoceles appear on US as anechoic fluid collections with septations. The size and effect on the kidney determine the need for treatment. Because lymphoceles are frequently located medial and inferior to the kidney, they are a common cause of

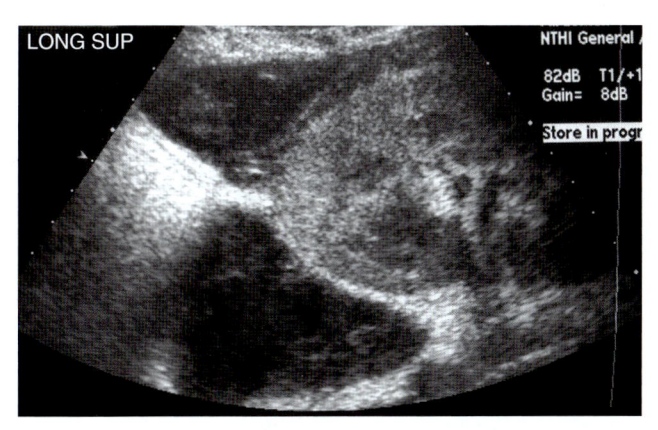

Figure 28.103 Renal transplant with hematoma: ultrasonography. Longitudinal image of the upper aspect of the transplanted kidney reveals two hypoechoic collections adjacent to the kidney. The heterogeneous hypoechoic nature of the collections suggests that they are hematomas, as opposed to urinomas or lymphoceles, which in general are anechoic.

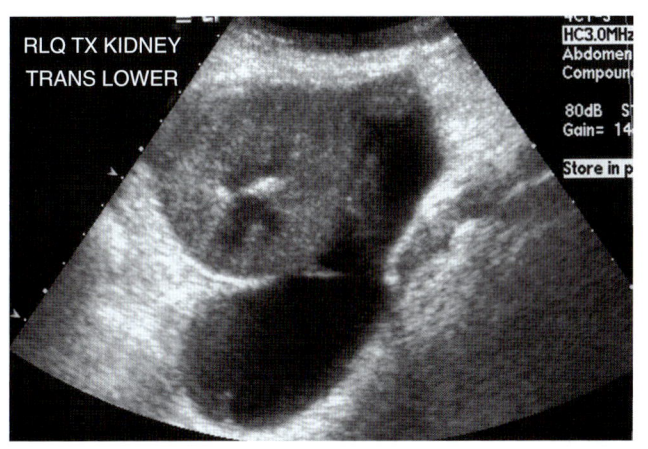

Figure 28.104 Renal transplant with urinoma: ultrasonography. Transverse image through the lower aspect of the transplanted kidney reveals a normal appearance with a large anechoic fluid collection adjacent to the kidney. This fluid was aspirated under US guidance, and the findings led to the diagnosis of urinoma. The patient was treated with catheter placement and drainage, also performed with US guidance.

obstruction to the kidney. US or CT guidance for drainage may be used. In a minority of cases, sclerotherapy may be needed to treat the lymphocele.[420]

Abscess near the transplanted kidney usually develops in association with renal infection or the infection of other fluid collections in the immunocompromised patient. On US examination, abscess appears as a complex fluid collection, possibly containing gas.[414] Fluid aspiration is usually necessary for the accurate characterization of fluid within a collection. Because blood products have characteristic signal intensities on T1- and T2-weighted sequences, MRI can provide specific diagnostic information that may help avoid an unnecessary interventional procedure in cases of hematoma.

Renal obstruction or hydronephrosis may be observed in the transplanted kidney with renal dysfunction and is reversible. US is the best means for assessment.[415] In the immediate posttransplantation period, mild caliectasis is common as a result of edema at the ureteral anastomosis site. Obstruction may also be caused by fluid collections around the transplanted kidney that may be visible also with US. Blood clots within the pelvicalyceal system may also lead to hydronephrosis. Later strictures may occur, primarily at the ureteral anastomosis site. Renal stones may also cause hydronephrosis during their passage to the bladder. A functional obstruction may be visible with an overdistended bladder. With bladder emptying, US demonstrates a resolution of the hydronephrosis.

Hypertension with or without renal dysfunction may be observed in many transplant recipients.[414] Vascular and nonvascular causes must be differentiated. Doppler US is the first step of evaluation. RAS may be found in up to 23% of patients.[421] The stenosis may occur before the anastomosis in the iliac artery, at the anastomosis site, or more distally. In more than half the cases, the stenosis is at the anastomotic site, and it is more common in end-to-end anastomosis. CT or MRA is used to determine the site and the degree of stenosis (Figure 28.105). Angioplasty is successful in managing most cases.[421]

Arteriovenous fistulas may occur in transplant recipients after kidney biopsy. Most close spontaneously within 4 to 6 weeks. Gray-scale images demonstrate only a simple- or complex-appearing cystic structure, whereas Doppler color-flow and duplex Doppler imaging demonstrate high-velocity and turbulent flow localized to a single segmental or interlobar artery and the adjacent vein. Arterialized flow is noted in the draining vein. If the structure is large and growing, embolization may become necessary.

Neoplasm occurs in transplant recipients with increased frequency, up to 100 times more frequently than in the general population.[414] Neoplasms develop as a result of prolonged immunosuppression. The risk for renal cell carcinoma in the transplanted kidney may be increased. Posttransplantation lymphoproliferative disorder may also occur in renal transplant recipients.[422] Although the transplanted kidney may be involved, the most frequent sites are the brain, liver, lungs, and gastrointestinal tract. The appearance is similar to that of conventional lymphomas with mass lesions in the organs, with or without associated adenopathy.

The MRI findings of renal transplant rejection are nonspecific (Figure 28.106; see Figures 28.34 and 28.35). Sadowski and colleagues demonstrated the feasibility of using BOLD MRI to evaluate the renal transplant oxygen status and presence of acute rejection.[121] The authors conclude that MRI may differentiate acute rejection from normal function and acute tubular necrosis, but further research is required. Animal research is being performed with the hope of using noninvasive diffusion MRI techniques as a tool for monitoring early renal graft rejection after transplantation.[118]

Nuclear medicine procedures are also employed in the renal transplant recipient and play a role in the assessment of the complications associated with transplantation. These include vascular compromise (arterial or venous thrombosis), lymphocele formation, urine extravasation, acute tubular necrosis, drug toxicity, and organ rejection. Scintigraphy provides important imaging information about these

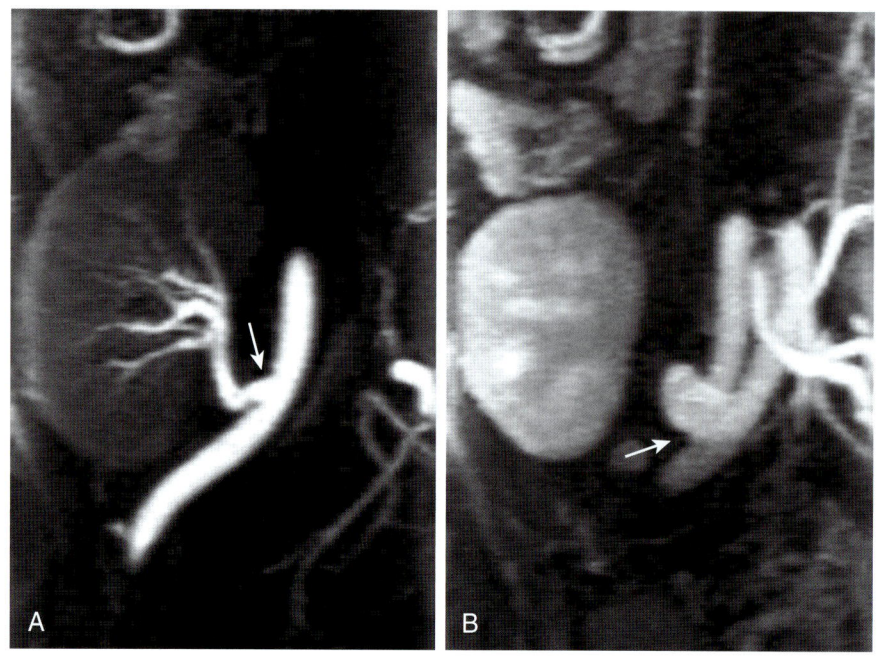

Figure 28.105 Renal transplant magnetic resonance angiogram, showing normal arterial (**A**) and normal venous (**B**) anastomoses (*arrows*).

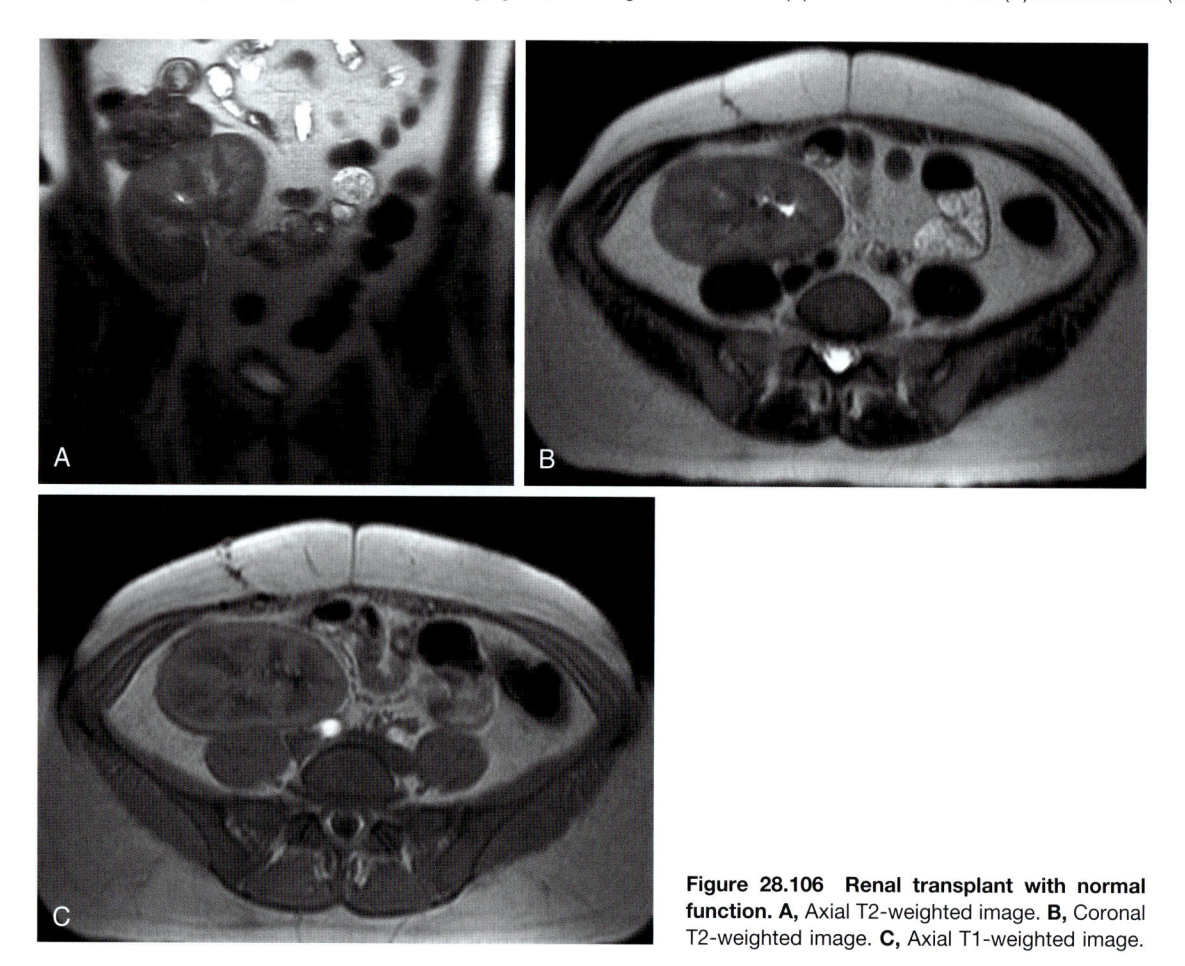

Figure 28.106 Renal transplant with normal function. A, Axial T2-weighted image. **B,** Coronal T2-weighted image. **C,** Axial T1-weighted image.

potential complications, which can then guide corrective intervention.[423]

An early complication may be hyperacute rejection, which is often apparent immediately after transplantation and is caused by preformed cytotoxic antibodies. Other early complications include sudden decline in urine output and acute urinary obstruction. Scintigraphy with ^{99m}Tc-DTPA or ^{99m}Tc-MAG3 demonstrates absence of perfusion and function with complete thrombosis in the renal artery or renal vein. A sensitive but nonspecific sign of acute rejection is

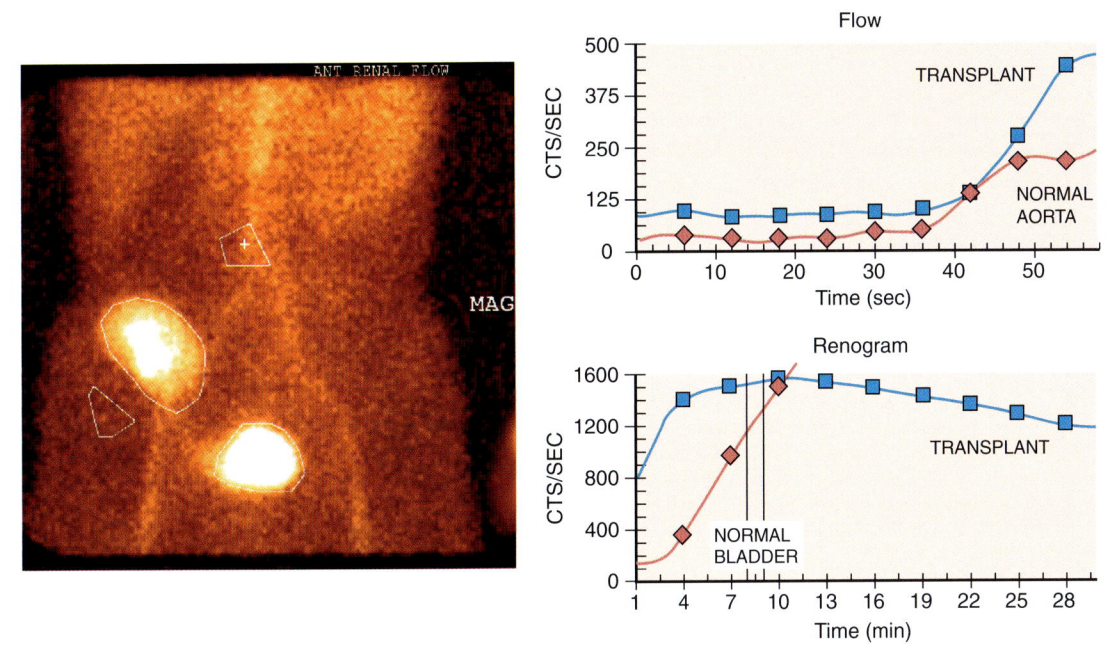

Figure 28.107 Abnormal technetium 99m–labeled mercaptoacetyltriglycine renogram. The pattern involving the right pelvic renal transplant from a living related donor is compatible with acute tubular necrosis.

the finding of more than a 20% decline in the ratio of renal activity to the aortic activity.[424]

Renal scintigraphy performed a few days after the transplantation often reveals intact perfusion but delayed and decreased excretion of the tracer and some cortical retention of the tracer. These findings are typically caused by acute tubular necrosis and are more common with cadaveric grafts than with grafts from living related donors (Figure 28.107). If both perfusion and function continue to decline, then the possibility of rejection should be considered. However, acute tubular necrosis, obstruction, drug (cyclosporine) toxicity, and rejection can produce relatively similar scintigraphic appearances. The differential diagnosis should be considered in the clinical context and with regard to the interval since transplantation, although two or more of these conditions may coexist. In one report a nonascending second phase of ^{99m}Tc-MAG3 renogram curve was predictive of graft dysfunction. However, patients with acute tubular necrosis were not significantly more likely to have a nonascending curve than were those with acute rejection. An ascending curve was nonspecific and could be observed in both normally and poorly functioning grafts.[425]

Urine extravasation may be noted on the renal scans as collections of excreted radiotracer outside of the transplanted kidney and the urinary bladder. Because of small urine leaks and impaired renal transplant function, it may be difficult to identify a leak on scintigraphy. However, a cold-appearing defect that becomes warmer in appearance with time on the sequential images usually represents a urinoma or a urinary leak. If the activity declines with voiding, then the finding probably represents a urinoma. A chronic photopenic defect may represent a hematoma or a lymphocele (or both).[426] For assessing potential obstructive disease, scintigraphy with a diuretic may be considered, as previously discussed. Results of an animal-based study also suggested that FDG-PET may have a role in early detection of graft rejection by demonstrating significantly elevated graft tracer uptake induced by inflammatory infiltrates.[46]

ACKNOWLEDGMENTS

Katherine To'o, VA Medical Center, Palo Alto, California, for work on the CIN section and Alicia Alvarez-McDermott and Sona Devedjian for manuscript preparation.

Complete reference list available at ExpertConsult.com.

KEY REFERENCES

3. *ACR appropriateness criteria*. Available at: <http://www.acr.org/~/media/ACR/Documents/AppCriteria/Diagnostic/Hematuria.pdf>. Accessed June 20, 2015.
4. Dyer RB, Chen MYM, Zagoria RF: Intravenous urography: technique and interpretation. *Radiographics* 21:799–824, 2001.
25. Park BK, Kim B, Kim SH, et al: Assessment of cystic renal masses based on Bosniak classification: comparison of CT and contrast-enhanced US. *Eur J Radiol* 61:310–314, 2007.
36. Lang EK, Macchia RJ, Thomas R, et al: Improved detection of renal pathologic features on multiphasic helical CT compared with IVU in patients presenting with microscopic hematuria. *Urology* 61:528–532, 2003.
38. Coursey CA, Nelson RC, Boll DT, et al: Dual-energy multidetector CT: how does it work, what can it tell us, and when can we use it in abdominopelvic imaging? *Radiographics* 30:1037–1055, 2010.
49. Kidney Disease: Improving Global Outcomes: *KDIGO clinical practice guideline for acute kidney injury*. Available at: <http://www.kdigo.org/clinical_practice_guidelines/AKI.php>. Accessed June 20, 2015.
50. Davenport MS, Khalatbari S, Dillman JR, et al: Contrast material-induced nephrotoxicity and intravenous low-osmolality iodinated contrast material. *Radiology* 267:94–105, 2013.
57. Thomsen HS: European Society of Urogenital Radiology guidelines on contrast media application. *Curr Opin Urol* 17:70–76, 2007.
59. Canadian Association of Radiologists: *Consensus guidelines for the prevention of contrast induced nephropathy*. Available at: <http://www.car.ca/uploads/standards%20guidelines/20110617_en_prevention_cin.pdf>. Accessed June 20, 2015.

74. Shellock FG: *Reference manual for magnetic resonance safety, implants and devices*, ed 2014, Los Angeles, 2014, Biomedical Research Publishing Company.
75. Rofsky NM, Weinreb JC, Bosniak MA, et al: Renal lesion characterization with gadolinium-enhanced MR imaging: efficacy and safety in patients with renal insufficiency. *Radiology* 180:85–89, 1991.
94. U.S. Food and Drug Administration: *Gadolinium-based contrast agents: class labeling change—risk of nephrogenic systemic fibrosis*. Available at: <http://www.fda.gov/Safety/MedWatch/SafetyInformation/SafetyAlertsforHumanMedicalProducts/ucm225375.htm>. Accessed August 7, 2013.
100. American College of Radiology Committee on Drugs and Contrast Media: *ACR manual on contrast media*, version 9, 2013. Available at: <http://www.acr.org/quality-safety/resources/contrast-manual>. Accessed June 20, 2015.
118. Zhang JL, Rusinek H, Chandarana H, et al: Functional MRI of the kidneys. *J Magn Reson Imaging* 37:282–293, 2013.
119. Thoeny HC, De Keyzer F, Oyen RH, et al: Diffusion-weighted MR imaging of kidneys in healthy volunteers and patients with parenchymal diseases: initial experience. *Radiology* 235:911–917, 2005.
122. He W, Fischman AJ: Nuclear imaging in the genitourinary tract: recent advances and future directions. *Radiol Clin North Am* 46:25–43, 2008.
136. Esteves FP, Taylor A, Manatunga A, et al: 99mTc-MAG3 renography: normal values for MAG3 clearance and curve parameters, excretory parameters, and residual urine volume. *AJR Am J Roentgenol* 187:W610–W617, 2006.
139. *ACR appropriateness criteria: renal failure*. Available at: <http://www.acr.org/Quality-Safety/Appropriateness-Criteria/Diagnostic/~/media/ACR/Documents/AppCriteria/Diagnostic/RenalFailure.pdf>. Accessed June 20, 2015.
158. Saremi F, Jadvar H, Siegel M: Pharmacologic interventions in nuclear radiology: indications, imaging protocols, and clinical results. *Radiographics* 22:477–490, 2002.
162. Dyer RB, Chen MYM, Zagoria RJ: Abnormal calcifications in the urinary tract. *Radiographics* 18:1405–1424, 1998.
171. *ACR appropriateness criteria: acute onset flank pain*. Available at: <http://www.acr.org/Quality-Safety/Appropriateness-Criteria/Diagnostic/Urologic-Imaging>. Accessed June 20, 2015.
178. Cheng PM, Moin P, Dunn MD, et al: What the radiologist needs to know about urolithiasis: part I: pathogenesis, types, assessment, and variant anatomy. *AJR Am J Roentgenol* 198:W540–W547, 2012.
179. Cheng PM, Moin P, Dunn MD, et al: What the radiologist needs to know about urolithiasis: part II: CT findings, reporting, and treatment. *AJR Am J Roentgenol* 198:W548–W554, 165, 2012.
195. Boll DT, Patil NA, Paulson EK, et al: Renal stone assessment with dual-energy multidetector CT and advanced postprocessing techniques: improved characterization of renal stone composition—pilot study. *Radiology* 250:813–820, 2009.
201. Takahashi N, Kawashima A, Ernst RD, et al: Ureterolithiasis: can clinical outcome be predicted with unenhanced helical CT? *Radiology* 208:97–102, 1998.
206. Kawashima A, Sandler CM, Goldman SM, et al: CT of renal inflammatory disease. *Radiographics* 17:851–866, 1997.
216. *ACR appropriateness criteria: acute pyelonephritis*. Available at: <http://www.acr.org/Quality-Safety/Appropriateness-Criteria/Diagnostic/Urologic-Imaging>. Accessed June 20, 2015.
222. Ziessman HA, Majd M: Importance of methodology on (99m)technetium dimercapto-succinic acid scintigraphic image quality: imaging pilot study for RIVUR (Randomized Intervention for Children with Vesicoureteral Reflux) multicenter investigation. *J Urol* 182:272–279, 2009.
229. Kenney PJ: Imaging of chronic renal infections. *AJR Am J Roentgenol* 155:485–494, 1990.
235. Bosniak Morton A: The use of the Bosniak classification system for renal cysts and cystic tumors. *J Urol* 157:1852–1853, 1997.
238. Israel GM, Hindman N, Bosniak MA: Evaluation of cystic renal masses: comparison of CT and MR imaging by using the Bosniak classification system. *Radiology* 231:365–371, 2004.
240. Hecht EM, Israel GM, Krinsky GA, et al: Renal masses: quantitative analysis of enhancement with signal intensity measurements versus qualitative analysis of enhancement with image subtraction for diagnosing malignancy at MR imaging. *Radiology* 232:373–378, 2004.
255. Hartman DS, Choyke PL, Hartman MS: From the RSNA refresher courses: a practical approach to the cystic renal mass. *Radiographics* 24:S101–S115, 2004.
259. Israel GM, Bosniak MA: Follow-up CT of moderately complex cystic lesions of the kidney (Bosniak category IIF). *AJR Am J Roentgenol* 181:627–633, 2003.
268. Patard JJ: Incidental renal tumours. *Curr Opin Urol* 19:454–458, 2009.
269. Berland LL, Silverman SG, Gore RM, et al: Managing incidental findings on abdominal CT: white paper of the ACR incidental findings committee. *J Am Coll Radiol* 7:754–773, 2010.
281. Bosniak M, Megibow AJ, Hulnick DH, et al: CT diagnosis of renal angiomyolipoma: the importance of detecting small amounts of fat. *AJR Am J Roentgenol* 151:497–501, 1988.
290. Davidson AJ, Hartman DS, Choyke PL, et al: Radiologic assessment of renal masses: implications for patient care. *Radiology* 202:297–305, 1997.
293. Suh M, Coakley FV, Qayyum A, et al: Distinction of renal cell carcinomas from high-attenuation renal cysts at portal venous phase contrast–enhanced CT. *Radiology* 228:330–334, 2003.
300. Kim JK, Kim TK, Ahn HJ, et al: Differentiation of subtypes of renal cell carcinoma on helical CT scans. *AJR Am J Roentgenol* 178:1499–1506, 2002.
306. Browne RFJ, Meehan CP, Colville J, et al: Transitional cell carcinoma of the upper urinary tract: spectrum of imaging findings. *Radiographics* 25:1609–1627, 2005.
321. Zukotynski K, Lewis A, O'Regan K, et al: PET/CT and renal pathology: a blind spot for radiologists? Part 1: primary pathology. *AJR Am J Roentgenol* 199:W163–W167, 2012.
331. Wang HY, Ding HJ, Chen JH, et al: Meta-analysis of the diagnostic performance of [18F] FDG PET and PET/CT in renal cell carcinoma. *Cancer Imaging* 12:464–474, 2012.
338. Kayani I, Avril N, Bomanji J, et al: Sequential FDG-PET/CT as a biomarker of response to sunitinib in metastatic clear cell renal cancer. *Clin Cancer Res* 17:6021–6028, 2011.
361. *ACR appropriateness criteria: renovascular hypertension*. Available at: <http://www.acr.org/~/media/ACR/Documents/AppCriteria/Diagnostic/RenovascularHypertension.pdf>. Accessed October 29, 2014.
378. Schoenberg SO, Knopp MV, Londy F, et al: Morphologic and functional magnetic resonance imaging of renal artery stenosis: a multireader tricenter study. *J Am Soc Nephrol* 13:158–169, 2002.
380. Soulez G, Oliva VL, Turpin S, et al: Imaging of renovascular hypertension: respective values of renal scintigraphy, renal Doppler US, and MR angiography. *Radiographics* 20:1355–1368, 2000.
392. Taylor A, Nally J, Aurell M, et al: Consensus report on ACE inhibitor renography for detecting renovascular hypertension. Radionuclides in Nephrourology Group. Consensus Group on ACEI Renography. *J Nucl Med* 37:1876–1882, 1996.
422. Patel NH, Jindal RM, Wilkin T, et al: Renal arterial stenosis in renal allografts: retrospective study of predisposing factors and outcome after percutaneous transluminal angioplasty. *Radiology* 219:663–667, 2001.

The Kidney Biopsy

Alan D. Salama | H. Terence Cook

CHAPTER OUTLINE

SAFETY AND COMPLICATIONS OF BIOPSIES, 915
PERFORMING THE BIOPSY, 918
BIOPSY SPECIMEN HANDLING, 919
LIGHT MICROSCOPY, 919
Staining for Light Microscopy, 919
Examination of the Biopsy Specimen by Light Microscopy, 920
Terminology for Description of Glomerular Disease, 920
IMMUNOHISTOCHEMICAL ASSAY, 921
ELECTRON MICROSCOPY, 922
OTHER STUDIES PERFORMED ON THE KIDNEY BIOPSY SPECIMEN, 923
BIOPSY SPECIMENS FROM TRANSPLANTED KIDNEYS, 923
SIZE OF THE BIOPSY SPECIMEN, 923
BIOPSY REPORT, 924
CONCLUSIONS, 924

The kidney biopsy has become a fundamental component in the management of renal disease. Before its routine use, only autopsy material was available to investigate the pathophysiology of kidney disease, limiting antemortem diagnosis. However, its development and refinement since the late 1950s has been fundamental for the diagnosis and definition of clinical syndromes and the discovery of new pathologic entities.[1] Through the critical analysis of kidney biopsies taken at different disease time points, key pathophysiologic features of kidney disease have been discovered, which have in turn helped to establish new paradigms in nephrology and have led to considerable alterations in patient management. This is true for biopsies of both native kidneys and renal transplants.[2] In addition, much is still being learned regarding disease pathogenesis through the study of kidney biopsy material, which not only remains a gold standard for disease diagnosis, but has allowed the development of novel biopsy markers, which have revolutionized our concepts of pathologic mechanisms.

The first percutaneous kidney biopsies were performed over 50 years ago using a liver biopsy needle and intravenous pyelograms for screening, with the patient either sitting or supine. Their success in obtaining renal tissue and in aiding management confirmed the benefit of the procedure.[1] Many innovations, including using real-time ultrasonography, which allows visualization of the needle entering the kidney, spring-loaded needles or needle holders, and careful preoperative evaluation of the patient,[3] have improved the rate of obtaining renal tissue while minimizing the risks of the procedure.[4] Consequently, this has placed percutaneous kidney biopsy at the very center of modern clinical nephrology. The range of diagnoses for a group of 2219 native kidney biopsies performed at the authors' institution over a 5-year period is shown in Figure 29.1.

SAFETY AND COMPLICATIONS OF BIOPSIES

Although generally considered safe, there is morbidity and a small, but measurable, mortality associated with the procedure, and it is therefore imperative to subject to these risks only those patients in whom there will be a potential benefit. Indications for kidney biopsy may vary from center to center, but accepted indications are listed in Table 29.1. The significant complications related to the procedure are hemorrhage, development of arteriovenous fistulas, and to a lesser extent sepsis.[5-7] Bleeding with macroscopic hematuria and the development of perinephric hematomas may be minor and self-resolving or major and require intervention in the form of blood transfusions, embolization, or rarely surgery. There is a risk for formation of arteriovenous fistulas, which may be asymptomatic and spontaneously resolve or lead to a significant vascular steal syndrome, compromising the rest of the kidney through ischemia. Finally, there is the risk for sepsis following the procedure, through the introduction of a septic focus or its dissemination. Overall, the risks for complication vary from center to center and between practitioners but can be estimated to be between 3.5% and 13%, with the majority being minor complications (approximately 3% to 9%).[5-7] Mortality from the procedure is generally as a result of undiagnosed bleeding with significant hematoma formation and was reported in up to 0.2% of cases from some of the larger biopsy series,[6,7] although other studies suggest that it represents an extremely rare adverse event.[4] Some degree of bleeding is common, with approximately half of patients showing a drop in hemoglobin level after biopsy and a third developing some hematoma, but bleeding is significant and requires intervention in only a minority (up to 7%).[4,7,8] Complications appear to

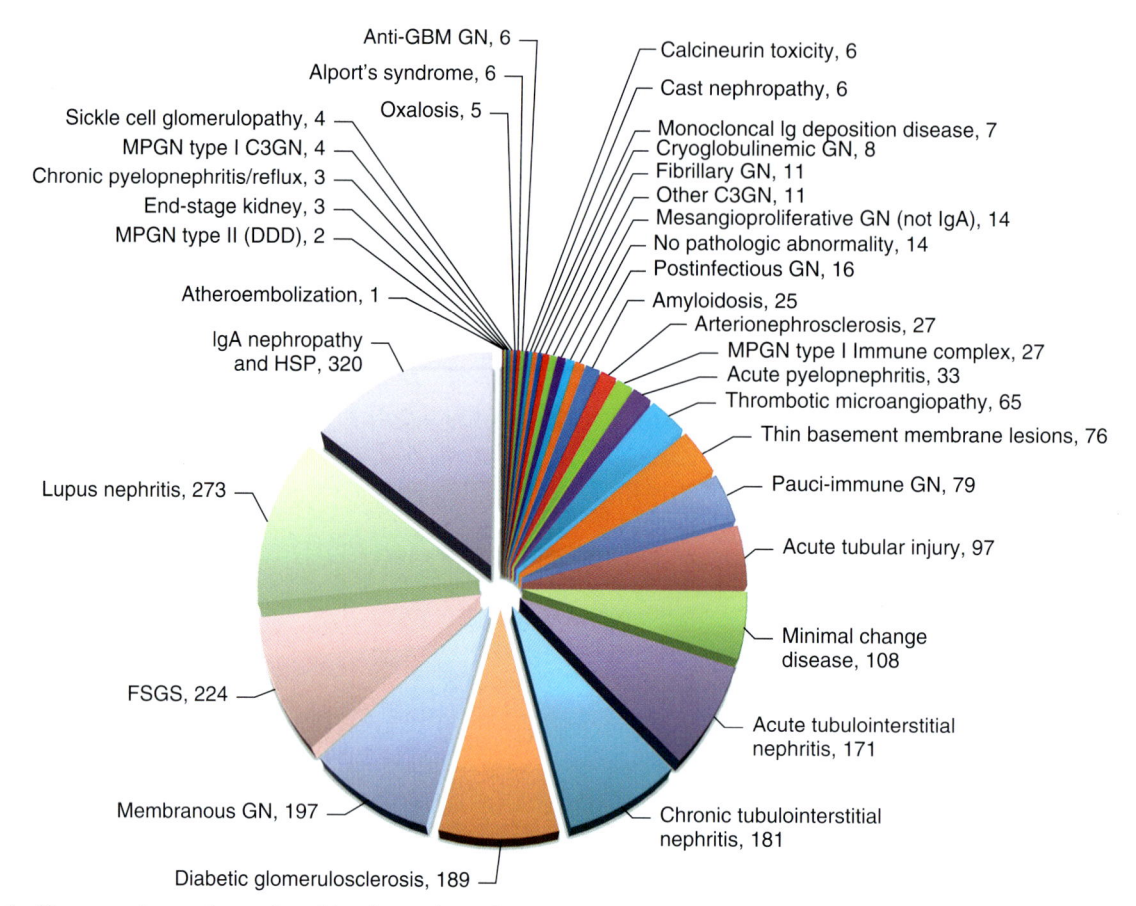

Figure 29.1 Diagnoses in specimens from biopsies performed on 2219 native kidneys at Hammersmith Hospital over a 5-year period. DDD, Dense deposit disease; FSGS, focal segmental glomerulosclerosis; GBM, glomerular basement membrane; GN, glomerulonephritis; HSP, Henoch-Schönlein purpura; Ig, immunoglobulin; IgA, immunoglobulin A; MPGN, membranoproliferative glomerulonephritis.

Pie chart values:
- IgA nephropathy and HSP, 320
- Lupus nephritis, 273
- FSGS, 224
- Membranous GN, 197
- Diabetic glomerulosclerosis, 189
- Chronic tubulointerstitial nephritis, 181
- Acute tubulointerstitial nephritis, 171
- Minimal change disease, 108
- Acute tubular injury, 97
- Pauci-immune GN, 79
- Thin basement membrane lesions, 76
- Thrombotic microangiopathy, 65
- Acute pyelonephritis, 33
- MPGN type I Immune complex, 27
- Arterionephrosclerosis, 27
- Amyloidosis, 25
- Postinfectious GN, 16
- No pathologic abnormality, 14
- Mesangioproliferative GN (not IgA), 14
- Other C3GN, 11
- Fibrillary GN, 11
- Cryoglobulinemic GN, 8
- Monoclonal Ig deposition disease, 7
- Cast nephropathy, 6
- Calcineurin toxicity, 6
- Anti-GBM GN, 6
- Alport's syndrome, 6
- Oxalosis, 5
- Sickle cell glomerulopathy, 4
- MPGN type I C3GN, 4
- Chronic pyelopnephritis/reflux, 3
- End-stage kidney, 3
- MPGN type II (DDD), 2
- Atheroembolization, 1

Table 29.1 Indications for Kidney Biopsy

- Significant proteinuria (>1 g/day or protein to creatinine ratio > 100 mg/mmol or > 1 g/g)
- Microscopic hematuria with any degree of proteinuria
- Unexplained renal impairment (native or transplanted kidney)
- Renal manifestations of systemic disease

---

be more common in biopsies of native than transplanted kidneys and in patients with more advanced renal impairment, prolonged bleeding times, or lower hemoglobin levels (11 ± 2 vs. 12 ± 2 g/dL).[6,7] One prospective study identified the only risk factors for bleeding complications as female gender, younger age (35 ± 14.5 years vs. 40.3 ± 15.4 years), and a prolonged partial thromboplastin time.[9] Interestingly, needle size, number of passes, blood pressure, and renal impairment were not different between those with bleeding complications and those without. However, in this study all patients with prolonged bleeding times received desmopressin (DDAVP) to correct the abnormality, and 75% of patients had serum creatinine values of less than 132 μmol. Conversely, others using retrospective univariate analysis have reported blood pressure greater than 160/100 mm Hg or a serum creatinine level of more than 2 mg/dL more than doubled the risk for bleeding.[7,10] Overall, however, no effective means has been established to identify those individuals at risk for developing clinically significant complications. In one small series, the results of ultrasonography performed within an hour after biopsy had a 95% negative predictive value for predicting clinically significant hemorrhagic complications,[8] meaning that the absence of a hematoma on the postbiopsy scan was very suggestive of an uncomplicated clinical course. Debate continues regarding the routine use of DDAVP to counteract uremic bleeding tendencies. In part this is because its use was previously reserved for only those patients with prolonged bleeding times, and numerous studies have since demonstrated that complication rates are no different if bleeding time estimation is omitted from the preoperative assessment,[11,12] because it does not predict clinical complications.[9] However, later data from a randomized double-blind trial suggested a significant benefit in preventing bleeding complications with few adverse events.[13] In this trial 162 low-risk adult patients undergoing biopsy were enrolled and randomized to subcutaneous DDAVP (0.3 μg/kg) or placebo. The patients were normotensive and had preserved renal function with serum creatinine levels of less than 1.5 mg/dL (estimated glomerular filtration rate > 60 mL/min). The patients given desmopressin demonstrated a significant reduction in postbiopsy bleeding from 30.5% to

13.7% (relative risk [RR], 0.45), a significant reduction in hematoma size in those who did hemorrhage, and a reduction in duration of hospital stay. However, the drop in hemoglobin level after biopsy was minimal, and there were no major complications, leading some to question the benefit of reduction in clinically unimportant hematomas, which can be frequently found following biopsy if looked for. No thrombotic, hyponatremic, or cardiovascular events were recorded. Whether these data, in patients with preserved renal function, could be translated to those higher-risk patients with greater renal impairment is unclear and is a question worthy of a randomized trial.

Guidelines on obtaining informed consent from patients and providing appropriate risk estimates have been produced by certain national renal groups, and one such example is provided in Table 29.2. These estimates may err on the conservative side and should be adapted to local practice if adequate complication data are available. In addition to patients' developing procedure-related complications, there is the chance that an inadequate core is obtained for diagnosis, containing too few glomeruli or insufficient cortical material, and this is reported in 1% to 5% of cases. The size requirements for accurate diagnosis are discussed later.

There are certain absolute contraindications that preclude percutaneous biopsy, whereas there are a number of relative contraindications (Table 29.3) that may be circumvented depending on the importance of the biopsy, the operator's experience, and the supportive facilities available. Ideally, all efforts should be made to deal with the relative contraindications; however, in the context of acute kidney injury this may not always be possible. The critical preoperative steps are to ensure that blood pressure is controlled, that the patient does not have a bleeding diathesis or a urinary tract infection, and that the kidneys are suitably imaged, with no evidence of obstruction, widespread cystic disease, or malignancy (although percutaneous biopsy is increasingly used to diagnose the nature of renal masses). As a result, preoperative assessment should allow those patients unsuitable for percutaneous biopsy to be referred for an alternative approach (Figure 29.2). In these patients there are other means of obtaining renal tissue, which include open biopsies,[14] laparoscopic biopsies, or transjugular biopsies.[15] Each is associated with certain complications and has particular merits depending on the clinical scenario (Table 29.4). Overall, these are generally required for only a minority of potential biopsy patients.

The safe duration of observation following kidney biopsy has been investigated in a number of studies. Findings suggest that early discharge (after only 4 hours of observation) will result in a number of missed complications, with many more occurring between 8 and 24 hours after the procedure. Even after 8 hours, 23% to 33% of complications will be missed. However, an overnight stay will allow an extra 20% of complications to be identified before discharge, with between 85% and 95% of complication being identified at 12 hours and 89% to 98% following 24-hour observation.[7,16] Some units practice a policy of day biopsies with a minimum 6-hour bed rest period, which is extended only if there is evidence of bleeding. Vigilant observation of blood pressure, pulse rate, and evidence of hematuria is required in all cases.

Table 29.2 Risks of Kidney Biopsy*

Complication	Risk
Macroscopic hematuria	1:10
Bleeding that requires a blood transfusion	Less than 1:50
Bleeding that may require urgent x-ray examination or even an operation to stop the bleeding	Less than 1:1500
Severe bleeding necessitating nephrectomy	Less than 1:3000
Deaths	Extremely rare

*According to UK Renal Association. Available at: http://www.renal.org/information-resources/procedures-for-patients.

Table 29.3 Contraindications to Kidney Biopsy

Absolute Contraindication	Relative Contraindication
Uncontrolled hypertension	Single kidney
Bleeding diathesis	Antiplatelet/clotting agents
Widespread cystic disease	Anatomic abnormalities
Hydronephrosis	Small kidneys
Uncooperative patient	Active urinary/skin sepsis
	Obesity

Table 29.4 Alternative Methods for Obtaining Real Tissue and Their Risks and Benefits Compared to a Percutaneous Approach

Method	Advantage	Disadvantage
Transjugular approach	Can be of use in those with a bleeding diathesis and in patients receiving artificial ventilation, or if combined liver and kidney biopsy is required	Carries risk for capsular perforation. Inadequate material retrieved in up to 24%
Open approach	Provides high yield of adequate tissue. Hemostasis is more secure	Requires general/spinal anesthesia; recovery period is longer
Laparoscopic approach	Provides high yield of adequate tissue. Hemostasis is more secure	Requires general/spinal anaesthesia; recovery period is longer

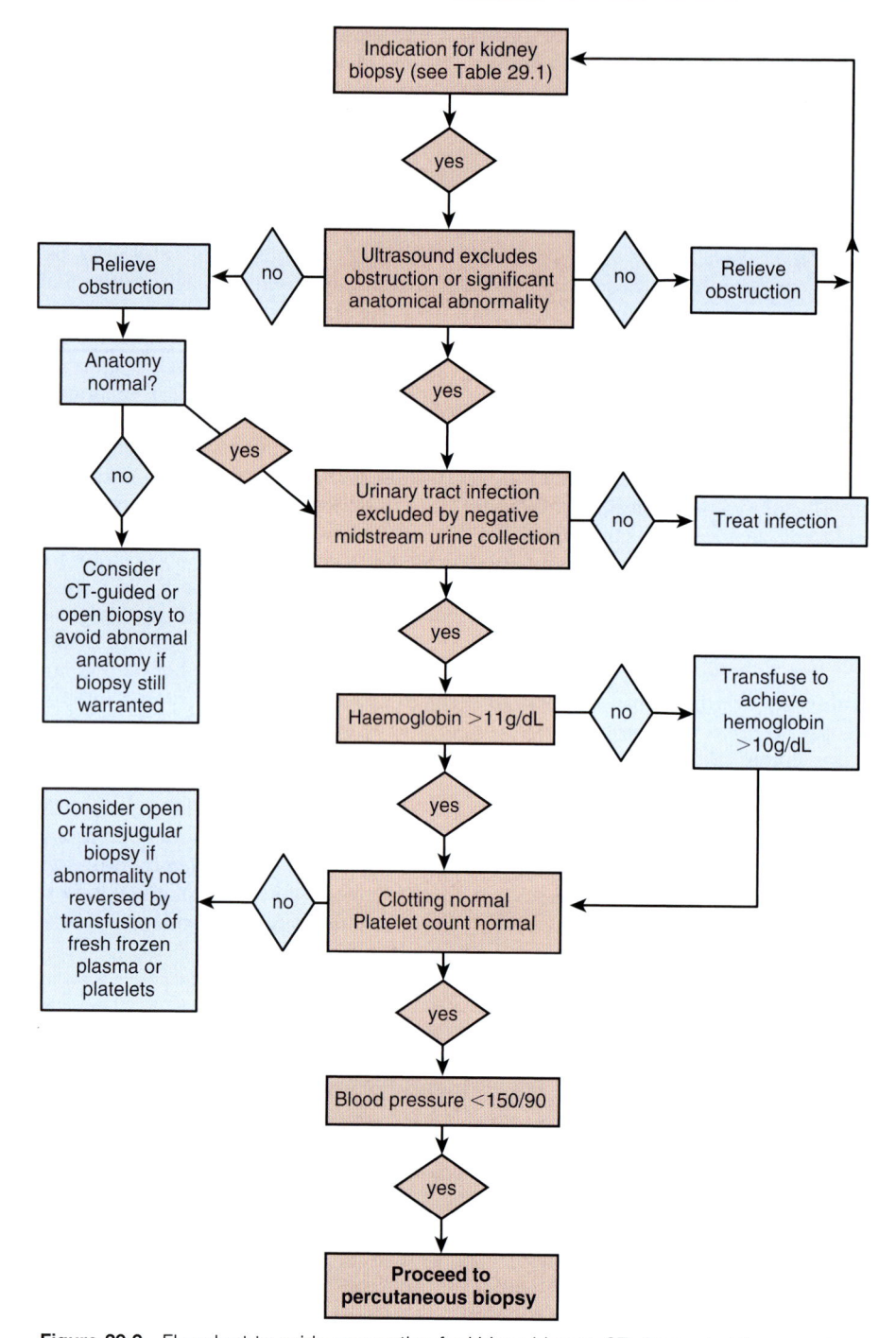

Figure 29.2 Flowchart to guide preparation for kidney biopsy. CT, Computed tomography.

PERFORMING THE BIOPSY

Following informed consent, the patient is positioned prone for biopsy of a native kidney or supine for biopsy of a renal transplant. A posterolateral approach is taken for biopsy of a native kidney. The procedure is performed under sterile conditions with disposable sterile ultrasonographic probe covers, allowing real-time visualization of the kidneys. The procedure is generally performed with the patient under light sedation and with local anesthesia. The lower pole of the left kidney is commonly the biopsy site, but the kidney that is best visualized and most accessible is preferable. After skin preparation, a small incision is made to accommodate the biopsy needle, which is advanced until it reaches the renal capsule. The patient is asked to hold his or her breath while the needle biopsy mechanism is deployed. Most operators now prefer spring-loaded Tru-cut needles or Biopty guns. Needle size varies from 14 gauge to 18 gauge, with many using 16 gauge as a compromise between obtaining a suitable core and increasing the risk for bleeding. Two cores are taken, which should be divided for different assessments as outlined later. In high-risk patients the needle tract may be plugged following the procedure with appropriate material such as Gelfoam. In these cases the biopsy is done through a coaxial introducer needle, and after biopsy the tract is plugged during removal of the coaxial introducer needle.

Careful postprocedure observations of vital signs are performed to detect early signs of bleeding, and all urine is tested by dipstick for blood.

BIOPSY SPECIMEN HANDLING

Detailed descriptions of methods of handling biopsies can be found in a number of publications including references.[17-19]

A full assessment of the kidney biopsy specimen requires examination by light microscopy, immunohistochemical methods, and electron microscopy (EM), with the use of other tests in some circumstances. Therefore it is necessary for the biopsy specimen to be divided to provide material for each of these methods of examination. During this process it is extremely important that the biopsy not be damaged by handling or by drying, and that the tissue be fixed using an appropriate fixative as quickly as possible, ideally within minutes. This is best achieved by dividing the biopsy specimen at the bedside. Examination of the biopsy specimen with a dissecting microscope allows cortex, containing glomeruli, to be distinguished from medulla and thus facilitates assessment of the adequacy of the cores and division of the biopsy specimen so that glomeruli are present in the samples for each modality of examination. If a dissecting microscope is not available, then a standard light microscope can be used with the biopsy specimen placed in a drop of normal saline on a microscope slide. If it is not possible to examine the biopsy specimen in this way, then a standard approach to obtain material for EM is to take small fragments (approximately 1 mm in length) from each end of each core. In that way if there is cortex in the core, glomeruli should be sampled. The remainder of the cores can then be divided for light microscopy and for immunofluorescence. The part of the biopsy specimen for light microscopy is then placed in appropriate fixative and that for immunofluorescence is either snap frozen or transported to the laboratory in suitable transport medium such as that described by Michel and colleagues[20]; tissue placed in this medium can remain for several days at room temperature without loss of antigens. During division of the biopsy specimen it is important not to introduce artifacts due to crushing or stretching. Forceps should not be used to pick up the specimen; this can be done using either a needle or a small wooden stick such as a toothpick. The biopsy specimen should be cut using a fresh scalpel.

If the biopsy specimen has to be taken to the histology laboratory for division, this should be done as quickly as possible with the biopsy specimen wrapped in saline-moistened gauze or in tissue culture medium. Artifacts may be produced if the biopsy specimen is placed on dry gauze or gauze moistened with water, or if it is placed in ice-cold saline.

If the amount of material obtained at biopsy is limited, then it may be necessary to adapt the way in which it is divided, and the decision as to how this is done must depend on the clinical question. In most cases it is possible to omit frozen material for immunofluorescence and instead perform immunohistochemical examination on paraffin sections. However, if there is a suspicion of crescentic glomerulonephritis due to anti–glomerular basement membrane (anti-GBM) disease, immunofluorescent testing is more reliable for detecting the linear capillary wall staining. It may be possible to omit EM and perform it if necessary on material reprocessed from the paraffin block, but if this is done, it is not possible to obtain accurate measurements of glomerular capillary membrane thickness.[21]

LIGHT MICROSCOPY

The most commonly used fixative for light microscopy is buffered 10% aqueous formaldehyde solution. This is actually a 10% solution of the 37% commercially available concentrated solution of formaldehyde, giving a final concentration of approximately 4%. This fixative is generally available in all histology laboratories, provides adequate fixation for light microscopy, and also allows the tissue to be used for immunohistochemical assay and EM.

Some more specialized fixatives such as Bouin's or Zenker's fixative provide better preservation of certain morphologic details, but in general the problems with handling these fixatives and the difficulties of subsequently using the material for immunohistochemical assay or EM, outweigh the advantages. For example, Bouin's contains picric acid, which is explosive when dry. However, the authors do commonly use Bouin's fixative for examination of mouse kidneys, in which the improvement in glomerular morphology is significant. Methacarn, a modified Carnoy's fixative, also provides good fixation for light microscopy and EM and may allow the immunohistochemical detection of antigens that are not detected in formalin-fixed tissue. Details of the preparation of various fixatives can be found in the appendix of Churg and associates.[17]

The standard method of processing tissue for light microscopy is by dehydration in graded alcohols, transfer to a clearing agent such as xylene, and embedding in paraffin wax. This is usually performed in an automated instrument but can be done by hand. Rapid processing schedules allow for same-day processing, and it is possible to obtain stained slides within 3 to 4 hours of receipt of the specimen in the laboratory.

It is important to have thin uniform sections for light microscopy. These should be cut as thin as possible—no more than 3 μm. It is often stated that kidney biopsy sections should be cut at 2 μm, but this may lead to problems in cutting with damage to the tissue. Because many pathologic lesions may be focal within glomeruli, interstitium, or vessels, it is essential that the biopsy be examined at multiple levels, and each laboratory will have its preferred way to achieve that. In general, serial sections should be cut with at least two placed on each slide. Multiple slides can then be stained with each stain, with some intervening unstained sections kept either for potential immunohistochemical examination or for other special stains as necessary.

STAINING FOR LIGHT MICROSCOPY

Most renal pathologists employ a number of stains for light microscopy. The commonly used stains are hematoxylin and eosin (H&E), periodic acid–Schiff (PAS), silver methenamine, and a trichrome stain. The H&E stain is a good general histologic stain for studying the overall architecture of the kidney. It is good for studying the morphology of tubular cells and the morphology of interstitial infiltrates. With experience the different staining characteristics of hyaline, fibrin, and amyloid, all of which are eosinophilic, can usually be distinguished. However, the H&E stain does not distinguish staining of glomerular matrix and basement membrane from cell cytoplasm and therefore is less useful for the assessment of glomerular architecture. In the PAS reaction the mesangial matrix and basement membrane are stained purple, and this allows a good assessment of the amount of matrix and the thickness of the GBM. PAS also stains the tubular basement membranes and hyaline deposits. The silver methenamine stain is the best stain for studying the detailed morphology of the GBM and for highlighting the membrane spikes seen in membranous glomerulonephritis and the double contours seen in membranoproliferative glomerulonephritis. Its only drawback is that a satisfactory result is more technically demanding than the other stains. A trichrome stain, such as Masson's trichrome, will stain the glomerular mesangial matrix and basement membrane and may also help in highlighting fibrin and immune complex deposits. Other stains are a matter of personal preference. The authors always use an elastin stain to demonstrate the elastic laminae of vessels, and this is counterstained with picrosirius red to stain fibrillar collagen in the interstitium. Amyloid is most specifically detected in a Congo red stain, and the authors feel it is prudent to perform this in all native kidney biopsy specimens. This is the exception to the requirement for thin sections; because the Congo red stain is relatively insensitive, a section cut at 10 μm should be used. Details of staining methods are given in the appendix of Churg and coworkers.[17] Other stains that may be employed when necessary include the von Kossa stain, which demonstrates calcium deposition, and the Perls Prussian blue stain for iron.

EXAMINATION OF THE BIOPSY SPECIMEN BY LIGHT MICROSCOPY

It is important to approach the examination of the biopsy systematically. Sections should first be assessed at low power to determine what parts of the kidney (or other structures in some cases) they contain, including whether there is cortex and/or medulla. A low-power view will also allow an assessment of the amount of chronic nephron damage, as demonstrated by tubular atrophy and interstitial fibrosis, and the presence of interstitial inflammatory infiltrates. It will also allow an assessment of interstitial expansion, most commonly due to either edema or fibrosis, but occasionally due to infiltration by, for example, amyloid. Examination should then proceed by studying the glomeruli, tubules, interstitium, and vessels, including arteries, arterioles, and veins, in more detail. Features that should be looked for in glomeruli and tubules are detailed in Tables 29.5 and 29.6. Arterioles should be examined for the presence of hyalinosis, thrombosis, and necrosis. Arteries should be assessed for intimal thickening and whether it is accompanied by reduplication of the internal elastic lamina, thrombosis, necrosis, inflammation, and cholesterol emboli.

Table 29.5 Features to Be Assessed by Light Microscopy in Glomeruli

- Size
- Cellularity: If increased, then are the extra cells mesangial, in capillary lumens (endocapillary), or in Bowman's space? (Normal mesangial areas contain two or three cells.)
- Capillary wall thickness (use PAS or silver stain): If thickened, are there double contours or spikes on the silver-stain section?
- Is the mesangium expanded? If so, are there nodules?
- Is there deposition of abnormal material (e.g., amyloid)?
- Is there segmental sclerosis?
- Is there thrombosis?
- Is there necrosis?

PAS, Periodic acid–Schiff.

Table 29.6 Features to Be Assessed by Light Microscopy in Tubules

- Percentage atrophy
- Signs of acute damage (e.g., dilatation, epithelial flattening, granular casts, mitoses)
- Tubulitis
- Casts: Granular casts suggest acute tubular injury; eosinophilic fractured casts suggest myeloma; neutrophil casts suggest acute pyelonephritis
- Crystals (e.g., oxalate)
- Viral inclusions (e.g., BK virus)

TERMINOLOGY FOR DESCRIPTION OF GLOMERULAR DISEASE

The involvement of glomeruli by a pathologic process can be defined either by the percentage of glomeruli involved by a lesion or by whether the lesion involves all or only part of any individual glomerulus. A lesion that involves all or nearly all glomeruli is described as *diffuse*, whereas one that involves some but not all glomeruli is described as *focal*. In the definitions given in the World Health Organization atlas of glomerular diseases, it was suggested that the cutoff for focal versus diffuse should be 80% of glomerular involvement. However, in later classifications of lupus glomerulonephritis and immunoglobulin A (IgA) nephropathy,[22,23] the cutoff is defined as 50%. If a lesion involves only part of a glomerulus (i.e., with some capillary lumens remaining uninvolved), it is called *segmental*, whereas if it involves the whole glomerulus, it is called *global*. In the classifications of lupus glomerulonephritis and IgA nephropathy,[22,23] the cutoff is set at 50% glomerular tuft involvement, except for segmental sclerosis in IgA nephropathy, in which any area of sclerosis that leaves some of the glomerulus unaffected is defined as segmental.

There are a number of other terms, such as sclerosis and hyalinosis, that have specific definitions in the glomerulus, and these are listed in Table 29.7.

Table 29.7 Definitions of Terms Used in Describing Glomerular Lesions

Term	Definition
Sclerosis	Lesion resulting from an increase in mesangial matrix and/or collapse and condensation of the basement membranes—the sclerotic material stains with eosin, PAS, and silver stains
Hyalinosis	Lesion containing an acellular structureless material consisting of glycoproteins and sometimes lipids—stains intensely with eosin and PAS but not with silver stains
Fibrosis	Lesion consisting of collagen fibers, which may be differentiated from sclerosis by not staining with PAS reagent or silver stains
Necrosis	Lesion characterized by fragmentation of nuclei and/or disruption of the basement membrane, often associated with the presence of fibrin-rich material
Extracapillary proliferation or cellular crescent	Extracapillary cell proliferation of more than two cell layers with >50% of the lesion occupied by cells
Extracapillary fibrocellular proliferation or fibrocellular crescent	Extracapillary lesion comprising cells and extracellular matrix, with <50% cells and <90% matrix
Extracapillary fibrosis or fibrous crescent	>10% of the circumference of Bowman's capsule covered by a lesion composed of >90% matrix

PAS, Periodic acid–Schiff.

IMMUNOHISTOCHEMICAL ASSAY

The understanding of renal pathology was transformed in the 1960s by the use of immunofluorescence microscopy. This allowed the detection and localization of immunoglobulins and complement components in glomeruli and the identification of new entities such as IgA nephropathy. It is mandatory to perform immunohistochemical testing for a full assessment of glomerular pathology in biopsy specimens of native kidneys. The use of immunohistochemical analysis in transplant biopsy specimens is discussed further later. There are a number of diagnoses that cannot be made on kidney biopsy without immunohistochemical testing, including IgA nephropathy, C1q nephropathy, anti-GBM disease, and light-chain deposition disease.

In native kidney biopsy specimens a minimum panel of immunohistochemical stains would include antibodies for IgA, IgG, IgM, C3c, and κ- and λ-light chains. Light-chain immunohistochemical assay is very important if diagnoses such as light-chain deposition disease or monoclonal immunoglobulin deposition disease are not to be missed. Many pathologists would also add antibodies for C1q, C4c, and fibrinogen to this routine panel. In transplanted kidney biopsy specimens staining for C4d is invaluable in assessing the activation of the classical pathway of complement by antibody and hence in the diagnosis of antibody-mediated rejection. There are a number of other antigens whose detection may be useful in particular circumstances. These include the following:

1. Microorganisms, including BK virus, cytomegalovirus, and Epstein-Barr virus.
2. Amyloid proteins. Antibodies are available to AA amyloid and many of the rarer inherited forms of amyloid.
3. α-Chains of type IV collagen. In suspected hereditary nephropathy of the Alport type, it may be helpful to stain for the $α_3$ and $α_5$ chains of type IV collagen.
4. IgG subclasses in cases of suspected monoclonal immunoglobulin deposition.
5. Myoglobin in suspected myoglobinuria.
6. Lymphocyte surface antigens, particularly in cases of suspected lymphoid neoplasia.
7. Type III collagen in collagenofibrotic glomerulopathy.
8. Fibronectin in fibronectin glomerulopathy

Immunohistochemical testing is performed either on cryostat sections of a piece of snap frozen tissue or on paraffin sections. Antigen detection on frozen sections is usually performed using an antibody labeled with a fluorochrome, and this is then viewed using a fluorescence microscope—commonly referred to as immunofluorescence or IF. The use of fluorescent-labeled antibodies on frozen sections is technically straightforward and very sensitive because the antigens have not been altered by fixation. There are some drawbacks. First, it requires a separate piece of tissue to have been obtained at the time of biopsy. Second, the morphology of frozen sections is never as good as that of paraffin sections, and so it may be more difficult to define the site of the antigen within the glomerulus. In addition, immunofluorescent sections will fade over time but if appropriately mounted and refrigerated in the dark will retain staining for weeks to months

If paraffin sections are used, then some form of antigen retrieval is essential for most antigens, because they become "masked" during fixation and processing. For the detection of immunoglobulins and complement the antigen retrieval that works best is some form of protease digestion. The length of time required for protease digestion is critically dependent on a number of factors such as the length of time the biopsy specimen has been in fixative and the particular processing schedule used; some of these may be difficult to control. This variability of the antigen retrieval process is the major drawback of immunohistochemical testing on paraffin sections and means that results are highly dependent on the skills of the technician performing the staining. After the antigen retrieval step, antigens are generally detected using a primary antibody followed by a detection system that leads to the deposition of a colored reaction product that is visible by light microscopy. Commonly this product is developed by a reaction that utilizes the enzyme horseradish peroxidase, and hence this method is often referred to as immunoperoxidase staining. However, it is also possible to use fluorescent antibody staining on paraffin sections after antigen retrieval.[24]

The major advantage of immunohistochemical testing on paraffin sections is that it is not necessary to take a separate piece of tissue for frozen section. In addition, it is possible to specifically localize antigens and compare these sections with adjacent sections examined by light microscopy. However, it is technically demanding, and also it is significantly less sensitive for some antigens. Direct comparison of the two methods showed that detection of IgG, IgA, and C3c by immunoperoxidase on protease-digested deparaffinized sections of formaldehyde-fixed tissue is, with few exceptions, equal to IF on frozen sections.[25] The authors' experience is that it is extremely difficult to get satisfactory staining for light chains using peroxidase techniques on paraffin sections (although fluorescence on paraffin sections may be more successful) and that detection of the linear capillary wall staining of anti-GBM antibodies is more difficult in paraffin sections. It may also be more difficult to detect very early deposits of membranous glomerulonephritis in paraffin as compared with frozen tissue.

In the authors' experience most renal pathologists find immunofluorescent testing on frozen sections the most satisfactory way to detect immunoglobulins and complement, but, regardless of preference, there will always be cases in which no material is available for frozen section, or the material is inadequate, and so laboratories should also be competent to carry out immunohistochemical analysis on paraffin sections.

In reporting immunohistochemical staining for immunoglobulins and complement, it is important to describe the site of staining in the glomerulus (e.g., mesangial or capillary wall), its nature (whether linear, finely or coarsely granular), and its intensity. For estimation of intensity most pathologists rely on a semiquantitative subjective scale from 0 to 3+, but formal quantitation by image analysis may be useful for research. In addition to the glomerulus, staining should also be assessed in the tubules, particular the tubular basement membrane, interstitium, and vessels.

ELECTRON MICROSCOPY

Electron microscopy is invaluable for assessing structural changes in the glomerulus and for identifying immune complexes, which are seen as areas of electron density. Although the importance of EM has become much reduced in other areas of surgical pathology, because of the development of immunohistochemical testing, it remains an invaluable technique for the examination of glomeruli in biopsy specimens from native kidneys and, increasingly, for the determination of causes of dysfunction in transplanted kidneys. The part of the kidney biopsy specimen on which EM is to be performed is usually placed in separate fixative, although entirely satisfactory results can be obtained using material fixed in formalin. Most laboratories prefer either ice-cold glutaraldehyde or paraformaldehyde. The material is then exposed to osmium tetroxide and processed into resin blocks. To select the areas to be studied, "semithin" 0.5-µm sections are first screened by light microscopy to select areas of interest that can then be examined further with the electron microscope. An ultramicrotome is then used to obtain the very thin sections required for the electron microscope. A permanent record of the electron microscopic appearances is kept either as photographs or, increasingly, as digital images. As with light microscopy, examination of the biopsy specimen by EM should be systematic, with assessment of the glomerular capillary basement membrane and its thickness; the endothelium and whether there is thickening or loss of fenestrations; the capillary lumen and particularly whether there is narrowing by cells or other material; and the podocytes, looking particularly at the preservation of the foot processes and whether the cell bodies show any vacuolation or microvillous change. The presence of any electron-dense deposits—most commonly due to immune complex deposition—should be noted, together with their distribution—mesangial, subendothelial, or subepithelial. Electron microscopy may also demonstrate a number of other structures, such as fibrils in amyloidosis or fibrillary glomerulonephritis, tubules in immunotactoid glomerulopathy, or the characteristic inclusion bodies of various storage diseases.

Although EM is most useful in the assessment of glomerular morphology, it may also be very helpful in demonstrating ultrastructural changes in other parts of the kidney. For example, it may help in demonstrating tubular basement membrane immune complexes, in elucidating the nature of tubular epithelial cell inclusions, and in examining the morphology of mitochondria in tubular epithelial cells, which may show abnormalities in inherited conditions or as a result of drugs.

Several studies have assessed the utility of EM in the assessment of native kidney biopsy specimens. Most studies suggest that EM provides useful information in approximately half of all native kidney biopsy specimens and is essential for diagnosis in approximately 20%.[26] Because it is impossible to know which these are at the time of biopsy, it is prudent to always have material available for EM even if, in some cases, it is not processed further after light microscopy and immunohistochemical analysis. Table 29.8 shows some conditions for which EM is essential for the diagnosis and others for which it is helpful. Also listed are some conditions in which the diagnosis may be reached without EM, but even in these cases it is important to remember that EM may allow a more detailed description of the morphology of these conditions or also reveal a totally unrelated pathologic condition.

Morphometric analysis of EM is mainly of importance for research. However, it is important to be able to measure the thickness of the GBM to quantitate the thinning that may be seen in thin basement membrane lesion or the thickening commonly seen in diabetic glomerulosclerosis. Accurate unbiased measurement of the GBM thickness requires complex morphometric techniques to avoid the bias introduced by tangential sectioning of capillary loops. However, in practice it is satisfactory to use direct measurement of GBM thickness (distance from endothelial to podocyte plasma membrane) and determination of the arithmetic mean of such measurements. Das and colleagues found that if 16 measurements from each of two glomeruli were made using this direct method, the results were reproducible.[27] Ideally, each laboratory should define a normal range using this method.

Table 29.8 Examples of the Use of Electron Microscopy in Diagnosis of Kidney Biopsies

EM Essential for Diagnosis

Thin membrane lesion
Fibrillary glomerulopathy
Immunotactoid glomerulopathy
Alport's syndrome
Fabry disease
LCAT deficiency
Nail patella syndrome

EM Very Helpful for Diagnosis

Dense deposit disease
Minimal change disease
Early diabetic glomerulopathy
Early membranous GN (particularly if only paraffin sections are available for immunohistochemical analysis)
Membranoproliferative GN
Postinfectious GN
HIV-associated nephropathy
Lipoprotein glomerulopathy
Collagenofibrotic glomerulopathy

Diagnosis May Be Made without EM

IgA nephropathy
Acute tubulointerstitial nephritis
Myeloma cast nephropathy
Pauci-immune crescentic GN
Amyloid disorder (although amyloid fibrils may be detected by EM when it has been missed on light microscopy)

EM, Electron microscopy; GN, glomerulonephritis; HIV, human immunodeficiency virus; IgA, immunoglobulin A; LCAT, lecithin-cholesterol acetyltransferase.

OTHER STUDIES PERFORMED ON THE KIDNEY BIOPSY SPECIMEN

In addition to examination by light microscopy, immunohistochemical testing, and EM, it may also be appropriate to consider other methods for studying the tissue. In cases of suspected infection, part of the biopsy specimen may be sent for culture or for polymerase chain reaction analysis for infective organisms. In biopsy specimens with lymphoid infiltrates, immunoglobulin gene rearrangement studies may allow the confirmation of clonality. The chemical composition of material in the biopsy specimen, for example crystalline material, may be determined by energy-dispersive x-ray spectroscopy.

There has been considerable interest in the possibilities of extracting messenger RNA from biopsy specimens, to study differences in gene expression in different pathologic conditions,[28] and in studying the range of proteins in the biopsy—the proteome.[29] These techniques have been applied to whole biopsy specimens or to parts of the biopsy specimen, for example glomeruli isolated either by simple dissection under a dissecting microscope or by laser capture microdissection. At present these remain promising research techniques and do not have a clear place in routine diagnostic practice, although in the future microarray data may provide additional diagnostic information.[30] For example, results from a group in Edmonton have suggested that transcript analysis of transplanted kidney biopsy specimens could have a role in diagnosis of acute antibody-mediated rejection.[31,32]

BIOPSY SPECIMENS FROM TRANSPLANTED KIDNEYS

The handling of transplant biopsy specimens differs in some respects from that of native kidney specimens. For biopsies taken to assess the cause of kidney dysfunction in the first few months after transplantation, it may not be necessary to carry out immunohistochemical testing with a full panel of antibodies to immunoglobulins and complement, or to perform EM, unless there is a clinical suspicion of glomerular disease. However, immunohistochemical assay for C4d may be helpful to assess antibody binding and complement activation on peritubular capillary endothelium. In later biopsy specimens EM is very useful in the diagnosis of chronic allograft glomerulopathy and its differentiation from recurrence of de novo glomerulonephritis. It is also helpful in identifying chronic rejection involving peritubular capillaries, which is associated with multilayering of the peritubular capillary basement membranes.[33] The recommendations from the Banff Conference on Allograft Pathology in 2013 are that ultrastructural studies should be performed in all biopsy specimens from patients who are sensitized, have documented donor-specific antibodies at any time after transplantation, and/or who have had a prior biopsy showing C4d staining, glomerulitis and/or peritubular capillaritis.[34] It is also advised that EM be considered in all specimens from biopsies performed more than 6 months after transplantation and from "for-cause" biopsies done more than 3 months after transplantation to determine if early changes of transplant glomerulopathy are present, prompting testing for donor-specific antibodies.

SIZE OF THE BIOPSY SPECIMEN

The kidney biopsy specimen is only a small sample of the renal parenchyma, and this always needs to be kept in mind when making inferences about the state of the whole kidney from changes seen in the biopsy specimen. Some diseases may affect the kidney only focally and therefore may be missed on biopsy (e.g., reflux nephropathy or arterial cholesterol emboli). Others may be segmental at the level of the glomerulus (e.g., focal segmental glomerulosclerosis or pauci-immune necrotizing glomerulonephritis), and therefore the chance of detecting them will depend on how many glomeruli are present in the biopsy specimen and how many sections are examined. Sampling is also a problem when extrapolating from the amount of disease seen in the biopsy specimen to the amount that affects the kidney. For example, if 20% of the glomeruli in a biopsy specimen have crescents, the examiner tends to assume that this is the percentage of the glomeruli in the kidney that have crescents. However, because of the small size of most biopsy specimens, the confidence limits that can be placed on the true involvement of glomeruli are usually very wide. An elegant mathematical description of the problems of glomerular sampling has been published by Corwin and associates.[35] This shows, for example, that to confidently exclude a segmental glomerular disease that is affecting approximately 5% of the glomeruli, a biopsy with 20 glomeruli is needed. The situation is worse if one considers the problem of comparing the amount of glomerular involvement in two different biopsy specimens, a question that often arises, for example, in patients with lupus glomerulonephritis who have repeat biopsies. In that case, to confidently detect a 10% difference in glomerular involvement between two biopsies would require over 100 glomeruli in each biopsy specimen. To detect differences of 25% to 40% glomerular involvement the minimum biopsy size is 20 to 25 glomeruli.

For some diseases, classification schemes have defined minimum sizes for biopsy adequacy. Thus for lupus glomerulonephritis it is suggested that a biopsy specimen should contain a minimum of 10 glomeruli.[22] In transplant biopsies the Banff group has suggested that the requirements for biopsy specimen adequacy are 10 or more glomeruli with at least two arteries.[36] It has been shown that examining two rather than one core of tissue increases the sensitivity for the diagnosis of acute rejection from 91% to 99%.[37] In acute cellular rejection, examining slides taken at only one level rather than at three, misses 33% of cases with intimal arteritis.[38]

BIOPSY REPORT

The biopsy report should include a morphologic description of the biopsy and an interpretation of the appearances in the light of the clinical presentation. The changes seen on light microscopy, immunohistochemical analysis, and EM must be integrated, and this is best done if a single person examines the biopsy specimen by each modality. A committee of the Renal Pathology Society has published recommendations for the essential elements that should be present in a kidney biopsy report.[39]

The description of the light microscopy should include the number of glomeruli present and the number that show global or segmental sclerosis. It is essential to provide a quantitative estimate of the amount of irreversible nephron damage in the biopsy specimen and, where appropriate, the severity of any active inflammatory process. The best way to estimate the irreversible damage is by specifying the number of globally sclerosed glomeruli and the amount of tubular atrophy and interstitial fibrosis. The estimate of activity will depend on the particular disease process but should include an indication of the proportion of glomeruli involved by crescents, necrosis, and endocapillary hypercellularity. For some diagnoses there are established classification schemes that should be applied to the biopsy specimen, for example the International Society of Nephrology/Renal Pathology Society classification of lupus nephritis,[22] the Oxford classification of IgA nephropathy,[40] and the Banff classification of allograft pathology.

The interpretation of kidney biopsy findings requires the pathologist to integrate the biopsy findings with detailed clinical information and therefore requires a thorough understanding of renal disease and the therapeutic implications of the biopsy diagnosis. Close communication between the clinician and pathologist is essential, and it is generally very helpful for the biopsy specimen to be viewed and discussed at a clinicopathologic conference so that full discussion of the implications of the biopsy specimen appearances for patient management can take place.

CONCLUSIONS

Percutaneous kidney biopsy is generally safe if care is taken to select and prepare the patients beforehand. It has become a cornerstone of nephrologic practice, and its handling and interpretation should be made by those experienced in renal pathology. The interpretation of the biopsy findings should be carried out with adequate clinical information for integrated clinicopathologic conclusions to be drawn.

KEY REFERENCES

1. Cameron JS, Hicks J: The introduction of kidney biopsy into nephrology from 1901 to 1961: a paradigm of the forming of nephrology by technology. *Am J Nephrol* 17:347–358, 1997.
2. Pascual M, Vallhonrat H, Cosimi AB, et al: The clinical usefulness of the renal allograft biopsy in the cyclosporine era: a prospective study. *Transplantation* 67:737–741, 1999.
3. Kim D, Kim H, Shin G, et al: A randomized, prospective, comparative study of manual and automated renal biopsies. *Am J Kidney Dis* 32:426–431, 1998.
4. Korbet SM: Percutaneous kidney biopsy. *Semin Nephrol* 22:254–267, 2002.
5. Hergesell O, Felten H, Andrassy K, et al: Safety of ultrasound-guided percutaneous kidney biopsy-retrospective analysis of 1090 consecutive cases. *Nephrol Dial Transplant* 13:975–977, 1998.
6. Preda A, Van Dijk LC, Van Oostaijen JA, et al: Complication rate and diagnostic yield of 515 consecutive ultrasound-guided biopsies of renal allografts and native kidneys using a 14-gauge Biopty gun. *Eur Radiol* 13:527–530, 2003.
7. Whittier WL, Korbet SM: Timing of complications in percutaneous kidney biopsy. *J Am Soc Nephrol* 15:142–147, 2004.
8. Waldo B, Korbet SM, Freimanis MG, et al: The value of post-biopsy ultrasound in predicting complications after percutaneous kidney biopsy of native kidneys. *Nephrol Dial Transplant* 24:2433–2439, 2009.
9. Manno C, Strippoli GF, Arnesano L, et al: Predictors of bleeding complications in percutaneous ultrasound-guided kidney biopsy. *Kidney Int* 66:1570–1577, 2004.
10. Shidham GB, Siddiqi N, Beres JA, et al: Clinical risk factors associated with bleeding after native kidney biopsy. *Nephrology (Carlton)* 10:305–310, 2005.
11. Stiles KP, Hill C, LeBrun CJ, et al: The impact of bleeding times on major complication rates after percutaneous real-time ultrasound-guided renal biopsies. *J Nephrol* 14:275–279, 2001.
12. Lehman CM, Blaylock RC, Alexander DP, et al: Discontinuation of the bleeding time test without detectable adverse clinical impact. *Clin Chem* 47:1204–1211, 2001.
13. Manno C, Bonifati C, Torres DD, et al: Desmopressin acetate in percutaneous ultrasound-guided kidney biopsy: a randomized controlled trial. *Am J Kidney Dis* 57:850–855, 2011.
14. Nomoto Y, Tomino Y, Endoh M, et al: Modified open kidney biopsy: results in 934 patients. *Nephron* 45:224–228, 1987.
15. Mal F, Meyrier A, Callard P, et al: Transjugular kidney biopsy. *Lancet* 335:1512–1513, 1990.
16. Marwah DS, Korbet SM: Timing of complications in percutaneous kidney biopsy: what is the optimal period of observation? *Am J Kidney Dis* 28:47–52, 1996.
17. Churg J, Bernstein J, Glassock RJ: *Renal disease: classification and atlas of glomerular diseases*, New York, 1995, Igaku-Shoin.
18. Walker PD, Cavallo T, Bonsib SM: Practice guidelines for the kidney biopsy. *Mod Pathol* 17:1555–1563, 2004.

19. Furness PN: Acp. Best practice no 160. Kidney biopsy specimens. *J Clin Pathol* 53:433–438, 2000.
20. Michel B, Milner Y, David K: Preservation of tissue-fixed immunoglobulins in skin biopsies of patients with lupus erythematosus and bullous diseases—preliminary report. *J Invest Dermatol* 59:449–452, 1972.
21. Nasr SH, Markowitz GS, Valeri AM, et al: Thin basement membrane nephropathy cannot be diagnosed reliably in deparaffinized, formalin-fixed tissue. *Nephrol Dial Transplant* 22:1228–1232, 2007.
22. Weening JJ, D'Agati VD, Schwartz MM, et al: The classification of glomerulonephritis in systemic lupus erythematosus revisited. *J Am Soc Nephrol* 15:241–250, 2004.
23. Roberts IS, Cook HT, Troyanov S, et al: The Oxford classification of IgA nephropathy: pathology definitions, correlations, and reproducibility. *Kidney Int* 76:546–556, 2009.
24. Nasr SH, Galgano SJ, Markowitz GS, et al: Immunofluorescence on pronase-digested paraffin sections: a valuable salvage technique for renal biopsies. *Kidney Int* 70:2148–2151, 2006.
25. Molne J, Breimer ME, Svalander CT: Immunoperoxidase versus immunofluorescence in the assessment of human renal biopsies. *Am J Kidney Dis* 45:674–683, 2005.
26. Haas M: A reevaluation of routine electron microscopy in the examination of native renal biopsies. *J Am Soc Nephrol* 8:70–76, 1997.
27. Das AK, Pickett TM, Tungekar MF: Glomerular basement membrane thickness—a comparison of two methods of measurement in patients with unexplained haematuria. *Nephrol Dial Transplant* 11:1256–1260, 1996.
28. Neusser MA, Lindenmeyer MT, Kretzler M, et al: Genomic analysis in nephrology—towards systems biology and systematic medicine? *Nephrol Ther* 4:306–311, 2008.
29. Sedor JR: Tissue proteomics: a new investigative tool for kidney biopsy analysis. *Kidney Int* 75:876–879, 2009.
30. Colvin RB: Getting out of flatland: into the third dimension of microarrays. *Am J Transplant* 7:2650–2651, 2007.
31. Sis B, Halloran PF: Endothelial transcripts uncover a previously unknown phenotype: C4d-negative antibody-mediated rejection. *Curr Opin Organ Transplant* 15:42–48, 2010.
32. Sellares J, Reeve J, Loupy A, et al: Molecular diagnosis of antibody-mediated rejection in human kidney transplants. *Am J Transplant* 13:971–983, 2013.
33. Ivanyi B, Fahmy H, Brown H, et al: Peritubular capillaries in chronic renal allograft rejection: a quantitative ultrastructural study. *Hum Pathol* 31:1129–1138, 2000.
34. Haas M, Sis B, Racusen LC, et al: Banff 2013 meeting report: inclusion of c4d-negative antibody-mediated rejection and antibody-associated arterial lesions. *Am J Transplant* 14:272–283, 2014.
35. Corwin HL, Schwartz MM, Lewis EJ: The importance of sample size in the interpretation of the kidney biopsy. *Am J Nephrol* 8:85–89, 1988.
36. Racusen LC, Solez K, Colvin RB, et al: The Banff 97 working classification of renal allograft pathology. *Kidney Int* 55:713–723, 1999.
37. Colvin RB, Cohen AH, Saiontz C, et al: Evaluation of pathologic criteria for acute renal allograft rejection: reproducibility, sensitivity, and clinical correlation. *J Am Soc Nephrol* 8:1930–1941, 1997.
38. McCarthy GP, Roberts IS: Diagnosis of acute renal allograft rejection: evaluation of the Banff 97 Guidelines for Slide Preparation. *Transplantation* 73:1518–1521, 2002.
39. Chang A, Gibson IW, Cohen AH, et al: A position paper on standardizing the nonneoplastic kidney biopsy report. *Clin J Am Soc Nephrol* 7:1365–1368, 2012.
40. Cattran DC, Coppo R, Cook HT, et al: The Oxford classification of IgA nephropathy: rationale, clinicopathological correlations, and classification. *Kidney Int* 76:534–545, 2009.

30 Biomarkers in Acute and Chronic Kidney Diseases

Chirag R. Parikh | Jay L. Koyner

CHAPTER OUTLINE

BIOMARKER DEFINITION, 927
PROCESS OF BIOMARKER DISCOVERY, ASSAY VALIDATION, AND QUALIFICATION IN A CLINICAL CONTEXT, 927
Phase 1: Discovery of Potential Biomarkers through Hypothesis-Generating Exploratory Studies, 927
Phase 2: Development and Validation of an Assay for the Measurement or Identification of the Biomarker in Clinical Samples, 928
Phase 3: Demonstration of the Biomarker's Potential Clinical Utility in Retrospective Studies, 928
Phase 4: Performance of Prospective Screening Studies, 928
Phase 5: Continued Assessment of the Validity of the Biomarker in Routine Clinical Practice, 929
ANALYSIS OF BIOMARKER PERFORMANCE, 929
CHARACTERISTICS OF AN IDEAL BIOMARKER FOR KIDNEY DISEASE, 930
ACUTE KIDNEY INJURY MARKERS, 930
GLOMERULAR INJURY MARKERS, 932
Serum Glomerular Filtration Markers, 932
Urinary Glomerular Cell Injury Markers, 936
URINARY TUBULAR INJURY MARKERS, 937
Urine Microscopy, 937
α_1-Microglobulin, 937
β_2-Microglobulin, 938
Glutathione S-Transferase, 938
Hepcidin-25, 939
Interleukin-18, 939
Kidney Injury Molecule-1, 941
Liver-Type Fatty Acid–Binding Protein, 942
Netrin-1, 943
Neutrophil Gelatinase–Associated Lipocalin, 943
N-Acetyl-β-D-Glucosaminidase, 947
Proteinuria, 947
Albuminuria, 948
Urinary Cystatin C, 948
TIMP-2 AND IGFBP-7, 949
CHRONIC KIDNEY DISEASE BIOMARKERS, 949
Plasma Asymmetric Dimethylarginine, 950
Fibroblast Growth Factor-23, 950
Urinary Monocyte Chemoattractant Protein-1, 950
URINARY RENAL FIBROSIS MARKERS, 951
Connective Tissue Growth Factor, 951
Transforming Growth Factor-β_1, 951
Collagen IV, 951
COMBINATIONS OF MULTIPLE BIOMARKERS, 952
FDA CRITICAL PATH INITIATIVE: A NEED FOR BETTER BIOMARKERS, 953
THE KIDNEY HEALTH INITIATIVE, 953
FUTURE OF BIOMARKERS, 954

Kidney disease is a global health problem. Acute kidney injury (AKI) and chronic kidney disease (CKD) are increasing in incidence.[1] In the U.S., it is clear that the incidence of AKI, regardless of its severity, has been steadily rising at a rate that is disturbingly high, and it is increasingly recognized that AKI predisposes to the progression of CKD toward end-stage kidney disease (ESKD), which ultimately requires dialysis or kidney transplantation.[2-4] According to the World Health Organization, approximately 850,000 patients develop ESKD every year.[5-7] Across the globe, treatment of ESKD poses a major challenge for health care systems and the global economy. The burden of kidney disease is most significant in developing countries and is adversely influenced by inadequate socioeconomic and health care infrastructures.[5,8,9] Importantly, kidney disease progression may be curtailed if the disease is diagnosed early. Hence, detection and management of kidney diseases, whether acute or chronic, in the early, reversible, and potentially treatable stages are of paramount importance. Biomarkers that will help diagnose kidney injury, predict progression of kidney disease, and provide information regarding the effectiveness of therapeutic intervention will be important adjuncts to our standard management strategies.

Many novel high-throughput technologies in the fields of genomics, proteomics, and metabolomics have now made it easier to interrogate hundreds or even thousands of potential biomarkers at once, without prior knowledge of the underlying biology or pathophysiology of the system being studied.[10-13] As a result, there is a renewed interest in discovering novel biomarkers for use in drug development and patient care. Despite notable achievements, however, only a few biomarkers—blood urea nitrogen (BUN) level, serum creatinine concentration, urinalysis results, albuminuria, and proteinuria—are routinely used to diagnose and monitor kidney injury. These commonly used "gold standard" biomarkers of kidney function are not optimal to detect injury or dysfunction early enough to allow prompt therapeutic intervention. Although additional candidate biomarkers have been reported, none has been adequately validated to justify its use in making patient care decisions, but a few look quite promising.

BIOMARKER DEFINITION

In 2001, the U.S. Food and Drug Administration (FDA) standardized the definition of a biomarker as "a characteristic that is objectively measured and evaluated as an indicator of normal biologic processes, pathogenic processes, or pharmacologic responses to therapeutic intervention."[14] The National Institutes of Health further classified biomarkers on the basis of their utility (see Table 30.1).[14] Biomarkers can potentially serve a wide range of functions in drug development, clinical trials, and therapeutic management strategies. There are many different classes of biomarkers: prognostic, predictive, pharmacodynamic, and surrogate. Of note, these categories are not mutually exclusive. Definitions of the different types of biomarkers can be found in Table 30.1. Examples of biomarkers are proteins, lipids, genomic or proteomic patterns, imaging determinations, electrical signals, and cells present in urine. Some biomarkers also serve as surrogate endpoints. A surrogate endpoint is a biomarker intended to substitute for a clinical endpoint. Furthermore, a surrogate endpoint biomarker is expected to predict clinical benefit (harm or lack of benefit) on the basis of epidemiologic, therapeutic, pathophysiologic, or other scientific evidence.[15] An ideal biomarker is easily measurable, reproducible, sensitive, cost effective, easily interpretable, and present in readily available specimens (blood and urine).

PROCESS OF BIOMARKER DISCOVERY, ASSAY VALIDATION, AND QUALIFICATION IN A CLINICAL CONTEXT

Primary challenges to the development of biomarkers for kidney injury and toxicity are discovery of candidate markers, design of an assay, validation of the assay, and

Table 30.1 Biomarker Definitions

Biomarker	A characteristic that is objectively measured and evaluated as an indicator of normal biologic process, pathogenic processes, or pharmacologic responses to therapeutic intervention.
Prognostic biomarker	A baseline patient or disease characteristic that categorizes patients by degree of risk for disease occurrence or progression, informing about the natural history of the disorder in the absence of a therapeutic intervention.
Predictive biomarker	A baseline characteristic that categorizes patients by their likelihood of response to a particular treatment, predicting either a favorable or unfavorable response.
Pharmacodynamic biomarker	A dynamic assessment that shows that a biologic response has occurred in a patient who has received a therapeutic intervention. Pharmacodynamic biomarkers may be treatment-specific or broadly informative of disease response, with the specific clinical setting determining how the biomarker is used and interpreted.
Clinical endpoint	A characteristic or variable that reflects how a patient fares or functions or how long a patient survives.
Surrogate endpoint biomarker (type 2 biomarker)	A marker that is intended to substitute for clinical endpoint. A surrogate endpoint is expected to predict clinical benefit, harm, lack of benefit, or lack of harm on the basis of epidemiologic, therapeutic, pathophysiologic, or other scientific evidence.

qualification of the biomarker for use in specific clinical contexts. The process of biomarker identification and development is arduous and involves several phases.[16,17] For the purpose of simplicity, this process can be divided into the following five phases (adapted and modified from Pepe and colleagues[16]).

PHASE 1: DISCOVERY OF POTENTIAL BIOMARKERS THROUGH UNBIASED OR HYPOTHESIS-GENERATING EXPLORATORY STUDIES

The primary goal of phase 1 is to identify potential leads using various technologies and to confirm and prioritize the identified leads. The search for biomarkers often begins with preclinical studies that compare either tissue or biologic fluids in diseased animals (e.g., animals with kidney injury) with those in healthy animals to identify genes or proteins that appear to be upregulated or downregulated in diseased tissue relative to control tissue. When biologic samples, such as blood and urine, are readily available from humans, it is possible to forgo the animal model stage. Innovative discovery technologies include microarray-based gene expression profiling that provides information regarding expression of genes, microRNA-based expression, and proteomic as well as metabolomic profiling of biologic fluids based on mass spectrophotometry and other technologies. The candidate marker approach, especially when informed by the pathophysiology of the disease for which the biomarker is being evaluated, should not be ignored.

Once a promising biomarker is discovered, the validation process begins. An assay has to be developed and validated. The validation process is laborious and expensive, requiring access to patient samples with complete clinical annotation and long-term follow-up, as described in the discussion of phase 2. In addition, each biomarker must be qualified for specific application. This statement is especially true in the case of kidney diseases, for which one biomarker alone may not satisfy the requirements of an ideal biomarker. This situation is described in the subsequent section on phase 4. Incorporation of several of these novel biomarkers into a biomarker panel may enable simultaneous assessment of site-specific kidney injury or several mechanisms contributing to clinical syndromes.

PHASE 2: DEVELOPMENT AND VALIDATION OF AN ASSAY FOR THE MEASUREMENT OR IDENTIFICATION OF THE BIOMARKER IN CLINICAL SAMPLES

The primary goal of phase 2 is to develop and validate a clinically useful assay for a biomarker that has the ability to distinguish a person with kidney disease/injury from persons with healthy kidneys in a high-throughput fashion. This phase involves development of an assay, optimization of assay performance, and evaluation of the reproducibility of the assay results within and among laboratories. Defining reference ranges of biomarker values is a crucial step before the biomarker can be used clinically.[18,19] It is important to characterize how the levels of these markers vary with patient age, sex, and race or ethnicity, and how biomarker values are related to known risk factors.[20]

PHASE 3: DEMONSTRATION OF THE BIOMARKER'S POTENTIAL CLINICAL UTILITY IN RETROSPECTIVE STUDIES

In phase 3 of biomarker development, the primary objectives are to (1) evaluate the biomarker potential in samples obtained from a completed clinical study, (2) test the diagnostic potential of the biomarker for early detection, and (3) determine the sensitivity and specificity of the biomarker using defined threshold values of the biomarker for utility in prospective studies. For instance, if the levels of biomarker differ significantly between subjects with acute or chronic kidney injury and control subjects only at the time of clinical diagnosis, then the biomarker shows little promise for population screening or early detection. In contrast, if levels differ significantly at hours, days, or years before clinical symptoms appear, then the biomarker's potential for early detection is increased. This phase also involves comparing the biomarker with several other novel biomarkers or existing "gold standard" biomarkers and defining the biomarkers' performance characteristics (i.e., sensitivity, specificity) using receiver operating characteristic curve analysis. This latter process is particularly challenging in kidney disease, given uncertainties in the sensitivity and specificity of the gold standard used.[21]

PHASE 4: PERFORMANCE OF PROSPECTIVE SCREENING STUDIES

The primary aim of phase 4 studies is to determine the operating characteristics of the biomarker in a relevant population by measuring detection rate and false referral rate. In contrast to phase 1, 2, and 3 studies, which are based primarily on stored specimens, studies in phase 4 involve screening subjects prospectively and demonstrating that clinical care is changed as a result of the information provided by the biomarker analysis.

BIOMARKER QUALIFICATION PROCESS

The application for FDA qualification of novel biomarkers requires the intended use of the biomarker in nonclinical and clinical contexts and collection of evidence supporting qualification. This can be a joint and collaborative effort among regulatory agencies, pharmaceutical companies, and academic scientists.

Steps involved in the biomarker qualification pilot process, as described by Dr. Federico Goodsaid when he was at the FDA, are as follows[22]: (1) submission to an FDA interdisciplinary pharmacogenomic review group of a request to qualify the biomarker for a specific use; (2) recruitment of a biomarker qualification review team (containing both nonclinical and clinical members); (3) assessment of the biomarker context and available data in a voluntary data submission; (4) evaluation of the qualification study strategy; (5) review of the qualification study results; and (6) acceptance or rejection of the biomarker for the suggested use.

Data are shared between the FDA and pharmaceutical industry or academic laboratories through voluntary exploratory data submissions (VXDSs).[22] Submission of exploratory biomarker data through VXDSs allows interaction between reviewers at the FDA and researchers in industry or academia regarding study designs, sample collection and storage protocols, technology platforms, and data analysis. This pilot process for biomarker qualification allowed the Predictive Safety Testing Consortium to apply to both U.S. and European drug authorities simultaneously for qualification of new nephrotoxic biomarkers (kidney injury molecule-1, albumin, total protein, cystatin C, clusterin, trefoil factor 3, and α_2-microglobulin) as predictors of drug-mediated nephrotoxicity.[22-24] The FDA and the corresponding European authority (European Medicines Agency, or EMA) reviewed the application separately and made decisions as to whether each would allow the new biomarkers to be "fit for purpose" in preclinical research.[23,24] Some of these markers were proposed to be qualified as biomarkers for clinical drug–induced nephrotoxicity once further supportive human data are submitted.

It is notable that the process described here is specific for the FDA and the United States and that the biomarker validation and approval process varies significantly around the world. As of June 2014, the FDA had not approved a new biomarker for the diagnosis or clinical management of acute or chronic renal dysfunction; however, several biomarkers have been approved for clinical use in several other countries throughout Europe and Asia.

PHASE 5: CONTINUED ASSESSMENT OF THE VALIDITY OF THE BIOMARKER IN ROUTINE CLINICAL PRACTICE

Phase 5 addresses whether measurement of the biomarker alters physician decision making and/or reduces mortality or morbidity associated with the given disease in the population.

ANALYSIS OF BIOMARKER PERFORMANCE

The widely accepted measure of biomarker sensitivity and specificity is the receiver operating characteristic (ROC) curve.[25] ROC curves display the proportion of subjects both with and without disease correctly identified at various cutoff points. An ROC curve is a graphic display of trade-offs between the true-positive rate (sensitivity) and the false-positive rate (1-specificity, where specificity is expressed as a value from 0 to 1) when the biomarker is a continuous variable (Figure 30.1).[26,27] Sensitivity is plotted along the ordinate, and the value of (1-specificity) is plotted on the abscissa. Each point on the curve represents the true-positive rate and false-positive rate associated with a particular test value. The diagonal, represented by the equation *true-positive rate (sensitivity) = false-positive rate (1-specificity)*, corresponds to the set of points for which there is no selectivity in predicting disease. The area under this line of "unity" is 0.5, which indicates no advantage relative to the flip of a coin. The performance of a biomarker can be quantified by calculating the area under the ROC curve (AUC). The AUC is the probability that a randomly sampled case has a larger biomarker value (or risk score) than the value for a randomly sampled control. Although this definition makes the AUC easily interpretable, the interpretation is not always clinically meaningful, because patients with the disease (cases) and controls do not present to clinicians in random pairs. Thus, although an ideal biomarker could supply an AUC of 1.0 (a clinical rarity), in actuality the AUC lacks true direct clinical relevance.[27] Despite these flaws, the AUC is widely reported and familiar to clinicians. The shortcomings of AUC extend into the assessment of the incremental change in AUC (Δ AUC) when a new marker is added to a group of previously established predictors. The clinical impact of a Δ AUC of 0.02 is often unclear, and the statistics and *P* values behind such calculations remain problematic.[28,29]

Other important parameters related to biomarker performance, primarily with respect to the testing of larger or specific populations, are positive and negative predictive values. The positive predictive value is the proportion of persons who test positive for a disease and truly have the disease, whereas negative predictive value represents the proportion of persons who test negative and do not have the disease. There is considerable interest in developing algorithms that use a composite of values of several biomarkers that are measured in parallel for the purpose of increasing diagnostic potential or predicting disease course and patient outcomes.

More recently the Net Reclassification Index (NRI) and the Integrated Discrimination Improvement Index (IDI) have been used to evaluate the ability of new biomarkers. They have gained popularity, in part, because of the aforementioned difficulty in interpreting the true clinical meaning of significant but small changes in AUC (e.g., a 0.04 increase). Additionally, new biomarkers often must have exceptional discriminatory powers to increase the AUC once it has reached a certain level.[30] Briefly, reclassification involves the use of predefined risk categories and then recalculates risk using the previously established predictors as well as the new biomarkers. The Reclassification Rate is simply the proportion of the population whose risk category changes with the new biomarker; a low reclassification rate means that treatment decisions will rarely be altered by the new biomarker. The categorical NRI expands on the reclassification rate and uses predefined risk strata but considers an improvement in reclassification as any increase in model-based predicted probabilities of an event (e.g., AKI) after the addition of the biomarker to a pre-existing clinical model as well as a decrease in the probabilities for the non-events (e.g., no AKI). By definition, the categorical NRI does not depend on the underlying performance of the clinical model and is very sensitive to the number and

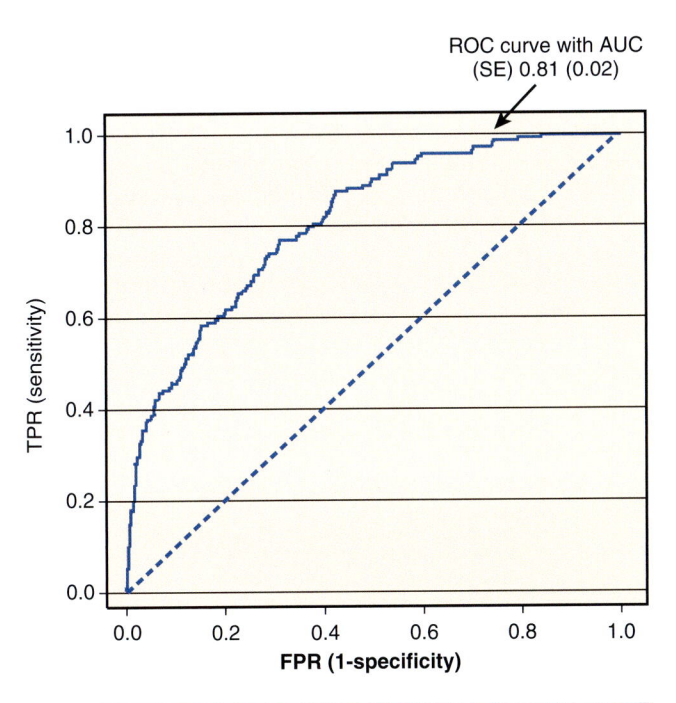

		True disease state	
		Diseased	Non-diseased
Biomarker test	Positive (diseased)	True positive (TP)	False positive (FP)
	Negative (non-disease)	False negative (FN)	True negative (TN)

Biomarker classification by disease status
True positive rate (TPR) = sensitivity = TP/(TP + FN)
False positive rate (FPR) = 1-specifity = FP/(FP + TN)

Figure 30.1 Receiver operator characteristic (ROC) curves. AUC, area under the curve.

thresholds set for the individual risk categories. A worsening in the reclassification is defined by a decrease in the probabilities for events and an increase in the probabilities for non-events. Pencina and colleagues have previously stated that medium effect sizes have an NRI between 0.4 and 0.6 and that large effect sizes have an NRI greater than 0.6.[31] It is worth noting that NRI values may fall between 0.0 and 2.0 with the ideal NRI being 2.0, consisting of 1.0 (100%) increased reclassification of events and 1.0 (100%) reclassification of non-events.

The use of a category-free NRI has been on the rise; this version of the NRI accounts for any upward or downward movement in predicted risk, regardless of risk strata thresholds. The Integrated Discrimination Improvement (IDI) is defined as the difference in discrimination slopes between the unadjusted and biomarker-adjusted clinic models, with large effect sizes having an IDI of 0.10 or greater and medium effect sizes having an IDI between 0.05 and 0.10.[31] The NRI and IDI have gained rapid acceptance in the renal and nonrenal biomarker literature and are potentially more sensitive metrics than AUC; however, we must use caution with the clinical utility because these metrics have not been widely accepted by all statisticians.[32]

CHARACTERISTICS OF AN IDEAL BIOMARKER FOR KIDNEY DISEASE

Characteristics of an ideal biomarker for kidney disease are described in Table 30.2. For AKI, the biomarker should be (1) organ specific and should allow differentiation among intrarenal, prerenal, and postrenal causes of AKI as well as acute glomerular injury; (2) able to detect AKI early in the course and to predict the course of AKI and, potentially, the future implications of AKI; (3) able to identify the cause of AKI; (4) site specific and able to inform pathologic changes in various segments of renal tubules during AKI as well as to correlate with the histologic findings in kidney biopsy specimens; (5) easily and reliably measured in a noninvasive or minimally invasive manner; (6) stable in its matrix; (7) rapidly and reliably measurable at the bedside; and (8) inexpensive to measure.

In CKD (unlike AKI), the timing and nature of the insult are very hard to estimate, making the search for early biomarkers for CKD very difficult. An ideal biomarker for CKD shares many of the requirements described earlier for AKI biomarkers, including providing insight into (1) the location of the injury (e.g., glomerular, interstitial, tubular), (2) the disease mechanism, (3) the progressive course of the disease, and (4) the risk of complications from comorbid conditions such as cardiovascular disease and diabetes.

ACUTE KIDNEY INJURY MARKERS

In the cardiac sciences, the discovery of biomarkers, such as troponins that reflect early cardiomyocyte damage rather than decreased cardiac function, has enabled the development and implementation of novel therapeutic strategies to reduce coronary insufficiency and associated morbidity and mortality.[33,34] By contrast, the delay in diagnosis that is associated with the use of kidney biomarkers, such as serum creatinine concentration, has impaired the ability of nephrologists to conduct interventional studies in which the intervention can be implemented early in the course of the disease process.[35] Although the last decade has seen a revolution in terms of diagnostic criteria for AKI with the RIFLE (Risk, Injury, Failure, Loss, End-Stage Kidney Disease) classification[36] and the Acute Kidney Injury Network (AKIN) definition of AKI[37] being harmonized into the Kidney Disease: Improving Global Outcomes (KDIGO) classification[38] (Table 30.3), these criteria remain limited by their reliance on the serum creatinine concentration on some level. This limitation stems from creatinine's role as a

Table 30.2 Characteristics of an Ideal Kidney Biomarker

Functional Properties	Physiochemical Properties
• Shows rapid and reliable increase in response to kidney diseases • Is highly sensitive and specific for acute and/or chronic kidney disease • Shows good correlation with degree of renal injury • Provides risk stratification and prognostic information (severity of kidney disease, need for dialysis, length of hospital stay, and mortality) • Is site-specific to detect early injury (proximal, distal, interstitium, or vasculature) and identify pathologic changes in specific segments of renal tubules • Is applicable across different races and age groups • Allows recognition of the cause of kidney injury or disease (e.g., ischemia, toxins, sepsis, cardiovascular disease, diabetic nephropathy, lupus, or combinations) • Is organ-specific and allows differentiation among intrarenal, prerenal, and extrarenal causes of kidney injury • Noninvasively identifies the duration of kidney failure (acute kidney injury, chronic kidney injury) • Is useful to monitor the response to therapeutic interventions • Provides information on the risk of complications from comorbid conditions (especially in chronic kidney disease)	• Is stable over time across different temperature and pH conditions, with clinically relevant storage conditions • Is rapidly and easily measurable • Is not subject to interference by drugs or endogenous substances

Table 30.3	Kidney Disease: Improving Global Outcomes (KDIGO) Staging of AKI	
Stage	Serum Creatinine Criteria*	Urine Output Criteria
1	1.5-1.9 times baseline Or ≥0.3 mg/dL (26.5 μmol/L) increase	<0.5 mL/kg/hr for 6-12 hr
2	2.0-2.9 times baseline	<0.5 mL/kg/hr for ≥12 hr
3	≥3.0 times baseline Or Increase in serum creatinine to ≥4.0 mg/dL (≥353.6 μmol/L) Or Initiation of renal replacement therapy Or In patients <18 years, decrease in estimated glomerular filtration rate (eGFR) to <35 mL/min/m²	<0.3 mL/kg/hr for ≥24 hr or anuria for 12 hr

Table 30.4	Potential Utilization for Biomarkers of AKI and CKD
AKI	• Early detection of AKI • Differential diagnosis of AKI (e.g., distinguishing between volume-mediated AKI [prerenal] and intrinsic tubular injury [ATN]) • Predicting outcomes of AKI at the time of clinical diagnosis (need for RRT, development of post-AKI CKD, short- and long-term mortality) • Predicting recovery from AKI • Ascertaining the nephron-specific location and etiology of renal injury • Monitoring the effects of an intervention
CKD	• Early detection and diagnosis of CKD • Predicting the progression of CKD (rapid vs. slow progression) • Predicting outcomes of CKD at the time of clinical diagnosis (development of ESKD, short- and long-term mortality) • Predicting cardiovascular disease/outcomes among patients with CKD • Monitoring the effects of an intervention

AKI, Acute kidney injury; ATN, acute tubular necrosis; CKD, chronic kidney disease; ESKD, end-stage kidney disease; RRT, renal replacement therapy.

functional biomarker; it can rise in cases of prerenal azotemia when there is no tubular injury and can be unchanged under conditions of significant tubular injury, particularly when patients have good underlying kidney function and significant kidney reserve. Nonetheless, these criteria have advanced our understanding of the epidemiology of AKI, and these standardized consensus definitions have allowed for comparisons and aggregation of data from a larger number of papers.[39] Biomarkers of AKI can serve several purposes and are no longer thought of as a replacement for serum creatinine. Table 30.4 summarizes several of the potential uses of AKI biomarkers. Figure 30.2 summarizes the kidney-specific locations of the AKI biomarkers discussed in this section.

Urine and serum biomarkers each have advantages and disadvantages. Serum biomarkers are often not stable and are difficult to measure because of interference with several serum proteins. By contrast, urinary biomarkers are relatively stable and easy to assess; however, their concentrations are greatly influenced by the hydration/volume status of the patient and other conditions that affect urinary volume. To overcome this challenge, urinary biomarker concentrations have often been normalized to urinary creatinine concentrations to eliminate the influence of urinary volume, on the assumption that urinary creatinine excretion rate is constant over time and that biomarker production or excretion has a linear relationship with urinary creatinine excretion rate. Waikar and colleagues have challenged this assumption, however, especially in AKI settings, in which urine creatinine excretion rate is not constant and changes over time, greatly influencing the normalized value of a putative urinary biomarker after normalization.[40] They suggested that the most accurate method to quantify biomarkers is the timed collection of urine samples to estimate the renal excretion rate[40]; however, this approach is not practical for routine clinical care. Ralib and colleagues further delved into this issue by demonstrating that the ideal method for quantitating biomarkers of urinary AKI depends on the outcome of interest; absolute biomarker concentrations best diagnosed AKI at the time of intensive care unit (ICU) admission, whereas normalization to urinary creatinine improved the prediction of incipient AKI.[41] A potential explanation of the failings of normalization is that it often amplifies the signal. For example, when the glomerular filtration rate (GFR) is reduced in immediate response to a tubular injury, the amount of biomarker produced increases, and urinary creatinine level decreases. The normalized value therefore increases by a greater amount in the short term than can be explained by the increase in the absolute level of biomarker production.

Because AKI and CKD share functional and structural aspects, there are overlapping as well as distinct classes of functional and structural biomarkers. Among the functional markers, the GFR is often used as the gold standard. Although the true GFR, as determined by agents that are freely filtered and undergo minimal handling by the tubule (iothalamate, iohexol, inulin), represents a sensitive measure for determining changes in kidney function, tests using these agents are invasive and laborious to perform. Moreover, because of the renal reserve, changes in GFR may not indicate structural injury until significant injury has occurred. On the other hand, structural markers of tubular injury are expressed by tubular cells, and subtle changes in epithelial cells lead to release of these markers into the urine. It is becoming increasingly clear that many of these biomarkers serve as signals for both acute and chronic kidney disease and also may be used to monitor progression from AKI to CKD. A challenge is to define at what level of release of these markers the injury is clinically significant in

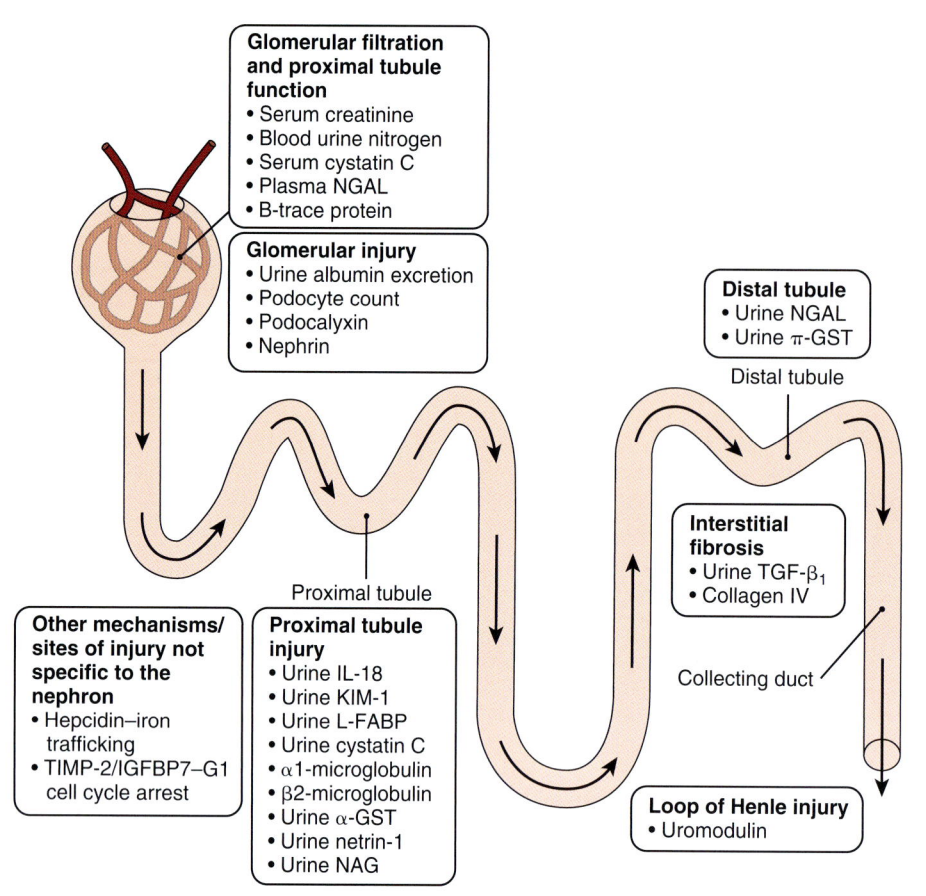

Figure 30.2 Biomarkers in relation to their site of injury in the nephron. GST, glutathione S-transferase; IGFBP7, insulin-like growth factor–binding protein-7; IL-18, interleukin-18; KIM-1, kidney injury molecule-1; L-FABP, liver-type fatty acid–binding protein; NAG, N-acetyl-β-D-glucosaminidase; NGAL, neutrophil gelatinase–associated lipocalin; TGF-β1, transforming growth factor-β1; TIMP-2, tissue inhibitor metalloproteinase-2. (Adapted from Koyner JL, Parikh CR: Clinical utility of biomarkers of AKI in cardiac surgery and critical illness. *Clin J Am Soc Nephrol* 8:1034-1042, 2013.)

either the acute or chronic setting. Failure to identify the separate impacts of CKD and AKI on these biomarker values will lead to inappropriate clinical decision and/or poor results in clinical studies.[42,43]

GLOMERULAR INJURY MARKERS

SERUM GLOMERULAR FILTRATION MARKERS

During the course of injury, kidney function may be impaired with reduction in the GFR and accumulation of several nitrogenous compounds in the blood. Serum creatinine and BUN concentrations are routinely used as markers of kidney injury, but it is important to recognize these parameters as markers of kidney dysfunction rather than as direct markers of injury.

As discussed elsewhere in this text, the estimated GFR (eGFR), using creatinine as a biomarker, is most reliable for CKD under steady-state conditions. In the acute setting, its use is more problematic for reasons that have already been discussed. In healthy persons, the GFR is in the range of 90 to 130 mL/min/1.73 m^2. By definition, patients with stage 4 or 5 CKD have GFRs that are below 30 mL/min/1.73 m^2.[44] Complications of CKD are more pronounced at lower GFRs, and mild to moderate CKD may progress to ESKD.

In AKI, the GFR is only indirectly linked to kidney injury, and changes in the GFR reflect a late consequence in a sequence of events associated with a primary insult to the kidney. Furthermore, because of renal reserve, a large amount of functioning renal tissue can be lost without significant changes in the GFR.[45,46] The functional effects of renal reserve on the GFR can be demonstrated in kidney donors, who often have only modest changes in serum creatinine levels and the GFR after donating one kidney, even though half of the renal mass is lost.[47]

Ideally, a serum GFR marker should be freely filtered with no reabsorption or secretion in the kidney and should maintain a constant plasma level when kidney function is stable. GFR can be determined using exogenous and endogenous markers of filtration. Evaluation of the GFR using the exogenous marker inulin, iothalamate, or iohexol provides reliable results and represents the gold standard; however, the process is time consuming and expensive and can be performed only in specialized settings.[44] Once the GFR level falls below 60 mL/min/1.73 m^2, renal functional impairment can be estimated adequately from the serum creatinine level, various equations being used to calculate the eGFR.[48-50] Although traditionally, these equations have been less accurate for patients with higher GFRs, newer formulas have been constructed utilizing more patients with normal and near normal GFRs.[50]

CREATININE (see also Chapter 26)

Determination of the eGFR using endogenous creatinine is cost effective but can be problematic. Creatinine is a breakdown product of creatine and phosphocreatine, which are involved in the energy metabolism of skeletal muscle. Creatinine is freely filtered by the glomerulus but is also to a lesser extent (10% to 30%) secreted by the proximal tubule. Under normal conditions, the daily synthesis of creatinine of approximately 20 mg per kg of body weight reflects muscle mass and varies little.[51]

Accumulated data from various studies indicate that the creatinine concentration is not an ideal marker for diagnosing AKI for a variety of reasons, including the following:[52-54]

1. Creatinine production and its release into the circulation vary greatly with age, gender, muscle mass, certain disease states, and, to a lesser extent, diet. For example, in rhabdomyolysis, serum creatinine concentrations may rise more rapidly, owing to the release of preformed creatinine from the damaged muscle. Also, body creatinine production, as measured by 24-hour urinary excretion, decreases with older age, falling from a mean of 23.8 mg per kg of body weight in men aged 20 to 29 years to 9.8 mg per kg of body weight in men aged 90 to 99 years, largely because of the reduction in muscle mass.[55]
2. Serum creatinine concentrations are not specific for renal tubular injury. For example, intravascular volume depletion/"prerenal" factors (severe dehydration, blood volume loss, altered vasomotor tone, or age-related decrease in renal blood flow) and postrenal factors (obstruction or extravasation of urine into the peritoneal cavity) may falsely elevate serum concentrations in the absence of parenchymal damage. Thus, a decrease in the eGFR inferred from an increase in serum creatinine level may not distinguish among prerenal, intrinsic renal, and postrenal causes of impaired kidney function; this may not be the case for some biomarkers of renal tubular injury.[56] Even in cases in which serum creatinine is elevated as a consequence of direct renal injury, it cannot be used to determine the location of the injury (glomerular vs. tubular, or proximal tubular vs. distal tubular).
3. Static measurement of serum creatinine level does not reflect the real-time changes in the GFR resulting from acute changes in kidney function because creatinine accumulates over time. Given the large amounts of functional kidney reserve in healthy persons and the variable amounts of kidney reserve in patients with mild to moderate disease, creatinine is not a sensitive marker.[57]
4. Drug-induced reduction in tubular secretion of creatinine might result in underestimation of kidney function. Medications such as cimetidine and trimethoprim inhibit creatinine secretion and increase the serum creatinine concentration without affecting the true GFR.[58,59]
5. The creatinine assay is subject to interference by intake of certain drugs or by certain pathophysiologic states, including hyperbilirubinemia and diabetic ketoacidosis.[58]

Similarly, the use of serum creatinine levels in CKD is also limited by several patient-dependent and patient-independent variables (including age, race, sex, and comorbid conditions). Serum creatinine concentration can significantly decrease in advanced kidney disease without relation to its renal clearance.[60] The sensitivity of serum creatinine levels in determining kidney function can be improved by serial measurements of timed creatinine clearance (usually, but not always, 24-hour collections). However, many individuals find this collection cumbersome, and errors (e.g., skipped voids) typically lead to underestimation of function.

Serum creatinine is stable during long-term storage, after repeated thawing and refreezing,[61] and for up to 24 hours in clotted whole blood at room temperature.[62] The Jaffé reaction–based assay (alkaline picrate assay) is routinely used in clinical laboratories to assess creatinine levels. However, Jaffé methods overestimate serum creatinine concentration by approximately 25% because of the interference of noncreatinine chromogens, particularly proteins. Interference from glucose[63,64] and acetoacetate[65] are particularly important because diabetic patients are particularly prone to development of CKD. As a result, eGFRs are higher when Jaffé methods are used than when other approaches are employed. Expert professional bodies have recommended that all methods of creatinine measurement should become traceable to a reference method based on isotope dilution mass spectrometry.[66] Several modifications of the Jaffé method have been made to improve the specificity by decreasing the influence of interfering substances.[67,68] Enzymatic methods of measuring creatinine are widely adopted by clinical laboratories as an alternative to alkaline picrate assays. Although various substances do interfere with enzymatic assays, the assays are reported to be subject to less interference than Jaffé methods.[69-71] The high-performance liquid chromatography (HPLC)–based assay has evolved as a potential alternative approach for the measurement of serum creatinine level.[72,73] Several studies have demonstrated that HPLC methods have greater analytical specificity than conventional methods.[74-76] This approach clearly has severe limitations with respect to throughput, however.

Finally, over the last decade, there has been a dedicated national effort (within the United States) to standardize serum creatinine assays by establishing calibration traceability to an isotope dilution mass spectrometry (IDMS) reference standard. Prior to standardization, there was a large variability in serum creatinine results among clinical laboratories, with roughly 10% to 20% bias being reported in the literature.[77] This process, which started in 2005, has led to standardization of assays, which has led to less variation in estimating renal function and more accurate eGFR measurements when used in conjunction with the IDMS-traceable MDRD (Modification of Diet in Renal Disease) study equation.[78,79]

BLOOD UREA NITROGEN

Blood urea is a low-molecular-weight waste product derived from dietary protein catabolism and tissue protein turnover, and its levels are inversely correlated with decline in the GFR.[80] Urea is filtered freely, and a variable amount (approximately 30% to 70%) is reabsorbed predominantly in the proximal tubule, with recycling between tubule and interstitium in the kidney medulla. The normal range of urea nitrogen in blood or serum is 5 to 20 mg/dL (1.8 to 7.2 mmol urea per liter).[80] The wide reference range reflects the influence on BUN of nonrenal factors, including dietary protein intake, endogenous protein catabolism, fluid intake, and hepatic urea synthesis.[80,81] BUN concentrations also increase with excessive tissue catabolism, especially in cases of fever, severe burns, trauma, high corticosteroid dosage, tetracyclines, chronic liver disease, and sepsis.[80] In addition, any factor that increases the tubular reabsorption of urea, including decreased effective arterial volume (i.e., impaired renal perfusion) and/or obstruction of urinary drainage, increases the BUN concentration.[80,82,83] Because of these limitations, BUN is a not sensitive and specific marker for acute or chronic kidney disease. However, for patients with advanced CKD (e.g., CKD 4-5), some authorities have suggested averaging urea clearance and creatinine clearance to serve as a more accurate estimate of the true GFR. This approach is suggested in part because at these lower levels of renal function, creatinine clearance overestimates the (secretion) GFR and urea clearance underestimates the GFR.[84] BUN is measured by spectrophotometry. Because of these undesirable limitations of creatinine and BUN as markers, there has been a great deal of interest in the identification of improved biomarkers for kidney injury.

CYSTATIN C

For the last 10 to 15 years, there has been a tremendous amount of research investigating serum cystatin C as a marker of GFR, and urinary cystatin C excretion has been proposed as a tubular injury marker. In 1961, Butler and Flynn studied the urine proteins of 223 individuals by starch gel electrophoresis and found a new urine protein fraction in the post–gamma globulin fraction.[85] They named this protein fraction *cystatin C*. Cystatin C is a low-molecular-weight protein produced at a constant rate by all nucleated cells and eliminated exclusively by glomerular filtration. It is small (13 kDa) and has a positive charge at physiologic pH. It is neither secreted nor reabsorbed by renal tubules but undergoes almost complete catabolism by proximal tubular cells, and thus, little, if any, appears in the urine under normal circumstances. Any impairment of reabsorption in proximal tubules can lead to marked increases in urinary levels of cystatin C in humans and animals. There have been a number of studies on the diagnostic potential of both serum and urinary cystatin C levels in acute and chronic kidney disease in humans.

Chronic Kidney Disease

Because of the short half-life (approximately 2 hours) and other properties described earlier, some researchers believe that serum cystatin C levels reflect the GFR better than creatinine concentration. Initially, it was thought that the serum levels of cystatin C would be unaffected by gender, age, population ancestry, and muscle mass, but over the last several years, multiple studies have demonstrated that these factors are in fact associated with altered levels of the biomarker.[86,87] Notably, cystatin C levels have been shown to be associated with factors similar to those associated with creatinine, namely that these levels may be elevated in males, taller and heavier patients, and those with higher lean body mass.[86-88] However, unlike serum creatinine, which is usually lower in older adults given their decreased muscle mass, a study investigating a subset of more than 7500 subjects from the third National Health and Nutrition Examination Survey (NHANES III) study demonstrated that cystatin C values were elevated in more than 50% of those older than 80 years.[88]

Despite these minor limitations, cystatin C remains an excellent biomarker of CKD and performs on par with, if not better than, serum creatinine in some instances. Equations for estimating GFR and CKD classification are discussed elsewhere in this text (see Chapter 26). In a prospective cohort study of 26,643 Americans enrolled in the Reasons for Geographic and Racial Differences in Stroke (REGARDS) study, Peralta and colleagues demonstrated that cystatin C–based eGFR improves CKD classification/definition as well as risk stratification (for development of ESKD and death) relative to creatinine-based eGFR.[89] This correlation with mortality was not novel because cystatin C demonstrated a stronger risk relationship with mortality than creatinine concentration or eGFR in older adults with cardiovascular disease.[90] In the Cardiovascular Health Study cohort of 4637 community-dwelling elderly, higher serum cystatin C concentrations were associated with a significantly elevated risk of death from cardiovascular causes (hazard ratio [HR], 2.27 [95% CI, 1.73 to 2.97]), myocardial infarction (HR, 1.48 [95% CI, 1.08 to 2.02]), and stroke (HR, 1.47 [95% CI, 1.09 to 1.96]) after multivariate adjustment. In the same study, higher serum creatinine values were not independently associated with any of these three outcomes.[91] Furthermore, a study in the general population suggests that cystatin C level has a stronger association with cardiovascular disease outcomes than creatinine concentration or estimated GFR, especially among the elderly.[91-93] Thus, serum cystatin C levels may be a better marker of kidney function than serum creatinine concentration, especially in older adults.

In addition to older adults, cystatin C has proved superior to serum creatinine in patients infected with human immunodeficiency virus (HIV). Choi and colleagues demonstrated that cystatin C–based eGFRs outperformed serum creatinine levels in the ability to predict 5-year all-cause mortality in a cohort of 922 HIV-infected individuals.[94] These findings are mirrored by those from a later study of 908 HIV-infected women, which demonstrated that CKD risk factors are associated with an overestimate of GFR by serum creatinine relative to cystatin C and that cystatin C significantly improves mortality risk prediction when added to a clinical model that already includes serum creatinine.[95]

This concept of using cystatin C in concert with, rather than in place of, serum creatinine has been gaining momentum. Using cross-sectional analyses and data from 5352 participants from 13 previously published studies, Inker and colleagues developed estimation equations using cystatin C alone and cystatin C and creatinine combined. They then went on to validate these equations in a cohort of 1119 participants from five different studies. They demonstrated that combined equations outperformed the creatinine-alone equations and in some instances led to an NRI of 0.194 ($P < 0.001$).[96] Although this study was performed predominantly in Caucasians, thus limiting its broad applicability, it demonstrates the potential of cystatin C (and other biomarkers) to be used to augment the diagnostic scope of serum creatinine rather than to replace it.[96] Given the mounting clinical evidence and the emergence of automated, relativity inexpensive assays, it is increasingly apparent that this biomarker should become a routine part of the nephrologist laboratory assessment of CKD and points to an increased role for cystatin C in the management of patients with CKD.[97]

Acute Kidney Injury

Given its success as a marker of glomerular filtration, several groups have investigated serum cystatin C as a potential biomarker of AKI. In a single-center mixed ICU population of 85 subjects (44 of whom had RIFLE-classified AKI), Herget-Rosenthal and colleagues demonstrated that serum cystatin C had excellent diagnostic value, predicting AKI 24 and 48 hours prior to serum creatinine (AUCs of 0.97 and 0.82, respectively).[98] These data were followed up by a study of 442 patients from two separate ICUs demonstrating that plasma cystatin C increased earlier than serum creatinine and was able to significantly predict several adverse patient outcomes, including sustained AKI, death, and dialysis.[99] Similarly, in a study of 202 diverse ICU patients, in 49 of whom development of AKI was based on urine output and/or serum creatinine RIFLE Failure criteria, serum cystatin C levels showed excellent predictive value for AKI. However, the serum cystatin C concentration did not rise earlier than the serum creatinine concentration.[100]

Outside the ICU, cystatin C levels were shown to be capable of detecting a decrease in the GFR after contrast agent administration earlier than the serum creatinine value in adult patients who underwent coronary angiography.[101] In a prospective study of 87 patients who underwent elective catheterization, contrast medium–induced nephropathy occurred in 18 patients, and ROC analysis showed a higher AUC for cystatin C level than for serum creatinine concentration (0.933 vs. 0.832; $P = 0.012$). When a cutoff value of more than 1.2 mg/L was used, cystatin C level before catheterization exhibited 94.7% sensitivity and 84.8% specificity for predicting contrast medium–induced nephropathy.[102]

Serum cystatin C has been studied as a biomarker for both early AKI (rising earlier than serum creatinine) and AKI severity, with several smaller studies providing mixed results.[103-106] The larger multicenter Translational Research Investigating Biomarker Endpoints in AKI (TRIBE-AKI) study investigated several aspects of serum cystatin C following both adult and pediatric cardiac surgery. In 1147 adults, Shlipak and colleagues demonstrated that preoperative serum cystatin C values outperformed serum creatinine and creatinine-based eGFRs in its ability to forecast postoperative AKI. After adjustment for clinical variables known to contribute to AKI, serum cystatin C had a C-statistic (a measure akin to the AUC of a ROC) of 0.70 and an NRI of 0.21 in comparison with serum creatinine ($P < 0.001$).[107] However, when this same group investigated sensitivity and rapidity of AKI detection (defined as 25%, 50%, and 100% increases from preoperative values) by postoperative changes in serum cystatin C, they did not find a clear advantage over changes in serum creatinine. In fact, they concluded that serum cystatin C was less sensitive for AKI detection; however, serum cystatin C did appear to identify a subset of patients with adverse outcomes.[108] This failure of postoperative serum cystatin C in adults contrasts starkly with the results in 288 children undergoing cardiac surgery.

Zappitelli and colleagues demonstrated that serum cystatin C measured within the first 6 postoperative hours was associated with both stage 1 and stage 2 pediatric AKI. Additionally, postoperative serum cystatin C values were associated with adverse patient outcomes, including duration of mechanical ventilation and length of ICU stay. However, unlike in the adult population, preoperative values were not associated with postoperative AKI.[109]

β-TRACE PROTEIN

β-Trace protein (BTP), also referred to as *prostaglandin D synthase*, has emerged as another promising biomarker for GFR. BTP is a small protein with a molecular weight of 23 to 29 kDa, depending on the size of the glycosyl moiety. BTP belongs to the lipocalin protein family, whose members are primarily involved in the binding and transport of small hydrophobic ligands. It is primarily produced in the cerebral fluid, where its concentrations are more than 40-fold higher than in the serum. BTP is primarily eliminated by glomerular filtration, and its concentrations in urine range from 600 to 1200 µg/L.[110]

The first observation of elevated BTP values in association with impaired kidney function was reported by Hoffman and associates in 1997.[111] Since then, several research studies have been conducted to evaluate the sensitivity and specificity of BTP as a marker of GFR and to compare it with serum creatinine in patients with CKD[112] and in kidney transplant recipients. In two separate cohort studies, one adult and one pediatric, serum cystatin C was shown to outperform BTP for the detection of decreased renal function (as measured by inulin clearance), and both markers were shown to outperform serum creatinine alone.[113,114]

Another study, by Donadio and colleagues, evaluated the relationship between serum concentration of BTP and GFR in comparison with cystatin C levels. Serum concentrations of BTP progressively increased with reduced GFR, and strong direct correlations were found between GFR and serum concentrations of BTP ($r = 0.918$) and cystatin C ($r = 0.937$). Importantly, no statistically significant difference was found between BTP and cystatin C as indicators of moderately impaired kidney function.[115]

In a later study, Foster and colleagues investigated the association of BTP, serum cystatin C, and creatinine-based eGFR with all-cause mortality in a subset of patients from the NHANES cohort. They analyzed data from 6445 adults (enrolled from 1988 to 1994) with follow-up through December 2006. All three markers were associated with increased mortality after adjustments were made for demographics. When the mortality risk of the fifth (highest) quintile was compared with that of the third (middle) quintile, however, only the associations with BTP (HR, 2.14; 95% CI, 1.56 to 2.94) and serum cystatin C (HR, 1.94; 95% CI, 1.43 to 2.62) remained statistically significant (creatinine-based eGFR: HR, 1.31; 95% CI, 0.84 to 2.04) (all HR comparing the 5th quintile to the middle quintile).[116] These effects remained significant for both cardiovascular disease– and coronary heart disease–associated mortality. Similarly, in data from the Atherosclerosis Risk in Communities (ARIC) study, BTP was shown to outperform creatinine-based eGFR (using the CKD-EPI [Chronic Kidney Disease Epidemiology Collaboration] equation) in the prediction of mortality and the development of kidney failure.[117]

Concentrations of BTP are not affected by commonly used immunosuppressive medications such as prednisone, mycophenolate mofetil, and cyclosporine.[118] This feature is especially useful in the evaluation of kidney function in kidney transplant recipients, in whom cystatin C concentrations may be falsely elevated as a result of steroid treatment.[119] Unlike with serum creatinine values, age and race were not associated with BTP concentrations. Several new GFR estimation equations based on BTP have been developed for use in kidney transplant recipients.[118,119] However, these equations require external validation in larger and more diverse patient groups. In contrast to creatinine, one limitation of using BTP is lack of widespread availability and standardization of the assay.

URINARY GLOMERULAR CELL INJURY MARKERS

Defects in podocyte structure have been reported in many glomerular diseases, which have been classified as "podocytopathies."[120,121] Injured podocytes have been reported in immunologic and nonimmunologic forms of human glomerular disease, including hemodynamic injury, protein overload states, injury from environmental toxins, minimal change disease, focal segmental glomerulosclerosis, membranous glomerulopathy, diabetic nephropathy, and lupus nephritis.[122-127] Podocytes may be injured in many forms of human and experimental primary glomerular disease and in secondary forms of focal segmental glomerulosclerosis, including that caused by hypertension, diabetes, and tubulointerstitial disease.[128-130] Before detachment from the glomerular basement membrane, podocytes undergo structural changes, including effacement of foot processes and microvillous transformation.[120,121,131,132]

PODOCYTE COUNT

After undergoing the aforementioned structural changes, podocytes detach from glomerular basement membrane and are excreted into the urine. Urinary levels of viable podocytes have been extensively studied in several renal diseases.[133-136] Numerous studies have reported that the number of podocytes shed is significantly higher in patients with active glomerular disease than in healthy controls and in patients with inactive disease. Importantly, podocyte number in urine correlates with disease activity (assessed by renal biopsy) and has been shown to decline with treatment. For example, Nakamura and colleagues found podocytes in the urine of patients with type 2 diabetes with microalbuminuria and macroalbuminuria, but not in the urine of patients with diabetes without albuminuria, suggesting that urinary podocytes may represent the active phase of diabetic nephropathy.[137] Numerous studies have linked podocytopenia and disease severity in immunoglobulin A (IgA) nephropathy[133,134] and diabetic nephropathy.[135,136] Additionally, in a study of 42 preterm neonates receiving indomethacin, the number of podocytes excreted in the urine was higher when compared to controls not receiving a known nephrotoxin, potentially linking podocytes and nephrotoxin-induced kidney injury.[138] Thus, urinary levels of podocytes may reflect real-time changes in disease activity.

The methods used to count urinary podocytes, however, are limited by several factors: (1) cytologists are needed to perform the counting, (2) the process is very time consuming, and (3) urine sediments contain whole viable podocytes as well as cell debris, and the latter may not necessarily reflect disease status. An improved and standardized laboratory method is urgently needed to facilitate measurement of urinary podocyte number. Alternative methods that indirectly assess the number of podocytes in urine include detection of messenger RNA (mRNA) and protein levels of podocyte-specific proteins by polymerase chain reaction (PCR) and enzyme-linked immunosorbent assay (ELISA), respectively.

PODOCALYXIN

Podocalyxin is the most commonly used marker protein for detecting podocytes in urine.[139] A highly O-glycosylated and sialylated type I transmembrane protein of approximately 140 kDa, podocalyxin is expressed in podocytes, hematopoietic progenitor cells, vascular endothelial cells, and a subset of neurons.[139] Podocalyxin participates in a number of cellular functions through its association with the actin cytoskeleton, ezrin, and Na^+-H^+-exchanger regulatory factors 1 and 2 (NHERF-1 and NHERF-2) proteins. Urinary podocalyxin has been reported as a marker of activity in a number of diseases, including IgA nephropathy, Henoch-Schönlein purpura, diabetic nephropathy, lupus nephritis, poststreptococcal glomerulonephritis, focal segmental glomerulosclerosis, and preeclampsia.[140-147] Podocalyxin has been reported to be the most reproducible marker for podocyte injury in the urine. Measurements of podocalyxin protein in the urine by ELISA also correlated with histologic changes and disease activity in children with IgA nephropathy, Henoch-Schönlein purpura, lupus nephritis, membranoproliferative glomerulonephritis, and poststreptococcal glomerulonephritis.[140,148,149] Several studies have also shown that the number of podocalyxin-positive cells in the urine falls after various therapeutic interventions in patients with focal segmental glomerulosclerosis, lupus nephritis, Henoch-Schönlein purpura, IgA nephropathy, poststreptococcal glomerulonephritis, and diabetic nephropathy.[136,140,148,149] Unfortunately, because podocalyxin is expressed on a number of cell types, the presence of podocalyxin in the urine is not always reflective of urinary podocytes.

NEPHRIN

Nephrin, a transmembrane protein of the immunoglobulin superfamily, is a component of the filtration slit diaphragm between neighboring podocytes.[150,151] Immunohistochemical analysis and in situ hybridization have shown that nephrin is primarily expressed in glomerular podocytes.[152] On the basis of these observations, it has been proposed that nephrin is a key component of the glomerular filtration barrier, which plays a pivotal role in preventing protein leakage. Various experimental models of diabetes and hypertension show alterations in nephrin mRNA or protein levels in glomeruli. In experimental models of diabetes, glomerular nephrin mRNA expression was reduced, but treatment with an angiotensin-converting enzyme (ACE) inhibitor or angiotensin II antagonist was able to abrogate this reduced expression.[153,154] Langham and associates examined renal biopsy specimens from 14 patients with type 2 diabetes and nephropathy who had been randomly assigned to receive treatment with either the ACE inhibitor perindopril (4 mg/day) or placebo for the preceding 2 years.[155] They reported that glomeruli from placebo-treated patients with diabetic nephropathy showed a significant reduction in nephrin expression compared with those from control subjects. This finding is in line with experimental models demonstrating that urinary nephrin excretion is increased in the setting of active podocyte/glomerular injury and that excretion is attenuated in the presence of RAAS (renin angiotensin aldosterone system) blockers.[156] In both placebo- and perindopril-treated patients, a close inverse correlation was observed between the magnitude of nephrin gene expression and the degree of proteinuria.[155] In accordance with these observations, nephrin has been reported in urine (nephrinuria) in several experimental and human proteinuric diseases, including hypertension, diabetes, and pre-eclampsia.[147,157-160] Because nephrin is known to be expressed in pancreatic β-cells, there was speculation that β-cells may release nephrin into the serum, which is ultimately excreted in the urine. However, Patari and colleagues demonstrated that nephrin was absent in the sera of nephrinuric patients.[161] Thus, urinary nephrin is most likely produced by the kidneys.

URINARY TUBULAR INJURY MARKERS

Microscopic examination of the urine has been used for many years to gain insight into the severity of glomerular and tubular injury. Other components of the urine have been used to quantitate tubular cell injury in a more specific and sensitive fashion. These markers have been demonstrated to be extremely valuable in detecting kidney injury in the setting of AKI. Moreover, some of these biomarkers, such as interleukin-18 (IL-18), kidney injury molecule-1 (KIM-1), neutrophil gelatinase–associated lipocalin (NGAL), and liver-type fatty acid–binding protein (L-FABP), have been shown to be potentially useful in a variety of contexts in both acute and chronic kidney injury. Here, the utility of urine microscopy is described briefly and some of the emerging biomarkers of tubular injury are discussed.

URINE MICROSCOPY

Urine microscopy with sediment examination is a time-honored test that is routinely used to assist in the diagnosis of kidney injury.[162-164] The urine from patients with tubular injury typically contains proximal tubular epithelial cells, proximal tubule epithelial cell casts, granular casts, and mixed cellular casts. Patients with predominantly prerenal azotemia occasionally have hyaline or fine granular casts in their urine.[165-167] Several studies have shown that the increase in urinary cast excretion correlates well with AKI.[166,168,169] Marcussen and associates demonstrated that patients with tubular injury had a high number of granular casts than those with prerenal azotemia.[168]

There has now been a resurgence in urinalysis sediment scoring systems for the diagnosis of AKI.[167,170] Several of these systems have shown excellent specificity for AKI and correlate well with severity of AKI.[170-172] However, their widespread acceptance has been hampered by the relatively modest sensitivity of urine microscopy for detecting AKI.[167,170,173,174] Urine microscopy remains a user-dependent tool that displays a tremendous amount of interphysician variability, a feature that likely contributes to its suboptimal sensitivity for AKI.[175] Three of the most widely reported urine microscopy scoring systems are reviewed in Table 30.5.

Table 30.5 Review of Urine Microscopy Scoring Systems

Study	Scoring System
Chawla et al 2008[170]	Grade 1: No casts or RTEs Grade 2: At least 1 cast or RTE but <10% of LPF Grade 3: Many casts or RTEs (between 10% and 90% of LPF) Grade 4: Sheet of muddy brown casts and RTEs in >90% of LPF
Perazella et al 2010[171]	0 points: No casts or RTEs seen 1 point each: 1-5 casts per LPF or 1-5 RTEs per HPF 2 points each: ≥6 casts per LPF or ≥6 RTEs per HPF
Bagshaw et al 2011[173]	0 points: No casts or RTEs seen 1 point each: 1cast or 1 RTE per HPF 2 points each: 2-4 casts or RTEs per HPF 3 points each: ≥5 casts or ≥5 RTEs per HPF

LPF, Low-power field; HPF, high-power field; RTE, renal tubule epithelial (cell).

Several later studies have looked at the potential of using urine microscopy in combination with other biomarkers for tubular injury with varying degrees of success.[171-173] In the near future, urine microscopy, a current mainstay in the clinical diagnosis of AKI, could be used in concert with markers of glomerular function and validated biomarkers of tubular injury to diagnose AKI.

α_1-MICROGLOBULIN

α-Microglobulin is a low-molecular-weight glycoprotein of approximately 27 to 30 kDa and a member of the lipocalin superfamily. It is primarily synthesized by the liver and is available both in free form and as a complex with IgA.[176] α_1-Microglobulin has been detected in human serum, urine, and cerebrospinal fluid. Urine and serum values have been found to be elevated in patients with renal tubular diseases. α_1-Microglobulin is freely filtered at the glomerulus and completely reabsorbed and catabolized by the normal proximal tubule. Megalin mediates the uptake of this protein in the proximal tubule. Therefore, an increase in the urinary concentration of α_1-microglobulin indicates proximal tubular injury or dysfunction. The urinary levels of α_1-microglobulin are influenced by age. The normal range in populations younger than 50 years is less than 13 mg per g of creatinine and in those 50 years or older is less than 20 mg per g of creatinine.[176] In comparison with β_2-microglobulin, α_1-microglobulin is more stable over a range of pH levels in the urine,[177] making it a more acceptable urinary biomarker.

ACUTE KIDNEY INJURY

α_1-Microglobulin quantitation in the urine has been reported as a sensitive biomarker for proximal tubule dysfunction in both adults and children.[176,178] In a small cohort, 73 patients, of whom 26 required renal replacement therapy (RRT), Herget-Rosenthal and colleagues compared levels of α_1-microglobulin, β_2-microglobulin, cystatin C, retinol-binding protein, α-glutathione S-transferase (α-GST), lactate dehydrogenase, and N-acetyl-β-D-glucosaminidase (NAG) early in the course of AKI. They found that urinary cystatin C and $α_1$-microglobulin had the highest ability to predict the need for RRT.[179] In this study, urinary $α_1$-microglobulin had an AUC of 0.86 for prediction of the need for RRT. This is similar to the results reported by Zheng and associates, who measured $α_1$-microglobulin levels in 58 children undergoing cardiac surgery and found that levels were higher in those in whom AKI developed (AKIN criteria). Four hours after cardiopulmonary bypass, $α_1$-microglobulin provided an AUC of 0.84 (95% CI, 0.72 to 0.95) with a value of 290 mg/g, providing a sensitivity of 90% and a specificity of 79%.[180] However, follow-up studies have reported mixed results, with Martensson and colleagues finding no difference in $α_1$-microglobulin levels between those with and those without AKI in the setting of sepsis and septic shock in a small, prospective, single-center study of 45 subjects.[181]

$α_1$-Microglobulin levels at the time of arrival at the emergency department (ED) have also demonstrated the ability to correlate with the development of AKI, with an AUC of 0.88 and a cutoff value of 35mg/g providing reasonable sensitivity (80%) and specificity (81%). However, $α_1$-microglobulin level did not remain an independent predictor of AKI in the multivariate model (odds ratio [OR] 1.85; 95% CI, 0.80 to 4.31).[182] In addition, $α_1$-microglobulin has been reported as a useful marker for proximal tubular damage and recovery in early infancy and has been shown to correlate with tubular atrophy and interstitial fibrosis on renal transplant biopsy 1 year after transplantation.[183,184]

CHRONIC KIDNEY DISEASE

There have been fewer studies investigating $α_1$-microglobulinin in the setting of CKD, and limited studies demonstrate that this condition may correlate with disease activity and proximal tubule damage in the setting of diabetic nephropathy as well as idiopathic membranous nephropathy.[185,186] Limitations associated with the use of $α_1$-microglobulin level include the variation in serum levels with age, gender,[187] and clinical conditions, including liver diseases,[176] ulcerative colitis,[188] HIV infection, and mood disorders,[176] as well as the lack of international standardization. Urinary $α_1$-microglobulin is measured by an immunonephelometric assay.

$β_2$-MICROGLOBULIN

$β_2$-Microglobulin is a low-molecular-weight polypeptide with a molecular weight of 11.8 kDa. It is present on the cell surfaces of all nucleated cells and in most biologic fluids, including serum, urine, and synovial fluid. $β_2$-Microglobulin is normally excreted by glomerular filtration, reabsorbed almost completely (approximately 99%), and catabolized by the normal proximal tubule in humans.[189,190] Megalin mediates the uptake of this protein in the proximal tubule.[190] In healthy individuals, approximately 150 to 200 mg of $β_2$-microglobulin is synthesized daily with a normal serum concentration of 1.5 to 3 mg/L. Any pathologic state that affects kidney function results in an increase in $β_2$-microglobulin levels in the urine because of the impeded uptake of $β_2$-microglobulin by renal tubular cells. For spot urine collections, the concentration of $β_2$-microglobulin in healthy individuals is typically 160 μg/L or less or 300 μg per g of creatinine or less. Unlike serum levels of urea, those of $β_2$-microglobulin are not influenced by food intake, making this polypeptide an attractive marker for malnourished patients with low serum urea levels. In patients with CKD, increases in serum $β_2$-microglobulin levels reflect the decrease in glomerular function. In patients with ESKD, serum levels of $β_2$-microglobulin are usually in the range of 20 to 50 mg/L. $β_2$-Microglobulin accumulation is linked to toxicity because the molecule precipitates and forms fibrillary structures and amyloid deposits, particularly in bone and periarticular tissue, leading to the development of carpal tunnel syndrome and erosive arthritis.[190,191] Elevations of $β_2$-microglobulin have been reported in several AKI and CKD clinical settings, including in cadmium toxicity[192] and following cardiac surgery,[193,194] liver transplantation,[195] and renal transplantation.[196] In idiopathic membranous nephropathy, $β_2$-microglobulin level was identified as a superior independent predictor of the development of renal insufficiency.[197] Other studies have reported that $β_2$-microglobulin performs as well as, if not better than, serum creatinine for the detection of acute kidney injury in critically ill children[198] or after cardiac surgery in adults.[194]

Serum concentrations of $β_2$-microglobulin should be interpreted cautiously because they are altered significantly in various diseases, including rheumatoid disorders and several types of cancers.[199,200] Initially, it was believed that the increase in $β_2$-microglobulin levels in CKD is solely due to declines in kidney function, but later studies have shown that other factors, including increased synthesis of $β_2$-microglobulin, may contribute in patients with ESKD.[201] Another significant drawback associated with the use of urinary $β_2$-microglobulin as a marker of kidney injury is its instability in urine at room temperature, particularly when the pH is less than 5.5; for this reason, the urine should be alkalinized and frozen at −80° C immediately after collection.[191,202]

GLUTATHIONE S-TRANSFERASE

Primarily two subtypes of the enzyme glutathione S-transferase (GST) are found in the kidney. α-GST is found mainly in the proximal tubular cells, whereas π-GST is found predominantly in the distal tubular epithelial cells. Elevation of urinary α-GST has been reported in several animal models treated with nephrotoxic drugs or after ischemic renal injury.[203,204] However, in a prospective study of patients with sepsis admitted to the ICU, α-GST levels were no different in patients in whom AKI developed and in patients without AKI. π-GST levels were higher in all patients with sepsis than in healthy volunteers but π-GST levels were not predictive of AKI as defined by the AKIN criteria.[205] In one prospective study, the value of tubular enzyme levels in predicting AKI was assessed in 26 critically ill adult patients admitted to the ICU. AKI developed in 4 patients, and ROC analysis showed that γ-glutamyl transpeptidase, π-GST, α-GST, alkaline phosphatase, and NAG had excellent discriminating power for AKI (AUCs = 0.950, 0.929, 0.893, 0.863, and 0.845, respectively).[206] Both α-GST and π-GST have demonstrated limited ability to detect AKI following adult cardiac surgery.[42,207] However, in a small single-center study of 123 subjects, π-GST did demonstrate the ability to detect which patients with AKIN stage 1 AKI would go on to progress to stage 3 or need RRT (AUC = 0.86; P = 0.002); however, to date, these data have not been validated in a larger cohort.[42]

In kidney transplant recipients, increased levels of α-GST were associated with cyclosporine A toxicity, whereas π-GST elevation was associated with acute allograft rejection.[208] In a cross-sectional study of patients with diabetes, the relationships between urine albumin/creatinine ratio and urinary levels of collagen IV, α-GST, and π-GST were assessed. Levels of all three markers were directly (albeit weakly) correlated with urine albumin/creatinine ratio, but a progressive increase in the proportion of patients with abnormal biomarker levels in those with normal urine albumin levels, microalbuminuria, and macroalbuminuria was observed only for collagen IV and π-GST.[209]

HEPCIDIN-25

Hepcidin-25, a 2.8-kDa hormonal regulator of iron metabolism, is produced in the liver, heart, and kidney. Hepcidin binds and induces the internalization and degradation of the transmembrane iron exporter ferroportin.[210] Hepcidin acts to downregulate iron uptake and reduce extracellular iron availability from stored iron.[211] Given its link to iron metabolism and the fact that free iron is known to be released in the setting of the ischemia reperfusion injury and oxidative stress that occurs with cardiopulmonary bypass, urinary hepcidin-25 has been investigated as a marker of kidney injury following cardiac surgery. Ho and colleagues identified urinary hepcidin-25 in a nested case-control study of 44 adults who underwent cardiac surgery. Using surface-enhanced laser desorption/ionization time-of-flight mass spectrometry (SELDI-TOF-MS) on urine samples from 22 individuals in whom at least RIFLE Risk category AKI developed and 22 individuals whose creatinine did not increase more than 10% from baseline during the postoperative period (no AKI), these researchers found that hepcidin-25 was dramatically upregulated in the urine of patients with no AKI.[212] Taking this a step further, the same group quantified the concentration of hepcidin in the urine (normalized to urine creatinine) and demonstrated that concentrations were higher in those who did not go on to have postoperative AKI (P < 0.0005). In a multivariate analysis, hepcidin-25 was significantly associated with the avoidance of AKI with urinary concentrations on postoperative day 1, providing an AUC of 0.80.[213] The data from this small study have been corroborated by those from another modest-sized cohort of 100 adults undergoing cardiopulmonary bypass. Haase-Fielitz and associates demonstrated that 6 hours after cardiopulmonary bypass, urinary hepcidin-25 levels were lower in the nine subjects in whom RIFLE-based AKI developed than in those with no AKI (AUC = 0.80; P = 0.004).[214] These results warrant further preliminary investigations in other AKI settings as well as prompt validation in a larger cohort of cardiac surgery patients.

INTERLEUKIN-18

IL-18 is an 18-kDa proinflammatory cytokine that is activated by caspase-1 and is produced by renal tubular cells and macrophages. Animal studies indicate that IL-18 is a mediator of acute tubular injury, including both neutrophil and monocyte infiltration of the renal parenchyma.[215,216] Studies have shown that caspase-1 knockout mice experienced the same degree of ischemic AKI as wild-type mice injected with an IL-18–neutralizing antiserum, demonstrating that IL-18 is an important mediator of ischemic AKI.[216] Others have shown that IL-18 plays a major role in macrophage activation, with mice engrafted with IL-18–deficient bone marrow experiencing less AKI than those with IL-18–replete marrow.[217] Similarly, in IL-18 knockout mice with AKI, tumor necrosis factor-α, inducible nitric oxide synthase, macrophage inflammatory protein-2, and monocyte chemoattractant protein-1 mRNA expression are all decreased, speaking to the deleterious impact of IL-18 in AKI. In the human kidney, IL-18 is induced and cleaved mainly in the proximal tubules and released into the urine. IL-18 has been shown to participate in a variety of renal disease processes, including ischemia-reperfusion injury, allograft rejection, infection, autoimmune conditions, and malignancy. IL-18 is easily and reliably measured in urine by commercially available ELISA and microbead-based assays.

ACUTE KIDNEY INJURY

Several studies have demonstrated the usefulness of IL-18 as a biomarker for detection of AKI. Originally, Parikh and associates studied a group of 72 patients and reported urinary IL-18 levels significantly higher in patients diagnosed with acute tubular necrosis (ATN) than in patients with prerenal azotemia or urinary infection and in healthy control subjects with normal renal function.[218] Since then, several large multicenter studies have gone on to investigate the ability of IL-18 to detect AKI in a variety of clinical settings.

The TRIBE-AKI Consortium measured IL-18 in 1219 adults who underwent cardiac surgery. Identification of those at high risk for postoperative AKI required the presence of one of the following: (1) emergency surgery, (2) preoperative serum creatinine higher than 2 mg/dL, (3) left ventricular ejection fraction < 35%, (4) New York Heart Association stage III or IV heart failure—left ventricular function, (5) age more than 70 years, (6) preexisting diabetes mellitus, (7) and concomitant coronary artery bypass grafting (CABG) and valve surgery or (8) repeat cardiac surgery. Those with preoperative AKI, kidney transplants, ESKD, or a preoperative serum creatinine higher than 4.5 mg/dL were excluded. After dividing the cohort into quintiles according to IL-8 level, compared to the lowest quintile, the highest quintile of IL-18 was associated with a 6.8-fold higher risk of AKI, defined as a postoperative doubling of serum creatinine or requirement for acute dialysis.[219] The first postoperative concentration of IL-18 (0-6 hours) provided an AUC of 0.74, which increased to 0.76 after IL-18 values were combined with a clinical model of factors known to impact AKI risk. The TRIBE-AKI pediatric cohort (311 children) reported results in line with the TRIBE adult study, in which the highest quintile of IL-8 values was associated with 9.4-fold increased risk of AKI (doubling of serum creatinine or dialysis) in comparison with the lowest quintile. The effect was slightly attenuated after adjustments were made for clinical factors known to impact AKI (adjusted OR, 28.8; 95% CI, 6.9 (1.7 to 28.8).[220]

In a secondary analysis of the adult cohort, Koyner and associates demonstrated that IL-18 value at the time of AKI can identify those with early AKI (AKIN stage 1) who will progress to more severe stages of AKI (AKIN stage 2 or 3). Of the 380 adults in whom at least stage 1 AKI developed, 45 went on to have stage 2 or 3 disease. In the entire cohort, those whose IL-8 values were in the fifth quintile were at increased risk for development of progressive AKI (OR, 3.63; 95% CI, 1.64 to 8.03) and this effect was only slightly attenuated after adjusting for the clinical model (OR, 3.00; 95% CI, 1.25 to 7.25).[221]

Finally, when investigated in a separate secondary analysis of this cohort, IL-18 concentrations collected in the immediate postoperative period were associated with long-term mortality following cardiac surgery. This later investigation provided a median follow-up of 3.0 years (interquartile range [IQR], 2.2 to 3.6), during which 139 of the 1199 subjects died (50 deaths per 1000 person-years). After adjustments were made for clinical factors known to affect mortality, in patients without AKI (n = 792), those whose IL-18 values were in the third tertile were at increased risk of long-term mortality in comparison with those whose values were in the first tertile (adjusted HR, 1.23; 95% CI, 1.02 to 1.48). This effect was magnified in those subjects with perioperative AKI (n = 407), in whom those with values in the third tertile had an adjusted hazard ratio of 3.16 (95% CI, 1.53 to 6.53) in comparison with the reference cohort. Thus IL-18 provides additional prognostic information about long-term postoperative mortality in patients with and without AKI.[222]

When investigated in the setting of critical illness and ICU admission, IL-18 has not demonstrated the same robust results. In a study of 451 critically ill subjects, in 86 of whom AKI developed within the first 48 hours, Siew and colleagues demonstrated that urine IL-18 did not reliably predict AKI. Although IL-18 levels at the time of ICU admission were higher in those who went on to have AKI, the AUC was 0.62 (95% CI, 0.54 to 0.69) and only marginally improved to 0.67 after the exclusion of those with prior known CKD (eGFR > 75 mL/min). Despite the inability to reliably detect AKI, urine IL-18 levels did correlate with other adverse patient outcomes, including the need for RRT and 28-day mortality.[223] This poor performance in the setting of critical illness has been corroborated by other studies, including a post hoc analysis of data from the EARLYARF trial. In this prospective observational study in two large general ICUs (n = 529), IL-18 provided an AUC of only 0.62 for the diagnosis of AKIN stage 1 AKI but once again performed much better at forecasting the need for RRT or death (within 7 days). Unlike other biomarker studies, this IL-18 study did not demonstrate improved predictive powers with the cohort stratified according to pre-admission CKD stage.[224] In a separate post hoc analysis of the same EARLYARF cohort, urinary IL-18 concentrations were shown to be significantly higher in patients with prerenal azotemia (defined as AKI that recovered within 48 hours of ICU admission and was associated with a fractional excretion of sodium < 1%; n = 61) than in those with no AKI (n = 285). There was a trend toward higher values in those with AKI (n = 114, non-prenal) than in those with prerenal AKI (P = 0.053).[225]

In a single-center study of 339 mixed surgical and medical ICU patients, Doi and colleagues demonstrated that IL-18 values were significantly elevated in those with both established and newly diagnosed AKI at the time of ICU arrival. Although biomarker concentrations and AUCs were higher in those with established AKI (AUC = 0.78) than in those with newly diagnosed AKI (AUC = 0.59), concentrations and AUCs in both of these subgroups were significantly different from those in the "no AKI" cohort. In this same study, IL-18 levels were significantly higher in nonsurvivors.[226] These results were fairly similar to those reported by Nikolas and colleagues, who measured urinary biomarkers in 1635 ED patients at the time of admission and compared the values with adjudicated AKI outcomes in which prerenal AKI was defined as RIFLE Risk category that returned to baseline within 72 hours and was in the clinical setting, suggesting decreased transient effective circulating volume. These researchers demonstrated that IL-18 values for patients with more severe intrinsic AKI were significantly higher than those for patients with prerenal AKI. However, there was no difference in values between those with prerenal AKI and those with no AKI.[227]

When measured at kidney transplantation, IL-18 level accurately predicted delayed graft function (AUC = 0.90) and predicted the rate of decline in serum creatinine concentration.[228] In patients with diabetic kidney disease and proteinuria, IL-18 levels in renal tubular cells are higher than in patients with nondiabetic proteinuric disease.[229] To understand the utility of IL-18 and urinary NGAL in predicting graft recovery after kidney transplantation, Hall and colleagues conducted a prospective, multicenter, observational cohort study of recipients of deceased-donor kidney transplants.[230] They collected serial urine samples from 91 patients for 3 days after transplantation. After adjustment for recipient and donor age, cold ischemia time, urine output, and serum creatinine concentration, NGAL and IL-18 concentrations accurately predicted the need for dialysis in transplant recipients. Furthermore, NGAL and IL-18 concentrations predicted graft recovery up to 3 months later.[230] In further follow-up of this cohort, urine IL-18 concentrations collected at the time of surgery were correlated with graft outcomes 1 year after transplantation. Upper median values of IL-18 on the first postoperative day had an adjusted OR of 5.5 (95% CI, 1.4 to 21.5) and poor graft function, defined as a GFR < 30 mL/min or return to RRT.[231]

In a study by Ling and associates involving patients who underwent coronary angiography, urinary IL-18 and NGAL concentrations were significantly increased at 24 hours after the procedure in those in whom contrast medium–induced nephropathy developed but not in the control group. ROC curve analysis demonstrated that both IL-18 and NGAL showed better performance in early diagnosis of contrast nephropathy than serum creatinine ($P < 0.05$). Importantly, elevated urinary IL-18 concentrations 24 hours after contrast administration were also found to be an independent predictive marker for later major cardiac events (relative risk [RR] = 2.1).[232]

CHRONIC KIDNEY DISEASE

There is promising data about IL-18 in the setting of CKD. In the Women's Interagency HIV study, urine IL-18 levels were independently associated with a more rapid loss of renal function after multivariate adjustment.[233] In this cohort study of 908 HIV-infected women, urine IL-18 was the only biomarker (KIM-1 and albumin to creatinine ratio [ACR] were also measured) that was associated with worsening renal function over time, as measured by eGFR–cystatin C. Urine IL-18 predicted an increased RR of renal function decline between 1.4 and 2.16, depending on the model used. In a follow-up study, the same group measured urine IL-18 in 908 HIV-infected and 289 noninfected women in the Women's Inter-agency HIV study.[234] This cross-sectional cohort study demonstrated that after multivariate adjusted linear regression analysis, IL-18 concentrations were significantly higher in subjects with HIV (38%; $P < 0.0001$). Additionally, these researchers found that urine IL-18 concentrations were significantly associated with higher HIV RNA levels and lower CD4 cell counts, hepatitis C infection, and high-density lipoprotein (HDL) cholesterol levels, thus pointing to a more extensive role for IL-18 in the setting of HIV-related kidney care.[234] These promising HIV results are in contrast to those of the Consortium for Radiologic Imaging for the Study of Polycystic Kidney Disease (CRISP), which measured IL-18 in 107 patients with autosomal dominant polycystic kidney disease and found that although there was an increased mean IL-18 over the 3-year follow-up period, there was no association between tertiles of IL-18 values and change in total kidney volume or eGFR.[235]

KIDNEY INJURY MOLECULE-1

Kidney injury molecule-1 (KIM-1 in humans, Kim-1 in rodents), which is also referred as *T cell immunoglobulin and mucin domains–containing protein-1* (*TIM-1*) and *hepatitis A virus cellular receptor-1* (*HAVCR-1*), is a type I transmembrane glycoprotein with an ectodomain containing a six-cysteine immunoglobulin-like domain, two N-glycosylation sites, and a mucin domain. In an effort to identify molecules involved in kidney injury, Bonventre's group originally discovered Kim-1 using representational difference analysis (a PCR-based technique) in rat models of acute ischemic kidney injury.[236,237] Importantly, KIM-1 was shown to be significantly expressed in kidneys, specifically in proximal tubular cells of humans after ischemic injury, whereas it was virtually absent or present at low levels in healthy kidneys. KIM-1 has evolved as a marker of proximal tubular injury, the hallmark of virtually all proteinuric, toxic, and ischemic renal diseases. KIM-1 has been shown to be a highly sensitive and specific marker of kidney injury in several rodent models, including models of injury due to ischemia,[236,238] cisplatin, folic acid, gentamicin, mercury, chromium,[239,240] cadmium,[241] contrast agents,[242] cyclosporine,[243] ochratoxin A, aristolochic acid, D-serine, and protein overload.[244]

In 2002, the Bonventre group published the first clinical study linking urinary levels of KIM-1 with AKI, demonstrating that tissue expression of KIM-1 is correlated with the severity of acute tubular necrosis and corresponding levels of KIM-1 ectodomain in the urine of patients with clinically significant AKI.[238] Since then, numerous other studies have been published on the ability of KIM-1 to detect AKI in a variety of settings, including cardiac surgery, critical illness, and general hospitalized AKI, which has been mixed.[42,224,225,245-251]

Later, KIM-1 was investigated in several multicenter larger trials. In the TRIBE-AKI adult and pediatric cardiac surgery cohorts, the fifth quintile of urinary KIM-1 values was associated with a risk of AKI (defined as postoperative doubling of serum creatinine concentration or need for acute dialysis) 6.2-fold greater than that for the lowest KIM-1 values. This risk remained significant (4.8-fold) after adjustment of data for the clinical model used (age, race, sex, cardiopulmonary bypass time, non-elective surgery, preoperative GFR, diabetes, hypertension, and study center). The effect was completely attenuated after urinary IL-18 and plasma and urine NGAL were included in the model.[250] As for the long-term mortality in the TRIBE cohort, the third tertile of perioperative KIM-1 concentrations was found to be associated with increased mortality. In patients without AKI (n = 792), the third tertile had an adjusted HR of 1.83 (95% CI, 1.44 to 2.33), whereas in the 407 subjects with AKI, the adjusted HR was slightly higher, at 2.01 (95% CI, 1.31 to 3.1).[222] In the pediatric cohort, those with KIM-1 values in the fifth quintile were at increased risk of AKI in the unadjusted analysis; however, this effect failed to remain significant after a pediatric adjustment model was applied.[250]

The data on KIM-1 in the setting of critical illness–related AKI have been just as mixed as the perioperative results, with KIM-1 providing an AUC of 0.66 (95% CI, 0.61 to 0.72) for the diagnosis of AKI in samples from the EARLYARF study. The results were less impressive with regard to the prediction of dialysis (AUC = 0.62) or death (AUC = 0.56) within the first week following ICU admission.[224] In the cohort of 529 mixed ICU patients, KIM-1 outperformed other biomarkers in its ability to detect AKI at the time of ICU admission in those with a preadmission GFR < 60 mL/min (AUC, 0.7; 95% CI, 0.58 to 0.82). In a separate post hoc analysis of this cohort, KIM-1 levels demonstrated a significant stepwise increase in the comparison of those with no AKI (median serum creatinine 170 µg/mmol [IQR, 69 to 445]), those with prerenal AKI (median serum creatinine 291 µg/mmol [IQR, 121 to 549]), and those with intrinsic AKI (lasting more than 48 hours) (serum creatinine 376 µg/mmol [IQR, 169 to 943]).[225] In addition, KIM-1 demonstrated the ability to forecast the development of intrinsic AKI at the time of ED arrival with an AUC of 0.71 (95% CI, 0.65 to 0.76; $P < 0.001$). KIM-1 values again increased in a stepwise fashion, values being lowest in those with no AKI or CKD and rising in other subjects in the following order: stable CKD, prerenal AKI, and intrinsic AKI. Additionally, KIM-1 values were able to forecast inpatient mortality and the need for RRT.[227]

The usefulness of KIM-1 has been demonstrated not only as a urinary marker but also as a tool for evaluating kidney injury in kidney biopsy specimens by immunohistochemical methods. For example, Van Timmeren and associates found that the level of KIM-1 protein expression in proximal tubular cells correlated with tubulointerstitial fibrosis and inflammation in kidney tissue specimens from 102 patients who underwent kidney biopsy for a variety of kidney diseases.[252] In a subset of patients whose urine was collected near the time of biopsy, urinary KIM-1 levels correlated with tissue KIM-1 expression in 100% of biopsy samples from patients with deterioration in kidney function and histologic changes indicative of tubular damage. In biopsy specimens from transplanted kidneys, greater KIM-1 staining was detected in 100% of patients with deterioration of kidney function and pathologic changes indicating tubular injury, in 92% of patients with acute cellular rejection, and in 28% of patients with normal biopsy findings.[253] In contrast, Hall and associates demonstrated that urinary KIM-1 levels did not correlate with peritransplantation or 1-year graft function.[231,248] Similarly, Schroppel and colleagues investigated KIM-1 RNA expression in perioperative samples collected from both living- and deceased-donor kidneys and found no significant correlation between KIM-1 staining and the occurrence of delayed graft function.[254]

CHRONIC KIDNEY DISEASE

KIM-1 also shows promise as a useful biomarker in CKD. In addition to its serving as a marker of proximal tubule dysfunction, animal data demonstrate that KIM-1 is upregulated in the later phases of AKI as well and plays an important role in renal repair; thus, it may be a major player in the pathophysiology of CKD/repair.[255] This ability to serve as a marker of CKD was evident in a nested case-control study involving 686 participants from the Multi-Ethnic Study of Atherosclerosis (MESA). Cases were defined as involving patients with a baseline eGFR higher than 60 mL/min in whom CKD stage 3 subsequently developed and/or who had a rapid drop in kidney function over the 5-year study period. Each doubling of KIM-1 level (pg/mL) was associated with a 1.15 (95% CI, 1.02 to 1.29) increased odds of development of CKD stage 3 or a rapid decline in GFR. Similarly, at study entry, patients in the highest decile for KIM-1 value had a twofold higher risk of this same end point than those in the other 90%. This ability of KIM-1 value to predict the development and progression of CKD was independent of the presence of albuminuria.[256] These results contrast with those of Bhavsar and associates, who measured KIM-1 in a similar case-control substudy of the ARIC study. New-onset CKD stage 3 developed in 143 of the 286 subjects, but KIM-1 did not display the ability to forecast or identify those at risk for CKD development or progression.[257]

Despite these mixed results in community studies of CKD, KIM-1 has been investigated and has shown promise in a variety of other clinical settings, including in children with chronic renal tubular damage from vesicoureteral reflux,[258] HIV, and in adults with nephropathy[233] or diabetic nephropathy.[259,260] In patients with IgA nephropathy, urinary KIM-1 levels were significantly higher than in healthy controls. Furthermore, the levels of urinary KIM-1 correlated positively with serum creatinine concentration and proteinuria and correlated inversely with creatinine clearance. Similarly, tubular KIM-1 expression as determined by immunohistochemical analysis correlated closely with urinary levels ($r = 0.553$; $P = 0.032$).[261] Sundaram and associates evaluated the potential of KIM-1, L-FABP, NAG, NGAL, and transforming growth factor-β_1 (TGF-β_1), together with conventional renal biomarkers (urine albumin level, serum creatinine concentration, and serum cystatin C–estimated GFR) to detect nephropathy early in patients with sickle cell anemia. Only KIM-1 and NAG showed correlations with albuminuria, which were strong; other markers did not show any association with albuminuria.[262]

LIVER-TYPE FATTY ACID–BINDING PROTEIN

Urinary fatty acid–binding protein 1 (FABP1) has been proposed to be a useful biomarker for early detection of AKI and monitoring of CKD. Also known as *L-type* or *liver-type fatty acid–binding protein* (L-FABP), which will be used in this book, FABP1 was first isolated in the liver as a binding protein for oleic acid and bilirubin. FABP1 binds selectively to free fatty acids and transports them to mitochondria or peroxisomes, where free fatty acids are β-oxidized and participate in intracellular fatty acid homeostasis. There are several different types of FABP, which are ubiquitously expressed in a variety of tissues. At this time, nine different FABPs have been reported: liver (L), intestinal (I), muscle and heart (H), epidermal (E), ileal (I1), myelin (M), adipocyte (A), brain (B), and testis (T). L-FABP is expressed in proximal tubules of the human kidney and localized in the cytoplasm. Increased cytosolic L-FABP in proximal tubular epithelial cells may derive not only from endogenous expression but also from circulating L-FABP that might be filtered at the glomeruli and reabsorbed by tubular cells.

Susantitaphong and associates published a meta-analysis reporting the performance of L-FABP from 15 prospective cohorts and two case-control studies.[263] Although the researchers were able to meta-analyze only 7 of the cohort studies, they demonstrated that L-FABP levels were 74.5% sensitive (95% CI, 60.4% to 84.8%) and 77.6% specific (95% CI, 61.5% to 88.2%) for the diagnosis of AKI. Additionally, they demonstrated that the results were more promising for the predication of in-hospital mortality. They concluded that on the basis of the low quality of many of the studies and the varied clinical settings, L-FABP may be a promising biomarker for the early detection of AKI.[263] In this discussion we highlight some of the larger and later clinical investigations of L-FABP.

Portilla and colleagues demonstrated that L-FABP predicts the development of AKI within 4 hours of surgery in children undergoing cardiac surgery.[264] Others have attempted to validate this finding in the setting of cardiac surgery, with mixed success.[249,265,266] The TRIBE-AKI Consortium published the results of the largest study investigating L-FABP in the setting of adult cardiac surgery, demonstrating that after adjustments were made for a clinical model that consisted of factors known to affect the development of AKI, L-FABP did not correlate with the development of AKI in their pediatric (n = 311) or adult (n = 1219) cohorts. The consortium demonstrated that although L-FABP levels were statistically higher in those adults with AKI than in those without AKI, the L-FABP concentration (ng/mL) measured up to 6 hours postoperatively provided an AUC of 0.61, and the performance was only marginally better with the 6- to 12-hour measurement. Similarly, in the pediatric cohort, although the fifth quintile of L-FABP concentrations at the earliest postoperative timepoint (0-6 hours) significantly associated with the development of AKI (OR, 2.9; 95% CI, 1.2 to 7.1), this effect disappeared after adjustment for the clinical model (OR, 1.8; 95% CI, 0.7 to 4.6).[250]

Siew and colleagues reported the performance of L-FABP in 380 critically ill subjects from medical, surgical, trauma, and cardiac ICUs, in 130 of whom AKI was defined as AKIN stage 1. L-FABP levels were higher in those with AKI ($P = 0.003$) and were able to discriminate incident AKI with an AUC of 0.59 (95% CI, 0.52 to 0.65). Although L-FABP was able to predict the composite endpoint of death or RRT, using multivariate regression L-FABP significantly predicted the need for acute RRT (HR, 2.36; 95% CI, 1.30 to 4.25).[267] These findings mirror those of Doi and associates, who published a prospective single-center observational cohort study examining the performance of L-FABP in 339 mixed ICU patients. In their study, L-FABP outperformed NGAL, IL-18, NAG, and other biomarkers in the detection of AKI, defined by RIFLE Risk category. Furthermore L-FABP predicted 14-day mortality with an AUC of 0.90.[226] This study, which followed a smaller study (n = 145) by this same group of investigators, has paved the way for L-FABP to be validated for clinical use in Japan.[268]

In a cross-sectional study of general hospitalized patients that included 92 participants with AKI and 68 control subjects (26 healthy volunteers and 42 hospitalized: 29 patients about to undergo coronary catheterization and 13 patients in the ICU with no AKI), Ferguson colleagues demonstrated that urinary levels of L-FABP were significantly higher in subjects with AKI than in hospitalized control patients without AKI, with an AUC of 0.93 (95% CI, 0.88 to 0.97); sensitivity was 83% and specificity was 90% at a cutoff value of 47.1 ng per mg of creatinine.[269] Nickolas and associates examined L-FABP at the time of ED arrival and found that it had only fair discriminatory power with regard to AKI. In their cohort of 1635 subjects, L-FABP provided an AUC of 0.70 (95% CI, 0.65 to 0.76); however, there was a clear and significant stepwise increase in L-FABP concentrations across the spectrum of AKI (normal < CKD < prerenal < intrinsic AKI).[227]

Because L-FABP is also expressed by the liver, liver injury can be a potential contributor to increased urinary levels of L-FABP during AKI. However, previous studies in patients with CKD, AKI, and sepsis have shown that serum L-FABP levels do not have an influence on urinary levels and that urinary L-FABP levels are not significantly higher in patients with liver disease than in healthy subjects.[264,270,271]

Urinary L-FABP levels have been investigated as an early diagnostic and predictive marker for contrast medium–induced nephropathy.[272,273] In a study of adult patients with normal serum creatinine concentrations who underwent percutaneous coronary intervention, serum NGAL level rose at 2 and 4 hours, whereas urinary NGAL and urinary L-FABP increased significantly after 4 hours and remained elevated up to 48 hours, after cardiac catheterization.[274] Nakamura and associates demonstrated that baseline urinary L-FABP levels were significantly higher in patients whom contrast medium–induced nephropathy developed after coronary angiography; however, the investigators did not evaluate the diagnostic performance of urinary L-FABP in predicting AKI.[273]

CHRONIC KIDNEY DISEASE

To date, there have been limited investigations of the role of L-FABP in the setting of CKD. Small studies investigating the excretion of L-FABP in the setting of diabetic nephropathy have been mixed, with some reporting a link between decreased urinary concentrations of L-FABP in the setting of renin angiotensin aldosterone system blockade and preserved GFR and others finding no correlation.[275,276] Further investigation is needed to elucidate the role of L-FABP in the setting of CKD.

NETRIN-1

Netrin-1 is a 50- to 75-kDa, laminin-like protein, initially recognized as a chemotropic factor, that plays an essential role in guiding neurons and axons to their targets. Studies have now revealed diverse roles of netrin-1 beyond axonal guidance, including development of various organs, angiogenesis, adhesion, tissue morphogenesis, inflammation, and tumorigenic processes.[277,278] Netrin-1 is expressed in several tissue types, including brain, lung, heart, liver, intestine, and kidney.[279]

A study by Wang and colleagues showed a rapid induction of netrin-1 in tubular epithelial cells in response to ischemia-reperfusion injury of the kidney in animal models.[280] In this study, netrin-1 was excreted in the urine as early as 1 hour after a kidney insult, increased more than fortyfold by 3 hours, and reached its peak levels (approximately fiftyfold) before the elevation of blood creatinine and BUN concentrations.[281] Importantly, this rapid increase in netrin-1 expression appeared to be regulated at the translational level because netrin-1 gene transcription was actually decreased after ischemia-reperfusion injury.[281] The researchers also tested the sensitivity and specificity of netrin-1 in animal models of toxin-induced kidney injury, using cisplatin, folic acid, and endotoxin (lipopolysaccharide). These kidney insults resulted in increases in the excretion of netrin-1 in urine, supporting a potential role as an early biomarker for hypoxic and toxic renal injuries. In a later study, through the exogenous administration of netrin-1 following a murine model of ischemia-reperfusion AKI, the same group demonstrated that netrin-1 regulates the inflammatory response in the setting of AKI via the inhibition of cyclo-oxygensase-2 (COX-2)–mediated prostaglandin E_2 production. They demonstrated that netrin-1 regulates COX-2 expression through the regulation of nuclear factor-kappaB (NF-κB) activation.[282]

Although most of the investigations of netrin have focused on cellular and animal models, netrin-1 has been increasingly investigated in humans.[283] Ramesh and colleagues also demonstrated significantly higher urine levels of netrin-1 in patients with established AKI due to various causes (n = 16) than in healthy volunteers. In a later study, the same group of scientists evaluated the potential of netrin-1 to predict AKI in patients undergoing cardiopulmonary bypass.[284] They included serial urine samples that were collected from 26 patients in whom AKI developed and 36 patients in whom it did not after cardiopulmonary bypass. By ROC analysis, the investigators demonstrated that netrin-1 could predict AKI at 2 hours, 6 hours, and 12 hours, with an AUC of 0.74 (95% CI, 0.86 to 0.89). The levels of urinary netrin-1 6 hours after cardiopulmonary bypass correlated with the severity of AKI, as well as the length of hospital stay, and remained a powerful independent predictor of AKI.[284]

Netrin-1 seems to be a promising early biomarker for AKI, but additional studies need to be conducted in larger cohorts with AKI due to various causes to further evaluate its potential.

NEUTROPHIL GELATINASE–ASSOCIATED LIPOCALIN

Neutrophil gelatinase–associated lipocalin (also known as *lipocalin 2* or *lcn2*) is one of the biomarkers of AKI that has been studied extensively. NGAL has many of the characteristics required for a good biomarker for AKI in comparison with serum creatinine measurement or urine output.[285] It is a 25-kDa protein with 178 amino acids belonging to the lipocalin superfamily. Lipocalins are extracellular proteins with diverse functions involving transport of hydrophilic substances through membranes, thereby maintaining cell homeostasis.[286] NGAL is a glycoprotein bound to matrix metalloproteinase-9 in human neutrophils. It is expressed in various tissues in the body, such as salivary glands, prostate, uterus, trachea, lung, stomach, and kidney,[287] and its expression is markedly induced in injured epithelial cells, including those in the kidney, colon, liver, and lung.

Transcriptome profiling studies in rodent models identified NGAL as one of the most upregulated genes in the kidney very early after tubular injury.[288,289] Mishra and associates demonstrated that NGAL values were significantly elevated within 2 hours after injury in mouse models of renal ischemia-reperfusion.[290] In addition, urinary NGAL was detectable after one day of cisplatin administration, suggesting its sensitivity in other models of tubular injury.[290]

ACUTE KIDNEY INJURY

Many clinical studies followed these important observations in animals. Mishra and associates first demonstrated the value of NGAL as a clinical marker in a prospective study of 71 children undergoing cardiopulmonary bypass. In this study, both serum and urinary NGAL levels were upregulated within 2 hours in patients in whom AKI developed. A cutoff NGAL value of 50 µg/L was 100% sensitive and 98% specific in predicting AKI.[291] Following this seminal study, several other groups investigated NGAL in the setting of cardiac surgery, with several demonstrating that both urine and serum NGAL values were able to predict AKI earlier than serum creatinine as well as to correlate with AKI severity.[42,43,103,104,219-221,249,251,292-297] However, no study was able to replicate the near-perfect results reported by Mishra and associates.[291] Given the wealth of studies that have reported on NGAL over the last decade, we have chosen to highlight the larger and multicenter trials that have studied NGAL.

URINE NGAL

In the setting of the ED, urine NGAL was originally shown to perform quite well with the first study by Nickolas and associates in 635 patients, demonstrating that a cutoff of 130 µg per g of creatinine carried a sensitivity of 90% and specificity of 99.5% for AKI, defined as RIFLE Risk category. In this single-center prospective study, urine NGAL also predicted the future need for nephrology consultation, admission to the ICU, as well as need for RRT.[60] In a follow-up multicenter study of 1635 subjects, urine NGAL provided an AUC of 0.81 (95% CI, 0.76 to 0.86) for the prediction of AKI (RIFLE Risk category) and provided an NRI of 26.1% while demonstrating the ability to improve the classification of both AKI events and non-events. Additionally, urine NGAL values were significantly different and increased in a stepwise fashion in the following order: patients with no AKI, patients with CKD, patients with prerenal AKI, patients with intrinsic AKI.[298]

Lieske and colleagues measured urine NGAL in 363 ED patients and determined that NGAL provided an AUC of 0.70 for the detection of AKIN AKI while providing only modest sensitivity (65%) and specificity (65%).[172] In addition to demonstrating that NGAL levels increased with severity of AKI, these researchers showed that pyuria and urinary white blood cells were associated with increased urinary NGAL levels. Urine NGAL has been studied less extensively in the pediatric ED but has demonstrated similar potential in a smaller study (n = 252) with a lower AKI incidence rate (n = 18, 7.1%).[247]

Urine NGAL has also been studied in the setting of critical illness by Siew and colleagues, who showed that urine NGAL was able to predict AKI within the first 24 (AUC = 0.71) and 48 (AUC = 0.64) hours of ICU admission. In this single-center prospective study of 451 critically ill adults, urine NGAL was independently associated with the development of AKI even after adjustment for factors known to be correlated with the development of AKI (including severity of illness and sepsis).[299] NGAL performed similarly when measured in a post hoc analysis of the EARLYARF trial. Data from this prospective observational study performed in two general (mixed) ICUs in New Zealand demonstrated that urine NGAL could modestly predict the development of AKI (AKIN stage 1) (AUC = 0.66) but was also able to forecast the need for RRT (AUC = 0.79) and death (AUC = 0.66) within the first 7 ICU days ($P < 0.001$ for all three). Additionally, urine NGAL performed better in predicting AKI on ICU arrival in those with higher baseline eGFRs (AUC = 0.70 for those with eGFRs of 90-120 mL/min vs. AUC 0.64 for those with eGFRs < 60 mL/min).[224] This improved ability to detect the future development of AKI in patients with higher eGFRs has been demonstrated by others in the setting of cardiac surgery.[42,43] In a separate post hoc analysis of the EARLYARF study, urine NGAL values again demonstrated a significant increase across the spectrum of AKI; values were lowest in subjects without AKI, and values for subjects with transient AKI that lasted less than 48 hours were in between levels in subjects with no AKI and subjects with AKI that lasted longer than 48 hours.[225] In the discovery phase of the multicenter prospective observational Sapphire trial with 522 participants, urine NGAL provided an AUC of 0.66 (95% CI, 0.60 to 0.71) for the development of RIFLE injury or failure within the first 36 hours of study enrollment; the AUC increased to 0.71 (05% CI, 0.66 to 0.76) for the development of RIFLE Injury or Failure disease within the first 12 hours.[300]

In the setting of cardiac surgery, urine NGAL has provided similar mixed results. In the TRIBE-AKI adult cohort, the highest quintile of urine NGAL values obtained 0 to 6 hours after surgery was associated with an increased risk of AKI (defined as doubling of serum creatinine or need for RRT); however, this effect was no longer significant after adjustment for factors known to contribute to AKI risk.[219] In addition to providing an AUC of 0.67 for the detection of AKI in this cohort of 1219 adults, urine NGAL levels were significantly associated with the composite endpoint of inpatient mortality or receipt of RRT, as well as length of ICU stay and length of hospitalization. Urine NGAL did not display the ability to detect AKI progression in the 380 adults in whom at least AKIN stage 1 developed. Although those subjects with urine NGAL values in the fifth quintile at the time of serum creatinine increase were at increased risk for more progressive AKI (e.g., going from AKIN stage 1 to AKIN stage 3), this effect was no longer significant in the adjusted analysis.[221] These results contrasted with those in the pediatric cohort (n = 311), in which patients with urine NGAL values in the fifth quintile remained at significantly increased risk for development of AKI (doubling of serum creatinine or need for RRT) even after adjustment for the clinical model (OR, 4.1; 95% CI, 1.0 to 16.3). Additionally, urine NGAL levels correlated with the length of mechanical ventilation, ICU stay, and hospitalization.[220]

In a separate secondary analysis that examined the long-term mortality of the adult TRIBE cohort, those subjects with urine NGAL values were in the third tertile (n = 407) were at increased risk of death during the median 3.0-year follow-up. The adjusted HR for this group (compared with those in the first tertile) was 2.52 (95% CI, 1.86 to 3.42). A similar effect was not seen in patients with values in the third tertile who did not have AKI (n = 792, (HR, 0.90; 95% CI, 0.50 to 1.63).[222]

Urine NGAL has been investigated in several other smaller studies in more niche cohorts and has demonstrated some promise in detecting AKI in critically ill neonates,[301] hepatic impairment or death in individuals with cirrhosis/hepatorenal syndrome,[302,303] and both delayed graft function[248,304] and 1-year graft survival[231] in kidney transplant recipients. However, these trials and others require validation in larger and multicenter investigations.

PLASMA NGAL

Plasma NGAL has been examined in many of the same studies with urine NGAL, including in the settings of the ED, the ICU, and following cardiac surgery. DiSomma and colleagues demonstrated that the plasma NGAL from a specimen drawn at the time of ED arrival provided an AUC value of 0.80 for the future development of AKI. In this multicenter prospective cohort study, the AUC improved to 0.90 when ED physician clinical judgment was added to plasma NGAL level. This combination of physician clinical judgment and NGAL outperformed both physician judgment alone and serum creatinine alone, leading to a significant NRI of 32.4%.[305]

In the setting of critical illness, plasma NGAL was measured as part of a post hoc analysis of the multicenter EARLYARF study (n = 528), in which it provided an AUC of 0.74 (95% CI, 0.69 to 0.79) for the development of AKIN stage 1 AKI (n = 147) during subsequent ICU stay. This study defined functional AKI according to the AKIN criteria but also defined structural AKI in terms of urine NGAL concentrations. Plasma NGAL performed even better (AUC = 0.79) at predicting urine NGAL–defined structural AKI (n = 213). In addition to strong associations with creatinine and urine NGAL–based definitions of AKI, plasma NGAL was associated with the need for RRT (n = 19) but not with inpatient mortality (n = 53).[306] In the Sapphire trial, which also examined the performance of plasma NGAL in the setting of ICU-associated AKI, NGAL provided an AUC of 0.64 (95% CI, 0.58-0.70) for the detection of RIFLE Injury or Failure disease within the first 12 hours of study enrollment; this significant ability to forecast more severe forms of AKI did not dramatically change when the ability to detect the same level of AKI over the first 36 hours was assessed (AUC = 0.64; 95% CI, 0.58 to 0.71).[300]

It has been postulated that NGAL's performance in the setting of critical illness is likely attenuated in part because of the preponderance of sepsis-related AKI in the ICU and that NGAL levels are inherently higher in those with sepsis because it is derived in part from neutrophils. De Gues and colleagues published a prospective observational cohort study of 663 patients admitted to the ICU in whom plasma NGAL was measured four times during the first 24 hours. These investigators demonstrated that plasma NGAL levels were significantly higher in patients with sepsis than in those without sepsis and that when the cohort was stratified according the presence of sepsis (n = 80, 12% of the cohort), plasma NGAL was able to detect AKI remarkably well in both cohorts (AUC of 0.76 in those with sepsis vs. 0.78 in those without sepsis).[307] These data corroborate the work of Noiri's group, which demonstrated in a prospective observational study of 139 critically ill patients that plasma NGAL levels are highest in those with sepsis associated with AKI, lower in those with non-sepsis AKI, and even lower in those with no AKI.[308] Future investigations of plasma NGAL will need to take this association with sepsis into account as we begin to construct normal ranges as well as clinically validated cutoffs to utilize NGAL in interventional trials to treat patients with the early stages of AKI.[309,310]

Although its ability to detect AKI in the setting of critical illness requires further investigation, plasma NGAL has been shown to predict recovery from AKI in preliminary studies. In 181 patients with community-acquired pneumonia and at least RIFLE Failure AKI, plasma NGAL measures on the first day that met Failure criteria were able to predict the failure of recovery of renal function. Individuals with high plasma NGAL levels were less likely to recover, with an AUC of 0.74. However, this performance was not significantly different from that of a clinical model consisting of age, serum creatinine, and severity of illness scores.[311] This potential ability to detect nonrecovery of AKI is yet another aspect of NGAL and other biomarkers that requires further investigation.

Plasma NGAL has also been extensively studied in the setting of cardiac surgery. In the TRIBE-AKI adult cohort (n = 1219), plasma NGAL levels were significantly higher in those in whom AKI developed (defined as doubling of serum creatinine or need for RRT) in the early postoperative period. Those in the fifth quintile of plasma NGAL values up to 6 hours after surgery (>293 ng/mL) were at a 7.8-fold higher risk for development of AKI than those in the first NGAL quintile (<105 pg/mL). This effect was attenuated after adjustment for factors known to associate with AKI but remained significant (OR, 5.0; 95% CI, 1.6 to 15.3), although it was no longer significant after adjustment for serum creatinine.[219] Additionally, plasma NGAL was significantly associated with increased length of ICU and hospital stays as well as with a composite of in-hospital death or dialysis. In this same adult cohort, plasma NGAL, measured at the time of a clinical AKI/serum creatinine increase, demonstrated a remarkable ability to detect those individuals with progressive AKI (e.g., going from AKIN stage 1 to stage 2 or 3) (n = 380). After adjustment for the clinical model, patients in the fifth quintile of plasma NGAL values (>322 ng/mL) were nearly eight times more likely to have progressive AKI (OR, 7.72; 95% CI, 2.65 to 22.49) than those in the first two quintiles. Plasma NGAL displayed the ability to improve the reclassification of both those with and those without progressive AKI (events and non-events), providing a category-free NRI of 0.69 ($P < 0.0001$).[221] The results in the TRIBE-AKI pediatric cohort were less promising, with plasma NGAL not displaying the ability to predict severe AKI (defined as doubling of serum creatinine or need for RRT) in the early postoperative period. However, the fifth quintile of NGAL (>259 ng/ml) measured within the first 6 postoperative hours was significantly associated with the development of RIFLE Risk AKI with an adjusted OR of 2.3 (95% CI, 1.0 to 5.5),[220] although falling well short of the near-perfect performance published in the original Mishra paper.[312]

In addition to large trials, smaller trials have also investigated NGAL in a variety of AKI settings, so much so that Haase and colleagues conducted a pooled prospective study (n = 2322; 1452 having had after cardiac surgery and 870 with critical illness) that designated subjects as NGAL$^+$ or NGAL$^-$ and as creatinine$^+$ or creatinine$^-$ (creatinine$^+$ was defined as RIFLE Risk AKI). After analyzing NGAL data from ten separate prospective observational studies, the group demonstrated that individuals who were NGAL$^+$ but creatinine$^-$ needed acute dialysis more than 16 times more often than those who were NGAL$^-$ creatinine$^-$ (OR, 16.4; 95% CI, 3.6 to 76.9; $P < 0.001$). The study also demonstrated incremental increases in ICU stay, hospital stay, and mortality among the four study groups in the following order: NGAL$^-$ creatinine$^-$, NGAL$^+$ creatinine$^-$, NGAL$^-$ creatinine$^+$, NGAL$^+$ creatinine$^+$.[39]

The function of NGAL as a diagnostic marker of contrast medium–induced nephropathy has also been evaluated. In a prospective study of 91 children undergoing coronary angiography, both urine and plasma NGAL levels were found to be significantly increased within 2 hours of contrast medium administration in the group in which contrast medium–induced nephropathy developed but not in the control group. By comparison, AKI detection using increases in serum creatinine concentration was possible only later, 6 to 24 hours after contrast agent administration. When a cutoff value of 100 ng/mL was used, both urine and serum NGAL levels at 2 hours predicted contrast medium–induced nephropathy, with AUCs of 0.91 and 0.92, respectively.[313] In several studies of adults undergoing procedures requiring contrast agents, early rises in both urine (4-hour) and plasma (2-hour) NGAL levels were documented, compared with a much later increase in plasma cystatin C levels, providing support for the use of NGAL as an early biomarker for contrast medium–induced nephropathy.[232,314] A meta-analysis found an overall AUC of 0.89 for prediction of AKI when NGAL was measured within 6 hours after contrast agent administration and AKI was defined as a 25% or greater increase in serum creatinine concentration.[315]

The origin of plasma and urinary NGAL rises after AKI requires further clarification. Gene expression and transgenic animal studies have demonstrated an upregulation of NGAL in the distal nephron segments, specifically in the thick ascending limb of Henle and the collecting ducts; however, most of the injury in AKI occurs in the proximal tubules.[316,317] On the other hand, the source of plasma NGAL in AKI is not well defined. For instance, in animal studies, direct ipsilateral renal vein sampling after unilateral ischemia indicates that NGAL synthesized in the kidney does not enter the circulation.[317] The increase in plasma NGAL observed in AKI may derive from the fact that NGAL is an acute phase reactant and may be released from neutrophils, macrophages, and other immune cells. Yndestad and colleagues reported strong immunostaining for NGAL in cardiomyocytes within the failing myocardium in experimental and clinical heart failure.[318] Furthermore, any impairment in GFR resulting from AKI would be expected to decrease renal clearance of NGAL, with subsequent accumulation in the systemic circulation. However, the contribution of these mechanisms to the rise in plasma NGAL concentration after AKI has yet to be investigated. NGAL levels are also influenced by various medical conditions, such as CKD, hypertension, anemia, systemic infections, hypoxia, inflammatory conditions, and cancers, making it relatively less specific for kidney injury.[319] Additionally, there is some evidence to suggest that NGAL concentrations degrade over time, with concentrations decreasing by nearly 50% within the first 6 months of storage at −80° C. These degradation issues also affect other biomarkers (including NAG and KIM-1), and their effects on clinical results remain unclear because this is an area of continued investigation.[320] Nevertheless, NGAL represents a very promising candidate as a biomarker for early diagnosis of AKI and potential prediction of outcome.

CHRONIC KIDNEY DISEASE

In addition to extensive investigation in the setting of AKI, NGAL has been increasingly investigated in the setting of CKD. Some of this work was inspired by animal data demonstrating that NGAL, like KIM-1, was highly upregulated by the persistent inflammation and late immune response following AKI and potentially contributes to the development of post-AKI CKD.[255] Moving this concept into humans, Nickolas and associates reported on the correlation of NGAL with histologic changes in native kidney biopsy specimens from subjects with CKD. The group demonstrated that NGAL levels were inversely correlated with eGFR while being directly correlated with both interstitial fibrosis and tubular atrophy.[298]

In a case-control substudy of the ARIC cohort (n = 286), urine NGAL did not initially correlate with baseline eGFR. However, the fourth quartile of urine NGAL was at a more than twofold higher risk for development of incident stage 3 CKD during the follow-up period. It should be noted, however, that this effect was attenuated after adjustments were made for urine creatinine and urine albumin.[257] These adjusted model data corroborate the findings from the MESA cohort, which was unable to find an association between urine NGAL levels and the development of incident CKD stage 3. In a 1:1 nested case-control study, NGAL levels were not associated with the development of CKD stage 3 or a decrease in eGFR of more than 3 mL/min per year, over a 5-year follow-up period.[256] Finally, in an analysis from the Chronic Renal Insufficiency Cohort (CRIC), Liu and colleagues demonstrated that there was a strong association between baseline urine NGAL and the risk of CKD progression (defined as a 50% reduction of MDRD-calculated eGFR or development of ESKD) over the mean follow-up of 3.2 years. However, although this effect was significant in an unadjusted analysis, urine NGAL offered no improved prediction after adjustment for baseline age, race, eGFR, proteinuria, diabetes, and other factors known to impact CKD progression (C-statistic of 0.847 for both). Thus, in this cohort of 3386 individuals with CKD, urine

NGAL was no better at predicting CKD outcomes than more traditional markers.[321]

These findings from ARIC, MESA, and CRIC contrast directly with those in a prospective observational cohort study of 158 white patients with baseline CKD stage 3 or 4, which demonstrated that urine NGAL (adjusted for urine creatinine) was associated with CKD progression. Forty patients reached the primary endpoint of all-cause mortality or need for RRT during the 2-year follow-up. The baseline urine NGAL was associated with this composite primary endpoint, with every increase in urine NGAL of 5 µg/mmol being associated with a 27% increase in risk of death or RRT.[322] These findings are similar to those of Bolignano and colleagues, who performed a prospective observational study of 96 subjects with CKD with a median follow-up of 18.5 months. They demonstrated that both urine and serum NGAL values were associated with a composite endpoint of either doubling of baseline serum creatinine or development of ESKD.[323] Conversely, in a 4-year follow-up study of 78 patients with type 1 diabetes conducted to evaluate the potential of urinary NGAL level to predict progression to diabetic nephropathy, NGAL levels were not associated with decline in GFR or development of ESKD and death after adjustment for known progression promoters.[324]

N-ACETYL-β-D-GLUCOSAMINIDASE

NAG is a lysosomal brush border enzyme that resides in the microvilli of tubular epithelial cells. Damage to these cells results in shedding of this enzyme into the urine. NAG has a high molecular weight, 130 kDa, and hence plasma NAG is not filtered by the glomeruli. Its excretion into urine correlates with tubular lysosomal activity. Increased urinary concentrations of NAG have been found in patients with AKI, chronic glomerular disease, diabetic nephropathy, exposure to nephrotoxic drugs, delayed renal allograft function, environmental exposure, contrast medium–induced nephropathy, and sepsis, and following cardiopulmonary bypass.[206,246,325-330] In a prospective study involving 201 hospitalized patients with AKI, patients with higher concentrations of urinary NAG and KIM-1 were more likely to die or require dialysis. The results of this study suggest the utility of NAG in combination with KIM-1 in predicting adverse clinical outcomes in patients with AKI.[246] In another study, urinary NAG concentrations were significantly higher in patients with contrast medium–induced nephropathy than in patients without such nephropathy within 24 hours of the administration of a contrast agent.[329]

Similarly, in a two-center Japanese study of 77 patients undergoing cardiac surgery, NAG values were elevated in those in whom postoperative AKI developed.[265] In this study, biomarker performance significantly improved when NAG was combined with L-FABP (an AUC improvement from 0.75 to 0.81). This same group published a single-center study investigating the performance of NAG in predicting the development of AKI (RIFLE) in a mixed, medical-surgical ICU. NAG did not perform as well in this cohort of 339 subjects, providing an AUC of 0.62 for the development of RIFLE Risk disease.[226] In a cohort of 635 ED patients, an NAG value over 1.0 units/g provided an AUC of 0.71 (95% CI, 0.62 to 0.81) for the development of AKI during the subsequent hospital admission. However, this effect was attenuated in a multivariate analysis that included other novel and traditional biomarkers of AKI (creatinine, BUN, NGAL, etc.).[182]

In the setting of CKD, one study of patients with type 1 diabetes and nephropathy by Vaidya and colleagues showed that lower levels of urinary KIM-1 and NAG were associated with the regression of microalbuminuria.[260] Similarly, in a nested-case-control study from the Diabetes Control and Compliance Trial, baseline NAG concentrations were shown to predict microalbuminuria and macroalbuminuria.[331] To date, there are little or no data on the role of NAG in CKD progression.

There are some limitations in the use of NAG as a marker of kidney injury. Inhibition of NAG enzyme activity has been reported in the presence of metal ions and at higher urea concentrations in the urine. Moreover, increased urinary levels of NAG have been reported in several nonrenal diseases, including rheumatoid arthritis and hyperthyroidism, as well as in conditions with increased lysosomal activity without cellular damage.[332,333] Because of concerns about its specificity, the clinical utility of NAG as a biomarker has been limited.

PROTEINURIA

In a healthy person, urinary protein excretion is less than 150 mg/day and consists mainly of filtered plasma proteins (60%) and tubular Tamm-Horsfall proteins (40%).[334,335] Proteinuria can result from at least three different pathophysiologic mechanisms, glomerular (increased permeability of glomerular filtration barrier to protein due to glomerulopathy, raised glomerular capillary hydrostatic pressure, or altered glomerular filtration coefficient), overflow (due to increased production of low-molecular-weight plasma proteins, e.g., immunoglobulin light chains in myeloma), and tubular processes (decreased tubular absorption of filtered proteins or increased production of tubular proteins by damaged tubules). Proteinuria mechanisms and consequences are discussed in Chapter 53.

Proteinuria is diagnosed when total urinary protein is greater than 300 mg/24 hour. Methods for detecting and monitoring proteinuria are discussed in Chapter 26.

Several publications highlight the diagnostic power of total protein for AKI in various drug-induced nephrotoxicities, including cisplatin and nonsteroidal antiinflammatory drugs.[336,337] Low eGFR is a known risk factor for AKI, but the utility of proteinuria in combination with the eGFR to predict the risk of this disease is now being investigated.[338] In a large cohort of nearly 1 million adult Canadians, James and colleagues demonstrated an independent association among eGFR, proteinuria, and incidence of AKI.[339] This group reported that patients with normal eGFR levels (≥60 mL/min per 1.73 m^2) and mild proteinuria (urine dipstick trace to 1+) have 2.5 times more risk of admission to hospital with AKI than do patients with no proteinuria. The risk was increased to 4.4-fold when patients with heavy proteinuria (urine dipstick ≥2+) were included. Adjusted rates of admission with AKI and kidney injury requiring dialysis remained high in patients with heavy dipstick proteinuria independent of the eGFR.[18] These findings confirm previous reports suggesting that eGFR and proteinuria are potent risk factors for subsequent AKI.[340,341]

ALBUMINURIA

Albuminuria is recognized as one the most important risk factors for progression of chronic kidney diseases. Albumin is a major serum protein slightly larger than the pores of the glomerular filtration membrane, so albuminuria is best known as a biomarker of glomerular dysfunction; the appearance of albumin in large amounts in urine represents compromised integrity of the glomerular basement membrane.[342] In smaller amounts, however, the presence of albumin in the urine may reflect tubular injury. Albuminuria is classified in the KDIGO classification system as stage A1 (urine AE [albumin excretion] < 30 mg/day or urine ACR [urine albumin to creatinine ratio] < 30 mg per g creatinine), stage A2 (previously termed microalbuminuria; urine AE 30-300 mg/day or uACR = 30-300 mg per g creatinine), and stage A3 (previously termed macroalbuminuria urine AE > 300 mg/day or urine ACR > 300 mg per g creatinine). In a number of clinical studies, albuminuria has been shown to be a sensitive biomarker of drug-induced tubular injury.[343,344] It is routinely used as a marker of kidney damage for making a CKD diagnosis at eGFRs above 60 mL/min/1.73 m^2.[335]

Guidelines of the National Kidney Foundation (NKF) and of the American Heart Association (AHA), respectively, include microalbuminuria and an increase in the urinary total protein excretion as risk factors for renal and cardiovascular diseases. Both NKF and AHA guidelines suggest measurement of urine ACR in an untimed spot urine sample. Ideally, urine ACR should be assessed in at least three different samples to decrease the intraindividual variation.[345] Albuminuria is a continuous risk factor for ESKD and cardiovascular mortality with no lower limit, even after adjustment for eGFR and other established risk factors.[346-348] Urine albumin value has been in use as a biomarker for monitoring CKD progression and to monitor potential therapeutic efficacy, although the FDA does not accept albuminuria as a surrogate marker.

Using microalbuminuria as a marker, Levin and colleagues demonstrated that N-acetylcysteine may attenuate contrast medium–induced glomerular and tubular injury.[349] In the last several years, there has been more investigation of urine albumin excretion as a biomarker for AKI. The TRIBE-AKI Consortium measured preoperative albuminuria in 1159 adult patients, organizing the cohort into clinical risk categories on the basis of the preoperative urine ACR: 10 mg/g or less (≤1.1 mg/mmol), 11 to 29 mg/g (1.2 to 3.3 mg/mmol), 30 to 299 mg/g (3.4 to 33.8 mg/mmol), and 300 mg/g or greater (≥33.9 mg/mmol). The incidence of AKI, defined as AKIN stage 1, increased across the ACR categories, with patients whose urine ACR was greater than 300 mg/g having a relative risk of 2.36 (95% CI, 1.85 to 2.82) in comparison with to the group whose urine ACR was less than 10 mg/g. This association was slightly attenuated after adjustments for variables known to affect proteinuria and AKI (RR, 2.21; 95% CI, 1.66 to 2.73).[350] These adult data contrast with pediatric TRIBE-AKI data (n = 294), which demonstrated no association between preoperative urine ACR and the development of postoperative AKI.[351]

The adult ACR data support use of an additional biomarker to aid in cardiac surgery AKI prediction models and supplement other data that point to the use of proteinuria/albuminuria as a biomarker of AKI both preoperatively and postoperatively.[352,353]

In the postoperative setting, the TRIBE-AKI cohort showed that urine albumin concentrations (mg/L) and dipstick proteinuria values obtained within 6 hours of adult cardiac surgery correlated with the future development of AKI. Compared with the lowest quintile, the highest quintile of albuminuria and highest group of dipstick proteinuria were associated with the greatest risk of AKI (adjusted RR, 2.97; 95% CI, 1.20 to 6.91, and adjusted RR, 2.46; 95% CI, 1.16 to 4.97, respectively). However, only postoperative urine albumin concentration (mg/L) was associated with improved risk stratification when added to the clinical model (AUC increased from 0.75 to 0.81; $P = 0.006$). Despite its known utility in other settings, a higher early postoperative urine ACR (mg/g) was not statistically associated with AKI risk. The poor performance of urine ACR in the context of adult cardiac surgery may be explained by variations in the urine creatinine excretion within and between individuals, which could be especially prominent when renal function is not in a steady state. Urinary albumin (mg/L) in the early postoperative period was highly predictive of long-term mortality in the TRIBE-AKI adult cohort. Specifically, of patients with perioperative AKI (n = 407), those in the second tertile of albuminuria values were at increased risk of death in the 3.0-year follow-up period (adjusted HR, 2.28; 95% CI, 1.06 to 4.88). Although this effect was further magnified in the third tertile of those with AKI (adjusted HR, 2.85; 95% CI, 1.36 to 5.99); there was no increased mortality across any of the tertiles of urine albumin concentration in the 792 subjects without perioperative AKI.[222]

In the TRIBE-AKI pediatric cohort, perioperative values of urine ACR (mg/g), and not albuminuria (mg/L), were found to be predictive of AKI. In children younger than 2 years, an absolute first postoperative urine ACR of 908 mg/g or higher (103 mg/mmol, highest tertile) predicted the development of AKIN stage 2 or 3 AKI with an adjusted RR of 3.4 (95% CI, 1.2 to 9.4) in comparison with the first tertile. In children 2 years or older, a postoperative urine ACR value of 169 mg/g or higher (19.1 mg/mmol, highest tertile), regardless of preoperative values, predicted stage 1 AKI after adjustments for clinical factors, such as age, race, sex, and preoperative eGFR, and type of cardiac surgery (adjusted RR, 2.1; 95% CI, 1.1 to 4.1).[351] Although urine albumin concentration and urine ACR remain established and readily available laboratory tests, the diversity of results in investigations of the development of postoperative AKI indicate that further studies are needed before either may be used in clinical practice.

URINARY CYSTATIN C

Urinary cystatin C tracks the function of proximal tubular cells. In healthy individuals, the urinary levels of cystatin C are almost undetectable and any damage to proximal tubular cells can impede the reabsorption and enhance the urinary excretion of cystatin C. Several clinical studies sought to understand the potential of urinary cystatin C levels for prediction of kidney injury and its prognosis. Herget-Rosenthal and associates analyzed data for 85 patients in the ICU who were at high risk for development of AKI and used the RIFLE classification to define AKI. The investigators reported that serum cystatin C level signaled AKI 1 to 2 days before changes in serum creatinine level, with AUC values of 0.82 and 0.97 on day 2 and day 1, respectively, as well as demonstrating that urine cystatin C served as a marker of AKI severity, correlating with future need for RRT.[354,355] Urinary cystatin C concentrations, normalized to urinary creatinine, of more than 11.3 mg/mmol were significantly associated with proteinuria. Attempts to validate urine cystatin C as a marker of ICU-associated AKI have provided mixed results. Siew and colleagues measured urine cystatin C in 380 ICU patients (mixed-surgical, medical, trauma, and cardiac) and demonstrated that there was no difference in concentrations between those with and those without AKI ($P = 0.87$).[267] More encouraging data from the EARLYARF trial showed that in a cohort of 529 subjects, urinary cystatin C may have the limited ability to detect AKI (AUC = 0.67 upon ICU arrival) with no significant difference in its ability to detect AKI in patients with GFRs above and below 60 mL/min.[224] Additionally, in a separate post hoc analysis of the same study, urinary cystatin C values exhibited a stepwise and significant ($P < 0.001$) increase in the following order: patients with no AKI, patients with prerenal AKI, patients with intrinsic AKI (which was defined as AKIN stage 1 > 48 hours).

In contrast to these mixed ICU-associated AKI data, several small studies investigating urinary cystatin C in the setting of cardiac surgery have demonstrated promise.[42,104,295,356] However, these results were not validated in the TRIBE-AKI study. In unadjusted analyses of the adult cohort, several quintiles of urine cystatin C were significantly associated with the development of either mild (AKIN stage 1) or severe (doubling of creatinine or need for RRT) AKI at both the 0- to 6-hour and 6- to 12-hour postoperative time points. However, the small associations were completely attenuated after adjustments for the clinical model. Similarly, in the TRIBE pediatric cohort, no quintile remained significantly associated with AKI (mild or severe) in the adjusted analyses.[357] Urinary cystatin C demonstrated similar results when measured in a cohort of 1635 ED patients, supplying an AUC of 0.65 (95% CI, 0.58 to 0.72) for the future development of AKI. However, utilizing a multivariate analysis that included traditional (creatinine) and more modern (urine NGAL, KIM-1, IL-18, and LFABP) biomarkers, urinary cystatin C was not a significant contributor to the prediction of the composite outcome of inpatient RRT or death.[227] Finally, when investigated in a prospective multicenter observation cohort study of deceased-donor kidney transplants, urinary cystatin C values from the first postoperative day were modestly correlated with 3-month allograft function, whereas the AUC for predicting delayed graft function at the 6-hour postoperative timepoint was 0.69.[358]

A number of studies have reported increased urinary cystatin C levels in patients with proteinuria, suggesting the possibility of tubular damage as a consequence of protein overload.[359-361] Currently, cystatin C level has several disadvantages as a biomarker, including lack of international standardization and expense of the assay. Although serum cystatin C level has been demonstrated as a reliable biomarker of eGFR, one must remember that cystatin C synthesis is increased in smokers, patients with hyperthyroidism, those receiving glucocorticoid therapy, and those with elevations of inflammatory markers such as white blood cell count and C-reactive protein level, and the impact of these factors on urinary cystatin C in the setting of AKI has not been fully investigated.[362,363] Furthermore, several different commercial assays are available to measure cystatin C. Advantages are that the commercially available immunonephelometric assay provides rapid, automated measurement of cystatin C, and results are available in minutes.[364] In addition, preanalytic factors, such as routine clinical storage conditions, freezing and thawing cycles, and interfering substances such as bilirubin and triglycerides, do not affect cystatin C measurement.[364,365]

TIMP-2 AND IGFBP-7

Tissue inhibitor metalloproteinase-2 (TIMP-2) and urine insulin-like growth factor-binding protein-7 (IGFBP-7) have been shown to serve as biomarkers of AKI in the setting of critical illness. They were originally discovered as part of a three-center discovery cohort of 522 subjects. These patients had AKI stemming from sepsis, shock, major surgery, and trauma. More than 300 potential markers were evaluated, with TIMP-2 and IGFBP-7 being the two that best predicted the development of KDIGO stage 2 or 3 AKI. This finding was then validated in a prospective international multicenter observational study of 728 subjects.[300] In this validation study, TIMP-2 and IGFBP-7 remained the top two performing biomarkers for the prediction of RIFLE Injury or Failure stage within the first 12 to 36 hours of study enrollment, providing AUCs of 0.77 and 0.75, respectively. When these two biomarker values were multiplied together, they demonstrated an improved ability to detect this same endpoint (AUC = 0.80). However, we are cautious about the interpretation of these data because the study did not supply information about the combination of TIMP-2 and IGFBP-7 with other biomarkers of AKI (e.g., NGAL, KIM-1, L-FABP, IL-18).[300] This is the first and only publication to demonstrate that either of these markers plays a role in diagnosing AKI and will require validation in follow-up studies. These biomarkers are unique in that they play a role in cell cycle arrest. Both IGFBP-7 (through p523 and p21) and TIMP-2 (through p27) block the effect of cyclin-dependent protein kinase complexes, resulting in short periods of G_1 cell cycle arrest.[366-368] A commercial assay for these biomarkers is currently available in Europe, but the TIMP-2 and IGFBP-7 test has not been approved for clinical use in the United States.

CHRONIC KIDNEY DISEASE BIOMARKERS

Currently, eGFR and proteinuria are used as markers of CKD progression because of the widespread availability of the tests and the ease of performing them. All forms of CKD are associated with tubulointerstitial injury. As described previously, markers of tubular injury, including KIM-1, IL-18, NGAL, and L-FABP, have been shown to predict outcomes in CKD associated with a variety of causes. In addition, systemic elevations of molecules that have impaired kidney clearance or increased production in CKD (e.g., asymmetric dimethylarginine, fibroblast growth factor-23) as well as chemokines (e.g., monocyte chemoattractant protein-1) and fibrotic markers (connective tissue growth factor, TGF-β1, and collagen IV) are discussed here.

PLASMA ASYMMETRIC DIMETHYLARGININE

Nitric oxide is synthesized by oxidation of the terminal guanidine nitrogen of L-arginine by nitric oxide synthase (NOS). This process can be reversibly inhibited by guanidine-substituted analogs of L-arginine, such as in asymmetric dimethylarginine (ADMA).[369,370] Three types of methylated arginines have been described in vivo: ADMA, N^G-monomethyl-L-arginine, and symmetric dimethylarginine, an inert isomer of ADMA. Of these, ADMA is the major type of endogenously generated methylated arginine that displays inhibitor activity of NOS. However, administration of ADMA to endothelial NOS knockout mice also induces vascular lesions, suggesting that ADMA may have actions independent of nitric oxide and NOS in vivo.[371] Vallance and associates first reported that plasma values of ADMA are elevated in patients with renal failure[372] and hypothesized that impaired renal clearance of ADMA may account for the rise. This assumption has been challenged by follow-up studies in animal models demonstrating that only a small portion of circulating ADMA is excreted in the urine.[373] Moreover, elevated plasma ADMA levels are also reported in patients with incipient renal disease but normal renal function.[374]

Elevated plasma levels of ADMA have been reported in patients with a variety of cardiovascular risk factors, such as hypertension, diabetes, and hyperlipidemia.[375-377] Among these groups, plasma ADMA levels are particularly high in patients with CKD, patients with ESKD undergoing hemodialysis or peritoneal dialysis, and kidney transplant recipients.[372,378,379] Plasma levels of ADMA are strongly associated with carotid intima-media thickness, left ventricular hypertrophy, cardiovascular complications, and mortality in patients with ESKD.[380-382] Plasma ADMA levels have been shown to prospectively correlate, in an inverse manner, with CKD progression in patients with and without diabetes-related CKD.[383,384] Similarly ADMA levels may also be associated with the presence of proteinuria/albuminuria.[385] Large longitudinal studies are needed to demonstrate the ability of ADMA to identify CKD and predict its progression in cohorts with CKD from multiple causes.

FIBROBLAST GROWTH FACTOR-23

Fibroblast growth factor-23 (FGF-23) is a 32-kDa protein consisting of 251 amino acids coded by a gene, which is located on chromosome 12 in the human genome. FGF-23 serves as an endocrine hormone that is secreted by osteoblasts and osteoclasts and that binds an FGF receptor and its co-receptor Klotho and stimulates phosphaturia.[386-388] In addition to promoting phosphaturia, FGF-23 decreases levels of 1,25 dihydroxy-vitamin D and of parathyroid hormone.[389,390] Several cross-sectional studies have demonstrated that FGF-23 values are elevated in both adult and pediatric patients with CKD.[391-393] In a prospective observational study of 3879 subjects in the CRIC, FGF-23 levels were shown to be increased in individuals with CKD stages 2 through 4, with FGF-23 elevation occurring in the absence of abnormalities in serum phosphate and PTH.[394] As such, FGF-23 has emerged as a candidate biomarker to detect CKD and abnormalities of bone-mineral metabolism in the absence of changes in serum phosphate and PTH.

FGF-23 is principally expressed in the ventrolateral thalamic nucleus in mice and is also known to be secreted in minimal amounts in liver, heart, thymus, and lymph node. Maintenance of phosphate homeostasis is carried out by the sodium-dependent phosphate cotransporters NaPi-IIa and NaPi-IIc at the brush border membrane of proximal tubular cells in kidney, and FGF-23 has been shown to regulate the activity of these transporters.[395,396]

FGF-23 is increased in CKD and is a prognostic indicator for cardiovascular disease in patients with CKD.[397] In an analysis of 3860 participants in the CRIC, FGF-23 levels in the highest quartiles (compared with the lowest) were independently associated with a graded risk of congestive heart failure (HR, 2.98; 95% CI, 1.97 to 4.52) and atherosclerotic events (HR, 1.76; 95% CI, 1.20 to 2.59) even after adjustment for eGFR, proteinuria, and other traditional cardiovascular risk factors.[398] Other studies have shown that elevated plasma FGF-23 concentrations are associated with cardiovascular events in patients not requiring dialysis as well as with mortality in patients receiving hemodialysis, with levels in those with ESKD reaching nearly 1000-fold above normal.[399] Interestingly, FGF-23 levels have also been shown to rapidly decline in individuals with prompt allograft function after renal transplantation.[400,401] It has been reported that serum FGF-23 concentrations may be a useful marker for predicting future development of refractory hyperparathyroidism and the response to vitamin D therapy in patients receiving dialysis.[402] Similarly, FGF-23 may be useful in the evaluation of calcium, phosphate, and vitamin D disorders in early-stage CKD in pediatric as well as adult patients.[403,404] Lowering FGF-23 levels (e.g., with oral phosphate binders) may reduce cardiovascular morbidity in patients with CKD,[405] although more studies are needed. For further discussion of FGF-23, see Chapter 55.

URINARY MONOCYTE CHEMOATTRACTANT PROTEIN-1

Monocyte chemoattractant protein-1 (MCP-1) is a chemotactic protein secreted by a variety of cells that attracts blood monocytes and tissue macrophages through interaction with the cell surface receptor CCR2 (chemokine C-C motif receptor 2).[406,407] Induction of MCP-1 at the transcript or protein level has been demonstrated in a variety of human cell types, including fibroblasts, endothelial cells, peripheral blood mononuclear cells, and epithelial cells, on proinflammatory stimuli.[407-411] Kidney cells also produce MCP-1 in response to proinflammatory cytokines, including tumor necrosis factor-α and IL-1β.[412] Expression of MCP-1 is induced in kidney diseases with significant inflammation, such as diabetic nephropathy and other glomerulonephropathies.[413-415] In particular, podocytes and tubular cells produce MCP-1 in response to high levels of glucose and advanced glycosylation end products.[416] Furthermore, urine values of MCP-1 are significantly increased in patients with diabetic nephropathy and correlate significantly with albuminuria and NAG levels in human as well as experimental diabetic nephropathy.[417-420] In a prospective observational study of patients with diabetic nephropathy, urine values of connective tissue growth factor (CTGF) were elevated in patients with microalbuminuria and macroalbuminuria, but urinary MCP-1 was elevated only in those with macroalbuminuria.[421] Urinary CTGF levels correlated with progression to macroalbuminuria, whereas urinary MCP-1 levels (but not CTGF levels) correlated with the subsequent rate of eGFR decline (at a median follow-up of 6 years). The investigators concluded that increased urinary CTGF concentration is associated with early progression of diabetic nephropathy, whereas MCP-1 level is associated with later-stage disease.[421]

The independent association of urine MCP-1 with the risk of CKD progression has been confirmed by others.[422,423] Elevations of urinary MCP-1 were reported in patients with lupus nephritis, and the presence of MCP-1 in urine reflected its intrarenal expression.[424,425] Serum concentrations of MCP-1 were also shown to be elevated in patients with diabetic nephropathy and lupus nephritis, but the serum levels did not correlate with disease progression.[424-426] Moreover, the lack of correlation between urinary and serum MCP-1 levels suggests that urinary MCP-1 is the result of local production of MCP-1 by the kidney rather than simply filtration of serum MCP-1. Vianna and colleagues demonstrated that plasma and urinary concentrations of MCP-1 were elevated in pediatric CKD (from either glomerular disease or congenital anomalies) but were not correlated with each other. MCP-1 levels were significantly higher in patients with CKD than in those without CKD and there were differences in MCP-1 concentration depending on the cause of the CKD.[415]

Munshi and associates demonstrated that urinary concentrations of both MCP-1 transcripts and protein were elevated in patients with AKI as well as in experimental models of AKI; however, these data have yet to be replicated in other AKI cohorts.[427]

URINARY RENAL FIBROSIS MARKERS

Excessive production of extracellular matrix (collagen IV) and profibrotic growth factors contributes to renal fibrosis, and CTGF as well as TGF-β1 are growth factors implicated in the progression of renal fibrosis.

CONNECTIVE TISSUE GROWTH FACTOR

Connective tissue growth factor (also known as *CCN2*), a member of the CCN family of matricellular proteins, was first discovered by Bradham and colleagues in 1991 as a secreted protein in the conditioned media of human umbilical vascular endothelial cells.[428] CTGF has been implicated in a variety of cellular functions, including proliferation, cell adhesion, angiogenesis, and wound healing.[380,429,430] Accumulated evidence on CTFG in the last few years indicates that it is both a marker and a mediator of tissue fibrosis.[431] CTGF is an immediate-early gene potently induced by TGF-β that has also been shown to promote fibrosis primarily through TGF-β.[432] CTGF is overexpressed in several fibrotic diseases, such as scleroderma and lung and hepatic fibrosis.[433-435]

In the kidney, CTGF expression has been shown to be upregulated in various forms of renal disease, including IgA nephropathy, focal and segmental glomerulosclerosis, and diabetic nephropathy.[434] CTGF has been found to be elevated in the glomeruli at early and late stages of diabetic nephropathy.[436] Riser and associates first reported that CTGF is elevated in the urine of diabetic rats and in diabetic patients.[437] Subsequently, several groups reported higher urinary levels of CTGF in diabetic patients than in healthy individuals,[438,439] indicating its potential as a marker for diabetic nephropathy. In patients with diabetes, plasma CTGF levels were shown to be higher in those with macroalbuminuria than in those with a normal urine albumin level. CTGF was an independent predictor of ESKD and correlated with the rate of decline in GFR.[440] In another study, both blood and urine levels of intact CTGF and the N-terminal fragment were measured in 1050 patients with type 1 diabetes from the Diabetes Control and Complications Trial/Epidemiology of Diabetes Interventions and Complication (DCCT/EDIC).[441] Patients with macroalbuminuria had higher plasma levels of CTGF N-terminal fragment than diabetic patients with or without microalbuminuria. Intact CTGF levels were associated with the duration of diabetes as well as common carotid artery intima-media thickness. Additionally, in regression analyses, log plasma CTGF N-terminal fragments concentrations were independently associated with the intima thickness of the common and internal carotid artery. Plasma CTGF levels, therefore, serve as a risk marker for diabetic renal and vascular disease.

TRANSFORMING GROWTH FACTOR-β_1

Transforming growth factor-β is essential for the development and differentiation of various tissues.[442] Three isoforms of TGF-β have been identified in mammalian species: TGF-β_1, TGF-β_2, and TGF-β_3. TGF-β_1 is the predominant isoform in humans.[443] It is mainly secreted as high-molecular-weight inactive complex and undergoes a cleavage process for its activation.[444] Several studies have demonstrated the association of urine levels of TGF-β_1 with the progression of CKD. Elevated urinary TGF-β_1 levels were found in patients with glomerulonephritis and diabetic nephropathy as well as in renal allograft recipients.[444-447] In addition, some of the profibrotic molecules induced by TGF-β_1, including TGF-β–inducible gene H3 (βig-H3) and plasminogen activator inhibitor-1 (PAI-1), were also detected at high levels in the urine.[448,449] Because TGF-β_1 is mostly secreted as an inactive complex that requires chemical modification for its activation, βig-H3 and PAI-1 can be used as surrogate markers for TGF-β_1 activity. Urine levels of both βig-H3 and PAI-1 have been shown to correlate with renal injury and fibrosis in patients with diabetic nephropathy.[448,449] However, in a study of 3939 participants from the CRIC study, TGF-β levels were not shown to be significantly associated with CKD progression or the presence of macroalbuminuria.[450] In a much smaller case-control study of TGF-β in the setting of pediatric obstructive nephropathy (posterior urethral valves), however, TGF-β levels were shown to be inversely correlated with GFR.[451]

COLLAGEN IV

Collagen IV is a component of the extracellular matrix, and excess deposition of collagen IV is present in renal fibrosis. Furthermore, elevation of urinary collagen IV has been

Table 30.6 Biomarker Performance in Detecting AKI from Multicenter Studies at a Variety of Clinical Timepoints

	Peri-operative AKI				Critically Ill			Emergency Room	
	Preop AKI Risk	Early Post-op AKI	AKI Progression	Long-Term Mortality	Early Diagnosis of AKI	Type of AKI (Transient vs. Intrinsic)	Need for RRT	Early Diagnosis of AKI	Type of AKI (Transient vs. Intrinsic)
Urine NGAL	N/A	+	−	+	+	+	+	+	+
Blood NGAL	−	+	+	?	−	?	−	?	?
Blood CysC	+	+	−	?	+	+	+	?	?
Urine CysC	N/A	−	−	−	+	+	+	+	+
Urine IL-18	N/A	+	+	+	+	+	+	+	+
Urine KIM-1	N/A	+	−	+	+	−	−	+	+
Urine L-FABP	N/A	−	−	+	?	?	−	+	+
TIMP-2/IGFBP-7	N/A	?	?	?	+	?	+	?	?
Urine protein/albumin	+	+	+	+	?	?	?	?	?

Adapted and expanded from Koyner JL, Parikh CR: Clinical utility of biomarkers of AKI in cardiac surgery and critical illness. Clin J Am Soc Nephrol 8:1034-1042, 2013.

+, Data published displays the ability to detect this aspect of AKI; −, data published does not display the ability to detect this aspect of AKI; ?, no large multicenter data published on this biomarker/aspect of AKI; N/A, not applicable, because biomarkers of tubular injury have no role in preoperative risk screening.

AKI, Acute kidney injury; CysC, cystatin C; IGFBP7, insulin-like growth factor–binding protein-7; IL-18, interleukin-18; KIM-1, kidney injury molecule-1; L-FABP, liver-type fatty acid–binding protein; NGAL, neutrophil gelatinase–associated lipocalin; postop, postoperative; preop, preoperative; RRT, renal replacement therapy; TIMP-2, tissue inhibitor metalloproteinase-2.

Table 30.7 Biomarker Performance in Detecting CKD from Multicenter Studies

	Diagnosis of CKD	Progression of CKD to ESKD	Cardiovascular/Mortality Risk Assessment in CKD	Progression of HIV-Associated CKD
Urine NGAL	?	−	?	?
Blood NGAL	?	−	?	?
Blood CysC	+	+	+	+
Urine IL-18	−	?	?	+
Urine KIM-1	?	?	?	−
β-Trace protein	−	?	+	?
Urine protein/albumin	+	+	+	+
FGF-23	−	+	+	?

+, Data published displays the ability to detect this aspect of CKD; −, data published does not display the ability to detect this aspect of CKD; ?, no large multicenter data published on this biomarker/aspect of CKD.

CKD, chronic kidney disease; CysC, Cystatin C; ESKD, end-stage kidney disease; FGF-23, fibroblastic growth factor-23; HIV, human immunodeficiency virus; IL-18, interleukin-18; KIM-1, kidney injury molecule-1; NGAL, neutrophil gelatinase–associated lipocalin.

reported in patients with IgA nephropathy as well as in those with diabetic nephropathy and has been correlated with declining renal function.[452,453] In a prospective observational cohort study of 231 normoalbuminuric and microalbuminuric patients with type 1 diabetes, collagen IV was significantly associated with decline in eGFR over time in both univariate and multivariate analyses, with collagen IV values being elevated in patients with lower GFRs.[454]

Tables 30.6 and 30.7 summarize the ability of biomarkers to detect clinical endpoints related to AKI and CKD in a variety of clinical settings.

COMBINATIONS OF MULTIPLE BIOMARKERS

In the classic biomarker paradigm, one biomarker detects one disease. However, acute and chronic kidney diseases are complex with multiple underlying causes. A single biomarker may not be optimal to make an early diagnosis and predict the longer-term outcome of the disease process. Different biomarkers provide different sets of information. As discussed in this chapter, some biomarkers excel at detecting AKI in different clinical settings (cardiac surgery vs. ICU vs. ED vs. other) whereas others detect different aspects of AKI (early diagnosis vs. AKI severity vs. prerenal disease). This same phenomenon is true of CKD biomarkers with some being more likely to detect CKD in the setting of diabetes or in obstruction or in other forms of glomerulonephritis. Thus, it is important to consider the clinical utility of a panel of biomarkers for acute and chronic kidney diseases.

It is becoming increasingly clear, in part on the basis of the evidence discussed here, that multiple biomarkers are already a viable option in the care of patients with CKD. Serum creatinine can be used in conjunction with cystatin C for the detection/diagnosis of CKD. Proteinuria/albuminuria can be used in combination with these two markers of glomerular function to further diagnose and risk-stratify individuals. Recall that in the setting of normal serum creatinine and serum cystatin C, the presence of albuminuria constitutes a diagnosis of CKD.

Utilization of multiple biomarkers in the setting of AKI has been an area of increased investigation, with several studies attempting to combine two or more biomarkers to improve their predictive capabilities.[249,250,265,300,308] Some studies have simply used the product of two biomarkers and then assessed the AUC, and others have used logistic regression models to assess the AUC for two or more biomarkers. There has not been a consensus about the statistical methods for combining biomarkers, and this remains an area of continued investigation. Later studies have acknowledged the aforementioned premise that individual biomarkers have their own specific kinetics and that combining biomarkers from different timepoints may improve their predictive capabilities.[250] However, the clinical implications and feasibility of collecting biomarker samples at several distinct timepoints following cardiac surgery or ICU admission remain untested. As more and more biomarker data are amassed, we anticipate advances in novel methods for assessing biomarker combinations. Table 30.8 summarizes a variety of rationales and approaches to combining biomarker results in the hope of achieving improved prediction of patient outcomes.

Table 30.8 Strategies for Biomarker Combination

Combine for different functions	Combine a marker of filtration with one of tubular injury
	Combine a marker of proximal tubular injury with a marker of distal tubular injury
Combine for kinetics	Combine biomarkers with different time courses to improve duration of diagnosis
Combine for improved accuracy	Use of two or more biomarkers in statistical equations
Strategic combinations	Combine a diagnostic biomarker with a prognostic biomarker
	Combine an extremely sensitive marker with an extremely specific marker

FDA CRITICAL PATH INITIATIVE: A NEED FOR BETTER BIOMARKERS

The Critical Path Initiative was launched in March 2004 by the FDA as a strategy for modernizing the sciences through which FDA-regulated products are developed, evaluated, manufactured, and used. The 2006 report of the Critical Path Initiative outlined specific key areas of Critical Path focus identified by FDA experts and the public. Commenting on a major initiative of the FDA that focuses on biomarkers, Janet Woodcock, MD, deputy commissioner for operations and head of the FDA's Critical Path Initiative, stated: "Most researchers agree that a new generation of predictive biomarkers would dramatically improve the efficiency of product development, help identify safety problems before a product is on the market (and even before it is tested in humans), and facilitate the development of new types of clinical trials that will produce better data faster."[455] The Critical Path Initiative is the FDA's attempt to stimulate and facilitate a national effort to modernize the scientific process through which a potential human drug, biologic product, or medical device progresses from the discovery or "proof of concept" stage into a medical product.[456] The FDA has provided guidelines stating that a biomarker can be considered "valid" only if (1) it is measured in an analytical test system with well-established performance characteristics, and (2) there is an established scientific framework or body of evidence that elucidates the physiologic, pharmacologic, toxicologic, or clinical significance of the test result.

The initial project hosted by Critical Path Institute, the Predictive Safety Testing Consortium (PSTC), brought together 16 pharmaceutical and biotechnology companies, one nonprofit patient organization, and advisors from academic institutions, the FDA, and the EMA to exchange data and methodologies with the goal of qualifying organ safety biomarkers for regulatory decision making in preclinical, translational, and clinical contexts.[23,24] Seven urinary proteins (KIM-1, albumin, total protein, β_2-microglobulin, cystatin C, clusterin, and trefoil factor 3) were evaluated for their utility to outperform current tests, including serum creatinine concentration and BUN concentration, in the detection of drug-induced kidney injury. The Predictive Safety Testing Consortium submitted the data to the FDA, EMA, and Japanese Pharmaceutical and Medical Devices Agency for evaluation.[24] In 2010, the FDA and EMA reached the formal conclusion that these biomarkers are considered qualified for use in regulatory decision making for drug safety to detect acute drug-induced kidney injury in preclinical studies and, on a case-by-case basis, in early clinical studies in combination with standard biomarkers.[23,24,457,458]

THE KIDNEY HEALTH INITIATIVE

In response to the epidemic of CKD and AKI and the limited number of randomized controlled trials, in 2013 the FDA, the American Society of Nephrology, and their industry partners announced the founding of the Kidney Health Initiative (KHI). This public-private partnership was designed to foster collaborations to optimize the evaluation of drugs, devices, biologics, and food products in the greater kidney community. This initiative is intended to facilitate the delivery of these products to the U.S. market in a safe and expeditious manner.[459] Despite the growing evidence of their ability to predict AKI, CKD progression, and other adverse patient outcomes, no new biomarkers have been approved in the United States for clinical use, so it remains to be seen how this new initiative will affect the biomarkers field.

FUTURE OF BIOMARKERS

Advances in molecular analysis and proteomics have resulted in the identification of a wide range of potential serum and urine biomarkers for assessing renal function and injury as well as predicting the development of kidney disease. Not only are many of these biomarkers sensitive, but some are site specific. A number of them have been reported to be predictive of an adverse outcome. For some, however, a great deal of additional work is still needed to bring these biomarkers successfully to clinical practice for kidney diseases.

Because kidney disease is complex with multiple causes and often manifests in the setting of systemic diseases, a single biomarker may be insufficient for early diagnosis, insight into pathophysiology, and prediction of clinical course and outcome. Different biomarkers will be useful in different contexts. In some circumstances, a single biomarker may suffice, but in others, benefit will come from the use of multiple biomarkers in plasma, urine, or both to provide early evidence of risk and injury and to distinguish among various types of kidney diseases. Many of these biomarkers can be grouped according to their association with a particular type of injury (e.g., podocyte or tubular injury) or mechanism of damage (e.g., oxidative stress, inflammation, fibrosis). Understanding the relationships among these different biomarker categories may help us to better understand disease processes.

These biomarkers are not only useful for assessing kidney injury in humans in early stages and predicting progression of disease but also crucial for translating novel therapeutic compounds from preclinical animal models to first human trials. In the past, the use of newly emerged biomarkers in preclinical and clinical studies and drug development has been hindered by lack of regulatory acceptance. It is hoped that in the future, biomarker measurements obtained using biomarker test panels will be used not only to diagnose kidney injury and predict outcome but also as surrogate endpoints in clinical trials, an approach that might speed up clinical evaluation of desperately needed therapies for kidney diseases.

ACKNOWLEDGEMENT

Dr. Koyner was supported by NIH grant K23DK081616. Dr. Parikh was supported by NIH grant RO1HL085757 to fund the TRIBE-AKI Consortium to study novel biomarkers of acute kidney injury in cardiac surgery. Dr. Parikh is also a member of the NIH-sponsored ASsess, Serial Evaluation, and Subsequent Sequelae in Acute Kidney Injury (ASSESS-AKI) Consortium (U01DK082185).

We wish to acknowledge and thank Drs. Joseph V. Bonventre and Venkata Sabbisetti, who wrote prior versions of this chapter.

DISCLOSURE

Dr. Koyner reports research grants from Abbott Laboratories, Abbvie, and Astute Medical for conducting observational biomarker studies. Dr. Koyner has received research funding from Argutus Medical and NxStage Medical. Dr. Koyner is named on a patent from EFK Diagnostics for the use of π-GST for the diagnosis of severe AKI following cardiac surgery.

Dr. Parikh is a named co-inventor on the IL-18 patent licensed to the University of Colorado (no financial value).

Complete reference list available at ExpertConsult.com.

KEY REFERENCES

1. Uchino S, et al: Acute renal failure in critically ill patients: a multinational, multicenter study. *JAMA* 294(16106006):813–818, 2005.
14. Biomarkers Definitions Working Group: Biomarkers and surrogate endpoints: preferred definitions and conceptual framework. *Clin Pharmacol Ther* 69(3):89–95, 2001.
16. Pepe MS, Etzioni R, Feng Z, et al: Phases of biomarker development for early detection of cancer. *J Natl Cancer Inst* 93(14):1054–1061, 2001.
21. Waikar SS, et al: Imperfect gold standards for kidney injury biomarker evaluation. *J Am Soc Nephrol* 23(22021710):13–21, 2012.
24. Dieterle F, et al: Renal biomarker qualification submission: a dialog between the FDA-EMEA and Predictive Safety Testing Consortium. *Nat Biotechnol* 28(20458315):455–462, 2010.
31. Pencina MJ, D'Agostino RB, Sr, Steyerberg EW: Extensions of net reclassification improvement calculations to measure usefulness of new biomarkers. *Stat Med* 30(1):11–21, 2011.
36. Bellomo R, et al: Acute renal failure—definition, outcome measures, animal models, fluid therapy and information technology needs: the Second International Consensus Conference of the Acute Dialysis Quality Initiative (ADQI) Group. *Crit Care* 8(4):R204–R212, 2004.
37. Mehta RL, et al: Acute Kidney Injury Network: report of an initiative to improve outcomes in acute kidney injury. *Crit Care* 11(2):R31, 2007.
38. Kidney Disease: Improving Global Outcomes (KDIGO) Acute Kidney Injury Work Group: KDIGO clinical practice guideline for acute kidney injury. *Kidney Int* (Suppl 2):1–138, 2012.
39. Haase M, et al: The outcome of neutrophil gelatinase-associated lipocalin-positive subclinical acute kidney injury: a multicenter pooled analysis of prospective studies. *J Am Coll Cardiol* 57(17):1752–1761, 2011.
49. Levey AS, et al: A more accurate method to estimate glomerular filtration rate from serum creatinine: a new prediction equation. Modification of Diet in Renal Disease Study Group. *Ann Intern Med* 130(6):461–470, 1999.
50. Levey AS, et al: A new equation to estimate glomerular filtration rate. *Ann Intern Med* 150(9):604–612, 2009.
56. Singer E, et al: Urinary neutrophil gelatinase-associated lipocalin distinguishes pre-renal from intrinsic renal failure and predicts outcomes. *Kidney Int* 80(4):405–414, 2011.
91. Shlipak MG, et al: Cystatin C and the risk of death and cardiovascular events among elderly persons. *N Engl J Med* 352(15901858):2049–2060, 2005.
96. Inker LA, et al: Estimating glomerular filtration rate from serum creatinine and cystatin C. *N Engl J Med* 367(1):20–29, 2012.
104. Koyner JL, et al: Urinary cystatin C as an early biomarker of acute kidney injury following adult cardiothoracic surgery. *Kidney Int* 74(8):1059–1069, 2008.
109. Zappitelli M, et al: Early postoperative serum cystatin C predicts severe acute kidney injury following pediatric cardiac surgery. *Kidney Int* 80(6):655–662, 2011.
147. Wang Y, et al: Increased urinary excretion of nephrin, podocalyxin, and βig-h3 in women with preeclampsia. *Am J Physiol Renal Physiol* 302(9):F1084–F1089, 2012.

150. Ruotsalainen V, et al: Nephrin is specifically located at the slit diaphragm of glomerular podocytes. *Proc Natl Acad Sci U S A* 96(10393930):7962–7967, 1999.
165. Perazella MA, et al: Urine microscopy is associated with severity and worsening of acute kidney injury in hospitalized patients. *Clin J Am Soc Nephrol* 5(20089493):402–408, 2010.
182. Nickolas TL, et al: Sensitivity and specificity of a single emergency department measurement of urinary neutrophil gelatinase-associated lipocalin for diagnosing acute kidney injury. *Ann Intern Med* 148(11):810–819, 2008.
216. Melnikov VY, et al: Impaired IL-18 processing protects caspase-1-deficient mice from ischemic acute renal failure. *J Clin Invest* 107(11342578):1145–1152, 2001.
218. Parikh CR, et al: Urinary interleukin-18 is a marker of human acute tubular necrosis. *Am J Kidney Dis* 43(14981598):405–414, 2004.
219. Parikh CR, et al: Postoperative biomarkers predict acute kidney injury and poor outcomes after adult cardiac surgery. *J Am Soc Nephrol* 22(9):1748–1757, 2011.
220. Parikh CR, et al: Postoperative biomarkers predict acute kidney injury and poor outcomes after pediatric cardiac surgery. *J Am Soc Nephrol* 22(9):1737–1747, 2011.
221. Koyner JL, et al: Biomarkers predict progression of acute kidney injury after cardiac surgery. *J Am Soc Nephrol* 23(5):905–914, 2012.
222. Coca SG, et al: Urinary biomarkers of acute kidney injury and mortality 3-years after cardiac surgery. *J Am Soc Nephrol* 25(5):1063–1071, 2013.
223. Siew ED, et al: Elevated urinary IL-18 levels at the time of ICU admission predict adverse clinical outcomes. *Clin J Am Soc Nephrol* 5(8):1497–1505, 2010.
224. Endre ZH, et al: Improved performance of urinary biomarkers of acute kidney injury in the critically ill by stratification for injury duration and baseline renal function. *Kidney Int* 79(10):1119–1130, 2011.
225. Nejat M, et al: Some biomarkers of acute kidney injury are increased in pre-renal acute injury. *Kidney Int* 81(12):1254–1262, 2012.
226. Doi K, et al: Evaluation of new acute kidney injury biomarkers in a mixed intensive care unit. *Crit Care Med* 39(11):2464–2469, 2011.
227. Nickolas TL, et al: Diagnostic and prognostic stratification in the emergency department using urinary biomarkers of nephron damage: a multicenter prospective cohort study. *J Am Coll Cardiol* 59(3):246–255, 2012.
230. Hall IE, et al: IL-18 and urinary NGAL predict dialysis and graft recovery after kidney transplantation. *J Am Soc Nephrol* 21(19762491):189–197, 2010.
231. Hall IE, et al: Association between peritransplant kidney injury biomarkers and 1-year allograft outcomes. *Clin J Am Soc Nephrol* 7(8):1224–1233, 2012.
238. Han WK, et al: Kidney Injury Molecule-1 (KIM-1): a novel biomarker for human renal proximal tubule injury. *Kidney Int* 62(12081583):237–244, 2002.
250. Parikh CR, et al: Performance of kidney injury molecule-1 and liver fatty acid-binding protein and combined biomarkers of AKI after cardiac surgery. *Clin J Am Soc Nephrol* 8(7):1079–1088, 2013.
251. Han WK, et al: Urinary biomarkers in the early detection of acute kidney injury after cardiac surgery. *Clin J Am Soc Nephrol* 4(5):873–882, 2009.
255. Ko GJ, et al: Transcriptional analysis of kidneys during repair from AKI reveals possible roles for NGAL and KIM-1 as biomarkers of AKI-to-CKD transition. *Am J Physiol Renal Physiol* 298(6):F1472–F1483, 2010.
263. Susantitaphong P, et al: Performance of urinary liver-type fatty acid-binding protein in acute kidney injury: a meta-analysis. *Am J Kidney Dis* 61(3):430–439, 2013.
281. Reeves WB, Kwon O, Ramesh G: Netrin-1 and kidney injury. II. Netrin-1 is an early biomarker of acute kidney injury. *Am J Physiol Renal Physiol* 294(18234954):731–738, 2008.
291. Mishra J, et al: Neutrophil gelatinase-associated lipocalin (NGAL) as a biomarker for acute renal injury after cardiac surgery. *Lancet* 365(15811456):1231–1238, 2005.
300. Kashani K, et al: Discovery and validation of cell cycle arrest biomarkers in human acute kidney injury. *Crit Care* 17(1):R25, 2013.
305. Di Somma S, et al: Additive value of blood neutrophil gelatinase-associated lipocalin to clinical judgement in acute kidney injury diagnosis and mortality prediction in patients hospitalized from the emergency department. *Crit Care* 17(1):R29, 2013.
321. Liu KD, et al: Urine neutrophil gelatinase-associated lipocalin levels do not improve risk prediction of progressive chronic kidney disease. *Kidney Int* 83(5):909–914, 2013.
339. James M, Hemmelgarn B, Wiebe N: Glomerular filtration rate, proteinuria, and the incidence and consequences of acute kidney injury: a cohort study. *Lancet* 376(9758):2096–2103, 2010.
340. Hsu CY, Ordonez JD, Chertow GM: The risk of acute renal failure in patients with chronic kidney disease. *Kidney Int* 74(1):101–107, 2008.
394. Isakova T, et al: Fibroblast growth factor 23 and risks of mortality and end-stage renal disease in patients with chronic kidney disease. *JAMA* 305(21673295):2432–2439, 2011.
398. Scialla JJ, et al: Fibroblast growth factor-23 and cardiovascular events in CKD. *J Am Soc Nephrol* 25(2):349–360, 2014.
460. Koyner JL, Parikh CR: Clinical utility of biomarkers of AKI in cardiac surgery and critical illness. *Clin J Am Soc Nephrol* 8(6):1034–1042, 2013.

DISORDERS OF KIDNEY STRUCTURE AND FUNCTION

SECTION V

31 Acute Kidney Injury

Asif A. Sharfuddin | Steven D. Weisbord | Paul M. Palevsky | Bruce A. Molitoris

CHAPTER OUTLINE

DEFINITION OF ACUTE KIDNEY INJURY, 958
INCIDENCE OF ACUTE KIDNEY INJURY, 962
CAUSES OF ACUTE KIDNEY INJURY, 963
Prerenal Acute Kidney Injury, 963
Intrinsic Acute Kidney Injury, 964
Postrenal Acute Kidney Injury, 968
PATHOPHYSIOLOGY OF ACUTE KIDNEY INJURY, 968
Experimental Models, 968
Acute Tubular Necrosis, 969
EVALUATION OF ACUTE KIDNEY INJURY, 983
Clinical Assessment, Urinary Findings, and Blood and Radiographic Evaluation, 983
Clinical Assessment of the Patient, 983
Urine Assessment, 986
Laboratory Evaluation, 988
Novel Biomarkers of Kidney Injury, 988
Radiologic Evaluation, 989
Kidney Biopsy, 990
DIFFERENTIAL DIAGNOSIS OF ACUTE KIDNEY INJURY IN SPECIFIC CLINICAL SETTINGS, 990
Acute Kidney Injury in the Setting of Cancer, 990
Acute Kidney Injury in Pregnancy, 990
Acute Kidney Injury Following Cardiac Surgery, 992
Acute Kidney Injury after Solid Organ or Bone Marrow Transplantation, 992
Acute Kidney Injury Associated with Pulmonary Disease, 993
Acute Kidney Injury Associated with Liver Disease, 993
Acute Kidney Injury and the Nephrotic Syndrome, 994
COMPLICATIONS OF ACUTE KIDNEY INJURY, 994
Complications of Potassium Homeostasis, 995
Complications of Acid-Base Homeostasis, 995
Complications of Mineral and Uric Acid Homeostasis, 996
Volume Overload and Cardiac Complications, 996
Hematologic Complications, 996
Nutritional and Gastrointestinal Complications, 996
Infectious Complications, 996
Other Sequelae of Acute Kidney Injury, 996
Complications during Recovery from Acute Kidney Injury, 996
PREVENTION AND MANAGEMENT OF ACUTE KIDNEY INJURY, 997
Prerenal Acute Kidney Injury, 997
Intrinsic Acute Kidney Injury, 999
Postrenal Acute Kidney Injury, 1002
Nondialytic Supportive Management of Acute Kidney Injury, 1003
Renal Replacement Therapy in Acute Kidney Injury, 1004
OUTCOMES OF ACUTE KIDNEY INJURY, 1008

DEFINITION OF ACUTE KIDNEY INJURY

Acute kidney injury (AKI) is a heterogeneous syndrome defined by rapid (hours to days) decline in the glomerular filtration rate (GFR) resulting in the retention of metabolic waste products, including urea and creatinine, and dysregulation of fluid, electrolyte, and acid-base homeostasis.[1] Although often considered a discrete syndrome, AKI represents a broad constellation of pathophysiologic processes of varied severity and cause. These include decreases in GFR as the result of hemodynamic perturbations that disrupt normal renal perfusion without causing parenchymal injury; partial or complete obstruction to urinary flow; and a spectrum of processes with characteristic patterns of glomerular, interstitial, tubular, or vascular parenchymal injury. AKI precipitating events are quite often multifactorial and occur in a heterogeneous patient population (genetics, age, kidney functional status, accompanying comorbid conditions). Added to this heterogeneity are the multiple pathophysiologic processes such as necrosis, apoptosis, mesenchymal transformation, cellular infiltration, coagulation, complement activation, and the multitude of cell types and processes within the innate and adaptive immune response.

The term AKI has largely supplanted the older term acute renal failure (ARF). This change reflects recognition of serious shortcomings of the older terminology. The term *acute renal failure* suggested a dichotomous relationship between normal kidney function and overt organ failure; in contrast, the term *acute kidney injury* captures the growing body of data associating small-to-modest acute and transient decrements in kidney function with serious, adverse outcomes. While the newer terminology does emphasize the graded aspect of acute kidney disease, it should be recognized that this terminology is also imperfect. The term "injury" can be construed to imply the presence of parenchymal organ damage, which may be absent in a variety of settings associated with an acute decline in kidney function, such as early obstructive disease and prerenal azotemia associated with volume depletion. Although the term acute kidney dysfunction might better characterize the entire spectrum of the syndrome, acute kidney injury is the term that has been adopted by consensus and is now increasingly utilized in the medical literature.[2,3] In this chapter the term AKI will be used to describe the entire spectrum of the syndrome, while ARF will be restricted to situations of organ failure requiring renal replacement therapy (RRT). Although in clinical practice the term acute tubular necrosis (ATN) is often used synonymously with AKI, these terms should not be used interchangeably. While ATN is the most common form of intrinsic AKI, particularly in critically ill patients, it represents only one of multiple forms of AKI. In addition, there may be a lack of concordance between the clinical syndrome and the classic histopathologic findings of ATN.[4,5]

Decreased urine output is a cardinal (though not universal) manifestation of AKI, and patients are often classified based on urine flow rates as nonoliguric (urine output > 400 mL/day), oliguric (urine output < 400 mL/day), or anuric (urine output < 100 mL/day).[6] Transient oliguria may occur in the absence of significant decrements in kidney function, as increased tubular salt and water reabsorption is a normal physiologic response to volume depletion. In contradistinction, persistent oliguria despite the presence of adequate intravascular volume is virtually always a manifestation of AKI, with lower levels of urine output typically associated with more severe initial renal injury. The categorization of AKI based on urine volume has clinical implications for the development of volume overload, severity of electrolyte disturbances, and overall prognosis. Although oliguric AKI is associated with higher mortality risk than nonoliguric AKI, therapeutic interventions to augment urine output (see later) have not been shown to improve patient outcomes.[7]

Acute kidney injury can develop de novo in the setting of intact kidney function or can be superimposed on underlying chronic kidney disease (acute-on-chronic kidney injury). In fact, the presence of underlying impaired kidney function has been shown to be one of the most important risk factors for the development of AKI.[8,9] Multiple mechanisms may contribute to this increased susceptibility, including diminished renal functional reserve, impaired salt and water conservation predisposing to intravascular volume contraction, decreased activity of detoxification mechanisms increasing susceptibility to cytotoxic injury, impaired clearance of potential nephrotoxins increasing the risk for and/or duration of exposure, and associated macrovascular and microvascular disease increasing the risk for ischemic injury.

The causes of AKI are usually divided into three broad pathophysiologic categories:

1. Prerenal AKI—diseases characterized by effective hypoperfusion of the kidneys in which there is no parenchymal damage to the kidney (Table 31.1)
2. Intrinsic AKI—diseases involving the renal parenchyma (Table 31.2)
3. Postrenal (obstructive) AKI—diseases associated with acute obstruction of the urinary tract (Table 31.3)

While these categories are useful for didactic purposes and help inform the initial clinical assessment of patients

Table 31.1 Causes of Prerenal Acute Kidney Injury

Intravascular Volume Depletion

Hemorrhage—trauma, surgery, post partum, gastrointestinal
Gastrointestinal losses—diarrhea, vomiting, nasogastric tube loss
Renal losses—diuretics, osmotic diuresis, diabetes insipidus
Skin and mucous membrane losses—burns, hyperthermia
Nephrotic syndrome
Cirrhosis
Capillary leak

Reduced Cardiac Output

Cardiogenic shock
Pericardial diseases—restrictive/constrictive/tamponade
Congestive heart failure
Valvular diseases
Pulmonary diseases—pulmonary hypertension; pulmonary embolism
Sepsis

Systemic Vasodilation

Sepsis
Cirrhosis
Anaphylaxis
Drugs

Renal Vasoconstriction

Early sepsis
Hepatorenal syndrome
Acute hypercalcemia
Drugs—norepinephrine, vasopressin, nonsteroidals, angiotension-converting enzyme, calcineurin inhibitors
Iodinated contrast media

Increased Intraabdominal Pressure

Abdominal compartment syndrome

Table 31.2 Major Causes of Intrinsic Acute Kidney Injury

Tubular Injury

Ischemia due to hypoperfusion	Hypovolemia, sepsis, hemorrhage, cirrhosis, CHF (see Table 31.1)
Endogenous toxins	Myoglobin, hemoglobin, paraproteinemia, uric acid (see Table 31.5)
Exogenous toxins	Antibiotics, chemotherapy agents, radiocontrast media, phosphate preparations (see Table 31.5)

Tubulointerstitial Injury

Acute allergic interstitial nephritis	Nonsteroidal antiinflammatory drugs, antibiotics
Infections	Viral, bacterial, and fungal infections
Infiltration	Lymphoma, leukemia, sarcoid
Allograft rejection	

Glomerular Injury

Inflammation	Anti-GBM disease, ANCA disease, infection, cryoglobulinemia, membranoproliferative glomerulonephritis, IgA nephropathy, SLE, Henoch-Schönlein purpura, polyarteritis nodosa
Hematologic disorders	Hemolytic uremic syndrome, thrombotic thrombocytopenic purpura, drugs

Renal Microvasculature

	Malignant hypertension, toxemia of pregnancy, hypercalcemia, radiocontrast media, scleroderma, drugs

Large Vessels

Arteries	Thrombosis, vasculitis, dissection, thromboembolism, atheroembolism, trauma
Veins	Thrombosis, compression, trauma

ANCA, Antineutrophil cytoplasmic antibody; CHF, congestive heart failure; GBM, glomerular basement membrane; IgA, immunoglobulin A; SLE, systemic lupus erythematosus.

Table 31.3 Causes of Postrenal Acute Kidney Injury

Upper Urinary Tract Extrinsic Causes

Retroperitoneal space—lymph nodes, tumors
Pelvic or intraabdominal tumors—cervix, uterus, ovary, prostate
Fibrosis—radiation, drugs, inflammatory
Ureteral ligation or surgical trauma
Granulomatous diseases
Hematoma

Lower Urinary Tract Causes

Prostate—benign prostatic hypertrophy, carcinoma, infection
Bladder—neck obstruction, calculi, carcinoma, infection (schistosomiasis)
Functional—neurogenic bladder secondary to spinal cord injury, diabetes, multiple sclerosis, stroke, pharmacologic side effects of drugs (anticholinergics, antidepressants)
Urethral—posterior urethral valves, strictures, trauma, infections, tuberculosis, tumors

Upper Urinary Tract Intrinsic Causes

Nephrolithiasis
Strictures
Edema
Debris, blood clots, sloughed papillae, fungal ball
Malignancy

presenting with AKI, there is often a degree of overlap between these categories. For example, renal hypoperfusion may cause a spectrum of renal injury ranging from prerenal azotemia to overt ATN depending on its severity and duration. As a result, precise categorization of the cause of AKI in these three groups may not always be possible, and there are often transitions between etiologic categories.

A prior absence of a uniform operational definition of AKI impeded epidemiologic studies and hampered clinical evaluations of preventive and therapeutic interventions. Older literature was characterized by a plethora of definitions utilizing varying absolute and/or relative changes in the serum creatinine concentration with or without associated decrements in urine output, which made it difficult to compare findings across studies. In 2002 the Acute Dialysis Quality Initiative (ADQI) proposed the first consensus definition of AKI. The ADQI work group proposed a classification scheme with three strata based on the magnitude of increase in serum creatinine concentration and/or duration of oliguria (Table 31.4).

Conceptually, the first strata would provide the greatest sensitivity for diagnosing AKI, while the higher strata would provide increasing specificity of diagnosis. These three strata were combined with two outcome stages defined by the need for and duration of RRT resulting in the five-tiered RIFLE classification (Risk for renal dysfunction, Injury to the kidney, Failure of kidney function, and the two outcome stages, Loss of kidney function and End-stage kidney disease).[10] Subsequently, the Acute Kidney Injury Network (AKIN) modified the RIFLE classification by adding an absolute increase in serum creatinine concentration of 0.3 mg/dL or more to the 50% relative increase in the serum creatinine concentration to the definition of AKI and specifying that these increments develop over no more than 48 hours (see Table 31.4).[2] This definition has been further modified in the Kidney Disease: Improving Global Outcomes (KDIGO) Clinical Practice Guideline for Acute Kidney Injury, which clarifies that while the 0.3-mg/dL increment in serum creatinine concentration needs to occur over 48 hours, from a known baseline value, the 50% increase may occur over a longer 7-day interval.[3]

The KDIGO Clinical Practice Guideline for Acute Kidney Injury recognized a gap in the nosology of acute and chronic kidney disease.[3] Based on the definitions provided earlier, AKI has an onset of less than 7 days while chronic kidney disease (CKD) is defined by the presence of impaired kidney

Table 31.4 RIFLE, Acute Kidney Injury Network, and Kidney Disease: Improving Global Outcomes Definitions and Staging of Acute Kidney Injury

Definitions			
	RIFLE	AKIN	KDIGO
Serum creatinine level	An increase of >50% developing over <7 days	An increase of ≥0.3 mg/dL or of >50% developing over <48 hr	An increase of ≥0.3 mg/dL developing over <48 hr; or an increase of >50% developing over <7 days
Urine output*	<0.5 mL/kg/hr for >6 hr	<0.5 mL/kg/hr for >6 hr	<0.5 mL/kg/hr for >6 hr

Staging Criteria							
RIFLE	Increase in Serum Creatinine Level	AKIN	Increase in Serum Creatinine Level	KDIGO	Increase in Serum Creatinine Level	Urine Output*	
Risk	≥50%	Stage 1	≥0.3 mg/dL; or ≥50%	Stage 1	≥0.3 mg/dL; or ≥50%	<0.5 mL/kg/hr for >6 hr	
Injury	≥100%	Stage 2	≥100%	Stage 2	≥100%	<0.5 mL/kg/hr for >12 hr	
Failure	≥200%	Stage 3	≥200%	Stage 3	≥200%	<0.5 mL/kg/hr for >24 hr or anuria for >12 hr	
Loss	Need for renal replacement therapy for >4 wk						
End-stage	Need for renal replacement therapy for >3 mo						

*The urine output criteria for both definition and staging of acute kidney injury are the same for the RIFLE, AKIN, and KDIGO criteria.
AKIN, Acute Kidney Injury Network; KDIGO, Kidney Disease: Improving Global Outcomes; RIFLE, Risk, Injury, Failure, Loss and End-stage kidney disease.

function or structural kidney damage with implications for health present for more than 3 months.[11] Recognizing that some patients develop kidney disease with a more subacute onset than that of AKI but of less than 3 months' duration, the KDIGO Acute Kidney Injury Workgroup proposed the concept of acute kidney disease, defined as AKI or a reduction in GFR to less than 60 mL/min/1.73 m², a decrease in GFR by 35% or more, an increase in serum creatinine concentration by more than 50%, or the presence of structural kidney damage of less than 3 months' duration.

Several limitations to these criteria for diagnosis and staging of AKI have been recognized.[12,13] First, while validation studies have demonstrated that AKI stage correlates with increasing mortality risk, it is not clear that this is the appropriate metric for assessing their validity. Second, there is poor correlation between AKI stage and GFR. Since the magnitude of change in serum creatinine concentration is time dependent, a patient may demonstrate progression over time from less severe (RIFLE-R or AKIN or KDIGO stage 1) to more severe AKI stage (RIFLE-F or AKIN or KDIGO stage 3) despite an improving GFR. Third, the definition of AKI by serum creatinine criteria relies on a referent baseline serum creatinine level, which is often unavailable. Furthermore, variations in specifications for this referent value (e.g., admission serum creatinine concentration versus most recent outpatient serum creatinine concentration before admission versus other definitions) can alter the classification of patients.[14] Fourth, both RIFLE and AKIN employ relative changes in serum creatinine concentration to stage AKI. Analyses of creatinine kinetics demonstrate that the time required to attain a fixed percentage change in serum creatinine concentration in the setting of severe AKI is dependent upon the baseline level of kidney function, while the initial rate of change in serum creatinine concentration is relatively independent of kidney function.[12] Thus, early in the course of AKI, absolute changes in serum creatinine concentration may be detected more readily than relative changes. Fifth, concordance between the serum creatinine and urine output criterion is poor, even with regard to mortality risk.[15] Transient changes in urine output may reflect variation in volume status or the administration of medications and do not necessarily correlate with other parameters of kidney function. Finally, it must be remembered that these classification systems are independent of the various causes of AKI (i.e., prerenal, intrinsic, obstructive). Despite these shortcomings, the use of standardized classification schemes has enhanced and will enhance further the interpretation of epidemiologic studies and design of clinical trials.

Conceptually, AKI comprises a spectrum of structural and functional kidney disease in which there may be an evolution from injury to organ dysfunction and finally overt organ failure (Figure 31.1). Reliance solely on changes in serum creatinine concentration and/or urine output to diagnose AKI has resulted in the inability to identify the incipient stages of intrinsic kidney damage, which may be the most opportune time for pharmacologic intervention.[16] In order to facilitate the early diagnosis of intrinsic injury, multiple biomarkers of tubular injury have been evaluated.[17-22] Biomarkers for AKI include N-acetyl-β-D-glucosaminidase,

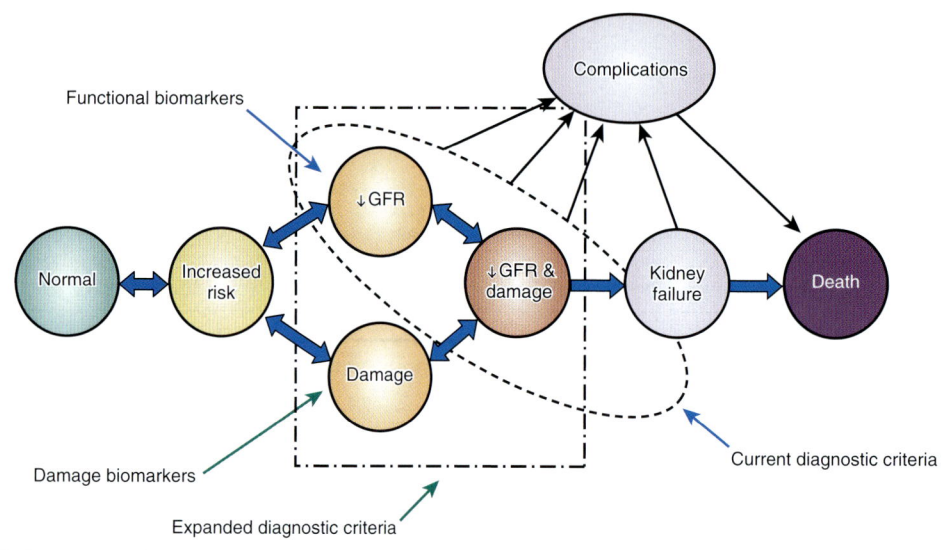

Figure 31.1 Modified conceptual model of acute kidney injury. The availability of specific biomarkers permits recognition of kidney damage separately from changes in kidney function. Kidney damage and changes in function may precede each other or occur concurrently. The time sequence of events depends on the nature and duration of the insult and the underlying state of health of the kidney. The timing of diagnosis will depend on the frequency with which specific biomarkers of kidney damage and function are assessed. GFR, Glomerular filtration rate. (From Murray PT, et al: Potential use of biomarkers in acute kidney injury: report and summary of recommendations from the 10th Acute Dialysis Quality Initiative consensus conference. Kidney Int 85:513-521, 2014.)

kidney injury molecule-1 (KIM-1), neutrophil gelatinase–associated lipocalin (NGAL), interleukin (IL)-18, liver-type fatty acid–binding protein (L-FABP), tissue inhibitor of metalloproteinase 2 (TIMP-2) and insulin-like growth factor–binding protein-7 (IGFBP-7), among others.[17-22] In addition, serum cystatin C level has been proposed as more sensitive (and in some settings more specific) than serum creatinine concentration for detecting changes in GFR, and urinary cystatin C level has been proposed as a marker of tubular injury.[17,23,24] While none of these biomarkers has yet been adequately validated for routine clinical use, they have the potential to provide an earlier diagnosis of intrinsic AKI than serum creatinine concentration, to differentiate volume-responsive (prerenal) AKI from intrinsic disease, to diminish confounding related to creatinine generation, and to provide prognostic information regarding the clinical course of an episode of AKI. One or more of these biomarkers may provide a means by which patients could be identified at the incipient stage of AKI in order to guide the implementation of specific therapy to ameliorate kidney damage or promote recovery of kidney function.

INCIDENCE OF ACUTE KIDNEY INJURY

Estimates of the incidence of AKI are highly dependent on the case definition used, with rates among hospitalized patients ranging from as high as 44% when defined based on a change in serum creatinine concentration of at least 0.3 mg/dL to as low as 1% using an increase in serum creatinine of at least 2.0 mg/dL.[25-28] Approximately 3% to 7% of hospitalized patients and 25% to 30% of intensive care unit (ICU) patients develop AKI, with 5% to 6% of the ICU population requiring RRT after developing AKI.[25-28] In a single-center analysis conducted in 1996 at an urban tertiary care hospital, AKI, defined as an increase in serum creatinine concentration of 0.5 mg/dL for patients with a baseline serum creatinine concentration of 1.9 mg/dL or less, of 1.0 mg/dL for patients with a baseline serum creatinine concentration of 2.0 to 4.9 mg/dL, and 1.5 mg/dL for patients with a baseline serum creatinine concentration greater than 5 mg/dL, developed in 7.2% of 4622 consecutive patients.[25] The overall incidence of AKI is approximately 21.6% for all hospitalized adults worldwide,[29] with known associations for accelerating CKD to end-stage kidney disease (ESKD).[30-32] This rate was higher than the 4.9% rate the investigators had observed in a similar study in 1979.[33] The most frequent cause of AKI was decreased renal perfusion, observed in 39% of episodes, followed by medication-associated AKI (16%), radiocontrast media–induced AKI (11%), postoperative AKI (9%), and sepsis-associated AKI (6.5%). Overall mortality was 19.4%, with higher mortality rates associated with larger maximal increments in serum creatinine concentration.

Although definition is less of an issue with regard to rates of AKI requiring RRT, reported rates vary considerably because of differences in characteristics of patient populations and variability in criteria for the initiation of RRT. In a multinational, multicenter observational study of 29,269 critically ill patients, 5.7% developed severe AKI and 4.3% received RRT.[34]

Many epidemiologic studies of AKI have relied on data from large administrative databases. Such data need to be interpreted with caution, however, as administrative coding for AKI is incomplete and may only capture 20% to 30% of all episodes of AKI.[35,36] Ascertainment of AKI requiring RRT using administrative data is substantially more complete. In an analysis of data from the National Hospital Discharge Survey in the United States, the Centers for Disease Control and Prevention observed an increase in hospital discharges with a diagnosis of AKI from 18 per 100,000 population in 1980 to 365 per 100,000 in 2005.[37] Similar trends have been observed in analyses of the U.S. National (Nationwide) Inpatient Sample (NIS) and a 5% sample of U.S. hospitalized Medicare beneficiaries. In an analysis that combined administrative and clinical data from a single integrated health care delivery system, the incidence of AKI that did not require the use of RRT increased from 322.7 to 522.4 cases per 100,000 person-years from 1996 to 2003.[38] Over the same period, AKI requiring RRT increased from 19.5 to 29.5 cases per 100,000 person-years.[38] AKI was more common among men and in older adults. In a more recent analysis using data from the NIS, a nationally representative administrative database of hospitalizations, the incidence of AKI requiring dialysis increased from 222 cases per million person-years in 2000 to 533 cases per million person-years in 2009 with the largest rise in incidence occurring in patients 65 to 74 years of age and 75 years of age or older.[39] While a portion of these temporal trends may be attributable to earlier initiation of dialysis and more frequent utilization of RRT in older patients, these changes are unlikely to account for the majority of the increase in incidence of severe AKI.

Preexisting kidney disease is one of the major risk factors for the development of AKI requiring dialysis.[40] Higher levels of risk are associated with more severe baseline CKD. Compared to patients with baseline estimated GFR (eGFR) above 60 mL/min/1.73 m^2, patients with eGFR values of 45 to 59 mL/min/1.73 m^2 have a nearly twofold increased risk for developing dialysis-requiring AKI. This risk increases to more than 40-fold among patients with baseline eGFR values of less than 15 mL/min/1.73 m^2.[40] Underlying diabetes mellitus, hypertension, and the presence of proteinuria are also associated with increased risk for hospital-acquired AKI.

CAUSES OF ACUTE KIDNEY INJURY

Although in the clinical setting AKI is often multifactorial, the cause should most often be evaluated based on the three major pathophysiologic categories, namely, prerenal, intrinsic, and postrenal (obstructive).

PRERENAL ACUTE KIDNEY INJURY

Prerenal azotemia is the most common cause of AKI, accounting for approximately 40% to 55% of all cases.[25,27,41] It results from kidney hypoperfusion due to reductions in actual or effective arterial blood volume (EABV; the volume of blood effectively perfusing the body organs). Common conditions causing true hypovolemia include hemorrhage (traumatic, gastrointestinal, surgical), gastroinrestnal (GI) losses (vomiting, diarrhea, nasogastric suction), renal losses (overdiuresis, diabetes insipidus), and third spacing (pancreatitis, hypoalbuminemia). In addition, cardiogenic shock, septic shock, cirrhosis, hypoalbuminemia, and anaphylaxis all are pathophysiologic conditions that decrease EABV, independent of total body volume status, resulting in reduced renal blood flow. Prerenal azotemia reverses rapidly if renal perfusion is restored because by definition the integrity of the renal parenchyma has remained intact. However, severe and prolonged hypoperfusion may result in tissue ischemia leading to ATN. Therefore prerenal azotemia and ischemic ATN are part of a continual spectrum of manifestations of renal hypoperfusion.

Prerenal azotemia has also been divided into volume responsive and volume nonresponsive. The former is easy to comprehend, while the latter is less straightforward. In volume nonresponsive forms, additional intravenous volume is of no help in restoring kidney perfusion and function. Disease processes such as congestive heart failure, liver failure, and sepsis may not respond to intravenous fluids as markedly reduced cardiac output or total vascular resistance, respectively, prevent improved kidney function (see Table 31.1).

True or effective hypovolemia causes a decrease in mean arterial pressure that activates baroreceptors and initiates a cascade of neural and humoral responses, leading to activation of the sympathetic nervous system and increasing production of catecholamines, especially norepinephrine. There is increased release of antidiuretic hormone mediated primarily by hypovolemia, resulting in vasoconstriction, water retention, and urea back diffusion into the papillary interstitium. In response to volume depletion or states of decreased EABV, there is increased intrarenal angiotensin II (Ang II) activity via activation of the renin angiotensin aldosterone system (RAAS). Ang II is a very potent vasoconstrictor, which preferentially increases efferent arteriolar resistance, preserving GFR in the setting of decreased renal perfusion through maintenance of glomerular hydrostatic pressure. In addition, Ang II increases proximal tubular sodium absorption through a combination of alterations in hydrostatic forces in the peritubular capillaries and through direct activation of sodium-hydrogen exchangers. During severe volume depletion, Ang II activity is even greater, leading to afferent arteriolar constriction that reduces renal plasma flow, GFR, and the filtration fraction and markedly augments proximal tubular sodium reabsorption in an effort to restore plasma volume.[42] Ang II has also been shown to have direct effects on transport in the proximal tubule through receptors located in the proximal tubule. It has also been postulated that the proximal tubule can locally produce Ang II. Hence, under conditions of volume depletion, the Ang II stimulates a larger fraction of the transport, whereas volume expansion will blunt this response.[43-47]

Renal sympathetic nerve activity is significantly increased in prerenal azotemia. Studies have shown that in the setting of hypovolemia, adrenergic activity independently constricts the afferent arteriole, as well as changing the efferent arteriolar resistance through Ang II. α-Adrenergic activity primarily influences kidney vascular resistance, whereas renal nerve activity is linked to renin release through β-adrenergic receptors on renin-containing cells. In contrast, α$_2$-adrenergic agonists primarily decrease the glomerular ultrafiltration coefficient via Ang II. Although vasodilation might be expected as a result of acute removal of adrenergic activity, a transient increase in Ang II is actually seen, maintaining GFR and renal blood flow. Even after subacute renal denervation, renal vascular sensitivity increased to Ang II as a result of major upregulation of Ang II receptors. Hence complex effects on renin-angiotensin activity occur within the kidney secondary to increased renal adrenergic activity during prerenal azotemia.[48]

All of these systems work together and stimulate vasoconstriction in musculocutaneous and splanchnic circulations, inhibit salt loss through sweat, and stimulate thirst, thereby causing retention of salt and water to maintain blood pressure and preserve cardiac output and cerebral perfusion. Concomitantly, there are various compensatory mechanisms to preserve glomerular perfusion.[49] Autoregulation is achieved by stretch receptors in afferent arterioles that cause vasodilation in response to reduced perfusion pressure. Under physiologic conditions autoregulation works until a mean systemic arterial blood pressure of 75 to 80 mm Hg. Below this level, the glomerular ultrafiltration pressure and GFR decline abruptly. Renal production of prostaglandins, kallikrein, and kinins, as well as nitric oxide (NO), is increased, contributing to the vasodilation.[50,51] Nonsteroidal antiinflammatory drugs (NSAIDs), by inhibiting prostaglandin production, worsen kidney perfusion in patients with hypoperfusion. Selective efferent arteriolar constriction, a result of Ang II, helps preserve the intraglomerular pressure and hence GFR. Angiotensin-converting enzyme (ACE) inhibitors inhibit synthesis of Ang II and so disturb this delicate balance in patients with severe reductions in EABV such as severe congestive heart failure or bilateral renal artery stenosis and thus can worsen prerenal azotemia. On the other hand, very high levels of Ang II, as seen in circulatory shock, cause constriction of both afferent and efferent arterioles, negating its protective effect.

Although these compensatory mechanisms minimize the progression toward AKI, they too are overcome in states of severe hypoperfusion. Renovascular disease, hypertensive nephrosclerosis, diabetic nephropathy, and older age predispose patients to prerenal azotemia[52] at lesser degrees of hypotension.[52] Prerenal azotemia also predisposes patients to radiocontrast media–induced AKI, and events such as anesthesia and surgery that are known to result in further decreases in renal blood flow. Therefore it is imperative to diagnose prerenal azotemia promptly and initiate effective treatment because it is a potentially reversible condition that can lead to ischemic ATN and/or nephrotoxic AKI if therapy is delayed or the severity of the condition increases. In patients with advanced liver disease and portal hypertension, the hepatorenal syndrome (HRS) represents an extreme form of prerenal disease, characterized by peripheral and splanchnic vasodilation with intense intrarenal vasoconstriction unresponsive to volume resuscitation.[53-55] AKI can also result from abdominal compartment syndrome (ACS), characterized by marked elevation in intraabdominal pressure resulting in a clinical presentation with features similar to those of prerenal AKI.[56,57]

INTRINSIC ACUTE KIDNEY INJURY

DISEASES OF LARGE VESSELS AND MICROVASCULATURE

Total occlusion of the renal artery or vein is an uncommon event but can be seen in certain scenarios such as trauma, instrumentation, thromboemboli, thrombosis, and dissection of an aortic aneurysm. Stenosis of the renal artery is a slow, chronic process with or without evidence of declining GFR and rarely presents as an acute event. Renal vein thrombosis has classically and frequently been associated with hypercoagulable states such as nephrotic syndrome, particularly when associated with membranous nephropathy. An atheroembolic source should be considered in patients who present with AKI after instrumentation with angiography, arteriography, or aortic surgery or after blunt trauma or acceleration-deceleration injury.[58] Cholesterol-laden atheroembolic plaques in the aorta or other larger arteries may become disrupted, and fragments may become trapped in smaller renal arteries, leading to hypoperfusion and an intense inflammatory reaction, akin to a vasculitis. Other organs may also be affected leading to gastrointestinal ischemia, peripheral gangrene, livedo reticularis, and acute pancreatitis. Patients frequently develop fevers and exhibit eosinophilia, elevated erythrocyte sedimentation rate, and hypocomplementemia, which sometimes help in differentiating this condition from other simultaneous insults (e.g., radiocontrast media administration).

Renal artery thrombosis is usually a posttraumatic or postsurgical complication, especially in the transplant setting, but can also occur in other hypercoagulable states such as antiphospholipid antibody syndrome.[59-61] Diseases affecting the small vessels generally termed vasculitides include polyarteritis nodosa, necrotizing granulomatous vasculitis, hemolytic uremic syndrome, thrombotic thrombocytopenic purpura, and malignant hypertension; they usually tend to occlude the vessels by fibrin deposition along with platelets. Endothelial cell damage leads to an inflammatory response in the renal microvasculature (and in other organs), leading to reduced microvascular blood flow and tissue ischemia, giving rise to superimposed ATN. One should keep in mind the intricate relationship between these inflammatory vasculitides and subsequent ischemic injury, as even though the origin of these disease processes is located at a site distant from the tubules, the final result is quite often ATN if not treated early. Hence virtually any disease that compromises blood flow within the renal microvasculature can induce AKI (see Table 31.2).

DISEASES OF THE TUBULOINTERSTITIUM

Ischemic and septic ATN are the most common causes of intrinsic AKI. These are discussed extensively in later sections of the chapter on ATN. Other disorders of the tubulointerstitium causing AKI, such as acute allergic interstitial nephritis, drug-induced tubular toxicity, and endogenous toxins, are presented in the sections that follow.

Interstitial Disease

Acute interstitial nephritis (AIN) results from an idiosyncratic allergic response to different pharmacologic agents, most commonly to antibiotics (e.g., methicillin and other penicillins, cephalosporins, sulfonamides, and quinolones) or NSAIDs (e.g., ibuprofen).[62] Other conditions such as leukemia, lymphoma, sarcoidosis, bacterial infections (e.g., *Escherichia coli*), and viral infections (e.g., cytomegalovirus) can also cause AIN leading to AKI. Systemic allergic signs such as fever, rash, and eosinophilia are often present in antibiotic-associated AIN but not usually present in NSAID-related AIN, where lymphocytes tend to predominate.[63] The presence of inflammatory infiltrates within the interstitium is the key hallmark of AIN. These inflammatory infiltrates are often patchy and present most commonly in the deep cortex and outer medulla. Interstitial edema is typically seen with the infiltrates, and sometimes patchy tubular necrosis may be present in close proximity to areas with extensive inflammatory infiltrates.[62] The majority of cases of AIN are probably induced by extrarenal antigens being produced by drugs or infectious agents that may be able to induce AIN by (1) binding to kidney structures, (2) modifying immunogenetics of native renal proteins, (3) mimicking renal antigens, or (4) precipitating as immune complexes and hence serving as the site of antibody- or cellular-mediated injury.[64] This reaction is triggered by many events, including activation of complements and release of inflammatory cytokines by T cells and phagocytes. Acute allograft rejection in the transplant recipient is by far the most common immunologic cause of AIN.

Tubular Disease—Exogenous Nephrotoxins

Nephrotoxic ATN is the second most common cause of intrinsic AKI. We shall briefly review the common drug nephrotoxicities in the context of AKI (Table 31.5). The kidneys are vulnerable to toxicity due to the high blood flow, and they are the major elimination/metabolizing route of many of these elements. Furthermore, concentration of drugs within the tubular lumen and the interstitium leads to a more intense level of exposure.

Radiocontrast Media–Induced Nephropathy. Iodinated radiocontrast medium–induced nephropathy (CIN) is a common complication of radiologic or angiographic procedures. The incidence varies from 3% to 7% in patients without any risk factors but can be as high as 50% in patients with moderate to advanced CKD. Other risk factors include diabetes mellitus, intravascular volume depletion, use of high-osmolality contrast media, advanced age, proteinuria, and anemia.[65,66] Unlike many other forms of intrinsic tubular injury, radiocontrast media–induced AKI is usually associated with urinary sodium retention and a fractional excretion of sodium (FE_{Na}) of less than 1%. AKI resulting from iodinated contrast media is typically nonoliguric and rarely requires dialysis. However, requirement for renal support, prolonged hospitalization, and increased mortality are associated with this condition.

The pathophysiology of CIN likely consists of combined hypoxic and toxic renal tubular damage associated with renal endothelial dysfunction and altered microcirculation.[67,68] The administration of radiocontrast media mediates vasoconstriction and markedly affects renal parenchymal oxygenation, especially in the outer medulla, as documented in various studies where the cortical PO_2 declined from 40 to 25 mm Hg, while the medullary PO_2 fell from 26 to 30 mm Hg to 9 to 15 mm Hg.[68-70] Radiocontrast media injection leads to an abrupt but transient increase in renal plasma flow, GFR, and urinary output.[71] This effect is due to the hyperosmolar radiocontrast medium enhancing solute delivery to the distal nephron and leads to increased oxygen consumption by enhanced tubular sodium reabsorption. Using video microscopy, it has also been documented that radiocontrast media markedly reduce inner medullary papillary blood flow, even to the extent of near cessation of red blood cell (RBC) movement in papillary vessels, associated with RBC aggregation within the papillary vasa recta.[72] However, it should be noted that there may be different patterns of response possibly related to the type, volume, and route of radiocontrast media administration. Numerous neurohumoral mediators may contribute to the changes in renal microcirculation caused by radiocontrast media injection. Intrarenal NO synthase activity, NO concentration, plasma endothelin, adenosine, prostaglandins, and vasopressin are all thought to play a role in altering the cortical and medullary microcirculation after radiocontrast media injection. Mechanical factors may also play a role as radiocontrast media increase blood viscosity and may affect the flow in the complex low-pressure medullary microcirculation.[70] An increased plasma viscosity after radiocontrast media administration can interfere with blood flow, particularly under the hypertonic conditions of the (inner) renal medulla, where the plasma viscosity is already

Table 31.5 Major Causes of Endogenous and Exogenous Toxins Causing Acute Tubular Injury

Endogenous Toxins	Exogenous Toxins
Myoglobulinuria	**Antibiotics**
Muscle breakdown—trauma, compression, electric shock, hypothermia, hyperthermia, seizures, exercise, burns	Aminoglycosides
	Amphotericin B
	Antiviral agents—acyclovir, cidofovir, indinavir, foscarnet, tenofovir
Metabolic—hypokalemia, hypophosphatemia,	Pentamidine
Infections—tetanus, influenza	Vancomycin
Toxins—isopropyl alcohol, ethanol, ethylene glycol, toluene, snake and insect bites, cocaine, heroin	**Chemotherapy**
	Cisplatin
	Ifosfamide
Drugs—HMG-CoA reductase inhibitors (statins), amphetamines, fibrates	Plicamycin
	5-Fluorouracil
	Cytarabine
Inherited disease—deficiency of myophosphorylase, phosphofructokinase, carnitine palmitoyltransferase	6-Thioguanine
	Methotrexate
	Calcineurin Inhibitors
Autoimmune—polymyositis, dermatomyositis	Cyclosporine
	Tacrolimus
Hemoglobinuria	**Organic Solvents**
Mechanical—prosthetic valves, microangiopathic hemolytic anemia, extracorporeal circulation	Toluene
	Ethylene glycol
	Poisons
Drugs—hydralazine, methyldopa	Snake venom
Chemicals—benzene, arsine, fava beans, glycerol, phenol	Paraquat
Immunologic—transfusion reaction	**Miscellaneous**
Genetic—G6PD deficiency, PNH	Radiocontrast media
Intratubular Obstruction from Crystalluria or Paraproteins	Intravenous immune globulin
Tumor lysis syndrome	Nonsteroidal antiinflammatory drugs
HGPT deficiency	Oral phosphate bowel preparations
Multiple Myeloma	
Oxalate (ethylene glycol)	

G6PD, Glucose-6-phosphate dehydrogenase; HGPRT, hypoxanthine-guanine phosphoribosyltransferase; HMG-CoA, 3-hydroxy-3-methylglutaryl–coenzyme A; PNH, paroxysmal nocturnal hemoglobinuria.

increased as a result of hemoconcentration. Indeed, there are several animal studies that have shown a correlation between experimental CIN and viscosity of the radiopaque compound.[73,74]

Evidence also suggests direct tubular toxicity from radiocontrast media. Early studies on isolated renal tubules in vitro have shown direct toxic effects of radiocontrast media on proximal tubular cells (PTCs).[75] Radiocontrast media (diatrizoate, iopamidol) induced a decline in tubule K^+, adenosine triphosphate (ATP), and total adenine nucleotide contents. At the same time, there was a decrease in the respiratory rate of the tubules and an increase in Ca^{2+} content. These changes were more pronounced with the very high-osmolality ionic compound diatrizoate than with the lower osmolality nonionic iopamidol. Importantly, the cytotoxic effects were aggravated by hypoxia, indicating interactions between direct cellular mechanisms and vasoconstriction-mediated hypoxia.[76] Andersen and coworkers have demonstrated the concentration-dependent radiocontrast media–mediated release of tubular marker enzymes, ultrastructural changes, and cell death in both Madin-Darby canine kidney (MDCK) and LLC-PK$_1$ cells.[77] Radiocontrast media–induced critical medullary hypoxia may lead to the formation of reactive oxygen species (ROS) with subsequent membrane and DNA damage. A vicious cycle of hypoxia, free radical formation, and further hypoxic injury may be activated after radiocontrast media exposure. Clinically, CIN presents with an acute decline in GFR within 24 to 48 hours of administration, with a peak serum creatinine concentration usually occurring in 3 to 5 days and return to baseline within 1 week, although patients with moderate to advanced CKD may take somewhat longer to return to baseline serum creatinine concentration. Existing CKD, diabetic nephropathy, advanced age, congestive heart failure, volume depletion, and coincident use of NSAIDs increase the risk for CIN. Although numerous agents have been shown to be protective in the experimental setting, only volume expansion with isotonic crystalloid is of proven clinical benefit with possible benefits associated with use of bicarbonate-containing fluids and administration of N-acetylcysteine (NAC). The renoprotective effects of NAC may be related to enhanced NO-dependent vasodilation and medullary oxygenation in addition to scavenging of free radicals.[67]

Aminoglycoside Nephrotoxicity. The nephrotoxicity of aminoglycosides has best been characterized for gentamicin, a polar drug, excreted by glomerular filtration. It is thought that cationic amino groups (NH_3^+) on the drug bind to anionic phospholipid residues on the brush border of proximal tubular cells and are then internalized by endocytosis. Although the precise subcellular mechanisms of the toxicity of aminoglycosides have not been fully elucidated, binding at the apical surface of proximal tubular cells is known to involve megalin.[78,79] A three-dimensional model has recently described the complex between megalin and gentamicin. Gentamicin binds to megalin with low affinity and exploits the common ligand-binding motif previously described utilizing the indole side chain of amino acids Trp-1126 and the negatively charged residues of Asp-1129, Asp-1131, and Asp-1133.[80] Once endocytosed, aminoglycosides inhibit endosomal fusion. They are also directly trafficked to the Golgi apparatus and, through retrograde movement, to the endoplasmic reticulum (ER). From the ER, gentamicin moves into the cytosol in a size- and charge-dependent manner.[81] Once in the cytosol, either from the ER[81] or via lysosomal rupture, aminoglycosides distribute to various intracellular organelles and mediate organelle-specific toxicity such as mitochondrial dysfunction.[81,82] Also, delivery to the ER via retrograde transport from the Golgi apparatus allows for binding of aminoglycosides to the 16S rRNA subunit,[83] resulting in a reduction of protein synthesis. The number of cationic groups on the molecules determines the facility with which these drugs are transported across the cell membrane and are an important determinant of toxicity.[84,85] Neomycin is associated with the most nephrotoxicity; gentamicin, tobramycin, and amikacin are intermediate, and streptomycin is the least nephrotoxic. Risk factors for aminoglycoside nephrotoxicity include the use of high or repeated doses or prolonged therapy, CKD, volume depletion, diabetes, advanced age, and the coexistence of renal ischemia or other nephrotoxins[86-88] (Figure 31.2).

Cisplatin Nephrotoxicity. Cisplatin (cis-platinum), a platinum-based compound widely used for chemotherapy, is commonly associated with nephrotoxicity. The pathophysiologic mechanism of cisplatin-induced tubular damage is complex and involves a number of interconnected factors, such as accumulation of cisplatin mediated by membrane transportation, conversion into nephrotoxins, DNA damage, mitochondrial dysfunction, oxidative stress, inflammatory response, activation of signal transducers and intracellular messengers, and activation of apoptotic pathways. The S3 segment of the proximal tubule in the corticomedullary region is the most common site of cisplatin nephrotoxicity in rats. More distal sites may be affected in humans, but glomeruli remain unaffected. Cisplatin causes a decrease in kidney function in a dose-dependant fashion and is usually reversible after cessation of the drug[89] (Table 31.6; see Table 31.5)

Acute Phosphate Nephropathy. AKI has been described as a complication following the administration of oral sodium phosphate solution as a bowel cathartic in preparation for colonoscopy and bowel surgery.[90-92] While the mechanism linking oral sodium phosphate administration with AKI remains incompletely understood, the pathogenesis likely relates to a transient and significant rise in serum phosphate concentration that occurs simultaneously with intravascular volume depletion.

When the urine is oversaturated and buffering factors such as pH, citrate, and pyrophosphate are overwhelmed, renal phosphorus excretion becomes compromised. This may lead to intratubular precipitation of calcium phosphate salts that obstruct the tubular lumen and cause direct tubular damage. ROS generated by binding of calcium phosphate crystals further promote tubular damage. Risk factors for acute phosphate nephropathy include preexisting volume depletion, the use of ACE inhibitors and angiotensin receptor blockers (ARBs), NSAIDs, CKD, older age, female sex, and higher dose of oral sodium phosphate.[91,92] Patients who develop acute phosphate nephropathy typically present with elevated serum creatinine concentrations days to months following the administration of oral sodium

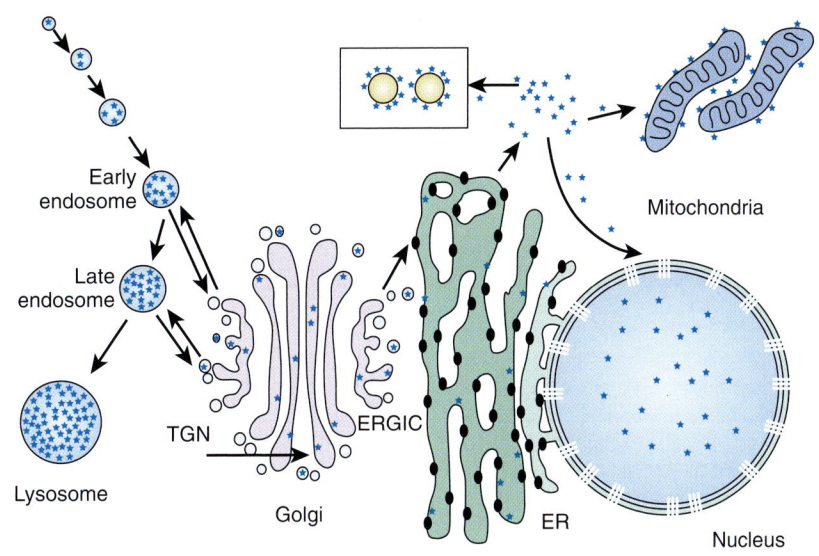

Figure 31.2 **Retrograde trafficking of gentamicin along the endocytic pathway in LLC-PK cells.** Internalization occurs via receptor-mediated endocytosis with approximately 90% of the internalized material accumulating within lysosomes. However approximately 10% is shuttled to the Golgi complex and is transported past the endoplasmic reticulum (ER)-Golgi intermediate compartment (ERGIC) to the ER. From there, translocation to the cytosol occurs. Once in the cytosol, association with various organelles such as the mitochondrial membranes and nuclei can initiate an additional cascade of events leading to renal proximal tubular injury. TGN, Trans-Golgi network. (From Sandoval RM, Molitoris BA: Gentamicin traffics retrograde through the secretory pathway and is released in the cytosol via the endoplasmic reticulum. *Am J Physiol Renal Physiol* 286:F617-F624, 2004.)

solution and can experience progression to chronic and end-stage kidney disease.

Tubular Disease—Endogenous Nephrotoxins

Myoglobin and hemoglobin are the endogenous toxins most commonly associated with ATN. Myoglobin, a 17.8-kDa heme protein released during muscle injury, is freely filtered and causes red-brown urine with a dipstick result positive for heme, in the absence of RBCs in the urine. Intravascular hemolysis results in circulating free hemoglobin, which when excessive is filtered, resulting in hemoglobinuria, hemoglobin-cast formation, and heme uptake by proximal tubular cells. The renal injury is due to a combination of factors, including volume depletion, renal vasoconstriction, direct heme protein–mediated cytotoxicity, and intraluminal cast formation. The heme center of myoglobin may directly induce lipid peroxidation and liberation of free iron. Iron is an intermediate accelerator in the generation of free radicals. Evidence suggests there is increased formation of H_2O_2 in rat kidney models of myohemoglobinuria.[93] The subsequent hydroxyl (OH^-) radical plays a vital role in oxidative stress–induced AKI through mechanisms discussed in detail later in the chapter. Various iron chelators such as deferoxamine and other scavengers of ROS such as glutathione have been shown to provide protection against myohemoglobinuric AKI.[94] Similarly, endothelin antagonists have also been shown to prevent hypofiltration and proteinuria in rats that underwent glycerol-induced rhabdomyolysis.[95] In addition, NO supplementation may be beneficial by preventing the heme-induced renal vasoconstriction, as heme proteins scavenge NO.[96,97] Finally, precipitation of myoglobin with Tamm-Horsfall protein and shed proximal tubular cells leads to cast formation and tubular obstruction, which is enhanced in acidic urine.[98] In human studies, volume expansion and perhaps alkalization of urine to limit cast formation are the preventive measures generally employed as none of the experimental agents used in animal studies has been convincingly beneficial. This emphasizes the multifactorial nature of these conditions. It is unlikely a single agent will be beneficial in this setting.[99]

Other endogenous nephrotoxins include uric acid and immunoglobulin light chains. Excessive immunoglobulin light chains, produced in diseases such as multiple myeloma, are filtered, absorbed, and then catabolized in proximal tubular cells. The concentration of light chains leaving the proximal portion of the nephron depends on both the concentration of light chains in the glomerular filtrate and the capacity of the proximal tubule to reabsorb and catabolize them. Certain light chains can be directly toxic to the proximal tubules themselves.[100] Light chain–induced cytokine release has been associated with nuclear translocation of nuclear factor κ light-chain enhancer of activated B cells (NF-κB), suggesting that light-chain endocytosis leads to production of inflammatory cytokines through activation of NF-κB.[101] Once the capacity for proximal tubule uptake is overwhelmed, a light-chain load is presented to the distal tubule, where, upon reaching a critical concentration, the light chains aggregate and coprecipitate with Tamm-Horsfall protein and form characteristic light-chain casts.[102] Recent studies have also shown that light chains, in the amount seen in plasma cell dyscrasia patients, are capable of catalyzing the formation of hydrogen peroxide in cultured HK-2 cells. Hydrogen peroxide stimulates the production of monocyte chemoattractant protein-1 (MCP-1), a key chemokine involved in monocytes/macrophage recruitment to proximal tubular cells.[103] Any process reducing GFR, such as volume depletion, hypercalcemia, or NSAIDs, will accelerate and aggravate light-chain cast formation. It has been proposed that acutely reducing the presented light-chain load by plasmapheresis or dialysis using high-cutoff

Table 31.6 Classification of Various Common Drugs Based on Pathophysiologic Categories of Acute Kidney Disease

1. Vasoconstriction/Impaired Microvasculature Hemodynamics (Prerenal)

NSAIDs, ACE inhibitors, angiotensin receptor blockers, norepinephrine, tacrolimus, cyclosporine, diuretics, cocaine, mitomycin C, estrogen, quinine, interleukin-2, COX-2 inhibitors

2. Tubular Cell Toxicity

Antibiotics—aminoglycosides, amphotericin B, vancomycin, rifampicin, foscarnet, pentamidine, cephaloridine, cephalothin
Radiocontrast media, NSAIDs, acetaminophen, cyclosporine, cisplatin, mannitol, heavy metals, IVIG, ifosfamide, tenofovir

3. Acute Interstitial Nephritis

Antibiotics—penicillins, cephalosporins, sulfonamides, quinolones, rifampicin, vancomycin
NSAIDs (aspirin, fenoprofen, naproxen, piroxicam, phenylbutazone), thiazide diuretics, phenytoin, furosemide, allopurinol, cimetidine, omeprazole

4. Tubular Lumen Obstruction

Sulfonamides, acyclovir, cidofovir, methotrexate, triamterene, methoxyflurane, protease inhibitors, ethylene glycol, indinavir, oral sodium phosphate bowel preparations

5. Thrombotic Microangiopathy

Clopidogrel, cocaine, ticlopidine, cyclosporine, tacrolimus, mitomycin C, oral contraceptives, gemcitabine, bevacizumab

6. Osmotic Nephrosis

IVIG, mannitol, dextrans, hydroxyethyl starch

ACE, Angiotensin-converting enzyme; COX-2, cyclo-oxygenase-2; IVIG, intravenous immune globulin; NSAID, nonsteroidal antiinflammatory drug.

---

membranes might be beneficial in limiting cast formation and reducing the extent of the AKI in certain select patients, allowing for initiation of chemotherapy to decrease bone-marrow dependent light-chain formation.[104,105]

Tumor cell necrosis following chemotherapy can release large amounts of intracellular contents such as uric acid, phosphate, and xanthine into the circulation, potentially leading to AKI. Acute uric acid nephropathy with intratubular crystallization leading to obstruction and interstitial nephritis is not seen as commonly as it was in the past, mainly due to prophylactic use of allopurinol or rasburicase before chemotherapy to acutely lower the serum uric acid levels. Several other well-known therapeutic agents such as amphotericin B, vancomycin, acyclovir, indinavir, cidofovir, foscarnet, pentamidine, and ifosfamide can all directly cause acute tubular injury and associated AKI.

POSTRENAL ACUTE KIDNEY INJURY

Postrenal azotemia occurs from obstruction of either the ureters or of the bladder outlet or urethra. AKI from ureteric obstruction requires that the blockage occur either bilaterally at any level of the ureters or unilaterally in a patient with a solitary functioning kidney or CKD. Ureteric obstruction can be either intraluminal or external. Bilateral ureteric calculi, blood clots, and sloughed renal papillae can obstruct the lumen, while external compression from tumor or hemorrhage can block the ureters as well. Fibrosis of the ureters intrinsically or from the retroperitoneum can narrow the lumen to the point of complete luminal obstruction. The most common cause for postrenal azotemia is structural or functional obstruction of the bladder neck. Prostatic conditions, therapy with anticholinergic agents, and a neurogenic bladder can all cause postrenal AKI. Relief of the obstruction usually causes prompt return of GFR if the duration of obstruction has not been excessive. The rate and magnitude of functional recovery is dependent on the extent and duration of the obstruction.[106]

AKI resulting from obstruction usually accounts for fewer than 5% of cases, although in certain settings (e.g., transplant), it can be as high as 6% to 10%. Clinically patients can present with pain and oliguria, though these are neither specific nor sensitive. Because of the availability of retroperitoneal imagining using either ultrasonography or computed tomography, the diagnosis is usually straightforward, although on occasions, a volume-depleted patient or a patient with severe reduction in GFR may not show hydronephrosis on radiologic assessment. Since GFR is typically not affected early in the course of obstructive AKI, volume repletion can increase the sensitivity of diagnosis by increasing GFR and urine production into the ureter, leading to dilation of the ureter proximal to the obstruction, enhancing ultrasonographic visualization. Early diagnosis and prompt relief of obstruction remain key goals in preventing long-term parenchymal damage as the shorter the period of obstruction, the better the chances for recovery and favorable long-term outcomes. The pathophysiology and treatment of obstructive uropathy are discussed extensively in Chapter 38 (see Table 31.3).

PATHOPHYSIOLOGY OF ACUTE KIDNEY INJURY

EXPERIMENTAL MODELS

There are a variety of animal and cell culture models of AKI designed to better understand the pathophysiology of acute kidney injury and to investigate novel therapeutic agents. However, there remains a need to develop in vivo experimental models of AKI that more closely resemble clinical AKI for the development of effective therapies.[4,107] Some of the important principles in studying the pathophysiology of AKI in various models include outcome measures at multiple time points and the ability to control physiologic functions known to affect kidney function (e.g., temperature, blood pressure, anesthesia, fluid status). Limitations in most experimental models include the lack of comorbid conditions (e.g., aged animals, impaired kidney function, multiorgan failure, preexisting vascular changes, or multiple renal insults) that often coexist in human AKI. We will briefly describe the pros and cons of using presently characterized experimental models (Table 31.7).

Table 31.7 Comparison of Models of Studying Acute Kidney Injury

	Humans	Animals							Cells	
		Ischemic			Septic		Toxic			
	Warm Ischemia-Reperfusion	Cold Ischemia-Warm Reperfusion	Hypoperfusion/Cardiac Arrest	Isolated Perfused Kidneys	Endotoxin	Cecal Ligation and Puncture	Bacterial Infusion	Contrast/Pigment/Glycerol/Drug	Isolated Proximal Tubular Cells	Cultured Tubular Cells
Simplicity	+	++	++	++	+++	++	++	+++	+++	++++
Reproducibility	++++	+++	+++	+++	+++	+++	+++	+++	+	+
Clinical relevance	++++	+++	++++	+++	++	++++	+++	+++	++	++
Therapeutic value	+++	++	+++	++	++	+++	+++	+++	+++	+++
Studying mechanisms	++	++	++	++	+	+++	+++	++	++++	++++
Controlling extrinsic factors	+	++	++	+++	++	++	++	++	++++	++++
Isolating single variables	++	++	+	+++	++	++	++	++	+++	+++
Standardization value	+	+++	++	++	++	++	++	++	++	++
Experimental limitation	+++	+++	+++	++	++	+++	++	+	+	+

Ratings are on a scale from +, minimally applicable to, ++++, very applicable.

The warm ischemia-reperfusion renal pedicle clamp model is one of the most widely used experimental models in rats and mice because of its simplicity and reproducibility. However, the inflammatory response differs greatly between mice and rats. Furthermore, tubular injury and repair and medullary congestion are difficult to compare to human ischemic ATN. In human AKI, "pure" ischemia alone is seen in the minority of cases and there is usually not complete cessation of blood flow to the kidneys. The parenteral delivery of prophylactic therapeutic agents is impossible in complete occlusion models. Since oxygen and metabolic substrates are unable to reach the kidney, generation of ROS and peroxynitrite species, considered to be important mediators of injury, might have a different or delayed role as compared to low oxygen states in hypoperfusion models. Total blood flow cessation also prevents the degradative products of the ischemic kidney from being washed out. Other factors playing a role in the pathophysiology of AKI, such as inflammatory mediators released from ischemic gut, endothelium, and vascular smooth muscle cells, need to be taken into consideration in any experimental model. Bowel proteins released into the circulation can act as inflammatory mediators and increase the susceptibility to AKI.[108] The S3 segment of the proximal tubule is almost completely necrosed in clamp models, a finding seen rarely in human AKI. In contrast to animal models, human AKI histologic biopsy data are lacking at early time points from the onset of insult.[4]

The cold ischemia–warm reperfusion model resembles the human transplant scenario but is inadequately studied and difficult experimentally. In the isolated perfused kidney model, the kidney is perfused ex vivo using perfusates with and without erythrocytes, and the model employs either ischemic (stopping perfusate) or hypoxic (reduced oxygen tension of erythrocytes) to induce functional impairment. The morphologic patterns are different in erythrocyte-free and erythrocyte-rich perfusates. The latter system is more comparable with what is observed histologically in animal models. Additionally, limitations include exclusion of various inflammatory mediators, neuroendocrine hemodynamic regulation, and systemic cytokine and growth factor interactions known to be present and play a pathophysiologic role in animal models and likely in human ischemia.

Cardiac arrest is a common scenario leading to human AKI. Recently Burne-Taney and colleagues described a whole-body ischemia-reperfusion injury model induced by 10 minutes of cardiac arrest, followed by cardiac compression resuscitation, ventilation, epinephrine, and fluids that lead to a significant rise in serum creatinine level and renal tubular injury at 24 hours.[109] One of the unique advantages of this model is the crosstalk between vital organs such as the brain, heart, lung, and the renal hemodynamics.[110] A hypoperfusion model of AKI using partial aortic clamping, first described by Zager,[111] may be more representative of human AKI, reflecting a state of reduced blood flow to the kidney with systolic blood pressure of approximately 20 mm Hg, resulting in reproducible AKI.[111,112] This was also recently adapted and refined in a study by Sharfuddin and associates where a novel compound, soluble thrombomodulin, was used to minimize ischemic injury in a partial aortic clamp AKI model.[113] It is less likely that AKI induced by clamping of the renal pedicle for 30 to 45 minutes in experimental animals is consistent with human AKI. The dissociation between animal and human AKI perhaps may be best reflected by data from the urology literature that reveal that clamping of the renal pedicle for 30 to 60 minutes is not associated with AKI or CKD in patients undergoing partial nephrectomy.[114] However, tissue samples were taken at the time of the clamp, and previous studies have shown worsening of injury after clamp removal in rodents.

Toxic models of kidney failure employ various known toxins, such as radiocontrast media, gentamicin, cisplatin, glycerol, and pigments, including myoglobin and hemoglobin. Septic models to study AKI include cecal ligation and puncture (CLP), endotoxin infusion, and bacterial infusion into the peritoneal cavity. The endotoxin model, which is simple, inexpensive, and suitable for studying new pharmacologic agents, has certain drawbacks as well. There is variability among sources of lipopolysaccharide (LPS) endotoxin, the rates and methods of administration vary, and it is usually of short duration due to the high mortality associated with the doses required to induce AKI. It also tends to be a vasoconstrictive model and does not recapitulate the early hemodynamics or inflammation of human sepsis.[115] Wichterman and colleagues were the first to describe a sepsis model in the early 1980s utilizing the CLP laboratory model.[116] In the CLP model there is considerable similarity to sepsis in humans with acute lung injury, metabolic derangement, and systemic vasodilation, accompanied initially by increased cardiac output. However, there is some variability depending on the mode and size of cecal perforation. Doi and coworkers have developed a new sepsis model keeping under consideration the following facts: (1) animals should receive the same supportive therapy that is standard for ICU patients (i.e., fluid resuscitation and antibiotics); and (2) age, chronic comorbid conditions, and genetic heterogeneity vary.[117] Complex animal models of human sepsis that introduce these disease-modifying factors are likely more relevant and may be more pharmacologically relevant than simple animal models.[117]

This description is intended to remind the reader of the potential pitfalls in each model when evaluating experimental studies or therapeutic interventions using these models. The lack of ability to demonstrate effectiveness of an agent in humans shown to be efficacious in animal models does not necessarily reflect a flaw with the model or the agent in question. Most often, the agent is administered late in the course of the human disease; patient heterogeneity and the difficulty in stratifying patients by severity of injury makes it even more difficult to establish efficacy.[118] It is also important to remember that experimental models of hypoxic acute kidney damage differ both conceptually and morphologically in the distribution of tubular cell injury. Tubular segment types differ in their capacity to undergo anaerobic metabolism and to mount hypoxia-adaptive responses mediated by hypoxia-inducible factors (HIFs), and in cell type-specific molecules shed into the urine, which may serve as early biomarkers for kidney damage.[119]

ACUTE TUBULAR NECROSIS

EPITHELIAL CELL INJURY

While all segments of the nephron may undergo injury during an ischemic insult, the major and most commonly injured epithelial cell involved in AKI related to ischemia, sepsis, and/or nephrotoxins is the PTC. Of the three segments (S1 to S3), the S3 segment of the proximal tubule in the outer stripe of the medulla is the cell most susceptible to ischemic injury for several reasons.[120] First, it has limited capacity to undergo anaerobic glycolysis. Second, due to its unique primarily venous capillary regional blood flow, there is marked hypoperfusion and congestion in this medullary region after injury that persists even though cortical blood flow may have returned to near-normal levels after ischemic injury. Endothelial cell injury and dysfunction are primarily responsible for this phenomenon, often referred to as the "extension phase" of AKI.[121] The other major epithelial cells of the nephron involved are those of the medullary thick ascending limb located more distally. The S1 and S2 segments are most commonly involved in toxic nephropathy due to their high rates of endocytosis, leading to increased cellular uptake of the toxin. PTCs and thick ascending limb of Henle (TAL) cells have been shown to be involved as sensors, effectors, and injury recipients of AKI stimuli.

PTC injury and dysfunction during ischemia or sepsis lead to a profound drop in GFR through afferent arteriolar vasoconstriction, mediated by tubular glomerular feedback and proximal tubular obstruction. This, along with tubular backleak, leads to a fall in effective GFR[122,123] (Figure 31.3).

Morphologic Changes

On histologic examination the classical hallmark of ATN is the loss of the apical brush border of the PTCs. Microvilli disruption and detachment from the apical cell surface forming membrane-bound blebs occurs early with release into the tubular lumen. Patchy detachment and subsequent loss of tubular cells exposing areas of denuded tubular basement and focal areas of proximal tubular dilation along with the presence of distal tubular casts are also major pathologic findings in ATN.[124] The sloughed tubular cells, brush border vesicle remnants, and cellular debris in combination with Tamm-Horsfall glycoprotein form the classical "muddy-brown granular" casts.[125] These distal casts have the potential to obstruct the tubular lumen. Frank necrosis itself is inconspicuous and restricted to the highly susceptible outer medullary regions. Alternatively, features of apoptosis are more commonly seen in both proximal and distal tubular cells. Glomerular epithelial cell injury in ischemic, septic, or nephrotoxic injury is not classically seen, although some studies have shown thickening and coarsening of foot processes, and recently Wagner and associates have shown podocyte-specific molecular and cellular changes.[126] The future morphologic course of the tubular cell alterations varies according to the type and extent of injury as discussed in the next section (Figure 31.4).

Cytoskeletal and Intracellular Structural Changes

Epithelial cellular structure and function are mediated in part by the actin cytoskeleton, which plays an integral role in surface membrane structure and function, cell polarity, endocytosis, signal transduction, cell motility, movement of organelles, exocytosis, cell division, cell migration, barrier function of the junctional complexes, cell-matrix adhesion, and, last but not least, signal transduction.[127] Based on its role in the multitude of processes, any disruption of the actin cytoskeleton results in changes and/or disruption of the functions mentioned earlier. This is especially important for PTCs, where amplification of the apical membrane by microvilli is essential for normal cell function.

Actin microfilaments are formed by self-assembly of globular or G-actin into filamentous F-actin. In PTCs the actin cytoskeleton forms a terminal web layer just below the apical plasma membrane, and a core of F-actin filaments extends from the terminal web into the tips of the microvilli to maintain the architectural integrity of the brush border. Ischemic insult results in cellular ATP depletion, which in turn leads

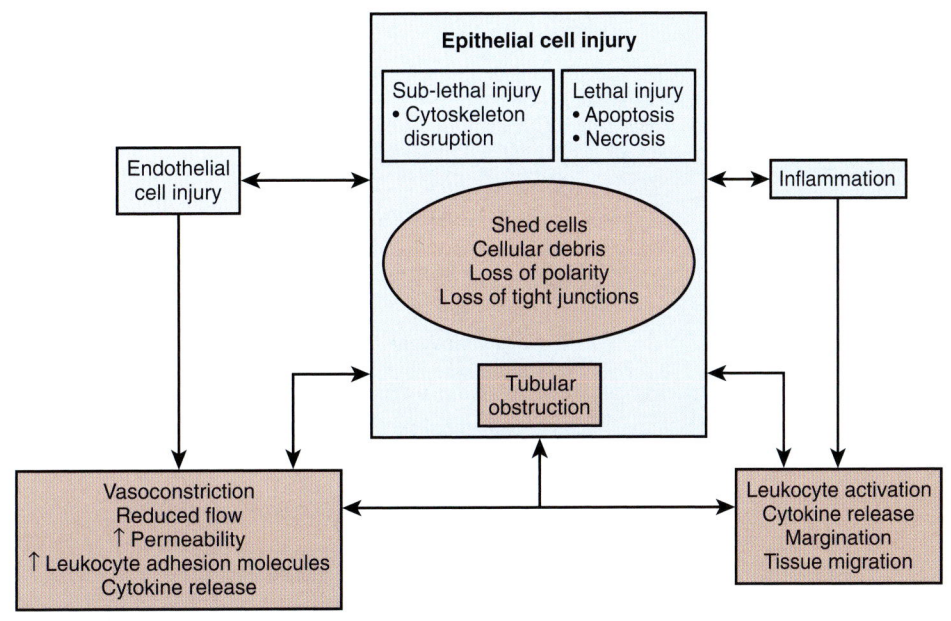

Figure 31.3 Overview of pathogenesis in acute kidney injury. The major pathways of impairment of glomerular filtration rate in ischemic acute tubular necrosis as a result of vascular and tubular injury (see text for details). (From Sharfuddin A, Molitoris B: Epithelial cell injury. In Vincent JL, Hall JB, editors: *Encyclopedia of intensive care medicine*, New York, 2012, Springer.)

to a rapid disruption of the apical actin and disruption and redistribution of the cytoskeleton F-actin core, resulting in formation of membrane-bound extracellular vesicles or blebs.[128] These can be either exfoliated into the tubular lumen or internalized with the capability of being recycled. The core mechanism of disruption is the depolymerization mediated by actin-binding protein known as actin depolymerizing factor (ADF) or cofilin.[129] This protein family is normally maintained in the inactive phosphorylated form where it cannot bind to actin. Ischemia results in ATP depletion, which has been shown to cause rho GTPase inactivation.[130] This can lead to activation and relocalization of ADF/cofilin to the apical membranes, where it can mediate different effects, including depolymerization, severing, capping, and nucleation of F-actin. This destroys the actin filament core structure of microvilli and results in surface membrane instability and blebbing[131,132] (Figure 31.5).

Concomitantly, the concentration of F-actin in the cell increases with the formation of large cytosolic aggregates in the perinuclear region and near the junctional complexes of the basolateral membranes. Other proteins involved in the depolymerization process are tropomyosin and ezrin. Specifically, it has been shown that during ischemia ezrin, an actin-binding phosphorylated protein, becomes dephosphorylated, and the attachment between the microvillar F-actin core and the plasma membrane is lost. Similarly, tropomyosins physiologically bind to and stabilize the F-actin microfilament core in the terminal web by preventing access to ADF. After ischemia, there is dissociation of tropomyosins from the microfilament core, resulting in access of the microfilaments in the terminal web to the binding, severing, and depolymerizing actions of ADF/cofilin.[133,134]

Another important consequence of disruption of the actin cytoskeleton is the loss of tight junctions and adherens junctions. These junctional complexes actively participate in numerous functions, including paracellular transport, cell polarity, and cellular shape. The tight junctions, also known as zonula occludens (ZO), are composed of a growing number of proteins such as occludin, claudin, ZO-1, and protein kinase C with numerous barrier functions, such as adhesion, permeability, and transport. The actin present in the terminal web is linked to ZO, and hence any disruption of the terminal web results in disruption of

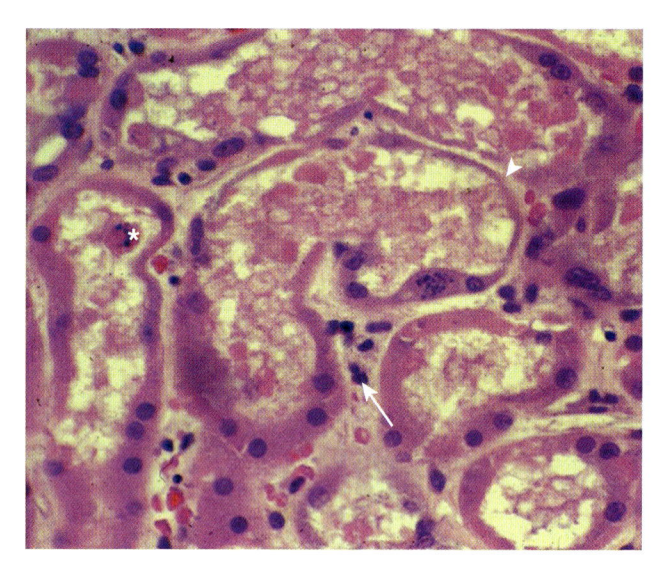

Figure 31.4 Morphology of acute tubular necrosis in human biopsy specimen. The biopsy specimen, obtained within 24 hours from a patient with exercise-induced rhabdomyolysis, revealed significant proximal tubular cell damage with intraluminal accumulation of apical membrane fragments and detached cell (*), thinning of proximal tubular cells to maintain monolayer tubule integrity (*arrowhead*), and dividing cells and accumulation of white cells within the microvascular space in the peritubular area (*arrow*). The patient required renal replacement therapy but did regain complete renal function eventually. (From Molitoris BA: Actin cytoskeleton in ischemic acute renal failure. *Kidney Int* 66:871-883, 2004.)

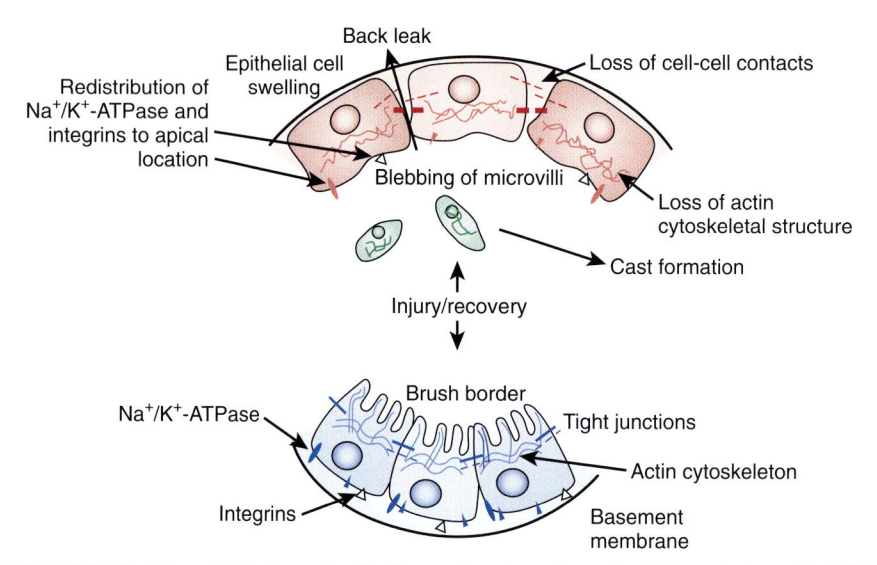

Figure 31.5 Overview of sublethally injured tubular cells. Sodium-potassium adenosine triphosphatase (Na^+-K^+-ATPase) pumps are normally located at the basolateral membrane. In sublethal ischemia the pumps redistribute to the apical membrane of the proximal tubule. Upon reperfusion, the pumps reverse back to their basolateral location. (From Sharfuddin A, Molitoris B: Epithelial cell injury. In Vincent JL, Hall JB, editors: *Encyclopedia of intensive care medicine*, New York, 2012, Springer.)

the tight junctions. Early ischemic injury results in "opening" of these tight junctions, leading to increased paracellular permeability causing further backleak of the glomerular filtrate into the interstitium.[127] Only recently has it been shown that in the glomerulus ischemia also induces rapid loss of interaction between slit diaphragm junctional proteins NEPH1 and ZO-1,[126] leading to podocyte damage, effacement, and proteinuria. The molecular mechanisms underlying these changes have been studied as well and show that ATP depletion that resulted in actin polymerization is followed by a reduction in cellular adhesion ability. Pretreatment with jasplakinolide, an actin stabilizer, prevented ATP depletion–induced actin polymerization and reduction of cell adhesion, indicating that the cytoskeleton reorganization decreased the cellular adhesion ability. Furthermore, the ATP depletion markedly increased the levels of p38 mitogen-activated protein (MAP) kinase and heat shock protein 27 (hsp27) phosphorylation with enhanced translocation of phosphorylated hsp27 from cytoskeleton to cytoplasm. The inhibition of p38 MAP kinase by specific inhibitor SB203580 blocked the ATP depletion to induce hsp27 phosphorylation and actin polymerization. These findings suggest that ischemia remodels F-actin leading to desquamation of proximal tubular epithelial cells through p38 MAP kinase–hsp27 signaling.[135]

During ischemia, epithelial cells also lose their attachment to the underlying extracellular matrix due to disruption of integrins. Integrins are transmembrane proteins normally responsible for the anchoring of epithelial cells to the substrate matrix via the actin cytoskeleton. It has been shown that ATP depletion results in relocalization of β-integrins from the basal membrane to the apical membrane, with subsequent detachment of the viable cells from the tubular basement membrane. The exfoliated cells can then exhibit abnormal adhesions within the tubular lumen among themselves, forming cellular casts within the tubular lumen as mentioned earlier. Extracellular signal–regulated kinases 1 and 2 (ERK1/2) have been shown to be activated at 24 hours after reperfusion in an in vivo model of ischemia as well as in in vitro models of rat proximal cells. ERK1/2 affect cytoskeletal organization and focal complex assembly during reperfusion, since a specific upstream ERK inhibitor, U0126, improved actin and tubulin cytoskeleton structure, reduced cell contraction, and prevented paxillin redistribution. This suggests that ERK1/2 signaling plays an essential role in ischemia-reperfusion–induced injury, mediating proximal cell adhesive alterations.[136]

Actin cytoskeleton alterations and dysfunction during ischemia result in changes in cell polarity and function. Normally, sodium-potassium adenosine triphosphatase (Na^+-K^+-ATPase) pumps reside in the basolateral membrane of the tubular epithelial cell, but under conditions of ischemia, they redistribute to the apical membrane as early as within 10 minutes.[137] This occurs due to the disruption of the pumps' attachment to the membrane via the spectrin/actin cytoskeleton. Postulated mediated mechanisms include hyperphosphorylation of the protein ankyrin, with consequent loss of the binding protein spectrin, and cleavage of spectrin by activation of proteases such as calpain. This redistribution of the Na^+-K^+-ATPase pump results in bidirectional transport of sodium and water across the epithelial cell apical membrane as well as the basolateral membrane. This results in transport of cellular Na back into the tubular lumen, one of the major mechanisms of the high FE_{Na} seen in patients with ATN,[138] and the inefficient use of cellular ATP, as it uncouples ATP use and effective Na transport.

An expanding role for the PTC as a sensor of both self and nonself danger-associated molecular patterns (DAMPs) and pathogen-associated molecular patterns (PAMPs) recognition signals utilizing pattern recognition receptors (PRRs) such as Toll-like receptor 4 (TLR4) has been delineated.[139] Proximal tubule TLR4 has been shown to upregulate and migrate to the apical domain in response to LPS in S1 PTCs, which are the earliest segments of epithelial cell postglomerular filtration.[140] Interestingly, the S1 cell internalizes and processes LPS via TLR4 receptors, which is inducible with preexposure to LPS but is protected from injury by upregulated defense mechanisms, including heme oxygenase-1 (HO-1) and sirtuin 1 (SIRT1), two cytoprotective proteins. However, S2 to S3 PTC cells undergo oxidative injury with minimal uptake of LPS, implying communication, crosstalk, and co-regulation between the segments following LPS exposure.[141] This injury is dependent on CD14, likely due to peroxisomal disruption, perhaps mediated by tumor necrosis factor-α (TNF-α), and the PTC injury was found to be independent of systemic cytokines.

Another important role for epithelial TLR4 in mediating ischemic injury was shown early on by Wu and colleagues using chimeric mice for TLR4 and MyD88.[142] A role for epithelial TLR2 during ischemic injury was also shown[143] by using TLR2 knockout mice. Cytokine and chemokine production was reduced and white blood cell (WBC) infiltration was minimized in chimeric mice with use of antisense therapy, and this effect was more consistent in proximal tubule effects via TLR2.

The PTCs release cytokines and chemokines in response to cell injury, and these agents have direct effects on endothelial function. Investigators directly studied these responses by using fluorescent cytopathologic E. coli, microinjected into early proximal tubule segments, by recording cellular and physiologic responses using two-photon microscopy.[144-146] Attachment to the apical membrane, but without penetration into or through the PTC monolayer barrier, resulted in rapid and selective termination of blood flow to the adjacent area and thus vascular isolation of the infected area with localized hypoxia, WBC migration, and necrosis. The same E. coli strain, missing only one virulence factor, required a far longer time to initiate this protective process. Tissue concentrations of cytokines, elevated in the affected area compared to none in the injected areas, revealed marked increases.[146] Finally, prevention of this microvascular response resulted in widespread organ dissemination of the injected E. coli and death of the rat within 24 hours, something not seen with the intact system.[146] Thus a line of communication among PTC and endothelial cells leads to localization of the infecting agent and prevention of systemic spread.

In recent years there has been considerable progress in understanding PTC repair following severe injury. Increasing durations of ischemia result in more severe cell injury and longer recovery periods. Pioneering work revealed PTC recovered rapidly and completely following mild ischemia. As the duration increased, the loss of PTC into the lumen, necrosis, and apoptosis increased, indicating that AKI recovery likely required new cells. With innovative approaches the possibility of extratubular stem or progenitor cell populations migrating into the tubule was minimized or eliminated using chimera and genetic fate–tracing strategies.[147,148] In a follow-up study[149] use of lineage and clonal behavior of fully differentiated PTC after injury using a CreER^{T2} cassette knocked into the Na-dependent PO$_4$ transporter locus showed that both regeneration and proliferation occurred and clonal growth was more pronounced with increased severity of injury. The authors also documented expression of putative epithelial stem cell markers on injured PTC. These data provide further evidence that terminally differentiated epithelia are able to proliferate, and there was no evidence for an intratubular stem cell population. These data indicate minimizing PTC injury, by either reducing initial injury or reducing injury subsequent to microvascular dysfunction during the extension phase, will minimize cellular death and cell detachment and loss and allow for a higher percentage of cells repairing by regeneration and not proliferation.

Tamm-Horsfall protein (also known as uromodulin) is a heavily glycosylated protein that is uniquely produced in the kidney by TALs.[150,151] Interestingly, uromodulin appears to be an essential effector produced during kidney injury to modulate innate immunity and inflammation.[139,150,152,153] Uromodulin knockout mice subjected to ischemia-reperfusion injury (IRI) showed increased S3 injury and necrosis compared to wild-type controls.[152,154] This was associated with increased neutrophil infiltration in the outer medulla and increased expression of TLR4 and CXCL2 by S3 segments.[152,154] Neutralization of CXCL2 was protective, suggesting that a TLR4-CXCL2 proinflammatory pathway may be important in the pathophysiology and supports uromodulin-dependent TAL-S3 crosstalk. Indeed, after IRI a shift of trafficking of uromodulin was demonstrated toward the interstitium and basolateral aspects of S3 segments,[153] where a putative receptor for uromodulin is expressed.[152] This translocation of uromodulin was not the result of altered polarity of TAL. Furthermore, a significant increase in uromodulin level was shown in the kidney at the onset of recovery, which was concomitant with suppression of tubular-derived cytokines and chemokines such as MCP-1, supporting the concept that the protective crosstalk mediated by uromodulin may be important in modulating recovery from AKI.[153]

Apoptosis and Necrosis

The fate of the epithelial cell after an injury ultimately depends on the extent of the injury. Cells undergoing sublethal or less severe injury have the capacity for functional and structural recovery if the insult is interrupted. Cells that suffer a more severe (or lethal) injury undergo apoptosis or necrosis, leading to cell death. Apoptosis is an energy-dependent, "programmed" cell death after injury that results in condensation of nuclear and cytoplasmic material, forming apoptotic bodies. These apoptotic bodies, which are plasma-membrane bound, are rapidly phagocytosed by macrophages and neighboring viable epithelial cells. In necrosis, there is cellular and organelle swelling, with loss of plasma membrane integrity, and release of cytoplasmic and nuclear material into the lumen or interstitium.[155]

Apoptotic mechanisms are complex with various interplaying and counteracting factors affecting a number of pathways. The caspase family of proteases has now been identified to be an important initiator as well as an effector of apoptosis.[156,157] Both the intrinsic (mitochondrial) and extrinsic (death receptor) apoptotic pathways are activated in human AKI. Specifically, activation of procaspase-9 primarily depends on intrinsic mitochondrial pathways regulated by the Bcl-2 family of proteins, while that of procaspase-8 results from extrinsic signaling via cell surface death receptors such as Fas and their ligand FADD (Fas-associated protein with death domain). There also exists considerable crosstalk between the intrinsic and extrinsic pathways. The other group of caspases, 3, 6, and 7, are effector caspases, which are more abundant and catalytically robust, cleaving many cellular proteins, resulting in the classical apoptotic phenotype. Caspase activation in epithelial cells occurs due to ischemic and other cytotoxic insults, whereas inhibition of caspase activity has been shown to be protective against such injury in cultured and in vivo renal epithelial tubular AKI[158,159] (Figures 31.6 and 31.7).

Several pathways, including the intrinsic (Bcl-2 family, cytochrome c, caspase-9), extrinsic (Fas, FADD, caspase-8), and regulatory (p53 and NF-κB), appear to be activated during ischemic renal tubular cell injury. It has also been shown that the balance between cell survival and death depends on the relative concentrations of the proapoptotic (Bax, Bcl-2–associated death promoter [Bad], and Bid) and antiapoptotic (Bcl-2 and Bcl-xL) members of the Bcl-2 family of proteins. Overexpression of proapoptotic or relative deficiency of antiapoptotic proteins may lead to formation of mitochondrial pores. Conversely, the inhibition of such pore formation may occur with the opposite imbalance.[160-162]

Other important proteins that have been shown to play a significant role in the apoptotic pathways include NF-κB and p53.[163,164] The central proapoptotic transcription factor p53 can be activated by hypoxia, via HIF-1α, as well as by other noxious stimuli such as certain drugs (e.g., cisplatin). The kinase-mediated pathways such as ERKs and c-Jun N-terminal kinases (JNKs) are responsible for mediating cellular responses involved in apoptosis, survival, and repair through their interaction with other signals from growth factors such as hepatocyte growth factor, insulin-like growth factor-I, epidermal growth factor, and vascular endothelial growth factor (VEGF).[165,166] These independent mechanisms can inhibit proapoptotic proteins such as Bad and activate the antiapoptotic transcription of CREB (cyclic adenosine monophosphate response element-binding) factors. More recent data indicate that there is rapid delivery of small interfering RNA (siRNA) to proximal tubular cells in AKI, and targeting siRNA to minimize p53 production leads to a dose-dependent attenuation of apoptotic signaling and kidney function, suggesting potential therapeutic benefit for ischemic and nephrotoxic kidney injury.[167] In vivo microRNA-24 (miR-24) also regulates HO-1 and H2A histone family, member X. Overall, these results indicate miR-24 promotes renal ischemic injury by stimulating apoptosis in endothelial and tubular epithelial cells.[168]

Overall, the therapeutic implications of apoptosis in preventing epithelial cell injury are significant, considering that various targets are available for blockade or modulation. It is also possible that the "window" to prevent lethal injury and prevent cells from progressing to necrosis is in the early

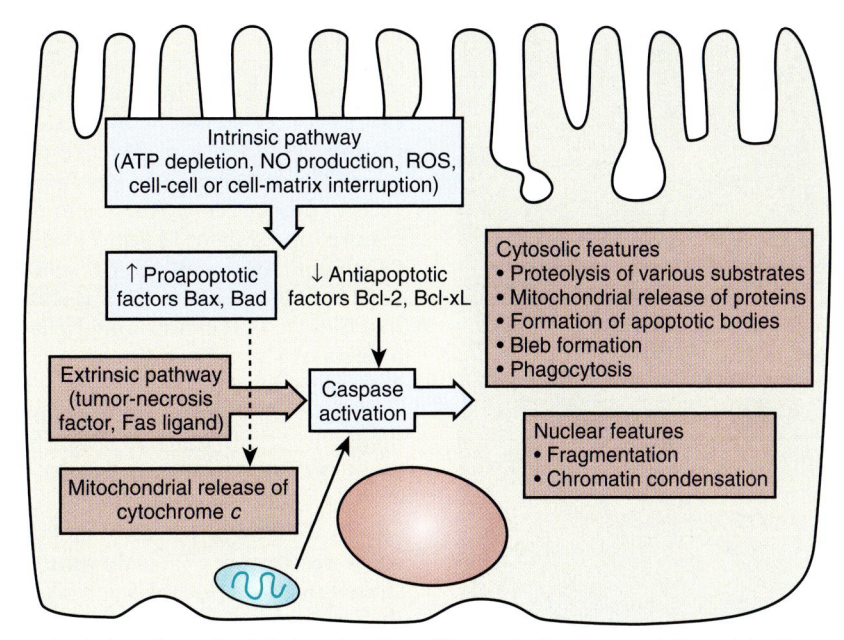

Figure 31.6 The cell injury or intrinsic pathway leads to translocation of Bax and other proapoptotic proteins from cytosol to the mitochondria, forming pores, causing the release of cytochrome c. Apoptosis-activating factor is activated by cytochrome c, which binds to and activates procaspase-9. Caspase-3 is activated by activated caspase-9, which along with other downstream caspases induces proteolysis of various cytosolic and nuclear proteins. The death receptor or extrinsic pathway functions primarily by binding of death ligands such as Fas or tumor necrosis factor-α (TNF-α) to their cell-surface receptor, resulting in the activation of procaspase-8 to its active form. This occurs through mediation with adaptor proteins such as FADD (Fas-associated protein with death domain) and TRADD (TNF receptor 1–associated death domain). Active caspase-8 activates caspase-3 and cleaves proapoptotic protein Bid to its truncated form tBid, which acts via Bax to induce cytochrome c from the mitochondria. Hence the extrinsic pathway also amplifies the events induced by the intrinsic pathway. ATP, Adenosine triphosphate; NO, nitric oxide; ROS, reactive oxygen species. (Adapted from Levine JS, Lieberthal W: Terminal pathways to cell death. In Molitoris BA, Finn WF, editors: *Acute renal failure: a companion to Brenner & Rector's the kidney*, Philadelphia, 2001, Saunders, p 43; and Sharfuddin A, Molitoris B: Epithelial cell injury. In Vincent JL, Hall JB, editors: *Encyclopedia of intensive care medicine*, New York, 2012, Springer.)

initiating apoptotic phases. Epithelial cell necrosis, on the other hand, is a "passive" non–energy dependent process that develops secondary to severe ATP depletion from toxic or ischemic insult. It is not dependent on caspase activation but rather results from a rise in intracellular calcium and the activation of membrane phospholipases.[169,170] Hence morphologically, necrotic cells do not exhibit the nuclear fragmentation or chromatin condensation seen in apoptosis, and they do not form apoptotic bodies. Functionally, severe ATP depletion results first in mitochondrial injury with subsequent arrest of oxidative phosphorylation, causing further depletion of energy stores, and robust formation of ROS that in turn mediate further cellular injury.

Numerous studies have shown that ATP depletion leads to a rise in intracellular calcium through impairment of calcium ATPases, while inhibition of the Na^+-K^+-ATPase activity potentiates calcium entry into the cell via the sodium-calcium exchanger. Increased cytosolic calcium causes further mitochondrial injury and cytoskeletal alterations.[171] This chain of events results in downstream activation of proteases such as calpain and phospholipases. Phospholipases such as phospholipase A_2 cause direct hydrolytic damage to membranes and also release toxic free fatty acids. They also cause release of eicosanoids that have vasoactive and hemokinetic activities, resulting in an intense surrounding inflammatory response. Calpain mediates plasma membrane permeability, as well as hydrolysis of the cytoskeleton proteins.[172,173] Finally, there is release of lysosomal enzymes and proteases that degrade histones, resulting in accessibility of the endonucleases to the entire segment, classically seen as the "smear" pattern on gel electrophoresis, in contrast to the typical "ladder" pattern seen in apoptosis.[174]

Parenchymal Inflammation

Recent attention has turned to understanding the role of the immune response to AKI from both sepsis and ischemia. Virtually all WBC types have been implicated in this response, and either deletion or enhancement of each cell's response has been shown to result in an improved short-term outcome.[175] In particular, the roles of polymorphonuclear cells,[176-178] monocytes/macrophages,[179-182] natural killer T,[183,184] natural killer,[185] regulatory T (T_{reg}),[186-188] and B cells[189,190] have been shown. The time course of involvement varies by the cell type[142,183] with polymorphonuclear cells leading the way followed by monocytes/macrophages in both rapidity of response and numbers of cells. Most invading cells are detrimental, but some are beneficial, such as T_{reg} cells.[186-188] Macrophages play a special role as type I macrophages arrive early and mediate cellular injury, but type II macrophages are essential for normal repair later in the process.[180,181,191] Numerous reviews cover the involvement of infiltrating cells in AKI, and therapeutic attempts are being undertaken to control this invasion and limit the damage done.[192] Early inflammation is classically characterized by margination of leukocytes to the activated vascular endothelium, via interactions between selectins and ligands

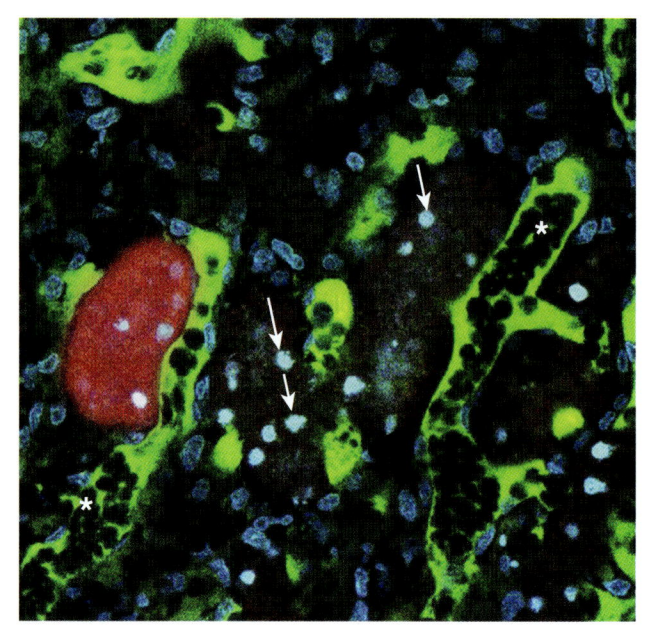

Figure 31.7 Live two-photon imaging of a Sprague-Dawley rat kidney 24 hours after cecal ligation and puncture. Nuclei are labeled *blue* with Hoechst stain. *Green* represents 500-kDa fluorescein isothiocyanate (FITC) dextran, which labels the vasculature. *Red* represents 3-kDa Texas Red dextran, which is filtered and labels the tubular lumens. Note apoptotic nuclei, which show intense Hoechst staining along with condensation and fragmentation (*arrows*). Many of these apoptotic nuclei are shed into the lumens of tubules with compromised urine flow. Also noted is the rouleaux formation and congestion in peritubular capillary with lack of blood flow (*). (Courtesy Pierre Dagher, MD, Division of Nephrology, Indiana University School of Medicine.)

that allows firm adhesion, followed by transmigration. A number of potent mediators are generated by the injured proximal epithelial tubular cell, including proinflammatory cytokines such as TNF-α, IL-6, IL-1β, MCP-1, IL-8, transforming growth factor-β (TGF-β), and RANTES (regulated on activation, normal T expressed, and secreted).[193] TLR2 has been shown to be an important mediator of endothelial ischemic injury, while TLR4 has been shown to play a similar role in animal models of both ischemic and septic injury,[194] especially in PTC.[142]

Neutrophils are the earliest to accumulate in ischemic injury in animal models but are rarely seen in human ATN. Blockade of neutrophil function or neutrophil depletion has been shown to provide only partial protection against injury. Hence other leukocytes also play an important role. These include macrophages, B lymphocytes, and T lymphocytes.[195] Selective deletion, knockout mice models, and specific blockade animal experiments have shown that all of these cells do mediate tubular injury at various phases and that these are synergistic interactions between different cellular types.[195] It is also known that during ischemic injury, complement receptor 5a (CR5a) expression is markedly upregulated on proximal tubule epithelial cells as well as interstitial macrophages. C5a is a powerful chemoattractant that recruits these inflammatory cells. Complement cascades are activated during sepsis, and C5a, a potent complement component with procoagulant properties, has been found to be elevated in rodent models of sepsis.

Blocking C5a or its receptor has shown some promise in improving survival with sepsis.[196] Whether released from the endothelium or the epithelial cell, numerous cytokines exert a concerted biochemical effort to augment the inflammatory response seen as a result of ischemic or septic injury.[197] Furthermore it has been shown that in culture, mouse tubular cells when stimulated with LPS cells in culture upregulate TLR2, TLR3, and TLR4 and secrete CC-chemokines such as CC motif chemokine ligand 2 (CCL2)/MCP-1 and CCL5/RANTES. These data suggest that tubular TLR expression might be involved in mediating interstitial leukocyte infiltration and tubular injury during bacterial sepsis.[198]

TLR2 and TLR4 are constitutively expressed on renal epithelium, and their expression is enhanced following renal IRI. El-Achkar and coworkers have shown that in a CLP rat model of sepsis, TLR4 expression increases markedly in all tubules (proximal and distal), glomeruli, and the renal vasculature.[140] Furthermore these authors demonstrated that in sepsis there is a TLR4-dependent increase in the expression of proinflammatory mediator cyclooxygenase-2 (COX-2), which was mostly restricted to cortical and medullary TALs, which characteristically express and secrete Tamm-Horsfall protein.[199] Tamm-Horsfall protein may stabilize the outer medulla in the face of injury by decreasing inflammation, possibly through an effect on TLR4.[154] Genetic deletion of either TLR2 or TLR4 protects from renal IRI,[142,200] thus indicating the prominent role TLR plays in AKI.

Macrophages produce proinflammatory cytokines that can stimulate the activity of other leukocytes. Day and associates have shown that depletion of kidney and spleen macrophages using liposomal clodronate before renal IRI prevented AKI, and adoptive transfer of macrophages reconstituted AKI.[179] There may also be a regulatory role for macrophages. Bone marrow–derived macrophages that overexpress the antiinflammatory interleukin IL-10 when adoptively transferred increase their intracellular iron pool, which in turn augments the expression of lipocalin-2 and its receptors. Infusion of these macrophages into rats after 1 hour of reperfusion resulted in localization of the cells to injured kidney tissue, caused increases in regenerative markers, and resulted in a notable reduction in levels of both blood urea nitrogen (BUN) and creatinine. Furthermore, IL-10 therapy decreased the local inflammatory profile and upregulated the expression of pro-regenerative lipocalin-2 and its receptors. Interleukin-10–mediated protection and subsequent renal repair were dependent on the presence of iron and lipocalin-2.[201]

Dendritic cells, a resident population of bone marrow–derived cells and macrophages, form a network between the basement membranes of tubular epithelia and peritubular endothelial cells.[202,203] While dendritic cells and macrophages are often considered as distinct cell types with characteristic functions, recent data have shown considerable overlap in cell surface markers and function between dendritic cells and macrophages.[204] Located in the interstitial space, dendritic cells have access to endogenous and exogenous DAMPs and PAMPs released by epithelial cells, invading organisms, and infiltrating cells and thus are key initiators, potentiators, and effectors of the innate immune system. Dendritic cells have enormous plasticity and can be either antiinflammatory or proinflammatory.[205,206] In ischemic AKI they lead to recruitment of inflammatory cells but also participate in recovery via IL-10 production.[207] They are known to be the earliest producers of IL-6, TNF-α, MCP-1, and RANTES.[208] They can also be involved in producing tolerance by inducing T cell anergy or depletion or induction of T_{reg} cells.[209] Deletion of dendritic cells using a human diphtheria toxin approach reduced IRI, and deletion of sphingosine 1-phosphate receptor 3 ($S1P_3R$) or inhibition of $S1P_2R$ resulted in protection from IRI.[210-212] Finally, dendritic cells migrate away from the kidney via the lymphatic system to present antigen and regulate lymphocytic responses. Thus dendritic cells serve at the crossroads of communication between the epithelium and endothelium regulating both innate and adaptive immunity, self-tolerance, and tissue injury and repair.

T_{reg} cells have also been recently shown to play a role in ischemic AKI. Liu and colleagues have shown that in a murine model of ischemic acute kidney injury there was a significant trafficking of T_{reg} cells into the kidneys after 3 and 10 days. Postischemic kidneys had increased numbers of TCR-β+CD4+ and TCR-β+CD8+ T cells with enhanced proinflammatory cytokine production. They also noted that T_{reg} depletion starting 1 day after ischemic injury using anti-CD25 antibodies increased renal tubular damage, reduced tubular proliferation at both time points, enhanced infiltrating T lymphocyte cytokine production at 3 days and TNF-α generation by TCR-β+CD4+ T cells at 10 days. In separate mice studies, infusion of CD4+CD25+ T_{reg} cells 1 day after initial injury reduced interferon (IFN)-γ production by TCR-β+CD4+ T cells at 3 days, improved repair, and reduced cytokine generation at 10 days. These studies demonstrate that T_{reg} cells infiltrate ischemic-reperfused kidneys during the healing process promoting repair, likely through modulation of proinflammatory cytokine production of other T cell subsets.[213] The role of T_{reg} cells has been further extended by Kinsey and coworkers, who have shown that partial depletion of T_{reg} cells with an anti-CD25 monoclonal antibody potentiated kidney damage induced by IRI and that reducing the number of T_{reg} cells resulted in more neutrophils, macrophages, and innate cytokine transcription in the kidney after IRI.[188] Furthermore FoxP3 (forkhead box P3)+ T_{reg} cell–deficient mice accumulated a greater number of inflammatory leukocytes after renal IRI than mice containing T_{reg} cells and that co-transfer of isolated T_{reg} cells and Scurfy lymph node cells significantly attenuated IRI-induced renal injury and leukocyte accumulation.[188] Finally, it has been shown that the anticoagulant function of activated protein C is responsible for suppressing LPS-induced stimulation of the proinflammatory mediators ACE-1, IL-6, and IL-18, perhaps accounting for its ability to modulate renal hemodynamics and protect against septic AKI.[214]

Heat shock protein 70 (hsp70) has been shown to have renoprotective effects that are partially mediated by T_{reg} cells as well.[215] The mechanisms elucidated by studying adoptively transferred T_{reg} cells have shown that IL-10 production, adenosine production through CD73, expression of the adenosine 2A receptor, and programmed cell death 1 on the cell surface are required by T_{reg} cells to protect recipient mice from IRI.[216] Taken together, these studies suggest that intrinsic T_{reg} cells traffic to the injured kidney to promote repair from ischemic injury.

While the myofibroblast is the cell type responsible for depositing collagen, investigators have been searching for its precursors. Other than interstitial fibroblasts that are known to transition, pericytes and dendritic, endothelial, and epithelial cells have been identified as potential contributors.[217] Fate-tracing studies by Humphreys and associates showed that while epithelial cells can obtain mesenchymal markers, they do not penetrate the basement membrane to enter into the interstitial space and differentiate into myofibroblasts.[218] Using lineage analysis it was the platelet-derived growth factor receptor (PDGFR)-β–positive pericytes that differentiated into myofibroblasts in a unilateral ureteral obstruction (UUO) model. Thus dissociation of pericytes from their endothelial partners seems to be an early step initiated by alterations in communication between these two cell types or interstitial signals generated by many potential cell types.[219]

Several studies now place the pericyte at the crossroads of microvascular dropout and therefore chronic hypoxia and CKD progression after AKI. Using an unbiased approach to identify upregulated and downregulated pericyte genes in injury, Schrimpf and colleagues found increased activation and expression of ADAMTS1 (a disintegrin-like and metalloprotease with thrombospondin type 1 repeats 1) and downregulation of its inhibitor metalloproteinase 3 (TIMP-3).[220] TIMP-3-stabilized pericytes maintained collagen capillary tube networks, while ADAMTS1-treated pericytes led to enhanced destabilization. TIMP-3 has many functions, including regulating VEGF signaling, pericyte migration, and matrix metalloproteinase 2 (MMP-2) and MMP-9 activity.[221] Furthermore, TGF-β$_1$ has recently been shown to activate the pericyte-myofibroblast transition, thus adding to the stimuli for pericyte involvement in fibrosis.[222] Injured epithelial cells reduce production of VEGF, a trophic factor for endothelial maintenance, and increase production of both TGF-β and PDGFR, which enhance pericyte dedifferentiation into myofibroblasts. Finally, PDGFR blockade on pericytes or vascular endothelial growth factor receptor 2 (VEGFR-2) on endothelial cells led to a reduction in fibrosis and stabilization of the microvasculature in the UUO model.[223] Thus numerous factors favor microvascular maladaptation after injury, including TGF-β production and lack of VEGF production by epithelial cells, reductions in PDGF production by endothelial cells, and increased ADAMTS1 expression with reduced TIMP-3 production by pericytes. These events also suggest several therapeutic targets that could limit microvascular dropout and loss of kidney function secondary to the fibrotic process. One cautionary note: much of the data generated with regard to pericytes comes from the UUO model and not typical AKI models. The UUO model is extremely fibrogenic, and so one has to be careful about interpretation of the data as they relate to AKI.

Intracellular Mechanisms—Role of Reactive Oxygen Species, Heme Oxygenase, and Heat Shock Proteins

ROS such as OH^-, peroxynitrite ($ONOO^-$), and hypochlorous acid (HOCl) are generated in epithelial cells during ischemic injury by catalytic conversion. These ROS can damage cells in a variety of ways (e.g., peroxidation of lipids in plasma and intracellular membranes). They can also destabilize the cytoskeletal proteins and integrins required to maintain cell-cell adhesion, as well as extracellular matrix. These ROS can also have vasoconstrictive effects by their capacity to scavenge NO.[224] Much of the previous discussion has been on proteins or mechanisms that promote injury. However, there are protective mechanisms that allow cells to have a defense against numerous stresses. The complex hsp system is induced to exceptionally high levels during stress conditions. The hsps are believed to facilitate the restoration of normal function by assisting in the refolding of denatured proteins, along with aiding the appropriate folding of newly synthesized proteins. They also help in degradation of irreparable proteins and toxins to limit their accumulation. Thus their role has been studied, and it was found that overexpression before injury has protective effects.[225-227] The proteins hsp90, hsp72, and hsp25 in particular have been extensively studied (e.g., overexpression of hsp25 has been shown to be protective against actin-cytoskeleton disruption).[228] After in vivo renal ischemia, hsp90 has been shown to be rapidly induced in cytosolic proximal tubular epithelial cells, particularly in late stages, leading to the conclusion that hsp90 may be crucial for disposition of damaged proteins and the assembly of newly formed peptides. Intrarenal transfection with hsp90 has been shown to be protective against IRI with restoration of endothelial nitric oxide synthase (eNOS)–hsp90 coupling, eNOS activating phosphorylation, and rho kinase levels, suggesting their implication in regulating the NO/eNOS pathway and the intrarenal vascular tone.[229] In nephrotoxic models, hsp72 has been shown to limit apoptosis through increased Bcl-2/Bax ratio, implicating the role of hsp72 in cell death as well.[228]

The enzyme HO-1 has also emerged as a prominent constituent in epithelial cell injury. Numerous observations have shown that the biologic actions of HO-1 include anti-inflammatory, vasodilatory, cytoprotective, antiapoptotic, and cellular proliferative effects in the setting of AKI. Its gene is arguably one of the most readily inducible genes, responding to numerous stressors, including, but not limited to, hypoxia, hyperthermia, oxidative stress, and exposure to LPS. Consequently, induction of HO-1 has been described in various forms of AKI, including ischemic, endotoxin, and nephrotoxic models. Following ischemia-reperfusion, aged mice, compared with young mice, exhibit worse renal injury and less renal induction of HO-1, especially in the medulla. A number of studies indicate a protective effect of induction of HO-1 in AKI.[230,231] Prior induction of HO-1 by hemoglobin can reduce endotoxemia-induced renal dysfunction and mortality. Inhibition of HO-1 activity in the intact, disease-free kidney reduces medullary blood flow without exerting any effect on cortical blood flow. Overexpression of HO-1 by hemin results in a significant reduction in cisplatin-induced cytotoxicity.[232] TNF-α–induced apoptosis in endothelial cells is also attenuated by induction of HO-1. These findings have been supported by studies in which HO-1–deficient mice, in the glycerol-induced AKI model, exhibited marked exacerbation of renal insufficiency and mortality.[233] The protective mechanisms of HO-1 have been extensively studied by Inguaggiato and coworkers, who showed overexpression of HO-1 in cultured renal epithelial cells induces upregulation of the cell cycle inhibitory protein p21 and confers resistance to apoptosis.[234] Macrophages in which HO-1 is upregulated by adenoviral strategies also protect against ischemic AKI. Fibroblasts from organs of transgenic pigs expressing HO-1 are resistant to proapoptotic stressors and exhibit a blunted proinflammatory response to LPS or TNF-α.

Pretreatment with hemin augments glomerular HO-1 expression and renal expression of thrombomodulin and endothelial cell protein C receptor (EPCR), while reducing renal dysfunction, glomerular thrombotic microangiopathy, and the procoagulant state; hemin also increases plasma levels of activated protein C in this model, suggesting its important role in the endothelial-epithelial axis of AKI. Perhaps more importantly, HO-1 might also contribute to the repair and regeneration of tubular cells.[96,231] Following an acute insult, HO-1 is rapidly induced, but its expression subsides before renal recovery fully occurs; such abatement in HO-1 expression may allow the continued expression of proinflammatory and fibrogenic genes. In this regard, HO-1 deficiency promotes epithelial-mesenchymal transition, a process that may underlie the transition of AKI to CKD.[235] Hence upregulation or overexpression of HO-1 may be an attractive protective strategy and therapeutic target against cellular injury.

Repair, Regeneration, and Role of Stem Cells

The renal tubular epithelial cells have the remarkable potential to regenerate functionally and structurally after ischemic or toxic insults. Once the insulting factors have been removed (e.g., reperfusion, cessation of toxic drugs, treatment of sepsis), minimally injured cells repair themselves without going through a "dedifferentiated" stage. More severely injured cells can, however, undergo this stage, which morphologically appears as flattened cells with an ill-defined brush border. Essentially there is proliferation of the viable cells that spread across the denuded basement membrane, after which they regain their differential character back into a normal tubular epithelial cell.

Functionally, there is reassembly of the cytoskeleton structure once ATP repletion occurs. It has been shown that the apical microvilli can be restored in as early as 24 hours after ATP depletion following mild injury. Similarly, Na^+-K^+-ATPase is lost from the apical location and relocates to the basolateral membranes within 24 hours. Lastly, although lipid polarity is eventually reestablished, it can lag behind reestablishment of protein polarity and is completed by approximately 10 days after injury.[236,237]

Growth factors and signals from injured cells are crucial at this stage to promote the timely and appropriate regenerative capacity of the viable cells. In animal models, administration of exogenous growth factors has been shown to accelerate renal recovery from injury. These include epidermal growth factor, insulin-like growth factor-I, α-melanocyte stimulating hormone, erythropoietin, hepatocyte growth factor, and bone-morphogenic protein-7 (BMP-7).[238-242] These effects have not yet been validated in human clinical trials of ATN.[243,244] They all likely increase GFR through direct hemodynamic effects and may therefore hasten tubular epithelial cell recovery.

There has been a major interest in studying the roles of progenitor/stem cells and mesenchymal stem cells in tubular epithelial cell injury. Investigators have now shown that different types of stem cells may reside in the renal architecture. In the human kidney, $CD133^+$ progenitor/

stem cells with regenerative potential have been identified.[245] These cells were able to differentiate in vitro toward renal epithelium and endothelium. When injected into mice with glycerol-induced AKI, they enhanced recovery from tubular damage, possibly by integrating into the proximal and distal tubules.[246] Mesenchymal stem cells are also present in the kidney and may have been derived from the embryonic tissue or bone marrow. Bone marrow cells are known to migrate to the kidney and participate in normal tubular epithelial cell turnover and repair after acute kidney injury.[247] Evidence of the kidney engraftment capacity of cells derived from male bone marrow is based on the presence of cells positive for the Y chromosome with epithelial cell markers in the tubules from kidneys of female recipient mice.[248,249] Although the evidence is not yet conclusive, there is evidence that stem cells as well as bone marrow–derived mesenchymal stem cells may contribute to structural and functional renal repair. Although the protective mechanisms have not yet been completely elucidated, they have been postulated to be less by direct differentiation into renal epithelial cells and more by paracrine effects such as supplying growth factors that stimulate the regeneration of tubular and resident stem cells. The "renotropism" exhibited by these cells may inform therapeutic options in the future once their roles are more fully defined.[250]

Further details of the role of stem cells in the kidney can be found in a separate chapter in this book (see Chapter 86).

Endothelial Dysfunction

Endothelial cells control vascular tone, regulation of blood flow to local tissue beds, modulation of coagulation and inflammation, and lastly permeability. Both ischemia and sepsis have profound effects on the endothelium. The renal vasculature and endothelium are particularly sensitive to these insults. When such an insult occurs, the endothelial bed becomes ineffective in performing its function, and the ensuing vascular dysregulation leads to continued ischemic conditions and further injury following the initial insult, which has been termed the extension phase of acute kidney injury.[121] Histopathologically this is seen as vascular congestion, edema formation, diminished microvascular blood flow, and margination and adherence of inflammatory cells to endothelial cells.

Vascular Tone

Conger and associates were among the first to demonstrate that postischemic rat kidneys manifest vasoconstriction in response to decreased renal perfusion pressure and hence cannot autoregulate blood flow even when total renal blood flow had returned to baseline values up to 1 week after injury.[251,252] Goligorsky and colleagues have extensively studied this increased constrictor response and found that it could be blocked by Ca^{2+} antagonists. They also demonstrated that the phenomenon of loss of normal eNOS function was due to a loss of vasodilator responses to acetylcholine and bradykinin. Selective inhibition, depletion, or deletion of inducible NOS (iNOS) has clearly shown renoprotective effects during ischemia.[253,254] Although still unclear, NO production from the endothelium (eNOS) may be impaired at the level of enzyme activity or modified by ROS to impair normal vasodilatory activity.[255] Hence overall, in ischemic AKI, *there is an imbalance of eNOS and iNOS.* Thus it is also proposed that due to a relative decrease in eNOS, secondary to endothelial dysfunction and damage, there is a loss of antithrombogenic properties of the endothelium, leading to increased susceptibility to microvascular thrombosis.[256]

Administration of L-arginine, the NO-donor molsidomine, or the eNOS co-factor tetrahydrobiopterin can preserve medullary perfusion and attenuate AKI induced by IRI; conversely the administration of N^ω-nitro-L-arginine methyl ester, an NO blocker, has been reported to aggravate the course of AKI following IRI injury. Although clearly important, these pharmacologic studies continue to assess the contribution of eNOS impairment in the overall course of reduced renal function following IRI.[257,258]

Cytoskeleton

The cytoskeletal structure of endothelial cells includes actin filament bundles that form a supportive ring around the periphery, along with the adhesion complexes that provide the integrity of the endothelial layer. The assembly and disassembly of actin filaments is regulated by a large family of actin-binding proteins, including ADF/cofilin. With ischemic injury the normal architecture of the actin cytoskeleton is markedly changed along with endothelial cell swelling, impaired cell-cell and cell-substrate adhesion, and loss of tight junction barrier functions. ATP depletion of cultured endothelial cells has been shown to induce dephosphorylation/activation of ADF/cofilin in a direct and concentration-dependant fashion. This activity results in depolymerized and severed actin filaments, seen as F-actin aggregates at the basolateral aspects of the cell.[259]

Recent studies also show a role of the sphingosine-1 phosphate receptor (S1PR) in maintaining structural integrity after AKI. Okusa and coworkers have shown that S1PRs in the proximal tubule are necessary for stress-induced cell survival, and $S1P_1R$ agonists are renoprotective via direct effects on tubular cells.[260]

Permeability

The endothelial barrier serves to separate the inner space of the blood vessel from the surrounding tissue and to control the exchange of cells and fluids between the two. It is defined by a combination of transcellular and paracellular pathways, the latter being a major contributor to the inflammation-induced barrier dysfunction.

Sutton and associates have studied the role of endothelial cells in acute kidney injury by a series of experiments utilizing florescent dextrans and two-photon intravital imaging. The increased microvascular permeability observed in AKI is likely a combination of numerous factors such as loss of endothelial monolayer, breakdown of perivascular matrix, alterations of endothelial cell contacts, and upregulated leukocyte-endothelial interactions. These investigators have shown that 24 hours after ischemic injury there was loss of localization in vascular endothelial cadherin immunostaining, suggesting severe alterations in the integrity of the adherens junctions of the renal microvasculature.[261] In vivo two-photon imaging demonstrated a loss of capillary barrier function within 2 hours of reperfusion as evidenced by leakiness of high-molecular-weight dextrans (>300,000 Da) into the interstitial space.

Critical constituents of the perivascular matrix, including collagen IV, are known to be substrates of MMP-2 and MMP-9, which are collectively known as gelatinases. Breakdown of barrier function may also be due to MMP-2 or MMP-9 activation, and this upregulation is temporally correlated with an increase in microvascular permeability.[121,262] MMP-9 gene deletion stabilizes microvascular density following ischemic AKI in part by preserving tissue VEGF levels.[263] In addition, minocycline, a broad-based MMP inhibitor and the gelatinase-specific inhibitor ABT-518 both ameliorated the increase in microvascular permeability in this model. Taken together, many findings indicate that the loss of endothelial cells following ischemic injury is not a major contributor to altered microvascular permeability, although renal microvascular endothelial cells are vulnerable to the initiation of apoptotic mechanisms following ischemic injury that can ultimately impact microvascular density[264] (Figure 31.8).

Coagulation

The endothelial cell plays a central role in coagulation via its interaction with protein C through the EPCR and thrombomodulin. The protein C pathway helps to maintain normal homeostasis and limits inflammatory responses. Protein C is activated by thrombin-mediated cleavage, and the rate of this reaction is further augmented 1000-fold when thrombin binds to the endothelial cell surface receptor protein thrombomodulin. The activation rate of protein C is further increased by approximately 10-fold when EPCR binds protein C and presents it to the thrombin-thrombomodulin complex. Activated protein C essentially then has antithrombotic actions and profibrinolytic properties and participates in numerous antiinflammatory and cytoprotective pathways to restore normal homeostasis.[265] Based on these properties, the endothelial cell plays an absolutely essential and critical role in maintaining a normal

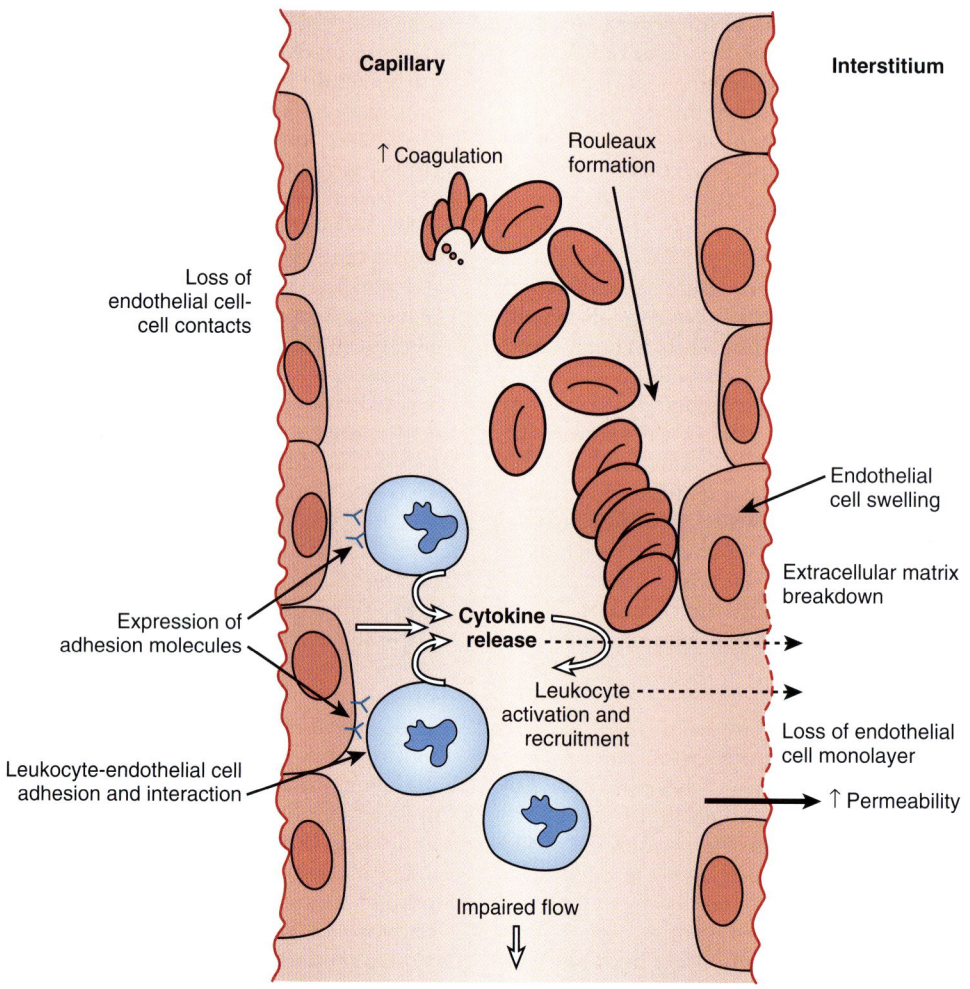

Figure 31.8 Key events in endothelial cell activation and injury. Ischemia causes upregulation and expression of genes coding for various cell surface proteins such as E-(endothelial) and P-(platelet) selectin, vascular cell adhesion molecule-1 (VCAM-1), intercellular adhesion molecule-1 (ICAM-1), and reduced thrombomodulin (TM). Activated leukocytes adhere to endothelial cells through these adhesion molecules. Endothelial injury increases the production of endothelin-1 and decreases endothelial nitric oxide synthase (eNOS), which serve to induce vasoconstriction and platelet aggregation. The combination of leukocyte adhesion and activation, platelet aggregation, and endothelial injury serves as the platform for vascular congestion of the medullary microvasculature. There are permeability defects between endothelial cells as a result of tight and adherens junctional alterations. (From Sharfuddin A, Molitoris B: Epithelial cell injury. In Vincent JL, Hall JB, editors: *Encyclopedia of intensive care medicine*, New York, 2012, Springer.)

and healthy vasculature and endothelial bed. In AKI, ultimately microvascular function is compromised, resulting in disseminated intravascular coagulation and microvascular thrombosis, decreased tissue perfusion, and hypoxemia leading to organ dysfunction/failure. It has been shown that both pretreatment and postinjury treatment with soluble thrombomodulin attenuates renal injury with minimization of vascular permeability defects with improvement in capillary renal blood flow.[113]

The leukocyte and the endothelial cell are dynamically involved in the process of adherence of leukocytes to the vascular endothelium. Leukocyte activation and its release of cytokines require signals through chemokines circulating in the bloodstream or through direct contact with the endothelium. Rolling leukocytes can be activated by chemoattractants such as complement C5a and platelet-activating factor. Once activated, leukocyte integrins bind to endothelial ligands to promote firm adhesion. β_2-integrin (CD18) seems to be the most important ligand for neutrophil adherence. These interactions with the endothelium are mediated through endothelial adhesion molecules that are upregulated during ischemic conditions.[266]

The initial phase starts with slow neutrophil migration mediated by tethering interactions between selectins and their endothelial cell ligands. Singbartl and colleagues have found that platelet P-selectin and not endothelial P-selectin was the main determinant in neutrophil-mediated ischemic renal injury.[266] There is also significant protection from both ischemic injury and mortality by blockade of the shared ligand to all three selectins (E-, P-, and L-selectin), which seems to be dependent on the presence of a key fucosyl sugar on the selectin ligand.[267,268] In a CLP model of septic azotemia, mice gene-deficient for E-selectin or P-selectin or both were completely protected. Furthermore, selectin-deficient mice demonstrated similar intraperitoneal leukocyte recruitment but altered cytokine levels when compared to wild-type mice.[269] Therefore it is possible that selectins exert their effects through modulation of systemic cytokine profiles rather than through engagement in leukocyte-endothelial cell interactions.[270]

Inflammation

Altered endothelial cell function also mediates inflammation, a hallmark of ischemic injury that has been the subject of numerous recent studies. Ischemia induces the increased expression of a number of leukocyte adhesion molecules such as P-selectin, E-selectin, and intercellular adhesion molecule (ICAM) and B7-1. Consequently, it has also been shown that strategies to pharmacologically block or genetically ablate the expression of these molecules are protective against ischemic or septic AKI.[177] Investigators have also shown that T cells also play a major role in vascular permeability during ischemic injury. Gene microarray analysis showed the production of TNF-α and IFN-γ protein was increased in CD3 and CD4 T cells from the blood and kidney after ischemia. Furthermore, it has also been demonstrated that in CD3, CD4, and CD8 T cell–deficient mice, there is a significantly attenuated rise in renal vascular permeability after ischemic injury. Hence T cells directly contribute to the increased vascular permeability, potentially through T cell cytokine production.[213,271] Another feature noted during inflammation and endothelial cell injury is the phenomenon of erythrocyte trapping with rouleaux formation, prolonging the reduction in renal blood flow and exacerbating tubular injury.[272]

DNA microarray analysis of ischemic kidneys from TLR4-sufficient and TLR4-deficient mice showed that pentraxin 3 (PTX3), an endothelial induced protein, was upregulated only on the former, while transgenic knockout of PTX3 ameliorated AKI. PTX3 was shown to be expressed predominantly on peritubular endothelia of the outer medulla of the kidney in control mice and increased PTX3 protein in the kidney and the plasma. Stimulation studies performed in primary renal endothelial cells suggest that endothelial PTX3 was induced by pathways involving TLR4 and ROS and demonstrated that these effects could be inhibited by conditional endothelial knockout of myeloid differentiation. Compared to wild-type mice, PTX3 knockout mice had decreased endothelial expression of cell adhesion molecules at 4 hours of reperfusion, possibly contributing to a decreased early maladaptive inflammation in the kidneys of knockout mice, whereas later at 24 hours of reperfusion, PTX3 knockout increased expression of endothelial adhesion molecules when regulatory and reparative leukocytes enter the kidney. Thus endothelial PTX3 plays a pivotal role in the pathogenesis of ischemic acute kidney injury.[273]

The role of glomerular endothelial injury is unclear in AKI. Recent work in a mouse model of LPS-induced sepsis showed decreased abundance of endothelial surface layer heparan sulfate proteoglycans and sialic acid, leading to albuminuria, likely reflecting altered glomerular filtration permselectivity and decreased expression of VEGF. LPS treatment also decreased the GFR, caused ultrastructural alterations in the glomerular endothelium, and lowered the density of glomerular endothelial cell fenestrae. These LPS-induced effects were diminished in TNF receptor 1 (TNFR1) knockout mice, suggesting the role of TNF-α activation of TNFR1, and intravenous administration of TNF also led to decreased GFR and led to loss of glomerular endothelial cell fenestrae, increased fenestrae diameter, and damage to the glomerular endothelial surface layer. Thus glomerular endothelial injury, mediated by TNF-α and decreased VEGF levels, extends the development and progression of AKI and albuminuria in the LPS model of sepsis in the mouse.[274]

Long-Term Effects of Endothelial Cell Injury

There is also evidence showing that acute injury to endothelial cells may have long-term chronic implications, as shown in a series of publications by Basile and coworkers, where the investigators have shown significant reduction in blood vessel density following ischemic injury, leading to the phenomenon of vascular dropout.[275] Vascular dropout was verified by Horbelt and associates, who found a drop in the vascular density by almost 45% at 4 weeks after an ischemic insult.[264] These findings suggest that unlike the renal epithelial tubular cells, the renal vascular system lacks comparable regenerative potential. It is not clear yet whether apoptosis and/or necrosis play a major role in endothelial cell dropout. Ischemia has been shown to inhibit the angiogenic protein VEGF while inducing ADAMTS1, thought to be a VEGF inhibitor.[276] It was then postulated that the lack of vascular repair could be due to lack of VEGF, as shown by experiments where administration of VEGF-121 preserved the microvascular density.[276] Reduction of the microvasculature density increases hypoxia-mediated fibrosis and alters usual hemodynamics, which may lead to hypertension. Thus loss of microvasculature density and its consequential effects may play a critical role in the progression of CKD following initial recovery from ischemia-reperfusion–induced AKI.[275]

Furthermore, renal oxidative stress has been shown to persist with resultant increased Ang II sensitivity in rats following recovery from ischemia-reperfusion–induced AKI after 5 weeks. Post-AKI rats showed significantly enhanced renal vasoconstrictor responses to Ang II, and treatment of AKI rats with apocynin normalized these responses. The renal messenger RNA (mRNA) expression for common reduced nicotinamide adenine dinucleotide phosphate (NADPH) oxidase subunits was not altered in kidneys following recovery from AKI; however, mRNA screening using polymerase chain reaction arrays suggested that post-AKI rats had decreased renal glutathione peroxidase 3 mRNA and an increased expression of other prooxidant genes such as lactoperoxidase, myeloperoxidase, and dual oxidase-1. Following infusion with Ang II, renal fibrosis was enhanced in post-AKI rats. The profibrotic response was significantly attenuated in rats treated with apocynin. These data suggest that there is sustained renal oxidant stress following recovery from AKI that alters the hemodynamic and fibrotic responses to Ang II and may contribute to the transition to CKD following AKI.[277] This also highlights the importance of managing recovering AKI very carefully to avoid further insults that may enhance ROS or sensitivity to Ang II.

Targets of Therapy—Role of Endothelial Progenitor Cells

Due to the numerous mechanisms in initiating and continuing existing injury, there are several targets available to reduce the effect of endothelial cell injury and potentially minimize actual endothelial cell damage itself. The concept of restoration of vascular supply to damaged or ischemic organs for accelerating their regeneration is well established. One therapeutic strategy based on this concept is the delivery of angiogenic factors. The current view is that endothelial progenitor cells (EPCs) are a heterogeneous group, which by latest count originates from hematopoietic stem cells or their angioblastic subpopulation and mesenchymal stem cells. In the bone marrow these cells are characterized by the combination of surface markers such as CD34, VEGFR-2 (Flk-1), and an early marker CD133; moreover, in the blood they may express markers of hematopoietic stem cells, c-kit and Sca-1. Upon further differentiation, these cells lose CD133 and acquire vascular endothelial cadherin and von Willebrand factor.[278]

There is a growing body of evidence that EPCs may improve vascular regeneration in different ischemic organs. Recent data also suggest that EPCs are mobilized after acute ischemic injury and are recruited in the ischemic kidney, where they can ameliorate AKI through paracrine effects and repair of the injured renal microvasculature.[279] Transplanting intact endothelial cells in injured ischemic vasculature has also shown promise in reduction of ischemic injury. Although the underlying mechanisms are not fully understood, replacement of damaged cells will mainly be generated by neighboring cells or cells recruited from the circulation.[279] Microvesicles derived from EPCs have also been shown to protect the kidney from ischemic acute injury by delivering their RNA content, the microRNA (miRNA) cargo of which contributes to reprogramming hypoxic resident renal cells to a regenerative program.[280]

In summary, the endothelial cell is now recognized as a major contributor to the initiation and extension of AKI, and targeting the mechanisms to block these dysfunctional intracellular processes may be of therapeutic value (see Figure 31.8).

Effects of Acute Kidney Injury on Distant Organs

There is accumulating evidence that in many cases AKI is a systemic condition that can potentially cause alterations in other organs of the body, clinically evidenced by the fact that patients experience an increase in mortality after AKI, much of which is due to extrarenal complications. Kelly and associates have demonstrated the effects of renal ischemia on cardiac tissues.[110] Induction of IL-1, TNF-α, and ICAM-1 mRNA was seen in cardiac tissues as early as 6 hours after renal ischemic injury and remained elevated up to 48 hours after renal ischemic injury. There was also a significant increase in myeloperoxidase activity in the heart and liver, apart from the kidneys. The increase in cardiac myeloperoxidase activity could be prevented by administration of anti–ICAM-1 antibody at the time of renal ischemia. At 48 hours, cardiac function evaluation by echocardiography also revealed increases in left ventricular end systolic and diastolic diameter and decreased fractional shortening. As little as 15 minutes of ischemia also resulted in significantly more apoptosis in cardiac tissue.[110] In transgenic sickle mice, bilateral renal IRI results in marked cardiac vascular congestion and increased serum amyloid P component (the murine equivalent of C-reactive protein). Kramer and colleagues have shown that renal ischemic injury leads to an increase in pulmonary vascular permeability defects that are mediated through macrophages.[281] Furthermore, they showed that in a rat model of bilateral renal ischemic injury or nephrectomy, there was downregulation of lung epithelial Na channel, Na^+-K^+-ATPase, and aquaporin-5 expression, but not in unilateral ischemic models, suggesting the role of uremic toxins in modulating these effects in the lung.[282] Lui and colleagues have also shown effects of AKI on functional changes in the brain. Mice with AKI had increased neuronal pyknosis and microgliosis in the brain, with increased levels of the proinflammatory chemokines keratinocyte-derived chemoattractant and granulocyte colony-stimulating factor in the cerebral cortex and hippocampus and increased expression of glial fibrillary acidic protein in astrocytes in the cortex and corpus callosum. In addition, extravasation of Evans blue dye into the brain suggested that the blood-brain barrier was disrupted in mice with AKI.[283]

Many of the same processes involved in kidney-lung, kidney-heart, and kidney-brain interactions have been observed in the liver: increased neutrophil infiltration, vascular congestion, and vascular permeability after AKI. Following experimental AKI, levels of hepatic TNF-α, IL-6, IL-17A, ICM-1, keratinocyte-derived chemoattractant, IL-10, and MCP-1 are increased. The presence of AKI before a "second-hit" ischemic hepatic injury further exacerbates liver injury as well, suggesting an ongoing crosstalk between kidney and liver.

Conversely, other organs also regulate ischemic renal injury. Imai and coworkers have demonstrated the role of lung injury in inducing renal damage. They found that in rabbits, injurious lung ventilatory strategies (high tidal volume and low peak end-expiratory pressure) alone were sufficient to induce renal epithelial cell apoptosis. This finding was further substantiated by the fact that plasma obtained from rabbits that underwent the injurious ventilation strategy induced greater apoptosis in cultured LLC-RK$_1$ cells in vitro, suggesting that circulating soluble factors associated with the injurious mechanical ventilation might be involved in this process.[284]

An example of extrarenal organs regulating ischemic AKI is evidenced by the effect of brain death on kidney transplants. Traumatic brain injury elicits a cytokine and inflammatory response. These cytokines result in renal inflammation in kidney transplants from brain-dead donors, distinct from living or cardiac-death donors.[285] Pretransplantation biopsies of brain-dead donor kidneys contain notably more infiltrating T lymphocytes and macrophages. Reperfusion of kidneys from brain-dead donors is associated with the instantaneous release of inflammatory cytokines, such as granulocyte colony-stimulating factor, IL-6, IL-9, IL-16, and MCP-1. In contrast, kidneys from living and cardiac-death donors show a more modest cytokine response with release of IL-6 and small amounts of MCP-1.[286] Since AKI is associated with high mortality and morbidity, these studies indicate that multiorgan crosstalk that occurs in the setting of AKI is likely to be a major contributor to nonrenal organ dysfunction that may mediate clinically observable events such as cardiac, pulmonary, and central nervous system events.

Last is the issue of unilateral AKI affecting contralateral kidney function. In a model where the ischemia-reperfusion–injured kidney was removed after 5 weeks to isolate effects on the untouched kidney, challenge with elevated dietary sodium levels manifested a significant increase in blood pressure relative to sham-operated controls. Similarly, contralateral kidneys had impaired pressure natriuresis and hemodynamic responses, but reductions in vascular density were observed in the contralateral kidney. However, contralateral kidneys contained interstitial cells, some of which were identified as activated (low CD62L/CD4$^+$) T lymphocytes. Taken together, these data suggest that the salt-sensitive features of AKI on hypertension and CKD can be segregated such that effects on hemodynamics and hypertension may develop independent of direct renal damage.[287]

EVALUATION OF ACUTE KIDNEY INJURY

CLINICAL ASSESSMENT, URINARY FINDINGS, AND BLOOD AND RADIOGRAPHIC EVALUATION

The assessment of the patient with AKI requires a meticulous history and physical examination; comprehensive review of medical records; evaluation of urinary findings, including the urinary sediment; review of laboratory tests; renal imaging; and, when appropriate, kidney biopsy.[288]

Analysis of serum creatinine concentration over time is invaluable for differentiating acute from chronic kidney disease and identifying the timing of events that precipitated the acute decline in kidney function. The presence of an acute process is easily confirmed if review of laboratory records reveals a sudden rise in BUN and serum creatinine concentrations from previously stable baseline values. Spurious causes of elevated BUN and serum creatinine levels must be excluded before a diagnosis of AKI is made. When prior BUN and serum creatinine measurements are not available, key findings that suggest that a chronic process is present include physical manifestations of hyperparathyroidism (resorption of distal phalangeal tufts or lateral aspect of clavicles), band keratopathy, "half-and-half" nails, and small echogenic kidneys on radiographic imaging. Enlarged kidneys do not necessarily rule out a chronic process as diabetic nephropathy, human immunodeficiency virus–associated nephropathy, amyloidosis, and polycystic kidney disease are characterized by increased kidney size even with moderate to advanced CKD. Anemia is a less useful differentiating feature as it is often present in both AKI and CKD. Once the presence of AKI has been confirmed, attention should focus on patient, urine, laboratory, and radiographic assessments to help differentiate among prerenal, intrinsic, and postrenal processes to permit identification of the cause of AKI and to guide treatment.

CLINICAL ASSESSMENT OF THE PATIENT

Prerenal AKI should be suspected in clinical settings associated with intravascular volume depletion, including hemorrhage, excessive gastrointestinal (e.g., vomiting or diarrhea), urinary, or insensible fluid losses and severe burns, or with reduced EABV due to congestive heart failure, liver disease, or nephrotic syndrome (Table 31.8). The risk for intravascular volume depletion is increased in comatose, sedated, or obtunded patients and in patients with restricted access to salt and water. Clinical clues to a prerenal cause of AKI on history include patient report of excessive thirst, orthostatic light-headedness or dizziness, significant diarrhea and/or vomiting, diuretic use, and recent use of medications that alter intrarenal hemodynamics, including NSAIDs, and inhibitors of the RAAS, including direct renin inhibitors, ACE inhibitors, and ARBs. Findings suggestive of volume depletion on physical examination may include orthostatic hypotension (postural fall in diastolic blood pressure greater than 10 mm Hg) and tachycardia (postural increase in heart rate greater than 10 beats/min), reduced jugular venous pressure, diminished skin turgor, dry mucous membranes, and the absence of axillary sweat. However, overt signs and symptoms of hypovolemia do not usually manifest until extracellular fluid volume has fallen by more than 10% to 20%. In addition, in patients with heart failure or liver disease, renal hypoperfusion may be present despite total body volume overload. Findings on physical examination of peripheral edema, pulmonary vascular congestion, pleural effusion, cardiomegaly, gallop rhythms, elevated jugular venous pressure, or hepatic congestion may point to a state of reduced cardiac output and decreased effective intravascular volume. The presence of acute or chronic liver disease is suggested by evidence of icterus, ascites, splenomegaly, palmar erythema, telangiectasia, and caput medusae.

Table 31.8 Useful Clinical Features, Urinary Findings, and Confirmatory Tests in the Differential Diagnosis of Acute Kidney Injury

Cause of Acute Kidney Injury	Some Suggestive Clinical Features	Typical Urinalysis Results	Some Confirmatory Tests
Prerenal azotemia	Evidence of true volume depletion (thirst, postural or absolute hypotension and tachycardia, low jugular venous pressure, dry mucous membranes and axillae, weight loss, fluid output greater than input) or decreased effective circulatory volume (e.g., heart failure, liver failure), treatment with NSAID, diuretic, or ACE inhibitor/ARB	Hyaline casts $FE_{Na} < 1\%$ $U_{Na} < 10$ mmol/L SG > 1.018	Occasionally requires invasive hemodynamic monitoring; rapid resolution of AKI with restoration of renal perfusion
Diseases Involving Large Renal Vessels			
Renal artery thrombosis	History of atrial fibrillation or recent myocardial infarction, nausea, vomiting, flank or abdominal pain	Mild proteinuria Occasionally RBCs	Elevated LDH level with normal transaminase levels, renal arteriogram, MAG3 renal scan, MRA*
Atheroembolism	Usually age > 50 yr, recent manipulation of aorta, retinal plaques, subcutaneous nodules, palpable purpura, livedo reticularis	Often normal Eosinophiluria Rarely casts	Eosinophilia, hypocomplementemia, skin biopsy, renal biopsy
Renal vein thrombosis	Evidence of nephrotic syndrome or pulmonary embolism, flank pain	Proteinuria, hematuria	Inferior venacavogram, Doppler flow studies, MRV*
Diseases of Small Renal Vessels and Glomeruli			
Glomerulonephritis or vasculitis	Compatible clinical history (e.g., recent infection), sinusitis, lung hemorrhage, rash or skin ulcers, arthralgias, hypertension, edema	RBC or granular casts, RBCs, white blood cells, proteinuria	Low complement levels; positive antineutrophil cytoplasmic antibodies, anti–glomerular basement membrane antibodies, anti–streptolysin O antibodies, anti-DNase, cryoglobulins; renal biopsy
HUS/TTP	Compatible clinical history (e.g., recent gastrointestinal infection, cyclosporine, anovulants), pallor, ecchymoses, neurologic findings	May be normal, RBCs, mild proteinuria, rarely RBC or granular casts	Anemia, thrombocytopenia, schistocytes on peripheral blood smear, low haptoglobin level, increased LDH, renal biopsy
Malignant hypertension	Severe hypertension with headaches, cardiac failure, retinopathy, neurologic dysfunction, papilledema	May be normal, RBCs, mild proteinuria, rarely RBC casts	LVH by echocardiography or ECG, resolution of AKI with BP control
Ischemic or Nephrotoxic Acute Tubular Necrosis			
Ischemia	Recent hemorrhage, hypotension, surgery often in combination with vasoactive medication (e.g., ACE inhibitor, NSAID)	Muddy-brown granular or tubular epithelial cell casts $FE_{Na} > 1\%$, $U_{Na} > 20$ mmol/L SG ≈ 1.010	Clinical assessment and urinalysis usually inform diagnosis
Exogenous toxin	Recent contrast medium–enhanced procedure; nephrotoxic medications; certain chemotherapeutic agents often with coexistent volume depletion, sepsis, or chronic kidney disease	Muddy-brown granular or tubular epithelial cell casts $FE_{Na} > 1\%$, $U_{Na} > 20$ mmol/L SG ≈ 1.010	Clinical assessment and urinalysis usually inform diagnosis
Endogenous toxin	History suggestive of rhabdomyolysis (coma, seizures, drug abuse, trauma)	Urine supernatant tests positive for heme in absence of RBCs	Hyperkalemia, hyperphosphatemia, hypocalcemia, increased CK, myoglobin
	History suggestive of hemolysis (recent blood transfusion)	Urine supernatant pink and tests positive for heme in absence of RBCs	Hyperkalemia, hyperphosphatemia, hypocalcemia, hyperuricemia, and free circulating hemoglobin
	History suggestive of tumor lysis (recent chemotherapy), myeloma (bone pain), or ethylene glycol ingestion	Urate crystals, dipstick-negative proteinuria, oxalate crystals, respectively	Hyperuricemia, hyperkalemia, hyperphosphatemia (for tumor lysis); circulating or urinary monoclonal protein (for myeloma); toxicology screen, acidosis, osmolal gap (for ethylene glycol)

Table 31.8	Useful Clinical Features, Urinary Findings, and Confirmatory Tests in the Differential Diagnosis of Acute Kidney Injury (Continued)		
Cause of Acute Kidney Injury	Some Suggestive Clinical Features	Typical Urinalysis Results	Some Confirmatory Tests
Diseases of the Tubulointerstitium			
Allergic interstitial nephritis	Recent ingestion of drug and fever, rash, loin pain, or arthralgias	White blood cell casts, white blood cells (frequently eosinophiluria), RBCs, rarely RBC casts, proteinuria (occasionally nephritic)	Systemic eosinophilia, renal biopsy
Acute bilateral pyelonephritis	Fever, flank pain and tenderness, toxic state	Leukocytes, occasionally white blood cell casts, RBCs, bacteria	Urine and blood cultures
Postrenal AKI	Abdominal and flank pain, palpable bladder	Frequently normal, hematuria if stones, prostatic hypertrophy	Plain abdominal radiography, renal ultrasonography, postvoid residual bladder volume, computed tomography, retrograde or antegrade pyelography

*Contrast-enhanced MRA and MRV should be used with extreme caution in patients with AKI.
ACE, Angiotensin-converting enzyme; AKI, acute kidney injury; ARB, angiotensin receptor blocker; BP, blood pressure; CK, creatine kinase; DNase, deoxyribonuclease; ECG, electrocardiography; FE_{Na}, fractional excretion of sodium; HUS, hemolytic uremic syndrome; LDH, lactate dehydrogenase; LVH, left ventricular hypertrophy; MAG3, mercaptoacetyltriglycine; MRA, magnetic resonance angiography; MRV, magnetic resonance venography; NSAID, nonsteroidal antiinflammatory drug; RBC, red blood cell; SG, specific gravity; TTP, thrombotic thrombocytopenic purpura; U_{Na}, urinary sodium concentration.

In select critically ill patients, invasive hemodynamic monitoring using central venous or pulmonary artery catheters or ultrasonography of the heart and central veins may assist in assessing intravascular volume status. Definitive diagnosis of prerenal AKI is usually based on prompt resolution of AKI after restoration of renal perfusion. In patients with underlying systolic heart failure, restoration of renal perfusion may be difficult and may require the use of inotropic support.

There is a high likelihood of ischemic ATN if AKI follows a period of severe renal hypoperfusion and the impairment in kidney function persists or worsens despite restoration of renal perfusion. It should be noted, however, that significant hypotension is evident in fewer than 50% of patients with postsurgical ATN.[289] Although septic shock is a common cause of ATN, ATN may also develop in sepsis in the absence of overt hypotension.[289,290] The diagnosis of nephrotoxic ATN requires a comprehensive review of all clinical, pharmacy, nursing, radiographic, and procedural notes for evidence of administration of nephrotoxic agents. Pigment-induced ATN may be suspected if the clinical assessment reveals risk factors for rhabdomyolysis (e.g., seizures, excessive exercise, alcohol or drug abuse, treatment with statins, prolonged immobilization, limb ischemia, crush injury) or hemolysis, as well as selected signs and symptoms of the former (e.g., muscle tenderness, weakness, evidence of trauma or prolonged immobilization).[291-294]

While most AKI is prerenal or ischemic, nephrotoxic, or septic ATN, patients should be carefully evaluated for other intrinsic renal parenchymal processes as their management and prognosis may differ substantially. Flank pain may be a prominent symptom of acute renal artery or renal vein occlusion, acute pyelonephritis, and rarely necrotizing glomerulonephritis.[295-297] Interstitial edema leading to distension of the renal capsule and flank pain may be seen in up to one-third of patients with AIN.[298] Dermatologic examination is also important as a maculopapular rash may accompany allergic interstitial nephritis; subcutaneous nodules, livedo reticularis, digital ischemia, and palpable purpura may suggest atheroembolism or vasculitis; a malar butterfly rash may be associated with systemic lupus erythematosus; and impetigo or needle tracks from intravenous drug use may underlie infection-associated glomerulonephritis. Ophthalmologic examination is useful to assess for signs of atheroembolism; hypertensive or diabetic retinopathy; the keratitis, uveitis, and iritis of autoimmune vasculitides; icterus; and the rare but nevertheless pathognomonic band keratopathy of hypercalcemia and flecked retina of hyperoxalemia. Uveitis may also be an indicator of coexistent allergic interstitial nephritis, sarcoidosis, and the TINU (tubulointerstitial nephritis and uveitis) syndrome.[299] Examination of the ears, nose, and throat may reveal conductive deafness and mucosal inflammation or ulceration suggestive of necrotizing granulomatous vasculitis or the neural deafness caused by aminoglycoside toxicity. Respiratory failure, particularly if associated with hemoptysis, suggests the presence of pulmonary renal syndrome, and the stigmata of severe chronic liver disease suggest the possibility of HRS. Cardiovascular assessment may reveal marked elevation in systemic blood pressure, suggesting malignant hypertension or scleroderma, or demonstrate a new arrhythmia or murmur, suggesting a potential source of thromboemboli or subacute bacterial endocarditis (acute glomerulonephritis), respectively. Chest or abdominal pain and reduced pulses in the lower limbs should suggest aortic dissection or, rarely, Takayasu arteritis. Abdominal pain and nausea are frequent clinical correlates of atheroembolic disease, commonly in patients who have recently undergone angiographic evaluation, particularly in the presence of widespread atheromatous disease. The presence of a tensely distended abdomen may indicate the presence of ACS and should prompt transduction of bladder pressure.[57] Pallor and recent bruising are important clues to the thrombotic microangiopathies, and the combination of bleeding and fever should raise the possibility of AKI resulting from viral hemorrhagic fevers. A recent jejunoileal bypass may be a vital clue to oxalosis, a rare but reversible cause of AKI following bariatric surgery.[300] Hyperreflexia and asterixis often portend the development of uremic encephalopathy or may, in the presence of focal neurologic signs, suggest a diagnosis of thrombotic microangiopathy (i.e., hemolytic uremic syndrome [HUS] or thrombotic thrombocytopenic purpura [TTP], see Chapter 35).

Postrenal AKI may be asymptomatic if obstruction to the drainage of urine develops gradually. While anuria will be seen in complete obstruction, urine volume may be normal or even increased in the setting of partial obstruction. A pattern of fluctuating urine output may also be seen in some patients with partial obstruction. Suprapubic or flank pain may be the presenting complaint if there is acute distension of the bladder or renal collecting system and capsule, respectively. Colicky flank pain radiating to the groin suggests acute ureteral obstruction, most commonly from renal stone disease. Prostatic disease should be suspected in older men with a history of nocturia, urinary frequency, urgency, or hesitancy and an enlarged prostate on rectal examination. Urinary retention may be exacerbated acutely in such patients by medications with anticholinergic properties, such as antihistamine agents and antidepressants. Rectal or pelvic examination may reveal obstructing tumors in female patients. Neurogenic bladder is a likely diagnosis in patients with spinal cord injury or autonomic insufficiency and should be suspected in patients with long-standing diabetes mellitus. Bladder distension may be evident on abdominal percussion and palpation in patients with bladder neck or urethral obstruction. Definitive diagnosis of postrenal AKI usually relies on examination of the postvoid bladder volume and radiographic evaluation of the upper urinary tract and is confirmed by improvement in kidney function following relief of the obstruction.

URINE ASSESSMENT

Urine volume is a relatively unhelpful parameter in differentiating the various forms and causes of AKI. Anuria can be seen with complete urinary tract obstruction but can also be seen with severe prerenal or intrinsic renal disease (e.g., renal artery occlusion, severe proliferative glomerulonephritis or vasculitis, bilateral cortical necrosis). Wide fluctuation in urine output may be suggestive of intermittent obstruction. Patients with partial urinary tract obstruction may present with polyuria caused by secondary impairment of urinary concentrating mechanisms.

Assessment of the urine is essential in patients with AKI and is an inexpensive and useful diagnostic tool.[301-303] Measured urine specific gravity above 1.015 to 1.020 often accompanies prerenal AKI, although impaired urinary concentration may be present in patients with underlying CKD or as a result of diuretic therapy. Acute glomerulonephritis may also present with concentrated urine. Isosthenuria (a urine specific gravity of 1.010, similar to that of plasma) is characteristic of ATN. Hematuria on dipstick may result from urologic trauma from catheterization, urologic disease, interstitial nephritis, acute glomerulonephritis, atheroembolic disease, renal infarction, or pigment (hemoglobinuric or myoglobinuric) nephropathy. The latter are suggested when the dipstick test for blood is positive but there are no RBCs seen on microscopic examination of the urinary sediment.

Examination of the urinary sediment of a centrifuged urine specimen complements the dipstick analysis and is highly valuable for distinguishing among the various forms of AKI. The sediment should be inspected for the presence of cells, casts, and crystals (Table 31.9). In prerenal AKI, the urine sediment is typically bland (i.e., devoid of cells or casts) but may contain transparent hyaline casts. Hyaline casts are formed in concentrated urine from normal urinary constituents, principally Tamm-Horsfall protein secreted by epithelial cells of the loop of Henle. Postrenal AKI may also present with a bland urine sediment, although hematuria is common in patients with intraluminal obstruction (e.g., stones, sloughed papilla, blood clot) or prostatic disease. Renal tubular epithelial cells, epithelial cell casts, and pigmented "muddy-brown" granular casts are characteristic of ischemic or nephrotoxic ATN. They may be found in association with microscopic hematuria and mild "tubular" proteinuria (<1 g/day). Casts may be absent in approximately 20% to 30% of patients with ischemic or nephrotoxic ATN and are not a requisite for diagnosis[301,304]; however, semiquantitative scoring systems have been developed to assess the presence of epithelial cells and casts in patients with AKI to assist in the diagnosis of ATN and correlate with the clinical course.[302,305,306] RBC casts are almost always indicative of acute glomerular disease but may be observed, albeit rarely, in AIN. Dysmorphic RBCs, best seen using phase-contrast microscopy, are a more common urinary finding in patients with glomerular injury but are a less specific finding than RBC casts. Urine sediment abnormalities vary in diseases involving preglomerular blood vessels, such as HUS, TTP, atheroembolic disease, and vasculitis involving medium-sized or large vessels, and range from benign to overtly nephritic. White blood cell casts and nonpigmented granular casts suggest interstitial nephritis, while broad granular casts are characteristic of CKD and probably reflect interstitial fibrosis and dilation of tubules. Eosinophiluria (between 1% and 50% of urine leukocytes) is a common finding (90%) in drug-induced allergic interstitial nephritis.[307,308] However, eosinophiluria has poor sensitivity and specificity for the diagnosis of AIN, with eosinophiluria of 1% to greater than 5% occurring in a variety of other diseases, including atheroembolization, ischemic and nephrotoxic AKI, proliferative glomerulonephritis, pyelonephritis, cystitis, and prostatitis. In a series of 566 patients who had urinary eosinophil testing and renal histology from kidney biopsy, eosinophiluria only had 31% sensitivity and 68% specificity for the diagnosis of interstitial nephritis.[309] Uric acid crystals (pleomorphic) may be seen in the urine in prerenal AKI but should raise the possibility of acute urate

Table 31.9	Urine Sediment in the Differential Diagnosis of Acute Kidney Injury

Normal or Few Red Blood Cells or White Blood Cells

Prerenal azotemia
Arterial thrombosis or embolism
Preglomerular vasculitis
HUS/TTP
Scleroderma crisis
Postrenal AKI

Granular Casts

Acute tubular necrosis
Glomerulonephritis or vasculitis
Interstitial nephritis

Red Blood Cell Casts

Glomerulonephritis or vasculitis
Malignant hypertension
Rarely interstitial nephritis

White Blood Cell Casts

Acute interstitial nephritis or exudative glomerulonephritis
Severe pyelonephritis
Marked leukemic or lymphomatous infiltration

Eosinophiluria (>5%)

Allergic interstitial nephritis (antibiotics ≫ NSAIDs)
Atheroembolism

Crystalluria

Acute urate nephropathy
Calcium oxalate (ethylene glycol intoxication)
Acyclovir
Indinavir
Sulfonamides
Methotrexate

HUS, Hemolytic uremic syndrome; NSAID, nonsteroidal antiinflammatory drug; TTP, thrombotic thrombocytopenic purpura.

---

nephropathy if seen in abundance. Oxalate crystalluria (either needle- or dumbbell-shaped monohydrate crystals or envelope-shaped dihydrate crystals) may suggest a diagnosis of ethylene glycol toxicity.[310]

Increased urinary protein excretion, characteristically less than 1 g/day, is a common finding in ischemic or nephrotoxic ATN and reflects failure of both injured proximal tubular cells to reabsorb normally filtered protein and excretion of cellular debris (tubular proteinuria). Proteinuria greater than 1 g/day suggests injury to the glomerular ultrafiltration barrier (glomerular proteinuria) or excretion of light chains.[100,311] The latter are not detected by conventional dipsticks (which detect albumin) and must be sought by other means (e.g., sulfosalicylic acid test). Heavy proteinuria is also a frequent finding (80%) in patients with allergic interstitial nephritis triggered by NSAIDs. In addition to acute interstitial inflammation, these patients have a glomerular lesion that is almost identical to minimal change disease.[312] A similar syndrome has been reported in patients receiving other agents such as ampicillin, rifampin, and interferon alfa.[313,314]

Hemolysis and rhabdomyolysis may often be differentiated by inspection of plasma, which is characteristically pink in hemolysis, but clear in rhabdomyolysis.

Analysis of urine biochemical parameters may be helpful in differentiating between prerenal and intrinsic ischemic or nephrotoxic AKI. Sodium is usually avidly reabsorbed from the glomerular filtrate in patients with prerenal AKI as a consequence of renal adrenergic activation, stimulation of the RAAS, suppression of atrial natriuretic peptide (ANP) secretion, and local changes in peritubular hemodynamics. In contrast, Na^+ reabsorption is impaired in ATN as a result of injury to the renal tubular epithelium. Renal sodium handling can be assessed based on the urinary sodium concentration (U_{Na}) with values of less than 10 mmol/L commonly seen in prerenal disease compared to greater than 20 mmol/L in ATN (Table 31.10). Normalizing sodium excretion to creatinine provides a more sensitive index. The FE_{Na} is the ratio between urinary sodium excretion ($U_{Na} \times V$, where U_{Na} is the urinary sodium concentration and V is the urine volume) and the filtered load of sodium (calculated as $P_{Na} \times CrCl$, where P_{Na} is the plasma sodium concentration and CrCl is the creatinine clearance, which can be calculated as $[(U_{Cr} \times V)/P_{Cr}]$, where V is the urine volume and U_{Cr} and P_{Cr} are the urine and plasma creatinine concentrations, respectively). Since urine volume is in both the numerator and denominator of this ratio, the FE_{Na} can be calculated as $[(U_{Na} \div P_{Na})/(U_{Cr} \div P_{Cr})] \times 100$ using an untimed (spot) urine sample and simultaneous serum creatinine determination. The FE_{Na} is usually less than 1% (frequently <0.5%) in the setting of prerenal azotemia, whereas it is typically greater than 2% in patients with ischemic or nephrotoxic AKI. The utility of the FE_{Na} is limited in a variety of clinical settings. Values greater than 1% are not uncommon in the setting of prerenal AKI in patients receiving diuretics, those with metabolic alkalosis and bicarbonaturia (in whom Na^+ is excreted with HCO_3^- to maintain electroneutrality), in the presence of adrenal insufficiency, and in the setting of underlying CKD.[315-317] Conversely, a FE_{Na} of less than 1% may be observed in the setting of ATN, particularly in the settings of radiocontrast media administration and rhabdomyolysis, although it has been reported in approximately 15% of patients with ATN from a variety of other causes, including ischemia, burns, and sepsis.[315,318,319] It has been postulated that this reflects a milder degree of intrinsic renal injury in which epithelial cell damage is probably localized to the corticomedullary junction and outer medulla with relative preservation of function in other Na^+-transporting segments and may represent a transition state between prerenal azotemia and ATN. It should be recognized that a FE_{Na} of less than 1% is not abnormal and reflects normal sodium homeostasis in patients on a moderate- to low-sodium diet. The FE_{Na} is also often less than 1% in AKI caused by urinary tract obstruction, glomerulonephritis, and diseases of the renal vasculature; other parameters must be employed to distinguish these conditions from prerenal AKI.

A variety of other indices have also been proposed to differentiate between causes of AKI. The renal failure index, calculated as $U_{Na}/(U_{Cr} \div P_{Cr})$, provides comparable information to the FE_{Na} because clinical variations in serum Na^+ concentration are relatively small. The fractional excretion of urea (FE_{urea}) has been proposed as an alternative to the

Table 31.10 Urine Indices Used in the Differential Diagnosis of Prerenal Acute Kidney Injury and Acute Tubular Necrosis

Diagnostic Index	Prerenal Acute Kidney Injury	Acute Tubular Necrosis
Fractional excretion of sodium (%)	<1*	>2*
U_{Na} (mmol/L)	<20	>40
Urine creatinine/plasma creatinine ratio	>40	<20
Urine urea nitrogen/plasma urea nitrogen ratio	>8	<3
Urine specific gravity	>1.018	≈1.010
Urine osmolality (mOsm/kg H_2O)	>500	≈300
Plasma BUN/creatinine ratio	>20	<10-15
Renal failure index, $U_{Na}/(U_{Cr}/P_{Cr})$	<1	>1
Urine sediment	Hyaline casts	Muddy-brown granular casts

*Fractional excretion of sodium (FE_{Na}) may be >1% in prerenal acute kidney injury associated with diuretic use and/or in the setting of bicarbonaturia or chronic kidney disease; FE_{Na} often <1% in acute tubular necrosis caused by radiocontrast media or rhabdomyolysis.

BUN, Blood urea nitrogen; P_{Cr}, plasma creatinine concentration; U_{Cr}, urine creatinine concentration; U_{Na}, urinary sodium concentration.

FE_{Na}, with particular utility in patients on diuretic therapy. Values of FE_{urea} calculated as $([U_{urea} \div P_{urea}]/[U_{Cr} \div P_{Cr}] \times 100)$ of less than 35% are suggestive of a prerenal state.[320-322] Similarly, indices of urinary concentrating ability such as urine specific gravity, urine osmolality, urine/plasma creatinine or urea ratios, and serum urea nitrogen/creatinine ratio are of limited value in differentiating between prerenal and intrinsic AKI. This is particularly true for older patients, in whom urinary concentrating mechanisms are frequently impaired while mechanisms for Na^+ reabsorption are typically preserved.

LABORATORY EVALUATION

The pattern and timing of change of BUN and serum creatinine levels often provide clues to the cause of AKI. Enhanced tubular reabsorption of filtered urea in parallel with sodium and water reabsorption in prerenal states commonly leads to a disproportionate elevation in BUN level relative to serum creatinine level (ratio > 20:1). Conversely, with intrinsic AKI the increase in BUN level usually parallels the rise in serum creatinine level, maintaining a ratio of approximately 10:1 (see Table 31.10). However, severe malnutrition and low dietary protein intake blunt the rise in BUN and creatinine levels, while gastrointestinal bleeding, steroid therapy, and hypercatabolic states may lead to increases in the BUN level that do not reflect prerenal physiology. In addition, aggressive volume resuscitation may rapidly expand the volume of distribution of urea and creatinine and may also obscure the acute rise in serum creatinine level. Sepsis and other forms of critical illness have also been associated with decreased creatinine generation.[323,324] The serum creatinine concentration typically begins to rise within 24 to 48 hours when ATN results from an ischemic insult. Although the clinical course can be highly variable, the serum creatinine concentration will generally peak within 7 to 10 days, and, depending on the severity of the insult and underlying comorbid illnesses, the AKI will resolve to varying degrees over the ensuing 1 to 2 weeks. Following iodinated contrast exposure, the peak in serum creatinine concentration generally occurs within 5 to 7 days. The time course of nephrotoxic ATN caused by aminoglycoside antibiotics or cisplatin is more variable, often with delayed onset of AKI (7 to 10 days).

Additional clues to the diagnosis can be obtained from biochemical and hematologic tests. The presence of marked hyperkalemia, hyperuricemia, and hyperphosphatemia point to cell lysis, which in the setting of elevated creatine kinase levels and hypocalcemia strongly suggests rhabdomyolysis.[325,326] Biochemical signs of cell lysis with very high levels of uric acid, normal or mildly elevated creatine kinase levels, and a urine uric acid/creatinine ratio greater than 1.0 are suggestive of acute urate nephropathy and tumor lysis syndrome.[327,328] Severe hypercalcemia can precipitate AKI, commonly in the form of prerenal AKI from concomitant hypovolemia and renal vasoconstriction. AKI associated with widening of both the serum anion ($Na^+ - [HCO_3^- + Cl^-]$) and osmolal (measured serum osmolality minus calculated osmolality) gaps suggests a diagnosis of ethylene glycol toxicity and should prompt a search for urine oxalate crystals. Severe anemia in the absence of hemorrhage may reflect the presence of hemolysis, multiple myeloma, or thrombotic microangiopathy (e.g., HUS, TTP, toxemia, disseminated intravascular coagulation, accelerated hypertension, systemic lupus erythematosus, scleroderma, radiation injury). Other laboratory findings suggestive of thrombotic microangiopathy include thrombocytopenia, dysmorphic RBCs on peripheral blood smear, a low circulating haptoglobin level, and elevated circulating levels of lactate dehydrogenase. Systemic eosinophilia suggests allergic interstitial nephritis but may also be a prominent feature in other diseases such as atheroembolic disease and polyarteritis nodosa, particularly eosinophilic granulomatosis with polyangiitis (formerly designated Churg-Strauss vasculitis). Depressed complement levels and high titers of anti–glomerular basement membrane antibodies, antineutrophil cytoplasmic antibodies, antinuclear antibodies, circulating immune complexes, or cryoglobulins are useful diagnostic tools in patients with suspected glomerulonephritis or vasculitis (see Table 31.8).

NOVEL BIOMARKERS OF KIDNEY INJURY

A number of novel biomarkers of kidney injury have been evaluated for potential roles in the early identification, differential diagnosis, and prognosis of AKI, including serum cystatin C, NGAL, KIM-1, IL-18, L-FABP, TIMP-2, and IGFBP-7, among others.[17-24] While none of these biomarkers has been adequately validated for routine clinical use, they have the potential to provide an earlier diagnosis of intrinsic AKI, to differentiate volume-responsive (prerenal) AKI from intrinsic disease, and to provide prognostic information regarding the clinical course of an episode of AKI.

CYSTATIN C

Cystatin C is a 13-kDa protein that is filtered by the glomerulus and completely reabsorbed and degraded by the proximal tubule. Cystatin C has been validated as an alternative marker of glomerular filtration.[329,330] As the result of its shorter serum half-life, serum cystatin C concentrations change more rapidly than serum creatinine concentrations in response to changes in kidney function, allowing changes in serum cystatin C concentration to be detected sooner than changes in serum creatinine concentration following the onset of AKI.[331] Under normal circumstances, urinary cystatin C is virtually undetectable; however, following tubular injury, tubular reabsorption of filtered cystatin is diminished and urinary cystatin C can be detected, raising the possibility of its use as an early marker of tubular injury.[332]

NEUTROPHIL GELATINASE–ASSOCIATED LIPOCALIN

NGAL is a 25-kDa protein whose expression by renal tubular epithelial cells is markedly upregulated following ischemic or nephrotoxic kidney injury.[333,334] NGAL is believed to enhance the trafficking of iron-siderophore complexes, enhancing the delivery of iron, upregulating HO-1, reducing apoptosis, and increasing the normal proliferation of renal tubule epithelial cells.[335] Urine and plasma NGAL have been evaluated in numerous clinical settings as an early biomarker of tubular injury.[336-346] Initial studies in children undergoing cardiac surgery demonstrated extremely high sensitivity and specificity for identification of AKI, with an area under the concentration-time curve (AUC) of greater than 0.99; however, these early results have not been reproduced across other clinical settings.

KIDNEY INJURY MOLECULE-1

KIM-1 is a transmembrane protein whose expression is markedly upregulated in the proximal tubule following tubular injury.[347-350] The extracellular component of the KIM-1 protein is shed into the urine following tubular injury, permitting its potential use as a marker of tubular damage; however, the time course of peak KIM-1 expression in the urine is later than seen with NGAL.[343,351-353]

INTERLEUKIN-18

IL-18 is a proinflammatory cytokine whose expression is increased in the kidney following ischemic and nephrotoxic injury.[354] Urinary IL-18 levels have been shown to rise within 6 hours following tubular injury following cardiac surgery and in critically ill patients.[345,346,355,356]

LIVER-TYPE FATTY ACID–BINDING PROTEIN

Despite its name, L-FABP is expressed in the proximal tubule.[357,358] Elevated L-FABP levels may be detected in the urine within 6 hours of ischemic or nephrotoxic injury, permitting its potential use as a marker of tubular injury.[353,359-361] In a meta-analysis of published studies, the sensitivity and specificity of urinary L-FABP for diagnosis of AKI were each approximately 75%.[362]

TISSUE INHIBITOR OF METALLOPROTEINASE 2 AND INSULIN-LIKE GROWTH FACTOR–BINDING PROTEIN-7

TIMP-2 and IGFBP-7 are expressed in epithelial cells and act in an autocrine and paracrine manner to arrest cell cycle in AKI.[363-365] In three discovery cohorts comprising 522 patients, these two biomarkers were identified as having the highest discriminant ability among 340 candidate biomarkers of AKI.[22] In a subsequent validation study of 728 patients, this pair of biomarkers had an AUC of 0.80, which was significantly better than the performance of other candidate biomarkers, including NGAL, KIM-1, IL-18, and L-FABP.[22]

RADIOLOGIC EVALUATION

Imaging of the abdomen is a highly useful adjunct to laboratory testing to determine the cause of AKI. In cases of suspected obstructive uropathy, postvoid residual volumes of greater than 100 to 150 mL suggest a diagnosis of bladder outlet obstruction. While plain films rarely provide definitive evidence of postrenal AKI, they may identify the presence of calcium-containing stones that can cause obstructive disease. Renal ultrasonography is the screening test of choice to assess cortical thickness, differences in cortical and medullary density, the integrity of the collecting system, and kidney size. Although pelvicalyceal dilation is usual in cases of urinary tract obstruction (98% sensitivity), dilation may not be observed in the volume-depleted patient during the initial 1 to 3 days after obstruction, when the collecting system is relatively noncompliant, or in patients with obstruction caused by ureteric encasement or infiltration (e.g., retroperitoneal fibrosis, neoplasia).[366] Alternatively, computed tomography may be used to visualize the kidneys and collecting system, although radiocontrast media administration should ideally be avoided in patients with AKI. Visualization of the collecting system may be suboptimal in the absence of contrast media enhancement; however, unenhanced computed tomographic scans are useful for the identification of obstructing ureteral stones.[367,368] Ultrasonography and computed tomography have essentially replaced the use of intravenous pyelography, which now has little or no role in the evaluation of AKI. Cystoscopic retrograde or percutaneous antegrade pyelography are useful tests for the precise localization of the site of obstruction and can be combined with placement of ureteral stents or percutaneous nephrostomy tubes to allow therapeutic decompression of the urinary tract. Radionuclide scans have been proposed as useful for assessing renal blood flow, glomerular filtration, tubule function, and infiltration by inflammatory cells in AKI; however, these tests lack specificity and yield conflicting or poor results in controlled studies.[369,370] Magnetic resonance angiography (MRA) of the kidneys is extremely useful for detecting renal artery stenosis and has been used in the evaluation of acute renovascular crises.[371] However, given the association of gadolinium-based contrast media administration with the development of nephrogenic systemic fibrosis, contrast media–enhanced MRA is contraindicated in the majority of patients with AKI.[372,373] Doppler ultrasonography and spiral computed tomography are also useful in patients with suspected vascular obstruction; however, contrast media angiography remains the gold standard for definitive diagnosis.

KIDNEY BIOPSY

Kidney biopsy in AKI is usually reserved for patients in whom prerenal and postrenal AKI have been excluded and the cause of intrinsic AKI is unclear.[374] Kidney biopsy is particularly useful when clinical assessment, urinalysis, and laboratory investigation suggest diagnoses other than ischemic or nephrotoxic injury that may respond to specific therapy. Examples include anti–glomerular basement membrane disease and other forms of necrotizing glomerulonephritis, vasculitis, HUS and TTP, allergic interstitial nephritis, and myeloma cast nephropathy.

DIFFERENTIAL DIAGNOSIS OF ACUTE KIDNEY INJURY IN SPECIFIC CLINICAL SETTINGS

The differential diagnosis of AKI in several common clinical settings warrants special mention (Table 31.11).

ACUTE KIDNEY INJURY IN THE SETTING OF CANCER

There are several potential causes of AKI in the patient with cancer. Prerenal AKI is common in the setting of underlying malignancy and may be related to tumor- or chemotherapy-induced vomiting or diarrhea, reduced oral intake secondary to anorexia, the use of NSAIDs for pain management, and malignancy-associated hypercalcemia.[375,376] Intrinsic AKI can be triggered by a variety of chemotherapeutic agents. Cisplatin is the classical chemotherapeutic medication associated with AKI.[377,378] The principal site of renal damage with cisplatin is the proximal tubule. The nephrotoxicity of cisplatin is dose dependent, yet AKI can result from a single exposure. Electrolyte disturbances, including hypomagnesemia and hypokalemia, are common following cisplatin administration. Other platinum-containing chemotherapy agents, such as carboplatin and oxaliplatin are less nephrotoxic than cisplatin but are not risk-free, particularly when high cumulative doses are administered. Ifosfamide, which has been used to treat germ cell tumors, sarcomas, other solid tumors, and occasionally lymphoma, is also associated with AKI in a dose-dependent fashion.[379-381] Methotrexate nephrotoxicity occurs following intravenous administration of high doses (>1 g/m²), primarily as the result of precipitation of the drug and metabolites within the tubular lumen.[382-384] Risk factors for methotrexate nephrotoxicity include volume depletion and the presence of acidic urine. Direct tubular toxicity may also contribute to the development of AKI.

Renal parenchymal invasion by solid and hematologic cancers is reported in 5% to 10% of autopsy studies but is an uncommon cause of AKI.[385,386] Infiltration of leukemic cells into the renal parenchyma can precipitate AKI and typically presents with hematuria, proteinuria, and enlarged kidneys on ultrasonographic imaging. Prompt diagnosis is important as the AKI may respond to chemotherapeutic intervention.

The tumor lysis syndrome, which is associated with hyperuricemia, hyperphosphatemia, and hypocalcemia, is a well recognized cause of AKI in patients with cancers.[387,388] Tumor lysis syndrome occurs most commonly following the initiation of chemotherapy for patients with poorly differentiated, rapidly growing lymphoproliferative malignancies (e.g., Burkitt's lymphoma or acute lymphoblastic or promyelocytic leukemia), yet it can occur spontaneously and in the setting of certain solid tumors that are highly sensitive to radiation and/or chemotherapy (e.g., testicular carcinoma). The Cairo-Bishop criteria, which include both laboratory and clinical criteria, have been utilized to provide a standard definition for the diagnosis of tumor lysis syndrome (Table 31.12).[388] AKI associated with the tumor lysis syndrome is triggered by direct tubular injury and luminal obstruction by uric acid and calcium phosphate crystals. Prophylactic therapy with aggressive volume administration and either xanthine oxidase inhibitors to inhibit uric acid synthesis or recombinant uricase to convert uric acid to allantoin has markedly reduced the incidence of this form of AKI.[389-392] Less common causes of AKI include tumor-associated glomerulonephritis and thrombotic microangiopathy induced by medications or irradiation. Chemotherapy-associated thrombotic microangiopathy is a well-recognized complication of several agents, including mitomycin C and gemcitabine.[393-395]

AKI is a common complication of multiple myeloma.[311,396] Causes of AKI in this setting include intravascular volume depletion, myeloma cast nephropathy, sepsis, hypercalcemia, ATN induced by drugs or tumor lysis during therapy, cryoglobulinemia, hyperviscosity syndrome, and plasma cell infiltration. Multiple myeloma may also result in impaired kidney function as the result of amyloidosis or light-chain deposition disease; however, these most commonly present with proteinuria and a more subacute decline in kidney function. Myeloma cast nephropathy results from the binding of filtered immunoglobulin Bence Jones proteins to Tamm-Horsfall glycoprotein forming casts that obstruct the tubular lumen. Higher excretion rates of free light chains, volume depletion, and hypercalcemia are associated with higher risks for development of myeloma cast nephropathy. Prompt treatment to lower free light-chain burden may result in recovery of kidney function. Studies of the effectiveness of plasmapheresis in the treatment of myeloma cast nephropathy have yielded conflicting results.[397-400] The use of dialysis membranes that are permeable to light chains and other proteins with molecular weights lower than albumin (high-cutoff membranes) has also been proposed as a potential therapeutic strategy; however, data from rigorously conducted trials evaluating the efficacy of this strategy are not available.[105,401]

ACUTE KIDNEY INJURY IN PREGNANCY

In the industrialized world the incidence of dialysis-requiring AKI in the setting of pregnancy is approximately 1 in 20,000 births.[402,403] The marked decline in this complication over the past 50 years is a result of improved prenatal care and advancements in obstetrics practice. In early pregnancy, ATN induced by nephrotoxic abortifacients remains a relatively common cause of AKI in developing countries but is rare in the developed world. Ischemic ATN, severe toxemia of

Table 31.11 Major Causes of Acute Kidney Injury in Specific Clinical Settings

AKI in the Cancer Patient

Prerenal azotemia
  Hypovolemia (e.g., poor intake, vomiting, diarrhea)
Intrinsic AKI
  Exogenous nephrotoxins: chemotherapy, antibiotics, contrast media
  Endogenous toxins: hyperuricemia, hypercalcemia, tumor lysis, paraproteins
  Other: radiation, HUS/TTP, glomerulonephritis, amyloid, malignant infiltration
Postrenal AKI
  Ureteric or bladder neck obstruction

AKI after Cardiac Surgery

Prerenal azotemia
  Hypovolemia (surgical losses, diuretics), cardiac failure, vasodilators
Intrinsic AKI
  Ischemic ATN (even in absence of hypotension)
  Atheroembolic disease after aortic manipulation/intraaortic balloon pump
  Preoperative or perioperative administration of contrast medium
  Allergic interstitial nephritis induced by perioperative antibiotics
Postrenal AKI
  Obstructed urinary catheter, exacerbation of voiding dysfunction

AKI in Pregnancy

Prerenal azotemia
  Acute fatty liver of pregnancy with fulminant hepatic failure
Intrinsic AKI
  Preeclampsia or eclampsia
  Postpartum HUS/TTP
  HELLP syndrome
  Ischemia: postpartum hemorrhage, abruptio placentae, amniotic fluid embolus
  Direct toxicity of illegal abortifacients
Postrenal AKI
  Obstruction with pyelonephritis

AKI after Solid Organ or Bone Marrow Transplantation

Prerenal azotemia
  Intravascular volume depletion (e.g., diuretic therapy)
  Vasoactive drugs (e.g., calcineurin inhibitors, amphotericin B)
  Hepatorenal syndrome, venoocclusive disease of liver (BMT)
Intrinsic AKI
  Postoperative ischemic ATN (even in absence of hypotension)
  Sepsis
  Exogenous nephrotoxins: aminoglycosides, amphotericin B, radiocontrast media
  HUS/TTP (e.g., cyclosporine or myeloablative radiotherapy related)
  Allergic tubulointerstitial nephritis
Postrenal AKI
  Obstructed urinary catheter

AKI and Pulmonary Disease (Pulmonary Renal Syndrome)

Prerenal azotemia
  Diminished cardiac output complicating pulmonary embolism, severe pulmonary hypertension, or positive-pressure mechanical ventilation
Intrinsic AKI
  Vasculitis
    Goodpasture's syndrome, ANCA-associated vasculitis, SLE, eosinophilic granulomatosis with polyangiitis, polyarteritis nodosa, cryoglobulinemia, right-sided endocarditis, lymphomatoid granulomatosis, sarcoidosis, scleroderma
  Toxins
    Ingestion of paraquat or diquat
Infections
  Legionnaires' disease, *Mycoplasma* infection, tuberculosis, disseminated viral or fungal infection
AKI from any cause with hypervolemia and pulmonary edema
Lung cancer with hypercalcemia, tumor lysis, or glomerulonephritis

AKI and Liver Disease

Prerenal azotemia
  Reduced true (GI hemorrhage, GI losses from lactulose, diuretics, large-volume paracentesis) circulatory volume or effective (hypoalbuminemia, splanchnic vasodilation)
  Hepatorenal syndrome type 1 or 2
  Tense ascites with abdominal compartment syndrome
Intrinsic AKI
  Ischemic (severe hypoperfusion—see earlier) or direct nephrotoxicity and hepatotoxicity of drugs or toxins (e.g., carbon tetrachloride, acetaminophen, tetracyclines, methoxyflurane)
  Tubulointerstitial nephritis plus hepatitis caused by drugs (e.g., sulfonamides, rifampin, phenytoin, allopurinol, phenindione), infections (leptospirosis, brucellosis, Epstein-Barr virus infection, cytomegalovirus infection), malignant infiltration (leukemia, lymphoma), or sarcoidosis
  Glomerulonephritis or vasculitis (e.g., polyarteritis nodosa, ANCA-associated glomerulonephritis, cryoglobulinemia, SLE, postinfectious hepatitis or liver abscess

AKI and Nephrotic Syndrome

Prerenal azotemia
  Intravascular volume depletion (diuretic therapy, hypoalbuminemia)
Intrinsic AKI
  Manifestation of primary glomerular disease
  Collapsing glomerulopathy (e.g., HIV, pamidronate)
  Associated ATN (older hypertensive males)
  Associated interstitial nephritis (NSAIDs, rifampin, interferon alfa)
Other—amyloid or light-chain deposition disease, renal vein thrombosis, severe interstitial edema

---

AKI, Acute kidney injury; *ANCA,* antineutrophil cytoplasmic antibody; *ATN,* acute tubular necrosis; *BMT,* bone marrow transplantation; *GI,* gastrointestinal; *HELLP,* hemolysis, elevated liver enzymes, low platelets; *HIV,* human immunodeficiency virus; *HUS,* hemolytic uremic syndrome; *NSAID,* nonsteroidal antiinflammatory drug; *SLE,* systemic lupus erythematosus; *TTP,* thrombotic thrombocytopenic purpura.

> **Table 31.12** Cairo-Bishop Definition of Tumor Lysis Syndrome
>
> **Diagnosis of Laboratory Tumor Lysis Syndrome**
>
> Requires at least two of the following criteria achieved in the same 24-hr interval from 3 days before to 7 days after chemotherapy initiation:
> - Uric acid level: ≥ 8.0 mg/dL or ≥ 25% increase from baseline
> - Potassium level: ≥ 6.0 mmol/L or ≥ 25% increase from baseline
> - Phosphorus level: ≥ 4.6 mg/dL (≥6.5 mg/dL in children) or ≥ 25% increase from baseline
> - Calcium level: ≤ 7.0 mg/dL or ≥ 25% decrease from baseline
>
> **Diagnosis of Clinical Tumor Lysis Syndrome**
>
> Laboratory tumor lysis syndrome plus at least one of the following:
> - Serum creatinine level ≥ 1.5 times the age-adjusted upper limit of normal
> - Cardiac arrhythmia/sudden death
> - Seizure
>
> Adapted from Cairo MS, Bishop M: Tumour lysis syndrome: new therapeutic strategies and classification. Br J Haematol 127:3-11, 2004.

pregnancy, and postpartum HUS and TTP are the most common causes of AKI in late term pregnancy.[402,404,405] Ischemic ATN is usually precipitated by placental abruption or postpartum hemorrhage, and less commonly by amniotic fluid embolism or sepsis. Glomerular filtration is usually normal in mild or moderate preeclampsia; however, AKI may complicate severe preeclampsia.[405,406] In this setting, AKI is typically transient and found in association with intrarenal vasospasm, marked hypertension, and neurologic abnormalities. A variant of preeclampsia, the HELLP syndrome (*H*emolysis, *E*levated *L*iver enzymes, *L*ow *P*latelets), is characterized by a benign initial course that can rapidly deteriorate with the development of thrombotic microangiopathy with hemolysis, coagulation abnormalities, derangement in hepatic function, and AKI.[406-408] Immediate delivery of the fetus is indicated in this setting. Thrombotic microangiopathy can also develop in the postpartum setting and typically occurs in patients who have had a normal pregnancy.[409] Postpartum thrombotic microangiopathy is characterized by thrombocytopenia, microangiopathic anemia, and normal prothrombin and partial thromboplastin times and frequently results in long-term impairment of renal function.

Acute fatty liver of pregnancy occurs in approximately 1 in 7000 pregnancies and is associated with AKI, likely as a result of intrarenal vasoconstriction, as occurs in HRS. Although the exact origin of acute fatty liver of pregnancy is unknown, the incidence is increased in women who carry a fetus with a defect in fatty acid oxidation and who are themselves carriers of a genetic mutation that compromises intramitochondrial fatty acid oxidation.[408] Acute bilateral pyelonephritis may also precipitate AKI in pregnancy and should be obvious from the patient's presentation (fever, flank pain), findings on urinalysis (bacteria, leukocytes), and laboratory test results (leukocytosis, elevated serum creatinine level).[404,407,410,411] The diagnosis of postrenal AKI in the pregnant patient is particularly challenging due to the physiologic dilation of the collecting system that normally occurs in the second and third trimesters. As a result, determining the presence of abnormal findings on renal ultrasonography is more difficult.

ACUTE KIDNEY INJURY FOLLOWING CARDIAC SURGERY

An acute deterioration in renal function is a common complication following cardiac surgery with an incidence of 7.7% to 42% depending on the criteria used to define AKI.[412-416] AKI requiring dialytic support occurs in up to 5% of patients following cardiac surgery.[412-416] AKI in the perioperative period is most commonly attributed to prerenal azotemia associated with decreased cardiac function or to ATN. Risk factors for cardiac surgery–associated AKI can be broadly categorized into presurgical patient-related factors, surgical factors, and postoperative events. The principal patient-related risk factors include underlying CKD, advanced age, left ventricular dysfunction, previous myocardial revascularization, diabetes mellitus, and peripheral vascular disease.[415-418] Operative factors include the need for emergent surgery, prolonged time on cardiopulmonary bypass, insertion of intraaortic balloon pump, the performance of concomitant valvular surgery, and redo coronary artery bypass graft (CABG). Several studies have compared the incidence of AKI following on-pump versus off-pump CABG, with some data suggesting that off-pump CABG is associated with a lower incidence of AKI.[419-423] Postoperative factors associated with an increased risk for AKI include reduced cardiac output, bleeding, vasodilatory shock, and the overzealous use of diuretics and afterload-reducing agents.

Additional potential causes of AKI following CABG include the administration of iodinated contrast media in the preoperative, perioperative and/or postoperative period, antibiotic-associated AIN, and atheroembolic disease.[58] Whereas prerenal azotemia and ATN typically occur within days of the surgical procedure, atheroembolic AKI may take longer to develop and can be distinguished by the characteristic clinical features of livedo reticularis, cyanosis, and gangrenous digital lesions, as well as the findings of eosinophilia, eosinophiluria, and hypocomplementemia.

ACUTE KIDNEY INJURY AFTER SOLID ORGAN OR BONE MARROW TRANSPLANTATION

Nonrenal solid organ transplant recipients have a particularly high risk for AKI from cardiopulmonary and hepatic failure, sepsis, and the nephrotoxic effects of antimicrobial and immunosuppressive agents. In a large retrospective multicenter study, 25% of all nonrenal solid organ transplant recipients developed AKI, with 8% requiring RRT.[424] The development of AKI requiring dialysis was associated with a 9- to 12-fold increase in mortality. AKI developed in 35% of heart transplant recipients and 15% of lung transplant recipients. As many as 30% of liver transplant recipients develop AKI, many of whom had CKD before transplantation.[425,426] There are conflicting data as to whether impaired kidney function before transplantation predicts outcomes in patients undergoing orthotopic liver transplantation; however, patients with impaired kidney function preoperatively have longer hospital and ICU stays and are more likely to need dialysis compared to patients with intact preoperative kidney function.[427-429]

AKI is a well-recognized complication of hematopoietic cell transplantation (HCT).[375,430,431] The three types of HCT are myeloablative autologous, myeloablative allogeneic, and nonmyeloablative allogeneic, and the incidence, severity, and outcomes of AKI following these forms of HCT vary considerably.[430,432,433] In a study of 272 patients who underwent myeloablative HCT (predominantly allogeneic), 53% developed AKI and 24% required dialysis.[434] Of patients with dialysis-requiring AKI, the mortality rate was 84%. A recent study found an incidence of severe AKI in this patient population of 73%.[435] AKI following nonmyeloablative allogeneic HCT is less common.[435,436] A study of 253 patients demonstrated an incidence of AKI within 3 months of HCT of 40.4%, with just 4.4% of patients requiring dialysis.[436] The incidence of AKI following myeloablative autologous HCT is considerably lower.[437,438] A study of 173 patients following autologous HCT reported an incidence of AKI of 21%, with 5% of patients requiring dialysis.[438] The absence of graft-versus-host disease and more rapid engraftment likely account for the lower incidence of AKI in this setting. Causes of HCT-associated AKI include hypovolemia, sepsis, tumor lysis syndrome, direct tubular toxicity from cytoreductive therapy, thrombotic microangiopathy, graft-versus-host disease, antibiotics, immunosuppressive agents, and hepatic venoocclusive disease (VOD). VOD results from acute radiochemotherapy-induced endothelial cell injury of hepatic venules.[434,439-441] This condition occurs most commonly in conditioning regimens that include total body irradiation and cyclophosphamide and/or busulphan and in the setting of myeloablative allogeneic HCT. The syndrome is characterized clinically by profound jaundice and avid salt retention with edema and ascites within the first month after engraftment and subsequently the development of AKI. Oliguric AKI is common in moderate VOD and certain in severe cases. The mortality rate for patients with severe VOD approaches 100%. BK virus is a human polyomavirus that is a common opportunistic infection in both solid organ transplant and HCT patients.[442] Detectable BK viruria may be seen in as many as 50% of patients undergoing HCT.[443] Reactivation of latent BK virus infection in immunosuppressed patients is associated with both hemorrhagic cystitis and with renal involvement with tubular atrophy and fibrosis with an inflammatory lymphocytic infiltrate with intranuclear BK virus inclusion bodies.[444] The diagnosis is suggested by rising viral titers in blood and/or urine, and the mainstay of treatment is minimization of immunosuppression.

ACUTE KIDNEY INJURY ASSOCIATED WITH PULMONARY DISEASE

The coexistence of AKI and pulmonary disease (pulmonary renal syndrome) classically suggests the presence of Goodpasture's syndrome, antineutrophil cytoplasmic antibody (ANCA)-associated vasculitis, or other vasculitides.[445-447] The detection of anti–glomerular basement membrane antibodies, antineutrophil cytoplasmic antibodies, or low serum complement concentrations can be helpful in differentiating among the various causes of pulmonary renal syndrome, although the urgent need for definitive diagnosis and treatment may mandate lung or kidney biopsy. Several toxic ingestions and infections may also precipitate simultaneous pulmonary and kidney injury that mimics vasculitis-associated pulmonary renal syndrome. Furthermore, AKI of any cause may be complicated by secondary hypervolemia and pulmonary edema. Severe lung disease and ventilator support with increased intrathoracic pressure may compromise cardiac output and induce prerenal AKI.

ACUTE KIDNEY INJURY ASSOCIATED WITH LIVER DISEASE

The differential diagnosis of AKI in patients with liver disease is broad. Common causes of AKI in this setting include intravascular volume depletion, gastrointestinal bleeding, sepsis, and nephrotoxins. Most cases of AKI in advanced liver disease are due to prerenal azotemia, ATN, or HRS, and differentiating these conditions can be clinically challenging.[53,55,448] Although a U_{Na} of less than 20 mmol/L and FE_{Na} of less than 1% are typical of prerenal AKI and HRS, high-dose diuretics, which are commonly prescribed in patients with advanced liver disease, may lead to higher sodium excretion rates. Differentiating ATN from other forms of AKI is further confounded by he fact that bile-stained casts, which can be seen in prerenal AKI and HRS, have a similar appearance to the classical "muddy-brown" granular casts of ATN.[449] Kidney disease in patients with liver disease may also result from acute glomerular disease, including immunoglobulin A nephropathy, hepatitis B virus–associated membranous nephropathy, and hepatitis C virus–associated membranoproliferative glomerulonephritis with cryoglobulinemia. Acetaminophen toxicity may cause nephrotoxic ATN in addition to being one of the most common causes of acute hepatotoxicity.

The term hepatorenal syndrome (HRS) is typically reserved for a clinical syndrome marked by irreversible AKI that develops in patients with advanced cirrhosis, although it has been described in the setting of fulminant viral and alcoholic hepatitis. HRS almost certainly represents the terminal stage of a state of hypoperfusion that begins early in the course of chronic liver disease. The precise pathophysiologic mechanisms underlying the hemodynamic alterations in HRS are incompletely understood. In the early stages of HRS, increased vascular capacitance as the result of splanchnic and systemic vasodilation is thought to trigger activation of the RAAS and sympathetic nervous system.[55] Renal perfusion is preserved in this stage by the local release of renal vasodilatory factors; however, these compensatory mechanisms are eventually overwhelmed, and progressive renal hypoperfusion ensues. An inadequate increase in cardiac output relative to the fall in vascular resistance is thought to also contribute to the development of HRS.

Clinically, the presentation of HRS closely resembles that of prerenal AKI. However, unlike prerenal AKI, HRS does not improve with aggressive expansion of the intravascular space. Criteria for the diagnosis of HRS (Table 31.13) include an increase in serum creatinine concentration above 1.5 mg/dL in the setting of cirrhosis with ascites; failure of kidney function to improve after at least 2 days

> **Table 31.13 Diagnostic Criteria for Hepatorenal Syndrome**
>
> **Diagnostic Criteria for Hepatorenal Syndrome**
> - Cirrhosis with ascites
> - Serum creatinine level > 1.5 mg/dL
> - No improvement of serum creatinine level (decrease to a level of ≤ 1.5 mg/dL) after at least 2 days of diuretic withdrawal and volume expansion with albumin (1 g/kg body weight per day to a maximum of 100 g/day)
> - Absence of shock
> - Absence of parenchymal kidney disease as indicated by:
>   - Proteinuria > 500 mg/day
>   - Microhematuria (>50 red blood cells per high-power field) and/or
>   - Abnormal renal ultrasonography findings
>
> **Type 1 Hepatorenal Syndrome**
>
> Rapid progressive AKI with doubling of the serum creatinine level to >2.5 mg/dL in < 2 wk
>
> **Type 2 Hepatorenal Syndrome**
>
> Moderate renal dysfunction (serum creatinine level of 1.5 to 2.5 mg/dL) with a steady or slowly progressive course
>
> AKI, Acute kidney injury.

with diuretic withdrawal and volume expansion with albumin; and the absence of shock, concurrent or recent treatment with nephrotoxic drugs, or parenchymal kidney disease (defined by proteinuria > 500 mg/day, hematuria [>50 RBCs per high-power field], and/or abnormal renal ultrasonography findings).[450]

Two subtypes of HRS have been described. Type 1 HRS is characterized by a rapid onset of AKI defined by at least a doubling of the serum creatinine concentration to a level of at least 2.5 mg/dL or a reduction in GFR of 50% or more to a level of less than 20 mL/min over a 2-week period.[451,452] Type 1 HRS typically develops in hospitalized patients and may be precipitated by variceal bleeding, overly rapid diuresis, the performance of paracentesis, or, most commonly, the development of spontaneous bacterial peritonitis. Other postulated triggers include infections, minor surgery, or the use of NSAIDs or other drugs. However, caution must be exerted in these cases to exclude reversible causes of AKI. Type 1 HRS is generally characterized by a fulminant course with oliguria, encephalopathy, marked hyperbilirubinemia, and death within 1 month of clinical presentation. However, advances in the management of HRS discussed later suggest that there may be a trend toward better survival in those patients who respond to therapy.[453,454] Type 2 HRS is typified by a more gradual decline in renal function that develops in the setting of diuretic-resistant ascites and avid sodium retention. The prognosis of type 2 HRS is considerably better than that of type 1 HRS, with a reported median survival of 6 months and a 1-year survival as high as 30%.[54,455] The development of a sudden deterioration in kidney function after a prolonged stable period may occur in patients with type 2 HRS, leading to outcomes similar to those of patients with type 1 HRS.

Definitive treatment of HRS is dependent upon recovery of hepatic function or successful liver transplantation. However, the use of vasoconstrictive agents combined with volume expansion with colloid has shown promise for improving kidney function.[456,457] It is postulated that by reversing the splanchnic and peripheral vasodilation, more normal renal perfusion can be restored. Vasoconstrictive regimens that have been utilized include norepinephrine, combination therapy with midodrine and octreotide, and the vasopressin agonist terlipressin.[458-461] Although vasoconstrictive therapy is associated with improvement in kidney function, and patients who respond have an improved prognosis, the use of vasoconstrictive therapy has not been shown to improve overall prognosis in patients with AKI, suggesting that survival remains limited by the underlying severity of liver disease.

ACUTE KIDNEY INJURY AND THE NEPHROTIC SYNDROME

AKI in the context of the nephrotic syndrome presents a unique array of potential diagnoses. Epithelial injury, if severe, can trigger both nephrotic-range proteinuria and acute or subacute kidney injury.[462,463] The epithelial injury typically occurs as a manifestation of primary glomerular diseases such as collapsing glomerulopathy or crescentic membranous nephropathy. Less dramatic visceral epithelial cell injury, in combination with proximal tubular injury (e.g., pan–epithelial cell injury induced by NSAIDs or possible undiagnosed viral illness) or interstitial nephritis (e.g., rifampicin induced) can also present as AKI complicating the nephrotic syndrome.[464-466] Massive excretion of light-chain proteins in patients with multiple myeloma may also present in this fashion.[467,468] ATN in association with nephrotic syndrome is seen in a subpopulation of older patients with minimal change disease, and in other patients with nephrosis and severe hypoalbuminemia, particularly if they have been overzealously diuresed. In general, patients with AKI complicating nephritic syndrome have higher blood pressure and urinary protein excretion than patients without AKI.[462] The higher incidence of arteriosclerosis in biopsy samples from these patients may point to preexisting hypertensive nephrosclerosis as a risk factor for the development of this complication. Renal vein thrombosis must always be considered in the differential diagnosis of the nephrotic syndrome and AKI, particularly in the pediatric population and in adults with membranous nephropathy in association with high-grade proteinuria and hypoalbuminemia.

COMPLICATIONS OF ACUTE KIDNEY INJURY

The acute loss of kidney function in AKI results in multiple derangements in fluid, electrolyte, and acid-base homeostasis and in hematologic, gastroenterologic, and immunologic function (Table 31.14).

COMPLICATIONS OF POTASSIUM HOMEOSTASIS

Hyperkalemia is a common and potentially life-threatening complication of AKI.[469,470] Serum K^+ typically rises by 0.5 mmol/L/day in oligoanuric patients and reflects

Table 31.14 Common Complications of Acute Kidney Injury

Metabolic	Cardiovascular	Gastrointestinal	Neurologic	Hematologic	Infectious	Other
Hyperkalemia	Pulmonary edema	Nausea	Neuromuscular irritability	Anemia	Pneumonia	Hiccups
Metabolic acidosis	Arrhythmias	Vomiting	Asterixis	Bleeding	Septicemia	Elevated parathyroid hormone level
Hyponatremia	Pericarditis	Malnutrition	Seizures		Urinary tract infection	Low total triiodothyronine and thyroxine levels
Hypocalcemia	Pericardial effusion	Hemorrhage	Mental status changes			Normal thyroxine level
Hyperphosphatemia	Hypertension					
Pulmonary embolism	Myocardial infarction					
Hypermagnesemia						
Hyperuricemia						

impaired excretion of K⁺ derived from a patient's diet, the administration of K⁺-containing solutions, and drugs administered as potassium salts, as well as the release of K⁺ from the injured tubular epithelium. Hyperkalemia may be compounded by coexistent metabolic acidosis and/or hyperglycemia or other hyperosmolar states that promote K⁺ efflux from cells. Hyperkalemia present at the time of diagnosis of AKI or the rapid development of severe hyperkalemia suggests massive tissue destruction such as rhabdomyolysis, hemolysis, or tumor lysis.[291,325,471] Hyperuricemia and hyperphosphatemia may accompany hyperkalemia in these settings. Mild hyperkalemia (<6.0 mmol/L) is usually asymptomatic. Higher levels are frequently associated with electrocardiographic abnormalities, including peaked T waves, prolongation of the PR interval, flattening of P waves, widening of the QRS complex, and intraventricular conduction defects.[472-474] These electrocardiographic findings may precede the onset of life-threatening cardiac arrhythmias such as bradycardia, heart block, ventricular tachycardia, ventricular fibrillation, and asystole. In addition, hyperkalemia may induce neuromuscular abnormalities such as paresthesias, hyporeflexia, weakness, ascending flaccid paralysis, and respiratory failure.

Hypokalemia is unusual in AKI but may complicate nonoliguric ATN caused by aminoglycosides, cisplatin, or amphotericin B, presumably because of impaired K⁺ reabsorption resulting from epithelial cell injury in the TAL.[475,476]

COMPLICATIONS OF ACID-BASE HOMEOSTASIS

Normal metabolism of dietary protein yields between 50 and 100 mmol/day of fixed nonvolatile acids (principally sulfuric and phosphoric acid) that are normally excreted by the kidneys to maintain acid-base homeostasis. Predictably, AKI is commonly complicated by metabolic acidosis, typically with a widening of the serum anion gap due to retention of phosphates, sulfates, and organic anions.[477] Acidosis may be severe (daily fall in plasma HCO_3^- > 2 mmol/L) when the generation of H⁺ is increased by additional mechanisms (e.g., diabetic or fasting ketoacidosis; lactic acidosis complicating generalized tissue hypoperfusion, liver disease, or sepsis; metabolism of ethylene glycol).[53,310,478] In contrast, metabolic alkalosis is an infrequent finding but may complicate overzealous correction of acidosis with HCO_3^-, overzealous use of combination loop plus thiazide diuretics, or loss of gastric acid by vomiting or nasogastric aspiration.

COMPLICATIONS OF MINERAL AND URIC ACID HOMEOSTASIS

Mild to moderate hyperphosphatemia (5 to 10 mg/dL) is a common consequence of AKI, and hyperphosphatemia may be severe (10 to 20 mg/dL) in highly catabolic patients or when AKI is associated with rapid cell death as in rhabdomyolysis, severe burns, hemolysis, tumor lysis, or exogenous administration.[479-482] Factors that potentially contribute to hypocalcemia include skeletal resistance to the actions of parathyroid hormone, reduced levels of 1,25-dihydroxyvitamin D, Ca^{2+} sequestration in injured tissues such as muscle in the setting of rhabdomyolysis, and metastatic deposition of calcium phosphate salts in the setting of severe hyperphosphatemia.[483-485] Hypocalcemia is usually asymptomatic, possibly because of the counterbalancing effects of acidosis on neuromuscular excitability. However, symptomatic hypocalcemia can occur in patients with rhabdomyolysis or acute pancreatitis or after treatment of acidosis with HCO_3^-.[483] Clinical manifestations of hypocalcemia include perioral paresthesias, muscle cramps, seizures, hallucinations, and confusion, as well as prolongation of the QT interval and nonspecific T-wave changes on electrocardiogram. The Chvostek (contraction of facial muscles on tapping of the jaw over the facial nerve) and Trousseau (carpopedal spasm after occlusion of arterial blood supply to the arm for 3 minutes with a blood pressure cuff) signs are useful indicators of latent tetany in high-risk patients.

Mild asymptomatic hypermagnesemia is common in oliguric AKI and reflects impaired excretion of ingested magnesium (dietary magnesium, magnesium-containing laxatives, or antacids).[486,487] More significant hypermagnesemia is usually the result of overzealous parenteral magnesium administration, as in the management of AKI associated with preeclampsia. Hypomagnesemia occasionally complicates nonoliguric ATN associated with cisplatin or amphotericin B and, as with hypokalemia, likely reflects injury to the TAL, a principal site for Mg^{2+} reabsorption.[476,488,489] Hypomagnesemia is usually asymptomatic but may occasionally manifest as neuromuscular instability, cramps, seizures, cardiac arrhythmias, or resistant hypokalemia or hypocalcemia.[486,490]

Uric acid is cleared from blood by glomerular filtration and secretion by proximal tubular cells, and mild to moderate asymptomatic hyperuricemia (12 to 15 mg/dL) is typical in established AKI. Higher levels suggest increased production of uric acid and may point to a diagnosis of acute urate nephropathy.[491-493] The urinary uric acid/creatinine ratio on a random specimen has been proposed as a means to distinguish between hyperuricemia caused by overproduction and impaired excretion. In a small series of patients, this ratio was less than 1 in five patients with acute uric acid nephropathy and was less than 1 in 27 patients with AKI due to other causes.[494] In a subsequent case series, elevations in the uric acid/creatinine ratio to values of greater than 1 were described in other causes of AKI, most notably patients with infections who were markedly hypercatabolic.[495]

VOLUME OVERLOAD AND CARDIAC COMPLICATIONS

Extracellular volume overload is an almost inevitable consequence of diminished salt and water excretion in AKI and may present clinically as mild hypertension, increased jugular venous pressure, pulmonary vascular congestion, pleural effusion, ascites, peripheral edema, increased body weight, and life-threatening pulmonary edema. Hypervolemia may be particularly troublesome in patients receiving multiple intravenous medications, high volumes of enteral or parenteral nutrition, and/or excessive volumes of maintenance intravenous fluids. Moderate or severe hypertension is unusual in ATN and should suggest other diagnoses such as hypertensive nephrosclerosis, glomerulonephritis, renal artery stenosis, and other diseases of the renal vasculature.[404,496-498] Excessive water ingestion or administration of hypotonic saline or dextrose solutions can trigger hyponatremia, which, if severe, may cause cerebral edema, seizures, and other neurologic abnormalities.[499] Cardiac complications include arrhythmias and myocardial infarction. Although these events may reflect primary cardiac disease, abnormalities in myocardial contractility and excitability may be triggered or compounded by hypervolemia, acidosis, hyperkalemia, and other metabolic sequelae of AKI.[500]

HEMATOLOGIC COMPLICATIONS

Anemia develops rapidly in AKI and is usually mild and multifactorial in origin. Contributing factors include inhibition of erythropoiesis, hemolysis, bleeding, hemodilution, and reduced RBC survival time.[501-503] Prolongation of the bleeding time is also common, resulting from mild thrombocytopenia, platelet dysfunction, and clotting factor abnormalities (e.g., factor VIII dysfunction).

NUTRITIONAL AND GASTROINTESTINAL COMPLICATIONS

Malnutrition remains one of the most frustrating and troublesome complications of AKI. The majority of patients have net protein breakdown, which may exceed 200 g/day in catabolic subjects.[504-506] Malnutrition is usually multifactorial in origin and may reflect inability to eat, loss of appetite, and/or inadequate nutritional support; the catabolic nature of the underlying medical disorder (e.g., sepsis, rhabdomyolysis, trauma); nutrient losses in drainage fluids or dialysate; and increased breakdown and reduced synthesis of muscle protein and increased hepatic gluconeogenesis, probably through the actions of toxins, hormones (e.g., glucagon, parathyroid hormone), or other substances (e.g., proteases) that accumulate in AKI.[507-511] Nutrition may also be compromised by the high incidence of acute gastrointestinal hemorrhage, which complicates up to 15% of cases of AKI. Mild gastrointestinal bleeding is common (10% to 30%) and is usually due to stress ulceration of gastric or small intestinal mucosa.[512,513]

INFECTIOUS COMPLICATIONS

Infection is the most common and serious complication of AKI, occurring in 50% to 90% of cases and accounting for up to 75% of deaths.[25,469,514-516] It is unclear whether this high incidence of infection is due to a defect in host immune responses or repeated breaches of mucocutaneous barriers (e.g., intravenous cannulae, mechanical ventilation, bladder catheterization) resulting from therapeutic interventions.

OTHER SEQUELAE OF ACUTE KIDNEY INJURY

Protracted periods of severe AKI or short intervals of catabolic, anuric AKI often lead to the development of the uremic syndrome. Clinical manifestations of the uremic syndrome, in addition to those already listed, include pericarditis, pericardial effusion, and cardiac tamponade; gastrointestinal complications such as anorexia, nausea, vomiting, and ileus; and neuropsychiatric disturbances, including lethargy, confusion, stupor, coma, agitation, psychosis, asterixis, myoclonus, hyperreflexia, restless leg syndrome, focal neurologic deficit, and/or seizures (see Table 31.14). The uremic toxin responsible for this syndrome has yet to be defined. Candidate molecules include urea, other products of nitrogen metabolism such as guanidine compounds, products of bacterial metabolism such as aromatic amines and indoles, and other compounds that are inappropriately retained in the circulation in AKI or are underproduced, such as NO.[517]

COMPLICATIONS DURING RECOVERY FROM ACUTE KIDNEY INJURY

A vigorous diuresis may complicate the recovery phase of AKI and precipitate intravascular volume depletion and a delay in recovery of renal function. This diuretic response probably reflects the combined effects of an osmotic diuresis induced by retained urea and other waste products, excretion of retained salt and water accumulated during AKI, and delayed recovery of tubular reabsorptive function relative to glomerular filtration leading to salt wasting.[518-521] Hypernatremia may also complicate this recovery phase if free water losses are not replenished or are inappropriately replaced by relatively hypertonic saline solutions. Hypokalemia, hypomagnesemia, hypophosphatemia, and hypocalcemia are rarer metabolic complications during recovery from AKI. Mild transient hypercalcemia is relatively frequent during recovery and appears to be a consequence of delayed resolution of secondary hyperparathyroidism. In addition, hypercalcemia may complicate recovery from rhabdomyolysis because of mobilization of sequestered Ca^{2+} from injured muscle.[522]

PREVENTION AND MANAGEMENT OF ACUTE KIDNEY INJURY

Specific treatment is not available for the majority of forms of AKI.[3] As a result, management focuses on interventions to prevent the development of AKI when possible and on providing supportive therapy to ameliorate derangements of fluid and electrolyte homeostasis and prevent uremic complications. In advanced AKI, RRT is often required. The ultimate goals of management are to prevent death, facilitate recovery of kidney function, and minimize the risk for subsequent development of CKD.

PRERENAL ACUTE KIDNEY INJURY

Prerenal AKI is defined as hemodynamically mediated kidney dysfunction that is rapidly reversible following normalization of renal perfusion.[48] In patients in whom prerenal AKI develops as the result of intravascular volume depletion, treatment consists of restoration of normal circulating blood volume. The optimal composition of administered fluids in these patients with hypovolemic prerenal AKI depends on the source of fluid loss and associated electrolyte and acid-base disturbances. The initial management usually consists of volume resuscitation with an isotonic electrolyte solution such as 0.9% saline. RBC transfusion should be used for hemorrhagic hypovolemia when there is ongoing bleeding, particularly if the patient is hemodynamically unstable, or if the blood hemoglobin concentration is dangerously low. The relative merits of colloid and crystalloid resuscitation fluids in the management of nonhemorrhagic renal, extrarenal, and third-space fluid losses have been controversial with advocates for the use of colloids positing that they are more effective at restoring circulating blood volume due to greater retention in the intravascular compartment. However, recent randomized controlled trials and meta-analyses comparing crystalloid with colloid replacement for resuscitation in critically ill patients have not confirmed this theoretical benefit and have demonstrated an increased need for RRT and other adverse outcomes associated with colloid formulations containing hydroxyethyl starch.[523-530] In a meta-analysis of 55 trials involving 3504 patients randomly assigned to treatment with albumin or crystalloid, there was no evidence of either improved outcomes or decreased mortality or other complications associated with albumin administration.[531] These results were subsequently confirmed in a multicenter randomized controlled trial of fluid resuscitation in nearly 7000 hypovolemic medical and surgical ICU patients in which 28-day survival, development of single or multiple organ failure, and duration of hospitalization were similar in both groups.[532] Although specific data on the development of AKI were not described, need for RRT was similar with saline versus albumin resuscitation. However, in a post hoc analysis of patients with traumatic brain injury, albumin resuscitation was associated with increased mortality risk.[533] The use of synthetic colloid solutions has been proposed as an alternative to albumin administration; however, hydroxyethyl starch preparations have been associated with an increased risk for AKI. In a multicenter randomized controlled trial comparing fluid resuscitation with hydroxyethyl starch to a 3% gelatin solution in 129 patients with sepsis, hydroxyethyl starch was associated with a more than twofold increased risk for AKI.[526] A subsequent meta-analysis confirmed the increased risk for AKI associated with hydroxyethyl starch across 34 studies that included 2604 individuals.[527] In a subsequent randomized controlled trial that included 7000 critically ill patients who were assigned to receive either 6% hydroxyethyl starch or isotonic saline, there was an approximately 20% increased risk for AKI treated with RRT associated with use of hydroxyethyl starch.[530] Based on these data demonstrating no benefit and potential increased risk for AKI along with the higher costs associated with colloid use, the routine use of colloids in volume resuscitation in hypovolemia and sepsis is not advisable. In particular, hydroxyethyl starch solutions should be used only sparingly, with regular monitoring of renal function, and the risk for hyperoncotic renal failure minimized by the concomitant use of appropriate crystalloid solutions.[3,526,527,529,530]

Experimental data have suggested that volume resuscitation with isotonic sodium chloride solutions, which contain supraphysiologic concentrations of chloride, may exacerbate renal vasoconstriction and diminish GFR as compared to isotonic crystalloid solutions with lower chloride content.[534-536] In healthy subjects, magnetic resonance imaging demonstrated that infusion of isotonic saline was associated with reduced renal blood flow velocity and renal cortical tissue perfusion as compared to administration of a reduced-chloride isotonic crystalloid solution.[537] In a subsequent open-label, sequential period study conducted in a single ICU, replacing use of high-chloride intravenous solutions with fluids with lower chloride content was associated with a reduction in the incidence of KDIGO stage 3 AKI from 14% to 8.4% and in the use of RRT from 10% to 6.3%.[538] These results need to be confirmed in prospective randomized controlled trials but are strongly suggestive that saline-based resuscitation protocols may need to be reassessed.

Following initial volume resuscitation, replacement of ongoing urine and gastrointestinal fluid losses should generally be with hypotonic crystalloid solutions (e.g., 0.45% saline); even though urinary and gastrointestinal losses may vary greatly in composition, they are usually hypotonic to plasma. Their volume and electrolyte content, as well as patients' serum electrolytes and acid-base status, should be closely monitored to guide adjustments in the composition of the replacement fluids. Although the potassium content in gastric juices tends to be low, concomitant urinary potassium losses may be quite high as the result of metabolic alkalosis.

HEART FAILURE

The management of prerenal AKI in the setting of heart failure is dependent upon the clinical setting and cause of the heart failure. In patients with congestive heart failure in whom AKI has developed in the setting of excessive diuresis, withholding of diuretics and cautious volume replacement may be sufficient to restore kidney function. In acute decompensated heart failure (ADHF), AKI may develop despite worsening volume overload; intensification of diuretic therapy is often required for treatment of pulmonary vascular congestion. Although diuretic therapy may exacerbate prerenal AKI, it can also result in improvement in kidney function via several postulated mechanisms: (1) decreasing ventricular distension resulting in a shift from the descending limb to the ascending limb of the Starling curve and improvement in myocardial contractility, (2) decreasing venous congestion,[535,539-542] and (3) diminishing intraabdominal pressure.[543] Additional therapies for ADHF in the setting of AKI include inotropic support, vasodilators for afterload reduction, and mechanical support, including intraaortic balloon pumps and ventricular assist devices. The use of invasive hemodynamic monitoring in ADHF has been controversial; although it is often used to guide pharmacologic management, clinical data have not demonstrated improved renal outcomes when management is guided by pulmonary artery catheters.[544] The role of isolated ultrafiltration in ADHF is also controversial. Although negative fluid balance can be achieved more readily using extracorporeal ultrafiltration as compared to conventional diuretic therapy, studies have not demonstrated differences in kidney function or survival.[545-547] In the Ultrafiltration versus Intravenous Diuretics for Patients Hospitalized for Acute Decompensated Heart Failure (UNLOAD) trial, hypervolemic patients with heart failure who were randomized to isolated ultrafiltration had more rapid fluid loss and decreased rehospitalizations within 90 days as compared to patients randomized to diuretic therapy, with no differences in kidney function.[546] In contrast, in the subsequent Cardiorenal Rescue Study in Acute Decompensated Heart Failure (CARRESS-HF) trial, ultrafiltration was inferior to diuretic therapy with respect to the bivariate end point of change in the serum creatinine level and body weight 96 hours after enrollment ($P = 0.003$), owing primarily to worsening of kidney function in the ultrafiltration group.[547] Based on these data, extracorporeal ultrafiltration cannot be recommended for primary management of patients with decompensated heart failure.

LIVER FAILURE AND HEPATORENAL SYNDROME

Although volume-responsive prerenal azotemia is common in patients with advanced liver disease, differentiation from HRS and intrinsic AKI may be difficult.[53,54,548-550] While patients with liver failure typically have total-body sodium overload, with peripheral edema and ascites, true hypovolemia or reduced effective systemic arterial blood volume is often an important contributory factor to the development of AKI. The underlying pathophysiology of salt and water retention in cirrhosis involves multiple pathways. Portal hypertension leads directly to ascites formation, while splanchnic and peripheral vasodilation result in a state of relative arterial underfilling, activating neurohumoral vasoconstrictors that produce intrarenal vasoconstriction, salt and water retention, and decreased GFR.[551] Volume-responsive AKI may develop in the setting of excessive diuresis, increased gastrointestinal losses (often as the result of therapy for hepatic encephalopathy), rapid drainage of ascites, or spontaneous bacterial peritonitis. Worsening hepatic function is often associated with diuretic resistance and progressive or precipitous worsening of kidney function. It has been postulated that an inadequate increase in cardiac output in response to the fall in peripheral vascular resistance may be central to the development of the HRS.[552]

Differentiation between volume-responsive prerenal AKI and HRS is based on the clinical response to volume loading. The optimal fluid for volume expansion in this setting has been controversial. Recent expert opinion has advocated the use of hyperoncotic (20% or 25%) albumin at a dose of 1 g/kg/day[450,553]; however there is an absence of rigorous data supporting this regimen as compared to volume expansion with isotonic crystalloid solutions. There are more data regarding the use of albumin infusion to prevent AKI in patients undergoing large-volume (>5 L) paracentesis[54,554,555] and in the treatment of spontaneous bacterial peritonitis.[556] In a randomized controlled trial, infusion of 10 g of albumin per liter of drained ascites was associated with less activation of the RAAS and a significantly lower rate of worsening of kidney function than in patients who did not receive albumin infusion.[554] In a subsequent study, albumin infusion was superior to administration of either dextran or gelatin solutions in preventing AKI following large-volume paracentesis.[555] Current recommendations are to infuse 6 to 8 g of albumin per liter of ascites drained when paracentesis volume exceeds 5 L. In a randomized controlled trial comparing antibiotics alone to antibiotics plus albumin, infusion of 1.5 g/kg of albumin at initiation of treatment and an additional 1 g/kg on the third day of treatment was associated with reduced rates of both AKI and mortality,[556] although the benefit appears to be restricted to patients in whom the serum creatinine level is greater than 1 mg/dL, the BUN level is above 30 mg/dL, or the total bilirubin level is greater than 4 mg/dL.[557]

Definitive therapy of HRS requires restoration of hepatic function, usually achieved through liver transplantation.[53,553] The role of peritoneovenous shunting (e.g., LeVeen and Denver shunts) in HRS has been inadequately studied. In a subset of 33 patients with HRS included in a randomized trial comparing peritoneovenous shunts to medical therapy, shunting was not associated with improved survival.[558] These data need to be interpreted with caution due to the small sample size and because data on improvement in kidney function were not reported. In addition, as a result of poor long-term patency rates and high rates of complications, particularly encephalopathy, the use of the peritoneovenous shunt has largely been supplanted by the transjugular intrahepatic portosystemic shunt (TIPS). TIPS has been demonstrated to provide better control of ascites than sequential paracentesis[559-562] and, in one series, lower rates of HRS,[560] albeit with a higher risk for encephalopathy.[563] In a small case series, TIPS has been reported to be effective as primary therapy for HRS,[564] but it has not been evaluated in a randomized trial.[553] Pharmacologic therapy with vasoconstrictors, when combined with albumin infusion, has been associated with improvement in kidney function in patients with HRS.[553,565] Agents that have shown benefit include norepinephrine,[566] the combination of octreotide and midodrine,[567-570] and the type 1 vasopressin receptor agonist terlipressin,[456,457,571] although only terlipressin has been evaluated in randomized controlled trials. In meta-analyses of published trials, terlipressin treatment was associated with a 3.5- to 4-fold increased odds of reversal of HRS.[572,573] Treatment of HRS with terlipressin was also associated with a modest short-term reduction in mortality;

however, longer-term outcomes are primarily a function of the underlying liver disease rather than treatment for HRS.[573] In addition, terlipressin was associated with markedly increased risk for adverse cardiovascular events. At present, terlipressin is not approved for use in the United States.

ABDOMINAL COMPARTMENT SYNDROME

AKI can result from elevations in intraabdominal pressure, resulting in a clinical presentation with features similar to those of prerenal AKI. ACS is defined by an intraabdominal pressure of 20 mm Hg or higher associated with dysfunction of one or more organ systems.[56] However, intraabdominal pressures lower than 20 mm Hg may be associated with ACS, while values higher than this threshold do not universally lead to the ACS.[574-577] ACS typically develops in critically ill patients, most commonly in the setting of trauma with abdominal hemorrhage, abdominal surgery, massive fluid resuscitation, liver transplantation, and gastrointestinal conditions, including peritonitis and pancreatitis. Mechanisms underlying the development of AKI in ACS are believed to involve renal vein compression and constriction of the renal artery from sympathetic system and RAAS activation and reduced cardiac output.[578-580] Oliguria, which can lead to anuria, often develops; as is true for other forms of AKI associated with impaired renal perfusion, U_{Na} is commonly reduced.

The diagnosis of ACS should be suspected in patients with acute abdominal distension, rapidly accumulating ascites, or abdominal trauma and can be made by simple transduction of bladder pressure.[56,57,574] Treatment is prompt abdominal decompression; if ascites is present, this may be achieved by performing large-volume paracentesis; however, surgical laparotomy is often required for definitive therapy.

INTRINSIC ACUTE KIDNEY INJURY

GENERAL PRINCIPLES

Strategies to prevent intrinsic AKI vary based on the specific cause of kidney injury. Optimization of cardiovascular function and restoration of intravascular volume status are key interventions to minimize the risk that prerenal AKI evolves into ischemic ATN. There is compelling evidence that aggressive intravascular volume expansion dramatically reduces the incidence of ATN after major surgery or trauma, burns, and cholera.[294,523,581,582] AKI due to sepsis is common and is associated with mortality rates as high as 80%.[34,516,583] The role of early goal-directed therapy (EGDT) utilizing resuscitation to defined hemodynamic targets (mean arterial pressure > 65 mm Hg, central venous pressure 10 to 12 mm Hg, urine output > 0.5 mL/kg/hr, central venous oxygen saturation >70%) using a combination of crystalloid solutions, RBC transfusion, and vasopressors guided by invasive hemodynamic monitoring in improving overall outcomes and decreasing the risk for AKI has been controversial. In a seminal single-center randomized controlled trial, EGDT resulted in a significant reduction in overall organ dysfunction and mortality in patients presenting with severe sepsis or septic shock, although specific data on the incidence of AKI were not reported.[584] However, these benefits were not confirmed in the Protocolized Care for Early Septic Shock (ProCESS) trial, a subsequent three-arm multicenter randomized controlled trial that compared EGDT to protocol-based standard therapy and usual care.[585] Although the benefits of EGDT were not confirmed, the results of these trials suggest that early recognition of sepsis, prompt initiation of antibiotic therapy and rapid volume resuscitation, and hemodynamic stabilization improve outcomes and are likely to minimize the risk for AKI.[586] The role of maintenance of normoglycemia in critically ill patients in minimizing the risk for AKI has also been controversial. Two single-center randomized controlled trials that utilized intensive insulin management to maintain blood glucose levels of 80 to 110 mg/dL as compared to conventional management maintaining the glucose concentration between 180 and 220 mg/dL each resulted in decreased rates of AKI, defined either on the basis of change in serum creatinine level or the need for RRT.[587-589] However, the benefits of tight glycemic control were not confirmed in the Normoglycemia in Intensive Care Evaluation—Survival Using Glucose Algorithm Regulation (NICE-SUGAR) trial, a 6104 patient multicenter trial that compared intensive therapy to achieve a target glucose level of approximately 80 to 110 mg/dL to more conventional therapy designed to maintain the blood glucose below 180 mg/dL.[590] In the NICE-SUGAR trial, intensive glycemic control was associated with an increased risk for hypoglycemia, an increased mortality risk (27.5% vs. 24.9%, $P = 0.02$), and no reduction in the need for RRT.

In surgical patients, avoidance of hypotension has been associated with a decreased risk for AKI. In a retrospective analysis of over 33,000 patients who underwent noncardiac surgery, episodes of intraoperative hypotension with a mean arterial blood pressure less than 55 mm Hg were associated with a marked increase in the probability of AKI.[591] The adjusted odds of AKI with intraoperative hypotension increased with duration of hypotension, from an odds ratio of 1.2 with less than 10 minutes of hypotension, to 1.3 with 10 to 20 minutes of hypotension, and 1.5 with more than 20 minutes of hypotension.

Intravascular volume depletion has been identified as a risk factor for ATN resulting from iodinated contrast material, rhabdomyolysis, hemolysis, cisplatin, amphotericin B, multiple myeloma, aminoglycosides, and other nephrotoxins; crystal-associated AKI related to acyclovir and acute urate nephropathy; and AKI stemming from hypercalcemia.[100,311,388,397,471,493,582,592-594] Restoration of intravascular volume status prevents the development of experimental and human ATN in many of these clinical settings.

Avoidance of potentially nephrotoxic medications or insults in high-risk patients and settings is also important to reduce the risk for ATN. Specifically, among patients with advanced cardiac and/or liver disease, in whom renal perfusion may be diminished, use of selective or nonselective NSAIDs that inhibit the production of vasodilatory prostaglandins may exacerbate intrarenal vasoconstriction and precipitate AKI.[595-599] Diuretics, NSAIDs (including selective COX-2 inhibitors), ACE inhibitors, ARBs, and other inhibitors of the RAAS should be used with caution in patients with suspected absolute or effective intravascular volume depletion or in patients with renovascular disease as these agents may convert reversible prerenal AKI to intrinsic ischemic ATN. The combined use of agents that block the RAAS, diuretics, and NSAIDs has been identified as a risk factor for AKI, particularly among patients with heart failure, liver failure, or other causes of reduced baseline renal perfusion.[600,601]

Careful monitoring of circulating drug levels appears to reduce the incidence of AKI associated with aminoglycoside antibiotics and calcineurin inhibitors.[602-604] The observation that the antimicrobial efficacy of aminoglycosides persists in tissues even after the drug has been cleared from the circulation (postantibiotic killing) has led to the use of once-daily dosing with these agents. Dosing regimens that provide higher peak drug levels but less frequent administration appear to provide comparable antimicrobial activity and less nephrotoxicity than older conventional dosing regimens.[88,604-606] Nephrotoxicity of drugs may also be reduced through changes in formulation. For example, the use of lipid-encapsulated formulations of amphotericin B may decrease the risk for amphotericin-induced AKI.[607]

PREVENTION OF CONTRAST MEDIUM–INDUCED ACUTE KIDNEY INJURY

The preventive role of intravascular volume resuscitation has been best demonstrated in the setting of AKI due to iodinated contrast medium administration. Administration of intravenous fluids to high-risk patients before and following exposure to intravascular iodinated contrast medium diminishes the risk for contrast medium–induced AKI (CIAKI), although the optimal regimen for fluid administration is unknown.[3,608,609] In a small clinical trial that was stopped early due to safety concerns, periprocedural intravenous isotonic saline was associated with a markedly lower rate of AKI after contrast medium exposure than oral fluid administration.[608] In a larger randomized trial, isotonic saline significantly reduced the incidence of CIAKI following coronary angiography compared with half-normal saline, with a particular benefit noted in patients with diabetes and those receiving large volumes of contrast.[609] Later clinical trials have compared the effects of isotonic sodium bicarbonate compared to isotonic saline for prevention of contrast medium–induced AKI.[610-619] These studies have generally been underpowered and have yielded conflicting results, although certain meta-analyses have concluded that there is an overall benefit associated with bicarbonate administration with regard to AKI defined by small changes in serum creatinine level. There has been no demonstrable benefit with bicarbonate with regard to the need for dialysis.[620-622] Clinical practice guidelines therefore recommend administration of intravenous isotonic sodium chloride or sodium bicarbonate to high-risk patients receiving iodinated contrast material.[3,623,624] For hospitalized patients, administration of isotonic fluids at a rate of 1 mL/kg/hr for 6 to 12 hours before and 6 to 12 hours following the procedure is recommended; for outpatients, an alternative regimen of 3 mL/kg/hr for 1 hour before the procedure followed by 6 mL/kg administered over 4 to 6 hours following the procedure may be more feasible.

NAC is an antioxidant with vasodilatory properties that has been investigated in numerous clinical trials for the prevention of contrast medium–induced AKI. The rationale for the use of NAC for the prevention of CIAKI relates to its capacity to scavenge ROS, reduce the depletion of glutathione, and stimulate the production of vasodilatory mediators including NO.[625,626] Clinical trials of oral and intravenous NAC have yielded conflicting findings.[627-636] Although initially utilized at a dose of 600 mg twice daily,[627] subsequent studies suggested greater efficacy with higher doses of up to 1200 mg twice daily.[634,635] In the largest trial evaluating the effectiveness of NAC, 2308 patients were randomized to receive 1200 mg of NAC or placebo twice daily beginning before the procedure and continuing for three doses after the procedure.[636] No differences were observed in the incidence of contrast medium–induced AKI at 48 to 96 hours after contrast administration or in the incidence of death or need for dialysis within 30 days; however, the overall study population had relatively well preserved kidney function, with a median serum creatinine level of 1.1 mg/dL, and fewer than 16% of patients had a baseline serum creatinine level greater than 1.5 mg/dL. There is an absence of consensus among clinical practice guidelines as to whether NAC is beneficial[3,623,624] with some guidelines concluding that, while its efficacy is uncertain, it is safe and inexpensive in its oral form. If NAC is administered, it should not be used in lieu of appropriate intravenous volume administration.[3]

Trials of other pharmacologic interventions, including furosemide, dopamine, fenoldopam, calcium channel blockers, and mannitol have failed to demonstrate significant benefit and in some cases have been associated with an increased risk for CIAKI.[637-643] Studies on the benefit of natriuretic peptides, aminophylline, theophylline, statins, and ascorbic acid have also yielded conflicting results.[644-653] Given the absence of convincing data on the efficacy of these interventions and potential safety concerns with the use of natriuretic peptides, aminophylline, and theophylline in patients with cardiovascular disease, their routine use is not recommended.[652] Although data with other statins have not shown a clear benefit, clinical trials have demonstrated a reduction in risk for contrast-induced AKI in patients treated with rosuvastatin as compared to controls.[654,655] RRTs for the prevention of CIAKI have been largely ineffective, and in some instances the use of "prophylactic" hemodialysis has been associated with harm.[656-658] The interpretation of studies of hemofiltration for prevention of CIAKI are confounded by their consideration of change in serum creatinine level as an end point, since hemofiltration lowers serum creatinine concentrations.[659,660] Given the risks associated with intravenous line placement and the procedures themselves, along with lack of definitive benefit, use of dialysis or hemofiltration to prevent CIAKI is not currently recommended.[3,661]

Over the past 25 years there has been considerable progress in developing less nephrotoxic contrast media.[662] The use of lower-osmolal contrast media in place of the older and more nephrotoxic high-osmolal media resulted in a decreased incidence of CIAKI.[663,664] Data regarding the added benefit associated with the isoosmolal radiocontrast medium iodixanol have been less consistent[665-671] and may reflect heterogeneity in the risk for CIAKI associated with specific lower-osmolal media.[672]

PREVENTION OF OTHER FORMS OF INTRINSIC ACUTE KIDNEY INJURY

Allopurinol (10 mg/kg/day in three divided doses, maximum 800 mg per day) is useful for limiting uric acid generation in patients at high risk for acute urate nephropathy; however, AKI can develop despite the use of allopurinol, probably through the toxic actions of hypoxanthine crystals on tubule function.[388,471,491,493,673,674] In the setting of high rates of uric acid generation such as tumor lysis syndrome, the use of recombinant urate oxidase (rasburicase, 0.05 to 0.2 mg/kg) may be more effective. Rasburicase catalyzes the degradation of uric acid to allantoin and has been shown to be effective both as prophylaxis and treatment for acute uric acid–mediated tumor lysis syndrome and to prevent the development of AKI due to tumor lysis syndrome–associated hyperuricemia.[392,471,674-677] In oligoanuric patients, prophylactic hemodialysis may be used to acutely lower uric acid levels.

Amifostine, an organic thiophosphate, has been demonstrated to ameliorate cisplatin nephrotoxicity in patients with solid organ or hematologic malignancies.[678-681] NAC limits acetaminophen-induced renal injury if given within 24 hours of ingestion, and dimercaprol, a chelating agent, may prevent heavy-metal nephrotoxicity.[682,683] Ethanol inhibits ethylene glycol metabolism to oxalic acid and other toxic metabolites, but its use has been largely replaced by fomepizole, an inhibitor of alcohol dehydrogenase that decreases production of ethylene glycol metabolites and prevents the development of AKI.[684-687]

PHARMACOLOGIC THERAPY FOR ACUTE TUBULAR NECROSIS

During the past 2 decades there has been extensive investigation into the pathogenesis of AKI using experimental animal models and cultured cells. These studies have resulted in substantial advances in our understanding of the pathophysiology of ATN in humans and led to the discovery of an array of potentially novel targets for the treatment of this common and serious disease. However, multiple interventions shown to ameliorate AKI in animals have failed to be effective in humans with ATN. There are many possible reasons for the lack of success in translating therapeutic successes for AKI from animal models to clinical practice. A principal obstacle relates to the difficulty in identifying the incipient stage of ATN before elevations in the serum creatinine concentration or clinical evidence of decreased urine output. Over the past decade, as previously reviewed, several novel serum and urinary biomarkers have been investigated for their ability to identify AKI in its earliest stages and differentiate ATN from volume-responsive AKI.[17] Work in this area may facilitate the identification of those patients most likely to respond to treatments that have been found to be effective in animal models.

Dopamine

Historically, low-dose dopamine ("renal-dose" dopamine; <2 mg/kg/min) was widely advocated for the management of oliguric AKI.[688-690] In experimental studies of animals and healthy human volunteers, low-dose dopamine increases renal blood flow and to a lesser extent GFR. However, low-dose dopamine has not been demonstrated to prevent or alter the course of ischemic or nephrotoxic ATN in prospective clinical trials.[691-695] This absence of clinical benefit may relate to differences in the hemodynamic response to low-dose dopamine in patients with renal disease as compared to healthy individuals. In contrast to the reduction in renal resistive index associated with low-dose dopamine in critically ill patients without kidney disease, dopamine infusion is associated with an increase in renal resistance in patients with AKI.[696] Moreover, dopamine, even at low doses, is potentially toxic in critically ill patients and can induce tachyarrhythmias, myocardial ischemia, and extravasation necrosis.[696] Thus the routine administration of low-dose dopamine to ameliorate or reverse the course of AKI is not justified based on the balance of experimental and clinical evidence.[697,698]

Fenoldopam

Fenoldopam is a selective postsynaptic dopamine agonist that acts on D_1 receptors and mediates more potent renal vasodilation and natriuresis than dopamine.[699] However, fenoldopam is a potent antihypertensive agent and causes hypotension by decreasing peripheral vascular resistance. Several small studies suggested that fenoldopam could reduce the incidence of AKI in high-risk clinical situations[700,701]; however, a subsequent larger randomized trial comparing fenoldopam to standard hydration in patients undergoing invasive angiographic procedures found no benefit in regard to decreasing the incidence of contrast medium–induced AKI.[640] In another large randomized controlled trial, fenoldopam administration failed to reduce mortality or the need for RRT in ICU patients with early ATN.[702] Therefore there is currently no clinical role for fenoldopam in the prevention or treatment of AKI.

Natriuretic Peptides

ANP is a 28–amino acid polypeptide synthesized in cardiac atrial muscle.[703,704] ANP augments GFR by triggering afferent arteriolar vasodilation and constriction of the efferent arteriole.[705,706] In addition, ANP inhibits sodium transport and lowers oxygen requirements in several nephron segments.[707,708] Synthetic analogs of ANP showed promise in the management of ATN in the laboratory setting; however, these benefits in animal models of AKI have failed to translate into clinical benefit in humans. A large multicenter, prospective, randomized placebo-controlled trial of anaritide, a synthetic analog of ANP, in patients with ATN failed to show clinically significant improvement in dialysis-free survival or overall mortality,[709] although there was an improvement in dialysis-free survival in oliguric patients. This benefit in oliguric patients was not confirmed in a subsequent prospective study.[710] It has been suggested that the absence of benefit may be related to both the relatively late initiation of therapy and to the effect of ANP on systemic blood pressure. In a subsequent pilot study, low-dose recombinant ANP administration in high-risk cardiac surgery patients was associated with a reduction in the requirement for postoperative RRT.[711] Until these results are confirmed in a larger, multicenter trial, the use of ANP in this setting cannot be recommended. Trials of ANP for the prevention of contrast medium–induced AKI have generated mixed results.[649,650] Ularitide (urodilantin) is a natriuretic pro-ANP fragment produced within the kidney. In a small randomized trial, ularitide did not reduce the need for dialysis in patients with AKI.[712] A recent meta-analysis of ANP for the treatment of AKI concluded that the paucity of high-quality studies precluded a determination of the effects of this therapy.[713]

Loop Diuretics

High-dose intravenous diuretics are commonly prescribed to increase urine output in patients with oliguric AKI.

Although this strategy assists in volume management and minimizes the risk for progressive volume overload, there is no evidence that diuretic therapy alters the natural history of AKI or improves mortality or dialysis-free survival. In a retrospective analysis, diuretic therapy was associated with an increased risk for death and nonrecovery of renal function.[714] These risks were restricted, however, to patients who did not respond to diuretic administration with increased urine volume; in patients responsive to diuretics, outcomes were similar to untreated patients. In a prospective randomized trial, high-dose intravenous furosemide augmented urine output but did not alter the outcome of established AKI.[715] In a posthoc analysis of data from the Fluid and Catheter Treatment Trial, a positive fluid balance after AKI in patients with acute lung injury was strongly associated with increased mortality while diuretic therapy was associated with improved 60-day patient survival.[716] Given the risks of loop diuretics in AKI, including irreversible ototoxicity and exacerbation of prerenal AKI, these agents should be used solely to facilitate the management of extracellular volume overload (see later).[717]

Mannitol

The osmotic diuretic mannitol, which also has renal vasodilatory and oxygen free radical scavenging properties, has been investigated as a preventive treatment for AKI.[718,719] No adequate data exist to support the routine administration of mannitol to oliguric patients. Moreover, when administered to severely oliguric or anuric patients, mannitol may trigger expansion of intravascular volume and pulmonary edema, as well as severe hyponatremia due to an osmotic shift of water from the intracellular to the intravascular space.[719-723]

MANAGEMENT OF OTHER CAUSES OF INTRINSIC ACUTE KIDNEY INJURY

Acute Vasculitis and Acute Glomerular Disease

The management of acute vasculitis involving the kidney and acute glomerular disease is covered in detail in Chapters 32 to 34. AKI caused by acute glomerulonephritis or vasculitis may respond to corticosteroids, alkylating agents, rituximab, and plasmapheresis depending on the primary cause of the disease. Plasma exchange is useful in the treatment of sporadic TTP and possibly sporadic HUS in adults.[724,725] The role of plasmapheresis in the drug-induced thrombotic microangiopathies is less certain, and removal of the offending agent is the most important initial therapeutic maneuver.[375,726,727] Postdiarrheal HUS in children is usually managed conservatively as evidence suggests that early antibiotic therapy may actually promote the development of HUS.[728] Treatment with eculizumab, a humanized monoclonal antibody that prevents cleavage of complement component C5 into C5a and C5b, inhibiting terminal complement activation, may be considered in patients with nondiarrheal (complement-mediated) HUS unresponsive to plasma exchange.[729] Hypertension and AKI associated with scleroderma may be exquisitely sensitive to treatment with ACE inhibitors.[730-732]

Acute Kidney Injury in Multiple Myeloma

Early studies suggested that plasmapheresis may be of benefit in AKI due to myeloma cast nephropathy.[104,397,733] Clearance of circulating light chains with concomitant chemotherapy to decrease the rate of production had been postulated to reverse renal injury in patients with circulating light chains, heavy Bence Jones proteinuria, and AKI. A subsequent randomized controlled trial compared plasma exchange and standard chemotherapy with chemotherapy alone. Although the study did not demonstrate improvement with plasma exchange with regard to a composite outcome of death, dialysis dependence, or GFR less than 30 mL/min at 6 months, the study was inadequately powered to definitively exclude a clinical benefit, and there was a trend toward improved outcomes with plasmapheresis.[398-400] It has been suggested that the use of dialysis membranes that are permeable to light chains and other proteins with molecular weights lower than albumin (high-cutoff membranes) may be an effective therapeutic strategy in patients with acute kidney injury due to light-chain cast nephropathy. However, until additional data are available on the benefit of high-cutoff membranes, their use should be considered experimental.[105]

Acute Interstitial Nephritis

AIN is a relatively common cause of AKI and in the majority of cases is due to an allergic response to a medication.[734] The initial therapeutic step in AIN is discontinuation of the offending medication or treatment of the probable inciting factor if AIN is not drug induced. Data on the efficacy of corticosteroids derive from small observational studies that have yielded highly discordant results. While some studies suggest that early use of corticosteroids (i.e., before significant renal damage and within 7 to 14 days of discontinuation of the offending medication)[735] may be beneficial, other studies demonstrate no clear evidence of efficacy.[298] There have been no large, prospective randomized clinical trials investigating the role of corticosteroids in the treatment of AIN. As corticosteroids are associated with a series of potentially serious side effects, their use should be considered on a case-by-case basis. If corticosteroid therapy is being considered and no patient-related contraindications exist, one potential regimen used in a recent study involves the intravenous administration of methylprednisolone (250 to 500 mg/day) for 3 to 4 days followed by oral prednisone at a dose of 1 mg/kg/day tapered over 8 to 12 weeks.[735] However, there are no data supporting the superiority of this specific approach over others. Mycophenolate mofetil has also been investigated as a therapeutic agent for AIN. In a study of eight patients with AIN, six experienced improvement in renal function with mycophenolate mofetil therapy, while two had stabilization in renal function.[736] While this small case series suggests a possible role for mycophenolate mofetil in the treatment of AIN, additional data are needed to confirm its efficacy for this indication.

POSTRENAL ACUTE KIDNEY INJURY

The principle underlying the management of postrenal AKI is the prompt relief of urinary tract obstruction. This topic is reviewed extensively in Chapter 38. Urethral or bladder neck obstruction may be relieved with the placement of a transurethral or suprapubic bladder catheter. Similarly, ureteric obstruction may be acutely relieved by placement of percutaneous nephrostomy tubes or by cystoscopically placed ureteral stents. Following the initial relief of obstruction, most patients experience a physiologic diuresis that resolves after several days as the result of excretion of volume and solutes retained during the period of renal obstruction; however, approximately 5% of patients may have a more prolonged diuretic phase because of delayed recovery of tubule function relative to GFR, resulting in a salt-wasting syndrome, which may require intravenous fluid replacement to maintain blood pressure.[520,521,737] Following initial relief of obstruction, urologic evaluation is required for definitive evaluation and management of the underlying cause of obstruction.

NONDIALYTIC SUPPORTIVE MANAGEMENT OF ACUTE KIDNEY INJURY

Metabolic complications such as intravascular volume overload, hyperkalemia, hyperphosphatemia, and metabolic acidosis are common in oliguric AKI, and preventive measures should be implemented beginning with initial diagnosis (Table 31.15). Adequate nutrition should be provided to meet caloric requirements and minimize catabolism. In addition, all medications that are normally excreted by the kidney need to be adjusted based on the severity of renal impairment.

INTRAVASCULAR VOLUME

After correction of intravascular volume deficits, salt and water intake should be adjusted to match ongoing losses (urinary, gastrointestinal, drainage sites, insensible losses). Extracellular volume overload can usually be managed by restriction of salt and water intake and by judicious use of diuretics. High doses of loop diuretics (e.g., the equivalent of 200 mg of furosemide administered as an intravenous bolus infusion or 20 mg/hr as a continuous infusion) or combination therapy with both thiazide and loop diuretics may be required. If an adequate diuresis cannot be attained, further use of diuretics should be discontinued to minimize the risk for complications such as ototoxicity. Fluid administration should be closely monitored to avoid progressive volume overload. Although there is a strong association between progressive fluid overload and mortality risk in patients with AKI,[738-740] a causal relationship has not been definitively established, and volume overload may be a surrogate for hemodynamic instability and capillary leak. Fluid conservative management has, however, been demonstrated to result in improved outcomes in critically ill patients with lung failure.[741] Ultrafiltration or dialysis may be required for volume management when conservative measures fail.

HYPONATREMIA

Hyponatremia associated with a fall in effective serum osmolality can usually be corrected by restriction of water intake. Conversely, hypernatremia is treated by administration of water, hypotonic saline solutions, or hypotonic dextrose-containing solutions (the latter are effectively hypotonic because dextrose is rapidly metabolized).

HYPERKALEMIA

Mild hyperkalemia (<5.5 mmol/L) should be managed initially by restriction of dietary potassium intake and the discontinuation of potassium supplements and potassium-sparing diuretics. More severe degrees of hyperkalemia (5.5 to 6.5 mmol/L) can usually be controlled with the aforementioned steps coupled with the administration of

Table 31.15 Supportive Management of Acute Kidney Injury

Management Issue	Treatment
Intravascular volume overload	Restriction of salt (<1-2 g/day) and water (<1 L/day) intake
	Diuretic therapy (if nonoliguric)
	Ultrafiltration
Hyponatremia	Restriction of oral and intravenous free water
Hyperkalemia	Calcium gluconate (10 mL of 10% solution over 5 min) if ECG changes present
	Glucose (50 mL of 50%) + insulin (10-15 U regular) IV
	Albuterol (10-20 mg by nebulizer or MDI)
	Renal replacement therapy
	Loop diuretics (if nonoliguric)
	K^+ binding resin
	Discontinue K^+ supplements or K^+-sparing diuretics
	Restriction of dietary potassium
Metabolic acidosis	Restriction of dietary protein
	Sodium bicarbonate (if HCO_3^- <15 mmol/L)
	Renal replacement therapy
Hyperphosphatemia	Restriction of dietary phosphate intake
	Phosphate-binding agents (aluminum hydroxide, calcium carbonate, calcium acetate, sevelamer carbonate, lanthanum carbonate)
Hypocalcemia	Oral or intravenous replacement (if symptomatic or sodium bicarbonate to be administered)
Hypermagnesemia	Discontinue magnesium-containing antacids
Nutrition	Caloric intake: 20-30 kcal/day
	Protein intake:
	Non–dialysis requiring: 0.8-1.0 g/kg/day
	Dialysis-requiring: 1.0-1.5 g/kg/day
	Continuous renal replacement therapy: up to 1.7 g/kg/day
	Enteral route of nutrition preferred
Drug dosage	Adjust all doses for GFR and renal replacement modality

ECG, Electrocardiography; GFR, glomerular filtration rate; IV, intravenously; MDI, metered-dose inhaler.

sodium polystyrene sulfonate, a potassium-binding resin, to enhance gastrointestinal potassium losses. While this resin has been widely used for decades, concerns have been raised regarding its safety, particularly when administered in 70% sorbitol, due to reports of bowel necrosis.[742,743] Loop diuretics can also increase potassium excretion in diuretic-responsive patients. Emergency measures need to be employed in patients with more severe hyperkalemia and in patients with electrocardiographic manifestations of hyperkalemia. In patients with severe hyperkalemia with concomitant electrocardiographic manifestations, the intravenous administration of calcium will antagonize the cardiac and neuromuscular effects of hyperkalemia and is a valuable emergency temporizing measure, allowing time for the additional measures described later to be implemented. Intravenous calcium must be used with caution, however, if there is concomitant severe hyperphosphatemia or evidence of digitalis toxicity. Intravenous insulin (10 to 15 U of regular insulin) promotes potassium entry into cells and lowers extracellular potassium concentration within 15 to 30 minutes, with an effect that lasts for several hours.[744,745] Concomitant administration of intravenous dextrose (25 to 50 g over 30 to 60 minutes) is required to prevent hypoglycemia in patients who do not have hyperglycemia. β-Adrenergic agonists, such as inhaled albuterol (10 to 20 mg by nebulizer), also promote rapid potassium uptake into the intracellular compartment.[744] Although sodium bicarbonate also stimulates potassium uptake into the intracellular compartment, this effect is not sufficiently rapid to be clinically useful for the emergent management of hyperkalemia.[745] Emergent dialysis is indicated if hyperkalemia is resistant to these measures.

METABOLIC ACIDOSIS

The treatment of metabolic acidosis is dependent upon the clinical setting and cause. As a general rule, metabolic acidosis does not require treatment unless the serum HCO_3^- concentration falls below 15 mmol/L or the pH is lower than 7.15 to 7.20. In patients with AKI in whom metabolic acidosis is due to the underlying renal failure, more severe acidosis can be corrected by either oral or intravenous bicarbonate administration. Initial rates of replacement should be based on estimates of HCO_3^- deficit and adjusted thereafter according to serum levels. In patients with underlying lactic acidosis, the role of bicarbonate therapy is controversial, and the primary focus of therapy should be on correction of the underlying cause.[746-749] Patients treated with intravenous bicarbonate need to be monitored for complications of therapy, including metabolic alkalosis, hypocalcemia, hypokalemia, hypernatremia, and volume overload.

CALCIUM, PHOSPHATE, MAGNESIUM, AND URIC ACID

Hypocalcemia does not usually require treatment unless it is severe, as may occur in patients with rhabdomyolysis or pancreatitis or after administration of bicarbonate. Hyperphosphatemia can usually be controlled by restricting dietary phosphate intake and the use of oral phosphate binders (e.g., aluminum hydroxide, calcium salts, sevelamer carbonate, or lanthanum carbonate). Caution must be employed when using aluminum-containing phosphate binders as prolonged use may result in aluminum intoxication, which can produce acute neurologic symptoms and bone disease; however short-term use is rarely associated with this complication. Hypermagnesemia can be prevented through avoidance of magnesium-containing medications, such as antacids, and limiting magnesium content of parenteral nutrition. Hyperuricemia is usually mild in AKI (<15 mg/dL) and does not require specific intervention. Severe hyperuricemia secondary to cell lysis may be managed by blocking xanthine oxidase with allopurinol or by enhancing degradation with recombinant uricase as previously described.

NUTRITION

Patients with AKI are clinically heterogeneous, and individualized nutritional management is required, especially in critically ill patients undergoing RRT, in whom protein catabolic rates can exceed 1.5 g/kg of body weight per day.[3,505,506,508,509,750,751] The objective of nutritional management in AKI is to provide sufficient calories to preserve lean body mass, avoid starvation ketoacidosis, and promote healing and tissue repair while minimizing production of nitrogenous waste. If the duration of renal insufficiency is likely to be short and the patient is not extremely catabolic and does not require RRT, then dietary protein should be approximately 0.8 to 1.0 g/kg of body weight per day.[3] Protein intake should not be restricted in patients in whom AKI is likely to be prolonged, who are hypercatabolic, or who are receiving RRT. Protein intake in these patients should generally be 1.0 to 1.5 g/kg of body weight per day.[505,506,750,751] There is no evidence of improved outcomes with protein intake greater than 1.7 g/kg of body weight per day, even in extremely hypercatabolic patients.[3] Total caloric intake should generally be 20 to 30 kcal/kg of body weight per day and should not exceed 35 kcal/kg of body weight per day.[3,505,506,750,751] Management of nutrition is easier in nonoliguric patients and after institution of dialysis. Vigorous parenteral hyperalimentation has been claimed to improve prognosis in AKI; however, a consistent benefit has yet to be demonstrated. The enteral route of nutrition is preferred because it avoids the morbidity associated with parenteral nutrition while providing support to intestinal function.[508] Water-soluble vitamins and trace elements should be supplemented in patients receiving RRT.[750,751]

Severe anemia is generally managed with blood transfusion. Transfusion is usually not required for patients with a hemoglobin level above 7 g/dL.[752] The role of erythropoiesis-stimulating agents in AKI has not been well studied.[753] Patients with AKI or other acute illness are relatively resistant to the effect of these agents. In randomized controlled trials in critically ill patients, recombinant human erythropoietin decreased transfusion requirement but had no effect on other outcomes.[754,755] Uremic bleeding usually responds to desmopressin, correction of anemia, estrogens, or dialysis.

Doses of drugs that are excreted by the kidney must be adjusted for renal impairment and the use of RRT.[756-759] Whenever possible, pharmacokinetic monitoring should be employed to ensure appropriate drug dosing, especially for agents with narrow therapeutic windows (see Chapter 64). In addition to careful monitoring for toxicity of agents that are normally excreted by the kidney, careful attention must be paid to dosing of antibiotics and other drugs removed by RRT to ensure that therapeutic drug levels are achieved, particularly in patients receiving augmented intensity of RRT.

RENAL REPLACEMENT THERAPY IN ACUTE KIDNEY INJURY

Renal replacement therapy (RRT) is the generic term for the multiple modalities of dialysis and hemofiltration employed in the management of kidney failure. Although kidney transplantation is also a form of RRT for end-stage kidney disease, transplantation does not play a role in the management of AKI. RRT facilitates the management of patients with AKI, allowing correction of acid-base and electrolyte disturbances, amelioration of volume overload, and removal of uremic waste products. Although RRT can forestall or reverse the life-threatening complications of uremia associated with severe and prolonged AKI, it does not hasten and can potentially delay the recovery of kidney function in patients with AKI[760] and can be associated with potentially life-threatening complications.[761] Despite more than 60 years of research and clinical experience,[762,763] numerous questions regarding the optimal application of RRT in AKI remain.[3,764-767]

INDICATIONS FOR RENAL REPLACEMENT THERAPY

In clinical practice there are wide variations in the initiation of RRT for patients with AKI.[768] Widely accepted indications for initiation of RRT include volume overload unresponsive to diuretic therapy, severe metabolic acidosis or hyperkalemia despite appropriate medical therapy, and overt uremic manifestations, including encephalopathy, pericarditis, or uremic bleeding diathesis (Table 31.16). However even these specific indications are subject to substantial clinical interpretation. In many patients, RRT is initiated in the absence of these specific indications in response to a clinical course marked by progressive azotemia or sustained oliguria. A precise correlation does not exist between the BUN level and the onset of uremic symptoms, although the longer the duration and the greater the severity of azotemia, the more likely that overt symptoms will develop. Observational series and small clinical trials dating from the 1950s through the 1980s suggested that initiating RRT when the BUN concentration approached 90 to 100 mg/dL was associated with improved survival as compared with more delayed initiation of therapy.[769-773] Later observational studies have suggested that initiation of RRT at even less severe degrees of azotemia may further improve survival.[774-777] These studies need to be interpreted with caution, however, as the outcomes associated with earlier initiation of RRT may reflect differences related to the reasons for initiation of therapy (e.g., volume overload or hyperkalemia versus progressive azotemia) rather than a benefit due to the earlier therapy per se. In addition, these observational series included only patients in whom RRT was actually initiated rather than the broader population of patients with AKI, including patients who either recovered kidney function or died without receiving RRT. There has been a paucity of prospective clinical trials evaluating timing of initiation of RRT in AKI. In a small randomized controlled trial of critically ill patients randomized to early high-volume hemofiltration, early low-volume hemofiltration, or late low-volume hemofiltration, there was no benefit associated with earlier initiation of treatment.[778] In a subsequent trial comparing earlier to later initiation of dialysis in patients with community-acquired AKI, mortality was lower in patients initiated on dialysis later than in the group of patients started earlier with no difference in recovery of kidney function between groups.[779] This latter trial needs to be interpreted with caution, however, as almost half of the patients admitted with community-acquired AKI were excluded due to urgent need for dialysis.

Although volume overload unresponsive to diuretic therapy is a widely accepted indication for initiation of RRT, wide variations in the degree of volume overload at initiation of therapy exist.[739,780,781] Observational studies have demonstrated a strong association between the degree of volume overload and mortality risk, leading to the suggestion that RRT should be initiated early, before the development of progressive volume overload.[738,782] It should be recognized, however, that the association between volume overload and mortality risk does not establish a causal relationship; disease processes that contribute to the development of volume overload may independently contribute to mortality risk in these patients. Prospective studies will therefore be required to demonstrate that preemptive RRT, before the development of more severe degrees of volume overload, decreases morbidity and mortality.

Given the current level of evidence, the KDIGO Clinical Practice Guideline for Acute Kidney Injury does not make strong recommendations for the timing of initiation of RRT.[3] The guideline suggests that RRT be "… initiated emergently when life-threatening changes in fluid, electrolyte, and acid-base balance exist"[3] and further suggests that "…the broader clinical context, the presence of conditions that can be modified by RRT, and trends of laboratory tests—rather than single BUN and creatinine thresholds alone—[be considered] when making the decision to start RRT."[3]

Renal replacement therapy should be continued until renal function recovers or because continued provision of renal support is no longer consistent with the overall goals of care for the patient.[3] Recovery of kidney function is usually heralded by increased urine volume; although no specific threshold of urine output correlates with sufficient recovery of kidney function, it is unlikely that a urine output of less than 1 L/day is sufficient to sustain dialysis independence. Although diuretics may increase daily urine volume, there is no evidence that diuretic therapy promotes recovery of kidney function.[783] Improved solute clearance is manifested by spontaneous fall in BUN and creatinine concentration or a persistent downward trend in predialysis values. The role of creatinine clearance measurement to assess recovery of kidney function is uncertain, with a paucity of data to define specific thresholds for recovery of kidney function. In the Acute Renal Failure Trial Network study, RRT was continued if measured creatinine clearance on a 6-hour timed urine collection was less than 12 mL/min; RRT was stopped if the clearance was greater than 20 mL/

Table 31.16 Indications for Renal Replacement Therapy

Absolute indications	Volume overload unresponsive to diuretic therapy
	Persistent hyperkalemia despite medical therapy
	Severe metabolic acidosis
	Overt uremic symptoms
	Encephalopathy
	Pericarditis
	Uremic bleeding diathesis
Relative indications	Progressive azotemia without uremic manifestations
	Persistent oliguria

min; and the decision was left to the discretion of the clinician if the creatinine clearance was between 12 and 20 mL/min.[784,785]

MODALITIES OF RENAL REPLACEMENT THERAPY

Multiple modalities of RRT are available for the management of patients with AKI, including conventional intermittent hemodialysis (IHD), peritoneal dialysis, multiple forms of continuous RRT (CRRT), and prolonged intermittent renal replacement therapy (PIRRT) such as sustained low-efficiency dialysis (SLED; also known as extended daily dialysis). Detailed descriptions of the technical aspects of these modalities are provided in Chapters 65 (hemodialysis), 66 (peritoneal dialysis), and 67 (CRRT and PIRRT). Objective data to guide the selection of modality for individual patients are limited, and the choice of modality is often guided by the resources of the health care institution and the technical expertise of the physician and nursing staff. The KDIGO Clinical Practice Guideline for Acute Kidney Injury suggests that for the majority of patients the available modalities of RRT are complementary, with the caveats that CRRT and PIRRT be used in hemodynamically unstable patients and that CRRT be used for patients with acute brain injury or other causes of increased intracranial pressure of generalized brain edema.[3]

Intermittent Hemodialysis

Acute IHD has been the mainstay of RRT in AKI for more than 5 decades. Patients typically undergo dialysis treatments for 3 to 5 hours on a thrice-weekly, alternate-day, or daily schedule depending on catabolic demands, electrolyte disturbances, and volume status. Just as with the timing of initiation of dialysis, the most appropriate dosing strategy for IHD in patients with AKI has been the subject of considerable investigation. The dose of IHD may be adjusted by altering the intensity of each individual dialysis session, usually quantified as the product of urea clearance (K) and treatment time (t) divided by body urea volume (V) (Kt/V), or by changing the frequency of the dialysis sessions. In an observational study, Paganini and colleagues demonstrated a survival benefit in patients with intermediate severity of illness scores when the delivered Kt/V was more than 1.0 per treatment as compared to a delivered Kt/V of less than 1.0 per treatment.[786] However, there have been no prospective clinical trials evaluating the relationship between the delivered Kt/V when dialysis is provided on a constant treatment schedule and outcomes. Schiffl and colleagues reported on a prospective trial of 160 patients with AKI assigned in an alternating fashion to alternate-day or daily IHD.[787] The more frequent treatment schedule was associated with a reduction in mortality at 14 days after the last dialysis session from 46% in the alternate-day dialysis arm to 28% in the daily treatment arm ($P = 0.01$). Duration of renal failure declined from 16 ± 6 days to 9 ± 2 days ($P = 0.001$). This study has been criticized, however, because the delivered dose of therapy per session was low in both treatment arms (Kt/V < 0.95), resulting in a high rate of symptoms in the alternate-day dialysis arm that may have been due to overtly inadequate dialysis.[788] The impact of frequency of IHD was also evaluated in the Acute Renal Failure Trial Network study.[784] In the study, 1124 critically ill patients were randomized to an intensive or less intensive strategy for the management of RRT. When patients were hemodynamically stable, they received IHD, and when hemodynamically unstable they received CRRT or SLED, regardless of treatment arm. Patients randomized to the less intensive treatment strategy received IHD on a thrice-weekly (alternate-day except Sunday) schedule while patients randomized to the intensive arm received six-times-per-week (daily except Sunday) IHD. Sixty-day all-cause mortality was 53.6% in the intensive treatment arm as compared to 51.5% in the less intensive arm ($P = 0.47$).[784] The mean delivered Kt/V was 1.3 per treatment after the first IHD session. Although the study was not designed to evaluate outcomes by individual modality of RRT, there were no differences in mortality between groups when evaluated based on percentage of time treated using IHD.[789] Based on these results, it does not appear that there is further benefit to routinely increasing the frequency of IHD treatments beyond three times per week so long as the delivered Kt/V is at least 1.2 per treatment. More frequent treatments may be necessary if the target dose per treatment cannot be achieved, in hypercatabolic patients, in patients with severe hyperkalemia or metabolic acidosis, and for issues related to volume management. The KDIGO Clinical Practice Guideline for Acute Kidney Injury recommends delivering a Kt/V of 3.9 per week when using IHD in AKI, calculating the weekly Kt/V as the arithmetic sum of the delivered dose per treatment.[3] It should be recognized, however, that this approach for calculating an equivalent weekly Kt/V is not consistent with urea kinetic principles and that rigorous data for the appropriate dose of therapy when treatments are delivered more frequently than three times per week are not available.[13]

The selection of IHD dialyzer membrane may also impact clinical outcomes. Exposure to cellulosic membranes results in greater leukocyte and complement activation and delayed recovery of kidney function in experimental models of AKI as compared to exposure to more biocompatible synthetic membranes.[790,791] Clinical trials comparing dialysis membranes have yielded conflicting results. Although some studies demonstrated delayed recovery of kidney function with cellulosic membranes,[792-794] other studies observed no benefit with synthetic membranes.[795-799] When these data have been aggregated in systematic reviews, a benefit of the synthetic membranes is not convincingly demonstrated.[800,801] While the effect of membrane type on humoral and cellular activation may still influence recovery of kidney function in AKI, the clinical importance of this issue has diminished as the cost differential between synthetic and cellulosic membranes has narrowed and the use of unsubstituted cellulosic membranes has decreased.

The major complications associated with acute dialysis are related to the need to access the vasculature, the need for anticoagulation to maintain patency of the extracorporeal circuit, and intradialytic hypotension primarily resulting from shifts in solute and volume.[784,787,802] Many of these issues, particularly the need for vascular access and anticoagulation, are similar for IHD, CRRT, and SLED.

Vascular access is usually obtained through insertion of a double-lumen catheter into a large-caliber central (internal jugular or subclavian) or femoral vein.[803] The major complications associated with vascular access include vascular and organ trauma during insertion; bleeding; catheter malfunction and thrombosis; and infection.[803] Although femoral catheters are generally associated with an increased risk for infection as compared to catheters in the subclavian or internal jugular veins, an increased risk for infection was observed only when femoral vein catheters were used in patients with a high body mass index in a randomized controlled trial involving patients undergoing acute RRT.[804] The use of tunneled dialysis catheters has been proposed as a means of decreasing the risk for infection in patients undergoing acute dialysis[805,806]; however, this strategy has not been rigorously evaluated in prospective clinical trials.

Anticoagulation is used to help maintain patency of the extracorporeal dialysis circuit in IHD, CRRT, and SLED.[807,808] The most commonly used anticoagulant for dialysis is unfractionated heparin; with multiple protocols used to attain sufficient anticoagulation of the dialysis circuit while minimizing systemic effects.[807,808] Regional heparinization, in which heparin is infused proximal to the dialyzer and protamine, to reverse its effect, is infused into the return line,[809] can be used but has generally been supplanted by low-dose heparin protocols.[810] Low-molecular-weight heparin may be used as an alternative to unfractionated heparin; however, the benefits of this approach are unclear as low-molecular-weight heparin is not associated with enhanced efficacy, drug half-life is variably prolonged in renal failure, and monitoring of the anticoagulant effect is more difficult.[807] In patients with heparin-induced thrombocytopenia, heparin administration is contraindicated. Alternative anticoagulation strategies include regional citrate[807,811-813]; the serine protease inhibitor nafamostat[814]; the direct thrombin inhibitors hirudin, lepirudin, and argatroban[815-819]; and, rarely, the prostanoids epoprostenol and iloprost.[807,808] In many patients, particularly those with underlying coagulopathy or thrombocytopenia, and in patients with active hemorrhage or recent postoperative status, acute RRT can be provided in the absence of anticoagulation.[784,820,821]

Intradialytic hypotension is common in patients undergoing acute IHD.[760,784,789,802,822] Episodes of hypotension may impair solute clearance and the efficiency of dialysis and can further compromise renal perfusion and delay recovery of kidney function.[760,823-825] Intradialytic hypotension is typically triggered by intercompartmental fluid shifts or excessive fluid removal, leading to decreased intravascular volume, and may be exacerbated by altered vascular responsiveness related to the underlying acute process.[802,826] Hypotension may be particularly problematic in critically ill patients in whom sepsis, cardiac dysfunction, hypoalbuminemia, malnutrition, or large third-space losses may accompany the development of AKI. Prevention of intradialytic hypotension requires careful assessment of intravascular volume, prescription of realistic ultrafiltration targets, extension of treatment time so as to minimize the ultrafiltration rate, increasing the dialysate sodium concentration, and decreasing the dialysate temperature.[822,826,827] Although there is a tendency to reduce the extracorporeal blood flow in patients prone to hypotension, there is little evidence that this provides any benefit; although reducing blood flow decreased the volume of the extracorporeal circuit in the past when parallel plate and coil dialyzers were used, there is little change in the volume of the extracorporeal circuit in response to changes in blood flow when hollow fiber dialyzers are used. Reducing blood flow may, however, result in reduction of the delivered dose of dialysis.

Continuous Renal Replacement Therapy

The CRRTs represent a spectrum of treatment modalities. In their initial description, the continuous therapies were provided using arteriovenous extracorporeal circuits.[828-832] While this approach provided technical simplicity, blood flow was dependent upon the gradient between mean arterial and central venous pressure, and there was an increased risk for complications from prolonged arterial cannulation.[833] As a result, the continuous arteriovenous therapies have largely been supplanted by pump-driven, venovenous CRRT.[834-837] The modalities of venovenous CRRT vary predominantly based on their mechanism of solute removal: in continuous venovenous hemofiltration (CVVH), solute transport occurs by convection; in continuous venovenous hemodialysis (CVVHD), by diffusion; and in continuous venovenous hemodiafiltration (CVVHDF), by a combination of the two.[837-839] Although, at the same level of urea clearance, convective therapies provide enhanced clearance of higher-molecular-weight solutes than diffusive therapies, no clear clinical benefit has been demonstrated for CVVH or CVVHDF as compared to CVVHD.

The clearance of urea and other small solutes during CRRT is generally proportional to the total effluent flow rate (the sum of ultrafiltrate and dialysate flow rates),[832,837,838] and dose of therapy is usually expressed as the effluent volume indexed to body weight. This approach to estimating solute clearance is based on the assumption of near-complete solute equilibration between blood and effluent and may overestimate the actual solute clearance.[840,841] Several single-center randomized controlled trials demonstrated an improvement in survival when doses of CVVH were increased from 20 to 25 mL/kg/hr to doses in excess of 35 to 45 mL/kg/hr[842,843]; however, other small studies did not find a similar benefit.[778,844] Two large multicenter randomized controlled trials also did not find a survival benefit associated with more intensive CRRT.[784,845] As described previously, in the Acute Renal Failure Trial Network study, 1124 patients were randomized to two intensities of RRT.[784] In both treatment arms, patients received IHD when hemodynamically stable and CVVHDF or SLED when hemodynamically unstable. In the less intensive arm, CVVHDF was provided at an effluent flow rate of 20 mL/kg/hr, and in the more intensive arm at 35 mL/kg/hr. Sixty-day all-cause mortality was 51.5% in the less intensive arm and 53.6% in the more intensive arm ($P = 0.47$).[784] In the Randomized Evaluation of Normal versus Augmented Level (RENAL) Replacement Therapy Study, 1508 patients were randomized to CVVHDF at either 25 mL/kg/hr or 40 mL/kg/hr.[845] Ninety-day all-cause mortality was 44.7% in both treatment arms ($P = 0.99$).[845] Based on these data, the KDIGO Clinical Practice Guideline for Acute Kidney Injury recommends delivering an effluent volume during CRRT of 20 to 25 mL/kg/hr, recognizing that a slightly higher dose may need to be prescribed to achieve the target delivered dose to compensate for interruptions in treatment.[3]

Given the greater hemodynamic tolerance of CRRT as compared to IHD, particularly in patients with underlying hemodynamic instability, it has been postulated that CRRT would be associated with improved clinical outcomes. Five randomized controlled trials comparing outcomes with CRRT and IHD have been published. In a multicenter randomized controlled trial of 166 patients with AKI, Mehta and colleagues observed ICU and hospital mortality rates of 59.5% and 65.5%, respectively, in patients randomized to CRRT as compared to 41.5% and 47.6%, respectively, in patients randomized to IHD ($P < 0.02$).[846] As the result of an imbalance in randomization, patients in the CRRT arm had greater severity of illness as measured by the Acute Physiology and Chronic Health Evaluation III (APACHE III) score and a higher rate of liver failure. Adjusting for the imbalanced randomization in a post hoc analysis, the investigators found no difference in mortality attributable to modality of RRT. In a single-center randomized trial involving 80 patients, Augustine and coworkers reported more effective fluid removal and greater hemodynamic stability associated with CVVHD as compared to IHD but observed no difference in survival.[847] Similarly, in another single-center randomized controlled trial from Switzerland, Uehlinger and colleagues observed no difference in survival in 70 patients randomized to CVVHDF as compared to 55 patients assigned to IHD.[848] In the Hemodiafe study, a multicenter randomized controlled trial conducted in 21 ICUs in France, Vinsonneau and associates reported 60-day survival rates of 31.5% in 184 patients randomized to IHD as compared to 32.6% in 175 patients randomized to CVVHDF ($P = 0.98$).[822] Similarly, Lins and colleagues observed hospital morality rates of 62.5% in 144 patients randomized to IHD and 58.1% in 172 patients randomized to CRRT ($P = 0.43$).[849] Multiple meta-analyses have concluded that there is no association between survival and either of these modalities of RRT.[850-852] Although several studies have suggested that CRRT is associated with improved rates of recovery of kidney function in surviving patients as compared to IHD,[846,853-856] all of these studies are notable for higher mortality rates in the CRRT group. When analyzed across studies in which there were no differences in mortality, rates of recovery of kidney function do not appear to be impacted by modality of RRT.[760,850,852,857]

Prolonged Intermittent Renal Replacement Therapy

PIRRT represents therapies in which conventional hemodialysis equipment is modified to provide extended-duration dialysis using lower blood flow rates and dialysate flow rates.[858,859] Various terms have been developed to describe these therapies, including SLED,[860,861] extended daily dialysis,[862] and sustained low-efficiency daily diafiltration.[863] By extending the duration of the dialysis treatment while providing slower ultrafiltration and solute clearance, these therapies are associated with enhanced hemodynamic tolerability as compared to IHD. The degree of metabolic control attained with these treatments is comparable to that observed with CRRT.[864] In an observational study performed in three ICUs in New Zealand, Australia, and Italy that changed from using CRRT to PIRRT, there was no change in outcomes following the change in modality of RRT.[859] Similarly, in a single-center prospective randomized controlled trial that included 232 patients, 90-day survival rates were similar in the PIIRT and CRRT groups (PIRRT, 50.4%; CRRT, 44.4%; $P = 0.43$), although overall resource utilization was lower with PIRRT.[865]

Peritoneal Dialysis

The use of peritoneal dialysis in the management of AKI has diminished as the use of continuous and hybrid therapies have increased.[866-868] Peritoneal dialysis has the advantage of requiring minimal technology, thus facilitating its use in remote or resource-constrained areas.[869] As a result, it is still used in the treatment of AKI in regions where access to IHD or CRRT is not possible. Access for acute peritoneal dialysis can be obtained either by percutaneous placement of an uncuffed temporary peritoneal catheter or through surgical placement of a tunneled cuffed catheter. Peritoneal dialysis has the advantage of avoiding the need for vascular access or anticoagulation. Solute clearance and control of metabolic parameters may be inferior to those achieved with other modalities of RRT.[870] Although systemic hypotension is less of an issue than with other modalities of RRT, ultrafiltration cannot be as tightly controlled. Other limitations include the relative contraindication in patients with acute abdominal processes or recent abdominal surgery, the risk for visceral organ injury during catheter placement, the risk for peritoneal dialysis–associated peritonitis, and an increased tendency toward hyperglycemia due to the high glucose concentrations in peritoneal dialysate, which is associated with adverse outcomes in acute illness. Several trials have compared outcomes using peritoneal dialysis to those of other modalities of RRT in AKI.[870-873] In a study of 70 patients with infection-associated AKI in Vietnam, 58 of whom had severe falciparum malaria, peritoneal dialysis was associated with less adequate metabolic control and higher mortality than continuous hemofiltration.[870] In contrast, in a study of 120 patients in Brazil who were randomized to high-volume peritoneal dialysis or daily hemodialysis, indices of metabolic control, recovery of kidney function, and survival were similar with both modalities of therapy.[871] In a meta-analysis that included eight observational studies and four clinical trials, Chionh and colleagues observed similar survival rates with peritoneal dialysis as compared to extracorporeal RRT in patients with AKI.[874]

OUTCOMES OF ACUTE KIDNEY INJURY

The crude short-term mortality rate among patients with intrinsic AKI approximates 50% and has changed little over the past 3 decades.[25,26,28,34,469,515,516,787,875-883] This lack of improvement in survival despite significant advances in supportive care may reflect a decrease in the proportion of patients with isolated AKI, and a corresponding increase in the number of patients with AKI complicating the multiple-organ dysfunction syndrome.[28,34,884,885] The risk for death differs considerably depending on the cause of AKI and clinical setting, with mortality estimates of approximately 15% in obstetric patients with AKI, 30% in toxin-related AKI, and 60% to 90% in patients with sepsis.[25,26,404,884,886,887] In two large randomized controlled trials of severe AKI, the overall 60-day mortality rate was 52.6% in the Acute Renal Failure Trial Network study, conducted in the United States,[784] and the 90-day mortality rate was 44.7% in the Randomized Evaluation of Normal versus Augmented Level (RENAL) Replacement Therapy Study, conducted in Australia and New Zealand.[845]

Factors that have been found to predict poor outcomes in AKI include male sex, advanced age, oliguria (<400 mL/day), a rise in the serum creatinine value of greater than 3 mg/dL, and coexistent sepsis or nonrenal organ failure, factors that reflect more severe renal injury and overall severity of illness. However, even mild decrements in renal function that do not necessitate dialytic support are recognized as being associated with poor patient outcomes. Lassnigg and associates demonstrated that increases in serum creatinine concentration of less than 0.6 mg/dL following cardiothoracic surgery were independently associated with a nearly twofold increase in 30-day mortality (hazard ratio [HR], 1.92; 95% confidence interval [CI], 1.34 to 2.77).[888] Furthermore, several studies of contrast medium–induced AKI have demonstrated that small increments in serum creatinine concentration, even if transient, are associated with increased short- and long-term mortality.[889-892] Whether such transient increases in serum creatinine concentration directly mediate adverse long-term outcomes or represent a biochemical marker of patients at higher risk for such outcomes remains unclear.[893]

While the development of AKI is associated with remarkably high short-term mortality rates, surviving an episode of AKI is also associated with an increased risk for serious longer-term morbidity and mortality. Although older data suggested that complete recovery of kidney function was common in patients surviving an episode of AKI with only 5% of patients having no recovery of kidney function and an additional 5% manifesting progressive deterioration in kidney function after an initial recovery phase, more recent data have challenged this teaching. Rates of recovery of kidney function in recent clinical trials of RRT in AKI have been highly variable, with less than 10% of surviving patients remaining dialysis dependent in the RENAL study[845] as compared to approximately 25% of surviving patients in the Acute Renal Failure Trial Network study[784] and approximately 40% in the Hannover Dialysis Outcome study.[894] The reason for this wide variation in recovery of kidney function across studies is not known.

In patients who recover kidney function, approximately half have subclinical functional defects in glomerular filtration, tubular solute transport, H^+ secretion, and urinary concentrating mechanisms or have tubulointerstitial scarring on kidney biopsy.[895-898] Epidemiologic studies have demonstrated that patients who survive an episode of AKI are at increased risk for progressive CKD and development of ESKD and have an increased long-term mortality risk. Using data from a 5% representative sample of older Medicare beneficiaries, Ishani and coworkers observed that AKI in the absence of underlying CKD was independently associated with a markedly increased risk for the development of ESKD at 2 years of follow-up (HR, 13.0; 95% CI, 10.6 to 16).[32] AKI that developed in the setting of preexistent CKD was associated with an even higher risk for ESKD (HR, 41.2; 95% CI, 34.6 to 49.1). Wald and associates conducted a population-based cohort study comparing long-term outcomes of 3769 patients who developed AKI that required temporary dialysis with 13,598 matched controls who were hospitalized but did not develop AKI.[899] At a median of 3 years of follow-up, the risk for ESKD was more than threefold higher among patients who required acute transient dialysis compared to severity-of-illness matched controls (adjusted HR, 3.23; 95% CI, 2.70 to 3.86). Lo and colleagues examined the association of AKI that required transient dialysis with long-term mortality.[900] Among 562,799 hospitalized patients who had a baseline eGFR of 45 mL/min/1.73 m² or higher, 703 sustained dialysis-requiring AKI, of whom 295 (42%) died, 65 (9%) remained chronically dialysis dependent, and 343 (49%) recovered sufficient kidney function to be able to discontinue dialysis by the time of hospital discharge. In multivariable analyses, AKI requiring transient dialysis was associated with a twofold increased risk for death over 6 years of follow-up.[900] In the same study, AKI requiring transient dialysis was associated with a 28-fold increased risk for developing progressive CKD, defined as a decline in kidney function to an eGFR of 30 mL/min/1.73 m² or less.[900] In a study of over 87,000 patients, Newsome and colleagues demonstrated that increases in serum creatinine concentration of 0.3 to 0.5 mg/dL following acute myocardial infarction were independently associated with an increased risk for ESKD (HR, 2.36; $P < 0.05$) and long-term mortality (HR, 1.26; $P <.05$).[901]

As part of an epidemiologic study of 11,249 patients in Alberta, Canada, James and coworkers demonstrated that mild AKI following coronary angiography, defined as an increase in serum creatinine concentration of 50% to 99% or 0.3 mg/dL or more was associated with a nearly fivefold increased risk for experiencing a sustained reduction in kidney function at 90 days (adjusted odds ratio [OR], 4.74; 95% CI, 3.92 to 5.74).[902] Patients who developed more severe AKI, defined by an increase in serum creatinine concentration of 100% or more had a greater than 17-fold increased risk for persistent renal injury at 90 days following angiography (adjusted OR, 17.3; 95% CI, 12.0 to 24.9), supporting a graded relationship between the severity of AKI and risk for sustained renal damage at 90 days. AKI was also associated with an increased risk for accelerated decline in kidney function, defined as a loss of eGFR of more than 4 mL/min/1.73 m² per year over 2 to 3 years of follow-up (OR, 2.9; 95% CI, 2.2 to 3.7), as well as a markedly increased risk for ESKD over this same period of follow-up (OR, 13.8; 95% CI, 7.4 to 25.9).[902] Even patients with baseline normal kidney function who have apparent complete recovery of kidney function appear to be at increased risk. In an analysis of over 30,000 hospital discharges, Bucaloiu and colleagues observed increased risks for subsequent CKD and long-term mortality in patients with normal baseline kidney function who sustained an episode of AKI and had recovery of kidney function to a serum creatinine concentration within 0.1 mg/dL of baseline.[903] In this study, long-term mortality risk was markedly attenuated after adjusting for development of CKD, suggesting that the mortality risk was mediated, at least in part, by the development of CKD. In addition, a recent analysis of longitudinal data from patients from Taiwan who recovered kidney function after an episode of dialysis-requiring AKI as compared to matched controls suggests that patients surviving an episode of AKI are at increased risk for cardiovascular disease, with an observed hazard of coronary events of 1.7 (95% CI, 1.4 to 2.0) after adjusting for development of CKD and ESKD.[904] Thus the development of AKI appears to accelerate the progression of CKD and the development of ESKD and places patients at increased risk for cardiovascular disease and longer-term mortality.

AKI also extends the length of hospitalization and is associated with substantial health resource utilization.[469,853,905-907] The U.S. cost of treating AKI was estimated in 1999 to be $50,000 per quality-adjusted life-year, a level that is important to consider regarding the cost-benefit analysis of potential interventions for this condition.[908] In a more recent analysis of long-term outcomes of 153 ICU survivors who had recovered from AKI, quality-adjusted survival was poor as compared to an age- and gender-matched community population.[909] Quality-adjusted survival in this cohort was poor (15 quality-adjusted years per 100 patient-years in the first year following discharge); however, despite the low health-related quality of life, the subject's self-perceived health satisfaction was not significantly different from that of the general population.[909] Similar poor health-related quality of life was also observed in follow-up of 415 subjects who participated in the Acute Renal Failure Trial Network study and survived at least 60 days, with 27% of respondents' health states corresponding to levels considered by the general population to be equivalent to or worse than death.[910]

The design of many of the clinical studies that have examined the efficacy of therapeutic interventions on hard outcomes of AKI has been problematic. Measurement of the benefit of interventions for the treatment of AKI has been confounded by the difficulty in accurately defining the onset and resolution of this condition. Furthermore, many human studies of AKI suffer from a lack of well-defined end points.[10] For example, although the need for dialysis has been used as an end point in many trials of AKI, uniform criteria for the initiation and discontinuation of dialysis have often not been established before the study, and among studies that do define specific criteria for dialysis, such criteria may differ across trials and study populations.[911-913] Finally, the necessary duration of follow-up to fully capture the sequelae of AKI remains uncertain.[914-916] The assessment of outcomes clearly needs to extend beyond ICU and hospital discharge, as accumulating data associate AKI with longer-term morbidity and mortality.[32,900,914]

Complete reference list available at ExpertConsult.com.

KEY REFERENCES

3. Kidney Disease: Improving Global Outcomes (KDIGO) Acute Kidney Injury Work Group: KDIGO clinical practice guideline for acute kidney injury. *Kidney Int Suppl* 2:1–138, 2012.
13. Palevsky PM, Liu KD, Brophy PD, et al: KDOQI US commentary on the 2012 KDIGO clinical practice guideline for acute kidney injury. *Am J Kidney Dis* 61:649–672, 2013.
19. Vanmassenhove J, Vanholder R, Nagler E, et al: Urinary and serum biomarkers for the diagnosis of acute kidney injury: an in-depth review of the literature. *Nephrol Dial Transplant* 28:254–273, 2013.
31. Coca SG, Singanamala S, Parikh CR: Chronic kidney disease after acute kidney injury: a systematic review and meta-analysis. *Kidney Int* 81:442–448, 2012.
34. Uchino S, Kellum JA, Bellomo R, et al: Acute renal failure in critically ill patients: a multinational, multicenter study. *JAMA* 294:813–818, 2005.
37. Hospitalization discharge diagnoses for kidney disease—United States, 1980-2005. *MMWR Morb Mortal Wkly Rep* 57:309–312, 2008.
38. Hsu CY, McCulloch CE, Fan D, et al: Community-based incidence of acute renal failure. *Kidney Int* 72:208–212, 2007.
39. Hsu RK, McCulloch CE, Dudley RA, et al: Temporal changes in incidence of dialysis-requiring AKI. *J Am Soc Nephrol* 24:37–42, 2013.
57. Kirkpatrick AW, Roberts DJ, De Waele J, et al: Intra-abdominal hypertension and the abdominal compartment syndrome: updated consensus definitions and clinical practice guidelines from the World Society of the Abdominal Compartment Syndrome. *Intensive Care Med* 39:1190–1206, 2013.
81. Sandoval RM, Molitoris BA: Gentamicin traffics retrograde through the secretory pathway and is released in the cytosol via the endoplasmic reticulum. *Am J Physiol Renal Physiol* 286:F617–F624, 2004.
83. Zingman LV, Park S, Olson TM, et al: Aminoglycoside-induced translational read-through in disease: overcoming nonsense mutations by pharmacogenetic therapy. *Clin Pharmacol Ther* 81:99–103, 2007.
105. Hutchison CA, Cockwell P, Stringer S, et al: Early reduction of serum-free light chains associates with renal recovery in myeloma kidney. *J Am Soc Nephrol* 22:1129–1136, 2011.
110. Kelly KJ: Distant effects of experimental renal ischemia/reperfusion injury. *J Am Soc Nephrol* 14:1549–1558, 2003.
113. Sharfuddin AA, Sandoval RM, Berg DT, et al: Soluble thrombomodulin protects ischemic kidneys. *J Am Soc Nephrol* 20:524–534, 2009.
114. Parekh DJ, Weinberg JM, Ercole B, et al: Tolerance of the human kidney to isolated controlled ischemia. *J Am Soc Nephrol* 24:506–517, 2013.
140. El-Achkar TM, Huang X, Plotkin Z, et al: Sepsis induces changes in the expression and distribution of Toll-like receptor 4 in the rat kidney. *Am J Physiol Renal Physiol* 290:F1034–F1043, 2006.
153. El-Achkar TM, McCracken R, Liu Y, et al: Tamm-Horsfall protein translocates to the basolateral domain of thick ascending limbs, interstitium and circulation during recovery from acute kidney injury. *Am J Physiol Renal Physiol* 304:F1066–F1075, 2013.
167. Molitoris BA, Dagher PC, Sandoval RM, et al: siRNA targeted to p53 attenuates ischemic and cisplatin-induced acute kidney injury. *J Am Soc Nephrol* 20:1754–1764, 2009.
182. Zhang MZ, Yao B, Yang S, et al: CSF-1 signaling mediates recovery from acute kidney injury. *J Clin Invest* 122:4519–4532, 2012.
184. Yang SH, Lee JP, Jang HR, et al: Sulfatide-reactive natural killer T cells abrogate ischemia-reperfusion injury. *J Am Soc Nephrol* 22:1305–1314, 2011.
212. Park SW, Kim M, Brown KM, et al: Inhibition of sphingosine 1-phosphate receptor 2 protects against renal ischemia-reperfusion injury. *J Am Soc Nephrol* 23:266–280, 2012.
217. Basile DP, Friedrich JL, Spahic J, et al: Impaired endothelial proliferation and mesenchymal transition contribute to vascular rarefaction following acute kidney injury. *Am J Physiol Renal Physiol* 300:F721–F733, 2011.
218. Humphreys BD, Lin SL, Kobayashi A, et al: Fate tracing reveals the pericyte and not epithelial origin of myofibroblasts in kidney fibrosis. *Am J Pathol* 176:85–97, 2010.
220. Schrimpf C, Xin C, Campanholle G, et al: Pericyte TIMP3 and ADAMTS1 modulate vascular stability after kidney injury. *J Am Soc Nephrol* 23:868–883, 2012.
260. Bajwa A, Jo SK, Ye H, et al: Activation of sphingosine-1-phosphate 1 receptor in the proximal tubule protects against ischemia-reperfusion injury. *J Am Soc Nephrol* 21:955–965, 2010.
263. Lee SY, Horbelt M, Mang HE, et al: MMP-9 gene deletion mitigates microvascular loss in a model of ischemic acute kidney injury. *Am J Physiol Renal Physiol* 301:F101–F109, 2011.
274. Xu C, Chang A, Hack BK, et al: TNF-mediated damage to glomerular endothelium is an important determinant of acute kidney injury in sepsis. *Kidney Int* 85:72–81, 2014.
277. Basile DP, Leonard EC, Beal AG, et al: Persistent oxidative stress following renal ischemia-reperfusion injury increases ANG II hemodynamic and fibrotic activity. *Am J Physiol Renal Physiol* 302:F1494–F1502, 2012.
280. Cantaluppi V, Gatti S, Medica D, et al: Microvesicles derived from endothelial progenitor cells protect the kidney from ischemia-reperfusion injury by microRNA-dependent reprogramming of resident renal cells. *Kidney Int* 82:412–427, 2012.
294. Sever MS, Vanholder R, Lameire N: Management of crush-related injuries after disasters. *N Engl J Med* 354:1052–1063, 2006.
384. Perazella MA, Moeckel GW: Nephrotoxicity from chemotherapeutic agents: clinical manifestations, pathobiology, and prevention/therapy. *Semin Nephrol* 30:570–581, 2010.

388. Cairo MS, Bishop M: Tumour lysis syndrome: new therapeutic strategies and classification. *Br J Haematol* 127:3–11, 2004.
392. Lopez-Olivo MA, Pratt G, Palla SL, et al: Rasburicase in tumor lysis syndrome of the adult: a systematic review and meta-analysis. *Am J Kidney Dis* 62:481–492, 2013.
450. Salerno F, Gerbes A, Gines P, et al: Diagnosis, prevention and treatment of hepatorenal syndrome in cirrhosis. *Gut* 56:1310–1318, 2007.
506. Druml W: Nutritional management of acute renal failure. *J Ren Nutr* 15:63–70, 2005.
538. Yunos NM, Bellomo R, Hegarty C, et al: Association between a chloride-liberal vs chloride-restrictive intravenous fluid administration strategy and kidney injury in critically ill adults. *JAMA* 308:1566–1572, 2012.
547. Bart BA, Goldsmith SR, Lee KL, et al: Ultrafiltration in decompensated heart failure with cardiorenal syndrome. *N Engl J Med* 367:2296–2304, 2012.
573. Gluud LL, Christensen K, Christensen E, et al: Terlipressin for hepatorenal syndrome. *Cochrane Database Syst Rev* (9):CD005162, 2012.
622. Jang JS, Jin HY, Seo JS, et al: Sodium bicarbonate therapy for the prevention of contrast-induced acute kidney injury—a systematic review and meta-analysis. *Circ J* 76:2255–2265, 2012.
636. Acetylcysteine for prevention of renal outcomes in patients undergoing coronary and peripheral vascular angiography: main results from the randomized Acetylcysteine for Contrast-induced nephropathy Trial (ACT). *Circulation* 124:1250–1259, 2011.
694. Friedrich JO, Adhikari N, Herridge MS, et al: Meta-analysis: low-dose dopamine increases urine output but does not prevent renal dysfunction or death. *Ann Intern Med* 142:510–524, 2005.
734. Perazella MA, Markowitz GS: Drug-induced acute interstitial nephritis. *Nat Rev Nephrol* 6:461–470, 2010.
784. Palevsky PM, Zhang JH, O'Connor TZ, et al: Intensity of renal support in critically ill patients with acute kidney injury. *N Engl J Med* 359:7–20, 2008.
808. Tolwani AJ, Wille KM: Anticoagulation for continuous renal replacement therapy. *Semin Dial* 22:141–145, 2009.
845. Bellomo R, Cass A, Cole L, et al: Intensity of continuous renal-replacement therapy in critically ill patients. *N Engl J Med* 361:1627–1638, 2009.
851. Bagshaw SM, Berthiaume LR, Delaney A, et al: Continuous versus intermittent renal replacement therapy for critically ill patients with acute kidney injury: a meta-analysis. *Crit Care Med* 36:610–617, 2008.
857. Schneider AG, Bellomo R, Bagshaw SM, et al: Choice of renal replacement therapy modality and dialysis dependence after acute kidney injury: a systematic review and meta-analysis. *Intensive Care Med* 39:987–997, 2013.
865. Schwenger V, Weigand MA, Hoffmann O, et al: Sustained low efficiency dialysis using a single-pass batch system in acute kidney injury—a randomized interventional trial: the REnal Replacement Therapy Study in Intensive Care Unit PatiEnts. *Crit Care* 16:R140, 2012.
874. Chionh CY, Soni SS, Finkelstein FO, et al: Use of peritoneal dialysis in AKI: a systematic review. *Clin J Am Soc Nephrol* 8:1649–1660, 2013.

32 Primary Glomerular Disease

William F. Pendergraft, III | Patrick H. Nachman | J. Charles Jennette | Ronald J. Falk

CHAPTER OUTLINE

GENERAL DESCRIPTION OF GLOMERULAR SYNDROMES, 1013
Isolated Proteinuria, 1013
Recurrent or Persistent Hematuria, 1014
GLOMERULAR DISEASES THAT CAUSE NEPHROTIC SYNDROME, 1016
Nephrotic Syndrome, 1016
Minimal Change Disease, 1016
Focal Segmental Glomerulosclerosis, 1024
C1q Nephropathy, 1034
Membranous Nephropathy, 1035
Membranoproliferative Glomerulonephritis and C3 Glomerulopathy, 1045
Membranoproliferative Glomerulonephritis Type I, 1046
Membranoproliferative Glomerulonephritis Type III 1050

C3 Glomerulopathies (Dense Deposit Disease and C3 Glomerulonephritis), 1050
Acute Poststreptococcal Glomerulonephritis, 1054
Immunoglobulin A Nephropathy, 1059
Fibrillary Glomerulonephritis and Immunotactoid Glomerulopathy, 1069
RAPIDLY PROGRESSIVE GLOMERULONEPHRITIS AND CRESCENTIC GLOMERULONEPHRITIS, 1072
Nomenclature and Categorization, 1072
Immune Complex–Mediated Crescentic Glomerulonephritis, 1075
Anti–Glomerular Basement Membrane Glomerulonephritis, 1076
Pauci-Immune Crescentic Glomerulonephritis, 1081

The underlying cause of many glomerular diseases remains an enigma; however, each edition of this chapter presents important discoveries that have been made since its previous editions that substantially increase our understanding of the causes and pathogenesis of a number of glomerular diseases—for example, idiopathic (primary) membranous nephropathy (MN), focal segmental glomerulosclerosis (FSGS), IgA nephropathy, antineutrophil cytoplasmic autoantibody (ANCA) glomerulonephritis, dense deposit disease, and C3 glomerulonephritis. Infectious agents, autoimmunity, legal and illegal drugs, inherited disorders, and environmental agents have been implicated as causes of certain glomerular diseases. Until the precise causes and pathogenesis of glomerular disorders are unraveled, we continue in the tradition of Richard Bright—studying the relationship of clinical, pathologic, and laboratory signs and symptoms of disease, and basing our diagnostic categorization on these features rather than on causes.

Glomerular diseases may be categorized into those that primarily involve the kidney (primary glomerular diseases) and those in which kidney involvement is part of a systemic disorder (secondary glomerular diseases). This chapter focuses on primary glomerular diseases. Some forms of glomerular disease occur not only as a renal-limited (primary) disease in some patients but also as a component of systemic disease in other patients, for example, anti–glomerular basement membrane (anti-GBM) glomerulonephritis with and without pulmonary disease, and ANCA glomerulonephritis with and without systemic vasculitis and granulomatosis. Chapter 33 concentrates on secondary glomerular diseases and Chapter 34 focuses on therapy for glomerular disease. The separation of glomerular disease into primary versus secondary is somewhat problematic because, in some instances, what are considered primary glomerular diseases are similar, if not identical, to secondary glomerular diseases. For example, immunoglobulin A (IgA) nephropathy, pauci-immune necrotizing and crescentic glomerulonephritis, anti-GBM glomerulonephritis, MN, and membranoproliferative glomerulonephritis (MPGN) can occur as primary kidney diseases or as components of systemic diseases such as IgA vasculitis, pauci-immune small vessel vasculitis, Goodpasture's syndrome, systemic lupus erythematosus (SLE), and cryoglobulinemic vasculitis, respectively. Of note, since the last edition there has been a successful shift, as in many settings, to phase out the nosologic use of eponyms and to substitute non-eponymous terms that more accurately reflect pathophysiologic specificity in the nomenclature of vasculitides. This nomenclature of vasculitides was formally revised in 2012 at the second international Chapel Hill Consensus Conference, and the following vasculitides with new names are relevant to this edition: IgA vasculitis (formerly designated Henoch-Schönlein purpura), granulomatosis with polyangiitis (GPA, formerly designated Wegener's granulomatosis), and eosinophilic granulomatosis with polyangiitis (EGPA, formerly designated Churg-Strauss syndrome).[1] This chapter focuses on the diagnosis and management of glomerular diseases that do not appear to be a component of a systemic disease.

When a patient presents with glomerular disease, the clinician not only must evaluate the clinical signs and symptoms but also must be vigilant for evidence of a systemic process or disease that could be causing the kidney disease. Clinical evaluation includes assessment of proteinuria, hematuria, the presence or absence of renal insufficiency, and the presence or absence of hypertension. Some glomerular diseases cause isolated proteinuria or isolated hematuria with no other signs or symptoms of disease. More severe glomerular disease often results in the nephrotic syndrome or nephritic (glomerulonephritic) syndrome. Glomerular disease may have an indolent course or begin abruptly, leading to acute or rapidly progressive glomerulonephritis. Although some glomerular disorders consistently cause a specific syndrome (e.g., minimal change disease [MCD] results in the nephrotic syndrome), most disorders are capable of causing features of both nephrosis and nephritis (Table 32.1). This sharing and variability of clinical manifestations among different glomerular diseases may not allow an accurate diagnosis based on clinical features alone. Therefore, kidney biopsy has an important role in the evaluation of many patients and remains the gold standard for definitive diagnosis of many glomerular diseases.

This chapter describes the clinical syndromes caused by glomerular diseases, including isolated proteinuria, isolated hematuria, and specific forms of primary glomerular disease that cause the nephrotic or nephritic syndrome, and reviews their distinctive pathologic features.

GENERAL DESCRIPTION OF GLOMERULAR SYNDROMES

ISOLATED PROTEINURIA

Proteinuria can be caused by systemic overproduction of proteins that cross glomerular capillary walls (e.g., multiple myeloma with Bence Jones proteinuria), tubular dysfunction (e.g., Fanconi's syndrome), or glomerular dysfunction. It is important to identify patients in whom proteinuria is a manifestation of substantial glomerular disease as opposed to patients who have benign functional, transient, postural (orthostatic), or intermittent proteinuria.

Plasma proteins larger than 70 kDa cross the basement membrane in a manner normally restricted by both size-selective and charge-selective barriers.[2,3] The functional characteristics of the glomerular capillary filter have been extensively studied by the evaluation of the fractional clearance of molecules of different size and charge.[4] The size-selective barrier is most likely a consequence of functional pores within the glomerular basement membrane (GBM) that restrict filtration of plasma proteins of more than 150 kDa. There is also a shape restriction of molecules that allows elongated molecules to cross the glomerular capillary wall more readily than molecules of the same molecular weight, and there is a charge-selective nature of the barrier that is largely a consequence of glycosaminoglycans arranged along the capillary wall. Loss of charge selectivity may be a defect in patients with MCD, whereas a loss of size selectivity may be the cause of proteinuria in, for instance, patients with MN.[3]

A number of factors have proven to be important in the disruption of the glomerular capillary wall as a consequence of tissue-degrading enzymes, complement components that assemble or deposit in it, and oxygen radicals that target both the GBM and the slit diaphragm. Heparanase and hyaluronidase alterations in the aminoglycan content of the glomerular capillary wall may play a role in increased protein excretion.[5,6] Genetic studies have provided exciting clues to the specific components of the glomerular capillary wall, including mutations in the podocyte or proteins in the slit diaphragm, that result in proteinuria (reviewed by Tryggvason and colleagues[7] and more recently by Garg and Rabelink.[8])

Another major mechanism resulting in proteinuria is impaired reabsorption of plasma proteins by proximal

Table 32.1 Manifestations of Nephrotic and Nephritic Features by Glomerular Diseases

	Nephrotic Features	Nephritic Features
Minimal change disease	++++	−
Membranous nephropathy	++++	+
Focal segmental glomerulosclerosis	+++	++
Fibrillary glomerulonephritis	+++	++
Mesangioproliferative glomerulopathy*	++	++
Membranoproliferative glomerulonephritis†	++	+++
Proliferative glomerulonephritis*	++	+++
Acute diffuse proliferative glomerulonephritis‡	+	++++
Crescentic glomerulonephritis§	+	++++

*Mesangioproliferative and proliferative glomerulonephritis (focal or diffuse) are structural manifestations of a number of glomerulonephritides, including IgA nephropathy and lupus nephritis.
†Both mesangiocapillary (type I) and dense deposit disease (type II).
‡Often a structural manifestation of acute poststreptococcal glomerulonephritis.
§Can be immune complex mediated, anti–glomerular basement membrane antibody mediated, or associated with antineutrophil cytoplasmic autoantibodies.

Modified with permission from Jennette JC, Mandal AK: The nephrotic syndrome. In Mandal AK, Jennette JC, editors: Diagnosis and management of renal disease and hypertension, Durham NC, 1994, Carolina Academic Press, pp 235-272.

tubular epithelial cells. A number of low-molecular-weight proteins, including albumin and β_1-, β_2-, and α_1- microglobulins, are filtered by the glomerulus and absorbed by tubular epithelial cells. When tubular epithelial cells are damaged, these proteins are excreted. Russo and colleagues have studied the critical importance of tubular absorption of proteins.[9] Glomerular capillary sieving coefficient for albumin was examined in normal and nephrotic rats by two-photon (laser) intravital microscopy. The glomerular capillary sieving coefficient for albumin was 3.4×10^2 rather than 6.2×10^4 as found by earlier micropuncture studies in rats.

Several important observations emanate from this study. First, there is a large amount of albumin filtered across the glomerular capillary bed daily in the normal rat. Second, investigators found no evidence for a charge-based restriction to the passage of albumin through the glomerular filter. Third, in normal and nephrotic animals, the vast majority of the filtered albumin was "reclaimed" from the filtrate by a high-capacity transcytotic pathway in the proximal tubule, which returns intact (unaltered) albumin to the peritubular capillary circulation. These are important concepts, because most nephrologists view albuminuria as resulting solely from enhanced glomerular permeability (recently reviewed by Vallon[10]).

The term *isolated proteinuria* is used in several conditions, including mild transient proteinuria of less than 1 g protein per day that typically accompanies physiologically stressful conditions such as fever in hospitalized patients, exercise, and congestive heart failure.[11] In other patients, transient proteinuria is a consequence of the overflow of proteins of low molecular weight due to overproduction of light chains, heavy chains, or other fragments of immunoglobulins. Additional examples of proteinuria caused by increased circulating proteins are β_2-microglobinuria, myoglobinuria, and hemoglobinuria.

The term *orthostatic proteinuria* is defined by the absence of proteinuria while the patient is in a recumbent posture and its appearance during upright posture, especially during ambulation or exercise.[12] The total amount of protein excretion in a 24-hour period is generally less than 1 g but may be as much as 2 g. Orthostatic proteinuria is more common in adolescents and is uncommon in individuals older than 30 years.[12,13] Some 2% to 5% of adolescents have orthostatic proteinuria. Among patients with orthostatic proteinuria who underwent kidney biopsy, 47% were found to have normal glomeruli by light microscopy, 45% to have minimal to moderate glomerular abnormalities of nonspecific nature, and the remainder to have evidence of a primary glomerular disease.[14]

Why is proteinuria increased during upright posture in individuals with normal glomeruli by light microscopy? Although the answer to this question is not fully known, there are several likely possibilities. Orthostatic proteinuria may occur as a consequence of alterations in glomerular hemodynamics. It is possible that even in histologically "normal" glomeruli in which there are no specific lesions, subtle glomerular abnormalities exist, including abnormal basement membranes or focal changes of the mesangium.[15] Alternatively, orthostatic proteinuria has been demonstrated with anatomic entrapment and subsequent obstruction of the left renal vein between the aorta and superior mesenteric artery (commonly referred to as "renal nutcracker").[16]

In addition, the observation that surgical correction of a kink in an allograft renal vein resulted in the disappearance of orthostatic proteinuria gives credence to venous entrapment as a cause for orthostatic proteinuria.[15]

There are several approaches to the diagnosis of orthostatic proteinuria. These include comparison of protein excretion in two 12-hour urine collections, one during recumbency and one during ambulation. Another approach is to compare protein level in a split collection of 16 hours during ambulation and 8 hours of overnight collection. It is important that patients be recumbent for at least 2 hours before their ambulatory collection is completed to avoid the possibility of contamination of the recumbent collection by urine formed during ambulation. The diagnosis of orthostatic proteinuria requires that protein excretion during recumbency be less than 50 mg during those 8 hours. Few convincing data exist on the usefulness of comparing urinary protein to creatinine ratio measurements during recumbency versus ambulation as a diagnostic test for orthostatic proteinuria.

Twenty-year follow-up of orthostatic proteinuria suggests a benign long-term course.[13] Orthostatic proteinuria resolves in most patients. It is present in 50% of patients after 10 years and only 17% of patients after 20 years.[13] In the absence of a kidney biopsy, an underlying glomerulopathy cannot be completely excluded, and an orthostatic component of proteinuria may be found in early glomerular disease. Thus, it is important to reassess patients after an interval of about 1 year to be certain that the degree or pattern of proteinuria has not changed.

Fixed proteinuria is present whether the patient is upright or recumbent. The proteinuria disappears in some patients, whereas others will have a more ominous glomerular lesion that portends an adverse long-term outcome. The prognosis depends on the persistence and severity of the proteinuria. If proteinuria disappears, it is less likely that the patient will develop hypertension or reduced glomerular filtration rate (GFR). These patients must be evaluated periodically for as long as proteinuria persists.

RECURRENT OR PERSISTENT HEMATURIA

Hematuria is the presence of an excessive number of red blood cells in the urine and is categorized as either microscopic (visible only with the aid of a microscope) or macroscopic (urine that is tea-colored or cola-colored, pink, or even red). Hematuria can result from injury to the kidney or to another site in the urinary tract.

Healthy individuals may excrete as many as 10^5 red cells in the urine in a 12-hour period. An acceptable definition of hematuria is more than two red cells per high-power field in centrifuged urine.[17] The approach to processing urine varies from laboratory to laboratory; therefore, the number of red cells per high-power field that is an accurate indicator of hematuria may vary slightly among different laboratories. The urine dipstick test detects one or two red cells per high-power field and is a very sensitive test. A negative result on dipstick examination virtually excludes hematuria.[18]

Hematuria is present in about 5% to 6% of the general population[19] and 4% of schoolchildren. In the majority of children, follow-up urinalyses are normal.[20] In most people, hematuria emanates from the lower urinary tract, especially in conditions affecting the urethra, bladder, and prostate. Less than 10% of cases of hematuria are caused by glomerular bleeding.[17] Persistent hematuria, especially in older individuals, should raise the possibility of malignancy. The incidence of malignancy, especially of the bladder, ranges from 5% in individuals with persistent microscopic hematuria to over 20% in individuals with gross hematuria.[21] Other causes of nonglomerular hematuria include neoplasms, trauma, metabolic defects such as hypercalciuria, vascular diseases including renal infarctions and renal vein thrombosis, cystic diseases of the kidney including polycystic kidney disease, medullary cystic disease and medullary sponge kidney, and interstitial kidney disease such as papillary necrosis, hydronephrosis, and drug-induced interstitial nephritis. In children with asymptomatic hematuria, hypercalciuria is the cause in 15% of cases, and 10% to 15% have IgA nephropathy. In up to 80% of children and 15% to 20% of adults with hematuria, no cause can be identified.[22]

Transient hematuria has been found in a number of settings. Transient hematuria is present in 13% of postmenopausal women.[23] Episodic hematuria in a cyclical pattern during a menstrual cycle is most likely a consequence of the invasion of the urinary tract by endometrial implants.[24] In 1000 males between the ages of 18 and 33, hematuria was present at least once in 39% and on two or more occasions in 16%. In patients with isolated asymptomatic hematuria without proteinuria or renal insufficiency, the hematuria resolves in 20% of cases; however, some of these patients will develop hypertension and proteinuria.[25] In older individuals, transient hematuria should raise a concern of malignancy.[17,26,27] In some individuals, transient hematuria may be a consequence of exercise.

Glomerular hematuria, in contrast to hematuria caused by injury elsewhere in the urinary tract, is characterized by misshapen red cells that have been distorted by osmotic and chemical stress as red blood cells pass through the nephron. Hematuria with dysmorphic cells, especially cells that have membrane blebs producing the picture of acanthocyturia, is strong evidence for glomerular bleeding.[21] The finding of protein (especially >2 g/day), hemoglobin, or red cell casts in the urine enhances the possibility that hematuria is of glomerular origin. Although brown or cola-colored urine is most commonly associated with glomerular hematuria, its absence does not exclude glomerular disease. Interestingly, clots do not occur in the urine with glomerular bleeding.

The differential pathologic diagnosis of glomerular hematuria without proteinuria, renal insufficiency, or red blood cell casts includes IgA nephropathy, thin basement membrane nephropathy, hereditary nephritis, and histologically normal glomeruli.[28] In a study in Europe,[29] 80 normotensive adults underwent kidney biopsy for evaluation of recurrent macroscopic hematuria or persistent microscopic hematuria. Approximately 30% of these patients had IgA nephropathy, 20% had thin basement membrane nephropathy, and 30% had no discernible lesion. Hematuria disappeared in 13 of the latter patients. The remaining patients had mesangioproliferative glomerulonephritis, interstitial nephritis, or focal glomerulosclerosis. In contrast, 216 Chinese adults with isolated hematuria who underwent a kidney biopsy were much more likely to have IgA nephropathy than any other lesion.[30]

Table 32.2 provides data from an analysis of native kidney biopsy specimens from patients with hematuria performed by the University of North Carolina Nephropathology Laboratory. Patients with SLE were excluded from the study. The patients selected for the study had a serum creatinine level of less than 1.5 mg/dL or more than 3 mg/dL. Patients with a serum creatinine level of less than 1.5 mg/dL were further divided into those with proteinuria less than 1 g protein per day and those with proteinuria of 1 to 3 g protein per day. The data showed that patients with a relatively normal serum creatinine level, hematuria, and proteinuria of less than 1 g protein per day were most likely to have thin basement membrane nephropathy, IgA nephropathy, or no identifiable renal lesion. When hematuria is accompanied by 1 to 3 g protein per day of proteinuria but no significant renal insufficiency, IgA nephropathy was the most likely cause. Patients with hematuria and a serum creatinine of more than 3 mg/dL most often had aggressive glomerulonephritis with crescents.

Table 32.2 Frequency of Kidney Disease in Patients with Hematuria Undergoing Renal Biopsy (in Percent)*

Biopsy Findings	Hematuria, Urinary Protein <1 g/day, Creatinine <1.5 mg/dL	Hematuria, Urinary Protein 1-3 g/day, Creatinine <1.5 mg/dL	Hematuria, Creatinine >3 mg/dL
No abnormality	30	2	0
Thin basement nephropathy	26	4	0
Immunoglobulin A nephropathy	28	24	8
Glomerulonephritis without crescents[†]	9	26	23
Glomerulonephritis with crescents[†]	2	24	44
Other kidney disease[‡]	5	20	25
Total	100 (n = 43)	100 (n = 123)	100 (n = 255)

*Based on an analysis of kidney biopsy specimens evaluated at the University of North Carolina Nephropathology Laboratory. Specimens from patients with systemic lupus erythematosus were excluded from the analysis.
[†]Proliferative or necrotizing glomerulonephritis other than immunoglobulin A nephropathy or lupus nephritis.
[‡]Includes causes of nephrotic syndrome such as membranous nephropathy and focal segmental glomerulosclerosis.
Data from Caldas MLR, Jennette JC, Falk RJ, et al: Immunoelectron microscopic documentation of the translocation of proteins reactive with ANCA to neutrophil cell surfaces during neutrophil activation. Third International Workshop on ANCA, 1990 [abstract].

Despite these overall tendencies, it is not possible to definitively determine the cause of asymptomatic hematuria without kidney biopsy, and even kidney biopsy specimen evaluation fails to reveal a cause in a minority of patients. Certain rules generally apply to the clinical prediction of the most likely cause. Gross hematuria is most commonly found in IgA nephropathy or hereditary nephritis. Patients with thin basement membrane nephropathy typically do not have substantial proteinuria.

The potential benefits of kidney biopsy in patients with isolated hematuria include reduction of patient and physician uncertainty by confirming a specific diagnosis. Nonetheless, the role of kidney biopsy in the evaluation of asymptomatic hematuria in patients without proteinuria, hypertension, or kidney insufficiency remains unclear. In biopsy series involving patients in whom asymptomatic hematuria is accompanied by low-grade proteinuria, specific glomerular diseases including IgA nephropathy and membranoproliferative glomerular disease may be discovered when there is no proteinuria, and IgA nephropathy and thin basement membrane disease or nondiagnostic minor changes remain the most common findings.[31,32] Confirmation of a glomerular cause eliminates the need for repeated urologic studies, and a more accurate long-term prognosis can be made (e.g., thin basement membrane nephropathy is less likely to progress than is IgA nephropathy). However, isolated glomerular hematuria without proteinuria or renal insufficiency may not warrant a kidney biopsy, because the findings often will not affect management. In one study of patients with isolated hematuria, the biopsy results altered patient management in only 1 of 36 patients.[33]

GLOMERULAR DISEASES THAT CAUSE NEPHROTIC SYNDROME

NEPHROTIC SYNDROME

Nephrotic syndrome results from proteinuria of more than 3.5 g protein per day and is characterized by edema, hyperlipidemia, hypoproteinemia, and other metabolic disorders (described in detail later). Nephrotic syndrome not only may be caused by primary (idiopathic) glomerular diseases but also may be secondary to a large number of identifiable disease states (Table 32.3). Despite the differences in these causes, the loss of substantial amounts of protein in the urine results in a shared set of abnormalities that comprise nephrotic syndrome (Tables 32.4, 32.5, and 32.6). We are likely to witness an explosion of new insights into primary glomerular diseases responsible for nephrotic syndrome with the recent establishment of the Nephrotic Syndrome Study Network (NEPTUNE) and Cure Glomerulonephropathy (CureGN), both funded by the National Institutes of Health (NIH). NEPTUNE is a North American multicenter collaborative translational research consortium geared toward longitudinal clinical monitoring and blood, urine, and kidney tissue sample collection from 450 adults and children with MCD, FSGS, and MN.[34] CureGN (https://curegn.org/) is a longitudinal multicenter cohort study that will study 2400 children and adults with MCD, FSGS, MN, and IgA nephropathy. Both NEPTUNE and CureGN provide the infrastructure for multiple ancillary studies that will advance our understanding and management of glomerular diseases.

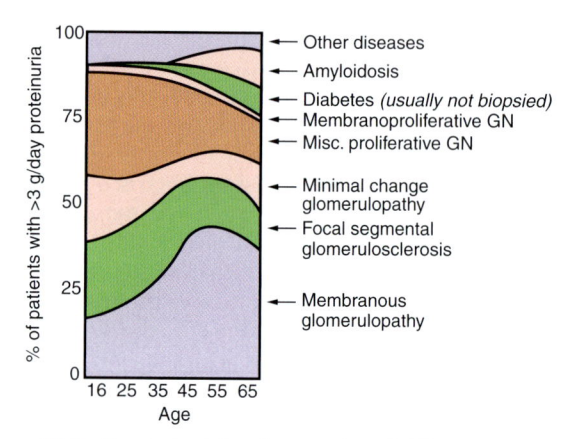

Figure 32.1 Graph depicting frequencies of different forms of glomerular disease identified in kidney biopsy specimens from patients with proteinuria of more than 3 g of protein per day evaluated at the University of North Carolina Nephropathology Laboratory. Some diseases that cause proteinuria are underrepresented because they are not always evaluated by kidney biopsy. For example, in many patients steroid-responsive proteinuria is given a presumptive diagnosis of minimal change disease and patients do not undergo biopsy, and most patients with diabetes and proteinuria are presumed to have diabetic glomerulosclerosis and do not undergo biopsy. GN, Glomerulonephritis.

MINIMAL CHANGE DISEASE

EPIDEMIOLOGY

Minimal change disease (MCD), was first described in 1913 by Munk, who called it *lipoid nephrosis* because of the presence of lipid in the tubular epithelial cells and urine.[35] MCD is most common in children, accounting for 70% to 90% of nephrotic syndrome in children younger than age 10 and 50% in older children. MCD also causes 10% to 15% of primary nephrotic syndrome in adults (Figure 32.1).

The incidence of MCD has geographic variations. MCD is more common in Asia than in North America or Europe.[36] This may be a consequence of differences in kidney biopsy practices or of differences in environmental or genetic influences. The disease may also affect older adult patients in whom there is a higher propensity for the clinical syndrome of MCD and Acute Kidney Injury (AKI) (discussed later). There appears to be a male preponderance of this process in some research series, especially in children, in whom the male/female ratio is 2:1 to 3:1[37]; however, data from the authors' institution do not support this finding.

PATHOLOGY

The effacement of podocyte foot processes is accompanied by increased density of the cytoskeleton, including actin filaments, in clumps near the basement membrane surface of the podocytes. However, the extent of effacement appears to correlate more with the duration of active nephrotic syndrome than with the magnitude of proteinuria.[38]

Light Microscopy

In MCD, no glomerular lesions are seen by light microscopy (Figure 32.2), or only a minimal focal segmental mesangial

Table 32.3 Classification of the Disease States Associated with the Development of Nephrotic Syndrome

Idiopathic Nephrotic Syndrome due to Primary Glomerular Disease
Nephrotic Syndrome Associated with Specific Causal Events or in Which Glomerular Disease Arises as a Complication of Other Diseases
1. Medications and other chemicals
    Organic, inorganic, elemental mercury*
    Organic gold
    Penicillamine, bucillamine
    Street heroin
    Probenecid
    Captopril
    Nonsteroidal antiinflammatory drugs
    Lithium
    Interferon-α
    Chlorpropamide
    Rifampin
    Pamidronate
    Paramethadione (Paradione), trimethadione (Tridione)
    Mephenytoin (Mesantoin)
    Tolbutamide[†]
    Phenindione[†]
    Warfarin
    Clonidine[†]
    Perchlorate[†]
    Bismuth[†]
    Trichloroethylene[†]
    Silver[†]
    Insect repellent[†]
    Contrast media
    Anabolic steroids
2. Allergens, venoms, immunizing agents
    Bee sting
    Pollens
    Poison ivy and poison oak
    Antitoxins (serum sickness)
    Snake venom
    Diphtheria, pertussis, tetanus toxoid
    Vaccines
3. Infections
    Bacterial: *poststreptococcal glomerulonephritis,* infective endocarditis, *shunt nephritis,* leprosy, syphilis (congenital and secondary), *Mycoplasma* infection, tuberculosis,[†] chronic bacterial pyelonephritis with vesicoureteral reflux
    Viral: hepatitis B, hepatitis C, cytomegalovirus infection, infectious mononucleosis (Epstein-Barr virus infection), herpes zoster, vaccinia, infection with human immunodeficiency virus-1
    Protozoal: *malaria* (especially quartan malaria), toxoplasmosis
    Helminthic: *schistosomiasis*, trypanosomiasis, filariasis
4. Neoplasms
    Solid tumors (carcinoma and sarcoma): tumors of the *lung, colon, stomach, breast,* cervix, kidney, thyroid, ovary, prostate, adrenal, oropharynx, carotid body[†]; melanoma, pheochromocytoma, Wilms' tumor, mesothelioma, oncocytoma
    Leukemia and lymphoma: *Hodgkin's disease*, chronic lymphocytic leukemia, multiple myeloma (amyloidosis), Waldenström's macroglobulinemia, lymphoma
    Graft-versus-host disease after bone marrow transplantation
5. Multisystem disease[‡]
    Systemic lupus erythematosus
    Mixed connective tissue disease
    Dermatomyositis
    Rheumatoid arthritis
    Goodpasture's syndrome
    IgA vasculitis (see also immunoglobulin A nephropathy, Berger's disease)
    Systemic vasculitis (including GPA)
    Takayasu's arteritis
    Mixed cryoglobulinemia
    Light- and heavy-chain disease (Randall type)
    Partial lipodystrophy
    Sjögren's syndrome
    Toxic epidermolysis
    Dermatitis herpetiformis
    Sarcoidosis
    Ulcerative colitis
    Amyloidosis (primary and secondary)
6. Hereditary-familial and metabolic disease[‡]
    Diabetes mellitus
    Hypothyroidism (myxedema)
    Graves' disease
    Amyloidosis (familial Mediterranean fever and other hereditary forms, Muckle-Wells syndrome)
    Alport's syndrome
    Fabry's disease
    Nail-patella syndrome
    Lipoprotein glomerulopathy
    Sickle cell disease
    α_1-Antitrypsin deficiency
    Asphyxiating thoracic dystrophy (Jeune's syndrome)
    Von Gierke's disease
    Podocyte/slit diaphragm mutation
    Nephrin mutation
    FAT2 mutation
    Podocin mutation
    CD2AP mutation
    Denys-Drash syndrome (*WT1* mutation)
    ACTN4 mutation
    Charcot-Marie-Tooth syndrome
    Congenital nephrotic syndrome (Finnish type)
    Cystinosis (adult)
    Galloway-Mowat syndrome
    Hurler's syndrome
    Familial dysautonomia
7. Miscellaneous
    Pregnancy associated (preeclampsia, recurrent, transient)
    Chronic renal allograft failure
    Accelerated or malignant nephrosclerosis
    Unilateral renal arterial hypertension
    Intestinal lymphangiectasia
    Chronic jejunoileitis[†]
    Spherocytosis[†]
    Renal artery stenosis
    Congenital heart disease[†] (cyanotic)
    Severe congestive heart failure[†]
    Constrictive pericarditis[†]
    Tricuspid insufficiency[†]
    Massive obesity
    Vesicoureteric reflux nephropathy
    Papillary necrosis
    Gardner-Diamond syndrome
    Castleman's disease
    Kartagener's syndrome
    Buckley's syndrome
    Kimura's disease
    Silica exposure

*Italics denote diseases and other agents that are the more commonly encountered causes of nephrotic syndrome.
[†]Based on single case reports or small series in which cause-and-effect relationship cannot be established. Other factors (e.g., use of mercurial diuretics in heart failure) may have been true inciting event.
[‡]See Chapter 33 for detailed discussion of the secondary forms of nephrotic syndrome.
ACTN4, α-Actinin-4; CD2AP, CD2-associated protein; FAT2, FAT tumor suppressor homolog 2 (*Drosophila*); GPA, granulomatosis with polyangiitis; WT1, Wilms' tumor 1.

Table 32.4 Alterations of Plasma Protein in Nephrotic Syndrome

Immunoglobulins (Ig)

Decreased IgG
Normal or increased IgA, IgM, or IgE
Increased α_2- and β-globulins
Decreased α_1-globulin

Metal-Binding Proteins

Loss of metal-binding proteins
    Iron
    Copper
    Zinc
Loss of erythropoietin
Depletion of transferrin
Transcortin deficiency

Complement

Decreased factor B
Decreased C3
Decreased C1q, C2, C8, Ci
Increased C3, C4bp
Normal C1s, C4, and C1 inhibitor

Coagulation Components

Decreased factors XI, XII, kallikrein inhibitor
Decreased factors IX, XII
Decreased α_2-antiplasmin, α_1-antitrypsin
Plasminogen activator, endothelial prostacyclin-stimulating factor
Decreased antithrombin III
Elevated β-thromboglobulin
Procoagulant

Data from references 465, 1344-1358.

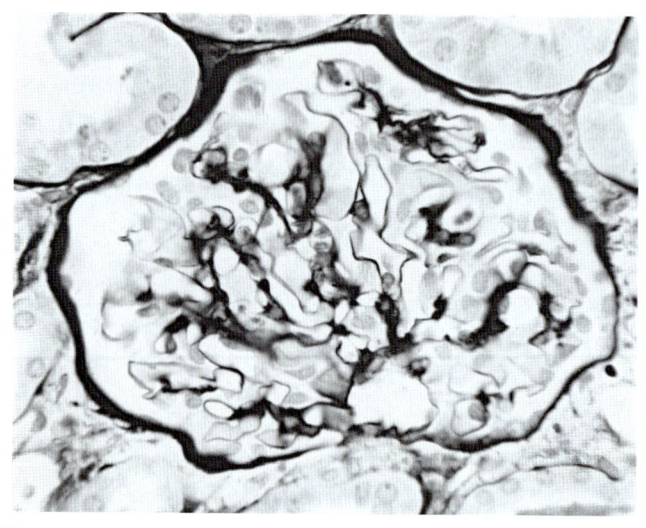

Figure 32.2 Unremarkable light microscopy appearance of a biopsy specimen from a patient with minimal change disease. Glomerular basement membranes are thin, and there is no glomerular hypercellularity or mesangial matrix expansion. (Jones' methenamine silver stain, ×300.)

Table 32.5 Coagulation Factors in Nephrotic Syndrome

Increased blood viscosity
Hemoconcentration
Increased plasma fibrinogen
Increased intravascular fibrin formation
Increased α_2-macroglobulins
Increased tissue-type plasminogen activator
Increased factors II, V, VII, VIII, X, XIII
Decreased factors IX, XI, XII
Decreased α-antitrypsin
Decreased fibrinolytic activity
Decreased plasma plasminogen
Decreased antithrombin III
Decreased protein S
Thrombocytosis
Increased platelet aggregability

Data from references 468, 1357, and 1359-1373.

Table 32.6 Diseases That Cause Nephrotic Syndrome*

Glomerular Lesion	N	Male/Female Ratio	White/Black Ratio
Minimal change disease	522	1.1:1.0	1.9:1.0
Focal segmental glomerulosclerosis (FSGS) (typical)	1103	1.4:1.0	1.0:1.0
Collapsing glomerulopathy FSGS	135	1.2:1.0	1.0:7.8
Glomerular tip lesion FSGS	94	1.0:1.0	4.7:1.0
Membranous nephropathy	1120	1.4:1.0	1.9:1.0
C1q nephropathy	114	1.0:1.0	1.0:4.8
Fibrillary glomerulonephritis	76	1.0:1.2	14.3:1.0

*Data from 9605 native kidney biopsies from the University of North Carolina Nephropathology Laboratory. This laboratory evaluates kidney biopsies from a base population of approximately 10 million throughout the southeastern United States and centered in North Carolina. The expected white/black ratio in this renal biopsy population is approximately 2:1.

prominence is noted.[39] This mesangial prominence should have no more than three or four cells embedded in the matrix of a segment, and the matrix should not be expanded to the extent that capillary lumens are compromised. Capillary walls should be thin and capillary lumens patent.

The most consistent tubular lesion is increased protein and lipid resorption droplets in tubular epithelial cells. These droplets stain with periodic acid–Schiff stain. Conspicuous resorbed lipid in epithelial cells prompted the designation *lipoid nephrosis* for this disease prior to the recognition of the ultrastructural glomerular lesion. Interstitial edema is rare, even in patients with severe nephrotic syndrome and anasarca. Focal proximal tubular epithelial flattening (simplification), which is histologically identical to that seen with ischemic AKI, occurs in patients who have the syndrome of MCD with AKI.[40]

Focal areas of interstitial fibrosis and tubular atrophy in a specimen that otherwise looks like MCD, especially in a young person, should raise the possibility of FSGS that was not sampled in the biopsy specimen. Examination of additional levels of section may reveal a sclerotic glomerulus.

Immunofluorescence Microscopy

Glomeruli usually show no staining with antisera specific for IgG, IgA, IgM, C3, C4, or C1q. The most frequent positive finding is low-level mesangial staining for IgM, sometimes accompanied by low-level staining for C3. If the IgM staining is not accompanied by mesangial electron-dense deposits by electron microscopy, it is consistent with a diagnosis of MCD. Patients whose specimens show mesangial IgM staining by immunofluorescence microscopy (in the absence of dense deposits by electron microscopy) do not have a worse prognosis than patients whose specimens are without IgM staining.[41,42] The presence of mesangial dense deposits identified by electron microscopy worsens the prognosis and thus justifies altering the diagnosis, for example to IgM mesangial nephropathy.[43] Anything more than trace staining for IgG or IgA casts substantial doubt on a diagnosis of MCD. Even when no sclerotic glomerular lesions are seen by light microscopy, well-defined irregular focal segmental staining for C3 and IgM should raise the possibility of FSGS because sclerotic lesions can be enriched for C3 and IgM. Glomerular and tubular epithelial cell cytoplasmic droplets and tubular casts may stain positively for immunoglobulins and other plasma proteins when there is substantial proteinuria.

Electron Microscopy

The pathologic sine qua non of MCD is effacement of podocyte foot processes observed by electron microscopy (Figures 32.3 and 32.4). However, this is not a specific feature, because it occurs in the glomeruli of patients with severe proteinuria due to any cause. During active nephrosis, the effacement often is very extensive, with only a few scattered intact foot processes. As the patient enters remission, the extent of foot process effacement diminishes. The effacement usually is accompanied by microvillous transformation, which is the development of numerous villous projections from the podocyte surface into the urinary space. These intracytoplasmic densities should not be confused with subepithelial immune complex dense deposits as a result of resorption of increased lipids and proteins in the urine. Glomerular and proximal tubular epithelial cells have increased clear and dense cytoplasmic droplets.

All of these ultrastructural glomerular changes occur in other glomerular disease when there is nephrotic-range proteinuria. Therefore, MCD is a diagnosis by exclusion that is made only when there is no evidence by light, immunofluorescence, and electron microscopy for any other glomerular disease.

PATHOGENESIS

Although the pathogenesis of MCD remains unclear, this disorder is most likely a consequence of abnormal regulation of a T cell subset[44-48] and pathologic elaboration of a circulating permeability factor. A role for the T cell is

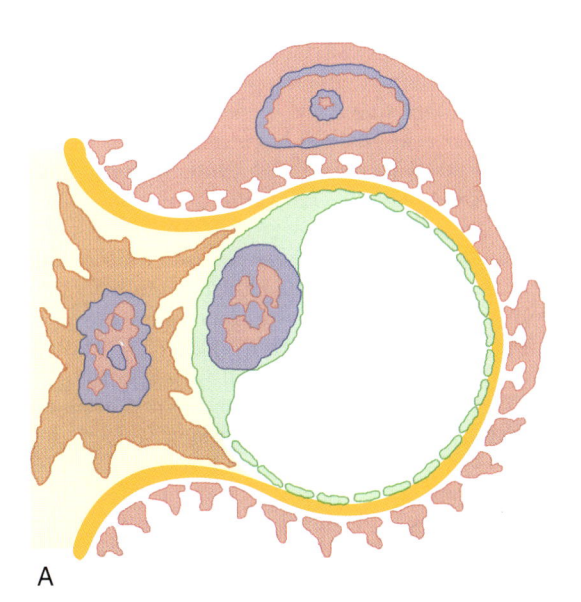

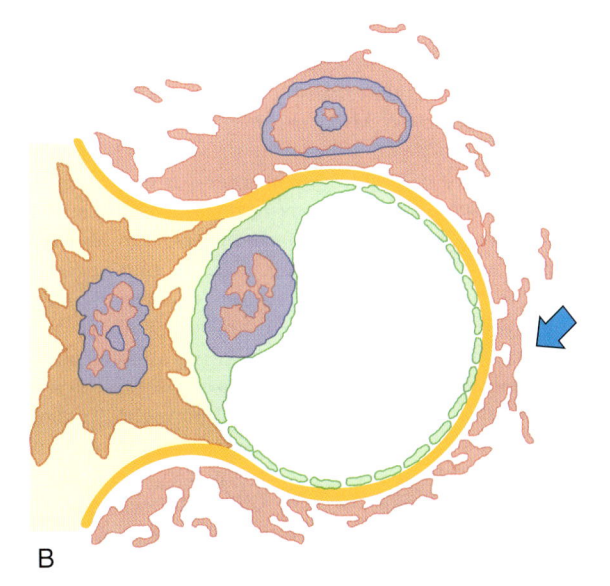

Figure 32.3 Diagrams depicting the ultrastructural features of a normal glomerular capillary loop **(A)** and a capillary loop with features of minimal change disease **(B)**. The latter has effacement of podocyte foot processes (*arrow*) and microvillous projections of podocyte cytoplasm. (Courtesy J. Charles Jennette.)

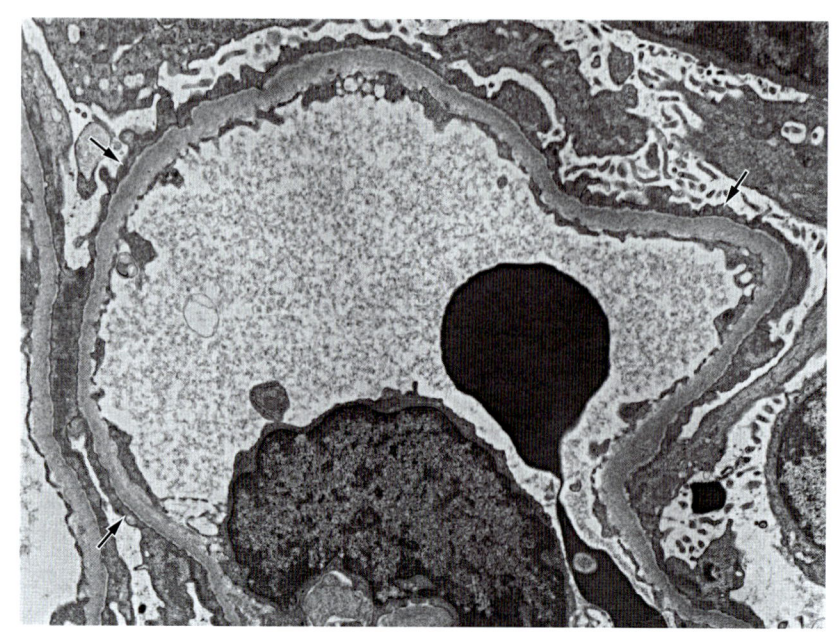

Figure 32.4 Electron micrograph of a glomerular capillary wall from a patient with minimal change disease showing extensive podocyte foot process effacement (*arrows*) and microvillous transformation. (×5000.)

supported by the effectiveness of corticosteroids and alkylating drugs in the induction of remission of MCD as well as by an association of MCD with Hodgkin's disease,[49,50] and remissions are associated with depression of cell-mediated immunity during viral infections such as measles. Specific evidence stems from the finding that a glomerular permeability factor is produced by human T cell hybridomas obtained from a patient with MCD. When this factor was injected into rodents, proteinuria occurred with partial fusion of glomerular epithelial cell foot processes.[51] Although there are no recognized abnormalities in T or B cell populations in patients with relapsing or quiescent MCD,[52-55] lymphocytes have depressed reactivity when challenged with mitogens.[56-64] T cells apparently produce a product, most likely a lymphokine, which increases glomerular permeability to protein. When the glomerular permeability factor is removed from the kidney, it functions normally. This is supported by the intriguing observation that transplantation of a kidney from a patient with refractory MCD resulted in rapid disappearance of proteinuria.[65]

A likely target of the pathogenic process is the podocyte, possibly a constituent of the slit pore membrane. Attention has focused on the role of plasma hemopexin in MCD.[66,67] Hemopexin is present in normal plasma, but an active isoform of the protein has been suggested to cause increased glomerular permeability due to enhanced protease activity.[66] Patients with MCD in relapse demonstrate altered isoforms of plasma hemopexin with increased protease activity compared with patients with MCD in remission, patients with other forms of nephrotic syndrome, and normal subjects.[67] It is not understood how and why the plasma hemopexin is altered in MCD or how the enhanced protease activity results in alterations in glomerular permeability.

Differential gene expression techniques have also suggested an alteration in tumor necrosis factor–related apoptosis-inducing ligand (TRAIL) in peripheral blood mononuclear cells in MCD during relapse compared with remission.[68] Many additional genes (at least 15 of the more than 20,000 examined) were upregulated during relapse, which demonstrates the complexity of events occurring in MCD. Included among these was the IgE-dependent histamine-releasing factor gene,[69] and the well-known association of MCD with atopic allergic states could be the reason for this finding.

This factor may have specificity for podocytes that results in loss of the charge-selective barrier of the GBM. The loss of charge selectivity has been assessed by dextran studies.[70,71] In these studies, there is less evidence for a defect in the size-selective barrier and more of an alteration of the basement membrane electrostatic charge. The glomerular negative charge is reduced in relapse.[72]

Genetic aspects of MCD are under intense investigation. Familial clustering of MCD has not generally been observed.[73] Heterozygous amino acid changes in nephrin and podocin are seen in about one third of patients with typical MCD, but no amino acid changes were observed for *NEPH1* and *CD2AP* in a study involving 104 adults who presented with childhood-onset MCD.[73] Thus, the genotype in MCD may be quite variable.

Polymorphisms in the genes encoding interleukins 4 and 13 (IL-4 and IL-13), activating transcription factor 6, and macrophage migration inhibitory factor have been described in MCD.[74-76] IL-13 polymorphisms may relate to phenotype, because they have been associated with relapsing forms of MCD. IL-13 has also been suggested as a potential permeability factor in MCD. The implication of IL-13 in the pathogenesis of MCD is further suggested by the rat model of Lai and colleagues,[77] in which IL-13–transfected Wistar rats (n = 41) showed significant albuminuria, hypoalbuminemia, and hypercholesterolemia compared with control rats (n = 17). No significant histologic changes were seen in glomeruli of IL-13–transfected rats; however, electron microscopy revealed up to 80% effacement of podocyte foot process.

A recent observation is that podocyte-specific angiopoietin-like 4 (ANGPTL$_4$) overproduction in transgenic rats results in ANGPTL$_4$ binding to GBM with subsequent loss of GBM charge, diffuse foot process effacement, and nephrotic-range proteinuria. Furthermore, ANGPTL$_4$ expression has been observed in serum, glomeruli, and urine of patients with MCD,[78,79] and further understanding of this pathway may prove to be fruitful.

CLINICAL FEATURES AND NATURAL HISTORY

The cardinal clinical feature of MCD in children is the relatively abrupt onset of proteinuria and development of nephrotic syndrome with heavy proteinuria, hypoalbuminemia, and hyperlipidemia.[39] The edematous picture is typically what prompts the parents of these children to seek medical attention. Hematuria is distinctly unusual, and in children, hypertension is uncommon. The clinical features of MCD in adults tend to be somewhat different. In a group of 89 adults older than age 60, hypertension, sometimes severe, as well as renal insufficiency, were more common.[80] Because individuals older than age 60 account for almost one quarter of adult patients with MCD, this presentation must be considered.

MCD has been associated with several other conditions, including viral infections, use of certain pharmaceutical agents, malignancy, and allergy (Table 32.7). In some patients, there is a history of a drug reaction before the onset of MCD. The use of nonsteroidal antiinflammatory drugs, and in particular fenoprofen, has been associated with and may cause MCD.[81] In this setting, most patients have not only proteinuria but also pyuria and renal insufficiency as a consequence of the simultaneous development of acute tubulointerstitial nephritis. This same process has also been described with other compounds, including interferon,[82] penicillins, and rifampin. In most of these patients, discontinuation of the offending drug leads to resolution of the proteinuria, but it may take weeks to months for complete amelioration of pyuria and renal insufficiency.

MCD has been associated with lymphoid malignancy, usually Hodgkin's disease or thymoma. In a retrospective study of adult patients,[83] MCD was associated with classic Hodgkin's lymphoma of the nodular sclerosis type. MCD appeared before the diagnosis of lymphoma in 40% of patients.

MCD has also been associated with a variety of underlying exposures such as nonsteroidal antiinflammatory drugs as mentioned earlier,[84] and with syndromes such as SLE[85,86]; it has also occurred after allogeneic stem cell transplantation for leukemia[87] and after hematopoietic cell transplantation.

There is an association of glomerular disease with simultaneous graft-versus-host disease. Nephrotic syndrome generally follows graft-versus-host disease within 5 months in approximately 60% of patients with either MCD or MN. Compared with MN, MCD occurred earlier after hematopoietic cell transplantation, was diagnosed soon after medication change, and exhibited a better prognosis because 90% of patients attained complete remission (vs. 27% of patients with MN).

MCD is also associated with food allergy. This is an important association because in some patients, removal of the allergen has resulted in the resolution of the proteinuria.

Table 32.7 Common Associations with Minimal Change Disease

Infections	Allergies
• Viral • Parasitic	• Food • Dust • Bee stings • Pollen • Poison ivy and poison oak • Dermatitis herpetiformis
Pharmaceutical Agents	**Disease and Other Associations**
• Nonsteroidal antiinflammatory drugs • Gold • Lithium • Interferon • Ampicillin • Rifampin • Trimethadione • Tiopronin	• Systemic lupus erythematosus • Following allogeneic stem cell transplantation for leukemia • Following hematopoietic cell transplantation
Tumors	
• Hodgkin's disease • Lymphoma/leukemia • Solid tumors	

Data from references 82, 99, 127-129, and 1374-1381.

Of 42 patients with idiopathic nephrotic syndrome, 16 had positive results on skin tests for food allergy. For 13 of 42, a minimally antigenic diet was prescribed that resulted in a significant reduction in proteinuria.[88] Thus, it is important to ask patients about potential allergens, especially those found in food.

A syndrome of MCD accompanied by a reversible AKI occurs at higher incidence in adults than in children.[80,89,90] This syndrome of adult MCD with AKI was studied in 21 patients who, on presentation, had a serum creatinine level of more than 177 µmol/L and who were compared with 50 adult patients with MCD who had a serum creatinine of less than 133 µmol/L. Patients who had AKI were older (59 years vs. 40 years), had a higher systolic blood pressure (158 mm Hg vs. 138 mm Hg), and had more proteinuria (13.5 vs. 7.9 g of protein per 24 hours). Importantly, kidney biopsy specimens showed evidence of focal tubular epithelial simplification compatible with ischemic AKI. Of the 18 patients with renal failure for whom follow-up data were available, all showed recovery of kidney function, but only after prolonged periods of dialytic renal replacement therapy.[40]

The complications of nephrotic syndrome in MCD have been well described. The development of AKI during the course of MCD, mostly in adults older than age 40, has been well recognized, but the underlying mechanisms are debated. Explanations for this phenomenon include marked decrease in glomerular permeability due to extensive foot process effacement, tubular obstruction from proteinaceous casts, and intrarenal hemodynamic changes. Increased endothelin-1 expression in the kidneys of patients with MCD and AKI could indicate a hemodynamic change that underlies the pathogenesis of renal failure in these circumstances,[91] but the true cause of AKI in MCD remains uncertain and is probably multifactorial.

Another complication of MCD with nephrotic syndrome is the development of reduced bone mineral density, possibly due to the effects of glucocorticoids and/or vitamin D deficiency.[92] Statins may have a beneficial effect on bone mineral density, but the most recent study in 2005 reported no beneficial effect of fluvastatin on bone mineral density of children with MCD, although it did have some effect in lowering proteinuria.[93]

LABORATORY FINDINGS

The ubiquitous laboratory feature of MCD is severe proteinuria.[39] Microscopic hematuria is seen in less than 15% of patients, with only rare episodes of macroscopic hematuria. The rapidity of the development of proteinuria in some patients is associated with evidence of volume contraction with increased hematocrit and hemoglobin level. The erythrocyte sedimentation rate is increased as a consequence of the hyperfibrinogenemia as well as hypoalbuminemia. The serum albumin concentration is usually depressed, whereas the total cholesterol, low-density lipoprotein (LDL), and triglyceride levels are increased. Total serum protein concentration is usually reduced to between 4.5 and 5.5 g/dL with a serum albumin concentration of generally less than 2 g/dL and, in more severe cases, less than 1 g/dL. Pseudohyponatremia has been observed in the setting of marked hyperlipidemia. Serum calcium may be low, largely due to hypoproteinemia.

Several abnormalities that promote thrombosis are frequent in patients with severe nephrosis, including increased plasma viscosity, increased red cell aggregation, low plasminogen levels, and low levels of antithrombin III.[94] Kidney function is usually normal, although the serum creatinine level may be slightly increased at the time of presentation. A minority of patients (usually older adults) have substantial AKI as discussed earlier.

The loss of albumin into the urine is largely a function of a loss of charge-selective permselectivity.[70,71,95,96] Consequently, the fractional excretion of albumin is proportionately greater than the fractional excretion of IgG. IgG levels may be profoundly decreased, however—a condition that occurs most notably during episodes of relapse. This low level of immunoglobulin may result in susceptibility to infections. IgM levels may be elevated after a remission.[97] Mean serum IgA levels may be substantially higher in patients with MCD than in those with other kidney disease[98] and are also elevated in association with relapse in children.[99] Among adult patients with MCD, over half have elevated levels of serum IgE and two thirds of patients have evidence of some allergic symptoms.[100] Elevation of IgE suggests a relationship between MCD and allergy. Complement levels are typically normal in patients with MCD.

TREATMENT

The general approach to treatment of patients with MCD has been to institute corticosteroid therapy. For children, the dose of prednisone is 60 mg/m^2/day. For adults, the dose of prednisone is 1 mg/kg of body weight, not to exceed 80 mg/day. In children, this form of therapy results in a complete remission with disappearance of proteinuria in over 90% of patients within 4 to 6 weeks of therapy. A response to prednisone therapy has occurred if the patient has had no proteinuria by dipstick analysis for at least 3 days.

It should be noted that the serum albumin and serum lipid levels might not return to normal for prolonged periods of time following resolution of proteinuria.[101]

Treatment is generally continued for at least 6 weeks after complete remission of proteinuria. During those 6 weeks, the dose should be changed to alternate-day administration of prednisone or to a stepwise reduction in the daily dose of prednisone. If the dose is changed to alternate-day dosing when remission has occurred, the dosage may be decreased in children from 60 mg/m^2/day to 40 mg/m^2/day.[48,102-106]

In adult patients with MCD, a response to corticosteroid treatment may take up to 15 weeks.[80] In a study of 89 adult patients given prednisolone, remission occurred in 60% after 8 weeks, in 76% after 16 weeks, and 81% over the course of the study. Of the 58 treated patients who showed a response, 24% never experienced relapse, 56% experienced relapse on a single occasion or infrequently, and only 21% had frequent relapses. Of these 89 patients, only 4 remained nephrotic, and 2 of these presented with AKI. Cyclophosphamide therapy was administered to 36 of the 89 patients, and in 66% of these patients the disease was in remission at 5 years.

In a large retrospective analysis of 95 patients with primary adult-onset MCD, AKI complicated the nephrotic syndrome in 20% of patients.[107] The cohort was largely middle-aged with a substantial prevalence of hypertension (45%) and microscopic hematuria (30%). Ninety-two percent of patients were initially treated with oral corticosteroids, two thirds were on a daily regimen, and one third were on an alternate-day regimen. The initial steroid dose was approximately 1 mg/kg on the daily regimen and approximately 2 mg/kg on the alternate-day regimen, so that cumulative doses were similar in the two groups. There were no significant differences in demographic features between the two groups, but patients treated with the alternate-day steroid regimen tended to have a lower serum albumin level at presentation than those treated with the daily regimen (1.91 ± 0.14 g/dL vs. 2.31 ± 0.1 g/dL, respectively; $P = 0.055$). No significant differences were seen between the daily and alternate-day treatment groups in the percentage of patients experiencing complete or partial remission (remissions in 76.8% and 73.9% of patients, respectively) or in the time to remission. It is interesting to note that the rate of relapse of nephrotic syndrome was quite elevated at 73% of those who showed an initial response. Of the patients who were treated with at least one additional course of corticosteroids, 92% achieved a remission (complete remission in 84.4%). This nonrandomized, uncontrolled study suggests that alternate-day and daily steroid regimens are of equivalent efficacy and safety in the treatment of MCD.

One of the most controversial issues with respect to treatment is the regimen for tapering the prednisone after the initial response. Sudden withdrawal of corticosteroids, or a rapid taper of prednisone immediately following complete remission, may prompt a relapse. Whether this is a consequence of adrenal insufficiency or depression of the hypothalamic-pituitary-adrenal axis has been a matter of debate.[106,108,109] At least in children, the likelihood of relapse is decreased with prolonged administration of corticosteroids over a 10- to 12-week period.[104,110,111] Once remission has been obtained, an alternate-day schedule should begin

Table 32.8 Patterns of Response of Minimal Change Disease to Corticosteroid Treatment

Primary responder, no relapse

Primary responder with only one relapse in the first 6 months after an initial response

Initial steroid response with two or more relapses within 6 months (frequent relapse)

Initial steroid-induced remission with relapses during tapering of corticosteroid, or within 2 weeks after their withdrawal (steroid dependent)

Steroid-induced remission, but no response to a subsequent relapse

No response to treatment (steroid resistant)

Data from references 104, 105, 121, and 1382.

---

within at least 4 weeks of the response to decrease steroid-induced side effects.

In children who have not undergone biopsy prior to treatment, a kidney biopsy is usually appropriate if there is failure to respond to a 4- to 6-week course of prednisone, particularly if changes have occurred in the clinical course during this period of time suggestive of another glomerular disease. Many pediatricians advocate a biopsy at the onset of the disease if there are clinical features suggesting a diagnosis other than MCD (e.g., hypertension, red blood cell casts in the urine, or hypocomplementemia), or if the nephrotic syndrome begins in the first year of life or after 6 years of age.

After the clinical response to initial treatment, as few as 25% experience a long-term remission,[90] 25% to 30% have infrequent relapses (no more than one a year), and the remainder experience frequent relapses, steroid dependence, or steroid resistance (Table 32.8). Nephrotic patients who are steroid dependent or experience frequent relapses require additional forms of therapy. The treatment is aimed at minimizing the complications of corticosteroid therapy. In general, induction of a remission with prednisone therapy followed by the institution of cyclophosphamide treatment results in higher urine flow rates and reduced risk of hemorrhagic cystitis. When cyclophosphamide is given in dosages of 2 mg/kg for 8 to 12 weeks, 75% of patients remain free of proteinuria for at least 2 years.[80,112-114] The response to cyclophosphamide may be predicted from the response to corticosteroids. Patients who have experienced an immediate relapse after the cessation of corticosteroid therapy have a greater chance of experiencing relapse immediately after the cessation of cyclophosphamide treatment. Those who have had longer remissions after corticosteroid therapy have a decreased risk of relapse after cyclophosphamide therapy.[115] In one study, in patients who were steroid dependent, the response to cyclophosphamide was improved by increasing the duration of therapy to up to 12 weeks.[112] In at least one other investigation, however, a 12-week course of cyclophosphamide was not proven efficacious.[116]

Cyclosporine is emerging as a reasonable alternative to cyclophosphamide.[117,118] Based on uncontrolled observations, complete remissions are common (over 80%), and cyclosporine resistance is seen in only about 10% to 15% of patients. Side effects such as a rise in serum creatinine, hypertrichosis, and gingival hyperplasia are quite common. Relapses are very common after cessation of cyclosporine treatment. The best method of monitoring cyclosporine levels is not agreed upon. Measurement of trough blood levels with twice-daily dosing, measurement of cyclosporine levels 1 to 2 hours after a once-daily dose (C1-C2), and abbreviated under-the-curve monitoring of cyclosporine have all been recommended.[118-120] Cyclosporine may be an acceptable alternative to cyclophosphamide therapy for relapsing or steroid-dependent MCD.

STEROID-RESISTANT MINIMAL CHANGE DISEASE

Approximately 5% of children with MCD appear to be steroid resistant. In those patients who never underwent kidney biopsy, resistance to corticosteroid therapy is an indication for kidney biopsy. Often, evaluation of the kidney biopsy specimen will demonstrate FSGS or other forms of glomerular injury other than MCD.[121]

If the diagnosis remains MCD after kidney biopsy specimen evaluation, there may be several reasons for steroid resistance. Some patients, especially those for whom corticosteroid therapy is overly toxic, may skip doses or not fully adhere to the therapy regimen. For other patients, especially some adults, alternate-day therapy may not provide sufficient amounts of corticosteroid to induce clinical remission. In very edematous patients, oral corticosteroid therapy may not be well absorbed, and intravenous administration of a dose of methylprednisolone may provide a more reliable route. Available data suggest that pulse methylprednisolone may induce remission in some corticosteroid-resistant children. In one study, five of eight corticosteroid-resistant children had a remission with pulse methylprednisolone,[122] although this experience is not universal.[123]

Patients with MCD may have an unrecognized lesion of focal and segmental glomerulosclerosis that requires longer courses of steroid therapy (usually >4 months) to achieve a lasting remission. A regimen of calcineurin inhibitor (cyclosporine or tacrolimus) followed by mycophenolate mofetil (MMF) and monthly intravenous pulse cyclophosphamide therapy was demonstrated in an uncontrolled study to result in a high frequency of complete remission.[124] There are anecdotal reports of the use of combinations of sirolimus and tacrolimus to treat steroid-resistant MCD,[125] but the overall safety and efficacy of this regimen is unknown. In a small nonrandomized trial, use of cyclosporine with steroids was associated with better outcomes in steroid-resistant MCD.[126]

Cyclosporine can be administered at a dose of approximately 5 mg/kg. Up to 90% of patients may experience either a partial or complete remission with cyclosporine.[99,104,127-129] Unfortunately, only rarely do patients experience long-term remission once cyclosporine is discontinued.[105] Two trials examined the use of cyclosporine in steroid-resistant nephrosis. A study conducted by the French Society of Pediatric Nephrology combined cyclosporine with prednisone. Prednisone was given at a dose of 30 mg/m^2/day for the first month and then changed to alternate-day dosing for 5 months. Cyclosporine was administered at a dosage of 150 to 200 mg/m^2/day.[130] In this study, 48% of patients with MCD experienced complete remission, some within the first month of therapy. A minority of those who showed a response became steroid sensitive when they later experienced relapse. In a study by Ponticelli and colleagues,[131] 13 of 45 patients had MCD and were treated with cyclosporine. In those patients with MCD, partial or complete remission occurred within 2 months of initiation of therapy. Unfortunately, in spite of the early positive results of this study, relapses occurred in all patients after cyclosporine was stopped.

In a summary of nine studies,[132] only 20% of children had complete remission with cyclosporine, and many, if not most, relapsed with cessation of therapy. Moreover, although cyclosporine and cyclophosphamide appear to have a similar degree of efficacy with respect to controlling nephrotic syndrome, one study found that cyclophosphamide-treated patients experience a more stable long-term remission.[133] In this study, the likelihood of a long-term remission was 63% in patients treated with cyclophosphamide but only 25% in those treated with cyclosporine.

To counteract the usual relapse of nephrosis when cyclosporine has been used for 6 months, an alternative approach to cyclosporine treatment relies on a long-term course of this drug, using gradually lower doses to maintain the patient in remission. In one study,[134] patients who had been in complete remission for longer than 1 year while taking cyclosporine remained in remission if the cyclosporine was gradually tapered and then stopped. Serial biopsy specimens from patients treated for as long as 20 months showed no overt sign of nephrotoxicity.

An emerging treatment option in adults for steroid-resistant and relapsing MCD reported in numerous case reports and series to date is the B lymphocyte–depleting agent, rituximab. Most recently, the Rituximab in Nephrotic Syndrome of Steroid-Dependent or Frequently Relapsing MCD or FSGS (NEMO) Study Group conducted a multicenter trial in Italy in 10 children and 20 adults with recurrent MCD, mesangial proliferative glomerulonephritis, or FSGS, who were treated with one or two doses of rituximab.[135] Interestingly, all patients were in remission at the 1-year mark, 18 were treatment free, and 15 never relapsed. There was also a significant decrease in the number of relapses and median prednisone dose across all disease groups over 1 year of follow-up, and rituximab was well tolerated. Although rituximab appears to be effective in some individuals, greater mechanistic understanding is needed.[136-138] Larger, prospective, randomized trials are needed to accurately assess the utility of rituximab in MCD.

FOCAL SEGMENTAL GLOMERULOSCLEROSIS

FSGS is not a single disease but rather a diagnostic term for a clinical-pathologic syndrome that has multiple causes and pathogenic mechanisms, as well as somewhat limited therapeutic options.[139-142] The ubiquitous *clinical* feature of the syndrome is proteinuria, which may be nephrotic or nonnephrotic. The ubiquitous *pathologic* feature is focal segmental glomerular consolidation or scarring, which may have several distinctive patterns (Figure 32.5). These patterns can

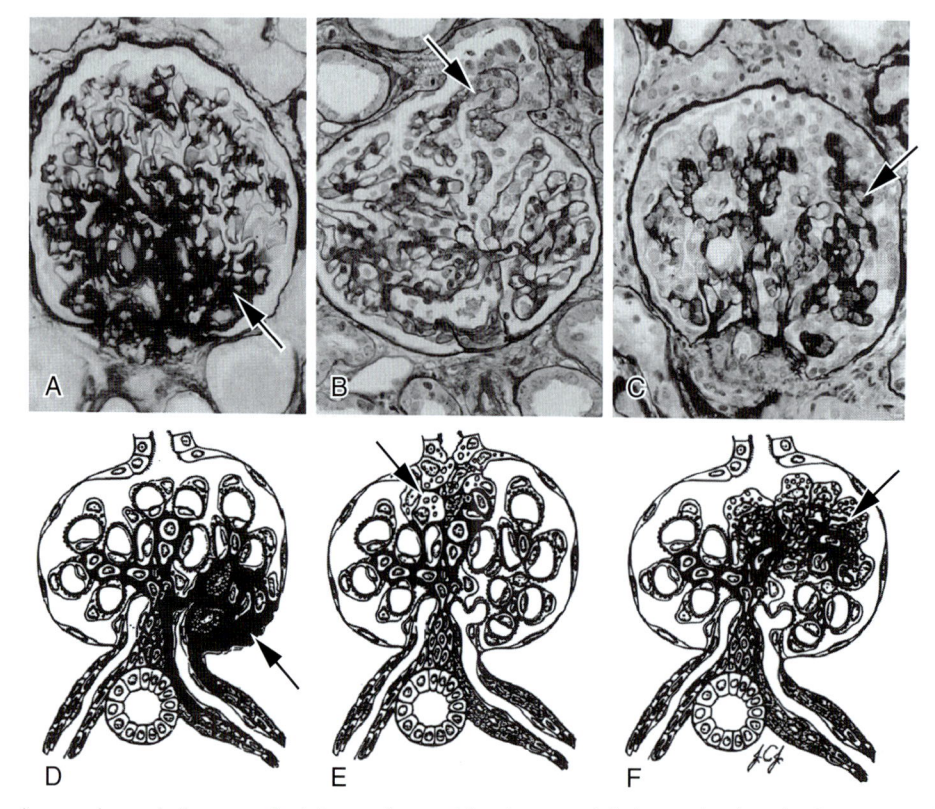

Figure 32.5 Light micrographs and diagrams depicting patterns of focal segmental glomerulosclerosis. One pattern has a predilection for sclerosis in the perihilar regions of the glomeruli (**A** and **D**). The glomerular tip lesion variant has segmental consolidation confined to the segment adjacent to the origin of the proximal tubule (**B** and **E**). The collapsing glomerulopathy variant has segmental collapse of capillaries with hypertrophy and hyperplasia of overlying podocytes (**C** and **F**). (Jones' methenamine silver stain, ×100.)

Table 32.9 Classification of Focal Segmental Glomerulosclerosis (FSGS)

Primary (Idiopathic) FSGS

FSGS not otherwise specified (NOS)
Glomerular tip lesion variant of FSGS
Collapsing variant of FSGS
Perihilar variant of FSGS
Cellular variant of FSGS

Secondary FSGS

With HIV disease
With IV drug abuse
With other drugs (e.g., pamidronate, interferon, anabolic steroids)
With identified genetic abnormalities (e.g., mutations in podocin, α-actinin-4, TRPC6)
With glomerulomegaly
   Morbid obesity
   Sickle cell disease
   Cyanotic congenital heart disease
   Hypoxic pulmonary disease
With reduced nephron numbers
   Unilateral renal agenesis
   Oligomeganephronia
   Reflux-interstitial nephritis
   After focal cortical necrosis
   After nephrectomy

TRPC6, Transient receptor potential cation channel, subfamily C, member 6.

---

enlargement. FSGS that is associated with human immunodeficiency virus (HIV) infection has a collapsing pattern.[143,144]

EPIDEMIOLOGY

Over the past two decades, the incidence of FSGS has increased, whether expressed as an absolute number of patients or as a proportion of the total incident population of patients with end-stage kidney disease (ESKD).[145] This trend appears to hold true even when one accounts for a possible increase in the rate of diagnosis resulting from an increase in the frequency of kidney biopsies. Although this trend was previously reported to be most significant among African Americans, it has now been confirmed among whites as well. A review of kidney biopsy findings performed between 1974 and 2003 in Olmsted County, Minnesota, in which 90% of the population are whites of northern European ancestry, FSGS was found to account for 17% of glomerulonephritides, second only to IgA nephropathy (22%), and was more frequent than MN (10%).[145] Over that period of time, the incidence of FSGS increased by 13-fold ($P < 0.001$), compared with a 2-fold increase in the incidence of all glomerular diseases ($P < 0.001$), and 2.5- to 3-fold increase in MN and IgA nephropathy, respectively.

PATHOLOGY

Light Microscopy

FSGS is characterized by focal and segmental glomerular sclerosis or consolidation.[139,140,146] The sclerosis may begin as segmental consolidation caused by insudation of plasma proteins causing hyalinosis, by accumulation of foam cells, by swelling of epithelial cells, and by collapse of capillaries resulting in obliteration of capillary lumens. These events are accompanied by increased extracellular matrix material that accounts for the sclerosis component of the lesion.

FSGS is, by definition, a focal process when it begins. The limited number of glomeruli in a kidney biopsy specimen may not include any of the segmentally sclerotic glomeruli that are present in the kidney. In this instance, focal tubulointerstitial injury or glomerular enlargement, which often accompanies FSGS, can be used as a surrogate marker. For example, FSGS should be considered in kidney biopsy specimens of patients with nephrotic syndrome when there is relatively well-circumscribed focal tubular atrophy and interstitial fibrosis with slight chronic inflammation, even when there are no light microscopic glomerular lesions, no immune deposits, and no ultrastructural changes other than foot process effacement. Segmental sclerosis that is adequate for diagnosis may be present only in the tissue examined by immunofluorescence or electron microscopy.

Focal segmental glomerular scarring is nonspecific. Many injurious processes can cause focal glomerular scarring and must be ruled out before making a diagnosis of FSGS. For example, hereditary nephritis causes progressive glomerular scarring that can mimic FSGS, as revealed by identification of ultrastructural changes that are characteristic of hereditary nephritis. Focal segmental glomerular sclerosis, caused by IgA nephropathy, lupus nephritis, or ANCA-associated glomerulonephritis, for example, can result in focal segmental glomerular scarring that is histologically indistinguishable from that caused by FSGS. Findings by immunofluorescence and electron microscopy, and by

---

be classified as collapsing FSGS, tip lesion FSGS, cellular FSGS, perihilar FSGS, and FSGS not otherwise specified (NOS).[139,140] The collapsing variant of FSGS is a clinically aggressive variant that is much more common in African Americans than in white populations and is characterized pathologically by segmental collapse of capillaries accompanied by hypertrophy and hyperplasia of epithelial cells, and accumulation of prominent protein resorption droplets in podocytes. The glomerular tip lesion variant of FSGS, which typically presents with marked nephrosis but often has a good outcome, is characterized by consolidation and sclerosis in the glomerular segment that is adjacent to the origin of the proximal tubule.[140] The term *cellular FSGS* is used when numerous cells, especially foam cells, are within consolidated segments. However, this term has been used in a number of ways in the literature, especially before the publication of the Columbia classification system. For example, this term has been used to describe the collapsing variant and the tip lesion variant of FSGS. Care must be taken when reading the literature to determine if this term is being used as defined by the Columbia classification system.[139] The perihilar variant of FSGS is characterized pathologically by sclerosis at the hilum of the glomerulus that typically contains foci of hyalinosis.[139]

As shown in Table 32.9, FSGS may appear to be a primary kidney disease, or it may be associated with, and possibly caused by, a variety of other conditions. When FSGS is secondary to obesity or reduced numbers of nephrons, it often has a perihilar pattern and is accompanied by glomerular

serology, can reveal a glomerulonephritic basis for focal glomerular scarring.

Based on the character and glomerular distribution of lesions, five major structural variants of FSGS can be recognized that correlate, at least in part, with outcome (prognosis) and that may have different causes and different pathogenic mechanisms.[139,140] As mentioned earlier, these five pathologic variants are collapsing FSGS, tip lesion FSGS, cellular FSGS, perihilar FSGS, and FSGS NOS.[139,140]

The characteristic feature of the collapsing variant of FSGS is focal segmental or global collapse of glomerular capillaries with obliteration of capillary lumens. Podocytes overlying collapsed segments are usually enlarged and contain conspicuous resorption droplets. Hyperplasia of podocytes raises the possibility of crescentic glomerulonephritis. The convention among most renal pathologists is not to refer to the epithelial hyperplasia of collapsing glomerulopathy as crescent formation, although the term *pseudocrescent* has been used by some. The degree of adhesion formation relative to the extent of glomerular sclerosis is much less in collapsing glomerulopathy than in typical FSGS. This may result in contracted (collapsed) tuft basement membranes and sclerotic matrix separated from Bowman's capsule by hypertrophied and hyperplastic epithelial cells. The collapsing glomerulopathy variant of FSGS is the major pathologic expression of HIV nephropathy[39,144,147,148] and also occurs with intravenous drug abuse and as an idiopathic process.[149,150] In kidney transplants, this phenotype of FSGS occurs as both recurrent and de novo disease.[151,152]

Relative to the extent of glomerular sclerosis, tubulointerstitial injury is more severe in collapsing glomerulopathy than in typical FSGS. Tubular epithelial cells have larger resorption droplets, extensive proteinaceous casts, and marked focal dilation of lumens (microcystic change). There is also more extensive interstitial infiltration by mononuclear leukocytes. Immunofluorescence microscopy findings are similar to those observed in typical FSGS except for the usual finding of larger protein resorption droplets in glomerular podocytes and tubular epithelial cells. Electron microscopy reveals the same structural changes as seen by light microscopy. In a specimen with the collapsing glomerulopathy variant of FSGS, an important ultrastructural assessment is for the presence or absence of endothelial tubuloreticular inclusions. Endothelial tubuloreticular inclusions are identified in more than 90% of patients with HIV infection and collapsing glomerulopathy but in less than 10% of patients with idiopathic collapsing glomerulopathy. Other settings in which endothelial tubuloreticular inclusions are numerous are in patients with SLE and in patients treated with interferon-α.

The glomerular tip lesion variant of FSGS was first described by Howie and colleagues and is characterized by consolidation of the glomerular segment that is adjacent to the origin of the proximal tubule and thus opposite the hilum (Figure 32.5B and E).[153-157] The initial consolidation usually has obliteration of capillary lumens by foam cells, swollen endothelial cells, and an increase in collagenous matrix material (sclerosis). Podocytes adjacent to the consolidated segment are enlarged and contain clear vacuoles and hyaline droplets. These altered podocytes often are contiguous to, if not attached to, adjacent parietal epithelial cells and tubular epithelial cells at the origin of the proximal tubule, which also have irregular enlargement and vacuolation. The tip lesion may project into the lumen of the proximal tubule. Some lesions are less cellular with a predominance of matrix and collagenous adhesions to Bowman's capsule at the origin of the proximal tubule.

The cellular variant of FSGS as defined by the Columbia classification system has lesions that resemble the cellular lesion for the tip variant, but they are distributed more widely in the glomerular tuft and not confined to the tip.[139] Perihilar FSGS is characterized by the perihilar predilection of lesions and the presence of hyalinosis. The FSGS NOS category is a nonspecific category with lesions that do not have the distinctive features of any of the other four variants.

As is discussed later, different pathologic variants of FSGS have distinctive demographic characteristics, clinical presentations, and outcomes.

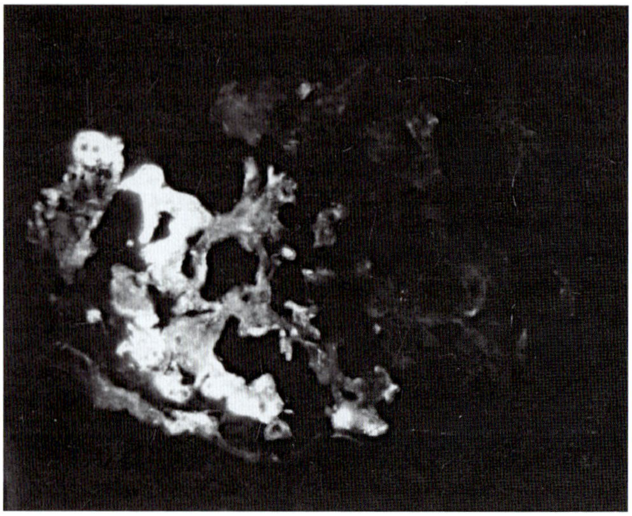

Figure 32.6 Immunofluorescence micrograph showing irregular segmental staining for C3 corresponding to a site of segmental sclerosis in a patient with focal segmental glomerulosclerosis. (Fluorescein isothiocyanate anti-C3 stain, ×3000.)

Immunofluorescence Microscopy

In all of the histologic variants, nonsclerotic glomeruli and segments usually show no staining for immunoglobulins or complement. As in patients with MCD, as well as individuals with no kidney dysfunction, a minority of patients with FSGS has low-level mesangial staining for IgM in nonsclerotic glomeruli. Low-level mesangial C3 staining is less frequent, and low-level IgG and IgA staining is uncommon. The presence of substantial staining of nonsclerotic glomeruli for immunoglobulins, especially if immune complex–type electron-dense deposits are present, points toward the sclerotic phase of a focal immune complex glomerulonephritis rather than FSGS.

Sclerotic segments typically show irregular staining for C3, C1q, and IgM (Figure 32.6). Other plasma constituents are less frequently identified in the sclerotic areas. Epithelial resorption droplets stain for plasma proteins.

Electron Microscopy

The ultrastructural features of FSGS are nonspecific. Electron microscopy plays an important role in the diagnosis of

Table 32.10 Gene Mutations with Causal Links to Focal Segmental Glomerulosclerosis

Gene	Protein	Mode of Inheritance
NPHS1	Nephrin	Autosomal recessive
NPHS2	Podocin	Autosomal recessive
CD2AP	CD2-associated protein	Autosomal dominant
TRPC6	Transient receptor potential cation channel, subfamily C, member 6	Autosomal dominant
PTPRO	Protein tyrosine phosphatase receptor type O (GLEPP1)	Autosomal recessive
LAMB2	Laminin-β_2	Autosomal recessive
ITGB4	β_4-Integrin	Autosomal recessive
CD151	Tetraspanin CD151	Autosomal recessive
ACTN4	α-Actinin-4	Autosomal dominant
PLCE1	Phospholipase Cε_1	Autosomal recessive
MYH9	Nonmuscle myosin heavy-chain A (NMMHC-A)	Autosomal dominant, de novo mutation
INF2	Inverted formin 2	Autosomal dominant
MYO1E	Myosin 1E	Autosomal recessive
WT1	Wilms' tumor suppressor protein	Autosomal dominant, de novo mutation
SMARCAL1	Smarca-like protein	Autosomal recessive
mtDNA-A3243G	tRNAleu	Maternal
COQ2	Coenzyme Q_2 4-hydroxybenzoate polyprenyltransferase	Autosomal recessive
COQ6	Coenzyme Q_{10} biosynthesis monooxygenase 6	Autosomal recessive
SCARB2	Lysosomal integral membrane protein (LIMP) type II	Autosomal recessive
APOL1	Apolipoprotein L-I	Autosomal recessive

FSGS by helping to identify other causes for glomerular scarring that can be mistaken for FSGS by light microscopy alone.

Foot process effacement in FSGS affects sclerotic and nonsclerotic glomeruli and usually is more focal than in MCD. Foot process effacement is less extensive in some forms of secondary FSGS than in idiopathic FSGS. Occasionally, glomerular capillaries have segmental denudation of foot processes. Podocytes adjacent to collapsed segments in collapsing FSGS are cuboidal and appear dedifferentiated. Nonsclerotic glomeruli and segments should have no immune complex–type electron-dense deposits. One must be careful not to confuse electron-dense "insudated" lesions with immune complex deposits. These lesions correspond to the hyalinosis seen by light microscopy and result from accumulation of plasma proteins within sclerotic areas. When electron-dense material is present in sclerotic but not in nonsclerotic glomerular segments, it should not be considered as evidence for immune complex–mediated glomerular disease. Conversely, well-defined mesangial or capillary wall electron-dense deposits in nonsclerotic segments indicate immune complex–mediated glomerulonephritis with secondary scarring, which should be confirmed and further characterized by immunofluorescence microscopy.

PATHOGENESIS

The past 20 years have witnessed an explosion of interest in the role of the podocyte in FSGS, in part due to concomitant rapidly advancing genomic technology that has revealed genetic abnormalities. Podocytes are highly differentiated postmitotic cells whose function requires a complex cellular architecture. Tremendous interest has centered on the genetics of familial FSGS, and podocyte defects have taken center stage (reviewed by D'Agati and colleagues[142] and Garg and colleagues[8]). This has led to the identification of several proteins important to the normal function of podocytes and the development of proteinuria. Mutations in several genes have been identified and linked to familial and sporadic cases of FSGS. These include, but are not limited to, genes coding for podocin (NPHS2),[158] nephrin (NPHS1),[159] α-actinin-4 (ACTN4),[160,161] transient receptor potential cation channel, subfamily C, member 6 (TRPC6),[162-164] and phospholipase Cε_1 (PLCE1).[165] In addition to mutations in genes encoding podocyte-specific proteins, mutations in other genes are associated with syndromes of which FSGS is often a part.[166] These include the COQ2 gene,[167] Wilms' tumor gene (WT1), and gene for LIM homeobox transcription factor 1β (LMX1B), which is a transcription factor required for the expression of CD2AP and NPHS2, associated with nail-patella syndrome. The genes implicated in the pathogenesis of FSGS are summarized in Table 32.10 and were recently reviewed by Rood and colleagues.[167]

Whereas these genetic mutations were primarily identified based on cases of familial forms of FSGS, their implication in sporadic FSGS in children and adults and their impact on treatment and outcome and recurrence after transplantation have been the focus of numerous investigations.

Mutations in NPHS2, the gene encoding podocin, are the most frequent genetic cause of steroid-resistant nephrotic syndrome and were initially described in early-onset disease (see recent review of all known mutations by Bouchireb and colleagues[168]). In a study of a large cohort of 430 patients from 404 different families with steroid-resistant nephrotic syndrome, recessive podocin mutations were present in 18.1%.[169] The R138Q mutation (a single nucleotide substitution of G to A at position 413 in the third exon of podocin gene) was found in 57% of families with two disease-causing mutations on each of the parental gene copies. Seventy percent of podocin mutations were nonsense, frameshift, or homozygous R138Q. Patients with these mutations manifested symptoms at a significantly earlier age (mean onset

<1.75 years) than any other patient group, with or without podocin mutations (mean onset >4.17 years). The sequence variant R229Q was found in 9% of families in the heterozygous mutation and 0.5% as a homozygous mutation.

The significance of the R229Q sequence variant as a cause of nephrotic syndrome was addressed in a study of 546 patients (from 455 families) with familial or sporadic FSGS, only 24% of whom developed nephrotic syndrome after age 18.[170] The R229Q allele frequency was significantly higher among European and South American patients than among control individuals (0.089 for European patients vs. 0.026 for controls, $P = 0.00001$; and 0.17 for South American patients vs. 0.007 for controls, $P = 0.000002$). Compared with individuals without a p.R229Q allele, those with a p.R229Q allele had a significantly higher likelihood of having a single pathogenic *NPHS2* mutation, which strongly suggests a pathogenic role of p.R229Q in the compound heterozygous state with a *NPHS2* mutation. Patients carrying p.R229Q and one *NPHS2* mutation developed nephrotic syndrome significantly later than those carrying two pathogenic mutations (median 19.0 vs. 1.1 years; $P < 0.01$). The frequency of *NPHS2* mutations in adults with treatment-resistant nephrotic syndrome was 11% in sporadic cases and 25% in familial cases. This study suggests that compound heterozygosity for p.R229Q is associated with adult-onset, steroid-resistant nephrotic syndrome. Furthermore, genetic analysis of *NPHS2* may identify individuals who are steroid-resistant prior to treatment initiation as well as those who are more likely to progress to ESKD and/or have low post-transplant recurrence risk.[171]

The role of *NPHS2* polymorphisms in sporadic cases of late-onset idiopathic or HIV-associated FSGS was studied in 377 biopsy-confirmed FSGS cases and 919 controls without known kidney disease.[172] No homozygotes or compound heterozygotes were observed for any of five missense mutations identified on gene sequencing. R138Q carriers were five times more frequent among FSGS cases than controls ($P = 0.06$), but heterozygosity for the other four missense mutations (including R229Q) was equally distributed among FSGS cases and controls. Genetic variation or mutation of *NPHS2* may therefore play a role in late-onset sporadic FSGS. However, given the very low frequency of R138Q (4 to 8 per 1000) and the lack of involvement of other mutations, the attributable risk of *NPHS2* for adult sporadic or HIV-associated FSGS is extremely small. The presence of the nonsynonymous variants of *NPHS2* (p.R229Q and p.A242V) did not significantly alter the risk of albuminuria in the Nurses' Health Study participants.[173]

In summary, *NPHS2* gene mutations are associated with familial and childhood-onset steroid-resistant nephrotic syndrome but may not contribute significantly to adult-onset sporadic FSGS. Heterozygosity for R138Q is associated with a fivefold increased risk of FSGS in adults. When combined with other pathogenic mutations of *NPHS2*, the R229Q variant appears to be associated with disease onset at older age.

Classically, mutations in *NPHS1*, which encodes nephrin, are associated with congenital nephrotic syndrome of the Finnish type presenting within the first 3 months of life. A study of 160 patients from 142 unrelated families who presented with nephrotic syndrome at least 3 months after birth identified *NPHS1* mutations in one familial case and in nine sporadic cases.[174] Kidney biopsy at presentation revealed mesangioproliferative lesions in one patient, MCD in six patients, and FSGS in three patients. This study broadens the spectrum of kidney disease related to nephrin mutations and raises the possibility that mutations in *NPHS1* may contribute to sporadic nephrotic syndrome in combination with mutations in other genes associated with this syndrome.[174,175]

Mutations in *ACTN4*, the gene encoding the actin-binding protein α-actinin-4, are a cause of familial FSGS with an autosomal dominant pattern of inheritance and may be associated with a distinctive ultrastructural feature of podocyte injury consisting of cytoplasmic electron-dense aggregates that may aid in identifying patients with *ACTN4* mutations.[176] Interestingly, recent mechanistic investigations revealed that ACTN4 protein mutants lack the ability to activate protective nuclear hormone receptors in podocytes.[177]

African Americans have a disproportionate risk for several forms of kidney disease, including a 4-fold increased risk for FSGS and an 18- to 50-fold increased risk for HIV-associated FSGS. The basis for that susceptibility is thought to be multifactorial, with a suspected genetic component. Two landmark studies, both of which used genomewide mapping by admixture linkage disequilibrium, identified a chromosome 22 region that was associated with kidney disease in subjects of African ancestry.[178,179] Initial efforts focused on *MYH9*, which encodes a nonmuscle myosin heavy-chain type IIA expressed in kidney podocytes and possibly mesangial cells, where it binds to actin to perform intracellular motor functions. Mutations in this gene were already known to cause a group of hereditary syndromes collectively known as the giant platelet syndromes, some of which also involve glomerular disease.[180] However, more recent studies have shown that the associations observed with *MYH9* were actually the result of linkage disequilibrium with variants in the adjacent gene *APOL1* (encoding the protein apolipoprotein L-I), which are most likely causally related to disease risk and which define a spectrum of *APOL1* nephropathies.[181] Two groups identified sequence variants in the *APOL1* gene that likely explain the genetic association of kidney disease in patients of African ancestry.[182,183] Reexamination of the interval surrounding *MYH9* led to these newer findings. Genovese and colleagues[182] and Tzur and colleagues[183] used data from the 1000 Genomes Project—which conducts the sequencing of genomic DNA derived from subjects around the globe, especially the Yoruba tribe of Western Africa—and identified sequence variants in the *APOL1* gene that were associated with kidney disease. A key clue to sorting this out was the observed discrepancy between absence of *APOL1* risk variants in the face of higher than expected allele frequencies of *MYH9* risk haplotypes in Ethiopian populations lacking a higher prevalence of these nephropathies.[184] The *APOL1* risk variants were found to be more strongly associated with ESKD than the previously reported *MYH9* variants.

In African Americans, Genovese and colleagues found that FSGS and hypertension-attributed ESKD were associated with two independent sequence variants in the *APOL1* gene on chromosome 22 (FSGS [odds ratio (OR), 10.5; 95% confidence interval (CI), 6.0 to 18.4]; hypertension-attributed ESKD [OR, 7.3; 95% CI, 5.6 to 9.5]). The two

APOL1 variants were common in African chromosomes but absent from European chromosomes, and both reside within haplotypes that harbor signatures of positive selection. The *APOL1* gene product, apolipoprotein L-1, has been studied for its role in trypanosomal lysis, autophagic cell death, and lipid metabolism, as well as for its vascular effects.

Apolipoprotein L-1 is a serum factor that lyses trypanosomes. Of interest, it was hypothesized that *APOL1* variants protect patients against *Trypanosoma brucei,* the parasite that causes sleeping sickness in thousands of people in Africa. Conversely, and with great irony, these same sequences are associated with kidney disease. In vitro assays revealed that only the kidney disease–associated apolipoprotein L-1 variants lysed *Trypanosoma brucei rhodesiense,* a particularly aggressive newer subspecies. Carrying two copies of the haplotype posed significantly more risk of kidney disease than carrying one copy. In some respects, therefore, kidney disease–associated *APOL1* variants and protection from tsetse flies mirrors sickle cell anemia and protection from malaria.

Risk variants in *MYH9* and *APOL1* are in strong linkage dysequilibrium, and genetic risk that was previously attributed to *MYH9* may reside in *APOL1*. More study is required to test whether more complex models of risk are operative. Nonetheless, this genetic association on chromosome 22 explains, at least in part, racial disparities in nondiabetic ESKD and HIV-associated kidney disease because of the high prevalence of these haplotypes in individuals of African ancestry.[185]

In addition to being the site of genetic anomalies, the podocyte may be the target of injury through several mechanisms.[186] These mechanisms include infections (e.g., HIV infection), exposure to certain drugs (e.g., pamidronate or interferon), metabolic disorders (e.g., diabetes), and deposition of abnormal protein (e.g., amyloid). Podocyte injury can lead to proteinuria through abnormalities of the slit diaphragm (e.g., due to genetic mutations); podocyte loss; loss of negative charges from loss of podocyte proteins (decreased podocalyxin or glomerular epithelial protein), decreased production of these proteins (decreased heparin sulfates), or destruction of the GBM (e.g., proteases); malformation of GBM; or podocyte-related endothelial cell dysfunction (e.g., decrease in vascular endothelial growth factor).[186] In addition, the response of the podocyte to injury may be expressed differently, depending on the nature of the insult, and result in different clinical syndromes. Thus, it has been proposed that various clinical and histologic variants of nephrotic syndromes depend on whether the podocyte injury results in apoptosis, podocyte loss, or podocyte dedifferentiation and reentry into the cell cycle and proliferation.[187] Indeed, this concept led to proposals to change the classification of nephrotic syndromes based on the understanding of the pathogenetic mechanisms of disease in addition to a description of histologic variants.[188]

In collapsing forms of FSGS, podocytes undergo changes in which mature podocyte markers disappear, which suggests a dysregulated podocyte phenotype in these diseases.[189-191] In fact, podocyte proliferation is seen in some examples of FSGS, which may be a consequence of the decrease in cyclin-dependent kinase inhibitors P27 and P57.[192] This has led to the concept that in collapsing FSGS, podocytes become dysregulated and proliferate.[193] However, the concept that the podocyte is a proliferating cell in collapsing FSGS has been challenged. In a mouse model of focal sclerosis, parietal epithelial and not podocytes were involved in the proliferative event.[194] This challenge is also supported from the findings of a study of two patients with HIV- and pamidronate-associated collapsing FSGS.[195]

The effacement of foot processes may be a consequence of the overproduction of oxygen radicals and accumulation of lipid peroxidase.[196] In theory, podocyte loss could result in focal areas of GBM denudation with diminished barrier function. Podocyte dropout may be a major factor in the development of glomerulosclerosis in general, and specifically in the development of collapsing FSGS.[197-200]

Some of the same pathogenic events that result in segmental scarring secondary to focal glomerular injury caused by a proliferative or necrotizing glomerulonephritis are probably operative in producing the sclerosis of FSGS. In this regard, the overproduction of transforming growth factor-β_1 (TGF-β_1) in glomeruli due to acute inflammatory lesions may cause glomerular sclerosis.[201] In experimental models of glomerular inflammation, the administration of antibodies to TGF-β or other inhibitors of TGF-β resulted in a decrease in matrix accumulation and a reduction in the severity of glomerular scarring.[202] Several mechanisms are associated with the fibrosis of kidney disease. Extracellular matrix, and proteoglycans such as decorin and biglycan, may have a pathogenic role in fibrosing diseases through regulation of TGF-β_1.[203]

FSGS also results from the loss of nephrons, which causes compensatory intraglomerular hypertension and enlargement in the remaining glomeruli. The compensatory capillary hypertension results in podocyte and endothelial cell injury, as well as mesangial alterations that lead to progressive focal and segmental sclerosis.[204-210] This process, at least in experimental animals, is made worse by increased dietary protein intake and is ameliorated by both protein restriction and antihypertensive therapy.

A permeability factor has been described in some patients with FSGS. In a seminal study, 33 patients with FSGS that recurred after transplantation had a higher mean value for permeability to albumin value than did normal subjects.[211] After plasmapheresis, the level of permeability factor in six patients was reduced, and proteinuria significantly decreased. The nature of the FSGS permeability factor continues to elude research efforts at identifying it. It is hypothesized to consist of low-molecular-weight anionic proteins or proteins that alter phosphorylation of glomerular proteins.[212] There is also a report of high affinity of the FSGS permeability factor to galactose, which appears to inhibit its activity in vitro.[213] Treatment with oral galactose is anecdotally reported to afford remission of nephrotic syndrome[214] and is the subject of a pilot study that has just been completed but not yet published (www.clinicaltrials.gov, NCT01113385). Another proposed permeability factor is circulating serum soluble urokinase receptor (suPAR), which has been reported to be elevated in two thirds of patients with primary FSGS as compared to patients with other glomerular diseases.[215] Furthermore, suPAR was shown in the same study in mice to activate podocyte β_3-integrin resulting in foot process effacement, proteinuria, and histopathologic changes akin to human FSGS.

Subsequently, serum suPAR levels were shown to be elevated in two cohorts of children and adults with FSGS and not disease controls[216]; however, more recent studies have reported an inverse correlation between estimated GFR (eGFR) and suPAR, and it is apparent that more studies are needed to clarify the role of suPAR.[217-224]

Regarding the role of a circulating permeability factor in the pathogenesis of the disease, it should be noted that in a minority of patients with steroid-resistant FSGS in native kidneys, plasmapheresis may diminish proteinuria and stabilize kidney function. In most patients, however, there is no improvement in proteinuria despite loss of the permeability factor following plasmapheresis.[225]

Glomerular enlargement accompanied by the development of FSGS occurs in the setting of hypoxemia, for example, in patients with sickle cell anemia, congenital pulmonary disease, or cyanotic congenital heart disease. Obesity predisposes to FSGS.[226,227] Weight loss and the administration of an angiotensin-converting enzyme (ACE) inhibitor decreased protein excretion by 80% to 85%.[228,229] Patients with sleep apnea may have proteinuria that is more functional in nature but with little or no evidence of glomerular scarring or epithelial injury observed in biopsy specimens.[230,231] The association between sleep apnea and proteinuria was examined in an analysis of 148 patients referred for polysomnography who were not diabetic and had not been treated previously for obstructive sleep apnea.[232] In this patient population, clinically significant proteinuria was uncommon; it was found to be associated with older age, hypertension, coronary artery disease, and arousal index by univariate analysis but only with age and hypertension by multiple regression analysis. Body mass index and apnea-hypopnea index were not associated with urine protein to creatinine ratio. The authors concluded that nephrotic-range proteinuria should not be ascribed to sleep apnea and deserves a more thorough nephrologic evaluation.

A number of infections cause FSGS. HIV-associated FSGS is pathologically identical to idiopathic collapsing FSGS, except that endothelial tubuloreticular inclusions are present in the former but not the latter. This close association of HIV infection with collapsing FSGS, as well as experimental evidence of focal glomerular sclerosis in mice transgenic for HIV-1 genes,[147,233-239] raise the possibility that the HIV virus can be a causal agent of FSGS in infected patients. Whether other viral diseases, including parvovirus B19 infection, cause the idiopathic collapsing variant of FSGS remains to be elucidated.[240,241] Parvovirus B19 has been found with greater frequency in patients with idiopathic and collapsing FSGS than in patients with other diagnoses.[240] The polyomavirus SV40 may also play a role.[242]

FSGS is associated with a number of malignant conditions that have been linked to lymphoproliferative disease. In one study,[243] an association of FSGS was found with monoclonal gammopathies of undetermined significance (MGUS) and multiple myeloma. When the lymphoproliferative disease was treated, the renal lesion improved.

Finally, FSGS has been linked to exposure to a number of medications, including pamidronate[194,244] and interferon,[245] and with the use of anabolic steroids.[246] Like pamidronate and interferon therapy, the latter may also be associated with collapsing FSGS. Discontinuation of the anabolic steroids may lead to reduced levels of protein in the urine.

CLINICAL FEATURES AND NATURAL HISTORY

Proteinuria is the hallmark feature of all forms of primary FSGS. The degree of proteinuria varies from nonnephrotic (1 to 2 g of protein per day) to over 10 g of protein per day, associated with all of the morbid features of nephrotic syndrome. Hematuria occurs in over half of FSGS patients, and approximately one third of patients present with some degree of renal insufficiency. Gross hematuria is more commonly seen in FSGS than in MCD.[247] Hypertension is a presenting feature in one third of patients. There are differences in the presentation of FSGS in adults and children.[248-251] More children than adults tend to have proteinuria, whereas hypertension is more common in adults.

Differences in clinical manifestations correlate with different pathologic phenotypes of FSGS.[252] Patients with perihilar FSGS accompanied by glomerular enlargement more commonly have nonnephrotic-range proteinuria than patients without glomerular hypertrophy. In addition, there are differences in the clinical presentation of the collapsing variant of FSGS and the glomerular tip lesion variant of FSGS.

Patients with collapsing FSGS have a substantially higher level of urine protein, a lower serum albumin level, and a higher serum creatinine level than patients with perihilar FSGS.[149,150,253] The development of proteinuria, edema, or hypoalbuminemia may occur rapidly over the course of days to weeks, in contrast to the more indolent development of proteinuria in most patients with typical FSGS. Moreover, patients with collapsing FSGS more frequently have extrarenal manifestations of disease a few weeks prior to onset of the nephrosis, such as episodes of diarrhea, upper respiratory tract infections, or lower respiratory tract–like symptoms that are usually ascribed to viral or other infectious processes. However, the systemic symptoms of fever, malaise, and anorexia occur in less than 20% of patients at the time of onset of nephrosis. Pamidronate, a bisphosphonate that prevents bone disease in patients with myeloma and metastatic tumors, has been reported to be associated with collapsing FSGS.[194,244] After discontinuation of the drug, kidney function stabilized in all patients except those with collapsing FSGS. Treatment with interferon has also been reported to be associated with the development of collapsing FSGS.[245]

The clinical presentation of glomerular tip lesion differs from that of both perihilar FSGS and collapsing FSGS.[214] Patients with glomerular tip lesion tend to be older white males, in contrast to the younger black male prevalence in collapsing FSGS. The proteinuria in these patients usually is severe and the onset is abrupt, with sudden development of edema and hypoalbuminemia. The rapidity of onset of the disease process is similar to the clinical presentation of MCD.[155,254,255] Patients with glomerular tip lesion may develop reversible AKI especially at the time of initial presentation when proteinuria, edema, and hypoalbuminemia are at their peak. This also is similar to the presentation of MCD but rarely occurs with other variants of FSGS.

Several studies have addressed the clinical applicability and implications of distinguishing the variants of FSGS. An analysis of data for 197 patients followed within the

Glomerular Disease Collaborative Network between 1982 and 2001 found the FSGS NOS variant in 42% of cases, the perihilar variant in 26%, the tip lesion in 17%, the collapsing lesion in 11%, and the cellular variant in 3% of patients.[140] African Americans accounted for 91% of patients with collapsing FSGS but only 15% of patients with the tip lesion variant. Both collapsing and tip variants were associated with significantly greater amounts of urine protein (10.0 ± 5.3 g protein per day and 9.7 ± 7.0 g protein per day, respectively) than perihilar or NOS variants of FSGS (4.4 ± 3.3 g protein per day and 5.5 ± 4.6 g protein per day, respectively; $P < 0.001$). In this retrospective, uncontrolled analysis, patients with the tip lesion variant of FSGS were significantly more likely to attain a complete remission even after adjustment for corticosteroid exposure ($P < 0.001$). Collapsing FSGS had the worst 1-year (74%) and 3-year renal survival rates of all other variants, regardless of differences in the histologic severity of injury, which suggests the possibility that the nature of the injury was inherently different.

Similarly, an analysis of data for 225 patients studied at Columbia University[252] confirmed the predilection of the tip lesion variant of FSGS for whites (86.2%), although the predominance of African Americans among patients with collapsing FSGS was less pronounced (53.6%). In this large cohort, 10% of patients had the cellular variant, of whom 32% were African American. The mean urine protein level (9.5 ± 1.2 g of protein per day) in these patients was comparable to that in patients with the collapsing or tip variant (8.8 ± 1.3 g of protein per day and 7.8 ± 0.6 g of protein per day, respectively). Patients with cellular FSGS showed intermediate rates of remission (44.5%) and ESKD (27.8%) compared to patients with collapsing FSGS (remission rate, 13.2%; ESKD rate, 65.3%) and tip FSGS (remission rate, 75.8%; ESKD rate, 5.7%).

A retrospective analysis of data for a cohort of 93 adult patients in the Netherlands confirms the improved renal survival of patients with the tip variant compared with patients with the other variants (5-year survival of 78% for tip vs. 63% for FSGS NOS and 55% for perihilar FSGS; $P = 0.02$).[256]

A major prospective FSGS study evaluated the clinical impact of these histopathologic variants among participants with steroid-resistant primary FSGS in the FSGS Clinical Trial.[257,258] As in prior retrospective studies, the tip variant and collapsing variant had the strongest association with whites (86%) and blacks (63%; $P = 0.003$), respectively. This study also confirmed poor renal survival in participants with the collapsing variant and better renal survival in participants with the tip variant, although the sample size was small for these groups.

The degree of proteinuria is a predictor of long-term clinical outcome. Nonnephrotic-range proteinuria correlates with a more favorable renal survival of over 80% after 10 years of follow-up.[259,260] In contrast, patients who have proteinuria of more than 10 g of protein per day have very poor long-term renal survival, with the majority of patients reaching ESKD within 3 years.[261,262] Patients with FSGS and protein excretion that measures between nonnephrotic range and massive proteinuria have variable long-term renal outcomes. In general, these patients have a relatively poor outcome, with half reaching ESKD by 10 years.[250,251,263]

One of the most useful prognostic indicators for patients with FSGS is whether remission of nephrotic syndrome is achieved.[249] Patients who experience remission of nephrosis have a substantially greater renal survival rate than those who do not.[249,259,260,264,265] According to Korbet and colleagues,[250,251] less than 15% of patients who achieve complete or partial remission progress to ESKD within 5 years of follow-up. Up to 50% of patients who do not experience remission progress to end-stage disease within 6 years of follow-up.

As in other forms of glomerular injury, entry serum creatinine level correlates with long-term renal survival.[259,261,266,267] Patients with a serum creatinine level of higher than 1.3 mg/dL have poorer renal survival than those with lower serum creatinine concentrations, irrespective of the level of urine protein (10-year renal survival of 27% vs. 100%).[251] Multivariate analysis indicates that entry serum creatinine level may be more important than urine protein level as a predictor of progression to ESKD.[259,260,262,263,266,267]

LABORATORY FINDINGS

Hypoproteinemia is common in patients with FSGS, with total serum protein reduced to varying extents. The serum albumin concentration may fall to below 2 g/dL, especially in patients with collapsing and glomerular tip variants of FSGS. As in other forms of nephrotic syndrome, levels of immunoglobulins are typically depressed and levels of lipids are increased, especially serum cholesterol level. Serum levels of complement components are generally in the normal range in FSGS. Circulating immune complexes have been detected in patients with FSGS,[268,269] although their pathogenic significance has not been determined. Serologic testing for HIV infection should be obtained for patients with FSGS, especially those with the collapsing pattern.

TREATMENT

Angiotensin Inhibitors

ACE inhibitors and angiotensin II receptor blockers (ARBs) have been evaluated in the treatment of FSGS. ACE inhibitors have been shown to decrease levels of urine protein and the rate of progression to ESKD in diabetic and nondiabetic kidney disease.[270-273] These results have been observed in the presence of diabetes as well as in cases of nondiabetic kidney disease. A systematic review of studies revealed that ACE inhibitors significantly reduce urine protein levels in children with steroid-resistant nephrotic syndrome.[274] In a randomized controlled trial involving normotensive children with steroid-resistant nephrotic syndrome, the addition of fosinopril to prednisone resulted in a greater reduction in urine protein levels than prednisone alone.[275]

In patients with glomerulomegaly and nonnephrotic-range proteinuria, an ACE inhibitor or ARB sufficiently decreases proteinuria and potentially decreases hyperlipidemia, edema, and other manifestations of persistent loss of protein in the urine with excellent long-term prognosis. Regardless of what other forms of antiinflammatory or immunosuppressive therapy are employed, the beneficial effects of these agents indicates that they should be added, despite the well-known side effects of hyperkalemia and reduction in GFR, especially in patients with serum creatinine levels of over 3 mg/dL.

Before immunomodulatory or immunosuppressive therapy is initiated in a patient with FSGS, a careful evaluation should be undertaken to exclude the possibility of an underlying cause as described in the section on pathogenesis. Patients with secondary FSGS are unlikely to benefit from immunosuppressive therapy and may be at particularly high risk of complications. In addition, an assessment of the risk and benefit of immunosuppressive therapy should be undertaken for each patient. Patients with subnephrotic-range proteinuria have a generally good prognosis, and the initial therapy should be focused on blood pressure control, preferentially using maximal tolerated dosages of renin angiotensin aldosterone system (RAAS) blockers. Glucocorticoids or immunosuppressive therapy should be targeted to patients with idiopathic FSGS and nephrotic syndrome.

Glucocorticoids

No randomized placebo-controlled trial has been conducted to formally assess the role of glucocorticoids in the treatment of FSGS. The available data are based on case series using different treatment protocols; different definitions of remission, response, relapse, and resistance; and different lengths of therapy.[249,259,264,276] One review of studies suggested that only 15% of patients with FSGS responded to treatment, in sharp contrast to those with MCD.[277] More optimistic reports have been obtained by groups in Toronto and Chicago[249,250] which suggest that 30% to 40% of adult patients may attain some form of remission with corticosteroid treatment. A compilation of these studies by Korbet and colleagues[251] suggests that of 177 patients who received a variety of different forms of therapy, 45% experienced complete remission, 10% experienced partial remission, and 45% showed no response.[249,259,264,276,278]

In children, the initial treatment of FSGS is similar to that of MCD because treatment is typically initiated without histologic confirmation of the disease process. Thus, the International Study of Kidney Diseases in Children recommended using an initial course of prednisone of 60 mg/m^2/day up to 80 mg/m^2/day, for 4 weeks. This is followed with 40 mg/m^2/day, up to 60 mg/m^2/day, administered in divided doses for 3 consecutive days out of 7, for 4 weeks, and then tapered off for 4 more weeks. As in adult patients with MCD, a longer course of therapy at higher doses of prednisone may be necessary to induce remission. Thus, in those series and retrospective analyses that showed an increased remission rate,[131,249,259,264,276,279,280] prednisone treatment was continued for 16 weeks to achieve remission. In adult patients, median time for complete remission was 3 to 4 months.[134]

A portion of patients showing a positive response to corticosteroid treatment will experience relapse. Guidelines for re-treatment of relapsing patients are similar to those for treatment of patients with relapsing MCD. In patients whose remission prior to relapse was prolonged (more than 6 months), a repeat course of corticosteroid therapy may again induce a remission. In steroid-dependent patients who develop frequent relapses, repeated rounds of high-dose corticosteroid therapy result in unacceptable cumulative toxicity. Thus, alternative strategies, such as the addition of cyclosporine, may be useful. In patients with the glomerular tip lesion variant of FSGS, a trial of corticosteroids is appropriate because many patients experience a decline in protein excretion.[154,255,281]

The practice of using higher dosages of corticosteroids to induce remission has resulted in the use of alternative therapeutic approaches.

Administration of very high doses of corticosteroids in children, and continuation of daily prednisone therapy for up to 6 to 9 months in adults, is not without enormous short- and long-term side effects. In studies in which long-term, high-dose corticosteroids are administered, few analyses have been undertaken to evaluate the development of osteoporosis, short- and long-term risk of infection, cataracts, diabetes, or other long-term sequelae. Thus, the available data do not allow for careful understanding of risk/benefit ratios. Until the use of high-dose methylprednisolone has been studied in controlled clinical trials, this potentially useful yet dangerous approach must be viewed with caution.

Attempts at alternate-day steroid therapy have not been successful except in older adult populations. The Toronto group[282] demonstrated that a 40% remission rate could be achieved in patients older than age 60 by administering up to 100 mg of prednisone on alternate days for 3 to 5 months. This therapy was well tolerated in this population, with no obvious side effects during the study period. Alternate-day prednisone most likely works in this population because of an increased susceptibility to the immunosuppressive effects of corticosteroids and altered glucocorticoid kinetics in older adults.

The benefit of corticosteroid therapy may differ among whites and African Americans. In a retrospective analysis[283] of renal survival in predominantly African American individuals with FSGS, renal survival was found to be higher when the initial serum creatinine level was lower and blood pressure was well controlled, but treatment with steroids had no effect on renal survival.

Cyclophosphamide

Several studies have failed to document the effectiveness of cytotoxic drugs in the treatment of FSGS.[264,284] In one review, only 23% of 247 children with FSGS showed a response to steroid therapy, and 70 patients were treated with cytotoxic drugs. Of these, 30% showed a response. In the final analysis, the disease was in remission in less than 20% of the 247 children. The use of cytotoxic drugs has been evaluated in only one series of adults.[264] Although their use correlated with longer remissions and fewer relapses, no other study has corroborated these results.

The International Study of Kidney Diseases in Children carefully examined the role of cyclophosphamide in the treatment of children with FSGS.[285] Daily oral cyclophosphamide (2.5 mg/kg) was administered in addition to prednisone (40 mg/m^2 every other day) for 12 months, and results were compared with those for prednisone alone. The addition of cyclophosphamide had no effect on the change in proteinuria or the likelihood of achieving complete resolution of proteinuria.[285] Similarly, in a nonrandomized comparative study involving children with FSGS or steroid-resistant or frequently relapsing nephrotic syndrome, the addition of oral cyclophosphamide to prednisone for 3 months had no statistically significant effect on the rate of complete or partial remission or progression to ESKD.[286] In summary, the limited currently available data do not support the use of cyclophosphamide in patients with FSGS.

Cyclosporine

FSGS that is resistant to prednisone may be induced into remission by cyclosporine. The effectiveness of cyclosporine in inducing remission of proteinuria in patients with FSGS has been demonstrated in two randomized controlled trials. In the study by Ponticelli and colleagues, 45 patients with steroid-resistant nephrotic syndrome were randomly assigned to receive supportive therapy or cyclosporine (5 mg/kg/day for adults, 6 mg/kg/day for children) for 6 months, with the drug then tapered off by 25% every 2 months.[131] Remission occurred in 13 of 22 patients receiving cyclosporine, compared with 3 of 19 patients in the control group ($P < 0.001$). Unfortunately, relapses occurred in 69% of patients after withdrawal of cyclosporine.

In the North America Nephrotic Syndrome Study Group trial, 49 patients were randomly assigned to treatment with low-dose prednisone alone or in combination with oral cyclosporine for 26 weeks.[287] At the end of 26 weeks of therapy, partial or complete remission of proteinuria occurred in 70% of patients in the cyclosporine-treated group compared to only 4% in the control group ($P < 0.001$); however, relapses occurred by 52 weeks in 40% of those experiencing remission. Treatment with cyclosporine was also associated with a 70% reduction in the risk that GFR would decline by 50%.[287]

A randomized controlled trial compared the efficacy of cyclosporine to intravenous cyclophosphamide in the initial treatment of 22 children with steroid-resistant nephrotic syndrome related to MCD, FSGS, or mesangial hypercellularity.[288] All patients were also receiving alternate-day prednisone therapy. Treatment with cyclosporine afforded a statistically significant higher rate of partial remission of proteinuria at both 12 weeks (60% of cyclosporine-treated patients vs. 17% in the cyclophosphamide group; $P < 0.05$). By study's end, 12 of the 14 patients who showed no response to cyclophosphamide were patients with FSGS. Of note, all six patients who were heterozygous for the NPHS2 R229Q variant or the R6QH mutation were assigned to the cyclophosphamide group, and only one of those showed a response to treatment. These results support the use of cyclosporine over cyclophosphamide in children with steroid-resistant nephrotic syndrome.

Results were recently reported from the FSGS Clinical Trial, the largest multicenter, randomized controlled trial of its kind, comparing a 12-month course of cyclosporine to a combination of oral pulse dexamethasone and MMF in 138 randomized children and young adults with biopsy-proven, steroid-resistant primary FSGS.[257] The trial was designed to determine whether treatment with MMF plus pulse steroids was superior to treatment with cyclosporine in inducing remission of proteinuria over 12 months. Partial or complete remission by the 12-month mark was achieved in only 22 MMF-treated patients and 33 cyclosporine-treated patients, and the odds ratio for achieving remission or better with MMF compared to cyclosporine was not significant (OR, 0.59; 95% CI, 0.30 to 1.18). Furthermore, remission by 26 weeks after treatment cessation was not significantly different between the two groups. The investigators concluded that the lack of signal difference may have been due to insufficient sample size and that the low rates of remission in the trial amplify the profound need for better and more targeted therapies.

How long should patients be treated with cyclosporine? In a study by Meyrier and colleagues,[134] when patients remained in remission for over 12 months, cyclosporine was slowly tapered and eventually removed without subsequent relapse.[134] Unfortunately, long-term treatment with cyclosporine was associated with increases in tubular atrophy and interstitial fibrosis, the degree of which was positively correlated with the initial serum creatinine level, the number of segmental scars on initial biopsy specimens, and a cyclosporine dose of more than 5.5 mg/kg/day. Thus, there is a clear trade-off with the use of cyclosporine over the long term given the risk of development of interstitial fibrosis and tubular atrophy.

Mycophenolate Mofetil

Data regarding the use of MMF in the treatment of FSGS has been largely anecdotal, with one small case series reporting transient improvement in proteinuria in 8 of 18 patients; however, two clinical trials have occurred within the past decade.

A randomized controlled trial compared the efficacy of an MMF-based regimen to treatment with corticosteroids with or without cyclophosphamide in adult patients with idiopathic MN (n = 21) or FSGS (n = 33).[289] MMF was given at a dosage of 2 g/day for 6 months along with prednisolone at 0.5 mg/kg/day for 2 to 3 months. Patients with FSGS in the comparison group received prednisolone 1 mg/kg/day for 3 to 6 months. There was no difference between the two groups with respect to the proportion of complete or partial remissions (70% vs. 69%) or the time to remission of proteinuria at any point. Remission was achieved faster in the MMF-treated FSGS patients than in the corticosteroid-only group (5.6 months vs. 10.2 months, respectively), and cumulative steroid dose was lower (1.9 ± 0.3 g vs. 7.3 ± 0.9 g, respectively). Although limited to a small number of patients and relatively short follow-up, this first controlled study suggests that the addition of MMF is steroid sparing and achieves rates of remission comparable to those for corticosteroids alone in patients with FSGS. The randomized controlled FSGS Clinical Trial, discussed in the cyclosporine section, showed no significant difference in outcomes when comparing cyclosporine to oral pulse dexamethasone and MMF.[257]

Other Therapies

The use of sirolimus in the management of FSGS is poorly supported. Several reports have emerged of new-onset proteinuria in kidney transplant recipients who were switched from calcineurin inhibitor–based therapy to sirolimus.[290-294]

In a study of 78 solid organ transplant recipients treated with sirolimus, 18 patients (23.1%) developed proteinuria in an average of 11.2 ± 2.1 months after starting sirolimus therapy.[295] Kidney biopsy specimens obtained after the onset of proteinuria revealed various degrees of mesangial proliferation and mesangial expansion commonly seen in patients who previously had a diagnosis of chronic allograft nephropathy but showed FSGS in only two patients (14.3%). There was no correlation between proteinuria levels and sirolimus dose or trough blood levels. In the six patients in whom sirolimus was withdrawn, a complete reversal of proteinuria and edema was observed. This study certainly raises significant concern about the induction of proteinuria by sirolimus in transplant recipients.

The data pertaining to the use of sirolimus in the management of FSGS in native kidneys is rather conflicting. In a prospective open-label trial of sirolimus in 21 patients with steroid-resistant FSGS, at 6 months 4 patients (19%) had achieved a complete remission, 8 (38%) had experienced a partial remission, and 1 patient had experienced a rapid decline in kidney function.[296] Sirolimus therapy was associated with a substantial number of adverse events, including hyperlipidemia and anemia in 43% of patients. In patients who showed no response to sirolimus, the mean serum creatinine level increased from 1.66 mg/dL at baseline to 2.2 mg/dL at 6 months and 3.24 mg/dL at 12 months (significantly different from baseline at the $P = 0.028$ level). In patients who showed a response to sirolimus, the mean serum creatinine level increased from 1.76 mg/dL at baseline to 1.91 mg/dL at 12 months.

In contrast, a phase II open-label clinical trial of sirolimus had to be interrupted for safety reasons after five out of six patients enrolled experienced a sharp decrease in GFR, and none achieved a complete remission.[297] Three patients had a more than twofold increase in proteinuria during sirolimus therapy. Similar deleterious effects were reported in a cohort of 11 patients with a variety of glomerular diseases.[298] Although inconclusive, the bulk of the data currently available suggest that sirolimus has a deleterious effect in FSGS and should be avoided.

Future approaches to the treatment of FSGS may come from the treatment of recurrent FSGS following transplantation. A recent study reported the use of CTLA-4-Ig (abatacept), an inhibitor of the T cell costimulatory molecule B7-1 (CD80), in four patients with recurrent FSGS and one with primary FSGS given that podocytes also express B7-1 in some individuals with proteinuric kidney disease, including FSGS.[299] Surprisingly, nephrotic-range proteinuria resolved in all patients; however, much larger, more controlled studies are needed to validate this encouraging result.

Intriguing cases of recurrent FSGS after transplantation have been published in which the proteinuria resolved after treatment with rituximab.[300] Interestingly, in one case[301] the diagnosis of posttransplant lymphoproliferative disease was established 5 months after the transplantation, even though recurrent nephrotic syndrome occurred within 2 weeks postoperatively. In addition, there are a few reports of recurrent FSGS after transplantation which responded to rituximab (after plasmapheresis or immunoadsorption) that are not related to posttransplant lymphoproliferative disease.[302-305] These patients may represent a specific category, and the lessons learned from their treatment may not necessarily apply to the general population of patients with FSGS. Anecdotal reports are emerging of treatment of primary and recurrent FSGS with rituximab, usually in combination with other immunomodulating therapies, but results show a mixed response to this treatment[306,307] with several reports of failures.[308] In the largest case series, five of eight adult patients with resistant FSGS failed to show a response to a course of rituximab, and two patients suffered a rapid deterioration of kidney function.[309] Only two patients had a clear and sustained improvement of kidney function and proteinuria. More recently, as discussed in the section on MCD, a small prospective trial in Italy of rituximab in 10 children and 20 adults with relapsing FSGS, MCD, and mesangial proliferative glomerulonephritis showed significant benefit, which warrants further investigation with larger randomized clinical trials.[135] It has also been shown in the setting of recurrent FSGS that rituximab can bind to podocyte-derived sphingomyelin phosphodiesterase acid–like 3b (SMPDL-3b) to preserve its expression as a regulator of acid sphingomyelinase activity to prevent disruption of the actin cytoskeleton and apoptosis.[310] It is becoming clear that the use of rituximab for the treatment of FSGS requires further evaluation in the setting of a randomized controlled trial.

Another potential future approach targets renal fibrosis, which represents a common final pathway of FSGS and other chronic kidney diseases.[311] The orally available antifibrotic agent pirfenidone was evaluated in an open-label pilot study to determine its effect on the rate of decline in GFR in 18 patients with FSGS selected for having a monthly rate of decline in eGFR of more than 0.35 mL/min/1.73 m^2.[312] The monthly change in GFR improved from a median of −0.61 mL/min/1.73 m^2 during the baseline period to −0.45 mL/min/1.73 m^2 with pirfenidone therapy, which represented a median of 25% improvement in the rate of decline ($P < 0.01$). Pirfenidone had no effect on blood pressure or proteinuria and was associated with frequent dyspepsia, sedation, and photosensitive dermatitis. These results provide a strong rationale for a larger placebo-controlled trial in patients with progressive chronic kidney disease.

Other forms of treatment have been used. Plasmapheresis and protein absorption strategies to remove circulating factors responsible for FSGS have led to remission of recurrent FSGS but do not appear to be beneficial in treating the primary disease.[225,313]

In summary, patients with primary FSGS remain frustrating patients to treat. Enthusiasm for the use of high-dose, prolonged corticosteroid therapy in adults and children has prompted the use of this therapy in many FSGS patients. Only a prospective randomized trial that carefully evaluates this approach will determine its effectiveness. The first step in therapy should be geared toward excellent blood pressure control using RAAS blockers. In those patients who have nephrotic-range proteinuria, careful supportive care and consideration of a trial of oral corticosteroids in adult patients may be an acceptable approach after patients are carefully informed about the risks and potential benefits of 12 to 16 weeks of daily corticosteroid therapy. Alternatively a trial of cyclosporine may be warranted for patients who have contraindications to corticosteroid therapy or in whom corticosteroid therapy fails to produce improvement.

C1q NEPHROPATHY

C1q nephropathy is a relatively rare cause of proteinuria and nephrotic syndrome that can mimic MCD or FSGS clinically and histologically, although the clinical and pathologic presentations are quite variable.[314,315] In a single-center retrospective analysis of kidney biopsy specimens from children and adolescents, C1q nephropathy was found in 6.6% of native kidney biopsy specimens.[316] In the largest case series at the University of Ljubljana, Slovenia, which included both children and adults, C1q nephropathy was identified in 1.9% of native kidney biopsy specimens.[317] There appears to be a slight male predominance (56% to 68%).[317,318] Depending on the case series, there may be an association with African American or Hispanic ethnicity.[318] Patients of all ages with C1q nephropathy have been described.

The diagnosis is based on the presence of mesangial immune complex deposits that show conspicuous staining for C1q in a patient with no clinical or laboratory evidence of SLE. The C1q staining usually is accompanied by staining for IgG, IgM, and C3. Electron microscopy demonstrates well-defined mesangial immune complex–type dense deposits. Light microscopic findings vary from no lesion (mimicking MCD), to focal glomerular hypercellularity, to proliferative glomerulonephritis with mesangial hypercellularity, to focal segmental sclerosing lesions that may be indistinguishable histologically from those of FSGS. Anecdotal case reports have described C1q nephropathy associated with a collapsing FSGS lesion.[319,320] The findings by immunofluorescence microscopy and electron microscopy, however, readily differentiate C1q nephropathy from MCD and FSGS. The findings by immunofluorescence and electron microscopy suggest an immune complex pathogenesis, but the details of the pathogenic mechanism and the causes are unknown.

Patients with C1q nephropathy generally have proteinuria, which may or may not be associated with nephrotic syndrome. Hematuria is present in at least 50% of patients and is more common among patients with a mesangial proliferative lesion found through use of light microscopy.[317] Likewise, hypertension affects a minority of patients with no discernible lesions on light microscopy (similar to MCD) but is much more prevalent among patients with mesangial proliferation (55%).[317] Interestingly, many patients are relatively asymptomatic, and proteinuria may first be detected at the time of a physical examination in connection with sports participation or induction into the armed forces. These patients, by definition, have no clinical or serologic evidence of SLE, despite the presence of C1q in the kidney biopsy specimen. C1q nephropathy may show spontaneous improvement.[321]

The renal outcome of patients with C1q nephropathy appears generally favorable,[316] especially in patients whose biopsy specimens show minimal change–like histologic features.[317,322] Studies suggest, however, that they may experience more frequent relapses and require additional immunosuppressants more often than patients with "pure" MCD.[316,317,322] Patients whose biopsy specimens show FSGS-like or mesangial proliferative lesions based on histologic analysis may show a less favorable response to immunosuppressive therapy although the data are rather limited.

MEMBRANOUS NEPHROPATHY

EPIDEMIOLOGY

Membranous glomerulopathy, also known as membranous nephropathy (MN), is one of the most common causes of nephrotic syndrome in adults.[323–326] MN occurs as a primary form of glomerular disease usually caused by antibodies specific for M-type phospholipase A_2 receptor (PLA_2R) or secondary to multiple nonrenal diseases, including autoimmune diseases (e.g., SLE, autoimmune thyroiditis), infection (e.g., hepatitis B, hepatitis C, malaria), drugs (e.g., penicillamine, gold), and malignancies (e.g., colon or lung cancer). Secondary MN, especially that caused by hepatitis B[327-331] and lupus, is more frequent in children than in adults. In patients older than age 60, MN is associated with a malignancy in 20% to 30% of patients.

MN is the cause of nephrotic syndrome in approximately 25% of adults with the syndrome.[323,332-340] A study of patients who had urinary excretion of more than 1 g of protein per 24 hours, conducted by the Medical Research Council in the United Kingdom from 1978 to 1990, determined that 20% had MN. The peak incidence of MN is in the fourth to fifth decade of life.[323,341-345] A pooled analysis of studies of patients with idiopathic MN found a 2:1 predominance of males (1190 males and 598 females).[346] The adult/child ratio was 26:1 (1734 adults and 67 children); however, this low proportion of children among MN patients was biased by the exclusion of children from some of the studies included in the analysis. MN affects all population groups.

Although most patients with MN present with nephrotic syndrome, 10% to 20% of patients have proteinuria that remains at less than 2 g of protein per day.[347] It is thus likely that the frequency of MN in the general population is underestimated, because asymptomatic individuals with subclinical proteinuria often do not come to diagnosis or undergo kidney biopsy.

There are geographic variations in the clinical manifestations of MN. In studies in Australia and Japan, lower percentages of patients have nephrotic syndrome at entry than in Europe or North America. The geographic differences may be related to differences in the prevalence of underlying causes of secondary MN, such as hepatitis B, malaria, and other infections.[327,329]

The association of MN with underlying malignancy is well recognized. In a large cohort study of 240 patients in France,[348] the incidence of cancer was significantly higher in patients with MN than in the general population (standardized incidence ratio, 9.8 [5.5 to 16.2] for men and 12.3 [4.5 to 26.9] for women). In almost half the patients, the tumor was asymptomatic and was detected only because of diagnostic procedures prompted by the diagnosis of MN. The most common malignancies were cancers of the lung and prostate. The frequency of malignancy increased with age. In a separate cohort study in Norway,[349] the incidence of cancer in 161 patients with MN was significantly higher compared with the age- and sex-adjusted general Norwegian population, corresponding to a standardized incidence ratio of 2.25 (95% CI, 1.44 to 3.35). The median time from diagnosis of MN to diagnosis of cancer was 60 months. Patients with MN who developed cancer were older (65 vs. 52 years; $P < 0.001$).[349]

Risk factors for malignancy in patients with MN include older age and a history of smoking, although the clinical presentation does not differ between patients with cancer-associated MN and those with primary MN.[348] In patients with cancer-associated MN, clinical remission of the cancer is associated with a reduction of proteinuria.[348] These studies highlight the importance of thorough cancer screening among older patients with MN, not only at the time of first diagnosis but also during subsequent long-term follow-up.

PATHOLOGY

Electron Microscopy

The pathologic sine qua non of MN is the presence of subepithelial immune complex deposits or their structural consequences.[350] Electron microscopy provides the most definitive diagnosis of MN, although a relatively confident diagnosis can be made based on typical light microscopic and immunofluorescence microscopic findings.

Figure 32.7 depicts the four ultrastructural stages of MN as described by Churg and Ehrenreich.[341] The earliest ultrastructural manifestation, stage I, is characterized by the presence of scattered or more regularly distributed small immune complex–type electron-dense deposits in the subepithelial zone between the basement membrane and the podocyte. Podocyte process effacement and microvillous transformation occur in all stages of MN when there is substantial proteinuria. Stage II is characterized by projections of basement membrane material around the subepithelial deposits. In three dimensions, these projections surround the sides of the deposits, but when observed in cross section, they appear as spikes extending between the deposits (Figures 32.7 and 32.8). In stage III, the new basement membrane material surrounds the deposits, and thus in cross section there is basement membrane material between the deposits and the epithelial cytoplasm. At this point the deposits are in essence intramembranous rather than subepithelial; however, the ultrastructural appearance allows the inference that they once were subepithelial and thus indicative of MN. Stage IV is characterized by loss of the electron density of the deposits, which often results in irregular electron-lucent zones within an irregularly thickened basement membrane. Although not described by Churg and Ehrenreich, some nephropathologists recognize stage V, which is characterized by a repaired outer basement membrane zone with the only residual basement membrane disturbance in the inner aspect of the basement membrane.

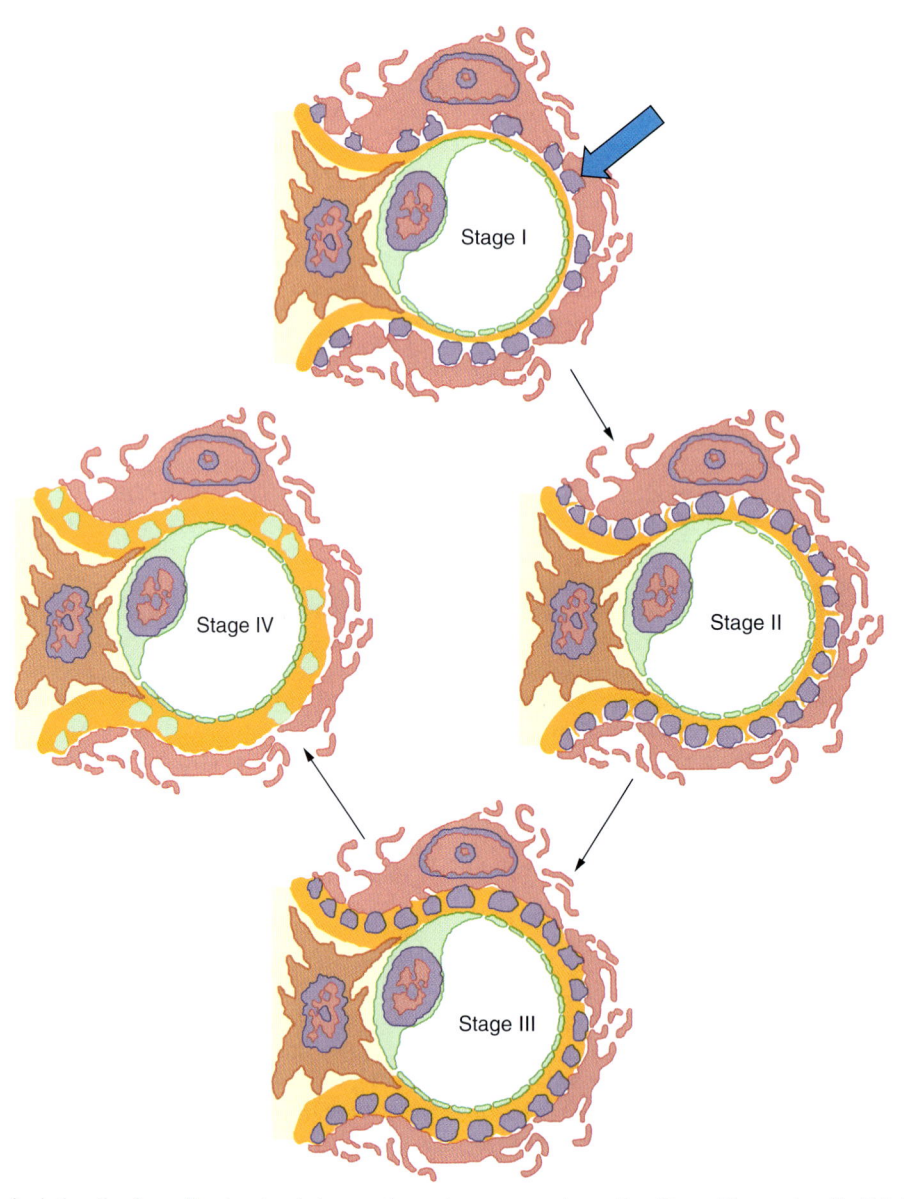

Figure 32.7 Diagram depicting the four ultrastructural stages of membranous nephropathy. Stage I has subepithelial dense deposits (*arrow*) without adjacent basement membrane reaction. Stage II has projections of basement membrane adjacent to deposits. Stage III has deposits surrounded by basement membrane. Stage IV has thickened basement membrane with irregular lucent zones. (Courtesy J. Charles Jennette, University of North Carolina at Chapel Hill, Chapel Hill, NC.)

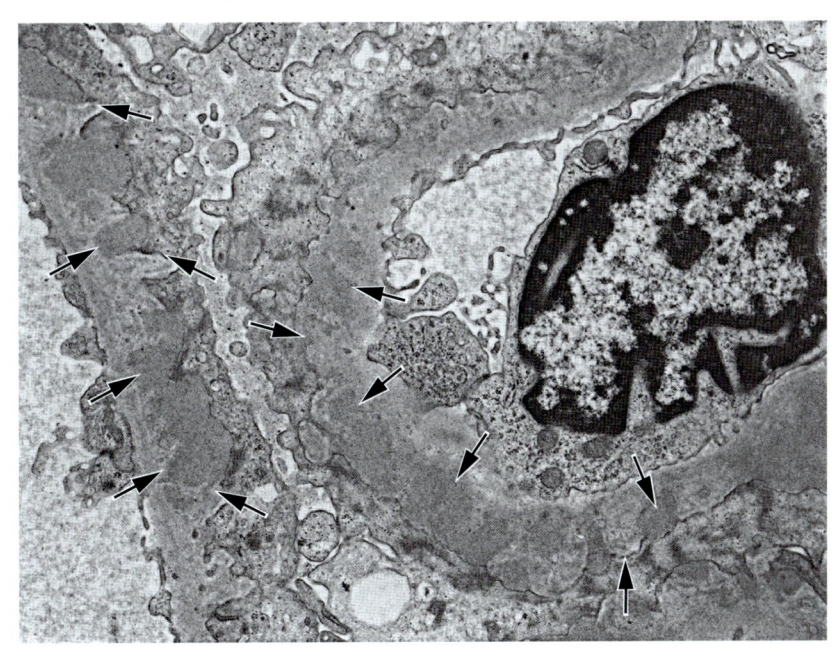

Figure 32.8 Electron micrograph showing features of stage II membranous nephropathy with numerous subepithelial dense deposits (*arrows*) and adjacent projections of basement membrane material. (×100.)

At the time of kidney biopsy, most patients in the United States have stage I or II disease (Table 32.11).

Mesangial dense deposits are rare in primary MN but are more frequent in secondary MN (see Table 32.11). This suggests, but does not prove, that primary MN is caused by subepithelial in situ immune complex formation with antibodies from the circulation complexing with antigens derived from the podocyte. Immune complexes formed only at this site could not go against the direction of filtration to reach the mesangium. Secondary forms of MN usually are caused by immune complexes that contain antigens that are in the circulation, such as antigens derived from infections (e.g., hepatitis B), tumor antigens (e.g., colon cancer), or autoantigens (e.g., thyroglobulin). With both the antigens and antibodies in the systemic circulation, it is likely that some immune complexes would form that would localize not only in the subepithelial zone but also in the mesangium or subendothelial zone. This is demonstrated in the secondary form of MN that occurs in patients with SLE. In over 90% of lupus MN specimens, mesangial dense deposits are identified by electron microscopy.[351] Therefore, the presence of mesangial dense deposits should raise the index of suspicion for secondary rather than primary MN.

Immunofluorescence Microscopy

The characteristic immunofluorescence microscopy finding in MN is diffuse global granular capillary wall staining for immunoglobulin and complement (Figure 32.9).[350] IgG is the most frequent and usually the most intensely staining immunoglobulin, although less pronounced staining for IgA and IgM is common (see Table 32.11). IgG4 is the most prominent IgG subclass in the capillary wall deposits of primary MN.[352,353] C3 staining is present over 95% of the time but typically is relatively low intensity. C1q staining is uncommon and of low intensity in primary MN but is

Table 32.11 Pathologic Features of Nonlupus Membranous Nephropathy*,†

	Feature Present (%)
Immunofluorescence Microscopy	
Immunoglobulin G	99 (3.5+)
Immunoglobulin M	95 (1.2+)
Immunoglobulin A	84 (1.1+)
C3	97 (1.6+)
C1q	34 (1.1+)
κ-light chain	98 (3.1+)
λ-light chain	98 (2.8+)
Electron Microscopy	
Subepithelial electron-dense deposits	99
Mesangial electron-dense deposits	16
Subendothelial electron-dense deposits	7
Endothelial tubuloreticular inclusions	3
Stage I	38
Stage II	32
Stage III	6
Stage IV	5
Stage V	1
Mixed stage	20

*Based on an analysis of 350 consecutive kidney biopsy specimens from patients with nonlupus membranous nephropathy evaluated at the University of North Carolina Nephropathology Laboratory.
†Values in parentheses indicate mean intensity of positive staining on a scale of 0 to 4+.

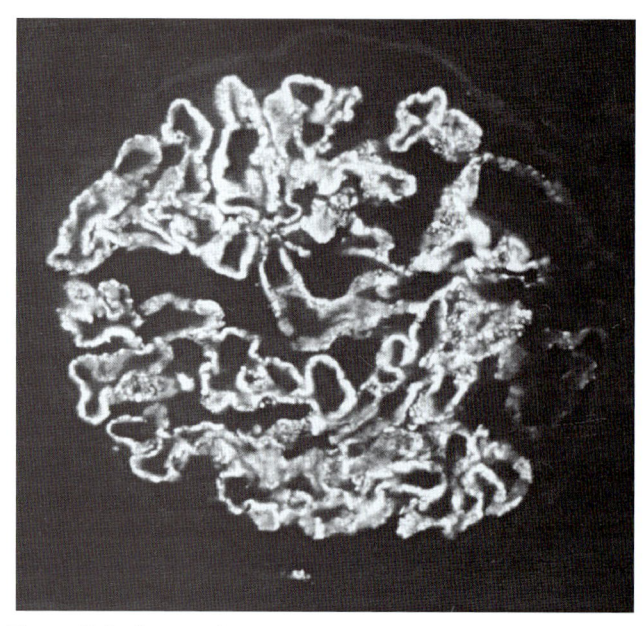

Figure 32.9 Immunofluorescence micrograph showing global granular capillary wall staining for immunoglobulin G (IgG) in a glomerulus with membranous nephropathy. (Fluorescein isothiocyanate anti-IgG stain, ×300.)

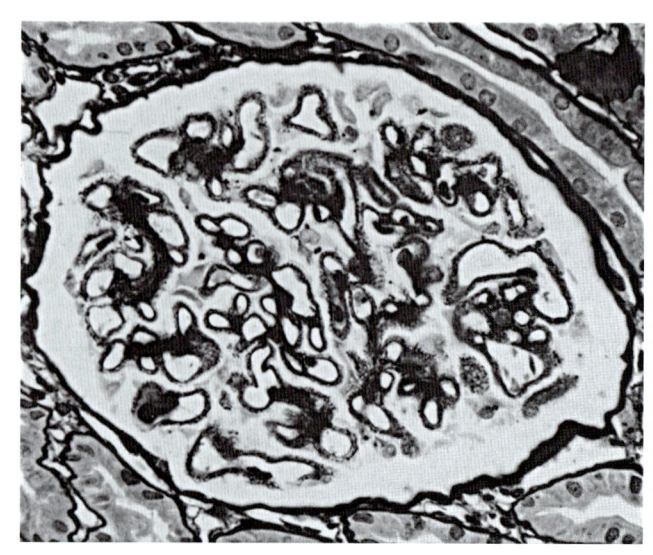

Figure 32.10 Light micrograph of a glomerulus with features of stage II membranous nephropathy demonstrating spikes along the outer aspects of the glomerular basement membrane (see Figure 32.2). These correspond to the projections of basement membrane material between the immune deposits. (Jones' methenamine silver stain, ×300.)

frequent and of high intensity in lupus MN.[351] Although terminal complement components (i.e., components of the membrane attack complex) are not usually evaluated in routine diagnostic preparations, there is very intense staining of the capillary walls for these components. In the rare patients who have concurrent anti-GBM glomerulonephritis and MN, linear staining for IgG can be discerned just below the granular staining.[354]

Tubular basement membrane staining for immunoglobulins or complement is rare in primary MN, but it is common in secondary MN, especially lupus MN.[351]

Light Microscopy

The characteristic histologic abnormality by light microscopy is diffuse global capillary wall thickening in the absence of significant glomerular hypercellularity.[355] The light microscopic features of MN, however, vary with the stage of the disease and with the degree of secondary chronic sclerosing glomerular and tubulointerstitial injury. Mild stage I lesions may not be discernible by light microscopy, especially when only a hematoxylin and eosin stain is used. Stage II, III, and IV lesions usually have readily discernible thickening of the capillary walls.

Masson trichrome stains may demonstrate the subepithelial immune complex deposits as tiny fuchsinophilic (red) grains along the outer aspect of the GBM. However, this is not a sensitive, specific, or technically reliable method for detecting glomerular immune complex deposits. Special stains that accentuate basement membrane material, such as the Jones' methenamine silver stain, may reveal the basement membrane changes that are induced by the subepithelial immune deposits. Spikes along the outer aspect of the GBM usually are seen in stage II lesions (Figure 32.10). Stage III and IV lesions have irregularly thickened and trabeculated basement membranes, which resemble changes that occur with MPGN and chronic thrombotic microangiopathy.

Overt mesangial hypercellularity is uncommon in primary MN, although it is more frequent in secondary MN.[351] Crescent formation is rare unless there is concurrent anti-GBM disease or ANCA disease.[356-362]

With disease progression, chronic sclerosing glomerular and tubulointerstitial lesions develop. Glomeruli become segmentally and globally sclerotic and develop adhesions to Bowman's capsule. Worsening tubular atrophy, interstitial fibrosis, and interstitial infiltration by mononuclear leukocytes parallels progressive loss of kidney function.[355]

PATHOGENESIS

MN is caused by immune complex localization in the subepithelial zone of glomerular capillaries. The nephritogenic antigens can be endogenous to the glomerulus itself (e.g., podocyte autoantigens) or can be exogenous (e.g., hepatitis B antigens). In the latter case, the antigen may be deposited in the subepithelial zone as part of preformed, circulating, immune complexes, or could be produced in or planted in the subepithelial zone as free antigen to which antibodies bind to form immune complexes in situ. In rat Heymann's nephritis, an animal model that closely resembles human primary MN, there is convincing evidence that the subepithelial immune deposits form in situ as a result of the binding of antibodies to glycoproteins produced by podocytes followed by accumulation of masses of the immune complexes in the subepithelial zone.[363-365]

The long-standing search for antigens targeted in a substantial proportion of patients with MN has recently witnessed significant breakthroughs. The podocyte neutral endopeptidase was identified as the endogenous target of autoantibodies in a neonate with nephrotic syndrome. This antibody crossed the placenta and was induced in the mother, who lacked the neutral endopeptidase epitope because of a mutational deletion. Sensitization to the nascent antigen was induced during a previous pregnancy.[366-368] Although this target antigen does not account for a significant proportion of MN cases, these findings provide direct support for the paradigm of in situ immune complex formation in the pathogenesis of human primary MN, and constitute an example of alloimmunization leading to the generation of immune complex–mediated glomerulopathy.[368,369]

The team of Beck and Salant identified M-type PLA_2R as a target antigen common to about 70% of patients with primary MN.[370] In contrast, none of the sera from normal controls, patients with MN secondary to SLE or hepatitis B, patients with proteinuric conditions other than MN, or other autoimmune disorders (n = 7) reacted with this antigen. Anti-PLA_2R autoantibodies in serum samples from patients with primary MN were predominantly of the IgG4 subclass, which is the predominant immunoglobulin subclass seen in glomerular deposits of patients with this disease. PLA_2R expression in podocytes was confirmed by immunofluorescence microscopy and in cultured immortalized human podocytes, indicating that this target antigen is intrinsic to glomeruli rather than deposited from sera of patients with primary MN. Analysis of serial samples from patients with MN also suggests a decline or disappearance of anti-PLA_2R antibodies with remission of proteinuria. These findings have since been confirmed in additional patients with primary MN by multiple independent groups throughout the world.[371-373]

Interestingly, given that only roughly 70% of patients with primary MN harbor autoantibodies to PLA_2R, another group identified antibodies to circulating cationic bovine serum albumin in 11 patients with MN, including 4 children, out of 50 MN patients and 172 controls tested.[374] Bovine serum albumin was also found to be present in glomerular immune deposits in all four of the children tested.

In separate studies, the team led by Prunotto detected specific anti–aldose reductase (AR) and anti–manganese superoxide dismutase (SOD2) IgG4 in sera of patients with MN.[375] Anti-AR IgG4 and anti-SOD2 IgG4 were also eluted from microdissected glomeruli of patients with MN but not from biopsy specimens of patients with lupus nephritis or MPGN. Anti-AR and anti-SOD2 co-localized with IgG4 and C5b-9 in electron-dense immune deposits. Interestingly, these antigens were detected in glomeruli of patients with MN but not in those with MCD or in those with normal kidneys. AR was minimally detected in biopsy specimens from patients with IgA nephropathy and type 2 diabetes mellitus, whereas SOD2 was not detected in these patients. The mechanism and trigger for the "neoexpression" of these antigens in podocytes are unknown but may be a result of an initial injury mediated by pathogenic antibody deposition such as anti-PLA_2R, possibly driven by oxidative stress. These important breakthroughs in identifying target antigens in human MN open the door to understanding the role of these autoantibodies and antibodies in the pathogenesis of primary MN.

Whereas the nature of the immune complex deposits in MN requires further study, the mechanisms leading to the proteinuric and nephrotic state are better understood. The current understanding of these mechanisms is largely based on data emerging from studies of passive Heymann's nephritis.[365,376] In this model, immune complex formation in the subepithelial zone initiates activation of the complement pathway leading to the formation of the C5b-C9 membrane attack complex. This results in complement-mediated injury to the epithelial cells.[377-379] The proposed sequence of events includes complement activation and sublytic complement C5b-9 attack on podocytes resulting in upregulated expression of genes for the production of oxidants, proteases, prostanoids, growth factors, connective tissue growth factor, TGF, and TGF receptors leading to overproduction of extracellular matrix.[367,368,380] C5b-9 also causes alterations of the cytoskeleton that lead to abnormal distribution of slit diaphragm proteins and detachment of viable podocytes. These events result in disruption of the functional integrity of the GBM and the protein filtration barrier of podocytes.

The characteristic findings of a predominance of IgG4 with less IgG3 and no IgG1 in subepithelial deposits,[352,353] and the paucity of C1q and C4 in these deposits,[381] argues against a predominant role for the classical or lectin pathways of complement activation in MN, and rather points to a role of the alternative pathway.[382] The fact that the alternative pathway is spontaneously active in turn points to the likely importance of the complement-regulatory proteins. Podocytes primarily rely on membrane complement receptor 1 (CR1; Crry in rodents) and decay-accelerating factor, and have the capability to make their own factor H. The importance of complement-mediated injury (at least in passive Heymann's nephritis) comes from evidence that nephritogenic serum contains antibodies to membrane complement-regulatory proteins (Crry).[383,384] In a model of active Heymann's nephritis, immunization with fraction 1A (Fx1A) lacking Crry leads to the formation of anti-Fx1A antibodies and subepithelial immune complex deposits but does not lead to complement activation or the development of proteinuria.[385] Conversely, the overexpression of Crry or treatment with exogenous Crry has a salutory effect on immune complex–mediated glomerulonephritis.[386,387] Subsequent injury to the epithelial cell membrane and to the GBM is hypothesized to be mediated, at least in part, by the production of reactive oxygen species and lipid peroxidation of cell membrane proteins and of type IV collagen.[388]

Proteinuria may also be mediated by mechanisms independent of the formation of the C5b-9 membrane attack complex as is suggested by the generation of proteinuria in passive Heymann's nephritis in PVG rats that are deficient in complement factor 6 (PVG/C6 rats). These rats are incapable of generating the membrane attack complex. In this study, PVG/C6 and normal PVG rats developed similar levels of proteinuria after injection of Fx1a antisera. Isolated glomeruli showed similar deposition of rat Ig and C3 staining in both groups of rats, but C9 deposition was not detected in the glomeruli of C6-deficient rats, which indicates that the C5b-9 membrane attack complex had not formed.[389] Furthermore, the alteration in the glomerular extracellular matrix seen in MN may be caused, at least in part, by a decrease in fibrinolytic activity, due to the stabilization of active plasminogen activator inhibitor I in conjunction with vitronectin in the subepithelial deposits.[390]

Complement activation also results in tubular epithelial cell injury and mediates progressive interstitial disease in MN.[391-393] Proteinuria itself may lead to tubulointerstitial damage through activation of the alternative complement pathway. Strong staining for properdin, a soluble complement regulator also known as *complement factor P*, on the luminal surface of the tubules was observed in kidney biopsy specimens from patients with primary MN but not from healthy kidney donors.[394] After spontaneous hydrolysis of C3, properdin binds to C3b and enhances complement activation by stabilizing C3 convertase. Target-bound properdin may serve as a focal point for amplification of C3 activation. Properdin was shown in vitro to bind proximal tubular epithelial cells. Exposure of proximal tubular epithelial cells with normal human serum as a source of complement, but not to properdin-depleted serum, resulted in complement activation with deposition of C3 and generation of C5b-9. This led to the hypothesis that in proteinuric kidney disease, filtered properdin may bind to proximal tubular epithelial cells and act as a focal point for alternative pathway activation.

The human leukocyte antigen (HLA) class II antigen DR3 has been linked with MN,[395-397] and its presence is associated with a relative risk of 12.[395] In a Japanese population, there is an increased frequency of HLA-DR2[398,399] and HLA-DQW1[400] in patients with MN. It is possible that a haplotype containing HLA-DR3 and specific HLA class I antigens may be common in these patients as well.[395] For instance, HLA-B18 and HLA-DR3 haplotypes may confer an even greater risk of the development of MN.[401] Also associated with an increased susceptibility to MN are polymorphisms of the tumor necrosis factor-α (TNF-α) gene.[402,403] C4-null alleles are also more frequently found in patients with MN, especially in white populations.[404] A recent genomewide association study of Caucasian patients with primary MN from the United Kingdom (n = 335), France (n = 75), and the Netherlands (n = 146) identified two significant genomic loci, namely, chromosome 2q24 containing the gene encoding the culprit autoantigen PLA_2R and chromosome 6p21 containing the gene encoding HLA-DQA1.[405] Despite the relative risk associated with some of these genetic markers, there are relatively few examples of familial MN.[406-411]

Recent studies have also suggested a possible role for APOL1 risk alleles in increasing risk or accelerating progression of PLA_2R-associated MN in association with collapsing nephropathy.[412]

CLINICAL FEATURES AND NATURAL HISTORY

Patients with MN usually have nephrotic syndrome with hypoalbuminemia, hyperlipidemia, peripheral edema, and lipiduria. This presentation occurs in 70% to 80% of patients.[343,413] The onset of nephrotic syndrome is usually not associated with any prodromal disease process or antecedent infections. Hypertension may be present at the outset of disease in 13% to 55% of patients.[345] Most patients present with normal or slightly decreased kidney function at presentation.

If progressive renal insufficiency develops, it is usually relatively indolent. An abrupt change to more acute renal insufficiency should prompt investigation of a superimposed condition, such as a crescentic glomerulonephritis.[414] One third of these patients have anti-GBM antibodies, and some have ANCAs.

Other causes of sudden deterioration of kidney function include acute bilateral renal vein thrombosis, and hypovolemia in the setting of massive nephrosis. The incidence of renal vein thrombosis in MN varies from 4% to 52%. The diagnosis of renal vein thrombosis may be clinically apparent based on the sudden development of macroscopic hematuria, flank pain, and reduction in kidney function, but a more insidious development is also common. Although ultrasonography with Doppler studies may demonstrate the renal thrombus,[415] venography with contrast remains the gold standard. Spiral computerized tomography[416] and magnetic resonance imaging with contrast have also been used.

Drug-induced kidney injury is another reason for the sudden deterioration in kidney function in a patient with MN. The use of nonsteroidal antiinflammatory drugs, diuretics, and antimicrobials has been linked to the occurrence of acute interstitial nephritis or acute tubular necrosis.

An estimate of renal survival in patients with MN can be obtained from a pooled analysis of outcomes in clinical studies.[346] In this analysis of 1189 pooled patients,[323,335,344,417-429] the probability of renal survival was 86% at 5 years, 65% at 10 years, and 59% at 15 years. Although 35% of patients may progress to ESKD by 10 years, 25% may experience a complete spontaneous remission of proteinuria within 5 years.[430] In a study in Italy of 100 untreated patients with MN who were followed for 10 years, 30% had progressive renal impairment after 8 years of follow-up. On the other hand, of the 62% who presented with nephrotic-range proteinuria, 50% underwent spontaneous remission in 5 years.[424]

In a retrospective study of 328 patients with MN who were not treated with immunosuppressive agents, spontaneous remission of proteinuria occurred in 32% of patients: partial remission (proteinuria ≤ 3.5 g/day) occurred in a mean of 14.7 ± 11.4 months, and the mean time to complete remission was 38.0 ± 25.2 months.[431] Importantly, severe proteinuria at onset of disease does not preclude the possibility of spontaneous remission, because it occurred in 26% of patients with baseline proteinuria of 8 to 12 g of protein per day and 21% of patients with baseline proteinuria of more than 12 g of protein per day. Multivariate analysis revealed that the best predictor of spontaneous remission was a decrease in proteinuria of more than 50% in the first year of follow-up (HR, 12.6; 95% CI, 5.2 to 30.5; $P < 0.0001$). Other predictors were the baseline serum creatinine level, baseline proteinuria, and the use of angiotensin II inhibitors.[431]

Persistent proteinuria is more predictive of renal insufficiency than proteinuria at a single time point. Thus, persistent proteinuria of 8 g or more of protein per day for at least 6 months was associated with a 66% probability of progressive chronic kidney disease (CKD). Patients with at least 6 g of protein per day for 9 months or longer had a 55% probability of developing CKD. Persistent proteinuria of 4 g or more of protein per day for longer than 18 months was associated with an even greater risk of CKD.[432] Patients with overtly declining kidney function are at higher risk for progressive kidney deterioration.[430]

In addition to decreased glomerular filtration rate (GFR) and proteinuria, other factors may be associated with an increased risk of progressive CKD. Male sex, advanced age (older than age 50), poorly controlled hypertension, and reduced GFR at presentation have been reported as risk factors for progressive decline in kidney function.[342,424,428,430,432-436] In addition to the clinical prognostic features, the presence of advanced MN on kidney biopsy specimens (stage III or IV), tubular atrophy, and interstitial fibrosis can also be associated with increased risk. In fact, chronic interstitial fibrosis and tubular atrophy have been shown to be independent predictors of progressive renal failure in primary MN.[423,437-439] The presence of crescents on kidney biopsy specimens may also portend a poor long-term prognosis. The stage of glomerular lesions detected by electron microscopy has also been suggested as a risk factor for poor prognosis in some[440-442] but not all studies.[332,428,437,443] Similarly, FSGS superimposed on MN may have a worse long-term renal prognosis than MN without sclerosis.[444,445] However, the importance of these demographic and histologic risk factors was not substantiated in a retrospective analysis of a large cohort of patients from the University of Toronto that examined the *rate* of progression (slope).[446] Of the histologic variables, only a greater degree of complement deposition appeared to be associated with a more rapid decline in GFR.[447]

In a prospective study, a urinary excretion of β_2-microglobulin level of more than 0.5 μg/min and a urinary IgG level of more than 250 mg/24 hr, assessed in a timed urine sample, were found to predict progressive loss of GFR in a prospective cohort of 57 patients with primary MN and normal kidney function.[448] In a multivariate analysis, urine β_2-microglobulin excretion was the strongest independent predictor of the development of renal insufficiency, with a sensitivity and specificity of 88% and 91%, respectively. Unfortunately, the measurement of urine β_2-microglobulin is cumbersome because it is unstable in urine and requires alkalinization of the urine prior to collection. More recently, there have been several studies from different groups demonstrating an association between high anti-PLA_2R autoantibodies and worse long-term outcomes in that there appears to be growing evidence for an inverse correlation between the level of the autoantibodies and disease.[372,373,449,450]

In summary, one of the strongest indicators of progressive disease appears to be *persistence* of moderate proteinuria.[435] Impaired kidney function, severe proteinuria at presentation, the presence of substantial interstitial infiltrates on biopsy specimen, superimposed crescentic glomerulonephritis, and segmental sclerosis also portend a poorer outcome.

LABORATORY FINDINGS

Proteinuria is the hallmark of MN. Well over 80% of MN patients excrete more than 3 g of protein per 24 hours. In some patients, the amount of urinary protein may exceed 20 g/day. A Medical Research Council study reported that 30% of patients with MN excreted more than 10 g of protein per day at the time of presentation.[347] Microscopic hematuria is present in 30% to 50% of patients at the time of presentation.[343,451,452] Macroscopic hematuria, on the other hand, is distinctly uncommon and occurs in less than 4% of adult patients,[453,454] although it may be common in children.[455] Most patients have either normal or only slightly decreased kidney function. In fact, impaired kidney function is found in less than 10% of patients at the time of presentation.[451,456]

In patients with severe nephrosis, hypoalbuminemia is common, as is the loss of other serum proteins, including IgG. Serum lipoprotein levels are characteristically elevated, as they are in other forms of nephrotic syndrome. Elevated levels of low-density and very low-density lipoproteins are common in MN. In one study, elevated levels of lipoprotein(a) normalized in patients whose disease was in remission.[457]

Levels of complement components C3 and C4 are typically normal in patients with MN. The complex of terminal complement components known as *C5b-9* is found in the urine of some patients with active MN. There is increased excretion of this complex in patients with active immune complex formation. The excretion may decrease during disease inactivity.[377-379,458-463]

To exclude common causes of secondary MN, one should order serologic tests for nephritogenic infections such as hepatitis B, hepatitis C, and syphilis, as well as tests for immunologic disorders such as lupus, mixed connective tissue disease, and cryoglobulinemia. MN has been associated with graft-versus-host disease following allogeneic stem cell transplant, and this should be considered as well.[464]

Although hypercoagulability appears to be present in patients with nephrosis in general, this tendency may be enhanced in patients with MN.[465-467] The exact mechanisms leading to thrombophilia in this group of patients are poorly understood. Patients with MN have hyperfibrinogenemia with increased levels of circulating procoagulants and decreased levels of anticoagulant factors such as antithrombin III.[468] The thrombotic tendency may be increased by the erythrocytosis that occurs in some patients, as well as by the effect of lipoprotein(a) to retard thrombolysis. Other possible contributors to the thrombophilic state include volume depletion, diuretic and/or steroid use, venous stasis, immobilization, and immune complex activation of the clotting cascade and anti–α-enolase antibodies.[469-471] Renal vein thrombosis is reported more frequently in patients with MN than in those with nephrotic syndrome due to other causes.[467,472-475] The prevalence of renal vein thrombosis in patients with MN ranges from approximately 5% to 63%, depending on what mode of diagnosis is used and whether or not systematic screening is performed. The prevalence of all forms of deep vein thrombosis in patients with MN ranges from 9% to 44%. The combined burden of deep vein and renal vein thrombosis has been estimated to be as high as 45%.[471] Renal vein thrombosis is often silent, with pulmonary embolism being the first presenting sign. The risk of venous thromboembolic events appears to be higher when the serum albumin concentration is less than 2.5 g/dL, and such events occur in as many as 40% of these patients.[471,476]

It is the concern for the morbidity and, at times, mortality associated with pulmonary embolism that has led to the use of prophylactic anticoagulation for patients with severe nephrotic syndrome and MN. A decision analysis suggested that the risk of life-threatening complications of pulmonary embolism outweighed the risks associated with anticoagulant therapy.[477] However, this analysis may be based on an overestimate of the true incidence of thromboses among patients with MN. No direct controlled data are available to support or refute such a contention. More recently, using data from an inception cohort of 898 patients with primary MN as well as literature review–based risk estimates of hemorrhage, a clinical tool to estimate the likelihood of benefit of anticoagulation, based primarily on bleeding risk and serum albumin concentration, was proposed as a way to begin to personalize prophylactic anticoagulation (www.gntools.com).[478] A retrospective analysis of a treatment regimen to prevent venous thromboembolism in 143 patients with nephrotic syndrome (low-molecular-weight heparin or low-dose heparin for patients with serum albumin less than 2.0 g/dL and aspirin 75 mg daily for patients with serum albumin 2.0 to 3.0 g/dL) appeared to be effective with very few complications.[479] Unfortunately, there is no direct controlled support for the routine use of prophylactic anticoagulation in patients with primary MN; however, the case could be made for the judicious use of warfarin in patients with severe nephrotic syndrome who have a profoundly decreased serum albumin level (probably <2 mg/dL) if no contraindications are present. Randomized, controlled trials are warranted.

TREATMENT

Corticosteroids

Despite numerous studies, the optimal treatment of MN remains incompletely defined. The difficulty in treating MN is a consequence of the chronic nature of the disease, the tendency for spontaneous remission and relapse, the variability of clinical severity, and the only partial efficacy of existing treatment protocols. The role of corticosteroids and alkylating agents in the treatment of this disease has been debated for decades. Common therapeutic approaches for new-onset disease include (1) conservative therapy with RAAS blockade, (2) corticosteroid therapy (usually prednisone or methylprednisolone), and (3) administration of alkylating agents, such as chlorambucil or cyclophosphamide, with or without concurrent corticosteroid treatment.

Numerous studies using corticosteroid treatment have demonstrated different outcomes.[323,334,335,344,417-424,427-430,443,480,481] In a pooled analysis of these studies, corticosteroid therapy was found to have no beneficial effect on renal survival.[346] Three large prospective randomized trials examined the efficacy of oral corticosteroid therapy in adult patients with MN with different results.[419,420,482] Findings of the U.S. Collaborative Study[334] suggested that 8 weeks of treatment with 100 to 150 mg of prednisone given on alternate days resulted in a transient decrease in urinary protein excretion to less than 2 g of protein compared to placebo. Prednisone was discontinued after 3 months unless proteinuria recurred after either a partial or complete remission. Relapses were treated by reinstitution of high-dose prednisone for 1 month followed by a taper. The results of this study suggested that patients treated with prednisone were less likely to experience a doubling of their entry serum creatinine level and were more likely to experience a transient decrease in proteinuria to less than 2 g of protein per day, and that even a partial remission of proteinuria was associated with well-preserved, long-term kidney function. This seminal study was criticized because the control group fared substantially worse than untreated patients in several other studies.

A British Medical Research Council study[419] utilized a similar regimen except that prednisolone was discontinued after 8 weeks without tapering and without treatment of the relapse of proteinuria. Patients with lower creatinine clearance (≤30 mL/min) were included in the study. Three to nine months after study entry, patients showed no improvement in kidney function, and the urine protein excretion and albumin level improved only transiently.

A third prospective randomized study of corticosteroid reported by Cattran and colleagues[420] included patients with relatively low levels of urine protein (≤0.3 g of protein per day). In this study, alternate-day prednisone (45 mg/m^2 of body surface area) afforded no benefit with regard to either proteinuria or renal function.

In a meta-analysis[346] of the U.S. Collaborative Study[334] and the studies by Cameron and colleagues,[419] Cattran and colleagues,[420] and Kobayashi and colleagues[421] comparing glucocorticoid to supportive therapy, corticosteroid therapy was associated with a trend toward achievement of complete remission at 24 to 36 months, but this result did not reach statistical significance. A pooled analysis of randomized trials and prospective studies again demonstrated a lack of benefit of corticosteroid therapy in inducing a remission of nephrotic syndrome or preserving kidney function.

An alternative to oral glucocorticoid therapy has been treatment with pulse methylprednisolone, largely in patients with deteriorating kidney function. Treatment of patients with renal insufficiency using pulse methylprednisolone at 1 g/day for 5 days followed by oral prednisone was associated with an improvement in kidney function for 6 months and a reduction in proteinuria.[483] The long-term outcomes for over half of these patients were discouraging: one third experienced renal failure and 13% developed myocardial infarction with kidney dysfunction. A similar study[484] combined pulse methylprednisolone with azathioprine or cyclophosphamide. Although there may have been some improvement in proteinuria and kidney function in a minority of patients, substantial side effects were experienced by almost the entire study population. The evidence to date does not support the use of oral corticosteroids alone for the treatment of primary MN.

Cyclophosphamide or Chlorambucil

Cytotoxic drugs, including cyclophosphamide and chlorambucil, have been used for the treatment of primary MN in conjunction with intravenous and/or oral corticosteroids. In a number of studies, Ponticelli and colleagues demonstrated that chlorambucil has a beneficial effect in the treatment of MN.[423,441,443,485] In these studies, patients with primary MN were treated initially with intravenous pulse methylprednisolone at 1 g/day for the first 3 days of each month, with daily oral glucocorticoid therapy (methylprednisolone at 0.4 mg/kg/day or prednisone 0.5 mg/kg/day), given on an alternating monthly schedule with chlorambucil at a dose of 0.2 mg/kg/day. In patients randomly assigned to the treatment group, nephrotic syndrome lasted for a significantly shorter duration, and a complete or partial remission of proteinuria occurred in 83% of MN patients compared with 38% of control patients.[485] The slope of the mean reciprocal plasma creatinine level remained stable in the treatment group but declined in the untreated patients beginning at 12 months. At the 10-year follow-up, the probability of having a functioning kidney was 92% in the treated patients and 60% in the control patients. In only 10% of patients was therapy discontinued because of side effects. Compared to treatment with glucocorticoids alone, treatment with a combination of chlorambucil and methylprednisolone was associated with an earlier remission of nephrotic syndrome and a greater stability of complete or partial remission of proteinuria.[443] Interestingly, the overall decline in kidney function was no different in the two treatment groups. Unfortunately, although a difference in favor of the chlorambucil-treated patients persisted for the first 3 years of follow-up, it was no longer statistically significantly different by 4 years (62% without nephrotic syndrome in the group receiving combination therapy vs. 42% in the steroid-only group, $P = 0.102$). In a study comparing cyclophosphamide with chlorambucil, cyclophosphamide was found to be at least as effective as chlorambucil when used in a similar dosing protocol and appeared to have somewhat fewer side effects.[486]

A prospective, open-label, randomized study in India[487] involving 93 patients followed for a median of 11 years (range, 10.5 to 12 years) compared supportive therapy (dietary sodium restriction, diuretics, and antihypertensive agents) with a 6-month course of alternate months of steroid and cyclophosphamide treatment similar to the Ponticelli protocol.[485,488] Unfortunately, angiotensin II blockade was withheld in all patients for at least 1 year. Study end points were doubling of serum creatinine, development of ESKD, or patient death. Of the 47 patients who received the immunosuppressive protocol, 34 experienced remission compared with 16 of 46 in the control group ($P < 0.0001$). The 10-year dialysis-free survival was 89% in the immunosuppression group and 65% in the supportive treatment group ($P = 0.016$), and the likelihood of survival without death, dialysis, or doubling of serum creatinine level was 79% and 44% ($P = 0.0006$), respectively. A significant divergence between the two groups in terms of proteinuria became apparent within the first year, and the eGFR was significantly lower in the control group than in the cyclophosphamide-treated group from 4 years onward. This study confirms, in a different patient population, the short- and long-term benefits associated with treatment with cyclophosphamide and corticosteroids according to the Ponticelli protocol.[485,488]

A more recent randomized controlled trial of 108 patients with biopsy-documented primary MN in the United Kingdom compared prednisolone in combination with chlorambucil to either cyclosporine or supportive therapy alone. The primary end point was a further 20% decline in excretory kidney function from baseline readings, which was significantly lower in the prednisolone and chlorambucil group (HR, 0.44; 95% CI, 0.24 to 0.78; $P = 0.0042$); however, this group also had a higher frequency of serious adverse events.[489]

Despite these reported benefits, there has been lack of corroboration in other trials regarding the salutary effects of alkylating agents combined with prednisone or other agents[422,426,429,490]; however, two meta-analyses suggested that the use of cytotoxic agents improved the chance of a complete remission of proteinuria by fourfold to fivefold but had no long-term protective effect on renal survival.[346,491] Furthermore, a recent meta-analysis of 36 clinical trials investigating the effects of immunosuppression on adults with idiopathic MN concluded that corticosteroids combined with alkylating agents significantly reduced all-cause mortality or ESKD (8 randomized controlled trials, 448 participants; risk ratio 0.44; 95% CI, 0.26 to 0.75; $P = 0.002$) and increased partial or complete remission (7 randomized controlled trials, 422 participants; risk ratio 1.46; 95% CI, 1.13 to 1.89; $P = 0.004$) but led to more adverse events (4 randomized controlled trials, 303 participants; risk ratio, 4.20; 95% CI, 1.15 to 15.32; $P = 0.03$).[492]

Calcineurin Inhibitors

Despite the most recent trial showing superiority of prednisolone in combination with chlorambucil over cyclosporine,[489] there has been interest in the use of cyclosporine, which has resulted in improvement in proteinuria and stability of kidney function in many patients.[493-495] In a randomized, controlled trial comparing 26 weeks of treatment with cyclosporine plus low-dose prednisone to treatment with placebo plus prednisone, 75% of the cyclosporine group but only 22% of the control group ($P < 0.001$) experienced a partial or complete remission of proteinuria by 26 weeks.[496] Relapse occurred in about 40% of patients achieving remission in both treatment groups. The fraction of patients achieving sustained remission remained significantly different between the groups until the end of the study (cyclosporine treatment 39%, placebo 13%, $P = 0.007$). Kidney function was unchanged and equal in the two groups over the test medication period.[496] This study was criticized for the rapid discontinuation of cyclosporine over 4 weeks at the end of the 26-week treatment period.

In a prospective study, treatment with cyclosporine alone (2 to 3 mg/kg/day) was compared to treatment with a combination of cyclosporine and oral prednisolone in 51 patients.[497] Prednisolone was started at 0.6 mg/kg/day, then gradually tapered to 10 to 15 mg/day at 6 months and continued to 12 months. Patients who experienced complete or partial remission then received long-term treatment with lower doses of cyclosporine (1 to 1.5 mg/kg/day) plus prednisolone (0.1 mg/kg/day) or cyclosporine alone. This study did not have a randomized design because patients with contraindications to corticosteroid use were assigned to the cyclosporine-only group. During the follow-up phase of the study, relapses were more common in patients treated with cyclosporine alone than in patients receiving cyclosporine plus oral prednisolone (47% vs. 15%, respectively; $P < 0.05$). However, the results suggest that the risk of relapse may be determined by the levels of cyclosporine, because patients in both groups who experienced relapse had lower cyclosporine trough levels than those who did not experience relapse (72 ± 48 ng/mL vs. 194 ± 80 ng/mL, respectively; $P < 0.03$).

A prospective randomized controlled trial was undertaken to evaluate monotherapy with tacrolimus versus supportive therapy alone in 48 patients with MN who had preserved kidney function and had persistent nephrotic syndrome for longer than 9 months despite treatment with an ACE inhibitor or ARB.[498] Treatment with tacrolimus consisted of 0.05 mg/kg/day divided into two daily doses and adjusted to achieve a whole-blood 12-hour trough level between 3 and 5 ng/mL if a remission was not obtained after the first 2 months of treatment. The target trough level was increased to between 5 and 8 ng/mL if a remission was not obtained after the first 2 months of treatment. Tacrolimus was continued for a total of 12 months followed by a 6-month taper. The probability of remission in the treatment group was 58%, 82%, and 94% after 6, 12, and 18 months but was only 10%, 24%, and 35%, respectively, in the control group. The decrease in proteinuria was significantly greater in the treatment group. Notably, six patients in the control group and only one in the treatment group reached the secondary end point of a 50% increase in serum creatinine level. Unfortunately, as in the previously published study of cyclosporine, almost half of the patients who had achieved remission experienced a recurrence of nephrotic syndrome by the eighteenth month after tacrolimus withdrawal.

An interesting pilot study from Spain[499] looked at combination therapy with corticosteroids, MMF, and tacrolimus in patients with persistent nephrotic syndrome after 6 months of treatment with full-dose RAAS blockers, and a creatinine clearance of more than 60 mL/min/1.73 m². The initial dose of prednisone was 0.5 mg/kg/day for the first month, and the drug was then tapered to 7.5 mg/day at month 6. The starting dose of tacrolimus was 0.05 mg/kg/day to achieve target whole-blood trough levels of 7 to 9 ng/mL. If the level of protein excretion was less than 1 g of protein per day at the end of 3 months of this therapy, the tacrolimus dosage was reduced to maintain blood levels between 5 and 7 ng/mL and continued for a period of 9 more months. If, however, the level of proteinuria was greater than 1 g of protein per day, the dose of tacrolimus was reduced and MMF was added at a dose of 0.5 g twice daily and adjusted to achieve target whole-blood trough levels of 2 to 4 mg/L. Triple therapy was then maintained for 9 additional months, after which immunosuppressants were tapered off over 3 months in all patients. Of the 21 adult patients enrolled, 11 had proteinuria of less than 1 g of protein per day at the end of 3 months and then received maintenance dosages of prednisolone plus tacrolimus. MMF was added after the third month in nine patients and was associated with complete or partial remission in five. Unfortunately, the relapse rate was very high in all groups of patients, whether treated with double or triple therapy. Clearly, additional controlled trials are required to determine the optimal duration of treatment and the benefit of adding MMF in patients who show only partial response to treatment with calcineurin inhibitors alone.

Adrenocorticotropic Hormone

The use of synthetic adrenocorticotropic hormone (ACTH) has been assessed in patients with nephrotic syndrome, including those with MN.[500] In one randomized control trial,[501] 32 patients were treated with either corticosteroids and chlorambucil or cyclophosphamide administered according to the Ponticelli protocol, or with ACTH (tetracosactide) administered intramuscularly twice weekly for a year. Eighty-seven percent of patients in the ACTH arm experienced complete or partial remission with a dramatic reduction in proteinuria and mean serum cholesterol, and remission at almost 3 years.[501] Few patients developed symptoms and signs of excess glucocorticoids.

Given the lack of availability of the synthetic, long-acting ACTH analog formulation in the United States, a retrospective case series examined the role of a natural ACTH gel formulation for nephrotic syndrome.[502] Eleven patients with primary MN out of 21 patients with nephrotic syndrome were treated with ACTH gel, and 9 of 11 (82%) MN patients achieved complete (3 of 11, 27%) or partial (6 of 11, 55%) remission. A subsequent prospective, open-label study evaluated the efficacy of ACTH gel (80 units subcutaneously twice weekly for 6 months) in patients with resistant glomerular disease defined as failure to achieve sustained remission of proteinuria off immunosuppressive therapy with at least two treatment regimens.[503] Five patients with primary MN out of 15 patients were treated; 2 patients achieved partial remission and 3 patients achieved immunologic remission. The mechanism responsible for the beneficial effect of ACTH is unknown. Recent evidence points to the expression of the melanocortin 1 receptor on podocytes, which suggests a possible direct effect of ACTH on these cells.[504]

Mycophenolate Mofetil

Interest has arisen in the use of MMF for the management of MN in a few small studies yielding disparate results. In an open-label study in the Netherlands, 32 patients with primary MN treated with MMF were compared with a historical matched control group treated with oral cyclophosphamide for 12 months.[505] Both groups received intermittent methylprednisolone and alternate-day prednisone. Although on average the degree of proteinuria decreased similarly in the MMF-treated group and in the cyclophosphamide-treated group, and although the cumulative incidence of remission of proteinuria at 12 months was comparable in the two groups, the percentage of patients who showed no response to therapy was statistically significantly higher in the MMF-treated group, as was the proportion of patients who experienced a relapse.

In a 1-year randomized controlled trial of 36 patients, treatment with MMF (target dose of 2 g/day) for 12 months was compared to conservative care alone.[506] The change in mean urine protein/creatinine ratio from baseline to month 12 was measured; the ratio decreased by 1834 mg/g in the control group and increased by 213 mg/g in the MMF group ($P = 0.3$). Complete or partial remission at month 12 was observed in 37% of patients in the MMF group and 41% in the control group.

In a separate prospective, randomized, controlled, open-label study involving 20 patients in Hong Kong and Shanghai,[507] treatment with MMF and prednisolone given for 6 months was compared with treatment that followed a modified Ponticelli regimen.[486] Over a total follow-up of 15 months, proteinuria decreased to a similar extent in both treatment groups; therefore, resultant overall remission rates were not statistically different (63.6% and 66.7% in the MMF and control groups, respectively, $P = 1.000$). However, there was more leukopenia in the chlorambucil group. Data from this pilot study indicate that more than 60% of patients with MN and nephrotic syndrome respond to combined MMF and prednisolone treatment, and suggest potential benefits of MMF as being steroid-sparing and having less adverse effects compared with other commonly used cytotoxic agents. These results are in marked distinction to those of the previously described study comparing MMF with conservative therapy.[506] These two studies differ in the makeup of the patient populations (whites vs. Asians) and by the concomitant use of prednisolone in the Hong Kong/Shanghai study. Overall, the results of studies of MMF have been disappointing, with the notable exception of those involving Chinese patients.

Rituximab

Given the high likelihood of antibody-mediated injury in patients with MN, there has been an explosion of interest in the use of rituximab, a humanized anti-CD20 monoclonal antibody. In an initial report of eight patients, treatment with rituximab (4 weekly doses of 375 mg/m² body surface area) was associated with prompt and sustained reduction in proteinuria.[508,509] There have been additional positive open-label studies,[510-514] but the effects of rituximab on long-term renal outcome are unproven. The available uncontrolled data suggest that rituximab, dosed either as 375 mg/m² once weekly for 4 weeks or at 1 g on days 1 and 15, achieves a 15% to 20% rate of complete remission and a 40% to 45% rate of partial remission.[515]

A cohort study reported on the effect of rituximab in 13 patients with MN deemed to be calcineurin inhibitor dependent (defined as the occurrence of at least four calcineurin inhibitor–responsive relapses of nephrotic proteinuria while the patient was being weaned off these drugs).[516] After rituximab therapy (375 mg/m² weekly for 4 weeks, with each dose preceded by 125 mg of methylprednisolone), proteinuria decreased significantly, and calcineurin inhibitors and other immunosuppressant drugs could be withdrawn in all patients.

Although the aggregate of these uncontrolled case series suggests a beneficial effect of rituximab in the management of MN, whether, when, and how (and how long) to use rituximab in treating MN remains to be determined. A large, pharmaceutical company–funded, randomizedcontrolled study comparing rituximab to calcineurin inhibitor therapy across 19 medical centers in the United States is now under way (www.clinicaltrials.gov, NCT01180036); however, results may be met with skepticism given prior unfavorable results seen with calcineurin inhibitors as compared to corticosteroids in combination with chlorambucil.[489]

Other Therapies

Other forms of therapy have been tried in primary MN with varying results. These include the use of azathioprine,[480,481] which demonstrated no positive effect either alone or in combination with prednisone. The use of pooled intravenous immunoglobulin has been evaluated only in a small case series[517] and a retrospective study.[518]

Based on the greater appreciation of the role of complement activation and especially that of complement-regulatory proteins in the pathogenesis of MN, a great deal of interest exists in targeting this pathway for therapy. Several compounds are under development. To date, human trials have been conducted only for eculizumab, a monoclonal antibody directed against the fifth component of complement (C5). In a randomized trial of patients with de novo MN, treatment with eculizumab was not associated with a statistically significant improvement in proteinuria or preservation of kidney function. These disappointing results were likely due to insufficient dosing, because consistent inhibition of complement was achieved only in a minority of patients.[519] Nevertheless, this general approach is thought to hold a great deal of promise based on early animal studies.

Summary of Therapies

In the absence of a full understanding of the pathogenesis of MN, and thus an effective targeted therapy, the current approach to the treatment of MN must rely on risk stratification. The indolent disease process that results in spontaneous remissions in one quarter of patients, coupled with the known adverse consequences of long-term treatment with oral glucocorticoids, alkylating agents, and calcineurin inhibitors, should prompt a careful analysis of the risk/benefit ratio in the treatment of any given patient. All patients should receive excellent supportive care, including the use of RAAS blockers[270,520-523] and lipid-lowering agents. Most patients should be observed for the development of adverse prognostic factors or the occurrence of spontaneous remissions. Adult patients with good prognostic features should be managed conservatively without the use of immunomodulatory or suppressive agents.

Patients at moderate risk (persistent proteinuria between 4 and 6 g of protein per day despite RAAS blockade and normal kidney function) or at high risk of progression (persistent proteinuria of more than 8 g of protein per day with or without renal insufficiency) should be considered for immunosuppressive therapy with either a combination of glucocorticoids and cyclophosphamide (or chlorambucil) in alternating monthly pulses (Ponticelli protocol). This decision must be individualized to each patient with consideration of the patient's comorbidities and assessment of the risk associated with each kind of therapy. The data currently available do not suggest that MMF alone is effective. Whether ACTH and/or rituximab are viable effective alternatives awaits further confirmation.

Individuals who have advanced chronic renal failure are best managed by supportive care while awaiting dialysis and kidney transplantation. Acute renal insufficiency in this population should prompt evaluation for interstitial nephritis, crescentic nephritis, and renal vein thrombosis.

MEMBRANOPROLIFERATIVE GLOMERULONEPHRITIS AND C3 GLOMERULOPATHY

Primary MPGN is a collection of morphologically similar but pathogenetically distinct disorders that have been traditionally classified into three subtypes, MPGN types I, II (dense deposit disease), and III. The primary basis for this classification was pathologic, namely, the appearance of the capillary wall by light microscopy and electron microscopy and the location of electron-dense deposits. Overall, MPGN is identified in approximately 10% of kidney biopsy specimens.[524,525]

Since the last edition of this text, advances in the understanding of the different pathogenetic mechanisms underlying the MPGN subtypes have resulted in a new classification system (Figure 32.11).[503,526-528] This new classification groups MPGN into two categories that can be separated by immunofluorescence microscopy: (1) immune complex–mediated (immunoglobulin-mediated) MPGN caused by deposition of immune complexes and classical pathway complement activation and (2) complement-mediated (non–immunoglobulin-mediated) MPGN caused by dysregulated activation of the alternative complement pathway. This modified classification system also includes a new category of diseases, termed *C3 glomerulopathy*, that includes dense deposit disease (formerly designated type II MPGN) and C3 glomerulonephritis, which comprises C3 glomerulopathy that does not have an MPGN pattern. Because most type I MPGN epidemiologic, clinical, and treatment outcome data were published using the old classification system, the

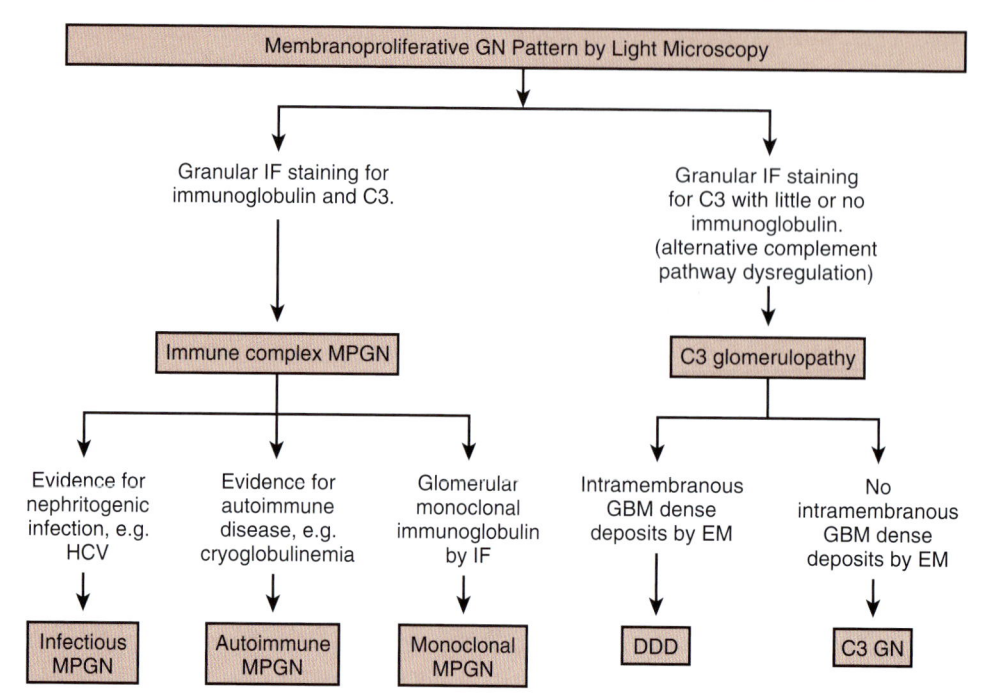

Figure 32.11 Algorithm for the histopathologic classification of membranoproliferative glomerulonephritis (MPGN) by immunofluorescence (IF) microscopy findings based on the presence of both immunoglobulin and C3 versus the presence of C3 with little or no immunoglobulin. This modified classification system also includes a new category of diseases termed *C3 glomerulopathy,* which includes dense deposit disease (formerly designated type II MPGN) and C3 glomerulonephritis, which comprises C3 glomerulopathy that does not have an MPGN pattern. DDD, Dense deposit disease; EM, electron microscopy; GBM, glomerular basement membrane; GN, glomerulonephritis; HCV, hepatitis C virus.

following review is based on type I MPGN data from heterogeneous patient cohorts that included both immune complex type I MPGN as well as C3 glomerulopathy type I MPGN. With time, refinement of cohorts will improve as these advances in pathogenetic mechanisms continue.

MEMBRANOPROLIFERATIVE GLOMERULONEPHRITIS TYPE I

PATHOLOGY

Light Microscopy

The typical histologic features of type I MPGN are diffuse global capillary wall thickening, increased mesangial matrix, and mesangial and endocapillary hypercellularity.[529,530] Infiltrating mononuclear leukocytes and neutrophils contribute to the glomerular hypercellularity. The consolidation of glomerular segments that results from these changes often causes an accentuation of the segmentation referred to as *hypersegmentation* or *lobulation.* As a consequence, an earlier name for this phenotype of glomerular injury was *lobular glomerulonephritis.* Markedly expanded mesangial regions may develop a nodular appearance with a central zone of sclerosis that may resemble that of diabetic glomerulosclerosis or monoclonal immunoglobulin deposition disease. However, the integration of light, immunofluorescence, and electron microscopy findings differentiates type I MPGN from other diseases that can mimic it by light microscopy.

A distinctive but not completely specific feature of type I MPGN is doubling or more complex replication of GBMs that can be seen with stains that highlight basement membranes, such as Jones' methenamine silver stain or periodic acid–Schiff stain (Figure 32.12). This change is caused by the production of basement membrane material between and around projections of mesangial cytoplasm that extend into an expanded subendothelial zone, probably in response to the presence of subendothelial immune complex deposits (Figure 32.13). The presence of "hyaline thrombi" within capillary lumens should raise the possibility of cryoglobulinemia or lupus as the cause for the MPGN. Hyaline thrombi are not true thrombi but rather are aggregates of immune complexes filling capillary lumens. A minority of patients with type I MPGN have crescents, but these rarely involve more than 50% of glomeruli.[531,532] As with other types of glomerulonephritis, substantial crescent formation correlates with a more rapid progression of disease.[530]

As noted earlier, C3 glomerulopathy is divided into dense deposit disease and C3 glomerulonephritis (see Figure 32.11). C3 glomerulonephritis in turn is divided into the C3 glomerulopathy variant of type I MPGN as well as other patterns of glomerulonephritis that do not fulfill the pathologic criteria for MPGN. Non-MPGN C3 glomerulonephritis often has focal or diffuse proliferative glomerulonephritis with varying degrees of endocapillary and mesangial hypercellularity (Figure 32.14).[528] Crescents may be present.

Immunofluorescence Microscopy

The characteristic pattern of immunofluorescence staining is peripheral granular to bandlike staining for complement, especially C3 (Figure 32.15). The C3 staining is accompanied by substantial immunoglobulin staining in patients with immune complex MPGN. This positive immunofluorescence corresponds to the prominent subendothelial immune deposits seen by electron microscopy. The staining

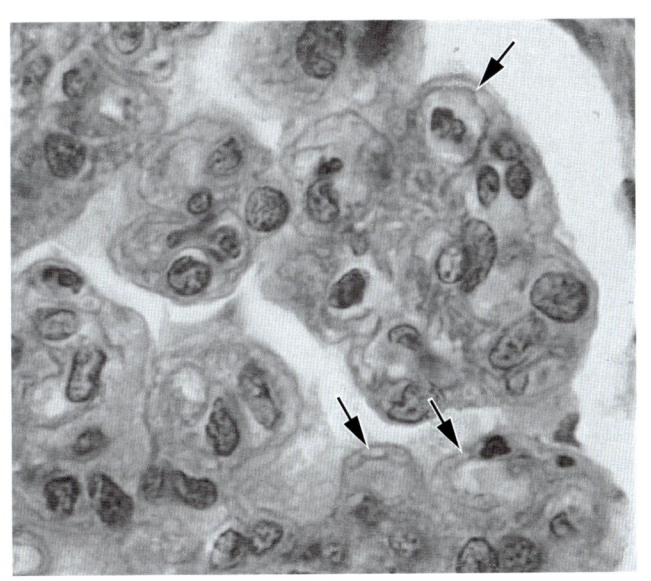

Figure 32.12 Light micrograph of a glomerular segment from a patient with type I membranoproliferative glomerulonephritis (MPGN) demonstrating doubling (*arrows*) and more complex replication of glomerular basement membranes. (Periodic acid–Schiff stain, ×1000.)

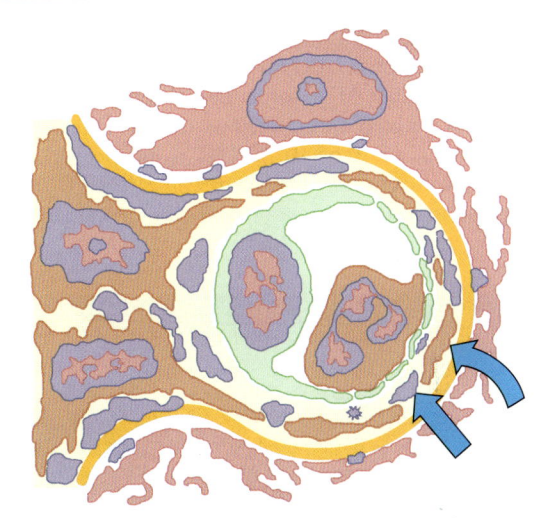

Figure 32.13 Diagram depicting the ultrastructural features of type I membranoproliferative glomerulonephritis (MPGN). Note the subendothelial dense deposits (*straight arrow*), subendothelial mesangial cytoplasm interposition (*curved arrow*), and production of new basement material (*asterisk*). (Courtesy J. Charles Jennette, University of North Carolina at Chapel Hill, Chapel Hill, NC.)

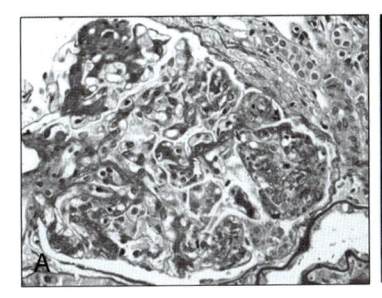

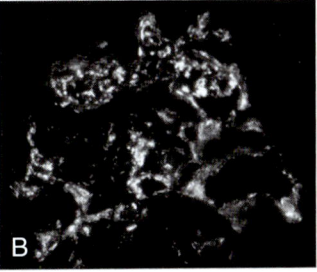

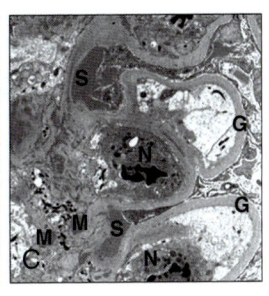

Figure 32.14 C3 glomerulonephritis variant of C3 glomerulopathy with **(A)** light microscopy showing segmental mesangial and endocapillary hypercellularity (PAS stain), **(B)** immunofluorescence microscopy showing granular capillary wall staining for C3 (there was no staining for immunoglobulin), and **(C)** electron microscopy demonstrating subepithelial electron-dense deposits (S), mesangial dense deposits (M), influx of capillary neutrophils (N), and no intramembranous dense deposits in glomerular basement membranes (G).

pattern is less granular and less symmetric than that seen in MN. Mesangial granular staining may be conspicuous or inconspicuous. The hypersegmentation or lobulation that is seen by light microscopy often can be discerned by immunofluorescence microscopy. A minority of patients with type I immune complex MPGN have staining along tubular basement membranes or in extraglomerular vessels, or both.

Most specimens with immune complex MPGN have more intense staining for C3 than for any immunoglobulin, but some specimens have more intense staining for IgG or IgM. Rare specimens have a predominance of IgA and can be considered an MPGN expression of IgA nephropathy. Intracapillary globular structures that stain intensely for immunoglobulin and complement correspond to the hyaline thrombi seen by light microscopy and raise the possibility of MPGN caused by lupus or cryoglobulinemia.

The C3 glomerulopathy variant of MPGN has little or no staining for immunoglobulin. However, Hou and colleagues[527] have noted that some specimens that seem appropriate for the C3 glomerulopathy category have minor staining for immunoglobulin rather than no staining. They propose a definition for C3 glomerulopathy that requires C3 dominant staining that is at least two orders of magnitude (on a scale of 0-3 or 0-4) more intense than any other immune reactant. In line with the evidence that C3 glomerulopathy is mediated by dysregulated activation of the alternative complement pathway, there is little or no staining for C4 or C1q in the C3 glomerulopathy variant of MPGN or in other histologic expressions of C3 glomerulonephritis.

Electron Microscopy

The ultrastructural hallmark of type I MPGN is mesangial interposition into an expanded subendothelial zone that contains electron-dense immune complex deposits (Figures 32.13 and 32.16). This distinct pattern of mesangial and capillary involvement has prompted a synonym for type I MPGN, *mesangiocapillary glomerulonephritis*. New basement membrane material is formed around the subendothelial deposits and around the projections of mesangial cytoplasm, which is the basis for the basement membrane replication seen by light microscopy (see Figure 32.12). Scattered mesangial dense deposits are usually found in association with mesangial hypercellularity and mesangial matrix expansion. Variable numbers of subepithelial electron-dense deposits occur. When they are numerous enough to resemble MN, some nephropathologists apply the diagnosis "mixed membranous and proliferative glomerulonephritis" or "type III MPGN" as proposed by Burkholder and colleagues.[533] The term *type III MPGN* also has been applied to a very rare pattern of glomerular injury that resembles type I MPGN by light microscopy and immunofluorescence microscopy but is characterized ultrastructurally by irregularly thickened GBMs with numerous intramembranous deposits of variable density.[534,535] Type III MPGN can be classified further as either immune complex disease or C3 glomerulopathy based on the presence or absence of staining for immunoglobulin. In the early application of the new classification system, type III MPGN as proposed by Burkholder tends to have an immune complex phenotype, whereas the other variant described by Strife tends to have a C3 glomerulopathy phenotype.

The hyaline thrombi seen by light microscopy appear as intraluminal spherical densities. When these structures, or any of the other electron-dense deposits, have a microtubular substructure, the possibility of cryoglobulinemic glomerulonephritis or immunotactoid glomerulopathy should be considered.

PATHOGENESIS

As noted earlier, two major pathogenic pathways can cause the pathology pattern of glomerular injury called MPGN, that is, immune complex localization and dysregulation of alternative pathway complement activation. A rare cause for this pattern is glomerular deposition of monoclonal immunoglobulin.

In the minority of patients with immune complex MPGN in whom the antigen has been identified, the sources have included infections, autoimmune diseases, neoplasms, and hereditary diseases (Table 32.12). The pathologic finding of intense immune complex deposition with hypercellularity suggests that the inflammation caused by the immune complexes has resulted in both the proliferation of mesangial and endothelial cells and the recruitment of inflammatory

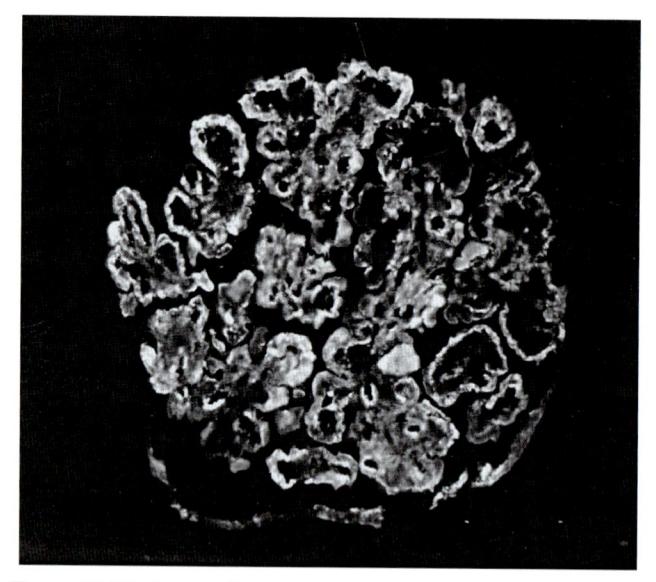

Figure 32.15 Immunofluorescence micrograph of a glomerulus with features of type I membranoproliferative glomerulonephritis (MPGN) showing global bandlike capillary wall staining for C3, as well as irregular mesangial staining. (Fluorescein isothiocyanate anti-C3 stain, ×300.)

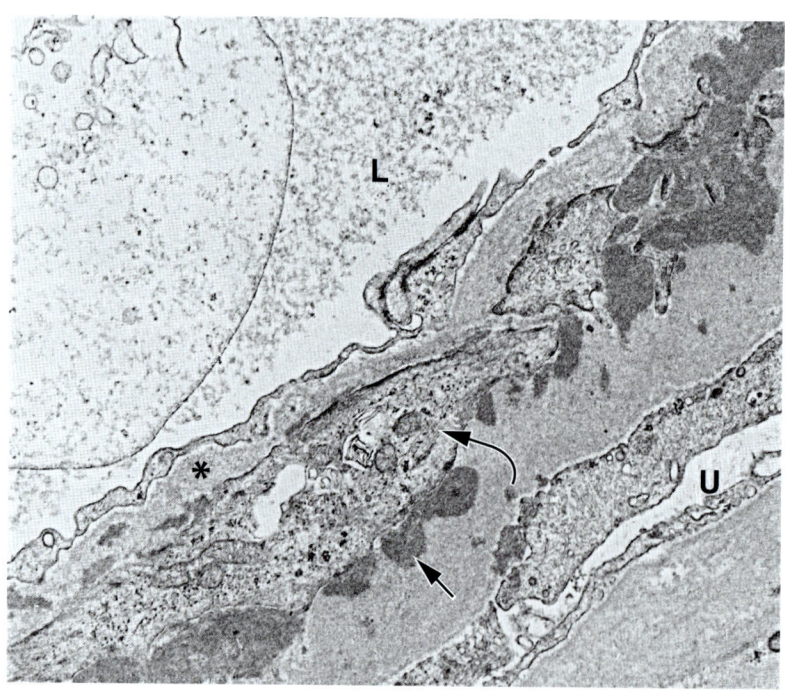

Figure 32.16 Electron micrograph of a capillary wall from a glomerulus with features of type I membranoproliferative glomerulonephritis (MPGN). The capillary lumen (L) is in the *upper left* and the urinary space (U) is in the *lower right*. In the subendothelial zone are dense deposits (*straight arrow*), extensions of mesangial cytoplasm (*curved arrow*), and new basement membrane material (*asterisk*) (see Figure 32.12). (×10,000.)

Table 32.12	Secondary Causes of Membranoproliferative Glomerulonephritis (MPGN)

Associated with Infection

Hepatitis B and C
Visceral abscesses
Infective endocarditis
Shunt nephritis
Quartan malaria
Schistosoma nephropathy
Mycoplasma infection

Associated with Rheumatologic Disease

Systemic lupus erythematosus
Scleroderma
Sjögren's syndrome
Sarcoidosis
Mixed essential cryoglobulinemia with or without hepatitis C infection
Anti–smooth muscle syndrome

Associated with Malignancy

Carcinoma
Lymphoma
Leukemia

Associated with an Inherited Disorder

α_1-Antitrypsin deficiency
Complement deficiency (C2 or C3), with or without partial lipodystrophy

Data from references 1047 and 1383-1391.

cells, including neutrophils and monocytes. These leukocytes are attracted to the glomerulus by activation of multiple mediator systems, including the complement system, cytokines, and chemokines.

Immune complex type I MGPN may be secondary to recognizable causes, such as cryoglobulinemia, hepatitis C, hepatitis B, osteomyelitis, subacute bacterial endocarditis, or infected ventriculoatrial shunt, malignancies,[536-538] autoimmune diseases (SLE or autoimmune thyroiditis[539]), light-chain nephropathy,[540] and celiac sprue.[541] Serologic and clinical evidence of these processes should be sought. The precise percentage of patients with MPGN due to hepatitis C may vary according to geographic area and cultural factors. The observation that upper respiratory tract infections precede the onset of MPGN in as many as one half of patients[542] raises the possibility that infectious agents contribute to the pathogenesis of many cases of type I MPGN.

When immune complex type I MPGN is secondary to other disease processes such as malignancy or a rheumatic condition, the laboratory results associated with the systemic disease (e.g., SLE) are positive (e.g., antibodies to double-stranded DNA). (See Chapter 33.) MPGN type I is also associated with underlying complement deficiency, notably of C2 and C3,[543] as well as deficiency in α_1-antitrypsin.

Even before recognition of the distinct C3 glomerulopathy variant of type I MPGN, alterations in circulating complement levels had been observed in MPGN patients (Table 32.13). C3 level is persistently depressed in approximately 75% of MPGN patients.[524,529,544-546] This is in contrast to poststreptococcal glomerulonephritis, in which depressed C3 levels typically return to normal within 2 months.[547-549] The persistent depression of C3 levels and the presence of nephritic syndrome should suggest type I MPGN. In some patients, activation of the alternative pathway is suggested by the observation that C3 levels are depressed, whereas levels of the classical pathway activators C1q and C4 are normal. Patients with this complement profile are likely to have a C3 glomerulopathy variant of MPGN. However, when MPGN is caused by cryoglobulinemia, which is an immune complex MPGN, there may be more depression of C4 than C3.[549]

EPIDEMIOLOGY

The majority of patients with MPGN are children between the ages of 8 and 16 years,[542] who account for 90% of patients with MPGN type I. The proportions of males and females are nearly equal.[524,525,529,534,550-556]

CLINICAL FEATURES

Type I MPGN (characterized by deposits of electron-dense material in the subendothelial zones of glomeruli) is a very heterogeneous disorder. Some combination of proteinuria (often nephrotic range), hematuria, hypertension, and renal failure is usually present.

TREATMENT

The prognosis of type I MPGN has been reviewed and described in several reports.[524,529,557,558] The 10-year renal survival appears to be between 40% in persistently nephrotic patients[529] and 65%.[524] Nonnephrotic patients have an improved 10-year renal survival of 85%.[529] A minority of patients may have a spontaneous remission.[524] The features suggestive of poor prognosis in MPGN type I include hypertension,[556,559] impaired GFR,[556,559-561] and the appearance of cellular crescents in biopsy specimens.[529,561,562]

The treatment of type I MPGN is based on the underlying cause of the disease process. Thus, the therapy for MPGN associated with cryoglobulinemia and hepatitis C should be aimed at treating hepatitis C virus infection, whereas the treatment of MPGN associated with lupus or scleroderma should be based on the principles of care for those rheumatologic conditions. Most recommendations for the treatment of type I MPGN are derived from studies involving children.[563-569] West touted the benefits of continuous prednisone therapy for improved renal survival.[565] Whether the benefit of low-dose prednisone therapy is seen only in children or whether similar effects can be achieved in adults has never been investigated in a prospective randomized trial. However, low-dose, alternate-day prednisone therapy may improve renal function.[567,568]

In addition to glucocorticoids, a number of other immunosuppressive and anticoagulant therapies have been used in the treatment of type I MPGN. Initial reports indicated that treatment with aspirin and dipyridamole had a positive effect in renal survival.[525] This approach was widely accepted; however, statistical design flaws led to a reanalysis of the data, which revealed no difference in the treatment and control groups with respect to long-term outcome.[544] A subsequent study using aspirin with dipyridamole demonstrated a slight decrease in urine protein excretion by 3 years but

Table 32.13 Selected Serologic Findings in Patients with Primary Glomerular Disease

Disease	C4	C3	ASO, ADNase B	Cryo Ig	Anti-GBM	ANCA
Minimal change disease	N	N	—	—	—	—
Focal glomerulosclerosis	N	N	—	—	—	—
Membranous nephropathy	N	N	—	—	—	—
Membranoproliferative GN*						
Type I	N or ↓↓	↓↓	+	++	—	—
Type II	N	↓↓↓	+	—	—	—
Fibrillary GN	N	N	—	—	—	—
IgA nephropathy	N	N	—	—	—	—
Acute poststreptococcal GN	N or ↓	↓↓	+++	++	—	—
Crescentic GN						
Anti-GBM	N	N	—	—	+++	±
Immune complex	N or ↓	N or ↓↓	—	N/++	—	±
ANCA small vessel vasculitis	N	N	—	—	±	+++

*Former membranoproliferative glomerulonephritis classification schema.
ANCA, Antineutrophil cytoplasmic autoantibody; ADNase B, anti–deoxyribonuclease B; ASO, anti–streptolysin O; cryo Ig, cryoglobulins; GBM, glomerular basement membrane; GN, glomerulonephritis; N, normal levels.

no effect on renal function.[570] Treatment with dipyridamole, aspirin, and warfarin, with or without cyclophosphamide, was examined in both controlled and uncontrolled studies.[422,525,569-574] A regimen of warfarin, dipyridamole, and cyclophosphamide[569] was suggested to improve long-term renal survival based on a retrospective analysis; however, a controlled trial in Canada demonstrated no benefit of this approach.[287]

The use of MMF and corticosteroids has been suggested based on uncontrolled and anecdotal observations.[575] In patients with a defined underlying disease (e.g., neoplasia or hepatitis B or C), treatment should be directed at the underlying condition.[576,577]

Type I MPGN is significantly ameliorated by the use of cyclosporine in the very rare condition known as *Buckley's syndrome*.[102,103,578]

MEMBRANOPROLIFERATIVE GLOMERULONEPHRITIS TYPE III

Type III MPGN occurs in a very small number of children and young adults. Regardless of the pathologic distinctions of MPGN type III of Burkholder and colleagues[533] and Strife and colleagues,[535] few distinguishing clinical characteristics are noted in these patients. These patients may have clinical features of disease quite similar to those of type I MPGN, and the long-term clinical course is quite similar as well. Patients with MPGN described by Strife and coworkers[534] have low C3 levels in the absence of C3 nephritic factor. Patients with nonnephrotic proteinuria do better than patients who have nephrotic syndrome.

C3 GLOMERULOPATHIES (DENSE DEPOSIT DISEASE AND C3 GLOMERULONEPHRITIS)

EPIDEMIOLOGY

Dense deposit disease accounts for about 25% of MPGN in children but is much less common in adults. The large majority of patients are children between the ages of 8 and 16 years,[542] who account for about 70% of cases. It is estimated to affect 2 to 3 persons per million. Males and females were reported to be similarly affected in some studies,[579] whereas other studies reported a female predominance.[529,580,581] A retrospective of 32 cases identified through the nephropathology laboratory at Columbia University between 1977 and 2007, reported that 43% of patients were children, of whom 65% were between the ages of 5 and 10 years, and 22% of patients were adults older than 60 years. The female/male ratio was 1.9, and 85% of patients were white.[582] It is unclear whether the unexpectedly high representation of older adults in this cohort reflects a change in the demographics of the disease, or a change in biopsy practices, or a selection or referral bias in this study or the older studies.

C3 glomerulonephritis includes all patients with C3 glomerulopathy who do not have intramembranous dense deposits that warrant a diagnosis of dense deposit disease and includes the C3 glomerulopathy variant of MPGN as well as other patterns of proliferative glomerulonephritis. There is a relative paucity of epidemiologic data given that this is a new diagnostic category; however, one study of 19 patients with C3 glomerulonephritis revealed a median age at onset of 29.9 years (range, 7 to 70 years).[583] A larger and more recent study of 88 patients with C3 glomerulopathy in the United Kingdom, including 59 patients with C3 glomerulonephritis and 21 with dense deposit disease, revealed that patients with C3 glomerulonephritis were significantly older (median age, 26 years vs. 12 years; $P = 0.002$).[584]

PATHOLOGY

The term *dense deposit disease* emphasizes the pathognomonic feature of discontinuous electron-dense bands within the GBM[528,530] (Figures 32.17 and 32.18). These are accompanied by spherical to irregular mesangial dense deposits and occasional subendothelial and subepithelial deposits, some of which resemble the "humps" seen in postinfectious

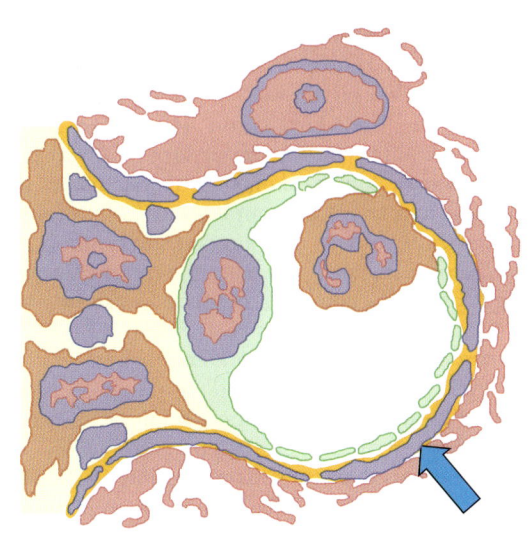

Figure 32.17 Diagram depicting a glomerular capillary loop with features of dense deposit disease with bandlike intramembranous dense deposits (*arrow*) and spherical mesangial dense deposits. (Courtesy J. Charles Jennette, University of North Carolina at Chapel Hill, Chapel Hill, NC.)

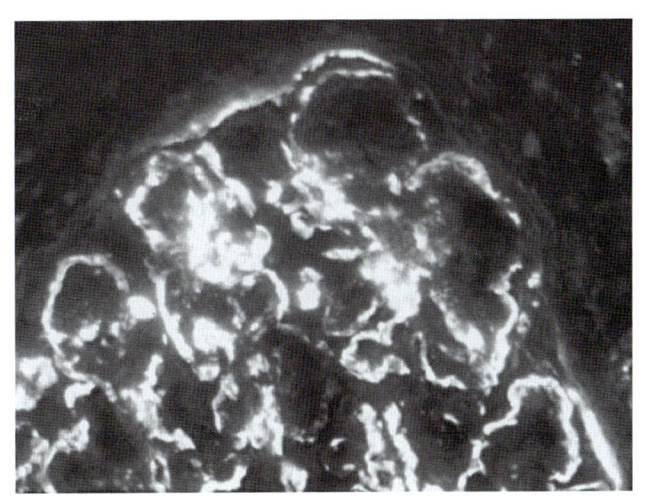

Figure 32.19 Immunofluorescence micrograph of a portion of a glomerulus with features of dense deposit disease demonstrating discontinuous bandlike capillary wall staining and granular mesangial staining for C3. (Fluorescein isothiocyanate anti-C3 stain, ×600.)

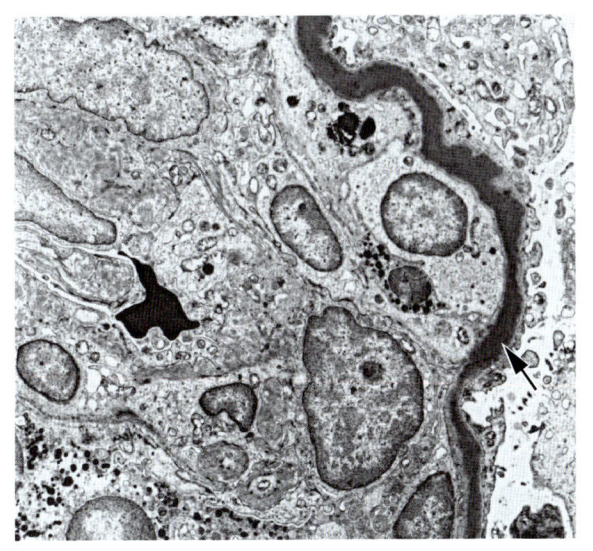

Figure 32.18 Electron micrograph of a glomerular capillary from a patient with dense deposit disease showing a bandlike intramembranous dense deposit (*arrow*) that has essentially replaced the normal glomerular basement membrane. Also note the endocapillary hypercellularity. (×5000.)

glomerulonephritis. Dense deposits also may be identified in Bowman's capsule and tubular basement membranes.

Immunofluorescence microscopy demonstrates intense capillary wall linear to bandlike staining for C3 (Figure 32.19), with little or no staining for immunoglobulin.[527,528,585,586] The capillary wall staining may have a fine double contour with outlining of the outer and inner aspects of the dense deposits. The mesangial deposits usually appear as scattered spherules or rings, with the latter resulting from staining of the outer surface but not the interior of the spherical deposits. There typically is intense staining for C3 with little or no staining for C4, C1q, or immunoglobulins.

The light microscopic appearance of dense deposit disease is much more variable than that of type I MPGN and often does not have a membranoproliferative appearance.[528] Thus, the term *dense deposit disease* is preferable to *type II MPGN*.[586,587] In a review of a large number of renal biopsy specimens obtained in North America, Europe, and Japan from patients with dense deposit disease, the light microscopy findings could be classified into five distinct patterns: (1) membranoproliferative pattern, (2) mesangioproliferative pattern, (3) crescentic pattern, (4) acute proliferative and exudative pattern, and (5) unclassified dense deposit disease. Of these, the mesangioproliferative lesion characterized by focal segmental and mesangial hypercellularity accounted for about 50% of the cases reviewed, with 28% presenting with a membranoproliferative pattern (type I) and 20% a crescentic lesion. Although the patients' ages ranged from 3 to 67 years, nearly 75% of the patients were younger than 20 years of age, and all patients with either crescentic dense deposit disease or acute proliferative dense deposit disease were between the ages of 3 and 18 years.[587] Therefore, the histologic appearance of dense deposit disease can mimic many other categories of glomerulonephritis, and the findings by immunofluorescence and especially electron microscopy are required for accurate diagnosis.

As described earlier in this chapter, the pathology of the non–dense deposit disease category of C3 glomerulopathy (i.e., C3 glomerulonephritis) is extremely variable by light microscopy but falls in the spectrum of type I MPGN, to focal or diffuse proliferative, to mesangial proliferative glomerulonephritis (see Figure 32.14).[528] As one of the variants of C3 glomerulopathy, C3 glomerulonephritis on immunofluorescence microscopy reveals C3 dominant staining with little or no staining for immunoglobulin, C4, or C1q. By definition, electron microscopy of C3 glomerulonephritis does not reveal the typical intramembranous dense deposits that are diagnostic for dense deposit disease. However, this is a somewhat subjective division, and borderline specimens are difficult to classify as dense deposit disease versus C3 glomerulonephritis. From a practical perspective, this may not be important because both are variants of C3 glomerulopathy and have a similar pathogenesis and clinical features.

PATHOGENESIS

As C3 glomerulopathies, dense deposit disease and C3 glomerulonephritis share a pathogenic mechanism that involves abnormal regulation of the alternative complement pathway (recently reviewed by Bomback and Appel).[528,588]

A porcine model of dense deposit disease suggests that there is massive deposition of C3 and the terminal C5b-9 complement complex (the membrane attack complex). In the circulation, there is extensive complement activation with very low C3 levels and high levels of circulating terminal complement components. No immunoglobulin deposits were detected in kidney tissue. In this animal model of dense deposit disease, the pathogenetic mechanism does not appear to involve immune complexes but rather utilizes some other mechanism for the activation of complement and the trapping of activating complement components within the GBM.[589]

The hypocomplementemia in dense deposit disease and other forms of C3 glomerulopathy reflects dysregulated activation of the alternative complement pathway (Figure 32.20). Under normal circumstances, the alternative complement pathway maintains low-level, basal activity termed *tickover*, which maintains C3 convertase. Any disruption in C3 convertase activity can thereby alter tickover and result in overactivation. Three distinct mechanisms result in uncontrolled activation of C3 convertase: (1) the development of an autoantibody, the C3 nephritic factor (C3NeF); (2) the absence of circulating regulators (e.g., factor H); and (3) the presence of a circulating inhibitor of factor H.[589] The most common of these is the presence of the autoantibody C3NeF. C3NeF is an antibody that protects C3 convertase (C3bBb) from dissociation by factor H and thus prolongs its half-life by 10-fold.[590] It does so in one of two ways—by binding either to C3bBb or to IgG-C3b-C3bBb of the assembled convertase. The stabilization of this complex results in perpetual C3 breakdown. It is tempting to incriminate this factor as central to the pathogenesis of MPGN, especially dense deposit disease, since most affected patients harbor C3NeF in their circulation. However, C3NeF does not always correlate with disease activity, and more importantly, progressive kidney damage still occurs in patients who have normal levels of complement.[591-593] Interestingly, autoantibodies to other complement components such as factor B, factor H, factor I, or a component of C3 convertase (C3b and/or CFB) can also be seen in some individuals.[588,594,595] More recently, reclassification of MPGN was strongly proposed by Sethi and colleagues, who found higher levels of alternative and terminal complement pathway components, as identified by mass spectrometry, directly within glomeruli of patients with dense deposit disease as compared to those from patients with immune complex–mediated forms of MPGN as well as healthy individuals.[596,597]

Normal protective, or regulatory, mechanisms control C3bBb levels and complement deposition, of which factor H is one of the most important. Factor H is a soluble glycoprotein that regulates complement in the fluid phase and on cell surfaces by binding to C3b.[598] Some mutations in factor H result in C3 glomerulopathy that does not have an MPGN pattern.[599,600]

The genetics of dense deposit disease are complex. Only a few families have been identified with more than one affected member, although families exist with one patient with dense deposit disease and other members affected by other autoimmune diseases. The most robust genetic association with dense deposit disease is a deficiency of factor H, associated with a mutation of the complement factor H (*CFH*) gene.[601,602] A more recent study identified a family with dense deposit disease in which a C3 convertase-resistant C3 gene mutation was identified in a mother and her identical twin sons, thereby resulting in alternative complement pathway activation.[603]

C3 glomerulonephritis is a result of overactivity of the alternative complement pathway due to autoantibodies to, and/or mutations in, critical regulators of the pathway.[528] The underlying genetic defect in C3 glomerulonephritis has been identified in some hereditary forms of the disease, such as CFHR5 nephropathy, and further insight is likely to occur rapidly given intense interest in this area.[604-606]

CLINICAL FEATURES

Patients with dense deposit disease may have hematuria, proteinuria, or both. They may have a nephrotic or acute nephritic syndrome. At least a third of patients have all of the components of the nephrotic syndrome on presentation. Microhematuria is present in the overwhelming majority of patients, whereas gross hematuria occurs only in about 15%.[582] Finally, one quarter of patients have acute nephritic syndrome associated with red cells and red cell casts in the urine, hypertension, and renal insufficiency.[524,529,544,545] Hypertension is typically mild but may be severe in some cases. Kidney dysfunction occurs in at least half of cases and is more common among adults than in children.[582] When present at the outset of disease, kidney dysfunction portends a poor prognosis.

Hypocomplementemia of the C3 factor is present in 80% to 90% of patients with dense deposit disease. In a

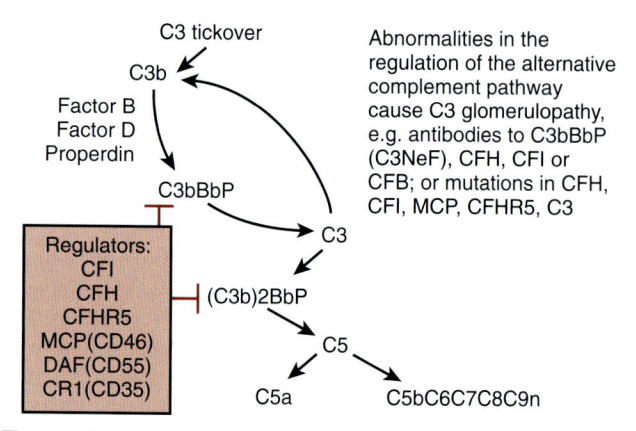

Figure 32.20 Regulators of the alternative complement pathway and abnormalities that cause C3 glomerulopathy. CF, Complement factor.

retrospective review from Columbia University, depressed C3 levels occurred in 100% of children but in only 41% of adults ($P = 0.001$).[582] Depressed C4 levels were very uncommon in both age groups. C3 hypocomplementemia is prolonged in patients with dense deposit disease[428] and is associated with decrements in terminal complement components C5b-9. C3NeF is present in more than 80% of patients.

Respiratory tract infections precede cases of MPGN in half of patients, especially in children.[582] On rare occasions, the onset can be triggered by a streptococcal infection, so that the disease mimics acute poststreptococcal glomerulonephritis except for the persistence of C3 hypocomplementemia beyond 8 weeks from onset.[607] Comorbid conditions may be seen in adult patients with dense deposit disease, including plasma cell dyscrasias, which were noted in 4 of 18 patients (22%) in the Columbia University review.[582]

Patients with dense deposit disease may have deposits in the retina, along Bruch's membrane, that are similar in structure and composition to the deposits in GBM. These whitish yellow drusen develop at an early age. Initially, drusen have little impact on visual acuity, but visual loss can occur in about 10% of patients.[608] A careful retinal exam is therefore indicated in all patients with proven dense deposit disease. There is no correlation between the severity of kidney and ocular involvement; however, patients with other forms of MPGN do not typically have drusen.[609]

Dense deposit disease may be associated with the syndrome of acquired partial lipodystrophy.[593] About 80% of patients with this syndrome have low C3 levels and C3NeF. About 20% of patients develop MPGN, although the lipodystrophy and glomerular disease may occur several years apart.[610] The link between acquired partial lipodystrophy and MPGN stems from the production by adipocytes of C3, factor B, and factor D (adipsin), whose function is the cleavage of factor B. In the presence of C3NeF, the alternative pathway of complement activation is dysregulated leading to the destruction of adipocytes.[610]

Patients with C3 glomerulonephritis, as also seen with dense deposit disease, can present with hypertension, azotemia, hematuria, and proteinuria with or without nephrotic syndrome. Interestingly, although C3 levels are usually low and C4 levels are normal, the large study of 59 patients with C3 glomerulonephritis in the United Kingdom found that C3 was more likely to be normal when compared to patients with dense deposit disease (52% vs. 11%, $P = 0.003$); therefore, a normal C3 level alone does not exclude C3 glomerulonephritis.[584,597] As with dense deposit disease, some patients may have C3NeF.[583,588,611]

TREATMENT

The prognosis for dense deposit disease is worse than that for type I MPGN. The less favorable prognosis is in accord with a higher frequency of crescentic glomerulonephritis and chronic tubulointerstitial nephritis at the time of biopsy in dense deposit disease.[559,612,613] In patients with dense deposit disease, clinical remissions are rare,[529,550] occurring in less than 5% in children. Patients generally reach ESKD in 8 to 12 years from onset of disease. In dense deposit disease, the prognosis is worse in adults than in children.[582]

There is currently no widely agreed upon treatment of dense deposit disease, and the available information remains based on small case series. Inhibition of angiotensin II may be helpful, but it has not been formally tested.[582] The use of corticosteroid therapy is probably not effective.[601] Immunosuppressive therapy with such agents as MMF and rituximab aimed at reducing C3NeF in dense deposit disease has been suggested.[614] It is not likely that immunosuppression with or without plasma exchange will be beneficial, except perhaps if an inhibitory autoantibody to complement factor H is present. There are reports of effective treatment of patients with defined deficiency of complement factor H with infusion of fresh-frozen plasma every 14 days to provide functionally intact factor H.[611,615-618] In a proof-of-concept study in mice genetically deficient in complement factor H, treatment with purified human complement factor H resulted in rapid normalization of plasma C3 levels and resolution of the GBM C3 deposition.[619] Based on the current understanding of the pathogenesis of dense deposit disease, inhibition of C5 activation and formation of the terminal component of complement activation (C5b-9) with the monoclonal antibody eculizumab would be theoretically beneficial, but evidence for this approach had been lacking[617] until a recent proof-of-concept efficacy and safety study in three patients with dense deposit disease and three patients with C3 glomerulonephritis treated in an open-label fashion with eculizumab. This resulted in reduced serum creatinine levels in two subjects, reduction in urine protein levels in one subject, and histopathologic improvement in one subject. It also appeared that elevated levels of the serum membrane attack complex might predict treatment response.[620]

Given that C3 glomerulonephritis represents a new diagnostic category, treatment protocols outside of supportive care are limited but will likely involve targeted therapies that correct complement dysregulation now that pathogenetic mechanisms are becoming increasingly understood.

Data are also limited with regard to prognosis; however, the study by Servais and colleagues found in a cohort of 134 patients with C3 glomerulopathy in France that roughly 25% of patients with C3 glomerulonephritis progress to ESKD over a follow-up period of 10 years.[621] Sethi and colleagues reported in 12 patients with C3 glomerulonephritis with a mean follow-up of 26.4 months that kidney function remained stable in every patient except for one who progressed to dialysis soon after presentation.[597] With regard to kidney transplantation, one group reported their experience with 21 patients with ESKD due to C3 glomerulonephritis who underwent kidney transplantation. Fourteen patients (68%) developed recurrent C3 glomerulonephritis in the allograft, which was typically manifested by hematuria and proteinuria, and median time to recurrence was 28 months. Furthermore, 50% of patients with recurrent C3 glomerulonephritis experienced graft failure with a median time to graft failure of 77 months.[622] Recurrences in kidney transplants of dense deposit disease are common (80% or higher),[550,623-625] especially in the presence of C3NeF or CFH mutations.[626] Prophylactic plasma infusions or simultaneous liver transplantation can be beneficial in the latter cases.[615,616] Levels of C3 in the serum do not seem to predict recurrences.[626] Figure 32.21 depicts a current framework for the diagnosis and management of C3 glomerulopathy, which is

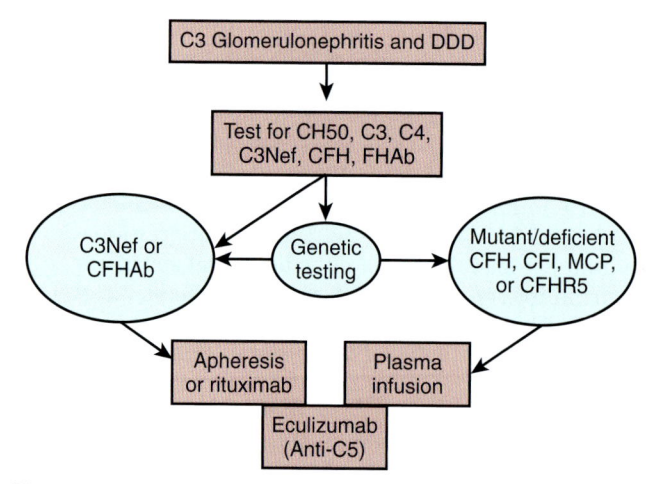

Figure 32.21 A framework for the diagnosis and management of C3 glomerulopathies: C3 glomerulonephritis and dense deposit disease (DDD). Ab, Antibody; CF, complement factor; C3Nef, C3 nephritic factor.

likely to be refined even further as additional pathogenetic insight occurs.

ACUTE POSTSTREPTOCOCCAL GLOMERULONEPHRITIS

EPIDEMIOLOGY

Acute poststreptococcal glomerulonephritis (PSGN) is a disease that affects primarily children, with a peak incidence between the ages of 2 and 6 years. Children younger than age 2 years and adults older than age 40 account for only about 15% of patients with acute PSGN. Interestingly, recent evidence points to acute PSGN as the cause of Wolfgang Amadeus Mozart's early death at the age of 35.[627] Subclinical microscopic hematuria may be four times more common than overt acute PSGN, as documented in studies of family members of affected patients.[628-630] Only rarely do PSGN and rheumatic fever occur concomitantly.[631] Males are more likely than females to have overt nephritis.

Acute PSGN may occur as part of an epidemic or sporadic disease. During epidemic infections of streptococci of proven nephrogenicity, the clinical attack rate appears to be about 12%,[632-634] but has been reported at 33%,[635] or even as high as 38% in certain affected families.[630]

Differences in incidence rates among different families argue for existence of host genetic susceptibility factors affecting the propensity for overt nephritis.[636] An association was found between PSGN and HLA-DRW4,[636] HLA-DPA*02-022 and DPB1*05-01,[637] and more recently DRB1*03011.[638]

The rate of acute PSGN after sporadic infections with group A streptococci of potentially nephritogenic types is quite variable,[639,640] which again points to an effect of ill-defined host factors. A minority of streptococcal infections lead to nephritic syndrome, which argues for the presence of certain nephritogenic characteristics of the offending agent. Indeed, in the 1950s Rammelkamp and colleagues[639,640] identified certain strains of streptococci within Lancefield group A, in particular type XII, that are capable of leading to an acute glomerulonephritis. Other nephritogenic serotypes include M types 1, 2, 3, 4, 18, 25, 31, 49, 52, 55, 56, 57, 59, 60, and 61. There are differences among these serotypes in their propensity to be associated with nephritis depending on the site of infection. Certain strains, such as types 2, 49, 55, 57 and 60, are usually associated with nephritis after pyoderma,[641,642] whereas M type 49 can lead to nephritis after either pharyngitis or pyoderma. In addition to occurring after infection with group A β-hemolytic streptococci, acute PSGN has also been described after infection with group C streptococci and possibly group G streptococci.[643,644]

Acute PSGN is on the decline in developed countries, but it continues to occur in developing communities.[645,646] Epidemic PSGN is frequently associated with skin infections, whereas pharyngitides are associated with sporadic PSGN in developed countries. Overt glomerulonephritis is found in about 10% of children at risk, but when one includes subclinical disease as evidenced by microscopic hematuria, about 25% of children at risk are found to be affected.[647,648] In some developing countries, acute PSGN remains the most common form of acute nephritic syndrome among children. The incidence rate appears to follow a cyclical pattern, with outbreaks occurring every 10 years or so.[649] A review of 11 published population-based studies estimated the median incidence of PSGN in children to be 24 cases per 100,000 patient-years based on studies that examined populations in less developed countries or included substantial minority populations in more developed countries; the incidence in adults was conservatively estimated to be 2 cases per 100,000 patient-years in less developed countries and 0.3 case per 100,000 patient-years in more developed countries.[650] The review authors estimated that more than 470,000 cases of acute PSGN occur annually, leading to approximately 5000 deaths (1% of total cases), 97% of which are in less developed countries.

Interestingly, the epidemiology of PSGN in Florida appears to have changed in the past two decades, compared to the 1960s and 1970s. Pharyngitis has replaced impetigo as the predominant underlying infection, a shift has occurred in racial distribution (now predominantly whites are affected) and in seasonal variation, and the severity of disease has decreased. These changes are thought to reflect a change in the causal agent of impetigo.[651]

PATHOLOGY

Light Microscopy

The pathologic appearance of acute PSGN varies during the course of the disease. The acute histologic change is influx of neutrophils, which results in diffuse global hypercellularity (Figure 32.22).[652-656] Endocapillary proliferation of mesangial cells and endothelial cells also contributes to the hypercellularity. The hypercellularity often is very marked and results in enlarged consolidated glomeruli. The description *acute diffuse proliferative glomerulonephritis* often is used as a pathologic designation for this stage of acute PSGN. A minority of patients have crescent formation, which usually affects only a small proportion of glomeruli.[657] Extensive crescent formation is rare.[658,659] Special stains that have differential reactions with immune deposits may demonstrate subepithelial deposits. For example, the

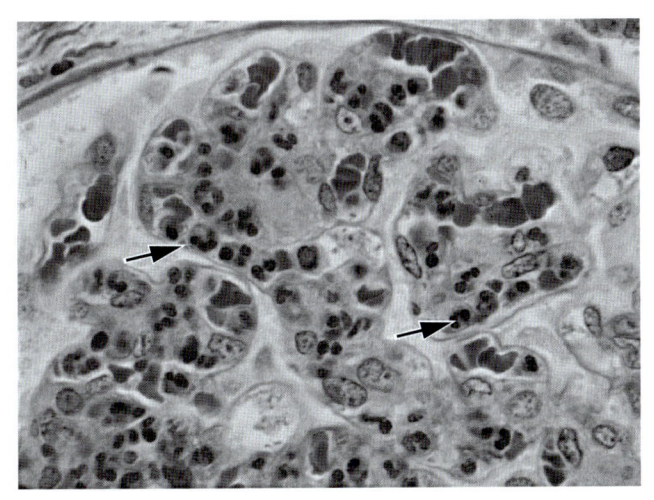

Figure 32.22 Light micrograph of a glomerulus with features of acute poststreptococcal glomerulonephritis demonstrating marked influx of neutrophils (*arrows*). (Masson trichrome stain, ×700.)

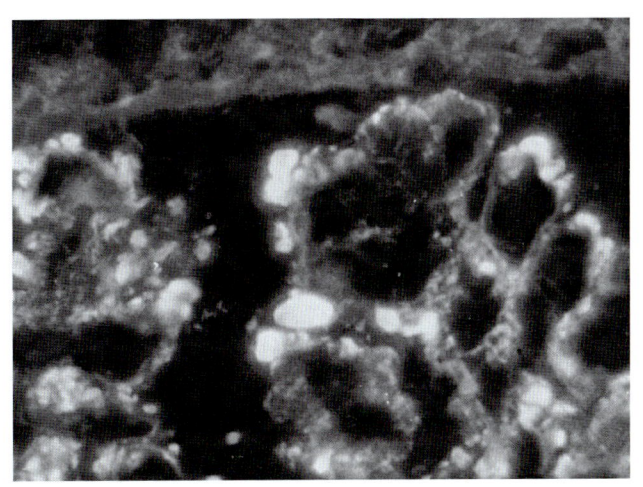

Figure 32.23 Immunofluorescence micrograph of a glomerular segment from a patient with acute poststreptococcal glomerulonephritis showing coarsely granular capillary wall staining for C3. Compare this to the finely granular capillary wall staining of membranous nephropathy in Figure 32.9. (Fluorescein isothiocyanate anti-C3 stain, ×800.)

subepithelial deposits may stain red (fuchsinophilic) with Masson trichrome stain.

Interstitial edema and interstitial infiltration of predominantly mononuclear leukocytes usually are present and occasionally are pronounced, especially with unusually severe disease associated with crescents. Focal tubular epithelial cell simplification (flattening) also may accompany severe disease. Arteries and arterioles typically have no acute changes, although preexisting sclerotic changes may be present in older patients.

During the resolving phase of self-limited PSGN, which usually begins within several weeks of onset, the infiltrating neutrophils disappear and endothelial hypercellularity resolves, leaving behind only mesangial hypercellularity.[653,660] This mesangioproliferative stage often is present in patients with PSGN who have had resolution of nephritis but have persistent isolated proteinuria, and it may persist for several months in patients who have complete clinical resolution. There may be focal segmental glomerular scarring as a sequela of particularly injurious inflammation, but this is seldom extensive except in the rare patients with crescentic PSGN. Ultimately, the pathologic changes of acute PSGN can resolve completely.[660,661]

Immunofluorescence Microscopy

Immunofluorescence microscopy demonstrates glomerular immune complex deposits in PSGN.[653,655,656,662] The pattern and composition of deposits change during the course of PSGN. During the acute diffuse proliferative phase of the disease, there is diffuse global coarsely granular capillary wall and mesangial staining that usually is very intense for C3 and of varying degrees for IgG from intense to absent (Figure 32.23). Staining for IgM and IgA is less frequent and usually less intense. In self-limited disease, biopsy should be performed later in the disease course because it is more likely that the staining will be predominantly or exclusively for C3 with little or no immunoglobulin staining. Because most patients with uncomplicated new-onset acute PSGN do not undergo kidney biopsy, most biopsy specimens are obtained later in the course when there is diagnostic uncertainty due to equivocal serologic confirmation or unusually aggressive or persistent clinical features. At this time, the immunofluorescence microscopy staining is usually predominantly for C3. This may reflect termination of nephritogenic immune complex localization in the kidney with masking of residual complexes by complement. An alternative explanation for the presence of C3 in the absence of immunoglobulin is activation of complement or blockade of complement regulatory mechanisms by factors released by the infection. This could initiate a pathogenic mechanism similar to that in C3 glomerulopathy. The continued presence of intense staining for IgG a month or more into the course of what otherwise looks like pathologically typical PSGN is cause for concern that the process will not be self-limited.

Several patterns of immune staining have been described but are of limited prognostic value.[653,656,663] The garland pattern is characterized by numerous large, closely apposed granular deposits along the capillary walls. Patients with this pattern usually have nephrotic-range proteinuria as a component of their disease. The starry sky pattern has more scattered granular staining, which corresponds somewhat to less severe disease. The mesangial pattern, especially when it is predominantly C3 staining, corresponds to the resolving phase with a mesangioproliferative light microscopic appearance.

Electron Microscopy

The hallmark ultrastructural feature of PSGN is the subepithelial humplike dense deposits (Figures 32.24 and 32.25).[655,660-662,664] However, small subendothelial and mesangial dense deposits can usually be identified with careful observation and theoretically may be more important in the pathogenesis of the disease, especially the neutrophilic influx and endocapillary proliferative response, than are the subepithelial humps. The subepithelial humps are covered

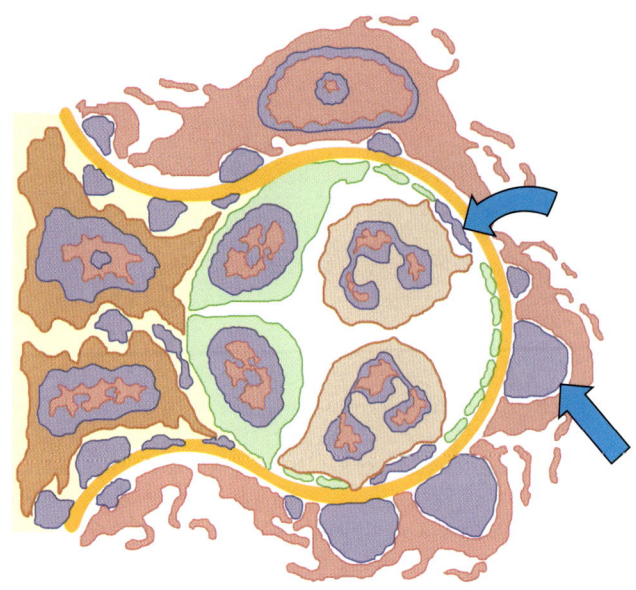

Figure 32.24 Diagram of the ultrastructural features of acute poststreptococcal glomerulonephritis (PSGN). Note the subepithelial humplike dense deposits (*straight arrow*), subendothelial deposits (*curved arrow*), and mesangial deposits. There is endocapillary hypercellularity caused by neutrophil infiltration, and endothelial and mesangial proliferation. (Courtesy J. Charles Jennette, University of North Carolina at Chapel Hill, Chapel Hill, NC.)

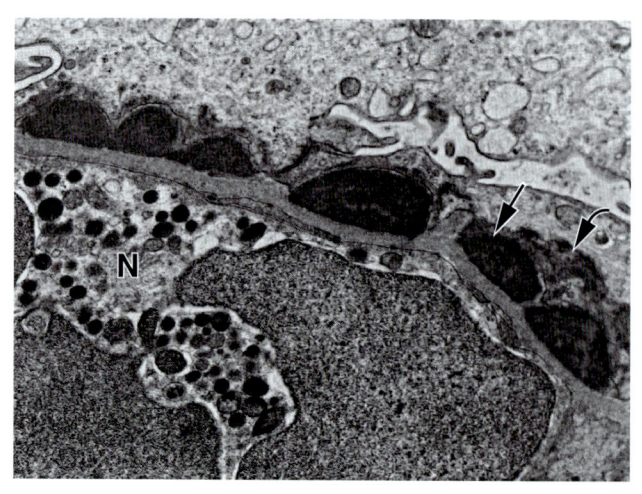

Figure 32.25 Electron micrograph of a portion of a glomerular capillary from a patient with acute poststreptococcal glomerulonephritis (PSGN) showing subepithelial dense deposits (*straight arrow*), condensation of cytoskeleton in adjacent podocyte cytoplasm (*curved arrow*), and a neutrophil (N) marginated against the basement membrane with no intervening endothelial cytoplasm. (×5000.)

by effaced epithelial foot processes, which usually contain condensed cytoskeletal filaments (including actin) that form a corona around the immune deposits (see Figure 32.25). Similar humps are observed in C3 glomerulopathy. During the acute phase, capillary lumens often contain marginated neutrophils, some of which are in direct contact with GBMs (see Figure 32.25). Lesser numbers of monocytes and macrophages contribute to the leukocyte influx.

Mesangial regions are expanded by increased numbers of mesangial cells and leukocytes as well as increased matrix material and varying amounts of electron-dense material.

During the resolution phase, usually 6 to 8 weeks into the course, the subepithelial humps disappear, leaving behind only mesangial and sometimes a few scattered subendothelial and intramembranous dense deposits. The subepithelial deposits first become electron lucent and then disappear completely. The humps in peripheral capillary loops disappear before the humps in the subepithelial zone adjacent to the perimesangial basement membrane.

PATHOGENESIS

Acute PSGN is the prototype disease of an acute glomerulonephritis associated with an infectious cause. The first description of this link dates back to the early 19th century after scarlet fever epidemics in Florence and Vienna. Richard Bright first described the association in 1836, reporting that scarlet fever was sometimes followed by hematuria and kidney disease.[665] In 1907, Schick described an asymptomatic interval of 12 days to 7 weeks between the onset of streptococcal infection and the onset of nephritis.[666] In the early 1950s, Rammelkamp and Weaver further defined the association of PSGN with specific serotypes of streptococci.[541,667]

Despite the early recognition of an association between streptococcal infection and acute glomerulonephritis, the pathogenic mechanism of disease remains incompletely understood. Conceptually, either acute PSGN could be secondary to a direct pathogenic effect of a streptococcal protein (e.g., a protein that activates or blocks regulation of the alternative complement pathway), or the streptococcal product could induce an immune complex–mediated injury. This could occur by a number of different mechanisms: (1) by introducing an antigen into the glomerulus (planted antigen), (2) by the deposition of circulating immune complexes, (3) by alteration of a normal renal antigen that causes it to become a self-antigen, or (4) by induction of an autoimmune response to a self-antigen by way of antigenic mimicry. It is conceivable that more than one streptococcal antigen may be involved in the pathogenesis of acute PSGN, and more than one pathogenic mechanism may be at play simultaneously.

Several streptococcal proteins have been implicated in the pathogenesis of acute PSGN.[668] M protein molecules protruding from the surface of group A streptococci contain epitopes that cross-react with glomerular antigens. Shared sequences of M protein types 5, 6, and 19 have been shown to elicit antibodies that react with several myocardial and skeletal muscle proteins.[669] Conversely, monoclonal antibodies raised against human kidney cortex have been shown to cross-react with types 6 and 12 M proteins, which provides evidence that certain M proteins may share antigenic determinants between all glomeruli.[670] The glomerular cross reactivity of the N-terminal region of type 1 M protein was further localized to a tetrapeptide sequence at position 23-26.[671] Antibodies raised against the N terminus of type 1 M protein were shown to cross-react with the cytoskeletal protein of glomerular mesangial cells, namely, the filament protein vimentin.[669] More recently, two antigens have been found within the glomerular deposits in kidney biopsy specimens from patients with PSGN and have been reported to induce an antibody response characteristic for nephritogenic streptococcal infections: streptococcal proteinase exotoxin B (SPEB, zymogen)[672] and the glycolytic enzyme glyceraldehyde 3-phosphate dehydrogenase (GAPDH), which shares exact homology with the nephritis-associated plasmin receptor (NaPlr) that binds plasminogen.[673] In a study that tested antigen deposition in 17 kidney biopsy specimens and circulating antibodies in sera from 53 patients, response to SPEB was more consistently found than deposits and antibody response to GAPDH.[674]

Currently, the spectrum of infectious agents associated with postinfectious or peri-infectious glomerulonephritis includes many more bacterial pathogens than streptococci. Other agents include staphylococci, gram-negative rods, and intracellular bacteria.[675,676] Likewise, the population at risk for peri-infectious glomerulonephritis has changed to include alcoholic individuals, intravenous drug users, and patients with ventricular atrial shunts and on immunosuppressive therapy.[676] However, PSGN remains one of the most extensively studied and documented infection-associated glomerulonephritides.

CLINICAL FEATURES AND NATURAL HISTORY

Classically, the syndrome of acute PSGN presents abruptly with hematuria, proteinuria, hypertension, and azotemia. This syndrome can show a wide spectrum of severity from asymptomatic disease to oliguric acute renal failure.[677] A latent period occurs from the onset of pharyngitis to the onset of nephritis. In postpharyngitic cases, the latent period averages 10 days with a range of 7 to 21 days. The latent period may be longer after a skin infection (from 14 to 21 days), although this period is harder to define after impetigo.[678] The latency period can exceed 3 weeks.[679] Short latency periods of less than 1 week are suggestive of a "synpharyngitic" syndrome corresponding typically to exacerbation of an underlying IgA nephropathy.

The hematuria is microscopic in more than two thirds of cases but may be macroscopic on occasion. Patients commonly report gross hematuria and transient oliguria. Anuria is infrequent, however, and if persistent, may indicate the development of crescentic glomerulonephritis.

Mild to moderate hypertension occurs in more than 75% of patients. It is most evident at the onset of nephritis and typically subsides promptly after diuresis.[631] Antihypertensive treatment is necessary in only about one half of patients. Signs and symptoms of congestive heart failure may occur and indeed may dominate the clinical picture. These include jugular venous distention, the presence of an S_3 gallop, dyspnea, and signs of pulmonary congestion.[679-682] Frank heart failure may be a complication in as many of 40% of older adult patients with PSGN.

Edema is the presenting symptom in two thirds of patients and is present in as high as 90% of cases.[628] The presence of edema is based on primary renal sodium and fluid retention. The edema typically appears in the face and upper extremities. Ascites and anasarca may occur in children.

Encephalopathy presenting as confusion, headache, somnolence, or even convulsion, is not common and may affect children more frequently than adults. Encephalopathy is not always attributable to severe hypertension but may be the result of central nervous system vasculitis instead.[679,681-683]

The clinical manifestations of acute PSGN typically resolve in 1 to 2 weeks as the edema and hypertension disappear after diuresis, and the patient typically remains asymptomatic. Hematuria and proteinuria may persist for several months but are usually resolved within a year. However, proteinuria may persist in those patients who initially had nephrotic syndrome.[62] The long-term persistence of proteinuria, and especially albuminuria, may be an indication of persistence of proliferative glomerulonephritis.[634]

The differential diagnosis of acute PSGN includes (1) IgA nephropathy[684] and IgA vasculitis, especially when the acute nephritic syndrome is associated with gross or rusty hematuria; (2) MPGN and C3 glomerulopathy; or (3) acute crescentic glomerulonephritis (rapidly progressive glomerulonephritis: immune complex mediated, anti-GBM mediated, or pauci-immune). The occurrence of acute nephritis in the setting of persistent fever should raise the suspicion of a peri-infectious glomerulonephritis, especially with persistence of an infection such as an occult abscess or infective endocarditis.

Although rheumatic fever and PSGN rarely occur together, their co-concurrence has been described.[685]

LABORATORY FINDINGS

Hematuria, microscopic or gross, is nearly always present in acute PSGN. There are, however, rare cases of documented acute PSGN with no associated hematuria.[630,686] Microscopic examination of urine typically reveals the presence of dysmorphic red blood cells[687] or red blood cell casts. Other findings on microscopy are leukocytes, renal tubular epithelial cells, and hyaline and granular casts.[631] When the hematuria is macroscopic, the urine typically has a rusty or tea color.

Proteinuria is nearly always present but typically in the subnephrotic range. In half of patients, urinary protein excretion may be less than 500 mg of protein per day.[688,689] Nephrotic-range proteinuria may occur in as many as 20% of patients and is more frequent in adults than in children.[628] The excreted proteins may include large amounts of fibrin degradation products and fibrinopeptides.[686,690]

A pronounced decline in GFR is common in older adult patients with acute PSGN, affecting nearly 60% of patients 55 years of age and older.[681] This profound decrease in GFR is uncommon in patients from childhood to middle age. Indeed, because of the accompanying fluid retention and increase in circulatory volumes, a mild decrease in GFR may not be accompanied by an increase in serum creatinine concentration above laboratory limits of normal. Renal plasma flow, tubular reabsorptive capacity, and concentrating ability are typically not affected. On the other hand, urinary sodium excretion and calcium excretion are greatly reduced.[691]

A transient hyporeninemic hypoaldosteronism may lead to mild to moderate hyperkalemia. This may be exacerbated by a concomitant decrease in GFR and reduced distal delivery of solute. This type 4 renal tubular acidosis may resolve with the resolution of nephritis in the event of diuresis but may be persistent beyond that point in some patients.[692] The suppressed plasma renin activity may be a consequence of the volume expansion present in those patients.[693]

Cultures of throat or skin samples frequently reveal group A streptococci.[631,694] The sensitivity and specificity of these tests are likely affected by the method of obtaining a culture specimen and the test used.[695] Such cultures may be less satisfactory than serologic studies to evaluate for the presence of recent streptococcal infection in patients suspected of having PSGN.[696] The antibodies most commonly studied for the detection of a recent streptococcal infection are anti–streptolysin O, antistreptokinase, antihyaluronidase, antideoxyribonuclease B, and anti–nicotinamide adenine dinucleotidase.[697] Of these, the most commonly used is the anti–streptolysin O test. An elevated anti–streptolysin O titer above 200 units may be found in 90% of patients with pharyngeal infection.[631] In the diagnosis of an acute PSGN, however, a rise in titer is more specific than the absolute level of the titer. The latter is likely affected by the geographic and socioeconomic prevalence of pharyngeal infections with group A streptococci. Increased anti–streptolysin O titers are present in about two thirds of patients with upper respiratory tract infection but in only about one third of patients following streptococcal impetigo.[628] Serial anti–streptolysin O titer determinations with a twofold or greater rise in titer are highly indicative of a recent infection.[628,631]

The streptozyme test combines several antistreptococcal antibody assays and may be a useful screening test.[696] Since certain strains of type 12 group A streptococci do not produce streptolysin S or O, and in patients in whom impetigo-associated PSGN is suspected, testing for anti–deoxyribonuclease B and antihyaluronidase is a useful procedure.[641] Antibodies to other streptococcal cell wall glycoproteins may also increase, including those for endostreptosin.[631,698-701] On occasion, autoantibodies to collagen and laminin may be detected.[631,702] Cultures of throat or skin specimens may yield positive results in as few as one fourth of patients.

The serial measurement of complement component levels is important in the diagnosis of PSGN. Early in the acute phase, the levels of hemolytic complement activity (CH-50 and C3) are reduced. These levels return to normal usually within 8 weeks.[631,679,703-708] The reduction in serum C3 levels is especially marked in patients with C3NeF, which is capable of cleaving native C3.[547-549] The finding of low properdin and C3 levels, and concomitant normal to modestly reduced levels of C1q, C2, and C4[703,704,709] all point to the importance of the activation of the alternate pathway of the complement cascade.[703] Immunohistochemical analysis of mannose-binding protein and mannose-binding protein–associated serine proteinase 1 suggests that the lectin pathway of complement activation is engaged in about a third of patients.[710] There is some evidence as well for activation via the classical pathway.[711] Another complement level abnormality is a mild depression of C5 levels, whereas levels of C6 and C7 are most often normal.[547,631,709] The plasma level of soluble terminal complement components (C5b-9) rises acutely and then falls to normal.[704] Because complement levels typically return to normal within 8 weeks, the presence of persistent depression of C3 levels may be indicative of another diagnosis, such as MPGN, endocarditis, occult sepsis, SLE, atheromatous emboli, or congenital chronic complement deficiency.[703]

Circulating cryoglobulins[712,713] as well as circulating immune complexes[714-717] may be detected in some patients with PSGN. The pathophysiologic importance of these circulating immune complexes for the development of acute nephritis is unclear.[716-718]

Abnormalities in blood coagulation systems may be detected in acute PSGN; thus thrombocytopenia may be seen.[719] Elevated levels of fibrinogen, factor VIII, plasmin activity, and circulating high-molecular-weight fibrinogen complexes may be seen and correlate with disease activity and an unfavorable prognosis.[720-724]

Although complement studies suggest that the alternative pathways are primarily involved in acute PSGN, there is some evidence also for activation via the classical pathway.[711]

TREATMENT

Treatment of acute PSGN is largely supportive care. Children almost invariably recover from the initial episode.[725-727] Of concern to clinicians are those patients who have acute renal failure at presentation. An initial episode of acute renal failure is not necessarily associated with a bad prognosis.[677] In a study of 20 adult patients with diffuse proliferative glomerulonephritis, 11 had acute renal failure and 9 had normal or mild renal insufficiency. There were no differences between these groups in clinical, immunologic, or histologic features. After 18 months of follow-up, outcome was similar in the two groups. Thus, there is little evidence to suggest the need for any form of immunosuppressive therapy. Because of the profound salt and water retention observed in these patients—and, in some, pulmonary congestion—it is important to use loop diuretics such as furosemide to avoid volume expansion and hypertension. When volume expansion does occur, antihypertensive agents are frequently useful to ameliorate the hypertension. Interestingly, plasma renin levels are reduced; however, captopril has been shown to lower blood pressure and improve GFR in patients with PSGN.[728]

Some patients with substantial volume expansion and marked pulmonary congestion show no response to diuretic therapy. In those individuals, dialytic support is appropriate, either hemodialysis or continuous venovenous hemofiltration in adults or peritoneal dialysis in children. Some patients develop substantial hyperkalemia. In those patients, treatment with exchange resins or dialysis may be useful. Importantly, so-called potassium-sparing agents, including triamterene, spironolactone, and amiloride, should not be used in this disease state. Usually, patients undergo a spontaneous diuresis within 7 to 10 days after the onset of their illness no longer require supportive care.[677,729] There is no evidence to date that early treatment of streptococcal disease, either pharyngitic or cellulitic, will alter the risk of PSGN. It has long been speculated that treatment with penicillin can control the spread of outbreaks of epidemic PSGN. In studies from aboriginal communities in Australia, the use of benzathine penicillin prevented new cases of PSGN, especially in children with skin sores and household contact with affected cases.[730]

The long-term prognosis of patients with PSGN is not as benign as previously considered. Widespread crescentic glomerulonephritis results in an increased number of obsolescent glomeruli associated with tubulointerstitial disease that results in progressive reduction of the renal mass over time.[731] A proportion of patients with streptococcal glomerulonephritis develop hypertension, proteinuria, and renal insufficiency 10 and 40 years after the illness.[731-733]

Nonetheless, it is most common that the long-term disease process is marked only by mild hypertension.

In some patients, there is evidence to suggest that the original diagnosis of PSGN may have been in error. This is especially true for individuals in whom a kidney biopsy was never performed. For instance, a patient who has an upper respiratory tract infection and then develops a glomerulonephritis may be considered to have PSGN when, in fact, the patient has another proliferative form of glomerulonephritis. In these patients, lack of resolution of the kidney disease should prompt a kidney biopsy to elucidate the underlying cause of the glomerular injury.

IMMUNOGLOBULIN A NEPHROPATHY

EPIDEMIOLOGY

IgA nephropathy remains one of most common forms, if not the most common form, of glomerulonephritis, especially in developed countries with low prevalence of infectious diseases.[734] Initially described in the late 1960s by Berger and Hinglais,[735,736] the disorder is characterized by deposition predominantly of IgA (and, to a lesser extent, of other immunoglobulins) in the mesangium with mesangial proliferation and with clinical features that span the spectrum from asymptomatic hematuria to rapidly progressive glomerulonephritis. Although it was previously considered a benign disease, it is now clear that up to 40% of patients may progress to ESKD. Moreover, it has become recognized that, in addition to a primary form of the disorder, IgA nephropathy is also associated with and may be secondary to a variety of disease processes (Table 32.14).

IgA nephropathy occurs in individuals of all ages, but it is most common in the second and third decades of life, and it is much more common in males than females (Table 32.15). IgA nephropathy is uncommon in children younger than 10 years of age. In fact, 80% of patients are between the ages of 16 and 35 at the time of kidney biopsy.[737-742] The male/female ratio has been described as anywhere from 2:1 to 6:1.[737-742]

The distribution of IgA nephropathy varies in different geographic regions throughout the world.[743] It is the most common form of primary glomerular disease in Asia, accounting for up to 30% to 40% of all biopsies performed for diagnosis of glomerular disease, and it accounts for 20% of all biopsies in Europe and 10% of all biopsies in North America.[743] This wide variation in incidence is partly attributable to the differing indications for kidney biopsy in Asia compared with those in North America. In Asia, urinalyses are performed routinely in school-aged children. Those with asymptomatic hematuria typically undergo biopsy, which may lead to an increased number of diagnoses of IgA nephropathy. Genetic issues may also be important in the

Table 32.14 Classification of Immunoglobulin A (IgA) Nephropathy

Primary IgA Nephropathy
Secondary IgA Nephropathy
Associated Disorders
IgA vasculitis
HIV infection
Toxoplasmosis
Seronegative spondyloarthropathy
Celiac disease
Dermatitis herpetiformis
Crohn's disease
Liver disease
Alcoholic cirrhosis
Ankylosing spondylitis
Reiter's syndrome
Neoplasia
Mycosis fungoides
Lung carcinoma
Mucin-secreting carcinoma
Cyclic neutropenia
Immunothrombocytopenia
Gluten-sensitive enteropathy
Scleritis
Sicca syndrome
Mastitis
Pulmonary hemosiderosis
Berger's disease
Leprosy
Familial IgA Nephropathy

Data from references 780, 802, 814, 925, 926, and 1392-1419.

Table 32.15 Diseases That Cause Glomerulonephritis*

Glomerular Lesion	N	Male/Female Ratio	White/Black Ratio
IgA nephropathy	693	2.0:1.0	14.0:1.0
MPGN type I	248	1.2:1.0	3.3:1.0
Anti-GBM	82	1.1:1.0	7.9:1.0
ANCA-GN	257	1.0:1.0	6.7:1.0
Fibrillary glomerulonephritis	76	1.0:1.2	14.3:1.0

*Based on the analysis of 9605 native kidney biopsy specimens evaluated at the University of North Carolina Nephropathology Laboratory. This laboratory evaluates kidney biopsy specimens from a base population of approximately 10 million throughout the southeastern United States and centered in North Carolina. The expected white/black ratio in this kidney biopsy population is approximately 3:2. ANCA-GN, Antineutrophil cytoplasmic antibody–associated glomerulonephritis; GBM, glomerular basement membrane; IgA, immunoglobulin A; MPGN, membranoproliferative glomerulonephritis.

geographic differences. A Japanese study of biopsy specimens obtained from kidney donors immediately before transplantation showed that 16% of donors had covert mesangial deposition of IgA.[744] IgA nephropathy has been reported to be rare in African Americans,[745,746] although population-based incidence rates of newly diagnosed IgA nephropathy have been found to be similar in African American and white populations.[747] IgA nephropathy is quite common in Native Americans of the Zuni and Navajo tribes.[748] The prevalence of IgA in the general population has been estimated to be between 25 and 50 cases per 100,000,[743,749] although notably, almost 5% of all patients undergoing kidney biopsy have at least some IgA deposits in their glomeruli.[750] Population studies in Germany and in France calculated an incidence of 2 cases per 10,000,[751-754] but autopsy studies performed in Singapore[755] suggested that 2.0% to 4.8% of the population had IgA deposition in their glomeruli.

GENETICS

IgA nephropathy is a histologically based diagnosis; it is unlikely to be related to a single genetic locus but rather is probably due to the interactions of multiple susceptibility and progression genes in combination with environmental factors.[756] A number of studies suggest that there are genes which render an individual susceptible to IgA nephropathy and genes that portend a more rapid progression of IgA nephropathy. Polymorphisms in a number of genes, including those coding for ACE, angiotensin, angiotensin II receptor, T cell receptor, IL-1 and IL-6, interleukin receptor antagonist, TGF, mannose-binding lectin, uteroglobin, nitric oxide synthase, and TNF, as well as major histocompatibility loci have been evaluated as possibly affecting both the susceptibility to and progression of disease.[730,757-763] A number of studies have examined the role of the ACE gene in IgA nephropathy with or without progressive disease. The D allele of the ACE gene may be associated with susceptibility to IgA nephropathy in Asians but not in whites.[764] The Polymorphism Research to Distinguish Genetic Factors Contributing to Progression of IgA Nephropathy (PREDICT-IgAN) study, which investigated associations between progression of IgA nephropathy and 100 atherosclerotic disease–related gene polymorphisms using a retrospective candidate gene approach, found significant associations between polymorphisms in the glycoprotein Ia and intercellular adhesion molecule-1 genes and progression of disease.[765] In this study, the association between the ACE I/D polymorphism and progression of disease was not found to be significant after adjustment for multiple comparisons.

Familial IgA nephropathy has been reported in multiple ethnic groups around the world, including Africa and Central America. Indeed, some studies suggest that 4% to 14% of patients with IgA nephropathy may have a family history of kidney disease,[751,766,767] and systematic screening of asymptomatic first-degree relatives has detected hematuria in more than 25% of them.[768] Disease findings in most pedigrees are consistent with autosomal dominant transmission with incomplete penetrance.[766] However, in some families, IgA nephropathy may aggregate with other glomerular diseases.[766,769]

Linkage studies have suggested an association of IgA nephropathy with genes at several loci.[766] Based on a genomewide linkage study of 30 kindreds with IgA nephropathy, a locus on chromosome 6q22-23 was identified with a logarithm of the odds ratio (LOD) score of 5.6[770]; and was named *IGAN1* (A LOD score of 3 or higher signifies odds of 1000:1 or higher in favor of linkage).[766]

Genomewide association studies have successfully identified candidate genes and single-nucleotide polymorphisms (SNPs) that may correlate with susceptibility to or protection against IgA nephropathy. A genomewide association study was first performed using DNA within the UK Glomerulonephritis DNA Bank from individuals with IgA nephropathy[771] and then later in Chinese cohorts.[772,773] These studies led to the identification of seven susceptibility loci (three loci within the MHC region on chromosome 6p21, DEFA locus on chromosome 8p23, TNFSF13 locus on chromosome 17p23, HORMAD2 locus on chromosome 22q12, and CFH/CFHR locus on chromosome 1q32), which implicate defects in innate immunity, adaptive immunity, and the alternative complement pathway.[774,775] Notably, the major histocompatibility complex has been implicated in every genomewide association study to date.

The prevailing hypothesis regarding the pathogenesis of IgA nephropathy focuses on defects in protein glycosylation, particularly in B cells secreting IgA1. Studies measuring serum levels of galactose-deficient IgA1 in patients with IgA nephropathy, their relatives, and unrelated controls found a higher level of aberrantly glycosylated IgA1 in patients with familial or sporadic IgA nephropathy and in their at-risk relatives than in unrelated individuals or control subjects.[776,777] This finding suggests that abnormal IgA1 glycosylation is an inherited rather than an acquired trait. Polymorphisms of the genes for the enzymes responsible for glycosylation of IgA1 may thus be associated with increased susceptibility to IgA nephropathy. Such genes include core 1β-galactosyltransferase gene (*C1GALT1*)[778,779] and the molecular chaperone COSMC (*C1GALT1C1*), although the findings are inconsistent across studies.

PATHOLOGY

Immunofluorescence Microscopy

IgA nephropathy can be definitively diagnosed only by the immunohistologic demonstration of glomerular immune deposits that stain dominantly or codominantly for IgA compared with IgG and IgM (Figure 32.26).[780-783] The staining is usually exclusively or predominantly mesangial, although a minority of specimens, especially from patients with severe disease, will have substantial capillary wall staining. By definition, 100% of IgA nephropathy specimens stain for IgA. On a scale of 0 to 4+, the mean intensity of IgA staining is approximately 3+.[782] IgM staining is observed in 84% of specimens with a mean intensity (when present) of only approximately 1+. IgG staining is observed in 62% of specimens, also with a mean intensity (when present) of approximately 1+. Early studies of IgA nephropathy described more frequent and more intense IgG staining than is seen today, but this probably was caused by the use of less specific antibodies that cross-react between IgA and IgG. Almost all IgA nephropathy specimens have substantial staining for C3. In contrast, staining for C1q is rare and weak when present. If there is intense staining in a specimen that shows substantial IgA and IgG, the possibility of lupus nephritis rather than

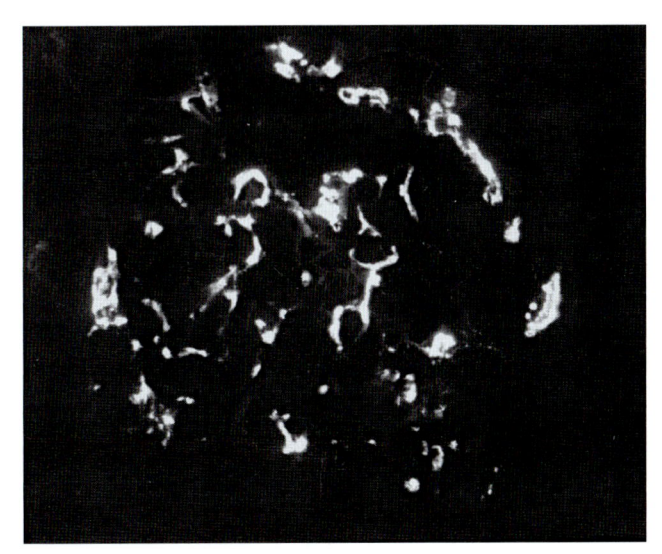

Figure 32.26 Immunofluorescence micrograph of a glomerulus with features of immunoglobulin A (IgA) nephropathy showing intense mesangial staining for IgA. (Fluorescein isothiocyanate anti-IgA stain, ×300.)

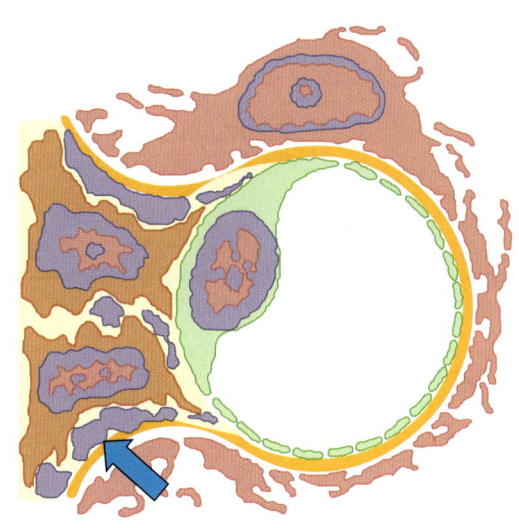

Figure 32.27 Diagram depicting the ultrastructural features of immunoglobulin A (IgA) nephropathy. Note the mesangial dense deposits (*arrow*) and mesangial hypercellularity. (Courtesy J. Charles Jennette, University of North Carolina at Chapel Hill, Chapel Hill, NC.)

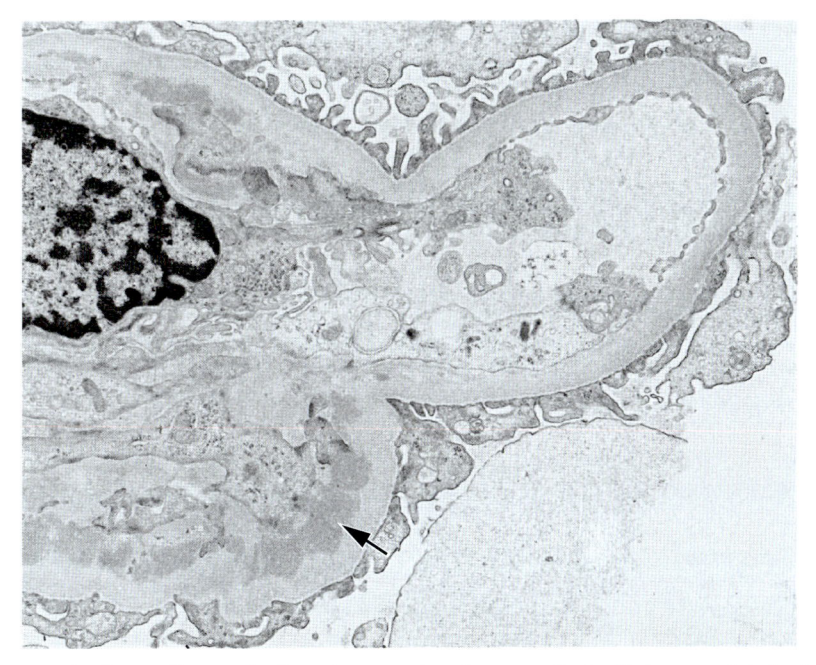

Figure 32.28 Electron micrograph of a capillary and adjacent mesangium from a patient with immunoglobulin A (IgA) nephropathy showing mesangial dense deposits (*arrow*) immediately beneath the perimesangial basement membrane. (×7000.)

IgA nephropathy should be considered.[782] An additional relatively distinctive feature of IgA nephropathy is that, unlike any other glomerular immune complex disease, the immune deposits usually have more intense staining for λ-light chains than κ-light chains.[780,782]

Electron Microscopy

The ubiquitous ultrastructural finding is mesangial electron-dense deposits that correspond to the immune deposits seen by immunohistologic analysis (Figures 32.27 and 32.28).[781] The mesangial deposits often are immediately beneath the perimesangial basement membrane. They are accompanied by varying degrees of mesangial matrix expansion and hypercellularity. Most specimens do not have capillary wall deposits, but a minority, especially from patients with more severe disease, show scattered subendothelial dense deposits, subepithelial dense deposits, or both. The extent of endocapillary proliferation and leukocyte infiltration parallels the pattern of injury observed by light microscopy. Epithelial foot process effacement is observed in those patients with substantial proteinuria.

Light Microscopy

IgA nephropathy can cause any of the light microscopic phenotypes of proliferative glomerulonephritis (Figure 32.29) or may cause no discernible histologic changes.[781-788]

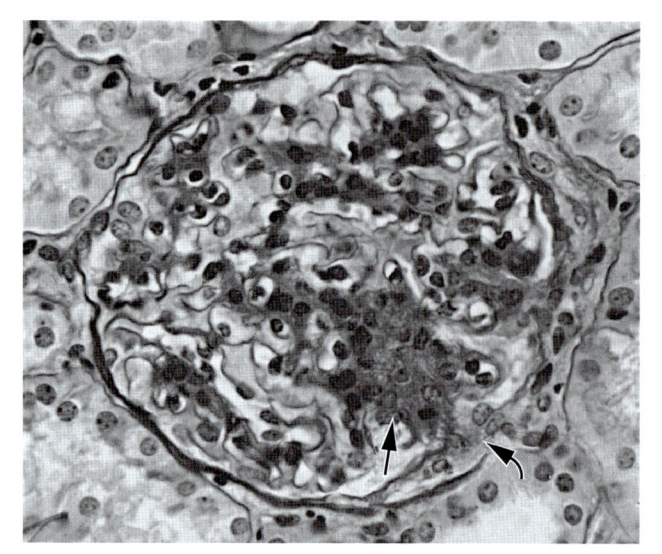

Figure 32.29 Light micrograph of a glomerulus with features of immunoglobulin A (IgA) nephropathy showing segmental mesangial matrix expansion and hypercellularity (*straight arrow*) and an adhesion to Bowman's capsule (*curved arrow*). (Periodic acid–Schiff stain, ×300.)

As depicted in Figure 32.30, this spectrum of glomerular inflammatory responses is shared by a variety of glomerulonephritides that have different causes but induce similar or identical light microscopic alterations in glomeruli. At the time of biopsy, IgA nephropathy usually manifests as a focal or diffuse mesangioproliferative or proliferative glomerulonephritis, although specimens from a few patients will have no lesion by light microscopy, those from a few will show aggressive disease with crescents, and occasional specimens will already demonstrate chronic sclerosing disease. Different criteria for performing kidney biopsy result in different frequencies of the various phenotypes of IgA nephropathy among distinct populations of patients. Of 668 consecutive native kidney IgA nephropathy specimens diagnosed in the University of North Carolina Nephropathology Laboratory, 4% showed no lesion by light microscopy, 13% had exclusively mesangioproliferative glomerulonephritis, 37% had focal proliferative glomerulonephritis (25% of these had <50% crescents), 28% had diffuse proliferative glomerulonephritis (45% of these had <50% crescents), 4% had crescentic glomerulonephritis (50% or more crescents), 6% had focal sclerosing glomerulonephritis without residual proliferative activity, 6% had diffuse chronic sclerosing glomerulonephritis, and 2% had lesions that did not fall into any of these categories.

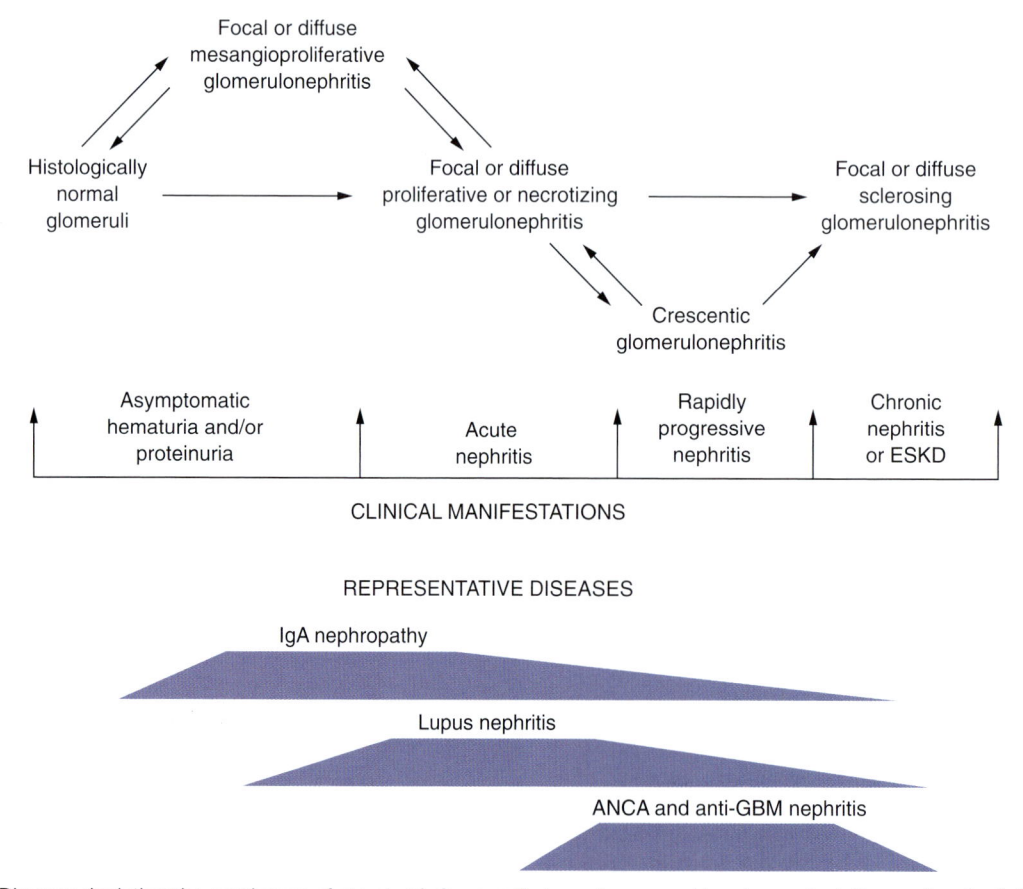

Figure 32.30 Diagram depicting the continuum of structural changes that can be caused by glomerular inflammation (*top*), the usual clinical syndromes that are caused by each expression of glomerular injury (*middle*), and the portion of the continuum that most often corresponds to several specific categories of glomerular disease (*bottom*). ANCA, Antineutrophil cytoplasmic autoantibody; ESKD, end-stage kidney disease; GBM, glomerular basement membrane; IgA, immunoglobulin A.

The mildest light microscopic expression of IgA nephropathy, other than no discernible lesion, is focal or diffuse mesangial hypercellularity without more complex endocapillary hypercellularity, such as endothelial proliferation or influx of leukocytes. This is analogous to International Society of Nephrology/Renal Pathology Service class II lupus nephritis. More severe inflammatory injury causes focal (involving less than 50% of glomeruli) or diffuse proliferative glomerulonephritis as the pathologic expression of IgA nephropathy, which is pathologically analogous to class III and class IV lupus nephritis. The lesions are characterized by not only mesangial hypercellularity but also some degree of endothelial proliferation or leukocyte infiltration that distorts or obliterates some capillary lumens. Extensive necrosis is rare in IgA nephropathy, although slight focal segmental necrosis with karyorrhexis can occur in severely inflamed glomeruli. With time, destructive glomerular inflammatory lesions progress to sclerotic lesions that may form adhesions to Bowman's capsule. Occasional patients with IgA nephropathy will have focal glomerular sclerosis by light microscopy that is indistinguishable from FSGS until the immunofluorescence microscopic findings are taken into consideration. Because of the episodic nature of IgA nephropathy, many patients have combinations of focal sclerotic lesions and focal active proliferative lesions. Patients with the most severe IgA nephropathy have crescent formation because of extensive disruption of capillaries.[788] Advanced chronic disease is characterized by extensive glomerular sclerosis associated with marked tubular atrophy, interstitial fibrosis, and interstitial infiltration by mononuclear leukocytes.

Whether histologic features detected on kidney biopsy can be used to predict the progression of IgA nephropathy has been studied for many years. Nephropathologic findings have previously provided limited prognostic value over and above that of simple clinical parameters such as blood pressure, serum creatinine level, and the degree of proteinuria. The Oxford classification of IgA nephropathy study is a seminal investigation that assessed the value of specific pathologic features in predicting the risk of progression of kidney disease in IgA nephropathy.[789,790] The study population was a multiethnic cohort of patients with IgA nephropathy that included children (n = 59) and adults (n = 206) who were followed for a mean of 69 months. By an iterative process, pathologic variables selected based on reproducibility, least susceptibility to sampling error, ease of scoring, and independent association with outcome were then correlated through multivariate analysis with three clinical outcomes: the rate of kidney function decline, survival from a 50% decline in kidney function or ESKD, and proteinuria during follow-up.[789]

Four parameters emerged as independently predictive of clinical outcomes: mesangial hypercellularity, endocapillary hypercellularity, segmental glomerulosclerosis, and tubular atrophy/interstitial fibrosis. Of these predictors, mesangial hypercellularity was significantly associated with ESKD or 50% reduction in GFR, segmental sclerosis was associated with the rate of decline in kidney function, and tubular atrophy/interstitial fibrosis was statistically associated with both the rate of decline and ESKD or 50% decline in kidney function. Endocapillary hypercellularity was not significantly predictive of the rate of decline of kidney function or survival from ESKD or 50% reduction in kidney function. However, patients with endocapillary (or extracapillary) hypercellularity were more likely to receive immunosuppressive therapy, and the relationship between this pathologic variable and the rate of decline in kidney function may have been influenced by the use of immunosuppression. This latter finding indirectly suggests that patients with this type of lesion are responsive to immunosuppressive therapy.

These conclusions led to a proposal to incorporate the following scoring of the four identified parameters (known as the *Oxford-MEST score*) into the pathology report for IgA nephropathy.[789]

Mesangial hypercellularity: score ≤0.5 = 0, or score >0.5 = 1
Endocapillary hypercellularity: absent = 0 or present = 1
Segmental glomerulosclerosis: absent = 0 or present = 1
Tubular atrophy/interstitial fibrosis: percentage of cortical area ≤25% = 0, 26% to 50% = 1, or >50% = 2

This scoring system was shown to be valid for both children and adults,[791] but true proof of its utility required validation in separate cohorts, especially in comparison to clinical features such as serum creatinine level and proteinuria.[792] Since the development of the Oxford classification of IgA nephropathy, a meta-analysis of 16 subsequent retrospective cohort studies between January 2009 and December 2012 assessing the utility of the scoring system found that M, S, T, and crescent (C) lesions (not E lesions) were strongly associated with progression to kidney failure defined as doubled serum creatinine level, 50% decline in eGFR, or ESKD.[793] A large validation study in Europe examined 1147 patients that had the whole spectrum of IgA nephropathy.[794] Over a median follow-up of 4.7 years, in patients with an eGFR less than 30 mL/min/1.73 m^2, M and T lesions independently predicted a poor survival, and in patients with urinary protein excretion less than 0.5 g/day, both M and E lesions were associated with a rise in proteinuria to 1 or 2 g/day or more. The combination of M, S, and T lesions with clinical parameters significantly increased the ability to predict progression in the absence of substantial immunosuppressive therapy. Studies to date have been retrospective and thus prospective studies using the Oxford classification are warranted.

PATHOGENESIS

A great deal of progress has been made in our understanding of the pathogenesis of IgA nephropathy.[730,795,796] The characteristic pathologic finding by immunofluorescence microscopy of granular deposits of IgA and C3 in the glomerular mesangium, as well as the dermal capillaries in IgA vasculitis, suggests that this disease is the result of the deposition of circulating immune complexes leading to the activation of the complement cascade via the alternate pathway. The deposited IgA is predominantly polymeric IgA1.[797-800] The fact that polymeric IgA1 is usually derived mainly from the mucosal immune system, as well as the association of clinical flare-ups in some cases of IgA nephropathy with syndromes that affect the respiratory tract or gastrointestinal tract, has led to the suggestion that IgA nephropathy is a consequence of defective mucosal immunity.[801] This concept was supported by the finding in some patients with IgA nephropathy of antibodies to dietary antigens or various infectious agents, both viral and bacterial,[802-815] and the clinical observation that hematuria increases acutely in some patients at the time of upper respiratory tract or gastrointestinal infections. However, it has now been determined that the elevation in polymeric IgA1 antibody synthesis does not occur in the mucosa, and polymeric IgA levels are increased after systemic immunization with tetanus toxoid.[798,816,817] In addition, an increase in IgA-secreting B cells was documented in both peripheral blood[818] and bone marrow[819] of patients.

Serum levels of IgA do not correlate with either disease activity or mesangial deposits; therefore, it is unlikely that the pathogenesis of IgA nephropathy is related to a quantitative increase in serum levels of polymeric IgA1. Rather, it relates to an anomaly in the IgA molecule itself, namely, in its glycosylation, as discussed earlier.[820] This is best exemplified by patients with IgA-secreting multiple myeloma, among whom only those patients with aberrant IgA glycosylation develop glomerulonephritis.

In humans, the heavy chain of IgA1, but not that of IgA2, contains an 18–amino acid hinge region that is rich in proline, serine, and threonine residues. O-linked monosaccharides or oligosaccharides consisting of N-acetylgalactosamine can be posttranslationally added to these amino acid residues. This N-acetylgalactosamine is usually substituted with a terminal galactose.[821] Lectin-binding studies and carbohydrate composition analysis have demonstrated that the IgA1 in patients with IgA nephropathy contains less terminal galactose than that of healthy control subjects.[798,822] The addition of a galactose residue to the glycosyl side chain is blocked by premature sialylation of the N-acetylgalactosamine residues on the hinge region of IgA1. The precise cause of this has not been fully elucidated. Three mechanisms have been postulated: excessive activity of α2,6-sialyltransferase, decreased activity of β1,3-galactosyltransferase, and decreased stability of β1,3-galactosyltransferase due to decreased activity of its chaperone (Cosmc).[823,824] Whether these abnormalities are acquired or genetically determined remains unclear.[779,825,826] IgA glycosylation may also be influenced by acquired abnormalities such as the polarity of the T cell cytokine milieu.[827]

Galactose-deficient IgA1 (Gd-IgA1) results in IgA1 hinge region exposure of N-acetylgalactosamine and neoepitope formation. This neoepitope is the target of IgG autoantibodies as demonstrated in studies of immortalized B cells from patients with IgA nephropathy,[824,828] and IgG autoantibodies specific for Gd-IgA1 are found in the circulation of such patients.[829] These autoantibodies were found to be of highly restricted heterogeneity directed at the unique epitopes present on the abnormally glycosylated IgA1.[828] The autoantibodies and target Gd-IgA1 form circulating immune complexes[830,831] that escape removal by the reticuloendothelial system and deposit in glomeruli via an interaction with a mesangial IgA receptor, possibly the transferrin receptor.[832-835] Once deposited in glomerular mesangium, these immune complexes provoke mesangial proliferation.[836] The deposition of IgA in glomeruli may also occur independently of immune complex formation[837] because abnormally glycosylated IgA1 also leads to an increased binding in the kidney.[820,831,838] However, aberrantly glycosylated IgA in isolation does not cause mesangial proliferation in tissue culture.[828] Mesangial Gd-IgA1 molecules induce a variety of phlogistic mediators, including cytokines, chemokines, and growth factors, as well as complement activation through the mannose-binding lectin pathway.[839-841]

Of particular interest is the clinical relevance of Gd-IgA1 and anti–Gd-IgA1 autoantibodies. A recent study demonstrated that serum levels of IgG- and IgA-based antiglycan autoantibodies from 97 patients with IgA nephropathy, compared to 30 patients with non-IgA nephropathy disease and 30 healthy controls, correlate with disease progression and poor prognosis.[842] A larger subsequent study followed 275 patients with IgA nephropathy for a median of 47 months (range, 12 to 96 months) and assessed renal survival. Not only was the level of Gd-IgA1 elevated compared to healthy controls, but higher levels were independently associated with a greater risk of renal failure (HR per standard deviation of natural log–transformed Gd-IgA1, 1.44; 95% CI, 1.11 to 1.88; $P = 0.006$).[843]

Another component of the pathogenesis of IgA nephropathy pertains to direct cytokine- or chemokine-induced podocyte injury, which is reflected by increased podocyturia. Podocyte damage may be the result of local complement activation and elevated levels of platelet-derived growth factor or TNF-α levels.[844-846]

It is hypothesized that a subsequent autoantibody response may be triggered by an environmental cross-reacting antigen and lead to in situ immune complex formation by interaction of circulating autoantibodies to the "planted" autoantigen. Formation of circulating immune complexes with abnormally glycosylated IgA and circulating IgA receptor molecules could also be involved.[847] Because IgA1 is normally cleared from the circulation by the liver via the asialoglycoprotein receptor,[848-850] it is also thought that the defective galactosylation of the hinge region in IgA1 may lead to decreased clearance of IgA1 molecules in patients with IgA nephropathy.[838,851]

The existence, nature, and role of other autoantibodies in IgA nephropathy is also under investigation. A number of autoantibodies to various putative autoantigens have been described in IgA nephropathy.[852] Such autoantigens include a mesangial cell membrane antigen,[853] endothelial cells (human umbilical vein endothelial cells),[803,852] single-stranded DNA,[803] and cardiolipin.[803,854] Most of these autoantibodies were found in subsets of patients that rarely exceeded 3% of patients with IgA nephropathy and may sometimes be the result of high circulating levels of IgA in these patients.[854] A more recent integrative "antibiomics" approach found 117 specific autoantibodies, many of which were directed to proteins within the kidney.[855] The presence of IgG ANCAs has been described to occur in a minority of patients with IgA nephropathy.[856] In addition, IgA ANCAs have been rarely associated with a systemic vasculitis, IgA vasculitis.[857-859] In the setting of IgA ANCAs, the autoantigen seems to be different from the major ANCA autoantigens, namely, myeloperoxidase (MPO) and proteinase 3 (PR3). Circulating IgA-fibronectin complexes have also been described in the circulation of patients with IgA nephropathy and HIV infection.[860] These complexes may not be true immune complexes, however, and may be directly related to increased IgA levels in patients with IgA nephropathy.[861] A special form of IgA-dominant immune complex glomerulonephritis that resembles postinfectious glomerulonephritis occurs secondary to staphylococcal infection, especially but not exclusively in patients with diabetes.[862]

CLINICAL FEATURES AND NATURAL HISTORY

Approximately 40% to 50% of patients have macroscopic hematuria at the time of their initial presentation. The episodes tend to occur in close temporal relationship to upper respiratory infection, including tonsillitis or pharyngitis. This synchronous association of pharyngitis and macroscopic hematuria has been given the name *synpharyngitic nephritis*. Much less commonly, episodes of macroscopic hematuria follow infections that involve the urinary tract or gastroenteritis. Macroscopic hematuria may be entirely asymptomatic but more often is associated with dysuria that may prompt the treating physician to consider bacterial cystitis. Systemic symptoms are frequently found, including nonspecific symptoms such as malaise, fatigue, myalgia, and fever. Some patients have abdominal or flank pain.[863,864] In a minority of patients (less than 5%), malignant hypertension may be an associated presenting feature.[865] In the most severe cases (less than 10%), acute glomerulonephritis results in acute renal insufficiency and failure.[866,867] Recovery typically occurs with resolution of symptoms, even in those patients who have been temporarily dialysis dependent.[867]

Macroscopic hematuria due to IgA nephropathy occurs more often in children than young adults. When it occurs in older individuals, it should raise the possibility of the more common causes of urinary tract bleeding, such as stones or malignancy.

A presentation with asymptomatic microscopic hematuria, with or without proteinuria, occurs in 30% to 40% of patients. Patients with IgA nephropathy come for evaluation of asymptomatic hematuria with or without the presence of proteinuria. In addition to having glomerulonephritis, these patients may commonly have hypertension. In fact, in white patients with hypertension and hematuria, IgA nephropathy is the most common form of hematuria.[868] Intermittent macroscopic hematuria occurs in 25% of these patients. Microscopic hematuria and proteinuria persist between episodes of macroscopic hematuria.

Patients with nephrotic syndrome at presentation may have widespread proliferative glomerulonephritis or coexisting IgA nephropathy and minimal change glomerulopathies.[869] Finally, some patients with IgA nephropathy have reached ESKD at the time of their first presentation. These individuals typically have had asymptomatic microscopic hematuria and proteinuria that has remained undetected.[866]

In addition to idiopathic IgA nephropathy, there is secondary IgA nephropathy that is the glomerular expression of a systemic disease (see Table 32.14). For example, patients with IgA vasculitis have abdominal pain, arthritis, a vasculitic rash, and a glomerulonephritis that is indistinguishable from that of primary IgA nephropathy. This condition is discussed more fully in Chapter 33.

Although IgA nephropathy was earlier thought to carry a relatively benign prognosis, it is estimated that, measured from the time of diagnosis, 1% to 2% of all patients with IgA nephropathy will develop ESKD each year. In a review encompassing 1900 patients derived from 11 separate series, long-term renal survival was estimated to be 78% to 87% at a decade after presentation.[870] Similarly, European studies have suggested that renal insufficiency may occur in 20% to 30% of patients within two decades of the original presentation.[741] In a study of the natural history of IgA nephropathy and "isolated" microscopic hematuria in 135 Chinese children,[30] spontaneous clinical remission occurred in 12%, whereas 88% had persisting hematuria. Almost 30% developed new onset of proteinuria, and hypertension developed in 32%. Eventually, 20% developed renal insufficiency of varying severity. A poor outcome was associated with persistent hematuria, microalbuminuria, and tubulointerstitial changes on the kidney biopsy specimen. This study clearly demonstrates that careful follow-up is required for all patients given the diagnosis of IgA nephropathy.

Overall, about 25% of patients develop ESKD within 10 to 25 years from diagnosis, depending on the initial severity of disease. Patients with episodes of gross (macroscopic) hematuria generally have a more favorable prognosis than those with persisting microhematuria; however, after an episode of microhematuria associated with acute renal failure a portion of patients (about 25%) may not recover normal kidney function.[871] The proliferative forms of IgA nephropathy seem to be associated with better outcomes in children than in adults.[872] It is unclear whether sex affects the prognosis of IgA nephropathy,[873] although some studies suggest that prognosis may be worse for males. Older age at disease onset may also connote a poor prognosis.[870,874-878]

Several studies have assessed features that predict a poor prognosis. Sustained hypertension, persistent proteinuria (especially proteinuria of >1 g protein per 24 hours), impaired kidney function, and nephrotic syndrome are markers of poor prognosis.[767,783,874] Controversy persists with respect to the issue of recurring bouts of macroscopic hematuria.[879] It is possible that macroscopic hematuria is an overt manifestation of disease and therefore identifies patients earlier in the course of their disease. Alternatively, macroscopic hematuria may represent an episodic process that results in self-limited inflammation, in contrast to persistent hematuria that represents ongoing, low-grade inflammation. In general, persistent microscopic hematuria is associated with a poor prognosis.[880] It is important to note that acute renal failure associated with macroscopic hematuria does not affect long-term prognosis. The fact that acute renal failure does occur during gross episodes of hematuria has been confirmed.[881-883] In these patients, the acute renal failure is most likely associated with acute tubular damage and not true crescentic disease. After the episodes of gross hematuria, kidney function typically returns to baseline and the long-term prognosis is good.

The degree of proteinuria is more than likely an additional marker of glomerular disease. Whether this is a consequence of the relationship between proteinuria and the tubular dysfunction found in many forms of glomerular disease or is specific to IgA nephropathy is not clear. In a study by Chen and colleagues,[884] mice that had been made proteinuric by various methods had enhanced deposition of administered IgA immune complexes. This suggests that these complexes might be more easily deposited in proteinuric states. More importantly, the amount of protein excretion 1 year after diagnosis was highly predictive of the development of ESKD within 7 years of subsequent follow-up. Individuals with urinary protein excretion of less than 500 mg/dL/24 hr had no renal failure within 7 years, whereas those with more than 3 g of protein excretion had approximately 60% chance of ESKD.[885]

Many formulas have been advanced to predict progression of IgA nephropathy in individual patients that yield different results for the same patient. The Toronto formula based on average mean arterial pressure and proteinuria during the first 2 years of observation is the best validated in white American and European subjects,[886] but a large fraction of the variation in progression remains unexplained by these two factors. Risk stratification for progression can be aided by algorithms employing a small set of variables (age, sex, family history of chronic kidney disease, reduced eGFR at diagnosis, proteinuria, serum albumin and total serum protein levels, hematuria, systolic or diastolic blood pressure, and histologic variables).[887-890] An absolute renal risk score to predict dialysis or death, developed by analysis of a prospective cohort of 332 patients with biopsy-proven IgA nephropathy followed for an average of 13 years, allowed for significant risk stratification ($P < 0.0001$) by counting the number of risk factors present at diagnosis: hypertension, proteinuria 1 g/day or more, and severe pathologic lesions.[891] One of the most recent risk prediction scores based on a large cohort of Chinese patients with IgA nephropathy, using four baseline variables (lower eGFR, serum albumin, hemoglobin, and higher systolic blood pressure) had a significant independent effect on risk of ESKD.[892] Treatment has also favorably influenced the long-term trends of progression in IgA nephropathy[893] and a postdiagnosis *decline* in the level of protein excretion to less than 1.0 g/day is a very reliable surrogate measure of a more favorable long-term prognosis.[894]

A large number of factors other than simple clinical assessment have been examined to predict outcomes. Some have been independently correlated with outcomes, whereas others have failed to demonstrate any added value in prognostication or therapeutic decision making.[895] Some of the more recently described factors include autophagy in podocytes,[896] CD19+CD5+ B cells in kidney biopsy specimens and in blood,[897] C5b-9 glomerular deposition,[898] extensive C4d deposition in the mesangium,[899] tubular $\alpha_3\beta_1$ integrin expression,[898] granule membrane protein of 17 kDa (GMP-17)-positive T cells in renal tubules,[900] glomerular density and size,[901] urinary epidermal growth factor/monocyte chemotactic peptide 1 ratios,[902,903] urinary growth arrest and DNA damage-45γ (GADD45γ) expression,[904] analysis of the urinary proteome (kininogen, trypsin-inhibitor chain-4, transthyretin)[905] and the fractional urinary excretion of IgG (in combination with assessment of nephron loss) in crescentic IgA nephropathy.[906] Likewise, hematuria associated with podocyturia may be associated with a poorer prognosis.[907] The clinical utility and applicability of these assays in prognostication and treatment decision making remains to be established and individual patient-level risk prediction still remains limited until risk scoring systems are validated in multiple diverse cohorts.

In addition to these variables, obesity,[908] elevated nocturnal blood pressure,[909] increased uric acid levels,[909] and elevated levels of C4-binding protein[910] have been associated with a poorer prognosis. Moderate alcohol consumption is associated with an improved prognosis in IgA nephropathy.[911] A mildly elevated serum bilirubin level (>0.6 mg/dL) was associated with an *improved* long-term outcome in Korean patients with IgA nephropathy,[912] a finding that has not been confirmed in a non-Asian population. Prolonged, high-level exposure to organic solvents may also confer a worse prognosis to patients with IgA nephropathy.[913]

Women with IgA tolerate pregnancy well. Only those women with uncontrolled hypertension, a GFR of less than 70 mL/min, or severe arteriolar or interstitial damage on kidney biopsy are at risk for kidney dysfunction.[914,915] Women with creatinine levels higher than 1.4 mg/dL have a greater propensity for hypertension and a progressive increase in creatinine level during the course of pregnancy, and pregnancy-related loss of maternal kidney function occurs in 43% of these patients. The infant survival rate was 93% in this study; preterm delivery occurred in almost two thirds and growth retardation in one third of infants.[916] A more recent study of 223 women (136 and 87 in the pregnancy and nonpregnancy groups) with biopsy-proven IgA nephropathy in Italy showed no difference in long-term outcomes of IgA nephropathy between the two groups over a minimum follow-up period of 5 years.

LABORATORY FINDINGS

To date, there are no specific serologic or laboratory tests diagnostic of IgA nephropathy or IgA vasculitis. The identification of abnormally galactosylated IgA1 has led to the development of a potential diagnostic test based on the detection of increased lectin binding in patients with IgA nephropathy.[917]

Although the serum IgA levels are elevated in up to 50% of patients, the presence of elevated IgA in the circulation is not specific for IgA nephropathy. The detection of IgA-fibronectin complexes was initially thought to be a marker in patients with IgA nephropathy, but it has not proven to be a useful clinical test.[918,919] As noted earlier, polymeric IgA also appears to be found in some patients with IgA nephropathy.[797,920-924] The polymeric IgA itself is of the IgA1 subclass. IgA may also be contained in circulating immune complexes that are not complement binding. Similar immune complexes have been described in IgA vasculitis.[925-942] The levels of circulating immune complexes wax and wane and may sometimes correlate with episodes of macroscopic hematuria. In one interesting study, the level of circulating immune complexes was increased after patients drank cow's milk. This phenomenon occurred in 10% to 15% of patients and possibly suggests sensitivity to bovine serum albumin. Unfortunately, none of these findings is pathognomonic of IgA nephropathy.

Antibodies to the GBM,[943] the mesangium,[944,945] glomerular endothelial cells,[802,855] neutrophil cytoplasmic constituents,[804,805] IgA rheumatoid factor,[946,947] and a number of infectious agents, bovine serum proteins, and soy proteins[807-814,948] have been found in patients with IgA nephropathy. Until studies demonstrate that certain patients have sensitivity to a particular pathogen or food allergen, it is difficult to know whether to perform antibody testing to identify certain foods that should be eliminated from the patient's diet. None of these antibody tests has been standardized in large patient populations. Therefore their applicability to all patients with IgA nephropathy is not known. Levels of complements, such as C3 and C4, are typically normal and, in some patients, even elevated,[949] as are complement components C1q, C2-C9.[739,925,926,949,950] The fact that these complement levels are normal may belie the fact that either the alternate or the classical pathway of complement may be activated. In this regard, C3 fragments are increased in 50% to 75% of patients,[951,952] and C4-binding protein concentrations are also increased.[950] It has also been suggested that both a decreased C3 level and an elevated IgA/C3 ratio may have diagnostic utility for IgA nephropathy[30] and may be associated with a higher risk of progression.[953,954] Interestingly, a large study in Korea of 343 patients with biopsy-proven IgA nephropathy also demonstrated an independently predictive correlation between decreased C3 and mesangial C3 deposition and renal outcomes.[955]

A typical finding is microscopic hematuria on urinalysis that may persist even at very low levels of macroscopic hematuria. The finding of dysmorphic erythrocytes in the urine is typical.[956] Proteinuria is found in many patients with IgA nephropathy, although in the majority, protein excretion is less than 1 g/day. Mesangial and endocapillary hypercellularity, segmental glomerulosclerosis, and extracapillary proliferation are strongly associated with proteinuria.[789]

Although older studies suggested that the detection of dermal capillary IgA deposits in the skin may be of diagnostic utility in IgA nephropathy,[957] this test has not gained widespread acceptance, largely because of the substantial variation in sensitivity and specificity of skin biopsy findings in IgA in patients with nephropathy.[958]

TREATMENT

In part because of the outcome variability of patients with IgA nephropathy, the best approach to therapy remains incompletely established.[959-961] Treatment is indicated for patients with urinary protein excretion of more than 0.5 g of protein per day.[962] Three major approaches have emerged and are supported by substantial direct evidence: (1) RAAS blockade, (2) oral and/or intravenous glucocorticoids, and (3) combined immunosuppressive (cytotoxic) therapy. The latter is usually reserved for those patients with documented progressive disease.[963] Combinations of these approaches are under intense evaluation, including in the Supportive versus Immunosuppressive Therapy of Progressive IgA Nephropathy (STOP-IgAN) trial, which is near completion (www.clinicaltrials.gov, NCT00554502).[964]

Angiotensin II Inhibition

In retrospective studies, angiotensin II inhibition has been associated with slower rate of loss of kidney function and a higher frequency of remission of proteinuria compared to either no therapy[965] or to the use of β-blockers.[966] Several randomized controlled trials of angiotensin II inhibition in patients with IgA nephropathy have been undertaken.[967-972]

A meta-analysis of 11 studies (totaling 585 subjects) revealed that the use of angiotensin II inhibition is associated with a reduction in proteinuria and preservation of GFR.[973] The antiproteinuric effects of the ACE inhibitor appear to be more profound in patients with the ACE gene DD genotype.[974] Observational studies of patients with IgA nephropathy suggest that an elevated fractional excretion of IgG is a powerful predictor of the renoprotective response to angiotensin II inhibition.[975] Higher doses of angiotensin II inhibitors may afford additional renoprotective effect. In a randomized controlled trial involving 207 patients, a high-dose ARB (losartan 200 mg/day) was compared with an ARB given at the usual dose (losartan 100 mg/day) as well as with a usual-dose ACE inhibitor and a low-dose ACE inhibitor (equivalent to enalapril 20 mg/day and 10 mg/day, respectively).[976] High-dose ARB therapy was most efficacious in reducing proteinuria and slowing the rate of loss of decline of eGFR. The current first line of treatment consists of escalating doses of an ARB to achieve a target urinary protein excretion of less than 1 g/day, along with dietary sodium restriction, for patients of any age with IgA nephropathy and proteinuria of more than 500 mg of protein excretion per day.

Glucocorticoids

Studies of glucocorticoid therapy for IgA nephropathy have been inconclusive. Although prednisone was initially considered to be without effect,[870] some cohort studies have suggested that corticosteroids may afford some benefit.[977,978] For instance, a randomized controlled trial demonstrated that a 6-month course of intravenous plus oral glucocorticoids may be useful in patients with IgA nephropathy who have well-preserved kidney function (serum creatinine level of <1.5 mg/dL and proteinuria of 1 to 3.5 g of protein per day).[979] After a 5-year follow-up, the risk of a doubling in plasma creatinine concentration was significantly lower in the corticosteroid-treated patients, who also showed a significant decrease in mean urinary protein excretion after 1 year that persisted throughout the follow-up.[980] This beneficial effect was maintained after 10 years of follow-up as reflected by a rate of renal survival (failure to double the serum creatinine level) of 97% in the treated group compared to 53% in the placebo group (log rank test $P = 0.0003$).[979] On the other hand, no benefit of corticosteroids over placebo could be demonstrated in the multicenter randomized controlled trial conducted by the Southwest Pediatric Nephrology Study Group,[981] although this negative result is mitigated by a statistically significant lower degree of proteinuria at baseline among placebo-treated patients. A meta-analysis of seven randomized controlled trials involving 366 patients suggested that glucocorticoid therapy was effective in reducing proteinuria and preventing loss of kidney function,[982] and a subsequent meta-analysis of 15 clinical trials that measured ESKD, doubling of serum creatinine, or urinary protein excretion as outcomes found that corticosteroid therapy was associated with a decrease of proteinuria and with a statistically significant reduction in ESKD risk.[983]

Another circumstance in which prednisone has demonstrated a substantial beneficial effect is in the treatment of patients with IgA nephropathy and concurrent MCD. These patients have nephrotic-range proteinuria and diffuse foot process effacement. They respond to prednisone in a manner very similar to that of patients with MCD.[127,869,984,985] Low doses of prednisone (20 to 30 mg/day tapered to 5 to 10 mg/day over 2 years) may also be effective in lowering proteinuria in patients with mild inflammatory glomerular lesions.[986] Conversely, poor response to glucocorticoids can be predicted in patients with extensive glomerular obsolescence, tuft adhesions, severe interstitial fibrosis, low serum albumin, low eGFR, and marked proteinuria.[987] A high number of fibroblast-specific protein 1 (FSP1)–positive cells in the interstitium (>33 FSP-1+ cells per high-power field) is highly predictive of a poor response to steroids.[988]

In summary, glucocorticoid therapy is a reasonable option for treatment of patients with adverse prognostic features with well-preserved kidney function (GFR > 60 mL/min/1.73 m^2) who remain proteinuric despite a 3- to 6-month trial of angiotensin II inhibitors or of patients with features of MCD and nephrotic syndrome.[989]

Combinations of Angiotensin II Inhibition and Glucocorticoid Therapy

Two randomized controlled trials in patients with IgA nephropathy have compared the combined use of glucocorticoids and angiotensin II inhibition to angiotensin II inhibition alone but not with glucocorticoids alone.[990,991] In the larger of the two studies,[991] (97 subjects with IgA nephropathy and urinary protein excretion of more than 1.0 g/day and eGFR of greater than 50 mL/min/1.73 m^2), 27% of the subjects receiving ramipril alone developed a doubling of baseline serum creatinine or ESKD, whereas only 4% of subjects in the ramipril plus steroid group developed these end points ($P = 0.003$) after a follow-up of 8 years. These studies demonstrate an added benefit of glucocorticoids over angiotensin II inhibitors alone. Whether such combined therapy should be instituted as initial therapy or only after a trial of angiotensin II inhibition alone remains to be investigated.

More aggressive treatment may be appropriate in patients with severe crescentic or progressive IgA nephropathy.[992-994] In a randomized controlled trial, patients with a serum creatinine concentration higher 1.5 mg/dL and a GFR declining at a rate of more than 15% per year either received no immunosuppression or were treated with oral prednisolone (initially at 40 mg/day) and cyclophosphamide (at 1.5 mg/kg/day) for 3 months followed by 2 years of treatment with azathioprine (1.5 mg/kg/day).[995] Over a follow-up of 2 to 6 years, 5-year renal survival was 72% in treated patients versus only 6% in untreated patients.[995] This approach of prednisone coupled with oral azathioprine for 2 years in patients with proteinuria of more than 2.5 g of protein per day was also observed in a retrospective survey.[996,997]

The use of pulse methylprednisolone, oral prednisone, and/or cyclophosphamide to treat patients who have rapidly progressive glomerulonephritis with widespread crescentic transformation has been reported.[998-1000] It is reasonable to treat crescentic disease in IgA nephropathy in a manner similar to other forms of crescentic glomerulonephritis (e.g., ANCA glomerulonephritis). Of concern, however, was the finding in 12 patients of the persistence of crescents on repeat biopsy, despite the early and aggressive treatment with pulse methylprednisolone and oral prednisone, and a short-term reversal of the acute crescentic glomerulonephritis.[1000] This study suggests that there was only a diminution in the rate of progression to ESKD.

Other Modalities

Aliskiren, a direct inhibitor of renin, has received attention of late as an antiproteinuric agent in IgA nephropathy. An open-label pilot study in 25 consecutive patients with IgA nephropathy in Hong Kong treated for 12 months with aliskiren resulted in a 26.3% (95% CI, 20.1 to 43.6; $P = 0.001$ vs. baseline) mean reduction in the urine protein to creatinine ratio and a significant reduction in plasma renin activity; however, there were mild allergic reactions in 2 patients (8%) and transient hyperkalemia in 6 patients (24%).[1001] A subsequent randomized crossover study using aliskiren or placebo in 22 patients in China with biopsy-proven IgA nephropathy and persistent proteinuria despite ACE inhibition or angiotensin receptor blockade demonstrated significant reductions in proteinuria at 4 weeks (1.76 ± 0.95 to 1.03 ± 0.69 g protein per g creatinine; $P < 0.0001$) and from 4 to 16 weeks, but there was a modest but statistically significant reduction in eGFR (57.2 ± 29.1 to 54.8 ± 29.3 mL/min/1.73 m^2; $P = 0.013$) (www.clinicaltrials.gov, NCT00870493).[1002]

In a 3-year prospective controlled trial of cyclophosphamide, dipyridamole, and low-dose warfarin, it is reasonably clear that treatment with the combination of oral cyclophosphamide, dipyridamole, and low-dose warfarin[1003] has very little long-term benefit in patients with IgA nephropathy. Five years after the end of a small controlled trial (N = 48), there was no significant difference in the rate of ESKD between patients previously treated with cyclophosphamide, dipyridamole, and warfarin (22%) and the control group (33%). Of note, it has since been proposed that the apparent lack of benefit of cyclophosphamide therapy may have been clouded by the potential risk of a recently recognized mechanism of acute kidney injury in study subjects, termed *warfarin-related nephropathy*.[1004] This observation warrants additional clinical trials utilizing combination therapy without this potential confounder.

Whether MMF is useful in the treatment of IgA nephropathy is currently unknown. Three randomized trials of MMF have shown conflicting results.[1005-1008] The studies based in China and Hong Kong reported a beneficial effect of MMF on proteinuria and hyperlipidemia[999,1009] but no effect on kidney function in the short term.[1005] Long-term follow-up of this cohort suggested better preservation of kidney function in the MMF-treated group.[1010] On the other hand, the two placebo-controlled studies of MMF in white populations of 32 and 34 patients failed to demonstrate a benefit of MMF on proteinuria or the preservation of kidney function.[1007,1008] It is noteworthy that in one study,[1007] patients had relatively advanced renal insufficiency (mean serum creatinine of 2.4 mg/dL). Collectively, these underpowered studies fail to establish a role for MMF in the treatment of IgA nephropathy and raise the question as to whether certain ethnic groups (Asians) may be more responsive to this form of therapy.

With regard to azathioprine use, a randomized controlled trial in Italy of 207 patients with biopsy-proven IgA nephropathy compared steroids alone or in combination with azathioprine for 6 months and found no difference in renal survival, defined as time to 50% increase in plasma creatinine from baseline over a median follow-up of 4.9 years. Five-year cumulative renal survival was not significantly different (88% vs. 89%, $P = 0.83$).[1011] A separate randomization list with a longer treatment course of 1 year in patients with impaired kidney function (plasma creatinine >2.0 mg/dL and proteinuria ≥1 g/day) involving 253 patients with biopsy-proven IgA nephropathy from the same group of investigators compared steroids alone or steroids in combination with azathioprine and similarly found no difference in renal survival at the 6-year mark.[1012]

There has been much discussion in the literature about the use of tonsillectomy in IgA nephropathy. Results of retrospective trials are inconsistent.[1013-1016] A single-center retrospective cohort study of 200 patients with biopsy-proven IgA nephropathy, 70 (35%) of whom received tonsillectomy, revealed by multiple regression modeling that tonsillectomy prevented GFR decline during the follow-up period (regression coefficient, 2.0; $P = 0.01$). This effect was also observed in non–steroid-treated patients.[1016] Based on a retrospective multivariate analysis[1014] of a large cohort of 329 patients from Japan, treatment with tonsillectomy and pulse glucocorticoid therapy (methylprednisolone 0.5 g/day for 3 days for three courses, followed by oral prednisolone at an initial dose of 0.6 mg/kg on alternate days, with a decrease of 0.1 mg/kg every 2 months) was associated with clinical remission. Similarly, in a multivariate analysis[1017] focusing on the subgroup of 70 patients from the same cohort with a baseline serum creatinine concentration of more than 1.5 mg/dL, treatment with the combination of tonsillectomy and pulse glucocorticoids was associated with improved long-term renal survival. Another retrospective analysis,[1013] however, showed no benefit of tonsillectomy on the clinical course of IgA nephropathy. Interestingly, a recent retrospective analysis of 365 patients with biopsy-proven IgA nephropathy in Japan revealed that tonsillectomy delayed disease progression to ESKD (OR, 0.09; 95% CI, 0.01 to 0.75; $P = 0.026$).[1018]

In a controlled nonrandomized trial, tonsillectomy plus pulse glucocorticoids was associated with a higher rate of remission of proteinuria and hematuria (but not kidney function) than pulse glucocorticoids alone.[1019] A very recent multicenter randomized controlled trial of patients with biopsy-proven IgA nephropathy randomly allocated patients to receive tonsillectomy with steroid pulses (n = 33) versus steroid pulses alone (n = 39). Although urinary protein excretion was significantly greater in the tonsillectomy group at the 12-month mark ($P < 0.05$), clinical remission (defined as disappearance of hematuria, proteinuria, or both) was not.[1020] Long-term follow-up results will possibly provide further clarity.

ω-3 Fatty Acids

Despite a great deal of interest in the past decade, the value of treatment with ω-3 long-chain polyunsaturated fatty acids (eicosapentaenoic and docosahexaenoic acids) in IgA nephropathy remains unproven. In a study by the Mayo Clinic[1021] 106 patients were randomly assigned to either 12 g of ω-3 fatty acids or olive oil for 2 years. Only 6% of patients treated with fish oil experienced a doubling of their plasma creatinine concentration, compared with 33% of those treated with olive oil. In the fish oil–treated patients, only 14% excreted more than 3.5 g of protein per day, in contrast to 65% of those treated with olive oil. The enthusiasm for this approach, however, was tempered by subsequent studies that showed no benefit of fish oil therapy.[1022,1023]

A meta-analysis of published trials on ω-3 fatty acids encompassing 17 trials and 626 subjects with a variety of kidney diseases, including 5 trials in IgA nephropathy,[1024] revealed no beneficial effects on proteinuria or slowing in the rate of GFR decline. In a recent randomized controlled trial involving 30 patients, the addition of ω-3 fatty acids to angiotensin II inhibition was more effective than angiotensin II inhibition alone in decreasing proteinuria and erythrocyturia over 6 months.[1025] A subsequent meta-analysis of five randomized controlled trials (N = 233) found a significant reduction in proteinuria with ω-3 fatty acid use, but there was no significant benefit in preservation of kidney function.[1026] Unfortunately, no benefit was found in a meta-analysis published the same year.[1027] In summary, if ω-3 fatty acids are used at all in the treatment of IgA nephropathy, they should be used adjunctively in combination with angiotensin II inhibition and not as monotherapy.

Summary of Recommended Treatment

In summary, patients with IgA nephropathy should be treated with maximally tolerated angiotensin II inhibition to a target protein excretion of less than 500 mg/day.[1028-1031] Should proteinuria persist despite angiotensin II inhibition, the addition of glucocorticoids (oral or intravenous plus oral) should be considered for patients with well-preserved kidney function (GFR ≥ 60 mL/min/1.73 m^2). In those patients with progressive renal insufficiency, the use of prednisone and cyclophosphamide followed by azathioprine should be considered.[995] This approach to therapy is the subject of an ongoing large multicenter randomized controlled trial in Germany, the STOP-IgAN study.[964] High-dose corticosteroids and/or cyclophosphamide should also be considered for patients with widespread crescentic glomerulonephritis, whereas patients with AKI associated with tubular necrosis and little glomerular damage should be treated conservatively, because these individuals have an excellent long-term response. Although there is no conclusive evidence of efficacy, the relatively benign side effect profile of ω-3 fatty acid therapy permits its use in patients who have an unfavorable prognosis. Those patients with nephrotic syndrome and MCD may benefit from oral glucocorticoids.

IMMUNOGLOBULIN A NEPHROPATHY AND KIDNEY TRANSPLANTATION

The recurrence of IgA deposits after kidney transplantation is common, and the rate may reach 75% to 80% with long-term (>20-year) survival of the patient and graft.[1032] Fortunately, most of these recurrences are clinically mild or are discovered incidentally at the time of an allograft biopsy to assess for possible rejection. Although graft loss due to recurrent IgA nephropathy is quite uncommon (<5%),[1033] a recurrence of IgA nephropathy worsens the overall prognosis for long-term survival of an allograft,[1034,1035] especially if crescentic disease is present. Nevertheless, overall graft survival in patients with IgA nephropathy is similar to that in patients with ESKD due to other causes.[1033] Suggested risk factors for recurrent IgA nephropathy after transplantation include a rapid course of the original disease due to crescentic glomerulonephritis, younger age, IgA deposits in the donor kidney at the time of grafting, and living related or "zero-mismatched" kidney donor.[1035,1036] Induction therapy with antithymocyte globulin appears to decrease the incidence of recurrent disease.[1037]

FIBRILLARY GLOMERULONEPHRITIS AND IMMUNOTACTOID GLOMERULOPATHY

NOMENCLATURE

Fibrillary glomerulonephritis and immunotactoid glomerulopathy are glomerular diseases that are characterized by patterned deposits seen by electron microscopy (Figure 32.31 and 32.32).[1038-1045] Most renal pathologists prefer to distinguish fibrillary glomerulonephritis from immunotactoid glomerulopathy based on the presence of fibrils of approximately 20 nm in diameter in fibrillary glomerulonephritis and larger 30- to 40-nm–diameter microtubular structures in immunotactoid glomerulopathy[1038,1040-1043] (see Figures 32.31 and 32.32). A minority of pathologists, however, advocate grouping glomerular diseases with either fibrillary deposits or microtubular deposits under the term *immunotactoid glomerulopathy*.[1042,1045]

FIBRILLARY GLOMERULONEPHRITIS PATHOLOGY
Electron Microscopy

The diagnosis of fibrillary glomerulonephritis requires the identification by electron microscopy of irregular accumulations of randomly arranged nonbranching fibrils of approximately 20 nm in diameter in glomerular mesangium, capillary walls, or both[1038-1044,1046] (Figure 32.31A). In capillary walls, the fibrillary deposits can be subepithelial, subendothelial, or intramembranous. The fibrillary deposits often contain blotchy electron-dense material but only rarely have

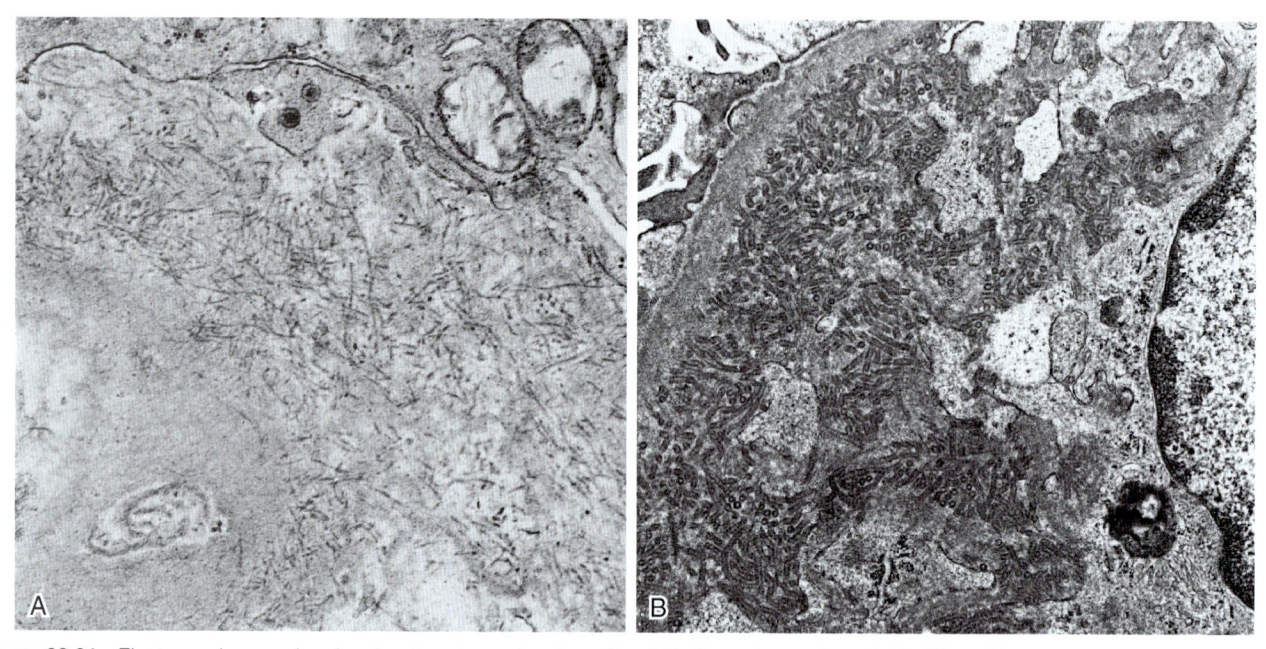

Figure 32.31 Electron micrographs showing the glomerular deposits of fibrillary glomerulonephritis **(A)** and immunotactoid glomerulopathy **(B)**. Note the random orientation of the former and the microtubular appearance and greater organization of the latter. (×20,000.)

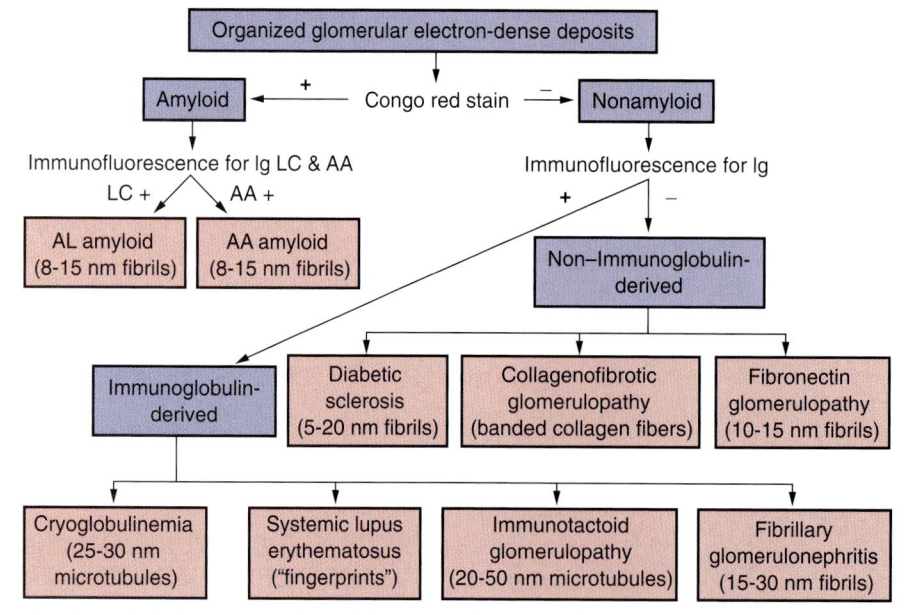

Figure 32.32 Algorithm for the pathologic categorization of glomerular diseases with patterned or organized deposits. The first division is into amyloid versus nonamyloid disease, and the second is into diseases that are caused by immunoglobulin molecule deposition and those that are not. By the approach illustrated, fibrillary glomerulonephritis is distinguished from immunotactoid glomerulopathy based on the ultrastructural characteristics of the deposits.

associated well-defined electron-dense deposits. The fibrils are distinctly larger than the actin filaments in adjacent cells, which is a useful observation that helps distinguish the fibrils of fibrillary glomerulonephritis from those of amyloidosis, which are only slightly larger than actin. The fibrils of fibrillary glomerulonephritis are not as large as the microtubular deposits of immunotactoid glomerulopathy or cryoglobulinemia, and they do not have the "fingerprint" configuration occasionally observed in lupus nephritis dense deposits. Most patients with fibrillary glomerulonephritis have substantial proteinuria, and therefore there usually is extensive effacement of visceral epithelial foot processes.

Light Microscopy

In fibrillary glomerulonephritis, extensive localization of fibrils in capillary walls causes capillary wall thickening. Mesangial localization causes increased mesangial matrix and usually stimulates mesangial hypercellularity. Varying distributions of the fibrillary deposits cause the light microscopic appearance of fibrillary glomerulonephritis to be extremely variable.[1038,1044] Therefore, fibrillary glomerulonephritis can mimic the light microscopic appearance of MPGN, proliferative glomerulonephritis, or MN. Crescents occur in the most aggressive phenotypes. Of 74 sequential fibrillary glomerulonephritis specimens evaluated at University of North Carolina, 28% had crescents with an average involvement of 29% of glomeruli (range, 5% to 80%). The fibrillary deposits typically have a moth-eaten appearance when stained with a Jones' methenamine silver stain. They do not show Congo red staining, which distinguishes them from amyloid deposits.

Immunofluorescence Microscopy

The deposits of fibrillary glomerulonephritis almost always stain more intensely for IgG than for IgM or IgA, and many specimens have little or no staining for IgM and IgA.[1038-1044] IgG4 is the dominant subclass. Only rare specimens have staining for only one light-chain type. C3 staining usually is intense. The immunofluorescence staining pattern of fibrillary glomerulonephritis is relatively distinctive (Figures 32.32 and 32.33). It is neither granular nor linear; instead, it has an irregular bandlike appearance in capillary walls and an irregular shaggy appearance in the mesangium.

IMMUNOTACTOID GLOMERULOPATHY PATHOLOGY

Electron Microscopy

The tubular substructure of the deposits of immunotactoid glomerulopathy is readily discerned at 5000 to 10,000 magnification (see Figure 32.31B). At this magnification, the deposits of fibrillary glomerulonephritis have no tubular structure. The microtubules of immunotactoid glomerulopathy also have a greater tendency to align in parallel arrays, whereas the fibrils of fibrillary glomerulonephritis always are randomly distributed.[781] The ultrastructural deposits of immunotactoid glomerulopathy resemble those seen in cryoglobulinemic glomerulonephritis, and thus the latter must be ruled out before making a diagnosis of immunotactoid glomerulopathy. However, cryoglobulinemic microtubules typically are shorter and less well designed than immunotactoid microtubules.

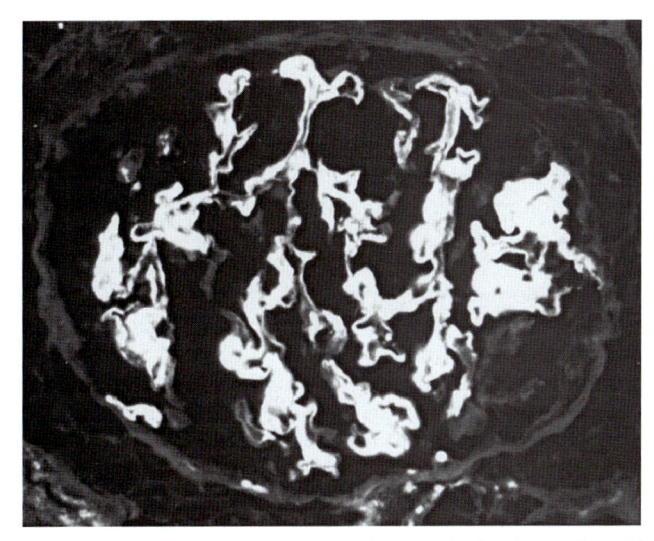

Figure 32.33 Immunofluorescence micrograph of a glomerulus with features of fibrillary glomerulonephritis showing mesangial and band-like capillary wall staining for immunoglobulin G (IgG). (Fluorescein isothiocyanate anti-IgG stain, ×300.)

Light Microscopy

Immunotactoid glomerulopathy has a varied light microscopic appearance. Combined capillary wall thickening and mesangial expansion is most common, which often gives a membranoproliferative appearance. Immunotactoid deposits may be massive, resulting in nodular mesangial expansion in some specimens.

Immunofluorescence Microscopy

The deposits of immunotactoid glomerulopathy usually are IgG dominant with staining for both κ- and λ-light chains; however, the immunoglobulin in the deposits of immunotactoid glomerulopathy is more often monoclonal than in fibrillary glomerulonephritis.[1040] Monoclonality warrants clinical workup for a B cell dyscrasia.

PATHOGENESIS

The causes and pathogenesis of fibrillary glomerulonephritis and immunotactoid glomerulopathy are not known. Fibrillary glomerulonephritis and immunotactoid glomerulonephritis have been associated with lymphoproliferative disease (e.g., chronic lymphocytic leukemia or B cell lymphomas).[1040,1046,1047] Immunotactoid glomerulonephritis is more frequently associated with a monoclonal gammopathy.[1048] On rare occasions, fibrillary glomerulonephritis can also be associated with a monoclonal gammopathy.[1049,1050] The possible oligoclonal character of the deposits of fibrillary glomerulonephritis may facilitate self-association and fibrillar organization in a fashion analogous to that of the monoclonal light chains of immunoglobulin light-chain (AL) amyloidosis.[1043] The resemblance of immunotactoid deposits to those of cryoglobulinemia, which often contain a monoclonal component, also raises the possibility that the presence of some type of uniformity of the immunoglobulin in the deposits may be causing the patterned organization in immunotactoid glomerulopathy. Rarely, fibrillary glomerulonephritis may be associated with concomitant hepatitis C virus infection[1051] or an unusual IgM glomerular deposit disease.[1052]

EPIDEMIOLOGY AND CLINICAL FEATURES

An analysis of 9085 consecutive native kidney biopsy specimens evaluated in the University of North Carolina Nephropathology Laboratory revealed a frequency of 0.8% for fibrillary glomerulonephritis and 0.1% for immunotactoid glomerulonephritis, compared with 14.5% for MN, 7.5% for IgA nephropathy, 2.6% for type I MPGN, 1.5% for amyloidosis, and 0.8% for anti-GBM glomerulonephritis. Thus, fibrillary glomerulonephritis is about as common as anti-GBM glomerulonephritis and much more frequent than immunotactoid glomerulopathy.

Patients with fibrillary glomerulonephritis present with a mixture of nephrotic and nephritic syndrome features.[1041,1042,1046] Patients may have microscopic or macroscopic hematuria, renal insufficiency (including rapidly progressive glomerulonephritis in a few patients), hypertension, and proteinuria, which may be in the nephrotic range. In a series of 28 patients with fibrillary glomerulonephritis seen at the University of North Carolina, the mean age was 49 years (range, 21 to 75 years), the ratio of males to females was 1:1.8, and the ratio of whites to blacks was 8.3:1.[1043] After 24 months of follow-up, renal survival was only 48%.[1043] In a subsequent series of 66 patients with fibrillary glomerulonephritis seen at Mayo Clinic in Rochester, Minnesota, between 1993 and 2010, the mean age at diagnosis was 53 years and the male/female ratio was 1:1.2. At presentation, 100% of patients had proteinuria, 52% had hematuria, 71% were hypertensive, and 66% had renal insufficiency. Underlying malignancy (23%), dysproteinemia (17%), and autoimmune disease (15%) were common. Of 61 patients with available data followed for an average of 52.3 months, 13% had complete or partial remission, 43% had persistent kidney dysfunction, and 44% progressed to ESKD. Not surprisingly, older age, higher creatinine and proteinuria at biopsy, and higher percentage of global glomerulosclerosis were independent predictors of ESKD by multivariate analysis.[1053] Overall, proteinuria is common at the time of presentation, as are hematuria, renal insufficiency, and hypertension. In patients in whom these disorders are diagnosed, malignancy, Crohn's disease, SLE, and cryoglobulinemia must be ruled out. Such patients have progressive renal failure in less than 5 years, although long-term patient survival is more than 80% at 5 years.[1048,1054]

In a group of six patients with immunotactoid glomerulopathy, the mean age was 62.[1041] At presentation, the clinical features in these patients looked very much like those in patients with fibrillary glomerulonephritis and included proteinuria, hematuria, and renal insufficiency. In the largest series to date, 16 patients with immunotactoid glomerulopathy were identified from the pathology archives at Mayo Clinic in Rochester, Minnesota. Proteinuria was present in 100% of patients; 80% had microhematuria, 69% had nephrotic syndrome, and 50% had renal insufficiency. Interestingly, 38% of patients had a hematologic malignancy. Over an average of 48 months of follow-up of 12 patients, 50% remitted, 33% had persistent kidney dysfunction, and 17% progressed to ESKD.[1055]

Importantly, patients with immunotactoid glomerular disease are more likely to have an associated hematopoietic process and poor long-term survival.[1041] In a review study of 67 patients presenting with fibrillary glomerulopathy (n = 61) or immunotactoid glomerulopathy (n = 6), all patients had proteinuria and half had nephrotic syndrome, whereas hematuria occurred in approximately two thirds of patients and hypertension in about three fourths of patients.[1056] Renal insufficiency was discovered in half the patient population. There were no statistically significant differences in clinical presentation between patients with fibrillary glomerulonephritis and those with immunotactoid glomerulonephritis. Etiologically, patients with immunotactoid glomerulonephritis were statistically more likely to have an underlying lymphoproliferative disease, a monoclonal spike on serum protein electrophoresis, and hypocomplementemia.[1056]

Fibrillary glomerulonephritis with associated pulmonary hemorrhage has been reported anecdotally.[1057] One patient with immunotactoid glomerulopathy also had extrarenal deposits in both the liver and bone.[1058]

TREATMENT

At this time, there is no convincingly effective form of treatment for patients with either fibrillary glomerulonephritis or immunotactoid glomerulopathy.[1046] The dismal prognosis in patients with either of these diseases has prompted physicians to search for some immunosuppressive form of treatment. Fully 40% to 50% of patients with these diseases develop ESKD within 6 years of presentation.[1038,1039,1041,1043] Efforts at treatment with either glucocorticoids or alkylating agents such as cyclophosphamide have typically shown either no response or, at best, some amelioration of proteinuria.[1059] In the authors' own experience, prednisone therapy alone has had no benefit. One small case series (three patients) reported significant improvement in proteinuria in response to rituximab (either alone or in combination with corticosteroids) or tacrolimus.[1060] In fibrillary glomerulonephritis and other forms of glomerulonephritis associated with chronic lymphocytic leukemia or other forms of lymphocytic lymphoma, there is a report of improvement in a minority of patients treated with chlorambucil. Thus, it is possible that the treatment of the underlying malignancy, if present, may improve the glomerulonephritis.[1047]

The recurrence rate of fibrillary glomerulonephritis after kidney transplantation is unclear. One report describes recurrent disease in three of four patients who had received five transplants.[1061] In a larger case series, recurrent disease occurred in none of five patients with fibrillary glomerulonephritis but in five of seven patients with monoclonal gammopathy and fibrillary deposits.[1062]

RAPIDLY PROGRESSIVE GLOMERULONEPHRITIS AND CRESCENTIC GLOMERULONEPHRITIS

NOMENCLATURE AND CATEGORIZATION

The term *rapidly progressive glomerulonephritis* (RPGN) refers to a clinical syndrome characterized by a rapid loss of kidney function, often accompanied by oliguria or anuria, and by features of glomerulonephritis, including dysmorphic erythrocyturia, erythrocyte cylindruria, and glomerular proteinuria.[1063] Aggressive glomerulonephritis that causes RPGN usually has extensive crescent formation.[1064] For this reason, the clinical term *rapidly progressive glomerulonephritis* is sometimes used interchangeably with the pathologic term *crescentic glomerulonephritis*. Crescentic glomerulonephritis is the most aggressive structural phenotype in the continuum of injury that results from glomerular inflammation (see Figure 32.30). This pathologic feature can be seen on light, immunofluorescence, and electron microscopy.[1064-1066] It is the result of focal rupture of glomerular capillary walls that allows inflammatory mediators and leukocytes to enter Bowman's space, where they induce epithelial cell proliferation and macrophage influx and maturation that together produce cellular crescents (Figure 32.34).[1067-1069]

Kidney diseases other than crescentic glomerulonephritis can cause the sign and symptoms of RPGN. Two examples are acute thrombotic microangiopathy and atheroembolic kidney disease. Although acute tubular necrosis and acute tubulointerstitial nephritis may cause rapid loss of kidney function and oliguria, these processes typically do not cause dysmorphic erythrocyturia, erythrocyte cylindruria, or substantial proteinuria.

A small minority of all patients with glomerulonephritis develop RPGN with the exception of patients with anti-GBM disease and ANCA disease who have a high frequency of crescents. The incidence of rapidly progressive glomerulonephritis has been estimated to be as low as seven cases per million population per year.[631,1070] The three major immunopathologic categories of crescentic glomerulonephritis have different frequencies in different age groups (Table 32.16).[1063-1065,1071] In a patient who has RPGN clinically and in whom crescentic glomerulonephritis is identified by light microscopy in a kidney biopsy specimen, the precise diagnostic categorization of the disease requires integration of clinical, serologic, immunohistologic, and electron microscopic data (Figure 32.35).

Immune complex crescentic glomerulonephritis is caused by immune complex localization within glomeruli. It is the most common cause of RPGN in children (see Table 32.16).[1064] The major clinical differential diagnosis in children is hemolytic uremic syndrome, which also can cause rapid loss of kidney function, hypertension, hematuria, and proteinuria. The presence of microangiopathic hemolytic anemia and thrombocytopenia are indicators that the rapid loss of kidney function is more likely caused by hemolytic uremic syndrome than crescentic glomerulonephritis. Pauci-immune crescentic glomerulonephritis, which shows little or no evidence of localization of immune complex or anti-GBM antibodies in glomeruli, is usually associated with the presence of ANCAs and is the most common cause for RPGN and crescentic glomerulonephritis in adults, especially older adults (Tables 32.16 and 32.17).[1063,1071-1073] In most patients, pauci-immune crescentic glomerulonephritis is a component of a systemic small vessel vasculitis, such as GPA or microscopic polyangiitis (MPA); however, some patients have renal-limited (primary) disease.[1064,1074] Anti-GBM disease is the least frequent cause of crescentic glomerulonephritis (see Tables 32.16 and 32.17).[1063,1064,1071,1072]

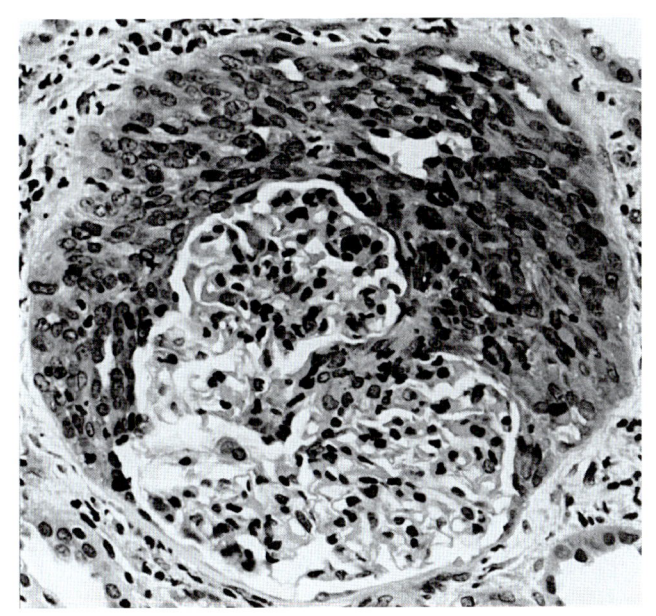

Figure 32.34 Light micrograph showing a large cellular crescent. (×500.)

Table 32.16 Relative Frequency of Immunopathologic Categories of Crescentic Glomerulonephritis (CGN) in Different Age Groups (in Percent)*

Immunopathologic Category	All Ages (N = 632)	Age in Years 1-20 (n = 73)	21-60 (n = 303)	>60 (n = 256)
Anti–glomerular basement membrane CGN	15	12	15	15
Immune complex CGN	24	45	35	6
Pauci-immune CGN†	60	42	48	79
Other	1	0	30	0

*CGN is defined as the presence of crescents in more than 50% of glomeruli. Frequency is determined with respect to age in patients whose kidney biopsy specimens were evaluated at the University of North Carolina Nephropathology Laboratory. Notice the very high frequency of pauci-immune disease (usually antineutrophil cytoplasmic antibody [ANCA] associated) in older adults.
†Approximately 90% associated with ANCA.
Data from Jennette JC, Nickeleit V: Anti-glomerular basement membrane glomerulonephritis and Goodpasture's syndrome. In Jennette JC, Olson JL, Silva FG, D'Agati V, editors, Heptinstall's Pathology of the kidney, ed 7, Philadelphia, 2015, Wolters Kluwer, pp 657-684.

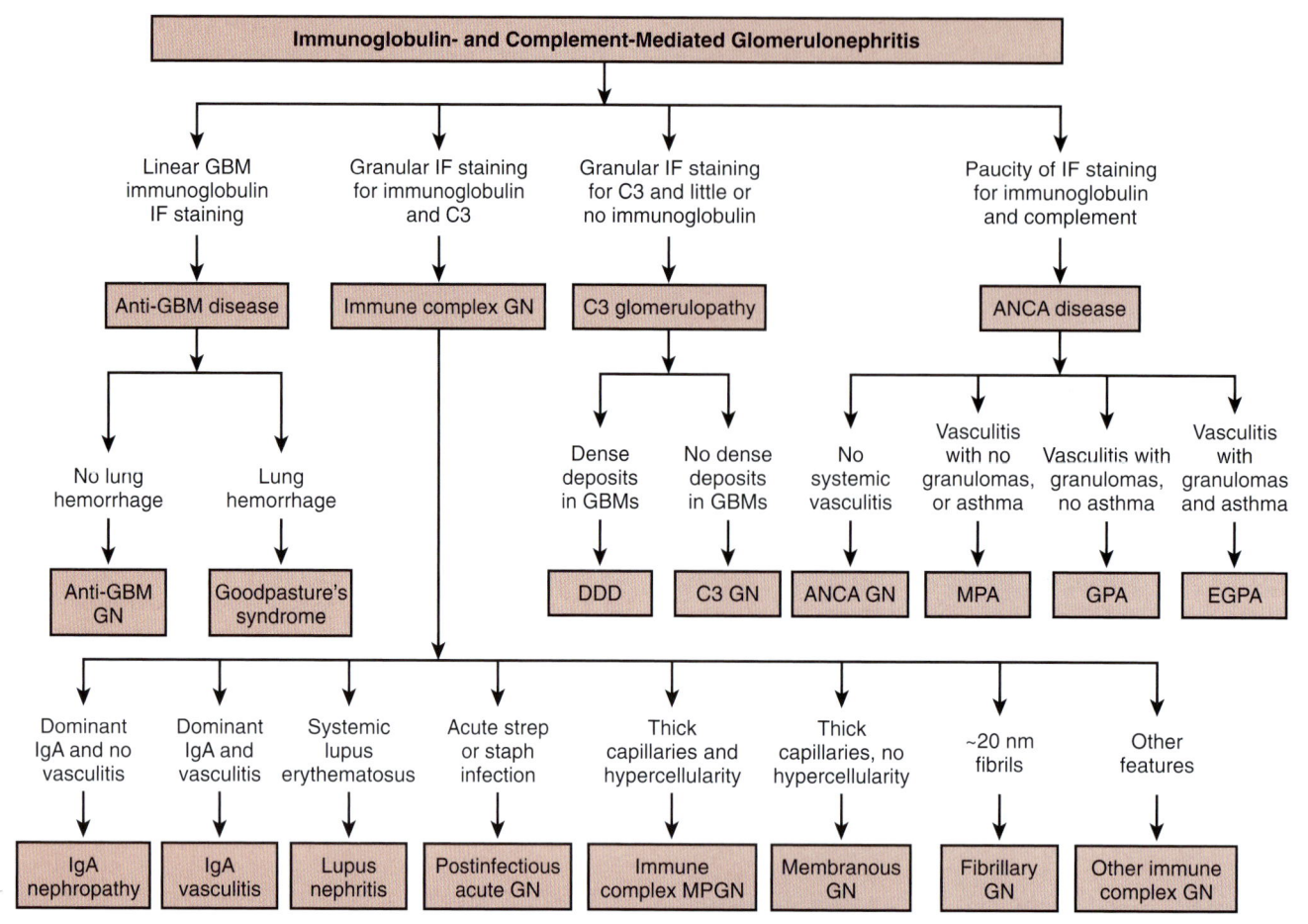

Figure 32.35 Algorithm for diagnostic classification of glomerulonephritis (GN) that is known or suspected of being mediated by antibodies and complement. Note that integration of light microcopy, immunofluorescence (IF) microscopy, electron microscopy, laboratory data, and clinical manifestations is required to precisely diagnose GN. ANCA, Anti-neutrophil cytoplasmic autoantibody; DDD, dense deposit disease; EGPA, eosinophilic granulomatosis with polyangiitis; GBM, glomerular basement membrane; GPA, granulomatosis with polyangiitis; IgA, immunoglobulin A; MPA, microscopic polyangiitis; MPGN, membranoproliferative glomerulonephritis.

Table 32.17 Frequency of Immunopathologic Categories of Glomerulonephritis (GN) in Kidney Biopsy Specimens Evaluated by Immunofluorescence Microscopy*

Immunohistology	All Proliferative GN (n = 1093)	Any Crescents (n = 540)	> 50% Crescents (n = 195)	Arteritis in Biopsy (n = 37)
Pauci-immune GN (<2+ immunoglobulin staining score)	45% (496/1093)	51% (227/540)	61% (118/195)[†]	84% (31/37)
Immune complex GN (≥2+ immunoglobulin staining score)	52% (570/1093)	44% (238/540)	29% (56/195)	14% (5/37)[‡]
Anti–glomerular basement membrane GN	3% (27/1093)	5% (25/540)[§]	11% (21/195)	3% (1/37)[¶]

*Based on the analysis of more than 3000 consecutive nontransplant renal biopsy specimens evaluated at the University of North Carolina Nephropathology Laboratory.
[†]Seventy of 77 patients (91%) tested positive for antineutrophil cytoplasmic antibody (ANCA) (44 for perinuclear ANCA [P-ANCA] and 26 cytoplasmic ANCA [C-ANCA]).
[‡]Four patients had lupus and one had poststreptococcal glomerulonephritis.
[§]Three of 19 patients (16%) tested positive for ANCA (2 for P-ANCA and 1 for C-ANCA).
[¶]This patient also tested positive for P-ANCA (myeloperoxidase ANCA).
Derived from Jennette JC, Nickeleit V: Anti-glomerular basement membrane glomerulonephritis and Goodpasture's syndrome. In Jennette JC, Olson JL, Silva FG, et al, editors: Heptinstall's pathology of the kidney, ed 7, Philadelphia, 2015, Wolters Kluwer, pp 657–684.

IMMUNE COMPLEX–MEDIATED CRESCENTIC GLOMERULONEPHRITIS

EPIDEMIOLOGY

Most patients with immune complex–mediated crescentic glomerulonephritis have clinical or pathologic evidence of a specific category of primary glomerulonephritis, such as IgA nephropathy, postinfectious glomerulonephritis, or MPGN, or they have glomerulonephritis that is a component of a systemic immune complex disease, such as SLE, cryoglobulinemia, or IgA vasculitis. A minority of patients with immune complex–mediated crescentic glomerulonephritis, however, do not have patterns of immune complex localization that readily fit into these specific categories of immune complex glomerulonephritis.[1075]

Immune complex–mediated crescentic glomerulonephritis accounts for the majority of crescentic glomerulonephritides in children but for only a minority of crescentic glomerulonephritides in older adults (see Table 32.16). The higher frequency in children and young adults reflects a similar trend in other types of immune complex glomerulonephritides such as IgA nephropathy, PSGN, MPGN, dense deposit disease, and lupus nephritis.

PATHOLOGY

Light Microscopy

The light microscopic appearance of immune complex–mediated crescentic glomerulonephritis depends on the underlying category of glomerulonephritis; for example, in their most aggressive expressions, MPGN, acute postinfectious glomerulonephritis, or proliferative glomerulonephritis, including IgA nephropathy, can all have crescent formation.[356,360,653,659,785,1000,1070,1076] This underlying phenotype of immune complex glomerulonephritis is recognized best in the intact glomeruli or glomerular segments. Immune complex–mediated glomerulonephritis and C3 glomerulopathy usually have varying combinations of capillary wall thickening and endocapillary hypercellularity in the intact glomeruli. This is in contrast to anti-GBM glomerulonephritis and ANCA glomerulonephritis, which tend to have surprisingly little alteration in intact glomeruli and segments in spite of the severe necrotizing injury in involved glomeruli and segments. In glomerular segments adjacent to crescents in immune complex glomerulonephritis, there usually is some degree of necrosis with karyorrhexis; however, the necrosis rarely is as extensive as that typically seen with anti-GBM or ANCA glomerulonephritis. In addition, there is less destruction of Bowman's capsule associated with crescents in immune complex glomerulonephritis, as well as less pronounced periglomerular tubulointerstitial inflammation. Crescents in immune complex glomerulonephritis have a higher proportion of epithelial cells to macrophages than crescents in anti-GBM or ANCA glomerulonephritis, which may be related to the less severe disruption of Bowman's capsule and thus less opportunity for macrophages to migrate in from the interstitium.[1075]

Immunofluorescence Microscopy

Immunofluorescence microscopy, as well as electron microscopy, provides the evidence that crescentic glomerulonephritis is immune complex or complement mediated versus anti-GBM antibody mediated or ANCA mediated. The pattern and composition of immunoglobulin and complement staining depend on the underlying category of immune complex glomerulonephritis or C3 glomerulopathy that has induced crescent formation.[357,658,1077] For example, crescentic glomerulonephritis with predominantly mesangial IgA-dominant deposits is indicative of crescentic IgA nephropathy; C3-dominant deposits with peripheral band-like configurations suggest crescentic MPGN; coarsely granular capillary wall deposits raise the possibility of crescentic postinfectious glomerulonephritis; and finely granular IgG-dominant capillary wall deposits suggest crescentic MN. The latter may be a result of concurrent anti-GBM disease, which also causes linear GBM staining beneath the granular staining, or concurrent ANCA disease, which can be documented serologically. About a quarter of all patients with crescentic immune complex glomerulonephritis are ANCA positive, whereas less than 5% of patients with noncrescentic immune complex glomerulonephritis are ANCA positive. This suggests that the presence of ANCAs in patients with immune complex glomerulonephritis may predispose to a disease that is more aggressive.

Electron Microscopy

As with the findings by immunofluorescence microscopy, the findings by electron microscopy in patients with crescentic immune complex glomerulonephritis depend on the type of immune complex disease that has induced crescent formation. The hallmark ultrastructural finding is immune complex–type electron-dense deposits. These deposits can be mesangial, subendothelial, intramembranous, subepithelial, or any combination of these. The pattern and distribution of deposits may indicate a particular phenotype of primary crescentic immune complex glomerulonephritis, such as postinfectious, membranous, membranoproliferative, or dense deposit disease.[357,658,1077] Ultrastructural findings also may suggest that the disease is secondary to some unrecognized systemic process. For example, endothelial tubuloreticular inclusions suggest lupus nephritis, and microtubular configurations in immune deposits suggest cryoglobulinemia.

In all types of crescentic glomerulonephritis, breaks in GBMs usually can be identified if looked for carefully, especially in glomerular segments adjacent to crescents. Dense fibrin tactoids occur in thrombosed capillaries, in sites of fibrinoid necrosis, and in the interstices between the cells in crescents. In general, the extent of fibrin tactoid formation in areas of fibrinoid necrosis is less conspicuous in crescentic immune complex glomerulonephritis than in crescentic anti-GBM or ANCA glomerulonephritis.

PATHOGENESIS

Crescentic glomerulonephritis is the result of a final common pathway of glomerular injury that results in crescent formation. Multiple causes and pathogenic mechanisms can lead to the final common pathway, including many types of immune complex disease. The general dogma is that immune complex localization in glomerular capillary walls and mesangium, by either deposition or in situ formation or both, activates multiple inflammatory mediator systems.[214,1063,1064] This includes humoral mediator systems, such as the coagulation system, kinin system, and complement system, as well as phlogogenic cells, such as neutrophils, monocytes/macrophages, lymphocytes, platelets, endothelial cells, and mesangial cells. The activated cells also release soluble mediators, such as cytokines and chemokines. If the resultant inflammation is contained internal to the GBM, a proliferative or membranoproliferative phenotype of injury ensues with only endocapillary hypercellularity. However, if the inflammation breaks through capillary walls into Bowman's space, extracapillary hypercellularity (crescent formation) results.

Complement activation has often been considered a major mediator of injury in immune complex glomerulonephritis; however, experimental data also indicate the importance of Fc receptors in immune complex–mediated injury.[1078,1079] For example, mice deficient for the FcγRI and FcγRIII receptors have a markedly reduced tendency to develop immune complex glomerulonephritis.[1080,1081]

TREATMENT

The therapy for immune complex–mediated crescentic glomerulonephritis is influenced by the nature of the underlying category of immune complex glomerulonephritis. For example, acute PSGN with 50% crescents might not prompt the same therapy as IgA nephropathy with 50% crescents. However, there is an inadequate number of controlled prospective studies to guide therapy for most forms of immune complex–mediated crescentic glomerulonephritis. Some nephrologists extrapolate from the lupus nephritis experience and choose to treat patients with crescentic immune complex disease with immunosuppressive drugs that they would not use if the glomerular lesions appeared less aggressive. For the minority of patients who have idiopathic immune complex crescentic glomerulonephritis, the most common treatment is immunosuppressive therapy with pulse methylprednisolone, followed by prednisone at a dosage of 1 mg/kg daily tapered over the second to third month to an alternate-day regimen until completely discontinued.[631,1082-1084] In patients with a rapid decline in kidney function, cytotoxic agents with or without plasma exchange in addition to corticosteroids may be considered. As with anti-GBM and ANCA disease, immunotherapy should be initiated as early as possible during the course of immune complex–mediated crescentic glomerulonephritis to reduce the likelihood of reaching the irreversible stage of advanced scarring. There is evidence, however, that crescentic glomerulonephritis with an underlying immune complex proliferative glomerulonephritis is less responsive to aggressive immunosuppressive therapy than is anti-GBM or ANCA crescentic glomerulonephritis.[1000,1075]

ANTI–GLOMERULAR BASEMENT MEMBRANE GLOMERULONEPHRITIS

EPIDEMIOLOGY

Anti-GBM disease accounts for about 10% to 20% of crescentic glomerulonephritides.[631] This disease is characterized by circulating antibodies to the GBM (anti-GBM) and deposition of IgG or, rarely, IgA along the GBM.[631,1075,1085-1097] Anti-GBM antibodies may be eluted from kidney tissue samples from patients with anti-GBM disease, which allows verification that the antibodies are specific to the GBM.[631,1091,1095] The antibodies eluted from kidney tissue bind to the same epitope of type IV collagen as the circulating anti-GBM antibodies from the same patient.[1098]

Anti-GBM disease occurs as a renal-limited disease (anti-GBM glomerulonephritis) and as a pulmonary-renal vasculitic syndrome (Goodpasture's syndrome).[631,1075,1085-1097,1099] The incidence of anti-GBM disease has two peaks with respect to age. The first peak is in the second and third decades of life, and anti-GBM disease in this age group shows a higher frequency of pulmonary hemorrhage (Goodpasture's syndrome). The second peak is in the sixth and seventh decades, and this later-onset disease is more common in women, who more often have renal-limited disease. Interestingly, anti-GBM autoantibodies were detected in multiple serum samples from the Department of Defense Serum Repository before diagnosis in a case-control study involving 30 patients with anti-GBM disease and 30 healthy controls (50% vs. 0%, $P < 0.001$),[1100] which suggests the development of the autoimmune response prior to onset of disease.

Genetic susceptibility to anti-GBM disease is associated with HLA-DR2 specificity.[1101] More detailed analysis of the association with HLA-DR2 revealed a link with the DRB1 alleles, DRB1*1501 and DQB*0602.[1102-1106] Further refinement of this association showed that polymorphic residues in the second peptide-binding region of the HLA class II antigen segregated with disease, supporting the hypothesis that the HLA association in anti-GBM disease reflects the ability of certain class II molecules to bind and present anti-GBM peptides to helper T (T_H) cells.[1102]

This concept is further supported by mouse models of anti-GBM disease in which crescentic glomerulonephritis and lung hemorrhage are restricted to only certain major histocompatibility complex (MHC) haplotypes, despite the ability of mice of all haplotypes to produce antibodies to the α3 NC1 (noncollagenous) domain of type IV collagen.[1107] Analysis of gene expression in the kidneys of mouse strains susceptible to anti-GBM antibody–induced nephritis, compared with those of control strains, revealed that one fifth of the underexpressed genes in these mice belonged to the kallikrein gene family, which encodes serine esterases implicated in the regulation of inflammation, apoptosis, redox balance, and fibrosis.[1108] Antagonizing the kallikrein pathway by blocking the bradykinin receptors B1 and B2 augmented disease, whereas bradykinin administration reduced the severity of anti-GBM antibody–induced nephritis in a susceptible mouse strain. Nephritis-sensitive mouse strains had kallikrein haplotypes that were distinct from those of control strains, including several regulatory polymorphisms. These results suggest that kallikreins are protective disease-associated genes in anti-GBM antibody–induced nephritis.[1108] Whether these findings pertain to susceptibility to or severity of anti-GBM disease in humans in unknown. It should also be noted that a more recent genomewide association study of 48 Chinese patients with anti-GBM disease compared to 225 matched healthy controls revealed a genetic association of an FCγRIIB polymorphism (I232T) with disease susceptibility.[1109] This same polymorphism has been identified in patients with SLE and is thought to alter this inhibitory receptor responsible for maintenance of B cell tolerance and activation thresholds.[1110]

PATHOLOGY

Immunofluorescence Microscopy

The pathologic finding of linear staining of the GBMs for immunoglobulin is indicative of anti-GBM glomerulonephritis (Figure 32.36).[1092,1096,1111-1114] The immunoglobulin is predominantly IgG; however, rare cases of patients with IgA-dominant anti-GBM glomerulonephritis have also been reported.[1093,1115] Linear staining for both κ- and λ-light chains typically accompanies the staining for γ-heavy chains. Linear staining for γ-heavy chains alone indicates γ-heavy-chain deposition disease. Most specimens with anti-GBM glomerulonephritis have discontinuous linear to granular capillary wall staining for C3, but a minority show little or no C3 staining. Linear staining for IgG may also occur along distal tubular basement membranes.[1096]

The linear IgG staining of GBMs frequently seen in patients with diabetic glomerulosclerosis and the less intense linear staining seen in older patients with hypertensive vascular disease must not be confused with that in anti-GBM disease. The clinical data and light microscopic findings should help make this distinction. Serologic confirmation should always be obtained to substantiate the diagnosis of anti-GBM disease.

Serologic testing for ANCAs should be ordered simultaneously, because a quarter to a third of patients with anti-GBM disease are also ANCA positive, and this may modify the prognosis and the likelihood of systemic small vessel vasculitis.[1116,1117]

Light Microscopy

At the time of biopsy, 97% of patients with anti-GBM disease have some degree of crescent formation, and 85% have crescents in 50% or more of glomeruli (Tables 32.17 and 32.18).[1064,1111] On average, 77% of glomeruli have crescents. Glomeruli with crescents typically have fibrinoid necrosis in adjacent glomerular segments. Nonnecrotic segments may look entirely normal by light microscopy or may have slight infiltration by neutrophils or mononuclear leukocytes. This differs from crescentic immune complex glomerulonephritis and C3 glomerulopathy, which typically have capillary wall thickening and endocapillary hypercellularity in the intact glomeruli. Special stains that outline basement membranes, such as Jones' methenamine silver stain or periodic acid–Schiff stain, often demonstrate focal breaks in GBMs in areas of necrosis and also show focal breaks in Bowman's capsule. The most severely injured glomeruli have global

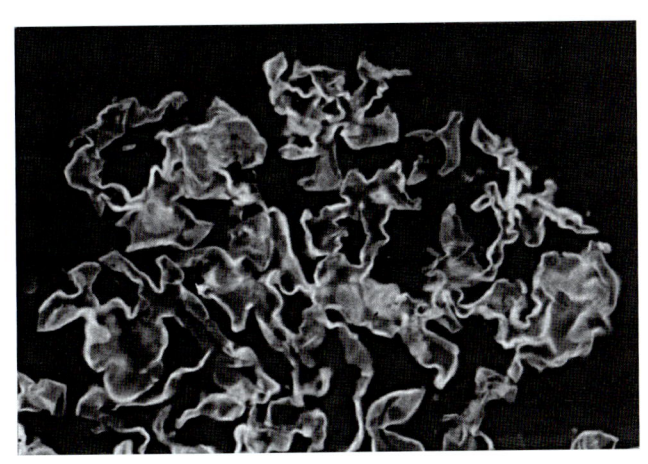

Figure 32.36 Immunofluorescence micrograph of a portion of a glomerulus with features of anti–glomerular basement membrane (anti-GBM) glomerulonephritis showing linear staining of GBMs for immunoglobulin G (IgG). (Fluorescein isothiocyanate anti-IgG stain, ×600.)

Table 32.18 Frequency of Crescent Formation in Various Glomerular Diseases*

Disease	Patients with Crescents (%)	Patients with ≥50% Crescents	Average % of Glomeruli with Crescents
Anti-GBM GN	97	85	77
ANCA-associated GN	90	50	49
Immune complex–mediated GN			
Lupus GN (classes III and IV)	56	13	27
IgA vasculitis[†]	61	10	27
IgA nephropathy[†]	32	4	21
Acute postinfectious GN[†]	33	3	19
Fibrillary GN	23	5	26
MPGN type I	24	5	25
Membranous lupus GN (class V)	12	1	17
Membranous GN (nonlupus)	3	0	15

*Based on the analysis of more than 6000 native kidney biopsy specimens evaluated at the University of North Carolina Nephropathology Laboratory. In general, diseases in which crescents are most often seen also have the largest percentage of glomeruli involved by crescents when they are present.

[†]Because more severe cases of immunoglobulin A nephropathy and postinfectious glomerulonephritis are more often evaluated by kidney biopsy, the extent of crescent involvement is higher in the patients included in this table than in the general group of patients with these diseases.

ANCA, Antineutrophil cytoplasmic antibody; GBM, glomerular basement membrane; GN, glomerulonephritis; IgA, immunoglobulin A; MPGN, membranoproliferative glomerulonephritis.

Derived from Jennette JC: Rapidly progressive crescentic glomerulonephritis. *Kidney Int* 63:1164-1172, 2003.

glomerular necrosis, circumferential cellular crescents, and extensive disruption of Bowman's capsule.

The acute necrotizing glomerular lesions and the cellular crescents evolve into glomerular sclerosis and fibrotic crescents, respectively.[1111] If the kidney biopsy specimen is obtained several weeks into the course of anti-GBM disease, the only lesions may be these chronic sclerotic lesions. There may be a mixture of acute and chronic lesions; however, the glomerular lesions of anti-GBM glomerulonephritis tend to be more in synchrony than those of ANCA glomerulonephritis, which more often show admixtures of acute and chronic injury.

Tubulointerstitial changes are commensurate with the degree of glomerular injury. Glomeruli with extensive necrosis and disruption of Bowman's capsule typically have intense periglomerular inflammation, including occasional multinucleated giant cells. There also is focal tubular epithelial acute simplification or atrophy, focal interstitial edema and fibrosis, and focal interstitial infiltration of predominantly mononuclear leukocytes. There are no specific changes in arteries or arterioles. If necrotizing inflammation is observed in arteries or arterioles, the possibility of concurrent anti-GBM and ANCA disease should be considered.

Electron Microscopy

The findings by electron microscopy reflect those seen by light microscopy.[1111,1118] In acute disease, there is focal glomerular necrosis with disruption of capillary walls. Bowman's capsule also may have focal gaps. Leukocytes, including neutrophils and monocytes, often are present at sites of necrosis but are uncommon in intact glomerular segments. Fibrin tactoids, which are electron-dense curvilinear accumulations of polymerized fibrin, accumulate at sites of coagulation system activation, including sites of capillary thrombosis, fibrinoid necrosis, and fibrin formation in Bowman's space (Figure 32.37). Cellular crescents contain cells with ultrastructural features of macrophages and epithelial cells. An important negative observation is the absence of immune complex–type electron-dense deposits. These occur only in specimens from patients with anti-GBM disease who have concurrent immune complex disease. Glomerular segments that do not have necrosis may appear remarkably normal, with only focal effacement of visceral epithelial foot processes. There may be slight lucent expansion of the lamina rara interna, but this is an inconstant and nonspecific feature. In chronic lesions, amorphous and banded collagen deposition distorts or replaces the normal architecture.

PATHOGENESIS

The landmark studies opening the way to an understanding of the pathogenesis of anti-GBM disease were those of Lerner, Glassock, and Dixon.[1091] In these studies, antibodies eluted from kidneys of patients with Goodpasture's syndrome and injected into monkeys led to the induction of glomerulonephritis, proteinuria, renal failure, and pulmonary hemorrhage along with intense staining of the GBM for human IgG.

The antigen to which anti-GBM antibodies react was initially found to be in the collagenase-resistant part of type IV collagen, the noncollagenous domain (NC1 domain).[1119-1121]

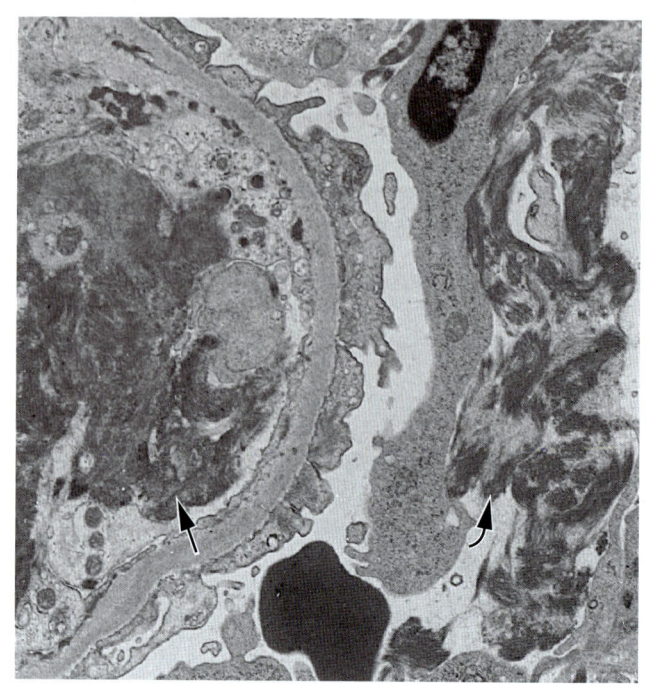

Figure 32.37 Electron micrograph of a portion of a glomerular capillary wall and adjacent urinary space from a patient with anti–glomerular basement membrane (anti-GBM) glomerulonephritis. Note the fibrin tactoids within a capillary thrombus (*straight arrow*) and in Bowman's space (*curved arrow*) between the cells of a crescent. Also note the absence of immune complex–type electron-dense deposits in the capillary wall. (×6000.)

The antigenic epitopes found in the NC1 domain are in a cryptic form, as evidenced by the fact that little reactivity is found against the native hexameric structure of the NC1 domain. However, when the hexameric NC1 domain is denatured and dissociates into dimers and monomers, the reactivity of antibodies increases 15-fold.[1121] About 90% of anti–type IV collagen antibodies are directed against the α3-chain of type IV collagen.[1083,1122] The Goodpasture epitopes in the native autoantigen are sequestered within the NC1 hexamers of the α3α4α5(IV) collagen network and are a feature of the quaternary structure of two distinct subsets of α3α4α5(IV) NC1 hexamers. Goodpasture antibodies breach only the quaternary structure of hexamers containing only monomer subunits, whereas hexamers composed of both dimer and monomer subunits (D-hexamers) are resistant to autoantibodies under native conditions.[1123,1124] The epitopes of D-hexamers are structurally sequestered by dimer reinforcement of the quaternary complex.[1124] Extensive work over the past several decades that focused on elucidating autoantibody-specific epitopes along the quaternary structure of the α3α4α5(IV) NC1 hexamer has reinforced the paradigm that this disease process is an autoimmune "conformeropathy."[1125] It is presumed that environmental factors, such as exposure to hydrocarbons,[1126] tobacco smoke,[1127] and endogenous oxidants,[1128] can also expose the cryptic Goodpasture epitopes. In patients with anti-GBM disease who do not have antibodies to the classic epitope on the α3-chain, antibodies to entactin have been detected.[1129] A small percentage of patients with anti-GBM disease may also have limited reactivity with the NC1 domains of the α1- or α4-chains of type IV collagen. These additional reactivities seem to be more frequent in patients with anti-GBM–mediated glomerulonephritis alone.[1130]

The majority of patients with anti-GBM disease express antibodies to two major conformational epitopes (E_A and E_B) located within the C-terminal noncollagenous (NC1) domain of the α3-chain of type IV collagen.[1131-1134] The immunodominant target epitope, E_A, is encompassed by α3 NC1 residues 17 to 31. A homologous region at α3 NC1 residues 127 to 141 encompasses the E_B epitope, recognized by the autoantibodies of only a small number of patients.[1135] In a large cohort of Chinese patients,[1136] the levels of antibody against E_A and E_B were strongly correlated with each other. Antibody levels against α3, E_A, and E_B correlated with serum creatinine level and with death or ESKD at 1 year but not with sex, age, presence of ANCAs, or hemoptysis. Interestingly, a more recent study found that autoantibodies against E_A and E_B were crucial for kidney dysfunction; multivariate Cox regression analysis revealed autoantibody reactivity to E_B was an independent risk factor for renal failure (HR, 6.91; $P = 0.02$).[1137] The stimuli and mechanism(s) leading to the formation of autoantibodies remain unclear, as does the mechanism by which the normally hidden target epitopes become accessible to circulating autoantibodies.

About one third of patients with anti-GBM/Goodpasture's syndrome also have circulating ANCAs, the majority being to MPO (MPO-ANCA).[1117,1130,1133,1138,1139] In a study of a large cohort of Chinese patients with anti-GBM disease with or without ANCAs, no differences in reactivity to the E_A, E_B, and S2 epitopes (a recombinant construct expressing the nine amino acid residues critical for the anti-GBM epitope)[1140] were detected between patients with anti-GBM antibodies plus ANCAs compared with anti-GBM antibodies alone.[1141] The mechanism by which some patients develop both anti-GBM antibodies and ANCAs is unknown. It is speculated that in such patients, ANCAs may appear first and cause damage to the GBM, thus exposing the normally hidden target epitopes of anti-GBM antibodies. Coexistence of ANCAs in patients with anti-GBM antibodies is associated with small vessel vasculitis in organs in addition to the lung and kidney. In experimental models, the presence of antibodies to MPO aggravates experimental anti-GBM disease.[1117,1142] Interestingly, analysis of sera stored in the Department of Defense Serum Repository from patients with anti-GBM disease revealed that multiple samples contained detectable anti-GBM autoantibodies prior to diagnosis compared to controls (50% vs. 0%, $P < 0.001$), and these same patients also had detectable PR3-ANCAs and/or MPO-ANCAs prior to diagnosis.[1100]

Unlike the autoantibodies seen in anti-GBM disease that are directed to the NC1 domain of the α3-chain of type IV collagen, the anti-GBM alloantibodies that cause posttransplant nephritis in some patients with X-linked Alport's syndrome are directed against conformational epitopes in the NC1 domain of α5(IV) collagen only.[1143] Allograft-eluted alloantibodies mainly targeted two epitopes accessible in the α3α4α5 NC1 hexamers of human GBM, unlike the sequestered α3 NC1 epitopes of anti-GBM autoantibodies.

A number of animal models of anti-GBM disease have been developed over the years, based on the immunization of animals with heterologous or homologous GBM.[1144] Alternatively, anti-GBM antibody–induced injury can be produced passively by the intravenous injection of heterologous anti-GBM antibodies. This leads to two phases of injury. The first, or so-called heterologous phase, occurs in the first 24 hours and is mediated by the direct deposition of the heterologous antibodies on the GBM with subsequent recruitment of neutrophils. This is usually followed by an autologous phase, depending on the host's immune response to the heterologous immunoglobulin bound to the GBM.[1144]

The rat model of anti-GBM disease induced by injection of heterologous anti-GBM antibodies has permitted the study of the roles of various inflammatory mediators in the development of anti-GBM disease.[1145-1148] Thus, in Wistar-Kyoto (WKY) rats injected with a rabbit antiserum to rat GBM, impairing leukocyte recruitment and monocyte/macrophage glomerular infiltrate by blocking the CXC motif chemokine ligand 16 (CXCL16) with a polyclonal anti-CXCL16 antiserum in the acute inflammatory phase or progressive phase of established glomerulonephritis significantly attenuated glomerular injury and improved proteinuria.[1149] Similarly, the depletion of $CD8^+$ cells prevented the initiation and progression of anti-GBM crescentic glomerulonephritis. In the same animal model, treatment with an antibody to perforin resulted in a significant reduction in the amount of proteinuria, frequency of glomerular crescents, and number of glomerular monocytes and macrophages, although the number of glomerular $CD8^+$ cells was not changed.[1150] These results suggest that $CD8^+$ cells play a role in glomerular injury as effector cells, in part through a perforin/granzyme-mediated pathway.

The more recent development of analogous murine models of anti-GBM disease opens the way for more specific evaluations of the inflammatory processes with the use of strains of mice with specific gene knockouts.[1107] For example, the role of protease-activated receptor 2 (PAR-2) in kidney inflammation was studied using PAR-2–deficient ($PAR-2^{-/-}$) mice.[1151] PAR-2 is a cellular receptor expressed predominantly on epithelial, mesangial, and endothelial cells in the kidney and on macrophages. PAR-2 is activated by serine proteases and coagulation factors VIIa and Xa. In the kidney, PAR-2 induces both endothelium-dependent and endothelium-independent vasodilation of afferent renal arteries and renal mesangial cell proliferation in vitro. Glomerulonephritis was induced in mice by intravenous injection of sheep anti-mouse GBM globulin. In this model, PAR-2–deficient mice had reduced crescent formation, proteinuria, and serum creatinine compared with wild-type mice, but this was not associated with a difference in glomerular accumulation of $CD4^+$ T cells or macrophages or in the number of proliferating cells in glomeruli. These results demonstrate a proinflammatory role for PAR-2 in crescentic glomerulonephritis that is independent of effects on glomerular leukocyte recruitment and mesangial cell proliferation.

Although anti-GBM disease is considered a prototypical antibody-mediated glomerulonephritis, several lines of evidence point to an important role for T cells in the initiation or pathogenesis of this disease. A role for T cells in the autoimmune response is suggested by the increased susceptibility to the disease associated with the presence of HLA class II antigens DRB1*1501 and DQB*0602.[1102-1106] Further evidence of the involvement of T cell activation in the development of the autoimmune response to the NC1 domain of the α3-chain of type IV collagen comes from studies of T cell proliferation in response to other monomeric components of the GBM[1152] and to synthetic oligopeptides.[1153] The transfer of CD4+ T cells specific to a recombinant GBM antigen into syngeneic rats resulted in a crescentic glomerulonephritis without linear anti-GBM IgG deposition.[1154] Furthermore, a single nephritogenic T cell epitope of type IV collagen α3 NC1 was demonstrated to induce glomerulonephritis in Wistar-Kyoto rats.[1155] More recently, CD4+ T cell clones generated from HLA-DRB*1501 transgenic mice immunized with a peptide corresponding to amino acids 3136-3146 of the NC1 domain of α3(IV) collagen were capable of transferring disease into HLA-DRB*1501 transgenic mice.[1156] Interestingly, cross-reactive peptides from human infection–related microbes could be identified that also induced severe proteinuria and moderate to severe glomerulonephritis in immunized rats.[1157] One peptide derived from *Clostridium botulinum* also induced pulmonary hemorrhage.[1157]

Upon immunization of mice with α3 NC1 domains of type IV collagen, the development of glomerulonephritis and lung hemorrhage depends on certain MHC haplotypes and the ability of mice to mount a T_H1 response.[1107] The role of T cells in this model was further documented by the fact that the passive transfer of lymphocytes or antibodies from nephritogenic strains to syngeneic recipients led to the development of nephritis, whereas the passive transfer of antibodies to T cell receptor–deficient mice failed to do so.[1107]

CD4+CD25+ regulatory T cells may play an important role in regulating the immune response in anti-GBM disease. Thus, the transfer of regulatory T cells into mice that were previously immunized with rabbit IgG, and before an injection of anti-GBM rabbit serum, significantly attenuated the development of proteinuria and dramatically decreased glomerular damage. On histologic analysis, there was reduced infiltration of CD4+ T cells, CD8+ T cells, and macrophages, but the deposition of immune complexes was not prevented.[1158] In humans, the action of regulatory T cells may explain, in part, the uncommon occurrence of disease relapses and the eventual disappearance of anti-GBM antibodies in patients even without the use of immunosuppressant medications.[1159] Thus, analysis of peripheral blood mononuclear cells from patients with Goodpasture's syndrome revealed the emergence of GBM-specific CD25+ regulatory T cells in the convalescent period, whereas they were undetected at the time of presentation.[1160]

The role of complement in the pathogenesis of anti-GBM disease is evidenced by the deposition of C3 along the GBM. The role of complement activation has been examined largely in studies of passive injection of heterologous antibodies to GBM. Investigations using this model suggest that the terminal components of the complement system are not involved in the pathogenesis of disease.[1161] Results of further studies in rabbits that are congenitally deficient in the sixth component of complement also suggested that the terminal components of complement do not play a major part in the pathogenesis of the disease except in leukocyte-depleted animals.[1162,1163] The role of complement cascade activation in a murine model of heterologous anti-GBM disease previously led to conflicting results as to the role of complement activation in this model.[1164] More recent studies involving the same model, using mice completely deficient of complement components C3 or C4, revealed a greater protective effect of C3 deficiency more than of C4 deficiency. Both protective effects could be overcome if the dose of nephritogenic antibodies was increased.[1165]

To further evaluate the role of complement activation and of Fcγ receptors, an "attenuated" mouse model of anti-GBM was developed using a subnephritogenic dose of rabbit anti-mouse GBM antibody followed 1 week later with an injection of mouse monoclonal antibody against rabbit IgG, which resulted in albuminuria.[1166] In this model, albuminuria was absent in Fcγ chain–deficient mice and reduced in C3-deficient mice, which indicates a role for both Fcγ receptors and complement. C1q- and C4-deficient mice did develop proteinuria, which is suggestive of involvement of the alternative complement pathway.[1166] The role of Fcγ receptors is also evidenced by the occurrence of severe lung hemorrhage in mice deficient in the inhibitory Fcγ 2b receptor that were treated with bovine type IV collagen.[1167]

Conclusions about the pathogenesis of human anti-GBM disease from animal models must be tempered because animal models may not accurately replicate human disease.

CLINICAL FEATURES AND NATURAL HISTORY

The onset of renal anti-GBM disease is typically characterized by an abrupt, acute glomerulonephritis with severe oliguria or anuria. There is a high risk of progression to ESKD if appropriate therapy is not instituted immediately. Prompt treatment with plasmapheresis, corticosteroids, and cyclophosphamide results in patient survival of approximately 85% and renal survival of approximately 60%.[1082,1168,1172]

Rarely, the disorder has a more insidious onset in which patients remain essentially asymptomatic until the development of uremic symptoms and fluid retention.[631,1099,1114,1173] The onset of disease may be associated with arthralgias, fever, myalgias, and abdominal pain; however, neurologic disturbances and gastrointestinal complaints are rare.

Goodpasture's syndrome is characterized by the presence of pulmonary hemorrhage concurrent with glomerulonephritis. The usual pulmonary manifestation is severe pulmonary hemorrhage, which may be life threatening; however, patients may have milder disease that can be focal. The absence of hemoptysis does not rule out diffuse alveolar hemorrhage. For patients with early or focal disease, a high level of suspicion is necessary to establish the diagnosis, especially in the presence of unexplained anemia. The diagnosis may be aided by measurements showing an increased diffusing capacity of carbon monoxide and by findings on computed tomography of the chest. Ultimately the diagnostic evaluation of alveolar hemorrhage usually includes bronchoscopic examination and bronchoalveolar lavage.[1174] This approach also allows exclusion of airway sources of bleeding and possible associated infections. In patients with anti-GBM disease, the occurrence of pulmonary hemorrhage is far more common in smokers than nonsmokers[1175] and may be associated with environmental exposures to hydrocarbons[1175-1178] or upper respiratory tract infections.[1179] Occupational exposure to petroleum-based mineral oils is a risk factor for the development of anti-GBM antibodies per se.[1180] The association of pulmonary hemorrhage with environmental exposures and infection raises the theoretical possibility that they expose the cryptic antigen in the alveolar basement membrane, thereby allowing its recognition by circulating anti-GBM antibodies.

LABORATORY FINDINGS

Kidney involvement by anti-GBM disease typically causes an acute nephritic syndrome with hematuria that includes dysmorphic erythrocytes and red blood cell casts. Although nephrotic-range proteinuria may occur, full nephrotic syndrome is rarely seen.[1096,1109,1111,1114,1173]

The diagnostic laboratory finding in anti-GBM disease is detection of circulating antibodies to GBM, and specifically to the α3-chain of type IV collagen. These antibodies are detected in approximately 95% of patients by immunoassays using various forms of purified or recombinant substrates.[1181] The anti-GBM antibodies are most often of the IgG1 subclass but may also be of the IgG4 subclass, with the latter being seen more often in females than in males.[1182]

TREATMENT

The standard treatment for anti-GBM disease is intensive plasmapheresis combined with corticosteroids and cyclophosphamide.[1082,1169,1183-1186] Plasmapheresis consists of removal of 2 to 4 L of plasma and its replacement with a 5% albumin solution continued on a daily basis until circulating antibody levels become undetectable. In those patients with pulmonary hemorrhage, clotting factors should be replaced by administering fresh-frozen plasma at the end of each treatment. Prednisone should be administered starting at a dose of 1 mg/kg of body weight for at least the first month and then tapered to alternate-day therapy during the second and third months of treatment. Cyclophosphamide is administered orally (at a dosage of 2 mg/kg/day, adjusted with consideration for the degree of impairment of kidney function and the white blood cell count) for 8 to 12 weeks. The role of high-dose intravenous methylprednisolone pulses remains unproven in the treatment of anti-GBM disease.[1187-1191] Nonetheless, the urgent nature of the clinical process prompts some nephrologists to administer methylprednisolone (7 mg/kg daily for 3 consecutive days) as part of induction therapy in this and other forms of crescentic glomerulonephritis.

When the regimen of aggressive plasmapheresis with corticosteroids and cyclophosphamide is used, patient survival is approximately 85% with 40% progression to ESKD.[1082,1168-1173] These results are better than those achieved before the introduction of plasmapheresis, when patient survival was less than 50% with a near 90% rate of ESKD. In a study at the Hammersmith Hospital in the United Kingdom, Gaskin and Pusey demonstrated that aggressive plasmapheresis, even in patients with severe renal insufficiency, may have an ameliorative effect and provide improved long-term patient and renal survival.[1192] In that cohort, among patients who had a creatinine concentration of 500 μmol/L or more (>5.7 mg/dL) at presentation but did not require immediate dialysis, patient and renal survival were 83% and 82% at 1 year and 62% and 69% at last follow-up, respectively. The renal prognosis of patients who presented with dialysis-dependent renal failure was poor—92% of patients had ESKD at 1 year. All patients who required immediate dialysis and whose kidney biopsy specimens had crescents involving 100% of glomeruli remained dialysis dependent.[1193]

The major prognostic marker for the progression to ESKD is the serum creatinine level at the time of initiation of treatment. Patients with a serum creatinine concentration higher than 7 mg/dL are unlikely to recover sufficient kidney function to discontinue renal replacement therapy.[1094] At issue is whether and for how long aggressive immunosuppression should persist in dialysis-dependent patients. Aggressive immunosuppression and plasmapheresis are warranted in patients with pulmonary hemorrhage. Aggressive immunosuppression should be withheld in patients with disease limited to the kidney whose kidney biopsy specimens show widespread glomerular and interstitial scarring and who have a serum creatinine concentration of higher than 7 mg/dL at presentation. In such patients, the risks of therapy outweigh the potential benefits. In patients who have an elevated serum creatinine level, yet whose biopsy specimens show active crescentic glomerulonephritis, aggressive treatment should continue for at least 4 weeks. If there is no restoration of kidney function without any evidence of pulmonary hemorrhage by 4 to 8 weeks, then, immunosuppression should be discontinued.

Patients who have both circulating anti-GBM antibodies and ANCAs, may have a better chance of recovery of kidney function than do patients with anti-GBM antibodies alone. In these patients, immunosuppressive therapy should not be withheld, even with serum creatinine levels higher than 7 mg/dL, because the concomitant presence of ANCAs was associated with a more favorable renal outcome in some studies[1191,1194] though not in all.[1195] In a retrospective analysis comparing patients with anti-GBM autoantibodies, MPO-ANCAs, and both, "double positive" patients and those with anti-GBM autoantibodies had significantly higher serum creatinine levels at presentation (10.3 ± 5.6 and 9.6 ± 8.1 mg/dL, respectively) than did patients with MPO-ANCAs alone (5.0 ± 2.9 mg/dL). One-year renal survival was better among patients with MPO-ANCAs alone (63%) than in the double-positive group (10.0%, $P = 0.01$) and the anti-GBM group (15.4%, $P = 0.17$).[1195]

Once remission of anti-GBM disease is achieved with immunosuppressive therapy, recurrent disease occurs only rarely.[1196-1199] Similarly, the recurrence of anti-GBM disease after kidney transplantation is also rare, especially when transplantation is delayed until after the disappearance or substantial diminution of anti-GBM antibodies in the circulation.[1200]

PAUCI-IMMUNE CRESCENTIC GLOMERULONEPHRITIS

EPIDEMIOLOGY

In pauci-immune crescentic glomerulonephritis, the characteristic feature of the glomerular lesion is focal necrotizing and crescentic glomerulonephritis with little or no glomerular staining for immunoglobulins by immunofluorescence microscopy.[1064,1086,1111,1184,1186] Pauci-immune crescentic glomerulonephritis usually is a component of a systemic small vessel vasculitis; however, some patients have renal-limited (primary) pauci-immune crescentic glomerulonephritis.[1116,1164,1174,1201] ANCA-associated small vessel vasculitis is also discussed in Chapter 33. Pauci-immune crescentic glomerulonephritis, including that accompanying small vessel vasculitis, is the most common category of RPGN in adults, especially older adults (see Table 32.16). The disease has a predilection for whites compared with blacks, and the prevalence of the disease is not significantly different in males compared with females (see Table 32.15).

PATHOLOGY

Light Microscopy

The light microscopic appearance of ANCA-associated pauci-immune crescentic glomerulonephritis is indistinguishable from that of anti-GBM crescentic glomerulonephritis.[357,657,1065,1075,1201-1204] Renal-limited (primary) pauci-immune crescentic glomerulonephritis also is indistinguishable from pauci-immune crescentic glomerulonephritis that occurs as a component of a systemic small vessel vasculitis, such as GPA, MPA, or EGPA. As illustrated in Figure 32.30, ANCA glomerulonephritis and anti-GBM glomerulonephritis most often manifest as crescentic glomerulonephritis.

At the time of biopsy, approximately 90% of kidney biopsy specimens with ANCA-associated pauci-immune glomerulonephritis have some degree of crescent formation, and approximately half of the specimens have crescents involving 50% or more of glomeruli (see Tables 32.17 and 32.18). Over 90% of specimens have focal segmental to global fibrinoid necrosis (Figure 32.38). As with anti-GBM disease, the intact glomerular segments often have no light microscopic abnormalities. The most severely injured glomeruli have not only extensive necrosis of glomerular tufts but also extensive lysis of Bowman's capsule with resultant periglomerular inflammation. The periglomerular inflammation contains varying mixtures of neutrophils, eosinophils, lymphocytes, monocytes, and macrophages, including occasional multinucleated giant cells. This periglomerular inflammation area may have a granulomatous appearance, especially when the glomerulus that was the nidus of inflammation has been destroyed or is not in the plane of section. This granulomatous appearance is a result of the periglomerular reaction to extensive glomerular necrosis and is not specific for a particular category of necrotizing glomerulonephritis.

This pattern of injury can be seen with anti-GBM glomerulonephritis, renal-limited pauci-immune crescentic glomerulonephritis, and crescentic glomerulonephritis secondary to MPA, GPA, and EGPA. Necrotizing granulomatous inflammation that is not centered on a glomerulus but, rather, is in the interstitium or centered on an artery raises the possibility of GPA or EGPA. The presence of arteritis in a biopsy specimen that has pauci-immune crescentic glomerulonephritis indicates that the glomerulonephritis is a component of a more widespread vasculitis, such as MPA, GPA, or EGPA.

The acute necrotizing glomerular lesions evolve into sclerotic lesions. During completely quiescent phases, a kidney biopsy specimen may have only focal sclerotic lesions that can mimic FSGS. ANCA-associated glomerulonephritis is also often characterized by many recurrent bouts of exacerbation. Therefore, combinations of active acute necrotizing glomerular lesions and chronic sclerotic lesions often occur in the same kidney biopsy specimen.

Immunofluorescence Microscopy

By definition, the distinguishing pathologic difference between pauci-immune crescentic glomerulonephritis and anti-GBM and immune complex–mediated crescentic glomerulonephritis is the absence or paucity of glomerular staining for immunoglobulins. How pauci-immune is pauci-immune crescentic glomerulonephritis? One basis for categorizing the disorder as pauci-immune crescentic glomerulonephritis is to determine whether the patient is likely to be ANCA positive, which increases the likelihood of certain systemic small vessel vasculitides.[363,1201,1205,1206] The likelihood of positivity for ANCAs is inversely proportional to the intensity of glomerular immunoglobulin staining by immunofluorescence microscopy in a specimen with crescentic glomerulonephritis.[1204] The likelihood of positive results on an ANCA serologic assay is approximately 90% if there is no staining for immunoglobulin, approximately 80% if there is trace to 1+ staining (on a scale of 0 to 4+), approximately 50% if there is 2+ staining, approximately 30% if there is 3+ staining, and less than 10% if there is 4+ staining. Thus, even patients with definite evidence for immune complex–mediated glomerulonephritis have a higher than expected frequency of the presence of ANCAs, but the highest frequency is in those patients with little or no evidence for immune complex– or anti-GBM–mediated disease.

The presence of ANCAs at higher than expected frequency in immune complex disease is intriguing and raises the possibility that ANCAs contribute to the pathogenesis of not only pauci-immune crescentic glomerulonephritis but also the most severe examples of immune complex disease.[363] Looking at this issue from a different perspective, approximately 25% of patients with idiopathic immune complex crescentic glomerulonephritis (i.e., immune complex glomerulonephritis that does not fit well into one of the categories of primary or secondary immune complex disease) are ANCA positive, compared to less than 5% of patients who have idiopathic immune complex glomerulonephritis with no crescents.[363]

Glomerular capillary wall or mesangial staining usually accompanies immunoglobulin staining and is present in

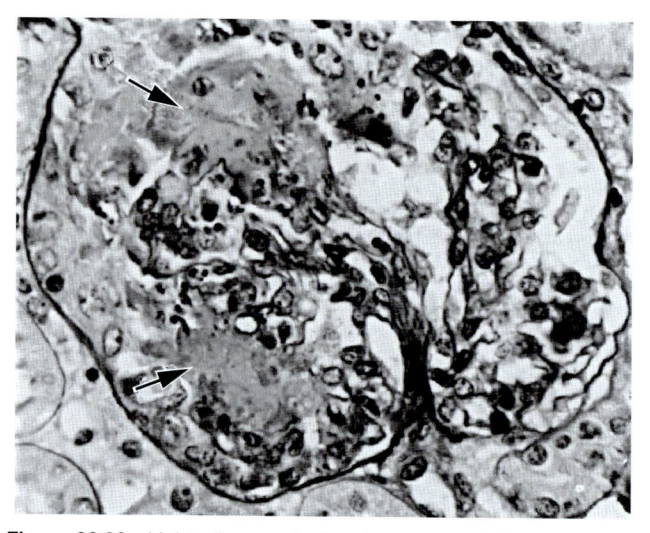

Figure 32.38 Light micrograph showing segmental fibrinoid necrosis in a glomerulus from a patient with antineutrophil cytoplasmic autoantibody–associated pauci-immune crescentic glomerulonephritis. (Periodic acid–Schiff stain, ×300.)

occasional specimens that do not have immunoglobulin staining. There is irregular staining for fibrin at sites of intraglomerular fibrinoid necrosis and capillary thrombosis and in the interstices of crescents. Foci of glomerular necrosis and sclerosis also may have irregular staining for C3 and IgM.

Electron Microscopy

The findings by electron microscopy are indistinguishable from those described earlier for anti-GBM glomerulonephritis.[1118] Specimens with pure pauci-immune crescentic glomerulonephritis have no or only a few immune complex–type electron-dense deposits. Foci of glomerular necrosis have leukocyte influx, breaks in GBMs, and fibrin tactoids in capillary thrombi and sites of fibrinoid necrosis.

PATHOGENESIS

The pathogenesis of pauci-immune crescentic glomerulonephritis is currently not fully understood, but there is strong evidence that ANCA IgG is a major pathogenic factor.[1207-1209] In the absence or paucity of immune complex deposition within glomeruli or other vessels, classical mechanisms of immune complex–mediated damage are not implicated in the pathogenesis of pauci-immune crescentic glomerulonephritis. On the other hand, the substantial accumulation of polymorphonuclear leukocytes at sites of vascular necrosis has led to examination of the role of neutrophil activation in this disease. There is now convincing evidence that ANCAs are directly involved in the pathogenesis of pauci-immune small vessel vasculitis or glomerulonephritis.[1209] Substantial in vitro data implicate a pathogenic role for ANCAs based on the demonstration that these autoantibodies activate normal human polymorphonuclear leukocytes.[1204,1207,1210-1212]

For anti-MPO autoantibodies, anti-PR3 autoantibodies, or autoantibodies to other neutrophil antigens contained within the azurophilic granules to interact with their corresponding antigens, either the antibodies must penetrate the cell or, alternatively, those antigens must translocate to the cell surface. Indeed, small amounts of cytokine (e.g., TNF-α and IL-1) at concentrations too low to cause full neutrophil activation are capable of inducing such a translocation of ANCA antigens to the cell surface.[1213] This translocation of ANCA antigens to the cell surface has been demonstrated in vivo on the neutrophils of patients with GPA and in patients with sepsis.[1214-1216] Patients with ANCA disease aberrantly express PR3 and MPO genes, and this expression correlates with disease activity.[1217] Despite the fact that these genes exist on different chromosomes, their expression appears coordinately upregulated during disease activity and downregulated during remission. Epigenetic changes occur as a result of increased unmethylated DNA at the MPO and PR3 loci and as a result of loss of recruitment of histone methylase PRC2 (Polycomb recessive complex 2) by RUNX3 (Runt-related transcription factor 3) in both MPO and PR3 genes with depressed gene transcription. In addition, JMJD3 (Jumonji domain–containing protein 3) appears to be expressed in these patients, which further diminishes histone H3K27me3 methylation status.[1218]

Regardless of whether the antigen is expressed on the surface of the cell as a consequence of cytokine stimulation or gene expression, in the presence of circulating ANCAs, the interaction of the autoantibody with its externalized antigen results in full activation of the neutrophil, which leads to the respiratory burst and degranulation of primary and secondary granule constituents.[1219,1220] The current hypothesis stipulates that ANCAs induce a premature degranulation and activation of neutrophils at the time of their margination and diapedesis, which leads to the release of lytic enzymes and toxic oxygen metabolites at the site of the vessel wall, thereby producing a necrotizing inflammatory injury. This view is supported by in vitro studies demonstrating that neutrophils activated by ANCAs lead to the damage and destruction of human umbilical vein endothelial cells in culture.[1221-1223]

Not only does neutrophil degranulation cause direct damage of the endothelium, but ANCA antigens released from neutrophils and monocytes enter endothelial cells and cause cell damage. PR3 can enter the endothelial cells by a receptor-mediated process[1224-1226] and result in the production of IL-8[1227] and chemoattractant protein-1. PR3 also induces an apoptotic event from both proteolytic and nonproteolytic mechanisms.[1228,1229] Interestingly, PR3-mediated apoptosis appears to be, in part, related to cleavage of the cell cycle inhibitor $p21^{CIP1/WAF1}$ and NF-κB.[1230,1231] Similarly, MPO enters endothelial cells by an energy-dependent process[1232] and transcytoses intact endothelium to localize within the extracellular matrix. There, in the presence of the substrates H_2O_2 and NO_2^-, MPO catalyzes nitration of tyrosine residues on extracellular matrix proteins,[1233] which results in the fragmentation of extracellular matrix protein.[1234] It also appears that endothelial cells inhibit superoxide generation by ANCA-activated neutrophils and that serine proteases may play a more important role than reactive oxygen species as mediators of endothelial injury during ANCA-associated systemic vasculitis.[1235]

Neutrophil activation by ANCAs is likely mediated by both the antigen-binding portion of the autoantibodies (F[ab′]$_2$) and by the engagement of their Fc fraction to Fcγ receptors on the surface of neutrophils.[1073,1222,1236,1237] Human neutrophils constitutively express the IgG receptors FcγRIIa and FcγRIIIb.[1238] Engagement of the Fc receptors results in a number of neutrophil-activation events, including respiratory burst, degranulation, phagocytosis, cytokine production, and upregulation of adhesion molecules. ANCAs have been shown to engage both types of receptors.[1222,1239] In particular, FcγRIIa engagement by ANCAs appears to increase neutrophil actin polymerization in neutrophils, which leads to distortion in their shape and possibly decreases their ability to pass through capillaries (the primary site of injury in ANCA vasculitis).[1240] Furthermore, polymorphisms of the FcγRIIIb receptors[1241,1242] (but not of FcγRII receptors[1243,1244]) appear to influence the severity of ANCA vasculitis.

In addition to the Fc receptor–mediated mechanism, substantial data support a role for the F(ab′)$_2$ portion of the antibody molecule in leukocyte activation. ANCA F(ab′)$_2$ portions induce oxygen radical production[1237] and the transcription of cytokine genes in normal human neutrophils and monocytes. Microarray gene chip analysis showed that ANCA IgG and ANCA-F(ab′)$_2$ stimulate transcription of a distinct subset of genes, some unique to whole IgG, some unique to F(ab′)$_2$ fragments, and some common to both.[1245] It is most likely that F(ab′)$_2$ portions of ANCA are capable of low-level neutrophil and monocyte activation.[1237] The Fc portion of the molecule almost certainly causes leukocyte activation once the F(ab′)2 portion of the immunoglobulin has interacted with the antigen, either on the cell surface or in the microenvironment.[1222] The signal transduction pathways of F(ab′)2 and Fc receptor activation through a specific p21ras (Kirsten-ras) pathway has also been elucidated.[1246]

Given the pathogenicity of ANCA, there has been considerable effort of late directed toward identifying specific epitope(s) on MPO that are recognized by ANCAs in an effort to begin to identify therapeutic avenues to eliminate this interaction in vivo. Using a highly sensitive epitope excision/mass spectrometry approach, investigators from the United States, the Netherlands, and Australia identified autoantibodies to specific epitopes of MPO in sera from patients with active disease that differed from those in remission. Furthermore, this same study reported what may be a seminal finding in that pathogenic MPO-ANCAs were found in patients with ANCA-negative disease, which were detected after IgG purification that eliminated ceruloplasmin (the natural inhibitor of MPO) contamination from serum.[1247]

The role of T cells in the pathogenesis of pauci-immune necrotizing small vessel vasculitis or glomerulonephritis, although suspected,[1248,1249] is less well defined. Such a role is suggested by the presence of CD4+ T cells in granulomatous[1250] and active vasculitic lesions[1251-1255] and by some correlation of the levels of soluble markers of T cell activation with disease activity,[1250,1256] specifically, soluble IL-2 receptor and sCD3.[1257,1258] Much is known about T cell responsivity in ANCA disease, including the recognition of PR3 and MPO by T cells.[1259,1260] The proportion of regulatory T cells in ANCA patients increases, although these regulatory T cells seem defective in their inability to suppress proliferation of effector cells in cytokine production. In addition, the percentage of T cells secreting IL-17 increases in the periphery, and serum levels of T_H17-associated cytokine IL-23 correlate with the propensity for disease activity.[1261] Although yet to be replicated and validated, gene expression profiling of purified CD8+ T cells from patients with ANCA-associated vasculitis identified a signature associated with poor prognosis and included an expanded CD8+ memory T cell population.[1262] A separate study examining purified CD4+ T cells from patients with ANCA-associated vasculitis found an increased frequency of regulatory T cells with decreased suppressive function in patients with active disease as well as a second T cell population that was resistant to regulatory T cell suppression.[1263]

It has long been proposed that patients with ANCA-associated vasculitis and glomerulonephritis have a genetic predisposition for disease. The first ever genomewide association study was performed recently using DNA samples from 1233 patients in the United Kingdom with ANCA-associated vasculitis and 5884 controls and a replication cohort of 1454 Northern European case patients and 1666 controls.[1264] Interestingly, genetic associations were made most strongly with respect to ANCA serotype rather than disease phenotype in that patients with PR3-ANCAs had significant associations with HLA-DP and genes encoding α_1-antitrypsin (SERPINA1, the endogenous inhibitor or PR3) and PR3 (PRTN3) itself ($P = 6.2 \times 10^{-89}$, $P = 5.6 \times 10^{-12}$, and $P = 2.6 \times 10^{-7}$, respectively). Patients with MPO-ANCAs had a significant genomewide association with HLA-DQ ($P = 2.1 \times 10^{-8}$). Of note, ANCA-associated vasculitis is notably rare in African Americans; however, an association of the HLA-DRB1*15 alleles with PR3-ANCA–positive disease has been found, conferring a 73.3-fold higher risk in African American patients than in community-based controls.[1265] Interestingly, the DRB1*1501 allelic variant, which is of Caucasian descent, was found in 50% of African American patients, whereas the DRB1*1503, of African descent, was underrepresented in this group.

Further establishment of a pathogenetic link between ANCAs and the development of pauci-immune necrotizing glomerulonephritis and small vessel vasculitis greatly benefited from the development of animal models of this disease.

Early models of disease were based on the finding of circulating anti-MPO antibodies in 20% of female MRL/lpr mice[1266] and in an inbred strain of mice, SCG/Kj, derived from the MRL/lpr mice and BXSB strains that develop a severe form of crescentic glomerulonephritis and systemic necrotizing vasculitis.[1267] Anti-MPO antibodies have been isolated from these strains of mice. Treatment of rats with mercuric chloride led to the development of widespread inflammation, including necrotizing vasculitis in the presence of anti-MPO antibodies and anti-GBM antibodies.[1268] A more convincing model points to a pathogenetic role for ANCAs. Aggravation of a mild anti-GBM–mediated glomerulonephritis in rats when the animals were previously immunized with MPO[1142] suggests that minor proinflammatory events could be driven to severe necrotizing processes in the presence of ANCAs.

More compelling models for ANCA small vessel vasculitis now exist. MPO-deficient mice were immunized with murine MPO, and splenocytes from these mice were transferred to immunoincompetent recombination-activating gene 2 (Rag2)–deficient mice. This resulted in the development of anti-MPO autoantibodies, severe necrotizing and crescentic glomerulonephritis, and, in some animals, vasculitis in the lung and other organ systems. In a separate but similar set of experiments, anti-MPO antibodies alone were transferred into $Rag2^{-/-}$ mice and induced pauci-immune necrotizing and crescentic glomerulonephritis.[1269] These studies indicate that anti-MPO antibodies cause pauci-immune necrotizing disease. The glomerulonephritis induced by anti-MPO antibodies is aggravated by the administration of lipopolysaccharide (LPS).[1270] Conversely, the disease is abrogated when the neutrophils of anti-MPO–recipient mice are depleted by a selective antineutrophil monoclonal antibody.[1271] In experiments to assess the role of T cells using this animal model, the transfer of T cell–enriched splenocytes (> 99% T cells) did not cause glomerular crescent formation or vascular necrosis. These data do not support a pathogenic role for anti-MPO T cells in the induction of acute injury.[1272] Furthermore, the role of genetic predisposition was investigated by inducing disease in 13 inbred mouse strains from the Collaborative Cross; however, a dominant quantitative trait locus was not identified, suggesting that differences in severity are likely polygenic in nature and possibly related to environmental milieu as well.[1273]

Using the same model described earlier, a previously unsuspected role of complement activation was demonstrated. Glomerulonephritis and vasculitis were abolished with administration of cobra venom factor and failed to develop in mice deficient in complement factors C5 and B, whereas C4-deficient mice developed disease comparable with that in wild-type mice.[1274] These results indicate that the alternative complement pathway is required for disease induction, but not the classical or lectin pathways. Using this same mouse model, glomerulonephritis was completely abolished or markedly ameliorated by treating the mice with a C5-inhibiting monoclonal antibody either 8 hours before or 1 day after disease induction with anti-MPO IgG and lipopolysaccharide.[1275] Thus, anti-C5 had a dramatic therapeutic effect on this mouse model of ANCA vasculitis. These results are corroborated by in vitro experiments demonstrating that blockade of the C5a receptor on human neutrophils abrogated their stimulation.[1276] More recent work confirmed the immunopathogenetic importance of the alternative complement pathway in that blockade of C5a receptor (C5aR) activity protects against disease development. Mice expressing human C5aR were protected from anti-MPO autoantibody–induced disease when given an oral small molecule antagonist of human C5aR called CCX168.[1277] In contrast, using the same mouse model, mice deficient in complement factor 6 were not protected from disease, thereby supporting the concept that formation of the membrane attack complex is not necessary for disease development. In aggregate, these results suggest an important role for complement activation in the pathogenesis of ANCA vasculitis and have implications for possible future therapeutic interventions using blockers of the complement cascade. Although yet to be confirmed, there is also preliminary evidence for this in humans, as abnormal levels of C3a, C5a, and soluble C5b-9 in plasma and urine have been identified in patients with active disease.[1278,1279] In fact, a human clinical trial is now under way to assess the safety and efficacy of CCX168 in patients with ANCA-associated glomerulonephritis (www.clinicaltrials.gov, NCT01363388). It is also important to note that all evidence for the role of the alternative complement pathway emanates from a model of anti-MPO autoantibody–mediated disease, and there is no direct evidence in mice or humans that this also applies to anti-PR3 autoantibody–mediated disease.

The pathogenic role of anti-MPO antibodies has also been documented in a second animal model in which rats immunized with human MPO developed anti-rat-MPO antibodies and necrotizing and crescentic glomerulonephritis, as well as pulmonary capillaritis.[1280] Using intravital microscopy, elegant studies have shown that anti-MPO–activated neutrophils undergo margination and diapedesis along the vascular wall.[1280,1281] These two animal models document that anti-MPO antibodies are capable of causing necrotizing and crescentic glomerulonephritis and a widespread systemic vasculitis.

A model of anti-PR3–induced vascular injury was developed in PR3/neutrophil elastase–deficient mice in which the passive transfer of murine anti-mouse PR3 was associated with a stronger localized cutaneous inflammation, and perivascular infiltrates were observed around cutaneous vessels at the sites of intradermal injection of TNF-α.[1272,1282] In summary, these animal studies document that both anti-MPO and PR3 antibodies are capable of causing disease.

As is true for most autoimmune responses, the inciting events in the breakdown of tolerance and the generation of anti-MPO or anti-PR3 antibodies are not known. Although genetic predispositions[1283] and environmental exposure to foreign pathogens,[1284] notably to silica,[1285,1286] have been implicated, no direct link between these exposures and the formation of ANCAs has been established. A serendipitous finding in ANCA vasculitis has spawned a theory of autoantigen complementarity.[1287,1288] This theory rests on evidence that proteins transcribed and translated from the sense strand of DNA bind to proteins that are transcribed and translated from the antisense strand of DNA. It has been demonstrated that some patients with PR3-ANCAs harbor antibodies to an antigen complementary to the middle portion of PR3. These anticomplementary PR3 antibodies form an anti-idiotypic pair with PR3-ANCAs. Moreover, cloned complementary PR3 proteins bind to PR3 and function as a serine proteinase inhibitor. Preliminary data suggest that the complementary PR3 antigens are found on a variety of microbes, some of which have been associated with ANCA vasculitis and have also been found in the genome of some patients with both PR3-ANCAs and MPO-ANCAs.[1288] Although these studies need to be confirmed and expanded to determine the source of the complementary PR3 antigens and their role (if any) in inducing vasculitis, these observations may provide a promising avenue for detection of the proximate cause of the ANCA autoimmune response.

CLINICAL FEATURES AND NATURAL HISTORY

The majority of patients with pauci-immune necrotizing crescentic glomerulonephritis and ANCAs have glomerular disease as part of a systemic small vessel vasculitis. The disease is clinically limited to the kidney in about one third of patients.[1289] When both renal-limited and vasculitis-associated pauci-immune crescentic glomerulonephritis are considered, this category of crescentic glomerulonephritis is the most common cause of RPGN in adults.[1064,1070,1116,1289,1290] When the disorder is part of a systemic vasculitis, patients have pulmonary-renal, dermal-renal, or a multisystem disease. Frequent sites of involvement are the eyes, ears, sinuses, upper airways, lungs, gastrointestinal tract, skin, peripheral nerves, joints, and central nervous system. The three major ANCA-associated syndromes are MPA, GPA, and EGPA.[1202,1291,1292] Even when patients have no clinical evidence of extrarenal manifestations of active vasculitis, systemic symptoms consisting of fever, fatigue, myalgias, and arthralgias are common.

Most patients with ANCA-associated pauci-immune necrotizing glomerulonephritis have RPGN with rapid loss of kidney function associated with hematuria, proteinuria, and hypertension. However, some patients follow a more indolent course of slow decline in function and less active urine sediment. In the latter group of patients, episodes of focal necrosis and hematuria resolve with focal glomerular scarring. Subsequent relapses result in cumulative damage to glomeruli.

It is important to note that patients who have only pauci-immune crescentic glomerulonephritis at presentation may later develop signs and symptoms of systemic disease with involvement of extrarenal organ systems.[1293] An autopsy study was conducted in deceased patients with ANCA-associated vasculitis. This study revealed the widespread presence of glomerulonephritis but also demonstrated the finding of clinically silent extrarenal vasculitis. Eight percent of patients died either from septic infections or from progressive recurrent vasculitis.[1293]

No studies currently available specifically examine the prognostic factors of pauci-immune crescentic glomerulonephritis in the absence of extrarenal manifestations of disease. In studies addressing the question of prognosis of patients with ANCA-related small vessel vasculitis in general,[1205,1293,1294] the presence of pulmonary hemorrhage was the most important determinant of patient survival. With respect to the risk of ESKD, the most important predictor of outcome is the entry serum creatinine level at the time of initiation of treatment.[1294] This parameter remained the most important predictive factor of renal outcome in a multivariate analysis that corrected for variables such as the presence or absence of extrarenal disease. Treatment resistance and progression to ESKD is also predicted by longer disease duration and vascular sclerosis on kidney biopsy specimens (presence of glomerular sclerosis, interstitial infiltrates, tubular necrosis, and atrophy),[1295] and the presence of clinical markers of chronic disease, including cumulative organ damage (measured by the Vasculitis Damage Index).[1296] A finding of vascular sclerosis on the biopsy was also found to be an independent predictor of treatment resistance[1297] and may be a reflection of chronic kidney damage due to hypertension or other atherosclerotic processes, with ANCA-associated nephritis providing an additional insult.

The impact of kidney damage as a predictor of resistance emphasizes the importance of early diagnosis and prompt institution of therapy. It is important to note that although the entry serum creatinine level is the most important predictor of renal outcome, there is no threshold of kidney dysfunction beyond which treatment is deemed futile, because more than half of patients who have a GFR of less than 10 mL/min at presentation reach a remission and experience a substantial improvement in kidney function.[1298] Therefore, aggressive immunosuppressive therapy is warranted in all patients with newly diagnosed disease.[1297] However, the risk of progression to ESKD is also determined by the change in GFR within the first 4 months of treatment. In the absence of other disease manifestations, the decision to continue immunosuppressive therapy in patients with a sharply declining GFR should be weighed against the diminishing chance of renal recovery.[1297]

Relapses of ANCA small vessel vasculitis occur in up to 40% of patients. Based on a large cohort study, the risk of relapse appears to be predicted by the presence of PR3-ANCAs (as opposed to MPO-ANCAs) and the presence of upper respiratory tract or lung involvement.[1297] Patients with glomerulonephritis alone who predominantly have MPO-ANCAs belong to the subgroup of patients with a relatively low risk of relapse, with a relapse rate of around 25% at a median of 62 months.

Pauci-immune necrotizing glomerulonephritis and small vessel vasculitis may recur after kidney transplantation.[1299,1300] The rate of recurrence for ANCA small vessel vasculitis in general, including pauci-immune necrotizing glomerulonephritis alone, is about 20%.[1301] The rate of recurrence in the subset of patients who have pauci-immune necrotizing glomerulonephritis alone without systemic vasculitis is unknown but may be lower than 20%. A positive ANCA test result at the time of transplantation does not seem to be associated with an increased risk of recurrent disease.

LABORATORY FINDINGS

Approximately 80% to 90% of patients with pauci-immune necrotizing and crescentic glomerulonephritis have circulating ANCAs.[362,1205,1208,1291,1302-1304] On indirect immunofluorescence microscopy of alcohol-fixed neutrophils, ANCAs cause two patterns of staining: perinuclear (P-ANCA) and cytoplasmic (C-ANCA).[1208,1304] The two major antigen specificities for ANCA are MPO and PR3.[1201,1304-1307] Both proteins are found in the primary granules of neutrophils and the lysosomes of monocytes. With rare exceptions, anti-MPO autoantibodies produce a P-ANCA pattern of staining on indirect immunofluorescence microscopy, whereas anti-PR3 autoantibodies produce a C-ANCA pattern of staining. About two thirds of patients with pauci-immune necrotizing crescentic glomerulonephritis without clinical evidence of systemic vasculitis will have MPO-ANCAs or P-ANCAs, and approximately 30% have PR3-ANCAs or C-ANCAs.[1202,1308] The relative frequency of MPO-ANCAs to PR3-ANCAs is higher in patients with renal-limited disease than in patients with MPA or GPA.[1202] A small percentage of patients will harbor both MPO- and PR3-ANCAs; however, this likely represents primarily those patients who have been exposed to levamisole-adulterated cocaine.[1309,1310]

As mentioned previously, about one third of patients with anti-GBM disease and approximately a quarter of patients with idiopathic immune complex crescent glomerulonephritis test positive for ANCAs; therefore, ANCA positivity is not completely specific for pauci-immune crescentic glomerulonephritis.[362] Maximal sensitivity and specificity with ANCA testing is achieved when both immunofluorescence and antigen-specific assays are performed. Antigen-specific assays may be either enzyme-linked immunosorbent assays or radioimmunoassays. A variety of commercial tests are now available, and their diagnostic specificity ranges from 70% to 90%, and sensitivity from 81% to 91%.[362,1311] Tests still do not provide the necessary sensitivity, specificity, and predictive power to allow their use as the basis for initiating or altering cytotoxic therapy.

The positive predictive value (PPV) of a positive ANCA test result (i.e., the percentage of patients with a positive result who have pauci-immune crescentic glomerulonephritis) depends on the signs and symptoms of disease in the patient who is tested. The signs and symptoms indicate the pretest likelihood of pauci-immune crescentic glomerulonephritis (predicted prevalence), which greatly influences predictive value. The PPV of a positive ANCA result in a patient with classic features of RPGN is 95%.[362] In patients with hematuria and proteinuria, the PPV of a positive ANCA result is 84% if the serum creatinine is greater than 3 mg/dL, 60% if the serum creatinine is 1.5 to 3.0 mg/dL, and only 29% if the serum creatinine is less than 1 mg/dL.[1312] Although the PPV is not good in this last setting, the negative predictive value is greater than 95%, and thus a negative result can allay any concerns that the patient has early or mild pauci-immune necrotizing glomerulonephritis.

Urinalysis findings in pauci-immune crescentic glomerulonephritis include hematuria with dysmorphic red blood cells, with or without red cell casts, and proteinuria. The proteinuria ranges from 1 g of protein per 24 hours to as much as 16 g of protein per 24 hours.[1293,1313] Serum creatinine concentration usually is elevated at the time of diagnosis and rising, although a minority of patients have relatively indolent disease. Erythrocyte sedimentation rate and C-reactive protein level are elevated during active disease. Serum complement component levels are typically within normal limits.

Whether a kidney biopsy is essential for the management of ANCA-associated pauci-immune glomerulonephritis depends on a number of factors, including the diagnostic accuracy of ANCA testing, the pretest probability of finding pauci-immune glomerulonephritis, the value of knowing the activity and chronicity of the renal lesions, and the risk associated with immunotherapy for ANCA-associated pauci-immune necrotizing glomerulonephritis. Based on a study of 1000 patients with proliferative and/or necrotizing glomerulonephritis and a positive test for either PR3-ANCA or MPO-ANCA, the PPV of ANCA testing was found to be 86% with a false-positive rate of 14% and a false-negative rate of 16%. Considering the serious risks inherent in treatment with high-dose corticosteroids and cytotoxic agents, it is prudent to confirm the diagnosis and characterize the activity and chronicity of ANCA-associated pauci-immune crescentic glomerulonephritis by kidney biopsy unless the patient is too ill to tolerate the procedure.[1312]

TREATMENT

Data on the treatment of ANCA-positive pauci-immune necrotizing and crescentic glomerulonephritis are derived from studies of ANCA-associated small vessel vasculitis, including GPA and MPA. There are scant data specifically addressing the treatment of patients with renal-limited pauci-immune necrotizing glomerulonephritis. The treatment of pauci-immune crescentic glomerulonephritis (with or without systemic vasculitis) remains based primarily on varying regimens of corticosteroids and cyclophosphamide.[1294,1314,1315]

In view of the potential explosive and fulminant nature of this disease, induction therapy should be instituted using pulse methylprednisolone at a dose of 7 mg/kg/day for three consecutive days in an attempt to halt the aggressive, destructive, inflammatory process. This is followed by the institution of daily oral prednisone, as well as cyclophosphamide, either orally or intravenously. Prednisone is usually started at a dosage of 1 mg/kg/day for the first month, then tapered to an alternate-day regimen, and then discontinued by the end of the fourth to fifth month. When a regimen of monthly intravenous doses of cyclophosphamide is used, the starting dose should be about 0.5 g/m^2 and should be adjusted upward to 1 g/m^2 based on the 2-week leukocyte count nadir.[1315,1316] A regimen based on daily oral cyclophosphamide should begin at a dose of 2 mg/kg/day[1314] and should be adjusted downward as needed to keep a nadir leukocyte count above 3000 cells/mm^3 as well as appropriate dose adjustment based on degree of reduction in GFR.

The optimal form of cyclophosphamide therapy (daily oral vs. intravenous pulse) has been the subject of investigation. In general, the intravenous regimen allows for an approximately twofold lower cumulative dose of cyclophosphamide than the oral regimen and is associated with a significant decrease in the rate of clinically significant neutropenia and other complications. In a meta-analysis of three randomized controlled trials, the rate of relapse associated with pulse cyclophosphamide was not statistically higher than the rate with a daily oral regimen, but the intravenous pulse regimen was associated with a statistically higher rate of remission and lower rates of leukopenia and infections.[1317] The final outcomes (death or ESKD) were no different for the two dosing regimens.

A large randomized controlled trial of pulse versus daily oral cyclophosphamide for induction of remission was conducted that included 149 patients with newly diagnosed generalized ANCA vasculitis with kidney involvement.[1318] Patients were randomly assigned to receive either pulse cyclophosphamide, 15 mg/kg every 2 weeks × 3 and then every 3 weeks, or daily oral cyclophosphamide, 2 mg/kg per day. Cyclophosphamide therapy was continued for 3 months beyond the time of remission. All patients were then switched to azathioprine (2 mg/kg/day orally) until month 18. All patients received prednisolone starting at 1 mg/kg orally, followed by a taper. Patients with a serum creatinine level of more than 500 μmol/L (5.7 mg/dL) were excluded from the study. Seventy-nine percent of patients achieved remission by 9 months (median time to remission was 3 months for both groups). The two treatment groups did not differ in time to remission or proportion of patients who achieved remission at 9 months (88.1% in the pulse group vs. 87.7% in the daily oral group). GFR did not differ between the two groups at any time point. By 18 months, 13 patients in the pulse group and 6 in the daily oral group had experienced a relapse (HR, 2.01; 95% CI, 0.77 to 5.30). Absolute cumulative cyclophosphamide dose in the daily oral group was almost twice that in the pulse group (15.9 g vs. 8.2 g, respectively; $P < 0.001$). The pulse group had a lower rate of leukopenia (HR, 0.41; 95% CI, 0.23 to 0.71), but the frequency of serious infections was not statistically different between the two treatment groups. Interestingly, the long-term results of this trial were recently reported with a median duration of 4.3 years' follow-up and data from 90% of patients in the original trial.[1319] There was no difference in survival between the two groups; however, risk of relapse was significantly lower in the daily oral cyclophosphamide arm (HR, 0.50; 95% CI, 0.26 to 0.93; $P = 0.029$) although kidney function was similar by the end of the study ($P = 0.82$), as were adverse events.

This randomized controlled trial confirms that the two cyclophosphamide regimens are associated with similar remission induction rates and time to remission induction, with the pulse cyclophosphamide regimen resulting in about one half the cumulative medication dose of the oral regimen and a significantly lower rate of leukopenia. The long-term results would suggest that the daily oral cyclophosphamide regimen portends less relapse risk, and there was a trend toward this in the original study. At this point, clinicians must weigh the risks and benefits of either regimen to determine which is most appropriate, and this decision may likely be based more heavily now on level of patient compliance.

The length of cyclophosphamide therapy has changed significantly, largely based on the results of a large controlled trial in which patients who attained a complete remission with cyclophosphamide after 3 months of therapy were randomly assigned to switch to azathioprine or to continue taking cyclophosphamide for a total of 12 months. After 12 months, both groups received azathioprine maintenance therapy for an additional year.[1145] Changing to azathioprine after 3 months of cyclophosphamide treatment appears as effective as receiving oral cyclophosphamide for 12 months followed by 12 months of azathioprine based on kidney function and the frequency of relapse. It is noteworthy that patients whose PR3-ANCA titers remained positive at the time of the switch had about a twofold increased risk of subsequent relapse compared with patients whose ANCA titers had reverted to negative.[1320]

In three relatively small randomized controlled trials addressing the role of plasmapheresis in the treatment of ANCA-associated small vessel vasculitis and glomerulonephritis,[1321-1323] plasmapheresis was not found to provide any added benefit over immunosuppressive treatment alone in patients with renal-limited disease or in patients with mild to moderate kidney dysfunction. However, the use of plasmapheresis in addition to immunosuppressive therapy appears to be beneficial in the subset of patients who require dialysis at the time of presentation.[1323,1324] In a study performed by the European Vasculitis Study Group of 137 patients with a new diagnosis of severe biopsy-confirmed ANCA-associated glomerulonephritis, the use of plasma exchange was found to be superior to pulse methylprednisolone in producing recovery of kidney function in patients with severe kidney dysfunction at the time of entry into the study (serum creatinine level of >5.8 mg/dL).[1325] Long-term follow-up of these patients did not show a significant difference in the proportion of patients free of ESKD or death; however, the small number of patients limited the power to detect differences.[1326] Because of the clinically observed increased risk of severe bone marrow suppression with the use of cyclophosphamide in patients receiving dialysis, such treatment should be pursued with extreme caution.

Patients who eventually are able to discontinue dialysis usually do so within 3 or 4 months of initiation of therapy.[1298,1316] For this reason, continuing immunosuppressive therapy beyond 4 months in patients who are still receiving dialysis is unlikely to be of added benefit (unless they continue to have extrarenal manifestations of vasculitis). In a retrospective analysis of 523 patients with ANCA vasculitis followed over a median of 40 months, 136 patients reached ESKD.[1327] Relapse rates of vasculitis were significantly lower in patients on long-term dialysis (0.08 episode/patient-year) than in the same patients before they reached ESKD (0.20 episode/patient-year) and in patients with preserved kidney function (0.16 episode/patient-year). Infections were almost twice as frequent among patients with ESKD receiving maintenance immunosuppressants and were an important cause of death. Given the lower risk of relapse with hemodialysis and the higher risk of infection and death with long-term immunosuppression, the risk/benefit ratio does not support the routine use of maintenance immunosuppression therapy in patients with ANCA small vessel vasculitis who are on long-term dialysis.

Although high-dose intravenous pooled immunoglobulin has been used in the treatment of systemic vasculitis resistant to usual immunosuppressive treatment,[1328-1332] there are no published reports of its use in patients with pauci-immune crescentic glomerulonephritis alone without systemic involvement.

Trimethoprim-sulfamethoxazole has been suggested to be of benefit in the treatment of patients with GPA.[1333,1334] Such beneficial effects, if any, seem to be limited to the upper respiratory tract, and this antibiotic is unlikely to have a role in the treatment of pauci-immune crescentic glomerulonephritis alone. Induction therapy with methotrexate has been compared with cyclophosphamide treatment in patients with "early" limited GPA and mild kidney disease.[1335-1339] The rate of remission at 6 months was comparable in the two treatment groups.[1337] However, the onset of remission was delayed in methotrexate-treated patients with more extensive disease or pulmonary involvement. Methotrexate was also associated with a significantly higher rate of relapse than was cyclophosphamide (69.5% vs. 46.5%, respectively), and 45% of relapses occurred while patients were receiving methotrexate. The dose of methotrexate must be reduced in patients whose creatinine clearance is less than 80 mL/min, and its use is contraindicated when creatinine clearances is less than 10 mL/min. Moreover, in our experience there are patients taking methotrexate who have progressive glomerulonephritis. Methotrexate is therefore unlikely to have any role in the treatment of pauci-immune crescentic glomerulonephritis alone.

Whether the use of cyclophosphamide can be reduced or avoided completely by the use of rituximab has been the subject of two randomized controlled trials. In the RITUX-VAS trial, 44 patients with newly diagnosed ANCA vasculitis were randomly assigned in a ratio of 3:1 to receive either rituximab (375 mg/m^2 weekly × 4) in addition to cyclophosphamide (15 mg/kg intravenously × 2, 2 weeks apart), or cyclophosphamide (15 mg/kg intravenously every 2 weeks × 3, then every 3 weeks for a maximum total of 10 doses) alone.[1339] Both groups received the same intravenous and oral prednisolone regimen. Patients in the rituximab group did not receive maintenance therapy, whereas those in the cyclophosphamide group were switched to azathioprine until the end of the trial. Minimum follow-up was 12 months. The rate of sustained remission was similar in the two treatment groups (76% in the rituximab group vs. 82% in the cyclophosphamide group, $P = 0.67$ for risk difference). Severe adverse events were common in both groups, affecting 45% of patients in the rituximab group and 36% in the cyclophosphamide group ($P = 0.60$). This study suggests that a combination of rituximab and reduced-dose cyclophosphamide may be no less effective than a "traditional" cyclophosphamide regimen, but it did not demonstrate a safety benefit of a rituximab-based approach. This study was not powered to establish equivalence or noninferiority.

In a large controlled trial designed to assess the noninferiority of rituximab compared to cyclophosphamide, 197 patients were randomly assigned to treatment with either rituximab (375 mg/m^2 infusions once weekly × 4) or cyclophosphamide (2 mg/kg/day orally) for months 1 to 3 followed by azathioprine (2 mg/kg/day orally) for months 4 to 6. All patients received methylprednisolone (1 g/day intravenously for up to 3 days) followed by prednisone (1 mg/kg/day, tapered off completely by 6 months). The induction phase of this trial revealed similar rates between the two treatment groups in complete remission at 6 months (64% in the rituximab group vs. 55% in the cyclophosphamide group, $P = 0.21$).[1340] No differences in relapse rates were observed between the groups. The 18-month efficacy of this single course of rituximab, as compared to cyclophosphamide followed by azathioprine, revealed persistent noninferiority; however, remission rates at the 18-month mark were 39% and 33% ($P = 0.32$), respectively signifying the critical and persistent need for more effective remission induction and maintenance strategies.[1341] Although these studies suggest that substitution of cyclophosphamide with rituximab may be effective, rituximab has not been formally evaluated in patients with severe renal failure requiring dialysis.

Studies pertaining to maintenance immunosuppression for relapse prevention are primarily geared to patients with GPA or MPA. Current data suggest that patients with pauci-immune glomerulonephritis alone and MPO-ANCAs are at a relatively low risk of relapse.[1297] The value of prolonged maintenance immunosuppression in this group of patients is unknown, and any benefit in preventing a relapse would have to be weighed against the potential toxicity of immunosuppressive agents and the risks associated with their use. Strategies for reducing treatment toxicity are being studied and are considered in greater detail in Chapter 34.

Complete reference list available at ExpertConsult.com.

KEY REFERENCES

1. Jennette JC, Falk RJ, Bacon PA, et al: 2012 Revised International Chapel Hill Consensus Conference nomenclature of vasculitides. *Arthritis Rheum* 65:1–11, 2013.
2. Brenner BM, Hostetter TH, Humes HD: Glomerular permselectivity: barrier function based on discrimination of molecular size and charge. *Am J Physiol* 234:F455–F460, 1978.
4. Brenner BM, Bohrer MP, Baylis C, et al: Determinants of glomerular permselectivity: Insights derived from observations in vivo. *Kidney Int* 12:229–237, 1977.
7. Tryggvason K, Patrakka J, Wartiovaara J: Hereditary proteinuria syndromes and mechanisms of proteinuria. *N Engl J Med* 354:1387–1401, 2006.
16. Mazzoni MB, Kottanatu L, Simonetti GD, et al: Renal vein obstruction and orthostatic proteinuria: a review. *Nephrol Dial Transplant* 26:562–565, 2011.
18. Schröder FH: Microscopic haematuria. *BMJ* 309:70–72, 1994.
34. Gadegbeku CA, Gipson DS, Holzman LB, et al: Design of the Nephrotic Syndrome Study Network (NEPTUNE) to evaluate primary glomerular nephropathy by a multidisciplinary approach. *Kidney Int* 83:749–756, 2013.
135. Ruggenenti P, Ruggiero B, Cravedi P, et al: Rituximab in steroid-dependent or frequently relapsing idiopathic nephrotic syndrome. *J Am Soc Nephrol* 25:850–863, 2014.
137. Hogan J, Radhakrishnan J: The treatment of minimal change disease in adults. *J Am Soc Nephrol* 24:702–711, 2013.
139. D'Agati VD, Fogo AB, Bruijn JA, et al: Pathologic classification of focal segmental glomerulosclerosis: a working proposal. *Am J Kidney Dis* 43:368–382, 2004.
140. Thomas DB, Franceschini N, Hogan SL, et al: Clinical and pathologic characteristics of focal segmental glomerulosclerosis pathologic variants. *Kidney Int* 69:920–926, 2006.
142. D'Agati VD, Kaskel FJ, Falk RJ: Focal segmental glomerulosclerosis. *N Engl J Med* 365:2398–2411, 2011.
181. Genovese G, Friedman DJ, Pollak MR: APOL1 variants and kidney disease in people of recent African ancestry. *Nat Rev Nephrol* 9:240–244, 2013.
370. Beck LH, Jr, Bonegio RG, Lambeau G, et al: M-type phospholipase A2 receptor as target antigen in idiopathic membranous nephropathy. *N Engl J Med* 361:11–21, 2009.
423. Ponticelli C, Zucchelli P, Passerini P, et al: A randomized trial of methylprednisolone and chlorambucil in idiopathic membranous nephropathy. *N Engl J Med* 320:8–13, 1989.
449. Beck LH, Jr, Fervenza FC, Beck DM, et al: Rituximab-induced depletion of anti-PLA2R autoantibodies predicts response in membranous nephropathy. *J Am Soc Nephrol* 22:1543–1550, 2011.
478. Lee T, Biddle AK, Lionaki S, et al: Personalized prophylactic anticoagulation decision analysis in patients with membranous nephropathy. *Kidney Int* 85:1412–1420, 2014.
489. Howman A, Chapman TL, Langdon MM, et al: Immunosuppression for progressive membranous nephropathy: a UK randomised controlled trial. *Lancet* 381:744–751, 2013.
526. Sethi S, Fervenza FC: Membranoproliferative glomerulonephritis—a new look at an old entity. *N Engl J Med* 366:1119–1131, 2012.
527. Hou J, Markowitz GS, Bomback AS, et al: Toward a working definition of C3 glomerulopathy by immunofluorescence. *Kidney Int* 85:450–456, 2014.
588. Bomback AS, Appel GB: Pathogenesis of the C3 glomerulopathies and reclassification of MPGN. *Nat Rev Nephrol* 8:634–642, 2012.
597. Sethi S, Fervenza FC, Zhang Y, et al: C3 glomerulonephritis: clinicopathological findings, complement abnormalities, glomerular proteomic profile, treatment, and follow-up. *Kidney Int* 82:465–473, 2012.
635. Rodriguez-Iturbe B, Musser JM: The current state of poststreptococcal glomerulonephritis. *J Am Soc Nephrol* 19:1855–1864, 2008.
676. Nasr SH, Radhakrishnan J, D'Agati VD: Bacterial infection-related glomerulonephritis in adults. *Kidney Int* 83:792–803, 2013.
734. Wyatt RJ, Julian BA: IgA nephropathy. *N Engl J Med* 368:2402–2414, 2013.
772. Gharavi AG, Kiryluk K, Choi M, et al: Genome-wide association study identifies susceptibility loci for IgA nephropathy. *Nat Genet* 43:321–327, 2011.
773. Yu XQ, Li M, Zhang H, et al: A genome-wide association study in Han Chinese identifies multiple susceptibility loci for IgA nephropathy. *Nat Genet* 44:178–182, 2012.
774. Kiryluk K, Li Y, Sanna-Cherchi S, et al: Geographic differences in genetic susceptibility to IgA nephropathy: GWAS replication study and geospatial risk analysis. *PLoS Genet* 8:e1002765, 2012.
789. Cattran DC, Coppo R, Cook HT, et al: The Oxford classification of IgA nephropathy: rationale, clinicopathological correlations, and classification. *Kidney Int* 76:534–545, 2009.
790. Roberts IS, Cook HT, Troyanov S, et al: The Oxford classification of IgA nephropathy: pathology definitions, correlations, and reproducibility. *Kidney Int* 76:546–556, 2009.
828. Suzuki H, Fan R, Zhang Z, et al: Aberrantly glycosylated IgA1 in IgA nephropathy patients is recognized by IgG antibodies with restricted heterogeneity. *J Clin Invest* 119:1668–1677, 2009.
979. Pozzi C, Andrulli S, Del VL, et al: Corticosteroid effectiveness in IgA nephropathy: long-term results of a randomized, controlled trial. *J Am Soc Nephrol* 15:157–163, 2004.
980. Pozzi C, Bolasco PG, Fogazzi GB, et al: Corticosteroids in IgA nephropathy: a randomised controlled trial. *Lancet* 353:883–887, 1999.
1043. Iskandar SS, Falk RJ, Jennette JC: Clinical and pathologic features of fibrillary glomerulonephritis. *Kidney Int* 42:1401–1407, 1992.
1054. Schwartz MM, Korbet SM, Lewis EJ: Immunotactoid glomerulopathy. *J Am Soc Nephrol* 13:1390–1397, 2002.
1055. Nasr SH, Fidler ME, Cornell LD, et al: Immunotactoid glomerulopathy: clinicopathologic and proteomic study. *Nephrol Dial Transplant* 27:4137–4146, 2012.
1056. Rosenstock JL, Markowitz GS, Valeri AM, et al: Fibrillary and immunotactoid glomerulonephritis: Distinct entities with different clinical and pathologic features. *Kidney Int* 63:1450–1461, 2003.
1100. Olson SW, Arbogast CB, Baker TP, et al: Asymptomatic autoantibodies associate with future anti-glomerular basement membrane disease. *J Am Soc Nephrol* 22:1946–1952, 2011.
1125. Pedchenko V, Bondar O, Fogo AB, et al: Molecular architecture of the Goodpasture autoantigen in anti-GBM nephritis. *N Engl J Med* 363:343–354, 2010.
1209. Jennette JC, Falk RJ: Pathogenesis of antineutrophil cytoplasmic autoantibody-mediated disease. *Nat Rev Rheumatol* 10:463–473, 2014.
1218. Ciavatta DJ, Yang J, Preston GA, et al: Epigenetic basis for aberrant upregulation of autoantigen genes in humans with ANCA vasculitis. *J Clin Invest* 120:3209–3219, 2010.

1247. Roth AJ, Ooi JD, Hess JJ, et al: Epitope specificity determines pathogenicity and detectability in ANCA-associated vasculitis. *J Clin Invest* 123:1773–1783, 2013.
1264. Lyons PA, Rayner TF, Trivedi S, et al: Genetically distinct subsets within ANCA-associated vasculitis. *N Engl J Med* 367:214–223, 2012.
1269. Xiao H, Heeringa P, Hu P, et al: Antineutrophil cytoplasmic autoantibodies specific for myeloperoxidase cause glomerulonephritis and vasculitis in mice. *J Clin Invest* 110:955–963, 2002.
1288. Pendergraft WF, Preston GA, Shah RR, et al: Autoimmunity is triggered by cPR-3(105-201), a protein complementary to human autoantigen proteinase-3. *Nat Med* 10:72–79, 2004.
1297. Hogan SL, Falk RJ, Chin H, et al: Predictors of relapse and treatment resistance in antineutrophil cytoplasmic antibody-associated small-vessel vasculitis. *Ann Intern Med* 143:621–631, 2005.
1304. Falk RJ, Jennette JC: Anti-neutrophil cytoplasmic autoantibodies with specificity for myeloperoxidase in patients with systemic vasculitis and idiopathic necrotizing and crescentic glomerulonephritis. *N Engl J Med* 318:1651–1657, 1988.
1307. Niles JL, McCluskey RT, Ahmad MF, et al: Wegener's granulomatosis autoantigen is a novel neutrophil serine proteinase. *Blood* 74:1888–1893, 1989.
1339. Jones RB, Tervaert JW, Hauser T, et al: Rituximab versus cyclophosphamide in ANCA-associated renal vasculitis. *N Engl J Med* 363:211–220, 2010.
1341. Specks U, Merkel PA, Seo P, et al: Efficacy of remission-induction regimens for ANCA-associated vasculitis. *N Engl J Med* 369:417–427, 2013.

Secondary Glomerular Disease

33

Gerald B. Appel | Jai Radhakrishnan | Vivette D'Agati

CHAPTER OUTLINE

SYSTEMIC LUPUS ERYTHEMATOSUS, 1092
Epidemiology, 1092
Pathogenesis of Systemic Lupus Erythematosus and Lupus Nephritis, 1093
Pathology of Lupus Nephritis, 1094
Tubulointerstitial Disease, Vascular Lesions, and Lupus Podocytopathy, 1097
Clinical Manifestations, 1098
Serologic Tests, 1098
Monitoring Clinical Disease, 1099
Drug-Induced Lupus, 1099
Pregnancy and Systemic Lupus Erythematosus, 1100
Dialysis and Transplantation, 1100
Course and Prognosis of Lupus Nephritis, 1100
Treatment of Lupus Nephritis, 1102
ANTIPHOSPHOLIPID SYNDROME, 1106
Treatment, 1107
MIXED CONNECTIVE TISSUE DISEASE, 1108
SMALL VESSEL VASCULITIS, 1109
Granulomatosis with Polyangiitis, 1109
Microscopic Polyangiitis, 1114
Eosinophilic Granulomatosis with Polyangiitis, 1116
GLOMERULAR INVOLVEMENT IN OTHER VASCULITIDES, 1118
Polyarteritis Nodosa (Classic Macroscopic Polyarteritis Nodosa), 1118
Temporal Arteritis (Giant Cell Arteritis), 1120
Takayasu Arteritis, 1120
HENOCH-SCHÖNLEIN PURPURA, 1121
Clinical Findings, 1121
Laboratory Features, 1121
Pathology, 1122
Pathogenesis, 1123
Course, Prognosis, and Treatment, 1123

ANTI–GLOMERULAR BASEMENT MEMBRANE DISEASE AND GOODPASTURE'S SYNDROME, 1124
Pathogenesis, 1124
Clinical Features, 1125
Laboratory Findings, 1125
Pathology, 1125
Course, Treatment, and Prognosis, 1126
SJÖGREN'S SYNDROME, 1127
SARCOIDOSIS, 1127
AMYLOIDOSIS, 1128
AL and AA Amyloidosis, 1128
End-Stage Kidney Disease in Amyloidosis, 1132
FIBRILLARY GLOMERULONEPHRITIS AND IMMUNOTACTOID GLOMERULONEPHRITIS, 1132
MONOCLONAL IMMUNOGLOBULIN DEPOSITION DISEASE, 1134
OTHER GLOMERULAR DISEASES AND DYSPROTEINEMIA, 1136
WALDENSTRÖM'S MACROGLOBULINEMIA, 1136
MIXED CRYOGLOBULINEMIA, 1137
HEREDITARY NEPHRITIS, INCLUDING ALPORT'S SYNDROME, 1138
Clinical Features, 1138
Pathology, 1139
Pathogenesis and Genetics, 1140
Course and Treatment, 1141
THIN BASEMENT MEMBRANE NEPHROPATHY, 1141
Clinical Features, 1141
Pathology, 1142
Pathogenesis, 1142
Differential Diagnosis of Familial Hematurias, 1142

NAIL-PATELLA SYNDROME (HEREDITARY OSTEO-ONYCHODYSPLASIA), 1142
Clinical Features, 1142
Pathology, 1143
Pathogenesis, 1143
Treatment, 1143
FABRY'S DISEASE (ANGIOKERATOMA CORPORIS DIFFUSUM UNIVERSALE), 1143
Clinical Features, 1143
Pathology, 1144
Pathogenesis, 1144
Diagnosis, 1144
Treatment, 1145
SICKLE CELL NEPHROPATHY, 1145
Clinical Features, 1145
Pathology, 1145
Pathogenesis, 1146
Treatment, 1146
LIPODYSTROPHY, 1146
LECITHIN-CHOLESTEROL ACYLTRANSFERASE DEFICIENCY, 1147
Clinical Features, 1147
Pathology, 1147
Pathogenesis, 1148
Diagnosis, 1148
Treatment, 1148
LIPOPROTEIN GLOMERULOPATHY, 1148
GLOMERULAR INVOLVEMENT WITH BACTERIAL INFECTIONS, 1148
Infectious Endocarditis, 1148
Shunt Nephritis, 1149
Visceral Infection, 1149
Other Bacterial Infections and Fungal Infections, 1149

GLOMERULAR INVOLVEMENT WITH PARASITIC DISEASES, 1150
Malaria, 1150
Schistosomiasis, 1150
Leishmaniasis, Trypanosomiasis, and Filariasis, 1150
Other Parasitic Diseases, 1151
GLOMERULAR INVOLVEMENT WITH VIRAL INFECTIONS, 1151
HIV-Related Glomerulopathies, 1151
HIV-Associated Nephropathy, 1151
Other Glomerular Lesions in Patients with HIV Infection, 1153
GLOMERULAR MANIFESTATIONS OF LIVER DISEASE, 1154
Hepatitis B, 1154
Hepatitis C, 1155
Autoimmune Chronic Active Hepatitis, 1156
Liver Cirrhosis, 1156
GLOMERULAR LESIONS ASSOCIATED WITH NEOPLASIA, 1157
Clinical and Pathologic Features, 1157
GLOMERULAR DISEASE ASSOCIATED WITH DRUGS, 1157
Heroin Nephropathy, 1157
Nonsteroidal Antiinflammatory Drug–Induced Nephropathy, 1158
Anti–Rheumatoid Arthritis Therapy–Induced Glomerulopathy, 1158
Other Medications, 1159
MISCELLANEOUS DISEASES ASSOCIATED WITH GLOMERULAR LESIONS, 1159

SYSTEMIC LUPUS ERYTHEMATOSUS

Lupus nephritis (LN) is a frequent and potentially serious complication of systemic lupus erythematosus (SLE).[1-6] Kidney disease influences morbidity and mortality both directly and indirectly through complications of therapy. Recent studies have more clearly defined the spectrum of clinical, prognostic, and renal histopathologic findings in SLE. Controlled randomized trials of induction therapy for severe LN have focused on achieving remissions of renal disease while minimizing adverse reactions to therapy. Maintenance trials have compared the efficacy of therapeutic agents in preventing renal flares and the progression of renal disease over several years. For patients who fail to respond to current treatment regimens, a number of newer immunomodulatory agents are being studied in resistant or relapsing disease.

EPIDEMIOLOGY

The incidence and prevalence of SLE depend on the age, gender, geographic locale, and ethnicity of the population studied as well as the diagnostic criteria for defining SLE.[1,6-9] Females outnumber males by about 10 to 1. However, males with SLE have the same incidence of renal disease as females. The onset of disease peaks between 15 and 45 years of age and more than 85% of patients are younger than 55 years of age. SLE is more often associated with severe nephritis in children and in males and is milder in older adults.[1,3,7,8] SLE and LN are more common and are associated with more severe renal involvement in African American, Asian, and

Hispanic populations although the precise roles of biologic-genetic versus socioeconomic factors have not been clearly defined.[1,10-12] The overall incidence of SLE ranges from 1.8 to 7.6 cases per 100,000 with a prevalence of from 40 to 200 cases per 100,000.[1,6,7] The incidence of renal involvement varies depending on the populations studied, the diagnostic criteria for kidney disease, and whether involvement is defined by renal biopsy or clinical findings. Approximately 25% to 50% of unselected lupus patients will have clinical renal disease at onset while as many as 60% of adults with SLE will develop renal disease during their course.[1,2,5,7,8]

A number of genetic, hormonal, and environmental factors clearly influence the course and severity of SLE.[1,2,6-9] A multiplicity of genes are involved in both SLE and LN. A genetic predisposition is supported by a higher concordance rate in monozygotic twins (25%) than fraternal twins (<5%), the greater risk of relatives of SLE patients developing SLE or other autoimmune disease, the association with certain HLA genotypes (e.g., HLA-B8, HLA-DR2, and HLA-DR3), inherited deficiencies in complement components (e.g., homozygous C1q, C2, and C4 deficiencies), and Fc receptor polymorphisms.[1,8] Genome-wide analyses have identified approximately 20 different genetic loci associated with an increased risk of SLE. These candidate susceptibility genes regulate diverse immune functions such as T cell activation, B cell signaling, Toll-like receptors, signal transduction, neutrophil function, and interferon (IFN) production.[1,8] Inbred spontaneous genetic murine models of SLE and LN include the NZB B/W F1 hybrid, the BXSB, and the MRL/lpr mouse. SLE is inducible in some murine strains through injection of autoantibodies against DNA or by injection of Smith antigen peptides. Evidence for the role of hormonal factors includes the strong predominance of SLE in females of childbearing age and the increased incidence of lupus flares during or shortly after pregnancy.[1,2,6,9-14] In the F1 NZB/NZW mice, females have more severe disease than males and disease severity is ameliorated by oophorectomy or androgen therapy. Environmental factors other than estrogens also modulate disease expression; these factors include immune responses to viral or bacterial antigens, exposure to sunlight and ultraviolet radiation, and certain medications.[1,6,9,14,15]

For study purposes, the diagnosis of SLE is established by the presence of certain clinical and laboratory criteria defined by the American College of Rheumatology (ACR).[1,5] Development of any 4 of the 11 criteria over a lifetime gives a 96% sensitivity and specificity for SLE. These criteria include malar rash, discoid rash, photosensitivity, oral ulcerations, nondeforming arthritis, serositis (including pleuritis or pericarditis), central nervous system disorder (such as seizures or psychoses), renal involvement, hematologic disorder (including hemolytic anemia, leukopenia, lymphopenia, or thrombocytopenia), immunologic disorder (including anti-DNA antibody, anti-Sm antibody, lupus anticoagulant, or antiphospholipid antibody), and antinuclear antibody (ANA). The criterion of renal involvement is defined by persistent proteinuria exceeding 500 mg/dL/day (or 3+ on the dipstick) or the presence of cellular urinary casts. Because some patients, especially those with mesangial or membranous LN, will present with clinical renal disease before they have fulfilled 4 of the 11 criteria, the diagnosis of SLE remains a clinical diagnosis with histopathologic findings supporting or confirming the presumed diagnosis.[1]

PATHOGENESIS OF SYSTEMIC LUPUS ERYTHEMATOSUS AND LUPUS NEPHRITIS

In patients with SLE, abnormalities of immune regulation lead to a loss of self-tolerance, autoimmune responses, and the production of a variety of autoantibodies and immune complexes.[1,2,14-20] SLE is associated with defective regulation of T cells with decreased numbers of cytotoxic and suppressor T cells, increased helper (CD4$^+$) T cells, dysfunctional T cell signaling, and abnormal T_H1, T_H2, and T_H17 cytokine production.[1,6,16-21] There is also polyclonal activation of B cells and defective B cell tolerance. The failure of apoptotic mechanisms to delete autoreactive B cell and T cell clones may promote their expansion and may trigger immune responses through interactions with Toll-like receptors with subsequent autoantibody production. The result of this loss of tolerance is the production of a wide range of autoantibodies, including those directed against nucleic acids, nucleosomes (double-stranded DNA in association with a core of positively charged histones), chromatin antigens, and nuclear and cytoplasmic ribonuclear proteins.[1,6,15,20,22] Viral or bacterial peptides containing sequences similar to native antigens may lead to "antigen mimicry" and stimulate autoantibody production.

In SLE, autoantibodies combine with self antigens to produce circulating immune complexes that deposit in the glomeruli, activate complement, and incite an inflammatory response. Immune complexes are also detectable in the skin at the dermal-epidermal junction, in the choroid plexus, pericardium, and pleural spaces. Renal involvement in SLE has been considered a human prototype of classic experimental chronic immune complex–induced glomerulonephritis.[23] The chronic deposition of circulating immune complexes plays a major role in the mesangial and the endocapillary proliferative patterns of LN. Immune complex size, charge, avidity, local hemodynamic factors, and the clearing ability of the mesangium influence the localization of circulating immune complexes within the glomerulus.[2,6,17,23] In diffuse proliferative LN, the deposited complexes consist of nuclear antigens (e.g., DNA) and high-affinity complement-fixing immunoglobulin G (IgG) antibodies.[1,2,23] In some SLE patients, the initiating event may be the local binding of cationic nuclear antigens such as histones to the subepithelial region of the glomerular capillary wall, followed by in situ immune complex formation. Once glomerular immune deposits form, the complement cascade is activated, leading to complement-mediated damage, activation of procoagulant factors, leukocyte Fc receptor activation with leukocyte infiltration, release of proteolytic enzymes, and production of various cytokines regulating glomerular cellular proliferation and matrix synthesis.

Neutrophils undergoing cell death may release chromatin meshworks (called neutrophil extracellular traps [NETs]). These NETs, which are detectable in LN biopsies, are not degraded properly in patients with lupus and are a source of autoantigen presentation and induction of IFN-α by plasmacytoid dendritic cells.[24] There is also evidence for intrarenal autoantibody production in patients with LN.[25]

Glomerular damage may be potentiated by mechanisms distinct from immune complex deposition, such as hypertension and coagulation abnormalities. Some lupus patients with associated antineutrophil cytoplasmic antibodies (ANCAs) have documented focal segmental necrotizing glomerular lesions without significant immune complex deposition, resembling a "pauci-immune" glomerulonephritis.[26,27] The presence of antiphospholipid antibodies, with their attendant alterations in endothelial and platelet function (including reduced production of prostacyclin and other endothelial anticoagulant factors, activation of plasminogen, inhibition of protein C or S, and enhanced platelet aggregation), can also potentiate glomerular and vascular lesions.[27]

PATHOLOGY OF LUPUS NEPHRITIS

The histopathology of LN is pleomorphic.[1-4,23] This diversity is evident when comparing biopsy findings from different patients or even adjacent glomeruli in a single biopsy. Moreover, the lesions have the capacity to transform from one pattern to another spontaneously or following treatment. Early classifications of LN simply divided glomerular changes into mild and severe forms.[2,23] The World Health Organization (WHO) classification system, used for almost 30 years,[28,29] classified LN by combining glomerular light microscopic, immunofluorescence, and electron microscopic findings. The 2003 International Society of Nephrology/Renal Pathology Society (ISN/RPS) classification of LN addressed limitations of the WHO classification system and is now widely accepted by nephrologists, pathologists, and rheumatologists[30] (Table 33.1). It has proven more reproducible and provides more standardized definitions for precise clinical pathologic correlations.[31,32]

ISN/RPS class I denotes normal-appearing glomeruli by light microscopy but with mesangial immune deposits by immunofluorescence and electron microscopy. Even patients without clinical renal disease often have mesangial immune deposits when studied carefully by the more sensitive techniques of immunofluorescence and electron microscopy.[30]

ISN/RPS class II is defined on light microscopy by mesangial hypercellularity, with mesangial immune deposits on immunofluorescence and electron microscopy (Figures 33.1, 33.2, and 33.3).[30] Mesangial hypercellularity is defined as more than three cells in mesangial regions distant from the vascular pole in 3-μm–thick sections. There may be rare minute subendothelial or subepithelial deposits visible by immunofluorescence or electron microscopy but not by light microscopy.

ISN/RPS class III, focal LN, is defined as focal segmental and/or global endocapillary and/or extracapillary glomerulonephritis affecting less than 50% of the total glomeruli sampled. Both active and chronic lesions are taken into account when determining the percentage of total glomeruli involved. There is typically focal segmental endocapillary proliferation, including mesangial cells and endothelial cells, with infiltrating mononuclear and polymorphonuclear leukocytes (Figures 33.4, 33.5, and 33.6).[30] Class III biopsies are classified as A (active, proliferative), C (inactive, chronic sclerosing), or A/C (active and inactive lesions). Active lesions may display cellular crescents, fibrinoid necrosis, nuclear pyknosis or karyorrhexis, and rupture of the glomerular basement membrane (GBM). Hematoxylin bodies, swollen basophilic nuclear material resulting from binding to ambient ANAs, are occasionally found within the necrotizing lesions. Subendothelial immune deposits may be visible by light microscopy as "wire loop" thickenings of the glomerular capillary walls or large intraluminal masses known as "hyaline thrombi." Chronic glomerular lesions consist of segmental and/or global glomerular sclerosis owing to scarred glomerulonephritis with or without fibrous crescents.[30] In class III biopsies, glomeruli adjacent to those with severe histologic changes may show only mesangial

Table 33.1 International Society of Nephrology/Renal Pathology Society (2003) Classification of Lupus Nephritis (LN)

Class	Description
I	Minimal mesangial LN
II	Mesangial proliferative LN
III	Focal LN* (<50% of glomeruli)
III (A)	Active lesions
III (A/C)	Active and chronic lesions
III (C)	Chronic lesions
IV	Diffuse LN† (≥50% of glomeruli)
	Diffuse segmental (IV-S) or global (IV-G) LN
IV (A)	Active lesions
IV (A/C)	Active and chronic lesions
IV (C)	Chronic lesions
V‡	Membranous LN
VI	Advanced sclerosing LN
	(≥90% globally sclerosed glomeruli without residual activity)

*Indicate the proportion of glomeruli with active and with sclerotic lesions.
†Indicate the proportion of glomeruli with fibrinoid necrosis and with cellular crescents.
‡Class V may occur in combination with III or IV, in which case both will be diagnosed.

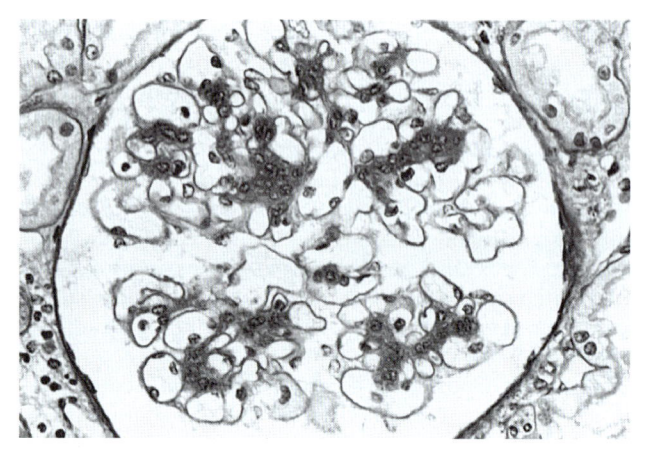

Figure 33.1 Lupus nephritis class II. There is mild global mesangial hypercellularity. (Periodic acid–Schiff stain, ×400.)

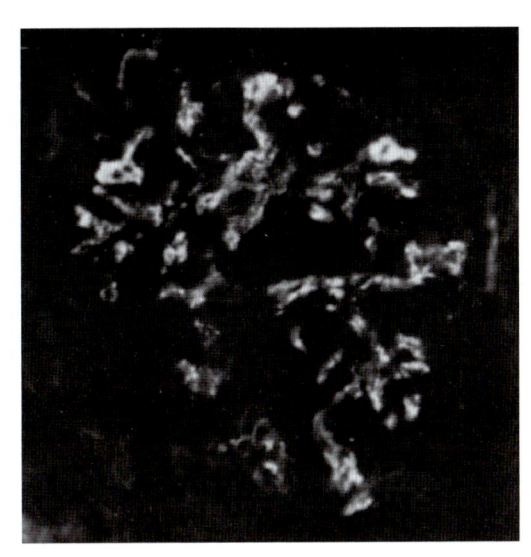

Figure 33.2 Lupus nephritis class II. Immunofluorescence photomicrograph showing deposits of C3 restricted to the glomerular mesangium. (×400.)

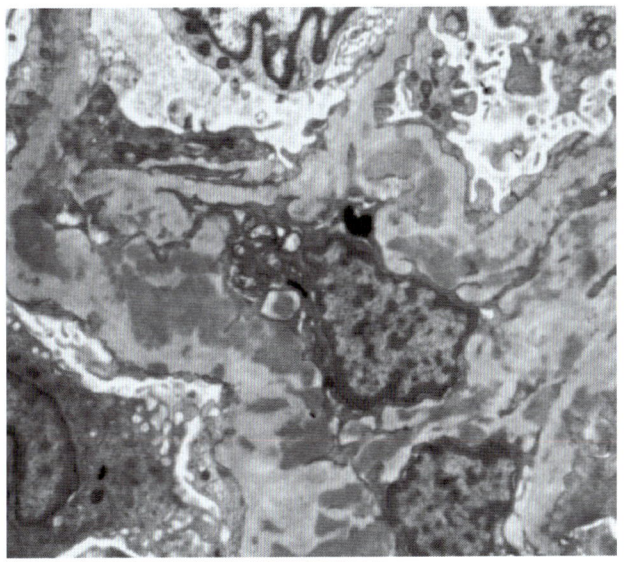

Figure 33.3 Lupus nephritis class II. Electron micrograph showing abundant mesangial electron-dense deposits (×12,000.)

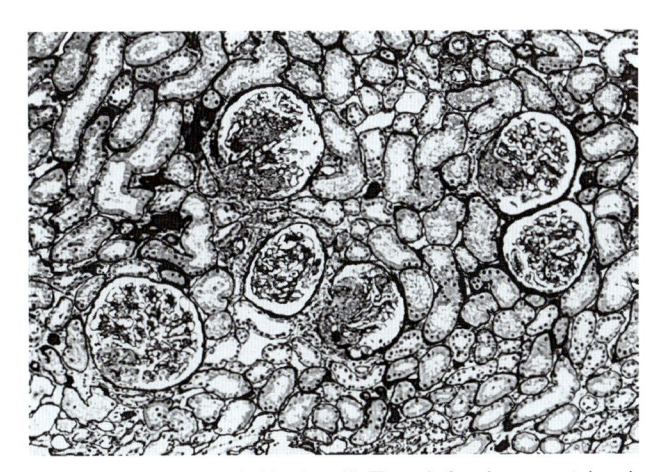

Figure 33.4 Lupus nephritis class III. There is focal segmental endocapillary proliferation. (Jones' methenamine silver stain, ×100.)

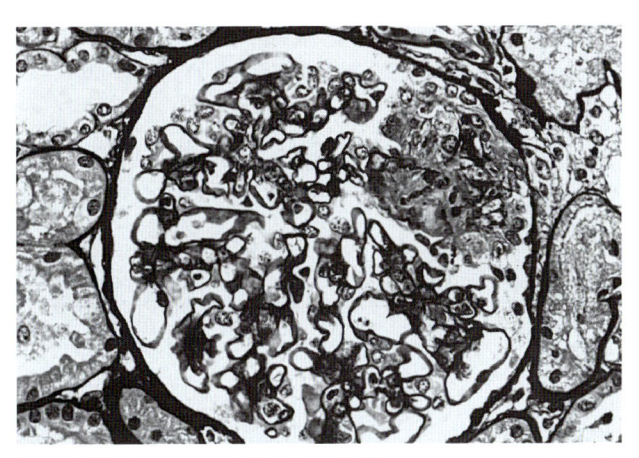

Figure 33.5 Lupus nephritis class III. The glomerular endocapillary proliferation is discretely segmental with necrotizing features and an early cellular crescent. (Jones' methenamine silver stain, ×400.)

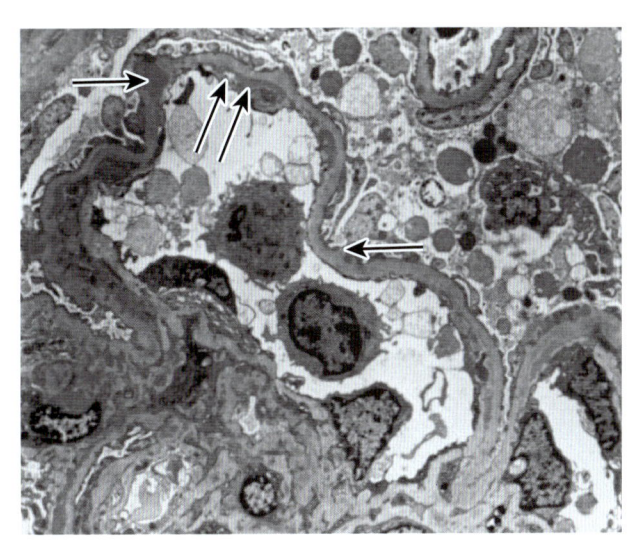

Figure 33.6 Lupus nephritis class III. Electron micrograph showing deposits in the mesangium as well as involving the peripheral capillary wall in subendothelial *(double arrow)* and subepithelial *(single arrows)* locations. (×4900.)

abnormalities by light microscopy. In class III, diffuse mesangial and focal and segmental subendothelial immune deposits are typically identified by immunofluorescence and electron microscopy. The segmental subendothelial deposits are usually present in the distribution of the segmental endocapillary proliferative lesions.

ISN/RPS class IV, diffuse LN, has qualitatively similar glomerular endocapillary and/or extracapillary lesions as class III but involves more than 50% of the total glomeruli sampled (Figures 33.7, 33.8, and 33.9).[28,30,33,34] Again, both active (proliferative) and chronic (sclerosing) lesions are included when determining the percentage of glomeruli affected. Class IV is subdivided into diffuse segmental proliferation, class IV-S, in which more than 50% of affected glomeruli have segmental lesions, and diffuse global proliferation, class IV-G, in which more than 50% of affected glomeruli have global lesions. All the active features described earlier for class III (including fibrinoid necrosis, leukocyte infiltration, wire loop deposits, hyaline thrombi, hematoxylin bodies, and crescents) may be encountered in

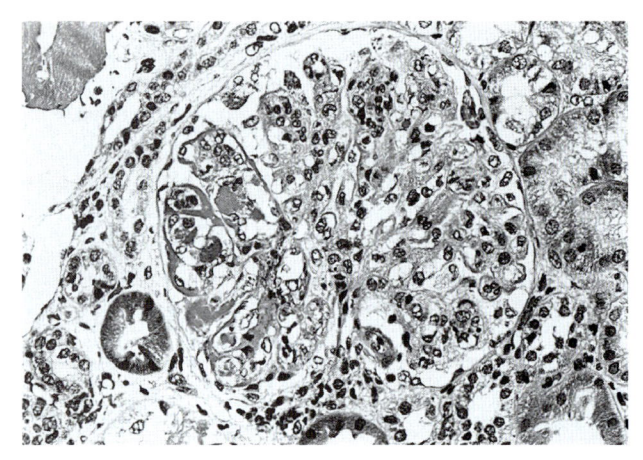

Figure 33.7 Lupus nephritis class IV. There is global endocapillary proliferation with infiltrating neutrophils and segmental wire loop deposits. (Hematoxylin and eosin stain, ×320.)

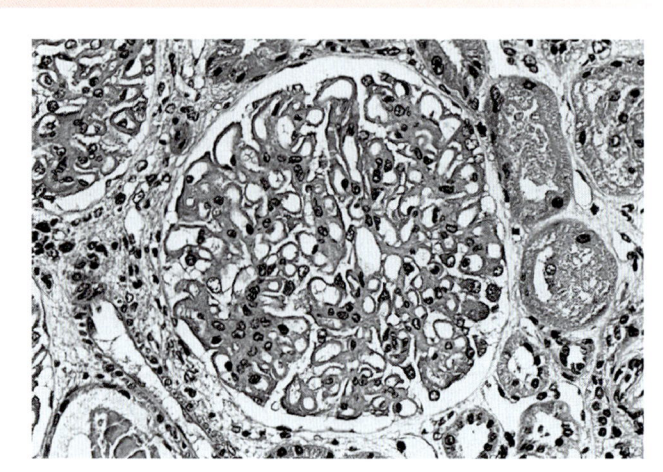

Figure 33.10 Lupus nephritis class V. There is diffuse uniform thickening of glomerular basement membranes accompanied by mild segmental mesangial hypercellularity. (Hematoxylin and eosin stain, ×320.)

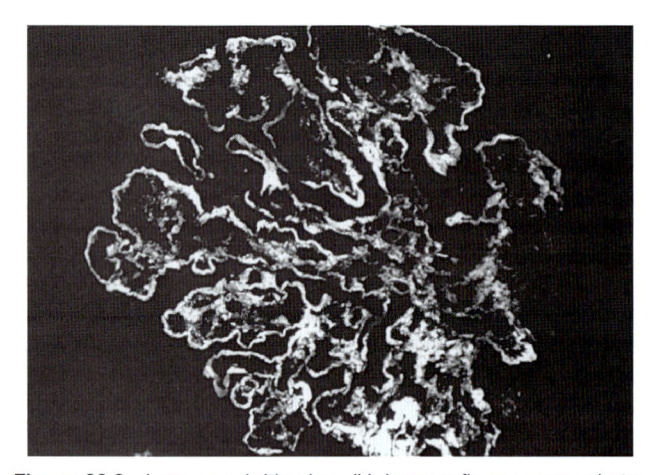

Figure 33.8 Lupus nephritis class IV. Immunofluorescence photomicrograph showing global deposits of IgG in the mesangial regions and outlining the subendothelial aspect of the peripheral glomerular capillary walls. (×600.)

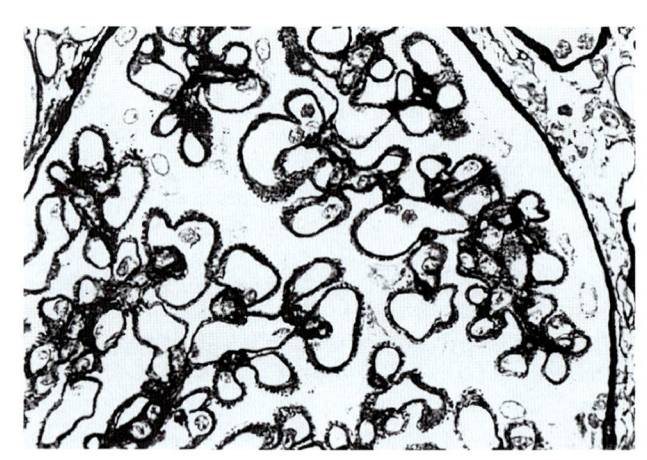

Figure 33.11 Lupus nephritis class V. Silver stain highlights glomerular basement membrane (GBM) spikes projecting outward from the GBMs toward the urinary space. (Jones' methenamine silver stain, ×800.)

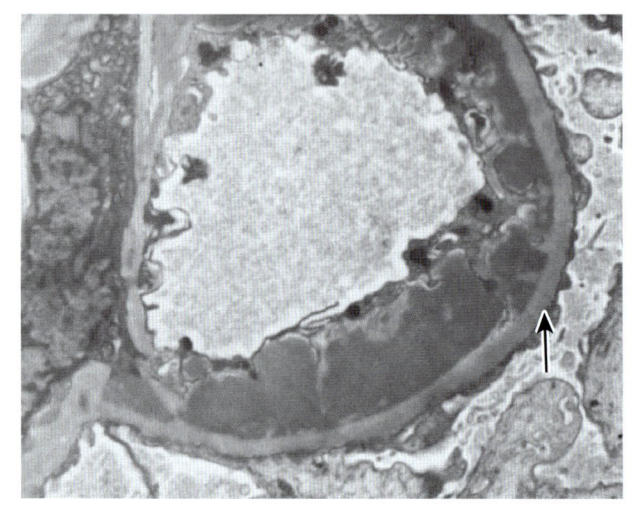

Figure 33.9 Lupus nephritis class IV. Electron micrograph showing a large subendothelial electron-dense deposit as well as a few small subepithelial deposits (arrow). (×1200.)

class IV LN. In general, there is more extensive peripheral capillary wall subendothelial immune deposition, and extracapillary proliferation in the form of crescents is not uncommon. Class IV lesions may have features similar to those of primary membranoproliferative glomerulonephritis (MPGN; also known as mesangiocapillary glomerulonephritis) with mesangial interposition along the peripheral capillary walls and double contours of the GBMs. Some class III and IV biopsies will have focal necrotizing and crescentic lesions akin to those seen in small vessel vasculitides. Some of these patients have had circulating ANCAs.[26,35]

ISN/RPS class V is defined by regular subepithelial immune deposits producing a membranous pattern (Figures 33.10, 33.11, and 33.12).[30,36-38] The coexistence of mesangial immune deposits and mesangial hypercellularity in most cases helps to distinguish membranous LN from primary membranous glomerulopathy.[39] Early membranous LN class V may have no identifiable abnormalities by light microscopy, but subepithelial deposits are detectable by immunofluorescence and electron microscopy. In well-developed

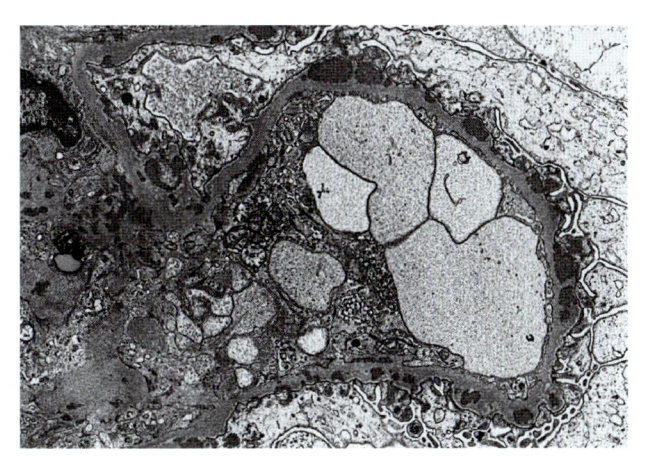

Figure 33.12 Lupus nephritis class V. Electron micrograph showing numerous subepithelial electron-dense deposits as well as mesangial deposits. (×5000.)

membranous lesions, there is typically thickening of the glomerular capillary walls and "spike" formation between the subepithelial deposits. Because sparse subepithelial deposits may also be encountered in other classes (III or IV) of LN, a diagnosis of pure lupus membranous LN should be reserved only for those cases in which the membranous pattern predominates. When the membranous alterations involve more than 50% of the total glomerular capillaries and are accompanied by focal or diffuse endocapillary proliferative lesions and subendothelial immune complex deposition, they are classified as class V + III or class V + IV, respectively.

ISN/RPS class VI, advanced sclerosing LN or end-stage LN, is reserved for biopsies with more than 90% of the glomeruli sclerotic and no residual activity.[30] In such cases, it may be difficult even to establish the diagnosis of LN without the identification of residual glomerular immune deposits by immunofluorescence and electron microscopy or a biopsy history of prior active LN.

IMMUNOFLUORESCENCE

In LN, immune deposits can be found in the glomeruli, tubules, interstitium, and blood vessels.[2-4,23,39] IgG is almost universal, with co-deposits of IgM, IgA, C3, and C1q common.[2,23,30] The presence of all three immunoglobulins (IgG, IgA, and IgM) along with the two complement components (C1q and C3) is known as "full house" staining and is highly suggestive of LN. Staining for fibrin-fibrinogen is common in crescents and segmental necrotizing lesions. The "tissue ANA"[39] (i.e., nuclear staining of renal epithelial cells in sections stained with fluoresceinated antisera to human IgG) is a frequent finding in any LN class. It results from the binding of patient's own ANA to nuclei exposed in the course of cryostat sectioning.

ELECTRON MICROSCOPY

The distribution of glomerular, tubulointerstitial, and vascular deposits seen by electron microscopy correlates closely with that observed by immunofluorescence microscopy.[2,6,23] Deposits are typically electron dense and granular. Some exhibit focal organization with a "fingerprint" substructure composed of curvilinear parallel arrays measuring 10 to 15 nm in diameter.[2,23] Tubuloreticular inclusions, intracellular branching tubular structures measuring 24 nm in diameter located within dilated cisternae of the endoplasmic reticulum of glomerular and vascular endothelial cells, are commonly observed in SLE biopsies.[2,4,23] Tubuloreticular inclusions are inducible on exposure to IFN-α (so-called interferon footprints) and are also present in biopsies of patients infected with human immunodeficiency virus (HIV) and those with some other viral infections.[40]

ACTIVITY AND CHRONICITY

Some investigators grade biopsies for features of activity (potentially reversible lesions) and chronicity (irreversible lesions). In the widely used National Institutes of Health (NIH) system, activity index is calculated by grading the biopsy on a scale of 0 to 3+ for each of six histologic features; these features are endocapillary proliferation, glomerular leukocyte infiltration, wire loop deposits, fibrinoid necrosis and karyorrhexis, cellular crescents, and interstitial inflammation.[41] The severe lesions of crescents and fibrinoid necrosis are assigned double weight. The sum of the individual components yields a total histologic activity index score of from 0 to 24. Likewise, a chronicity index of 0 to 12 is derived from the sum of glomerulosclerosis, fibrous crescents, tubular atrophy, and interstitial fibrosis, each graded on a scale of 0 to 3+. Studies at the NIH correlated both a high activity index (>12) and especially a high chronicity index (>4) with a poor 10-year renal survival rate.[41] However, in several other large studies, neither the activity index nor the chronicity index correlated well with long-term prognosis.[28,42,43] Other NIH studies concluded that a combination of an elevated activity index (>7) and an elevated chronicity index (>3) predicts a poor long-term outcome.[41] A major value of calculating the activity and chronicity indices is in the comparison of sequential biopsies in individual patients. This provides useful information about the efficacy of therapy and the relative degree of reversible versus irreversible lesions.[2-4,23,44,45]

TUBULOINTERSTITIAL DISEASE, VASCULAR LESIONS, AND LUPUS PODOCYTOPATHY

Some SLE patients have major changes in the tubulointerstitial compartment.[46-49] Active tubulointerstitial lesions include edema and inflammatory infiltrates, including T lymphocytes (both CD4+ and CD8+ cells), monocytes, and plasma cells.[49] Tubulointerstitial immune deposits of immunoglobulin and/or complement may be present along the basement membranes of tubules and interstitial capillaries. Severe acute interstitial changes and tubulointerstitial immune deposits are most commonly found in patients with active proliferative class III and IV LN. The degree of interstitial inflammation does not correlate well with the presence or quantity of tubulointerstitial immune deposits.[46,47] Interstitial fibrosis, tubular atrophy, or both are commonly encountered in the more chronic phases of LN. One study documented a strong inverse correlation between the degree of tubular damage and renal survival.[47] In addition, the renal survival rate was higher for patients with less expression on their renal biopsy of the intercellular adhesion molecule-1 (ICAM-1).[48]

Vascular lesions are not included in either the ISN/RPS classification or in the NIH activity and chronicity indices despite their frequent occurrence and clinical significance.[27,50-52] The most frequent vascular lesion is simple vascular immune deposition, most common in patients with active class III and IV biopsies. Vessels may be normal by light microscopy, but by immunofluorescence and electron microscopy there are granular immune deposits in the media and intima of small arteries and arterioles. Noninflammatory necrotizing vasculopathy, most common in arterioles in active class IV LN, is a fibrinoid necrotizing lesion without leukocyte infiltration that severely narrows or occludes the arteriolar lumen. True inflammatory vasculitis resembling polyangiitis is extremely rare in SLE patients. It may be renal limited or part of a more generalized systemic vasculitis.[27,51,52] Thrombotic microangiopathy involving vessels and glomeruli may be associated with anticardiolipin/antiphospholipid antibody or a hemolytic uremic/thrombotic thrombocytopenic purpura (HUS/TTP)–like syndrome.[27,51,52]

A number of other renal diseases have been documented on biopsy in SLE patients, including podocytopathies with features of minimal change disease, focal segmental glomerulosclerosis (FSGS), or collapsing glomerulopathy.[53-55] In some, the relationship between SLE and the podocytopathy suggests this is not a coincidental occurrence but perhaps related to SLE-induced cytokine effects on podocyte function. A collapsing pattern of focal sclerosis in SLE patients of African descent has been associated with APOL1 risk alleles.[56]

CLINICAL MANIFESTATIONS

Although SLE predominantly affects young females, the clinical manifestations are similar in both sexes and in adults and children.[5-8] Organ systems commonly affected include the kidneys, joints, serosal surfaces (including pleura and pericardium), central nervous system, and skin. In addition, cardiac, hepatic, pulmonary, hematopoietic, and gastrointestinal involvement is not infrequent.

Renal involvement often develops concurrently or shortly after the onset of SLE and may follow a protracted course with periods of remissions and exacerbations. Clinical renal involvement usually correlates well with the degree of glomerular involvement. However, some patients may have disproportionately severe vascular or tubulointerstitial lesions that dominate the clinical course.[27,46,52]

Patients with ISN/RPS class I biopsies often have little evidence of clinical renal disease. Likewise, most patients with mesangial lesions (ISN/RPS class II) have mild or minimal clinical renal findings.[1-4,21,28] They may have active lupus serology (a high anti-DNA antibody titer and low serum complement), but the urinary sediment is inactive, hypertension is infrequent, proteinuria is usually less than 1 g/day, and the serum creatinine concentration and glomerular filtration rate (GFR) are usually normal. Nephrotic-range proteinuria is extremely rare unless there is a superimposed podocytopathy.[53,54]

Class III, focal proliferative LN, is often associated with active lupus serologies, although the degree of serologic activity does not necessarily correlate with the histologic severity.[28,33] Hypertension and active urinary sediment are common. Proteinuria is often more than 1 g/day, and one quarter to one third of patients with focal LN have nephrotic syndrome at presentation. Many patients have an elevated serum creatinine concentration at presentation. Patients with less extensive glomerular proliferation, fewer necrotizing features, and no crescents are more likely to be normotensive and have preserved renal function.

Patients with ISN/RPS class IV, diffuse proliferative LN, typically present with the most active clinical features. They often have high anti-DNA antibody titers, low serum complement levels, and very active urinary sediment, with erythrocytes, and cellular casts on urinalysis.[1-4,28,30,32,34] Virtually all have proteinuria and as many as 50% of the patients will have nephrotic syndrome. Hypertension and renal dysfunction are typical. Even when the serum creatinine level is in the "normal range," the GFR is usually depressed.

Patients with membranous LN, ISN/RPS class V, typically present with proteinuria, edema, and other manifestations of nephrotic syndrome.[1-4,28,30,36-38] However, as many as 40% will have proteinuria of less than 3 g/day, and 16% to 20% less than 1 g/day. Only about 60% of membranous LN patients have a low serum complement concentration and an elevated anti-DNA antibody titer at presentation.[28] However, hypertension and renal dysfunction may occur without superimposed proliferative lesions. Patients with membranous LN may present with nephrotic syndrome before developing other clinical and laboratory manifestations of SLE.[28,36-38] In addition, they are predisposed to thrombotic complications such as renal vein thrombosis and pulmonary emboli.[27,51] Patients with mixed membranous and proliferative biopsies have clinical features that reflect both disease components.

End-stage LN, ISN/RPS class VI, is usually the result of "burned-out" LN of long duration.[30] Some renal histologic damage may represent nonimmunologic progression of sclerosis mediated by hyperfiltration in remnant nephrons. Although the lesions are sclerosing and inactive, class VI patients may still have microhematuria and proteinuria. Virtually all have hypertension and a decreased GFR. Levels of anti-DNA antibodies and serum complement levels often normalize at this late stage of disease.

"Silent LN"[1,22,57] has been described in patients without clinical evidence of renal involvement despite biopsy evidence of active proliferative LN. Some define silent LN as active biopsy lesions without active urinary sediment, proteinuria, or a depressed GFR, whereas others require negative lupus serologies as well. Although silent LN is well described in some studies, others have been unable to find even isolated examples.[1,21] It appears to be uncommon, and it is highly likely that even patients with true "silent disease" will manifest clinical renal involvement when followed into their course.

SEROLOGIC TESTS

The presence of antibodies directed against nuclear antigens (ANAs) and especially against DNA (anti-DNA) antibodies are included in the ACR criteria for SLE and are commonly used to monitor the disease course.[1,6,15] ANAs are a highly sensitive screen for SLE, being found in more than 90% of untreated patients, but they are not specific for SLE and occur in many other rheumatologic and non-rheumatologic conditions.[1,6,15,23] Neither the particular pattern of ANA fluorescence (homogeneous, speckled, nucleolar, or rim) nor the titer correlates well with the presence or the severity of renal involvement in SLE.

Autoantibodies directed against double-stranded DNA (anti-dsDNA) are a more specific but less sensitive marker of SLE and are found in almost three fourths of untreated active SLE patients.[1,6,15] Anti-dsDNA IgG antibodies of high avidity that fix complement have correlated best with the presence of renal disease,[1,6,15] and such anti-dsDNA antibodies have been found in the glomerular immune deposits of murine and human LN.[1,15,58,59] High anti-dsDNA antibody titers correlate well with clinical activity.[1,6,15] Anti–single-stranded DNA antibodies (anti-ssDNA), commonly found in SLE and other collagen vascular diseases, do not correlate with clinical lupus activity.

Autoantibodies directed against ribonuclear antigens are commonly present in lupus patients and include anti-Sm and anti-nRNP against extractable nuclear antigen (ENA).[1,6,15,20] Anti-Sm antibodies, although very specific for SLE, are found in only about 25% of lupus patients and are of unclear prognostic value. Anti-nRNP antibodies, found in over one third of SLE patients, are also present in many other rheumatologic diseases, particularly mixed connective tissue disease.[15,20,60] Anti-Ro/SSA antibodies are directed against the protein complex of a cytoplasmic RNA and are present in 25% to 30% of SLE patients. Anti-La/SSB autoantibodies, directed against a nuclear RNP antigen, are present in from 5% to 15% of lupus patients. Neither of the latter two antibodies is specific for SLE and both are found in other collagen vascular diseases, especially Sjögren's syndrome. Maternal anti-Ro antibodies are important in the pathogenesis of neonatal lupus and the development of cardiac conduction abnormalities in the newborn.[61] Anti-Ro antibodies are also associated with a unique dermal psoriasiform type of lupus, with SLE patients who are homozygous C2 deficient, and with a vasculitic disease associated with central nervous system involvement and cutaneous ulcers.[62,63] In addition, lupus patients may develop antibodies directed against histones, endothelial cells, phospholipids, the N-methyl-D-aspartate receptor (associated with central nervous system disease in SLE) and neutrophil cytoplasmic antigens (ANCAs).[64-66]

Levels of total hemolytic complement (CH50) and complement components are usually decreased during active SLE and especially active LN.[1,4,6] Levels of C4 and C3 often decline before a clinical flare of SLE. Serial monitoring of complement levels, with a decline in levels predicting a flare, is considered more useful clinically than an isolated depressed C3 or C4 value.[4] Likewise, normalization of depressed serum complement levels is often associated with improved renal outcome.[67] Levels of total complement and C3 may be decreased in the absence of active systemic or renal disease in patients with extensive dermatologic involvement by SLE. Several heritable complement deficiency states (including C1r, C1s, C2, C4, C5, and C8) have been associated with SLE, and such patients may have depressed total complement levels despite inactive disease.[68]

Other immunologic test results commonly found in lupus patients include elevated levels of circulating immune complexes, a positive lupus band test, and the presence of cryoglobulins. None correlates well with SLE or LN activity.[69-71] In both SLE and isolated discoid lupus, immune complex deposits containing IgG antibody and complement are found along the dermal-epidermal junction of involved skin lesions.[8,70] The presence of granular deposits in clinically unaffected skin (the lupus band test) is usually found only in patients with systemic disease. However, the specificity and sensitivity of this test is debated, and it requires immunofluorescence microscopy of the dermal biopsy.[1] Patients with SLE commonly have a false-positive Venereal Disease Research Laboratory (VDRL) test result due to the presence of antiphospholipid antibodies.[1]

MONITORING CLINICAL DISEASE

It is important to be able to predict systemic and renal relapses and prevent their occurrence through the judicious use of immunosuppressive agents. Serial measurements of many serologic tests (including complement components, autoantibodies, erythrocyte sedimentation rate [ESR], C-reactive protein [CRP], circulating immune complexes, and, recently, levels of cytokines and interleukins) have been used to predict lupus flares. Although there is controversy regarding the value of serum C3 and C4 levels and anti-DNA antibody titers in predicting clinical flares of SLE or LN, these have yet to be replaced by new biomarkers.[3,6,71] Serum levels of anti-dsDNA typically rise and serum complement levels typically fall as the clinical activity of SLE increases, often preceding clinical renal deterioration. In patients with active renal involvement, the urinalysis frequently reveals dysmorphic erythrocytes, red blood cell casts, and other formed elements. An increase in proteinuria from levels of less than 1 g/day to more than this amount, and certainly from low levels to nephrotic levels, is a clear indication of either increased activity or a change in renal histologic class.[3,28]

DRUG-INDUCED LUPUS

A variety of medications may induce a lupus-like syndrome or exacerbate an underlying predisposition to SLE. Those medications metabolized by acetylation, such as procainamide and hydralazine, have been common causes.[72,73] This occurs more commonly in patients who are slow acetylators due to a genetic decrease in hepatic N-acyltransferase. Diltiazem, minocycline, penicillamine, isoniazid, methyldopa, chlorpromazine, and practolol are other potential causes of drug-induced lupus.[72-75] Other drugs that have been associated less frequently with this syndrome include phenytoin, quinidine, propylthiouracil, sulfonamides, lithium, β-blockers, nitrofurantoin, PAS, captopril, glyburide, hydrochlorothiazide, interferon alfa, carbamazepine, sulfasalazine, rifampin, and TNF-α blockers.[72,76,77] Clinical manifestations of drug-induced lupus include fever, rash, myalgias, arthralgias and arthritis, and serositis. Central nervous system and renal involvement are relatively uncommon.[72,78,79] While elevated anti-DNA antibodies and depressed serum complement levels are less common in drug-induced lupus, antihistone autoantibodies are present in more than 95% of patients.[72] These are usually formed against a complex of the histone dimer H2A-H2B and DNA and other histone components.[72,80] Antihistone antibodies are also present in the vast majority of idiopathic, non–drug-related SLE patients, but they are directed primarily against different histone antigens (H1 and H2B).[72]

The presence of antihistone antibodies in the absence of anti-DNA antibodies and other serologic markers for SLE is also indicative of drug-induced disease. The diagnosis of drug-induced lupus depends on documenting the offending agent and achieving a remission following withdrawal of the drug. The primary treatment consists of discontinuing the offending drug.

PREGNANCY AND SYSTEMIC LUPUS ERYTHEMATOSUS

Because SLE occurs so commonly in women of childbearing age, the issue of pregnancy arises often in the care of this population. Independent but related issues are the health of the mother (in terms of both flares of lupus activity and progression of renal disease) and the fate of the fetus. It is unclear whether flares of lupus activity occur more commonly during pregnancy or shortly after delivery.[81-84] Some controlled studies found no increase in lupus flares in pregnant patients versus nonpregnant lupus controls.[81,83,84] Patients with quiescent lupus at the time of pregnancy are less likely to experience an exacerbation of SLE. However, in two small retrospective studies, flares of lupus activity including renal involvement occurred in more than 50% of the pregnancies.[81,84] This was significantly greater than the rate of flare after delivery and in nonpregnant lupus patients.

Pregnancy in patients with preexisting LN has also been associated with worsening of renal function.[85,86] This is less likely to occur in patients who have been in remission for at least 6 months. Patients with hypertension are likely to develop higher blood pressure levels, and those with proteinuria are likely to have increased levels during pregnancy. Patients with elevated serum creatinine levels are most likely to suffer worsening of renal function and to be at highest risk for fetal loss. Although high-dose corticosteroids, cyclosporine, tacrolimus, and azathioprine have all been used in pregnant lupus patients, their safety is unclear. Cyclophosphamide is contraindicated due to its teratogenicity, and newer agents such as mycophenolate and rituximab are not recommended, thus making the treatment of severe LN difficult.

The rate of fetal loss in all SLE patients in most series is 20% to 40% and may approach 50% in some series.[81,83,85,86] While fetal mortality is increased in SLE patients with renal disease, it may be decreasing in the modern treatment era.[85-88] Patients with anticardiolipin or antiphospholipid antibodies, hypertension, or heavy proteinuria are at higher risk for fetal loss.[84] One review of 10 studies in more than 550 women with SLE found fetal death occurred in 38% to 59% of all pregnant SLE patients with antiphospholipid antibodies compared to 16% to 20% of those without these antibodies.[89]

DIALYSIS AND TRANSPLANTATION

The percentage of patients with severe LN who progress to dialysis or transplantation varies from 5% to 50% depending on the population studied, the length of follow-up, and the response to therapy.[1,4,6,28,90-93] Many with slow progressive renal failure have a resolution of their extrarenal disease manifestations and serologic activity.[94,95] With more prolonged time on dialysis, the incidence of clinically active patients declines further, decreasing in one study from 55% at the onset of dialysis to less than 10% by the fifth year and 0% by the tenth year of dialysis.[95] Patients with end-stage kidney disease (ESKD) due to LN have increased mortality during the early months of dialysis due to infectious complications of immunosuppressive therapy.[94,95] Long-term survival of SLE patients on chronic hemodialysis or continuous ambulatory peritoneal dialysis is similar to that of nonlupus patients, with the most common cause of death being cardiovascular.[94-96]

Most renal transplant programs suggest that patients with active SLE undergo a period of dialysis for from 3 to 12 months to allow clinical and serologic disease activity to become quiescent before transplantation.[95] Allograft survival rates in patients with LN are comparable to the rest of the transplant population.[1,4,96-100] The rate of recurrent SLE in the allograft has been low, less than 4% in most series,[96-100] although in several recent reports a higher recurrence rate has been noted.[98] The prevalence of recurrent LN was only 2.44% in a 20-year study of nearly 7000 lupus transplant recipients and was more common in black, female, and younger patients.[99] When surveillance biopsies were used, however, recurrences could be detected in as many as 54% of a small cohort of lupus transplant recipients, although this was mostly subclinical mild mesangial LN.[100] The low rate of clinically important recurrence may be due, in part, to the immune suppressant action of the renal failure prior to transplantation and, in part, to the immunosuppressive regimens used following transplantation. Lupus patients with an antiphospholipid antibody may benefit from anticoagulation therapy during the posttransplant period.[101,102]

COURSE AND PROGNOSIS OF LUPUS NEPHRITIS

The course of patients with LN is extremely varied, with from less than 5% to more than 60% of patients developing progressive renal failure.[1,2,4,28,33,44,90-93,103] This course is defined by the initial pattern and severity of renal involvement as modified by therapy, exacerbations of the disease, and complications of treatment. The prognosis has clearly improved in recent decades with wider and more judicious use of new immunosuppressive medications. Most studies have found additional prognostic value of renal biopsy over clinical data in patients with LN.[33,104-106]

Patients with lesions limited to the renal mesangium generally have an excellent course and prognosis.[1-4,23] Patients with lesions that do not transform into other patterns are unlikely to develop progressive renal failure, and mortality is due to extrarenal manifestations and complications of therapy. Patients with focal proliferative disease have an extremely varied course. Those with mild proliferation involving a small percentage of glomeruli respond well to therapy and less than 5% progress to renal failure over 5 years.[1-4,28,106,107] Patients with more proliferation, necrotizing features, and/or crescent formation have a prognosis more akin to patients with class IV diffuse LN. Class III patients may transform into class IV over time. Some patients with very active segmental proliferative and necrotizing lesions resembling ANCA-associated small vessel vasculitis have a worse renal prognosis than other patients with focal proliferative lesions.[26,35,108]

Patients with diffuse proliferative disease have the least favorable prognosis in most older series.[1-4,23,28,33,34] Nevertheless, the prognosis for this group has markedly improved, with renal survival rates now exceeding 90% in some series of patients treated with modern immunosuppressive agents.[4,34,107,109] In trials from NIH, the risk of doubling the serum creatinine concentration, a surrogate marker for progressive renal disease, at 5 years in patients with diffuse proliferative lupus treated with cyclophosphamide-containing regimens ranged from 35% to less than 5%.[91,92,109] In an Italian study of diffuse proliferative LN, survival was 77% at 10 years and more than 90% if extrarenal deaths were excluded.[34] In a U.S. study of 89 patients with diffuse proliferative LN, renal survival was 89% at 1 year and 71% at 5 years.[110] It is unclear whether the improved survival rates in these recent series are largely due to improved immunosuppression or better supportive care and clinical use of these medications.

In the past, some studies have found age, gender, and race to be as important prognostic variables as clinical features in patient and renal survival in SLE.[1,3,10-12,41,105,110-113] However, a consistent finding is that African Americans have a greater frequency of LN and a worse renal and overall prognosis.[1,3,11,12,41,110-114] This worse prognosis appears to relate to both biologic/genetic and socioeconomic factors.[11,12] In a study from NIH of 65 patients with severe LN, clinical features at study entry associated with progressive renal failure included age, black race, hematocrit less than 26%, and serum creatinine concentration greater than 2.4 mg/dL.[41] Patients with combined activity index (>7) plus chronicity index (>3) on renal biopsy, as well as those with the combination of cellular crescents and interstitial fibrosis also had a worse prognosis. In another U.S. study of 89 patients with diffuse proliferative LN, none of the following features affected renal survival: age, gender, SLE duration, uncontrolled hypertension, or any individual histologic variable.[110] Entry serum creatinine level higher than 3.0 mg/dL, combined activity and chronicity indices on biopsy, and black race predicted a poor outcome. Five-year renal survival rate was 95% for the Caucasian patients but only 58% for the black patients. In a study of more than 125 LN patients with WHO class III or IV from New York, both racial and socioeconomic factors were associated with the worse outcomes in African Americans and Hispanics.[11] An evaluation of 203 patients from the Miami area confirmed worse renal outcomes in African Americans and Hispanics related to both biologic and economic factors.[12]

More rapid and more complete renal remissions are associated with improved long-term prognosis.[115,116] Renal flares during the course of SLE also may predict a poor renal outcome.[103,117,118] Relapses of severe LN over 5 to 10 years of follow-up occur in up to 50% of patients and usually respond less well and more slowly to repeated course of therapy.[3,103,119-121] A retrospective analysis of 70 Italian patients in which more than half had diffuse proliferative disease found excellent patient survival (100% at 10 years and 86% at 20 years) as well as preserved renal function with probability of not doubling the serum creatinine concentration to be 85% at 10 years and 72% at 20 years.[103] Most patients in this study were Caucasian, which likely influenced the excellent long-term prognosis. Multivariate analysis in the Italian study showed males, those more anemic, and especially those with flare-ups of disease, to have a worse outcome. Patients with renal flares of any type had 7 times the risk of renal failure, and those with rapid rises in creatinine had 27 times the chance of doubling their serum creatinine concentration. Another Italian study of 91 patients with diffuse proliferative LN showed more than 50% having a renal flare, which correlated with a younger age at biopsy (<30 years old), higher activity index, and karyorrhexis on biopsy.[117] The number of flares, nephritic flares, and flares with increased proteinuria correlated with a doubling of the serum creatinine. The role of relapses in predicting progressive disease has been documented by others as well, although relapse does not invariably predict a bad outcome.[122]

While an elevated anti-DNA antibody titer and low serum complement levels may correlate with active renal involvement, they do not correlate with long-term renal prognosis.[1,28,90,103,110] In several studies anemia has been a poor prognostic finding regardless of the underlying cause.[41,103] Severe hypertension has also been related to renal prognosis in some studies but not others.[28] Renal dysfunction, as noted by an elevated serum creatinine or decreased GFR or by heavy proteinuria, and nephrotic syndrome are indicative of a poor renal prognosis in the vast majority of series.[1-4,6,33] However, not all studies have found an elevation of the initial serum creatinine to predict a poor long-term prognosis, and in some the initial serum creatinine only predicted short-term renal survival.[110] Other renal features, such as duration of nephritis and rate of decline of GFR, may also predict prognosis.[90,107]

Finally, histologic features such as the class, the degree of activity and chronicity, and the severity of tubulointerstitial damage have also predicted prognosis. In a number of studies, the pattern of renal involvement, especially when using the ISN/RPS or older WHO classification, has been a useful guide to prognosis.[1,2,28,31,32] In NIH trials, patients with severe proliferative LN with a higher activity index or chronicity index were more likely to have progressive renal failure.[107] Other studies with different referral populations could not confirm this.[2,3,23,28,43] Regardless, the contribution of chronic renal scarring to a poor long-term outcome has been confirmed by many studies.[48,90,117,122,123] Some studies have found the initial renal biopsy to have little predictive value; rather, certain features on a repeat biopsy at 6 months proved to be a strong predictor of doubling the serum creatinine or progression to renal failure.[47,124] These include ongoing inflammation with cellular crescents, macrophages in the tubular lumens, persistent immune deposits (especially C3) on immunofluorescence microscopy, and persistent subendothelial and mesangial deposits. Other studies suggest that reversal of interstitial fibrosis and glomerular segmental scarring along with remission of initial inflammation and immune deposition is an important favorable prognostic finding on the 6-month biopsy.[122] Thus, chronic changes on biopsy are not always cumulative or immutable, and their reversal may be crucial in preventing ultimate renal failure when new acute lesions develop.

The natural history of membranous LN is less clear. In early studies, its course appeared far better than that for active proliferative disease.[21] Subsequent studies with longer follow-up suggested a worse outcome for membranous LN with persistent nephrotic syndrome.[28] Retrospective analyses show 5-year renal survival rates largely depend on whether patients have pure membranous lesions (class V) or superimposed proliferative lesions in a focal (class III + V) or diffuse (IV + V) distribution.[37,38] One U.S. study found the 10-year survival rate was 72% for patients with pure membranous lesions but only 20% to 48% for those with superimposed proliferative lesions.[37] Black race, elevated serum creatinine, higher degrees of proteinuria, hypertension, and transformation to another WHO pattern all portended a worse outcome.[1,3] The poor survival in blacks with membranous LN may explain the excellent results in retrospective Italian studies, which follow largely Caucasian cohorts. One such Italian study found the 10-year survival rate of membranous LN patients to be 93%.[38] Even in this Italian population, survival for pure membranous LN was far better than in patients with superimposed proliferative lesions. Thus, at least in part, the variability of prognosis in older studies can be explained by the differences in racial background, histology, and therapy.

TREATMENT OF LUPUS NEPHRITIS

The treatment of severe LN remains controversial.[1,3,6] Although recent controlled studies have better defined the course and therapy for this group, the most effective and least toxic regimen for any given patient is often less clear. While cyclophosphamide has been effective therapy for many patients with severe LN, newer regimens have been developed in the hope of attaining equal or greater efficacy with less toxicity. The concept of more vigorous initial therapy during an "induction" treatment phase followed by more prolonged lower dose therapy during a "maintenance phase" is now widely accepted.[1,2,125,126]

Patients with ISN/RPS class I and II biopsies have an excellent renal prognosis and need no therapy directed to the kidney. Transformation to another histologic class is usually heralded by increasing proteinuria and activity of the urinary sediment. At this point, repeat renal biopsy may serve as a guide to therapy.[1] ISN/RPS class III patients with only few mild proliferative lesions and no necrotizing features or crescent formation have a good prognosis and will often respond to a short course of high-dose corticosteroid therapy or a brief course of other immunosuppressive agents. Patients with greater numbers of affected glomeruli and those with necrotizing features and crescents usually require more vigorous therapy similar to therapy for patients with diffuse proliferative LN.

Patients with diffuse proliferative disease, ISN/RPS class IV lesions, require aggressive treatment to avoid irreversible renal damage and progression to ESKD.[1,2,6,107,109,115] The ideal immunosuppressive regimen should be individualized and based on the patient's prior therapy, risk and concern over potential side effects, compliance, and tolerability. Initial regimens may include combinations of the following: oral or intravenous corticosteroids, oral or intravenous cyclophosphamide, mycophenolate mofetil, cyclosporine, tacrolimus, and/or rituximab. A number of other treatments are currently being studied for resistant or relapsing disease and for maintenance therapy.

Prednisone, despite the lack of controlled trials, is included in most treatment regimens for LN. In retrospective studies, higher initial doses of corticosteroids appeared more effective than lower dose therapy (<30 mg prednisone daily).[1,3,4,6] Initial use of high-dose corticosteroid treatment alone is still used by some clinicians for limited focal proliferative disease. However, for severe proliferative LN, either class III or class IV, corticosteroids along with other immunosuppressive agents are required.[4] Common regimens use 1 mg/kg/day of prednisone, tapering after 4 to 6 weeks of treatment so that patients are on 30 mg/day or less by the end of 3 months of therapy. Other clinicians start with daily pulses of IV methylprednisolone for 1 to 3 days followed by the oral corticosteroids.

Despite initial favorable results with pulse methylprednisolone followed by oral corticosteroids in treating severe LN, there have been few randomized trials using this regimen versus other immunosuppressive therapy.[1,91,92] Two NIH trials have found pulse corticosteroids to be less effective than intravenous cyclophosphamide in preventing progressive renal failure.[91,92] In one trial, 48% of the pulse steroid–treated patients doubled their serum creatinine at 5 years compared to only 25% of the cyclophosphamide-treated group.[92]

Controlled randomized trials at the NIH and elsewhere have helped establish the role of cyclophosphamide in the treatment of severe LN.[44,91,92,109,125-127] In one seminal trial, patients were randomly assigned to regimens of high-dose corticosteroids for 6 months or oral cyclophosphamide, oral azathioprine, combined oral azathioprine plus cyclophosphamide, or intravenous cyclophosphamide every third month, all given with low-dose corticosteroids.[109] Evaluation at 120 months showed superior renal survival in the intravenous cyclophosphamide group versus the steroid group. At longer follow-up to 200 months, the renal survival of the azathioprine group was statistically no better than that of the corticosteroid group.[109] A subsequent Dutch collaborative trial found remission rates comparable between oral azathioprine and cyclophosphamide, but more relapses and worse long-term outcome with azathioprine.[128] Thus, for a number of years, cyclophosphamide was the most effective immunosuppressive agent for LN. Since side effects in the NIH trial appeared least severe when cyclophosphamide was used intravenously, subsequent NIH protocols utilized the drug in this manner given once monthly. Other trials at NIH and elsewhere have also used monthly pulses of intravenous cyclophosphamide for 6 consecutive months as opposed to the original every third month regimen.[119,125-127]

These studies and others have confirmed the benefits and response rate of intravenous cyclophosphamide regimens in severe LN.[44,110,119] In most patients treated with intravenous cyclophosphamide, side effects such as hemorrhagic cystitis, alopecia, and neoplasms have been infrequent.[1,6] Exceptions are menstrual irregularities and premature menopause, which are most common in women older than 25 years of age who have received intravenous cyclophosphamide for more than 6 months.[129] The dose of intravenous cyclophosphamide must be reduced for significant renal impairment and adjusted for some removal by hemodialysis. The cytoprotective agent Mesna has been used successfully by some to reduce bladder complications from cyclophosphamide.

A three-armed controlled randomized trial at NIH of 1 year of monthly doses of intravenous methylprednisolone, versus monthly intravenous cyclophosphamide for 6 months and then every third month, versus the combination of both therapies found the remission rate was highest with the combined treatment regimen (85%) as opposed to cyclophosphamide alone (62%) and methylprednisolone alone (29%).[91] Mortality was low and similar in all groups. Long follow-up indicated drug toxicity was not different between the cyclophosphamide group and the combined cyclophosphamide-methylprednisolone group.[127] It is likely that through higher sustained remissions and fewer relapses, fewer patients required repeated treatments in the combined cyclophosphamide-steroid–treated group. Moreover, the long-term efficacy, especially in terms of renal outcomes, was greatest for the combination therapy group. Thus, combined treatment with intravenous methylprednisolone pulses and intravenous cyclophosphamide pulses became a standard therapy for severe LN. However, it should be noted that some groups have achieved equal efficacy and few side effects using short courses of oral cyclophosphamide followed by other immunosuppressive medications.[130]

Studies showing that oral maintenance immunosuppressive agents other than cyclophosphamide were more effective and safer than cyclophosphamide have led to the search for equally effective but safer regimens as induction therapy. One approach to obtain efficacy with less toxicity uses lower induction doses of the cytotoxic agent. The Euro Lupus Nephritis Trial, a multicenter prospective trial of 90 patients with severe LN, compared low-dose versus "conventional" high-dose intravenous cyclophosphamide.[131] Patients were randomized to either 6-monthly intravenous pulses of 0.5 to 1 g/m^2 cyclophosphamide followed by two quarterly pulses or only 500 mg intravenously every 2 weeks for a total of six doses, both followed by oral azathioprine as maintenance therapy. At 40 months, follow-up, there were no statistically significant differences in treatment failures, renal remissions, or renal flares, but twice as many infections occurred in the high-dose group. Although this trial may have included some patients with milder renal disease (mean creatinine, 1 to 1.3 mg/dL; mean proteinuria, 2.5 to 3.5 g/day for both groups) and a predominantly Caucasian patient population, it supported the use of shorter duration and lower total dose cyclophosphamide for induction therapy. Longer follow-up of this population confirms these data and suggests that early response to therapy is predictive of a good long-term outcome and that the long-term results are excellent.[115] A recent trial of this regimen as standard care in both arms of an investigational study of Abatacept in patients with severe LN confirms that this regimen is effective in black as well as Caucasian populations.

Mycophenolate mofetil (MMF) has proven to be an effective immunosuppressive in transplant patients and a variety of other immunologic renal diseases.[132] It is a reversible inhibitor of inosine monophosphate dehydrogenase required for purine synthesis and blocks B and T cell proliferation, inhibits antibody formation, and decreases expression of adhesion molecules, among other effects. MMF is effective in treating murine LN.[132] MMF was shown to have good efficacy and reduced complications when compared to standard treatment regimens in a number of uncontrolled trials in LN.[132] In one 6-month Chinese trial of patients randomized to either MMF or intravenous pulse cyclophosphamide for induction therapy of severe LN,[133] proteinuria and microhematuria decreased more in the MMF-treated patients than in the cytotoxic group, with renal impairment before and after therapy, activity index on biopsy before and after therapy, and serologic improvement equivalent. MMF was better tolerated with fewer gastrointestinal side effects and fewer infections. In another randomized controlled trial of patients given either a regimen of prednisone plus oral MMF or a regimen of prednisone plus cyclophosphamide orally for 6 months followed by oral azathioprine for another 6 months, both regimens proved similar in efficacy.[134] Of the MMF group 81% achieved complete and 14% partial remission versus 76% complete and 14% partial remission for the cyclophosphamide-prednisone group. Treatment failures, relapses following therapy, discontinuations of therapy, mortality, and time to remission were similar. Longer follow-up at 4 years with the addition of more patients showed MMF to have comparable efficacy to cyclophosphamide with no significant difference in complete or partial remissions, doubling of baseline creatinine, or relapses. Significantly fewer MMF-treated patients developed severe infections, leukopenia, or amenorrhea, and all deaths and renal failure were in the cyclophosphamide group.[135]

A multicenter U.S. study comparing induction therapy in 140 patients with severe class III and class IV LN included more than 50% blacks, most with heavy proteinuria and active urinary sediment.[136] Patients were randomized to monthly pulses of intravenous cyclophosphamide 0.5 to 1 g/m^2 or oral MMF 2 to 3 g/day, both with tapering corticosteroid doses for 6 months. Although designed as an equivalency study, MMF proved superior in attaining both complete remissions and complete and partial remissions. The side effect profile also appeared better with MMF. At the 3-year follow-up, there was a trend to less renal failure and mortality with MMF. Thus, in a patient population at high risk for poor renal outcomes, MMF proved superior to intravenous cyclophosphamide. A subsequent international multicenter randomized controlled trial compared similar regimens of MMF to intravenous cyclophosphamide for induction therapy in 370 LN patients with ISN/RPS classes III, IV, or V.[10] This study found virtually identical rates of complete and partial remission (over 50%), improvement of renal function and proteinuria, and mortality rates between the two regimens. Diarrhea and gastrointestinal side effects were most common in the MMF group, whereas nausea, vomiting, and alopecia were more common in the cyclophosphamide group. In the small group of about 30 patients with a greatly reduced GFR (<30 mL/min), MMF proved at least as effective if not more so than intravenous cyclophosphamide.[137] In an analysis of different geographic and ethnic backgrounds, MMF proved uniformly more effective across different groups.[138] In another study of 52 patients with crescentic LN (>50% crescents on biopsy) randomized to induction therapy with MMF or intravenous cyclophosphamide, the MMF group had a higher remission rate and a lower relapse rate.[139] Thus, taken together, these two large, randomized controlled trials and a variety of other analyses support the use of MMF as a first-line treatment of severe LN. Both ACR and Kidney Disease: Improving Global Outcomes (KDIGO) guidelines support either a cyclophosphamide- or a mycophenolate-based regimen as first-line therapy for severe LN.[140] For patients who fail to achieve remission with either initial regimen at 6 months of therapy, use of the other regimen is recommended.

A number of studies have focused on the optimal maintenance therapy for LN with the goal of avoiding relapse and flares while minimizing the long-term immunosuppressive toxicity. One randomized controlled trial examined LN patients who had successfully completed induction of remission with 4 to 7 monthly pulses of intravenous cyclophosphamide and were then randomized to either continue with intravenous cyclophosphamide every third month, oral azathioprine, or oral MMF.[1,2,141] The 54 LN patients randomized were largely composed of blacks (50%) and Hispanics and included many patients with nephrotic syndrome (64%), reduced GFR, and severe proliferative LN. Fewer patients in the azathioprine and the MMF groups reached the primary end points of death and chronic renal failure compared to the group that continued to receive cyclophosphamide. The cumulative probability of remaining relapse free was higher with MMF (78%) and azathioprine (58%) compared with cyclophosphamide (43%), and there was increased mortality in patients given continued cyclophosphamide. Complications of therapy were also reduced in the MMF and azathioprine groups, including days of hospitalization, amenorrhea, and infections. Thus, maintenance therapy with either oral MMF or azathioprine was superior to intravenous cyclophosphamide and had less toxicity.

The results of two large randomized trials further delineate the role of these oral agents in the maintenance of patients with proliferative LN.[142,143] In the European MAINTAIN trial, 105 patients were randomized to either azathioprine or MMF for at least 3 years of maintenance (mean, 53 months).[142] There was no difference between these medications in the time to renal flares or to renal remission. In the worldwide Aspreva Lupus Management Study (ALMS) maintenance trial, 227 patients who achieved remission after induction therapy with either intravenous cyclophosphamide or MMF were re-randomized in double-blind fashion to either MMF or azathioprine maintenance for 3 years.[143] MMF proved superior to azathioprine with respect to the primary end point of time to treatment failure (death, ESKD, doubling of serum creatinine, LN flare, or requirement for rescue therapy).[143] Differences between the two studies likely explain the differing results. The MAINTAIN trial was prerandomized from day 1, included smaller numbers of patients who were largely Caucasian, and used the end point of renal flare since few patients in this population progress to renal failure. Even so, there were 26% flares in the azathioprine group compared to only 19% in the MMF group, although this difference was not statistically significant. The ALMS maintenance trial included only those patients who achieved remission after induction; was international, including multiracial and diverse populations; and used harder end points for response (doubling creatinine, ESKD, etc.). At present, both the ACR and KDIGO recommend either agent, azathioprine or MMF, as maintenance therapy.

The calcineurin inhibitors cyclosporine and tacrolimus have been proven to increase the induction remission rate in a number of uncontrolled and controlled trials.[1] Tacrolimus has been successful in increasing remissions as part of a multidrug regimen for severe LN patients with combined ISN/RPS class IV and V lesions.[144] Intravenous cyclophosphamide resulted in complete remission in 5% and partial remissions in 40% at 6 months versus a "multitargeted regimen" of tacrolimus, MMF, and corticosteroids, which led to a 50% complete and a 40% partial remission rate in this time period. A recent large multicenter trial from China of more than 350 patients showed equally good results with this multitargeted therapy.

Rituximab, a chimeric monoclonal antibody targeting CD20 B cells, depletes them through multiple mechanisms, including complement-dependent cell lysis; FcRγ-dependent, antibody-dependent, cell-mediated cytotoxicity; and induction of apoptosis. Rituximab, which is approved by the U.S. Food and Drug Administration (FDA) for the treatment of rheumatoid arthritis, granulomatosis with polyangiitis (formerly designated Wegener's granulomatosis), and microscopic polyangiitis, has been utilized with varying success in many other immunologic and autoimmune diseases, including a variety of primary glomerular diseases.[140] In LN it has been used in more than 300 patients, mostly in case reports and open-label uncontrolled trials.[1,4] However, two large randomized controlled trials have given disappointing results.[1,4,145,146] In one trial of 257 SLE patients without severe renal disease, patients were randomized to receive rituximab or placebo.[145] Although subgroup analyses suggested a beneficial effect in the African American and Hispanic subgroups, there were no significant differences between the placebo and the rituximab arms of therapy. In the Lupus Nephritis Assessment with Rituximab (LUNAR) trial, 140 patients with class III and IV LN were randomized to rituximab or placebo in addition to an induction regimen of MMF (goal 3 g/day) and tapering corticosteroids.[146] Although the rituximab group had a greater fall in anti-DNA antibody titers and rise in serum complement levels, there was no statistically significant difference in the primary renal response between treatment groups at 1 year.[147] At present, rituximab is not a first-line agent for induction therapy of most patients with severe LN. It continues to be used in patients resistant to other treatments and in those who do not tolerate conventional treatment.[148,149] A recent study of the use of rituximab and MMF in 50 LN patients without use of oral corticosteroids has given excellent complete and partial remission results.[150] A large multicenter controlled randomized trial of the use of rituximab as a steroid-sparing agent for the induction of LN is now under way.

Other monoclonal antibodies directed at B cells have been or are being studied. Ocrelizumab, a fully humanized anti-CD20 monoclonal antibody had the advantages of avoiding first-dose infusion reactions and the development of human antichimeric antibodies (HACAs) that were potential problems with rituximab therapy.[140] A controlled randomized trial using this agent in patients with LN was terminated early due to adverse events. Atacicept, a soluble fully humanized recombinant fusion protein that inhibits B cell stimulating factor (BLISS) and a proliferation-inducing ligand (APRIL), also failed in initial trials with patients with LN.[151] Epratuzumab, a humanized monoclonal antibody against CD22, a marker of mature B cells but not plasma cells, is currently being studied.[152]

T lymphocyte activation requires two signals.[140,153] The first occurs when the antigen is presented to the T cell receptor in the context of MHC class II molecules on antigen-presenting cells and the second by the interaction of costimulatory molecules on T lymphocytes and antigen-presenting cells. Disruption of costimulatory signals interrupts the (auto)immune response. Two clinical trials using different humanized anti-CD40L monoclonal antibodies in LN patients to block B and T cell costimulation have not been successful.[154,155] Another costimulatory pathway is mediated through the interaction of CD28CD80/86.[1] CTLA-4 Ig, Abatacept, a fusion molecule that combines the extracellular domain of human CTLA4 with the constant region (Fc) of the human IgG1 heavy chain, interrupts the CD28CD80/86 interaction. It is FDA approved for the treatment of rheumatoid arthritis. Two major randomized controlled trials in patients with severe LN treated with intravenous cyclophosphamide and steroids have now given negative results.[1,156,157] Recently belimumab, a humanized monoclonal antibody against BLys (B lymphocyte stimulator), has been FDA approved for the treatment of lupus based on two trials.[158,159] Although some patients with renal disease were included in these trials, few patients had true severe LN.[160] An ongoing trial is testing the use of this agent in LN.

Other therapies studied in controlled trials in LN have included plasmapheresis and intravenous γ-globulin administration. Plasmapheresis was studied in a multicenter controlled trial of 86 patients with severe LN.[161] This study found no benefit in terms of clinical remission, progression to renal failure, or patient survival beyond a more rapid lowering of anti-DNA antibody titers. Likewise, plasmapheresis synchronized to intravenous cyclophosphamide pulse therapy has not proven effective.[162] At present, plasmapheresis should be reserved for only certain LN patients (e.g., those with severe pulmonary hemorrhage, those with a TTP-like syndrome, and those with antiphospholipid antibodies and a clotting episode who cannot be anticoagulated due to hemorrhage, etc.).

Intravenous immune globulin has been used successfully in a number of SLE patients to treat thrombocytopenia as well as LN, leading to clinical and histologic improvement in some patients.[163,164] One controlled trial included only 14 patients but showed stabilization of the plasma creatinine, creatinine clearance, and proteinuria when intravenous immune globulin was used as maintenance therapy after successful induction of remission with intravenous cyclophosphamide.[165]

Other therapies that have been studied in small numbers of LN patients include the proteasome inhibitor bortezomib, adrenocorticotropic hormone (ACTH), total lymphoid irradiation, bone marrow ablation with stem cell rescue, laquinimod therapy, and use of tolerance molecules.[4,93,165-168] All are still experimental since none has yet undergone large successful controlled clinical trials. Immunoablative therapy with high-dose cyclophosphamide with and without stem cell transplantation has been used successfully in a limited number of SLE patients with only a short period of follow-up and relatively high risks. One new tolerance molecule, Abetimus, despite efficacy in animal models and encouraging early trials, failed to prevent flares of LN in the largest controlled randomized trial.[168]

For patients with class V membranous LN, there have been conflicting data regarding the course, prognosis, and response to treatment.[1,4] The degree of superimposed proliferative lesions greatly influences outcome in class V patients, and it is unclear if older trials included only pure membranous LN patients. Thus, early trials reported low and inconsistent response rates with oral corticosteroids.[36] Excellent long-term results with intensive immunosuppressive regimens from Italian studies and others raise questions of whether the results are related to the therapeutic intervention or to the population studied and better supportive treatments.[38] A retrospective Italian trial found better remission with a regimen of chlorambucil and methylprednisolone than with corticosteroids alone.[169] In a small non-randomized trial of cyclosporine in membranous LN, there was an excellent remission rate of nephrotic syndrome with mean proteinuria decreasing from 6 to 1 or 2 g/day by 6 months.[45] At long-term follow-up and re-biopsy, there was no evidence of cyclosporine-induced renal damage, but two patients had developed superimposed proliferative lesions over time. An NIH trial of 42 nephrotic patients with membranous LN compared cyclosporine, prednisone, and intravenous cyclophosphamide and found superior remission rates for the cyclosporine and cyclophosphamide regimens but a trend toward more relapses when the cyclosporine was withdrawn.[170] Tacrolimus has also been used for class V LN with good results. A study of 38 patients with pure membranous LN evaluated long-term treatment with prednisone plus azathioprine.[133] At 12 months 67% of the patients had experienced a complete remission and 22% a partial remission. At 3 years only 12% had relapsed, at 5 years only 16%, and at 90 months only 19% had relapsed. At the end of follow-up, no patient had doubled serum creatinine. Clearly in this population a regimen of steroids plus azathioprine was highly effective. The response of patients with membranous LN to MMF has been varied.[171-173] There were 84 patients with pure ISN class V membranous LN among the 510 patients enrolled in two similarly designed randomized controlled trials comparing MMF and intravenous cyclophosphamide induction therapy.[173] Rates of remissions, relapse, and course were similar in both treatment groups. Thus, MMF can also be considered a first-line therapy for certain patients with membranous LN.

Given limited data, the treatment of membranous LN should be individualized.[1,4] Patients with pure membranous LN and a good renal prognosis (subnephrotic levels of proteinuria and preserved GFR) may benefit from a short course of cyclosporine with low-dose corticosteroids along with inhibitors of the renin angiotensin aldosterone system and statins. For those at higher risk of progressive disease (African Americans, those fully nephrotic), options include cyclosporine, monthly intravenous pulses of cyclophosphamide, MMF, or azathioprine plus corticosteroids. Patients with mixed membranous and proliferative LN are treated in the same way as those with proliferative disease alone.

As effective and safer therapies for LN have evolved, greater attention has been directed to other causes of morbidity and mortality in the SLE population. Lupus patients have accelerated atherogenesis and a disproportionate rate of coronary vascular disease, leading to a high mortality rate.[174] The high cardiovascular risk rate has been attributed to concurrent hypertension, hyperlipidemia, nephrotic syndrome, prolonged corticosteroid use, antiphospholipid syndrome, and, in some, the added vascular risks of chronic kidney disease (CKD).[175,176] Despite limited data on therapeutic interventions in this population, aggressive management of modifiable cardiovascular risk factors may alter the morbidity and mortality of this population. Extrapolating from other proteinuric CKD populations, closely monitored blood pressure control (<130/80), the use of angiotensin-converting enzyme inhibitors (ACEIs) and/or angiotensin receptor blockers (ARBs), and correction of dyslipidemia with statins are all reasonable in LN patients. In addition, use of calcium, vitamin D supplements, and bisphosphonates to prevent glucocorticoid-induced osteoporosis may be useful.

Some form of antiphospholipid antibodies is present in 40% to 75% of lupus patients.[177-179] Since most do not experience thrombotic complications, they require no special treatment. However, some would recommend low-dose aspirin and hydroxychloroquine for prophylaxis of asymptomatic patients with antiphospholipid antibodies. In patients with evidence of a clinical thrombotic event, most investigators use chronic anticoagulation with warfarin as long as the antibody persists. While the standard practice has been not to anticoagulate other patients, in one recent series of more than 100 SLE patients, over one fourth had antiphospholipid antibodies, of whom almost 80% had a thrombotic event. The antibody-positive patients also had a greater incidence of chronic renal failure than the antibody-negative patients.[179] (See discussion of anticardiolipin antibodies and glomerulonephritis in the following section.)

ANTIPHOSPHOLIPID SYNDROME

Antiphospholipid syndrome (APS) may be associated with glomerular disease, small and large vessel renal involvement, as well as coagulation problems in dialysis and renal transplant patients.[177-180] Patients with APS have autoantibodies directed against plasma proteins bound to phospholipids. They may include IgG and/or IgM anticardiolipin antibodies, antibodies to β_2-glycoprotein I of IgG or IgM isotype, or lupus anticoagulant activity.[181-183] In some studies the presence of specific β_2-glycoprotein I antibodies has been correlated with an increased risk of thrombotic events in patients with APS.[184] Antiphospholipid antibodies may cause a false-positive VDRL. In addition to having one of these autoantibodies, patients with APS must have one or more episodes of venous, arterial, or small vessel thrombosis, or fetal morbidity. Thrombocytopenia and prolonged partial thromboplastin time are frequent laboratory findings. The presence of antiphospholipid antibodies should be documented on two or more occasions at least 12 weeks apart and within 5 years of clinical manifestations.

The pathogenesis of the APS remains unclear.[185-191] Susceptible individuals may develop antiphospholipid antibodies after exposure to infectious or other noxious agents. Among SLE patients there may be a genetic predisposition associated with HLA-DRB1 loci.[192] However, despite the presence of antiphospholipid antibodies, a "second hit" (such as pregnancy, contraceptive use, nephrotic syndrome, or hyperlipidemia) may be necessary for them to produce thrombotic events and the APS. The mechanism(s) of the procoagulant effect is likely to be multifactorial. Antiphospholipid antibodies exert procoagulant effects at multiple sites in the clotting cascade, including prothrombin, protein C, annexin V, coagulation factors VII and XII, platelets, serum proteases, and tissue factor procoagulant. They may also impair fibrinolysis through inhibition of such factors as tissue type plasminogen activator. The result is endothelial damage and intravascular coagulation.

Among patients with antiphospholipid antibodies, 30% to 50% have the primary APS in which there is no associated autoimmune disease.[177-179,181-183] Antiphospholipid antibodies are found in from 25% to 75% of SLE patients, although most patients never experience clinical features of the APS.[177-179,181-183] In an analysis of 29 published series with more than 1000 SLE patients, 34% were positive for the lupus anticoagulant and 44% for anticardiolipin antibodies.[189] Most studies have found a higher incidence of thrombotic events in SLE patients positive for antiphospholipid antibodies.[190,193-195] A European study of almost 575 SLE patients found the prevalence of IgG anticardiolipin antibodies to be 23% and of IgM 14%.[196] Patients with IgG antibodies had a clear association with thrombocytopenia and thromboses. A multicenter European analysis of 1000 SLE patients found thromboses in 7% of patients over 5 years. Patients with IgG anticardiolipin antibodies again had a higher incidence of thromboses, as did those with a lupus anticoagulant.[197] Antiphospholipid antibodies are also found in up to 2% of normal individuals and in those with a variety of infections (commonly in patients with HIV or hepatitis C virus [HCV]) and drug reactions, but these are not usually associated with the clinical features of the APS.[198-200]

The clinical features of APS relate to thrombotic events and consequent ischemia. Among 1000 APS patients the most common features were deep vein thrombosis (32%), thrombocytopenia (22%), livedo reticularis (20%), stroke (13%), pulmonary embolism (9%), and fetal loss (9%).[197] Patients may also experience pulmonary hypertension, cardiac involvement, memory impairment and other neurologic manifestations, fever, malaise, and constitutional symptoms.[177-180,194] Patients who test positive for all three diagnostic tests (lupus anticoagulant, anticardiolipin antibodies, and β_2-glycoprotein antibodies) are at higher risk for thromboembolic events. Catastrophic APS, a rare event (occurring in 0.8% of APS patients), is associated with rapid thromboses in multiple organ systems and has a high fatality rate.[201,202]

Renal involvement, so-called antiphospholipid nephropathy, occurs in as many as 25% of patients with primary APS and is characterized by thrombosis of blood vessels ranging from the glomerular capillaries to the main renal artery and vein.[177,180,203,204] Lesions involving the arteries and arterioles often have both a thrombotic component and a reactive or proliferative one with intimal mucoid thickening, subendothelial fibrosis, and medial hyperplasia (Figure 33.13).[204,205] Interstitial fibrosis and cortical atrophy may occur due to tissue ischemia. Glomerular lesions include glomerular capillary thrombosis with associated mesangiolysis, mesangial interposition and duplication of GBMs, and subendothelial accumulation of electron-lucent, flocculent material, resembling the changes in other forms of glomerular thrombotic microangiopathy such as HUS and TTP.

A retrospective renal biopsy study found antiphospholipid nephropathy in almost 40% of antiphospholipid-positive patients versus only 4% of patients without antiphospholipid antibody. When antiphospholipid nephropathy was present, it was associated with both lupus anticoagulant and anticardiolipin antibodies.[206] Among antiphospholipid-positive SLE

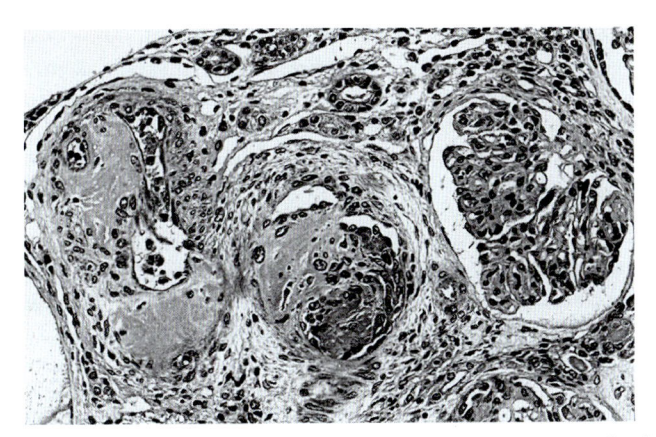

Figure 33.13 Antiphospholipid syndrome. Organizing recanalized thrombi narrow the lumens of two interlobular arteries. The adjacent glomerulus displays ischemic-type retraction of its tuft. (Hematoxylin and eosin stain, ×200.)

patients, antiphospholipid nephropathy was found in two thirds of those with APS and in one third of those without APS. Although patients with antiphospholipid nephropathy had a higher frequency of hypertension and elevated serum creatinine levels at biopsy in this series, they did not have a higher frequency of progressive renal insufficiency, ESKD, or death at follow-up.[207] This is in contrast to another series of more than 100 SLE patients which found the presence of antiphospholipid antibodies to be associated with both thrombotic events and a greater progression to renal failure.[179] In patients with antiphospholipid nephropathy, renal biopsies with thrombotic microangiopathy may be misclassified as FSGS, membranous nephropathy, and MPGN.[208] However, a recent study reports that some patients with APS may develop a number of other glomerular histologic patterns on light microscopic examination, including membranous nephropathy, minimal change/focal sclerosis, mesangial proliferative glomerulonephritis, and pauci-immune rapidly progressive glomerulonephritis (RPGN).[209]

The most frequent clinical renal findings are proteinuria, at times in the nephrotic range, active urinary sediment, hypertension, and progressive renal dysfunction.[177,178,203,205,206,208,209] Some patients present with an acute deterioration in renal function.[208] With major renal arterial involvement there may be renal infarction, and renal vein thrombosis may be silent or present with sudden flank pain and a decrease in renal function. Renal artery stenosis has been reported with and without malignant hypertension.[210-212]

About 10% of biopsied lupus patients have glomerular microthromboses as the major histopathologic finding. Therapy of this glomerular lesion clearly differs from that of immune complex–mediated glomerulonephritis.[51] One study of 114 biopsied SLE patients found vaso occlusive lesions in one third of biopsies, which correlated with both hypertension and an increased serum creatinine level.[213] In SLE, features that correlate well with high titers of IgG antiphospholipid antibodies are thrombocytopenia, the presence of a false-positive VDRL for syphilis (FTA negative), and a prolonged activated partial thromboplastin time.[177,178,213] Neither the titer of anti-DNA antibodies nor the serum complement levels correlate well with the antiphospholipid antibody levels. In SLE, high titers of IgG anticardiolipin antibody usually correlate well with the risk of thrombosis. However, in one study of 114 biopsied SLE patients, renal thrombi were related to lupus anticoagulant but not anticardiolipin antibodies.[213] The clinical features of APS in SLE patients are identical to those of primary APS. An important study documents the prevalence of antiphospholipid antibodies in 26% of 111 LN patients followed for a mean of 173 months.[179] Of the antiphospholipid antibody–positive patients, 79% developed a thrombotic event or fetal loss, and the presence of antibodies was strongly correlated with the development of progressive CKD.

There is a high prevalence of antiphospholipid antibodies (10% to 30%) in hemodialysis patients irrespective of patient age, gender, or duration of the dialysis.[214,215] In contrast, patients with renal insufficiency and those on peritoneal dialysis have a much lower incidence of antiphospholipid antibodies.[177] One hemodialysis study found more patients with arteriovenous (AV) grafts than native fistulas to have a raised titer of IgG anticardiolipin antibody.[215,216] There was a significant increase in the odds of having two or more episodes of AV graft thrombosis in patients with raised anticardiolipin titer. Whether AV grafts induce anticardiolipin antibodies or whether patients with anticardiolipin antibodies require AV grafts remains unclear.[177] In another study, of 230 hemodialysis patients, titers of IgG anticardiolipin antibodies were elevated in 26% of the patients as opposed to elevated titers of IgM antibodies in only 4%.[216] The mean time to AV graft failure was significantly shorter in the group with elevated IgG antibodies, and the use of warfarin increased graft survival in these patients.

In several studies 20% to 60% of SLE patients with antiphospholipid antibodies who received renal transplants had problems related to APS, such as venous thromboses, pulmonary emboli, or persistent thrombocytopenia.[101,102,217,218] In one large study of non-SLE patients, 28% of 178 transplant patients had antiphospholipid antibodies which were associated with a three- to fourfold increased risk of arterial and venous thromboses.[217] However, another study of 337 renal transplant recipients found the 18% who were IgG or IgM anticardiolipin antibody positive had no greater allograft loss or reduction in GFR than did patients who were anticardiolipin antibody negative.[219] Although most patients with antiphospholipid antibodies who have tested positive for HCV do not have evidence of increased thromboses and APS, when they receive a transplant, they appear to have a higher risk of allograft thrombotic microangiopathy.[220] In many of these transplant studies, treatment with anticoagulation has proven successful in preventing recurrent thromboses and graft loss.[101,102,218]

TREATMENT

The optimal treatment of patients with antiphospholipid antibodies and APS remains to be defined.[177,178,221] Many patients with antiphospholipid antibodies do not experience thrombotic events. In asymptomatic patients with antiphospholipid antibodies but no evidence of thrombotic events or APS, low-dose aspirin may be beneficial based on limited data.[222]

Since patients with higher titers of IgG antiphospholipid antibody have a greater incidence of thrombotic events, they may benefit from anticoagulation.[196,197] In patients with full APS, anticoagulation with heparin followed by warfarin has proven more effective than no therapy, aspirin, or low-dose anticoagulation in preventing recurrent thrombosis.[177,180,221] A retrospective analysis of 147 APS patients (including 62 primary disease, 66 SLE, and 19 lupus-like syndrome) reported 186 recurrent thrombotic events in 69% of the patients.[221] The median time between the initial thrombosis and the first recurrence was 12 months but with a broad range (0.5 to 144 months). Treatment with higher dose warfarin (international normalized ratio [INR] > 3) was more effective than treatment with low-dose warfarin (INR < 3) or treatment with aspirin. The highest rate of thrombosis (1.3 per patient-year) occurred in patients within 6 months after discontinuing anticoagulation. Bleeding complications occurred in 29 of the 147 patients but were severe in only 7 patients. The role of immunosuppression has been uncertain in APS.[177,178,198] In SLE patients the anti-DNA antibody titer and the serum complement may normalize with immunosuppression without a significant change in a high titer of IgG antiphospholipid antibody.[177] In pregnant patients with APS, heparin and low-dose aspirin have been successful, whereas prednisone therapy has not.[223,224] In rare patients who cannot tolerate anticoagulation due to recent bleeding, who have thromboembolic events despite adequate anticoagulation, or who have catastrophic APS, plasmapheresis with corticosteroids and other immunosuppressives have been used with some success.[224,225] It is uncertain whether hydroxychloroquine, used mostly in SLE patients, can prevent thromboembolic events in APS.[222,226,227] There is insufficient and conflicting data whether newer agents such as rituximab lower the levels of antiphospholipids or decrease the risk of thromboembolism.[228,229] The use of other treatments, such as eculizumab, intravenous γ-globulin, and stem cell transplant are only reported in isolated patients.[230,231]

MIXED CONNECTIVE TISSUE DISEASE

Mixed connective tissue disease (MCTD) is defined by a combination of clinical and serologic features.[60,232,233] Patients share overlapping features of SLE, scleroderma, and polymyositis.[232-234] They also typically have distinct serologic findings with a very high ANA titer, often with a speckled pattern, and antibodies directed against a specific ribonuclease-sensitive ENA, U1RNP.[233,234] MCTD has a low incidence and prevalence, a high female-to-male sex ratio, and linkage to HLA-DR4 and DR2 genotypes.[235,236] Not all patients with clinical features of MCTD have a positive ENA, and not all ENA-positive patients have the clinical features of MCTD.[234] Since over time some patients fulfill diagnostic criteria for other connective tissue diseases, investigators have questioned whether MCTD is a distinct syndrome and have developed specific criteria to categorize patients as having MCTD.[237] The term *undifferentiated autoimmune rheumatic and connective tissue disorder* or *overlap syndrome* has also been used.[234,235] One study of 161 MCTD patients followed for 8 years found 60% with unclassified MCTD, 17% systemic sclerosis, 9% SLE, 2.5% rheumatoid arthritis, and 11.5% with undifferentiated connective tissue disease.[237] A positive anti-DNA antibody predicted the development of SLE while hypomotility of the esophagus or sclerodactyly predicted the development of systemic sclerosis.

In early stages of MCTD, patients usually manifest nonspecific symptoms such as malaise, fatigue, myalgias, arthralgias, and low-grade fever. Over time features similar to other rheumatologic connective tissue diseases appear, including arthralgias, deforming arthritis, myalgias and myositis, Raynaud's phenomenon, swollen hands and fingers, restrictive pulmonary disease and pulmonary hypertension, esophageal dysmotility, pericarditis and myocarditis, serositis, oral and nasal ulcers, digital ulcers and gangrene, discoid lupus-like lesions, malar rash, alopecia, photosensitivity, and lymphadenopathy.[233,234,238] However, patients with MCTD, especially those documented to have anti-U1RNP antibodies, infrequently have major central nervous system disease or severe proliferative glomerulonephritis.[233,234,238] Low-grade anemia, lymphocytopenia, and hypergammaglobulinemia are all common in MCTD.

The most widely used serologic test to confirm a diagnosis of MCTD is the ENA with anti-U1RNP antibodies.[234,239] The diagnosis of MCTD is even firmer in those patients with IgG antibodies against an antigenic component of U1RNP, the 68kD protein.[239,240] Antibodies to other nuclear antigens have been found in MCTD and some correlate better with some clinical features of specific rheumatologic diseases.[233] Antibodies against dsDNA, Sm antigen, and Ro are infrequently positive in MCTD, but up to 70% of patients will have a positive rheumatoid factor.

The incidence of renal involvement has varied from 10% to 26% of adults and from 33% to 50% of children with MCTD.[234,240] Many patients have mild clinical manifestations with only microhematuria and less than 500 mg proteinuria daily. However, heavier proteinuria, severe hypertension, and acute kidney injury (AKI) reminiscent of "scleroderma renal crisis" may occur.[238,241,242] Although the titer of anti-RNP does not correlate with renal involvement, the presence of serologic markers of active SLE (e.g., high anti-dsDNA antibody titers, anti-Sm antibody) are more common with renal disease.[234] Low serum complement levels have not always correlated with the presence of renal involvement.[238] Children with MCTD more often have glomerular involvement with few clinical or urinary findings.[243]

The pathology of MCTD is diverse with the glomerular lesions resembling the spectrum found in SLE and the vascular lesions resembling those in scleroderma. Glomerular disease is most common and is usually superimposed on a background of mesangial deposits and hypercellularity as in SLE.[238,241,243-246] Up to 30% of biopsied patients have mesangial deposits of IgG and C3. Other patients have focal proliferative glomerulonephritis with both mesangial and subendothelial deposits, but fibrinoid necrosis and crescents are rare. The most common pattern of glomerular involvement is membranous nephropathy, reported in up to 35% of cases,[241,243-245] with typical peripheral capillary wall granular immunofluorescence staining for IgG, C3, and, at times, IgA and IgM. Some patients will have a mixed pattern of membranous plus mesangial proliferative glomerulonephritis.[243] Renal biopsy findings may transform over time from one pattern of glomerular involvement to another, similar to SLE patients. By ultrastructure analysis, lupus-like findings have been reported, including endothelial tubuloreticular inclusions, deposits with "fingerprint" substructure, and tubular basement membrane deposits.[238] In a review of 100 biopsied patients with MCTD, 12% had normal biopsies, 35% mesangial lesions, 10% proliferative glomerular lesions, and 36% membranous nephropathy.[247] In addition, 15% to 25% of patients had interstitial disease and vascular lesions. In autopsy series, in which two thirds of patients had clinical renal disease, a similar distribution of glomerular lesions was found.[246] Other renal pathology findings in MCTD include secondary renal amyloidosis,[248] vascular sclerosis ranging from intimal sclerosis to medial hyperplasia, and vascular lesions resembling those in scleroderma kidney with involvement of the interlobular arteries by intimal mucoid edema and fibrous sclerosis.[238]

Therapy of MCTD with corticosteroids is effective in treating the inflammatory features of joint disease and serositis.[234,238] Steroids are less effective in treating sclerodermatous features such as cutaneous disease, esophageal involvement, and especially pulmonary hypertension. Intravenous immunoglobulin has been used to treat thrombocytopenia and hemolytic anemia.[249] Treatment of the glomerular lesions is similar to that for LN.

Originally MCTD was felt to have a good prognosis with low mortality and few patients developing other distinct connective tissue disorders. The longer patients with MCTD are followed, the greater the percentage who evolve more clearly into a specific connective tissue disorder.[234] In some series, almost half of the patients with a short duration of follow-up were still felt to have true MCTD, but in those with longer follow-up the percentage had dropped to 15% or less.[234,238] Most patients evolve toward a picture of either SLE or systemic sclerosis, but some develop features of rheumatoid arthritis.[237,238] Mortality rates have been found to range from 15% to 30% at 10 to 12 years with patients with more clinical features of scleroderma and polymyositis faring worse.[234,238] The presence of anticardiolipin antibodies and anti–β_2-glycoprotein antibodies increases the mortality risk. In a recent study, 5-, 10-, and 15-year survival rates were 98%, 96%, and 88%.[250] The leading causes of mortality in MCTD are pulmonary hypertension and cardiovascular disease.[234,250] Other causes include vascular lesions of the coronary and other vessels, hypertensive scleroderma crisis, and chronic renal failure. Clearly MCTD is not a benign disorder but rather a disease with significant morbidity and mortality.

SMALL VESSEL VASCULITIS

Granulomatosis with polyangiitis (GPA; formerly designated Wegener's granulomatosis), microscopic polyangiitis (MPA), and eosinophilic granulomatosis with polyangiitis (EGPA; formerly designated Churg-Strauss syndrome or Churg-Strauss vasculitis) are usually classified together as three small vessel vasculitides.[125,251-260] All may affect the arterioles, capillaries, and venules. There is considerable overlap in the clinical, histologic, and laboratory features of these entities. Moreover, all may be associated with a positive serologic test for ANCA. However, genetic analyses are defining differences between these entities, and differences in the course and response to therapy are being noted.[261]

GRANULOMATOSIS WITH POLYANGIITIS

GPA has been traditionally defined by the triad of vasculitis associated with necrotizing, granulomatous inflammation of the upper and lower respiratory tracts and by glomerulonephritis.[252] Subsequent descriptions of "limited" upper respiratory tract disease, of multiorgan system involvement, and of the nature and pathogenesis of the serologic marker, ANCA, have enhanced our understanding of this disease.[253-257] Even in the pre-ANCA era these clinical criteria yielded a sensitivity of 88% and a specificity of 92% for the diagnosis of GPA. Adding ANCA to the diagnostic criteria increases these percentages.[258-260]

GPA has a slight male predominance and a peak incidence in the fourth to sixth decade of life.[252,255,262,263] Pauci-immune RPGN (including GPA and MPA) are the most common forms of crescentic glomerulonephritis at all ages, and especially in older adults.[259,260] Most patients have been Caucasian, although with use of ANCA screening, patients of all races are being diagnosed.[262] The occurrence of GPA in more than one family member has rarely been noted.[263] Certain HLA frequencies such as HLA-DR2, HLA-B7, and HLA-DR1 and DR1-DQW1 have been reported more commonly.[263,264]

PATHOLOGY

The classic histopathologic finding in GPA is a focal segmental necrotizing and crescentic glomerulonephritis (Figure 33.14).[256] Although the percentage of affected glomeruli can vary widely, the necrotizing changes are usually segmental in distribution.[256,265] Unaffected glomeruli typically appear normal. Global proliferation and necrotizing glomerular tuft involvement are more common in the more severe cases. The earliest lesions are "intracapillary thrombosis" with deposition of eosinophilic "fibrinoid" material associated with endothelial cell swelling, infiltration by polymorphonuclear leukocytes, and pyknosis or karyorrhexis.[256,265] In areas of active necrotizing glomerular lesions, there are ruptures in the GBM and formation of overlying cellular crescents that range from segmental to circumferential. Crescents are frequently associated with breaks in or broad destruction of Bowman's capsule.[266] Granulomatous crescents containing epithelioid histiocytes and giant cells

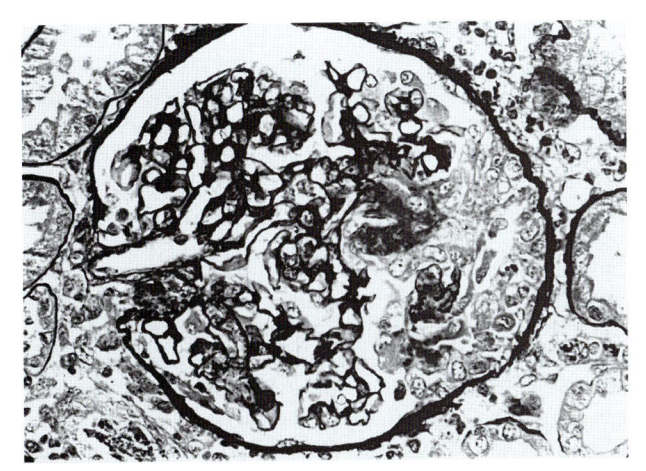

Figure 33.14 Granulomatosis with polyangiitis. A representative glomerulus displays segmental fibrinoid necrosis with rupture of glomerular basement membrane, fibrin extravasation into the urinary space, and an overlying segmental cellular crescent. (Jones' methenamine silver stain, ×500.)

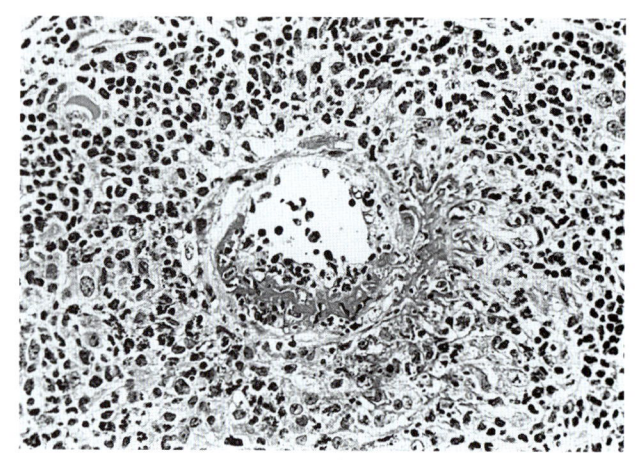

Figure 33.15 Granulomatosis with polyangiitis. An interlobular artery displays necrotizing vasculitis with intimal fibrin deposition and transmural inflammation by neutrophils and lymphocytes. (Hematoxylin and eosin stain, ×375.)

may involve from less than 15% to more than 50% of cases, and the finding of large numbers of them is more typical of GPA and cytoplasmic ANCA (C-ANCA) positivity than other vasculitides. Chronic segmental or global glomerulosclerosis with fibrous crescents often occur side by side with more active glomerular lesions. Although there is much overlap in the histologic findings between MPA and GPA, some differences have been noted. Patients with MPA and those who have anti-myeloperoxidase (anti-MPO) ANCA are more likely to have a greater degree and severity of glomerulosclerosis, interstitial fibrosis, and tubular atrophy on initial biopsy.[267]

The true vasculitis in GPA may affect small- and medium-sized renal arteries, veins, and capillaries.[256,265] It is focal in nature and has been reported in 5% to 10% of GPA biopsies.[252,255,256] It is more commonly found at autopsy with availability of larger tissue sampling and when serial sectioning and a directed search for the lesions have been performed. The necrotizing arteritis consists of endothelial cell swelling and denudation, intimal fibrin deposition, and mononuclear and polymorphonuclear leukocyte infiltration of the vessel wall with mural necrosis (Figure 33.15). In some cases, the arteritis displays granulomatous features. Tubules show focal degenerative and regenerative changes, and cortical infarcts may occur.[252,256] Interstitial inflammatory infiltrates of lymphocytes, monocytes, plasma cells, and polymorphonuclear leukocytes are common. Granulomas containing giant cells may form in the interstitium of the cortex and medulla in 3% to 20% of cases. Some of these cortical granulomas represent foci of glomerular destruction by granulomatous crescents. Papillary necrosis, often bilateral and affecting most papillae, has been reported, usually in those with necrotizing interstitial capillaritis of the vasa recta. Biopsy of extrarenal tissue may show necrotizing and granulomatous inflammation or evidence of vasculitis.[255,256]

There is no specific glomerular or vascular immune staining in most cases of GPA. Low-level staining for immunoglobulins and complement likely represents nonimmunologic trapping in areas of necrosis and sclerosis. This negative or only focal low-intensity immunofluorescence staining pattern is referred to as "pauci-immune."[252-256] Positivity for fibrin/fibrinogen is common in the distribution of the necrotizing glomerular lesions, crescents, and vasculitic lesions. By electron microscopy the glomeruli affected by necrotizing lesions often show areas of intraluminal and subendothelial fibrin deposition associated with endothelial necrosis and gaps in the GBM through which fibrin and leukocytes extravasate into Bowman's space.[252-256] There may be subendothelial accumulation of electron-lucent flocculent material associated with intravascular coagulation. True electron-dense immune-type deposits are not usually identified and, when present, are sparse and ill-defined.[252-256] Electron microscopy of the vessels in GPA may show swelling and denudation of endothelial cells, and subendothelial accumulation of fibrin, platelets, and amorphous electron-dense material, but no typical immune-type electron-dense deposits.

PATHOGENESIS

The pathogenesis of GPA remains unknown with abnormalities of both humoral and cell-mediated immunity described.[253,255,256] A recent genome wide association study found that GPA and MPA are genetically distinct diseases with the genetic markers strongly associated with the antigenic specificity of the ANCA rather than the clinical syndrome.[261] In vitro and animal experiments strongly support a role for ANCA in the pathogenesis of the disease.[268-271] ANCA production may relate to infectious, genetic, environmental, and other risk factors.[268] Both molecular mimicry to infectious pathogens and formation of antibody to antisense peptide have been proposed in the development of ANCA. Patients with proteinase 3 (PR3)–positive ANCA have been shown to have antibodies to complementary PR3, a protein encoded by the antisense RNA of the PR3 gene, and $CD4^+$ T_H1 memory cells responsive to the complementary PR3 peptide.[269] In Rag-2 mice, transfer of anti-MPO IgG causes glomerulonephritis with necrosis and crescent formation that appears identical to human ANCA-associated glomerulonephritis by light microscopy and immunofluorescence.[271] This can occur in the absence of antigen-specific T lymphocytes strongly suggesting a pathogenetic role for the antibodies themselves. In humans, neonatal MPA with pulmonary hemorrhage and renal disease has occurred secondary to the transfer of maternal MPO-ANCA.[272] One study has found a unique subgroup of ANCA directed against lysosomal associated membrane protein 2 (LAMP2) as opposed to MPO or PR3, to be present in more than 90% of ANCA-positive pauci-immune necrotizing glomerulonephritis.[273] Others have not been able to confirm a high incidence of anti-LAMP2 antibodies in this population.[274]

Cell-mediated mechanisms of tissue injury in GPA are supported by a predominance of $CD4^+$ T lymphocytes and monocytes in the inflammatory respiratory tract infiltrates, high levels of T_H1 cytokines, defects in delayed hypersensitivity, a rise in soluble markers of T cell activation as soluble interleukin-2 (IL-2) receptor and CD30, impaired lymphocyte blastogenesis, and T cell response to PR3.[257,275-277] Despite prominent respiratory tract involvement, no inhaled pathogen or environmental allergen has been identified as the initiator of the disease process. However, respiratory infections may allow the release of cytokines such as tumor necrosis factor (TNF) from cells that can "prime" neutrophils to express PR3 and other antigens on their cell surfaces. The expression of granule proteins on the surface of neutrophils and monocytes allows for the interaction with circulating ANCA, leading to a respiratory burst in the cell, degranulation and local release of damaging proteases and reactive oxygen species, release of chemoattractant products, and neutrophil apoptosis.[255-257,278-280] Endothelial injury, fibrinoid necrosis, and inflammation ensue. In the presence of ANCA, neutrophils exhibit exaggerated adhesion and transmigration through endothelium.[280]

A spectrum of glomerular and vascular disease reaction is seen depending on antigen expression, host leukocyte activation, circulating and local cytokines and chemokines, the condition of the endothelium, and the nature of T and B cell interactions.[255-257,278-280] The membranes of leukocytes from GPA patients may be primed to express PR3 molecules on their surfaces, making them ripe for activation of the disease process.[257,279,281,282] This priming phenomenon might explain the exacerbations of disease activity associated with respiratory infections as well as the potential benefits of prophylaxis with trimethoprim-sulfamethoxazole.[282,283]

CLINICAL AND LABORATORY FEATURES

Patients with GPA may present with an indolent, slowly progressive involvement of the respiratory tract and mild renal findings or with fulminant acute glomerulonephritis. Despite greater awareness of the disease, more extensive use of renal biopsy, and the widespread availability of ANCA serologic testing, diagnosis is still often delayed. Most patients will have constitutional symptoms, including fever, weakness, and malaise at presentation.[252-255,284,285] From 70% to 80% of patients have upper respiratory findings at presentation and more than 90% eventually develop upper respiratory problems over time.[252-255,284,285] There may be rhinitis, purulent or bloody nasal discharge and crusting, and sinusitis, typically involving the maxillary sinus and less commonly the sphenoid, ethmoid, and frontal sinuses.[252-255,284,285] Radiographs show sinus opacification, air-fluid levels, mass lesions, or rarely bony erosions. Upper respiratory tract involvement can also be manifest by tinnitus and hearing loss, otic discharge, earache, perforation of the tympanic membrane, and hoarseness and throat pain.[252-255] Chronic sequelae include deafness, chronic sinusitis, and nasal septal collapse with saddle nose deformity.[254]

Lower respiratory tract disease, found at presentation in up to 75% of patients and eventually in 85%, leads to symptoms of cough (often with sputum production), dyspnea on exertion and shortness of breath, alveolar hemorrhage and hemoptysis, and pleuritic pain.[252-256,286] Chest radiographs and computed tomographic scans may reveal single or multiple nodules, some with areas of cavitation, alveolar infiltrates, and interstitial changes, and less commonly small pleural effusions and atelectatic areas.

GPA is a multisystem disease with many organs involved by the vasculitic process and its sequelae.[252-256] Cutaneous involvement, present in 15% to 50% of patients, occurs with a variety of macular lesions, papules, nodules, or purpura, usually on the lower extremities. Patients with rheumatologic involvement have arthralgias of large and small joints as well as nondeforming arthritis of the knees and ankles or, more rarely, a myopathy or myositis. Up to 65% of patients have ophthalmologic disease with conjunctivitis, episcleritis and uveitis, optic nerve vasculitis, or proptosis due to retro-orbital inflammation. Nervous system involvement is most typically manifested as a mononeuritis multiplex but may involve cranial nerves or the central nervous system. Other organs involved include the liver, parotids, thyroid, gallbladder, and the heart.[252-256] Recent reports have emphasized the risks of thromboembolism, especially during active disease, perhaps related to endothelial injury and hypercoagulability induced by the vasculitis and its treatment.[287]

Abnormal laboratory tests in GPA include a normochromic, normocytic anemia and a mild leukocytosis and thrombocytosis.[252,256] Nonspecific markers of an inflammatory disease process such as elevated ESR and CRP levels, and rheumatoid factor tests are often positive and correlate with the general disease activity. Other serologic test results, including those for ANA, serum complement levels, and cryoglobulins, are normal or negative.[252]

ANCA has been detected in from 85% to more than 95% of GPA patients.[253-255,257,288] Patients with granulomatous lesions are more likely to be C-ANCA positive with antibody directed against PR3, a 228–amino acid serine proteinase found in the azurophilic granules of neutrophils and the lysosomes of monocytes.[251,253-255,288] However, many patients fitting the clinical and histologic definition of GPA will be perinuclear ANCA (P-ANCA) positive with antibodies directed against MPO, a highly cationic 140-kDa dimer located in a similar cellular distribution to PR3.[251,253-255,257] ANCA may also be directed to other antigens (e.g., lactoferrin, cathepsin, elastase, etc.), but these antibodies are not usually associated with vasculitis and are usually found in other immune-mediated diseases. In a study of 89 patients from China who fulfilled clinical and histopathologic criteria for GPA, 61% were MPO-ANCA positive and only 38% PR3-ANCA positive.[262] Although the specificity of C-ANCA for GPA has been as high as 98% to 99% by different assays, the sensitivity may be low in certain populations with inactive or limited disease.[289] Some patients with pauci-immune crescentic glomerulonephritis will be ANCA negative and may have a somewhat distinct disease from the more common ANCA-positive patients.[290] In a series of 141 Chinese patients with RPGN, 27% were ANCA negative and had more upper airway disease than the ANCA-positive group.[290] However, they had no difference in other clinical manifestations. Other patients with crescentic glomerulonephritis will be positive for both ANCA and anti-GBM antibodies (see "Anti–Glomerular Basement Membrane Disease and Goodpasture's Syndrome" section). "False-positive" C-ANCA tests have been reported in patients with certain infections (e.g., HIV, tuberculosis, subacute bacterial endocarditis) and neoplastic diseases. A number of medications have also been associated with ANCA, usually anti-MPO, and at very high titers. The strongest association is with the antithyroid drugs, including propylthiouracil, methimazole, and carbimazole. Hydralazine, minocycline, penicillamine, allopurinol, clozapine, rifampin, cefotaxime, isoniazid, and a number of other drugs have also been associated with ANCA-positive vasculitis.[291] Levamisole as an adulterant in cocaine has been associated with unique ANCA positivity, often with a positive P-ANCA and PR3-ANCA but negative MPO-ANCA.[292] While there has been debate whether the ANCA levels parallel the clinical and histologic activity in GPA, many patients will normalize their ANCA titer during periods of quiescence.[259,289,293-297] A subsequent rise in ANCA titer from low titer has been suggested to be predictive of renal and systemic flares.[293-297] Most clinicians prefer to use the ANCA level in the context of other clinical findings and often with other markers of active inflammation such as ESR and CRP. At times, renal biopsy is the only way to be certain of the clinical significance of a change in ANCA titer.

RENAL FINDINGS

Renal findings in GPA are extremely variable and usually occur together with other systemic manifestations.[252-256,285] The degree of renal involvement in ANCA-associated vasculitis is highly predictive of patient survival. Patients with active urinary sediment but normal GFR have a twofold increased risk of death, while those with impaired renal function have a fivefold greater risk of dying.[298] A number of studies confirm that severe renal disease is a negative prognostic feature. Many patients have some evidence of renal disease at presentation, and from 50% to 95% eventually develop clinical renal involvement. Proteinuria and urinary sediment abnormalities, including microscopic hematuria and red cell casts, are common. Patients with more severe glomerular involvement have a decrease in GFR and greater levels of proteinuria, but nephrotic syndrome is uncommon. The level of proteinuria may be higher in those with less severe renal insufficiency and may actually increase during therapy as the GFR improves.[285] The degree of renal failure and serum creatinine do not always correlate well with the percentage of glomerular necrotizing lesions, the percentage of glomerular crescent formation, or the presence of interstitial granulomas or vasculitis. The incidence of both acute oliguric renal failure and significant hypertension varies among reports but is higher in reports from renal centers. Intravenous pyelograms are typically normal, and by angiography vascular aneurysms are not usually present.

Other renal conditions found in GPA include pyelonephritis and hydronephrosis due to vasculitis, causing ureteral stenosis, papillary necrosis, perirenal hematoma from arterial aneurysm rupture, and lymphoid malignancies with neoplastic infiltration of the renal parenchyma in patients treated with immunosuppression.[299]

COURSE AND TREATMENT

The course of the active glomerulonephritis in GPA is typical of RPGN with progression to renal failure over days to months.[252-256] Patients with severe necrotizing, granulomatous glomerulonephritis are more likely to develop renal failure, and patients with more global glomerulosclerosis are more likely to develop ESKD. Greater degrees of glomerulosclerosis and interstitial fibrosis predict a poor renal outcome.[300] Even with immunosuppressive therapy, a significant number of patients will eventually progress over the long term to renal failure.

The introduction of effective cytotoxic immunosuppressive therapy dramatically changed the course of GPA. Initial studies of untreated or corticosteroid-treated patients documented survivals of only 20% to 60% at 1 year.[252,256] Both renal and extrarenal lesions may progress during corticosteroid therapy.[252] Long-term survival with cyclophosphamide-based regimens ranges from 87% at 8 years to 64% at 10 years.[252-256,301,302] Using a regimen of combined cyclophosphamide (1.5 to 2 mg/kg/day) and corticosteroids, remissions were achieved in 85% to 90% of 133 GPA patients.[252] Although many patients eventually relapsed, others remained in long-term remission off immunosuppression. Other studies have confirmed these results.[254-257,301] Complete remissions of renal and extrarenal symptoms, including severe pulmonary disease and renal failure requiring dialysis, have been described. More than 50% of dialysis-dependent patients will be able to discontinue dialysis and remain stable for years. Although resistance to therapy is well documented, some patients do not benefit from treatment for reasons of noncompliance, intercurrent infection requiring decreased treatment, or inadequate duration of therapy.

The optimal dose, duration of treatment, route of administration, and concomitant therapy to be given with cyclophosphamide is still debated for patients with ANCA-positive small vessel vasculitis.[254-257] Many recent trials have included both GPA and MPA patients. Cyclophosphamide is usually administered with corticosteroids initially, with the dose of the steroids tapered or changed to alternate-day therapy. Some regimens include intravenous high-dose "pulse" corticosteroids initially, and others have used plasmapheresis in critically ill patients. A typical regimen for induction therapy of severe GPA or MPA RPGN might include intravenous pulse methylprednisolone (7 mg/kg, to a maximum dose of 500 mg to 1000 mg) for 3 consecutive days followed by oral prednisone 1 mg/kg/day (to a maximum of 60 to 80 mg/day) for the first month, with subsequent tapering of the dose along with either intravenous or oral cyclophosphamide given for approximately 6 months.[253-256] Doses are adjusted for leukopenia and other side effects as well as for treatment response. Several studies have evaluated the role of pulse intravenous cyclophosphamide versus oral cyclophosphamide in ANCA-positive small vessel vasculitis.[303-306] In one study of 50 GPA patients randomly assigned to either 2 years of intravenous or oral cyclophosphamide, remissions at 6 months occurred in 89% of the intravenous group versus 78% of the oral group.[303] At the end of the study, remissions had occurred in 67% of the intravenous group and 57% of the oral group, but relapses were more common in the intravenous group (60% versus 13%). In a meta-analysis of 11 nonrandomized studies including more than 200 ANCA-associated vasculitis patients, complete remissions occurred in more than 60% of patients and partial remissions in another 15%.[304] Intravenous pulse cyclophosphamide was more likely to induce remission and less likely to cause infection than oral cyclophosphamide. However, relapses may be more frequent with intravenous use of the drug. This is clarified by a recent large multicenter trial that randomized 149 ANCA-positive vasculitis patients to either Solu-Medrol plus pulsed intravenous cyclophosphamide (15 mg/kg every 2 to 3 weeks) or plus oral cyclophosphamide (2 mg/kg/day).[304] There was no difference in time to remission or percentage of patients who achieved remission by 9 months (88% of both groups) and no difference in improvement of GFR over time. Although there were more relapses in the intravenous group, this was not statistically significant. The total dose of cyclophosphamide was approximately half as much in the intravenous group versus the oral group, and infections were more common with oral cyclophosphamide. Thus both regimens are effective, relapses appear more common with intravenous therapy, but total dose and adverse effects of the cytotoxic agent are reduced by intravenous usage. It is unclear how frequent the initial intravenous "pulses" of cyclophosphamide should be given; some investigators use monthly doses and others start with smaller doses every 2 to 3 weeks. It is clear that early application of an intensive immunosuppressive regimen helps prevent long-term morbidity and end-organ damage. Since the total dose of the cyclophosphamide is far less in patients receiving pulsed intravenous therapy, many prefer to use it as a less toxic regimen and try to enhance maintenance therapy to avoid relapse.

Methotrexate has been used for both induction and maintenance therapy in patients with GPA and other ANCA-associated vasculitides.[305-308] The largest trial, the NORAM trial, compared methotrexate (20 to 25 mg/wk orally) to oral cyclophosphamide (2 mg/kg/day), both for 1 year with corticosteroids in 95 ANCA-positive vasculitis patients (89 GPA, 6 MPA).[305] Although an equal percentage of both groups achieved remission, the time to remission was longer in the methotrexate group and the relapse rate much higher (70% vs. 47%). Given these data, methotrexate is rarely used for induction therapy in ANCA-positive vasculitis unless the disease is very mild and rapidly controllable.

The addition of plasmapheresis to therapy for GPA appears to benefit patients with severe renal failure, those with pulmonary hemorrhage, those with coexistent anti-GBM antibodies, and those failing all other therapeutic agents.[300,309] In one study of 20 ANCA-positive small vessel vasculitis patients with massive pulmonary hemorrhage treated with methylprednisolone, intravenous cyclophosphamide, and plasmapheresis, all 20 patients had resolution of pulmonary hemorrhage.[309] A trial of 137 patients with ANCA-positive glomerulonephritis, the Methylprednisolone versus Plasma Exchange (MEPEX) trial, evaluated patients with a marked elevation of the serum creatinine (higher than 500 µmol/L or 5.7 mg/dL) treated with induction therapy with either plasma exchange or intravenous pulsed methylprednisolone, both with oral corticosteroids and cyclophosphamide.[310] While both groups had an equal and high 1-year mortality rate, the plasma exchange group had an improved short-term patient survival and a greater likelihood of not reaching renal failure at 1 year (19% vs. 43%). The addition of etanercept, a TNF-α blocker, to a standard induction regimen for GPA was evaluated in 174 patients and provided no additional benefit in terms of sustained remissions or time to achieve remission.[311] Disease flares and adverse events were common in both treatment groups, and solid tumors developed in six of the etanercept group. The use of infliximab, another TNF-α blocker, in four uncontrolled trials was associated with an 80% remission rate but a high rate of infectious complications.[312] Likewise, a study of alemtuzumab, an anti-CD52 monoclonal antibody, in 70 patients gave a remission rate of 83% but was associated with high rates of relapse, infection, and mortality.[313]

Small uncontrolled trials initially found a role for rituximab in ANCA-positive vasculitis, with sustained remissions in many of the patients studied.[314,315] Two controlled randomized studies support the use of rituximab as a first-line therapy comparable in efficacy to cyclophosphamide for the treatment of ANCA-associated vasculitis.[316,317] In the RITUXIVAS study, 44 patients (mean age, 68 years old) were randomized with two thirds receiving four doses of intravenous rituximab and only two doses of intravenous cyclophosphamide and one of intravenous pulse Solu-Medrol versus the remaining one third of patients receiving 6 to 10 pulses of intravenous cyclophosphamide.[316] Both received steroids in tapering doses. The number of remissions, time to remission, and side effects were similar in the two groups. Mortality and morbidity were high in both groups due to the age of the patients and their renal dysfunction. In the Rituximab in ANCA Associated Vasculitis (RAVE) trial, 197 patients with severe ANCA-associated vasculitis (75% GPA) were randomized to steroids plus either four weekly doses (375 mg/m^2) of rituximab or oral cyclophosphamide (2 mg/kg/day) with replacement by azathioprine maintenance only in the cyclophosphamide group.[317] Among those in the rituximab group, 64% reached remission, whereas only 53% of the cyclophosphamide group did. More patients in the rituximab arm had resolution of active vasculitis by activity scores. Adverse events were similar in both arms of the study. The subgroups with renal involvement and pulmonary hemorrhage also fared the same. Those with relapsing disease had a significantly higher remission rate with rituximab compared with cyclophosphamide therapy. Recent long-term follow-up of this population confirms the equivalency of a steroid plus rituximab regimen to that of steroids plus cyclophosphamide followed by azathioprine maintenance in leading to a complete remission in ANCA-associated vasculitis.[318] There was no difference in adverse events in terms of infections or malignancies between the groups. While this does not mean rituximab will replace cyclophosphamide as standard treatment for ANCA-positive vasculitis, it does allow it to be used as an initial treatment option for many patients.[319]

Relapse rates from 20% to 50% have been reported often when infectious complications have led to a discontinuation of immunosuppressive therapy.[293,296,301,320] Predictors of relapse in a cohort of 350 patients with ANCA-positive vasculitis included C-ANCA or PR3 positivity, lung involvement, and upper respiratory involvement, as opposed to factors not predicting relapse, such as age, gender, race, and a clinical diagnosis of GPA rather than MPA or renal-limited vasculitis.[315,320] Most patients respond to another course of cyclophosphamide therapy.[301] In patients whose ANCA level has declined during remission, a major rise in titer may predict a relapse, although ANCA levels and clinical disease activity do not always correlate.[293-297]

Because of the potential for severe complications with cyclophosphamide therapy (infections, infertility, hemorrhagic cystitis, and an increased risk of long-term malignancy), once an initial remission has been achieved, patients have usually been switched to less toxic immunosuppressives such as azathioprine, low-dose methotrexate, or MMF.[320-323] A study of 155 patients with ANCA-positive vasculitis treated patients with cyclophosphamide and steroids to induce a remission and then randomized patients to either oral azathioprine or continued cyclophosphamide maintenance therapy.[323] Of the 155 patients, 144 entered remission and were randomized. There was no difference in the relapse rate in the two groups or in the adverse event rate. Relapse rates were lower in patients with MPA than in the GPA group. A controlled randomized trial of MMF versus azathioprine for remission maintenance found more relapses with MMF.[324] Rituximab, timed to prevent B cell repopulation and rise in the ANCA titer, and cyclosporine have also been used successfully for maintenance therapy.[325,326] Since respiratory infections, perhaps through priming of neutrophils or activation of ANCA, may be associated with flares of disease activity, prophylactic use of trimethoprim-sulfamethoxazole has been advocated.[327] Methotrexate has also been used as maintenance therapy in GPA.[307] Supportive measures for GPA patients such as sinus drainage procedures, hearing aids, and corrective surgery for nasal septal collapse may be helpful in individuals with chronic sequelae of upper respiratory involvement.[252-256] Attention to cardiovascular risks is important since patients with ANCA-associated vasculitis and renal disease have more than a twofold increased risk of cardiovascular events when compared to matched controls with CKD.[328]

ESKD occurs in about 25% of patients at 3 to 4 years after presentation. Dialysis and transplantation have been performed in increasing numbers of ANCA-associated vasculitis patients.[329-334] Many patients' disease activity diminishes with onset of renal failure, and relapses are significantly less frequent for patients who reach ESKD.[332] However, some patients still require intensive immunosuppression, and relapses have been reported well after onset of ESKD. Fatality rates may be high in some ESKD populations due to slow recognition of relapses of the vasculitic process or, more often, infectious complications. Most patients receiving allografts have been maintained on prednisone and cyclosporine or tacrolimus with or without mycophenolate with very good patient and allograft survival rates.[329-334] Patients should not receive a transplant until after a prolonged period of remission.[335,336] Recurrent active glomerulonephritis in the allograft occurs in 15% to 37% of patients and may respond to cyclophosphamide or rituximab therapy or other more intensive therapies.[329-334] There is no evidence that regimens including MMF or tacrolimus have advantages over older immunosuppressive regimens in preventing recurrences of ANCA-associated vasculitis.[333] There is only limited experience with sirolimus and other newer transplant immunosuppressives.[337]

MICROSCOPIC POLYANGIITIS

The incidence of renal disease associated with this ANCA-positive small vessel vasculitis appears to be increasing.[253-256] While this may be due to wider use of ANCA testing and renal biopsy, many investigators feel the absolute incidence has increased. In one large series ANCA-associated crescentic glomerulonephritis made up almost 10% of all glomerular diseases diagnosed by renal biopsy in a 2-year period. In very old adults this was the most common etiologic diagnosis.[258] Vasculitis and glomerulonephritis similar to those seen in MPA have been noted in relapsing polychondritis[338] and ANCA-positive polyangiitis induced by use of a number of medications, most notably the antithyroid medication propylthiouracil.[339]

PATHOLOGY
Light Microscopy

The most typical histologic finding is focal segmental necrotizing glomerulonephritis with crescents affecting from few to many glomeruli (Figure 33.16).[253-257,340] There is segmental rupture of the GBM associated with polymorphonuclear infiltration, karyorrhexis, and fibrin deposition within the glomerular tuft and the adjacent Bowman's space. Crescents characteristically overlie areas of segmental tuft necrosis and may be segmental or circumferential. Cellular and fibrous crescents often coexist. Some crescents are voluminous with a "sunburst" appearance due to massive circumferential destruction of Bowman's capsule. Uninvolved glomeruli are typically normocellular. In the chronic or healing phase of the disease there is segmental and global glomerulosclerosis with focal fibrocellular and fibrous crescents. While there are many similarities, one study documents biopsy differences between MPA and GPA patients. Biopsies from patients with MPA and patients who are MPO-ANCA positive were more likely to show glomerulosclerosis, interstitial fibrosis, and tubular atrophy.[267] This suggests a more prolonged, less fulminant course in patients with MPA compared to GPA. An international classification differentiates glomerular lesions depending on whether they are focal, crescentic, mixed, or sclerotic and found correlates with clinical outcome.[341]

Patients with MPA infrequently have a true arteritis identified on renal biopsy. The frequency ranges from 11% to 22% with predominant involvement of interlobular arteries and arterioles.[340] Involvement is circumferential, lesions are generally of the same age, and aneurysm formation is rare. The acute vasculitis is usually necrotizing with fibrinoid necrosis of the vessel wall and infiltration by neutrophils and mononuclear leukocytes. Vasculitis with granulomatous features is uncommon. In later stages of the disease there may be narrowing of the lumens of small arteries due to concentric intimal fibroplasia and elastic reduplication, but medial scarring is less frequent and severe than in classic polyarteritis nodosa (PAN). In MPA there is often a diffuse interstitial inflammatory cell infiltrate with plasma cells, lymphocytes, polymorphonuclear leukocytes, and sometimes eosinophils especially around glomeruli and vessels.

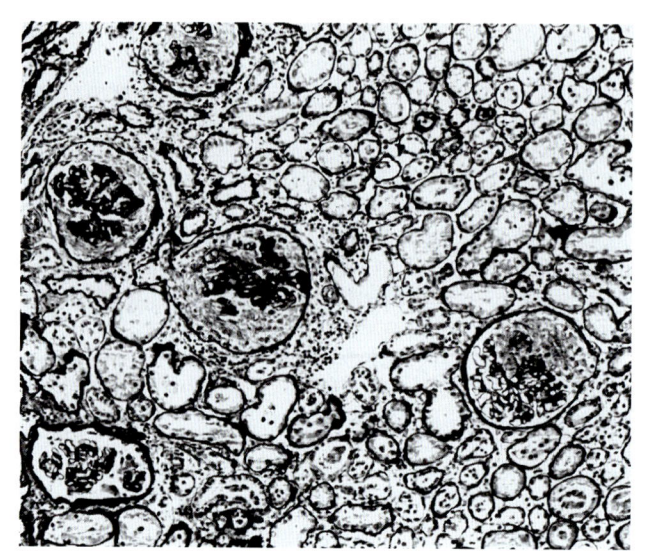

Figure 33.16 Microscopic polyangiitis. There are diffuse crescents with focal segmental necrosis of the glomerular tuft. (Jones' methenamine silver stain, ×125.)

Interstitial inflammatory cells may penetrate the tubular basement membrane causing tubulitis.[340] In more chronic stages there is patchy tubular atrophy with interstitial fibrosis that parallels the distribution of the glomerular and vascular damage.

Immunofluorescence and Electron Microscopic Findings

In most cases the glomeruli show no or only weak immunofluorescence staining consistent with the designation "pauci-immune" glomerulonephritis.[340,341] A review of a number of large series reported positivity for one or another immunoglobulin in 3% to 35% of cases with great heterogeneity and variability of intensity.[340] Fibrin/fibrinogen was the most common and intensely staining reactant identified in the glomeruli, followed by C3 with relatively sparse and weak IgG and C1q.[340,341] The pattern is thought to be consistent with "nonspecific trapping" rather than immune complex deposition. Vascular staining is similar.

By electron microscopy, the glomeruli in most patients with MPA have no or rarely sparse irregular, glomerular electron-dense deposits.[340,341] Glomeruli may show endothelial swelling, subendothelial accumulation of "fluffy" electron-lucent material, and subendothelial and intracapillary fibrin deposition. Through gaps in the GBM, fibrin tactoids and neutrophils exude into Bowman's space associated with epithelial crescents. Vascular changes have included swelling and focal degeneration of the endothelium; separation of the endothelium from its basement membrane with subendothelial fibrin deposition; and, with severe damage, intraluminal and intramural fibrin deposition, edema, and inflammatory infiltration of the intima and media by leukocytes.[340,341] No discrete electron-dense deposits are found in the vessels. In vessels with chronic changes, there may be expansion of the intima by concentric layers of fibrous or fibroelastic tissue, with focal scarring of the media.

PATHOGENESIS

ANCA is felt to play a pathogenetic role in ANCA-associated MPA and glomerulonephritis in a manner similar to GPA[268,270,271] (see "Anti–Glomerular Basement Membrane Disease and Goodpasture's Syndrome" section). There is initial priming of the neutrophil with cytokines and other mediators of inflammation, perhaps in response to infection, leading to expression of MPO-ANCA antigens on the surface of the neutrophil. These exposed antigens are then poised to react with circulating ANCAs. Neutrophils become activated and undergo a respiratory burst, with degranulation and release of reactive oxygen species onto endothelial surfaces. In drug-induced MPA, although ANCAs develop in relation to many different antigens (elastase, cathepsin G, lactoferrin, etc.), only patients with high titers of high avidity and complement-binding specific anti-MPO antibodies develop the disease.[339]

CLINICAL FEATURES

Patients with ANCA-negative pauci-immune focal segmental necrotizing glomerulonephritis and ANCA-positive RPGN have similar clinical findings and presentations regardless of whether vasculitis has been documented on renal biopsy.[253-256] Likewise, the extrarenal findings in many patients with ANCA-positive RPGN have been similar whether the patients are P-ANCA or C-ANCA positive.[253-256,342] Since MPA is a multisystem disease with various organs involved, many of the clinical findings are similar to those of ANCA-positive GPA, including the development of cutaneous disease, rheumatologic involvement, and neurologic disease. Pulmonary disease is common and presents with shortness of breath, dyspnea, cough, and wheezing.[253-256]

LABORATORY TESTS

Abnormal laboratory tests may include a normochromic, normocytic anemia, thrombocytopenia, and a mild leukocytosis, at times with eosinophilia.[253-257] Nonspecific inflammatory markers such as the ESR and CRP are often elevated. ANA, serum complement levels, and cryoglobulins are normal or negative.

The widespread use of accurate assays for ANCA has facilitated the clinical diagnosis of MPA.[253-257] There is considerable clinical overlap between patients with MPA, GPA, and EGPA, and all may have high rates of ANCA positivity. Although C-ANCA–positive patients are more likely to have biopsy-proven necrotizing vasculitis or granulomatous inflammation of the sinuses or lower respiratory tract, there is a large overlap in the clinical manifestations between C-ANCA–positive and P-ANCA–positive patients. For example, in a recent clinical trial of 198 patients with ANCA-positive disease, 75% of patients were clinically GPA, but only 67% were anti-PR3 positive.[317] Likewise, 25% of patients were clinically MPA, but 33% were anti-MPO positive. ANCA titers vary considerably among patients with similar clinical manifestation, and the role of the titer in predicting flares of the disease is not fully defined (see the "Granulomatosis with Polyangiitis" section under "Small Vessel Vasculitis"). Some patients will retain high ANCA levels despite clinical remission, and some patients are positive for anti-GBM antibodies as well as ANCA (see "Anti–Glomerular Basement Membrane Disease and Goodpasture's Syndrome" section).

RENAL FINDINGS

Most MPA patients will have laboratory evidence of renal involvement at presentation with urinary sediment changes of microscopic hematuria and erythrocyte casts.[253-257] Proteinuria is common but nephrotic syndrome is not. A decreased GFR is common in unselected series, and even more common in those selected for renal involvement. Severe renal insufficiency may be found at presentation. These renal findings are similar in patients with ANCA-positive RPGN, whether or not it is associated with systemic involvement.[253-257,267,343] In MPA the severity of the clinical renal findings generally correlates with the degree of glomerular involvement, similar to patients with GPA. Patients with normal serum creatinines or normal creatinine clearances are likely to have greater numbers of normal glomeruli on biopsy, while patients with reduced or deteriorating renal function are more likely to exhibit more glomeruli with severe segmental necrotizing glomerulonephritis or diffuse proliferative features.[343,344] Extensive crescent formation correlates with oliguria, severe renal failure, and a residual decrease in GFR after therapy.

PROGNOSIS AND TREATMENT

Standard treatment for MPA has included cyclophosphamide and corticosteroids in a fashion similar to the treatment of GPA (see the "Granulomatosis with Polyangiitis" section under "Small Vessel Vasculitis"). Controlled trials of the use of intravenous versus oral cyclophosphamide, anti–TNF-α agents, methotrexate, and rituximab have all been examined in populations of ANCA-positive vasculitis patients, including those with GPA and MPA.[304,305,309,310,312,316-319,323] These regimens are discussed extensively in the section on GPA. In most studies both MPO- and PR3-ANCA–positive patients have responded equally. Likewise, the presence or absence of systemic symptoms has not dictated the response. However, even patients with a good initial response to therapy may suffer residual glomerular damage and progress to ESKD.[344] Thus, aggressive, vigorous early therapy to turn off the disease process is thought to be crucial in preventing residual organ damage. Therapeutic intervention in addition to immunosuppressive therapy includes measures to prevent nonimmunologic glomerular disease progression such as the use of renin angiotensin aldosterone blockade, hyperlipidemia control, and low-protein diets in some patients.

EOSINOPHILIC GRANULOMATOSIS WITH POLYANGIITIS

EGPA (formerly designated Churg-Strauss syndrome or allergic granulomatosis and angiitis) is an uncommon multisystemic disease characterized by vasculitis, asthma, allergic rhinitis, organ infiltration by eosinophils, and peripheral eosinophilia.[345-348] Although there may be some overlap with other vasculitic and allergic processes such as GPA, MPA, polyarteritis nodosa, Loeffler's syndrome, and chronic eosinophilic pneumonitis, the clinical and pathologic features of EGPA are distinct.[345-348]

EGPA is the least frequent of the ANCA-positive small vessel vascultitides.[345-358] In a review of almost 185,000 asthmatic patients taking medications, only 21 cases of EGPA were identified.[349] The low incidence may reflect, in part, underrecognition. There is no gender predominance in EGPA, and the mean age at diagnosis is around 40 years.[345-351] Clinical renal involvement is clearly less prevalent than morphologic renal involvement. In autopsy series, the kidney is affected in more than 50% of patients, while clinical renal disease has been described in 25% to more than 90% of patients.[346-351]

A number of studies describe the rare occurrence of EGPA in steroid-dependent asthmatic patients taking leukotriene receptor antagonists (such as montelukast, zafirlukast, pranlukast) especially during reduction of the steroid therapy.[352-355] While not all investigators have been able to document this association, analysis of published reports does support it.[356,357] This may occur via unmasking of the vasculitic syndrome as the leukotriene receptor antagonist permits the steroid withdrawal. Similar cases have been reported in asthmatic patients following a change from oral to inhaled steroids. Rarely, substitution of a leukotriene receptor antagonist for inhaled steroids has also led to EGPA.[355-357]

PATHOLOGY

Histologic findings suggestive of EGPA in any organ include a number of the following features: eosinophilic infiltrates, areas of necrosis, an eosinophilic giant cell vasculitis of small arteries and veins, and interstitial and perivascular granulomas. Renal biopsies in EGPA vary from normal kidney tissue to severe glomerulonephritis, vasculitis, and interstitial inflammation.[339,345,346,358] There may be a focal segmental necrotizing glomerulonephritis, sometimes with small crescents. In most cases the glomerulonephritis is mild, affects only a minority of glomeruli, and involves the tuft segmentally. The glomerulonephritis rarely may be diffuse and global with severe necrotizing features and crescents. In some cases, there is only mesangial hypercellularity without endocapillary proliferation or necrosis.

In the original autopsy studies by Churg and Strauss, vasculitis was found in the kidney in more than one half of cases, and it has been noted on renal biopsy as well.[340] It may involve any level of the renal arterial tree from arterioles to large arcuate or interlobar arteries and may vary from fibrinoid necrotizing to granulomatous. Although resembling other forms of vasculitis, the arteritis is characterized by eosinophilic granulocytes within the arterial wall and in the surrounding connective tissue (Figure 33.17). Vascular lesions may display destruction of elastic membrane, aneurysms, and luminal thrombosis with recanalization, as well as epithelioid cells and multinucleated giant cells in the media, adventitia, and perivascular connective tissue. Active and healed lesions may coexist. Less commonly, venules and small veins of interlobular size are affected, typically with granulomatous features. The tubulointerstitial region is involved by an inflammatory infiltrate containing many eosinophils and some lymphocytes, plasma cells, and polymorphonuclear leukocytes in association with interstitial edema.[340] In some cases there are interstitial granulomas composed of a core of eosinophilic or basophilic necrotic material surrounded by a rim of radially oriented macrophages, giant cells of the Langhans type, and numerous eosinophils. Interstitial nephritis may be present without glomerular pathology.

By immunofluorescence, areas of segmental necrosis in the glomeruli may contain IgM, C3, and fibrinogen.[347] The presence of IgE in renal or other tissues has not been adequately investigated.[359] Electron microscopy of the glomeruli, pulmonary granulomas, venules, and capillaries reveals no electron-dense deposits.[340,346-348]

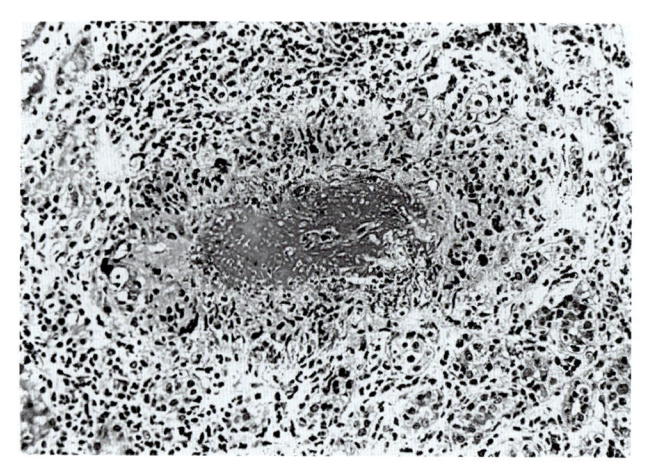

Figure 33.17 Eosinophilic granulomatosis with polyangiitis. Granulomatous vasculitis involves an arcuate artery. There is granulomatous transmural inflammation with focal giant cells and superimposed luminal thrombosis. (Hematoxylin and eosin stain, ×125.)

PATHOGENESIS

Although the pathogenesis of EGPA remains unclear, allergic or hypersensitivity mechanisms are supported by the presence of asthma, hypereosinophilia, and elevated plasma levels of IgE.[345-348,357,359] Eosinophils in patients with EGPA have prolonged survival due to inhibition of CD95-mediated apoptosis and T cell secretion of eosinophil-activating cytokines. Human eosinophil cationic proteins (ECPs), which are capable of tissue destruction in a variety of hypereosinophilic syndromes, have been found in granulomatous tissue from patients with EGPA.[360,361] Higher serum levels of ECP, soluble IL-2 receptor, and soluble thrombomodulin levels have been associated with disease activity.[362,363] The number of peripheral T regulatory cells producing IL-10 is reduced in EGPA and the number increases during clinical remission.[364] Hypocomplementemia and circulating immune complexes have rarely been observed, and the negative immunofluorescence and electron microscopy findings do not support an immune complex mechanism. Cell-mediated immunity is likely involved, and high helper-to-suppressor ratios in the peripheral blood during active disease, as well as a preponderance of helper T cells in the granulomas of skin biopsies, have been reported.[346] In those patients with positive ANCA, the ANCA antibody likely plays a pathogenic role akin to GPA and MPA.[278,279,282]

CLINICAL AND LABORATORY FEATURES

Patients may have initial constitutional symptoms such as weight loss, fatigue, malaise, and fever.[345-348] Characteristic extrarenal features include asthma (present in more than 95% of cases), an allergic diathesis, allergic rhinitis, and peripheral eosinophilia.[345-347,351] Asthmatic disease typically precedes the onset of the vasculitis by years, but it may occur simultaneously. The severity of the asthma does not necessarily parallel the severity of the vasculitis. Many patients subsequently develop eosinophilia in the blood along with eosinophilic infiltrates in multiple organs. Disease often involves the heart, with pericarditis, heart failure, and/or ischemic disease; the gastrointestinal tract, with abdominal pain, ulceration, diarrhea, or bowel perforation; and the skin, with subcutaneous nodules, petechiae, and/or purpuric lesions.[345-347,364,365] Peripheral neuropathy with mononeuritis multiplex is common, but migrating polyarthralgias and/or arthritis occur less frequently.[366] The eye, prostate, and genitourinary tract may be involved. Some patients with EGPA have overlapping features with PAN- or other ANCA-positive vasculitides.[347,345-348]

Laboratory evaluation may reveal anemia, leukocytosis, hypergammaglobulinemia, and elevated ESR and CRP levels.[345-348,350,351] Eosinophilia is universally present and may reach 50% of the total peripheral leukocyte count. The degree of eosinophilia and the ESR may correlate with disease activity as may the level of ECP, soluble IL-2 receptor, and soluble thrombomodulin levels.[362] Rheumatoid factor is often positive, but serum complement, hepatitis markers, circulating immune complexes, ANAs, and cryoglobulins are usually negative or normal.[345-347,350,351] Elevated serum IgE levels and IgE-containing circulating immune complexes are frequently found.[345-347,362] Chest radiography may show patchy infiltrates, nodules, diffuse interstitial disease, and pleural effusion.[345-347,367] Pleural effusions may be exudative and contain large numbers of eosinophils.[367] On angiography visceral aneurysms may be present in patients with both PAN overlap syndromes and classic EGPA.

ANCA levels are elevated in 40% to 60% of EGPA patients.[345-348,363,368,369] Most are P-ANCA and anti-MPO positive, but some are C-ANCA and anti-PR3 positive. In one analysis of almost 100 patients 35% were ANCA positive by indirect immunofluorescence with a perinuclear pattern and anti-MPO specificity in about three quarters.[363] Patients with clinically active vasculitis and those with active glomerulonephritis are likely to be ANCA positive.[358] Some investigators have found a good correlation between ANCA positivity or ANCA titers and clinical activity, whereas others have not.[363,364] Clearly in some, ANCA titers may remain positive despite clinical remissions. In EGPA, ANCA positivity has often correlated with active glomerulonephritis, pulmonary hemorrhage, neuropathy, and the presence of small vessel vasculitis.[345-348,368,369]

Clinical renal involvement in EGPA is quite variable. In one series of 383 patients with EGPA, renal involvement was found in 22%.[370] In another series of 116 patients, many patients had isolated urinary findings and approximately half had AKI.[358] Microscopic hematuria and mild proteinuria are common, but nephrotic-range proteinuria is infrequent. Hypertension is found in 10% to 30% of patients. In one study of patients undergoing renal biopsy, almost 70% had a necrotizing crescentic glomerulonephritis while others had an interstitial eosinophilic nephritis.[358] ANCA was positive in 75% of the patients with nephropathy as opposed to 25% of patients without nephropathy.

PROGNOSIS, COURSE, AND TREATMENT

Patients may have several phases of the syndrome over many years.[345-347,350,351,370] There may be a prodromal phase of asthma or allergic rhinitis followed by a phase of peripheral blood and tissue eosinophilia that is remitting and relapsing over months to years before the development of systemic vasculitis. A shorter duration of asthma prior to the onset of vasculitis has been associated with a worse prognosis. The correlation between ANCA levels and disease activity has been variable. In general, renal disease is mild, with only 7% of patients in one large literature review having renal failure as a cause of death, even including untreated patients.[347] However, cases progressing to severe renal failure and dialysis have certainly been reported.[351] Most patients surviving the initial insult fare well with survival rates in treated patients of approximately 90% at 1 year and 70% at 5 years.[345-347,350,351,370] Patients with significant cardiac, central nervous system, and gastrointestinal involvement, and those with greater degrees of renal damage have a poorer long-term survival.

Corticosteroid therapy is the primary treatment for many patients with EGPA with mild disease and those with interstitial disease.[345-347,350,351,370] Patients may respond rapidly to high daily oral prednisone therapy, and even relapses respond to re-treatment. Extrarenal disease often responds as well. In patients with multisystem disease, with necrotizing glomerulonephritis, and other signs of severe organ involvement, or for those with resistant or relapsing disease, other immunosuppression has been used together with corticosteroids.[371] Other agents have included cyclophosphamide, azathioprine, methotrexate, MMF, rituximab, or plasma exchange.[345-347,350,351,370,372,373] Intravenous immunoglobulin, interferon alfa, TNF blocking agents, mepolizumab (a humanized monoclonal antibody to IL-5), and omalizumab (a monoclonal anti-IgE) have also been used successfully in a few resistant patients.[374,375] Although the prognosis for recovery is good, some patients progress to dialysis and others relapse or have chronic sequelae such as permanent peripheral neuropathy, chronic pulmonary changes, and hypertension.

GLOMERULAR INVOLVEMENT IN OTHER VASCULITIDES

POLYARTERITIS NODOSA (CLASSIC MACROSCOPIC POLYARTERITIS NODOSA)

PAN, also called periarteritis nodosa, was first described in the mid-19th century.[376] Classic PAN is a systemic necrotizing vasculitis primarily affecting medium-sized, muscular arteries, often at branch points, producing lesions of varying ages with focal aneurysm formation.[288] A second, "microscopic" form was originally described as manifesting necrotizing inflammation of small arteries, veins, and capillaries associated with glomerulonephritis. The microscopic form is now understood to represent ANCA-positive MPA and should clearly be considered as part of the spectrum of ANCA-associated small vessel vasculitides (see the "Microscopic Polyangiitis" section under "Small Vessel Vasculitis").[288] This section will discuss only "classic" macroscopic PAN.

PAN is more common in males than females and occurs most often in the fifth and sixth decades of life. Incidence studies and prevalence studies show that PAN is uncommon and has a major regional variation.[377] Reduced rates have been noted in parallel to the reduction of hepatitis B viral (HBV) infections.[378] Clinically, the prevalence of renal disease in patients with PAN varies from 64% to 76% in unselected series and virtually 100% in nephrology-based series.[378-381] The prevalence of pathologic renal involvement exceeds that of clinically evident disease. True idiopathic PAN is a primary vasculitis. Classic polyarteritis has also been associated with abuse of amphetamines and other illicit drugs, but it is unclear how many of these patients had associated viral infectious hepatitis.[382] The most common associated illness found in patients with classic PAN is HBV infection. The incidence ranges from 0 to 55% in different series but is probably less than 10% of all cases.[378] PAN associated with HBV has similar clinical features to idiopathic PAN and often occurs early in the course of HBV infection. It is unclear how many of these patients have had concomitant HCV infection. In one series of 1200 patients with systemic autoimmune disorders who tested positive for HCV, 78 had PAN.[383] Hairy cell leukemia has also been reported in association with PAN.

PATHOLOGY

In classic PAN the glomeruli are usually unaffected. Some glomeruli may show ischemic retraction of the tuft and sclerosis of Bowman's capsule. Rarely, patients with large vessel vasculitis may also have a focal necrotizing glomerulonephritis akin to that seen in MPA.[288,340,381] The vasculitis in classic PAN affects the medium-sized to large arteries (i.e., those of subarcuate, arcuate, and interlobar caliber) in a segmental distribution, often producing lesions of different ages, including acute, healing, and chronic lesions.[288,381] Segments of arterial involvement are interspersed with normal areas producing "skip lesions," and even the involved portions of the vessel wall have eccentric inflammation. In areas of active vasculitis there is inflammation of the vessel wall by infiltrates of lymphocytes, polymorphonuclear leukocytes, monocytes, and occasionally eosinophils, which may involve the intima alone, the intima and media, or all three layers of the vessel wall. Lesions are often necrotizing with mural fibrin deposition and rupture of the elastic membranes. Areas of necrosis may lead to aneurysm formation particularly in larger arteries (i.e., arcuate, interlobar), which can be associated with rupture and hemorrhage into the renal parenchyma. Superimposed thrombosis with luminal occlusion is not uncommon. In the healing phase, inflammation subsides and the vessel wall is thickened by concentric cellular proliferation of myointimal cells separated by a loose ground substance. Localized destruction of elastic lamellae is demonstrable with elastic stains. Eventually the media is replaced by areas of broad fibrous scars. There may be almost total occlusion of the vessel lumen by intimal fibroplasia with areas of concentric reduplication and discontinuity of the internal elastic membrane. Wedge-shaped, macroscopic cortical infarcts are common and are usually caused by thrombotic occlusion of the vasculitic lesions.[381] In more chronic phases, tubular atrophy and interstitial fibrosis develop.

Autopsy studies in PAN describe the kidneys as being the most commonly affected organ (65%), followed by the liver (54%), periadrenal tissue (41%), pancreas (39%), and, less commonly, muscle and brain.[379-381] Other tissues giving high yields when biopsied for diagnostic vasculitic lesions include the testes, sural nerve, skin, rectum, and skeletal muscle.

PATHOGENESIS

PAN patients are typically ANCA negative; therefore, this form of vasculitis is not thought to be mediated by ANCA. The vasculitis of PAN may involve diverse pathogenetic factors, including humoral vascular immune deposits, cellular immunity, and endothelial cytopathic factors. An immune complex pathogenesis of vasculitis is suggested by experiments of acute serum sickness in which an acute glomerulonephritis is produced alongside a systemic vasculitis resembling PAN.[381] The vasculitis can be largely prevented by complement or neutrophil depletion. The experimental Arthus reaction can also induce a vasculitis resulting from in situ vascular immune complex formation with vessel injury preventable by neutrophil or complement depletion.[384] MRL1 mice develop an immune complex glomerulonephritis with necrotizing vasculitis similar to PAN in association with high levels of circulating immune complexes, predominantly with autoantibodies containing anti-DNA.[385] Viral infection of the muscle cells of the vessel media by murine leukemia virus is also associated with a necrotizing vasculitis and lupus-like syndrome with vascular deposits of immunoglobulin and complement.[386] However, glomerular and vascular immune deposits are rarely found in human PAN despite significant levels of circulating immune complexes.

Two models of cell-mediated vasculitis have been produced experimentally in mice.[387] There is no evidence in these models for vascular immune deposits, and some have a granulomatous form of vasculitis similar to that of PAN in multiple organs. In Kawasaki's vasculitis, IgM antiendothelial antibodies directed against endothelial surface antigens inducible by cytokines have been found.[388] Likewise, several viral infections in humans are capable of inducing direct cytopathic injury to arterial endothelium.[381]

CLINICAL FEATURES

The clinical features of PAN are quite variable. In classic PAN, patients are ANCA negative and typically have findings related to visceral organ infarction and ischemia, including abdominal, cardiac, renal, and neurologic involvement. The most common clinical features relate to constitutional symptoms of fever, weight loss, and malaise. Gastrointestinal involvement may include nausea, vomiting, abdominal pain, gastrointestinal bleeding, bowel infarcts, and perforations.[381,389,390] Liver involvement may be associated with HBV or HCV, and vasculitis of the mesenteric vessels, hepatic arteries, and of the gallbladder leading to cholecystitis have all been found.[378,390] Patients may develop heart failure, coronary artery ischemia with angina or myocardial infarction, and, less commonly, pericarditis and conduction abnormalities. Disease of the nervous system may be central, with seizures and cerebrovascular accidents, or related to peripheral nerves, with mononeuritis multiplex and peripheral neuropathies.[391-393] Patients may develop muscle weakness, myalgias or myositis, and arthralgias, but frank arthritis is uncommon.[381,394] Other clinical findings relate to disease in the gonads, salivary glands, pancreas, adrenals, ureter, breast, and eyes. In general, with the exception of liver manifestations and arthralgias, there is little difference between the clinical findings of patients who are HBV positive or negative. Cutaneous disease may present with "palpable purpura" owing to leukocytoclastic angiitis, or with petechiae, nodules, papules, livedo reticularis, and skin ulcerations.

LABORATORY TESTS

No laboratory test is diagnostic of PAN. Abnormal laboratory tests commonly include an elevated ESR, anemia, leukocytosis at times with eosinophilia, and thrombocytosis.[343,378,381] Patients with classic PAN are usually ANCA negative, and the finding of a positive ANCA should suggest the diagnosis of small vessel vasculitis such as MPA, GPA, or EGPA.[378] ANA testing is negative, and patients have normal serum complement values. Tests for rheumatoid factor are often positive. Although cryoglobulins have often been reported to be positive, it is unclear what percentage of cases have had associated viral hepatitis.[381] The incidence of hepatitis B antigenemia has ranged from 0 to 40% of PAN patients, as opposed to less than 10% of unselected patients.[347,378]

RENAL FINDINGS

The renal manifestations in classic PAN reflect renal ischemia and infarction due to predominant involvement of the larger vessels. Hypertension, which may be mild or severe, is found initially in up to one half of patients and can develop at any time during the course of the disease.[336,378-380,389,395] Presenting renal symptoms are uncommon in PAN but may include hemorrhage from a renal artery aneurysm, flank pain, and gross hematuria. Although mild proteinuria and microhematuria may be found, signs of glomerulonephritis such as erythrocyte casts and nephritic syndrome are absent.

Angiographic examination of the vasculature in PAN often reveals evidence of vasculitis and wedge-shaped areas of ischemia. Angiograms demonstrate multiple rounded, saccular aneurysms of medium-sized vessels in about 70% of cases, as well as thromboses, stenoses, and other luminal irregularities.[389,397] Aneurysms most commonly involve the hepatic, splanchnic, and renal vessels, are usually bilateral, multiple, and vary in size from 1 to 12 mm.[397] There is no way to clinically predict the presence of aneurysms. Vasculitic changes and even aneurysms can heal over time as documented by angiography, usually correlating with the clinical response of the patient.[395,397] Similar aneurysms have been documented in GPA, SLE, TTP, bacterial endocarditis, and EGPA.[381]

PROGNOSIS AND TREATMENT

In older studies, untreated patients with PAN had a dismal survival rate.[381] Many patients had a fulminant course with a high early mortality due to acute vasculitis leading to renal failure, gastrointestinal hemorrhage, or acute cardiovascular events. Late mortality has been attributed to chronic vascular changes with chronic renal failure and congestive heart failure.[379,398] In one series of more than 300 PAN patients, there were 20 deaths in the first year among the 109 HBV-positive patients and only 18 deaths among 200 non–HBV-positive PAN patients.[399] Risk factors for early mortality included older age, renal involvement, central nervous system disease, and gastrointestinal involvement. Treatment had no effect on this early mortality, which was due to vasculitis and infection.

Corticosteroid use improved the survival rate of PAN patients significantly, with a 5-year survival rate of approximately 50%.[379] Nevertheless, some patients achieved only partial remissions with long-term morbidity and mortality. Even recent attempts to use corticosteroids alone only in patients with mild disease have led to high relapse rates.[400] The use of cytotoxic immunosuppression in idiopathic PAN has improved the 5-year survival rate to well over 80%.[344,378,397,401,402] While a number of immunosuppressive medications have been used, cyclophosphamide is widely accepted as the most effective agent.[344,397,401,402] Initial therapy of idiopathic PAN usually consists of high doses of cyclophosphamide (e.g., 2 mg/kg/day), commonly given along with high doses of corticosteroids (e.g., prednisone, 1 mg/kg/day), which are then tapered over time. Many use another less toxic immunosuppressive (e.g., azathioprine) for maintenance therapy. Successful treatment can lead to complete inactivity of the vasculitic process and even reversal of severe renal failure. For PAN associated with HBV the following regimen has been effective. A short 2-week course of corticosteroids with or without plasma exchange followed by antiviral agents has been used in the treatment of PAN associated with HBV and hairy cell leukemia leading to reduced rates of relapse and mortality.[378] Hypertension control is an important part of therapy. For those patients with ESKD, immunosuppressive therapy should be continued for 6 to 12 months after the disease appears inactive. Transplantation has been performed in only a limited number of patients with PAN.

TEMPORAL ARTERITIS (GIANT CELL ARTERITIS)

Temporal arteritis, or giant cell arteritis, is a systemic vasculitis with giant cell involvement targeting medium-sized and large arteries.[403-406] It is characterized by segmental transmural inflammation of medium-sized and large elastic arteries by a mixed infiltrate of lymphocytes, monocytes, polymorphonuclear leukocytes, scattered eosinophils, and giant cells.[403-405]

The disease is the most common form of arteritis in Western countries.[403-405,407,408] Temporal arteritis is primarily a disease of older adults, the average age being 72 years, with more than 95% of patients exceeding 50 years of age.[407,408] Extracranial vascular involvement occurs in 10% to 15% of patients with giant cell arteritis.[403-405] Temporal arteritis should be suspected in older individuals who present with persistent headaches, abrupt visual disturbances, jaw claudication, symptoms of polymyalgia rheumatica, or unexplained fevers and malaise along with anemia and elevated levels of ESR and CRP. Temporal artery biopsy is the definitive diagnostic test and other techniques such as temporal artery ultrasonography are not sensitive.[409] Renal manifestations are rare and generally mild, although significant renal involvement has been reported.[403-405,408,410]

Some patients may have positive serology for P-ANCA or less commonly C-ANCA. The renal pathology has been described as a focal segmental necrotizing glomerulonephritis with focal crescents and vasculitis, primarily affecting small arteries and arterioles. Rarely visceral aneurysms are demonstrable angiographically. Whether these cases represent true manifestations of temporal arteritis or forms of "overlap" with small vessel vasculitis is not clear. There are also reports of LN, membranous nephropathy, and renal amyloidosis in patients with temporal arteritis.[410,411]

The most common renal manifestations of mild proteinuria and microhematuria are present in less than 10% of patients. Renal insufficiency is uncommon. Hypertension is infrequent and most often mild to moderate when present. Rare cases of renal failure have been attributed to renal arteritis affecting the main renal artery or its major intraparenchymal branches.[410] In some cases the pathology has been inadequate to diagnose the precise cause of the renal failure. Nephrotic syndrome has been reported in a patient with temporal arteritis and membranous nephropathy, with steroid therapy producing a reduction in proteinuria.[410]

The treatment of temporal arteritis with corticosteroids usually causes rapid and dramatic improvement in general well-being, specific symptomatology, and laboratory abnormalities.[403-405,408] Use of intravenous pulse steroids and a number of corticosteroid-sparing and secondary immunosuppressives have been used successfully.[408,412-415] There are conflicting results as to whether any agent such as methotrexate is equivalent to corticosteroids in efficacy, and some agents such as infliximab do not appear useful.[404,405,408,414] Some, such as cyclophosphamide, have led to good efficacy in steroid-dependent patients.[415,416] Recent studies have found tocilizumab to be effective.[417,418] With corticosteroid use, abnormalities of the urinary sediment disappear, and there is resolution of extracranial large vessel involvement. However, once established, visual loss is often permanent, despite resolution of the active disease process. Exacerbation of systemic vasculitis may occur if corticosteroids are tapered too rapidly.

TAKAYASU'S ARTERITIS

Takayasu's arteritis is a rare giant cell arteritis of unknown pathogenesis characterized by inflammation and stenosis of medium-sized and large arteries, with a predilection for the aortic arch and its branches.[419] The disease most commonly affects young women between the ages of 10 and 40, and Asians are much more commonly affected. Although findings are typically confined to the aortic arch (including the subclavian, carotid, and pulmonary arteries), the abdominal aorta and its branches may be affected. The histopathologic findings of the vessels include arteritis with transmural infiltration by lymphocytes, monocytes, polymorphonuclear leukocytes, and multinucleated giant cells. In the chronic phase of the disease, intimal fibroplasia and medial scarring may result in severe vascular stenoses or total luminal obliteration.

Although in the past, renal disease was thought to be uncommon, it is now reported more frequently.[420-422] This is usually due to an obliterative arteritis of the main renal artery or narrowing of the renal ostia by abdominal aortitis leading to renovascular hypertension. Arteriography is useful to diagnose Takayasu's arteritis although computerized tomography, MRI, and PET scan imaging also have been used.[423-425] Laboratory abnormalities reveal mild anemia, elevated ESR, increased levels of CRP, and elevated γ-globulin levels, but other serologic tests such as ANA, VDRL, anti–streptolysin O (ASLO), and serum complement levels are normal. Some patients have antiendothelial cell antibodies and others have elevated levels of pentraxin 3, a product of immune and vascular cells produced in response to inflammation.[421,426] Hypertension, which may be severe, occurs in 40% to 60% of patients and has been attributed to decreased elasticity of the aorta, increased renin secretion due to stenosis of major renal arteries, and other mechanisms.[427,428] Although mild proteinuria and hematuria are found in some patients, nephrotic-range proteinuria is uncommon.[429] The serum creatinine is usually normal but may be mildly elevated or associated with a high BUN-to-creatinine ratio suggestive of "prerenal" azotemia. Progressive renal failure is uncommon.[419]

A mild mesangial proliferative glomerulonephritis may occur in patients with Takayasu arteritis.[420-422] Mesangial deposits of IgG, IgM, IgA, C3, and C4 have been reported and mesangial electron-dense deposits are found. Most patients have normal renal function and only mild hematuria and proteinuria. Some patients have had glomerular involvement typical of IgA nephropathy.[419,420] Whether this is coincidental or part of the disease process is unclear. One series of patients with Takayasu's arteritis had unusual glomerular histopathology with mesangial sclerosis and nodules, as well as mesangiolysis and glomerular microaneurysms resembling a chronic thrombotic microangiopathy or diabetic glomerulosclerosis.[420] Immunofluorescence and electron microscopy in these cases of "centrolobular mesangiopathy" did not support an immune pathogenesis. There are also reports of renal amyloidosis, MPGN, crescentic glomerulonephritis, and proliferative glomerulonephritis.[430,431]

TREATMENT

In the majority of patients, corticosteroids are effective therapy for the vasculitis and systemic symptoms.[429,432] Other medications, including azathioprine, methotrexate, leflunomide, cyclophosphamide, and MMF, and anti-TNF therapy have also been used successfully in some individuals, as have anticoagulants, vasodilators, and acetylsalicylic acid.[433-436] Recent reports of the use of tocilizumab, a monoclonal antibody against the Il-6 receptor, have been promising.[417,418] Residual morbidity and mortality may result from the progressive fibrosis and stenosis of previously inflamed arteries.[437]

HENOCH-SCHÖNLEIN PURPURA

Henoch-Schönlein purpura (HSP), also called IgA vasculitis, is a systemic vasculitic syndrome with involvement of the skin, gastrointestinal tract, and joints in association with a characteristic glomerulonephritis.[288,438-440] In HSP, IgA-containing immune complexes deposit in association with an inflammatory reaction of the vessels. In the skin this leads to a leukocytoclastic angiitis with petechiae and purpura. In the gastrointestinal tract, there may be ulcerations, pain, and bleeding. In the kidney an immune complex–mediated glomerulonephritis is found.[438-440]

Males are slightly more commonly affected with HSP than are females, and children are far more frequently affected than are adults.[438,439,441-446] HSP is the most common vasculitis of childhood. The peak age of patients with HSP is approximately 5 years old as opposed to IgA nephropathy, which has a broad age distribution.[438,439,441-444] HSP may account for up to 15% of all glomerulonephritis in young children. More severe renal disease occurs in older children and adults.[445,447] HSP is uncommon in blacks. Familial occurrence has rarely been reported, and the frequency of HLA-Bw35 is increased in some series.[439-442] About one fourth of patients will have a history of allergy, but exacerbations related to a specific allergen are rare. Relapses of the syndrome have occurred after exposure to allergens or the cold, and seasonal variations show peak occurrence in the winter months.

HSP may be mistaken for systemic illnesses such as SLE and MPA, with ongoing infections such as meningococcemia, gonococcemia, and *Yersinia* enterocolitis, with certain medications and vaccination-related hypersensitivity, and with some postinfectious glomerulonephritides associated with systemic manifestations. Although an upper respiratory infection precedes HSP in 30% to 50% of patients, serologic evidence of streptococcal infection is often lacking.

CLINICAL FINDINGS

The classic tetrad of findings in HSP is dermal involvement, gastrointestinal disease, joint involvement, and glomerulonephritis, but not all patients will have clinical involvement of all organ systems.[438-440,448] Constitutional symptoms may include fever, malaise, fatigue, and weakness. Skin lesions are almost universal with HSP and are commonly found on the lower and upper extremities but may also be on the buttocks or elsewhere.[438-440,447] They are characterized by urticarial macular and papular reddish-violaceous lesions that do not blanch. Lesions may be discrete or may coalesce into palpable purpura associated with lower extremity edema. New crops of lesions may recur over weeks or months. On skin biopsy there is a leukocytoclastic angiitis with evidence of IgA-containing immune complexes along with IgG, C3, properdin but not C4 or C1q. Gastrointestinal manifestations are present in from 25% to 90% of patients and may include colicky pain, nausea and vomiting, melena, and hematochezia.[438-440,447-450] Abdominal pains may be mistaken for appendicitis, cholecystitis, or surgical emergencies, leading to exploratory laparotomy. One study of more than 260 patients found that 58% had abdominal pain and 18% evidence of gastrointestinal bleeding.[450] Endoscopy may reveal purpuric lesions, and rarely patients may develop areas of intussusception or perforation. Rheumatologic disease involves the larger joints, usually the ankles and knees, and less commonly the elbows and wrists. There may be arthralgias or frank arthritis with painful, tender effusions, but patients do not develop joint deformities or erosive arthritis.[438-440] Rarely patients will have evidence of involvement of other organs (e.g., lungs, central nervous system, or ureters).[438-440,447]

Renal involvement at presentation varies from 20% to 50% of patients with HSP.[438-440,447] Renal disease is more frequent and of greater severity in older children and adults.[446,447,451] In studies routinely examining the urine, renal involvement ranges from 40% to 60% of patients. The onset of active renal disease usually follows within days to weeks after the onset of the systemic manifestations and is characterized by microscopic hematuria, active urinary sediment, and proteinuria.[438,440,447,452] In one series of more than 200 children, HSP nephritis occurred in 46% of patients at a mean of 14 days and within 1 month in the majority.[452] In a series of 250 adults with HSP, 32% had renal insufficiency, usually with proteinuria (97%) and hematuria (93%).[447] Some patients will develop nephrotic syndrome and some will have a nephritic picture. There is no relationship between the severity of extrarenal organ involvement and the severity of the renal lesions.

LABORATORY FEATURES

In HSP, platelet counts and serum complement levels and other serologic tests are all usually normal.[438,440,448] Serum albumin may be low due to renal or gastrointestinal losses.[448] Serum IgA levels are elevated in up to one half of patients during active illness but do not correlate well with the severity of clinical manifestations or the course of the disease.[438-440,453] Patients with both IgA nephropathy and HSP have high levels of galactose-deficient IgA in their circulation.[454,455] A number of abnormal IgA antibodies have been noted, including IgA rheumatoid factor, circulating immune complexes with IgA and IgG, IgA anti-cardiolipin antibodies, IgA fibronectin aggregates, IgA anti–α-galactosyl antibodies, and IgA ANCA.[453,456-459] The relationship of these to active renal or systemic disease remains unclear, although concentrations of IgA and IgG immune complexes, IgA rheumatoid factor, and IgG and

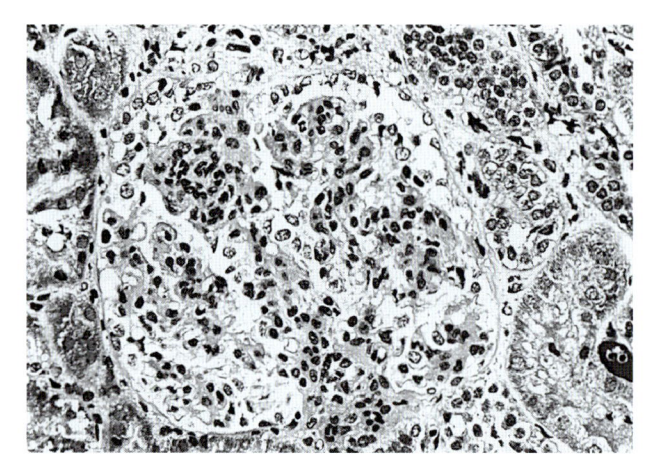

Figure 33.18 Henoch-Schönlein purpura nephritis. An example with global mesangial proliferation and focal infiltrating neutrophils. (Hematoxylin and eosin stain, ×500.)

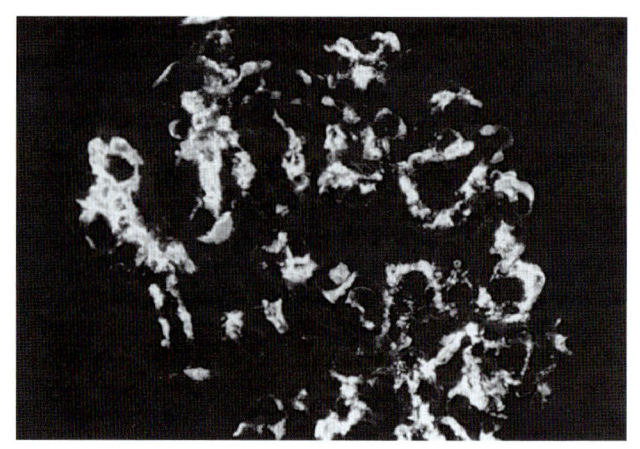

Figure 33.20 Henoch-Schönlein purpura nephritis. Immunofluorescence photomicrograph showing intense deposits of IgA distributed throughout the mesangium and also extending into a few peripheral glomerular capillary walls. (×600.)

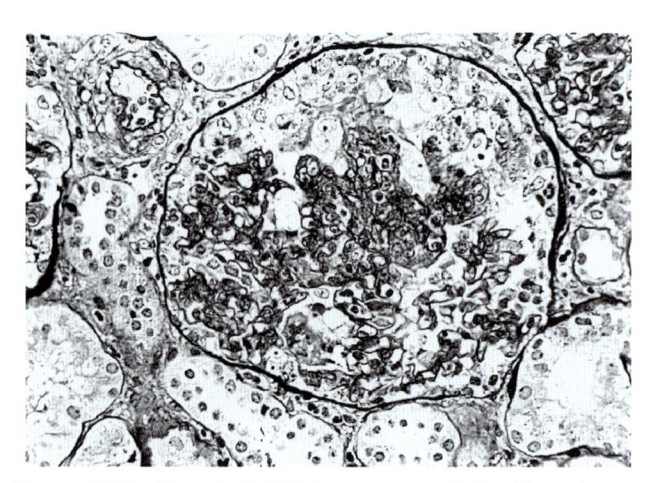

Figure 33.19 Henoch-Schönlein purpura nephritis. There is segmental endocapillary proliferation with an overlying segmental cellular crescent. (Periodic acid–Schiff, ×475.)

IgA anti-galactosyl antibodies have been correlated with clinical renal disease manifestations.[453,458,460] Recent studies suggest IgG and IgA autoantibodies against galactose-deficient IgA correlate with clinical outcome.[458]

PATHOLOGY

The renal biopsy findings of HSP overlap with those of IgA nephropathy. The typical glomerular pathology of HSP is a mesangial and endocapillary proliferative glomerulonephritis with variable crescent formation.[438-440,461] The mesangial changes include both increased mesangial cellularity and matrix expansion that may be focal or diffuse (Figure 33.18). In severe cases, polymorphonuclear cells and mononuclear cells also infiltrate the glomerular tufts in areas of endocapillary proliferation, often accompanied by fibrinoid necrosis. Increased numbers of monocyte/macrophages and CD4 and CD8 T cells are found.[462,463] Some cases have a well-developed membranoproliferative pattern with double contours of the GBM. Crescents are common and vary from segmental to circumferential, with evolution from cellular to fibrous crescents over time (Figure 33.19). Tubulointerstitial changes of atrophy and interstitial fibrosis are consistent with the degree of glomerular damage. In general, endocapillary and extracapillary proliferation as well as glomerular fibrin deposition are more frequent and severe in HSP than in IgA nephropathy. The histopathologic classification system proposed by the International Study of Kidney Disease of Childhood correlates the glomerular lesions with clinical manifestations as well as prognosis.[464] These categories include class I, with minimal glomerular alterations; class II, with mesangial proliferation only; class III, with either focal (a) or diffuse (b) mesangial proliferation but less than 50% of glomeruli containing crescents or segmental lesions of thrombosis, necrosis, or sclerosis; class IV, with similar mesangial proliferation as classes IIIa and IIIb but 50% to 75% of glomeruli with crescents; class V, with similar changes and more than 75% crescents; and class VI, a "pseudo" membranoproliferative pattern. While hematuria is common to all groups, and proteinuria of some degree may be found in all, nephrotic syndrome is present in only 25% of groups I, II, and III. Likewise, groups IIIb, IV, and V tend to have a more progressive course toward renal failure.[465] Even by light microscopy, deposits may be seen in the mesangial regions and rarely along the capillary walls. It is unusual to find the presence of vasculitis on renal biopsy.

By immunofluorescence, IgA is the dominant or codominant immunoglobulin. Co-deposits of IgG and IgM, C3, and properdin are common. Deposits are typically found in the mesangium, especially involving the paramesangial regions, and often extend segmentally into the subendothelial areas (Figure 33.20).[438-440] Some cases may have more abundant peripheral capillary wall than mesangial deposits. Early classical complement components of C1q and C4 are rarely present. These findings contrast with LN in which IgG usually predominates and C1q is almost always present. The deposited IgA is usually IgA1 subclass and may have the J-chain indicating its polymeric nature, but secretory piece is not found.[438-440,466,467] Fibrin-related antigens are also commonly present. IgA may be deposited along with C3 and C5 in both involved and uninvolved skin in the small vessels similar to the findings in IgA nephropathy.[468,469] Similar IgA deposits may also occur in the skin in dermatitis herpetiformis and in SLE along with early and late complement components. IgA is also found in vasculitic lesions in the intestinal tract.[449,450]

By electron microscopy, characteristic immune-type electron-dense deposits are found predominantly in the mesangial regions, accompanied by increase in mesangial cellularity and matrix.[438-440,464] In some capillaries, the deposits extend subendothelially from the adjacent mesangial regions. Occasionally, scattered subepithelial deposits are also present and may resemble the humps of poststreptococcal disease. Evidence of coagulation with fibrin and platelet thrombi may be found in capillary lumens. In cases with severe crescent involvement there may be focal rupture of the GBM. Immunoelectron microscopy has confirmed the predominance of IgA in association with some C3 and IgG in the deposits.[461]

PATHOGENESIS

The pathogenesis of HSP remains unknown. Patients with HSP and their blood relatives, like those with IgA nephropathy, have high circulating levels of galactose-deficient IgA.[454,455] HSP is clearly a systemic immune complex disease with IgA-containing deposits that are associated with small vessel vasculitis and capillary damage. The deposits contain polymeric IgA of the IgA1 subclass and late-acting complement components. This composition suggests alternate pathway complement activation. Patients with IgA nephropathy have increased levels of IgG and IgA antibodies directed against galactose-deficient IgA molecules.[458] They also have evidence of oxidative stress on proteins in their circulation along with the high levels of galactose-deficient IgA.[465] This combination may trigger autoantibody and immune complex formation. It is unclear whether IgA immune complexes trigger complement activation and what the ultimate role of complement participation is. The presence of circulating polymeric IgA complexes, the deposition of IgA in the kidney as well as the skin, intestines, and other organs, and recurrence of disease in the allograft point to the systemic nature of the disease process. The precise mechanism(s) whereby IgA deposition causes tissue injury is unclear because IgA is deposited in some diseases such as celiac disease and chronic liver disease without causing major clinical glomerular damage.[470] Complement activation, platelet activation and coagulation, vasoactive prostanoids, cytokines, and growth factors are thought to play a role. Impaired T cell activity has also been implicated in the pathogenesis of HSP.[471] HSP has also been reported in rare patients with IgA monoclonal gammopathy.[472]

The relationship of HSP to IgA nephropathy is obscure with some investigators considering the diseases separate entities and most describing them as opposite ends of a pathogenetic spectrum.[444] Similar renal histologic findings and similar immunologic abnormalities such as elevated circulating galactose-deficient IgA levels, IgA fibronectin aggregates, and antimesangial cell antibodies suggest a common mechanism of renal injury. IgG autoantibodies against mesangial cells parallel the course of the renal disease. Both IgA nephropathy and HSP have occurred in different members of the same families and in monozygotic twins after adenovirus infection.[444] Infectious agents associated with the occurrence of HSP have included varicella, measles, adenovirus, HBV and/or HCV, *Yersinia* spp., *Shigella* spp., *Mycoplasma*, HIV infection, and staphylococci including methicillin-resistant organisms, but none has been proven to be a causal agent.[439,473-475] Likewise, HSP has been reported to occur in association with vaccinations, insect bites, cold exposure and trauma, although causal relation is unproven.[476]

COURSE, PROGNOSIS, AND TREATMENT

In most patients HSP is a self-limited disease with a good long-term outcome.[438,439,447-449] Patients may have recurrences of the rash, joint symptoms, and gastrointestinal symptoms for months or years, but most patients have a benign short-term and long-term renal course. In general there is a good correlation between the clinical renal presentation and the ultimate prognosis.[438-440,449] Patients with focal mesangial involvement and only hematuria and mild proteinuria tend to have an excellent prognosis. In one recent large pediatric study, renal survival was 100%.[452] In another series of 150 patients with 50% renal involvement, only 2 patients had residual hematuria and no patients had abnormal renal function at 2.5 years.[438] In most series at several years from presentation, more than 50% of the patients had no renal abnormalities, less than 25% had urinary sediment abnormalities or proteinuria, and only 10% had decreased GFR. Less than 10% of patients with severe clinical renal involvement at onset had persistent hypertension or declining GFR over the long term. A review of more than 50 patients followed over 24 years after childhood-onset HSP found 7 of 20 with severe HSP at onset with residual renal impairment as adults as opposed to only 2 of 27 patients with mild initial renal disease.[477] In a long-term follow-up of more than 1100 children with HSP in a retrospective review of published series, no patients with a normal urinalysis developed renal impairment.[478] Renal impairment developed in less than 2% of patients with isolated urinary abnormalities and in 20% of those with full nephritic or nephrotic syndrome. Long-term renal function is not as good in adults with HSP.[447,460,477,479,480] In a series of more than 250 adults with HSP followed almost 15 years, 11% developed ESKD, 13% severe renal impairment with a clearance less than 30 mL/min, and 15% moderate renal insufficiency.[447] A poor renal prognosis is predicted by an acute nephritic presentation, older age, and especially by larger amounts of proteinuria and more severe nephrotic syndrome.[460,479-481] In one retrospective analysis of 219 patients with HSP and nephritis, no data at diagnosis were predictive of ultimate functional decline, but higher proteinuria levels at follow-up did correlate with this decline.[460] On renal biopsy, a poor prognosis is predicted by IgA deposits extending from the mesangium into the peripheral capillary walls, increased interstitial fibrosis, glomerular fibrinoid necrosis, and especially the presence of greater percentage of crescents.[447,460,480] In one study of more than 150 children with HSP, those with greater than 50% of glomeruli containing crescents had progression to ESKD in more than one third of cases and chronic renal insufficiency developed in another 18%. Repeat biopsies in patients with HSP who have clinically improved show decreased mesangial deposits and hypercellularity. Markers of oxidative stress on plasma proteins, circulating levels of galactose-deficient IgA, and the level of IgG and IgA antibodies directed against galactose-deficient IgA have correlated with renal prognosis.[455,458,469] While complete clinical recovery occurs in 95% of affected children and many adults with HSP have a lower recovery rate, those with nephritic syndrome, renal insufficiency, hypertension, a large percentage of glomeruli with crescents, and tubulointerstitial fibrosis are likely to have progressive disease.[460,480] More than one third of HSP patients who become pregnant have associated hypertension or proteinuria. Mortality in HSP is less than 10% at 10 years.

Therapy for the majority of patients with HSP has been mostly supportive.[438-440] Most fare well despite the lack of any immunosuppressive intervention. The use of corticosteroids is controversial, and although they are associated with decreased abdominal and rheumatologic symptoms, they have not clearly been proven to ameliorate the renal lesions in any controlled fashion.[448,482-484] On the other hand, several controlled randomized trials have shown benefit in terms of reductions of proteinuria and preservation of renal function after a short course of corticosteroids in patients with IgA nephropathy.[485,486] Since the renal pathology is the same, one might extrapolate to HSP patients. HSP patients with more severe clinical features, and especially those with nephrotic syndrome or more crescents on biopsy, have also been treated with anticoagulants, azathioprine, cyclophosphamide, chlorambucil, other immunosuppressives, and even plasma exchange.[487-489] Although these reports have shown anecdotal success in reversing the renal progression, controlled trials have not yet shown benefits of using cytotoxic immunosuppressive therapy.[481] For example, in one controlled trial of 54 adults with HSP, proliferative glomerulonephritis, and severe systemic manifestations, the addition of cyclophosphamide added no benefit over steroids alone in terms of remissions, renal outcome, or mortality.[490] Cyclosporine has been used successfully in a number of patients to control severe proteinuria.[491] Intravenous immune globulin has been used in several patients with nephrotic syndrome and decreased GFR in an uncontrolled nonrandomized but apparently successful fashion.[492]

ESKD occurs in 10% to 30% of adults with HSP at 15 years of follow-up.[445,447] Renal disease due to HSP may recur in the renal allograft.[493-495] As in IgA nephropathy, histologic recurrence is far more common than clinical recurrence. However, graft recurrence may lead to allograft loss in as many as 8% to 14% of patients.[494,495] This may be more common in patients who are transplanted either with living related donors or while still active clinically within the first few years of developing ESKD. Although the severity of original disease is not correlated with recurrent disease outcome, many would suggest waiting before transplanting a patient with active disease who has reached ESKD. Patient survival after renal transplantation is excellent and reaches 95% at 15 years.[494] Overall 5- and 10-year graft survival is similar to that of patients with IgA nephropathy and other disease leading to transplantation.[493-495]

ANTI–GLOMERULAR BASEMENT MEMBRANE DISEASE AND GOODPASTURE'S SYNDROME

Anti-GBM disease is caused by circulating antibodies directed against an antigenic site on type IV collagen in the GBM.[496-498] Although the original description of pulmonary hemorrhage and glomerulonephritis long antedated the discovery of the pathogenesis of anti-GBM disease, true Goodpasture's syndrome should consist of the triad of (1) proliferative, usually crescentic, glomerulonephritis; (2) pulmonary hemorrhage; and (3) the presence of anti-GBM antibodies.[496-499] In anti-GBM disease the pulmonary hemorrhage may precede, occur concurrently with, or follow the glomerular involvement.[498,500] Some patients with anti-GBM antibodies and glomerulonephritis and hence "anti-GBM" disease never experience pulmonary involvement and thus do not have true Goodpasture's syndrome. Documentation of anti-GBM antibody–induced disease may be via renal biopsy, or by establishing the presence of circulating anti-GBM antibodies.[496,498,500] Indirect immunofluorescence, although highly specific for diagnosis, requires an experienced pathologist.[501,502] Radioimmunoassay, enzyme-linked immunosorbent assay, and immunoblotting for the antibodies are highly specific and sensitive and readily available.[496,502]

PATHOGENESIS

Anti-GBM autoantibodies, produced in response to an unknown inciting stimulus, react with epitopes on the non-collagenous domain of the α3- and α5-chains of type IV collagen.[496-499] The antigenic epitope has been localized between amino acids 198 and 237 of the terminal region of the α3-chain.[496,497,500,503] The α3-chain of type IV collagen is found predominantly in the GBM and alveolar capillary basement membranes, which correlates with the limited distribution of disease involvement in Goodpasture's syndrome.[496,497,499] Goodpasture's syndrome is now considered an autoimmune "conformeropathy" involving perturbation of the quaternary structure of the α345 NC1 hexamer of type IV collagen.[496,497,503] In Goodpasture's disease autoantibodies to both the α3 NC1 and the α5 NC1 domains bind to the kidneys and lungs. These autoantibodies bind to epitopes encompassing the Ea region in the α5 NC1 domain and the Ea and Eb region of the α3 NC1 domain, but they do not bind to non-denatured native cross-linked α345 NC1 hexamers.[503] The epitope is identical in the glomeruli and the alveolar basement membranes and may require partial denaturation for full autoantigen exposure. Eluates of antibody from lung and kidney of patients with Goodpasture's syndrome cross-react with GBM and the alveolar basement membrane and can produce disease in animal models.[496,498-500] Antibody reacting with autoantigen(s) and perhaps aided by autoreactive T cells leads to an inflammatory response, the formation of proliferative glomerulonephritis, breaks in the GBM, and the subsequent extracapillary proliferation with exuberant crescent formation.[496,499] A role for T cells in Goodpasture's syndrome is supported by the T cell infiltrates on biopsy, patient T cell proliferation in vitro in response to α3 (IV) NC1 domain, the correlation of autoreactive T cells with disease activity, the role of $CD4^+CD25^+$ regulatory cells controlling the autoreactive T cell response, and a role for T cell epitope mimicry in disease induction.[496,504] An initial insult to the pulmonary vascular integrity may be required to produce damage to the basement membranes of the pulmonary capillaries, since alveolar capillaries are not normally permeable to passage of anti-GBM antibodies.[498,505-507] Exacerbations of disease and especially pulmonary disease with hemoptysis have been related to exposure to hydrocarbon fumes, cigarette smoking, hair dyes, metallic dust, D-penicillamine, and cocaine inhalation.[507-509] Although smokers with anti-GBM disease have a higher incidence of pulmonary hemorrhage, circulating anti-GBM antibody levels are no higher than in nonsmokers with the disease.[507,508] Goodpasture's syndrome has occasionally been reported in more than one family member. Certain HLA alleles may predispose to the syndrome and perhaps more severe disease.[510] Influenza A2 infection may be associated with Goodpasture's syndrome. Anti-GBM disease can also occur in patients with typical membranous nephropathy and in 5% to 10% of patients with Alport's syndrome receiving allografts.[511] However, in Alport's syndrome patients post transplantation, the alloantibodies, in contrast to those in anti-GBM disease, bind to the Ea region of the α5 NC1 domain of the intact α345 NC1 hexamer (rather than to denatured hexamer)[499] (see "Hereditary Nephritis, Including Alport's Syndrome" section).

CLINICAL FEATURES

Anti-GBM disease is rare.[496,498-500] Although some studies suggested occurrences as high as 3% to 5% of all glomerular diseases, most reduce this to 1% to 2%. The disease has two peaks of occurrence, the first in younger males, often associated with pulmonary hemorrhage, and the second in older females, often with isolated glomerulonephritis. Despite these trends, anti-GBM disease can occur at any age and in either gender.[496,498,499,507,512] Anti-GBM disease limited to the kidney may be more common in older patients. Goodpasture's syndrome is less common in blacks, perhaps due to less frequent occurrence of certain predisposing HLA antigens in this population. An upper respiratory infection precedes the onset of disease in 20% to 60% of cases.[496,498,499,507]

The most common extrarenal findings are pulmonary, including cough, dyspnea, and shortness of breath, and hemoptysis, which may vary from trivial amounts to life-threatening amounts associated with exsanguination and suffocation.[288,498,507,512] In almost three fourths of cases pulmonary hemorrhage precedes or is coincident with the glomerular disease.[496,498,507] Patients infrequently have constitutional symptoms of weakness, fatigue, weight loss, chills, and fevers. Others may have skin rash, hepatosplenomegaly, nausea and vomiting, and arthralgias at onset.[498]

The clinical renal presentation is usually an acute nephritic picture with hypertension, edema, hematuria and active urinary sediment, and reduced renal function. However, only 20% of patients are hypertensive at onset and in some series 15% to 35% have normal urinary sediment and GFR.[496,498,500,512] Renal function is usually already reduced at presentation and may deteriorate from normal to requiring dialysis in a matter of days to weeks.[496,498,512-514] There is a good correlation between the serum creatinine level and the percentage of glomeruli involved by severe crescent formation.

LABORATORY FINDINGS

Laboratory evaluation typically shows active urinary sediment with red cells and red cell casts.[498] Proteinuria, although common, is usually not in the nephrotic range. Serologic tests such as ASLO, ANA, serum complement levels, rheumatoid factor, and cryoglobulins are all either negative or normal.[498,507,512-514] Circulating anti-GBM antibodies are present in more than 90% of patients although the antibody titer does not always correlate well with the manifestations or course of either the pulmonary or renal disease.[499] From registry samples of plasma, anti-GBM antibodies have been found in the plasma of patients who eventually develop anti-GBM disease prior to the presentation of clinical disease.[515] Most patients have a decrease in serum antibody titer with time. From 10% to 38% of patients will have both positive anti-GBM antibodies and ANCA usually directed against MPO, but occasionally against PR3.[498,499,515,516] The anti-GBM antibodies in patients who are ANCA positive have the same antigenic specificity as in patients who are ANCA negative.[517] Some studies suggest that the course of patients double positive for anti-GBM antibodies and ANCA parallels that of patients with anti-GBM antibody disease, such that these patients are more likely to develop severe renal failure than those with purely ANCA-positive vasculitis.[516,518] Some patients have a clinical systemic vasculitis with purpura and arthralgias and arthritis, findings rarely seen in isolated Goodpasture's syndrome without coexistent ANCA.[516,517] In Goodpasture's syndrome a microcytic, hypochromic anemia is common even without overt pulmonary hemorrhage. Other patients may have leukocytosis. Iron deposition in the lungs may be documented by Fe59 scanning, bronchopulmonary lavage, or expectorated sputum showing hemosiderin-laden macrophages.[512] In patients with pulmonary involvement the chest radiograph is abnormal in more than 75% and typically shows infiltrates corresponding to areas of pulmonary hemorrhage. It may also demonstrate atelectasis, pulmonary edema, and areas of coexistent pneumonia.[498,500,512] Lung function discloses restrictive ventilatory defects and hypoxemia, and an increased arterial alveolar gradient is present in severe cases.[498,500,512,514]

PATHOLOGY

By light microscopy, patients with mild clinical involvement often have a focal, segmental proliferative glomerulonephritis associated with areas of segmental necrosis and overlying small crescents.[498,499,514] However, the most common biopsy picture is diffuse crescentic glomerulonephritis involving more than 50% of glomeruli, with exuberant, predominantly circumferential crescents (Figure 33.21).[266,500] The underlying tuft is compressed but displays focal necrotizing features. Disruption and destruction of large portions of the GBM and the basal lamina of Bowman's capsule may be seen on silver stain.[266] Early crescents are formed by proliferating glomerular epithelial cells and infiltrating T lymphocytes, monocytes, and polymorphonuclear leukocytes, while older ones are composed predominantly of spindled fibroblast-like cells, with few if any infiltrating leukocytes.[266] An associated tubulointerstitial nephritis with inflammatory cells and edema is common. Multinucleated giant cells may be present in the crescents or tubulointerstitial regions. Some patients, especially those who are ANCA positive, have necrotizing vasculitis of small arteries and arterioles. In biopsies taken later in the disease, there is progressive global and segmental glomerulosclerosis and interstitial fibrosis. Pulmonary histology reveals intraalveolar hemorrhage with

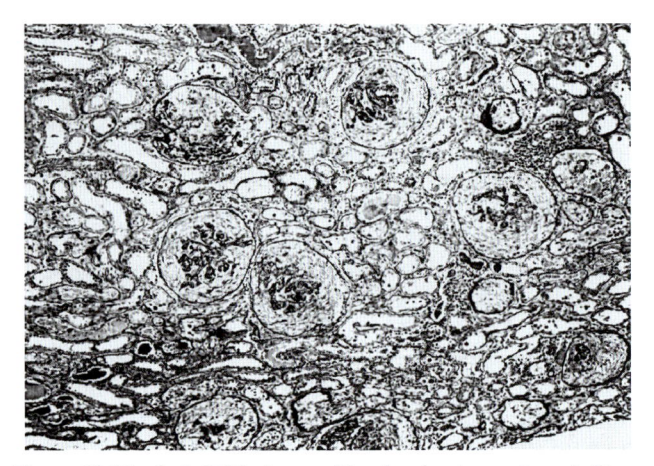

Figure 33.21 Anti-GBM disease (Goodpasture's syndrome). There is diffuse crescentic glomerulonephritis with large circumferential cellular crescents and severe compression of the glomerular tuft. (Periodic acid–Schiff stain, ×80.)

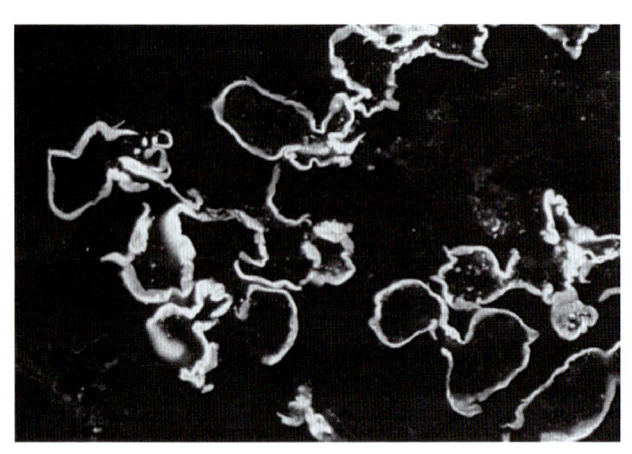

Figure 33.22 Anti-GBM disease (Goodpasture's syndrome). Immunofluorescence photomicrograph showing linear glomerular basement membrane (GBM) deposits of IgG. Some of the GBMs are discontinuous, indicating sites of rupture. (×800.)

widening and disruption of the alveolar septa and accumulations of hemosiderin-laden macrophages.[498,500]

The immunofluorescence findings define the disease process in Goodpasture's syndrome and differentiate it from both pauci-immune—and immune complex–mediated forms of crescentic glomerulonephritis. The diagnostic finding is an intense and diffuse linear staining for IgG, especially IgG1 and IgG4, involving the GBMs (Figure 33.22).[519,520] Rarely has IgM or IgA been identified in a linear distribution. C3 deposits are found in a more finely granular GBM distribution in many patients. C1q is typically absent. Linear immunofluorescence staining for IgG may also be found along some tubular basement membranes, particularly distal tubules. Fibrin-related antigens are commonly present within the crescents and segmental necrotizing lesions. In the lungs, similar linear deposition of IgG occurs along the alveolar capillary walls.

Electron microscopic findings typically do not reveal immune-type electron-dense deposits. There may be widening of the subendothelial space by fibrin-like material, and gaps in the GBM and in Bowman's capsule are commonly present.[266] Rare patients have coexistent membranous glomerulopathy with typical findings by light microscopy, immunofluorescence, and electron microscopy.

COURSE, TREATMENT, AND PROGNOSIS

The course of untreated Goodpasture's syndrome is one of progressive renal dysfunction leading to uremia.[499,500,516] In early studies almost all patients died from either pulmonary hemorrhage or progressive renal failure. In recent studies mortality is less than 10%, probably related to improved supportive care and more rapid diagnosis and treatment.[498,521] Once the disease is quiescent, relapses are rare in anti-GBM disease as opposed to GPA-, MPA-, and other ANCA-positive vasculitides. Spontaneous remission of the renal disease is rare, although with therapy many patients will have a stable course and some dramatic improvement.[498,521,522] If treatment is started early, patients may regain considerable kidney function. The plasma creatinine correlates fairly well with the degree of crescentic involvement, and if the plasma creatinine is markedly elevated and the patient requires dialysis, most such cases will develop ESKD.[498,499] A recent study from China in more than 100 patients with anti-GBM antibodies noted a poorer prognosis in patients with creatinine levels higher than 600 µmol/L, oligo-anuria at presentation, more than 85% crescents on biopsy, and renal involvement before pulmonary hemorrhage.[520] Anti-GBM autoantibodies against different target antigens may influence the disease severity.

There are no large randomized studies defining the benefits of any therapy for anti-GBM disease. While pulmonary hemorrhage and even renal disease have abated in some patients with high-dose oral or intravenous corticosteroids, combination therapy with steroids, cyclophosphamide, and plasmapheresis is now standard.[498,522] A typical treatment regimen might include a combination of oral prednisone (1 mg/kg/day) or intravenous pulse methylprednisolone (30 mg/kg/day up to 1000 mg/day) for several days followed by high-dose oral corticosteroid therapy along with cyclophosphamide (2 mg/kg/day) and plasmapheresis. Plasmapheresis may have a dramatic effect in reversing pulmonary hemorrhage and renal disease when used early in the course in combination with immunosuppressive agents.[498,518] Plasmapheresis removes the circulating anti-GBM antibodies while immunosuppressive therapy prevents new antibody formation and controls the ongoing inflammatory response. One uncontrolled study found that 40% of patients had stabilized or improved renal function with plasmapheresis.[522] Patients with severe renal failure who are already on dialysis or who have serum creatinine levels greater than 5 to 8 mg/dL are less likely to respond to therapy, but some have recovered. In one series, patients who were positive for both anti-GBM antibodies and ANCA behaved similarly to those with anti-GBM antibodies alone with a 1-year renal survival rate of 73% in those with a plasma creatinine concentration of less than 500 µmol/L and 0% in those on dialysis.[522] In other series dialysis-dependent patients who are both anti-GBM antibody and ANCA positive are still more likely to recover than patients who are dialysis dependent with only anti-GBM antibody positivity.[516] Although daily plasmapheresis is often maintained for weeks, its frequency can be determined by the rapidity of clinical response. Exacerbations of disease may occur with intercurrent infections. Immunosuppressive therapy is usually continued for 6 months with a tapering regimen to allow spontaneous cessation of autoantibody production. Some patients with early disappearance of circulating anti-GBM antibodies may respond to shorter therapy or tolerate change to less toxic maintenance immunosuppression such as azathioprine. There are limited data on other immunosuppressive regimens in Goodpasture's syndrome.[522-525] Rituximab has been used successfully in a small number of patients.[525] Immunoadsorption has also been used to remove the anti-GBM antibodies in Goodpasture's syndrome.[526] Even in patients with initial improvement of renal function, some with severe crescentic glomerular involvement will progress to renal failure over time, perhaps related to nonimmunologic progression of disease. The incidence of ESKD in patients with significant glomerular involvement is more than 50%, and the renal outcome is usually progressively downhill unless vigorous prompt therapy is instituted.

Anti-GBM–mediated renal disease may rarely recur in the renal allograft.[527-529] De novo anti-GBM disease may appear in patients with hereditary nephritis (see "Hereditary Nephritis, Including Alport's Syndrome" section). As with a number of other forms of glomerulonephritis, evidence of histologic recurrence (i.e., linear staining for IgG along GBMs) is far higher than clinical involvement and may be as high as 50%. The low recurrence rate recently reported in transplants probably reflects a combination of waiting sufficient time to document the absence of anti-GBM antibodies, the use of immunosuppressive medications and plasmapheresis to remove current antibody, and the "one-shot" nature of the disease.[528-530] Graft loss secondary to recurrent disease is rare. Patients should not be transplanted during the acute phase of their illness when autoantibody levels are high, and prophylactic pretransplant immunosuppression has been recommended for those receiving allografts from living related donors. Although patients with resolving pulmonary disease may have residual diminished gas exchange, most pulmonary function tests return to normal and do not limit the renal transplant process.[530]

SJÖGREN'S SYNDROME

Sjögren's syndrome is characterized by a chronic inflammatory cell infiltration of the exocrine salivary and lacrimal glands and is associated with the "sicca complex" of xerostomia and xerophthalmia.[531-533] Some patients may have involvement by a systemic inflammatory disease of the kidneys, lungs, esophagus, thyroid, stomach, and pancreas.[531-533] Others have manifestations of a connective tissue disease, most commonly rheumatoid arthritis, and less frequently SLE, scleroderma, polymyositis, or MCTD. Still other patients have different immunologic disorders such as chronic active hepatitis, primary biliary cirrhosis, Crohn's disease, and fibrosing alveolitis or develop lymphoma or Waldenström's macroglobulinemia. Serologic abnormalities in Sjögren's syndrome include hypergammaglobulinemia, rheumatoid factor, cryoglobulins, a homogeneous or speckled pattern ANA, anti-Ro/SSA and anti-La/SSB, but serum complement levels are generally normal unless the patient has associated SLE.[531-533]

The major clinical renal manifestations of patients with Sjögren's syndrome usually relate to tubulointerstitial involvement of the kidneys with tubular defects such as a distal renal tubular acidosis, impaired concentrating ability, hypercalciuria, and, less frequently, proximal tubular defects.[531-535] Most patients have no evidence of glomerular disease. In an analysis of more than 470 patients with primary Sjögren's syndrome followed for a mean of 10 years, only 20 patients (4%) developed overt renal disease.[532] Ten patients had interstitial nephritis, eight patients had glomerular lesions, and two had both interstitial nephritis and lesions. In those infrequent patients with glomerular lesions, hematuria, proteinuria, nephrotic syndrome, and renal insufficiency are found. Others may develop renal vasculitis with hypertension and renal insufficiency.

In most cases the renal pathology shows a chronic active interstitial inflammation by a predominantly lymphocytic infiltrate admixed with plasma cells, with variable interstitial fibrosis and tubular atrophy.[531-533,535] A nonspecific glomerulosclerosis with mesangial sclerosis and GBM thickening and wrinkling is found in those with chronic and severe tubulointerstitial damage. Infrequent patients will have immune complex–mediated glomerular involvement.[57,532-539] In one series of biopsied patients with primary Sjögren's syndrome, patients had either mesangial proliferative glomerulonephritis or MPGN.[532] Other series have had SLE features with the similar spectrum of glomerular involvement ranging from mesangial proliferative to focal proliferative, diffuse proliferative, and membranous glomerulonephritis.[57,536-539] A membranoproliferative pattern of glomerulonephritis has been reported in patients with associated cryoglobulinemia.[532,537-539] By immunofluorescence and electron microscopy, immune deposits have been localized in the various patterns to the mesangial region or the subendothelial or subepithelial aspect of the GBM. Some patients with Sjögren's syndrome have a necrotizing arteritis of the kidney occasionally with extrarenal involvement.[540] Most Sjögren's patients with tubulointerstitial disease respond to treatment with corticosteroids.[531-533,535] Patients with immune complex glomerulonephritis and Sjögren's syndrome are generally treated in a similar fashion to those with SLE, and those with vasculitis generally receive cytotoxic therapy similar to other necrotizing vasculitides.[535]

SARCOIDOSIS

Most manifestations of sarcoidosis are not related to the kidney.[541] The most common renal findings are granulomatous interstitial nephritis, nephrolithiasis, and tubular functional abnormalities.[542,543] Glomerular disease is infrequent and may be coincidental. Glomerular lesions described include minimal change disease, FSGS, membranous nephropathy, IgA nephropathy, MPGN, and proliferative and crescentic glomerulonephritis with and without a positive ANCA serology.[542-550] The immunofluorescence and electron microscopy features conform to the various histologic patterns. Some patients have granulomatous renal interstitial nephritis in addition to the glomerular lesions. Glomerular disease in sarcoidosis presents with proteinuria, active urinary sediment at times, and most commonly nephrotic syndrome. Some degree of proteinuria, usually

0.5 to 1 g/day is common in sarcoid patients with tubulointerstitial disease and no evidence of glomerular lesions.[551] Sarcoid patients have been treated with various forms of immunosuppression, including steroids, depending on their glomerular lesions.[544-550]

AMYLOIDOSIS

Amyloidosis comprises a diverse group of systemic and local diseases characterized by the extracellular deposition of fibrils in various organs.[552-555] Although more than 25 different proteins can produce amyloid fibrils, all share an antiparallel β-pleated sheet configuration on x-ray diffraction, leading to their amyloidogenic properties. All amyloid fibrils bind Congo red (leading to diagnostic apple green birefringence under polarized light) and thioflavin T, and have a characteristic ultrastructural appearance with randomly oriented 8- to 12-nm nonbranching fibrils. All amyloids also contain a 25-kDa glycoprotein, serum amyloid P component (SAP), a member of the pentraxin family. Amyloid deposits may also contain restricted sulfated glycosaminoglycans and proteoglycans noncovalently linked to the amyloid fibrils.[552-555] Only some amyloid proteins deposit in the kidney. Most renal amyloidoses are due to either AL amyloidosis or AA amyloidosis. In one recent series from a referral center for amyloidosis 1.3% of 21,500 renal biopsies over an 8.5-year period were found to have amyloidosis with 86% AL amyloid, 7% AA amyloid, and the remainder being a variety of types of "hereditary" amyloids.[556] In another single center series of 474 amyloidosis patients evaluated from 2007 to 2011, 85% were AL amyloid, 7% AA amyloid, and 4% hereditary amyloid.[552] In AL amyloidosis, the deposited fibrils are derived from the variable portion of immunoglobulin light chains produced by a clonal population of plasma cells or plasmacytic B cells. AA amyloid results from the deposition of serum amyloid A (SAA) protein in chronic inflammatory states.[552,553,557] A small fraction of renal amyloidoses are due to rare hereditary forms of amyloidosis, such as those caused by inherited gene mutations encoding transthyretin (ATTR), fibrinogen A α-chain (AFib), apolipoprotein A-I (apo A-I) or A-II (apo A-II), lysozyme (ALys), gelsolin (A Gel), and leukocyte chemotactic factor 2 (LECT2) peptide.[554,556,558-560] Laser microdissection and mass spectrometry were necessary to determine the origin of some of these unusual amyloid subtypes.[552,556,561,562] Difficulty in immunofluorescence diagnosis of AL amyloid occurs in as many as 14% to 35% of cases.[552,561,562]

It is unclear what factors confer the propensity for amyloidogenic proteins to fold into amyloid fibrils.[563-566] Cofactors such as amyloid P component may have an important role in the pathogenesis of tissue deposition. These may act by promoting fibrillogenesis, stabilization of the fibrils, binding to matrix proteins, or inhibiting denaturation and proteolysis. It is also possible that stabilizing co-factors are deposited after fibrillogenesis.[554,557,563-566] Amyloid fibrils generally resist biodegradation and accumulate in the tissues, resulting in organ dysfunction. However, amyloid deposits do exist in a dynamic state and have been shown to regress by radiolabeled SAP scintigraphy.[567] It is clear a critical mass of an abnormal protein is necessary to produce clinically significant amyloid of any type.[568] In SAA amyloid the SAA concentration has correlated with amyloid burden and reduction in circulating SAA with regression of amyloid deposits. Patients with AA amyloidosis have levels of circulating SAA protein no greater than those patients with inflammatory diseases who do not have amyloid deposition. Therefore, some additional unknown stimulus is required for amyloid fibrils to form and precipitate. In AL amyloid biochemical characteristics of the light chain, such as an aberrant amino acid composition at certain sites, appear important in determining amyloid formation.[569] This may account for the reproducibility of a given form of renal disease (cast nephropathy versus amyloid) in animal models infused with monoclonal light chains from affected patients.[569] Certain light chains may also form high-molecular-weight aggregates in vitro. Patients with AL amyloid more frequently produce abnormal excessive λ-than κ-light chains, and among AL amyloid patients with renal disease λ-light chains predominate over κ-light chains (by ratio of 12 : 1) as opposed to patients without renal disease (4 : 1).[552-554] Macrophage-dependent generation of preamyloid fragments with chemical properties allowing aggregation may also play a role. Mesangial cells have receptors for light chains and may modify them as well. Amyloid P component may also prevent degradation of amyloid fibrils once formed.[570]

AL AND AA AMYLOIDOSIS

In AL amyloidosis, fibrils are composed of the N-terminal amino acid residues of the variable region of an immunoglobulin light chain. λ-Light chains predominate over κ-light chains, and there is an increased incidence of monoclonal λ subtype VI.[552-554] The diagnosis of AL amyloidosis may be suspected on clinical grounds but requires biopsy documentation. The kidneys are the most common major organ involved by AL amyloid and most patients eventually develop renal amyloid.[552-554,571] In the past, up to 10% to 20% of patients older than 60 years with presumed idiopathic nephrotic syndrome had amyloidosis on renal biopsy.[572] Multiple myeloma occurs in up to 20% of primary amyloidosis cases. Amyloidosis should be suspected in all patients with circulating serum monoclonal M proteins, and approximately 90% of primary amyloid patients will have a paraprotein spike in the serum or urine by immunofixation,[552,553,571] and a greater percentage will have an elevation and predominance of one circulating light chain. While all AL amyloid patients will have an increased production of amyloidogenic light chains, not all patients with renal disease and a monoclonal protein in the serum will have amyloid. This is especially true in older patients, since 5% of patients older than 70 years of age will have a benign monoclonal gammopathy.

The incidence of AL amyloid is about 8 per million annually but varies greatly in different locations.[553] Most patients with AL amyloidosis are older than 50 years (median age, 59 to 63) and less than 1% are younger than 40 years of age. Men are affected twice as often as women.[552,553,571] Presenting symptoms include weight loss, fatigue, lightheadedness, shortness of breath, peripheral edema, pain due to peripheral neuropathy, and orthostatic hypotension. Patients may have cardiomyopathy, hepatosplenomegaly, macroglossia, or rarely enlarged lymph nodes. Multisystem organ involvement is typical with most commonly affected organs being the kidney (50%), heart (40%), and peripheral nerves (up to 25%).[552,553,571] In one series 25% of AL amyloid patients had one major organ system involved, 36% had two organ systems involved, and 38% had three or more involved.[573]

AA amyloidosis occurs in chronic inflammatory diseases and is composed of the N-terminal end of the acute phase reactant SAA protein.[552,554,565,567,574,575] SAA is produced in the liver and circulates in association with high-density lipoprotein. While in Westernized countries AA amyloid is most commonly found in association with rheumatoid arthritis and other inflammatory arthritides, it is also seen with inflammatory bowel disease, familial Mediterranean fever, quadriplegics with chronic urinary infections and decubitus ulcers, bronchiectasis, poorly treated osteomyelitis, and in chronic heroin addicts who inject drugs subcutaneously.[552,554,565,575-578] In one large multicenter study of 374 patients with AA amyloid, 60% had chronic inflammatory arthritis, 15% chronic infections, 9% periodic fever syndromes, 5% inflammatory bowel disease, 6% other etiologies, and in 6% no etiology was found.[574] In an autopsy study of 150 addicts, 14% of subcutaneous and 26% of those with chronic suppurative infections had renal amyloidosis.[577] AA amyloid typically occurs in older addicts with a long history of substance abuse who have exhausted sites of intravenous access and resorted to "skin popping."[578]

The diagnosis of amyloid is usually established by tissue biopsy of an affected organ.[552-554] Liver and kidney biopsy are positive in as many as 90% of clinically affected cases. A diagnosis may be made less invasively with fat pad aspirate (60% to 90%), rectal biopsy (50% to 80%), bone marrow aspirate (30% to 50%), gingival biopsy (60%), or dermal biopsy (50%).[579] Serum amyloid P whole body scintigraphy following injection of radiolabeled SAP allows the noninvasive diagnosis of amyloidosis as well as allowing a quantification of the extent of organ system involvement and assessment of the response to treatment.[580] This test may be positive even when tissue biopsy has been negative and may be more accurate in AA than in AL amyloidosis. In AL amyloidosis detection of an abnormal ratio of free κ- to λ-light chains in the serum is a technique to detect plasma cell dyscrasias which has a higher sensitivity than either serum or urinary protein electrophoresis and immunofixation.[581] It also allows assessment of response to therapy by following the level of abnormal free light chain in the serum.[576] Patients with hereditary amyloidosis due to deposition of abnormal transthyretin, apolipoproteins, lysozyme, or fibrinogen Aa may present in a fashion similar to AL amyloid. In one series 10% of 350 cases of hereditary amyloidosis were misdiagnosed as having AL amyloid.[559]

Although hereditary amyloidoses may present at any age, most patients are adults and present with higher serum creatinines and less proteinuria than those with AL or AA amyloidosis.[552] Some hereditary types lead to amyloid deposition in the tubulointerstitial and medullary compartment (e.g., amyloid due to apo A-I, A-II, A-IV) while others are associated with massive glomerular obliteration (AFib),[552] and still others such as LECT2 deposit in all compartments of the kidney.[556] Although the course of hereditary amyloid is often more prolonged and more benign than that of AL amyloid, presentation can be identical. Establishing the correct diagnosis is crucial since the treatment of hereditary amyloid may include liver transplantation rather than chemotherapy or stem cell transplantation as in AL amyloid.[556] Laser dissection of involved glomeruli and proteomic analysis by mass spectrometry, a test currently available in few specialized centers, can accurately diagnose all types of glomerular amyloid.[561]

Clinical manifestations of renal disease depend on the location and extent of amyloid deposition. Renal involvement predominates in AL amyloidosis with one third to one half of patients having renal manifestations at presentation.[552-554] Most patients have proteinuria, approximately 25% have nephrotic syndrome at diagnosis, and others present with varying degrees of azotemia.[552-554,571] Over time as many as 40% will develop nephrotic syndrome while others will have lesser degrees of proteinuria or azotemia. Urinalysis is typically bland, but microhematuria and cellular casts have been reported. Proteinuria is typically nonselective and almost 90% of patients with more than 1 g/day urinary protein will have a monoclonal protein in the urine. Hypercholesterolemia is less common than in other forms of nephrotic syndrome. The amount of glomerular amyloid deposition by light microscopy does not correlate well with the degree of proteinuria or renal dysfunction.[552,553] Despite the literature's suggestion of enlarged kidneys in AL amyloid, by ultrasonography most patients have normal-sized kidneys.[552] Hypertension is found in from 20% to 50% of patients, but many will have orthostatic hypotension due to peripheral neuropathy, autonomic neuropathy, and/or nephrotic syndrome. Patients with AA amyloid typically also have proteinuria and renal dysfunction with a progressive course. Patients with predominantly vascular involvement may have little proteinuria but rather renal insufficiency due to decreased renal blood flow. Infrequently patients will have predominantly tubulointerstitial deposition of amyloid with renal insufficiency and tubular defects such as distal renal tubular acidosis, Fanconi's syndrome, and nephrogenic diabetes insipidus.[552,553,571]

PATHOLOGY

In patients with clinical renal disease, the diagnostic sensitivity of an adequate renal biopsy approaches 100%.[553,557,582,583] Renal biopsy distinguishes AL amyloid from AA amyloid and excludes involvement by other renal disease in patients with known amyloidosis of other organs.

By light microscopy there is glomerular deposition of amorphous hyaline material that usually begins in the mesangium and extends into the peripheral capillary walls (Figure 33.23). Affected glomeruli appear hypocellular and may have a nodular aspect. This deposited material is lightly eosinophilic, weakly PAS positive, and nonargyrophilic in contrast to the findings in diabetic nodular glomerulosclerosis. In the peripheral GBM, amyloid deposits form spicular hairlike projections (Figure 33.24). Congo red stain gives an orange staining reaction and diagnostic apple green birefringence under polarized light (Figure 33.25). Amyloid deposits stain metachromatically with crystal or methyl violet and fluoresce under ultraviolet light following thioflavin T staining. Amyloid deposition may be confined to the glomeruli or involve tubular basement membranes, interstitium, and blood vessels, as well. The immunofluorescence in AL amyloidosis gives strong staining with antisera to the

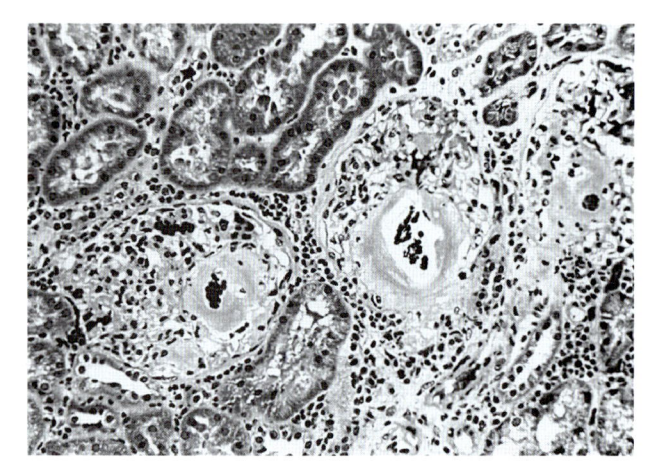

Figure 33.23 Amyloidosis. The glomerular tuft contains segmental deposits of amorphous eosinophilic hyaline material involving the vascular pole and some mesangial regions. (Hematoxylin and eosin stain, ×375.)

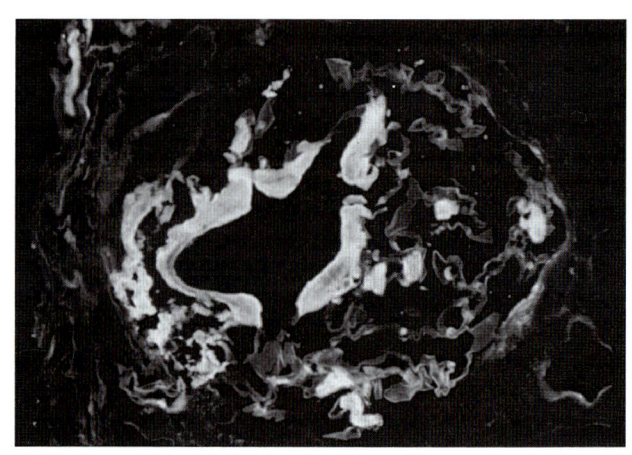

Figure 33.26 Amyloidosis. Immunofluorescence photomicrograph showing glomerular staining for λ-light chain in the distribution of the glomerular amyloid deposits in a patient with AL amyloidosis and plasma cell dyscrasia. (×600.)

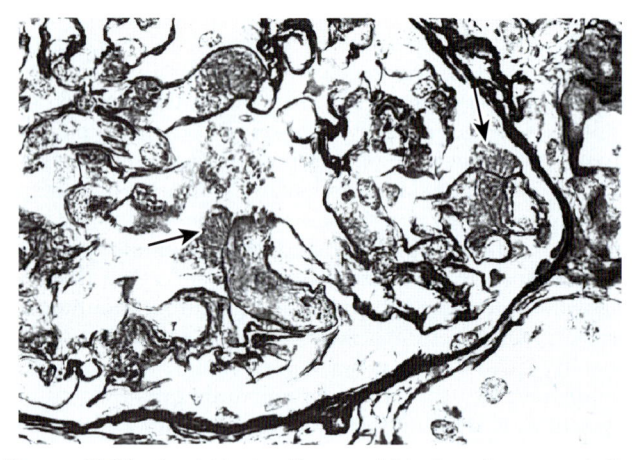

Figure 33.24 Amyloidosis. The amyloid deposits expand the mesangium and form focal spicular projections through the glomerular capillary walls, resembling spikes *(arrows)*. (Jones' methenamine silver stain, ×800.)

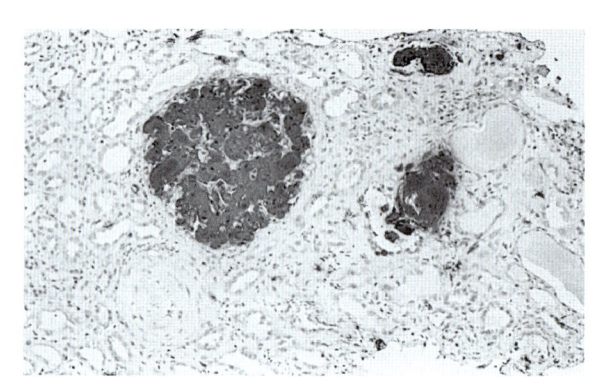

Figure 33.27 Amyloidosis. Immunoperoxidase staining for SAA protein stains the amyloid deposits in the glomeruli and arteries of a patient with secondary (AA) amyloidosis due to rheumatoid arthritis. (×125.)

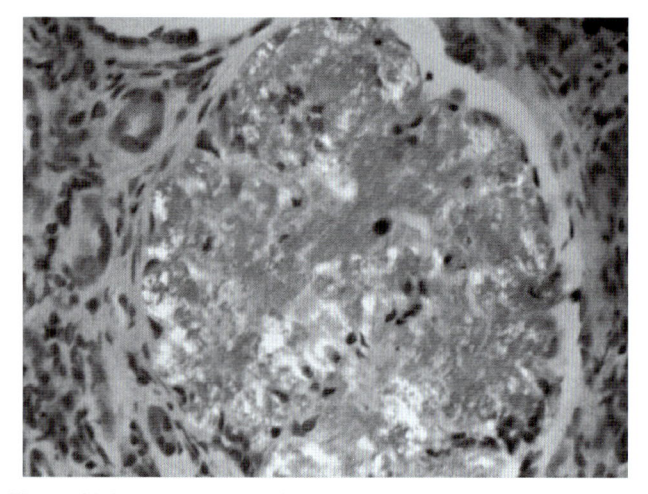

Figure 33.25 Amyloidosis. Congo red stain of a glomerulus that is largely replaced by amyloid demonstrates the characteristic birefringence under polarized light. (×450.)

pathogenic light chain, usually λ (Figure 33.26). Some less common forms of amyloid derived from Ig precursor proteins contain only Ig heavy chain (AH amyloid) or both heavy and light chain (AHL amyloid). The heavy chain is usually γ (derived from IgG), with less frequent α (IgA) and μ (IgM) forms. In AA amyloidosis, immunostaining for immunoglobulins and complement components is usually negative or gives a generalized weak reactivity due to nonspecific trapping. Diagnosis depends on the demonstration of strong reactivity for SAA protein by immunofluorescence or immunoperoxidase staining (Figure 33.27). Hereditary amyloidoses neither stain selectively for a single light chain nor for AA protein, but stain with antisera to the particular precursor protein. Nonspecific trapping of circulating proteins, including Ig and light chains, may lead to equivocal immunofluorescence results. In difficult cases, mass spectrometry–based proteomic analysis of the amyloid deposits extracted by laser capture microdissection from renal biopsy sections is required to identify the amyloid subtype.[561] By electron microscopy in all glomerular amyloidosis, typical nonbranching 8- to 12-nm-wide fibrils are

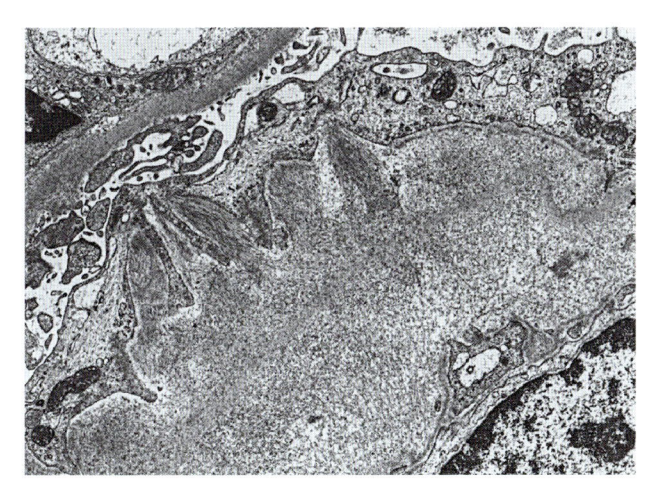

Figure 33.28 Amyloidosis. Electron micrograph showing extensive infiltration of the glomerular basement membrane by 10-nm fibrils that project toward the urinary space. (×8000.)

randomly distributed in the mesangium and frequently along the GBM in the subepithelial, intramembranous, and subendothelial locations (Figure 33.28). Mild cases may have deposition limited to the mesangium. More severe cases usually have more extensive deposition in the peripheral capillary walls and obliterating the lumina. By electron microscopy glomerular capillary wall infiltration by amyloid may form characteristic spicular, cockscomb-like projections along the subepithelial aspect of the GBMs.

COURSE, PROGNOSIS, AND TREATMENT

The prognosis of patients with AL amyloidosis in the past has been poor with some series having a median survival rate of less than 2 years.[552,553,571] The serum creatinine and the degree of proteinuria at baseline as well as hematologic response are predictive of the progression to ESKD. In older series, the median time from diagnosis to dialysis was 14 months, and from dialysis to death only 8 months.[552,553,571] Recent data suggest improved survival. Factors associated with decreased patient survival include evidence of cardiac involvement, renal dysfunction, and interstitial fibrosis on renal biopsy.[552,553,571] Cardiac involvement with associated heart failure and arrhythmias is the primary cause of death in amyloidosis, followed by renal disease.[552,553,571,584]

The course of AA amyloidosis has recently been defined in a study of 374 patients followed for a median time of more than 7 years.[576] Therapy to suppress the inflammatory disease was used whenever possible. The predominant manifestation and influence on the course of the disease was renal dysfunction and the median survival was more than 10 years. The SAA concentration correlated with overall mortality, amyloid burden, and renal prognosis. Amyloid deposits regressed (as assessed by SAP scans) in patients whose SAA concentration was kept low, and patient survival was superior in this group compared to those with no amyloid regression.[576]

The optimal treatment for AL amyloid depends on patient's age, organ system involvement, and overall health.[553,571,585] Treatment strategies focus on methods to decrease the production of monoclonal light chains. Promising chemotherapeutic agents used successfully in conjunction with dexamethasone include a number of agents used in myeloma, including melphalan, lenalidomide, thalidomide, bortezomib, and cyclophosphamide.[586-592] In some patients there is resolution of proteinuria, stabilization of renal function, improvement of symptoms, and occasionally evidence of decreased organ involvement such as reduced hepatosplenomegaly. In an older review of 153 AL amyloid patients treated with melphalan and prednisone only, 18% of the patients had a regression of organ manifestations of amyloidosis with responders having a 5-year survival of 78% versus only 7% in the nonresponders.[587] Patients with renal amyloidosis fared best with 25% having a 50% resolution in nephrotic-range proteinuria and stable or improved GFR. Other therapies used experimentally to treat AL amyloid, including dimethyl sulfoxide, colchicine, 4′-iodo-4′-deoxydoxorubicin, fludarabine, vitamin E, high-dose dexamethasone monotherapy, and interferon alfa-2, have not been effective.[585,588,592]

Reports using high-dose melphalan followed by allogeneic bone marrow transplant or stem cell transplant have given promising results.[593,594] Such regimens have led to resolution of nephrotic syndrome and biopsy-proven improvement of amyloid organ involvement in some cases. However, a renal complication of autologous stem cell transplantation (AKI) developed in 20% of one series of 173 amyloid patients. Although there was a high mortality in early reports (20% in the first 3 months), many survivors had a complete hematologic response, and many with renal involvement survived with a major decrease in proteinuria without a worsening of GFR. One retrospective study analyzed 65 AL amyloid patients with more than 1 g/day proteinuria treated with dose-intensive ablative chemotherapy followed by autologous blood stem cell transplantation.[595] Three fourths of the patients survived the first year, and among those, a good renal response was found in 36% at 1 year and 52% at 2 years. Patients with a complete hematologic response were more likely to have a good renal response, and patient survival was superior in younger patients with fewer than three organ systems involved and those able to tolerate higher doses of the ablative therapy. Toxicities included mucositis, edema, elevated liver function tests, pulmonary edema, gastrointestinal bleeding, and, in 23%, transient acute renal failure. Thus, for some younger patients with predominantly renal involvement stem cell transplantation is currently a reasonable alternative therapy. Some studies have supported stem cell transplantation as a beneficial therapy for some AL amyloid patients.[596] Even patients with ESKD due to amyloidosis may undergo this form of therapy with results no different from non-ESKD patients with AL amyloidosis.[597] However, the only large randomized trial of stem cell transplantation for amyloid found this treatment to be inferior to standard chemotherapy.[598] In this multicenter French trial, 100 patients were randomized to hematopoietic cell transplantation or melphalan plus dexamethasone. The chemotherapeutic group had a better overall survival. Although this study has been criticized for patient selection and the high subsequent mortality, it is the only large randomized trial. Regardless of whether chemotherapy or marrow transplant is used, the treatment of nephrotic amyloid patients requires supportive care. This may include judicious use of diuretics and salt restriction in those with edema, and treatment of orthostatic hypotension with compression stockings, fludrocortisone, and, in some, midodrine, an oral α-adrenergic agonist.

The treatment of AA amyloid focuses on the control of the underlying inflammatory disease process.[567,574,576,599] This has included surgical debridement of inflammatory tissue, antibiotic therapy of infectious processes, and antiinflammatory and immunosuppressive agents in rheumatoid arthritis and inflammatory bowel disease. Therapy may lead to stabilization of renal function, reduction in proteinuria, and resolution of amyloid deposits.[567,574,576,599] Prognosis may be good if the underlying disease can be controlled and there is not already extensive amyloid deposition. Immunosuppressives, antiinflammatory agents, and anticytokine therapy have been used in rheumatologic diseases and Crohn's disease, with evidence of increased GFR and decreased proteinuria, and in some cases with regression of renal amyloid deposits.[574,576,599,600] In familial Mediterranean fever (FMF)—an autosomal recessive disease caused by pyrin mutation primarily found in Sephardic Jews, Turks, Armenians, and Arabs—recurrent attacks of fever and serositis lead to the development of AA amyloidosis in up to 90% of untreated patients.[574] Colchicine can prevent effectively the febrile attacks and stabilize or reduce the development of proteinuria. However, renal function did deteriorate in patients with nephrotic syndrome at presentation. A retrospective analysis of FMF patients with milder renal clinical involvement and at least 5 years' follow-up concluded that high doses of colchicine were more effective in preventing renal dysfunction and that patients with lower levels of serum creatinine at presentation responded better to therapy. Once the serum creatinine level was elevated, however, increasing the dose of colchicine did not prevent progression. AA amyloidosis seen in drug abusers and patients with inflammatory states such as Behçet's disease and inflammatory bowel disease have occasionally responded to colchicine therapy, although it is unclear if this was due to cessation of drug abuse or treatment of the underlying inflammatory disease process.[578,601]

A multicenter randomized controlled trial compared a glycosaminoglycan mimetic (used to block fibrillogenesis) to placebo in 183 patients with AA amyloid. Although the drug had no significant effect on preventing progression to ESKD or risk of death, the glycosaminoglycan mimetic did reduce the rate of progression of the renal disease.[602] This study clearly shows the need for newer therapies for amyloidosis and the value of controlled trials in studying these agents. Several promising experimental therapies for treating amyloid include the use of anti-amyloid antibodies and the use of an inhibitor of the binding of amyloid P component to amyloid fibrils.[599]

END-STAGE KIDNEY DISEASE IN AMYLOIDOSIS

In most series the median survival of amyloid patients with ESKD is less than 1 year with the primary cause of death being complications of cardiac amyloid.[603,604] However, for patients who survive the first month of ESKD replacement therapy, the survival rate is more than 50% at 2 years and 30% at 5 years.[604] There is no survival difference between peritoneal dialysis or hemodialysis.[604] A report of survival data in 19 dialysis patients with AL amyloid found an 80% mortality at 35 months' follow-up, while 20 AA amyloid dialysis patients had a 15% mortality in this time period.[605] Likewise, another series found a shorter than 1 year median survival for hemodialysis patients with AL amyloidosis.

Experience with renal transplantation in AL amyloid is limited, but transplantation may be performed either before or after autologous stem cell transplantation.[596,597] An earlier series on transplantation in amyloid included 45 patients (42 with AA amyloid) and found an overall low patient survival, particularly in the early posttransplant period in older patients because of infectious and cardiovascular complications.[606] Graft survival, however, was not decreased despite rates of recurrence of amyloidosis in the allograft as high as 20% to 33%.[606,607] Survival rates at 5 and 10 years of renal transplant patients with AA amyloid, largely FMF patients, who received living related allografts have been as high as 80% and 66%, respectively. In hereditary amyloidosis due to fibrinogen A α-chain disease, recurrence occurred in 50% of allografts with frequent graft loss. Better results are reported with combined liver and kidney transplantation.

FIBRILLARY GLOMERULONEPHRITIS AND IMMUNOTACTOID GLOMERULONEPHRITIS

Some uncommon glomerular diseases have fibrillar deposits differing in size from those of amyloid.[608,609] Many investigators subdivide these patients into two major groups depending on clinical associations and fibril size.[608-611] In fibrillary glomerulonephritis the fibrils are approximately 16 to 24 nm (mean, 20 nm) in diameter, and in immunotactoid glomerulonephritis the deposits form larger hollow microtubules of 30 to 50 nm in diameter. Both of these fibrillar organized deposits may represent a slow-acting cryoprecipitate of polyclonal or monoclonal immunoglobulin. A third, rare form of fibrillary renal disease is fibronectin glomerulopathy in which the glomeruli are infiltrated by massive deposits of fibronectin.[612,613]

Although some classify both fibrillary glomerulonephritis and immunotactoid glomerulonephritis as a single disease entity, most clinicians and nephropathologists divide them into distinct disorders.[341,608-611] Almost 90% of cases have the smaller 20-nm fibrils of fibrillary glomerulonephritis. Fibrillary glomerulonephritis occurs mostly in adults, in both sexes, in all age groups, and most commonly in Caucasians. Although usually considered an isolated idiopathic renal entity, it has been associated in some series with malignancies, monoclonal gammopathies, and autoimmune disorders.[613] Patients with immunotactoid glomerulonephritis tend to be older, may have a less rapidly progressive course, and in all series are more likely to have underlying lymphoproliferative disease, (e.g., chronic lymphocytic leukemia or B cell lymphoma), often with a circulating paraprotein and sometimes with hypocomplementemia.[608-611] Patients with both diseases usually have proteinuria, and most have hypertension and hematuria. About 70% to 75% have nephrotic syndrome at biopsy. At presentation renal insufficiency is common and most patients progress to ESKD. Fibrillary glomerulonephritis and immunotactoid glomerulonephritis may be associated with HCV infection.[611]

Diagnosis of these disorders requires a renal biopsy to demonstrate the defining ultrastructural features.[608-611] Light microscopic findings in fibrillary glomerulonephritis

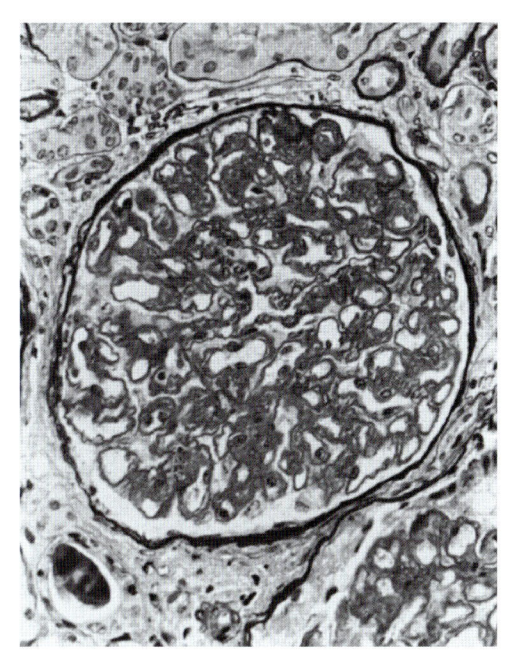

Figure 33.29 Fibrillary glomerulonephritis. The mesangium is mildly expanded and the glomerular capillary walls appear thickened with segmental double contours. (Periodic acid–Schiff stain, ×300.)

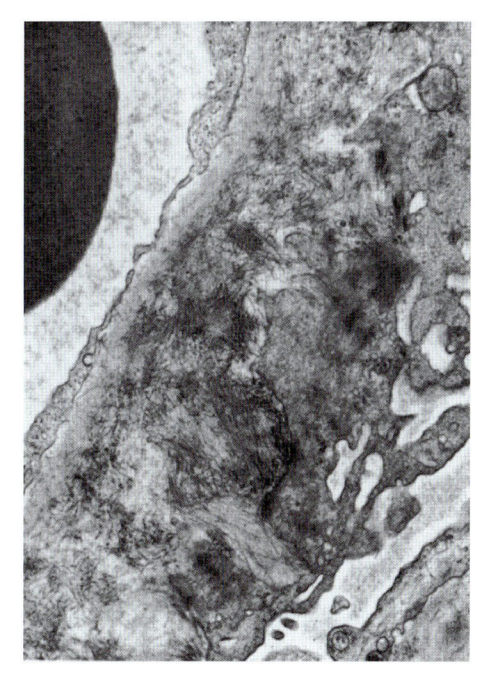

Figure 33.31 Fibrillary glomerulonephritis. Electron micrograph showing the characteristic randomly oriented fibrils, measuring 16-20 nm within the glomerular basement membrane. The foot processes are effaced. (×8000.)

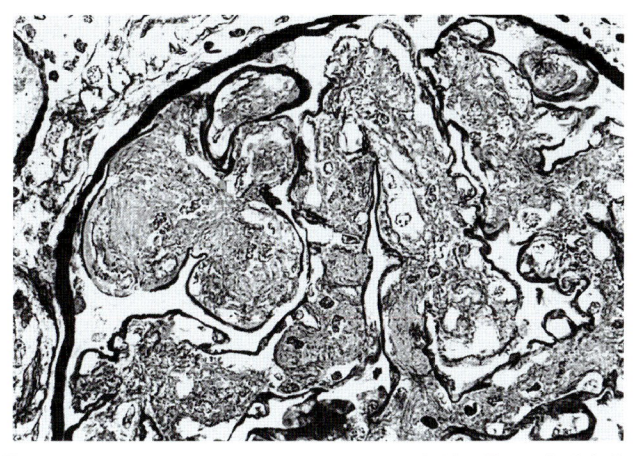

Figure 33.30 Immunotactoid glomerulonephritis. There is lobular expansion of the glomerular tuft by abundant mesangial deposits of silver-negative material. Segmental extension of deposits into the subendothelial aspect of some glomerular capillaries is also seen. (Jones' methenamine silver stain, ×500.)

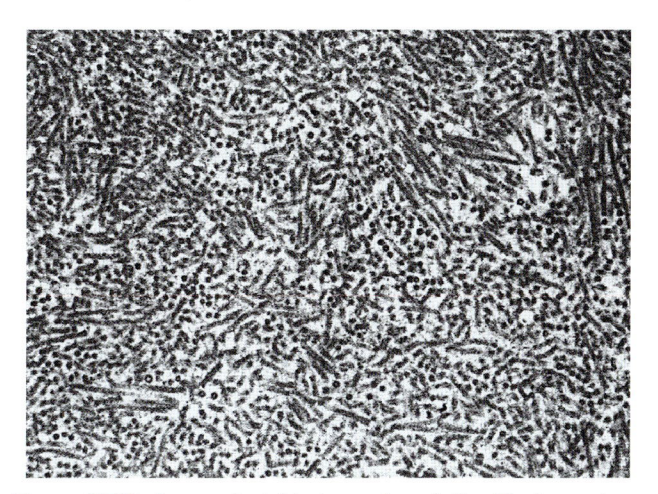

Figure 33.32 Immunotactoid glomerulonephritis. Electron micrograph showing abundant mesangial deposits of microtubular structures measuring approximately 35 nm in diameter. (×10,000.)

are highly variable and include mesangial proliferation; mesangial expansion by amorphous amyloid-like material; membranous, membranoproliferative, and crescentic glomerulonephritis (Figure 33.29).[608] In immunotactoid glomerulonephritis, glomerular lesions are often nodular and sclerosing, whereas others are proliferative or membranous (Figure 33.30). The pathognomonic findings seen on electron microscopy consist of nonbranching fibrils of 16 to 24 nm diameter in fibrillary glomerulonephritis (as opposed to 8 to 12 nm for amyloid) (Figure 33.31) and hollow microtubules of 30 to 50 nm in immunotactoid glomerulonephritis (Figure 33.32). In fibrillary glomerulonephritis, fibrils are arranged randomly in the mesangial matrix and GBMs.

By contrast, the microtubules of immunotactoid glomerulonephritis are often arranged in parallel stacks in the mesangium, subendothelial, and/or subepithelial regions. The fibrils and microtubules do not stain with Congo red or thioflavin T. In fibrillary glomerulonephritis, immunofluorescence is almost always positive for IgG (Figure 33.33) (especially subclasses IgG1 and IgG4), C3, and both κ- and λ-chains, indicating polyclonal deposits.[608-611] Staining for IgM, IgA, and C1 has been reported in a minority of cases. In immunotactoid glomerulonephritis, the immunoglobulin deposits are often monoclonal, consisting of IgG with a restricted light-chain isotype (either κ or λ). IgG subtypes IgG1 and IgG3 are most common and have the capacity to

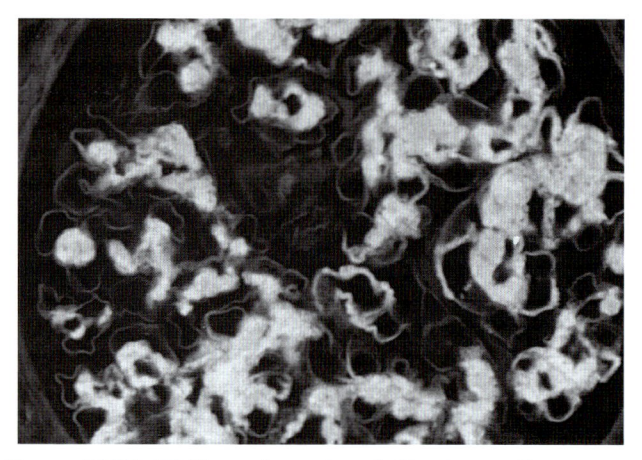

Figure 33.33 Fibrillary glomerulonephritis. Immunofluorescence photomicrograph showing smudgy deposits of IgG throughout the mesangium, with segmental extension into the peripheral glomerular capillary walls. (×800.)

fix complement, leading to glomerular co-deposits of C1q and C3. In both diseases, the deposits are usually limited to the glomerulus. In fibrillary glomerulonephritis, the fibrils may be focally admixed with more granular immune-type electron-dense deposits.[608] Rare patients with fibrillary glomerulonephritis have been reported to have extrarenal deposits involving alveolar capillaries and, in the case of immunotactoid glomerulonephritis, the bone marrow.[614,615]

Almost half of patients with fibrillary glomerulonephritis or immunotactoid glomerulonephritis develop ESKD within 2 to 6 years of presentation.[608,610] Those with crescentic lesions, sclerosing glomerulonephritis, and diffuse proliferative glomerulonephritis fare worse than those with mesangioproliferative glomerulonephritis and those with a membranous pattern. Younger patients, patients with a normal GFR, and those with subnephrotic-range proteinuria have a more benign renal course.[608]

Although there is no proven therapy for fibrillary glomerulonephritis, some clinicians choose to treat the light microscopy pattern observed on renal biopsy (e.g., membranous, membranoproliferative, crescentic, etc.).[608] Prednisone, cyclophosphamide, and colchicine have not led to consistent benefit in most patients.[608] However, in some with crescentic glomerulonephritis, cyclophosphamide and corticosteroid therapy has led to a dramatic improvement in GFR and proteinuria. Cyclosporine has also been used successfully in some patients with fibrillary glomerulonephritis and a membranous pattern on light microscopy. Rituximab has been used in those with MPGN pattern although recent larger series have given less promising results.[320,608,616,617] In some patients with associated chronic lymphocytic leukemia, treatment with chemotherapy has been associated with improved renal function and decreased proteinuria.[608,610] Dialysis and transplantation have been performed in both fibrillary glomerulonephritis and immunotactoid glomerulonephritis, but there is a significant recurrence rate in the allograft in both diseases.[608,618,619] Some have found a higher recurrence rate in those with an associated monoclonal gammopathy.[619]

Fibronectin glomerulopathy is a familial disease with autosomal dominant inheritance that presents with proteinuria and hematuria usually in adolescents and eventually progresses to nephrotic syndrome and slowly deteriorating renal function.[612,613] It is caused by an inherited mutation in the gene encoding fibronectin-1.[613] Patients who progress to ESKD may develop recurrent fibronectin glomerulopathy in the allograft.

MONOCLONAL IMMUNOGLOBULIN DEPOSITION DISEASE

Monoclonal immunoglobulin deposition disease (MIDD) includes light-chain deposition disease (LCDD), combined light- and heavy-chain deposition disease (LHCDD), and heavy-chain deposition disease (HCDD). MIDD is a systemic disease caused by the overproduction and extracellular deposition of a fragment of monoclonal immunoglobulins.[620-622] LCDD is by far the most common pattern. As opposed to amyloidosis, in LCDD the deposits in more than 80% of cases are composed of κ-light chains, most often of the VkIV subgroup, rather than λ-light chains.[620-623] In LCDD the deposits are granular in nature, do not have the biochemical properties necessary to form fibrils or β-pleated sheets and thus do not bind Congo red stain or thioflavin T, and are not associated with amyloid P protein.[620-623] In amyloid the fibrils are usually derived primarily from the variable region of the light chains, while in LCDD the deposits are predominantly composed of the constant region of the light chain. This may explain the far brighter immunofluorescence staining for light chains found in LCDD as opposed to amyloidosis. The nature of the light chains may also explain the far more common occurrence of light-chain cast nephropathy in LCDD than in amyloidosis.[620-623] The pathogenesis of the glomerulosclerosis in LCDD involves promotion of a profibrotic mesangial cell phenotype with production of transforming growth factor-β, which acts as an autacoid to stimulate mesangial cell synthesis of extracellular matrix proteins such as type IV collagen, laminin, and fibronectin.[624]

Patients with MIDD are generally older than 45 years.[620-623] However, in one recent series with a median age of 56 years, more than one third of the patients were younger than 50 years of age.[621] Many such patients develop frank myeloma, and some may have a lymphoplasmacytic B cell disease such as lymphoma or Waldenström's macroglobulinemia.[620-622] As in amyloidosis, the clinical features vary with the location and extent of organ deposition of the monoclonal protein. Patients typically have cardiac, neural, hepatic, and renal involvement, but other organs such as the skin, spleen, thyroid, adrenal glands, and gastrointestinal tract may be involved.[620-623] Patients with renal disease usually have significant glomerular involvement and present with proteinuria, nephrotic syndrome, and hypertension. Renal insufficiency is present in most, and some require dialysis. While by serum protein electrophoresis (SPEP) or urine protein electrophoresis (UPEP) 15% to 30% of patients may have no identifiable M spike, by analysis of serum-free light-chain assay, 100% have an abnormal protein and 80% have high levels of production.[621] Some patients may have greater tubulointerstitial involvement and less proteinuria along with renal insufficiency.[624]

The glomerular pattern by light microscopy is most often nodular sclerosing with mesangial nodules of acellular

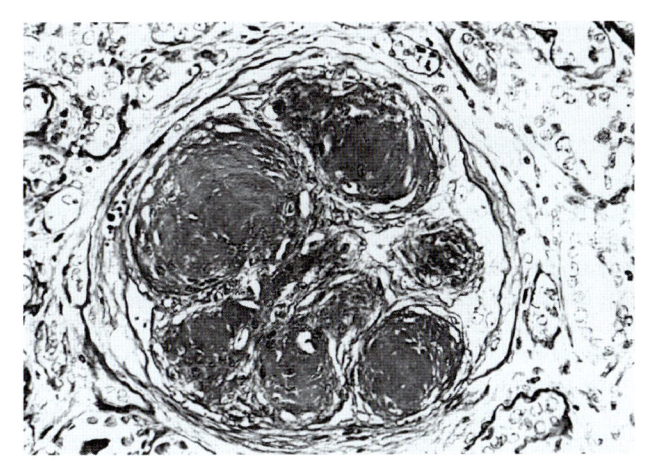

Figure 33.34 Light-chain deposition disease. There is nodular glomerulosclerosis with marked global expansion of the mesangium by intensely periodic acid–Schiff—positive material but without appreciable thickening of the glomerular capillary walls. (Periodic acid–Schiff stain, ×375.)

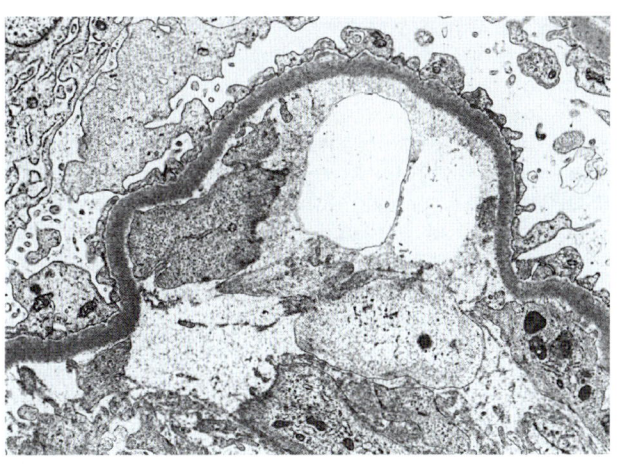

Figure 33.36 Heavy-chain deposition disease. Electron micrograph showing bandlike, finely granular electron-dense deposits involving the glomerular basement membrane, with greatest concentration along the inner aspect (×5000.)

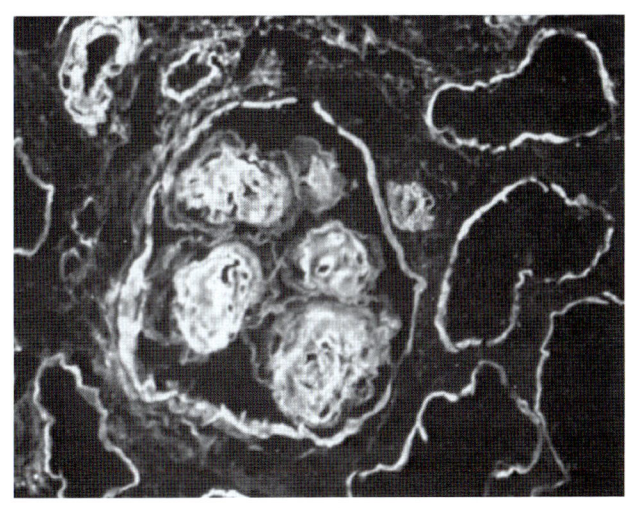

Figure 33.35 Light-chain deposition disease. Immunofluorescence photomicrograph showing linear staining for κ-light chain involving glomerular and tubular basement membranes, the mesangial nodules, Bowman's capsule, and vessel walls. (×250.)

eosinophilic material resembling the nodular glomerulosclerosis seen in diabetic patients (Figure 33.34).[620-622] Glomerular capillary microaneurysms also may occur.[625] Some glomeruli have associated membranoproliferative features. In LCDD the nodules are more strongly PAS positive and less argyrophilic than in diabetes, and the GBMs in LCDD are not usually visibly thickened by light microscopy.[620,621] Other glomeruli may be entirely normal or have only mild mesangial sclerosis. Immunofluorescence is usually diagnostic by demonstration of a monoclonal light chain (κ in 80%) staining in a diffuse linear pattern along the GBMs, in the nodules, and along the tubular basement membranes and vessel walls (Figure 33.35).[620,621] Staining for complement components is usually negative. By electron microscopy, deposition of a finely granular punctate, highly electron-dense material occurs along the lamina rara interna of the GBM, in the mesangium, and along tubular and vascular basement membranes.[620-623]

The prognosis for patients with LCDD is variable. Death is often attributed to heart failure, infectious complications, or the development of frank myeloma and renal failure.[620-623] In one series of 63 MIDD patients, 65% of patients developed myeloma and 36 patients developed uremia.[622] In another series of 64 patients with MIDD, including 51 with LCDD, with a median follow-up of over 2 years, 57% had stable or improved renal function, 4% worsening of renal function, and 39% progression to ESKD.[621] Patient survival is about 90% at 1 year and 70% at 5 years, with renal survival 67% and 37% at 1 and 5 years, respectively.[620-622,626,627] Predictors of worse renal outcome included increased age, associated light-chain cast nephropathy, and elevated serum creatinine at presentation.[620-622] Predictors of worse patient survival included increased age, occurrence of myeloma, higher initial serum creatinine, and extrarenal deposition of light chains.[620-622]

Treatment, akin to the treatment of myeloma or amyloidosis, has been with dexamethasone in combination with other agents, including melphalan, cyclophosphamide, bortezomib, thalidomide, and lenalidomide, and has led to stabilized or improved renal function in some MIDD patients.[620-622] However, this therapy is not usually successful in patients with significant renal dysfunction and a plasma creatinine above 4 mg/dL at initiation of treatment.[627] In one series of 32 patients treated with chemotherapy, 34% progressed to ESKD.[622] Marrow or stem cell transplantation is a therapeutic option for some patients with LCDD.[620,622] Although there are little data on dialysis and renal transplantation in LCDD, patients appear to fare as well as those with amyloidosis. Recurrences in the renal transplant have been reported[620,621,626-628] and recurrence rates in some series are as high as 70% to 75%.[596,621,628] Thus, suppression of the abnormal paraprotein producing cell clone is crucial prior to renal transplantation.

In some patients with a plasma cell dyscrasia, monoclonal light and heavy immunoglobulin chains combined (LHCDD) or short monoclonal truncated heavy chains alone (HCDD) are deposited in the tissue (Figure 33.36).[620,623,629,630] As in LCDD, the electron microscopy deposits are granular and biopsies are Congo red negative. The clinical features are similar to those of LCDD and amyloidosis.[630] Most patients are middle age or older. They present with renal insufficiency, hypertension, proteinuria, and often nephrotic syndrome. In most patients a monoclonal protein is detected in the serum or urine. In contrast to amyloid and LCDD, HCDD may be associated with hypocomplementemia if the heavy chain avidly binds complement (especially γ–heavy-chain subtypes G1 and G3).[630] All patients with HCDD have a deletion of the CH1 domain of the heavy chain, which causes the heavy chain to be secreted prematurely by the plasma cell.[630,631,643-645] The characteristic light microscopic finding in HCDD is a nodular sclerosing glomerulopathy at times with small crescents.[620,630-632] The diagnosis is made by immunofluorescence with linear positivity for the heavy chain of immunoglobulin (usually γ) and negativity for both κ- and λ-light chains.[630] The distribution is diffuse involving glomerular, tubular, and vascular basement membranes. Treatment has been similar to LCDD, and many patients have progressed to renal failure.[630,633] Recurrence in the renal transplant has been documented.[620]

OTHER GLOMERULAR DISEASES AND DYSPROTEINEMIA

Recent series have described patients with a proliferative glomerulonephritis resembling immune complex glomerulonephritis in association with a monoclonal gammopathy.[634,635] This newly described entity is known as proliferative glomerulonephritis with monoclonal IgG deposits (PGNMID). These patients presented with renal insufficiency and proteinuria, sometimes associated with nephrotic syndrome, but no evidence of cryoglobulinemia. Light microscopy shows an MPGN pattern in more than one half and an endocapillary proliferative pattern with membranous features in more than one third. All had ordinary-appearing granular nonorganized electron-dense deposits in the mesangial, subendothelial, and subepithelial sites, but by immunofluorescence these were restricted to a single monoclonal γ subclass and light-chain isotype (e.g., IgG1κ, IgG2λ, or IgG3κ). Although infrequent patients have had a pure membranous pattern by light microscopy and electron microscopy, they still have the same monoclonal restriction by immunofluorescence microscopy. M spike was identified in the serum in 30% of cases, but no patient developed overt myeloma or lymphoma during the follow-up period. In one large series at 2.5 years of follow-up, 38% of patients had had a complete recovery, 38% had persistent renal dysfunction, and 22% had progressed to ESKD.[635] Higher presenting serum creatinine, higher percentage of glomerulosclerosis, and more interstitial fibrosis on biopsy predicted progression to ESKD. Proliferative glomerulonephritis with monoclonal IgG deposits commonly recurs in the transplant and may in some cases be amenable to either rituximab or cyclophosphamide therapy.[636,637]

Other rare patients with dysproteinemia have had intracellular glomerular crystals within the podocytes, sometimes in association with tubular epithelial crystalline deposits.[638] Pamidronate-induced collapsing focal sclerosis has been noted in myeloma,[639] as has crescentic glomerulonephritis. MPGN has been reported rarely, particularly in patients with associated cryoglobulinemia (see "Mixed Cryoglobulinemia" section).

WALDENSTRÖM'S MACROGLOBULINEMIA

In Waldenström's macroglobulinemia, patients have an abnormal circulating monoclonal IgM protein in association with a B cell lymphoproliferative hematologic disorder.[640-643] This slowly progressive disorder occurs in older patients (median age, 60) who present with constitutional symptoms of fatigue and weight loss, bleeding, visual disturbances, neurologic symptoms, hepatosplenomegaly, lymphadenopathy, anemia, and often hyperviscosity syndrome.[640-643] Although renal involvement occurs in less than 5% of patients, glomerular lesions can present with microscopic hematuria, proteinuria, and nephrotic syndrome.[643,644] Patients may have enlarged kidneys. The renal pathology in Waldenström's macroglobulinemia is varied.[643-645] Some patients will have invasion of the renal parenchyma by neoplastic lymphoplasmacytic cells. Others have AKI with intraglomerular occlusive thrombi of the IgM paraprotein. These cases have large eosinophilic, amorphous, PAS-positive deposits occluding the glomerular capillary lumens with little or no glomerular hypercellularity (Figure 33.37). By immunofluorescence these glomerular "thrombi" stain for IgM and a single light-chain isotype, consistent with monoclonal IgM deposits, but complement components are usually negative or only weakly positive. By electron microscopy the deposits contain nonamyloid fibrillar or amorphous electron-dense material. Some patients develop MPGN with an associated type I or type II cryoglobulinemia (Figure 33.38). Cases of LCDD with intratubular casts similar to those of light-chain cast nephropathy and examples of renal amyloidosis have also been reported in patients with Waldenström's macroglobulinemia. Treatment of Waldenström's macroglobulinemia is directed against the lymphoproliferative disease with alkylating agents, melphalan, corticosteroids, rituximab, bone marrow transplantation, and at times plasmapheresis for hyperviscosity signs and symptoms.[646-648]

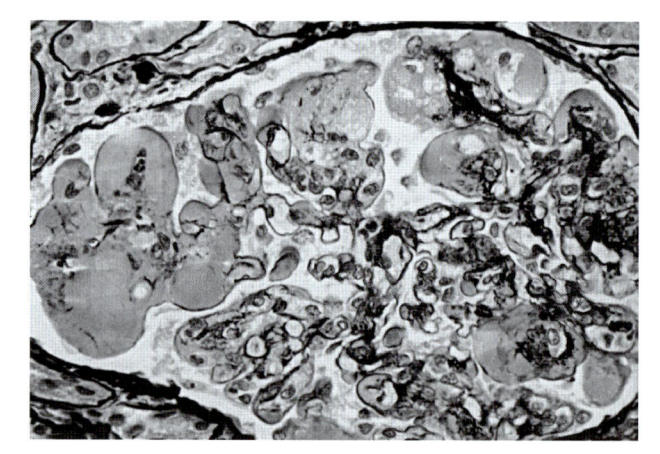

Figure 33.37 Waldenström's macroglobulinemia. Large "protein thrombi" corresponding to the monoclonal immunoglobulin M deposits fill the glomerular capillary lumens, with minimal associated glomerular hypercellularity. (Jones' methenamine silver stain, ×600.)

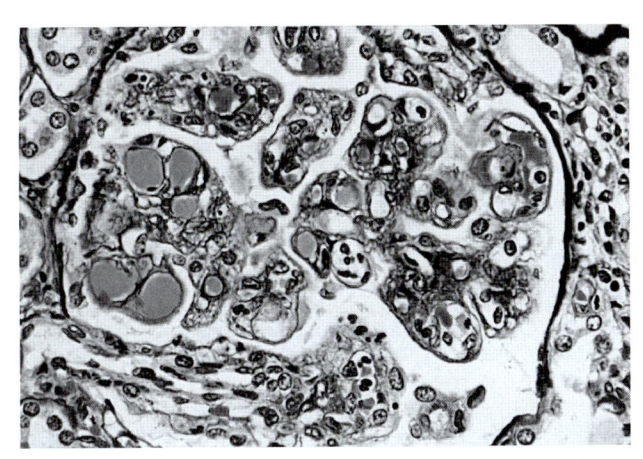

Figure 33.38 Waldenström's macroglobulinemia. An example with cryoglobulinemic glomerulonephritis showing the characteristic intraluminal deposits, infiltrating leukocytes, and double-contoured glomerular basement membranes. (Jones' methenamine silver stain, ×600.)

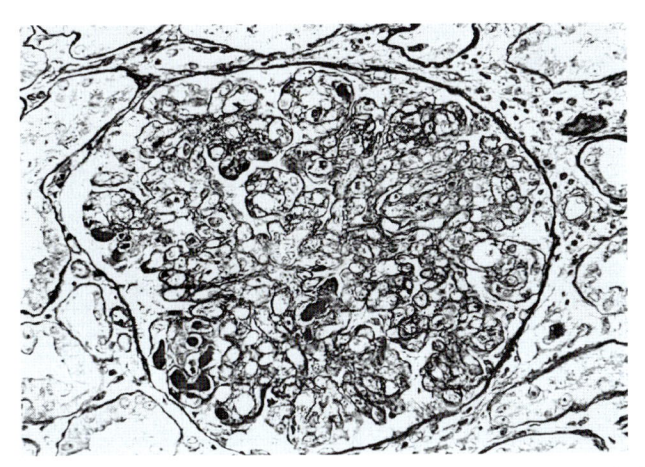

Figure 33.39 Cryoglobulinemic glomerulonephritis. There is global endocapillary proliferative glomerulonephritis with membranoproliferative features and focal intraluminal cryoglobulin deposits, forming "immune thrombi." (Periodic acid–Schiff stain, ×375.)

MIXED CRYOGLOBULINEMIA

Cryoglobulinemia is caused by circulating immunoglobulins that precipitate on cooling and resolubilize on warming.[649] Cryoglobulinemia is associated with a variety of infections, especially HCV, as well as collagen-vascular disease, and lymphoproliferative diseases.[383,649] Cryoglobulins have been divided into three major groups based on the nature of the circulating immunoglobulins.[649] In type I cryoglobulinemia, the cryoglobulin is a single monoclonal immunoglobulin often found associated with Waldenström's macroglobulinemia or myeloma. Type II and type III cryoglobulinemia are defined as mixed cryoglobulins, containing at least two immunoglobulins. In type II, a monoclonal immunoglobulin (IgMκ in more than 90%) is directed against polyclonal IgG and has rheumatoid factor activity. In type III, the antiglobulin is polyclonal in nature with both polyclonal IgG and IgM in most cases. The majority of patients with type II and III mixed cryoglobulins have now been shown to have HCV infection.[622,650-655] To establish a diagnosis of cryoglobulinemia, the offending cryoglobulins or the characteristic renal tissue involvement must be demonstrated.

In the past, there was often no obvious cause of cryoglobulinemia and the name "essential mixed cryoglobulinemia" was appropriate.[650] It is now clear that many such patients had HCV-related disease.[652,656,657] Systemic manifestations of mixed cryoglobulinemia include weakness, malaise, Raynaud's phenomenon, arthralgias-arthritis, hepatosplenomegaly with abnormal liver function tests in two thirds to three fourths of patients, peripheral neuropathy, and purpuric-vasculitic skin lesions.[383,649] Hypocomplementemia, especially of the early components (low C4 level), is a characteristic and often helpful finding. Renal disease occurs at presentation in less than 25% of patients but develops in as many as 50% over time.[650,658,659] In one review of 279 patients with severe life-threatening HCV-associated cryoglobulinemic vasculitis, 205 had AKI.[653] In those renal patients who died, sepsis was the most common cause of death, while for other patients, vasculitis of the gastrointestinal tract, central nervous system, and pulmonary system led to death. These causes of death are similar to those of 242 patients in a review of noninfectious mixed cryoglobulinemic vasculitis.[654] In most, an acute nephritic picture with hematuria, hypertension, proteinuria, and progressive renal insufficiency develops, and 20% of patients have nephrotic syndrome. Few patients develop RPGN with oliguria. The majority of patients with renal disease have a slow, indolent renal course characterized by proteinuria, hypertension, hematuria, and renal insufficiency.

Many older studies of type II cryoglobulinemia have shown evidence of HBV infection or other viral infections (e.g., Epstein-Barr virus).[655] However, recent studies have clearly documented HCV as a major cause of cryoglobulin production in most patients previously thought to have essential mixed cryoglobulinemia. Antibodies to HCV antigens have been documented in the serum, and HCV RNA and anti-HCV antibodies are enriched in the cryoglobulins of these patients.[652,656,658,659] This is true even for patients with normal levels of aminotransferases and no clinical evidence of hepatitis. HCV antigens have also been localized by immunohistochemistry to the glomerular deposits.[656]

In cryoglobulinemia, immunoglobulin complexes deposit in the glomeruli and small- and medium-sized arteries, binding complement and inciting a proliferative response.[652,658] The serum cryoglobulin participates in the formation of the glomerular immune complex deposits. In vitro studies have shown that IgM-κ rheumatoid factor from patients with type II cryoglobulinemia is much more likely to bind to cellular fibronectin (a component of the glomerular mesangium) than IgM from normal controls or IgM-containing rheumatoid factor from rheumatoid arthritis patients.[660] The particular physicochemical characteristics of the variable region of the immunoglobulin cryoglobulin may be important in the localization of the renal deposits.

Although by light microscopy the glomerular lesions of cryoglobulinemia may show a variety of proliferative and sclerosing features (Figure 33.39), certain features help to distinguish cryoglobulinemic glomerulonephritis from other proliferative glomerulonephritides.[650,658,659] These features include massive glomerular exudation of monocytes/

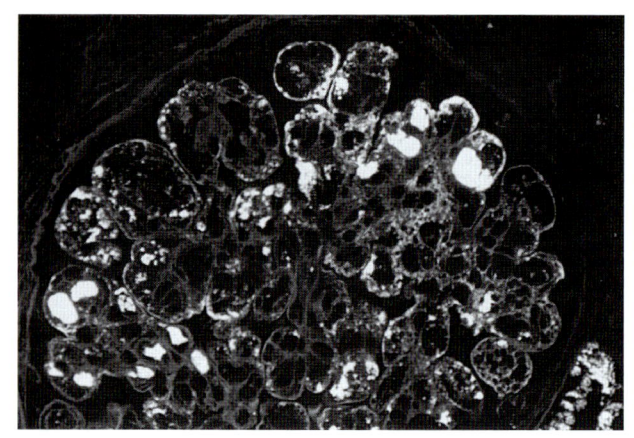

Figure 33.40 Cryoglobulinemic glomerulonephritis. Immunofluorescence photomicrograph showing deposits of immunoglobulin M corresponding to the large glomerular intracapillary deposits, with more finely granular subendothelial deposits outlining the glomerular capillary walls. (×900.)

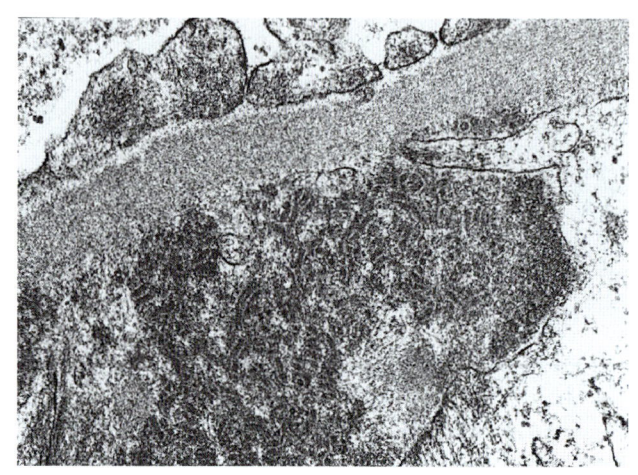

Figure 33.41 Cryoglobulinemic glomerulonephritis. Electron micrograph showing organized subendothelial deposits with an annular-tubular substructure. These curvilinear tubular structures measure approximately 30 nm in diameter. (×30,000.)

macrophages and, to a lesser degree, polymorphonuclear leukocytes; amorphous eosinophilic PAS-positive, Congo red negative deposits along the subendothelial aspect of the glomerular capillary wall and focally filling the capillary lumens, forming "immune thrombi"; membranoproliferative features with double-contoured GBMs and interposition of deposits, mesangial cells, and monocytes; and the rarity of extracapillary proliferation (crescents) despite the intense intracapillary proliferation. The glomerular lesions may be accompanied by an acute vasculitis of small- or medium-sized vessels. The monocytes of patients with active cryoglobulinemia and associated nephritis have been shown to phagocytose cryoglobulins but to be unable to catabolize them efficiently. By immunofluorescence (Figure 33.40), the glomeruli in type II or type III cryoglobulinemia contain deposits of both IgM as well as IgG, κ- and λ-light chains, and C3 and C1q in the distribution of subendothelial and mesangial deposits and the intracapillary "thrombi." Staining for both IgM and κ are often dominant, reflecting the deposition of type II cryoglobulins containing a monoclonal IgM-κ component. By electron microscopy (Figure 33.41), deposits in the subendothelial location or filling the capillary lumens often appear as either amorphous electron-dense deposits or organized deposits of curvilinear parallel fibrils or annular-tubular curvilinear structures with a diameter of 20 to 35 nm.[650,658] The infiltrating macrophages are in close contact with the subendothelial deposits and contain prominent phagolysosomes, suggesting active phagocytosis of the immune deposits. In some cases, the phagocytosis is so effective that immune deposits are difficult to detect by both immunofluorescence and electron microscopy.

Some patients with mixed cryoglobulinemia will have a partial or total remission of their disease while most have episodic exacerbations of their systemic and renal disease.[650,658] Before the association between mixed cryoglobulinemia and HCV was discovered, many patients were treated successfully with prednisone and cytotoxic agents such as cyclophosphamide and chlorambucil.[651] Treatments were not used in a controlled fashion. In patients with severe renal disease, in those with digital necrosis from the cryoglobulins, and in those with life-threatening organ involvement, plasmapheresis was used in combination with steroids and cytotoxics.[651,661] Most patients with cryoglobulinemia in the past did not die of renal disease but rather of cardiac or other systemic disease and infectious complications.[651] Currently, most patients with HCV-associated cryoglobulinemia are treated with antiviral agents[662] (see the "Hepatitis C" section under "Glomerular Manifestations of Liver Disease"). Aggressive immunosuppressive therapy carries the risk of promoting HCV replication in HCV-infected patients and of lymphoma in others. Rituximab has recently been used successfully for treatment of type II mixed cryoglobulinemia in patients with or without evidence of HCV infection and with and without prior antiviral therapy.[663-666] Rituximab has also been used successfully in small numbers of patients with HCV-related glomerulonephritis and mixed cryoglobulinemia.[667,668] Dialysis and transplantation in cryoglobulinemia have been used, but recurrences in the allograft have been reported.[669]

HEREDITARY NEPHRITIS, INCLUDING ALPORT'S SYNDROME

Alport's syndrome is an inherited (usually X-linked) disorder with characteristic glomerular pathology, frequently associated with hearing loss and ocular abnormalities. Guthrie first reported a family with recurrent hematuria.[670] Alport reported additional observations on this family, the occurrence of deafness associated with hematuria, and the observation that affected males died of uremia, whereas affected females lived to an old age.[671] Alport's syndrome and other hereditary and familial disease account for 0.4% of adults with ESKD in the United States.[672]

CLINICAL FEATURES

The disease usually manifests in children or young adults.[673-675] Males have persistent microscopic hematuria, with episodic gross hematuria, which may be exacerbated by respiratory infections or exercise. There may be flank pain or abdominal discomfort accompanying these episodes. Proteinuria is usually mild at first and increases progressively with age. Nephrotic syndrome has also been described.[676] Hypertension is a late manifestation. Slowly progressive renal failure is common in males. ESKD usually occurs in males between the ages of 16 and 35. In some kindred, the course may be more delayed, with renal failure occurring between 45 and 65 years of age. In most females, the disease is mild and only partially expressed; however, some females have experienced renal failure.[677] In the European Community Alport Syndrome Concerted Action (ECASCA) cohort, hematuria was observed in 95% of female carriers and consistently absent in the other 5%. Proteinuria, hearing loss, and ocular defects developed in 75%, 28%, and 15%, respectively.[678] This variability in disease severity in females can be explained by the degree of random inactivation of the mutated versus wild type X chromosome during lyonization.

High-frequency sensorineural deafness occurs in 30% to 50% of patients. Hearing impairment is always accompanied by renal involvement. The severity of hearing loss is variable, and there is no relation between the severity of hearing loss and of the renal disease. Based on brainstem auditory evoked responses, the site of the aural lesion is in the cochlea.[679,680] Families with hereditary nephritis but without sensorineural hearing loss have been described.[680,681]

Ocular abnormalities occur in 15% to 30% of patients.[682] Anterior lenticonus, which is the protrusion of the central portion of the lens into the anterior capsule, is virtually pathognomonic of Alport's syndrome. Other ocular abnormalities include keratoconus, spherophakia, myopia, retinal flecks, cataracts, retinitis pigmentosa, and amaurosis.[673,674,683] Aortic disease, including dissections, aneurysms, dilation, and aortic insufficiency, may be an unusual feature in some patients.[684]

Other variants of presumed Alport's syndrome, now known to be distinct entities with different genetic bases, include the association of hereditary nephritis with thrombocytopathia (megathrombocytopenia; so-called Epstein's syndrome),[685,686] diffuse leiomyomatosis,[687] ichthyosis and hyperprolinuria,[688] and Fechtner's syndrome (nephritis, macrothrombocytopenia, Döhle-like leukocyte inclusions, deafness, and cataract).[689]

PATHOLOGY

The light microscopic appearance of biopsies is nonspecific. The diagnosis rests on the electron microscopy findings. By light microscopy most biopsies have glomerular and tubulointerstitial lesions. In the early stages (<5 years of age), the kidney biopsy may be normal or nearly normal. The only abnormality may be the presence of superficially located fetal glomeruli involving 5% to 30% of the glomeruli or interstitial foam cells.[690,691] In the older child (5 to 10 years of age), mesangial and glomerular capillary wall lesions may be visible. These consist of segmental to diffuse mesangial cell proliferation, matrix increase, and thickening of the glomerular capillary wall.[692] Special stains such as Jones' methenamine silver or periodic acid–Schiff may reveal thickening and lamellation of the GBM. Segmentally or globally sclerosed glomeruli may be present.

Tubulointerstitial changes may include interstitial fibrosis, tubular atrophy, focal tubular basement membrane thickening, and interstitial foam cells. The glomerular and tubular lesions progress over time. A pattern of focal segmental and global glomerulosclerosis with hyalinosis is common in advanced cases, especially those with nephrotic-range proteinuria. Tubulointerstitial lesions progress from focal to diffuse involvement.[690,693]

By immunofluorescence many specimens are negative,[690,694] but some may have nonspecific granular deposits of C3 and IgM within the mesangium and vascular pole and along the glomerular capillary wall in a segmental or global distribution.[673,680] The finding in rare cases of nonspecifically trapped electron-dense material with positivity for IgG and C1q within the lamellated GBMs and paramesangial regions may lead to an erroneous diagnosis of immune complex glomerulonephritis.[695] With segmental sclerosis, subendothelial deposits of IgM, C3, properdin, and C4 are found.[673,690] The GBM of males with Alport's syndrome frequently lacks reactivity with sera from patients with anti-GBM antibody disease, or with monoclonal antibodies directed against the Goodpasture epitope.[696,697] This abnormality can help in diagnosing equivocal cases where the electron microscopic findings are not specific.[698]

In the mature kidney, collagen IV is composed of heterotrimers made up of six possible α-chains. Chains composed of α1, α1, and α2 are distributed in all renal basement membranes. Collagen IV chains composed of α3, α4, and α5 are present in mature GBM and some distal thin basement membrane. Chains of α5, α5, and α6 are distributed in Bowman's capsule and collecting duct thin basement membrane, as well as in epidermal basement membrane. Commercially available antisera to the subunits of collagen IV reveal preservation of the $α_1$- and $α_2$-subunits but loss of immunoreactivity for the $α_3$-, $α_4$-, and $α_5$-subunits from the GBM of affected males with X-linked disease. In addition, there is loss of $α_5$ staining from Bowman's capsule, distal tubular basement membranes, and skin in affected males with X-linked disease. Females are chimeras with segmental loss of $α_5$ in glomerular and epidermal basement membranes due to random inactivation of the mutated X chromosome in podocytes and basal keratinocytes. Patients with autosomal recessive forms of Alport's disease typically lack the $α_3$-, $α_4$- and $α_5$-subunits in GBM but retain $α_5$ immunoreactivity in Bowman's capsule, collecting ducts, and skin (where α5 forms a heterotrimer with α6). Thus, absence of $α_5$ staining in skin biopsies is highly specific for the diagnosis of X-linked Alport's syndrome.[699]

On electron microscopy the earliest change in young males is thinning of the GBM (which is not specific for hereditary nephritis and can occur in thin basement membrane disease). The cardinal ultrastructural abnormality is the variable thickening, thinning, basket weaving, and lamellation of the GBM (Figure 33.42). These abnormalities may also be seen in some patients without a family history of nephritis[700]; these patients may be offspring of asymptomatic carriers or may represent new mutations. The endothelial cells are intact, and foot process effacement may be seen overlying the altered capillary walls. The mesangium may be normal in early cases, but with time, matrix and cells increase and mesangial interposition into the capillary wall may be observed.[673,694] In males, the number of glomeruli showing lamellation increases from about 30% by age 10 to more than 90% by age 30. In females with mild disease, less than 30% of the glomeruli may be affected.[701] Some affected females have a predominantly thin basement membrane phenotype with only rare segmental areas of lamellation.

The specificity of the GBM findings has been questioned.[702] Foci of lamina densa lamellation and splitting have been seen in 6% to 15% of unselected renal biopsies. These changes also may be seen focally in other glomerulopathies. Thus clinical correlation and immunofluorescence examination are essential when the ultrastructural features suggest Alport's syndrome. Although diffuse thickening and splitting of the GBM strongly suggests Alport's syndrome, not all Alport kindreds show these characteristic features. Thick, thin, normal, and nonspecific changes have also been described.

PATHOGENESIS AND GENETICS

There are three genetic forms of hereditary nephritis (Table 33.2). In the majority of cases, the disease is transmitted via an X-linked inheritance (i.e., father-to-son transmission does not occur), and women tend to be carriers because of lyonization. Autosomal dominant and recessive inheritance have also been described, as has sporadic occurrence.[673,703,704] The frequency of the Alport gene has been estimated to be 1 : 5000 in Utah[705] and 1 : 10,000 in the United States.[706]

Hereditary nephritis is caused by defects in type IV collagen. Six genes for type IV collagen have been characterized. Mutations in the *COL4A5* gene (encoding the α_5-subunit of collagen type IV) on the X chromosome are responsible for the more frequent X-linked form of hereditary nephritis.[707] The identified mutations include deletions, insertions, substitutions, and duplications.[707-711] However, there are other abnormalities that are not encoded by the *COL4A5* gene. Other type IV collagen peptides are abnormally distributed. The α_1 and α_2 peptides, which are normally confined to the mesangial and subendothelial regions of the mature glomerulus, become distributed throughout the full thickness of the GBM in hereditary nephritis. With progressive glomerular obsolescence, these peptide chains disappear, with an increase in collagen types V and VI.[712] Moreover, the basement membranes of these patients do not react with anti-GBM antibodies. This implies that the NC1 domain of the α_3-subunit of type IV collagen is not incorporated normally into the GBM, probably because the α_5-subunit is required for normal assembly of the minor α-chains of collagen type IV into heterotrimers.[713] Cationic antigenic components are also absent.[714] The reason why these GBM abnormalities occur is not known but may be due to alteration in the

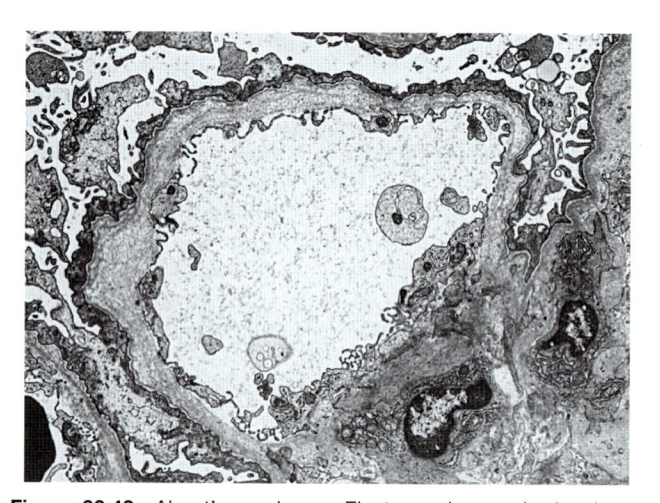

Figure 33.42 Alport's syndrome. Electron micrograph showing a thickened, lamellated glomerular basement membrane with the characteristic "split and splintered" appearance. (×4000.)

Table 33.2 Classification of Familial Hematurias

	Locus	Progressive Nephropathy	Deafness	Ocular Changes	GBM Changes	Hematologic Features
Type IV Collagen Disorders						
Alport's syndrome						
X-linked	COL4A5	+	+	+	Thickening	–
X-linked + diffuse Leiomyomatosis	COL4A5 + COL4A6	+	+	+	Thickening	–
Autosomal recessive	COL4A3 or COL4A4	+	+	+	Thickening	–
Autosomal dominant	COL4A3 or COL4A4	+	+	–	Thickening	–
Thin basement membrane nephropathy*	COL4A3 or COL4A4	–	–	–	Thinning	–
Noncollagen Disorders						
Fechtner's syndrome	MYH9	+	+	+	Thickening	Thrombocytopenia May-Hegglin anomaly
Epstein's syndrome	MYH9	+	+	+	Thickening	Thrombocytopenia

*Some families with thin basement membrane disease have mutations at loci other than the type IV collagen genes.
From Kasthan CE: Familial hematurias: what we know and what we don't. Pediatr Nephrol 20:1027-1035, 2005.

incorporation of other collagens into the GBM.[715] Autosomal recessive and autosomal dominant hereditary nephritis have been shown to involve the α_3- or α_4-chain. The genes for these proteins are encoded on chromosome 2. An abnormality of any of these chains could impair the integrity of the basement membranes in the glomerulus and cochlea, leading to similar clinical findings.

According to "Expert Guidelines for the Management of Alport Syndrome and Thin Basement Membrane Nephropathy,"[716] the term *Alport's syndrome* should be reserved for patients with the characteristic clinical features and a lamellated GBM with an abnormal collagen IV composition, and in whom a *COL4A5* mutation (X-linked disease) or two *COL4A3* or two *COL4A4* mutations in trans (autosomal recessive disease) are identified or expected. The term *thin basement membrane nephropathy* (TBMN) should be reserved for individuals with persistent isolated glomerular hematuria who have a thinned GBM due to a heterozygous *COL4A3* or *COL4A4* (but not *COL4A5*) mutation. This distinction is to ensure patients who have X-linked Alport's syndrome are not falsely reassured by the usually benign prognosis seen in TBMN. In those patients with renal impairment together with a heterozygous *COL4A3* or *COL4A4* mutation, there is likely to be a coincidental renal disease, such as IgA glomerulonephritis, or autosomal recessive Alport's syndrome, or a second, undetected *COL4* mutation. The correct diagnosis may be adjudicated after discussions among the nephrologist, pathologist, clinical geneticist, ophthalmologist, and audiologist, and interpretation of the relevant test results.[716] Genetic testing may be utilized when the diagnosis of Alport's syndrome is suspected but cannot be confirmed with other techniques and when TBMN is suspected but X-linked Alport's syndrome must be excluded. With current genetic techniques, the mutation detection rate is over 90% and more likely to be identified in individuals with early-onset renal failure and extrarenal manifestations.[716]

Minor causes of familial hematuria (Fechtner's syndrome and Epstein's syndrome), along with two other genetic conditions featuring macrothrombocytes (Sebastian's syndrome and May-Hegglin anomaly), result from heterozygous mutations in the gene *MYH9*, which encodes nonmuscle myosin heavy-chain II isoform A (NMMHC-IIA).[717]

COURSE AND TREATMENT

Recurrent hematuria and proteinuria may be present for many years, followed by the insidious onset of renal failure. Virtually all affected males reach ESKD, but there is considerable interkindred variability in the rate of progression. The rate of progression within male members of an affected family is usually but not always relatively constant.[673,718,719] The presence of gross hematuria in childhood, nephrotic syndrome, sensorineural deafness, anterior lenticonus, and diffuse GBM thickening are indicative of an unfavorable outcome in females.[677] In the ECASCA, a 90% probability rate of progression to end-stage renal failure by age 30 years in patients with large deletions, nonsense mutations, or frameshift mutations was noted. The same risk was of 50% and 70%, respectively, in patients with missense or splice site mutations. The risk of developing hearing loss before 30 years of age was approximately 60% in patients with missense mutations, compared to 90% for the other types of mutations.[720] Female carriers with the *COL4A5* mutation generally have less severe disease. In the ECASCA cohort described earlier, the probability of developing ESKD before the age of 40 years was 12% in females versus 90% in males. The risk of progression to ESKD appears to increase after the age of 60 years in women. Risk factors for renal failure in women included the development and progressive increase in proteinuria and the occurrence of a hearing defect.[678]

There is no proven therapy for Alport's syndrome. Proteinuria-reduction strategies, such as aggressive control of hypertension and use of ACEIs, might slow the rate of progression in patients with hereditary nephritis.[721-723] The addition of an aldosterone antagonist may further reduce proteinuria.[724] A small number of patients showed apparent stabilization when treated long term with cyclosporine[725]; however, calcineurin inhibitor toxicity can occur with long-term use.[726]

Renal replacement therapy (either dialysis or transplantation) may be performed in patients with hereditary nephritis. Allograft and patient survival rates were comparable to survival rates in the United Network for Organ Sharing (UNOS) database.[727] In approximately 2% to 4% of male patients receiving a renal transplant, anti-GBM antibody disease may develop.[728] These antibodies are directed against the α-5 noncollagenous (NC1) subunit of the intact α345 hexamer of collagen IV.[729] This antigen, which presumably does not exist in the native kidney of patients with hereditary nephritis, is present in normal donor kidneys and is thus recognized as foreign.[730,731] A profile of these patients has been compiled.[698] The patients are usually male, always deaf, and likely to have reached ESKD before the age of 30. There is a suggestion that certain mutations in the *COL4A5* gene, such as deletions (which account for 11% to 12% of Alport's cases), may predispose patients to the development of allograft anti-GBM nephritis.[731] In 75% of cases, the onset of anti-GBM nephritis occurs within the first year after transplantation, and 76% of the allografts were lost.

THIN BASEMENT MEMBRANE NEPHROPATHY

TBMN (also known as benign familial hematuria and thin GBM nephropathy) describes a condition that differs from Alport's disease in its generally benign course and lack of progression. The typical finding on renal pathology is diffuse thinning of the GBM. However, thin GBM may be found in other conditions as well (including early Alport's disease and IgA nephropathy).[732] The true incidence of TBMN is unknown but is estimated to affect at least 1% of the population; reports evaluating patients with isolated hematuria suggest that 20% to 25% of such patients have TBMN.[733-735]

CLINICAL FEATURES

Patients usually present in childhood with microhematuria. Hematuria is usually persistent but may be intermittent in some patients. Episodic gross hematuria may occur, particularly with upper respiratory infections.[736,737] Patients do not typically have overt proteinuria, but when present, this may suggest progression of disease.[733,738]

Table 33.3 Immunostaining Patterns for α_5-Subunit of Type IV Collagen in Kidney and Epidermal Basement Membranes

	Glomerular Basement Membrane	Bowman's Capsule	Epidermal Basement Membrane
Normal	Present/normal	Present/normal	Present/normal
X-linked Alport's syndrome males	Absent	Absent	Absent
X-linked Alport's syndrome female carriers	Present segmentally/mosaic	Present segmentally/mosaic	Present focally/mosaic
Autosomal recessive Alport's syndrome	Absent	Present/normal	Present/normal
Thin basement membrane disease	Present/normal	Present/normal	Present/normal

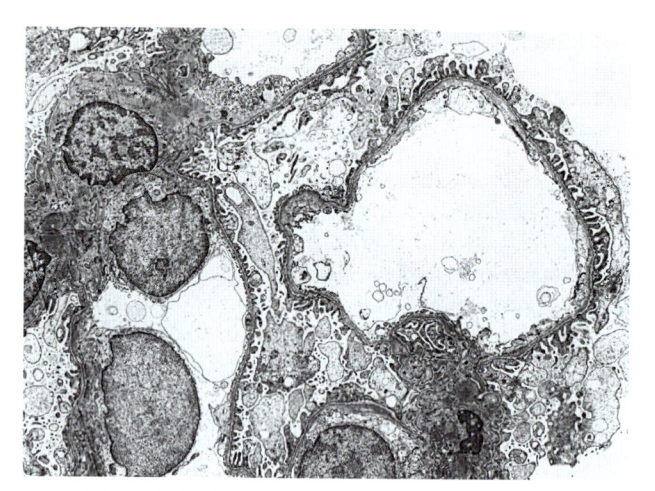

Figure 33.43 Thin basement membrane disease. By electron microscopy, the glomerular basement membranes are diffusely and uniformly thinned, measuring less than 200 nm in thickness. (×2500.)

PATHOLOGY

Renal biopsies typically show no histologic abnormalities with the exception of focal erythrocyte casts. By immunofluorescence, no glomerular deposits of immunoglobulins or complement are found. By electron microscopy, there is diffuse and relatively uniform thinning of the GBM (Figure 33.43). The normal thickness of the GBM is age and gender dependent. Vogler[739] has defined normal ranges for children: birth, 169 ± 30 nm; 2 years of age, 245 ± 49 nm; 11 years, 285 ± 39 nm. Steffes[740] has defined normal ranges for adults: males, 373 ± 42; females, 326 ± 45 nm. Each laboratory should attempt to establish its own normals for GBM thickness. A cutoff value of 250 nm has been reported by some authors,[741-743] whereas other groups have used a cutoff of 330 nm.[738] There is often accentuation of the lamina rara interna and externa. Focal GBM gaps may be identified ultrastructurally. Immunostaining for the α-subunits of collagen IV reveals a normal distribution in the GBM.

PATHOGENESIS

About 40% of TBMN disease has been linked to mutations of the *COL4A3* and *COL4A4* genes.[744] In most kindreds with TBMN, the disorder appears to be transmitted in an autosomal dominant pattern. In a few families with several affected children and apparently unaffected parents, the findings suggest a recessive mode of inheritance or that one parent was an asymptomatic carrier.[735,736,745] There appears to be a reduction or loss of the subepithelial portion of the basement membrane, which apparently contains normal relative amounts of type IV collagen.[746] The degree of GBM thinning does not appear to affect the clinical presentation or outcome.[747]

DIFFERENTIAL DIAGNOSIS OF FAMILIAL HEMATURIAS

Type IV collagen defects can cause both TBMN and Alport's syndrome. Patients with TBMN can be considered carriers of autosomal recessive Alport's syndrome.[748,749] With advances in molecular biology and immunopathology, hereditary forms of hematuria have been better characterized. Table 33.2 shows a summary of the clinical, pathologic, and genetic features of the various forms of hereditary nephritis.[750]

Since GBM thinning may be seen in early cases of Alport's syndrome, immunohistochemical analysis of α_3, α_4, and α_5-subunits should be undertaken (since genetic tests are not always practical). Table 33.3 shows the typical immunostaining patterns in the kidney and skin basement membranes.

NAIL-PATELLA SYNDROME (HEREDITARY OSTEO-ONYCHODYSPLASIA)

Nail-patella syndrome (NPS) is an autosomal dominant condition affecting tissues of both ectodermal and mesodermal origin, manifested as symmetric nail, skeletal, ocular, and renal anomalies.

CLINICAL FEATURES

The classical tetrad of anomalies of the nails, elbows, knees, and iliac horns was described by Mino and coworkers in 1948.[751] Nail dysplasia and patellar aplasia or hypoplasia are essential features for the diagnosis of NPS. The presence of triangular nail lunulae is a pathognomonic sign for NPS. Other skeletal abnormalities include dysplasia of the elbow joints, posterior iliac horns, and foot deformities. Various ocular anomalies have sporadically been found in NPS patients, including microcornea, sclerocornea, congenital cataract, iris processes, pigmentation of the inner margin of the iris, and congenital glaucoma.[752]

Renal involvement is variable, being present in up to 38% of patients. Renal manifestations first appear in children and young adults and may include proteinuria, hematuria,

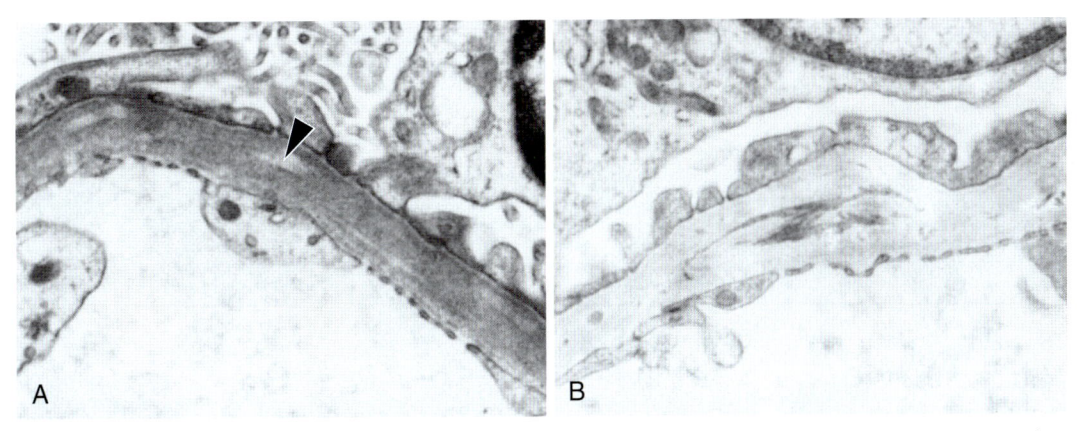

Figure 33.44 Nail-patella syndrome. **A,** Routine electron micrograph showing thickening of a glomerular basement membrane (GBM) with focal irregular internal lucencies. (×15,000.) **B,** Phosphotungstic acid–stained electron micrograph demonstrating the characteristic banded collagen fibrils within the rarefied segments of GBM. (×15,000.)

hypertension, or edema. Nephrotic syndrome and progressive renal failure may occasionally occur. The course is generally benign with renal failure being a late feature.[753,754] Congenital malformations of the urinary tract and nephrolithiasis are also more frequent in these patients. Cases with renal lesions typical of NPS but without skeletal abnormalities have been reported.[755]

PATHOLOGY

The findings on light microscopy are nonspecific and include focal and segmental glomerular sclerosis, segmental thickening of the glomerular capillary wall, and mild mesangial hypercellularity.[756] Immunofluorescence microscopy is nonspecific, and IgM and C3 have been observed in sclerosed segments. Ultrastructural studies show a thickened basement membrane that contains irregular lucencies, imparting a "moth-eaten" appearance (Figure 33.44A). The presence of intramembranous fibrils with the periodicity of collagen is revealed by phosphotungstic acid stains in electron microscopic sections, corresponding to the distribution of the intramembranous lucencies (see Figure 33.44B). These must be distinguished from the occasional collagen fibrils that can accumulate nonspecifically in the sclerotic mesangium in a variety of sclerosing glomerular conditions.[756]

PATHOGENESIS

The genetic locus for this syndrome is on chromosome 9 and results from mutations in the LIM homeodomain protein *LMX1B* gene, which is transmitted in an autosomal dominant pattern. Lmx1b plays a central role in dorsoventral patterning of the vertebrate limb.[757,758] The mechanism of disease-causing mutations is not fully elucidated, but haploinsufficiency may be associated with expression of podocyte structural proteins such as CD2AP.[755]

TREATMENT

There is no specific treatment for this condition; occasional patients with renal failure have been successfully transplanted.[759]

FABRY'S DISEASE (ANGIOKERATOMA CORPORIS DIFFUSUM UNIVERSALE)

Fabry's disease[760] is an X-linked inborn error of glycosphingolipid metabolism involving a lysosomal enzyme, α-galactosidase A (also known as ceramide trihexosidase). The enzyme deficiency leads to the accumulation of globotriaosylceramide (ceramide trihexoside) and related neutral glycosphingolipids, leading to multisystem involvement and dysfunction. Clinical guidelines for the diagnosis and treatment of Fabry's disease have been published.[761]

CLINICAL FEATURES

Fabry's disease has been reported in all ethnic groups, and the estimated incidence in males is 1 in 40,000 to 1 in 60,000. In male hemizygotes, the initial clinical presentation usually begins in childhood with episodic pain in the extremities and acroparesthesias. Renal involvement is common in male hemizygotes and is occasional in female heterozygotes. The disease presents with hematuria and proteinuria, which often progresses to nephrotic levels. In men, progressive renal failure generally develops by the fifth decade. Data from the Fabry Registry suggest that proteinuria is a strong determinant of renal outcome.[762] In the United States, Fabry's disease accounts for 0.02% of patients who began renal replacement therapy.[763]

The skin is commonly involved with reddish-purple macules (angiokeratomas) typically found "below the belt" on the abdomen, buttocks, hips, genitalia, and upper thighs. Other findings include palmar erythema, conjunctival and oral mucous membrane telangiectasia, and subungual splinter hemorrhages. The nervous system is involved with peripheral and autonomic neuropathy. Premature arterial disease of coronary vessels leads to myocardial ischemia and arrhythmias at a young age. Similarly, cerebrovascular involvement leads to early onset of strokes. In the heart, valvular disease and hypertrophic cardiomyopathy have also been reported. Corneal opacities are seen in virtually all hemizygotes and most heterozygotes. Posterior capsular cataracts, edema of retina and eyelids, and tortuous retinal and conjunctival vessels also may occur. Generalized

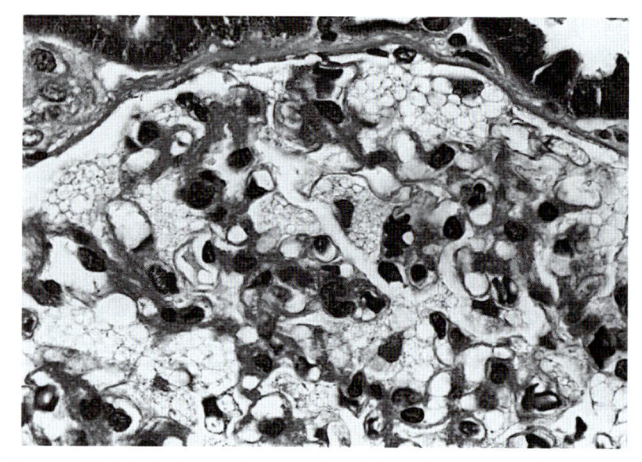

Figure 33.45 Fabry's disease. By light microscopy, the visceral epithelial cells (podocytes) are markedly enlarged with foamy-appearing cytoplasm. (Trichrome stain, ×800.)

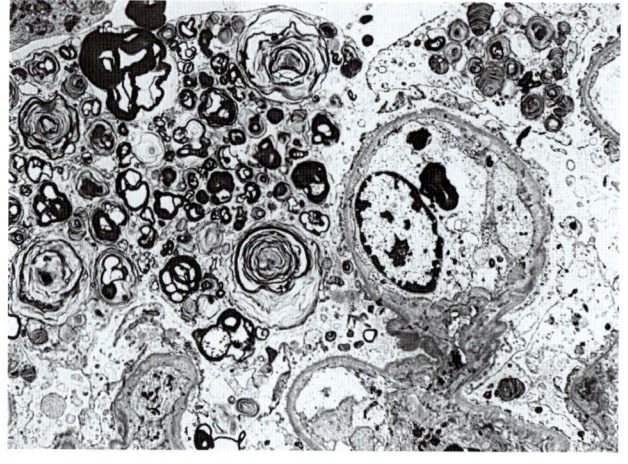

Figure 33.46 Fabry's disease. Electron micrograph showing abundant whorled myelin figures within the cytoplasm of the podocytes. A few similar inclusions are also identified within the glomerular endothelial cells. (×2000.)

lymphadenopathy, hepatosplenomegaly, aseptic necrosis of the femoral and humeral heads, myopathy, hypoalbuminemia, and hypogammaglobulinemia have been reported.

In carrier females, clinical manifestations may range from asymptomatic to severe disease similar to male hemizygotes. Up to one third of female carriers have been reported to have significant disease manifestations.[764]

PATHOLOGY

Glycosphingolipid accumulation begins early in life,[765] and the major renal site of accumulation is the podocyte (visceral epithelial cells). By light microscopy, these cells are enlarged with numerous clear, uniform vacuoles in the cytoplasm causing a foamy appearance (Figure 33.45). These vacuoles can be shown to contain lipids when fat stains (such as Oil Red O) are used or when viewed under the polarizing microscope, where they exhibit a double refractile appearance before being processed with lipid solvents. All renal cells may accumulate the lipid. These include (in addition to podocytes) parietal epithelial cells, glomerular endothelial cells, mesangial cells, interstitial capillary endothelial cells, distal convoluted tubular cells, and to a lesser extent, cells of the loops of Henle and proximal tubular cells. Indeed, vascular endothelial cells are involved in virtually every organ and tissue.[766] In the kidney, the myocytes and endothelial cells of arteries also are commonly involved. In heterozygotes, similar changes are present but with less severity.[767] Characteristic findings are noted on electron microscopy (Figure 33.46). The major finding is large numbers of "myelin figures" or "zebra bodies" within the cytoplasm of the podocytes and, to a variable extent, in other renal cell types. These intracytoplasmic vacuoles consist of single membrane-bound dense bodies with a concentric whorled or multilamellar appearance. Glomerular podocytes exhibit variable foot process effacement. The GBMs are initially normal, but with progression of disease, there may be thickening and collapse of the GBM, focal and segmental glomerular sclerosis, with accompanying tubular atrophy and interstitial fibrosis.[768] Findings on immunofluorescence microscopy are usually negative except in areas of segmental sclerosis, where IgM and complement may be demonstrated. Orange autofluorescence corresponding to the lipid inclusions may be found in podocytes and other renal cells.

PATHOGENESIS

The mutations in the *GLA* gene generally are "private," with specific molecular defects that vary from family to family, and include rearrangements, deletions, and point mutations.[769] Deficiency of the enzyme leads to accumulation of globotriaosylceramide especially in the vascular endothelium, with subsequent ischemic organ dysfunction. Patients with blood groups B and AB have earlier and more severe symptoms, likely related to accumulation of the terminal α-galactose substance during the synthesis of the B antigen on red blood cell membranes.[770] Globotriaosylceramide accumulation in podocytes may lead to proteinuria and renal dysfunction, but functional abnormalities are not always noted, especially in female heterozygotes. A gene-knockout mouse model of Fabry's disease has been produced, which shows the characteristic changes.[771]

DIAGNOSIS

The diagnosis in affected males can be established by measuring levels of α-galactosidase A in plasma or peripheral blood leukocytes followed by mutation analysis when positive. Hemizygotes have almost no measurable enzyme activity. Female carriers may have enzyme levels in the low to normal range; to diagnose female carriers, the specific mutation in the family must be demonstrated.[716] The measurement of urinary ceramide digalactoside and trihexoside levels may also be of use to identify the carrier state. Prenatal diagnosis can be made by measuring amniocyte enzyme levels in amniotic fluid. Screening of dialysis and renal transplant patients with undiagnosed renal failure, patients with hypertrophic cardiomyopathy, and patients with strokes has yielded the diagnosis of Fabry's disease in 1% to 5%.[772]

TREATMENT

Two forms of recombinant α-galactosidase A are available: agalsidase alfa (Replagal; Shire Human Genetic Therapies, Boston, MA) and agalsidase beta (Fabrazyme; Genzyme, Cambridge, MA). Agalsidase alfa is produced in a continuous human cell line and is administered as an intravenous infusion over 40 minutes at a dose of 0.2 mg/kg body weight every 2 weeks. Agalsidase beta is produced in Chinese hamster ovary (CHO) cells and is given as an intravenous infusion over a 4-hour period at a dose of 1.0 mg/kg body weight every 2 weeks.[761] Two pivotal randomized controlled trials have shown that recombinant human α-galactosidase A enzyme replacement therapy (ERT) is safe and can improve clinical parameters. In one short-term study, α-galactosidase A treatment was associated with improved neuropathic pain, decreased mesangial widening, and improved creatinine clearance.[773] In the second study, repeat renal biopsies showed decreased microvascular endothelial deposits of globotriaosylceramide.[766,774] However, a systematic review that included five trials and 187 patients did not provide robust evidence for the use of replacement therapy.[775] From a renal standpoint, open-label extension studies showed that renal function remained stable in the long term in most patients with normal renal function at baseline.[776,777] However, patients with impaired baseline renal function may show continued decline despite ERT.[777] Since there is a paucity of data showing hard outcomes (ESKD, doubling of creatinine, death), the recommendation is to start ERT only in patients with CKD stages 1 and 2 and only in the context of a clinical trial (interventional or observational).[761] Dose reduction of ERT or a switch from agalsidase beta to agalsidase alfa (which occurred during a shortage of agalsidase beta) has been associated with worsening albuminuria, decline in eGFR (in the switch group), and worsening pain scores (in the dose reduction group).[778] The experience with ERT in female carriers is limited. Clinical recommendations for the treatment of Fabry's disease have been published.[761]

The ERA–EDTA Registry in Europe reported that patient survival on dialysis was 41% at 5 years; cardiovascular complications (48%) and cachexia (17%) were the main causes of death. Graft survival at 3 years in 33 patients was not inferior to that of other nephropathies (72% vs. 69%), and patient survival after transplantation was comparable to that of patients younger than 55 years of age.[779] In the U.S. population, survival of patients with Fabry's disease was lower than nondiabetic renal failure patients.[763] Long-term allograft function in patients with Fabry's disease has been reported. Glycosphingolipid deposits recur in allografts but have not been reported to cause graft failure.[780]

SICKLE CELL NEPHROPATHY

Renal disease associated with sickle cell disease includes gross hematuria, papillary necrosis, nephrotic syndrome, renal infarction, inability to concentrate urine, renal medullary carcinoma, and pyelonephritis.[781,782] Microscopic or gross hematuria is likely the result of microinfarcts in the renal medulla.[783] Glomerular lesions, however, are less commonly encountered and may be seen in patients with sickle cell hemoglobin (HbSS) disease, sickle–hemoglobin C (HbSC) disease, and sickle cell thalessemia.[784]

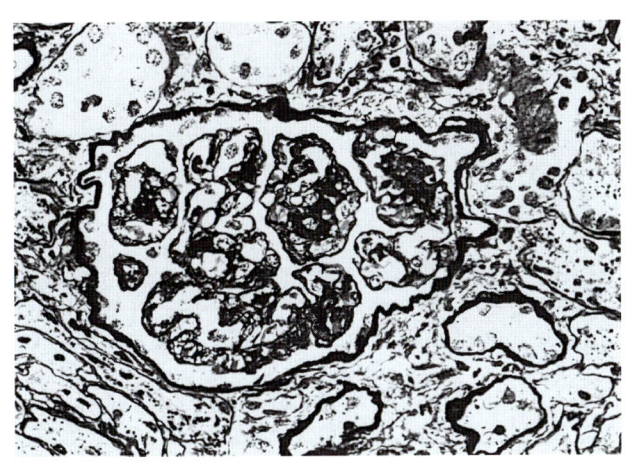

Figure 33.47 Sickle cell disease. An example of sickle cell glomerulopathy with membranoproliferative features. There are double contours of the glomerular basement membrane associated with segmental mesangiolysis. (Jones' methenamine silver stain, ×500.)

CLINICAL FEATURES

In one study, the prevalence of proteinuria (>1+ on a dipstick) in HbSS disease was 26%.[784] The majority of proteinuric patients had less than 3 g/day and elevated serum creatinine levels were present in 7% of patients. In another study, 4.2% with HbSS disease and 2.4% with HbSC disease developed renal failure. The median age of disease onset for these patients was 23.1 and 49.9 years, respectively. Survival time for patients with HbSS anemia after the diagnosis of renal failure, despite dialysis, was 4 years, and the median age at the time of death was 27 years. The risk for renal failure was increased in patients with the Central African Republic β S–gene cluster haplotype, hypertension, proteinuria, and severe anemia.[785] The course of HbSS renal disease is progressive; in one series, 18% of patients with HbSS disease progressed to ESKD.[786]

PATHOLOGY

Early glomerular lesions in patients with HbSS include enlarged glomeruli and dilated and congested capillaries containing sickled erythrocytes (some of these patients may have nephrotic proteinuria).[787] Heterogeneous patterns of glomerular injury have been reported. A membranoproliferative pattern exhibits mesangial proliferation with mild to moderate capillary wall thickening due to GBM reduplication and mesangial interposition (Figure 33.47). Some of these patients also exhibit features of chronic thrombotic microangiopathy, with narrow double contours of the GBM and mesangiolysis. A pattern of membranous glomerulonephritis has also been described. On immunofluorescence microscopy, irregular granular deposits of IgG and C3 have been reported in those cases with membranous features and in a subgroup of cases with membranoproliferative pattern on light microscopy.[787,788] Ultrastructural studies show granular dense deposits in the mesangial and subepithelial area. More commonly, those cases with membranoproliferative

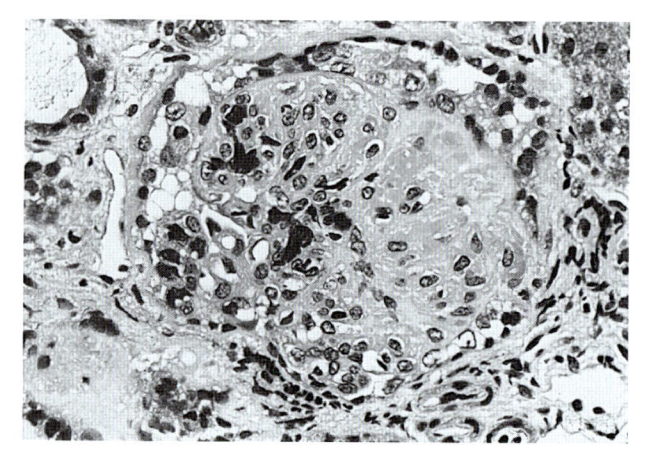

Figure 33.48 Sickle cell disease. An example with focal segmental glomerulosclerosis. The nonsclerotic glomerular capillaries are congested with sickled erythrocytes. (Hematoxylin and eosin stain, ×500.)

features have no detectable deposits but exhibit subendothelial accumulation of electron lucent "fluff" resembling the changes in chronic thrombotic microangiopathies. Mild mesangial proliferation and peripheral mesangial interposition are frequently seen. Sickled erythrocytes containing paracrystalline inclusions may be identified within glomerular capillaries.[788-792]

In the second form of sickle glomerulopathy, FSGS occurs in association with glomerulomegaly (Figure 33.48). Two patterns of FSGS may be observed: a "collapsing" pattern and an "expansive" pattern.[781,784,793-795] Using the modern classification of FSGS, collapsing, perihilar, tip, and not otherwise specified (NOS) variants have been reported.[787] On immunofluorescence, nonspecific IgM and C3 are seen in sclerosed segments. In all these forms, there may be prominent intracapillary erythrocyte sickling and congestion.

PATHOGENESIS

The mechanism(s) for glomerular abnormalities in HbSS patients is not fully understood. One theory proposes that mesangial cells are activated by the presence of fragmented red blood cells in glomerular capillaries. Activated mesangial cells promote synthesis of matrix proteins and migrate into the peripheral capillary wall, leading to GBM reduplication.[796] In another study, renal tubular epithelial antigens and complement components were detected in a granular pattern along the GBM, leading the authors to hypothesize that glomerulonephritis was mediated by glomerular deposition of immune complexes containing renal tubular epithelial antigen and specific antibody to renal tubular epithelial antigen (the antigen possibly released after tubular damage secondary to decreased oxygenation and hemodynamic alterations related to HbSS disease).[788]

In patients with the FSGS pattern, it is proposed that there is an initial but progressive obliteration of the glomerular capillary bed by red blood cell sickling that cannot be compensated by further glomerular hypertrophy. Hemodynamic glomerular injury ensues from the sustained or increasing hyperfiltration in a diminishing capillary bed, manifesting morphologically as the expansive pattern of sclerosis.[784,793] According to one report, the hyperfiltration observed in 51% of HbSS patients correlated positively with lower hemoglobin levels and reticulocyte counts, implying that the hemolysis-related vasculopathy may be contributing.[797] A role for reactive oxygen species as mediator of chronic vascular endothelial injury has also been proposed.[798]

Recently, polymorphisms in the *MYH9* and *APOL1* genes have been associated with risk for proteinuria in patients with HbSS disease. GFR was negatively correlated with proteinuria ($P < 0.0001$) and was significantly predicted by an interaction between *MYH9* and *APOL1* in a multivariable model.[799]

TREATMENT

The treatment of renal disease has generally been unsatisfactory. Treatment of patients with sickle cell nephropathy with ACEIs reduces the degree of proteinuria.[784,800] However, their effectiveness in preserving renal function remains to be established.[801] Hematopoietic stem cell transplantation in selected patients with sickle cell disease was found to be effective in preventing renal function decline compared to nontransplanted patients.[802]

HbSS nephropathy accounts for 0.1% of ESKD patients in the United States, with a higher mortality compared to other causes of ESKD (including diabetes).[803] Renal transplantation has been performed in HbSS patients. One-year graft survival in HbSS patients was similar to other transplanted patients; however, long-term renal outcome was worse, as was short- and long-term mortality.[804] Transplanted HbSS patients commonly experience sickle crises.[805,806] Recurrent sickle cell nephropathy has been reported in the transplanted kidney.[794,807] Patient survival has improved compared to previously, with survival rates comparable to diabetic recipients.[808]

LIPODYSTROPHY

Lipodystrophies are rare diseases associated with insulin resistance in which there is loss of fat, which may be localized to the upper part of the body in partial lipodystrophy (PLD) or more diffuse in generalized lipodystrophy (GLD).[809,810]

A majority of patients with GLD (both genetic and acquired) are proteinuric and have an elevated GFR (reflecting hyperfiltration). Renal biopsy showed FSGS as the most common finding, followed by MPGN type I and only rarely diabetic nephropathy.[811]

PLD is commonly associated with dense deposit disease. PLD most often presents in girls between ages 5 and 15 years. In addition to the loss of fat, the lipodystrophies are associated with a wide variety of metabolic and systemic abnormalities. Hyperinsulinism, insulin resistance, and diabetes are common. Other metabolic abnormalities include hyperlipidemia, hyperproteinemia, and euthyroid hypermetabolism. Clinical findings may include tall stature, muscular hypertrophy, hirsutism, macroglossia, abdominal distension, subcutaneous nodules, acanthosis nigricans, hepatomegaly, cirrhosis, clitoral or penile enlargement, febrile adenopathy, cerebral atrophy, cerebral ventricular dilation, hemiplegia, mental retardation, and cardiomegaly.[809,810] Renal disease occurs in 20% to 50% of patients with PLD,[809,810] and PLD occurs in 10% of patients with dense deposit disease.[812,813] Patients usually have asymptomatic proteinuria and microhematuria, but some may develop nephrotic syndrome.[814,815] Diminished C3 levels in association with the C3 nephritic factor (C3NeF) is the most prominent serologic abnormality. The course of glomerular disease is fairly rapid progression to ESKD, and the prognosis of PLD is determined mainly by renal disease.[810]

In GLD, nephrotic syndrome, nonnephrotic proteinuria, and hypertension have been reported.[809] A total of 88% of these patients had albumin excretion greater than 30 mg/24 hr, 60% had macroalbuminuria (>300 mg/24 hr), and 20% had nephrotic-range proteinuria greater than 3500 mg/24 hr.[816]

The pathogenesis of PLD and GLD is poorly understood. Acquired forms of lipodystrophy are believed to be autoimmune disorders. Most patients with PLD possess an IgG autoantibody, C3 nephritic factor (C3NeF), which binds to and stabilizes the alternate pathway convertase C3 convertase–C3bBb. In the presence of C3NeF, C3bBb becomes resistant to its regulatory proteins, factors H and I. Although the majority of patients with partial dystrophy have low serum C3, not all patients will exhibit nephritis.[817] There is no effective therapy for PLD, and although renal transplantation is the treatment of choice when ESKD ensues, recurrence in transplants has been reported.[810,818,819] In GLD, leptin therapy has been associated with improvement of renal parameters.[820] A single GLD patient has undergone renal transplantation.[821]

LECITHIN-CHOLESTEROL ACYLTRANSFERASE DEFICIENCY

Gjone and Norum reported a familial disorder characterized by proteinuria, anemia, hyperlipidemia, and corneal opacity.[822,823] Most of the initial patients were of Scandinavian origin; subsequently lecithin-cholesterol acyltransferase (LCAT) deficiency was reported from other countries.[824,825]

CLINICAL FEATURES

The triad of anemia, nephrotic syndrome, and corneal opacities suggests this disorder. Renal disease is a universal finding with albuminuria noted early in life. Proteinuria increases in severity during the fourth and fifth decades, often with development of nephrotic syndrome. The latter is accompanied by hypertension and progressive renal failure. Most patients are mildly anemic with target cells and poikilocytes on the peripheral smear. There is evidence of low-grade hemolysis. During childhood, corneal opacities appear as grayish spots over the cornea, accompanied by a lipoid arcus. Visual acuity is unimpaired. Fish eye disease results from a partial deficiency of LCAT and presents with corneal disease and without renal manifestations. Patients have reduced plasma high-density lipoprotein cholesterol concentrations (usually <0.3 mmol/L; 11.6 mg/dL) and plasma levels of apo A-I below 50 mg/dL. Premature atherosclerosis is unusual in complete LCAT deficiency but may occur from unknown reasons in fish eye disease.[826]

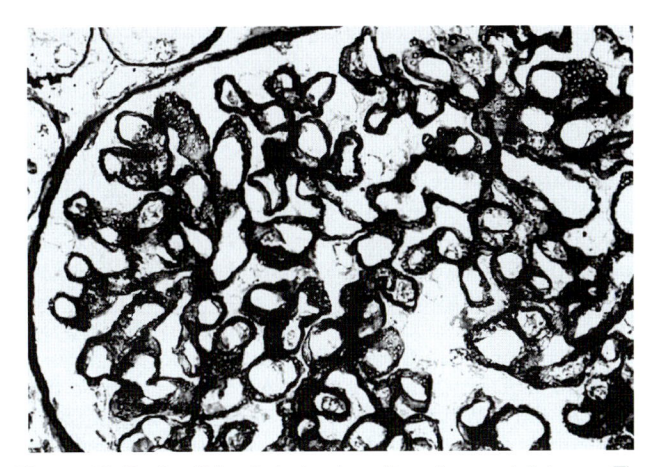

Figure 33.49 Lecithin-cholesterol acyltransferase deficiency. The glomerular basement membranes and mesangium have a vacuolated appearance, resembling stage 3 membranous glomerulopathy. (Jones' methenamine silver stain, ×800.)

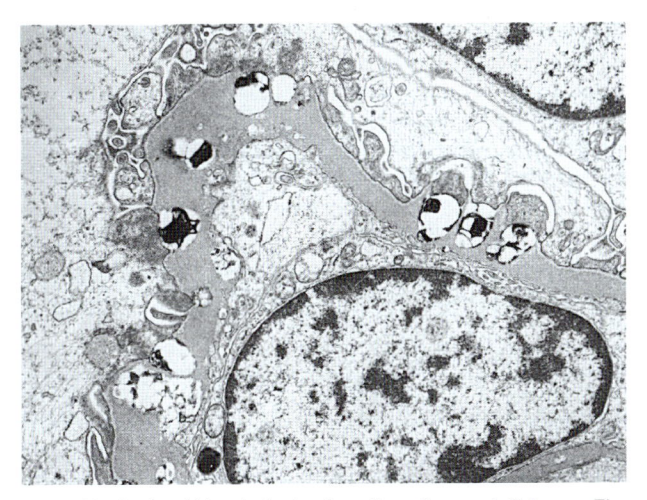

Figure 33.50 Lecithin-cholesterol acyltransferase deficiency. Electron micrograph showing intramembranous lacunae with rounded structures containing an electron-dense membranous core and electron-lucent periphery. (×5000.)

PATHOLOGY

Abnormalities are found mainly in the glomeruli, but arteries and arterioles may also be affected.[822,823,827,828] By light microscopy (Figure 33.49), the glomerular capillary walls are thickened and there is mesangial expansion. Basement membranes are irregular and often appear to contain vacuoles, resembling stage 3 membranous alterations. Double contouring of capillary walls is occasionally present. Similar vacuoles in the mesangium impart a honeycomb appearance. There is no associated glomerular hypercellularity, with the exception of occasional endocapillary foam cells. By immunofluorescence microscopy, there is typically negative staining for all immunoglobulin and complement components. On electron microscopy (Figure 33.50), the vacuolated areas seen by light microscopy correspond to extracellular irregular lucent zones (lacunae) in the mesangial matrix and GBM containing lipid inclusions. These inclusions consist of rounded, small, structures, either solid or with a lamellar substructure containing electron-lucent and electron-dense zones.

PATHOGENESIS

The disorder is inherited in an autosomal recessive pattern. Patients have little or no LCAT activity in their blood circulation because of mutations in the *LCAT* gene.[829,830] LCAT is an enzyme that circulates in the blood primarily bound to high-density lipoprotein and catalyzes the formation of cholesteryl esters via the hydrolysis and transfer of the sn-2 fatty acid from phosphatidylcholine to the 3-hydroxyl group of cholesterol. Thus patients with LCAT deficiency have high levels of phosphatidylcholine and unesterified cholesterol, with corresponding low levels of lysophosphatidylcholine and cholesteryl ester in the blood. An abnormal lipoprotein, lipoprotein-X (Lp-X) is present in patients' plasma. Lp-X is thought to arise from the surface of chylomicron remnants that are not further metabolized due to the absence of active LCAT. Accumulation of lipid component occurs in both intra- and extracellular sites. Lipid accumulation in the GBM results in proteinuria. Endothelial damage and resulting vascular insufficiency may contribute to renal insufficiency. It has been proposed that Lp-X stimulates mesangial cells, leading to the production of MCP-1 (monocyte chemoattractant protein-1), promoting monocyte infiltration, foam cell formation, and progressive glomerulosclerosis in a manner similar to atherosclerosis.[831] Rarely, acquired autoimmune LCAT deficiency may occur, with renal biopsy findings similar to familial LCAT deficiency with coexisting lesion of membranous nephropathy.[832]

DIAGNOSIS

In patients suspected of having LCAT deficiency, measurements of plasma enzyme should be performed. The enzyme levels and activity vary among kindreds[833]; thus, enzyme measurements should include activity as well as mass.

TREATMENT

Neither a low-lipid diet nor lipid-lowering drugs have shown to be of benefit.[827] Plasma infusions may provide reversal of erythrocytic abnormalities, but long-term benefits have yet to be demonstrated.[834] The lesions may recur in the allograft, but renal function is adequately preserved.[835]

LIPOPROTEIN GLOMERULOPATHY

Lipoprotein glomerulopathy (LPG) is characterized by dysbetalipoproteinemia and lipid deposition in the kidney, leading to glomerulosclerosis and renal failure. The majority of patients have been from Japan.[836,837]

The histologic hallmark of LPG is the presence of laminated thrombi consisting of lipids within the lumina of dilated glomerular capillaries. The pathogenesis of LPG is unknown, but the presence of thrombi consisting of lipoproteins suggests a primary abnormality in lipid metabolism.[838] Indeed type III hyperlipidemia (elevated LDL and high apo E levels) have been reported in Japanese patients, associated with apo E variants (commonly apo E-II as opposed to apo E-III).[837,839-843] Other genetic variants, such as apo E (Las Vegas), have been reported in Caucasians of European descent in the United States.[844] Furthermore, LPG-like deposits were detected in apo E–deficient mice transfected with apo E (Sendai), one of the apo E variants associated with LPG.

There is no uniformly effective therapy for LPG; however, intensive lipid-lowering therapy has been reported to be effective in one patient with LPG.[845] Recurrence of lesions of LPG have occurred in renal allografts.[846,847]

GLOMERULAR INVOLVEMENT WITH BACTERIAL INFECTIONS

INFECTIOUS ENDOCARDITIS

The natural history of endocarditis-associated glomerulonephritis has changed significantly in parallel with the changing epidemiology of infectious endocarditis and the advent of antibiotics.[848] In the pre-antibiotic era, *Streptococcus viridans* was the commonest organism and glomerulonephritis occurred in 50% to 80% of endocarditis cases.[849] During that era, glomerulonephritis was less common in association with acute endocarditis.[850,851] With the use of prophylactic antibiotics in patients with valvular heart disease, and an increase in intravenous drug use, *Staphylococcus aureus* has replaced *S. viridans* as the primary pathogen. Glomerulonephritis in these patients with acute infectious endocarditis occurs as commonly as in subacute endocarditis.[849,852-854] The incidence of glomerulonephritis with endocarditis with *S. aureus* ranges from 22% to 78%,[852,855] being higher in those series consisting predominantly of intravenous drug users.[855,856]

CLINICAL FEATURES

Renal complications of infectious endocarditis include infarcts, abscesses, and glomerulonephritis (all of which may coexist). In focal glomerulonephritis, mild asymptomatic urinary abnormalities, including hematuria, pyuria, and albuminuria, may be noted. Infrequently, with severe focal glomerulonephritis, renal insufficiency or uremia may be present. Renal dysfunction, microhematuria or gross hematuria, and nephrotic-range proteinuria may be present with diffuse glomerulonephritis.[849,852,857] Rapidly progressive renal failure with crescents has been reported.[849,858] Rarely, patients may present with vasculitic features (including purpura).[859] Although hypocomplementemia is frequent, it is neither invariable (occurring in 60% to 90% of patients with glomerulonephritis) nor specific for renal involvement.[854,855] The majority of patients demonstrate activation of the classical pathway.[855,860] Alternate pathway activation has been described in some cases of *S. aureus* endocarditis.[855] The degree of complement activation correlates with the severity of renal impairment,[855] and the complement levels normalize with successful therapy of the infection. Circulating immune complexes have been found in the serum in up to 90% of patients.[860,861] Mixed cryoglobulins and rheumatoid factor may also be present in the serum of patients.[854,862] ANCA positivity has been occasionally reported in biopsy-proven immune complex glomerulonephritis associated with infectious endocarditis, some of which have necrotizing and crescentic features.[863] Anti-GBM antibody in eluates from diseased glomeruli has been reported rarely.[864]

PATHOLOGY

On light microscopy, focal and segmental endocapillary proliferative glomerulonephritis with focal crescents is the most typical finding. Necrotizing lesions may be present. Some patients may exhibit a more diffuse endocapillary proliferative and exudative glomerulonephritis with or without crescents.[849,850,852,865,866] Immunofluorescence reveals granular capillary and mesangial deposits of IgG and C3, C3 alone, or varying combinations of IgM, IgG, and C3.[849,852,865] The finding of predominant IgM staining may be associated with *Bartonella* endocarditis.[867] Electron microscopy shows electron-dense deposits in mesangial, subendothelial, and occasionally subepithelial locations, with varying degrees of mesangial and endocapillary proliferation.[849,852,865,868] Rarely, patients with endocarditis may be ANCA positive with renal biopsy showing concomitant necrotizing lesions and proliferative lesions with relatively scant immune complex deposition.[869]

PATHOGENESIS

The diffuse deposition of immunoglobulin, the depression of complement, and electron-dense deposits supports an immune complex mechanism for the production of this form of glomerulonephritis. The demonstration of specific antibody in kidney eluates and the detection of bacterial antigen in the deposits further support this view. Both *S. aureus*[870] and hemolytic *Streptococcus*[871] antigens have been identified.

TREATMENT

With the initiation of antibiotic therapy, the manifestations of glomerulonephritis begin to subside. Rarely, microhematuria and proteinuria may persist for years.[849] Plasmapheresis and corticosteroids have been reported to promote renal recovery in some patients with renal failure.[858,872] However, this approach should be taken cautiously because of the risk of promoting infectious aspects of the disease while ameliorating the immunologic manifestations. Immunosuppression has also been used to treat patients with concomitant ANCA and immune complex–associated glomerulonephritis.[869]

SHUNT NEPHRITIS

Ventriculovascular (ventriculoatrial, ventriculojugular) shunts (which are rarely used nowadays) for the treatment of hydrocephalus were colonized commonly with microorganisms, particularly *Staphylococcus albus* (75%).[873] Less often, other bacteria (e.g., *Propionibacterium acnes*) have been implicated.[874,875] Ventriculoperitoneal shunts are more resistant to infection. However, glomerulonephritis has been reported with these shunts as well.[876]

Patients commonly present with fever. Anemia, hepatosplenomegaly, purpura, arthralgias, and lymphadenopathy are found on examination. Renal manifestations include hematuria (microscopic or gross), proteinuria (nephrotic syndrome in 30% of patients), azotemia, and hypertension. Laboratory abnormalities include presence of rheumatoid factor, cryoimmunoglobulins, elevated sedimentation rate and CRP levels, hypocomplementemia, and presence of circulating immune complexes.[877,878] Shunt nephritis usually presents within a few months of shunt placement, but delayed manifestations as late as 17 years have been reported.[879] By light microscopy, glomeruli exhibit mesangial proliferation or membranoproliferative pattern of glomerulonephritis. Immunofluorescence reveals diffuse granular deposits of IgG, IgM, and C3. IgM is often the predominant Ig deposited in shunt nephritis. Electron-dense mesangial and subendothelial deposits are found by electron microscopy.[875,880] Antibiotic therapy and prompt removal of the infected catheter usually lead to remission of the glomerulonephritis.[881] However, cases progressing to chronic renal failure have been reported.[882] Rarely, patients have elevated PR3-specific ANCA titers, which also improved after removal of the infected shunt, with or without corticosteroid therapy.[883]

VISCERAL INFECTION

Visceral infections in the form of abdominal, pulmonary, and retroperitoneal abscesses are known to be associated with glomerulonephritis.[884] The clinical and pathologic features of the syndrome resemble those of infective endocarditis. Beaufils and colleagues reported on 11 patients who had visceral abscesses and in whom acute renal failure developed. Circulating cryoglobulins, decreased serum complement levels, and circulating immune complexes were found in some of these patients. All renal biopsies showed a diffuse proliferative and crescentic glomerulonephritis. The evolution of the glomerulonephritis, documented by serial biopsies, closely paralleled the course of the infection. A complete recovery of renal function occurred in those cases in which a rapid and complete cure of the infection was obtained. For those patients in whom the infection was not cured or in whom therapy was delayed, chronic renal failure also developed.[885] Outcome is worse in older patients and in diabetics.[848]

OTHER BACTERIAL INFECTIONS AND FUNGAL INFECTIONS

Congenital, secondary, and latent forms of syphilis rarely may be complicated by glomerular involvement. Patients are typically nephrotic, and proteinuria usually responds to penicillin therapy.[886-890] Membranous nephropathy with varying degrees of proliferation and with granular IgG and C3 deposits is the commonest finding on biopsies. Treponemal antigen and antibody have been eluted from deposits. Rarely minimal change lesions[891] and crescentic glomerulonephritis[892] or amyloidosis may be seen.

Bartonella henselae is the organism responsible for bartonellosis (cat scratch disease), which typically manifests as a skin papule followed by regional lymphadenopathy. Rarely, endocarditis, central nervous system involvement (encephalopathy), generalized skin rash, and the Parinaud oculoglandular syndrome (fever, regional lymphadenopathy, and follicular conjunctivitis) may occur. Renal manifestations are rare and can include IgA nephropathy,[893] postinfectious glomerulonephritis with IgM dominance,[867,894] or necrotizing glomerulonephritis.[895] In general, spontaneous recovery may occur with control of infection; however, end-stage renal failure has been reported with aggressive renal disease.[895]

Renal involvement, including azotemia, proteinuria, nephrotic syndrome, renal tubular defects, and hematuria, is not uncommon in leprosy, especially with the lepra reaction.[896-901] Rarely, patients present with RPGN[902] or ESKD.[903] Mesangial proliferation, diffuse proliferative glomerulonephritis, crescentic glomerulonephritis, membranous nephropathy, MPGN, microscopic angiitis, and amyloidosis may all be seen in kidney biopsies. Organisms consistent with *Mycobacterium leprae* have been found in glomeruli.

Aspergillosis has been associated with immune complex–mediated glomerulonephritis.[904] Membranous nephropathy, MPGN, crescentic glomerulonephritis, and amyloidosis have been associated with *Mycobacterium tuberculosis*.[905,906-908] *Mycoplasma* has been reported to be associated with nephrotic syndrome and RPGN. Antibiotics do not seem to alter the course of the disease. Mycoplasmal antigen has been reported to be present in the glomerular lesions.[909-913] Acute glomerulonephritis with hypocomplementemia has been reported with pneumococcal infections. Proliferative glomerulonephritis with deposition of IgG, IgM, complements C1q, C3, and C4, and pneumococcal antigens have been observed in renal biopsies.[914,915] Nocardiosis has been associated with mesangiocapillary glomerulonephritis.[916] In infections with *Brucella*, patients may present with hematuria, proteinuria (usually nephrotic), and varying degrees of renal functional impairment. There usually is improvement after antibiotics, but histologic abnormalities, proteinuria, and hypertension may persist. Glomerular mesangial proliferation, focal and segmental endocapillary proliferation, diffuse proliferation, and crescents may be found in renal biopsies. Immunofluorescence may show no deposits, IgG, or occasionally IgA.[917-921] Asymptomatic urinary abnormalities may be seen in up to 80% of patients infected with *Leptospira*. Patients usually present with acute renal failure due to tubulointerstitial nephritis. Rarely, mesangial or diffuse proliferative glomerulonephritis may be seen.[922,923] From 1% to 4% of patients with typhoid fever secondary to *Salmonella* experience glomerulonephritis. Asymptomatic urinary abnormalities may be more frequent. Renal manifestations are usually transient, resolving within 2 to 3 weeks. Serum C3 may be depressed. Mesangial proliferation with deposits of IgG, C3, and C4 is the commonest finding. IgA nephropathy has also been reported.[924-926]

GLOMERULAR INVOLVEMENT WITH PARASITIC DISEASES

MALARIA

Four strains of malaria parasite cause human disease: *Plasmodium vivax, Plasmodium falciparum, Plasmodium malariae* (causing quartan malaria), and *Plasmodium ovale*. Of these, renal involvement has been extensively documented and studied in *P. malariae* and *P. falciparum*. In *P. falciparum* malaria, clinically overt glomerular disease is uncommon. Asymptomatic urinary abnormalities may occur with subnephrotic-range proteinuria and hematuria or pyuria. Renal function is usually normal. Renal biopsies show mesangial proliferation or membranoproliferative lesions.[927] Severe malaria may be manifest with hemoglobinuric acute renal failure.[928] In initial reports, quartan malaria was strongly associated with nephrotic syndrome in infected children. There was progression to end-stage renal failure within 3 to 5 years with no improvement following antimalarial treatment or steroids.[929] Renal biopsies in Ugandan adults and children with quartan malaria showed some form of proliferative glomerulonephritis (diffuse, focal, lobular, or minimal). Membranous nephropathy had also been described in these patients.[930] However, in Nigerian children, the most common lesion was a localized or diffuse thickening of glomerular capillary walls with focal or generalized double-contouring and segmental glomerular sclerosis.[931] Immunofluorescence examination revealed deposits of IgG, IgM, C3, and *P. malariae* antigen in the glomeruli. By electron microscopy, electron-dense material was observed within the irregularly thickened GBM.[932] Of note, a recent report from endemic areas in Nigeria has not found any cases of childhood nephrotic syndrome associated with quartan malaria.[933] The propensity of malaria to cause glomerular disease may be related to impaired clearance of immune complexes owing to reduced expression of complement receptor 1 (CR1) on monocytes/macrophages by the parasite. CR1 binds complement-bound immune complexes, which is critical to their clearance from the circulation.[934]

SCHISTOSOMIASIS

Schistosomiasis is a visceral parasitic disease caused by the blood flukes of the genus *Schistosoma*. *Schistosoma mansoni* and *Schistosoma japonicum* cause cirrhosis of the liver and *Schistosoma hematobium* causes cystitis. Glomerular involvement in *S. mansoni* includes mesangial proliferation, focal sclerosis, membranoproliferative lesions, crescentic changes, membranous nephropathy, amyloidosis, and eventually end-stage kidney disease.[935-937] Schistosomal antigens have been demonstrated in renal biopsies in such patients.[938] Treatment with antiparasitic agents does not appear to influence progression of renal disease.[939] *S. hematobium* is occasionally associated with nephrotic syndrome, which may respond to treatment of the parasite.[935] In some patients with schistosomiasis, renal involvement may be related to concomitant *Salmonella* infection.[940]

LEISHMANIASIS, TRYPANOSOMIASIS, AND FILARIASIS

Leishmaniasis, also known as kala-azar, is caused by *Leishmania donovani*. Renal involvement in kala-azar appears to be mild and reverts with anti-leishmanial treatment. Renal biopsies show glomerular mesangial proliferation or focal endocapillary proliferation. IgG, IgM, and C3 may be observed in areas of proliferation. Amyloidosis may also complicate kala-azar.[941,942] In trypanosomiasis, *Trypanosoma brucei, Trypanosoma gambiense,* and *Trypanosoma rhodesiense* cause African sleeping sickness and have rarely been associated with proteinuria.[943] Filariasis is caused by organisms in the genera *Onchocerca, Brugia, Loa,* and *Wuchereria*. Hematuria and proteinuria (including nephrotic syndrome) have been described. Renal manifestations may appear with treatment of infection. Renal biopsy findings have included mesangial proliferative glomerulonephritis with C3 deposition, diffuse proliferative glomerulonephritis, and collapsing glomerulopathy with loiasis.[944-949] In patients with lymphatic filariasis of the renal hilus, chyluria (the passage of milky white urine containing lymphatic fluid) may mimic nephrotic syndrome by producing nephrotic-range proteinuria but is distinguished by the absence of hypoalbuminemia or glomerular disease on biopsy.[950]

OTHER PARASITIC DISEASES

Trichinosis, caused by *Trichinella spiralis*, may be associated with proteinuria and hematuria, which abated after specific treatment. Renal biopsies in patients with loiasis have shown mesangial proliferative glomerulonephritis with C3 deposition.[951,952] *Echinococcus granulosus* and *Echinococcus multilocularis* cause hydatid disease, or echinococcosis, in humans. Mesangiocapillary glomerulonephritis and membranous nephropathy have occasionally been associated with hepatic hydatid cysts.[953,954] Toxoplasmosis may be associated with nephrotic syndrome in infants and, rarely, in adults. Mesangial and endothelial proliferation may be found, with deposition of IgG, IgA, IgM, C3, and fibrinogen in areas of proliferation.[955-957]

GLOMERULAR INVOLVEMENT WITH VIRAL INFECTIONS

Viruses have been postulated to cause glomerular injury by various mechanisms, including direct cytopathic effects, the deposition of immune complexes, or by initiation of autoimmune mechanisms.

In a study of previously healthy people with nonstreptococcal upper respiratory infections, 4% had erythrocyte casts and glomerulonephritis on biopsy. A reduction in serum complement and serologic evidence of infection with adenovirus, influenza A, or influenza B were observed in some. Initial renal biopsy showed either focal or diffuse mesangial proliferation in all nine specimens, with mesangial C3 deposits in six specimens. Sequential creatinine clearances were reduced in about half these patients during follow-up.[958]

Nephrotic syndrome has been described with Epstein-Barr virus (EBV) infections.[959] Renal biopsies in patients with urinary abnormalities have shown immune complex–mediated glomerulonephritis with tubulointerstitial nephritis,[960] minimal glomerular lesions with IgM deposition,[961] membranous nephropathy,[962] and widespread glomerular mesangiolysis sometimes admixed with segmental mesangial sclerosis.[963] In addition, the presence of EBV DNA in the glomerulus is thought to worsen glomerular damage in chronic glomerulopathies.[964] Other viruses have rarely been associated with glomerulonephritis, including herpes zoster, mumps, adenovirus, echovirus, coxsackievirus, and influenza A and B.[965]

HIV-RELATED GLOMERULOPATHIES

An estimated 35.3 million people are living with HIV worldwide, with more than 2 million new infections appearing each year.[966] A variety of glomerular lesions—and in particular, a unique form of glomerular damage, HIV-associated nephropathy (HIVAN)—are associated with HIV-infected patients.[967,968] Following the introduction of combination antiretroviral therapy (cART) in 1996, patients with acquired immunodeficiency syndrome (AIDS) are living longer with a concomitant change in the epidemiology of renal diseases.[969] The incidence of ESKD from HIVAN appears to have plateaued at 800 to 900 new cases each year, with an accompanying rise in prevalence on account of patients surviving longer because of cART.[672] Corresponding to this observation, the histologic diagnosis of HIVAN decreased from 80% to 20% from 1997 to 2004 in HIV-infected patients. However, in resource-poor countries, HIVAN remains a common cause of ESKD.[969]

HIV-ASSOCIATED NEPHROPATHY

CLINICAL FEATURES

In 1984, the first detailed account of a new pattern of sclerosing glomerulopathy in HIV-infected patients was reported.[970] Subsequent studies largely from large urban centers confirmed the occurrence and described the features of HIVAN.[970-980] In these largely urban East Coast centers, the prevalence of HIVAN approached 90% in nephrotic HIV-positive patients in contrast to a prevalence of only 2% in San Francisco where most seropositive patients were white homosexuals.[981-983]

There is a strong predilection for HIVAN among black HIV-infected patients. The black-to-white ratio among patients with HIVAN is 12 : 1.[984] HIVAN is the third leading cause of ESKD among black Americans aged 20 to 64, following diabetes and hypertension.[977,985] Racial factors may influence rates of mutations in HIV receptors, which may in part explain some differences in the racial predisposition to HIV infection and HIVAN.[986-988] Mapping by admixture linkage disequilibrium has linked HIVAN and sporadic FSGS to variants in the *MHY9* gene and in a subsequent study showed a stronger association to the closely linked *APOL1* gene on chromosome 22, thereby explaining most of the strong black racial predominance in these conditions.[989,990]

Although intravenous drug use has been the most common risk factor for HIVAN, the disease has been seen in all groups at risk for AIDS, including homosexuals, perinatally acquired disease, heterosexual transmission, and exposure to contaminated blood products.[967] HIVAN usually occurs in patients with a low CD4 count, but full-blown AIDS is certainly not a prerequisite for the disease. In one New York study, the onset of HIVAN was most common in otherwise asymptomatic HIV-infected patients (i.e., 12 of 26 were asymptomatic patients).[970,974] There is no relationship between the development of HIVAN and patient age and duration of HIV infection or types of opportunistic infections or malignancies.[967] The prevalence of HIVAN in patients who test positive for HIV is reported to be 3.5% in patients screened in the clinic setting[991]; the same investigative group reported that HIVAN was found in 6.9% of autopsies in HIV-infected patients.[992]

The clinical features of HIVAN include presenting features of proteinuria (typically in the nephrotic range and often massive) and renal insufficiency. Other manifestations

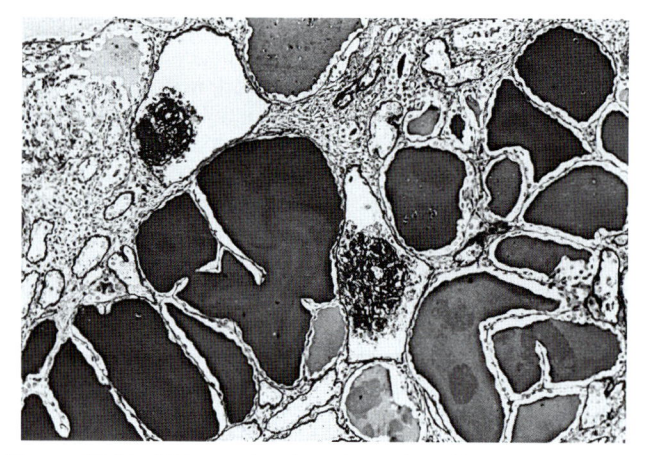

Figure 33.51 HIV-associated nephropathy. Glomeruli have collapsed tufts with capping of the overlying podocytes and dilation of the urinary space. The tubules are dilated, forming microcysts with abundant proteinaceous casts. (Periodic acid–Schiff stain, ×125.)

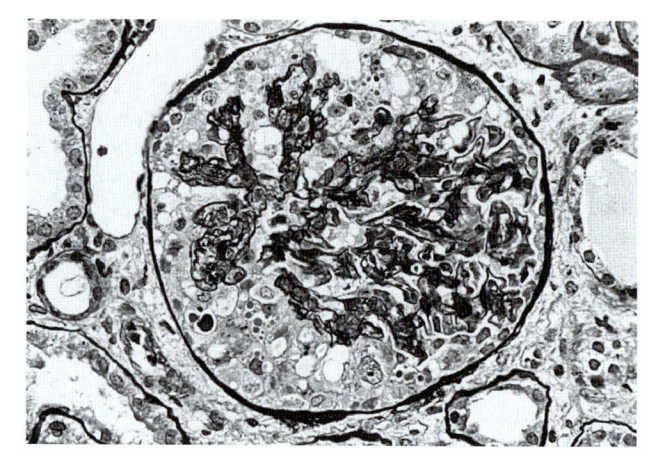

Figure 33.52 HIV-associated nephropathy. The characteristic pattern of collapsing glomerular sclerosis is depicted. Glomerular capillary lumens are occluded by wrinkling and retraction of the glomerular capillary walls associated with marked hypertrophy and hyperplasia of the visceral epithelial cells, forming a pseudocrescent. (Periodic acid–Schiff stain, ×325.)

of nephrotic syndrome, including edema, hypoalbuminemia, and hypercholesterolemia, have been common in some series but less so in others despite the heavy proteinuria.[967,970,973,974,978,980,993] Likewise, the incidence of hypertension has been variable even in patients with severe renal failure. Some patients, however, present with subnephrotic-range proteinuria and urinary sediment findings of microhematuria and sterile pyuria.[994] The renal sonograms in HIVAN show echogenic kidneys with preserved or enlarged size with an average of larger than 12 cm in spite of the severe renal insufficiency.[974,978] Echogenicity may correlate with the histopathologic tubulointerstitial changes better than the glomerular changes.[978]

PATHOLOGY

The term *HIVAN* is reserved for the characteristic light microscopy pattern of FSGS of the "collapsing" type with retraction of the glomerular capillary walls and luminal occlusion either in a segmental or global distribution[968,972,995] (Figure 33.51). There is striking hypertrophy and hyperplasia of the visceral epithelial cells, which form a cellular crown over the collapsed glomerular lobules (Figure 33.52). In one study analyzing the expression pattern of podocyte differentiation and proliferation markers, there was disappearance of all podocyte differentiation markers from collapsed glomeruli, associated with cell proliferation, suggesting that the podocyte phenotype is dysregulated.[996] Subsequent studies have emphasized the proliferation of parietal epithelial cells to replace lost podocytes.[997] Patients with HIVAN have a higher percentage of glomerular collapse, less hyalinosis, and greater visceral cell swelling than patients with classic idiopathic FSGS or heroin nephropathy even when matched for serum creatinine and degree of proteinuria.[972] The tubulointerstitial disease is also more severe in HIVAN, including tubular degenerative and regenerative features, interstitial edema, fibrosis, and inflammation.[968,972] Tubules are often greatly dilated into microcysts containing proteinaceous casts (see Figure 33.51). By immunofluorescence, IgM and C3 are present; however, by electron microscopy, immune deposits are not detected (Figure 33.53). In almost all biopsies of untreated HIVAN, there are numerous tubuloreticular inclusions within the glomerular and vascular endothelial cells (Figure 33.54).[967,968,972,995] These 24-nm interanastomosing tubular structures are found within the dilated cisternae of the endoplasmic reticulum. Of note, patients who develop HIVAN while receiving cART usually lack collapsing features but display classic FSGS lesions on biopsy.[998]

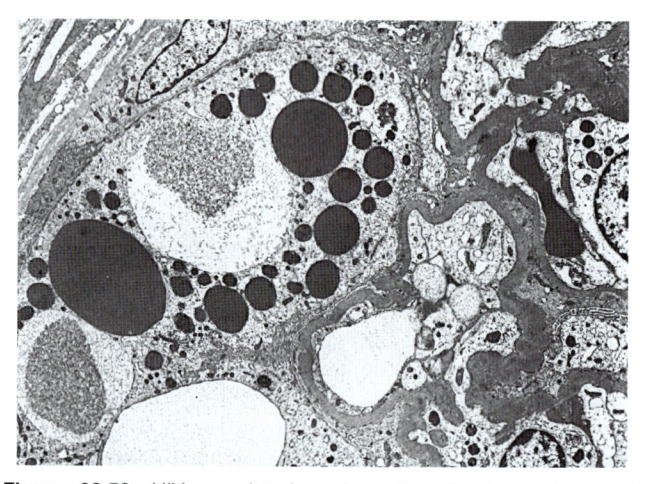

Figure 33.53 HIV-associated nephropathy. Electron micrograph showing wrinkling of glomerular basement membranes with marked podocyte hypertrophy, complete foot process effacement, and numerous intracytoplasmic protein resorption droplets. (×2500.)

PATHOGENESIS

Experimental evidence strongly supports a role for direct HIV-1 infection of renal parenchymal cells. By in situ hybridization, HIV-1 RNA was detected in renal tubular epithelial cells, glomerular epithelial cells (visceral and parietal), and interstitial leukocytes.[999] Renal epithelial cells may be an important reservoir for HIV because HIV RNA was found in the kidney of patients with undetectable viral loads in peripheral blood.[999] Moreover, HIV-infected tubular epithelium can support viral replication, as evidenced by the

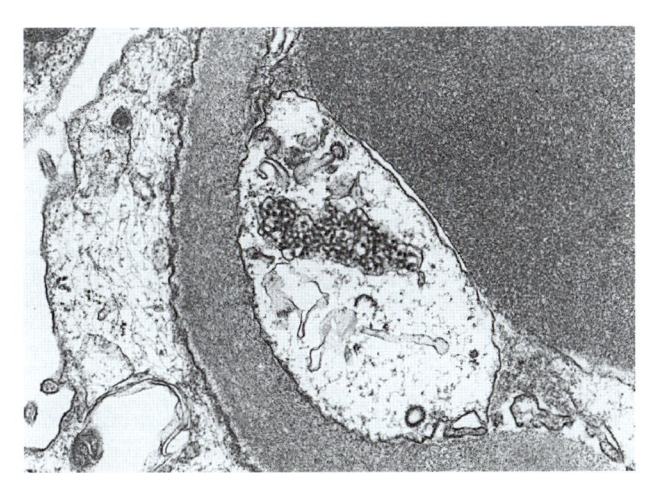

Figure 33.54 HIV-associated nephropathy. Electron micrograph showing a typical tuboloreticular inclusion within the endoplasmic reticulum of a glomerular endothelial cell. (×6000.)

detection of different HIV quasispecies in kidney epithelial cells compared to peripheral blood mononuclear cells of the same patient.[1000]

A replicative-deficient transgenic mouse model of HIVAN has been developed with lesions identical to HIV nephropathy,[1001-1003] suggesting that expression of viral gene products in renal epithelium underlies the development of nephropathy.

The lesions of collapsing glomerulopathy are associated with podocyte proliferation and dedifferentiation.[996] The expression of two cyclin-dependent kinase inhibitors (which regulate cell cycle), p27 and p57, were decreased in podocytes from HIVAN biopsies while expression of another inhibitor, p21, was increased.[1004] The specific HIV gene(s) required to produce these changes have been investigated. The *nef* gene (which is thought to act by activation of tyrosine kinases) was found to be essential in producing HIV-induced changes in podocyte cultures[1005] and in one murine model of HIVAN.[1006] There appears to be a synergistic role for *nef* and *vpr* on podocyte dysfunction and progressive glomerulosclerosis.[1007] *Vpr* has a role in G_2 cell cycle arrest and possibly the induction of apoptosis.[1008] There are several other abnormalities seen in the podocyte that are associated with an immature phenotype and subsequent loss of podocyte function. Synthesis of retinoic acid (an important differentiation factor) is impaired, associated with reduced expression of the enzyme retinol dehydrogenase 9.[1009] The expression of TERT, a telomerase protein, is increased in HIVAN podocytes. TERT increases upregulation of the Wnt pathway, which also is associated with podocyte dedifferentiation. Suppressing TERT or Wnt signaling led to amelioration of podocyte lesions.[1010]

The *APOL1* gene, which encodes apolipoprotein L-1, in a recessive model, is associated with a 29-fold higher odds for HIVAN in black patients. The lifetime risk of developing HIVAN is 50% in untreated HIV-infected black patients with two APOL1 risk alleles.[1011] Furthermore, the majority of patients with two APOL1 risk alleles had FSGS on kidney biopsies, whereas with one or no risk alleles, immune complex glomerulonephritis was more common.[1012] The mechanism whereby APOL1 variants associate with HIVAN is currently unknown.

COURSE AND TREATMENT

The natural history of HIVAN during the early part of the AIDS epidemic was characterized by rapid progression to ESKD. Case series from the United States that were published during the years that HIVAN was first described demonstrated an almost universal requirement for dialysis within 1 year of diagnosis.[970] The role of combined antiviral therapies and the use of newer agents in the treatment of HIVAN have been associated with beneficial effects.[998,1013-1015] The development of HIVAN is now considered an indication for antiretroviral therapy. Corresponding to the introduction of highly active antiretroviral therapy (HAART), the rise in new cases of ESKD due to HIVAN slowed markedly.[1016]

There have been a few studies using corticosteroids in HIVAN. In an early study, prednisone was not associated with improvement in children with HIVAN.[1017,1018] Remissions in HIV-infected children with the minimal change pattern (seen on biopsy) who were treated with steroids have been noted but not in children with sclerosing or collapsing lesions.[967] In adults, however, several retrospective studies have shown short-term improvement in clinical parameters.[1019-1021]

Three pediatric patients with HIVAN on biopsy had sustained remissions of nephrotic syndrome when treated with cyclosporine.[1017] They eventually developed opportunistic infections, requiring the cyclosporine to be discontinued and subsequently experienced relapses of the nephrotic proteinuria and renal failure.

In isolated patients and in several small trials, use of ACEIs has been shown to decrease proteinuria in HIVAN and to slow the progression to renal failure.[1022-1024] Serum angiotensin-converting enzyme levels are elevated in HIV patients, and ACEIs may prevent proteinuria and glomerulosclerosis by either hemodynamic mechanisms or through modulation of matrix production and mesangial cell proliferation or even by affecting HIV protease activity.[1022-1024] Although some of these studies used control groups of untreated HIV patients of similar age, sex, race, and degree of renal insufficiency and proteinuria, the studies were not randomized, blinded trials. Nevertheless, in each study the ACEI-treated group had less proteinuria, less rise in serum creatinine, and less progression to ESKD.

At present the therapy of HIVAN should include use of multiple antiviral agents as in HIV-infected patients without nephropathy. Use of ACEIs or perhaps angiotensin II receptor blockers, with careful attention to hyperkalemia and acute rises in the serum creatinine, may be beneficial. Several studies have documented favorable outcomes in HIVAN patients who received renal transplants.[1025-1027] The current opinion is that renal transplantation is no longer a contraindication in HIV-positive patients who have undetectable viral loads and a CD4 count greater than 200 cells/μL for at least 6 months.[1028]

OTHER GLOMERULAR LESIONS IN PATIENTS WITH HIV INFECTION

In the pre-HAART era, HIVAN was the most common form of glomerulopathy found in HIV-infected patients, but other lesions had been reported as well. In one series of more than 100 biopsies for glomerular disease in HIV-positive patients, 73% were classic HIVAN, but other lesions included MPGN in 10%, minimal change disease in 6%, amyloid in 3%, lupus-like nephritis in 3%, acute postinfectious glomerulonephritis in 2%, membranous nephropathy in 2%, and 1% each of focal and segmental necrotizing glomerulonephritis, thrombotic microangiopathy, IgA nephropathy, and immunotactoid nephropathy.[968] Collapsing FSGS is most common in urban centers with large black populations, while higher rates of immune complex glomerulonephritis are found in other cities and especially among European white populations.[1029,1030] In a study from Paris, immune complex glomerulonephritis was found in more than 50% of the white HIV-seropositive patients but in only 21% of the blacks.[1029,1030] Likewise, in a study from northern Italy of 26 biopsies on HIV-infected patients, most cases were of immune complex glomerulonephritis but none of classic HIVAN.[1031] In the present era with the availability of HAART, a renal biopsy in an HIV-positive patient with viral loads of less than 400 copies/mL is more likely to show hypertensive nephrosclerosis[1032] or diabetic nephropathy.[1033]

IgA nephropathy has been reported in a number of investigative series of HIV-infected patients.[1034-1038] This has occurred in both whites and blacks despite the rarity of typical IgA nephropathy in black populations. The clinical features usually include hematuria, proteinuria, and some renal insufficiency. Cases with leukocytoclastic angiitis of the skin (consistent with HSP) have also been noted. The histology shows a variety of changes from mesangial proliferative glomerulonephritis to collapsing glomerulosclerosis with mesangial IgA deposits. IgA anti-HIV immune complexes have been eluted from the kidneys of several such patients, and several patients have had circulating immune complexes containing IgA idiotypic antibodies directed against viral proteins, either anti-HIV p24 or HIV gp41.[1037]

MPGN may be the most common pattern of immune complex–mediated glomerulonephritis seen in HIV-infected patients. Two series document a high occurrence in intravenous drug abusers coinfected with HIV and HCV.[1039,1040] Most patients have had microscopic hematuria, nephrotic-range proteinuria, and renal insufficiency at biopsy. Cryoglobulins are commonly positive, as is hypocomplementemia, and some have had both HBV and HCV infection. The pathology of the glomerulopathy may be similar to idiopathic MPGN type I or type III although some patients also have segmental membranous or mesangioproliferative features.[1041]

A lupus-like immune complex glomerulonephritis has been reported in a number of patients.[977,1042-1045] Most of these patients have had positive serology for SLE with positive ANA, anti-DNA, and low complement levels. This contrasts with a low incidence of ANA positivity and almost no anti-DNA positivity in the general HIV-infected population.[1046] These patients are generally treated with corticosteroids with or without mycophenolate and concomitant HAART therapy. The results have been variable.[1045]

An occasional association in both white and black HIV-infected patients has been TTP. Most have been in an advanced stage of HIV infection and had renal involvement with hematuria, proteinuria, and variable renal insufficiency. Other typical findings of TTP, such as fever, neurologic symptoms, thrombocytopenia, and microangiopathic hemolytic anemia, are often present. The initiation/reinitiation of cART and plasma exchange with or without adjunctive immunosuppression can lead to remission.[1047] ADAMTS13 may be decreased (as in idiopathic TTP) and may be associated with a better prognosis.[1048] Other entities such as malignant hypertension, angioinvasive infections such as Kaposi's sarcoma, and direct HIV-associated hemolytic uremic syndrome need to be excluded.[1049]

GLOMERULAR MANIFESTATIONS OF LIVER DISEASE

HEPATITIS B

Hepatitis B antigenemia has been associated with glomerulonephritis for more than 30 years. Hepatitis B has a worldwide distribution. In countries where the virus is endemic (sub-Saharan Africa, Southeast Asia, and Eastern Europe), there is vertical transmission from mother to infant and horizontal transmission between siblings. Hepatitis B–associated nephropathy occurs in these children with a 4:1 male preponderance.[1050-1052] In the United States and Western Europe, where hepatitis B is acquired by parenteral routes or sexually, the nephropathy affects mainly adults and has a different clinical course from the endemic form.[1053-1055] However, hepatitis B–associated nephropathy is rare in hepatitis B carriers.[1056] PAN has also been associated with hepatitis B.[1057]

CLINICAL FEATURES

Most patients present with proteinuria or nephrotic syndrome. In endemic areas, there may not be a preceding history of hepatitis. The majority of patients have normal renal function at time of presentation. There may be urinary erythrocytes, but the majority have a bland sediment. Liver disease may be absent (carrier state) or chronic, and clinically mild. Serum aminotransferases may be normal or modestly elevated (between 100 and 200 IU/L). Liver biopsies in these patients often show chronic active hepatitis. Some patients ultimately develop cirrhosis. There is often spontaneous resolution of the carrier state with resolution of renal abnormalities. Spontaneous resolution of HBV-associated nephropathy is particularly common in children from endemic areas. The probability of a spontaneous remission may be as high as 80% after 10 years.[1058,1059]

PATHOLOGY

Most cases of hepatitis B–associated nephropathy manifest membranous nephropathy, although mesangial proliferation and sclerosis have also been reported.[1050,1051,1053-1055,1060,1061] In a cohort of Chinese patients with membranous nephropathy, HBV was found in 12%. There are fewer reports of MPGN with mesangial cell interposition, reduplication of the GBM, and subendothelial glomerular deposits.[1053,1055,1060] In a few series, cases of type III MPGN have been reported in which there are electron-dense subepithelial deposits in addition to the changes seen in type I MPGN.[1055] Crescentic glomerulonephritis in association with membranous changes and primary crescentic glomerulonephritis have also been described.[1062,1063]

The glomerular lesions appear to be immune complex mediated. HBsAg, HBcAg, and HBeAg[1064] have all been demonstrated in glomerular lesions, as has HBV DNA.[1052,1065]

TREATMENT

In children with the mild endemic form of hepatitis B–associated nephropathy, no treatment other than supportive care is advocated. In patients with progressive renal dysfunction, interferon has been used with mixed results.[1066-1069] Steroids that do not significantly improve proteinuria may potentially enhance viral replication.[1070,1071] Nucleoside analogs, including lamivudine, telbivudine, adefovir, entecavir, or tenofovir, that suppress HBV replication by inhibiting viral DNA polymerase have demonstrated clinical utility in treating hepatitis B infection; lamivudine was shown to reduce proteinuria and lead to a lesser incidence of ESKD in 10 patients with hepatitis B–associated nephropathy.[1072] Preemptive lamivudine therapy in renal transplant recipients has shown improved survival compared to historical controls.[1073,1074] A recent meta-analysis confirmed that corticosteroids did not ameliorate proteinuria, but antiviral therapy was associated with HBeAg clearance and improvement of proteinuria.[1075] Current recommendations for HBV treatment discourage the use of lamivudine in view of a high rate of drug resistance; tenofovir, entecavir, and pegylated interferon alfa-2a are suggested.[1076] However, there are no data on the response of hepatitis B–related glomerulonephritis to these newer regimens.

HEPATITIS C

Renal disease associated with HCV infection includes MPGN with or without associated mixed cryoglobulinemia and membranous glomerulopathy. The MPGN is most often type I, with fewer cases of type III.[1077-1079] Rare cases of diffuse proliferative and exudative glomerulonephritis, polyarteritis, and fibrillary and immunotactoid glomerulopathy have also been described in association with HCV.[1080,1081] Most patients have evidence of liver disease as reflected by elevated plasma transaminase levels. However, transaminase levels are normal in some cases and a history of acute hepatitis is often absent.

PATHOGENESIS

The pathogenesis of HCV-related nephropathies is immune complex mediated. A clonal expansion of B cells secreting IgM rheumatoid factors has been seen in patients with chronic HCV infection. HCV-specific proteins have been isolated from glomerular lesions.[1082] The disappearance of viremia in response to interferon (see later) is associated with a diminution of proteinuria; a relapse of viremia is accompanied by rising proteinuria.

CLINICAL AND PATHOLOGIC FEATURES

Mixed cryoglobulinemia is associated with HCV and may cause systemic vasculitis; patients may exhibit constitutional systemic symptoms, palpable purpura, peripheral neuropathy, and hypocomplementemia. The renal manifestations include hematuria, proteinuria (often in the nephrotic range), and renal insufficiency. The histologic findings resemble those in idiopathic MPGN type I or type III (Figures 33.55 and 33.56) except for intraluminal protein "thrombi" on light microscopy and the organized annular-tubular substructure of the electron-dense deposits on electron microscopy. Prior to the advent of hepatitis C serologic tests, mixed cryoglobulinemia was considered an idiopathic disease ("essential" mixed cryoglobulinemia). Up to 95% of these patients show signs of HCV infection.[1083] Few patients with thrombotic microangiopathy associated with cryoglobulinemia have been described.[1084] MPGN without associated cryoglobulinemia may occur but is much less common.[1078]

Rarely, membranous nephropathy may be associated with HCV infection. Patients present with nephrotic syndrome or proteinuria. Complement levels tend to be normal, and neither cryoglobulins nor rheumatoid factors are present in HCV-associated membranous nephropathy.[1085] Now that staining for phospholipase A_2 receptor (PLA$_2$R), the major target antigen in primary membranous nephropathy, is being performed on renal biopsies, it has become evident that some HCV-infected patients with membranous nephropathy actually have a primary form.[1086]

Both type I MPGN (with and without cryoglobulinemia) and membranous nephropathy may recur in the allograft after renal transplantation, sometimes leading to graft

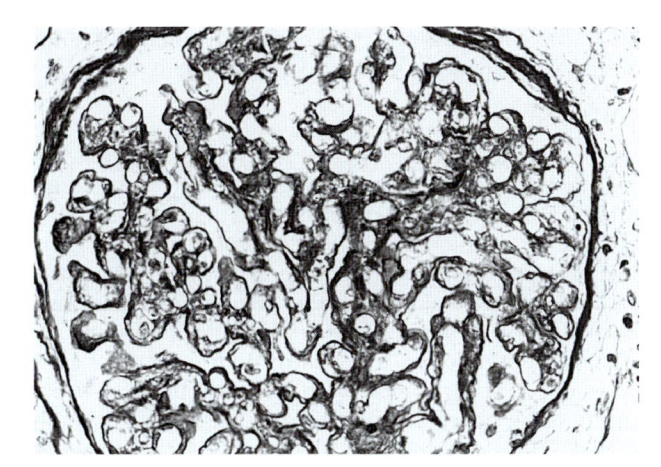

Figure 33.55 Hepatitis C–associated membranoproliferative glomerulonephritis type I. The mesangium is expanded by global mesangial hypercellularity associated with numerous double contours of the glomerular basement membranes. (Periodic acid–Schiff stain, ×500.)

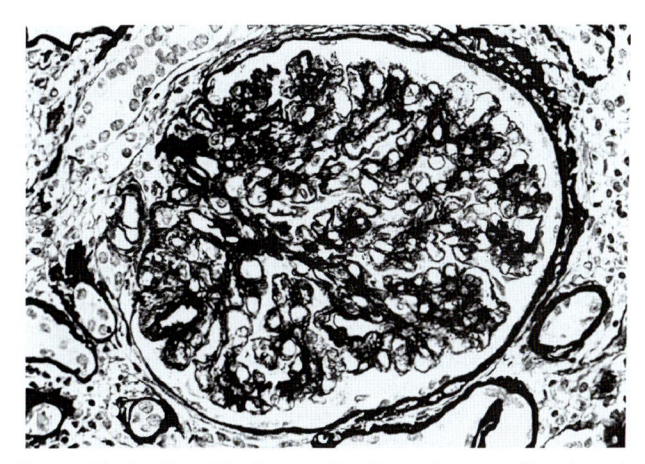

Figure 33.56 Hepatitis C–associated membranoproliferative glomerulonephritis (MPGN) type III. There are mixed features of MPGN type I (with mesangial proliferation and duplication of glomerular basement membrane [GBM]) and membranous glomerulopathy (with GBM spikes). (Jones' methenamine silver stain, ×325.)

loss.[1087-1090] Similar lesions have occurred in native kidneys after liver transplantation in HCV-positive patients.[1091,1092]

TREATMENT

The treatment of HCV-associated renal disease is limited to case reports and small randomized trials.[1093] Although a number of early reports demonstrated a beneficial response to α-interferon therapy,[1085,1094,1095] cessation of interferon therapy was associated with recurrence of viremia and cryoglobulinemia in a majority of patients in these studies. Interferon therapy may paradoxically exacerbate proteinuria and hematuria that appears to be unrelated to viral antigenic effects.[1096] Currently combination therapy with ribavirin and pegylated interferon is considered to be standard therapy for HCV.[1097] Combination therapy appeared to improve biochemical parameters of renal dysfunction in 20 HCV-glomerulonephritis patients, which was not accompanied by a significant virologic response.[1098] Another report on 18 patients showed sustained virologic responses in two thirds of patients, a finding that was associated with improvement in renal parameters.[1099] Combination therapy (especially ribavirin) may not be well tolerated in the presence of significant renal dysfunction.[1100] Interferon alfa treatment of renal transplant patients with HCV has been associated with acute renal failure[1101] and acute humoral rejection[1102] and is not recommended. Recent groundbreaking trials using interferon-free oral direct antiviral regimens have shown dramatic sustained viral remission rates over the short term.[1103]

In patients with symptomatic cryoglobulinemia, immunosuppressive therapy may provide symptomatic relief prior to the use of antiviral therapy. Cyclophosphamide treatment has been used successfully in HCV-glomerulonephritis,[1104] even if interferon resistant.[1105] Cyclophosphamide treatment may be associated with a temporary, reversible increase in viral load and a change of quasispecies.[1106] Fludarabine has been reported to decrease proteinuria in HCV-associated cryoglobulinemic MPGN.[1107] Rituximab has been associated with remissions of proteinuria in HCV-glomerulonephritis.[1108-1110] In renal transplant patients with HCV-glomerulonephritis, similar improvements in renal parameters have been reported, albeit with a higher incidence of infectious complications.[1111] It has been suggested that in patients with moderate proteinuria and slowly progressive renal dysfunction, interferon with or without ribavirin should be considered. When there is an acute flare of disease with nephrotic proteinuria or RPGN, treatment with plasma exchange and immunosuppressive drugs (rituximab or cyclophosphamide, with corticosteroids) followed by antiviral therapy may be considered.[1093]

AUTOIMMUNE CHRONIC ACTIVE HEPATITIS

Autoimmune chronic hepatitis is a distinctive progressive necrotic and fibrotic disorder of the liver with clinical and/or serologic evidence of a generalized autoimmune disorder.[1112] Two distinct clinical lesions have been associated with this disorder: glomerulonephritis and interstitial nephritis. Patients with the glomerular lesion present with nephrotic syndrome or renal insufficiency. On renal biopsy they have membranous glomerulonephritis or MPGN. In two patients with membranous nephropathy, circulating immune complexes containing U1RNP (ribonucleoprotein) and IgG have been reported. Eluates from the kidney tissue revealed higher concentrations of anti-U1RNP antibody. It is not known whether immunosuppressive therapy ameliorates the renal disorder.[1112] It is unclear if coexistent HCV infection had been present in many of these patients.

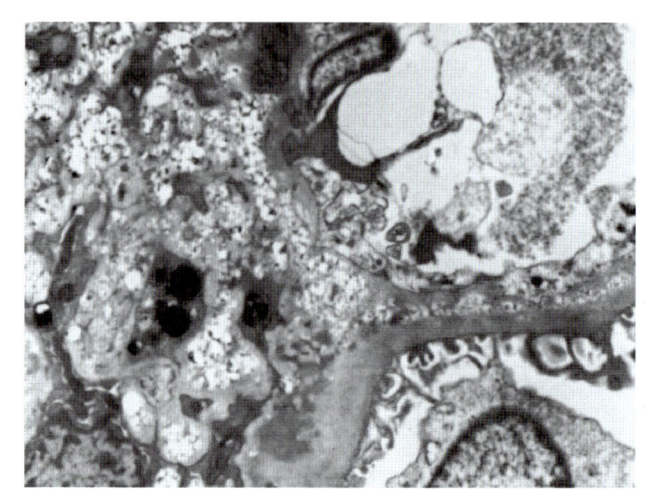

Figure 33.57 Hepatic glomerulopathy. A paramesangial electron-dense deposit corresponding to immune staining for IgA is seen. In addition, there are irregular lucencies containing dense granular and rounded membranous structures within the mesangial matrix and extending into the subendothelial space. (×6000.)

LIVER CIRRHOSIS

Glomerulonephritis is a rare manifestation of liver cirrhosis. Glomerular morphologic abnormalities with IgA deposition have been noted in more than 50% of patients with cirrhosis at both necropsy and biopsy,[1113,1114] although this has also been found in some autopsies of noncirrhotic kidneys.[1115] Clinically, there may be mild proteinuria and/or hematuria. There are two patterns on histology: a mesangial sclerosis ("cirrhotic glomerular sclerosis") or MPGN. The latter may be associated with more severe renal symptoms and a depression of serum complement C3 levels.[1116] Again, it is unclear if some patients had coexistent HCV infection. Rarely, HSP with RPGN has been described in association with cirrhosis.[1117]

Renal biopsies of patients with cirrhosis on light microscopy show an increase in mesangial matrix with little or no increase in mesangial cellularity, a lesion known as "hepatic glomerulopathy." Less commonly, the distinctive pathologic findings consist of mesangial proliferative glomerulonephritis with mesangial IgA deposits, usually accompanied by complement deposition and less intense IgG and/or IgM.[1113,1118,1119] By electron microscopy, the mesangium and subendothelial regions contain lucencies with dense granular and rounded membranous structures consistent with lipid inclusions (Figure 33.57). Increased serum IgA levels are found in more than 90% of cirrhotic patients with glomerular IgA deposition. Other authors have reported IgM as the dominant immunoglobulin.[1114] Cirrhotic glomerulonephritis is usually a clinically silent disease; however, the diagnosis can be suspected by finding proteinuria or abnormalities of the urine sediment. Kidney biopsies in cirrhotic patients at the time of liver transplantation may show glomerular lesions (predominantly IgA nephropathy or diabetic nephropathy) even if there is no clinical evidence of renal involvement. Diabetic lesions were associated with significantly worse renal function 5 years after transplantation compared to patients with IgA nephropathy.[1120]

The pathogenesis may relate to defective hepatic clearance of IgA as well as altered processing and/or portacaval shunting of circulating immune complexes.[1121] This theory is bolstered by the finding of increased deposits of IgA in skin and hepatic sinusoids in cirrhotic patients.[1122] Moreover, in patients with noncirrhotic portal fibrosis who underwent portal-systemic bypass procedures, there was an increase in the incidence of clinically overt glomerulonephritis (from 78% to 32%) associated with deposition of IgA after the procedure. In the latter group, there was also a significant incidence of renal failure (50% after 5 years).[1123] Similar findings were noted in children with end-stage liver disease from α_1-antitrypsin deficiency or biliary atresia, which resolved after liver transplantation.[1124]

GLOMERULAR LESIONS ASSOCIATED WITH NEOPLASIA

The occurrence of glomerular syndromes, both nephrotic and nephritic, may be associated with malignancy but is rare (<1%). Glomerular disease may be seen with a wide variety of malignancies. Carcinomas of the lung, stomach, breast, and colon are most frequently associated with glomerular lesions.[1125] Membranous nephropathy is the most common lesion associated with carcinoma.[1125] Patients older than age 50 presenting with nephrotic syndrome should be reviewed for the presence of a malignancy.[1126,1127]

CLINICAL AND PATHOLOGIC FEATURES

Clinically, the glomerulopathy of neoplasia may be manifested by proteinuria or nephrotic syndrome, an active urine sediment, and/or diminished glomerular filtration. Significant renal impairment is uncommon and is usually associated with the proliferative forms of glomerulonephritis. In evaluating an ESR in patients with nephrotic syndrome, it should be noted that most such patients have an ESR above 60 mm/hr, with roughly 20% being above 100 mm/hr. As a result, an elevated ESR alone in a patient with nephrotic syndrome (or with ESKD) is not an indication to evaluate the patient for an occult malignancy or underlying inflammatory disease.[1128,1129]

Membranous nephropathy may be associated with malignancies in 10% to 40% of cases.[1125,1127,1130,1131] These include carcinoma of the bronchus,[1132] breast,[1133] colon,[1134,1135] stomach, ovary,[1136] kidney,[1137] pancreas,[1138] and prostate,[1139,1140] as well as testicular seminoma,[1141] parotid adenolymphoma, carcinoid tumor,[1142,1143] Hodgkin's disease, and carotid body tumor.[1144] In some cases of membranous nephropathy associated with malignancy, tumor antigens have been detected within the glomeruli. It is postulated that tumor antigen deposition in the glomerulus is followed by antibody deposition, causing "in situ" immune complex formation, and subsequent complement activation.[1145,1146] Immune complexes and complement have been found in cancer patients without overt renal disease.[1145] Antibody to phospholipase A$_2$ receptor (PLA$_2$R), the target antigen in primary membranous nephropathy, has not been identified in the sera of patients with membranous nephropathy secondary to malignancy. Removal of the tumor may lead to remission of nephrotic syndrome, which may then recur, following the development of metastasis. In many instances successful treatment of the neoplasm has induced a partial or complete remission of the associated glomerulopathy.

Minimal change disease or focal glomerulosclerosis may occur in association with Hodgkin's disease,[1147-1149] less often with non-Hodgkin's lymphoma or leukemia,[1148] and rarely with thymoma,[1125,1150] mycosis fungoides,[1151] renal cell carcinoma,[1152] or other solid tumors.[1153-1155] Secretion of a lymphokine by abnormal T cells may underlie glomerular injury in these disorders.[1130,1156,1157]

Secondary amyloidosis (AA type) has been described with a number of malignancies, particularly renal cell carcinoma, Hodgkin's disease, and chronic lymphocytic leukemia.[1,2,4] In Hodgkin's disease, for example, renal amyloidosis is generally a late event resulting from a chronic inflammatory state; by comparison, minimal change disease most often occurs at the time of initial presentation.[5]

Both MPGN and RPGN have been described in patients with solid tumors and lymphomas, although the causal relationship between these conditions is not proven.[1155,1158] The association is probably strongest for MPGN and chronic lymphocytic leukemia and may be associated with circulating cryoglobulins or glomerular deposition of monoclonal immunoglobulins.[1159,1160] Mesangial proliferation with IgA deposition has been associated with mucosa-associated lymphoid tissue lymphoma, which resolved following treatment of the malignancy with chlorambucil.[1161] Although the association between crescentic glomerulonephritis and vasculitis with tumors may be coincidental, it has been suggested that the malignancy may act as a trigger for the vasculitis.[1162-1164] In contrast to the nephrotic states described earlier in which renal function is generally well preserved at presentation and the urine sediment is usually benign, patients with proliferative glomerulonephritis often have an acute decline in renal function and an active urine sediment.

Both HUS and the related disorder TTP can occur in patients with malignancy. An underlying carcinoma of the stomach, pancreas, or prostate may be associated with HUS. More commonly, however, antitumor therapy is implicated: mitomycin, gemcitabine, the combination of bleomycin and cisplatin, and radiation plus high-dose cyclophosphamide prior to bone marrow transplantation all can lead to HUS, which may become apparent months after therapy has been discontinued.[1165] Anti-VEGF agents are newly identified causes of glomerular thrombotic microangiopathy, leading to proteinuria, renal insufficiency, and hypertension.[1130,1166]

GLOMERULAR DISEASE ASSOCIATED WITH DRUGS

HEROIN NEPHROPATHY

In the 1970s, reports began to appear linking heroin abuse to nephrotic syndrome and renal biopsy findings of lesions of FSGS. This syndrome was referred to as heroin-associated nephropathy (HAN).[1167-1172] Similar lesions were seen in users of intravenous pentazocine (Talwin), and tripelennamine (Pyribenzamine), so-called Ts and Blues.[1173] This syndrome occurred almost exclusively in blacks; it has been suggested that blacks may have a genetic predisposition for developing HAN.[1174,1175] The mean age was younger than 30 years old with 90% of the patients being males. The duration of drug abuse varied from 6 months to 30 years (mean, 6 years) prior to the onset of renal disease. Most patients presented with nephrotic syndrome. The course of HAN was relentless progression to ESKD over many years in those addicts who continued to use heroin, whereas a regression of abnormalities was seen in patients who were able to stop using the drug. Kidney biopsies of these patients showed lesions of focal segmental and global sclerosis. Nonspecific trapping leads to the deposition of IgM and C3 in areas of sclerosis. There was usually significant interstitial inflammation associated with the glomerular lesion. The pathogenesis of HAN is unknown. Abnormalities of cellular and humoral immunity have been well described in heroin addicts.[1176] It has been suggested that morphine itself could act as an antigen and that contaminants used to "cut" the heroin could contribute to the pathogenesis. Morphine (the active metabolite of heroin) has been shown to stimulate proliferation and sclerosis of mesangial cells and fibroblasts.[1177,1178] The syndrome of HAN has almost disappeared among drug addicts presenting with renal failure; for example, there has been a sharp decline in incident cases of HAN and there were no reported cases of HAN-associated ESKD from Brooklyn, New York, during the period from 1991 to 1993.[1179,1180] In part this trend coincides with the rise of HIV infection and HIVAN.

NONSTEROIDAL ANTIINFLAMMATORY DRUG–INDUCED NEPHROPATHY

NSAIDs are being used by approximately 50 million of the general public in the United States at any point in time. Approximately 1% to 3% of patients exposed to NSAIDs will manifest one of the renal abnormalities associated with its use, which include fluid and electrolyte disturbances, acute renal failure, nephrotic syndrome with interstitial nephritis, and papillary necrosis.[1181] The combination of acute interstitial nephritis and nephrotic syndrome is characteristic of this group of compounds. Essentially all NSAIDs can cause this type of renal disease,[1182-1184] including the cyclo-oxygenase-2 inhibitors.[1185,1186]

CLINICAL AND PATHOLOGIC FEATURES
Minimal Change Disease with Interstitial Nephritis

The onset of NSAID-induced nephrotic syndrome is usually delayed, with a mean time of onset of 5.4 months (range, 2 weeks to 18 months) after initiation of NSAID therapy. Patients may present with edema and oliguria. Systemic signs of allergic interstitial nephritis are usually absent. The urine exhibits microhematuria and pyuria. Proteinuria is usually in the nephrotic range. The extent of renal dysfunction may be mild to severe. On light microscopy the findings consist of minimal change disease with interstitial nephritis. A focal or diffuse interstitial infiltrate consists predominantly of cytotoxic T lymphocytes (also other T cell subsets, B cells, and plasma cells).[1187,1188] The syndrome usually reverses after discontinuing therapy, and the time to recovery may be between 1 month and 1 year.[1184] Complete remission is usually seen.[1189] Relapse of proteinuria has been reported.[1190] Treatment of nephrotic syndrome is usually unnecessary, since the disorder is self-limiting. However, a short course of corticosteroids may be beneficial in patients in whom no response is seen after several weeks of discontinuation of the drug.[1191] Plasma exchange was reported with being associated with rapid recovery of renal function in two patients.[1192]

Other Patterns

Minimal change nephrotic syndrome without interstitial disease has been occasionally reported.[1193] Granulomatous interstitial disease without glomerular changes has also been described.[1194] Membranous nephropathy has also been reported in association with NSAID use,[1195] including the newer cyclo-oxygenase-2 inhibitors.[1186] As in minimal change nephrotic syndrome, there is rapid recovery after drug withdrawal in NSAID-induced membranous nephropathy.

PATHOGENESIS

The mechanism of NSAID-induced nephrotic syndrome has not been defined. It has been proposed that inhibition of cyclo-oxygenase by NSAIDs inhibits prostaglandin synthesis and shunts arachidonic acid pathways toward the production of leukotrienes. These by-products of arachidonic acid metabolism may promote T lymphocyte activation and enhanced vascular permeability, leading to minimal change disease.[1182-1184]

ANTI–RHEUMATOID ARTHRITIS THERAPY–INDUCED GLOMERULOPATHY

GOLD SALTS

Proteinuria and nephrotic syndrome have been reported to occur in association with both oral and parenteral gold.[1196,1197] Dermatitis may occur concurrently. Membranous nephropathy and, rarely, minimal change disease have been reported.[1198] A higher incidence of nephropathy has been reported in patients with HLA-B8/DR3.[1199,1200]

D-PENICILLAMINE

Proteinuria in association with membranous nephropathy is the most common lesion reported. Less commonly, minimal change disease and mesangial proliferative lesions have been reported.[1200] Goodpasture-like syndrome,[1201] minimal change nephrotic syndrome,[1202] and membranous nephropathy concurrently with vasculitis[1203] have been described rarely. HLA-B8/DR3 haplotypes are also associated with penicillamine nephropathy.[1204] Tiopronin and bucillamine (a penicillamine-like compound) have also been associated with the same renal lesions described for penicillamine.[1205,1206] The onset of proteinuria with gold or penicillamine therapy is usually between 6 and 12 months after starting therapy. Proteinuria usually resolves after withdrawing the offending agent; persistent renal dysfunction is uncommon.[1200,1204,1207] Under close supervision, gold and penicillamine have been continued in patients with nephropathy with no obvious adverse effect on renal function.[1208] Anti–TNF-α agents have been reported to promote the development of lupus-like nephritis and ANCA-associated glomerulonephritis in patients with rheumatoid arthritis.[1209]

OTHER MEDICATIONS

Organic mercurial exposure can occur with diuretics, skin lightening creams, gold refining, and industrial exposure. Proteinuria and nephrotic syndrome have been reported.[1210-1212] Renal biopsy in such patients has shown membranous nephropathy[1213,1214] or minimal change disease.[1215] Nephrotic syndrome has been associated with the anticonvulsants ethosuccimide,[1216] trimethadione,[1217] and paradione.[1218] Diffuse proliferative glomerulonephritis may be seen with mephenytoin (Mesantoin).[1219] ANCA-associated vasculitis as well as a lupus-like nephritis has been reported with propylthiouracil[1220-1223] and hydralazine.[1224] Captopril has been associated with the development of proteinuria and nephrotic syndrome due to membranous nephropathy.[1225] Substituting enalapril for captopril has been reported to ameliorate nephrotic syndrome.[1226] IFN-α has been associated with interstitial nephritis, minimal change disease, FSGS, and acute renal failure.[1227,1228] In patients with collapsing FSGS due to interferon therapy, discontinuation of therapy usually leads to improvement in both renal function and proteinuria.[1229] Cases of thrombotic microangiopathy[1230,1231] and crescentic glomerulonephritis[1232] have also been reported. Mercaptopropionylglycine (2-MPG) used in the treatment of cystinuria has been associated with membranous glomerulopathy.[1233] Lithium use has been associated with minimal change disease,[1234,1235] membranous nephropathy,[1236] and FSGS.[1237,1238] The use of high-dose pamidronate in patients with malignancies has been associated with HIV-negative collapsing FSGS.[1239] Cocaine may be contaminated with levamisole, a veterinary antihelmintic that is a known immunomodulator. This combination may result in a ANCA-positive systemic vasculitis with a predilection for skin necrosis and arthralgia; renal and pulmonary involvement may occur.[1240] Abuse of anabolic steroids in conjunction with a body-building regimen may produce FSGS with variable histologic subtypes. Roles for both increased glomerular filtration demand and potential direct toxic effects of anabolic steroids on glomerular cells have been proposed.[1241] Treatment of C3 glomerulopathies with eculizumab, a humanized monoclonal antibody directed to C5, may lead to binding of the drug to C5 deposits in renal tissue, producing de novo positivity for IgG-κ that mimics.[1242]

MISCELLANEOUS DISEASES ASSOCIATED WITH GLOMERULAR LESIONS

Well-documented cases exist of nephrotic syndrome associated with unilateral renal artery stenosis, which improved after correction of the stenosis. The mechanism of proteinuria presumably relates to high levels of angiotensin II.[1243-1245]

Acute silicosis has been associated with a proliferative glomerulonephritis with IgM and C3 deposits, leading to renal failure.[1246] A patient with dense lamellar inclusions in swollen glomerular epithelial cells, similar to those seen in Fabry's disease, has also been described.[1247]

Membranous nephropathy and MPGN[1248] have been described in association with ulcerative colitis.[1249]

Kimura's disease and angiolymphoid hyperplasia with eosinophilia (ALHE) produce skin lesions that appear as single or multiple red-brown papules or as subcutaneous nodules with a predilection for the head and neck region. Other associated features include eosinophilia and elevated IgE levels. Both Kimura's disease and the similar ALHE are frequently associated with glomerular disease. Mesangial proliferative glomerulonephritis[1250] and minimal change disease[1251] have been described.

Renal complications of Castleman's disease (angiofollicular lymph node hyperplasia) are uncommon. The reported cases are very heterogeneous, and their renal pathology includes minimal change disease, mesangial proliferative glomerulonephritis,[1252] membranous nephropathy,[1253] MPGN,[1254] crescentic glomerulonephritis,[1255] fibrillary glomerulonephritis,[1256] and amyloidosis.[1257] Serum IL-6 levels appear to be elevated and they decline with corticosteroid therapy.[1252] Removal of tumor mass or treatment with steroids appears to ameliorate the renal manifestations in some cases.

Angioimmunoblastic lymphadenopathy has been associated with diffuse proliferative glomerulonephritis with necrotizing arteritis and minimal change disease.[1148,1258]

Hemophagocytic syndrome related to infections or lymphoproliferative disease has been associated with collapsing FSGS.[1259]

Complete reference list available at ExpertConsult.com.

KEY REFERENCES

3. Bomback AS, Appel GB: Updates on the treatment of lupus nephritis. *J Am Soc Nephrol* 21(12):2028–2035, 2010.
10. Appel GB, et al: Mycophenolate mofetil versus cyclophosphamide for induction treatment of lupus nephritis. *J Am Soc Nephrol* 20(5):1103–1112, 2009.
21. Appel GB, et al: Renal involvement in systemic lupus erythematosus (SLE): a study of 56 patients emphasizing histologic classification. *Medicine (Baltimore)* 57(5):371–410, 1978.
30. Weening JJ, et al: The classification of glomerulonephritis in systemic lupus erythematosus revisited. *Kidney Int* 65(2):521–530, 2004.
91. Gourley MF, et al: Methylprednisolone and cyclophosphamide, alone or in combination, in patients with lupus nephritis. A randomized, controlled trial. *Ann Intern Med* 125(7):549–557, 1996.
109. Steinberg AD, Steinberg SC: Long-term preservation of renal function in patients with lupus nephritis receiving treatment that includes cyclophosphamide versus those treated with prednisone only. *Arthritis Rheum* 34(8):945–950, 1991.
131. Houssiau FA, et al: Immunosuppressive therapy in lupus nephritis: the Euro-Lupus Nephritis Trial, a randomized trial of low-dose versus high-dose intravenous cyclophosphamide. *Arthritis Rheum* 46(8):2121–2131, 2002.
141. Contreras G, et al: Sequential therapies for proliferative lupus nephritis. *N Engl J Med* 350(10):971–980, 2004.
142. Houssiau FA, et al: Azathioprine versus mycophenolate mofetil for long-term immunosuppression in lupus nephritis: results from the MAINTAIN Nephritis Trial. *Ann Rheum Dis* 69(12):2083–2089, 2010.
143. Dooley MA, et al: Mycophenolate versus azathioprine as maintenance therapy for lupus nephritis. *N Engl J Med* 365(20):1886–1895, 2011.
170. Austin HA, 3rd, et al: Randomized, controlled trial of prednisone, cyclophosphamide, and cyclosporine in lupus membranous nephropathy. *J Am Soc Nephrol* 20(4):901–911, 2009.

173. Radhakrishnan J, et al: Mycophenolate mofetil and intravenous cyclophosphamide are similar as induction therapy for class V lupus nephritis. *Kidney Int* 77(2):152–160, 2010.
213. Daugas E, et al: Antiphospholipid syndrome nephropathy in systemic lupus erythematosus. *J Am Soc Nephrol* 13(1):42–52, 2002.
252. Hoffman GS, et al: Wegener granulomatosis: an analysis of 158 patients. *Ann Intern Med* 116(6):488–498, 1992.
288. Jennette JC, et al: 2012 revised International Chapel Hill Consensus Conference Nomenclature of Vasculitides. *Arthritis Rheum* 65(1):1–11, 2013.
304. de Groot K, et al: Pulse versus daily oral cyclophosphamide for induction of remission in antineutrophil cytoplasmic antibody-associated vasculitis: a randomized trial. *Ann Intern Med* 150(10):670–680, 2009.
305. de Groot K, et al: Randomized trial of cyclophosphamide versus methotrexate for induction of remission in early systemic antineutrophil cytoplasmic antibody-associated vasculitis. *Arthritis Rheum* 52(8):2461–2469, 2005.
310. Jayne DR, et al: Randomized trial of plasma exchange or high-dosage methylprednisolone as adjunctive therapy for severe renal vasculitis. *J Am Soc Nephrol* 18(7):2180–2188, 2007.
311. Wegener's Granulomatosis Etanercept Trial Research, G.: Etanercept plus standard therapy for Wegener's granulomatosis. *N Engl J Med* 352(4):351–361, 2005.
316. Jones RB, et al: Rituximab versus cyclophosphamide in ANCA-associated renal vasculitis. *N Engl J Med* 363(3):211–220, 2010.
317. Stone JH, et al: Rituximab versus cyclophosphamide for ANCA-associated vasculitis. *N Engl J Med* 363(3):221–232, 2010.
323. Jayne D, et al: A randomized trial of maintenance therapy for vasculitis associated with antineutrophil cytoplasmic autoantibodies. *N Engl J Med* 349(1):36–44, 2003.
324. Hiemstra TF, et al: Mycophenolate mofetil vs azathioprine for remission maintenance in antineutrophil cytoplasmic antibody-associated vasculitis: a randomized controlled trial. *JAMA* 304(21):2381–2388, 2010.
378. Guillevin L, et al: Hepatitis B virus-associated polyarteritis nodosa: clinical characteristics, outcome, and impact of treatment in 115 patients. *Medicine (Baltimore)* 84(5):313–322, 2005.
439. Rai A, Nast C, Adler S: Henoch-Schonlein purpura nephritis. *J Am Soc Nephrol* 10(12):2637–2644, 1999.
447. Pillebout E, et al: Henoch-Schonlein Purpura in adults: outcome and prognostic factors. *J Am Soc Nephrol* 13(5):1271–1278, 2002.
487. Niaudet P, Habib R: Methylprednisolone pulse therapy in the treatment of severe forms of Schonlein-Henoch purpura nephritis. *Pediatr Nephrol* 12(3):238–243, 1998.
498. Pusey CD: Anti-glomerular basement membrane disease. *Kidney Int* 64(4):1535–1550, 2003.
522. Levy JB, et al: Long-term outcome of anti-glomerular basement membrane antibody disease treated with plasma exchange and immunosuppression. *Ann Intern Med* 134(11):1033–1042, 2001.
535. Maripuri S, et al: Renal involvement in primary Sjogren's syndrome: a clinicopathologic study. *Clin J Am Soc Nephrol* 4(9):1423–1431, 2009.
571. Kyle RA, Gertz MA: Primary systemic amyloidosis: clinical and laboratory features in 474 cases. *Semin Hematol* 32(1):45–59, 1995.
574. Lachmann HJ, et al: Natural history and outcome in systemic AA amyloidosis. *N Engl J Med* 356(23):2361–2371, 2007.
602. Dember LM, et al: Eprodisate for the treatment of renal disease in AA amyloidosis. *N Engl J Med* 356(23):2349–2360, 2007.
608. Rosenstock JL, et al: Fibrillary and immunotactoid glomerulonephritis: Distinct entities with different clinical and pathologic features. *Kidney Int* 63(4):1450–1461, 2003.
621. Nasr SH, et al: Renal monoclonal immunoglobulin deposition disease: a report of 64 patients from a single institution. *Clin J Am Soc Nephrol* 7(2):231–239, 2012.
635. Nasr SH, et al: Proliferative glomerulonephritis with monoclonal IgG deposits. *J Am Soc Nephrol* 20(9):2055–2064, 2009.
716. Savige J, Gregory M, Gross O, et al: Expert guidelines for the management of Alport syndrome and thin basement membrane nephropathy. *J Am Soc Nephrol* 24(3):364–375, 2013.
758. Vollrath D, Jaramillo-Babb VL, Clough MV, et al: Loss-of-function mutations in the LIM-homeodomain gene, LMX1B, in nail-patella syndrome. *Hum Mol Genet* 7:1091–1098, 1998.
761. Terryn W, Cochat P, Froissart R, et al Fabry nephropathy: indications for screening and guidance for diagnosis and treatment by the European Renal Best Practice. *Nephrol Dial Transplant* 28(3):505–517, 2013.
783. Kiryluk K, Jadoon A, Gupta M, et al: Sickle cell trait and gross hematuria. *Kidney Int* 71(7):706–710, 2007.
809. Senior B, Gellis SS: The syndromes of total lipodystrophy and partial lipodystrophy. *Pediatrics* 33:593–612, 1964.
848. Nasr SH, Radhakrishnan J, D'Agati VD: Bacterial infection-related glomerulonephritis in adults. *Kidney Int* 83(5):792–803, 2013.
998. Wyatt CM, Klotman PE, D'Agati VD: HIV-associated nephropathy: clinical presentation, pathology, and epidemiology in the era of antiretroviral therapy. *Semin Nephrol* 28(6):513–522, 2008.
1093. KDIGO Clinical Practice Guidelines for the Prevention, Diagnosis, Evaluation, and Treatment of Hepatitis C in Chronic Kidney Disease. *Kidney Int Suppl* 109:S1–S99, 2008.
1125. Lien YH, Lai LW: Pathogenesis, diagnosis and management of paraneoplastic glomerulonephritis. *Nat Rev Nephrol* 7(2):85–95, 2011.
1130. Jhaveri KD, Shah HH, Calderon K, et al: Glomerular diseases seen with cancer and chemotherapy: a narrative review. *Kidney Int* 84(1):34–44, 2013.

34 Overview of Therapy for Glomerular Disease

Daniel Cattran | Heather N. Reich | Michelle A. Hladunewich

CHAPTER OUTLINE

THE GLOBAL IMPACT AND CHALLENGES, 1161
OUTCOME MEASURES AND CLINICAL TRIALS IN GLOMERULONEPHRITIS, 1163
QUANTIFICATION OF THE BENEFITS OF PROTEINURIA REDUCTION, 1163
Membranous Glomerulonephritis, 1164
Focal Segmental Glomerulosclerosis, 1164
Immunoglobulin A Nephropathy, 1164
Remission in Lupus Nephritis and Vasculitis, 1165
INDIVIDUALIZING THERAPY: MECHANISM OF ACTION AND TOXICITIES OF THERAPY, 1166
Corticosteroids, 1166

Calcineurin Inhibitors, 1167
Alkylating Agents, 1168
Azathioprine, 1170
Mycophenolate Mofetil, 1170
Rituximab and Ocrelizumab, 1171
Eculizumab, 1171
Adrenocorticotropic Hormone, 1171
Treatment Algorithms and Considerations, 1172
CONCLUSION, 1173

THE GLOBAL IMPACT AND CHALLENGES

The societal burden of glomerulonephritis (GN) to both the individual and the health care system is grossly underappreciated and the costs underestimated due to the lack of national or international registries of GN at the level of renal pathologic processes. The full disease impact is also substantially discounted if assessed solely from figures derived from end-stage kidney disease (ESKD) registries, as GN is not only a common cause of ESKD that can affect patients at any age, but also treatment strategies for the disease are chronic and not without significant morbidity and mortality even in patients who never reach ESKD.

With respect to ESKD, there are significant global variations in the percentage of incident and prevalent patients secondary to GN. According to the United States Renal Data System, GN accounts for approximately 30% of the cases receiving pre-ESKD care and 10% to 20% of incident patients undergoing dialysis.[1] Very similar data have been reported from the Canadian Organ Replacement Registry, wherein GN accounted for 11% of ESKD cases, ranking second among identifiable causes behind diabetes.[2] In the countries belonging to the European Renal Association–European Dialysis and Transplant Association ESKD Registry, significant variations are noted with much higher GN incidence rates in Eastern European countries, ranging from 8.6% in Denmark to 19.6% in Romania, wherein GN is the most common identifiable cause of ESKD.[3] In the past, GN had dominated causation of ESKD in the Australia and New Zealand Registry, but current reports suggest the same trends as those observed in North American databases, wherein GN is now behind diabetes as a cause of ESKD (27% versus 30%, respectively).[4] In registries from Pacific Asian regions, however, GN continues to account for the majority of cases of incident ESKD.[5] These differences have been attributed to various factors, including genetic background as well as environmental and infectious exposures, but additional factors such as differences in health care policies and disparities in access to ESKD programs may also exist.[6] In contrast to data describing incident ESKD populations, GN dominates as the cause of ESKD among prevalent patients on renal replacement therapy or with a functioning renal transplant, but these numbers are likely to be biased, reflecting the younger age on average as well as the enhanced survival of the patient population with GN compared to patients with diabetes.[5] Regardless, the full burden of GN as an incident or prevalent cause of ESKD remains underestimated in ESKD registries due to the high likelihood that cases of ESKD categorized as "hypertensive nephrosclerosis" or "unknown" may very likely also represent undiagnosed GN given the often-asymptomatic course in many patients.

As a significant number of patients will live with GN for many years before they ultimately progress to dialysis or will

Table 34.1 Trends in Selected Kidney Biopsy Diagnoses Captured in the Regional Toronto Glomerulonephritis Registry, between 1975 and 2004 (Total Number of Biopsies during This Period, 9256)

	1975-79	1980-84	1985-90	1990-94	1995-99	2000-04	Total
IgA	129	215	227	262	309	356	1498
FSGS	141	164	163	239	311	271	1289
Membranous	134	172	171	164	129	143	913
MPGN	90	67	33	46	37	31	304
Lupus	170	191	143	174	136	100	914
Vasculitis	29	66	76	93	76	68	408
Total	693	875	813	978	998	969	5326

FSGS, Focal segmental glomerulosclerosis; IgA, immunoglobulin A; MPGN, membranoproliferative glomerulonephritis.

die before reaching that stage, an estimate of the global extent of these diseases may therefore be better approximated by imputing incidence rates from countrywide registries of renal pathologic conditions. Further, these broadly inclusive local registries based on pathologic processes that capture all biopsies performed in a large and defined geographic region can provide important insights regarding potential shifts in the distribution of histologic subtypes of GN. Such a registry from Finland, for example, reported an incidence of GN that ranged from 8.7 to 25.4 per 100,000 population in the central hospitals and the university center, respectively, which was remarkably higher than the rates reported by European biopsy registries (between 1 and 6.9).[7] Such variations are seen throughout the world, undoubtedly biased by biopsy practice patterns. However, if one were to assume an average crude incidence of GN to be between 100 and 200 per million population, this would indicate an annual incident rate of GN in North America (population 400 million) of between 40,000 and 80,000 cases.

Data from our own linked clinical and pathology regional registry that have captured GN cases from the greater Toronto area since 1975 have noted that the annual absolute number of biopsy-proven cases of GN has not substantially changed, but shifts within the specific histologic groups have occurred (Table 34.1).[8] There has been a 2- to 3-fold increase in immunoglobulin A (IgA) nephropathy (IgAN) and focal segmental glomerulosclerosis (FSGS), a 2-fold reduction in idiopathic membranoproliferative GN (MPGN), and virtually no change in the incidence of membranous glomerulonephritis (MGN) over the past 3 decades. Although similar shifts over time have been reported from other large North American centers, it is not entirely clear if this represents true changes in incidence patterns, variations in biopsy practice patterns or reporting, and/or changes to the ethnic composition of the study population through immigration. Geographic and ethnic variation clearly influences diagnostic patterns. In a large retrospective review of 600 biopsies from China, IgAN accounted for 40% of all diagnoses and was three times more common than FSGS and 30 times more common than membranous nephropathy.[9] The recognition of "new" treatable causative factors, such as hepatitis C virus producing the injury pattern of MPGN, is another possible explanation for variation and changes in histologic subtypes.[10] Still, changes in histologic subtypes of GN, if real, may reflect fundamental shifts in biologic and environmental factors underlying the pathogenesis of these diseases and is another substantive reason for the creation of national and international GN registries.

These crude estimates of the population incidence of GN are not informative with respect to describing the natural history of these disorders over the critical period between biopsy and registration as an ESKD statistic. Despite this limitation, during the past decade there have been important changes in our approach to the treatment of patients with GN driven by prospectively collected natural history data and therapeutic studies. There has also been an important shift in the treatment of GN to a more evidence-based approach with the publication of a new set of evidence-based recommendations for management of patients with GN developed under the auspices of Kidney Disease: Improving Global Outcomes (KDIGO).[11] Although this endeavor will assist with the standardization of practice, the paucity of high quality (level 1) evidence remains a significant obstacle in the treatment of glomerular disease.

The randomized controlled trial remains the gold standard for the assessment of therapeutic efficacy, but there are important limitations to both the interpretation and execution of such studies in patients with GN. Even the currently available clinical trials have limitations in regard to their generalizability, with existing trials excluding many patients such as those with atypical presentations and comorbid conditions, and often represent a skewed ethnic composition given that most are small single-center experiences. Furthermore, major changes in nonspecific treatment (such as introduction of inhibitors of the renin angiotensin aldosterone system for blood pressure control) and in our understanding of the pathogenesis of these diseases (such as the recognition of the causal link between MPGN and hepatitis C), have reduced the external validity of previously completed trials even though they may have been well-designed, randomized controlled studies. Larger randomized controlled trials in GN are not appealing to funding agencies (either in the private or public sector), as the target population is relatively small and the cost of such studies is high. Part of the financial burden relates to the size and duration of studies required to demonstrate "clinical benefit" in patients with GN. A major disincentive for the development of such studies is a lack of consensus regarding the clinical relevance of surrogate outcome measures. In general, only "hard outcomes" such as patient and/or renal survival are acceptable to granting agencies, government policy regulators, and the pharmaceutical industry.[12] Since the great majority of patients with GN, regardless of the specific subtype, will have slowly progressive disease, this limits the capacity to organize, fund, or even properly interpret clinical trials.

Assessment and follow-up of large cohorts of patients with GN during the trajectory of their chronic kidney disease though has yielded new and important information that has influenced patient management and altered how we assess treatment benefit. These efforts have allowed a more accurate identification of modifiable predictors of clinical outcome, thus allowing physicians to alter the course of the patient's disease. Although renal and patient survival remains the gold standard of benefit in the treatment of GN, surrogate markers of these end points have emerged during the past decade, and a significant contribution to this domain of practice has been a better understanding of the importance of proteinuria on renal injury and the recognition that its reduction has a substantial impact on both the rate of progression of kidney disease and ultimately on renal survival. It is generally accepted that complete remission of proteinuria does lead to significant improvement in quality of life (e.g., improvement of edema), as well as in renal survival.[12] A quantitative assessment of the value of proteinuria reduction is also emerging and will be a crucial element in the decision making of nephrologists in terms of balancing the risks and benefits of treatment. However, the quantitative impact of a partial remission in proteinuria, including its definition and duration on renal survival, requires further clarification before its universal acceptance as a surrogate indicator of long-term survival.

A series of publications on the most common primary and secondary progressive GNs has provided a more comprehensive framework focused on a more uniform definition and an improved estimate of the benefits of achieving a partial remission of proteinuria. This body of literature is described later. This should provide practicing nephrologists with a critical piece of information to assist them in both their therapeutic decisions and patient counseling. The capacity to translate proteinuria reduction into a semi-quantifiable estimate of improvement in long-term outcome provides an important element of the benefit in the risk/benefit equation, not only in terms of whether to initiate treatment, but more commonly today to provide help in the decision about prolonging treatment or retreating a patient to maintain or reestablish a partial remission.

OUTCOME MEASURES AND CLINICAL TRIALS IN GLOMERULONEPHRITIS

During the past decade there have been important changes in our approach to the treatment of patients with GN driven by prospectively collected natural history data, therapeutic studies, and the evolution toward a more evidence-based approach to clinical care. Central to this process is the identification of surrogate outcomes of kidney disease progression that indicate risk for kidney failure and morbidity attributable to kidney disease. This process is not only critical for design of clinical trials and regulatory drug approval processes, but also essential for defining treatment goals for patients.

A significant contribution to this domain of practice has been a better understanding of the importance of proteinuria in renal injury and the recognition that its reduction has a substantial impact on both the rate of progression of kidney disease and ultimately on renal survival.[13] Although this has significantly improved our capacity to assess the benefits of treatment, our evaluation of risks of therapy requires further refinement. Furthermore, while complete remission of proteinuria is accepted as a surrogate marker of favorable patient and kidney outcome in patients with GN, the relationship between partial remission of proteinuria in GN and reduction of kidney failure and mortality appears to be highly clinically relevant but requires further validation and refinement.

The shift in the treatment of GN to a more evidence-based approach is supported by the publication of clinical practice guidelines to help the nephrologist in the management of patients with these disorders.[14] While the randomized controlled trial remains the gold standard for the assessment of therapeutic efficacy, there are important limitations to both the execution and interpretation of such studies in patients with GN. Randomized controlled trials in GN are not appealing to funding agencies (either in the private or public sector), as the target population is relatively small and the diseases are most often slowly progressive, requiring longer observation periods to reach hard end points such as kidney failure, and therefore the cost of such studies is high. The lack of consensus regarding the clinical relevance of surrogate outcome measures limits design and feasibility of randomized controlled studies in GN.

The currently available clinical trials have limitations in regard to their generalizability. To design statistically and financially viable studies, investigators must select a relatively homogeneous population to ensure that the required sample size is achievable and that the study can be completed within an acceptable time frame. A homogeneous population, by definition, excludes many patients, such as those with atypical presentations and comorbid conditions, and often represents a skewed ethnic composition due to language fluency requirements for participation. Furthermore, major changes in nonspecific treatment (such as introduction of inhibitors of the renin angiotensin aldosterone system for blood pressure control) and in our understanding of the pathogenesis of these diseases (e.g., the causal link between MPGN and hepatitis C) have reduced the external validity of previously completed trials, even though they may have been well-designed, randomized controlled studies.[15,16]

QUANTIFICATION OF THE BENEFITS OF PROTEINURIA REDUCTION

Renal and patient survival remain the gold standard of measurement of benefit in the treatment of GN; however, few clinical trials in GN consider these definitive end points directly. The rare nature and relatively slow rate of progression of these diseases make the identification of surrogate end points of hard outcomes a necessity. A series of publications has focused on estimating the benefits of achieving a partial remission of proteinuria. This provides nephrologists with a critical piece of information to assist them in both their therapeutic decisions and patient counseling. The capacity to translate proteinuria reduction into a semiquantifiable estimate of improvement in long-term outcome remains a challenge; however, these studies suggest strongly that proteinuria should inform decisions regarding initiation and duration of immunosuppressive treatment.

MEMBRANOUS GLOMERULONEPHRITIS

Natural history studies in MGN have demonstrated the value of complete remission of proteinuria and the unfavorable outcome in patients with persistent high-grade proteinuria. Although a variety of definitions of partial remission have been applied to membranous nephropathy over the past 25 years, the great majority of studies required reduction to subnephrotic-range proteinuria (<3.5 g/day). A study of a prospective cohort of 348 nephrotic patients with MGN assessed the benefit of a complete or partial remission of proteinuria on both renal survival and rate of progression.[17] Partial remission required both a reduction to less than 3.5 g/day and a 50% decrease from peak proteinuria. Over a median follow-up of 60 months, 30% of patients had a complete remission, 40% had a partial remission, and the remaining 30% had no remission. At 10 years, renal survival in those with a complete remission was 100% with little disease progression over the same time frame as measured by the slope of the creatinine clearance (−1 mL/min/yr). Those achieving a partial remission had a 90% renal survival at 10 years and a more rapid rate of progression compared to those with complete remission, although still limited to a loss of −2 mL/min/yr of creatinine clearance. In comparison, those with no remission had a renal survival of only 50% at 10 years and a very significant increase in progression rate that was five times the rate seen in the partial remission group (−10 mL/min/yr). Achieving a partial remission was an independent predictor both of renal survival and rate of progression. Kidney survival from renal failure for partial remission was significantly improved (hazard ratio [HR] for ESKD compared to the reference group of no remission, 0.08; 95% confidence interval [CI], 0.03 to 0.19; $P < 0.001$). In addition, the value of a partial remission was also analyzed using time-dependent variables to ensure attribution of any benefit on survival to the time *after* partial remission has been achieved. Indeed the adjusted hazard ratio for the risk for ESKD in patients achieving a partial remission (expressed as a time-dependent variable) was 0.17 in comparison to those not achieving a remission of proteinuria (95% CI, 0.09 to 0.33; $P <0.001$). Additional important information gleaned from the study included the observation that treatment-induced partial remissions had the same favorable long-term outcome as those acquired spontaneously, and although the rate of relapse was high (47%), the relapses were often reversible with repeat treatment. These data strongly support the contention that partial remission is an important therapeutic target in patients with membranous GN with measurable and clinically relevant benefits for both progression rate and renal survival. This study did not identify the intervention required for achievement of partial remission of proteinuria; partial remission of proteinuria is also associated with favorable outcome when achieved spontaneously.[18] Nonetheless, the findings allow a better assessment of treatment benefits by attributing a quantitative value to partial remission. This in turn facilitates the assessment of the balance between benefits and risk of treatment of patients with MGN.

FOCAL SEGMENTAL GLOMERULOSCLEROSIS

The same estimates of benefit of proteinuria reduction in regard to the long-term outcome are available for patients with FSGS. It has been appreciated for some time that complete remission of proteinuria is the best predictor of favorable renal survival.[19,20] However, a standardized definition of partial remission and an assessment of its benefit would improve the physician's ability to balance the benefits of intense immunosuppressive treatment versus the well-recognized risks of the current available treatment regimens for FSGS.[21,22] Factors that have been previously associated with a poor outcome in FSGS have included the severity of initial proteinuria, the initial creatinine clearance, and the extent of tubulointerstitial disease on histologic examination.[18,23] Histologic variant is an important consideration; however, reduction of proteinuria is likely an independent determinant of outcome.[24]

The impact of proteinuria reduction on disease course was addressed in a long-term cohort study of 281 nephrotic patients with biopsy-proven primary FSGS followed over an average of 65 months.[25] A partial remission, defined by both a reduction of proteinuria to subnephrotic range (<3.5 g/day) and a 50% reduction from peak proteinuria, provided the best discrimination among the patients in terms of both renal survival and progression rate. During the observation period 55 patients had a complete remission, 117 patients achieved a partial remission, and 109 had no remission of proteinuria. Partial remission was independently predictive of both renal survival and rate of decline in renal function by multivariate analysis and was associated with more favorable outcome even in the context of a future disease relapse. Partial remission was associated with improved renal survival with a time-adjusted hazard ratio of 0.48 (95% CI, 0.24 to 0.96; $P = 0.04$). Ten-year renal survival was 75% in the partial remission group compared to 35% in those with no remission. Similar to MGN, this information on the quantitative benefits of partial remission is important in the assessment of the FSGS patient because it provides equipoise to the risks of treatment.

IMMUNOGLOBULIN A NEPHROPATHY

The importance of proteinuria in IgAN has been long recognized, but its relative value compared to FSGS and membranous nephropathy is quite distinct. There are important quantitative differences in the impact of proteinuria in patients with IgAN compared with those with FSGS and MGN. Proteinuria, at far lower levels compared to MGN and FSGS, is tightly correlated with renal outcome.[26]

Treatment studies and observational data support the importance of proteinuria reduction in mitigating risk for progressive disease in IgAN. Analyzing patients with IgAN enrolled in a series of randomized controlled trials of fish oils, Donadio and associates demonstrated an association between proteinuria reduction and both improved renal survival and prolonged time to doubling of serum creatinine clearance.[27] A study of a prospectively enrolled cohort of more than 500 patients with primary IgAN followed for an average of 78 months evaluated the clinical relevance of achieving a partial remission of proteinuria to less than 1 g/day. In the almost 200 patients who achieved and sustained partial remission of proteinuria (either spontaneously or through treatment), the mean rate of decline in renal function was only 10% of the rate in those who did not. Furthermore, regardless of the level of presenting proteinuria, those who attained a partial remission had the same long-term prognosis and slow rate of disease progression as those subjects whose peak proteinuria never exceeded 1 g/day. Although there were other modifiable factors identified in the multivariate analysis associated with kidney function decline (time-averaged mean arterial pressure and exposure to agents that blocked the renin angiotensin aldosterone system), the level of sustained proteinuria was the dominant modifiable risk. The differential in both progression rate and renal failure risk was dramatic, and understanding the impact of even a small but sustained improvement in proteinuria is extremely valuable information for the practicing physician. Occasionally IgAN presents with the nephrotic syndrome and preserved renal function. In this subset of patients, partial or complete remission of the nephrotic syndrome is also associated with a favorable outcome.[28]

Proteinuria has strong links to cardiovascular mortality in patients without GN.[29] A longitudinal study of nearly 1400 patients with IgAN followed in Korea suggested that this disease—particularly when associated with proteinuria of less than 1 g/day—may be associated with a higher standardized mortality rate.[30] The potential independent benefit of proteinuria reduction on mortality certainly merits further study.

REMISSION IN LUPUS NEPHRITIS AND VASCULITIS

Similar to the primary progressive variants of GN, complete absence of active renal disease has been associated with excellent long-term renal survival in systemic lupus erythematosus (SLE), although even this status does not guarantee freedom from ever developing chronic kidney disease.[31] Quantitation of the effect of partial remission of proteinuria on long-term outcome has been estimated in a long-term observational study of 86 patients with biopsy-proven diffuse proliferative lupus nephritis followed for a decade.[32] The authors defined complete remission as absence of significant proteinuria and a serum creatinine of less than 1.4 mg/dL and a partial remission as a 50% reduction in baseline proteinuria with a nadir in proteinuria of less than 1.5 g/day and no more than a 25% rise in baseline serum creatinine clearance. Patient and renal survival were strongly influenced by whether the patient achieved a complete remission, partial remission, or no remission in proteinuria. At 10 years the patient survival and renal survival in subjects achieving a complete remission were 95% and 94%, respectively; in those reaching a partial remission, they were 76% and 45%; and, in those who never met criteria for a partial or complete remission, they were only 46% and 13%. The clinical value of a reduction in proteinuria in terms of amelioration of long-term outcome was confirmed in a 10-year follow-up of a clinical trial comparing immunosuppressive regimens[33] and in pediatric and adolescent patients with SLE.[34]

Studies have indicated that long-term evaluation of proteinuria reduction and remission statistics is important for purposes of prognostication. At 6 months of evaluation, less than half of patients with severe lupus nephritis enrolled in therapeutic trials will have reached a complete remission.[35] A review of long-term outcomes of patients with severe lupus nephritis treated in a prior randomized controlled study indicated that halving of proteinuria at 6 months was an important predictor of both long-term renal and patient survival.[36] The finding of an association between polymorphic kidney disease risk variants at the apolipoprotein 1 gene (APOL1) and more rapid progression to ESKD in sub-Saharan African ancestry populations[37] may lead to genetically guided individualization of therapies, and certainly future clinical studies that include populations of African ancestry will need to take this variable into account.

Rapid deterioration in renal function is a severe and relatively common manifestation of vasculitis, a systemic disorder that commonly terminates in ESKD or death of the patient without appropriate therapy. The rapidity of kidney disease progression and the significant risk for either disease-associated or drug-related mortality distinguish vasculitis from the previously described primary GNs. The significant benefits in terms of both kidney and patient survival with treatment compared to no treatment is countered by the current potent drug regimens required that have their own significant life-threatening consequences; significant adverse effects are described in up to 90% of treated patients.[38-41] This confluence of severe disease and toxic therapy is aggravated by the more advanced average age at presentation of vasculitis compared to other types of GN. This further emphasizes the importance of accurate and early assessment of the predictive markers of outcome for both patient and renal survival.[42] The need for considering both risk and benefits was demonstrated in a review of 100 patients with vasculitis, whose presenting creatinine clearance was above 500 μmol/L (5.6 mg/dL).[43] Fifty-five percent of the deaths were attributed to the adverse effects of treatment, almost exclusively related to opportunistic infections, including *Pneumocystis jirovecii* (formerly *Pneumocystis carinii*) pneumonia and cytomegalovirus infections. In contrast, only 25% of the deaths were attributed to active uncontrolled vasculitic disease, with the remaining 25% related to the underlying advanced age and/or comorbid conditions of the patients. The authors determined that in patients presenting with vasculitis and severe renal failure, predictors of the need for permanent renal replacement therapy were limited. The only indicators identified were age at onset of the disease and pathologic process, the degree of arteriosclerosis, and the proportion of segmental crescents and/or eosinophilic infiltrates. No clinical parameters were independently predictive of death. Even within these limited predictive indices, the variation was wide and the sensitivity low.

In a prospective study in patients with mild to moderate renal involvement at presentation (i.e., serum creatinine concentration <500 μmol/L), the authors noted that the level of renal function at onset and renal pathologic lesions suggestive of chronicity were indicators of a poor prognosis. In contrast, the presence of active lesions such as crescents and necrosis was the only indicator that predicted a treatment response and improved renal outcome at 18 months.[44] A semiquantitative assessment of prognosis based on any one individual factor or a combination of them was not performed, likely related to the acuity of the condition and the wide deviations in these predictive indices. A systematic review of studies in vasculitis, including patients with minimal renal involvement, identified similar predictors of outcome in regard to remission, relapse, and renal and overall patient survival.[45]

Against this background, a heightened awareness of the risks of our current therapies needs to be considered in every patient by the practicing nephrologist. The real dangers associated with these therapies mandate repeated reviews of the patient, including a critical analysis of the response likelihood versus the accumulating risks of ongoing therapy. This assessment should include the possibility of a repeat renal biopsy to assess activity versus irreversible chronic damage. In addition, when evaluating potential benefit of immunosuppressive therapy, improvement in organ and patient survival should still be paramount, but the integration of the benefits of proteinuria reduction and improved quality of life should now also be counted. Often not considered in this balance of risks and benefits of treatment is the risk of inadequate treatment of the GN, forgetting that renal replacement modalities (i.e., dialysis or transplantation) have their own attendant high rate of morbidity and mortality.

INDIVIDUALIZING THERAPY: MECHANISM OF ACTION AND TOXICITIES OF THERAPY

With every one of the immunosuppressive agents used in the treatment of GN, the risks of treatment versus potential benefits must be assessed on the basis of drug exposure (a composite of dose and duration) and individual patient factors, including gender, age, and comorbid conditions such as obesity, diabetes mellitus, and cardiac disease. Further, there is not universal availability of many of the newer drugs and biologic agents due to the paucity of controlled data and the high costs of many of these agents. Thus careful attention must be paid to potential side effects from the therapeutic choices made by practicing clinicians with side effect profiles often dominating the choice of therapy.

CORTICOSTEROIDS

Glucocorticoids are the most common antiinflammatory and immunosuppressive drugs used in the treatment of both primary and secondary GN. They have protean effects on immune responses mediated by T and B cells, including reversibly blocking T cell and antigen-presenting cell–derived cytokine and cytokine-receptor expression. Their hydrophobic structure permits them to easily diffuse into cells and bind to specific cytoplasmic proteins, facilitating translocation of these proteins into the cell nucleus, where they bind to a highly conserved glucocorticoid receptor DNA-binding domain (the glucocorticoid response element) and modulate gene transcription.[46] Some of the downstream effects accounting for the antiinflammatory activity of glucocorticoids include the inhibition of synthesis of proinflammatory cytokines implicated in glomerular and tubulointerstitial injury, such as interleukin-2, interleukin-6, interleukin-8, and tumor necrosis factor.[47,48] Glucocorticoids also exert a host of nontranscriptional immunomodulatory effects on immune effector cells, including alteration of leukocyte trafficking and chemotactic properties and modulation of endothelial function, vasodilation, and vascular permeability.[46] Evidence suggests a potential role in modulating production of putative leukocyte-derived permeability factors that contribute to proteinuria.[49,50]

MAJOR ADVERSE EFFECTS

Infection is a potential risk common to all immunosuppressant medications. Pronounced suppression of cell-mediated immunity results from the protean effects of corticosteroids on the immune system. Glucocorticoid exposure poses a significant short- and long-term risk for infection, particularly in older patients. A nested case-control analysis indicated a rate of serious infection as high as 46% with 6 months of continuous use of greater than 5 mg/day in patients with rheumatoid arthritis.[51] In addition to the potential to cause infection, glucocorticoids have widespread systemic side effects, including, but not limited to, impaired glucose tolerance, cardiovascular and gastrointestinal toxicity, and potentially severe musculoskeletal damage, as well as a large array of cosmetic, ophthalmologic, and psychiatric side effects.

Glucocorticoids affect glucose metabolism by increasing hepatic gluconeogenesis and decreasing peripheral tissue insulin sensitivity. These changes in glucose homeostasis may be ameliorated by dose reduction.[52] However, the metabolic effects of these drugs may not be completely reversible, even when the dose is reduced to physiologic range or discontinued entirely.[53] While higher doses of glucocorticoids are associated with a higher risk for hyperglycemia, additional risk factors for steroid-induced hyperglycemia include African American and Hispanic ancestry, obesity (defined as a body mass index > 30 kg/m^2), older age, a family history of diabetes, and the presence of other components of the metabolic syndrome.[53]

Given the elevated risk for cardiovascular disease in patients with kidney disease, the added cardiovascular toxicity of glucocorticoids is also an important consideration. A large cohort study of 68,781 glucocorticoid users demonstrated that high-dose steroids are independently associated with cardiovascular events after adjustment for other traditional risk factors,[54] including hypertension, glucose intolerance, and obesity. Gastrointestinal effects of glucocorticoids include induction of gastritis and gastrointestinal bleeding.

Glucocorticoids have important musculoskeletal effects. Muscle injury associated with chronic steroid treatment with glucocorticoid produces a pattern of proximal weakness, atrophy, and myalgia. The ideal management includes discontinuation of steroid administration, although recovery can take weeks or months. Steroid myopathy is more common when the patient has been exposed to the potent fluorinated steroids (dexamethasone, betamethasone, triamcinolone), but similar patterns of muscle injury have been described with the nonfluorinated steroids such as prednisone.[55] Osteopenia is commonly seen in patients with chronic steroid exposure. A retrospective study of a quarter of a million oral corticosteroid users over 18 years of age suggested relative rate of nonvertebral fracture during oral corticosteroid treatment increased even at doses as low as 2.5 to 7.5 mg/day.[56] Fracture risk rapidly declined toward baseline after stopping treatment. The European League Against Rheumatism released recommendations regarding chronic prednisone dosing and avoidance of loss of bone density.[57] Avascular necrosis is a different type of bone injury. It is a devastating condition associated with destruction of the head of the femur or other long bones. The relationship between development of avascular necrosis and dose of prednisone is less clear.[58]

Vision may be affected by cataract formation and increased intraocular pressure. Thinning of the skin, easy bruising, development of striae, and impaired wound healing may also be potentiated by glucocorticoids. Mood lability and insomnia induced by glucocorticoids also contribute to their relatively poor patient tolerance.

STRATEGIES FOR REDUCING TOXICITY

There are several strategies available for minimizing steroid exposure. In minimal change disease and some cases of FSGS, for instance, alternate-day prednisone therapy may be considered in lieu of daily regimens. This alternate-day approach is, however, not supported with evidence suggesting equal efficacy in adults with the nephrotic syndrome. An alternate strategy is shortening the course and/or a more rapid taper of the prednisone, and this approach is currently being investigated in the context of vasculitis (Plasma Exchange and Glucocorticoids for Treatment of Anti-Neutrophil Cytoplasm Antibody (ANCA)–Associated Vasculitis [PEXIVAS] study, www.clinicaltrials.gov). More commonly, a second nonglucocorticoid immunosuppressive agent is introduced for its "steroid-sparing" potential. The introduction of these agents has allowed the total exposure to corticosteroids in many of these disorders to be limited by allowing a shorter initial total exposure to the drug.

Alternate strategies specifically focus on reducing or preventing the complications related to corticosteroid treatment. Such prophylactic strategies include the use of antibiotics such as trimethoprim-sulfamethoxazole to prevent *P. jirovecii* pneumonia. Retrospective studies indicate that a corticosteroid dose equivalent to 16 mg of prednisone for a period of 8 weeks was associated with a significant risk for pneumocystis pneumonia.[59,60] Ongoing surveillance for diabetes is required along with regular eye examinations. Antihypertensive regimens may require adjustment while on high-dose therapy, and gastric protection in the form of a proton pump inhibitor should be prescribed. In relationship to the risk for fracture, if daily corticosteroids (0.5 to 1 mg/kg) are expected to be used in excess of 8 to 12 weeks in adults, consideration should be given to adding vitamin D 1000 U/day and 1 g/day of calcium, or consider the addition of bisphosphonate therapy while on the steroids. Other high-risk indicators for fractures should also trigger preventive treatment such as previously documented osteoporosis, advanced age, or likelihood of inactivity/immobility during the use of steroids. Bisphosphonates may have more potent effects to prevent reduction in bone density during corticosteroid use; however, it is important to note that bisphosphonates remain in mineralized bone for months to years, posing a theoretical risk for teratogenicity when administered to women of childbearing potential.[61]

CALCINEURIN INHIBITORS

Cyclosporine and tacrolimus are calcineurin inhibitors (CNIs) that suppress the immune response by downregulating T cell activation. They specifically block calcium-dependent T cell receptor signaling transduction, thereby inhibiting the transcription of interleukin-2, as well as other proinflammatory cytokines, in both T cells and antigen-presenting cells.[62] Interleukin-2 serves as the major activation factor for T cells and a key modulator of both T and B cell activity in numerous immunologic processes.[63] Tacrolimus and cyclosporine have a common mechanism of action (i.e., inhibition of calcineurin phosphatase), though they bind different intracellular proteins. These intracellular proteins belong to the immunophilin family with cyclosporine binding cyclophilin and tacrolimus binding FKBP12.[64] The role of differential immunophilin binding in the mechanism of toxicity is not clear, but it may allow for the unique side effect profile of each of these drugs. An alternative mechanism of action of these agents has been suggested relating to their capacity to stabilize the internal cytoskeletal structure of the glomerular podocyte.[65] This is an intriguing possibility and may help explain the efficacy of CNI therapy in some of the glomerular-based diseases at lower drug levels compared to those required in solid organ transplantation.[66]

MAJOR ADVERSE EFFECTS

The CNI agents have significant adverse effects with the most concerning being their nephrotoxicity. This is particularly relevant when prolonged therapy is being contemplated. These longer treatment courses are usually given to prevent or modify the well-recognized risk for relapse of nephrotic syndrome that does occur upon treatment withdrawal. CNI-associated nephrotoxicity can be severe, and reports indicate a significant risk for chronic kidney disease if the drug is given in high doses for prolonged periods, such as occurred in early recipients of nonrenal solid organ transplants.[67] However, the cyclosporine dose and duration used in these studies are no longer considered appropriate,[68] and lower doses in the glomerular-based diseases versus solid organ transplantation are currently advocated.[69] In addition, modifications have occurred in drug formulation of cyclosporine, which have resulted in more consistent and predictable pharmacokinetics, allowing at least potentially even lower drug exposure regimens.[69]

New-onset or worsening of hypertension is another important and common dose-dependent adverse effect of CNI use and likely contributes to their long-term nephrotoxic potential. The reported incidence of hypertension in patients with glomerular diseases treated with CNIs varies from 10% to 30%.[70] An additional significant adverse effect is the induction of glucose intolerance and even overt diabetes.[71] This seems to be specific to CNIs and is somewhat more common with tacrolimus.[72] The transplantation literature highlights the potential contributions of CNIs to development of hyperglycemia, which is thought to be a result of both impaired insulin secretion and increased insulin resistance. The higher rate of hyperglycemia associated with tacrolimus use may reflect differential effects on pancreatic β-cell insulin transcription and release. Even when CNIs are used as monotherapy, the risk for new-onset diabetes has been reported to be as high as 4%.[73]

As with all immunosuppressive agents, CNIs affect immune surveillance and are associated with an increased rate of infections and malignancy. The incidence of malignancy induced by CNIs in the glomerular diseases is very hard to determine from the literature. Very few of the GN treatment studies have been long enough to assess CNI exposure as an independent risk factor. Cyclosporine, however, has been used in the long-term management of other autoimmune diseases, including rheumatoid arthritis and psoriasis. When patients with rheumatoid arthritis treated with cyclosporine were compared to control patients (who received placebo, D-penicillamine, or chloroquine), an increased cancer risk was not seen.[74] A review of patients with psoriasis did find an increase in the standardized incidence ratio of cancer in patients treated with cyclosporine compared to the general population. However, when examined more closely and skin malignancies, known to be more common in patients with psoriasis, were excluded, the incidence was not significantly higher in the CNI-treated patients.[75] As such, though not well described, the incidence of drug-associated malignancy specifically in the context of GN therapy is considered to be relatively low.[76] The underlying risks for infection associated with untreated nephrotic syndrome and the potential for malignancy associated with membranous nephropathy further complicate the assessment of risk for these complications with CNI treatment.

Other common adverse effects of CNIs are cosmetic and include gum hypertrophy and hypertrichosis (less frequent with tacrolimus than cyclosporine). The excess hair growth can be severe and can contribute to poor drug adherence. A cohort of approximately 200 pediatric nephrotic patients treated with cyclosporine for an average of 22 months[77] was reviewed; reported side effects of such prolonged therapy included hypertrichosis (52.3%), gum hyperplasia (25.4%), hypertension (18.8%), and renal impairment (9.1%). Close examination of the subgroup of patients with renal impairment in this study is revealing. In the small number (n = 18 patients) that demonstrated renal impairment, 12 recovered completely after the cyclosporine was stopped, 3 experienced stable but continued renal impairment, and only 3 (1.5% of the total number exposed) had slow progression of their renal disease. On multivariate analysis, resistance to the cyclosporine treatment was the only factor predictive of renal impairment

STRATEGIES FOR REDUCING TOXICITY

In contrast to transplantation, long-term low-dose therapy with cyclosporine (1.0 to 2 mg/kg/day) with or without low-dose steroids, has been shown to be both safe and effective at maintaining remission. The lower toxicity of CNIs in patients with GN is at least in part related to the lower daily maintenance dose required and the capacity to gradually increase the dose over days or weeks to achieve a therapeutic effect versus the need for a much more rapid dose escalation following solid organ transplantation.[69] Although higher doses of cyclosporine may be required for the induction phase in membranous nephropathy, the initial dose can usually be reduced during the maintenance phase.[78] In renal transplant patients, CNI dose has been safely reduced after the first year with renal function remaining stable even after 20 years of exposure to this agent.[79] Nevertheless, nephrotoxicity is a risk with this therapy, and careful monitoring of drug levels, a constant awareness of drug interactions (which may either increase or decrease drug levels), and frequent monitoring of renal function are mandatory.

One of the mechanisms of the nephrotoxicity that is attributable to these agents is their renal vasoconstrictive properties. This hemodynamic effect is both dose dependent and reversible[80] but may still result in dangerous episodes of acute kidney injury. Therefore patients should be cautioned as to what to do in the event of unanticipated volume contraction secondary to dehydration. The more delayed chronic damage in the tubulointerstitial compartment and the small arterioles is less well understood but may also be ameliorated at least in part by a dose reduction or discontinuation of the agent. Toxicity may be more evident when CNIs are used in patients with more advanced renal impairment and/or those with significant tubulointerstitial and/or vascular changes noted on histologic evaluation. However, with careful monitoring and the slow escalation of dosage, even patients with significant renal dysfunction can be safely treated with CNIs.[81]

The hypertension that commonly accompanies treatment with CNIs is another adverse effect that requires attention. However, the adjustments in antihypertensive medication are usually straightforward, and the presence of hypertension does not generally preclude or limit CNI usage. The vasoconstrictive effects of cyclosporine, in addition to their effects on renal potassium secretion, may limit the ability to use higher doses of inhibitors of the renin angiotensin aldosterone system to control blood pressure in patients on cyclosporine. With respect to the risk for diabetes, ongoing vigilance by the prescribing physician is required. In patients at highest risk for developing glucose intolerance, including obese individuals, those with a strong family history of diabetes, older adults, and those with metabolic syndrome,[53] strategies for preventing this adverse effect include preferential use of cyclosporine over tacrolimus and/or the use of CNI monotherapy, thereby at least avoiding the additive risk of corticosteroid exposure.

ALKYLATING AGENTS

Cyclophosphamide is the most common alkylating agent used in the treatment of GN. It is a cytotoxic agent that acts largely through the alkylation of purine bases. This DNA damage induces apoptosis or altered function of both B cells and T cells.[82] Chlorambucil is the other drug of this class that is used, although less commonly than cyclophosphamide because of significant differences in both the short- and long-term adverse effect profile and drug tolerability.

MAJOR ADVERSE EFFECTS

Infertility in both men and women has been reported with these agents, most commonly following cyclophosphamide, and is likely the most concerning long-term side effect given the often younger age of patients with glomerular disease. This effect is closely related to total exposure but is also strongly impacted by the age of the patient.[83] One early series indicated that the rate of permanent ovarian failure was 26% in those who received between 10 and 20 g of cyclophosphamide but was greater than 70% in those whose cumulative dose was more than 30 g.[84] This effect is of particular concern in women during the later part of their reproductive life. It has been estimated that women who receive a single course of cyclophosphamide therapy (10 to 20 g exposure) before the age of 25 years are at significantly less risk for permanent sterility (0% to 15% risk) compared to the same exposure after the age of 30 (30% to 40% risk).[84-86] An even higher risk has been estimated by Ioannidis and colleagues, who calculated the risk for permanent ovarian failure for a standard dose of 12 g/m^2 to be 90% in women when treated after the age of 32.[87] This combined effect of age and exposure on fertility can be expressed as an odds ratio. These authors suggest an odds ratio for permanent ovarian failure of 1.48 per 100 mg/kg of cumulative dose and 1.07 per patient-year of age.[87,88] Although more difficult to estimate, there is certainly a substantial risk for infertility in men as well. However, the age effect has not been as clearly demonstrated as in women. Studies have indicated that long-term gonadal toxicity was not evident until the cumulative exposure to cyclophosphamide was greater than 300 mg/kg, but later information suggests a substantial risk at a cumulative dose of less than 168 mg/kg (equivalent to 12 g for a 70-kg patient),[89,90] and gonadal toxicity, as indicated by a reduction in sperm count, has been documented with exposures as low as 100 mg/kg.[83] Various approaches have been examined to preempt loss of ovarian function and to preserve fertility during exposure to cytotoxic agents. Among these, the use of gonadotropin-releasing hormone agonists to induce a prepubertal state during exposure has been examined with promising effects, but no universal consensus.[91-93]

The other major adverse effect is the risk for malignancy. It is suspected that this has been underestimated in the past at least in part due to the delay between exposure to the drug and the appearance of the cancer. This latent period may be many years. Data from an epidemiologic study of 293 Danish patients with antineutrophil cytoplasmic antibody–associated vasculitis treated with cyclophosphamide suggested a much lower safety limit for exposure than previously indicated.[94] The authors concluded that patients who received a cumulative dose of more than 36 g of cyclophosphamide (equivalent to 2 mg/kg for 8 months in a 70-kg patient) had a substantial increased risk for the development of a malignancy compared to the normal age- and sex-controlled population. Their standardized incidence ratio of acute myelocytic leukemia was 59.0, bladder cancer was 9.5, and nonmelanoma skin cancer was 5.2 above this cumulative cyclophosphamide exposure. They also confirmed the substantial delay between exposure and malignancies with a latent period of 6.9 to 18.5 years. This exposure of 36 g is a much lower threshold for these serious complications than previously estimated and needs to be validated in an independent data set.[95,96] In the meantime, however, the potential for toxicity at much lower exposure limit should be kept in mind when considering the more prolonged course of cyclophosphamide as a treatment option in membranous nephropathy, lupus nephritis, or vasculitis.

An additional well-recognized, short-term adverse effect of the alkylating agents is bone marrow suppression, particularly the white cell line. A meta-analysis reported significant leukopenia in 25% of patients with lupus nephritis who were treated with cyclophosphamide.[97] Another short-term adverse effect of cyclophosphamide is an increased susceptibility to infections. These infections can be severe and resistant to therapy and in combination with leukopenia can be overwhelming. Additional less serious but disconcerting side effects that can affect compliance include alopecia and hemorrhagic cystitis. This long list of potentially serious complications makes monitoring, for both short-term and long-term effects of these agents, a critical and necessary component of management.

Chlorambucil is an alternative alkylating agent used in the treatment of membranous nephropathy. The original regimen developed by Ponticelli and coworkers with this agent cycled it monthly with corticosteroids over 6 months.[98] The adverse effects of chlorambucil are similar to cyclophosphamide, although it has not been associated with the bladder toxicity with associated gross hematuria. Even so, chlorambucil may be less well tolerated overall than cyclophosphamide and has the added associated risk for acute myelogenous leukemia.[99]

STRATEGIES FOR REDUCING TOXICITY

Strategies to limit exposure focus on limiting duration of therapy rather than modifying the dose. The exception to this is the use of intravenous cyclophosphamide in lupus and vasculitis, wherein less frequent and smaller doses of intravenous cyclophosphamide appear to be as effective as the earlier higher-dose regimens with fewer adverse events.[100] A shorter-duration regimen of exposure is an established option in membranous nephropathy. The two published effective regimens vary dramatically in terms of cyclophosphamide exposure (see earlier chapters). In the original classic 6-month regimen, for example, cyclophosphamide exposure is limited to 3 months[98] compared to the later-published routine that employs a full year of exposure.[99]

Substitution of other agents less toxic than cyclophosphamide is another option. Mycophenolate mofetil (MMF) or azathioprine for maintenance therapy in lupus nephritis are well-established options and appear to have similar efficacy with significantly fewer adverse effects. Data from a randomized controlled trial in patients with diffuse proliferative lupus nephritis confirmed that MMF (3 g/day) was associated with fewer pyogenic infections than a cyclophosphamide-based regimen (relative risk, 0.36).[101] Similarly, long-term therapy with azathioprine has been proven to be as efficacious as cyclophosphamide in the maintenance phase of vasculitis, with less toxicity.[102] Similar results in terms of complete and partial remissions were obtained when MMF was substituted for the year of cyclophosphamide in membranous nephropathy, but a significantly lower incidence of serious side effects was observed. This study was not a randomized controlled trial since the cyclophosphamide-treated patients were a historical control group. Unfortunately, the relapse rate was very much higher than in the cyclophosphamide group.[103] Replacement of the cyclophosphamide with CNIs is another option. This substitution strategy could be employed when initial therapy with cyclophosphamide has failed, in the situation where the patient has relapsed, and/or when repeated exposure to alkylating agents was being considered. This strategy can be used in the management of patients with membranous nephropathy, lupus nephritis, or FSGS.

Monitoring the other potential adverse effects of cyclophosphamide by frequent blood counts and adjusting the dose relative to degree of renal impairment, age, and other comorbid conditions are additional tools to minimize cyclophosphamide toxicity. The likelihood of inducing opportunistic infections such as *P. jirovecii* pneumonia and/or cytomegalovirus can also be reduced by the use of prophylactic antibiotics or antivirals as described earlier in the discussion of corticosteroids. With respect to the potential to cause infertility in young patients, young men might consider sperm banking, while there are also data to suggest a gonadotropin-releasing hormone analog may provide ovarian protection, decreasing the rates of premature ovarian failure from 30% to 5% in one study.[104]

AZATHIOPRINE

Azathioprine is an inhibitor of inosine monophosphate dehydrogenase, a critical enzyme involved in de novo purine synthesis, required for lymphocyte division resulting in depressed levels of both B and T lymphocytes as well as immunoglobulin synthesis. Its metabolite 6-Thio-GTP causes immunosuppression by blockade of GTPase activation in T lymphocytes specifically by blocking activation of Rac proteins.[105]

MAJOR ADVERSE EFFECTS

Gastrointestinal side effects, including nausea and vomiting, are common and remain the primary reason for treatment interruptions.[106] Liver toxicity with a significant increase in serum transaminase levels has also been described as has pancreatitis.[107] Dose-related bone marrow suppression primarily affects white blood cells but can affect all cell lines and can be severe in patients with low levels of thiopurine methyltransferase. This genetic abnormality affects approximately 0.3% of the population, in whom the enzyme is lacking, while 11% of individuals are heterozygous for a variant low-activity allele with intermediate activity,[108] causing diminished azathioprine metabolism. Similarly, allopurinol causes drug accumulation and can result in severe myelosuppression.[109] As with all immunosuppressive agents, bacterial and viral infections do occur, particularly in the setting of leukopenia, and increased rates of malignancies, in particular skin cancers, have been noted.[110,111]

STRATEGIES FOR REDUCING TOXICITY

There is no consensus among physicians treating glomerular disease with respect to the assessment for thiopurine methyltransferase deficiency. Both genetic testing and functional assays are available, but it is common practice to simply slowly escalate the dose while surveying for toxicity. Myelosuppression will typically improve with dose reductions, and allopurinol should be avoided.

MYCOPHENOLATE MOFETIL

MMF is a relatively new immunosuppressive agent. It is hydrolyzed into mycophenolic acid, the active moiety of the drug. Similar to azathioprine, MMF is a reversible inhibitor of inosine monophosphate dehydrogenase, a critical enzyme involved in de novo purine synthesis, required for lymphocyte division.[112] Several factors contribute to the lymphocyte-specific effects of MMF on purine metabolism. First, unlike other cells, lymphocytes are uniquely dependent upon de novo purine synthesis to generate RNA and DNA since they do not have a salvage pathway for purine generation. Inhibition of this pathway by MMF therefore predominantly affects lymphocyte metabolism. MMF also is a highly potent inhibitor of the isoform of inosine monophosphate dehydrogenase that is expressed in activated lymphocytes (the type II isoform), contributing to its specificity.[113,114] The selectivity of MMF for inhibiting lymphocyte proliferation is the concept that underlies the reduced toxicity of MMF compared to other alkylating agents that affect all dividing cells. In addition to its effects on T and B cells, MMF may also affect fibroblast proliferation or activity[115] and endothelial function.[116]

MAJOR ADVERSE EFFECTS

The principal adverse effects of MMF relate to gastrointestinal symptoms, including both upper gastrointestinal irritation with nausea and vomiting and lower tract involvement with diarrhea. This is more common with MMF than with cyclophosphamide.[117] These symptoms tend to occur early in the course of treatment and can improve over time.

As with all antimetabolites, MMF can cause hematologic complications, including leukopenia and anemia. The myelosuppressive effects of MMF contribute to the risk for infection associated with its use, and, while some data suggest a lower infection risk than with cyclophosphamide in lupus nephritis, several studies indicate similar risk for serious infection, and serious infections have been reported.[97,118-120] Furthermore, the transplantation literature suggests an increased risk for viral infections with MMF, particularly in the context of multidrug regimens.[121] It is too early to determine whether there is a difference with respect to risks for late-onset malignancy with MMF when used for the treatment of lupus or other variants of GN.

Although there is no fertility impact, MMF has now clearly emerged as a human teratogen with an identifiable pattern of malformations—craniofacial (microtia or anotia, absent auditory canal, cleft palate, hypertelorism) and limb anomalies. In women who become pregnant while on MMF, manufacturer's data notes a 33% increased miscarriage rate and a 22% rate of teratogenicity. Therefore some informed women may elect to terminate the pregnancy.

STRATEGIES FOR REDUCING TOXICITY

Unlike the transplantation context, the dose of MMF can frequently be titrated up over the course of days to weeks to minimize development of gastrointestinal symptoms. Splitting the dosage into four times per day versus the standard two doses per day also reduces gastrointestinal problems. Temporarily reducing the dose also may be tried. The predominant effect on the bone marrow is leukopenia and is usually corrected by a temporary dose reduction. If the full dose is still not tolerated, the addition of MMF-sparing agents such as a low dose of steroid or a CNI may be considered. Sexually active women initiating MMF should have a negative pregnancy test before initiating the therapy, and those who desire pregnancy should be off MMF at least 6 weeks before conception.

RITUXIMAB AND OCRELIZUMAB

Rituximab is a genetically engineered, chimeric, murine/human monoclonal antibody directed against the CD20 antigen found on the surface of normal and malignant pre-B and mature B cells. The CD20 antigen is not expressed on hematopoietic stem cells, pro-B cells, normal plasma cells, or other normal tissues. Thus it has an impressive safety record when compared to classic cytotoxic agents. The precise mechanism of action of anti-CD20 antibodies in autoimmune disease and in particular GN is unclear. It is known that B cells play an important role as immunoregulatory cells by both antigen presentation and cytokine release. Their elimination could have dampening effects on other immune cells such as T lymphocytes, dendritic cells, and macrophages. In vitro studies have demonstrated that the Fc portion of rituximab binds human complement and can lead to cell lysis of the targeted cell through complement-dependent cytotoxicity, and it has been demonstrated that rituximab mediates antibody-dependent cellular cytotoxicity. Rituximab has been shown to be effective in the treatment of idiopathic membranous nephropathy and may work at least in part by depletion of the autoantibody to the podocyte-located antigen phospholipase A_2 receptor.[122] Further, rituximab may have a direct podocyte-modulating effect via cross reactivity with sphingomyelin phosphodiesterase acid-like 3b (SMPDL-3b) protein and regulation of acid sphingomyelinase essential for the lipid-raft compartmentalization of the podocyte plasma membrane, as well as for the organization and signaling of podocytes in general.[123] This potential direct effect on podocytes independent of its known effect on selective depletion of the B cell clone may make it a very effective option to consider for the treatment of idiopathic glomerular diseases.

Ocrelizumab is a genetically engineered, fully humanized monoclonal antibody directed against the same CD20 antigen found on the surface of normal B cells, with the same mode of action as rituximab. Due to its fully humanized nature, this anti-CD20 antibody can be infused more rapidly and has less immediate infusion-related reactions than rituximab. In addition, due to the fully humanized construct, formation of autoantibodies directed against the drug are unlikely, thereby enhancing the potential efficacy and safety of repeated treatments.

MAJOR ADVERSE EFFECTS

Acute infusion-related reactions can vary from minor symptoms to severe life-threatening reactions. Minor reactions occur in up to 10% of exposed individuals and include skin rash, pruritus, flushing, nausea, vomiting, fatigue, headache, flulike symptoms, dizziness, hypertension, and/or runny nose. Anaphylaxis and shock can occur but are fortunately rare (<1%). Other rare side effects that have been seen with the use of rituximab include anemia, cardiac arrhythmias, respiratory failure, and acute kidney injury (occurring in <0.1.%).[124-128] The latter severe reactions have been seen primarily—though not exclusively—with the use of ocrelizumab in the treatment of hematologic malignancies where the tumor cell burden is high and an acute tumor lysis syndrome can develop. More delayed adverse effects include serum sickness and an increased incidence of infection, including reactivation of latent viral infections, including hepatitis B and several cases of pneumocystis pneumonia.[129] There have been several reports of the development of progressive multifocal leukoencephalopathy in patients treated with this agent. This devastating syndrome is due to the activation of latent JC polyomavirus and is associated with progressive neurologic impairment and ultimately death within months of diagnosis. In the majority of reported cases, progressive multifocal leukoencephalopathy developed when rituximab was used in combination with chemotherapy.[130] Given the impact of rituximab on antibody formation, vaccinations that contain live organisms should be avoided during treatment with rituximab.

Formation of human antichimeric antibodies (HACAs) does occur, although their clinical significance is unclear. Despite the appearance of HACAs in patients treated with rituximab and their theoretical consequences, these sequelae have not been uniformly observed in the small studies in GN.[131] The new fully humanized version of the anti-CD20 agent should either ameliorate or eliminate the problem of HACA formation.

STRATEGIES FOR REDUCING TOXICITY

The precise dose and/or regimen to use in patients with autoimmune disorders are unknown. Although the relationship between peripheral CD20-positive cell depletion and response is poor, it has been suggested that a single dose, in membranous nephropathy, is adequate for B cell depletion and provides a similar response in proteinuria as multiple doses of the agent.[132]

ECULIZUMAB

Eculizumab is an anti-C5 monoclonal antibody designed for use in diseases characterized by functional impairment of endogenous inhibitors of the activation of the alternative complement pathway. The activation of this cascade has classically been implicated in atypical hemolytic uremic syndrome, thus providing a potential rationale for this agent in these diseases.[133,134] Emerging evidence suggests that complement dysregulation may be a critical contributor to many forms of progressive glomerular injury traditionally attributed to classical or lectin-activated complement pathways. Activation of these pathways and their potential inhibition by eculizumab may have relevance in the context of MPGN,[135] SLE,[136] and other forms of GN.

MAJOR ADVERSE EFFECTS

Overall eculizumab is well tolerated, but there is the potential for an increased risk for *Neisseria meningitidis* infections associated with blocking the alternate complement pathway. Therefore vaccination and careful surveillance are recommended based on its use in patients with paroxysmal nocturnal hemoglobinuria.[137]

STRATEGIES FOR REDUCING TOXICITY

The precise dose and/or regimen to use in patients with glomerular diseases is presently unknown.

ADRENOCORTICOTROPIC HORMONE

Synthetic formulations of adrenocorticotropic hormone (ACTH) have previously proven effective in patients with nephrotic syndrome, and the use of ACTH for the treatment of elevated cholesterol and proteinuria dates back many decades.[138,139] In Europe the synthetic formulation of ACTH, tetracosactide (Synacthen), which is not available in North America, has proven similarly effective in both uncontrolled series and a small randomized controlled trial in which it was compared to cytotoxic therapy.[140-142] To date there are limited data to also suggest natural ACTH (H.P. Acthar Gel), which is currently the only available ACTH preparation in North America, may also have a beneficial effect in patients with nephrotic syndrome by lowering proteinuria and improving serum albumin and cholesterol profiles.[143]

The active ingredients of H.P. Acthar Gel are part of the family of structurally related peptides known as melanocortin peptides. Melanocortin peptides, which include ACTH and the α-, β-, and γ-melanocyte-stimulating hormones, are derived from the natural protein pro-opiomelanocortin, which binds to the cell surface G protein–coupled receptors known as melanocortin receptors (MCRs).[144] To date, five forms of MCRs have been cloned, each with different tissue distributions, affinities, and physiologic roles. As such, their potential therapeutic mechanisms are numerous and complex.[145] Potential renoprotective mechanisms include corticosteroid-mediated systemic immunosuppression and antiinflammatory actions subsequent to ACTH-induced steroidogenesis through MC2R interaction, as well as direct MCR-mediated immunomodulation and antiinflammatory effects (MC1R, MC3R, and MC5R). Correction of dyslipidemia mediated by MC1R and MC5R on hepatic cells and neurogenic antiinflammatory effects mediated by MC3R and MC4R expressed in the central nervous system are likely also beneficial to the kidneys. Finally, a direct MCR-mediated protective effect on kidney cells, particularly the podocytes, has been described. MCRs are expressed in glomerular podocytes, and receptor stimulation has been demonstrated to reduce oxidative stress and improve glomerular morphology by diminishing podocyte apoptosis, injury, and loss in the remnant kidney animal model.[146]

MAJOR ADVERSE EFFECTS

In a pilot study, side effects were noted to be dose dependent.[143] Reported side effects associated with the use of ACTH include steroid-like effects, including a cushingoid appearance, weight gain, and worsening of edema or bloating. Potential skin changes include acne, flushing, and bronzing. With respect to potential psychologic effects of the treatment, increased irritability, depression, and improved mood have been noted, along with transient insomnia, tremulousness, dizziness, muscle aches or pain, headaches, gastrointestinal symptoms, and blurred vision, as well as generalized weakness or fatigue. Glucose intolerance and frank diabetes are also potential rare side effects that tend to improve with the cessation of treatment.

STRATEGIES FOR REDUCING TOXICITY

The precise dose and/or regimen to use in patients with glomerular diseases is presently unknown.

TREATMENT ALGORITHMS AND CONSIDERATIONS

Treatment recommendations are reviewed in other chapters of this book. A rigorous effort to promote evidence-based therapy for GN has been published by the KDIGO group.[11] This has been an outstanding addition to guide nephrologists regarding therapeutic algorithms. The purpose of these guidelines is to assist in decision making and to highlight the evidence underlying each therapeutic algorithm.[14] However, guidelines cannot account for all of the variations in patient comorbid conditions or individual nuances in potential treatment toxicity (e.g., desire to preserve fertility). Therefore application of these guidelines to the individual patient requires careful consideration. In practice, we consider the following questions before making guideline-based treatment recommendations:

1. What is the risk for progression to kidney failure in this individual patient?

    The critical question is whether the risks of the medication outweigh the risks of progression of the kidney disease. Complementary considerations are the morbidity and mortality associated with dialysis or with transplantation, where many of the same medications will be used to prevent rejection.

    Proteinuria is one of our main considerations when we decide whether or not there is an advantage to addition of immunomodulatory treatment to conservative therapy for treatment of patients with primary idiopathic GN. While the threshold of proteinuria associated with highest risk for disease progression varies according to disease (Figure 34.1), this measure is a more important contributor to our treatment decisions than histologic diagnosis. For example, membranous nephropathy may be a lesion that is very amenable to immunologic therapy. However, patients with membranous GN with persistent subnephrotic-range proteinuria have an excellent long-term prognosis.[147] The added advantage of immunotherapy versus conservative therapy alone is not established in this subpopulation. Renal insufficiency at presentation and progression of renal insufficiency during observation should also be considered. While this may argue for a more aggressive approach to care, side effects of immunosuppressive therapy are often more frequent in patients with impaired clearance and additional susceptibility to infections. Pathologic indices of kidney injury, in particular tubulointerstitial fibrosis, are also informative to address chronicity and prognosis. Indeed, a common clinical error is to put patients with irreversible kidney injury at risk with little chance of benefit.[148] Advanced tissue injury with impaired clearance may change the risk/benefit ratio of immunotherapy.

2. What are the patient's comorbid conditions?

    Ideally the choice of therapy should be tailored to the individual patient, considering comorbid conditions that may place patients at risk for medication toxicity. For example, guidelines suggest that a trial of a minimum of 4 weeks of corticosteroid therapy should be considered as first-line treatment for idiopathic FSGS associated with clinical features of the nephrotic syndrome. However, in a patient with significant obesity, weight gain and glucose intolerance induced by steroids are important potential toxicities. A CNI may be a better first choice. Important comorbid conditions to consider include personal or family history of glucose intolerance, obesity, cancer history, and prior immunosuppression exposure.

3. What are plans for childbearing?

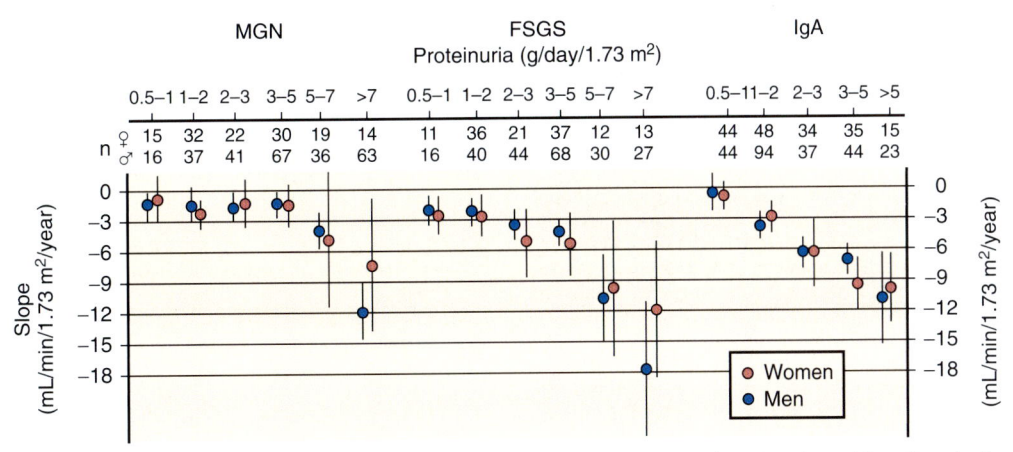

Figure 34.1 Differential impact of proteinuria according to sex and histologic subtype on the rate of renal function decline in membranous glomerulonephritis (MGN), focal segmental glomerulosclerosis (FSGS), and immunoglobulin A (IgA) nephropathy. (From Cattran DC, Reich HN, Beanlands HJ, et al: The impact of sex in primary glomerulonephritis. *Nephrol Dial Transplant* 23:2247-2253, 2008.)

Important considerations in patients contemplating future pregnancy include the teratogenicity of drugs, the effects of the medications on fertility, and the optimization of renal health before pregnancy.

CONCLUSION

GN remains a leading cause of chronic kidney disease and kidney failure. New data regarding clinically relevant surrogate end points and therapeutic goals will hopefully facilitate the development and study of novel agents to treat patients with GN and prevent loss of kidney function. The toxicity of immunotherapeutic agents requires careful consideration by clinicians; the risks of these drugs must always be weighed against the potential benefits in each individual patient, considering patient, disease, and drug-specific characteristics.

Complete reference list available at ExpertConsult.com.

KEY REFERENCES

6. Prakash S, Kanjanabuch T, Austin PC, et al: Continental variations in IgA nephropathy among Asians. *Clin Nephrol* 70:377–384, 2008.
7. Wirta O, Mustonen J, Helin H, et al: Incidence of biopsy-proven glomerulonephritis. *Nephrol Dial Transplant* 23:193–200, 2008.
12. Levey AS, Cattran D, Friedman A, et al: Proteinuria as a surrogate outcome in CKD: report of a scientific workshop sponsored by the National Kidney Foundation and the US Food and Drug Administration. *Am J Kidney Dis* 54:205–226, 2009.
14. Kidney Disease: Improving Global Outcomes (KDIGO) Glomerulonephritis Work Group: KDIGO Clinical Practice Guideline for Glomerulonephritis. *Kidney Int Suppl* 2:139–274, 2012.
15. Pozzi C, Bolasco PG, Fogazzi GB, et al: Corticosteroids in IgA nephropathy: a randomised controlled trial. *Lancet* 353:883–887, 1999.
17. Troyanov S, Wall CA, Miller JA, et al: Idiopathic membranous nephropathy: definition and relevance of a partial remission. *Kidney Int* 66:1199–1205, 2004.
18. Polanco N, Gutierrez E, Covarsi A, et al: Spontaneous remission of nephrotic syndrome in idiopathic membranous nephropathy. *J Am Soc Nephrol* 21:697–704, 2010.
25. Troyanov S, Wall CA, Miller JA, et al: Focal and segmental glomerulosclerosis: definition and relevance of a partial remission. *J Am Soc Nephrol* 16:1061–1068, 2005.
26. Berthoux F, Mohey H, Laurent B, et al: Predicting the risk for dialysis or death in IgA nephropathy. *J Am Soc Nephrol* 22:752–761, 2011.
28. Kim JK, Kim JH, Lee SC, et al: Clinical features and outcomes of IgA nephropathy with nephrotic syndrome. *Clin J Am Soc Nephrol* 7:427–436, 2012.
29. Weir MR: Microalbuminuria and cardiovascular disease. *Clin J Am Soc Nephrol* 2:581–590, 2007.
31. Contreras G, Pardo V, Cely C, et al: Factors associated with poor outcomes in patients with lupus nephritis. *Lupus* 14:890–895, 2005.
32. Chen YE, Korbet SM, Katz RS, et al: Value of a complete or partial remission in severe lupus nephritis. *Clin J Am Soc Nephrol* 3:46–53, 2008.
34. Gibson KL, Gipson DS, Massengill SA, et al: Predictors of relapse and end stage kidney disease in proliferative lupus nephritis: focus on children, adolescents, and young adults. *Clin J Am Soc Nephrol* 4:1962–1967, 2009.
35. Rovin BH, Parikh SV, Hebert LA, et al: Lupus nephritis: induction therapy in severe lupus nephritis—should MMF be considered the drug of choice? *Clin J Am Soc Nephrol* 8:147–153, 2013.
36. Korbet SM, Lewis EJ: Severe lupus nephritis: the predictive value of a (50% reduction in proteinuria at 6 months. *Nephrol Dial Transplant* 28:2313–2318, 2013.
37. Freedman BI, Langefeld CD, Andringa KK, et al: End-stage renal disease in African Americans with lupus nephritis is associated with APOL1. *Arthritis Rheumatol* 66:390–396, 2014.
40. de Groot K, Harper L, Jayne DR, et al: Pulse versus daily oral cyclophosphamide for induction of remission in antineutrophil cytoplasmic antibody-associated vasculitis: a randomized trial. *Ann Intern Med* 150:670–680, 2009.
41. Jayne D, Rasmussen N, Andrassy K, et al: A randomized trial of maintenance therapy for vasculitis associated with antineutrophil cytoplasmic autoantibodies. *N Engl J Med* 349:36–44, 2003.
43. de Lind van Wijngaarden RA, Hauer HA, Wolterbeek R, et al: Clinical and histologic determinants of renal outcome in ANCA-associated vasculitis: a prospective analysis of 100 patients with severe renal involvement. *J Am Soc Nephrol* 17:2264–2274, 2006.
45. Mukhtyar C, Flossmann O, Hellmich B, et al: Outcomes from studies of antineutrophil cytoplasm antibody associated vasculitis: a systematic review by the European League Against Rheumatism systemic vasculitis task force. *Ann Rheum Dis* 67:1004–1010, 2008.
49. McCarthy ET, Sharma M, Savin VJ: Circulating permeability factors in idiopathic nephrotic syndrome and focal segmental glomerulosclerosis. *Clin J Am Soc Nephrol* 5:2115–2121, 2010.
50. Audard V, Pawlak A, Candelier M, et al: Upregulation of nuclear factor-related kappa B suggests a disorder of transcriptional regulation in minimal change nephrotic syndrome. *PLoS One* 7:e30523, 2012.
51. Dixon WG, Abrahamowicz M, Beauchamp ME, et al: Immediate and delayed impact of oral glucocorticoid therapy on risk of

serious infection in older patients with rheumatoid arthritis: a nested case-control analysis. *Ann Rheum Dis* 71:1128–1133, 2012.
66. Cattran D: Management of membranous nephropathy: when and what for treatment. *J Am Soc Nephrol* 16:1188–1194, 2005.
73. Praga M, Barrio V, Juarez GF, et al: Tacrolimus monotherapy in membranous nephropathy: a randomized controlled trial. *Kidney Int* 71:924–930, 2007.
76. Anderka MT, Lin AE, Abuelo DN, et al: Reviewing the evidence for mycophenolate mofetil as a new teratogen: case report and review of the literature. *Am J Med Genet A* 149A:1241–1248, 2009.
77. Sheashaa H, Mahmoud I, El Basuony F, et al: Does cyclosporine achieve a real advantage for treatment of idiopathic nephrotic syndrome in children? A long-term efficacy and safety study. *Int Urol Nephrol* 39:923–928, 2007.
78. Alexopoulos E, Papagianni A, Tsamelashvili M, et al: Induction and long-term treatment with cyclosporine in membranous nephropathy with the nephrotic syndrome. *Nephrol Dial Transplant* 21:3127–3132, 2006.
97. Moore RA, Derry S: Systematic review and meta-analysis of randomised trials and cohort studies of mycophenolate mofetil in lupus nephritis. *Arthritis Res Ther* 8:R182, 2006.
98. Ponticelli C, Zucchelli P, Passerini P, et al: A 10-year follow-up of a randomized study with methylprednisolone and chlorambucil in membranous nephropathy. *Kidney Int* 48:1600–1604, 1995.
101. Ginzler EM, Dooley MA, Aranow C, et al: Mycophenolate mofetil or intravenous cyclophosphamide for lupus nephritis. *N Engl J Med* 353:2219–2228, 2005.
102. Contreras G, Pardo V, Leclercq B, et al: Sequential therapies for proliferative lupus nephritis. *N Engl J Med* 350:971–980, 2004.
109. Min MX, Weinberg DI, McCabe RP: Allopurinol enhanced thiopurine treatment for inflammatory bowel disease: safety considerations and guidelines for use. *J Clin Phar Ther* 39:107–111, 2014.
110. Gomez-Garcia M, Cabello-Tapia MJ, Sanchez-Capilla AD, et al: Thiopurines related malignancies in inflammatory bowel disease: local experience in Granada, Spain. *World J Gastroenterol* 19:4877–4886, 2013.
111. Pedersen EG, Pottegard A, Hallas J, et al: Risk of non-melanoma skin cancer in myasthenia patients treated with azathioprine. *Eur J Neurol* 21:454–458, 2014.
115. Morath C, Schwenger V, Beimler J, et al: Antifibrotic actions of mycophenolic acid. *Clin Transplant* 20(Suppl 17):25–29, 2006.
117. Appel AS, Appel GB: An update on the use of mycophenolate mofetil in lupus nephritis and other primary glomerular diseases. *Nat Clin Pract Nephrol* 5:132–142, 2009.
120. Walsh M, James M, Jayne D, et al: Mycophenolate mofetil for induction therapy of lupus nephritis: a systematic review and meta-analysis. *Clin J Am Soc Nephrol* 2:968–975, 2007.
123. Fornoni A, Sageshima J, Wei C, et al: Rituximab targets podocytes in recurrent focal segmental glomerulosclerosis. *Sci Transl Med* 3:85ra46, 2011.
124. Fervenza FC, Cosio FG, Erickson SB, et al: Rituximab treatment of idiopathic membranous nephropathy. *Kidney Int* 73:117–125, 2008.
126. Rovin BH, Furie R, Latinis K, et al: Efficacy and safety of rituximab in patients with active proliferative lupus nephritis: the Lupus Nephritis Assessment with Rituximab study. *Arthritis Rheum* 64:1215–1226, 2012.
132. Cravedi P, Ruggenenti P, Sghirlanzoni MC, et al: Titrating rituximab to circulating B cells to optimize lymphocytolytic therapy in idiopathic membranous nephropathy. *Clin J Am Soc Nephrol* 2:932–937, 2007.
133. Legendre CM, Licht C, Loirat C: Eculizumab in atypical hemolytic-uremic syndrome. *N Engl J Med* 369:1379–1380, 2013.
134. Nurnberger J, Philipp T, Witzke O, et al: Eculizumab for atypical hemolytic-uremic syndrome. *N Engl J Med* 360:542–544, 2009.
135. Smith RJ, Alexander J, Barlow PN, et al: New approaches to the treatment of dense deposit disease. *J Am Soc Nephrol* 18:2447–2456, 2007.
140. Berg AL, Arnadottir M: ACTH-induced improvement in the nephrotic syndrome in patients with a variety of diagnoses. *Nephrol Dial Transplant* 19:1305–1307, 2004.
141. Ponticelli C, Passerini P, Salvadori M, et al: A randomized pilot trial comparing methylprednisolone plus a cytotoxic agent versus synthetic adrenocorticotropic hormone in idiopathic membranous nephropathy. *Am J Kidney Dis* 47:233–240, 2006.
143. Hladunewich MA, Cattran D, Beck LH, et al: A pilot study to determine the dose and effectiveness of adrenocorticotrophic hormone (H.P. Acthar® Gel) in nephrotic syndrome due to idiopathic membranous nephropathy. *Nephrol Dial Transplant* 29:1570–1577, 2014.
144. Gong R: The renaissance of corticotropin therapy in proteinuric nephropathies. *Nat Rev Nephrol* 8:122–128, 2012.

Microvascular and Macrovascular Diseases of the Kidney

35

Piero Ruggenenti | Paolo Cravedi | Giuseppe Remuzzi

CHAPTER OUTLINE

MICROVASCULAR DISEASES, 1175
Thrombotic Microangiopathies: Hemolytic-Uremic Syndrome and Thrombotic Thrombocytopenic Purpura, 1175
Atheroembolic Renal Disease, 1191
Radiation Nephropathy, 1193
Renal Involvement in Systemic Diseases: Scleroderma, Sickle Cell Disease, and the Antiphospholipid Syndrome, 1195

MACROVASCULAR DISEASES, 1201
Occlusion of the Renal Artery, 1201
Aneurysms of the Renal Artery, 1203
Dissecting Aneurysms of the Renal Artery, 1204
Thrombosis of the Renal Vein, 1204

MICROVASCULAR DISEASES

Injury to endothelial cells is the primary event in many microvascular diseases of the kidney, including thrombotic microangiopathies, radiation nephropathy, scleroderma, and the antiphospholipid syndrome. Moreover, physiologic conditions in the medulla predispose to erythrocyte deformation and occlusion of the microvasculature in patients with sickle cell disease, whereas in patients with atherosclerosis, small renal arteries and arterioles can be injured and occluded by cholesterol-containing emboli dislodged from atherosclerotic plaques lining the main arteries. Independent of the initiating events, diseases that occlude the renal microvasculature invariably impair kidney perfusion and function. Early diagnosis and effective interventions to restore the integrity of the kidney microvasculature are instrumental to prevent irreversible tissue damage and kidney failure.

THROMBOTIC MICROANGIOPATHIES: HEMOLYTIC-UREMIC SYNDROME AND THROMBOTIC THROMBOCYTOPENIC PURPURA

The term *thrombotic microangiopathy* (TMA) defines a lesion of arteriolar and capillary vessel wall thickening, with intraluminal platelet thrombosis and partial or complete obstruction of the vessel lumina. Depending on whether renal or brain lesions prevail, two pathologically indistinguishable, but somehow clinically different, entities have been described, the hemolytic-uremic syndrome (HUS) and thrombotic thrombocytopenic purpura (TTP). In HUS and TTP, microvascular thrombosis is associated with thrombocytopenia, hemolytic anemia, and dysfunction of affected organs. Advances in our understanding of the molecular pathology have led to the recognition of three different diseases—typical HUS caused by Shiga toxin–producing *Escherichia coli* (Stx-HUS), atypical HUS (aHUS), associated with genetic or acquired disorders of regulatory components of the complement system, and TTP that results from a deficiency of ADAMTS13, a plasma metalloprotease that cleaves von Willebrand factor (Table 35.1). Complement hyperactivation appears to be a common pathogenetic effector that leads to endothelial damage and microvascular thrombosis in all three diseases.[1] In Stx-HUS, the toxin triggers endothelial complement deposition through the upregulation of P-selectin and possibly interferes with the activity of complement regulatory molecules. In aHUS, mutations in the genes coding for complement components predispose to hyperactivation of the alternative pathway of complement. In TTP, severe ADAMTS13 deficiency leads to the generation of massive platelet thrombi, which might contribute to complement activation (Figure 35.1). More importantly, evidence is emerging that pharmacologic targeting of complement with the anti-C5 monoclonal antibody eculizumab can effectively treat not only aHUS for which it is indicated, but in some cases, also Stx-HUS and TTP (see Figure 35.1).[1]

CLINICAL FEATURES
Hemolytic-Uremic Syndrome

The term *hemolytic-uremic syndrome* was introduced in 1955 by Gasser and coworkers in their description of an acute

Table 35.1	Classification of Hemolytic Uremic Syndrome and Thrombotic Thrombocytopenic Purpura*
Clinical Presentation	**Cause**
Hemolytic-Uremic Syndrome (HUS)	
Stx-associated	Infection by Shiga toxin–producing bacteria
Neuraminidase-associated	Infection by *Streptococcus pneumoniae*
Atypical: Familial	Mutations: *CFH*, 40%-45%; *CFI*, 5%-10%; *C3*, 8%-10%; *MCP*, 7%-15%; *THBD*, 9%; *CFB*, 1%-2%.
Atypical: Sporadic	
Idiopathic	Mutations: *CFH*, 15%-20%; *CFI*, 3%-6%; *C3*, 4%-6%; *MCP*, 6%-10%; *THBD*, 2%; *CFB*, two cases; anti-CFH antibodies: 6%-10%
Pregnancy-associated	Mutations: *CFH*, 20%; *CFI*, 15%
HELLP syndrome	Mutations: *CFH*, 10%; *CFI*, 20%; *MCP*, 10%
Drugs	Mutations: Rare *CFH* mutations; large majority unknown
Transplantation (de novo aHUS)	Mutations: *CFH*, 15%; *CFI*, 16%
HIV	Unknown†
Malignancy	Unknown†
Thrombotic Thrombocytopenic Purpura (TTP)	
Congenital	Homozygous or compound heterozygous mutations in *ADAMTS13* gene
Idiopathic	Anti-ADAMTS13 autoantibodies
Secondary	
Ticlopidine, clopidogrel	Anti-ADAMTS13 autoantibodies (ticlopidine, 80%-90%; clopidogrel, 30%)
HSC transplantation	Unknown; rarely, low ADAMTS13 levels
Malignancies	Unknown; rarely, low ADAMTS13 levels
HIV	HIV virus; rarely, low ADAMTS13 levels

*According to clinical presentation and underlying cause.
†No published data on frequency of complement gene mutations or anti-CFH autoantibodies; antiphospholipid syndrome, systemic lupus erythematosus, and other autoimmune diseases—depends on the specific primary disease.
HSC, Hematopoietic stem cell transplantation; HELLP, hemolytic anemia, elevated liver enzymes, and low platelet count.

fatal syndrome in children characterized by hemolytic anemia, thrombocytopenia, and severe renal failure.[2] HUS occurs most frequently in children younger than 5 years (incidence, 6.1 children/100,000/yr compared to an overall incidence of 1 to 2 children/100,000/yr). Most cases (>90% of those in children) are associated with infection by Shiga toxin (Stx)–producing *E. coli* (Stx-HUS).[3] Stx-HUS in 90% of cases is preceded by diarrhea, often bloody. Usually, patients are afebrile. *Streptococcus pneumoniae* causes a distinctive form of HUS, accounting for 40% of cases not associated with Stx-producing bacteria.[4]

Approximately 10% of HUS cases are classified as atypical, caused neither by Stx-producing bacteria nor by *Streptococcus*.[5] Atypical HUS occurs at any age, can be familial or sporadic, and has a poor outcome; 50% progress to end-stage renal disease (ESRD), and 25% may die in the acute phase.[4,6] Neurologic symptoms and fever can occur in 30% of patients. Pulmonary, cardiac, and gastrointestinal manifestations can also occur.[4,6]

Thrombotic Thrombocytopenic Purpura

Thrombotic thrombocytopenic purpura is a rare disease, with an incidence of approximately two to four cases/1 million persons/yr.[7,8] It is more common in women (female/male ratio, 3:2 to 5:2) and in whites (white/black ratio, 3:1). The peak incidence is in the third and fourth decades of life, but TTP can affect any age group.[8,9] TTP typically presents with the pentad of thrombocytopenia, microangiopathic hemolytic anemia, fever, and neurologic and renal dysfunction.[10] Thrombocytopenia is essential for the diagnosis; most patients present with a platelet count below 60,000/μL.[8,9] Purpura is minor and can be absent. Retinal hemorrhages can be present, but bleeding is rare. Neurologic symptoms can be seen in over 90% of patients during the entire course of the disease. Central nervous system involvement mainly represents thromboocclusive disease of the grey matter, but can also include headache, cranial nerve palsies, confusion, stupor, and coma. These features are transient but recurrent. Up to 50% of patients who present with neurologic involvement may be left with sequelae. Renal insufficiency may occur. One group has reported 25% of patients to have creatinine clearance less than 40 mL/min. Low-grade fever is present in 25% of patients at diagnosis, but can often be seen as a consequence of plasma exchange. Less common manifestations include acute abdomen, pancreatitis, and sudden death.[9]

LABORATORY FINDINGS

Laboratory features of thrombocytopenia and microangiopathic hemolytic anemia are almost invariably present in patients with TMA lesions and reflect the consumption and disruption of platelets and erythrocytes in the microvasculature (Figure 35.2).[5,9,11] Hemoglobin levels are low (<10 g/dL in >90% of patients). Reticulocyte counts are uniformly elevated. The peripheral smear reveals increased schistocyte numbers (see Figure 35.2), with polychromasia and, often, nucleated red blood cells. The latter may represent not only a compensatory response, but also damage to the bone marrow–blood barrier resulting from intramedullary vascular occlusion. Detection of fragmented erythrocytes is crucial to confirm the microangiopathic nature of the hemolytic anemia, provided heart valvular disease and other anatomic artery abnormalities that may cause erythrocyte fragmentation are excluded. Other indicators of intravascular hemolysis include elevated lactate dehydrogenase (LDH), increased indirect bilirubin, and low haptoglobin levels.[5,9,11] The Coombs test is negative. Moderate leukocytosis may accompany the hemolytic anemia. Thrombocytopenia is uniformly present in HUS and TTP. It may be severe but is usually less so in patients with predominant renal

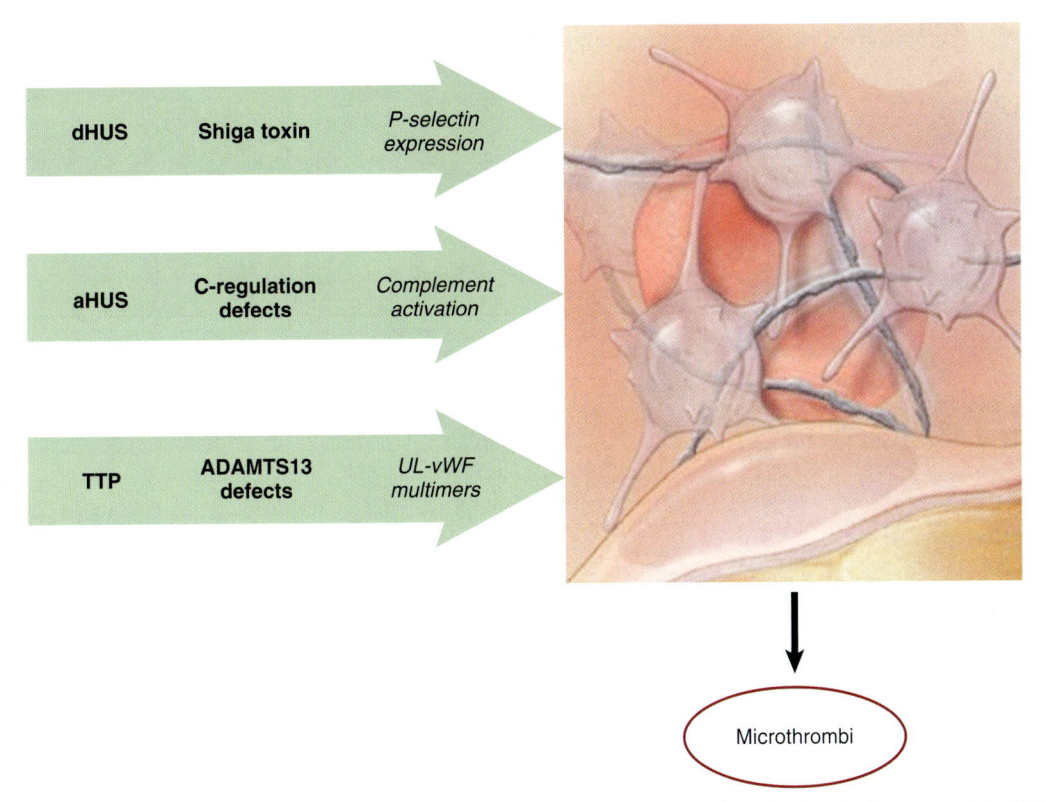

Figure 35.1 Pathways of thrombus formation in different forms of thrombotic microangiopathy. In diarrhea-associated HUS (dHUS), the microangiopathic process is initiated by endothelial exposure to Shiga toxin (Stx), with consequent up regulation of P-selectin expression and other adhesion molecules. In atypical HUS (aHUS), the process is mediated by genetic or acquired defects in different modulators of the complement system, with secondary uncontrolled complement activation, and in TTP by genetic or acquired defects in ADAMTS13 activity with abnormal von Willebrand factor (vWF) cleavage and persistency in the circulation of ultra-large vWF multimers. Independent of the initial event, microvascular occlusion by intravascular thrombi is the final event common to different forms of thrombotic microangiopathy.

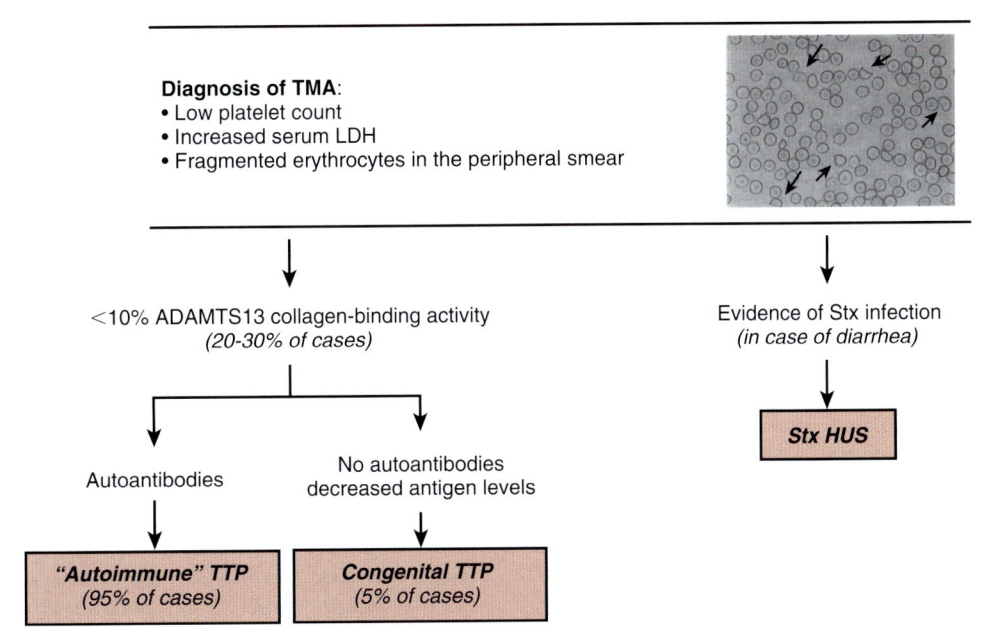

Figure 35.2 Diagnostic algorithm for TMA. A peripheral blood smear from a patient with thrombotic microangiopathy is shown **(upper right)**. The presence of fragmented red blood cells that may assume the appearance of a helmet (fragmented erythrocytes with the shape of a helmet are identified by the *black arrows*) is pathognomonic for microangiopathic hemolysis in patients with no evidence of heart valvular disease.

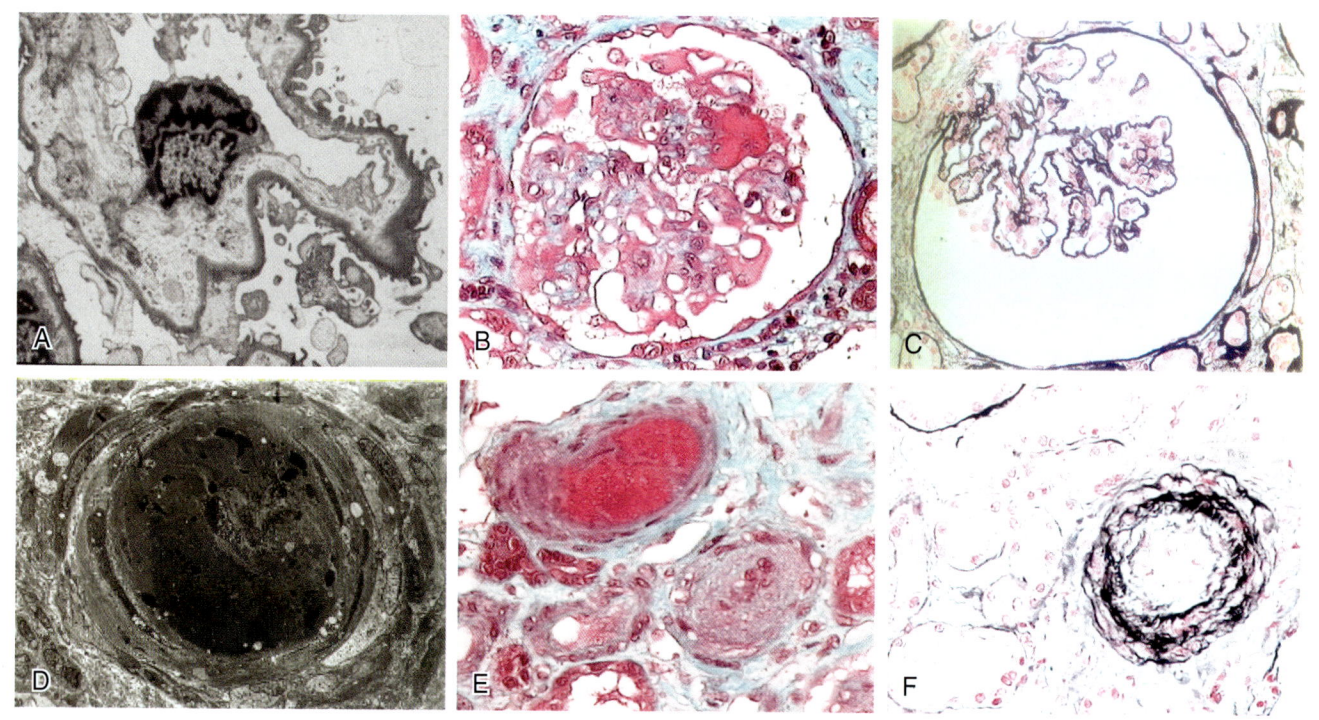

Figure 35.3 Micrographs of renal biopsy samples from patients with thrombotic microangiopathy. **A,** Electron micrograph of a glomerular capillary. The endothelium is detached from the glomerular basement membrane. Beneath the endothelium is a thin layer of newly formed glomerular basement membrane. The subendothelial space is widened and occupied by electron-lucent fluffy material and cell debris. **B,** By light microscopy, a glomerular capillary shows an intraluminal thrombus (Periodic acid–Schiff). **C,** Light micrograph of an ischemic and markedly retracted glomerulus with wrinkled capillary tuft (Silver stain). **D,** Electron micrograph of a renal arteriole. The vascular lumen is completely occluded by thrombotic material and the wall contains several myointimal cells. **E,** One small renal artery is occluded by a thrombus **(upper left).** A nearby arteriole **(middle right)** shows an extremely narrowed lumen that appears to be surrounded by a swollen intimal layer (Periodic acid–Schiff). **F,** An arteriole shows intimal thickening and multilayering of the vascular wall (Silver stain). (**A** from Remuzzi G, Ruggenenti P, Bertani T: Thrombotic microangiopathy. In Tisher C, Brenner B, editors: *Renal pathology with clinical and functional correlations,* ed 2, 1989, pp 1154–1184; **D** from Pisoni R, Ruggenenti P, Remuzzi G: Thrombotic microangiopathies including the hemolytic-uremic syndrome. In Johnson R, Feehally J, editors: *Comprehensive clinical nephrology,* ed 2, 2003, pp 413–423.)

involvement.[12] The presence of giant platelets in the peripheral smear, reduced platelet survival time, or both is consistent with peripheral consumption. In children with Stx-HUS, the duration of thrombocytopenia is variable and does not correlate with the course of renal disease.[13] Bone marrow biopsy specimens usually show erythroid hyperplasia and an increased number of megakaryocytes. Prothrombin time (PT), partial thromboplastin time (PTT), fibrinogen level, and coagulation factors are normal, thus differentiating HUS and TTP from disseminated intravascular coagulation (DIC). Mild fibrinolysis, with minimal elevation in fibrin degradation products, however, may be observed.

Evidence of renal involvement is present in all patients with HUS (by definition) and in about 25% of patients with TTP.[11,14,15] Microscopic hematuria and subnephrotic proteinuria are the most consistent findings. In a retrospective study of 216 patients with a clinical picture of TTP, the following features were noted[15]:

- Hematuria was detected in 78% and proteinuria in 75% of cases.
- Sterile pyuria and casts were present in 31% and 24% of cases, respectively.
- Gross hematuria was rare.

PATHOLOGY

The diagnostic histologic lesions of TMA consist of widening of the subendothelial space and microvascular thrombosis (Figure 35.3). Electron microscopy best identifies the characteristic lesions of swelling and detachment of the endothelial cells from the basement membrane and the accumulation of fluffy material in the subendothelium (see Figure 35.3*A*), intraluminal platelet thrombi, and partial or complete obstruction of vessel lumina (see Figure 35.3*B, D,* and *E*).[16-18] These lesions are similar to those seen in other renal diseases, such as scleroderma, malignant nephrosclerosis, chronic transplant rejection, and calcineurin inhibitor nephrotoxicity. In HUS, microthrombi are present primarily in the kidneys, whereas in TTP they mainly involve the brain, where thrombi may repeatedly form and resolve, producing intermittent neurologic deficits. In pediatric patients, particularly in those younger than 2 years and in those with HUS secondary to gastrointestinal infection with Stx-producing strains of *E. coli,* the glomerular injury is predominant. Thrombi and leukocyte infiltration are common in the early phases of the disease and usually resolve after 2 to 3 weeks. Patchy cortical necrosis may be present in severe cases; crescent formation is uncommon. In idiopathic and familial forms, and in adults, the injury

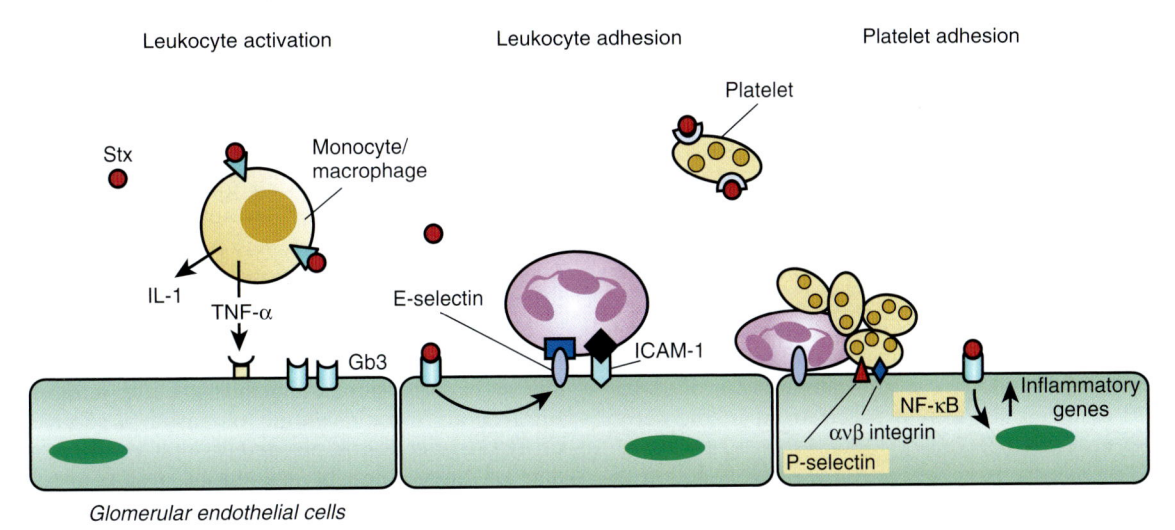

Figure 35.4 Pathways mediating microvascular thrombosis and inflammation on Shiga toxin (Stx) exposure. Stx binds specific receptors on circulating leukocytes that are activated and release interleukin-1 (IL-1) and tumor necrosis factor-α (TNF-α).

mostly involves arteries and arterioles with thrombosis and intimal thickening (see Figure 35.3F), secondary glomerular ischemia, and retraction of the glomerular tuft (see Figure 35.3C). The prognosis is good in patients with predominant glomerular involvement, but is more severe in those with predominant preglomerular injury. Focal segmental glomerulosclerosis may be a long-term sequela of acute cases of HUS and is usually seen in children with long-lasting hypertension and progressive chronic renal function deterioration.[16-18]

The typical pathologic changes of TTP are the thrombi that occlude capillaries and arterioles in many organs and tissues. These thrombi consist of fibrin and platelets, and their distribution is widespread. They are usually detected in kidneys, pancreas, heart, adrenals, and brain. Compared to HUS, pathologic changes of TTP are more extensively distributed, probably reflecting the more systemic nature of the disease.[16-18]

MECHANISMS, CLINICAL COURSE, AND THERAPY FOR DIFFERENT FORMS OF THROMBOTIC MICROANGIOPATHY

Hemolytic-Uremic Syndrome

Shiga Toxin–Associated Hemolytic-Uremic Syndrome

Mechanisms. Stx-HUS may follow infection by certain strains of *E. coli* or *Shigella dysenteriae*, which produce a powerful exotoxin (Shiga toxin, or Stx).[3] The term *Shiga toxin* was initially used to describe the exotoxin produced by *Shigella dysenteriae* type 1. Then some strains of *E. coli* (mostly the serotype O157:H7, but also other serotypes—e.g., O111:H8, O103:H2, O123, and O26) isolated from human cases with diarrhea were found to produce a toxin similar to the one of *S. dysenteriae*. After food contaminated by Stx-producing *E. coli* or *S. dysenteriae* is ingested, the toxin is released in the gut and may cause watery or usually bloody diarrhea because of a direct effect on the intestinal mucosa. Stx-producing *E. coli* organisms adhere closely to the epithelial cells of the gastrointestinal mucosa, causing destruction of brush border villi.[19] These toxins are picked up by polarized gastrointestinal cells via transcellular pathways and translocate into the circulation, probably facilitated by the transmigration of neutrophils (PMN), which increase paracellular permeability.[20,21] Circulating human blood cells, such as erythrocytes platelets, and monocytes express Stx receptors on their surface and have been suggested to serve as Stx carriers from the intestine to the kidney and other target organs (Figure 35.4).[22-25]

Recently, evidence has been provided that Stx interacts with von Willebrand factor (vWF), a multimeric plasma glycoprotein that mediates platelet adhesion, activation, and aggregation.[26] In vitro experiments have shown that Stx binds to ultra-large vWF (UL-vWF) secreted from, and anchored to, stimulated human umbilical vein endothelial cells (HUVECs) and to immobilized vWF-rich HUVEC supernatant. This Stx binding reduces the rate of ADAMTS-13–mediated cleavage of vWF. The resulting delay in cleavage of endothelial cell–anchored UL-vWF multimers, by increasing the time available for platelet adhesion, activation, and aggregation, provides a possible explanation for thrombotic microangiopathy in diarrhea associated (D)+HUS.

Diagnosis rests on detection of *E. coli* O157:H7 and other Stx-producing bacteria in sorbitol-MacConkey stool cultures. Serologic tests for antibodies to Stx and O157 lipopolysaccharide can be done in research laboratories, and tests are being developed for rapid detection of *E. coli* O157:H7 and Stx in stools.

Over the last decades, *E. coli* O157:H7 and, less frequently, other Stx-producing *E. coli* strains, have been responsible for multiple outbreaks throughout the world, becoming a public health problem in developed and developing countries. Contaminated undercooked ground beef, meat patties, raw vegetables, fruit, milk, and recreational or drinking water have all been implicated in the transmission of *E. coli*. A recent widespread outbreak associated with spinach in North America had dramatically higher than typical rates of hospitalization (52%) and HUS (16%) due to the emergence of a new variant of O157:H7 serotype that had acquired several gene mutations, which likely contributed to more severe disease.[27]

Secondary person-to-person contact is an important way of spread in institutional centers, particularly daycare centers and nursing homes. Infected patients should be excluded from daycare centers until two consecutive stool cultures are negative for Stx-producing *E. coli* to prevent further transmission. However, the most important preventive measure in childcare centers is supervised hand washing.

Clinical Course. Following exposure to Stx-*E.coli*, 38% to 61% of individuals develop hemorrhagic colitis and 3% to 9% (in sporadic infections) and up to 20% (in epidemic forms) progress to overt HUS.[28,29] Stx-*E.coli* hemorrhagic colitis not complicated by HUS is self-limiting and is not associated with an increased long-term risk of high blood pressure or renal dysfunction, as shown by a 4-year follow-up study in 951 children who were exposed to a drinking water outbreak of *E.coli* O157:H7.[30]

Stx-HUS is characterized by prodromal diarrhea followed by acute renal failure. The average interval between *E.coli* exposure and illness is 3 days. Illness typically begins with abdominal cramps and nonbloody diarrhea; diarrhea may become hemorrhagic in 70% of cases, usually within 1 or 2 days.[31] Vomiting occurs in 30% to 60% and fever in 30% of cases. The leukocyte count is usually elevated, and a barium enema may demonstrate thumbprinting, suggestive of edema and submucosal hemorrhage, especially in the region of the ascending and transverse colon. HUS is usually diagnosed 6 days after the onset of diarrhea.[3] After infection, Stx-*E.coli* may be shed in the stools for several weeks after the symptoms are resolved, particularly in children younger than 5 years.[3]

Bloody diarrhea, fever, vomiting, elevated leukocyte count, extremes of age, and female gender, as well as the use of antimotility agents, have been associated with an increased risk of HUS following *E.coli* infection.[28,32] Stx-HUS is not a benign disease. Of patients who develop HUS, 70% require red blood cell transfusions, 50% need dialysis, and 25% have neurologic involvement, including stroke, seizure, and coma.[28,33,34] Although mortality for infants and young children in industrialized countries decreased when dialysis became available, and after the introduction of intensive care facilities, still 3% to 5% of patients die during the acute phase of Stx-HUS.[33] A meta-analysis of 49 published studies (3476 patients; mean follow-up, 4.4 years) describing the long-term prognosis of patients who survived an episode of Stx-HUS, has reported death or permanent ESRD in 12% of patients and a glomerular filtration rate (GFR) below 80 mL/min/1.73 m^2 in 25%.[34]

Disease presentation and outcome were particularly severe during the Shiga toxin–producing *Escherichia coli* (STEC) O104:H4 German outbreak, in which 53 of 855 HUS patients died in Germany by its end.[35] Compared to previous STEC epidemics, there was a higher incidence of dialysis-dependent kidney failure (20% vs. 6%) and death (6% vs. 1%).[35] Almost 50% of patients presented with neurologic symptoms, and 20% of patients suffered seizures. The severe clinical phenotype was explained by lack of previous immunity to this novel STEC strain and also by its exceptional virulence.[35] *E. coli* O104:H4 not only produces the same Stx as STEC enterohemorrhagic strains, but also has 93% of the genomic sequence of enteroaggregative *E. coli* strains that form fimbriae, which facilitates adhesion to the intestinal wall. The evolution of *E.coli* O104:H4 is likely the result of the acquisition by an enteroaggregative strain of *E.coli* of a Stx-encoding phage from a Stx-producing enterohemorrhagic strain of *E.coli*. The combination of these two virulence factors would lead to increased gut colonization and thus the release of increased quantities of toxin into the circulation. Moreover, although enterohemorrhagic *E. coli* are found in the gastrointestinal tract of ruminants, enteroaggregative *E. coli* appear to have their reservoir in humans. This might explain why this strain has acquired new resistances to antibiotics most commonly used in human disease.

Therapy. Typical treatment of Stx-associated HUS of children is based on supportive management of anemia, renal failure, hypertension, and electrolyte and water imbalances. Intravenous isotonic volume expansion as soon as an *E. coli* O157:H7 infection is suspected—that is, within the first 4 days of illness, even before culture results are available—may limit the severity of kidney dysfunction and the need for renal replacement therapy.[36] Bowel rest is important for the enterohemorrhagic colitis associated with Stx-HUS. Antimotility agents should be avoided because they may prolong the persistence of *E. coli* in the intestinal lumen and therefore increase the patient's exposure to its toxin. The use of antibiotics should be restricted to the very limited number of patients presenting with bacteremia[37] because, in children with gastroenteritis, they may increase the risk of HUS by 17-fold.[38] A possible explanation is that antibiotic-induced injury to the bacterial membrane might favor the acute release of large amounts of preformed toxin. Alternatively, antibiotic therapy might give *E. coli* O157:H7 a selective advantage if these organisms are not as readily eliminated from the bowel as normal intestinal flora. Moreover, several antimicrobial drugs, particularly the quinolones, trimethoprim, and furazolidone, are potent inducers of the expression of the Stx2 gene and may increase the level of toxin in the intestine. Although the possibility of a cause-and-effect relationship between antibiotic therapy and increased risk of HUS has been challenged by a meta-analysis of 26 reports,[39] there is no reason to prescribe antibiotics because they do not improve the outcome of colitis, and bacteremia is only exceptionally found in Stx-associated HUS. However, when hemorrhagic colitis is caused by *S. dysenteriae* type 1, early and empirical antibiotic treatment shortens the duration of diarrhea, decreases the incidence of complications, and reduces the risk of transmission by shortening the duration of bacterial shedding. Thus, in developing countries where *S. dysenteriae* is the most frequent cause of hemorrhagic colitis, antibiotic therapy should be started early, even before the involved pathogen is identified.

Careful blood pressure control and renin angiotensin aldosterone system (RAAS) blockade may be particularly beneficial in the long term for patients who suffer chronic renal disease after an episode of Stx-HUS. A study of 45 children with renal sequelae of HUS followed for 9 to 11 years has documented that early restriction of proteins and use of angiotensin-converting enzyme inhibitors (ACEIs) may have a beneficial effect on long-term renal outcome, as documented by a positive slope of 1/creatinine (1/Cr) values over time in treated patients.[40] In another study, 8- to 15-year treatment with ACEIs after severe Stx-HUS normalized blood pressure, reduced proteinuria, and improved GFR.[41]

Table 35.2 Specific Therapies Used in Thrombotic Microangiopathy

Therapy	Dosing	Efficacy
Antiplatelet		Anecdotal efficacy in TTP
Aspirin	325-1300 mg/day	
Dipyridamole	400-600 mg/day	
Dextran 70	500 mg twice daily	
Prostacyclin	4-20 mg/kg/min	Anecdotal efficacy in HUS
Antithrombotic		
Heparin	5000-U bolus followed by 750- to 1000-U/hr infusion	
Streptokinase	250,000-U bolus followed by 100,000-U/hr infusion	
Shiga toxin–binding (Synsorb)	500 mg/kg/day for 7 days	Not effective in preventing or treating Stx-associated HUS
Antioxidant (vitamin E)	1000 mg /m^2/day	Anecdotal efficacy in HUS
Immunosuppressive		Probably effective in addition to plasma exchange in patients with TTP and anti-ADAMST13 autoantibodies or in aHUS with antifactor H autoantibodies and in forms associated with autoimmune diseases; lack of evidence from controlled trials for immune-mediated HUS or TTP
Prednisone	200 mg tapered to 60 mg/day, then 5-mg reduction/wk	
Prednisolone	200 mg tapered to 60 mg/day, then 5-mg reduction/wk	
Immunoglobulins	400 mg/kg/day	
Vincristine	1.4 mg/m^2 followed by 1 mg every 4 days	
CD20 cell depletion (rituximab)	375 mg/m^2/wk up to CD20 depletion	Effective in treatment or prevention of TTP associated with immune-mediated ADAMTS13 deficiency resistant to, or relapsing after, immunosuppressive therapy
Fresh-frozen plasma		
Exchange	1-2 plasma volumes/day	First-line therapy for aHUS and TTP; unproven efficacy in childhood Stx-HUS
Infusion	20-30 mL/kg followed by 10-20 mL/kg/day	To be considered if plasma exchange not available
Cryosupernatant	See plasma infusion, exchanges	To replace whole plasma in case of plasma resistance or sensitization
Solvent detergent–treated plasma	See plasma infusion, exchanges	To limit the risk of infections
Liver-kidney transplantation		To prevent FH-associated HUS recurrence posttransplantation; ≈30% mortality risk
Complement inhibition (eculizumab)	600 mg/wk for first 4 wk; 900 mg every 14 days, up to 6 mo	Reported efficacy in FH-associated HUS

FH, Factor H; *HUS*, hemolytic-uremic syndrome; *TTP*, thrombotic thrombocytopenic purpura.

An oral Stx-binding agent that may compete with endothelial and epithelial receptors for Stx in the gut (Synsorb PK) has been developed with the rationale of limiting target organ exposure to the toxin (Table 35.2). However, a prospective, randomized, double-blind, placebo-controlled clinical trial of 145 children with diarrhea-associated HUS failed to demonstrate any beneficial effect of treatment on disease outcome.[42]

Heparin and antithrombotic agents may increase the risk of bleeding and should be avoided.

The efficacy of specific treatments in adult patients is difficult to evaluate because most information has been derived by uncontrolled series, which may include also atypical HUS cases. In particular, no prospective randomized trials are available to establish definitively whether plasma infusion or exchange may offer some specific benefit as compared to supportive treatment alone. However, comparative analyses of two large series of patients treated or not treated with plasma have suggested that plasma therapy may dramatically decrease overall mortality of Stx-*E. coli* 0157:H7–associated HUS.[43,44] These findings lead to the consideration of plasma infusion or exchange suitable for adult patients, in particular those with severe renal insufficiency and central nervous system involvement, such as patients involved in *E. coli* O104:H4 HUS outbreaks.[45] In this context, immunoglobulin G (IgG) depletion, through immunoadsorption rescue therapy added on to plasma exchange, has been reported to achieve complete neurologic recovery in 10 of 12 critically ill patients with delirium, epileptic seizures, or requirement for mechanical ventilation.[46]

Kidney transplantation should be considered as an effective and safe treatment for children who progress to ESRD. Indeed, recurrence rates range from 0% to 10%, and graft survival at 10 years is even better than in control children with other diseases.[47-49] Importantly, genetic screening performed in a young woman with history of Stx-HUS and early graft failure, before planning a second transplantation, revealed a complement factor I (CFI) mutation.[50] This case indicates that screening of HUS-associated genes should be performed in patients on dialysis following severe episodes of Stx-HUS because they may be undiagnosed cases of HUS precipitated by STEC infection on a genetic background of impaired complement regulation.

Evidence that uncontrolled complement activation may contribute to microangiopathic lesions of STEC-HUS provided the background for complement inhibitor therapy in three children with severe STEC-HUS who fully recovered with the anti-C5 monoclonal antibody eculizumab.[51-53] These encouraging results prompted nephrologists to use eculizumab therapy in HUS patients involved in the STEC O104:H4 outbreak in Germany (see Table 35.2). However, data are largely inconclusive because they were substantially biased by the retrospective and nonrandomized design of the studies. Although uncontrolled reports have suggested that eculizumab is associated with prompt and complete recovery, in particular if treatment is started early after disease onset,[54,55] evidence from controlled studies—that disease outcome was similar between patients who received eculizumab together with plasma exchange and those who received plasma exchange alone—has strongly questioned the benefit of eculizumab added on as best available therapy, including plasma exchange.[45,56] However, these findings are difficult to interpret because they were most likely biased by the preferential administration of eculizumab to patients with more severe disease. Thus, whether eculizumab is a useful adjunct to treating the most severe forms of STEC-HUS needs to be clarified by prospective, randomized, controlled trials.[35]

Streptococcus pneumoniae–Associated Hemolytic-Uremic Syndrome

Mechanisms. This is a rare but potentially fatal disease that may complicate pneumonia or, less frequently, meningitis caused by *Streptococcus pneumoniae*.[57] Neuraminidase produced by *S. pneumoniae*, by removing sialic acid from the cell membranes, exposes Thomsen-Friedenreich antigen (T-antigen).[58] T-antigen exposure on red cells is detected using the lectin *Arachis hypogaea*. An immunoglobulin M cold antibody occurring naturally in human serum causes the polyagglutination of red blood cells in vitro. This is why, unlike in other forms of HUS, there is a positive Coombs test result in neuraminidase-associated HUS. T–anti-T interaction on red cells, platelets, and endothelium was thought to explain the pathogenesis, whereas the pathogenic role of the anti-T cold antibody in vivo is uncertain.[59]

Recently, a study investigating the complement system in five patients with *S. pneumoniae* HUS (SP-HUS) found a decrease in components of the classical and alternative pathways during the acute phase of the disease.[60] This indicates early severe activation and consumption of complement, and most of these alterations normalized later in remission. In addition, three of the five SP-HUS patients carried mutations and/or risk haplotypes in genes previously reported to associate with complement-mediated aHUS—a previously described variant of factor I (PC50A) and two new mutations in factor H (R1149X) and thrombomodulin (T44I). These observations suggest that severe complement dysregulation and consumption, in addition to neuraminidase action, accompany the progression of SP-HUS, and genetic variations of complement genes may contribute to the development of this complication in some affected patients.

Clinical Course. Patients, usually younger than 2 years, present with severe microangiopathic hemolytic anemia. The clinical picture is severe, with respiratory distress, neurologic involvement, and coma. The acute mortality is about 25%.

Therapy. The outcome is strongly dependent on the effectiveness of antibiotic therapy. In theory, plasma, infused or exchanged, is contraindicated, because adult plasma contains antibodies against the Thomsen-Friedenreich antigen that may accelerate polyagglutination and hemolysis.[58] Thus, patients should be treated only with antibiotics and washed red cells. In some cases, however, plasma therapy, occasionally in combination with steroids, has been associated with recovery. Evidence that complement activation plays a role in the pathogenesis of SP-HUS might provide a background for the possible benefits of complement inhibitor therapy in this context.

Atypical Hemolytic-Uremic Syndrome. Atypical HUS includes a number of associations and presentations. It can occur sporadically or within families. Research in the last 10 years has linked aHUS to uncontrolled activation of the complement system (Figure 35.5).[61]

Fewer than 20% of atypical HUS cases are familial. Reports date back to 1965, when Campbell and Carre described hemolytic anemia and azotemia in concordant monozygous twins.[62] Since then, familial HUS has been reported in children and, less frequently, in adults. Although some cases were in siblings, suggesting autosomal recessive transmission, others were across two or three generations, suggesting an autosomal dominant mode.[63,64] The prognosis is poor (cumulative incidence of death or ESRD, 50% to 80%).

Sporadic aHUS encompasses cases without a family history of the disease. Triggering conditions for sporadic aHUS[65] include HIV infection, anticancer drugs (e.g., mitomycin, cisplatin, bleomycin, gemcitabine), immunotherapeutic agents (e.g., cyclosporine, tacrolimus, OKT3, interferon, quinidine), antiplatelet agents (e.g., ticlopidine, clopidogrel), malignancies, transplantation, and pregnancy.[11,66]

De novo posttransplantation HUS has been reported in patients receiving renal transplants or other organs due to calcineurin inhibitors or humoral rejection. It has been reported in up to 5% to 15% of renal transplantation patients who receive cyclosporine and in approximately 1% of those who are given tacrolimus.[67-69] Dose reduction or changing one calcineurin inhibitor for another sometimes results in recovery and suggests a causative role.

In 10% to 15% of female patients, aHUS manifests during pregnancy or postpartum.[6,65] Atypical HUS may present at any time during pregnancy, but mostly in the last trimester and about the time of delivery. It is sometimes difficult to distinguish it from preeclampsia. The HELPP syndrome (**he**molytic anemia, elevated **l**iver enzymes, and low **p**latelets) is a life-threatening disorder of the last trimester or parturition with severe thrombocytopenia, microangiopathic hemolytic anemia, renal failure, and liver involvement. These forms are always an indication for prompt delivery, which is usually followed by complete remission.[65] Postpartum HUS manifests within 3 months of delivery in most cases. The outcome is usually poor. About 50% of sporadic aHUS cases show no clear trigger (idiopathic HUS).

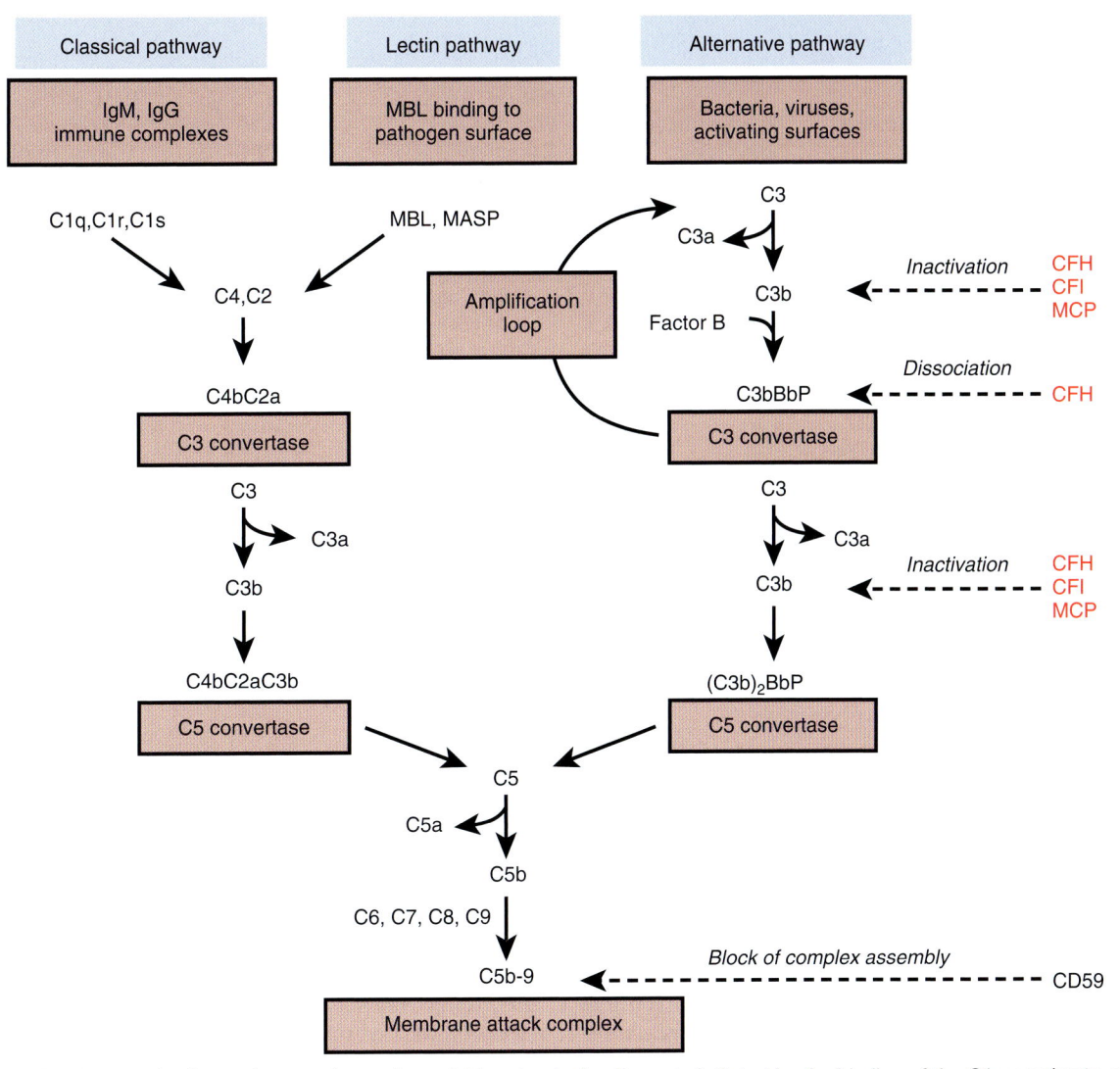

Figure 35.5 The three activation pathways of complement. The classical pathway is initiated by the binding of the C1 complex to antibodies bound to an antigen on the surface of a bacterial cell, leading to the formation of a C4b2a enzyme complex, the C3 convertase of the classical pathway. The mannose-binding lectin pathway is initiated by binding of the complex of mannose-binding lectin (MBL) and the serine proteases mannose-binding, lectin-associated proteases 1 and 2 (MASP1 and MASP2) to mannose residues on the surface of a bacterial cell; this leads to the formation of the C3 convertase enzyme C4bC2a. The alternative pathway is initiated by the covalent binding of a small amount of C3b generated by spontaneous hydrolysis in plasma to hydroxyl groups on cell surface carbohydrates and proteins. This C3b binds factor B to form the alternative pathway C3 complex C3bBb. The C3 convertase enzymes cleave many molecules of C3 to form the anaphylatoxin C3a and C3b, which binds covalently around the site of complement activation. Some of this C3b binds to C4b and C3b in the convertase enzymes of the classical and alternative pathways, respectively, forming C5 convertase enzymes that cleave C5 to form the anaphylatoxin C5a and C5b, which initiates the formation of the membrane attack complex. The human complement system is highly regulated to prevent nonspecific damage to host cells and limit the deposition of complement to the surface of pathogens. This fine regulation occurs through a number of membrane-anchored and fluid phase regulators (in *red*) that inactivate complement products formed at various levels in the cascade and protect host tissues. CD59, Protectin (prevents the terminal polymerization of the membrane attack complex); CFB, complement factor B; CFH, complement factor H; CFI, complement factor I; MCP, membrane cofactor protein.

Mechanisms. Complement Abnormalities. Reduced serum levels of C3 with normal C4 in aHUS patients have been recognized since 1974.[70,71] In cases of familial aHUS, serum C3 was low, even during remission, hinting to genetic defects.[70,72] A low C3 reflected complement activation and consumption with high levels of activated products, C3b, C3c, and C3d.[73]

The complement system is part of innate immunity and consists of several plasma- and membrane-bound proteins protecting against invading organisms.[74] Three activation pathways—classical, lectin, and alternative pathways—produce protease complexes, termed *C3* and *C5 convertases*, that cleave C3 and C5, respectively, eventually leading to the membrane attack complex (MAC) lytic complex (Figure 35.5). The alternative pathway is initiated spontaneously in plasma by C3 hydrolysis responsible for the covalent deposition of a low amount of C3b onto almost all plasma-exposed surfaces (see Figure 35.5). On bacterial surfaces, C3b leads to opsonization for phagocytosis by neutrophils and macrophages. Without regulation, a small initiating stimulus is

Table 35.3 Outcomes of Atypical Hemolytic-Uremic Syndrome (aHUS)*

Affected Gene(s)	Affected Protein and Main Effect	Frequency in aHUS (%)	Rate of Remission With Plasma Exchange†	5- to 10-yr Rate of Death or ESRD (%)	Rate of Recurrence after Kidney Transplantation (%)
CFH	Factor H (no binding to endothelium)	20-30 (dose- and timing-dependent)	60	70-80	80-90‡
CFHL1, CFHL3	Factor HR1, R3 (anti–factor H antibodies)	6	70-80 (combined with immunosuppression)	30-40	20‡
MCP	Membrane cofactor protein (no surface expression)	10-15	No indication for plasma exchange	<20	15-20§
	Factor I (low levels, low cofactor act)	4-10	30-40	60-70	70-80
	Factor B (C3 convertase stabilization)	1-2	30	70	One case reported
	Complement C3 (resistance to C3b inactivation)	5-10	40-50	6%	40-50
	Thrombomodulin (reduced C3b inactivation)	5	60	60	One case reported

*According to the associated genetic abnormality.
†Complete remission or hematologic remission with renal sequelae.
‡Kidney or combined liver and kidney transplantation.
§Single kidney transplantation.

quickly amplified to a self-harming response until the consumption of complement components (see Figure 35.5). On host cells, such a dangerous cascade is controlled by membrane-anchored and fluid phase regulators (see Figure 35.5). They both favor the cleavage of C3b to inactive iC3b by the plasma serine-protease factor I (CFI, cofactor activity) and dissociate the multicomponent C3 and C5 convertases (decay acceleration activity). Foreign targets and injured cells that lack membrane-bound regulators or cannot bind soluble regulators are attacked by complement.

The C3 convertases of the classical and lectin pathways are formed by C2 and C4 fragments, whereas the alternative pathway convertase requires cleavage of C3 only (see Figure 35.5).[74] Thus, low serum C3 levels in aHUS with normal C4 indicated selective AP activation.[72]

Genetic Abnormalities. A variety of genetic abnormalities in members of the alternative pathway of complement have been described in aHUS, which account for about 60% of cases (see Table 35.1). Of note, different genetic abnormalities account for different patterns of dysfunction of the complement system with different outcomes, response to therapy, and risk of recurrence after kidney transplantation (Table 35.3).

COMPLEMENT FACTOR H. Complement factor H (CFH) regulates the alternative pathway by competing with complement factor B (CFB) for C3b recognition by acting as a cofactor for CFI, and enhancing dissociation of C3 convertase.[75] In 1998, Warwicker and coworkers demonstrated linkage of aHUS to the chromosome 1q32 locus, containing genes for CFH and other complement regulators.[76] Since then, over 80 *CFH* mutations (interactive FH-HUS mutations database, http://www.FH-HUS.org) have been identified in aHUS patients (mutation frequency—40% to 45% familial forms, 10% to 20% sporadic forms).[77-83] These mutations usually do not result in a quantitative CFH deficiency, but result in normal levels of a protein that is unable to bind to and regulate complement on endothelial cells and platelets.[84] A high degree of sequence identity between *CFH* and the genes *CFHR1-5* for five factor H–related proteins (CFHRs) located in tandem to *CFH* may predispose to nonallelic recombinations.[85] In 3% to 5% of patients with aHUS, a heterozygous hybrid gene derived from an uneven crossover between *CFH* and *CFHR1* contained the first 21 *CFH* exons and the last two *CFHR1* exons, resulting in a gene product with decreased complement regulatory activity on endothelial surfaces.[85] Additional forms of CFH and CFHR hybrid genes have been recently described.

Acquired defects of CFH function are also seen in the form of inhibitory antibodies that are reported in 5% to 10% of aHUS patients.[86] Analogous to the genetic defect seen in CFH, these autoantibodies also predominantly target the C-terminal end of the protein, thereby impairing complement regulation on host cell surfaces. The development of CFH autoantibodies in aHUS has a genetic predisposition, being strongly associated with a deletion of the *CFHR1* and *CFHR3* genes.

MEMBRANE COFACTOR PROTEIN. Membrane cofactor protein (MCP) is pivotal against C3 activation on glomerular endothelium. Anti-MCP antibody completely blocked cofactor activity in cell extracts.[87] In 2003, two groups described mutations in *MCP* encoding the widely expressed transmembrane regulator, membrane cofactor protein, in affected individuals of four families. MCP serves as a cofactor for CFI to cleave C3b and C4b on cell surfaces.[88-90] *MCP* mutations account for 10% to 15% of aHUS cases.[81] Most are heterozygous, about 25% are homozygous or compound heterozygous (http://www.FH-HUS.org). Most cluster in critical extracellular modules for regulation. Expression on blood leukocytes was reduced for about 75% of mutants, causing quantitative defects. Conversely, others have low C3b-binding capability and decreased cofactor activity.[81,91]

COMPLEMENT FACTOR I. CFI is a plasma serine protease that regulates the three complement pathways by cleaving C3b and C4b in the presence of cofactor proteins. *CFI* mutations affect 4% to 10% of aHUS patients.[81,92-94] All mutations are heterozygous; 80% cluster in the serine-protease domain. Approximately 50% of mutations result in low CFI levels. Others disrupt C3b and C4b cleavage.[81,92-94]

COMPLEMENT FACTORS B AND C3. Gain-of-function mutations can affect genes encoding the alternative pathway C3 convertase components, CFB and C3.[95,96] *CFB* mutations are rare in aHUS (1% to 2%).[96] Patients have chronic alternative pathway activation, with low C3 and, usually, normal C4.[96] *CFB* mutants have excess C3b affinity and form a hyperactive C3 convertase resistant to dissociation. C3b formation is thereby enhanced in vivo.[96]

About 4% to 10% of aHUS patients have heterozygous mutations in *C3*, usually with low C3 levels. Most mutations reduce C3b binding to CFH and MCP, severely impairing degradation of mutant C3b.[95]

THROMBOMODULIN. Mutations in the *THBD* gene encoding thrombomodulin, a membrane-bound glycoprotein with anticoagulant properties that modulates complement activation on cell surfaces, have been associated with aHUS.[97] About 5% of aHUS patients carry heterozygous *THBD* mutations. Cells expressing these variants inactivate C3b less efficiently than cells expressing wild-type thrombomodulin.[97] These data document a functional link between complement and coagulation, opening new perspectives for candidate gene research in aHUS.

DIACYLGLYCEROL KINASE-ε. Homozygous or compound heterozygous mutations in diacylglycerol kinase-ε *(DGK-ε)* were recently reported in nine unrelated children with aHUS and autosomal recessive inheritance.[98] Mutation carriers presented with aHUS before the age of 1 year, had persistent hypertension, hematuria, and proteinuria, and developed chronic kidney disease as they got older. *DGK-ε* encodes diacylglycerol kinase-ε, which is expressed in endothelium, platelets, and podocytes. Diacylglycerol kinase-ε is apparently unrelated to the complement cascade, and the mechanism whereby *DGK-ε* mutations cause aHUS remains to be elucidated.

Determinants of Disease Penetrance. Two other factors are thought to determine the development of aHUS. First, in most patients, there is a trigger. Infection and pregnancy are the most frequently described triggers.[99] Second, a further genetic variant (modifier) can increase the risk of developing the disease. This can be in the form of an additional mutation in one of the aforementioned genes and/or the presence of a common at-risk genetic variant. It is now recognized that about 10% of aHUS patients will have mutations in more than one gene.[50] Common at-risk genetic variants (single-nucleotide polymorphisms [SNPs] and haplotype blocks) in *CFH, CD46,* and *CFHR1* have been shown to act as susceptibility factors for development of the disease.[50]

Clinical Course. Of aHUS patients, irrespective of mutation type, 67% are affected during childhood, and almost all patients with anti-CFH antibodies develop the disease before 16 years.[81,100,101] Acute episodes manifest with severe hemolytic anemia, thrombocytopenia, and acute renal failure. Extrarenal involvement (central nervous system or multivisceral) occurs in 20% of cases.[5,81,100]

Short- and long-term outcomes vary according to the underlying complement abnormality (see Table 35.3). About 60% to 70% of patients with *CFH, CFI,* and *C3* mutations and one third of children with anti-CFH autoantibodies lose renal function, die during the presenting episode, or develop ESRD following relapses.[5,81,100] *CFB* mutations are associated with poor renal outcome (renal function loss in seven of eight patients).[96]

Chronic complement dysregulation may lead to atheroma-like lesions. About 20% of patients with *CFH* mutations have cardiovascular complications (e.g., coronary or cerebrovascular disease, myocardial infarction) and excess mortality. Long-term survival is worse in patients with *CFH* mutations (50% at 10 years) than in those with *CFI* and *C3* mutations or anti-CFH autoantibodies (80% to 90% at 10 years).[5,81,100]

MCP mutation carriers have a good prognosis (complete remission, 80% to 90%). Recurrences are frequent but the long-term outcome is good, and 80% of patients remain dialysis free.[5,81,100] However, rare patients with *MCP* mutations have severe disease, immediate ESRD, intractable hypertension, and coma, possibly because of concurrent genetic abnormalities.[81]

Therapy. *Fresh-Frozen Plasma.* Guidelines suggest that plasma therapy (plasma exchange, one or two plasma volumes/day; plasma infusion, 20 to 30 mL/kg/day) should be started within 24 hours of diagnosis.[5] Plasma exchange allows supplying larger amounts of plasma than would be possible with infusion while avoiding fluid overload (see Table 35.2). Trials of plasma therapy in HUS are scanty and not current. The only two published trials in HUS comparing supportive therapy alone with supportive therapy plus plasma infusion did not demonstrate significant benefit for plasma in inducing remission.[102,103] However, neither trial examined outcomes separately for Stx-HUS versus aHUS, which invariably weakened the potential benefits of plasma for aHUS.[104,105] Because CFH is a plasma protein, plasma infusion or exchange provides normal CFH to patients carrying *CFH* mutations.[81,100,106,107] Long-term treatment, however, may fail due to the development of plasma resistance.[108] Heterozygous *CFH* mutation carriers usually have normal levels of CFH, half of which is dysfunctional. The beneficial effect of plasma is strongly dependent on amount, frequency, and modality of administration, with plasma exchange being superior to plasma infusion for remission and prevention of recurrences by removal of mutant *CFH* that could antagonize the normal protein.[109,110] Overall, published data in patients with *CFH* mutations show complete or partial (hematologic normalization with renal sequelae) remission of 60% of plasma-treated episodes (see Table 35.3).[5,81,100] Plasma exchange is used to remove anti-CFH antibodies, but the effect is usually transient.[86,100] Immunosuppressants (corticosteroids and azathioprine or mycophenolate mofetil) and rituximab, an anti-CD20 antibody, combined with plasma exchange allows long-term, dialysis-free survival in 60% to 70% of patients.[86,101,111,112]

Patients with *CFI* mutations show only a partial response, with remission in about 30% to 40% of plasma-treated episodes.[5,81,100,113] Because MCP is a cell-associated protein, effects of plasma are unlikely in patients with *MCP* mutations. Indeed, 80% to 90% of patients undergo remission independently of plasma treatment (see Table 35.3).[5,81,100,113]

Thirty-forty percent of patients with *CFB* mutations and 50% of those with *C3* mutations respond to plasma infusion or exchange.[5,95,96] Possibly, these patients need abundant and frequent plasma exchanges to clear the hyperfunctional mutants *CFB* and *C3*.[5]

Transplantation. Whether kidney transplantation is appropriate for aHUS patients with ESRD has been long debated. Disease recurred in about 50% of transplant patients with *CFH, CFI, CFB,* and *C3* mutations, and graft failure occurred in 80% to 90% of them.[92,95,96,100,114-116] Living related donation is contraindicated by a high risk of recurrence and may be risky to donors.[116,117] A man with a heterozygous *CFH* mutation developed de novo HUS after donating a kidney to his child.[117]

Intensive chronic plasma prophylaxis prevented recurrence in one patient with a *CFH* mutation but failed in another patient.[118,119] Simultaneous kidney and liver transplantation was performed in two children with aHUS and *CFH* mutations, with the rationale of correcting the genetic defect and preventing recurrences.[120,121] However, both cases were complicated by premature liver failure. The first child recovered after a second liver transplantation. The child had no symptoms of HUS for 3 years but died from sequelae of hepatic encephalopathy.[120] This case offered the proof of concept that transplantation could cure HUS associated with *CFH* mutations by correcting the genetic defect. The second case was also complicated by liver failure, with widespread microvascular thrombosis and complement deposition.[121] It was reasoned that the surgical stress with ischemia and reperfusion induced complement activation in the liver that could not be regulated because of functional *CFH* deficiency. A modified approach to the combined transplantation was applied to eight cases, including extensive plasma exchange before surgery to provide a timely enough normal CFH until the liver graft recovered synthetic function.[122,123] This procedure was successful in seven patients. However, another child developed severe hepatic thrombosis and fatal encephalopathy.[122] The risks of kidney and liver transplantation require a careful assessment of benefits for candidate patients.

The outcome of kidney transplantation is favorable in patients with *MCP* mutations. More than 80% did not experience HUS recurrence, with long-term graft survival comparable to that of patients transplanted for other causes.[5,100,114,115] The theoretical rationale is strong. MCP is a transmembrane protein that is highly expressed in the kidney. Not surprisingly, a kidney graft corrects the defect of *MCP*-mutated recipients.

Screening for mutations should allow patients and clinicians to make informed decisions regarding listing for transplantation based on the risk of recurrence (Figure 35.6). Algorithms have been developed to optimize the cost-effectiveness of screening programs for genetic defects in patients with aHUS (see Figure 35.6). A position paper has defined the groups of patients in whom isolated kidney transplantation is extremely risky, where a combined kidney-liver transplantation is recommended, and those eligible to isolated kidney transplantation.[122]

Complement Inhibitors. Identifying complement gene abnormalities has paved the way for tailored treatments aimed at specifically hampering complement activation. In particular, the humanized anti-C5 monoclonal antibody eculizumab is going to change short- and long-term prognosis of aHUS radically. More than 25 aHUS patients treated with eculizumab have been reported in the literature thus far.[124] Some patients were treated for aHUS on native kidneys, and others received eculizumab to treat or prevent posttransplantation aHUS recurrence. Most patients treated during acute episodes achieved remission with eculizumab, including dramatic cases with severe neurologic involvement or peripheral gangrene. The efficacy of eculizumab in aHUS has been definitely proven in two open-label controlled trials of adult and adolescent patients with plasma therapy–sensitive or plasma therapy–resistant aHUS.[125] Based on these results, in late 2011, eculizumab received the approval for the treatment of aHUS in the United States and Europe.

How long eculizumab therapy should be continued and which is the ideal treatment regimen to be administered, however, remains to be established. Conceivably, chronic lifelong treatment with eculizumab at doses able to block the complement cascade persistently might be needed to prevent disease recurrence, at least in a subgroup of patients. However, whether and to what extent this applies to all patients with aHUS and complement intrinsic abnormalities are unknown. Reasonably, different underlying genetic defects, different clinical courses before eculizumab therapy, and different residual complement activity while on eculizumab therapy should be taken into consideration when strategies of chronic eculizumab therapy are planned. Prospective studies titrating eculizumab dosing to reliable markers of complement activation are needed to explore the possibility of gradual back titration and possible withdrawal of chronic treatment, at least in a subset of affected patients. This should reduce the risk of possible and still unknown long-term adverse effects and, considering the tremendous costs of eculizumab therapy, would have major implications for health care providers.

Liver Transplantation. In the pre-eculizumab era, liver transplantation had been suggested to correct the complement abnormality and prevent disease recurrence in patients with defects in genes encoding circulating complement proteins that are synthesized in the liver.[120] In patients with aHUS and ESRD, combined liver-kidney transplantation was found to restore renal function and prevent recurrence of aHUS related to a CFH mutation. The outcome, however, was complicated by early liver failure in 15% to 30% of cases.[126] Evidence of widespread microvascular thrombosis with diffuse deposition of complement MAC in liver sinusoids consistent with complement activation was taken to suggest that the surgical stress with liver ischemia and reperfusion might induce intense local complement activation that could not be regulated, as occurs normally, because of the deficiency in functional CFH.[121]

Because the risk of premature liver failure does not appear to be solely affected by perioperative intensified plasma therapy, combined liver-kidney transplantation to prevent aHUS recurrence is still a risky procedure. Availability of eculizumab, however, has led to reconsider this therapeutic option. Eculizumab has been used to

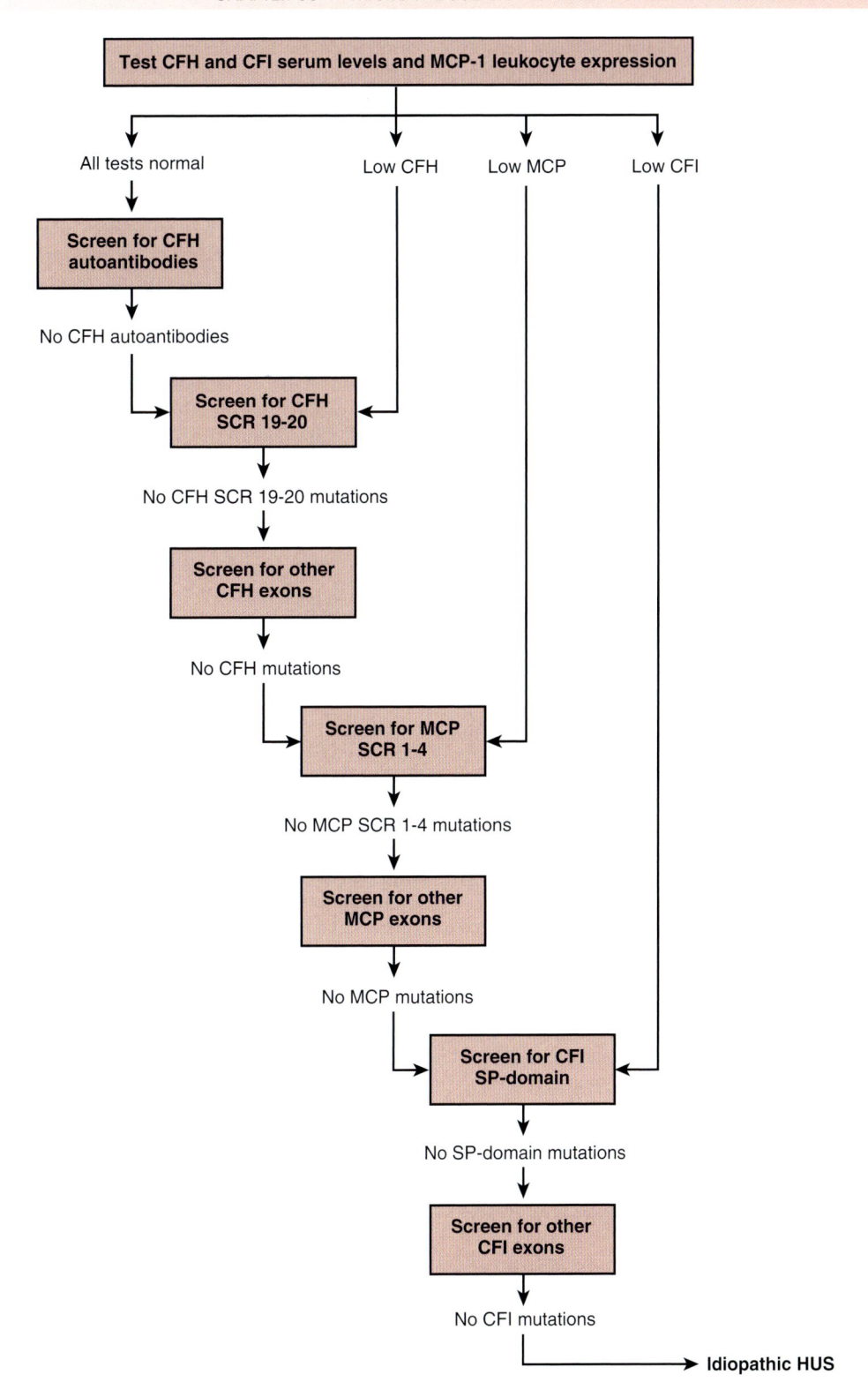

Figure 35.6 Flow diagram of the steps suggested to optimize the cost-effectiveness of screening for genetic defects in patients with aHUS and suspected genetically determined abnormalities in complement regulatory proteins. A preliminary screen for serum CFH and CFI levels by enzyme-linked immunosorbent assay (ELISA) or radial immunodiffusion (RID), and for MCP expression in peripheral blood leukocytes by flow cytometry (FACS), is recommended to identify which is the candidate gene to evaluate. If no abnormalities are detected, we suggest screening for anti-CFH autoantibodies and then, if none are detected, to look for mutations of candidate genes starting with the CFH gene; this is more frequently affected by pathogenic mutations, followed by MCP1 and CFI genes, respectively. Within each gene, the exons where the mutations tend to localize more frequently should be studied first. CFH, Complement factor H; CFI, complement factor I; MCP, membrane cofactor protein.

prevent and treat aHUS recurrence after solitary kidney transplantation.[127] This approach is safe and effective as long as treatment is continued. In some cases, eculizumab might have the additional benefit of reducing the risk of antibody-mediated rejection.[128] On the other hand, the risk of sensitization associated with chronic drug exposure and the enormous costs that could be unbearable in resource-limited settings suggest that careful treatment tapering up to withdrawal, whenever possible, should be attempted in most cases under tight control of disease and complement activity. In this context, a successful liver transplantation might allow safely withdrawing eculizumab therapy by restoring the bioavailability of liver-produced complement modulators such as factor H or factor I. On the other hand, perioperative eculizumab therapy might protect the liver from thrombotic microangiopathy and protect against early failure by preventing uncontrolled complement activation precipitated by surgical stress and revascularization damage. Thus, liver transplantation, under the umbrella of perioperative eculizumab therapy, might be a valuable option when chronic eculizumab therapy is unfeasible because of safety concerns or resource restriction.[129]

Hemolytic-Uremic Syndrome Associated with Inborn Abnormal Cobalamin Metabolism

Mechanisms. This is a rare autosomal recessive form of HUS associated with an inborn abnormality of cobalamin C metabolism.[130] The biochemical features of cobalamin C deficiency are hyperhomocysteinemia and methylmalonic aciduria.

Clinical Course. Patients with cobalamin C deficiency usually present in the early days and months of life with failure to thrive, poor feeding, and vomiting.[65,130] Rapid deterioration occurs due to metabolic acidosis, gastrointestinal bleeding, hemolytic anemia, thrombocytopenia, severe respiratory and hepatic failure, and renal insufficiency. Children may present neurologic symptoms of fatigue, delirium, psychosis, and seizures. In cases with early onset, the disease has a fulminant evolution and occasionally involves the pulmonary vasculature, but when it ensues later in childhood it may follow a more chronic course. The hallmarks of defective cobalamin C metabolism are hyperhomocysteinemia and methylmalonic aciduria, and the extremely high homocysteine levels (up to tenfold higher than normal) have been suggested to have a role in the pathogenesis of the vascular lesions. Without treatment, the disease is fatal, and some children likely die undiagnosed.

Therapy. Daily intramuscular administrations of hydroxycobalamin may reduce homocysteine levels and methylmalonic aciduria, whereas oral hydroxycobalamin and cyanocobalamin are ineffective. Oral betaine helps reduce serum homocysteine levels further by activating betaine homocysteine methyltransferase. Folic acid supplementation to avoid folate deficiency induced by methyltetrahydrofolate trapping and L-carnitine to increase propionyl carnitine excretion have been suggested, but their role in improving disease outcome is unclear.[131]

Despite treatment, most children with early-onset disease die or have severe neurologic sequelae. Intensified treatment in older children with less acute disease may achieve remission of the microangiopathic process and amelioration of the other clinical manifestations of the metabolic disorder. Whether plasma therapy has a role in improving disease outcome is unknown.

Thrombotic Thrombocytopenic Purpura

In the microvasculature of patients with TTP, systemic platelet thrombi are developed, mainly formed by platelets and vWF. This protein plays a major role in primary hemostasis by forming platelet plugs at the sites of vascular injury under high shear stress. vWF is a large glycoprotein synthesized in vascular endothelial cells and megakaryocytes. On stimulation, vWF is secreted by endothelial cells as ultra-large multimers that form stringlike structures attached to the endothelial cells, possibly through interaction with P-selectin.[132] Under fluid shear stress, the UL-vWF strings are cleaved to generate the range of vWF multimer sizes that normally circulate in the blood, from approximately 500 kDa to 20 million Da.[133] The proteolytic cleavage of vWF multimers appears to be critical to prevent thrombosis in the microvasculature (Figure 35.7, *right upper panel*).

ADAMTS13 is the protease, predominantly expressed by the liver, that cleaves vWF; it is deficient in most patients with TTP, leading to the accumulation of UL-vWF multimers that are highly reactive with platelets (see Figure 35.7, *right lower panel*).[134-136] Two mechanisms for the deficiency of ADAMTS13 activity have been identified in patients with idiopathic TTP—an acquired deficiency caused by the formation of anti-ADAMTS13 autoantibodies (acquired TTP) and a genetic deficiency due to homozygous or compound heterozygous mutations in the *ADAMTS13* gene (congenital TTP; see Table 35.1).

Immune-Mediated Deficiency of ADAMTS13 Associated with Thrombotic Thrombocytopenic Purpura

Mechanisms. This is an immune-mediated, nonfamilial form of TTP that most likely accounts for most cases (from 60% to 90%) so far reported as acute idiopathic or sporadic TTP (see Table 35.2). The disease is characterized by a severe deficiency of ADAMTS13; its activity is inhibited by specific autoantibodies that develop transiently and tend to disappear during remission.[8,134,135,137,138] These inhibitory anti-ADAMTS13 antibodies are mainly IgG, although IgM and IgA anti-ADAMTS13 antibodies have also been described.[134,135,139]

Patients with TTP secondary to hematopoietic stem cell transplantation, malignancies, or HIV infection rarely have severe ADAMTS13 deficiency and inhibitory IgG antibodies.[140-147] TTP associated with ticlopidine and clopidogrel (thienopyridine drugs that inhibit platelet aggregation) represent interesting exceptions of secondary TTP consistent with a drug-induced autoimmune disorder. Severe ADAMTS13 deficiency and ADAMTS13 inhibitory antibodies were detected in 80% to 90% of patients with ticlopidine-associated TTP and in two patients with clopidogrel-induced TTP.[148] The deficiency resolved after the drugs were discontinued.

Evidence of the pathogenic role of TTP-associated, anti-ADAMTS13 autoantibodies has been derived by the finding that they usually disappear from the circulation when remission is achieved by effective treatment; this occurs in parallel with the normalization of ADAMTS13 activity. In patients with acquired ADAMTS13 deficiency, a risk as high as 50% to develop a relapse has been reported, and undetectable

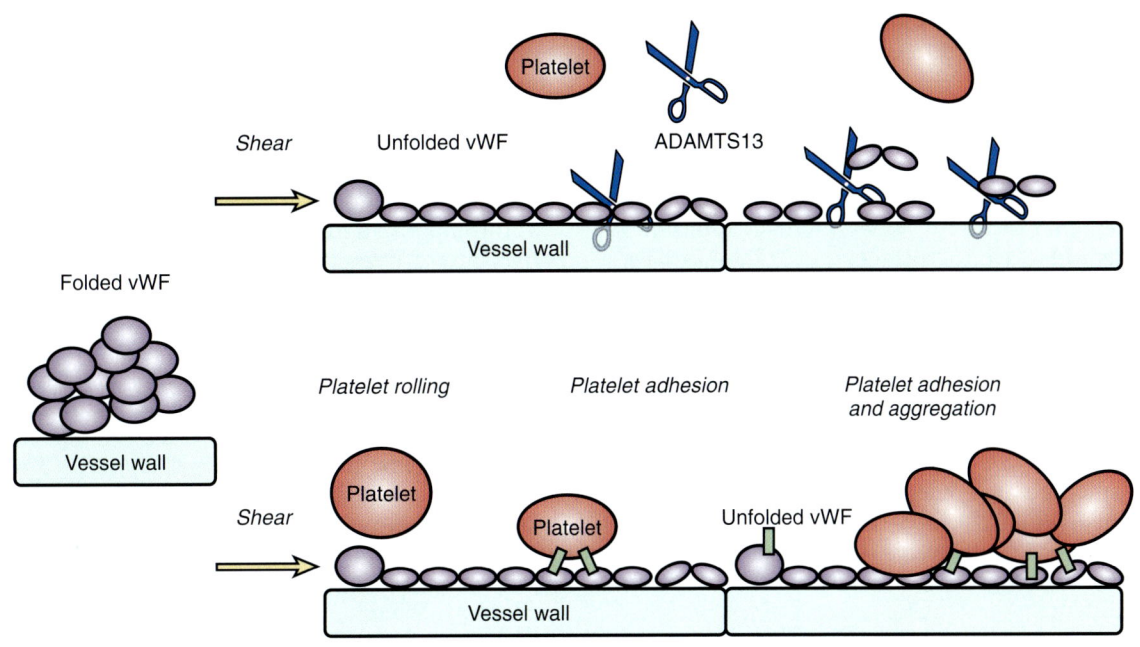

Figure 35.7 Pathophysiology of platelet aggregation in thrombotic thrombocytopenic purpura. Von Willebrand factor (vWF) is synthesized and stored as ultra-large (UL) multimers in endothelial cells and megakaryocytes. On stimulation, UL-vWF multimers are secreted by endothelial cells into the circulation in a folded structure. On exposure to enhanced shear stress, UL multimers form stringlike structures that adhere to endothelial cells. Normally, UL-vWF strings are cleaved by ADAMTS13 to generate vWF multimers from 500 kDa to 20 million Da in size to prevent thrombosis in the microvasculature **(upper panel)**. When the ADAMTS13 proteolytic activity is defective because of the inhibitory effect of anti-ADAMTS13 autoantibodies or congenital defective synthesis of the protease, UL-vWF multimers accumulate and interact with activated platelets to facilitate platelet adhesion and aggregation, with thrombus formation and occlusion of the vascular lumen **(lower panel)**.

ADAMTS13 activity and the persistence of anti-ADAMTS13 antibodies during remission predict recurrences.[139,149,150]

Clinical Course. Patients with anti-ADAMTS13 antibodies experience a more severe manifestation of the disease and have a higher mortality rate than patients without these antibodies.[151] Neurologic symptoms usually dominate the clinical picture and may be fleeting and fluctuating, probably because of continuous thrombus formation and dispersion in the brain microcirculation. Coma and seizures complicate the most severe forms. The detection of high titers of anti-ADAMTS13 antibodies correlates with relapsing disease and poor prognosis.

TTP has been reported in 1 in 1600 to 5000 patients treated with ticlopidine. Eleven cases have been reported during treatment with clopidogrel, a new antiaggregating agent that has achieved widespread clinical use for its safety profile. Most patients had neurologic involvement. The overall survival rate is 67% and is improved by early treatment withdrawal and plasma therapy.

Therapy. Plasma manipulation is a cornerstone in the therapy of the acute episode (see Table 35.2). Plasma may serve to induce remission of the disease by replacing defective protease activity. In theory, as compared to infusion, exchange may offer the advantage of also rapidly removing anti-ADAMTS13 antibodies but this needs to be proven in controlled trials. Corticosteroids might be of benefit in autoimmune forms of TTP by inhibiting the synthesis of anti-ADAMTS13 autoantibodies. In a series of 33 patients with undetectable ADAMTS13 activity and anti-ADAMTS13 antibodies, combined treatment with plasma exchange and prednisone was associated with disease remission in about 90% of cases.[139] The rationale of combined treatment is that plasma exchange will have only a temporary effect on the presumed autoimmune basis of the disease, and additional immunosuppressive treatment may cause a more durable response. Of 108 patients with TTP or HUS, 30 were reported to have recovered after treatment with corticosteroids alone. All of them, however, had mild forms, and none of them were tested for ADAMTS13 activity.[152]

Some prospective studies have successfully and safely used rituximab in patients who had failed to respond to standard daily plasma exchange and methylprednisolone and in patients with relapsed acute TTP who had previously demonstrated antibodies to ADAMTS13 (see Table 35.2).[153,154] Treatment was associated with clinical remission in all patients, disappearance of anti-ADAMTS13 antibodies, and an increase of ADAMTS13 activity to levels higher than 10%. Rituximab has been also used electively to prevent relapses in patients with autoantibodies and recurrent disease.[8,154-156] In one study, five patients with persistent undetectable ADAMTS13 activity and high autoantibody titers were treated with rituximab preemptively during remission. ADAMTS13 activity ranging from 15% to 75% and the disappearance of inhibitors were achieved after 3 months in all patients, and activity was still more than 20% at 6 months. Three patients maintained a disease-free status after 29, 24, and 6 months, respectively.[156,157] Relapses were documented at 13 and 51 months in the remaining two patients during follow-up. Longitudinal evaluation of ADAMTS13 activity and autoantibody levels may help monitor patient response to treatment. Retreatment with rituximab should be considered to prevent a relapse when

ADAMTS13 activity decreases and inhibitors reappear into the circulation (see Table 35.2).

Congenital Deficiency of ADAMTS13 Thrombotic Thrombocytopenic Purpura

Mechanisms. This rare form is associated with a genetic defect of ADAMTS13 and accounts for about 5% of all cases of TTP (see Table 35.2).[134,137] Emerging data also indicate that patients with a clinical diagnosis of HUS may have a complete lack of ADAMTS13 activity, albeit less frequently.[120,138,158-160] Thus, on clinical grounds, a possible congenital defect of ADAMTS13 cannot be excluded only on the basis of predominantly renal localization of disease manifestations. TTP associated with congenital ADAMTS13 deficiency has been found in families or patients with no familial history of the disease.[134,136,138] In both cases the disease is inherited as a recessive trait, as documented by the fact that ADAMTS13 levels in unaffected relatives of patients fell into a bimodal distribution, one group had half-normal levels, consistent with carriers, and the other had normal values.

To date, more than 80 *ADAMTS13* mutations have been identified in patients with TTP.[136,161] Most patients are carriers of compound heterozygous mutations; only 15 mutations have been observed in homozygous form. Studies on secretion and activity of the mutated forms of the protease have shown that most of these mutations lead to an impaired secretion from cells and, when the mutated protein is secreted, the proteolytic activity is greatly reduced.[162]

Clinical Course. Approximately 60% of patients with a congenital deficiency of ADAMTS13 experience their first acute episode of disease in the neonatal period or during infancy, but a second group (10% to 20%) manifests the disease after the third decade of life. TTP recurrences are common but their frequency varies widely. Although some patients with congenital ADAMTS13 deficiency depend on frequent chronic plasma infusions to prevent recurrences, many patients who achieved clinical remission after plasma treatment remain in a disease-free status for long periods after plasma discontinuation, despite the absence of protease activity.[157]

Emerging data have suggested that the type and location of *ADAMTS13* mutations may influence the age of onset of TTP and penetrance of the disease in mutation carriers.[157] One of the most frequently reported *ADAMTS13* mutations, the 4143-4144insA in the second CUB domain, leading to a frameshift and loss of the last 49 amino acids of the protein, is associated with neonatal and childhood onset; only one out of 16 reported carriers, homozygous or compound heterozygous with other *ADAMTS13* mutations, reached adulthood without developing TTP.[157,163] In vitro expression studies have revealed that the mutation causes a severe impairment of protein secretion, combined with a strongly reduced specific protease activity. On the other hand, mutations in the sixth and seventh TSP1 appear to lead to adult onset and a milder course of TTP.[157,164] Expression studies have revealed that these mutations result in severe defects in secretion of the metalloprotease, although a small fraction of the mutant protein is released in the supernatant, but the mutants maintain normal specific protease activity.[157,165] It is possible that in carriers of these mutations, low ADAMTS13 activity may be present in the circulation, which is enough to prevent onset of the disease in childhood or even in adulthood. The latter possibility is supported by descriptions of asymptomatic carriers of these mutations who never developed TTP.[157,162,164]

Environmental factors may contribute to induce full-blown manifestation of the disease. According to this two-hit model, deficiency of ADAMTS13 predisposes to microvascular thrombosis, and thrombotic microangiopathy supervenes after a triggering event that activates microvascular endothelial cells and causes the secretion of UL-vWF multimers and P-selectin expression. Potential triggers of these phenomena are infections and pregnancy. Six women with congenital ADAMTS13 deficiency developed late-onset TTP during pregnancy.[162,166] Also, genetic modifiers may be implicated in the susceptibility to develop thrombotic microangiopathy in a condition of ADAMTS13 deficiency, which may include genes encoding proteins involved in the regulation of the coagulation cascade, vWF, or platelet function, components of the endothelial vessel surface or of the complement cascade.

Therapy. When a critically ill patient is admitted because of severe anemia and thrombocytopenia with renal failure and/or neurologic signs, and the microangiopathic nature of the anemia is confirmed by detection of fragmented erythrocytes in the peripheral blood smear in association with increased serum LDH levels (see Figure 35.2), therapy with plasma exchange should be immediately started. If the clinical history, screening for Stx-producing *E. coli* infection, and evaluation of ADAMTS13 activity allow reasonably excluding Stx HUS and TTP, eculizumab should be started as soon as possible on the basis of the assumption that the patient could be affected by aHUS (see Figure 35.2). In most cases, eculizumab will achieve prompt remission of signs and symptoms of the microangiopathic process, and plasma exchange will no longer be required. However, should more exchange sessions be indicated, additional eculizumab doses should be administered shortly after each procedure because the drug is fully cleared from the circulation during the exchange.

If less than 10% ADAMTS13 activity orients the diagnosis toward TTP, plasma exchange should be continued to restore ADAMTS13 bioavailability and to remove anti-ADAMTS13 autoantibodies in patients with immune-mediated disease. Fresh-frozen plasma, 1 or 2 L, should be exchanged daily until complete and sustained remission of the microangiopathic process has been obtained (see Table 35.2).[167] Plasma cryosupernatant—plasma without the cryoprecipitate—may supply the same amount of ADAMTS13 as fresh-frozen plasma, with a reduced risk of acute infusion reactions. Moreover, at least according to some uncontrolled reports, it also appears to be effective in patients who failed to respond to exchange with fresh-frozen plasma.[168,169] These findings could be explained by less vWF content and less ADAMTS13 in complex with larger vWF multimers, which might translate into increased ADAMTS13 bioavailability as compared to that of fresh-frozen plasma.[170]

In immune-mediated cases, add-on therapy with steroids or other immunosuppressants is indicated to inhibit the production of anti-ADAMTS13 autoantibodies. Prospective studies have successfully and safely used rituximab (see Table 35.2), an anti-CD20 monoclonal antibody depleting B lymphocytes, in patients who had failed to respond to standard daily plasma exchange and methylprednisolone and in patients with relapsed acute TTP who had previously demonstrated antibodies to ADAMTS13. Treatment was associated with clinical remission in all patients, disappearance of anti-ADAMTS13 antibodies, and an increase of ADAMTS13 activity to levels higher than 10%.[171] Of the approximately 100 rituximab-treated patients reported in the literature so far, normalization of platelets and LDH have been noted in about 95% of cases, but time to remission has been variable, from 1 to 4 weeks after the first dose. The duration of remission has ranged from 9 months to 4 years, with relapses reported in approximately 10%. Rituximab has been also used electively to prevent relapses in patients with autoantibodies and recurrent disease.[156] Longitudinal evaluation of ADAMTS13 activity and autoantibody levels may help monitor response to treatment. Retreatment with rituximab should be considered when ADAMTS13 activity decreases and inhibitors reappear in the circulation to prevent a relapse.

After plasma exchange has effectively restored a stable clinical and laboratory state in patients suffering from TTP associated with congenital ADAMTS13 deficiency, disease remission might be maintained by plasma infusion alone. Providing sufficient ADAMTS13 to achieve 5% normal enzymatic activity is sufficient to degrade large vWF multimers, which translates into induced remission of the microangiopathic process, and this effect is sustained over time. Infused ADAMTS13 has a plasma half-life of 2 or 3 days in vivo and, although plasma levels fall below 5% within 3 to 7 days after plasma administration, the effect of plasma on the platelet count and clinical parameters may last up to 3 weeks, suggesting that ADAMTS13 remains available (e.g., on platelets and endothelial cells).[172] Patients with congenital ADAMTS13 deficiency tend to relapse. Patients with frequent relapses, a severe clinical course with neurologic sequelae, renal insufficiency, and patients who have siblings who have died of TTP, should be put on regular prophylactic plasma infusions every 2 to 3 weeks, a regimen that has been shown to be effective in preventing acute TTP bouts and maintaining the patient in good health for years.

Although complement activation appears to play a role also in the pathogenesis of TTP, at this stage there is no controlled evidence in support of eculizumab therapy in this context.[1]

ATHEROEMBOLIC RENAL DISEASE

Atheroembolic renal disease (ARD) is part of a systemic syndrome of cholesterol crystal embolization. Renal damage results from the embolization of cholesterol crystals from atherosclerotic plaques present in large arteries, such as the aorta (see Figure 35.3), to small arteries in the renal vasculature.[173] The prevalence appears to depend on sampling bias; it has ranged from 0.8% in a series of 2126 autopsies in patients older than 60 years to 36% in a cohort of patients undergoing surgical revascularization for atherosclerotic renal artery stenosis.[174,175] In two large renal biopsy studies, a 1% prevalence was reported.[176,177] However, in people older than 60 years, the prevalence was 4.0% to 6.5%.[178,179] In clinical practice, Mayo and Swartz have estimated that 5% to 10% of all cases of acute renal failure could be due to atheroembolism.[180]

CLINICAL FEATURES

The disease may ensue suddenly, few days after a precipitating factor, or insidiously, over weeks or months.[181] General systemic manifestations occur in fewer than 50% of patients and include fever, myalgias, headaches, and weight loss.[182] The rate of cutaneous manifestations such as livedo reticularis, purple toes, and toe gangrene varies widely, from 35% to 90%, in parallel with the heterogeneous accuracy of data reporting.[181,182] Cutaneous symptoms constitute the most common extrarenal findings and may herald renal involvement, but other regions, such as the eyes, musculoskeletal system, nervous system, and abdominal organs, can be affected.[181] An autopsy review of 121 cases of ARD noted the kidney to be the most commonly involved internal organ, with 75% of patients showing evidence of renal cholesterol emboli.[183] In other series, the kidneys were affected in approximately 50% of patients.[184]

Almost 50% of patients manifest with mild or accelerated, and occasionally malignant, hypertension.[184] Renal function loss is usually progressive but, in a few cases, renal failure can be acute and oliguric.[181,184] The clinical course of renal failure can be variable. Dialysis is needed in 28% to 61% of patients with acute or subacute disease, with 20% to 30% recovering some kidney function after a variable period of dialytic support.[180,181,185-187] Renal infarction is rare.

The differential diagnosis includes systemic vasculitis, subacute bacterial endocarditis, polymyositis, myoglobinuric renal failure, drug-induced interstitial nephritis, and renal artery thrombosis or thromboembolism.[188] The time course of renal dysfunction may help differentiate atheroembolic renal disease that manifests over 3 to 8 weeks after angiographic procedures from radiocontrast-induced nephropathy, which manifests earlier and often resolves within 2 to 3 weeks after appropriate intervention.[185] Definitive diagnosis is based on the histologic demonstration of cholesterol crystals in small arteries and arterioles of target organs.

Atheroembolic renal disease can also occur in renal allografts, with a frequency ranging from 0.39% to 0.47%.[189,190] Atheroemboli causing injury to the renal allograft can arise from the donor or recipient vessels. Two distinct clinical presentations have been described. The first is an early atheroembolic renal disease, with emboli frequently released from the donor's arteries before or during organ harvesting. More rarely, early embolization originates from the recipient's atheromatous vessels during the anastomosis. The early form is usually associated with primary nonfunction, and the embolic disease is confined to the allograft. The second form is a late clinical presentation, which can arise years after transplantation in stable grafts. In these cases, emboli originate from the recipient's vessels. The disease is usually associated with precipitating factors, and in some cases shows features of a systemic disorder.[173]

Outcomes differ significantly. Early presentation is frequently associated with poor prognosis, whereas late manifestations generally have a more benign course.[181,189-191] This difference could be attributable to extensive embolization in an atherosclerotic donor during organ procurement. Because the use of donors and recipients older than 60 years and of marginal donors with advanced atherosclerosis has increased, atheroembolic renal disease in renal allografts

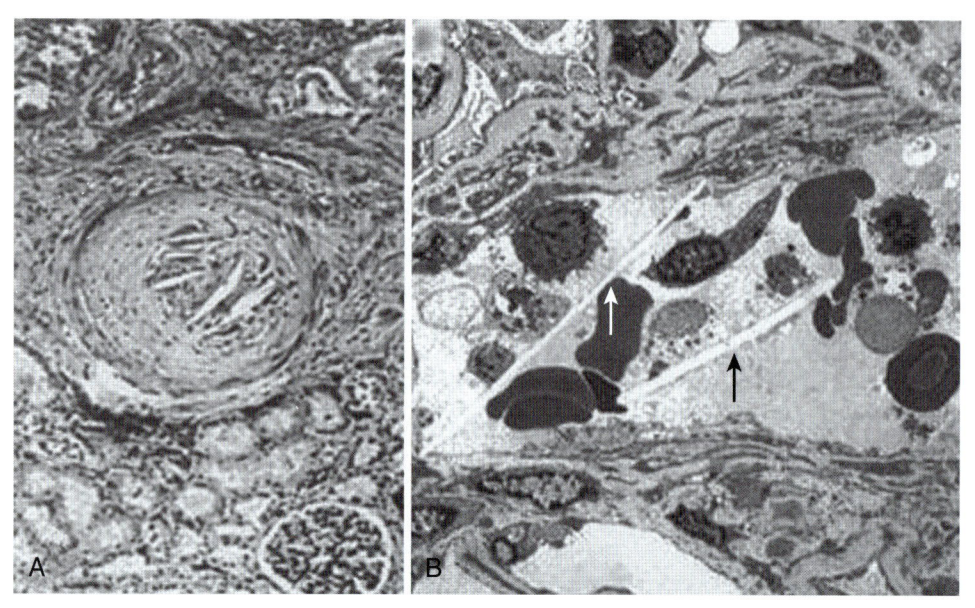

Figure 35.8 **A,** Atheroemboli lodged in an interlobular artery of a kidney obtained postmortem. The elongated clefts are actually voids where cholesterol crystals were located before fixation and staining. Note the exuberant intimal thickening and the cellular proliferation, which completely occlude the lumen. **B,** Electron micrograph showing needle-like clefts from atheroemboli to afferent arterioles. Both *arrows* indicate needle-like clefts. (**A** courtesy W. Margaretten; **B** from Polu KR, Wolf M: Clinical problem-solving. Needle in a haystack. *N Engl J Med* 354:68-73, 2006.)

will probably be encountered more often than previously. To reduce the risk of atheroemboli, an accurate assessment of organ donors should be done. At the time of organ procurement, manipulation of the aorta should be kept to a minimum, mobilizing the kidneys without cross-clamping the aorta, as done for living related donors.[173]

LABORATORY FINDINGS

Laboratory test findings are nonspecific, such as anemia, leukocytosis, thrombocytopenia, and raised concentrations of inflammatory markers (e.g., erythrocyte sedimentation rate [ESR], C-reactive protein). Hypocomplementemia has also been reported but is not a consistent finding.[184,181,192] At diagnosis, as many as 25% of patients have a serum creatinine level higher than 5 mg/dL, and in about 80% it is higher than 2 mg/dL.[182] Changes in the urinary sediment are frequent but nonspecific.[181] Granular and hyaline casts occur in approximately 40% of cases, whereas microscopic hematuria or pyuria are observed in fewer than 30%.[182] Eosinophiluria was observed in one third of patients with renal biopsy–proven atheroembolic renal disease. Proteinuria is present in more than 50% of patients and may occasionally be in the nephrotic range.[181,182] Eosinophilia is reported in up to 60% to 80% of patients and is usually transient.[181,182,184,186] An increased ESR, leukocytosis, and anemia are frequent, but usually transient. Antineutrophilic cytoplasmic antibodies (ANCAs) have been found in a few cases, but not in large series, and their relevance is uncertain.[181,193] A few studies have reported cholesterolemia in patients with atheroembolic renal disease, with total cholesterol levels higher than 5.2 mmol/L, ranging from 23% to 64%.[180,194]

PATHOLOGY

The histologic hallmark of the disease is the presence of elongated, biconvex, transparent needle-shaped clefts, which represent the cholesterol crystals that are dissolved during tissue processing. These crystals are usually small and may not completely occlude the vessel lumen; however, they frequently induce an endothelial inflammatory response, which leads to complete obstruction of the vessel within weeks or months (Figure 35.8). Cholesterol crystals are birefringent under polarized light. The subsequent intravascular inflammatory reaction has been studied in experimental models of atheroembolism and in human biopsy and autopsy samples.[181] The early phase is characterized by a variable polymorphonuclear (PMN) and eosinophil infiltrate, followed by the appearance of macrophages and multinucleated giant cells in the lumens of affected vessels within 24 to 48 hours after atheroembolism. In the chronic phase, tissue ischemia is perpetuated by marked endothelial proliferation, intimal thickening, concentric fibrosis of the vessel wall, and persistence of cholesterol crystals and giant cells in the lumens of affected arteries. Hyalinization of glomeruli, atrophy of renal tubules, and multiple wedge-shaped infarcts in the kidney result in reduced kidney size.[181]

MECHANISMS

Male gender, older age, hypertension, and diabetes mellitus are important predisposing factors.[192,195] Patients with cholesterol embolization syndrome often have a history of ischemic cardiovascular disease, aortic aneurysm, cerebrovascular disease, congestive heart failure, or renal insufficiency.[182,192] A significant association between renal artery stenosis and atheroembolic renal disease has also been reported.[181,192] At least one of the precipitating factors, which include vascular surgery, arteriography, angioplasty, anticoagulation, and thrombolytic therapy, can be identified in most patients.[187,192,196] Arteriographic procedures constitute the most common intervention reported to incite cholesterol embolization.[182] The most common is coronary angiography, which has a rate of cholesterol embolism of 0.1% to 1.4%.[192,197] An estimated 15% of patients with atheroembolism do not have any of the known risk factors.[182]

The molecular mechanisms of crystal-induced inflammation have been only rather recently identified and involve crystal uptake by tubular cells into intracellular lysosomes and, eventually, lysosomal leakage.[198] Crystal uptake activates the NLRP3 (NOD-like receptor family, pyrin domain containing 3) inflammasome and triggers caspase-1–dependent interleukin-1β (IL-1β) and IL-18 secretion. These events induce a general inflammatory response, including the recruitment of neutrophils and macrophages to the site of crystal formation. Although these enhance local inflammation, macrophages may also contribute to crystal clearance or progressive scarring, respectively.

TREATMENT

Various treatments have been suggested to improve the outcome of atheroembolic renal disease, but none has been found to be appreciably effective, with probably the only exception being chronic therapy with cholesterol-lowering agents.[187] A plausible explanation is that statins have a plaque-stabilizing effect, perhaps as a result of their cholesterol-lowering effect, as well as their antiinflammatory and immunomodulatory properties. The use of steroids is controversial and, in some series, does not appear to be beneficial, whereas in other series it has been associated with improved outcomes, independent of the doses administered.[181,182,199-203] The therapeutic efficacy of low-density lipoprotein (LDL) apheresis is also uncertain, whereas anticoagulants should be avoided because of the risk of precipitating more atheroembolization.[184] Surgical excision of atheromatous plaques in the suprarenal region of the aorta is not advocated because of significant postoperative mortality, worsening renal function, and lower limb loss.[204]

Altogether, improved outcomes that have been observed appear to be largely explained by better supportive therapy, including immediate withdrawal of anticoagulants, postponement of aortic procedures, reduction of blood pressure to less than 140/80 mm Hg, careful treatment of heart failure, dialysis therapy, and adequate nutritional support.[181,186] On the other hand, lack of effective specific treatments that can appreciably improve the outcome of the disease are thought to emphasize the importance of preventive measures aimed at limiting the risk of arterial thromboembolism—in particular, during angiographic studies. Also, the brachial approach for aortography or coronary angiography appears to be burdened by less morbidity than the femoral approach. Interest has arisen about the use of distal protection devices (DPDs) to prevent embolization of material during interventional procedures. They have been most widely used in the coronary and carotid vascular beds, where they have demonstrated the capacity to trap embolic materials and, in some cases, reduce complications. Early experience with DPDs in the renal arteries in patients with suitable anatomy has suggested retrieval of embolic materials in approximately 70% of cases and renal function improvement or stabilization in 98%; the combination of platelet inhibition and a DPD may provide even greater benefit.[205]

There are isolated reports of successful therapy in small numbers of patients given iloprost, pentoxifylline, and LDL apheresis. However, these approaches have yet to be tested in controlled studies.[206-208]

RADIATION NEPHROPATHY

Following the original description in 1904 by Baerman and Linser, a great number of studies have indicated that external kidney radiation causes progressive tissue injury, resulting in organ dysfunction and fibrosis.[209] This process is an example of tissue response to radiation that may affect any organ exposed to therapeutic irradiation. Because kidney inflammation is minimal or absent on radiation exposure, the term *radiation nephritis* originally introduced to describe this clinical entity has been progressively replaced with the more appropriate term, *radiation nephropathy*. This is the terminology we will use throughout this review.

CLINICAL FEATURES

Typically, exposure of the kidneys to x-rays or gamma rays in a dose higher than 2000 cGy (rad) is required to cause radiation nephropathy. However, a 10-Gy, single-fraction dose is sufficient to cause chronic renal failure after bone marrow transplantation (BMT), and with many years of follow-up, a 1-Gy, single-fraction dose is associated with the development of chronic kidney disease.[210,211] Although these effects are not immediate, as is the case for radiation injury to the bone marrow or gastrointestinal tract, kidney injury at these doses indicates that the kidneys are quite radiosensitive.

Modern radiation therapy is sharply focused on the area to be treated; therefore, it is very unlikely that the kidneys would be irradiated in a case of irradiation for uterine cervical cancer or prostate cancer. In patients who have undergone BMT, partial renal shielding reduces, but does not abolish, the risk of BMT nephropathy.

TYPES

Acute Radiation Nephropathy

Radiation nephropathy may ensue abruptly 6 to 12 months after exposure to ionizing radiation with headache, vomiting, fatigue, hypertension, and edema. Patients manifest arteriovenous nicking on funduscopic examination, normochromic normocytic anemia, microscopic hematuria, proteinuria, and urinary casts. Worsening of renal function may accompany these symptoms.[212] The outcome may range from complete or partial recovery of renal function to terminal kidney failure and can be complicated by malignant hypertension.[212]

Acute BMT nephropathy (BMTN) is one of the most frequent forms of acute radiation nephropathy and may follow total-body irradiation of candidates for bone marrow transplantation. Acute BMTN presents with an HUS-like picture, with severe hypertension, peripheral edema, microangiopathic hemolytic anemia, and thrombocytopenia. Renal function decreases progressively, with significant proteinuria and microscopic hematuria, with or without casts. In a retrospective analysis of 363 recipients of allogeneic, myeloablative BMT, the incidence of severe renal failure (grades 2 and 3 combined) was approximated 50%.[213] In this study, acute renal failure did not appear to affect patient survival, but in another study it was associated with increased mortality.[213,214]

Chronic Radiation Nephropathy

Occasionally, the disease manifests with hypertension, proteinuria, and gradual loss of renal function, with a latency period that from 18 months to years after the initial exposure.[212] Hypertension, isolated or occasionally associated with proteinuria, and isolated low-level proteinuria may ensue 2 to 5 and 5 to 19 years after exposure, respectively. These are expressions of a mild disease, with a benign outcome in most cases.[212]

Chronic BMTN presents with mild to moderate hypertension and mild hemolytic anemia. Kidney function decreases slowly, with a biphasic pattern in most patients, with persistent decline in the first 12 to 24 months, followed by a period of stabilization.[215] Also present is proteinuria higher than 1 g/day and microscopic hematuria, with or without casts. A period of 8 years is generally necessary for chronic renal failure to occur.[215] In a long-term study of 103 adult survivors of BMT, Lawton and colleagues reported late renal dysfunction in 14 patients.[216] All of them had received 1400 rad prior to transplantation, whereas none of the patients receiving lower doses of irradiation developed late hypertension or decreased GFR.

Late Malignant Hypertension

This condition arises 18 months to 11 years after irradiation in patients with chronic radiation nephropathy or benign hypertension.[212] High-renin hypertension resulting from irradiation of one kidney and recovery after removal of the affected kidney have been described.[212] Irradiation to one kidney and the ipsilateral renal artery may produce renovascular hypertension, mostly in infants and children.

PATHOLOGY

Early changes following renal irradiation include atypia, endothelial microvascular damage, as observed on light microscopy, with mild endothelial cell swelling, and basement membrane splitting in the glomerular capillaries. With scanning (e.g., computed tomography [CT], magnetic resonance imaging [MRI]), marked subendothelial expansion, with deposition of basement membrane-like material adjacent to the endothelial cells, is evident. The endothelial cell lining may be absent in some capillary loops.[212] Immunofluorescence studies do not show specific staining patterns. Similar glomerular endothelial injury was observed in kidney biopsy specimens from patients who developed renal insufficiency and hypertension after total body irradiation (TBI) and BMT.[217] Some patients also showed arteriolar intimal thickening and tubular atrophy. Glomerular capillary endothelial cell loss and mesangiolysis are observed within weeks after irradiation.[218] After initial injury, the endothelial injury resolves, but mesangial lesions progress. Late changes include reduction in total renal mass, with prominent and sclerosed interlobar and arcuate arteries, glomerular capillary loop occlusion and hyalinization, with progressive tubular atrophy, increased mesangial matrix, mesangial sclerosis and, finally, glomerulosclerosis.[212,218]

MECHANISMS

Renal tissue damage and dysfunction are a direct consequence of ionized radiation. The effect of radiation is dose-dependent, and pathogenic doses exceed by at least 1000-fold the dose to which a patient can be exposed for a radiologic examination, such as a standard abdominal CT scan. Irradiation for neoplastic diseases of the pelvis, in particular for the treatment of malignant seminomas, has historically been the major cause of radiation nephropathy. This explains why, in parallel with the progressive replacement of irradiation with pharmacologic therapy for this disease, the incidence of radiation nephropathy has been progressively declining over time. In more recent years, however, the incidence of the disease again began to increase, along with the rapidly increasing use of total body irradiation of candidates for bone marrow transplantation. It has been suggested that chemotherapy administered as part of the preparative regimen could potentiate the effects of irradiation on the kidneys.[212] Actinomycin enhances the effects of irradiation on many tissues (e.g., gut, lung, skin). Whether this also applies to the kidney is controversial. Cisplatin and carmustine (BCNU) are toxic, mainly when radiation precedes platinum administration.

Most of the theories proposed to explain the pathogenesis of radiation nephropathy are based on murine studies. These studies have consistently shown that endothelial, mesangial, and tubular cells are the major targets of radiation injury and that double-stranded DNA breaks are the initial cause of radiation-induced cell apoptosis and death.[219] Damage to the endothelial cell may impair the physiologic thromboresistance of the capillary vascular wall, which, in more severe cases, may cause intravascular clotting, with pathologic patterns typical of thrombotic microangiopathy.[219] Impaired generation of prostacyclin by endothelial cells and increased production of plasminogen-activator inhibitor mRNA have been suggested to explain the microangiopathic processes that often complicate radiation nephropathy.[219] On the other hand, mesangial cells might acquire a myofibroblast phenotype, which may further contribute to progressive fibrosis and scarring of the kidney tissue. Diffuse apoptosis and lysis of tubular cells, with different degrees of proliferation of the residual cells, is another characteristic pattern of radiation nephropathy. Apoptosis early after 5-Gy, single-dose, total body irradiation has been demonstrated in rats, followed by a late proliferative response.[219] The net balance between cell death and replication will eventually determine the extent of residual tubular atrophy and loss.

Activation of RAAS may also contribute to sustain and amplify the initial injury induced by radiation exposure. Angiotensin II infusion from 4 to 8 weeks after total body irradiation causes more azotemia than irradiation alone. This effect was associated with the induction of arteriolar fibrinoid necrosis, which, in combination with increased transforming growth factor-β (TGF-β) production and enhanced oxidative stress, may contribute to progressive tissue fibrosis and scarring.[220] Finding that this sequence of events is attenuated by concomitant treatment with an inhibitor of RAAS has provided additional evidence for the central role of angiotensin II in the pathogenesis and progression of renal damage in radiation injury.[219]

THERAPY

No specific therapies are available for radiation nephropathy, and the disease is often progressive, independent of treatment. Thus, preventive measures to be observed during the administration of radiation therapy are of paramount importance to limit or prevent adverse effects on the kidney. These include selective shielding of the kidneys and the use of minimum effective doses of fractionated radiation, when possible.[216] The use of radioprotectors such as glutathione or cysteine concomitant with irradiation is still in the experimental phase.[221]

Treatment of hypertension may help slow the progression of established nephropathy. As in chronic proteinuric nephropathies, ACEIs appear to have a specific protective effect against progression of radiation nephropathy that exceeds the benefit expected solely on the basis of achieving blood pressure control.[216,222-224] In a study randomizing 55 subjects exposed to total body irradiation to ACEI therapy or placebo, ACE inhibition consistently slowed serum creatinine level increases over time, a finding taken to indicate that RAAS blockade may be renoprotective in this population.[166,225] Radiation-induced renovascular hypertension may require angioplasty or surgical repair.[212] Uncontrolled hypertension in patients with radiation nephropathy who progress to ESRD may warrant bilateral nephrectomy.

RENAL INVOLVEMENT IN SYSTEMIC DISEASES: SCLERODERMA, SICKLE CELL DISEASE, AND THE ANTIPHOSPHOLIPID SYNDROME

SCLERODERMA

Scleroderma is a complex disease of extensive fibrosis, vascular changes, and autoantibodies against various cellular antigens. The reported incidence ranges from 2.3 to 22.8 cases/million population with a 3 to 14 times higher incidence in women than men.[226,227]

Clinical Features

The pattern of presentation may range from limited to diffuse cutaneous involvement. In limited cutaneous scleroderma, fibrosis is mainly restricted to the hands, arms, and face. Raynaud's phenomenon affects approximately 95% of patients and usually is the first manifestation of the disease. Diffuse cutaneous scleroderma is a rapidly progressing disease that in addition to affecting a large area of the skin, compromises one or more internal organs. The kidneys, along with the esophagus, heart, and lungs, are the most frequent targets (Figure 35.9), although any internal organ can be involved. In rare cases, skin can be spared by scleroderma. Systemic lupus erythematosus, rheumatoid arthritis, polymyositis, or Sjögren's syndrome may accompany scleroderma in the context of an overlap syndrome.[228]

Renal Involvement

Renal involvement typically manifests with malignant hypertension and acute renal failure (scleroderma renal crisis). The crisis may occur de novo or may complicate a preexisting chronic kidney involvement. Less frequently, renal involvement manifests with slowly progressing kidney dysfunction and occasionally as rapidly progressive kidney disease.[228-230]

Renal Crisis. The prevalence of renal crises is decreasing, perhaps related to early therapy with ACEIs. However, in the United States, renal crisis affects approximately 10% of patients with diffuse scleroderma and 2% of patients with limited disease.[231] Studies from the European League Against Rheumatism (EULAR) Scleroderma Trials and Research (EUSTAR) database have suggested a lower prevalence (5% of diffuse scleroderma and 2% of limited), and a retrospective cohort study from Japan has reported a

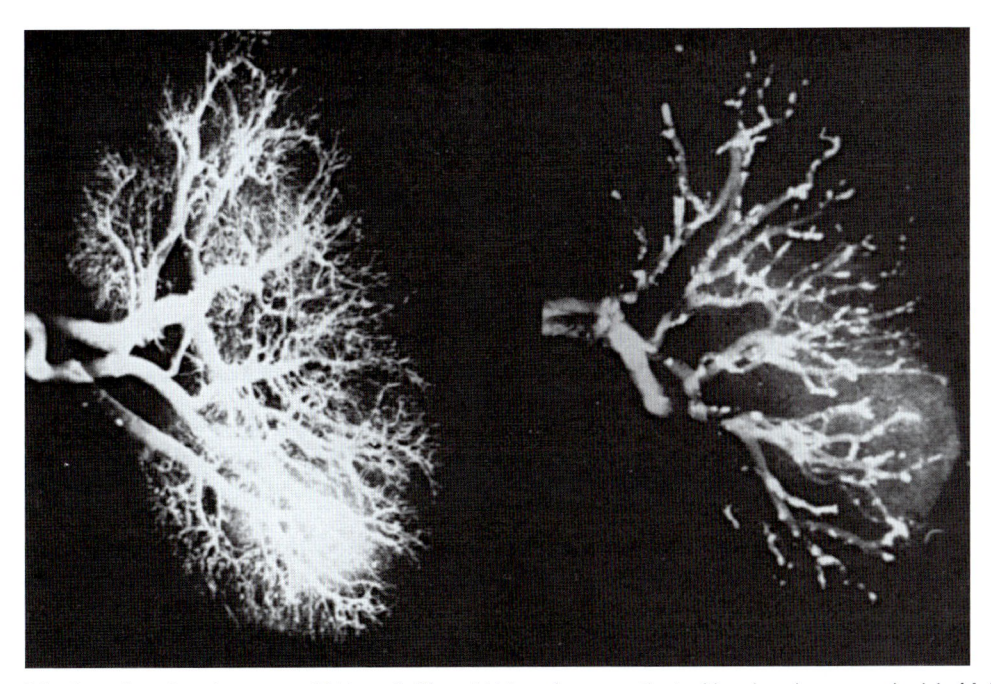

Figure 35.9 Latex injection of postmortem normal kidney **(left)** and kidney from a patient with scleroderma renal crisis **(right)**. Note obstruction to flow at the level of the medium-sized interlobular arteries.

prevalence of 3.2%.[232,233] Geographic differences in autoantibody profiles, particularly anti-RNA polymerase III antibodies, likely contribute to these prevalence variations.

The renal crisis resembles a Raynaud-like phenomenon in the kidney.[234] Severe vasospasm leads to cortical ischemia and enhanced production of renin and angiotensin II, which in turn sustain renal vasoconstriction. Hormonal changes (e.g., pregnancy), physical and emotional stress, or cold temperature may trigger the Raynaud-like arterial vasospasm.[235] The role of the RAAS in perpetuating renal ischemia is underscored by the significant benefit of ACEIs in treating this potentially fatal complication.

Affected patients typically present with severe hypertension and acute renal impairment. Hypertension, however, is not universal and normotensive crises, usually with poor outcome, have been described.[236,237] Nonnephrotic proteinuria and hematuria, often with granular casts, are common findings. Oliguria is an ominous sign, but is unusual in patients diagnosed and treated appropriately.[238,239] Other clinical features include hypertensive retinopathy and encephalopathy.[240] Evidence that retinal and central nervous system involvement may also affect patients with seemingly mild hypertension or even normal blood pressure confirms that endothelial dysfunction may play a central role in the pathogenesis of vascular lesions of scleroderma, independently of blood pressure levels. Microangiopathic hemolytic anemia is common, although significant coagulopathy is rare.[238,239] Pericarditis, myocarditis, and arrhythmias may supervene and are associated with a poorer prognosis.[241-243]

Chronic Kidney Disease. Kidney function can be decreased in patients with scleroderma, even without renal crisis.[244] In these cases, a decreased GFR reflects a chronic kidney disease that may also reflect chronic kidney hypoperfusion due to concomitant cardiac and pulmonary arterial involvement or concomitant treatment with nephrotoxic drugs; it is normally characterized by a benign prognosis.[243,245]

Laboratory Findings

Detection of autoantibodies against topoisomerase (Scl-70), centromere-associated proteins, and nucleolar antigens is crucial for the diagnosis of the disease and may help predict clinical manifestations and prognosis. Antibodies against centromeres are associated with limited cutaneous involvement and risk for pulmonary hypertension, whereas those targeting topoisomerase I are associated with diffuse progressive disease and severe interstitial lung disease. Patients with anti-Th/To antibodies normally have limited skin involvement but are at high risk for lung fibrosis and pulmonary artery hypertension, with severe involvement of kidneys and other internal organs, whereas those with anti-RNA polymerase I/III antibodies have an almost selective renal involvement.[228]

Pathology

Renal Crisis. Biopsy samples from patients with scleroderma crisis show intimal and medial vessel proliferation, with luminal narrowing that typically occurs in arcuate arteries and are indistinguishable from changes of accelerated or malignant hypertension (Figure 35.10). Fibrinoid necrosis and thrombosis are also common. A study of 58 biopsies has shown that acute vascular changes, including mucoid

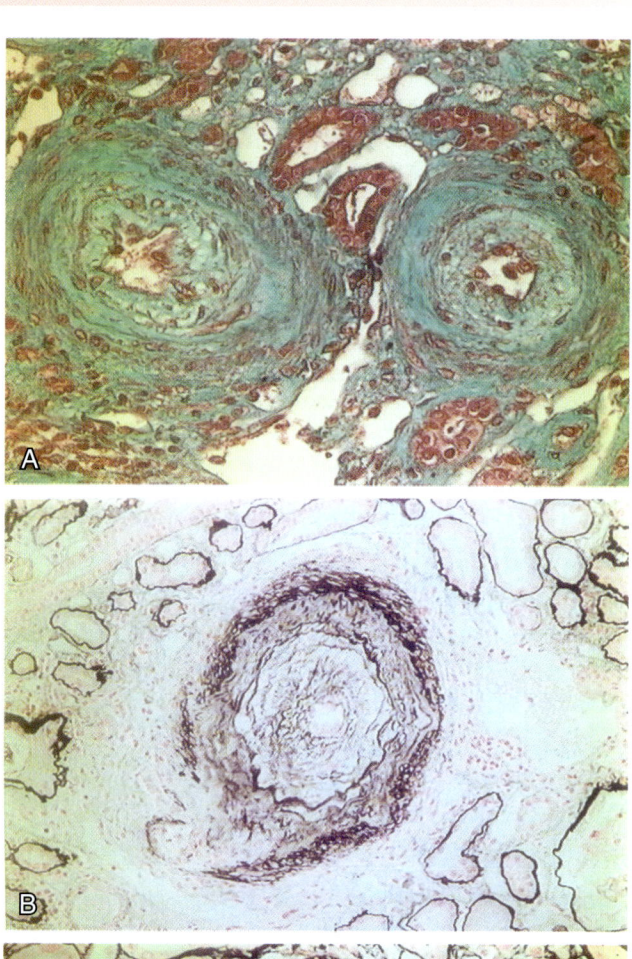

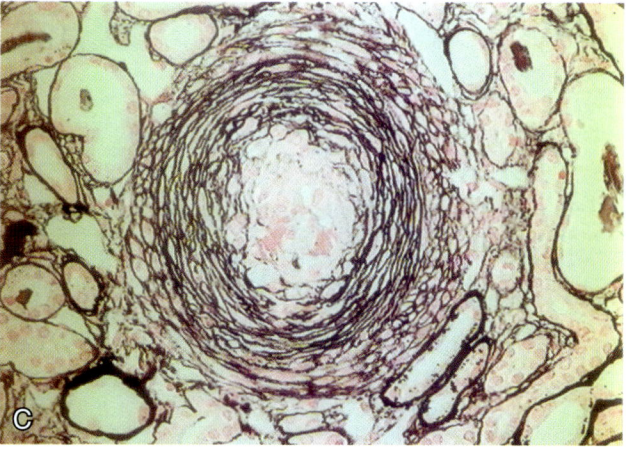

Figure 35.10 Micrographs of renal biopsy samples from patients with scleroderma renal crisis. **A,** Lumina of interlobular arteries are narrowed because of intimal thickening (Trichrome stain). **B,** The thickened intima has a mucoid appearance and is associated with severe luminal narrowing (Silver stain). **C,** The arterial wall shows multilayering of the internal elastic lamina and medial hyperplasia (Silver stain).

intimal thickening and thrombosis, invariably predict a poor outcome, with 50% of affected subjects progressing to terminal kidney failure compared to only 13% of those with predominantly chronic changes.[238,239]

Chronic Kidney Disease. As in other affected organs, the histologic pattern of chronic kidney involvement is characterized by an extensive interstitial fibrosis that is invariably associated with glomerular sclerosis and tubular atrophy. Patterns of glomerulonephritis are occasionally reported but are rare, even in patients with concomitant connective diseases.[148,246]

Mechanisms

The pathogenesis of scleroderma is still unclear, with multiple cells and mediators taking part in the different phases of the microangiopathic process.[228] Microvascular injury is an early event most likely initiated by endothelial cell damage, with secondary proliferation of basal lamina layers. Entrapment of peripheral blood mononuclear cells in the vessel wall, as well as perivascular mononuclear cell infiltrates, are occasionally observed. Activated endothelial cells, in turn, release endothelin-1, which induces chemotaxis, proliferation, extracellular matrix production, and the release of cytokines and growth factors that amplify the inflammatory focus. The next phase is characterized by fibrosis, organ architecture disruption, rarefaction of blood vessels, and eventually, hypoxia, which fuels fibrosis.[228]

Microvascular Injury. Patients with scleroderma often display early signs of vasculopathy, with many experiencing Raynaud's phenomenon, often for many years before developing overt signs of skin fibrosis.[247] Consistent with this, morphologic changes in capillaries are detectable before or at disease onset, which can be used for early diagnosis using nail fold capillaroscopy. Endothelial injury, whether caused by immunologic stimuli, ischemia-reperfusion injury, or other factors results in increased production of endothelin.[248] Endothelin 1 (ET-1) is involved in the regulation of vascular function under normal physiologic conditions and plays a key role in vascular disease by promoting hypertrophy of the vascular smooth muscle cells, vascular permeability, and activating leukocytes through the induction of cytokine and adhesion molecule expression.[248] The effects of endothelin are transmitted on binding to two cognate receptors, endothelin type A (ET-A) and endothelin type B (ET-B), which are mainly expressed on endothelial cells, smooth muscle cells, and fibroblasts.[247] Endothelial dysfunction has been found to be ameliorated by therapy with the ET-1 antagonist bosentan, which provides additional, although indirect, evidence of the pathogenic role of the ET system in the vascular damage of scleroderma.[247]

Increased Collagen Production. Fibroblast secretion of collagen, the main extracellular matrix component of connective tissue, is markedly increased in scleroderma.[235,249] Cytokines and growth factors, such as TGF-β, connective tissue growth factor (CTGF), platelet-derived growth factor (PDGF), and ET-1, secreted in the skin and lungs, activate resident fibroblasts, promoting the accumulation of collagen, proteoglycans, fibronectin, tenascin, and elastin.[250,251] Furthermore, TGF-β induces the differentiation of fibroblasts into smooth muscle cell-like myofibroblasts in situ. Myofibroblasts elaborate matrix molecules and profibrotic cytokines that increase the stiffness of the extracellular matrix (ECM). Moreover, they are relatively resistant to apoptosis and accumulate and persist in affected tissues, where they contribute to further progression of the fibrosis.

Bone marrow–derived mesenchymal progenitor cells fuel expansion of the fibroblast population in affected tissue, which then further contributes to connective tissue accumulation. The signals inducing the bone marrow to mobilize progenitor cells and govern their homing and engraftment in lesional tissue remain unknown. Intriguingly, patients with scleroderma have circulating antibodies directed against the PDGF receptor that activates fibroblasts.[252] Once collagen is secreted into the extracellular space, it undergoes cross-linking and maturation, resulting in a highly stable matrix that accounts for the stiffness of fibrotic skin and other tissues. The stiff matrix may itself serve as a strong stimulus for integrin-mediated TGF-β activation and increasing fibrosis.[252]

Immunologic Mediators. A wide spectrum of autoantibodies have been recently discovered that may have a major role in the pathogenesis of the disease—such as autoantibodies against extracellular matrix components such as metalloproteinases and fibrillin-1, fibroblasts and endothelial cells, and the PDGF receptor—and have been associated with different clinical manifestations and outcomes. Thus, a careful evaluation of circulating autoantibodies is instrumental to predict individual risk and guide treatment. Thus, patients with anticentromere antibodies (ACAs) have limited cutaneous involvement and good outcome, provided pulmonary hypertension is detected early and treated adequately.[253,254]

Cytokines. In addition to autoantibodies, immune injury is sustained by the release of cytokines such as IL-1, IL-2, IL-8, tumor necrosis factor-α (TNF-α), PDGF, TGF-β, interferon-γ (IFN-γ), and endothelin.[248] Moreover, intercellular adhesion molecules and soluble IL-2 receptors have been demonstrated in patients.[255-257] Skin fibroblasts from patients with scleroderma produce much higher levels of IL-6 than normal fibroblasts and may contribute to T cell activation.[258] IL-6 and PDGF-A were shown to be elevated through the action of endogenous IL-1α in fibroblasts from patients with scleroderma.[259]

Therapy

Although there is no evidence for any effective strategy to prevent renal crises, it is common practice to advise patients and physicians of the risk of renal crisis to expedite rapid diagnosis and therapy. A major advancement in the treatment of scleroderma renal crises has been achieved with the introduction of ACEIs in clinical practice (Table 35.4).[47,234,241,248] In the pre-ACEI era, the 1-year survival rate did not exceed 10%, whereas with the use of ACEIs, up to 65% of patients survive the crisis.[47,241] A prospective cohort study evaluating short-term and long-term outcomes of 154 patients with renal crises treated with ACEIs found that 61% were free from chronic dialysis, and 80% to 85% were alive at 8 years after the event, a survival rate similar to that of patients with diffuse scleroderma without renal crises.[241-243] Angiotensin II receptor blockers are less effective than ACEIs and can be considered as add-on therapy when full-dose ACEI therapy is not sufficient to control blood pressure.[260,261] α-Blockers and calcium antagonists are also helpful for refractory hypertension, whereas diuretics are best avoided because of their ability to stimulate renin

Table 35.4 Therapies Used for Scleroderma

Therapy	Dose	Efficacy
Antimetabolites: Methotrexate	10-25 mg/wk	Disappointing results, with only mild effect on skin disease
Antioxidants*	1 tablet/day	Not effective
Corticosteroids: Dexamethasone	100 mg/mo for 6 mo	Improvement in skin scores
Endothelin receptor antagonists: Bosentan	62.5 mg for 4 wk, then 125 mg for 12 wk	Improvement in pulmonary function
Hormones: Relaxin	25/100 µg/kg/day (IV)	Improvement in skin scores
Immunosuppressives: Cyclophosphamide	600 mg/m^2	Significant, albeit modest, improvement in lung function
Interferons		
Interferon-2α	13.5 × 10^6 units/wk	Disappointing results with interferon-α, improved organ involvement with interferon-γ
Interferon-γ	300 mg/wk	
RAAS inhibitors		
ACE inhibitors	Up to maximal tolerated doses	Improved renal and patient survival in renal crisis, slowed progression in chronic renal involvement
Angiotensin II inhibitors		
Prostacyclin analogue		
Iloprost	960 ng/kg/day (IV)	Improvement in pulmonary function
Beraprost	60 µg three times daily	
Nonpharmacologic treatment—photopheresis		Not effective

*Selenium, beta-carotene, vitamin E, vitamin C, and methionine.
ACE, Angiotensin-converting enzyme; RAAS, renin angiotensin adosterone system.
From Henness S, Wigley FM. Current drug therapy for scleroderma and secondary Raynaud's phenomenon: evidence-based review. Curr Opin Rheumatol 19:611-618, 2007.

release.[262] Plasma exchange is also indicated when the renal crisis is accompanied by a microangiopathic process.

With this therapy, it is estimated that approximately two thirds of patients with renal crisis presenting to an experienced center will require renal replacement therapy. However, about 50% of them will eventually recover sufficiently to discontinue dialysis and be maintained on conservative therapy and remain dialysis free. Patients treated appropriately when experiencing a scleroderma renal crisis (SRC) may recover renal function for up to 2 years. This should be taken into consideration before including patients on a waiting list for kidney transplantation.[238]

Renal transplant recipients who have progressed to ESRD because of renal crises have a lower graft and patient survival rate as compared to those with diabetic renal disease.[263] One of the causes of premature graft or patient loss is the recurrence of the disease in the transplanted kidney, in particular in those with more aggressive disease process before transplantation.[264-266] In a cohort of 260 patients with scleroderma renal crisis who developed ESRD and underwent kidney transplantation, the overall 5-year graft survival rate was 56.7%. Among those, the recurrence of disease after transplantation was 6.7% in a report of the United Network of Organ Sharing (UNOS).[265] Based on the finding that cyclosporine A (CsA) may be responsible for acute renal failure in patients with scleroderma and systemic sclerosis (SSc), calcineurin inhibitors are not generally recommended as immunosuppressants after kidney transplantation.[267] The use of high-dose steroids should be also limited as much as possible due to studies supporting an association between doses higher than 15 to 30 mg/day and the onset of renal crisis.[268,269] Several groups have tested continuous low doses of prostacyclin, with no strong beneficial evidence.[270] Plasma exchange or immunosuppressive drugs have shown no beneficial effect in the treatment of SRC.[241] As noted, because of their deleterious effects, corticosteroids are contraindicated in SRC.

Endothelin receptor blockers have been proposed as first-line therapy in addition to ACEIs.[271] In a small open-label trial, six patients within 6 weeks of confirmed SRC received bosentan, 62.5 mg for 1 month, and then 125 mg twice daily for 5 months. Bosentan seemed safe and well-tolerated when combined with ACEI therapy for SRC, with no difference in mortality and dialysis rates between the two study groups.[272] This evidence formed the basis for a larger prospective study testing the effect of bosentan on renal crisis (NCT01241383; see Table 35.4).

SICKLE CELL DISEASE

Sickle cell anemia, and occasionally the heterozygous forms of sickle cell disease, can lead to multiple renal abnormalities, which include hematuria, proteinuria, tubular dysfunction, or a combination of these, eventually resulting in renal function impairment.

Clinical Features

Hematuria and Renal Papillary Necrosis. Gross and often painless hematuria is one of the most frequent features of sickle cell anemia, sickle cell trait (HbSA) disease, and HbSC disease.[273] Hematuria in sickle cell disease can occur at any age and is reported most often with HbSA.[274] A total of 15% to 36% of patients with sickle cell disease develop renal papillary necrosis, which could manifest as an episode of gross hematuria or as a silent finding. Papillary necrosis

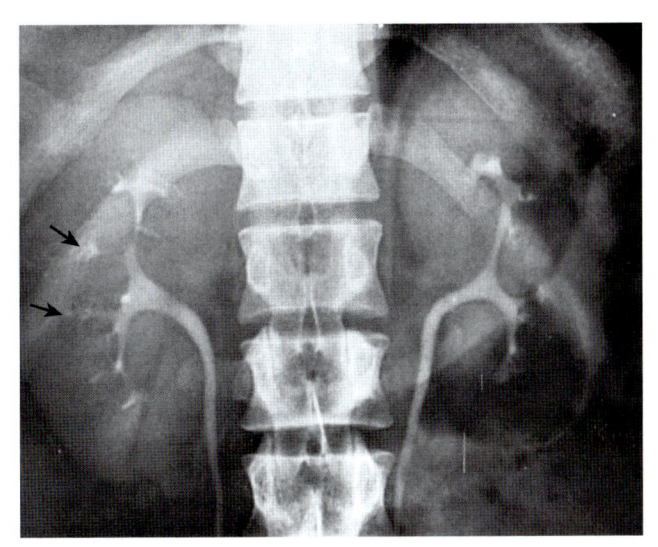

Figure 35.11 Renal papillary necrosis with various forms of cavitation in a 33-year-old man with sickle cell hemoglobinopathy and hematuria. Kidneys are normal size and smooth in contour. Central cavitation is present in many papillae, particularly in right interpolar areas *(arrows)*. (From Davidson AJ, Hartman DS: *Radiology of the kidney and urinary tract,* ed 2, Philadelphia, 1994, WB Saunders, p 184.)

occurs in both the homozygous and the heterozygous forms of sickle cell disease and is best diagnosed by intravenous pyelography (Figure 35.11).[273] Microscopic hematuria is present in most patients with sickle cell anemia. The origin of blood is usually the left kidney, but either kidney may be involved.[273]

Proteinuria. Proteinuria occurs in 20% to 30% of patients with sickle cell disease, more commonly in homozygous HbSS than in heterozygous HbSA, with HbSC in between.[274] Proteinuria can be in the nephrotic or nonnephrotic range. Nephrotic patients have a poorer prognosis and tend to progress to renal failure.[274]

Tubular Dysfunction. Patients with homozygous and heterozygous forms of sickle cell disease fail to concentrate the urine maximally because of erythrocyte sickling in the medullary microcirculation, with secondary medullary ischemia and dysfunction. This abnormality is reversible with multiple transfusions for children younger than 15 years, but becomes irreversible later in life.[275] Patients with sickle cell anemia are capable of diluting their urine normally. Another renal defect seen in patients with sickle cell disease, particularly those with the HbSS or HbSC phenotype, is an incomplete form of distal renal tubule acidosis characterized by the inability to achieve minimal urinary pH during acid loading because of impairment of titratable acid excretion. This defect, however, is not severe enough to cause systemic acidosis. Patients with sickle cell trait (HbSA) do not have evidence of impaired urinary acidification. Other tubular defects in sickle cell anemia (SCA) include mild impairment of K^+ excretion that does not lead to clinical hyperkalemia.[274] Fractional excretion of creatinine is increased, which necessitates the use of inulin clearance to measure the GFR accurately.[275] However, Herrera and colleagues have demonstrated an impaired tubular secretion of creatinine in SCA patients with a normal GFR.[276] In addition, there is increased phosphorus reabsorption in the proximal tubule, which could account for the hyperphosphatemia observed in SCA patients.[275]

Pathology

In 1923, Sydenstricker and colleagues described enlarged glomeruli distended with blood in the kidneys of patients with sickle cell disease.[277] Necrosis and pigmentation of tubular cells were also observed.[273] Medullary lesions are the most prominent finding in the kidneys of these patients. Edema, focal scarring, interstitial fibrosis, and tubule atrophy are observed. Cortical infarction has also been reported in patients with sickle cell disease or sickle cell trait.[273] In Hb-SS patients without renal insufficiency, renal pathology includes glomerular hypertrophy characterized by open, dilated, glomerular capillary loops.[278] Enlarged glomeruli are most commonly found in the juxtamedullary region of the kidney. In patients with proteinuria and mild renal insufficiency, Falk and coworkers reported glomerular hypertrophy and focal segmental glomerulosclerosis (FSGS).[279] FSGS is thought to be the most common cause of renal failure in sickle cell disease.[280] In a study of 240 adult patients with sickle cell anemia and the nephrotic syndrome, Bakir and associates reported the presence of mesangial expansion and glomerular basement membrane duplication by electron microscopy, as well as effacement of epithelial cell foot processes.[281] These changes suggest hyperfiltration injury and often are referred to in these patients as sickle cell glomerulopathy. Membranoproliferative pathology was observed in some sickle cell anemia patients, most of whom had no immune deposits.[273,280]

Mechanisms

The underlying biologic defect in sickle cell disease is a single amino acid substitution of valine for glutamic acid at the sixth position in the hemoglobin β-chain. This alteration leads to the aggregation of deoxygenated sickle cell hemoglobin (HbSS) molecules, resulting in a deformation of the shape and decreased flexibility of red blood cells.[282] HbSS polymer formation is promoted by higher degrees of deoxygenation, increased intracellular hemoglobin concentration, and the absence of hemoglobin F.[282] As red blood cells from sickle cell patients flow through arterioles and capillaries, HbSS polymerization may occur, increasing the adherence of Hb-SS erythrocytes to the vascular endothelium. Gee and Platt have found that sickle reticulocytes adhere to the endothelium via vascular cell adhesion molecule-1 (VCAM-1).[283,284] Kumar and coworkers have reported that increased sickle erythrocyte adherence to the endothelium involves $\alpha_4\beta_1$-integrin receptors.[285] $\alpha_4\beta_1$-Integrins on the cell surface of red blood cells (RBCs) bind to fibronectin and vascular cell adhesion molecule-1 (VCAM-1) on endothelial cells. This is induced by the presence of inflammatory cytokines such as TNF-α.[274]

Platelet activation has also been suggested to play a role in sickle cell–mediated vasoocclusion.[286] Thrombospondin from activated platelets promotes sickle erythrocyte adherence to the microvascular endothelium.[286] Increased concentration of intracellular sickle hemoglobin may promote polymerization and trigger the sickling process.

The pathogenesis of medullary renal lesions in sickle cell disease is the result of microvascular occlusion by erythrocytes that carry the mutant hemoglobin β-chain. Erythrocytes passing through the vessels of the inner renal medulla and renal papillae are most vulnerable to sickling because of the high osmolality of the blood, which leads to cell shrinkage and increased hemoglobin concentration.

The pathogenesis of sickle cell glomerulopathy is generally attributed to hyperfiltration, which is common in children affected by the disease. Later in life, the GFR often declines, despite persistently high renal blood flow rates.[274] Guasch and associates have described a distinct pattern of glomerular dysfunction in patients with sickle cell anemia that consists of a generalized increase in permeability to dextrans secondary to an increased pore radius in the glomerular basement membrane.[287,288] With progression to chronic renal failure, the number of pores is reduced and a size-selective defect occurs.[287] This abnormality may account for the proteinuria observed in patients with sickle cell glomerulopathy. Schmitt and colleagues found that in early dysfunction, the ultrafiltration coefficient is increased.[289]

Hypoxia and decreased blood flow, with a secondary increase in ET-1 secretion, have been suggested in the pathogenesis of sickle nephropathy.[290,291] In addition, the roles of nitric oxide (NO) and the activation of NO synthase have been studied in the mechanism of glomerular hyperfiltration, and in ischemia-reperfusion–mediated apoptosis of cells.[292,293]

Therapy

The management of patients with sickle cell disease is targeted at limiting sickle cell crises and end-organ damage. Factors that trigger sickling, such as infection and dehydration, should be treated aggressively. Exposure to hypoxia, cold, or medications that may induce sickle cell crisis should be avoided. Treatment options include transfusion therapy and, more recently, BMT.[294] Interestingly, multiple transfusions may restore the urine-concentrating capacity in very young children with sickle cell anemia.[275]

A conservative approach for hematuria is suggested, considering its generally benign course. Maintaining high urinary flow through adequate fluid intake and the use of diuretics is helpful in clearing clots from the bladder. Alternative approaches targeting pathogenic mechanisms have been proposed. The use of hydroxyurea in patients with sickle cell anemia aims at increasing the formation of HbF instead of HbSS. Studies in adults and children have shown a reduction in the incidence of acute sickling episodes, and this allows normal growth and development in children.[274] In some reports, the use of ACEIs significantly reduced proteinuria, and combined therapy with ACEIs and hydroxyurea may prevent progression from microalbuminuria to frank proteinuria.[273-275,295]

Patients with sickle cell disease who reach ESRD have a 60% survival rate at 2 years after the administration of renal replacement therapy. Dialysis is the most common form of renal replacement therapy used. Kidney transplantation as a possible alternative to dialysis has been attempted, with reported success. One study demonstrated a 1-year survival rate adjusted for age in kidney transplant recipients that was similar between groups, with or without sickle cell disease.[296] However, graft loss increased significantly with the duration of follow-up in transplanted patients with sickle cell disease compared to patients without sickle cell disease. Scheinman analyzed U.S. Renal Data System (USRDS) data up to the year 2000.[297] A total of 237 transplant patients with sickle cell disease had a survival rate of 56%, whereas 1419 sickle cell disease patients on dialysis had a survival rate of 14%. As such, we believe that the best option for renal replacement therapy in patients with ESRD is kidney transplantation, although a greater frequency of posttransplantation crises has been described in correlation with anemia correction. Moreover, sickle cell nephropathy can recur in the graft, even within 3.5 years, although graft loss due to this cause is rare. Hydroxyurea has been suggested to prevent recurrence. There is no place for the use of nonsteroidal antiinflammatory drugs (NSAIDs) or steroids in the management or prevention of sickle cell nephropathy.[273] Because of the high rate of hyperimmune individuals among sickle cell disease patients, identification of novel immunosuppressive strategies able to control the anti-HLA humoral response will be instrumental in improving the prognosis of kidney transplant recipients with sickle cell disease.[298]

ANTIPHOSPHOLIPID SYNDROME

The antiphospholipid syndrome (APS) is an autoimmune disorder characterized by hypercoagulability, arterial and venous thromboses, and pregnancy morbidity.[299] The diagnosis rests on the detection of lupus anticoagulant (LA), anticardiolipin (aCL), or anti-β$_2$–glycoprotein I antibodies persisting in the circulation for a minimum of 12 weeks. The syndrome can be an isolated idiopathic entity or is found in subjects with other immune diseases, in particular systemic lupus erythematosus (SLE).[299] When APS is associated with SLE, morbidity and mortality are remarkably increased. Antiphospholipid antibodies can also be found in otherwise healthy subjects, with a prevalence of less than 1% in the general population and up to 5% of older subjects. In those with SLE, the prevalence is much higher, and IgG aCL, IgM aCL, and LA have been observed in 24%, 13%, and 15% of patients, respectively.[300] Notably, subjects with persistently moderate-to-high aCL levels and/or LA who had previous thrombotic events are at higher risk of future events.[301]

Clinical Features

The most common manifestations of APS include deep vein thrombosis, pulmonary embolism, stroke, myocardial infarction, and renal macrovascular and microvascular thrombosis. Livedo reticularis is a hallmark of the disease that almost invariably predicts a severe outcome. Hypertension is frequent.[302] It affects more than 90% of those with renal involvement and is often associated with vascular lesions, including arteriosclerosis, fibrous intimal hyperplasia, arterial and arteriolar fibrous and fibrocellular occlusions, and TMA.[303] Poorly controlled hypertension often reflects renal artery stenosis, a disease that may affect up to 26% of hypertensive patients with antiphospholipid antibodies as compared to only 8% of young patients attending a hypertension clinic and 3% of living related renal donors with stenosis.[304] The stenotic lesions are generally smooth noncritical stenoses in the midportion of the renal artery, quite distinct from fibromuscular dysplasia or atherosclerosis.

Thrombotic Microangiopathy. This is one of the more serious manifestations of the syndrome. It can be isolated or may be a component of catastrophic APS, a rare but devastating disease that manifests in approximately 1% of patients with AP antibodies, in most cases following a triggering event such as infection, trauma, or surgery. Hypertension and proteinuria are almost invariable findings often associated with renal impairment, even in the early phases of the disease. Proteinuria is mild, and the sudden onset of nephrotic-range proteinuria may reflect a concomitant thrombosis of the renal veins and inferior vena cava. Outcome is poor, in particular in the context of lupus nephritis and catastrophic APS.[305] In catastrophic APS, three or more target organs are involved, multiorgan failure is frequent, and the mortality rate approximates 50%.[306]

Pathology

Kidney biopsy samples from patients with APS-associated thrombotic microangiopathy show focal or diffuse microangiopathic changes affecting the whole intrarenal vascular tree and glomerular tufts, with fresh or old recanalizing thrombi.[307] Ultrastructure findings pathognomonic for APS nephropathy include a combination of glomerular basement membrane wrinkling and reduplication and redundant wrinkled segments of basement membrane, with straighter thin basement membrane sections adjacent to the endothelium.[307] Small arterioles can also be affected by a noninflammatory and frequently thrombotic vasculopathy. These changes, however, are less specific because they can be observed in a wide variety of conditions, including TTP, HUS, scleroderma renal crisis, malignant hypertension, preeclampsia, postpartum renal failure, cyclosporine or chemotherapy toxicity, and renal transplant rejection.[299,307]

Mechanisms

A two-hit hypothesis has been suggested to explain the clinical observation that thrombotic events occur only occasionally, in spite of the persistent presence of antiphospholipid antibodies.[308] According to this principle, the antibody (representing the first hit) induces a thrombophilic state, but clotting takes place only in the presence of another thrombophilic condition (the second hit).[309] Providing support for this mechanism, the administration of a small amount of lipopolysaccharide (LPS) was required for human β_2-glycoprotein I (β_2-GPI)–specific antiphospholipid antibody IgG to produce a thrombogenic effect in rat mesenteric microcirculation.[310] In line with this observation, it has been suggested that infectious processes might constitute the second hit because they frequently precede full-blown APS and might be the initiator of the catastrophic subtype.[311] This hypothesis fits well with the potential involvement of pattern recognition receptors (e.g., Toll-like receptors [TLRs]) in sensing microbes and triggering an inflammatory response. Because TLR2 and TLR4 have been reported to contribute to endothelial cell and monocyte activation by β_2-GPI–dependent antiphospholipid antibodies, one can speculate that the combination of the effect of infection plus the perturbation of TLR function mediated by the autoantibodies overcomes the threshold for triggering thrombosis.[312,313] Alternatively, infections or inflammation might increase expression of the antiphospholipid antibodies' target antigen or the expression of antigenic epitopes that are hidden in resting conditions.[314] Accordingly, preliminary data have shown that LPS can upregulate β_2-GPI expression in mice.[315]

Therapy

Risk factors for atherosclerosis and cardiovascular disease, including obesity, smoking, hypertension, diabetes, and hyperlipidemia, should be addressed with lifestyle measures and appropriate pharmacologic therapy. Oral contraceptives and estrogen replacement therapy are absolutely contraindicated, given their association with thromboembolic complications. Aspirin, heparin, warfarin, and immunosuppressive drugs are key elements of the pharmacologic therapy of APS. Effective anticoagulation may help prevent worsening of hypertension, stent re-occlusions, and progressive renal impairment and should be considered, even in the absence of previous thrombotic events.[316] Treatment with rituximab, an anti-CD20 monoclonal antibody, achieved persistent disappearance of AP antibodies from the circulation in isolated case reports.[317] However, whether this may translate into improvements in clinical outcomes remains to be addressed in adequately designed trials.[318] TMA is an indication for plasmapheresis with fresh-frozen plasma. In secondary forms of APS, treatment will also be aimed at the underlying renal disease. Thus, steroids and immunosuppressants, including cyclophosphamides, may be indicated for patients with SLE and renal involvement.[299]

Case reports have documented the use of the C5 inhibitor eculizumab to prevent APS-associated thrombotic microangiopathy that complicates renal transplantation and to treat patients with acute catastrophic antiphospholipid syndrome.[319,320] In vivo murine studies implicating the activation of the classical complement pathway in thrombosis associated with APS were the basis for the use of eculizumab in these case reports.[310,321] Activation of complement by antiphospholipid autoantibodies generates C5a, which binds and activates neutrophils, leading to tissue factor expression.[322] On the basis of murine studies, C3 and C5 have been proposed as possible therapeutic targets for treating obstetric APS.[323,324]

MACROVASCULAR DISEASES

Macrovascular diseases of the kidney include acute occlusion, aneurysms, and dissecting aneurysms of the renal artery and thrombosis of the renal artery. Stenosis of the renal artery is discussed in Chapter 47.

OCCLUSION OF THE RENAL ARTERY

THROMBOEMBOLISM OF THE RENAL ARTERY

Different conditions may predispose to artery thrombus formation, including atherosclerosis, renal artery aneurysm, fibrinoid dysplasia, and aortic dissection, as well as the presence of endothelial injury secondary to the use of substances such as cocaine.[325,326] Infectious and inflammatory states are also known to predispose to renal artery thrombosis, with cases reported in patients with polyarteritis nodosa, Takayasu's arteritis, and Behçet's disease.[327-329]

Although inherited hypercoagulable states are typically associated with venous rather than arterial thrombosis, acquired hypercoagulable states can lead to arterial thrombosis, including APS, factor V Leiden mutation, antithrombin, methylenetetrahydrofolate reductase (NAD(P)H) (MTHFR), hyperhomocysteinemia, and nephrotic syndrome.[330-335]

Clinical Features

The clinical presentation of renal artery thromboembolism is variable and depends on the extent of renal injury and overall clinical picture.[336] Although anuria is characteristic of bilateral renal artery and solitary kidney renal artery involvement, it has been reported in unilateral renal artery thromboembolism, probably because of reflex vasospasm of the contralateral kidney.[337] Patients usually present with unexplained abdominal pain, gross hematuria, abdominal or flank tenderness, fever, and hypertension.[338] There may be signs of involvement of other end-organs by thromboembolic or recent cardiac events, such as atrial fibrillation or myocardial infarction. Most patients have an elevated serum LDH level and hematuria, and leukocytosis is common.[339]

Doppler ultrasound with contrast agents may represent the first-line investigation, although it is operator dependent and is burdened by the possibility of false-negative results.[340,341] In case of high clinical suspicion (despite negative Doppler), a contrast-enhanced CT scan readily demonstrates the absence of enhancement in the affected renal tissue although there is concern about further damage to the kidney with the use of iodinated contrast material.[342] Contrast-enhanced three-dimensional magnetic resonance angiography (MRA) displays sharp images of the renal arteries and perfusion abnormalities.[343] Isotopic flow scans show absent or markedly reduced perfusion of the affected kidney.[340] Although angiography is considered the gold standard for diagnosis, its use is reserved for situations in which intervention is contemplated.

Mechanisms

The heart is the main source of peripheral thromboemboli, including those to the renal arteries.[338] Men and women with atrial fibrillation have a fourfold and almost sevenfold risk, respectively, of developing peripheral thromboemboli compared to those without atrial fibrillation, but only 2% of peripheral emboli secondary to atrial fibrillation target the kidney.[344] Myocardial infarction and heart failure may predispose to the formation of thromboemboli. Valvular heart disease, bacterial endocarditis, heart tumors, and dilated cardiomyopathy are other predisposing factors. The aorta can be a source of renal artery thromboemboli, especially following endovascular repair of aortic aneurysms.[345] The incidence of renal infarcts after such a procedure is about 9%.[345] Endovascular revascularization of renal artery stenosis may also be complicated by distal emboli.[346] However, the use of angioplasty and stenting with distal protection baskets may decrease the rate of complications.[336]

Therapy

The human kidney is believed to tolerate the absence of blood flow for 60 to 90 minutes.[347] The presence of adequate collateral circulation from lumbar, suprarenal, or ureteral vessels may allow the kidney a longer ischemia time.[348] The duration and extent of ischemia are major determinants of the prognosis of an ischemic kidney.[340]

Treatment options for an acutely occluded renal artery are surgical embolectomy, percutaneous interventional techniques, and intraarterial thrombolysis.[348] Despite the restoration of kidney function in up to 64% of patients with surgical intervention, the mortality rate ranges between 15% and 20%.[349] The outcome of surgical embolectomy has been reported to be worse regarding kidney function.[350] The use of intraarterial thrombolytic agents has been associated with a high rate of renal artery recanalization, but the success of the procedure does not always translate into recovery of renal function.[351] Patients who sustain a complete occlusion or receive delayed treatment have a generally worse prognosis. Nevertheless, there are several case reports that describe favorable outcomes with intraarterial thrombolysis, even in cases of prolonged ischemia (20 to 72 hours) and in renal transplantation patients.[340] Successful results have also been reported with the use of systemic thrombolysis. Percutaneous aspiration thrombolectomy and rheolytic thrombectomy have been performed, with some success.[349]

TRAUMATIC THROMBOSIS OF THE RENAL ARTERY

Renal artery thrombosis is an uncommon sequela of blunt abdominal trauma. Motor vehicle accidents are the main cause of this injury.[352] Renal vessels can be affected by stretch injury, contusion, or avulsion, all of which may lead to thrombosis.[352] The left renal artery is slightly more affected than the right, but bilateral injury may be present as well.[352] Patients with traumatic renal artery thrombosis are usually critically ill and have other associated injuries, usually abdominal. The prognosis is poor, with the mortality rate reaching 44%.[353]

Clinical Features

Patients present with a history of major trauma and have flank and abdominal pain, nausea, vomiting, and fever. They may develop severe hypertension. Patients with bilateral renal artery thrombosis or thrombosis of a solitary functioning kidney develop anuria.[340] Hematuria is present in the majority, but may be absent in about 25% of patients. Mild proteinuria is often present. Blood analyses show elevation of serum lactate dehydrogenase, creatinine phosphokinase, serum transaminase, and alkaline phosphatase levels.[340] CT is the preferred diagnostic modality in patients with suspected renal artery thrombosis. It has the advantage of speed, accuracy, and the ability to detect other associated injuries.[352] Patients with renal artery thrombosis usually have absent parenchymal enhancement in the affected kidney. There is also abrupt termination of the renal artery just beyond its origin.[342] There might be enhancement of the cortex due to perfusion from peripheral and collateral arteries; this is referred to as the rim sign on CT.[354] The gold standard for the diagnosis of renal artery injury is renal artery angiography, which shows intimal flaps with partial stenosis or complete occlusion.[352] Angiography has the advantage of detecting the location of the injury with high accuracy; however, angiography is not usually necessary for confirmation if the CT scan is diagnostic and is associated with an increased risk of contrast-induced nephropathy.[342] Ultrasonography is unreliable.[355]

Therapy

Ischemia time is a major determinant of the outcome of revascularization in patients with traumatic renal artery thrombosis; 80% of renal artery revascularizations performed within 12 hours are successful. The success rate decreases with time, reaching zero for revascularizations performed after more than 18 hours.[356] However, there are case reports of late successful revascularizations.[357] Other determinants of the outcome are the extent of renal injury, presence of collateral circulation, technical difficulties of the surgical procedure, and injury to other organs.[340]

A significant number of patients who have had successful surgical revascularization develop hypertension. Many of them eventually require nephrectomy.[358] The outcome of surgical revascularization in patients with unilateral traumatic renal artery thrombosis may be no better than observation and medical management.[340] Nevertheless, revascularization is indicated for patients with bilateral renal artery thrombosis and patients with a solitary kidney.[358] Late revascularization may be considered if the kidney size is normal on imaging studies and if preserved glomerular architecture is noted on renal biopsy.[359]

Several surgical procedures can be performed for the repair of a renal pedicle injury, including thrombectomy, resection of the injured arterial segment and replacement with a venous or graft bypass, and autotransplantation with ex vivo repair of the vascular lesions.[340] Endovascular stent placements for traumatic intimal tears have been described.[360] Nephrectomy is required at times to control renal hemorrhage.[340]

ANEURYSMS OF THE RENAL ARTERY

Large autopsy studies have suggested that the incidence of renal artery aneurysms (RAAs) is 0.01% in the general population, but in patients undergoing renal arteriography primarily for the evaluation of renovascular hypertension, RAAs are observed in 1%.[340] Many RAAs remain asymptomatic. However, the clinical concerns of RAAs are their potential to rupture, thrombose (causing distal embolization), or lead to renovascular hypertension. Intrarenal aneurysms may erode into adjacent veins to produce arteriovenous fistulae.[340]

Clinical Features

Renal artery aneurysms are classified as saccular, fusiform, dissecting, or intrarenal. They may be located anywhere along the vascular tree, but most of them are found at the bifurcation of the renal artery or in the first-order branch arteries.[361] Saccular aneurysms, the most common type, constitute 60% to 90%. They are diagnosed typically at about 50 years of age, but can be seen in those from 13 to 78 years of age. In approximately 20% of cases, RAAs are bilateral. Renal artery stenosis may be associated.

Renal artery aneurysms are frequently asymptomatic and are diagnosed as part of a workup for renovascular hypertension. Occasionally, patients may complain of flank pain, which should raise the concern of an expanding aneurysm, rupture and hemorrhage, thrombosis, thromboemboli with impending renal infarction, or dissection.[340] Rupture of an RAA, a potentially catastrophic event, may present with vascular collapse and hemorrhagic shock. Aneurysm size is a factor in the potential for rupture. The incidence of rupture of RAAs smaller than 2.0 cm in diameter is low. Large aneurysms, especially those larger than 4.0 cm in diameter, have a greater tendency to rupture and usually require surgical intervention.[250] Pregnant women constitute a disproportionate number of cases of RAA rupture. In a review of 43 cases of rupture, 18 (42%) occurred in pregnant women.[362] Most of these occurred during the last trimester of pregnancy, but rupture and hemorrhage also occurred earlier in pregnancy and during the postpartum period.[361] Pathogenic factors include increased renal blood flow, particularly during the last trimester, the effect of female hormones on the vasculature, and increased intraabdominal pressure.[340] Emergency nephrectomy is usually required in this setting to control the hemorrhage. Maternal mortality decreased to 6% and fetal mortality to 25% if the pregnancy reached the third trimester.[363] If rupture occurs before the third trimester, fetal mortality approaches 100%.

Rupture of an RAA manifests with flank pain, vascular collapse, and shock. Abdominal distention or a flank mass may be detected. Hematuria may be a helpful finding in some patients, but its absence does not exclude the diagnosis. Renal angiography and MRA will diagnose RAAs, and CT and radionuclide scanning may be useful screening techniques.

Mechanisms

Renal artery aneurysms are sometimes attributed to atherosclerosis, but marked atherosclerotic changes are found in only 16% of patients and may be secondary.[361] Fusiform aneurysms are often seen in medial fibromuscular dysplasia and usually arise distal to a focal stenotic segment, giving the appearance of a poststenotic dilation.[364] Occasionally, several small aneurysms in sequence give the string of beads appearance seen in fibromuscular dysplasia. Fusiform aneurysms are typically found in young hypertensive patients who undergo renal angiography for the evaluation of renovascular hypertension. As with fibromuscular dysplasia, fusiform aneurysms are more common in women. Renal artery aneurysms have been described in polyarteritis nodosa, Takayasu's arteritis, Behçet's disease, Ehlers-Danlos syndrome, and mycotic aneurysms.[329,365-367] Intraparenchymal renal aneurysms make up 10% to 15% of RAAs and are frequently multiple. They may be congenital, posttraumatic (e.g., after renal biopsy), or associated with polyarteritis nodosa.

Therapy

Various authors have attempted to provide criteria for elective surgical intervention for RAAs.[340] Most agree that an aneurysm larger than 4.0 cm in diameter should be resected, and one smaller than 2.0 cm in diameter can be safely followed with periodic imaging studies. There is uncertainty about the midsized aneurysms, those between 2.1 and 4.0 cm. It may be prudent to recommend repair of RAAs larger than 3.0 cm in diameter in patients with surgical risks if there is reasonable certainty that nephrectomy will not be required.[340] In addition to large size of the aneurysm, other factors are considered in the choice for elective surgical intervention, including the presence of lobulations, expansion over time, presence of signs and symptoms, women of childbearing age, localization in a solitary kidney with the potential for embolization or dissection, or secondary renovascular hypertension.[340]

Several surgical techniques for the treatment of RAAs have been described, but the most commonly used approach is in situ aneurysmectomy and revascularization. When carefully done, this surgery carries the least risk of damage to the kidney and ureter. However, even at experienced centers, almost 5% of patients eventually undergo an unplanned nephrectomy because of technical complications encountered during the attempted revascularization.[361]

DISSECTING ANEURYSMS OF THE RENAL ARTERY

Dissecting aneurysms of the renal artery are rare but severe disorders of the renal artery. Acute dissections may manifest in an explosive manner, with malignant hypertension, flank pain, and renal infarction. Chronic dissection usually manifests as renovascular hypertension.[364] Acute dissection can occur spontaneously and can be precipitated by strenuous physical activity or trauma.[368] Fibromuscular dysplasia and atherosclerosis are common predisposing factors that lead to intimal tears, medial necrosis of the artery wall, and dissection. Iatrogenic dissection due to angiographic procedures may occur from trauma induced by guidewires, catheters, or angioplasty balloons.[340] Dissections have also been found as incidental autopsy findings, apparently without clinical symptoms during life.[340] Renal artery dissections are about three times more common in men, and there is a predilection toward involvement of the right side. Approximately 20% to 30% are bilateral. Dissection is most common in 40- to 60-year-olds, although younger patients with fibromuscular dysplasia may be affected.

Patients with acute dissection may present with new-onset, accelerated, or worsening hypertension.[369] Flank pain is frequent, and headache may occur, perhaps as a result of hypertension. In some cases, especially with lesions that develop from an angiographic procedure, the patient may be asymptomatic except for worsening hypertension. Selective angiography is necessary for the diagnosis.[340] The clinical course is variable. Some patients have persistent, severe renovascular hypertension that may be resistant to medical therapy. These patients may benefit from revascularization or nephrectomy if they suffered renal infarction, and many show improvement or complete resolution of hypertension after these procedures.[369] Endovascular interventions have also been reported.[370] Appropriate therapy depends on the severity of the hypertension and its response to therapy. Edwards and colleagues have noted adequate responses to medical management in most patients.[368] Dissecting aneurysms can be managed with open surgery, endovascular repair, or a combination of both.[371]

THROMBOSIS OF THE RENAL VEIN

In adults, renal vein thrombosis (RVT) is usually associated with nephrotic syndrome but can also occur in a variety of other clinical settings, such as tumors, aneurysm, or abscesses resulting in direct compression or from hypovolemic or hypercoagulable states.[372] The overall incidence in nephrotic syndrome ranges from 5% to 62%, and is highest in patients affected with membranous nephropathy or membranoproliferative glomerulonephritis.[373,374]

Clinical Features

Rapidity of the venous occlusion and the development of a venous collateral circulation determine the clinical presentation and resultant renal function.

Acute Renal Vein Thrombosis. An acute presentation is usually seen in young patients with a short history of nephrotic syndrome. RVT manifests with acute flank pain, macroscopic hematuria, and loss of renal function and may mimic a renal colic or acute pyelonephritis.[372,375] The physician should have a high index of suspicion, especially in patients with predisposing risk factors for hypercoagulability. In these cases, imaging reveals an enlarged kidney and pyelocalyceal irregularities.[372]

Chronic Renal Vein Thrombosis. A chronic presentation is usually seen in older patients with the nephrotic syndrome who have little or no accompanying symptoms except for peripheral edema, increase in proteinuria, and gradual decline in renal function.[376] They also have a greater incidence of pulmonary emboli and other thromboembolic events.[372]

Diagnostic Procedures

Doppler ultrasonography can visualize the actual venous flow, increased blood velocity, and turbulence in a narrowed vein or complete cessation of flow if the lumen is totally occluded. Ultrasonography with Doppler color flow should be the initial noninvasive diagnostic study. However, sonography is highly operator dependent and has a low specificity (56%), despite a high sensitivity (85%) in experienced hands.[377]

A characteristic radiographic finding of RVT is notching of the ureter, which usually occurs when collateral veins in close relation to the ureters become tortuous as they dilate to form an alternative drainage route. Originally, the notching of the ureters was interpreted as representing mucosal edema; however, more detailed radiographic studies have shown indentation of the ureters by the collateral venous circulation. Notching of the ureter is a very infrequent finding in nephrotic patients with RVT and usually occurs only in a minority of patients with chronic rather than acute RVT.[378] Retrograde pyelography may demonstrate a rectangular, linear mucosal pattern, with irregular renal pelvic outlines.

Inferior venacavography with selective catheterization of the renal vein establishes the diagnosis of RVT. If the inferior vena cava is patent and free of filling defects, and if a good streaming of unopacified renal blood is demonstrated to wash out contrast from the vena cava, a diagnosis of RVT is unlikely. The Valsalva maneuver is useful during venacavography; when the intraabdominal pressure is increased, the transit of contrast agent and blood from the inferior vena cava is slowed, the proximal part of the main renal vein may be opacified, and the patency of the lumen or even the outline of the thrombus may be demonstrated.[340]

Often, the inferior venacavogram is not diagnostic, and selective catheterization of the renal vein must be performed. A normal renal venogram demonstrates the entire intralobular venous system to the level of the arcuate vein. In general, the use of epinephrine for better visualization of the smaller vessels is not necessary. However, in the presence of normal renal blood flow, all contrast material is washed out of the renal vein within 3 seconds or less, and occasionally only the main renal vein and major branches are visualized. In this situation, there may be uncertainty about thrombi in major or smaller branches. Then the use of intrarenal arterial epinephrine, by decreasing blood flow,

```
↑ Prothrombotic factors              ↓ Antithrombotic factors
• Increased fibrinogen                • Reduced antithrombin
  and factor VII levels                 III levels
• Increased platelet                  • Reduced protein C and
  adhesiveness                          S levels or activity

              → Renal vein thrombosis ←

Impaired thrombolytic activity        Concomitant factors
• Decreased plasminogen levels        • Blood volume depletion
• Elevated plasminogen activator        (Hypoalbuminemia,
  inhibitor-1                           diuretic therapy)
• Impaired plasminogen-fibrin         • Immobilization
  interaction due to albumin          • Slowed venous blood flow
  deficiency
• Anti-enolase antibodies in MN
  patients (possibly interfering
  with fibrinolysis)
```

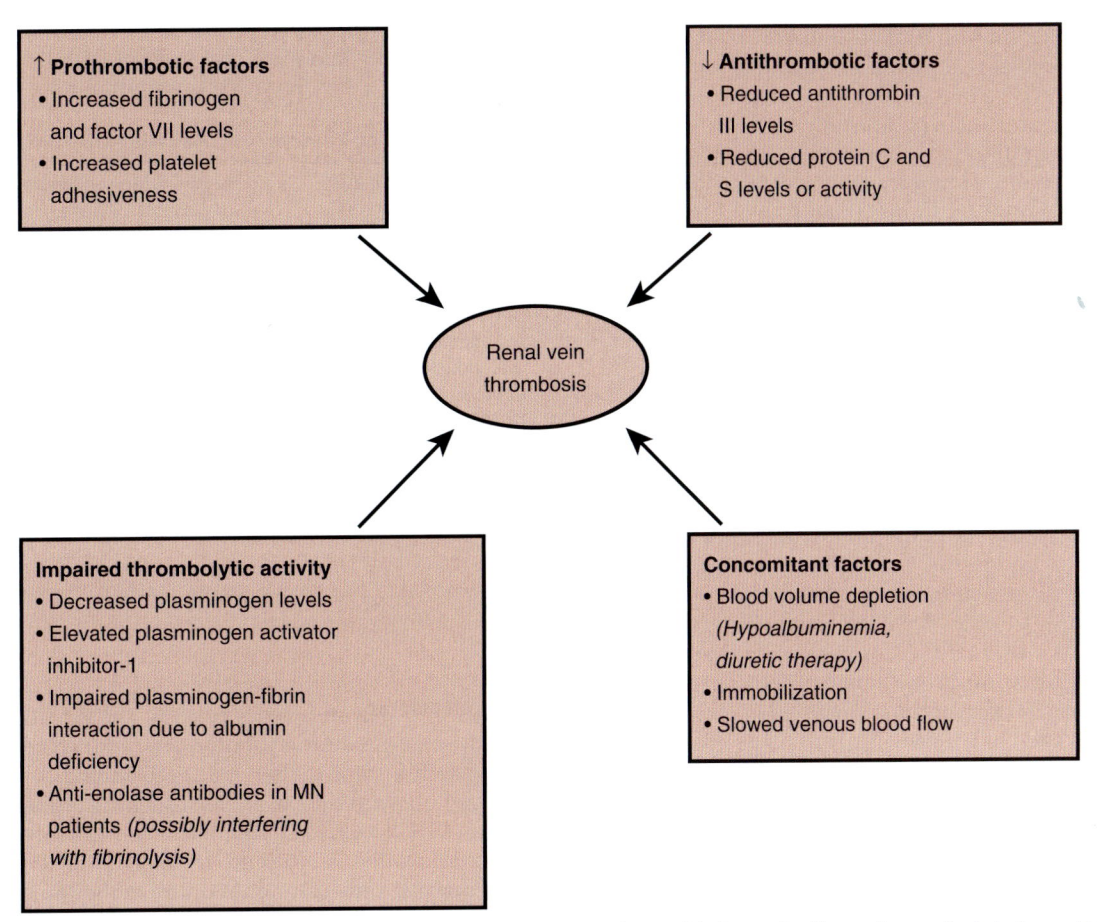

Figure 35.12 Pathogenic factors predisposing to renal vein thrombosis in patients with the nephrotic syndrome. An imbalanced bioavailability of prothrombotic and antithrombotic factors in favor of prothrombotic factors predisposes to intravascular clotting. Impaired thrombolysis and concomitant factors such as volume depletion, hypoalbuminemia, impaired venous blood flow, and immobilization may contribute to precipitate renal vein thrombosis.

enhances retrograde venous filling and allows later visualization of the smaller intrarenal veins. An abnormal renal venogram usually demonstrates a thrombus within the lumen as a filling defect surrounded by contrast material. In the presence of partial thrombosis, extensive collateral circulation can be demonstrated. The presence of such collaterals usually reflects the chronicity of the RVT and may explain the lack of renal functional deterioration.[340]

Both contrast-enhanced CT and MRI have been used for the diagnosis of RVT. Both are less invasive than venography; CT uses ionizing radiation and iodinated contrast agent, so MRI has significant advantages over CT.[377] Because MRI produces highly contrasting images of flowing blood, vascular walls, and surrounding tissues, vascular patency may be best determined by this technique. However, a low signal from the renal veins and pseudofilling defects due to slow flow, mimicking a thrombus, makes interpretation of the image difficult.[377] Gadolinium-enhanced MRI can overcome the limitation of poor signal from the renal vessels and, by performing a delayed second scan, the venous anatomy is well demonstrated, and an occult renal artery stenosis can also be disclosed.[377]

Mechanisms

Nephrotic Syndrome. Multiple hemostatic abnormalities have been described in patients with nephrotic syndrome that can increase the risk of RVT (Figure 35.12); these abnormalities vary in intensity in proportion to the degree of albuminuria and hypoalbuminemia.[379] The underlying mechanisms of the so-called thrombophilia of the nephrotic syndrome are essentially related to an imbalance of pro-thrombotic factors (e.g., increased fibrinogen levels, increased factor VIII levels, increased platelet adhesiveness) and antithrombotic factors (e.g., reduced antithrombin III levels, reduced protein C and S levels or activity) and impaired thrombolytic activity (e.g., decreased plasminogen levels, elevated plasminogen activator inhibitor-1 levels, or albumin deficiency–related impairment of the interaction of plasminogen and fibrin). An additional mechanism sustaining the procoagulant state is thrombocytosis, which has been found in a number of nephrotic adults and children. Moreover, platelets of nephrotic patients seem to display a tendency to hyperaggregability.[380] Hypoalbuminemia results in a higher availability of arachidonic acid for the synthesis of the proaggregant thromboxane A2 within platelets. Platelet activation may also be enhanced by high levels of cholesterol, fibrinogen, and vWF and by thrombin and immune complexes.[374] Volume depletion, diuretic and/or steroid therapy, venous stasis, immobilization, or immune complex activation of the clotting cascade may also participate in the thrombophilia of the nephrotic syndrome. It remains a mystery why only certain conditions have such a strong (but variable) association with RVT. The discovery of the association of antienolase autoantibodies with membranous nephropathy offers a tantalizing clue, because these autoantibodies could interfere with fibrinolysis.[381] The coexistence of another thrombophilic state with nephrotic syndrome, such as hereditary resistance to the activation of protein C (Leiden trait), could be another factor involved in the generation of thrombotic events in selected patients.[379,382]

Other Predisposing Factors. In addition to the hemostatic abnormalities associated with the nephrotic syndrome, other causative factors include amyloidosis, oral contraceptives, steroid administration, and genetic procoagulant defects.[375] Thrombosis can occur secondary to trauma (e.g., blunt, surgical), neoplasms (e.g., hypernephroma, Wilms' tumor), extrinsic compression (e.g., retroperitoneal tumors, pregnancy, lymphoma), arterial diagnostic puncture, placement of central catheters, and functional states of hypoperfusion, such as congestive heart failure.[376] Hypovolemia, a cause of RVT in neonates, has also been reported in adults. Morrissey and associates have reported a case of bilateral RVT in a previously healthy 22-year-old man that resulted in a moderate proteinuria without underlying glomerular pathology and with a normal coagulation profile.[376] The RVT was preceded by a 3-day history of nausea and vomiting as the only precipitating event. Treatment with fibrinolytics followed by heparin was successful.[376]

Renal vein thrombosis triggered by hypovolemia has also been suggested in other studies.[380] Steroids aggravate hypercoagulable states by increasing factor VIII and other serum protein levels and by decreasing fibrinolytic activity.[383] Historically, the advent of steroid therapy coincided with an increase in thromboembolic complications.[384] The use of oral contraceptives has been implicated as an additional cause of RVT and may unmask underlying hypercoagulable disorder.[375]

Acute RVT has been noted with increasing frequency in the transplanted kidney, which, unlike the native kidney, has a single drainage system.[385] In this setting, RVT may be accompanied by thrombosis of extrarenal sites.[335] RVT usually leads to permanent damage of the graft within hours. Predisposing factors are muromonab-CD3 (OKT3) and cyclosporine therapy.[385] Neonatal RVT accounts for 15% to 20% of systemic thromboembolic events in neonates and results in significant long-term morbidity.[386] Maternal and patient risk factors for RVT are presented in Table 35.5.

Therapy: Treatment of Overt Thrombotic or Embolic Events

Treatment of established renal vein thrombosis can be divided into measures targeting the specific cause of the occlusion (primary renal disease, tumors, systemic disease) and those aimed at the thrombus itself and/or its complications. The latter includes volume resuscitation, dialysis as necessary, but first and primarily anticoagulation. Current management of renal vein thrombosis has shifted from surgical to medical treatment.[387]

Anticoagulation and Thrombolysis. Anticoagulation is the mainstay of therapy, and is intended to prevent further propagation of the thrombus and thromboembolic complications while permitting recanalization of occluded vessels.[372,373] Thrombolytics provide the possibility of more rapid and complete resolution than anticoagulants but at the expense of a higher risk of bleeding.[372] The relative efficacy of anticoagulation versus fibrinolytics in the treatment of RVT is not well defined.[372] Thrombolytic therapy is likely warranted in patients with bilateral RVT, extension into inferior vena cava, pulmonary embolism, acute kidney injury (AKI), acute renal failure (ARF), or severe flank pain.[372]

Choice of systemic versus local administration depends on the evaluation of risk-benefit factors. Systemic administration is safe and effective if no obvious contraindications exist and avoids the need for invasive procedures.[388] Anticoagulation is indicated for nephrotic patients who experience a thromboembolic event. Heparin should be given, although its effect may be attenuated in the presence of low antithrombin III (ATIII) levels. ATIII deficiency in nephrotic patients rarely causes heparin resistance.[383] If ATIII levels are extremely low, fresh-frozen plasma or ATIII concentrates can be administered.[389]

Following heparin, oral vitamin K antagonists should be used. The optimal duration of warfarin therapy is unknown, but given the risk of recurrence, it is reasonable to maintain anticoagulation as long as the patient is nephrotic and has significant hypoalbuminemia. Treatment with heparin warrants monitoring of the anticoagulation response and is associated with some complications, such as thrombocytopenia and osteoporosis.[390] Low-molecular-weight heparin (LMWH) has been suggested as an alternative for the treatment of RVT.[390]

Prophylactic Anticoagulation of Asymptomatic Patients with Nephrotic Syndrome. No randomized controlled trials have been conducted to assess the risk-benefit profile of anticoagulation therapy in patients with nephrotic syndrome. However, a Markov-based decision analysis model has found that the number of fatal emboli prevented by prophylactic anticoagulation exceeds that of fatal bleeding in nephrotic patients with idiopathic membranous nephropathy.[391]

Table 35.5 Maternal and Patient Risk Factors for Renal Vein Thrombosis

Maternal Risk Factors	Patient Risk Factors
Fetal distress, 26%	Respiratory distress, 30%
Diabetes, traumatic birth, 17%	Cardiac disease, diarrhea/dehydration, hypotension, polycythemia, factor V Leiden heterozygosity, 13%
Steroids, preeclampsia, 13%	
Polyhydramnios, amphetamine, protein C deficiency, 4%	Femoral-umbilical catheter, protein C deficiency, twin-twin transfusion, 4%
No maternal risk factors, 35%	No patient risk factors, 26%

From Zigman A, Yazbeck S, Emil S, et al: Renal vein thrombosis: a 10-year review. J Pediatr Surg 35:1540-1542, 2000.

However, before formal evidence from a properly designed randomized trial is available, indications for anticoagulant therapy should be decided on an individual basis. Patients who have severe nephrotic syndrome, regardless of underlying cause, and a history of a thromboembolic event (DVT or pulmonary embolus) should be offered prophylactic anticoagulants if no contraindications exist. Patients with severe nephrotic syndrome (serum albumin level <2.0 to 2.5 g/dL) should also be considered candidates for prophylactic anticoagulation if they have other risk factors for thrombosis (e.g., congestive heart failure, prolonged immobilization, morbid obesity, abdominal, orthopedic, or gynecologic surgery). Patients with a family history of thrombophilia might also be considered for prophylactic therapy.

An alternative therapeutic approach is represented by low-dose aspirin, considering the increased platelet function in nephrotic patients.[392] A retrospective study to assess the influence of low-dose aspirin on the incidence of RVT in deceased and living related renal transplant recipients receiving cyclosporine-based triple immunosuppression has shown that although not abolished, the incidence of RVT decreases significantly with the addition of low-dose aspirin.[393]

ACKNOWLEDGMENTS

The authors are grateful to Marina Noris for her invaluable contribution to the paragraph on thrombotic microangiopathies and to Franco Marchetti and Mauro Abbate for their help in preparing the iconography of the manuscript.

Complete reference list available at ExpertConsult.com.

KEY REFERENCES

61. Noris M, Remuzzi G: Atypical hemolytic-uremic syndrome. *N Engl J Med* 361:1676–1687, 2009.
81. Caprioli J, Noris M, Brioschi S, et al: Genetics of HUS: the impact of MCP, CFH, and IF mutations on clinical presentation, response to treatment, and outcome. *Blood* 108:1267–1279, 2006.
86. Dragon-Durey MA, Loirat C, Cloarec S, et al: Anti-factor H autoantibodies associated with atypical hemolytic uremic syndrome. *J Am Soc Nephrol* 16:555–563, 2005.
96. Goicoechea de Jorge E, Harris CL, Esparza-Gordillo J, et al: Gain-of-function mutations in complement factor B are associated with atypical hemolytic uremic syndrome. *Proc Natl Acad Sci U S A* 104:240–245, 2007.
97. Delvaeye M, Noris M, DeVriese A, et al: Mutations in thrombomodulin in hemolytic-uremic syndrome. *N Engl J Med* 361:345–357, 2009.
98. Lemaire M, Fremeaux-Bacchi V, Schaefer F, et al: Recessive mutations in DGKE cause atypical hemolytic-uremic syndrome. *Nat Genet* 45:531–536, 2013.
100. Loirat C, Noris M, Fremeaux-Bacchi V: Complement and the atypical hemolytic uremic syndrome in children. *Pediatr Nephrol* 23:1957–1972, 2008.
104. Noris M, Remuzzi G: Thrombotic microangiopathy: what not to learn from a meta-analysis. *Nat Rev Nephrol* 5:186–188, 2009.
105. Michael M, Elliott EJ, Craig JC, et al: Interventions for hemolytic uremic syndrome and thrombotic thrombocytopenic purpura: a systematic review of randomized controlled trials. *Am J Kidney Dis* 53:259–272, 2009.
107. Licht C, Weyersberg A, Heinen S, et al: Successful plasma therapy for atypical hemolytic uremic syndrome caused by factor H deficiency owing to a novel mutation in the complement cofactor protein domain 15. *Am J Kidney Dis* 45:415–421, 2005.
108. Nathanson S, Fremeaux-Bacchi V, Deschenes G: Successful plasma therapy in hemolytic uremic syndrome with factor H deficiency. *Pediatr Nephrol* 16:554–556, 2001.
114. Bresin E, Daina E, Noris M, et al: Outcome of renal transplantation in patients with non-Shiga toxin-associated haemolytic uremic syndrome: prognostic significance of genetic background. *Clin J Am Soc Nephrol* 1:88–99, 2006.
123. Saland JM, Emre SH, Shneider BL, et al: Favorable long-term outcome after liver-kidney transplant for recurrent hemolytic uremic syndrome associated with a factor H mutation. *Am J Transplant* 6:1948–1952, 2006.
124. Schmidtko J, Peine S, El-Housseini Y, et al: Treatment of atypical hemolytic uremic syndrome and thrombotic microangiopathies: a focus on eculizumab. *Am J Kidney Dis* 61:289–299, 2013.
125. Legendre CM, Licht C, Muus P, et al: Terminal complement inhibitor eculizumab in atypical hemolytic-uremic syndrome. *N Engl J Med* 368:2169–2181, 2013.
133. Sadler JE: Von Willebrand factor, ADAMTS13, and thrombotic thrombocytopenic purpura. *Blood* 112:11–18, 2008.
134. Furlan M, Robles R, Galbusera M, et al: von Willebrand factor-cleaving protease in thrombotic thrombocytopenic purpura and the hemolytic-uremic syndrome. *N Engl J Med* 339:1578–1584, 1998.
135. Tsai HM, Lian EC: Antibodies to von Willebrand factor-cleaving protease in acute thrombotic thrombocytopenic purpura. *N Engl J Med* 339:1585–1594, 1998.
136. Levy GG, Nichols WC, Lian EC, et al: Mutations in a member of the ADAMTS gene family cause thrombotic thrombocytopenic purpura. *Nature* 413:488–494, 2001.
139. Ferrari S, Scheiflinger F, Rieger M, et al: Prognostic value of anti-ADAMTS 13 antibody features (Ig isotype, titer, and inhibitory effect) in a cohort of 35 adult French patients undergoing a first episode of thrombotic microangiopathy with undetectable ADAMTS 13 activity. *Blood* 109:2815–2822, 2007.
148. Zheng XL, Sadler JE: Pathogenesis of thrombotic microangiopathies. *Annu Rev Pathol* 3:249–277, 2008.
153. Scully M, Cohen H, Cavenagh J, et al: Remission in acute refractory and relapsing thrombotic thrombocytopenic purpura following rituximab is associated with a reduction in IgG antibodies to ADAMTS-13. *Br J Haematol* 136:451–461, 2007.
156. Bresin E, Gastoldi S, Daina E, et al: Rituximab as pre-emptive treatment in patients with thrombotic thrombocytopenic purpura and evidence of anti-ADAMTS13 autoantibodies. *Thromb Haemost* 101:233–238, 2009.
157. Galbusera M, Noris M, Remuzzi G: Inherited thrombotic thrombocytopenic purpura. *Haematologica* 94:166–170, 2009.
159. Remuzzi G, Galbusera M, Noris M, et al: von Willebrand factor cleaving protease (ADAMTS13) is deficient in recurrent and familial thrombotic thrombocytopenic purpura and hemolytic uremic syndrome. *Blood* 100:778–785, 2002.
164. Palla R, Lavoretano S, Lombardi R, et al: The first deletion mutation in the TSP1-6 repeat domain of ADAMTS13 in a family with inherited thrombotic thrombocytopenic purpura. *Haematologica* 94:289–293, 2009.
167. George JN: How I treat patients with thrombotic thrombocytopenic purpura: 2010. *Blood* 116:4060–4069, 2010.
171. Ireland R: Thrombotic microangiopathy: rituximab in severe autoimmune TTP. *Nat Rev Nephrol* 8:131, 2012.
173. Scolari F, Ravani P: Atheroembolic renal disease. *Lancet* 375:1650–1660, 2010.
194. Scolari F, Ravani P, Gaggi R, et al: The challenge of diagnosing atheroembolic renal disease: clinical features and prognostic factors. *Circulation* 116:298–304, 2007.
198. Duewell P, Kono H, Rayner KJ, et al: NLRP3 inflammasomes are required for atherogenesis and activated by cholesterol crystals. *Nature* 464:1357–1361, 2010.
228. Gabrielli A, Avvedimento EV, Krieg T: Scleroderma. *N Engl J Med* 360:1989–2003, 2009.
233. Hashimoto A, Endo H, Kondo H, et al: Clinical features of 405 Japanese patients with systemic sclerosis. *Mod Rheumatol* 22:272–279, 2012.
246. Penn H, Denton CP: Diagnosis, management and prevention of scleroderma renal disease. *Curr Opin Rheumatol* 20:692–696, 2008.
250. Fonseca C, Lindahl GE, Ponticos M, et al: A polymorphism in the CTGF promoter region associated with systemic sclerosis. *N Engl J Med* 357:1210–1220, 2007.
253. Allanore Y, Avouac J, Wipff J, et al: New therapeutic strategies in the management of systemic sclerosis. *Expert Opin Pharmacother* 8:607–615, 2007.

266. Zandman-Goddard G, Tweezer-Zaks N, Shoenfeld Y: New therapeutic strategies for systemic sclerosis—a critical analysis of the literature. *Clin Dev Immunol* 12:165–173, 2005.
271. Dhaun N, MacIntyre IM, Bellamy CO, et al: Endothelin receptor antagonism and renin inhibition as treatment options for scleroderma kidney. *Am J Kidney Dis* 54:726–731, 2009.
272. Penn H, Burns A, Black CM, et al: An open label trial of the endothelin receptor antagonist bosentan in scleroderma renal crisis (BIRD-1). *Arthritis Rheum* 60(Suppl 10):451, 2009 [abstract].
305. Erkan D, Lockshin MD: New approaches for managing antiphospholipid syndrome. *Nat Clin Pract Rheumatol* 5:160–170, 2009.
307. Fakhouri F, Noel LH, Zuber J, et al: The expanding spectrum of renal diseases associated with antiphospholipid syndrome. *Am J Kidney Dis* 41:1205–1211, 2003.
314. Agar C, van Os GM, Morgelin M, et al: Beta2-glycoprotein I can exist in 2 conformations: implications for our understanding of the antiphospholipid syndrome. *Blood* 116:1336–1343, 2010.
319. Lonze BE, Singer AL, Montgomery RA: Eculizumab and renal transplantation in a patient with CAPS. *N Engl J Med* 362:1744–1745, 2010.
324. Girardi G, Berman J, Redecha P, et al: Complement C5a receptors and neutrophils mediate fetal injury in the antiphospholipid syndrome. *J Clin Invest* 112:1644–1654, 2003.
361. Henke PK, Cardneau JD, Welling TH, 3rd, et al: Renal artery aneurysms: a 35-year clinical experience with 252 aneurysms in 168 patients. *Ann Surg* 234:454–462, 2001.
378. Llach F, Papper S, Massry SG: The clinical spectrum of renal vein thrombosis: acute and chronic. *Am J Med* 69:819–827, 1980.
379. Glassock RJ: Prophylactic anticoagulation in nephrotic syndrome: a clinical conundrum. *J Am Soc Nephrol* 18:2221–2225, 2007.
380. Robert A, Olmer M, Sampol J, et al: Clinical correlation between hypercoagulability and thrombo-embolic phenomena. *Kidney Int* 31:830–835, 1987.
382. Price DT, Ridker PM: Factor V Leiden mutation and the risks for thromboembolic disease: a clinical perspective. *Ann Intern Med* 127:895–903, 1997.
388. Hussein M, Mooij J, Khan H, et al: Renal vein thrombosis, diagnosis and treatment. *Nephrol Dial Transplant* 14:245–247, 1999.

Tubulointerstitial Diseases

36

Carolyn J. Kelly | Eric G. Neilson

CHAPTER OUTLINE

HISTORICAL VIEW, INCLUDING STRUCTURE-FUNCTION RELATIONSHIPS, 1209
MECHANISMS OF TUBULOINTERSTITIAL INJURY, 1210
Genetic Diseases, 1210
Glomerular-Related Events, 1210
Glomerular Filtered Growth Factors and Cytokines, 1212
Activation of Complement Components, 1213
Tubulointerstitial Antigens, 1214
Cellular Infiltrates, 1215
Interstitial Fibrosis, 1216
ACUTE INTERSTITIAL NEPHRITIS, 1218
Causes, 1218
Pathology, 1219
Clinical Features, 1219
Prognosis and Management, 1220
CHRONIC TUBULOINTERSTITIAL NEPHRITIS, 1221
Pathology, 1221
Clinical Features, 1221
Causes, 1221

Tubulointerstitial injury is always present when kidney disease progresses clinically. As a final common pathway, its presence correlates with impaired renal function and the presence of renal fibrosis on biopsy.[1,2] Tubulointerstitial disease may be the primary inciting event or secondary to glomerulonephritis or cystic renal diseases. The effects of common systemic conditions such as hypertension, diabetes, and atherosclerosis likely damage glomerular and interstitial compartments at the same time and, of course, the aging kidney gradually alters glomerular and interstitial tissues, making it even more sensitive to new injury in older individuals.[3,4]

HISTORICAL VIEW, INCLUDING STRUCTURE-FUNCTION RELATIONSHIPS

For much of the nineteenth century, the kidney was considered a tubulosecretory organ[5]; with Bowman's description of the malpighian bodies connecting to tubules,[6] the interstitial compartment was initially considered a separate anatomic region of the kidney.[7] In 1860, the finding of interstitial infiltrates at autopsy and the development of experimental models of interstitial injury[8] raised the possibility that the tubulointerstitium was not only relevant to renal physiology, but also a key feature of kidney disease. Based on previous observations of the presence of fibroblast-like cells in the renal interstitium,[9] Traube hypothesized in 1870 that interstitial changes documented in Bright's disease were responsible for kidney scarring and shrinkage associated with end-stage kidney failure.[10] Cellular and fluid exudation in the interstitial tissue was observed in the kidneys of patients dying with scarlet fever and diphtheria by Councilman in 1898.[11] In particular, the organs were sterile, thus raising the possibility of an allergic-type phenomenon. The entity was termed *acute tubulointerstitial nephritis*. This report, and insights from several models of tubulointerstitial injury developed across the century, provided the rationale to Volhard and Fahr[12] for the inclusion of interstitial nephritis in their 1914 classification of kidney diseases. Suggestions of an association between drugs and interstitial nephritis in humans emerged in the 1940s with the observation that antibiotics and analgesics could damage the interstitial compartment.[13] This opened the way to consider a variety of other drugs for risk of interstitial nephritis.

After the early evidence in 1913 that injection of heterologous proteins into rabbits led to lymphocyte infiltration in the renal interstitium,[14] attention to the immunologic basis of interstitial injury was only renewed in 1971 by Steblay and Rudofsky,[15] who described a model of tubulointerstitial nephritis induced by antibodies reactive with the tubular basement membrane (TBM) in guinea pigs. Since then, autoimmune tubulointerstitial disease has been seen in a number of species, including mice, rats, and rabbits following immunization with heterologous TBM.[16] Although all these models illustrate immune mechanisms that have been reported in humans with interstitial nephritis, none of them offered the intrinsic value of a spontaneously occurring renal lesion. In 1984, Neilson and coworkers[17] characterized a model of spontaneous interstitial nephritis in kdkd mice. Absent renal antibodies, they found that this inheritable model of interstitial nephritis, due to mutations in mitochondrial prenyltransferase,[18] involves the cellular and regulatory T cell limb of the immune system.

In almost all forms of progressive experimental and human chronic kidney disease, a prominent inflammatory infiltrate exists within the interstitial compartment. The extent of these infiltrates,[19] number of fibroblasts present,[20] and area of fibrosis all correlate[18] with progressive decline in renal function. The concept of tubulointerstitial damage mediating impaired renal function is not new.[13] Several studies have pointed out the prognostic significance of severe injury of the tubulointerstitium in lupus nephritis,[21] membranous nephropathy,[22] and IgA nephropathy.[23] About 50 years ago, Risdon and colleagues[22] first described an association between the degree of renal impairment and extent of tubulointerstitial damage in patients with glomerular disease. In 50 cases of persistent glomerulonephritis, the correlation between creatinine clearance, plasma creatinine concentration, ability of the kidney to concentrate the urine, and glomerular changes were less striking than those documented between the extent of tubular lesions and alterations in renal function. These findings suggested, in chronic glomerulonephritis, that interstitial damage across multiple tubules has much more effect on the glomerular filtration rate (GFR) than structural injury in the glomeruli. Bohle and coworkers also studied tubulointerstitial changes in a wide variety of glomerulopathies.[24] As urine osmolality decreased, the renal function dropped. Conversely, decreasing maximal urine osmolality correlated best with increasing interstitial volume, lowering the cross-sectional area of proximal tubular epithelium or epithelium from the thick segment of the loop of Henle. This was not a unique feature because other key interstitial changes documented by light microscopy, immunofluorescence, or histochemistry—which include the presence of immune inflammatory cells, activated fibroblasts, extracellular matrix (ECM) components, antibodies, and complement—also predict the long-term prognosis in chronic glomerulonephritis.[24,25]

Several mechanisms may explain how tubulointerstitial disease affects renal function. The simplest explanation is that tubular obstruction from interstitial inflammation and fibrosis impedes urine flow, increases intratubular pressure, and eventually lowers glomerular filtration.[24] Although no direct measurements are available, tubular atrophy and cell debris within tubules would represent a hurdle to draining fluid.[26] A second possible mechanism implicates reduction in the volume of peritubular capillaries[27] and, in this setting, the tubulointerstitial compartment becomes relatively avascular and ischemic. As a result of the increase in vascular resistance in the postglomerular region, the hydrostatic pressure in glomerular capillaries also increases, impairing glomerular arteriolar outflow. Perhaps more significant would be alterations in tubuloglomerular feedback as a third explanation. The presence of edema and inflammation in the renal interstitium, by increasing the interstitial pressure, may lower the sensitivity of the feedback mechanism,[28] possibly through local control of production of vasoactive substances such as angiotensin II (Ang II), nitric oxide, and prostaglandins.[29] When tubulointerstitial fibrosis develops, the autoregulation of renal blood flow is also disrupted permanently.[30] Fourth, glomerular-tubular disconnection, or finding atrophic tubules and glomeruli no longer connected to each other, is a well-recognized consequence of tubulointerstitial injury.[31] This is in harmony with evidence from human studies showing a positive correlation between the fractional volume of the interstitium, percentage of proximal tubuli without connection to a glomerulus, and decline of renal function in patients with chronic pyelonephritis.[32] Collectively, all these pathophysiologic processes are interrelated and may apply in some combinatorial fashion. It is difficult to make clean comparisons between experimental animals and humans because almost all that is known about this process in humans comes from detailed work in experimental models.

MECHANISMS OF TUBULOINTERSTITIAL INJURY

The mechanisms of tubulointerstitial injury share many components.[1,33] Typically, there are primary innate and adaptive immune injuries in the tubulointerstitium driving inflammation and, in the case of glomerulonephritis, there are secondary downstream effects from proteinuria leading to tubulointerstitial nephritis. Persistent inflammation always leads to destructive progression with fibrosis. Sometimes the inflammatory process is propelled by genotypic variations among hosts.

GENETIC DISEASES

A small number of genetic diseases producing interstitial nephritis have been identified in the last several years. Of particular note are the multiple genetic defects seen in ciliopathies associated with nephronophthisis,[34] karyomegaly associated with altered DNA repair,[35] prenyltransferase mutations,[18] mitochondrial cytopathies,[36] and mutations in uromodulin.[37] There are also new HLA associations with tubulointerstitial nephritis with uveitis (DQA1*01:04 and DRB1*14) or without (DQA1*04:01, DQB1*04:02, and DRB1*08).[38] Another recent study has identified different HLA associations (HLA-DRB1*01 and DQB1*05) with tubulointerstitial nephritis with uveitis, suggesting that current findings may be study population–dependent.[39]

GLOMERULAR-RELATED EVENTS

Glomerular diseases incite tubulointerstitial injury through multiple pathways, such as the following[40]: (1) impaired glomerular permselectivity allows the escape into the urinary space of substances that are morphogenic to tubuli[2,40]; (2) altered glomerular hemodynamics can damage nephrons by intraglomerular hypertension[41] and, alternatively, glomerular hypoperfusion may diminish postglomerular blood flow, provoking tubular ischemia; (3) immunologic mechanisms in glomeruli may incur the loss of tolerance and thereby instigate tubulointerstitial injury[42]; and (4) inflammatory mediators may seep from glomeruli into the urinary space or percolate into the interstitium through the juxtaglomerular apparatus.[43] In addition, leukocytes may migrate into the interstitium through the mesangial stalk and vascular pole of the glomerulus.[44] Nephron loss caused by the destruction of glomeruli and attached tubules may facilitate metabolic adaptations in surviving nephrons that induce tubulointerstitial injury through the renin angiotensin system.[2,45]

Two additional hypotheses to explain the interstitial damage associated with chronic glomerular disease have been proposed.[46] Based on histology studies of the development and progression in animal and human renal disease, these two new mechanisms are the notions of misdirected filtration and crescentic cell proliferation (Figure 36.1). According to the misdirection mechanism, there is an extension of a proteinaceous crescent into the outer aspect of the proximal tubule. As a consequence of persistent misdirected filtration, a proteinaceous filtrate near the glomerulotubular junction expands into the space between the tubular epithelial and TBM and may spread along the entire proximal convolution within this space. This process is predominantly associated with degenerative glomerular disease[47] but may also be contributory along individual nephrons in inflammatory disease.[48] A more direct approach to the tubulointerstitial compartment, however, may simply be passage through the juxtaglomerular apparatus.[43]

The other mechanism is the encroachment of a growing cellular crescent on the glomerulotubular junction, where the initial segment of the proximal tubule is incorporated into the crescent. This process is more characteristic of the inflammatory models.[48,49] However, cellular proliferation is complemented frequently in inflammatory models by misdirected filtrate spreading, leading to mixed crescents. In both cases, this results in the loss of nephrons and subsequent fibrosis, which some consider a reparative process important for the maintenance of renal structure rather than a determinant of further injury.[46] Although this hypothesis does not exclude a direct effect of proteins filtered into the tubular lumen, it underlines the fact that therapeutic intervention to prevent renal progression of disease should target these glomerular changes, as well as processes activating proximal tubular cells.

This loss of containment of injury within the confines of the glomerulus opens up inflammation to a very large tubulointerstitial compartment. Chronic injury and the accompanying fibrosis, driven by glomerular processes, provide a conduit for the easy transmission of more inflammation into areas previously uninvolved by original disease. Tubulointerstitial disease can thus bridge areas that separate injured and noninjured nephrons.

PROTEINURIA-INDUCED TUBULAR CELL ACTIVATION AND DAMAGE

One important mechanism of glomerular-tubulointerstitial interaction is through proteinuria. Although proteinuria has been considered historically as simply a surrogate marker of the severity of underlying glomerular damage, clinical and experimental data have indicated that proteinuria is an independent risk factor and plays an important role in the progression of renal disease.[50]

In 1932, Chanutin and Ferris[51] observed that removing 75% of the total renal mass in the rat led to a slowly progressive deterioration in the function of the remaining nephrons, with progressive azotemia and glomerulosclerosis. The glomerular lesions of the remnant kidneys were associated with abnormal glomerular permeability and proteinuria. At that time, proteinuria was considered solely as a marker of the extent of the glomerular damage, despite the fact that Volhard and Fahr in 1914[12] and von Mollendorrf and Stohr in 1924[52] had already found that renal damage might be pathogenically related to exuberant protein excretion in the urine. In 1954, Oliver and associates[53] recognized protein droplets in the cytoplasm of tubular cells, possibly the result of impaired reabsorption of plasma proteins normally carried out by renal tubules, and proposed that proteinuria could damage nephrons.

The mechanisms whereby increased urinary protein concentration leads to nephrotoxic injury are certainly multifactorial and involve numerous pathways of cellular damage. Obstruction of tubular lumens by casts and obliteration of the tubular neck by glomerular tuft adhesions may contribute to tubulointerstitial damage from proteinuria. Accumulating evidence, however, has emphasized the direct effects of filtered macromolecules on tubular cells.[54] Proteins escaping into the glomerular filtrate and reaching the tubular urine are largely reabsorbed in the proximal segments at the apical poles of tubular epithelium. This involves receptor-mediated endocytosis, followed by clustering of the ligand-receptor complex into clathrin-coated pits, giving rise to endocytic vesicles. On endocytic uptake, progress to the lysosome requires endosomal acidification to dissociate proteins from the receptors, permitting their degradation in lysosomes by the action of specific enzymes. The tandem endocytic receptors megalin and cubilin, which are abundantly expressed at the brush border of proximal tubular cells, interact to mediate the reabsorption of a large amount of proteins, including carrier proteins important for transport and cellular uptake of vitamins and lipids.[55]

Insights into specific mechanisms linking the excess traffic of plasma proteins and tubulointerstitial injury have come from in vitro studies using polarized proximal tubular cells to assess the effect of apical exposure to proteins. Protein overload activates proximal tubular cells into acquiring a proinflammatory phenotype,[56] perhaps through the

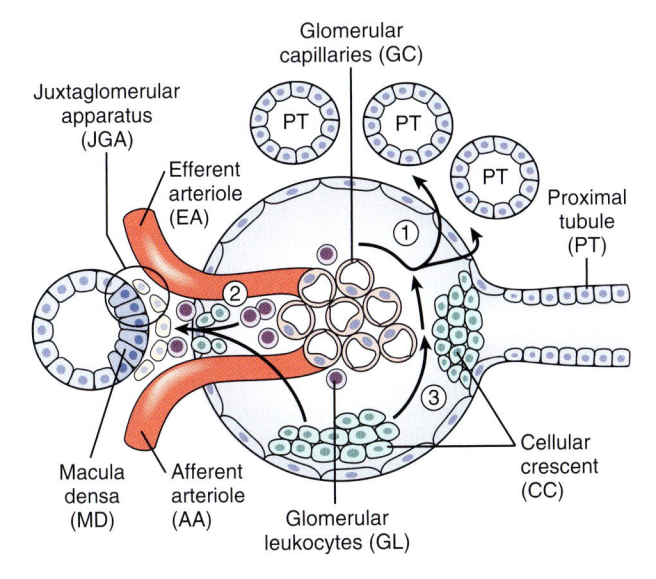

Figure 36.1 New mechanisms of interstitial damage in glomerular disease. **1.** Intraglomerular hypertension producing pressure disruption of Bowman's capsule or downstream along the tubular nephron, causing filtrate leak carrying inflammatory mediators to the tubulointerstitium. **2.** Escape of glomerular capillary leukocytes or expansion of cellular crescent causing inflammatory disruption of Bowman's capsule, including the macula densa. **3.** Proliferative migration of a cellular crescent that clogs the proximal tubule, causing misdirected filtration. There is misdirected filtration at the glomerular-tubular junction, producing filtrate leak behind the tubular epithelium and then into the interstitium. AA, Afferent arteriole; CC, cellular crescent; EA, efferent arteriole; GC, glomerular capillary; GL, glomerular leukocytes; JGA, juxtaglomerular apparatus; MD, macula densa; PT, proximal tubule.

lipocalin-2/24p3 receptor.[57] Indeed, upregulation of inflammatory and fibrogenic genes, and production of related proteins, have been reported on challenge of proximal tubular cells with plasma proteins. These include cytokines and chemokines such as monocyte chemoattractant protein-1 (MCP-1), RANTES (regulated on activation, normal T cell expressed and secreted), interleukin-8 (IL-8),[58-60] and fractalkine.[61] Moreover, the profibrogenic cytokine transforming growth factor-β (TGF-β) and its type II receptor,[62] as well as tissue inhibitors of metalloproteinase, TIMP-1 and TIMP-2, and membrane surface expression of the αvβ5 integrin,[63] are also highly increased in vitro by plasma proteins. These events are triggered by protein kinase C–dependent generation of reactive oxygen species,[64] nuclear translocation of nuclear factor-κB (NF-κB),[65] and the engagement of mitogen-activated protein kinase (MAPK/ERK).[61,66]

Extrapolation from such in vitro data to the in vivo situation in humans is difficult, considering the somewhat conflicting data observed with different proteins in different cell systems,[67,68] as well as the reported changes in the expression of several genes of still unknown function.[69] One of these concerns relates to the possibility that in vitro evidence of phenotypic changes induced in the proximal tubular cells by protein overload cannot adequately reflect the in vivo proteinuric conditions in animals and humans—in particular, the fact that concentrations of albumin used to challenge proximal tubular cells in culture (~10 mg/mL) have usually been much higher than one would expect in human disease.

The hypothesis of proteinuria-induced tubulointerstitial changes, however, is supported by attempts to interfere specifically with the cascade of events leading to renal damage, particularly by blocking the renin angiotensin system.[70-74] Angiotensin-converting enzyme (ACE) inhibitors given to animals with experimental chronic nephropathies have markedly reduced urinary protein excretion and, at the same time, attenuated interstitial inflammation and fibrosis. Further evidence has suggested that inhibition of the renin angiotensin system, in addition to reducing proteinuria, may also attenuate albumin-induced signaling in tubular cells.[75] Moreover, transfection with a monocyte chemotactic protein-1 antagonist or a truncated form of IκBα, thereby inhibiting NF-κB, inhibits albumin-overload induced tubulointerstitial injury.[1,65]

PROTEINURIA-INDUCED TUBULAR CELL APOPTOSIS

Apoptosis[76] and autophagy[77] are mechanisms that underlie protein-induced tubular cell injury. Protein overload causes a dose- and duration-dependent induction of apoptosis in cultured proximal tubular cells, as disclosed by evidence of internucleosomal DNA fragmentation, morphologic changes (e.g., cell shrinkage, nuclear condensation), and plasma membrane alterations.[67] Apoptosis in this setting is associated with the activation of the Fas-FADD-caspase 8 pathway.[76,77] Evidence of apoptotic responses to protein load is not confined to cultured tubular epithelial cells. Persistent proteinuria is associated with increased numbers of terminal deoxyuridine triphosphate (dUTP) nick end labeling positive apoptotic cells, both in the tubulointerstitial compartment and in the glomeruli in a rat model of albumin overload.[78] In tubuli, most of the positive cells belonged to those expressing Ang II type 2 receptors. Findings of reduced phosphorylation of MAPK/ERK and Bcl-2 reflect an AT_2 receptor–mediated mechanism underlying tubular cell apoptosis.[78]

Proximal tubular cell apoptosis, which may contribute to glomerular-tubular disconnection and atrophy,[31] was also found in response to proteinuria in passive Heymann nephritis.[79] Apoptotic cells were detected in proximal and distal tubular profiles in biopsy specimens of patients with primary focal segmental glomerulosclerosis.[80] In support of the pathophysiologic significance of such observation, a strong positive correlation was found between proteinuria and the incidence of tubular cell apoptosis, which was identified as a strong predictor of outcome in these patients.

GLOMERULAR FILTERED GROWTH FACTORS AND CYTOKINES

Plasma contains many growth factors and cytokines at considerable concentrations, usually in high-molecular-weight precursor forms or bound to specific binding proteins that regulate their biologic activity. They are present in nephrotic tubular fluid.[81] Insulin-like growth factor-1 (IGF-1) is present in serum at a concentration of 20 to 40 nM, which is more than 1000-fold of its biologic activity. Almost all the circulating IGF-1 is present in higher molecular weight complexes at about 50 and 150 kDa, normally preventing glomerular ultrafiltration. However, in experimental proteinuria, there is translocation of this growth factor into tubular fluid (primarily as the 50-kDa complex), as shown by micropuncture collection of early proximal tubular fluid.[82] Tubular fluid from nephrotic rats activates IGF-1 receptors in cultured tubular cells that are expressed in basolateral and apical membranes in some tubular segments.[82]

Hepatocyte growth factor (HGF) is largely of hepatic origin and is present in serum in an inactive monomeric form (97 kDa) and as heterodimeric HGF (80 to 92 kDa, depending on glycosylation). Its specific signaling receptor, the $p190^{mer}$ protein, is expressed in apical membranes in proximal tubuli in normal rats and at increased levels in diabetic animals. HGF is present in early proximal tubular fluid from rats with streptozotocin-induced diabetic nephropathy and is excreted with urine in diabetic animals.[83] Circumstantial evidence has suggested that HGF undergoes glomerular ultrafiltration in proteinuric states, probably as the mature bioactive form of the molecule.

TGF-β is a pluripotent cytokine (25 kDa) that is also present in serum at considerable levels and in high concentrations in platelets. In these reservoirs, almost all the peptide is maintained in inactive complexes by binding to latency-associated protein (LAP), which is further bound to latent TGF-β–binding protein (LTBP), forming a high-molecular-weight LAP-LTBP complex (220 kDa). TGF-β is also associated in serum with $α_2$-macroglobulin (900 kDa). The high-molecular-weight TGF-β complexes prevent glomerular ultrafiltration under physiologic conditions. However, in proteinuric glomerular diseases, TGF-β is present in early proximal tubular fluid, and at least a portion is bioactive. The remainder is likely activated during downstream tubular flow by the acidification of tubular fluid, perhaps by increasing urea concentrations and the presence of enzymes such as plasminogen activator inhibitor-1 (PAI)-1. The concentration of TGF-β in glomerular ultrafiltrate from rats with diabetic nephropathy is approximately 30 pM, which is one to two orders of magnitude greater than that required for biologic responses.[83]

TGF-β receptors are expressed in most tubular segments.[83,84] IGF-1, HGF, and TGF-β are also present in urine in patients with proteinuric diseases.[85,86] Urinary excretion of these proteins, however, does not prove glomerular ultrafiltration of IGF-1 and TGF-β because they are also expressed along tubular segments in some renal diseases; nevertheless, the presence of these cytokines in the urine of patients with proteinuric diseases is certainly compatible with their glomerular ultrafiltration. Ultrafiltered IGF-1, HGF, and TGF-β appear to act on tubular cells through their apical signaling receptors. There are several biochemical responses to these cytokines by tubular cells, which collectively resemble activation and moderate change in phenotype. This includes a moderate increase in the production of collagen types I and IV in response to IGF-1.[82] Incubation of proximal tubular cells with pooled early proximal tubular fluid, collected by micropuncture from rats with diabetic nephropathy, increases fibronectin expression.[83] TGF-β also increases the transcription of the genes encoding Col3A1 and Col1A, as well as fibronectin in proximal tubular cells. Thus, ultrafiltered growth factors induce moderately increased expression of matrix proteins by tubular cells that most likely contribute to interstitial fibrosis. HGF signals a mixed message by increasing the expression of fibronectin in tubular cells[83] blocking the expression of Col3A1,[83] which is consistent with an antifibrogenic role.

GLOMERULAR FILTERED LIPIDS

In addition to proteins themselves, fatty acids carried by filtered proteins can trigger tubulointerstitial injury. In rats with overload proteinuria, a potent chemotactic lipid was isolated from the urine, which attracted monocytes, but not neutrophils.[87] Similar results were observed in mice transgenic for human liver–type fatty acid–binding protein, which in human proximal tubular cells binds free fatty acids in the cytoplasm and carries them to mitochondria or peroxisomes for metabolism by β-oxidation.[88] These mice developed less macrophage infiltration and a tendency toward reduced tubulointerstitial damage, possibly suggesting that intracellular accumulation of free fatty acids modulates proliferative activity. Attempts have also been made to differentiate the effects of individual fatty acids (palmitate, stearate, oleate, and linoleate) on cellular toxicity and fibronectin production in cultured proximal tubular cells.[89] Oleate and linoleate were identified as the most profibrogenic and tubulotoxic fatty acids.

An additional pathogenic pathway has been linked to a form of low-density lipoprotein (LDL) modified by hypochlorous acid (HOCl) that accumulates in tubular epithelial cells in settings of injury.[90] Hypochlorous acid/hypochlorite is a major oxidant generated from hydrogen peroxide (H_2O_2) by myeloperoxidase during an oxidative burst. In the HK-2 proximal tubular cells, hypochlorite-modified LDL causes a rapid increase in the expression of several genes encoding for proteins engaged in the control of cellular proliferation and apoptosis (Gadd153), production of reactive oxygen species (hemeoxygenase 1, cytochrome $β_5$ reductase), tissue remodeling and inflammation (connective tissue growth factor, vascular cell adhesion molecule-1, IL-1β, matrix metalloproteinase-7, and vascular endothelial growth factor [VEGF]). Hypochlorite-modified LDL, but not naive LDL also has antiproliferative and proapoptotic effects in these cells. Comparable changes in gene expression were also found in renal biopsy samples microdissected from proteinuric patients with declining renal function. The presence of hypochlorite-modified LDL in damaged tubular cells was confirmed by immunohistochemistry.[90] These observations seem to mirror altered patterns of gene expression that occur selectively in response to oxidative LDL modifications and enhance inflammatory and fibrogenic processes in chronic proteinuric conditions.

ACTIVATION OF COMPLEMENT COMPONENTS

Among specific components of proteinuria, serum or tubular-derived complement factors can be harmful, especially on activation by the proximal tubules.[91] Renal tubular epithelial cells appear most susceptible to luminal attack by C5b-9 because of the relative lack of membrane-bound complement regulatory proteins, such as membrane cofactor protein (CD46), decay-accelerating factor, or CD55 and CD59 on the apical surface,[92] as opposed to other cell types, such as endothelium or circulating cells that are routinely exposed to complement.

C3 is an essential factor of the classic and alternative pathways of complement activation that lead to the formation of C5b-9 membrane attack complexes. Engagement of C3a receptors seems more important than C5a receptors in modulating tubulointerstitial injury.[93] Proximal tubular cells exposed to human serum in vitro activate complement by the alternative pathway, leading to fixation of the C5b-9 membrane attack complex neoantigen on their cell surface.[94] These events are followed by marked cytoskeletal alterations, with disruption of the network of actin stress fibers, formation of blebs, and cytolysis. Increased production of superoxide anion and H_2O_2 and synthesis of proinflammatory cytokines such as IL-6 and tumor necrosis factor-α (TNF-α) are also present.[95]

Within the kidney, complement proteins form deposits along the luminal side and are internalized by proximal tubular cells in rats with protein overload proteinuria,[96] renal mass ablation,[97] and aminonucleoside nephrosis,[98] a pattern commonly observed in kidneys of patients with nonselective proteinuria. C6-deficient rats with 5/6 nephrectomy show marked improvement in tubulointerstitial injury and function,[99] which suggests that treatments to reduce C5b-9 attack complexes on tubular cells may slow disease progression and facilitate functional recovery independently of initial incitement by glomerular injury.

Intracellular C3 staining is also evident in proximal tubules early after renal mass ablation in a stage closely preceding the appearance of inflammation. C3 co-localizes with immunoglobulin G (IgG) in the same tubules in adjacent sections. These accumulations in proximal tubular cells are followed by local recruitment of infiltrating mononuclear cells that concentrate almost exclusively in regions containing C3-positive proximal tubuli.[100]

The amidation of C3 by ammonia in the presence of high protein catabolism may also contribute to the luminal formation of C5b-9 complexes[101] and the generation of a monocyte-activating factor.[102] Treatment with an ACE inhibitor, although preventing proteinuria, limited both the tubular accumulation of C3 and IgG and interstitial inflammation at the same time.[97] These results suggest that the pivotal role of complement as a mediator of progressive tubulointerstitial damage requires an environment of protein-enriched ultrafiltrate, something that has been substantiated by showing that in the absence of proteinuria, C5b-9 does not exert significant pathogenic potential as a mediator of chronic tubulointerstitial disease.[103] In three distinct models of nonproteinuric tubulointerstitial disease in PVG rats, an increased deposition of C5b-9 at peritubular sites is associated with tubular and interstitial changes.[103] In each model, the severity of the disease is equivalent, regardless of whether the animals are from breeding pairs with normal complement activity or C6 deficiency. Finding that C6 deficiency does not alter the severity and progression of structural damage, despite the upregulation of C5b-9 on basolateral membranes of tubuli also suggests, in contrast to proteinuric states, that C5b-9 does not have a significant impact on the progression of chronic nonglomerular kidney disease. Renal parenchymal tissues express a limited repertoire of complement receptors, including CR1, CR3, and CD88, that directly bind complement proteins present in the ultrafiltrate. Whether the stimulation of complement receptors on tubular cells has functional consequences in progressive renal disease is unknown.

In addition to activating exogenous complement, proximal tubular epithelial cells synthesize a number of complement components, including C3, C4, factor B, and C5.[104] The exposure of cultured tubular epithelial cells to total serum proteins at the apical surface upregulates mRNA encoding C3 and protein biosynthesis.[105] The enhanced secretion of C3 is predominantly basolateral, providing in vitro evidence for locally synthesized complement in the process of tubulointerstitial damage. Serum fractionation experiments have identified the substance(s) responsible for such effects in the molecular size range of 30 to 100 kDa. This fraction contains proteins that pass through the glomerular barrier in proteinuric states, including transferrin. After incubation with apical transferrin, C3 mRNA is overexpressed, increasing apical and basolateral C3 secretion.[106] A similar degree of C3 upregulation is obtained when iron-poor transferrin or apotransferrin is used, indicating that the synthesis of C3 in proximal tubular cells is upregulated by transferrin, suggesting that protein, rather than the iron moiety, accounts for the observed effects.

These findings raise the potential roles of intrarenal C3 synthesis in progressive renal disease and the relative contribution of locally synthesized versus ultrafiltered complement components in promoting inflammation and fibrosis. C3-deficient mice significantly attenuate the interstitial accumulation of cells expressing the F4/80 marker of monocytes-macrophages and dendritic cells in response to protein overload with serum albumin. The latter causes significant upregulation of mRNA encoding C3 in whole kidney.[107] Finally, complement activation may directly regulate the renal immunologic response. Of great interest is the observation that local synthesis of C3 stimulates the transmigration of T cells across tubular epithelial cell barriers.[108] This pathway involves the direct action of tissue C3 with infiltrating T cells expressing C3 receptors and is a potential target for lymphocyte inhibitor agents such as mycophenolate mofetil, which is effective if combined with antiproteinuric therapy against primary nonimmune disease characterized by the tubular deposition of complement.[97,109]

TUBULOINTERSTITIAL ANTIGENS

When the immune system targets the interstitial compartment of the kidney as a primary process, the target antigens are derived from endogenous renal cells, tubular basement membrane, or other extracellular matrix components, or are exogenous antigens processed and presented by native renal cells or minor populations of professional antigen-presenting cells, such as dendritic cells, within the interstitium. Drugs may also become nephritogenic antigens by acting as haptens.

ANTIGENS FROM RENAL CELLS AND TUBULE BASEMENT MEMBRANE

The antigen that is the target of anti-TBM antibody-mediated interstitial nephritis (TIN) in humans has been identified.[110] Immunofluorescent staining using sera from patients with anti-TBM nephritis or monoclonal antibodies specific to TIN antigen revealed its localization in the basement membrane of the proximal and, to a lesser extent, distal tubules and Bowman's capsule in the kidney.[111] Glycoprotein isoforms of 54 to 58 and 40 to 50 kDa have been identified as the TIN antigen recognized by anti-TBM antibodies.[110,111] This glycoprotein has affinity for type IV collagen and laminin[112] and likely serves to stabilize the tubular basement membrane. The human TIN antigen has been mapped to chromosome 6p 11.2-12, and cDNAs encoding rabbit TIN antigen and its human homolog have been cloned and sequenced.[111,113] The antigen of anti-TBM disease in rodent models has been named 3M-1.[114] Polymorphic expression of TIN antigen has been observed in humans and in inbred rat strains. The absence of TIN antigen does not appear to impair renal function in rodents. A recent case report of a child with chronic renal failure and without detectable TIN antigen and a large genomic deletion in the corresponding location on chromosome 6 raises the possibility that its absence may lead to chronic renal failure.[115] The absence of TIN antigen may rarely result in anti-TBM disease following renal transplantation and is one reason for resistance to anti-TBM disease in some inbred rat strains.[116]

Tamm-Horsfall glycoprotein (uromodulin), along with antibodies directed at this large glycoprotein, are frequently seen within the interstitium in a variety of renal diseases, including chronic interstitial nephritis and reflux nephropathy.[117] Such immune deposits can also be seen in experimental models when animals are immunized with this protein.[118] Although there is insufficient evidence that abnormal Tamm-Horsfall protein (THP) deposits in the kidney have a critical role in the inflammatory process,[118] a role in the progression of chronic kidney disease (CKD) has been suggested from variant genotypes.[119] Recent data from experimental models, including the remnant kidney and unilateral ureteral obstruction, have implicated oxidized LDL as a neoantigen recognized by renal parenchymal T cells in these models.[120] Some presumably autoimmune forms of interstitial nephritis have concomitant inflammation in a separate organ. The tubulointerstitial nephritis and uveitis syndrome may result from an immune response to modified C-reactive protein.[121]

Drugs and/or drug-hapten complexes can also serve as nephritogenic antigens. These antigens, along with antibodies recognizing them, can form immune deposits in situ within the interstitium or precipitate as a circulating complex. Examples of this include members of the penicillin family, cephalosporins, and phenytoin. In some cases, antibodies directed against microorganisms may discover cross-reactive epitopes on interstitial components, as in the antibodies to nephritogenic streptococci, which cross-react with type IV collagen. Some anti-DNA antibodies also react with laminin and heparin sulfate, extracellular matrix components.

EXOGENOUS AND ENDOGENOUS ANTIGEN PRESENTATION BY TUBULAR CELLS

T cells recognize foreign antigens only when they are properly digested into small fragments and presented on the surface of antigen-presenting cells (APCs) bound to major histocompatibility antigen (MHC) molecules.[122] The recognition of this bimolecular complex on the surface of APCs leads to activation of T cells. $CD4^+$ T cells typically recognize antigens exogenous to an APC following the processing and presentation of that antigen in conjunction with class II MHC molecules. In contrast, $CD8^+$ T cells typically recognize antigens synthesized by the APC in conjunction with class I MHC molecules. Activation of T cells by APCs expressing processed antigen is also optimized by a number of cell-cell interactions involving cell surface costimulatory molecules and their ligands. In general, recognition of class II MHC molecules by $CD4^+$ T cells results in proliferation and cytokine expression by these cells, whereas in comparison, $CD8^+$ T cells cause target cell death on encountering antigen–class I complex-bearing cells.

Tubular epithelial cells activated by inflammatory circumstance have the capacity to release proinflammatory cytokines and $CD4^+ T_H1$ chemokines, but not T_H17 chemokines.[123] Renal tubular epithelial cells in culture also have the ability to process and present exogenous and self-proteins to T lymphocytes.[124-126] In addition to processing multiple potentially immunogenic peptides, proximal tubular cells could also be exposed to filtered low-molecular-weight proinflammatory cytokines such as interferon-γ (IFN-γ), IL-1, and TNF-α. Such cells are also exposed to cytokines secreted by immune cells infiltrating the interstitium. Ultimately, the ability of renal epithelial cells to present antigen or serve as a target for $CD8^+$ T cells will depend on the cytokine milieu and whether the net effect of those mediators is proinflammatory or antiinflammatory. Proinflammatory cytokines would typically augment the expression of class II MHC molecules on epithelial cells. Expression of class II is typically seen in less than 5% of tubular epithelial cells in normal kidney but is markedly augmented in interstitial nephritis, as is the expression of adhesion molecules such as intercellular adhesion molecule-1 (ICAM-1).[127]

In addition to requiring upregulation of class II molecules, renal tubule cells require the augmented expression of co-stimulatory molecules, which are required for full activation of T cells.[128] The interaction of the co-stimulatory molecular pair (a T cell receptor and an APC ligand) can result in activation or inhibition of the immune response. Many of the receptors on T cells are members of the Ig superfamily, including CD28, CTLA-4, ICOS, and PD-1. The ligands for these receptors are members of the B7 family. Proinflammatory cytokines can induce the expression of B7.1 and B7.2 on tubular epithelial cells.[129] Tubular epithelial cells can also be induced to express other accessory molecules, such as CD40, ICAM-1, VCAM-1, and ICOS-L, which are involved in T cell activation.[130,131] In the adriamycin nephropathy model of chronic proteinuric renal disease, treatment of mice with a monoclonal antibody directed to the CD40 ligand protects against renal structural and functional injury.[132] On the other hand, renal tubule cell expression of PD-L1, the receptor for PD-1 (programmed death 1), may have inhibitory effects on T cell proliferation and/or effector functions.[133,134] In renal biopsies from patients with IgA nephropathy, interstitial nephritis, or lupus nephritis, there is significant staining of tubules for B7-H1 (PD-L1),[135] suggesting that the expression of this co-stimulatory molecule is also upregulated in vivo. Thus, the number of receptor ligand pairs that potentially regulate the outcome of renal tubule cell interactions with T cells is large; the net effect of the interaction is difficult to predict without functional studies.

CELLULAR INFILTRATES

Cell-mediated immune responses were historically implicated in the pathogenesis of interstitial nephritis because of in vivo (delayed-type hypersensitivity) and in vitro (lymphoblast transformation) evidence of hypersensitivity to specific inciting antigens. Tubulointerstitial inflammation may result from antigen-specific stimulation, but may also occur in the absence of antigenic stimulation.[136] In the latter case, there is growing evidence for the role of innate immune sensors (TLR-2, TLR4, and MyD88 signaling) and the inflammasome complex in initiating tubulointerstitial injury.[137,138]

The interstitial infiltrate of most human chronic renal diseases consists of a number of different effector cells, including macrophages and $CD4^+$ and $CD8^+$ T cells. Most studies have reported that T cells predominate, and most of these are $CD4^+$ cells, although there is considerable variation between these analyses.[139] The predominant T cell population may also be altered by immunosuppressive therapy before biopsy or by the stage of disease at the time of biopsy. Corticosteroids can markedly deplete the number of lymphocytes seen in interstitial nephritis.

Studies in animal models have also described an important role for monocytes and macrophages in the initiation and progression of injury in chronic renal disease. Conditional in vivo expression of KIM-1, an epithelial phosphatidylserine receptor in renal tubular cells, induces interstitial fibrosis, apparently by triggering the renal expression of monocyte chemotactic protein-1 (MCP-1), which attracts interstitial monocytes.[140] Collecting duct epithelial cells express Kruppel-like factor 5, and the expression of this transcription factor is directly linked to the accumulation of discrete subsets of macrophages, thus affecting local inflammation and the balance between inflammation and fibrosis.[141] Notch3 receptors may also play a role in monocytic infiltration.[142] Direct damage to resident cells is caused through the generation by macrophages of radical oxygen species (ROS), nitric oxide (NO), complement factors, and proinflammatory cytokines.[136] Macrophages can also affect supporting matrix and vasculature through the expression of metalloproteinases and vasoactive peptides. Depletion of macrophages by treating animals with a monoclonal antibody directed against the CD11b/CD18 integrin, which is expressed by macrophages, depletes renal cortical macrophages by almost 50% in adriamycin nephropathy and reduces structural and functional injury if animals are treated prophylactically prior to adriamycin administration.[143] Macrophages may also have a beneficial role in interstitial injury. They may serve as markers of disease remission[144] or have an antifibrotic role, as documented in mice with unilateral ureteric obstruction reconstituted with bone marrow of Ang II type 1 receptor gene knockout or wild-type mice.[145] Clearly, interstitial macrophages in a number of interstitial injury models have phenotypic and functional heterogeneity.[146]

In most cases, B and T lymphocytes accompany macrophages to varying degrees. This is the case regardless of whether the form of injury is viewed as immune-mediated, leading to curiosity about the role of infiltrating lymphocytes or whether their presence implies antigen-specific recognition or effector function. In fact, the composition of the interstitial infiltrate is similar, whether the initiating cause of injury is chronic ischemia induced by unilateral renal artery stenosis,[147] autoimmune tubulointerstitial nephritis,[148] aminonucleoside nephrosis,[149] cyclosporine nephrotoxicity,[150] or protein overload proteinuria.[96] It is possible that immune responses to neoantigens expressed by interstitial cells damaged by ischemia or toxins are a final common pathway for such interstitial injury. This concept is supported by the known expression of neoantigens, such as vimentin, in animals with overload proteinuria.[96] Heat shock proteins, which can be induced in response to a number of cellular stresses, can also be recognized by T cells. Earlier studies have demonstrated that the heat shock protein HSP70 is expressed in renal tubules following chronic exposure of mice to cadmium chloride. T cells infiltrating the interstitial compartment were reactive to HSP70 and could induce interstitial nephritis in cadmium chloride–treated animals following adoptive transfer, suggesting a general mechanism whereby a toxic nephropathy might induce chronic injury through an antigen-specific immune response.[151] In remnant kidney models, an infiltration of the interstitium with macrophages and lymphocytes correlates with functional parameters of renal failure, and improvement in these parameters is obtained with immunosuppressive treatment[152]; this provides intriguing support for the importance of immune-mediated injury in the progressive interstitial disease seen in nonimmune forms of primary injury.

The histologic appearance of human interstitial disease can vary from granulomatous interstitial nephritis with an intense cellular infiltrate to sparse infiltrates with striking microcystic changes. Although this type of variable appearance may reflect different stages of an immune-mediated lesion or different target antigens, it may also reflect the biologic activity of discrete populations of activated T cells.[153] Some experimental interstitial lesions are histologically analogous to a cutaneous, delayed-type hypersensitivity reaction. This type of lesion is frequently seen in experimental anti-TBM disease, in which the interstitial compartment displays focal aggregates of mononuclear cells. In the murine form of this disease, this histologic appearance can be largely reproduced after adoptive transfer of a T cell clone that mediates delayed-type hypersensitivity to the target antigen and cytotoxic injury to renal tubule cells.[154] Although such interstitial injury can be induced by a single T cell clone, the resultant damage to interstitial and tubular cells is the end result of interactions among many cell types. The cytotoxic activity of renal antigen-reactive T cell clones may account for tubular cell destruction and resultant tubule atrophy. Cultured cytotoxic T cell clones that express pore-forming proteins such as perforin and serine esterase granzymes elicit interstitial nephritis following adoptive transfer, and maneuvers that decrease the expression of these mediators abrogate the ability of the T cells to mediate interstitial inflammatory lesions.[155-157] The nature of the variable genes used to assemble T cell antigen receptors expressed on cells in interstitial nephritis has been examined in human kidney tissue and in experimental models, with results varying from the use of multiple V regions to an oligoclonal usage in a case of drug-associated interstitial nephritis.[158,159]

There is functional diversity among CD4+ T cells, and it is clear that certain subpopulations suppress rather than initiate or augment immune responses. The most well-characterized example of an inhibitory subpopulation is CD4+CD25+, which plays an active role in downregulating pathogenic autoimmune responses.[160] More recent work suggested that Foxp3 expression, regardless of CD25 expression, identifies regulatory T cells.[161] CD4+CD25+ T cells suppress T cell proliferation in vitro but also have the capacity to suppress immune responses to autoantigens, alloantigens, tumor antigens, and infectious antigens in vivo.[162] The regulatory activity of these cells has been examined in the adriamycin nephropathy model, in which SCID mice reconstituted with CD4+CD25+ T cells had significantly reduced glomerulosclerosis, tubular injury, and interstitial expansion.[143] In the same model, adoptive transfer of Foxp3-transduced T cells led to decreased urine protein excretion, reduction in serum creatinine level, less tubular and glomerular damage, and diminution in the interstitial infiltrate.[163] It is likely that much of the earlier work with suppressor T cells conducted in rodent models of interstitial nephritis represented the activity of cells that are now defined by Foxp3 expression.[156,164-168]

INTERSTITIAL FIBROSIS

Fibrosis is the final common pathway leading to end-stage kidney disease (ESKD), irrespective of initiating events.[1] The process of tubulointerstitial fibrosis involves the loss of renal tubules and the accumulation of fibroblasts and matrix proteins, such as collagen (types I to V and VII), fibronectin, and laminin.[169] Sirius red staining to assess the degree of fibrosis quantitatively may be helpful.[23] Cells infiltrating the renal interstitium have long been thought to play a role in the initiation and progression of tubulointerstitial fibrosis[170] because the degree to which a number of cell types, macrophage, lymphocytes, and fibroblasts accumulate in the renal interstitium parallels the extent of fibrogenesis.[1] Moreover, it has been difficult to distinguish harmful cells from beneficial cells without functional analyses.[171] Recent advances in molecular technology, however, now enable cell types to be analyzed separately, and fibroblasts have been identified as the principal effector mediating tubulointerstitial fibrosis.[172]

EPITHELIAL-MESENCHYMAL TRANSITIONS IN FIBROSIS

Since the identification of fibroblast-specific protein-1 (FSP-1) as a marker of tissue fibroblasts,[173] they have been found to originate or multiply from a variety of sources, including local epithelial-mesenchymal transition (EMT), bone marrow, resident fibroblasts, or myofibroblasts.[174] We also know now that EMT is also a robust source of tissue fibroblasts.[175,176] Fibroblasts derived from EMT play a critical role in tubulointerstitial fibrosis.[177]

Epithelial and endothelial cells that line tubes and ducts have plasticity.[178,179] Midway through development, these cells can transition into fibroblasts by EMT as part of organ growth.[177] Of seven lineage tracing studies, all but two have confirmed these events in adult tissue.[1] Tubular epithelia[180] and endothelia[175] undergoing EMT during persistent injury in the kidney produce new renal fibroblasts, as well as resident and new fibroblasts that proliferate to expand numbers. Approximately 12% to 14% of kidney fibroblasts likely derive from EMT events that occur in bone marrow,[180] and fibroblasts from this niche circulate to peripheral tissue; more recent studies have suggested that this number may be higher.[181] Some have also suggested that pericytes are also a source of fibroblasts,[182] but they also would have to undergo a transition for this to occur. Recent comprehensive comparisons of the mechanisms of renal fibroblast formation using various fate mapping and ablative studies have indicated that new renal fibroblasts are derived through a combination of nonproliferative production in bone marrow (35%), followed by migration to the site of injury in the kidney, and from proliferating resident fibroblasts (50%), some of which form by endothelial-epithelial EMT (15%), with no contribution from vascular pericytes.[181] This latter finding concerning pericytes is consistent with recent observations that renal pericytes do not produce collagen type I.[183]

Kindlin-2 activation of ERK1/2 expression in tubular epithelium is a key mediator of tubular plasticity, interstitial inflammation and fibrosis.[184] The transcription factor inhibitor known as inhibitor of differentiation-1 (Id1) also potentiates NF-kB and Snail1 expression and EMT in tubular cells, leading to the accumulation of interstitial inflammatory cells. Absence of Id1 in vivo reduces interstitial inflammation and myofibroblast activation, and collagen deposition in mice.[185] Epithelial TGF-β is perhaps the strongest link to interstitial inflammation and fibrosis[1,186]; low levels of Klotho enhance TGF-β expression, which aggravates fibrogenesis.[187] Persistent cytokine activity during renal inflammation and disruption of the underlying basement membrane by local proteases initiates the process of EMT.[188]

Rather than falling into the tubular lumen to be washed away, some epithelial cells transition into fibroblasts while translocating back into the interstitial space, behind decondensating tubules through rents in the basement membrane.[189] Wnt proteins, integrin-linked kinases, IGF-1 and IGF-2, epidermal growth factor (EGF), fibroblast growth factor-2 (FGF-2), and TGF-β are among the archetypal modulators of EMT by outside-inside signaling.[177] For example, FGF-2 promotes the transition of tubular epithelia by inducing the release of matrix metalloproteinase 2 (MMP-2) and MMP-9, which eventually damages the underlying basement membranes.[189,190] FGF-2 also synergizes with TGF-β and EGF in mediating EMT by reducing cytokeratin expression and stimulating the movement of transitioning cells across damaged basement membranes.

Together, TGF-β and EGF provide the strongest stimulus for completion of epithelial transitions.[1] During EMT, FGF-2 activates its receptor FGFR-1 on the cell surface. These growth factors or their intermediates are imported into the nucleus, where they engage a variety of sequence-specific transcription factors (e.g., CBF-A, Snail, Smad3, Twist).[191,192] The net result is the emergence of the EMT proteome, which represses epithelial proteins.[188] Loss of E-cadherins and cytokeratins, rearrangement of actin stress fibers, and expression of FSP1, vimentin, interstitial collagens, and occasionally α-smooth muscle actin, mark the morphologic transition of epithelial cells into fibroblasts. EMT also operates in human tubular cells[193,194] and pathologic renal tissues.[20,195,196]

Of note, HGF and bone morphogenetic protein-7 (BMP-7) antagonize the epithelial transitions driven by FGF-2 and TGF-β.[197,198] At which stage antifibrotic modulators are most effective is not yet known. The transcriptional modulators for signaling in EMT or its reversal involve intracellular Smad/β-catenin activity.[1,192] EMT is also regulated by TRAP proteins,[199] accessory molecules that circulate in interstitial spaces as soluble moieties to block receptor activation by free ligand.[200] This control mechanism favors a state of differentiation in epithelia, which preserves organ structure and function. What is becoming increasingly clear is that mature epithelia are in a dynamic but not terminal state of differentiation.[179] Morphogenic forces that normally maintain epithelial phenotypes are pitted against countervailing forces trying to weaken that stability. Chronic inflammation into the interstitium destabilizes epithelial tissues by favoring fibrogenesis.

CHRONIC HYPOXIA IN FIBROSIS

One of the most important contributors to the development of tubulointerstitial fibrosis is chronic ischemia.[201-203] Production of Ang II and inhibition of production of nitric oxide underlie chronic vasoconstriction, which may contribute to tissue ischemia and hypoxia,[204] and hypoxia stimulates EMT.[201] In vitro, such hypoxia induces fibroblast proliferation and matrix production by tubular epithelial cells.[205] Histologic studies of animal models and human kidney have indicated that there is often a loss of peritubular capillaries in areas of tubulointerstitial fibrosis.[1,204] Downregulation of VEGF is implicated in the progressive rarefaction of peritubular capillaries.[206] Moreover, given that the size of the interstitial compartment determines the diffusion distance between peritubular capillaries and tubular cells, interstitial fibrosis likely makes tubular oxygen supply worse. This interstitial reduction of capillary blood flow, leading to starvation of tubules, may underlie tubular atrophy and loss. Under these conditions, the remaining tubules are subject to functional hypermetabolism, with increased oxygen consumption, which further promotes the hypoxic environment.

ACUTE INTERSTITIAL NEPHRITIS

Acute interstitial nephritis (AIN) is a pattern of primary renal injury usually associated with an abrupt deterioration in renal function and characterized histopathologically by inflammation and edema in the renal interstitium. The term was first used by Councilman[11] in 1898 to note the histopathologic changes in autopsy specimens of patients with diphtheria and scarlet fever. Although the term *acute interstitial nephritis* is more commonly used, acute tubulointerstitial nephritis more accurately describes the injury because lesions involve the tubules and interstitium. AIN is an important cause of acute renal failure, largely due to drug hypersensitivity reactions as a result of the increasing use of antibiotics and other medications that might induce an allergic response in the interstitium. AIN occurs in approximately 1% of renal biopsies during the evaluation of hematuria or proteinuria. In some studies of patients with acute renal failure, approximately 5% to 15% had AIN.[207] In recent decades, its prevalence has increased in those older than 65 years, perhaps because of their more frequent exposure to prescribed drugs.[208]

CAUSES

The most frequent cause of AIN is generally found in one of two categories: drugs and infections. Spontaneous autoimmune interstitial lesions occur but are uncommon (Table 36.1). Pharmaceutical exposures are reported most commonly, in up to 60% to 70% of cases.[209]

DRUGS

The list of drugs implicated in causing AIN continues to expand. Drugs are more frequently recognized as causative factors in AIN because of the increased use of renal biopsy and the characteristic clinical presentation. Although proton pump inhibitors[210] and a growing number of chemotherapeutic agents[211] used in cancer treatment are now recognized as causing tubulointerstitial injury, antibiotics still remain the major cause of drug-related renal toxicity; they produce acute renal failure and tubulointerstitial disease, depending on the drug. Tubulointerstitial disease is more commonly seen with β-lactam antibiotics (including cephalosporins), but other antibiotics (e.g., sulfonamides, rifampin,[212] vancomycin,[213] ciprofloxacin) are also involved. Clarithromycin[214] (the newer ketolide, a semisynthetic erythromycin A derivative) and telithromycin[215] are implicated in renal, biopsy-proven AIN. Approximately one third of cases of drug-related AIN are caused by antibiotics.[216]

Two complicating factors make the nephrotoxicity of antibiotics more common than other categories of drugs. First, many of these drugs are given in combination. Consequently, the toxicity of one agent may be aggravated by another, as exemplified by the co-administration of aminoglycosides and nonsteroidal anti-inflammatory drugs (NSAIDs). Second, many antimicrobials are removed from the body essentially, or at least predominantly, through a renal route. The serum levels of these drugs will therefore increase as renal function declines, either as a consequence of drug toxicity itself or because of concomitant renal damage caused by another drug or another cause of nephrotoxicity. β-Lactams produce interstitial nephritis because they behave like haptens, which may bind to serum or cellular proteins to be subsequently processed and presented by MHC molecules as hapten-modified peptides.[217] The most common form of haptenization for penicillin is the penicilloyl configuration, which arises from the opening of a strained β-lactam ring, yielding an additional carboxylic function that allows the molecule to bind covalently to the lateral and terminal amino terminus of proteins. Serum molecules thus facilitate haptenization. This reaction occurs with the prototype benzylpenicillin and almost all semisynthetic penicillins, but other derivatives (termed *minor determinants*) can be formed in small quantities and will stimulate variable immune responses. Because β-lactams share the same basic structure, they are all disposed to haptenization. Variation in the side chains and corresponding differences in the chemical nature of the haptens, however, explain why clinical consequences are variable from one class of β-lactams to another. Cross-reactivity between penicillins and cephalosporins is accordingly rare.

Approximately 1% to 5% of patients exposed to NSAIDs develop a variety of nephrotoxic syndromes.[218] Whereas this relatively low prevalence is apparently not alarming, the extensive use profile of analgesic, antiinflammatory, and

Table 36.1 Acute Interstitial Nephritis: Causative Factors

Cause	Specific Agent
Drugs	
Antibiotics	Cephalosporins, ciprofloxacin, ethambutol, isoniazid, macrolides, penicillins, rifampin, sulfonamides, tetracycline, vancomycin
NSAIDs	Almost all agents
Diuretics	Furosemide, thiazides, triamterene
Miscellaneous	Acyclovir, allopurinol, amlodipine, azathioprine, captopril, carbamazepine, clofibrate, cocaine, creatine, diltiazem, famotidine, indinavir, mesalazine, omeprazole, phenteramine, phenytoin, pranlukast, propylthiouracil, quinine, ranitidine
Infectious Agents	
Bacteria	*Corynebacterium diphtheriae*, *Escherichia coli*; *Legionella*, *Staphylococcus*, *Streptococcus*, *Yersinia*, *Brucella*, *Campylobacter* species
Viruses	Cytomegalovirus, Epstein-Barr virus, hantaviruses, hepatitis C, herpes simplex virus, HIV, mumps, polyoma virus
Others	*Leptospira*, *Mycobacterium*, *Mycoplasma*, *Chlamydia* species; rickettsia, syphilis, toxoplasmosis
Idiopathic	
Immune	Spontaneous tubulointerstitial nephritis

antipyretic agents suggests that an enormous number of individuals are at risk for kidney dysfunction. For example, approximately one in seven patients with rheumatologic disorders is likely to be given such a prescription, and approximately one in five (50 million) U.S. citizens have reported that they use an NSAID for other acute complaints.[219] Thus, it is possible to estimate that some type of renal abnormality is likely to develop among the 0.5 to 2.5 million U.S. individuals exposed to NSAIDs on a regular or intermittent basis anually.[218] The problem takes on an added dimension in that 20% of patients taking NSAIDs are predisposed to the development of renal toxicity because of volume contraction, low cardiac output, or other conditions compromising renal perfusion.

The combination of AIN with moderate or heavy proteinuria and minimal-change glomerulopathy is characteristically seen in fewer than 0.2/1000 subjects who take NSAIDs other than aspirin.[220] Preexisting renal impairment does not appear to be a factor. Advancing age is a risk factor, and this relationship may simply reflect the prevailing use of NSAIDs by older adults. Almost all NSAIDs have been reported to cause the nephrotic syndrome. The onset of proteinuria, combined with interstitial nephritis, manifests after several days or months of NSAID exposure (range, 0.5 to 18 months).[218] The AIN lesion may be the result of a toxic effect of NSAIDs on the immune system resulting from the blockade of cyclo-oxygenase (COX), causing arachidonic acid metabolism to favor the alternative lipoxygenase pathway, thus increasing the production of proinflammatory leukotrienes or epoxy and hydroxy eicosanoids.[220] However, the fact that some cases of NSAID-related interstitial disease are allergic has been suggested by the presence of tissue eosinophils or other manifestations of IgE-mediated hypersensitivity. The risk factors for this latter form of NSAID-induced nephropathy are unknown.

INFECTIONS

AIN is associated with primary renal infections such as acute bacterial pyelonephritis, renal tuberculosis, and fungal nephritis. *Streptococcus*,[221] leptospirosis,[222] cryptococcosis,[223] *Legionella*,[224] histoplasmosis,[225] and viruses such as cytomegalovirus,[222,226] hantavirus,[227,228] and Epstein-Barr virus[229,230] are classic risks for AIN. Systemic infections can cause direct injury because of pathologic processes in the kidney or can be associated with the medications used in the treatment of infection. HIV, for example, can underlie interstitial nephritis caused by opportunistic infections by using drugs such as indinavir or sulfonamide antibiotics, or perhaps the virus itself.[231,232]

PATHOLOGY

The hallmark of AIN is the infiltration of inflammatory cells with associated edema, usually sparing glomeruli and blood vessels.[207] The predominant pathology is interstitial, cortical more than medullary, and comprises edema and inflammatory infiltrates, which may be sparse, focal, or intense. The most numerous cells are lymphocytes, with CD4+ T cells rather more frequent than CD8+ T cells, B lymphocytes, plasma cells, natural killer cells, or macrophages.[233] Polymorphonuclear granulocytes, usually eosinophils, are often present early. The inflammatory reaction may be concentrated around and seen invading the tubular epithelium (so-called tubulitis). In more severe cases, tubulitis is associated with epithelial cell degeneration resembling patchy tubular necrosis, with some disruption of the TBM. Granulomas may occur in the interstitium, but vasculitis is uncommon. An increased matrix, followed by destructive fibrogenesis, may appear as early as the second week of acute inflammation.[233] Immunofluorescence microscopy or immunoperoxidase staining may show the following, with diminishing frequency: (1) no complement or immunoglobulin; (2) immune complexes, occasionally with complement along the TBM; or (3) linear IgG and complement on the TBM.[233] Thus, the pathology indicates a cell-mediated, delayed-type hypersensitivity reaction against tubular cells or nearby interstitial structures. However, dimethoxyphenyl-penicilloyl radicals may attach to TBM as hapten in β-lactam–associated nephritis,[217] and antibody to this combination is occasionally present. In AIN with minimal-change glomerulopathy induced by NSAIDs, the interstitial inflammatory exudate resembles that of acute allergic interstitial nephritis, except that cytotoxic T cells predominate, and eosinophils are uncommon.[234] There is no evidence of antibody-mediated injury in this latter form of interstitial nephritis.

CLINICAL FEATURES

The clinical presentation is comprised of local and systemic manifestations of acute inflammation of the kidneys. Patients with AIN typically present with nonspecific symptoms of declining renal function, including oliguria, malaise, anorexia, or nausea and vomiting, with an acute or subacute onset.[235] The clinical features range from an asymptomatic elevation in creatinine or blood urea nitrogen levels and an abnormal urinary sediment to generalized hypersensitivity syndrome, with fever, rash, eosinophilia, and oliguric renal failure. The classic triad of low-grade fever, skin rash, and arthralgias was primarily described with methicillin-induced AIN, but only about one third of the time. Pooled analyses of three large series have yielded a total of 128 patients with AIN.[216,236,237] These series spanned a period from 1968 to 2001 and consisted of 72 of 128 males (56.3%), with a mean age of 46.6 years. At presentation, rash was present in 14.8%, fever in 27.3%, and eosinophilia in 23.3%. The classic triad of fever, rash, and arthralgias was present in only 10% of patients for whom information was available. Nevertheless, this finding is in stark contrast to earlier series, in which allergic features were more robust.[216] This collection of signs and symptoms in the setting of drug reaction is known today as the DRESS syndrome (*d*rug *r*ash, *e*osinophilia, and *s*ystemic *s*ymptoms), which is associated with interstitial nephritis in up to 40% of patients with persistent exposure to selected drugs.[238] Blood pressure in AIN is usually not high, except with oliguric renal failure. Nonoliguric patients typically have a fractional excretion of sodium of more than 1 and usually have modest proteinuria (<1 g/day) but are not nephrotic unless injury is secondary to NSAIDs.

AIN should be considered in any patient with a rising serum creatinine level but little or no evidence of glomerular or arterial disease, no prerenal factors, and no dilation of the urinary collecting system on ultrasonography. The clinical history of exposure to a high-risk drug such as an

NSAID or susceptibility to ascending urinary infection, without a recent or coexisting condition causing shock or associated exposure to contrast media, will usually suggest the diagnosis. The most difficulty in arriving at the correct diagnosis is seen in patients exposed to a nephritogenic or nephrotoxic agent at about the same time as a major operation, serious infection, or other significant illness that may itself have caused acute tubular necrosis. The presence of features such as a hypersensitivity reaction, significant eosinophiluria in the case of β-lactam antibiotics, or moderate or heavy albuminuria after exposure to NSAIDs indicates a drug-related cause. Urine eosinophils are often sought to provide confirmatory evidence of AIN. Early studies[239] found that Hansel stain for eosinophils was more sensitive than Wright stain but did not conclusively demonstrate that urine eosinophils were diagnostically useful in confirming or excluding AIN. One study[240] found a positive predictive value of 38% and a negative predictive value of 74% among 51 patients for whom urine eosinophils were tested to help diagnose an acute renal disease; of these patients, 15 were suspected of having AIN, although biopsies were not performed in all patients. Other conditions such as cystitis, prostatitis, and pyelonephritis can also be associated with eosinophiluria. The finding of eosinophils in the urine supports the diagnosis of allergic interstitial nephritis, but the positive predictive value is low, even with more than 5% eosinophils in the urine, and the absence of eosinophiluria does not exclude the diagnosis of AIN.[241] Thus, the diagnostic value of urine eosinophils remains unclear.

Renal ultrasonography may demonstrate kidneys that are normal to enlarged in size with increased cortical echogenicity, but no ultrasonographic findings will reliably confirm or exclude AIN versus other causes of acute renal failure. Gallium-67 (^{67}Ga) scanning has been proposed as a useful test to diagnose AIN[242]; experimentally, uptake intensity can distinguish AIN from acute tubular necrosis.[243] In one small series, nine patients with AIN had positive ^{67}Ga scans, whereas six patients with acute tubular necrosis had negative scans. Nonrenal disorders such as iron overload or severe liver disease, can also result in a positive ^{67}Ga scan. Similarly, patients with biopsy-proven acute tubulointerstitial disease have had negative ^{67}Ga scans. Therefore, the predictive value of this test may hinge on the degree of uptake and may not supersede the value of a renal biopsy in making the correct diagnosis.

Renal biopsy is the gold standard for the diagnosis of AIN, with the typical histopathologic findings of lymphocytic infiltrates in the peritubular areas of the interstitium, usually with interstitial edema. Renal biopsy, however, is not needed in all patients for whom a probable precipitating drug can be easily withdrawn or who improve readily after withdrawal of a potentially offending drug. Patients who do not improve after withdrawal of likely precipitating medications, who have no contraindications to renal biopsy, and who are being considered for steroid therapy are good candidates for renal biopsy.

PROGNOSIS AND MANAGEMENT

The detailed treatment of acute interstitial nephritis has been reviewed elsewhere.[244] Most patients with AIN in whom offending medications are withdrawn early can expect to recover normal or near-normal renal function within a few weeks. Patients who discontinue offending medications within 2 weeks of the onset of AIN (measured by increased serum creatinine levels) are more likely to recover almost baseline renal function than those who remain on the precipitating medication for 3 weeks or longer. On the other hand, reviewing the three modern series of AIN, only 64.1% of patients made a full recovery (serum creatinine < 132 µmol/L), whereas 23.4% gained a partial recovery (serum creatinine > 132 µmol/L), and 12.5% remained on renal replacement therapy.[216] This relatively poor outcome may reflect a different case mix in recent series, with fewer patients having traditional allergic-type AIN. Clearly, it would be useful to have prognostic indicators for AIN, and it had been suggested previously that the long-term outcome is worse if renal failure lasts for longer than 3 weeks.[216] Two series have shown worse prognoses with increasing age, but there appears to be no correlation with peak creatinine concentration.[216] Attempts have also been made to gain prognostic information from the renal biopsy. Some authors have reported that patchy cellular infiltrates predict a better outcome than diffuse disease.[216] However, other studies have not supported a correlation between the degree of cellular infiltration or tubulitis and outcome.[245] The degree of interstitial fibrosis is correlated with outcome,[23,245] as has the number of interstitial fibroblasts.[20] These conflicting observations may be due to the patchy nature of the disease, random sampling on renal biopsy and, most importantly, too few patients under study.

Withdrawal of medications that are likely to cause AIN is the most significant step in the early management of suspected or biopsy-proven AIN.[235] If multiple potentially precipitating medications are being used by a patient, it is reasonable to substitute other medications for as many of these as possible and to withdraw the most likely causative agent among medications that cannot be substituted. Most patients with early AIN improve spontaneously after the withdrawal of medications. Other supportive care includes fluid and electrolyte management, maintenance of adequate extracellular volume, symptomatic relief for fever and systemic symptoms, and symptomatic relief for rash. Indications for dialysis in the management of acute renal failure include uncontrolled hyperkalemia, azotemia with mental status changes, and other symptomatic fluid or electrolyte derangements.

The role of steroids in the treatment in AIN is uncertain. Some have continued to question the use of or indications for steroid therapy. It is true that there are no robust randomized trials supporting its use.[216] However, small case reports and limited retrospective studies have demonstrated rapid diuresis, clinical improvement, and return of normal renal function within 72 hours after starting steroid treatment, although some case reports also indicated lack of efficacy, especially in NSAID-induced AIN.[246] In nonrandomized observational series, patients treated with steroids tended to do somewhat better.[247] The decision to use steroids should be guided by the clinical course following withdrawal of offending medications. A role for steroid therapy in tubulointerstitial nephritis with uveitis, the so-called TINU syndrome, is widely accepted, particularly in children (see later).[248] Clearly, steroids are not to be used in cases caused by infectious agents, in which proper therapy is directed at eliminating infection. If steroid therapy is started, a reasonable dosage is prednisone, 1 mg/kg/day orally for 2 or 3 weeks, followed by a gradually tapering dose over 3 to 4 weeks.[249] The merits of immunosuppressive agents, specifically cyclophosphamide or cyclosporine, are even less certain. They can be used as steroid-sparing agents, and consideration should be given to patients who fail to respond to a 2-week course of steroid therapy.[244] A 4-week course of cyclophosphamide (2 mg/kg body weight/day) while monitoring renal function and white blood cell count should suffice to determine response. Therapy for longer than 4 to 6 weeks is not indicated. Of interest is a case of granulomatous interstitial nephritis successfully treated with mycophenolate mofetil.[250] Plasmapheresis has been used in patients with circulating anti-TBM antibodies, similar to patients treated for anti–glomerular basement membrane (GBM) disease.

CHRONIC TUBULOINTERSTITIAL NEPHRITIS

PATHOLOGY

The pathologic features of chronic tubulointerstitial nephritis are largely conserved across a wide variety of presumed distinct causes. These features include atrophy of tubular cells with flattened epithelial cells and tubule dilation, interstitial fibrosis, and areas of mononuclear cell infiltration within the interstitial compartment and between tubules. Tubular basement membranes are frequently thickened. The cellular infiltrate in chronic interstitial disease is composed of lymphocytes, macrophages, and B cells, with only occasional neutrophils, plasma cells, and eosinophils. This infiltrate is typically less marked than in AIN. If immunofluorescent studies are performed on biopsy specimens, they might occasionally reveal immunoglobulin or C3 along the tubular basement membranes.

In chronic interstitial disease, the glomeruli may remain remarkably normal by light microscopy, even when marked functional impairment is present. As chronic interstitial injury progresses, glomerular abnormalities are more evident and consist of periglomerular fibrosis, segmental sclerosis and, ultimately, global sclerosis. Small arteries and arterioles show fibrointimal thickening of variable severity, but vasculitis is not a feature of chronic interstitial disease.

CLINICAL FEATURES

Unless a patient is found to have an abnormal urinalysis or elevated serum creatinine level from a screening test, patients with chronic interstitial disease present because of systemic symptoms of a primary disease or because of nonspecific symptoms of renal insufficiency. These nonspecific symptoms depend on the severity of the renal insufficiency but may include nocturia, lassitude, weakness, nausea, and sleep disturbances. In a series of patients with biopsy-documented chronic interstitial disease, the creatinine clearance at presentation was below 50 mL/min in 75% of cases and below 15 mL/min in about 33% of cases. Typical laboratory findings in these patients included non–nephrotic range proteinuria, microscopic hematuria and pyuria, glycosuria (25% of cases) and, surprisingly, positive urine cultures in 28% of patients.[251] Acidifying and concentrating defects are common. Some causes of chronic interstitial disease display characteristic patterns of tubular dysfunction (proximal or distal renal tubular acidosis) or marked early concentrating defects (primary medullary dysfunction). More typically, the pattern of tubular dysfunction is not highly restricted. Serum uric acid levels are usually lower than expected for the degree of renal failure, presumably because of tubular defects in the reabsorption of uric acid. Anemia occurs relatively early in the course of certain forms of chronic interstitial disease, presumably because of early destruction of erythropoietin-producing interstitial cells. Approximately 50% of patients presenting with chronic interstitial disease have hypertension.[251]

CAUSES

The pathologic and clinical scenarios outlined can occur in association with a number of diseases of presumably diverse causes. Distinguishing features of several of these are discussed individually here. For many of these entities, biopsies are infrequently performed, which limits clinicopathologic correlations. Table 36.2 provides a more exhaustive list of common and rare causes of chronic interstitial disease.

ANALGESICS

Long-term ingestion of large quantities of analgesics is associated in epidemiologic studies with chronic interstitial nephritis and papillary necrosis. The incidence of analgesic nephropathy varies among different countries and among different U.S. geographic areas. Before the removal of phenacetin from analgesic mixtures, it had been reported as a more common cause of chronic renal failure in Scotland, Belgium, and Australia, accounting for 10% to 20% of patients with ESKD in those countries.[251a] In the United States, case-control studies from the Philadelphia area did not detect an excess risk of renal disease in daily users of analgesic, whereas this was apparent in North Carolina. These two populations differed in the degree of regular analgesic use, consistent with previous suggestions that variations in the frequency of analgesic nephropathy track with patterns of analgesic use. In the 1990s, there was a clear decrease in the prevalence and incidence of analgesic nephropathy among patients undergoing dialysis in several European countries and Australia. Most authors associated this decrease with the removal of phenacetin from analgesic mixtures.[252]

The compound analgesic mixtures implicated in analgesic nephropathy contain aspirin or antipyrine in combination with phenacetin, acetaminophen (paracetamol), or salicylamide and caffeine or codeine in over-the-counter proprietary mixtures.[253] Generalities that have emerged from epidemiologic studies include the following. The development of analgesic nephropathy requires prolonged regular ingestion of combination analgesics (at least six tablets daily for >3 years). Most of the clinical features displayed by patients with analgesic nephropathy are consistent with the general features outlined previously. However, some distinctions are worth noting. This entity is recognized far more frequently in women than in men (five to seven times). The patients typically give a history of chronic

Table 36.2	Causes of Chronic Interstitial Nephritis
Cause	Examples
Drugs and toxins	Combination analgesics
	5-Aminosalicylic acid
	NSAIDs
	Chinese herbs
	Lithium
	Lead
	Cadmium
	Balkan endemic nephropathy
	Calcineurin inhibitors
Metabolic disorders	Abnormal uric acid metabolism
	Hypokalemia
	Hypercalcemia
	Hyperoxaluria
	Cystinosis
Immune-mediated	Sarcoidosis
	Behçet's syndrome
	Sjögren's syndrome
	Inflammatory bowel disease
	TINU
	IgG4-related systemic disease
	Allograft rejection
	Systemic lupus erythematosus
Infection	Bacterial pyelonephritis
	Hantavirus
	Leptospirosis
	Xanthogranulomatous pyelonephritis
Hematologic disorders	Sickle cell disease
	Light chain nephropathy
	Amyloidosis
	Myeloma
Obstructive	Tumors
	Stones
	Outlet obstruction
	Vesicoureteral reflux
Miscellaneous	Radiation nephritis
	Progressive glomerular disease
	Ischemia
	Hypertension

headaches, joint pain, and/or abdominal pain. Flank pain with or without associated hematuria may indicate a sloughed and potentially obstructing papilla. It is thought that the caffeine component of combination analgesics contributes to dependence on the drugs. Because these drugs are available over the counter, many patients may not come to the attention of health care professionals until CKD has reached an advanced stage. At that point, renal functional abnormalities attributable to chronic interstitial nephritis are nonspecific, including nocturia, sterile pyuria, and azotemia.[254] Anemia is common. Discontinuation of heavy analgesic use can slow or arrest progression of the renal disease.[255]

The late course of analgesic nephropathy may be complicated by urinary tract malignancy. The major presenting symptom of this complication is microscopic or gross hematuria. New-onset hematuria should be evaluated with urinary cytology and, if indicated, cystoscopy with retrograde pyelography.[256] It has been estimated that a urinary tract malignancy will develop in as many as 8% to 10% of patients with analgesic nephropathy, typically after 15 to 25 years of heavy analgesic use.[257] Some of these patients may not have been previously diagnosed with analgesic nephropathy.[258] Up to 50% of nephrectomy specimens from patients with analgesic nephropathy progressing to transplantation show evidence of atypical uroepithelial cells within the renal pelvis.[256] Some have proposed that these patients should have prophylactic nephrectomies of their native kidneys at the time of transplantation. The pathogenesis of these uroepithelial malignancies presumably relates to the concentration and accumulation of phenacetin metabolites with alkylating capabilities within the renal medulla and lower urinary tract.[258] Whether NSAIDs and acetaminophen are associated with these kidney tumors remains controversial.[255,259] A recent meta-analysis of epidemiologic studies has suggested that both classes of drugs are associated with a significant increase in the risk of developing kidney cancer, regardless of the presence of analgesic nephropathy.[260]

The likelihood that regular and sustained ingestion of single classes of nonnarcotic analgesics, as opposed to combination analgesics, can lead to chronic renal insufficiency has been the subject of a number of epidemiologic and case-control studies.[261-265] In a case-control study examining the relative risk of end-stage renal failure after regular analgesic intake, the authors found increased risks, varying from 2.6 to 4.8 for analgesic combination drugs, but no significant increased risk for single nonnarcotic analgesics.[266] This study did identify increased risks for combination analgesics lacking phenacetin. This has also been observed by others; that is, classic analgesic nephropathy can occur in the absence of phenacetin, which was withdrawn from analgesic mixtures in the United States, Australia, and Western Europe in the early 1980s.[267] However, in the past decade, the preponderance of epidemiologic studies has supported the conclusion that the classic form of analgesic nephropathy has greatly diminished, if not disappeared, following the removal of phenacetin from combination analgesics.[268-270] However, these studies have not directly addressed the issue of whether nonphenacetin analgesics could contribute to the progression of other forms of renal disease.

In the classic analgesic nephropathy secondary to dose- and time-dependent ingestion of combination analgesics containing phenacetin, most experimental work has supported a mechanism of injury dependent on several drug components and their metabolites (Figure 36.2). Phenacetin and its metabolites, including acetaminophen, can injure cells through lipid peroxidation.[271] These drugs and metabolites are present in highest concentration in the medulla and papillary tip, which is where the initial lesions of capillary sclerosis are seen.[272] In the presence of aspirin, there is competition for glutathione within the cortex and papillae of the kidney. If cellular glutathione is depleted, there is the possibility of potentiation of the renal toxicity of phenacetin, acetaminophen, and their reactive metabolites.[272,273] In addition, because aspirin and other NSAIDs can suppress the production of vasodilatory prostaglandins, renal blood flow to the medulla may be compromised, adding a hemodynamic contribution to injury.

Given the high prevalence of analgesic nephropathy in Western Europe during the 1980s, attempts have been made to develop diagnostic criteria for the entity. Findings on noncontrast computer tomography (CT) scans of small

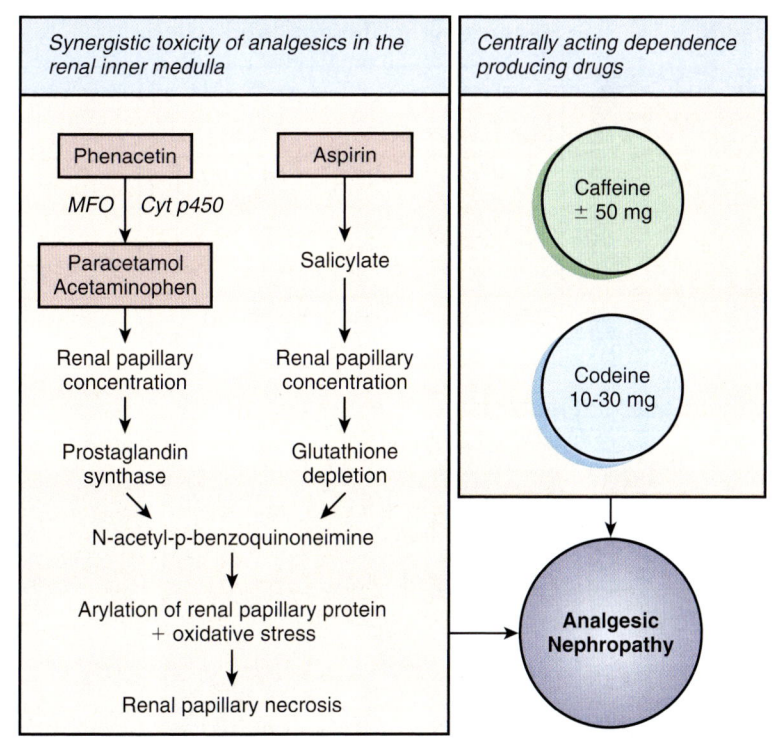

Figure 36.2 Synergistic toxicity of analgesics in the inner medulla and centrally acting dependence-producing drugs lead to analgesic nephropathy. Acetaminophen undergoes oxidative metabolism by prostaglandin H synthase to a reactive quinone imine that is conjugated to glutathione. If acetaminophen is present alone, sufficient glutathione is generated in the papillae to detoxify the reactive intermediate. If the acetaminophen is ingested with aspirin, the aspirin is converted to salicylate, and salicylate becomes highly concentrated in the cortex and papillae of the kidney. Salicylate depletes stores of glutathione. With the cellular glutathione depleted, the reactive metabolite of acetaminophen then produces lipid peroxidases and arylation of tissue proteins, ultimately resulting in necrosis of the papillae. MFO, mixed function oxidases. (Redrawn from Kincaid-Smith P, Nanra RS: Lithium-induced and analgesic-induced renal diseases. In Schrier RW, Gottschalk CW [editors]: *Diseases of the kidney,* ed 5, Boston, 1993, Little Brown, pp 1099-1129; and Duggin GG: Combination analgesic-induced kidney disease: the Australian experience, *Am J Kidney Dis* 28[Suppl 1]:S39-S47, 1996.)

kidneys, with bumpy renal contours and papillary calcifications, were found to diagnose analgesic nephropathy with greater sensitivity and specificity than clinical signs and symptoms (Figure 36.3).[274,275] One study has found that these CT findings are infrequent in the ESKD population in the United States and do not occur frequently enough among those patients with heavy and sustained analgesic use to make it a sensitive tool to detect analgesic nephropathy.[276]

CHINESE HERBS—ARISTOLOCHIC ACID NEPHROPATHY

In the early 1990s, there first appeared published reports from Belgium of patients, frequently women, presenting with an unusually rapidly progressive form of renal failure. Renal biopsies from these patients revealed findings consistent with those of chronic interstitial nephritis.[277] Initial reports noted that affected patients shared a history of chronic ingestion of the same preparation of Chinese slimming herbs as part of a weight loss regimen.[278] The number of case reports grew throughout the 1990s to over 120 cases by early 2000. With growing numbers of case reports came the recognition that the spectrum and severity of the disease were heterogeneous and more common but not consistently as severe as the initial reports had suggested.[279-282] Clinical subtypes have been defined, including acute kidney injury, tubular dysfunction with normal serum creatinine levels, and chronic interstitial nephropathy.[283] Growing evidence from clinical investigation and animal models has suggested that this lesion is attributable, at least in part, to the presence of aristolochic acid in the slimming herb preparations.[284,285] More recent studies have focused on the significant contribution of the cumulative ingestion of herbal medications containing aristolochic acid to the epidemiology of CKD and ESKD in Taiwan and mainland China.[286,287] Aristolochic acid now appears to be the common factor underlying the development of the nephropathy associated with Chinese herbs and Balkan nephropathy.[288]

The diagnosis of chronic TIN secondary to aristolochic acid ingestion relies on an accurate history. Typically, these patients present clinically because of mild-to-moderate renal insufficiency. As in many case of chronic interstitial nephritis, hypertension is not a prominent finding. Anemia is typically more pronounced at the same level of GFR than with glomerular diseases. The urine sediment is typically bland, although evidence of tubular dysfunction may be present on chemical analysis, including low-grade, nonnephrotic proteinuria (including albumin and low-molecular-weight filtered proteins) and occasionally glycosuria.[289] CT scans of the retroperitoneum may reveal bilaterally small kidneys with irregular contours in the setting of advanced azotemia. The clinical course is variable. Some patients demonstrate a rapid progression over weeks to months to renal failure, whereas others demonstrate slowly progressive

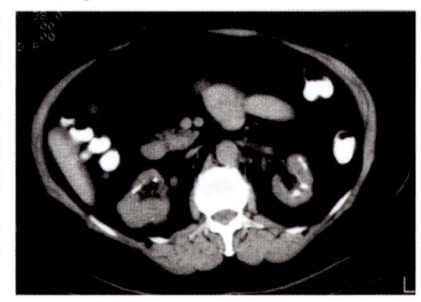

Figure 36.3 Renal imaging criteria of analgesic nephropathy (AN) as observed in a postmortem kidney and in computed tomography (CT) scans without contrast material. These criteria include a decreased renal size, bumpy contours, and papillary calcifications. RA, Renal artery; RV, renal vein; SP, spine. (Adapted from De Broe ME, Elseviers MM: Analgesic nephropathy. *N Engl J Med* 338:446-452, 1998.)

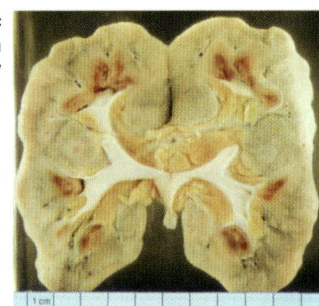

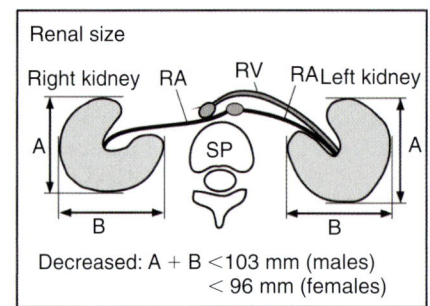

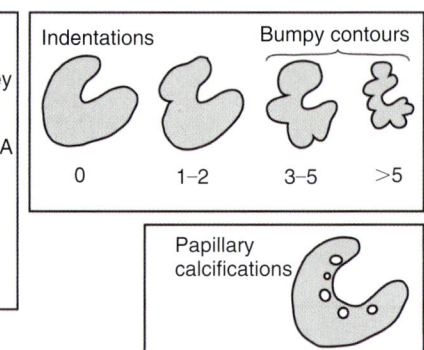

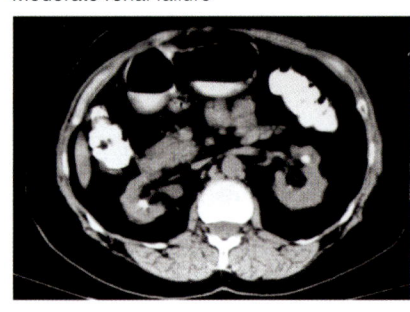

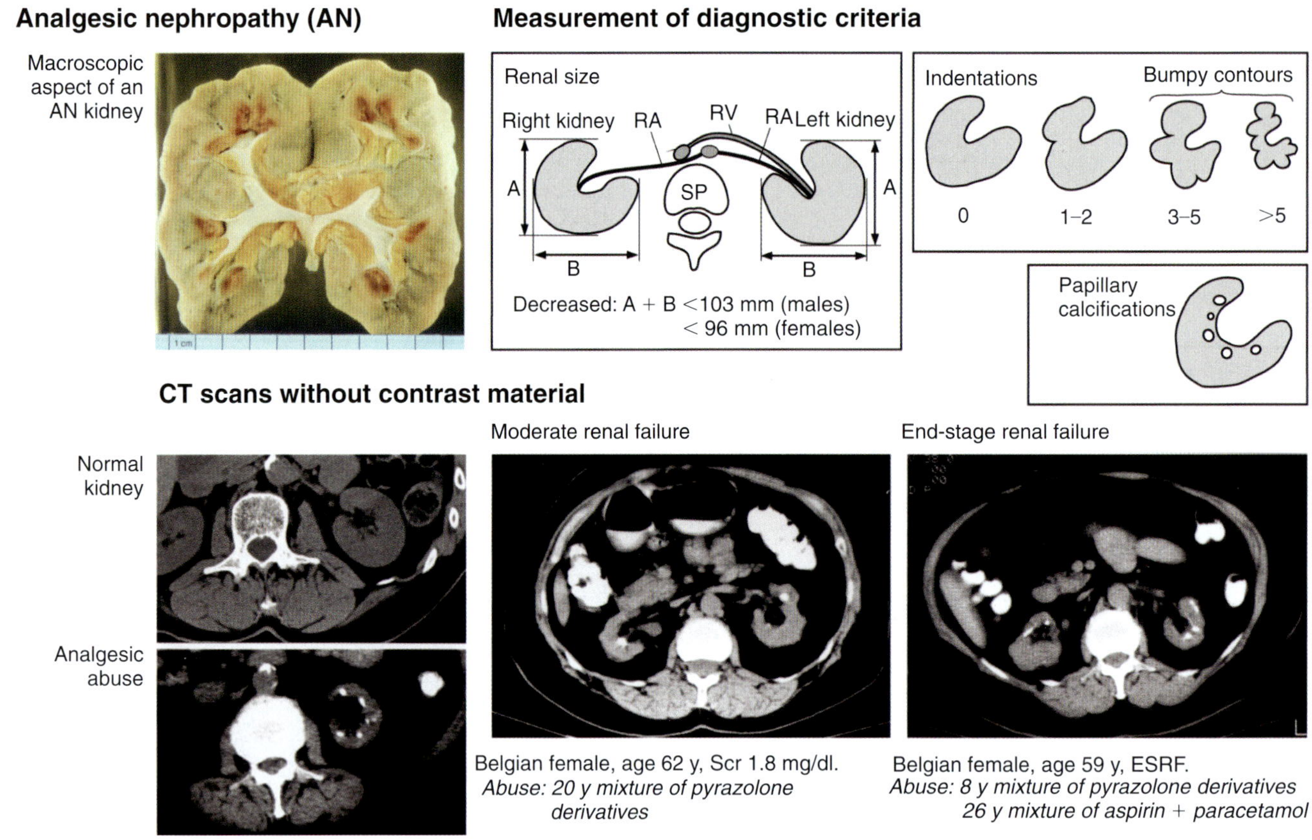

or relatively stable degrees of azotemia. Although there is no guarantee that discontinuation of ingestion of the herbal medication will arrest disease progression, it is the prudent recommendation. Other than the ingestion history, the clinical and laboratory findings are nonspecific. No specific therapies have been described to arrest the progression of this disease process reliably. The susceptibility of some but not all individuals exposed to the same herbal preparations is not well understood, although gender, toxin dose, and toxin metabolism may all play a role.[279]

Renal biopsies from these patients can demonstrate significant cortical fibrosis, with atrophy and dropout of tubules. Fibrosis has historically been reported as a more dominant feature than cellular infiltration (Figure 36.4).[280] Thickening of the interlobular arteriolar walls has been described. There are no immune deposits.[290] Research techniques may demonstrate aristolochic acid–related DNA adducts within the kidneys. A more recent study has demonstrated significant infiltration of the medullary rays and outer medulla by monocytes and macrophages, as well as T and B lymphocytes, even in kidneys removed from patients with ESKD.[285]

The role of aristolochic acid in producing this lesion has been supported by the creation of a similar renal lesion in rabbits and rats to which aristolochic acid was administered regularly over weeks to months.[291,292] Kidneys from these animals display interstitial fibrosis, tubular atrophy, and some cellular infiltration, along with some atypical and/or malignant uroepithelial cells. Renal functional abnormalities, such as a decreased GFR, may vary, depending on volume depletion or other exogenous factors. In genetically manipulated mice, the absence of the Smad3 signaling system abrogates the expression of aristolochic acid nephropathy. In vitro, aristolochic acid elicits EMT and augmented collagen production, which are dependent on TGF-beta/Smad3– and JNK/MAP kinase–dependent mechanisms.[293]

The potential for uroepithelial malignancies in patients exposed to aristolochic acid is well documented. For example, in a study of 39 patients with Chinese herbal nephropathy and ESKD who underwent removal of their native kidneys and ureters, urothelial carcinoma was discovered in 18 and mild-to-moderate urothelial dysplasia in 19 patients. Malignant transformation may be related to p53 mutations.[294] The occurrence of malignancy correlated with the cumulative amount of Chinese herbs ingested. Current thinking links the presence of aristolactam-DNA adducts to p53 mutations, specifically A:T to T:A transversions at acceptor splice sites.[295] Such findings have led to recommendations that these patients should undergo regular surveillance for abnormal urinary cytology and, perhaps in high-risk patients, bilateral nephrectomies.[296]

BALKAN ENDEMIC NEPHROPATHY

Balkan endemic nephropathy (BEN) is a chronic tubulointerstitial disease seen largely in families residing on the

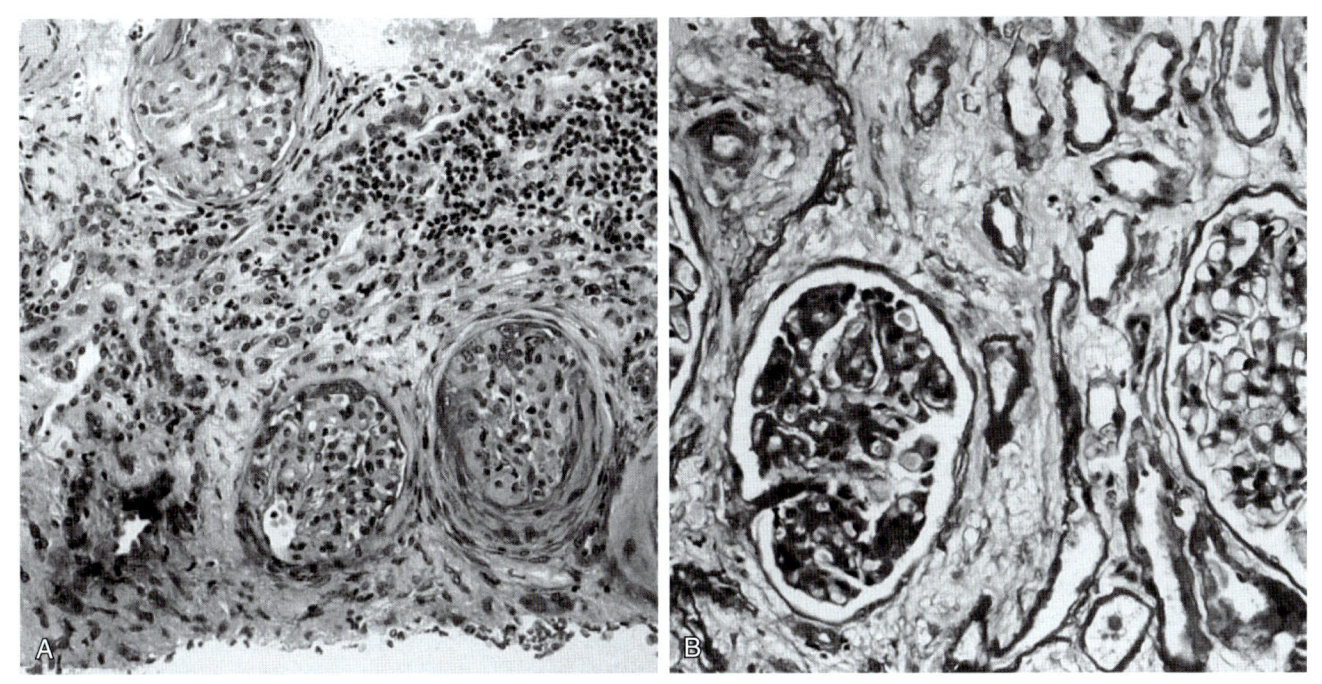

Figure 36.4 Case of Chinese herb nephropathy. The kidney biopsy shows tubular atrophy, widening of the interstitium, cellular infiltration, important fibrosis, and glomeruli surrounded by a fibrotic ring. **A,** Masson stain. **B,** Hematoxylin-eosin stain.

alluvial plains of the Danube River in Serbia, Bosnia, Herzegovina, Croatia, Romania, and Bulgaria. The prevalence is high in these areas, ranging from 0.5% to 5%.[297] Although historically genetic and environmental factors have been suspected to play a role in its pathogenesis, current evidence suggests that environmental factors are dominant, but may only lead to disease in those with certain genetic backgrounds.[298]

Patients with BEN share the clinical features common to many chronic tubulointerstitial diseases. Renal and urinary abnormalities first appear after residing in an endemic area for at least 15 years. Affected individuals are not usually hypertensive. Initial renal abnormalities include tubular dysfunction characterized by tubular proteinuria, glycosuria, aminoaciduria, and impaired acid excretion. This is temporally followed by impaired concentrating ability and slowly progressive (over years) azotemia, which can result in ESKD. A normochromic normocytic anemia is typical as well. Kidneys are of normal size early in the course of the disease, but kidney size diminishes with time (Figure 36.5). The diagnosis is presumptive, based on renal abnormalities consistent with chronic interstitial disease in a patient residing in an endemic area.[299] There is no specific therapy for this form of interstitial disease.

Renal pathology demonstrates cortical tubular atrophy, interstitial fibrosis, and sparse mononuclear cell infiltrates. Glomerular sclerosis is seen in more advanced cases. There is an extremely high incidence of cellular atypia and urothelial carcinoma of the genitourinary tract.[300] Like several other forms of chronic tubulointerstitial disease, BEN is also associated with uroepithelial malignancies, in particular transitional cell carcinoma of the renal pelvis or ureter.[297] For this entity as well, periodic screening of urine for abnormal cytology has been recommended.

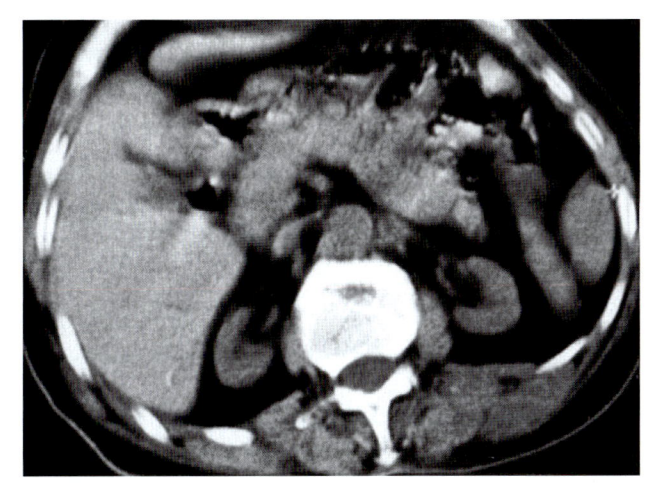

Figure 36.5 Computed tomography (CT) scan without contrast media in a patient with Balkan endemic nephropathy, creatinine clearance of 15 mL/min, no hypertension, and proteinuria, with values less than 1 g/24 hr. Of importance are the bilateral atrophy of the kidneys and absence of intrarenal calcifications.

Three major environmental factors are currently considered as potential contributors to the pathogenesis of BEN. Aristolochic acid has been proposed as a toxin underlying this disease, in addition to Chinese herb nephropathy. The pathologic changes in the kidney are similar, and both are associated with a high prevalence of uroepithelial malignancies. Aristolochic acid DNA adducts are found in the kidneys of patients with Chinese herb nephropathy as well as BEN. The same specific A:T and T:A transversions in p53 are also seen in these patients.[301] The other environmental causes that have been considered include ochratoxin A, a mycotoxin, and polycyclic hydrocarbons, which leach into drinking water from low-rank coal present in endemic areas.[302] Exposure to the environmental factors has changed over the past several decades in that the dominant population now affected by BEN are older than 60 years.[298]

LITHIUM

Patients who take lithium for the treatment of bipolar affective disorder commonly have a nephrogenic diabetes insipidus. This is a predictable side effect of therapeutic levels of the drug and is slowly reversible following discontinuation of the medication. The nephrogenic diabetes insipidus is reproducible in animals treated with lithium, where it is associated with diminished expression of the vasopressin-regulated water channel aquaporin-2.[303] Hyperparathyroidism can also be observed in patients treated with lithium, and the associated hypercalcemia is an additional contributor to abnormalities in urinary concentration. Whether chronic ingestion of lithium is associated with a form of chronic tubulointerstitial nephritis and progressive azotemia has been more controversial.[304,305] Current prevailing views are that lithium is associated with the development of chronic tubulointerstitial nephritis (Figure 36.6). In some patients, focal segmental glomerular sclerosis has also been reported.[306]

Support for the hypothesis that chronic lithium ingestion can lead to chronic interstitial nephritis and functional impairment was bolstered by the development of an animal model in rabbits. When the kidneys from rabbits fed lithium were examined over a 12-month period, clear differences were seen compared to control rabbits. Epithelial cells lining the distal convoluted tubules and collecting ducts displayed cytoplasmic vacuolation with accompanying histologic changes of focal interstitial nephritis, including tubular atrophy, interstitial fibrosis, and distal tubular dilation and microcyst formation. Glomerular sclerosis and azotemia also occurred by 12 months.[307]

In a study of patients treated chronically with lithium (mean duration of therapy > 13 years), the authors examined renal biopsies from 24 patients. Biopsies were performed because of the presence of azotemia and, in some of the patients, abnormal proteinuria (>1.0 g/24 hr).[308] In this selected population, all the patients had findings consistent with chronic TIN on biopsy. Tubular dilation and cysts were also present in the cortex and medulla. A number of patients also had focal or global glomerulosclerosis. A serum creatinine value of greater than 2.5 mg/dL at the time of biopsy was the most powerful predictor of ultimate progression to ESKD, which occurred even if lithium was discontinued. Lepkifker and coworkers[309] found that approximately 20% of long-term lithium patients demonstrated slowly rising serum creatinine values, but this did not correlate with duration of therapy or cumulative dose. A more recent study from Sweden has described a sixfold increase in prevalence for ESKD in patients taking lithium compared with the general population. The prevalence of CKD in the lithium-treated population was about 1.2%, with duration of therapy as the only identified risk factor.[310]

The clinical management of patients on chronic lithium who develop azotemia requires judgment and a risk-benefit analysis. The polyuria and polydipsia that are common to most patients on lithium, because of the nephrogenic diabetes insipidus, will be resolved if the drug is withdrawn, but are frequently symptoms that are tolerated because of the efficacy of the drug in treating mania and/or bipolar disorder. Lithium levels should be carefully monitored and maintained at the lowest level that controls symptoms. Given the more recent development and testing of additional drugs (e.g., olanzapine, quetiapine, lamotrigine) for first-line treatment of bipolar disorder, it is reasonable to try these agents instead in patients with a stable elevated creatinine level, preferably before irreversible interstitial damage has occurred.

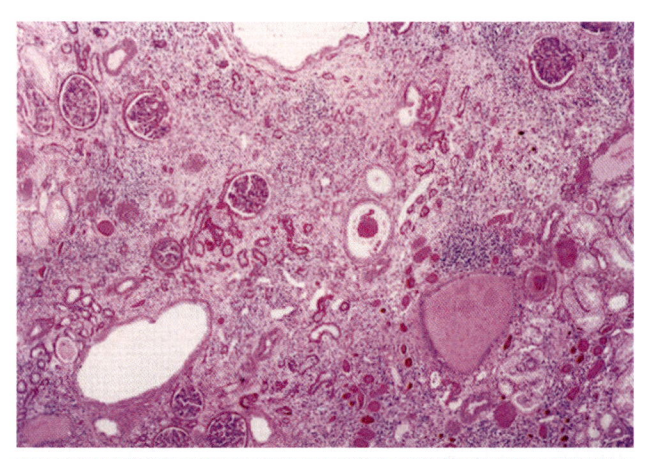

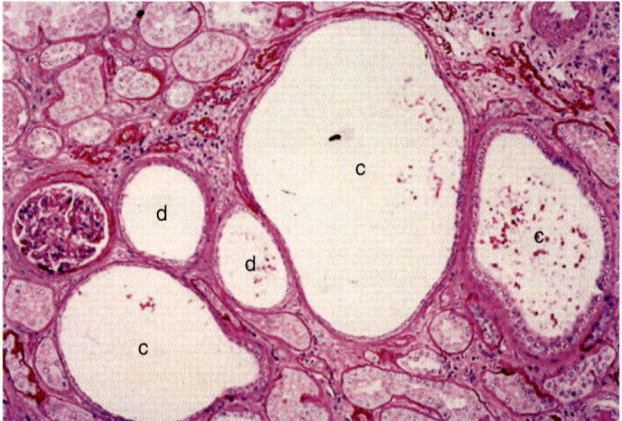

Figure 36.6 Top, Severe lithium-associated chronic tubulointerstitial nephropathy, with the additional finding of focal tubular cysts arising in a background of severe interstitial fibrosis and tubular atrophy. (Periodic acid–Schiff [PAS] stain, ×40.) **Bottom,** High-power view of tubular cysts lined by simple cuboidal epithelium (c). Adjacent tubules show tubular dilation (d). (PAS stain, ×100.) (From Markowitz GS, Radhakrishnan J, Kambham N, et al: Lithium nephrotoxicity: a progressive combined glomerular and tubulointerstitial nephropathy, *J Am Soc Nephrol* 11:1439-1448, 2000.)

LEAD

Epidemiologic studies have strongly implicated excessive exposure to lead as a cause of chronic tubulointerstitial nephritis leading to renal failure.[311] Despite restriction of occupational exposure to lead and banning of lead-based paints, continuing exposure to low levels of lead occurs through old water pipes, pottery, crystal, and lead-based paint in older dwellings. The current focus is on whether low-level sustained exposure to lead contributes, solely or in combination with other factors, to the development of ESKD. Determining whether there has been significant lead exposure requires a careful history and, optimally, the use of a screening questionnaire. Part of the challenge in ascertaining the relationship between low-level lead exposure and kidney function relates to the accurate measurement of body lead burden (ethylenediaminetetraacetic acid [EDTA] mobilization test), which is required because blood lead levels only indicate recent, not chronic, lead exposure. Several studies have now demonstrated correlations between elevated blood levels and/or body lead burden with the presence of kidney disease and/or accelerated rates of progression of chronic renal disease.[312,313] Using data from the Third National Health and Nutrition Examination Survey (NHANES III), Muntner and colleagues concluded that among the adult U.S. population with hypertension, even low-level exposure to lead is associated with chronic kidney disease.[313] The same study also showed that in U.S. adolescents, higher blood lead levels correlated with lower GFRs.[314] This relationship has also been demonstrated using the cystatin C–based estimated GFR (eGFR).[315] Experimental studies in the rat remnant kidney model have supported the hypothesis that ingestion of lead can accelerate chronic kidney disease in association with hypertension and accentuated vascular and interstitial injuries.[316]

The pathogenesis of chronic lead nephropathy is related to the reabsorption of filtered lead by the proximal tubule, with preferential deposition within the S3 segment of the proximal tubule. Lead exposure can thus lead to defects in proximal tubule function, especially in children, including aminoaciduria, glycosuria, and phosphaturia representing Fanconi's syndrome. These defects can also occur individually. Renal biopsies in adult patients with subclinical lead nephropathy and a mild to moderate decrease in GFR primarily show chronic interstitial nephritis, tubular atrophy, and interstitial fibrosis.

Adults who develop chronic interstitial nephritis in association with lead exposure typically have hypertension and frequently gout as well. Progression to ESKD develops slowly over years. Such slow progression has encouraged clinical investigators to examine whether chelation of lead might slow or reverse the progression of this disease. Earlier studies with small numbers of patients suggested that chronic injections of EDTA in patients with mild renal insufficiency and industrial exposure to lead could improve the GFR.[317] Two larger prospective studies in patients with nondiabetic chronic renal disease, no lead exposure history, and normal or low-normal total body lead burdens demonstrated that chronic EDTA chelation can improve GFR over a 24-month period relative to the control group.[318,319] Although EDTA chelation may be exerting a benefit through processes other than lead removal, it is intriguing to consider that lead may adversely affect the progression of other forms of renal disease and that this may be positively affected by EDTA chelation. The use of EDTA chelation therapeutically for chronic lead nephropathy still requires confirmation in larger studies.

CADMIUM

Cadmium accumulates in the body after gastrointestinal absorption or inhalation. Cadmium nephropathy can develop in those with prolonged low-level exposure to excess cadmium, such as with zinc smelter workers, or in the setting of massive environmental contamination, as occurred in Japan in the early part of the twentieth century. In the latter case, water contaminated with cadmium from mining operations was ultimately used for drinking water and for the irrigation of rice fields, entering the food chain and leading to an epidemic of cadmium poisoning. Prominent features of this poisoning were bone pain (itai-itai or ouch-ouch disease), osteopenia, and renal failure.[320] Cadmium is bound to metallothionein, and proximal tubular cells take up the complexes. Cadmium induces a tubular proteinuria.[321] Other proximal tubule defects, including renal glycosuria, aminoaciduria, hypercalciuria, and phosphaturia, are also observed. The functional tubular defects that ensue may relate to apoptosis secondary to the activation of calpains and caspases.[322] Uncommonly, such renal damage may progress to an irreversible reduction in glomerular filtration.[323]

The high levels of environmental contamination with cadmium related to mining in Japan were an unusual event. The extent to which chronic, low-level environmental exposure to cadmium affects renal function is much less clear. The CadmiBel Study recruited over 2000 adults from different areas of Belgium in an attempt to compare the relationships among hypertension, cardiovascular disease, and renal abnormalities with urinary cadmium excretion. The results demonstrated that although hypertension and cardiovascular risk were not associated with urinary cadmium excretion, there was a direct correlation with alkaline phosphatase activity, urinary excretion of retinol-binding protein, N-acetyl-β-glucosaminidase, β2-microglobulin, amino acids, and calcium with urinary cadmium excretion.[323] Interestingly, a 5-year follow-up study of individuals with the highest urinary cadmium excretion did not demonstrate evidence of progressive renal damage or loss of function.[324] Although this is somewhat reassuring, it is still prudent to limit nutritional and occupational exposure to cadmium.[325] The increased urinary calcium excretion seen in those exposed to cadmium is associated with an increased prevalence of calcium phosphate kidney stones.[326]

HYPERURICEMIA AND URATE NEPHROPATHY

As the major organ responsible for the excretion of uric acid, the kidney can be affected in a number of ways by abnormal uric acid metabolism. In general, problems arise following the crystallization of uric acid in the tubules, collecting system, or outflow tract or the deposition of uric acid within the interstitium, with attendant inflammation. Uric acid solubility is pH and concentration dependent. Thus, because uric acid in the tubular lumen is concentrated and exposed to a lower pH in the distal nephron, the likelihood of precipitation increases. Uric acid stones are a well-recognized entity and are discussed elsewhere in this text. Acute uric acid nephropathy, typically seen as an acute kidney injury phenotype following cell breakdown, is also a recognized entity for which prophylactic treatment can usually be given.

Whether sustained and chronic hyperuricemia leads to chronic interstitial nephritis has been historically a controversial issue. Claims in the 1970s that up to 11% of chronic interstitial disease could be attributed to disorders of uric acid metabolism[327] were challenged in the 1980s because of the difficulty in identifying effects of hyperuricemia, which could not be attributed to hypertension, vascular disease, stones, or aging.[328] An additional controversy was related to the possibility that patients with coexisting gout and chronic interstitial nephritis might have chronic lead intoxication as a cause of both disturbances. It is likely that only a minority of patients with sustained chronic hyperuricemia (with or without clinical gout) have chronic interstitial nephritis. These are typically patients with serum urate levels greater than 13 mg/dL (men) or more than 10 mg/dL (women). Clearly, the coexistence of hypertension, diabetes mellitus, abnormal lipid metabolism, and nephrosclerosis are frequently confounding variables.[329] An autosomal dominant disease in children, familial juvenile hyperuricemic nephropathy, is characterized by sustained hyperuricemia and chronic interstitial nephritis leading to progressive renal failure.[330]

Sustained hyperuricemia could also contribute to progressive azotemia in a number of forms of CKD. Thus, it seems reasonable to recommend dietary restriction of protein and purines in patients with gout and interstitial disease or patients with CKD and a similarly elevated serum urate level.[331] In studies seeking to understand how hyperuricemia may relate to the progression of renal disease, this abnormality has been shown to induce endothelial dysfunction. Uric acid regulates critical proinflammatory pathways in vascular smooth muscle cells, potentially having a role in the vascular changes associated with hypertension and vascular disease.[332,333] Studies in rats in which hyperuricemia was induced by uricase inhibitor oxonic acid show resultant hypertension, intrarenal vascular disease, and renal injury. Hyperuricemia accelerates renal progression in the remnant kidney model via a mechanism linked to high systemic blood pressure and COX-2–mediated, thromboxane-induced vascular disease.[334] Mice with systemic knockout of the glut9 urate transporter (typically expressed in liver and kidney) have moderate hyperuricemia, significant hyperuricosuria, and renal injury, with interstitial inflammation, uric acid stones, and progressive interstitial fibrosis.[335] Taken in aggregate, these studies provide strong evidence that uric acid may be a true mediator of renal disease and progression.

SARCOIDOSIS

Sarcoidosis[336] usually affects the kidney through disordered Ca^{2+} metabolism.[337] Of patients with sarcoidosis, 10% to 15% have hypercalcemia, with even more affected by normocalcemic hypercalciuria. These abnormalities can lead to concentrating defects, depress glomerular filtration, and result in nephrocalcinosis or nephrolithiasis.[338] Nephrolithiasis occurs in approximately 1% to 14% of patients with sarcoidosis and may be the presenting feature. Nephrocalcinosis, observed in over 50% of those with renal insufficiency, is the most common cause of chronic renal failure in sarcoidosis.[339] Some patients may develop granulomatous interstitial disease, glomerular disease, obstructive uropathy and, very rarely, ESKD. Rarely, renal disease can be the most prominent manifestation of the disease.[340,341]

Autopsy and renal biopsy series have suggested that 15% to 30% of patients with sarcoidosis may have noncaseating granulomas in the renal interstitium. In many cases, these lesions are not clinically apparent. Typically, biopsy findings reveal interstitial noncaseating granulomas composed of giant cells, histiocytes, and lymphocytes. The extent of these granulomas is variable, but they may replace the bulk of the cortical volume. Focal lymphocytic infiltrates and periglomerular fibrosis are commonly seen.[342] Immunofluorescent and electron microscopic studies typically show no immune deposits.

Other diseases characterized by granuloma formation, including tuberculosis, silicosis, and histoplasmosis, can cause hypercalcemia and renal insufficiency but are only rarely associated with granulomatous interstitial nephritis. Allergic interstitial nephritis related to drugs can result in a granulomatous interstitial nephritis. It is unusual to see glomerular abnormalities in sarcoidosis. Membranous nephropathy and focal glomerulosclerosis have been described but would be distinguishable clinically by heavy proteinuria, which is not seen in the granulomatous interstitial nephritis of sarcoidosis.

Patients with granulomatous interstitial nephritis caused by sarcoidosis often have an impressive therapeutic response to corticosteroid therapy, with improvement in the GFR and, on repeat biopsy, loss of granulomas and lymphocytic infiltrate. Failure to respond to steroids at 1 month correlates with more severe chronic kidney disease.[343] There have been no controlled trials of corticosteroid therapy. The often concomitant hypercalcemia is also corticosteroid-responsive, typically to lower doses. Healing of the granulomatous interstitial nephritis can lead to interstitial fibrosis. Ketoconazole, an inhibitor of steroidogenesis, has been used in a single patient who could not tolerate corticosteroids and was effective in decreasing the level of active vitamin D, as well as serum and urinary calcium levels.[344] One study has described successful treatment of interstitial nephritis with infliximab in a patient with sarcoidosis.[341]

AUTOIMMUNE DISEASES

Immunologic diseases such as Behçet's disease, Sjögren's syndrome, sarcoidosis, systemic lupus erythematosus, inflammatory bowel diseases, IgG4-related systemic disease, and vasculitides may also produce chronic interstitial nephritis.[345-349] Most of these diseases are lingering multifaceted illnesses, which obfuscates the recognition of a complication such as AIN—is it acute or the acute recognition of chronicity? Most patients have elements of chronicity on renal biopsy by the time the disease is diagnosed, but some patients with these systemic diseases will develop AIN following a drug reaction.

Anti-TBM nephritis occasionally manifests in association with membranous nephropathy.[350] The characteristics of patients with this combination include a predominance of males, onset in early childhood, microscopic hematuria, and nephrotic-range proteinuria. In addition, patients show tubular dysfunction (complete or incomplete Fanconi's syndrome), circulating anti-TBM antibodies, and progression to ESKD.[350] Circulating anti-TBM antibodies from these patients react exclusively with the proximal TBM, not with GBM, exhibiting binding to tubular antigens. The precise mechanisms of combined immune complex deposition in glomeruli and antibody formation against idiopathic tubulointerstitial antigens are unclear. Soluble tubulointerstitial antigen binding to its relevant antibody may participate in the formation of immune complexes in the glomerular lesions. However, tubulointerstitial antigens are not detected within the immune complex deposits. The patients showing membranous nephropathy preceding anti-TBM nephritis have suggested that anti-TBM antibodies are formed by tubulointerstitial antigens modified by certain components or exposed to enzymes present within the massive proteinuria. The role of human leukocyte antigens in the evolution of these autoimmune disorders has also been suggested.

In 1975, Dobrin and associates described a new syndrome characterized by anterior uveitis, bone marrow granulomas, hypergammaglobulinemia, increased erythrocyte sedimentation rate, and renal failure, with renal histologic features of interstitial nephritis.[351] The renal failure caused by tubulointerstitial nephritis associated with uveitis was thus termed *TINU syndrome*.[352] TINU syndrome is particularly common in children; among adults, it occurs predominantly in females (3:1). Familial occurrence has suggested that a genetic influence may play some role in pathogenesis.[248,353] A significant association has been reported in the frequency of selected HLA haplotypes. The anterior uveitis may precede, concur with, or follow the nephropathy. These patients generally suffer from weight loss and anemia and have a raised erythrocyte sedimentation rate. Although associations with chlamydia and mycoplasma infections have been suggested, the cause remains obscure.[354] The syndrome appears immune-mediated, with T cell proliferation in the kidney.[355] Moreover, the possibility of a delayed-type hypersensitivity reaction is also suggested on the basis of the 2:1 ratio of $CD4^+/CD8^+$ interstitial lymphocytes. Prolonged steroid therapy usually leads to improvement in renal function and uveitis, although the latter may relapse.[352]

Complete reference list available at ExpertConsult.com.

KEY REFERENCES

1. Zeisberg M, Neilson EG: Mechanisms of tubulointerstitial fibrosis. *J Am Soc Nephrol* 21:1819–1834, 2010.
2. Harris RC, Neilson EG: Toward a unified theory of renal progression. *Annu Rev Med* 57:365–380, 2006.
4. Yang H, Fogo AB: Cell senescence in the aging kidney. *J Am Soc Nephrol* 21:1436–1439, 2010.
26. Chevalier RL, Forbes MS, Thornhill BA: Ureteral obstruction as a model of renal interstitial fibrosis and obstructive nephropathy. *Kidney Int* 75:1145–1152, 2009.
31. Chevalier RL, Forbes MS: Generation and evolution of atubular glomeruli in the progression of renal disorders. *J Am Soc Nephrol* 19:197–206, 2008.
33. Tanaka T, Nangaku M: Pathogenesis of tubular interstitial nephritis. *Contrib Nephrol* 169:297–310, 2011.
34. Hildebrandt F, Attanasio M, Otto E: Nephronophthisis: disease mechanisms of a ciliopathy. *J Am Soc Nephrol* 20:23–35, 2009.
37. Rampoldi L, Scolari F, Amoroso A, et al: The rediscovery of uromodulin (Tamm-Horsfall protein): from tubulointerstitial nephropathy to chronic kidney disease. *Kidney Int* 80:338–347, 2011.
40. Eddy AA: Proteinuria and interstitial injury. *Nephrol Dial Transplant* 19:277–281, 2004.
45. Ruggenenti P, Cravedi P, Remuzzi G: Mechanisms and treatment of CKD. *J Am Soc Nephrol* 23:1917–1928, 2012.
56. Abbate M, Zoja C, Remuzzi G: How does proteinuria cause progressive renal damage? *J Am Soc Nephrol* 17:2974–2984, 2006.
76. Sanz AB, Santamaria B, Ruiz-Ortega M, et al: Mechanisms of renal apoptosis in health and disease. *J Am Soc Nephrol* 19:1634–1642, 2008.
93. Bao L, Wang Y, Haas M, et al: Distinct roles for C3a and C5a in complement-induced tubulointerstitial injury. *Kidney Int* 80:524–534, 2011.
119. Bleyer AJ, Zivná M, Kmoch S: Uromodulin-associated kidney disease. *Nephron Clin Pract* 118:c31–c36, 2011.
137. Anders HJ, Muruve DA: The inflammasomes in kidney disease. *J Am Soc Nephrol* 22:1007–1018, 2011.
140. Humphreys BD, Xu F, Sabbisetti V, et al: Chronic epithelial kidney injury molecule-1 expression causes murine kidney fibrosis. *J Clin Invest* 123:4023–4035, 2013.
141. Fujiu K, Manabe I, Nagai R: Renal collecting duct epithelial cells regulate inflammation in tubulointerstitial damage in mice. *J Clin Invest* 121:3425–3441, 2011.
153. Liu L, Kou P, Zeng Q, et al: CD4+ T lymphocytes, especially Th2 cells, contribute to the progress of renal fibrosis. *Am J Nephrol* 36:386–396, 2012.
155. Bailey NC, Kelly CJ: Nephritogenic T cells use granzyme C as a cytotoxic mediator. *Eur J Immunol* 27:2302–2309, 1997.
165. Kelly CJ: T cell regulation of autoimmune interstitial nephritis. *J Am Soc Nephrol* 1:140–149, 1990.
177. Liu Y: New insights into epithelial-mesenchymal transition in kidney fibrosis. *J Am Soc Nephrol* 21:212–222, 2010.
178. Zeisberg M, Neilson EG: Biomarkers for epithelial-mesenchymal transitions. *J Clin Invest* 119:1429–1437, 2009.
179. Neilson EG: Plasticity, nuclear diapause, and a requiem for the terminal differentiation of epithelia. *J Am Soc Nephrol* 18:1995–1998, 2007.
186. Gentle ME, Shi S, Daehn I, et al: Epithelial cell TGFbeta signaling induces acute tubular injury and interstitial inflammation. *J Am Soc Nephrol* 24:787–799, 2013.
188. Kalluri R, Neilson EG: Epithelial-mesenchymal transition and its implications for fibrosis. *J Clin Invest* 112:1776–1784, 2003.
199. Lin J, Patel SR, Cheng X, et al: Kielin/chordin-like protein, a novel enhancer of BMP signaling, attenuates renal fibrotic disease. *Nat Med* 11:387–393, 2005.
203. Haase VH: Mechanisms of hypoxia responses in renal tissue. *J Am Soc Nephrol* 24:537–541, 2013.
207. Michel DM, Kelly CJ: Acute interstitial nephritis. *J Am Soc Nephrol* 9:506–515, 1998.
210. Blank ML, Parkin L, Paul C, et al: A nationwide nested case-control study indicates an increased risk of acute interstitial nephritis with proton pump inhibitor use. *Kidney Int* 86:837–844, 2014.
211. Shirali AC, Perazella MA: Tubulointerstitial injury associated with chemotherapeutic agents. *Adv Chronic Kidney Dis* 21:56–63, 2014.
220. Murray MD, Brater DC: Renal toxicity of the nonsteroidal anti-inflammatory drugs. *Annu Rev Pharmacol Toxicol* 33:435–465, 1993.
231. Parkhie SM, Fine DM, Lucas GM, et al: Characteristics of patients with HIV and biopsy-proven acute interstitial nephritis. *Clin J Am Soc Nephrol* 5:798–804, 2010.
238. Criado PR, Criado RF, Avancini JM, et al: Drug reaction with eosinophilia and systemic symptoms (DRESS)/drug-induced hypersensitivity syndrome (DIHS): a review of current concepts. *An Bras Dermatol* 87:435–449, 2012.
241. Muriithi AK, Nasr SH, Leung N: Utility of urine eosinophils in the diagnosis of acute interstitial nephritis. *Clin J Am Soc Nephrol* 8:1857–1862, 2013.
244. Smith J, Neilson EG: Treatment of acute interstitial nephritis. In Wilcox CA, editor: *Therapy of renal disease*, Philadelphia, 2008, WB Saunders.
247. Raza MN, Hadid M, Keen CE, et al: Acute tubulointerstitial nephritis, treatment with steroid and impact on renal outcomes. *Nephrology (Carlton)* 17:748–753, 2012.
248. Jahnukainen T, Saarela V, Arikoski P, et al: Prednisone in the treatment of tubulointerstitial nephritis in children. *Pediatr Nephrol* 28:1253–1260, 2013.
254. Murray TG, Goldberg M: Analgesic-associated nephropathy in the U.S.A.: epidemiologic, clinical and pathogenetic features. *Kidney Int* 13:64–71, 1978.
282. Gokmen MR, Cosyns JP, Arlt VM, et al: The epidemiology, diagnosis, and management of aristolochic acid nephropathy: a narrative review. *Ann Intern Med* 158:469–477, 2013.
288. De Broe ME: Chinese herbs nephropathy and Balkan endemic nephropathy: toward a single entity, aristolochic acid nephropathy. *Kidney Int* 81:513–515, 2012.
310. Bendz H, Schon S, Attman PO, et al: Renal failure occurs in chronic lithium treatment but is uncommon. *Kidney Int* 77:219–224, 2010.
312. Yu CC, Lin JL, Lin-Tan DT: Environmental exposure to lead and progression of chronic renal diseases: a four-year prospective longitudinal study. *J Am Soc Nephrol* 15:1016–1022, 2004.

322. Lee WK, Torchalski B, Thevenod F: Cadmium-induced ceramide formation triggers calpain-dependent apoptosis in cultured kidney proximal tubule cells. *Am J Physiol Cell Physiol* 293:C839–C847, 2007.
334. Kang DH, Nakagawa T, Feng L, et al: A role for uric acid in the progression of renal disease. *J Am Soc Nephrol* 13:2888–2897, 2002.
336. Valeyre D, Prasse A, Nunes H, et al: Sarcoidosis. *Lancet* 383:1155–1167, 2014.
345. Neilson EG: Tubulointerstitial nephritis. In Goldman LA, Schafer AI, editors: *Goldman-Cecil medicine*, ed 25, Philadelphia, 2015, WB Saunders.
348. Zaidan M, Lescure FX, Brocheriou I, et al: Tubulointerstitial nephropathies in HIV-infected patients over the past 15 years: a clinico-pathological study. *Clin J Am Soc Nephrol* 8:930–938, 2013.
349. Raissian Y, Nasr SH, Larsen CP, et al: Diagnosis of IgG4-related tubulointerstitial nephritis. *J Am Soc Nephrol* 22:1343–1352, 2011.
352. Neilson EG, Farris AB: Case records of the Massachusetts General Hospital. Case 21-2009. A 61-year-old woman with abdominal pain, weight loss, and renal failure. *N Engl J Med* 361:179–187, 2009.

37
Urinary Tract Infection in Adults

Lindsay E. Nicolle

CHAPTER OUTLINE

DEFINITIONS, 1231
GENERAL CONCEPTS, 1232
Host Defenses of the Normal Urinary Tract, 1232
Immune and Inflammatory Responses to Urinary Tract Infection, 1232
Urine Culture, 1233
Pharmacokinetic and Pharmacodynamic Considerations for Treatment, 1234
USUAL PRESENTATIONS OF URINARY TRACT INFECTION, 1236
Acute Uncomplicated Urinary Tract Infection: Cystitis, 1236
Acute Nonobstructive Pyelonephritis, 1240
Complicated Urinary Tract Infection, 1242
Asymptomatic Bacteriuria, 1245
Prostatitis, 1247
URINARY TRACT INFECTION IN UNIQUE PATIENT POPULATIONS, 1248

Renal Transplant Recipients, 1248
Persons with Renal Failure, 1249
Persons with Urinary Stones, 1249
OTHER INFECTIONS OF THE URINARY TRACT, 1250
Renal and Perinephric Abscesses, 1250
Infected Renal Cysts, 1250
Emphysematous Cystitis and Pyelonephritis, 1251
Xanthogranulomatous Pyelonephritis, 1251
Pyocystis, 1252
UNCOMMON ORGANISMS, 1252
Genitourinary Tuberculosis, 1252
Bacille de Calmette-Guérin Infection, 1254
Fungal Urinary Tract Infection, 1254
Viral Infections, 1255
Parasitic Infestations of the Urinary Tract, 1255

Urinary tract infection of the bladder, the kidney, or (in men) the prostate is one of the most common human infections. Infecting organisms are usually bacteria; fungi also contribute. Much less frequently, infection is caused by viruses or parasites. Other manifestations of genitourinary tract infection are renal and perinephric abscesses, emphysematous cystitis and pyelonephritis, xanthogranulomatous pyelonephritis, and pyocystitis. Disseminated viral infections (e.g., mumps, cytomegalovirus [CMV], and other herpes viruses) and fungal infections (e.g., blastomycosis, histoplasmosis) may also involve the urinary tract but are not discussed in this chapter. Polyomavirus BK infection in kidney transplant recipients and urinary tract infection in children, including vesicoureteral reflux, are addressed in Chapters 71 and 74, respectively.

DEFINITIONS

Urinary tract infection is the presence of bacteria or other microorganisms in the urine or genitourinary tissues, which are normally sterile. The term *bacteriuria* describes isolation of any bacteria in the urine, although in practice it usually refers to isolation of organisms in concentrations that meet standard quantitative criteria. Infection is asymptomatic when the urine culture result meets quantitative criteria for bacteriuria without signs or symptoms attributable to infection. Symptomatic urinary tract infection may manifest as bladder infection (cystitis or lower tract infection), kidney infection (pyelonephritis or upper tract infection), or prostate infection (acute or chronic bacterial prostatitis). Acute uncomplicated urinary tract infection occurs in women with a normal genitourinary tract, usually manifesting as cystitis.[1,2] Pyelonephritis, also referred to as *acute nonobstructive* or *acute uncomplicated pyelonephritis*, also occurs in such women but much less frequently.[2] Complicated urinary tract infection occurs in individuals with functional or structural abnormalities of the genitourinary tract (Table 37.1).[3,4] In healthy postmenopausal women without genitourinary abnormalities and diabetic women without nephropathy or neurologic bladder impairment, urinary tract infection should be considered uncomplicated. Acute uncomplicated

1231

Table 37.1 Abnormalities of the Urinary Tract That May Be Associated with Complicated Urinary Tract Infection

Abnormality	Example(s)
Obstruction	Pelvicalyceal junction obstruction, ureteric or urethral strictures, prostate hypertrophy, urolithiasis, tumor, extrinsic compression
Neurologic impairment	Neurogenic bladder
Urologic devices	Indwelling catheter, ureteric stent, nephrostomy tube
Urologic abnormalities	Vesicoureteral reflux, bladder diverticuli, cystoceles, urologic procedures, ileal conduit, augmented bladder, neobladder
Metabolic/congenital diseases	Nephrocalcinosis, medullary sponge kidney, urethral valves, polycystic kidneys
Immunologic impairment	Renal transplantation

Table 37.2 Host Defenses Other Than Voiding That Contribute to Maintaining Sterility of Urine

Defense	Example(s)
Urine characteristics	pH, osmolality, concentration of organic acids
Urine proteins	Tamm-Horsfall protein, secretory immunoglobulins, lactoferrin, lipocalin, cationic peptides (defensins, cathelicidins)
Inflammatory cells	Polymorphonuclear leukocytes
Uroepithelium	Mucopolysaccharide layer, chemokines/cytokine production, uroplakin barrier
Prostate secretions	Chemokines, immunoglobulins

urinary tract infection rarely occurs in men. A urinary tract infection in a man should be considered complicated until underlying abnormalities have been ruled out.

Urinary tract infection commonly recurs. *Reinfection* is infection that recurs after entry of an organism into the genitourinary tract, usually from the periurethral flora. Reinfection characteristically occurs with a different organism. However, when periurethral colonization with a potential uropathogen persists, the same strain may be isolated from reinfection. *Relapse* occurs when an infecting organism persists in the urinary tract despite antimicrobial therapy; the same organism is isolated from recurrent infection after therapy.

GENERAL CONCEPTS

HOST DEFENSES OF THE NORMAL URINARY TRACT

The urine and genitourinary tract are normally sterile, apart from the distal urethra. The normal flora of the distal urethra plays an important role in host defense by preventing colonization at this site by potential uropathogens. The flora includes aerobic bacteria that are common skin commensals, such as coagulase-negative staphylococci, viridans group streptococci, and *Corynebacterium* species.[5,6] There is also a large and complex anaerobic flora.[6] Molecular investigations have revealed that multiple additional, as yet unclassified bacteria are also present.[7] Urine is a good nutrient source for most bacterial species, and common uropathogens grow well in urine. The most important host defense that maintains sterility of the urine is normal, unobstructed voiding. An array of urine and uroepithelial cell components also contributes to maintenance of sterile urine in the normal genitourinary tract (Table 37.2).[8,9] Inhibitors of bacterial adherence to uroepithelial cells prevent persistence of bacteria once they have entered the urinary tract. Tamm-Horsfall protein, the most abundant protein in the urine, appears to have an important role in this regard.[9] This protein prevents attachment of *Escherichia coli* to uroepithelial cell receptors by binding to the type 1 fimbria adhesin (FimH) and also removes other uropathogens such as *Klebsiella pneumoniae* and *Staphylococcus saprophyticus*.[10] It may have an immunomodulatory role through activation of the innate immune response by a Toll-like receptor-4–dependent mechanism.[9]

Adherence of bacteria to uroepitheal cells is also prevented by the surface mucopolysaccharide-glycosaminoglycan layer of the uroepithelium, by urine immunoglobulin G (IgG) and secretory immunoglobulin A (IgA), and by some low-molecular-weight oligosaccharides present in the urine. The relative importance of any of these specific components in vivo is not yet established. Despite this array of components contributing to sterility of the urine, bacteriuria is readily established once normal voiding is impaired. In the complicated urinary tract, infection occurs through increased entry of organisms into the bladder or kidney, which may be attributed to the use of urologic devices, turbulent urine flow, or reflux. Organisms may then persist, despite other host defenses, as infected urine is retained if voiding is incomplete or in biofilm on urologic devices.

IMMUNE AND INFLAMMATORY RESPONSES TO URINARY TRACT INFECTION

Urinary tract infection induces a wide spectrum of local and systemic inflammatory and immune responses. The intensity of response is determined by the interactions of microbial pathogenicity, individual genetic regulation, and the site of infection.[11,12] Unique *E. coli* strains have a variable capacity to stimulate or evade activation of the innate immune response. Uropathogenic strains that cause symptomatic infection induce a strong innate immune response, whereas strains isolated from asymptomatic bacteriuria evoke a limited response.[13,14] Strains that successfully evade immune activation probably have a pathogenetic advantage for establishing bladder colonization and persistent infection.[15,16] Host genetic polymorphisms affecting the innate immune response may predispose to acute pyelonephritis or asymptomatic bacteriuria.[12,17]

Infecting organisms in the urinary tract activate uroepithelial cells through Toll-like receptors, resulting in cytokine production, particularly of interleukin-6 (IL-6) and IL-8 (CXCL8). These cytokines recruit neutrophils and other immunocompetent cells to the kidney and bladder.[9,12] Chemokine and cytokine elaboration follow both direct stimulation of uroepithelial cells by bacterial lipopolysaccharide and bacterial adherence to epithelial cells.[18] The chemotactic cytokine IL-8 is released at the mucosal site and recruits polymorphonuclear leukocytes, resulting in pyuria. Urine and serum IL-6 concentrations are correlated with the severity of infection. The highest levels occur in patients with pyelonephritis. Systemic elaboration of IL-1β and IL-6 produces fever and activation of the acute phase response. The acute inflammatory infiltrate of polymorphonuclear leukocytes that develops in renal tissue during pyelonephritis limits bacterial spread and persistence within the kidney but also contributes to tissue damage and renal scarring.

Both IL-6 and IL-8 are also secreted by the bladder urothelium in direct response to bacterial antigens, including lipopolysaccharide.[19] IL-8 induces a rapid influx of neutrophils into the bladder, with subsequent phagocytosis and clearance of bacteria. This innate immune response rapidly clears most uropathogenic *E. coli* organisms from the bladder, but it does not produce a sterilizing immunity in murine models.[19] In humans, bacteriuria often persists despite marked pyuria. A vigorous local and systemic humoral immune response occurs in patients with pyelonephritis.[8,13] The antibody response is directed against surface antigens of the infecting bacteria, including O antigens, and surface proteins such as the type 1 (FimH) and P fimbriae, which are major adhesins of *E. coli*.[19,20] IgM antibodies dominate the systemic humoral response in the first episode of infection in the upper urinary tract, but subsequent episodes are characterized by an IgG response. In pyelonephritis, elevations of IgG antibodies to lipid A are correlated with severity of renal infection and parenchymal destruction. There is also a substantial urinary IgG and secretory IgA antibody response. Despite this robust response, the protective role, if any, of the antibody response in pyelonephritis is not clear. Bacteria often persist in the renal parenchyma despite very high levels of specific antibodies. In addition, in women who do not produce secretory IgA, the frequency of urinary tract infection is not increased.

IgA-producing plasma cells are found in higher numbers in the bladder submucosa of patients with bacterial cystitis than in healthy controls. However, acute cystitis is associated with a reduced or undetectable serologic response, presumably reflecting the superficial nature of the infection. The local immune response is of short duration and is reactivated for each infection. This limited immunologic response to bladder infection may explain why early reinfection with the same *E. coli* strain is observed in some women with acute cystitis. However, animal studies have reported some protection against same-strain reinfection by systemic and local antibodies.[19]

Cell-mediated immunity appears to have a limited role in the host defense against urinary tract infection. A small number of mucosal T lymphocytes are present throughout the urinary tract, and both CD4+ and CD8+ T cells can be found in the submucosa and lamina propria of the bladder and urethra. Recruitment of B and T lymphocytes to the bladder wall is observed with secondary infections. T cell–derived proinflammatory cytokines also stimulate renal tubular epithelial cells to produce IL-6, which may increase IgA secretion of committed B cells.[19] However, women infected with human immunodeficiency virus (HIV) who have very low CD4+ counts do not appear to have an increased susceptibility to or severity of urinary tract infection[21]; this finding suggests that cell-mediated immunity is not an essential defense against such infection.

URINE CULTURE

The definitive diagnosis and appropriate management of urinary tract infection usually require microbiologic confirmation by urine culture. Urine specimens for culture should always be obtained before antimicrobial therapy is initiated because urinary excretion of antimicrobial agents rapidly sterilizes urine. Once collected, the specimen should be forwarded promptly to the laboratory. Organisms present in small quantitative counts (i.e., contaminants) grow readily in urine at room temperature and reach high quantitative counts within a few hours. If the specimen is delayed in reaching the laboratory, it should be refrigerated at 4° C until transported.

A urine specimen for culture must be collected with a method that minimizes contamination. For both men and women, a clean-catch voided specimen without additional periurethral cleaning is usually appropriate. When patients cannot cooperate for the collection of a voided specimen, urine may be collected by an in-and-out catheter. For men, a specimen may be obtained in an external condom catheter after application of a clean condom catheter and collecting bag.[22] Urine samples may also be collected by suprapubic aspiration or directly from the renal pelvis when percutaneous drainage of an obstructed urinary tract is necessary. Specimens obtained from patients with short-term indwelling catheters should be collected by puncture of the catheter port. For a long-term indwelling catheter, two to five organisms are present in the catheter biofilm at any time, so urine collected through the catheter will be contaminated by organisms present in the biofilm.[23] The long-term indwelling catheter should be removed and replaced by a new catheter, and a specimen of bladder urine obtained through the newly placed catheter.[22,23]

The standard quantitative criterion for diagnosis of urinary tract infection with voided specimens is an organism count of 10^5 colony-forming units (CFU) or more per milliliter. Women usually have low numbers of contaminating organisms from vaginal or periurethral flora isolated from voided specimens, and this quantitative criterion distinguishes bacteriuria from contamination. Application of this quantitative standard is always appropriate for the diagnosis of asymptomatic bacteriuria, but for symptomatic cases, the quantitative urine culture results must be interpreted in the context of the clinical presentation and with consideration of the method of specimen collection (Table 37.3). Bacteria require several hours of incubation in bladder urine to achieve a concentration of 10^5 CFU/mL or higher. Some patients with frequency or diuresis may not retain urine in the bladder for a sufficient time to achieve

Table 37.3 Quantitative Counts of Bacteria in the Urine for Microbiologic Diagnosis of Urinary Tract Infection in Patients Not Receiving Antimicrobial Therapy

Collection Method	Quantitative Criteria (CFU/mL)
Voided specimen:	
Asymptomatic women or men	$\geq 10^5$*
Women: acute uncomplicated	
Cystitis	$\geq 10^3$
Pyelonephritis	$\geq 10^4$†
Men: Symptomatic	$\geq 10^3$
External condom collection	$\geq 10^5$
Catheter:	
In-and-out	$\geq 10^2$
Indwelling‡	
Asymptomatic	$\geq 10^5$
Symptomatic	$\geq 10^2$
Suprapubic or percutaneous aspiration	Any growth

*Two consecutive specimens are recommended for women.
†In 95% of cases, values $\geq 10^5$ colony-forming units (CFU) per milliliter.
‡A long-term catheter should be replaced and the specimen collected through a new catheter.

renal tissue, which are correlated with serum levels, determine outcome for pyelonephritis.[24] Treatment of urinary tract infection is unique in some respects because of the exceptionally high urine concentrations achieved by many antimicrobial agents excreted into the urine (Table 37.4). The urine concentration is determined by the interplay of glomerular filtration, active tubular secretion, and tubular reabsorption, all influenced by pH, protein binding, and the molecular structure of the drug. Cystitis and pyelonephritis may be successfully treated with antimicrobial agents at minimum inhibitory concentrations (MICs) to which the infecting organism would not usually be considered susceptible. The "intermediate" susceptibility designation reported by the clinical microbiology laboratory implies clinical efficacy in body sites where antimicrobial agents are physiologically concentrated, such as the urine, and is relevant to treatment of urinary tract infection. Thus, when an organism isolated from the urine is reported to have intermediate susceptibility to an antimicrobial agent, the drug is usually appropriate for treatment of urinary tract infection with that organism. The urine bactericidal activity of some antimicrobial agents is modified by the urine pH. Penicillins, tetracyclines, and nitrofurantoin are more active in acidic urine, and aminoglycosides, fluoroquinolones, and erythromycin are more active in alkaline urine. This pH variability has not, however, been shown to be relevant for therapeutic outcomes, with the exception of methenamine salts, for which an acidic pH is necessary to release formaldehyde, the active component.

The prostate is a unique compartment for consideration of antimicrobial efficacy. There are no active antibiotic transport mechanisms for the gland and most antibiotics penetrate poorly into prostate tissue and fluid.[25,26] The interior of the gland is an acidic environment. Drug entry and activity depend on concentration gradient, protein binding, lipid solubility, molecular size, local pH, and pK_a of the antimicrobial agent. Alkaline drugs such as trimethoprim diffuse into the prostate and are trapped, and high concentrations are thus achieved, but the drug remains in an inactive, ionized form. Fluoroquinolones and macrolides, however, penetrate well and remain active.

Current pharmacodynamic models for antimicrobial treatment of infection distinguish between time-dependent and concentration-dependent bacterial killing. Bacterial killing by β-lactam antimicrobial agents is time dependent; the therapeutic efficacy depends on how long the concentration of the antimicrobial agent remains above the MIC of the infecting organism. Bacterial killing by fluoroquinolones and aminoglycosides is concentration dependent; the therapeutic efficacy is measured by the ratio of peak antimicrobial concentration to MIC, or the ratio of the area under the curve to MIC. A pharmacodynamic model in which the urine bactericidal titer replaces the MIC has been applied to predict optimal dosing regimens for antimicrobial treatment of urinary tract infection.[24,27] The validity of these models for urinary tract infection, however, still requires confirmation in clinical trials.[28,29] In particular, the relevance to treatment of complicated urinary tract infection is uncertain because impaired renal function, voiding abnormalities, and the presence of biofilms introduce variability that may affect antimicrobial efficacy.[27]

the concentration of 10^5 CFU/mL or higher. Quantitative counts may also be lower when infection is caused by some fastidious organisms or if the patient is receiving a urinary antiseptic. For symptomatic men, a single urine specimen in which 10^3 CFU/mL or more of a uropathogen is isolated is diagnostic for bladder bacteriuria, on the basis of paired comparisons of voided specimens and suprapubic aspirates.

A urine specimen obtained by suprapubic aspiration or other percutaneous collection method such as renal pelvis drainage is assumed to be a sterile specimen, and any quantitative count of an organism represents true bacteriuria. However, in specimens collected by an in-and-out catheter, contaminating organisms are introduced from the periurethral area, and a quantitative criteria of 10^2 CFU/mL or higher is recommended. Other relevant considerations in interpreting a urine culture result include the number and type of organisms isolated. A single infecting organism is usual, but in patients with complicated urinary tract infection, particularly those with indwelling urinary devices, more than one organism is frequently present. Commensal bacteria of the normal skin flora, such as diphtheroids and coagulase-negative staphylococci, usually represent contaminants when they are isolated from voided urine specimens. In young healthy women, group B streptococci and *Enterococcus* species isolated in any quantitative count are also usually contaminants.

PHARMACOKINETIC AND PHARMACODYNAMIC CONSIDERATIONS FOR TREATMENT

Therapeutic success in the treatment of cystitis depends on antimicrobial levels in the urine. Antimicrobial levels in

Table 37.4 Urinary Excretion of Antimicrobial Agents in Persons with Normal Renal Function

Antimicrobial Agent	% of Absorbed Drug Excreted Renally as Parent Metabolites (Active Metabolites)*	Usual Dosage for Normal Renal Function†
Penicillins		
Penicillin G	80	1-2 million U IV q4-6h
Amoxicillin	90	500 mg PO tid
Amoxicillin/clavulanic acid	Clavulanate: 20-60	500 mg PO tid or 875 mg PO bid
Ampicillin	90 (10)	1-2 g IV q6h
Cloxacillin	35-50	1-2 g IV q4-6h
Piperacillin	50-80	200-300 mg/kg/day IV qid
Piperacillin/tazobactam	Tazobactam: 60-80	3.375 g IV q6h
Pivmecillinam	45	200-400 mg bid or tid
Cephalosporins		
Cephalexin	>80 (18)	500 mg PO qid
Cefazolin	>80	1 g IV q8h
Cefuroxime	>80	250-500 mg PO bid
Cefotaxime	50-60 (30)	1 g IV q8h
Ceftriaxone	50	1-2 g IV q24h
Cefepime	85	1-2 g PO q12h
Cefixime	15-20	400 mg PO qd
Cefpodoxime	20-35	100-200 mg PO q12h
Cefprozil	60	250-500 mg PO q12h
Ceftazidime	80-90	1-2g IV q8-12h
Ceftaroline	50	600 mg I V q12h
Macrolides, Lincosamides		
Erythromycin	5-15	500 mg PO qid or 1g IV q6h
Clindamycin	≤6 (some active metabolites)	150-300 mg PO tid or 600-900 mg IV q6-8h
Clarithromycin	20-30 (10-15)	250-500 mg PO q12h
Azithromycin	6	500 mg PO qd
Aminoglycosides		
Gentamicin	99	5 mg/kg/day IV in 1-3 divided doses
Tobramycin	99	5 mg/kg/day IV in 1-3 divided doses
Amikacin	99	15 mg/kg/day IV in 1-3 divided doses
Carbapenems		
Imipenem/cilastatin	70-76	500 mg IV q6h
Meropenem	70-80	500 mg to 1 g IV q6-8h
Ertapenem	40	1g IV q24h
Doripenem	70 (15)	500 mg q8h
Fluoroquinolones		
Norfloxacin	25-40 (10-20)	400 mg bid
Ciprofloxacin	40 (10-20)	250-750 mg PO or 400 mg IV bid
Levofloxacin	70-80	250-750 mg PO or IV q24h
Moxifloxacin	20	400 mg PO or IV q24h
Other Antibacterials		
Vancomycin	>90	1 g IV q12h
Teicoplanin	>90	6-12 mg/kg IV q12h
Dalbavancin	42	1g IV
Daptomycin	54	4 mg/kg IV q24h
Linezolid	35	600 mg PO or IV q12h
Tigecycline	32	250-500 mg IV q6h div q12h
Colistin	64-70	1.5-2.5 mg/kg/day
Trimethoprim	66-95	100 mg PO q12h
Sulfamethoxazole	20-40	
Trimethoprim/sulfamethoxazole		180/800 mg PO bid
Nitrofurantoin monohydrate/macrocrystals	40-60	50-100 mg PO q6h

Continued on following page

Table 37.4 Urinary Excretion of Antimicrobial Agents in Persons with Normal Renal Function (Continued)

Antimicrobial Agent	% of Absorbed Drug Excreted Renally as Parent Metabolites (Active Metabolites)*	Usual Dosage for Normal Renal Function†
Fosfomycin tromethamine	30-60	3g, one dose
Doxycycline	20-30	100 mg PO bid
Aztreonam	66	1-2 g IV q6-8h
Metronidazole	15 (30-60)	500 mg PO or IV tid
Rifampin	<10/50	600 mg PO qd
Antifungals		
Amphotericin B deoxycholate	<10	0.5-1 mg/kg IV qd
Amphotericin B lipid formulations	<1	1-5 mg/kg/day IV
5-Flucytosine	90	100-150 mg/kg/day PO in 4 divided doses
Ketoconazole	<10	400 mg PO qd
Fluconazole	80	100-400 mg PO or IV q24h
Itraconazole	<1	200 mg bid PO or IV × 2 days, then 200 mg PO qd
Voriconazole	<1	6 mg/kg IV × 1 dose, then 200 mg IV bid; 200-mg PO bid × 1 day, then 100 mg bid
Posaconazole	<1	400 mg PO bid
Caspofungin	<1	70-mg loading dose, then 50 mg IV q24h
Micafungin	<1	50-100 mg IV q24h
Anidulafungin	<1	100- to 200-mg IV loading dose, then 50-100 mg IV q24h

*Except where noted, values are the proportion of dose renally excreted unchanged.
†Not all antimicrobial agents have an indication for urinary tract infection.
bid, Twice a day; IV, intravenous; PO, by mouth; qd, once a day; qid, four times a day; tid, twice a day.

USUAL PRESENTATIONS OF URINARY TRACT INFECTION

ACUTE UNCOMPLICATED URINARY TRACT INFECTION: CYSTITIS

EPIDEMIOLOGY

Acute uncomplicated urinary tract infection manifesting as acute cystitis is a common syndrome that affects otherwise healthy women.[1] About 10% of young, sexually active, premenopausal women experience a urinary tract infection each year, and 60% of all women have one or more such infections in their lifetimes.[30] From 2% to 5% of women experience frequent recurrent infection for at least some period. After a first episode of cystitis, 21% of female college students in one study reported a second infection within 6 months.[31] Among postmenopausal women aged 55 to 75 years who were enrolled in a Seattle health group, the incidence was seven infections per 100 patient-years; in 24 months, 7% of women had one infection, 1.6% had two infections, and 1% had three or more infections.[32] Despite the frequency of this condition, there has been little systematic evaluation of the impact on quality of life.[33] Acute cystitis is associated with considerable short-term morbidity, with female college students reporting that symptoms persisted for an average of 6.1 days.[2] In another survey of ambulatory women with cystitis, the mean duration of symptoms was reported to be 4.9 days, and for 63% of patients, their usual activities were compromised by the infection.[34] However, despite the large number of women affected, including many with frequent recurrence of infection, there is no long-term morbidity. Acute uncomplicated urinary tract infection is uncommon in healthy young men, with an estimated incidence of less than 0.1% per year.

PATHOGENESIS

Microbiology

Acute uncomplicated urinary tract infection is primarily a disease of extraintestinal pathogenic *E. coli*, also referred to as *uropathogenic E. coli*. These organisms are isolated in 80% to 85% of episodes of acute cystitis.[32,35] Infection occurs via the ascending route after bacterial strains that usually originate in the gut flora colonize the vagina or periurethral area.[6] Although urethral colonization with a potential uropathogen appears to be a prerequisite for infection, cystitis does not subsequently develop in most women with periurethral colonization.[6] Strains of *E. coli* that colonize the periurethral area and subsequently cause urinary tract infection belong to a restricted number of phylogenetic *E. coli* groups and more frequently express diverse virulence factors than do periurethral strains that do not cause symptomatic infection.[36,37] A necessary characteristic for establishing bladder infection is production of FimH, an adhesin attaching to receptors on uroepithelial cells.[38] This surface protein, however, is common on *E. coli* strains, regardless of whether they cause infection. Other potential urovirulence characteristics include adhesins, iron sequestration systems, and toxins.[37] However, the putative virulence factors produced by strains isolated from symptomatic infection overlap with those produced in asymptomatic infection, and no single characteristic is uniquely correlated with symptomatic infection.[39] Uropathogenic *E. coli* strains may be acquired during travel and from ingestion of food or water, and are transmitted among household members, including pets, and between sexual partners.[40,41] Clonal outbreaks may occur with transmission of a single strain within a community or larger geographic area.[42]

S. saprophyticus, a coagulase-negative staphylococcal species, is an organism virtually unique to acute cystitis. It is the second most frequently isolated species (in 5% to 10% of episodes), and there is a seasonal variation of infection, with isolation more common in late summer or fall. Genetic elements described in the *S. saprophyticus* genome that may promote urovirulence include adhesins, transport systems to support growth in urine, and urease production.[43] Other Enterobacteriaceae, most commonly *K. pneumoniae*, are isolated in fewer than 5% of premenopausal women but in 10% to 15% of postmenopausal women.[32,44] Gram-positive organisms such as *Enterococcus* species and group B streptococci are uncommon pathogens in premenopausal women. *Salmonella* species and bacteria associated with sexually transmitted infections, such as *Ureaplasma urealyticum*, *Gardnerella vaginalis*, and *Mycoplasma hominis*, are occasionally isolated.[45]

Acute uncomplicated urinary tract infection recurs frequently and is characteristically reinfection. In as many as 30% of early reinfections—those occurring within 1 month of treatment of an episode of acute cystitis—an *E. coli* strain similar to the pretherapy strain is isolated. This finding is assumed to be a consequence of failure of the antimicrobial therapy to eliminate virulent strains from the gut or vaginal flora reservoirs.[2] Intracellular persistence of *E. coli* in uroepithelial cells is an alternative mechanism proposed to explain same-strain recurrence, on the basis of observations in animal studies.[46,47] However, prospective studies in women document periurethral colonization prior to infection onset for most episodes,[48] and the contribution of an intracellular reservoir to recurrent acute uncomplicated cystitis in humans remains uncertain.

Host Factors

Acute, uncomplicated urinary tract infection is a consequence of the interaction of a virulent organism with host genetic susceptibility and behavioral variables.[8,11] The notion of genetic propensity is supported by two consistent observations: (1) an increased frequency of urinary tract infection in first-degree female relatives of women with recurrent infection[1,49] and (2) the fact that infection at a younger age is a major risk factor for recurrent cystitis in women of any age.[1,32,49] One well-characterized genetic association is being a nonsecretor of the ABH blood-group antigens.[49,50] Women with recurrent urinary tract infection are at least three times more likely to be nonsecretors than are those without recurrent infection. Nonsecretors express cell-surface glycosphingolipids on the vaginal epithelium and, presumably, urethral mucosa that differ from those expressed by secretors and that bind uropathogenic *E. coli* more avidly.[11] Other potential genetic determinants include genetic polymorphisms of the IL-8 receptor CXCR1, Toll-like receptors, and the tumor necrosis factor promoter.[11]

The most important behavioral association of urinary tract infection in premenopausal women is sexual intercourse.[1,2,51] In young, sexually active women, 75% to 90% of episodes are attributable to intercourse, and there is a correlation between frequency of intercourse and frequency of infection.[50] Intercourse appears to promote infection by facilitating ascension of organisms from the periurethral area into the bladder. Spermicide use for birth control is another independent behavioral risk factor for acute cystitis in premenopausal women. The frequency of recurrent infection is at least twice as high among women who use spermicides as among women who do not.[50] Spermicides are bactericidal for the hydrogen peroxide–producing lactobacilli of the normal vaginal flora, which maintain the acidic pH. If these bacteria are not present, elevation of vaginal pH facilitates colonization with potential uropathogens, such as *E. coli*. Case-control studies have consistently demonstrated that behavioral variables popularly identified as risks for cystitis—such as type of underwear, bathing rather than showering, postcoital voiding, frequency of voiding, perineal hygiene practices, vaginal douching, and tampon use—are not associated with an increased risk of infection.[52]

A history of prior urinary tract infection at a younger age is the strongest association of recurrent acute cystitis in postmenopausal women.[53-55] Sexual intercourse is not an important contributor.[55,56] Estrogen deficiency has been proposed to promote recurrent urinary tract infection in these women through alterations in vaginal flora, including replacement of lactobacilli by potential uropathogens. However, prospective cohort studies and case-control studies uniformly demonstrate no association of oral or topical estrogen use with recurrent urinary tract infection, regardless of restoration of vaginal lactobacilli and acid pH.[57] Acute uncomplicated urinary tract infection in men is uncommon, but reported risk factors have included intercourse with a female partner with recurrent urinary tract infection, not being circumcised, and anal intercourse.

DIAGNOSIS

The classic clinical manifestation of symptomatic lower urinary tract infection is the acute onset of one or more irritative bladder symptoms, such as urgency, frequency, dysuria, stranguria, and hesitancy.[1] Gross hematuria is also common. The differential diagnosis includes sexually transmitted infections, vulvovaginal candidiasis, and noninfectious syndromes such as interstitial cystitis. The combination of new-onset frequency, dysuria, and urgency, together with the absence of vaginal discharge and pain, has a positive predictive value for acute cystitis of 90%.[58] Women who experience recurrent infection also have more than 90% accuracy in self-diagnosis on the basis of symptoms.[2]

A urine culture is not recommended routinely for women with a clinical presentation consistent with acute uncomplicated cystitis.[45,59] The utility of the urine culture is limited by the reliability of the clinical diagnosis, predictable microbiology, and prompt clinical response with short-course empirical antimicrobial therapy. Final culture results are often not available until therapy is completed, and quantitative bacterial counts of less than 10^5 CFU/mL are isolated in as many as 30% of women with acute cystitis.[60] Therefore, interpretation of culture results may be problematic.[1,45] In fact, urine culture results are negative in as many as 10% of women with a characteristic clinical presentation, and these women have a clinical response to antimicrobial therapy similar to that of women with positive cultures.[60] This high proportion of women who have low quantitative counts of organisms in the urine culture has been suggested to reflect urethritis, rather than cystitis. However, both urinary frequency and increased fluid intake are characteristic of patients with acute cystitis. Thus, the limited dwell time of urine in the bladder seems the likely explanation for the observation of a high frequency of urine cultures with lower quantitative counts. Culture results may be negative because organisms are present in quantitative counts below the level of detection by standard laboratory procedures (usually <10^3 CFU/mL) or because fastidious organisms may not be identified by routine laboratory procedures used in processing urine specimens.

A urine specimen for culture should be obtained, however, from selected women with possible acute uncomplicated urinary tract infection. When the clinical presentation is not characteristic, a urine culture may help confirm or exclude the diagnosis of urinary tract infection. Failure to respond to appropriate empirical antimicrobial therapy or an early (<1 month) symptomatic recurrence after therapy is suggestive of infection with a resistant organism. In these situations, a urine culture should be obtained to confirm whether antimicrobial resistance is present and to facilitate selection of an effective alternative regimen.

The presence of pyuria, identified by routine urinalysis or leukocyte esterase dipstick testing, is a consistent accompaniment of acute cystitis.[1,59] The absence of pyuria is suggestive of an alternative diagnosis but does not rule out urinary tract infection in women with a consistent clinical presentation.[1,61-63] Thus, routine screening for pyuria is not recommended in the management of women presenting with presumed acute cystitis.[1,59] A urine nitrite dipstick test screens for the presence of bacteria, rather than leukocytes, and results are usually positive in women with infection.[63] False-negative nitrite test results may occur when there is infection with bacteria that do not reduce nitrate, such as *Enterococcus* species, or when urine has not been retained in the bladder a sufficient time to allow bacteria to convert nitrate to nitrite. Nitrite tests uncommonly have false-positive results, but these may occur when blood, urobilinogen, or some dyes are present in the urine.

TREATMENT

For many women, the natural history of acute uncomplicated cystitis is spontaneous clinical and microbiologic resolution within a few days or weeks. In a clinical trial in which subjects were randomly assigned to receive antibiotic therapy or placebo, 28% of 277 women who received placebo were asymptomatic by 1 week, and 45% had negative culture results by 6 weeks.[64] In another study, 54% of women who received placebo were asymptomatic by 3 days and 52% at 7 days.[65] However, antimicrobial treatment is associated with a significantly shorter duration of symptoms. The rates of clinical cure were 77% with nitrofurantoin, in comparison with 54% with placebo at 3 days, and 88% and 52%, respectively, at 7 days.[65] After initiation of antimicrobial therapy, 54% of women reported symptom improvement by 6 hours, 87% by 24 hours, and 91% by 48 hours. In another case series, 72% of women reported complete symptom resolution by the fourth day of effective treatment.[34]

Many antimicrobial agents are effective for treatment of acute cystitis (Table 37.5). The anticipated cure rate for recommended first-line empirical regimens is 80% to 95%.[66] Trimethoprim/sulfamethoxazole (TMP/SMX) has been a mainstay of empirical treatment of acute cystitis for decades and remains highly effective against susceptible organisms.[66,67] However, increasing rates of TMP/SMX resistance in community *E. coli* isolates compromise the use of this agent as first-line empirical therapy. Some antimicrobial

Table 37.5 Preferred Antimicrobial Regimens for Treatment or Prevention of Acute Uncomplicated Urinary Cystitis in Women with Normal Renal Function

First-Line Therapy	Other Therapy
Acute Cystitis	
TMP/SMX, 160/800 mg bid × 3 days	Norfloxacin, 400 mg bid × 3 days
Nitrofurantoin, 50-100 mg qid, or monohydrate/macrocrystals, 100 mg bid × 5 days*	Ciprofloxacin, 250 mg bid, or extended-release preparation, 500 mg qd × 3 days
Pivmecillinam, 400 mg bid × 5 days or 200 mg bid × 7 days*	Levofloxacin, 250-500 mg qd × 3 days
Fosfomycin trometanol, 3 g single dose*	Trimethoprim, 100 mg bid × 3 days
	Amoxicillin 500 mg tid × 7 days*
	Amoxicillin/clavulanic acid, 500 mg tid or 875 mg bid × 7 days*
	Cephalexin, 250-500 mg qid × 7 days*
	Cefpodoxime proxetil, 100 mg bid × 3 days
	Cefuroxime axetil, 500 mg bid × 7 days*
	Cefixime, 400 mg qd × 7 days*
	Doxycycline, 100 mg bid × 7 days
Prophylaxis	
Long-Term Low-Dose Regimens (at Bedtime)	
Nitrofurantoin, 50 mg qd, or monohydrate/macrocrystals, 100 mg qd	Cephalexin, 500 mg qd*
	Norfloxacin, 200 mg every other day
TMP/SMX, 40/200 mg od or every other day	Ciprofloxacin, 125 mg qd
	Trimethoprim, 100 mg qd
Postcoital (Single-Dose) Regimen	
TMP/SMX, 40/200 mg or 80/400 mg	Cephalexin, 250 mg*
Trimethoprim, 100 mg	Norfloxacin, 200 mg
Nitrofurantoin, 50 or 100 mg*	Ciprofloxacin, 125 mg

*Recommended for pregnant women.
bid, Twice a day; PO, by mouth; qd, once a day; qid, four times a day; tid, twice a day; TMP/SMX, trimethoprim/sulfamethoxazole.

agents—nitrofurantoin, pivmecillinam, and fosfomycin—have indications largely restricted to acute cystitis. These drugs do not induce cross-resistance with other classes of antimicrobial agents and to date, limited resistance has been observed in community uropathogens. Thus, they are ecologically attractive for treatment of acute cystitis.[66] Fosfomycin and pivmecillinam, however, are not available in all countries, and results of clinical trials suggest that these agents may be 5% to 10% less effective than TMP/SMX or fluoroquinolones. The fluoroquinolones—norfloxacin, ciprofloxacin, and levofloxacin—are not generally recommended as first-line therapy because of concerns that their widespread use will lead to the emergence of resistance. Fluoroquinolones with limited urinary excretion, such as moxifloxacin, are not indicated for treatment of urinary tract infection.

β-Lactam antimicrobial agents, including amoxicillin, amoxicillin/clavulanic acid, and cephalosporins, are reported to be 10% to 15% less effective than first-line agents.[66,68] The β-Lactam agents are useful, however, for treatment in pregnant women because they are safe for the fetus.[45] To limit adverse effects, cost, and emergence of bacterial resistance, the shortest effective duration of antimicrobial therapy should be prescribed. For TMP/SMX and the fluoroquinolones, 3 days is optimum.[66] The duration of nitrofurantoin therapy is 5 days.[69] For β-lactam antimicrobial agents, 7 days is recommended; shorter courses are less effective. Fosfomycin is given as a single dose; multiple doses of this antimicrobial are associated with rapid emergence of resistance. Single-dose therapy is not recommended for other agents because a single dose is generally 5% to 10% less effective than the recommended longer regimens.[45,66]

The antimicrobial susceptibility of uropathogenic *E. coli* strains acquired in the community evolves continually in response to antimicrobial pressure.[35,70,71] Resistance in community isolates has compromised the efficacy of ampicillin, cephalosporins, and TMP/SMX for use as empirical therapy, and growing resistance to fluoroquinolones has been reported.[35] Recent prior antimicrobial therapy is most strongly associated with isolation of a resistant organism.[72] Treatment of cystitis with an antimicrobial agent to which the infecting organism is resistant is associated with a high failure rate, despite very high urinary levels of the drug.[73,74] In fact, cure rates when the organism is resistant to the antimicrobial agent are similar to those reported with placebo: about 50%. If the local prevalence of resistance to an antimicrobial agent in community *E. coli* strains exceeds 20%, that agent should not be used for first-line empirical therapy.[66] The current expansion of extended-spectrum β-lactamase (ESBL)–producing *E. coli* in community-acquired infections is of particular concern because these strains are usually also resistant to TMP/SMX and fluoroquinolones.[75] Optimal treatment of infection with ESBL-producing *E. coli* is not yet well defined. Nitrofurantoin, fosfomycin trometanol, and pivmecillinam currently remain effective for many of these strains. Amoxicillin/clavulanic acid may also be effective for some strains.[76]

A 2010 pilot study reported similar resolution of cystitis symptoms whether treatment was given with an antimicrobial, with ciprofloxacin, or with only the nonsteroidal anti-inflammatory ibuprofen.[77] This preliminary observation suggests that symptom treatment alone may be as effective as antimicrobial therapy for managing acute episodes but requires confirmation in further clinical trials.

OTHER INVESTIGATIONS

Young women with a characteristic clinical presentation and prompt response following appropriate empirical therapy do not require further diagnostic imaging or urologic investigation.[78] Fewer than 5% of these women have urologic abnormalities, and the few women in whom abnormalities are identified usually do not require further intervention. However, investigation may be appropriate to rule out alternative pathologic processes when the diagnosis is uncertain or clinical presentation is atypical.

RECURRENT INFECTION

Episodes of acute cystitis recur frequently in many women. Effective control can be achieved with low-dose prophylactic antimicrobial therapy given either daily or every other day at bedtime or after intercourse (see Table 37.5). This strategy is recommended for women who experience more than two episodes in 6 months. The initial course of prophylaxis lasts 6 or 12 months. Antimicrobial prophylactic therapy decreases recurrent symptomatic episodes by about 95% while the agent is being taken, but it does not alter the frequency of recurrent infection once prophylaxis is discontinued. About 50% of women experience reinfection within 3 months of discontinuing prophylaxis. Reinstitution of prophylaxis for as long as 2 years is appropriate for these women. Self-treatment is another effective strategy for managing recurrent infections; this approach is often preferred by women who are traveling or who experience less frequent recurrences.[2] A 3-day course of TMP/SMX or ciprofloxacin has been shown to be effective for empirical self-treatment in clinical trials, but other regimens are also probably effective.

The only feasible behavioral intervention to prevent recurrent urinary tract infection is to avoid spermicide use. Other proposed nonantimicrobial approaches for prevention include daily intake of cranberry products, oral or vaginal probiotics to reestablish normal vaginal flora, and estrogen replacement for postmenopausal women.[79,80] Initial studies reported that daily intake of cranberry juice or tablets decreased episodes of recurrent cystitis by 30% in comparison with placebo.[81] The proposed mechanism for this effect is inhibition of the P fimbria–mediated adherence of *E. coli* to uroepithelial cells by the proanthocyanidins present in cranberry products and excreted in the urine. However, later large clinical trials reported no benefit of daily cranberry juice in comparison with placebo[82] and that cranberry capsules were less effective than TMP/SMX prophylaxis.[83] Although one clinical trial reported some efficacy of a *Lactobacillus crispatus* probiotic to prevent recurrent infection,[84] other trials of oral or vaginal *Lactobacillus* probiotics have reported no efficacy of these products in preventing urinary tract infection.[85,86] The role of estrogen replacement to prevent urinary tract infection in postmenopausal women is controversial.[2,87] In prospective clinical trials, researchers have uniformly reported no benefit of systemic estrogen over placebo, despite restoration of an acidic vaginal pH and increased vaginal colonization with lactobacilli in subjects who received estrogen.[57] Two small clinical trials comparing vaginal estrogen with placebo in postmenopausal women with frequent, recurrent infection demonstrated a decreased frequency of symptomatic episodes in women treated with topical estrogen therapy, but in a comparative trial, an estrogen-containing pessary was substantially less effective than nitrofurantoin prophylaxis.[57,88] Currently, topical vaginal estrogen should only be considered for use to prevent infection in selected women with a very high frequency of recurrent infection.

Several other potential nonantimicrobial approaches for prevention of recurrent urinary tract infection are under investigation.[46,89,90] These include strategies to block bacterial FimH adhesion, vaccination using FimH or iron receptors, and immune stimulation with heat-killed whole bacteria.[90] The clinical efficacy of any of these interventions remains uncertain.

ACUTE NONOBSTRUCTIVE PYELONEPHRITIS

EPIDEMIOLOGY

Pyelonephritis is a less common manifestation of acute uncomplicated urinary tract infection than cystitis. The ratio of pyelonephritis to cystitis episodes is reported to be between 18:1 and 29:1 in women with recurrent infection.[2] The highest incidence is among women aged 20 to 30 years. Pyelonephritis is associated with substantial morbidity; hospitalization is required for as many as 20% of affected nonpregnant women.[91] Severe manifestations such as sepsis syndrome are, however, uncommon. Acute pyelonephritis complicates 1% to 2% of pregnancies. When this complication occurs at the end of the second trimester or early in the third trimester, preterm labor and delivery may occur and lead to poor fetal outcomes, as with any febrile illness in later pregnancy.[92]

Acute nonobstructive pyelonephritis is rarely a direct cause of renal failure. In the few reports of renal failure attributed to pyelonephritis, the patients were elderly[93] or had comorbid conditions such as diabetes and HIV infection.[94] Renal scarring is a complication of pyelonephritis in some women with more severe clinical presentations. An Italian study reported renal scars identified by computed tomography (CT) or magnetic resonance imaging (MRI) at a 6-month follow-up in 29% of women who required hospitalization for pyelonephritis.[95] In an Israeli study, 30% of a cohort of 203 women admitted for acute pyelonephritis were reassessed 10 to 20 years after admission; renal scars were detected in 46% of these women on technetium Tc 99m–labeled dimercaptosuccinic acid scanning. However, the renal scars were not associated with hypertension or renal impairment.[96] The histologic finding of "chronic pyelonephritis" in patients with renal failure was formerly attributed to infection. However, this condition is now recognized as an end stage of many chronic inflammatory conditions of the kidney, and it is attributable to infection in only a few patients in whom there is a clear history of renal infection.

PATHOGENESIS

E. coli is isolated in 85% to 90% of women who present with acute uncomplicated pyelonephritis.[2,97] Infecting strains are characterized by production of the P fimbria adhesin Gal(α1-4) Galβ disaccharide galabiose. This surface protein appears to have a direct role in the pathogenesis of pyelonephritis through induction of mucosal inflammation.[37,98] A familial susceptibility to pyelonephritis has been reported and attributed to polymorphisms with decreased expression of the IL-8 receptor.[99] Other genetic and behavioral risk factors for pyelonephritis in healthy women are similar to those described for acute uncomplicated cystitis.[97] For premenopausal women, these associations are frequency of sexual intercourse, history of urinary tract infection, history of urinary tract infection in the patient's mother, a new sexual partner, and recent spermicide use. The strongest association is with recent sexual intercourse. Diabetes is also an independent risk factor for pyelonephritis. Young diabetic women are 15 times more likely to be hospitalized for pyelonephritis than age-matched nondiabetic women. Behavioral risk factors associated with pyelonephritis in postmenopausal women have not yet been described.

DIAGNOSIS

The classic clinical manifestation of renal infection is costovertebral angle pain or tenderness, often accompanied by fever and variable lower urinary tract symptoms. There is a wide spectrum of severity, however, from mild irritative symptoms with minimal costovertebral angle tenderness to severe symptoms that may include high fever, nausea and vomiting, and severe pain. Acute cholecystitis, renal colic, and pelvic inflammatory disease are occasionally confused with pyelonephritis. When patients present with severe symptoms, underlying complicating factors such as obstruction and abscess must be excluded. A urine specimen for culture should be obtained before initiation of antimicrobial therapy in every case of suspected pyelonephritis. The culture will confirm the diagnosis of urinary tract infection and identify the specific infecting organism and susceptibilities so that antimicrobial therapy can be optimized. In 95% of women with pyelonephritis, 10^5 CFU/mL of organisms or more are isolated from the urine culture.

Bacteremia is identified in 10% to 25% of women presenting with acute pyelonephritis if blood culture specimens are collected routinely. However, the clinical utility of routine blood cultures is limited because bacteremia does not alter therapy, nor is it predictive of outcome.[100,101] Thus blood cultures should be obtained selectively, usually only if the diagnosis is uncertain or the clinical presentation is severe. Growth of the same organism from both blood and urine usually confirms a urinary source for the infection. However, bacteria isolated from the urine are occasionally attributable to bacteremia from a source outside the urinary tract. This finding may reflect hematogenous seeding with development of renal microabscesses, which is well described for *Staphylococcus aureus* in particular.[102] The proportion of cases in which *S. aureus* bacteriuria has a nonurinary source, however, is controversial.[102,103]

Additional investigations recommended for most patients presenting with acute pyelonephritis are measurements of peripheral leukocyte count and serum creatinine level. The leukocyte count is usually elevated and may be useful as a parameter to monitor the response to therapy. C-reactive protein and procalcitonin values are elevated in most women with acute pyelonephritis and tend to correlate with severity of presentation.[2,104,105] The serum procalcitonin value at presentation is a marker for bacteremia[106] and septic shock,[107] but it does not reliably discriminate between patients requiring inpatient therapy and those who can undergo outpatient therapy[108] and is not predictive of outcome.[104] An elevated C-reactive protein value at discharge has been associated with prolonged hospitalization and postdischarge recurrence.[105]

DIAGNOSTIC IMAGING

When the clinical presentation of pyelonephritis is mild or moderate and the clinical response after initiation of antimicrobial therapy is prompt, routine diagnostic imaging is not indicated.[45,109] Women whose clinical presentations are severe, in whom treatment fails, or who experience early posttreatment recurrent infection should undergo prompt imaging to rule out obstruction or abscesses and to determine whether intervention is necessary. Ultrasonography is often the initial imaging modality because it is safe and widely accessible.[110] The ultrasound examination in women with uncomplicated pyelonephritis usually yields normal results, but enlargement and edema in one or both kidneys are observed in 20% of patients.[111] Ultrasonography is less sensitive or specific for pyelonephritis than is either CT or MRI.

The optimal diagnostic imaging is contrast-enhanced CT.[111] Abnormalities observed on CT are characterized as unilateral or bilateral, focal or diffuse, focal swelling or no focal swelling, and renal enlargement or no renal enlargement.[110] In addition to renal enlargement and edema, dilation of the collecting system in the absence of obstruction, wedge-shaped areas of decreased attenuation, and rounded low-attenuation masses with delayed enhancement may be observed. Obstruction of the renal tubules by inflammatory debris or impaired function with tubular ischemia may result in a "striated nephrogram."[110] Abnormalities within the renal cortex and medulla, inflammatory changes in Gerota's fascia or the renal sinuses, and thickening of the urothelium are sometimes observed. *Acute focal pyelonephritis* (or acute lobar nephronia) is infection confined to a single lobe and may be more common in women who have diabetes or are immunocompromised. The response to treatment is similar, however, for patients with or without this imaging finding.[111] In one study the presence of a focal lesion characterized by peripheral ring enhancement without central uptake of contrast material on CT or MRI at presentation was the only imaging finding that was correlated with subsequent development of renal scars.[95]

TREATMENT

The majority of women with uncomplicated pyelonephritis receive treatment as outpatients.[45,66] Indications for hospitalization include pregnancy, hemodynamic instability, uncertain gastrointestinal absorption or compliance with oral therapy, the need to exclude complicating factors such as obstruction and abscess, and the necessity of monitoring or treatment of associated medical illnesses. Appropriate supportive management for hypotension, nausea and vomiting, and pain should be initiated promptly. When oral tolerance is uncertain because of nausea and vomiting, a strategy frequently used in emergency department management is to provide a single parenteral dose of ceftriaxone, 1 g, or of gentamicin, 120 mg, followed by oral therapy once gastrointestinal symptoms are controlled.

Many parenteral antimicrobial regimens are effective for pyelonephritis (Table 37.6). Options for empiric parenteral therapy include aminoglycosides, extended-spectrum cephalosporins such as cefotaxime and ceftriaxone, and fluoroquinolones such as ciprofloxacin or levofloxacin.[2,66] Aminoglycosides have unique efficacy for the treatment of renal infection in that they are bound in high concentrations in the renal cortex.[2] Ceftriaxone therapy is the preferred empirical regimen for pregnant women. Although it is suggested that gentamicin be avoided in pregnancy because of potential fetal ototoxicity, excess otologic impairment has not been reported in large cohorts of newborn infants stratified by gentamicin exposure in utero.[112] Thus, when cephalosporins cannot be used because of antimicrobial resistance or patient intolerance, gentamicin remains an alternate antimicrobial for treatment of pregnant women.

A satisfactory clinical response is usually observed by 48 to 72 hours after initiation of antimicrobial therapy. Oral therapy selected on the basis of urine culture results can then be prescribed to complete the antimicrobial course. In most young, nonpregnant women, acute pyelonephritis is effectively managed with outpatient oral therapy (see Table 37.6).[45,66] The recommended empirical antimicrobial choice

Table 37.6 Antimicrobial Regimens for Treatment of Acute Uncomplicated Pyelonephritis in Women with Normal Renal Function and Susceptible Organisms

First-Line Therapy	Other Therapy
Oral	
Ciprofloxacin, 500 mg bid or 1000 mg extended-release preparation, qd × 7 days	TMP/SMX, 160/800 mg bid × 7-14 days
Levofloxacin, 750 qd × 5 days	Amoxicillin, 500 mg PO tid × 14 days*
	Amoxicillin/clavulanic acid, 500 mg tid or 875 mg PO bid × 14 days*
	Cephalexin, 500 mg qid × 14 days*
	Cefuroxime axetil, 500 mg bid × 14 days*
	Cefixime, 400 mg qd × 14 days*
Parenteral†	
Ciprofloxacin, 400 mg q12h × 7 days	Ertapenem, 1 g qd
Levofloxacin, 750 mg qd × 5 days	Meropenem, 500 mg q6h
Gentamicin or tobramycin, 3-5 mg/kg qd, ± ampicillin, 1 g q4-6h	Piperacillin/tazobactam, 3.375 g q6h
Ceftriaxone, 1-2 g qd*	Doripenem 500 mg q8h
Cefotaxime, 1 g q8h*	

*Recommended for pregnant women.
†Change to oral therapy to complete course once condition is clinically stable.
bid, Twice a day; PO, by mouth; qd, once a day; qid, four times a day; tid, twice a day; TMP/SMX, trimethoprim/sulfamethoxazole.

is either ciprofloxacin or levofloxacin.[66] Oral TMP/SMX is effective, but because of the high prevalence of TMP/SMX-resistant *E. coli* in many communities, this agent is recommended only when the infecting organism is known to be susceptible. Other oral regimens are also effective and may be appropriate, depending on organism susceptibility and the patient's tolerance. The usual duration of treatment is 10 to 14 days, but ciprofloxacin, 500 mg twice daily given for 5 or 7 days, is effective,[113,114] and levofloxacin 750 mg daily for 5 days is also effective.[115]

As previously discussed, women with pyelonephritis are usually afebrile with substantial improvement or resolution of other symptoms by 48 to 72 hours after initiation of effective therapy. Risk factors predictive of a poor outcome are hospitalization, isolation of a resistant organism, concurrent diabetes mellitus, and history of renal stones.[116] All these variables are suggestive of greater severity of illness at presentation or of a complicated infection. Prophylactic antimicrobial strategies similar to those for recurrent cystitis are effective for prevention of recurrent uncomplicated pyelonephritis.

COMPLICATED URINARY TRACT INFECTION

EPIDEMIOLOGY

The frequency of complicated urinary tract infection varies, depending on the underlying genitourinary abnormality (see Table 37.1).[3,4] Some individuals with a transient abnormality, such as pyelonephritis that complicates passage of a ureteric stone, may experience only a single infection. Other patients, including those with indwelling devices or persistent obstruction, may experience frequent recurrent infections. For instance, in men with spinal cord injury in whom voiding is managed with an indwelling catheter, the incidence is 2.72 infections/1000 days; when voiding is managed with intermittent catheterization, the incidence is 0.41/1000 days.[117] In residents of long-term care facilities with long-term indwelling urethral catheters, the incidence of symptomatic infection is 3.2/1000 catheter days.[118]

Complicated urinary tract infection is a frequent cause of hospitalization. The urinary tract is the most common source of community-acquired bacteremia,[119,120] and most bacteremic episodes of urinary tract infection are attributable to complicated infection.[121] Patients who have obstruction or an indwelling catheter or who have undergone recent manipulation of the urinary tract with mucosal bleeding are at greatest risk of bacteremia and severe sepsis. The genitourinary tract is the source of infection in 10% of patients admitted to critical care units with septic shock.[122]

These patients are also at risk for local suppurative complications, such as renal or perinephric abscess, or metastatic infection after bacteremia, such as septic arthritis, osteomyelitis, or endocarditis. Serious complications are more common in patients who are diabetic, are immunocompromised, or have long-term urologic devices or obstruction. Renal functional impairment in patients with complicated urinary tract infection is usually attributable to the underlying abnormality or to organ failure complicating septic shock, rather than being a direct consequence of infection. For instance, introduction of voiding strategies to maintain low bladder pressure and to prevent reflux have almost eliminated the complication of chronic renal failure in persons with spinal cord injury, despite a continued high incidence of urinary tract infection in these patients.[123]

PATHOGENESIS

Microbiology

Host impairment rather than organism virulence is the major determinant of infection. *E. coli* remains the organism most frequently isolated in complicated urinary tract infection.[3,4] The *E. coli* strains are characterized by a low frequency of expression of virulence factors in comparison with strains isolated in acute uncomplicated infection.[39] Many other bacteria and yeast species are also isolated.[4,124,125] Enterobacteriaceae such as *Klebsiella* species, *Enterobacter* species, *Serratia* species, *Citrobacter* species, *Proteus mirabilis*, *Morganella morganii*, and *Providencia stuartii* are common. Other gram-negative organisms that may be isolated include *Pseudomonas aeruginosa*, *Stenotrophomonas maltophilia*, and *Acinetobacter* species. Gram-positive organisms are also frequently isolated, including group B streptococci, *Enterococcus* species, and coagulase-negative staphylococci. *S. aureus* is less commonly isolated. *Candida* species may be isolated, usually from patients who have diabetes or indwelling urologic devices or who are undergoing broad-spectrum antimicrobial therapy.[126]

Organisms isolated from patients with complicated urinary tract infection often have increased antimicrobial resistance.[127] Risk factors for isolation of a resistant organism include a history of recent antimicrobial therapy or of health care interventions, such as an indwelling urethral catheter or an invasive urologic procedure. Uncommon bacteria are occasionally a cause of infection. Some of these organisms may not be identified with standard laboratory procedures for processing urine specimens. *Corynebacterium urealyticum* is a urease-producing gram-positive rod associated with the unique clinical manifestations of encrusted cystitis or pyelonephritis.[128] This infection is characterized by ulcerative inflammation and struvite encrustations on the bladder or renal pelvis wall. Pyelitis, if untreated, may lead to destruction of the kidney. *U. urealyticum* is another urease-producing bacterium that may cause cystitis or pyelonephritis, often with urolithiasis. Healthy persons may become infected with this organism, but case reports suggest a predisposition in immunocompromised individuals, particularly those with hypogammaglobulinemia. *Aerococcus sanguinicola* is a rare cause of complicated urinary tract infection; the diagnosis is usually made by isolation of the organism in the blood culture.[129] *Aerococcus urinae* was isolated in 0.3% to 0.8% of urine specimens in one clinical microbiology laboratory, usually from older persons with underlying abnormalities and bacteremia.[130] Anaerobic organisms are seldom identified in the absence of suppurative complications such as abscess.[131]

Host Factors

Genitourinary abnormalities facilitate infection through increased entry of organisms into the bladder (e.g., by intermittent catheterization, urologic procedures) and subsequent persistence due to incomplete voiding (e.g., as a result of obstruction, urolithiasis, diverticula, reflux) or in biofilm on urologic devices.[3,4] Asymptomatic bacteriuria is the usual outcome in patients with persistent abnormalities.[132] The determinants that lead to symptomatic infection in chronically bacteriuric individuals are not well characterized. However, obstruction and mucosal trauma with bleeding are well-recognized risk factors for bacteremia and sepsis in patients with preexisting bacteriuria.

CLINICAL PRESENTATIONS

Complicated urinary tract infection manifests across a wide clinical spectrum of signs and symptoms, from mild, irritative symptoms of lower tract infection to pyelonephritis and bacteremia, including septic shock.[3,4,133] Localizing signs and symptoms consistent with cystitis or pyelonephritis are usually present. Patients with indwelling urethral catheters or other indwelling devices usually present with fever alone, although costovertebral angle pain or tenderness, hematuria, or catheter obstruction, if present, identifies a genitourinary source. Patients with chronic neurologic impairment sometimes report symptoms that are not classic for urinary tract infection. For instance, spinal cord–injured patients experience increased bladder and leg spasms or autonomic dysreflexia,[123] whereas patients with multiple sclerosis may present with fatigue or deterioration in neurologic function.[4]

The clinical diagnosis of symptomatic infection is often problematic in older populations with cognitive impairment.[134,135] These patients frequently have chronic genitourinary symptoms and impaired communication, which limits the assessment of signs and symptoms. Because bacteriuria is very common in elderly individuals with functional impairment, nonlocalizing clinical deterioration is frequently attributed to urinary tract infection because the urine culture has positive results.[136] However, nonlocalizing clinical manifestations, including fever, are unlikely to have a urinary source in elderly persons without a long-term indwelling catheter.[22,135] Changes in character of the urine, such as cloudiness and odor, are also frequently interpreted as symptoms of urinary tract infection. Cloudiness may be attributed to pyuria, which usually accompanies bacteriuria, and an unpleasant odor is suggestive of production of polyamines by bacteria in the urine. However, alterations in characteristics of the urine are neither sensitive nor specific for the diagnosis of infection. They may be attributable to other causes, such as precipitation of crystals and dehydration. Thus, changes in character of the urine should not be interpreted as symptoms of urinary tract infection.

LABORATORY DIAGNOSIS

A urine specimen for culture should be obtained before initiation of antimicrobial therapy for every patient with suspected complicated urinary tract infection. Because of the wide variety of potential infecting organisms and increased likelihood of resistant strains, definitive microbiologic characterization is necessary to optimize antimicrobial management.

Contamination from biofilm on devices within the urinary tract complicates interpretation of the urine culture in some patients with complicated infection. In the patient with a long-term indwelling catheter, the catheter should be replaced, and the new catheter should be used to sample bladder urine and avoid contamination by organisms present in the biofilm of the old catheter.[22,23] When intestine is interposed into the urinary tract through creation of an ileal conduit, continent cutaneous diversion, or neobladder, urine collected through the conduit or reservoir is often bacteriuric, regardless of symptoms.[137] The organisms isolated represent mixed gram-positive flora, including streptococcal species and *Staphylococcus epidermidis*, but uropathogenic strains such as *E. coli*, *P. mirabilis*, *P. aeruginosa*, and *Enterococcus faecalis* may also be present. Similar urine culture findings are reported in 30% to 60% of patients with orthoptic bladder substitution or augmentation cystoplasty[138]; individuals with these reservoirs who practice clean intermittent catheterization are more likely to have positive culture findings.[137] Thus, when symptomatic urinary tract infection is suspected, results of a urine culture in such a patient must be interpreted in the context of this usual bacteriuria.

Infection with a fastidious organism should be considered when the clinical presentation suggests symptomatic urinary tract infection but urine culture results are repeatedly negative, particularly when pyuria is present. These organisms may include *C. urealyticum*, *U. urealyticum*, and *Haemophilus* species. A persistently alkaline pH with pyuria but a negative urine culture suggests a urease-producing organism such as *C. urealyticum* or *U. urealyticum*. The laboratory should be consulted if a fastidious organism is considered, and appropriate specimens should be collected for additional laboratory evaluation to maximize the likelihood of isolating potential infecting organisms.

Patients with genitourinary abnormalities frequently have pyuria, whether or not they have bacteriuria or symptomatic infection, and so pyuria by itself is not diagnostic for urinary tract infection.[4] The absence of pyuria, however, has a high negative predictive value for ruling out urinary tract infection in some populations, such as elderly patients.[22] The severity of clinical manifestations determines whether additional investigation, such as blood culture or a peripheral leukocyte count, is indicated. Renal function should be assessed in every patient with complicated urinary tract infection. A second urine culture after antimicrobial therapy is not recommended if the patient remains asymptomatic.

ANTIMICROBIAL TREATMENT

The principles of management for individuals with complicated urinary tract infection include prompt specimen collection to identify the specific infecting organism; characterization of renal function and underlying abnormalities; and early institution of appropriate antimicrobial therapy. The antimicrobial regimen selected is individualized on the basis of site of infection, severity of manifestations, known or presumed infecting organism and susceptibility, and the patient's tolerance.[4] When the presenting symptoms are mild, it is preferable to delay initiation of antimicrobial therapy until results of the urine culture are available. This approach allows selection of a narrow-spectrum agent specific for the infecting organism and minimizes antimicrobial pressure, which promotes resistance.

When patients present with severe symptoms, empirical antimicrobial therapy is initiated pending urine culture results. Previous urine culture results, if available, and recent antimicrobial therapy received by the patient should be considered in the selection of empirical regimen.[4] Parenteral therapy is indicated for patients who present with hemodynamic instability, who cannot tolerate or absorb oral medications, or who are known or suspected to have an infecting organism resistant to available oral options. Patients with presentation of severe sepsis, including septic shock, should receive initial empirical antimicrobial therapy that provides broad coverage for both gram-positive and gram-negative bacteria, including resistant organisms.[133] Appropriate regimens for these patients may include an aminoglycoside, with or without ampicillin; piperacillin/tazobactam; piperacillin with an aminoglycoside; a carbapenem (ertapenem, imipenem, meropenem); or an extended-spectrum cephalosporin.

Fluoroquinolones with good urinary excretion and broad gram-negative coverage—norfloxacin, ciprofloxacin, and levofloxacin—are often used in empirical oral therapy.[4] Many other oral agents are effective and may be appropriate, depending on patient tolerance and the specific infecting organism.[4] These include TMP/SMX, amoxicillin, amoxicillin/clavulanic acid, oral cephalosporins, and doxycycline. Nitrofurantoin is effective for treatment of some episodes of bladder infection, but it is not effective for renal or prostate infection. It is contraindicated for treatment of patients with renal failure because peripheral neuropathy has been reported to occur with accumulation of this agent's toxic metabolites. *K. pneumoniae*, *P. aeruginosa*, and *P. mirabilis* strains are uniformly resistant to it. Nitrofurantoin remains effective, however, for some resistant organisms such as vancomycin-resistant *Enterococcus* and extended-spectrum β-lactamase–producing *E. coli*.

Substantial clinical improvement is expected by 48 to 72 hours after initiation of effective antimicrobial therapy. Empirical therapy is reassessed at this time, with consideration of the clinical response and urine culture results. Therapy is usually modified to an appropriate narrow-spectrum parenteral or oral agent to complete a 7- to 14-day course. If an organism isolated in the pretherapy urine culture specimen is resistant to the empirical antimicrobial, therapy should be altered to include an antimicrobial agent to which the infecting organism is susceptible, even if clinical improvement has occurred.

OTHER INTERVENTIONS

The optimal management of complicated urinary tract infection requires characterization of the underlying genitourinary abnormality and appropriate urologic or other interventions to assist in resolution of the current infection and prevention of subsequent infections. Urgent diagnostic imaging or urologic investigation is indicated for patients who have severe systemic symptoms or whose symptoms do not respond to appropriate antimicrobial therapy despite isolation of a susceptible organism. The goal of early imaging is to identify obstruction or abscesses, for which immediate drainage may be necessary for source control.[133] When the underlying abnormality is already well characterized—as in the case of a patient with an indwelling catheter or a neurogenic bladder managed with intermittent catheterization—further investigations may still be appropriate if the patient has experienced a recent change in frequency or severity of infections. Such a patient remains at risk for development of urolithiasis, tumors, and suppurative complications.

The approach to diagnostic imaging and urologic investigation is determined by the clinical presentation and the patient's previous history. A plain radiograph of the abdomen may identify emphysematous infections and some stones. CT is the imaging modality of choice. It identifies calculi, gas, hemorrhage, calcification, obstruction, renal enlargement, and inflammatory masses. Contrast media–enhanced scans are recommended, with helical and multislice CT to study different phases of contrast excretion.[109-111] Ultrasound examination is less sensitive and specific than other imaging modalities such as spiral CT and MRI, but it may be more accessible.[111]

Appropriate supportive care must be initiated promptly. The removal and replacement of a long-term indwelling catheter before institution of antimicrobial therapy are associated with a more rapid defervescence and a lower risk of early relapse after therapy, as well as facilitating collection of a more valid urine culture specimen.[23] The clinical benefits of catheter replacement are presumed to result from removal of the high concentration of organisms in the biofilm, which are often not eradicated by antimicrobial therapy and remain a source for relapse. Urologic investigations such as cystoscopy, retrograde pyelography, and urodynamic studies should be obtained as appropriate. If encrusted *C. urealyticum* infection is present, surgical resection of the encrustations is required together with antimicrobial therapy. *C. urealyticum* strains are generally susceptible to vancomycin, tetracyclines, and fluoroquinolones.[128]

MANAGEMENT OF RECURRENT INFECTION

When symptoms recur early after antimicrobial treatment, the susceptibility of the pretherapy infecting organism should be reviewed to confirm that the antimicrobial agent prescribed is effective. If the organism is susceptible, underlying genitourinary abnormalities should be reviewed and further evaluation obtained, if appropriate, to identify abnormalities such as abscesses that may necessitate drainage. Even if the abnormalities cannot be fully corrected, interventions to improve urine drainage may decrease the frequency of episodes of symptomatic infection.[3,4] Indwelling devices should be removed whenever possible. Evidence-based infection control guidelines provide recommendations for prevention of catheter-acquired urinary tract infection.[139-141] Specific practices include appropriate catheter use, limiting duration of use, appropriate practices for insertion and care, and selection of size. Interventions that have been shown not to be effective and that are not recommended include use of different catheter materials, antimicrobial coating of catheters, antiseptic or antimicrobial meatal care, and instillation of antiseptics into the drainage bag. Patients with long-term indwelling catheters and other indwelling devices experience infection because of biofilm formation on these devices; therefore, the prevention of catheter-acquired infection will ultimately require development of biofilm-resistant biomaterials.[142]

Long-term prophylactic antimicrobial therapy is not recommended.[4,123,143] When patients with impaired voiding or indwelling devices are given prophylactic antimicrobial agents, there is little, if any, decrease in symptomatic infection, but rapid reinfection with resistant organisms is uniformly observed.[4] For the selected patient with a persistent abnormality and symptomatic relapsing infection that cannot be eradicated, suppressive therapy may be considered. The goal of suppressive therapy is not to prevent reinfection but either to control symptomatic episodes when infecting bacteria cannot be eradicated or to prevent stone enlargement when inoperable infection stones are present. The antimicrobial regimen is selected on the basis of the infecting organism and is prescribed initially at a full therapeutic dose. If the patient remains clinically stable and the urine is sterile, this dose is usually decreased to about half after 4 to 6 weeks. Suppressive therapy is not appropriate for patients with indwelling devices because biofilm formation facilitates rapid reinfection and emergence of resistant organisms. However, short-term use of such therapy (several weeks or months) for patients with complex urologic abnormalities and indwelling devices may occasionally be considered as part of a palliative care strategy.

A novel approach currently being evaluated for control of recurrent infection in patients with impaired bladder emptying is "bacterial interference."[144] This strategy establishes asymptomatic bacteriuria with a nonpathogenic E. coli strain in patients with impaired voiding. The avirulent strain in the bladder then prevents infection by other, potentially more virulent, strains. The proposed mechanisms for this protective effect include blocking of bacterial receptors present on uroepithelial cells, competition for nutrients in the urine, and toxin production. Preliminary clinical trials have demonstrated some efficacy of this approach in a small number of carefully selected patients.[145]

ASYMPTOMATIC BACTERIURIA

EPIDEMIOLOGY

Asymptomatic bacteriuria is a common finding, particularly in women, older persons, and some patients with persistent genitourinary abnormalities (Table 37.7).[132] The prevalence of bacteriuria among sexually active young women ranges from 3% to 5% but is less than 1% among age-matched controls who are not sexually active. Bacteriuria is present in 5% to 10% of healthy postmenopausal women[132] and in 20% of women older than 80 years living in the community.[146] Asymptomatic bacteriuria is uncommon in younger men, but the prevalence increases in men older than 65 years, presumably concurrently with age-related prostate hypertrophy. Bacteriuria occurs in 10% of healthy men older than 80 years living in the community.[146] Among residents of nursing homes who do not have indwelling catheters, 20% to 50% of women and 15% to 40% of men are bacteriuric. The prevalence among persons with long-term indwelling catheters is 100%.[135] Among spinal cord–injured patients with impaired voiding and no indwelling catheter, the prevalence of bacteriuria is 50%, regardless of the method used for bladder emptying.[123]

Patients with an increased prevalence of asymptomatic bacteriuria also have a higher incidence of symptomatic urinary tract infection. However, this higher frequency of symptomatic infection is not attributable to bacteriuria. The same biologic determinants promote both asymptomatic and symptomatic infection. Bacteriuria in healthy young women is usually transient, but up to 8% have acute cystitis within 1 week of initial identification of a positive urine culture result.[147] In women with diabetes[148] and female or male residents of nursing homes,[135] persistent bacteriuria for months or years, frequently with the same strain, is often observed. No long-term negative outcomes have been attributed to asymptomatic bacteriuria.[132,148] Bacteriuric individuals are not more likely to experience hypertension or chronic renal failure, and survival is similar to that for persons without bacteriuria.

Harmful short-term outcomes attributable to asymptomatic bacteriuria are recognized in only two distinct populations: pregnant women and patients who undergo traumatic genitourinary procedures.[132] The prevalence of bacteriuria during early pregnancy is 3% to 7%, similar to that among age-matched nonpregnant women. The physiologic changes that accompany the increased progesterone levels in pregnancy include smooth muscle relaxation and decreased peristalsis, which result in dilation of the renal pelvis and ureters. In later pregnancy, ureteric obstruction may result from pressure of the uterus at the pelvic brim. In 20% to 35% of pregnant women with bacteriuria that is not treated, acute pyelonephritis develops later in pregnancy, usually at the end of the second trimester or early in the third trimester. This incidence of pyelonephritis is twenty- to thirtyfold

Table 37.7 Asymptomatic Bacteriuria in Normal Populations and in Selected Patients with Underlying Genitourinary Abnormalities

Population/Patients	Prevalence of Bacteriuria (%)
Healthy Women	
Aged 20-50 years:	
Sexually active	3-5
Not sexually active	<1
Aged 50-70 years	3-9
Aged ≥80 years	14-22
Healthy Men	
Aged <65 years	<1
Aged ≥80 years	6-10
Patients with Complicated Genitourinary Abnormalities	
Spinal cord injury:	
Bladder retrained	25
Intermittent catheterization	23-89
Sphincterotomy/condom	58
Ileal neobladder	30-60
Residence in long-term care facility:	
Women	25-57
Men	19-37
Indwelling urethral catheter:	
Short term	5%-7% acquisition/day
Long term	100
Urethral stents:	
Temporary	45
Permanent	100

Data from Nicolle LE, Bradley S, Colgan R, et al: Infectious Diseases Society of America guidelines for the diagnosis and treatment of asymptomatic bacteriuria in adults, Clin Infect Dis 40:643-654, 2005; and Rodhe N, Mölstad S, Englund L, et al: Asymptomatic bacteriuria in a population of elderly residents living in a community setting: prevalence, characteristics, and associated factors, Fam Pract 23:303-307, 2006.

higher among untreated women with bacteriuria than among women whose initial screening urine cultures yielded negative results or in whom bacteriuria was treated. Acute pyelonephritis in later pregnancy is associated with premature delivery and poorer fetal outcomes. The second group of bacteriuric patients at risk are those who undergo traumatic urologic procedures. If bacteriuria remains untreated, bacteremia develops in as many as 60% after the procedure, and in 5% to 10% progresses to severe sepsis or septic shock.

PATHOGENESIS

Microbiology

E. coli is isolated from 80% of healthy women with asymptomatic bacteriuria.[147] Most of the remaining bacterial strains are *K. pneumoniae*, *Enterococcus* species, and coagulase-negative staphylococci. For men older than 65 years, coagulase-negative staphylococci are isolated most frequently, followed by *E. coli* and *Enterococcus* species. In patients with underlying genitourinary abnormalities, a wider variety of organisms are isolated. *E. coli* and other organisms associated with asymptomatic bacteriuria are characterized by the relative absence of or lack of expression of recognized virulence factors.[149] Some strains that are strongly adherent but unable to stimulate an epithelial cell IL-6 cytokine response have been described. These relatively avirulent *E. coli* strains may originate from nonvirulent commensal strains or may evolve from virulent strains by attenuation of virulence genes.[150,151] Other organisms that are frequently isolated, such as coagulase-negative staphylococci and *Enterococcus* species, are relatively nonpathogenic and seldom associated with symptomatic infection.

Biofilm formation is responsible for the universal development of bacteriuria in patients with indwelling urinary devices.[152] After a device is inserted, a conditioning layer composed of proteins and other host components immediately coats it. This coat provides a surface for subsequent attachment of bacteria or yeast that originate from the periurethral flora or drainage bags or are introduced after disruption of the closed drainage system. Organisms grow along the device, elaborating an extracellular polysaccharide substance, and colonies of microorganisms persist within this relatively protected environment. Urine components such as Tamm-Horsfall protein and magnesium or calcium ions are also incorporated into the biofilm. Organisms ascend in the biofilm along the interior and exterior surfaces of the device and reach the bladder within days. The initial infection is usually with a single organism, but a polymicrobial flora is invariably present on long-term indwelling devices.[23,152-154] Urease-producing organisms such as *P. mirabilis*, *K. pneumoniae*, *M. morganii*, and *P. stuartii* are isolated more frequently from individuals with long-term indwelling catheters and persist longer than other organisms, such as *Enterococcus* species. Complications attributed to biofilm formation with urease-producing organisms include development of renal or bladder stones and obstruction of the device.[155] Although the most common device is the urethral catheter, the process of biofilm formation is similar with other indwelling devices, such as ureteric stents and nephrostomy tubes.[153,154] From 34% to 42% of ureteral stents are found at removal to be colonized with bacteria or yeast species, often with multiple organisms. More than 50% of organisms identified by stent biofilm analysis are not isolated from culture of urine specimens collected at the same time.

HOST FACTORS

The genetic and behavioral risk factors and genitourinary abnormalities associated with asymptomatic bacteriuria are similar to those described for uncomplicated and complicated symptomatic urinary tract infection. For younger women, behavioral risks are sexual activity and spermicide use.[147] Bacteriuric women older than 80 years who reside in the community have reduced mobility and urinary incontinence and are receiving estrogen treatment; and men older than 80 years with bacteriuria are characterized by prostate disease, history of stroke, and residence in supervised housing.[146] Functional impairment is the major risk factor associated with asymptomatic bacteriuria in the long-term care facility population without indwelling catheters.[135] Higher residual urine volume is not associated with increased bacteriuria in elderly populations but has been associated with bacteriuria in patients referred to an ambulatory urology clinic.[135]

DIAGNOSIS

The quantitative criterion for identification of asymptomatic bacteriuria is an organism quantitative count of 10^5 CFU/mL or higher. For women, two consecutive urine specimens with similar culture results are recommended, but a single specimen is sufficient for men.[132] When an initial urine culture in a young woman yields positive results, a second positive result in a specimen obtained within 2 weeks confirms bacteriuria in 85% to 90% of women. If the second specimen result is negative, the initial positive culture result may have been contaminated; however, bacteriuria may also have resolved spontaneously. If a voided specimen has a low quantitative count of a single potential uropathogen, and if it is essential to rule out bacteriuria, a second urine specimen should be collected as a first morning void.

Pyuria accompanies bacteriuria in most patients, but there is variability in the frequency of pyuria observed in different populations. Pyuria is present in only 50% of bacteriuric pregnant women; therefore, screening for pyuria is not a reliable method to rule out bacteriuria in pregnancy.[156] Pyuria is present in about 75% of diabetic women with bacteriuria, in 90% of bacteriuric patients undergoing hemodialysis, and in more than 90% of elderly persons with bacteriuria.[132] Pyuria also occurs in 30% to 70% of bacteriuric patients with short-term indwelling catheters and in 100% of those with long-term indwelling catheters.

TREATMENT

Screening for and treatment of asymptomatic bacteriuria is recommended only for pregnant women or for patients who will undergo a traumatic genitourinary tract procedure.[132] For other patients, treatment does not improve short- or long-term clinical outcomes, but negative consequences, such as reinfection with organisms of increased antimicrobial resistance and adverse drug effects, do occur.[132,157] In girls and women, an increased frequency of symptomatic infection has been reported after treatment of asymptomatic bacteriuria.[132,158] This finding may be attributable to alteration of vaginal flora by antimicrobial therapy or to replacement of a benign organism by a more virulent organism. Studies suggest no benefits of treatment of asymptomatic bacteriuria for patients with complicated infection, including renal transplant recipients.[159,160] The benefits, if any, of screening for or treatment of bacteriuria in patients with neutropenia are not well characterized, and further clinical evaluation is required for these patients.

Identification and treatment of asymptomatic bacteriuria early in pregnancy reduces the risk of pyelonephritis from between 25% and 30% to between 1% and 2%.[132] All pregnant women should be screened for bacteriuria by urine culture at the end of the first trimester and treated if bacteriuria is found.[156] Recommended regimens include a 5- or 7-day course of nitrofurantoin[161] or a 7-day course of amoxicillin, amoxicillin/clavulanic acid, or a cephalosporin. The specific regimen is chosen on the basis of the organism isolated and the patient's tolerance. Shorter antimicrobial courses are sometimes prescribed, but these abbreviated courses are likely less effective.[162] TMP/SMX should be avoided, especially in the first trimester, and fluoroquinolones are contraindicated during pregnancy. After treatment for asymptomatic or symptomatic urinary tract infection, urine cultures should be performed at least monthly. If infection recurs, prophylactic antimicrobial therapy should be initiated and continued for the duration of the pregnancy. Nitrofurantoin and cephalexin are the preferred prophylactic regimens because both are safe for the fetus.

Initiation of effective antimicrobial treatment immediately before a traumatic urologic procedure prevents bacteremia and sepsis in a bacteriuric patient.[132,163] Conceptually, this approach is surgical prophylaxis rather than treatment of asymptomatic bacteriuria. A single dose of an antimicrobial agent is usually adequate, although some guidelines recommend that the antimicrobial agent be continued after transurethral resection of the prostate until the indwelling catheter is removed.[132] Antimicrobial agents are not recommended for minor urologic procedures such as cystoscopy and urodynamic studies or before replacement of a long-term urethral catheter, because the risk of bacteremia and sepsis with these procedures is low and clinical outcomes are not improved when prophylactic antimicrobial agents are given prior to these interventions.[4,140,164]

PROSTATITIS

The development of the National Institutes of Health (NIH) classification of prostatitis syndromes (Table 37.8) and subsequent application of this classification in clinical trials and patient care have greatly advanced the understanding and appropriate management of this common problem.[165] Only bacterial prostatitis, either acute or chronic, is considered attributable to infection and has indications for antimicrobial therapy.[25,166]

Acute bacterial prostatitis is a severe infection, which is a urologic emergency.[25] This syndrome is usually community acquired, although health care–associated infection may occur, particularly after prostate biopsy.[167] Affected patients present with severe systemic manifestations including fever and marked urinary symptoms of dysuria and frequency. Urinary obstruction and intense suprapubic pain are often present. Bacteremia is reported in 27% of episodes. A digital rectal examination is not recommended because it may precipitate bacteremia.[25]

E. coli is isolated in 70% of episodes. These strains are characterized by the presence of multiple virulence factors.[168] *Proteus* species, *Klebsiella* species, *Enterococcus* species, *P. aeruginosa*, and *S. aureus* are each isolated in fewer than 10% of cases.[167] Management includes bladder drainage by insertion of a urethral or suprapubic catheter, blood and urine cultures to characterize the infecting organism, and initiation of empirical parenteral antimicrobial therapy. Most antimicrobial agents are active in the acutely inflamed prostate. A combination of a β-lactam and an aminoglycoside is considered first-line therapy, although other broad-spectrum parenteral antibiotics, such as piperacillin/tazobactam and carbapenems, are also effective.[26] After confirmation of the infecting organism and an adequate clinical response, antibiotic therapy is modified to oral therapy to complete a 6-week course. A fluoroquinolone, either ciprofloxacin or levofloxacin, is recommended as oral therapy if the infecting organism is susceptible. When there is not a prompt clinical response following bladder drainage and initiation of effective antimicrobial therapy, CT or MRI is indicated to search for the uncommon complication prostate abscess. When an abscess is identified, transrectal ultrasonography-guided aspiration is usually effective for drainage. Only a small proportion of patients, 10% to 15%, have chronic bacterial prostatitis following acute prostatitis.[168]

Chronic bacterial prostatitis occurs in men with persistent prostate infection.[25,166,169] Bacteria enter the prostate from the urethra and persist because of limited antimicrobial diffusion or activity in the gland as well as the frequent presence of infected prostate stones in older men. A common clinical presentation is recurrent acute cystitis because bacteria in the prostate intermittently enter the bladder. The same organism is often repeatedly isolated, but the intervals between symptomatic episodes may last months or even years. Other symptoms are generally mild, such as irritative voiding symptoms and discomfort localized to the testicles,

Table 37.8 National Institutes of Health Classification of Prostatitis Syndromes

Class	Description
I	Acute bacterial prostatitis
II	Chronic bacterial prostatitis
III	Chronic pelvic pain syndrome (CPPS)
IIIa	Inflammatory CPPS
	Leukocytes present in semen, in urine after prostate massage, or in expressed prostate secretions
IIIb	Noninflammatory CPPS
	Absence of leukocytes in specimens
IV	Asymptomatic inflammatory prostatitis
	Leukocytes in specimens similar to those in inflammatory CPPS, but no symptoms

Data from Krieger JN, Nyberg L, Nickel JC: NIH consensus definition and classification of prostatitis, JAMA 281:236-237, 1999.

lower back, or perineum. Results of the prostate examination are usually normal, but tenderness may occasionally be elicited.

In only 10% of men who present with the clinical syndrome of chronic prostatitis or chronic pelvic pain syndrome is chronic bacterial prostatitis subsequently documented microbiologically. The diagnosis requires paired cultures of midstream and post–prostatic massage urine specimens.[26] The midstream specimen confirms negative results of a urine culture, and the post–prostatic massage specimen reveals pyuria and organisms of presumed prostate origin.[25,169] Gram-negative organisms, including Enterobacteriaceae and *P. aeruginosa*, and gram-positive *Enterococcus* species, *S. aureus*, coagulase-negative staphylococci, and group B streptococci are the bacteria most commonly isolated.[168] Sexually transmitted organisms such as *Chlamydia trachomatis*, *U. urealyticum*, *Mycoplasma genitalium*, and *Trichomonas vaginalis* are uncommon and, when present, are usually identified in younger men.[26] The clinical relevance of post–prostatic massage cultures, however, remains controversial. In one study of 463 patients and 121 age-matched controls, 70% of subjects were found to harbor at least one organism in a post–prostatic massage specimen, and uropathogens such as *E. coli* were isolated from 8% of patients and 8.3% of controls.[170] In another study, gram-positive organisms were isolated from 6% of 470 men after prostatic massage, but 97% of these organisms were not confirmed on second culture.[171]

Despite this uncertainty, chronic bacterial prostatitis does respond to appropriate antimicrobial treatment, although relapse after treatment is common. Ciprofloxacin and levofloxacin are the first choices for antimicrobial treatment of chronic bacterial prostatitis when susceptible organisms are isolated. These agents penetrate well into the prostate and seminal fluid, and they remain active in the acidic environment of the prostate. Cure rates at 6 months after a 4-week course are 75% to 89%,[26,166] although late relapses may still occur. Doxycycline and macrolides are considered second-line drugs but are preferred for gram-positive infections.[166] Men who present for the first time with chronic pelvic pain syndrome, and with evidence of inflammation (i.e., leukocytes) in expressed prostatic secretions, but in whom cultures are negative, should be prescribed a 4-week trial of antimicrobial therapy if they have not previously received a prolonged antimicrobial course.[166,172] In reported case series, as many as 10% of men with such findings show response to antimicrobial therapy despite negative culture results; however, comparative clinical trials in treatment-naive men with negative culture results have not been reported. If symptoms persist or recur after this 4-week antimicrobial trial, and if results of post–prostatic massage cultures remain negative, further antimicrobial therapy is not indicated.[169,173]

URINARY TRACT INFECTION IN UNIQUE PATIENT POPULATIONS

RENAL TRANSPLANT RECIPIENTS

Urinary tract infection accounts for 45% to 60% of infections that occur in patients after renal transplantation.[174-177] By 6 months after transplantation, 17% of recipients have experienced at least one urinary tract infection, and by 3 years, posttransplantation infection has occurred in 60% of female recipients and 47% of male recipients.[178] The incidence is highest in the first 3 months after transplantation, when infection complicates surgical intervention and the use of urologic devices such as urinary catheters and ureteric stents.[179-181] The clinical manifestation may be either cystitis or pyelonephritis; 3% to 14% of episodes are associated with bacteremia.[175,177,180,182] Early posttransplantation infections tend to be more severe and to manifest more frequently as pyelonephritis or with bacteremia.[183]

Risk factors for urinary tract infection are (1) patient specific, such as female gender, diabetes mellitus, pretransplantation urinary tract infections, prolonged prior dialysis, and polycystic kidney disease, or (2) transplant related, such as allograft trauma, microbial contamination of cadaveric kidneys, technical complications related to ureteral anastomosis, the presence of urinary catheters and ureteric stents, immunosuppression, reimplantation, and vesicoureteric reflux.[181,184] Independent risk factors for any symptomatic or asymptomatic infection in the first year after transplantation are reported to be older age, female gender, higher number of days of indwelling catheter after transplant, anatomical genitourinary abnormalities, and urinary infection within 1 month prior to the procedure.[185] For acute pyelonephritis at any time after transplantation, independent risk factors are female gender, experiencing acute rejection episodes, higher number of urinary infections, and receiving mycophenolate mofetil.[186] Following transplantation, the risk for development of urinary tract infection correlates with the duration of perioperative catheterization or ureteral stent.[175,176,187,188] The routine use of ureteric stents at transplantation decreases the overall transplantation complication rate, but stent implantation is associated with a small, but significant, increased risk of urinary tract infection.

Asymptomatic bacteriuria is not a risk factor for impaired graft survival.[132] Transplant recipients with asymptomatic bacteriuria who progress to graft failure invariably also experience symptomatic infection. Graft failure in these patients is usually attributable to urologic abnormalities that promote infection rather than a direct consequence of infection. Antimicrobial therapy for asymptomatic bacteriuria does not improve graft survival.[159] Symptomatic urinary tract infection has also not been independently associated with graft survival.[182,189-192] However, case reports have described transplant recipients receiving stable immunosuppressive regimens who experience deterioration in graft function that is coincident with an episode of acute pyelonephritis.[193] This occurrence may be attributable to activation of the immune system by the infection.

The principles of management are similar to those for any patient with complicated urinary tract infection. They include prompt clinical diagnosis and initiation of antimicrobial therapy, obtaining appropriate specimens for culture, and evaluating for underlying genitourinary abnormalities that may promote infection. Enterobacteriaceae, particularly *E. coli*, are the most common infecting organisms, but a variety of other bacteria or yeasts may be isolated. The choice of antimicrobial agent is determined by the susceptibility of the infecting organism and the patient's tolerance. A 2-week course of antimicrobial agents is recommended. The effect of type and intensity of immunosuppressive therapy on antimicrobial efficacy has not been reported. Screening for and treatment of asymptomatic bacteriuria is not recommended. Bacteriuria does not compromise renal function,[184,190] and its treatment does not prevent subsequent symptomatic episodes but may, in fact, increase the frequency of symptomatic infection.[159,160] Current guidelines do not recommend screening for bacteriuria.[194] Treatment of asymptomatic candiduria in renal transplant recipients has also not been shown to be beneficial and is not recommended.[195]

Urinary tract infection after transplantation can be prevented by optimal surgical technique, which includes minimizing the perioperative duration of indwelling urinary devices. TMP/SMX prophylaxis given for the first 6 months after transplantation decreases the risk of both symptomatic and asymptomatic urinary tract infection as well as other infections.[132] When urinary tract infection is diagnosed in patients receiving TMP/SMX prophylaxis, the organisms isolated are invariably resistant to TMP/SMX. Frequent recurrent symptomatic infection after transplantation may be attributable to an inadequate duration of antimicrobial treatment, resistance of the infecting organism, the presence of urologic abnormalities such as obstruction and stones, or infection of native kidneys. When infection recurs shortly after treatment, previous urine culture results should be reviewed to establish whether reinfection or relapse is occurring and to confirm that the infecting organism is susceptible to the antimicrobial therapy given. If relapse with a susceptible organism occurs after a 2-week course of therapy, re-treatment with a 4- to 6-week course is recommended, although the effectiveness of such prolonged retreatment has not been critically evaluated.[182] Repeated relapse after prolonged antimicrobial therapy in patients without identified urologic abnormalities is often caused by infection localized to the native kidneys. Such patients usually have a history of recurrent urinary tract infection before transplantation. The organisms frequently cannot be eradicated, presumably because of failure of antibiotics to achieve effective levels in the nonfunctioning kidney. Long-term suppressive therapy may be necessary to prevent further symptomatic episodes in these patients.

PERSONS WITH RENAL FAILURE

Urinary tract infections in patients with mild to moderate renal failure usually respond adequately to antimicrobial therapy.[196] When renal impairment is severe, however, adequate urine or renal levels of antimicrobial agents may not be achieved because of limited kidney perfusion. If renal failure occurs with acute pyelonephritis, the response following initiation of antimicrobial therapy may be delayed or the risk of relapse after therapy may be increased. Systematic evaluation of antimicrobial efficacy for treatment of urinary tract infection in patients with renal failure has been limited.[4] Aminoglycosides have little penetration into nonfunctioning kidneys and are not recommended for treatment. Fluoroquinolones, TMP/SMX, ampicillin, and cephalosporins have all been effective for treatment in individual case reports.

Another therapeutic problem arises when infection is localized to a unilateral nonfunctioning kidney. Antimicrobial therapy sterilizes the urine and often ameliorates symptoms because high urine levels are achieved by antimicrobial excretion through the functioning kidney. However, organisms persist in the kidney with impaired function because antimicrobial penetration to the site of infection is inadequate. When antimicrobial therapy is discontinued, a prompt relapse of infection occurs. Localization of infection to one kidney can be documented in a patient not receiving antibiotics, by culture of urine collected directly from the ureter after bladder irrigation with normal saline to remove the infected bladder urine before ureteric catheterization. For symptomatic relapsing infection when a nonfunctioning kidney is known or suspected to be infected, management options include a trial of a more prolonged course of antimicrobial therapy, continuous suppressive therapy, and surgical removal of the nonfunctioning kidney.

PERSONS WITH URINARY STONES

Urinary tract infection complicates urolithiasis through several different mechanisms; infection may be the cause of stone formation, noninfected metabolic stones may become colonized with bacteria which persist in biofilm, and obstructing noninfected stones may precipitate infection proximal to the obstruction.[197] In any patient with urolithiasis and infection, the infection should be controlled with appropriate antimicrobial therapy before urologic manipulations.[198]

Infection stones, also called *struvite stones,* are a complication of infection with urease-producing organisms such as *P. mirabilis.* Urease catalyzes the hydrolysis of urea in the urine. This process produces ammonia and alkalinity of the urine, favoring precipitation of magnesium ammonium phosphate, carbonate apatite, and monoammonium urate.[199] These crystals are incorporated into bacterial biofilm, creating the infection stone.[152] Infection stones continue to enlarge, sometimes rapidly, and ultimately cause obstruction and renal failure if not adequately treated. Patients at increased risk for development of infection stones are those with long-term indwelling catheters, urinary tract obstruction, neurogenic voiding dysfunction, distal renal tubular acidosis, and medullary sponge kidney.

Management of infection stones requires complete removal of the stone, together with sterilization of the urine.[198] Percutaneous ultrasonic lithotripsy is effective in removing 60% to 90% of these stones, whereas extracorporeal shock wave lithotripsy is 30% to 60% effective. Multiple stone fragments are passed after lithotripsy. Antimicrobial therapy, selected on the basis of urine culture results, is continued until all fragments are passed. The optimal duration of antimicrobial therapy after lithotripsy is controversial. Currently, 4 weeks is recommended, although some writers suggest a shorter duration. When percutaneous lithotripsy is not effective or is contraindicated, open surgery or nephrectomy may be necessary for stone removal. For selected elderly or debilitated patients with complex urologic or medical problems, stone removal may not be possible. In such patients, continuous suppressive antimicrobial therapy is recommended to limit stone enlargement and preserve renal function. The antimicrobial agent is selected on the basis of urine culture results, and therapy is continued indefinitely if effective and tolerated.

Bacteria may adhere to the surface of a stone that is not initially infected and may subsequently persist in biofilm.[152] Culture of a voided urine specimen in such cases often does not reflect the bacteriology of the stone. In a series of 75 patients with renal stones that were not infection stones, 36 (49%) of the stones were colonized, but only 19 (53%) of the patients also had bacteriuria.[200] Organisms isolated from the colonized stones included *E. coli* (75%), *Enterococcus* species (100%), *P. aeruginosa* (19%), *Klebsiella* species (31%), *P. mirabilis* (8.3%), *Streptococcus* species (31%), *Citrobacter* species (8.3%), *S. saprophyticus* (19%), *M. morganii* (8.3%), and *Gemella* species (8.3%). Larger stones were more likely to be colonized. Patients with stones colonized with bacteria are at increased risk for postprocedure sepsis, even when the voided urine specimen culture has negative results.[201] Perioperative antimicrobial agents are recommended for all patients with stones who have indwelling catheters or stents, because they are at increased risk of stone colonization. Even with antimicrobial prophylaxis, 10% of patients undergoing percutaneous nephrolithotomy experience postoperative fever; positive urine bacterial culture results, diabetes, staghorn calculi, and preoperative nephrostomy are risk factors for fever.[202]

A noninfected stone may cause ureteric obstruction complicated by infection of the undrained urine proximal to the stone. Complete obstruction is associated with a high risk for bacteremia and sepsis, and prompt drainage is essential.[203] When a ureter is obstructed, the voided urine specimen culture may not accurately reflect the microbiology of urine sampled directly from the renal pelvis. Among patients with obstruction and a positive culture result for urine sampled from the renal pelvis, the voided urine specimen culture had positive results in only 16.4% of cases in one report, and the organisms isolated were concordant between the two specimens in only 23% of patients.[204] Thus, a urine specimen should be obtained for culture by percutaneous aspiration of the renal pelvis in patients with obstruction whenever possible.

OTHER INFECTIONS OF THE URINARY TRACT

RENAL AND PERINEPHRIC ABSCESSES

Renal and perinephric abscesses are uncommon suppurative complications associated with substantial morbidity and mortality. Renal abscesses are located entirely within the renal parenchyma, whereas perinephric abscesses occupy the retroperitoneal fat and fascia surrounding the kidney. Abscesses may involve both the renal and perinephric tissues: 25% to 39% of abscesses are intranephric, 19% to 25% are both intranephric and perinephric, and 42% to 51% are perinephritic alone.[205,206] These abscesses develop after ascending urinary tract infection and pyelonephritis, or after hematogenous spread to the renal cortex or retroperitoneum of bacteremia from another site. Multiple bilateral cortical microabscesses suggest hematogenous spread. Complicating factors such as diabetes, urolithiasis, and obstruction are present in most cases. A population-based study from Taiwan reported an incidence of hospitalization for renal and perinephric abscess of 4.6/10,000 person-years for diabetic patients and 1.1/10,000 for nondiabetic patients.[207]

The organisms most commonly isolated from abscesses are *E. coli*, *K. pneumoniae*, *P. mirabilis*, *S. aureus*, and anaerobes. *S. aureus* abscesses are most likely to have originated with hematogenous spread from another site of infection. The clinical manifestations of both renal and perinephric abscesses mimic those of acute pyelonephritis. The characteristic findings are fever and costovertebral angle pain or tenderness. Despite appropriate antimicrobial therapy for pyelonephritis, however, clinical failure, delayed response, and early symptomatic relapse are observed. In a multivariate analysis, patients subsequently found to have renal abscess rather than pyelonephritis were more likely to have diabetes mellitus, hypotension, acute renal impairment, and a peripheral leukocyte (white blood cell [WBC]) count greater than 20,000 WBC/mL.[208]

CT is the preferred imaging modality for diagnosing the presence of an abscess; it also characterizes the extent of infection and may identify the potential source.[110] Ultrasonography identifies most perinephric abscesses, but it may not be able to distinguish an inflammatory lobar mass from a true renal abscess.[111]

The management goals for renal and perinephric abscesses include prompt diagnosis, early institution of effective antimicrobial therapy, and, in selected patients, abscess drainage for both therapeutic and diagnostic purposes. Culture of the abscess fluid identifies the specific infecting organisms and directs antimicrobial choice. If abscess fluid cannot be sampled for culture, organisms isolated from blood or urine culture should be considered in the selection of antimicrobial therapy. Initial antimicrobial administration is usually intravenous. Once the patient's condition is stabilized, therapy can be continued with an appropriate oral antimicrobial agent that has good bioavailability. Small renal abscesses (up to 5 cm in diameter) often respond to antimicrobial therapy without drainage, but for larger abscesses, drainage is usually required for resolution of infection.[205,206,209-211] Renal abscesses tend to be smaller, and about 70% of these have been reported to resolve with medical therapy alone.[206] Perinephric or mixed abscesses are larger, and drainage is usually required. The current initial approach is to attempt percutaneous drainage and, if this is not effective, to proceed to open drainage or nephrectomy. Resolution of the abscess is monitored by repeated imaging studies. Antimicrobial therapy is continued until the abscess has completely resolved or until there is only a residual, stable scar.

INFECTED RENAL CYSTS

The frequency of occurrence and risk factors for development of cyst infection are not well described. A French series reported that 8.4% of 389 patients with autosomal dominant polycystic kidney disease admitted to the nephrology department over a 10-year period had definite or likely cyst infection[212]; 24% of the episodes were associated with bacteremia, and two patients had more than one episode. Infected cysts complicating polycystic kidney disease may be problematic to diagnose.[213] Fever and abdominal pain or tenderness, often with bacteremia, are the usual clinical manifestations. However, the differential diagnosis includes pyelonephritis, infected kidney stones, perinephric abscess, cyst hemorrhage, and other intraabdominal pathology. Most patients with infected cysts also have peripheral leukocytosis and elevated C-reactive protein values. *E. coli*, *K. pneumoniae*, *Enterococcus* species, and group B streptococci are the most common infecting organisms, but *Salmonella* spp, *P. aeruginosa*, *Clostridium* species, *Candida* species, and *Aspergillus* species have also been reported. In view of the wide spectrum of potential pathogens, the specific infecting organism should be confirmed by cyst aspiration whenever possible. Imaging studies are usually necessary to confirm the diagnosis and identify the implicated cyst. Ultrasonography and CT are not useful.[214] MRI[214] and white blood cell–labeled scans[214,215] were successful in localizing the infected cyst in individual case reports. Positron emission tomography with fludeoxyglucose F-18 is reported to be most effective in localizing the infected cyst, but access to this technology is limited.[213,216-218]

Once the potential infected cyst is identified, a cyst aspiration, if possible, can confirm the presence of infection and provide therapeutic drainage.[219] Antimicrobial penetration into the cyst is presumed to be transepithelial. Effective concentrations of TMP/SMX, chloramphenicol, and fluoroquinolones are achieved in the cyst.[196] Cyst and serum levels of levofloxacin are similar, whereas cyst levels reported with ciprofloxacin are only 40% of serum levels.[220] Therapeutic antimicrobial levels are achieved in cysts with therapy with penicillins, cephalosporins, aminoglycosides,[196] and amphotericin B.[221] Prolonged antimicrobial therapy, for at least 4 weeks, is recommended, although clinical trials defining the optimal duration of therapy have not been reported. In the French case series described previously, the mean duration of antibiotic therapy was 5 weeks, and the initial course of therapy was successful for 71% of cases.[212] Nephrectomy is occasionally necessary when cyst drainage and appropriate antimicrobial therapy are not successful in controlling the infection.

EMPHYSEMATOUS CYSTITIS AND PYELONEPHRITIS

Emphysematous cystitis and pyelonephritis are acute necrotizing infections characterized by gas formation. Gas within the urinary collecting system can be seen after many interventional procedures, but emphysematous infection is characterized by gas in the tissues.[111] Gas is localized to the bladder wall and lumen in cystitis[222] and in and around the kidney in pyelonephritis.[223] Emphysematous pyelitis is a gas-forming infection restricted to the collecting system; the renal parenchyma is spared. Affected patients usually have diabetes with poor glucose control. Obstruction is another common predisposing factor for emphysematous pyelonephritis. *E. coli* and *K. pneumoniae* are the organisms most commonly isolated. High levels of glucose in the urine serve as a substrate for these bacteria, and large amounts of gas are generated through natural fermentation. In affected patients who are not diabetic, protein fermentation is a proposed source of gas formation.[222] CT is considered the optimal imaging technique for confirming emphysematous infection and characterizing the extent of involvement.[110,111]

A review of 135 cases of emphysematous cystitis identified over a period of 50 years reported that the median patient age was 66 years (range, <1 to 90 years), 64% of patients were women, and 67% had diabetes.[222] Presenting symptoms ranged from pneumaturia alone through irritative lower tract voiding symptoms to severe illness suggestive of acute abdominal disease or sepsis; 7% of cases were asymptomatic. *E. coli* was isolated from 58%, *K. pneumoniae* from 21%, and *Clostridium* species and *Enterobacter aerogenes* each from 7% of cases. The diagnosis was apparent on a plain radiograph of the abdomen in 84% of cases. Medical management—including antimicrobial therapy, bladder drainage, and glycemic control—was usually effective. Surgical intervention was required for only 10% of cases and included cystectomy, partial cystectomy, and surgical debridement when concomitant emphysematous pyelonephritis was present. The overall mortality rate was only 7%.

Emphysematous pyelonephritis is a more serious infection with a substantially higher mortality rate.[224] In case series of patients with emphysematous pyelonephritis, 62% to 100% were diabetic, and the majority were women.[225-227] Serum glucose levels are often very high in the diabetic patients, and serum C-reactive protein was generally elevated. *E. coli* was isolated from 45% to 54% of episodes, and bacteremia occurred in 20% to 50% of subjects in whom blood cultures were performed. Plain abdominal radiographs identified gas in the kidney in only 50% of cases. Ultrasonography of the kidneys usually showed some abnormalities but was less accurate than CT in identifying emphysematous infection. Management includes antimicrobial therapy together with percutaneous or open drainage of abscesses and correction of obstruction.[223,224,226-228] Aggressive glucose control and supportive care are also necessary. The mortality rate ranges from 7% to 20% in patients with less severe manifestations to 70% in patients with a fulminant course characterized by necrosis, intravascular thrombosis, and microabscess formation.

Emergency nephrectomy was traditionally considered necessary for any patient presenting with emphysematous pyelonephritis. Currently, percutaneous drainage is the recommended initial approach, and it is associated with lower mortality rates than either emergency nephrectomy or medical management alone.[224,228,229] In a retrospective case series describing a relatively small number of patients, the mortality rates were 50% with medical management alone, 25% with medical management and emergency nephrectomy, and 13.5% with medical management combined with initial percutaneous drainage.[225] Later elective nephrectomy may subsequently be required for some patients.

XANTHOGRANULOMATOUS PYELONEPHRITIS

Xanthogranulomatous pyelonephritis is an uncommon, severe, subacute or chronic suppurative process characterized by destruction and replacement of the renal parenchyma by granulomatous tissue containing histocytes and foamy cells.[230,231] The inflammatory process may extend into perinephric structures such as Gerota's fascia, the posterior perirenal space, the psoas muscle, the diaphragm, and the spleen. Less than 1% to 8% of kidneys removed or subjected to biopsy for inflammatory conditions are reported to show evidence of xanthogranulomatous pyelonephritis.[231] The pathogenesis of this process is unknown, but potential contributing factors include chronic urinary tract infection, abnormal lipid metabolism, lymphatic obstruction, impaired leukocyte function, and vascular occlusion. Urine culture results are positive in 62% to 89% of cases. The organisms most commonly isolated from renal tissue are *P. mirabilis* (38%), *E. coli* (33%), *Klebsiella/Enterobacter* species (8%), *P. aeruginosa* (8%), and *S. aureus* (10%).

In a single-center experience covering 1994 through 2005, 35 (85%) of 41 cases occurred in women.[232] Xanthogranulomatous pyelonephritis was responsible for 19% of 214 nephrectomies performed at this facility during the review period. The most common presenting symptoms were fever, flank or abdominal pain, weight loss, lower urinary tract symptoms, and gross hematuria. All patients had renal calculi. Of 17 cases in which urine culture specimens were obtained, *E. coli* was isolated in 35% and *P. mirabilis* in 18%; in 35% there was no growth.

In a second single-center review from Greece of 39 cases occurring between 1980 and 1999, the female/male ratio was 2:1.[230] The presenting history included urolithiasis or renal colic, recurrent urinary tract infections, and previous urologic procedures. All patients were symptomatic at presentation; symptoms included complaints of fever, flank or abdominal pain, chills, and malaise. Anorexia, weight loss, lower tract symptoms, and gross hematuria were also reported. *E. coli* was isolated in 15 cases and *P. mirabilis* in 12. Plain radiographs or intravenous pyelography (IVP) showed a nonfunctioning kidney in 63% of cases, single or multiple calculi in 52%, staghorn calculus in 48%, calyceal deformity in 26%, and hydronephrosis in 23%.

CT is considered the optimal imaging modality; it identifies the abnormality in 74% to 90% of cases.[110,111,233] Because of the current widespread access to CT, the diagnosis is now usually made preoperatively. Characteristic findings include an enlarged kidney, frequently with replacement of renal parenchyma and multiple fluid-filled cavities, together with urolithiasis. Ultrasonography identifies nonspecific abnormalities, including renal enlargement with relative preservation of renal contour and multiple hypoechoic round masses.[111] MRI shows abnormalities similar to those observed with CT.[233] The differential diagnosis includes malignancy and tuberculosis. The usual management is nephrectomy; antimicrobial therapy has only a secondary role.[231] If the diagnosis is made early, when there is only focal renal involvement, partial nephrectomy may be curative.

PYOCYSTIS

Pyocystis, also called *vesicle empyema*, is an infection characterized by a purulent fluid collection in the bladder of a patient with a nonfunctioning bladder. In effect, the bladder becomes an undrained abscess. This is a rare complication diagnosed in patients with anuric renal failure or surgically bypassed bladders. The clinical presentation includes suprapubic pain or distension, abdominal pain, foul-smelling urethral discharge, and fever or sepsis.[234,235] Organisms isolated have included *E. coli*, *P. mirabilis*, *P. aeruginosa*, *Serratia marcescens*, *Streptococcus* species, *Enterococcus* species, and *Candida* species. Mixed cultures are common. It is not known whether anaerobic organisms may also contribute.

When the condition is suspected, a specimen of bladder fluid should be obtained for diagnosis and culture. The laboratory should be requested to identify all organisms isolated, so that the specimen is processed as abscess fluid rather than urine. The treatment approach involves systemic antimicrobial agents and urethral catheterization for bladder drainage. Antimicrobial therapy is directed by the specific organisms isolated. Bladder irrigation with either saline or an antibiotic solution is sometimes recommended, but whether irrigation provides an additional therapeutic benefit is not clear.[236] Surgical intervention to achieve adequate drainage is necessary in rare recalcitrant cases.

UNCOMMON ORGANISMS

GENITOURINARY TUBERCULOSIS

Genitourinary tuberculosis is diagnosed in 1.1% to 1.5% of all tuberculosis cases, and 5% to 6% of cases of extrapulmonary tuberculosis.[237-239] This infection is usually a consequence of local reactivation following hematogenous dissemination of *Mycobacterium tuberculosis* to the renal cortex during primary pulmonary infection. The renal cortex is also frequently involved with miliary disease, when multiple granulomas are usually present. The high oxygen tension of the renal cortex is favorable for renal localization. Men are infected twice as often as women. The latent period, from the time of initial pulmonary infection to diagnosis of clinical urogenital tuberculosis, is 22 years on average with a range of 1 to 46 years.[240] Reactivation of tuberculosis usually occurs in only one kidney; thus disease is characteristically unilateral. Contiguous involvement of the collecting system leads to *M. tuberculosis* bacilluria with subsequent ureteric and bladder infection. Prostate and epididymis infection may result directly from hematogenous dissemination rather than contiguous spread. The kidneys are affected in 60% to 100% of cases, the ureters in 19% to 41%, the bladder in 15% to 20%, and the prostate or epididymis in 20% to 50% of men.[240]

Substantial morbidity is attributed to urogenital tuberculosis. Severe calyceal clubbing and dilation of the renal pelvis and ureters leading to total destruction of the kidney and autonephrectomy occur in 23% to 33% of cases, and renal failure occurs in 1% to 10%.[240] A summary of cases reported worldwide noted that 27% of patients had a nonfunctioning unilateral kidney at presentation, but this proportion varied from 8% to 72% in different countries, presumably reflecting the timeliness of diagnosis.[241]

Presenting genitourinary symptoms are often vague or nonspecific but may include back or flank pain, dysuria, and urinary frequency. As many as 50% of patients have no localizing genitourinary symptoms. About 25% to 33% of patients have systemic complaints, usually pulmonary symptoms, fever, and weight loss.[240,242] The subacute presentation and results of the initial evaluation can mimic those of xanthogranulomatous pyelonephritis. In men, additional features suggestive of tuberculosis include an enlarged, hard, and nontender epididymis; thickened or beaded vas deferens; indurated or nodular prostate; and nontender testicular mass.[238] Tuberculous granulomatous prostatitis may manifest as a nodular prostate with an elevation of prostate-specific antigen that is clinically indistinguishable from that in prostate carcinoma. Most patients with renal tuberculosis have evidence of concomitant extragenital disease. The most common site is the lungs, but the pulmonary disease is usually inactive. The chest radiograph is abnormal in 67% to 75% of patients, and the tuberculin skin test result positive in 60% to 90%.

The urinalysis findings are abnormal in more than 90% of patients with genitourinary tuberculosis.[237] Sterile pyuria with hematuria is present in 51% of cases, sterile pyuria alone in 26%, and gross or microscopic hematuria alone in 13%. For patients with HIV infection, an algorithm that incorporates negative results of routine urine culture and the presence of pyuria, albuminuria, or hematuria has good predictive value for detecting genitourinary tuberculosis.[243,244] As many as half of HIV-positive patients, however, have concomitant bacteriuria with other organisms at presentation, and this finding may obscure the initial assessment of the urinalysis.

IVP was traditionally the standard imaging approach, but CT is now preferred.[240] Imaging studies identify unilateral disease in 75% of cases of renal tuberculosis (Figure 37.1). The characteristic early finding is erosions of the renal calyx; the erosions subsequently progress to papillary necrosis, hydronephrosis, renal parenchymal cavitation, and dilated calyces. Ureteric tuberculosis is characterized by a thickened ureteric wall and strictures. Lesions are most common in the distal third of the ureter. Bladder tuberculosis may manifest as reduced bladder volume with wall thickening, ulceration, and filling defects resulting from granulomatous involvement. In advanced disease, scarring results in permanent loss of volume and a residual small, irregular, calcified bladder. The most common finding on CT is renal calcification, present in 50% of cases.[245] Other characteristic findings are hydrocalyx secondary to infundibular stenosis and cavity formation. In advanced disease, cortical loss, uroepithelial thickening, and dystrophic calcification are present.

The diagnosis is confirmed by growth of *M. tuberculosis* in urine or tissue culture. Appropriate specimens for mycobacterial culture should be obtained whenever this diagnosis is considered. Three sequential early morning urine specimens for mycobacterial culture are recommended. Urine cultures have positive results in 75% to 90% of affected patients. A positive acid-fast bacillus smear of urine usually signifies *M. tuberculosis,* but culture confirmation is essential to rule out colonization with nonpathogenic mycobacteria and for susceptibility testing of the infecting strain.[246,247] If a suggestive renal abnormality is present but urine culture results are negative, tissue biopsy may be necessary to confirm the diagnosis. Polymerase chain reaction (PCR) nucleic acid antigen testing of urine specimens has been reported to be more sensitive than culture and, if available, provides a more rapid diagnosis.[239,244] However, culture is still necessary to isolate the organism for susceptibility testing.

The treatment of genitourinary tuberculosis is similar to that of extrapulmonary tuberculosis at other sites. The initial regimen consists of four drugs (isoniazid, rifampin, pyrazinamide, and ethambutol) for 2 months, followed by two drugs (isoniazid, rifampin) for 4 months if the isolate is susceptible to first-line therapy. Antimycobacterial treatment should be provided under the supervision of a physician with expertise in tuberculosis management. Follow-up IVP every 6 months has been recommended to monitor healing, because ureteral scarring and obstruction may develop or progress during therapy as part of the

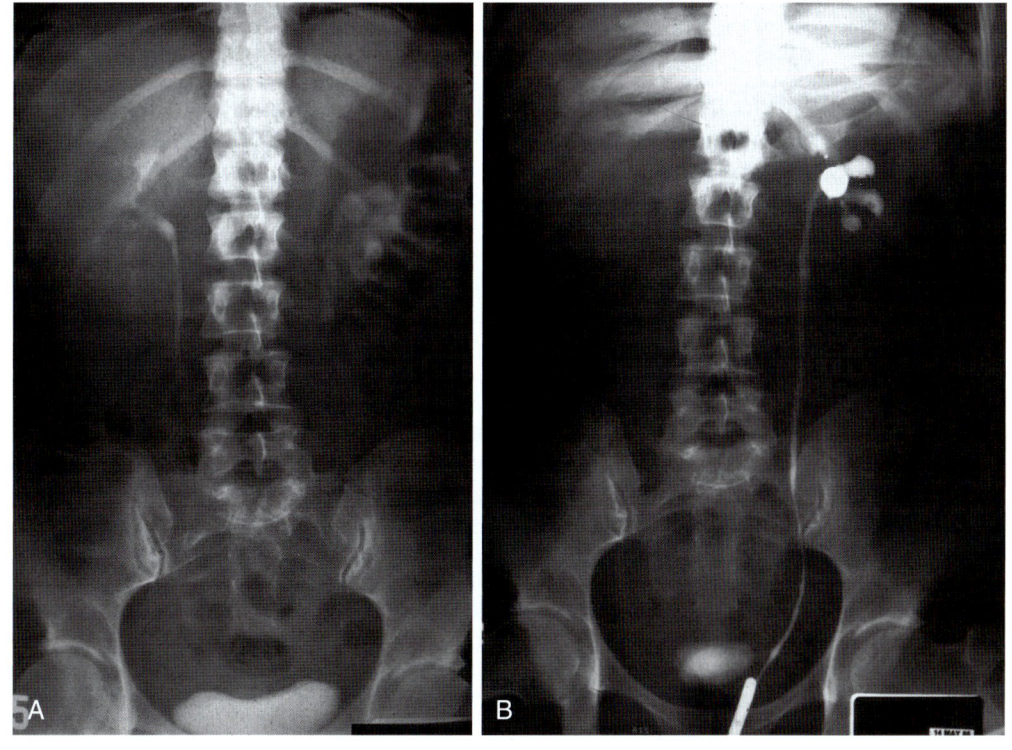

Figure 37.1 Renal tuberculosis. **A,** Intravenous pyelogram, showing unilateral hydronephrosis and calyceal distension. **B,** Retrograde pyelogram in the same patient, showing distal ureteric narrowing.

healing process. Corticosteroid therapy does not prevent this complication.[237] Ureteral reimplantation, endoscopic balloon dilation, or implantation of ureteral stents may be necessary if progressive obstruction develops. Nephrectomy is rarely required but may be indicated for intractable pain, untreatable infection proximal to a stricture, uncontrollable hematuria or hypertension, or drug resistance. Bladder augmentation surgery may be required if the bladder is scarred and contracted after tuberculosis infection.[248]

BACILLE DE CALMETTE-GUÉRIN INFECTION

Intravesical vaccine instillation of bacille de Calmette-Guérin (BCG) is considered first-line treatment for superficial bladder tumors and carcinoma in situ. Treatment with this biologic therapy may be complicated by systemic or local BCG infection.[249-251] BCG bladder instillation is followed by local irritative symptoms such as dysuria in 80% of cases, but these symptoms do not usually persist beyond 48 hours.[252] If symptoms do persist, isoniazid for 14 days is recommended, and if symptoms continue despite isoniazid therapy, a full course of antituberculous therapy is recommended.[253] Other, less common genitourinary infections that accompany BCG instillation include prostatitis in 1% to 3% of patients, epididymitis in 0.2%,[250] and, in rare cases, testicular abscesses, bladder ulcers, local skin infections, or renal infection. Reflux may be a risk factor for the rare complication of BCG pyelonephritis.[254] Localized genitourinary infection tends to have a delayed onset and is usually not apparent clinically until more than 3 months after BCG treatment.[249,251] BCG may not be isolated from urine or tissue cultures.[249] Tissue biopsy usually shows necrotizing granulomatous inflammation, and this finding in the context of prior BCG therapy is sufficient for diagnosis even if subsequent culture results are negative.

FUNGAL URINARY TRACT INFECTION

Fungal urinary tract infection is usually caused by *Candida* species, which have an extensive array of virulence factors that may facilitate successful colonization and invasion of the urinary tract.[255] Infection may be either antegrade, following candidemia, or retrograde via the urethra.[255] Clinical manifestations are asymptomatic candiduria, cystitis, and pyelonephritis. Bladder or renal fungus balls and systemic fungemia are rare complications.[256]

Candida albicans is isolated from more than 50% of episodes, followed by *Candida glabrata*, *Candida tropicalis* and *Candida parapsilosis*.[257,258] Candiduria is usually identified in patients who are seriously ill with multiple comorbid conditions, and most infections are asymptomatic.[256] The most important risk factors for candiduria are the presence of an indwelling catheter or other indwelling urologic device, diabetes mellitus, and exposure to broad-spectrum antimicrobial agents.[258] Treatment of asymptomatic candiduria is not beneficial and is currently recommended only for selected patients with neutropenia or before a traumatic urologic procedure.[259-261] Indwelling devices should be removed whenever possible to facilitate resolution of candiduria. Imaging studies to exclude fungus balls should be considered in patients who have recurrent symptomatic infection or urinary obstruction.[262] If fungus balls are present, their surgical removal is required for cure of the infection.

Fluconazole is the treatment of choice for *Candida* urinary tract infection because it is excreted in the urine in active form and high urinary levels are achieved.[260,261] A 2-week course of fluconazole, 200 to 400 mg daily, is recommended (Table 37.9). Amphotericin B deoxycholate, 0.3 to 0.6 mg/kg daily, is the alternative treatment recommended for fluconazole-resistant strains, including most *C. glabrata* organisms, as well as in patients who are allergic to fluconazole or in whom treatment fails despite optimal fluconazole therapy and urologic management. Treatment duration with amphotericin B is 1 to 7 days for cystitis and 2 weeks for pyelonephritis. Amphotericin B may also be effective for treatment of fungal cystitis when administered as a bladder washout, but this approach is not generally recommended because it requires several days of urethral catheterization and the optimal dose, frequency, and duration are not well established.[263] With the lipid formulations of amphotericin B, concentrations of active drug achieved in renal tissue and urine are very low, so these formulations are not recommended.

The antifungal 5-flucytosine is excreted in the urine and is indicated for treatment of *Candida* urinary tract infection as a single agent or in combination with amphotericin B for renal infection.[260,261] Resistance to 5-flucytosine develops rapidly when this drug is used as a single agent, and the frequent adverse effects of bone marrow suppression and enterocolitis also limit its use, particularly in patients with renal failure. Echinocandins such as caspofungin, micafungin, and anidulafungin and other azoles such as itraconazole, voriconazole, and posaconazole, which are not excreted into the urine, are not recommended for treatment of urinary tract infection.[260,261] There are, however, case reports of successful treatment of *C. glabrata* urinary tract infection with caspofungin.[264]

Table 37.9 Recommended Treatment of Candiduria

	Cystitis	Pyelonephritis
Fluconazole (if isolate is susceptible)	200-400 mg daily, 14 days	200-400 mg daily, 14 days
Amphotericin B deoxycholate	0.3-0.6 mg/kg daily, 1-7 days	0.5-0.7 mg/kg daily, 14 days
Amphotericin B bladder irrigation	5-50 mg/L continuous irrigation for 2-7 days	Not indicated
Flucytosine	25 mg/kg qid; 7-10 days	25 mg/kg qid, 14 days*

From Pappas PG, Kauffman CA, Andes D, et al: Clinical practice guidelines for the management of candidiasis 2009: Update by the Infectious Diseases Society of America, Clin Infect Dis 48:503-535, 2009.
*May be used in combination with amphotericin B.
qid, Four times a day.

VIRAL INFECTIONS

Viral urinary tract infections are uncommon in adults and occur largely in immunocompromised patients.[265-268] Clinical manifestations of viral infection generally follow reactivation of latent infection in immunocompromised patients, although de novo infection may occur. The usual clinical manifestation is hemorrhagic cystitis, but nephropathy has also been described.[265,269-271] The most common viruses are adenovirus, parvovirus B19, and CMV. More than one viral infection may coexist. Most adult cases occur in recipients of hematopoietic stem cell transplants, particularly those with severe graft-versus-host disease, and in renal transplant recipients. Infection has also been reported in other immunosuppressed patients, such as HIV-infected patients with low $CD4^+$ cell counts.[267,272] HIV-associated nephropathy (HIVAN) as a distinct clinical entity, including consideration of the role of host genetic background, glomerular cell viral entry and replication, is considered in Chapter 33.

Management of parvovirus B19 infection in the transplanted kidney is discussed in Chapter 72. Adenovirus or CMV infection is diagnosed by viral culture or PCR of the urine. Management includes minimization of immunosuppressive therapy if possible. For HIV-infected patients, antiretroviral therapy to increase the $CD4^+$ cell count should be initiated. CMV infection responds to treatment with ganciclovir or foscarnet.[265] Treatment of adenovirus infection employs cidofovir, although some efficacy has been reported with vidarabine.[265] There have also been case reports of successful treatment of adenovirus with ganciclovir and ribavirin.[265,273]

PARASITIC INFESTATIONS OF THE URINARY TRACT

The most common and important parasitic infestation of the urinary tract is with *Schistosoma hematobium*.[274,275] This parasite is acquired after exposure to contaminated water. *Schistosoma* larvae penetrate the intact skin and migrate in the blood to the liver, where they transform into young worms (schistosomulae) that mature in 4 to 6 weeks and then further migrate to the perivesical venules. The life span of the adult worm in the venule is usually 3 to 5 years but can be longer. Most eggs produced by the adult worms enter the bladder lumen and are removed in the urine. However, some eggs are retained locally in the bladder wall, where they incite an eosinophilic inflammatory and granulomatous immune response that causes progressive fibrosis.

The functional abnormality early in the disease is obstruction of the bladder neck. Late complications include recurrent bacterial urinary tract infection, bladder or ureteric stone formation, renal functional abnormalities, and, ultimately, kidney failure.[275,276] *Schistosoma* infestation is also a risk factor for squamous cell carcinoma of the bladder. The relative risk of cancer for persons with schistosomiasis varies from 1.8 to 23.5; the incidence is highest in the 30- to 50-year age group.[277]

The prevalence of infection in endemic areas is high. Surveys from rural Zimbabwe revealed that 60% of women younger than 20 years of age and 29% of those aged 45 to 49 years have eggs in the urine; HIV-infected women older than 35 years had a significantly higher prevalence of infestation.[278] Travelers to endemic areas may acquire infection with only minimal exposure to contaminated water.[279,280]

Acute genitourinary symptoms occur in up to 50% of cases following acquisition of infection and include hematuria, which is often terminal, together with dysuria and urinary frequency. Microhematuria is reported in 41% to 100% and gross hematuria in 0% to 97% of patients with chronic schistosomal infestation. Radiologic abnormalities are present in the upper urinary tract in 2% to 62% of chronic cases.[275] Ultrasonography of the urinary tract demonstrates thickening of the bladder wall, granulomatous changes, hydronephrosis, and, on occasion, bladder or ureteric calcification. The diagnosis is established by identification of parasite eggs in the urine or biopsy specimens or by serologic findings. Urine specimens collected for identification of eggs should be obtained on consecutive days between 1100 and 1300 hours because egg passage is maximal at this time. Sedimentation or filtration of the urine before examination increases the sensitivity of egg detection.[275,281]

Treatment with one dose of praziquantel, 40 mg per kg body weight, leads to cure in 80% of cases. Follow-up urine specimens for parasite examination are recommended 3 months after treatment to identify patients in whom treatment has failed and must be repeated. Bladder wall thickening and hydroureters may be reversed if treatment is given early in the course of infestation. However, when chronic disease is established and fibrotic lesions are present, changes may not be reversible, and corrective surgery or management of end-stage renal disease is required.[281]

The protozoal parasite *T. vaginalis* is commonly transmitted sexually and is occasionally identified on microscopy with routine urinalysis. In women, the parasite may originate from contamination of the urine by vaginal secretions, but the organism is a well-described cause of urethritis for both men and women. Whenever *T. vaginalis* is identified, treatment of the patient and his or her sexual partners is indicated, regardless of symptoms. The recommended treatment is a single dose of metronidazole, 2 g, or tinidazole, 2 g.[282]

Echinococcus granulosus infestation occasionally involves the kidneys.[274] Renal cysts are reported in 2% to 3% of cases of hydatid disease.[283,284] The diagnosis is usually made after an incidental finding of a cyst in the kidneys, ureters, bladder, or testes. On occasion, flank pain or a mass is present. Hydatid cysts are not excreted in the urine. Treatment consists of surgical cyst removal or marsupialization; nephrectomy is occasionally necessary. Perioperative albendazole therapy is also usually recommended for patients with hydatid disease. A less common helminthic infestation is *Wucheria bancrofti* (filariasis), which may cause lymphatic obstruction and rupture into the urinary collecting system, producing chyluria.[274]

Complete reference list available at ExpertConsult.com.

KEY REFERENCES

1. Hooton TM: Uncomplicated urinary tract infection. *N Engl J Med* 366:1028–1037, 2012.
4. Nicolle LE, AMMI-Canada Guidelines Committee: Complicated urinary tract infection in adults. *Can J Infect Dis Med Microbiol* 16:349–360, 2005.

11. Finer G, Landau D: Pathogenesis of urinary tract infections with normal female anatomy. *Lancet Infect Dis* 4:631–635, 2004.
12. Ragnarsdottir B, Svanborg C: Susceptibility to acute pyelonephritis or asymptomatic bacteriuria: Host-pathogen interaction in urinary tract infections. *Pediatr Nephrol* 27:2017–2029, 2012.
13. Wullt B, Bergsten G, Fischer H, et al: The host response to urinary tract infection. *Infect Dis Clin North Am* 17:279–302, 2003.
22. High KP, Bradley SF, Gravenstein S, et al: Clinical practice guideline for the evaluation of fever and infection in older adult residents of long term care facilities. *Clin Infect Dis* 48:149–171, 2009.
26. Lipsky BA, Byren I, Hoey CT: Treatment of bacterial prostatitis. *Clin Infect Dis* 50:1641–1652, 2010.
33. Bermingham SL, Ashe JF: Systematic review of the impact of urinary tract infections on health-related quality of life. *BJU Int* 110:e830–e836, 2012.
37. Johnson JR: Microbial virulence determinants and the pathogenesis of urinary tract infection. *Infect Dis Clin North Am* 17:261–278, 2003.
57. Perrotta C, Aznar M, Mejia R, et al: Oestrogens for preventing recurrent urinary tract infection in postmenopausal women. *Cochrane Database Syst Rev* (2):CD005131, 2008.
59. Bent S, Saint S: The optimal use of diagnostic testing in women with acute uncomplicated cystitis. *Am J Med* 113(Suppl 1A):20S–28S, 2002.
66. Gupta K, Hooton TM, Naver KG, et al: International clinical practice guidelines for the treatment of acute uncomplicated cystitis and pyelonephritis in women: A 2010 update by the Infectious Diseases Society of America and the European Society for Microbiology and Infectious Diseases. *Clin Infect Dis* 52:e103–e120, 2011.
80. Beerepoot MAJ, Geerlings SE, van Haarst EP, et al: Nonantibiotic prophylaxis for recurrent urinary tract infections: A systematic review and meta-analysis of randomized controlled trials. *J Urol* 190:1981–1989, 2013.
81. Jepson RG, Craig JC: Cranberries for preventing urinary tract infections. *Cochrane Database Syst Rev* (1):CD001321, 2008.
90. Naber KG, Cho YH, Matsumoto T, et al: Immunoactive prophylaxis of recurrent urinary tract infections: a meta-analysis. *Int J Antimicrob Agents* 33:111–119, 2009.
92. Hill JB, Sheffield JS, McIntire DD, et al: Acute pyelonephritis in pregnancy. *Obstet Gynecol* 105:18–23, 2005.
97. Scholes D, Hooton TM, Roberts PL, et al: Risk factors associated with acute pyelonephritis in healthy women. *Ann Intern Med* 142:20–27, 2005.
110. Demetzis J, Menias CD: State of the art: imaging of renal infections. *Emerg Radiol* 14:13–22, 2007.
114. Sandberg T, Skoog G, Hermansson AB, et al: Ciprofloxacin for 7 days versus 14 days in women with acute pyelonephritis: a randomized, open-label and double-blind, placebo controlled non-inferiority trial. *Lancet* 380:484–490, 2012.
123. D'Hondt F, Everaert K: Urinary tract infections in patients with spinal cord injuries. *Curr Infect Dis Rep* 13:544–551, 2011.
126. Kauffman CA, Vazquez JA, Sobel JD, et al: National Institute for Allergy and Infectious Diseases Mycoses Study Group: prospective, multicenter surveillance study of funguria in hospitalized patients. *Clin Infect Dis* 30:14–18, 2000.
132. Nicolle LE, Bradley S, Colgan R, et al: Infectious Diseases Society of America guidelines for the diagnosis and treatment of asymptomatic bacteriuria in adults. *Clin Infect Dis* 40:643–654, 2005.
133. Nicolle LE: Urinary tract infection. *Crit Care Clin* 3:699–715, 2013.
134. Loeb M, Bentley DW, Bradley S, et al: Development of minimum criteria for the initiation of antibiotics in residents of long term care facilities: results of a consensus conference. *Infect Control Hosp Epidemiol* 22:120–124, 2001.
137. Wullt B, Agace W, Mansson W: Bladder, bowel and bugs—bacteriuria in patients with intestinal urinary diversion. *World J Urol* 22:186–195, 2004.
140. Hooton TM, Bradley SF, Cardenas DD, et al: Diagnosis, prevention, and treatment of catheter-associated urinary tract infections in adults: 2009 international clinical practice guidelines from the Infectious Diseases Society of America. *Clin Infect Dis* 50(5):625–663, 2010.
141. Gould CV, Umscheid CA, Agarwal RK, et al: Health Care Infection Control Practices Advisory Committee: Guidelines for prevention of catheter-associated urinary tract infections 2009. *Infect Control Hosp Epidemiol* 31(4):319–326, 2010.
142. Siddiq DM, Darouiche RO: New strategies to prevent catheter-associated urinary tract infections. *Nature Rev Urol* 9:305–314, 2012.
152. Marcus RJ, Post JC, Stoodley P, et al: Biofilms in nephrology. *Expert Opin Biol Ther* 8:1159–1166, 2008.
158. Cai T, Mazzoli S, Mondaini N, et al: The role of asymptomatic bacteriuria in young women with recurrent urinary infections: To treat or not to treat? *Clin Infect Dis* 55:771–777, 2012.
159. Green H, Rahamimov R, Golbert E, et al: Consequences of treated versus untreated asymptomatic bacteriuria in the first year following kidney transplantation: retrospective observational study. *Eur J Clin Microbiol Infect Dis* 32:127–131, 2012.
162. Widmer M, Gulmezoglu AM, Mignini L, et al: Duration of treatment of asymptomatic bacteriuria during pregnancy. *Cochrane Database Syst Rev* (12):CD000491, 2011.
165. Krieger JN, Nyberg L, Nickel JC: NIH consensus definition and classification of prostatitis. *JAMA* 281:236–237, 1999.
167. Etienne M, Chavanet P, Sibert L, et al: Acute bacterial prostatitis: heterogenicity in diagnostic criteria and management. Retrospective multicentric analysis of 371 patients diagnosed with acute prostatitis. *BMC Infect Dis* 8:12, 2008.
174. de Souza RM, Olsburgh J: Urinary tract infection in the renal transplant patient. *Nature Clin Pract* 4:252–264, 2008.
196. Gilbert DN: Urinary tract infections in patients with chronic renal failure. *Clin J Am Soc Nephrol* 1:327–331, 2006.
198. Zanetta G, Paparella S, Trinchieri A, et al: Infections and urolithiasis: current clinical evidence in prophylaxis and antibiotic therapy. *Arch Ital di Urol Androl* 80:5–12, 2008.
206. Coelho RF, Schneider-Montero ED, Mesquita JLB, et al: Renal and perinephric abscess. Analysis of 65 consecutive cases. *World J Surg* 31:431–436, 2007.
210. Hung C-H, Liou J-D, Yan M-Y, et al: Immediate percutaneous drainage compared with surgical drainage of renal abscess. *Int Urol Nephrol* 39:51–55, 2007.
212. Saller M, Rafat C, Zahar J-R, et al: Cyst infections in patients with autosomal dominant polycystic kidney disease. *Clin J Am Soc Nephrol* 4:1183–1189, 2009.
213. Jouret F, Lhommel R, Devuyst O, et al: Diagnosis of cyst infection in patients with autosomal dominant polycystic kidney disease: attributes and limitations of the current modalities. *Nephrol Dial Transplant* 27:3746–3756, 2012.
222. Thomas AA, Lane BR, Thomas AZ, et al: Emphysematous cystitis: a review of 135 cases. *BJU Int* 100:17–20, 2007.
224. Pontin AR, Barnes RD: Current management of emphysematous pyelonephritis. *Nat Rev Urol* 6:272–279, 2009.
226. Bjurlin MA, Hurley SD, Kim DY, et al: Clinical outcomes of nonoperative management in emphysematous urinary tract infections. *Urol* 79:1281–1285, 2012.
240. Figuerido AA, Lucon AM: Urogenital tuberculosis: update and review of 8961 cases from the world literature. *Rev Urol* 10:207–217, 2008.
249. Gonzalez DY, Musher DM, Brar I, et al: Spectrum of bacille Calmette-Guérin (BCG) infection after intravesical BCG immunotherapy. *Clin Infect Dis* 36:140–148, 2003.
256. Kauffman CA, Fisher JF, Sobel JD, et al: *Candida* urinary tract infections: diagnosis. *Clin Infect Dis* 52(Suppl 6):S452–S456, 2011.
260. Pappas PG, Kauffman CA, Andes D, et al: Clinical practice guidelines for the management of candidiasis 2009: update by the Infectious Diseases Society of America. *Clin Infect Dis* 48:503–535, 2009.
262. Sadegi BJ, Patel BK, Wilbur AC, et al: Primary renal candidiasis: importance of imaging and clinical history in diagnosis and management. *J Ultrasound Med* 28:507–514, 2009.
265. Paduch DA: Viral lower urinary tract infections. *Curr Urol Rep* 8:324–335, 2007.
276. Khalaf I, Shokeir A, Shalaby M: Urologic complications of genitourinary schistosomiasis. *World J Urol* 30:31–38, 2012.

Urinary Tract Obstruction

38

Jørgen Frøkiær

CHAPTER OUTLINE

PREVALENCE AND INCIDENCE, 1257
CLASSIFICATION, 1258
ETIOLOGY, 1258
Congenital Causes of Obstruction, 1258
Acquired Causes of Obstruction, 1259
CLINICAL ASPECTS, 1262
DIAGNOSIS, 1262
History and Physical Examination, 1262
Biochemical Evaluation, 1263
Evaluation by Medical Imaging, 1263
PATHOPHYSIOLOGY OF OBSTRUCTIVE NEPHROPATHY, 1268
Effects of Obstruction on Renal Blood Flow and Glomerular Filtration, 1269

Effects of Obstruction on Tubular Function, 1271
PATHOPHYSIOLOGY OF RECOVERY OF TUBULAR EPITHELIAL CELLS FROM OBSTRUCTION OR TUBULOINTERSTITIAL FIBROSIS, 1277
Fetal Urinary Tract Obstruction, 1279
TREATMENT OF URINARY TRACT OBSTRUCTION AND RECOVERY OF RENAL FUNCTION, 1279
Estimating Renal Damage and Potential for Recovery, 1280
Recovery of Renal Function after Prolonged Obstruction, 1280
POSTOBSTRUCTIVE DIURESIS, 1281

In adults 1.5 to 2.0 L of urine flows daily from the renal papillae through the ureter, bladder, and urethra in an uninterrupted, unidirectional flow. Any obstruction of urinary flow at any point along the urinary tract may cause retention of urine and increased retrograde hydrostatic pressure, leading to kidney damage and interference with waste and water excretion, as well as fluid and electrolyte homeostasis. Because the extent of recovery of renal function in obstructive nephropathy is related inversely to the extent and duration of obstruction, prompt diagnosis and relief of obstruction are essential for effective management. Fortunately, urinary tract obstruction in most cases is a highly treatable form of kidney disease.

Several terms describe urinary tract obstruction, and definitions may vary.[1-3] In the following discussion *hydronephrosis* is defined as a dilation of the renal pelvis and calyces proximal to the point of obstruction. *Obstructive uropathy* refers to blockage of urine flow due to a functional or structural derangement anywhere from the tip of the urethra back to the renal pelvis that increases pressure proximal to the site of obstruction. Obstructive uropathy may or may not result in renal parenchymal damage. Such functional or pathologic parenchymal damage is referred to as *obstructive nephropathy*. It should be noted that hydronephrosis and obstructive uropathy are not interchangeable terms—dilation of the renal pelvis and calyces can occur without obstruction, and urinary tract obstruction may occur in the absence of hydronephrosis.

PREVALENCE AND INCIDENCE

The incidence of urinary tract obstruction varies widely among different populations, and depends on concurrent medical conditions, sex, and age. Unfortunately, epidemiologic reports have been based on the studies of selected "populations," such as women with high-risk pregnancies and data from autopsy series. In the United States it has been estimated that 166 patients per 100,000 population had a presumptive diagnosis of obstructive uropathy on admission to hospitals in 1985.[4] The introduction of routine prenatal ultrasound scanning resulted in an increasing number of infants suspected with urinary tract obstruction,[5] and with the increasing age of the population during the past 25 years the incidence of obstructive uropathy may be expected to increase even more.

A review of 59,064 autopsies of individuals varying in age from neonate to 80 years noted hydronephrosis as a finding in 3.1% (3.3% in males and 2.9% in females). In individuals younger than 10 years, representing 1.5% of all autopsies, the principal causes of urinary tract obstruction were ureteral or urethral strictures or neurologic abnormalities. It is unclear how frequently these abnormalities represented incidental findings, as opposed to being recognized clinically. Until the age of 20, there was no substantial sex difference in frequency of abnormalities (for details please also see Chapter 73). Between the ages of 20 and 60, urinary tract obstruction was more frequent among women than among men, mainly due to the effects of uterine cancer and pregnancy. Above the age of 60, prostatic disease raised the frequency of urinary tract obstruction among men above that observed among women.

In children younger than age 15, obstruction occurred in 2% of autopsies. Hydronephrosis was found in 2.2% of the boys and 1.5% of the girls; 80% of the hydronephrosis that did occur was found in individuals younger than 1 year.[6] Consistent with this, another autopsy series of 3172 children identified urinary tract abnormalities in 2.5%. Hydroureter and hydronephrosis were the most common findings, representing 35.9% of all cases.[7] However, it was not clear what proportion of cases was diagnosed clinically before death.

Because a high proportion of these autopsy-detected cases of obstruction likely went undetected during life, the overall prevalence of urinary tract obstruction is very likely far greater than reports suggest. This conclusion is reinforced by the fact that there are several common but temporary causes of obstruction, such as pregnancy and renal calculi.

CLASSIFICATION

Classification of urinary tract obstruction can be by duration (acute or chronic),[8] by whether it is congenital or acquired, and by its location (upper or lower urinary tract, supravesical, vesical or subvesical, and so on). Acute obstruction may be associated with sudden onset of symptoms. Upper urinary tract (ureter or ureteropelvic junction [UPJ]) obstruction may present with renal colic. Lower tract (bladder or urethra) obstruction may present with disorders of micturition. By contrast, chronic urinary tract obstruction may develop insidiously and present with few or only minor symptoms, and with more general manifestations. For example, recurrent urinary tract infections, bladder calculi, and progressive renal insufficiency may all result from chronic obstruction. Congenital causes of obstruction arise from developmental abnormalities, whereas acquired lesions develop after birth, either due to disease processes or as a result of medical interventions.[9]

ETIOLOGY

Because congenital and acquired urinary tract obstructions differ to a great degree in cause and clinical course, they will be described separately.

CONGENITAL CAUSES OF OBSTRUCTION

Congenital anomalies may obstruct the urinary tract at any level from the UPJ to the tip of urethra, and the obstruction may damage one or both kidneys (Table 38.1). Although some lesions occur rarely, as a group they represent an important cause of urinary tract obstruction, because in younger patients they often lead to severe renal impairment and may result in catastrophic end-stage kidney disease.[10] Thus this condition is also presented in detail in Chapter 73.

Table 38.1 Congenital Causes of Urinary Tract Obstruction

Ureteropelvic Junction
Ureteropelvic junction obstruction

Proximal and Middle Ureter
Ureteral folds
Ureteral valves
Strictures
Benign fibroepithelial polyps
Retrocaval ureter

Distal Ureter
Ureterovesical junction obstruction
Vesicoureteral reflux
Prune-belly syndrome
Ureteroceles

Bladder
Bladder diverticula
Neurologic conditions (e.g., spina bifida)

Urethra
Posterior urethral valves
Urethral diverticula
Anterior urethral valves
Urethral atresia
Labial fusion

The widespread use of fetal ultrasonography, and its increasing sensitivity, has led to early detection in an increasing number of cases. With an estimated prevalence of 2% to 5.5%, dilation of the renal collecting system is the most common ultrasonographic abnormality found in the fetal urinary tract.[11] In cases of severe obstruction, early detection may lead to termination of the pregnancy or attempts to ameliorate the obstruction in utero.[10,12,13] However, ultrasonography may detect mild obstruction of unknown clinical significance.[10,12] In brief, UPJ obstruction is the most common cause of hydronephrosis in fetuses[14] and young children,[15] with a reported incidence of 5 cases per 100,000 population per year,[16] and it may affect adults as well.[17] There is considerable controversy as to whether all cases of obstruction early in life are clinically significant. The widespread use of fetal ultrasonography has resulted in detection of many cases that remain asymptomatic and may resolve spontaneously with simple follow-up of the child.[3,18] Despite the numerous cases there is a lack of consistency with respect to the nomenclature and grading systems used in the clinical risk assessment of infants with antenatal hydronephrosis.[5] Although most cases of congenital UPJ obstruction are diagnosed prenatally by ultrasonography,[19] the most common neonatal clinical presentation is a flank or abdominal mass.[20] By contrast, adults generally present with flank pain.[17] Because intermittent obstruction may produce symptoms that mimic those of gastrointestinal disease, diagnosis may be delayed. At any age, UPJ obstruction may be associated with kidney stones, hematuria, hypertension, or recurrent urinary tract infection.[16,17] A detailed presentation of the different causes of UPJ obstruction is provided in Chapter 73, where a thorough presentation of the pathophysiology of proximal and distal congenital ureteral obstruction is discussed.

Congenital bladder outlet obstruction may be caused by mechanical or functional factors and will also be discussed in Chapter 73.

Because operative complications may be high,[21] the use of fetal[13,22] or neonatal[22,23] surgery for the relief of obstruction remains controversial.[10,12,13] Although bilateral obstruction requires intervention, patients with unilateral hydronephrosis are often followed without surgery, but with aggressive observation to identify the approximately 20% of patients with congenital hydronephrosis who require pyeloplasty.[23,24] Indications for surgery in unilateral hydronephrosis include symptoms of obstruction or impaired function in a presumably salvageable hydronephrotic kidney.

ACQUIRED CAUSES OF OBSTRUCTION

INTRINSIC CAUSES

Acquired causes of obstruction may be intrinsic to the urinary tract (i.e., resulting from intraluminal or intramural processes) or may arise from causes extrinsic to it (Table 38.2). Intrinsic causes of obstruction may be considered according to anatomic location.

Intrinsic intraluminal causes of obstruction may be intrarenal or extrarenal. Intrarenal causes arise from formation of casts or crystals within the renal tubules. These include uric acid nephropathy[25]; deposition of crystals of drugs that

Table 38.2 Acquired Causes of Urinary Tract Obstruction

Intrinsic processes
  Intraluminal
    Intrarenal
      Uric acid nephropathy
      Sulfonamides
      Acyclovir
      Indinavir
      Multiple myeloma
    Intraureteral
      Nephrolithiasis
      Papillary necrosis
      Blood clots
      Fungus balls
  Intramural
    Functional
      Diseases
        Diabetes mellitus
        Multiple sclerosis
        Cerebrovascular disease
        Spinal cord injury
        Parkinson's disease
      Drugs
        Anticholinergic agents
        Levodopa (α-adrenergic properties)
    Anatomic
      Ureteral strictures
        Schistosomiasis
        Tuberculosis
        Drugs (e.g., nonsteroidal antiinflammatory agents)
        Ureteral instrumentation
      Urethral strictures
      Benign or malignant tumors of the renal pelvis, ureter, bladder
Extrinsic processes
  Reproductive tract
    Females
      Uterus
        Pregnancy
        Tumor (fibroids, endometrial or cervical cancer)
        Endometriosis
        Uterine prolapse
        Ureteral ligation (surgical)
      Ovary
        Tubo-ovarian abscess
        Tumor
        Cyst
    Males
      Benign prostatic hyperplasia
      Prostate cancer
  Malignant neoplasms
    Genitourinary tract
      Tumors of kidney, ureter, bladder, urethra
    Other sites
      Metastatic spread
      Direct extension
  Gastrointestinal system
    Crohn's disease
    Appendicitis
    Diverticulosis
    Chronic pancreatitis with pseudocyst formation
    Acute pancreatitis
  Vascular system
    Arterial aneurysms
      Abdominal aortic aneurysm
      Iliac artery aneurysm
    Venous
      Ovarian vein thrombophlebitis
    Vasculitides
      Systemic lupus erythematosus
      Polyarteritis nodosa
      Granulomatosis with polyangiitis (formerly designated Wegener's granulomatosis)
      Henoch-Schönlein purpura
  Retroperitoneal processes
    Fibrosis
      Idiopathic
      Drug-induced
      Inflammatory
        Ascending lymphangitis of the lower extremities
        Chronic urinary tract infection
        Tuberculosis
        Sarcoidosis
      Iatrogenic (multiple abdominal surgical procedures)
    Enlarged retroperitoneal nodes
    Tumor invasion
    Tumor mass
    Hemorrhage
    Urinoma
  Biologic agents
    Actinomycosis

precipitate in the urine, including sulfonamides,[26] acyclovir,[27] indinavir,[28] and ciprofloxacin[29]; and multiple myeloma.[30] Uric acid nephropathy usually results from the large uric acid load released when alkylating agents abruptly kill large numbers of tumor cells in the treatment of patients with malignant hematopoietic neoplasms. The risk for uric acid nephropathy relates directly to plasma uric acid concentrations.[25] Uric acid nephropathy may also occur in the setting of disseminated adenomatous carcinoma of the gastrointestinal tract.[31] Sulfonamide crystal deposition, once a common occurrence, became rare with the introduction of sulfonamides that are more soluble in acid urine than earlier drugs. Sulfadiazine has been used as antiretroviral therapy, because it is relatively lipophilic and penetrates the brain well, making it an excellent treatment for toxoplasmosis in patients with acquired immunodeficiency syndrome (AIDS). However, the same lipophilicity makes the drug prone to the formation of intrarenal crystals, which can lead to acute kidney injury when the drug is given in large doses.[26,32] Ciprofloxacin may also precipitate in the tubule fluid, resulting in crystalluria with stone formation and urinary tract obstruction.[29] A common renal complication of multiple myeloma is "myeloma kidney," a condition also known as myeloma cast nephropathy. The renal lesions (casts) are directly related to the production of monoclonal immunoglobulin free light chains (FLCs), which coprecipitate with Tamm-Horsfall protein (THP) in the lumen of the distal nephron, obstructing tubule fluid flow.[33,34] Promising experiments have identified the determinants of the molecular interaction between FLCs and THP, which permitted development of a peptide that demonstrated strong inhibitory capability in the binding of FLCs to THP in vitro.[34]

Several intrinsic intraluminal, extrarenal, or intraureteral processes may also cause obstruction. Nephrolithiasis represents the most common cause of ureteral obstruction in younger men.[35] In the U.S. population the prevalence of symptomatic kidney stone of adult ages 20 to 74 was estimated from self-reported incidents between 1988 and 1994 to afflict 5.2% of adults (6.3% males and 4.1% females).[36] The significance of this number is also reflected by the large number of hospital admissions due to calculus of kidney and ureters, amounting to 166,000 hospital stays in 2006.[37] Calcium oxalate stones occur most commonly. Obstruction caused by such stones occurs sporadically, and tends to be acute and unilateral, and usually without a long-term impact on renal function. Of course, when a stone obstructs a solitary kidney, the result can be anuric or oliguric acute kidney injury. Less common types of stones, such as struvite (ammonium-magnesium-sulfate) and cysteine stones, more frequently cause significant renal damage because these substances accumulate over time and often form staghorn calculi. Stones tend to lodge and to obstruct urine flow at narrowings along the ureter, including the UPJ, the pelvic brim (where the ureter arches over the iliac vessels), and the ureterovesical junction.

Other processes that cause ureteral obstruction include papillary necrosis, blood clots, and cystic inflammation. Papillary necrosis[38] may result from sickle cell disease or trait, amyloidosis,[39] analgesic abuse, acute pyelonephritis, or diabetes mellitus. Renal allografts may develop papillary necrosis as well.[40] Acute obstruction may even require surgical intervention.[41] Blood clots secondary to a benign or malignant lesion of the urinary tract or cystic inflammation of the ureter (ureteritis cystica) can also lead to obstruction and hydronephrosis.[42]

Intrinsic intramural processes that cause obstruction include failure of micturition or more rarely of ureteral peristalsis. Bladder storage of urine and micturition require complex interplay of spinal reflexes, midbrain, and cortical function.[43] Neurologic dysfunction[44] occurring in diabetes mellitus, multiple sclerosis, spinal cord injury, cerebrovascular disease, and Parkinson's disease can result from upper motor neuron damage. These can produce a variety of forms of bladder dysfunction. If the bladder fails to empty properly, it can remain filled most of the time, resulting in chronic increased intravesical pressure, which is transmitted retrograde into the ureters and to the renal pelvis and kidney. In addition, failure of coordination of bladder contraction with the opening of the urethral sphincter may lead to bladder hypertrophy. In this setting, bladder filling requires increased hydrostatic pressures to stretch the hypertrophic detrusor muscle. Again the increased pressure in the bladder is transmitted up the urinary tract to the ureters and renal pelvis. Lower spinal tract injury may result in a flaccid, atonic bladder and failure of micturition, as well as recurrent urinary tract infections.

Various drugs may cause intrinsic intramural obstruction by disrupting the normal function of the smooth muscle of the urinary tract. Anticholinergic agents[45] may interfere with bladder contraction, whereas levodopa[46] may mediate an α-adrenergic increase in urethral sphincter tone, resulting in increased bladder outlet resistance. Chronic use of tiaprofenic acid (Surgam) can cause severe cystitis with subsequent ureteral obstruction.[47] In all circumstances when the bladder does not void normally, renal damage may develop as a consequence of recurrent urinary tract infections and back pressure produced by the accumulation of residual urine.

Acquired anatomic abnormalities of the wall of the urinary tract include ureteral strictures and benign as well as malignant tumors of the urethra, bladder, ureter, or renal pelvis.[48] Ureteral strictures may result from radiation therapy in children[49] and in adults[50] treated for pelvic or lower abdominal cancers, such as cervical cancer, or rarely as a result of analgesic abuse.[51] Strictures may also develop as a complication of ureteral instrumentation or surgery.

Infectious organisms may also produce intrinsic obstruction of the urinary tract. *Schistosoma haematobium* afflicts nearly 100 million people worldwide. Though active infection can be treated and obstructive uropathy may resolve, chronic schistosomiasis (bilharziasis) may develop in untreated cases, leading to irreversible ureteral or bladder fibrosis and obstruction.[52] Of other infections, the incidence of genitourinary tuberculosis has remained constant over the past 30 years, amounting to 3% to 5% of patients with tuberculosis.[53] Mycoses such as *Candida albicans* or *Candida tropicalis* infection may also result in obstruction due to intraluminal obstruction (fungus ball) or invasion of the ureteral wall.[54]

EXTRINSIC CAUSES

Acquired extrinsic urinary tract obstruction occurs in a wide variety of settings. The relatively high frequency of obstructive uropathy from processes in the female reproductive tract such as pregnancy and pelvic neoplasms results in higher rates of urinary tract obstruction in younger women than in younger men.[2] The advent of routine abdominal and fetal ultrasonography in pregnant women has revealed that more than two thirds of women entering their third trimester demonstrate some degree of dilation of the collecting system,[55] most often resulting from mechanical ureteral obstruction.[55] This temporary form of obstruction is usually observed above the point at which the ureter crosses the pelvic brim and affects the right ureter more often than the left.[55] The vast majority of these cases are subclinical and appear to resolve completely soon after delivery.[56] Clinically significant obstructive uropathy in pregnancy almost always presents with flank pain.[57] In these cases, ultrasonography serves as a useful initial screening test,[20] and magnetic resonance imaging (MRI) can be used if the ultrasonography is not conclusive.[57] Of course, the diagnostic evaluation must be tailored to minimize fetal radiation exposure. If the obstruction is significant, a ureteral stent can be placed cystoscopically, and its efficacy can be monitored with repeated follow-up ultrasonography.[58] The stent can be left in place for the duration of pregnancy, if needed. Clinically significant ureteral obstruction is rare in pregnancy, and bilateral obstruction leading to acute kidney injury is exceptionally rare.[57] Conditions in pregnancy that may predispose to obstructive uropathy and acute kidney injury include multiple fetuses, polyhydramnios, an incarcerated gravid uterus, or a solitary kidney.[56]

Pelvic malignancies, especially cervical adenocarcinomas, represent the second most common cause of extrinsic obstructive uropathy in women.[59] In older women, uterine prolapse and other failures of normal pelvic floor tone may cause obstruction, with hydronephrosis developing in 5% of patients.[60] In this setting prolapse may lead to compression of the ureter by uterine blood vessels. In addition, prolapse has been associated with urinary tract infection, sepsis, pyonephrosis, and renal insufficiency. Prolapse of other pelvic organs due to weakening of the pelvic floor may also result in obstruction.[60] Various benign pelvic abnormalities may cause ureteral obstruction, including uterine tumors or cystic ovary and pelvic inflammatory disease, particularly a tubo-ovarian abscess. Pelvic lipomatosis, a disease with an unclear etiology that is seen more often in men, is another rare reason for compressive urinary tract obstruction.[61]

Although endometriosis only rarely results in ureteral obstruction,[62] it should be included in the differential diagnosis any time a premenopausal woman presents with unilateral obstruction. The onset of obstruction may be insidious, and the process is usually confined to the pelvic portion of the ureter.[62] Ureteral involvement may be intrinsic or extrinsic, with extrinsic compression arising principally from adhesions associated with the endometriosis. Because ureteral involvement may come on slowly and may be unilateral, it is important to screen for obstructive uropathy in advanced cases of endometriosis,[62] preferably using computed tomography (CT) because ultrasonography may not reveal hydronephrosis if adhesions are preventing dilation of the ureter above the site of obstruction.[63] When surgery of any kind is contemplated in patients with endometriosis, it is all the more important to image the ureters, because they cross the anticipated surgical field and may well be near, or attached to, adhesions.[62,63] It is important to note that 52% of inadvertent ligations of the ureter in abdominal and retroperitoneal operations occur in gynecologic procedures.[64]

Above age 60 obstructive uropathy occurs more commonly in men than in women. Benign prostatic hyperplasia, which is by far the most common cause of urinary tract obstruction in men, produces some symptoms of bladder outlet obstruction in 75% of men aged 50 years and older.[65,66] It is likely that the proportion of affected older men would be higher if physicians routinely took a detailed history for symptoms.[65,66] Presenting symptoms of bladder outlet obstruction include difficulty initiating micturition, weakened urinary stream, dribbling at the end of micturition, incomplete bladder emptying, and nocturia. The diagnosis may be established by history and urodynamic studies, as well as imaging in some cases.[65-67]

Malignant genitourinary tumors occasionally cause urinary tract obstruction. Bladder cancer is the second most common cause (after cervical cancer) of malignant obstruction of the ureter.[2] Despite stage migration to more organ-confined disease in the era of prostate-specific antigen, obstruction due to prostate cancer compressing the bladder neck and invading the ureteral orifices is still relatively common.[68] Urinary tract obstruction in advanced and metastatic prostate cancer can have a varied presentation, because it may occur in multiple anatomic locations, including the ureter and pelvic lymph nodes.[69] Although urothelial tumors of the renal pelvis, ureter, and urethra are very rare, they also may lead to urinary obstruction.[70]

Several gastrointestinal processes may rarely cause obstructive uropathy. Inflammation in Crohn's disease may extend into the retroperitoneum, leading to obstruction of the ureters,[71] usually on the right side.[72] In addition, several gastrointestinal diseases may cause oxalosis, leading to nephrolithiasis.[73] Appendicitis may lead to retroperitoneal scarring or abscess formation in children and young adults,[74] leading to obstruction of the right ureter. Diverticulitis in older patients[75] may rarely cause obstruction of the left ureter. Fecaloma is another rare cause of bilateral ureteral obstruction.[76] Chronic pancreatitis with pseudocyst formation sometimes causes left ureteral obstruction[77] and may very rarely cause bilateral obstruction.[78] Acute pancreatitis may result in right-sided obstruction.[79]

Vascular abnormalities or diseases may also lead to obstruction. Abdominal aortic aneurysm is the most common vascular cause of urinary obstruction,[80] which may be caused by direct pressure of the aneurysm on the ureter or associated retroperitoneal fibrosis. Aneurysms of the iliac vessels may also cause obstruction of the ureters as they cross over the vessels.[80] Rarely, the ovarian venous system may cause right ureteral obstruction.[81] In addition, and also rarely, vasculitis caused by systemic lupus erythematosus,[82] polyarteritis nodosa,[83] granulomatosis with polyangiitis (formerly designated Wegener's granulomatosis),[84] and Henoch-Schönlein purpura[85,86] have been reported to cause obstruction.

Retroperitoneal processes, such as tumor invasion leading to compression, as well as retroperitoneal fibrosis, can result in obstruction. The major extrinsic causes of retroperitoneal obstruction, accounting for 70% of all cases, are due to tumors of the colon, bladder, prostate, ovary, uterus, or cervix.[2,87,88] When idiopathic, retroperitoneal fibrosis[87,88] usually involves the middle third of the ureter and affects men and women equally, predominantly those in the fifth and sixth decades of life.[88] Retroperitoneal fibrosis may also be induced by drugs (e.g., methysergide), or it may occur as a consequence of scarring from multiple abdominal surgical procedures.[88] It may also be associated with conditions as varied as gonorrhea, sarcoidosis, chronic urinary tract infections, Henoch-Schönlein purpura, tuberculosis, biliary tract disease, and inflammatory processes of the lower extremities with ascending lymphangitis.[88]

Malignant neoplasms can obstruct the urinary tract by direct extension or by metastasis,[89] which may be managed by retrograde stenting as a practical but guarded treatment and should be tailored to each patient.[89] As noted earlier, cervical cancer is the most common obstructing malignant neoplasm, followed by bladder cancer.[2,90,91] Rare childhood tumors such as pelvic neurofibromas can induce upper urinary tract obstruction in up to 60% of patients.[92] Wilms' tumor may obstruct via local compression of the renal pelvis.[93] Miscellaneous inflammatory processes can also result in obstruction. These include granulomatous causes such as sarcoidosis[94] and chronic granulomatous disease of childhood.[95] Amyloid deposits may produce isolated involvement of the ureter. Furthermore, a pelvic mass or inflammatory process associated with actinomycosis may cause external ureteral compression.[96,97] Retrovesical echinococcal cyst can also impede urine flow.[98] Retroperitoneal malacoplakia can also be a rare cause of urinary obstruction.[99] Polyarteritis nodosa associated with hepatitis B has also been reported to result in bilateral hydronephrosis.[100]

Hematologic abnormalities induce obstruction of the urinary tract by a variety of mechanisms. In the retroperitoneum, enlarged lymph nodes or a tumor mass may compress the ureter.[33,101] Alternatively, precipitation of cellular breakdown products such as uric acid (see earlier) and paraproteins, as in multiple myeloma, may cause intrinsic obstruction. In patients with clotting abnormalities, blood clots or hematomas may obstruct the urinary tract, as can sloughed papillae in patients with sickle cell disease or analgesic nephropathy (see earlier). Although leukemic infiltrates rarely cause obstruction in adults, in children they cause obstruction in 5% of patients.[102] Lymphomatous infiltration of the kidney occurs relatively commonly, but obstruction related to ureteral involvement in lymphoma is rarer.[103]

CLINICAL ASPECTS

Urinary tract obstruction may cause symptoms referable to the urinary tract. However, even patients with severe obstruction may be asymptomatic, especially in settings where the obstruction develops gradually or in patients with spinal cord injury.[104] The clinical presentation often depends on the rate of onset of the obstruction (acute or chronic), the degree of obstruction (partial or complete), whether the obstruction is unilateral or bilateral, and whether the obstruction is intrinsic or extrinsic. Pain in obstructive uropathy is usually associated with obstruction of sudden onset, as from a kidney stone, blood clot, or sloughed papillae, and appears to result from abrupt stretching of the renal capsule or the wall of the collecting system, where C-type sensory fibers are located. The severity of the pain appears to correlate with the rate, rather than the degree, of distension. The pain may present as typical renal colic (sharp pain that may radiate toward the urethral orifice), or, in patients with reflux, the pain may radiate to the flank only during micturition. With UPJ obstruction, flank pain may develop or worsen when the patient ingests large quantities of fluids or receives diuretics.[105] Early satiety and weight loss may be another symptom.[106] Ileus or other gastrointestinal symptoms may be associated with the pain, especially in cases of renal colic, so that it can be difficult to differentiate obstruction for gastrointestinal disease.

Sometimes patients notice changes in urine output as obstruction sets in. Urinary tract obstruction is one of the few conditions that can result in anuria, usually because of bladder outlet obstruction or obstruction of a solitary kidney at any level. Obstruction may also occur with no change in urine output. Alternatively, episodes of polyuria may alternate with periods of oliguria. Recurrent urinary tract infections may be the only sign of obstruction, particularly in children. As mentioned earlier, prostatic disease with significant bladder outlet obstruction often presents with difficulty initiating urination, decreased size or force of the urine stream, postvoiding dribbling, and incomplete emptying.[107] Spastic bladder or irritative symptoms such as frequency, urgency, and dysuria may result from urinary tract infection. The appearance of obstructive symptoms synchronous with the menstrual cycle may also be a sign of endometriosis.[108]

On physical examination, several signs may suggest urinary obstruction. A palpable abdominal mass, especially in neonates, may represent hydronephrosis, or, in all age-groups, a palpable suprapubic mass may represent a distended bladder. On laboratory examination, proteinuria, if present, is generally less than 2 g/day. Microscopic hematuria is a common finding, but gross hematuria may develop occasionally such as in rare cases with appendiceal granuloma.[109] The urine sediment is often unremarkable. Less common manifestations of urinary tract obstruction include deterioration of renal function without apparent cause, hypertension,[110] polycythemia, and abnormal urine acidification and concentration capacity.

DIAGNOSIS

Careful history taking and physical examination represent the cornerstone of diagnosis, often leading to detection of urinary tract obstruction and suggesting the reason for it. The findings of the history and physical examination should focus the evaluation, so that minimal amount of time and expense are incurred in determining the cause of the obstruction.

HISTORY AND PHYSICAL EXAMINATION

Important information in the history includes the type and duration of symptoms (voiding difficulties, flank pain, decreased urine output), presence or absence of urinary tract infections and their number and frequency (especially in children), pattern of fluid intake and urine output, as well as any symptoms of chronic kidney disease (such as fatigue, sleep disturbance, loss of appetite, pruritus). In addition, relevant past medical history should be reviewed in detail, looking for predisposing causes, including stone disease, malignancies, gynecologic diseases, history of recent surgery, AIDS, and drug use.

The physical examination should focus first on vital signs, which may provide evidence of infection (fever, tachycardia) or of frank volume overload (hypertension). Evaluation of the patient's volume status will guide fluid therapy. The abdominal examination may reveal a flank mass, which may represent hydronephrosis (especially in children), or a suprapubic mass, which may represent a distended bladder. Features of chronic kidney disease, such as pallor (anemia), drowsiness (uremia), neuromuscular irritability (metabolic abnormalities), or pericardial friction rub (uremic pericarditis), may also be noted. A thorough pelvic examination in women and a rectal examination for all patients are mandatory. A careful history and a well-directed and complete physical examination often reveal the specific cause of urinary obstruction. Coexistence of obstruction and infection is a urologic emergency, and appropriate studies (ultrasonography, CT, MRI) must be performed immediately, so that the obstruction can be relieved promptly. Intravenous urography (IVU) is now less common to use in the diagnostic workup of these patients.

BIOCHEMICAL EVALUATION

The laboratory evaluation includes urinalysis and examination of the sediment on a fresh specimen by an experienced observer. Unexplained kidney failure with benign urinary sediment should suggest urinary tract obstruction. Microscopic hematuria without proteinuria may suggest calculus or tumor. Pyuria and bacteriuria may indicate pyelonephritis; bacteriuria alone may suggest stasis. Crystals in a freshly voided specimen should lead to consideration of nephrolithiasis or intrarenal crystal deposition.

Hematologic evaluation includes the hemoglobin level, hematocrit, and mean corpuscular volume (to identify anemia of chronic kidney disease), and white blood cell count (to identify possible hematopoietic system neoplasm or infection). Serum electrolyte levels (Na^+, Cl^-, K^+, and HCO_3^-), blood urea nitrogen concentration, creatinine concentration, and levels of Ca^{2+}, phosphorus, Mg^{2+}, uric acid, and albumin should be measured. These will help identify disorders of distal nephron function (impaired acid excretion or osmoregulation) and uremia. Urinary chemistry panels may also suggest distal tubular dysfunction (high urine pH, isosthenuric urine), inability to reabsorb sodium normally (urinary Na^+ > 20 mEq/L, fractional excretion of sodium [FE_{Na}] > 1%, and osmolality < 350 mOsm). Alternatively, in acute obstruction urinary chemistry values may be consistent with prerenal azotemia (urinary Na^+ < 20 mEq/L, FE_{Na} < 1%, and osmolality < 500 mOsm).[8]

Novel biomarkers relevant for the functional as well as cellular and molecular changes are being developed as an index of renal injury and to predict renal reserve or recovery after reconstruction. Simple tests examining the value of risk-proteins have suggested that elevated levels of neutrophil gelatinase–associated lipocalin (NGAL) and $β_2$-microglobulin are present in the urine from obstructed kidneys.[111] Attempts to predict the clinical outcome of congenital unilateral UPJ obstruction in newborns by urine proteome analysis reveals an example of this powerful new technology. Polypeptides in the urine were identified and enabled diagnosis of the severity of obstruction. When this technique was used, the clinical evolution was predicted with 94% precision in neonates,[112] whereas the precision was only 20% in older children with UPJ obstruction.[113] Thus far, application of large-scale urinary proteomic analysis holds promise for better classification of individuals with hydronephrosis for early selection of surgical candidates,[114] but long-term follow-up studies are warranted to determine the true clinical value of this diagnostic approach.[115]

EVALUATION BY MEDICAL IMAGING

The history, physical examination, and initial laboratory study results should guide the medical imaging evaluation. Pain, degree of renal dysfunction, and the presence of infection dictate the speed and nature of the evaluation. Numerous imaging techniques are available; each has advantages and disadvantages, including the ability to identify the site and cause of the obstruction and to separate functional obstruction from mere dilation of the urinary tract. Patient-specific factors, such as the risk of radiocontrast in the setting of renal insufficiency or the risk of exposure to radiation in pregnant women, must also be weighed.[20]

ULTRASONOGRAPHY

Ultrasonography is the preferred screening modality when obstruction is suspected[116,117] because it is highly sensitive for hydronephrosis,[116,117] is safe and can be repeated frequently, is readily available at low cost, and avoids ionizing radiation, making it ideal for pregnant patients,[20] infants, and children.[116,118] Moreover, because ultrasonography requires no radiographic contrast, it is well suited to patients in whom contrast is contraindicated, including those with an elevated or rising serum creatinine level,[116,117] to rule out obstruction as a cause of renal insufficiency, as well as in patients allergic to contrast material, in patients with nephrogenic fibrosis, and in pediatric patients.[119] In addition to detecting hydronephrosis, ultrasonography can reveal dilation of the renal pelvis and calyces. It may also determine the size and shape of the kidney and may demonstrate thinned cortex in case of severe long-standing hydronephrosis (Figure 38.1). Finally, ultrasonography may detect perinephric abscesses, which may complicate some forms of obstructive nephropathy. Importantly, in a multicenter comparative-effectiveness trial in patients with suspected nephrolithiasis subjected to point-of-care ultrasonography (emergency ultrasonography), ultrasonography performed by a radiologist, or abdominal CT, it was concluded that using ultrasonography as the initial test resulted in no need for CT in most patients, lower cumulative radiation exposure, and no significant differences in the risk for subsequent serious adverse events, pain scores, return emergency department visits, or hospitalizations.[120]

Ultrasonography is both highly sensitive and highly specific in detecting hydronephrosis, with the rates approaching 90%.[116,117,121,122] Importantly, ultrasonography works equally well in patients with azotemia, in whom radiocontrast studies are contraindicated.[122] Hydronephrosis is detected as a dilated collecting system—an anechoic central area surrounded by echogenic parenchyma.

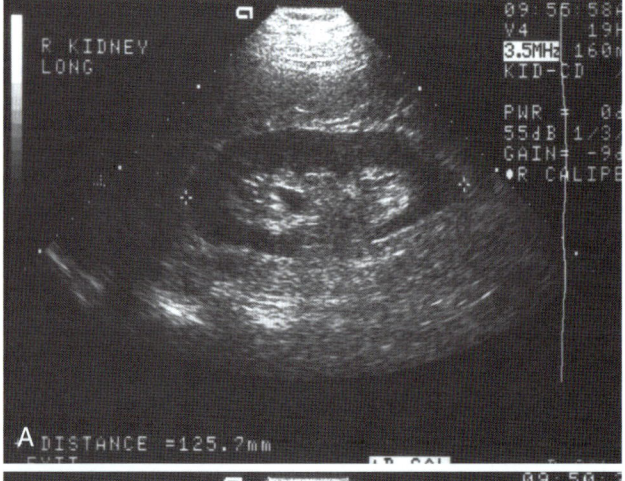

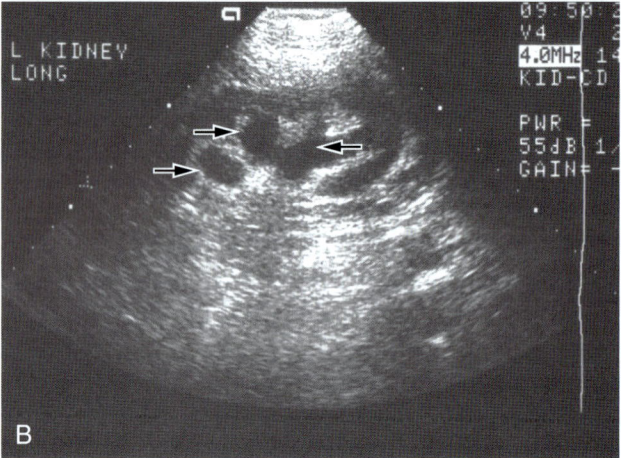

Figure 38.1 Renal ultrasonography. **A,** Normal kidney. **B,** Hydronephrotic kidney: dilated calyces and pelvis (*arrows*).

However, in some cases of acute urinary obstruction, ultrasonography may fail to detect pathologic processes. During the first 48 hours of obstruction[116,117,121,122] or when hydronephrosis is absent despite obstruction evaluated by CT, ultrasonography may reveal no abnormality.[123] False-negative results also occur in cases of dehydration, staghorn calculi, nephrocalcinosis,[122] retroperitoneal fibrosis,[124] misinterpretation of caliectasis as cortical cysts,[125] and in cases of tumor encasement of the collecting system.[126] A dilated collecting system without obstruction may be observed in up to 50% of patients with urinary diversion through ileal conduits.[127] To enhance the sensitivity and specificity of ultrasonography, some investigators have developed special obstructive scoring systems, which grade increased echogenicity, parenchymal rims greater than 5 mm, contralateral hypertrophy, resistive index (RI) ratio of 1.10 or higher, and other features to differentiate between obstructing and nonobstructing hydronephrosis.[118] False-positive studies may result from a large extrarenal pelvis, parapelvic cysts,[128] vesicoureteral reflux, or high urine flow rate.[122] In addition, ultrasonography may only suggest, but not reveal, the presence or cause of the obstruction. Renal ultrasound elastography provides measurement of kidney elasticity by the Shearwave technique.[129] This new imaging technique provides information about renal stiffness related to fibrosis (i.e., chronic obstruction). However, elastography is also sensitive to mechanical and functional parameters such as hydronephrosis and external pressure.[129]

Importantly, although ultrasonography is a useful screening test, it does not define renal function and cannot completely rule out obstruction, especially when prior clinical suspicion is high. Every experienced nephrologist has seen cases of obstruction with negative ultrasonographic study results. Therefore the diagnosis of obstruction must still be considered in patients with worsening renal function, chronic azotemia, or acute changes in renal function or urine output, even in the absence of hydronephrosis on ultrasonography.[130]

ANTENATAL ULTRASONOGRAPHY

Prenatal diagnosis of renal pathologic processes was first described in the 1970s.[131] After that, routine maternal ultrasonography using devices of ever-increasing resolution resulted in a fourfold increase in antenatal detection of congenital urinary tract obstruction.[132] Prenatal hydronephrosis is diagnosed with an incidence of between 1 in 100 and 1 in 500 maternal-fetal ultrasonographic studies.[10,12,102] Either obstructive or nonobstructive processes can cause dilation of the urinary tract. Overall the causes of urinary tract obstruction are as follows: UPJ obstruction (44%), ureterovesical junction obstruction (21%), multicystic dysplastic kidney, ureterocele or ureteral ectopia, duplex kidney (12%), posterior urethral valves (9%), urethral atresia, sacrococcygeal teratoma, and hydrometrocolpos (fluid distension of the uterus).[103,133-135] Nonobstructive causes include vesicoureteral reflux (VUR, 14%), physiologic dilation, prune-belly syndrome, renal cystic disease, and megacalycosis (massive dilation of the renal calyces).[103,133-135] Increased renal echogenicity and oligohydramnios (inadequate quantities of amniotic fluid) in the setting of bladder distension are highly predictive (87%) of an obstructive cause. This finding is important in the prenatal counseling and treatment of boys with bilateral hydronephrosis and marked bladder dilation.[136]

Determining which cases require intervention and which can be treated conservatively remains a major issue in prenatal ultrasonographic diagnosis of urinary tract obstruction. Persistent postnatal renal abnormalities appear likely when the anteroposterior diameter of the fetal renal pelvis measures more than 6 mm at less than 20 weeks, more than 8 mm at 20 to 30 weeks, and more than 10 mm at more than 30 weeks of gestation. The long-term morbidity of mild hydronephrosis (pelviectasis without calyceal dilation) is low.[10,12] Moderate hydronephrosis (dilated pelvis and calyces without parenchymal thinning) may be associated with gradual improvement in severity of dilation, without loss of anticipated relative renal function. Cases of severe hydronephrosis (pelvicalyceal dilation with parenchymal thinning) may require surgical intervention for declining renal function, infection, or symptoms. Overall, because only approximately 5% to 25% of patients with antenatal hydronephrosis will ultimately require surgical intervention,[102,137] careful long-term follow-up of these patients is required throughout childhood and into adulthood. Almost all patients with antenatal hydronephrosis will have postnatal ultrasonography performed in the first days of life, keeping in mind that most cases of the mild hydronephrosis will resolve without intervention.[138] Functional imaging is required to define residual renal function of patients with hydronephrosis and to monitor its course over postnatal life. However, in the absence of bilateral hydronephrosis, a solitary kidney, or suspected posterior urethral valve, functional imaging can be deferred until the first 4 to 6 weeks of life.[102] Otherwise, nuclear medicine examination with radioisotope renography should be performed.

In the United States most infants with prenatally detected hydronephrosis that is confirmed with postnatal studies are placed on antibiotic prophylaxis pending the outcome of further evaluation.[102] This is not the routine treatment in Europe. However, an infection in the setting of ureteral obstruction can cause significant morbidity, resulting in an infant with sepsis, and renal damage is a potential comorbid condition. Oral amoxicillin is the most commonly used prophylactic antibiotic.[102]

DUPLEX DOPPLER ULTRASONOGRAPHY

Ultrasonography has emerged as the primary imaging modality in conditions in which either renal obstruction or renal medical disease is suspected on the basis of clinical and laboratory findings. In urinary tract obstruction, pathophysiologic changes affecting the pressure in the collecting system and kidney perfusion are well imaged and form the basis for the correct interpretation of real-time ultrasonography and color duplex Doppler ultrasonography. As detailed earlier, ultrasonography is very sensitive for the detection of collecting system dilation ("hydronephrosis"); however, obstruction is not synonymous with dilation, because either obstructive or nonobstructive dilation may be present. To differentiate these conditions, color duplex Doppler ultrasonography with measurement of the RI in the intrarenal arteries may be helpful, because obstruction (except in the acute and subacute stages) leads to intrarenal vasoconstriction with a consecutive increase of the RI above the upper limit of 0.7, whereas nonobstructive dilation does not.[103,133] Diuretic challenge to the kidney may further enhance these differences in RI between obstruction and dilation.[134] Of clinical relevance, renal colic patients constitute 30% to 35% of all urologic emergencies, and color Doppler predicted the onset of acute dilation with higher sensitivity, specificity, accuracy, and diagnostic efficiency than ultrasonography in patients with renal colic.[139]

INTRAVENOUS UROGRAPHY

IVU, also known as intravenous pyelography (IVP), was for many years state-of-the-art when a patient suspected with a history of urinary tract obstruction was referred for imaging (Figure 38.2). IVU has now been replaced by ultrasonography, CT, and MRI.

COMPUTED TOMOGRAPHY

CT was initially used mainly in cases with a high index of clinical suspicion in which ultrasonography or IVU had failed to identify obstruction.[140] With the advance to higher resolution of multidetector CT scanners, the CT scan has supplanted IVU for evaluation of the upper urinary tract.[140,141] CT has a particular advantage because it can visualize a dilated collecting system without the requirement for contrast enhancement. It can also be performed much more quickly than IVU, especially when renal impairment

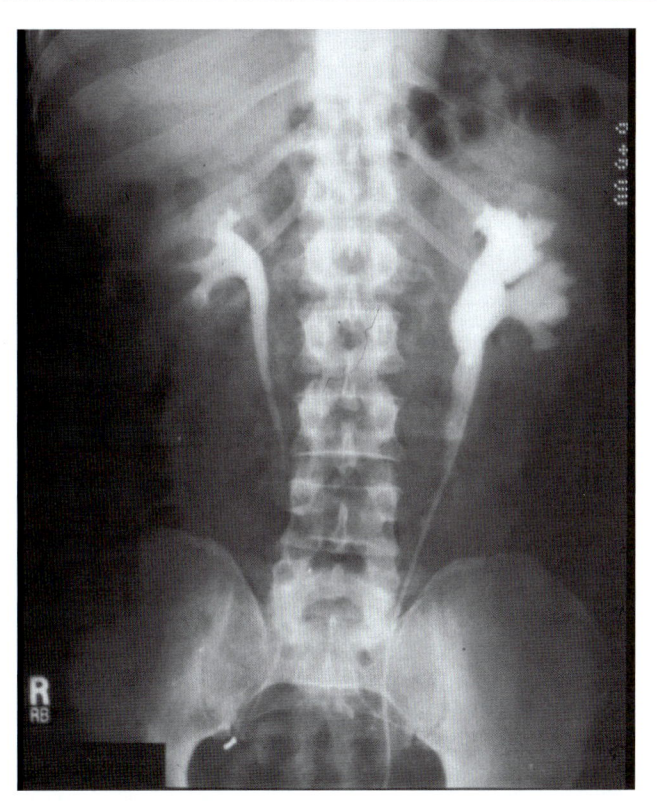

Figure 38.2 Intravenous pyelography. Normal right kidney and dilated collecting system on the left. The obstruction was relieved with a stent.

or obstruction would delay contrast excretion by the affected kidney in an IVU (Figure 38.3). Non–contrast-enhanced CT identifies ureteral stones more effectively than IVU and detects the presence or absence of ureteral obstruction as effectively as IVU.[142,143] Because of its exquisite sensitivity to density, CT can identify even radiolucent stones, because even uric acid stone density is at least 100 Hounsfield units (HU), which is higher than soft tissue density on CT (usually 10 to 70 HU). CT is especially effective in identifying extrinsic causes of obstruction (e.g., retroperitoneal fibrosis, lymphadenopathy, hematoma). The use of CT for the diagnosis of stones has increased by a factor of 10 over the past 15 years in the United States,[144] probably because of its greater sensitivity and because it can be performed at will in most emergency departments in the United States.[145] This was highlighted in a multicenter comparative-effectiveness trial in patients with suspected nephrolithiasis subjected to either point-of-care ultrasonography (emergency ultrasonography), ultrasonography performed by a radiologist, or abdominal CT demonstrated that CT has a higher sensitivity than ultrasonography, whereas ultrasonography has higher specificity than CT.[120] Along this line it must be emphasized that although the cancer risk from radiation exposure to CT scans is very low, CT scans might produce a small additional cancer risk,[146] especially when children are subjected to CT scans.[147]

Helical CT has also proven to be an accurate and noninvasive method of demonstrating crossing vessels in UPJ obstruction.[148] CT can detect extraurinary pathologic conditions and can establish nonurogenital causes of pain. All of these advantages establish non–contrast-enhanced helical

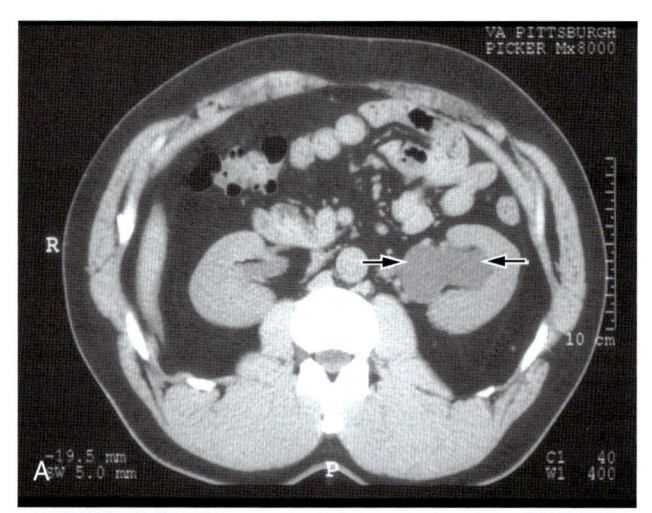

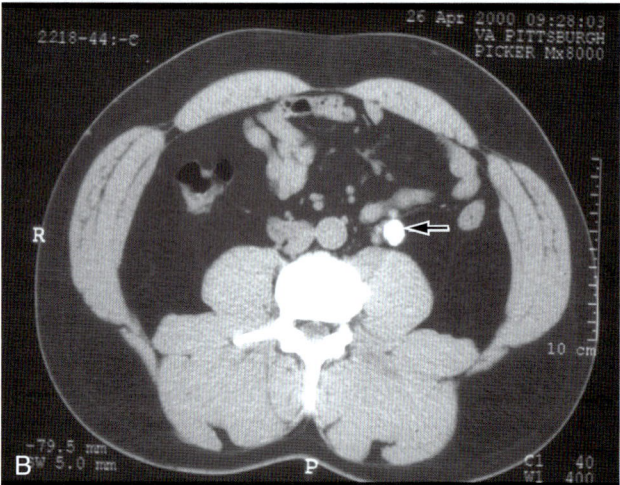

Figure 38.3 Computed tomography, noncontrast study. **A,** Left hydronephrosis: dilated renal pelvis (*arrows*), with normal kidney on right. **B,** Reason for obstruction: left midureteral stone (*arrow*).

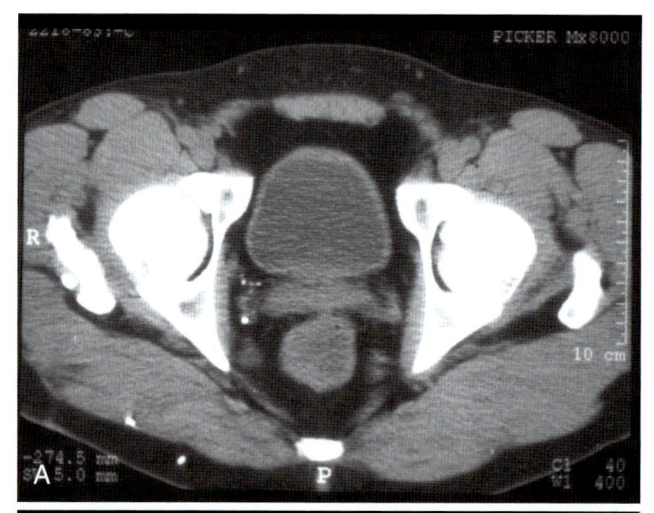

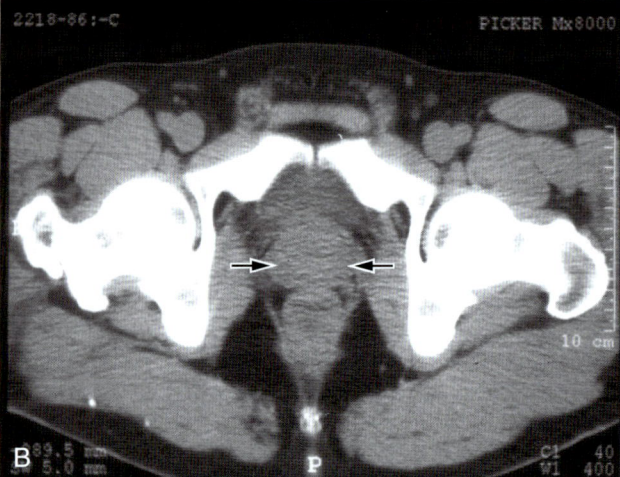

Figure 38.4 Computed tomography of the pelvis. **A,** Large post-voiding residual urine in the bladder. **B,** Enlarged prostate (*arrows*), leading to urinary retention.

CT as the diagnostic study of choice for the evaluation of the patient with acute flank pain.[123] CT is very useful in delineating the pelvic organs, such as the bladder and prostate, and may demonstrate abnormalities such as an obstructed and distended bladder (Figure 38.4) secondary to an enlarged prostate. Ultrasonography may be the first method of diagnosis in this setting (Figure 38.5), but CT resolution and depiction of details are usually superior to those of ultrasonography.[140] An exception to using a noncontrast CT is nephrolithiasis secondary to HIV protease inhibitors, primarily indinavir. These stones are not radiopaque, and signs of obstruction may be minimal or absent; thus the diagnosis may be missed with ultrasonography and noncontrast CT scan. Contrast-enhanced CT scanning may be required to establish the diagnosis in this circumstance.[149]

ISOTOPIC RENOGRAPHY

Isotopic renography, or renal scintigraphy, is helpful in diagnosing upper urinary tract obstruction and providing information on the differential renal function (DRF) of both kidneys, while avoiding the risk of radiocontrast agents.[150,151] Radioisotope is injected intravenously, and its dynamic uptake and excretion by the kidneys is followed using imaging with a gamma camera. Although this method gives a functional assessment of the obstructed kidney, anatomic definition is suboptimal compared with CT. Isotopic renography is typically used to estimate the fractional contribution of each kidney to overall renal function. The noninvasive character of this examination with its high reproducibility makes it excellent for monitoring patients, and it helps the urologist to decide whether to perform surgical intervention or watchful waiting.[23] In addition, the test can be repeated after the relief of obstruction to gauge the extent to which relief of the obstruction has restored renal function.

Diuretic renography was introduced into clinical practice in 1978[152] and may be used to distinguish between hydronephrosis or pelvic dilation with obstruction and dilation without obstruction. The method was developed, applied, and validated in adults.[152] In particular this is important when applying diuretic renography in children and infants, in whom it is not always easy to distinguish between dilation and obstruction. Following administration of radioisotope, when the isotope appears in the renal pelvis, a loop diuretic such as furosemide is given intravenously. If stasis is causing the dilation, the induced diuresis may result in prompt washout of the tracer from the renal pelvis. By contrast,

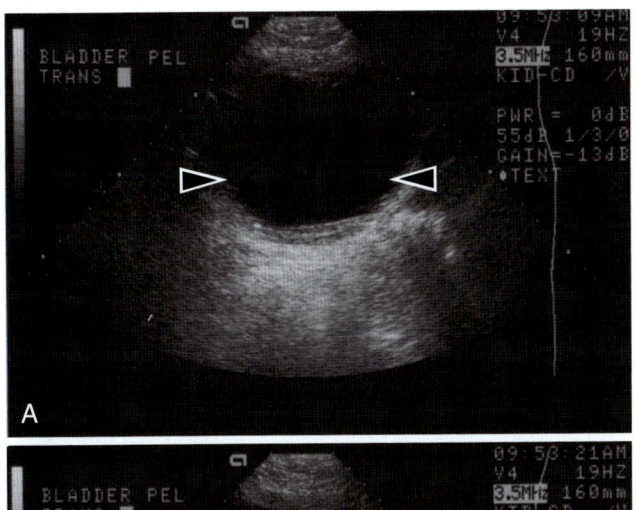

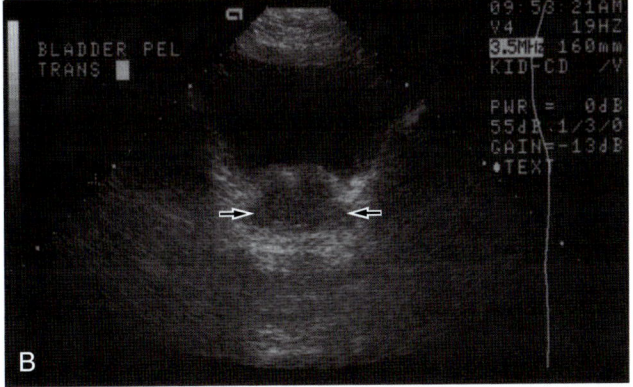

Figure 38.5 Pelvic ultrasonography. A, Distended bladder (*arrowheads*). **B,** Enlarged prostate (*arrows*), causing infravesical urinary obstruction.

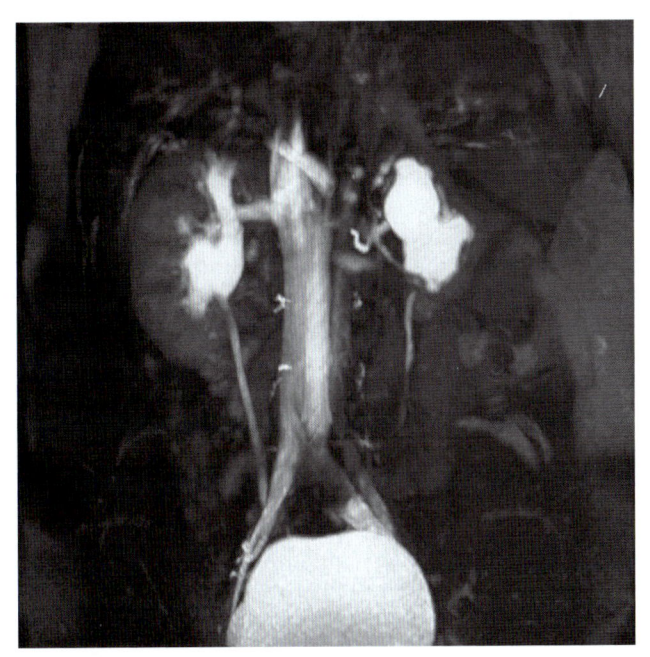

Figure 38.6 Magnetic resonance urography of left-sided hydronephrosis with parenchymal thinning. Magnetic resonance urographic image shows large dilation of the left pelvicalyceal system and narrowing of the left ureteropelvic junction segment.

when dilation is caused by obstruction, the washout does not occur.[153] Data should be interpreted visually and by quantitative measurement, including the half-life ($t_{1/2}$) for the excretion of the tracer from the collecting system.[154] It is generally accepted that the clearance of the isotope from the collecting system with $t_{1/2}$ less than 15 minutes is normal, and a $t_{1/2}$ of more than 20 minutes may indicate obstruction in adults. Renal excretion of the tracer with a $t_{1/2}$ between 15 and 20 minutes is considered equivocal. An absent or blunted diuretic response resulting from decreased renal function or grossly dilated pelvis makes interpretation of the test difficult and limits its usefulness and may require support tools to increase the diagnostic performance.[155] Moreover, in children diuretic renography is also a very important method for guiding the management of asymptomatic congenital hydronephrosis. From this examination the DRF can be obtained, which is a robust measure provided there is adequate background subtraction. Pitfalls are related to the drawing of regions of interest, particularly in infants, to estimating the interval during which DRF is calculated, and to an adequate signal-to-noise ratio. There is no definition of a "significant" reduction in DRF. The classical variables of the diuretic renogram may not allow an estimate of the best drainage. Poor pelvic emptying may be apparent because the bladder is full and because the effect of gravity on drainage is incomplete. Estimating the drainage as residual activity rather than any parameter on the slope might be more adequate, especially if the time of furosemide administration is changed. Renal function and pelvic volume can influence the quality of drainage. Misinterpretation can easily take place if the renal pelvis is very large and does not allow proper drainage within the study time, and drainage may be better estimated using new tools.[156]

MAGNETIC RESONANCE IMAGING

New MRI systems and specific MRI contrast agents provide significant developments in the evaluation of renal performance (glomerular filtration rate [GFR] measurement), in the search for prognostic factors (hypoxia, inflammation, cell viability, degree of tubular function, and interstitial fibrosis), and for monitoring new therapies.[141,157] New developments that have provided higher signal-to-noise ratio and higher spatial and/or temporal resolutions have the potential to direct new opportunities for obtaining morphologic and functional information on tissue characteristics that are relevant for various renal diseases, including urinary tract obstruction, with respect to diagnosis, prognosis, and treatment follow-up.[141,157] MRI can be used to explore the urinary tract when obstruction is suspected. MRI provides improved spatial resolution, and it is superior to IVU in detecting obstruction in the presence of severe kidney failure.[141] MRI has very limited application for the evaluation of stone disease because it cannot directly detect calcifications or stone material.[158]

Depending on local conditions, MRI may be more expensive than other modalities. In children, MR urography (Figure 38.6) may replace conventional uroradiologic methods, and a study suggests that functional MRI plays an important potential role in identifying those who will benefit most from pyeloplasty and those who are probably best observed.[159] Promising experimental studies have demonstrated that MRI may provide valuable information regarding renal function, including energy consumption from blood oxygenation level–dependent (BOLD) MRI; this kind of data may be helpful in the future in predicting the level of return of renal function following obstruction.[160,161] Of interest, functional MRI using BOLD imaging demonstrated the ability to identify pathophysiologic changes in patients with acute obstruction due to calculi in the ureter.[162] Concern related to MRI in renal patients was highlighted by the increased risk for developing nephrogenic systemic fibrosis (NSF) induced by the toxicity of gadolinium in patients with severely impaired renal function, whereas patients with normal or moderate renal function impairment do not develop NSF. It is recommended that gadolinium contrast media should be avoided in patients with stage 4 or 5 chronic kidney disease because of the risk for NSF.[163]

WHITAKER TEST

The Whitaker test traditionally ideally defines the functional effect of upper urinary tract dilation by measuring the hydrostatic pressures in the renal pelvis and bladder during infusion of a saline and contrast mixture into the renal pelvis via a catheter.[164] With a bladder catheter in place, the patient is placed in the prone position on the fluoroscopic table, and a cannula is inserted percutaneously into the renal pelvis and connected to a pressure transducer. A mixture of saline and contrast material is infused through the renal cannula at a rate of 10 mL/min, and pressures are monitored. The urinary tract is considered nonobstructed if renal pelvic pressure is less than 15 cm H_2O, equivocal at a pressure between 15 and 22 cm H_2O, and obstructed if pressure exceeds 22 cm H_2O.[164] With the advent of noninvasive imaging techniques, the test should be reserved for assessing potential upper urinary tract obstruction only in the following circumstances: equivocal results from less invasive tests, suspected obstruction with poor kidney function, loin pain with negative diuresis renogram findings, suspected intermittent obstruction, and gross dilation with positive diuresis renogram findings.[165] The test is used only rarely, and interpretations rely on solid experience with the method.

RETROGRADE AND ANTEGRADE PYELOGRAPHY

When other tests do not provide adequate anatomic detail, or when obstruction must be relieved (e.g., obstruction of a solitary kidney, bilateral obstruction, or symptomatic infection in the obstructed system), more invasive investigation, with a combination of treatments, may be necessary. When retrograde pyelography rarely is performed, this takes place during cystoscopy, by cannulating the ureteral orifice and injecting contrast.[61,166,167] In some cases of complete obstruction, contrast may not reach the kidney, but the procedure will define the lower level of the obstruction. Retrograde pyelography can be combined with placement of a ureteral stent to relieve an obstruction, or with possible stone extraction. Because the procedure passes through the bladder to reach the upper urinary tract, the risk for introducing infection proximal to the obstruction must be kept in mind, and the obstruction should be relieved immediately after retrograde pyelography. Antegrade pyelography is performed by percutaneous cannulation of the renal pelvis and injection of the contrast material into the kidney and ureter.[166,167] This procedure should establish the proximal level of obstruction and may also serve as a first step in relieving obstruction by means of percutaneous nephrostomy (Figure 38.7).

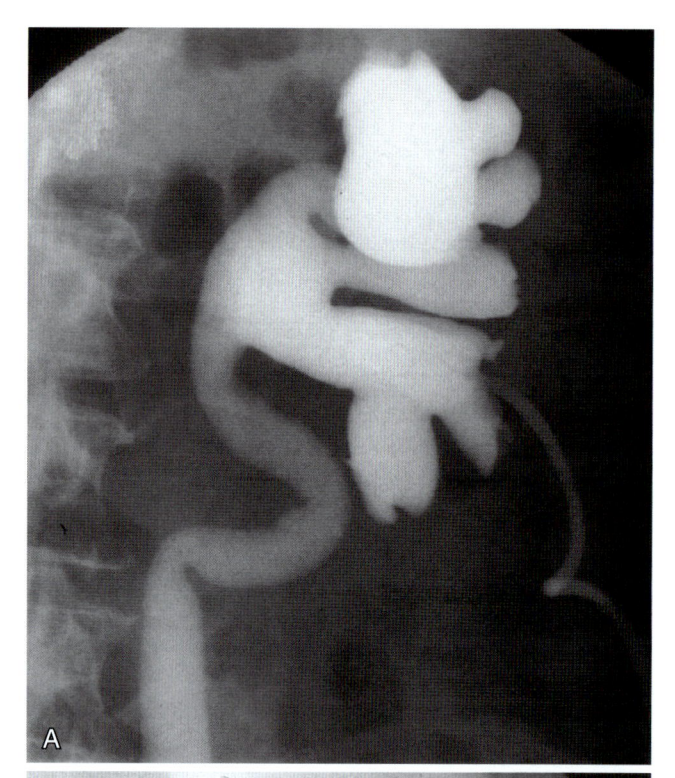

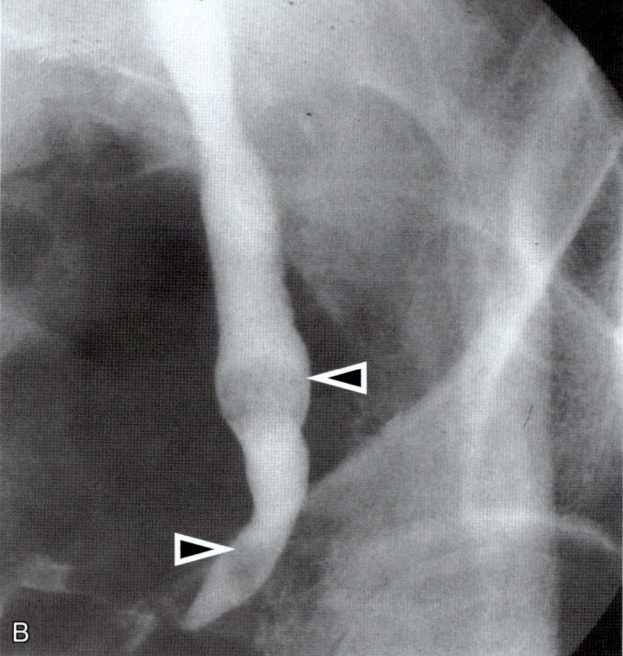

Figure 38.7 Antegrade pyelography. **A,** Dilated renal pelvis and calyces on left. **B,** Stones (*arrowheads*) as filling defects in the distal ureter (not seen on plain film). Intravenous pyelography was unsuccessful owing to the obstructed and malfunctioning kidney.

PATHOPHYSIOLOGY OF OBSTRUCTIVE NEPHROPATHY

Despite the fact that acquired obstructive nephropathy in humans usually results from partial urinary tract obstruction and is generally prolonged in its time course, most mechanistic studies of renal dysfunction in acquired obstruction use models of acute complete obstruction, usually for 24 hours. In these animal models the extent of obstruction is clear and reproducible, and, if the kidneys are studied soon after the obstruction is performed or released, the results are not confounded by changes in renal structure brought on by inflammation or fibrosis. Complete obstruction of short duration strikingly alters renal blood flow, glomerular filtration, and tubular function, while producing minimal anatomic changes in blood vessels, glomeruli, and tubules.[2]

EFFECTS OF OBSTRUCTION ON RENAL BLOOD FLOW AND GLOMERULAR FILTRATION

Obstruction profoundly alters all components of glomerular function. The extent of the disturbance in GFR depends on the severity and duration of the obstruction, whether it is unilateral or bilateral, and the extent to which the obstruction has been relieved or persists.[2] To describe the effects of obstruction on glomerular filtration, we must review aspects of normal GFR. Whole-kidney GFR depends on the filtration rate of all functioning glomeruli and the proportion of glomeruli actually filtering. As detailed in Chapter 3, single nephron GFR (SNGFR) is determined by the blood flow in the glomerulus, the net ultrafiltration pressure across the glomerular capillary, and the glomerular ultrafiltration coefficient (K_f). Glomerular blood flow and the glomerular capillary hydraulic pressure (P_{GC}) are determined by the resistances of the afferent (R_A) and efferent (R_E) arterioles. Net ultrafiltration pressure is determined by P_{GC}, the hydraulic pressure of Bowman's space (which equals the proximal tubule hydraulic pressure, P_T), and the differences in oncotic pressure between the glomerular capillary and Bowman's space. K_f is determined by the permeability properties of the filtering surface and the surface area available for filtration. Obstruction can alter one or all of these determinants of GFR.

THE EARLY, HYPEREMIC PHASE

In the 2 to 3 hours immediately following the onset of unilateral ureteral obstruction, blockade of antegrade urine flow markedly increased P_T. This increase in pressure in Bowman's space would be expected to halt GFR immediately.[168-170] However, during this early phase of obstruction, the afferent arterioles dilate, decreasing R_A, increasing P_{GC}, and counteracting the increase in P_T.[168,169] Because this vasodilator or "hyperemic" response occurs in denervated kidneys in situ and in isolated perfused kidneys,[171,172] it must result from intrarenal mechanisms. In fact, glomeruli of individual nephrons exhibit the same response in in vivo micropuncture experiments when antegrade urine flow is blocked by placement of a wax block in the tubule of the nephron.[173]

Many mechanisms may mediate this afferent vasodilation, including increases in vasodilator hormones such as prostaglandins, regulation by the macula densa, and a direct myogenic reflex. This hyperemic response is not attenuated by renal nerve stimulation or infusion of catecholamines,[174] and it may be linked to changes in interstitial pressure.[172]

In the tubuloglomerular feedback response, reduced distal tubular flow past the macula densa induces reductions in R_A and increases in P_{GC}, so that SNGFR rises. Similarly, because obstruction reduces urine flow past the macula densa, this structure induces afferent vasodilation.[173] However, elegant micropuncture studies separated the stoppage in flow from increases in P_T by placing an additional puncture in the tubule that was proximal to the blockage of flow to the macula densa. In this setting, flow past the macula densa was halted, but P_T remained normal, because accumulating tubule fluid was permitted to leak out.[169] In such nephrons the increase in P_{GC} observed in obstructed tubules did not occur, which indicates that the obstruction itself and not the macula densa stimulates afferent vasodilation.[169]

Renal prostaglandins and renal nerves play important roles in the hyperemic response. Indomethacin blocks the hyperemic response, which indicates that vasodilator prostaglandins are critical to afferent vasodilation.[170,175] A renorenal reflex mechanism in the hemodynamic response to obstruction can be discerned from studies in bilateral obstruction, in which the afferent vasodilation response is absent or markedly attenuated.[2,172] Obstruction of the left kidney augments afferent renal nerve activity from the left kidney and efferent nerve activity to the right kidney. Increased efferent nerve activity to the right kidney was accompanied by reduced blood flow to that kidney. This vasoconstrictor response was ablated by denervation of either the left or right kidney before induction of left ureteral obstruction, which suggests that increased afferent renal nerve traffic triggers vasoconstrictive renorenal reflex activity that counteracts the early intrinsic renal vasodilator effects of obstruction in bilateral ureteral obstruction.[172]

THE LATE, VASOCONSTRICTIVE PHASE

Because obstruction results in cessation of glomerular filtration, efforts to study the regulation of SNGFR later in obstruction have measured determinants of GFR immediately after release of obstruction.[2,176] Using this approach, investigators have shown that renal blood flow declines progressively after 3 hours of unilateral obstruction and through 12 to 24 hours of obstruction.[177,178] Interestingly, although tubular pressures rise initially after obstruction, they then decline, so that by 24 hours renal plasma flow, GFR, and intratubular pressures have all dropped below normal values.[168,170,178,179] At 24 hours into the obstruction, examination of regional blood flow in the kidney by injections of silicone rubber reveals large areas of the cortical vascular bed that are either underperfused or not perfused at all.[2,170,178] Depending on the species, the different vascular beds in the outer and juxtamedullary cortex receive differing proportions of the renal blood flow under basal conditions and following obstruction. However, it is clear that at 24 hours of obstruction, reduced whole-kidney GFR is due, in large part, to nonperfusion of many glomeruli.

Beyond 24 hours of obstruction, SNGFR of glomeruli that remain perfused is decreased markedly, both because of reduced blood flow to the afferent arteriole and because of afferent vasoconstriction, which in turn reduces P_{GC}.[179,180] Because P_{GC} responds in the same manner when the individual nephron is blocked with oil for 24 hours before micropuncture measurements are performed, it is clear that afferent arteriolar vasoconstriction plays an important role in attenuating SNGFR during the established phase of obstruction.[181] These results indicate that, as in the early hyperemic response, intrarenal mechanisms play the major

Table 38.3 Glomerular Hemodynamics in Ureteral Obstruction*

Stage of Obstruction	P_T	R_A	P_{GC}	SNGFR
1-2 hr unilateral	↑↑	↓	↑	=
24 hr unilateral	=	↑↑	↓	↓↓
24 hr bilateral	↑↑	=	=	↓↓
After release: 24 hr unilateral	↓	↑↑	↓↓	↓↓
After release: 24 hr bilateral	=	↑↑	↓	↓↓

*See text for discussion and references.
=, Unchanged; ↑, increased; ↑↑, markedly increased; ↓, reduced; ↓↓, markedly reduced; P_{GC}, glomerular capillary hydraulic pressure; P_T, proximal tubule hydraulic pressure; R_A, afferent arteriole resistance; SNGFR, single nephron glomerular filtration rate.

role in the late vasoconstrictive response to unilateral obstruction. In bilateral obstruction, renal blood flow is reduced to levels 30% to 60% below normal[179,180,182] (Table 38.3). In both unilateral and bilateral obstruction, SNGFR falls to a similar degree. However, the mechanisms involved are different in the two conditions. In unilateral obstruction, reduced P_{GC} lowers the driving pressure for filtration when set against a nearly normal P_T. By contrast, in bilateral obstruction, P_{GC} remains normal and GFR is halted by a highly elevated P_T.[179] These results suggest that systemic factors, such as accumulation of extracellular fluid volume and urea, increases in natriuretic substances, and alterations in renal nerve activity modulate the vasoconstrictive effect of obstruction on the affected kidney.[182]

REGULATION OF THE GLOMERULAR FILTRATION RATE IN RESPONSE TO OBSTRUCTION

The level to which renal blood flow and GFR are reduced after release of obstruction varies with the species studied and the duration of obstruction.[2] Following release of a 24-hour complete unilateral obstruction, the GFR remains below 50% of normal in dogs and 25% of normal in rats; renal blood flow remains markedly reduced in both species.[2] After release of bilateral ureteral obstruction, renal blood flow reaches levels higher than that observed following unilateral obstruction, likely due to systemic natriuretic influences such as volume accumulation, reduced sympathetic tone, or increased circulating atrial natriuretic peptide (ANP), but the GFR remains markedly attenuated. Despite the fact that renal blood flow is increased, GFR remains low in part because of nonperfusion or underperfusion of many glomeruli as shown in silicone rubber injections.[170,178] Where glomeruli remain perfused, intense afferent vasoconstriction reduces P_{GC}, so that even though P_T also falls with release of the obstruction, the driving force for glomerular filtration remains low.[179,180] In addition, a sharp reduction in K_f also augments the fall in GFR at this point following release of unilateral and bilateral obstruction.[179,180]

Several mechanisms contribute to afferent vasoconstriction and a reduced K_f. First, release of obstruction strikingly augments the flow of tubule fluid past the macula densa. Although the absolute rate of flow is still far below normal, the macula densa likely senses the dramatic change in the rate of flow, and this may lead to intense vasoconstriction.[2] In favor of this view, the sensitivity of the tubuloglomerular feedback mechanism is enhanced in unilateral, as compared with bilateral, obstruction, which suggests that the ability of the mechanism to regulate afferent arteriolar tone is modulated by the extrarenal hormonal milieu.[183]

There is substantial evidence that increased intrarenal secretion of angiotensin II participates actively in afferent vasoconstriction and reduced K_f following release of ureteral obstruction. Ureteral obstruction rapidly increases renal vein renin levels at a time when renal blood flow is normal or elevated, but at later time points, renal vein renin levels return to normal.[184-186] In addition, infusion of captopril attenuated the declines in renal blood flow and GFR observed in both unilateral and bilateral obstruction.[184,186] Because inhibition of angiotensin-converting enzyme can also increase kinin activity, infusions of either carboxypeptidase B, which destroys kinins, or aprotinin, which blocks kinin generation, were used to eliminate the kinin effect. Captopril remained equally effective in the presence of either agent, which indicates that captopril reduced R_A primarily by blocking generation of angiotensin II.[2] The significance of the renin-angiotensin-aldosterone system as an important contributor to vasoconstriction has been highlighted in studies in which treatment with angiotensin subtype 1 receptor blocker (ARB1) attenuated the reduction in GFR in the postobstructive period in both adult rats[187] and rats with neonatally induced unilateral partial obstruction.[188]

Thromboxane A_2 (TXA_2) plays a role in the obstruction-induced vasoconstriction.[184,189] Chronically hydronephrotic kidneys exhibit increased TXA_2 accumulation, as measured by accumulation of its more stable metabolite, TXB_2.[189] Furthermore, whole-kidney GFR and renal blood flow were increased in response to thromboxane synthase inhibitor treatment,[184,190] likely by reducing afferent arteriolar resistance and thereby increasing K_f.[191] From these results, TXA_2 appears to be generated in the kidney following release of obstruction and mediates afferent vasoconstriction and reductions in K_f.

Although the source of TXA_2 generation remains unclear, in some cases,[192] but not all,[193] glomeruli isolated from obstructed kidneys have shown increased ability to synthesize TXA_2, and other studies have suggested inflammatory cells as the source of TXA_2. This is consistent with the observations that suppressor T cells and macrophages migrate to the renal cortex and medulla during the first 24 hours of obstruction, reaching levels 15-fold higher than those observed in normal kidneys[194] and a parallel rise in TXA_2 release and the fall in GFR.[194] These changes can be attenuated by renal irradiation, which indicates that obstruction stimulates migration of inflammatory leukocytes, which in turn generate vasoconstrictors such as TXA_2.[195] The role of angiotensin II for this is highlighted because glomeruli isolated from obstructed kidneys showed increased eicosanoid synthesis after angiotensin II stimulation and treatment of obstructed animals with angiotensin-converting enzyme inhibitors enhanced GFR and reduced TXA_2 generation by glomeruli isolated from these animals.[196] Thus these vasoconstrictors may contribute to regulating R_A and GFR following release of obstruction.

Because vasoconstriction is less severe in animals with bilateral ureteral obstruction, as noted earlier, it is likely that extrarenal factors play a major role in modulating the hemodynamic response of the kidney to obstruction and release of obstruction. In addition to renorenal reflexes already mentioned, various other factors, including accumulation of volume and solutes such as urea, ANP and its congeners, and other natriuretic substances may ameliorate the vasoconstrictive effects of obstruction when both ureters are ligated.[197,198] Following 24 hours of obstruction, GFR is preserved to some degree if the contralateral kidney is also obstructed or removed.[197] In addition, in animals following release of 24 hours of unilateral obstruction, if the urea, salt, and water content of the urine from the contralateral kidney is reinfused into the animal, a striking increase in GFR over standard unilateral obstruction is observed,[197,199] which suggests that ANP, urea, and other excreted urine solutes have a protective effect and can ameliorate vasoconstriction following release of ureteral obstruction by direct vasodilation of afferent arterioles, constriction of efferent arterioles, and an increase in K_f.

Additional studies in dogs and rats have implicated endothelins as contributors to reduced GFR in obstruction and have suggested that prostaglandin E_2 (PGE_2) and nitric oxide (NO) may play an ameliorating role in glomerular vasoconstriction in chronic obstructed kidneys.[200,201] Renal PGE_2 levels increase markedly in obstruction (see later) and in states of extracellular volume expansion, as occurs in bilateral ureteral obstruction. Given the vasodilator effects of PGE_2, it appears likely that increased levels could ameliorate falls in GFR in obstruction. Bilateral obstruction may reduce generation of NO, leading to a net vasoconstrictive effect.[196]

In summary, both intrarenal and extrarenal factors combine to decrease GFR profoundly during and immediately after release of obstruction. The decrease in GFR is caused by a sharp reduction in the number of perfused glomeruli and by a reduction in the SNGFR of functioning nephrons. Decreased K_f and increased R_A reduce SNGFR. Increases in various vasoconstrictors, such as angiotensin II and TXA_2, as well as other vasoconstrictors, some coming from inflammatory cells, augment these hemodynamic effects. In the setting of bilateral obstruction, retention of urea and other solutes, as well as volume expansion and increases in circulating levels of vasodilators such as ANP, help to offset these vasoconstrictive effects, but only partially.

RECOVERY OF GLOMERULAR FUNCTION AFTER RELIEF OF OBSTRUCTION

The extent of recovery of glomerular filtration following release of obstruction depends on several factors, including the duration and extent of obstruction, the presence or absence of a functioning contralateral kidney, the presence or absence of associated infection, and the level of preobstruction renal blood flow.[2,202] In a classic experiment in dogs subjected to a 1-week period of complete unilateral ureteral obstruction, GFR fell to 25% of normal on release of the obstruction and recovered gradually to 50% of normal levels 2 years later, which indicates persisting irreversible changes.[203] In rats, release of unilateral ureteral obstruction of 7 and 14 days' duration left residual GFR at 17% and 9% of control levels, respectively, when the contralateral kidney was left in place, and 31% and 14% when the animals underwent contralateral nephrectomy at the time of release of the obstruction.[204] A similar beneficial effect on the obstructed kidney of contralateral nephrectomy was observed in rats subjected to chronic partial obstruction.[204] As discussed earlier, this beneficial effect likely results from the accumulation of urea and other solutes and increased levels of ANP when the functioning contralateral kidney is absent.

The partial recovery of total GFR following release of obstruction masks a very uneven distribution of blood flow and nephron function. In micropuncture studies, some nephrons never regain filtration function, whereas others reveal striking hyperfiltration.[202] It appeared in some studies that surface nephrons exhibited normal SNGFR, whereas the whole-kidney GFR was reduced to 18% of normal.[205] These results suggest that chronic partial obstruction causes selective damage to juxtamedullary and deep cortical nephrons.[178,202,205] Similarly, studies of the long-term outcome of complete 24-hour ureteral obstruction revealed that total renal GFR recovered to normal levels by 14 and 60 days after release of obstruction. However, 15% of the glomeruli were not filtering in recovered kidneys, and other nephrons were hyperfiltering. In this model of complete obstruction, there appeared to be no selective advantage for surface glomeruli over deep cortical and juxtamedullary glomeruli.[202]

Similarly, in the developing kidney, the duration of obstruction and timing of release have a striking impact on long-term renal function. Release after 1 week of obstruction completely prevented development of hydronephrosis and reduction in renal blood flow and GFR in rats subjected to partial unilateral ureteral obstruction (UUO) at birth, whereas release after 4 weeks resulted in little or no renal function in the obstructed kidney. This demonstrates that early release of neonatal obstruction provides dramatically better protection of renal function than release of obstruction after the maturation process is completed.[206] Consistent with this, studies in pigs subjected to neonatal unilateral partial obstruction demonstrated impaired nephrogenesis with a reduced number of glomeruli in the obstructed kidney.[207] With an intact kidney function this is suggestive of some degree of glomerular hyperfiltration. In line with the hypothesis that hyperfiltration is associated with an increased risk for systemic hypertension,[208] studies in pigs and rats have demonstrated that renal expressions of neuronal nitric oxide synthase (NOS) and endothelial NOS proteins were lower in animals with hydronephrosis.[209,210] These findings suggest that the reduced NO response in the obstructed hydronephrotic kidney in hydronephrosis, and subsequent resetting of the tubuloglomerular feedback mechanism, plays an important role in the development of hypertension in hydronephrosis.

EFFECTS OF OBSTRUCTION ON TUBULAR FUNCTION

Obstruction severely impairs the ability of renal tubules to transport Na^+, K^+, and H^+, and reduces their ability to concentrate and dilute the urine (Table 38.4).[2,211-217] The resulting inability to reabsorb water and solutes facilitates postobstructive diuresis and natriuresis. As is the case with glomerular filtration, the extent of disruption of tubular

Table 38.4 Segmental Reabsorption in Superficial and Juxtamedullary Nephrons and in Collecting Ducts in Normal Rats after Release of Bilateral or Unilateral Obstruction

Site	Normal		After Unilateral Obstruction		After Bilateral Obstruction	
	Water Remaining (%)	Na+ Remaining (%)	Water Remaining (%)	Na+ Remaining (%)	Water Remaining (%)	Na+ Remaining (%)
S_1	100	100	100	100	100	100
S_2	44	44	26	26	45	45
S_3	26	14	21	12	40	22
S_4	9.4	5	3.2	1.9	25	7
J_1	100	100	100	100	100	100
J_2	12	40	42	52	42	62
CD_1	3.3	2	4.2	3.8	8	6
CD_2	0.4	0.6	2.9	2.5	16.7	12

S_1 to S_4 are values found in superficial nephrons: S_1, Bowman's space; S_2, end of proximal convoluted tubule; S_3, earliest portion of distal tubule; S_4, end of distal tubule/beginning of collecting duct. J_1 to J_2 are values found in juxtamedullary nephrons: J_1, Bowman's space; J_2, tip of loop of Henle. CD_1 and CD_2 are values found in the collecting duct: CD_1, collecting duct at base of papilla, first accessible portion of inner medullary collecting duct; CD_2, end of collecting duct as it opens into renal pelvis.

In obstruction, increased proportions of filtered salt and water are delivered to the loop of Henle in juxtamedullary nephrons J_1 and J_2, which indicates decreased reabsorption. Delivery of salt and water to the first accessible portion of the inner medullary collecting duct, labeled CD_1, was also increased, and net salt and water reabsorption along the inner medullary collecting duct (between CD_1 and CD_2) was diminished in both bilateral and unilateral obstruction. In bilateral obstruction, there was net addition or secretion of salt and water into the lumen of the inner medullary collecting duct, which suggests that in this setting the inner medullary collecting duct secretes salt and water.[195]

---

transport depends directly on the duration and severity of the obstruction.

Pathologically, prolonged obstruction leads to profound tubular atrophy and chronic interstitial inflammation and fibrosis (see later), whereas at early time points following the onset of obstruction, such as at 24 hours, there are only slight structural and ultrastructural changes, including mitochondrial swelling, modest blunting of basolateral interdigitations in the thick ascending limb and proximal tubule epithelial cells, as well as flattening of the epithelium and some widening of the intercellular spaces in the collecting ducts.[2,218,219] The only cell death at early time points is observed at the very tip of the papilla, where focal necrosis may be observed.[218]

Because there is so little cell damage, and because of the simplicity of the model, most investigators have examined the effect of 24 hours of complete ureteral obstruction on tubular function. As discussed later, regulation of tubular transport is complex and is due to both direct damage of epithelial cells and the action of extratubular mediators, arising from both the kidney and extrarenal sources.

EFFECTS OF OBSTRUCTION ON TUBULAR SODIUM REABSORPTION

Following release of 24 hours of unilateral ureteral obstruction, volume excretion from the postobstructed kidney is normal or slightly increased[2,182,197,220] (see Table 38.4). However, as discussed earlier, normal volume excretion occurs in the setting of a markedly reduced (20% of normal) GFR. Consequently, FE_{Na} is markedly elevated in the postobstructed kidney. After release of bilateral obstruction, salt and water excretion jumps up to five to nine times normal.[2,182,211,212] Because GFR is also decreased in this setting, FE_{Na} may be 20-fold higher than normal.

The micropuncture studies summarized in Table 38.4 demonstrate that the reabsorption defect following release of obstruction is localized similarly in both unilateral and bilateral ureteral obstruction. Obstruction reduced net salt and water reabsorption in the medullary thick ascending limb (MTAL), the distal convoluted tubule, and the entire length of the collecting duct, including its cortical, outer medullary, and inner medullary segments.[211]

These studies in whole animals were confirmed and extended by a series of studies from multiple laboratories using isolated perfused tubule and cell suspension preparations (Table 38.5). As shown in the table, the segments, including proximal straight tubule, MTAL, and cortical collecting duct isolated from unilaterally or bilaterally obstructed animals, exhibited profound impairment of reabsorptive capacity.[212,213] This finding was confirmed in studies of freshly prepared suspensions of MTAL cells from obstructed kidneys, in which transport-dependent oxygen consumption, a measure of salt reabsorptive capacity, was markedly reduced.[214] Given the major regulatory role of mineralocorticoid in the collecting duct, it is important to note that these decreases in collecting duct reabsorptive capacity occurred in tubules taken from obstructed kidneys, whether or not the animal had been pretreated with mineralocorticoid.[213,215,216] Because it is highly branched and difficult to perfuse reliably in vitro, transport in the inner medullary collecting duct has been studied in cell suspensions. In these preparations, transport-dependent oxygen consumption was markedly reduced in cells isolated from animals with bilateral obstruction.[217]

Taken together, the data derived from micropuncture, tubule perfusion, and cell suspension studies reveal a striking impairment of volume reabsorption in the proximal straight tubule, the MTAL, and the entire collecting duct.

Table 38.5 Function of Isolated Perfused Tubules in Obstructive Nephropathy

	J$_v$ SPCT (nL/mm/min)	J$_v$ PST (nL/mm/min)	ΔCl⁻ MTAL (mEq/L)	J$_v$ CCT (AVP) (nL/mm/min)
Control	0.75 ± 0.08	0.25 ± 0.02	−37 ± 3	0.90 ± 0.08
Unilateral obstruction	0.73 ± 0.11	0.12 ± 0.03	−9 ± 1	0.22 ± 0.04
Bilateral obstruction	0.80 ± 0.08	0.16 ± 0.02	−10 ± 1	0.23 ± 0.04

The J$_v$ in the SPCT was not affected by obstruction, whereas J$_v$ in PST decreased by 52% in unilateral obstruction (0.12 ± 0.03 vs. 0.25 ± 0.02 nL/mm/min) and similarly in response to bilateral obstruction. In MTAL the ability to lower the perfusate chloride ion concentration was reduced by 76% (−9 ± 1 vs. −37 ± 3 mEq/L) and similarly in response to bilateral ureteral obstruction. Following relief of unilateral obstruction, the ability of the CCT to respond to ADH was reduced by 76% (0.22 ± 0.04 vs. 0.90 ± 0.08 nL/mm/min), and similarly following relief of bilateral obstruction.

AVP, Antidiuretic hormone; CCT, cortical collecting tubule; ΔCl⁻ MTAL, change in Cl⁻ concentration per length of the medullary thick ascending limb; J$_v$, net fluid reabsorption rate per length of the tubule segment; PST, proximal straight tubule; SPCT, superficial proximal convoluted tubule.

Data from Buerkert J, Martin D, Head M, et al: Deep nephron function after release of acute unilateral ureteral obstruction in the young rat. J Clin Invest 62:1228-1239, 1978; and Hanley MJ, Davidson K: Isolated nephron segments from rabbit models of obstructive nephropathy. J Clin Invest 69:165-174, 1982.

Because these functional derangements occur in the absence of clear-cut ultrastructural damage to the epithelial cells, obstruction likely induces a selective impairment in the regulation of active cellular transport mechanisms. Unlike the situation with glomerular filtration, the functional impairment appears similar in both unilateral and bilateral obstruction.[213,216,217] Thus it appears that a major component of impaired active transport is likely due to direct tubular cell injury, rather than to the continuous action of natriuretic substances. Added onto this intrinsic injury, natriuretic substances may be responsible for the apparent secretion of salt and water in the inner medullary collecting duct of animals following release of bilateral obstruction (see Table 38.4).

A combination of studies of cell suspensions and antibody-based targeted proteomics in which long-term regulation renal transporters and channels can be examined in intact animals to understand the integrated response to obstruction has improved the molecular understanding of mechanisms by which tubular epithelial cell salt reabsorption is impaired in the setting of obstruction. Active tubular Na$^+$ transport requires an apical entry step (e.g., Na$^+$-K$^+$-2Cl$^-$-cotransporter type 2 [NKCC2] in MTAL or epithelial sodium channels [ENaCs] in the collecting duct) coupled to the basolateral sodium-potassium adenosine triphosphatase (Na$^+$-K$^+$-ATPase). In addition, the cell must generate sufficient adenosine triphosphate (ATP) to fuel active transport by adenosine triphosphatase (ATPase). Suspensions of MTAL cells from obstructed kidneys exhibited markedly reduced furosemide-sensitive oxygen consumption,[214] which indicates striking decreases in apical NKCC2 activity in these cells. Isotopic bumetanide binding revealed a marked reduction in the number of cotransporter protein molecules available for binding on the membrane, with no change in affinity of binding, which indicates that obstruction downregulates the expression of the cotransporter protein on the membrane surface.[214] Later studies using antibody-based targeted approaches clearly showed that obstruction diminishes expression of the cotransporter protein on the MTAL cell apical membrane.[221] Similar approaches demonstrated downregulation of Na$^+$-K$^+$-ATPase of both α- and β-subunits at the transcriptional and posttranscriptional level.[221,222]

In the inner medullary collecting duct similar studies demonstrated downregulation of ENaC.[223] Consistent with this, suspensions from obstructed kidneys showed marked decreases in amiloride-sensitive oxygen consumption as well as amiloride-sensitive isotopic sodium entry into hyperpolarized cells.[217]

As occurred in MTAL cells, the rates of ouabain-sensitive oxygen consumption and of ouabain-sensitive ATPase were markedly diminished in inner medullary collecting duct cells from obstructed animals, and the levels of both pump subunits were also reduced in these preparations.[217] Patterns of mRNA expression were also similar to those in MTAL, which indicates transcriptional and posttranscriptional downregulation of pump subunit expression. Using the targeted antibody–based approach demonstrated that in both unilateral and bilateral ureteral obstruction, the expression of Na$^+$-H$^+$-exchanger isoform 3 (NHE$_3$) and the Na$^+$-PO$_4^{3-}$-exchanger type 2 were strikingly decreased in the proximal tubule.[221,224] These changes in sodium transporter expression occurred in both the proximal convoluted and proximal straight tubule, even though the micropuncture and tubule perfusion studies cited earlier revealed preserved proximal convoluted tubule salt reabsorption and inhibition of proximal straight tubule reabsorption.[224,225] The same studies demonstrated significant downregulation of total transporter protein and apical membrane expression of the distal convoluted tubule Na$^+$-Cl$^-$-cotransporter, which indicates that obstruction likely reduces distal convoluted tubule Na$^+$ reabsorption by mechanisms similar to those observed in the MTAL and collecting duct.[221,224]

Taken together, these results demonstrate that obstruction downregulates membrane expression of transporter proteins responsible for apical sodium entry and basolateral sodium exit. Interestingly, metabolic studies reveal that obstruction reduces activities as well of several enzymes of the oxidative and glycolytic pathways, consistent with a downregulation of metabolic capacity for energy generation in these cells. This may also be enhanced by the observed reductions in the extent of basolateral infolding and in the density of mitochondria in tubules of obstructed kidneys.[218] Interestingly, in MTAL and collecting duct suspension, obstruction reduces transport-dependent but not transport-independent oxygen consumption, which indicates that the rate of ATP generation (oxygen consumption) is not rate limiting for active transport in these cells. On this basis, it appears more likely that obstruction-induced reduction of epithelial sodium transport is a regulated process as a result of reduced metabolic demands during obstruction.

The mechanisms and pathways responsible for downregulation of transport proteins in tubular epithelial cells by obstruction remain to a large extent incomplete. Possible signals include the halting of urine flow, increased hydrostatic pressure on tubular epithelial cells, changes in blood flow to the tubules or in interstitial pressure, and generation of natriuretic substances in the kidney that result in long-term inhibition of transporter function. Powerful mass spectrometry analysis of tissue from obstructed rat kidneys and mpkCCD cells has led to proteomic identification of significant changes in more than 100 proteins, including proteins belonging to the cytoskeleton. These findings suggest that obstruction induces acute molecular changes in the renal cytoskeleton, in part mediated by increased stretch of the renal tubular cells during obstruction.[226]

Obstruction impairs glomerular filtration, and urine production is dramatically reduced (stopped in occlusion). Consequently, sodium delivery to each tubular segment is reduced, and apical membrane Na^+ entry slows dramatically because the electrochemical gradients for Na^+ entry between the stationary apical fluid and the cell interior become increasingly unfavorable for continued sodium transport. Reduced Na^+ entry might then directly stimulate downregulation of transporter activity and expression. In both MTAL and inner medullary collecting duct cells, blocking Na^+ entry by furosemide or amiloride, respectively, promptly reduces ouabain-sensitive oxygen consumption,[214,227] which indicates acute downregulation of Na^+-K^+-ATPase. In addition, in mineralocorticoid-clamped animals, chronic blockade of Na^+ entry at the MTAL or cortical collecting duct by administration of furosemide or amiloride, respectively, reduced the levels of ouabain-sensitive ATPase in microdissected tubule segments.[228,229]

These results suggest that the halt in urine flow might represent a major signaling mechanism by which obstruction downregulates Na^+ transport.[227] To test this hypothesis, apical Na^+ entry was inhibited for 24 hours in a cell line that mimics cortical collecting duct cells, A6 cells, grown on permeable supports. When apical Na^+ entry was blocked either by substituting another cation for sodium in the apical solution, or by adding amiloride to the apical solution, apical sodium entry was markedly reduced for some hours after the blockade was removed.[230] This downregulation is accompanied by selective reduction in the levels of expression of the β-subunit, but not the α- or γ-subunits of ENaC in the apical membranes of the A6 cells, but not in whole cell content of these subunits.[231] At the integrated level, rats with urinary tract obstruction demonstrated downregulation of α-, β-, and γ-subunits of ENaC which indicates that downregulation of all three subunits may play a role in the impaired sodium reabsorption in obstruction.[223] Interestingly, and in contrast to the results in cell suspensions or whole kidney,[214,217,221,224] inhibition of apical

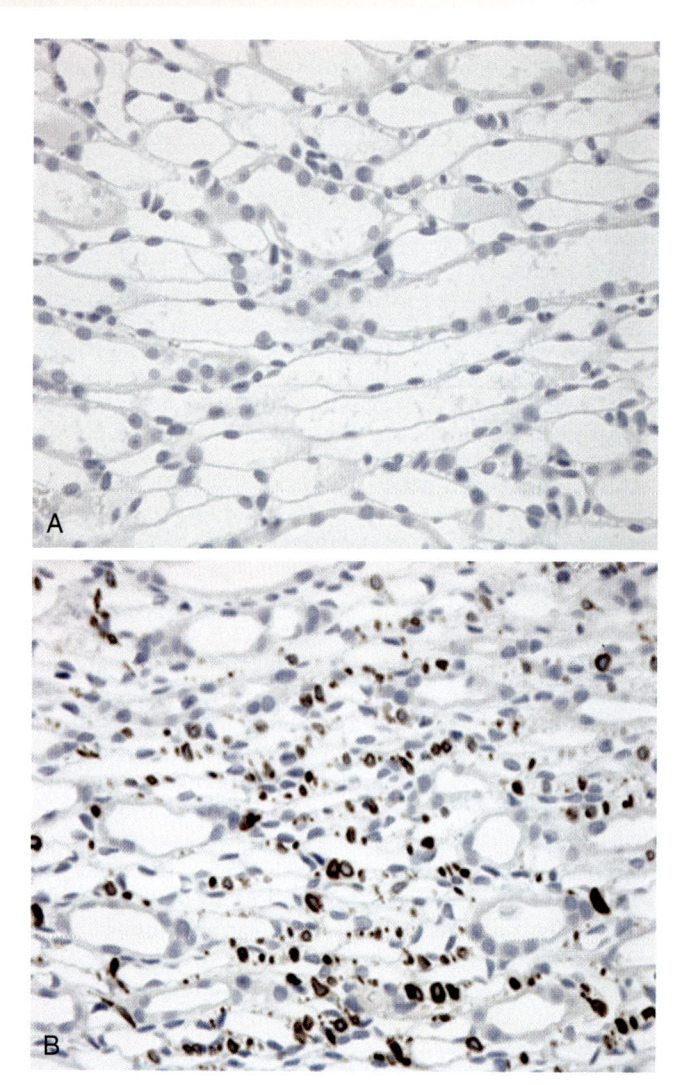

Figure 38.8 Immunohistochemistry for cyclo-oxygenase-2 (COX-2) in kidney inner medulla of sham-operated rats (**A**) and rats subjected to 24 hours of bilateral ureteral obstruction (**B**). There is a strong labeling at the base of the inner medulla in obstructed kidneys located exclusively in the interstitial cells (**B**). Labeling is not detectable in sham-operated kidneys (**A**).

sodium entry had no effect on expression of either subunit of Na^+-K^+-ATPase.[231] These results provide direct evidence that reductions in the rate of Na^+ entry, which may occur when urine flow is blocked, can directly downregulate Na^+ transport in renal epithelial cells.

In addition to the direct effects of halting urine flow, changes in intrarenal mediators and subcellular pathways likely play a critical role in the reduction of salt transport observed with obstruction. Obstruction markedly accelerates the already-rapid generation of PGE_2 in the renal medulla.[189,190,193,232] The molecular basis for this is a dramatic medullary cyclo-oxygenase-2 (COX-2) induction (Figure 38.8).[232,233] Consistent with the known effect of PGE_2 to markedly inhibit Na^+ reabsorption in the MTAL, as well as in the cortical and inner medullary collecting ducts,[234-236] COX-2 inhibition in rats with obstruction and release of obstruction attenuated the downregulation of NHE2, NKCC2, and Na^+-K^+-ATPase.[233,237] From these results, obstruction likely reduces apically localized sodium cotransport proteins in the tubular epithelium and sodium pump activity in tubular epithelia in part by increasing renal levels of PGE$_2$.

As discussed earlier, obstruction brings on a monocellular infiltrate in the kidney[194]; and this infiltrate tends to follow a peritubular distribution.[194] When obstructed kidneys were irradiated, the level of medullary inflammation was diminished, and there was a modest decrease in the FE$_{Na}$.[195] In addition, it has been shown that obstruction causes an enhanced renal angiotensin II generation. This may have important implications for regulation of renal sodium handling. Blockade of the angiotensin II subtype 1 receptor (AT$_1$R) was associated with a marked attenuation of downregulation of NHE3 and NKCC2, which was paralleled by a reduction in renal sodium loss.[57]

In summary, obstruction reduces net reabsorption of salt in several nephron segments, including the proximal straight tubule, the MTAL, and the cortical and inner medullary collecting ducts, by downregulating the expression and activities of specific transporter proteins. Several signals mediate this downregulation, including the cessation of urine flow with its attendant reduction of the rate of Na$^+$ entry across the apical membrane, increased levels of natriuretic substances such as PGE$_2$, and infiltration of the obstructed kidney by mononuclear cells.

When both ureters are obstructed, extrarenal factors markedly enhance the sodium-wasting tendency already present in the obstructed kidney. One mechanism involves the volume expansion that occurs when bilateral obstruction ablates all renal function. Volume expansion impairs activity in the sympathetic nervous system, reduces circulating levels of aldosterone, and, along with reduced renal clearance, increases levels of ANP. Reduced sympathetic tone and aldosterone levels, coupled with increased ANP levels, markedly stimulate sodium excretion. ANP likely represents a particularly important mediator of salt wasting in bilateral obstruction. Levels of ANP are markedly elevated in bilateral, but not unilateral, obstruction.[238] ANP enhances salt wasting at several nephron segments. By blocking renin release in the macula densa and angiotensin action in the proximal tubule, ANP reduces proximal tubule sodium reabsorption.[198,238,239] ANP also reduces aldosterone release and directly inhibits sodium reabsorption in the collecting ducts.[198,238,239] In agreement with this mechanism, infusion of ANP into animals in which obstruction has just been released leads to marked increases in sodium and water excretion.[238] Moreover, efforts to reduce circulating ANP levels following bilateral obstruction attenuated sodium excretion somewhat.[238]

In addition, accumulation of urea and other solutes enhances sodium wasting by obstructed kidneys. Following release of 24 hours of unilateral obstruction, removal or obstruction of the contralateral kidney markedly enhances salt wasting by the obstructed kidney.[197] If the contralateral kidney is left in place but amounts of urea, salt, and water equivalent to what the contralateral kidney is excreting are infused into the animal, there is a striking increase in sodium excretion in both the obstructed and the contralateral kidney.[197,199] On this basis, bilateral obstruction induces hormonal changes and promotes accumulation of solutes and volume that together enhance natriuresis from the obstructed kidney.

EFFECTS OF OBSTRUCTION ON URINARY CONCENTRATION AND DILUTION

Because obstruction eliminates the ability of the renal tubules to concentrate and dilute the urine, urine osmolality following release of obstruction in humans and experimental animals approaches that of plasma.[2,240,241] Dilution of the urine requires that the thick ascending limb reabsorb sodium without water and that the collecting duct maintain the dilute urine by not reabsorbing water along its length, despite the presence of a concentrated medullary interstitium.[242] Concentration of the urine requires active sodium reabsorption in the thick limb and the action of the countercurrent multiplier to generate a concentrated medullary interstitium, as well as the ability of the collecting duct to insert the vasopressin-regulated water channel aquaporin-2 (AQP2) into the apical membrane.[243,244]

Obstructive nephropathy disrupts several of these mechanisms.[224,240,241,245] As noted earlier, obstruction also markedly reduces MTAL sodium reabsorption, limiting this segment's ability to dilute the urine and to generate a high medullary interstitial osmolality. Indeed, interstitial osmolality has been shown to be reduced in obstructed kidneys.[2] In addition, collecting ducts isolated from obstructed kidneys reveal normal basal water permeabilities, but a marked reduction in their ability to increase water permeability in response to antidiuretic hormone or other stimulants of cyclic adenosine monophosphate (cAMP) accumulation in the cells. As was the case with sodium transport, the effects were similar in unilateral and bilateral obstruction.[240,245] Detailed mechanistic studies show that obstruction markedly reduces transcription of mRNA encoding AQP2, as well as synthesis of AQP2 protein, and that collecting duct cells in obstructed kidneys do not traffic AQP2-containing vesicles effectively to the apical surface in response to vasopressin or increased cAMP.[240,244-246] Part of this failure in trafficking results from a decrease in phosphorylation of AQP2 in obstructed kidneys[224] and likely also to the fact that vasopressin type 2 receptor (V$_2$R) protein expression is downregulated.[247] Redistribution of AQP2 and AQP2 phosphorylated at ser261 to more intracellular localizations after bilateral obstruction and co-localization with early endosomal antigen 1 (EEA1) and the lysosomal marker cathepsin D suggest that early downregulation of AQP2 could in part be caused by degradation of AQP2 through a lysosomal degradation pathway.[248]

In addition, UUO markedly decreases synthesis and deployment to the basolateral membrane of AQP3 and AQP4; when AQP2 is in the apical membrane, these aquaporins mediate the water flux across the basolateral membrane.[224] Enhancing the causal relationship of the changes in aquaporin activity and ability to concentrate the urine, expression of AQP2 remains suppressed for 7 days following relief of the obstruction, and the rise in urinary concentration parallels the recovery in AQP2 expression.[224,240,241,245]

The fact that collecting ducts from obstructed kidneys do not respond to cAMP indicates that the lesion also involve sites beyond the receptor for antidiuretic hormone.[247] Consistent with the idea that PGE$_2$-mediated inhibition of collecting duct water permeability does not directly affect cAMP levels but may have post-cAMP effects rather than actions via cAMP regulation,[249] experiments have shown that

COX-2 inhibition prevented dysregulation of AQP2 in obstructed kidneys in which COX-2 protein expression was markedly increased.[233,250]

On the basis of these results, the defect in urinary dilution in obstruction is due to reduced ability of the thick ascending limb to dilute the urine by transporting salt from the lumen of the tubule to its basolateral side. The collecting duct in obstructed kidneys maintains its low water permeability in the absence of antidiuretic hormone, so that the failure to dilute the urine is not due to collapse of osmotic gradients in the collecting duct. The inability to concentrate the urine results from the failure of the thick limb to generate a concentrated interstitium, as well as the inability of the collecting duct to synthesize and to traffic AQP2 and other water channels in response to antidiuretic hormone.

EFFECTS OF RELIEF OF OBSTRUCTION ON URINARY ACIDIFICATION

Obstruction dramatically reduces urinary acidification in both experimental animals and humans. In humans, release of obstruction does not lead to bicarbonate wasting, which indicates that proximal tubule bicarbonate reclamation is maintained. By contrast, in both experimental animals and patients following release of obstruction, the urine pH does not decrease in response to an acid load, which indicates that obstruction impairs the ability of the distal nephron to acidify the urine.[251-253] This defect likely involves proton transport proteins both in the collecting duct[251,252] and in the proximal tubule and thick ascending limb of Henle.[253,254]

Reduced collecting duct acid secretion could result from defects in H^+ (H^+-ATPase, or H^+-K^+-ATPase) or HCO_3^- (e.g., Cl^--HCO_3^- exchange) transport pathways, backleak of protons down their electrochemical gradient from the lumen to the basolateral side of the tubule, or, in the cortical collecting duct, the failure to generate a sufficiently lumen-negative transepithelial voltage.[251,252,255] As described in detail earlier, obstruction reduces the activity of apical ENaC in the cortical collecting duct; the resulting loss of luminal negativity may attenuate acid secretion in these segments.[251,252]

In the rat inner medullary collecting duct (studied by micropuncture) and in isolated perfused rat and rabbit outer medullary collecting duct, obstruction markedly reduces luminal acidification rates.[251] Because Na^+ transport does not play a major role in acidification in these segments, the defect must be due to direct inhibition of acid or HCO_3^- transport pathways, or backleak of protons from lumen to interstitium.[255] At low perfusion rates, outer medullary collecting ducts from obstructed animals maintain the ability to generate steep pH gradients,[251] which indicates that obstruction does not block the ability of the tubule to prevent back flux of protons. By contrast, at high perfusion rates, acidification was markedly lower in tubules from obstructed, as opposed to normal, kidneys,[251] which demonstrates that obstruction inhibits activity or expression of H^+ or HCO_3^- transport pathways.

Antibody-based targeted studies examining the Cl^--HCO_3^--exchanger and subunits of H^+-ATPase revealed reduced expression of these transporters in collecting ducts of unilaterally obstructed kidneys compared with contralateral and control kidneys.[253,255] Two possible mechanisms of reduced acid secretion were explored.[255] One was that the intercalated cells in obstructed kidneys would exhibit a high proportion of "reverse" orientation, with the proton pump in the basolateral membrane and the Cl^--HCO_3^--exchanger in the apical membrane. The other possibility was that the orientation of intercalated cells would not change, but there would be reduced expression of the H^+ or HCO_3^- transporter. The orientation of the intercalated cells was not altered by obstruction. However, obstruction did reduce the appearance of H^+-ATPase along the apical membranes of intercalated cells, without altering the total content of H^+-ATPase in extracts of renal cortex or medulla, in unilaterally obstructed as compared with contralateral kidneys.[255] In obstructed kidneys, fewer intercalated cells exhibited an apical labeling pattern, and many that did showed discontinuities or gaps in apical membrane labeling,[255] which suggests that obstruction inhibits trafficking of H^+-ATPase to the apical membranes of intercalated cells. However, this disorder alone cannot account for the entire acidification defect in obstructive nephropathy, because the labeling pattern returns to control levels as the obstruction persists, whereas the acidification defect remains.[255] In addition, the extent of the decrease in labeling appears to be too small to account for the profound defect in acidification.

In addition to defective collecting duct H^+ transport, reduced generation of the main buffer that carries acid equivalents in the urine, ammonia, has also been observed in kidneys released from obstruction. Cortical slices of obstructed kidneys exhibit reduced glutamine uptake and oxidation, reduced gluconeogenesis, and reduced total oxygen consumption, all adding up to a reduced ability to generate ammonia from glutamine.[256,257]

EFFECTS OF RELIEF OF OBSTRUCTION ON EXCRETION OF POTASSIUM

As with sodium excretion, potassium excretion increases markedly following release of bilateral obstruction.[258,259] Micropuncture and microcatheterization studies show that proximal potassium reabsorption is unchanged by obstruction, whereas potassium is more rapidly secreted in the collecting duct, likely due to increased distal delivery and therefore more rapid distal luminal flux of sodium and volume following release of obstruction.[211,258] By contrast, following release of unilateral obstruction, potassium excretion falls roughly in proportion to the reduction in GFR,[260] an effect that may be related to reduced distal delivery of sodium. However, administration of sodium sulfate in this state does not stimulate potassium excretion in obstructed kidneys as it does in controls, which suggests that collecting ducts in unilateral obstructed kidneys have an intrinsic defect in potassium secretion.[261] This intrinsic defect may represent a response similar to the downregulation of sodium transporters in obstructed kidneys described in detail earlier. The kaliuretic effect observed in bilateral obstruction may be due as well to the influence of elevated levels of ANP, which, at high levels, can stimulate potassium secretion in the distal nephron.

EFFECTS OF RELIEF OF OBSTRUCTION ON EXCRETION OF PHOSPHATE AND DIVALENT CATIONS

When bilateral ureteral obstruction is released, phosphate excretion rises in proportion to sodium excretion.[221,224,262,263] Phosphate restriction before the release of the obstruction prevents phosphate accumulation during bilateral obstruction, thereby blocking the increase in phosphate excretion.[262] This can also be achieved by blockade of angiotensin II–mediated effects, which highlights the importance of enhanced renal angiotensin II levels in the obstructed kidney.[57] In addition, phosphate wasting of similar magnitude to that observed following release of bilateral obstruction can be duplicated by phosphate loading of normal animals.[262] By contrast, release of unilateral obstruction results in phosphate retention, likely due to reduced GFR and avid proximal phosphate reabsorption.[264] Calcium excretion may be increased or decreased, depending on whether the obstruction is unilateral or bilateral and depending on the species studied.[262,264] Magnesium excretion is markedly increased following release of either bilateral or unilateral obstruction. This magnesium wasting probably occurs because both forms of obstruction markedly attenuate thick ascending limb sodium reabsorption, leading to reduced positive luminal transepithelial voltages and therefore a reduced driving force for lumen-to-basolateral magnesium flux across the paracellular pathway.[265]

PATHOPHYSIOLOGY OF RECOVERY OF TUBULAR EPITHELIAL CELLS FROM OBSTRUCTION OR TUBULOINTERSTITIAL FIBROSIS

An important focus of many experimental studies in obstructive nephropathy has been devoted to the renal effects of longer-term obstruction.[266] In part these studies use UUO as a convenient model for chronic renal damage, because the timing of the injury is clear and because the extent of injury should be reproducible from animal to animal.[266] These studies, which have been conducted almost entirely in rodents, have elucidated an overall pathway for renal tubular epithelial damage and have identified several potential targets for intervention. Obstruction inhibits oxidative metabolism and promotes anaerobic respiration, leading to decreased ATP levels and increased levels of adenosine diphosphate and adenosine monophosphate.[257,267,268] In addition, obstruction alters a wide variety of metabolic enzymes, as well as the expression of many different gene products.[257,268-270] These changes are summarized in Table 38.6. Many of these changes are difficult to link mechanistically with changes in GFR or tubular transport function observed in obstruction. It is possible, however, that reduced ability to generate ATP, along with reductions in Na+-K+-ATPase expression, contributes to the natriuresis observed following release of obstruction (see earlier discussion).

It is thought that chronic obstruction damages tubular epithelial cells by increasing hydrostatic pressure, reducing blood flow (due to the renal vasoconstriction that occurs in obstruction, see earlier), and increasing oxidative stress.[266] In response, tubular epithelial cells release a number of autocrine factors and cytokines, including angiotensin II,[266,271] transforming growth factor-β (TGF-β),[271,272] platelet activator inhibitor,[273] and tumor necrosis factor (TNF).[274] These factors, along with the presence and increase in levels of adhesion factors, lead to the infiltration of the renal interstitium with inflammatory cells, including macrophages. These in turn release additional cytokines.

Table 38.6 Effects of Urinary Tract Obstruction on Renal Enzymes and Renal Gene Expression

Changes in Energy and Substrate Metabolism

Decreased oxygen consumption
Decreased substrate uptake
Increased anaerobic glycolysis
Decreased ATP/(ADP + AMP)
Decreased ammoniagenesis

Changes in Enzyme Activity

Decreased

Alkaline phosphatase
Na+-K+-ATPase
Glucose-6-phosphatase
Succinate dehydrogenase
NADH/NADPH dehydrogenase

Increased

Glucose-6-phosphate dehydrogenase
Phosphogluconate dehydrogenase
Mitogen-activated protein kinases
Matrix metalloproteinase 2 or 9
Mast cell protease 1 (chymase)

Changes in Gene Expression

Reduction in glomerular $G_{\alpha s}$ and $G_{\alpha q/11}$ proteins
Reduction in prepro–epidermal growth factor and Tamm-Horsfall protein
Transient induction of growth factors FOS and MYC
Striking induction of cellular damage (TRPM2) genes
Induction of plasminogen activator gene

ADP, Adenosine diphosphate; AMP, adenosine monophosphate; ATP, adenosine triphosphate; ATPase, adenosine triphosphatase; FOS, FBJ murine osteosarcoma viral oncogene homolog; MYC, myelocytomatosis viral oncogene homolog; NADH, reduced form of nicotinamide adenine dinucleotide; NADPH, reduced form of nicotinamide adenine dinucleotide phosphate; TRPM2, transient receptor potential cation channel, subfamily M, member 2.

All these factors accelerate the development of interstitial fibrosis by increased extracellular matrix, cell infiltration, apoptosis, and accumulation of activated myofibroblasts.[275] In addition, there is upregulation of various receptors that are targeted by autocrine factors and cytokines, including both type 1 and type 2 angiotensin receptors (AT$_1$R and AT$_2$R).[276] The complex cellular migration process may become amplified by epithelial-mesenchymal transition (EMT),[277] which is characterized by downregulation of epithelial marker proteins such as E-cadherin, zonula occludens 1, and cytokeratin; loss of cell-to-cell adhesion; upregulation of mesenchymal markers, including vimentin, α-smooth muscle actin, and fibroblast-specific protein 1; basement membrane degradation; and migration to the interstitial compartment.[277] The entire cascade leads to tubulointerstitial fibrosis and permanent loss of renal function, which may continue to progress after the obstruction has been relieved (Figure 38.9).

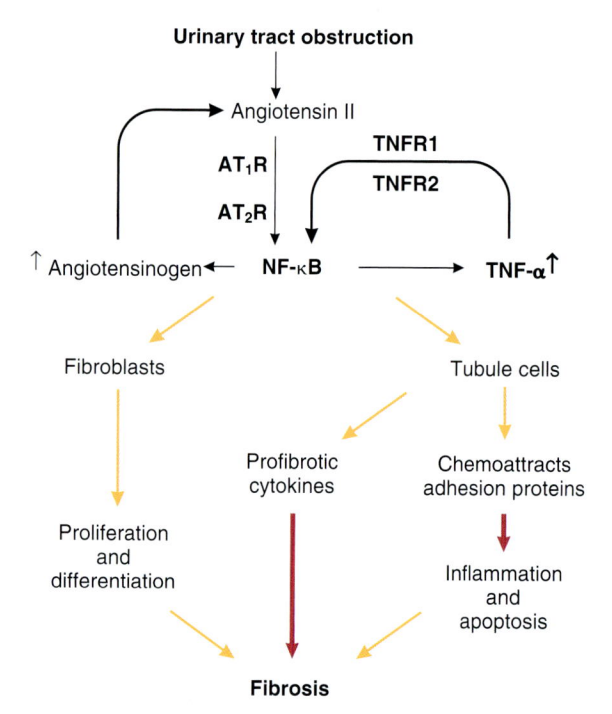

Figure 38.9 Urinary tract obstruction causes an enhanced expression of angiotensin II. The regulation of gene expression by angiotensin II occurs through specific receptors that are ultimately linked to changes in the activity of transcription factors within the nucleus of target cells. In particular, members of the nuclear factor-kappaB (NF-κB) family of transcription factors are activated, which in turn fuels at least two autocrine-reinforcing loops that amplify angiotensin II and tumor necrosis factor-α (TNF-α) formation. TNFR1 and TNFR2, TNF-α receptors.

It has been hypothesized that changes in the intratubular dynamic forces—so-called tubular stretch—in urinary tract obstruction also are an important determinant for development of tubulointerstitial fibrosis in the kidney.[278] Thus both in vivo[272] and in vitro models[279,280] of obstructive uropathy demonstrate that tubular stretch induces robust expression of TGF-β$_1$, activation of tubular apoptosis, and induction of nuclear factor-kappaB signaling, which contribute to the inflammatory and fibrotic milieu.[278,281] Because fibrosis is absent in mast cell–deficient mice with UUO, this suggests that mast cells play an important role in induction of the inflammation and development of tubulointerstitial fibrosis in obstruction.[282] Furthermore, the importance of the renin angiotensin aldosterone system for the development of fibrosis was also underscored by the observation that mast cells release renin, possibly stimulated by autocrine histamine release.[282]

Thus the pathogenesis of renal fibrosis is a progressive and complicated process involving multiple molecular pathways and cellular targets, including angiotensin II as highlighted already.[4,184] Because angiotensin II is known to stimulate production of TGF-β, which is critical for tubulointerstitial development,[283] this has been highlighted by the in vivo documentation of a relationship between angiotensin II and TGF-β in genetically defined mouse models of Marfan syndrome.[284] Interestingly, studies show that selected manifestations of Marfan syndrome reflect excessive signaling by TGF-β.[285] Moreover, systemic antagonism of TGF-β through administration of a TGF-β–neutralizing antibody or treatment with losartan prevented aortic aneurysm[284] and normalized muscle architecture, repair, and function in Marfan-like fibrillin-1–deficient mice.[285] Collectively these studies propose that mast cells' release of renin and local angiotensin II formation in the obstructed kidney may lead to both vasoconstriction, which causes reduction in renal blood flow, as well as GFR and fibroblast and macrophage activation, which increases TGF-β levels and causes fibrosis of the kidney. Along this line, data suggest that mast cells also have the capacity to release chymase, a protease, which may limit development of tubulointerstitial fibrosis by decreasing infiltration of inflammatory cells and release of proinflammatory and profibrotic chemokines and cytokines.[286]

Several studies have shown that antagonism of angiotensin II, TGF-β, TNF, or factors that attract inflammatory cells may ameliorate postobstructive renal damage.[266,271-275,287-289] Similarly, augmentation of expression of factors that favor epithelial growth and differentiation, such as hepatocyte growth factor,[290] insulin-like growth factor, or bone morphogenic protein-7,[266] may also have a protective effect.

From multiple studies, it has been suggested that the main mechanism that is responsible for the onset of the pathophysiologic cascades is the increased pressure in the renal pelvis, which leads to increased pressure in the parenchyma and subsequently mechanical stress, which leads to activation of stretch and swelling-activated cation channels within focal adhesions of the epithelial cells, causing subsequent influx of Ca^{2+}.[280,281] This causes oxidative stress and stimulates migration of macrophages to the obstructed kidney. However, the complexity of the process and the experience from multiple studies demonstrating that there is no single pathway that is responsible for the cellular changes was highlighted by the potential role of infiltrating macrophages in the pathophysiology of inflammation during UUO. It was demonstrated that activation of AT$_1$R on macrophages in UUO is prerequisite for suppression of their release of proinflammatory cytokine interleukin-1 (IL-1).[291] This indicates that a key role of AT$_1$R on macrophages is to protect the kidney from fibrosis by limiting activation of IL-1 receptors in the obstructed kidney. Further, this finding may show implications for the design of novel potent therapies to overcome the shortcomings of global angiotensin receptor blockade. Thus the process leading to kidney fibrosis is complex, and numerous processes contribute to regulating the cellular changes that are responsible for these pathophysiologic changes.

Given species differences and the fact that obstruction in humans is often partial, the animal models may not predict entirely the behavior of postobstructive kidneys in humans. However, if the studies are relevant to human obstructive nephropathy, they suggest that patients undergoing release of obstruction may benefit from therapies that block proapoptotic, proinflammatory, or profibrotic mediators or from treatments that stimulate epithelial cell growth and differentiation.[266,271-275,287-289]

Experimentally, protection from obstruction-induced detrimental effects on renal function can also be achieved by NO supplementation. This can be accomplished either by angiotensin-converting enzyme inhibition, which increases kinin levels and subsequently increases NO formation, or by stimulation of endogenous NOS with L-arginine.[292] L-Arginine is a semi-essential amino acid and is also substrate and the main source for generation of NO via NOS. Importantly, chronic unilateral obstruction in mice leads to significant reduction in inducible NOS (iNOS) activity, and the obstructed kidney of iNOS knockout mice exhibited significantly more apoptotic renal tubules than controls, which underscores the important role NO plays for protecting the cellular functions in the obstructed kidney.[293] Dietary L-arginine supplementation attenuated renal damage of a 3-day unilateral ureteral obstruction in rats, which indicates that L-arginine treatment may be a useful pharmacologic avenue in obstructive nephropathy.[266] It was also shown that several of the detrimental effects of obstruction can be attenuated by treatment with the α-melanocyte–stimulating-hormone (α-MSH), which is a potent antiinflammatory hormone. These results support the view that inflammation is a crucial determinant for the onset of renal deterioration in urinary tract obstruction.[294] Interestingly, it has been demonstrated that recombinant human erythropoietin (rhEPO) treatment inhibits the progression of renal fibrosis in the obstructed kidney and attenuates the TGF-β_1–induced EMT, which suggests that the renoprotective effects of rhEPO could be mediated, at least partly, by inhibition of TGF-β_1–induced EMT.[295]

FETAL URINARY TRACT OBSTRUCTION

Obstructive uropathy constitutes the largest fraction of identifiable causes of renal insufficiency and kidney failure in infants and children. Compared with adult obstructive nephropathy, fetal obstructive nephropathy is particularly devastating because renal growth and continued nephron development are impaired by the progression of fibrosis. Several studies have examined aspects of obstructive nephropathy in the newborn using a neonatal rat model of unilateral obstruction, and the pathophysiology involved in fetal urinary tract obstruction will be discussed in Chapter 73. Briefly, fetal urinary obstruction may lead to changes in tissue differentiation. At the time of birth, the rodent kidney is not fully developed and is representative of human renal development at approximately the midtrimester, and animal models reveal that fetal obstruction causes aberrations of morphogenesis, gene expression, cell turnover, and urine composition.[296,297] The earlier the kidney is obstructed in utero, the greater will be the changes in renal tissue.[296,297] After birth, obstruction may affect renal growth, especially in neonates and during the first year of life, but the obstruction will not cause tissue dedifferentiation.

Studies have demonstrated the upregulation of the renin angiotensin aldosterone system, as well as involvement of other substrates (TGF-β_1, endothelin-1, and many other mediators) in obstructed kidneys.[296-299] The exact mechanisms of action of these molecules in the alteration of renal morphogenesis are not fully understood. It is not well known either if obstruction alone is enough to induce renal dysplasia,[296,297] or if the latter results from secondary obstruction-induced mesenchymal disruption. To know the exact role of obstruction in the kidney malformation is very important clinically, because, as mentioned earlier, it is now possible to detect and potentially relieve obstruction in utero. The critical role of AT$_2$R in stimulating the process of ureteric bud branching in kidney development has been highlighted.[300] Along this line, polymorphisms in the AT$_2$R gene have been shown to be associated with UPJ obstruction.[301]

If urinary obstruction is not the cause of subsequent renal impairment, then some may question whether it is worthwhile to relieve the obstruction in utero. However, in experimental models, obstruction in utero can cause pulmonary hyperplasia and renal impairment directly or indirectly, leading to significant morbidity and mortality.[296,297,302] In addition, shunting of urinary outflow from obstructed kidneys in animals before the end of nephrogenesis may allow reversal of the arrest of glomerulogenesis seen in this setting,[303] which favors early intervention.[302-305] The changes in renal gene expression and protein production afford many potential biomarkers of disease progression and targets for therapeutic manipulation.[306]

TREATMENT OF URINARY TRACT OBSTRUCTION AND RECOVERY OF RENAL FUNCTION

Once the presence of obstruction is established, intervention is usually strongly indicated to relieve it. The type of intervention depends on the location of the obstruction, its degree, and its cause, as well as the presence or absence of concomitant diseases and complications, and the general condition of the patient.[307] The initial emphasis focuses on prompt relief of the obstruction, followed by the definitive treatment of its cause. Obstruction below the bladder (e.g., benign prostatic hyperplasia or urethral stricture) is easily relieved with placement of a urethral catheter. If the urethra is impassable, suprapubic cystostomy may be needed. For obstruction above the bladder, insertion of a nephrostomy tube or ureteral stent may be indicated. The urgency of the intervention depends on the degree of renal function, the presence or absence of infection, and the overall risk of the procedure.[296] The presence of infection in an obstructed urinary tract, or urosepsis, represents a urologic emergency that requires immediate relief of the obstruction, in addition to antibiotic treatment. Acute kidney injury, associated with bilateral ureteral obstruction or with the obstruction of single functioning kidney, also calls for emergent intervention.

Calculi, the most common form of acute unilateral urinary obstruction, can usually be managed conservatively with analgesics for control of pain and intravenous fluids to increase urine flow. Ninety percent of stones smaller than 5 mm pass spontaneously, but as stones get larger, spontaneous stone passage becomes progressively less probable. Active efforts to fragment or remove the stone are indicated for persistent obstruction, uncontrollable pain, or urinary tract infection. Current possibilities for treatment include extracorporeal shock wave lithotripsy (which may require ureteral stent placement if the patient is symptomatic),[308] ureteroscopy with stone fragmentation (usually with laser lithotripsy), and, in rare cases, open excision of the stone.[166,167,309] In general, a combination of lithotripsy and endourologic procedures will succeed in removing the stone. In the past, complex stones high up in the ureter or in the renal pelvis have been difficult to remove without open surgery. However, improved methods of lithotripsy, including the use of laser lithotripsy through the ureteroscope, have made more stones amenable to fragmentation, whereas miniaturization of flexible ureteroscopes has made the entire upper urinary tract accessible in nearly all patients, except those with severe anatomic abnormalities.[166,167] Once the stone has been removed, of course, appropriate medical therapy is needed to prevent recurrence.[167]

Intramural or extrinsic ureteral obstruction may be relieved by placement of a ureteral stent through the cystoscope.[308] If this cannot be accomplished or is ineffective (especially in cases of extrinsic ureteral compression by tumor), then nephrostomy tubes will need to be inserted to effect prompt relief of the obstruction.[308]

For infravesical obstruction due to benign prostatic hyperplasia, surgery can be safely delayed or completely avoided in patients with minimal symptoms, lack of infection, and an anatomically normal upper urinary tract.[310] If needed, transurethral resection of the prostate, laser ablation, or other techniques can be used for definitive treatment. Internal urethrotomy with direct visualization may be effective in the treatment of urethral strictures, because dilation usually has only a temporary effect. Suprapubic cystostomy may be necessary in patients with impassable urethral strictures, followed by open urethroplasty to restore urinary tract continuity, when possible.

Patients with neurogenic bladder require a variety of approaches, including frequent voiding, often by external compression or Credé's method; medications to stimulate bladder activity or relax the urethral sphincter; and intermittent catheterization using meticulous technique to avoid infection.[44,311] Long-term indwelling bladder catheters should be avoided because they increase the risk for infection and renal damage. If more conservative measures such as frequent voiding or intermittent catheterization are not effective, ileovesicostomy or other forms of urinary diversion should be considered. Electrical stimulation has also been attempted with varying success.[312]

In many forms of obstruction, initial stabilization of the patient's condition is followed by a decision as to whether to continue observation or to move on to definitive surgery or nephrectomy. The actual course chosen depends on the likelihood that renal function will improve with the relief of obstruction. Factors that help decide whether to operate and what form of surgical intervention to use include the age and general condition of the patient, the appearance and function of the obstructed kidney and the contralateral one, the cause of the obstruction, and the absence or presence of infection.[313] As noted earlier, the extent of recovery of renal function depends on the extent and duration of the obstruction.

Robotic surgery has evolved from simple extirpative surgery to complex reconstructions, including hydronephrosis, which is feasible and safe.[314,315] A detailed discussion of the indications and surgical techniques for intervention to treat urinary tract obstruction is beyond the scope of this chapter and may be found in other sources.[307,316]

ESTIMATING RENAL DAMAGE AND POTENTIAL FOR RECOVERY

As noted earlier, when deciding whether to bypass or reconstruct drainage of an obstructed kidney rather than excise it, the potential for meaningful recovery of function in the affected kidney represents a critical issue. In many cases, obstruction may be partial, so that it is difficult on the basis of the history alone to predict the outcome. In addition, imaging studies that reveal both anatomy and function of the obstructed kidney predict the extent of functional recovery poorly (see earlier), because the extent of anatomic distortion during obstruction correlates poorly with the extent of recovery once the obstruction is relieved.[317] Isotopic renography with a variety of isotopes can be used to examine renal function, as outlined earlier. This approach is a far more reliable indicator of potential renal function when applied well after temporary drainage of the obstructed kidney (e.g., by nephrostomy tubes) has been achieved than if it is performed while the obstruction is still present.[317] Imaging of the anatomy will provide information on the size and volume of the kidney but does not demonstrate reliable information on kidney function. All of these considerations figure into the clinical judgment as to whether attempts should be made to salvage the kidney. However, there are presently no methods available to predict reliably the functional potential recovery of an obstructed kidney.

In cases of prenatal urinary tract obstruction, clinical decision making is complex because the risks of not intervening can be very high, as can the risks of prenatal surgery. Because fetal intervention can be associated with frequent complications and a high rate of fetal wastage, patients for the intervention should be carefully chosen. Fetal renal biopsy, which demonstrated a 50% to 60% success rate, correlates well with outcome and has few maternal complications.[10,12,13,296,304] It may be used as one of the methods to determine treatment strategy. Studies demonstrate that antenatal intervention may help fetuses with the most severe forms of obstructive uropathy, otherwise usually associated with a fatal neonatal course.[10,12,13,302]

RECOVERY OF RENAL FUNCTION AFTER PROLONGED OBSTRUCTION

In patients the potential for renal recovery depends primarily on the extent and duration of the obstruction. However, other factors, such as the presence of other illnesses and the presence or absence of urinary tract infection, play an important role as well. In dogs subjected to 40 days of ureteral ligation, release of the obstruction led to no recovery of renal function. However, recovery of renal function in humans has been documented following release of obstruction of 69 days or longer.[318,319] Because it is difficult to predict whether renal function will recover when temporary relief of obstruction has been achieved, it makes sense to measure function repeatedly with isotopic renography over time, before deciding on a definitive surgical course. Chronic bilateral obstruction, as seen in benign prostatic hyperplasia, can cause chronic kidney disease, especially when the obstruction is of prolonged duration and when it is accompanied by urinary tract infections.[319,320] Progressive loss of renal function can be slowed or halted by relieving the obstruction and treating the infection.

When obstruction has been relieved and there is poor return of renal function, interstitial fibrosis and inflammation may have supervened. To ensure that there is no other process hampering recovery of renal function, renal biopsy may be indicated. As noted earlier, studies in experimental animals have implicated a variety of factors in chronic kidney disease due to prolonged obstruction, including excessive production of renal vasoconstrictors such as renin and angiotensin, growth factors that may enhance fibrosis. Based on these findings, inhibitors such as captopril,[308] angiotensin receptor antagonists,[298] NO supplementation,[292] α-MSH,[294] and EPO[295] have been shown experimentally to ameliorate to some degree the long-term damage of kidney functions observed following prolonged obstruction.

POSTOBSTRUCTIVE DIURESIS

Release of obstruction can lead to marked natriuresis and diuresis with the wasting of potassium, phosphate, and divalent cations. It is notable that clinically significant postobstructive diuresis usually occurs only in the setting of prior bilateral obstruction, or unilateral obstruction of a solitary functioning kidney. The mechanisms involved have been described in detail earlier and involve the combination of intrinsic damage to tubular salt, solute, and water reabsorption, as well as the effects of volume expansion, solute (e.g., urea) accumulation, and attendant increases in natriuretic substances such as ANP. When the obstruction is unilateral and there is a functioning contralateral kidney, the volume expansion, solute accumulation, and increases in natriuretic substances do not occur, and the contralateral kidney may retain salt and water, resulting in some compensation for the natriuresis and diuresis occurring in the postobstructive kidney. Management of the patient with postobstructive diuresis focuses on avoiding severe volume depletion due to salt wasting, and other electrolyte imbalances, such as hypokalemia, hyponatremia, hypernatremia, and hypomagnesemia.

Postobstructive diuresis is usually self-limited. It usually lasts for several days to a week but may, in rare cases, persist for months. Acute massive polyuria or prolonged postobstructive diuresis may deplete the patient of Na^+, K^+, Cl^-, HCO_3^-, and water, as well as divalent cations and phosphate. Volume or free water replacement is appropriate only when the salt and water losses result in volume depletion or a disturbance of osmolality. In many cases, excessive volume or fluid replacement prolongs the diuresis and natriuresis. Because the initial urine is isosthenuric, with an initial Na^+ of approximately 80 mEq/L, an appropriate starting fluid for replacement may be 0.45% saline, given at a rate somewhat slower than that of the urine output. During this period, meticulous monitoring of vital signs, volume status, urine output, and serum and urine chemistry values and osmolality is imperative. This will determine the need for ongoing replacement of salt, free water, and other electrolytes. With massive diuresis, these measurements will need to be repeated frequently, up to four times daily, with frequent adjustment of replacement fluids, as needed. With relief of uncomplicated obstruction, the kidney function usually returns to normal with adequate hormonal responses. However, some cases, especially in infants with bilateral obstructive nephropathy, have been described in which the distal tubule remains refractory to aldosterone (pseudohypoaldosteronism) and the patient develops paradoxical hyperkalemia despite a returning kidney function and a falling plasma creatinine level.[321] In such cases during postobstructive diuresis, plasma potassium levels must be monitored carefully.

Complete reference list available at ExpertConsult.com.

KEY REFERENCES

2. Yarger WE: Urinary tract obstruction. In Brenner BM, Rector FC, editors: *The kidney*, Philadelphia, 1991, Saunders, pp 1768–1808.
4. Klahr S: Obstructive nephropathy. *Intern Med* 39:355–361, 2000.
9. Chevalier RL, Klahr S: Therapeutic approaches in obstructive uropathy. *Semin Nephrol* 18:652–658, 1998.
23. Ulman I, Jayanthi VR, Koff SA: The long-term followup of newborns with severe unilateral hydronephrosis initially treated nonoperatively. *J Urol* 164:1101–1105, 2000.
36. Stamatelou KK, Francis ME, Jones CA, et al: Time trends in reported prevalence of kidney stones in the United States: 1976-1994. *Kidney Int* 63:1817–1823, 2003.
43. de Groat WC, Yoshimura N: Pharmacology of the lower urinary tract. *Annu Rev Pharmacol Toxicol* 41:691–721, 2001.
44. Wein AJ: Lower urinary tract dysfunction in neurologic injury and disease. In Wein AJ, Kavoussi LR, Novick AC, et al, editors: *Campbell-Walsh urology*, ed 9, Philadelphia, 2007, Saunders Elsevier, pp 2011–2045.
62. Deprest J, Marchal G, Brosens I: Obstructive uropathy secondary to endometriosis. *N Engl J Med* 337:1174–1175, 1997.
89. Chung SY, Stein RJ, Landsittel D, et al: 15-Year experience with the management of extrinsic ureteral obstruction with indwelling ureteral stents. *J Urol* 172:592–595, 2004.
102. Roth JA, Diamond DA: Prenatal hydronephrosis. *Curr Opin Pediatr* 13:138–141, 2001.
108. Akcay A, Altun B, Usalan C, et al: Cyclical acute renal failure due to bilateral ureteral endometriosis. *Clin Nephrol* 52:179–182, 1999.
112. Decramer S, Wittke S, Mischak H, et al: Predicting the clinical outcome of congenital unilateral ureteropelvic junction obstruction in newborn by urinary proteome analysis. *Nat Med* 12:398–400, 2006.
116. Shokeir AA: The diagnosis of upper urinary tract obstruction. *BJU Int* 83:893–900, 1999.
129. Grenier N, Gennisson JL, Cornelis F, et al: Renal ultrasound elastography. *Diagn Interv Imaging* 94:545–550, 2013.
138. Feldman DM, DeCambre M, Kong E, et al: Evaluation and follow-up of fetal hydronephrosis. *J Ultrasound Med* 20:1065–1069, 2001.
140. Sheth S, Fishman EK: Multi-detector row CT of the kidneys and urinary tract: techniques and applications in the diagnosis of benign diseases. *Radiographics* 24:e20, 2004.
141. Grenier N, Hauger O, Cimpean A, et al: Update of renal imaging. *Semin Nucl Med* 36:3–15, 2006.
155. Taylor A, Manatunga A, Garcia EV: Decision support systems in diuresis renography. *Semin Nucl Med* 38:67–81, 2008.
157. Grenier N, Basseau F, Ries M, et al: Functional MRI of the kidney. *Abdom Imaging* 28:164–175, 2003.
160. Prasad PV: Functional MRI of the kidney: tools for translational studies of pathophysiology of renal disease. *Am J Physiol Renal Physiol* 290:F958–F974, 2006.
173. Wright FS, Briggs JP: Feedback control of glomerular blood flow, pressure, and filtration rate. *Physiol Rev* 59:958–1006, 1979.
176. Harris RH, Gill JM: Changes in glomerular filtration rate during complete ureteral obstruction in rats. *Kidney Int* 19:603–608, 1981.
177. Moody TE, Vaughan ED, Jr, Gillenwater JY: Relationship between renal blood flow and ureteral pressure during 18 hours of total unilateral ureteral occlusion. *Invest Urol* 13:246–251, 1975.
178. Harris RH, Yarger WE: Renal function after release of unilateral ureteral obstruction in rats. *Am J Physiol* 227:806–815, 1974.
182. Yarger WE, Aynedjian HS, Bank N: A micropuncture study of postobstructive diuresis in the rat. *J Clin Invest* 51:625–637, 1972.
184. Yarger WE, Schocken DD, Harris RH: Obstructive nephropathy in the rat: possible roles for the renin-angiotensin system, prostaglandins, and thromboxanes in postobstructive renal function. *J Clin Invest* 65:400–412, 1980.
188. Topcu SO, Pedersen M, Norregaard R, et al: Candesartan prevents long-term impairment of renal function in response to

neonatal partial unilateral ureteral obstruction. *Am J Physiol Renal Physiol* 292:F736–F748, 2007.
211. Sonnenberg H, Wilson DR: The role of the medullary collecting duct in postobstructive diuresis. *J Clin Invest* 57:1564–1574, 1976.
214. Hwang SJ, Haas M, Harris HW, Jr, et al: Transport defects of rabbit medullary thick ascending limb cells in obstructive nephropathy. *J Clin Invest* 91:21–28, 1993.
224. Li C, Wang W, Knepper MA, et al: Downregulation of renal aquaporins in response to unilateral ureteral obstruction. *Am J Physiol Renal Physiol* 284:F1066–F1079, 2003.
227. Zeidel ML: Hormonal regulation of inner medullary collecting duct sodium transport. *Am J Physiol* 265:F159–F173, 1993.
231. Lebowitz J, An B, Edinger RS, et al: Effect of altered Na+ entry on expression of apical and basolateral transport proteins in A6 epithelia. *Am J Physiol Renal Physiol* 285:F524–F531, 2003.
233. Norregaard R, Jensen BL, Li C, et al: COX-2 inhibition prevents downregulation of key renal water and sodium transport proteins in response to bilateral ureteral obstruction. *Am J Physiol Renal Physiol* 289:F322–F333, 2005.
240. Frokiaer J, Marples D, Knepper MA, et al: Bilateral ureteral obstruction downregulates expression of vasopressin-sensitive AQP-2 water channel in rat kidney. *Am J Physiol* 270:F657–F668, 1996.
253. Wang G, Li C, Kim SW, et al: Ureter obstruction alters expression of renal acid-base transport proteins in rat kidney. *Am J Physiol Renal Physiol* 295:F497–F506, 2008.
266. Docherty NG, O'Sullivan OE, Healy DA, et al: Evidence that inhibition of tubular cell apoptosis protects against renal damage and development of fibrosis following ureteric obstruction. *Am J Physiol Renal Physiol* 290:F4–F13, 2006.
271. Ma LJ, Yang H, Gaspert A, et al: Transforming growth factor-beta-dependent and -independent pathways of induction of tubulointerstitial fibrosis in beta6(-/-) mice. *Am J Pathol* 163:1261–1273, 2003.
274. Misseri R, Meldrum DR, Dinarello CA, et al: TNF-alpha mediates obstruction-induced renal tubular cell apoptosis and proapoptotic signaling. *Am J Physiol Renal Physiol* 288:F406–F411, 2005.
277. Grande MT, Lopez-Novoa JM: Fibroblast activation and myofibroblast generation in obstructive nephropathy. *Nat Rev Nephrol* 5:319–328, 2009.
279. Broadbelt NV, Stahl PJ, Chen J, et al: Early upregulation of iNOS mRNA expression and increase in NO metabolites in pressurized renal epithelial cells. *Am J Physiol Renal Physiol* 293:F1877–F1888, 2007.
281. Quinlan MR, Docherty NG, Watson RW, et al: Exploring mechanisms involved in renal tubular sensing of mechanical stretch following ureteric obstruction. *Am J Physiol Renal Physiol* 295:F1–F11, 2008.
282. Veerappan A, Reid AC, O'Connor N, et al: Mast cells are required for the development of renal fibrosis in the rodent unilateral ureteral obstruction model. *Am J Physiol Renal Physiol* 302:F192–F204, 2012.
285. Cohn RD, van Erp C, Habashi JP, et al: Angiotensin II type 1 receptor blockade attenuates TGF-beta induced failure of muscle regeneration in multiple myopathic states. *Nat Med* 13:204–210, 2007.
289. Anders HJ, Vielhauer V, Frink M, et al: A chemokine receptor CCR-1 antagonist reduces renal fibrosis after unilateral ureter ligation. *J Clin Invest* 109:251–259, 2002.
291. Zhang JD, Patel MB, Griffiths R, et al: Type 1 angiotensin receptors on macrophages ameliorate IL-1 receptor-mediated kidney fibrosis. *J Clin Invest* 124:2198–2203, 2014.
292. Morrissey JJ, Ishidoya S, McCracken R, et al: Nitric oxide generation ameliorates the tubulointerstitial fibrosis of obstructive nephropathy. *J Am Soc Nephrol* 7:2202–2212, 1996.
295. Park SH, Choi MJ, Song IK, et al: Erythropoietin decreases renal fibrosis in mice with ureteral obstruction: role of inhibiting TGF-beta-induced epithelial-to-mesenchymal transition. *J Am Soc Nephrol* 18:1497–1507, 2007.
297. Chevalier RL: Pathogenesis of renal injury in obstructive uropathy. *Curr Opin Pediatr* 18:153–160, 2006.
303. Edouga D, Hugueny B, Gasser B, et al: Recovery after relief of fetal urinary obstruction: morphological, functional and molecular aspects. *Am J Physiol Renal Physiol* 281:F26–F37, 2001.
306. Chevalier RL: Obstructive nephropathy: towards biomarker discovery and gene therapy. *Nat Clin Pract Nephrol* 2:157–168, 2006.

Diabetic Nephropathy

39

Peter Rossing | Paola Fioretto | Bo Feldt-Rasmussen | Hans-Henrik Parving

CHAPTER OUTLINE

PATHOLOGY OF THE KIDNEY IN DIABETES, 1283
Structural-Functional Relationships in Type 1 Diabetic Nephropathy, 1288
Microalbuminuria and Renal Structure, 1289
Risk Factors for Nephropathy Intrinsic to the Kidney, 1290
Comparisons of Nephropathy in Types 1 and 2 Diabetes, 1290
Structural-Functional Relationships in Type 2 Diabetic Nephropathy, 1291
Other Renal Disorders in Diabetic Patients, 1291
Reversibility of Diabetic Nephropathy Lesions, 1292
EPIDEMIOLOGY OF MICROALBUMINURIA AND DIABETIC NEPHROPATHY, 1292
Prevalence and Incidence, 1292
Microalbuminuria as a Predictor of Nephropathy, 1294
Prognosis of Microalbuminuria, 1294
Prognosis of Diabetic Nephropathy, 1295
CLINICAL COURSE AND PATHOPHYSIOLOGY, 1296

Diabetic Nephropathy, 1298
Extrarenal Complications In Diabetic Nephropathy, 1300
TREATMENT, 1300
Glycemic Control, 1301
Blood Pressure Control, 1303
Lipid-Lowering Therapy, 1312
Dietary Protein Restriction, 1312
New Treatment Options, 1312
END-STAGE KIDNEY DISEASE IN DIABETIC PATIENTS, 1313
Epidemiology, 1313
Management of the Patient with Advanced Renal Failure, 1314
TRANSPLANTATION, 1318
Kidney Transplantation, 1318
Combined Kidney-Pancreas Transplantation, 1319
Islet Cell Transplantation, 1319
New-Onset Diabetes After Transplantation, 1320
Bladder dysfunction, 1320
Urinary Tract Infection, 1320

Persistent albuminuria (>300 mg/24 hr or 200 µg/min) is the hallmark of diabetic nephropathy that can be diagnosed clinically if the following additional criteria are fulfilled—presence of diabetic retinopathy and absence of clinical or laboratory evidence of other kidney or renal tract disease. This clinical definition of diabetic nephropathy is valid in types 1 and 2 diabetes.[1]

Since the 1990s, several longitudinal studies have shown that raised urinary albumin excretion (based on a single measurement) that is below the level of clinical albuminuria (by reagent strip), so-called microalbuminuria, strongly predicts the development of diabetic nephropathy in types 1 and 2 diabetes.[2-4] Microalbuminuria is defined as urinary albumin excretion of more than 30 mg/24 hr (20 µg/min), and 300 mg/24 hr (200 µg/min) or less, irrespective of how the urine is collected.

Nephropathy is a major cause of illness and death in diabetes. Indeed, the excess mortality of diabetes occurs mainly in proteinuric diabetic patients and results not only from end-stage kidney disease (ESKD), but also from cardiovascular disease, with the latter being particularly common in type 2 diabetic patients.[5-7] Diabetic nephropathy is the single most common cause of ESKD in Europe, Japan, and the United States, with diabetic patients accounting for 25% to 45% of all patients enrolled in ESKD programs.

PATHOLOGY OF THE KIDNEY IN DIABETES

This section outlines the renal pathology in type 1 diabetes, followed by a comparison of the similarities and differences in renal pathology in type 2 diabetes. When its features are taken together, diabetic nephropathology in type 1 diabetes is unique to this disease (Table 39.1).[8-10] Thickening of the glomerular basement membrane (GBM) is the first change

Table 39.1 Pathology of Diabetic Nephropathy in Patients with Type 1 Diabetes and Proteinuria

Always Present	Often or Usually Present	Sometimes Present
Glomerular basement membrane thickening*	Kimmelstiel-Wilson nodules (nodular glomerulosclerosis)*; global glomerular sclerosis; focal-segmental glomerulosclerosis, atubular glomeruli	Hyaline "exudative" lesions (subendothelial)†
Tubular basement membrane thickening*		Capsular drops†
Mesangial expansion with predominance of increased mesangial matrix (diffuse glomerulosclerosis)*		Atherosclerosis
	Foci of tubular atrophy	Glomerular microaneurysms
Interstitial expansion with predominance of increased extracellular matrix material	Afferent and efferent arteriolar hyalinosis*	
Increased glomerular basement membrane, tubular basement membrane, and Bowman's capsule staining for albumin and IgG*		

*In combination, diagnostic of diabetic nephropathy.
†Highly characteristic of diabetic nephropathy.

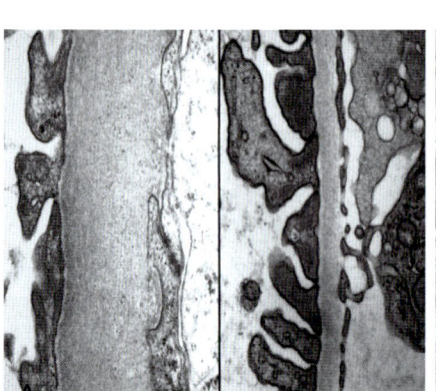

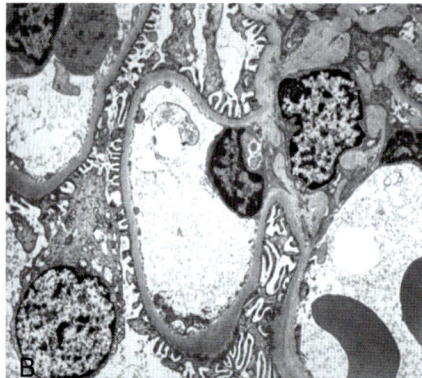

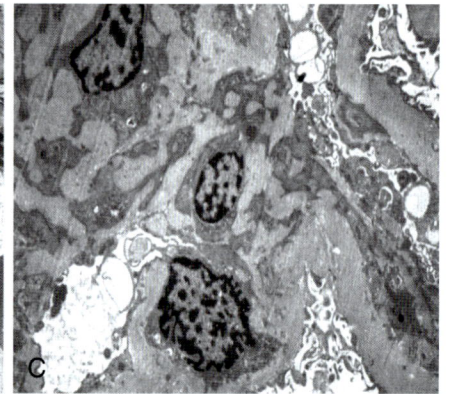

Figure 39.1 Electron microscopic photomicrographs. **A,** Normal glomerular basement membrane (GBM; **left**) compared to thickened GBM from a proteinuric type 1 diabetic patient (**right**). **B,** Normal glomerular capillary loops and mesangial zone. **C,** Thickened glomerular basement membrane (GBM), mesangial expansion (predominantly with mesangial matrix), and capillary luminal narrowing in a proteinuric type 1 diabetic patient.

that can be quantitated (Figure 39.1A and C).[11] Thickening of tubular basement membranes (TBMs) parallels this GBM thickening (Figure 39.2).[12,13] Afferent and efferent glomerular arteriolar hyalinosis can also be detected within 3 to 5 years after the onset of diabetes or following transplantation of a normal kidney into the diabetic patient.[14] This can lead to the total replacement of the smooth muscle cells of these small vessels by waxy, homogeneous, translucent-appearing material that is positive for the periodic acid–Schiff (PAS)–positive material (Figure 39.3A and B) and consists of immunoglobulins, complement, fibrinogen, albumin, and other plasma proteins.[15,16] Arteriolar hyalinosis, glomerular capillary subendothelial hyaline (hyaline caps), and capsular drops along the parietal surface of Bowman's capsule (see Figure 39.3C) represent the so-called exudative lesions of diabetic nephropathy. Progressive increases in the fraction of glomerular afferent and efferent arterioles occupied by the extracellular matrix (ECM) and medial thickness have also been reported in young type 1 diabetes mellitus (T1DM) patients.[17]

Increases in the fraction of the volume of the glomerulus occupied by the mesangium or mesangial fractional volume

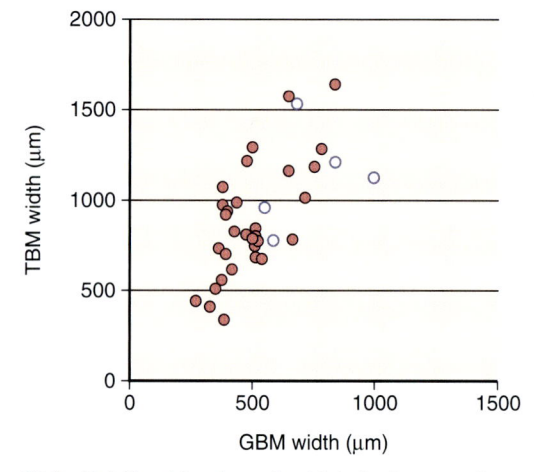

Figure 39.2 Relationship of proximal tubular basement membrane (TBM) width and glomerular basement membrane (GBM) width in 35 type 1 diabetic patients, 25 of whom were normoalbuminuric. The hypertensive patients are represented by the open circles (correlation coefficient $r = 0.64$; $P < 0.001$). (From Brito PL, Fioretto P, Drummond K, et al: Proximal tubular basement membrane width in insulin-dependent diabetes mellitus. *Kidney Int* 53:754-761, 1998.)

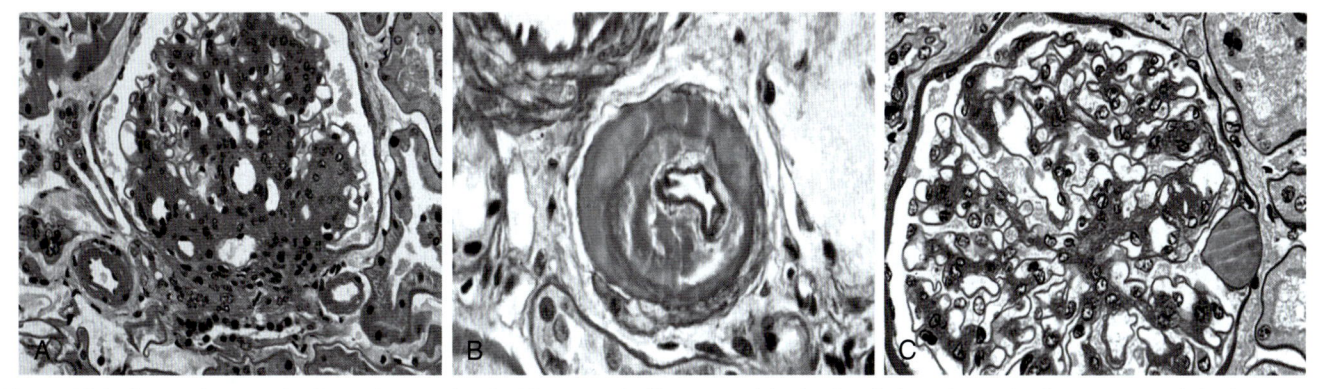

Figure 39.3 Light microscopic photomicrographs. **A,** Afferent and efferent arteriolar hyalinosis in a glomerulus from a type 1 diabetic patient. The glomerulus shows diffuse and nodular mesangial expansion (periodic acid–Schiff stain, ×120). **B,** Glomerular arteriole showing almost complete replacement of the smooth muscle wall by hyaline material and lumeral narrowing (periodic acid–Schiff stain, ×300). **C,** Glomerulus with minimal mesangial expansion and a capsular drop at 3 o'clock (periodic acid–Schiff stain, ×120).

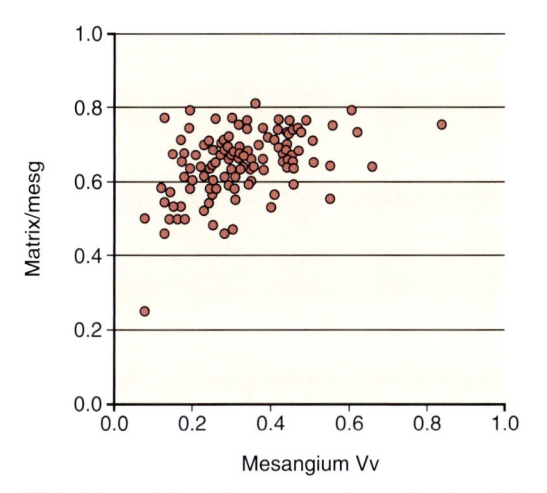

Figure 39.4 Mesangial matrix expressed as a fraction of the total mesangial (Matrix/mesg) plotted against the mesangial fractional volume (Mesangium Vv) in long-standing type 1 diabetic patients. The normal value for Matrix/mesg is approximately 0.5. Note that most diabetic patients have elevated values for Matrix/mesg whether or not there is an increase in Mesangium Vv (i.e., values above 0.24). (From Steffes MW, Bilous RW, Sutherland DER, Mauer SM: Cell and matrix components of the glomerular mesangium in type I diabetes. *Diabetes* 41:679-684, 1992.)

(Vv[Mes/glom]) can be documented as early as 4 to 5 years after the onset of type 1 diabetes.[11] In many cases, this may take 15 or more years to manifest, possibly because the relationship of mesangial expansion to diabetes duration is nonlinear, with slow development earlier and more rapid development later in the disease.[18] This mesangial expansion is due, in major part, to absolute and relative increases in mesangial matrix, with lesser contributions from fractional increases in mesangial cell volume (Figure 39-4; see Figure 39.1C).[19] The first change in the volume fraction of cortex that is interstitium, or Vv(Int/cortex), is a decrease in this parameter, perhaps due to the expansion of the tubular compartment of the cortex. In contrast to the mesangium expansion, initial interstitial expansion is primarily due to an increase in the cellular component of this renal compartment.[20,21] An increase in interstitial ECM fibrillar collagen is a relatively late finding in this disease, measurable only in patients with an already established decline in the glomerular filtration rate (GFR).[21]

Abnormalities of the glomerulotubular junction with focal adhesions, obstruction of the proximal tubular takeoff from the glomerulus, and detachment of the tubule from the glomerulus (atubular glomerulus) (Figure 39.5) are also late disease manifestations, largely restricted to patients with overt proteinuria (Figure 39.6).[21]

These various lesions of diabetic nephropathy can progress at varying rates in type 1 diabetic patients and, as discussed later, this is even more the case in type 2 diabetes.[22,23] For example, GBM width and Vv(Mes/glom) are not highly correlated with one another; some patients have relatively marked GBM thickening without much mesangial expansion and others have the converse (Figure 39.7).[22] Marked renal extracellular basement membrane accumulation resulting in extreme mesangial expansion and GBM thickening are present in the vast majority of type 1 diabetic patients who develop overt diabetic nephropathy manifesting as proteinuria, hypertension, and declining GRF (see later).[22,23] Ultimately, focal and global glomerulosclerosis, tubular atrophy, interstitial expansion and fibrosis, and glomerulotubular junction abnormalities are evident when rates of functional loss are marked.[21]

The diffuse and generalized process of mesangial expansion has been termed *diffuse diabetic glomerulosclerosis* (Figure 39.8). Nodular glomerulosclerosis (Kimmelstiel-Wilson nodular lesions) represents areas of marked mesangial expansion appearing as large, round, fibrillar mesangial zones, with palisading of mesangial nuclei around the periphery of the nodule, often with extreme compression of the adjacent glomerular capillaries (Figure 39.9C). This is typically a focal and segmental change likely resulting from glomerular capillary wall detachment from a mesangial anchoring point with consequent microaneurysm formation (see Figure 39.9A) and subsequent filling of the increased capillary space with mesangial matrix material (see Figure 39.9B).[24] Approximately 50% of type 1 diabetic patients with proteinuria have at least a few glomeruli with nodular lesions. Typically, this occurs in patients with moderate to severe diffuse diabetic glomerulosclerosis. However, there are some patients who have occasional nodular lesions and little diffuse mesangial expansion, which suggests that

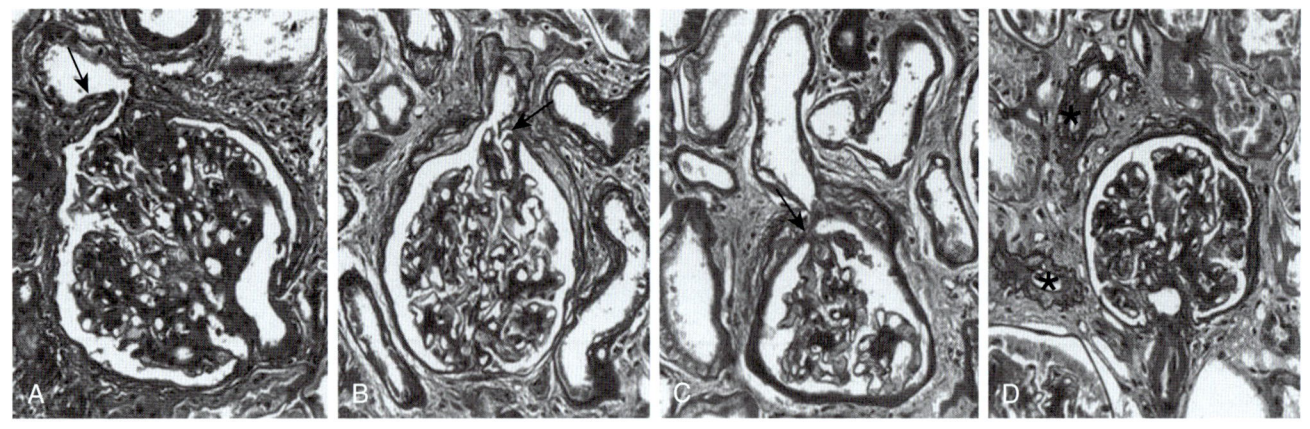

Figure 39.5 Glomerulotubular junction abnormalities. **A,** Glomerulus attached to a short atrophic tubule (SAT). The *arrow* points to the atrophic segment. **B,** Glomerulus attached to a long atrophic tubule (LAT). The *arrow* points to the atrophic segment and tuft adhesion. **C,** Glomerulus attached to an atrophic tubule with no observable opening (ATNO) and a tip lesion (*arrow*). **D,** Atubular glomerulus (AG). *Tubular remnants that possibly belonged to the AG. (From Najafian B, Crosson JT, Kim Y, Mauer M: Glomerulotubular junction abnormalities are associated with proteinuria in type 1 diabetes. *J Am Soc Nephrol* 17:S53-S60, 2006.)

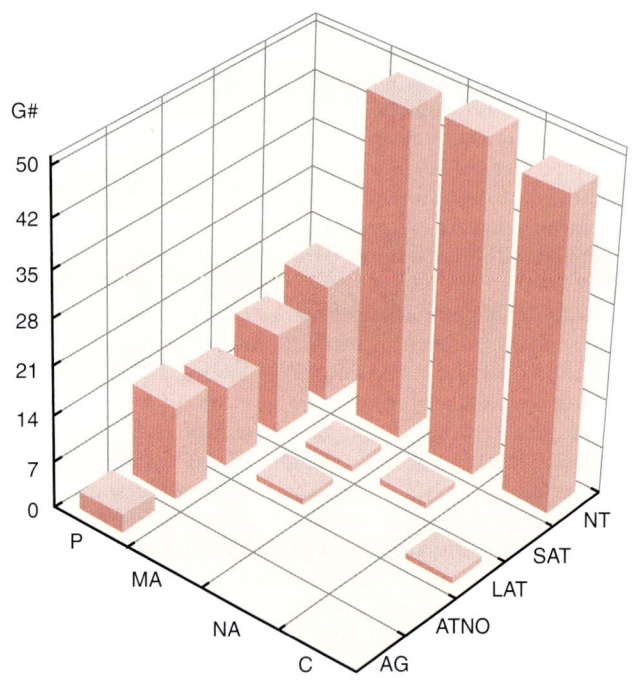

Figure 39.6 Frequency of glomerulotubular junction abnormalities in normoalbuminuric (NA), microalbuminuric (MA), and proteinuric (P) patients and control subjects (C). ATNO, Atrophic tubule with no observable opening; G#, number of glomeruli; LAT, long atrophic tubule; NT, normal tubules; SAT, short atrophic tubule . (From Najafian B, Crosson JT, Kim Y, Mauer M: Glomerulotubular junction abnormalities are associated with proteinuria in type 1 diabetes. *J Am Soc Nephrol* 17:S53-S60, 2006.)

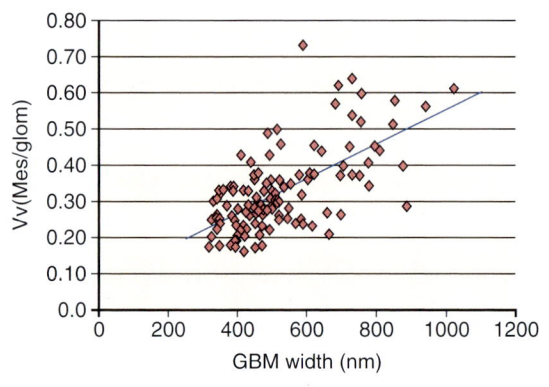

Figure 39.7 Relationship between glomerular basement membrane (GBM) width and mesangial fractional volume (Vv[Mes/glom]) in 125 long-standing type 1 diabetic patients, 88 of whom were normoalbuminuric, 17 microalbuminuric, and 18 proteinuric ($r = 0.58$; $P < 0.001$).

these two forms of diabetic mesangial change may, at least in part, have a different pathogenesis.

As mentioned earlier, most (about two thirds) of the mesangial expansion in diabetes is due to an increased mesangial matrix and one third is due to mesangial cell expansion. Thus, the matrix fraction of mesangium, as opposed to the cellular fraction, is increased in diabetic patients, often even in those in whom Vv(Mes/glom) is still within the normal range (see Figure 39.4).[18]

Clinical diabetic nephropathy is primarily the consequence of ECM accumulation, which presumably results from an imbalance in renal ECM dynamics. In this setting, which occurs over many years, the rate of ECM production exceeds the rate of removal. The accumulation of mesangial, GBM, TBM, and ECM materials represents the accumulation of the intrinsic ECM components of these structures, including types IV and VI collagen, laminin, fibronectin and, perhaps, additional ECM components not yet identified. However, not all renal ECM components change in parallel. Thus, α_3 and α_4 chains of type IV collagen increase in density in the GBM of patients with diabetic renal lesions, whereas α_1 and α_2 type IV collagen chains and type IV collagen decrease in density in the mesangium and subendothelial space.[25,26] However, the absolute amount of these ECM components per glomerulus is increased due to the marked absolute increase in mesangial matrix material. The glomerular expression of so-called scar collagen is very late in the evolution of diabetic glomerulopathy, occurring primarily in association with global glomerulosclerosis.

As the disease progresses toward renal insufficiency, more glomeruli become totally sclerosed or have capillary closure

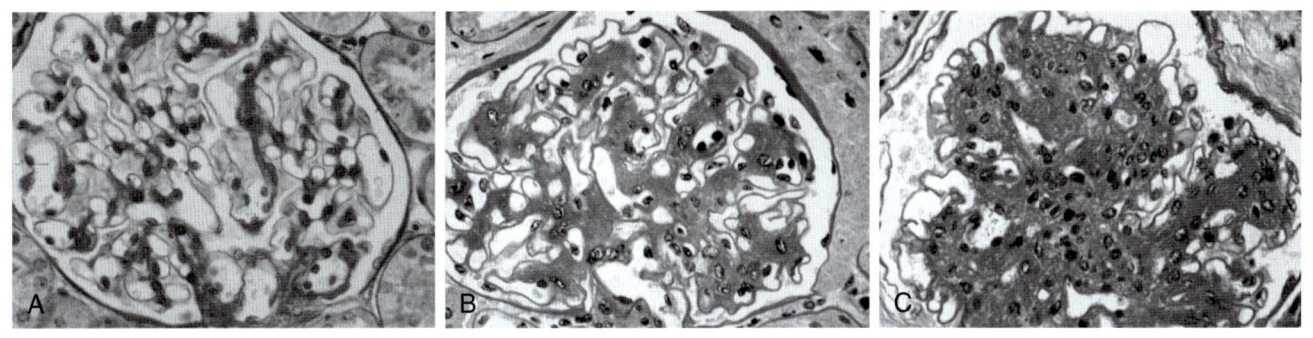

Figure 39.8 Light microscopic photomicrographs (PAS stain). **A,** Normal glomerulus. **B,** Glomerulus from a normoalbuminuric type 1 diabetic patient with glomerular basement membrane (GBM) thickening and moderate mesangial expansion. **C,** Glomerulus from a type 1 diabetic patient with overt diabetic nephropathy and severe diffuse mesangial expansion (periodic acid–Schiff stain, ×120).

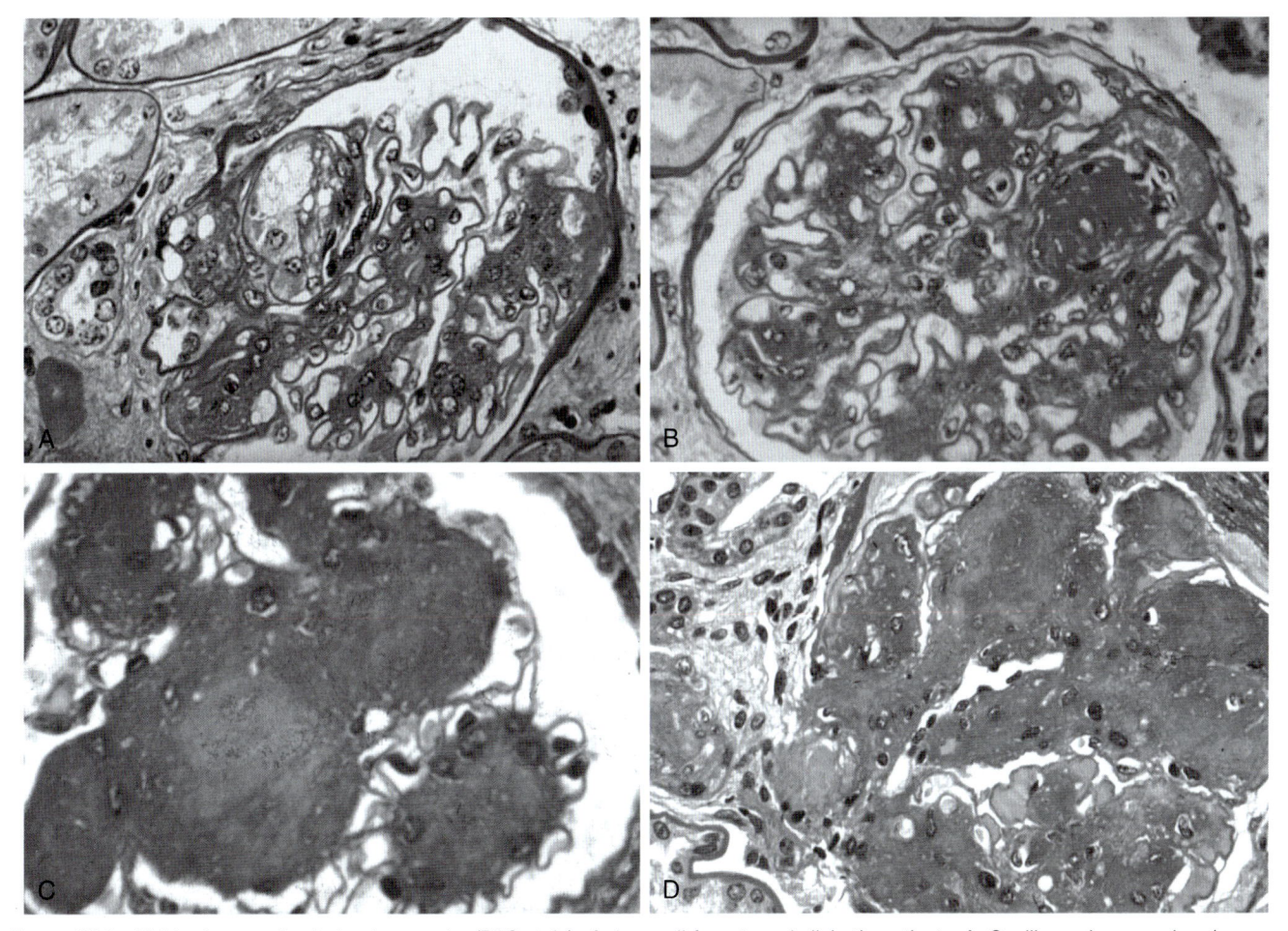

Figure 39.9 Light microscopic photomicrographs (PAS stain) of glomeruli from type 1 diabetic patients. A, Capillary microaneurism (mesangiolysis) at 11 o'clock. **B,** Nodule formation within a capillary microaneurism. **C,** Nodular glomerulosclerosis (Kimmelstiel-Wilson nodules). **D,** End-stage diabetic glomerular changes with almost complete capillary closure (periodic acid–Schiff stain, ×180).

within incompletely scarred glomeruli due to massive mesangial expansion (see Figure 39.7D). However, an increased fraction of glomeruli may become globally sclerosed in diabetic patients when other glomeruli do not show marked mesangial changes.[27] Hørlyck and colleagues[28] found that the distribution pattern of scarred glomeruli in type 1 diabetic patients was more often in the plane vertical to the capsule of the kidney than chance would dictate. This finding suggests that glomerular scarring results, at least in part, from obstruction of medium-sized renal arteries.[28] In fact, patients with increased numbers of globally sclerosed glomeruli have more severe arteriolar hyalinosis lesions.[27] In general, global glomerular sclerosis and mesangial expansion are correlated in type 1 diabetic patients, but this may be less often the case in type 2 diabetes (see later).[27]

Podocyte number and/or numeric density (number, volume) are reportedly reduced in types 1 and 2 diabetes.[29-32] These changes may be associated with albuminuria and disease progression. Podocyte detachment from GBM may be an early phenomenon in type 1 diabetes, appears to worsen with increasing albuminuria, and could be responsible for podocyte loss.[33] However, the experimental techniques used currently to quantify podocyte number are problematic and unstandardized, and more work is needed.

When research renal biopsies were performed in patients with diabetes of at least 10 years' duration who were selected using no other criteria, significant but only imprecise relationships were found between renal pathology and duration of diabetes.[22] This is consistent with the marked variability in glycemia and susceptibility to diabetic nephropathy, with some patients in renal failure after 15 years of diabetes and others without renal complications, despite having had type 1 diabetes for many decades.

Renal extracellular membranes, including GBM, TBM, and Bowman's capsule, demonstrate increased intensity of immunofluorescent linear staining for plasma proteins, especially albumin and immunoglobulin G (IgG).[15] Because these changes are seen in all diabetic patients and appear unrelated to disease risk, their only clinical importance is that they should not be confused with other entities, such as anti-GBM antibody disorders.

Immunohistochemical studies have also revealed decreased nephrin expression in association with decreased nephrin messenger RNA expression in podocytes of albuminuric diabetic patients, which opens up interesting research avenues for study of these associations and diabetic nephropathy pathogenesis.[32,34-36]

STRUCTURAL-FUNCTIONAL RELATIONSHIPS IN TYPE 1 DIABETIC NEPHROPATHY

Mesangial expansion is the major lesion leading to renal dysfunction in type 1 diabetes patients.[22] Mesangial expansion out of proportion to increases in glomerular volume—that is, increased Vv(Mes/glom)—is strongly correlated with decreased peripheral GBM filtration surface density, Sv(PGBM/glom) (Figure 39.10), and filtration surface per glomerulus (S/G) is strongly correlated with GFR in type 1 diabetes.[22,37] Vv(Mes/glom) is also closely related to the urinary albumin excretion rate (AER; Figure 39.11A) and is a strong concomitant of hypertension.[22,23] Thus, all the clinical manifestations of diabetic nephropathy are associated with mesangial expansion and consequent restriction of the filtration surface. Although GBM width is also directly correlated with blood pressure and AER (Figure 39.12A) and inversely correlated with GFR, the relationships are somewhat weaker than those seen with Vv(Mes/glom).[22,23] However, Vv(Mes/glom) and GBM width, together, explain almost 60% of AER variability in type 1 diabetic patients over the full range of proteinuria, with AERs ranging from normoalbuminuria to proteinuria.[23]

As noted earlier, decreased glomerular podocyte number and detachment have been related to glomerular permeability alterations in diabetes. In addition, changes in podocyte shape, including increases in foot process width and decreases in filtration slit length density, correlate with AER increases in types 1 and 2 diabetic patients.[30,32,38,39]

Heparan sulfate proteoglycans, presumed to represent an epithelial cell product important in glomerular charge-based permselectivity, are decreased in density in the lamina rara externa in proportion to the increase in AER in type 1 diabetic patients.[40] Whether the addition of podocyte cell structural variables would reduce the residual unexplained variability in AER or GFR in diabetic nephropathy (see later) has not yet been tested. If true, this would support the idea that podocyte alterations contribute to proteinuria and renal insufficiency. Moreover, confirmation that reduced podocyte numbers predict diabetic nephropathy development or progression would add further credence to the importance of this cell in this disease.[41]

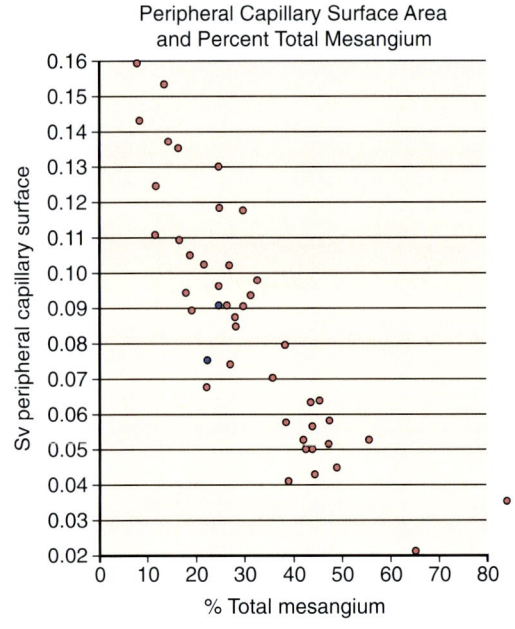

Figure 39.10 Relationship of mesangial fractional volume (% total mesangium) and filtration surface density (Sv peripheral capillary surface) in type 1 diabetic patients.

The total peripheral capillary filtration surface is directly correlated with GFR across the spectrum, from hyperfiltration to renal insufficiency.[38,42] Nonetheless, as already noted, diabetic glomerulopathy structural parameters, examined in linear regression models, explain only a minority of GFR variability in type 1 diabetic patients.[23] The percentage of global sclerosis and interstitial expansion are also linearly correlated with the clinical manifestations of diabetic nephropathy and are, to some extent, independent predictors of renal dysfunction and hypertension in type 1 diabetes.[9,27] Some have argued that renal dysfunction in diabetes is primarily consequent to interstitial rather than glomerular lesions.[43,44] However, the conclusion that the interstitium is more closely related to renal dysfunction in diabetes than glomerular changes was derived from studies in which most, if not all, patients already had elevated serum creatinine values and in which the interstitium was carefully measured but the glomerular structure was only subjectively estimated.[43,44] Throughout most of the natural history of diabetic nephropathy, glomerular parameters are more important determinants of renal dysfunction, whereas interstitial changes may become stronger determinants of the rate of progression from established renal insufficiency to terminal uremia.[45] Furthermore, as mentioned earlier, in the first decade of diabetes, Vv(Int/cortex) is decreased,

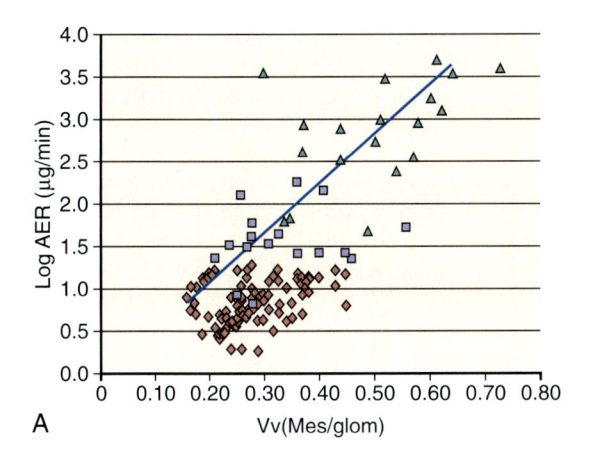

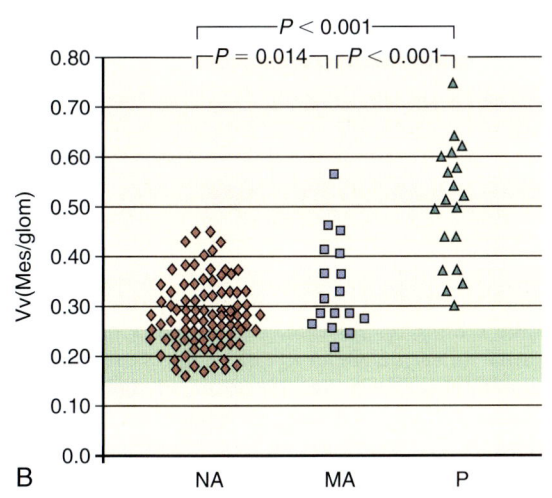

Figure 39.11 A, Correlation between mesangial fractional volume (Vv[Mes/glom]) and albumin excretion rate (AER) in 124 patients with type 1 diabetes. **B,** Vv(Mes/glom) in 88 normoalbuminuric (NA), 17 microalbuminuric (MA), and 19 proteinuric (P) patients with type 1 diabetes. The hatched area represents the mean ± 2 SD in a group of 76 age-matched normal control subjects. All groups are different from control subjects. ♦, Normoalbuminuric patients; □, microalbuminuric patients; △, proteinuric patients ($r = 0.75$; $P < 0.001$). (From Caramori, ML, Kim Y, Huang C, et al: Cellular basis of diabetic nephropathy: 1. Study design and renal structural-functional relationships in patients with long-standing type 1 diabetes. *Diabetes* 51:506-513, 2002.)

whereas Vv(Mes/glom) and GBM width are already increased. Moreover, early interstitial expansion in type 1 diabetes is mainly due to expansion of the cellular component of this compartment, and increased interstitial fibrillar collagen is seen in patients whose GFR is already reduced.[20] These and other findings suggest that the interstitial and glomerular changes of diabetes have somewhat different pathogenetic mechanisms and that advancing interstitial fibrosis generally follows the glomerular processes in type 1 diabetes.

Through much of the natural history of diabetic nephropathy, lesions develop in complete clinical silence. When microalbuminuria and proteinuria initially manifest, lesions are often far advanced, and a decreased GFR may then progress relatively rapidly toward ESKD. This typical clinical story is best mirrored by nonlinear analyses of structural-functional relationships.[21] When piecewise regression models were used, glomerular structural variables alone (e.g., Vv[Mes/glom], GBM width, and total S/G) explained 95% of the variability in AER, ranging from normoalbuminuria to proteinuria; this leaves little room for improvement in predictive models by adding nonglomerular structural variables to the parameters. These same glomerular structures, however, explained only 78% of GFR variability. With the addition of indices of glomerulotubular junction abnormalities and Vv(Int/cortex), this increased to 92%.[21]

In summary, most of the AER and GFR changes in type 1 diabetes are explained by diabetic glomerulopathy changes. These structural-functional relationships are largely driven by more advanced lesions, however; structural changes are highly variable (from almost none to moderately severe) in patients without functional abnormalities. Predictive tools for the first decade of type 1 diabetes are needed. In a cohort of 94 long-term, normoalbuminuric, type 1 diabetic patients followed for 11 ± 7 years after kidney biopsy was performed, the structural parameters predictive of the subsequent progression to proteinuria and/or GFR loss were GBM width, percentage of global glomerular sclerosis, and index of arteriolar hyalinosis. Multiple logistic regression analysis indicated that GBM width and hemoglobin A_{1c} (HbA_{1c}) values were the only independent predictors of progression.[46]

MICROALBUMINURIA AND RENAL STRUCTURE

As discussed elsewhere in this chapter, persistent microalbuminuria is a predictor of the development of clinical nephropathy, whereas the absence of microalbuminuria in patients with long-standing type 1 diabetes indicates a lower nephropathy risk. Proteinuria in type 1 diabetes of 10 or more years' duration is typically associated with advanced diabetic glomerular pathology.[22,23] One might reason that microalbuminuria is therefore associated with underlying renal structural changes that are predictive of the ultimate progression of this pathology. However, the relationship of renal structural changes to these low levels of albuminuria (i.e., normoalbuminuria or microalbuminuria) is complex and incompletely understood.

As a group, normoalbuminuric patients with a mean of 20 years of type 1 diabetes have increased GBM width and Vv(Mes/glom). The structural parameters in this group vary from within the normal range to advanced abnormalities that overlap those of patients with proteinuria (see Figures 39.11B and 39-12B). Patients with microalbuminuric AERs (20 to 200 μg/min) have, on average, even greater GBM and mesangial expansion, with almost no values in the normal range, but these values overlap with those of normoalbuminuric and proteinuric patients (see Figures 39-11B and 39-12B). The incidence of hypertension and reduced GFR is greater in patients with microalbuminuria. Thus, microalbuminuria is a marker of more advanced lesions as well as other functional disturbances.[23,47] Studies have suggested that greater GBM width in baseline biopsy specimens of normoalbuminuric patients is predictive of later clinical progression to microalbuminuria.[47] Furthermore, microalbuminuric patients with greater GBM width are more likely to progress to proteinuria.[48,49] Curiously, some normoalbuminuric patients with long-standing type 1 diabetes have a reduced GFR, which is associated with worse diabetic

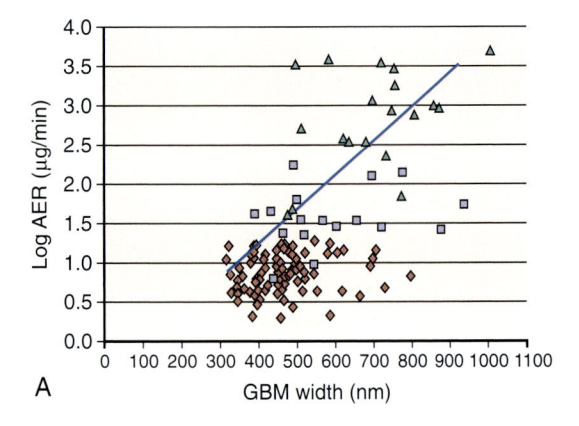

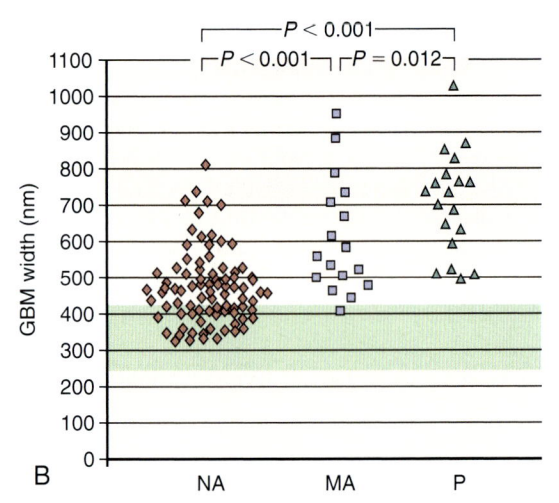

Figure 39.12 **A,** Correlation between glomerular basement membrane (GBM) width and albumin excretion rate (AER) in 124 patients with type 1 diabetes. **B,** GBM width in 88 normoalbuminuric (NA), 17 microalbuminuric (MA), and 19 proteinuric (P) patients with type 1 diabetes. The *hatched area* represents the mean ±2 SD in a group of 76 age-matched normal control subjects. All groups are different from control subjects. ♦, Normoalbuminuric patients; □ microalbuminuric patients; ∆, proteinuric patients ($r = 0.62$; $P < 0.001$). (From Caramori, ML, Kim Y, Huang C, et al: Cellular basis of diabetic nephropathy: 1. Study design and renal structural-functional relationships in patients with long-standing type 1 diabetes. *Diabetes* 51:506-513, 2002.)

glomerulopathy lesions.[50,51] This is particularly evident in females with retinopathy or hypertension, Thus, an increased AER is not always the initial clinical indicator of diabetic nephropathy. GFR measurements may be indicated for normoalbuminuric female patients with the aforementioned characteristics.[51]

RISK FACTORS FOR NEPHROPATHY INTRINSIC TO THE KIDNEY

In nondiabetic members of identical twin pairs discordant for type 1 diabetes, glomerular structure is within the normal range.[12] In every pair studied, the diabetic twin had higher values for GBM and TBM width and Vv(Mes/glom) than the nondiabetic twin. Several diabetic members of these discordant diabetic twins had values for GBM width and Vv(Mes/glom) that were within the range of normal, yet had so-called lesions when compared with their nondiabetic twin, whereas others had more severe lesions.[12] Thus, given sufficient duration, probably all type 1 diabetic patients have structural changes that are similar in direction, but the rate at which these lesions develop varies markedly among individuals.

There is a growing body of information, discussed elsewhere in this chapter, which supports the view that not only is glycemia a risk factor, but genetic variables also confer susceptibility or resistance to diabetic nephropathy. This is also suggested by the marked variability in the rate of development of kidney lesions of diabetic nephropathy in transplanted kidneys, despite the fact that the recipients all had ESKD secondary to diabetic nephropathy.[52] This variability, only partially explained by glycemic control, argues for genetically determined renal tissue responses as being important in determining nephropathy clinical outcomes.[52]

Glomerular volume and number could be structural determinants of nephropathy risk. Mean glomerular volumes were higher in patients developing diabetic nephropathy after 25 years of type 1 diabetes compared with a group developing nephropathy after only 15 years.[53] These studies suggest that as mesangial expansion develops, glomerular volume increases, and argue that patients unable to respond to mesangial expansion with glomerular enlargement will more quickly develop overt nephropathy than those whose glomeruli enlarge to provide compensatory preservation of glomerular filtration surface. The number of glomeruli per kidney can vary markedly among nondiabetic individuals and among diabetic patients and it has been suggested that fewer glomeruli per kidney could be a risk factor for diabetic nephropathy.[54,55] However, studies of transplant recipients with type 1 diabetes have indicated that having a single kidney does not result in accelerated lesion development compared with having two kidneys.[56] Diabetic patients with advanced renal failure have reduced numbers of glomeruli, but this likely results from resorption of sclerotic glomeruli.[54] If reduced glomerular number were a risk factor, it would be predicted that proteinuric patients without advanced renal failure would have fewer glomeruli, but this was not the case.[54] Although probably not important in the initiation phase of diabetic nephropathology, reduced glomerular numbers could be associated with more rapid progression to ESKD once advanced lesions and overt diabetic nephropathy have developed.

COMPARISONS OF NEPHROPATHY IN TYPES 1 AND 2 DIABETES

Renal pathology and structural-functional relationships have been less well studied in type 2 diabetic patients, despite the fact that 80% or more of diabetic patients with ESKD have type 2 diabetes. Proteinuric white Danish patients with type 2 diabetes were reported to have structural changes similar to those of proteinuric patients with type 1 diabetes, and the severity of these changes was strongly correlated with the subsequent rate of decline of GFR; however, the study reporting these findings also noted that some proteinuric patients with type 2 diabetes had little or no diabetic glomerulopathy.[57] A study of 52 type 2 diabetic patients from Northern Italy who underwent biopsy for clinical indications described greater heterogeneity in renal structure, with one third having nondiabetic renal diseases.[58] In a Danish study, 75% of unselected proteinuric type 2 diabetic patients had diabetic nephropathology but 25% had a variety of nondiabetic glomerulopathies, including minimal lesions, glomerulonephritis, mixed diabetic and glomerulonephritis changes, and chronic glomerulonephritis.[59] All patients with proteinuria and diabetic retinopathy had diabetic nephropathy; only 40% of patients without retinopathy had diabetic nephropathy.[59]

It is very likely that these high incidences of diagnoses—other than or in addition to diabetic nephropathy—represent a significant selection bias because a number of patients in these studies had clinical indications for kidney biopsy, many because of atypical clinical presentations or findings. In fact, the likelihood of finding nondiabetic renal disease among type 2 diabetic patients is highly influenced by a center's clinical indications for renal biopsy in type 2 diabetic patients.[60]

When renal biopsies are performed for research and not for diagnostic purposes, definable renal diseases other than those secondary to diabetes are distinctly uncommon.[60] However, marked heterogeneity in renal structure is present in type 2 diabetic patients with an increased AER.[61] Only a minority of patients have histopathologic patterns resembling those typically present in patients with type 1 diabetes; the typical pattern is 30% of patients with microalbuminuria and 50% of those with proteinuria (P. Fioretto, personal communication, 2014).[61] The remainder have minimal renal abnormalities or tubulointerstitial, vascular, and global glomerulosclerotic changes, which are disproportionally severe relative to the diabetic glomerulopathy lesions (atypical pattern, about 40% of patients with microalbuminuria and proteinuria).[61]

In type 2 diabetes, a reduced GFR in the presence of a normal albumin excretion rate is a common finding. Ekinci and colleagues[62] have recently described that among normoalbuminuric type 2 diabetic patients with impaired renal function, only a subset had typical diabetic glomerulopathy, whereas the remaining patients had predominantly tubulointerstitial and vascular changes. Similarly, in Japanese type 2 diabetic patients with a reduced GFR and normal albumin excretion rate, Shimizu and associates[63] have reported that tubulointerstitial and vascular are more severe than glomerular lesions.

STRUCTURAL-FUNCTIONAL RELATIONSHIPS IN TYPE 2 DIABETIC NEPHROPATHY

Renal structural-functional relationships in Japanese patients with type 2 diabetes were initially reported to be similar to those in type 1 patients.[64] However, a more recent study indicated greater heterogeneity in Japanese patients with type 2 diabetes, with some microalbuminuric and proteinuric patients having normal glomerular structural parameters.[65] Østerby and coworkers found less advanced glomerular changes in type 2 than type 1 diabetic patients with similar AERs; however, the type 1 patients had lower GFR levels than type 2 patients with similar AERs.[57] These findings could reflect much larger glomerular volumes in the type 2 patients, with associated preservation of filtration surface. In fact, GFR and S/G were correlated in these patients.[57] Also, the proteinuria in these type 2 patients was, at least in part, unexplained. Vv(Mes/glom) increased progressively from early to long-term diabetes, with clinical findings ranging from normoalbuminuria to microalbuminuria to clinical nephropathy in Pima Indian patients with type 2 diabetes, and global glomerular sclerosis correlated inversely with GFR in these patients.[30] The authors of this study also suggested, as noted earlier, that glomerular podocyte loss was related to proteinuria in these patients, although this was not seen in microalbuminuric patients. However, a study performed in type 2 diabetic white patients demonstrated a significant reduction in podocyte density in the microalbuminuric compared to the normoalbuminuric patients.[32] Significant relationships were described between albumin excretion levels and both podocyte density and foot process width.

The imprecise correlation between glomerular structure and renal function in patients with type 2 versus type 1 diabetes may be related to the more complex patterns of renal injury seen in type 2 diabetic patients (see earlier).[64] These considerations are relevant to prognosis in that the patients with more typical diabetic glomerulopathy morphometric findings of mesangial expansion on electron microscopy were more likely to have progressive loss of GFR over the next 4 years of follow-up.[66] This was confirmed in a study of proteinuric Danish patients with type 2 diabetes in which those whose biopsy specimens showed changes of diabetic glomerulopathy on light microscopy experienced a much more rapid decline in the GFR over a median of 7.7 years of follow-up.[67]

In summary, it appears that in patients with type 2 diabetes, renal structural changes are more heterogeneous and diabetic glomerulopathy lesions less severe than in type 1 patients with similar urine albumin levels. Approximately 40% of patients showed atypical renal injury patterns, and these patterns were associated with a higher body mass index and less diabetic retinopathy.[64] Further cross-sectional and longitudinal studies in type 2 diabetic patients are required before these complexities can be better understood.

It is possible that the atypical manifestations of renal injury in type 2 diabetes could be related to the pathogenesis of type 2 diabetes per se. Obesity, hypertension, increased plasma triglyceride levels, decreased high-density lipoprotein cholesterol concentrations, and accelerated atherosclerosis accompany hyperglycemia in many type 2 diabetic patients. Renal dysfunction in these patients could be the consequence of hypertensive nephrosclerosis, hyperlipidemic renal vascular atherosclerosis, renal hypoperfusion due to congestive heart failure, or the synergistic effects of these multiple risk factors for renal disease, which could simulate nephropathy clinically in type 2 diabetes. The increased risk of clinical renal disease in distinct populations, such as African American, American Indian, or Hispanic patients, could represent variability in the renal consequence of one or more of these pathogenetic influences. For example, there are differences in the renal structural consequences of hypertension in African American compared with white patients.[68]

OTHER RENAL DISORDERS IN DIABETIC PATIENTS

It has been reported that renal disorders, such as minimal change nephrotic syndrome and membranous nephropathy, occur with greater frequency in patients with type 1 diabetes than in nondiabetic persons.[69,70] In fact, when biopsies are performed for research purposes only and not for clinical indications, fewer than 1% of patients with type 1 diabetes for 10 years or longer and fewer than 4% of those with proteinuria and long duration of diabetes will be found to have conditions other than, or in addition to, diabetic nephropathy (M. Mauer, personal communication, 2014). As already discussed, proteinuric type 2 diabetic patients without retinopathy may have a high incidence of atypical renal biopsy findings or other diseases. Proteinuric patients with type 1 diabetes of less than 10 years' duration and type 2 diabetic patients without retinopathy should be thoroughly evaluated for other renal diseases, and a renal biopsy should be strongly considered for diagnosis and prognosis.

REVERSIBILITY OF DIABETIC NEPHROPATHY LESIONS

Mesangial expansion present after 7 months of diabetes reversed within 2 months after normoglycemia was induced by islet transplantation in rats with streptozotocin-induced diabetes.[71] It was thus disappointing that no improvement in diabetic nephropathy lesions in their native kidneys was found after 5 years of normoglycemia following successful pancreatic transplantation in type 1 patients with a diabetes duration of approximately 20 years.[72] After 10 years of normoglycemia, however, these same patients showed marked reversal of diabetic glomerulopathy lesions. Thus, GBM and TBM width were reduced at 10 years compared with the baseline and 5-year values, with several patients having values at 10 years that had returned to the normal range (Figure 39.13A and B).[73] Similar results were obtained with Vv(Mes/glom), primarily due to a marked decrease in mesangial matrix fractional volume (see Figure 39.13C and D). Remarkable glomerular architectural remodeling was seen by light microscopy, including the complete disappearance of Kimmelstiel-Wilson nodular lesions (Figure 39.14).[73] The reason for the long delay in this reversal process is not understood but could include epigenetic memory of the diabetic state, the slow process of replacement of glycated by nonglycated ECM, or other as yet undetermined processes. Regardless of the mechanism, relevant renal or circulating cells must be able to recognize the abnormal ECM environment and to initiate and sustain a state of imbalance in which the rate of ECM removal exceeds that of ECM production. This is clearly not the normal situation because, throughout adult life, GBM width and mesangial matrix remain quite constant, consistent with balanced ECM production and removal.[74] More recently, remodeling and healing in the tubulointerstitium has also been demonstrated in these same patients.[75] These studies have demonstrated reduction in total cortical interstitial collagen and underscore the remarkable potential for healing of kidney tissue that has been damaged by long-standing diabetes.[75]

Blockade of the renin angiotensin aldosterone system (RAAS) for 5 years did not lead to regression or slowing of the progression of diabetic glomerulopathy lesions in young patients with type 1 diabetes and normoalbuminuria. Whether healing can be induced by treatments other than cure of the diabetic state is currently unknown.[76]

EPIDEMIOLOGY OF MICROALBUMINURIA AND DIABETIC NEPHROPATHY

PREVALENCE AND INCIDENCE

Table 39.2 displays the prevalence, incidence, and cumulative incidence of abnormally elevated urinary albumin excretion in types 1 and 2 diabetes. The overall prevalence of microalbuminuria and macroalbuminuria is around 30% to 35% in both types of diabetes. However, the range in prevalence of diabetic nephropathy is much wider in type 2 diabetic patients. Clearly, the inability to define the onset of disease in type 2 diabetes is a confounding issue. However, ethnic differences are also a major influence. The highest prevalence, exceeding 50%, is found in Native Americans, followed by Asians, Mexican Americans, blacks, and European white patients.[77] It should be stressed that a good agreement has been documented between the result of clinic- and population-based studies. The cumulative incidence of persistent proteinuria in patients whose type 1 diabetes was diagnosed before 1942 was about 40% to 50% after diabetes of 25 to 30 years' duration, but it declined to 15% to 30% in patients receiving a diagnosis of type 1 diabetes after 1953.[2,78] Unfortunately, this so-called calendar effect has not been seen in white European patients with type 2 diabetes. The reason for the declining cumulative incidence of proteinuria

Table 39.2 Prevalence, Incidence and Cumulative Incidence of Microalbuminuria and Nephropathy In Diabetes

Parameter	Clinic-Based		Population-Based
	Type 1	Type 2	Type 2
Prevalence (%) of:			20 (17-21)
Microalbuminuria[80,94,574,575]	13 (9-20)	25 (13-27)	
Macroalbuminuria[2,80,574]	15 (8-22)	14 (5-48)	16 (9-46)
Incidence of macroalbuminuria (%/yr)[6]	1.2 (0-3)	1.5 (1-2)	—
Cumulative incidence of macroalbuminuria (%/25 yr)[2,6,78,576]	31 (22-34)	28 (25-31)	—

Median and range indicated.

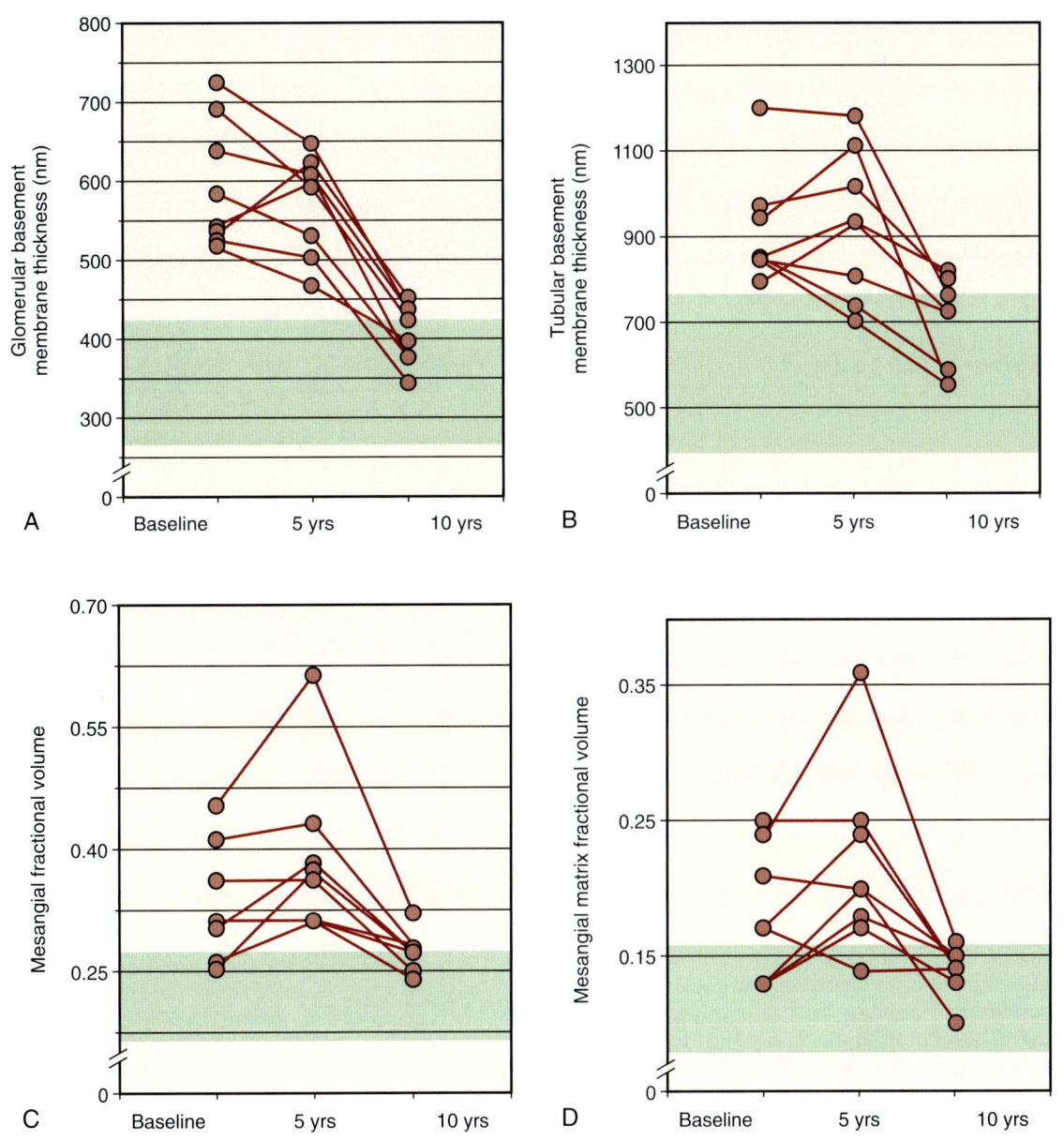

Figure 39.13 **A,** Thickness of the glomerular basement membrane (GBM). **B,** Thickness of the tubular basement membrane (TBM). **C,** Mesangial fractional volume and mesangial-matrix fractional volume at baseline and 5 and 10 years after pancreas transplantation **(D)**. The *shaded area* represents the normal ranges obtained in the 66 age- and sex-matched normal controls (mean ± 2 SD). Data for individual patients are connected by lines. (From Fioretto P, Steffes MW, Sutherland DER, et al: Reversal of lesions of diabetic nephropathy after pancreas transplantation. *N Engl J Med* 339:69-75, 1998.)

in type 1 diabetic patients is unknown, but improved diabetes care and blood pressure control,[79] in addition to a decline in the prevalence of smoking and a general decline in nondiabetic glomerulopathies, have been suggested as factors.

Diabetic nephropathy rarely develops in patients with type 1 diabetes before 10 years after diagnosis, whereas approximately 3% of patients with newly diagnosed type 2 diabetes already have overt nephropathy.[80] The incidence peak (3%/year) is usually found in those who have had diabetes for 10 to 20 years. Thereafter, a progressive decline in incidence takes place. Thus, the risk of developing diabetic nephropathy is reduced for a normoalbuminuric patient who has had diabetes for longer than 30 years.[81] This changing pattern of risk indicates that the magnitude of exposure to diabetes is not sufficient to explain the development of diabetic nephropathy. This suggests that kidney complications occur in only a subset of patients.

Studies have demonstrated impaired renal function (chronic kidney disease [CKD] stage 3—estimated GFR < 60 mL/min/1.73 m^2) in many patients with normoalbuminuria.[82,83] It has been discussed whether this is the result of aging, rather than kidney disease, because it is often seen in older women (and frequently is nonprogressive), or whether it is due to treatment-induced remission of albuminuria in patients with diabetic nephropathy or even a nonalbuminuric phenotype of diabetic nephropathy.[84,85] In addition, the estimated GFR (eGFR) underestimates the GFR and decline in GFR, depending to some extent on the

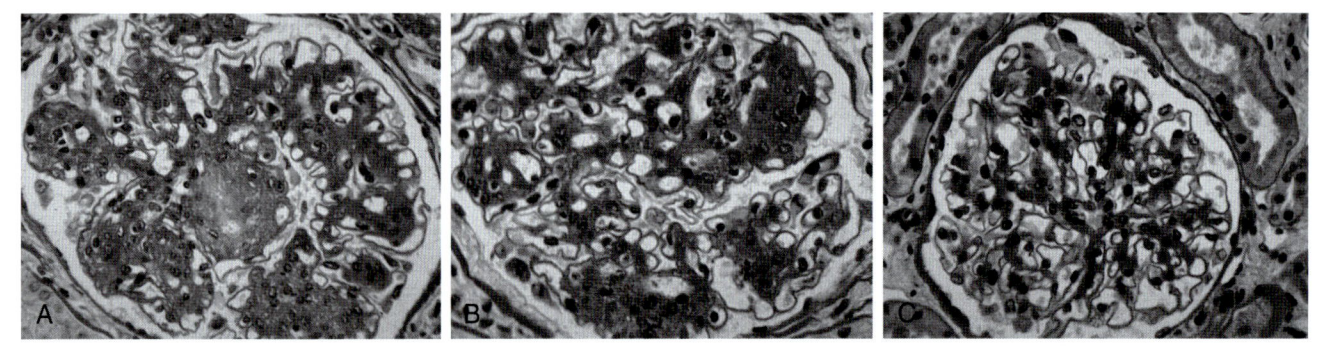

Figure 39.14 Light microscopic photomicrographs of renal biopsy specimens obtained before and after pancreas transplantation from a 33-year-old woman with type 1 diabetes of 17 years' duration at the time of transplantation. **A,** Typical glomerulus from the baseline biopsy specimen, which is characterized by diffuse and nodular (Kimmelstiel-Wilson) diabetic glomerulopathy. **B,** Typical glomerulus 5 years after transplantation, with persistence of the diffuse and nodular lesions. **C,** Typical glomerulus 10 years after transplantation, with marked resolution of diffuse and nodular mesangial lesions and more open glomerular capillary lumina (periodic acid–Schiff stain, ×120). (From Fioretto P, Steffes MW, Sutherland DER, et al: Reversal of lesions of diabetic nephropathy after pancreas transplantation. *N Engl J Med* 339:69-75, 1998.)

marker—for example, creatinine or cystatin C—and equation applied.[86-88] In a 19-year follow-up of the Diabetes Control and Complications Study in type 1 diabetic patients, 24% of patients developing an eGFR below 60 mL/min/1.73 m² had normoalbuminuria, as determined by all prior measurements.[89] Presently, sufficient longitudinal data to clarify this are lacking.

MICROALBUMINURIA AS A PREDICTOR OF NEPHROPATHY

The subpopulation of patients with type 1 diabetes who are at risk for nephropathy may be identified fairly accurately by the detection of microalbuminuria.[3] Several longitudinal studies have shown that microalbuminuria strongly predicts the development of diabetic nephropathy in type 1 diabetic patients, with a predictive power of 80%.[90,91] It has been suggested that 58% of microalbuminuric patients revert to normoalbuminuria, but in contrast to treatment-induced regression, long-lasting spontaneous normalization is seen in 16% of microalbuminuric patients with type 1 diabetes.[4,92]

Type 1 diabetic patients with microalbuminuria have a median risk ratio of 21 for developing diabetic nephropathy, whereas the risk ratio for developing diabetic nephropathy ranges from 4.4 to 21 (median, 8.5) in type 2 diabetic patients with microalbuminuria.[93] In addition to microalbuminuria, several other risk factors or markers for the development of diabetic nephropathy have been documented or suggested, as discussed in detail later (Table 39.3).

PROGNOSIS OF MICROALBUMINURIA

Microalbuminuria is a strong predictor of total and cardiovascular mortality and cardiovascular morbidity in diabetic patients, as confirmed by meta-analyses.[94,95] Similarly, microalbuminuria predicts coronary and peripheral vascular disease and death from cardiovascular disease in the general nondiabetic population.[95-97] Microalbuminuria and proteinuria were also linked to stroke in recent metaanalysis.[98] In recent guidelines from the Kidney Disease: Improving Global Outcome (KDIGO) for CKD, elevated albuminuria was included as a marker of ESKD and death.[99] The Chronic Kidney Disease Epidemiology Consortium also demonstrated that an increase in albuminuria conferred the same increase in relative risk for death and ESKD in patients with and without diabetes, although at a higher level in diabetic patients.[100]

Table 39.3 Risk Factors and Markers for Development of Diabetic Nephropathy in Types 1 and 2 Diabetic Patients

Risk Factor, Marker	Type 1	Type 2
Normoalbuminuria (above median)[162,163,577]	+	+
Microalbuminuria[81,92,177,578,579]	+	+
Gender[5,80]	M > F	M > F
Familial clustering[580-583]	+	+
Predisposition to arterial hypertension[201-203]	+/−	+
Increased sodium-lithium countertransport[201,202,584-589]	+/−	−
Ethnic conditions[77,590]	+	+
Onset of insulin-dependent diabetes mellitus before 20 yr[5,81]	+	?
Glycemic control[3,4,158,579,591]	+	+
Hyperfiltration[157-159,161]	+/−	+/−
Prorenin[397,592-594]	+	?
Smoking[217,595]	+	+
Cholesterol[162,163,596]	+	+
Presence of retinopathy[57,162,163,207,597]	+	+
Use of oral contraceptive[598]	+	?
Inflammation[143,599,600]	+	+
Adiponectin[601]	+	+
Nocturnal hypertension[602]	+	+
Uric acid[168]	+	?
Mannose-binding lectin[600]	+	?
Tubular damage[603]	+	?
Obesity[266]	?	+
Tumor necrosis factor receptors 1 and 2[604,605]	+	+

+, Present; −, not present; ?, no relevant information.

The mechanisms linking microalbuminuria to death from cardiovascular disease are poorly understood. Microalbuminuria has been proposed to be a marker of widespread endothelial dysfunction, which might predispose to enhanced penetrations of atherogenic lipoprotein particles into the arterial wall, and as a marker of established cardiovascular disease.[101,102] In addition, microalbuminuria is associated with an excess of both well-accepted Framingham and nontraditional cardiovascular risk factors.[102] Raised blood pressure, dyslipoproteinemia, increased platelet agreeability, endothelial dysfunction, insulin resistance, and hyperinsulinemia have all been demonstrated in microalbuminuric diabetic patients, as previously reviewed.[3,94,103] Autonomic neuropathy, which is also associated with microalbuminuria, predicts death (often sudden) from cardiovascular disease in diabetic patients.[104-106] Surprisingly, the prevalence of coronary heart disease, as inferred from a Minnesota-coded electrocardiogram, is not increased in microalbuminuric patients with type 2 diabetes.[80] Echocardiographic studies have revealed impaired diastolic function and cardiac hypertrophy in microalbuminuric patients with type 1 or type 2 daibetes.[107-110] Left ventricular hypertrophy predisposes the individual to ischemic heart disease, ventricular arrhythmia, heart failure, and sudden death.[111] It has been demonstrated that a high level of N-terminal pro-brain natriuretic peptide (NT-proBNP) is a major risk marker for cardiovascular disease in type 2 diabetes patients with microalbuminuria.[112] In type 2 patients without a history of cardiovascular disease (CVD), 35% of patients had significant CVD when thoroughly investigated following the findings of elevated NT-proBNP and coronary calcium values.[113]

PROGNOSIS OF DIABETIC NEPHROPATHY

In a cohort of 1030 patients in whom type 1 diabetes was diagnosed between 1933 and 1952, patients who did not develop proteinuria had a low and constant relative mortality, whereas patients with proteinuria had a 40 times higher relative risk of mortality.[5] Type 1 diabetic patients with proteinuria were found to have the characteristic bell-shaped relationship between diabetes duration and age and relative mortality, with a maximal relative mortality of 110 in females and 80 in males in the age interval of 34 to 38 years. Several other studies have confirmed the poor prognosis for type 1 diabetic patients with diabetic nephropathy.[5] In three early studies that described the natural course of diabetic nephropathy patients with type 1 diabetes, the cumulative death rate 10 years after the onset of nephropathy ranged from 50% to 77%.[103,114] The 50% figure represents a minimal value because the study included only death caused by ESKD. More recent studies have demonstrated how excess mortality in type 1 diabetes compared to the background population is almost entirely seen in patients with elevated albumin excretion.[115-117]

The overall decrease in relative mortality from 1933 to 1972 was 40%, which is partly explained by the decrease in the cumulative incidence of proteinuria. Unfortunately, this calendar effect is less well described in proteinuric type 2 diabetic patients, but data from a cohort followed from 2000 to 2010 demonstrated a 50% reduction in mortality compared to patients followed from 1983 to 2000.[6,118] The prognostic importance of proteinuria in type 2 diabetic patients is considerably less than in type 1 diabetes. Proteinuria confers a 3.5 times higher risk of death, and the concomitant presence of arterial hypertension increases this relative risk to 7 in Pima Indians with type 2 diabetes.[119] Part of the issue may be the typically increased age of type 2 diabetic patients relative to type 1 diabetic patients. The lower baseline risk of death in young patients in the general population magnifies the relative risk for type 1 diabetic patients. Among European patients with type 2 diabetes, those with proteinuria had a fourfold excess of premature death compared with patients without proteinuria.[120] The cumulative death rate 10 years after the onset of abnormally elevated urinary albumin excretion in European patients with type 2 diabetes was 70% compared with 45% in normoalbuminuric type 2 diabetic patients.[121] It is important to note that among patients with type 2 diabetes, approximately 90% of the proteinuric patients will die from cardiovascular or nonrenal causes before developing ESKD. Thus, the 10% who develop ESKD can be regarded as survivors, and improvement in cardiovascular prognosis will subsequently increase the number of patients developing ESKD. This is a key issue.

ESKD is the major cause of mortality and accounts for 59% to 66% of all deaths in type 1 diabetic patients with nephropathy.[5] The cumulative incidence of ESKD 10 years after the onset of persistent proteinuria in type 1 diabetic patients is 50%, compared with 3% to 11% in proteinuric European patients with type 2 diabetes and 65% in proteinuric Pima Indians with type 2 diabetes. However, renal insufficiency was defined as a serum creatinine level of 2.0 mg/dL or more in the Pima study. Some studies have suggested that the increase in ESKD due to diabetic nephropathy has been leveling off in several countries, including the United States and Spain.[122-124] In addition, the survival of diabetic patients with ESKD has also improved.[125] Of the excess mortality associated with type 2 diabetes in the Pima population, 97% is found in patients with proteinuria; 16% of the deaths were ascribed to ESKD, whereas 22% were due to CVD.[119]

CVD is also a major cause of death (15% to 25%) in type 1 diabetic patients with nephropathy, despite the relatively low age at death.[5] Borch-Johnsen and Kreiner[126] studied a cohort of 2890 patients with type 1 diabetes and demonstrated that the relative mortality from cardiovascular disease was 37 times higher in proteinuric type 1 diabetic patients than in the general population. Abnormalities related to well-established cardiovascular risk factors alone cannot account for this finding. Data from the RENAAL (Reduction of Endpoints in NIDDM with the Angiotensin II Antagonist Losartan) study have shown that type 2 diabetic patients with diabetic retinopathy have a poor prognosis.[127] Several studies have shown abnormally raised levels of serum apolipoprotein A to be an independent risk factor for premature ischemic heart disease in nondiabetic subjects. However, studies in types 1 and 2 diabetic patients with diabetic nephropathy have yielded conflicting results.[128-131] Most studies have demonstrated that a familial predisposition to CVD is present in type 1 diabetic patients with diabetic nephropathy.[132-134]

Increased left ventricular hypertrophy, an established CVD risk factor, and a decrease in diastolic function occur early in the course of diabetic nephropathy.[106,135,136] Left ventricular hypertrophy is a well-established risk factor for CVD. It has been shown that cardiac autonomic neuropathy predicts cardiovascular morbidity and mortality in type 1 diabetic patients with diabetic nephropathy.[105,106] An increased plasma homocysteine concentration is also a CVD risk factor and predicts mortality in type 2 diabetic patients with albuminuria.[137]

It has been demonstrated that increased urinary albumin excretion, endothelial dysfunction, and chronic inflammation are interrelated processes that develop in parallel, progress with time, and are strongly and independently associated with risk of death in type 2 diabetes.[138] Early multifactorial intervention to target glycemia, block the RAAS, reduce blood pressure, correct dyslipidemia, improve coagulation (aspirin), and address lifestyle factors is therefore important and has been demonstrated to reduce the development of microvascular and macrovascular complications and mortality by approximately 50% (see later).[139] Tarnow and associates have demonstrated that an elevated level of circulating NT-proBNP is a new independent predictor of the excess overall and cardiovascular mortality in types 1 and 2 diabetic patients with proteinuria but without symptoms of heart failure (see Chapter 13).[140,141] In addition, several new circulating biomarkers of cardiovascular risk in diabetic nephropathy have been identified, including asymmetric dimethylarginine, mannose-binding lectin, osteoprotegerin, connective tissue growth factor, high sensitive troponin T, and adiponectin.[142-147] Finally, it should be reiterated that reduced kidney function is a major independent cardiovascular risk factor.[148-150]

CLINICAL COURSE AND PATHOPHYSIOLOGY

A preclinical phase of diabetic nephropathy consisting of a normoalbuminuric and microalbuminuric stage and a clinical phase characterized by albuminuria has been well documented in both types 1 and 2 diabetic patients.

NORMOALBUMINURIA

Approximately one third of type 1 diabetic patients will have a GFR above the upper normal range for age-matched healthy nondiabetic subjects.[151] The degree of hyperfiltration is less in type 2 diabetic patients, and hyperfiltration is even reported to be lacking in some studies.[152-154] The GFR elevation is particularly pronounced in patients with newly diagnosed diabetes and during other intervals with poor metabolic control. Intensified insulin treatment and control to near-normal blood glucose levels reduce the GFR toward normal levels after a period of days to weeks in types 1 and 2 diabetic patients.[152] Additional metabolites, vasoactive hormones, and increased kidney and glomerular size have been suggested as mediators of hyperfiltration in diabetes.[151]

Four factors regulate GFR. First, the glomerular plasma flow influences the mean ultrafiltration pressure and thereby GFR. Enhanced renal plasma flow has been demonstrated in types 1 and 2 diabetic patients with elevated GFR.[152] Second, GFR is also regulated by the systemic oncotic pressure, which is reported to be normal in diabetes as calculated from plasma protein concentrations. The third determinant of GFR is the glomerular transcapillary hydraulic pressure difference, which cannot be measured in humans. However, the demonstrated increase in filtration fraction is compatible with an enhanced transglomerular hydraulic pressure difference. The last determinant of GFR is the glomerular ultrafiltration coefficient, Kf, which is determined by the product of the hydraulic conductance of the glomerular capillary and the glomerular capillary surface area available for filtration. Total glomerular capillary surface area is clearly increased at the onset of human diabetes.

Studies of rats with experimentally induced diabetes treated with insulin have revealed hyperfiltration, hyperperfusion, enhanced glomerular capillary hydraulic pressure, reduced proximal tubular pressure, unchanged systemic oncotic pressure, and unchanged or slightly elevated Kf.[155] Several studies have suggested that insulin-like growth factor-1 plays a major role in the initiation of renal and glomerular growth in diabetic animals.[156]

Longitudinal studies have suggested that hyperfiltration is a risk factor for subsequent increase in urinary albumin excretion and development of diabetic nephropathy in type 1 diabetic patients, but conflicting results have also been reported.[157-159] A meta-analysis based on 10 cohort studies following 780 patients has found a hazard ratio (HR) of 2.71 (95% confidence interval [CI], 1.20 to 6.11) for progression to microalbuminuria in patients with hyperfiltration. The authors also found evidence of heterogeneity.[160]

The prognostic significance of hyperfiltration in type 2 diabetic patients is still debated.[161] Six prospective cohort studies following normoalbuminuric types 1 and 2 diabetic patients for 4 to 10 years revealed that slight elevation of urinary albumin excretion, which remained in the normal range, poor glycemic control, hyperfiltration, elevated arterial blood pressure, retinopathy, and smoking contribute to the development of persistent microalbuminuria and overt diabetic nephropathy.[158,162-166] Because several of these risk factors are modifiable, intervention is feasible (see later). It has been suggested that uric acid level is related to hypertension, metabolic syndrome, and renal disease.[167] Recently, an elevated serum uric acid level was found to be a predictor of the development of diabetic nephropathy in type 1 diabetic patients, and a multicenter study has been initiated to study whether lowering uric acid in patients with early diabetic nephropathy preserves renal function.[168,169]

MICROALBUMINURIA

In 1969, Keen and colleagues demonstrated elevated urinary albumin excretion in patients with newly diagnosed type 2 diabetes.[170] This abnormal but subclinical AER has been termed *microalbuminuria* and can be normalized by improving glycemic control. Recently, for CKD in general, it has been suggested to use the term *moderately increased albuminuria* instead of microalbuminuria.[99] In addition to hyperglycemia, many other factors can induce microalbuminuria in diabetic patients, such as hypertension, massive obesity, heavy exercise, various acute or chronic illnesses, and cardiac failure.[171,172] The daily variation in urinary AER is high, 30% to 50%. Consequently, more than one urine sample is needed to determine whether an individual patient has persistent microalbuminuria. Urinary albumin excretion in the microalbuminuric range (30 to 300 mg/24 hr) in at least two of three consecutive nonketotic sterile urine samples is the generally accepted definition of persistent microalbuminuria. For convenience, it has been recommended to use early morning spot urine samples for screening and monitoring. The urinary albumin creatinine ratio is measured; microalbuminuria is defined as 30 to 300 mg/g creatinine (×0.1131 for mg/mmol).[173] It has been suggested that adjusting the urinary albumin concentration for urinary creatinine concentration may not only correct for diuresis, but elevated ratios may reflect two independent risk factors—elevated albumin excretion, reflecting renal and vascular damage, and reduced creatinine excretion, associated with reduced muscle mass.[174,175] Persistent microalbuminuria has not been detected in children with type 1 diabetes younger than 12 years and, in general, is exceptional in the first 5 years of diabetes.[176] The annual rate of increase in urinary albumin excretion is about 20% in type 2 diabetes and type 1 diabetic patients with persistent microalbuminuria.[177,178]

The excretion of albumin in the urine is determined by the amount filtered across the glomerular capillary barrier and the amount reabsorbed by the tubular cells. A normal urinary β_2-microglobulin excretion rate in microalbuminuria suggests that albumin is derived from enhanced glomerular leakage rather than from reduced tubular reabsorption of protein. The transglomerular passage of macromolecules is governed by the size- and charge-selective properties of the glomerular capillary membrane and hemodynamic forces operating across the capillary wall. Alterations in glomerular pressure and flow influence the diffusive and convective driving forces for transglomerular passage of proteins. Studies using renal clearance of endogenous plasma proteins or dextrans have not detected a simple size-selective defect.[179-181] Determination of the IgG/IgG$_4$ ratio suggests that loss of glomerular charge selectivity precedes or accompanies the formation of new glomerular macromolecular pathways in the development of diabetic nephropathy.[179] Reduction in the negatively charged moieties of the glomerular capillary wall, particularly sialic acid and heparin sulfate, has been suggested, but not all studies have confirmed these findings.[40,102,182] It has also been suggested that the glycocalyx, which is located on the apical surface of endothelial cells in capillaries and large vessels, is part of the glomerular barrier for filtration. Reduction in the glycocalyx above the endothelial cell may represent the first abnormality in the development of albuminuria.[183] The glycocalyx is reduced in diabetes, particularly in poorly controlled diabetes and may link microalbuminuria and cardiovascular disease.[184,185]

Long-term diabetes in spontaneously hypertensive rats is associated with a reduction in messenger RNA and protein expression of nephrin within the kidney.[186] As discussed earlier, changes in podocyte number and morphology have been implicated in the pathogenesis of proteinuria and progression of diabetic kidney disease.[30,187-189] The filtration fraction is presumed to reflect the glomerular hydraulic pressure, and microalbuminuric type 1 diabetic patients have elevated filtration at rest and during exercise compared with normal controls. A close correlation between filtration fraction and urinary albumin excretion has also been shown. The demonstration that microalbuminuria diminishes promptly with acute reduction in arterial blood pressure argues that reversible hemodynamic factors play an important role in the pathogenesis of microalbuminuria. Imanishi and colleagues have demonstrated that glomerular hypertension is present in type 2 diabetic patients with early nephropathy and is closely correlated with increased urinary albumin excretion.[190] In addition, it should be mentioned that increased pressure has been demonstrated in the nail fold capillaries of microalbuminuric type 1 diabetic patients.[191]

The GFR, measured using the single-injection, chromium-51–radiolabeled ethylenediaminetetraacetic acid (^{51}Cr-EDTA) plasma clearance method or renal clearance of inulin is normal or slightly elevated in type 1 diabetic patients with microalbuminuria. Prospective studies have demonstrated that GFR remains stable at normal or supranormal levels for at least 5 years if clinical nephropathy does not develop.[192] Nephromegaly is still present and is even more pronounced in microalbuminuric than in normoalbuminuric type 1 diabetic patients.[193] In microalbuminuric type 2 patients, GFR declines at rates of about 3 to 4 mL/min/yr.[194]

Changes in tubular function take place early in diabetes and are related to the degree of glycemic control. The proximal tubular reabsorption of fluid, sodium, and glucose is enhanced.[195] This process could diminish distal sodium delivery and thereby modify tubuloglomerular feedback signals, which would result in enhancement of the GFR. A direct effect of insulin on increasing distal sodium reabsorption has also been demonstrated.[195,196] The consequences of these alterations in tubular transport for overall kidney function are unknown. Markers of acute tubular damage have also been investigated in relation to prediction and progression of diabetic nephropathy. In some studies, elevated markers, such as liver fatty acid–binding protein, were slightly elevated in normo- or microalbuminuric patients who later progressed to diabetic nephropathy.[197,198]

Several studies have demonstrated blood pressure elevation in children and adults with type 1 diabetes and microalbuminuria.[103,114] The prevalence of arterial hypertension (*Seventh Report of the Joint National Committee on Prevention, Detection, Evaluation, and Treatment of High Blood Pressure* criterion of ≥140/90 mm Hg) in adult patients with type 1 diabetes increases with urine albumin level, and prevalence rates are 42%, 52%, and 79% in those with normoalbuminuria, microalbuminuria, and macroalbuminuria, respectively.[199] The prevalence of hypertension in those with type 2 diabetes (mean age, 60 years) was higher—71%, 90%, and 93% in the normoalbuminuria, microalbuminuria, and macroalbuminuric groups, respectively.[80,199] A genetic predisposition to hypertension in type 1 diabetic patients who develop diabetic nephropathy has been suggested, but other studies did not confirm the concept.[200-202] The original finding was confirmed by applying 24-hour blood pressure monitoring in a large group of parents of type 1 diabetic patients, with and without diabetic nephropathy.[203] The cumulative incidence of hypertension was found to be higher among parents of proteinuric patients, with a shift toward a younger age at the onset of hypertension in this parental group. However, the difference in prevalence of parental hypertension was not evident when office blood pressure measurements were used. Several studies have reported that sodium and water retention play a dominant role in the initiation and maintenance of systemic hypertension in patients with microalbuminuria and diabetic nephropathy, whereas the contribution of the RAAS is smaller.[204]

DIABETIC NEPHROPATHY

Diabetic nephropathy is a clinical syndrome characterized by persistent albuminuria (>300 mg/24 hr, or 300 mg/g creatinine), a relentless decline in GFR, raised arterial blood pressure and enhanced cardiovascular morbidity and mortality.[103,114] Although albuminuria is the first sign, peripheral edema is often the first symptom of diabetic nephropathy. Fluid retention is frequently observed early in the course of this kidney disease—that is, at a stage characterized by well-preserved renal function and only modest reduction in serum albumin level. Some studies have suggested that capillary hypertension, increased capillary surface area, and reduced capillary reflection coefficient for plasma proteins contribute to the edema formation, whereas the washdown of subcutaneous interstitial protein tends to prevent the progressive edema formation in diabetic nephropathy.[205,206]

Most studies dealing with the natural history of diabetic nephropathy have demonstrated a relentless, often linear rate of decline in GFR. Importantly, this rate of decline is highly variable across individuals, ranging from 2 to 20 mL/min/yr, with a mean of about 12 mL/min/yr.[3,103,114] Type 2 diabetic patients with nephropathy display the same degree of loss in filtration function and in variability of GFR.[207,208] Morphologic studies in types 1 and 2 diabetic patients have demonstrated a close inverse correlation between the degree of glomerular and tubulointerstitial lesions on the one hand and the GFR level on the other, as earlier. Myers and colleagues have demonstrated a reduction in the number of restrictive pores resulting in loss of ultrafiltration capacity (Kf) and impairment of glomerular barrier size-selectivity leading to progressive albuminuria and increases in urine levels of IgG in diabetic nephropathy.[209,210] Furthermore, the extent to which ultrafiltration capacity is impaired appears to be related to the magnitude of the defect in the barrier size-selectivity. A defect in the glomerular barrier size-selectivity has also been demonstrated in type 2 diabetic patients with diabetic nephropathy.[211] The reduction in renal plasma flow is proportional to the reduction in GFR (filtration fraction unchanged), and the impact on GFR is partially offset by the diminished systemic colloid osmotic pressure.

Several putative promoters of progression in kidney dysfunction have been studied in types 1 and 2 diabetic patients who have nephropathy (Figure 39.15).[207,212-218] A close correlation between blood pressure and the rate of decline in GFR has been documented in types 1 and 2 diabetic patients.[45,214,216,217,219-221] This suggests that systemic blood pressure accelerates the progression of diabetic nephropathy. Previously, the adverse impact of systemic hypertension on renal function and structure was thought to be mediated through vasoconstriction and arteriolar nephrosclerosis.[222] However, evidence from rat models has shown that systemic hypertension is transmitted to the single glomerulus, which results in increases in glomerular hydrostatic pressure in such a way as to lead to hyperperfusion and increased capillary pressure.[223] Intraglomerular hypertension has also been documented directly in rats with streptozotocin-induced diabetes and has been estimated to prevail in human diabetic patients, particularly those whose diabetes is complicated by kidney disease.[190,223] Impaired or abolished renal autoregulation of GFR and renal plasma flow, as demonstrated in types 1 and 2 diabetic patients with nephropathy, increases vulnerability to hypertension or ischemic injury of glomerular capillaries.[224] Defective autoregulation of GFR has been demonstrated in rats with streptozotocin-induced diabetes during hyperglycemia.[225] In contrast, studies in humans with type 2 diabetes have revealed no effect of glycemic control on GFR autoregulation.[226]

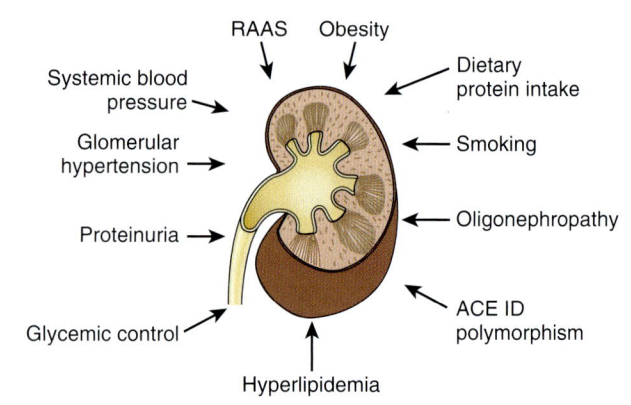

Figure 39.15 Putative promoters for progression of diabetic nephropathy.

Several components of the RAAS are elevated and considered to contribute to the progression of diabetic nephropathy.[227] Accordingly, blocking the RAAS has been demonstrated to be renoprotective (see later). Experimental studies have suggested that succinate, formed by the tricarboxylic acid cycle, provides a direct link between high glucose and renin release in the kidney through the G protein–coupled receptor for succinate GPR91, which functions as a detector of cell metabolism.[228] Initially, focus was on the damaging effect of angiotensin II. Recently, a kidney biopsy study revealed increased angiotensin-converting enzyme (ACE) activity and reduced expression of ACE2 in patients with diabetic nephropathy compared with controls and patients with nondiabetic kidney disease.[229] Aldosterone represents another component of the RAAS that should be considered important in the pathophysiology of diabetic nephropathy. Aldosterone is a hormone that, in addition to regulating electrolyte and fluid homeostasis, has widespread actions through genomic and nongenomic effects, both in the kidney and in tissues not originally considered target tissue for aldosterone, such as the vasculature, central nervous system, and heart.[230,231] This includes upregulation of the prosclerotic growth factors plasminogen activator inhibitor-1 and transforming growth factor-β_1 (TGF-β_1), as well as promotion of macrophage infiltration, which consequently leads to renal fibrosis.[232,233]

A longitudinal observational study involving a heterogeneous group of types 1 and 2 diabetic patients with microalbuminuria has demonstrated that systolic blood pressure, hyperangiotensinemia, and hyperaldosteronemia act as independent predictors of more rapidly declining kidney function (measured as 1/Cr, the reciprocal creatinine slope).[234] Increasing levels of aldosterone during long-term treatment with the angiotensin II receptor antagonist losartan were demonstrated to be associated with a faster decline in GFR.[235]

Originally, Remuzzi and Bertani[236] suggested that proteinuria itself may contribute to renal damage. Type 1 diabetic patients with diabetic nephropathy and nephrotic range proteinuria (>3 g/24 hr) had the worst prognosis. Several observational studies and treatment trials have confirmed and extended these findings to include also subnephrotic range proteinuria.[45,119,219,237]

For many years, it was believed that once albuminuria had become persistent, glycemic control had lost its beneficial impact on kidney function and structure, and consequently the concept of "point of no return" was advocated by many investigators.[103] This misconception was based on studies involving a limited number of patients and those that used inappropriate methods for monitoring kidney function (e.g., serum creatinine level) and glycemic control (e.g., random blood glucose level). Several more recent studies encompassing large numbers of type 1 diabetic patients have documented the important impact of glycemic control on the progression of diabetic nephropathy.[216,221,238] In contrast, most of the studies involving proteinuric patients with type 2 diabetes have failed to demonstrate any significant impact, with two exceptions.[206,207,217,239,240]

Almost all studies in types 1 and 2 diabetic patients have demonstrated a correlation between serum cholesterol concentration and progression of diabetic nephropathy, at least in univariate analyses, but some have failed to demonstrate cholesterol level as an independent risk factor in multiple regression analyses.[206,207,214,216,217,219-221]

Dietary protein restriction retards the progression of renal disease in almost every experimental animal model tested.[222] Surprisingly, all major observational studies in types 1 and 2 diabetic patients with diabetic nephropathy have failed to demonstrate an effect of dietary protein intake on the rate of decline.[206-208,219-221] Some but not all studies have suggested that smoking may act as a progression promoter in types 1 and 2 diabetic patients with proteinuria.[241,242] However, some larger, long-term studies have not been able to confirm these initial findings.[217,243]

Several gene variants have been investigated as candidate genes for risk factors for diabetic nephropathy. One of the most intensively studied is the insertion/deletion (I/D) polymorphism of the ACE gene (ACE/ID). The deletion (D)-allelic variant is strongly associated with the level of circulating ACE and increased risk of coronary heart disease in nondiabetic and diabetic patients.[244,245] The I/D polymorphism represents a common allelic variant in the sequence of the human ACE gene that reflects the insertion (I genotype) or deletion (D genotype) of a 282-nucleotide Alu repetitive element within a downstream intron of the gene. The plasma ACE level in DD homozygous individuals is about twice that of II homozygous individuals, with ID heterozygous individuals having intermediate levels.[246] Yoshida and colleagues followed 168 proteinuric type 2 diabetic patients for 10 years.[247] Analysis of the clinical course of individuals with the three ACE genotypes revealed that most patients with the DD genotype (95%) progressed to ESKD within 10 years. Moreover, the DD genotype appeared to be associated with increased mortality once dialysis was initiated. Three observational studies have confirmed that the D allele has a deleterious effect on kidney function.[248-250] Finally, more severe diabetic glomerulopathy lesions have been documented during the development and progression of renal disease in type 2 diabetic patients with the D allele.[251] Furthermore, microalbuminuric type 1 diabetic patients carrying the D allele show increased progression of diabetic glomerulopathy, based on the findings in renal biopsy specimens obtained at baseline and after 26 to 48 months of follow-up.[252]

In a large, double-blind, placebo-controlled randomized study (RENAAL) examining the renoprotective effects of losartan administered along with conventional blood pressure–lowering drugs in proteinuric type 2 diabetic patients, Parving and colleagues demonstrated that the associations of kidney disease measured mortality and end-stage renal disease in individuals with and without diabetes: a meta-analysis presence of the D allele of the ACE gene had a harmful impact in terms of the likelihood of reaching the composite end point of a doubling of baseline creatinine concentration, ESKD, or death.[254] The impact was more pronounced in the white and Asian patient group than the black and Hispanic group. The beneficial effects of losartan were greatest in the ACE/DD group and intermediate in the ID group for almost all end points, a trend that suggests a quantitative interaction between treatment and ACE genotype in the progression of renal disease. Such an interaction was most significant for the reduction of risk of reaching the ESKD end point.[254]

Parving and colleagues showed an accelerated initial and sustained loss of GFR during ACE inhibitor treatment of albuminuric type 1 patients homozygous for the DD polymorphism of the ACE gene.[254] The DD genotype independently influenced the sustained rate of decline in GFR; in other words, it acted as a progression promoter. Three other studies have demonstrated that the D allele is a risk factor for an accelerated course of diabetic nephropathy in patients with type 1 diabetes.[255-257] A potential contribution from other candidate genes in relation to the RAAS has also been suggested.[257] Another gene that was suggested to influence the outcome in type 2 diabetic patients and have an effect on RAAS blocking treatment was the ADAMTS13 gene (involved in the proteolysis of highly thrombogenic von Willebrand factor [vWF] ultrahigh-weight multimers). One variant (the 618Ala variant) was associated with less proteolytic activity, higher risk of chronic renal and cardiovascular complications, and better response to ACE inhibitor (ACWI) therapy in a substudy of the BErgamo NEphrologic DIabetes Complications Trial (BENEDICT).[258]

Recently, genome-wide association studies have been performed in the search for genes linked to diabetic nephropathy and, although some areas of the genome have attracted attention, no major susceptibility genes have been identified so far.[259-262] For example, genetic heterogeneity at the apolipoprotein L-1 gene on chromosome 19 explains an important component of the susceptibility of those with African ancestry to nondiabetic CKD. This genetic variant does not predict diabetic nephropathy risk.

A common feature in severe CKD is anemia. Anemia seems to occur at an earlier stage in diabetic nephropathy than in other kidney diseases, so anemia is a frequent finding in patients with diabetic nephropathy and moderately reduced renal function.[263] Furthermore, the degree of anemia has been found to be an independent risk factor associated with the decline in GFR or development of ESKD in type 2 diabetic patients with diabetic nephropathy.[217,218] Importantly, the Trial to Reduce Cardiovascular Events with Aranesp Therapy (TREAT) has revealed that correction of anemia with erythropoiesis-stimulating agents, specifically darbepoetin, does not improve the prognosis of CKD in iron-replete diabetic patients with mild anemia and modest impairments of GFR.[264]

Obesity is an increasing problem in the general and diabetic population. Several studies have indicated that severe obesity (body mass index [BMI] > 40 kg/m^2) enhances ESKD risk sevenfold.[265] Even a BMI higher than 25 kg/m^2 was found to increase ESKD risk.[265] This effect is independent of the effects of hypertension and diabetes, the prevalence of which is increased in individuals with obesity. An effect of obesity on renal hemodynamics leading to increased glomerular pressure and hyperfiltration has been suggested as the mechanism.[266]

As discussed in Chapter 49, pregnancy in women with diabetic nephropathy is accompanied by an increase in complications such as hypertension and proteinuria and by increases in premature birth and fetal loss. The impact of pregnancy on the long-term course of renal function in women with diabetic nephropathy has not been clarified until rather recently. A study by Rossing and associates has suggested that pregnancy has no adverse long-term impact on kidney function and survival in type 1 diabetic patients with diabetic nephropathy who have well-preserved kidney function (serum creatinine concentration < 100 μmol/L at the start of pregnancy), and similar data for type 2 diabetes patients have also been presented.[256,257]

Nondiabetic glomerulopathy is very seldom seen in proteinuric type 1 diabetic patients, although this condition is common in proteinuric type 2 diabetic patients without retinopathy.[59] A prevalence of biopsy specimens with normal glomerular structure or nondiabetic kidney diseases of approximately 30% was demonstrated. Furthermore, a more rapid decline in GFR and a progressive rise in albuminuria in type 2 diabetic patients with diabetic glomerulopathy compared with type 2 diabetic patients without diabetic glomerulopathy has been demonstrated.[67,267]

Systemic blood pressure elevation to a hypertensive level is an early and frequent phenomenon in diabetic nephropathy.[80,103,114] Furthermore, nocturnal blood pressure elevation (nondipping) occurs more frequently in types 1 and 2 diabetic patients with nephropathy.[268,269] An exaggerated blood pressure response to exercise has also been reported in patients with long-standing type 1 diabetes with microangiopathy. Finally, the increase in glomerular pressure consequent to nephron adaption may be accentuated with concomitant diabetes, as suggested in animal studies.[270]

Recently, several new biomarkers associated with renal and cardiovascular outcome have been identified (see later). Connective tissue growth factor (CTGF) has been recognized as a key factor in ECM production and other profibrotic activity mediated by TGF-β_1. CTGF is induced in renal cells by elevated glucose levels and is upregulated in diabetic nephropathy. Elevated levels were found to be independently associated with faster decline in the GFR and development of ESKD in type 1 diabetic patients with diabetic nephropathy.[145]

Osteoprotegerin is a 120-kDa secretory glycoprotein belonging to the tumor necrosis factor receptor superfamily. It was first discovered in bone but is also present in the arterial wall. Osteoprotegerin may be involved in the development of vascular calcification. In cross-sectional studies, the osteoprotegerin level was elevated in types 1 and 2 diabetic patients with microvascular and macrovascular complications.[271,272] A prospective study has demonstrated that elevated levels of osteoprotegerin predict increased all-cause and cardiovascular mortality, as well as enhanced decline in GFR in type 1 diabetic patients with nephropathy.[144]

Adiponectin is secreted by adipocytes and has been shown to possess antiinflammatory, antiatherogenic, and cardioprotective properties in type 2 diabetic patients. Paradoxically, elevated levels were found in type 1 diabetic patients with diabetic nephropathy, and these increased levels were associated with an enhanced rate of decline in GFR and development of ESKD.[147] Experimental studies have suggested that adiponectin affects podocytes and thereby could link obesity and kidney disease.[273]

Urinary proteomic profiles characteristic for diabetic nephropathy have been identified.[274] These changes are partly normalized during renoprotective intervention.[275] Furthermore, this metabolomics-based profile (Figure 39.16) was also able to identify normoalbuminuric patients with elevated risk for later development of diabetic nephropathy, independent of other risk factors.[276,277]

EXTRARENAL COMPLICATIONS IN DIABETIC NEPHROPATHY

Diabetic retinopathy is present in almost all type 1 diabetic patients with nephropathy, whereas only 50% to 60% of proteinuric type 2 diabetic patients have retinopathy.[80] The absence of retinopathy should prompt further investigation for nondiabetic glomerulopathies.[1] Blindness due to severe proliferative retinopathy or maculopathy is approximately five times more frequent in types 1 and 2 diabetic patients with nephropathy than in normoalbuminuric patients.[80] Macroangiopathies (e.g., stroke, carotid artery stenosis, coronary heart disease, peripheral vascular disease) are two to five times more common in patients with diabetic nephropathy and, as stated earlier, macroangiopathy is the major cause of mortality rather than ESKD for patients with diabetic nephropathy.[80,118]

Peripheral neuropathy is present in almost all patients with advanced nephropathy. Foot ulcers with sepsis leading to amputation occur frequently (>25% of cases), probably due to a combination of neural and arterial diseases. Autonomic neuropathy may be asymptomatic and manifest simply as abnormal cardiovascular reflexes, or it may result in debilitating symptoms. Almost all patients with nephropathy have grossly abnormal results on autonomic function tests.[105]

TREATMENT

The major therapeutic interventions that have been investigated include control of blood glucose to near-normal levels, antihypertensive treatment, lipid-lowering therapy,

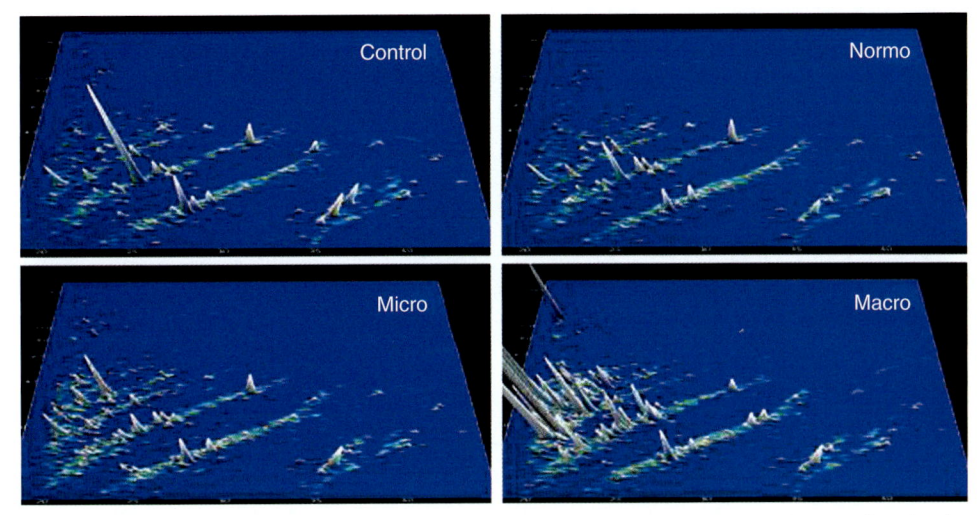

Figure 39.16 Protein patterns of patients with diabetes with normoalbuminuria, microalbuminuria, and macroalbuminuria and control subjects examined. The molecular mass (0.7 to 25 kDa, on a logarithmic scale) is plotted against normalized migration time (17 to 47 min). Signal intensity is encoded by peak height and color. (From Rossing K, Mischak H, Dakna M, et al: Urinary proteomics in diabetes and CKD. *J Am Soc Nephrol* 19:1283-1290, 2008.)

Table 39.4 RENAAL and IDNT Results: Comparison of Primary Composite End Point and Components

Composite End Point	Risk Reduction (% [95% CI])			
	Losartan vs. Placebo (80)	Irbesartan vs. Placebo (81)	Irbesartan vs. Amlodipine (81)	Amlodipine vs. Placebo (81)
DsCr, ESKD, death	16 (2, 28)	20 (3, 34)	23 (7, 37)	−4 (14, −25)
Doubling of sCr	25 (8, 39)	33 (13, 48)	37 (19, 52)	−6 (16, −35)
ESKD	28 (11, 42)	23 (−3, 43)	23 (−3, 43)	0 (−32, 24)
Death	−2 (−27, 19)	8 (−31, 23)	−4 (23, −40)	12 (−19, 34)
ESKD or death	20 (5, 32)	—	—	—

DsCr, Doubling of serum creatinine; ESKD, end-stage kidney disease; IDNT, Irbesartan Diabetic Nephropathy Trial; RENAAL, Reduction of End Points in NIDDM with the Angiotensin II Antagonist Losartan study; sCR, serum creatinine.

and restriction of dietary proteins. The impact of these four treatment modalities on progression from normoalbuminuria to microalbuminuria (primary prevention), microalbuminuria to diabetic nephropathy (secondary prevention), and diabetic nephropathy to ESKD will be described and discussed. Newer treatment options that are in development or have been tested and failed recently are subsequently discussed.

GLYCEMIC CONTROL

PRIMARY PREVENTION

Strict metabolic control achieved by insulin treatment or islet cell transplantation normalizes hyperfiltration, hyperperfusion, and glomerular capillary hypertension and reduces the rate of increase in urinary albumin excretion in experimental diabetic animals.[103] This treatment also mitigates the development of diabetic glomerulopathy, although the glomerular enlargement remains unaffected. Risk factors for progression from normoalbuminuria to microalbuminuria and macroalbuminuria have been identified (Table 39.4). Short-term blood glucose control to near-normal levels in normoalbuminuric type 1 diabetic patients reduces GFR, renal plasma flow, urinary AER, and observed increases in kidney size. Increased kidney size is associated with an exaggerated renal response to amino acid infusion, and studies have suggested that both abnormalities can be corrected by 3 weeks of intensified insulin treatment.[278] A meta-analysis of long-term intensive blood glucose control (8 to 60 months) documented a beneficial effect on the progression from normoalbuminuria to microalbuminuria in type 1 diabetic patients.[279] The odds ratios for progressing from normoalbuminuria to microalbuminuria ranged from 0.22 to 0.40 in the intensified treatment groups. A worsening of diabetic retinopathy was observed during the initial months of intensive therapy but, in the longer term, the rate of deterioration was slower than in the type 1 diabetic patients receiving conventional treatment.[280]

Side effects are a major concern with intensive therapy. The frequency of severe hypoglycemic episodes and diabetic ketoacidosis was found to be greater in several studies.[279] In the Diabetes Control and Complications Trial (DCCT),[281] intensive therapy reduced the occurrence of microalbuminuria by 39% (95% CI, 0.21 to 0.52), and that of albuminuria by 54% (95% CI, 0.19 to 0.74) when the primary and secondary prevention cohorts were combined

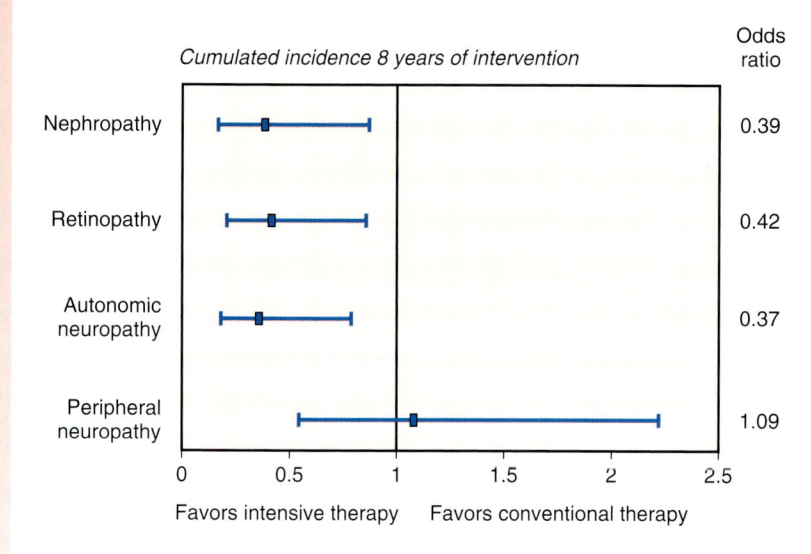

Figure 39.17 Odds ratio for progression of microvascular complications in microalbuminuric type 2 diabetic patients from the STENO-2 trial, including 160 patients treated with multifactorial intensive therapy compared to standard therapy. (From Gaede P, Vedel P, Larsen N, et al: Multifactorial intervention and cardiovascular disease in patients with type 2 diabetes. *N Engl J Med* 348:383-393, 2003.)

for analysis. With further follow-up of DCCT patients in the Epidemiology of Diabetes Interventions and Complications (EDIC) study, it was demonstrated that the reduction in the development of microalbuminuria and albuminuria translated into a 50% reduced risk (95% CI, 0.18 to 0.69; $P = 0.006$) of development of impaired renal function (eGFR < 60).[282] Despite this, however, 16% in the primary prevention cohort and 26% in the secondary prevention cohort developed microalbuminuria during the 9 years of intensive treatment. This clearly documents the need for additional treatment modalities to reduce the burden of diabetic nephropathy.

In Japanese type 2 diabetic patients, a beneficial impact of strict glycemic control on the progression of normoalbuminuria to microalbuminuria and macroalbuminuria was demonstrated in a small study with a design similar to that of the DCCT.[283] Results of this study have been confirmed and extended by data from the UK Prospective Diabetes Study (UKPDS) documenting a progressively beneficial effect of intensive metabolic control on the development of microalbuminuria and overt proteinuria, and a 10-year poststudy follow-up demonstrated a long-lasting beneficial effect.[284,285] This beneficial effect was confirmed in the Action in Diabetes and Vascular Disease: Preterax and Diamicron Modified-Release Controlled Evaluation (ADVANCE) study, in which 11,140 patients with type 2 diabetes were followed for a median of 5 years and a 21% reduction in the development of nephropathy (95% CI, 0.07 to 0.34) was seen in patients randomly assigned to strict glycemic control.[286] The same trend was seen in the smaller Veterans Affair Diabetes Trial, but the values did not reach statistical significance.[287]

It has been suggested that newer classes of glucose-lowering agents in type 2 diabetes have a beneficial effect on the kidney, apart from lowering glucose. Thus, it has been found that rosiglitazone, which is a thiazolidinedione, reduces microalbuminuria independently of glycemia in a study by Bakris and coworkers.[288] Treatment with dipeptidyl peptidase 4 inhibitors (DPP4 inhibitors) also provided evidence suggesting that they reduced albumin excretion compared to placebo as a secondary outcome.[289,290] Experimental data have suggested that the effect could be linked to effects on B-type natriuretic peptide and CXC chemokine receptor type 4 (CXCR4). The glucagon-like peptide 1 (GLP-1) analogue exenatide has also been found to reduce albumin excretion by 15% in a clinical study.[291] For most of these studies, there has been a difference in glucose levels between groups, in addition to treatment differences, and albumin excretion has been a secondary end point in all studies. Therefore, further evaluation is needed to confirm whether these agents have a renoprotective effect above and beyond their effect on lowering blood glucose levels.

SECONDARY PREVENTION

Several modifiable risk factors for progression from microalbuminuria to overt diabetic nephropathy (including the level of urinary albumin excretion, HbA_{1c} level, smoking, blood pressure, and serum cholesterol concentration) have been identified in clinical trials and observational studies of types 1 and 2 diabetic patients.[3,4,177,292-295]

Data regarding the renal impact of intensive diabetic treatment versus conventional diabetic treatment on the progression or regression of microalbuminuria in type 1 diabetic patients have been conflicting.[103] These disappointing results might be due, in part, to the relatively short length of the follow-up period, because the UKPDS with 15 years of follow-up documented a progressive beneficial effect over time on the development of proteinuria and a twofold increase in plasma creatinine level.[284] Furthermore, pancreatic transplantation was found to reverse glomerulopathy in patients with type 1 diabetes and normoalbuminuria ($N = 3$) or microalbuminuria ($N = 4$), but reversal required more than 5 years of normoglycemia.[73] It has been demonstrated that intensified multifactorial intervention (pharmacologic therapy targeting hyperglycemia, hypertension, dyslipidemia, and microalbuminuria) in patients with type 2 diabetes and microalbuminuria substantially slows progression to overt nephropathy, retinopathy, and autonomic neuropathy (Figure 39.17).[104,296] Also, a follow-up study has demonstrated that the rate of development of ESKD is significantly reduced by intensive multifactorial intervention after 13 years (Figure 39.18).[297] A Japanese study has confirmed the effect of multifactorial intervention by showing a 54% regression of microalbuminuria, with aggressive reduction in multiple risk factors.[298]

NEPHROPATHY

The impact of improved metabolic control on the progression of kidney function in type 1 diabetic patients with nephropathy has been disappointing. Studies have not found the rate of decline in GFR and the rise in proteinuria and systemic blood pressure to be affected by improved glycemic control. However, it should be stressed that none of the trials was randomized, and the number of patients included was small. In contrast, most major prospective observational studies have indicated an important role for glycemic control in the progression of diabetic nephropathy (see earlier).[103,219,221,237] The renal outcomes from the ADVANCE trial showed a 65% reduced risk for ESKD in addition to a reduced risk for development of microalbuminuria and macroalbuminuria.[299] However, only 27 of 11,140 patients enrolled in the study developed ESKD. Therefore, the event rate was very low. If 37 patients developing renal death was combined with patients with ESKD, the HR for a reduction with intensive glucose control was not significant (HR, 0.85; 95% CI, 0.45 to 1.63; $P = 0.63$), and there was no effect on doubling of the serum creatinine level to at least 200 μmol/L (HR, 1.15; 95% CI, 0.82 to 1.63; $P = 0.42$; Figure 39.19). This is in accordance with a recent meta-analysis.[300] Thus, there are still no data to demonstrate the prevention of renal failure with improved glucose control.

BLOOD PRESSURE CONTROL

PRIMARY PREVENTION

Originally, Zatz and colleagues[301] showed that prevention of glomerular capillary hypertension in normotensive, insulin-treated rats with streptozotocin-induced diabetes effectively protects against the subsequent development of proteinuria and focal and segmental glomerular structural lesions. Other studies have confirmed the beneficial effect of ACE inhibition in uninephrectomized rats made diabetic by streptozotocin. Anderson and associates have demonstrated that antihypertensive therapy slows the development of diabetic glomerulopathy but found that ACEIs provide better long-term protection than triple therapy with reserpine, hydralazine, and hydrochlorothiazide or a calcium channel blocker (nifedipine).[302,303] Some observations are consistent with the concept that glomerular hypertension is a major factor in the pathogenesis of experimental diabetic glomerulopathy and indicate that a lowering of systemic blood pressure without concomitant reduction of glomerular capillary pressure may be insufficient to prevent glomerular injury.[302-304] Reduction of systemic blood pressure by ACEIs or conventional antihypertensive treatment affords significant renoprotection in spontaneously hypertensive rats with streptozotocin-induced diabetes.[305] No specific added

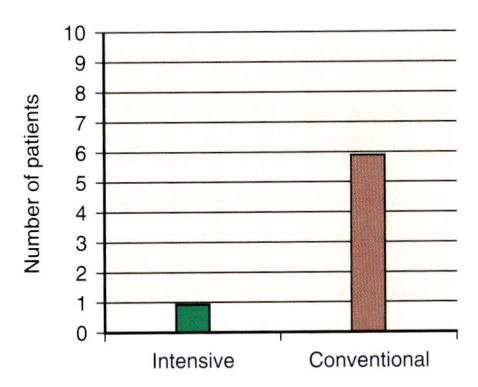

Figure 39.18 Development of ESKD in microalbuminuric type 2 diabetic patients from the STENO-2 trial, including 160 patients. One patient had progression to ESKD in the intensive group compared to six patients in the conventional group ($P = 0.04$). (From Gaede P, Vedel P, Larsen N, et al: Multifactorial intervention and cardiovascular disease in patients with type 2 diabetes. *N Engl J Med* 348:383-393, 2003.)

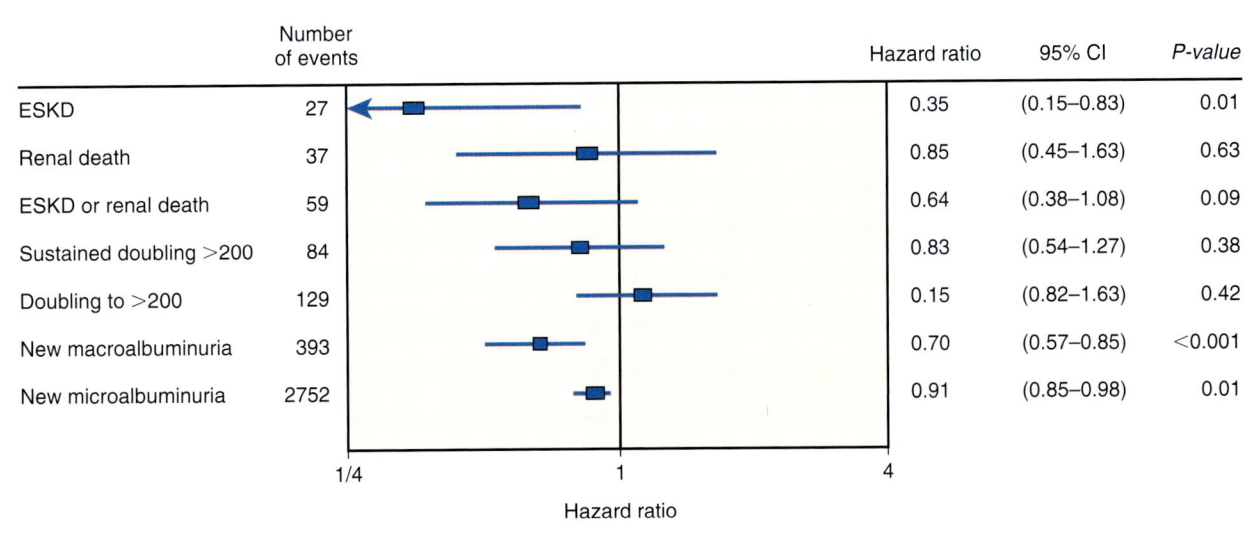

	Number of events	Hazard ratio	95% CI	P-value
ESKD	27	0.35	(0.15–0.83)	0.01
Renal death	37	0.85	(0.45–1.63)	0.63
ESKD or renal death	59	0.64	(0.38–1.08)	0.09
Sustained doubling >200	84	0.83	(0.54–1.27)	0.38
Doubling to >200	129	0.15	(0.82–1.63)	0.42
New macroalbuminuria	393	0.70	(0.57–0.85)	<0.001
New microalbuminuria	2752	0.91	(0.85–0.98)	0.01

Figure 39.19 Summary plot showing the effects of intensive glucose lowering compared with standard glucose lowering on renal outcomes in the ADVANCE trial. Doubling to >200, adjudicated doubling of serum creatinine to a value over 200 μmol/L; sustained doubling >200, doubling of creatinine as above that remained at least doubled at the final available follow-up reading; ESKD, end-stage kidney disease. (From Perkovic V, Heerspink HL, Chalmers J, et al: Intensive glucose control improves kidney outcomes in patients with type 2 diabetes. *Kidney Int* 83:517-523, 2013.)

benefit of ACE inhibition was observed in this hypertensive model in contrast to the normotensive models.

Three randomized, placebo-controlled trials in normotensive types 1 and 2 diabetic patients with normal AER have suggested a beneficial effect of ACEIs on the development of microalbuminuria.[306-308] In contrast to these three studies, which were carried out as placebo-controlled trials, subsequent studies compared the effect of ACEIs versus a long-acting dihydropyridine calcium antagonist or versus a β-blocker in hypertensive type 2 diabetic patients with normoalbuminuria.[309,310] All three of the latter studies reported a similar beneficial renoprotective effect of blood pressure reduction, with and without ACE inhibition. Furthermore, the UKPDS study reported that by 6 years, a smaller proportion of patients in the group in whom blood pressure was tightly controlled had developed microalbuminuria, and those in the tight control group had a 29% reduction in risk for microalbuminuria ($P < 0.009$), with a nonsignificant 39% reduction in the risk for proteinuria ($P = 0.061$).[311]

Aggressive blood pressure control in normotensive type 2 diabetic patients (blood pressure < 160/90 mm Hg) has been demonstrated to have beneficial effects on albuminuria, retinopathy, and incidence of stroke.[312] The results were the same whether enalapril or nisoldipine was used as the initial blood pressure–lowering drug. The Renin Angiotensin System Study (RASS) compared the effects of ACE inhibition, angiotensin II receptor blockade, and placebo on the primary renal structural end point of mesangial volume fraction in type 1 diabetic patients who were normotensive (blood pressure < 135/85 mm Hg) and normoalbuminuric (median AER, 5 μg/min). This 5-year randomized controlled trial did not find any benefit of RAAS blockade on the progression of nephropathy as measured in terms of the primary end point and other secondary renal structural parameters.[76] Also, RAAS blockade did not prevent an increase in AER.[76] In contrast, the odds for progression of retinopathy were significantly reduced by 65% to 70% with the RAAS blocking agents compared with placebo. Originally, the EUCLID study group demonstrated a significant beneficial effect of ACE inhibition on progression of diabetic retinopathy and development of proliferative retinopathy in type 1 diabetic patients.[313] The DIRECT study evaluated the effect of angiotensin II receptor blockade with candesartan versus placebo on the development or progression of retinopathy in a randomized controlled trial lasting 5 years involving 3326 patients with type 1 diabetes and 1905 patients with type 2 diabetes.[314,315] Most patients were normotensive, and all had normoalbuminuria (median urinary AER, 5.0 μg/min). The development of microalbuminuria was also evaluated.[316] In type 1 diabetic patients, the incidence of retinopathy was reduced by candesartan treatment but progression was not affected, whereas significant regression of retinopathy was seen in type 2 diabetic patients. The DIRECT study did not show any significant effect on the incidence of microalbuminuria.[316] The BENEDICT study has demonstrated that use of an ACE inhibitor, alone or in combination with a calcium channel blocker, decreases the incidence of microalbuminuria in hypertensive type 2 diabetic patients with normoalbuminuria. The effect of the calcium channel block verapamil alone was similar to that of placebo.[317] In the ADVANCE study, which included type 2 diabetic patients with or without hypertension, the fixed combination of perindopril and the diuretic indapamide also reduced blood pressure, and the development of new-onset microalbuminuria was reduced by 21% (95% CI, 0.14 to 0.27).[318]

The Randomized Olmesartan and Diabetes Microalbuminuria Prevention (ROADMAP) study tested whether the angiotensin II receptor blocker olmesartan could reduce development of microalbuminuria in 4447 mostly hypertensive type 2 diabetic patients with normoalbuminuria. Development of microalbuminuria was seen in 8.2% of the patients in the olmesartan group and 9.8% in the placebo group; the time to onset of microalbuminuria was increased by 23% with olmesartan (HR for onset of microalbuminuria, 0.77; 95% CI, 0.63 to 0.94; $P = 0.01$). Overall, there were slightly fewer cardiovascular events with olmesartan but more fatal events, although numbers were very small (15 vs. 3).[319]

In the ONTARGET study, 25,620 patients with atherosclerotic disease or diabetes (38% with diabetes) who had end-organ damage were randomly assigned to treatment with an ACEI, angiotensin receptor blocker (ARB), or both and were followed for a median of 56 months. The mean urinary albumin/creatinine ratio was 7.2 mg/g, and the sustained rate of decline in GFR was less than 1 mL/min/yr. Although the combination treatment reduced the increase in urinary AER, the number of events for the composite primary outcome of doubling of the serum creatinine level, need for dialysis, or death was similar for telmisartan ($N = 1147$ [13.4%]) and ramipril ($N = 1150$ [13.5%]; HR, 1.00; 95% CI, 0.92 to 1.09) but was increased with combination therapy ($N = 1233$ [14.5%]; HR, 1.09; 95% CI, 1.01 to 1.18; $P = 0.037$).[320] It is important to stress that the ONTARGET study did not include important numbers of patients with overt diabetic nephropathy. Therefore, the therapeutic risk or benefit for RAAS combination therapy in patients with diabetic nephropathy could not be addressed by this study. Patients intolerant to ACE inhibition ($N = 5927$), but otherwise similar at baseline to patients enrolled in the ONTARGET study, were randomly assigned to receive a placebo or ARB in the TRANSCEND study. Albuminuria increased less in patients receiving the ARB than in those receiving the placebo (32% [95% CI, 0.23 to 0.41] vs. 63% [95% CI, 0.52 to 0.76]). Very few patients (<2%) reached the prespecified renal end points, which were identical to those of the ONTARGET study, and no difference was seen between treatment groups with regard to these end points.[321]

In conclusion, RAAS blockade has been effective in reducing the frequency of development of microalbuminuria in hypertensive normoalbuminuric patients, whereas the effect has not been significant in normotensive patients. This would correspond clinically to a beneficial effect in most type 2 diabetic patients but not type 1 diabetic patients with normoalbuminuria (Figure 39.20). Possibly, the intrarenal RAAS is not enhanced in normotensive patients in contrast to hypertensive patients. However, the studies have used variable end points, intermittent or persistent microalbuminuria. Furthermore, the studies typically enrolled patients with very low levels of urinary albumin excretion. The use of ACEIs or other antihypertensive agents for the primary prevention of nephropathy in normotensive normoalbuminuric patients is not recommended in published guidelines.[322]

Odds ratio for development of microalbuminuria with RAS blockade

Trial	Odds ratio (95% CI)
Type 2 diabetes	
HOPE	0.80 (0.67; 0.95)
BENEDICT	0.57 (0.31; 1.05)
ADVANCE	0.79 (0.72; 0.86)
DIRECT	0.91 (0.70; 1.20)
ROADMAP	0.77 (0.63; 0.94)
Type 1 diabetes	
EUCLID	0.75 (0.63; 1.58)
DIRECT	1.04 (0.76; 1.44)
RASS-enalapril	0.66 (0.18; 2.42)
RASS-losartan	2.97 (1.11; 7.95)

Odds ratio (±95% CI)

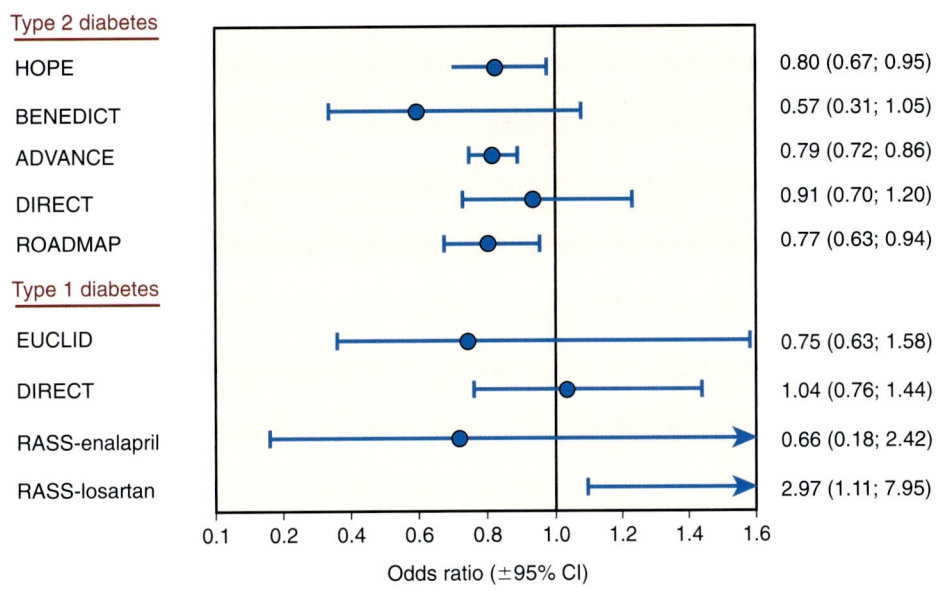

Figure 39.20 Odds ratios from various trials for progression from normoalbuminuria to microalbuminuria in patients with type 1 or type 2 diabetes treated with RAAS blocking agents.[313,316]

SECONDARY PREVENTION

A meta-analysis of 12 trials of 698 type 1 diabetic patients with microalbuminuria who were followed for at least 1 year has revealed that treatment with ACEIs reduces the risk of progression to macroalbuminuria compared with placebo (odds ratio [OR], 0.38; 95% CI, 0.25 to 0.57).[323] The rate of regression to normoalbuminuria was three times higher than in patients receiving placebo. At 2 years, the urinary AER was 50% lower in patients taking ACEIs than in those receiving placebo. Furthermore, it has been shown that the beneficial effect of ACEIs in preventing progression from microalbuminuria to overt nephropathy is long-lasting (8 years) and, more importantly, is associated with preservation of normal GFR.[324] Data from a 3-year, double-blind, randomized study found that long-acting dihydropyridine calcium antagonists are as effective as ACEIs in delaying the occurrence of macroalbuminuria in normotensive patients with type 1 diabetes with persistent microalbuminuria.[325] Finally, agents blocking the effect of the RAAS have a beneficial impact on glomerular structural changes in types 1 and 2 diabetic patients with early diabetic glomerulopathy.[326-328]

Borch-Johnsen and colleagues have analyzed the cost versus benefit of screening and antihypertensive treatment of early renal disease indicated by microalbuminuria in type 1 diabetic patients.[178] They concluded that screening and intervention programs are likely to have lifesaving effects and lead to considerable economic savings.

The impact of ACE inhibition in microalbuminuric type 2 diabetic patients has also been evaluated. A randomized study was conducted in which diabetic patients with microalbuminuria were treated with perindopril or nifedipine for 12 months.[329] Both treatments significantly reduced mean arterial blood pressure and urinary AER. Unfortunately, the study enrolled a heterogeneous group of hypertensive and normotensive patients with either type 1 or type 2 diabetes. Ravid and associates conducted a double-blind randomized study of 94 normotensive microalbuminuric type 2 diabetic patients who received enalapril or placebo for 5 years.[177] In the actively treated group, kidney function remained stable, and only 12% of patients developed diabetic nephropathy, whereas in the group receiving placebo, kidney function declined by 13%, and 42% of the patients developed nephropathy. These data have been confirmed in other studies.[294,295,312,330]

Antihypertensive treatment has a renoprotective effect in hypertensive patients with type 2 diabetes and microalbuminuria, although evidence has been conflicting regarding the existence of a specific renoprotective effect that is beyond the hypotensive effect of agents that block the RAAS in patients with type 2 diabetes and microalbuminuria.[296,308-311,331-336] The inconclusive nature of the previous evidence may have been due in part to the small size of the patient groups studied and the short duration of antihypertensive treatment in most previous trials. An exception is the long-lasting UKPDS, which suggested the equivalence of a β-blocker and an ACEI.[311]

To address this issue, Parving and coworkers have evaluated the renoprotective effect of the angiotensin II receptor antagonist irbesartan in hypertensive patients with type 2 diabetes and microalbuminuria in a study known as the IRMA 2 trial.[337] A total of 590 hypertensive patients with type 2 diabetes and microalbuminuria were enrolled in this multinational, randomized double-blind, placebo-controlled study of irbesartan at a dosage of 150 or 300 mg daily and were followed for 2 years. The primary outcome was the time to onset of diabetic nephropathy, defined by persistent albuminuria in overnight specimens, with a urinary AER higher than 200 μg/min and at least 30% higher than baseline level. The baseline characteristics in the three subject groups were similar (placebo, irbesartan at 150 mg daily, and irbesartan at 300 mg daily). Ten of 194 patients in the 300-mg group (5.2%) and 19 of 195 patients in the 150-mg group (9.7%) reached the primary end point as compared

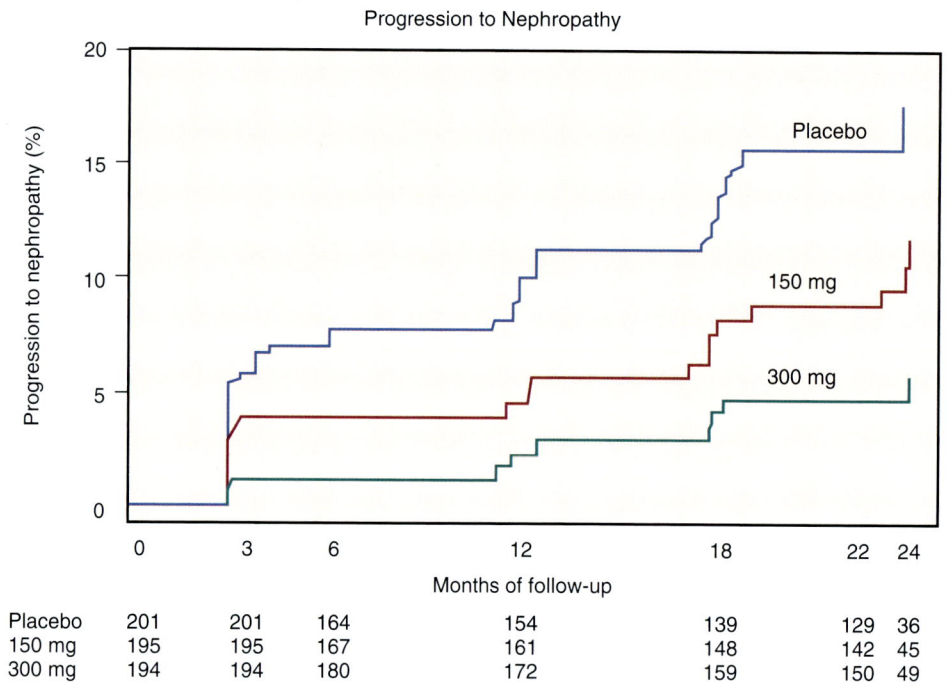

Figure 39.21 Probability of progression to diabetic nephropathy during treatment with irbesartan, 150 mg daily (*red line*), 300 mg daily (*green line*), or placebo (*blue line*) in hypertensive type 2 diabetic patients with persistent microalbuminuria. The difference between placebo and irbesartan 150 mg daily was not significant ($P = 0.08$ by log-rank test) but significant when compared to irbesartan 300 mg daily ($P < 0.001$ by log-rank test).

with 30 of 201 patients receiving placebo (14.9%; HR, 0.30; 95% CI, 0.14 to 0.61; $P < 0.001$ and HR, 0.61; 95% CI, 0.34 to 1.08; $P = 0.08$ for the two irbesartan groups, respectively; Figure 39.21). The average blood pressure during the course of the study was 144/83 mm Hg in the placebo group, 143/83 mm Hg in the 150-mg group, and 141/83 mm Hg in the 300-mg group ($P = 0.004$ for the comparison of systolic blood pressure between the placebo group and combined irbesartan groups). Serious adverse events were less frequent among the patients treated with irbesartan ($P = 0.02$). The IRMA 2 study demonstrated that irbesartan is renoprotective independently of its blood pressure–lowering effect in patients with type 2 diabetes and microalbuminuria. In a substudy of IRMA 2, irbesartan was found to be renoprotective independently of its beneficial effect in lowering 24-hour blood pressure.[338]

Another substudy has shown a persistent reduction of microalbuminuria after withdrawal of all antihypertensive treatment, which suggested that the dosage of 300 mg of irbesartan daily confers long-term renoprotection.[339] In addition, irbesartan treatment diminished inflammatory markers such as highly sensitive C-reactive protein, fibrinogen, and interleukin-6 when compared with placebo. The changes in interleukin-6 were associated with the changes in albumin excretion.[340] Remission to normoalbuminuria was more common in the irbesartan-treated patients than in those treated with placebo.[337] The importance of this finding is a slower decrease in GFR, as also demonstrated in the STENO-2 study.[194] Another study has demonstrated an enhanced renoprotective effect of ultrahigh dosages of irbesartan (900 mg daily) in patients with type 2 diabetes and microalbuminuria.[341] Finally, the cost-effectiveness of early irbesartan treatment versus placebo, in addition to standard conventional blood pressure–lowering treatment, has been demonstrated.[342] The beneficial effect of RAAS blockade in microalbuminuric patients was also shown in the INNOVATION study in an Asian population.[343]

Cardiovascular morbidity is a major burden in patients with type 2 diabetes. The STENO-2 study enrolled patients with type 2 diabetes and microalbuminuria and evaluated the effect on cardiovascular and microvascular diseases of an intensified, targeted, multifactorial intervention. This was comprised of behavior modification and polypharmacologic therapy aimed at several modifiable risk factors (hyperglycemia, hypertension, dyslipidemia, microalbuminuria), along with secondary prevention of cardiovascular disease with aspirin. This approach was compared with a conventional intervention addressing multiple risk factors.[104] Patients receiving intensive therapy had a significantly lower risk of cardiovascular disease (HR, 0.47; 95% CI, 0.24 to 0.73), nephropathy (HR, 0.39; 95% CI, 0.17 to 0.87), retinopathy (HR, 0.42; 95% CI, 0.21 to 0.86) and autonomic neuropathy (HR, 0.37; 95% CI, 0.18 to 0.79). In conclusion, a target-driven, long-term, intensified intervention aimed at multiple risk factors in patients with type 2 diabetes and microalbuminuria reduces the risk of cardiovascular and microvascular events by about 50%. In a poststudy follow-up, the effects were maintained after an additional 5 years. As noted, the incidence of ESKD was significantly reduced in the intensively treated group. Even more importantly, mortality was reduced in the intensively treated group (HR, 0.54; 95% CI, 0.32 to 0.89), which corresponded to an absolute risk reduction of 20% (Figure 39.22).[139] The cost-effectiveness of treatment was assessed after 8 years, and intensive therapy was found to be more cost-effective than conventional treatment. On the assumption that patients in both

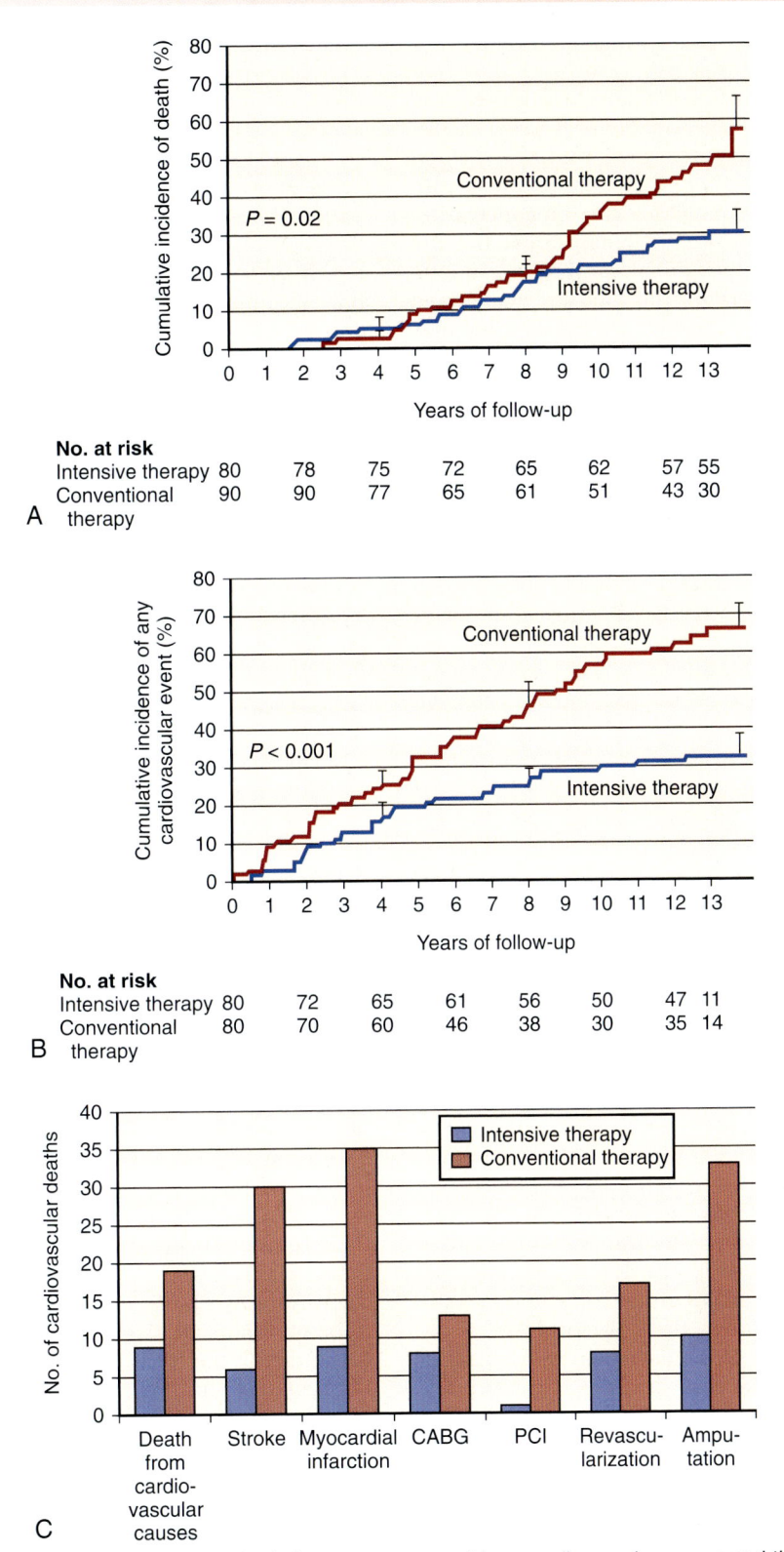

Figure 39.22 Kaplan-Meier estimates of the risk of death from any cause and from cardiovascular causes and the number of cardiovascular events, according to treatment group. **A,** Cumulative incidence of the risk of death from any cause (the study's primary end point) during the 13.3-year study period. **B,** Cumulative incidence of a secondary composite end point of cardiovascular events, including death from cardiovascular causes, nonfatal stroke, nonfatal myocardial infarction, coronary artery bypass grafting (CABG), percutaneous coronary intervention (PCI), revascularization for peripheral atherosclerotic artery disease, and amputation. **C,** Number of events for each component of the composite end point. **A** and **B**, I bars represent standard errors. (From Gaede P, Lund-Andersen H, Parving HH, Pedersen O: Effect of a multifactorial intervention on mortality in type 2 diabetes. *N Engl J Med* 358:580-591, 2008.)

arms are treated in a primary care setting, intensive therapy is cost saving and lifesaving.[344]

In 1995, a consensus report on the detection, prevention, and treatment of diabetic nephropathy with special reference to microalbuminuria was published.[345] Improved blood glucose control (HbA$_{1c}$ < 7.5% to 8%) and treatment with an ACEI is recommended. An audit of the implementation of this strategy in clinical practice has demonstrated that the beneficial outcome found in the initial, short-term, randomized clinical trial results could be confirmed and maintained for 10 years.[346] The American Diabetes Association has now stated that "Either ACE inhibitors or ARBs (but not both in combination) are recommended for the treatment of the nonpregnant patient with modestly elevated (30 to 299 mg/24 hr) or higher levels (>300 mg/24 hr) of urinary albumin excretion."[322]

NEPHROPATHY

From a clinical point of view, the ability to predict the long-term effect on kidney function of a recently initiated treatment modality (e.g., antihypertensive therapy) would be of great value because this could allow for early identification of patients in need of an intensified or alternative therapeutic regimen. In two prospective studies dealing with conventional antihypertensive treatment and ACE inhibition, Rossing and colleagues found that the initial reduction in albuminuria (surrogate end point) predicted a beneficial long-term treatment effect on the rate of decline in GFR (principal end point) in diabetic nephropathy.[347,348] These findings have been confirmed and extended.[221,349] Furthermore, similar findings have been demonstrated in nondiabetic nephropathies.[350,351]

The antiproteinuric effect of ACE inhibition in patients with diabetic nephropathy varies considerably. Individual differences in the RAAS may influence this variation. Therefore, the potential role of an ID polymorphism of the ACE gene on this early antiproteinuric responsiveness was tested in an observational follow-up study of young type 1 diabetic patients with hypertension and diabetic nephropathy.[352] The study found that type 1 diabetic patients with the homozygous II genotype are particularly likely to benefit from commonly advocated renoprotective treatment. The EUCLID Study demonstrated that urinary AER during lisinopril treatment was 57% lower in the II group, 19% lower in the ID group, and 19% higher in the DD group compared with the placebo group.[306] Furthermore, the polymorphism of the ACE gene predicts therapeutic efficacy of ACEIs against the progression of nephropathy in type 2 diabetic patients.[250] All previous observational studies in patients with diabetic and nondiabetic nephropathies had demonstrated that the deletion polymorphism of the ACE gene, particularly the DD genotype, is a risk factor for an accelerated loss of kidney function.[248,249,254,255,353-358] Furthermore, the ACE deletion polymorphism reduces the long-term beneficial effects of ACE inhibition on progression of diabetic and nondiabetic kidney disease.[254,356] These findings suggest that patients with the DD genotype should be offered more aggressive ACE inhibition, treatment with ARBs, or dual blockade of the RAAS. Further studies of appropriate therapy in patients with the DD genotype are warranted to test this hypothesis.

In an attempt to overcome a potential interaction between ACEI therapy and ACE deletion polymorphism, two studies evaluated the short- and long-term renoprotective effect of losartan in type 1 diabetic patients with diabetic nephropathy who were homozygous for the insertion or deletion allele.[359,360] The results suggested that this ARB offers similar short- and long-term renoprotective and blood pressure lowering effects in albuminuric, hypertensive, type 1 diabetic patients with the ACE II and DD genotypes. Also, data from the RENAAL study (see earlier) indicated that proteinuric type 2 diabetic patients with the D allele of the ACE gene have an unfavorable renal prognosis that can be mitigated and even improved by treatment with losartan.[361] In addition to the interaction between ACE inhibition and the *ADAMTS13* gene in the BENEDICT study, another example of pharmacogenetic interaction is the relationship between losartan and CYP2C9 of the cytochrome P450 superfamily.[258] This encodes an enzyme that metabolizes losartan and forms the active metabolite E-3174, responsible for the antihypertensive effect of losartan. The CYP2C9*3 polymorphism could modulate the blood pressure–lowering response to optimal monotherapy losartan treatment in hypertensive type 1 diabetic patients with diabetic nephropathy.[362] This illustrates the future potential of individualized therapy based on pharmacogenomic profiling.

Direct comparisons of ACEIs and ARBs have suggested that these drugs have a similar ability to reduce albuminuria and blood pressure in diabetic patients with elevated urinary albumin excretion.[363-365] These results indicate that the reduction in albuminuria and blood pressure induced by ACE inhibition is primarily caused by interference with the RAAS. Because reduction of proteinuria is a prerequisite for successful long-term renoprotection, one study investigated whether individual patient factors are determinants of antiproteinuric efficacy.[366] The results suggested that patients responding favorably to one class of antiproteinuric drugs also respond favorably to other classes of available drugs. Dose escalation studies of different ARBs have demonstrated that the optimal renoprotective dosage is 100 mg daily for losartan, 16 mg daily for candesartan, 900 mg daily for irbesartan, and 320 to 640 mg for valsartan.[341,367-369] In the SMART study, which included patients with urine protein levels of more than 1 g/day, of which 54% had diabetes, 128 mg of candesartan had a higher antiproteinuric effect than 16 mg of candesartan.[370] Unfortunately, less information is available about the optimal renoprotective dosage of the various ACEIs. At least for lisinopril, 40 mg daily seems to be the optimal dose.[371] A comparison of the antiproteinuric effect of the ARBs telmisartan and losartan in diabetic nephropathy has suggested that telmisartan is more effective.[372]

Initial short-term studies have indicated that the combination of ACE inhibition and angiotensin II receptor blockade may offer additional renal and cardiovascular protection in diabetic patients with elevated AERs.[373-379] A meta-analysis has suggested that the combination might be expected to reduce albuminuria by approximately 25% more than monotherapy.[380] These findings were consistent with results in experimental animal studies, suggesting that low-dose dual blockade of RAAS might achieve a more important reduction in kidney tissue angiotensin II activity than high doses of captopril or losartan.[381] However, as discussed earlier, the ONTARGET study of patients with low renal risk who had a mean urinary albumin/creatinine ratio of

7.2 mg/g and a sustained decline in GFR of less than 1 mL/min/yr but high cardiovascular risk demonstrated a salutary effect of dual blockade with telmisartan and ramipril on urinary AER within the normal range; this was accompanied by an increase in the composite primary end point of doubling of the creatinine level, need for dialysis, or death.[320] Importantly, a post hoc analysis demonstrated that changes in albuminuria were predictive of outcome in the study.[382]

In the Olmesartan Reducing Incidence of Endstage Renal Disease in Diabetic Nephropathy Trial (ORIENT), 577 type 2 diabetic patients with macroalbuminuria were randomized to the ARB olmesartan or placebo on top of the usual treatment (77% were treated with ACE inhibition). The study found that there was no significant effect on the primary end point—development of ESKD, death, or doubling of the serum creatinine level. In the olmesartan group, 116 patients developed the primary outcome (41.1%) compared with 129 (45.4%) in the placebo group (HR, 0.97; 95% CI, 0.75 to 1.24; $P = 0.791$).[383] The Veterans Affair Nephron Diabetes study (VA Nephron D) randomized 1448 patients with type 2 diabetes and macroalbuminuria and a eGFR of 30 to 90 mL/min/1.73 m^2 to lisinopril or placebo on top of 100 mg losartan once daily. The primary end point was first occurrence of a change in the eGFR (decrease ≥ 30 mL/min/1.73 m^2 if the initial eGFR was ≥60 mL/min/1.73 m^2 or higher or decrease ≥ 50% if the initial eGFR was <60 mL/min/1.73 m^2), ESKD, or death. The study was stopped early because of safety concerns. Among 1448 randomly assigned patients with a median follow-up of 2.2 years, there were 152 primary end point events in the monotherapy group and 132 in the combination therapy group (HR with combination therapy, 0.88; 95% CI, 0.70 to 1.12; $P = 0.30$). Combination therapy increased the risk of hyperkalemia (6.3 vs. 2.6 events/100 person-years with monotherapy; $P < 0.001$) and acute kidney injury (12.2 vs. 6.7 events/100 person-years; $P < 0.001$).[384] Thus, it has not been possible to demonstrate long-term benefits of dual RAAS blockade with ACE inhibition and ARBs.

In recent years, it has become clear that aldosterone should be considered a hormone with widespread unfavorable effects on the vasculature, heart, and kidneys.[233,385-387] It has been demonstrated that an elevated plasma aldosterone level during long-term treatment with losartan is associated with an enhanced decline in GFR in type 1 diabetic patients with diabetic nephropathy.[235] Consequently, aldosterone blockade could be considered for patients with suboptimal renoprotection during conventional RAAS blockade. Short-term studies in types 1 and 2 proteinuric diabetic patients have demonstrated that spironolactone safely adds to the renal and cardiovascular protective benefits of treatment with maximally recommended dosages of ACEIs or ARBs by reducing albuminuria and blood pressure.[388-390] The selective aldosterone blocker eplerenone has also been demonstrated to reduce proteinuria by 48% when added to an ACEI in type 2 diabetic patients with albuminuria (urine protein level > 50 mg/g).[391]

Recently, aliskiren, the first oral direct renin inhibitor, has been developed for treatment of hypertension, which makes it feasible to block the RAAS at the first rate-limiting step in the RAAS cascade. This occurs without an increase in plasma renin activity. In transgenic (mRen-2) 27 rats, the ACEI perindopril was compared with aliskiren. The drugs had similar effects on albuminuria and glomerular structural changes, but the amount of interstitial fibrosis was attenuated to a greater extent with aliskiren.[392] Another study of aliskiren using the same rat model demonstrated reduced expression of the prorenin receptor described by Nguyen and associates in 2002, and it has been suggested to be important for the development of renal and cardiac fibrosis.[393-396] The prorenin level has been demonstrated to predict diabetic microvascular complications, but whether aliskiren has specific protective effects remains to be established.[397,398] In type 2 diabetic patients with albuminuria, a significant reduction in urinary AER was seen after 2 to 4 days of treatment with aliskiren, 300 mg daily, with a maximal reduction of 44% after 28 days. Systolic blood pressure was significantly lowered after 7 days, with no further reduction after 28 days.[399] Another study of type 2 diabetic patients with elevated albumin excretion demonstrated a similar antiproteinuric effect of aliskiren and the ARB irbesartan. Importantly, a further antiproteinuric effect was seen when the agents were combined.[400] Increasing the aliskiren dosage to 600 mg daily did not significantly increase the antiproteinuric effect.[401]

The renoprotective effect of adding of a renin inhibitor to optimal renoprotective treatment with losartan 100 mg was demonstrated in the AVOID study, in which patients receiving optimal standard therapy were randomly assigned to receive aliskiren or placebo for 6 months. The study included 599 patients with type 2 diabetes. After 6 months, a reduction in albuminuria of 20% (95% CI, 0.09 to 0.30) was seen in the aliskiren-treated patients compared with those receiving only standard therapy. Side effects were few; in particular, hyperkalemia was not more frequent in the intervention group.[402] The long-term effects of combined therapy with aliskiren plus conventional antihypertensive treatment on cardiovascular and renal morbidity and mortality in type 2 diabetic patients were subsequently evaluated in the Aliskiren Trial in Type 2 Diabetes Using Cardio-Renal Endpoints (ALTITUDE) study, which included 8561 patients. The study was stopped prematurely after the second interim analysis. After a median follow-up of 32.9 months, the primary end point had occurred in 783 patients (18.3%) assigned to aliskiren as compared with 732 (17.1%) assigned to placebo (HR, 1.08; 95% CI, 0.98 to 1.20; $P = 0.12$).[403] Effects on secondary renal end points were similar. The mean reduction in the urinary albumin/creatinine ratio was 14%, which was less than in the AVOID trial. Hyperkalemia was significantly more common in the aliskiren group than in the placebo group (11.2% vs. 7.2%), as was the proportion with reported hypotension (12.1% vs. 8.3%; $P < 0.001$ for both comparisons). Thus, addition of aliskiren to RAAS-blocking treatment was not supported by the study and discouraged by the investigators and regulatory agencies.

Initiation of antihypertensive treatment usually induces an initial drop in GFR that is three to five times higher per unit of time than that during the sustained treatment period.[404] This phenomenon occurs with conventional antihypertensive treatment, β-blockers, and diuretics and when ACEIs are used. Whether this initial phenomenon is reversible (hemodynamic effect) or irreversible (structural damage) with prolonged antihypertensive treatment has been investigated in type 1 diabetic patients with diabetic nephropathy. The results supported the hypothesis that the faster initial decline in GFR is due to a functional (hemodynamic) effect of antihypertensive treatment that does not attenuate over time, whereas the subsequent slower decline reflects the beneficial effect on the progression of nephropathy.[404] A similar effect has been demonstrated in nondiabetic glomerulopathies.[405] In contrast, results of another study have suggested that the faster initial decline in GFR after initiation of antihypertensive therapy in hypertensive type 2 diabetic patients with diabetic nephropathy is due to an irreversible effect.[406]

In 1982, Mogensen described a beneficial effect of long-term antihypertensive treatment in five hypertensive men with type 1 diabetes and nephropathy.[407] A prospective study initiated in 1976 by Parving and coworkers demonstrated that early and aggressive antihypertensive treatment reduces albuminuria and the rate of decline in GFR in young men and women with type 1 diabetes and nephropathy.[408-410]

Figure 39.23 shows the mean values for arterial blood pressure, GFR, and albuminuria in nine patients undergoing long-term treatment (>9 years) with metoprolol, furosemide, and hydralazine.[410] Note that the data are consistent with a time-dependent renoprotective effect of antihypertensive treatment that in the long term might lead to regression of the disease (ΔGFR $\leq$ 1 mL/min/yr), at least in some patients. The same progressive benefit in ΔGFR over time has also been demonstrated in patients with nondiabetic renal diseases.[411] Regression of kidney disease (ΔGFR $\leq$ 1 mL/min/yr) has been documented in a sizable fraction (22%) of type 1 diabetic patients receiving aggressive antihypertensive therapy for diabetic nephropathy.[412] Remission of proteinuria for at least 1 year (urine protein excretion $\leq$ 1 g/24 hr) has been described in patients with type 1 diabetes participating in the captopril collaborative study.[413] Of 108 patients, 8 experienced remission during long-term

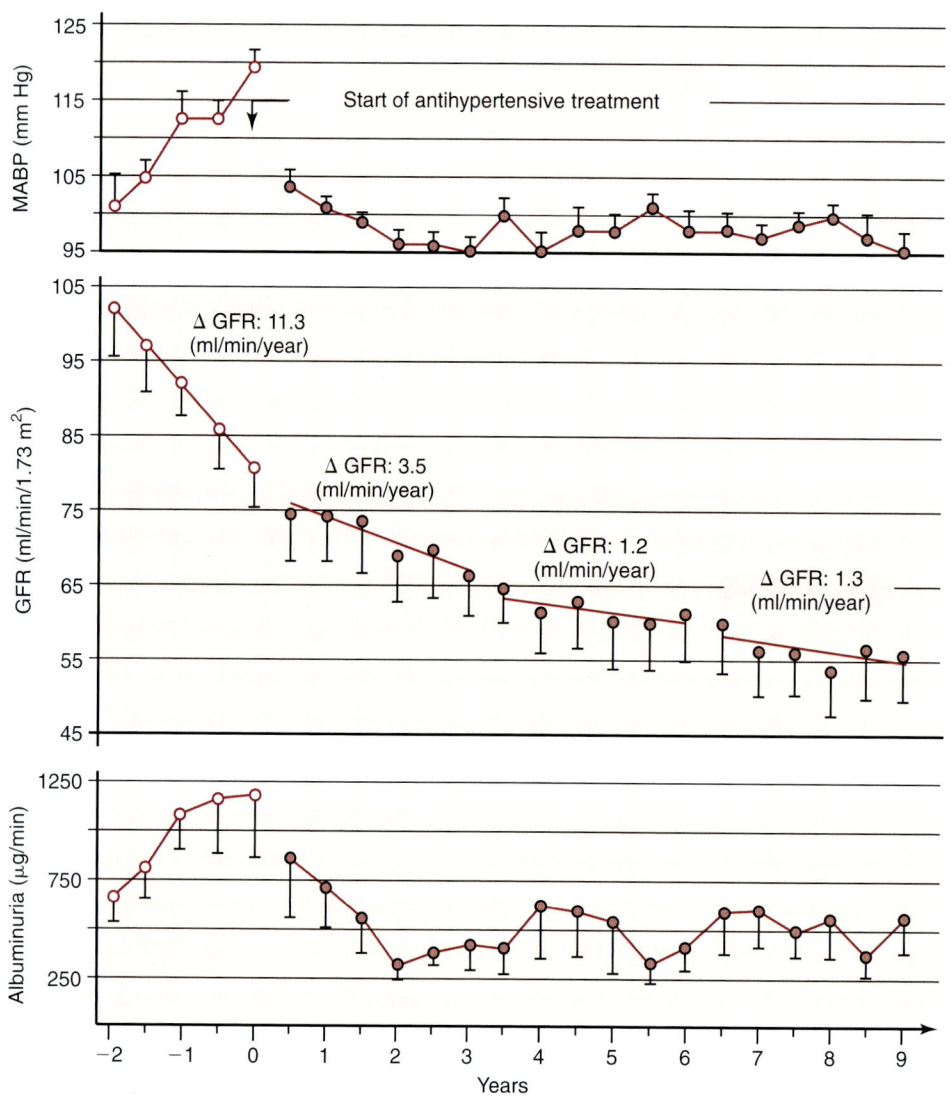

Figure 39.23 Average course of mean arterial blood pressure, GFR, and albumin before (*open circles*) and during (*solid circles*) long-term effective antihypertensive treatment on nine type 1 patients with diabetic nephropathy. (From Parving HH, Rossing P, Hommel E, Smidt UM: Angiotensin-converting enzyme inhibition in diabetic nephropathy: ten years' experience. *Am J Kidney Dis* 26:99-107, 1995.)

follow-up.[413] These findings were confirmed and extended in a long-term prospective observational study of 321 patients with type 1 diabetes and nephropathy.[414] The remission group, not surprisingly, was characterized by a slow progression of diabetic nephropathy and improved cardiovascular risk profile. More importantly, the prospective study suggested that remission of nephrotic-range albuminuria in types 1 and 2 diabetic patients, induced by aggressive antihypertensive treatment with and without the use of ACEIs, is associated with a slower progression in diabetic nephropathy and a substantially improved survival.[415,416]

In 1992, Björck and colleagues suggested that the use of ACEIs in patients with diabetic nephropathy confers renoprotection; that is, it has a beneficial effect on renal function and structure above and beyond that expected from the blood pressure–lowering effect alone.[417] Their investigation was a prospective, open, randomized study lasting for 2.2 years that included patients with type 1 diabetes. In 1993, the Captopril Collaborative Study Group demonstrated a significant reduction (48%; 95% CI, 0.16 to 0.69) in the risk of doubling serum creatinine levels in patients with type 1 diabetes and nephropathy who received captopril.[418] In comparison, the placebo-treated patients received conventional antihypertensive therapy, excluding calcium channel blockers. Long-term treatment (4 years) with an ACEI or long-acting dihydropyridine calcium channel antagonist was observed to have similar beneficial effects on the progression of diabetic nephropathy in hypertensive patients with type 1 diabetes.[419]

Thus, it was initially demonstrated that pharmacologic interruption of the RAAS slows the progression of renal disease in patients with type 1 diabetes, but similar data were not available for patients with type 2 diabetes.[103] Against this background, two large multinational, double-blind, randomized, placebo-controlled trials of ARBs—the RENAAL study and Irbesartan Diabetic Nephropathy Trial (IDNT)—were carried out in comparable populations of hypertensive patients with type 2 diabetes, proteinuria, and elevated serum creatinine levels.[420,421] In both trials, the primary outcome was the composite of a doubling of the baseline serum creatinine concentration, ESKD, or death.

A comparison of the benefits obtained in the RENAAL and IDNT studies is shown in Table 39.4. Side effects were low, and fewer than 2% of the patients had to stop taking an ARB because of severe hyperkalemia. The number of sudden deaths was not significantly different in the various treatment groups. Taken together, the results of these two landmark studies led to the following conclusion: "Losartan and irbesartan conferred significant renal benefits in patients with type 2 diabetes and nephropathy. This protection is independent of the reduction in blood pressure it causes. The ARBs are generally safe and well tolerated." A meta-analysis of the IRMA study and the two ARB trials revealed a significant reduction (15%) in the risk of cardiovascular events in the experimental groups compared with the control groups.[337,420-422] Based on these three outcome trials of ARBs, the American Diabetes Association now states that "in patients with type 2 diabetes, hypertension macroalbuminuria and renal insufficiency (serum creatinine > 1.5 mg/dL), ARBs have been shown to delay the progression of nephropathy."[322]

Early studies describing the prognosis for overt diabetic nephropathy observed a median patient survival time of 5 to 7 years after the onset of persistent proteinuria. End-stage renal failure was the primary cause of death in 66% of patients. When deaths attributed only to ESKD were considered, the median survival time was 10 years. All this was before patients were offered antihypertensive therapy.[103] Long-term antihypertensive therapy was evaluated prospectively from 1974 to 1978 in 45 type 1 diabetic patients who developed overt diabetic nephropathy. The cumulative death rate was 18% at 10 years after the onset of diabetic nephropathy, and the median survival time was longer than 16 years.[423,424] Rossing and associates went on to examine whether antihypertensive therapy also improved survival in an unselected cohort of 263 patients with diabetic nephropathy who were followed for up to 20 years; they observed a median survival time of 13.9 years, and only 35% of patients died because of ESKD (serum creatinine level > 500 μmol/L).[425] Fortunately, survival continues to improve; a median survival time of 21 years after the onset of diabetic nephropathy has been demonstrated (Figure 39.24).[426] A

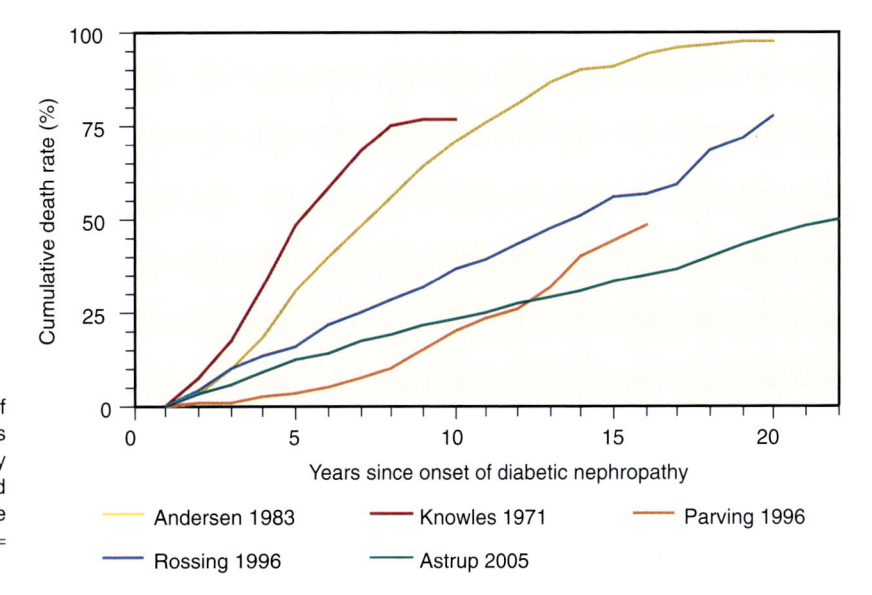

Figure 39.24 Cumulative death rate from onset of diabetic nephropathy in type 1 diabetic patients during the natural history of diabetic nephropathy (red line, N = 45,[572]; yellow line, N = 360[573]) compared with patients who had effective antihypertensive treatment (orange line, N = 45[424]; black line, N = 263[120]; green line, N = 199[426]).

recent study has confirmed an improved prognosis, with a further 50% reduction in age-adjusted mortality.[238]

The first information regarding the effect of antihypertensive treatment on the progression of nephropathy to come from a randomized, double-blind, placebo-controlled trial was presented by the Collaborative Study Group of Angiotensin-Converting Enzyme Inhibition, which examined the use of captopril in type 1 diabetic patients with diabetic nephropathy.[418] In this study, which lasted on average for 2.7 years, the risk of death or progression to dialysis or transplantation was reduced by 61% (95% CI, 0.26 to 0.80, $P = 0.002$) in the subgroup of 102 captopril-treated patients with a baseline serum creatinine concentration of more than 133 µmol/L and by 46% (95% CI, 0.22 to 0.76; $P = 0.14$) in the 307 patients with a baseline serum creatinine concentration below 133 µmol/L compared with placebo-treated patients. An economic analysis of the use of captopril in patients with diabetic nephropathy has revealed that ACE inhibition will provide significant savings in health care costs.[427]

In conclusion, the prognosis for diabetic nephropathy in type 1 diabetic patients has improved during the past decades, largely because of effective antihypertensive treatment with conventional drugs (β-blockers, diuretics) and ACEIs. Less information on this important issue is available for type 2 diabetic patients with diabetic nephropathy. The IDNT and RENAAL studies have demonstrated that there is a need for further improvement in prognosis for these patients.[420,421] Andresdottir and colleagues have demonstrated that multifactorial intervention with RAAS blockade and aggressive control of risk factors, including blood pressure, glycemic control, lipids and smoking, has also improved the prognosis significantly in type 2 diabetic patients with nephropathy, with a 50% reduction in age-adjusted mortality after 2000.[118]

LIPID-LOWERING THERAPY

In albuminuric patients with diabetes, the risk of cardiovascular disease is enhanced. Consequently, these patients should be treated with statins according to current guidelines for patients at high risk.[428] The renoprotective effect of 3-hydroxy-3-methylglutaryl-coenzyme A reductase inhibitors in patients with type 1 or 2 diabetes who have microalbuminuria or macroalbuminuria appears to be highly variable.[148] However, all nine studies examining this effect were of short duration, enrolled a small number of patients, and evaluated only a surrogate end point—namely, urinary albumin excretion. The effect of fenofibrate on macrovascular and microvascular outcome was evaluated in the FIELD study, which included 9795 type 2 diabetic patients.[429] The study also evaluated the effect on urinary albumin excretion. There was no effect on progression of urinary albumin excretion alone, but when data were combined for a slightly improved regression from microalbuminuria to normoalbuminuria and a reduced progression of albuminuria, it was observed that 2.6% more patients treated with fenofibrate showed no progression or a regression of albuminuria. This result was significantly different from that for the placebo group ($P = 0.002$).

The Study of Heart and Renal Protection (SHARP) investigated the effect of LDL lowering using a combination of simvastatin 20 mg and ezetimibe in 9270 patients with advanced CKD (3023 on dialysis and 6247 not on dialysis).[430] About 20% had diabetes. The combination therapy was used to reduce LDL cholesterol using a low dose of simvastatin (which should not be used in high doses for CKD due to side effects). The treatment reduced the incidence of major atherosclerotic events in a wide range of patients, including diabetic patients, with advanced CKD. There was no effect on mortality. On these grounds, most recent guidelines recommend the initiation of lipid-lowering treatment in all diabetic patients with CKD stages 1 to 4, which is in accordance with guidelines of the American Diabetes Association (ADA). The new guidelines also recommend not discontinuing treatment when patients progress to CKD stage 5 and ESKD. Controversy exists about whether statins should be initiated in these patients if they are already on renal replacement therapy.

DIETARY PROTEIN RESTRICTION

Short-term studies in type 1 diabetic patients with normoalbuminuria, microalbuminuria, or macroalbuminuria have shown that a low-protein diet (0.6 to 0.8 g/kg/day) reduces urinary albumin excretion and hyperfiltration independently of changes in glucose control and blood pressure.[431,432] Longer term trials in type 1 patients with diabetic nephropathy have suggested that protein restriction reduces the progression of kidney function, but this interpretation has been challenged.[433-436] Pedrini and colleagues have performed a meta-analysis and concluded that dietary protein restriction effectively slows the progression of diabetic renal disease, but their conclusion has been disputed.[437-439] A 4-year prospective randomized controlled trial with concealed randomization compared the effects of a low-protein diet with a usual-protein diet in 82 type 1 diabetic patients with progressive diabetic nephropathy. The end point of ESKD or death occurred in 27% of patients consuming a usual-protein diet compared with 10% consuming a low-protein diet (log-rank test, $P = 0.04$).[440] The relative risk of ESKD or death was 0.23 (95% CI, 0.07 to 0.72) for patients assigned to a low-protein diet after an adjustment for the presence of cardiovascular disease at baseline. Currently, a dietary protein intake of 0.8 g/kg body weight/day is recommended in the Kidney Disease Outcomes Quality Initiative guidelines for patients with diabetes and chronic renal disease stages 1 through 4.[428]

NEW TREATMENT OPTIONS

New options are needed to treat diabetic nephropathy, despite the success of the treatment modalities discussed. A number of new options have been suggested by experimental and clinical studies (Table 39.5).

Vitamin D (1,25-dihydroxyvitamin D_3) or activation of the vitamin D receptor with vitamin D analogues has recently been suggested to play a role in inhibiting the development of diabetic nephropathy. In addition, vitamin D is a negative regulator of the RAS.[441] In experimental studies, the combination of an ARB and a vitamin D analogue was more effective than either agent alone in preventing renal injury.[442] In three short-term studies evaluating the safety of the vitamin D analogue paricalcitol in patients with CKD, an

> **Table 39.5 Major Microvascular and Macrovascular Complications in Patients with Diabetic Nephropathy**
>
> Microvascular complications
> - Retinopathy
> - Polyneuropathy, including autonomic neuropathy (gastroparesis, diarrhea, obstipation, detrusor paresis, painless myocardial ischemia, erectile dysfunction; supine hypertension, orthostatic hypotension)
>
> Macrovascular complications
> - Coronary heart disease, left ventricular hypertrophy, congestive heart failure
> - Cerebrovascular complications (stroke)
> - Peripheral artery occlusive disease
>
> Mixed complications
> - Diabetic foot (neuropathic, vascular)

antiproteinuric effect was observed.[443] This therapy was evaluated in type 2 diabetic patients with microalbuminuria or macroalbuminuria in the Selective Vitamin D Receptor Activator for Albuminuria Lowering (VITAL) study, including 288 patients for 6 months, which found an 18% to 28% reduction in albuminuria with 2 μg paricalcitol, but no long-term data are available.[444]

Soludexide, a glycosaminoglycan mixture of heparin sulfate and dermatan sulfate, was found to reduce albuminuria in a pilot study but subsequently failed to reduce albuminuria in microalbuminuric or macroalbuminuric type 2 diabetic patients.[445] Tranilast is an antifibrotic agent that has been shown to suppress collagen synthesis in experimental models. Small studies in human patients found reduced albuminuria and type IV collagen excretion with tranilast treatment.[446] Analogues are now being developed because of concerns about potential adverse effects related to tranilast use.[447] Other antifibrotic approaches have been used with antibodies against growth factors, including CTGF and TGF-β, as well as the antifibrotic agent pirfenidone, which in a small study was demonstrated to reduce a decrease in GFR in low doses, whereas higher doses had more adverse events, leading to dropouts.[448,449]

As discussed earlier, several of the new glucose-lowering agents used for type 2 diabetes, including glitazones, dipeptidyl dipeptidase 4 inhibitors, glucagon-like peptide 1 receptor agonists, and sodium glucose transporter 2 inhibitors, have been suggested to be renoprotective. Although it is not clear if the effects are independent of the glucose-lowering action, most end points have been secondary, and studies on hard end points are lacking.

Endothelin receptor A antagonism was tested with avosentan because preclinical data demonstrated an albuminuria-lowering effect. The study was stopped early due to excess cardiovascular events with treatment.[450] Atrasentan is a selective antagonist with the same antiproteinuric effect but with less fluid retention in type 2 diabetic patients based on a short-term study of 211 patients.[451] This agent is now being tested in a phase 3 study that plans to enroll over 4000 participants, currently the only ongoing phase 3 study of diabetic nephropathy.

Experimental studies have suggested antiinflammatory agents or agents affecting oxidative stress to be potentially renoprotective. Bardoxolone methyl is an agent that reduces oxidative stress through the activation of nuclear factor (erythroid-derived 2)–like 2 (Nrf2). Short-term studies have demonstrated an increase in eGFR in type 2 diabetic patients with impaired renal function without affecting proteinuria.[452] Subsequently, a phase 3 study, including 2185 type 2 diabetic patients, aimed to show the effect on hard end points, but was stopped prematurely due to cardiovascular events.[453]

Pentoxifylline (PTF) is another antiinflammatory agent that was recently tested in 169 patients with type 2 diabetes for 2 years in an open-label study. The study demonstrated a between-group difference in decrease in GFR of 4.3 mL/min/1.73 m^2 (95% CI, 3.1 to 5.5 mL/min/1.73 m^2; $P < 0.001$) in favor of pentoxifylline.[454]

END-STAGE KIDNEY DISEASE IN DIABETIC PATIENTS

EPIDEMIOLOGY

Diabetic nephropathy is the leading cause of ESKD in most Western countries.[455] For many years, there has been a progressive increase in the total number of patients with ESKD. This has, to some extent, been driven by the increasing number of ESKD patients with diabetic nephropathy. In the 2005 report of the U.S. Renal Data System (USRDS; http://www.usrds.org), diabetes was reported as a comorbid condition in 159 patients/million, corresponding to 44.8% of incident ESKD patients (4.3%, type 1 diabetes; 40.5%, type 2 diabetes). It is very encouraging that first in Europe, and then in the United States, the rate of new ESKD cases due to diabetes has been plateauing. In 2011, in the United States, it was 4.2% lower than in the previous year and it has now fallen to a level not seen since 1998.[455a] In Europe, the proportion of diabetic individuals varies considerably among countries.[456] An average of 117 diabetic patients/million population/year develop ESKD and, again, the rate of new cases was plateauing in the European Renal Association–European Dialysis and Transplant Association (ERA-EDTA) registry in 2012 (www.ERA-EDTA-REG.org).[123] This is very important because the treatment of ESKD patients is very costly and the prognosis very poor, with a 5-year survival of patients with type 2 diabetes being only 20%.

The reason for the stabilized incidence of patients with diabetes and ESKD is basically unknown but may relate to the implementation of multifactorial intervention in patients with microalbuminuria and early stages of diabetic nephropathy, according to current clinical guidelines.[457] The number of patients with ESKD and diabetes reflects not only the number of patients with diabetic nephropathy. Many patients with type 2 diabetes will have a renal diagnosis different from diabetic nephropathy, and diabetes in these patients is a comorbid condition. One study has found that diabetes is present in no fewer than 48.9% of patients admitted for renal replacement therapy; and 90% of these had type 2 diabetes.[458] However, clinical features of classic Kimmelstiel-Wilson disease (large kidneys, heavy proteinuria) were evident only in 60% of these patients; 13% had an atypical presentation consistent with ischemic nephropathy (shrunken kidneys with no major proteinuria), and 27%

had a known primary kidney disease (e.g., polycystic disease, analgesic nephropathy, primary or secondary glomerulonephritis) with concomitant or superimposed diabetes. At the time of admission, diabetes had not been diagnosed in 11% of these patients. Although many factors may account for this, it has been argued that because patients often lose weight with advanced CKD secondary to anorexia, self-correction of hyperglycemia occurs.[459] Patients with diabetic nephropathy may completely lose hyperglycemia after weight loss in the preterminal stage and regain weight following refeeding on dialysis. Therefore, new-onset diabetes developing while patients are receiving dialysis may represent changes in dietary caloric intake because appetite improves with improvement in the uremic diathesis.

A diabetic patient with ESKD has several options for renal replacement therapy:

1. Transplantation (kidney only, pancreas plus kidney simultaneously, pancreas after kidney)
2. Hemodialysis (center, limited care, self-care or home dialysis)
3. Peritoneal dialysis (continuous ambulatory peritoneal dialysis [CAPD]), assisted, automated peritoneal dialysis (AAPD)

Currently, there is consensus that medical rehabilitation and survival are best after transplantation, particularly after transplantation of the pancreas plus kidney.[460,461] Survival on peritoneal dialysis and hemodialysis are inferior to transplantation, but comparable between peritoneal dialysis and hemodialysis.

MANAGEMENT OF THE PATIENT WITH ADVANCED RENAL FAILURE

The diabetic patient with advanced renal failure in CKD stage 4 or 5 has a much higher burden of microvascular and macrovascular complications (Table 39.6) than the diabetic patient without proteinuria or in the earliest stages of diabetic nephropathy. Measures of morbidity in diabetic patients with CKD exceed overall morbidity for all ambulatory clinic diabetics. Consequently, even when such patients are asymptomatic, they must be monitored at regular intervals for timely detection of complications (ophthalmologic examination at half-yearly intervals, cardiac and vascular status yearly, foot inspection at each visit), and they must be closely monitored for the need of conservative intervention against anemia and calcium metabolic abnormalities.

The physician who acts as a case manager for a diabetic patient with impaired kidney function has to face a spectrum of therapeutic challenges (Table 39.7). The most vexing clinical problems are related to coronary heart disease and autonomic polyneuropathy, but collaboration between diabetologists and nephrologists are mandatory in stages 3b, 4, and 5 to optimize conservative treatment of the uremic condition and planning of dialysis and transplantation.

HYPERTENSION

At any given level of the GFR, blood pressure tends to be higher in diabetic than in nondiabetic patients with CKD. Because of their beneficial effects on cardiovascular complications and progression of CKD, ACEIs or ARBs are obligatory unless there are temporary or persistent absolute or relative contraindications.[337,418,420,421,462] For example, there could be an acute major increase in serum creatinine concentration (e.g., renal artery stenosis, hypovolemia) or hyperkalemia resistant to corrective maneuvers (e.g., loop diuretics, dietary potassium restriction, omission of β-blockers, correction of metabolic acidosis). Because of their marked propensity to retain salt, patients with diabetic nephropathy have a tendency to develop hypervolemia and edema.[463] Therefore, dietary salt restriction and the use of loop diuretics are usually indicated. Thiazides are no longer

---

Table 39.6 Frequent Therapeutic Challenges in the Diabetic Patient with Renal Failure

Hypertension (blood pressure amplitude, circadian rhythm)
Hypervolemia
Glycemic control (insulin half-life, accumulation of oral hypoglycemic agents, HbA1c is falsely too low)
Cardiovascular comorbidities
Malnutrition—protein-energy wasting
Bacterial infections (e.g., diabetic foot)

And in Close Collaboration Between Diabetologists and Endocrinologists

Diagnosis and treatment of renal anemia
Diagnosis and treatment of calcium / phosphate metabolic changes
Timely creation of vascular access
Evaluation for preemptive transplantation of kidney and, in some cases, pancreas

---

Table 39.7 Potential New Treatment Modalities for Diabetic Nephropathy

Tested in Humans*

Vitamin D receptor stimulation[443,606]
Tranilast and analogues[446,447]
Protein kinase C inhibition[607]
Advanced glycation end product cross-link breakers[608]
Pyridoxamine[609]
Growth hormone inhibition (L. Tarnow, personal communication, 2011.)
Benfothiamine[610]
Pentoxifylline (MCP-1 inhibition?)[454,611]
Thiozolidinediones[288]
Endothelin antagonist[451,612]
Connective tissue growth factor inhibition[613]
Pirfenidone[449]

Tested in Experimental Models

Tissue transglutaminase inhibition[614]
Monocyte chemoattractant CC chemokine ligand 2 (MCP-1)[615]
Uric acid lowering (allopurinol)[616]
Nox 1/4 inhibition[617]

*Most of the studies are preliminary, dealing with small numbers of patients and surrogate end points.
MCP-1, Monocyte chemoattractant protein-1.

sufficient, at least in monotherapy, once GFR falls below 30 to 45 mL/min (CKD 3b and worse). When the creatinine concentration is elevated, multidrug antihypertensive therapy and dietary salt restriction are indicated. To normalize blood pressure it is necessary to administer, on average, three to five antihypertensive agents. In these patients, hypertension is also characterized by a high blood pressure amplitude (as a result of increased aortic stiffness) and by an attenuated nighttime decrease in blood pressure (non-dipping), which in itself is a potent risk predictor of cardiovascular events and accelerated progression to CKD.[464,465]

GLUCOSE CONTROL

Insulin resistance is often present in the early stages of CKD, and the prevalence of impaired glucose tolerance and fasting hyperglycemia is high. Insulin resistance is improved after dialysis is instituted. On the other hand, the biologic half-life of insulin is prolonged, and renal gluconeogenesis is impaired, which may cause a tendency to develop hypoglycemic episodes. More importantly, these patients often have lost or reduced their ability to sense low blood glucose levels because of the concomitant autonomic neuropathy. This risk is further compounded by the anorexia of ESKD patients.

Monitoring of glycemic control in ESKD is difficult due to the reduced life span of the erythrocyte and treatment with erythrocyte-stimulating agents (ESAs), leading to artificially low Hb_{A1c} values and a too-optimistic evaluation of the glycemic level. At the same time, many patients have difficulties in frequent measurements of glucose because of impaired vision and defective vascularization of fingers caused by their vasculopathy.

Antidiabetic treatment should be carefully considered. Most patients with type 2 diabetes will be treated with metformin according to all treatment guidelines. Metformin is totally metabolized through the kidneys via excretion in the urine. Therefore, the treatment must be stopped or carefully monitored once the GFR is below 45 mL/min, or earlier. If the patient continues the use of metformin into stage 3b or worse, she or he should be instructed to stop treatment and consult the endocrinologist if dehydrated due to fever, vomiting, or diarrhea, in which case he or she is at high risk of acute kidney injury (AKI) and lactic acidosis. Alternative treatments are glimepiride or DPP-4 inhibitors (dipeptidyl dipeptidase inhibitors), which are not metabolized or cleared by the kidneys. Many centers avoid glitazones because of their sodium retention effects and their cardiovascular risk profile. Hypoglycemia is feared by the patient but insulin is feasible, in particular if the patient can respond to hypoglycemia adequately. Insulin is also advantageous due to its universally anabolic actions in these often protein energy–wasted patients. For details on dosing contraindications and pharmacokinetics, refer to the recent report of the National Kidney Foundation.[466]

MALNUTRITION—PROTEIN-ENERGY WASTING

Patients with diabetes are predisposed to develop malnutrition and protein-energy wasting (PEW), particularly during periods of intercurrent illness and fasting. They may also have been given an ill-advised, aggressive recommendation of a protein-restricted diet, without attention to the potential risk of concomitant reduction of energy intake in anorectic patients. Malnutrition is a potent independent predictor of mortality, and its presence justifies an early start of renal replacement treatment.[467] Anorectic obese patients with type 2 diabetes and advanced CKD often undergo massive weight loss, leading to normalization of fasting and even postloading glycemia.

Wasting with accompanying low muscle mass is an important dilemma for treating physicians. The severity of renal failure may be underappreciated at any given level of GFR because serum creatinine concentrations can be spuriously low in such patients. This contributes to errors in dosing of drugs that accumulate in renal failure, and may also result in a belated start of renal replacement therapy. In advanced CKD (GFR < 60 mL/min/1.73 m^2), it is advisable to estimate the GFR using the Modification of Diet in Renal Disease equation, but even this estimate may overestimate the kidney function in diabetic patients with PEW.[468] Direct measurements of GFR may be superior to eGFR in this setting. It is important to make a total analysis of the clinical and biochemical situation, including an evaluation of calcium, phosphate, parathyroid hormone (PTH), and renal anemia to classify the true clinical stage of CKD and identify the medical needs of these patients.

ACUTE AND "ACUTE-ON-CHRONIC" RENAL FAILURE

Diabetic patients with diabetic nephropathy, especially those with multiple comorbid conditions, are particularly prone to develop acute renal failure (AKI) on top of chronic kidney disease.[469] In one series, 27% of patients with AKI had diabetes.[458] The most common causes of AKI were emergency cardiologic interventions involving the administration of radiocontrast agents, septicemia, low cardiac output, and shock. Prevention of radiocontrast-induced AKI necessitates adequate preparation of the patient with saline and temporary interruption of diuretic (and metformin) treatment.[470] The high susceptibility of the kidney to ischemic injury, at least in experimental diabetes, may be a contributory factor.[471] Not infrequently, AKI necessitates hemodialysis and carries a high risk of leading to irreversible chronic renal failure. This mode of presentation—as irreversible acute renal failure—has a particularly poor prognosis.[472] Even when the patient recovers from AKI, the risk of developing delayed CKD is high.[473]

VASCULAR ACCESS

Timely creation of vascular access is of overriding importance. It should be considered when the eGFR is approximately 20 to 25 mL/min. Although venous runoff problems are not unusual (due to venous occlusion from prior injections, infusions, or infections, as well as hypoplasia of veins, particularly in older female diabetic patients), inadequate arterial inflow has been increasingly recognized as the major cause of fistular malfunction.[474] If distal arteries are severely sclerotic, anastomosis at a more proximal level may be necessary. The use of native vessels is clearly the first choice, and results of grafts are definitely inferior. It is often necessary to create an upper arm native arteriovenous fistula or use a more sophisticated approach.[475-478] Arteriosclerosis of arm arteries not only jeopardizes fistula flow, but also predisposes to the steal phenomenon, with the potential for distal neurovascular compromise and the serious complications of finger gangrene or Volkmann's ischemic contracture.[479]

ANEMIA

Anemia is more frequent and more severe at any given level of GFR in diabetic patients with renal failure than in nondiabetic patients.[480] The major cause of anemia is an inappropriate response of the plasma erythropoietin (EPO) concentration to anemia. Inhibition of the RAAS may be an additional factor. In patients whose serum creatinine concentration is still normal, the EPO concentration predicts the future rate of loss of GFR.[481] Interestingly, a single-nucleotide polymorphism in the EPO gene promoter is associated with a higher risk of nephropathy and retinopathy.[482] There had been some concern that correction of anemia by erythrocyte-stimulating agents (ESAs), including classic EPO administration, may accelerate the rate of loss of GFR, but this has not been confirmed.[483] There is no controlled evidence concerning the effect of reversal of anemia by ESAs on diabetic end-organ damage. Although ESAs are retinal proangiogenic factors in diabetes, uncontrolled observations have indicated some improvement of diabetic retinopathy after ESA therapy, in line with experimental observations showing a protective role for EPO in retinal ischemia and diabetic polyneuropathy.[484-487] The TREAT study in type 2 diabetic patients in the early stages of CKD found no significant survival benefit from treatment with an ESA beyond guideline recommendations and noted an increased risk of hemorrhagic strokes. This study provided evidence to influence treatment strategies. Taken together with prior observations, current KDIGO guidelines for treating renal anemia recommend aiming for lower hemoglobin levels than previously used in asymptomatic, iron-replete patients.[487a]

INITIATION OF RENAL REPLACEMENT THERAPY

Many, but not all, nephrologists think that renal replacement therapy should be started earlier in diabetic than in nondiabetic patients (eGFR ≅ 15 mL/min). An even earlier start may be justified when hypervolemia and blood pressure become uncontrollable, the patient is anorectic and cachectic, and the patient's upper GI motility dysfunction complicates uremia and gastroparesis.

HEMODIALYSIS

In recent years, survival of diabetic patients receiving hemodialysis has tended to improve; the 2014 USRDS reported that 34% of patients with diabetes and ESKD were alive at 5 years following the initiation of hemodialysis.[456] Astonishingly high survival rates—for example, 50% at 5 years for diabetic patients undergoing dialysis—have been reported in East Asia. To a large extent, the differences among countries may reflect the frequency of cardiovascular death in the background population.

Intradialytic Blood Pressure

Diabetic patients undergoing dialysis tend to be more hypertensive than nondiabetic patients undergoing dialysis. Blood pressure is exquisitely volume-dependent in diabetic patients. The problem is compounded by the fact that patients are predisposed to intradialytic hypotension so that it is difficult to reach the target dry weight by ultrafiltration during a dialytic session. Although reduced dietary salt intake, long, slow dialysis, nocturnal hemodialysis, and added ultrafiltration may permit control of hypertension without medication, antihypertensive agents are required in almost all patients. The main causes of intradialytic hypotension are, on the one hand, disturbed counterregulation (autonomous polyneuropathy) and, on the other hand, disturbed left ventricular compliance, so that cardiac output decreases abruptly when left ventricular filling pressure is reduced by ultrafiltration.[488] One or more of the following approaches are useful to avoid intradialytic hypotension: daily dialysis with home-hemodialysis; long dialysis sessions; omission of antihypertensive agents immediately before dialysis sessions; and prescription or modelled ultrafiltration. If none of these methods works, however, alternative treatment modalities, such as hemofiltration, nocturnal hemodialysis, or peritoneal dialysis, should be considered. Intradialytic hypotension increases the risk of cardiac death by a factor of three.[489] It also predisposes to myocardial ischemia, arrhythmia, deterioration of maculopathy, and nonthrombotic mesenteric infarction, especially in older adults.

Elevated pulse pressure, impaired elasticity, and calcification of central arteries are major predictors of death and cardiovascular events in nonuremic patients. They are also significant predictors of death in nondiabetic patients. Paradoxically, for unknown reasons, these factors are not predictive in diabetic patients on hemodialysis.[490]

Cardiovascular Problems

Patients with diabetic nephropathy evidence high cardiovascular morbidity and mortality.[101] The survival of diabetic patients undergoing hemodialysis (and CAPD) is inferior to that of nondiabetic patients because of the high rate of cardiovascular death in diabetic hemodialysis patients. Stack and Bloembergen have examined the prevalence of congestive heart failure in a national random sample of patients entering renal replacement programs; they noted that the prevalence of congestive heart failure was significantly higher in diabetic than in nondiabetic patients, with the difference between these two groups even exceeding the difference observed between genders.[491]

Diabetic patients are at a greater risk of acquiring cardiovascular disease in the predialytic phase. The OR for the development of new cardiovascular disease was 5.35 for diabetic patients with established kidney disease who were not yet undergoing dialysis.[492] This explains the high prevalence of cardiovascular complications when diabetic patients enter dialysis programs. The rate of onset of ischemic heart disease is strikingly and significantly higher in diabetic patients than in nondiabetic patients on hemodialysis.[491-493]

When coronary complications supervene, the prognosis is also worse for diabetic patients than for nondiabetic patients. If myocardial infarction occurs, short-term and long-term survivals are poor in all hemodialysis patients. However, it is poorest in diabetic patients on hemodialysis, with a mortality of 62.3% in diabetic patients versus 55.4% in nondiabetic patients after 1 year and 93.3% versus 86.9% after 5 years.[494] Diabetic patients are also more prone to develop sudden cardiac death during dialysis sessions and more likely to die from sudden death in the interdialytic interval.[495] In diabetic patients undergoing dialysis, coronary calcification is more pronounced, and complex triple-vessel lesions are more frequent, but the high mortality rate is not fully explained by the severity of stenosing coronary lesions. The impact of ischemic heart disease is presumably amplified by further cardiac abnormalities such as congestive heart failure, left ventricular hypertrophy, and disturbed sympathetic innervations.[496,497] Fibrosis of the heart and microvessel disease with diminished coronary reserve and deranged cardiomyocyte metabolism with reduced ischemia tolerance may also be contributory factors.[498] Such functional abnormalities, particularly insufficient nitric oxide–dependent vasodilator reserve and perturbed sympathetic innervation, have been documented, even in the earliest stages of diabetes, and are especially frequent in diabetic patients undergoing dialysis.[499]

Therapeutic challenges include prevention in the asymptomatic patient and intervention in the symptomatic patient. With respect to prevention, unfortunately, little evidence-based information is available, but it is sensible to reduce afterload (by controlling blood pressure) and preload (by reducing hypervolemia). Despite the evidence of benefit from statin therapy in diabetic patients without renal failure, the 4D study (Die Deutsche Diabetes Dialyse Studie) found no reduction of the composite cardiac end point with atorvastatin therapy in type 2 diabetic patients undergoing dialysis.[500,501] The SHARP study was a bit more optimistic but also showed no effect on mortality in dialysis patients.[430] Diabetic patients with renal failure are characterized by the development of premature and more pronounced anemia. No controlled data are available regarding which target hemoglobin value is protective. In view of the outcome of the TREAT study, it is prudent to follow the guidelines strictly.

There is limited controlled evidence for the efficacy of ACEIs in diabetic patients undergoing dialysis. One controlled study in patients on hemodialysis treated with fosinopril showed no significant beneficial effect on outcome but, based on pathophysiologic reasoning, the administration of ACEIs or ARBs appears to be logical.[502] In view of the importance of disturbed sympathetic innervation, it is surprising that β-blockers are only sparingly administered to diabetic patients undergoing dialysis, although β-blockers have been shown to lead to better survival in observational studies, and carvedilol therapy resulted in substantially better survival in heart failure patients undergoing dialysis in a controlled interventional study.[503-505] It has been recommended to use the metabolically more advantageous β-blockers in this situation.[506]

In a very small series of diabetic patients with symptomatic coronary heart disease, active intervention, percutaneous transluminal coronary angioplasty (PTCA), or coronary artery bypass grafting (CABG) was superior to medical treatment alone.[507] In another series, only 15% of the surgically managed patients had experienced a cardiovascular end point after 8.4 months of follow-up compared with 77% of those in the medically managed group.[508] Because patients often fail to complain of pain, and because screening tests such as exercise electrocardiography and thallium scintigraphy are notoriously poor predictors, one should resort directly to coronary angiography if there is any suspicion of coronary heart disease. The use of gadolinium-enhanced magnetic resonance imaging is contraindicated at that stage of renal function.[509]

No dogmatic statements concerning the type of intervention are possible in the absence of controlled prospective evidence. Retrospective interventional studies have consistently shown more adverse outcomes in diabetic than in nondiabetic patients who were treated with CABG or PTCA.[508-511] After PTCA, the coronary reocclusion rate had been devastating in the past—for example, reaching 70% at 1 year in some series, even in nondiabetic hemodialysis patients. Results have improved considerably in recent years. More recent series have suggested markedly better outcomes after PTCA plus stenting than after PTCA alone.[512] However, the frequency of diffuse three-vessel disease with heavy calcification in diabetic patients undergoing dialysis remains a major problem.[513] A retrospective analysis of data for diabetic patients undergoing dialysis has suggested that CABG using internal mammary artery grafts, rather than CABG using venous grafts, yields superior outcome compared with PTCA, with or without stenting.[511] In view of the fact that renal failure per se aggravates insulin resistance, and that in uremia insulin-mediated glucose uptake of the heart is reduced, normalization of blood glucose levels by insulin and glucose infusion is presumably important for uremic patients with diabetes and ischemic heart disease.[514,515]

Glycemic Control

Dialysis partially reverses insulin resistance so that insulin requirements often become lower than before dialysis. In other patients, however, insulin requirements increase, presumably because anorexia is reversed, so that appetite and food consumption increase. It is conventional to use dialysates that contain glucose, usually about 200 mg/mL. This allows insulin to be administered at the usual times of day, reduces the risk of hyperglycemic or hypoglycemic episodes, and causes fewer hypotensive episodes.[516]

Adequate control of glycemia is important because hyperglycemia causes thirst and high fluid intake, as well as an osmotic shift of water and potassium from the intracellular to the extracellular space. This leads to circulatory congestion and hyperkalemia. Diabetic patients with poor glucose control are also more susceptible to infection.

Observational studies have suggested that good glycemic control in patients entering dialysis programs, as well as patients already undergoing dialysis, reduces overall and cardiovascular mortality.[517,518] As an indicator for monitoring glycemic control, glycated albumin is theoretically superior to HbA_{1c}, but this test is not routinely available; HbA_{1c} level may be falsely low because of a shortened erythrocyte half-life or EPO use and, in some assays, is confounded by carbamylation of hemoglobin.[519]

Type 1 diabetic patients obviously continue treatment with insulin in ESKD. In type 2 diabetic patients, alternative treatments are glimepiride or DPP-4 inhibitors which are not metabolized or cleared via the kidneys. Many centers would avoid glitazones due to their effects on sodium retention and their cardiovascular risk profile. Hypoglycemia is feared by the patients but insulin is feasible, in particular if the patients can adequately respond to hypoglycemia. Insulin is also advantageous due to its universally anabolic actions in these often protein energy–wasted patients.

Malnutrition—Protein-Energy Wasting During Dialysis

Because of anorexia and prolonged habituation to dietary restriction, the dietary intake of energy in diabetic patients on hemodialysis (recommended to be 30 to 35 kcal/kg/day) and protein (recommended to be 1.3 g/kg/day) often falls short of the target. It is of concern that indicators of malnutrition and microinflammation are more commonly found in diabetic patients than in nondiabetic patients undergoing hemodialysis.[520] PEW and high mortality remain a challenge in the treatment of ESKD patients. The challenge of treating PEW is even more complex in patients with diabetes who may be obese but yet protein energy–wasted. Several treatment modalities are available, including dietary intervention, intradialytic parenteral nutrition, and anabolic steroids in severe cases, but they are often of limited efficacy and not without compliance problems and adverse effects. Surprisingly, conventional indicators of malnutrition were not predictive of survival in diabetic hemodialysis patients, possibly because of the burden of the other serious comorbidities seen in these patients.[521]

Retinopathy

In the distant past, the visual prognosis for diabetic dialysis patients was extremely poor, and a high proportion of patients were blind after several months. Despite the use of heparin (which in the past had been accused of being a culprit), de novo amaurosis in patients on hemodialysis has become very rare.

Amputation

At the start of hemodialysis, 16% of diabetic patients have undergone amputation, most frequently above-ankle amputation.[522] The distinction between neuropathic and vascular foot lesions is crucial to improve outcomes because the treatment of the two conditions is quite different, and major amputation can be prevented by making the right diagnosis.[522-524] The presence of diabetic foot lesions is the most powerful predictor of survival in diabetic dialysis patients, possibly as a result of the associated microinflammatory state.[523]

PERITONEAL DIALYSIS

Peritoneal dialysis (PD) is not the most common treatment modality, at least in the United States. According to the 2013 USRDS report, as of 2011, some 45,750 incident diabetic patients were treated with hemodialysis, 2985 were treated with PD, and 437 underwent renal transplantation.[455a] The proportion of diabetic patients treated with PD varies greatly among countries, which illustrates that the selection of treatment modality not only is based on medical considerations, but also is strongly influenced by logistics, physician experience, and reimbursement policies. There are very good a priori reasons to offer CAPD treatment to diabetic patients with ESKD at the outset. For example, forearm vessels are often sclerosed, so that it is not possible to create a fistula. The alternative of hemodialysis via intravenous catheters (instead of arteriovenous fistulas or grafts) yields unsatisfactory long-term results because blood flow is low and the risk of infection is high. Long-term dialysis via catheter was identified as one major predictor of poor survival of patients undergoing hemodialysis.[525] There are additional reasons for offering PD to the diabetic patient, at least as the initial mode of renal replacement therapy. According to Heaf and associates, during the first 2 years, survival is better for patients treated with PD than for those treated with hemodialysis, and this was also true for diabetic patients, except for much older patients.[526,527] A survival advantage is no longer demonstrable beyond the second year (presumably because residual renal function has decayed by then). Moreover, PD provides slow and sustained ultrafiltration without rapid fluctuations of fluid volumes and electrolyte concentrations, facilitating blood pressure control and prevention of heart failure.

An interesting concept has been proposed by van Biesen and coworkers.[528] Patients who started treatment with PD and were transferred to hemodialysis after residual renal function had decayed had better long-term survival than patients who started treatment with hemodialysis and remained on hemodialysis throughout. As a potential explanation, it has been proposed that an early start on CAPD prevents the organ damage that accumulates in the terminal stage of uremia. Survival of patients who remained on CAPD longer than 48 months was inferior to that of patients on hemodialysis, presumably because CAPD is no longer sufficiently effective when residual renal function is gone, at least in heavier patients. It is also relevant that CAPD treatment presents no surgical contraindications to renal transplantation.

Although protein is lost across the peritoneal membrane, the main nutritional problem in PD is gain of glucose and calories because of the high glucose concentrations in the dialysate, which are necessary for osmotic removal of excess body fluid. This leads to weight gain and obesity. Daily glucose absorption is 100 to 150 g, and the CAPD patient is exposed to 3 to 7 tons of fluid containing 50 to 175 kg of glucose/year. The use of glucose-containing fluids causes another problem. Heat sterilization of glucose under acid conditions creates highly reactive glucose degradation products, such as methylglyoxal, glyoxal, formaldehyde, 3-deoxyglucosone, and 3,4-dideoxyglucosone-3-ene.[529] Glucose degradation products are cytotoxic and cause formation of advanced glycation end products (AGEs). Even in nondiabetic patients on CAPD, deposits of AGEs are found in the peritoneal membrane. AGEs trigger fibrogenesis and neoangiogenesis, presumably by interaction with RAGE, one of the receptors for AGEs.[530] The products also enter the systemic circulation, most likely contributing to systemic microinflammation.[531] These findings have led many to apply the term *local diabetes mellitus*.[532] Heat sterilization of two-compartment bags circumvents the generation of toxic glucose degradation products. In prospective studies, CAPD fluid produced using this sterilization technique was much less toxic than conventional CAPD fluid, despite the high glucose concentration.[533]

TRANSPLANTATION

KIDNEY TRANSPLANTATION

There is consensus that medical rehabilitation of the diabetic patient with uremia is best after transplantation.[460] Survival of a diabetic patient with a kidney graft is worse than that of a nondiabetic patient with a kidney graft. Nevertheless, because survival of a diabetic patient is so much poorer on dialysis, the percentage gain in life expectancy of a diabetic patient with a graft, compared with a diabetic patient undergoing dialysis who is on the waiting list, is much greater than that of a nondiabetic patient. Wolfe and colleagues calculated an adjusted relative risk of death in transplant recipients compared with patients on the waiting list.[460] The adjusted relative risk was 0.27 in patients with diabetes and 0.39 in patients with glomerulonephritis. Unfortunately, the perioperative risk is higher in diabetic than in nondiabetic patients. Nevertheless, in diabetic patients, the predicted survival after transplantation is substantially higher than the survival on dialysis (i.e., on the waiting list). Currently, patients with type 1 diabetes constitute the majority of diabetic patients receiving a transplant. Graft and patient survival were found to be acceptable in carefully selected type 2 diabetic patients without macrovascular complications who received kidney grafts, but transplantation of kidneys into type 2 diabetic patients violates current transplant criteria of the Eurotransplant International Foundation.[534] Diabetic patients must be subjected to rigorous pretransplantation evaluation which in most centers includes routine coronary angiography. Patients should also undergo Doppler ultrasonography of pelvic arteries and, if necessary, angiography to avoid attachment of a renal allograft to an iliac artery with compromised arterial flow and the attendant risk of ischemia of an extremity and amputation. Preemptive transplantation, (i.e. transplantation before initiation of dialysis), provides some modest long-term benefit.[535]

COMBINED KIDNEY-PANCREAS TRANSPLANTATION

After the seminal double transplantation by Lillehei in Minneapolis, the results of simultaneous pancreas and kidney transplantation (SPK) remained disappointing for a long time.[90] The breakthrough came with the introduction of calcineurin inhibitors and low-steroid protocols. Current regimens usually include initial induction therapy (antithymocyte globulin, alemtuzumab, or interleukin-2 receptor antagonists) and mycophenolate mofetil, tacrolimus, and steroids. This regimen reduces acute rejections after combined kidney-pancreas transplantation from 30% to 18%.[536] The bladder drainage of the exocrine pancreas secretion has been abandoned and has been substituted by enteric drainage. Efforts to anastomose the pancreatic graft vein to the portal vein have been abandoned.

There are four transplantation strategies:

1. Kidney only
2. Simultaneous pancreas plus kidney (SPK)
3. Pancreas after kidney (PAK)
4. Pancreas transplantation alone (PTA)

The graft survival has improved considerably, and the 5-year survival in 2010 was about 70%, according to the United Network for Organ Sharing.[536a] In 2010, 1200 U.S. pancreas transplantations were performed. Of these, about 900 were SPK and about 300 were PAK or PTA.

Reversal of established microvascular complications after SPK, at least in the short term, is minor, with the important exception of improvement in autonomic polyneuropathy and some improvement in nerve conduction.[537,538] SPK is associated with superior quality of life, better metabolic control, and improved survival.[461] It has recently been shown that excessive cardiovascular risk is also reduced by pancreas transplantation, but it takes approximately 10 years for the difference to become apparent.[539] This is analogous to the time span necessary for reversal of glomerular lesions in the kidney, presumably another example of so-called metabolic or epigenetic memory.[73] Survival of patients undergoing SPK was equal to and later surpassed by that of patients undergoing isolated cadaver-donor and even live-donor kidney transplantation. Beyond the 10th year, the HR was 0.55 for pancreas plus kidney transplantation compared with live-donor kidney transplantation alone.

There is an increasing tendency for early or even preemptive SPK.[540] Because graft outcome is progressively more adverse with increasing time spent on hemodialysis, this strategy may make sense.[541] In the United States, diabetic patients younger than 55 years are usually considered for SPK when GFR has become less than 40 mL/min, whereas in Europe the criteria are more conservative, requiring a GFR of less than 20 mL/min.[542]

An alternative strategy must be considered in the diabetic patient who has a live kidney donor; in a first step, the living donor kidney can be transplanted and, subsequently, once stable renal function has been achieved (GFR $\geq$ 50 mL/min), a cadaver donor pancreas is transplanted (PAK). The outcomes are quite satisfactory.[543]

Oral glucose tolerance normalizes after SPK unless the pancreas graft is damaged by ischemia or by subclinical rejection related to HLA-DR mismatch.[544] Most investigators find normalization of insulin sensitivity or some impairment of insulin-stimulated, nonoxidative glucose metabolism, possibly related to insulin delivery into the systemic circulation (as opposed to physiologic delivery into the portal circulation).[545-547] Impressive normalization of lipoprotein lipase activity and the lipid spectrum have also been reported, consistent with reduced atherogenic risk.[548]

An interesting issue is whether graft rejection affects kidney and pancreatic grafts in parallel. Although this is usually the case, which permits the use of renal function as a surrogate marker of rejection in the pancreas, it is by no means obligatory. Pancreatic biopsies are increasingly used. Pancreatic graft biopsy findings are also able to distinguish graft pancreatitis from immune injury to the graft. Pancreatic grafts are usually lost because of alloimmunity reactions but, in rare cases, graft loss resulting from destruction by autoimmune mechanisms has been described.[549] Recurrence of autoimmune inflammation (insulitis) in the recipient with lymphocytic infiltration and selective loss of insulin-producing β-cells (while glucagon, somatostatin, and pancreatic polypeptide-secreting cells were spared) was often seen in the pioneering era, when segmental pancreatic grafts were exchanged between monozygotic twins. Today this has become rare, presumably because immunosuppression keeps autoimmunity under control. Rejection of the pancreas responds poorly to steroid therapy. Its treatment should always include administration of T cell antibodies.

ISLET CELL TRANSPLANTATION

Sophisticated procedures such as transplantation of stem cells or precursor cells, transplantation of encapsulated islet cells, islet xenotransplantation, and insulin gene therapy are still beyond the horizon. Only islet cell transplantation has been tested so far. The initial enthusiasm raised by the Edmonton protocol waned after the long-term results were not confirmed by a multicenter study, which possibly reflected single-site expertise or the effect of the heavy immunosuppression regimens.[550,551] Therefore, this approach currently has been largely abandoned, but there are ongoing clinical trials testing various aspects of this treatment approach. It is noteworthy that recent reports have raised the promise of stem cell–based approaches to β-cell regeneration.[552]

NEW-ONSET DIABETES AFTER TRANSPLANTATION

An increasingly serious problem of solid organ transplantation, including renal transplantation, is the de novo appearance of diabetes (also called new-onset diabetes after transplantation [NODAT] or posttransplantation diabetes mellitus [PTDM]). This was seen in 17.4% of recipients in Spain and in up to 21% of recipients in the United States at 10 years.[553,554] It was previously reported to be even higher, mainly because there were no valid data on glucometabolic characteristics before transplantation. The diagnosis was often based on the use of insulin postoperatively, oral agents used, random glucose monitoring, and a fasting glucose value of 7 to 13 mmol/L (126 to 234 mg/dL).

There is a huge variation in the literature regarding risk factors for developing NODAT. They can be divided into factors related to glucose metabolism or patient demographics and into modifiable and nonmodifiable factors. Screening for risk factors should start early and be reevaluated while the patient is on the waiting list. Patients on the waiting list for renal transplantation and transplanted patients share many characteristics in having hyperglycemia, disturbed insulin secretion, and increased insulin resistance. Predictors of de novo diabetes are a family history of diabetes, older age, African American ethnicity, obesity, hepatitis C, and treatment with steroids and calcineurin inhibitors.[553,555] The DIRECT study found a significantly lower incidence of new-onset diabetes and impaired fasting glucose level in patients treated with cyclosporine (26.0%) than in those receiving tacrolimus (33.6%), but currently the difference between these two drugs is still debated.[556] Reduction of the steroid dosage improves glycemic control, but complete withdrawal provides no metabolic benefit compared with 5 mg/day prednisolone and increases the risk of graft rejection.[557,558] Complications include increased cardiovascular events and even delayed graft loss from allograft diabetic nephropathy.[559,560] More recently, new guidelines on NODAT have been published, based on experience in Scandinavian countries.[561]

BLADDER DYSFUNCTION

Bladder dysfunction as a sequela of autonomic diabetic polyneuropathy is frequent in diabetic patients. In males, this is often combined with erectile dysfunction.[562] Disabling symptoms are rare, however. Bladder dysfunction is frequently associated with other features of autonomic polyneuropathy, such as postural hypotension, gastroparesis, constipation, and nocturnal diarrhea.

URINARY TRACT INFECTIONS

It has been long controversial whether the frequency of bacteriuria is higher in diabetic patients, but there has never been any doubt that symptomatic urinary tract infections (UTIs) are more severe and more aggressive. A higher prevalence of UTIs, usually asymptomatic, was initially found by Vejlsgaard in female diabetic patients (18.8% vs. 7.9% in controls), but not in males with diabetes.[563] The results of prospective studies remained controversial. A more recent prospective study in diabetic and nondiabetic women has shown that the incidence of UTIs and asymptomatic bacteriuria is twice as high in diabetic than in nondiabetic women.[564] UTIs may also pose problems after renal transplantation.[565]

The spectrum of bacterial isolates as well as the resistance rates to antibiotics did not differ between diabetic and nondiabetic individuals.[566] Symptomatic UTIs definitely run a more aggressive course in diabetic patients. By multivariate analysis, diabetes and poor glycemic control were found to be independent factors associated with upper urinary tract involvement.[567] UTIs in diabetic patients may also lead to complications such as prostatic abscess, emphysematous cystitis, pyelonephritis, intrarenal abscess formation, renal carbuncle and penile necrosis (Fournier's disease).[122,568,569] Renal papillary necrosis was common in the past but has virtually disappeared, according to one autopsy series.[570] Extrarenal bacterial metastases (e.g., endophthalmitis, spondylitis, endocarditis, iliopsoas abscess formation) are common in patients with UTIs and septicemia, particularly UTIs caused by methicillin-resistant staphylococci.[571]

The reasons for the possibly higher frequency and definitely higher severity of UTIs in diabetic patients are not known, but may include more favorable conditions for bacterial growth (glucosuria), defective neutrophil function, increased adherence to uroepithelial cells, and impaired bladder evacuation (detrusor paresis).

In regard to the management of UTI, no clear benefits of antibiotic therapy have been demonstrated for the treatment of asymptomatic bacteriuria in diabetic patients. Community-acquired, symptomatic, lower UTIs may be managed with trimethoprim, trimethoprim sulfamethoxazole, or gyrase inhibitors. For nosocomially acquired UTIs, sensitivity testing and sensitivity-directed antibiotic intervention are necessary. Invasive candiduria can be managed with amphotericin by irrigation or systemic administration of fungicidal agents.

Complete reference list available at ExpertConsult.com.

KEY REFERENCES

3. Rossing P: Prediction, progression and prevention of diabetic nephropathy. The Minkowski Lecture 2005. *Diabetologia* 49:11–19, 2006.
8. Fioretto P, Mauer M: Histopathology of diabetic nephropathy. *Semin Nephrol* 27:195–207, 2007.
51. Caramori ML, Fioretto P, Mauer M: Enhancing the predictive value of urinary albumin for diabetic nephropathy. *J Am Soc Nephrol* 17:339–352, 2006.
57. Østerby R, Gall MA, Schmitz A, et al: Glomerular structure and function in proteinuric type 2 (non-insulin-dependent) diabetic patients. *Diabetologia* 36:1064–1070, 1993.
61. Fioretto P, Mauer SM, Brocco E, et al: Patterns of renal injury in NIDDM patients with microalbuminuria. *Diabetologia* 39:1569–1576, 1996.

67. Christensen PK, Larsen S, Horn T, et al: Renal function and structure in albuminuric type 2 diabetic patients without retinopathy. *Nephrol Dial Transplant* 16:2337–2347, 2001.
73. Fioretto P, Steffes MW, Sutherland DER, et al: Reversal of lesions of diabetic nephropathy after pancreas transplantation. *N Engl J Med* 339:69–75, 1998.
100. Fox CS, Matsushita K, Woodward M, et al: Associations of kidney disease measures with mortality and end-stage renal disease in individuals with and without diabetes: a meta-analysis. *Lancet* 380:1662–1673, 2012.
101. Deckert T, Feldt-Rasmussen B, Borch-Johnsen K, et al: Albuminuria reflects widespread vascular damage. The Steno hypothesis. *Diabetologia* 32:219–226, 1989.
114. Parving HH: Diabetic nephropathy: Prevention and treatment. *Kidney Int* 60:2041–2055, 2001.
115. Groop PH, Thomas MC, Moran JL, et al: The presence and severity of chronic kidney disease predicts all-cause mortality in type 1 diabetes. *Diabetes* 58:1651–1658, 2009.
118. Andresdottir G, Jensen ML, Carstensen B, et al: Improved survival and renal prognosis of patients with type 2 diabetes and nephropathy with improved control of risk factors. *Diabetes Care* 37:1660–1667, 2014.
139. Gaede P, Lund-Andersen H, Parving HH, et al: Effect of a multifactorial intervention on mortality in type 2 diabetes. *N Engl J Med* 358:580–591, 2008.
155. Hostetter TH, Troy JL, Brenner BM: Glomerular hemodynamics in experimental diabetes mellitus. *Kidney Int* 19:410–415, 1981.
173. American Diabetes Association: Standards of medical care in diabetes—2009. *Diabetes Care* 32:S13–S61, 2009.
174. Lambers Heerspink HJ, Gansevoort RT, Brenner BM, et al: Comparison of different measures of urinary protein excretion for prediction of renal events. *J Am Soc Nephrol* 21:1355–1360, 2010.
208. Nelson RG, Bennett PH, Beck GJ, et al: Development and progression of renal disease in Pima Indians with non-insulin-dependent diabetes mellitus. *N Engl J Med* 335:1636–1642, 1996.
216. Hovind P, Rossing P, Tarnow L, et al: Progression of diabetic nephropathy. *Kidney Int* 59:702–709, 2001.
217. Rossing K, Christensen PK, Hovind P, et al: Progression of nephropathy in type 2 diabetic patients. *Kidney Int* 66:1596–1605, 2004.
218. Keane WF, Brenner BM, de Zeeuw D, et al: The risk of developing end-stage renal disease in patients with type 2 diabetes and nephropathy: the RENAAL study. *Kidney Int* 63:1499–1507, 2003.
223. Hostetter TH, Rennke HG, Brenner BM: The case for intrarenal hypertension in the initiation and progression of diabetic and other glomerulopathies. *Am J Med* 72:375–380, 1982.
238. Andresdottir G, Jensen ML, Carstensen B, et al: Improved prognosis of diabetic nephropathy in type 1 diabetes. *Kidney Int* 87(2):417–426, 2014.
264. Pfeffer MA, Burdmann EA, Chen CY, et al: A trial of darbepoetin alfa in type 2 diabetes and chronic kidney disease. *N Engl J Med* 361:2019–2032, 2009.
274. Rossing K, Mischak H, Dakna M, et al: Urinary proteomics in diabetes and CKD. *J Am Soc Nephrol* 19:1283–1290, 2008.
282. de Boer IH, Sun W, Cleary PA, et al: Intensive diabetes therapy and glomerular filtration rate in type 1 diabetes. *N Engl J Med* 365:2366–2376, 2011.
286. ADVANCE Collaborative Group, Patel A, MacMahon S, et al: Intensive blood glucose control and vascular outcomes in patients with type 2 diabetes. *N Engl J Med* 358:2560–2572, 2008.
301. Zatz R, Dunn BR, Meyer TW, et al: Prevention of diabetic glomerulopathy by pharmacological amelioration of glomerular capillary hypertension. *J Clin Invest* 77:1925–1930, 1986.
308. Heart Outcomes Prevention Evaluation (HOPE) Study Investigators: Effects of ramipril on cardiovascular and microvascular outcomes in people with diabetes mellitus: results of the HOPE study and MICRO-HOPE substudy. *Lancet* 355:253–259, 2000.
319. Haller H, Ito S, Izzo JL, Jr, et al: Olmesartan for the delay or prevention of microalbuminuria in type 2 diabetes. *N Engl J Med* 364:907–917, 2011.
322. American Diabetes Association: Standards of medical care in diabetes—2014. *Diabetes Care* 37:S14–S80, 2014.
323. ACE Inhibitors in Diabetic Nephropathy Trialist Group: Should all patients with type 1 diabetes mellitus and microalbuminuria receive angiotensin-converting enzyme inhibitors? A meta-analysis of individual patient data. *Ann Intern Med* 134:370–379, 2001.
324. Mathiesen ER, Hommel E, Hansen HP, et al: Randomised controlled trial of long-term efficacy of captopril on preservation of kidney function in normotensive patients with insulin dependent diabetes and microalbuminuria. *BMJ* 319:24–25, 1999.
349. de Zeeuw D, Remuzzi G, Parving HH, et al: Proteinuria, a target for renoprotection in patients with type 2 diabetic nephropathy: lessons from RENAAL. *Kidney Int* 65:2309–2320, 2004.
361. Parving HH, de Zeeuw D, Cooper ME, et al: ACE gene polymorphism and losartan treatment in type 2 diabetic patients with nephropathy. *J Am Soc Nephrol* 19:771–779, 2008.
382. Schmieder RE, Mann JF, Schumacher H, et al: Changes in albuminuria predict mortality and morbidity in patients with vascular disease. *J Am Soc Nephrol* 22:1353–1364, 2011.
384. Fried LF, Emanuele N, Zhang JH, et al: Combined angiotensin inhibition for the treatment of diabetic nephropathy. *N Engl J Med* 369:1892–1903, 2013.
389. Schjoedt KJ, Rossing K, Juhl TR, et al: Beneficial impact of spironolactone in diabetic nephropathy. *Kidney Int* 68:2829–2836, 2005.
403. Parving HH, Brenner BM, McMurray JJ, et al: Cardiorenal end points in a trial of aliskiren for type 2 diabetes. *N Engl J Med* 367:2204–2213, 2012.
418. Lewis E, Hunsicker L, Bain R, et al: The effect of angiotensin-converting enzyme inhibition on diabetic nephropathy. *N Engl J Med* 329:1456–1462, 1993.
420. Brenner BM, Cooper ME, de Zeeuw D, et al: Effects of losartan on renal and cardiovascular outcomes in patients with type 2 diabetes and nephropathy. *N Engl J Med* 345:861–869, 2001.
421. Lewis EJ, Hunsicker LG, Clarke WR, et al: Renoprotective effect of the angiotensin-receptor antagonist irbesartan in patients with nephropathy due to type 2 diabetes. *N Engl J Med* 345:851–860, 2001.
451. de Zeeuw D, Coll B, Andress D, et al: The endothelin antagonist atrasentan lowers residual albuminuria in patients with type 2 diabetic nephropathy. *J Am Soc Nephrol* 25:1083–1093, 2014.
453. de Zeeuw D, Akizawa T, Audhya P, et al: Bardoxolone methyl in type 2 diabetes and stage 4 chronic kidney disease. *N Engl J Med* 369:2492–2503, 2013.
462. Yusuf S, Sleight P, Pogue J, et al: Effects of an angiotensin-converting enzyme inhibitor, ramipril, on cardiovascular events in high-risk patients. The Heart Outcomes Prevention Evaluation Study Investigators. *N Engl J Med* 342:145–153, 2000.
466. National Kidney Foundation: KDOQI clinical practice guideline for diabetes and CKD: 2012 update. *Am J Kidney Dis* 60:850–886, 2012.
494. Herzog CA, Ma JZ, Collins AJ: Poor long-term survival after acute myocardial infarction among patients on long-term dialysis. *N Engl J Med* 339:799–805, 1998.
500. Colhoun HM, Betteridge DJ, Durrington PN, et al: Primary prevention of cardiovascular disease with atorvastatin in type 2 diabetes in the Collaborative Atorvastatin Diabetes Study (CARDS): multicentre randomised placebo-controlled trial. *Lancet* 364:685–696, 2004.
501. Wanner C, Krane V, Marz W, et al: Atorvastatin in patients with type 2 diabetes mellitus undergoing hemodialysis. *N Engl J Med* 353:238–248, 2005.
561. Hornum M, Lindahl JP, von Zur-Muhlen B, et al: Diagnosis, management and treatment of glucometabolic disorders emerging after kidney transplantation: a position statement from the Nordic Transplantation Societies. *Transpl Int* 26:1049–1060, 2013.
604. Niewczas MA, Gohda T, Skupien J, et al: Circulating TNF receptors 1 and 2 predict ESKD in type 2 diabetes. *J Am Soc Nephrol* 23:507–515, 2012.

Index

A

AA amyloidosis, 1128-1132, 1157, 2485
Abatacept, 1104-1105
ABCG2, 221, 221*t*
Abdomen, plain radiograph of, 846, 847*f*, 873
Abdominal aortic aneurysm, 1261
Abdominal compartment syndrome, 999, 2138
ABO blood group antigens, 2236-2237, 2581-2582
ABO-incompatible renal transplantation, 2156-2157, 2423
Aboriginal Australians. *See* Australia, indigenous (Aboriginals) population of
Abscess, renal. *See* Renal abscess
Absolute hypovolemia. *See* Hypovolemia, absolute
Acanthocytes, 756, 756*f*
Accountable care organizations, 2631-2632
Accuracy, of estimating glomerular filtration rate equations, 785
Acebutolol, 1656*t*-1657*t*, 1658
Acellular tissue matrices, 2610
Acetaminophen poisoning, 2187-2188
Acetazolamide, 450, 541, 629, 1704
Acetoacetic acid, in ketoacidosis, 247
Acetylcholine, 101-102, 110
Acetylcholine receptor, 587-588
N-Acetyl-seryl-lysyl-proline, 1887-1888
Acid(s)
   dietary sources of, 517
   excretion of, diurnal variation in, 256
   production of, 514-515
   protein catabolism for generation of, 517
   renal excretion of, 518-519
Acid/alkali-sensing receptors, 256
Acid-base balance
   age-related changes in, 740-741, 740*f*
   in children, 2382-2383, 2382*t*
   in elderly, 740-741, 740*f*
   hyperkalemia and, 537
   renal regulation of, 514-515
Acid-base disorders. *See also specific disorder*
   cellular adaptations to, 245-246
   compensatory mechanisms for, 513-514, 516, 517*f*
   diagnosis of, 511, 521-525, 521*t*, 524*t*
   management of, 511
   mixed, 521-523, 525, 550-552
   urinary tract infection and, 778
Acid-base homeostasis, 512-514
   buffer systems in, 512-514
   citrate excretion in, 247-248
   description of, 5, 512
   hepatic role in, 517

Acid-base homeostasis *(Continued)*
   organic anion excretion in, 247-248
   pulmonary involvement in, 512
   renal role in, 517
   sensors involved in, 256
   soluble adenylyl cyclase in, 256
   type B intercalated cell in, 241
Acid-base nomogram, 522, 522*f*
Acid-base regulation, 331, 1749
Acid-base status, 237, 563, 1336-1337
Acid-base transport, 244
Acid-base transporters, 238, 1454-1457
Acidemia, 518, 522, 2177
Acidosis
   adverse effects of, 1758-1759
   causes of, 526*t*
   of chronic kidney disease, 549-550, 684-685, 1758-1759
   collecting duct's response to, 244
   in elderly, 740
   high anion gap. *See* High anion gap acidosis
   hyperkalemic, 572
   insulin resistance and, 1816-1817
   lactic. *See* Lactic acidosis
   metabolic. *See* Metabolic acidosis
   normal anion gap, 525*t*
   of progressive renal failure, 541-543
   respiratory. *See* Respiratory acidosis
   uremic, 549-550
Acquired immunodeficiency syndrome, 883
Acquired perforating dermatosis, 1944, 1944*f*
Acromegaly, 609, 627, 1550
Actin cytoskeleton, 294
Actin-associated proteins, 294-295
Actinin-4, 113
α-Actinin-4, 113, 1430
Action myoclonus-renal failure syndrome, 1432
Activating protein-1, 1787
Activity product ratio, 1327-1328
ACTN4 mutations, 1028
ActRIIB, 1967
Acute allergic interstitial nephritis, 2270
Acute coronary syndrome, 1721-1722
Acute cortical necrosis, 2499, 2501-2502
Acute decompensated heart failure, 997-998, 1719-1722, 2139, 2140*f*
Acute Dialysis Quality Initiative, 960
Acute fatty liver of pregnancy, 992, 1617*t*, 1632
Acute glomerular disease, 1002
Acute interstitial nephritis
   causes of, 1218-1219, 1218*t*
   clinical features of, 1219-1220
   definition of, 1218
   description of, 964-965, 1002
   drugs that cause, 1218-1220, 1218*t*

Acute interstitial nephritis *(Continued)*
   infections associated with, 1219
   kidney biopsy of, 1220
   management of, 1220-1221
   pathology of, 1219
   prognosis for, 1220-1221
   proteinuria and, 1219
   after renal transplantation, 2270
   serum creatinine levels in, 1219-1220
   after thiazide diuretic therapy, 1732
   ultrasonography of, 1220
Acute kidney injury (AKI)
   in acute respiratory distress syndrome, 2138-2139
   in Africa. *See* Africa, acute kidney injury in
   anemia associated with, 983
   animal model for, 299
   atheroembolic, 744
   bee stings as cause of, 2500, 2525
   biologic agent and, 1398
   biomarkers for
      cystatin C, 935, 989
      description of, 930-932, 931*t*
      glutathione S-transferase, 938-939
      hepcidin-25, 939
      insulin-like growth factor-binding protein-7, 989
      interleukin-18, 939, 989
      kidney injury molecule-1, 941, 989
      liver-type fatty acid-binding protein, 942-943, 989
      β_1-microglobulin, 937-938
      β_2-microglobulin, 938
      multiple, 953
      N-acetyl-β-D-glucosaminidase, 947
      netrin-1, 943
      neutrophil gelatinase-associated lipocalin, 943-946, 989
      performance data on, 952*t*
      tissue inhibitor of metalloproteinase 2, 989
   after bone marrow transplantation, 991*t*, 992-993
   in *Bothrops* envenomations, 2447
   in cancer, 990, 991*t*, 1390
   cardiac arrest as cause of, 970
   cardiac surgery-related, 991*t*, 992
   cardiac tissues affected by, 982
   causes of, 770, 770*t*, 959, 959*t*-960*t*, 963-968
   characteristics of, 1390
   chronic kidney disease secondary to, 678, 691, 747, 926-927, 1777-1778, 1778*f*
   cold ischemia–warm reperfusion model of, 970
   complications of, 994-997, 995*t*
      acid-base homeostasis, 995
      cardiac, 996
      extracellular volume overload, 996

Page numbers followed by "f" indicate figures, and "t" indicate tables.

Acute kidney injury (AKI) *(Continued)*
    gastrointestinal, 996
    hematologic, 996
    hyperkalemia, 994-995, 2140
    hypermagnesemia, 995
    hyperphosphatemia, 995
    hypocalcemia, 995
    hypokalemia, 995
    hypomagnesemia, 995
    infectious, 996
    malnutrition, 996
    nutritional, 996
    potassium homeostasis, 994-995
    recovery-related, 996-997
    uremic syndrome, 996
    volume overload, 996
conceptual model of, 962*f*
continuous renal replacement therapy for, 2417-2418
contrast media-induced nephropathy as cause of, 853, 964-966, 1000
after coronary angiography, 1009
after coronary artery bypass grafting, 992
COX metabolites in, 377
critical illness-related, 941
in *Crotalus* envenomations, 2446-2447
cytochrome P450 in, 385
definition of, 648, 649*t*, 769-770, 958-962
dengue fever as cause of, 2441, 2498-2499
in diabetic nephropathy, 1315
diagnostic approach, 771-773, 772*t*, 961
dialysis for, 652*f*, 744, 990-992
distant organs affected by, 982-983
diuretics for, 1725-1726
drug disposition affected by, 2035-2040
drug dosing in, 2046, 2051*t*-2054*t*, 2145-2146
in elderly, 742-744, 2513-2514
end-stage kidney disease as risk factor for, 744, 1009, 1777-1778
epidemiology of, 647-648
evaluation of
    biomarkers. *See* Acute kidney injury, biomarkers for
    blood urea nitrogen, 988
    clinical assessment, 983-986, 984*t*-985*t*
    imaging, 989-990
    kidney biopsy, 772-773, 990
    laboratory tests, 988
    magnetic resonance angiography, 989-990
    radiologic, 989-990
    ultrasonography, 989-990
    urine assessments, 986-988, 987*t*-988*t*
experimental models of, 968-983, 969*t*
in Far East. *See* Far East, acute kidney injury in
glomerular filtration rate in, 788, 932, 947-948, 963, 2043, 2145
hantavirus as cause of, 2515-2516, 2517*f*
health resource utilization for, 1010
hematopoietic stem cell transplantation and, 1394
hepatorenal syndrome and, 993-994, 994*t*, 998-999
hornet stings as cause of, 2500
hospital-acquired, 744
hospitalization costs for, 1010
hyperphosphatemia caused by, 627
imaging of, 863*f*864*f*, 866-871, 866*f*-871*f*
incidence of, 648, 650*t*, 652*f*, 770, 926-927, 962-963, 1390, 2495
in Indian subcontinent. *See* Indian subcontinent, acute kidney injury in
insect stings as cause of, 2525

Acute kidney injury (AKI) *(Continued)*
in intensive care unit patients, 2137, 2458-2459
intermittent hemodialysis for, 1006-1007, 1315, 2141*t*
intrinsic
    acute glomerular disease as cause of, 1002
    acute phosphate nephropathy as cause of, 966-967
    acute tubular necrosis as cause of, 964
    acute vasculitis as cause of, 1002
    aminoglycoside nephrotoxicity as cause of, 966
    causes of, 960*t*, 964-968
    cisplatin nephrotoxicity as cause of, 966, 968*t*, 990
    contrast media-induced nephropathy as cause of, 853, 964-966, 965*t*, 1000
    description of, 744, 771, 772*t*
    early-goal directed therapy for, 999
    endogenous nephrotoxins that cause, 967-968
    general principles of, 999-1000
    hypotension and, 999
    interstitial disease as cause of, 964-965
    iron chelators as cause of, 967
    mortality rates for, 1008
    myoglobin as cause of, 967
    nephrotoxins that cause, 965-968
    prevention of, 999-1002
    renal artery occlusion as cause of, 964
    tubulointerstitial diseases as cause of, 964-968
    uric acid as cause of, 967-968
kidney function in, 994
in Latin America, 2440-2444
in leptospirosis, 2444, 2497-2498
liver disease and, 991*t*, 993-994
loading drug dose in, 2046
Lonomia caterpillar stings as cause of, 2446
in loxoscelism, 2445
maintenance drug dose in, 2046
malaria as cause of, 2443, 2470-2472, 2496-2497, 2517-2520, 2519*f*2521*f*
mesenchymal stem cells in, 2611-2613
in Middle East, 2469-2472
mortality rates for, 742, 1008-1009, 1390
multifactorial causes of, 771
in multiple myeloma, 990, 1002, 2152
nephrolithiasis and, 1632-1633
nephrotic syndrome and, 991*t*, 994
neutrophil gelatinase-associated lipocalin levels in, 772
nondialytic supportive management of, 1002-1004, 1003*t*
    hypermagnesemia, 1003*t*, 1004
    hypernatremia, 1003-1004, 1003*t*
    hyperuricemia, 1003*t*, 1004
    hypocalcemia, 1003*t*, 1004
    hyponatremia, 1003, 1003*t*
    intravascular volume, 1003
    metabolic acidosis, 1003*t*, 1004
nonsteroidal antiinflammatory drugs as cause of, 362-363, 743-744
nutrition management in, 1003*t*, 1004
obstruction as cause of, 968
obstructive nephropathy as cause of, 2496
obstructive uropathy and, 1632-1633
oliguric, 959, 995, 1001-1002
outcomes of, 1008-1010
pathophysiology of, 769-770, 1396
    acute tubular necrosis, 970-983
    algorithm for, 971*f*
    apoptosis in, 974-975
    coagulation, 980-981

Acute kidney injury (AKI) *(Continued)*
    cytoskeleton, 971-974, 979
    endothelial dysfunction, 979
    endothelial progenitor cells, 982
    epithelial cell injury, 970-983
    experimental models, 968-983, 969*t*
    heat shock proteins, 977-978
    heme oxygenase, 977-978
    inflammation, 981
    intracellular skeletal changes, 971-974
    necrosis in, 974-975
    parenchymal inflammation, 975-977
    reactive oxygen species, 977-978
    stem cells, 978-979
    T_{reg} cells, 977
    vascular tone, 979
peritoneal dialysis for, 2120
polyuria in, 299
porphyria cutanea tarda in, 1946, 1946*f*
postrenal
    asymptomatic presentation of, 986
    causes of, 960*t*, 968
    clinical features of, 984*t*-985*t*
    diagnosis of, 984*t*-985*t*
    management of, 1002-1003
    prevention of, 1002-1003
    urine sediment evaluations, 986-987
in pregnancy, 990-992, 991*t*, 1631-1633
prematurity as risk factor for, 711-712
prerenal
    in abdominal compartment syndrome, 999
    in acute decompensated heart failure, 997-998
    in cancer, 990
    causes of, 959*t*, 963-964
    clinical assessment, 983-985
    clinical features of, 984*t*-985*t*
    definition of, 997
    description of, 959
    diagnosis of, 983-985
    in heart failure, 997-998
    hepatorenal syndrome and, 998
    hypovolemia in, 963
    in liver failure, 998-999
    management of, 997-999
    prevention of, 997-999
    renal replacement therapy for, 997
    urine sediment evaluations, 986-987
prerenal azotemia as cause of, 963
prevalence of, 648
pulmonary disease and, 991*t*, 993
recovery from, complications during, 996-997
renal function assessments in, 2043-2044
renal replacement therapy for, 962-963
    continuous, 1007-1008
    in critically ill patients, 2137, 2139-2140
    definition of, 1004-1005
    duration of, 1005-1006
    indications for, 1005-1006, 1005*t*, 2140
    in intensive care unit, 2139-2140
    intermittent hemodialysis, 1006-1007, 1315
    modalities of, 1006-1008
    peritoneal dialysis, 1008
    prolonged intermittent, 1008
in renal transplantation, 2271*t*
RIFLE criteria for, 648, 770, 770*t*, 930-931, 960, 961*t*, 2138
risk factor for, 959
scleroderma associated with, 1002
in sepsis, 338, 999, 2137-2138
severe fever with thrombocytopenia syndrome virus as cause of, 2516-2517, 2518*f*

Acute kidney injury (AKI) *(Continued)*
  snakebites as cause of, 2499-2500
  after solid organ transplantation, 991*t*, 992-993
  sphingosine-1 phosphate receptor, 979
  staging of, 961, 2043
  toxins that cause, 965-968, 2458
  tumor lysis syndrome and, 990, 992*t*, 1395-1397
  ultrasonography of, 866-867
  urinary microscopy evaluations, 937, 937*t*
  urine output in, 959
  wasp stings as cause of, 2500, 2525
  zygomycosis as cause of, 2498, 2498*f*
Acute Kidney Injury Network, 930-931
Acute liver failure, 2139
Acute mountain sickness, 1704
Acute myelogenous leukemia, 1390
Acute myocardial infarction, 623, 1721
Acute phase reactant proteins, 1970
Acute phosphate nephropathy, 966-967
Acute poststreptococcal glomerulonephritis
  in children, 1054, 2331-2333
  clinical features of, 1057, 2332
  coagulation abnormalities in, 1058
  complement levels in, 1058
  cryoglobulins in, 1058
  in developing communities, 1054
  diagnosis of, 2332
  differential diagnosis of, 1057, 2332-2333
  in elderly, 1057
  electron microscopy findings, 1055-1056, 1056*f*
  epidemic, 1054
  epidemiology of, 1054, 2331-2332
  hematuria in, 1057
  hypertension in, 1057
  immunofluorescence microscopy findings, 1055, 1055*f*
  incidence of, 1054
  infectious agents associated with, 1057
  laboratory findings in, 1057-1058
  light microscopy findings, 1054-1055, 1055*f*
  natural history of, 1057
  nephrotic syndrome caused by, 1054-1059
  pathogenesis of, 1056-1057, 2332
  pathology of, 1054-1056, 1055*f*-1056*f*
  prognosis for, 1058-1059, 2333
  pyoderma and, 2331-2332
  streptococcal proteins in, 1056-1057
  streptozyme test for, 1058
  treatment of, 1058-1059, 2333
  ultrastructural features of, 1056*f*
Acute pyelonephritis. *See* Pyelonephritis, acute
Acute radiation nephropathy, 1193
Acute renal failure, 1021. *See also* Acute kidney injury
Acute renal ischemia, 141-142
Acute respiratory distress syndrome, 2138-2139
Acute thrombotic microangiopathy, after renal transplantation, 2269
Acute tubular necrosis (ATN), 2139
  atrial natriuretic peptide for, 1001
  clinical features of, 984*t*-985*t*
  description of, 744
  diagnosis of, 984*t*-985*t*
  dopamine for, 1001
  fenoldopam for, 1001
  intravascular volume depletion as risk factor for, 999
  intrinsic acute kidney injury and, 999

Acute tubular necrosis (ATN) *(Continued)*
  ischemic, 984*t*-985*t*, 985, 2263-2264, 2263*t*
  loop diuretics for, 1001-1002
  magnetic resonance imaging of, 870*f*
  mannitol for, 1002
  morphologic changes in, 971, 972*f*
  natriuretic peptides for, 1001
  nephrotoxic medications as cause of, 999-1000
  pathophysiology of, 970-983
  pharmacologic therapy for, 1001-1002
  pigment-induced, 985
  in pregnancy, 1631-1632
  renal transplantation with, 910*f*
  risk factors for, 999
  snakebite as cause of, 2499
  urinary protein excretion in, 987
Acute tubulointerstitial nephritis, 1209
Acute vasculitis, 1002
ADAM17, 360-361
ADAMTS1, 977
ADAMTS13, 1154, 1175, 1188-1189, 2356
  deficiency of, thrombotic thrombocytopenia purpura associated with, 1188-1191, 2154-2155
Adamts1, 30
Adamts4, 30
Addison's disease, 315, 538, 588-589
Adenine nucleotide translocase, 126-127
Adenine phosphoribosyl transferase deficiency, 1347
Adenohypophysitis, 475-476
Adenosine, 108-109, 135, 136*f*
Adenosine diphosphate, 124
Adenosine monophosphate-activated protein kinase (AMPK), 140-142, 141*f*, 732-733
Adenosine triphosphatases, 124
Adenosine triphosphate, 124, 129, 130*f*
Adenosine triphosphate-binding cassette, subfamily B, 2486
Adenosine type 1 receptor antagonists, 1714
Adenovirus infection, 1404
Adhesion proteins, 25
AdiC, 230*t*
Adiponectin, 1300, 1770-1771
Adipsic hypernatremia, 477-478
Adjuvant therapy, 1381-1382
ADMTS13, 1299
Adrenal adenomas, 575-576, 576*f*
Adrenal cortex, 305
Adrenal glands, 2-3, 852-853, 1919-1920
Adrenal hypoplasia congenita, 588
Adrenal insufficiency, 493, 495, 588-589
α2-Adrenergic agonist, 1629
α-Adrenergic antagonists, 456, 562, 1698
β-Adrenergic antagonists
  airway disease and, 1661
  calcium channel blockers and, 1669, 1691
  central adrenergic agonists and, 1692
  central nervous system effects of, 1661
  in coronary artery disease patients, 1660
  description of, 1564-1565, 1629
  dosing of, 1649*t*-1650*t*
  efficacy of, 1660-1661
  in elderly, 1685
  hyperkalemia treated with, 594-595
  hypertensive urgencies and emergencies treated with, 1698
  indications for, 1660
  lipid levels affected by, 1661
  mechanism of action, 1656-1659
  nonselective, 1656-1659, 1657*t*, 1661

β-Adrenergic antagonists *(Continued)*
  pharmacodynamic properties of, 1657*t*
  pharmacokinetics properties of, 1657*t*
  pharmacologic properties of, 1656*t*
  plasma renin activity affected by, 1659-1660
  potassium concentration affected by, 563*t*
  renal effects of, 1659-1660
  in renal insufficiency patients, 1649*t*-1650*t*
  renin-angiotensin-aldosterone inhibitors and, 1692
  safety of, 1660-1661
  selective, 1656, 1658
  sympathoadrenal drive affected by, 1688
  with vasodilatory properties, 1658-1659, 1658*t*-1659*t*
  withdrawal of, 1661
α_2-Adrenergic receptors, 1673
β_1-Adrenergic receptors, 1656, 1661
β_2-Adrenergic receptors, 1656, 1661
Adrenocorticotropic hormone (ACTH)
  aldosterone levels affected by, 575
  in chronic kidney disease, 1919
  deficiency of, 474
  ectopic, 577
  glomerular disease treated with, 1171-1172
  membranous nephropathy treated with, 1044
  secretion of, 463
  vasopressin 3 receptor's role in release of, 410
Adrenomedullin, 418, 437
Advance directives, 2561-2562, 2599
Advanced care planning, 2599-2600
Advanced glycosylation end products, 730-732, 1318, 1815, 2126-2127
Advanced glycosylation end receptor 1, 730-731, 731*f*
Advanced oxidation protein products, 1909
Adynamic bone disease, 1843
Aedes aegypti, 2441, 2520
Afferent arterioles, 85*f*, 138
Affordable Care Act, 2584, 2631-2632
Africa
  acute kidney injury in, 2457-2459, 2457*t*
  autosomal dominant polycystic kidney disease in, 2459
  children in, nephrotic syndrome in, 2463
  cholera in, 2455-2456
  chronic kidney disease in, 2459-2461, 2465
  diabetes mellitus in, 2463
  diabetic nephropathy in, 2463
  dialysis in, 2463-2464, 2464*f*-2465*f*
  diarrheal diseases in, 2455-2456
  end-stage kidney disease in, 2460*f*, 2461-2462, 2465-2466
  fluid and electrolyte abnormalities in, 2455-2457
  glomerular diseases in
    description of, 2461
    focal segmental glomerulosclerosis, 2463
    hepatitis B virus nephropathy as cause of, 2461-2462
    HIV-associated, 2462-2463
    malaria as cause of, 2462
    poststreptococcal glomerulonephritis, 2461
    schistosomiasis as cause of, 2462
  glomerular filtration rate estimations in, 2459

Africa *(Continued)*
  hemodialysis in, 2463-2464
  hepatitis B virus nephropathy in, 2461-2462
  human immunodeficiency virus in, 2455-2458, 2462-2463
  hypertension in, 2459-2461
  leading causes of death in, 2454, 2455f
  malaria in, 2462
  nephrology-specific challenges for, 2465
  nephrotoxic agents in, 2458
  population of, 2454
  renal replacement therapy in, 2456t, 2463-2465, 2464f
  renal transplantation in, 2464
  sickle cell anemia in, 2463
  snakebites in, 2458
  sub-Saharan, 2454-2455
  urbanization of, 2454
African American Study of Kidney Disease and Hypertension, 679, 1553, 1553f
African Americans
  antihypertensive drug therapy in, 1686, 1686t
  chronic kidney disease in, 666, 674
  end-stage kidney disease in, 663, 665-666, 674, 1028-1029, 1770
  focal segmental glomerulosclerosis in, 1028, 1769-1770
  thiazide diuretics in, 1686
Agalsidase alfa, 1145
Agalsidase beta, 1145
Age/aging. *See also* Elderly
  acid-base balance affected by, 740-741, 740f
  aldosterone levels affected by, 738
  ammonia excretion affected by, 740
  atrial natriuretic peptide levels affected by, 738-739
  calcium balance affected by, 741-742
  coronary heart disease and systolic blood pressure by, 1527f
  creatinine levels affected by, 737
  glomerular filtration rate affected by, 736-737, 737f, 2586-2587
    estimated, 2586-2587
  hypertension and, 1525
  membrane cholesterol in, 742
  phosphate balance affected by, 742
  potassium balance affected by, 741, 741f
  renal function affected by, 1878
  renal plasma flow affected by, 735-736, 736f
  sodium conservation in, 737-738
  sodium excretion affected by, 738-739
  urinary concentration affected by, 739-740
  urinary dilution affected by, 740
Agonistic Ang II type I receptor autoantibody, 1623
AGT1, 229
Agtr1a, 35
Agtr1b, 35
Air embolism, in hemodialysis, 2075
A-kinase anchoring proteins, 292-293
AL amyloidosis, 1128-1132
Alagille syndrome, 2297t
Albright's hereditary osteodystrophy, 616
Albumin
  catabolism of, in hypoalbuminemia, 1796
  excretion rate for, 1288, 1291, 1296-1297
  fragments of, 794
  free fatty acids binding to, 1761
  hepatic synthesis of, 1796

Albumin *(Continued)*
  loop diuretic binding to, 1707-1708
  normal levels of, 791, 1796
  plasma, 602, 791, 1798
  as plasmapheresis replacement fluid, 2162
  podocyte function for, 112-113
  in proximal tubule, 1784-1785, 1785f
  reabsorption of, by proximal tubular cells, 1791
  serum, 683, 1969-1970, 2099
  urinary
    acute kidney injury and, 948
    albumin-to-creatinine ratios, 792, 795-796
    excretion of, 1288, 1291, 1296-1297
    high-performance liquid chromatography measurement of, 794
    hypoalbuminemia secondary to loss of, 1796
    laboratory methods for measurement of, 794-795
    low-protein diet effects on, 1312
    measurement of, 793-795
    in minimal change disease, 1022
    timed versus random collection of, 795
Albumin dialysis, 2171, 2172t
Albumin-to-creatinine ratio, 792, 795-796, 2587, 2588f
Albuminuria, 1556-1557. *See also* Hypoalbuminemia
  angiotensin receptor blockers for, 1308
  angiotensin-converting enzyme inhibitors for, 1308
  cannabinoid receptor 1 blockade as cause of, 120
  cardiovascular disease and, 1860-1861
  chronic kidney disease progression, 948
  in diabetic nephropathy, 1283
  hypertension as risk factor for, 1765
  metabolic control for, 2592-2593
  mortality risks associated with, 673
  in older adults, 2587
  thromboxane A_2's role in, 378
Albuterol, 594-595
Alcohol consumption, 685-686
Alcoholic ketoacidosis, 547
Alcoholism, 633
Aldh1a2, 23
Aldolase B deficiency, 1445
Aldosterone
  action of, 310-311
  adrenal cortex synthesis of, 305
  adrenal release of, 569
  age-related changes in, 738
  angiotensin II in production of, 305-306, 408-409, 2366-2367
  apical sodium channels affected by, 179
  basolateral membrane effects of, 312
  calcium channel blockers effect on, 1662
  chemical structure of, 304f
  in chronic kidney disease, 1919-1920
  collagen synthesis stimulated by, 1757
  collecting duct bicarbonate reabsorption regulated by, 244
  colon and, 316-317
  in congestive heart failure, 322
  diuretic-induced secretion of, 1728
  epithelial sodium channels affected by, 172-173, 311-312, 409, 565-566, 1800, 2366-2367
  glomerulus secretion of, 305
  heart failure and, 431
  hyperkalemia effects on, 182, 2366-2367
  ion transport effects of, 321

Aldosterone *(Continued)*
  kaliuresis affected by, 588
  lung and, 317
  mineralocorticoid receptor binding of, 310
  nonepithelial actions of, 322-323
  nongenomic effects of, 321
  potassium chloride effects on, 741f
  potassium loading affected by, 179-180
  potassium secretion regulation by, 312-314, 317, 564-566
  in primary aldosteronism, 321-322
  in principal cells, 567
  production of, 408-409
  renin effects on secretion of, 568, 568f
  renovascular effects of, 101
  serum- and glucocorticoid-regulated kinase induction by, 317-318
  SGK-1 induction by, 173
  sodium absorption regulation by, 310-315
  sodium chloride transport affected by, 171-173
  sodium-retaining effect of, 409
  synthesis of, 304f-305f, 305-306, 588
  systemic effects of, 1309
Aldosterone antagonists
  chronic kidney disease progression affected by, 2003
  description of, 1564
  epithelial sodium channel inhibitors and, 1692
  indications for, 451
  selective aldosterone receptor antagonists, 1678-1679
Aldosterone receptors, 304-305
Aldosterone-producing adenomas, 575
Aldosterone/renin ratio, 1529f
Aldosterone-sensitive distal nephron, 311f, 314-315, 316f, 318-320
Alemtuzumab, 2248, 2255-2256
Alfacalcidol, 2026, 2032
Alginate, 2610
Aliphatic amines, 1812-1813
Aliskiren
  characteristics of, 1677
  combination therapy using, 1678
  efficacy of, 1678
  immunoglobulin A nephropathy treated with, 1068
  proteinuria caused by, 1678
  renal effects of, 1677-1678
  renin-angiotensin-aldosterone system blockade using, 1309
  safety of, 1678
Alkalemia, 186, 523
Alkali gain, 519-520
Alkali therapy, 535-536, 542, 546, 1362-1364, 1363t
Alkalosis
  causes of, 526t
  metabolic. *See* Metabolic alkalosis
  respiratory. *See* Respiratory alkalosis
Alkylating agents
  adverse effects of, 1168-1169
  bone marrow suppression caused by, 1169
  glomerular disease treated with, 1168-1170
  malignancy risks, 1169
  ovarian failure caused by, 1168-1169
  steroid-sensitive nephrotic syndrome treated with, 2329
  toxicity of, 1169-1170
Allergic interstitial nephritis, 984t-985t, 1158
Alloantibodies, 1903

Allograft rejection, 378
Allopurinol, 1363t, 1364
Allostatic load, 2576
Alpert syndrome, 2297t
Alport's syndrome, 1421-1424
    clinical features of, 1138-1139
    course of, 1141
    definition of, 1138
    description of, 755, 761, 872
    diagnosis of, 1423-1424
    electron microscopy of, 1139-1140, 1140f
    end-stage kidney disease secondary to, 1138
    genetics of, 1140-1141, 1421-1422, 1782
    high-frequency sensorineural deafness in, 1139
    immunofluorescence microscopy of, 1139
    light microscopy of, 1139
    manifestations of, 1423
    ocular abnormalities in, 1139
    pathogenesis of, 1140-1141, 1421-1422
    pathology of, 1139-1140, 1140f, 1423-1424
    proteinuria in, 1141
    skin manifestations of, 1953
    treatment of, 1141
    variants of, 1139
Alström's syndrome, 1509
Altered nuclear transfer, 2606
Almandine, 333
Aluminum, 1843, 1844f, 1887, 1935
Aluminum-containing binders, 2022
Amatoxin, 2525-2526
Ambulatory blood pressure monitoring. *See* Blood pressure, ambulatory monitoring of
American Joint Committee on Cancer staging system, 1378
Amifostine, for cisplatin nephrotoxicity, 1001
Amiloride, 489, 590, 1712-1713, 1726
Amiloride-sensitive sodium channel, 125
Amino acid(s)
    anionic, 228-229
    branched-chain, 1971
    catabolism of, 1963-1964, 2084
    in chronic kidney disease, 1972
    D–, 1809-1810
    essential, 1971-1972
    metabolism of, uremia effects on, 1817
    metabolites of, 1972
    neutral, 222-226
    in peritoneal dialysis solutions, 2125
    plasma, 1971-1973, 1972f
    reabsorption of, 222, 223f
    transepithelial flux of, 222
Amino acid decarboxylase, 152-153
Amino acid reabsorption, 1445, 1446f
Amino acid transport, 222-229, 1445-1450
Amino acid transporters
    anionic, 228-229
    apical, 222-228
    basolateral, 228
    cationic, 226-228
    5 + 5 inverted repeat fold of, 229
    heteromeric, 225-227, 226f, 231-232
    neutral, 222-226
    SLC6 transporters, 229-230
    structure of, 229-232
Aminoaciduria, 223t, 1436-1437, 1445, 1612
ε-Aminocaproic acid, 587
Aminoglycosides, 621-622, 966, 1235t-1236t
Aminophylline, 1714

Amlodipine besylate, 1665
Ammonia
    assessment of, 840f
    bicarbonate reabsorption affected by, 245
    blood levels of, 1962
    chemistry of, 248
    collecting duct secretion of, 252, 252f
    formation of, 2036
    hyperkalemia effects on, 537-538, 537t, 571
    impaired excretion of, 1344, 1344f
    interstitial, sulfatide binding of, 251-253
    molecular forms of, 248
    production of, 248-249, 250f, 515f, 517, 1344-1345
    secretion of, 1344-1345
    synthesis of, 537f, 1749
    transport of, 251-253, 1706
    urinary concentrations of, 529
Ammonia excretion
    age-related changes in, 740
    hyperkalemia effects on, 537t
    impaired, 538
    in metabolic acidosis response, 246f
    pathways of, 537f
    Rhbg's role in, 255
    Rhcg's role in, 255
    urinary, 528-529, 538, 840
Ammonia metabolism
    aquaporins in, 254
    in bicarbonate generation, 248-255
    carbonic anhydrase in, 254-255
    description of, 248
    glutamate dehydrogenase in, 253
    H^+-K^+-ATPase in, 254
    Na^+-K^+-ATPase in, 254
    Na^+-K^+-$2Cl^-$ cotransport in, 254
    phosphate-dependent glutaminase in, 253
    potassium channels in, 254
    proteins involved in, 253-255
    Rh glycoproteins in, 255
    schematic diagram of, 249f
    sulfatides in, 255-256
Ammoniagenesis, 248-251, 251f, 840
Amniotic fluid- and placental-derived stem cells, 2607
Amphotericin B, 621, 2131
Amphotericin B deoxycholate, 1254, 1254t
Amyloid light-chain amyloidosis, 1392
Amyloidosis
    AA, 1128-1132, 1157, 2485
    AL, 1128-1132
    characteristics of, 1128
    course of, 1131-1132
    diagnosis of, 1129
    dialysis-related, 1949
    in elderly, 746-747
    end-stage kidney disease progression of, 1131-1132
    hereditary, 1129-1131
    immunofluorescence microscopy of, 1130f
    melphalan for, 1131-1132
    multiple myeloma in, 1128
    nephrotic syndrome in, 1129
    pathology of, 1129-1131, 1130f-1131f
    prognosis for, 1131-1132
    renal disease in, 1129
    renal transplantation in, 1132
    serum amyloid A in, 1128-1129, 1130f
    serum amyloid P in, 1128
    treatment of, 1131-1132

Anabolic hormones, for anorexia, 2125
Anabolic steroids, 1159
Anakinra, 1913, 2486
Analgesic nephropathy, 686, 1221-1223, 1223f-1224f, 2544-2546
Analgesics, 686, 1222t, 2595
Anasarca, 1798
Andersen's syndrome, 573
Androgen deprivation therapy, 1923
Androgens, 152
Anemia
    adverse outcomes of, 1888
    in autosomal dominant polycystic kidney disease, 1888
    blood transfusion for, 1004
    in children, 2405-2406, 2434
    of chronic disease, 1885-1887
    in chronic kidney disease
        adverse outcomes of, 1888, 2013
        algorithm for, 1900f
        causes of
            aluminum overload, 1887
            blood loss, 1885, 1962
            drugs, 1887-1888
            erythropoietin production, 1884, 2013, 2089
            folic acid deficiency, 1887
            inflammation, 1887
            iron metabolism abnormalities, 1885-1887
            shortened red blood cell survival, 1884-1885, 2013
            uremic erythropoiesis inhibitors, 1885
            vitamin D deficiency, 1887
            zinc deficiency, 1887
        definition of, 1875-1878
        description of, 683, 983, 1299-1300, 1776, 1863-1864, 1871-1872, 2593-2594
        in elderly, 2593-2594
        flowchart for, 1900f
        management of, 2013-2014, 2610-2611
        menses associated with, 1921
        pathobiology of, 1878-1884
        prevalence of, 1875-1878, 1876f-1877f, 2626
        red blood cell transfusion for, 1902-1904, 1903f
        stroke risks, 1930
    definition of, 1875-1878
    in diabetes mellitus, 1877-1878
    in diabetic nephropathy, 1299-1300, 1316
    diabetic retinopathy and, 1888
    drugs that affect, 1887-1888
    in elderly, 2593-2594
    in end-stage kidney disease, 1875-1876, 1879f, 2405-2406
    erythropoietin response to, 1316, 1871
    in maintenance hemodialysis, 2097-2098
    megaloblastic, 1883
    pathobiology of, 1878-1884
    prevalence of, 1875-1878, 1876f-1877f
    racial predilection of, 1876-1877
    after renal transplantation, 2434
    stroke risks associated with, 1930
    treatment of, 1871-1872
        erythropoiesis-stimulating agents, 1889-1892, 1900-1902, 2405-2406, 2626-2628
        iron in, 1892-1904, 2098
            intravenous, 1896-1900, 1897t
            markers of, 1893-1896

Anemia *(Continued)*
    parenteral, 1898
      safety of, 1900-1902
    recombinant human erythropoietin, 1906, 2097
    red blood cell transfusion, 1902-1904, 1903f
    trials of, 1901-1902
    uremic platelet dysfunction and, 1905, 1907f
  in women, 1876-1877
Aneurysmectomy, for renal artery aneurysms, 1203-1204
Angioedema, 1648
Angiogenesis, 6, 32, 34
Angiogenic imbalance, 1621-1623
Angiography
  central vein stenosis, 2212f-2213f
  magnetic resonance. *See* Magnetic resonance angiography
  renal artery, 1202
Angioimmunoblastic lymphadenopathy, 1159
Angiokeratoma corporis diffusum universale. *See* Fabry's disease
Angiolymphoid hyperplasia with eosinophilia, 1159
Angiomyolipomas, 891, 893f, 1368-1369, 1375-1376, 1500
Angioplasty, 2198-2202, 2198t, 2200f, 2208-2210, 2209t
Angiopoietin 1, 34-35
Angiopoietin 2, 34-35
Angiopoietin-like 4, 1021
Angiotensin, 1568-1569
Angiotensin-(1-7), 333, 408, 445, 1644
Angiotensin-(1-12), 333
Angiotensin-(2-10), 333
Angiotensin A, 333
Angiotensin I, 35, 326, 1530-1531
Angiotensin II, 35, 139, 183, 1580
  AT_1 receptors for, 152
  acid-base regulation and, 331
  in aldosterone production, 305-306, 408-409, 2366-2367
  angiotensin receptor blockers effect on, 1653-1654
  apelin and, 420
  atrial natriuretic peptide inhibition of, 154
  bicarbonate reabsorption affected by, 237-238, 408
  blockade of, 1598f
  blood pressure levels affected by, 1532f, 1640-1641
  calcium channel blockers effect on, 1662
  chloride absorption activated by, 174
  in chronic kidney disease progression, 1764-1765
  collecting ducts affected by, 244-245
  efferent arterioles affected by, 99
  epidermal growth factor receptor transactivation by, 329f
  formation of, 1530-1531
  functions of, 333
  glomerular capillary hypertension and, 1738
  glomerular filtration rate affected by, 408
  hemodynamic effects of, 331
  juxtaglomerular granular cell expression of, 53
  juxtaglomerular nephrons affected by, 99, 100f
  K_f affected by, 99
  mediation of, 407

Angiotensin II *(Continued)*
  medullary blood flow affected by, 90
  mesangial cells affected by, 99
  in nephron injury after renal mass ablation, 1756-1757
  nitric oxide release stimulated by, 99
  nonhemodynamic effects of, 1763-1764
  norepinephrine effects on, 110
  nuclear factor-κB activation by, 334
  oxidative stress and, 982
  as paracrine agent, 407
  peritubular carbon dioxide effects on, 237
  physiologic effects of, 330-331, 409
  podocytes affected by, 1788
  potassium intake effects on, 567-568
  pregnancy and, 1613f
  profibrotic effects of, 729
  proximal sodium chloride reabsorption affected by, 152, 153f
  proximal tubule bicarbonate reabsorption affected by, 237
  proximal tubule synthesis and secretion of, 152
  proximal tubule transport affected by, 408
  in renal artery stenosis, 907
  renal fibrosis in aging kidneys, 728-729
  renal hemodynamics affected by, 407-408
  renal hypoperfusion, role in, 1577-1578
  in renal metabolism, 139
  renal vascular responses to, 384
  ROMK activity affected by, 566-567
  sodium chloride absorption affected by, 155
  sodium reabsorption affected by, 407-408
  sodium transport affected by, 331
  transforming growth factor-β expression induced by, 334
  in tubuloglomerular feedback, 399
  urinary tract obstruction effects on expression of, 1278f
  vasoconstrictive effects of, 99-100, 409, 963, 1270, 1645
Angiotensin II inhibitors, 1067-1068
Angiotensin II receptors, 1530-1531, 1623-1624, 1652t, 1653, 2236
Angiotensin III, 332
Angiotensin IV, 332-333
Angiotensin peptides, 332-333
Angiotensin receptor(s), 35, 1569-1570
Angiotensin receptor blockers
  acute kidney injury after initiation of therapy with, 2006t
  adverse effects of, 1655
  albuminuria treated with, 1308
  angiotensin II affected by, 1653-1654
  angiotensin-converting enzyme inhibitors and, 1654, 1764-1765, 2002-2003
  biphenyl tetrazoles, 1651-1653
  cancer risks and, 1655-1656
  in children, 2362
  chlorthalidone and, 1681
  in chronic kidney disease patients, 1654
  description of, 1563-1564, 1598f
  direct renin inhibitors and, 1764-1765
  dosing of, 1649t-1650t, 1654-1655
  drug interactions with, 1656
  efficacy of, 1654-1656
  focal segmental glomerulosclerosis treated with, 1031
  in hypertensive patients, 1653-1654
  mechanism of action, 1651
  metabolic effects of, 1655
  neutral endopeptidase inhibitors and, combination therapy using, 345-346
  nonbiphenyl tetrazoles, 1653
  nonheterocyclic derivatives, 1653

Angiotensin receptor blockers *(Continued)*
  nonsteroidal anti-inflammatory drugs effect on, 1656
  in pregnancy, 1647, 1655
  renal effects of, 1653-1654
  renal function affected by, 1655
  in renal insufficiency patients, 1649t-1650t
  renin-angiotensin-aldosterone system inhibition by, 591f, 1642f, 1651, 2000-2003, 2001f
  renoprotection using, 729, 1757, 1764-1765, 1995, 1998t, 2000-2003, 2001f
  safety of, 1654-1656
  thiazide diuretics and, 1655
  urinary protein excretion affected by, 1654
Angiotensin receptor–neprilysin inhibitor, 345-346
Angiotensin type 1 receptor, 328-330, 1277
  angiotensin II effects mediated by, 328-329
  dimerization of, 330
  expression of, 328-329
  G protein-mediated signaling and, 329
  internalization of, 330
  ligand-independent activation of, 330
  reactive oxygen species and, 329
  regulation of, 330f
  tyrosine kinases and, 329-330
Angiotensin type 2 receptor, 331, 1277
Angiotensin type 1 receptor-associated protein 1, 330, 330f
Angiotensin-(2-B), 332
Angiotensin-(3-B), 332
Angiotensin-converting enzyme, 27, 100-101, 328, 1308
Angiotensin-converting enzyme 2, 332
Angiotensin-converting enzyme escape, 1644
Angiotensin-converting enzyme inhibitors, 1563, 1569-1570, 1598f, 1630. *See also specific drug*
  acute kidney injury after initiation of therapy with, 2006t
  adverse effects of, 1648
  albuminuria treated with, 1308
  anaphylactoid reactions caused by, 1650
  angioedema caused by, 1648
  angiotensin peptide levels affected by, 1644
  angiotensin receptor blockers and, 1654, 1764-1765, 2002-2003
  antiproteinuric effects of, 1308
  blood pressure control using, 1303-1305, 1928-1929
  calcium channel blockers and, 1669, 1681-1682, 1684f
  carboxyl, 1641-1644, 1643t
  in children, 2362
  cough caused by, 1648, 1685
  cutaneous reactions to, 1650
  diabetic nephropathy treated with, 1308, 1998-1999
  dosing of, 1649t-1650t
  drug interactions with, 1650
  efficacy of, 1646-1650
  focal segmental glomerulosclerosis treated with, 1031
  glomerular filtration rate affected by, 1299, 1645
  glucose metabolism affected by, 1648
  hyperkalemia caused by, 591-592, 1650
  hypertension treated with, 2592
  hypertensive urgencies and emergencies treated with, 1697t, 1698
  hyponatremia and, 497

Angiotensin-converting enzyme inhibitors (Continued)
- hypotension caused by, 1648
- indications for, 1647
- leukopenia caused by, 1650
- mechanism of action, 1640-1641, 1641t, 1642f
- metabolic effects of, 1647-1648
- microalbuminuria treated with, 1305-1306, 1999
- pharmacodynamics of, 1643t
- pharmacokinetics of, 1643t
- phosphinyl, 1644
- plasmapheresis in patients receiving, 2164
- in pregnancy, 1647, 1685
- renal artery stenosis treated with, 907
- renal effects of, 1644-1646, 1644t
- renal function affected by, 1645-1646
- in renal insufficiency patients, 1649t-1650t
- renal protective effects of, 729
- renin-angiotensin-aldosterone system inhibition by, 591f, 1642f, 1998-2000
- renograms enhanced with, 908
- renoprotection using, 1995, 1998, 1998t
- safety of, 1646-1650
- scleroderma renal crises treated with, 1197-1198
- stroke risk reduction using, 1928-1929
- sulfhydryl, 1641, 1643t
- tissue specificity of, 1645

Angiotensinogen, 35, 326
Angptl, 34
Anion exchanger(s), 238, 243, 1339, 1339f
Anion gap, 523-524, 524t, 837
Anionic amino acids, 228-229
Annexin II, 1836-1837
Anorexia, 2099, 2125, 2357
Antegrade pyelography, 1268, 1268f
Anthropometrics, 1971
Antiangiogenic therapy, 1382
Anti–B cell therapy, 119
Antibacterial agents, 1235t-1236t
Antibiotics, 1218, 1365
Antibodies
- anti-ADAMTS13, 1189
- anti-glomerular basement membrane, 1124
- anti-glomerular basement membrane glomerulonephritis, 1079
- anti-MPO, 1083-1085
- antineutrophil cytoplasmic. See Antineutrophil cytoplasmic antibodies
- antinuclear, 1098-1099
- antiphospholipid, 1106-1107
- anti-Ro/SSA, 1099
- anti-U1RNP, 1108

Antibody-mediated rejection, 2423
Anti-CD20 monoclonal antibody, 2256
Anticoagulation
- antiphospholipid syndrome treated with, 1107-1108
- atrial fibrillation treated with, 1932
- extracorporeal dialysis circuit patency maintained using, 1007
- during hemodialysis, 2091-2092, 2092t
- in membranous nephropathy, 1041-1042
- plasmapheresis use of, 2162
- regional, 2092
- in renal replacement therapy, 2144
- renal vein thrombosis treated with, 1206

Antidiuretic hormone. See Arginine vasopressin
Antifungal agents, 1235t-1236t
Antigens
- human leukocyte. See Human leukocyte antigens
- tubulointerstitial, 1214-1215, 1228-1229

Anti-glomerular basement membrane antibodies, 1124
Anti-glomerular basement membrane autoantibodies, 1124-1125
Anti-glomerular basement membrane disease. See also Goodpasture's syndrome
- clinical features of, 1125
- corticosteroids for, 1126-1127
- course of, 1126-1127
- electron microscopy of, 1126
- etiology of, 1124
- immunofluorescence microscopy of, 1126, 1126f
- kallikrein-kinin system in, 350
- laboratory findings in, 1125
- methylprednisolone for, 1126-1127
- pathogenesis of, 1124-1125
- pathology of, 1125-1126, 1126f
- plasmapheresis for, 1126-1127, 2149-2150, 2149t-2150t
- prognosis for, 1126-1127
- recurrence of, in renal allograft, 1127, 2270
- renal transplantation after, 2150
- rituximab for, 1126-1127
- treatment of, 1126-1127

Anti-glomerular basement membrane glomerulonephritis, 746
- animal models of, 1079-1080
- antibodies in, 1079
- antigens in, 1078-1079
- autoantibodies in, 1079
- characteristics of, 1076
- clinical features of, 1080-1081
- complement in, 1080
- electron microscopy of, 1078, 1078f
- end-stage kidney disease progression of, 1080-1081
- epidemiology of, 1076
- genetic susceptibility to, 1076
- immunofluorescence microscopy of, 1077, 1077f
- laboratory findings in, 1081
- light microscopy of, 1077-1078
- mouse models of, 1076
- natural history of, 1080-1081
- pathogenesis of, 1078-1080
- pathology of, 1077-1078, 1077f-1078f, 1077t
- plasmapheresis for, 1081
- prednisone for, 1081
- T cells in, 1079-1080
- treatment of, 1081
- tubulointerstitial changes in, 1078

Antihypertensive drug therapy, 1563-1565, 1563t
- β-adrenergic antagonists. See β-Adrenergic antagonists
- in African Americans, 1686, 1686t
- angiotensin receptor blockers. See Angiotensin receptor blockers
- angiotensin-converting enzyme inhibitors. See Angiotensin-converting enzyme inhibitors
- bedtime dosing of, 1692
- blood pressure goals, 1680-1681

Antihypertensive drug therapy (Continued)
- during breastfeeding, 1631
- calcium channel blockers. See Calcium channel blockers
- cardiovascular protection using, 2009-2011
- central adrenergic agonists. See Central adrenergic agonists
- central and peripheral adrenergic neuronal blocking agents, 1673
- combination therapies, 1681-1682, 1683t, 1689-1692, 1690f
- direct-acting vasodilators, 1673-1674, 1674t
- dosing of, 1692
- drug interactions, 1694
- in elderly, 1682-1685, 1684t
- endothelin receptor antagonists, 1675
- gender-based, 1685, 1686t
- history of changes to, 1587
- hypotension risks during hemodialysis secondary to, 2106
- morning dosing of, 1692
- new types of, 1696f
- nonadherence to, 1695
- in obese patients, 1686-1688, 1688t
- in older adults, 1682-1685
- peripheral α$_1$-adrenergic antagonists. See Peripheral α$_1$-adrenergic antagonists
- in pregnancy, 1629f, 1630t, 1685, 1687f
- rapid-acting oral drugs, 1699
- in renal insufficiency patients, 1649t-1650t
- in renal transplantation recipients, 2284t
- renin inhibitors, 1677-1678
- selective aldosterone receptor antagonists, 1678-1679
- for slowing chronic kidney disease progression, 1995-1998
- therapeutic effect with, 1684f
- tyrosine hydroxylase inhibitor, 1679-1680

Anti-IL$_2$-R antibodies, 2248
Antimicrobial agents, 1234, 1235t-1236t, 1238-1239, 1238t, 1243-1244, 1247
Anti-MPO antibodies, 1083-1085
Antimycin A, 133
Antineoplastic drugs, 497
Antineutrophil cytoplasmic antibodies
- in anti-glomerular basement membrane glomerulonephritis, 1079
- crescentic glomerulonephritis induced by, 2150-2151
- cytoplasmic, 1086, 1111-1112, 1120
- in eosinophilic granulomatosis with polyangiitis, 1117
- in granulomatous with polyangiitis, 1111-1112
- in immunoglobulin A nephropathy, 1064
- laboratory tests for, 1115
- in microscopic polyangiitis, 1114-1115
- in pauci-immune crescentic glomerulonephritis, 1082
- perinuclear, 1086, 1111-1112, 1120
- in systemic lupus erythematosus, 1093-1094
- in temporal arteritis, 1120

Antineutrophil cytoplasmic antibody–associated vasculitides, 2351-2352, 2532
Antineutrophil cytoplasmic antibody–associated vasculitis, 350, 1084, 1086, 2150-2151
Antinuclear antibodies, in systemic lupus erythematosus, 1098-1099
Antioxidants, 1626

Antiphospholipid syndrome, 1106-1108, 1107f
Anti-phospholipase A_2 receptor antibodies, 746-747
Antiphospholipid antibodies, 1106-1107
Antiphospholipid nephropathy, 1106-1107
Antiphospholipid syndrome
  bilateral adrenal hemorrhage caused by, 588-589
  catastrophic, plasmapheresis for, 2158-2159
  clinical features of, 1200-1201
  definition of, 1200
  mechanisms of, 1201
  pathology of, 1201
  thrombotic microangiopathy caused by, 1200-1201
  treatment of, 1201
Antiplatelet therapy, 1625, 1625f, 1873, 1931-1932, 2012-2013
Anti-rheumatoid arthritis therapy-induced glomerulopathy, 1158-1159
Anti-Ro/SSA antibodies, 1099
Antisense oligonucleotides, 7-9
Anti-thin basement membrane nephritis, 1228-1229
Antithrombin III, 1206, 1803
Antithymocyte globulins, 1637t, 2247-2248, 2255, 2423-2424
Anti-U1RNP antibodies, 1108
Aorta, coarctation of, 1550, 1571f
Aortic baroceptors, 396
Aortic valve calcification, 1859, 2408
Aortoarteritis, 2506-2507
ApcT, 230t
Apelin, 419-420, 438, 446-447
Apical organic anion transporters, 219
Apical potassium channels, 159-160, 176-177, 564
Apical sodium channels, 179
Apical sodium hydrogen exchange, 154-155
Aplasia, 2294
Apnea, sleep, 1939-1940
Apo calbindin D28K, 192
APOL1, 674-676, 1153, 1165, 1429, 1770
Apolipoprotein-1, 693-694
Apolipoprotein A-1, 1801
Apolipoprotein B100, 2159
Apolipoprotein C, 1801
Apolipoprotein L-1, 1029
Apolipoprotein(a), 2100
Apoptosis
  in acute kidney injury pathophysiology, 974-975
  description of, 718
  of endothelial cells, 4-5, 1789
  erythropoietin suppression of, 1882-1883, 1882f
  of podocytes, 1788
  of proximal tubular cells, 1212, 1791
  tumor necrosis factor-like weak inducer of, 743
  in vascular calcification, 1836-1837
Apparent mineralocorticoid excess syndrome, 577-578, 1463
Appetite, loss of, 1819
Aquaporin(s)
  in ammonia metabolism, 254
  description of, 1468
  in nonepithelial cells, 288
  permeability properties of, 286
  in principal cells, 289, 289f
  in *Xenopus* oocytes, 288
Aquaporin-1, 147-148, 234, 254, 260-261, 273-276, 299, 805, 805f

Aquaporin-2
  basolateral, in cell migration and tubule morphogenesis, 290
  in cirrhosis, 300
  in cirrhosis-related water retention, 446
  clathrin-coated pits' role in recycling of, 291
  connecting tubule expression of, 69
  definition of, 286
  description of, 805, 805f, 1275
  in elderly, 739
  endocytosis of, phosphorylation's role in, 293
  endocytotic proteins and, 293-294
  endogenous, 289
  in endosomes, 287-288
  exocytosis of, phosphorylation's role in, 293
  exogenous, 288-289
  expression of, 286, 287f, 481f, 498, 1712
  in hypercalcemia, 299, 481
  in hypokalemia, 299
  in hyponatremia, 299-300
  impermeability of, 286
  in intracellular compartments, 291
  knockout mice model of, 276, 290f
  lithium effects on, 297-299, 298f
  membrane topology of, 286f
  methyl-β-cyclodextrin effects on, 292f
  nephrogenic diabetes insipidus and, 285, 298f, 481-482, 2338
  phosphorylation of, 293-294
  physiologic and pathophysiologic conditions associated with, 297t
  plasma membrane accumulation of, S256 residue's role in, 293
  plasma membrane expression of, 286, 287f
  in polyuria, 297
  in principal cells, 173, 289
  as recycling membrane protein, 291
  recycling of, 291
  S256 and, 293-294
  statins effect on, 301
  vasopressin effects on, 410, 805
Aquaporin-2 protein, 1472f
Aquaporin-2 trafficking
  actin cytoskeleton's role in, 294
  actin-associated proteins involved in, 294-295
  collecting duct used to examine, 289
  intracellular pathways of, 291
  kidney tissue slices used to examine, 289
  microtubules and, 295
  regulation of, 283f, 291-296, 296f
  SNARE proteins and, 295-296
  vasopressin-regulated, 287-288
Aquaporin-3, 254, 276, 289
Aquaporin-4, 276, 289, 299
Aquaporin-8, 254
Arachidonic acid
  cytochrome P450 metabolism of, 382, 382f-383f
  de-esterification of, 355
  definition of, 355
  epoxygenase metabolites of, 383
  esterification of, 355
  lipoxygenase metabolism of, 379f
  metabolism of, 355, 356f, 375, 382, 382f-383f
  metabolites of, 355
Arachnoid membrane cyst, 1491
ARAP1. See Angiotensin type 1 receptor-associated protein 1
Arcuate arteries, 84
Area cribrosa, 43, 44f

Arginine vasopressin receptor antagonists, 504-506, 509
Aristolochic acid, 755
Aristolochic acid nephropathy, 1223-1226, 2534
β-Arrestin, 282-284
Arrestin-receptor complexes, 283-284
Arrhythmias, 569-571, 598, 2107
Artemisinin, 2497
Arterial blood gas measurement, 521, 521t
Arterial calcification
  bone calcification and, 1836
  in chronic kidney disease, 1856-1857, 1857f, 1864, 1866
  clinical manifestations of, 1850
  detection of, 1847
  histology of, 1835f
Arterial stiffness, 1535, 1856
Arterial tone, 1856
Arterial wall thickening, in chronic kidney disease, 1855-1856
Arteriohyalinosis, 728f
Arteriosclerosis, 1315, 1855
Arteriovenous fistulas
  accessory vein ligation in, 2208-2209, 2209f
  angioplasty of, 2208-2210, 2209t
  blood flow rate, 2413
  digital subtraction angiography of, 2210f
  in elderly, 747-748, 2598
  failure of, 2206-2207
  hemodialysis vascular access using, 2064-2065, 2065f
  immature, 2206-2209, 2207t, 2209f
  maturation of, 2207, 2208f
  native, 2207
  neointimal hyperplasia in, 2194, 2195f
  preoperative vascular mapping of, 2203-2206, 2206f, 2206t
  quality improvement and, 2629-2631
  after renal transplantation, 911
  side-to-side, 2064-2065
  sonographic vascular mapping of, 2205-2206, 2206f
  stenotic lesions, angioplasty of, 2208, 2209t
  thrombosis of, 2210-2212
  tunneled catheters versus, 2629-2631
  vascular access stenosis in, 2194
  vascular mapping of, 2203-2206, 2206f, 2206t
Arteriovenous grafts
  failure of, 2194-2195
  hemodialysis using, 2065-2067, 2066f
  mortality associated with, 2542-2543
  percutaneous thrombectomy of, 2199-2202, 2199t, 2201f-2202f
  primary patency of, 2198, 2198t
  stenosis of
    angioplasty for, 2198-2202, 2198t, 2200f
    detection methods, 2195, 2196t
    monitoring of, 2196t
    pathophysiology of, 2197-2198
    stent deployment for, 2202-2203, 2204f-2205f
    surveillance for, 2194-2198, 2196t-2198t
    thrombosis secondary to, 2194-2195, 2196t, 2197
  thrombectomy of, 2199-2202, 2199t, 2201f-2202f
  thrombosis of, 2194-2195, 2196t, 2197
  vascular access stenosis, 2194
Arteriovenous shunt, 1949, 2558
Ascites, cirrhotic, 449, 1712, 1723
Ascorbic acid, 1361
ASCT2, 225

ASKP1240, 2259
Aspergillosis, 1150
Aspirin, 380, 2012
Aspirin, phenacetin, and caffeine, 2545
Asymmetric dimethylarginine, 443, 735
   as chronic kidney disease biomarker, 685, 950, 1811, 1934-1935
   endothelial dysfunction in chronic kidney disease and, 1856
   plasma levels of, 950
Asymptomatic bacteriuria, 1633
   antimicrobial treatment of, 1247
   biofilm formation as cause of, 1246
   description of, 749, 777
   diagnosis of, 1246
   epidemiology of, 1245-1246, 1245t
   Escherichia coli as cause of, 1246
   host factors associated with, 1246
   in men, 1245t
   microbiology of, 1246
   pathogenesis of, 1246
   in pregnancy, 1245-1247
   prevalence of, 1245
   pyuria associated with, 1246
   in renal transplantation recipients, 1248
   risk factors for, 1246
   treatment of, 1246-1247
Asymptomatic microscopic hematuria, 754-755
AT_1 receptor, 382, 407
AT_2 receptor, 407
Atenolol, 1656t-1657t, 1658
Atheroembolic acute kidney injury, 744
Atheroembolic renal disease, 1191-1193, 1192f
   cholesterol-lowering agents for, 1193
   clinical features of, 1191-1192
   differential diagnosis of, 1191
   distal protection devices for, 1193
   hypertension in, 1191
   hypocomplementemia in, 1192
   laboratory findings, 1192
   mechanisms of, 1192-1193
   outcomes of, 1191-1192
   pathology of, 1192, 1192f
   in renal allografts, 1191
   renal artery stenosis and, 1192-1193
   treatment of, 1193
Atherosclerosis
   calcifications associated with, 1833-1835, 1855
   in children, 2407-2408
   description of, 1855, 1859-1860
   fibromuscular disease versus, 1581-1582
   malnutrition and, 1930
   natural history of, 1802
   progression of, 1585, 1598-1599
   renal artery aneurysms caused by, 1203
   risk factor for, 1201
Atherosclerotic plaque, 1604
Atherosclerotic renal artery stenosis, 1580, 1583-1584
   angioplasty and stenting for, 1600-1602
   concurrent diseases associated with, 1587
   hypertension and, 1595-1596
   medical versus interventional therapy trials for, 1596t
   percutaneous transluminal renal angioplasty for, 1602-1603
   prevalence of, 1581t
   progression of, 1586f
   stenting and, 1600-1602
Atherosclerotic renovascular disease, 1568f, 1582f

ATPase, H^+ transporting, lysosomal accessory protein 2, 332
ATPases. *See* Adenosine triphosphatases
ATP6V1B1, 2385
Atrial fibrillation
   anticoagulation for, 1932
   in chronic kidney disease, 1859, 1908
   in end-stage kidney disease, 1929-1930
   in hemodialysis, 2107
   stroke risks associated with, 1928t, 1929-1930, 1932
   valvular heart disease and, 1929-1930
Atrial natriuretic peptide (ANP)
   acute tubular necrosis treated with, 1001
   age-related changes in, 738-739
   aldosterone levels affected by, 305-306
   angiotensin II inhibition by, 154
   atrial pressure effects on, 395
   blood pressure affected by, 342
   brain natriuretic peptide versus, 340
   cardiovascular effects of, 342
   in cirrhosis-related sodium retention, 447, 448f
   description of, 339, 413
   as disease biomarkers, 343
   in effective arterial blood volume regulation, 413-414
   furosemide effects on, 1717
   growth regulatory properties of, 414
   half-life of, 340
   in heart failure, 433
   natriuretic action of, 1799
   natriuretic effects of dopamine modulated by, 154
   plasma levels of, 414
   in portal hypertension, 447
   proANP, 340
   prostaglandins effect on, 436-437
   recombinant, 344
   renal effects of, 342
   smooth muscle affected by, 413-414
   sodium retention and, 447, 448f
   structure of, 339-340, 339f, 413
   synthesis of, 339-340
   therapeutic uses of, 344
   volume expansion effects on, 589
Atrial sensors, 394-395
Atrium, 395
Atypical hemolytic-uremic syndrome. *See* Hemolytic-uremic syndrome, atypical
Australia
   analgesic nephropathy in, 2544-2546
   chronic kidney disease in, 2544
   dialysis in, 2540f, 2542-2544
   end-stage kidney disease in, 2539-2540, 2541t
   health care access in, 2539-2540
   hemodialysis in, 2540f, 2542-2543
   indigenous (Aboriginals) population of
      chronic kidney disease in, 2549
      description of, 2538
      end-stage kidney disease in, 2547
      renal disease in, 2546-2549
      renal replacement therapy in, 2546
      renal transplantation in, 2548, 2548f
   peritoneal dialysis in, 2540f
   population of, 2540t
   renal replacement therapy in, 2540-2544, 2540f2543f, 2545f, 2545t
   renal supportive care in, 2544
   renal transplantation in, 2540f, 2543-2544, 2543f
   Torres Strait Islanders, 2538, 2546

Australia and New Zealand Dialysis and Transplant Registry, 2538-2539
Australian and New Zealand Society of Nephrology, 2539, 2541-2542
Autacoids, 52
Autoantibodies, 1064, 1093, 1099, 1124-1125
Autoimmune chronic active hepatitis, 1156
Autoimmune diseases, 1228-1229
Autoimmune hypoparathyroidism, 617
Autonephrectomy, 882
Autonomic diabetic polyneuropathy, 1320
Autonomic nervous system, 54-55
Autonomic neuropathy, 1939
Autophagy, 734-735, 735f, 1837
Autoregulation, renal, 104-110, 396, 1740-1741
Autosomal diabetes insipidus, 1473
Autosomal dominant distal renal tubular acidosis, 1456f
Autosomal dominant early-onset hypertension with severe exacerbation during pregnancy, 1463
Autosomal dominant hypocalcemia with hypercalciuria, 2345
Autosomal dominant hypomagnesemia, 2388-2389
Autosomal dominant hypophosphatemic rickets, 630-631, 1452
Autosomal dominant polycystic kidney disease, 1371, 1416
   in Africa, 2459
   anemia in, 1888
   in children, 2319-2321
   computed tomography of, 869f, 1486f, 1491f
   cyst in, 1484f
   description of, 885
   diagnosis of, 1485-1487
   diverticular disease and, 1492
   epidemiology of, 1479
   gender differences in, 658
   genetics of, 1479-1480, 1486f
   genotype-phenotype correlations for, 1417
   glomerular filtration rate and, 1490f
   hypertension and, 1487-1489
   imaging of, 885-888, 888f889f, 1486f
   magnetic resonance imaging of, 1486f
   manifestations of, 1487-1492
   in Middle East, 2477
   pain in, 1489, 1493
   pathogenesis of, 1480-1483
   progression of, 658, 1488f
   renal cyst infection associated with, 1250-1251
   renal failure and, 1489-1491
   tolvaptan for, 505
   treatment of, 1492-1496
   ultrasound of, 1485f, 1485t
Autosomal dominant polycystic kidney disease in situ, 1483f
Autosomal dominant tubulointerstitial kidney disease, 1504-1505
Autosomal recessive Alport's syndrome, 1423
Autosomal recessive ciliopathies with interstitial nephritis and renal cystic disease, 1505-1509, 1507t
Autosomal recessive distal renal tubular acidosis, 1456f
Autosomal recessive hypercholesterolemia, 179-180
Autosomal recessive hypophosphatemic rickets, 631, 1452, 1830

Autosomal recessive polycystic kidney disease, 1416-1417, 1496-1500, 1497f-1498f, 2319-2321
Autosomal recessive pseudohypoaldosteronism type I, 539, 539f
Avosentan, 338
Axial osmolality gradient, 265
Axitinib, 1383-1384, 1383f
Azathioprine
 adverse effects of, 1170, 2425
 in children, 2425
 definition of, 1170
 immunoglobulin A nephropathy treated with, 1068
 immunosuppressive uses of, 2245, 2254t, 2257, 2425
 lupus nephritis treated with, 1169-1170
 membranous nephropathy treated with, 1045
 prednisone and, 2257
 during pregnancy, 1637, 1637t
 toxicity of, 1170
Azilsartan medoxomil, 1651, 1652t
Azotemia, 1727. See also Prerenal azotemia
Azotemic renovascular disease, 1567-1568, 1577-1579

B

B7-1, 116
B cells, 1793
Bacille de Calmette-Guérin, 1254
Bacteremia, 1240, 2220
Bacterial peritonitis, 2128
Bacterial prostatitis, 750, 1247-1248
Bacteriuria
 asymptomatic. See Asymptomatic bacteriuria
 definition of, 1231-1232
 in elderly, 1243
Bad, 1791
Balkan endemic nephropathy, 1224-1226, 1225f
Bangladesh. See Indian subcontinent
Barbiturates, 2183
Bardet-Biedl syndrome, 1417, 1509, 2322, 2322t
Bardoxolone methyl, 1313
Bariatric surgery, 1342f
Baroreceptors, 396, 468
Bartonella henselae, 1149-1150
Bartter's syndrome, 176, 189-190, 554, 1417-1418, 1457-1459
 antenatal, 578, 2334-2335, 2336f
 in children, 2333-2335, 2344, 2376-2378, 2377f, 2377t
 classic, 578, 2334, 2378
 clinical manifestations of, 578, 2377-2378
 clinical presentation of, 1458-1459, 2333-2334
 hypocalcemia with, 2335
 metabolic alkalosis caused by, 551-552, 554
 in Middle East, 2479
 pathogenesis of, 1457-1458
 prevalence of, 2333
 pseudo-, 579-583
 renal magnesium wasting in, 622
 thick ascending limb and, 579f
 treatment of, 1459, 2335, 2377-2378
 types of, 578-579, 2334-2335, 2377f, 2377t
Barttin, 157, 161
Base, 517
Basement membrane. See also Glomerular basement membrane
 of Bowman's capsule, 52-53

Basement membrane (Continued)
 epithelial, 25
 of peritubular capillaries, 89-90
 plasma protein passage across, 1013
 proximal tubule, 1284f
 of thin limbs of loop of Henle, 62
Basolateral intercellular space, 55-56
Basolateral organic anion transporters, 219
B^0AT1, 222-225
B^0AT3, 224-225
Beckwith-Wiedemann syndrome, 2297t
Bee stings, 2500, 2525
Beer potomania, 496
Beers criteria, 2594
Belatacept, 2248, 2254t, 2258-2259
Belimumab, 1104-1105
Benazepril hydrochloride, 1641-1642, 1643t
Bence Jones proteins, 990
Benidipine, 1665
Benign cystic neoplasm, 1369-1370
Benign epithelial tumor, 1368
Benign mesenchymal tumor, 1368-1369
Benign neoplasm, 1368-1370
Benign prostatic hyperplasia, 1261, 1280
β-trace protein, 935-936
Betaxolol, 1656t-1657t, 1658
Betel nut chewing, 2534
Bevacizumab, 1383f, 1384, 1398
BGT1, 226
Bias, of estimating glomerular filtration rate equations, 785
Bicarbonate
 cytosolic, 234-235
 diarrhea effects on, 528-529
 excretion of, 551
 in extracellular fluid, 514, 519, 830f
 gain of, systemic response to, 519-520
 gastrointestinal loss of, 529, 529t
 generation of
  ammonia metabolism in, 248-255
  carbon dioxide retention effects on, 516
  citrate excretion in, 247-248
  organic anion excretion in, 247-248
  titratable acid excretion in, 246-247
 in hemodialysis dialysate, 2094-2095
 hydrogen removal by, 835
 luminal, 234, 241
 metabolic alkalosis caused by, 552-553
 in paracellular sodium chloride transport, 147
 in peritoneal dialysis solutions, 2119, 2125
 plasma concentration of
  arterial blood gas values and, 521
  chloride repletion for, 520
  description of, 513-514
  in high anion gap acidosis, 524-525
  increase in, renal response to, 520
 proximal tubule excretion of, 519
 regeneration of, 515
 secretion of, 244-245
 serum, 684-685
 supplementation of, 684-685, 2004
 urine, 2382
Bicarbonate reabsorption
 ammonia effects on, 245
 angiotensin II effects on, 408
 carbonic anhydrase for, 1703-1704
 carbonic anhydrase inhibitors effect on, 136
 in chronic kidney disease, 1749
 in collecting ducts
  aldosterone regulation of, 244
  anion exchangers in, 243
  carbonic anhydrase's role in, 243
  cells involved in, 239-241, 239f-241f
  chloride channel's role in, 243

Bicarbonate reabsorption (Continued)
 cortical, 242
 H^+-ATPase's role in, 242
 H^+-K^+-ATPase's role in, 242-243
 hormonal regulation of, 244-245
 inner medullary, 242
 intercalated cells involved in, 239-241, 239f-241f
 kidney anion exchanger 1's role in, 243
 outer medullary, 242
 paracrine regulation, 245
 principal cells involved in, 241
 proteins involved in, 242-244
 segments of, 239
 sodium-bicarbonate cotransporters in, 243-244
 in connecting tubules, 241-242
 in distal convoluted tubule, 238-239
 diuretics effect on, 1703-1704
 intercalated cells involved in, 239-241, 239f-241f
 in loop of Henle, 238
 metabolic acidosis effects on, 236-238, 244
 metabolic alkalosis effects on, 244
 osmotic gradient caused by, 147-148
 proximal, 151
 in proximal tubule
  acid-base effects on, 237
  angiotensin II effects on, 237
  calcium-sensing receptor effects on, 238
  carbonic anhydrase in, 237
  description of, 530
  electroneutral sodium-bicarbonate cotransporter in, 236-237
  endothelin effects on, 237
  general mechanisms of, 234-235
  H^+-ATPase in, 235-236
  luminal flow rate effects on, 237
  metabolic acidosis effects on, 236-237
  Na^+-H^+ exchangers in, 235
  parathyroid hormone effects on, 237-238
  potassium effects on, 237
  regulation of, 237-238
  schematic diagram of, 236f, 2384f
 sites of, 234, 235f
 in thick ascending limb, 238
Bikunin, 1330-1331
Bilateral cortical necrosis, 1631-1632
Bilateral disease, 1570t
Bilateral renal artery stenosis, 1595
Bilateral ureteral obstruction, 299
Bile acid metabolism, 734
Bile salts, 2508
Bilirubin, 790
Biochemical hypoparathyroidism, 1453
Bioelectrical impedance analysis, 2079, 2096, 2099
Bioethics, 2558-2562
Biofilms, catheter-related bacteremia caused by, 2220
Bioflavonoids, 2036
Biomarkers
 acute kidney injury, 930-932, 931t
 candidate markers, 927
 chronic kidney disease. See Chronic kidney disease, biomarkers for
 chronic kidney disease–mineral bone disorder, 1840t
 clinical utility of, retrospective studies of, 928
 Critical Path Initiative for, 953
 definition of, 927, 927t
 development of, 927-930

Biomarkers *(Continued)*
  diabetic nephropathy, 1294t
  discovery of, 927-930
  exploratory studies for, 927-928
  future of, 954
  glomerular filtration, 932-936
  ideal, 930, 930t
  Integrated Discrimination Improvement Index for, 929-930
  Kidney Health Initiative on, 953-954
  multiple, combination of, 952-953, 953t
  natriuretic peptides as, 343-344
  Net Reclassification Index for, 929-930
  performance analysis of, 929-930, 929f
  pharmacodynamic, 927t
  predictive, 927t
  prognostic, 927t
  prospective screening studies for, 928-929
  qualification process for, 928-929
  receiver operator characteristic curve for, 929, 929f
  serum, 931
  surrogate endpoint, 927t
  urinary
    albuminuria as, 948
    cystatin C, 948-949
    description of, 931
    glomerular cell injury, 936-937
    glutathione S-transferase, 938-939
    hepcidin-25, 939
    insulin-like growth factor-binding protein-7, 949
    interleukin-18, 939-941
    kidney injury molecule-1, 941-942
    liver-type fatty acid-binding protein, 942-943
    β_1-microglobulin, 937-938, 1041
    β_2-microglobulin, 938
    N-acetyl-β-D-glucosaminidase, 947
    nephrin, 936-937
    netrin-1, 943
    neutrophil gelatinase-associated lipocalin, 943-947
    podocalyxin, 936
    podocyte count, 936
    proteinuria as, 947-948
    for renal fibrosis, 951-952
    tissue inhibitor metalloproteinase-2, 949
    tubular injury, 937-949
  urinary tract obstruction, 1263
  validation process for, 928
Biomaterials, 2602, 2609-2610
Biopsy
  bone, 1842-1846, 1845t
  kidney. *See* Kidney biopsy
Biotin, 1983-1984
Biphenyl tetrazoles, 1651-1653
Birth weight
  blood pressure affected by, 706-709, 707f-708f
  categories of, 694t
  chronic kidney disease and, 712
  end-stage kidney disease and, 712, 713f
  fetal drug exposure effects on, 719
  gestational hyperglycemia effects on, 717-718
  glomerular characteristics by, 696t
  glomerular filtration rate affected by, 709-710
  low. *See* Low birth weight
  nephron number and, 703-705
  proteinuria and, 710-711
  renal function affected by, 709-712

Birt-Hogg-Dube syndrome, 1374, 1951-1952, 1952f, 1952t
Bisoprolol, 1656t-1657t, 1658
Bisphosphonates, 611, 627, 1399, 2396
BK channels, 179, 564, 574
BK virus, 1404-1405, 2272, 2428, 2430
Bladder cancer, 755, 1261
Bladder dysfunction, 1320, 2314
Bladder tumors, 862f
Blood
  arterial, pH of, 2382
  loss of, 1885, 1962
  phosphorus in, 196, 197t, 626
Blood pressure. *See also* High blood pressure; Hypertension
  ambulatory monitoring of, 1538, 1540-1542, 1541t-1542t, 1693, 1694f
  angiotensin II and, 1532f, 1640-1641
  atrial natriuretic peptide effects on, 342
  birth weight effects on, 706-709, 707f-708f
  catch-up growth effects on, 721-722
  in children, 2360
  chronic kidney disease and, 679, 1563f
  classification of, 765, 765t
  control of, 1527-1528, 1552-1553
    angiotensin-converting enzyme inhibitors for, 1303-1305, 1317, 1928-1929
    antihypertensive drug therapy goals for, 1680-1681. *See also* Antihypertensive drug therapy
    cardiovascular disease risk prevention through, 1867-1868, 2009
    in chronic kidney disease management, 1867, 1975, 2009, 2283
    in diabetic nephropathy, 1303-1312
    dietary modifications for, 1931
    during hemodialysis, 1316, 2103
    intravenous agents, 1630-1631
    in kidney disease patients, 1689, 1689t
    kidney's role in, 1861
    nighttime ventilation techniques for, 1694
    renoprotection through, 1765-1767
  developmental programming of, 709, 709f
  diastolic, 1524, 1524t, 1526f, 1681
  in elderly, 745, 745f, 2010f, 2592
  endothelium and, 1534-1535
  EP4 receptor's role in regulation of, 372
  glomerular volume and, 709, 709f
  goals for, 1680-1681
  hepatocyte growth factor effects on, 1741
  homeostasis of, 393f
  kidney function decline and, 1562f
  left ventricular hypertrophy and, 1688-1689
  low birth weight effects on, 707, 1627f
  magnesium and, 623
  measurement of, 766, 1525t, 1538-1542, 1539f
  metabolic capacity and, 722f
  metabolic load and, 722f
  mortality in veterans with chronic kidney disease, 1559f
  nephron number and, 697t-698t, 709, 709f
  in patients undergoing dialysis, 1561-1562
  physiology of, 1528
  plasmapheresis effects on, 2163
  preeclampsia prevention and, 1626
  prematurity effects on, 706-709, 707f-708f
  rapid reduction of, 1699-1700

Blood pressure *(Continued)*
  soluble epoxide hydrolase in regulation of, 385
  stroke risks and, 1929f
  sudden reduction in, 1700
Blood urea nitrogen, 123, 933-934, 988, 1808, 1959, 1968-1969
BMAL1 gene, 256
Bmp4, 31
BMP4, 2297-2298
Bmp1ra, 27
Body fluids, 391f-392f, 460-462, 461f, 486, 2365, 2414
Body lead burden, 686-687
Body mass index, 1323f, 1343f, 1771
Bohr effect, 527
BOLD magnetic resonance imaging, 864, 1271
Bone
  biology of, 1831-1833
  calcification of, 1836
  calcium-sensing receptor's role in, 1826
  cellular components of, 1832
  composition of, 1831-1832
  histology of, 1844f
  hyperparathyroid, 1844f
  immunosuppressive agents effect on, 1851-1852
  magnesium in, 193, 193t
  mineralization of, 1845
  phosphorus in, 196
  postrenal transplantation changes in, 1851-1852
  remodeling of, 1830, 1832, 1833f-1834f, 1845, 1849
  resorption of, 611-612
  trabecular, 1831-1832, 1842
  turnover of, 1845-1846, 1845t
  volume of, 1845
Bone disease, 1352-1355, 1437, 1843
Bone formation rate, 1845
Bone marrow transplantation (BMT), 991t, 992-993, 1193, 2249-2250
Bone marrow-derived fibrocytes, 1793
Bone marrow-derived mesenchymal progenitor cells, 1197
Bone marrow-derived mesenchymal stem cells, 2611
Bone mineral density (BMT)
  fractures and, 1852, 2283
  minimal change disease effects on, 1022
  posttransplantation reductions in, 2282-2283
  stone formers and, 1353t
  thiazide diuretics effect on, 1726-1727
Bone morphogenetic proteins (BMPs), 28-29, 34, 1217, 1757-1758, 1843
Bone pain, 2282
Bone-specific alkaline phosphatase, 1842
Bortezomib, 1105, 2248-2249
Bosniak renal cyst classification, 1375, 1376t
Bothrops snakebites, 2447
Bouin's fixative, 919
Bowel dysfunction, 2314
Bowman's capsule, 4-5, 45-46, 52-53
Bowman's space, 45-46, 47f, 94-96, 95f, 1789
BQ-123, 338
Brachyury, 2603
Bradford-Hill criteria, of causality, 670, 670t
Bradykinin, 417, 1740
Bradykinin receptors, 347, 350
Brain herniation, 503

Brain natriuretic peptide (BNP)
    antifibrotic effects of, 342
    atrial natriuretic peptide versus, 340
    as biomarker, 343-344
    in cirrhosis, 447
    description of, 339
    in effective arterial blood volume
        regulation, 414
    half-life of, 340
    in heart failure, 433-434
    nephrectomy effects on levels of, 1739
    NT-proBNP, 343, 433-434, 453
    plasma levels of, 414, 434
    preproBNP, 340
    pro-, 1800
    recombinant, 344
    renal effects of, 342
    secretion of, 414
    structure of, 339f, 340, 413
    synthesis of, 340
    therapeutic uses of, 344
Branched-chain amino acids, 1971
Branching morphogenesis, 5
Branchio-oto-renal syndrome, 2297t, 2299, 2318
Brazil, 2451. *See also* Latin America
Breast cancer, 607-608, 1670
Breastfeeding, 1631, 1638
Brescia-Cimino procedure, 2064
Bright's disease, 1855
Bromodeoxyuridine, 2608
Bronchiectasias, 1492
Bronchogenic carcinoma, 499-500
Brugada sign, 570-571
Brush border
    of pars convoluta cells, 56-59
    of proximal tubule, 55, 57f
Brush border membrane vesicles, 211
Brushite, 1323, 1328, 1342f
Buckley's syndrome, 1050
Bufadienolide, 419
Buffer systems
    in acid-base homeostasis, 512-514
    open, 513
    physicochemical, chemical equilibria of, 512-513
    regulation of, 513-514
Buffering, 512, 519
Bumetanide, 1707
Bundled prospective payment system, 2628-2629
Burst-forming units–erythroid, 1882-1883
bZIP transcription factor, 2483

C

C fibers, 1942
C3, 1761, 1792
C3 convertases, 1183-1184
C5 convertase, 1183-1184
C3 glomerulonephritis, 1046, 1046f-1047f, 1050, 1053
C3 glomerulopathies
    algorithm for, 1054f
    classification of, 1046, 1046f
    dense deposit disease. *See* Dense deposit disease
    description of, 1045-1046
    diagnosis of, 1054f
    eculizumab for, 1159
    epidemiology of, 1050
    immunofluorescence microscopy findings, 1051
    nephrotic syndrome caused by, 1045-1046
    pathogenesis of, 1052, 1052f
    pathology of, 1050-1052, 1051f

C3 nephritic factor, 1146-1147
Cadmium nephropathy, 1227
Caenorhabditis elegans, 19
Cairo-Bishop criteria, 990, 992t
Calbindin, 2390-2391
Calbindin-D28K, 66-67, 192
Calcidiol, 1828, 1841, 1848
Calcific uremic arteriolopathy. *See* Calciphylaxis
Calcifications
    aortic valve, 1859
    arterial. *See* Arterial calcification
    in atherosclerosis, 1855
    extraskeletal, 1850
    metastatic, 1945-1946
    mitral valve, 1859
    renal, 871-878
    renal parenchymal, 1775
    vascular. *See* Vascular calcification
Calcimimetics
    for chronic kidney disease–mineral bone disorder, 1873, 2026-2028
    definition of, 2026
    for secondary hyperparathyroidism, 2032
Calcineurin, 189
Calcineurin inhibitors, 1398-1399
    adverse effects of, 1167-1168
    bone pain caused by, 2282
    glomerular disease treated with, 1167-1168
    hyperkalemia associated with, 541, 2281
    hypertension caused by, 1167-1168
    hypomagnesemia caused by, 622
    immunosuppressive uses of, 2256, 2271, 2424-2425
    lupus nephritis treated with, 1104
    malignancies induced by, 1168
    membranous nephropathy treated with, 1043-1044
    nephrotoxicity caused by, 378, 1167, 2259, 2268-2269, 2272-2275
    podocytes affected by, 119
    renal transplantation uses of, 2256, 2271
    steroid-resistant nephrotic syndrome treated with, 2330-2331
    steroid-sensitive nephrotic syndrome treated with, 2329-2330
    toxicity of, 1168
    vasoconstriction caused by, 2265
Calciphylaxis, 1944-1945, 1945f, 2103
Calcitonin, 1400
    bicarbonate reabsorption stimulated by, 245
    bone resorption inhibition using, 612
    in children, 2390-2391
    nephrogenic diabetes insipidus treated with, 301
Calcitonin gene-related peptide, 110
Calcitriol, 1830, 1872-1873, 1923-1924, 2025, 2089
Calcium
    absorption of, 185-187, 1824-1825
    blood forms of, 602
    bound form of, 186
    calcimimetics effect on, 1873, 2027
    in cellular processes, 185-186
    in children. *See* Children, calcium in
    in chronic kidney disease–mineral bone disorder, 1847
    citrate association with, 219
    components of, 186f
    daily ingestion of, 601-602
    dosage of, 1361
    excretion of, 1334f
        in Bartter's syndrome, 578
        in chronic kidney disease, 2031

Calcium (*Continued*)
    diuretics effect on, 1726
    hypocalcemia prevention goals for, 2393
    in proximal renal tubular acidosis, 533
    fibroblast growth factor-23 effects on levels of, 2019-2020
    filtered, 188f
    forms of, 186
    fractional excretion of, 1706, 1749-1750
    free, 186, 602
    globulin binding of, 602
    glomerulus filtration of, 187
    in hemodialysis dialysate, 2094, 2106
    homeostasis of
        age-related changes in, 741-742
        description of, 1824-1825
        disorders of. *See* Hypercalcemia; Hypocalcemia
        hormones involved in, 1838-1839
        modulation of, 601
        parathyroid hormone effects on, 601, 1826-1827, 1923-1924
        parathyroid hormone–vitamin D endocrine system regulation of, 187, 187f
        schematic diagram of, 186f
        whole-body, 601-602
    hyperkalemia treated with, 593-594
    insulin effects on deposition of, 1914
    intestinal hyperabsorption of, 1331-1333
    intracellular, 306
    ionized, 1824
    kidney stones and, 1324
    measurement of, 2028-2029
    monitoring of, 2014
    nephron loss-specific adaptations in metabolism of, 1749-1750
    oxalate concentration versus, 1325-1327
    parathyroid hormone and, 606f, 1827f, 2023
    preeclampsia prevention use of, 1626
    protein-bound, 186, 187f, 602
    reabsorption of, 187-189
        in distal tubule, 189, 190f
        intestinal, 741-742
        in loop of Henle, 188-189
        metabolic acidosis effects on, 191
        metabolic alkalosis effects on, 191
        parathyroid hormone effects on, 1828
        in proximal tubule, 188, 188f
        in thick ascending limb, 188
    renal parenchymal deposits of, 1775
    serum, 186, 186f, 1822, 1824, 1851
    transport of. *See* Calcium transport
    whole-body amount of, 601-602
Calcium acetate, 2022
Calcium antagoist, 1560
Calcium carbonate, 2022
Calcium channel blockers (CCBs), 1564, 1629, 1995
    adverse effects of, 1668
    angiotensin II affected by, 1662
    angiotensin-converting enzyme inhibitors and, 1669, 1681-1682, 1684f
    antiproteinuric effects of, 1667
    atherogenesis inhibition by, 1669
    benzothiazepines, 1663-1664
    β-blockers and, 1669, 1691
    breast cancer and, 1670
    contraindications for, 1668
    dihydropyridines, 1662, 1664-1670, 1668t, 1699
    diphenylalkylamine, 1664
    diuresis caused by, 1662

Calcium channel blockers (CCBs) (Continued)
  diuretics and, 1691
  dosing of, 1649t-1650t
  drug interactions with, 1669-1670, 1670t
  dual therapy using, 1691
  efficacy of, 1668-1671
  in elderly, 1685
  hemodynamic effects of, 1666-1667, 1668t
  hypertensive urgencies and emergencies treated with, 1697t, 1698-1699
  indications for, 1662
  long-term effects of, 1667
  mechanism of action, 1662
  nondihydropyridines, 1662
  nonhemodynamic effects of, 1667
  pharmacodynamics of, 1663t
  pharmacokinetics of, 1663t
  renal autoregulation blockade by, 105
  renal effects of, 1666-1667, 1667t
  in renal insufficiency patients, 1649t-1650t
  in renal transplantation recipients, 1667
  renin-angiotensin-aldosterone inhibitors and, combination therapy using, 1690-1691
  safety of, 1668-1671
  side effects of, 1689-1690
  types of, 1662-1666, 1663t
  vasodilatory properties of, 1662, 1685
Calcium channels, 1662
Calcium chloride, 593-594
Calcium citrate, 1758-1759
Calcium gluconate, 593-594, 618
Calcium oxalate, 1324-1325, 1328, 1338f. See also Oxalate
Calcium oxalate stones, 873, 1260, 1323, 1323f, 1325, 1326f, 1633, 2507
Calcium phosphate stones, 873, 1323f, 1325, 1326f, 1633
Calcium stone, 1323, 1323f, 1331-1341, 1352-1355, 1633
Calcium transport
  in distal nephron, 190f
  in distal tubule, 192f
  epithelial, 1826f
  parathyroid hormone effects on, 187
  proteins involved in, 191-193
  regulation of, 189-191
    calcium-regulating hormones involved in, 189
    diuretics in, 189-191
    estrogens in, 191
    extracellular calcium in, 189
    Klotho in, 191
    metabolic acidosis effects on, 191
    novel proteins involved in, 191
    proteins involved in, 191
    sclerostin in, 191
  renal, 1825
  transcellular, 188
  transepithelial, 1706
Calcium-binding protein 39, 163
Calcium-containing binders, 2022, 2031, 2094
Calcium/magnesium-sensing receptor-associated disorder, 1466
Calcium–parathyroid hormone–fibroblast growth factor-23 loop, 1839
Calcium-phosphate deposition, in end-stage kidney disease, 1775
Calcium-regulating hormones, 189

Calcium-sensing receptor (CaSR)
  activation of
    in hypercalcemia, 609-610
    parathyroid hormone secretion affected by, 2026
    phospholipase C stimulation secondary to, 1827f
  apical, 574
  bicarbonate reabsorption affected by, 238, 245
  in bone, 1826
  calcimimetic agent interaction with, 2020
  calcimimetic targeting of, 2026-2027
  description of, 164, 164f, 189, 448, 601-602, 1825
  expression of, 1825-1826
  gain-of-function mutations in, 614-616
  gene expression, 1334
  mutations of, 579, 2378
  in vascular calcification, 1826
Calculated panel reactive antibody, 2260
Caloric intake, in chronic kidney disease, 1973
Calorie restriction, 732-733
Calyceal cyst, 1518
Calyceal diverticulum, 889
Camptomelic dysplasia, 2297t
Cancer
  acute kidney injury and, 990, 991t, 1390
  angiotensin receptor blockers and, 1655-1656
  renal failure and, 1390t
  in renal transplantation recipients, 2284-2286, 2285t, 2543-2544
  viral infections associated with, 2285t
Candesartan cilexetil, 1651-1652, 1652t
Candida species, 1254, 1404, 2129
Candidate gene, 1348
Candiduria, 1254, 1254t
Cannabinoid receptor 1 blockade, albuminuria caused by, 120
Cannabinoid receptors, in cirrhosis, 443-444
Capillarization of sinusoids, 441
Capillary hydraulic pressure, 426
Captopril
  adverse effects of, 1648
  characteristics of, 1641
  dosage of, 1641
  hypertensive urgencies and emergencies treated with, 1697t
  proteinuria associated with, 1159, 1645
  renography enhanced with, 908
  sodium excretion affected by, 444-445
Captopril challenge test, 1546
Captopril trial, 1555
Carbamazepine, 471, 497, 2182-2183
Carbapenems, 1235t-1236t
Carbenoxolone, 577
Carbohydrates, 128f, 1816
Carbon dioxide, 255, 513-514
Carbon dioxide load, 512
Carbon dioxide tension, 515-516
Carbon dioxide–bicarbonate system, 513
Carbon monoxide poisoning, 545
Carbonic acid, 234
Carbonic anhydrase
  in ammonia secretion, 253-255
  in bicarbonate reabsorption, 237, 243
  collecting duct ammonia secretion affected by, 253
  deficiency of, 531-532
  description of, 1702

Carbonic anhydrase (Continued)
  II, 237
  intercalated cell levels of, 71-72
  IV, 237, 243, 254-255
  metabolic acidosis effects on, 244
  in proximal tubule bicarbonate reabsorption, 237
  XII, 243
Carbonic anhydrase II, 530-532, 1455
Carbonic anhydrase inhibitors
  adverse effects of, 1704
  bicarbonate reabsorption affected by, 136
  bicarbonate wasting caused by, 532
  in elderly, 1704
  indications for, 1704
  long-term administration of, 1703-1704
  mechanism of action, 1702-1704
  metabolic acidosis caused by, 1730
  pharmacokinetics of, 1704
  site of action, 1702-1704
  urine alkalization using, 2168
Carboxyl angiotensin-converting enzyme inhibitors, 1641-1644, 1643t
3-Carboxy-4-methyl-5-propyl-2-furanpropionic acid, 2037
Carboxypeptidase G_2, 2188
Cardenolide, 419
Cardiac arrest, 970, 2107
Cardiac dysfunction, 2139
Cardiac filling sensors, 394-396
Cardiac output, 83, 85, 133, 393-394, 396
Cardiac remodeling, 342
Cardiac surgery, 991t, 992
Cardioembolic stroke, 1927
Cardiorenal syndrome, 2139
Cardiovascular calcification index, 1847
Cardiovascular disease
  albuminuria and, 1860-1861
  antihypertensive drug therapy for, 1688-1689
  in children, 2406-2409, 2421-2422, 2432-2433
  in chronic kidney disease. See Chronic kidney disease, cardiovascular disease associated with
  clinical manifestations of, 1859-1860
  in diabetes nephropathy, 1295, 1316-1317
  diagnosis of, 2101-2102
  in elderly, 2590
  estimated glomerular filtration rate and, 1855, 1866, 2008
  hyperlipidemia and, 1802
  in kidney disease, 1166
  kidney function and, 1860
  microalbuminuria and, 1295
  mortality caused by, 2409
  occlusive, antiplatelet therapy for, 1873
  in peritoneal dialysis, 2127-2128
  preeclampsia and, 1618, 1618f
  premature, 1855
  in renal transplantation recipients, 2283-2284
  risk factors for, 1201
    anemia, 1863-1864, 1930
    chronic kidney disease–mineral bone disorder, 1864-1865, 1872-1873
    coagulation defects, 1863
    congestive heart failure, 1862t
    diabetes mellitus, 1865
    dyslipidemia, 1863, 2011
    fibroblast growth factor-23, 2101
    in hemodialysis patients, 2100-2101

Cardiovascular disease *(Continued)*
  homocysteine, 1864, 1970
  hypertension, 1861, 1862t, 1873, 2127, 2421-2422
  inflammation, 1865, 2100
  left ventricular hypertrophy, 1295-1296, 1857-1858, 2101-2102, 2421-2422
  list of, 1862t
  obesity, 1865-1866
  oxidative stress, 1865, 2100-2101
  phosphate retention, 1978-1979
  stroke, 1862t
  vitamin D levels, 1864-1865
  treatment of, 2101-2102
  in type 1 diabetes mellitus, 1295
  urolithiasis and, 1351, 1351f
Cardiovascular system
  bradykinin effects on, 417
  COX-2 inhibitor effects on, 363-364
  hypermagnesemia manifestations of, 625
  hypomagnesemia manifestations of, 622-623
  natriuretic peptides effect on, 342
Caribbean, 2442f
Caroli's disease, 1496-1497
Carotid baroceptors, 396
Carotid endarterectomy, 1932
Carotid-femoral pulse wave velocity, 1535
Carp bile, raw, 2525
Carperitide, 344
Carteolol, 1656t-1657t, 1657
Carvedilol, 1658t-1659t, 1659
Case-control studies, 671
Casein kinase 2, 154
CASK, 29
Caspase-1, 2485-2486
Caspase-3, 1817, 1965
Cast nephropathy, 1391-1393
Castleman's disease, 1159
Casts, in urine, 800, 800t, 801f
Cat scratch disease, 1149-1150
Catabolism
  amino acid, 1963-1964
  fats, 128f
  muscle, 1967
  myostatin activation caused by, 1967
  protein, 128f, 517, 1959-1960
Catastrophic antiphospholipid antibody syndrome, 2158-2159
Catch-up growth, 721-723
Catecholamines
  arginine vasopressin effects on, 1717
  hypokalemic effect of, 562
  myocardial infarction effects on, 1729
  phosphate transport affected by, 200-201
  thermogenic effect of, 137
Catecholamine-secreting tumor, 1548
β-Catenin, 28-29, 1832-1833, 1834f
Caterpillar stings, 2445-2446, 2446f
Catestatin, 438, 1533
Catheters
  bacteremia associated with, 2220
  hemodialysis. *See* Hemodialysis, catheters for
  infection of, 2068f
  peritoneal dialysis. *See* Peritoneal dialysis, catheters used in
  subclavian, 2145
  tunneled. *See* Tunneled catheters
Cation exchange resins, 596-597
Causality, Bradford-Hill criteria of, 670, 670t
ClC-K1 channel, 156-157, 157f, 161, 278
CD28, 2240-2241

CD133+ cells, 2609
CD4+ T cells, 1216, 1795
Cd2ap, 38
CD2AP disease, 1430
CD2-associated protein, 113
Cdc42, 38, 39f
CDX2 gene, 2606
CE45, 2611
Cefotaxime, 1241t
Ceftazidime, 2041
Ceftriaxone, 1241, 1241t
Celiprolol, 1658t-1659t, 1659
Cell membrane, 125
Cell-mediated immunity, 1233
Central α₂-adrenergic agonist, 1698
Central adrenergic agonists
  dosing of, 1649t-1650t
  efficacy of, 1672
  mechanism of action, 1671
  pharmacodynamics of, 1671, 1672t
  pharmacokinetics of, 1671, 1671t
  receptor binding of, 1671t
  renal effects of, 1672
  in renal insufficiency patients, 1649t-1650t
  safety of, 1672
  types of, 1671-1672
Central and peripheral adrenergic neuronal blocking agents, 1673
Central diabetes insipidus. *See* Diabetes insipidus, central
Central hypervolemia, 394-395
Central nervous system, 342, 419, 501-502
Central vein stenosis, 2212-2214, 2212f-2214f
Central venous catheters, 2412-2413, 2542-2543
Centrifugation, 2160, 2161f
Cephalosporins, 1235t-1236t
Cerebral blood flow, 1700
Cerebral edema, 813, 1619-1620, 1705
Cerebral hypoperfusion, 1930
Cerebral salt wasting, 493
Cetuximab, 575, 1398
CHADS₂ score, 1932
Channel-activating protease-1, 565-566
Charcot-Marie Tooth neuropathy-associated glomerulopathy, 1429
CHARGE syndrome, 2300
CHD7, 2300
Chemokine(s), 1794, 2241, 2243
Chemokine C-C motif receptor 1, 1754-1755
Chemokine ligand 2, 976
Chemokine ligand 8, 1233
Chemotherapy, 1385
  cast nephropathy and, 1392
  hyperuricemia and, 1396
  nephrotoxic injury and, 1397
  tumor cell necrosis after, 968
  volume expansion before, 628
  for Wilms' tumor, 1387
Childbirth, 1617
Children. *See also* Infants
  acid-base equilibrium in, 2382-2383, 2382t
  acute postinfectious glomerulonephritis in, 2331-2333
  Bardet-Biedl syndrome in, 2322, 2322t
  Bartter's syndrome in, 2333-2335, 2344, 2376-2378, 2377f, 2377t
  blood pressure screening in, 2360
  calcitonin in, 2390-2391
  calcium in
    balance of, 2389-2390, 2389f/2390f
    disorders of, 2391-2396
    distribution of, 2389, 2389f
    intestinal absorption of, 2390
    regulation of, 2389

Children *(Continued)*
  chronic kidney disease in
    angiotensin receptor blockers for, 2362
    angiotensin-converting enzyme inhibitors for, 2362
    cardiovascular comorbidities, 2359-2361
    demographics of, 2309
    description of, 2308
    development effects of, 2357-2359
    glomerular filtration rate assessments, 2309
    growth failure secondary to, 1918, 2357-2359, 2358f/2359f
    hypertension caused by, 2360, 2421-2422
    intima-media thickness changes associated with, 2361, 2361f
    left ventricular hypertrophy with, 2360-2361, 2421-2422, 2432
    metabolic acidosis with, 2359
    neurodevelopment dysfunctions secondary to, 2309
    nutrition effects of, 2357-2359
    progression of, 2361-2362, 2362f
    pubertal delay caused by, 2357, 2435-2436
    recombinant growth hormone therapy for, 2359, 2359f
    renal function changes, 2361
    renal transplantation for, 2422
    vitamin D deficiency associated with, 2434
  chronic kidney disease–mineral bone disorder in, 2361, 2406
  congenital anomalies of the kidney and urinary tract in. *See* Congenital anomalies of the kidney and urinary tract (CAKUT)
  continuous renal replacement therapy in, 2417-2418
  creatinine concentration in, 2341f
  cystinosis in, 2339-2340, 2341f
  cystinuria in, 2345-2346, 2346f
  dehydration in, 2367-2368, 2373-2374, 2373t
  Dent's disease in, 2344-2345
  dialysis in
    hemodialysis. *See* Children, hemodialysis in
    long-term, renal transplantation advantages over, 2410-2411, 2410f
    modality changes, 2417
    peritoneal. *See* Children, peritoneal dialysis in
  diuretic renography in, 1266-1267
  EAST syndrome in, 167, 2379
  end-stage kidney disease in, 2308-2309, 2321
    anemia secondary to, 2405-2406
    arrhythmias associated with, 2408
    atherosclerosis associated with, 2407-2408
    cardiovascular diseases associated with, 2406-2409, 2421-2422
    chronic kidney disease–mineral bone disorder associated with, 2406
    clinical consequences of, 2404-2409
    congenital anomalies of the kidney and urinary tract as cause of, 2361, 2404, 2421
    description of, 2308-2309, 2321
    diastolic dysfunction associated with, 2408
    electrolyte imbalance secondary to, 2405
    epidemiology of, 2403, 2419t

Children (Continued)
 etiology of, 2404, 2404t
 growth effects, 2405
 hyperkalemia associated with, 2405
 hypertension secondary to, 2406-2407
 left ventricular hypertrophy associated with, 2408, 2421-2422
 life expectancy of, 2404
 linear growth effects, 2405
 metabolic acidosis secondary to, 2405
 mortality rate for, 2409
 neurodevelopment effects of, 2408-2410, 2408f
 nutrition effects, 2404-2405
 renal osteodystrophy associated with, 2407f
 renal replacement affected by, 2409
 renal replacement therapy for. See Children, renal replacement therapy in
 valvular disease associated with, 2408
 vascular calcification associated with, 2407-2408
 weight effects, 2404-2405
extracellular fluid in, 2365-2366, 2368, 2414
familial hypomagnesemia with hypercalciuria and nephrocalcinosis in, 2345
fibroblast growth factor-23 in, 2390-2391, 2400
focal segmental glomerulosclerosis in, 1030, 1032
Gitelman's syndrome in, 2335, 2378-2379
glomerular diseases in, 2322-2340
glomerular filtration rate in, 787, 787t, 2309-2310
growth in
 end-stage kidney disease effects on, 2405
 failure of, chronic kidney disease as cause of, 2357-2359, 2358f-2359f
hematuria in, 1014-1015
hemodialysis in
 apparatus for, 2413-2414
 blood flow, 2413-2414
 complications of, 2414-2415
 continuous renal replacement therapy versus, 2418
 costs of, 2411
 dialyzer for, 2413
 dose of, 2414
 fluid removal, 2414
 machine for, 2413
 peritoneal dialysis versus, 2411, 2412t, 2417
 renal transplantation versus, 2410
 tubing for, 2413
 vascular access for, 2412-2414
hemolytic-uremic syndrome in
 atypical, 2354t, 2355-2362
 clinical features of, 2354t
 cobalamin C synthase deficiency as cause of, 2356-2357
 complement disorders as cause of, 2355-2356, 2355f
 definition of, 2352
 diacyl glycerol kinase ε mutations as cause of, 2356
 diagnosis of, 2353
 epidemiology of, 2352-2353
 pathogenesis of, 2353
 prognosis for, 2354-2355
 Shiga toxin-associated, 2352-2357

Children (Continued)
 Streptococcus pneumoniae-associated, 2355
 treatment of, 2353-2354
 von Willebrand factor-cleaving protease deficiency as cause of, 2356
hereditary hypophosphatemic rickets with hypercalciuria in, 2345
hospitalized, hyponatremia in, 2372
hypercalcemia in, 608, 2393-2396, 2394t, 2396f, 2397t
hypercalciuria in, 2340, 2344, 2344f
hyperkalemia in, 2380-2382, 2380t-2381t
hypernatremia in, 2367-2370
hypernatremic dehydration in, 2367-2368, 2374
hyperosmolality in, 2367-2370, 2367t
hyperphosphatemia in, 2398-2400, 2399f, 2399t
hypertension in, 2329, 2421-2422
hypocalcemia in
 citrate blood product infusions as cause of, 2391
 diagnostic workup for, 2392
 early neonatal, 2391
 late neonatal, 2391
 lipid infusions as cause of, 2391
 monitoring of, 2393
 respiratory alkalosis as cause of, 2392
 treatment of, 2392-2393, 2394t
hypokalemia in, 2375-2379, 2375t, 2376f-2378f, 2377t
hypomagnesemia in
 autosomal dominant, 2388-2389
 causes of, 2387t
 description of, 2387
 familial
  with hypercalciuria and nephrocalcinosis, 2387-2388
  with secondary hypocalcemia, 2388, 2388f
 isolated autosomal recessive, with normocalciuria, 2389
hyponatremia in, 2370-2372, 2371t
hypo-osmolality in, 2370-2371, 2371t
hypophosphatemia in, 2396-2398, 2397t-2398t, 2398f
immune complex-mediated crescentic glomerulonephritis in, 1073
inborn errors of metabolism in, renal replacement therapy in, 2417
intracellular fluid in, 2365-2366
intrinsic renal failure in, 2368t
Joubert's syndrome in, 2322, 2322t
kidney malformation in, 2294-2295, 2295f
kidney stones in, 2340-2342
left ventricular hypertrophy in, 2360-2361, 2421-2422, 2432
Liddle's syndrome in, 2379
linear growth in, 2405, 2434-2435
lower urinary tract abnormalities in, 2296
magnesium in
 disorders involving, 2386-2389
 metabolism of, 2386-2389
Meckel-Gruber syndrome in, 2322, 2322t
medications in, 2409-2410
membranoproliferative glomerulonephritis type I in, 1049
membranous nephropathy in, 1041
metabolic acidosis in, 2382-2383, 2382t
minimal change disease in, 1021
nephritic syndrome in, 2331-2333
nephrocalcinosis in, 2340

Children (Continued)
 nephrogenic diabetes insipidus in, 2338-2339, 2368-2370, 2370t
 nephrogenic syndrome of inappropriate diuresis in, 2372-2373
 nephrolithiasis in
  clinical features of, 2342-2343
  diagnosis of, 2343
  genetic, 2344-2348
  hypercalciuria in, 2340, 2344-2345, 2344f
  hyperoxaluria in, 2340, 2346-2348, 2422
  hyperuricosuria in, 2342, 2343t
  hypocitraturia in, 2340-2342
  interventional treatment of, 2343-2344
  nonhypercalciuric, 2345-2348
  risk factors for, 2340-2342
  treatment of, 2343-2344
  urinary tract infections associated with, 2342
 nephronophthisis in, 2321-2322
 nephronophthisis-related ciliopathies in, 2321
 nephrotic syndrome in, 2322-2333
  in Africa, 2463
  classification of, 2323
  congenital, 1414, 2324t, 2325-2326
  definition of, 2323
  early-onset, 2324t, 2325-2326
  hereditary, 2323-2327, 2324t, 2325f
  idiopathic
   allergic responses associated with, 2327
   classification of, 2328-2329
   clinical features of, 2328
   definition of, 2327
   epidemiology of, 2327
   glucocorticoids for, 2329
   incidence of, 2327
   mesangioproliferative glomerulonephritis with, 2327-2328
   microscopic hematuria in, 2328
   pathogenesis of, 2327-2328
   proteinuria in, 2327
   renal biopsy for, 2328-2329
   treatment of, 2329-2331
  infantile and childhood, 2324t, 2326-2327
  juvenile, 2324t, 2327
  late-onset, 2324t, 2327
  pathogenesis of, 2323
  plasma exchange for, 2331
  steroid-resistant
   calcineurin inhibitors for, 2330-2331
   description of, 2323
   focal segmental glomerulosclerosis in, 2328
   molecular genetic screening for, 2326f
   mycophenolate mofetil for, 2331
   renin-angiotensin-aldosterone antagonists for, 2331
   rituximab, 2331
   syndromic forms of, 2323
   treatment of, 2330-2331
  steroid-sensitive, 2329-2330
 neurodevelopment of, 2408-2410, 2408f
 nutrition in, 2357-2359, 2404-2405
 obesity in, 2576-2577
 obstructive uropathy in, 1279
 oculocerebrorenal syndrome in, 2345
 parathyroid hormone in, 2390-2391

Children (Continued)
  peritoneal dialysis in
    access for, 2415
    adequacy of, 2416
    adherence to, 2417
    automated, 2415
    complications of, 2416-2417
    continuous ambulatory, 2415
    continuous renal replacement therapy versus, 2418
    contraindications, 2415
    dwell time for, 2416
    exchange volume of, 2416
    global disparities in, 2417
    hemodialysis versus, 2411, 2412t, 2417
    Kt/V assessments, 2416
    nocturnal intermittent, 2415
    prescription for, 2415-2416
    renal transplantation versus, 2410
    solutions for, 2415-2416
    termination of, 2417
    tidal, 2415
  phosphate in
    balance of, 2389-2390, 2389f-2390f
    dietary intake of, 2390
    disorders of, 2396-2399, 2397t-2400t, 2398f-2399f
    distribution of, 2389, 2390f
    fractional excretion of, 2397
    homeostasis of, 2391f
    regulation of, 2389
  polycystic kidney disease in, 2319-2321, 2320f
  polydipsia in, 2369, 2370t
  polyuria in, 2369, 2370t
  potassium in
    disorders involving, 2374-2382
    metabolism of, 2374-2382
  prerenal failure in, 2368t
  proteinuria in, 798, 2310-2311
  pseudohypoaldosteronism in, 2380-2382
  racial-ethnic disparities, 2583
  recurrent focal segmental glomerulosclerosis in, 2156
  renal disorders in, 2308-2309, 2309f
  renal function in, 2309-2311, 2361
  renal replacement therapy in
    continuous, 2417-2418
    costs of, 2411
    inborn errors of metabolism, 2417
    quality of life effects of, 2409-2410
    renal transplantation versus, 2410-2411, 2410f
  renal transplantation in
    ABO compatibility in, 2423
    acute rejection of, 2428
    advantages of, over long-term dialysis, 2410-2411, 2410f
    allocation of, 2419-2420
    allografts
      artery stenosis, 2432
      delayed function of, 2427-2428
      failure of, 2432
      loss of, 2427
      survival of, 2432
      vesicoureteral reflux to, 2435
    anemia after, 2434
    blood pressure monitoring after, 2432
    bone health and growth after, 2434-2435, 2435f
    cancer after, 2433-2434
    cardiovascular disease after, 2432-2433
    chronic allograft nephropathy after, 2431
    in chronic kidney disease patients, 2422

Children (Continued)
  complications of
    acute rejection, 2428
    BK virus infection, 2430
    cutaneous warts, 2430
    cytomegalovirus infection, 2429
    delayed graft function, 2427-2428
    Epstein-Barr virus infection, 2429-2430
    infections, 2428-2431
    Pneumocystis jiroveci pneumonia, 2430-2431
    primary kidney disease recurrence, 2431
    respiratory viruses, 2430
    ureteral obstruction, 2435
    urinary tract infection, 2429
    urologic, 2435
    varicella infection, 2430
  contraindications, 2420
  cost-effectiveness of, 2411
  demographics of, 2419, 2419t
  HLA matching and sensitization for, 2422-2423
  hypertension after, 2432
  immunosuppression for
    antimetabolites, 2425-2426
    azathioprine, 2425
    calcineurin inhibitors, 2424-2425
    combination therapies, 2426-2427
    corticosteroids, 2426
    cyclosporine, 2424-2425
    induction, 2423-2424
    maintenance, 2424-2427, 2424f
    mammalian target of rapamycin inhibitors, 2426
    mycophenolate mofetil, 2425-2426
    sirolimus, 2426
    tacrolimus, 2425
  incidence of, 2419-2420
  metabolic syndrome after, 2433
  patient nonadherence after, 2436
  postoperative period, 2427
  posttransplantation lymphoproliferative disorder after, 2433
  preoperative management of, 2427
  prevalence of, 2419-2420
  puberty after, 2435-2436
  quality of life after, 2410, 2436
  recipient preparation, 2420-2422, 2421t
  rehabilitation after, 2436
  rejection of, 2428
  reproduction effects of, 2435-2436
  survival benefits of, 2410, 2431-2432
  timing of, 2420
  transition after, 2436
  urologic complications of, 2435
  renal tubular acidosis in, 2335-2338, 2337t, 2383-2386
  socioeconomic disparities, 2583
  sodium in
    disorders involving, 2365-2374
    metabolism of, 2365-2367
  solute urinary excretion rates in, 2343t
  statural growth in
    chronic kidney disease effects on, 2357-2359, 2358f-2359f
    end-stage kidney disease effects on, 2405
  syndrome of inappropriate antidiuretic hormone secretion in, 2372
  thirst in, 2366
  thrombosis in, 1805
  total body water in, 2365, 2414
  urinary calculi in, 2340
  urinary protein excretion in, 2310-2311

Children (Continued)
  urinary tract disorders in
    posterior urethral valves, 2316, 2317f, 2435
    primary megaureter, 2315-2316
    spectrum of, 2308-2309, 2309f
    ureteropelvic junction obstruction, 2311, 2314-2315, 2315f
    vesicoureteral reflux, 2311, 2313-2314, 2314f
  urinary tract infection in, 2313-2314
  urinary tract obstruction in, 1258
  urolithiasis in, 2340-2348
  vascular calcification in, 2407-2408
  vasculitides in
    antineutrophil cytoplasmic antibody–associated, 2351-2352
    eosinophilic granulomatosis with polyangiitis, 2351
    granulomatosis with polyangiitis, 2351
    Henoch-Schönlein purpura, 2348-2350
    microscopic polyangiitis, 2351
    polyarteritis nodosa, 2350-2351
    Takayasu's arteritis, 2352
  vitamin D in, 2390-2391
  water metabolism in, 2365-2367
Chimerism, 2249
China
  diabetes mellitus in, 2529, 2529f
  end-stage kidney disease in, 2535
  hemodialysis in, 2535
  idiopathic membranous nephropathy in, 2531
  peritoneal dialysis in, 2535
  primary glomerular diseases in, 2529-2531, 2530f
  renal replacement therapy in, 2535
  scientific publications in, 2536
Chinese herb nephropathy, 1223-1224, 1225f, 2534
Chlorambucil, for membranous nephropathy, 1042-1043, 1169
Chloride
  deficiency of, in metabolic alkalosis, 520
  fractional excretion of, 814-815
  in urine, 816
Chloride channels, 161-162, 243
Chloride formate exchange, 148
Chloride oxalate exchange, 148
Chloride transport, 156-158, 157f, 163, 314
Chloride-bicarbonate exchanger mutation, 1457
Chlorine, 144
Chlorpropamide, 487, 497
Chlorthalidone, 1681, 1685, 1710
Chloruresis, 553
CHOIR study, 1901-1902
Cholecalciferol, 1923, 2025, 2390
Cholera, 2455-2456
Cholesterol, 1801, 1828
Cholesterol embolization syndrome, 1192-1193
Cholesterol ester transfer protein, 1802
Cholesterol feeding, 1578
Cholinesterase inhibitors, 1938
Chondrocalcinosis, 580, 2379
Chromodomain helicase DNA binding protein 1-like protein, 2300
Chromophilic carcinoma, 1371, 1371t
Chromophobe tumors, 892
Chromophobic carcinoma, 1371, 1371t, 1372f
Chronic allograft glomerulopathy, 923

Chronic allograft nephropathy, 2244, 2273, 2425, 2431
Chronic antibody-mediated rejection, 2274
Chronic bacterial prostatitis, 750, 1247-1248
Chronic heart failure, 1722
Chronic hypertension, 1627-1631, 1629f
Chronic hyponatremia, 502-504, 815
Chronic hypoxia, in interstitial fibrosis, 1217-1218
Chronic inflammatory demyelinating polyneuropathy, 2158
Chronic ischemia, 1794
Chronic kidney disease (CKD)
  acidosis of, 549-550, 1758-1759
  acute kidney injury as cause of, 652, 678, 691, 747, 926-927, 1777-1778, 1778f
  acute phase reactant proteins in, 1970
  adrenal androgens in, 1920
  adrenal glands in, 1919-1920
  adrenocorticotropic hormone in, 1919
  advanced care planning in, 2599-2600
  in Africa. See Africa, chronic kidney disease in
  in African Americans, 666, 2577
  aldosterone in, 1919-1920
  alkali therapy for, 542
  amino acids in, 1972
  ammonia synthesis, 1749
  anemia associated with. See Anemia, in chronic kidney disease
  animal models of, 1835-1836
  anthropometrics in, 1971
  atrial fibrillation in, 1859, 1908
  in Australia, 2544, 2549
  bicarbonate reabsorption in, 1749
  biomarkers for
    anemia, 683, 1299-1300, 1776, 1863-1864, 2594
    asymmetric dimethylarginine, 685, 950, 1811
    bicarbonate, 684-685
    creatinine, 933
    cystatin C, 934-935, 2043
    dyslipidemia, 683-684, 1863, 2011
    fibroblast growth factor-23, 950, 1864
    interleukin-18, 940-941
    kidney injury molecule-1, 942
    liver-type fatty acid-binding protein, 943
    β_1-microglobulin, 938
    β_2-microglobulin, 938
    monocyte chemoattractant protein-1, 950-951
    N-acetyl-β-D-glucosaminidase, 947
    neutrophil gelatinase-associated lipocalin, 946-947
    performance data on, 952t
    phosphate, 685
    serum albumin, 683
    serum bicarbonate, 684-685
    serum phosphate, 685
    serum uric acid, 684
    symmetric dimethylarginine, 1811
    uric acid, 684
    urinary protein excretion, 682-683, 947
  birth weight and, 712
  bleeding in, 1885
    desmopressin for, 1906
    diagnosis of, 1906
    pathophysiology of, 1904-1906
    risk factors for, 1905f
    treatment of, 1906
  blood pressure and, 1559f, 1563f, 1867-1868, 1975, 2283
  blood urea nitrogen in, 1959

Chronic kidney disease (CKD) (Continued)
  bradykinin receptors in, 350
  caloric requirements in, 1973
  cardiovascular disease associated with, 681-682
    antihypertensive agents for, 2010
    antiplatelet therapy for, 2012-2013
    arterial calcification, 1856-1857, 1857f, 1864, 1866
    arterial disease, 1855-1857, 1855t
    arterial stiffening, 1856
    arterial wall thickening, 1855-1856
    arteriosclerosis, 1855
    atrial fibrillation, 1859, 1908
    cardiac disease, 1857-1859
    characteristics of, 1855t
    clinical manifestations of, 1859-1860
    congenital heart disease, 2421-2422
    description of, 681-682, 2008-2009
    dietary factors, 1970
    dysrhythmias, 1859
    in elderly, 2593
    endothelial dysfunction, 1856, 2407
    epidemiology of, 1860-1861, 1860f
    interventions for, 2008-2013
    left ventricular function changes, 1859
    left ventricular hypertrophy, 1295-1296, 1857-1858
    myocardial disease, 1858f
    myocardial fibrosis, 1858-1859
    overview of, 1854-1855
    relationship between, 1861-1865
    risk factors for
      anemia, 1863-1864
      chronic kidney disease–mineral bone disorder, 1864-1865, 1872-1873
      coagulation defects, 1863
      congestive heart failure, 1862t
      diabetes mellitus, 1865
      dyslipidemia, 1863, 2011
      homocysteine, 1864, 1970
      hypertension, 1861, 1862t, 1873, 2421-2422, 2461
      inflammation, 1865
      list of, 1862t
      obesity, 1865-1866
      oxidative stress, 1865, 2100-2101
      phosphate retention, 1978-1979
      stroke, 1862t
      vitamin D levels, 1864-1865
    risk prediction, 1866-1867
    risk prevention in
      anemia correction, 1871-1872
      antiplatelet therapy, 1873
      blood pressure reductions, 1867-1868, 2009
      glycemic control, 1871
      homocysteine levels, 1872
      low-density lipoprotein cholesterol reductions, 1868-1871, 1869f-1870f
      smoking cessation, 1867, 1991
      uncertainties regarding, 1855
    summary of, 1873-1874
    valvular diseases, 1859
  cardiovascular events and, 670
  carotid endarterectomy in, 1932
  causes of, 1414t, 1415-1416
  in children. See Children, chronic kidney disease in
  chronic cognitive impairment in, 1936-1938, 1937f-1938f
  chronic kidney disease–mineral bone disorder in, 2030f

Chronic kidney disease (CKD) (Continued)
  classification of, 1989f
  clinics for, 2632, 2633f, 2633t
  cognitive impairment in, 1818-1819
  computed tomography of, 869, 869f
  cortisol in, 1919-1920
  costovertebral tenderness in, 776
  creatinine excretion in, 1961
  cytochrome P450 in, 385, 2038-2039
  deep vein thrombosis in, 1906-1907, 1908f
  definition of, 773, 1927, 1987
  dehydroepiandrosterone in, 1920
  dehydroepiandrosterone sulfate in, 1920
  demographics of, 2578-2579
    age, 673-674
    ethnicity, 660-662, 674
    gender, 655-660, 673-674
    race, 660-663, 666
  description of, 652
  diagnostic approach, 774-776, 2621
  dialysis for, 1971, 2016
  dietary modifications in, 1982-1983
  dietary support during
    justification for, 1956-1959
    low-protein diet, 1977, 1981-1982, 1994
    modified diets, 1982-1983
    potassium intake, 1975
    randomized controlled trials of, 1979-1981
    salt intake, 1974-1975
    summary of, 1984-1985
  1,25-Dihydroxyvitamin D levels in, 1913, 2014
  disordered mineral metabolism in, 2019-2023
  disparities in treatment of, 2580
  drug disposition affected by, 2035-2040
  drug dosing in, 2044-2046, 2045t, 2051t-2054t
  dyslipidemia in, 683-684, 1863, 2011
  early-stage, 669-670
  economic costs of treating, 2134, 2582
  in elderly, 747, 2568-2569, 2594-2596
  electrolyte balance alterations in, 1968
  endometrial hyperplasia in, 1921
  endothelin in, 337
  endothelin-1 in, 337-338
  endothelin-A receptors in, 337-338
  endothelin-B receptors in, 337-338
  end-stage kidney disease progression of, 671, 776, 962, 1737, 2007-2008
  energy intake in, 1973
  energy requirements in, 1973
  environmental exposures as cause of, 665
  epidemiology of, 643-647
  erectile dysfunction in, 1921-1922
  estimated glomerular filtration rate in, 1989-1990
  ethnicity and, 660-662, 674, 1769-1770
  extracellular fluid in, 775-776, 1747-1748
  in Far East. See Far East, chronic kidney disease in
  fibrinogen levels in, 1863, 1905-1906
  fibroblast growth factor-23 concentrations in, 950, 1749-1750, 1775, 1831, 1864, 2019
  follicle-stimulating hormone in, 1920-1921
  gender differences in, 655-660, 673-674
  genetic factors, 674-675
  genomewide association studies, 676
  global incidence of, 655, 656f
  glomerular filtration rate in, 681, 773, 932, 1749

Chronic kidney disease (CKD) *(Continued)*
  glomerulonephritis as cause of, 775
  gonadal dysfunction in, 1920-1923
  gonadotropic hormone axis in, 2358
  graft-versus-host disease-related, 1395
  growth hormone in, 1916-1919
  health-related quality of life in patients with, 1818
  hematopoietic stem cell transplantation and, 1394
  hemodynamic factors, 676-681
    acquired nephron deficit, 676-678
    blood pressure, 679
    nephron endowment, 676
    nephron loss, 676-678
    nephron number, 676-678
  hepatocyte growth factor in, 1757
  hepcidin concentrations in, 1886
  hereditary factors, 674-676
  high-density lipoprotein cholesterol in, 1863
  1α-hydroxylase deficiency in, 617
  hyperaldosteronism in, 1919
  hyperammonemia in, 1962
  hypercholesterolemia in, 1970
  hypercoagulability in, 1906-1909, 1908f
  hypercortisolism in, 1919
  hyperkalemia in, 585
  hyperphosphatemia caused by, 627, 1774-1775
  hyperprolactinemia in, 1919
  hypertension and, 1544-1545, 1559-1560
  hypoactive sexual desire disorder in, 1921
  hypocalciuria in, 1749-1750
  hypogonadism in, 1921-1922
  hypothalamic-pituitary-gonadal axis disturbances in, 1920
  hypothyroidism in, 1916
  hypoxia in, 139
  imaging of, 863f-864f, 866-871, 866f-871f
  incidence of, 645, 926-927
    in Africa, 2459
    disparities in, 2575, 2578
    ethnicity-based, 660-662
    gender-based, 655, 656f
    in Indian subcontinent, 2502
    in Middle East, 2474
    race-based, 660-662, 2584
    socioeconomic factors, 664-665, 664f, 2578, 2584
  inflammation and, 1865, 1909, 1969-1970
  inflammatory cell infiltration in, 334
  insulin resistance in, 1315, 1912-1916, 1913t
  interdisciplinary clinics for, 2632-2634, 2633f
  international comparisons of, 647
  intraarterial volume status assessments in, 775-776
  intrauterine growth restriction and, 665
  iodide retention in, 1915
  iron balance in, 1893
  iron therapy in, 1898-1900, 1899t
  kallikrein-kinin system in, 350
  Kidney Disease Improving Global Outcomes classification of, 773, 774t
  Kidney Disease Outcomes Quality Initiative for, 773, 773t
  kidney stones and, 1352
  klotho in, 1831, 1832t
  in Latin America, 2447-2449
  leukocytes in, 1909
  low birth weight and, 712, 2576
  luteinizing hormone in, 1920-1921
  malnutrition in, 1971

Chronic kidney disease (CKD) *(Continued)*
  metabolic acidosis in, 542, 1913, 2004, 2357, 2359
  micronutrients in, 1983
  in Middle East patients. *See* Middle East, chronic kidney disease in
  mineralocorticoid receptor blockade in, 322
  monitoring of, 2005-2006
  mortality rates in, 773
  muscle mass losses in, 1968
  musculoskeletal complications of, 775
  mutation analysis for, 1412
  National Kidney Foundation classification system for, 773, 773t, 1736, 1957-1958, 1958t
  nephron losses in, 676-678, 1991f
  neurologic aspects of
    cerebrovascular disease, 1926
    cognitive function disorders. *See* Cognitive function disorders
    description of, 1926
    neuropathy, 1939
    sleep apnea, 1939-1940
    stroke, 1926-1934. *See also* Stroke
  in New Zealand, 2550-2551
  nitrogenous products turnover in
    ammonia, 1962
    creatinine, 1961
    fecal nitrogen, 1962
    nonurea nitrogen, 1962-1963
    overview of, 1959
    urea, 1959-1961
    uric acid, 1961-1962
  nonurea nitrogen levels in, 1962
  nutritional counseling in, 1985f
  obesity in, 679-680, 1770-1771, 1992
  25(OH)D levels and, 2031-2032
  in older adults, 747, 2568-2569, 2586-2588
  ophthalmic complications of, 775
  orthostatic hypotension and, 776
  outcome of, by stages, 645
  oxidative stress and, 1758, 1865
  palliative care for, 2563
  parathyroid hormone in, 2014, 2019
  phosphate in, 1977-1979, 2019
  phosphorus retention in, 1977-1978
  plasma protein binding in, 2037
  potassium intake in, 1975
  preeclampsia effects on, 680-681
  pregnancy effects on, 680-681, 1633-1638
  prematurity and, 712
  prevalence of, 645, 655, 656f, 669-670, 2108-2109
    in Africa, 2459
    age-based, 673, 747
    ethnicity-based, 661-662
    in Far East, 2526, 2527t
    income-based, 665
    in Indian subcontinent, 2502
    in Latin America, 2448
    in Middle East, 2474
    race-based, 661-662
    socioeconomic factors, 665
    trends in, 646t
  primary care provider recognition of, 2622
  primary hypertension and, 1562-1565
  prognosis for, 1972-1973
  progression of, 1552-1553
    acidosis effects on, 684-685, 1963-1964, 2004
    acute kidney injury effects on, 678, 1777-1778
    in African Americans, 674
    albuminuria as risk factor for, 948

Chronic kidney disease (CKD) *(Continued)*
    anemia as predictor of, 683, 1776, 2013
    angiotensin II in, 1764-1765
    asymmetric dimethylarginine as risk factor for, 685
    biomarkers of, 949-950
    blood pressure in, 679, 2009
    body mass index and, 1771
    calcium channel blockers effect on, 1995
    calcium metabolism and, 1774-1775
    in children, 2361-2362, 2362f
    description of, 671, 776
    diabetic nephropathy effects on, 681
    dietary protein intake and, 1767-1768
    dihydropyridine calcium channel blockers effect on, 1995-1996
    dyslipidemia as predictor of, 683-684, 1772-1774
    to end-stage kidney disease, 671, 776, 962, 1737, 2007-2008
    ethnic differences in, 662
    fibroblast growth factor-23 in, 1775
    gender differences in, 657, 1768-1769
    hyperlipidemia in, 1802-1803
    hyperparathyroidism and, 1775
    hypertension effects on, 673, 679, 1765-1767
    hyperuricemia in, 684, 1228, 2004
    low-protein diet effects on, 1981-1982, 1994
    male sex hormones in, 1923
    mechanism of, 1990
    metabolic syndrome effects on, 679-680, 1770-1771, 1992
    obesity effects on, 679-680, 1770-1771, 1992
    phosphate metabolism and, 1774-1775
    podocyte injury in, 1753-1754
    preeclampsia effects on, 680-681
    in pregnancy, 680-681
    primary renal disease effects on, 681
    proteinuria as predictor of, 2361-2362
    racial differences in, 662
    renal calcium deposition and, 1775
    renal risk scores for, 691
    renin-angiotensin-aldosterone system inhibition, 1764-1765
    risk factors for, 673, 1990, 2361-2362
    slowing of. *See* Chronic kidney disease, slowing progression of
    smoking effects on, 685, 1776-1777
    socioeconomic factors, 665-666
    sympathetic nervous system overactivity in, 1771-1772
    total protein measurements used in, 793
    unified hypothesis of, 1763-1764, 1764f
    uric acid-lowering therapy effects on, 684
  prolactin, 1919
  prolactinemia in, 1919
  protein in
    intake of, 1975-1976
    losses of, 1965, 1967
    low-protein diet, 1977, 1994
    randomized controlled trials of, 1979-1980
    requirements for, 1976, 1976t
  protein stores in, assessment of
    anthropometrics for, 1971
    complement, 1970-1971
    insulin-like growth factor-1, 1970-1971
    nitrogen balance for, 1968-1969, 1975

Chronic kidney disease (CKD) *(Continued)*
  overview of, 1968
    plasma amino acids, 1971-1973, 1972*f*
    prealbumin, 1970-1971
    serum albumin, 1969-1970
    serum transferrin, 1970-1971
    urea nitrogen appearance rate, 1969
  protein-energy wasting in, 1817, 1913, 1994-1995
  proteinuria associated with, 682-683, 947-948, 2361-2362
  pulmonary embolism in, 1906-1907
  quality initiatives in, 2632-2635, 2633*f*, 2633*t*-2634*t*
  race and, 660-663, 666
  recombinant human growth factor in, 1918
  renal replacement therapy for, in stage 5 patients, 2016
  renal risk scores, 687-691, 688*t*-689*t*
  renal transplantation for, 2016
  renoprotection in
    angiotensin receptor blockers for, 2000-2003, 2001*f*
    angiotensin-converting enzyme inhibitors for, 1995, 1998-2000, 1998*t*
    strategies for, 2006-2008, 2008*t*
  risk factors for, 773, 774*t*, 1849
    alcohol consumption, 685-686
    analgesics, 686
    asymmetric dimethylarginine, 685
    cadmium, 687
    childhood obesity, 679-680
    cocaine use, 686
    epidemiologic studies for identifying, 670-671
    heavy metal exposure, 686-687
    high dietary protein intake, 680
    hypertension, 679, 1861, 1868, 1873, 1974-1975, 2461, 2590-2591
    hyperuricemia, 684, 1228, 2004
    initiation, 673
    in Latin America, 2448
    lead exposure, 686-687
    list of, 672*t*
    maternal, 2576
    nephron number, 676-678
    nephrotoxins, 685-687
    obesity, 679-680, 1771
    postnatal environment, 2576
    prenatal environment, 2575-2576
    protein intake, high dietary, 680
    racial-ethnic disparities in, 2583
    recreational drug use, 686
    serum bicarbonate levels, 684-685
    serum phosphate levels, 685
    serum uric acid levels, 684
    smoking, 685, 1776-1777, 1867
    social contribution of, 2576
    socioeconomic conditions, 2576-2577
    susceptibility, 671-673
  risk stratification for, 786, 1990
  in scleroderma, 1196-1197
  screening for, 669-670, 2587-2588
  secondary hyperparathyroidism in, 2024*f*
  sex hormones in, 1921, 1923
  sexual function in, 1920-1921
  sleep disorders in
    periodic limb movements of sleep, 1939-1940
    prevalence of, 1939
    restless legs syndrome, 1940, 1940*t*
    sleep apnea, 1939-1940

Chronic kidney disease (CKD) *(Continued)*
  slowing progression of
    antihypertensive therapy for, 1995-1998
    bicarbonate supplementation for, 684-685, 2004
    blood pressure lowering for, 1996-1998, 2009
    dietary protein restriction for, 1767-1768, 1994-1995
    glycemic control for, 1995
    hyperuricemia correction, 2004
    initiation of therapies for, 2006-2007
    lifestyle interventions for, 1990-1995
    metabolic acidosis treatment for, 2004
    monitoring for, 2005-2006
    proteinuria treatment for, 2004-2005
    rationale for, 1990
    renin-angiotensin-aldosterone system inhibition for, 1764-1765, 1998-2004, 2127
    smoking cessation for, 1776-1777, 1991-1992
    sodium restriction for, 1993-1994, 1993*f*
    strategies for, 2006-2008, 2008*t*
    weight loss for, 1992-1993
  socioeconomic factors, 663-666, 664*f*, 2576
  somatotropic axis in, 1917*f*
  stage 1 and 2
    abdominal ultrasonography in, 2015
    diagnosis of, 2014
    glomerular filtration rate reductions in, 2029-2031
    management of, 1988*t*
    monitoring guidelines in, 2015*t*
    phosphate restriction in, 2031
    stepped care approach in, 2014-2015
    treatment of, 2029-2031
  stage 3
    calcium monitoring in, 2014
    glomerular filtration rate in, 2015
    glomerular filtration rate reductions in, 2029-2031
    management of, 1988*t*
    monitoring guidelines in, 2015*t*
    parathyroid hormone monitoring in, 2014
    phosphate restriction in, 2031
    phosphorus monitoring in, 2014
    stepped care approach in, 2015
    vitamin D analogues in, 2031-2032
  stage 4
    cardiovascular events in, 2015
    dialysis preparations in, 2016
    glomerular filtration rate in, 2015-2016, 2029-2031
    hepatitis B vaccination in, 2016
    management of, 1988*t*
    monitoring guidelines in, 2015*t*
    preemptive renal transplantation indications in, 2016
    stepped care approach to, 2015-2016
    vitamin D analogues in, 2031-2032
  stage 5
    glomerular filtration rate in, 2016
    hyperphosphatemia in, 2020
    hypocalcemia in, 2020
    management of, 1988*t*
    monitoring guidelines in, 2015*t*
    pericarditis in, 2107-2108
    renal replacement therapy in, 2016
    stepped care approach to, 2016
    transition from, to end-stage kidney disease, 2063-2064

Chronic kidney disease (CKD) *(Continued)*
  systemic complications of, 773-774
  targeted programs for, 2582
  testosterone deficiency in, 1921
  thyroid hormone disturbances in, 1915-1916, 1915*t*
  thyrotropin levels in, 1915-1916
  trace elements in, 1983-1984
  treatment of, 2013, 2580
  trials in nondiabetic, 1553
  ubiquitin-protease system in, 1964-1965
  urea in, 1959-1961, 1968-1969
  uric acid excretion in, 1813, 1961
  vascular calcifications in, 1850, 2102-2103
  vitamin D in
    actions of, 1923-1924
    deficiency of, 1775, 1849, 1912, 1924
    metabolism of, 1923-1924
    supplementation of, 1924, 2406
  vitamins in, 1983-1984
  volume overload in, 776
  white cell function in, 1909-1910
Chronic Kidney Disease Epidemiology Collaboration, 645, 677-678, 759, 784*t*, 785-786, 2005
Chronic Kidney Disease Hard Point Trials in Diabetes, 1555-1556
Chronic kidney disease–mineral bone disorder (CKD–MBD)
  biochemical abnormalities in
    bone-specific alkaline phosphatase, 1842
    calcium, 1847-1848
    clinical consequences of, 1847-1850
    collagen-based bone biomarkers, 1842
    fibroblast growth factor-23, 1841, 1848
    fracture secondary to, 1849
    klotho, 1841-1842
    parathyroid hormone, 1839-1841, 1840*f*, 1848
    phosphorus, 1847-1848
    sclerostin, 1842
    tartrate-resistant acid phosphatase 5B, 1842
    vitamin D, 1841, 1848-1849
  biomarkers for, 1840*t*
  bone assessments in
    bone biopsy for, 1842-1846, 1845*t*
    dual-energy x-ray absorptiometry for, 1846
    high-resolution peripheral computerized tomography for, 1846
    histomorphometry for, 1842-1845, 1844*f*
    micro-computed tomography for, 1846-1847
    micro-magnetic resonance imaging for, 1846-1847
    noninvasive, 1846-1847
    quantitative computed tomography for, 1846
  bone formation in, 1843, 1845*t*
  calcimimetics for, 1873, 2026-2028
  calcium-sensing receptor in, 1825-1826
  cardiovascular disease and, 1864-1865, 1872-1873
  in children, 2361, 2406
  in chronic kidney disease, 2030*f*
  clinical management of, 2028-2029
  definition of, 2020
  1,25-dihydroxycholecalciferol, 2024*f*, 2025
  in end-stage kidney disease, 2029

Chronic kidney disease–mineral bone disorder (CKD–MBD) *(Continued)*
  fracture in, 1849
  hormonal regulation of
    fibroblast growth factor-23, 1830-1831
    Klotho, 1830-1831
    parathyroid hormone, 1826-1828
    vitamin D, 1828-1830
  hyperphosphatemia and, 1977, 2021
  management of, 2013-2014
  in Middle East, 2488
  pathophysiology of, 1822-1839
  phosphate concentrations in, 1864, 1872, 1923
  in renal transplantation recipients, 1850-1852
  treatment of, 2028-2029
    cinacalcet and vitamin D analogues for, 2029
    overview of, 2021*t*
    phosphate-binding agents, 2020-2023
    principles of, 2020-2021
    vitamin D analogues, 2020
  vitamin D metabolism abnormalities in, 2025
  vitamin D sterols for, 2026
Chronic pain, 2569
Chronic radiation nephropathy, 1194
Chronic renal injury, polyuria in, 299
Chronic tubulointerstitial nephritis
  Balkan endemic nephropathy, 1224-1226, 1225*f*
  causes of
    analgesics, 1221-1223, 1222*t*
    aristolochic acid, 1223-1226
    autoimmune diseases, 1228-1229
    cadmium, 1227
    Chinese herbs, 1223-1224
    hyperuricemia, 1227-1228
    lead, 1226-1227
    lithium, 1226, 1226*f*
    overview of, 1222*t*
    sarcoidosis, 1228
    urate nephropathy, 1227-1228
  clinical features of, 1221
  pathology of, 1221
Churg-Strauss syndrome. *See* Eosinophilic granulomatosis with polyangiitis
Chvostek's sign, 612-613, 623, 995
Chylomicrons, 1801-1802
Chyluria, 1255
Cicaprost, 377
Cigarette smoking. *See* Smoking
Cilazapril, 1642, 1643*t*
Ciliopathies, 2319-2322, 2320*f*, 2322*t*
Cilioprotein, 1506*f*
Cinacalcet, 612, 631, 1873, 2026-2027, 2029, 2032
Ciprofloxacin, 1405
  crystalluria caused by, 1259-1260
  for pyelonephritis, 1241-1242, 1241*t*
  for urinary tract infection, 1244
Cirrhosis
  apelin in, 446-447
  aquaporin-2 protein abundance in, 300
  ascites with, 449, 1712, 1723
  brain natriuretic peptide in, 447
  carbon tetrachloride-induced, 494
  COX metabolites in, 378
  C-type natriuretic peptide in, 447
  diuretics for, 1722-1724
  extracellular fluid expansion associated with, 299-300
  fluid retention in, 1724*f*
  glomerulonephritis caused by, 1156

Cirrhosis *(Continued)*
  hyponatremia associated with, 494
  intrahepatic vascular pressure in, 439
  norepinephrine levels in, 445
  prostaglandins in, 378
  renal biopsy of, 1156-1157
  sinusoidal pressure in, 439
  sodium retention in
    apelin in, 446-447
    arginine vasopressin in, 446
    atrial natriuretic peptide in, 447, 448*f*
    brain natriuretic peptide in, 447
    C-type natriuretic peptide in, 447
    Dendroaspis natriuretic peptides in, 447
    effector mechanisms, 444-449
    endothelin in, 446
    natriuretic peptides in, 447-449
    overflow hypothesis, 449
    pathogenesis of, 449
    prostaglandins in, 448-449
    renin-angiotensin-aldosterone system in, 444-445, 452
    sympathetic nervous system in, 445-446
    treatment of
      α-adrenergic agonists, 456
      liver transplantation, 458
      midodrine, 456
      pharmacologic, 455-457
      PROMETHEUS, 458
      renal replacement therapy, 457-458
      somatostatin analogues, 456
      systemic vasoconstrictors, 455-456
      terlipressin, 455-456
      transjugular intrahepatic portosystemic shunt, 457
      vasoconstrictor antagonists, 455
      vasodilators, 455
      vasopressin 2 receptor antagonists, 456-457
      vasopressin-1 receptor analogues, 455-456
    tubular sodium reabsorption and, 444
    underfilling hypothesis of, 449
    volume-sensing abnormalities as cause of, 439-444, 447
  sympathetic nervous system in, 445-446
  vasopressin levels in, 446
  water retention in, 439, 446
Cirrhotic cardiomyopathy, 441
Cisplatin, 621, 966, 968*t*, 990, 1001, 1397
Cited1, 29
Cited1-EGFP transgene, 19
Citrate
  acid-base homeostasis role of, 247-248
  actions of, 1337
  basolateral transport of, 248
  bicarbonate generation secondary to excretion of, 247-248
  calcium affinity for, 219
  excretion of, 247-248, 841, 2385
  functions of, 219
  as kidney stone inhibitor, 1330, 1337*f*
  proximal tubule absorption and metabolism of, 217*f*, 248
Citrate transport disorders, 219
Citric acid cycle, 126
Class I HLA molecules, 2231-2233, 2232*f*
Class II HLA molecules, 2233
Classical congenital adrenal hyperplasia, 1547
Clathrin, 56-59
Clathrin-coated pits, 291

Claudins
  -2, 55-56
  -10, 55-56
  -14, 189
  -16, 160, 161*f*, 195-196, 195*f*
  -19, 160, 194-196, 195*f*
  description of, 147, 188-189
CLC-K2, 161, 243
CLDN19, 2388
Clear cell carcinoma, 890*f*, 1371-1374, 1371*t*, 1372*f*, 1377
Clevidipine, 1665, 1695*t*, 1698-1699
Clinical endpoint, 927*t*
CLINITEK system, 797
Clock gene, 256
$CL^−$-OH exchange, 148
Clonidine
  with diuretics, 445-446
  hypertensive urgencies and emergencies treated with, 1697*t*
  indications for, 1629, 1671-1672, 1671*t*-1672*t*
Clopidogrel, 1932, 2012
c-Met, 1757
Coagulation, 980-981, 1863
Coagulation factors, 1018*t*, 1803
Coated pits, 56-59
Cobalamin C deficiency, 1188, 2356-2357
Cocaine, 686
Cockcroft-Gault equation, 784*t*, 786, 2042-2044, 2064, 2587*f*
Cognitive function disorders
  delirium syndromes. *See* Delirium syndromes
  dialysis dementia, 1935-1936
  uremic encephalopathy, 1934-1935
Cognitive impairment, 1935-1938, 1937*f*, 1938*f*, 2590
Cohort studies, 671
Col3A1, 1213
COL4A3, 1141-1142
COL4A4, 1141-1142
Colchicine
  adverse effects of, 2486
  familial Mediterranean fever treated with, 2485-2486
  gout treated with, 2282
  polymorphonuclear cell accumulation of, 2485-2486
Cold ischemia time, 2265, 2278
Collagen, 1757, 2610
Collagen IV, 951-952, 1139
Collapsing focal segmental glomerulosclerosis, 1026, 1029-1031, 1159, 2328
Collapsing glomerulopathy, 1153
Collecting duct (CD)
  acid secretion, 1276
  acid-base transport in, 244-245
  alkalosis and, 244
  ammonia secretion by, 252, 252*f*
  anatomy of, 44-45, 45*f*, 69-75, 262, 263*f*, 269*f*
  angiotensin II effects on, 244-245
  carbonic anhydrase in, 243
  cells of, 30, 69-70, 239-241, 239*f*-241*f*, 282
  cortical. *See* Cortical collecting duct
  EETs in, 385
  elongation of, 25-26
  embryology of, 5, 6*f*
  endothelin-1 synthesis by, 245
  EP3 receptor mRNA in, 371
  HKα expression in, 242-243
  HKα$_2$ expression in, 242-243
  HKβ expression in, 242-243

Collecting duct (CD) (Continued)
  hydrogen in, 242, 1276
  initial, 239
  inner medullary, 44-45, 45f, 69-70, 74-75
  intercalated cells involved in, 239-241, 239f-241f
  lithium in, 297-298
  metabolic acidosis and, 244
  metabolic alkalosis and, 244
  outer medullary, 44-45, 45f, 69-70, 73-74
  papillary, 27, 75f
  potassium in, 178, 540-541, 1729f
  regions of, 69-70
  respiratory acidosis and, 244
  segments of, 239, 262
  sodium absorption in, 73
  sodium transport in, 374
  tubulopathy of, 1417-1418
  tumor of, 1371, 1371t
  urea accumulation, 268-269, 268f
  vasopressin effects on, 296-297
  water absorption in, 269f, 270-271
  water impermeability of, 491
  water permeability in, prostaglandins' effect on, 301
Collecting system
  composition of, 5
  duplicated, 864f, 2296, 2303, 2303f, 2313
  formation of, 25-27
  water absorption in, 271
Colloid osmotic pressure, 94-96, 95f, 98
Colloid solutions, for hypovolemia, 425
Colon, 316-317
Colonic isoform, 242
Columns of Bertin, 850
"Comet tail" sign, 874-876
Complement
  activation of, 1183f, 1213-1214
  in acute poststreptococcal glomerulonephritis, 1058
  in anti-glomerular basement membrane glomerulonephritis, 1080
  in atypical hemolytic-uremic syndrome, 1183-1185
  genetic abnormalities in, 1184
  hemolytic-uremic syndrome caused by disorders of, 2355-2356, 2355f
  in membranoproliferative glomerulonephritis, 1049
  in membranous nephropathy, 1041
  nephritic syndrome levels of, 759-760, 759t
Complement factor 1, 1185
Complement factor B, 1185
Complement factor D, 1788
Complement factor H, 1184-1185, 2355-2357
Complement factor H-related proteins, 1184
Complement inhibitors, 1186
Complement protein D, 1810
Computed tomography angiography, 853f, 904, 904f-905f
Computed tomography angiography (CTA), 853f, 904, 904f-905f
Computed tomography (CT), 851-856
  anatomy on, 852-853, 852f/855f
  angiomyolipomas on, 891, 893f
  autosomal dominant polycystic kidney disease on, 869f, 885-888, 888f, 1486f
  chronic kidney disease on, 869, 869f
  contrast-enhanced
    acute pyelonephritis on, 878-880, 880f
    description of, 851

Computed tomography (CT) (Continued)
  emphysematous pyelonephritis on, 882f
  hydronephrosis on, 872f
  nephropathy caused by, 853-856
  obstructive urography evaluations, 871, 873f
  pyelonephritis on, 882f, 1241
  renal abscess on, 880, 881f
  renal cysts on, 883-885, 886f-887f, 891f
  renal masses on, 883-885, 886f, 890, 892f
  after renal transplantation, 910
  renal tuberculosis on, 884f
  renal vein thrombosis on, 909, 1205
  xanthogranulomatous pyelonephritis on, 881, 883f
  corticomedullary phase on, 853f
  definition of, 851
  description of, 851
  dual-energy, 852f
  excretory phase on, 854f
  helical, 1265-1266
  history of, 851
  kidney stones on, 873, 875f, 1359
  multidetector, 851
  nephrographic phase on, 854f
  polycystic kidney disease on, 869f
  renal cell carcinoma on, 894f, 898f
  renal colic on, 873
  renal cysts on, 883-885, 886f-887f
  renal mucormycosis on, 2498f
  renal parenchymal disease on, 880-881
  ureteral stone on, 875f-876f
  urinary tract obstruction on, 1265-1266, 1266f
  xanthogranulomatous pyelonephritis on, 1252
Computed tomography scanners, 851
Computed tomography urography
  intravenous urography versus, 852
  normal findings on, 855f
  technique for, 851-852
Conception, 1635
Conflicts of interest, 2562
Congenital adrenal hyperplasia, 1461, 1547
Congenital anomalies of the kidney and urinary tract (CAKUT), 713, 1415-1416
  branchio-oto-renal syndrome, 2297t, 2299, 2318
  ciliopathies, 2319-2322, 2320f, 2322t
  clinical management of, 2304-2305
  clinical presentation of, 2302-2304
  copy number variants in, 2300
  definitions, 2311
  description of, 2294
  DSTYK in, 2300
  ectopic kidney, 2295, 2295f, 2305, 2311
  end-stage kidney disease progression of, 2361, 2404, 2421
  epidemiology of, 2296, 2311
  fetal presentation of, 2302
  functional consequences of, 2301-2302
  genetics of, 2296, 2297t
  genotype-phenotype correlations for, 1416
  GLI3 repressor, 2299
  hedgehog signaling, 2299
  horseshoe kidney, 2295, 2296f, 2303-2304, 2311
  in utero environment effects on, 2300-2301, 2301t
  in utero management of, 2304-2305
  Kallmann's syndrome, 2297t, 2318
  long-term outcomes of, 2305

Congenital anomalies of the kidney and urinary tract (CAKUT) (Continued)
  molecular pathogenesis of, 2297-2300
  multicystic dysplastic kidney, 889, 2294-2296, 2295f, 2303, 2305, 2312-2313
  mutant alleles associated with, 2297
  neuropsychiatric disorders and, 2300
  outcomes of, 2305
  pathogenesis of, 1416, 2296-2302
  posterior urethral valves, 2316, 2317f, 2435
  postnatal management of, 2304-2305
  primary megaureter, 2315-2316
  prune-belly syndrome, 2318-2319
  renal agenesis, 2302, 2311-2312
  renal collecting system duplication, 2296, 2303, 2303f, 2313
  renal coloboma syndrome, 2297t, 2317-2318
  renal cyst and diabetes syndrome, 2316-2317
  renal dysplasia. See Renal dysplasia
  renal ectopy, 2295, 2295f, 2303, 2305, 2311
  renal fusion, 2303-2305, 2311
  sporadic forms of, 2299-2300
  syndromic forms of, 2316-2322
  Townes-Brocks syndrome, 2318
  ureteric budding, 2297-2298
  ureteropelvic junction obstruction, 2314-2315, 2315f
  VACTERL association, 2318
  VATER association, 2318
  vesicoureteral reflux, 2311, 2313-2314, 2314f
Congenital chloridorrhea, 553
Congenital heart disease, 2421-2422
Congenital hydronephrosis, 1259
Congenital lipoid adrenal hypoplasia, 588
Congenital nephrotic syndrome of the Finnish, 1426-1428
Congestive heart failure. See Heart failure
Conivaptan, 504, 1713-1714
Connecting segment cell, 239
Connecting tubules
  anatomy of, 68-69
  aquaporin-2 expression by, 69
  bicarbonate reabsorption in, 241-242
  cells of, 68-69
  chloride absorption in, 170
  functional role of, 241-242
  intercalated cells in, 68-69
  potassium secretion by, 176-178
  in rat, 68-69
  sodium chloride transport in, 169-171
  in sodium reabsorption, 69
  water absorption in, 271
Connective tissue growth factor, 951, 1300
Connexin 40, 400
Connexins, 55-56
Conn's syndrome, 321
Continuous ambulatory peritoneal dialysis (CAPD)
  antibiotic administration in, 2130t
  azotemia treated with, 2486
  in children, 2415
  description of, 1318, 1963-1964, 2049, 2117, 2119-2120
  frequency of exchanges, 2122
  residual kidney function affected by, 2126
Continuous cyclic peritoneal dialysis, 2119
Continuous flow centrifugation, 2160

Continuous hemodiafiltration, 598
Continuous positive airway pressure, for sleep apnea, 1940
Continuous quality improvement, 2623
Continuous renal replacement therapy (CRRT)
　acute kidney injury treated with, 1007-1008
　administration of, 2141
　in children, 2417-2418
　critically ill patients treated with, 2141, 2141t
　drug dosing in, 2048-2049
　hepatorenal syndrome treated with, 457
　metformin clearance during, 2185
　poison removal using, 2171
　renal function estimations in, 2044
Continuous venovenous hemodiafiltration, 1007, 2142
Continuous venovenous hemodialysis, 1007-1008
Continuous venovenous hemofiltration, 1007, 2142
Contrast media
　computed tomography enhanced with. See Computed tomography (CT), contrast-enhanced
　in elevated creatinine patients, 854-856
　estimated glomerular filtration rate and, 854-856
　high osmolar, 847-848
　intravenous, 849, 854
　iodinated, 847-848
　low osmolar, 847-848, 855-856
　magnetic resonance angiography using, 859-861, 862f
　magnetic resonance urography using, 861-863, 862f
　nephropathy caused by, 853-854, 964-966, 1000
　nephrotoxicity of, 1000, 2273
Convection, 2068-2069, 2068f, 2078, 2112
Cooperative Study of Renovascular Hypertension, 1569
Copper, 1444
Copper sulfate poisoning, 2500
Copy number variants, 2300
Core binding factor α-1, 1835
Cori cycle, 132
Corin, 340, 1800
Coronary artery bypass grafting, acute kidney injury after, 992
Coronary artery calcification, 1850
Coronary artery disease, 1660
Coronary heart disease, 1527f
Cortical blood flow, 87
Cortical collecting duct (CCD)
　AE1 immunoreactivity in, 72-73
　apical potassium channels in, 564
　autosomal recessive type I pseudohypoaldosteronism in, 539
　bicarbonate reabsorption in, 242, 245
　cells of, 70, 70f
　characteristics of, 44-45, 45f, 69-70
　chloride absorption in, 170
　initial collecting tubule/duct, 65-66, 68, 69f, 70
　intercalated cells of, 70-71, 72f, 239, 239f
　luminal surface of, 71f
　medullary ray collecting duct, 70
　metabolism, 133
　parts of, 70
　potassium secretion by, 73, 176-178, 563-564, 1748-1749
　principal cells of, 70, 70f, 74
　prostaglandin synthesis in, 365

Cortical collecting duct (CCD) (Continued)
　SK channels in, 180f
　sodium chloride transport in, 169-171
　vasopressin effects on, 819
　voltage defects in, 539f
　water absorption in, 569
Cortical interstitium, 77-78
Cortical labyrinth, 261-262
Cortical nephrons, 45
Cortical stromal cells, 5-6
Cortical tubules, 89, 90f
Cortical-medullary junction, 91
Corticomedullary arcades, 6
Corticosteroids. See also specific drug
　acute interstitial nephritis treated with, 1002
　adverse effects of, 1166-1167, 2426
　anti-glomerular basement membrane disease treated with, 1126-1127
　in children, 2426
　eosinophilic granulomatosis with polyangiitis treated with, 1117-1118
　fracture risks, 1167
　glomerulonephritis treated with, 1166-1167
　gout treated with, 2282
　Henoch-Schönlein purpura treated with, 1124
　immunosuppressive uses of, in renal transplantation, 2245, 2254t, 2259, 2426
　linear growth affected by, 2434-2435
　membranous nephropathy treated with, 1042
　minimal change disease treated with, 1022-1023, 1023t
　mixed connective tissue disease treated with, 1109
　osteopenia caused by, 1166-1167
　perinatal exposure to, 717
　polyarteritis nodosa treated with, 1119-1120
　during pregnancy, 1637
　pruritus treated with, 1943
　Takayasu arteritis treated with, 1121
　temporal arteritis treated with, 1120
　toxicity of, 1167
Corticosterone, 309
Cortisol, 305, 309, 1919-1920
Costimulatory signal blockers, 2258-2259
Costovertebral angle pain, 1240, 1250
Coulomb's law, 124
Countercurrent multiplication paradigm, 266, 267f
COX-1, 355, 360f, 361f, 361, 411-412
COX-2
　description of, 355
　expression of, 357-361
　　acute ischemic injury effects on, 377
　　in cirrhosis, 448
　　cyclosporine A effects on, 378
　　in developing kidney, 363
　　in diabetes mellitus, 378
　　glomerular, 376
　　in loop of Henle, 373-374
　　in macula densa, 357-358, 359f, 360
　　in medullary interstitial cells, 360-361
　　in renal cortex, 357-361
　　in renal medulla, 360-361, 360f
　glucocorticoids effect on, 357
　immunohistochemistry for, 1274f
　knockout mice model of, 358-360
　prostaglandin synthesis in renomedullary interstitial cells mediated by, 80
　prostanoids from, 357-358

COX-2 (Continued)
　reactive oxygen species as mediator of, 379
　renin release and, 568
　sodium intake effects on, 412
COX-2 inhibitors
　acute kidney injury caused by, 362-363
　cardiovascular effects of, 363-364
　heart failure and, 437
　hyperkalemia caused by, 590
　nephrogenesis affected by, 719
　proteinuria treated with, 377-378
　renin production affected by, 360
　thrombotic events and, 363-364
　vascular tone affected by, 363
C1q nephropathy, 1034-1035
C-reactive protein, 1910, 1969-1970, 2100
CREATE trial, 1901
Creatine phosphate, 1961
Creatine–creatine phosphate, 1961
Creatinine
　in children, 2341f
　contrast media administration in patients with elevated levels of, 854-856
　cystatin C and, 934-935
　degradation of, 1961
　excretion of
　　age of patient and, 1961
　　in chronic kidney disease, 1961
　　factors that affect, 1961
　　fractional, 1199
　　variability in, 796
　formation of, 1961
　glomerular filtration rate and, 678, 782-783, 933, 2309-2310, 2587, 2587f
　Jaffe method for measuring, 782, 787
　measurement of, 782-783
　plasma
　　glomerular filtration rate estimations using, 782-783, 783f
　　in hypovolemia diagnosis, 423
　　trimethoprim-sulfamethoxazole effects on, 2273
　secretion of, 782
　serum
　　acute interstitial nephritis levels of, 1219-1220
　　age-related changes in, 737
　　angiotensin receptor blockers effect on, 2006
　　angiotensin-converting enzyme inhibitors effect on, 2006
　　degradation and, 1961
　　as glomerular filtration rate biomarker, 933
　　glomerular filtration rate effects on, 782, 933
　　renal function assessments using, 783
　　storage of, 933
　in titratable acid excretion, 247
　in uremia, 1808
Creatinine clearance, 736, 783, 2544
　estimated, 2042, 2042t, 2044
　peritoneal dialysis dosage based on, 2120-2121
Creatol, 1811
Crescentic glomerulonephritis
　definition of, 1072-1073
　diagnostic classification of, 1074f
　immune complex-mediated
　　in children, 1073
　　electron microscopy findings, 1075
　　epidemiology of, 1075
　　immunofluorescence microscopy findings, 1075

Crescentic glomerulonephritis (Continued)
light microscopy findings, 1075
methylprednisolone for, 1076
pathogenesis of, 1075-1076
pathology of, 1075
treatment of, 1076
immunopathologic categories of, 1073t-1074t
pauci-immune
anti-MPO antibodies in, 1083-1085
antineutrophil cytoplasmic autoantibodies in, 1082-1084, 1086-1087
anti-PR3 autoantibodies in, 1083
clinical features of, 1085-1086
crescent formation in, 1082
cyclophosphamide for, 1087-1088
electron microscopy of, 1083
end-stage kidney disease progression of, 1086
epidemiology of, 1081-1082
immunofluorescence microscopy of, 1082-1083
laboratory findings in, 1086-1087
light microscopy of, 1082, 1082f
methylprednisolone for, 1087-1089
natural history of, 1085-1086
pathogenesis of, 1083-1085
pathology of, 1082-1083, 1082f
plasmapheresis for, 1088
PR3 in, 1083
prognostic factors for, 1086
relapse prevention in, 1089
after renal transplantation, 1086
rituximab for, 1088-1089
segmental fibrinoid necrosis in, 1082f
T cells in, 1084
treatment of, 1087-1089
urinalysis findings in, 1086-1087
Crescentic immunoglobulin A nephropathy, 1068
c-ret receptor, 719
Critical care nephrology. See Critically ill patients
Critical Path Initiative, 953
Critically ill patients
acute kidney injury in, 2137-2139
acute respiratory distress syndrome, 2138-2139
cardiac dysfunction, 2139
cardiorenal syndrome, 2139
drug dosing in, 2145-2146
fluid management for, 2138
hemodialysis in, 2142
hypocalcemia caused by, 618
liver dysfunction, 2139
outcomes in, 2142
pulmonary dysfunction, 2138-2139
renal replacement therapy in
anticoagulation during, 2144
continuous renal replacement therapy, 2141-2142, 2141t
drug dosing considerations, 2145
euvolemia, 2144
fluid balance, 2144
hemodynamic stability, 2144
intensity of, 2142-2144
intermittent hemodialysis, 2140-2142, 2141t
subclavian catheters used in, 2145
sustained low-efficiency dialysis, 2141t, 2142, 2145-2146
ultrafiltration, 2144
vascular access, 2145

Critically ill patients (Continued)
sepsis, 2137-2138
volume overload in, 2144
Crossed renal ectopy, 2295, 2295f, 2304
Cross-reactive groups, 2236
Cross-sectional studies, 670
Crotalus snakebites, 2446-2447
Crotoxin, 2447
Cryoglobulin(s), 1058, 1137, 2152
Cryoglobulinemia, 1071, 2152
Cryoglobulinemic glomerulonephritis, 1137-1138, 1137f-1138f
Cryoplasty balloon, for stenotic lesions, 2212
Cryoprecipitate, 1906
Crystals, 1327
agglomeration of, 1329
aggregation assessments, 1329
growth of, 1327f, 1329
nucleation of, 1327f, 1328-1329
in urine, 800-802, 801t
CTLA-4-Ig, 1034, 1104-1105, 2248
C-type natriuretic peptide (CNP)
in cirrhosis, 447
description of, 339
in effective arterial blood volume regulation, 414-415
functions of, 340
in heart failure, 342, 434-435
knockout mouse models of, 343
plasma concentrations of, 340
preproCNP, 340
structure of, 339f, 340
synthesis of, 340
Cullin 3, 168
Cushing's disease, 556
Cushing's syndrome, 766, 1549
Cutaneous metastases, 1949
Cutting balloons, for stenotic lesions, 2212
CXCL13, 1793
CXCR4, 34
CXCR7, 34
Cyclic adenosine monophosphate (cAMP)
apical sodium hydrogen exchange affected by, 154-155
description of, 463
hormones that stimulate, 1706
soluble adenylyl cyclase production of, 256
vasopressin effects on, 282-283
Cyclic GMP, 101, 398
Cyclical pulsatile load, 1535
Cyclin-dependent kinase, 1745
Cyclooxygenases (COX), 355, 357
-1. See COX-1
-2. See COX-2
in arachidonic acid metabolism, 355, 356f
description of, 355
enzymatic chemistry of, 357
expression of, antiinflammatory steroids' regulation of, 357
gene expression, 357
metabolites
in acute kidney injury, 377
in cirrhosis, 378
in diabetes mellitus, 378
in glomerular inflammatory injury, 375-376
in glomerular noninflammatory injury, 376-377
in hepatorenal syndrome, 378
in sodium transport, 373-374
in urinary tract obstruction, 377-378
in water transport, 373-374

Cyclooxygenases (COX) (Continued)
molecular biology of, 355
nephronal distribution of, 364-366
reactive oxygen species generated by, 379
sources of, 364-366
Cyclophosphamide, 1397-1398
adverse effects of, 1168-1169
focal segmental glomerulosclerosis treated with, 1032
glomerular disease treated with, 1168-1170
granulomatous with polyangiitis treated with, 1112-1114
lupus nephritis treated with, 1102-1103
malignancy risks, 1169
membranous nephropathy treated with, 1042-1043
microscopic polyangiitis treated with, 1112-1113, 1115-1116
minimal change disease treated with, 1023
ovarian failure caused by, 1168-1169
pauci-immune crescentic glomerulonephritis treated with, 1087-1088
polyarteritis nodosa treated with, 1119-1120
side effects of, 1113-1114
steroid-sensitive nephrotic syndrome treated with, 2329
toxicity of, 1169-1170
Cyclosporin A, 378, 1398-1399, 1637, 1637t. See also Cyclosporine
Cyclosporine
adverse effects of, 2330
in children, 2424-2425
fibrillary glomerulonephritis treated with, 1134
focal segmental glomerulosclerosis treated with, 1033
glomerular disease treated with, 1167-1168
hyperkalemia caused by, 590
hypomagnesemia caused by, 622
immunosuppressive uses of, 2246-2247, 2254t, 2256-2257
lupus nephritis treated with, 1104
membranous nephropathy treated with, 1043
minimal change disease treated with, 1023-1024
nephrogenesis affected by, 719
nephrotoxicity of, 2264
renal transplantation uses of, 2246-2247, 2254t, 2256-2257, 2269
side effects of, 1023
steroid-sensitive nephrotic syndrome treated with, 2329-2330
CYP24A1, 2390
CYP11B2, 305
CYP27B1, 1830, 2390
Cyst. See Renal cyst
Cyst hemorrhage, 1493
Cystatin C
as acute kidney injury biomarker, 935, 989
as chronic kidney disease biomarker, 934-935, 2043
Chronic Kidney Disease Epidemiology Collaboration equation for measuring, 786
clearance of, 1810
creatinine and, 934-935

Cystatin C (Continued)
  description of, 678, 737
  glomerular filtration rate estimations using, 783-784, 934-935, 2310
  urinary, 948-949
Cysteamine, 1441f, 2339
Cysteine, 1346f
Cysteinyl leukotriene receptors, 380
Cystic disease of renal sinus, 1517
Cystic fibrosis transmembrane regulator protein, 160
Cystic kidney disease, 1416, 1514-1516, 1515f-1516f
Cystic neoplasm, 1516-1517
Cystic nephroma, 1517
Cystic partially differentiated nephroblastoma, 1517
Cystic renal cell carcinoma, 1515f, 1516
Cystic renal mass, 1375. *See also* Bosniak renal cyst classification
Cystine, 1346f, 1441f, 1817
Cystine chelation therapy, 1365
Cystine stone, 1345-1346, 1448
Cystinosis, 1439-1441, 1440t, 2339-2340, 2341f
Cystinuria, 1445
  characteristics of, 223t, 227
  in children, 2345-2346, 2346f
  classification of, 228, 1448
  dietary intervention in, 1361-1362
  in Middle East, 2478-2479
  mutations in, 227
  rBAT/b$^{0,+}$AT in, 227-228
Cystitis, 1633
  antimicrobial agents for, 1238-1239, 1238t
  description of, 1231-1232
  diagnosis of, 1237-1238
  emphysematous, 1251
  epidemiology of, 1236
  Escherichia coli as cause of, 749-750, 778, 1233
  host factors, 1237
  microbiology of, 1236-1237
  pathogenesis of, 1236-1237
  prophylaxis for, 1239
  pyuria associated with, 1238
  recurrence of, 1237, 1239-1240
  reinfection of, 1237
  sexual intercourse as cause of, 1237
  spermicides and, 1237, 1239-1240
  Staphylococcus saprophyticus as cause of, 1237
  treatment of, 1238-1239, 1238t
  urine culture for, 1237-1238
Cytapheresis, 2160-2161
Cytochrome P450
  4A2 gene, 385
  in acute kidney disease, 385, 2038-2039
  alterations in, 2038-2039
  in chronic kidney disease, 385, 2038-2039
  CYP3A4, 2039
  description of, 355
  metabolites of, from arachidonic acid metabolism
    description of, 382, 382f-383f
    in hypertension, 385
    in renal blood flow autoregulation, 384
    as second messengers, 383-384
    in tubuloglomerular feedback, 384
  monooxygenases, 382-383
  parathyroid hormone effects on, 2019
  in proximal tubule, 384
  vasculature affected by, 383-384
Cytofolds, 47

Cytokines
  bicarbonate transport regulation by, 238
  macrophage production of, 976
  prostaglandin E$_2$ synthesis stimulated by, 376
  renal transplantation and, 2241
  in scleroderma, 1197
  suppressors of cytokine signaling, 1913
  therapeutic uses of, 1382
  tubular epithelial cell release of, 1215
  in tubulointerstitial injury, 1212-1213
Cytology, urine, 799
Cytomegalovirus, 1255, 2278, 2287-2288, 2429
Cytoplasmic antineutrophil cytoplasmic antibody, 759-760, 1109-1110
Cytoreductive nephrectomy, 1381
Cytotoxic lymphocyte activation antigen 4, 2240
Cytotoxic nephropathy, 1402-1403

D

Daclizumab, 2256
D–amino acids, 1809-1810
Dark cells, 70, 72f
Dcn, 31
Dead in bed syndrome, 572-573
Decorin, 31
Deep vein thrombosis (DVT)
  in chronic kidney disease, 1906-1907, 1908f
  in membranous nephropathy, 1041
  in nephrotic syndrome, 1804
  risk of, factors that affect, 1908f
Dehydration, 2367-2368
  description of, 2367-2368
  fluid therapy for, 2373-2374, 2373t
  hypernatremic, 2367-2368, 2374
  hypertonic, 478-480
  urinary concentrating ability affected by, 296-297
7-Dehydrocholesterol, 1828
Dehydroepiandrosterone, 1920
Dehydroepiandrosterone sulfate, 1920
Delirium syndromes
  definition of, 1934
  depression and, 1937-1938
  dialysis dysequilibrium, 1935
  differential diagnosis of, 1934t
  uremic encephalopathy, 1934-1935
Delta1, 30
Delta gap, 837
Dementia, 1935-1936, 1938
Dendritic cells, 976-977, 1792-1793
Dendroaspis natriuretic peptide, 339-341, 339f, 415, 447
Dengue fever
  acute kidney injury caused by, 2498-2499, 2520-2521, 2522t
  in Far East, 2520-2521, 2522t
  in Indian subcontinent, 2498-2499
  in Latin America, 2440-2441
Dengue hemorrhagic fever, 2520-2521
Dengue shock syndrome, 2520-2521
Denosumab, 612
Dense deposit disease
  classification of, 1046f
  clinical features of, 1052
  description of, 1046
  epidemiology of, 1050
  genetics of, 1052
  hypocomplementemia in, 1052-1053
  light microscopy findings in, 1051, 1051f
  lipodystrophy associated with, 1053

Dense deposit disease (Continued)
  microhematuria in, 1052
  pathogenesis of, 1052
  pathology of, 1050-1051
  retinal deposits associated with, 1053
  treatment of, 1053
Dentin matrix protein, 1830
Dent's disease, 1437-1438, 2344-2345
Denys-Drash syndrome, 1431, 2325
Deoxycorticosterone, 304f
Depletional hyponatremia, 503-504
Depression, 1937-1938, 2063
Dermatitis, arteriovenous shunt, 1949
Dermatosis, acquired perforating, 1944, 1944f
Desferrioxamine, 1887
Desmopressin
  central diabetes insipidus treated with, 487-488
  description of, 162-163, 175, 279, 282
  hyponatremia caused by, 488, 496-497
  kidney biopsy-related bleeding complications treated with, 915-917
  nephrogenic diabetes insipidus applications of, 484, 487, 2338
  renal response to, 808-809
  uremic bleeding treated with, 1906
  urine flow rate affected by, 806, 810-811
  vasopressin deficiency treated with, 285
Developmental origins of health and disease, 694
Developmental programming
  birth weight and, 694, 694t
  of blood pressure, 709, 709f
  definition of, 694
  mechanisms of, 713-723, 715t, 725f
    apoptosis, 718
    catch-up growth, 721-723
    congenital urinary tract obstruction, 719-720
    c-ret receptor function, 719
    fetal exposures
      to drugs, 719
      to glucocorticoids, 717
      to hyperglycemia, 717-718
    gender, 720
    glial cell line-derived neurotrophic factor, 719
    maternal nutrient restriction, 715-717
  nephron endowment, 696-701
  nephron number, 695-696, 695t
  prematurity and, 694, 694t
  of renal function and disease, 703-712
  renin-angiotensin-aldosterone system and, 703, 704t-705t
  transgenerational effects of, 722-723
Dexamethasone, 696-699
D1g1, 29
DHA (2,8-dihydroxyadenine) stone, 1347
Diabetes Control and Complications Trial, 1301-1302
Diabetes insipidus (DI), 1467-1473
  acquired, 285
  acute traumatic, 488-489
  calcium stones and uric acid stones, 1343f
  causes of, 808-809
  central
    adenohypophysitis and, 475-476
    arginine vasopressin for, 488
    causes of, 473-476, 473t
    clinical manifestations of, 483
    description of, 285, 809, 2369-2370
    desmopressin for, 487-488
    familial, 474-475, 475f
    idiopathic, 475-476

Diabetes insipidus (DI) *(Continued)*
    partial, 809-810, 810*f*
    pathophysiology of, 476-477, 478*f*
    polyuria in, 810-811
    treatment of, 487-489
  characteristics of, 285
  clinical manifestations of, 483
  definition of, 282
  dipsogenic, 482
  familial, 285
  fluid deprivation test for diagnosis of, 485, 485*t*
  magnetic resonance imaging of, 485-486
  nephrogenic. *See* Nephrogenic diabetes insipidus
  partial, 477
  postsurgical, 488
  of pregnancy, 1612
  thiazide diuretics for, 1727
  thirst mechanisms in, 484
  treatment of
    arginine vasopressin, 486
    chlorpropamide, 487
    desmopressin, 487
    goals for, 486
    natriuretic agents, 487
    options for, 486*t*
    prostaglandin synthase inhibitors, 487
    thiazide diuretics, 487
Diabetes mellitus (DM)
  in Africa, 2463
  anemia in, 1877-1878
  in China, 2529, 2529*f*
  chronic kidney disease progression affected by, 681, 1865
  COX-2 in, 378
  Diabetes Outcome Clinical Trial, blood pressure levels achieved in, 1554*t*
  dipeptidyl peptidase-4 inhibitors for, 2593
  in elderly, 2590, 2592-2593
  end-stage kidney disease caused by, 2060, 2280
  in Far East, 2529
  glucagon-like peptide-1 analogues for, 2593
  glyburide for, 2593
  glycemic control in, 1301-1303, 1995
  hemoglobin A_{1c} in, 2593
  hyperkalemia in, 586-587
  hypoglycemic agents for, 2593
  hypomagnesemia in, 620
  malnutrition associated with, 1315
  maternal, 2301
  maturity-onset diabetes type 5, 2299-2300
  mesangial expansion in, 1288, 1292
  in Middle East, 2472
  in New Zealand, 2550-2551
  new-onset, after transplantation, 1320
  oral hypoglycemic agents for, 2593
  osmotic diuresis in, 812-813
  plasma renin levels in, 334-335
  posttransplantation, 1320, 2283
  pregnancy and, 1634
  prevalence of, 1865
  renal disorders in, 1291-1292, 2592
  renal failure in, 1314-1318, 1314*t*
  after renal transplantation, 2433
  renal transplantation in patients with, 1318-1319, 2288-2289
  repaglinide for, 2593
  stroke risks associated with, 1928*t*, 1929, 1931
  telmisartan versus losartan trial, 1557

Diabetes mellitus (DM) *(Continued)*
  thiazide diuretics and, 1730
  transplantation for
    islet cell, 1319-1320
    new-onset diabetes after, 1320
    renal, 1318-1319, 2288-2289
    renal-pancreas, 1319
  type 1
    blood pressure in, 1297-1298
    cardiovascular disease in, 1295
    chronic kidney disease in, 1981
    diabetic nephropathy in, 1285, 1293, 1294*t*, 1299, 1312
    end-stage kidney disease in, 1295
    glomerular filtration rate in, 1296
    glomerular structure in, 1291
    glomeruli in, 1287*f*
    hypertension in, 1297-1298
    mesangial expansion in, 1288, 1292
    microalbuminuria in, 1283, 1292-1294
    nephropathy in, 1290-1291
    peripheral capillary filtration surface in, 1288-1289
    podocyte number in, 1287-1288
    proteinuria in, 1292-1293, 1300
    structural-functional relationships in, 1288-1289, 1289*f*
    urinary kallikrein excretion in, 350
  type 2
    blood pressure in, 1298
    cardiovascular morbidity in, 1306-1308
    diabetic nephropathy in, 1293, 1294*t*
    glomerular structure in, 1291
    glucose-lowering therapies for, 1313
    metformin for, 1315
    microalbuminuria in, 1283, 1292-1293
    nephropathy in, 1290-1291
    podocyte number in, 1287-1288
    structural-functional relationships in, 1291
    telmisartan versus losartan trial, 1557
  urinary tract infections in, 1320
  urolithiasis and, 1350-1351
Diabetic ketoacidosis (DKA), 525, 546-547, 570, 628, 633, 2398
Diabetic nephropathy, 1556-1557
  acute kidney injury in, 1315
  "acute-on-chronic" renal failure in, 1315
  in Africa, 2463
  albuminuria in, 1283
  amputations in patients with, 1318
  anemia in, 1299-1300, 1316
  biomarkers for, 1294*t*
  bladder dysfunction in, 1320
  cardiovascular disease in, 1295, 1316-1317
  characteristics of, 1298
  chronic kidney disease caused by, 2503, 2592
  complications of, 1300, 1313*t*
  course of, 1296-1300
  description of, 112, 378
  diabetic retinopathy associated with, 1300
  electron microscopy of, 1284*f*
  endothelin system in, 337-338
  end-stage kidney disease caused by, 681, 1295, 1313-1314, 2592
  extracellular matrix accumulation in, 1286
  extrarenal complications in, 1300
  fluid retention in, 1298*f*
  genes associated with, 1299
  glycemic control in, 1301-1303
  hemodialysis for, 1316-1318
  hypertension in, 1314-1315, 1667

Diabetic nephropathy *(Continued)*
  kallikrein-kinin system in, 349-350
  light microscopy of, 1285*f*
  malnutrition associated with, 1315
  mesangial matrix fraction in, 1285-1286, 1285*f*
  microalbuminuria in, 1289-1290, 1292*t*, 1294-1298, 1301-1302
  mortality rates for, 1295
  natural history of, 1298
  normoalbuminuria, 1293-1294, 1296
  in Pacific Islands, 2553
  pathology of, 1284*t*
  pathophysiology of, 1298-1300, 1865
  peripheral neuropathy associated with, 1300
  podocytes in, 115*t*, 116-117, 120
  pregnancy in patients with, 1300, 1634
  prognosis for, 1295-1296, 1311-1312
  progression of, 658-659, 1298-1299, 1298*f*
  proteinuria in, 1295, 2004-2005
  reactive oxygen species in, 337
  recurrence of, after renal transplantation, 2275-2276
  renal replacement therapy for
    hemodialysis, 1316-1318
    initiation of, 1316
    peritoneal dialysis, 1318
  reversibility of, 1292
  risk factors for, 1290, 1294*t*, 1299
  transplantation for
    islet cell, 1319-1320
    new-onset diabetes after, 1320
    renal, 1318-1319
    renal-pancreas, 1319
  treatment of
    angiotensin receptor blockers, 2002
    angiotensin-converting enzyme inhibitors, 1308, 1998-1999, 2002
    blood pressure control, 1303-1312
    description of, 1300-1301
    dietary protein restriction, 1312
    glycemic control, 1301-1303
    lipid-lowering therapy, 1312
    new modalities for, 1312-1313, 1314*t*
    vitamin D, 1312-1313
  type 1, 1288-1289, 1289*f*
  type 2, 1291, 1999
  in type 1 diabetes mellitus, 1290-1291, 1312
  in type 2 diabetes mellitus, 1290-1291
  urinary proteomic profiles for, 1300
  urinary tract infections in, 1320
  urotensin II levels in, 352
  vascular access in, 1315
Diabetic retinopathy, 1300, 1318, 1888
Diacylglycerol, 355
Dialysance, 2071
Dialysate pump, 2078
Dialysis
  acute kidney injury treated with, 744
  advance directives and, 2561-2562
  in Africa, 2463-2464, 2464*f*2465*f*
  albumin, 2171
  amyloidosis associated with, 1949
  in Australia, 2540*f*, 2542-2544
  blood pressure management in patients undergoing, 1561-1562
  cardioembolic stroke in, 1927
  cessation of, 2560-2561, 2561*t*
  chronic inflammation in, 1969-1970
  chronic kidney disease treated with, 1971
  "difficult" patients undergoing, 2567-2568, 2568*t*

Dialysis *(Continued)*
  drug clearance during, 2047
  early initiation of, 1971
  in elderly, 744, 2568-2569, 2590, 2591*f*, 2596-2598
  energy expenditure during, 1973
  epidemiology of, 2191-2192
  ethical dilemmas
    access, 2560
    advance directives, 2561-2562
    age-based rationing, 2572
    cessation of treatment, 2560-2561, 2561*t*
    conflicts of interest, 2562
    denial of treatment, 2559
    "difficult" patients, 2567-2568, 2568*t*
    older patients, 2568-2569
    patient selection, 2559-2561
    rationing, 2559-2561, 2572
    reimbursement, 2562
    shared decision-making, 2563*t*-2566*t*
    withdrawal of treatment, 2560-2567, 2561*t*, 2563*t*
    withholding of treatment, 2562-2567
  folate deficiency associated with, 1887
  goals of, 2069
  health disparities in, 2580-2581
  hemodialysis. *See* Hemodialysis
  history of, 2059
  hyperkalemia treated with, 598-599
  hypermagnesemia treated with, 626
  hypoalbuminemia in patients receiving, 1969-1970
  isothermic, 2095
  life expectancy after initiation of, in elderly, 2596, 2597*f*
  lupus nephritis treated with, 1100
  Medicare costs for, 2627*f*
  in Middle East, 2487-2489
  muscle wasting in, 1817
  in New Zealand, 2551-2552
  in older adults, 2596-2598
  payment for, 1902
  peritoneal. *See* Peritoneal dialysis
  physical functioning in patients receiving, 1818
  potassium removal with, 598-599
  pregnancy and, 1635-1636
  protein intake after, 1983
  reimbursement for, 2562
  renal function assessments in, 2044
  shared decision-making, 2563*t*-2566*t*, 2597
  skin manifestations of, 1944
  steal syndrome associated with, 1948
  stroke risks associated with, 1927-1928, 1930
  sustained low-efficiency, 2141*t*, 2142, 2145-2146, 2171, 2459
  taste acuity reductions secondary to, 1819
  uremia treated with, 2083
  uremic platelet dysfunction affected by, 1905
  vascular access for, 2191-2192
  vascular calcification in, 1850
  withdrawal of, 2560-2561, 2561*t*
Dialysis dementia, 1935-1936
Dialysis disequilibrium syndrome, 1935, 2106-2107, 2414
Dialysis Outcomes and Practice Patterns Study, 643
Dialysis Outcomes Quality Initiative, 2621-2622, 2631
Diarrhea
  acute kidney injury in Indian subcontinent patients caused by, 2496
  bicarbonate levels affected by, 528-529

Diarrhea *(Continued)*
  fluid therapy for, 2496
  magnesium deficiency caused by, 620
Diastolic blood pressure, 1524, 1524*t*, 1526*f*
Diastolic dysfunction, 1688*t*, 2408
Diazoxide, 1696-1697
Dibasic aminoaciduria, 226-227
Dicarboxylate-sulfate transporters. *See* NaDC transporters
Dicarboxylic aminoaciduria, 223*t*, 229, 1450
Dicer1, 39
Dichloroacetate, for lactic acidosis, 546
Diet
  low-protein. *See* Low-protein diet
  phosphorus-restricted, 2031
  sodium-restricted, 450
  uremic solutes affected by, 1814-1815
Dietary potassium, 559-560, 566, 584*t*, 1975
Dietary reference intake, 2405
Dietary sodium. *See* Sodium, dietary
Diffuse diabetic glomerulosclerosis, 1285-1286, 1287*f*
Diffusion, 2068-2069, 2068*f*, 2078, 2112
Diffusion-weighted imaging, 863-864, 871*f*
Digitalis-like factors, 419
Digoxin, 587, 2073
Dihydropyridine calcium channel blockers, 1662, 1664-1667, 1699, 1995-1996
1,25-Dihydroxycholecalciferol, 2024*f*, 2025, 2032
Dihydroxyeicosatrienoic acids, 382-383
1,25-Dihydroxyvitamin D
  absorptive hypercalciuria independent of, 1332-1333
  calcitriol as replacement for, 2089
  catabolism of, 2390
  chronic kidney disease levels of, 1913, 2014
  dependence, 1331-1332
  description of, 1864-1865
  fibroblast growth factor-23 suppression of, 2031-2032
  functions of, 2023-2024
  hemodialysis replacement of, 2089
1,25-Dihydroxyvitamin D3, 1632-1633
1α25-Dihydroxyvitamin D
  description of, 187*f*
  humoral hypercalcemia of malignancy and, 607
  osteoclastic bone resorption caused by, 603
  phosphate transport regulation by, 200
Diltiazem hydrochloride, 1663-1664, 1663*t*, 1668*t*, 1697*t*
Dilutional acidosis, 529-530
Dimethylamine, 1812-1813
Dimethylarginine dimethylaminohydrolase, 443, 685
Dipeptidyl peptidase-4 inhibitors, 2593
Dipsogenic diabetes insipidus, 482
Direct renin inhibitors, 1564, 1764-1765, 2003-2004
Direct-acting vasodilators
  combination therapies using, 1692
  dosing of, 1649*t*-1650*t*
  efficacy of, 1674
  hypertensive urgencies and emergencies treated with, 1695*t*, 1696-1699
  indications for, 1565
  mechanism of action, 1673
  renal effects of, 1674
  in renal insufficiency patients, 1649*t*-1650*t*
  safety of, 1674
  types of, 1673-1674, 1674*t*

Disasters, 2472, 2473*f*
Discoid lupus erythematosus, 1950, 1950*f*
Disease management organizations, 2631
Disequilibrium pH, 253
Dissecting renal artery aneurysms, 1204
Disseminated histoplasmosis, 1405
Dissolution therapy, 1365
Distal calcium, 1334*f*
Distal convoluted tubule (DCT)
  anatomy of, 65-68, 165, 261-262
  bicarbonate reabsorption in, 238-239
  cells of, 65-66, 67*f*, 167, 238-239
  11-β-hydroxysteroid dehydrogenase in, 66-67
  loop diuretics effect on, 1715
  luminal surface of, 68*f*
  magnesium reabsorption in, 194
  magnesium transport in, 195*f*
  microprojections on, 65-66
  mineralocorticoid receptor expression in, 315
  Na^+K^+-ATPase activity in, 66
  NCC expression by, 165-166
  pars convoluta of, 68*f*
  potassium secretion by, 176-178
  sodium absorption in, 566-568
  sodium pump activity in, 129
  thiazide and thiazide-like diuretics action on, 1710, 1711*f*
  water impermeability of, 67-68
  water transport pathways in, 274*f*
Distal potassium-sparing diuretics
  adverse effects of, 1713
  drug interactions, 1713
  hyperkalemia caused by, 1713, 1732
  indications for, 1713
  loop diuretics and, 1719
  magnesium excretion affected by, 1730
  mechanism of action, 1712
  pharmacokinetics of, 1712-1713
  sites of action, 1712
  thiazide diuretics and, 1719
Distal protection devices, 1193
Distal renal tubular acidosis, 1456*f*, 1457
  alkali therapy for, 535-536
  classical, 534, 534*t*-535*t*
  clinical spectrum of, 534-535, 535*t*
  in Far East, 2533
  features of, 534-535
  generalized, 534*t*
  H^+K^+-ATPase's involvement in, 534
  hyperkalemic, 540, 589
  hypokalemic, 534, 581
  pathophysiology of, 533-534
  pyelonephritis caused by, 534-535
  treatment of, 535-536, 536*t*
  type A intercalated defects, 534
Distal tubule
  adaptations of, to nephron loss, 1746
  ammonia secretion in, 252
  anatomy of, 63
  calcium in, 189, 190*f*, 192*f*
  embryology of, 5
  macula densa of, 54
  potassium secretion measurements, 569
  segments of, 63
  water absorption in, 271
Diuresis, postobstructive, 1281
Diuretic renography, 1266-1267
Diuretics, 1564, 1629-1630
  acute kidney injury treated with, 1725-1726
  adenosine type 1 receptor antagonists, 1714
  adverse drug interactions, 1732

Diuretics (Continued)
  adverse effects of
    azotemia, 1727
    drug allergy, 1732
    extracellular volume depletion, 1727
    hypercalcemia, 1730
    hyperglycemia, 1730-1731
    hyperkalemia, 1730
    hyperlipidemia, 1731
    hyperuricemia, 1731
    hypokalemia, 1728-1730, 1729f
    hypomagnesemia, 1730
    hyponatremia, 492-493, 1727-1728, 1727f
    impotence, 1731-1732
    malignancies, 1732
    metabolic alkalosis, 1730
    ototoxicity, 1732
    skin-related, 1732
    vitamin B deficiency, 1732
  bicarbonate reabsorption affected by, 1703-1704
  β-blockers and, combination therapy using, 1691
  braking phenomenon, 1714-1716, 1715f-1716f, 1716t
  breast milk transmission of, 1732
  calcium channel blockers and, combination therapy using, 1691
  calcium excretion affected by, 1726
  calcium transport regulation by, 189-191
  carbonic anhydrase inhibitors. See Carbonic anhydrase inhibitors
  chloruresis induced by, 553
  clonidine added to, 445-446
  combination therapies, 1719
  distal potassium-sparing. See Distal potassium-sparing diuretics
  dopaminergic agents as, 1713
  edematous conditions treated with, 1719-1725
  heart failure treated with, 1719-1722
  hypercalcemia treated with, 1726
  hypervolemia treated with, 450-451
  hypokalemia caused by, 574
  hypovolemia caused by, 502
  idiopathic edema treated with, 1725
  liver cirrhosis treated with, 1722-1724
  loop. See Loop diuretics
  mechanism of action, 1703f
  metabolic alkalosis caused by, 553, 1704
  modulators of response to
    arginine vasopressin, 1717
    atrial natriuretic peptide, 1717
    catecholamines, 1717
    eicosanoids, 1716-1717
    renin angiotensin aldosterone system, 1716
  nephrolithiasis treated with, 1726
  nephrotic syndrome treated with, 1723f, 1724-1725
  neprilysin inhibitors, 1714
  nesiritide, 1714
  osmotic. See Osmotic diuretics
  osteoporosis treated with, 1726-1727
  pharmacokinetics of, 1720
  potassium excretion affected by, 595
  potassium-sparing. See Potassium-sparing diuretics
  proximal tubule, for hypervolemia, 450
  renal tubular acidosis treated with, 1726
  renin-angiotensin-aldosterone inhibitors and, combination therapy using, 1691

Diuretics (Continued)
  resistance to, 451, 1717-1719, 1718f, 1724, 1797
  sites of action, 1703f
  thiazide. See Thiazide diuretics
  thiazide-like. See Thiazide-like diuretics
  urea channel inhibitors, 1714
  vasopressin receptor antagonists, 1713-1714
  volume depletion caused by, 422
Diverticular disease, 1492
Djenkol beans, 2525
DNA microarrays, 2249
Dominant inheritant disease, 1411-1412, 1411t
Donor-specific anti-HLA antibody, 2260, 2422
Dopamine
  acute tubular necrosis treated with, 1001
  natriuretic effects of, 152-154
  phosphate transport affected by, 201
  renal toxicity prevention using, 1398
Dopamine D_1-like receptor agonist, 1699
Doppler color-flow ultrasonography, 848-849, 850f
Doppler ultrasonography
  description of, 848-849, 850f
  renal artery stenosis evaluations, 903-904
  renal transplantation assessments using, 910
  renal vein thrombosis evaluations, 1204
  urinary tract obstruction evaluations, 1265
Double-antibody radioimmunoassay, for urinary albumin measurement, 794
Double-filtration plasmapheresis, 2160
Doxazosin, 1676, 1676t
Doxercalciferol, 2032
Doxycycline, for leptospirosis prophylaxis, 2444
DP receptors, 369
D-Penicillamine, 1158-1159, 1445
Drosophila, 20
Drug(s). See also specific drug
  absorption of, 2035-2036
  acute interstitial nephritis caused by, 1218-1220, 1218t
  clearance of, 2039, 2039t
  distribution of, 2036-2037
  in elderly patients, 2594-2596, 2595t
  high anion gap acidosis caused by, 543, 547-550
  hypercalcemia caused by, 609
  hyperkalemia caused by, 540, 540t, 590-592
  hypocalcemia caused by, 617-618
  hypophosphatemia caused by, 632
  intraperitoneal administration of, 2049
  lactic acidosis caused by, 545
  malabsorption of, 2036
  metabolism of, 2037-2039
  metabolites of, 2038t
  potassium loss caused by, 574-575
  renal excretion of, 2039, 2039t
  systemic lupus erythematosus caused by, 1099-1100
  tubulointerstitial diseases caused by, 1218-1219, 1218t
  urinary tract obstruction caused by, 1260
Drug disposition
  absorption, 2035-2036
  distribution, 2036-2037, 2036t
  intravenous administration effects on, 2035, 2035f
  metabolism, 2037-2039

Drug dosing
  in acute kidney injury, 2046, 2051t-2054t, 2145-2146
  in chronic kidney disease, 2044-2046, 2045t, 2051t-2054t
  Cockcroft-Gault equation for, 2042-2044
  in continuous renal replacement therapy, 2048-2049
  in hemodialysis, 2046-2048, 2048t
  intravenous administration, 2035, 2035f
  in peritoneal dialysis, 2049
  pharmacodynamics, 2040-2041
  pharmacogenomics, 2039-2040
  pharmacokinetic considerations, 2035-2039, 2036t
  recommendations for, 2051t-2054t
  renal function assessments, 2041-2044
  renal replacement therapy considerations for, 2145
Drug resistance transporters, 211
Dry weight, 2095-2096
DSTYK, 2300
Dual energy x-ray absorptiometry (DEXA), 1846, 2099
Duane-radial ray syndrome, 2297t
Ducts of Bellini, 43, 44f, 74, 264
Dutch Renal Artery Stenosis Intervention Cooperative (DRASTIC), 1596t, 1602-1603
Dynactin, 295
Dyneins, 295
Dyslipidemia, 1442
  chronic kidney disease and, 683-684, 1772-1774, 1863, 2011
  in elderly, 2593
  renal injury and, 1772-1773
  statins for, 1773-1774, 1931, 2011, 2593
  treatment of, 1773-1774, 2011
Dysnatremias, 2137
Dyspigmentation, 1943f
Dysplasia, renal. See Renal dysplasia
Dyspnea, 434
Dysrhythmias, 1859

E

EAAT3, 228-229
Eagle-Barrett syndrome. See Prune-belly syndrome
Early endosomal antigen 1, 1275
EAST syndrome, 167, 2379
Eating disorders, 581-583
E-Cadherin, 36
Echinococcus granulosus, 1255
Echocardiography, 1866
Eclampsia, 1616-1617
Ectonucleotide pyrophosphatase/ phosphodiesterase 1, 631
Ectopic adrenocorticotropic hormone, 577
Ectopic kidneys, 850-851, 2295, 2295f, 2305, 2311
Eculizumab
  antiphospholipid-associated thrombotic microangiopathy treated with, 1201
  atypical hemolytic-uremic syndrome treated with, 1186, 2356
  C3 glomerulopathies treated with, 1159
  description of, 1045, 2269
  glomerular diseases treated with, 1171
Edema
  blood volume alterations and, 1798-1799
  cerebral, 813, 1619-1620, 1705
  formation of, 1798-1800, 1798f-1799f

End-stage kidney disease (ESKD) (Continued)
  global prevalence of, 643, 644f, 2060, 2574
  glomerulonephritis progression to, 1161
  glycemic control in, 1315
  granulomatous with polyangiitis
      progression to, 1114
  hazard ratios for, 675f
  health disparities in, 2577-2578
  hematocrit target for, 2628t
  hemodialysis for, 2097
  hemoglobin target for, 2098, 2628t
  Henoch-Schönlein purpura progression
      to, 1123-1124
  heroin nephropathy progression to,
      1157-1158
  historical description of, 2403
  in Hong Kong, 2535
  human immunodeficiency virus
      nephropathy as cause of, 1153
  hyperkalemia in, 585, 2405
  hyperprolactinemia in, 1919
  hypertension in, 1765, 1770, 2406-2407
  hypogonadism in, 1921-1922
  immunoglobulin A nephropathy
      progression to, 1065
  immunotactoid glomerulopathy
      progression to, 1072
  incidence of, 638-641, 639f-640f, 656,
      926-927, 1479, 2007-2008, 2059-2060,
      2059f-2060f, 2575, 2577, 2597f
  in Indonesia, 2536
  insulin resistance in, 1816
  international comparisons of, 643, 644f
  interstitial fibrosis as cause of, 1216-1217
  in Japan, 2534-2535
  kidney stones and, 1352
  in Korea, 2535
  in Latin America, 2449-2451, 2449f,
      2450t
  lead exposure and, 1226-1227
  lupus nephritis progression to, 1100
  magnetic resonance imaging of, 889f
  in Malaysia, 2535-2536
  in Maori population, 2552-2553
  Medicare costs and, 1524
  Medicare program, 2558-2559, 2562, 2572,
      2625
  in microalbuminuria, 1303f
  in Middle East, 2473-2474, 2476
  mortality rates for, 641, 642f, 645, 773,
      2061-2063, 2062f
  in Native Americans, 2583
  in New Zealand, 2550, 2552-2553
  obesity as risk factor for, 679, 1300
  obstructive uropathy progression to,
      764
  25(OH)D levels and, 1872-1873
  palliative care for, 2563
  parathyroid hormone levels in, 2023-2026
  pauci-immune crescentic
      glomerulonephritis progression to,
      1086
  pericardial disease secondary to,
      2107-2108
  in Philippines, 2536
  phosphorus measurements in, 2028-2029
  potassium in, 174-175, 2093
  poverty and, 666
  preeclampsia as risk factor for, 681
  prevalence of, 641-642, 2059-2060, 2574
  quality improvement in, 2625-2626
  Quality Initiative for, 2626
  race and, 1769f, 2577, 2597f
  rapidly progressive glomerulonephritis
      progression to, 2150
  renal risk scores for, 690-691, 690f

End-stage kidney disease (ESKD) (Continued)
  renal transplantation for, 1181-1182
  scleroderma renal crisis progression to,
      1198
  sickle cell disease progression to, 1200
  in Singapore, 2536
  skin manifestations of, 1942-1945, 1943f,
      1945f
  smoking and, 1992
  in Social Security Amendments to
      Medicare bill, 2558-2559, 2562
  stroke in, risk factors for, 1928-1933
  in Taiwan, 2534
  testosterone supplementation in,
      1922-1923
  in Thailand, 2535
  treatment of, 1424, 1493-1494
    dialysis. See Dialysis
    disparities in, 2580-2582
    economic considerations in, 2025-2026
    renal transplantation. See Renal
        transplantation
    vitamin D sterols, 2026
  trends in, 639f
  ultrasonography of, 868, 868f
  vascular calcification in, 2128
  in Vietnam, 2536
  X-linked Alport's syndrome and, 1424
End-stage liver disease, 610
End-stage renal disease. See End-stage kidney
    disease
Energy-based tissue ablation, 1380
Enteric hyperoxaluria, 1325, 1340, 2340
Enterohemorrhagic Escherichia coli, 2154
Eosinophil(s), 799-800
Eosinophilia, 988
Eosinophilic granulomatosis with
    polyangiitis (EGPA), 1012-1013
  antineutrophil cytoplasmic antibodies in,
      1117
  in children, 2351
  clinical features of, 1117
  corticosteroids for, 1117-1118
  course of, 1117-1118
  description of, 1116-1118
  laboratory features of, 1117
  pathogenesis of, 1117
  pathology of, 1116, 1116f
  prognosis for, 1117-1118
  symptoms of, 1117
  treatment of, 1117-1118
Eosinophiluria, 799-800, 986-987
EP receptors
  EP1 receptors, 370, 379
  EP2 receptors, 370-371, 373
  EP3 receptors, 371-372
  EP4 receptors, 372-373
  renal cortical hemodynamics affected by,
      372
  renal function regulated by, 372-373
Epac, 294-295
Ephedrine, 1347
Ephrin-Eph family, 34
Ephrins, 34
Epidermal basement membranes, 1142t
Epidermal growth factor, 24-25, 1217
Epidermal growth factor receptor, 329f,
    621
Epistaxis, 1328-1329
Epithelial angiomyolipoma, 1501
Epithelial basement membranes, 25
Epithelial calcium channel, 580
Epithelial cells
  injury to, 970-983
  parietal, 4-5, 52-53, 52f-53f, 1789-1790
  plasticity of, 1217

Epithelial sodium channel(s)
  aldosterone effects on, 172-173, 311-312,
      409, 565-566, 1800, 2366-2367
  amiloride effects on, 565, 590, 1712
  composition of, 1462f
  description of, 166-167, 169
  inhibitors of, 590-591, 1692
  knockout mice model, 278
  lithium and, 297-298
  localization of, 278
  pentamidine effects on, 591
  potassium secretion affected by, 313
  proteolytic cleavage activation of, 312
  serum- and glucocorticoid-regulated
      kinase stimulation of, 318, 319f
  SGK-1 effects on, 172-173
  sodium absorption via, 175
  sodium reabsorption via, 169-170, 310-311,
      314-317, 319-320
  tissue kallikrein effects on, 349
  triamterene effects on, 1712
  vasopressin activation of, 173-174
Epithelial-to-mesenchymal transition, 1217,
    1793-1794
Epithelioid angiomyolipoma, 1368-1369
Eplerenone, 322, 540-541, 1678-1679, 1692
Epoetin, 1890, 2626-2627
Epoxides, 383-384
Epoxygenases, 383
Epratuzumab, 1104
Eprosartan, 1652, 1652t
Epstein-Barr virus, 1151, 1404, 2429-2430
Epstein's syndrome, 1140t
Equilibrative nucleoside transporter 1, 399
Equilibrium solubility product, 1325-1327
Erectile dysfunction, 1921-1922
Ergocalciferol, 1923, 2025, 2032, 2390
ERK1/2, 1217
Eruptive xanthomas, 1946-1947, 1946f
Erythrocytes. See also Red blood cell(s)
  dysmorphic, 798
  erythropoietin production by, 1878
  ferritin concentration, 1894
  uremic, 1884-1885
  in urine, 798-799, 799f
  zinc protoporphyrin concentration, 1894
Erythrocytosis, 1375
  definition of, 1888
  in hemodialysis, 1888
  polycystic kidney disease as cause of,
      1888
  posttransplantation, 1888-1889
  in renal artery stenosis, 1889
  in renal tumors, 1889
Erythroferrone, 1885
Erythropoiesis
  burst-forming units–erythroid, 1882-1883
  description of, 1878-1884
  erythropoietin regulation of, 1875,
      1878-1883
  folate in, 1883-1884
  hypoxia-inducible factors, 1880-1881,
      1880f
  inefficient, in megaloblastic anemia, 1883
  inflammation effects on, 1887
  iron in, 1883-1884, 1893
  model of, 1882f
  parathyroid hormone effects on, 1887
  testosterone effects on, 1922
  uremic inhibitors of, 1885
  vitamin B_{12} in, 1883-1884
Erythropoiesis-stimulating agents (ESA)
  anemia treated with, 1889-1892, 2405-
      2406, 2626
  ascorbic acid added to, 1900
  darbepoetin alfa, 1890-1892

Erythropoiesis-stimulating agents (ESA) *(Continued)*
  epoetin, 1890
  during hemodialysis, 2098
  hemoglobin concentration affected by, 1892, 1902
  hypoxia-inducible factor stabilizers, 1892
  initiation of, 1892
  maintenance of, 1892
  methoxypolyethylene glycol epoetin beta, 1892
  prolactin levels affected by, 1919
  resistance to, 2098
  risk/benefit relationship for, 1902
  route of administration, 2098
  trials of, 1901-1902
Erythropoietin
  anemia in chronic kidney disease and, 1884, 2013, 2089, 2097-2098, 2610-2611
  apoptosis suppression by, 1882-1883, 1882f
  bone marrow clearance of, 1881
  carbohydrate chains of, 1881
  clearance of, 1881
  definition of, 1878
  description of, 1316, 1871
  endogenous production of, 1887-1888
  erythropoiesis regulation by, 1875, 1878-1883
  hyperparathyroidism and, 1887
  hypoxia-inducible factor stabilizers effect on, 1892
  identification of, 1881
  liver production of, 1881
  in posttransplantation erythrocytosis, 1889
  production of, 1884, 1887-1888, 2602-2603
  protein intake effects on, 1980
  purification of, 1881
  recombinant human, 1888-1890, 1895, 1906, 1922, 2097
  serum levels of, 1883
  stroke risk prevention using, 1932-1933
Erythropoietin receptors, 1881, 1887
Escherichia coli
  asymptomatic bacteriuria caused by, 1246
  enterohemorrhagic, 2154
  0157:H7, 1179, 2154
  prostatitis caused by, 1247
  urinary tract infection caused by, 749-750, 778, 1233, 1236-1237, 1240
  uropathogenic, 1236-1237, 1239
Esmolol hydrochloride, 1695t, 1698
ESRD Amendment to Public Law, 2559
Essential amino acids, 1971-1972
Essential fatty acid deficiency, 355, 375
Essential hypertension, 336-337
Estimated creatinine clearance, 2042, 2044
Estimated glomerular filtration rate. *See* Glomerular filtration rate, estimated
Estradiol, 191
Estrogens, 191, 1906
Et-B receptor, 256
Ethacrynic acid, 1732
Ethanol-induced high anion gap acidosis, 548
Ethical dilemmas
  bioethics, 2558-2562
  chronic pain, 2569
  conflicts of interest, 2562
  dialysis-related. *See* Dialysis, ethical dilemmas

Ethical dilemmas *(Continued)*
  end-of-life care, 2567
  fiscal crisis in nephrology, 2572
  hospice referral, 2569-2570
  palliative care, 2569-2570
  reimbursement, 2562, 2572
  renal transplantation access, 2570-2572
Ethnicity
  chronic kidney disease and, 660-662, 1769-1770
  definition of, 660
  end-stage kidney disease and, 1769
  hypertension and, 693-694, 1526-1527
  kidney stones and, 1348
Ethylene dibromide poisoning, 2501
Ethylene glycol
  acute kidney injury caused by, 2500-2501
  extracorporeal treatments for, 2173-2178, 2174t, 2176t
  fomepizole for, 548
  high anion gap acidosis caused by, 548
Eukaryotes, 36
Euvolemia, 2141, 2144
Euvolemic hyponatremia, 504-505, 507f
Everolimus, 1383f, 1384, 2247, 2258, 2426
Excitation, 856
Expanded polytetrafluoroethylene, 2064-2066
Experimental atherosclerosis, 1578f
Explant cultures, 8f, 9
Extended-spectrum β-lactamase, 1239
External magnetic field, 856
Extracapillary proliferation, 921t
Extracellular fluid (ECF)
  bicarbonate in, 514, 519, 830f
  calcium concentration in, 601
  in children, 2365-2366, 2368, 2414
  chlorine in, 144
  description of, 390-391
  homeostasis of, 1748
  mannitol distribution in, 1704
  osmotic pressure of, 461
  potassium in, 174-175
  sodium in, 144
  solute composition of, 461
  total body water in, 460
Extracellular fluid volume (ECFV)
  assessment of, 835
  depletion of, 492-493, 1727
  description of, 391-393
  effective arterial blood volume and, 393, 813
  expansion of, 621
  in heart failure, 431f
  hematocrit for estimating of, 814t
  nephron loss-specific adaptations in, 1747-1748
Extracellular matrix 1, 31-32
Extracellular matrix (ECM)
  biomaterials as substitute for, 2609-2610
  connective tissue growth factor in production of, 1300
  diabetic nephropathy accumulation of, 1286
  myofibroblast production of, 1763
Extracorporeal shock wave lithotripsy, for urinary calculi, 1279-1280
Extracorporeal ultrafiltration, 451, 2139
Extraglomerular mesangium, 53-54
Extraskeletal calcifications, 1850
Extrauterine pregnancy, preeclampsia and, 1618
Eya1, 21
EYA1, 22, 2298-2299, 2318

Ezetimibe, 1869, 1869f, 2593
Ezrin, 155

F

Fabry's disease, 1143-1145, 1144f, 1952, 2479
F-actin, 972
Factitious hyperkalemia, 585
Factitious hyponatremia, 490
Factor VIII, 1803
Familial clustering, 1348
Familial diffuse mesangial sclerosis, 1429-1430
Familial hyperaldosteronism, 575, 1464
Familial hypercholesterolemia, 2159
Familial hypertension with hyperkalemia, 179-180, 183, 589-590, 2381-2382
Familial hypocalcemia with hypercalciuria, 614-616
Familial hypocalciuric hypercalcemia, 608, 622, 2391, 2395
Familial hypokalemic alkalosis, 578-580
Familial hypomagnesemia
  description of, 193-194
  with hypercalciuria and nephrocalcinosis, 1466, 2345, 2387-2388
  with secondary hypocalcemia, 2388, 2388f
  with secondary hypocalciuria, 1466
Familial iminoglycinuria, 1450
Familial Mediterranean fever (FMF)
  AA amyloidosis associated with, 2485-2486
  clinical spectrum of, 2479, 2484-2485
  colchicine for, 2485-2486
  description of, 1132, 2479
  end-stage kidney disease and, 2486
  genetics of, 2479, 2481t-2482t
  genotype-phenotype correlations, 2481t-2482t
  interferon-α for, 2486
  MEFV mutation in, 2479, 2484-2485
  pyrin's role in, 2479-2483, 2483f-2484f, 2486
  renal diseases associated with, 2484-2485
  treatment of, 2485-2486
Familial neurohypophyseal diabetes insipidus, 1469
Familial renal glucosuria, 1454
Familial renal hamartomas associated with hyperparathyroidism-jaw tumor syndrome, 1503
Familial renal hypouricemia, 1453
Familial tumoral calcinosis, 627, 1453
Fanconi syndrome, 530-531
  acquired versus inherited, 1435, 1435t
  causes of, 1439
  characteristics of, 580-581, 1435
  clinical presentation of, 1436-1437
  description of, 209
  GLUT2 mutations in, 207
  hypophosphatemia caused by, 632
Fanconi-Bickel syndrome, 209
Far East
  acute kidney injury in
    dengue fever as cause of, 2520-2521, 2522t
    djenkol beans as cause of, 2525
    hantavirus as cause of, 2515-2516, 2517f
    infections as cause of, 2511-2523, 2511f, 2512t
    insect stings as cause of, 2525
    leptospirosis as cause of, 2511-2513, 2511f, 2512t

Far East *(Continued)*
    malaria as cause of, 2517-2520, 2519f/2520f
    melamine as cause of, 2526
    mushrooms as cause of, 2525-2526
    opisthorchiasis as cause of, 2522-2523
    raw carp bile as cause of, 2525
    scrub typhus as cause of, 2513-2515
    severe acute respiratory syndrome as cause of, 2521-2522, 2523f
    severe fever with thrombocytopenia syndrome virus as cause of, 2516-2517, 2518f
    snakebites as cause of, 2523-2525, 2524t
    star fruit as cause of, 2525
  ANCA-associated vasculitides in, 2532
  betel nut chewing in, 2534
  China. *See* China
  chronic kidney disease in
    description of, 2526
    diabetes mellitus as cause of, 2529
    diagnostic criteria for, 2526
    etiology of, 2527
    infectious causes of, 2527-2529
    leptospirosis as cause of, 2528f
    prevalence of, 2526, 2527t
  countries of, 2510
  demographics of, 2510
  diabetes mellitus in, 2529
  distal renal tubular acidosis in, 2533
  end-stage kidney disease in, 2534-2536
  glomerulonephritis in, 2527-2532, 2528t, 2530f
  granulomatous with polyangiitis in, 2532
  hepatitis B/hepatitis C virus-associated glomerulonephritis in, 2532-2533
  herbal medicines in, 2533-2534
  Hong Kong, 2535
  human immunodeficiency virus infection in, 2533
  immunoglobulin A nephropathy in, 2530-2531, 2530f/2531f
  Indonesia, 2536
  Japan. *See* Japan
  Korea, 2535
  lupus nephritis in, 2531-2532
  Malaysia, 2535-2536
  microscopic polyangiitis in, 2532
  Philippines, 2536
  renal replacement therapy in, 2534-2536
  scientific publications in, 2536
  Singapore, 2536
  systemic lupus erythematosus in, 2531-2532
  Taiwan, 2534
  Thailand, 2535
  Vietnam, 2536
Farnesoid X receptor, 728, 733-734
Fat catabolism, 128f
Fat malabsorption syndromes, 617
Fat-soluble vitamins, 1984
Fatty acid-binding protein 1, 942
Fatty acids, 1967
Febuxostat, 1363t, 1364-1365, 2282
Fecal elimination enhancement techniques, for poison removal, 2168-2169
Fecal nitrogen, 1962
Fechtner's syndrome, 1140t
Felodipine, 1665
Female sex hormones, 1921
Fenoldopam mesylate, 1001, 1695t, 1699, 1713
Ferric carboxymaltose, 1896, 1897t
Ferric citrate, 1896, 2023
Ferric gluconate, 1896, 1897t, 1898-1899
Ferritin, 50f, 1893-1894

Fertility, 1635
Ferumoxytol, 1896-1898, 1897t
"Fetal programming" hypothesis, 2575-2576
Fetuin-A, 1836-1838
Fetus
  congenital anomalies of the kidney and urinary tract in, 2302
  exposures in
    to drugs, 719
    to glucocorticoids, 717
    to hyperglycemia, 717-718
  hydronephrosis in, 2314-2315
  loss of, in systemic lupus erythematosus, 1100
  sodium transport maturation in, 2302
  urinary tract obstruction in, 1258-1259, 1279
FGF9, 29
FGF20, 29
FHHt, 589-590
Fibrillary glomerulonephritis
  characteristics of, 1069-1070, 1132
  clinical features of, 1072
  cyclosporine for, 1134
  electron microscopy findings, 1070-1071, 1070f, 1133f
  end-stage kidney disease progression of, 1072, 1134
  epidemiology of, 1072
  fibrils in, 1132
  hematuria in, 1072
  immunofluorescence microscopy findings, 1071, 1071f, 1134f
  immunotactoid glomerulopathy versus, 1069-1070
  light microscopy findings, 1071
  monoclonal gammopathy and, 1071
  nephrotic syndrome caused by, 1069-1072
  pathogenesis of, 1071
  pathology of, 1070-1071, 1070f, 1133f
  pulmonary hemorrhage associated with, 1072
  recurrence of, after renal transplantation, 1072
  renal biopsy for, 1132-1134
  treatment of, 1072, 1134
Fibrinogen, 1863, 1905-1906, 2163
Fibroblast growth factor-7, 202
Fibroblast growth factor-23
  assays for, 1841f
  calcium levels affected by, 2019-2020
  cardiovascular disease and, 2101
  in children, 2390-2391, 2400
  in chronic kidney disease, 950, 1749-1750, 1775, 1831, 1864, 1977-1979, 2019
  in chronic kidney disease–mineral bone disorder, 1830-1831, 1841, 1841f, 1848
  definition of, 1830
  description of, 191, 197-198, 198f, 201, 627, 631
  1,25-dihydroxyvitamin D, 2031-2032
  phosphate concentration affected by, 1749-1750, 1775, 1776f, 1872, 1978, 2281, 2390-2391
  postrenal transplantation levels of, 1851
  receptors for, 1749-1750
  vitamin D activation affected by, 1774, 1864-1865
Fibroblastic growth factor signaling pathways, 24-25
Fibroblast-specific protein 1, 1067, 1217
Fibrocytes, bone marrow-derived, 1793
Fibrofolliculoma, 1374
Fibromuscular disease, 1580-1582, 1599-1600

Fibromuscular dysplasia, 907, 907f, 1580-1581
Fibronectin glomerulopathy, 1134
Fibrosarcoma, 1386
Fibrosis
  definition of, 921t
  renal. *See* Renal fibrosis
  renin-angiotensin-aldosterone system in, 334
  tubulointerstitial, 729f, 1754-1755, 1763, 1793
Fibrous intimal thickening, 728f
Fick's law, 2112
Filariasis, 1150-1151
Filtration barrier, 5
Filtration fraction, 138-139, 415-416, 738f
Filtration slit, 49-51, 1782-1783, 1783f
Filtration slit membrane, 51. *See also* Slit diaphragm
Fish oil, 376, 1069, 1803
Fistula
  arteriovenous. *See* Arteriovenous fistulas
  dialysis-associated steal syndrome secondary to, 1948
Fixatives, for light microscopy, 919
FK506-binding proteins, 2247
FKHRL1, 730-731
Flexner, Abraham, 2621
Flow cytometric cross-match, 2260
Flt1, 39
Fluconazole, 1254, 1254t
5-Flucytosine, 1254, 1254t
Fludrocortisone, 539
Fludrocortisone suppression test, 1546
Fluid deprivation test, 485
Fluid overload, 1726, 2138, 2144
Fluid restriction, for hyponatremia, 504, 504t
Fluid therapy, 1361, 2138
Fluorine 18 2-fluoro-2-deoxy-D-glucose, 865, 900, 1377
Fluoroquinolones, 1235t-1236t
Focal adhesion kinase, 120
Focal necrotizing glomerulonephritis, 2151
Focal segmental glomerulonephritis (FSGN), 657
Focal segmental glomerulosclerosis (FSGS), 1429
  ACTN4 mutations in, 1028
  in Africa, 2463
  in African Americans, 1028, 1769-1770
  APOL1 gene and, 1429
  APOL1 in, 1028-1029
  in Australia, 2544
  cause of, 1430
  cellular variant of, 1026
  in children, 1030, 1032
  classification of, 1025t
  clinical features of, 1024-1025, 1030-1031
  collapsing, 1026, 1029-1031, 1159, 2328
  electron microscopy findings, 1026-1027
  end-stage kidney disease progression from, 2155, 2404
  epidemiology of, 1025
  gene mutations associated with, 1027t
  glomerular enlargement associated with, 1030
  glomerular scarring in, 1025-1026
  glomerular tip lesion variant of, 1026, 1030-1031
  glomerulomegaly associated with, 1146, 1146f
  HIV-associated, 1028, 1030
  immunofluorescence microscopy findings, 1026, 1026f
  infections that cause, 1030

Focal segmental glomerulosclerosis (FSGS) (Continued)
  laboratory findings in, 1031, 1050t
  light microscopy findings, 1024f, 1025-1026
  malignant conditions associated with, 1030
  mechanism of action, 116
  medications associated with, 1030
  natural history of, 1030-1031
  nephron loss as cause of, 1029
  nephrotic syndrome caused by, 1024-1035
  NPHS2 mutations in, 1027-1028
  pamidronate and, 1030
  parietal epithelial cell activation in, 1789-1790
  pathogenesis of, 1027-1030, 1027t
  pathology of, 1024f, 1025-1027, 1026f, 1027t
  perihilar, 1026, 1030
  permeability factor associated with, 1029-1030
  podocytes in, 115t, 116, 118-119, 1027, 1029
  prednisone for, 1167
  primary, 1025, 1025t
  prognostic indicators for, 1031
  proteinuria in, 1024-1025, 1030-1031, 1164, 1750-1752
  recurrent
    in children, 2156, 2422, 2431
    description of, 1034, 2270
    immunosuppressive drugs for, 2155-2156
    plasmapheresis for, 2155-2157
    risk factors for, 2155, 2270
  renal fibrosis secondary to, 1034
  after renal transplantation, 1034
  secondary, 1025, 1025t
  in sickle cell disease, 1199
  in steroid-resistant nephrotic syndrome, 2328
  treatment of
    angiotensin II receptor blockers, 1031
    angiotensin inhibitors, 1031-1032
    angiotensin-converting enzyme inhibitors, 1031
    CTLA-4-Ig, 1034
    cyclophosphamide, 1032
    cyclosporine, 1033
    glucocorticoids, 1032
    mycophenolate mofetil, 1033
    prednisone, 1032
    sirolimus, 1033-1034
  tubulointerstitial injury in, 1026, 1763
  variants of, 1026, 1029-1031
Folate, 1883-1884
Folic acid, 1887, 1983
Follicle-stimulating hormone, 1920-1921
Folliculin gene, 1374
Fomepizole, 548, 2177-2178
Food allergy, 1021
Foot processes, of podocytes. *See* Podocyte(s), foot processes of
Forced diuresis, 2167
Forearm loop graft, 2065-2066, 2066f
Formic acid, 2174
Forward genetics, 9
Foscarnet, 618
Fosinopril sodium, 1644
4F2hc/LAT2, 225-226, 231
4F2hc/y⁺LAT1, 228
Foxc1, 27

Foxd1, 31
FOXO3, 733
FP receptors, 369-370
Fractional excretion
  of calcium, 1749-1750
  of chloride, 814-815
  of creatinine, 1199
  of magnesium, 619-621
  of organic anions, 216
  of potassium, 2375-2376
  of sodium, 814-815, 987, 1659, 1708-1710, 1747
Fracture
  bone mineral density reductions associated with, 1852
  in chronic kidney disease–mineral bone disorder, 1849
  hip, 1849
  after renal transplantation, 1851
  risks of, 1846
Frailty, 2590
Fras1, 22-23
Fraser's syndrome, 22-23, 26f, 1431, 2297t, 2325
Free calcium, 602
Free fatty acids, 1761
Free ionized calcium, 1325-1327
Free light chains, 1391-1393
Fresh-frozen plasma (FFP), 1185, 2155, 2162
Frizzled receptor, 28-29
Fructose intolerance, 531
Fuhrman grading system, 1378
Fumarate hydratase gene, 1373-1374
Fumarylacetoacetate hydrolase, 1443
Fungal peritonitis, 2129
Fungal urinary tract infection, 1254
Fungemia, 1805
Furin, 340
Furosemide
  albumin and, 1708
  arginine vasopressin levels affected by, 1717
  atrial natriuretic peptide affected by, 1717
  bioavailability of, 1720
  in cirrhosis patients, 1723
  description of, 871, 1706
  hyponatremia treated with, 506
  left ventricular hypertrophy treated with, 1721-1722
  metabolism of, 1709f
  natriuretic response to, 1715-1717, 1723-1724
  pharmacokinetics of, 1709f
  plasma protein binding of, 1724-1725
  potassium loss caused by, 1716
  proximal secretion of, 1708
  renin-angiotensin-aldosterone system activation by, 1714
  sodium excretion and, 1710f
  thick ascending limb receptor for, 1725
FXYD2, 2388-2389

G

G protein-coupled receptor kinases, 283
G protein-coupled receptors
  4, 256
  illustration of, 367f
  vasopressin 2 receptor as. *See* Vasopressin 2 receptor
G protein-mediated signaling, 329
GadC, 230t

Gadolinium-chelate contrast media, for magnetic resonance imaging. *See* Magnetic resonance imaging, gadolinium-chelate contrast media
Galactose-deficient IgA1, 1064
Galactosemia, 1444
α-Galactosidase A, 1145, 2479
Gallium nitrate, 612
Galloway-Mowat syndrome, 1431
GALNT3, 627
Gamble phenomenon, 277-278
Ganglionic blocking agent, 1698
Gap junctions, 53-54, 56
Gap programs, 2583
Gastric aspiration, 553
Gastrointestinal fistula, 620
Gastrointestinal therapeutic system, 1665
Gastroparesis, 2125
Gender differences
  antihypertensive drug therapy, 1685, 1686t
  autosomal dominant polycystic kidney disease progression and, 658
  chronic kidney disease, 655-660, 673-674, 1768-1769
  developmental programming and, 720
  diabetic nephropathy progression and, 658-659
  end-stage kidney disease, 656-657, 659, 2060f
  focal segmental glomerulonephritis and, 657
  glomerular disease and, 657
  glomerular filtration rate and, 655, 736
  glomerulonephritis and, 657
  hormone replacement therapy and, 659-660
  hypertension and, 1525
  immunoglobulin A nephropathy and, 657
  lupus nephritis and, 658
  membranous nephropathy and, 657
  oral contraceptives and, 659-660
  primary glomerular disease progression and, 657
Gene panel, 1413
Generalized lipodystrophy, 1146-1147
Genetic hypercalciuric stone-forming rat, 1333
Genetic mapping, 1410, 1412
Genetic testing, for autosomal dominant polycystic kidney disease, 1486f
Genetics
  of Alport's syndrome, 1140-1141, 1421-1422, 1782
  of autosomal dominant polycystic kidney disease, 1479-1480, 1486f
  of hypertension, 1529-1530
  of kidney stones, 1348-1350
  of nephrocalcinosis, 1349f
  of urolithiasis, 1349f
  of Wilms' tumor, 1387
Genitourinary tract. *See* Urinary tract
Genitourinary tuberculosis, 1252-1254, 1260
Genodermatoses, 1951-1953, 1952f, 1952t
Genomewide association study, 1348-1349
Genomics, 2249
Genotyping, 2039-2040
Gentamicin
  acute pyelonephritis treated with, 1241, 1241t
  nephrogenesis affected by, 719
  nephrotoxicity of, 966, 967f
Geophagia, 586
Gerota's fascia, 852-853

Gestational diabetes insipidus, 471, 480, 489
Gestational hypertension, 1627-1631
Ghrelin, 420, 2125
Giant cell arteritis, 1120
Gibbs-Donnan effect, 391-392
Gitelman's syndrome, 67-68, 1417-1418, 1457-1459, 1459f, 2379
  characteristics of, 580, 2333
  in children, 2335, 2378-2379
  chondrocalcinosis in, 2379
  clinical presentation of, 1459
  hypocalciuria in, 580
  management of, 2379
  metabolic alkalosis caused by, 551-552, 554-555
  in Middle East, 2479
  pathogenesis of, 1459
  plasma renin levels in, 580
  potassium-sparing diuretics for, 1727
  prevalence of, 2333
  prognosis for, 2335
  renal magnesium wasting in, 622
  treatment of, 1459
GLEPP1 disease, 1431
Glial-derived neurotrophic factor (GDNF), 22-23, 701-702, 719
Globotriaosylceramide, 1143-1144
Globulin, calcium binding to, 602
Glomerular basement membrane (GBM)
  anatomy of, 48-49
  anionic sites in, 48-49
  anti-GBM disease. *See* Anti-glomerular basement membrane disease
  composition of, 48
  electron microscopy analysis of, 922
  embryology of, 4-5, 118
  glomerular filtration barrier and, 48-49, 50f
  histology of, 48f
  hydraulic connectivity of, 98
  inherited disorders affecting, 1421-1426
  layers of, 48, 48f
  maturation of, 39-40
  morphologic nature of, 1424f
  organization of, 1782
  permeability of, 48-49
  podocytes effect on, 118
  proteinuria and, 2323
  in rat models, 48, 48f
  surface area of, 2301-2302
  thickness of, 922, 1285, 1293f
Glomerular capillaries
  description of, 46, 84
  function of, 1780
  histology of, 93f
  hydraulic pressures in, 94-96, 95f
  loss of, 1790
  mesangial cells and, 1753
  pressures of, 94, 95f
  scanning electron microscopy of, 1751f
  ultrafiltration coefficient of, 98
  wall of, 46, 1781
Glomerular capillary membrane
  endothelial cell layer of, 1781-1782
  epithelial filtration slits, 1782-1783, 1783f
  filtering surface of, 1781
  organization of, 1781
  ultrastructure of, 1781-1783
Glomerular diseases, 1404
  acute, 1002
  bacterial infections associated with, 1149-1150
  categorization of, 1012-1013
  cause of, 1421
  crescent formation in, 1077t

Glomerular diseases *(Continued)*
  drugs associated with, 1157-1158
  in elderly, 746-747
  filariasis and, 1150-1151
  gender differences in, 657
  global, 920
  heroin nephropathy and, 1157-1158
  interstitial damage in, 1211f
  leishmaniasis and, 1150-1151
  miscellaneous diseases associated with, 1159
  neoplasia associated with, 1157
  nephritic features of, 1013t
  nephrotic features of, 1013t
  parasitic diseases associated with, 1150-1151
  pathogenesis of, 1012
  podocytes involved in, 113, 115t
  primary
    algorithm for, 1070f
    C3 glomerulopathies. *See* C3 glomerulopathies
    categorization of, 1070f
    crescent formation in, 1077t
    definition of, 1012-1013
    in elderly, 746
    in Far East, 2529-2531, 2530f
    focal segmental glomerulosclerosis. *See* Focal segmental glomerulosclerosis
    hematuria in, 1014-1016, 1015t
    immune complex-mediated crescentic glomerulonephritis. *See* Immune complex-mediated crescentic glomerulonephritis
    membranoproliferative glomerulonephritis. *See* Membranoproliferative glomerulonephritis
    membranous nephropathy. *See* Membranous nephropathy
    minimal change disease. *See* Minimal change disease
    nephrotic syndrome caused by. *See* Nephrotic syndrome, glomerular diseases that cause
    proteinuria in, 1013-1014
    serologic findings in, 1050t
  schistosomiasis and, 1150
  secondary
    antiphospholipid syndrome, 1106-1108, 1107f
    definition of, 1012-1013
    in elderly, 746
    Fabry's disease, 1143-1145, 1144f
    fibrillary glomerulonephritis. *See* Fibrillary glomerulonephritis
    granulomatous with polyangiitis. *See* Granulomatous with polyangiitis
    heavy-chain deposition disease, 1134-1136, 1135f
    Henoch-Schönlein purpura, 1121-1124
    immunotactoid glomerulopathy. *See* Immunotactoid glomerulopathy
    lecithin-cholesterol acyltransferase deficiency, 1147-1148, 1147f
    light-chain deposition disease, 1134-1136, 1135f
    lipodystrophy, 1146-1147
    lipoprotein glomerulopathy, 1148
    lupus nephritis. *See* Lupus nephritis
    mixed connective tissue disease, 1108-1109
    mixed cryoglobulinemia, 1137-1138
    monoclonal immunoglobulin deposition disease, 1134-1136, 1135f

Glomerular diseases *(Continued)*
    nail-patella syndrome, 1142-1143, 1143f
    polyarteritis nodosa, 1118-1120
    sarcoidosis, 1127-1128
    sickle cell nephropathy, 1145-1146, 1145f
    Sjögren's disease, 1127
    systemic lupus erythematosus. *See* Systemic lupus erythematosus
    Takayasu arteritis, 1120-1121
    temporal arteritis, 1120
    Waldenström's macroglobulinemia, 1136, 1136f-1137f
  segmental, 920
  terminology used to describe, 920, 921t
  treatment of
    adrenocorticotropic hormone, 1171-1172
    algorithms for, 1172-1173
    alkylating agents, 1168-1170
    azathioprine, 1170
    calcineurin inhibitors, 1167-1168
    considerations for, 1172-1173
    corticosteroids, 1166-1167
    cyclophosphamide, 1168-1170
    cyclosporine, 1167-1168
    eculizumab, 1171
    mycophenolate mofetil, 1170
    ocrelizumab, 1171
    rituximab, 1171
    tacrolimus, 1167-1168
  trypanosomiasis and, 1150-1151
  tubulointerstitial injury caused by, 1210
  ultrafiltration capacity affected by, 1797
  visceral infections associated with, 1149
Glomerular endothelial cells, 46-48, 46f
  apoptosis of, 1789
  description of, 1781-1782
  glycocalyx of, 47
  injury to, 1789
  intermediate filaments in, 47
  maturation of, 39-40
  vascular endothelial growth factor receptor expression by, 47-48
Glomerular endotheliosis, preeclampsia and, 1619, 1621f
Glomerular filtration
  determinants of, 94-98
    alterations in, 97-98
    colloid osmotic pressure, 98
    glomerular plasma flow rate, 97
    transcapillary hydraulic pressure difference, 97-98
  obstructive nephropathy effects on, 1269-1271
  regulation of, 98-110
  urinary tract obstruction effects on, 1269-1271
Glomerular filtration barriers, 1436f
  anatomy of, 791
  functional properties of, 1780
  glomerular basement membrane and, 48-49, 50f
  illustration of, 50f
  schematic of three layers of, 1427f
  vascular endothelial growth factor-A for, 32-34, 33f
Glomerular filtration coefficient, 96-97
Glomerular filtration rate (GFR), 1575f, 1576f, 1598f
  in acute kidney injury, 788, 932, 1390, 2043, 2145
  age-related changes in, 736-739, 737f
  angiotensin II effects on, 408
  angiotensin-converting enzyme inhibitors effect on, 1299, 1645

Glomerular filtration rate (GFR) (Continued)
  autoregulation of, 105
  autosomal dominant polycystic kidney disease and, 1490f
  biomarkers for, 781-787
    blood urea nitrogen, 933-934
    creatinine, 782-783, 933
    creatinine clearance, 783
    cystatin C, 783-784, 934-935, 2310
    EDTA, 786-787
    endogenous, 782-786
    exogenous, 786-787, 932
    inulin, 786
    radiolabeled markers, 786-787
    serum, 932-936
    β-trace protein, 935-936
    unlabeled radiocontrast agents, 787
    urea, 782, 933-934
  birth weight effects on, 709-710
  calculation of, 781
  in children, 787, 787t, 2309-2310
  in chronic kidney disease, 681, 773, 932, 1749, 2029-2031
  creatinine as marker of, 678, 2309-2310
  decline in
    hypothyroidism associated with, 496
    polycystic kidney disease as cause of, 681
    renal risk scores to predict, 690-691
  definition of, 781, 1797
  description of, 780-781
  drug dosing considerations, 788
  in effective arterial blood volume regulation, 398-421
  endogenous markers of, 737
  estimated
    in acute kidney injury, 788, 947-948, 963
    in adolescents, 787, 787t
    in Africa, 2459
    age-related changes in, 2586-2587
    biomarkers for. See Glomerular filtration rate, biomarkers for
    cardiovascular disease and, 1855, 1866, 2008
    in children, 787, 787t, 2043
    in chronic kidney disease, 1989-1990
    Chronic Kidney Disease Epidemiology Collaboration equation for, 784t, 785-786
    Cockcroft-Gault equation for, 784t, 786, 2587f
    contrast media risks and, 854-856
    creatinine as biomarker for, 932-933, 2309-2310
    cystatin C as biomarker of, 783-784, 934-935, 2310
    description of, 677-678
    in drug dosing, 788
    equations for, 784-786, 784t, 2042t, 2310, 2502
    hemoglobin affected by, 2405-2406
    MDRD equation for, 645, 677-678, 782, 784t, 785-786, 788, 2526
    measurement of, 2587
    in pediatrics, 2043
    in pregnancy, 788
    reduced, adverse outcomes associated with, 2588-2590
  expression of, 781
  filtration-reabsorption system, 204
  gender differences in, 655, 736
  homocysteine levels and, 1864
  hyperphosphatemia caused by reductions in, 627

Glomerular filtration rate (GFR) (Continued)
  leukotriene A_4 effects on, 380
  liver transplantation effects on, 458
  in low birth weight, 710
  measurement of, 677-678, 781, 2041-2042, 2042t
  neural regulation of, 110
  normal, 781
  oxygen consumption rate and, 134-135
  parathyroid hormone levels affected by, 1865
  physiology of, 781
  polycystic kidney disease effects on, 681
  during pregnancy, 1611-1612, 1612f
  prematurity effects on, 709-710
  reduction of, 1582-1583
  regulation of
    factors involved in, 1296
    glomerular transcapillary hydraulic pressure difference in, 1296
    glomerular ultrafiltration coefficient in, 1296
    oncotic pressure in, 1296
    renal plasma flow in, 1296
    in urinary tract obstruction setting, 1270-1271
  renal blood flow and, 134, 138, 401-402
  renal function assessments using, 2041-2042
  renal plasma flow effects on, 1296
  renin-angiotensin system's role in control of, 99
  single-nephron, 1269, 1271, 1737-1738, 1743, 1746-1747, 1785
  size of, 1819-1820
  sodium chloride reabsorption affected by, 150
  technetium 99m-labeled diethylenetriaminepentaacetic assessments of, 865
  total, for single nephron, 94, 96
  tubuloglomerular feedback control of, 108-109, 209-210
  in type 1 diabetes mellitus, 1296
  in uremia, 1819-1820
Glomerular hematuria, 756-757, 757t, 798, 1015
Glomerular hyperfiltration, 1737-1738
Glomerular hypertension, 1737-1738
Glomerular injury
  biomarkers of
    blood urea nitrogen, 933-934
    cystatin C, 934-935
    description of, 932-936
    podocalyxin, 936
    podocyte count, 936
    β-trace protein, 935-936
  cyclooxygenase metabolites in, 375-377
  progressive, 1787f
Glomerular permselectivity, 1783-1784
Glomerular plasma flow rate, 97
Glomerular proteinuria, 791
Glomerular sclerosis, 1578
Glomerular ultrafiltrate, 1784
Glomerular volume, 696, 709, 709f
Glomerulogenesis, 699
Glomerulomegaly, 705, 1146, 1146f
Glomerulonephritis, 1403-1404
  acute poststreptococcal. See Acute poststreptococcal glomerulonephritis
  anti-glomerular basement membrane, 746
  C3, 1046, 1046f-1047f
  calcineurin inhibitors for, 1167-1168
  cardiovascular mortality in, 1165

Glomerulonephritis (Continued)
  chronic kidney disease caused by, 775
  cirrhosis as cause of, 1156
  clinical trials in, 1163
  corticosteroids for, 1166-1167
  crescentic. See Crescentic glomerulonephritis
  cryoglobulinemic, 1137-1138, 1137f-1138f
  diagnostic classification of, 1074f
  diseases that cause, 1059t
  in elderly, 746
  end-stage kidney disease caused by, 1161
  fibrillary. See Fibrillary glomerulonephritis
  gender differences in, 657
  global impact of, 1161-1163, 1162t
  in granulomatous with polyangiitis, 1112
  IgA, 2275, 2544
  immunopathologic categories of, 1073t-1074t
  immunotactoid. See Immunotactoid glomerulopathy
  incidence of, 1161-1162
  in Indian subcontinent, 2506, 2506t
  infection-related, 2527, 2528t
  kidney biopsy for, 2544
  malignancy and, 1403t
  mesangiocapillary, 1047-1048
  in New Zealand, 2550
  outcome measures in, 1163
  pauci-immune necrotizing, 1084-1085
  poststreptococcal, 757
  proliferative glomerulonephritis with monoclonal IgG deposits, 1136
  rapidly progressive. See Rapidly progressive glomerulonephritis
  societal burden of, 1161
  in Takayasu arteritis, 1120-1121
Glomerulopathy
  anti-rheumatoid arthritis therapy-induced, 1158-1159
  collapsing, 1153
  fibronectin, 1134
  hepatic, 1156f
  HIV-associated, 1151
  lipoprotein, 1148
  nondiabetic, 1300
  obesity as cause of, 679-680, 1770-1771
  sickle, 1146, 1146f
  sickle cell, 1200
Glomerulosclerosis
  age-related decreases in, 728-729
  in Balkan endemic nephropathy, 1225
  characteristics of, 1786-1787
  focal segmental. See Focal segmental glomerulosclerosis
  glomerular hypertrophy and, 1759
  illustration of, 728f
  nodular, 1285-1286, 1287f
Glomerulotubular balance
  description of, 150, 1736-1737
  in effective arterial blood volume regulation, 400-407
  illustration of, 152f
  luminal composition in, 402
  maintenance of, 1747
  nephron loss adaptations, 1746
  peritubular capillary Starling forces in, 400-402
  peritubular factors in, 151-152
  in proximal tubule sodium chloride transport, 150-152, 151f
Glomerulotubular junction abnormalities, 1286f

Glomerulus
  aldosterone secretion by, 305
  anatomy of, 46f-47f, 107f
  calcium filtration by, 187
  capillary loops of, 46f, 92-93, 92f, 1019f
  capillary wall of, 1020f
  cells of, 4-5, 46-53, 46f, 52f. See also Podocyte(s)
  classification of, 84
  cross-section of, 107f
  development of, 4-5, 33f, 36-39, 37f
  function of, 46
  histology of, 47f
  hypertrophy of, after nephron loss, 1742-1743, 1759
  inherited systemic syndromes affecting, 1431-1432
  juxtamedullary, 45-46
  low-glycotoxin diet effects on, 732f
  magnesium filtration by, 194
  mesangium of, 98-99
  microcirculation of, 92-94, 92f
  mineralocorticoid receptor expression in, 315
  murine model of, 36f
  nephrectomy-related changes in, 1751f
  nephron loss responses by, 1737-1741
  nephron number and, 696
  permselective dysfunction, 1786
  proteinuria-induced damage to, 1786-1790, 1787f
  variations in, 45-46
  vascular pathways in, 93, 93f
  volume of, 45-46
GlpT, 213-214, 230t
GltPh, 230t
Glucagon, 1767
Glucagon-like peptide-1, 420
Glucocorticoid(s)
  adverse effects of, 1166
  angiotensin II inhibitors and, for IgA nephropathy, 1068
  bicarbonate reabsorption affected by, 238
  COX-2 expression regulated by, 357
  deficiency of, 495
  description of, 1400
  fetal exposure to, 717
  focal segmental glomerulosclerosis treated with, 1032
  glomerulonephritis treated with, 1166
  hypercalcemia treated with, 612
  idiopathic nephrotic syndrome treated with, 2329
  immunoglobulin A nephropathy treated with, 1067-1068
  membranoproliferative glomerulonephritis type I treated with, 1049-1050
  musculoskeletal effects of, 1166-1167
  podocytes affected by, 119
Glucocorticoid-remediable hyperaldosteronism, 555-556, 575, 1463-1464
Gluconeogenesis, 130-132
Glucose
  absorption of, 206f, 1730
  endothelin synthesis affected by, 337
  insulin and, 594
  lactate conversion to, 132
  metabolism of, angiotensin-converting enzyme inhibitors effect on, 1648
  in peritoneal dialysis solutions, 2117-2119
  plasma concentration of, 204-205
  reabsorption of, in proximal tubule, 129-130, 205
  renal handling of, 205

Glucose (Continued)
  sources of, 812
  transport of. See Glucose transport
  urinary excretion of, 205f
  in urine, 790
Glucose degradation products, 2117-2119, 2126-2127
Glucose transport, 204-215
  characteristics of, 206f
  inherited disorders of, 1453-1454
  maximal rate of, 205
  monogenic defects of, 207-210
  physiology of, 204-205
  proteins involved in
    cell model of, 205-207
    GLUT1, 207
    GLUT2, 207
    SGLT1, 205-206
    SGLT2, 206-207
  proximal tubule, 205-207
Glucose transporter diseases, 209
Glucose-galactose malabsorption, 206-207, 1454
Glucose-6-phosphate dehydrogenase deficiency, 2494, 2501
Glucosuria, 206-207, 1437, 1454, 1454t, 1612
GLUT1, 207, 208t
GLUT2, 207, 208t
GLUT4, 207, 208t
GLUT9, 221, 221t
Glutamate, 253, 623
Glutamate dehydrogenase, 248, 253
Glutamine, 129-130, 249-251, 517
τ-Glutamyl transpeptidase, 253
Glutathione, 549
Glutathione S-transferase, 938-939, 1898, 1909
Glyburide, 2593
Glycemic control
  cardiovascular disease risk prevention through, 1871
  in chronic kidney disease, 1871, 1995
  in diabetic nephropathy, 1301-1303
  in end-stage kidney disease, 1315
  during hemodialysis, 1317
Glycinuria, 223t
Glycogen, 1442f
Glycogen storage disease type 1, 1442
Glycogenosis (von Gierke's disease), 1442-1443
Glycolysis, 132
β_2-glycoprotein I-specific antiphospholipid antibody IgG, 1201
Glycosaminoglycan, 1331
Glycosuria, 205, 207-209, 790
Glycosylated hemoglobin, 1931
Glycyrrhetinic acid, 556, 596
Glycyrrhizinic acid, 577
Glyoxylate reductase/hydroxypyruvate reductase (GRHPR), 1337-1338, 2347-2348
Glypican-3, 2299
Gold salts, 1158
Goldblatt hypertension, 1568-1569
Goldmann voltage equation, 124-125
Golgi apparatus, 56
Gonadal dysfunction
  in chronic kidney disease, 1920-1923
  in men, 1921-1923
  in women, 1920-1921
Gonadal dysgenesis, 2-3
Gonadotropin-releasing hormone, 2318
Goodpasture's syndrome. See also Anti-glomerular basement membrane disease
  clinical features of, 1125

Goodpasture's syndrome (Continued)
  components of, 1124
  course of, 1126-1127
  description of, 759-760, 1076, 1080-1081
  laboratory findings in, 1125
  pathogenesis of, 1124-1125
  prognosis for, 1126-1127
  treatment of, 1126-1127
Gordon's syndrome, 179-180, 539-540, 589-590, 827, 2381-2382. See also Pseudohypoaldosteronism
Gout, 1442, 1731, 2282
Graft-versus-host disease (GVHD)
  chronic kidney disease related to, 1395
  description of, 2249-2250
  glomerulonephritis associated with, 1404
  nephrotic syndrome after, 1021
  transplantation-associated thrombotic microangiography and, 1395
Granular casts, 800, 800t, 801f
Granular cells, juxtaglomerular, 53, 54f, 55
Granulomatous disease, 610
Granulomatous interstitial nephritis, 1228
Granulomatous with polyangiitis (GPA)
  antineutrophil cytoplasmic antibodies in, 1111-1112
  in children, 2351
  clinical features of, 1111-1112
  course of, 1112-1114
  cyclophosphamide for, 1112-1114
  definition of, 1109
  end-stage kidney disease progression of, 1114
  eosinophilic, 1116-1118, 2351
  in Far East, 2532
  glomerulonephritis in, 1112
  immunosuppressive agents for, 1112
  incidence of, 1109
  laboratory features of, 1111-1112
  lower respiratory tract disease associated with, 1111
  methotrexate for, 1113
  mycophenolate mofetil for, 1113-1114
  organ involvement in, 1111
  papillary necrosis in, 1110
  pathogenesis of, 1110-1111
  pathology of, 1109-1110, 1109f-1110f
  plasmapheresis for, 1113
  recurrence of, after renal transplantation, 2275
  relapse of, 1113
  renal findings in, 1112
  rituximab for, 1113
  survival rates in, 1112
  tissue injury in, 1110-1111
  treatment of, 1088-1089, 1112-1114
Greater splanchnic nerve, 80-81
Grip1, 25
Growth arrest-specific gene 6, 1932
Growth differentiating factor 8. See Myostatin
Growth differentiation factor 15, 1887
Growth factors, 1212-1213, 1744, 1792
Growth hormone
  in chronic kidney disease, 1916-1919
  definition of, 1917-1918
  functions of, 1916-1917
  hypercalcemia caused by, 609
  phosphate excretion affected by, 200
  recombinant, for pediatric chronic kidney disease, 2359, 2359f
  uninephrectomy effects on, 1744
Guaifenesin, 1347
Guanabenz, 1671t-1672t, 1672
Guanfacine, 1671t-1672t, 1672

Guanidinoacetic acid, 1810-1811
Guanidinosuccinic acid, 1904
Guanylate cyclase A, 395
Guanylin peptides, 397-398
Guillain-Barré syndrome, 2158
Gynecomastia, 1713

H

Haber-Weiss-Fenton reaction, 1892-1893
Hairy cell leukemia, 1118-1120
Half-and-half nails, 1949-1950, 1949f
Half-maximum effect, 2040, 2040f
HANAC syndrome, 1425
Hand ischemia, vascular access-induced, 2214
Hantavirus, 2515-2516, 2517f
Hartnup's disorder, 222-224, 223t, 1449-1450
H^+-ATPase, 331
   acquired defects in, 534
   in bicarbonate reabsorption, 235-236, 242
   genetic defects in, 242
   in hydrogen secretion, 239
   in proximal tubule bicarbonate reabsorption, 235-236
   P-type, 239
   vacuolar, 242
Health care
   in Australia, 2539-2540
   equitable, 2582-2583
   gap programs, 2583
   in Latin America, 2451-2452
   in Middle East, 2471f
   in New Zealand, 2549
   socioeconomic gradients in, 2583-2584
   targeted programs, 2582
   wastes in, 2623-2624
Health disparities
   biologic origins of, 2578
   in chronic kidney disease treatment, 2580
   definition of, 2574
   in end-stage kidney disease, 2577-2578
   health system access and surveillance, 2578-2579
   health system structure, 2579-2580
   in nephrology, 2578-2580
   postnatal environment, 2576
   prenatal environment, 2575-2576
   race and, 2577-2578
   social determinants of, 2575f
   social origins of, 2575-2578, 2584
   strategies to reduce, 2582-2584
Health justice, 2575
Health status disparity, 2574
Heart failure (HF)
   acute decompensated, 997-998, 1719-1722, 2139, 2140f
   adrenomedullin in, 437
   aldosterone and, 322, 431
   antinatriuretic systems in, 429-433
   apelin in, 438
   atrial natriuretic peptide in, 433
   baroreceptor reflex impairment in, 427
   brain natriuretic peptide in, 343, 433-434
   cardiac output decrease in, 393
   cardiopulmonary reflex impairment in, 427
   catestatin in, 438
   chronic, 1722
   COX-2 inhibitors and, 437
   C-type natriuretic peptide in, 342, 434-435

Heart failure (HF) (Continued)
   diuretics for, 1719-1722, 1720f
   dyspnea caused by, 434
   extracellular fluid, 299-300, 431f
   glomerular hemodynamic alterations in, 429
   high blood pressure and, 1522-1524
   hypertension and, 1660-1661
   hyponatremia in, 432, 493-494
   natriuretic peptide receptors in, 435
   natriuretic peptides in, 433-435, 453
   nesiritide for, 453, 1720-1721
   neuropeptides in, 438
   nitric oxide in, 435-436
   norepinephrine levels in, 432
   NT-proBNP as biomarker of, 343
   peroxisome proliferator-activated receptors in, 438-444
   prerenal acute kidney injury in, 97-998
   progression of, 1722
   prostaglandins in, 436-437
   renal blood flow decreases in, 429-430
   renin-angiotensin-aldosterone system in, 429-431, 451-452
   sodium balance in, 435
   sodium reabsorption in, 429, 431
   sodium retention in, 427-429, 428f, 431
   sympathetic nervous system in, 432, 435
   treatment of
      β-blockers, 452
      endothelin antagonists, 452-453
      natriuretic peptide blockers, 453
      nesiritide, 453
      neutral endopeptidase inhibitors, 453-454
      nitric oxide donor, 452
      omapatrilat, 453-454
      reactive oxygen species, 452
      renin-angiotensin-aldosterone system inhibition, 451-454
      vaptans, 454
      vasopeptidase inhibitors, 453-454
      vasopressin receptor antagonists, 454-455
   urotensin in, 437-438
   vasoconstrictor systems in, 429-433
   vasopressin in, 432-433
Heat shock protein 70, 977
Heat shock protein 90, 301-302, 977-978
Heavy-chain deposition disease, 1134-1136, 1135f
Hedgehog signaling, 2299
HELLP syndrome, 480, 990-992, 1182, 1613-1627, 1617t
Hemangioma, 1369
Hemangiopericytoma, 1369
Hematomas
   magnetic resonance imaging of, 876-878, 878f-879f
   perirenal, 2253
   renal transplantation with, 911f
   subcapsular, 878f-879f, 910, 911f
Hematopoietic stem cell transplantation (HSCT), 1392
   acute kidney injury after, 993
   cast nephropathy and, 1392
   chronic kidney disease and, 1394
   complications of, 1393
   purpose of, 1393-1394
   renal syndromes associated with, 1393t, 1394
   total-body irradiation and, 1400-1401
   types of, 993

Hematuria
   in acute poststreptococcal glomerulonephritis, 1057
   algorithm for, 758f
   causes of, 800t
   in children, 1014-1015
   definition of, 754-755, 798, 1014
   diagnostic approach, 755-757, 756f, 758f
   in elderly, 1014-1015
   familial
      Alport's syndrome. See Alport's syndrome
      differential diagnosis of, 1142
      renal replacement therapy for, 1141
      thin basement membrane nephropathy, 1141-1142
   in fibrillary glomerulonephritis, 1072
   glomerular, 756-757, 757t, 798, 1015
   glomerular disease in, 1014-1016, 1015t
   gross, 754-756
   history-taking, 755-756
   in immunoglobulin A nephropathy, 1065
   kidney biopsy evaluations, 1016
   macroscopic, 1065
   malignancy risks in, 759f
   microscopic, 754-755, 799, 1022, 1065, 1198-1199
   proteinuria and, 758-759
   pyuria and, 756
   in sickle cell disease, 1198-1200
   transient, 798, 1015
   urinary tract infection as cause of, 755
Hematuria-associated deafness, 1421-1422
Heme oxygenase, 977-978
Heme oxygenase 1, 2194
Hemodialysis (HD)
   acute coronary syndromes in patients receiving, 2102
   acute kidney injury treated with, 1006-1007, 1315
   adequacy of
      blood urea nitrogen measurements, 2084
      clearance monitoring as indicator of, 2079
      historical perspectives on, 2082-2083
      measurements of, 2083-2087, 2109
      urea reduction ratio, 2085-2087, 2087f
   advances in, 2109
   in Africa, 2463-2464
   air embolism prevention in, 2075
   anticoagulation during, 2091-2092, 2092t
   antiphospholipid antibodies in patients receiving, 1107
   in Australia, 2540f, 2542-2543
   barbiturate poisoning treated with, 2183
   blood clotting during, 2091-2092
   blood flow in, 2080, 2091
   blood leaks during, 2108
   blood loss caused by, 1885
   blood pressure management in, 1316, 2103
   blood urea nitrogen measurements, 2084
   cardiovascular disease in patients receiving, 2101-2102
   cardiovascular problems during, 1316-1317
   catheters for
      description of, 2067-2068
      nontunneled temporary, 2214-2216
      temporary, 2214-2216
      tunneled
         bacteremia of, 2220
         complications of, 2217, 2217f-2218f

Hemodialysis (HD) (Continued)
    description of, 2216
    dysfunction of, 2219-2220
    exchange of, 2219-2220
    femoral, 2218
    insertion of, 2216-2217, 2217f-2218f
    less common locations for, 2218-2219, 2219f
    prevalence of use, 2629-2630
    transhepatic, 2219
    translumbar, 2218-2219, 2219f
  cerebral hypoperfusion associated with, 1930
  in China, 2535
  cognitive impairment in, 1937f
  comorbid conditions associated with, 2063
  complications of
    arrhythmias, 598, 2107
    atrial fibrillation, 2107
    cardiac arrest, 2107
    central vein stenosis, 2212-2214, 2212f-2214f
    disequilibrium syndrome, 2106-2107, 2414
    hemolysis, 2108
    hemorrhage, 2108
    hypoglycemia, 2108, 2415
    hypophosphatemia, 2415
    hypotension, 2105-2106, 2170, 2414
    hypothermia, 2414
    muscle cramps, 2107
    myocardial stunning, 2107
    pericardial disease, 2107-2108
    pulmonary hypertension, 2413
    ventricular arrhythmias, 2107
  conductivity clearance in, 2087
  coronary artery calcification associated with, 1850
  coronary artery disease in patients receiving, 2102
  in critically ill patients, 2142
  depression in patients receiving, 2063
  diabetic nephropathy treated with, 1316-1318
  dialysance, 2071
  dialysate
    bicarbonate concentration of, 2094-2095
    calcium concentration in, 2094, 2106
    composition of, 2092-2095
    computer controls for, 2079-2080
    delivery system for, 2075, 2078
    flow rate for, 2091
    glucose concentration in, 2092, 2095
    hypotension concerns, 2105-2106
    magnesium concentration in, 2094
    potassium concentration in, 2093
    sodium concentration in, 2092-2093
    sodium ramping of, 2079-2080, 2092-2093
    solutes in, 2080t
    temperature of, 2095
    ultrapure, 2082
  dialysate pump, 2078
  dialyzers
    biofeedback systems used with, 2080
    clearance by, 2072-2074
    definition of, 2075
    description of, 2413
    functions of, 2076-2077
    high-efficiency, 2077-2078
    high-flux, 2077-2078, 2092-2093
    hollow-fiber, 2075-2076
    membranes, 2076-2077, 2091, 2108
    monitoring by, 2079-2080
    reactions to, 2108

Hemodialysis (HD) (Continued)
    reuse of, 2096-2097
    selection of, 2090-2091
    ultrafiltration coefficient, 2091
    values for, 2077t
  discomforts during, 2085
  dose of, 2087, 2414, 2627f
  drugs during, 2046-2048, 2048t
  dry weight, 2095-2096
  duration of, 2085, 2088-2090
  in elderly, 747-748, 2598
  end-stage kidney disease treated with, 2097
  erythrocytosis in, 1888
  erythropoiesis-stimulating agents during, 2098
  ethical dilemmas. See Dialysis, ethical dilemmas
  ethylene glycol poisoning treated with, 2178
  extracorporeal circuit
    air detector, 2075
    arterial pressure monitor, 2075
    blood circuit, 2075
    components of, 2074-2082
    dialysate circuit, 2078-2079
    monitoring by, 2079-2080
    pressure monitors, 2075
    venous air trap, 2075
    venous pressure monitor, 2075
  frequency of, 2090
  future of, 2108-2109
  glycemic control during, 1317
  goals of, 2069, 2089-2090
  hematocrit monitoring during, 2079
  hepatitis B vaccination in, 2016, 2104
  hepatitis C in, 2504
  history of, 2059, 2074-2075, 2082-2083, 2558
  home-based, 2542-2543
  homocysteine levels in, 2100
  hormone replacement uses of, 2089
  hypermagnesemia treated with, 626
  hyperpigmentation associated with, 1944
  hypokalemia during, 2093
  hypophosphatemia during, 2074, 2415
  incidence of, 2059-2060
  in Indian subcontinent, 2503-2504
  infections in patients receiving, 2061, 2104-2105
  inflammation in, 1913
  insulin resistance affected by, 1317
  intermittent, 1006-1007, 2140-2141, 2181
  intravenous iron in, 1891f
  isopropanol poisoning treated with, 2178
  KT/V for, 2088, 2109
  in Latin America, 2450t
  left ventricular hypertrophy, 2100-2102
  lipid abnormalities in, 2100
  maintenance
    anemia during, 2097-2098
    anorexia associated with, 2099
    cardiovascular disease risks, 2100-2102
    end-stage kidney disease during, 2097
    hepatitis B management during, 2104
    hepatitis C management during, 2104
    hypertension management during, 2103-2104
    immune disorders in patients receiving, 2104-2105
    nutrition during, 2098-2100
    primary care management during, 2105
    protein-energy wasting in, 2099
    vascular access for, 2066-2067, 2192
    vitamin supplementation during, 2099-2100

Hemodialysis (HD) (Continued)
  in Malaysia, 2535-2536
  malnutrition during, 1317-1318, 2089-2090, 2098t, 2504
  metabolic acidosis correction during, 2094-2095
  methanol poisoning treated with, 2178
  in Middle East, 2475t, 2487-2488
  mineral metabolism-related issues in patients receiving, 2102-2103
  mortality caused by, 2060-2063, 2062f, 2063t, 2085f-2086f
  native kidney in, 2069, 2089
  nephrologist referral in, 2063
  nocturnal, 1936, 2088, 2542
  nutrition during, 1817-1818, 2089-2090
  outcome determinants, 2109
  paraquat poisoning treated with, 2186
  peritoneal dialysis versus, 2087, 2134-2135, 2411
  pneumonia in patients receiving, 2105
  poison removal using, 2169-2170, 2170t, 2172t
  pressure monitors used in, 2075
  prevalence of, 2059-2060
  principles of, 2068-2074, 2068f
  protein binding effects, 2073f
  protein-energy wasting in, 1317-1318, 2098-2099
  psychologic support during, 2063
  pyrogenic reactions during, 2082
  rebound after, 2093
  short daily, 2088-2089
  skin manifestations of, 1944
  sleep apnea in patients receiving, 2101
  solute clearance in
    description of, 2069-2070
    determinants of, 2072, 2072t
    dialyzer, 2072-2074
    dose increase effects on, 2089f
    factors that affect, 2070-2071
    flow-limited, 2071f, 2073f
    membrane-limited, 2072f-2073f
    mode of, 2142
    monitoring of, 2079
    removal rate versus, 2070
    standard, 2088
    urea, 2070
    whole body, 2072-2074
  solute sequestration, 2072-2073, 2074f
  sudden death risks in, 2093, 2101
  survival rates for, 2060-2061, 2062f
  theophylline poisoning treated with, 2187
  toxin removal by, 2069
  treatment time for, 2085, 2088-2090
  tubing used in, 2413
  ultrafiltration, 2068-2069, 2080, 2095, 2105
  ultrafiltration rate, 2095-2096
  urea in, 2083-2087, 2083f-2084f
  uremia treated with, 2083
  vaccination recommendations, 2105
  vascular access for
    arteriovenous fistulas, 2064-2065, 2065f, 2075, 2412-2413, 2598
    arteriovenous grafts, 2065-2067, 2066f, 2075, 2412-2413, 2542-2543
    background on, 2064
    catheters, 2067-2068, 2075, 2412-2413
    central venous catheters, 2412-2413, 2542-2543
    in children, 2412-2413
    in elderly, 2598
    expanded polytetrafluoroethylene materials used in, 2064-2066
    health care costs based on, 2064, 2072t

Hemodialysis (HD) *(Continued)*
   ideal characteristics of, 2064t
   infection risks, 2104
   loss of, 2067
   maintenance of, 2066-2067
   monitoring of, 2066-2067
   prophylactic therapy for, 2067
   surveillance of, 2066-2067
   top-ladder technique, 2066
   in Vietnam, 2536
   water used in
      bacteria in, 2081-2082
      endotoxins in, 2081-2082
      hazards associated with, 2080-2081
      microbiology of, 2081-2082
      quality monitoring of, 2082
      treatment systems for, 2080-2082, 2081f
   zinc deficiency in, 1887
Hemofiltration, 2142, 2170, 2172t
Hemoglobin
   end-stage kidney disease levels of, 2098
   erythropoiesis-stimulating agents effect on, 1892, 1902
   glycosylated, 1931
   health-related quality of life affected by, 1902
   in hypovolemia, 423
   recombinant human erythropoietin effects on, 2097
   reticulocyte, 1895
   in urine, 790
Hemoglobin A$_{1c}$, 2593
Hemoglobin SC disease, 1198-1199
Hemoglobin SS, 1145-1146, 1199
Hemolytic disease of the fetus and newborn, 2159
Hemolytic-uremic syndrome (HUS)
   acute kidney injury in Indian subcontinent patients, 2496
   atypical, 1175
      C3 convertases in, 1183-1185
      characteristics of, 2154
      cobalamin C synthase deficiency as cause of, 1188, 2356-2357
      complement abnormalities in, 1183-1185, 2355-2356, 2355f
      complement factor B in, 1185
      complement factor H in, 1184-1185, 2154, 2355-2357
      complement inhibitors for, 1186
      course of, 1185
      diacylglycerol kinase-ε in, 1185, 2356
      eculizumab for, 1186, 2356
      end-stage kidney disease caused by, 2431
      fresh-frozen plasma for, 1185-1186
      genetic forms of, 2422
      genetic screening in, 1187f
      liver transplantation for, 1186-1188
      mechanisms of, 1183-1185
      membrane cofactor protein in, 1184-1185
      outcomes of, 1184t, 1185
      plasmapheresis for, 2154, 2354
      in pregnancy, 1182
      prognosis for, 2356-2357
      renal transplantation for, 1186, 2357
      sporadic, 1182
      thrombomodulin in, 1185
      treatment of, 1185-1188, 2356-2357
      von Willebrand factor-cleaving protease deficiency as cause of, 2356
   in children. *See* Children, hemolytic-uremic syndrome in

Hemolytic-uremic syndrome (HUS) *(Continued)*
   classification of, 1176t
   clinical features of, 1175-1176, 2154
   cobalamin C metabolism abnormality associated with, 1188
   de novo posttransplantation, 1182
   description of, 990-992, 1157
   laboratory findings, 1176-1178
   mechanism of action, 1179-1191
   plasmapheresis for, 2154-2155
   postpartum, 1182
   prognosis for, 2354-2355
   recurrence of, after renal transplantation, 2270
   Shiga toxin-associated, 1179-1182, 2352-2357
   Shiga-like toxin, 1175-1176
   Streptococcus pneumoniae-associated, 1182, 2355
Hemolytic-uremic syndrome/thrombotic thrombocytopenic purpura, 1617t, 1632
Hemoperfusion, 2169-2170, 2172t, 2183
Hemopexin, 1020
Hemophagocytic syndrome, 1159, 1402-1403
Hemorrhage
   cyst, 1493
   during hemodialysis, 2108
   intracerebral, 1927
   pulmonary, 1072
Hemorrhagic cystitis, 1405
Hemorrhagic fever with renal syndrome, 2515-2516
Hemorrhagic stroke, 1927, 1931
Hemostasis, 1804
Henderson equation, 521-522
Henderson-Hasselbalch equation, 521-522, 2382
Henoch-Schönlein purpura (HSP)
   in children, 2348-2350
   clinical findings in, 1121
   corticosteroids for, 1124
   course of, 1123-1124
   end-stage kidney disease progression of, 1123-1124
   epidemiology of, 2348
   gender predilection of, 1121
   histopathologic features of, 2348, 2349f
   imaging of, 2349f
   immunoglobulin A nephropathy and, 1122-1123
   immunoglobulins in, 1122-1123
   laboratory findings in, 1121-1122
   pathogenesis of, 1123, 1951
   pathology of, 1122-1123, 1122f
   prognosis for, 1123-1124, 2350
   renal manifestations of, 1121, 2348-2350
   skin manifestations of, 1951, 1951f
   symptoms of, 1121
   treatment of, 1123-1124, 1951, 2350
Henry's law, 513
Heparan sulfate, 1288
Heparin, 2091-2092, 2144, 2162
Heparinase, 1013
Heparin-induced thrombocytopenia, 1909
Hepatic glomerulopathy, 1156f
Hepatitis B
   in Africa, 2461-2462
   cryoglobulinemia associated with, 1137
   in dialysis patients, 2504
   end-stage kidney disease and, 2488
   in Far East, 2532-2533
   glomerular manifestations of, 1154-1157

Hepatitis B *(Continued)*
   glomerulonephritis associated with, in Far East patients, 2532-2533
   nephropathy associated with, 1154-1155, 2461-2462
   nucleoside analogs for, 1155
   in polyarteritis nodosa, 1118-1120
   proteinuria in, 1154
   treatment of, 1155
   vaccination for, 2016, 2104
Hepatitis B antigenemia, 1154
Hepatitis B surface antigen, 2532
Hepatitis C
   clinical features of, 1155-1156
   cryoglobulinemia associated with, 1138
   end-stage kidney disease and, 2488
   in Far East, 2533
   glomerulonephritis associated with, in Far East patients, 2532-2533
   in hemodialysis patients, 2104, 2504
   immunosuppressive therapy for, 1156
   membranoproliferative glomerulonephritis associated with, 1155f, 2273
   membranous nephropathy associated with, 1155
   mixed cryoglobulinemia associated with, 1155
   pathogenesis of, 1155
   pathologic features of, 1155-1156, 1155f
   pegylated interferon for, 1156
   proteinuria in, 1156
   renal allograft dysfunction caused by, 2273, 2280
   renal disease associated with, 1155-1156
   ribavirin for, 1156
Hepatocellular jaundice, 2508
Hepatocyte growth factor (HGF), 120, 1212, 1741, 1757
Hepatocyte nuclear factor-1β, 1503-1504, 2316-2317
Hepatointestinal reflexes, 397
Hepatoportal receptors, 397
Hepatopulmonary syndrome, 442
Hepatorenal reflexes, 397, 440
Hepatorenal syndrome (HRS), 2139
   acute kidney injury and, 993-994, 994t, 998-999
   COX metabolites in, 378
   endothelin-1 in, 338, 446
   mortality rate for, 455
   peripheral arterial vasodilation and, 442
   prerenal acute kidney injury and, 998
   prognosis for, 455
   sodium retention in, 378
   treatment of, 998-999
      α-adrenergic agonists, 456
      liver transplantation, 458
      midodrine, 456
      peritoneovenous shunting, 998-999
      pharmacologic, 455-457
      PROMETHEUS, 458
      renal replacement therapy, 457-458
      somatostatin analogues, 456
      systemic vasoconstrictors, 455-456
      terlipressin, 455-456, 998-999
      transjugular intrahepatic portosystemic shunt, 457, 998-999
      vasoconstrictor antagonists, 455
      vasodilators, 455
      vasopressin 1 receptor analogues, 455-456
      vasopressin 2 receptor antagonists, 456-457

Hepatorenal syndrome (HRS) (Continued)
  type 1, 449, 455
  type 2, 449, 455
Hepcidin, 1885-1886, 1886f
Hepcidin-25, 939
Herbal medicine, 2507-2508, 2533-2534
Hereditary angiopathy nephropathy, aneurysm and muscle cramp (HANAC syndrome), 1425
Hereditary cystic kidney disorder, 1479-1505
Hereditary fructose intolerance, 1445
Hereditary hypokalemic salt-losing tubulopathy, 1473
Hereditary hypophosphatemic rickets with hypercalciuria, 631-632, 1453, 2345
Hereditary leiomyomatosis and renal cell carcinoma syndrome, 1373-1374, 1952, 1952f, 1952t
Hereditary nephritis, 1140-1141. See also Alport's syndrome
Hereditary osteo-onychodysplasia. See Nail-patella syndrome
Hereditary polycystic kidney disease, 1371
hERG, 569
Hernia, 2132
Heroin nephropathy, 686, 1157-1158
Herpes zoster vaccination, 2105
Heteromeric amino acid transporters, 225-227, 226f, 231-232
Heterotrimeric G proteins, 282-284
Hexokinase, 790
High anion gap acidosis, 543, 2382t
  causes of, 524, 525t, 543, 543t
  definition of, 523
  description of, 528
  drugs as cause of, 543, 547-550
  ethanol as cause of, 548
  ethylene glycol as cause of, 548
  features of, 524-525
  isopropyl alcohol as cause of, 549
  ketoacidosis as cause of, 543, 546-547
  lactic acidosis as cause of, 543t, 544-546
  methanol as cause of, 548-549
  paraldehyde as cause of, 549
  propylene glycol acid as cause of, 549
  pyroglutamic acid as cause of, 549
  salicylate as cause of, 547-548
  screening of, 543
  toxins as cause of, 543, 548-550, 2181
  uremia as cause of, 549-550
  uremic acidosis as cause of, 543
High blood pressure, 1522-1524, 1527f. See also Blood pressure; Hypertension
High osmolar contrast media, 847-848
High-cutoff dialyzers, 2153
High-cutoff hemodialysis, 1393
High-density lipoprotein, 1761, 1863, 2100
High-efficiency dialyzers, 2077-2078
High-flux dialyzers, 2077-2078, 2092-2093
Highly active antiretroviral therapy, 1153, 2455-2456
High-molecular-weight plasma proteins, 791
High-resolution peripheral computerized tomography, 1846
Hill coefficient, 2040-2041
Hill equation, 2040
Hilus cyst, 1517
Hip fractures, 1849, 2282-2283
Hippurate, 1809f, 1811-1812
Histomorphometry, in chronic kidney disease–mineral bone disorder, 1842-1843, 1844f
HKα, 242
HKβ, 242
H^+-K^+-ATPase, 178, 254, 534
HLA-DR, 2233

HLA-DR3, 1040
HMG-CoA reductase inhibitors, for dyslipidemia, 1931
HO-1, 978
hOCT2A, 212
Hodgkin's disease, 1021, 1157
Hodgkin's lymphoma, 1404
Hollow-fiber dialyzers, 2075-2076
Home blood pressure monitoring, 1538, 1540-1542, 1541t-1542t
Homeostasis model assessment, 1912, 1914f
Homocysteine, 1817, 1864, 1872, 1930, 1938, 1970, 2100
Homocystinuria, 1864
Homogeneous population, 1163
Hong Kong, 2535
Hopewell hypothesis, 1470-1471
Hormone(s). See also specific hormone
  replacement therapy, 659-660
  sodium reabsorption regulation by, 126
Hornet stings, 2500
Horseshoe kidney, 2295, 2296f, 2303-2304, 2311
Hospice referral, 2569-2570
Hounsfield unit, 851
Hox11, 22
Hoxa11, 22
HoxB7-EGFP, 19, 20f
Hoxc11, 22
H.P. Acthar Gel, 1172
Human antichimeric antibodies, 1171
Human Development Index, 2470t
Human embryonic stem cells, 2603-2607
Human immunodeficiency virus (HIV)
  in Africa. See Africa, human immunodeficiency virus in
  in Far East, 2533
  focal segmental glomerulosclerosis associated with, 1028, 1030
  glomerular lesions in, 1153-1154
  glomerulopathies associated with, 1151
  in hemodialysis patients, 2104-2105
  immunoglobulin A nephropathy in, 1154
  renal transplantation in patients with, 2289
Human immunodeficiency virus nephropathy
  in Africa, 2462
  clinical features of, 1151-1152
  course of, 1153
  electron microscopy of, 1152f
  end-stage kidney disease caused by, 1153
  pathogenesis of, 1152-1153
  pathology of, 1152, 1152f-1153f
  podocytes in, 116
  treatment of, 1153
Human leukocyte antigens (HLA)
  class I, 2231-2233, 2232f
  class II, 2233
  inheritance of, 2233-2234, 2234f
  loci strengths, 2235-2236
  racial differences in, 2582
  sensitization, 1903, 2422-2423
  typing of, 2234-2235
Human polyomavirus infection, 2272-2273
Humoral hypercalcemia of malignancy, 603, 607-608
Hungry bone syndrome, 616, 620
Hyaline casts, 800, 800t
Hyalinosis, 921t
Hyaluronidase, 1013
Hyaluronan, 273
Hydralazine, 1673-1674, 1674t, 1695t
Hydration, 854-855

Hydraulic pressure, 94-96, 95f
Hydraulic pressure gradient, 94
Hydraulic pressure profile, 85, 85f
Hydrogen, 835, 841, 844, 1758-1759
Hydrogen gradient, 126-127
Hydronephrosis
  bilateral, 862f
  calyces in, 867-868
  congenital, 1259
  contrast-enhanced computed tomography of, 872f
  definition of, 764, 1257
  fetal, 2314-2315
  grading of, 867-868
  mild, 867-868, 867f
  moderate, 867-868, 867f
  morbidity of, 1264-1265
  nonobstructive, 765, 868
  renal cystic disease versus, 868
  severe, 867-868, 868f
  in transplanted kidney, 911
  ultrasonography of, 867-869, 867f-868f, 1263
  unilateral, 1259
Hydrostatic pressure, 813
Hydroureter, 764-765
Hydroxyapatite, 196
β-Hydroxybutyric acid, 247
Hydroxyeicosatetraenoic acids
  12(S)-, 380, 382
  15-, 380-381
  19-, 382-384
  20-, 382-384
  description of, 355, 380
1α-Hydroxylase, 1829f
11β-Hydroxylase deficiency, 1461
17α-Hydroxylase deficiency, 1461
11β-Hydroxysteroid dehydrogenase, 66-67, 577, 1919-1920
11β-Hydroxysteroid dehydrogenase type 2
  in blood vessels, 320-321
  defective, 320
  description of, 304-305, 717
  expression of, 320
  mineralocorticoid receptor activity affected by, 320
  mineralocorticoid specificity and, 320
  pharmacologic inhibition of, 577, 596
  roles of, 321
25-Hydroxyvitamin D, 1924, 2014, 2390
25-Hydroxyvitamin D 1α-hydroxylase, 187
Hyperaldosteronism
  in chronic kidney disease, 1919
  glucocorticoid-remediable, 555-556
  idiopathic, 575-577
  kaliuresis in, 576-577
  potassium loss caused by, 575-577, 576f
  primary, 575, 576f, 1545-1547
  sleep-disordered breathing and, 1547
  sodium reabsorption reinforced by, 1724-1725
Hyperammonemia, 1962, 2181
Hyperbicarbonatemia, 520
Hypercalcemia, 1375
  algorithm for, 605f
  aquaporin-2 membrane targeting affected by, 299, 481
  bisphosphonates for, 611, 2396
  bone resorption inhibition in, 611-612
  calcium-sensing receptor activation by, 609-610
  causes of, 602-603, 603t
    1,25 $(OH)_2$ vitamin D, 608
    acromegaly, 609
    acute kidney disease, 610
    breast cancer, 607-608

Hypercalcemia *(Continued)*
    chronic kidney disease, 610
    estrogens, 609
    familial primary hyperparathyroidism syndromes, 608
    granulomatous disease, 610
    growth hormone, 609
    immobilization, 610
    lithium, 609
    liver disease, 610
    malignancy, 603-604, 607-608
    medications, 609
    milk-alkali syndrome, 609-610
    nonparathyroid endocrinopathies, 608-609
    pheochromocytoma, 609
    primary hyperparathyroidism, 604-607
    selective estrogen receptor modifiers, 609
    thiazide diuretics, 609, 1730
    vitamin A, 609
    vitamin D, 609
  in children. *See* Children, hypercalcemia in
  clinical features of, 604*t*, 2393-2394
  description of, 185-186
  diagnosis of, 604-605, 605*f*, 2396, 2396*f*
  familial hypocalciuric, 608, 2391, 2395
  glucocorticoids for, 612
  humoral hypercalcemia of malignancy, 603, 607-608
  hypercalciuria induced by, 604
  hypertension and, 1549
  idiopathic infantile, 2394
  incidence of, 602
  laboratory findings in, 604
  loop diuretics for, 610-611
  of malignancy, 1399-1400, 1399*t*
  management of, 610-612, 611*t*
  mild, 608-609
  neonatal, 2394*t*
  pathophysiology of, 602-603
  in peritoneal dialysis patients, 2132
  pharmacologic therapy for, 611*t*
  in renal transplantation recipients, 2281
  sarcoidosis and, 1228
  signs and symptoms of, 603-604
  treatment of, 2396, 2397*t*
  vitamin D-mediated, 609
  volume repletion for, 610-611
  Williams-Beuren syndrome as cause of, 2394-2395
Hypercalcemia-hypercalciuria of malignancy, 767-768
Hypercalciuria, 1331-1335, 1437
  absorptive, 1331-1333, 1333*f*
  autosomal dominant hypocalcemia with, 2345
  in children, 2340, 2344, 2344*f*
  familial hypomagnesemia with, 1466
  familial hypomagnesemia with hypercalciuria and nephrocalcinosis, 2345, 2387-2388
  genetic hypercalciuric rat model of, 1333-1334
  hereditary hypophosphatemic rickets with, 631-632, 2345
  hypercalcemia-induced, 604
  in hypophosphatemia, 629
  metabolic acidosis associated with, 191
  in nephrolithiasis, 2340, 2344, 2344*f*
Hypercalciuric calcium nephrolithiasis, 1364*t*

Hypercapnia
  acute, 526-527
  arginine vasopressin secretion affected by, 470
  chronic, 516
  metabolic alkalosis secondary to, 553-554
  positive end-expiratory pressure as cause of, 526
Hyperchloremic metabolic acidosis, 1437, 2382-2383
  algorithm for, 842*f*
  assessment of, 840-841
  case study of, 840-844
  clinical approach to, 841-844, 842*f*, 842*t*
  description of, 528-530, 529*t*, 764, 768
  toluene metabolism as cause of, 843*f*
Hypercholesterolemia, 301, 1129, 1970
Hypercoagulability
  in chronic kidney disease, 1906-1909, 1908*f*
  clinical consequence of, 1804-1805
  in membranous nephropathy, 1041
  in nephrotic syndrome, 1803-1805, 1803*f*
  pathogenesis of, 1803-1804
Hypercortisolism, 1549, 1919
Hyperdibasic aminoaciduria, 223*t*
Hyperglycemia, 1454*t*
  diuretics as cause of, 1730, 1731*f*
  fetal exposure to, 717-718
  gestational, 717-718
  glycosuria caused by, 790
  maternal, 717*f*
  in peritoneal dialysis patients, 2132
  thiazide diuretics as cause of, 1730, 1731*f*
Hyperhomocysteinemia, 2284
Hyperkalemia
  acid-base balance and, 537
  in acute kidney injury, 994-995, 2140
  in Addison's disease, 589
  aldosterone affected by, 182, 2366-2367
  algorithm for, 593*f*, 826*f*
  ammonia production and excretion affected by, 537-538, 537*t*
  angiotensin-converting enzyme inhibitors as cause of, 591-592, 1650
  Brugada sign associated with, 570-571
  calcineurin inhibitors associated with, 541, 2281
  cardiac arrhythmias associated with, 570-571
  cardiac effects of, 570-571, 593-594
  causes of, 825-827, 826*t*
  in children, 2380-2382, 2380*t*-2381*t*
  chronic, 828-830, 829*f*
  in chronic kidney disease, 585
  clinical approach to, 592, 825-828
  clinical sequelae of, 592
  consequences of, 570-572
  COX-2 inhibitors as cause of, 590
  cyclosporine as cause of, 590
  definition of, 585, 2380
  description of, 818
  in diabetes mellitus, 586-587
  distal potassium-sparing diuretics as cause of, 1713, 1732
  diuretics as cause of, 1730, 1732
  drug-induced, 540, 540*t*
  electrocardiographic abnormality associated with, 571, 571*t*
  in end-stage kidney disease, 585, 2405
  epidemiology of, 585
  epithelial sodium channel inhibition as cause of, 590-591, 591*f*

Hyperkalemia *(Continued)*
  excessive potassium intake as cause of, 586
  factitious, 585
  familial hypertension with, 179-180, 183, 2381-2382
  hereditary tubular defects as cause of, 589-590
  hospitalization for, 592
  hyperphosphatemia and, 1003-1004
  hyperuricemia and, 994-995
  hyporeninemic hypoaldosteronism and, 589
  impaired net acid excretion disorders with, 536-541
  medications that cause, 590-592
  mineralocorticoid antagonists as cause of, 591-592
  mortality rate for, 585
  muscle effects of, 570-571
  non-anion gap metabolic acidosis and, 536
  nonsteroidal antiinflammatory drugs as cause of, 362
  potassium excretion in, 827
  potassium redistribution as cause of, 586-588
  potassium shift out of cells as cause of, 825-827, 826*t*
  potassium-sparing diuretics as cause of, 451
  of primary mineralocorticoid deficiency, 538
  proximal tubule bicarbonate reabsorption affected by, 237
  pseudohyperkalemia, 585-586, 827, 829, 2380
  red cell transfusion as cause of, 586
  renal consequences of, 571-572
  in renal transplantation recipients, 2281
  renin and, 814*t*
  renin-angiotensin-aldosterone system inhibitors as cause of, 591-592, 741, 2005-2006
  tacrolimus as cause of, 590
  tissue necrosis as cause of, 586
  treatment of, 1003-1004, 2381*t*
    β_2-adrenergic agonists, 594-595
    albuterol, 594-595
    algorithm for, 593*f*
    calcium, 593-594
    cation exchange resins, 596-597
    dialysis, 598-599
    insulin in, 594
    mineralocorticoids in, 595-596
    potassium binders, 597-598
    potassium redistribution in, 594-595
    potassium removal agents in, 595-596
    sodium bicarbonate, 595, 595*f*
    sodium polystyrene sulfonate, 596-597
  trimethoprim as cause of, 590, 828
Hyperkalemic acidosis, 572
Hyperkalemic hyperchloremic metabolic acidosis, 536*t*, 538, 541
Hyperkalemic periodic paralysis, 567*f*, 571
Hyperkalemic renal tubular acidosis, 540, 1726, 2337*t*, 2338
Hyperlactatemia, 545
Hyperlipidemia
  cardiovascular disease and, 1802
  causes of, 2284
  clinical consequences of, 1802-1803
  description of, 2127

Hyperlipidemia (Continued)
  nephrotic, 1801-1803, 1801f, 1803f, 1816-1817
  in peritoneal dialysis patients, 2132
  renal injury secondary to, 1773
  in renal transplantation recipients, 2284
  thiazide diuretics as cause of, 1731
Hypermagnesemia
  in acute kidney injury, 995, 1003t, 1004
  cardiovascular system manifestations of, 625
  causes of, 625
  in chronic renal failure, 616
  clinical manifestations of, 625-626
  description of, 193
  dialysis for, 626
  hemodialysis for, 626
  nervous system manifestations of, 625
  progressive, 625
  renal insufficiency and, 625
  treatment of, 625
Hypermineralocorticoidism, 551
Hypernatremia
  in acute kidney injury, 1003-1004, 1003t
  adipsic, 477-478
  in children, 2367-2370
  in elderly, 742
  osmoreceptor dysfunction as cause of, 489
  prevention of, in nephrogenic diabetes insipidus, 2338
Hyperosmolality, 478-479, 483, 2367-2370, 2367t
Hyperoxaluria, 1337-1340, 1338f, 1342f, 2340, 2346-2348, 2422, 2431, 2478
Hyperparathyroidism, 603
  in chronic kidney disease, 1912
  erythropoietin and, 1887
  hypertension and, 1549
  hypophosphatemia caused by, 630
  hypophosphaturia caused by, 630
  left ventricular hypertrophy and, 1924
  lithium and, 1226
  maternal, 2391
  neonatal severe, 608, 2395-2396
  posttransplantation, 2282
  primary, 603-604
  in renal transplantation recipients, 2282
  secondary, 1797-1798, 1827-1828, 1835-1836, 1887, 2023, 2026, 2031-2032
Hyperparathyroidism–jaw tumor syndrome, 608
Hyperphosphatemia
  in acute kidney injury, 1004
  causes of, 626-627, 627t, 2399, 2399t
    acromegaly, 627
    acute kidney injury, 627, 995
    bisphosphonates, 627
    chronic kidney disease, 627, 1774-1775
    exogenous phosphate load, 627-628
    familial tumoral calcinosis, 627
    glomerular filtration rate reductions, 627
    hypoparathyroidism, 627
    metabolic acidosis, 628
    pseudohypoparathyroidism, 627
    respiratory acidosis, 628
    rhabdomyolysis, 628
    tumor lysis syndrome, 628
  in children, 2398-2400, 2399f, 2399t
  in chronic kidney disease stage 5, 2020
  chronic kidney disease–mineral bone disorder secondary to, 1977, 2021
  clinical manifestations of, 628-629
  definition of, 626
  diagnosis of, 2399, 2399f

Hyperphosphatemia (Continued)
  hyperkalemia and, 1003-1004
  imaging of, 2399
  in intensive care unit settings, 628
  neonatal, 2389
  phosphate-binding agents for, 2029. See also Phosphate-binding agents
  pseudo-, 628
  treatment of, 628-629, 2021, 2399, 2400t
  tumor lysis syndrome and, 1396
Hyperprolactinemia, 1919
Hyperprostaglandin E syndrome, 2376-2377
Hypertension, 1549. See also Blood pressure; High blood pressure; Secondary hypertension
  in acute poststreptococcal glomerulonephritis, 1057
  in Africa, 2459-2461
  African American study of kidney disease and hypertension, 1553
  age and, 1525
  albuminuria risks, 1765
  angiotensin II-dependent mouse model of, 369
  antihypertensive treatment, 1563t
  in antiphospholipid syndrome, 1200
  arterial stiffness and, 1535
  in atheroembolic renal disease, 1191
  atherosclerotic renal artery stenosis and, 1595-1596
  autosomal dominant early-onset hypertension with severe exacerbation during pregnancy, 1463
  autosomal dominant polycystic kidney disease and, 1487-1489, 1492-1493
  bevacizumab causing, 1398
  blood pressure measurement and, 1539f
  calcineurin inhibitors as cause of, 1167-1168
  cardiovascular disease and, 1688-1689, 1861, 1868, 2127
  in children, 2329, 2360, 2406-2407, 2421-2422
  chronic kidney disease and, 673, 679, 1544-1545, 1765-1767, 1861, 1868, 1873, 1974-1975, 2360, 2421-2422, 2590-2591
  clinical outcome trials for, 1552-1562
  congenital adrenal hyperplasia and, 1547
  definition of, 1680
  in diabetic nephropathy, 1314-1315
  diagnostic approach, 765-767
  drug-resistant, 1974-1975
  economics of, 1528
  effects of, 1522, 1523f
  in elderly, 744-746, 745f, 1557-1560, 1558t, 2590-2592
  endothelin's role in, 336-337
  in end-stage kidney disease, 1765, 1770, 2406-2407
  epidemiology of, 1524-1527
  ethnicity and, 662f, 693-694, 1526-1527
  evaluation of, 1536-1543, 1537t
  familial, with hyperkalemia, 179-180, 183
  fractional excretion of sodium affected by, 1747-1748
  gender and, 662f, 1525
  genetics of, 1529-1530
  gestational, 1627-1631
  glomerular, 1737-1738
  glomerular hematuria and, 758
  heart failure and, 1660-1661
  in hemodialysis patients, 2103-2104
  immune system and, 1535-1536
  inherited disorders with, 1459-1464
  intraabdominal, 2138

Hypertension (Continued)
  intrahepatic, 441
  isolated systolic, 1685
  kallikrein-kinin system in, 349
  laboratory tests for, 1542-1543, 1543t
  lifestyle factors, 693-694, 745-746
  malignant, 758, 1194-1195, 1765
  masked, 2360
  medical versus interventional therapy trials for, 1596t
  metabolic acidosis caused by, 555
  in New Zealand, 2550
  nonsteroidal antiinflammatory drugs as cause of, 361-362
  obesity and, 766, 1533-1534, 1694
  peripheral vasoconstriction and, 1572
  in polyarteritis nodosa, 1119
  potassium intake and, 1542
  preeclampsia and, 1615-1618, 1615t
  in pregnancy, 681
  pressure-natriuresis curve in, 701
  prevalence of, 765, 1487, 1528f
  pseudohypertension, 766
  race and, 662f, 1526-1527
  after radiation nephropathy, 1194-1195
  refractory, 1695
  renal artery stenosis and, 1582
  in renal transplantation recipients, 911, 1637, 2283-2284, 2284t, 2432
  resistant, 1691t, 1693-1695
  salt-sensitive, 1974-1975
  in scleroderma renal crisis, 1196
  secondary, 766t, 1694
  sleep-disordered breathing and, 766
  sodium intake and, 1542, 1993
  stroke risks associated with, 1522, 1928-1931, 1928t, 1933-1934
  sympathetic nervous system activation effect on, 1533f
  symptoms of, 766
  systemic hemodynamics and extracellular fluid volume, 1543
  telmisartan versus losartan trial, 1557
  thyroid dysfunction and, 1549
  traditional cut points of blood pressure for, 1524t
  treatment of
    β-adrenergic antagonists, 1660. See also β-Adrenergic antagonists
    angiotensin receptor blockers, 1654, 2592
    angiotensin-converting enzyme inhibitors, 2592
    description of, 1195, 1314-1315, 1930-1931, 2283-2284
    in elderly, 2591-2592
    intravenous agents, 1630-1631
    in older adults with chronic kidney disease, 1559-1560
    during pregnancy, 1629
  treatment-resistant, 1580
  in type 1 diabetes mellitus, 1297-1298
  urolithiasis and, 1351-1352
  volume overload as cause of, 2127
  weight loss benefits for, 1992
  in Williams-Beuren syndrome, 2395
Hypertensive emergencies, 1550-1552
  definition of, 1695
  diazoxide for, 1696-1697
  direct-acting vasodilators for, 1695t, 1696-1699
  drug treatment of, 1695-1700, 1697t
  parenteral drugs for, 1695t, 1696-1699
  treatment of, 1551t
  types of, 1551t, 1693t
Hypertensive nephropathy, 2459

INDEX

Hypertensive nephrosclerosis, 639-641, 775, 1765
Hypertensive urgencies
  definition of, 1695
  direct-acting vasodilators for, 1695t, 1696-1699
  drug treatment of, 1695-1700
Hypertonic dehydration, 478-480
Hypertonic saline, 503
Hypertriglyceridemia, 2284
Hyperuricemia, 994-995, 1396, 1962
  in acute kidney injury, 1003t, 1004
  cause of, 1442
  chronic kidney disease progression affected by, 684, 1228, 2004
  chronic tubulointerstitial nephritis caused by, 1227-1228
  protease inhibitors as cause of, 2456-2457
Hyperuricosuria, 1335-1336, 1336f, 1342-1343, 2342, 2343t
Hyperventilation, 527
Hypervolemia
  arterial volume overload in, 449
  clinical manifestations of, 449
  definition of, 425
  diagnosis of, 449-450
  edema in, 426
  etiology of, 425-426
  interstitial fluid accumulation in, 449
  pathophysiology of, 426-429
  prerenal azotemia and, 450
  sodium retention in. See also Sodium retention
    effective arterial blood volume reductions and, 426-427
    pathophysiology of, 426
    primary, 425-426, 449
    secondary, 426, 449
    systemic factors that stimulate, 426-433
    treatment of, 450-451
  treatment of, 450-451
    collecting duct diuretics, 451
    distal tubule diuretics, 451
    diuretics, 450-451
    extracorporeal ultrafiltration, 451
    loop diuretics, 450-451
    proximal tubule diuretics, 450
Hypoactive sexual desire disorder, 1921
Hypoalbuminemia
  consequences of, 1797-1798
  description of, 1041, 1969-1970, 2169
  drug toxicity risks secondary to, 1797
  in nephrotic-range proteinuria, 1796-1798, 1796f
  pathogenesis of, 1796-1797, 1796f
  venous thromboembolism and, 1805
Hypoaldosteronism
  hyporeninemic, 538, 538t, 588-589, 1057
  isolated, in critically ill patients, 538-539, 539t
  primary, 588
Hypocalcemia
  in acute kidney injury, 1003t, 1004
  algorithm for, 614f
  autosomal dominant hypocalcemia with hypercalciuria, 2345
  Bartter's syndrome and, 2335
  calcium gluconate for, 618
  cataracts secondary to, 613
  causes of, 613t, 2392t
    acute kidney injury, 995
    acute pancreatitis, 618
    alcohol consumption, 616

Hypocalcemia (Continued)
    critical illness, 618
    drugs, 617-618
    foscarnet, 618
    hypoparathyroidism, 614-617
    magnesium disorders, 616-617
    medications, 617-618
    regional citrate anticoagulation, 617
    vitamin D, 617
  in children. See Children, hypocalcemia in
  chronic, 618
  in chronic kidney disease stage 5, 2020
  Chvostek's sign in, 612-613
  cinacalcet dosing and, 2027
  clinical features of, 612t
  definition of, 612
  diagnosis of, 613-614, 2392, 2393f
  familial, with hypercalciuria, 614-616
  familial hypomagnesemia with secondary hypocalcemia, 2388, 2388f
  hypomagnesemia and, 624
  laboratory findings, 613
  management of, 618
  monitoring of, 2393
  neonatal, 2391-2393, 2392t, 2394t
  in nephrotic syndrome, 1797-1798
  in plasmapheresis, 2163
  signs and symptoms of, 612-613
  treatment of, 2163, 2392-2393, 2394t
  Trousseau's sign in, 612-613
  tumor lysis syndrome and, 1396
  workup for, 2392, 2393f
Hypocalciuria
  in chronic kidney disease, 1749-1750
  in Gitelman's syndrome, 580
  isolated dominant hypomagnesemia with, 1466
  thiazide diuretics as cause of, 190-191
Hypocapnia, 516, 527
Hypochromic red blood cells, 1894-1895
Hypocitraturia, 1336-1337, 1337t, 2340-2342
Hypocomplementemia, 1052-1053, 1137, 1148-1149, 1192
Hypodipsia, 480
Hypogastric plexus, 80-81
Hypoglycemia
  arginine vasopressin secretion affected by, 470
  cause of, 1442
  during glucose treatment of hyperkalemia, 594
  during hemodialysis, 2108, 2415
  in renal insufficiency, 1816
Hypogonadism, 1920-1923
Hypokalemia
  in acute kidney injury, 995
  adverse effects of, 1729
  aquaporin-2 and, 299
  arrhythmias secondary to, 569
  cardiovascular consequences of, 570
  causes of, 822t
    Bartter's syndrome, 578-580
    Gitelman's syndrome, 580
    magnesium deficiency, 581
    nonrenal, 574
    renal tubular acidosis, 580-581
  in children, 2375-2379, 2375t, 2376f-2378f, 2377t
  citrate excretion in, 247
  clinical approach to, 581-583, 582f, 821-825
  description of, 299, 818
  diagnostic algorithm for, 2376f
  diuretics as cause of, 1728-1730, 1729f

Hypokalemia (Continued)
  in eating disorders, 581-583
  emergencies associated with, 821
  epidemiology of, 572
  during hemodialysis, 2093
  high potassium excretion and, 825
  hyperpolarization caused by, 570
  in hypomagnesemia, 624
  hypovolemia and, 424-425
  inherited disorders with, 1459-1464
  low potassium excretion and, 823-825
  magnesium deficiency and, 823
  metabolic acidosis and, 821, 1723
  in metabolic alkalosis, 550-551, 821-823
  in peritoneal dialysis patients, 2132
  polyuria in, 570
  potassium shift into cells as cause of, 821, 824
  in primary hyperaldosteronism, 576-577
  proximal tubule bicarbonate reabsorption affected by, 237
  rebound hyperkalemia in, 583
  redistribution and, 572-573
  refeeding syndrome and, 572-573
  renal consequences of, 570
  renin and, 814t
  rhabdomyolysis associated with, 586
  sodium polystyrene sulfonate for, 2168-2169
  spurious, 572
  in thyrotoxic periodic paralysis, 573-574
  transtubular potassium concentration gradient in, 569
  treatment of, 583-585, 824-825
  ventricular arrhythmia risks, 569
  volume expansion in, 584
Hypokalemic alkalosis, familial, 578-580
Hypokalemic nephropathy, 2375
Hypokalemic periodic paralysis, 569, 571, 573-574, 1704
Hypomagnesemia, 1465-1466
  in acute kidney injury, 995
  aminoglycosides as cause of, 621-622
  amphotericin B as cause of, 621
  autosomal dominant, 2388-2389
  calcineurin inhibitors as cause of, 622
  calcium-sensing disorders as cause of, 622
  cardiovascular manifestations of, 622-623
  causes of, 2387t
  in children, 2387-2389, 2387t
  clinical manifestations of, 622-624
  cutaneous losses as cause of, 620
  description of, 618-625, 2387
  in diabetes mellitus, 620
  diuretics as cause of, 1730
  electrolyte homeostasis and, 624
  epidermal growth factor receptor blockers as cause of, 621
  familial
    description of, 193-194
    with hypercalciuria and nephrocalcinosis, 2387-2388
    with secondary hypocalcemia, 2388, 2388f
  hypocalcemia and, 624
  hypokalemia in, 624
  incidence of, 619
  intestinal malabsorption as cause of, 620
  intravenous magnesium replacement for, 624
  isolated autosomal recessive, with normocalciuria, 2389
  loop diuretics as cause of, 621

Volume 1 pp. 1-1321 • Volume 2 pp. 1322-2636

Hypomagnesemia (Continued)
  neuromuscular system manifestations of, 623
  oral magnesium replacement for, 624-625
  parathyroid hormone resistance caused by, 617
  in parenteral nutrition patients, 620
  pentamidine as cause of, 622
  potassium-sparing diuretics for, 625
  proton pump inhibitors as cause of, 620
  refeeding syndrome as cause of, 620
  renal magnesium wasting as cause of, 620-622
  in renal transplantation recipients, 2281
  skeletal system manifestations of, 623-624
  tetany of, 193
  treatment of, 624-625
  tubule nephrotoxins as cause of, 621
Hyponatremia
  in acute kidney injury, 1003, 1003t
  acute symptomatic, 501
  aquaporin-2 in, 299-300
  brain herniation caused by, 503
  case studies of, 816-817
  causes and pathogenesis of
    angiotensin-converting enzyme inhibitors, 497
    antineoplastic drugs, 497
    carbamazepine, 497
    chlorpropamide, 497
    congestive heart failure, 493-494
    desmopressin, 488, 496-497
    diuretics, 492-493, 1727-1728, 1727f
    drugs, 496-497
    endurance exercise, 496
    extracellular fluid volume depletion, 492-493
    extracellular fluid volume excess, 493-495
    glucocorticoid deficiency, 495
    heart failure, 432, 493-494
    hepatic failure, 494
    hypothyroidism, 495-496
    narcotics, 497
    nephrotic syndrome, 494-495
    oxcarbazepine, 497
    primary polydipsia, 496
    psychotropic drugs, 497
    renal failure, 495
  central nervous system symptoms in, 501-502
  in children, 2370-2372, 2371t
  chronic, 502-504, 508, 815, 817
  cirrhosis and, 494
  classification of, 501t, 815
  clinical manifestations of, 500-501
  definition of, 815
  depletional, 503-504
  diagnosis of, 492f
  edema and, 495
  in elderly, 497, 501, 742
  euvolemic, 504-505, 507f
  factitious, 490
  hospital-acquired, 496
  in hospitalized children, 2372
  hypo-osmolality and, 490-491
  hypovolemic, 492-493
  incidence of, 490
  laboratory tests for, 816
  morbidity and mortality associated with, 500-503
  in osmoreceptor dysfunction, 480
  in peritoneal dialysis patients, 2132
  postoperative, 496
  prevalence of, 490
  in psychosis, 496

Hyponatremia (Continued)
  sodium concentration monitoring in, 508
  spontaneous correction of, 507-508
  symptoms of, 500-503, 506-508
  syndrome of inappropriate antidiuretic hormone secretion as cause of, 497-498
  thiazide diuretics and, 817-818
  transient, 477
  translocational, 491
  treatment of
    arginine vasopressin receptor antagonists, 504-506, 509
    fluid restriction, 504, 504t
    furosemide, 506
    future of, 508-509
    guidelines for, 506-508
    hypertonic saline, 503
    isotonic saline, 503-504
    neurologic outcomes secondary to, 503
    urea, 506
Hyponatremic encephalopathy, 500-501, 2371
Hyponatremic hypertensive syndrome, 575
Hypo-osmolality, 490-491, 2370-2371, 2371t
Hypoparathyroidism
  acquired, 616-617
  algorithm for, 614f
  autoimmune, 617
  in children, 613
  genetic causes of, 614-616
  genetic syndromes with, 615t
  hyperphosphatemia caused by, 627
  hypocalcemia caused by, 614-617
  incidence of, 614
  after thyroid surgery, 616
Hypoparathyroidism, sensorineural deafness, and renal anomalies syndrome, 2297t
Hypophosphatemia
  in acute leukemia, 633
  causes of, 629-633, 2397, 2397t
    alcoholism, 633
    autosomal dominant hypophosphatemic rickets, 630-631
    autosomal recessive hypophosphatemic rickets, 631
    description of, 629-630
    diabetic ketoacidosis, 633, 2398
    drugs, 632
    Fanconi's syndrome, 632
    hereditary hypophosphatemic rickets with hypercalciuria, 631-632
    hyperparathyroidism, 630
    kidney transplantation, 632
    malabsorption, 632-633
    malnutrition, 632
    phosphate redistribution, 633
    phosphatonins, 630-631
    refeeding syndrome, 633
    respiratory alkalosis, 633
    tumor-induced osteomalacia, 631
    vitamin D, 633
    X-linked hypophosphatemia, 630
  in children, 2396-2398, 2415
  chronic, 629
  clinical manifestations of, 629
  definition of, 629
  diagnosis of, 629
  drug-induced, 632
  in heat stroke, 633
  hematologic effects of, 629
  in hemodialysis, 2074, 2415
  1α-hydroxylase system stimulated by, 2390
  25-hydroxyvitamin D$_3$ 1α-hydroxylase induced by, 200

Hypophosphatemia (Continued)
  hypercalciuria in, 629
  imaging of, 2398
  intravenous phosphorus for, 634
  isoproterenol and, 200-201
  metabolic consequences of, 629
  mild, 2396-2397
  moderate, 629
  neuromuscular abnormalities secondary to, 629
  phosphate replacement therapy for, 633-634
  in renal transplantation recipients, 2281
  skeletal abnormalities secondary to, 629
  in toxic shock syndrome, 633
  treatment of, 633-634, 2398, 2398t
Hypophosphatemic rickets, 630-632
Hypophosphaturia, 630
Hypopituitarism, 495
Hypoplasia, 10t-17t
Hyporeninemic hypoaldosteronism, 538, 538t, 586, 588-589, 1057
Hypotension
  angiotensin-converting enzyme inhibitors as cause of, 1648
  during hemodialysis, 2105-2106, 2170
  orthostatic, 1538-1539
Hypothalamic gonadotropin-releasing hormone, 1635
Hypothermia, 2414
Hypothyroidism, 495-496, 1916
Hypotonic polyuria, 473t, 482-484
Hypouricemia, 498
Hypovolemia, 963
  absolute, 421-422, 424-425
  arginine vasopressin secretion by, 467-468
  clinical manifestations of, 423
  colloid solutions for, 425
  definition of, 421
  diagnosis of, 423-425
  diuretic-induced, 502
  etiology of, 421
  hemoglobin findings in, 423
  hypoalbuminemia and, 441
  hypokalemia and, 424-425
  laboratory findings in, 423-424
  metabolic acidosis and, 424
  in nephrotic syndrome, 422-423
  plasma potassium concentration in, 423
  plasma sodium concentration in, 423
  potassium chloride for, 424-425
  relative, 422-423, 425, 439
  renal allograft dysfunction caused by, 2265-2266
  renal vein thrombosis caused by, 1206
  replacement fluids for, 424-425
  signs and symptoms of, 423
  treatment of, 424-425
  urea levels in, 423
  urine biochemical parameters for, 423-424
Hypovolemic thirst, 472
Hypoxia
  arginine vasopressin secretion affected by, 470
  in chronic kidney disease, 139
  intrarenal, 139-140
  postglomerular, 1790
Hypoxia-inducible factors, 1373
  -1α, 1888
  -2α, 1888
  anemia and, 1880-1881, 1880f
  description of, 140, 970
  in postglomerular hypoxia, 1790
  preeclampsia and, 1619
  stabilizers, 1892
  von Hippel-Lindau gene and, 1373f

I

Ibandronate, 611-612
I-BOP, 367-368
Ichthyosis, 1943-1944
Icodextrin peritoneal dialysis solution, 2118, 2415-2416
Idiopathic calcium oxalate intake, 1325
Idiopathic hypercalciuria, 1331
Idiopathic infantile hypercalcemia, 2394
Idiopathic rapidly progressive glomerulonephritis, 2151
Ifosfamide, 1397
IgA glomerulonephritis, 2275, 2544
IgA nephropathy. *See* Immunoglobulin A nephropathy
Imaging
   acute kidney injury, 863*f*-864*f*, 866-871, 866*f*-871*f*
   acute pyelonephritis, 878-880
   angiography. *See* Angiography
   angiomyolipomas, 891, 893*f*
   autosomal dominant polycystic kidney disease, 885-888, 888*f*-889*f*
   captopril-enhanced renography, 908
   chronic kidney disease, 863*f*-864*f*, 866-871, 866*f*-871*f*
   computed tomography. *See* Computed tomography
   fibromuscular dysplasia, 907, 907*f*
   iodinated contrast media used in, 847-848
   kidney development studies using, 19
   lymphoma, 899, 902*f*
   magnetic resonance imaging. *See* Magnetic resonance imaging
   malacoplakia, 881-882
   medullary sponge kidney, 888-889
   metastases, 899, 902*f*
   multicystic dysplastic kidney, 889
   obstructive urography evaluations, 871
   pyelonephritis, 1241
      acute, 878-880
      chronic, 882-883
      emphysematous, 881, 882*f*
      xanthogranulomatous, 881, 883*f*
   renal abscess, 880, 881*f*-882*f*
   renal calcifications, 871-878
   renal cell carcinoma, 892, 894*f*-899*f*
   renal function evaluations, 865-866, 866*f*
   renal hamartomas, 891, 893*f*
   renal masses, 883-899, 884*f*-899*f*
   renal neoplasms, 891
   renal transplantation assessments, 909-910, 909*f*-913*f*
   renal tuberculosis, 882, 884*f*
   renal tubular ectasia, 888-889
   renal vascular disease, 903-907, 904*f*-907*f*
   renal vein thrombosis, 908-909
   transitional cell carcinoma, 898-899, 900*f*-901*f*
   ultrasonography. *See* Ultrasonography
Imidapril, 1643, 1643*t*
Imidazole receptor agonists, 1649*t*-1650*t*
IMINO^B, 224-225
Iminoglycinuria, 223*t*, 224, 1450
Immobilization, hypercalcemia caused by, 610
Immune complex-mediated crescentic glomerulonephritis
   aspergillosis associated with, 1150
   in children, 1073
   electron microscopy findings, 1075
   epidemiology of, 1075
   in HIV-infected patients, 1154

Immune complex-mediated crescentic glomerulonephritis *(Continued)*
   immunofluorescence microscopy findings, 1075
   light microscopy findings, 1075
   methylprednisolone for, 1076
   pathogenesis of, 1075-1076
   pathology of, 1075
   treatment of, 1076
Immune disorders, 2104-2105
Immune system, 1535-1536
Immune tolerance, 2229-2230
Immunity, 334, 1233
Immunofluorescence microscopy
   acute poststreptococcal glomerulonephritis findings, 1055, 1055*f*
   Alport's syndrome findings, 1139
   amyloidosis findings, 1130*f*
   anti-glomerular basement membrane disease findings, 1126, 1126*f*
   anti-glomerular basement membrane glomerulonephritis findings, 1077, 1077*f*
   C3 glomerulonephritis findings, 1051-1052
   dense deposit disease findings, 1051, 1051*f*
   fibrillary glomerulonephritis findings, 1071, 1071*f*, 1134*f*
   focal segmental glomerulosclerosis findings, 1026, 1026*f*
   immune complex-mediated crescentic glomerulonephritis findings, 1075
   immunoglobulin A nephropathy findings, 1060-1061
   immunotactoid glomerulopathy findings, 1071
   lupus nephritis findings, 1095*f*-1096*f*, 1097
   membranoproliferative glomerulonephritis findings, 1046-1047, 1048*f*
   membranous nephropathy findings, 1037-1038, 1037*t*, 1038*f*
   microscopic polyangiitis findings, 1115
   minimal change disease findings, 1019
   nail-patella syndrome findings, 1143
   pauci-immune crescentic glomerulonephritis findings, 1082-1083
   sickle cell nephropathy findings, 1145-1146, 1145*f*
   Waldenström's macroglobulinemia findings, 1136
Immunoglobulin A, 1233. *See also* Henoch-Schönlein purpura
Immunoglobulin A nephropathy
   antineutrophil cytoplasmic autoantibodies in, 1064
   autoantibodies in, 1064
   in children, 1059
   classification of, 920, 1059*t*
   clinical features of, 1065-1066
   crescentic, 1068
   description of, 355
   end-stage kidney disease secondary to, 1065
   familial, 1060
   in Far East, 2530-2531, 2530*f*-2531*f*
   galactose-deficient IgA1 in, 1064
   gender differences in progression of, 657
   genetics of, 1060
   genomewide association studies of, 1060
   geographic distribution of, 1059-1060

Immunoglobulin A nephropathy *(Continued)*
   hematuria in, 758, 1065
   Henoch-Schönlein purpura and, 1122-1123
   in HIV-infected patients, 1154
   idiopathic, 1065
   IgA1 in, 1063-1064
   IgA levels in, 1066-1067
   immunofluorescence microscopy findings, 1060-1061
   in Japan, 2531*f*
   laboratory findings in, 1066-1067
   linkage studies of, 1060
   macroscopic hematuria in, 1065
   magnetic resonance imaging of, 870*f*
   microscopic hematuria in, 1065, 1067
   minimal change disease and, 1404
   mycophenolate mofetil for, 1068, 2531
   natural history of, 1065-1066
   nephrotic syndrome caused by, 1059-1069
   outcomes of, 1063, 1066
   Oxford-MEST score, 1063
   pathogenesis of, 1063-1064, 1431
   pathology of, 1060-1063
   podocyte injury in, 1064
   in pregnancy, 1066
   prognostic factors, 1065-1066
   progression of, 1063, 1065-1066, 1068
   proteinuria in, 1065-1066, 1069, 1164-1165
   after renal transplantation, 1069
   secondary, 1065
   treatment of
      aliskiren, 1068
      angiotensin II inhibitors, 1067-1068
      azathioprine, 1068
      cyclophosphamide, dipyridamole, and warfarin combination therapy, 1068
      fish oil, 1069
      glucocorticoids, 1067-1068
      mycophenolate mofetil, 1068
      omega-3 fatty acids, 1069
      prednisone, 1067
      summary of, 1069
      tonsillectomy, 1068-1069
   upper respiratory tract infection and, 755
Immunoglobulins
   G, in membranous nephropathy, 1037-1039, 1038*f*
   in Henoch-Schönlein purpura, 1122-1123
   light chains, 967-968
   M, in minimal change disease, 1018*t*, 1019
Immunohistochemical assay, 921-922
Immunologic intolerance, 1620-1621
Immunophilins, 2247
Immunosuppression
   allograft survival rates with, 2236
   breastfeeding and, 1638
   cancer risks secondary to, 2284, 2433
   future of, 2290
   history of, 2229
   during pregnancy, 1637-1638, 1637*t*
Immunosuppressive agents
   alemtuzumab, 2248, 2255-2256
   allograft survival rates with, 2236
   anti-CD20 monoclonal antibody, 2256
   antiproliferative, 2257-2258
   antithymocyte globulins, 2255
   azathioprine, 2245, 2254*t*, 2257
   belatacept, 2248, 2254*t*, 2258-2259
   bone histology affected by, 1851-1852
   calcineurin inhibitors, 2256
   cessation of, 2290
   corticosteroids, 2245, 2254*t*, 2259

Immunosuppressive agents (Continued)
  costimulatory signal blockers, 2258-2259
  cyclosporine, 2246-2247, 2254t, 2256-2257
  daclizumab, 2256
  in elderly, 749
  everolimus, 2247, 2258
  genomics for, 2249
  granulomatous with polyangiitis treated with, 1112
  hepatitis C treated with, 1156
  history of, 2229
  interleukin-2 receptor antagonist, 2256
  JAK3 inhibitor, 2258
  lupus nephritis treated with, 1103, 1105
  maintenance types of, 2256-2257
  mammalian target of rapamycin inhibitors, 2247, 2258
  mechanism of action, 2246f, 2253-2255, 2254f
  monoclonal antibodies, 2248-2249, 2255-2256
  muromonab-CD3, 2255-2256
  mycophenolate mofetil, 2245-2246, 2246f, 2254t, 2257-2258
  mycophenolic acid, 2245-2246, 2246f
  overview of, 2253-2255, 2254t
  polyclonal immune globulins, 2247-2248, 2255
  proteomics, 2249
  protocols for, 2259
  rapamycin, 2247
  rituximab, 2256
  sirolimus, 2254t, 2258
  tacrolimus, 2247, 2254t, 2257-2258
  tofacitinib, 2258
  voclosporin, 2257
Immunotactoid glomerulopathy
  characteristics of, 1069-1070, 1132
  clinical features of, 1072
  cryoglobulinemia and, 1071
  electron microscopy findings, 1070f, 1071, 1133f
  end-stage kidney disease progression of, 1072, 1134
  epidemiology of, 1072
  fibrillary glomerulonephritis versus, 1069-1070
  immunofluorescence findings, 1071
  light microscopy findings, 1071
  nephrotic syndrome caused by, 1069-1072
  pathogenesis of, 1071
  pathology of, 1070f, 1071, 1133f
  proteinuria in, 1072, 1132
  renal insufficiency in, 1072
  treatment of, 1072
Immunotherapy, 1385
Immunoturbidimetric technique, 794
Impetigo, 1953
Importin-α, 306-307
Impotence, 1731-1732
Inborn errors of metabolism, 2417
Incidentaloma, 766-767
India. See Indian subcontinent
Indian subcontinent
  acute kidney injury in
    acute cortical necrosis as cause of, 2501-2502
    bee stings as cause of, 2500
    causes of, 2495, 2495t
    chemical toxins as cause of, 2500-2501
    chromic acid poisoning as cause of, 2501
    copper sulfate poisoning as cause of, 2500
    demographics of, 2495
    dengue fever as cause of, 2498-2499

Indian subcontinent (Continued)
    diarrheal diseases as cause of, 2496
    ethylene dibromide poisoning as cause of, 2501
    ethylene glycol poisoning as cause of, 2500-2501
    glucose-6-phosphate dehydrogenase deficiency as cause of, 2501
    hair dye as cause of, 2501
    hemolytic uremic syndrome as cause of, 2496
    hornet stings as cause of, 2500
    infections as cause of, 2496-2499
    intravascular hemolysis as cause of, 2501
    leptospirosis as cause of, 2497-2498
    malaria as cause of, 2496-2497
    snakebites as cause of, 2499-2500
    surgical causes of, 2496
    wasp stings as cause of, 2500
    zygomycosis as cause of, 2498, 2498f
  aortoarteritis in, 2506-2507
  chronic kidney disease in
    causes of, 2502-2503, 2502t
    demographics of, 2502-2503
    diabetic nephropathy as cause of, 2503
    financial issues, 2503
    hemodialysis for, 2503-2504
    incidence of, 2502
    peritoneal dialysis for, 2504
    prevalence of, 2502
    reimbursement issues, 2503
  development indicators in, 2495t
  economic indicators in, 2495t
  end-stage kidney disease in, 2503
  geography of, 2494
  glomerulonephritis in, 2506, 2506t
  hemodialysis in, 2503-2504
  herbal medicine toxicity in, 2507-2508
  indigenous therapies of, 2507-2508
  nephrolithiasis in, 2507
  nephrotic syndrome in, 2506t
  renal calculi in, 2507
  renal replacement therapy in, 2503-2504
  renal transplantation in, 2504-2506
  renovascular hypertension in, 2506-2507
  Takayasu arteritis in, 2506
Indoles, 1812
Indomethacin, 1269
Indonesia, 2536
Indoxyl sulfate, 1812
Induced pluripotent stem cells, 2606-2607
Inducible nitric oxide synthases, 416, 979, 1739
INF2 disease, 1429
INF2 protein, 1429
Infants. See also Children
  hypocalcemic, 2392
  renal transplantation in, 2420
  syndrome of inappropriate antidiuretic hormone secretion in, 499
Infection(s)
  acute interstitial nephritis caused by, 1219
  in acute kidney injury, 996
  acute kidney injury caused by
    in Far East, 2511-2523, 2511f, 2512t
    in Indian subcontinent, 2496-2499
  catheter-related, 2068f, 2128, 2131
  focal segmental glomerulosclerosis caused by, 1030
  glomerulonephritis caused by, 2527, 2528t
  in hemodialysis patients, 2061, 2104-2105
  renal transplantation complicated by, 2286-2288, 2287t, 2420-2421, 2505-2506
  susceptibility to, in nephrotic syndrome, 1805

Infection stone, 1323f, 1346-1347, 1365-1366
Infectious endocarditis, 1148-1149
Inferior vena cava occlusion, 440
Inferior venacavography, 1204-1205
Inflammation
  in acute kidney injury pathophysiology, 981
  anemia of chronic disease and, 1887
  cardiovascular disease risks, 1865, 2100
  in chronic kidney disease, 1865, 1909, 1969-1970
  erythropoiesis affected by, 1887
  in hemodialysis, 1913
  markers of, 1942
  oxidative stress affected by, 1758
  in peritoneal dialysis, 2125-2126
  protein wasting and, 1817
  in proteinuria, 1792-1794
  renal parenchymal, 975-977
  renin-angiotensin-aldosterone system and, 334
  tubulointerstitial, 1215
Inflammatory bowel disease, hyperoxaluria in, 1342f
Informed consent, for kidney biopsy, 917-919
Infusion equilibrium technique, 1332
Inherited Fanconi's syndrome, 1435, 1435t
Inherited primary glomerular disorder of unknown cause, 1431
Inherited renal tubulopathy, 1417-1418
Inhibition of crystal agglomeration, 1329
Inhibitory factor 1, 140
Initial collecting tubules, 65-66, 68, 69f, 70, 241-242
Innate inflammatory immune response, 1791-1792
Inner medulla
  concentrating mechanism of, 271-273
  description of, 45, 45f, 91-92, 91f
  sodium chloride concentration in, 271-273
  urea accumulation in, 268-270
Inner medullary collecting duct (IMCD)
  anatomy of, 44-45, 45f, 74, 75f, 166, 239, 262
  bicarbonate reabsorption in, 242
  cell of, 241
  eNOS activation in, 417
  Na^+-K^+-ATPase in, 254
  portions of, 74, 77f
  potassium transport in, 133
  principal cells of, 75, 76f
  terminal portion of, 77f
Inositol 1,4,5-triphosphate, 1825
Insect stings, 2525
Institute of Medicine, 2620
Insulin
  diabetic ketoacidosis treated with, 547
  glucose and, 594
  hypokalemic effect of, 562, 570
  Na^+-H^+ exchanger activation by, 818
  phosphate excretion affected by, 200
  potassium distribution affected by, 562, 587, 594
Insulin receptor substrate 1, 1913
Insulin receptor-related receptor, 256
Insulin resistance
  adverse effects of, 1816
  cardiovascular risk and, 1914
  causes of, 1913, 1913t
  in chronic kidney disease, 1315, 1912-1916, 1913t
  definition of, 1912
  in end-stage kidney disease, 1816

Insulin resistance *(Continued)*
  hemodialysis effects on, 1317
  homeostasis model assessment-estimated, 1912, 1914f
  in peritoneal dialysis, 1913
  thiazolidinediones for modulating of, 2127
  treatment of, 1914-1915
  uremic, 1816, 1913-1915
  vitamin D in, 1913
Insulin-like growth factor-binding proteins
  -1, 718
  -7, 949, 989
  description of, 1917-1918
Insulin-like growth factors
  -1, 181, 197-198, 200, 1212, 1967, 1970-1971, 2099, 2612
  -2, 1744
  description of, 718
Intact nephron hypothesis, 1736-1737
Integrated Discrimination Improvement Index, 929-930
$\alpha_8\beta_1$-Integrin, 25
β-Integrin receptors, on mesangial cells, 51-52
Intensive care unit, 628, 2137, 2139-2140, 2458-2459
Intercalated cells
  acid-base perturbations and, 245-246
  basolateral anion exchanger in, 243
  bicarbonate secretion by, 519
  carbonic anhydrase levels in, 71-72
  collecting ducts
    bicarbonate reabsorption, 239-241, 239f-241f
    description of, 30, 69-71, 72f
  in connecting tubules, 68-69
  of cortical collecting duct, 70-71, 72f
  of distal convoluted tubule, 238-239
  of inner medullary collecting duct, 75
  kidney anion exchanger 1 in, 243
  mineralocorticoid receptor, 314
  non-A, non-B, 241
  of outer medullary collecting duct, 74f
  transcellular chloride absorption across, 171
  type A, 70-72, 72f, 239-241, 240f-241f, 533-534
  type B, 70-72, 72f, 240f-241f, 241, 519
  type C, 241
Intercellular adhesion molecule-1, 1097, 1215
Intercellular junctions, 4-5
Interdisciplinary clinics, 2632-2634, 2633f
Interferon, 1385
Interferon-α, 1159, 1398, 2486
Interleukin-2, 1385, 1398, 2248
Interleukin-2 receptor antagonist, 2256
Interleukin-6, 1197, 1233, 2100
Interleukin-8, 1233
Interleukin-13, 1020
Interleukin-18, 939-941, 989
Interlobar arteries, 84
Interlobular arteries, 84, 84f
Intermesenteric plexus, 80-81
Intermittent centrifugation, 2160
Intermittent hemodialysis, 1006-1007
International Verapamil-Trandolapril Study (INVEST), 1553-1554
Internist's tumor, 1374
Interpodocyte space, 1781
Interstitial calcium plaque, 1325
Interstitial cells, 77-80, 78f

Interstitial fibrosis, 728f. *See also* Renal fibrosis
  chronic hypoxia in, 1217-1218
  end-stage kidney disease caused by, 1216-1217
  epithelial-mesenchymal transitions in, 1217
  pathophysiology of, 1277
  tubulointerstitial injury caused by, 1216-1218
Interstitial fibrosis and tubular atrophy, 2244
Interstitial nephritis, 363, 1158, 1505-1509, 1507t, 2476
Interstitial pressure, 761
Interventional nephrologists, 2193, 2193t
Interventional nephrology
  access-induced hand ischemia, 2214
  arteriovenous fistulas. *See* Arteriovenous fistulas
  arteriovenous grafts. *See* Arteriovenous grafts
  central vein stenosis treated with, 2212-2214, 2212f-2214f
  hemodialysis catheters. *See* Hemodialysis, catheters for
  percutaneous kidney biopsy, 2222-2224, 2223t, 2224f
  peritoneal dialysis catheters, 2220-2222
  personal safety in, 2194
  procedures performed in, 2193t
  radiation safety in, 2194
  rationale for, 2192-2194
  stenotic lesions treated with, 2212
Intestine
  calcium absorption in, 185-187, 1824-1825
  magnesium homeostasis by, 193-194, 193f
  phosphorus secretion into, 196
  potassium loss in, 574
Intraabdominal hypertension, 2138
Intracellular adhesion molecule-1, 728
Intracellular fluid
  in children, 2365-2366
  description of, 390-391
  osmotic pressure of, 461
  potassium in, 174
  solute composition of, 461
  total body water in, 460
Intracerebral hemorrhage, 1619-1620, 1927
Intracranial aneurysm, 1494-1495
Intracranial pressure, 2139
Intradialytic hypotension, 1007
Intrahepatic hypertension, 441
Intrarenal progenitor cells, 2608-2609
Intrauterine growth restriction, 665, 700f, 2300
Intravenous immune globulin, 1105, 2157
Intravenous pyelography, 1253, 1253f, 1265, 1265f, 1359
Intravenous urography
  computed tomography urography versus, 852
  description of, 846-847
  excretory phase of, 847f
  kidney stone disease evaluations, 873
  medullary sponge kidney on, 888-889
  nephrogram, 846-847, 847f
  renal masses on, 883
  transitional cell carcinoma evaluations, 898-899, 900f
Intrinsic acute kidney injury. *See* Acute kidney injury (AKI), intrinsic
Intrinsic kidney disease, 1544-1550
Inulin, 786
Iodide, 1915

Iodinated contrast media, 847-848
Iodine 131-labeled ortho-iodohippurate, 865
Iodocholesterol scintigraphy, 1546
Iododerma, 1947, 1947f
Iohexol, 736, 787, 2310
Ion exchange resins, 596
Ion trapping, 2168
Ionized calcium, 1824
Iothalamate, 787
IP receptors, 369
IQGAP1, 113
Iran. *See* Middle East
Irbesartan, 1305-1306, 1652, 1652t
Iron
  anemia treated with, 1892-1904, 2098
    intravenous iron, 1896-1900, 1897t
    markers of, 1893-1896
    parenteral administration, 1898
    safety of, 1900-1902
  balance of, 1896
  bone marrow, 1895
  chronic kidney disease treated with, 1898-1900, 1899t
  deficiency of, 1887, 1893, 1940
  description of, 1892-1900
  in erythropoiesis, 1883-1884, 1893
  intravenous, for anemia, 1891f, 1896-1900, 2098
  liver magnetic resonance imaging of, 1895
  markers of, 1893-1896
    bone marrow, 1895
    erythrocyte ferritin concentration, 1894
    erythrocyte zinc protoporphyrin concentration, 1894
    hypochromic red blood cells, 1894-1895
    reticulocyte hemoglobin content, 1895
    serum ferritin, 1893
    serum transferrin receptor, 1893-1894
  maternal restriction from, 716
  metabolism of, 1885-1887, 1886f
  parenteral administration of, 1898
  serum, 1893
Iron chelators, 967
Iron dextran, 1896, 1897t
Iron isomaltoside 1000, 1897t, 1898
Iron sucrose, 1896, 1897t
Ischemia-reperfusion injury, 1786
Ischemic nephropathy, 1567-1568
  diagnosis and evaluation of, 1588-1594, 1588t
  endovascular renal angioplasty and stenting, 1599
  management of, 1608f
  mechanism of, 1574-1575
  pathophysiology of, 1570-1580
  surgical treatment of, 1604-1607
  therapy goals for, 1588
Ischemic renal injury, 350
Ischemic stroke, 1927
Islet cell transplantation, 1319-1320
Isolated dominant hypomagnesemia with hypocalciuria, 1466
Isolated hypoaldosteronism, 538-539, 539t
Isolated office hypertension, 1540
Isolated proteinuria, 1013-1014
Isolated recessive hypomagnesemia, 1466-1467
Isolated renal hypoplasia, 2297t
Isolated systolic hypertension, 1685
Isopropanol, 2173-2178, 2174t, 2176t
Isopropyl alcohol-induced high anion gap acidosis, 549
Isoproterenol, 200-201, 245
Isosmotic sodium storage, 1530

Isosthenuria, 986
Isothermic dialysis, 2095
Isotonic saline, 503-504
Isotopic renography, 1266-1267, 1280
Isradipine, 1665, 1669-1670
Israel, 2477t

J

Jaffe method, 782, 787
JAK3 inhibitor, 2258
Janus tyrosine kinases-2, 1881-1882
Japan, 2531f, 2534-2535
Joubert's syndrome, 1508-1509, 2322, 2322t
Juxtaglomerular apparatus (JGA)
    anatomy of, 53
    angiotensin I secretion by, 326
    autonomic innervation of, 54-55
    composition of, 35
    definition of, 106
    description of, 35-36
    histology of, 54f
    noradrenergic nerve endings in, 327
    renin secretion by, 334-335, 360, 568
    vascular component of, 53
Juxtaglomerular cell tumor, 1369
Juxtaglomerular granular cells, 53, 54f, 55
Juxtaglomerular nephrons, 99, 100f
Juxtamedullary arterioles, 88f

K

Kaliuresis, 181-182, 574-577, 588
Kallikrein, 245, 346-350
Kallikrein-kinin system
    in anti-glomerular basement membrane disease, 350
    in antineutrophil cytoplasmic antibody-associated vasculitis, 350
    bradykinin receptors, 347
    in chronic kidney disease, 350
    components of, 346-347
    definition of, 346
    description of, 417
    in diabetic nephropathy, 349-350
    discovery of, 346
    enzymatic cascade of, 348f
    genetic mutations of, 349
    in hypertension, 349
    in ischemic renal injury, 350
    kallikrein, 346-347
    kallistatin, 347
    kininases, 347
    kininogen, 346
    in lupus nephritis, 350
    plasma, 347-348
    renal, 348-349
    renal blood flow regulation by, 348
    renin-angiotensin-aldosterone system and, 418
    tissue, 347-348
Kallistatin, 347
Kallmann's syndrome, 2297t, 2318
Kaposi's sarcoma, 2285, 2492
Kayser-Fleisher ring, 1444-1445
KCC4, 243
KCC proteins, 150
KCNJ5, 568-569, 575
KCNJ1, 2334
KCNQ1, 177
Ketoacidosis
    acetoacetic acid excretion in, 247
    alcoholic, 547
    diabetic, 525, 546-547, 628, 633, 2398
    high anion gap acidosis caused by, 543, 546-547

Ketoacidosis (Continued)
    β-hydroxybutyric acid excretion in, 247
    starvation, 547
    treatment of, metabolic acidosis after, 555
Ketoconazole, 1332-1333
15-Ketodehydrogenase, 374
α-Ketoglutarate, 218-219, 517
Ketones, 790
K_f, 99
Kidney
    afferent nerve supply to, 81
    agenesis of, 2302
    anatomy of, 42-82, 260f, 849f. See also specific anatomy
    in animals, 43
    arteries of, 83-85
    bisected, 43f-44f
    blood flow to. See Renal blood flow
    congenital anomalies of. See Congenital anomalies of the kidney and urinary tract
    dysplasia of. See Renal dysplasia
    efferent nerve supply to, 80-81
    embryology of, 2603
    function of. See Renal function
    gluconeogenesis by, 130-132
    gross features of, 42-43
    horseshoe, 2295, 2296f, 2303-2304, 2311
    in utero development of, 2302
    innervation of, 80-81
    length of, 42-43
    lymphatic system of, 80, 80f
    malformation of, in children, 2294-2295, 2295f, 2311. See also Congenital anomalies of the kidney and urinary tract
    microcirculations of. See Microcirculations
    outer cortical region of, 5
    peptide clearance by, 1810
    regeneration of, developmental approaches to, 2613
    regions of, 43
    size of, 850
    ultrasonography of, 850-851, 850f
    vascular-tubule relations in, 87
    vasculature of, 42, 43f
    veins of, 83-85
    weight of, 42
Kidney anion exchanger, 239-241
Kidney anion exchanger 1, 243
Kidney biopsy
    acute cortical necrosis diagnosis using, 2501-2502
    acute interstitial nephritis evaluations, 1220
    acute kidney injury diagnosis using, 772-773, 990
    algorithm for, 918f
    bleeding complications of, 915-917, 2223
    cirrhosis evaluations, 1156-1157
    complications of, 915-917, 2223
    contraindications for, 917, 917t, 2223
    description of, 915
    diagnoses obtained from, 916f
    electron microscopy analysis, 922, 923t
    fetal, 1280
    for fibrillary glomerulonephritis, 1132-1134
    flowchart for, 918f
    glomerular disease on, 920
    glomerulonephritis evaluations, 2544
    hematuria evaluations, 1016
    history of, 915
    idiopathic nephrotic syndrome, 2328-2329
    immunohistochemical assay, 921-922
    indications for, 915-917, 916t

Kidney biopsy (Continued)
    informed consent for, 917-919
    laparoscopic, 917, 917t
    light microscopy in
        biopsy report details about, 924
        fixative for, 919
        specimen examination, 920, 920t
        staining for, 919-920
        thin sections for, 919
    nephritic syndrome evaluations, 760
    nephrotic syndrome evaluations, 763-764
    open approach, 917, 917t
    percutaneous, 2222-2224, 2223t, 2224f
    performing of, 918-919
    real-time ultrasound guidance during, 2223-2224, 2223t, 2224f
    report from, 924
    risks of, 917t
    safety of, 915-917
    specimens, 919-920, 920t, 923-924
    transjugular, 917, 917t
    ultrasonography uses during, 850
Kidney development
    adhesion proteins in, 25
    collecting system, 5
    fetal, maternal single kidney effects on, 721
    genetic analysis of, 21-40, 22f
        adhesion proteins, 25
        collecting system, 25-27
        juxtaglomerular apparatus, 35-36
        nephron development, 30-31
        non-GDNF pathways in metanephric mesenchyme, 23
        stromal cell lineage, 31-32
        tubulogenesis, 30-31
        ureteric bud and metanephric mesenchyme interaction, 21-25
        ureteric bud positioning, 27-28
        vascular formation, 32-35, 33f
    imaging studies of, 19
    interstitial cells, 5-6
    lineage tracing studies of, 19
    metanephros, 3, 3f-4f
    model systems for studying
        antisense oligonucleotides, 7-9
        Caenorhabditis elegans, 19
        conditional mouse lines, 18t
        Drosophila, 20
        knockout mouse models, 9-19, 10t-17t
        mutant phenotypic analyses, 7
        nonmammalian, 19-21
        organ culture, 6-9
        transgenic mouse models, 9-19, 10t-17t
        Xenopus laevis, 21
        zebrafish, 20-21
    nephrogenic zone, 5
    nephron, 4-5
    overview of, 4f
    programming of, 713-723, 715t
    renal stroma, 5-6
    stages of, 2-3, 3f
    urogenital system, 2-3
    vasculature, 6, 7f
Kidney disease
    acute. See Acute kidney injury
    advanced care planning for, 2599-2600
    African American study of kidney disease and hypertension, 1553
    cardiovascular disease in, 1166
    causes of, 1410-1411
    chronic. See Chronic kidney disease
    genetic approaches to, 1410
    lymphoma and, 1401-1402
    preeclampsia and, 1617-1618
    uromodulin-associated, 165

Kidney Disease: Improving Global Outcomes, 669-670, 773, 774t, 792t, 930-931, 931t, 960-961, 1005, 1839-1841, 1846, 1868-1871, 1902, 1989-1990, 1989f, 2025, 2028, 2191-2192, 2404-2405, 2474, 2587, 2621-2622, 2632, 2634t
Kidney Disease Outcomes Quality Initiative, 643-645, 669-670, 773, 773t
Kidney donor profile index, 2279
Kidney Health Australia, 2539
Kidney Health Initiative, 953-954
Kidney injury molecule-1, 941-942, 989
Kidney size, 700-701, 700f, 713-715
Kidney stones. See also Calcium oxalate stones; Calcium stone; Urolithiasis
　analysis of, 1359
　calcium oxalate, 1260
　causes of
　　calcium intake, 1324
　　dietary factors, 1354
　　melamine, 1348
　　over-the-counter drugs, 1347
　　protein consumption, 1324
　in children, 2340-2342
　chronic kidney disease and, 1352
　diagnostic approach
　　computed tomography, 873, 875f-876f
　　history-taking, 767-768
　　imaging, 768-769, 871-878, 874f-878f
　　intravenous urography, 873
　　laboratory tests, 768
　　magnetic resonance imaging, 876, 876f
　　magnetic resonance urography, 876-878, 877f
　　physical examination, 768
　　plain radiographs, 874f
　　review of systems, 767-768
　　ultrasonography, 873, 875f
　　urine studies, 768
　differential diagnosis of, 769, 769t
　enteric hyperoxaluria and, 1325
　environment, lifestyle, and medical history for, 1355
　epidemiology of, 1322-1324
　family history of, 1355-1356
　genetics and, 1348-1350
　histopathology of, 1325
　imaging studies of, 1359-1360
　incidence of, 1324
　inhibitors of, 1329-1331, 1329t, 1337f
　interstitial calcium plaque and, 1325
　laboratory evaluation for, 1356-1360
　management of, 1360-1366, 1360f
　medications associated with, 767
　nonsteroidal anti-inflammatory drugs for, 769
　occurrence of, 1323f
　pharmacotherapeutic trial for, 1363t
　predisposing medical conditions for, 767-768
　prevalence of, 767, 1260, 1322-1323
　in renal fusion, 2304
　risk factors for, 767
　risk of, 1327f
　Roux-en-Y gastric bypass and, 1340, 1341t
　in sarcoidosis, 1228
　signs and symptoms of, 767, 1355
　treatment of, 769
　types of, 1323f
　ureteral obstruction caused by, 1260
　urinary tract cancer and, 1352
　vertebral bone loss and, 1354-1355

Kidney transplantation. See Renal transplantation
Kidneys, ureters, and bladder x-ray, 846, 847f, 1359
Kidney-specific chloride channel 1 knockout mice model, 278
Kidney-specific protein, 2603-2604
Kif26b, 22-23
Killer inhibitory receptors, 2243
Kimmelstiel-Wilson nodular lesions, 1285-1286
Kimura's disease, 1159
Kinases, in aquaporin-2 trafficking, 292-293
Kindlin-2, 1217
Kininases, 347
Kininogen, 346
Kinins, 346-347, 417-418
Kir1.1, 278
Kir3.4, 306
KIR4.1 protein, 167
KIR4.2 protein, 167
Klotho, 191, 1822, 1830-1831, 1832t, 1841-1842, 1978-1979, 2390
KLOTHO, 627, 632, 732, 734
Knockout mice models
　aquaporin-1, 273-276
　aquaporin-2, 276
　aquaporin-3, 276
　aquaporin-4, 276
　epithelial sodium channel, 278
　kidney development studies using, 9-19, 10t-17t
　kidney-specific chloride channel 1, 278
　Na$^+$-H$^+$-exchanger isoform 3, 278
　Na$^+$-K$^+$-2Cl cotransporter type 2, 278
　prostanoid receptors, 368f
　renal outer medullary potassium, 278
　type 2 vasopressin receptor, 278-279
　UT-A1/3 urea transporter, 276-278
Korea, 2535
Korotkoff phase V disappearance of sound, 1524
Kussmaul's sign, 761-762

L

Labetalol, 1629, 1630t, 1658, 1658t, 1695t, 1697t
Lacidipine, 1666
Lacis, 53
β-Lactams, 719, 1234, 1239
Lactate
　handling of, 130-132
　L-lactic acidosis and, 544-545
　metabolism of, 544
　in peritoneal dialysis solutions, 2117
　in renal metabolism, 131f
Lactic acid, 544
Lactic acidosis, 543t, 544-546
　alkali therapy for, 546
　carbon monoxide poisoning as cause of, 545
　case study of, 839-840
　clinical features of, 545
　clinical spectrum of, 545
　D-, 544
　diagnosis of, 545
　dichloroacetate for, 546
　drugs that cause, 545
　hyperphosphatemia caused by, 628
　inborn errors of metabolism as cause of, 545
　L-, 544-546
　medical conditions associated with, 545

Lactic acidosis *(Continued)*
　metformin-associated, 2184-2185
　physiology of, 544-545
　toxins that cause, 545
　treatment of, 545-546, 555
Lactobacillus crispatus probiotic, 1239-1240
LacY, 213-214
Lama5, 25
Lamb2, 25
LAMB2 gene, 1426
Lamc1, 25
Laminin disease. See Pierson's syndrome
Lanthanum carbonate, 2021-2022
Laparoscopic kidney biopsy, 917, 917t
Large vessel renovascular disease, 1578f
L-arginine, 979
Latency-associated protein, 1212-1213
Latin America
　acute kidney injury in, 2440-2444
　brain death criteria in, 2451
　chronic kidney disease in, 2447-2449
　demographic changes in, 2447-2448
　dengue fever, 2440-2441
　end-stage kidney disease in, 2449-2451, 2449f, 2450t
　health care coverage in, 2451-2452
　hemodialysis in, 2450t
　leptospirosis, 2443-2444, 2443f
　life expectancy in, 2440
　Lonomia caterpillar stings, 2445-2446, 2446f
　malaria, 2442-2443
　nephropathy in, 2448-2449
　peritoneal dialysis in, 2450t
　population of, 2440
　renal replacement therapy in, 2449, 2450t
　renal transplantation in, 2451
　snakebites, 2446-2447
　spider bites, 2445-2446, 2445f
　trends in, 2451-2452
　yellow fever, 2441-2442, 2442f
Laws of thermodynamics, 123
L-Carnitine, 2107, 2125
LCAT gene, 1148
LCZ696, 345-346
Lead
　chronic kidney disease risks, 686-687
　chronic tubulointerstitial nephritis caused by, 1226-1227
　end-stage kidney disease secondary to exposure to, 1226-1227
Lead nephropathy, 686-687, 1227
Lean principles, 2623-2624, 2623t, 2624f
Lecithin-cholesterol acyltransferase (LCAT), 1147-1148, 1147f, 1802
Lecticans, 30
Left ventricle, 434, 1857, 1859
Left ventricular ejection fraction, 434
Left ventricular hypertrophy (LVH)
　blood pressure and, 1688-1689
　as cardiovascular disease risk factor, 1295-1296, 1857-1858, 1924, 1978-1979, 2100-2102, 2421-2422
　in children, 2360-2361, 2421-2422, 2432
　in chronic kidney disease, 2360-2361
　description of, 1295-1296, 1857-1858
　furosemide for, 1721-1722
　in pediatric end-stage kidney disease, 2408, 2421-2422, 2432
　treatment of, 1721
Leiomyoma, 1369
Leishmaniasis, 1150-1151
Leptin, 1819

Volume 1 pp. 1-1321 • Volume 2 pp. 1322-2636

Leptospira spp., 2443, 2497-2498, 2511
Leptospirosis
  acute kidney injury caused by, 2443-2444, 2443f, 2497-2498, 2511-2513, 2511f, 2512t
  clinical features of, 2497-2498
  clinical manifestations of, 2511, 2512t-2513t
  diagnosis of, 2498, 2513
  in Far East, 2511-2513, 2511f, 2512t, 2528f
  histologic features of, 2498
  in Indian subcontinent, 2497-2498
  pathogenesis of, 2498
  pathology of, 2511f, 2513f
  penicillin for, 2513, 2514f
  treatment of, 2498, 2513, 2514f
Lercanidipine, 1666
Lesch-Nyhan syndrome, 1347
Leucovorin, 2188
Leukemia, 1401-1403
Leukocyte(s)
  activation of, 1909-1910
  functional impairment of, 1909
  in urine, 799-800
  vascular endothelium adherence of, 981
Leukocyte esterase, 790
Leukocytoclastic angiitis, 1154
Leukocytoclastic vasculitis, 1950-1951, 1951f
Leukopenia, 1650, 2434
Leukotriene A_4, 379-381
Leukotriene B_4, 381-382
Leukotriene B_4 receptor, 380
Leukotriene C_4, 381
LeuT fold, 229, 230t, 231f
Levamisole, 2330
Levodopa, 1940
Levofloxacin, 1241t
Lgr5-EGFP transgene, 19
Lhx1, 23
Licorice, 556
Liddle's syndrome, 311-312, 556, 565, 578, 1462-1463, 1463t, 2379
Lifestyle modifications
  chronic kidney disease progression affected by, 1990-1995
  hypertension treated with, 745-746
  restless legs syndrome managed with, 1940
Light- and heavy-chain deposition disease, 1134-1136
Light microscopy
  acute poststreptococcal glomerulonephritis findings, 1054-1055, 1055f
  Alport's syndrome findings, 1139
  anti-glomerular basement membrane glomerulonephritis findings, 1077-1078
  biopsy analysis using, 919-920, 920t, 924
  dense deposit disease findings, 1051
  diabetic nephropathy findings, 1285f
  Fabry's disease findings, 1144, 1144f
  fibrillary glomerulonephritis findings, 1071
  focal segmental glomerulosclerosis findings, 1024f, 1025-1026
  immune complex-mediated crescentic glomerulonephritis findings, 1075
  immunotactoid glomerulopathy findings, 1071
  membranoproliferative glomerulonephritis findings, 1046, 1047f
  membranous nephropathy findings, 1038, 1038f

Light microscopy *(Continued)*
  microscopic polyangiitis findings, 1114-1115, 1114f
  minimal change disease findings, 1015t, 1016-1019
  pauci-immune crescentic glomerulonephritis findings, 1082, 1082f
Light-chain deposition disease, 1134-1136, 1135f, 1391-1393
LIM homeobox transcription factor 1 beta, 1431
Limulus amoebocyte lysate assay, 2082
Lincosamides, 1235t-1236t
Lindsay's nail, 1949-1950, 1949f
Lineage tracing, kidney development studies using, 19
Lip cancer, 2285
Lipid(s)
  β-adrenergic antagonist therapy effects on, 1661
  glomerular-filtered, 1213
  metabolism of, 733-734, 1816-1817
  peroxidation of, 375
  in renal disease, 1773
  uremia effects on metabolism of, 1816-1817
Lipid rafts, 37-38
Lipid-lowering therapy, 1312
Lipiduria, 762-763, 763f
Lipocalin 2. *See* Neutrophil gelatinase-associated lipocalin
Lipodystrophy, 1053, 1146-1147
Lipofuscin, 728f
Lipoid nephrosis, 1016, 1019
Lipoma, 1369
Lipopolysaccharides, 238
Lipoprotein
  high-density, 1761, 1863, 2100
  low-density. *See* Low-density lipoprotein
  in nephrotic syndrome, 1802
  synthesis of, 1801
  very-low-density, 1801-1802
Lipoprotein glomerulopathy, 1148
Lipoprotein lipase, 1802
Lipoprotein(a), 1863, 2100
Lipoprotein-X, 1148
Lipotoxicity, 1344-1345, 1345f
Lipoxins, 380
Lipoxygenases
  5-, 379-380
  10-, 379-380
  15-, 379-380
  arachidonic acid metabolism by, 379f
  biologic activities of, 381
  description of, 355, 379-380
  enzymes, 379-380
  in renal pathophysiology, 381-382
Lisinopril, 1643, 1643t
Lithium
  aquaporin-2 expression affected by, 297-299, 298f
  chronic tubulointerstitial nephropathy caused by, 1226, 1226f
  hypercalcemia caused by, 609
  hyperparathyroidism associated with, 1226
  loop diuretics effect on, 1732
  minimal change disease caused by, 1159
  nephrogenic diabetes insipidus caused by, 297-299, 298f, 379, 482, 1226
  nephrotoxicity of, 379
  overdose of, 2180-2181
  polyuria caused by, 379
  renal cysts caused by, 889, 890f
  toxicokinetics of, 2180

Lithogenesis, 1325-1329
Lithotripsy, 878f
Live donor nephrectomy, 2252
Live donor renal transplantation, 2252, 2278, 2582
Liver
  cancer of, acute kidney injury and, 1390
  dysfunction of, 2139
  tyrosinemia and, 1443
  Wilson's disease and, 1444
Liver cyst, 1484
Liver disease, 991t, 993-994, 998-999
Liver flukes, 2522-2523
Liver transplantation
  atypical hemolytic-uremic syndrome treated with, 1186-1188
  glomerular filtration rate after, 458
  hepatorenal syndrome treated with, 458
  Model of End-stage Liver Disease scores, 458
Liver-type fatty acid-binding protein, 942-943, 989, 1213
Lixivaptan, 454, 456-457
LLC-PK1 cells, 160, 161f
Localized renal cystic disease, 1512-1513
Long QT syndrome, 569
Lonomia caterpillars, 2445-2446, 2446f
Loop diuretics
  absorption of, 1707
  acute kidney injury treated with, 1725-1726
  acute tubular necrosis treated with, 1001-1002
  adverse effects of, 1710
  calcium transport regulation by, 189-190
  ceiling doses of, 1726t
  distal convoluted tubule hypertrophy caused by, 1715
  distal potassium-sparing diuretics and, 1719
  dose-response curve for, 1721f
  drug interactions, 1732
  hypercalcemia treated with, 610-611
  hyperlipidemia caused by, 1731
  hypervolemia treated with, 450-451
  hypokalemia caused by, 1728
  hypomagnesemia caused by, 621
  idiopathic nephrotic syndrome treated with, 2329
  indications for, 1710
  lithium plasma concentrations affected by, 1732
  magnesium reabsorption affected by, 1730
  mechanism of action, 1705-1707, 1705f
  metabolic alkalosis caused by, 1704, 1730
  metabolism of, 1707-1708
  in nephrotic syndrome, 1725
  ototoxicity caused by, 1732
  pharmacokinetics of, 1707-1710
  proximal fluid reabsorption affected by, 1706
  renin secretion stimulation by, 1706-1707
  resistance to, 1718f, 1797
  sites of action, 1705-1707
  thiazide diuretics and, 1712-1713
  thromboxane A_2 excretion affected by, 1717
Loop of Henle, 1458f
  adaptations of, to nephron loss, 1746
  anatomy of, 45, 259-261
  bicarbonate reabsorption in, 238
  calcium reabsorption in, 188-189
  computer-assisted reconstruction of, 261f
  descending portion of, 259-260, 260f
  description of, 2302
  diuretic action on, 1705f

Loop of Henle (Continued)
  length of, 45
  potassium transport in, 175-176, 563-564
  sodium reabsorption by, 1747
  thick ascending limb of. See Thick ascending limb
  thin limbs of, 61-63, 63f-64f
Losartan potassium, 1309, 1652-1653, 1652t
Loss of appetite, 1819
Low birth weight
  acute kidney injury in, 711-712
  blood pressure in patients with, 707
  catch-up growth, 721
  chronic kidney disease in, 712, 2576
  congenital anomalies of the kidney and urinary tract and, 2300
  description of, 694, 694t
  dexamethasone and, 696-699
  glomerular filtration rate in, 710
  preeclampsia and, 1617-1618
  proteinuria and, 710-711
  risk factors for, 722
  treatment-induced decrease in blood pressure and, 1627f
Low osmolar contrast media, 847-848, 855-856
Low-density lipoprotein
  apheresis, 2159
  catabolism of, 1802
  description of, 1213, 1863
  mesangial cells affected by, 1761-1762
  in nephrotic syndrome, 1761, 1801
  normalization of, 1970
  oxidized, 1773
  reductions in, for cardiovascular disease prevention, 1868-1871, 1869f-1870f
  statins for reduction of, 1868-1869
Low-density lipoprotein receptor-related proteins 5 and 6, 1832-1833
Lower urinary tract abnormalities, 2296, 2311
Lower-molecular-weight iron dextran, 1896
Lowe's syndrome, 1438-1439, 2345
Low-molecular-weight proteins, 791, 1810t
Low-protein diet
  chronic kidney disease progression affected by, 1977, 1981-1982, 1994
  meta-analyses of, 1981-1982, 1982f
  after renal transplantation, 1977
  serum albumin affected by, 1312
  transforming growth factor-β affected by, 1958
Loxosceles spider bites, 2444, 2445f
Loxoscelism, 2444
LP1, 223t
L-type calcium channels, 1662
Luminal carbonic acid, 234
Luminal flow rate, 237
Lung, 317
Lupus erythematosus
  discoid, 1950, 1950f
  systemic. See Systemic lupus erythematosus
Lupus glomerulonephritis, 920
Lupus nephritis
  activity and chronicity, 1097
  azathioprine for, 1169-1170
  bortezomib for, 1105
  calcineurin inhibitors for, 1104
  classification of, 1094, 1094f-1096f, 1094t
  clinical manifestations of, 1098
  course of, 1100-1102
  cyclophosphamide for, 1102-1103
  cyclosporine, 1104
  description of, 1092

Lupus nephritis (Continued)
  dialysis for, 1100
  diffuse proliferative, 1098, 1102
  electron microscopy of, 1095f-1096f, 1097
  end-stage, 1098
  epidemiology of, 1092-1093
  in Far East, 2531-2532
  focal proliferative, 1098
  gender differences in, 658
  immunofluorescence microscopy of, 1095f-1096f, 1097
  immunosuppressive agents for, 1103, 1105
  intravenous immune globulin for, 1105
  kallikrein-kinin system in, 350
  membranous, 1098, 1101-1102, 1105
  methylprednisolone for, 1102-1103
  mycophenolate mofetil for, 1103-1104, 1169-1170
  natural history of, 1101-1102
  neutrophil extracellular traps in, 1093-1094
  ocrelizumab for, 1104
  pathogenesis of, 1093-1094
  pathology of, 1094-1097, 1094f-1096f, 1094t
  plasmapheresis for, 1105, 2151-2152
  prednisone for, 1102
  pregnancy and, 1100, 1634-1635
  prognosis for, 1100-1102
  proteinuria remission in, 1165-1166
  recurrence of, after renal transplantation, 2275
  renal transplantation for, 1100
  rituximab for, 1104
  serologic tests for, 1098-1099
  silent, 1098
  survival rates, 2532
  T cell activation therapies for, 1104-1105
  tacrolimus for, 1104-1105
  treatment of, 1102-1106, 2532
Lupus podocytopathy, 1097-1098
Luteinizing hormone, 1920-1921
Lymph node dissection, 1380-1381
Lymphangioleiomyomatosis, 1368-1369
Lymphatic capillaries, 80
Lymphatic system, 80, 80f
Lymphoceles, 910-911
Lymphocytes, 1793
Lymphoma, 899, 902f, 1401-1402
Lysinuric protein intolerance, 228, 1449
Lysosomal associated membrane protein 2, 1110
Lysosomes, 59-60, 61f, 284-285

M

Macroalbuminuria, 791-792
Macrolides, 1235t-1236t
Macromolecule, 1330-1331
Macrophages
  B cells and, 1216
  cytokines production by, 976, 1215-1216
  infiltrating, 1754-1755
  in proteinuria, 1793-1795
  T cells and, 1216
  in tubulointerstitial injury, 1794
Macrovascular diseases, 1201-1204
Macula densa
  anatomy of, 53-54
  basement membrane of, 54
  cells of, 106
  COX-2 expression in, 357-358, 359f, 360
  neuronal nitric oxide synthases in, 109
  nitric oxide production by, 108-109

Macula densa (Continued)
  renin release regulated by, 358-360, 359f
  in renin secretion, 1706
Magnesium
  absorption of, 2387
  blood pressure and, 623
  in bone, 193, 193t
  in cellular processes, 193
  in children, 2386-2389
  concentrations of, 186t, 193, 193t
  cytoplasmic, 581
  dietary intake of, 193-194
  disorders of
    hypermagnesemia. See Hypermagnesemia
    hypocalcemia caused by, 616-617
    hypomagnesemia. See Hypomagnesemia
  fractional excretion of, 619-621, 1706
  functions of, 193
  glomerulus filtration of, 194
  in hemodialysis dialysate, 2094
  homeostasis of, 193-194, 193f
  inherited disorders of processing of, 1465-1467
  intravenous replacement of, 624
  as kidney stone inhibitor, 1329-1330
  oral replacement of, 624-625
  in plasma, 193
  preeclampsia prevention and, 1626-1627
  reabsorption of, 194, 194f, 1468f, 1730
  recommended daily allowance of, 624
  regulation of, 2387
  renal wasting of, 620-622
  role of, 1465-1466
  serum, 193, 619, 2387
  serum concentration of, 193, 619, 2387
  tissue concentrations of, 193t
  transport of, 195-196, 195f, 195t, 1467t
  uptake of, factors that affect, 195t
  urinary excretion of, 194
Magnesium deficiency
  in acute myocardial infarction, 623
  bone compartment redistribution as cause of, 620
  bone mass decreases in, 623-624
  causes of, 619-622, 619f
  description of, 618-625
  diarrhea as cause of, 620
  dietary causes of, 620
  electrolyte homeostasis and, 624
  extrarenal causes of, 620
  hypokalemia and, 581, 823
  intravenous magnesium replacement for, 624
  metabolic acidosis caused by, 555
  migraine headache and, 624
  oral magnesium replacement for, 624-625
  potassium-sparing diuretics for, 625
  prevention of, 624
  treatment of, 624-625
Magnesium tolerance test, 618-619
Magnetic resonance angiography (MRA)
  acute kidney injury evaluations, 989-990
  contrast-enhanced, 859-861, 862f, 904-905, 906f, 1202
  fibromuscular dysplasia on, 907, 907f
  limitations of, 905-906
  motion artifacts associated with, 905-906
  phase-contrast, 859-861, 906
  renal artery stenosis on, 904-906
  renal artery stents on, 906-907, 906f
  renal transplantation applications of, 911, 912f

Magnetic resonance imaging (MRI), 856-864
  acute pyelonephritis on, 880
  acute tubular necrosis on, 870f
  autosomal dominant polycystic kidney disease on, 885-888, 889f, 1486f
  BOLD, 864, 1271
  clear cell carcinoma in von Hippel–Lindau disease, 890f
  contraindications for, 857
  corticomedullary differentiation on, 860f
  definition of, 856
  description of, 846
  diabetes insipidus diagnosis using, 485-486
  diffusion-weighted imaging, 863-864, 871f
  end-stage kidney disease on, 889f
  external magnetic field, 856
  gadolinium-chelate contrast media, 857-859, 878
    acute tubular necrosis imaging using, 870f
    adverse reactions to, 857
    applications of, 857
    chemical structure of, 858f
    description of, 857
    in nephrogenic systemic fibrosis, 858-859
    paramagnetic effects of, 858f
    recommendations for, 859
    in renal disease, 858-859
    technique for, 859, 861f
  hematoma evaluations, 876-878, 878f-879f
  immunoglobulin A nephropathy on, 870f
  implanted medical devices as contraindication for, 857
  kidney stone evaluations, 876, 876f, 1359-1360
  liver, for iron deposition evaluations, 1895
  lymphoma, 899, 902f
  principles of, 856
  pulse repetition time, 856-857
  pulse sequences, 856-857
  pyelonephritis on, 880, 882-883, 883f
  renal abscess on, 880, 882f
  renal cell carcinoma on, 892, 895f-897f
  renal cysts on, 883-885, 886f-887f, 889f
  renal function evaluations using, 863-864
  renal parenchymal disease on, 869, 870f, 880-881
  after renal transplantation, 910
  renal transplantation applications of, 870f, 911, 912f
  renal tuberculosis on, 884f
  renal vein thrombosis on, 909, 1205
  signal characteristics, 857f
  T1 weighting, 856-857
  T2 weighting, 856-857, 860f
  technique for, 859-863, 860f-863f
  tissue signal intensity, 856
  transitional cell carcinoma on, 898-899, 902f
  ureteral stone evaluations, 877f
  urinary tract obstruction on, 1267-1268, 1267f
  urine on, 857f-858f
  xanthogranulomatous pyelonephritis on, 883f
Magnetic resonance renography, 863
Magnetic resonance urography
  applications of, 863, 864f
  contrast media-enhanced, 861-863, 862f
  kidney stone evaluations, 876-878, 877f
  technique for, 861-863
  T2-weighted, 863
  ureteropelvic junction obstruction findings, 2315, 2315f
  urinary tract obstruction on, 1267-1268

Magnetic resonance urography (Continued)
MAGUK, 29
Major histocompatibility complex, 2230-2231, 2230f
Malabsorption syndromes, 620, 632-633
Malacoplakia, 881-882, 1262
Malaria, 1150. See also Plasmodium falciparum
  acute kidney injury caused by, 2496-2497, 2517-2520, 2519f2521f
  in Africa, 2462
  clinical features of, 2496-2497
  clinical manifestations of, 2520f
  diagnosis of, 2497, 2519
  in Far East, 2517-2520, 2519f2521f
  histologic features of, 2497
  in Indian subcontinent, 2496-2497
  in Latin America, 2442-2443
  in Middle East, 2470-2472
  nephropathy caused by, 2520f
  pathogenesis of, 2497
  renal lesions associated with, 2521f
  symptoms of, 2518
  treatment of, 2497, 2519-2520
Malaysia, 2535-2536
Malignancies
  alkylating agents and, 1169
  calcineurin inhibitors as cause of, 1168
  cyclophosphamide and, 1169
  diuretics as cause of, 1732
  glomerulonephritis associated with, 1403t
  hematuria and, 759f
  humoral hypercalcemia of, 603, 607-608
  hypercalcemia of, 1399-1400, 1399t
  membranous nephropathy, 1035, 1157
  pelvic, obstructive uropathy caused by, 1261
  syndrome of inappropriate antidiuretic hormone secretion associated with, 499
Malignant hypertension, 758, 1194-1195, 1765
Malignant neoplasm, 1370-1387
Malnutrition
  in acute kidney injury, 996
  atherosclerosis and, 1930
  in chronic kidney disease, 1971
  definition of, 1969
  in diabetes mellitus, 1315
  in hemodialysis, 1317-1318, 2089-2090, 2098t, 2504
  hypophosphatemia caused by, 632
  maternal. See Maternal malnutrition
  in peritoneal dialysis, 2504
  serum albumin levels used to diagnose, 1969
Malnutrition, inflammation, and atherosclerosis syndrome, 1970
Mammalian target of rapamycin, 1374
  description of, 238, 732-733
  inhibitors of, 2247, 2258, 2426. See also Everolimus; Sirolimus
Mammary-ulnar syndrome, 2297t
Manidipine, 1665
Mannitol, 1002, 1704, 1717
Maori. See New Zealand
Marrow infusion syndrome, 1394
Masked hypertension, 1540, 1540f
Mass transfer area coefficient, 2070-2071, 2112-2113
Masson's trichrome stain, 919-920
MATE1, 212t, 214-215
MATE2-K, 212t, 214-215
Maternal endothelial dysfunction, 1619
Maternal malnutrition, 715-717
Maternal obesity, 2576
Maternal overnutrition, 2576

Matrix extracellular phosphoglycoprotein, 201-202
Matrix gamma-carboxyglutamate protein, 1838
Matrix metalloproteinases, 977, 1794
Matrix vesicles, 1836-1837
Matrix-Gla protein, as kidney stone inhibitor, 1331
Maturity-onset diabetes type 5, 2299-2300, 2317
May-Hegglin anomaly, 1141
MDR1, 211, 212t
MDRD equation, 645, 677-678, 782, 784t, 785-786, 788, 2042-2043, 2526, 2544
MDRD study, 1553, 1979-1980, 1982-1983, 1994
Mechanical ventilation, 526
Meckel-Gruber syndrome, 1417, 1509, 2322, 2322t
Medial calcification, 1850
Medial fibroplasia, 1580-1581, 1580f
Medical expulsive therapy, 1360, 1360f
Medicare coverage, for end-stage kidney disease, 1524, 2558-2559, 2562, 2572, 2625, 2627f
Medicare Improvement for Patients and Providers Act of 2008, 2628-2629
Mediterranean diet, 1957
Medullary blood flow, 90, 362f
Medullary capillaries, 92
Medullary circulation, 105
Medullary collecting ducts
  functions of, 73-74
  inner, 44-45, 45f, 69-70, 74-75
  outer, 44-45, 45f, 69-70, 73-74, 133
  prostaglandin synthesis in, 365
  sodium absorption modulation by, 314
  solute transport in, 133
  water absorption in, 569
Medullary cystic kidney disease, 1504, 1504f
Medullary fibroma, 1369
Medullary interstitial cells, COX-2 expression in, 360-361
Medullary interstitium, 78-80, 79f, 262-264, 269f, 273
Medullary microcirculation, 86f, 90-92
Medullary osmotic gradient, 238
Medullary plasma flow, 403-404
Medullary potassium recycling, 175-176
Medullary ray collecting duct, 70
Medullary rays of Ferrein, 43
Medullary renal cell carcinoma, 1372
Medullary sponge kidney, 888-889, 1513-1514, 1513f
Medullary stromal cells, 5-6
Megalin, 56-59, 1791
Megalin-25, 2390
Megaloblastic anemia, 1883
Megaureter, primary, 2315-2316
Megestrol acetate, 1920
Melamine, 1348, 2526
Melphalan, 1131-1132
Membrane cofactor protein, 1184-1185, 2356
Membrane permeability constant, 2070-2071
Membrane-associated C-terminal fragment, 1791
Membranoproliferative glomerulonephritis
  algorithm for, 1046f
  C3 glomerulopathy variant of, 1047. See also C3 glomerulopathies; Dense deposit disease
  characteristics of, 2328-2329
  classification of, 1045-1046, 1046f
  complement alterations in, 1049
  complement-mediated, 1045-1046, 1046f

Membranoproliferative glomerulonephritis *(Continued)*
  hepatitis C-associated, 1155*f*, 2273
  immune complex-mediated, 1045-1046, 1046*f*, 1048-1049
  neoplasia associated with, 1157
  nephrotic syndrome caused by, 1045-1050
  primary, 1045
  recurrence of, after renal transplantation, 1155-1156, 2275, 2422, 2431
  respiratory tract infections associated with, 1053
  secondary causes of, 1049*t*
  subtypes of, 1045
  type I
    in children, 1049
    clinical features of, 1049
    electron microscopy findings of, 1047-1048, 1048*f*
    epidemiology of, 1049
    glomerular capillary wall findings in, 1048*f*
    glucocorticoids for, 1049-1050
    hyaline thrombi associated with, 1046, 1048
    immunofluorescence findings, 1046-1047, 1048*f*
    laboratory findings in, 1050*t*
    light microscopy findings, 1046, 1047*f*
    mesangial dense deposits in, 1047-1048
    mycophenolate mofetil for, 1050
    pathogenesis of, 1048-1049, 1049*t*
    pathology of, 1046-1048, 1047*f*-1048*f*, 1051*f*
    prognosis for, 1049
    treatment of, 1049-1050
    ultrastructural findings of, 1047-1048, 1047*f*
  type II, 1050*t*, 1051. *See also* Dense deposit disease
  type III, 1047-1048, 1050
  types of, 2328-2329
Membranous glomerulonephritis, 1164
Membranous nephropathy
  anticoagulation prophylaxis in, 1041-1042
  carcinoma associated with, 1157
  in children, 1041
  chlorambucil for, 1042-1043, 1169
  clinical features of, 1040-1041
  complement in, 1041
  deep vein thrombosis in, 1041
  electron microscopy findings, 1035-1037, 1036*f*-1037*f*, 1037*t*
  epidemiology of, 1035
  gender differences in, 657
  geographic variations in, 1035
  glomerular capillary wall findings in, 1037-1038, 1038*f*
  hepatitis C associated with, 1155
  HLA-DR3 and, 1040
  hypercoagulability associated with, 1041
  immune complex deposits in, 1039
  immunofluorescence microscopy findings, 1037-1038, 1037*t*, 1038*f*
  immunoglobulin G in, 1037-1039, 1038*f*
  interstitial disease in, 1039-1040
  laboratory findings in, 1041-1042, 1050*t*
  light microscopy findings, 1038, 1038*f*
  malignancies associated with, 1035, 1157
  mesangial dense deposits in, 1037, 1037*t*
  mesangial hypercellularity in, 1038
  natural history of, 1040-1041
  nephritogenic antigens in, 1038-1039
  nephrotic syndrome caused by, 1035-1045

Membranous nephropathy *(Continued)*
  pathogenesis of, 1038-1040
  pathology of, 1035-1038, 1036*f*-1038*f*, 1037*t*
  phospholipase A_2 receptors in, 1035, 1039
  podocytes in, 115*t*, 116
  progression of, 1038, 1040-1041, 1045
  proteinuria in, 1035, 1039-1041, 1158-1159
  recurrence of, 2275
  renal failure progression of, 1040-1041
  renal insufficiency associated with, 1040
  renal vein thrombosis in, 1041
  survival estimations in, 1040
  in systemic lupus erythematosus, 1037
  treatment of
    adrenocorticotropic hormone, 1044
    azathioprine, 1045
    calcineurin inhibitors, 1043-1044
    chlorambucil, 1042-1043
    corticosteroids, 1042
    cyclophosphamide, 1042-1043
    cyclosporine, 1043
    eculizumab, 1045
    methylprednisolone, 1042
    mycophenolate mofetil, 1044
    prednisolone, 1043
    rituximab, 1044-1045
    summary of, 1045
    tacrolimus, 1043-1044
  ultrastructural stages of, 1036-1037, 1036*f*
Mendelian disease, 1411
Mendelian randomization, 671
Mental health conditions, 2621
Meperidine, 2038, 2038*t*
Mercaptopropionylglycine, 1159
α-Mercaptopropionylglycine, 2346
6-Mercaptopurine, 2425
Mesangial advanced glycosylation end receptor 1, 730-731
Mesangial cells
  angiotensin II effects on, 99
  autacoid generation by, 52
  COX-1 localization to, 361*f*
  description of, 5
  extraglomerular, 53-54
  glomerular, 46*f*, 51-52
  glomerular function role of, 1744-1745, 1788
  β-integrin receptors on, 51-52
  low-density lipoprotein effects on, 1761-1762
  matrix of, 51-52
  microfilaments of, 51
  morphology of, 51
  in nephron development, 36
  nephron loss-related hemodynamic injury, 1753
  phagocytic properties of, 52
  platelet-derived growth factor-B effects on, 1789
  prostanoids effect on, 377
  proteinuria effects on, 1788-1789
  in renal hypertrophy, 1744-1745
  survival factors for, 1788
Mesangiocapillary glomerulonephritis, 1047-1048
Mesangioproliferative glomerulonephritis, 2327-2328
Mesenchymal stem cells (MSC)
  acute kidney injury applications of, 2611-2613
  in amniotic fluid and placenta, 2607
  bone marrow-derived, 2611

Mesenchymal stem cells (MSC) *(Continued)*
  description of, 2607
  differentiation of, into renal tissue, 2611
  immunosuppressive capabilities of, 2612-2613
Mesoamerican nephropathy, 2448-2449, 2451*t*
Mesonephros, 2-3, 3*f*, 20-21
Messenger RNA, 1738-1739, 2604-2605
Metabolic acidosis
  in acute kidney injury, 1003*t*, 1004
  added acids as cause of, 835-841
  ammonia excretion in, 246*f*
  anion gap in, 528
  anorexia caused by, 2125
  assessment of, 835-837, 836*t*
  bicarbonate reabsorption affected by, 238, 830
  calcium reabsorption affected by, 191
  carbonic anhydrase inhibitors as cause of, 1730
  causes of, 834*t*-835*t*
  characteristics of, 522
  in children, 2382-2383, 2382*t*, 2405
  in chronic heart failure patients, 556-557
  in chronic kidney disease, 542, 1913, 2004, 2357, 2359
  citrate excretion in, 247
  clinical approach to, 833-841
  collecting duct's response to, 244
  compensatory responses for, 518*t*
  Cushing's disease as cause of, 556
  definition of, 833
  distal renal tubular acidosis. *See* Distal renal tubular acidosis
  drugs that cause, 547-548
  extracellular volume expansion as cause of, 555
  glucocorticoid-remediable hyperaldosteronism as cause of, 555-556
  glutamate dehydrogenase activity affected by, 253
  glutamine transport affected by, 251
  hemodialysis for correction of, 2094-2095
  high anion gap. *See* High anion gap acidosis
  high-protein diet and, 1971
  hypercalciuria associated with, 191
  hyperchloremic, 528-530, 529*t*, 764, 768, 2382-2383
  hyperkalemic hyperchloremic, 536*t*, 538, 541
  hyperphosphatemia caused by, 628
  hypertension as cause of, 555
  hypokalemia and, 821, 1723
  hypovolemia with, 424
  after ketoacidosis treatment, 555
  after lactic acidosis treatment, 555
  licorice ingestion as cause of, 556
  Liddle's syndrome as cause of, 556
  magnesium ion deficiency as cause of, 555
  non-anion gap, 528-530, 529*t*, 532, 536
  nonreabsorbable anions as cause of, 555
  pathophysiology of, 528
  peritoneal dialysis for correction of, 2125
  phosphate excretion increases in, 247
  potassium ion deficiency as cause of, 555
  primary aldosteronism as cause of, 555
  proximal tubule bicarbonate reabsorption affected by, 236-237
  proximal tubule phosphate-dependent glutaminase activity affected by, 253
  in renal transplantation recipients, 2281

Volume 1 pp. 1-1321 • Volume 2 pp. 1322-2636

Metabolic acidosis (Continued)
  renin levels and, 555-556
  salicylates as cause of, 547-548
  symptoms of, 556
  titratable acid in, 246f
  toluene metabolism as cause of, 843f
  treatment of, 556-557, 2004
Metabolic alkalosis
  acid-base transport changes secondary to, 244
  assessment of, 831
  Bartter's syndrome as cause of, 551-552, 554
  bicarbonate administration as cause of, 552-553
  calcium reabsorption affected by, 191
  case studies of, 831-833
  causes of, 551-552, 551t, 832t
  characteristics of, 522
  chloride deficiency in, 520
  citrate administration as cause of, 2163
  citrate excretion in, 247
  clinical approach to, 831
  compensatory responses for, 518t
  congenital chloridorrhea as cause of, 553
  diagnosis of, 550-552, 552f, 552t
  diuretics as cause of, 553, 1704
  edematous states as cause of, 553
  gastric aspiration as cause of, 553
  gastrointestinal causes of, 553
  Gitelman's syndrome as cause of, 551-552, 554-555
  hypercapnic response to, 519
  hypokalemia in, 550-551, 821-823
  hypoventilation caused by, 519
  after ketoacidosis treatment, 555
  after lactic acidosis treatment, 555
  loop diuretics as cause of, 1704, 1730
  milk-alkali syndrome as cause of, 553
  mixed, 550-552
  pathophysiology of, 550f
  posthypercapnia as cause of, 553-554
  potassium deficiency in, 520
  respiratory compensation for, 550
  simple, 550-552
  villous adenoma as cause of, 553
  vomiting as cause of, 525, 553
Metabolic evaluation, 1356, 1357t-1358t
Metabolic substrates, 126-132
Metabolic syndrome, 679-680, 1350-1351, 1770-1771, 1992, 2284, 2433
Metabolism
  angiotensin II's role in, 139
  basics of, 126-127
  cortical collecting duct, 133
  definition of, 122
  natriuretic peptides effect on, 342-343
  renal autoregulation mediation by, 109-110
  thermodynamic approach to, 123
Metal-binding proteins, 1018t
Metanephric adenoma, 1368
Metanephric blastema, 44-45
Metanephric mesenchyme
  bone morphogenetic protein-7 expression in, 29
  cell populations in, 7f
  condensing, 29, 31
  description of, 3
  early lineage determination of, 21
  endothelial progenitors within, 6
  gene expression in, 2298-2299
  non-GDNF pathways in, 23
  stromal cells from, 5-6
  ureteric bud and, 4f, 5-6, 21-25

Metanephros, 2-3, 3f, 6-7, 7f-8f, 22f, 2603, 2613-2615
Metastases
  cutaneous, 1949
  imaging of, 899, 902f
  recurrence rate of, 1381
  renal cell carcinoma, 896f, 1949
  resection of, 1381
  treatment of, 1385
Metastatic calcifications, 1945-1946
Metformin, 1315, 1915, 2184-2185
Methanol, 548-549, 2173-2178, 2174t, 2176t
Methotrexate, 990, 1113, 1398, 2188-2189
Methoxypolyethylene glycol epoetin beta, 1892
Methylcobalamin, 2100
Methyl-β-cyclodextrin, 292f
Methyldopa, 1629, 1630f, 1671-1672, 1671t-1672t, 1695t, 1698
Methylguanidine, 1810-1811
Methylprednisolone
  anti-glomerular basement membrane disease treated with, 1126-1127
  immune complex-mediated crescentic glomerulonephritis treated with, 1076
  lupus nephritis treated with, 1102-1103
  membranous nephropathy treated with, 1042
  pauci-immune crescentic glomerulonephritis treated with, 1087-1089
Metolazone, 450
Metoprolol, 1656t-1657t, 1658, 1660-1661
Metyrosine, 1679-1680
Microalbuminuria, 1556
  angiotensin-converting enzyme inhibitors for, 1305-1306, 1999
  as biomarker, 948
  cardiovascular disease and, 1295
  course of, 1296-1298
  criteria for, 1785-1786
  definition of, 791-792, 1296-1297, 1785-1786
  in diabetic nephropathy, 1289-1290, 1292t
  end-stage kidney disease in, 1303f
  hormone replacement therapy and, 659-660
  as hyperfiltration sign, 710
  incidence of, 1292-1294, 1292t
  microvascular complications in, 1302f
  in New Zealand, 2550
  oral contraceptives and, 659-660
  pathophysiology of, 1296-1298
  prevalence of, 1292-1294, 1292t
  primary prevention of, 1301-1302
  prognosis for, 1294-1295
  renin-angiotensin-aldosterone system blockade for prevention of, 1304
  secondary prevention of, 1302
  smoking and, 1777, 1991-1992
Microcirculations
  description of, 6
  glomerular, 92-94, 92f
  medullary. See Medullary microcirculation
  types of, 83
  vasomotor properties of, 98-99
Micro-computed tomography, 1846-1847
$β_1$-microglobulin, 937-938, 1041
$β_2$-microglobulin, 938, 1810, 1949
Micro-magnetic resonance imaging, for bone assessments, 1846-1847
Micronutrients, 1983
Microorganisms, in urine, 802
MicroRNA-21, 729-730

Microscopic agglutination test, for leptospirosis, 2444
Microscopic hematuria, 754-755, 799, 1022, 1065, 1198-1199
Microscopic polyangiitis
  antineutrophil cytoplasmic antibodies in, 1114-1115
  in children, 2351
  clinical features of, 1115
  cyclophosphamide for, 1112-1113, 1115-1116
  electron microscopy of, 1115
  in Far East, 2532
  immunofluorescence microscopy of, 1115
  laboratory tests for, 1115
  light microscopy of, 1114-1115, 1114f
  pathogenesis of, 1110, 1115
  pathology of, 1114-1115, 1114f
  prognosis for, 1115-1116
  proteinuria in, 1115
  recurrence of, after renal transplantation, 2275
  renal findings in, 1115
  treatment of, 1115-1116
Microtubules, 295, 296f
Microvascular diseases
  antiphospholipid syndrome. See Antiphospholipid syndrome
  atheroembolic renal disease, 1191-1193, 1192f
  chronic cognitive impairment secondary to, 1936
  endothelial cell injury in, 1175
  glycemic control for, 1871
  hemolytic-uremic syndrome. See Hemolytic-uremic syndrome
  overview of, 1175-1201
  radiation nephropathy, 1193-1195
  scleroderma. See Scleroderma
  sickle cell disease. See Sickle cell disease
  thrombotic microangiopathies. See Thrombotic microangiopathies
  thrombotic thrombocytopenia purpura. See Thrombotic thrombocytopenia purpura
Microvascular injury, 1197
Microvascular rarefaction, 1578f
Microvascular thrombosis, 1179f
Microvilli, 56-59, 2111
Micturition cystourethrography, 2313
Middle East
  acute kidney injury in, 2469-2472
  Bartter's syndrome in, 2479
  chronic kidney disease in, 2472-2486, 2477t, 2480t-2482t, 2483f
  chronic kidney disease–mineral bone disorder in, 2488
  consanguinity rates in, 2476
  countries of, 2468, 2469f
  cystinuria in, 2478-2479
  definition of, 2468
  demographics of, 2470t
  diabetes mellitus in, 2472, 2476
  dialysis in, 2487-2489
  disasters in, 2472, 2473f
  earthquakes in, 2472
  end-stage kidney disease in
    diabetes mellitus as cause of, 2476
    familial Mediterranean fever and, 2486
    hemodialysis for, 2487-2488
    hepatitis with, 2488-2489
    management of, 2486-2492
    peritoneal dialysis for, 2487
    statistics regarding, 2473-2474

Middle East (Continued)
  Fabry's disease in, 2479
  familial Mediterranean fever in. See Familial Mediterranean fever
  genetic kidney diseases in, 2476-2486, 2477t, 2480t-2482t, 2483f
  Gitelman's syndrome in, 2479
  health care expenditures in, 2471f
  health indicators in, 2470t
  hemodialysis in, 2475t, 2487-2488
  Human Development Index in, 2470t
  life expectancy in, 2468, 2470t
  malaria in, 2470-2472
  map of, 2469f
  mortality rate in, 2468, 2470t
  nephrolithiasis in, 2478-2479
  peritoneal dialysis in, 2475t, 2487
  population of, 2468
  primary hyperoxaluria type 1 and 2 in, 2478
  renal hypoplasia in, 2479
  renal parenchymal disease in, 2469-2470
  renal replacement therapy in
    hemodialysis, 2475t, 2487-2488
    peritoneal dialysis, 2475t, 2487
    statistics regarding, 2475t
  renal transplantation in, 2475t, 2489-2492
  summary of, 2492
  wealth in, 2471f
Midodrine and octreotide, for hepatorenal syndrome, 456
Milk-alkali syndrome, 553, 609-610
Mineral metabolism, 2102-2103
  disordered, 1850-1851, 2019-2023
  in peritoneal dialysis patients, 2132
Mineralocorticoid(s)
  antagonists of, 591-592
  bicarbonate reabsorption affected by, 238
  excess of, 320, 1547
  hyperkalemia treated with, 595-596
  resistance, 540
Mineralocorticoid receptors
  aldosterone action and, 306f
  aldosterone binding to, 310
  cortisol binding by, 309
  description of, 304-305, 1679
  distal convoluted tubule expression of, 315
  DNA-binding domain of, 307-308, 308f
  domain structure of, 307-310, 308f-309f
  expression sites for, 315
  functioning of, 306-310
  glomerulus expression of, 315
  as hormone-regulated transcription factor, 306-307
  11β-hydroxysteroid dehydrogenase type 2 effects on, 320
  intercalated cell, 314
  ligand/hormone-binding domain of, 307-309, 309f
  N-terminal domain of, 310
  nuclear translocation of, 307f
  preinitiation complex, 310
  proximal convoluted tubule expression of, 315
  thick ascending limb expression of, 315
  transcription initiation, 310
Minimal change disease
  acute renal failure associated with, 1021
  bone mineral density reductions in, 1022
  in children, 1021, 1023
  clinical features of, 1021-1022, 1021t
  conditions associated with, 1021, 1021t
  corticosteroids for, 1022-1023, 1023t

Minimal change disease (Continued)
  cyclophosphamide for, 1023
  cyclosporine for, 1023-1024
  in elderly, 746
  electron microscopy findings in, 1019, 1019f1020f
  epidemiology of, 1016-1024
  food allergy and, 1021
  genetic findings in, 1020
  hemopexin in, 1020
  in Hodgkin's disease, 1021, 1157
  Hodgkin's lymphoma and, 1404
  IgA nephropathy and, 1404
  immunofluorescence microscopy findings in, 1019
  incidence of, 1016
  interleukin-13 in, 1020
  laboratory findings in, 1022, 1050t
  light microscopy findings in, 1015t, 1016-1019
  lithium as cause of, 1159
  mesangial dense deposits in, 1019
  natural history of, 1021-1022
  nephrotic syndrome caused by, 1016-1034, 1158
  nonsteroidal anti-inflammatory drugs that cause, 1021, 1021t
  pathogenesis of, 1019-1021
  pathology of, 1016-1019
  podocyte foot process effacement in, 1019, 1020f
  prednisone for, 1022-1024, 1167
  proteinuria in, 1022
  steroid-resistant, 1023-1024
  T cell abnormalities in, 1019-1020
  treatment of, 1022-1024
  tumor necrosis factor-related apoptosis-induced ligand alterations in, 1020
Minimal change nephropathy, 114-116, 115t
Minimal inhibitory concentrations, 2041
Mini-Mental State Examination, 1936-1937
Minoxidil, 1674, 1674t, 1692
Minute ventilation, 1612
miRNAs, 36
Mithramycin, 1400
Mitochondria, 142
Mitochondrial diseases, 142
Mitochondrial disorder, 1432
Mitral valve calcification, 1859
Mitral valve prolapse, 1492
Mixed acid-base disorders, 521-523, 525, 550-552
Mixed chimerism, 2249
Mixed connective tissue disease, 1108-1109
Mixed cryoglobulinemia, 1137-1138, 1155, 2152
Mixed epithelial stromal tumor, 1369-1370, 1517
Mixed lymphocyte reaction, 2235
Mixed metabolic-respiratory disturbance, 522
Mixed uremic osteodystrophy, 1843, 1844f
Mixed-bed ion-exchange system, 2081
Mixing entropy, 122
Model of End-stage Liver Disease, 458
Modification of Diet in Renal Disease study. See MDRD study
Moexipril hydrochloride, 1643, 1643t
Molecular Adsorbent Recirculating System, 457-458, 2171
Mönckeberg's calcification, 1833-1835
Mönckeberg's sclerosis, 1855-1856
Moncrief-Popovich catheter, 2115-2116

Monoclonal antibodies, 2248-2249, 2255-2256
Monoclonal gammopathies, 1030, 1071
Monoclonal immunoglobulin deposition disease, 1134-1136, 1135f
Monocyte chemoattractant protein-1, 729, 950-951, 967-968, 1148, 1215-1216
Monocytes, 1792-1793
Monogenic disease, 1411, 1411t
Monogenic hypercalciuria, rodent models for, 1350t
Monomethylamine, 1812-1813
Mononeuropathy, 1939
Moxonidine, 1671-1672, 1671t-1672t
Mucormycosis, 1405
Muehrcke's lines, 762
Muir-Torre syndrome, 1952-1953, 1952t
Multicystic dysplastic kidney, 889, 1510-1511, 2294-2296, 2295f, 2303, 2305, 2312-2313, 2312f
Multidetector computed tomography, 851
Multidrug resistance protein, 375
Multilocular cystic nephroma, 1369-1370, 1517
Multimedia depth filters, for hemodialysis water treatment, 2081
Multiple cutaneous and uterine leiomyoma, 1373-1374
Multiple endocrine neoplasia, 608, 1548
Multiple myeloma
  acute kidney injury and, 990, 1002, 1390, 2152
  cast nephropathy and, 1391
  diagnosis of, 1391
  in elderly, 746
  free light chains in, 2152, 2153f
  incidence of, 1390-1391
  kidney involvement and, 1391
  manifestations of, 1392
  plasmapheresis for, 2153t
  presentation of, 1391
  treatment of, 1392-1393
Multiple-dose activated charcoal, 2168, 2183
Multipotent adult progenitor cell, 2607-2608
Multivesicular bodies, 59-60
Muromonab-CD3, 1637t, 2248, 2255, 2423
Muscle
  atrophy of, 1965-1968
  catabolism of, 1967
  potassium depletion in, 1968
  protein losses, 1965, 1966f, 1970
Muscle cramps, 2107
Muscle wasting, 1817
Mushrooms, 2525-2526
Myasthenia gravis, 2158
Mycobacterium tuberculosis, 1150, 1252-1253
Mycophenolate mofetil (MMF)
  adverse effects of, 1170, 2257-2258, 2330
  in children, 2425-2426
  focal segmental glomerulosclerosis treated with, 1033
  glomerular disease treated with, 1170
  granulomatous with polyangiitis treated with, 1113-1114
  hematologic complications of, 1170
  immunoglobulin A nephropathy treated with, 1068, 2531
  immunosuppressive uses of, 2245-2246, 2246f, 2254t, 2257-2258, 2425-2426
  lupus nephritis treated with, 1103-1104, 1169-1170
  membranoproliferative glomerulonephritis type I treated with, 1050

Mycophenolate mofetil (MMF) (Continued)
  membranous nephropathy treated with, 1044
  during pregnancy, 1637-1638, 1637t
  steroid-resistant nephrotic syndrome treated with, 2331
  steroid-sensitive nephrotic syndrome treated with, 2330
  toxicity of, 1170
Mycophenolate sodium, 2258
Mycophenolic acid, 2245-2246, 2246f, 2426
Mycophenolic acid glucuronide, 2245-2246
Myeloma cast nephropathy, 990, 1002. See also Cast nephropathy
Myeloma cells, 603
Myeloperoxidase, 1910
MYH9, 1028
Myocardial disease, 1858f
Myocardial fibrosis, 1858-1859
Myocardial infarction, 1351f
Myocardial stunning, 2079, 2107
MYO1E, 2326
MYO1E disease, 1430-1431
Myoepithelial cells, 53
Myofibrillar proteins, 1965
Myofibroblasts, 977, 1763
Myogenic mechanism, for renal autoregulation, 105-106
Myoglobin, 790, 967
Myoinositol, 1813
Myosin I, 294-295
Myosin light-chain kinase, 294-295
Myostatin, 1967-1968

N

N-Acetylcysteine, 856, 1000
N-acetyl-β-D-glucosaminidase, 947
NaDC transporters, 217-218, 217f, 218f, 218t
NADH, 132
Nadolol, 1656t-1657t, 1657
Na^+-H^+ exchangers
  ammonia metabolism and, 253
  insulin effects on, 818
  isoform 3, 136, 1273
  knockout mice model of, 278
  in proximal tubule bicarbonate reabsorption, 235
Nail-patella syndrome, 762, 1142-1143, 1143f, 1431
Na^+-K^+-ATPase. See Sodium pump
Na^+-K^+-ATPase enzyme, 560
Na^+-K^+-$2Cl^-$ cotransporter, 254, 278, 299
Nandrolone decanoate, 1922
National Cooperative Dialysis Study, 2082-2083
National Health Service Corps, 2583-2584
National Institutes of Health prostatitis classification, 1247, 1247t
National Kidney Foundation Kidney Disease Outcomes Quality Initiative, 773, 773t, 1736, 1818, 1957-1958, 1958t
Native kidney, 2069, 2089, 2610
Natriuresis, 342, 410-411
Natriuretic hormones, 152-153
Natriuretic peptide(s), 1534
  actions of, 342-343
  acute tubular necrosis treated with, 1001
  antifibrotic effects of, 342
  atrial. See Atrial natriuretic peptide
  brain. See Brain natriuretic peptide
  in cardiac remodeling, 342
  cardiovascular effects of, 342
  central nervous system effects of, 342
  in cirrhosis, 447-449
  C-type. See C-type natriuretic peptide

Natriuretic peptide(s) (Continued)
  definition of, 339
  Dendroaspis. See Dendroaspis natriuretic peptide
  as disease biomarkers, 343-344
  in effective arterial blood volume regulation, 413-415
  in heart failure, 433-435, 453
  metabolism mediation by, 342-343
  nephron loss adaptations and, 1739
  neutral endopeptidase, 341-342, 345, 413
  as renal disease biomarkers, 343-344
  renal effects of, 342
  in sodium retention, 447-449
  structure of, 339-341, 339f
  synthesis of, 339-341
  therapeutic uses of, 344-345
  types of, 339
  urodilatin. See Urodilatin
Natriuretic peptide precursor type A, 339-341
Natriuretic peptide precursor type C, 340-341
Natriuretic peptide receptors
  -A, 341
  -B, 341-342
  biologic effects of, 341
  -C, 341
  description of, 341
  kinase homology domain of, 341
Nausea, 469-470, 469f
NBC3, 243-244
NBCe.1, 530
NBCe1-A, 234-237
NCC, 66-68, 580
Nck1, 38
Nck2, 38
Near and Middle East. See Middle East
Nebivolol, 1658t-1659t, 1659
Necrosis, 586, 921t, 974-975
Necrotizing pancreatitis, 1732
Nedd4-2, 172-173, 312, 318-319, 565
Neoadjuvant therapy, 1382
Neointimal hyperplasia, 2194, 2195f, 2202
Neonatal severe hyperparathyroidism, 608, 2395-2396
Neonates
  hypercalcemia in, 2394t
  hyperphosphatemia in, 2389
  renal vein thrombosis in, 1206
Neoplasia, 1157
Neoplasms
  angiomyolipomas, 891, 893f
  benign, 1368-1370
  benign cystic, 1369-1370
  cystic, 1516-1517
  imaging of, 891
  malignant, 1370-1387
  oncocytoma, 891-892
  after renal transplantation, 911
Neph1, 38
Nephelometry, 794-795
Nephrectomy, 1379. See also Partial nephrectomy
  adjuvant therapy after, 1381
  allograft, 2290
  cytoreductive, 1381
  for emphysematous pyelonephritis, 1251
  glomerulus changes after, 1751f
  inferior vena caval involvement with tumor thrombus and, 1381
  proteinuria after, 1752f
  renal hypertrophy after, 1742
  whole-kidney responses to, 1741-1742, 1742f

Nephrin, 37-38, 113, 936-937, 1413-1414, 1414t, 1426, 2323
Nephrin disease, 1426-1428
Nephritic syndrome
  characteristics of, 757
  in children, 2331-2333
  complement levels in, 759-760, 759t
  diagnostic approach, 757-760, 759t-760t
  glomerular hematuria associated with, 758-759
Nephritis
  acute interstitial. See Acute interstitial nephritis
  allergic interstitial, 984t-985t, 1158
  anti-thin basement membrane, 1228-1229
  granulomatous interstitial, 1228
  interstitial, 1158
  shunt, 1149
  tubulointerstitial, 1220-1221
Nephroblastoma, 1386-1387
Nephrocalcinosis, 1417
  in children, 2340
  description of, 534-535, 871-873, 2385
  familial hypomagnesemia with, 1466
  familial hypomagnesemia with hypercalciuria and, 2387-2388
  genetic causes of, 1349f
  hypercalcemia and dehydration as cause of, 2393-2394
Nephrogenesis
  COX-2 inhibitors effect on, 719
  cyclosporine effects on, 719
  gentamicin effects on, 719
  β-lactam effects on, 719
  onset of, 699
  penicillin effects on, 719
  tripartite inductive interactions regulating, 28f
Nephrogenic diabetes insipidus (NDI), 1470
  acquired causes of, 285, 297
  amiloride for, 489
  aquaporin-2 and, 285, 298f, 481-482, 2338
  calcitonin for, 301
  causes of, 285, 297, 480-482
  in children, 2338-2339, 2368-2370, 2370t
  congenital, 285, 480-481, 2338, 2369-2370
  definition of, 2338, 2368
  description of, 285
  desmopressin test for, 484, 2338
  diagnosis of, 809, 2338
  heat shock protein 90 for, 301-302
  hereditary, 285, 297
  history of, 480-481
  hypernatremia prevention in, 2338
  knockout mouse models of, 282
  lithium as cause of, 297-299, 298f, 379, 482, 1226
  molecular therapies for, 2338-2339
  pathophysiology of, 482
  phosphodiesterase inhibitors for, 300-301
  prostaglandins for, 301
  secretin for, 301
  statins for, 301
  treatment of, 285, 300-302, 489-490, 2338-2339
  type II, 285
  X-linked, 278-279, 300, 1470-1473, 2338
Nephrogenic syndrome of inappropriate antidiuresis, 499
Nephrogenic syndrome of inappropriate diuresis, 2372-2373
Nephrogenic systemic fibrosis, 858-859, 1947-1948, 1948f, 1949f
Nephrogenic zone, 4f-5f, 5, 28-29
Nephrogram, 847f

Nephrolithiasis, 1417, 1419
  acetazolamide as risk factor for, 1704
  in children. See Children, nephrolithiasis in
  diagnostic approach, 767-769
  differential diagnosis of, 769, 769t
  diuretics for, 1726
  hypercalciuric, 2340, 2344-2345, 2344f
  in Indian subcontinent, 2507
  medications associated with, 767
  metabolic syndrome and, 1350-1351
  in Middle East, 2478-2479
  nonsteroidal anti-inflammatory drugs for, 769
  obesity and, 1351f
  predisposing medical conditions for, 767-768
  prevalence of, 767, 1260
  risk factors for, 767
  risk of developing, 873
  in sarcoidosis, 1228
  symptoms of, 767
  treatment of, 769, 1493
  ureteral obstruction caused by, 1260
Nephrologist referral, 2063, 2595-2596
Nephromegaly, 2320f
Nephron, 44-69
  active transport along, 126-132
  anatomy of, 44-69, 45f
  autonomic innervation of, 54-55
  components of, 44-45
  cortical, 45
  development of, 4-5, 30-31, 36-39, 44-45, 2309
  distal
    aldosterone-sensitive, 311f, 314-315, 316f, 319-320
    calcium transport mechanisms in, 190f
    cortical, potassium secretion in, 819
    development of, 30
    intercalated cells in, 166
    potassium in, 563-564
    potassium secretion by, vasopressin effects on, 182
    sodium chloride and potassium transport in, 182-183
  diuretics site of action in, 1703f
  generalized dysfunction of, 541t
  gluconeogenic enzymes along, 131f
  high-affinity adrenergic receptors in, 405
  juxtaglomerular, angiotensin II effects on, 99, 100f
  juxtamedullary, 45, 45f, 85, 89f, 90-91, 93
  lactate production along, 130-132
  long-looped, 259
  low mass, knockout and transgenic models for studying, 10t-17t
  maturation of, 5
  number of, 44-45
  phosphorus reabsorption along, 198-199, 199f
  secretory nature of, 204
  short-looped, 259
  sodium pump activity along, 142, 146f
  substrates along, 131f
  tight junctions in, 147f
  types of, 259
Nephron endowment
  chronic kidney disease risks, 676, 1769
  development programming of, 696-701
  kidney transplantation affected by, 723-724
  low, 1769

Nephron loss
  chronic kidney disease risks, 676-678, 1991f
  focal segmental glomerulosclerosis caused by, 1029
  glomerular hemodynamic adaptations to
    bradykinin, 1740
    description of, 1737-1738
    eicosanoids in, 1740
    endothelins in, 1739
    mediators of, 1738-1741
    natriuretic peptides in, 1739
    nitric oxide in, 1740
    renin angiotensin aldosterone system in, 1738-1739
    urotensin II, 1740
  injury after
    acidosis, 1758-1759
    aldosterone, 1757
    angiotensin II, 1756-1757
    bone morphogenetic protein-7, 1757-1758
    cellular infiltration in remnant kidneys, 1754-1755
    description of, 1755
    endothelial cells in, 1752-1753
    hepatocyte growth factor, 1757
    hypertrophy, 1759
    mechanical stress in, 1752
    mesangial cells in, 1753
    microRNAs, 1758
    oxidative stress, 1758
    podocytes, 1753-1754
    proteinuria, 1760-1763
    transforming growth factor-β, 1755-1756
  long-term adverse consequences of adaptations to, 1750-1752, 1751f-1752f
  mesangial cell response to, 1744-1745
  renal autoregulatory mechanism adjustments to, 1740-1741
  renal hypertrophic responses to
    algorithm for, 1745f
    description of, 1741
    endocrine effects, 1744
    glomerular enlargement, 1742-1743
    growth factors, 1744
    mechanisms involved in, 1745f
    mechanisms of, 1743-1745
    mesangial cells, 1744-1745
    renotropic factors, 1743-1744
    solute load, 1743
    tubular cell responses, 1745
    whole-kidney, 1741-1742, 1742f
  tubule function adaptations to
    acid-base regulation, 1749
    calcium metabolism, 1749-1750
    description of, 1745
    distal nephron, 1746
    glomerulotubular balance, 1746-1747
    loop of Henle, 1746
    phosphate metabolism, 1749-1750
    potassium excretion, 1748-1749
    proximal tubule solute handling, 1745-1746
    sodium excretion, 1747-1748
    urinary concentration and dilution, 1748
Nephron mass, 724, 2278
Nephron number
  birth weight and, 703-705
  blood pressure and, 697t-698t, 709, 709f
  congenital deficit in, 701
  genetic variants associated with, 713-715
  glomerular volume and, 696

Nephron number (Continued)
  glomerulomegaly associated with, 705
  intrauterine growth restriction effects on, 700f
  kidney size as correlate of, 700-701, 700f
  low, 705, 705t, 721
  maternal hyperglycemia effects on, 717f
  maternal nutrient restrictions that affect, 716
  maternal vitamin A restriction effects on, 716
  plausibility of, 695-696
  postnatal augmentation of, 701
  prematurity and, 703-705
  programming of, in humans, 699-701
  renal size and, 697t-698t
  rescue of, 720-721
  variability of, 676, 695t, 699, 724
  vitamin A deficiency effects on, 716, 721
Nephronectin gene, 25
Nephronophthisis, 1508-1509, 2321-2322
Nephronophthisis-related ciliopathies, 1416-1417, 2321
Nephron-sparing surgery, 1379-1380
Nephropathy
  acute phosphate, 966-967
  analgesic, 686, 1221-1223, 1223f-1224f, 2544-2546
  antiphospholipid, 1106-1107
  aristolochic acid, 1223-1226, 2534
  Balkan endemic, 1224-1226, 1225f
  BK virus-associated, 2428-2429
  bone marrow transplantation, 1193-1194
  cadmium, 1227
  Chinese herb, 1223-1224, 1225f, 2534
  chronic allograft, 2244, 2273, 2425, 2431
  contrast media-induced, 853-856
  C1q, 1034-1035
  hepatitis B-associated, 1154-1155
  heroin, 1157-1158
  hypertensive, 2459
  hypokalemic, 2375
  in Latin America, 2448-2449
  lead, 686-687, 1227
  malarial, 2520f
  Mesoamerican, 2448-2449, 2451t
  myeloma cast, 990, 1002
  nonsteroidal antiinflammatory drug-induced, 1158
  obstructive. See Obstructive nephropathy
  salt-losing, 493
  sickle cell, 1145-1146, 1145f
  urate, 1227-1228
  warfarin-related, 1068
Nephrotic syndrome, 1435
  acute kidney injury in, 991t, 994
  albumin stores in, 1796-1797
  in amyloidosis, 1129
  anticoagulant abnormalities in, 1803-1804
  anticoagulation prophylaxis in, 1206-1207
  anticonvulsants that cause, 1159
  antithrombin III deficiency in, 1206, 1803
  biochemical findings in, 760
  characteristics of, 1016
  in children. See Children, nephrotic syndrome in
  coagulation factors in, 1018t
  deep vein thrombosis in, 1804
  diagnostic approach, 761-764
  diuretics for, 1723f, 1724-1725
  edema associated with, 761, 1798-1800, 1798f-1799f
  in elderly, 746-747
  in Epstein-Barr virus infection, 1151

Nephrotic syndrome (Continued)
etiology of, 1016
glomerular diseases that cause
acute poststreptococcal glomerulonephritis, 1054-1059
C3 glomerulopathies, 1045-1046, 1050-1054
C1q nephropathy, 1034-1035
fibrillary glomerulonephritis, 1069-1072
focal segmental glomerulosclerosis, 1024-1035
immunoglobulin A nephropathy, 1059-1069
immunotactoid glomerulopathy, 1069-1072
list of, 1017t-1018t
membranoproliferative glomerulonephritis, 1045-1050
membranous nephropathy, 1035-1045
minimal change disease, 1016-1034
gold salts and, 1158
after graft-versus-host disease, 1021
high-density lipoprotein in, 1801
hypercoagulability in, 1803-1805, 1803f
hyperlipidemia associated with, 1801-1803, 1801f, 1803f, 1816-1817
hypoalbuminemia caused by, 1796-1798, 1796f
hypocalcemia in, 1797-1798
hyponatremia in, 494-495
hypovolemia in, 422-423
in Indian subcontinent, 2506t
infection susceptibility in, 1805
intrarenal sodium retention in, 1801
lipiduria associated with, 762-763, 763f
lipoprotein in, 1802
loop diuretics in, 1725
low-density lipoprotein in, 1761, 1801
mechanisms of, 761
nail-patella syndrome with, 762
nonsteroidal antiinflammatory drugs as cause of, 363, 1158
plasma protein alterations in, 1018t
plasmin-induced fibrinolysis reduction in, 1804
platelet aggregation in, 1804
protein requirements in, 1976-1977
in proteinuria, 1796
pulmonary embolism in, 1805
renal artery stenosis associated with, 1159
renal vein thrombosis in, 1204-1206, 1804
renal water handling defects associated with, 1800
renin-angiotensin-aldosterone system inhibition in, 1799
secondary, 760, 760t
skin findings, 762
steroid-resistant, 1413-1415, 1414t
calcineurin inhibitors for, 2330-2331
characteristics of, 1428-1429
description of, 2323
focal segmental glomerulosclerosis in, 2328
genetics of, 1428
GLEPP1 disease and, 1431
manifestations of, 1428-1429
molecular genetic screening for, 2326f
monogenic causation of, 1413-1414
mutations causing, 1414
mycophenolate mofetil for, 2331
pathogenesis of, 1415, 1428
renin-angiotensin-aldosterone antagonists for, 2331
rituximab, 2331
single-gene causes of, 1415, 1415f

Nephrotic syndrome (Continued)
syndromic forms of, 2323
treatment of, 1429, 2330-2331
steroid-sensitive, 2329-2330
thromboembolism risks in, 1804
venous thromboembolism in, 1805
vitamin D-binding protein loss in, 1797
Nephrotoxic medications, 999-1000
Nephrotoxins, 685-687, 965-968
Neprilysin inhibitors, 1714
Nernst equation, 569-570
Nesiritide, 344, 453, 1714, 1720-1721
Net acid excretion, 1344f
Net Reclassification Index, 929-930
N-Ethyl-N-nitrosourea, 9-17
Netrin-1, 943
Neurogenic bladder, urinary tract obstruction in, 1280
Neurohypophyseal neurons, 477
Neurohypophysis, 463, 467, 467f, 474
Neuromuscular system, 623
Neuronal nitric oxide synthases, 109-110, 399
Neuronal Wiskott-Aldrich syndrome protein, 38
Neuropathy, 1939
Neuropeptides
in heart failure, 438
Y, 81, 419, 429, 438
Neutral endopeptidase, 341-342, 345, 413
Neutral endopeptidase inhibitors, 345-346, 453-454
Neutropenia, 2434
Neutrophil extracellular traps, 1093-1094
Neutrophil gelatinase-associated lipocalin, 772, 943-947, 989, 1263
New Zealand
chronic kidney disease in, 2550-2551
diabetes mellitus in, 2550-2551
dialysis in, 2551-2552
end-stage kidney disease in, 2550, 2552-2553
geography of, 2549
glomerulonephritis in, 2550
health care access in, 2549
hypertension in, 2550
life expectancy in, 2549
Maori population of
description of, 2538
end-stage kidney disease in, 2552-2553
health status of, 2549-2550
leading causes of death in, 2549
life expectancy in, 2549
renal replacement therapy in, 2552
renal transplantation in, 2553
statistics regarding, 2549
microalbuminuria in, 2550
population of, 2540t
renal replacement therapy in, 2541f, 2551-2552, 2551f
renal transplantation in, 2552
New-onset diabetes mellitus after transplantation, 1320, 2283
Next-generation sequencing technique, 1412
NH_3, 248, 249f, 252-253, 384, 570
NH_4^+, 248, 249f, 253
NHE2, 238-239
NHE3, 154-155, 159, 235, 251, 254, 2302
NHE8, 235
NHE proteins, 148-150
NHERF, 155f
NHERF-1, 155
NHERF-2, 155
Niacin, 1872
Nicardipine hydrochloride, 1663t, 1665-1666, 1695t, 1698

Nicotinamide adenine dinucleotide phosphate-oxidase, 1758
Nicotinamide mononucleotide, 1788
Nicotinic acetylcholine receptor, 2158
Nifedipine, 1663t, 1664-1665, 1669-1670
Nisoldipine, 1663t, 1666
Nitric oxide, 1578
acetylcholine effects on, 101-102
angiotensin II-induced release of, 99
cyclic guanosine monophosphate mediation of, 139
in effective arterial blood volume regulation, 416-417
endothelial production of, 1856
glomerular filtration regulation by, 101-102
in heart failure, 435-436
inhibitors of, 101-102, 1740
macula densa production of, 108-109
nephron loss adaptations and, 1740
platelet-activating factor effects on production of, 1741
renal fibrosis in aging kidney, 730
in renal hemodynamics, 416-417
renal hemodynamics regulation by, 101-102
in sodium balance, 417
soluble guanylate cyclase effects on, 416
vasodilatory effects of, 417
Nitric oxide synthases
description of, 101, 138-139
endothelial, 442-443, 728, 730, 979
inducible, 416, 979
isoforms of, 416
neuronal, 109-110, 399, 416
nitric oxide inhibition by, 400
Nitrites, 790
Nitroflurbiprofen, 377
Nitrofurantoin, 750, 1238t, 1244
Nitrogen, 1962-1963
Nitrogen balance, 1959, 1960f, 1968-1969, 1975
Nitroglycerin, 1695t, 1697
NKCC1, 177, 254, 562
NKCC2, 64, 125, 141, 158, 162-163, 188, 251, 254, 278, 396-397, 399, 450-451, 560, 702-703, 1705
NKCC2A, 55
NKCC2B, 55
NLRP3, 1193
Nodular glomerulosclerosis, 1285-1286, 1287f
Non-A, non-B intercalated cell, 241
Non-anion gap metabolic acidosis, 528-530, 529t, 536
Nonbiphenyl tetrazoles, 1653
Noncaseating granulomas, 1228
Noncontrast computed tomography, 1359
Nondiabetic chronic kidney disease, 1553
Nondiabetic glomerulopathy, 1300
Nonequilibrium thermodynamics, 123
Nonobstructive hydronephrosis, 765, 868
Nonobstructive intrahepatic bile duct dilatation, 1496-1497
Nonosmotic sodium storage, 1530
Nonreabsorbable anions, 555
Nonspecular reflectors, 848
Nonsteroidal antiinflammatory drugs (NSAIDs)
acute kidney injury caused by, 362-363, 743-744
angiotensin receptor blocker natriuretic effects affected by, 1656
Bartter's syndrome treated with, 2335
complications of, 361-363
edema caused by, 361-362

Nonsteroidal antiinflammatory drugs (NSAIDs) *(Continued)*
 hyperkalemia caused by, 362
 hypertension caused by, 361-362
 interstitial nephritis caused by, 363
 minimal change disease caused by, 1021, 1021t
 nephrolithiasis analgesia using, 769
 nephropathy caused by, 1158
 nephrotic syndrome caused by, 363, 1158
 nephrotoxic syndromes caused by, 1218-1219
 papillary necrosis caused by, 362
 prostaglandin E_2 blockade by, 371
 renal dysgenesis caused by, 363
 renal insufficiency associated with, 362-363
 sodium retention caused by, 361-362
Nonurea nitrogen, 1962-1963
Nordihydroguaiaretic acid, 385
Norepinephrine, 432, 445
Normeperidine, 2038, 2038t
Normoalbuminuria, 1293-1294, 1296
North American Pediatric Renal Trials and Collaborative Studies, 2403, 2419, 2434-2435
Norverapamil, 1664
Notch group, 30
Notch3 receptors, 1215-1216
Notch signaling pathway, 36
Novel erythropoiesis-stimulating protein, 1881
NPHP1, 2321
NPHS1, 1413-1414, 1414t, 1419, 1786, 2325, 2478
NPHS2, 118, 1027-1028, 1413-1414, 1414t, 2422, 2477-2478
NT-proBNP, 343-344
Nuclear factor of activated T cells, 2239
Nuclear factor-κB, 334, 603, 730, 974
Nuclear medicine. *See also* Radiopharmaceuticals
 acute pyelonephritis evaluations, 880
 description of, 864-865
 obstructive urography evaluations, 871
 renal cell carcinoma imaging using, 900-901
 after renal transplantation, 911-912
Nutrition. *See also* Malnutrition
 disease affected by, 1957
 health affected by, 1957
 during hemodialysis, 1817-1818, 2089-2090, 2098-2100
 during peritoneal dialysis, 1817-1818, 2124-2126
 preeclampsia prevention through, 1626
 status markers for, 2099
 uremia effects on, 1817-1818

O

OAT1, 1712
OAT3, 1712
OATPs, 218t, 219
Obesity
 antihypertensive drug therapy in patients with, 1686-1688, 1688t
 cardiovascular disease risks, 1865-1866
 childhood, 2576-2577
 chronic kidney disease progression affected by, 679-680, 1770-1771, 1865-1866, 1992-1993
 end-stage kidney disease risks, 679, 1300

Obesity *(Continued)*
 glomerulopathy caused by, 679-680, 1770-1771
 hypertension and, 766, 1533-1534, 1694
 maternal, 2576
 mortality risks, 1866
 nephrolithiasis and, 1351f
 renal plasma flow increases secondary to, 1771
 urolithiasis and, 1350-1351
Obstructive nephropathy
 acute kidney injury caused by, 2496
 description of, 1257
 glomerular filtration affected by, 1269-1271
 isolated perfused tubules in, 1273t
 pathophysiology of, 1268-1277
 renal blood flow affected by, 1269-1271
 urine concentration affected by, 1275-1276
 urine dilution affected by, 1275-1276
Obstructive uropathy
 acute kidney injury and, 1632-1633
 in children, 1279
 contrast-enhanced computed tomography of, 871
 definition of, 764, 1257
 diagnostic approach, 764-765, 871
 end-stage kidney disease progression from, 764
 extrinsic causes of, 1260-1261
 gastrointestinal processes that cause, 1261
 imaging of, 871
 in men, 1261
 nuclear medicine of, 871
 pain in, 1262
 pelvic malignancies as cause of, 1261
Occlusive, 1598-1599
Oceania
 Australia. *See* Australia
 demographics of, 2538
 history of, 2538
 map of, 2539f
 New Zealand. *See* New Zealand
 Pacific Islands, 2538, 2540t, 2553-2554
 population of, 2540t
 summary of, 2554
Ocrelizumab, 1104, 1171
OCT1, 211-214, 212t
OCT2, 211-214, 212t, 213f
OCT3, 211-214, 212t
Octreotide, 456
Oculocerebrorenal dystrophy, 1438-1439
Oculocerebrorenal syndrome, 2345
Ogilvie's syndrome, 574
$1,25(OH)D$, 617, 742, 1829-1830
$1,25(OH)_2D$, 1830, 1841, 1848
Older adults. *See* Elderly
Oligomeganephronia, 1759
Oliguric renal failure, 425-426
Olive oil, 1957
Olmesartan medoxomil, 1309, 1652t, 1653, 1655
Omapatrilat, 345, 453-454
Omega-3 fatty acids, 1069
Oncocytic carcinoma, 1371, 1371t, 1372f
Oncocytoma, 891-892, 1368, 1501
Oncotic pressure, plasma, 1798
One-kidney renal clip hypertension, 1568-1569, 1570t, 1573f
One-kidney renovascular hypertension, 1571-1572
OPC 31260, 299-300
Opioids, 1942-1943, 2595

Opisthorchiasis, 2522-2523
Oral contraceptives, 659-660
Oral glucose tolerance test, 1912
Orellanine, 2525-2526
Organ perfusion sensors, 396-398
Organic acids, 516-517
Organic anion(s)
 classes of, 216t
 definition of, 216
 description of, 215-216
 excretion of, 247-248
  in acid-base homeostasis, 247-248
  in bicarbonate generation, 247-248
 fractional excretion of, 216
 proximal tubule secretion of, 216
 transport of, 215-216, 216t
Organic anion transporters
 characteristics of, 218t
 clinical relevance of, 219
 description of, 125
 NaDC family of, 217-218, 218f, 218t
 OAT family of, 218-219, 218t
 OATP family of, 218t, 219
 types of, 218t
Organic anion transporting polypeptide, 211
Organic cation(s)
 apical exit of, 211
 peritubular uptake of, 210
 reabsorption of, 211
 secretion of, 210, 210f
 transport of, 210-215, 210f
 type I, 210
 type II, 210
Organic cation transporters
 apical, 212t, 214-215
 basolateral, 211-214
 MATE1, 212t, 214-215
 MATE2-K, 212t, 214-215
 OCT1, 211-214, 212t
 OCT2, 211-214, 212t, 213f
 OCT3, 211-214, 212t
 regulation of, 214
 single-nucleotide polymorphisms in, 214
 structure of, 213-214
Organum vasculosum of the lamina terminalis, 464-465
Orientia tsutsugamushi, 2513
Ornipressin, 455
Oro-facial-digital syndrome type 1, 1504
Orthostatic hypotension, 776, 1538-1539, 1677, 1939
Orthostatic proteinuria, 1014
Osmolal gap, 840
Osmolality
 definition of, 461, 2366
 effective, 461
 plasma, 461, 466f, 468f, 2366
 total, 461
 urine, 465, 789, 1748
Osmolar gap, 490-491
Osmole excretion rate, 807-808, 811-812
Osmolytes, 502, 502f
Osmoreceptor dysfunction
 causes of, 477-478
 clinical manifestations of, 483
 hypernatremia caused by, 489
 hyponatremia in, 480
 pathophysiology of, 478-480
 patterns of, 478
 treatment of, 489
Osmoreceptor neuron, 466-467
Osmotic demyelination syndrome, 504-505, 505f, 505t

Osmotic diuresis
    case studies of, 812-813
    clinical approach to, 812
    description of, 811-813
    in diabetes mellitus patient, 812-813
    evaluation of, 811-812
Osmotic diuretics
    adverse effects of, 1705
    dosage of, 1704
    indications for, 1705
    mechanism of action, 1704
    pharmacokinetics of, 1704
    sites of action, 1704
    sodium reabsorption affected by, 422
Osmotic pressure, 461, 464-467
Osmotic thirst, 471-472
OSR1, 163, 714-715
Osr1, 21
Osteitis fibrosa cystica, 606, 2020-2021
Osteoblasts, 1832, 1842
Osteocalcin, 1726-1727
Osteocytes, 1832
Osteodystrophy
    mixed uremic, 1843, 1844*f*
    renal, 1842, 1845, 1845*t*, 2407*f*, 2434
Osteomalacia, aluminum-induced, 1843, 1844*f*
Osteonecrosis, 2282
Osteopenia, 2282
Osteopontin, 1330
Osteoporosis, 1352, 1726-1727, 2282-2283
Osteoprotegerin, 1300, 1832, 1833*f*, 1838
Ouabain, 721
Outer medulla
    anatomy of, 45, 45*f*, 65*f*, 91, 91*f*
    axial sodium chloride gradient in, 265-268
    concentrating mechanism in, 268*f*
    osmolality gradient of, 266, 267*f*
Outer medullary collecting duct (OMCD), 44-45, 45*f*, 73-74, 133, 166, 178, 242
Ovarian cyst, 1491
Ovarian dysfunction, 1920
Overflow hypothesis, 494
Overflow proteinuria, 791
Overt nephropathy, 1557
Oxalate, 1813. See also Calcium oxalate
    absorption of, 1339, 1339*f*
    calcium concentration versus, 1325-1327
    hepatic metabolism and, 1337-1338
    homeostasis of, 1340
    kidney stones and, 1324, 1337-1340
    recommended dosage of, 1361
    role of, 1339
Oxaloacetic acid, 248-249
Oxalobacter formigenes, 1339-1340, 2347
Oxalosis, 985-986
Oxcarbazepine, 497
Oxford-MEST score, 1063
Oxidant stress, 1815, 1817
Oxidative stress, 1579
    angiotensin II and, 982
    cardiovascular disease risks, 2100-2101
    chronic kidney disease and, 1758, 1865
    definition of, 1865
    preeclampsia and, 1620
2-Oxoglutarate, 245, 248-249
Oxygen, 126, 131*f*
Oxygen consumption, 133-135, 137*f*
Oxygen consumption rate, 134-135
Oxygen transport, 134
Oxytocin, 463

P

p53, 974
Pacific Islands, 2538, 2540*t*, 2553-2554

Pain, 1262, 1489, 1493, 2569
Pakistan. *See* Indian subcontinent
Palliative care, 2563, 2569-2570
Pallister-Hall syndrome, 2297*t*, 2299
Pamidronate, 1030
p-Aminohippurate, 216, 216*f*
p-Aminohippuric acid, 86
Pancreas-kidney transplantation, 1319, 2289
Pancreatic cyst, 1491
Panel reactive antibody, 2157
Pantothenic acid, 1983-1984
Papillary collecting ducts, 27, 75*f*
Papillary necrosis
    in granulomatous with polyangiitis, 1110
    nephrolithiasis versus, 769
    nonsteroidal antiinflammatory drugs as cause of, 362
    in sickle cell disease, 1198-1199, 1199*f*
Papillary renal cell carcinoma, 892, 897*f*, 1372*f*, 1373
Paracellin-1, 160
Paraldehyde-induced high anion gap acidosis, 549
Paramembranous cisternal system, 56
Paraneoplastic glomerular disease, 1403-1404
Paraoxonase, 2101
Parapelvic cyst, 1517
Paraphenylenediamine, 2501
Paraproteinemia, 628, 746, 1435
Paraquat, 2185-2186
Parasitic diseases, 1150-1151, 1255
Parathormone, 1453
Parathyroid carcinoma, 607
Parathyroid gland disease, 2019-2020
Parathyroid hormone. *See also* Hyperparathyroidism
    assays for, 1839-1841, 1840*f*
    bone remodeling and, 1834*f*, 1849, 2020-2021
    calcimimetics effect on, 1873
    calcium and
        description of, 606*f*, 1827*f*
        homeostasis, 601, 1826-1827, 1923
        transport, 187
    calcium-sensing receptor activation effects on, 2026
    in children, 2390-2391
    in chronic kidney disease–mineral bone disorder, 1826-1828, 1839-1841, 1840*f*, 1848
    cinacalcet effects on, 2027, 2032
    cleavage of, 1827
    cytochrome P450 enzymes affected by, 2019
    deficiency of, 601
    erythropoiesis affected by, 1887
    functions of, 1826-1827, 1923
    glomerular filtration rate effects on, 1865
    magnesium depletion effects on, 2387
    monitoring of, in stage 3 chronic kidney disease, 2014
    mortality and, 2020
    net acid excretion and, 740-741
    NH3 activity affected by, 235
    phosphate excretion affected by, 197-198, 1838-1839, 1977-1978
    phosphate wasting and, 199*f*
    phosphate-binding agents effect on, 2031
    phosphorus homeostasis affected by, 197-198
    proximal tubule bicarbonate reabsorption affected by, 237-238
    systemic effects of, 1847
    TRPV5 channels affected by, 189
    urea production affected by, 1968

Parathyroid hormone *(Continued)*
    urinary phosphate excretion increased by, 200
    vitamin D analogues effect on, 2027-2029
Parathyroid hormone(1-34), 618
Parathyroid hormone(1-84), 1839
Parathyroid hormone receptors, 603, 1749-1750, 1775, 1827, 1833
Parathyroid hormone-dependent resorptive hypercalciuria, 1335
Parathyroid hormone–fibroblast growth factor-23–1,25(OH)2D loop, 1838-1839
Parathyroid hormone-independent resorptive hypercalciuria, 1335
Parathyroid hormone-related protein, 607, 1399
Parathyroidectomy, 607, 2282
Paraventricular nuclei, 463
Parenteral nutrition, 620
Paricalcitol, 1312-1313, 2025-2026, 2029, 2032
Parietal epithelial cells, 4-5, 52-53, 52*f*53*f*, 1789-1790
Parinaud oculoglandular syndrome, 1149-1150
Pars convoluta
    anatomy of, 55-60, 58*f*
    basolateral intercellular space of, 55-56
    cells of, 55-56
    illustration of, 59*f*
    lateral cell processes of, 56, 58*f*
    vacuolar-lysosomal system in, 59-60
Pars recta, 60-61, 62*f*
Partial lipodystrophy, 1146-1147
Partial nephrectomy, 1380, 1380*t*
Partial pressure of carbon dioxide, 515-516
Parvovirus B19 infection, 1255
Passive countercurrent multiplier mechanism, 272
Passive Heymann nephritis, 377
PAT2, 224
Patient Self-Determination Act, 2561
Patiromer, 597
Pauci-immune crescentic glomerulonephritis
    anti-MPO antibodies in, 1083-1085
    antineutrophil cytoplasmic autoantibodies in, 1082-1084, 1086-1087
    anti-PR3 autoantibodies in, 1083
    clinical features of, 1085-1086
    crescent formation in, 1082
    cyclophosphamide for, 1087-1088
    electron microscopy of, 1083
    end-stage kidney disease progression of, 1086
    epidemiology of, 1081-1082
    immunofluorescence microscopy of, 1082-1083
    laboratory findings in, 1086-1087
    light microscopy of, 1082, 1082*f*
    methylprednisolone for, 1087-1089
    natural history of, 1085-1086
    pathogenesis of, 1083-1085
    pathology of, 1082-1083, 1082*f*
    plasmapheresis for, 1088
    PR3 in, 1083
    prognostic factors for, 1086
    relapse prevention in, 1089
    after renal transplantation, 1086
    rituximab for, 1088-1089
    segmental fibrinoid necrosis in, 1082*f*
    T cells in, 1084
    treatment of, 1087-1089
    urinalysis findings in, 1086-1087
Pauci-immune necrotizing glomerulonephritis, 1084-1085

PAX2, 2298
Pax2, 23, 27
Pax8, 23
Pazopanib, 1383, 1383f
p-cresol, 1812
p-cresyl sulfate, 1963, 2097
PDGF-B, 36
Pediatrics. *See* Children; Infants
Pegylated interferon, 1156
Pelvic malignancies, 1261
Pelvic neurofibromas, 1262
Penbutolol, 1656t-1657t, 1657-1658
Pendrin, 243-244
Penicillamine, 1448
Penicillin(s), 719, 1235t-1236t, 2513, 2514f
Pentamidine, 540-541, 591, 622
Pentoxifylline, 1313
Peptides, 1810
Peptidyl leukotrienes, 380
Percutaneous angioplasty/stent, 1569-1570
Percutaneous kidney biopsy, 2222-2224, 2223t, 2224f
Percutaneous mechanical thrombectomy
  of arteriovenous fistulas, 2210-2212
  of arteriovenous graft, 2199-2202, 2199t, 2201f-2202f
Percutaneous transluminal renal angioplasty, 1600
  arteriovenous fistulas treated with, 2208-2210, 2209t
  atherosclerosis renal artery stenosis treated with, 1602-1603
  central vein stenosis treated with, 2213-2214
  complications after, 1603t
Pericardial disease, 2107-2108
Pericytes, 5-6, 1777-1778, 1794
Perihilar focal segmental glomerulosclerosis, 1026
Perindopril, 1643-1644, 1643t
Perinephritic abscess, 1250
Perinuclear antineutrophil cytoplasmic antibody, 759-760
Periodic limb movements of sleep, 1939-1940
Peripheral α_1-adrenergic antagonists
  combination therapies using, 1692
  efficacy of, 1677
  mechanism of action, 1676
  moderately selective, 1675-1676, 1676t
  orthostatic hypotension caused by, 1677
  pharmacodynamics of, 1676t
  pharmacokinetics of, 1676t
  renal effects of, 1677
  safety of, 1677
  types of, 1676-1677, 1676t
Peripheral adrenergic neuronal blocking agents, 1649t-1650t
Peripheral arterial vasodilation, 439
Peripheral neuropathy, 1300
Peripolar cells, 53
Perirenal hematomas, 2253
Perirenal lymphangioma, 1517
Perirenal urinoma, 1517
Peritoneal dialysis (PD)
  access for, 2114-2116, 2415
  acute kidney injury treated with, 1008, 2120
  adequacy of
    in children, 2416
    clearance targets, 2122-2124, 2123t
    considerations for, 2120t
    definition of, 2120
    indicators for evaluating, 2120-2121

Peritoneal dialysis (PD) *(Continued)*
    solute clearance determinants used in, 2121-2122
    targets, 2122-2124, 2123t
    urea clearance as indicator of, 2120
  anorexia secondary to, 2125
  automated, 2049, 2114, 2117, 2119, 2130t, 2415
  cardiovascular disease in, 2127-2128
  catheters used in
    bowel perforation during placement of, 2221
    complications associated with, 2116-2117
    description of, 2114-2116
    diaphragmatic leaks, 2132
    entrapment of, 2116-2117
    fluoroscopic insertion of, 2220-2221
    impaired drainage of, 2116
    infections associated with, 2116, 2128, 2131
    insertion of, 2220-2221
    leaks from, 2132, 2416
    Moncrief-Popovich, 2115-2116
    nonrigid, 2116
    peritoneoscopic insertion technique for, 2221-2222
    presternal, 2115, 2222
    removal of, 2131
    rigid, 2116
    segments of, 2114-2115
    surgical placement of, 2116
    swan-neck, 2115, 2115f, 2221
    Tenckhoff, 2114-2115, 2115f, 2221, 2415
  in China, 2535
  complications of
    catheter-related, 2116-2117, 2416
    encapsulating peritoneal sclerosis, 2133, 2416-2417
    fluid leaks, 2416
    hernia, 2132
    hypercalcemia, 2132
    hyperglycemia, 2132
    hyperlipidemia, 2132
    hypokalemia, 572, 2132
    hyponatremia, 2132
    infections, 2116, 2128, 2131, 2416
    intraabdominal pressure, 2131
    intraperitoneal pressure increases, 2131
    mechanical, 2131-2132
    metabolic, 2132
    noninfectious, 2131-2133
    peritonitis. *See* Peritonitis
    ultrafiltration failure, 2416
  continuous ambulatory. *See* Continuous ambulatory peritoneal dialysis (CAPD)
  continuous cyclic, 2119
  cost-effectiveness of, 2134-2135
  definition of, 2220-2221
  in developing countries, 2135
  diabetic nephropathy treated with, 1318
  dialysate, 2117, 2121
  dose of, 2087, 2120-2121, 2121t
  drug dosing in, 2049
  economics of, 2134-2135
  ethical dilemmas. *See* Dialysis, ethical dilemmas
  exchanges, frequency of, 2122
  fluid removal in, 2121-2122
  gastroparesis associated with, 2125
  hemodialysis versus, 2087, 2134-2135, 2411
  in Hong Kong, 2535
  in Indian subcontinent, 2504

Peritoneal dialysis (PD) *(Continued)*
  inflammation during, 2125-2126
  insulin resistance in, 1913
  intraabdominal pressure in, 2112
  intravenous iron in, 1891f
  Kt/V assessments, 2416
  in Latin America, 2450t
  L-carnitine and, 2125
  malnutrition in, 2504
  mass transfer area coefficient, 2112-2113
  in Middle East, 2475t, 2487
  mineral metabolism abnormalities in patients receiving, 2132
  modalities for, 2119-2120
  nocturnal intermittent, 2119, 2122, 2415
  nutrition during, 1817-1818, 2124-2126
  outcomes of, 2122-2124, 2133-2134
  peritonitis associated with. *See* Peritonitis
  poison removal using, 2171, 2172t
  prescription for, 2119, 2122, 2415-2416, 2504
  protein-energy wasting in, 2124, 2124t
  reasons for reduced use of, 2134-2135
  residual kidney function after, 2126-2127
  in Singapore, 2536
  solutes, 2112-2114, 2121-2122
  solutions
    amino acids in, 2125
    bicarbonate-based, 2119, 2125
    biocompatible, 2126-2127
    composition of, 2117-2118, 2117t
    dextrose in, 2117
    dosage calculations, 2121t
    electrolytes in, 2117-2118
    glucose-containing, 2117-2119, 2127, 2132
    glucose-sparing, 2119
    icodextrin, 2118, 2415-2416
    lactate as buffer in, 2117
    osmolality of, 2122
    pediatric, 2415-2416
  survival rates affected by, 2134
  in Thailand, 2535
  tidal, 2415
  volume exchange, 2122
  water transport during, 2113-2114
Peritoneal equilibration test, 2113-2114
Peritoneal membrane, 2111-2112, 2113t, 2133, 2416-2417
Peritoneovenous shunting, 998-999
Peritoneum
  capillaries of, 2111-2112
  definition of, 2111
  interstitium of, 2112
  mesothelial cells of, 2111-2112
  microvessels of, 2111
  surface area of, 2111
Peritonitis
  bacterial, 2128-2129
  catheter removal in patients with, 2131
  in children, 2416
  clinical course of, 2128-2129
  definition of, 2128-2129
  diagnosis of, 2128-2129
  fungal, 2129, 2131
  gram-negative bacteria that cause, 2128-2131, 2504
  gram-positive bacteria that cause, 2128-2130, 2504
  in Indian subcontinent, 2504
  mycobacterial, 2129, 2131
  polymicrobial, 2131
  prevention of, 2131
  Pseudomonas aeruginosa, 2128-2131

Peritonitis *(Continued)*
  refractory, 2131
  relapsing, 2131
  Staphylococcus aureus, 2128, 2130
  treatment of, 2129-2131, 2130*t*
Peritubular capillaries
  anatomy of, 88*f*
  basement membrane of, 89-90
  density, 727-728
  dynamics of, 89-90
  efferent vessels as source of, 90
  fenestrations, 89
  surface of, 89
Peritubular capillary Starling forces, 400-402
Peritubular interstitial cells, 5-6
Peritubular protein, 151-152
Perivascular matrix, 980
Permeability factor, 1029-1030
Permissive hypercapnia, 2138-2139
Peroxisome proliferator-activated receptor τ
  angiotensin receptor blockers effect on, 733
  description of, 174
  fatty acid oxidation affected by, 733, 1761
  fluid retention induced by, 438-439
Peroxisome proliferator-activated receptors, 374-375, 438-444
Peroxisomes, in pars recta, 60-61
Peroxynitrite scavengers, 452
PGI. *See* Prostacyclin
pH
  buffering, 512
  description of, 512
  disequilibrium, 253
  NH_3 affected by, 249*f*
  NH_4^+ affected by, 249*f*
  plasma potassium levels affected by, 563
  urine. *See* Urinary pH
Phallotoxin, 2525-2526
Pharmacodynamic biomarker, 927*t*
Pharmacodynamics, 2040-2041
Pharmacogenomics, 2039-2040
Pharmacokinetics, 2035-2037, 2036*t*
Pharmacotherapeutic trial, 1363*t*
Phase-contrast magnetic resonance angiography, 859-861
Phenformin-induced lactic acidosis, 545
Phenobarbital, 2183
Phenols, 1811-1812
Phenoxybenzamine, 1675-1676
Phentolamine mesylate, 1675-1676, 1695*t*, 1698
Phenytoin, 2183-2184
Pheochromocytoma, 1547-1549
Philippines, 2536
Phleboliths, 874-876
Phlorizin, 206-207
Phosphate. *See also* Hyperphosphatemia; Hypophosphatemia
  additives, 1979
  age-related changes in, 742
  in blood, 196, 197*t*, 626
  in bone, 196
  in cellular processes, 196
  in children
    balance of, 2389-2390, 2389*f*2390*f*
    dietary intake of, 2390
    disorders of, 2396-2399, 2397*t*-2400*t*, 2398*f*2399*f*
    distribution of, 2389, 2390*f*
    fractional excretion of, 2397
    homeostasis of, 2391*f*
    regulation of, 2389
  in chronic kidney disease, 1977-1979, 2019
  in chronic kidney disease–mineral bone disorder, 1864, 1872

Phosphate *(Continued)*
  concentrations of, 197*t*
  dietary
    fibroblast growth factor-23 affected by, 1978
    intake of, 196, 2390
    parathyroid hormone affected by, 1978
    phosphate-binding agents for, 2021-2022
    restriction of, 1774-1775
  dietary protein intake and, 1977
  distribution of, 197*t*
  excretion of, 1450-1451
    acetazolamide effects on, 629
    insulin effects on, 200
    in metabolic acidosis, 247
    parathyroid hormone effects on, 197-198, 1977-1978
    urinary, 199-200
    urinary tract obstruction relief effects on, 1276-1277
  fibroblast growth factor-23 effects on concentration of, 1749-1750, 1775, 1776*f*, 1872, 1978, 2281, 2390-2391
  filtered, 246-247
  homeostasis of, 196-198, 196*f*197*f*, 1924
  intestinal absorption of, 2021
  metabolism of, 626, 1749-1750, 1774-1775
  niacin effects on, 1872
  redistribution of, 633
  replacement therapy, 633-634
  serum, 685, 1978-1979
  as titratable acid, 246-247
  transport of, 1450-1451
    catecholamines effect on, 200-201
    dietary, 199-200
    dopamine effects on, 201
    growth hormone effects on, 200
    inherited disorders of, 1450-1453
    insulin effects on, 200
    insulin-like growth factor-1 effects on, 200
    intestinal, 1824*f*
    parathyroid hormone effects on, 200
    phosphatonins effect on, 201-202
    regulation of, 199-202
    renal nerves and, 200-201
    serotonin effects on, 201
    sodium-mediated, 1749-1750
    transporters involved in, 247
    vitamin D metabolites, 200
  urinary excretion of, 199-201
Phosphate binders, 1872, 1945
Phosphate wasting
  Fanconi's syndrome and, 1437
  matrix extracellular phosphoglycoprotein and, 201-202
  renal, 631
  tumors associated with, 201-202
  urinary, inherited disorders of, 631*f*
Phosphate-binding agents
  aluminum-containing binders, 2022
  calcium-containing binders, 2022, 2031, 2094
  chronic kidney disease–mineral bone disorder treated with, 2020-2023, 2031
  lanthanum carbonate, 2021-2022
  magnesium, 2023
  parathyroid hormone levels affected by, 2031
Phosphate-binding resins, 2022-2023
Phosphate-dependent glutaminase, 248, 251*f*, 253
Phosphate–parathyroid hormone–fibroblast growth factor-23 loop, 1839

Phosphatidylinositol-3-kinase, 312, 1964
Phosphatonins, 197-198, 1830
  fibroblast growth factor-23, 191, 197-198, 198*f*, 201
  hypophosphatemia as cause of increased production or activity of, 630-631
  phosphate transport affected by, 201-202
Phosphaturia, 1437
Phosphinyl angiotensin-converting enzyme inhibitors, 1644
Phosphocreatine, 782
Phosphodiesterase inhibitors, 300-301
Phosphoenolpyruvate, 248-249
Phospho*enol*pyruvate carboxykinase, 248-249, 253
Phosphofructokinase, 514
Phospholipase A_2, 164, 355
Phospholipase A_2 receptor, 1035, 1039, 1155
Phospholipase C, 399, 1827*f*
Phospholipase Cε1, 1413-1414, 1414*t*
Phospholipase Cε1 disease, 1429-1430
Phosphoric acid, 247, 517
Phosphorus
  absorption of, 1823
  balance of, 1823-1824
  in blood, 196, 197*t*, 626
  in bone, 196
  in cellular processes, 196
  in chronic kidney disease, 1977-1978
  in chronic kidney disease–mineral bone disorder, 1847
  concentrations of, 197*t*
  daily intake of, 626
  dietary intake of, 196
  distribution of, 197*t*
  in end-stage kidney disease, 2028-2029
  homeostasis of, 196-198, 196*f*197*f*, 1822-1824, 1838-1839
  hormonal feedback systems that regulate, 197, 197*f*
  in hydroxyapatite, 196
  inorganic, 1822-1823
  intravenous repletion of, for hypophosphatemia, 634
  metabolism of, 1979
  monitoring of, 2014
  in plasma, 196
  reabsorption of, 198-199, 199*f*
  secretion of, 196
  serum, 196, 1822, 1839*f*
  sodium-phosphate cotransporters and, 198-199
  transport of, proteins involved in, 202
Phospho-specific antibodies, 154-155
Physiologic hydronephritis, 1633
Pierson's syndrome, 1426, 1782, 2325
Pindolol, 1656*t*-1657*t*, 1658
Pirfenidone, 1034
Pivmecillinam, 1238*t*
Placenta, 1618, 2607
Placental growth factor, 1623*f*
Placental protein 13, 1624
Placental vascular remodeling, 1618-1619
Placentation, 1614*f*
Plain radiographs, 846, 873, 874*f*
Planar cell polarity, 30-31
Plan-Do-Study-Act, 2623, 2623*t*, 2624*f*
Plant toxins, 2458
Plasma
  albumin concentrations in, 602, 791
  arginine vasopressin concentrations in, 466*f*
  atrial natriuretic peptide levels in, 414
  bicarbonate concentration in, 513-514, 520
  brain natriuretic peptide levels, 414

Plasma (Continued)
  filtration of, 781
  growth factors in, 1212
  kallikrein, 346
  kallikrein-kinin system, 347-348
  magnesium in, 193
  neutrophil gelatinase-associated lipocalin, 945-946
  phosphorus in, 196
  renin concentration in, 328
  urotensin II levels, 352
  vasoactive hormones effect on, 1799
  vasopressin levels in, 282
Plasma aldosterone concentration/plasma renin activity, 576
Plasma amino acids, 1971-1973, 1972f
Plasma cells, 1135-1136, 1233
Plasma membrane, 286, 287f
Plasma membrane calcium pump A1, 192-193, 192f
Plasma oncotic pressure, 1798
Plasma osmolality
  description of, 461, 468f, 2366
  measurement of, 484, 490
  plasma vasopressin and, 500f
  reduction in, 486
  thirst and, 471-472
Plasma proteins
  abnormal filtration of, 1786
  basement membrane passage of, 1013
  bicarbonate reabsorption affected by, 238
  binding of, in chronic kidney disease, 2037
  description of, 89
  furosemide binding to, 1724-1725
  glomerular ultrafiltration of, 1790
  high-molecular-weight, 791
  in nephrotic syndrome, 1018t
  podocytes effect on, 118
  poison binding to, 2169
  in proteinuria, 1013-1014
Plasma renin concentration assay, 328
Plasma renin concentration immunologic assay, 328
Plasmapheresis
  adverse events during, 2162-2163
  albumin as replacement fluid for, 2162
  angiotensin-converting enzyme inhibitors and, 2164
  anticoagulation for, 2162
  anti–glomerular basement membrane disease treated with, 1126-1127, 2149-2150, 2149t-2150t
  anti–glomerular basement membrane glomerulonephritis treated with, 1081
  antineutrophil cytoplasmic antibody-associated vasculitis treated with, 2150-2151
  atypical hemolytic-uremic syndrome treated with, 2154, 2354
  blood pressure reductions caused by, 2163
  catastrophic antiphospholipid antibody syndrome treated with, 2158-2159
  chronic inflammatory demyelinating polyneuropathy treated with, 2158
  clotting factor decreases after, 2164t
  colloidal starch as replacement fluid for, 2162
  complications of, 2162-2164, 2163t
  cryoglobulinemia treated with, 2152
  definition of, 2148
  double-filtration, 2160
  familial hypercholesterolemia treated with, 2159

Plasmapheresis (Continued)
  fibrinogen levels affected by, 2163
  fresh frozen plasma for, 2155
  general principles of, 2148-2149
  granulomatous with polyangiitis treated with, 1113
  Guillain-Barré syndrome treated with, 2158
  hematologic disorders treated with, 2152-2154
  hemolytic uremic syndrome treated with, 2154-2155
  history of, 2148
  hypocalcemia during, 2163
  idiopathic rapidly progressive glomerulonephritis treated with, 2151
  intravenous immunoglobulin and, 2157
  lupus nephritis treated with, 1105, 2151-2152
  mixed cryoglobulinemia treated with, 2152
  multiple myeloma treated with, 2153t
  myasthenia gravis treated with, 2158
  myeloma cast nephropathy treated with, 1002
  pathologic factors removed using, 2149, 2149t
  pauci-immune crescentic glomerulonephritis treated with, 1088
  poison removal using, 2171
  in pregnancy, 2159
  premature delivery secondary to, 2159
  rapidly progressive glomerulonephritis treated with, 2150-2151
  renal transplantation applications of, 2155-2157
  replacement fluids for, 2162
  techniques of, 2159-2162, 2161f
  thrombotic thrombocytopenic purpura treated with, 2154-2155
  toxin removal using, 2159
  venous access for, 2161-2162
Plasminogen activator inhibitor-1, 378, 729, 1212-1213
Plasmodium falciparum, 1150, 2442-2443, 2470-2472, 2496, 2517-2518, 2519f. See also Malaria
Platelet(s)
  aggregation of, 1189f, 1804
  hyperaggregability of, hypoalbuminemia's role in, 1798, 1804
  thromboxane modulation of, 368
  in uremia, 1904-1905
  uremic, 1905, 1907f
Platelet-activating factor, 1741
Platelet-derived growth factor receptor, 330
Platelet-derived growth factor-B, 1789
PLCE1, 1413-1414, 1414t
PLCE1 disease, 1429-1430
Plicamycin, 612, 1400
PMCA. See Plasma membrane calcium pump A1
Pneumocystis jiroveci pneumonia, 2430-2431
Pneumocystosis, 2288
Pneumonia, 2105
Podocalyxin, 118, 936
Podocin, 37-38, 1413-1414, 1414t
Podocin disease. See Nephrotic syndrome, steroid-resistant
Podocyte(s)
  albumin passage affected by, 112-113
  angiopoietin-like 4 overproduction in, 1021
  angiotensin II effects on, 1788

Podocyte(s) (Continued)
  anti–B cell therapy effects on, 119
  apoptosis of, 1788
  biologic functions of, 112-113
  calcineurin inhibitors effect on, 119
  Cdc42 inactivation in, 38, 39f
  characteristics of, 49
  COX-2 overexpression in, 376
  cytoskeleton of, 113
  definition of, 791, 2609
  depletion of, 118-119
  in diabetic nephropathy, 115t, 116-117, 120
  disease-induced injury of, 117-119
  endocytosis by, 49
  filtration slit, 49-51, 1782-1783, 1783f
  in focal segmental glomerulosclerosis, 115t, 116, 118-119
  foot processes of
    description of, 36, 38, 49, 51f, 113
    effacement of
      in congenital nephrotic syndrome, 2325
      in Fabry's disease, 1144
      in focal segmental glomerulosclerosis, 1027, 1029
      in membranous nephropathy, 1036-1037
      in minimal change disease, 1016, 1019, 1020f
    function of, 2325f
    maintenance of, 2325f
  future therapeutic approaches for, 120
  glomerular basement membrane and, 4-5, 118
  in glomerular diseases, 113, 115t
  glucocorticoids effect on, 119
  in human immunodeficiency virus nephropathy, 116
  hypertrophy of, 1754
  in immunoglobulin A nephropathy, 1064
  inherited disorders affecting, 1426-1431
  injury of
    in chronic kidney disease progression, 1753-1754
    effacement after, 117-118, 117f
    glomerulosclerosis secondary to, 118-119
    hepatocyte growth factor effects on, 120
    after nephron loss, 1753-1754
    proteinuria affected by, 118
  in membranous nephropathy, 115t, 116
  in minimal change nephropathy, 114-116, 115t
  molecular anatomy of, 113, 115f
  morphologic features of, 36
  parathyroid hormone receptor expression by, 1775
  plasma protein passage affected by, 118
  protein uptake by, 1787
  proteinuria effects on, 1787-1788
  regeneration of, 2609
  renin-angiotensin-aldosterone inhibitors effect on, 119-120
  slit diaphragm in, 38-39, 51, 118, 1782-1783, 1782f
  structure of, 113, 114f
  summary of, 120
  transcription factors expressed by, 36-37
  ultrastructure of, 38f, 113, 114f, 1788
  vascular endothelial growth factor expression by, 1752-1753
  vascular endothelial growth factor-A, 32
Podocyte count, 936

Podocytopathy, 114-116
Poison removal/poisonings
  chromic acid, 2501
  copper sulfate, 2500
  corporeal treatments for, 2167-2169, 2168t
  description of, 2166-2167
  elimination enhancement techniques for, 2166-2167, 2167f
  ethylene dibromide, 2501
  extracorporeal treatments for
    acetaminophen, 2187-2188
    albumin dialysis, 2171, 2172t
    barbiturates, 2183
    carbamazepine, 2182-2183
    combination therapies, 2171
    continuous renal replacement therapy, 2171
    criteria for, 2169
    duration of, 2173
    endogenous clearance effects on, 2169
    ethylene glycol, 2173-2178, 2174t, 2176t
    exchange transfusion, 2171, 2172t
    extraction ratio, 2169
    factors that affect, 2169
    hemodialysis, 2169-2170, 2170t, 2172t
    hemofiltration, 2170, 2172t
    hemoperfusion, 2169-2170, 2172t
    heparinization, 2173
    indications for, 2172-2173
    isopropanol, 2173-2178, 2174t, 2176t
    lithium, 2180-2181
    metformin, 2184-2185
    methanol, 2173-2178, 2174t, 2176t
    methotrexate, 2188-2189
    paraquat, 2185-2186
    peritoneal dialysis, 2171, 2172t
    phenytoin, 2183-2184
    plasmapheresis, 2171
    poison-related factors that affect, 2169
    rebound after discontinuation of, 2173
    salicylic acid, 2178-2180
    technical considerations, 2173
    theophylline, 2186-2187
    therapeutic plasma exchange, 2171
    toxic alcohols, 2173-2178, 2174t, 2176t
    valproic acid, 2181-2182
    vascular access for, 2173
  hair dye, 2501
  multiple-dose activated charcoal for, 2168
  rebound after extracorporeal treatment discontinuation, 2173
  statistics regarding, 2167t
Polar cushion, 53
Polyarteritis nodosa
  angiographic findings in, 1119
  in children, 2350-2351
  classic, 1118-1119
  clinical features of, 1119, 2350
  corticosteroids for, 1119-1120
  cyclophosphamide for, 1119-1120
  diagnosis of, 2350
  gender predilection of, 1118
  hairy cell leukemia associated with, 1118-1120
  hepatitis B virus associated with, 1118-1120
  hypertension in, 1119
  incidence of, 1118
  laboratory tests, 1119, 2350
  microscopic, 1118
  pathogenesis of, 1118-1119, 2350
  pathology of, 1118
  prognosis for, 1119-1120
  renal findings in, 1119
  survival rate for, 1119-1120
  treatment of, 1119-1120, 2350-2351

Polychronotropism, 1385
Polyclonal immune globulins, 2247-2248, 2255
Polycystic kidney disease, 1416, 1479
  adult-acquired, 888, 889f
  in children. See Children, polycystic kidney disease in
  classification of, 885
  computed tomography of, 869f, 1489f, 1491f
  extrarenal manifestations of, 775
  glomerular filtration rate declines secondary to, 681
  hypothetical pathways upregulated and downregulated in, 1482f, 1483
  infantile, 885
  organomegaly associated with, 885
Polycystic liver disease, 1491, 1491f, 1494
Polycystin, 1477-1478, 1478f
Polycystin protein, 1481f
Polydipsia
  in children, 2369, 2370t
  primary. See Primary polydipsia
  psychogenic, 482
Polygenic disease, 1411t, 1412, 1419
Polygenic hypercalciuria, 1349-1350
Polygenic kidney disease, 1410
Polyols, 1813
Polyomavirus infection, 1404-1405, 2272-2273
Polyuria, 1437
  in acute renal injury, 299
  aquaporin-2 dysregulation in, 297
  in children, 2369, 2370t
  in chronic renal injury, 299
  classification of, 804
  definition of, 804
  differential diagnosis of, 483-486
  effects of, 1473
  in hereditary hypokalemic salt-losing tubulopathy, 1473
  in hypokalemia, 570
  hypotonic, 473t, 483-484
  lithium-induced, 379
Poorly differentiated renal cell carcinoma, 899f
Porphyria cutanea tarda, 1946, 1946f
Portal hypertension, 446-447
Port-wine stain, 1952
Positron emission tomography, 899-903
Positron emission tomography–computed tomography, 899-903
Posterior urethral valves, 2316, 2317f, 2435
Postglomerular hypoxia, 1790
Postobstructive diuresis, 1281
Postpartum recovery, 1617
Postrenal azotemia, 968
Postrenal failure, 770
Postrenal proteinuria, 791
Poststenotic renal perfusion pressure (iliac), 1570-1571, 1571f
Poststreptococcal glomerulonephritis
  acute. See Acute poststreptococcal glomerulonephritis
  in Africa, 2461
  description of, 757
  in New Zealand, 2550
Posttransplantation diabetes mellitus, 1320, 2283
Posttransplantation lymphoproliferative disorder (PTLD), 2285-2286, 2286t, 2423-2424, 2426, 2429, 2433
Potassium
  adrenal sensing, 568-569
  assessment of, 820-821
  balance of, 174, 741, 741f

Potassium (Continued)
  cell membrane permeability to, 125
  in children, 2374-2382
  connecting tubule secretion of, 176-178
  cortical collecting duct secretion of, 176-178
  deficiency of, 481, 520
  depletion of, 547, 1968
  deprivation of, 180-182
  dietary intake of, 559-560, 566, 584t, 1975
  distal convoluted tubule secretion of, 176-178
  distal nephron secretion of, vasopressin effects on, 182
  distribution of
    acid-base status effects on, 563
    factors that affect, 562-563, 562t-563t, 563f
    hyperkalemia caused by, 586-588
    illustration of, 560f
    insulin effects on, 562, 587, 594
    sympathetic nervous system effects on, 562
  diuretics effect on, 1728
  efflux of, 560-562
  in end-stage kidney disease, 174-175, 2093
  excessive intake of, 586
  excretion of
    abnormal rate of, 821
    in acquired tubular defects, 589
    diuretics effect on, 595, 1711-1712
    fractional, 2375-2376
    in hereditary tubular defects, 589-590
    high, 825
    in hyporeninemic hypoaldosteronism, 589
    low, 823-825
    nephron loss-specific adaptations in, 1748-1749
    reductions in, 588-590
    regulation of, 536-537
    thiazide diuretics effect on, 1711-1712
    urinary, 564f, 569, 595, 820
    urinary tract obstruction relief effects on, 1276
  extracellular, 174-175, 568f
  fractional excretion of, 2375-2376
  in hemodialysis dialysate, 2093
  hemodialysis effects on, 599
  homeostasis of, 565-567, 579, 587, 1748-1749
  intracellular, 174, 560
  loading of, 179-180
  loss of
    apparent mineralocorticoid excess, 577-578
    Bartter's syndrome and, 578-580
    diuretics as cause of, 574-575
    drugs as cause of, 574-575
    familial hypokalemic alkalosis as cause of, 578-580
    fecal, 574
    gastric, 574
    Gitelman's syndrome and, 580
    hyperaldosteronism as cause of, 575-577, 576f
    intestinal, 574
    Liddle's syndrome as cause of, 578
    minimization strategies for, 585
    nonrenal causes of, 574
    renal tubular acidosis as cause of, 580-581
  medullary recycling of, 175-176
  monocarboxylic acids effect on, 818f
  normal levels of, 559-563
  oral supplementation of, 583-585

Potassium *(Continued)*
  parenteral administration of, 583-584
  plasma, in hypovolemia, 423
  proximal tubule bicarbonate reabsorption affected by, 237
  reabsorption of
    by collecting duct, 178
    in distal nephron, 564
    in loop of Henle, 563-564
    in proximal tubule, 175, 563-564
  redistribution of, 586-588, 594-595
  renal excretion of, 818-819
  secretion of
    aldosterone in, 312-314, 317, 565-566
    in aldosterone-sensitive distal nephron, 319-320
    arginine vasopressin effects on, 1717
    connecting tubule's role in, 69
    cortical connecting tubule's role in, 73, 563-564, 1748-1749
    in cortical distal nephron, 819
    in distal colon, 174-175
    distal sodium absorption and, 566-568
    epithelial sodium channel activity effects on, 313
    pathways of, 563f
    potassium intake effects on, 566
  serum, 564f, 596, 1728
  in skeletal muscle, 174-175, 560
  sodium polystyrene sulfonate effects on, 596
  succinylcholine-induced efflux of, 587-588, 587f
  transcellular distribution of, 818-830
  transtubular potassium concentration gradient, 569, 573-574, 820-821, 2380
  urinary excretion of, 180, 564f, 2302
Potassium binders, 597-598
Potassium channels
  in ammonia metabolism, 254
  apical, 159-160, 313
  drugs that affect, 588
Potassium chloride
  description of, 424-425, 583
  oral preparations of, 584-585, 585t
  transport of, 162, 178
Potassium ion deficiency, 555
Potassium transport
  aldosterone effects on, 179-180, 564
  distal, 179-182
  in distal nephron, 563-564
  in inner medullary collecting duct, 133
  in loop of Henle, 175-176
  mechanisms of, 560-563, 561f
  in proximal tubule, 175, 175f
  sodium chloride transport and, in distal nephron, 182-183
  transepithelial, 175-176
Potassium wasting, 569, 1437
Potassium-chloride cotransporter, 150, 564
Potassium-sparing diuretics
  distal. *See* Distal potassium-sparing diuretics
  Gitelman's syndrome treated with, 1727
  hypervolemia treated with, 451
  hypomagnesemia treated with, 625
  mechanism of action, 451
  side effects of, 451
Potting compound, 2075-2076
POU domain-containing transcription factor, 30
Pou3f3, 30
Poverty, 666
Power Doppler ultrasonography, 850f

Pramipexole, 1940
Praziquantel, 1255
Prazosin, 1676t, 1677, 1697t, 1714
Prealbumin, 1970-1971
Predictive biomarker, 927t
Predictive Safety Testing Consortium, 953
Prednisolone, 1043, 2329
Prednisone
  anti-glomerular basement membrane glomerulonephritis treated with, 1081
  azathioprine and, 2257
  focal segmental glomerulosclerosis treated with, 1032, 1167
  immunoglobulin A nephropathy treated with, 1067
  lupus nephritis treated with, 1102
  minimal change disease treated with, 1022-1024, 1167
  during pregnancy, 1637, 1637t
Preeclampsia. *See also* Pregnancy
  acute kidney injury and, 1632
  angiogenic imbalance and, 1621-1623
  cardiovascular disease and, 1618, 1618f
  cerebral changes with, 1619-1620
  characteristics and effect of, 1613-1627
  chronic kidney disease progression affected by, 680-681
  clinical features of, 1616
  diabetes and, 1634
  diagnosis of, 1615t
  edema and, 1616
  endothelin-1 in, 338
  extrauterine pregnancy and, 1618
  glomerular endotheliosis and, 1619, 1621f
  hemodynamic and vascular changes with, 1619
  hypertension and, 1615-1618, 1615t
  hypoxia-inducible factor and, 1619
  immunologic intolerance and, 1620-1621
  incidence of, 1613
  intracerebral parenchymal hemorrhage and, 1619-1620
  kidney disease and, 1617-1618
  long-term cardiovascular and renal outcomes from, 1617-1618
  low birth weight and, 1617-1618
  management and treatment of, 1626-1627
  maternal and neonatal mortality during, 1617
  maternal endothelial dysfunction and, 1619
  medical conditions associated with, 1614
  oxidative stress and, 1620
  pathogenesis of, 1618-1624, 1620f
  placenta role in, 1618
  placental growth factor and, 1623f
  placentation in, 1614f
  plasma renin levels in, 1623-1624
  postpartum recovery and, 1617
  prevention of, 1625-1626
  proteinuria in, 798, 1615t, 1616, 1618
  renal changes with, 1619
  risk factors for, 1614-1615, 1615t
  screening for, 1624-1625
  seizures and, 1616
  sickle cell disease and, 1618
  soluble fms-like tyrosine kinase-1 and, 1621, 1622f
  uric acid levels and, 1616
  vascular endothelial growth factor and, 1619, 1621-1623
  vascular endothelial growth factor receptor 1 and, 1621

Pregnancy, 1617-1618. *See also* Preeclampsia
  acute fatty liver of, 992, 1632
  acute kidney injury in, 990-992, 991t, 1631-1633, 2458
  acute tubular and bilateral cortical necrosis in, 1631-1632
  angiotensin II and, 1613f
  angiotensin receptor blockers in, 1647, 1655
  angiotensin-converting enzyme inhibitors during, 1647, 1685
  antihypertensive treatment during, 1629f, 1630t, 1685, 1687f
  asymptomatic bacteriuria in, 1245-1247
  atypical hemolytic-uremic syndrome in, 1182
  characteristics of, 1610
  chronic kidney disease and, 680-681, 1633-1638
  diabetes insipidus of, 1612
  in diabetic nephropathy patients, 1300, 1634
  1,25-dihydroxyvitamin d3 levels during, 1632-1633
  drug classification for, 1637
  glomerular filtration rate estimations in, 788
  hemodynamic and vascular changes during, 1610-1611, 1611f
  hypertension in, 681, 1627-1631
  immunoglobulin A nephropathy during, 1066
  immunosuppressive therapy during, 1637-1638, 1637t
  kidney stones during, 1633
  long-term dialysis and, 1635-1636
  lupus nephritis and, 1100, 1634-1635
  maternal and neonatal mortality, 1617
  maternal nutrient restriction in, 715-717
  mean arterial pressure changes during, 1611f
  mechanism of vasodilation in, 1612-1613
  mycophenolic acid exposure during, 2426
  physiologic changes during, 1611t
  plasmapheresis in, 2159
  preeclampsia in, 680-681
  prostaglandin synthesis in, 378-379
  proteinuria in, 798
  pyelonephritis in, 1245-1246
  renal adaptation to, 1611-1612
  renal allograft function effect on, 1636-1637
  renal donation and, 1638
  renal transplantation in, 2289-2290
  in renal transplantation recipient, 1636-1638, 1636f, 2435-2436
  respiratory alkalosis of, 1612
  soluble fms-like tyrosine kinase-1 levels in, 1623
  systemic lupus erythematosus and, 1100
  thiazide diuretics during, 1732
  thrombotic microangiopathy during, 1632
  uric acid levels and, 1612, 1616
Prehypertension, 2360
Prematurity
  acute kidney injury risks, 711-712
  blood pressure affected by, 706-709, 707f-708f
  categories of, 694t
  chronic kidney disease and, 712
  glomerular filtration rate affected by, 709-710
  nephron number and, 703-705
  risk factors for, 722

PreproBNP, 340
PreproCNP, 340
Prepro-urotensin II, 418-419
Prerenal azotemia, 450, 770
  acute kidney injury caused by, 963
  in liver disease, 998
  radiocontrast media-induced acute kidney injury, 964
  renal sympathetic nerve activity in, 963
  volume-nonresponsive, 963
  volume-responsive, 963
Pressor kidney, 1568-1569
Pressure monitors, 2075
Pressure natriuresis, 373, 402-405, 1528-1529, 1529f
Presternal catheter, 2115
Preterm infants, sodium retention in, 2366-2367
Pretubular aggregates, 3, 28, 30
Primary aldosteronism, 322-323, 555, 1546
Primary cilium, 1477-1478, 1478f, 1505-1506, 1506f
Primary hyperaldosteronism, 575, 576f, 1545-1547
Primary hyperoxaluria, 1337-1338, 2346-2348, 2422, 2431, 2478
Primary hyperparathyroidism
  age of onset, 606
  clinical presentation of, 606
  diagnosis of, 606
  familial syndromes, 608
  hypercalcemia caused by, 604-607
  osteitis fibrosa cystica in, 606
  parathyroid carcinoma as cause of, 607
  parathyroidectomy for, 607
  surgery for, 606-607
Primary hypertension, 1562-1565
Primary hypoaldosteronism, 588
Primary megaureter, 2315-2316
Primary mineralocorticoid deficiency, 538
Primary polydipsia
  causes of, 482, 497-498
  definition of, 482
  hyponatremia in, 496
  pathophysiology of, 482-483
  treatment of, 490
Principal cells
  aldosterone in, 567
  aquaporin expression in, 289, 289f
  bicarbonate reabsorption affected by, 241
  in collecting ducts, 30, 69-70, 241
  in cortical collecting duct, 70, 70f, 74
  in inner medullary collecting duct, 75, 76f
  in outer medullary collecting duct, 73-74
ProANP, 340
Pro-brain natriuretic peptide, 1800
Progenitor cells, 1795, 2608-2609
Prognostic biomarker, 927t
Programmed death 1, 1215, 2240-2241
Progressive hypermagnesemia, 625
Progressive renal failure, acidosis of, 541-543
Progressive vascular occlusion, 1585-1587, 1598
PROK2, 2318
Prolactin, 1919
Prolactinemia, in chronic kidney disease, 1919
Proliferative glomerulonephritis, 1136, 1159
Prolonged intermittent renal replacement therapy, 1008
Prolyl-4-hydroxylase domains, 140
PROMETHEUS, 458
Pronephric duct, 2-3
Pronephric tubules, 2-3
Pronephros, 2-3, 3f, 20-21
Propranolol, 1656t-1657t, 1657

Propylene glycol-induced high anion gap acidosis, 549
Prorenin, 327-328, 327f
(Pro)renin receptor, 331-332
Prospective payment system, 2628-2629
Prostacyclin
  age-related changes in, 735-736
  description of, 364-365
  metabolism of, 374
  renal epithelial effects of, 369
  vasodilator role of, 369
Prostacyclin synthase, 364-365
Prostaglandin(s)
  angiotensin II effects on production of, 99
  aspirin effects on, 380
  atrial natriuretic peptide and, 436-437
  in cirrhosis, 378, 448-449
  classification of, 375
  COX-2–derived, 568
  cyclopentenone, 374-375
  description of, 1579
  in effective arterial blood volume regulation, 411-413
  as fatty acids, 375
  half-life of, 374
  in heart failure, 436-437
  metabolism of, 374-375
  nephrogenic diabetes insipidus treated with, 301
  PGD_2, 99
  in pregnancy, 378-379
  sodium retention and, 448-449
  synthesis of, 80, 360, 742
  transport of, 375
  as vasodilators, 411-412
  vasodilatory, 359f
  in volume homeostasis, 411
  w/w-1 hydroxylation of, 374
Prostaglandin A_2, 374
Prostaglandin D_2, 365
Prostaglandin D synthase, 365
Prostaglandin E_2, 412
  cytokines that stimulate synthesis of, 376
  hydroxylation of, 374
  medullary blood flow affected by, 362f
  metabolism of, 374
  nonsteroidal anti-inflammatory drug-induced blockade of, 371
  prohypertensive effects of, 372
  proximal tubule effects of, 373
  renal function by, 372
  salt excretion and, 362f
  sodium absorption affected by, 361-362
  sodium reabsorption affected by, 1716-1717
  vasoconstrictive effects of, 372
  water excretion and, 362f
Prostaglandin E synthases, 366
Prostaglandin $F_{2\alpha}$, 365, 374
Prostaglandin $F_{2\alpha}$ receptor, 369-370
Prostaglandin H_2, 364, 364f
Prostaglandin 9-ketoreductase, 365-366
Prostaglandin receptors, 367f
Prostaglandin synthase inhibitors, 487
Prostaglandin synthases, 357, 358f, 364f
Prostaglandin transporter, 375
Prostanoid receptors
  DP receptors, 369
  EP1 receptors, 370
  EP2 receptors, 370-371
  EP3 receptors, 371-372
  EP4 receptors, 372
  FP receptors, 369-370
  intrarenal distribution of, 367f
  IP receptors, 369

Prostanoid receptors (Continued)
  knockout mice models of, 368f
  mRNA, 366f
  tissue distribution of, 366f
  TP receptors, 366-369
Prostanoids
  cyclooxygenase-2–derived, 357-358
  degradation of, 411
  glomerular damage mediated by, 376
  mesangial cells affected by, 377
  transport of, 375
  vasodilatory, 376-377
Prostate cancer, 1261
Prostate gland, 1234, 1677
Prostatitis
  acute bacterial, 1247
  bacille de Calmette-Guérin as cause of, 1254
  chronic bacterial, in elderly, 750
  Escherichia coli as cause of, 1247
  National Institutes of Health classification of, 1247, 1247t
Protease inhibitors, 2456-2457
Protein
  catabolism of, 128f, 517, 1959-1960
  dietary
    albumin synthesis affected by, 1796
    caspase-3 effects on, 1965
    in chronic kidney disease, 1767-1768, 1975-1977, 1976t
    in diabetic kidney disease, 1981
    hemodynamic responses to changes in, 1958
    high intake of, chronic kidney disease risks associated with, 680
    hypermetabolism and, 1958
    low-protein diet, 1312, 1970, 1976-1977
    maternal, restriction of, 723
    metabolic acidosis effects on, 1963-1964
    myostatin effects, 1967-1968
    in nephrotic syndrome, 1976-1977
    oxidative stress and, 1958
    phosphates and, 1977
    proteinuria increases associated with, 1962
    renal function affected by, 1767-1768, 1958-1959, 1981
    requirements for, factors that affect, 1963-1968
    restriction of, 1312, 1767-1768, 1980-1981, 1994-1995
    transforming growth factor-β affected by, 1958
    transforming growth factor-β levels affected by, 1958
    ubiquitin-protease system effects on, 1964-1965
    urinary albumin affected by, 1312
  DNA variation, 1435t
  external losses of, 1968
  high-molecular-weight, 791
  kidney stones and, 1324, 1354
  low-molecular-weight, 791, 1810t
  metabolism of, uremia effects on, 1817
  muscle, 1965, 1966f, 1970
  normal levels of, 791
  physiology of, 791
  podocyte uptake of, 1787
  proximal tubule reabsorption of, 1784-1786
  slit diaphragm, 113
  Tamm-Horsfall, 791, 947
  tissue, loss of, 1817
  total, 793, 794t
  as uremic solute, 1810

Protein *(Continued)*
  urinary
    in acute tubular necrosis, 987
    in children, 2310-2311
    description of, 112, 682-683
    diurnal variation in excretion of, 796
    excretion of, 682-683, 947, 1654, 1784
    factors that affect, 792*t*
    fluctuations in excretion of, 796
    postural effects on excretion of, 796
    protein-to-creatinine ratios, 792, 795-796
    reagent strip testing for, 797
    timed versus random collection of, 795
    24-hour testing of, 795-796
  water homeostasis and, 1468
  in Western diets, 740-741
Protein C, 980-981
Protein kinase A, 154-155, 214, 292-293
Protein kinase C, 292-293
Protein kinase G, 292-293
Protein overload, 1212, 1792
Protein-bound calcium, 602
Protein-bound solutes, 1814
Protein-energy wasting
  in chronic kidney disease, 1817, 1913, 1994-1995
    during hemodialysis, 1317-1318, 2098-2099
  insulin-like growth factor-1 as biomarker of, 2099
  megestrol acetate for, 1920
  in peritoneal dialysis, 2124, 2124*t*
Protein-restricted diet, 1984
Protein-to-creatinine ratios, 792, 795-796
Proteinuria, 1398
  acute interstitial nephritis and, 1219
  aliskiren as cause of, 1678
  bevacizumab causing, 1398
  birth weight and, 710-711
  bone marrow-derived fibrocytes in, 1793
  captopril and, 1159, 1645
  categorization of, 791-792
  causes of, 1013-1014
  changes after long-term treatment, 1556*t*
  in children, 798, 2310-2311
  in chronic kidney disease, 682-683, 947-948, 2004-2005, 2361-2362
  COX-2 inhibitors effect on, 377-378
  C1q nephropathy as cause of, 1034-1035
  criteria for, 1785-1786
  definition of, 1785-1786
  dendritic cells in, 1792-1793
  description of, 790
  in diabetic nephropathy, 1295, 2004-2005
  diagnosis of, 947
  dietary proteins and, 1959, 1994-1995
  experimental models of, 1761-1762
  Fanconi's syndrome and, 1437
  fixed, 1014
  in focal segmental glomerulosclerosis, 1024-1025, 1030-1031, 1164, 1750-1752
  glomerular, 791, 1780, 1785-1786
  glomerular basement membrane and, 2323
  glomerular damage caused by, 1786-1790, 1787*f*
  as glomerular disease, 1013-1014
  as glomerular injury marker, 1760-1761
  gold salts and, 1158
  hematuria and, 758-759
  in hepatitis B, 1154
  in hepatitis C, 1156
  hereditary syndromes, 2323-2325

Proteinuria *(Continued)*
  in immunoglobulin A nephropathy, 1065-1066, 1069, 1164-1165
  in immunotactoid glomerulopathy, 1072, 1132
  interstitial inflammation and injury in, 1792-1794
  in ischemia-reperfusion injury, 1786
  isolated, 1013-1014, 2311
  Kidney Disease Improving Global Outcomes categories of, 792*t*
  in kidney transplantation, 798
  kidney-derived progenitor cells in, 1795
  lipid-lowering therapy effects on, 1774
  low birth weight and, 710-711
  in lupus nephritis, 1165-1166
  lymphocytes in, 1793
  macrophages in, 1793-1795
  measurement of, 792-793, 792*t*, 794*t*
  mechanisms of
    glomerular capillary wall, 1780-1784
    glomerular permselectivity, 1783-1784
  in membranous glomerulonephritis, 1164
  in membranous nephropathy, 1035, 1039-1041, 1158-1159
  mesangial cells affected by, 1788-1789
  in microscopic polyangiitis, 1115
  in minimal change disease, 1022
  monocytes in, 1792-1793
  after nephrectomy, 1752*f*
  nephrotic syndrome in, 1796
  nephrotic-range
    description of, 1796
    edema caused by, 1798-1800, 1798*f*-1799*f*
    hypercoagulability associated with, 1803-1805, 1803*f*
    hyperlipidemia associated with, 1801-1803, 1801*f*, 1803*f*, 1816-1817
    hypoalbuminemia caused by, 1796-1798, 1796*f*
    infection susceptibility, 1805
  orthostatic, 1014
  overflow, 791
  parietal epithelial cells in, 1789-1790
  plasma proteins in, 1013-1014
  podocytes affected by, 118, 1787-1788
  postglomerular hypoxia in, 1790
  postrenal, 791
  posttransplantation recurrence of, 1427-1428
  preeclampsia and, 798, 1615*t*, 1616, 1618
  proximal tubular cells in, 1791-1792
  reagent strip testing for, 797
  reduced, benefits of, 2010*f*
  regulatory T cells in, 1795
  renal allograft survival affected by, 2280
  renal artery stenosis and, 1584
  renal damage and, 1762-1763
  renal function affected by, 1645
  renin-angiotensin-aldosterone system in, 334
  serum albumin levels affected by, 683
  in sickle cell disease, 1199
  smoking and, 1991-1992
  statins effect on, 2011
  stroke risks associated with, 1928*t*, 1930
  in temporal arteritis, 1120
  treatment of, 1141, 1163-1166, 1429, 2004-2005
  tubular, 791, 793
  tubular cell activation and damage induced by, 1211-1212

Proteinuria *(Continued)*
  tubular damage caused by, 1790-1792, 1790*f*
  tubuloglomerular disconnection in, 1791
  in type 1 diabetes mellitus, 1292-1293, 1300
  types of, 791
  urinary cystatin C associated with, 949
  urinary protein in
    description of, 112, 682-683
    diurnal variation in excretion of, 796
    excretion of, as chronic kidney disease biomarker, 682-683
    factors that affect, 792*t*
    fluctuations in excretion of, 796
    postural effects on excretion of, 796
    protein-to-creatinine ratios, 792, 795-796
    reagent strip testing for, 797
    timed versus random collection of, 795
    24-hour testing of, 795-796
  urine studies for, 762-763
Proteomics, 2249
Proteus infections, 778
Proton ATPase subunit mutation, 1457
Proton pump inhibitors, 620
Proximal convoluted tubule (PCT)
  cells of, 59-60
  embryology of, 5
  filtered glutamine reabsorption in, 249
  fractional reabsorption of sodium in, 816
  illustration of, 58*f*
  mineralocorticoid receptor expression in, 315
Proximal renal tubular acidosis, 1455, 1456*t*
  acquired, 530-532
  calcium excretion in, 533
  carbonic anhydrase deficiency, 531-532
  clinical spectrum of, 532, 532*t*
  diagnosis of, 532-533, 533*f*
  features of, 532-533, 532*t*
  inherited, 530-532
  model of, 531-532
  pathogenesis of, 530-532
  physiology of, 530
  vitamin D deficiency and, 531
Proximal tubular cells
  activation of, 1791-1792
  albumin reabsorption by, 1791
  apoptosis of, 1212, 1791
  gene upregulation in, 1762
  histology of, 1784*f*
  megalin effects on, 1791
  protein filtration effects on, 1786
  protein overload of, 1790*f*
  in proteinuria, 1791-1792
Proximal tubule, 1440*f*, 1447*f*
  albumin degradation in, 1784, 1785*f*
  amino acid reabsorption in, 223*f*
  ammonia reabsorption in, 251
  ammoniagenesis in, 248
  anatomy of, 55
  angiotensin II in, 152, 384
  basement membrane, 1284*f*
  bicarbonate in
    excretion of, 519
    reabsorption of. *See* Bicarbonate reabsorption, in proximal tubule
  brush border of, 55, 57*f*
  calcium reabsorption in, 188, 188*f*
  citrate absorption and metabolism in, 217*f*, 248
  claudin expression in, 147
  cytochrome P450 in, 384

Proximal tubule (Continued)
  diuretics mechanism of action in, 1703f
  dopamine in, natriuretic effects of, 154
  electrolyte reabsorption functions of, 61
  enlargement of, 1745-1746
  filtered protein handling by, 1786
  fluid delivery from, 491
  functions of, 61, 144-145
  gap junctions in, 56
  glucose in, 129-130, 205, 206f
  glutamine synthetase expression by, 251
  as glyconeogenic organ, 204-205
  inherited disorders associated with dysfunction of, 1435-1445
  lateral cell processes of, 58f
  length of, 55
  lysosomes from, 59-60, 61f
  magnesium reabsorption in, 194, 194f
  microvilli of, 1784, 1784f
  natriuretic hormone targeting of, 152-153
  organic anion in, 216, 216t
  organic cation transport by, 210-211, 210f
  pars convoluta of. See Pars convoluta
  pathogenesis of, 1435-1436
  phosphate reabsorption in, 199f, 247
  phosphate-dependent glutaminase activity in, 253
  potassium channels in, 254
  potassium in, 175, 175f
  prostaglandin E_2 effects on, 373
  protein reabsorption by, 1784-1786
  in rat, 55, 56f-57f
  segments of, 55, 56f-57f, 145f. See also Pars convoluta; Pars recta
  serotonin synthesis in, 201
  sodium in, 132, 430f
  solutes, 132, 145f, 403f, 1745-1746
  ultrafiltered protein receptors in, 1792
  uric acid transport by, 220f
  water transport pathways in, 274f
Proximal tubule defect, 1417-1418
Proximal tubulopathy, GLUT2 mutation in, 209
Prune-belly syndrome, 2318-2319
Pruritus, 1942-1943, 1943f
Prussian blue, 2168-2169
Psen1, 30
Psen2, 30
Pseudoaneurysm, 2253
Pseudohyperkalemia, 585-586, 827, 829, 2380
Pseudohyperphosphatemia, 628
Pseudohypertension, 766, 1685, 1693
Pseudohypoaldosteronism, 179-180, 827, 2377-2378
  in children, 2380-2382
  type I, 539, 539f, 589, 1464, 2380-2381
  type II, 539-540, 589-590, 1464, 1465f, 2381-2382
Pseudohypocalcemia, 617
Pseudohyponatremia, 490, 816
Pseudohypoparathyroidism, 627, 1453
Pseudo-Kaposi's sarcoma, 1947
Pseudomonas aeruginosa peritonitis, 2128-2131
Pseudo-obstruction, 574
Pseudoporphyria, 1946
Pseudopseudohypoparathyroidism, 616
Psychogenic polydipsia, 482
Psychosis, 496
Psychotropic drugs, 497
Pubertal delay, 2357, 2435-2436
Pulmonary dysfunction, 2138-2139
Pulmonary embolism, 1805, 1906-1907
Pulmonary hemorrhage, 1072
Pulmonary hypertension, 2413
Pulmonary sensors, 395-396

Pulse pressure, 1681
Pulse repetition time, 856-857
Pulsus paradoxus, 761-762
Pure red cell aplasia, 2097
Pyelocalyceal cyst, 1518
Pyelocalyceal diverticula, 1518
Pyelonephritis
  acute, 1240-1242
    ciprofloxacin for, 1241-1242, 1241t
    clinical presentation of, 1241
    contrast-enhanced computed tomography of, 878-880, 880f, 1241
    imaging of, 878-880
    magnetic resonance imaging of, 880
    nuclear medicine of, 880
    treatment of, 1241-1242, 1241t
    ultrasonography of, 878, 880f
    vesicoureteral reflux associated with, 878
  bacille de Calmette-Guérin, 1254
  chronic, 882-883
  emergent interventions for, 778
  emphysematous, 881, 1251
  in pregnancy, 1245-1246
  xanthogranulomatous, 881, 883f, 1251-1252
Pyelorenal cyst, 1518
Pyk2, 256
Pyocystis, 1252
Pyoderma, 2331-2332
Pyrin, 2479-2483, 2483f, 2486
Pyrogenic reactions, 2082
Pyroglutamic acid-induced high anion gap acidosis, 549
Pyrophosphate, 1330, 1838
Pyuria, 756, 1238, 1246

Q

Quality, 2620-2622
Quality improvement
  arteriovenous fistulas and, 2629-2631
  continuous, 2623
  in end-stage kidney disease, 2625-2626
  erythropoiesis-stimulating agents in catalyzing, 2626-2628
  history of, 2621
  in kidney disease, 2625-2626
  lean principles, 2623-2624, 2623t, 2624f
  in nephrology, 2625
  overview of, 2620-2625
  Plan-Do-Study-Act, 2623, 2623t, 2624f
  prospective payment system, 2628-2629
  rationale for measuring, 2623
  Six Sigma, 2625, 2625f
  vascular access and, 2629-2631
Quality incentive program, 2628-2629
Quality of life, 2410, 2436, 2570
Quinapril hydrochloride, 1643t, 1644
Quinton-Scribner shunt, 2064

R

Race. See also specific race
  chronic kidney disease and, 660-663, 666
  definition of, 660
  end-stage kidney disease and, 1769f, 2577, 2597f
  health disparities and, 2577-2578
  hypertension and, 1526-1527
  renal function differences based on, 661t
Radiation, 2194
Radiation nephropathy
  acute, 1193
  chronic, 1194
  clinical features of, 1193

Radiation nephropathy (Continued)
  definition of, 1193
  malignant hypertension after, 1194-1195
  mechanisms of, 1194
  pathogenesis of, 1194
  pathology of, 1194
  renin-angiotensin-aldosterone system activation in, 1194
  treatment of, 1194-1195
  types of, 1193-1194
Radiation-associated kidney injury, 1400-1401
  clinical presentation of, 1401
  diagnosis of, 1401
  epidemiology of, 1400
  laboratory findings, 1401
  pathogenesis of, 1400
  prognosis for, 1401
  treatment of, 1401
Radiologist's tumor, 1374
Radiopharmaceuticals, 864-865
  fluorine 18 2-fluoro-2-deoxy-D-glucose, 865, 900
  iodine 131-labeled ortho-iodohippurate, 865
  technetium 99m-labeled diethylenetriaminepentaacetic acid, 864-866
  technetium 99m-labeled dimercaptosuccinic acid, 865, 880
  technetium 99m-labeled mercaptoacetyltriglycine, 865, 866f, 869-871, 874f, 913f
Ramipril, 1553, 1643t, 1644, 1650, 2362
Randall's plaque, 873-874, 1325, 1326f, 1329
Randomized controlled trials, 671
RANK, 1832, 1833f
RANKL, 603, 607, 1832, 1833f
RANTES, 729, 976-977, 1791
Rapalog, 1496
Rapamycin, 2247
Rapidly progressive glomerulonephritis (RPGN)
  categorization of, 1072-1073, 2150
  characteristics of, 2150
  definition of, 1072-1073
  end-stage kidney disease secondary to, 2150
  idiopathic, 2151
  neoplasia associated with, 1157
  nomenclature of, 1072-1073
  plasmapheresis for, 2150-2151
Ras-related C3 botulinum toxin substrate 1, 1753-1754
Raw carp bile, 2525
Rayer, Pierre, 2621
Raynaud's phenomenon, 1195
rBAT/b$^{0,+}$AT, 227-228
Rbpj, 35
Reactive oxygen species (ROS)
  in acute kidney injury, 977-978
  angiotensin type 1 receptor and, 329
  COX-2 actions mediated by, 379
  in diabetic nephropathy, 337
  in heart failure treatment, 452
  mitochondrial generation of, 732
Recalcification syndrome, 616
Receiver operator characteristic curve, 929, 929f
Receptor tyrosine kinase, 256
Receptor-mediated endocytosis, 341, 1791
Recessive disease, 1411, 1411t
Recluse spider bites, 2444-2445, 2445f
Recombinant atrial natriuretic peptide, 344
Recombinant growth hormone, 2125

Recombinant human erythropoietin, 1888-1890, 1895, 1906, 1922, 2097
Recombinant human growth factor, 1918
Recombinant tissue plasminogen activator, 1933
Recreational drugs, 686
Red blood cell(s). See also Erythrocytes
  in dialyzer, 2074
  erythropoiesis-stimulating agents effect on, 1892
  hypochromic, 1894-1895
  shortened survival of, anemia in chronic kidney disease secondary to, 1884-1885, 2013
  transfusion of, 586, 1902-1904, 1903f
  uremic, 1884-1885
Red blood cell casts, 756, 756f
Refeeding syndrome, 572-573, 620, 633
Refractory hypertension, 1695
Regional anticoagulation, 2092
Regional citrate anticoagulation, 2092, 2144
Regulated intramembrane proteolysis, 1791
Regulatory T cells, 1795, 2240, 2250
Reimbursement, 2503, 2562, 2572
Relative density of urine, 789
Relaxin, 465-466, 729-730
Remediable hypertension. See Secondary hypertension
Renal abscess
  contrast-enhanced computed tomography of, 880, 881f
  imaging of, 880, 881f-882f
  magnetic resonance imaging of, 880, 882f
  management of, 1250
  in transplanted kidney, 911
  urinary tract involvement of, 1250
Renal acidification, 1455f
Renal amyloidosis, 588-589
Renal anlagen, 2613-2616
Renal aplasia, 10t-17t
Renal artery
  angiography of, 1202
  description of, 42
  occlusion of, 964, 1201-1204
  stenosis of. See Renal artery stenosis
  stents in, magnetic resonance angiography of, 906-907, 906f
  thromboembolism of, 1201-1202
  thrombosis of, 964, 1202-1203, 2253, 2266
Renal artery aneurysms
  atherosclerosis as cause of, 1203
  classification of, 1203
  clinical features of, 1203
  dissecting, 1204
  incidence of, 1203
  mechanisms of, 1203
  rupture of, 1203
  saccular, 1203
  treatment of, 1203-1204
Renal artery angioplasty, 1595t, 1604
Renal artery stenosis, 1547
  acute kidney injury caused by, 964
  angiotensin II in, 907
  angiotensin-converting enzyme inhibitors for, 907
  arterial pressure and blood flow, 1570f
  atheroembolic renal disease and, 1192-1193
  atherosclerotic. See Atherosclerotic renal artery stenosis
  clinical features of, 1584f
  computed tomography angiography of, 904, 904f-905f
  Doppler ultrasonography of, 903-904

Renal artery stenosis (Continued)
  endovascular revascularization of, 1202
  epidemiology of, 1580-1581
  erythrocytosis associated with, 1889
  in Indian subcontinent, 2507, 2507f
  Kaplan-Meier survival for, 1585f
  magnetic resonance angiography of, 904-906, 906f
  management of, 1586t
  nephrotic syndrome associated with, 1159
  noninvasive assessment of, 1589t
  progression of, 1598-1599
  proteinuria and, 1584
  renin-angiotensin-aldosterone system activation in, 1574f
  renovascular hypertension and, 903, 1570-1571
  tissue hypoxia and, 139-140
  transplantation, 2272
Renal autoregulation, 104-110, 104f
  cellular mechanisms involved in, 105
  factors involved in, 110
  metabolic mechanisms that mediate, 109-110
  myogenic mechanism for, 105-106
  tubuloglomerular feedback mediation of, 106-109
Renal baroreceptor, 327
Renal biopsy. See Kidney biopsy
Renal blood flow
  adrenomedullin effects on, 418
  angiotensin II effects on, 407-408
  autoregulation of, 104-110, 104f, 384, 396-397
  calculation of, 85-86
  as cardiac output, 83, 85, 133
  characteristics of, 440f
  cortical, 87
  effective, 2614
  endothelin effects on, 336
  epoxygenase metabolites effect on, 383
  formula for calculating, 85
  glomerular filtration rate determination by, 134, 138, 401-402
  heart failure-related decreases in, 429-430
  intrarenal distribution of, 87-98
  kallikrein-kinin system regulation of, 348
  leukotriene A_4 effects on, 380
  medullary, 90
  obstructive nephropathy effects on, 1269-1271
  oxygen consumption and, 133-135
  oxygen delivery by, 126
  prostaglandins effect on, 436
  rate of, 83
  renal plasma flow used to estimate, 86
  renin-angiotensin system's role in control of, 99-101
  total, 85-87
  tubuloglomerular feedback control of, 108-109
  urinary tract obstruction effects on, 1269-1271
  urine formation from, 83
  vasomotor properties of, 98
  vasopressin effects on, 410
Renal calcifications, 871-878
Renal calcium excretion, 1334f
Renal candidiasis, 1404
Renal cell carcinoma, 1370
  acquired cystic kidney disease and, 1515f
  biologic pathways in, 1383f
  calcifications associated with, 871-872
  classification of, 1371, 1371t

Renal cell carcinoma (Continued)
  clear cell, 892, 895f-896f
  clinical features of, 1374-1375
  computed tomography of, 1376f-1377f
  epidemiology of, 1370-1371
  Fuhrman grading system for, 1378
  hormones produced by, 1375
  imaging of, 892, 894f-899f
    computed tomography, 894f, 898f
    magnetic resonance imaging, 892, 895f-897f
    positron emission tomography, 899-903
    positron emission tomography–computed tomography, 899-903
  laboratory features of, 1374-1375
  metastasis of, 896f, 1377-1378, 1377t, 1381
  molecular biology and hereditary disorders, 1372-1374
  nuclear medicine of, 900-901
  oncocytic, 891-892
  papillary, 892, 897f
  pathology for, 1371-1372, 1371t
  poorly differentiated, 899f
  prognosis for, 1375
  pseudocapsule with, 897f
  radiologic diagnosis of, 1375-1377
  staging of, 892-898, 895f, 1377-1379
    American Joint Committee on Cancer staging system, 1378
    survival rate and, 1378t
    TNM staging system, 1378, 1378t
  survival rate for, 1378-1379, 1379f
  symptoms of, 1374
  treatment of, 1375
    chemotherapy, 1385
    immunotherapy, 1385
    surgical, 1379-1381
    systemic therapy, 1381-1385
    vaccine, 1384-1385
  vascular thrombosis in, 898, 899f
Renal colic, 769, 873, 1360
Renal collecting system. See Collecting system
Renal coloboma syndrome, 2297t, 2317-2318
Renal corpuscle, 45-46, 46f-47f, 89f
Renal cortex
  anatomy of, 43, 43f
  calcification of, 872
  COX-2 expression in, 357-361
  cysts of, 889, 890f
  direct tubule innervation in, 81
  hemodynamics of, EP receptor regulation of, 372
  infarction of, in sickle cell disease, 1199
  interstitial cells in, 77-78, 78f
  medullary rays of, 90-91
  necrosis of, 2499, 2501-2502
  reabsorption in, 87
  ultrasonography of, 850
  venous drainage of, 93-94
Renal cortical adenoma, 1368
Renal crisis, scleroderma, 1195-1198, 1195f-1196f
Renal cyst(s), 1490f
  in autosomal dominant polycystic kidney disease, 1484f
  category I, 890
  category II, 890, 891f
  category III, 890
  category IV, 890, 891f-892f
  complex, 883-885, 887f
  contrast-enhanced computed tomography of, 883-885, 886f, 891f
  cortical, 889, 890f

Renal cyst(s) (Continued)
  in elderly, 750
  evolution of, 1477f
  hydronephrosis versus, 868
  imaging of, 883-885, 885f-887f
  infected, 1250-1251
  knockout and transgenic models for studying, 10t-17t
  lithium as cause of, 889, 890f
  magnetic resonance imaging of, 883-885, 887f, 889f
  nontubular origin, 1517-1518
  occurrence of, 1501
  in other organs, 1491
  simple, 886f, 1511-1512, 1512f
  treatment of, 1493
  ultrasonography of, 883, 885f
Renal cyst and diabetes syndrome, 2316-2317, 2389
Renal cystic ciliopathy, 1416-1417
Renal cystic disease. See also Cystic kidney disease
  autosomal recessive ciliopathies with, 1505-1509, 1507t
  classification of, 1475, 1476t
  evolution of cyst in renal tubules, 1477f
  localized or unilateral, 1512-1513
  pathogenesis of, 1417
Renal cystic dysplasia, 1510-1511, 1510f-1511f
Renal cystic neoplasm, 1516-1517
Renal dysgenesis, 363
Renal dysplasia
  clinical features of, 2302
  clinical presentation of, 2303
  definition of, 2294-2295
  description of, 2312
  diagnosis of, 2312
  histology of, 2295f
  management of, 2305
  multicystic, 889, 2294-2296, 2295f, 2303, 2305, 2312-2313
  prognosis for, 2305
Renal ectopy, 2295, 2295f, 2303, 2305, 2311
Renal epithelial cells, 128
Renal epithelial cyst, 1475-1479
Renal epithelium, 126, 137f
Renal fibrosis. See also Interstitial fibrosis
  biologic mediators and modulators of, in elderly
    advanced glycosylation end products, 730-732
    angiotensin II, 728-729
    autophagy, 734-735
    bile acid metabolism, 734
    calorie restriction, 732-733
    description of, 728
    farnesoid X receptor, 734
    Klotho, 734
    lipid metabolism, 733-734
    nitric oxide, 730
    oxidative stress, 732
    transforming growth factor-β, 729-730
  biomarkers for, 951-952
  focal segmental glomerulosclerosis progression to, 1034
  microRNAs in, 1758
  microvascular rarefaction and, 1578f
  pathogenesis of, 1278
  urinary biomarkers for, 951-952
Renal function
  in acute kidney injury, 2043-2044
  age-related changes in, 1878, 2034
  angiotensin receptor blockers effect on, 1655

Renal function (Continued)
  angiotensin-converting enzyme inhibitors effect on, 1645-1646
  assessment of, 2005, 2034
  birth weight effects on, 709-712
  cardiovascular disease and, 1860
  in children, 2309-2311
  in continuous renal replacement therapy, 2044
  creatinine clearance in, 2042t
  developmental programming of, 703-712
  in dialysis, 2044
  dietary modification effects on, 1957
  dietary protein influences on, 1767-1768, 1958-1959, 1981
  in drug dosing, 2041-2044
  early growth effects on, 722
  glomerular filtration rate as indicator of, 2041-2042
  imaging of, 865-866, 866f
  magnetic resonance imaging evaluation of, 863-864
  in nephrotic hypoalbuminemia, 1797
  thermodynamic analysis of, 123
  tubulointerstitial disease effects on, 1210
  after urinary tract obstruction, 1280-1281
Renal fusion, 2303-2305, 2311
Renal gluconeogenesis, 130-132
Renal glucosuria, 1454. See also Glucosuria
Renal hamartomas, 891, 893f
Renal hemodynamics, 101-104
Renal hilum, 42
Renal hypercalciuria, 1334-1335
Renal hypoperfusion, 436, 1570t, 1577-1578
Renal hypoplasia
  definition of, 2311
  description of, 2311-2312
  isolated, 2297t
  maternal diabetes and, 2301
  in Middle East, 2479
Renal infection, 878-883, 880f-885f, 1404-1405. See also specific type of infection
Renal insufficiency
  angiotensin-converting enzyme inhibitor dosing in, 1649t-1650t
  hypermagnesemia caused by, 625
  hypoglycemia secondary to, 1816
  in immunotactoid glomerulopathy, 1072
  in membranous nephropathy, 1040
  salt-losing nephropathy associated with, 493
  stents for, 1603-1604
  urinary concentration affected by, 1748
Renal interstitium
  anatomy of, 75-80
  composition of, 75-77
  cortical, 77-78
  inflammation and injury to, in proteinuria, 1792-1794
  medullary, 78-80, 79f
Renal ischemia, acute, 141-142
Renal kallikrein-kinin system, 348-349
Renal lobus, 43
Renal lymphangioma, 1369
Renal masses
  ablation of, 1741t, 1755-1757. See also Nephron loss
  contrast-enhanced computed tomography of, 883-885, 886f
  cystic, 890, 891f
  imaging of, 883-899, 884f-899f
  intravenous urography of, 883
Renal medulla
  adenosine effects on, 136f
  anatomy of, 43
  axial osmolality gradient in, 265

Renal medulla (Continued)
  blood supply of, 91
  calcifications in, 872
  countercurrent multiplication paradigm of, 266, 267f
  COX-2 expression in, 360-361, 360f
  glypican-3 and, 2299
  growth of, 2301-2302
  inner, 45, 45f, 91-92, 91f
  interstitium of, 75-77, 262-264
  lactate concentrations in, 132
  outer, 45, 45f, 65f, 91, 91f
  prostaglandin synthesis in, 360
  in tubular reabsorption of sodium, 404f
  urea accumulation in, 269, 269f
  urea recycling in, 270, 270f
  uric acid deposits in, 1961
  vascular-tubule relations, 92
  zones of, 45
Renal metabolism, 131f
Renal neoplasms
  angiomyolipomas, 891, 893f
  imaging of, 891
  oncocytoma, 891-892
  after renal transplantation, 911
Renal nerve stimulation, 110
Renal osteodystrophy, 1842, 1845, 1845t, 2407f, 2434
Renal outer medullary potassium. See ROMK
Renal oxygenation, 133-137, 134f
Renal papilla, 43, 44f
Renal parenchyma
  calcifications in, 1775
  calcium deposits in, 1775
  dendritic cell accumulation in, 1792
  inflammation of, 975-977
Renal parenchymal disease, 868-869, 870f, 880-881, 2469-2470
Renal pelvis
  anatomy of, 44f, 264
  description of, 42
  transitional epithelium of, 43
  tumors of, 1352, 1385-1386
Renal perfusion injury, 1579-1580
Renal perfusion pressure, 396, 402-405, 1570-1571, 1571f, 1575-1576
Renal phosphate excretion, 1450-1451
Renal phosphate transport, 1450-1453
Renal plasma flow
  age-related changes in, 735-736, 736f
  "effective", 86, 87f
  glomerular filtration rate affected by, 1296
  hypothyroidism and, 496
  obesity effects on, 1771
  rate of, 86
  renal blood flow estimated using, 86
  technetium 99m-labeled diethylenetriaminepentaacetic assessments of, 865-866
Renal proximal tubule. See Proximal tubule
Renal pyramids, 43, 872-873
Renal replacement therapy (RRT)
  acute kidney injury treated with. See Acute kidney injury (AKI), renal replacement therapy for
  in Africa, 2456t, 2463-2465, 2464f
  in Australia, 2540-2544, 2540f-2543f, 2545f, 2545t
  in China, 2535
  chronic kidney disease stage 5 treated with, 2016
  continuous. See Continuous renal replacement therapy
  in elderly, 747-748, 2597-2598
  familial hematuria treated with, 1141
  in Far East, 2534-2536

Renal replacement therapy (RRT) (Continued)
  future of, 2108-2109
  global uses of, 643
  hemodialysis. See Hemodialysis
  hepatorenal syndrome treated with, 457-458
  in Hong Kong, 2535
  hybrid, 2048-2049
  in Indian subcontinent, 2503-2504
  in Indonesia, 2536
  intensity of, 2142-2144
  in intensive care unit, 2139-2140
  intermittent hemodialysis, 2140-2141
  in Japan, 2534-2535
  in Korea, 2535
  in Latin America, 2449, 2450t
  in Malaysia, 2535-2536
  metformin poisoning treated with, 2185
  in Middle East, 2475t
  modalities, 2140-2142
  in New Zealand, 2541f, 2551-2552, 2551f
  in older adults, 2544
  in Philippines, 2536
  in Singapore, 2536
  sustained low-efficiency dialysis, 2141t, 2142, 2145-2146
  in Taiwan, 2534
  in Thailand, 2535
  uremic solute removal using, 1813-1814
  uremic syndrome caused by, 1926
  in Vietnam, 2536
Renal revascularization. See Revascularization
Renal risk scores
  for chronic kidney disease, 687-691, 688t-689t
  for end-stage kidney disease, 690-691, 690f
Renal salt wasting, 828
Renal sarcoma, 1386
Renal scarring, 1240
Renal sensors, 396-397
Renal sinus, 84, 1517
Renal stones. See Kidney stones; Nephrolithiasis
Renal transplantation
  ABO-incompatible, 2156-2157, 2423
  in Aboriginal Australians, 2548, 2548f
  abscess after, 911
  access to, 2570-2572
  acute tubular necrosis after, 910f, 2263-2264, 2263t
  in African Americans, 2581
  allogenic immune response in
    antigen recognition, 2229
    characteristics of, 2228-2230
    definition of, 2228-2229
    description of, 2253-2255
    immune tolerance, 2229-2230
    self–nonself discrimination, 2229
    self-tolerance, 2230
  allografts
    alloantibody response against, 2243
    biopsies of, 2267t, 2272
    delayed function of
      algorithm for, 2263f
      allograft survival affected by, 2277
      causes of, 2263-2264, 2427-2428
      in children, 2427-2428
      cold ischemia time and, 2265, 2278
      cyclosporine nephrotoxicity as cause of, 2264
      definition of, 2427-2428
      diagnosis of, 2262
      hyperacute rejection as cause of, 2264

Renal transplantation (Continued)
  incidence of, 2262
  induction regimens effect on, 2265t
  ischemic acute tubular necrosis as cause of, 2263-2264, 2263t
  outcome of, 2264-2265
  patient survival affected by, 2277
  risk factors for, 2262, 2263t
  significance of, 2264-2265
  tacrolimus nephrotoxicity as cause of, 2264
  dysfunction of
    biopsy diagnosis of, 2267t, 2269
    calcineurin inhibitor nephrotoxicity as cause of, 2268-2269, 2272, 2274-2275
    chronic antibody-mediated rejection as cause of, 2274
    description of, 2244-2245
    drug-related nephrotoxicity as cause of, 2273
    in early posttransplantation period, 2265-2271, 2266f
    hepatitis C virus as cause of, 2273
    human polyomavirus infection as cause of, 2272-2273
    hypovolemia as cause of, 2265-2266
    in immediate posttransplantation period, 2261-2265
    intrarenal, 2266-2271
    late, 2271-2276
    in late posttransplantation period, 2271-2273
    postrenal, 2270-2271
    radiocontrast nephrotoxicity as cause of, 2273
    renal vessel thrombosis as cause of, 2266
    sclerosing/chronic allograft nephropathy, 2273, 2274t
  failure of, 2432
  human leukocyte antigen matching effects on, 2277-2278
  immune response to, 2237
  late loss of, 2273-2276
  nephrectomy of, 2290
  placement of, 2251-2252, 2252f
  in pregnant patients, 2289-2290
  proteinuria effects on survival of, 2280
  rejection of. See Renal transplantation, rejection of
  renal artery thrombosis of, 2253
  survival of, 2235-2236, 2235f, 2276-2280, 2432
allorecognition in, 2237, 2238f
in amyloidosis, 1132
anatomy of, 2251-2252, 2252f
antigen(s)
  ABO blood group, 2236-2237
  blood transfusion effects on, 2237
  human leukocyte antigens (HLA)
    class I, 2231-2233, 2232f
    class II, 2233
    inheritance of, 2233-2234, 2234f
    loci strengths, 2235-2236
    typing of, 2234-2235
  major histocompatibility complex, 2230-2231, 2230f
  non-human leukocyte antigens, 2236
  nonself, 2230
  recognition of, 2229
antigen-presenting cells
  description of, 2229, 2253-2255

Renal transplantation (Continued)
  T cells and, interactions between, 2237-2241, 2253-2255
anti-glomerular basement membrane disease, 1127, 2150, 2270
arteriovenous fistulas after, 911
atheroembolic renal disease after, 1191
atypical hemolytic-uremic syndrome treated with, 1186, 2357
in Australia, 2540f, 2543-2544, 2543f
B cells, 2229, 2242-2243
biochemical changes after, 1851
biomarkers after, 939-940
biopsy specimens after, 923
bone changes after, 1851-1852
brain death effects on, 983
calcium monitoring after, 2283
chemokines, 2241, 2243
in children. See Children, renal transplantation in
in chronic kidney disease, 2016
commercial, in Middle East, 2491
complications of
  acute allergic interstitial nephritis, 2270
  acute pyelonephritis, 2269-2270
  acute thrombotic microangiopathy, 2269
  BK virus infection, 2430
  bone mineral density reductions, 2282-2283
  cutaneous warts, 2430
  cytomegalovirus, 2287-2288, 2288t, 2429
  hemorrhagic, 2253
  infectious, 2286-2288, 2287t, 2505-2506
  lymphocele, 2253
  in Middle East patients, 2492
  opportunistic infections, 2287, 2505-2506
  parvovirus B19 infection, 1255
  perirenal hematomas, 2253
  Pneumocystis jiroveci pneumonia, 2430-2431
  renal artery stenosis, 2272
  renal artery thrombosis, 2253
  renal vein thrombosis, 2253
  respiratory viruses, 2430
  surgical, 2253
  tuberculosis, 2505
  urinary tract infections, 2269-2270, 2429
  urinary tract obstruction, 2271
  urine leaks, 2270-2271
  varicella infection, 2430
  vascular, 2253
contrast-enhanced computed tomography after, 910
cost-effectiveness of, 2411
cytokines, 2241
diabetes mellitus after, 1320, 2283, 2433
in diabetes mellitus patients, 2288-2289
diabetic nephropathy treated with, 1318-1319, 2275-2276
donor kidney
  age of donor, 2278
  allograft survival affected by, 2278-2279
  from cardiac death donor, 2279, 2571
  cold storage preservation of, 2252
  from deceased donors, 2278, 2490, 2571, 2571t
  directed donation, 2570
  ethical dilemmas, 2570
  gender of donor, 2278
  handling of, 2252-2253
  imaging assessment of, 909-910
  kidney donor profile index, 2279

Renal transplantation (Continued)
    live, 2252, 2278, 2582
    in Middle East patients, 2490
    multidetector computed tomography of, 909-910
    nephron endowment effects on, 723
    nephron mass in, 2278
    nondirected donation, 2570
    pregnancy and, 1638
    preservation of, 2252-2253
    race and ethnicity of donor, 2278
    radiologic assessment of, 909
    solicitation of, 2570
  Doppler ultrasonography evaluations, 910
  in Egypt, 2490
  in elderly, 748-749, 748t, 2598-2599
  end-stage kidney disease treated with, 1181-1182, 2581-2582
  erythrocytosis after, 1888-1889
  ethical dilemmas, 2570-2572
  in failing kidney patients, 2290
  failure of, 723, 2277f
  fetal and neonatal outcomes in, 1636
  fibrillary glomerulonephritis recurrence after, 1072
  fibrosis after, 2245
  focal segmental glomerulosclerosis recurrence after
    in children, 2156, 2422, 2431
    description of, 1034, 2270
    immunosuppressive drugs for, 2155-2156
    plasmapheresis for, 2155-2157
    risk factors for, 2155, 2270
  fractures after, 1851
  future of, 2290
  granulomatous with polyangiitis recurrence after, 2275
  health disparities in, 2581-2582
  hematoma after, 911f
  hemolytic-uremic syndrome recurrence after, 2270
  history of, 2229, 2602
  in HIV-infected patients, 2289
  hydronephrosis after, 911
  hypophosphatemia caused by, 632
  IgA glomerulonephritis recurrence after, 2275
  imaging assessments before, 909-910, 909f-913f
  immune monitoring in, 2269
  immune tolerance in, 2229-2230, 2249
  immunoglobulin A nephropathy after, 1069
  immunosuppressive agents used in. See Immunosuppressive agents
  in Indian subcontinent, 2504-2506
  in infants, 2420
  infectious complications of, 2286-2288, 2287t
  in Iran, 2490-2491
  ischemic acute tubular necrosis after, 2263-2264, 2263t
  laboratory testing after, 2260t
  in Latin America, 2451
  live donor nephrectomy, 2252
  low-protein diet after, 1977
  lupus nephritis treated with, 1100, 2275
  lymphoceles after, 910-911
  magnetic resonance angiography after, 911, 912f
  magnetic resonance imaging of, 870f, 910
  in Maori population, 2553
  membranoproliferative glomerulonephritis recurrence after, 1155-1156, 2275, 2422, 2431

Renal transplantation (Continued)
  membranous nephropathy recurrence after, 2275
  metabolic syndrome after, 2284, 2433
  metanephros, 2614-2615
  microscopic polyangiitis recurrence after, 2275
  in Middle East, 2475t, 2489-2492
  mineral metabolism changes after, 1851
  neoplasms after, 911
  nephron endowment effects on, 723-724
  in New Zealand, 2552-2553
  nuclear medicine after, 911-912
  outcomes of
    allograft survival, 2276
    disparities in, 2582
    fetal, 1636
    improvements in, 2280-2281
    neonatal, 1636
    patient survival, 2276
    racial-ethnic disparities in, 2582
    short-term, 2276
  pancreas transplantation and. See Renal-pancreas transplantation
  parathyroid hormone monitoring after, 2283
  pauci-immune crescentic glomerulonephritis recurrence after, 1086
  phosphate monitoring after, 2283
  plasma cells, 2242
  positive T cell cross-match, 2157
  preemptive, in stage 4 chronic kidney disease, 2016
  pregnancy and, 1636-1638, 1636f, 2435-2436
  prevalence of, 642-643
  procedure for, 2251-2253
  quality of life after, 2410, 2436, 2570
  racial-ethnic disparities in, 2581-2582
  recipients
    acute kidney injury in, 2271t
    age of, 2279
    allograft survival affected by, 2279-2280
    anogenital cancers in, 2285
    antihypertensive agents in, 2284t
    body size of, 2280
    bone disorders in, 2281-2283
    calcidiol levels in, 1851
    calcineurin inhibitor-associated bone pain in, 2282
    calcium channel blockers in, 1667
    calcium levels in, 1851
    cancer in, 2284-2286, 2285t, 2433-2434, 2543-2544
    cardiovascular disease in, 2283-2284
    chronic kidney disease–mineral bone disorder in, 1850-1852
    cinacalcet use in, 2032
    compliance by, 2280
    cross-match of, 2260-2261
    cytomegalovirus disease in, 2287-2288, 2288t
    desensitization of, 2261
    diabetes mellitus in, 2283
    electrolyte disorders in, 2281
    ethnicity of, 2279
    flow cytometric cross-match of, 2260
    gender of, 2279-2280
    α-glutathione S-transferase levels in, 939
    gout in, 2282
    hip fractures in, 2282-2283
    hospitalization of, 2290
    hypercalcemia in, 2281
    hyperhomocysteinemia in, 2284
    hyperkalemia in, 2281

Renal transplantation (Continued)
    hyperlipidemia in, 2284
    hyperparathyroidism in, 2282
    hypertension in, 911, 2280, 2283-2284, 2284t
    hypertriglyceridemia in, 2284
    hypomagnesemia in, 2281
    hypophosphatemia in, 2281
    immunizations in, 2288, 2288t
    immunologic status of, 2260-2261
    immunosuppression of, 2280. See also Immunosuppressive agents
    Kaposi's sarcoma in, 2285, 2492
    leukopenia in, 2434
    lip cancer in, 2285
    medical status of, 2259-2260
    metabolic acidosis in, 2281
    metabolic syndrome in, 2284
    in Middle East, 2491
    neoplasia in, 2492
    nephron endowment effects on, 723-724
    neutropenia in, 2434
    osteonecrosis in, 2282
    osteoporosis in, 2282-2283
    pediatric, 2420-2422, 2421t
    pneumocystosis in, 2288
    posttransplant care of, 2261
    posttransplantation lymphoproliferative disorder, 2285-2286, 2286t
    pregnant, 2289-2290
    proteinuria measurement in, 798
    race of, 2279
    rejection risk factors in, 2260t
    sensitization of, 2280
    skin cancer in, 2285, 2285t, 2433-2434, 2492, 2543-2544
    surgery in, 2290, 2290t
    urinary tract infection in, 1248-1249
    vaccinations in, 2288, 2288t
    vascular calcification in, 1852
  rejection of
    accelerated, 2264
    acute
      allograft loss risks, 2280
      antibody-mediated, 2268
      cellular, 2244, 2266-2268, 2267t, 2276f, 2428
      in children, 2428
      humoral, 2157, 2244, 2266-2268, 2267t, 2276f
    acute calcineurin inhibitor nephrotoxicity versus, 2268-2269, 2272, 2274-2275
    chronic, 2244-2245, 2244f, 2268
    chronic antibody-mediated, 2274
    corticosteroids for, 2268
    effector mechanisms of, 2242-2244
    hyperacute, 912-913, 2264
    immune monitoring for prevention of, 2269
    immunosuppression for prevention of. See Immunosuppressive agents
    immunosuppressive agent cessation as precipitate of, 2290
    late acute, 2271-2272
    magnetic resonance imaging of, 911, 912f
    plasmapheresis for, 2157
    risk factors for, 2260t
  scintigraphy after, 913
  skin conditions after, 1947t
  small vessel vasculitis recurrence after, 1086
  socioeconomic factors and, 2581
  stroke in, 1927-1928

Renal transplantation (Continued)
  survival rates, 2410
  T cell(s)
    activation of, 2254f
    adhesion molecules on, 2239-2240
    allorecognition, 2237, 2238f
    anergic, 2240
    antigen-presenting cells and, interactions between, 2237-2241, 2253-2255
    CD4+, 2239, 2242
    CD8+, 2239, 2243f
    costimulatory molecules, 2240-2241
    cross-match, 2157
    cytotoxic CD8+, 2239
    description of, 2229
    helper, 2241-2242
    immune response, 2253-2255
    interleukin-17–producing lineage of, 2243-2244
    receptor complex of, 2237-2239
    regulatory, 2240, 2250
  thrombotic thrombocytopenia purpura recurrence after, 2270
  timing of, 2278
  tissue remodeling after, 2245
  tolerogenic protocols in, 2249-2250
  tumor necrosis factor, 2241
  ultrasonography evaluations, 910
  urinary tract infection after, 1248-1249
  urine extravasation after, 913
  urinoma after, 910, 911f
  vascular calcification after, 1852
Renal tuberculosis, 882, 884f, 1253f
Renal tubular acidosis, 1437
  characteristics of, 2335
  in children, 2335-2338, 2337t, 2383-2386, 2383t
  distal
    alkali therapy for, 535-536
    autosomal recessive, 2335
    causes of, 2335
    in children, 2384-2386
    classical, 534, 534t-535t
    clinical spectrum of, 534-535, 535t
    in Far East, 2533
    features of, 534-535
    generalized, 534t
    H^+-ATPase defects in, 242
    H^+-K^+-ATPase's involvement in, 534
    hyperkalemic, 540, 589
    hypokalemic, 534, 581
    pathophysiology of, 533-534
    primary type 1, 2384-2386
    pyelonephritis caused by, 534-535
    treatment of, 535-536, 536t
    type A intercalated defects, 534
  diuretics for, 1726
  hyperkalemic, 1726, 2337t, 2338
  inherited, 1456t
  mixed, 2338
  nephrocalcinosis in, 872
  proximal, 1455, 1456t
    acquired, 530-532
    autosomal dominant, 2383
    calcium excretion in, 533
    carbonic anhydrase deficiency, 531-532
    causes of, 2335-2336
    characteristics of, 580-581
    in children, 2383-2384
    clinical spectrum of, 532, 532t
    diagnosis of, 532-533, 533f
    features of, 532-533, 532t
    inherited, 530-532

Renal tubular acidosis (Continued)
    model of, 531-532
    NBCe1 defects as cause of, 236-237
    pathogenesis of, 530-532
    physiology of, 530
    vitamin D deficiency and, 531
  treatment of, 2338
  type 1, 2386t
  type 2, 2386t
  type 4, 2386, 2386t
  types of, 542t, 2337t
Renal tubular assist device, 2617
Renal tubular dysgenesis, 2294-2295, 2297t, 2300
Renal tubular ectasia, 888-889
Renal tumors
  erythrocytosis in, 1889
  pelvic, 1352, 1385-1386
Renal ultrasonography
  acute kidney injury diagnosis using, 772
  chronic kidney disease diagnosis using, 776
  obstructive uropathy diagnosis using, 765
  urinary tract infection evaluations, 778
Renal vascular disease, 903-907, 904f-907f
Renal vein thrombosis
  acute, 1204, 1206, 1804
  anticoagulation for, 1206
  chronic, 1204, 1804
  clinical features of, 1204
  contrast-enhanced computed tomography of, 1205
  description of, 994
  diagnosis of, 1204-1205
  Doppler ultrasonography of, 1204
  hypovolemia as cause of, 1206
  imaging of, 908-909
  inferior venacavography of, 1204-1205
  magnetic resonance imaging of, 1205
  manifestations of, 1804
  mechanisms of, 1205-1206
  in membranous nephropathy, 1041
  in neonates, 1206
  in nephrotic syndrome, 1204-1206, 1804
  predisposing factors, 1205f, 1206
  renal allograft dysfunction caused by, 2266
  in renal transplantation allograft, 2253
  risk factors for, 1206t
  thrombolysis for, 1206
  treatment of, 1206-1207
  warfarin for, 1206
Renalase, 1533
Renal-pancreas transplantation, 1319, 2289
Renin
  age-related changes in, 737-738
  aldosterone secretion affected by, 568, 568f
  COX-2 inhibitors effect on production of, 360
  description of, 326-327
  drug-induced impairments in, 540
  EP4 receptor effects on release of, 372-373
  expression of, 53, 55, 370
  glucocorticoid-remediable hyperaldosteronism effects on, 555-556
  hyperkalemia and, 814t
  hypokalemia and, 814t
  juxtaglomerular apparatus secretion of, 334-335, 360, 568
  juxtaglomerular granular cell expression of, 53, 55
  loop diuretics effect on, 1706-1707

Renin (Continued)
  macula densa's role in release of, 358-360, 359f
  metabolic acidosis and, 555-556
  metabolic control of, 327-328
  neural control of, 327
  plasma
    β-adrenergic antagonist therapy effects on, 1659-1660
    age-related changes in, 737-738
    description of, 328
    in diabetes mellitus, 334-335
    diuretic therapy effects on, 1716
    edema formation and, 1798-1799
    in Gitelman's syndrome, 580
    in hyporeninemic hypoaldosteronism, 592
    plasma aldosterone concentration/plasma renin activity, 576
  primary aldosteronism effects on, 555
  regulation of, 568-569
  secretion of, 327-328, 1706, 2603
  structure of, 326
  tubular control of, 327-328
Renin inhibitors, 568, 1677-1678, 1764-1765
Renin lineage cells, 2609
Renin profiling, 1542-1543
Renin-angiotensin system, 99-102, 139
Renin-angiotensin-aldosterone system (RAAS), 1401
  activation beyond renal artery stenotic lesion, 1574f
  activation of, 1716
  aliskiren for blockade of, 1309
  almandine, 333
  angiotensin-(1-7), 333, 408, 445
  angiotensin-(1-12), 333
  angiotensin-(2-10), 333
  angiotensin A, 333
  angiotensin III, 332
  angiotensin IV, 332-333
  angiotensin peptides, 332-333
  angiotensin type 1 receptor. See Angiotensin type 1 receptor
  angiotensin type 2 receptor, 331
  angiotensin-(2-B), 332
  angiotensin-(3-B), 332
  angiotensin-converting enzyme, 328
  angiotensin-converting enzyme 2, 332
  angiotensinogen, 326
  arginine vasopressin secretion affected by, 470
  blockade of, 1180, 1304, 1309, 1311, 1889
  blood pressure regulation and, 1530-1532
  in cirrhosis-related sodium retention, 444-445
  components of, 326f
  description of, 27, 35-36, 100-101, 325
  in developing kidney, 703
  developmental programming of, 703, 704t-705t
  in diabetic nephropathy progression, 1298
  disordered regulation of, 1645
  diuretic therapy affected by, 1716
  in effective arterial blood volume regulation, 407-409
  elements of, 1531f
  in fibrosis, 334
  furosemide effects on, 1714
  in heart failure, 429-431, 451-454
  identification of, 1568-1569

Renin-angiotensin-aldosterone system (RAAS) *(Continued)*
  immunity and, 334
  inflammation and, 334
  inhibition of
    acute kidney injury secondary to, 2006, 2006t
    dual, 1691-1692
    inflammation managed with, 2126
    in nephrotic syndrome, 1799
    renoprotective effects of, 639, 1752
    for slowing chronic kidney disease progression, 1646, 1998-2004, 2127
  inhibitors of
    aldosterone antagonism, 2003
    angiotensin receptor blockers, 591f, 1642f, 1651, 1681, 1689, 1764-1765, 2000-2003, 2001f
    angiotensin-converting enzyme inhibitors, 591f, 1642f, 1681, 1689, 1764-1765, 1998-2000
    β-blockers and, 1692
    calcium channel blockers and, 1681-1682, 1690-1691
    description of, 1778
    direct renin inhibitors, 2003-2004
    diuretics and, 1691
    heart failure treated with, 451-454
    hyperkalemia caused by, 591-592, 741, 2005-2006
    podocytes affected by, 119-120
    steroid-resistant nephrotic syndrome in children treated with, 2331
    thiazide diuretics with, 1681
  intracrine, 333-334
  intrarenal, 333-334
  kallikrein-kinin system and, 418
  mutations of, 2300
  nephron loss and, 1738-1739
  in one-kidney and two-kidney renovascular hypertension, 1571-1572
  physiologic and functional studies of, 1588-1589, 1589t
  potassium homeostasis affected by, 568
  prorenin in, 327-328, 327f
  (pro)renin receptor, 331-332
  in proteinuria, 334
  in radiation nephropathy, 1194
  renin, 326-328
  schematic diagram of, 326f
  in sodium retention, 444-445, 452
  sympathetic nervous system and, 703, 1533f
  in tubuloglomerular feedback, 400
  in urinary tract obstruction, 1279
Reninoma, 1369
Renomedullary interstitial cells, 78-80, 1369
Renoprotection
  aldosterone antagonists for, 2003
  amniotic fluid- and placental-derived stem cells for, 2607
  angiotensin receptor blockers for, 1764-1765, 1995, 1998t
  angiotensin-converting enzyme inhibitors for, 1757, 1995, 1998-2000, 1998t
  after nephrectomy, 1763-1764
  rationale for interventions for, 1990
  renin-angiotensin-aldosterone system inhibition for, 1752, 1998-2004
  spironolactone for, 2003
  strategies for, 2006-2008, 2008t
  weight loss for, 1992-1993
Renorenal reflex, 1269
Renovascular disease, 1567-1568. *See also* Renovascular hypertension
  in elderly, 746

Renovascular disease *(Continued)*
  medical therapy for, 1595-1599
  milestones in, timeline for, 1569f
  progressive vascular occlusion with, 1598
  reconstructed views of, 1592f
  secondary hypertension and, 1568-1569
  treatment of, 746
Renovascular hypertension, 1547, 1568-1569, 1595t. *See also* One-kidney renal clip hypertension; Renovascular disease; Two-kidney renal clip hypertension
  clinical features of, 1581-1582, 1583t
  development of, phases of, 1574, 1574f
  diagnosis and evaluation of, 1588-1594, 1588t
  endovascular renal angioplasty and stenting, 1599
  epidemiology of, 1580-1581
  in Indian subcontinent, 2506-2507
  management of, 1608f
  mechanism sustaining, 1572-1574
  pathophysiology of, 1570-1580
  prospective trials for, 1602-1603
  renal artery aneurysms associated with, 1203
  renal artery stenosis and, 903, 1570-1571
  renin-angiotensin-aldosterone system's role in, 1571-1572
  surgical treatment of, 1604-1607, 1605t
  syndromes associated with, 1583t
  therapy goals for, 1588
  vascular lesions producing, 1570t
Repaglinide, 2593
Reproductive cloning, 2604
Reserpine, 1673
Residual bodies, 59-60
Residual syndrome, 1807-1808
Resistant hypertension, 1691t, 1693-1695
Resistin, 1816
Resistive index, 849-850
Resorptive hypercalciuria, 1335
Respiratory acidosis
  carbon dioxide tension changes and, 515-516
  causes of, 525-526, 526t
  chronic, 527
  clinical features of, 526
  collecting duct's response to, 244
  compensatory responses for, 518t
  diagnosis of, 527
  hyperphosphatemia caused by, 628
  mechanical ventilation as cause of, 526
  proximal tubule bicarbonate reabsorption affected by, 237
  treatment of, 527
Respiratory alkalosis
  in alcoholics, 633
  carbon dioxide tension changes and, 515-516
  causes of, 526t, 527-528
  compensatory responses for, 518t
  description of, 527
  diagnosis of, 528
  effects of, 527
  hypocalcemia caused by, 2392
  hypophosphatemia caused by, 633
  plasma potassium affected by, 563
  of pregnancy, 1612
  treatment of, 528
Respiratory center depression, 526
Restenosis, 1603-1604
Resting energy expenditure (REE), 1815-1816, 1973
Resting membrane potential, 569-570, 818
Restless legs syndrome, 1818-1819, 1939-1940, 1940t

Ret, 23-24, 24f
RET, 2297-2298
Ret-GFRα1, 22
Reticulocyte hemoglobin content, 1895
Retinitis pigmentosa, 2321
Retinoic acid response element, 1795
Retinoids, 31-32
Retinol binding protein, 1816
Retrograde pyelography, 1268
Retroperitoneal fibrosis, 1261-1262
Revascularization, 1585f, 1586t, 1607t
  atheroembolism risks, 746
  benefits of, 1607
  of kidneys, 1599
  renal artery stenosis and, 1592f
  renal functional outcomes after, 1606f
Reverse causality, 1861
Reverse osmosis water treatment system, 2081f
Reversible posterior leukoencephalopathy, 1619-1620
Rh glycoproteins
  in ammonia metabolism, 255
  carbon dioxide transport by, 255
  RhAG/Rhag, 255
  RhBG/Rhbg, 255
  RhCG/Rhcg, 255
Rhabdomyolysis, 586, 628
Rh-associated glycoprotein, 586
Rheumatoid arthritis, 1168
Rhpj, 30
Ribavirin, 1156
Riboflavin, 1983
Ribosomal protein S6 kinase 1A, 732-733
Rickets, 630-631
RIFLE criteria, 770, 770t, 930-931, 960, 961t, 1390, 2138
Right ventricular failure, 1722
Rilmenidine, 1671-1672, 1671t-1672t
Rilonacept, 2486
Risk factors
  Bradford-Hill causality criteria, 670, 670t
  definition of, 670
  identification of, 670-671
Rituximab
  adverse effects of, 1171
  anti-glomerular basement membrane disease treated with, 1126-1127
  glomerular disease treated with, 1171
  granulomatous with polyangiitis treated with, 1113
  immunosuppressive uses of, 2256
  lupus nephritis treated with, 1104
  membranous nephropathy treated with, 1044-1045
  nephrotic syndrome treated with, 2330-2331
  pauci-immune crescentic glomerulonephritis treated with, 1088-1089
  podocytes affected by, 119
  toxicity of, 1171
Robo2, 27
ROBO2, 2297-2298
Rofecoxib, 437
Rolipram, 300-301
ROMK, 159-160, 163, 176, 179-181, 278, 310-311, 541, 564, 566, 578-579, 581, 1728, 2334
Ropinirole, 1940
Roux-en-Y gastric bypass, 1340, 1341t
Rubinstein-Taybi syndrome, 2297t
Rumack-Matthew nomogram, 2187-2188
Runx-2, 1835

S

S256, 293
Salicylates
　high anion gap acidosis caused by, 547-548
　metabolic acidosis caused by, 547-548
　poisoning, 2178-2180
Saline, 855-856
Sall1, 22-23
SALL1, 2298-2299
Salt, 258-259, 1354. *See also* Sodium
Salt sensitivity, 1528-1529, 1533-1534
Salt substitutes, 584-585
Salt-induced hypercalciuria, 1354
Salt-losing nephropathy, 493
Salt-losing tubulopathies, 1460*f*, 2334*t*. *See also* Bartter's syndrome; Gitelman's syndrome
Salt-sensitive hypertension, 1974-1975
Samoa, 2553-2554
Saponification, 620
Sarcoidosis, 762, 1127-1128, 1228
Sarcopenia, 1922
Satavaptan, 457
Saudia Arabia. *See* Middle East
Scar collagen, 1286
SCARB2 disease, 1432
Schimke's immuno-osseous dysplasia, 1432
Schistosoma haematobium, 755, 1255, 1260, 2462
Schistosomiasis, 1150, 1260, 2462
Schwartz equation, 2043, 2310
Scintigraphy, 913, 1266
Scleroderma
　acute kidney injury associated with, 1002
　chronic kidney disease in, 1196-1197
　clinical features of, 1195
　collagen production in, 1197
　cytokines in, 1197
　definition of, 1195
　immunologic mediators in, 1197
　laboratory findings in, 1196
　microvascular injury in, 1197
　pathogenesis of, 1197
　pathology of, 1196-1197
　Raynaud's phenomenon, 1195
　renal crisis, 1195-1198, 1195*f*-1196*f*
　renal involvement in, 1195-1196
　treatment of, 1197-1198, 1198*t*
Sclerosing/chronic allograft nephropathy, 2273
Sclerosis, 921*t*
Sclerosteosis, 191
Sclerostin, 191, 610, 1842
Scriber, Belding, 2558
Scrub typhus, 2513-2515
Sebastian's syndrome, 1141
Secondary hyperparathyroidism, 1827-1828, 1835-1836, 1887, 2023, 2026, 2031-2032
Secondary hypertension, 766*t*, 1543-1550, 1568-1569, 1628
Secondary tubulopathy, 1417-1418
γ-Secretase inhibitor, 30
Secreted procollagen type 1C propeptide, 1842
Secretin, for nephrogenic diabetes insipidus, 301
Sedatives, 2595
Seizure, 1616, 1626-1627
Selective aldosterone receptor antagonists, 1678-1679
Selenium supplementation, 2099-2100
Self-tolerance, 2230
Seminal vesicle cyst, 1491

Senior-Loken syndrome, 2321
Sensorimotor neuropathy, 1819
Sepsis, 2137-2138
Sequestered solutes, 1814
Serine 552, 235
Serine-threonine kinase, 565
Serotonin, 201
Serum amyloid A, 1128-1129, 1130*f*, 1969-1970, 2485
Serum amyloid P, 1128
Serum- and glucocorticoid-regulated kinase
　aldosterone induction of, 317-318
　in aldosterone-sensitive distal nephron, 318
　epithelial sodium channel stimulation by, 318, 319*f*
　molecular mechanisms of action, 318-320
　Nedd4-2 inhibition by, 318-319
　in sodium transport, 319
Serum chemistry, 1356
Serum frizzled-related protein 4, 197-198, 198*f*, 201
SeSAME syndrome, 167
Sevelamer hydrochloride, 563, 627, 2031
Seventh sickly cell nephrology, 1372
Severe acute respiratory syndrome, 2521-2522, 2523*f*
Severe fever with thrombocytopenia syndrome virus, 2516-2517, 2518*f*
Sex hormones, 400, 1921, 1923
Sexual intercourse, 1237
sFlt1, 39
SGK-1, 172-173, 567
SGLT1, 205-206
SGLT2, 206-207
SGLT3, 207
SGLT2, 207-209
Shear stress, 1578
Shh, 27
Shiga toxin-associated hemolytic-uremic syndrome, 1179-1182, 2352-2357
Shunt nephritis, 1149
Shwartzman reaction, 2502
Sickle cell disease
　in Africa, 2463
　clinical features of, 1198-1199
　cortical infarction in, 1199
　end-stage kidney disease secondary to, 1200
　focal segmental glomerulosclerosis in, 1199
　hematuria in, 1198-1200
　hemoglobin SS in, 1199
　mechanisms of, 1199-1200
　medullary lesions in, 1199
　pathogenesis of, 1199-1200
　pathology of, 1199
　preeclampsia and, 1618
　proteinuria in, 1199
　renal papillary necrosis in, 1198-1199, 1199*f*
　treatment of, 1200
　tubular dysfunction in, 1199
　vasoocclusion mediated by, 1199
Sickle cell glomerulopathy, 1146, 1146*f*, 1200
Sickle cell nephropathy, 1145-1146, 1145*f*
Sieving coefficient, 2170
Signal transducers and activators of transcription, 1760-1761, 1882
Signal-induced proliferation-associated gene 1, 295
Sildenafil citrate, 300-301
Silicosis, 1159

Simple cyst, 1511-1512, 1512*f*
Simple hypoplasia, 2294
Simpson-Golabi Behmel syndrome, 2297*t*
Simultaneous pancreas-kidney transplantation, 1319
Singapore, 2536
Single-gene kidney disorder, 1411-1412, 1413*t*, 1418
Single-nephron glomerular filtration rate, 1269, 1271, 1737-1738, 1743, 1746-1747, 1785
Single-pass albumin dialysis, 2171
Sinusoidal occlusion syndrome, 1394-1395
Sinusoidal pressure, 439-440
Sir2, 733
siRNA, 7-9
Sirolimus
　adverse effects of, 2426
　in children, 2426
　focal segmental glomerulosclerosis treated with, 1033-1034
　immunosuppressive uses of, 2254*t*, 2258, 2426
　during pregnancy, 1637, 1637*t*
SIRT1, 733
Sirtuins, 732-733, 1788
SITS, 146-147
Six1, 21
Six2, 29
SIX1, 2298-2299
Six Sigma, 2625, 2625*f*
Six2-EGFP transgene, 19
Size-exclusion high-performance liquid chromatography, 795
Sjögren's disease, 1127
S6K1, 733
SK channels, 180*f*, 564-565
Skeletal ciliopathy, 1509
Skeletal muscle, 174-175, 560, 1967
Skeletal system, 623-624
Skin
　cancer of, 2285, 2285*t*, 2433-2434, 2492, 2543-2544
　diuretics-related adverse effects of, 1732
　nitrogen losses from, 1963
Skin conditions and disorders, 1943*t*, 1947*t*, 1949*t*-1950*t*, 1952*t*-1953*t*
　acquired perforating dermatosis, 1944, 1944*f*
　in Alport's syndrome, 1953
　arteriovenous shunt dermatitis, 1949
　in Birt-Hogg-Dube syndrome, 1951-1952, 1952*f*, 1952*t*
　calciphylaxis, 1944-1945, 1945*f*
　cutaneous metastases, 1949
　dialysis-associated steal syndrome, 1948
　dyspigmentation, 1943*f*
　eruptive xanthomas, 1946-1947, 1946*f*
　in Fabry's disease, 1952
　genodermatoses, 1951-1953, 1952*f*, 1952*t*
　in Henoch-Schönlein purpura, 1951, 1951*f*
　in hereditary leiomyomatosis and renal cell carcinoma syndrome, 1952, 1952*f*, 1952*t*
　ichthyosis, 1943-1944
　impetigo, 1953
　iododerma, 1947, 1947*f*
　leukocytoclastic vasculitis, 1950-1951, 1951*f*
　Lindsay's nail, 1949-1950, 1949*f*
　metastatic calcification, 1945-1946
　in metastatic renal cell carcinoma, 1949
　in Muir-Torre syndrome, 1952-1953, 1952*t*

Skin conditions and disorders *(Continued)*
  nails, 1949-1950, 1949*f*
  in nephrogenic systemic fibrosis, 1947-1948, 1948*f*-1949*f*
  porphyria cutanea tarda, 1946, 1946*f*
  port-wine stain, 1952
  post-renal transplantation, 1947*t*
  pruritus, 1942-1943, 1943*f*
  pseudo-Kaposi's sarcoma, 1947
  pseudoporphyria, 1946
  streptococcal skin infection, 1953
  in systemic lupus erythematosus, 1950, 1950*f*
  in tuberous sclerosis, 1952
  in von Hippel–Lindau disease, 1952, 1952*t*
  xerosis, 1943, 1943*f*
SLC6 transporters, 229-230
SLC22, 375
SLC1A1, 228-229
SLC1A5, 225
SLC3A1/SLC7A9, 227-228
SLC3A2/SLC7A7, 228
SLC3A2/SLC7A9, 225-226
SLC5A1, 205-206
SLC6A6, 224-225
SLC6A18, 224
SLC6A19, 222-224
SLC6A20, 224
SLC7A13, 229
SLC16A10, 225
Slc26A6, 148-149
Slc26A7, 243
SLC36A2, 224
SLC3A1, 2345
SLC7A9, 2345
SLC12A1, 158-159
SLC12A3, 2378-2379
SLC22A, 218-219
Sleep apnea, 1533*f*, 1939-1940, 2101
Sleep disorders
  periodic limb movements of sleep, 1939-1940
  prevalence of, 1939
  restless legs syndrome, 1940, 1940*t*
  sleep apnea, 1939-1940
Sleep-disordered breathing, 766
Slit2, 27
Slit diaphragm
  definition of, 4-5, 51, 791
  in podocytes, 38-39, 51, 118, 791, 1782-1783, 1782*f*
  proteins, 113
  studies of, 51
  topologic organization of, 38
Slit pote, 49-51
SMAD1, 27
Small vessel vasculitis
  eosinophilic granulomatosis with polyangiitis, 1116-1118
  granulomatous with polyangiitis. *See* Granulomatous with polyangiitis
  microscopic polyangiitis. *See* Microscopic polyangiitis
  after renal transplantation, 1086
Smith, Homer, 1568-1569
Smith-Lemli-Opitz syndrome, 2297*t*
Smoking
  cessation of, 1867, 1991-1992, 2102
  chronic kidney disease risks, 685, 1776-1777, 1867
  fibromuscular dysplasia and, 1580-1581
  renal allograft survival affected by, 2283
  sympathetic nervous system affected by, 1776-1777
Smooth muscle, 371, 413-414

Snakebites
  acute kidney injury caused by, 2499-2500, 2523-2525, 2524*t*
  in Africa, 2458
  Bothrops, 2447
  Crotalus, 2446-2447
  in Far East, 2523-2525, 2524*t*
  in Indian subcontinent, 2499-2500
  in Latin America, 2446-2447
SNARE hypothesis, 295-296, 311
SNARE proteins, 295-296
SNAT3, 251
Sodium
  absorption of
    aldosterone-sensitive distal nephron and, 313-314
    in collecting ducts, 73
    distal, 566-568
    electrogenic, 316-317
    epithelial sodium channels, 175
    medullary collecting ducts in regulation of, 314
    prostaglandin E_2 effects on, 361-362
    regulation of, 310-315
  altered handling of, by kidney, 701-703
  balance of, 2366-2367
  in children, 2365-2374
  daily filtration of, 422
  deficit of, 323, 2374
  dietary
    in chronic kidney disease, 1974-1975
    diuretic braking phenomenon affected by, 1714, 1715*f*
    in edematous patients, 1719, 1725
    renal hypertrophy inhibition of, 1759
    restriction of, 566, 1716, 1725, 1993-1994
    stroke risks associated with, 1928*t*, 1930
    thromboxane A_2 expression regulated by, 365
  excretion of
    age-related changes in, 738-739, 738*f*
    captopril effects on, 444-445
    description of, 391, 395
    in elderly, 738-739, 738*f*
    endothelin effects on, 416
    furosemide and, 1710*f*
    interstitial pressure in control of, 402-405
    intrarenal control of, 402
    nephron loss-specific adaptations in, 1747-1748
    prostaglandin synthesis inhibition effects on, 412
    sympathetic nervous system in, 405, 432
  in extracellular fluid, 144
  fractional excretion of, 814-815, 987, 1659, 1708-1710, 1747
  in hemodialysis dialysate, 2092-2093
  metabolism of, 2365-2367
  monitoring of, 508
  nonsteroidal antiinflammatory drug-induced retention of, 361-362
  plasma, 423, 816, 2371
  restriction of, 1993-1994
  serum concentration of, 491, 523
  transport of
    angiotensin II effects on, 331
    in collecting duct, 374
    COX-1 metabolite effects on, 373-374
    COX-2 metabolite effects on, 373-374
    maturation of, in fetus and infant, 2302
    metabolic cost of, 135-136
    in proximal tubule, 132
    serum- and glucocorticoid-regulated kinase in, 319

Sodium *(Continued)*
    in thick ascending limb, 132-133
    transepithelial, 420
    urinary tract obstruction effects on, 1274
  in urine, 492, 816
Sodium balance, 1530
  arginine vasopressin effects on, 498
  central nervous system sensors of, 397
  disorders of
    hypernatremia. *See* Hypernatremia
    hyponatremia. *See* Hyponatremia
  nitric oxide in, 417
  physiology of, 390-421
  two-compartmental model of, 391*f*
Sodium bicarbonate, 595, 595*f*, 855-856, 1364, 2168
Sodium chloride
  absorption of
    angiotensin II effects on, 155
    description of, 144
    neurohumoral influences on, 152, 153*f*
    paracellular, 145-146
  dietary, 1993-1994
  hyponatremia treated with, 506
  in inner medulla, 271-273
  reabsorption of
    angiotensin II effects on, 152, 153*f*
    by thick ascending limb, 158
    description of, 145*f*, 146-147
    epithelial sodium channels' role in, 169-170
    glomerular filtration rate effects on, 150
    proximal, 152
Sodium chloride transport
  aldosterone effects on, 171-173
  apical, 158-159, 169-170
  in connecting tubules
    aldosterone effects on, 171-173
    arachidonic acid metabolites effects on, 174
    mechanisms of, 169-171
    regulation of, 171-174
  in cortical connecting duct
    aldosterone effects on, 171-173
    arachidonic acid metabolites effects on, 174
    mechanisms of, 169-171
    regulation of, 171-174
    vasopressin effects on, 173
  in cortical connecting tubules, 566
  in distal convoluted tubule
    description of, 148, 165-174
    mechanisms of, 166-167, 167*f*
    NCC expression, 165-166
    regulation of, 167-169
  electroneutral, 171
  in loop of Henle, 156-165
    thin ascending limb, 156-158, 157*f*
    thin descending limb, 156
  overview of, 144-174
  paracellular, 147-148, 160
  potassium transport and, in distal nephron, 182-183
  in proximal tubule, 144-156
    glomerulotubular balance in, 150-152, 151*f*
    neurohumoral influences on, 152-154, 153*f*
    paracellular, 147-148
    regulation of, 150-156
    transporters, regulation of, 154-156
  thiazide-sensitive electroneutral, 182-183
  in thick ascending limb
    activating influences on, 162-164
    apical mechanisms of, 158-160

Sodium chloride transport *(Continued)*
    basolateral mechanisms of, 160-162
    calcium-sensing receptor effects on, 164-165
    inhibitory influences on, 164-165, 164f
    paracellular mechanisms of, 160
    regulation of, 162-165
    ROMK protein effects on, 159-160
    transepithelial, 162
  in thin ascending limb, 156-158, 157f
  in thin descending limb, 156
  transcellular, 148-150
  transepithelial
    apical potassium channels for, 159
    by intercalated cells, 170f
    by principal cells, 170f
    calcium-sensing receptor inhibitory effects on, 164f
    cAMP-generating hormone stimulation of, 164
    description of, 148-149
    in proximal tubule, 149f
    stimulation of, 164
    in thick ascending limb, 158f, 162-164
  vasopressin effects on, 162-163
Sodium cotransporter, 69
Sodium hydrogen exchange, 148, 154, 154f
Sodium intake, 1528-1529
Sodium nitroprusside, 1575f, 1695t, 1697
Sodium phosphate-IIa transporter, 202f
Sodium polystyrene sulfonate, 596-597, 2168-2169
Sodium potential, 124-125
Sodium pump, 1729
  abundance of, 128-129
  adenosine triphosphatases, 124
  adenosine triphosphate and, 124
  in ammonia metabolism, 254
  basolateral, 150, 154-156, 160-161, 1800
  in bicarbonate reabsorption, 242-243
  bile salts and, 2508
  in collecting duct bicarbonate reabsorption, 242-243
  description of, 123, 1277
  digoxin effects on, 587
  in distal convoluted tubule, 129
  electrochemical gradients created using, 310
  energy and, 124-126
  kinetics of, 126
  metabolic substrates, 129
  nephron distribution of, 146f
  in nephron segments, 129, 129f
  ouabain inhibition of, 132
  physiologic conditions that affect, 243
  potassium uptake activated by, 573
  protein expression and activity, 129
  pump-leak processes, 124-125
  renal sodium transport effects on, 135
  sodium reabsorption and, 142
  structure of, 124, 124f
  in transcellular calcium transport, 188
  transport activity of, 1800
  in uremia patients, 1819
Sodium reabsorption
  age-related changes in, 737
  aldosterone-stimulated, 318
  angiotensin II effects on, 407-408
  connecting tubule's role in, 69
  efficiency of, 136
  electrogenic, 313
  electroneutral, 313
  fractional, 1726
  in heart failure, 429, 431

Sodium reabsorption *(Continued)*
  hormones that regulate, 126
  hyperaldosteronism effects on, 1724-1725
  hypocalciuria and, 190-191
  loop of Henle, 1747
  metabolic cost of, 135-137
  osmotic diuretics effect on, 422
  prostaglandin E_2 effects on, 1716-1717
  proximal tubule, 430f
  regulation of, 1800
  sodium pump and, 142
  in thick ascending limb, 135, 137
  transport systems in, 2378f
  tubular
    in cirrhosis, 444
    renal medulla's role in, 404f
    ureteral obstruction effects on, 1272
    urinary tract obstruction effects on, 1272-1275
  tubular disorders that affect, 422
  vasopressin effects on, 282
Sodium retention
  in cirrhosis. *See* Cirrhosis, sodium retention in
  in heart failure. *See* Heart failure, sodium retention in
  in hepatorenal syndrome, 378
  renin-angiotensin-aldosterone system in, 444-445, 452
Sodium wasting, 1437
Sodium-bicarbonate cotransporters, 243-244
Sodium-bicarbonate symporter mutation, 1455
Sodium-glucose cotransport, 205
Sodium-glucose-linked cotransporters, 209-210
Sodium-hydrogen exchanger regulatory factor, 155f
Sodium-hydrogen exchanger regulatory factor 1, 632
Sodium-phosphate cotransporters, 198-199, 626, 1450-1451, 1451f
Sodium-restricted diet, 450
Solid organ transplantation, 991t, 992-993
Solitary fibrous tumor, 1369
Soluble adenylyl cyclase, 256, 1348-1349
Soluble epoxide hydrolase, 385
Soluble fms-like tyrosine kinase-1, 1621, 1622f, 1623
Soluble guanylate cyclase, 416
Soluble urokinase receptor, 2327-2328
Solute disequilibrium, 2072-2073
Solute load hypothesis, 1743
Solute sequestration, 2072-2073
Solute transport
  active transport along nephron, 126-132
  cell polarity, 126
  in medullary collecting ducts, 133
  metabolic efficiency regulation during, 138-142
  in proximal tubule, 132
  sodium potential for, 124-125
  sodium pump for. *See* Sodium pump
  in thick ascending limb, 132-133
  vectorial, 126
Somatic cell nuclear transfer, 2604-2606
Somatostatin, 1916-1917
Somatostatin analogues, 456, 1495-1496
Somatotropic axis, 1917f
Sorafenib, 1382-1383, 1383f
Sorbitol, 596-597
SOST gene, 191, 1832-1833
South America. *See* Latin America
Sox17, 35

Sox18, 35
SPAK, 163, 168-169
Specific gravity of urine, 789
Specimens
  kidney biopsy, 919-920, 920t, 923-924
  urine, 788
Specular reflectors, 848
Spermicides, 1237, 1239-1240
Sphingomyelin phosphodiesterase acid-like 3b, 119, 1171
Sphingosine-1 phosphate receptor, 979
Spider venom, 2445-2446, 2445f
Spinal meningeal diverticula, 1491
Spironolactone
  adverse effects of, 1713
  Gitelman's syndrome treated with, 1727
  indications for, 1713
  magnesium excretion affected by, 1730
  pharmacokinetics of, 1713
  potassium secretion in collecting duct inhibited using, 540-541
  renoprotection using, 2003
Splanchnic vasodilation, 442
Spot urinalysis, 1356
Sprouty, 24-25
Spry1, 24-25, 27
Spurious hypokalemia, 572
SQSTM1, 734-735
Squamous cells, 800
Sri Lanka. *See* Indian subcontinent
SRY gene, 2611
SSIGN scoring system, 1379
Staghorn calculus, 877f, 879f, 883f, 2507
Staphylococcus aureus, 1148, 2128, 2351
Staphylococcus epidermidis, 2128
Staphylococcus saprophyticus, 1237
Star fruit, 2525
STAR trial, 1590, 1597t
Starling equation, 94, 400
Starling forces, 89, 426, 1799
Starvation ketoacidosis, 547
Statins
  dyslipidemia treated with, 1773-1774, 1931, 2011, 2593
  nephrogenic diabetes insipidus treated with, 301
  proteinuria effects, 2011
Steal syndrome, dialysis-associated, 1948, 2216f
Steatosis, 1344-1345, 1345f
Stem cells
  in acute kidney injury pathophysiology, 978-979
  adult, 2607-2608
  amniotic fluid- and placental-derived, 2607
  bromodeoxyuridine retention by, 2608
  description of, 2603
  embryonic, 2603-2607
  identification of, 2608-2609
  induced pluripotent, 2606-2607
  mesenchymal. *See* Mesenchymal stem cells
  transplantation. *See* Hematopoietic stem cell transplantation
  in tubular epithelial cell injury, 978-979
Stent/stenting
  angioplasty and, 1602-1604
  for arteriovenous graft stenosis, 2202-2203
  atherosclerotic renal artery stenosis and, 1600-1602
  complications after, 1603t
  endovascular renal angioplasty and, 1599-1602
  for renal insufficiency, 1603-1604

INDEX

Steroid biosynthesis pathway, 1461, 1461f
Steroidogenic acute regulatory protein, 306
Steroidogenic factor-1, 588
Steroid-resistant minimal change disease, 1023-1024
Sterol regulatory element binding protein-1, 733
Stokes-Einstein radius, 791
Stone former, 1328, 1344f, 1351f-1352f, 1353t-1354t
Streptococcal skin infection, 1953
Streptococcus pneumoniae, 1175-1176, 1182, 2355
Streptococcus viridans, 1148
Streptozyme test, 1058
Stress, 470
Stroke
  antiplatelet therapy for prevention of, 1931-1932
  characteristics of, 1926-1927
  in chronic kidney disease, 1926-1934
  classification of, 1927
  in dialysis, 1927-1928
  in elderly, 2590
  epidemiology of, 1927-1928, 1927t
  erythropoietin for, 1932-1933
  hemorrhagic, 1927, 1931
  hospitalization for, 1927f
  hypertension and, 1522
  intracranial stenosis as cause of, 2395
  ischemic, 1927
  management of, 1933-1934
  prevention of, 1930-1933
  recombinant tissue plasminogen activator effects on, 1933
  in renal transplantation, 1927-1928
  risk factors for
    anemia, 1928t, 1930
    atrial fibrillation, 1928t, 1929-1930, 1932
    diabetes mellitus, 1928t, 1929, 1931
    dialysis-associated factors, 1930
    homocysteine, 1930
    hypertension, 1928-1931, 1928t, 1929f, 1933-1934
    modifiable, 1928t
    nutrition, 1928t, 1930
    proteinuria, 1928t, 1930
  subtypes of, 1927t
  symptoms of, 1926-1927
  thrombolytic therapy for, 1933
  transient ischemic attack versus, 1926-1927
  vitamin B supplementation for, 1932
Stroma, 5-6, 31-32
Stromal cell-derived factor 1, 2353
Stromal cells, 5-6, 31-32
Struvite, 768
Struvite stones, 1249
Subcapsular hematoma, 878f-879f, 910, 911f
Subcapsular urinoma, 1517
Subclavian artery stenosis, 2214, 2215f
Subclavian catheters, 2145
Subclinical hypothyroidism, 1916, 2395
Subfornical organ, 470
Subpodocyte space, 1781
Substance P, 110
Succinate, 328
Succinate dehydrogenase complex, 139
Succinylcholine, 587-588, 587f
Sucroferric oxyhydroxide, 2023
Sudden death, 2093, 2101
Sulfadiazine, 1259-1260
Sulfatides, 252, 255-256
Sulfhydryl angiotensin-converting enzyme inhibitors, 1641, 1643t
Sulfuric acid, 516
Sulodexide, 1313
Sunitinib, 1382, 1383f
Superior vena cava occlusion, 2214f
Superoxide dismutase, 732, 1758
Suppressors of cytokine signaling, 1913, 2357-2358
Surgery, 606-607, 1366
Surgical revascularization, 1203
Surrogate endpoint biomarker, 927t
Surveillance, 1380
Sylvatic yellow fever, 2441
Symmetric dimethylarginine, 1811
Sympathetic nervous system, 1532-1533
  in cirrhosis, 445-446
  in effective arterial blood volume regulation, 405-407, 407f
  functions of, 703
  in heart failure, 432, 435
  hyperactivity, 1532-1533
  overactivity of, in chronic kidney disease progression, 1771-1772
  potassium distribution affected by, 562
  renin-angiotensin-aldosterone system regulation by, 703
  smoking effects on, 1776-1777
  in sodium excretion, 405, 432
  vasopressin and, 406
Syndrome of inappropriate antidiuretic hormone (SIADH) secretion
  clinical settings of, 498-500
  description of, 816, 2372
  disorders associated with, 499t
  hyponatremia caused by, 497-498
  hypouricemia associated with, 498
  in infants, 499
  long-term treatment of, 509f
  malignancy-associated, 499
  pathophysiology of, 498
  urea for, 506
Syngeneic, 2228-2229
Synpaptopodin, 113
Synpharyngitis nephritis, 1065
Syntaxin 4, 295-296
Syphilis, 1149
Systemic arterial pressure (carotid), 1570-1571, 1571f
Systemic inflammatory response syndrome, 2444
Systemic lupus erythematosus (SLE)
  anti-DNA antibodies in, 1098-1099, 1107-1108
  anti-dsDNA antibodies in, 1099
  antineutrophil cytoplasmic antibodies in, 1093-1094
  anti-nRNP antibodies in, 1099
  antinuclear antibodies in, 1098-1099
  antiphospholipid antibodies in, 1106-1107
  antiphospholipid syndrome in, 1200
  anti-Ro/SSA antibodies in, 1099
  atherogenesis in, 1105-1106
  autoantibodies in, 1093, 1099
  clinical manifestations of, 1098
  diagnosis of, 1093
  drug-induced, 1099-1100
  endothelin-1 in, 338
  epidemiology of, 1092-1093
  factors that affect, 1093
  in Far East, 2531-2532
  fetal loss in, 1100
  gender predilection of, 1092-1093, 1098
  genetic predisposition to, 1093
  hemolytic complement in, 1099
  incidence of, 1092-1093
  lupus nephritis. *See* Lupus nephritis
  lupus podocytopathy in, 1097-1098
Systemic lupus erythematosus (SLE) *(Continued)*
  malar rash associated with, 1950
  medications that cause, 1099-1100
  membranous nephropathy in, 1037
  monitoring of, 1099
  pathogenesis of, 1093-1094
  pregnancy and, 1100
  renal flares, 1101
  serologic tests of, 1098-1099
  skin manifestations of, 1950, 1950f
  T cells in, 1093
  tubulointerstitial disease in, 1097-1098
  vascular lesions in, 1097-1098
  in women, 1092-1093, 1098
Systemic therapy, 1381-1385
Systemic vasculitis, 1088
Systolic blood pressure, 1680-1681
  before and after two-kidney renal clip hypertension placement, 1572f
  before and after two-kidney renal clip placement for hypertension, 1572f
  coronary heart disease and, 1527f
  hypertension and, 1524, 1524t
  importance of, 1524
  Joint National Committee classifications for, 1526f
Systolic hypertension, 1554f

T

T cell(s)
  adhesion molecules on, 2239-2240
  allorecognition, 2237, 2238f
  anergic, 2240
  antigen recognition by, 1215
  antigen-presenting cells and, 2237-2241
  in anti-glomerular basement membrane glomerulonephritis, 1079-1080
  CD4+, 1216, 1795, 2239, 2242
  CD8+, 2239, 2243f
  costimulatory molecules, 2240-2241
  cytotoxic CD8+, 2239
  description of, 2229
  helper, 2241-2242
  interleukin-2 activation of, 2247
  interleukin-17–producing lineage of, 2243-2244
  macrophages and, 1216
  in minimal change disease, 1019-1020
  monoclonal antibody activation of, 2247
  in pauci-immune crescentic glomerulonephritis, 1084
  receptor complex of, 2237-2239
  regulatory, 1795, 2240, 2250
  in systemic lupus erythematosus, 1093
  in tubulointerstitial infiltrate, 1793
T cell cross-match, 2157
T cell immunoglobulin and mucin domains-containing protein-1, 941
T cell immunoglobulin mucin-1, 2243-2244
Tacrolimus, 1398-1399
  in children, 2425
  glomerular disease treated with, 1167-1168
  hyperkalemia caused by, 590
  hypomagnesemia caused by, 622
  immunosuppressive uses of, 2247, 2254t, 2257-2258, 2425
  lupus nephritis treated with, 1104-1105
  membranous nephropathy treated with, 1043-1044
  nephrotic syndrome treated with, 2329-2330
  nephrotoxicity of, 2264
  during pregnancy, 1637, 1637t

Taiwan, 2534
Takayasu arteritis, 1120-1121, 2352, 2506
Tamm-Horsfall protein, 791, 800, 947, 967, 1214-1215, 1232, 1259-1260, 1330, 1391
Tamoxifen, 2133
Targeted agent, 1382
Tartrate-resistant acid phosphatase 5B, 1842
TASK-1, 568
TASK-3, 568
TAT1, 225
TauT, 224-225
Taxus celebica, 2534
T-box transcription factor, 34-35
Tbx18, 34-35
Tcf21, 31
TCF2, 2299-2300, 2317
Technetium 99m-labeled diethylenetriaminepentaacetic acid, 864-865
Technetium 99m-labeled dimercaptosuccinic acid, 865, 880
Technetium 99m-labeled mercaptoacetyltriglycine, 865, 866f, 869-871, 874f, 913f
Telmisartan, 1652t, 1653
Tempol, 732
Temporal arteritis, 1120
Temsirolimus, 1383f, 1384
Tenckhoff catheters, 2114-2115, 2115f, 2221, 2415
Terazosin, 1676t, 1677
Teriparatide, 618
Terlipressin, 455-456, 998-999
Terminal web, 56-59
Terry's nails, 762
TERT, 1153
Testosterone deficiency, 1921
Tetany, 523, 554
Tezosentan, 338
Thailand, 2444, 2535
The Joint Commission, 2632-2633
Theophylline poisoning, 2186-2187
Therapeutic cloning, 2604-2606, 2605f
Therapeutic plasma exchange, 1393, 2171. *See also* Plasmapheresis
Thermofiltration, 2160-2161
Thiazide diuretics
 absorption of, 1712
 acute interstitial nephritis after initiation of, 1732
 adverse effects of, 1712
  hypercalcemia, 609, 1730
  hyperglycemia, 1730
  hyperlipidemia, 1731
  hyperuricemia, 1731
  hypocalciuria, 190-191
  hypokalemia, 1728
  impotence, 1731-1732
 in African Americans, 1686
 angiotensin receptor blockers and, 1655
 bone mineral density affected by, 1726-1727
 central diabetes insipidus treated with, 487
 description of, 1362, 1363t, 1560, 1564
 diabetes insipidus treated with, 487, 1727
 diabetes mellitus and, 1730
 differences among, 1712
 distal convoluted tubule action of, 1710, 1711f
 distal potassium-sparing diuretics and, 1719
 in elderly, 1682-1685, 1684t

Thiazide diuretics *(Continued)*
 extracellular fluid volume affected by, 190-191
 hypercalcemia caused by, 609, 1730
 hyperglycemia caused by, 1730, 1731f
 hyperlipidemia caused by, 1731
 hyperuricemia caused by, 1731
 hypervolemia treated with, 451
 hypocalciuria caused by, 190-191
 hypokalemia caused by, 1728
 hyponatremia and, 817-818
 indications for, 1712
 loop diuretics and, 1712-1713
 mechanism of action, 451, 1710-1712
 nephrogenic diabetes insipidus treated with, 2370
 osteocalcin inhibition by, 1726-1727
 pharmacokinetics of, 1712
 potassium excretion affected by, 1711-1712
 in pregnancy, 1732
 side effects of, 1689-1690
 sites of action, 1710-1712
 vasodilation using, 1685
 water clearance affected by, 1728, 1728f
Thiazide-like diuretics, 1710-1712, 1711f
Thiazolidinediones, 174, 2127
Thick ascending limb. *See also* Loop of Henle
 acid-base transporters in, 238
 ammonia in, 245, 251
 anatomy of, 45, 61, 63-65, 158
 apical potassium channels in, 159-160
 Bartter's syndrome and, 579f
 bicarbonate reabsorption in, 238
 calcium reabsorption in, 188
 cells of, 63-64, 158, 164-165, 1273
 chloride channels in, 161-162
 claudins expressed in, 160
 defect in, hypokalemia as indication of, 815
 EP3 receptor mRNA in, 371
 20-HETE and, 385
 innervation of, 81
 luminal surface of, 66f
 magnesium in, 194, 194f
 mineralocorticoid receptor expression in, 315
 mitochondria of, 63-64
 NKCC2 function in, 163
 reabsorptive processes in, 64-65
 sodium chloride transport in
  activating influences on, 162-164
  apical mechanisms of, 158-160
  basolateral mechanisms of, 160-162
  calcium-sensing receptor effects on, 164-165
  inhibitory influences on, 164-165, 164f
  paracellular mechanisms of, 160
  regulation of, 162-165
  ROMK protein effects on, 159-160
  transepithelial, 162
 sodium reabsorption in, 135, 137, 1272-1273
 sodium transport in, 132-133
 solute transport in, 132-133
 transepithelial resistance in, 160
 tumor necrosis factor-α expression in, 164
 urea recycling in, 270
Thin ascending limb
 apical chloride transport in, 156-157
 basolateral chloride transport in, 156-157
 osmolality in, 272

Thin ascending limb *(Continued)*
 passive countercurrent multiplier mechanism, 272
 sodium chloride transport in, 156-158, 157f
Thin basement membrane nephropathy, 1141-1142, 1424-1425
Thin descending limb, 156, 263f
Thin limbs of loop of Henle
 anatomy of, 61-63, 63f-64f
 early descending, 64f
 epithelium of, 65f
 types of, 61-62, 64f
Thiopurine methyltransferase, 2257, 2425
Thirst, 471-473, 2366
Thomsen-Friedenreich antigen, 1182
Thrombectomy, 2199-2202, 2199t, 2201f-2202f
Thrombin, 1904, 1907
Thrombin-activable fibrinolysis inhibitor, 1803-1804
Thromboembolism
 in nephrotic syndrome, 1804
 renal artery, 1201-1202
 venous, hypoalbuminemia and, 1805
Thrombolytic therapy, 1206, 1933
Thrombomodulin, 1185
Thrombosis
 arteriovenous fistula, 2210-2212
 arteriovenous graft, 2194-2195, 2196t
 in children, 1805
 deep vein. *See* Deep vein thrombosis
 renal artery, 964, 1202-1203, 2253, 2266
 renal vein. *See* Renal vein thrombosis
Thrombospondin-1, 1752-1753
Thrombotic events, COX-2 inhibitors and, 363-364
Thrombotic microangiopathies, 1405-1406
 acute, 2269
 antiphospholipid syndrome as cause of, 1200-1201
 causes of, 1405t
 description of, 1175
 electron microscopy of, 1178f
 hemolytic-uremic syndrome. *See* Hemolytic-uremic syndrome
 pathology of, 1178-1179, 1178f
 during pregnancy, 1632
 thrombotic thrombocytopenia purpura. *See* Thrombotic thrombocytopenia purpura
 treatment of, 1181t
Thrombotic thrombocytopenia purpura (TTP)
 ADAMTS13 deficiency associated with, 1188-1191, 2154-2155
 classification of, 1176t
 clinical features of, 1176, 2154
 description of, 990-992, 1157
 hematopoietic stem cell transplantation and, 1188
 laboratory findings, 1176-1178
 pathogenesis of, 2154-2155
 pathology of, 1179
 plasmapheresis for, 2154-2155
 platelet aggregation in, 1189f
 recurrence of, after renal transplantation, 2270
Thromboxane A$_2$, 364-365, 367-368, 1579
 in albuminuria, 378
 allograft rejection and, 378
 biosynthesis of, 376
 half-life of, 374
 loop diuretics effect on, 1717

Thromboxane A$_2$ *(Continued)*
  synthesis of, 1270
  vasoconstriction induced by, 377, 411, 1270
Thromboxane A$_2$ receptor, 368
Thromboxane A$_2$ synthase, 378-379
Thromboxane synthase, 364-365
Thrombus, 1177f
Thyroid dysfunction, 1549
Thyroid hormone disturbances, 1915-1916, 1915t
Thyroid hormone-binding globulin, 1915-1916
Thyroid surgery, 616
Thyroid-stimulating hormone, 1915-1916
Thyrotoxic periodic paralysis, 573
Thyrotropin, 1915-1916
Thyroxine, 1915-1916
Ticlopidine, 1189
Tie2 receptor, 34
Tight junctions, 147f, 188-189
Timolol, 1656t-1657t, 1657
TINU syndrome, 1229
Tiopronin, 1365
Tissue engineering
  definition of, 2602
  goal of, 2602-2603
  intrarenal progenitor cells, 2608-2609
  renal anlagen, 2613-2616
  renal units, 2616-2617
  stem cells used in
    adult, 2607-2608
    amniotic fluid- and placental-derived, 2607
    bromodeoxyuridine retention by, 2608
    description of, 2603
    embryonic, 2603-2607
    identification of, 2608-2609
    induced pluripotent, 2606-2607
    mesenchymal
      acute kidney injury applications of, 2611-2613
      bone marrow-derived, 2611
      description of, 2607
      differentiation of, into renal tissue, 2611
  therapeutic cloning, 2604-2606, 2605f
Tissue factor pathway inhibitor, 1803-1804, 1904
Tissue inhibitors of metalloproteinases (TIMP), 949, 989, 1757, 1794
Tissue ischemia, 1579
Tissue kallikrein, 181-182
Tissue kallikrein-kinin system, 347-348
Tissue necrosis, 586
Tissue plasminogen activator, 1804
Tissue-nonspecific alkaline phosphatase, 1838
Titratable acid excretion, 246-247
  buffers involved in, 246, 246f
  creatinine in, 247
  as phosphate, 246-247
  as phosphoric acid, 247
  uric acid in, 247
  urinary buffers involved in, 246-247, 246f
TMP, 540-541
TNM staging system, 1378, 1378t
Tobacco smoking. *See* Smoking
Tofacitinib, 2258
Toll-like receptor-2, 976, 1201
Toll-like receptor-4, 238, 976, 1201
Toluene-induced metabolic acidosis, 843f
Tolvaptan, 454, 504-505, 508, 1495, 1713-1714
Tonicity balance, 807-808, 808f

Tonicity-responsive enhancer-binding protein, 392
Tonsillectomy, 1068-1069
Topiramate-induced non-anion gap metabolic acidosis, 532
Torres Strait Islanders, 2538, 2546
Torsades de pointes, 569
Torsemide, 1707
Total body water, 460, 486, 2365, 2414
Total iron binding capacity, 1893
Total osmolality, 461
Total-body irradiation, 1400
Townes-Brock syndrome, 2297t, 2298-2299, 2318
Toxic alcohols, 839
Toxic gain of function, 1469-1470
Toxins. *See also* Poison removal/poisonings
  acidosis caused by, 543, 548-550
  acute kidney injury caused by, 2500-2501
  plasmapheresis for removal of, 2159
TP receptors, 366-369
Trabecular bone, 1831-1832, 1842
Trace elements, 1983-1984, 2099-2100
Trandolapril, 1643t, 1644
Tranexamic acid, 1906
Transcapillary hydraulic pressure difference, 97-98
Transcapillary hydrostatic pressure difference, 1760f
Transcription factor, 7
Transcription factor 3, 1372
Transepithelial potassium transport, 175-176
Transepithelial potential difference, 145-146
Transepithelial sodium chloride transport
  apical potassium channels for, 159
  by intercalated cells, 170f
  by principal cells, 170f
  calcium-sensing receptor inhibitory effects on, 164f
  cAMP-generating hormone stimulation of, 164
  description of, 148-149
  in proximal tubule, 149f
  stimulation of, 164
  in thick ascending limb, 158f, 162-164
Transferrin, serum, 1970-1971
Transferrin receptor, serum, 1893-1894
Transferrin saturation, 1893, 1894f
Transforming growth factor-β
  angiotensin II's role in expression of, 334
  definition of, 1212-1213
  low-protein diet effects on, 1958
  α$_2$-macroglobulin and, 1212-1213
  in nephron injury after renal mass ablation, 1755-1756
  renal fibrosis in aging kidney, 729-730
  role of, 1579
  stimulation of, 729-730
Transforming growth factor-β$_1$, 951
Transgenic mouse models, kidney development studies using, 9-19, 10t-17t
Transient hematuria, 1015
Transient hyponatremia, 477
Transient ischemic attack, 1926-1927
Transient receptor potential cation channel, 113, 1753-1754
Transient receptor potential channel melastatin 6, 1711-1712
Transient receptor potential vanilloid channels, 467, 1825
Transitional cell carcinoma, 898-899, 900f-902f
Transjugular intrahepatic portosystemic shunt, 457, 998-999
Translocation carcinoma, 1372
Translocational hyponatremia, 491

Transmembrane domains, of LeuT fold, 229
Transmembrane serine protease 6, 1887
Transmural pressure, 110
Transplant tourism, 2505
Transplantation
  hematopoietic stem cell, 1392
    acute kidney injury after, 993
    chronic kidney disease and, 1394
    complications of, 1393
    purpose of, 1393-1394
    renal syndromes associated with, 1393t
      acute kidney injury and, 1394
      total-body irradiation and, 1400-1401
    types of, 993
  islet cell, 1319-1320
  renal. *See* Renal transplantation
  renal-pancreas. *See* Renal-pancreas transplantation
Transplantation renal artery stenosis, 2272
Transplantation-associated thrombotic microangiopathy, 1395
Transtubular potassium concentration gradient, 569, 573-574, 820-821, 2380
Transtubular potassium gradient, 536-537
Treatment-resistant hypertension, 1580
Triamterene, 1712-1713
Tribonat, 546
Tricarboxylic acid cycle, 328
Trichomonas vaginalis, 1255
Trichorhinophalangeal syndrome, 29
Trichrome stain, 919-920
Triiodothyronine, 1915-1916
Trimethaphan camsylate, 1695t, 1698
Trimethoprim-sulfamethoxazole, 590, 750, 1238t, 2456-2457
Trimethylamine, 1812-1813
Triple phosphate, 768
Triple-helical type IV collagen molecule, 1421
TROP2, 25
Tropical diseases
  dengue fever. *See* Dengue fever
  leptospirosis. *See* Leptospirosis
  malaria. *See* Malaria
  yellow fever, 2441-2442, 2442f
Troponin I, 2101
Troponin T, 2101
Trousseau's sign, 612-613, 623, 995
Trpc6, 39
TRPC6 disease, 1430
TRPM6 channel, 196, 620
Trpm6 protein, 193-194
TRPV5, 189, 190f, 191-192, 741
Trypanosome spp., 1150-1151
Trypanosomiasis, 1150-1151
Tryptophan, 1812, 1983-1984
Tsutsugamushi disease, 2513-2515
T-type calcium channels, 1662
Tuberculosis, 882, 884f, 1252-1254, 1253f, 1260, 2505
Tuberous sclerosis, 1952, 1952t
Tuberous sclerosis complex, 1368-1369, 1374, 1500-1502
Tubular atrophy, 728f
Tubular epithelial cells, 1215, 1274, 1277-1279
Tubular proteinuria, 791, 793
Tubular stretch, 1278
Tubule fluid, 265-273
Tubuloglomerular feedback, 55, 135, 209-210, 1269
  adenosine's role in mediation of, 108-109, 135
  angiotensin II antagonists effect on, 109
  angiotensin II in, 399
  definition of, 106

Tubuloglomerular feedback (Continued)
  in effective arterial blood volume regulation, 399-400
  mechanism of action, 108f
  renal autoregulation mediation by, 106-109
  renal blood flow controlled by, 108-109
  renin-angiotensin-aldosterone system in, 400
  responses of, 109
  sex hormones that regulate, 400
Tubulointerstitial antigens, 1214-1215, 1228-1229
Tubulointerstitial diseases
  acute interstitial nephritis. See Acute interstitial nephritis
  chronic tubulointerstitial nephritis. See Chronic tubulointerstitial nephritis
  drugs that cause, 1218-1219, 1218t
  in HIV-related nephropathy, 1152
  renal function affected by, 1210
  structure-function relationships in, 1209-1210
  in systemic lupus erythematosus, 1097-1098
Tubulointerstitial fibrosis, 729f, 1754-1755, 1763, 1793
Tubulointerstitial inflammation, 1215
Tubulointerstitial injury
  antigens in, 1214-1215
  cellular infiltrates in, 1215-1216
  complement components in, 1213-1214
  cytokines associated with, 1212-1213
  description of, 1209
  in focal segmental glomerulosclerosis, 1026
  genetic diseases that cause, 1210
  glomerular diseases that cause, 1210
  glomerular-filtered lipids associated with, 1213
  growth factors associated with, 1212-1213
  interstitial fibrosis, 1216-1218
  macrophages in, 1794
  mechanisms of, 1210-1218
  tubulointerstitial antigens in, 1214-1215
Tubulointerstitial nephritis, 622, 1209, 1220-1221, 2511-2513
Tumor lysis syndrome, 990, 992t
  characteristics of, 1395-1397
  classification of, 1396, 1396t
  definition of, 628
  hyperphosphatemia caused by, 628
  prevention of, 628
  risk factors for, 1396t
  treatment of, 1396-1397
Tumor necrosis factor, 2241
Tumor necrosis factor-α-converting enzyme, 329
Tumor necrosis factor-like weak inducer of apoptosis, 743
Tumor necrosis factor-related apoptosis-induced ligand, 1020
Tumor vaccine, 1384-1385
Tumor-induced osteomalacia, 197-198, 631
Tunneled catheters
  arteriovenous fistulas versus, 2629-2631
  bacteremia of, 2220
  complications of, 2217, 2217f-2218f
  description of, 2216
  dysfunction of, 2219-2220
  exchange of, 2219-2220
  femoral, 2218
  insertion of, 2216-2217, 2217f-2218f

Tunneled catheters (Continued)
  less common locations for, 2218-2219, 2219f
  transhepatic, 2219
  translumbar, 2218-2219, 2219f
Turkey. See Middle East
Turnover, mineralization, and volume classification system, 1845, 1845t
Twin study, 1348
Two-kidney renal clip hypertension, 1568-1569, 1570t, 1571-1572, 1572f-1573f
Type 1 diabetes mellitus. See Diabetes mellitus, type 1
Type 2 diabetes mellitus. See Diabetes mellitus, type 2
Type 2 vasopressin receptor, 278-279
Type A intercalated cells, 70-72, 72f
Type AB cystinuria, 1448
Type B cystinuria, 1448
Type B intercalated cells, 70-72, 72f
Type IV collagen, 1421
Type IV collagen disease, 1421-1425
Type IV collagen gene, 1422f
Tyrosine hydroxylase inhibitor, 1679-1680
Tyrosine kinases, 329-330
Tyrosinemia, 1443-1444

U

Ub-activating enzyme, 1964
Ubiquitin-protease system, 1964-1965, 1970
UFP-803, 352
Ularitide, 344-345, 1001
Ulnar-mammary syndrome, 2297t
Ultrafiltration
  convection during, 2112
  extracorporeal, 2139
  failure of, 2416
  in hemodialysis, 2068-2069, 2080, 2095, 2105
Ultrafiltration coefficient, 1797
Ultrafiltration rate, 2095-2096
Ultrasonography, 848-851
  acute interstitial nephritis evaluations, 1220
  acute kidney injury evaluations, 866-867, 989-990
  acute pyelonephritis evaluations, 878, 880f
  anatomy on, 849f, 850-851
  angiomyolipomas on, 891
  antenatal, 1264-1265
  arteriovenous fistula vascular mapping using, 2205-2206, 2206f
  autosomal dominant polycystic kidney disease, 1485f, 1485t
  contrast-enhanced, 849-850
  description of, 848
  diagnostic, 848
  end-stage kidney disease diagnosis using, 868, 868f, 888
  equipment used in, 848
  fetal, for urinary tract obstruction diagnosis, 1258-1259
  hydronephrosis diagnosis using, 867-869, 867f-868f, 1263
  increased through-transmission, 848
  intravenous contrast agents used with, 849
  kidney biopsy uses of, 850, 2223-2224, 2223t, 2224f
  for kidney stones, 1359
  lymphoceles on, 910-911
  nonspecular reflectors, 848
  obstruction evaluations, 871

Ultrasonography (Continued)
  power Doppler, 850f
  pyelonephritis evaluations, 878, 880f, 881-883
  renal colic on, 873
  renal cysts on, 883, 885f
  renal parenchymal disease on, 868
  renal transplantation assessments using, 910
  resistive index, 849
  specular reflectors, 848
  ureteropelvic junction obstruction findings, 2315
  urinary tract obstruction findings, 1263-1265, 1264f, 1267f
  urinoma after renal transplantation on, 910, 911f
Uncoupling protein isoforms, 127
Unilateral renal artery stenosis, 1595-1598
Unilateral renal cystic disease, 1512-1513, 1570t
Upper limit of metastability, 1327
Upper tract urothelial carcinoma, 1386
Urantide, 352
URAT1, 221, 221t
Urate, 816, 1453
Urate nephropathy, 1227-1228
Urate-induced calcium oxalate stone, 1336f
Urban yellow fever, 2441
Urea
  blood urea nitrogen, 123, 933-934, 988, 1808, 1959, 1968-1969
  in chronic kidney disease, 1959-1961, 1968-1969
  clearance of, 2070
  degradation of, 1960-1961
  excretion of, 1808
  fractional clearance of, 2120
  glomerular filtration rate estimations using, 782
  hemodialysis generation of, 2083-2084, 2083f-2084f
  hyponatremia treated with, 506
  in inner medulla, 268-270
  intrarenal recycling of, 820f
  osmotic diuresis evaluations, 811-812
  parathyroid hormone effects on production of, 1968
  peritoneal dialysis clearance of, 2120
  plasma, 423, 816, 2036
  production of, 1960-1961, 1968
  recycling of, in renal medulla, 270, 270f
  serum concentration of, 2070
Urea channel inhibitors, 1714
Urea nitrogen
  blood, 123, 933-934, 988, 1959, 1968-1969
  serum, 2072
Urea nitrogen appearance rate, 1969
Urea reduction ratio, 2085-2087, 2087f
Urea transporters, 276-278, 277f, 410, 740
Ureaplasma urealyticum, 1242
Urease inhibitor, 1365
Uremia, 1421-1422
  amino acid metabolism affected by, 1817
  carbohydrate metabolism affected by, 1816
  chronic, nitrogenous product turnover in
    ammonia, 1962
    creatinine, 1961
    fecal nitrogen, 1962
    nonurea nitrogen, 1962-1963
    overview of, 1959
    urea, 1959-1961
    uric acid, 1961-1962

Volume 1 pp. 1-1321 • Volume 2 pp. 1322-2636

Uremia *(Continued)*
  clinical features of, 1807
  creatinine accumulation in, 1808
  glomerular filtration rate in, 1819-1820
  growth failure in children caused by, 2358-2359
  hemodialysis for, 2083
  high anion gap acidosis caused by, 549-550
  immune disorder induced by, 2104
  insulin resistance in, 1816, 1914-1915
  lipid metabolism affected by, 1816-1817
  loss of appetite associated with, 1819
  metabolic effects of, 1808t, 1815-1818
  neurologic function in, 1818-1819
  nutrition affected by, 1817-1818
  platelets in, 1904
  protein metabolism affected by, 1817
  protein-binding defect in, 2037f
  resting energy expenditure affected by, 1815-1816
  sensorimotor neuropathy in, 1819
  signs and symptoms of, 1808t, 1818-1820
  sleep-wake cycle disruptions in, 1939
  sodium pump inhibition in, 1819
  solutes retained in. *See* Uremic solutes
Uremic acidosis, 549-550
Uremic cardiomyopathy, 1858-1859
Uremic encephalopathy, 1934-1935
Uremic platelet dysfunction, 1905, 1907f
Uremic polyneuropathy, 1939
Uremic solutes, 1808t
  aliphatic amines, 1812-1813
  aromatic compounds, 1811-1812
  chemical structure of, 1809f
  D–amino acids, 1809-1810
  description of, 1807
  dietary effects on, 1814-1815
  gastrointestinal function effects on, 1814-1815
  guanidines, 1810-1811
  hippurate, 1809f, 1811-1812
  indoles, 1812
  organic transport systems for clearance of, 1815
  oxalate, 1813
  peptides, 1810
  phenols, 1811-1812
  polyols, 1813
  protein-bound, 1814
  proteins, 1810
  renal replacement therapy for removal of, 1813-1814
  sequestered, 1814
  tryptophan metabolites, 1812
  urea, 1808-1809
  uric acid, 1813
Uremic syndrome, 773, 996, 1926, 1969
Ureter(s), 43, 2303f, 2313
Ureteral jets, 850, 850f
Ureteral mesenchyme, 34-35
Ureteral obstruction
  causes of, 1260
  endometriosis as cause of, 1261
  glomerular hemodynamics in, 1270t
  nephrolithiasis as cause of, 1260
  after pediatric renal transplantation, 2435
  sodium reabsorption affected by, 1275
  tubular sodium reabsorption affected by, 1272
  urinary calculi as cause of, 1280
Ureteral stents, 1246, 2429
Ureteral stones, 873, 875f-877f
Ureteral strictures, 1260

Ureteric bud
  BMP7 expression in, 29
  branching of, 5, 25, 28f, 2298
  collecting duct from, 44-45
  congenital anomalies of the kidney and urinary tract and, 2297-2298
  ectopic, 10t-17t
  epithelial, 3
  epithelial cells, 25
  genes required by, 23-25
  glial-derived neurotrophic factor transcriptional regulation and, 22-23
  induction of, 22-23
  metanephric mesenchyme and, 4f, 5-6, 21-25
  outgrowth of, 2297-2298
  positioning of, 27-28
  Spry1 deficiency effects on, 24-25
Ureteric stones, 873
Ureteropelvic junction, 43, 1258-1259, 1262, 2298, 2311, 2314-2315, 2315f
Uric acid
  in chronic kidney disease, 1813, 1961
  drugs that affect, 221
  fractional clearance of, 1961
  functions of, 1228
  glomerular filtration of, 220
  metabolism of, 996
  nephrotoxicity of, 967-968
  physiochemistry of, 1341-1342
  pregnancy and, 1612, 1616
  reabsorption of, 221
  renal handling of, 220-221, 220f
  secretion of, 221
  serum levels of, 1962
  in titratable acid excretion, 247
  transport of, 220-221, 220f, 221t
  in uremia, 1813
Uric acid nephropathy, 1259-1260
Uric acid stones, 1227, 1323f-1324f, 1324, 1341-1345, 1342t, 1351
Uric acid transporters, 220-221, 220f, 221t
Uricase deficiency, 1341
Uricosuria, 1653
Uricosuric drugs, 220f, 221
Uridine triphosphate, 174
Urinalysis
  chronic kidney disease evaluations, 776
  ethylene glycol exposure determined with, 2177
  hematuria evaluations, 756
  pauci-immune crescentic glomerulonephritis findings, 1086-1087
  renal tuberculosis findings, 1253
  urinary tract infection evaluations, 777-778
  urine properties on, 788-790, 789t
  urine specimen for, 788
Urinary buffers, 246-247, 246f
Urinary calculi
  characteristics of, 1279-1280
  in children, 2340
  composition of, 873
  extracorporeal shock wave lithotripsy for, 1279-1280
  obstruction caused by, 1279-1280. *See also* Urinary tract obstruction
  passage of, 873
Urinary dilution, 740
Urinary microscopy, 937, 937t
Urinary pH, 789-790, 841f, 1327, 1341-1344, 2168
Urinary pole, 89f
Urinary prothrombin fragment 1, 1330
Urinary space. *See* Bowman's space

Urinary supersaturation estimation, 1357-1359
Urinary tract
  congenital anomalies of. *See* Congenital anomalies of the kidney and urinary tract
  emphysematous cystitis, 1251
  emphysematous pyelonephritis of, 1251
  host defenses of, 1232, 1232t
  infected renal cyst involvement of, 1250-1251
  obstruction of. *See* Urinary tract obstruction
  perinephric abscess involvement of, 1250
  pyocystis of, 1252
  renal abscess involvement of, 1250
  xanthogranulomatous pyelonephritis of, 1251-1252
Urinary tract cancer, 1352
Urinary tract infection (UTI)
  acid-base disorders associated with, 778
  acute pyelonephritis and, 1633
  acute uncomplicated
    antimicrobial agents for, 1238-1239, 1238t
    description of, 1231-1232
    diagnosis of, 1237-1238
    epidemiology of, 1236
    Escherichia coli as cause of, 749-750, 778, 1233
    host factors, 1237
    microbiology of, 1236-1237
    pathogenesis of, 1236-1237
    prophylaxis for, 1239
    pyelonephritis in, 1240
    pyuria associated with, 1238
    recurrence of, 1237, 1239-1240
    reinfection of, 1237
    sexual intercourse as cause of, 1237
    spermicides and, 1237, 1239-1240
    Staphylococcus saprophyticus as cause of, 1237
    treatment of, 1238-1239, 1238t
    urine culture for, 1237-1238
  in AIDS patients, 883
  anatomic abnormalities associated with, 777
  asymptomatic, 1231-1232
  asymptomatic bacteriuria. *See* Asymptomatic bacteriuria
  as autonomic diabetic polyneuropathy sequelae, 1320
  bacteria that cause, 777-778
  bacteriuria, 1231-1232
  Candida albicans, 1254
  in children, 2313-2314, 2429
  clinical presentation of, 777
  complicated
    antimicrobial treatment of, 1243-1244
    clinical presentation of, 1243
    description of, 1231-1232
    epidemiology of, 1242
    Escherichia coli as cause of, 1242
    hospitalization for, 1242
    host factors associated with, 1242-1243
    imaging of, 1244
    laboratory diagnosis of, 1243
    microbiology of, 1242
    pathogenesis of, 1242-1243
    recurrent, 1244-1245
    sequelae of, 1242
    supportive care for, 1244
    treatment of, 1243-1244
    urinary tract abnormalities associated with, 1232t, 1242-1243

Urinary tract infection (UTI) *(Continued)*
  cystitis. *See* Urinary tract infection, acute uncomplicated
  definition of, 1231-1232
  description of, 1231
  in diabetes mellitus, 1320
  diagnosis of, 777-778, 1233-1234, 1234t
  in elderly, 749-750
  Escherichia coli as cause of, 749-750, 778, 1233, 1240, 1242
  fungal, 1254
  hematuria caused by, 755
  immune responses to, 1232-1233
  inflammatory responses to, 1232-1233
  in men, 777
  nephrolithiasis and, 2342
  parasitic infestations as cause of, 1255
  prevalence of, 777
  pyelonephritis
    acute nonobstructive, 1240-1242
    bacteremia in, 1240
    ciprofloxacin for, 1241t
    costovertebral angle pain or tenderness associated with, 1240
    description of, 1231-1232
    diagnosis of, 1240-1241
    epidemiology of, 1240
    imaging of, 1241
    pathogenesis of, 1240
    renal scarring caused by, 1240
  recurrent, 777, 1239-1240
  reinfection, 1232, 1237
  relapse of, 1232
  in renal failure patients, 1249
  renal function assessments in, 778
  in renal transplant recipients, 1248-1249, 2269-2270, 2429
  risk factors for, 777, 1248, 2269-2270
  signs and symptoms of, 749
  stones associated with, 1249
  symptomatic, 1231-1232
  treatment of
    antimicrobial agents, 1234, 1235t-1236t, 1238-1239, 1238t
    β-lactams, 1239
    nitrofurantoin, 750, 1238t
    pharmacokinetic and pharmacodynamic considerations for, 1234
    pivmecillinam, 1238t
    trimethoprim-sulfamethoxazole, 750, 1238t
  urinary frequency associated with, 777
  urinary tract abnormalities associated with, 1232t
  urine culture of, 1233-1234, 1234t, 1237-1238
  uroepithelial cells, 1232-1233
  in urolithiasis patients, 1249-1250
  vaginitis and, 777
  viral causes of, 1255
  voiding symptoms associated with, 777
Urinary tract obstruction
  abdominal aortic aneurysm as cause of, 1261
  acquired causes of, 1259-1262, 1259t
  acute, 1258
  angiotensin II expression in, 1278f
  benign prostatic hyperplasia as cause of, 1261, 1280
  biomarkers of, 1263
  bladder cancer as cause of, 1261
  in children, 1258
  chronic, 1258
  classification of, 1258

Urinary tract obstruction *(Continued)*
  clinical aspects of, 1262
  congenital, 719-720, 1258-1259, 1258t
  COX metabolites in, 377-378
  description of, 299
  diagnosis of, 1262-1268, 1264f-1268f
  diuresis after, 1281
  divalent cations excretion affected by relief of, 1276-1277
  drugs that cause, 1260
  etiology of, 1258-1262, 1258t, 1264
  extrinsic causes of, 1260-1262
  fetal, 1258-1259, 1279-1280
  glomerular filtration affected by, 1269-1271
  glomerular filtration rate regulation during, 1270-1271
  hematologic abnormalities that cause, 1262
  imaging of
    antegrade pyelography, 1268, 1268f
    antenatal ultrasonography, 1264-1265
    computed tomography, 1265-1266, 1266f
    Doppler ultrasonography, 1265
    intravenous pyelography, 1265, 1265f
    isotopic renography, 1266-1267, 1280
    magnetic resonance imaging, 1267-1268, 1267f
    magnetic resonance urography, 1267-1268
    retrograde pyelography, 1268
    ultrasonography, 1263-1265, 1264f, 1267f
    Whitaker test, 1268
  incidence of, 1257-1258
  intrinsic causes of, 1259-1260, 1259t
  malignant neoplasms as cause of, 1262
  in neurogenic bladder, 1280
  partial, 1280
  pathophysiology of, 1268-1277
  pelvic neurofibromas as cause of, 1262
  phosphate excretion affected by relief of, 1276-1277
  potassium excretion affected by relief of, 1276
  prenatal, 1258-1259, 1279-1280
  prevalence of, 1257-1258
  in prostate cancer, 1261
  relief of
    diuresis after, 1281
    divalent cations excretion affected by, 1276-1277
    kidney biopsy after, 1280-1281
    phosphate excretion affected by, 1276-1277
    potassium excretion affected by, 1276
    renal function after, 1280-1281
    urine acidification affected by, 1276
  renal blood flow affected by, 1269-1271
  renal damage caused by, 1280
  renal enzymes affected by, 1277t
  renal function recovery after, 1280-1281
  renal gene expression affected by, 1277t
  in renal transplantation recipients, 2271
  renin-angiotensin-aldosterone system in, 1279
  retroperitoneal processes that cause, 1261-1262
  signs and symptoms of, 1262
  sodium reabsorption affected by, 1272-1275
  sodium transport affected by, 1274
  terms associated with, 1257

Urinary tract obstruction *(Continued)*
  treatment of, 1279-1281
  tubular epithelial cells after resolution of, 1277-1279
  tubular function affected by, 1271-1277
  unilateral, 1281
  ureteropelvic junction, 1258-1259
  uric acid nephropathy as cause of, 1259-1260
  urine acidification affected by relief of, 1276
  urine concentration affected by, 1275-1276
  urine dilution affected by, 1275-1276
  urine flow affected by, 1274-1275
  urine output affected by, 1262
Urinary trefoil factor 1, 1331
Urine
  acidification of, 74, 1276, 1365-1366
  alkalinization of, 2168, 2180
  ammonia excretion in, 528-529, 538, 840, 841f
  assessment of, in acute kidney injury evaluations, 986-988, 987t-988t
  bilirubin in, 790
  casts in, 800, 800t, 801f
  cells in, 798-800.
  chloride concentration in, 816
  citrate excretion in, 219
  cloudy, 788-789
  color of, 788-789, 789t
  crystals in, 800-802, 801t, 1329
  cytology of, 799
  daily volume of, 1257
  eosinophils in, 799-800
  erythrocytes in, 798-799, 799f
  extravasation of, after renal transplantation, 913
  fetal, 2302
  fluorine 18 2-fluoro-2-deoxy-D-glucose excretion in, 865
  formation of, 83, 94, 122
  gadolinium effects on, 858f
  glucose in, 205f, 790
  hemoglobin in, 790
  ketones in, 790
  leukocyte esterase in, 790
  leukocytes in, 799-800
  lipids in, 800
  low volume and uric acid stones, 1343
  magnesium excretion in, 194
  magnetic resonance imaging of, 857f-858f
  microorganisms in, 802
  microscopy evaluation of, 798-802, 799f, 800t-801t, 801f
  myoglobin in, 790
  neutrophil gelatinase-associated lipocalin, 944-945
  nitrites in, 790
  nitrogenous compounds in, 1962
  odor of, 789
  osmolality of, 789, 807
  phosphate excretion in, 199-200
  potassium excretion in, 180, 569, 820
  protein in, 112, 793, 947
  relative density of, 789
  sodium concentration in, 816
  specific gravity of, 789
  squamous cells in, 800
  sterility of, 1232, 1232t
  Tamm-Horsfall protein in, 1232
  urobilinogen in, 790
  urothelial cells in, 800

Urine chemistry, 1356-1359
Urine concentration
  ability, 271
  age-related changes in, 739-740
  aquaporins in, 274f
  assessment of, 789
  in elderly, 739-740
  knockout mice models of, 273-279
  loop of Henle in, 259-261
  mechanisms of, 92, 270
  nephron loss-specific adaptations in, 1748
  renal insufficiency effects on, 1748
  sites of, 264-265
  specific gravity, 789
  statins effect on, 301f
  urinary tract obstruction effects on, 1275-1276
  vasopressin in, 282
  water reabsorption effects on, 1748
Urine culture, 1233-1234, 1234t, 1237-1238
Urine dilution, 264-265, 1275-1276, 1748
Urine dipstick tests, 762-763, 777-778
Urine flow rate, 806, 810-811
Urine formation product ratio, 1328-1329
Urine leaks, 2270-2271
Urine osmolality, 465, 476, 479f
Urine osmoles, 811-812
Urine output, 959, 1262
Urine saturation, 1327
  factors influencing, 1327
  measurement of, 1327
  oxalate and calcium role in, 1340
  in stone formers, 1328
Urine sediment, 986-987, 987t
Urine specimen, 788
Urine studies, 762-763, 768
Urine volume, 476
Uriniferous pseudocyst, 1517
Urinoma, 910, 911f
Urobilinogen, 790
Urodilatin, 339, 339f, 341, 344-345
Uroepithelial cells, 1232-1233
Urogenital ridge, 2-3
Urogenital system, 2-3
Uroguanylin, 398
Urolithiasis. See also Kidney stone
  body mass index and, 1323f
  cardiovascular disease and, 1351, 1351f
  causes of, 1349, 1349f
  definition of, 1322
  diabetes mellitus and, 1350-1351
  differential diagnosis of, 769t
  epidemiology of, 1322-1324
  hypertension and, 1351-1352
  obesity and, 1350-1351
  polygenic animal model for, 1349-1350, 1350t
  prevalence by gender and weight, 1323f
  risk factors for, 1350-1351
  as systemic disorder, 1350-1355
  urinary tract infection in, 1249-1250
Uromodulin, 165, 800, 1214-1215, 1348-1349
Uromodulin-associated kidney disease, 165
Uropathogenic *Escherichia coli*, 1236-1237, 1239
Urotensin, 437-438
Urotensin I, 351
Urotensin II
  definition of, 351
  in diabetic nephropathy, 352
  in effective arterial blood volume regulation, 418-419
  in heart failure, 437-438
  interventional studies of, 352
  in kidney, 352

Urotensin II *(Continued)*
  nephron loss adaptations and, 1740
  physiologic role of, 351-352
  plasma levels of, 352
  prepro–U-11 mRNA, 351
  in renal disease, 352
  secretion of, 351
  synthesis of, 351, 351f
  urinary concentrations of, 352
  urine levels of, 352
  vasoconstrictive properties of, 351-352, 419
Urotensin II receptor, 352, 418-419
Urothelial cells, in urine, 800
Urothelial tumor, 1385
UT-A1/3 urea transporter knockout mice, 276-278
Uteroplacental insufficiency, 696-699

V

Vaccinations
  in hemodialysis patients, 2105
  in renal transplantation recipients, 2288, 2288t
  yellow fever, 2442
Vaccine, 1384-1385
VACTERL association, 2318
Vaginitis, 777
Valganciclovir, 2429-2430
Valproic acid, 2181-2182
Valsalva maneuver, 1204
Valsartan, 1652t, 1653
Valvular heart disease, 1859, 1929-1930, 2408
VAMP-2, 295-296
Vaptans
  adverse effects of, 455
  heart failure treated with, 454
  hyponatremia treated with, 504-505, 508
  loop diuretic-sparing effect of, 454-455
Vasa recta
  ascending, 92, 267, 269-270
  counterflow arrangement of, 262
  definition of, 262
  descending, 92, 269-270
  description of, 6, 87
  oxygen shunting, 133
  urea recycling through, 270
Vascular access
  in critically ill patients, for renal replacement therapy, 2145
  in diabetic nephropathy, 1315
  dialysis, 2191-2192
  for extracorporeal treatments for poisoning, 2173
  hand ischemia induced by, 2214
  hemodialysis. See Hemodialysis, vascular access for
  international trends in, 2630f
  quality improvement and, 2629-2631
Vascular calcification
  in adults, 2102-2103, 2128
  apoptosis in, 1836-1837
  assessment of, 1847
  atherosclerotic disease in, 1833-1835
  calcium-sensing receptor in, 1826
  cellular transformation in, 1835-1836
  in children, 2407-2408
  in chronic kidney disease, 1850, 2102-2103
  coronary artery, 1850
  in dialysis patients, 1850
  inhibitors of
    fetuin-A, 1837-1838
    matrix gamma-carboxyglutamate protein, 1838

Vascular calcification *(Continued)*
    osteoprotegerin, 1838
    pyrophosphate, 1838
  matrix vesicles in, 1836-1837
  pathophysiology of, 1833-1839, 1836f
  pathways in, 1837f
  prevalence of, 1837
  after renal transplantation, 1852
Vascular dementia, 1938
Vascular endothelial growth factor receptor 1, 1621
Vascular endothelial growth factor (VEGF)
  COX-2 inhibition effects on, 378
  downregulation of, 1794
  endothelial cell expression of, 47-48
  insulin-like growth factor-1 effects on production of, 1744
  podocyte expression of, 1752-1753
  preeclampsia and, 1619, 1621-1623
Vascular endothelial growth factor-A, 32-34, 33f
Vascular endothelial growth factor-C, 392
Vascular endothelium, 1752-1753
Vascular smooth muscle cells, 1835, 2102-2103
Vascular thrombosis, 898, 899f
Vascular tone, 363, 383f, 979
Vasculature, renal
  arteries, 83-85
  description of, 262
  development of, 6, 32-35, 33f
  EP2 receptor effects on, 373
  hydraulic pressure profile of, 85, 85f
  illustration of, 7f
  innervation of, 110
  molecular genetics of, 32-35, 33f
  vasoconstrictors that affect, 99
  veins, 83-85
Vasculitis, 1165-1166, 1950-1951, 1951f
Vasculogenesis, 6, 32
Vasodilation, 422, 1612-1613
Vasodilators
  direct-acting. See Direct-acting vasodilators
  parenteral, 1695t, 1696-1699
Vasohibin-1, 120
Vasopeptidase inhibitors, 345, 453-454
Vasopressin
  apical chloride transport affected by, 163
  aquaporin-2 phosphorylation sites modified by, 293, 805
  aquaporin-2 trafficking in collecting duct principal cells regulated by, 287-288
  bicarbonate reabsorption affected by, 238
  in bronchogenic carcinoma, 499
  cardiac function effects of, 432-433
  central diabetes insipidus treated with, 285, 488
  chloride transport affected by, 157-158
  cirrhosis-related water retention affected by, 446
  clearance of, 471
  copeptin fragment of, 463
  cortical collecting duct affected by, 819
  deficiency of, 474-477
  description of, 409-410, 2366
  diabetes insipidus treated with, 486
  distal nephron potassium secretion affected by, 182
  distribution of, 471
  diuretic therapy response affected by, 1717
  in effective arterial blood volume regulation, 415
  epithelial sodium channel activation by, 173-174

Vasopressin (Continued)
  fluid deprivation test for, 485, 485t
  functions of, 410
  furosemide levels affected by, 1717
  gene, 463, 465f
  in gestational diabetes insipidus, 471
  in heart failure, 432-433
  hemodynamic stimuli that affect, 467-468
  hypothalamic pathways that regulate, 464f
  inactivation of, 471
  natriuresis effects of, 410-411
  nephrogenic diabetes insipidus and, 285
  neurohypophysis production of, 463, 474
  neurophysin peptide fragment of, 463
  nonosmotic regulation of, 467-471
  osmotic regulation of, 464-467, 478
  plasma levels of, 282, 466f, 479f
  precursors of, 463
  prostaglandin E_2 effects on, 373-374
  renal blood flow affected by, 410
  renal response to, 808-809
  secretion of, 282
    baroreceptor mechanisms involved in, 468, 469t
    blood volume effects on, 468
    description of, 462-471
    drinking effects on, 468-469
    drugs that affect, 469t, 471
    hormones that affect, 469t
    hypercapnia effects on, 470
    hypoglycemia effects on, 470
    hypovolemia effects on, 467-468
    hypoxia effects on, 470
    nausea effects on, 469-470, 469f
    opioid inhibition of, 471
    renin-angiotensin-aldosterone system effects on, 470
    stress effects on, 470
    thirst and, 472-473
  sodium balance affected by, 498
  sodium chloride transport affected by, 162-163, 173
  sodium reabsorption affected by, 278, 282
  structure of, 463-464
  sympathetic nervous system and, 406
  synthesis of, 462-471, 474
  transepithelial sodium chloride transport affected by, 163-164
  in urinary concentration, 282
  water balance affected by, 498
  in water excretion, 258-259, 259f, 270-271
  water permeability effect on, 1469f
  water retention affected by, 446
  water transport regulation by, 374
Vasopressin 1A receptor, 245, 410
Vasopressin 1 receptor, 282, 455-456
Vasopressin 2 receptor, 282-285
  antagonists, for hepatorenal syndrome, 456-457
  arginine vasopressin activation of, 2366
  β-arrestin and, 282-284
  description of, 282
  downregulation, accessory proteins involved in, 282-283
  heterotrimeric G proteins and, 282-284
  internalization effects on, 284-285, 291
  lysosome degradation of, 284-285
  messenger RNA, 282-283
  trafficking of, 284f
  in urine concentration, 282
Vasopressin 3 receptor, 410
Vasopressin disorders
  description of, 473
  diabetes insipidus. See Diabetes insipidus

Vasopressin disorders (Continued)
  hyponatremia. See Hyponatremia
  hypotonic polyuria, 473t
  pathophysiology of, 473
Vasopressin receptor, 1471f
Vasopressin receptor antagonists, 454-455, 504-506, 509, 1713-1714
Vasopressin-vasopressin receptor antagonist, 1495
Vasopressin-vasopressin receptor mutation, 1471f
Vasopressin-vasopressin receptor shuttle pathway, 1468-1470
VATER association, 2318
Vectorial transport, 126
Venacavography, 1204-1205
Venoocclusive disease, 993, 1394-1395
Venous thromboembolism, 1805
Ventricular sensors, 395-396
Ventriculoperitoneal shunts, 1149
Verapamil hydrochloride, 1663t, 1664, 1668-1669, 1668t, 1697t
Vertebral fracture, 1352f
Vertical nystagmus, 623
Very-low-density lipoprotein, 1801-1802
Vesicoureteral reflux
  antibiotic prophylaxis in, 2314
  bladder and bowel dysfunction as risk factor for, 2314
  in children, 2311, 2313-2314, 2314f, 2435
  definition of, 2313
  diagnosis of, 2313
  epidemiology of, 2313
  grading of, 2313, 2314f
  management of, 2314
  prognosis for, 2313-2314
  in pyelonephritis, 878, 882-883
  in renal agenesis, 2302
  in renal ectopy, 2311
Vibrio sodium-galactose symporter, 207, 208f
Vietnam, 2536
Villous adenoma, 553
Viral urinary tract infection, 1255
Visceral epithelial cells, 49-51, 52f. See also Podocyte(s)
Visceral infections, 1149
Vitamin A
  hypercalcemia caused by, 609
  maternal restriction of, nephron number affected by, 716
  nephron number affected by, 721
  teratogenicity of, 716-717
Vitamin B, 1732, 1932, 1938
Vitamin B_6, 1983
Vitamin B_{12}, 1883-1884, 1983
Vitamin C, 1983
Vitamin D
  absorptive hypercalciuria and, 1331
  in children, 2390-2391
  in chronic kidney disease, 1912, 1923-1924
  in chronic kidney disease–mineral bone disorder, 1828-1830, 1841, 1848-1849
  deficiency of
    acquired, 1775
    anemia in chronic kidney disease and, 1887
    calcitriol for, 1872-1873, 1923-1924
    cardiovascular mortality risks, 2099-2100
    in chronic kidney disease, 1775, 1849, 1912, 1924, 2434
    in chronic kidney disease–mineral bone disorder, 1848-1849

Vitamin D (Continued)
    diseases and disorders associated with, 1848-1849, 1923-1924
    hypophosphatemia caused by, 633
    1,25(OH)D levels, 617, 1872-1873
    populations with, 617
    proximal renal tubular acidosis and, 531
  description of, 617
  diabetic nephropathy treated with, 1312-1313
  dietary supplementation of, 617
  forms of, 2390
  health benefits of, 1848-1849
  hypercalcemia caused by, 609, 2132
  hypertension and, 1549
  hypocalcemia caused by, 617
  in insulin resistance, 1913
  metabolism of, 1828f
  parenteral, 2026
  renal 1-hydroxylation of, 1749-1750
  rickets prevention using, 2394
  supplementation of, 1849, 1924, 2406
  types of, 1923
Vitamin D_2, 2390
Vitamin D_3, 2390
Vitamin D analogues
  in chronic kidney disease, 2032
  cinacalcet and, 2029, 2032
  description of, 2023-2026
  parathyroid hormone affected by, 2027-2029
Vitamin D receptor, 1333, 1831f
Vitamin D receptor mutant mice, 200-201
Vitamin D response elements, 2023-2025
Vitamin D sterols, 2026, 2029
Vitamin D-binding protein, 1797, 1828-1829, 1923-1924, 2390
Vitamin D-dependent rickets type 1, 617
Vitamin E, 1984
Vitamin K_2, 1838
Voclosporin, 2257
Voiding cystourethrogram, 2317f
Voltage-dependent calcium channels, 108
Volume overload
  clinical manifestations of, 776
  in critically ill patients, 2144
  extracorporeal ultrafiltration for, 2139
  in hypervolemia, 449
  resistant hypertension caused by, 1693
Volume repletion, 610-611
Voluntary exploratory data submissions, 928
Vomiting, 553
von Gierke's disease, 1442-1443
von Hippel–Lindau disease, 889, 890f, 1952, 1952t
von Hippel-Lindau disease type 2, 1548
von Hippel-Lindau gene, 1372-1373, 1373f
von Hippel–Lindau protein, 1881
von Hippel-Lindau syndrome, 1373, 1380, 1502-1503
von Willebrand factor, 1179, 1188, 1904-1906
von Willebrand factor-cleaving protease deficiency, 2356
V_2R. See Vasopressin 2 receptor
V_2R gene, 279

W

WAGR syndrome, 1387
Waldenström's macroglobulinemia, 1136, 1136f-1137f, 2153-2154

Warfarin, 1068, 1206, 1908, 2040
Wasp stings, 2500, 2525
Water
　collecting duct absorption sites, 269f, 270-271
　evaporative loss of, 462
　excretion of
　　arginine vasopressin's role in, 270-271
　　decreases in, 815
　　endothelin effects on, 416
　　factors that affect, 491
　　free, 462-463
　　insensible loss, 462
　　regulation of, 258-259
　homeostasis of, 1468
　insensible loss of, 462
　metabolism of, 462-473, 2365-2367
　permeability of, vasopressin effect on, 1469f
Water balance
　acquired disorders of, 297
　arginine vasopressin effects on, 498
　calculation of, 811
　electrolyte-free, 807
　long-term regulation of, 296-302
Water channels, 805
Water deprivation, 110
Water diuresis, 805-813
　assessment of
　　electrolyte-free water balance, 807
　　osmole excretion rate, 807-808
　　tonicity balance, 807-808, 808f
　　urine flow rate for, 806
　　urine osmolality, 807
　clinical approach to, 808-809
　desalination of luminal fluid, 806
　description of, 271
　driving force for, 805
　in elderly, 743, 743f
　filtrate, distal delivery of, 805-806
　urine volume during, 805
　water channels, 805
　water permeability, residual, 806

Water retention
　aquaporin-2 in, 446
　in cirrhosis. See Cirrhosis, water retention in
Water softener, 2081
Water transport, 373-374
Water-soluble vitamins, 1983-1984
Weak acid, 512
Weak base, 512
Wegener's type antineutrophil cytoplasmic antibody-associated vasculitis, 350
Weigert-Meyer rule, 2313
Weight loss, 1992-1993
Weil's disease, 2443-2444
Whitaker test, 1268
White cell function, 1909-1910
White coat hypertension, 1540, 1540f
Whittam model, 127-128, 127f
Whole-exome sequencing technique, 1410, 1418
Williams-Beuren syndrome, 2394-2395
Wilms' tumor, 1386-1387
Wilms' tumor 1, 2603
Wilms' tumor-1 gene, 7-9, 1413-1414, 1414t
Wilms' tumor oncogene, 1431
Wilson's disease, 1444-1445
With-no-lysine kinases, 819
WNK1, 179-180, 590, 1712
WNK4, 163, 183, 313, 539-540, 590
WNK kinases, 168, 180, 566
WNK-dependent signaling, 183
WNK-SPAK/OSR1 signaling cascade, 181f
Wnt4, 28
Wnt11, 28
Wnt9b, 28
Wolffian duct, 2-3
Wolframin, 475
Wolfram's syndrome, 475
WT1, 36-37
WT1, 2326

X

Xanthelasma palpebrarum, 762
Xanthine dehydrogenase, 1347

Xanthine oxidase inhibitors, 1364-1365, 2425
Xanthine stone, 1347
Xanthinuria, 1347
Xanthogranulomatous pyelonephritis, 881, 883f, 1251-1252
Xanthomas, eruptive, 1946-1947, 1946f
Xenogeneic, 2228-2229
Xenopus oocytes, 21, 288
Xerosis, 1943, 1943f
X-linked Alport's syndrome, 1423-1424
X-linked diabetes insipidus, 1473
X-linked hypophosphatemia, 630
X-linked hypophosphatemic rickets, 201-202, 1437, 1451-1452, 1830
X-linked nephrogenic diabetes insipidus, 278-279, 300, 1470-1473
X-linked recessive nephrolithiasis, 1437
Xp11.2 translocation carcinoma, 1372
X-ray, 1359

Y

Yellow fever, 2441-2442, 2442f

Z

Zebrafish, 20-21
Zellweger's syndrome, 2297t
Zenker's fixative, 919
Zero-order processes, 2069
Zinc
　deficiency of, 1887, 2099-2100
　supplementation of, 1984
Zinc-dependent metalloproteinases, 2447
Zoledronate, 611
Zonula adherens, 55-56
Zonula occludens, 972-973
Zonula occludens 1, 113
ZS-9, 597-598
Zucker diabetic fatty rat, 1344-1345, 1345f
Zygomatosis, 1405
Zygomycosis, 2498, 2498f